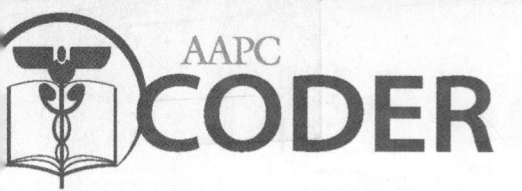

AAPC CODER

Accurate Coding Results, Best Encoder Value

W9-BRO-775

Offering Three Product Packages to Best Fit Your Needs

Pro Fee	Facility	Complete

Balance trusted accuracy with increased productivity using AAPC Coder, the highest value medical coding encoder on the market.

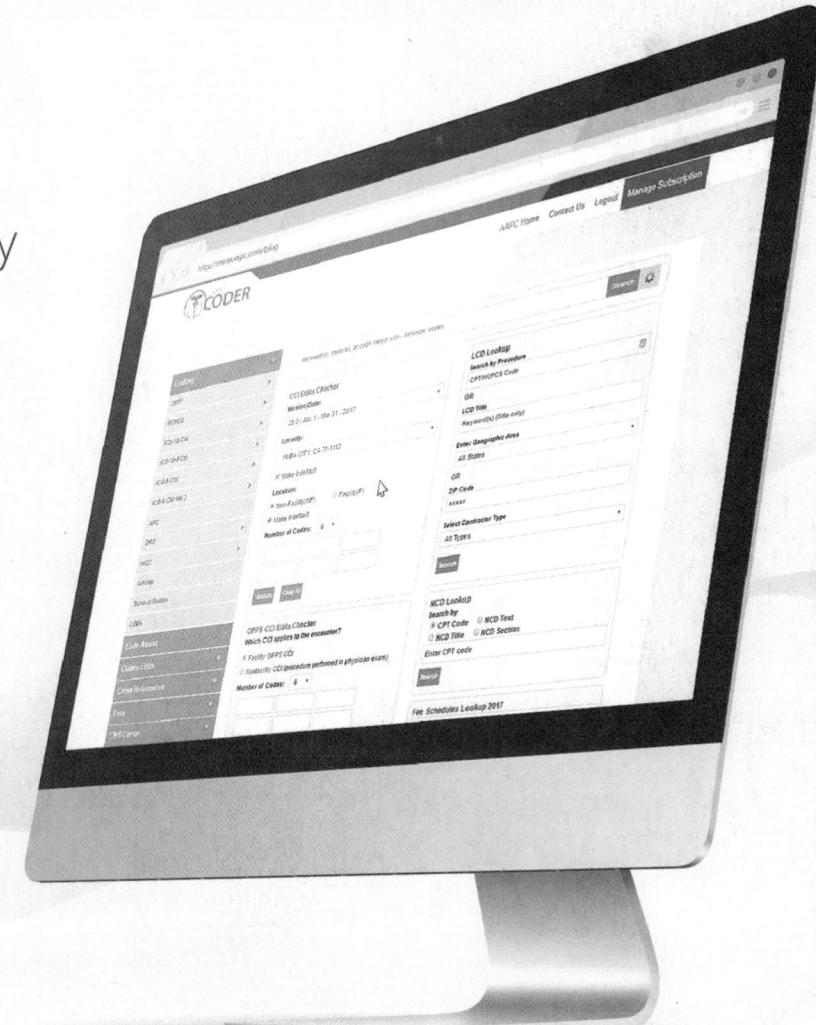

Get your Free 14-Day Trial at **aapc.com/coder**

Join the growing field of
Medical Documentation

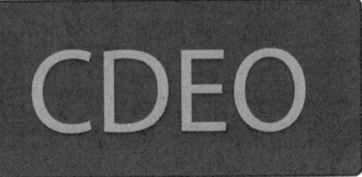
CDEO

Become a Certified Outpatient Documentation Expert Today!

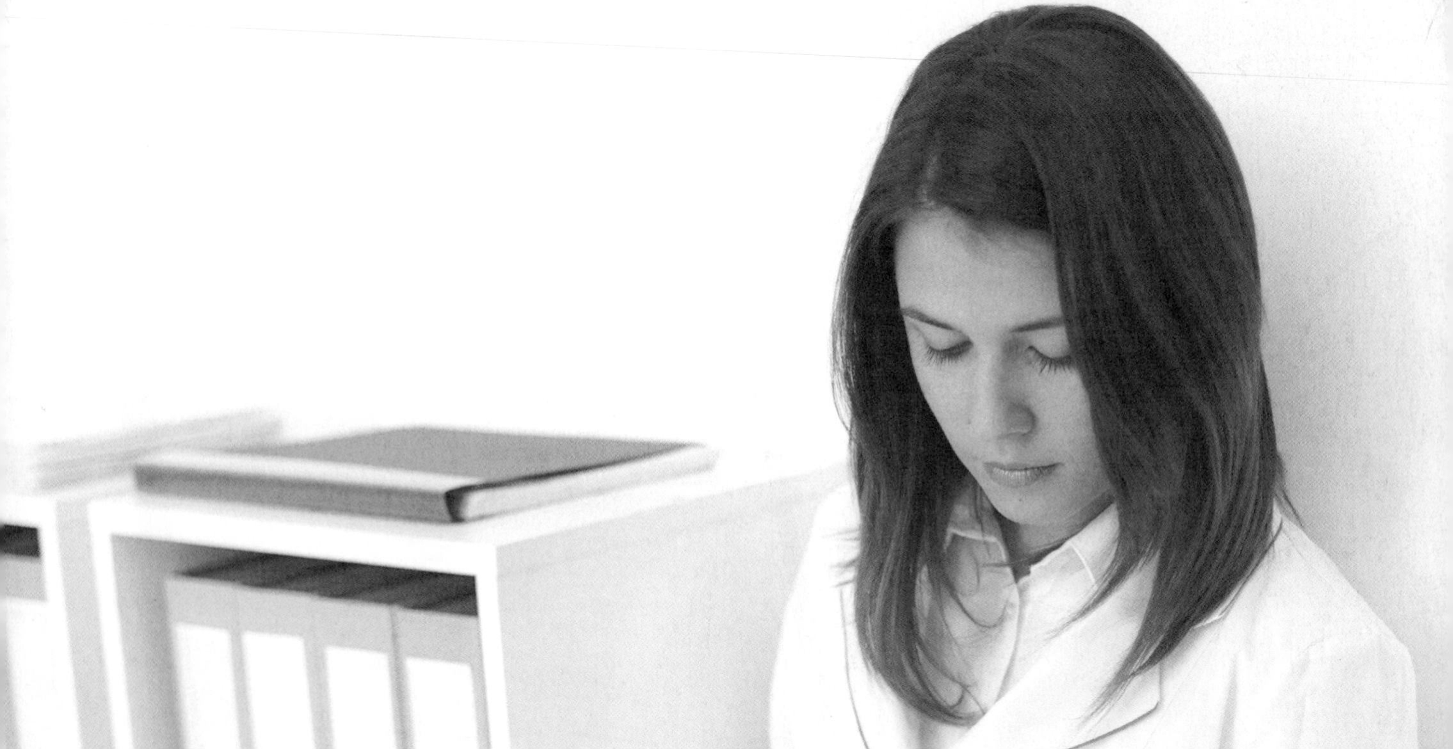

Visit **aapc.com/CDEO** to learn more about this new certification

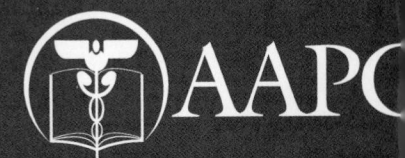
AAPC

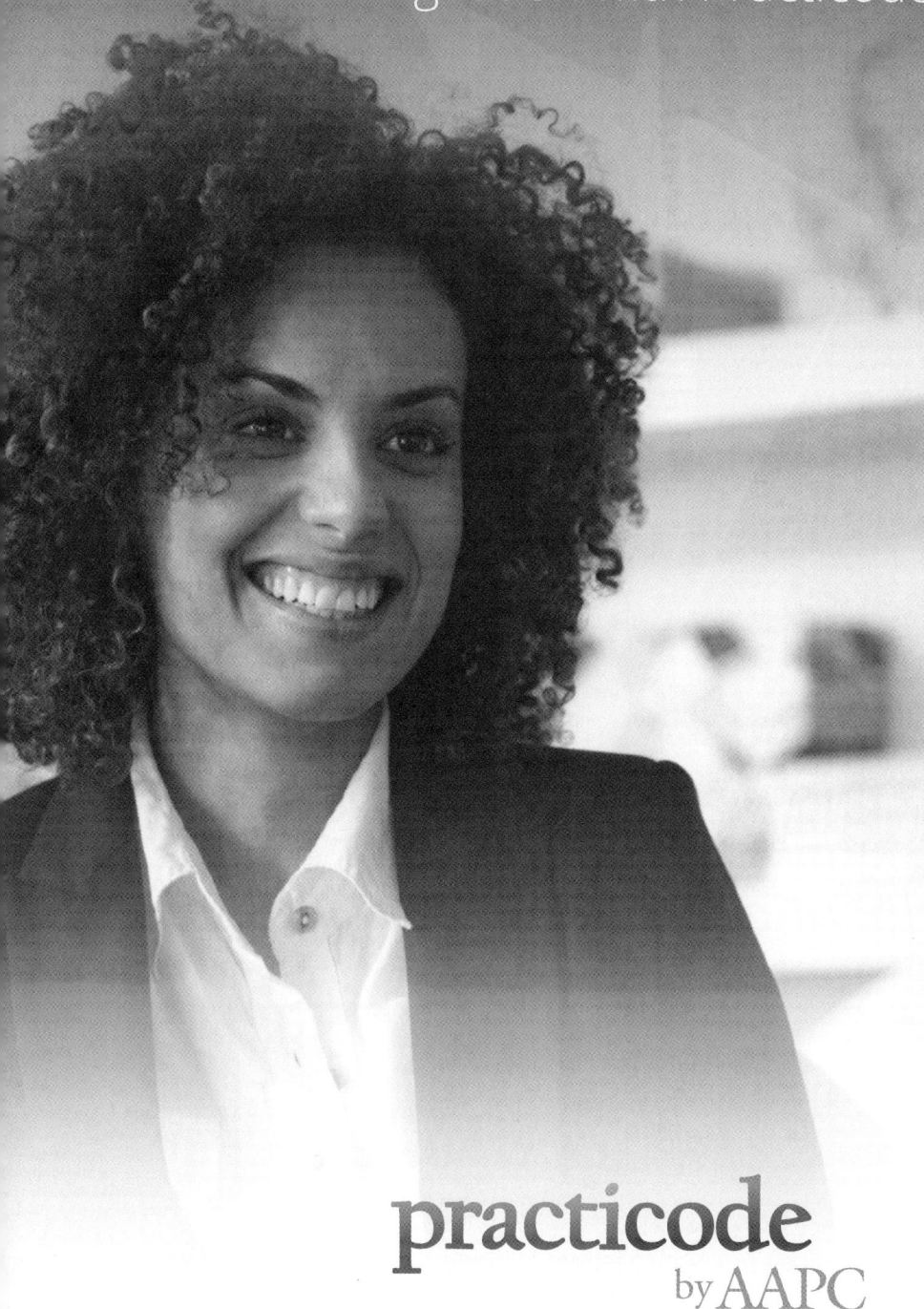

Land Your Dream Job

Accelerate your career and remove your apprentice designation with Practicode.

practicode
by AAPC

acticode gives you the experience you need to get the job you want. With over 600 al-world coding exercises, you'll earn one year of coding experience and get closer to removing your apprentice status. It's your career. Take control of it.

aapc.com/practicode

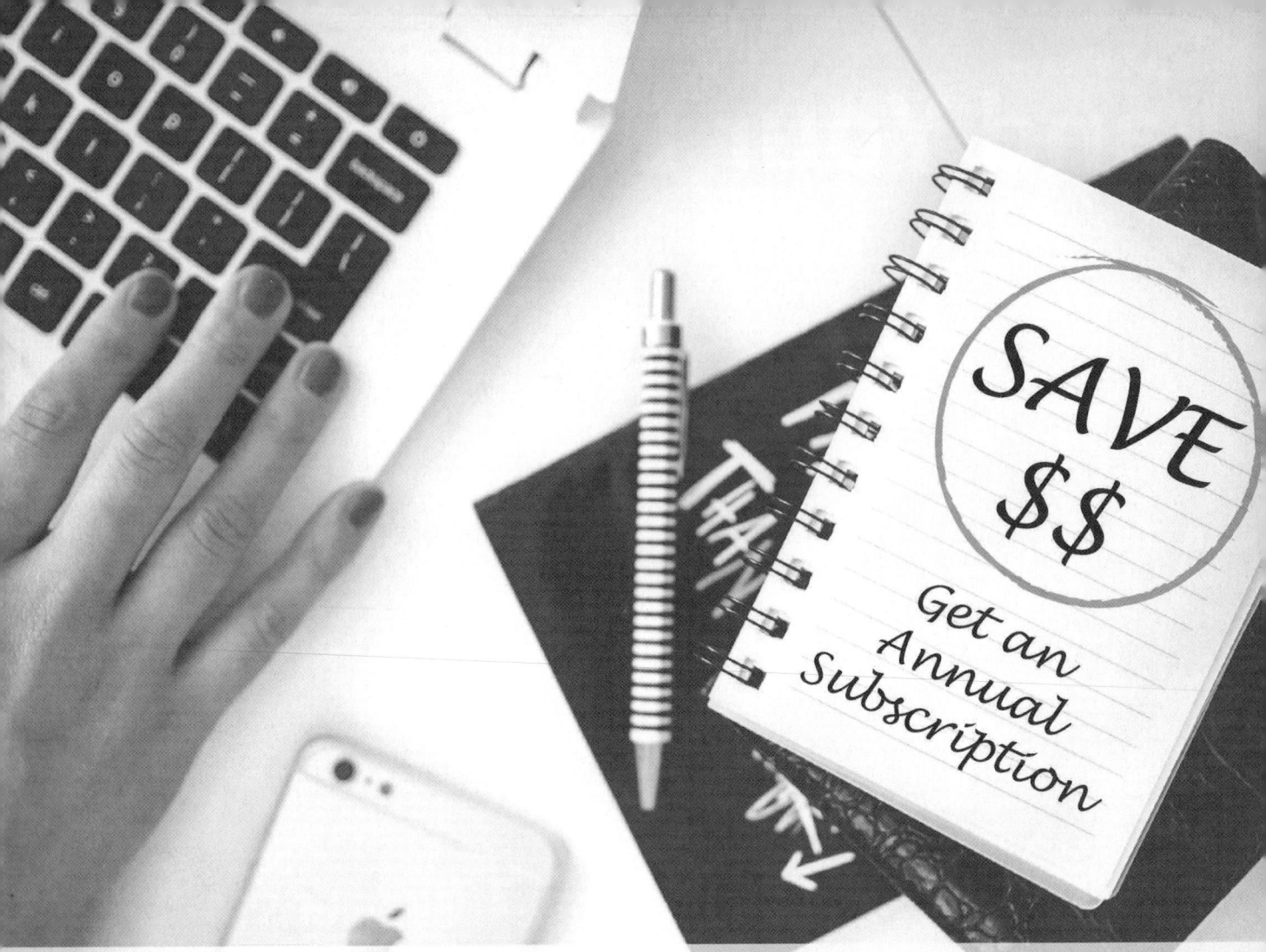

AAPC Annual Webinar Subscription

Healthcare Education You Can Afford

- 12 Months of Access to 40+ Live Events
  & Entire Library of 100+ On-Demand Webinars

- Receive 2 CEUs per Webinar (Live & On-Demand)

- Topics Cover 21+ Specialties

- 12-Month Subscription Starting at $295
  (Volume Discounting Available for Your Office)

Visit **aapc.com/webinars** for details

Where will YOU be next spring?

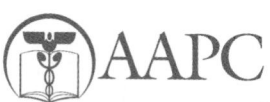

AAPC
HEALTHCON.com

NOTES

2018

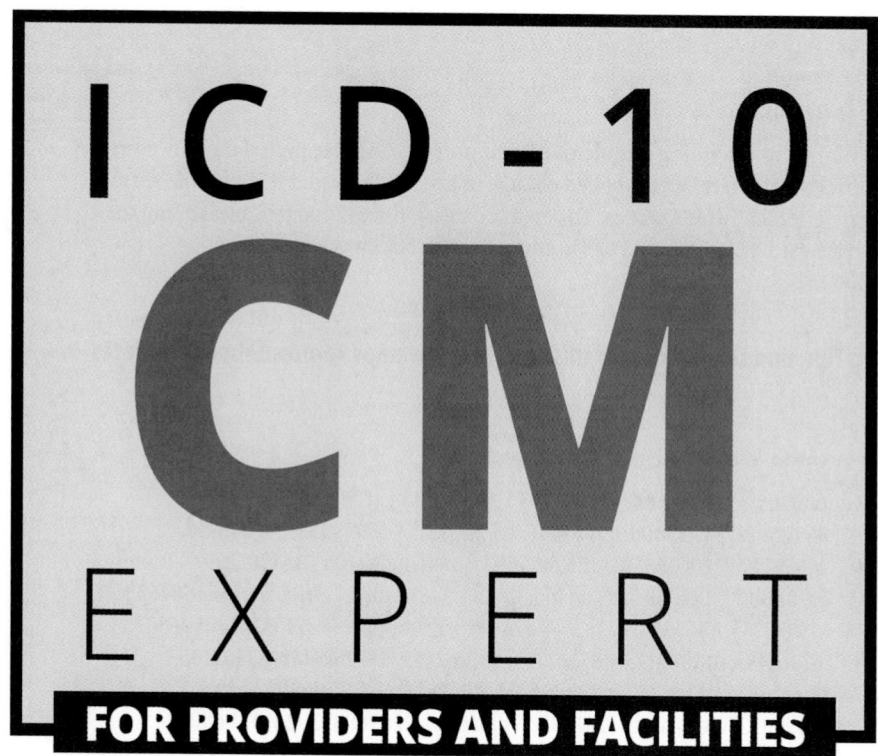

ICD-10
CM
EXPERT

FOR PROVIDERS AND FACILITIES

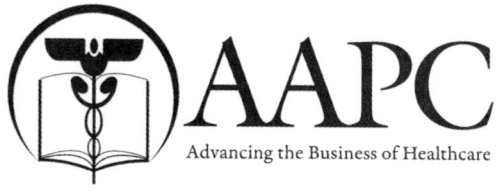

AAPC

Advancing the Business of Healthcare

PUBLISHER'S NOTICE

Coding, billing, and reimbursement decisions should not be made based solely upon information within this ICD-10-CM code book. Application of the information in this book does not imply or guarantee claims payment. Make inquiries of your local carriers' bulletins, policy announcements, etc., to resolve local billing requirements. Finally, the law, applicable regulations, payers' instructions, interpretations, enforcement, etc., of ICD-10-CM codes may change at any time in any particular area. Information in this book is solely based on ICD-10-CM rules and regulations.

This ICD-10-CM is designed to be an accurate and authoritative source regarding coding, and every reasonable effort has been made to ensure accuracy and completeness of content. However, this publisher makes no guarantee, warranty, or representation that this publication is complete, accurate, or without errors. It is understood that this publisher is not rendering any legal or professional services or advice in this code book and bears no liability for any results or consequences arising from use of this ICD-10-CM book.

AAPC'S COMMITMENT TO ACCURACY

This publisher is committed to providing our members accurate and reliable materials. However, codes and the guidelines by which they are applied change or are reinterpreted through the year. Check www.aapc.com periodically for updates. To report corrections and updates, please contact AAPC Customer Service via 1-800-626-2633 or via email to code.books@aapc.com.

Get Updates, Coding Tips, and Corrections for this book at www.aapc.com/codebook_updates.

Images/Illustrations by the following artists at shutterstock.com

miucci - 119473492 | ducu59us - 104022683, 125200733 | Alila Medical Media - 228843262, 155445686, 101696095, 96426923, 97755608, 97755611, 147943922, 125899358, 147943910, 155445662, 147943874, 108567068, 106263593, 106263560 | BlueRingMedia - 141162229, 141161560, 141161404 , 149006000, 145028440 | snapgalleria - 142194094 | okili77 - 156466463 | Designua - 180938618, 135935735, 186535475, 165084413 | stockshoppe - 99671552, 180896807, 180896810, 187162247, 187162193, 187162175, 187162163, 187162142, 187162118, 187162106, 187162070, 180896873, 180896855, 180896738, 180896720, 177791516, 177790997 | lotan - 186878060 | sciencepics - 199873508| Blamb - 24129706 | joshya - 226909492, 261971498 | Della_Liner - 324447776 | Marochkina Anastasiia - 414103342 | Alexander_P - 404964388

Front/Back cover photos: iStock

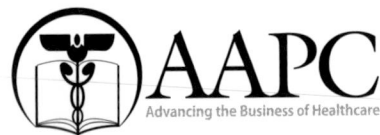

Copyright 2017 © AAPC
ISBN: 978-1-626884-717

Table of Contents

This page intentionally left blank

Preface

ICD-10-CM Official Preface

This FY 2018 update of the International Statistical Classification of Diseases and Related Health Problems, 10th revision, Clinical Modification (ICD-10-CM) is being published by the United States government in recognition of its responsibility to promulgate this classification throughout the United States for morbidity coding. The International Statistical Classification of Diseases and Related Health Problems, 10th Revision ICD-10, published by the World Health Organization (WHO), is the foundation of ICD-10-CM. ICD-10 continues to be the classification used in cause-of-death coding in the United States. The ICD-10-CM is comparable with the ICD-10. The WHO Collaborating Center for the Family of International Classifications in North America, housed at the Centers for Disease Control and Prevention's National Center for Health Statistics (NCHS), has responsibility for the implementation of ICD and other WHO-FIC classifications and serves as a liaison with the WHO, fulfilling international obligations for comparable classifications and the national health data needs of the United States. The historical background of ICD and ICD-10 can be found in the Introduction to the International Classification of Diseases and Related Health Problems (ICD-10), 2010, World Health Organization, Geneva, Switzerland.

ICD-10-CM is the United States' clinical modification of the World Health Organization's ICD-10. The term "clinical" is used to emphasize the modification's intent: to serve as a useful tool in the area of classification of morbidity data for indexing of health records, medical care review, and ambulatory and other health care programs, as well as for basic health statistics. To describe the clinical picture of the patient the codes must be more precise than those needed only for statistical groupings and trend analysis.

Characteristics of ICD-10-CM

ICD-10-CM far exceeds its predecessors in the number of concepts and codes provided. The disease classification has been expanded to include health-related conditions and to provide greater specificity at the sixth and seventh character level.

The sixth and seventh characters are not optional and are intended for use in recording the information documented in the clinical record. ICD-10-CM extensions, interpretations, modifications, addenda, or errata other than those approved by the Centers for Disease Control and Prevention are not to be considered official and should not be utilized. Continuous maintenance of the ICD-10-CM is the responsibility of the aforementioned agencies. However, because the ICD-10-CM represents the best in contemporary thinking of clinicians, nosologists, epidemiologists, and statisticians from both public and private sectors, when future modifications are considered, advice will be sought from all stakeholders. All official authorized addenda since the last complete update have been included in this revision. For more detailed information please see the complete official authorized addenda to ICD-10-CM, including the "ICD-10-CM Official Guidelines for Coding and Reporting," and a description of the ICD-10-CM updating and maintenance process.

Features of 2018 ICD-10-CM

This *2018 ICD-10-CM* edition includes the following features, designed in consultation with coding consultants and ICD-10 trainers, to provide a comprehensive and easy-to-use reference manual:

- A table of contents page
- The complete 2018 ICD-10-CM code set
- Full code descriptions
- Special color coding throughout to highlight instructional notes, bilateral and unilateral indicators, and other features
- Color coding and symbols for Medicare code edits to highlight age, sex, manifestation, other specified and unspecified codes, and MACRA codes required for quality and cost measures reporting under the Merit-based Incentive Payment System (MIPS)
- Illustrations at the beginning of the book and throughout the Tabular List
- ICD-10-CM conventions
- ICD-10-CM Official Guidelines for Coding and Reporting
- Official Index to Diseases and Injuries
- Official Index to External Causes of Injuries
- Table of Drugs and Chemicals
- Table of Neoplasms
- Extension "X" symbol to alert readers to the ICD-10-CM placeholder "x" convention
- Anatomy and physiology for various body systems, including illustrations and pathologies
- Trimester icon for applicable codes
- HCC and RxHCC icons
- Vertical yellow rule in the Alphabetic Index to Diseases and Injuries and Index to External Causes of Injuries

List of Features

ICD-10-CM is essential to documenting medical necessity for services rendered, and accurate codes mean better outcomes for the patient, your claims, and your practice or facility.

Count on this manual to help you choose and report the right ICD-10-CM code. Unique features, intuitive design, and expert features that coders developed assure this manual will keep your coding on target.

This manual includes the ICD-10-CM complete code set for 2018, including the Tabular List, Alphabetic Index to Diseases and Injuries, Table of Neoplasms, Table of Drugs and Chemicals, and Index to External Causes of Injuries, effective October 1, 2017.

To help you make the most of *2018 ICD-10-CM*, this manual also includes the following features:

- ICD-10-CM Official Guidelines for Coding and Reporting for 2018. The Health Insurance Portability and Accountability Act (HIPAA) requires all entities assigning ICD-10-CM codes to follow these guidelines.

- Guideline Tips for each chapter of the relevant ICD-10-CM Official Guidelines in easy-to-understand lay language are located on the publisher's website

- Anatomy and physiology descriptions before Tabular List chapters containing codes pertaining to specific body anatomy

- Full illustrations of body systems at the front of the book so you don't have to search the manual for these large color images of body systems

- Illustrations of anatomy and conditions throughout the Tabular List to help you to better understand how to assign specific codes

- AHA *Coding Clinic*® article references from the quarterly publication of the American Hospital Association

- Symbols indicating "Additional character required" so you know when a code requires an additional character for code specificity and validity (provided in both the Alphabetic Index and Tabular List)

- Age and sex edits showing which codes have restrictions on use based on age or sex of the patient

- Highlighted coding instructional and informational notes help you recognize important code usage guidance for specific sections including Includes, Excludes1, and Excludes2 notes

- Z code as first-listed diagnosis symbol to alert you when you can only assign a Z code as the first-listed diagnosis

- HCC and RxHCC symbols to alert you to HCC and RxHCC diagnoses

- Intuitive color-coded symbols and alerts identify critical coding and reimbursement issues quickly, such as "Other Specified" and "Unspecified" diagnosis alerts, along with MACRA codes shown in red

- Manifestation code alerts so you properly use codes that represent manifestations of an underlying disease and know when you must use two codes

- A user-friendly page design, including dictionary-style headers, color bleed tabs, and legend keys

- Key word green font is used to differentiate key words that appear in similar code descriptions in a given category.

- Symbols indicating new code, revised code, or revised text

- Stick-on tabs to use for main sections of the book, including each Tabular List chapter

- Appendix including Z codes for long-term use of drugs organized by drug name

- Appendix including 7-character codes for symbols throughout the book

- Notes pages following each Tabular List chapter to record important coding notes

Practical Steps for Using the ICD-10-CM Book

This manual includes the diagnosis code set from the International Classification of Diseases, 10th Revision, Clinical Modification (ICD-10-CM) 2018.

Understand Code Structure to Choose the Most Specific Code

ICD-10-CM codes are made up of a minimum of three characters and a maximum of seven characters:

- Character 1 – capital letter A-Z, except the letter U, which is not used
- Character 2 – number
- Character 3 – number
- Character 4 – number or letter – capital or lowercase
- Character 5 – number or letter – capital or lowercase
- Character 6 – number or letter – capital or lowercase
- Character 7 – number or letter – capital or lowercase; character 7 is only used in specific chapters, including pregnancy, musculoskeletal, injuries, and external causes of morbidity

Each Tabular List chapter is divided into subchapters, which are also called blocks. Subchapters are divided into groups of categories (3 characters).

Subchapters are divided into:

Categories (3 characters) – Represents one disease or a group of diseases or related conditions. If a category does not have a further subdivision, it is called a code.

Categories are divided into:

Subcategories (4-5 characters) – Represents greater specificity of one disease or a group of diseases.

Subcategories are divided into:

Codes (4-7 characters) – Codes are the final level which cannot be subdivided further. Codes that are 7 characters are always called "codes" because 7 is the maximum number of characters in a code.

Review the ICD-10-CM Volumes Included in This Manual

This manual includes:

- Tabular List, includes diagnosis codes in numerical order and their official descriptors in 21 chapters
- Alphabetic Index, includes three sections:
  - Index to Diseases and Injuries, which you'll use to search for the vast majority of codes

  - Two tables you'll find at the end of the Index to Diseases:
    - Table of Neoplasms
    - Table of Drugs and Chemicals
  - Alphabetic Index to External Cause of Injuries

This manual follows the industry standard of placing the Alphabetic Index before the Tabular List because when you search for a code, you should always check the Index first to make a preliminary code choice and then check the Tabular List for confirmation.

Code Diagnoses With Confidence Following This Approach

- ➢ The first step in choosing the proper ICD-10-CM code is reading the medical documentation to identify the diagnosis the provider documents and confirms. If there is no confirmed diagnosis, look for the sign or symptom that brought the patient in or other reason for the encounter.
  - Be sure to check online or hard copy references, such as medical dictionaries and anatomy resources to look up unfamiliar terms.
- ➢ Next, decide which main term you will search in the Index based on the patient's specific case. ICD-10-CM doesn't use body sites as main terms. Instead, look for the disease, sign, symptom, etc. You can find the body site as a subterm. For neoplasm diagnoses, review the Table of Neoplasms for the appropriate diagnosis. Search for the neoplasm histology as a main term (carcinoma, leukemia, glioblastoma) and the body site as a subterm. The histology will take you to a code to cross-reference to the Tabular or direct you to the Table of Neoplasms. If you cannot find the histology as a main term, or cannot find a code to cross-reference for the histology and body site, then go directly to the Table of Neoplasms to search for the body site of the neoplasm. You will also need to go directly to the Table of Neoplasms if the provider does not document the histology.
- ➢ Once you find the main term in the Index, note the recommended code. Start with the main term and review any available subterms. Also note whether the Index offers any other clues to proper coding, such as the need for additional characters or the need for an additional code.
- ➢ Turn to that code in the Tabular List, and read the full code descriptor. Keep in mind that you may need to read the subcategory and category titles as well as the code descriptor to get the full meaning of the code.
- ➢ Check to see whether ICD-10-CM requires additional characters for that code. If so, review the code definitions of any available categories and subcategories.

- Remember, if a code has seven characters available, you must report all seven characters, both to comply with coding rules and to prevent insurers from denying your claim. Similarly, if a code has four characters, with no fifth character available, you must report all four characters rather than a three-character code. This manual will alert you to the need for an additional character using easily identifiable symbols.

➢ If the Index points you to a code that includes the terms other, unspecified, NOS (not otherwise specified), or NEC (not elsewhere classifiable), double check that a more specific code isn't available. Always report the most specific code the medical record supports.

➢ Before making your final code decision, review all applicable notes and instructions to be sure they don't affect your choice. You'll find these notes and instructions on every level, from the chapter to the code itself. You will find many notes highlighted and color coded for easy reference in the Tabular List. You can find the meaning of the highlights in the legend at the bottom of each page in the Tabular List. Also review the surrounding codes to be sure there isn't a more appropriate code available.

➢ Finally, take a moment to confirm that your code choice complies with the philosophy of ethical coding. Never report an ICD-10-CM code simply because it will support reimbursement from a payer. Report only those codes the documentation supports.

Factor In the Other Resources in This Manual

In addition to the Alphabetic Index and Tabular List, you'll find the following materials in this manual:

Symbols and Conventions Specific to This ICD-10-CM Manual: To be sure you make the most of all of the resources and instructional symbols this manual includes, read this section.

ICD-10-CM Official Guidelines for Coding and Reporting: No coder should let a year go by without reviewing the Official Guidelines. These authoritative rules provide many instructions not available in the Tabular List.

Additional Content in Tabular List Chapters: At the beginning of specific Tabular List chapters, you'll find anatomy descriptions and the publisher's website also includes a useful breakdown of the relevant Official Guidelines specific to codes in that chapter.

Symbols and Conventions

Additional Characters Required

- [4th] This red symbol cautions that the code requires an additional fourth character.
- [5th] This red symbol cautions that the code requires an additional fifth character.
- [6th] This red symbol cautions that the code requires an additional sixth character.
- [7th] This red symbol cautions that the code requires an additional seventh character.

Extension "X" Alert

- [x7th] This blue symbol cautions that the code requires an additional seventh character following the placeholder X.

Medicare Code Edits Symbols and Colors

Code edit symbols and colors in this manual are based on the Medicare Code Editor (MCE) and Medicare's Integrated Outpatient Code Editor (I/OCE). The code edit information in this manual is based on MCE v34 with the addition of FY 2018 Inpatient Prospective Payment System (IPPS) Proposed Rule updates for the most current information available at the time of printing.

Age Conflict

Medicare's MCE and I/OCE code editors detect inconsistencies between a patient's age and any diagnosis on the patient's record. Examples include: a five-year-old patient with benign prostatic hypertrophy or a 78-year-old patient coded with a delivery.

[N]	Newborn	Age of 0 years; a subset of diagnoses intended only for newborns and neonates (e.g., fetal distress, perinatal jaundice).
[P]	Pediatric	Age range is 0–17 years inclusive (e.g., Reye's syndrome, routine child health exam).
[M]	Maternity	Age range is 12–55 years inclusive (e.g., diabetes in pregnancy, antepartum pulmonary complication).
[A]	Adult	Age range is 18–124 years inclusive (e.g., senile delirium, mature cataract).

Sex Conflict

Medicare's MCE and I/OCE code editors detect inconsistencies between a patient's sex and any diagnosis or procedure on the patient's record. Examples include: a male patient with cervical cancer (diagnosis) or a female patient with a prostatectomy (procedure).

In both instances, the indicated diagnosis or the procedure conflicts with the stated sex of the patient. Therefore, either the patient's diagnosis, procedure or sex is presumed to be incorrect.

- ♂ Male code symbol
- ♀ Female code symbol

Manifestation Codes

The code description is highlighted with a light blue color. Manifestation codes describe the manifestation of an underlying disease, not the disease itself, and therefore should not be used as a primary diagnosis.

Other Symbols and Color Coding

Key Terms

Bold green font is used in code descriptions throughout the Tabular List to quickly identify key terms in a given category.

MACRA code

MACRA codes are identified in pink

Other Specified Codes

The code description is highlighted with gray color. These codes are assigned when the documentation indicates a specified diagnosis, but the ICD-10-CM code set does not have a specific code that describes the condition.

Unspecified Codes

The code description is highlighted with yellow color. These codes are assigned when neither the diagnostic statement nor the documentation provides enough information to assign a more specific code.

Sequencing, Admission, Complication, and Comorbidity

When relevant, you'll see the following symbols to the right of the code descriptor:

[PDx]	Unacceptable principal diagnosis; based on Medicare code edits
[POA]	Code exempt from diagnosis present on admission requirement; based on ICD-10-CM Official Guidelines
[CC]	Complication or comorbidity; based on CMS data
[MCC]	Major complication or comorbidity; based on CMS data
[CC/MCC Exc]	Complications or comorbidities/Major complications or comorbidities (CC/MCC) exclusions; based on CMS data; please refer to the MS-DRG manual v. 34.0 Appendix C to review the links of principal diagnoses for each CC/MCC exclusion
[HAC]	Hospital-acquired condition (HAC) alert; based on CMS data
[PDx CC]	Principal diagnosis as its own complication or comorbidity; based on CMS data
[PDx MCC]	Principal diagnosis as its own major complication or comorbidity; based on CMS data
[?]	Questionable admission when used as principal diagnosis symbol; based on Medicare code edits
[HCC]	HCC diagnosis codes
[RxHCC]	RxHCC diagnosis codes
[Z-1]	Z code as first-listed diagnosis; certain codes may only be reported as the primary/first-listed diagnosis, except when there are multiple encounters on the same day and the medical records for the encounters are combined.

EXCLUDES 1	Not coded here Excludes1 notes are highlighted in black to alert you to NEVER assign codes listed under Excludes1 along with the code that you cross-referenced, with some exceptions.
EXCLUDES 2	Not included here Excludes2 notes are highlighted in gray to alert you that you most likely will not assign codes listed under Excludes2 along with the code that you cross-referenced. However, you could assign both an Excludes2 code with the cross-referenced code, as long as the provider documents both conditions.
INCLUDES	The word "Includes" appears immediately under certain categories to further define, or give examples of, the content of the category
NOTES	Notes appear throughout the Tabular List to provide additional coding information.
Code first	Code first notes appear throughout the Tabular List to provide the code to assign first.
Use additional code	Use additional code notes appear throughout the Tabular List to identify when to assign a code in addition to the principal or primary diagnosis.
1st	The 1st trimester symbol appears with applicable codes that apply to the first trimester.
2nd	The 2nd trimester symbol appears with applicable codes that apply to the second trimester.
3rd	3rd trimester symbol appears with applicable codes that apply to the third trimester.
● New Code	The new code symbol appears with a code that is new for the current year.
▲ Revised Code Title	A revised code title symbol appears with a code title that is revised for the current year.
▶◀ Revised Text	The revised text facing triangles symbol appears before and after text that is revised for the current year.

Citations to AHA's *Coding Clinic®* for ICD-10-CM

AHA's *Coding Clinic®*, a quarterly newsletter, is the official publication for coding guidelines and advice as designated by the four Cooperating Parties (American Hospital Association, American Health Information Management Association, Centers for Medicare and Medicaid Services (CMS), and National Center for Health Statistics) and the Editorial Advisory Board.

AHA   We've marked codes with related *Coding Clinic®* articles with a citation that includes the quarter and year of the issue.

Anatomical Illustrations

Circulatory System — Arteries and Veins

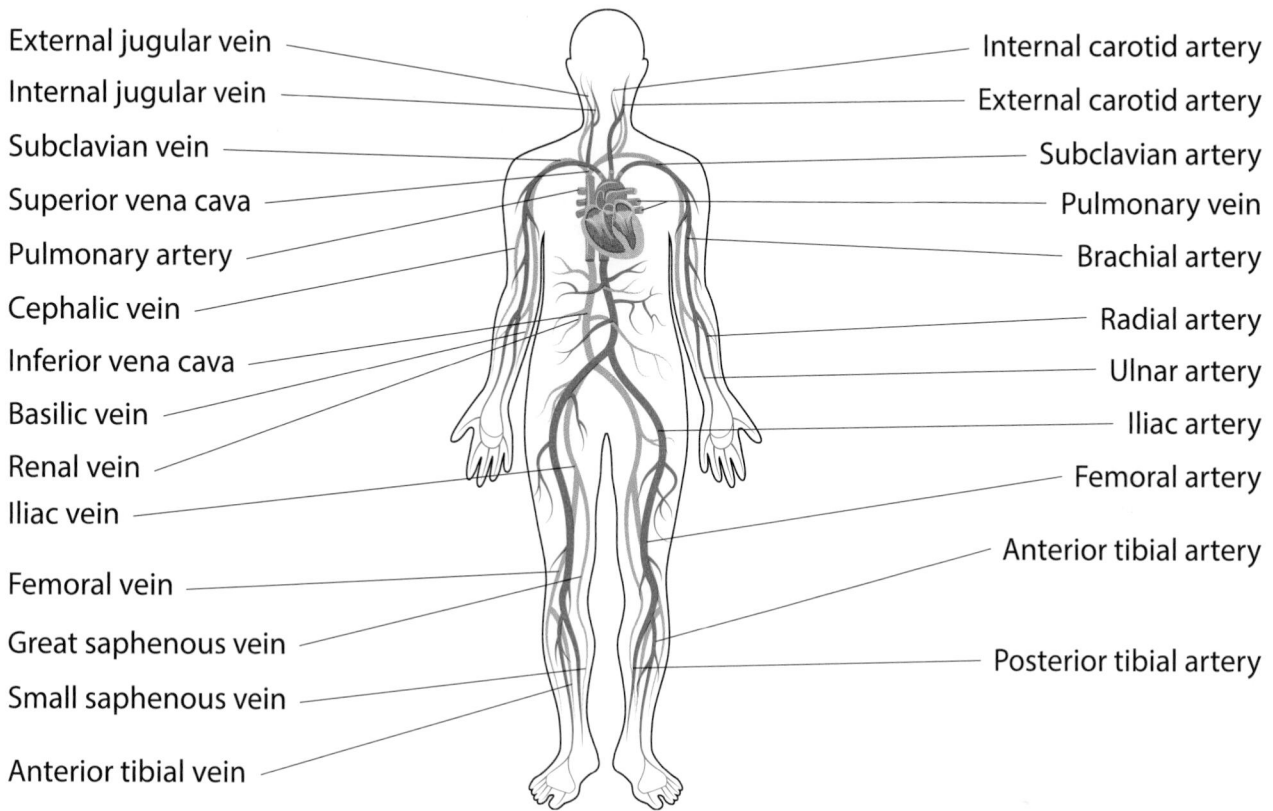

External jugular vein

Internal jugular vein

Subclavian vein

Superior vena cava

Pulmonary artery

Cephalic vein

Inferior vena cava

Basilic vein

Renal vein

Iliac vein

Femoral vein

Great saphenous vein

Small saphenous vein

Anterior tibial vein

Internal carotid artery

External carotid artery

Subclavian artery

Pulmonary vein

Brachial artery

Radial artery

Ulnar artery

Iliac artery

Femoral artery

Anterior tibial artery

Posterior tibial artery

Circulatory System — Artery and Vein Anatomy

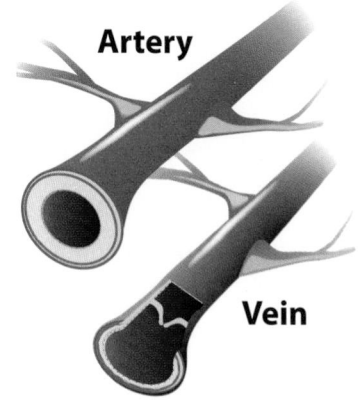

Artery

Vein

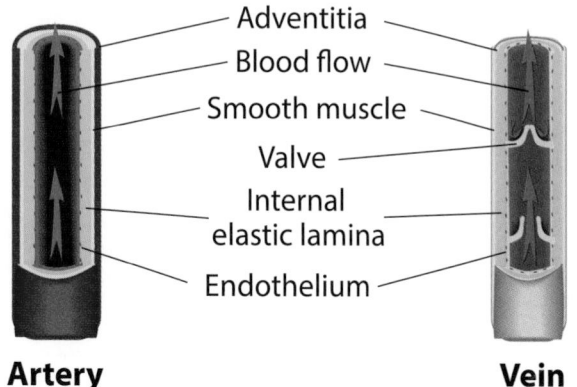

Adventitia

Blood flow

Smooth muscle

Valve

Internal elastic lamina

Endothelium

Artery

Vein

Circulatory System — Heart Anatomy and Cardiac Cycle

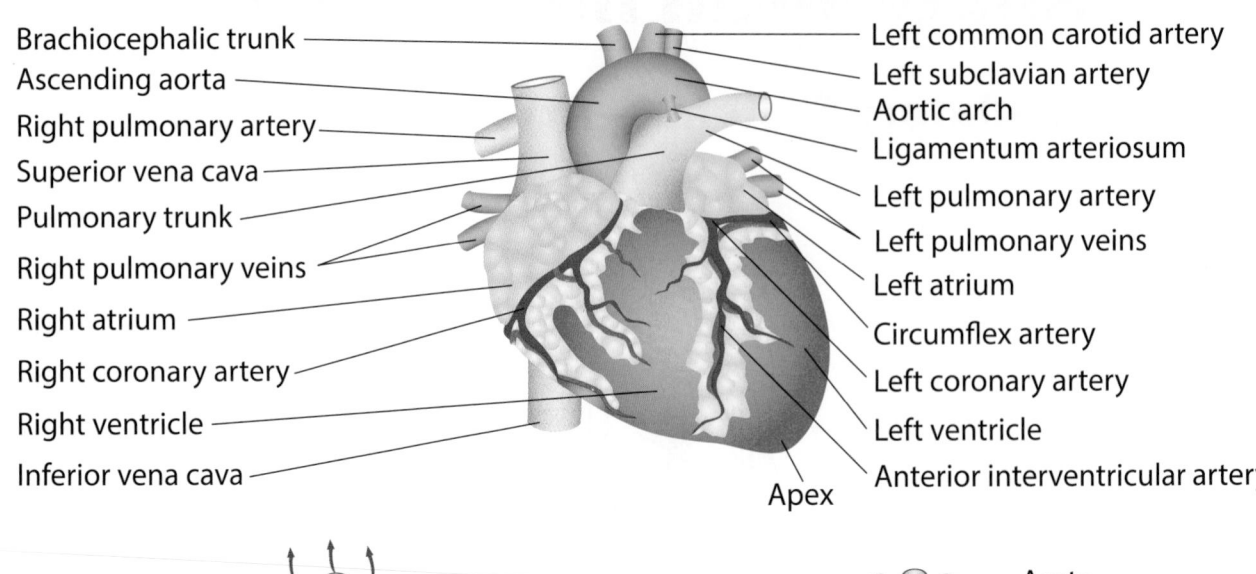

Brachiocephalic trunk
Ascending aorta
Right pulmonary artery
Superior vena cava
Pulmonary trunk
Right pulmonary veins
Right atrium
Right coronary artery
Right ventricle
Inferior vena cava

Left common carotid artery
Left subclavian artery
Aortic arch
Ligamentum arteriosum
Left pulmonary artery
Left pulmonary veins
Left atrium
Circumflex artery
Left coronary artery
Left ventricle
Anterior interventricular artery
Apex

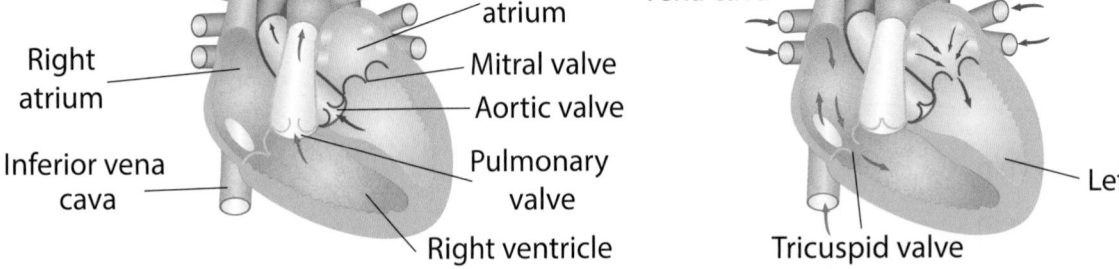

Right atrium
Inferior vena cava

Left atrium
Mitral valve
Aortic valve
Pulmonary valve
Right ventricle

**Diastole Ventricular
Relaxation and Filling**

Superior vena cava

Aorta
Pulmonary artery

Tricuspid valve

Left ventricle

**Systole Ventricular
Contraction and Ejection**

Digestive System — Digestive Organs

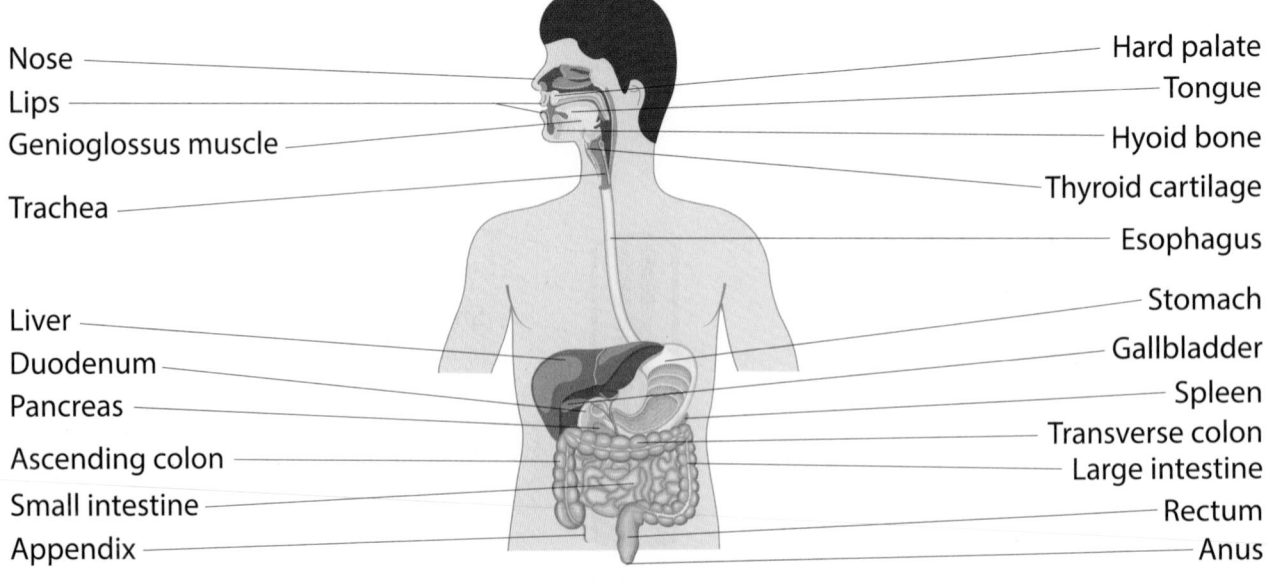

Nose
Lips
Genioglossus muscle
Trachea

Liver
Duodenum
Pancreas
Ascending colon
Small intestine
Appendix

Hard palate
Tongue
Hyoid bone
Thyroid cartilage
Esophagus
Stomach
Gallbladder
Spleen
Transverse colon
Large intestine
Rectum
Anus

ANATOMICAL ILLUSTRATIONS

Digestive System — Large Intestine Anatomy

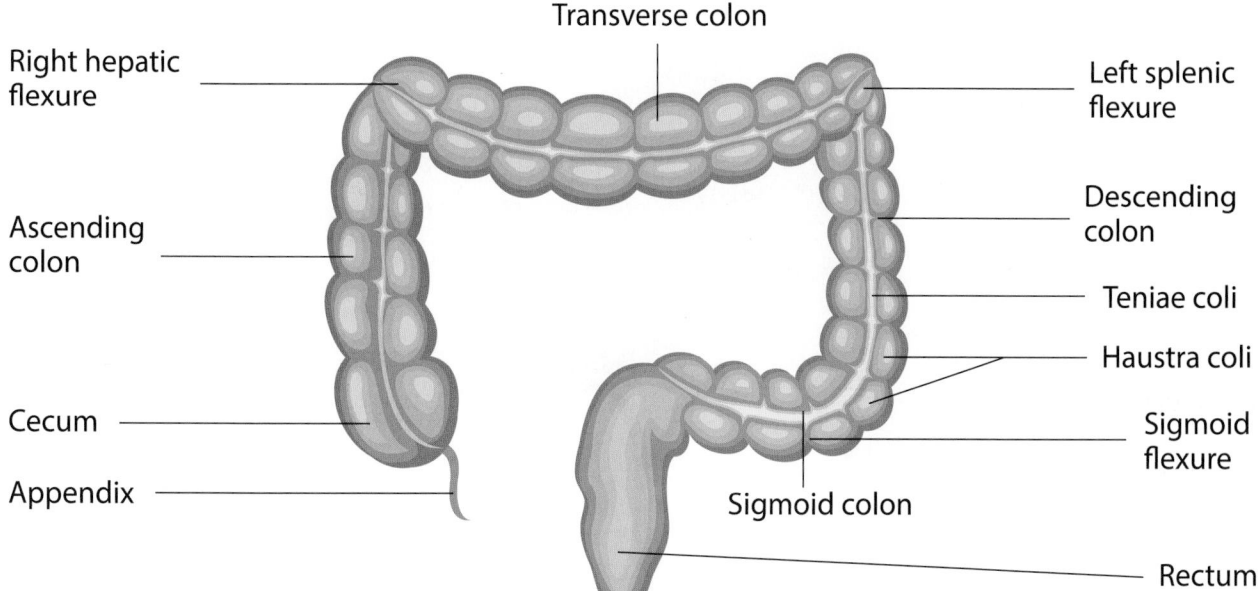

Transverse colon

Right hepatic flexure

Left splenic flexure

Ascending colon

Descending colon

Teniae coli

Haustra coli

Cecum

Sigmoid flexure

Appendix

Sigmoid colon

Rectum

Digestive System — Rectum Anatomy

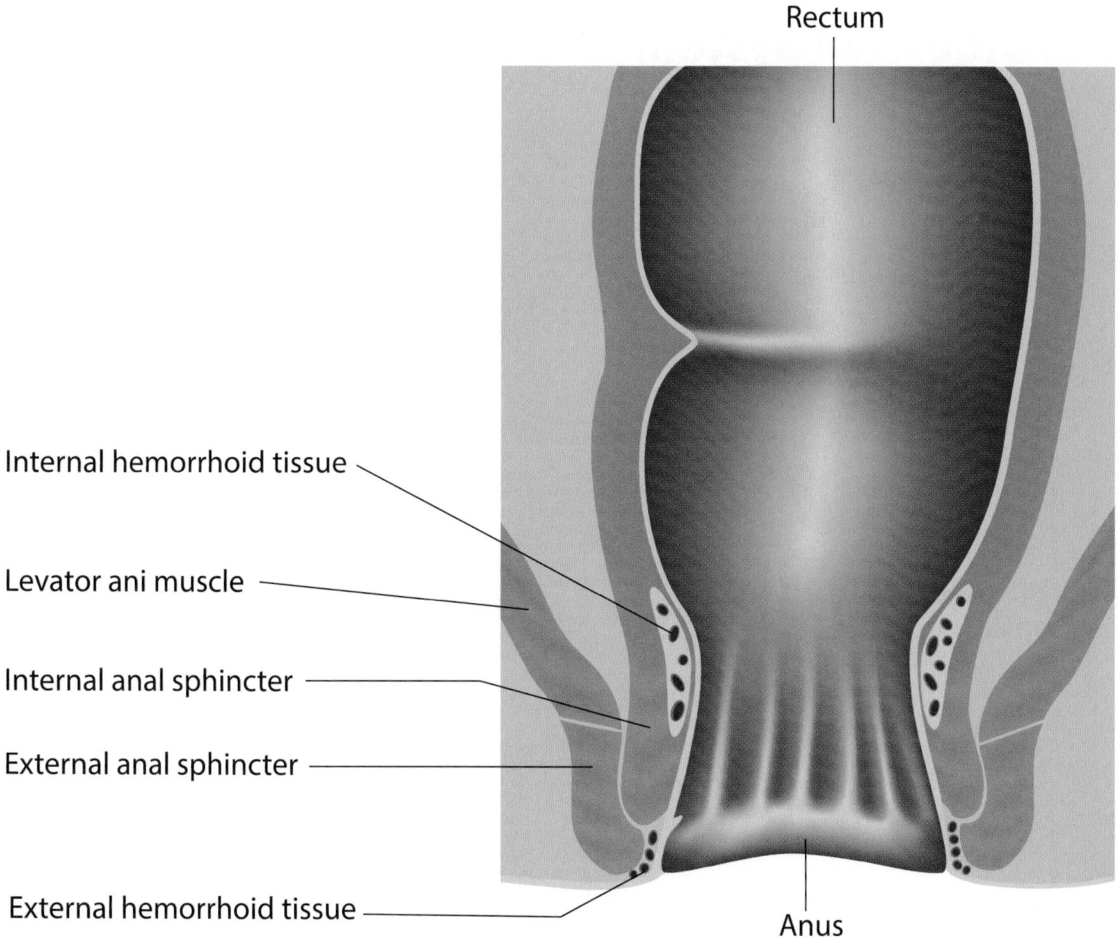

Rectum

Internal hemorrhoid tissue

Levator ani muscle

Internal anal sphincter

External anal sphincter

External hemorrhoid tissue

Anus

Digestive System — Liver Anatomy

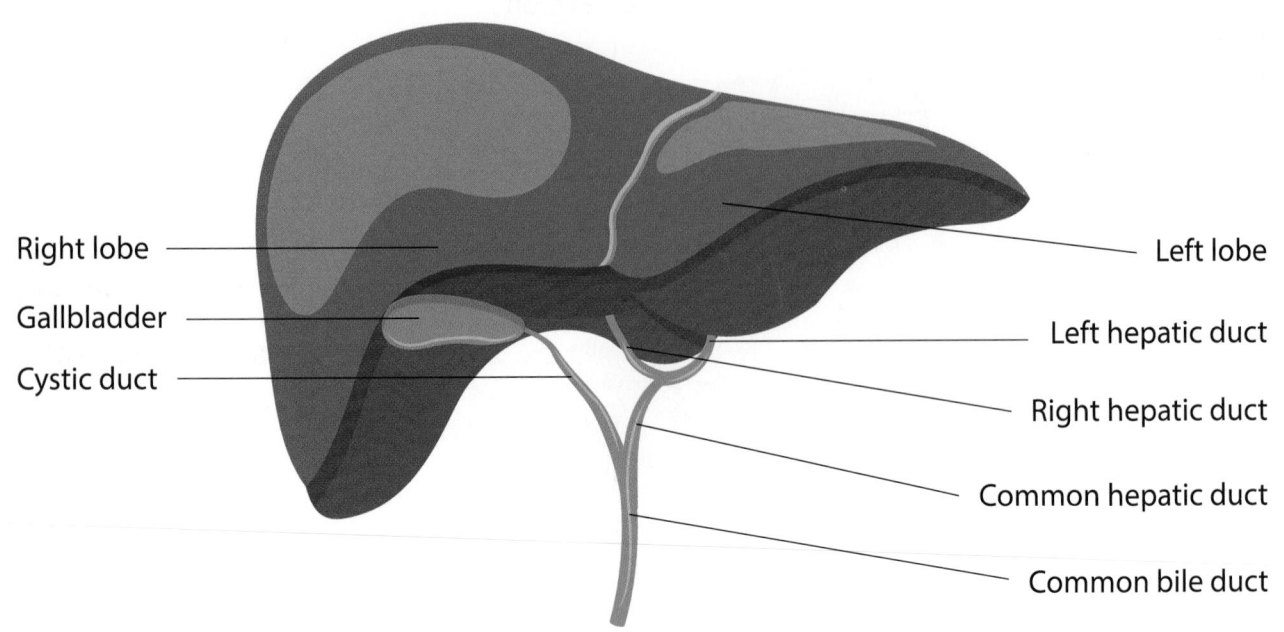

Right lobe

Gallbladder

Cystic duct

Left lobe

Left hepatic duct

Right hepatic duct

Common hepatic duct

Common bile duct

Digestive System — Pancreas Anatomy

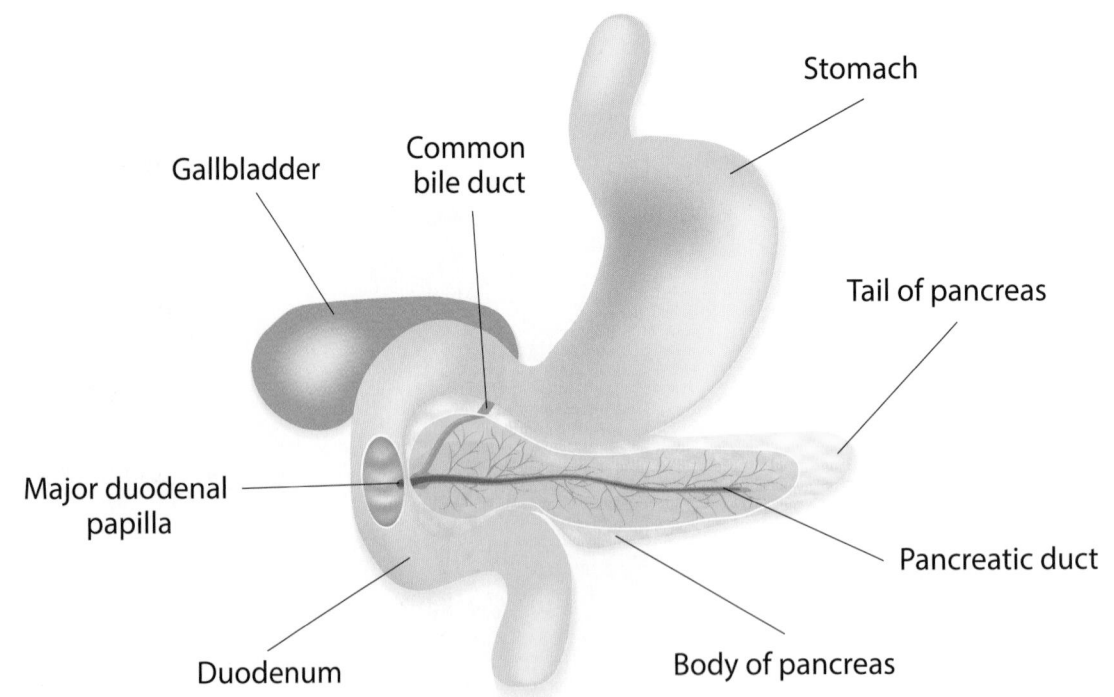

Gallbladder

Common bile duct

Stomach

Tail of pancreas

Major duodenal papilla

Duodenum

Pancreatic duct

Body of pancreas

Digestive System — Mouth Anatomy

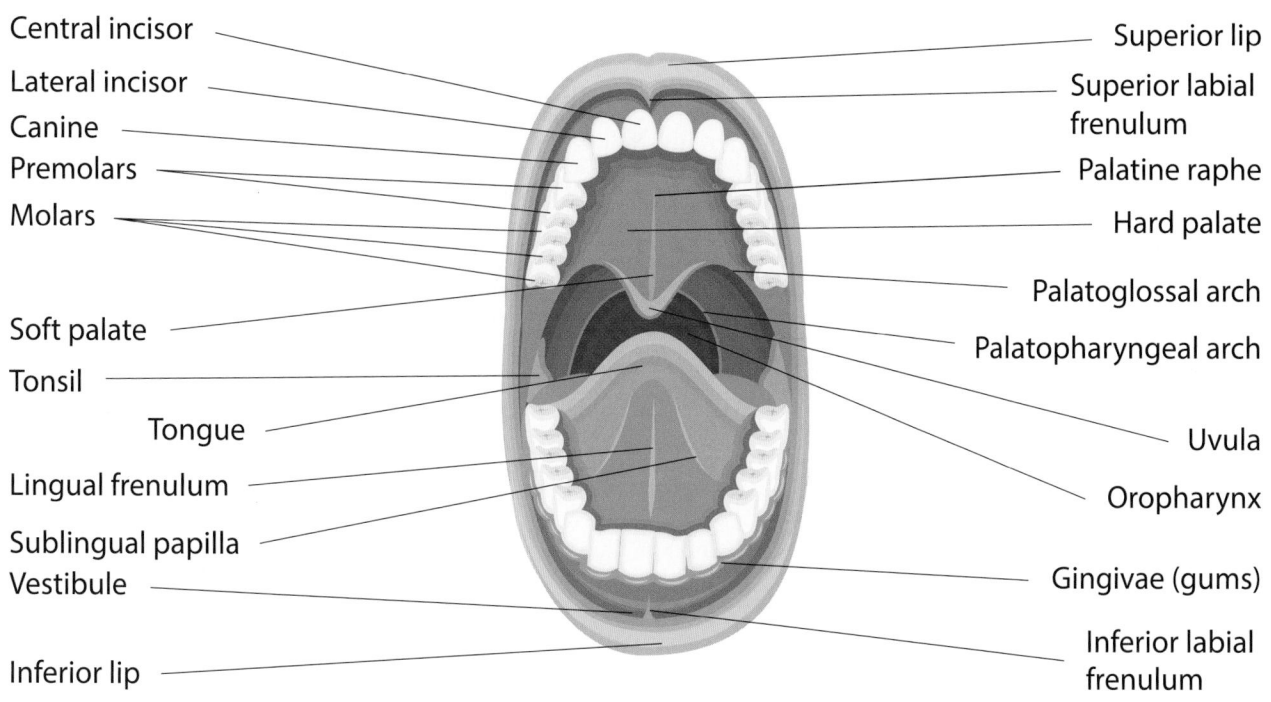

Central incisor
Lateral incisor
Canine
Premolars
Molars

Soft palate
Tonsil
Tongue
Lingual frenulum
Sublingual papilla
Vestibule

Inferior lip

Superior lip
Superior labial frenulum
Palatine raphe
Hard palate
Palatoglossal arch
Palatopharyngeal arch

Uvula
Oropharynx

Gingivae (gums)

Inferior labial frenulum

Digestive System — Tongue Anatomy

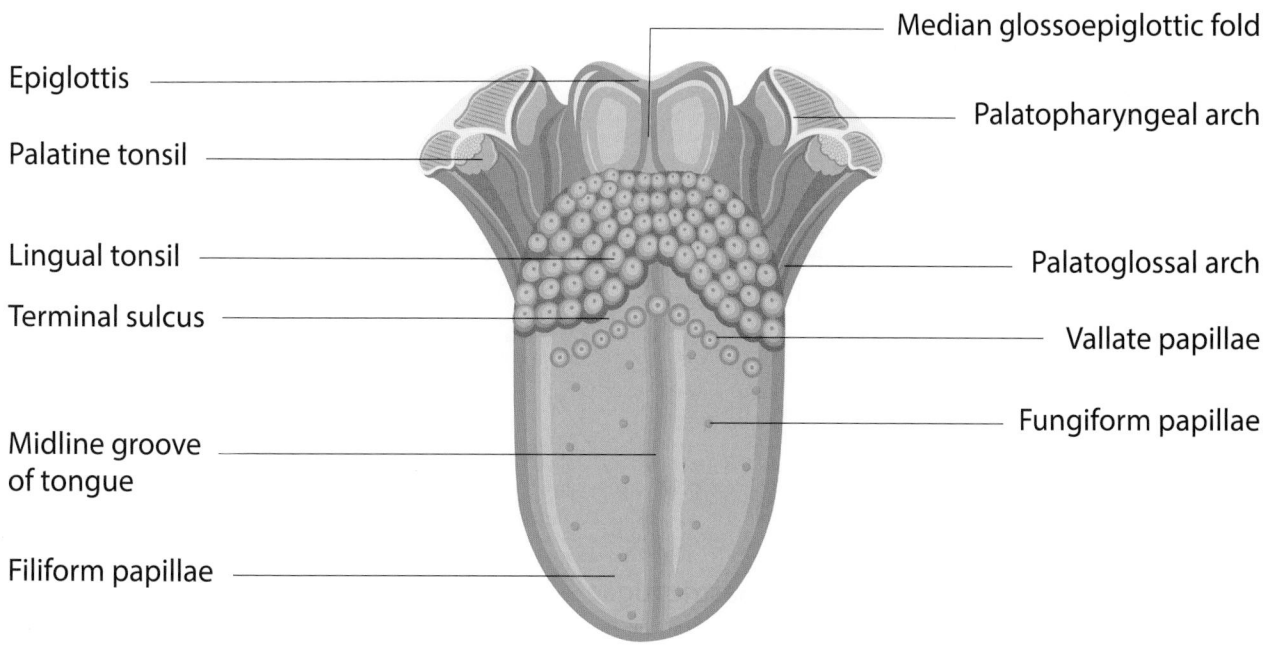

Epiglottis
Palatine tonsil

Lingual tonsil
Terminal sulcus

Midline groove of tongue

Filiform papillae

Median glossoepiglottic fold
Palatopharyngeal arch

Palatoglossal arch
Vallate papillae
Fungiform papillae

ANATOMICAL ILLUSTRATIONS

Digestive System — Small Intestine Anatomy

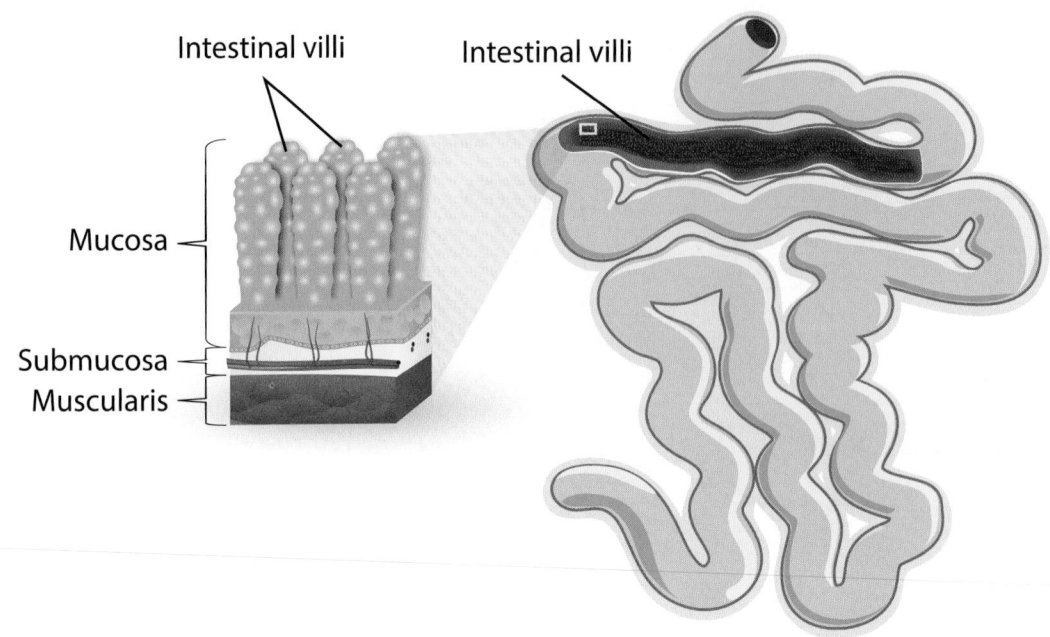

Intestinal villi

Intestinal villi

Mucosa

Submucosa

Muscularis

Digestive System — Stomach Anatomy

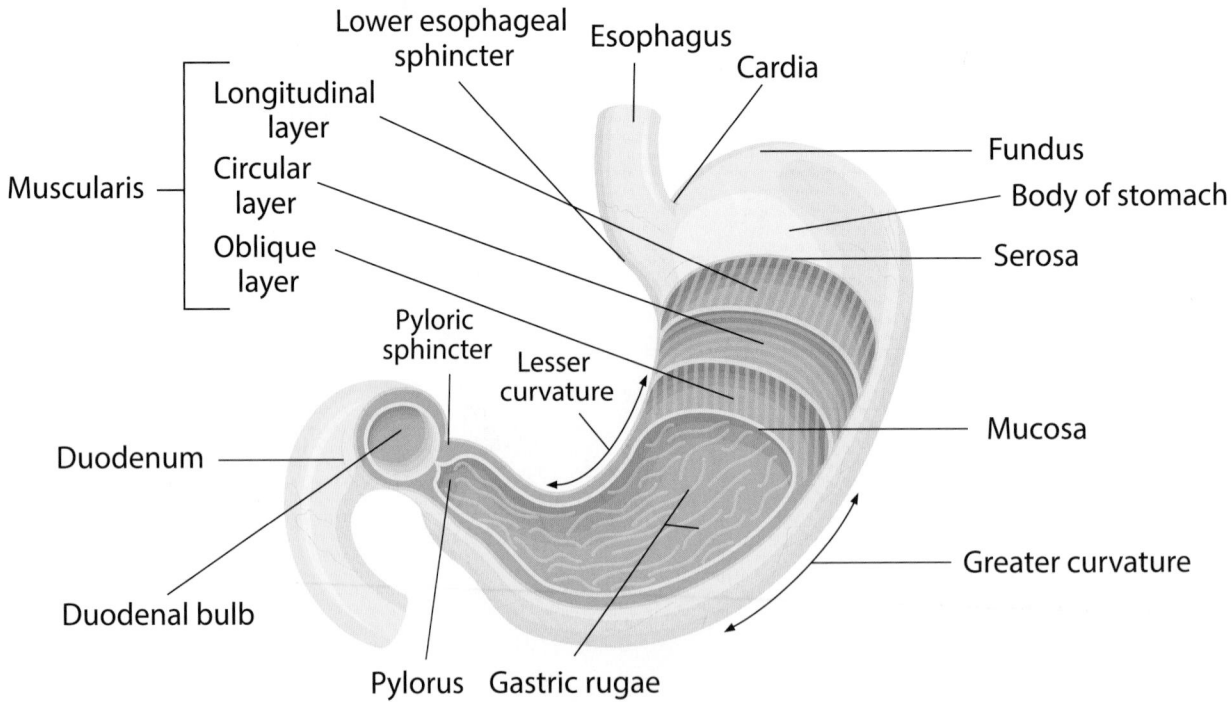

Lower esophageal sphincter

Esophagus

Cardia

Longitudinal layer

Circular layer

Oblique layer

Muscularis

Fundus

Body of stomach

Serosa

Pyloric sphincter

Lesser curvature

Duodenum

Mucosa

Duodenal bulb

Greater curvature

Pylorus   Gastric rugae

Ear Anatomy

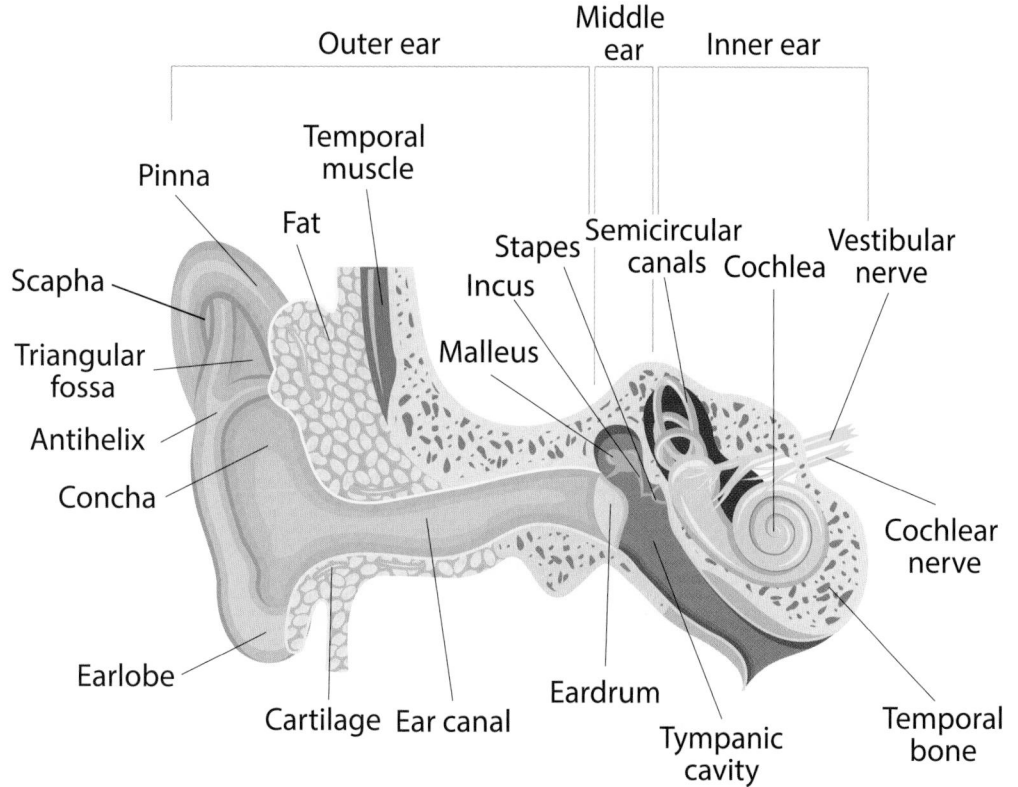

Cochlea Anatomy (Inner Ear)

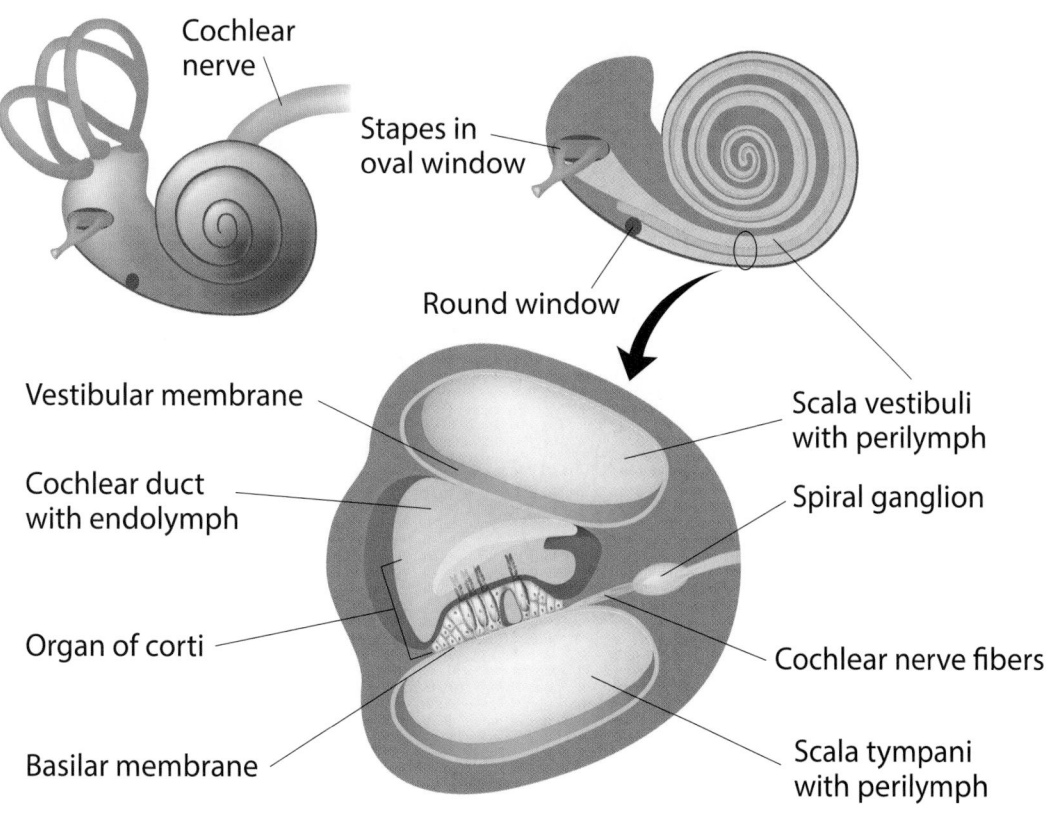

Endocrine System Anatomy

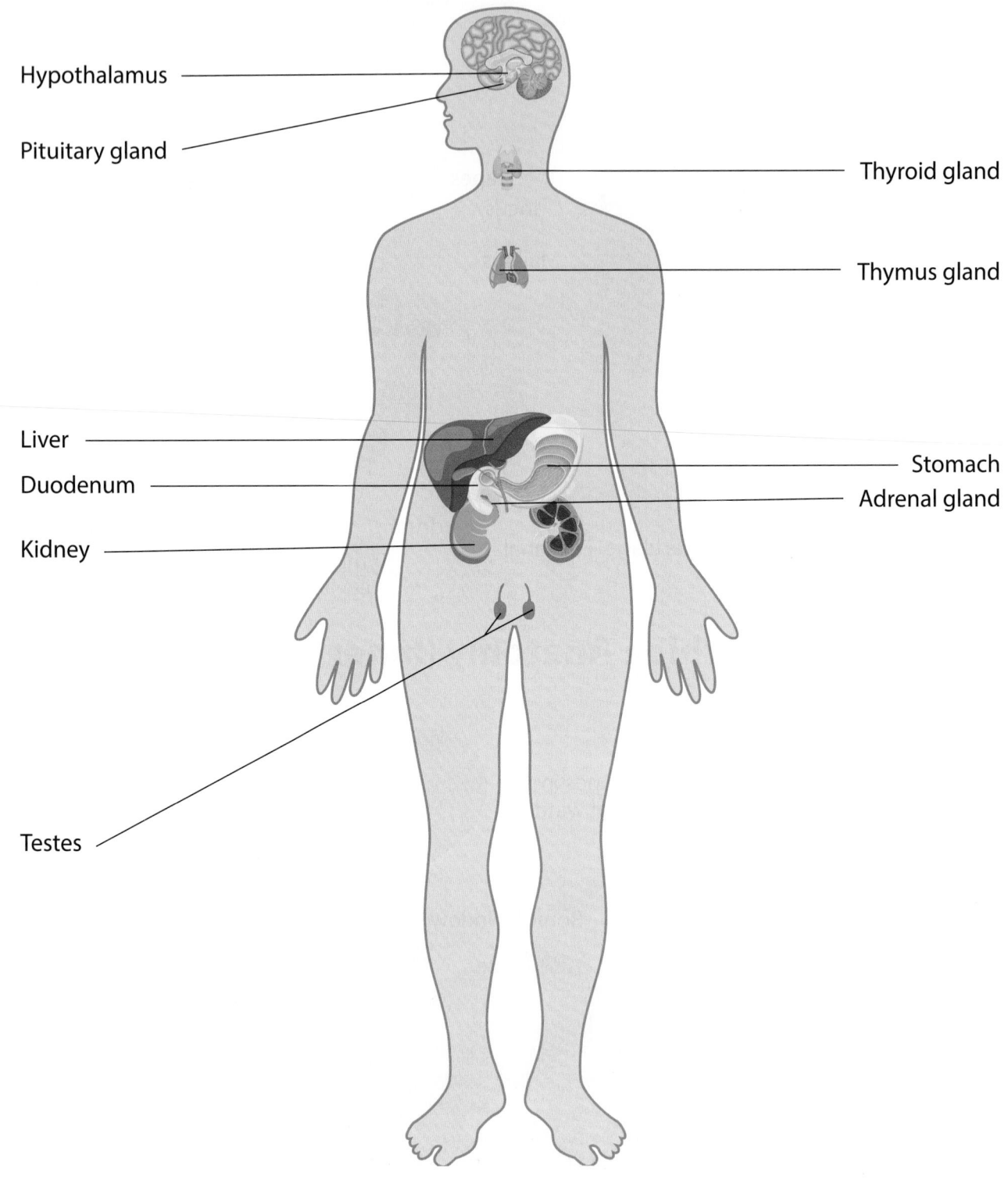

Hypothalamus

Pituitary gland

Thyroid gland

Thymus gland

Liver

Stomach

Duodenum

Adrenal gland

Kidney

Testes

Eye Anatomy

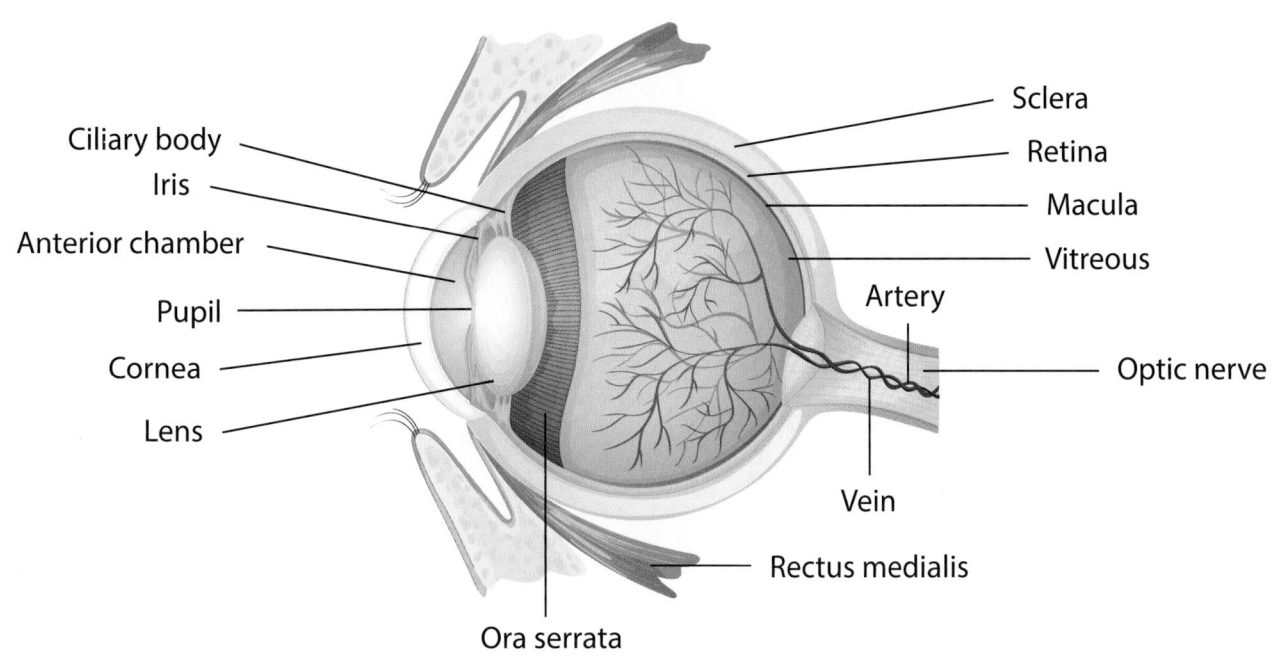

Ciliary body
Iris
Anterior chamber
Pupil
Cornea
Lens

Sclera
Retina
Macula
Vitreous
Artery
Optic nerve

Vein
Rectus medialis

Ora serrata

Muscles of the Eye

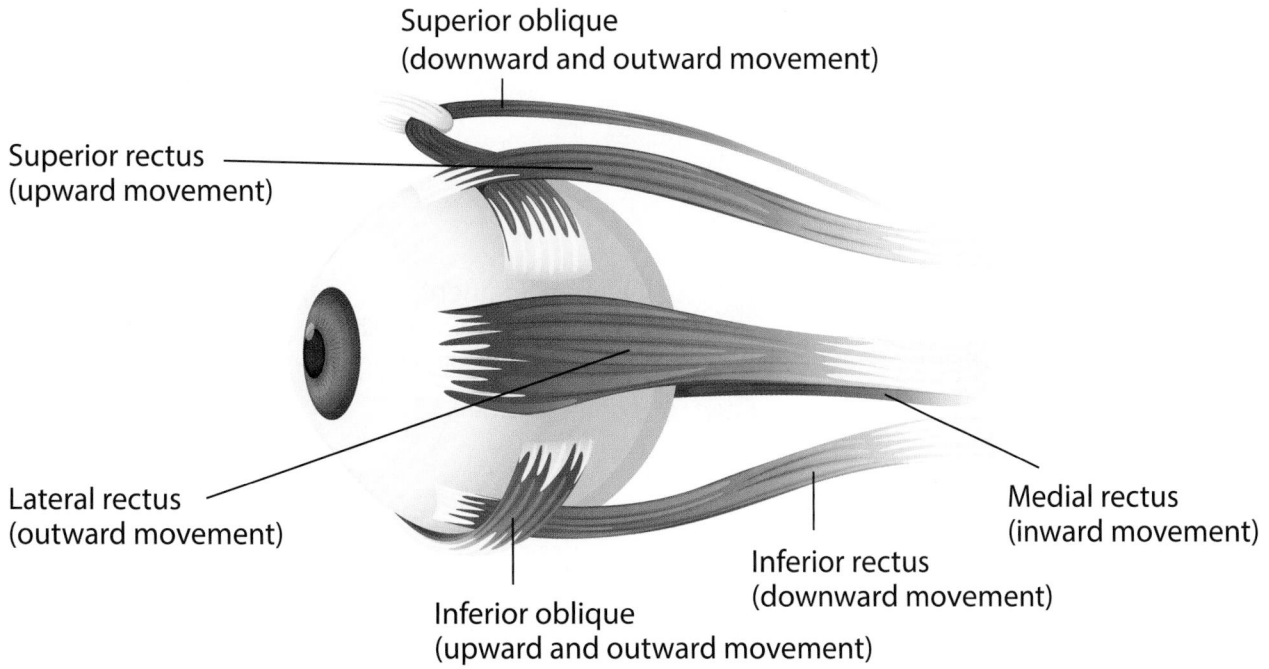

Superior oblique
(downward and outward movement)

Superior rectus
(upward movement)

Lateral rectus
(outward movement)

Inferior oblique
(upward and outward movement)

Inferior rectus
(downward movement)

Medial rectus
(inward movement)

Female Reproductive System Anatomy

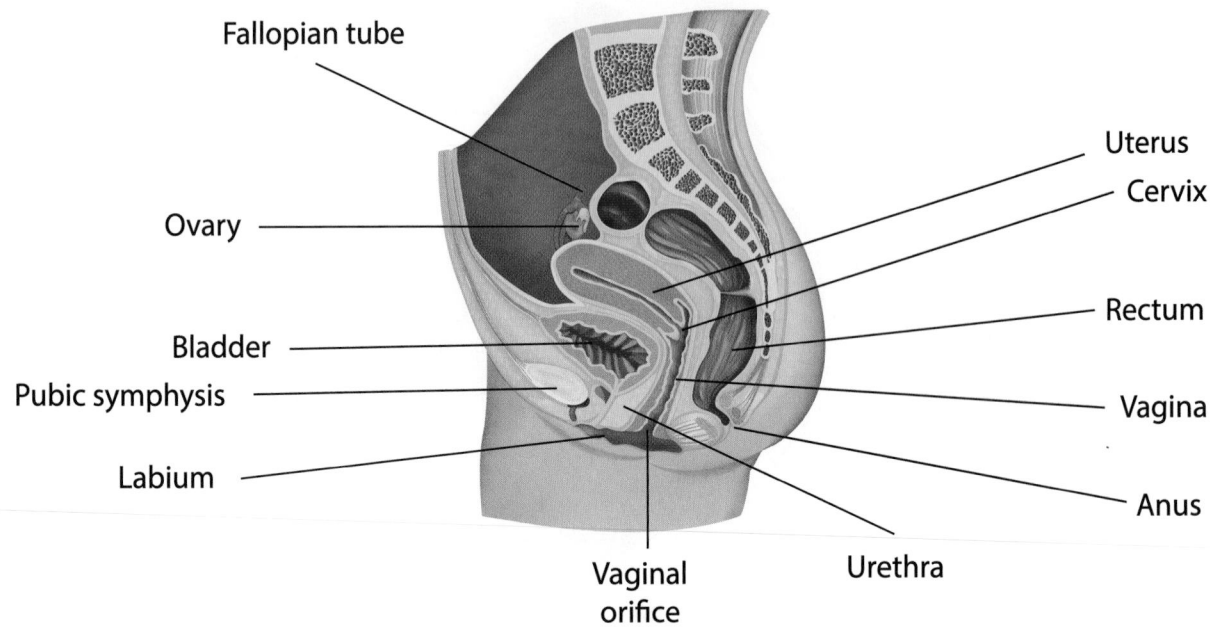

Fallopian tube

Ovary

Bladder

Pubic symphysis

Labium

Uterus

Cervix

Rectum

Vagina

Anus

Vaginal orifice

Urethra

Female Reproductive System — Uterus and Adnexa Anatomy

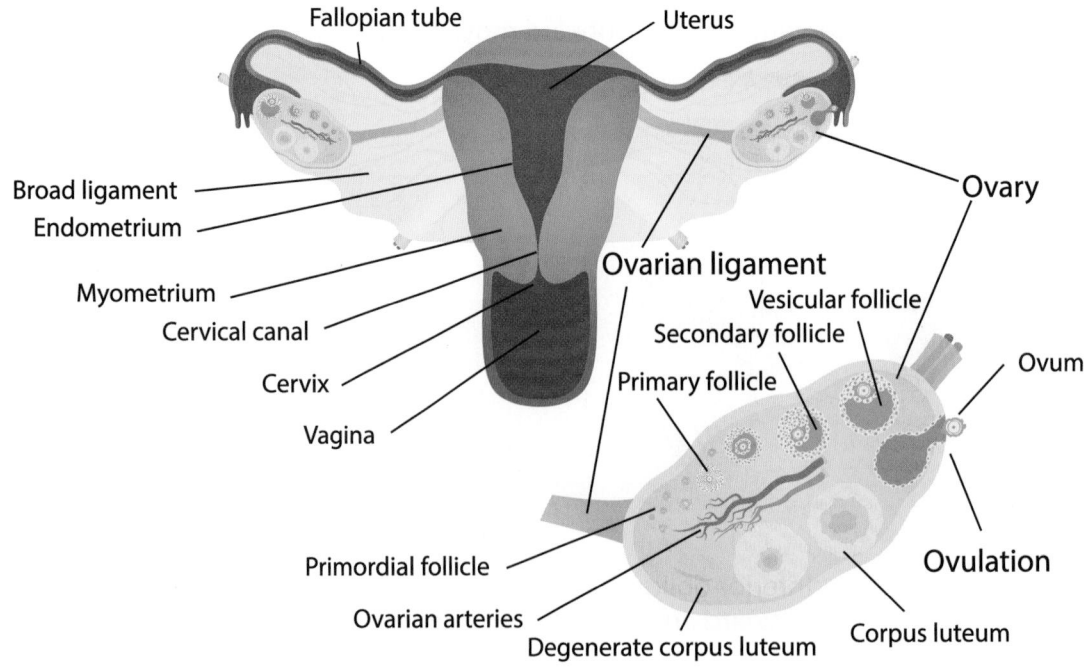

Fallopian tube

Uterus

Broad ligament

Endometrium

Myometrium

Cervical canal

Cervix

Vagina

Ovary

Ovarian ligament

Vesicular follicle

Secondary follicle

Primary follicle

Ovum

Primordial follicle

Ovarian arteries

Degenerate corpus luteum

Ovulation

Corpus luteum

ANATOMICAL ILLUSTRATIONS

Female Reproductive System — Breast Anatomy

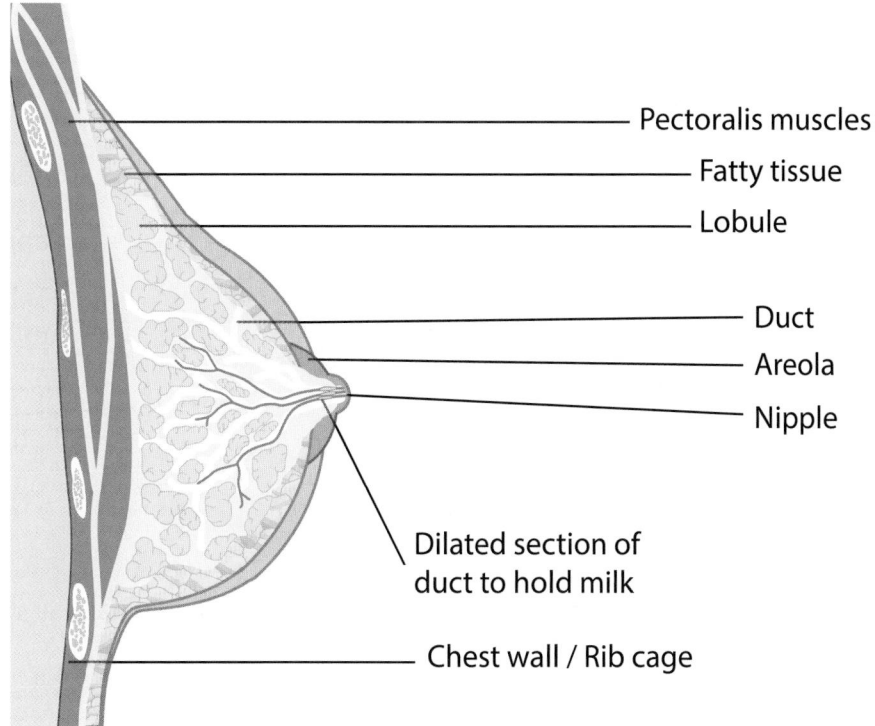

- Pectoralis muscles
- Fatty tissue
- Lobule
- Duct
- Areola
- Nipple
- Dilated section of duct to hold milk
- Chest wall / Rib cage

Female Reproductive System — Perineum Anatomy

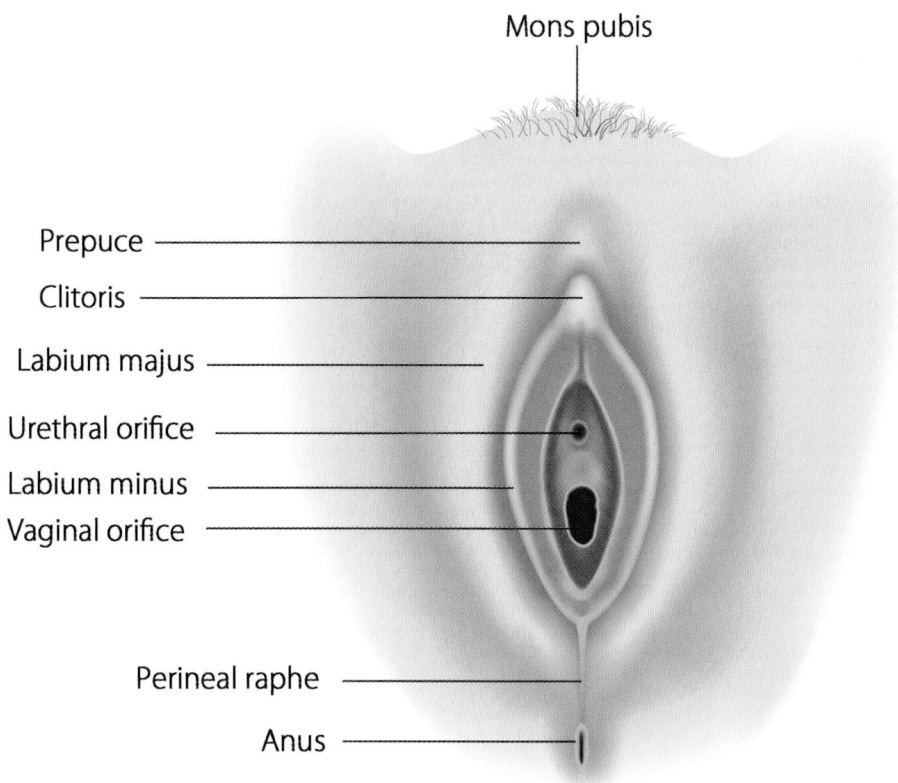

Mons pubis

- Prepuce
- Clitoris
- Labium majus
- Urethral orifice
- Labium minus
- Vaginal orifice
- Perineal raphe
- Anus

ANATOMICAL ILLUSTRATIONS

Integumentary System Anatomy

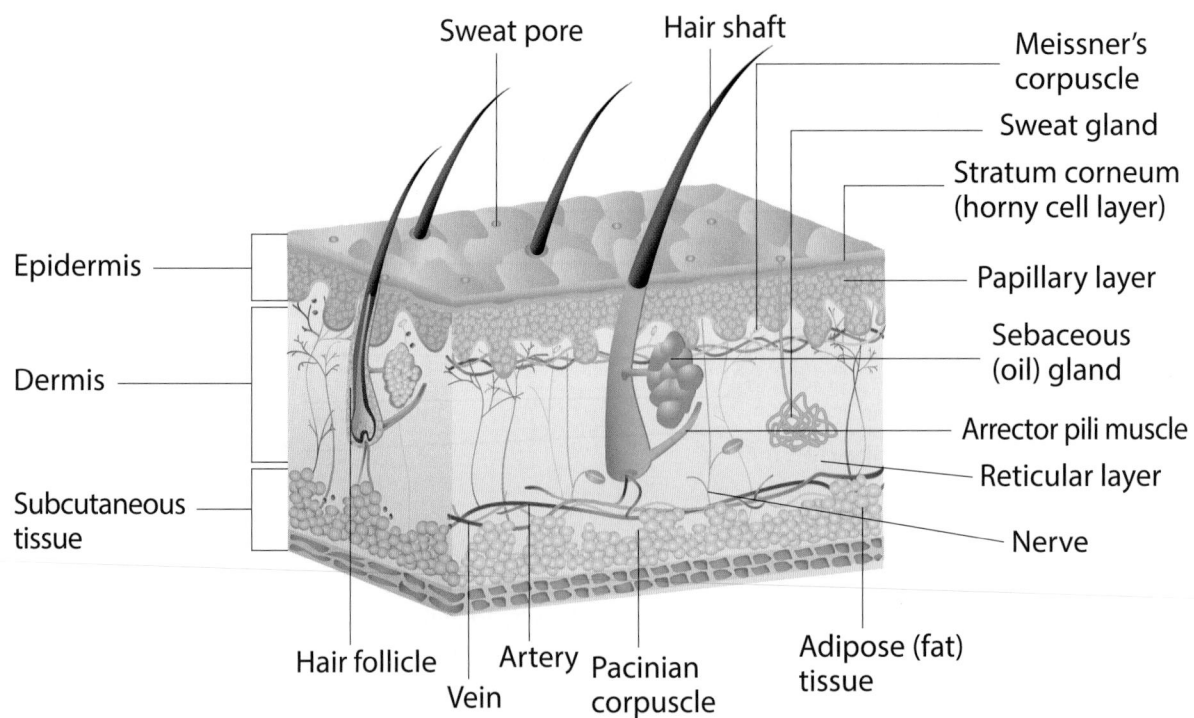

Sweat pore

Hair shaft

Meissner's corpuscle

Sweat gland

Stratum corneum (horny cell layer)

Papillary layer

Sebaceous (oil) gland

Arrector pili muscle

Reticular layer

Nerve

Epidermis

Dermis

Subcutaneous tissue

Hair follicle

Vein

Artery

Pacinian corpuscle

Adipose (fat) tissue

Lymphatic System Anatomy

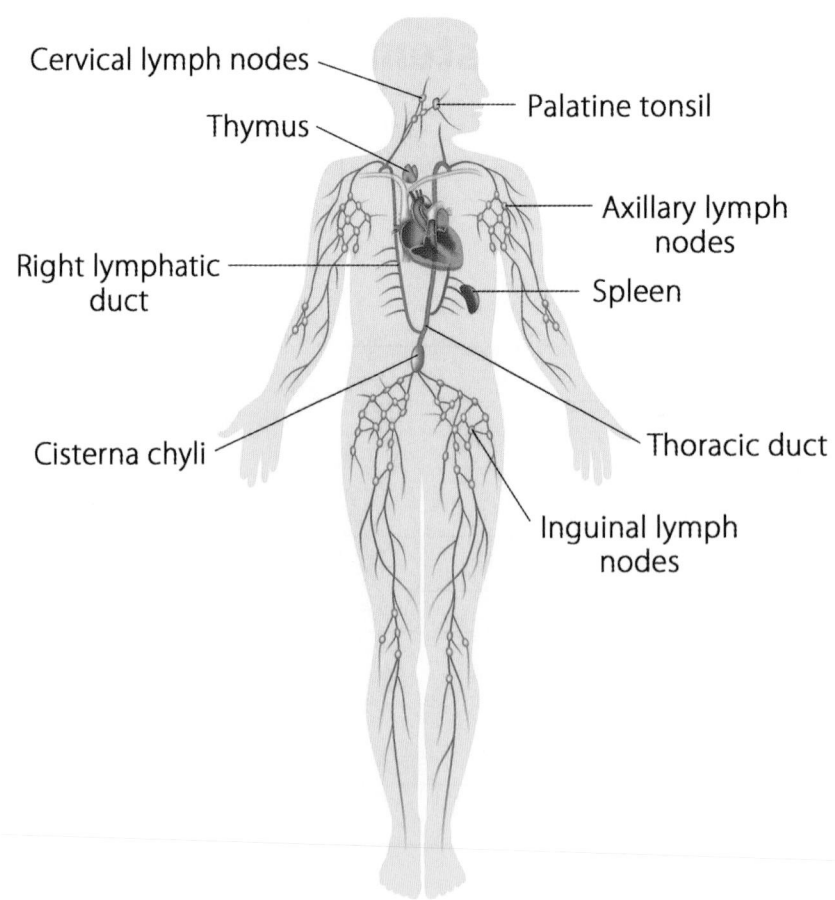

Cervical lymph nodes

Palatine tonsil

Thymus

Axillary lymph nodes

Right lymphatic duct

Spleen

Cisterna chyli

Thoracic duct

Inguinal lymph nodes

Lymphatic System — Humoral Immunity

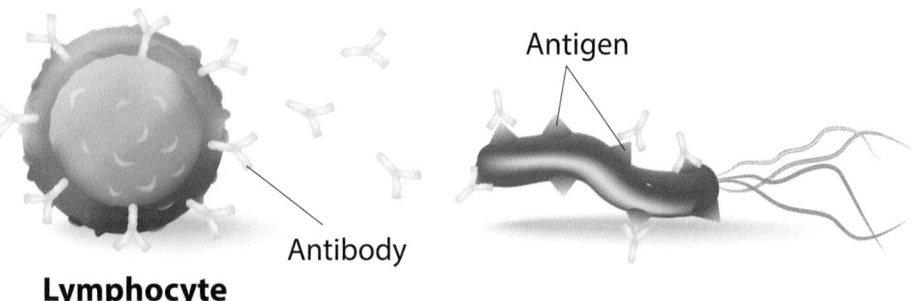

Antigen

Antibody

Lymphocyte

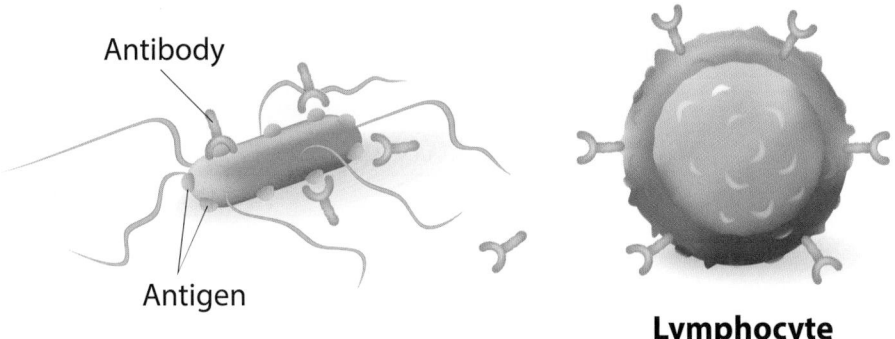

Antibody

Antigen

Lymphocyte

Lymph Node Anatomy

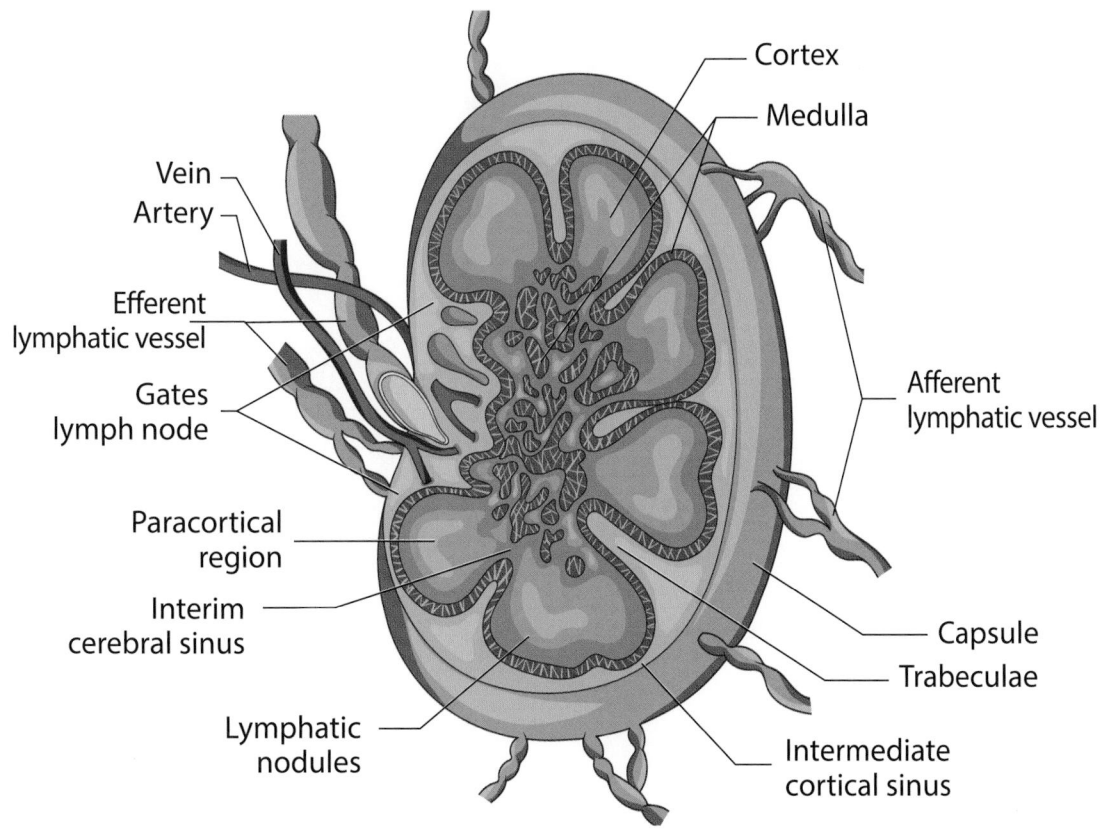

Cortex

Medulla

Vein

Artery

Efferent
lymphatic vessel

Gates
lymph node

Afferent
lymphatic vessel

Paracortical
region

Interim
cerebral sinus

Capsule

Trabeculae

Lymphatic
nodules

Intermediate
cortical sinus

Male Reproductive System Anatomy

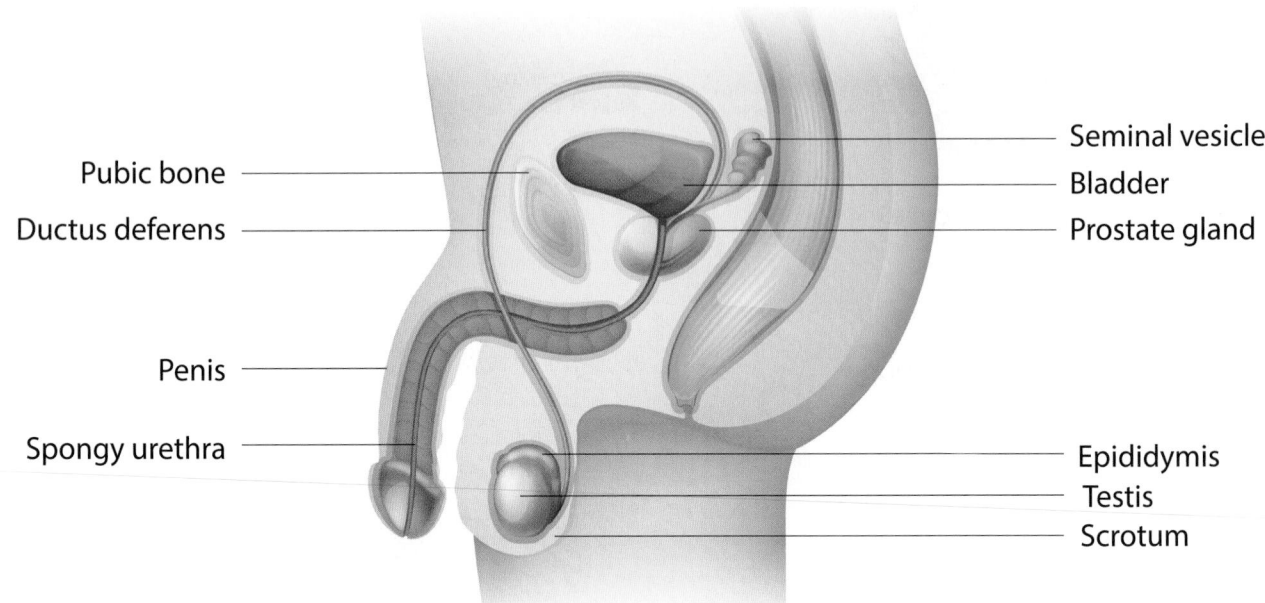

Pubic bone

Ductus deferens

Penis

Spongy urethra

Seminal vesicle

Bladder

Prostate gland

Epididymis

Testis

Scrotum

Male Reproductive System — Testicle Anatomy

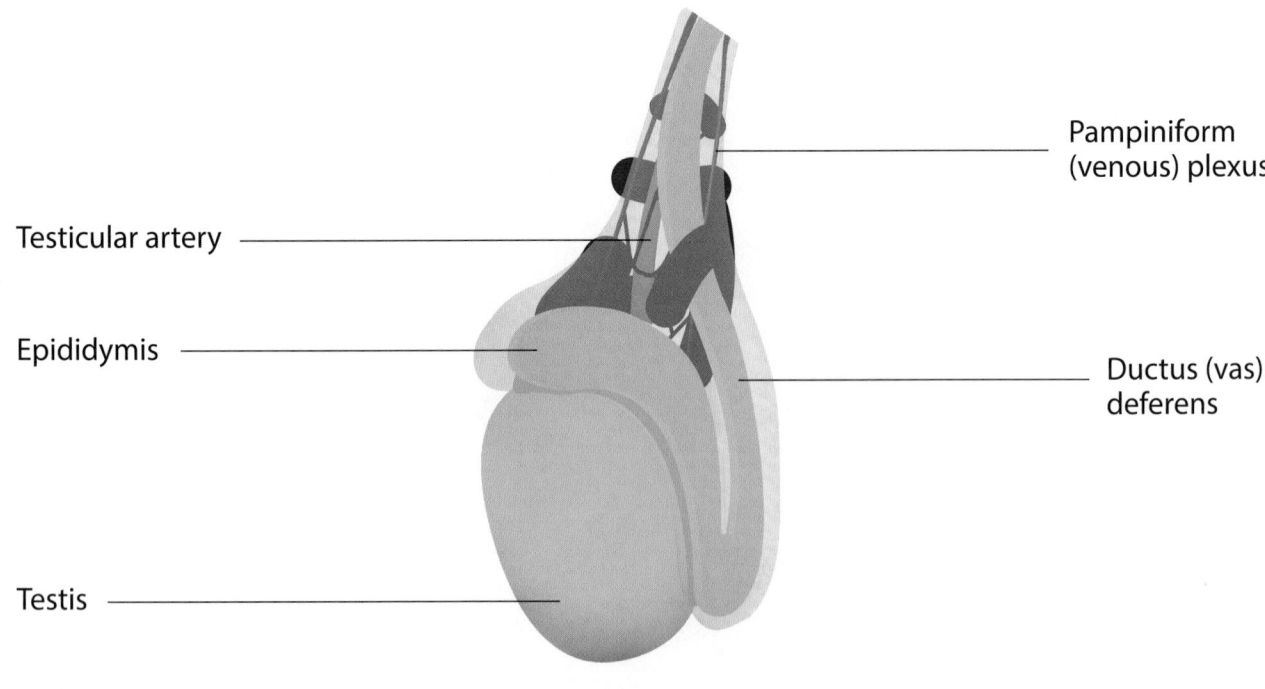

Testicular artery

Epididymis

Testis

Pampiniform (venous) plexus

Ductus (vas) deferens

ANATOMICAL ILLUSTRATIONS

Male Reproductive System — Penis Anatomy

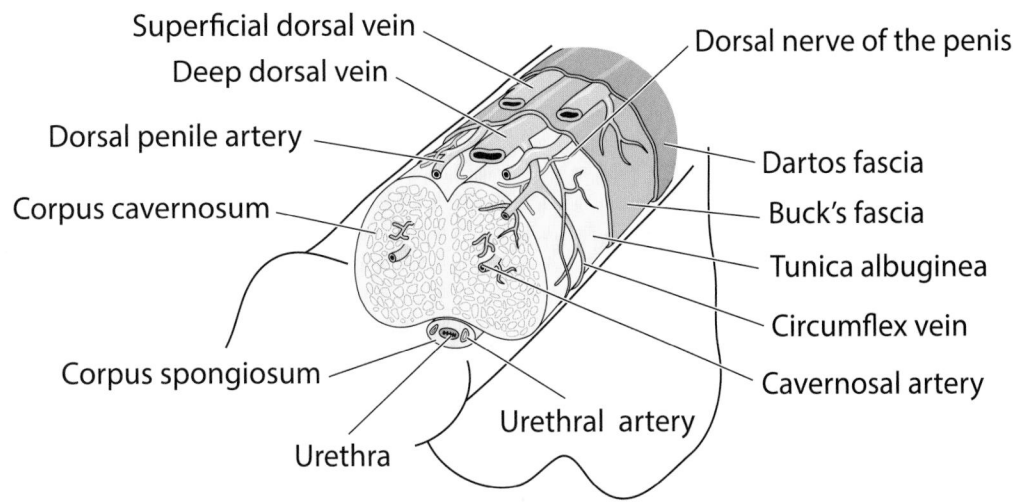

Superficial dorsal vein
Deep dorsal vein
Dorsal penile artery
Corpus cavernosum
Corpus spongiosum
Urethra
Urethral artery
Dorsal nerve of the penis
Dartos fascia
Buck's fascia
Tunica albuginea
Circumflex vein
Cavernosal artery

Muscular System Anatomy

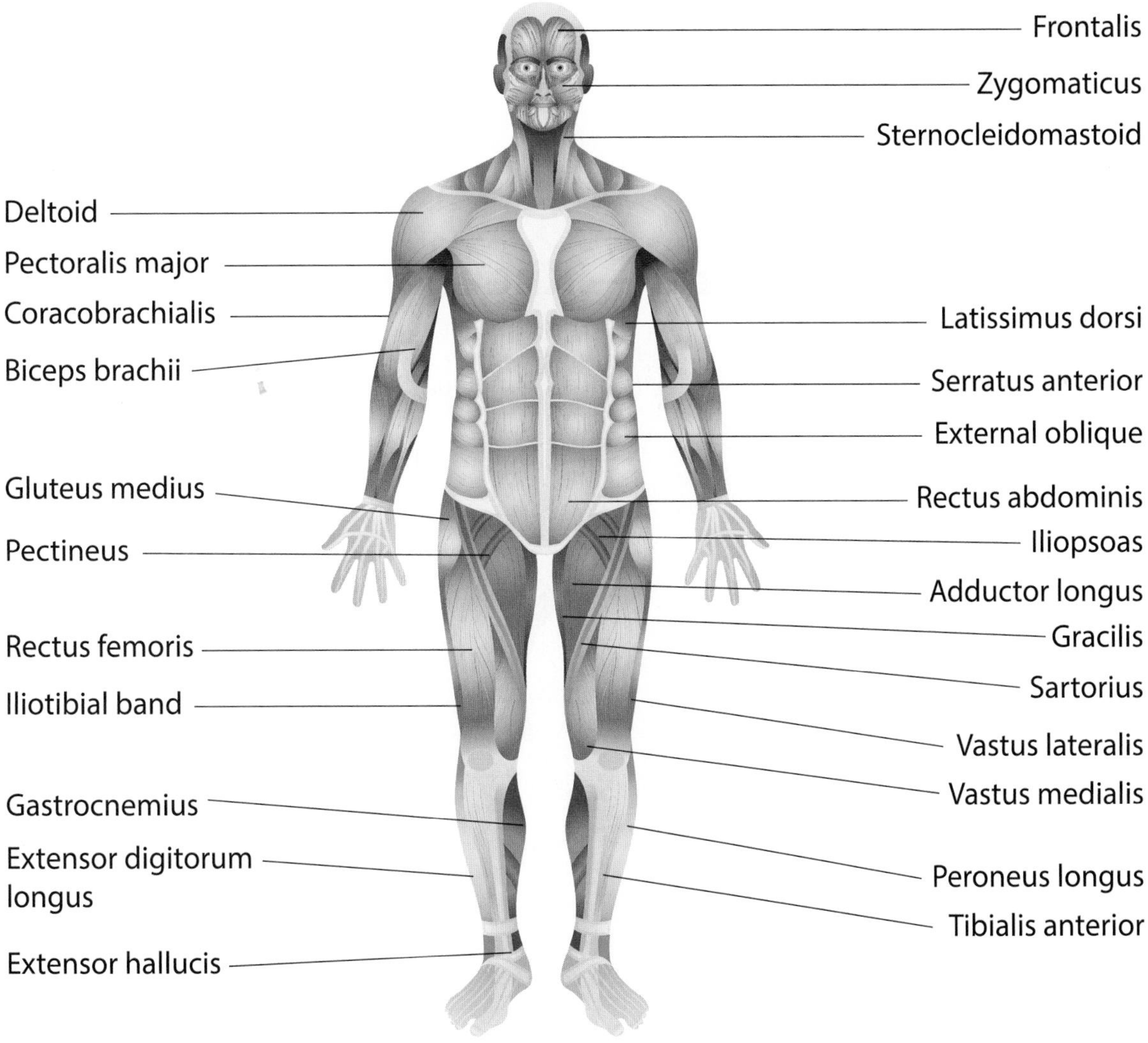

Frontalis
Zygomaticus
Sternocleidomastoid
Deltoid
Pectoralis major
Coracobrachialis
Biceps brachii
Latissimus dorsi
Serratus anterior
External oblique
Gluteus medius
Pectineus
Rectus abdominis
Iliopsoas
Adductor longus
Gracilis
Sartorius
Rectus femoris
Iliotibial band
Vastus lateralis
Vastus medialis
Gastrocnemius
Extensor digitorum longus
Peroneus longus
Tibialis anterior
Extensor hallucis

Muscular System — Forearm Muscles
(Right Arm, Posterior Compartment)

Superficial

Deep

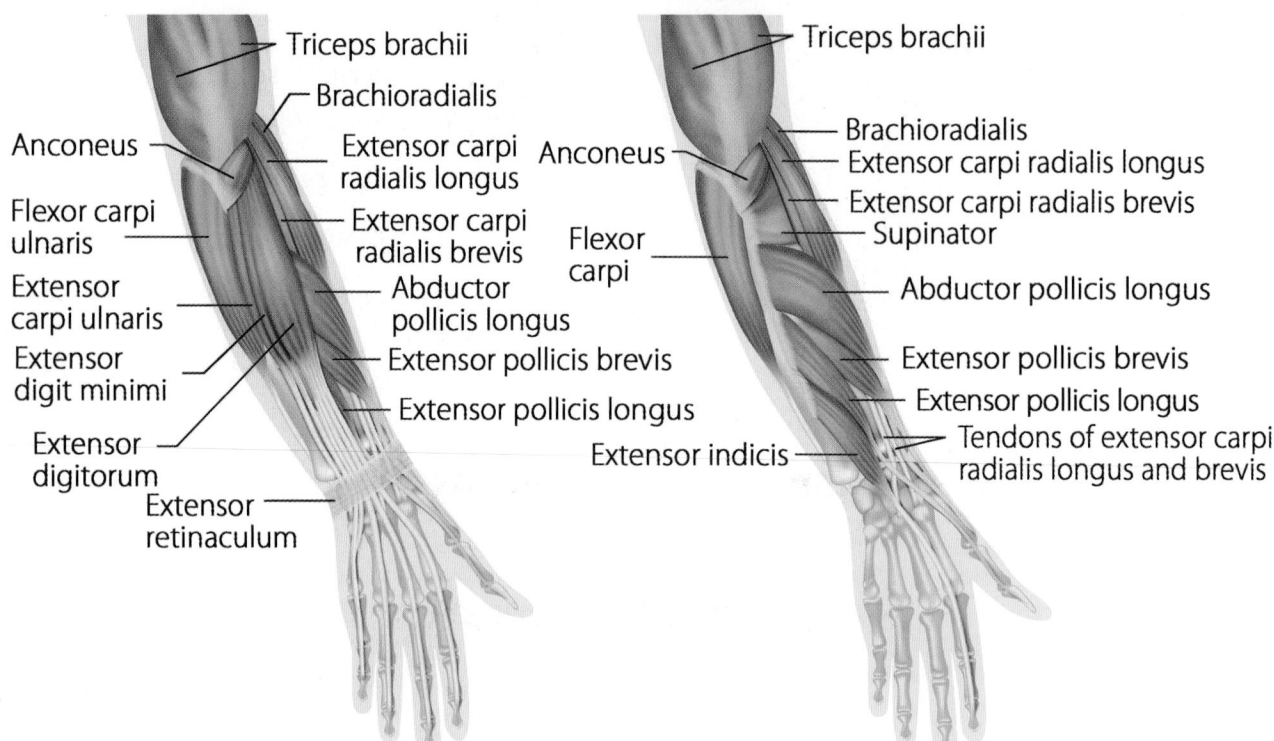

Superficial labels:
- Triceps brachii
- Brachioradialis
- Anconeus
- Extensor carpi radialis longus
- Flexor carpi ulnaris
- Extensor carpi radialis brevis
- Extensor carpi ulnaris
- Abductor pollicis longus
- Extensor digit minimi
- Extensor pollicis brevis
- Extensor pollicis longus
- Extensor digitorum
- Extensor retinaculum

Deep labels:
- Triceps brachii
- Anconeus
- Brachioradialis
- Extensor carpi radialis longus
- Extensor carpi radialis brevis
- Supinator
- Flexor carpi
- Abductor pollicis longus
- Extensor pollicis brevis
- Extensor pollicis longus
- Extensor indicis
- Tendons of extensor carpi radialis longus and brevis

Muscular System — Knee Joint Anatomy

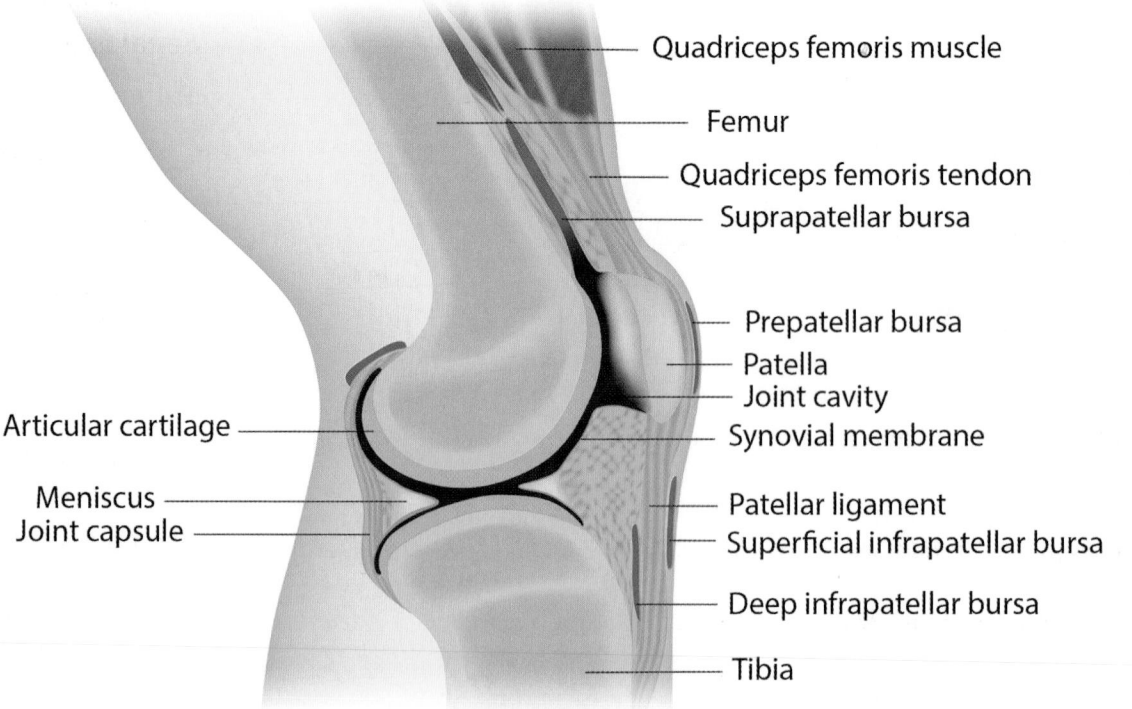

- Quadriceps femoris muscle
- Femur
- Quadriceps femoris tendon
- Suprapatellar bursa
- Prepatellar bursa
- Patella
- Joint cavity
- Articular cartilage
- Synovial membrane
- Meniscus
- Patellar ligament
- Joint capsule
- Superficial infrapatellar bursa
- Deep infrapatellar bursa
- Tibia

ANATOMICAL ILLUSTRATIONS

Muscular System — Shoulder (Rotator Cuff) Muscles

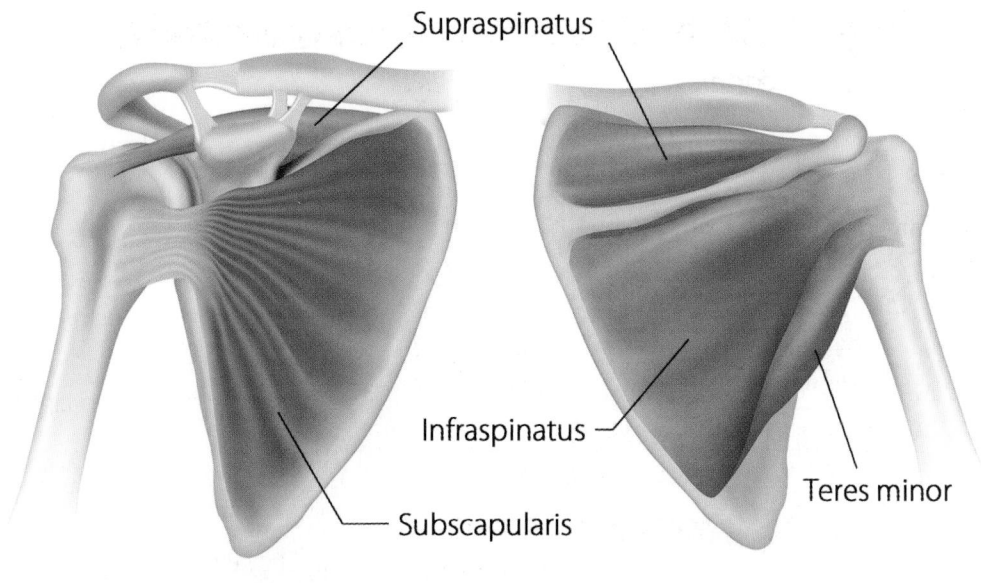

Supraspinatus

Infraspinatus

Teres minor

Subscapularis

Anterior view

Posterior view

Nervous System Anatomy

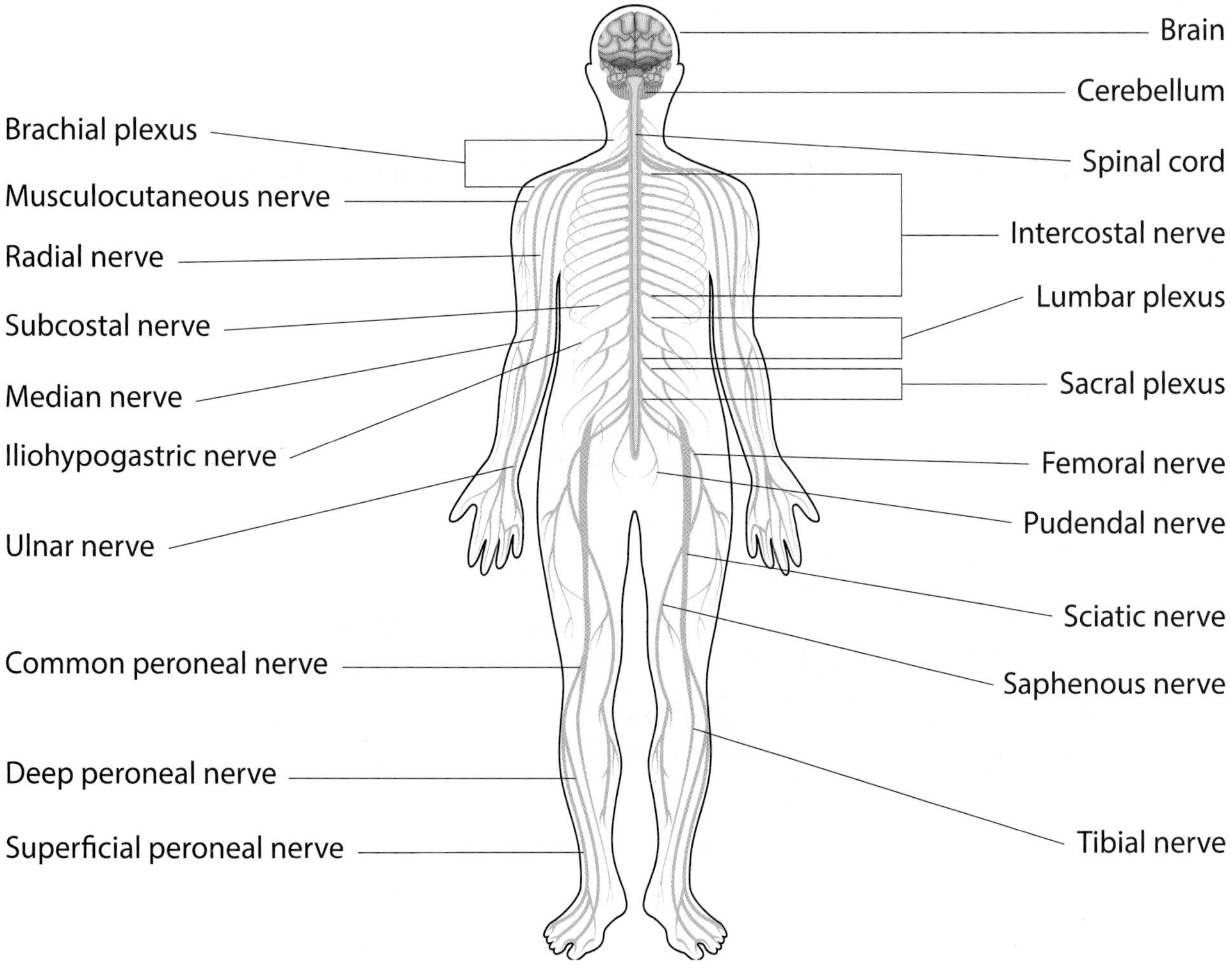

Brachial plexus

Musculocutaneous nerve

Radial nerve

Subcostal nerve

Median nerve

Iliohypogastric nerve

Ulnar nerve

Common peroneal nerve

Deep peroneal nerve

Superficial peroneal nerve

Brain

Cerebellum

Spinal cord

Intercostal nerve

Lumbar plexus

Sacral plexus

Femoral nerve

Pudendal nerve

Sciatic nerve

Saphenous nerve

Tibial nerve

ANATOMICAL ILLUSTRATIONS

Nervous System — Brain Anatomy

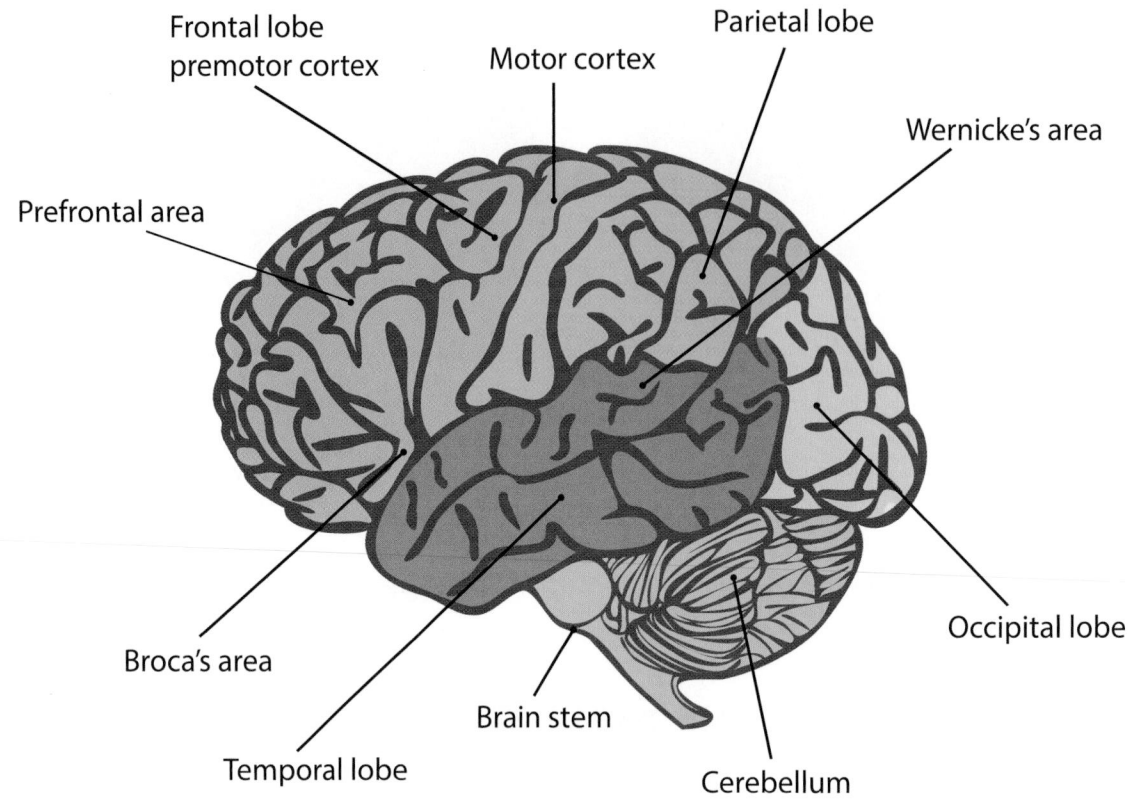

Frontal lobe premotor cortex

Motor cortex

Parietal lobe

Wernicke's area

Prefrontal area

Occipital lobe

Broca's area

Brain stem

Temporal lobe

Cerebellum

Nervous System — Cranial Nerves

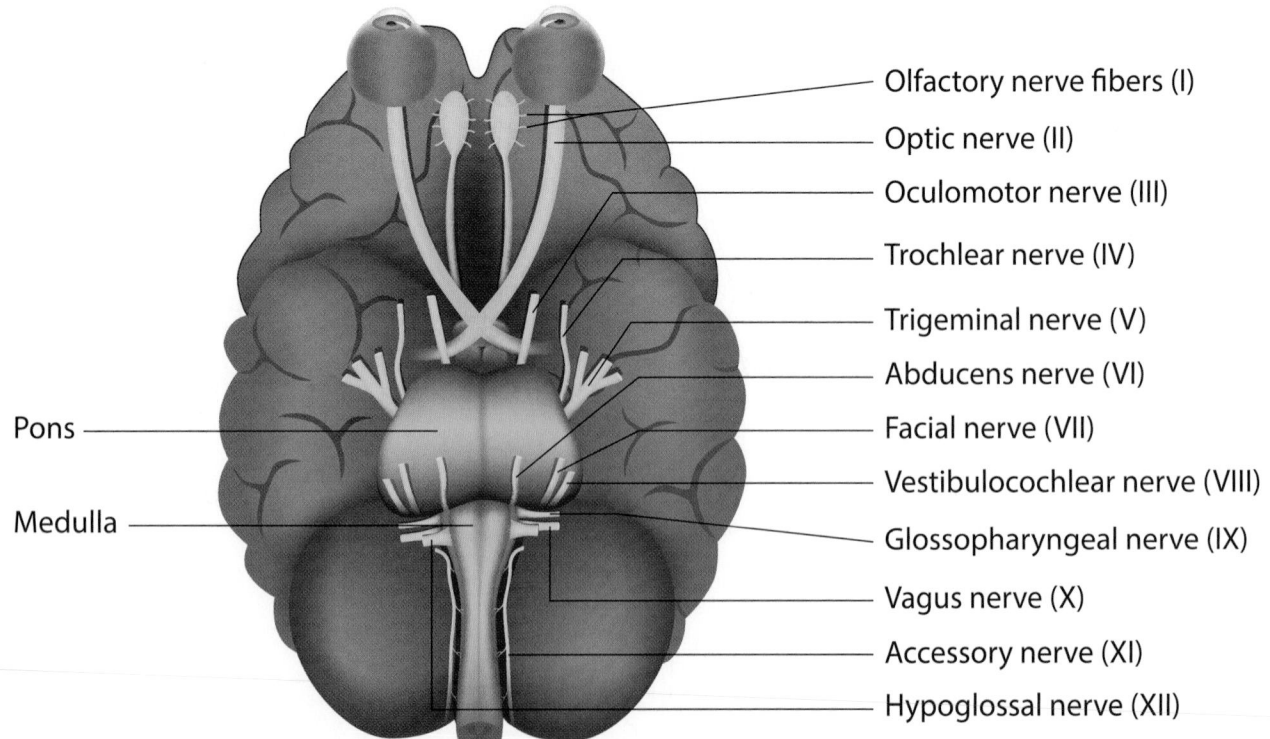

Olfactory nerve fibers (I)

Optic nerve (II)

Oculomotor nerve (III)

Trochlear nerve (IV)

Trigeminal nerve (V)

Abducens nerve (VI)

Facial nerve (VII)

Vestibulocochlear nerve (VIII)

Glossopharyngeal nerve (IX)

Vagus nerve (X)

Accessory nerve (XI)

Hypoglossal nerve (XII)

Pons

Medulla

ANATOMICAL ILLUSTRATIONS

Nervous System — Nerve Anatomy

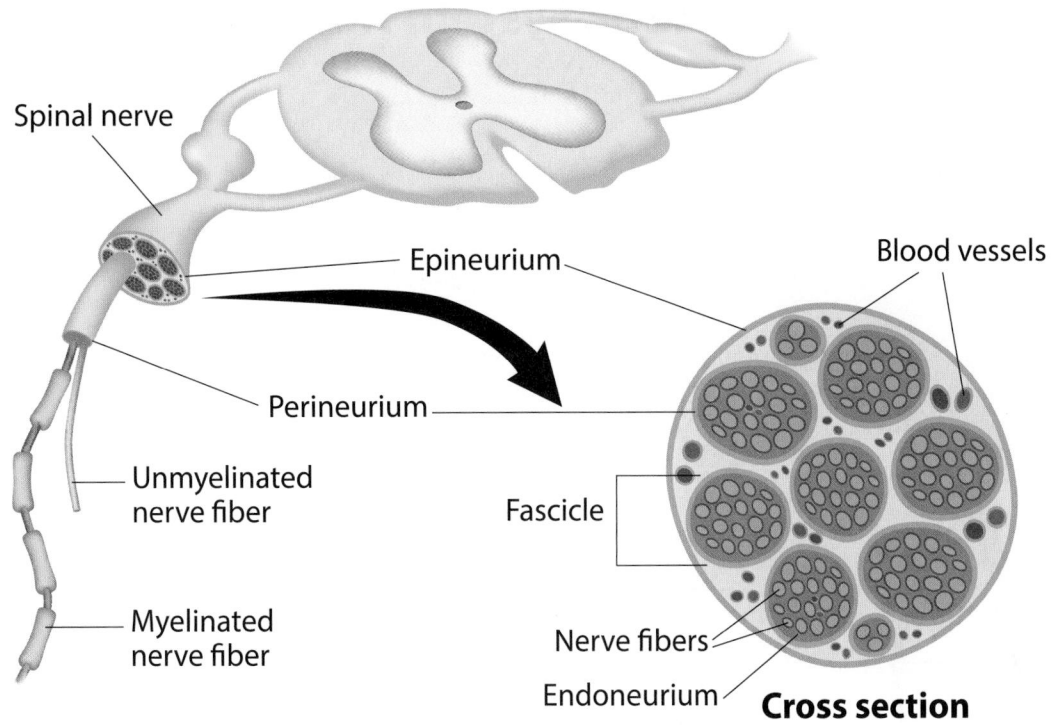

Spinal nerve

Epineurium

Blood vessels

Perineurium

Unmyelinated nerve fiber

Myelinated nerve fiber

Fascicle

Nerve fibers

Endoneurium

Cross section

Nervous System — Parasympathetic System Anatomy

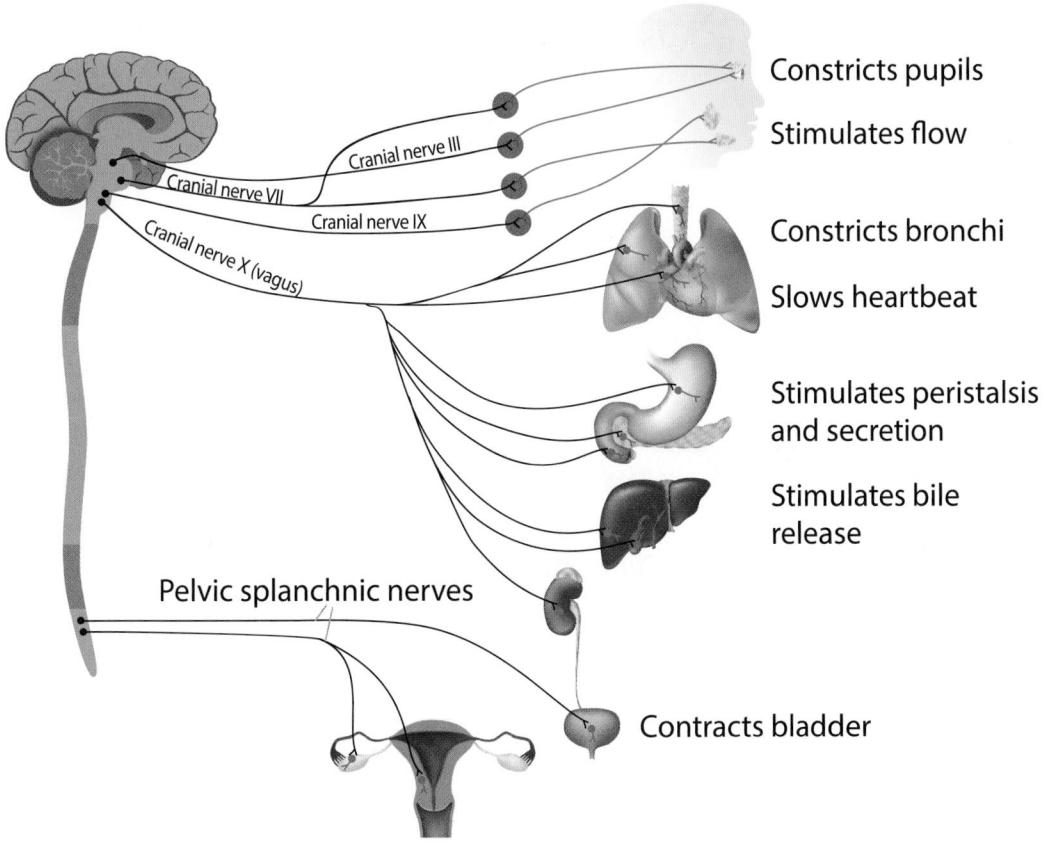

Constricts pupils

Stimulates flow

Cranial nerve III

Cranial nerve VII

Cranial nerve IX

Cranial nerve X (vagus)

Constricts bronchi

Slows heartbeat

Stimulates peristalsis and secretion

Stimulates bile release

Pelvic splanchnic nerves

Contracts bladder

Nervous System —
Sympathetic System Anatomy

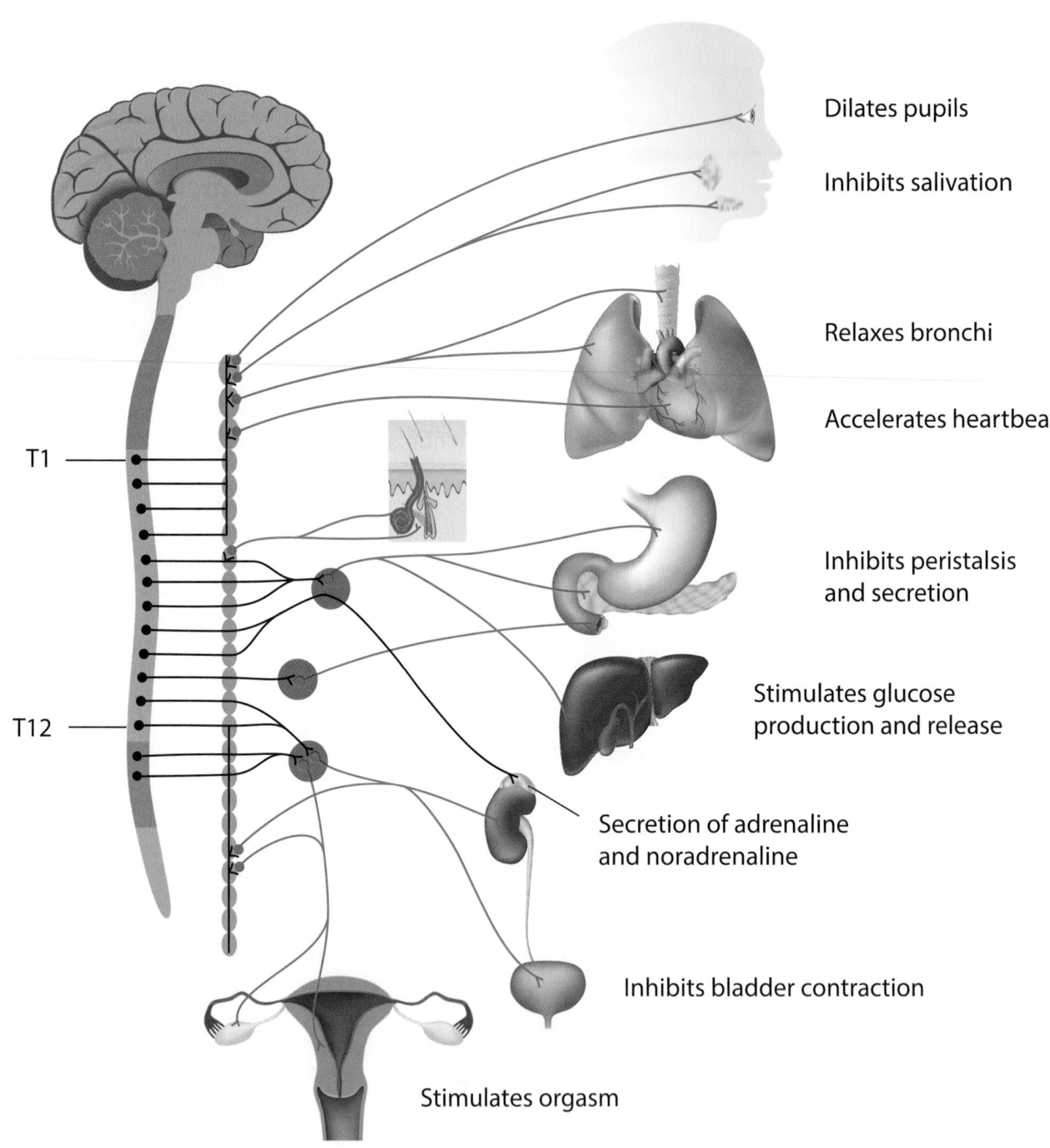

Dilates pupils

Inhibits salivation

Relaxes bronchi

Accelerates heartbeat

Inhibits peristalsis and secretion

Stimulates glucose production and release

Secretion of adrenaline and noradrenaline

Inhibits bladder contraction

Stimulates orgasm

T1

T12

ANATOMICAL ILLUSTRATIONS

Respiratory System Anatomy

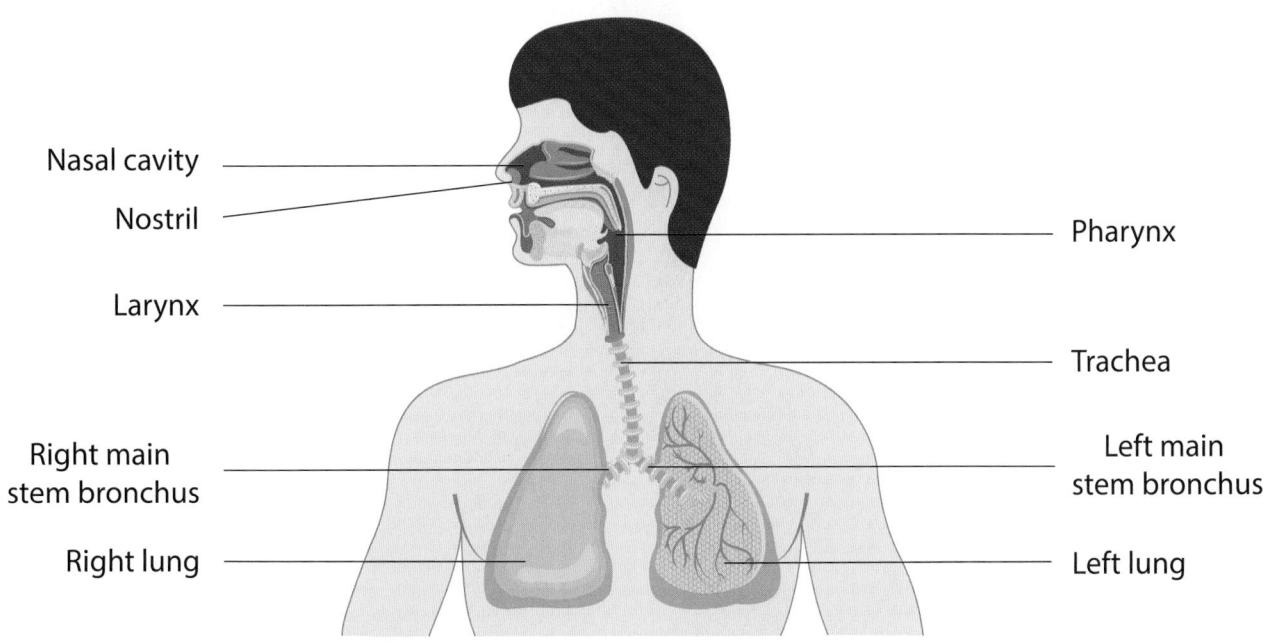

Respiratory System — Larynx Anatomy

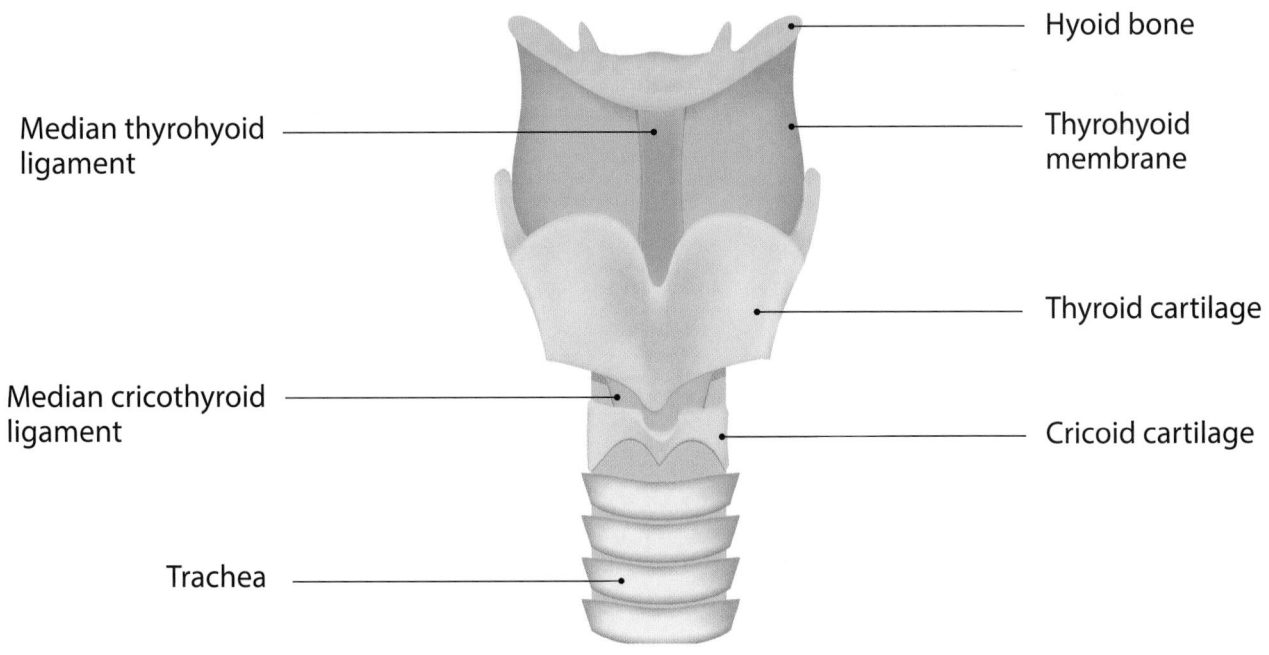

Respiratory System — Lung Anatomy

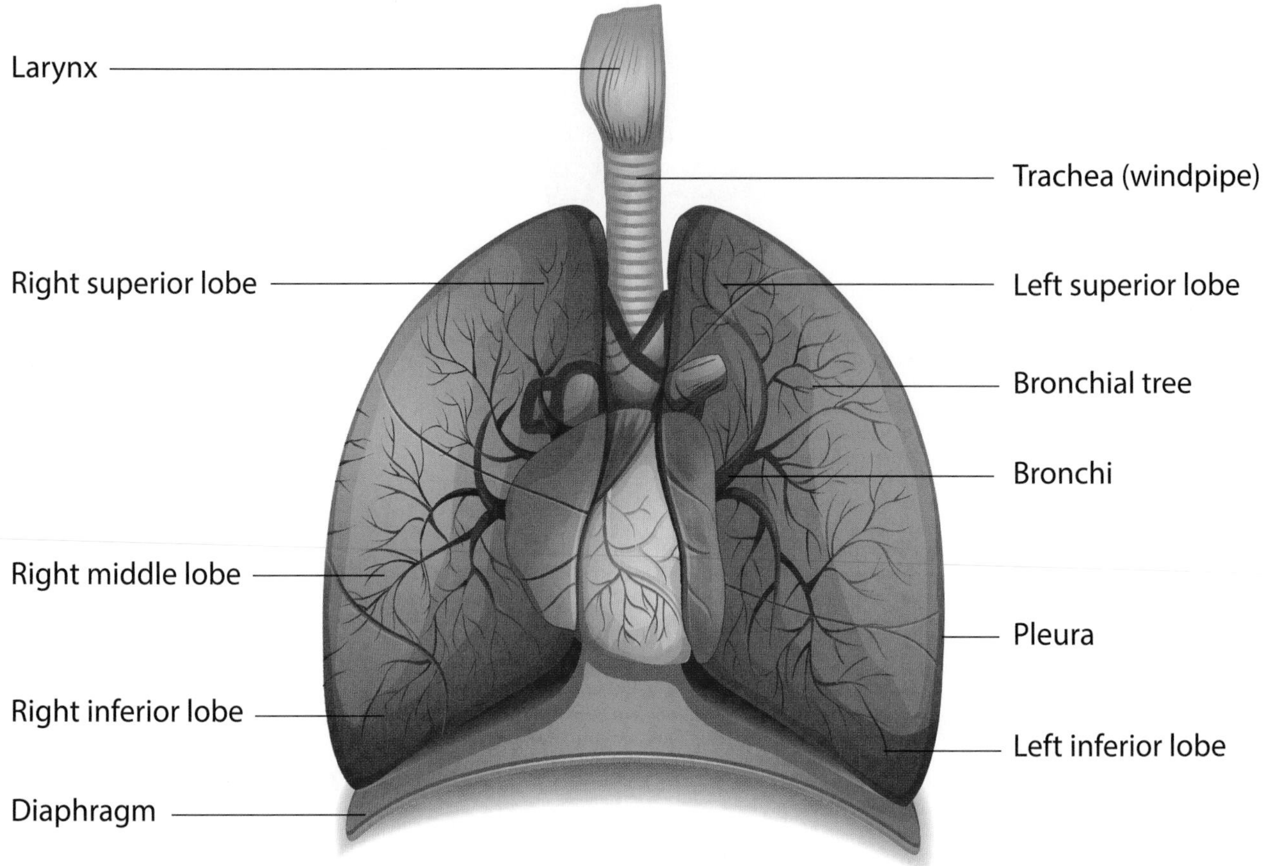

Larynx

Trachea (windpipe)

Right superior lobe

Left superior lobe

Bronchial tree

Bronchi

Right middle lobe

Right inferior lobe

Pleura

Left inferior lobe

Diaphragm

Respiratory System Function

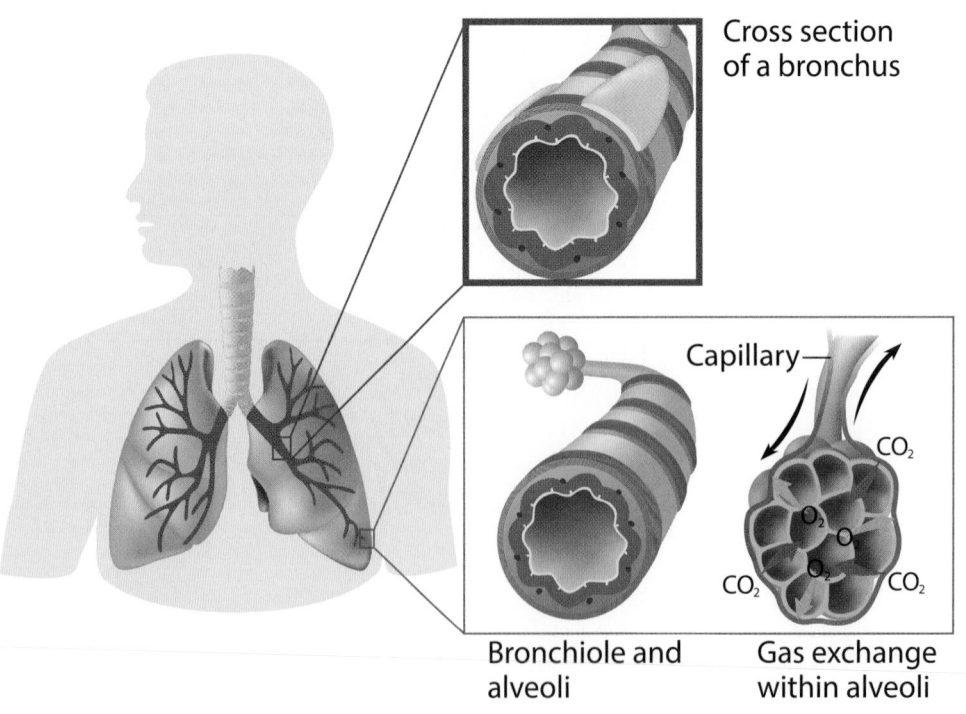

Cross section of a bronchus

Capillary

CO_2

O_2

CO_2

O_2

CO_2

Bronchiole and alveoli

Gas exchange within alveoli

Respiratory System — Nose Anatomy

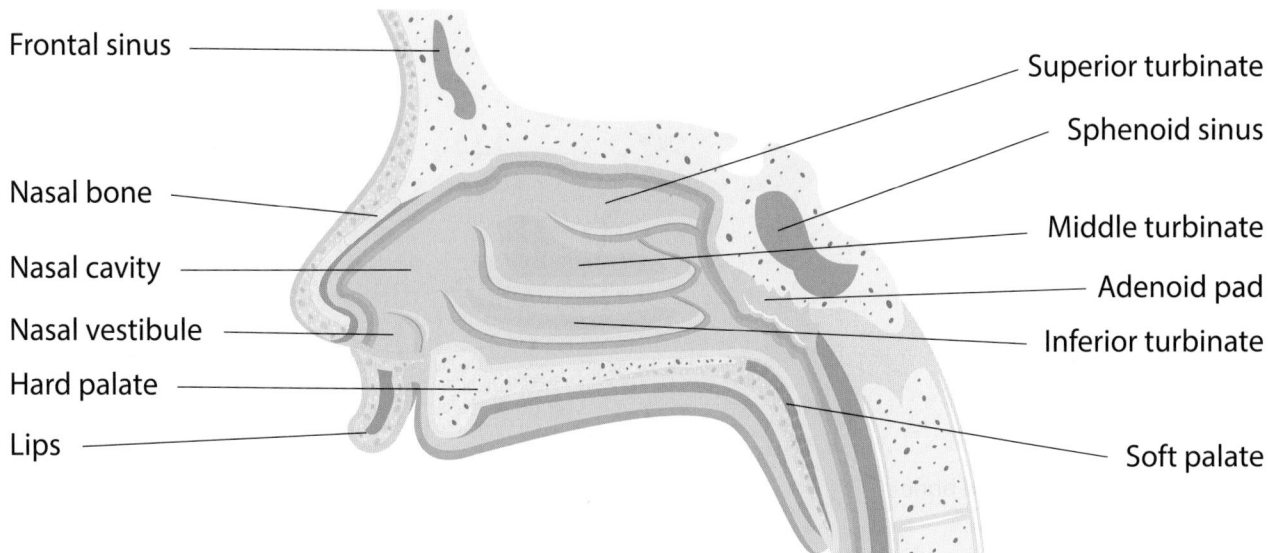

Frontal sinus

Nasal bone

Nasal cavity

Nasal vestibule

Hard palate

Lips

Superior turbinate

Sphenoid sinus

Middle turbinate

Adenoid pad

Inferior turbinate

Soft palate

Respiratory System — Sinus Anatomy

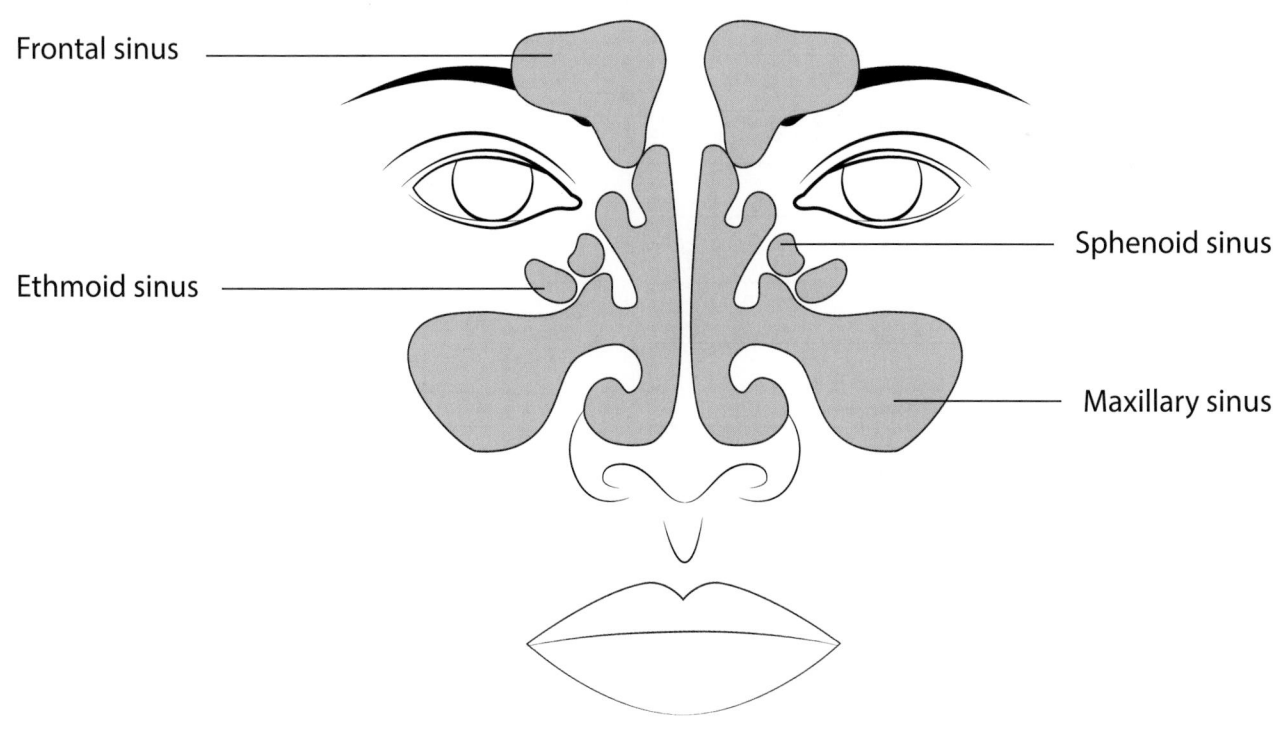

Frontal sinus

Ethmoid sinus

Sphenoid sinus

Maxillary sinus

Respiratory System — Throat Anatomy

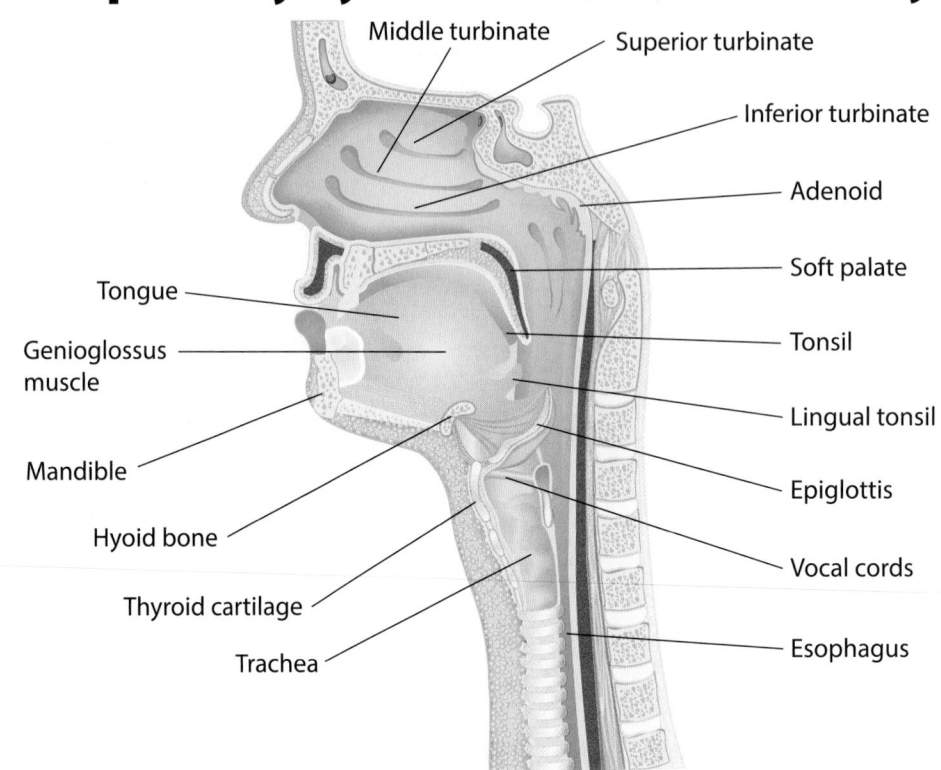

Middle turbinate
Superior turbinate
Inferior turbinate
Adenoid
Soft palate
Tongue
Genioglossus muscle
Tonsil
Lingual tonsil
Mandible
Epiglottis
Hyoid bone
Vocal cords
Thyroid cartilage
Esophagus
Trachea

Skeletal System Anatomy

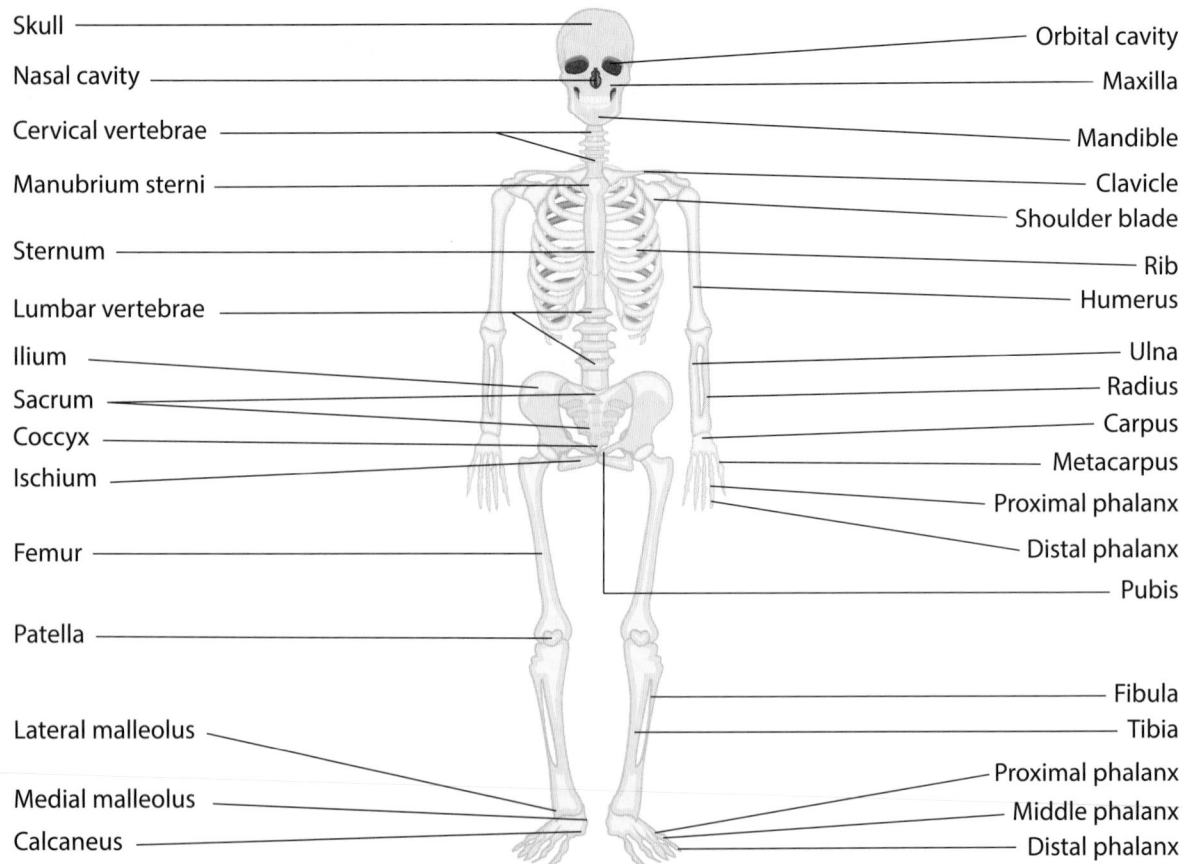

Skull
Orbital cavity
Nasal cavity
Maxilla
Cervical vertebrae
Mandible
Manubrium sterni
Clavicle
Shoulder blade
Sternum
Rib
Lumbar vertebrae
Humerus
Ilium
Ulna
Sacrum
Radius
Coccyx
Carpus
Ischium
Metacarpus
Proximal phalanx
Distal phalanx
Femur
Pubis
Patella
Fibula
Tibia
Lateral malleolus
Proximal phalanx
Medial malleolus
Middle phalanx
Calcaneus
Distal phalanx

ANATOMICAL ILLUSTRATIONS

Skeletal System — Bone Structure

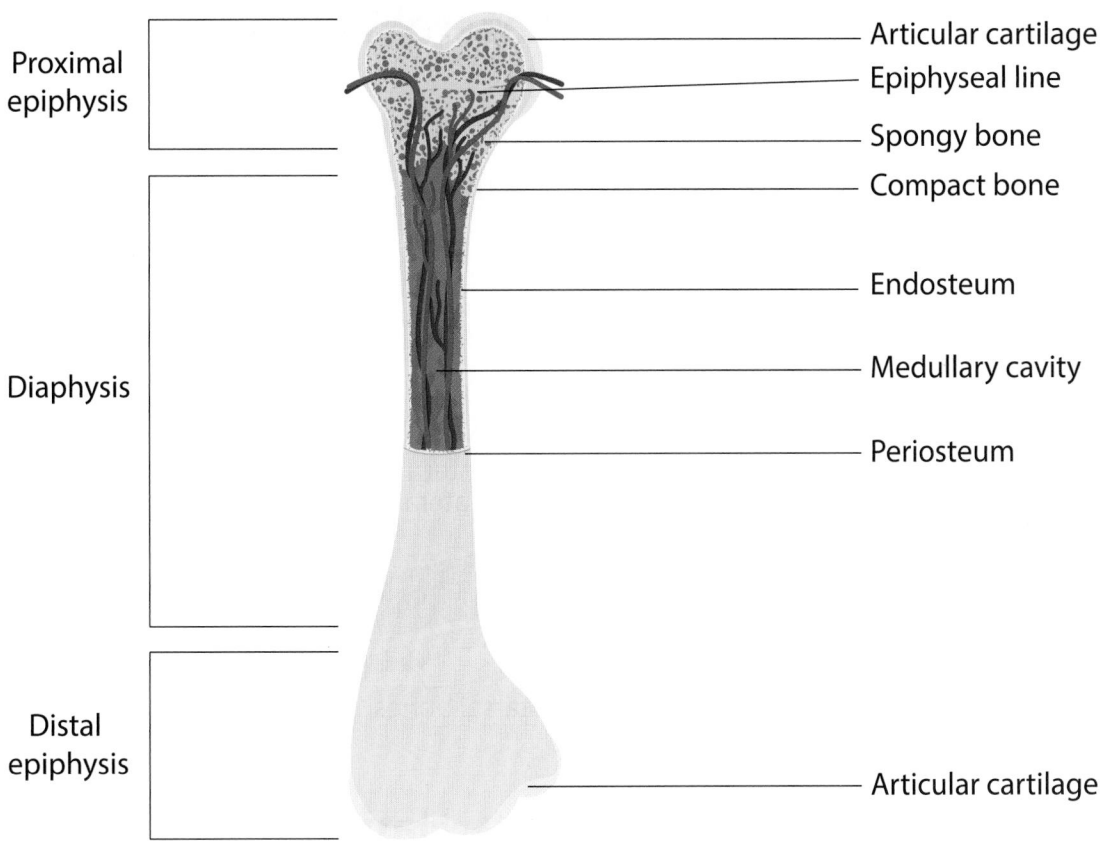

Proximal epiphysis

Diaphysis

Distal epiphysis

Articular cartilage

Epiphyseal line

Spongy bone

Compact bone

Endosteum

Medullary cavity

Periosteum

Articular cartilage

Skeletal System — Cervical, Thoracic, and Lumbar Spine

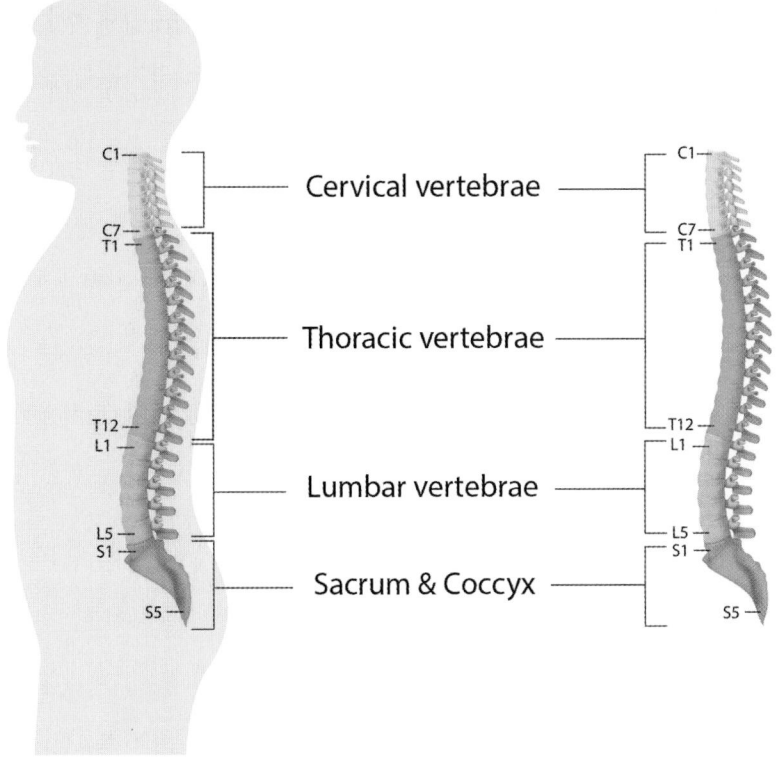

Cervical vertebrae

Thoracic vertebrae

Lumbar vertebrae

Sacrum & Coccyx

C1

C7
T1

T12
L1

L5
S1

S5

Skeletal System — Foot Bones
(Right Foot, Lateral View)

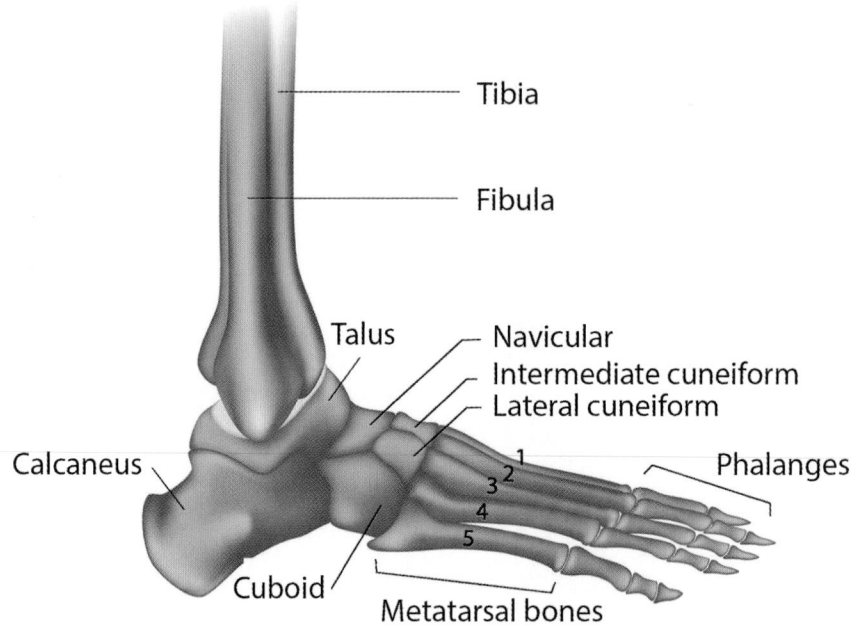

Tibia

Fibula

Talus

Navicular
Intermediate cuneiform
Lateral cuneiform

Calcaneus

1
2
3
4
5

Phalanges

Cuboid

Metatarsal bones

Skeletal System — Hand Bones

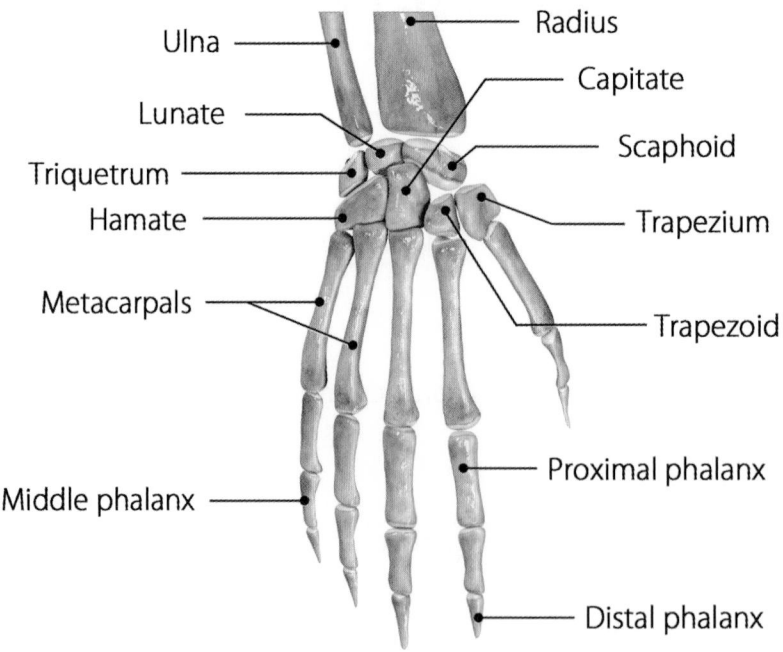

Ulna

Radius

Lunate

Capitate

Triquetrum

Scaphoid

Hamate

Trapezium

Metacarpals

Trapezoid

Proximal phalanx

Middle phalanx

Distal phalanx

ANATOMICAL ILLUSTRATIONS

Skeletal System — Skull Anatomy

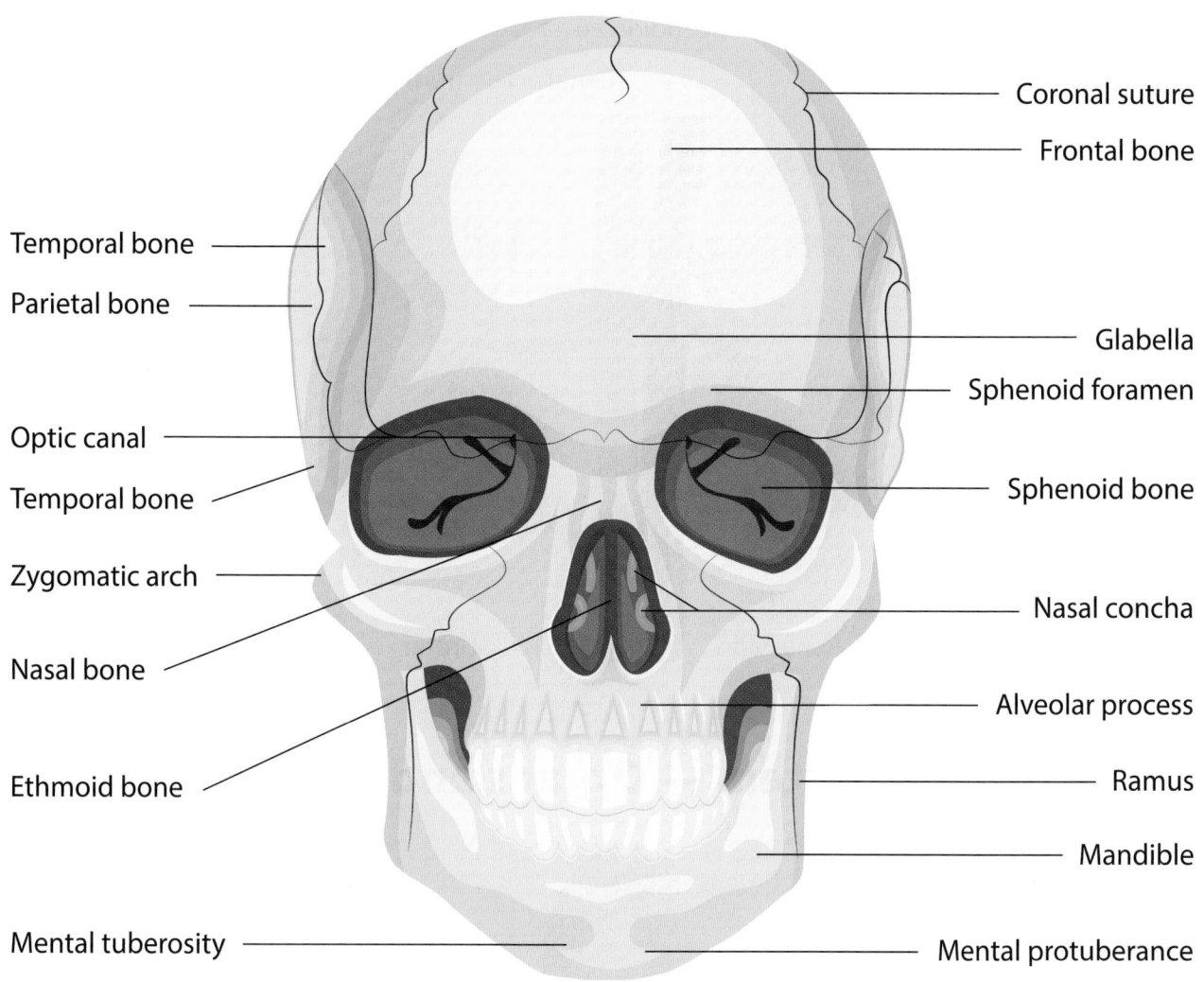

Coronal suture

Frontal bone

Temporal bone

Parietal bone

Glabella

Sphenoid foramen

Optic canal

Temporal bone

Sphenoid bone

Zygomatic arch

Nasal concha

Nasal bone

Alveolar process

Ethmoid bone

Ramus

Mandible

Mental tuberosity

Mental protuberance

Urinary System — Kidney Anatomy

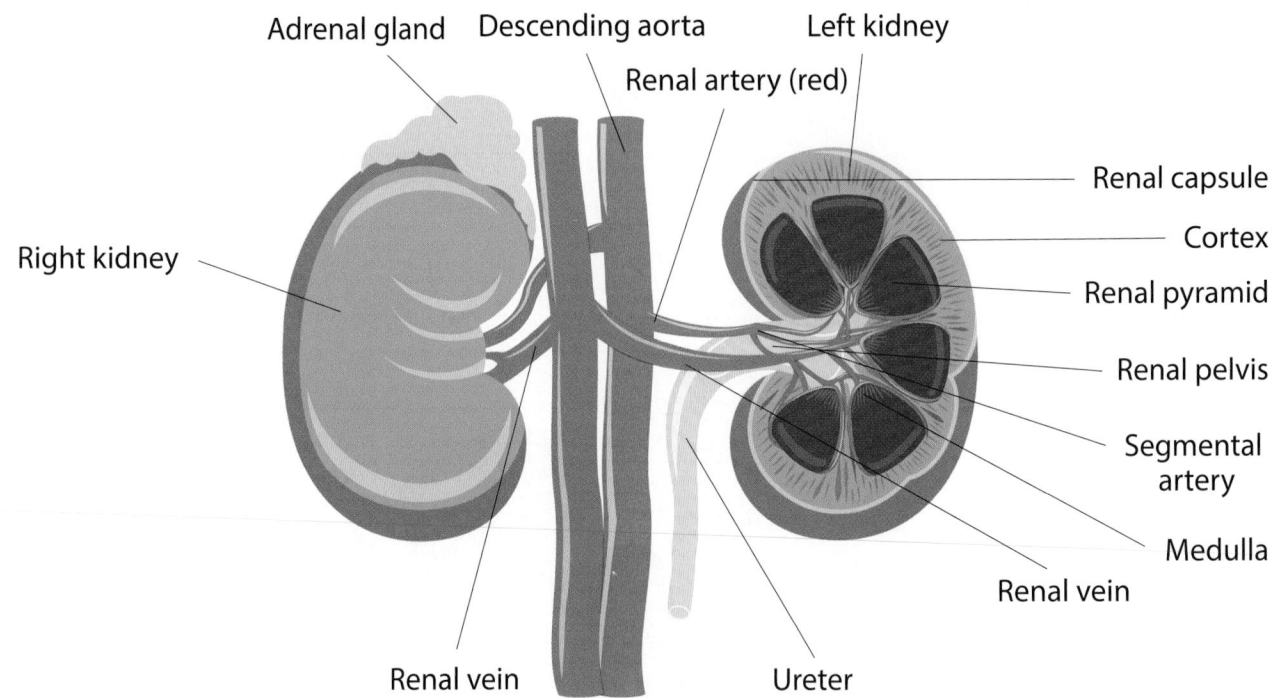

Adrenal gland Descending aorta Left kidney
Renal artery (red)
Renal capsule
Cortex
Renal pyramid
Right kidney
Renal pelvis
Segmental artery
Medulla
Renal vein
Renal vein Ureter

Urinary System — Organs and Structures

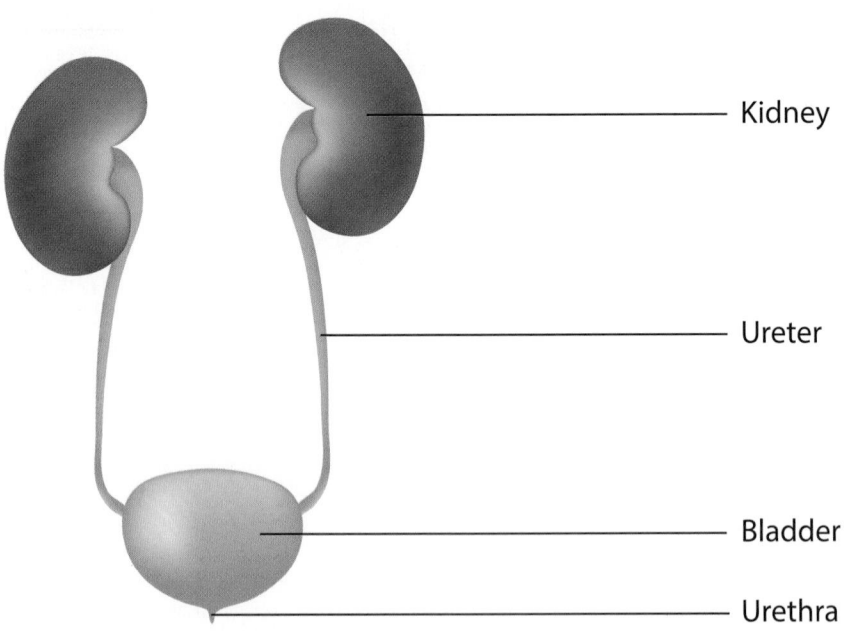

Kidney

Ureter

Bladder

Urethra

ICD-10-CM Index to Diseases and Injuries

The vertical yellow line appears at the 2nd and 4th indentations throughout the index.

A

Aarskog's syndrome Q87.1
Abandonment — *see* Maltreatment
Abasia (-astasia) (hysterical) F44.4
Abderhalden-Kaufmann-Lignac syndrome (cystinosis) E72.04
Abdomen, abdominal (*see also* condition)
  acute R10.0
  angina K55.1
  muscle deficiency syndrome Q79.4
Abdominalgia — *see* Pain, abdominal
Abduction contracture, hip or other joint — *see* Contraction, joint
Aberrant (congenital) (*see also* Malposition, congenital)
  adrenal gland Q89.1
  artery (peripheral) Q27.8
    basilar NEC Q28.1
    cerebral Q28.3
    coronary Q24.5
    digestive system Q27.8
    eye Q15.8
    lower limb Q27.8
    precerebral Q28.1
    pulmonary Q25.79
    renal Q27.2
    retina Q14.1
    specified site NEC Q27.8
    subclavian Q27.8
    upper limb Q27.8
    vertebral Q28.1
  breast Q83.8
  endocrine gland NEC Q89.2
  hepatic duct Q44.5
  pancreas Q45.3
  parathyroid gland Q89.2
  pituitary gland Q89.2
  sebaceous glands, mucous membrane, mouth, congenital Q38.6
  spleen Q89.09
  subclavian artery Q27.8
  thymus (gland) Q89.2
  thyroid gland Q89.2
  vein (peripheral) NEC Q27.8
    cerebral Q28.3
    digestive system Q27.8
    lower limb Q27.8
    precerebral Q28.1
    specified site NEC Q27.8
    upper limb Q27.8
Aberration
  distantial — *see* Disturbance, visual
  mental F99
Abetalipoproteinemia E78.6
Abiotrophy R68.89
Ablatio, ablation
  retinae — *see* Detachment, retina
Ablepharia, ablepharon Q10.3
Abnormal, abnormality, abnormalities (*see also* Anomaly)
  acid-base balance (mixed) E87.4
  albumin R77.0
  alphafetoprotein R77.2
  alveolar ridge K08.9
  anatomical relationship Q89.9
  apertures, congenital, diaphragm Q79.1
  auditory perception H93.29 ☑
    diplacusis — *see* Diplacusis
    hyperacusis — *see* Hyperacusis
    recruitment — *see* Recruitment, auditory
    threshold shift — *see* Shift, auditory threshold
  autosomes Q99.9
    fragile site Q95.5
  basal metabolic rate R94.8
  biosynthesis, testicular androgen E29.1
  bleeding time R79.1
  blood-gas level R79.81
  blood level (of)
    cobalt R79.0
    copper R79.0
    iron R79.0
    lithium R78.89
    magnesium R79.0
    mineral NEC R79.0
    zinc R79.0

Abnormal — *continued*
  blood pressure
    elevated R03.0
    low reading (nonspecific) R03.1
  blood sugar R73.09
  bowel sounds R19.15
    absent R19.11
    hyperactive R19.12
  brain scan R94.02
  breathing R06.9
  caloric test R94.138
  cerebrospinal fluid R83.9
    cytology R83.6
    drug level R83.2
    enzyme level R83.0
    hormones R83.1
    immunology R83.4
    microbiology R83.5
    nonmedicinal level R83.3
    specified type NEC R83.8
  chemistry, blood R79.9
    C-reactive protein R79.82
    drugs — *see* Findings, abnormal, in blood
    gas level R79.81
    minerals R79.0
    pancytopenia D61.818
    PTT R79.1
    specified NEC R79.89
    toxins — *see* Findings, abnormal, in blood
  chest sounds (friction) (rales) R09.89
  chromosome, chromosomal Q99.9
    with more than three X chromosomes, female Q97.1
    analysis result R89.8
      bronchial washings R84.8
      cerebrospinal fluid R83.8
      cervix uteri NEC R87.89
      nasal secretions R84.8
      nipple discharge R89.8
      peritoneal fluid R85.89
      pleural fluid R84.8
      prostatic secretions R86.8
      saliva R85.89
      seminal fluid R86.8
      sputum R84.8
      synovial fluid R89.8
      throat scrapings R84.8
      vagina R87.89
      vulva R87.89
      wound secretions R89.8
    dicentric replacement Q93.2
    ring replacement Q93.2
    sex Q99.8
      female phenotype Q97.9
        specified NEC Q97.8
      male phenotype Q98.9
        specified NEC Q98.8
      structural male Q98.6
    specified NEC Q99.8
  clinical findings NEC R68.89
  coagulation D68.9
    newborn, transient P61.6
    profile R79.1
    time R79.1
  communication — *see* Fistula
  conjunctiva, vascular H11.41 ☑
  coronary artery Q24.5
  cortisol-binding globulin E27.8
  course, eustachian tube Q17.8
  creatinine clearance R94.4
  cytology
    anus R85.619
      atypical squamous cells cannot exclude high grade squamous intraepithelial lesion (ASC-H) R85.611
      atypical squamous cells of undetermined significance (ASC-US) R85.610
      cytologic evidence of malignancy R85.614
      high grade squamous intraepithelial lesion (HGSIL) R85.613
      human papillomavirus (HPV) DNA test
        high risk positive R85.81
        low risk positive R85.82
      inadequate smear R85.615
      low grade squamous intraepithelial lesion (LGSIL) R85.612

Abnormal — *continued*
  cytology — *continued*
      satisfactory anal smear but lacking transformation zone R85.616
      specified NEC R85.618
      unsatisfactory smear R85.615
    female genital organs — *see* Abnormal, Papanicolaou (smear)
  dark adaptation curve H53.61
  dentofacial NEC — *see* Anomaly, dentofacial
  development, developmental Q89.9
    central nervous system Q07.9
  diagnostic imaging
    abdomen, abdominal region NEC R93.5
    biliary tract R93.2
    bladder R93.41
    breast R92.8
    central nervous system NEC R90.89
    cerebrovascular NEC R90.89
    coronary circulation R93.1
    digestive tract NEC R93.3
    gastrointestinal (tract) R93.3
    genitourinary organs R93.8
    head R93.0
    heart R93.1
    intrathoracic organ NEC R93.8
    kidney R93.42 ☑
    limbs R93.6
    liver R93.2
    lung (field) R91.8
    musculoskeletal system NEC R93.7
    renal pelvis R93.41
    retroperitoneum R93.5
    site specified NEC R93.8
    skin and subcutaneous tissue R93.8
    skull R93.0
    urinary organs specified NEC R93.49
    ureter R93.41
  direction, teeth, fully erupted M26.30
  ear ossicles, acquired NEC H74.39 ☑
    ankylosis — *see* Ankylosis, ear ossicles
    discontinuity — *see* Discontinuity, ossicles, ear
    partial loss — *see* Loss, ossicles, ear (partial)
  Ebstein Q22.5
  echocardiogram R93.1
  echoencephalogram R90.81
  echogram — *see* Abnormal, diagnostic imaging
  electrocardiogram [ECG] [EKG] R94.31
  electroencephalogram [EEG] R94.01
  electrolyte — *see* Imbalance, electrolyte
  electromyogram [EMG] R94.131
  electro-oculogram [EOG] R94.110
  electrophysiological intracardiac studies R94.39
  electroretinogram [ERG] R94.111
  erythrocytes
    congenital, with perinatal jaundice D58.9
  feces (color) (contents) (mucus) R19.5
  finding — *see* Findings, abnormal, without diagnosis
  fluid
    amniotic — *see* Abnormal, specimen, specified
    cerebrospinal — *see* Abnormal, cerebrospinal fluid
    peritoneal — *see* Abnormal, specimen, digestive organs
    pleural — *see* Abnormal, specimen, respiratory organs
    synovial — *see* Abnormal, specimen, specified
    thorax (bronchial washings) (pleural fluid) — *see* Abnormal, specimen, respiratory organs
    vaginal — *see* Abnormal, specimen, female genital organs
  form
    teeth K00.2
    uterus — *see* Anomaly, uterus
  function studies
    auditory R94.120
    bladder R94.8
    brain R94.09
    cardiovascular R94.30
    ear R94.128
    endocrine NEC R94.7
    eye NEC R94.118
    kidney R94.4
    liver R94.5
    nervous system

Abnormal

Abnormal — *continued*
  function studies — *continued*
    central NEC R94.09
    peripheral NEC R94.138
  pancreas R94.8
  placenta R94.8
  pulmonary R94.2
  special senses NEC R94.128
  spleen R94.8
  thyroid R94.6
  vestibular R94.121
  gait — *see* Gait
    hysterical F44.4
  gastrin secretion E16.4
  globulin R77.1
    cortisol-binding E27.8
    thyroid-binding E07.89
  glomerular, minor (*see also* N00-N07 with fourth character .0) N05.0
  glucagon secretion E16.3
  glucose tolerance (test) (non-fasting) R73.09
  gravitational (G) forces or states (effect of) T75.81 ☑
  hair (color) (shaft) L67.9
    specified NEC L67.8
  hard tissue formation in pulp (dental) K04.3
  head movement R25.0
  heart
    rate R00.9
      specified NEC R00.8
    shadow R93.1
    sounds NEC R01.2
  hemoglobin (disease) (*see also* Disease, hemoglobin) D58.2
    trait — *see* Trait, hemoglobin, abnormal
  histology NEC R89.7
  immunological findings R89.4
    in serum R76.9
      specified NEC R76.8
  increase in appetite R63.2
  involuntary movement — *see* Abnormal, movement, involuntary
  jaw closure M26.51
  karyotype R89.8
  kidney function test R94.4
  knee jerk R29.2
  leukocyte (cell) (differential) NEC D72.9
  liver function test R94.5
  loss of
    height R29.890
    weight R63.4
  mammogram NEC R92.8
    calcification (calculus) R92.1
    microcalcification R92.0
  Mantoux test R76.11
  movement (disorder) (*see also* Disorder, movement)
    head R25.0
    involuntary R25.9
      fasciculation R25.3
      of head R25.0
      spasm R25.2
      specified type NEC R25.8
      tremor R25.1
  myoglobin (Aberdeen) (Annapolis) R89.7
  neonatal screening P09
  oculomotor study R94.113
  palmar creases Q82.8
  Papanicolaou (smear)
    anus R85.619
      atypical squamous cells cannot exclude high grade squamous intraepithelial lesion (ASC-H) R85.611
      atypical squamous cells of undetermined significance (ASC-US) R85.610
      cytologic evidence of malignancy R85.614
      high grade squamous intraepithelial lesion (HGSIL) R85.613
      human papillomavirus (HPV) DNA test
        high risk positive R85.81
        low risk positive R85.82
      inadequate smear R85.615
      low grade squamous intraepithelial lesion (LGSIL) R85.612
      satisfactory anal smear but lacking transformation zone R85.616
      specified NEC R85.618
      unsatisfactory smear R85.615
    bronchial washings R84.6
    cerebrospinal fluid R83.6
    cervix R87.619

Abnormal — *continued*
  Papanicolaou — *continued*
    atypical squamous cells cannot exclude high grade squamous intraepithelial lesion (ASC-H) R87.611
    atypical squamous cells of undetermined significance (ASC-US) R87.610
    cytologic evidence of malignancy R87.614
    high grade squamous intraepithelial lesion (HGSIL) R87.613
    inadequate smear R87.615
    low grade squamous intraepithelial lesion (LGSIL) R87.612
    non-atypical endometrial cells R87.618
    satisfactory cervical smear but lacking transformation zone R87.616
    specified NEC R87.618
    thin preparation R87.619
    unsatisfactory smear R87.615
    nasal secretions R84.6
    nipple discharge R89.6
    peritoneal fluid R85.69
    pleural fluid R84.6
    prostatic secretions R86.6
    saliva R85.69
    seminal fluid R86.6
    sites NEC R89.6
    sputum R84.6
    synovial fluid R89.6
    throat scrapings R84.6
    vagina R87.629
      atypical squamous cells cannot exclude high grade squamous intraepithelial lesion (ASC-H) R87.621
      atypical squamous cells of undetermined significance (ASC-US) R87.620
      cytologic evidence of malignancy R87.624
      high grade squamous intraepithelial lesion (HGSIL) R87.623
      inadequate smear R87.625
      low grade squamous intraepithelial lesion (LGSIL) R87.622
      specified NEC R87.628
      thin preparation R87.629
      unsatisfactory smear R87.625
    vulva R87.69
    wound secretions R89.6
  partial thromboplastin time (PTT) R79.1
  pelvis (bony) — *see* Deformity, pelvis
  percussion, chest (tympany) R09.89
  periods (grossly) — *see* Menstruation
  phonocardiogram R94.39
  plantar reflex R29.2
  plasma
    protein R77.9
      specified NEC R77.8
    viscosity R70.1
  pleural (folds) Q34.0
  posture R29.3
  product of conception O02.9
    specified type NEC O02.89
  prothrombin time (PT) R79.1
  pulmonary
    artery, congenital Q25.79
    function, newborn P28.89
    test results R94.2
  pulsations in neck R00.2
  pupillary H21.56 ☑
    function (reaction) (reflex) — *see* Anomaly, pupil, function
  radiological examination — *see* Abnormal, diagnostic imaging
  red blood cell (s) (morphology) (volume) R71.8
  reflex — *see* Reflex
  renal function test R94.4
  response to nerve stimulation R94.130
  retinal correspondence H53.31
  retinal function study R94.111
  rhythm, heart (*see also* Arrhythmia)
  saliva — *see* Abnormal, specimen, digestive organs
  scan
    kidney R94.4
    liver R93.2
    thyroid R94.6
  secretion
    gastrin E16.4
    glucagon E16.3
  semen, seminal fluid — *see* Abnormal, specimen, male genital organs
  serum level (of)
    acid phosphatase R74.8

Abnormal — *continued*
  serum level — *continued*
    alkaline phosphatase R74.8
    amylase R74.8
    enzymes R74.9
      specified NEC R74.8
    lipase R74.8
    triacylglycerol lipase R74.8
  shape
    gravid uterus — *see* Anomaly, uterus
  sinus venosus Q21.1
  size, tooth, teeth K00.2
  spacing, tooth, teeth, fully erupted M26.30
  specimen
    digestive organs (peritoneal fluid) (saliva) R85.9
      cytology R85.69
      drug level R85.2
      enzyme level R85.0
      histology R85.7
      hormones R85.1
      immunology R85.4
      microbiology R85.5
      nonmedicinal level R85.3
      specified type NEC R85.89
    female genital organs (secretions) (smears) R87.9
      cytology R87.69
        cervix R87.619
          human papillomavirus (HPV) DNA test
            high risk positive R87.810
            low risk positive R87.820
          inadequate (unsatisfactory) smear R87.615
          non-atypical endometrial cells R87.618
          specified NEC R87.618
        vagina R87.629
          human papillomavirus (HPV) DNA test
            high risk positive R87.811
            low risk positive R87.821
          inadequate (unsatisfactory) smear R87.625
        vulva R87.69
      drug level R87.2
      enzyme level R87.0
      histological R87.7
      hormones R87.1
      immunology R87.4
      microbiology R87.5
      nonmedicinal level R87.3
      specified type NEC R87.89
    male genital organs (prostatic secretions) (semen) R86.9
      cytology R86.6
      drug level R86.2
      enzyme level R86.0
      histological R86.7
      hormones R86.1
      immunology R86.4
      microbiology R86.5
      nonmedicinal level R86.3
      specified type NEC R86.8
    nipple discharge — *see* Abnormal, specimen, specified
    respiratory organs (bronchial washings) (nasal secretions) (pleural fluid) (sputum) R84.9
      cytology R84.6
      drug level R84.2
      enzyme level R84.0
      histology R84.7
      hormones R84.1
      immunology R84.4
      microbiology R84.5
      nonmedicinal level R84.3
      specified type NEC R84.8
    specified organ, system and tissue NOS R89.9
      cytology R89.6
      drug level R89.2
      enzyme level R89.0
      histology R89.7
      hormones R89.1
      immunology R89.4
      microbiology R89.5
      nonmedicinal level R89.3
      specified type NEC R89.8
    synovial fluid — *see* Abnormal, specimen, specified
    thorax (bronchial washings) (pleural fluids) — *see* Abnormal, specimen, respiratory organs
    vagina (secretion) (smear) R87.629
    vulva (secretion) (smear) R87.69

☑ **Additional character required**

Abnormal   ICD-10-CM INDEX TO DISEASES AND INJURIES

Abnormal — *continued*
specimen — *continued*
wound secretion — *see* Abnormal, specimen, specified
spermatozoa — *see* Abnormal, specimen, male genital organs
sputum (amount) (color) (odor) R09.3
stool (color) (contents) (mucus) R19.5
bloody K92.1
guaiac positive R19.5
synchondrosis Q78.8
thermography (*see also* Abnormal, diagnostic imaging) R93.8
thyroid-binding globulin E07.89
tooth, teeth (form) (size) K00.2
toxicology (findings) R78.9
transport protein E88.09
tumor marker NEC R97.8
ultrasound results — *see* Abnormal, diagnostic imaging
umbilical cord complicating delivery O69.9 ☑
urination NEC R39.198
urine (constituents) R82.90
bile R82.2
cytological examination R82.8
drugs R82.5
fat R82.0
glucose R81
heavy metals R82.6
hemoglobin R82.3
histological examination R82.8
ketones R82.4
microbiological examination (culture) R82.79
myoglobin R82.1
positive culture R82.79
protein — *see* Proteinuria
specified substance NEC R82.99
chromoabnormality NEC R82.91
substances nonmedical R82.6
uterine hemorrhage — *see* Hemorrhage, uterus
vectorcardiogram R94.39
visually evoked potential (VEP) R94.112
white blood cells D72.9
specified NEC D72.89
X-ray examination — *see* Abnormal, diagnostic imaging
Abnormity (any organ or part) — *see* Anomaly
Abocclusion M26.29
hemolytic disease (newborn) P55.1
incompatibility reaction ABO — *see* Complication (s), transfusion, incompatibility reaction, ABO
Abolition, language R48.8
Aborter, habitual or recurrent — *see* Loss (of), pregnancy, recurrent
Abortion (complete) (spontaneous) O03.9
with
retained products of conception — *see* Abortion, incomplete
attempted (elective) (failed) O07.4
complicated by O07.30
afibrinogenemia O07.1
cardiac arrest O07.36
chemical damage of pelvic organ (s) O07.34
circulatory collapse O07.31
cystitis O07.38
defibrination syndrome O07.1
electrolyte imbalance O07.33
embolism (air) (amniotic fluid) (blood clot) (fat) (pulmonary) (septic) (soap) O07.2
endometritis O07.0
genital tract and pelvic infection O07.0
hemolysis O07.1
hemorrhage (delayed) (excessive) O07.1
infection
genital tract or pelvic O07.0
urinary tract O07.38
intravascular coagulation O07.1
laceration of pelvic organ (s) O07.34
metabolic disorder O07.33
oliguria O07.32
oophoritis O07.0
parametritis O07.0
pelvic peritonitis O07.0
perforation of pelvic organ (s) O07.34
renal failure or shutdown O07.32
salpingitis or salpingo-oophoritis O07.0
sepsis O07.37
shock O07.31
specified condition NEC O07.39
tubular necrosis (renal) O07.32
uremia O07.32

Abortion — *continued*
attempted — *continued*
urinary tract infection O07.38
venous complication NEC O07.35
embolism (air) (amniotic fluid) (blood clot) (fat) (pulmonary) (septic) (soap) O07.2
complicated (by) (following) O03.80
afibrinogenemia O03.6
cardiac arrest O03.86
chemical damage of pelvic organ (s) O03.84
circulatory collapse O03.81
cystitis O03.88
defibrination syndrome O03.6
electrolyte imbalance O03.83
embolism (air) (amniotic fluid) (blood clot) (fat) (pulmonary) (septic) (soap) O03.7
endometritis O03.5
genital tract and pelvic infection O03.5
hemolysis O03.6
hemorrhage (delayed) (excessive) O03.6
infection
genital tract or pelvic O03.5
urinary tract O03.88
intravascular coagulation O03.6
laceration of pelvic organ (s) O03.84
metabolic disorder O03.83
oliguria O03.82
oophoritis O03.5
parametritis O03.5
pelvic peritonitis O03.5
perforation of pelvic organ (s) O03.84
renal failure or shutdown O03.82
salpingitis or salpingo-oophoritis O03.5
sepsis O03.87
shock O03.81
specified condition NEC O03.89
tubular necrosis (renal) O03.82
uremia O03.82
urinary tract infection O03.88
venous complication NEC O03.85
embolism (air) (amniotic fluid) (blood clot) (fat) (pulmonary) (septic) (soap) O03.7
failed — *see* Abortion, attempted
habitual or recurrent N96
with current abortion — *see* categories O03-O04
without current pregnancy N96
care in current pregnancy O26.2 ☑
incomplete (spontaneous) O03.4
complicated (by) (following) O03.30
afibrinogenemia O03.1
cardiac arrest O03.36
chemical damage of pelvic organ (s) O03.34
circulatory collapse O03.31
cystitis O03.38
defibrination syndrome O03.1
electrolyte imbalance O03.33
embolism (air) (amniotic fluid) (blood clot) (fat) (pulmonary) (septic) (soap) O03.2
endometritis O03.0
genital tract and pelvic infection O03.0
hemolysis O03.1
hemorrhage (delayed) (excessive) O03.1
infection
genital tract or pelvic O03.0
urinary tract O03.38
intravascular coagulation O03.1
laceration of pelvic organ (s) O03.34
metabolic disorder O03.33
oliguria O03.32
oophoritis O03.0
parametritis O03.0
pelvic peritonitis O03.0
perforation of pelvic organ (s) O03.34
renal failure or shutdown O03.32
salpingitis or salpingo-oophoritis O03.0
sepsis O03.37
shock O03.31
specified condition NEC O03.39
tubular necrosis (renal) O03.32
uremia O03.32
urinary infection O03.38
venous complication NEC O03.35
embolism (air) (amniotic fluid) (blood clot) (fat) (pulmonary) (septic) (soap) O03.2
induced (encounter for) Z33.2
complicated by O04.80
afibrinogenemia O04.6
cardiac arrest O04.86
chemical damage of pelvic organ (s) O04.84
circulatory collapse O04.81
cystitis O04.88

Abortion — *continued*
induced — *continued*
defibrination syndrome O04.6
electrolyte imbalance O04.83
embolism (air) (amniotic fluid) (blood clot) (fat) (pulmonary) (septic) (soap) O04.7
endometritis O04.5
genital tract and pelvic infection O04.5
hemolysis O04.6
hemorrhage (delayed) (excessive) O04.6
infection
genital tract or pelvic O04.5
urinary tract O04.88
intravascular coagulation O04.6
laceration of pelvic organ (s) O04.84
metabolic disorder O04.83
oliguria O04.82
oophoritis O04.5
parametritis O04.5
pelvic peritonitis O04.5
perforation of pelvic organ (s) O04.84
renal failure or shutdown O04.82
salpingitis or salpingo-oophoritis O04.5
sepsis O04.87
shock O04.81
specified condition NEC O04.89
tubular necrosis (renal) O04.82
uremia O04.82
urinary tract infection O04.88
venous complication NEC O04.85
embolism (air) (amniotic fluid) (blood clot) (fat) (pulmonary) (septic) (soap) O04.7
missed O02.1
spontaneous — *see* Abortion (complete) (spontaneous)
threatened O20.0
threatened (spontaneous) O20.0
tubal O00.10 ☑
with intrauterine pregnancy O00.11 ☑
Abortus fever A23.1
Aboulomania F60.7
Abrami's disease D59.8
Abramov-Fiedler myocarditis (acute isolated myocarditis) I40.1
Abrasion T14.8 ☑
abdomen, abdominal (wall) S30.811 ☑
alveolar process S00.512 ☑
ankle S90.51 ☑
antecubital space — *see* Abrasion, elbow
anus S30.817 ☑
arm (upper) S40.81 ☑
auditory canal — *see* Abrasion, ear
auricle — *see* Abrasion, ear
axilla — *see* Abrasion, arm
back, lower S30.810 ☑
breast S20.11 ☑
brow S00.81 ☑
buttock S30.810 ☑
calf — *see* Abrasion, leg
canthus — *see* Abrasion, eyelid
cheek S00.81 ☑
internal S00.512 ☑
chest wall — *see* Abrasion, thorax
chin S00.81 ☑
clitoris S30.814 ☑
cornea S05.0 ☑
costal region — *see* Abrasion, thorax
dental K03.1
digit (s)
foot — *see* Abrasion, toe
hand — *see* Abrasion, finger
ear S00.41 ☑
elbow S50.31 ☑
epididymis S30.813 ☑
epigastric region S30.811 ☑
epiglottis S10.11 ☑
esophagus (thoracic) S27.818 ☑
cervical S10.11 ☑
eyebrow — *see* Abrasion, eyelid
eyelid S00.21 ☑
face S00.81 ☑
finger (s) S60.41 ☑
index S60.41 ☑
little S60.41 ☑
middle S60.41 ☑
ring S60.41 ☑
flank S30.811 ☑
foot (except toe (s) alone) S90.81 ☑
toe — *see* Abrasion, toe
forearm S50.81 ☑
elbow only — *see* Abrasion, elbow
forehead S00.81 ☑

Abrasion - Abscess

Abrasion - Abscess

ICD-10-CM INDEX TO DISEASES AND INJURIES

Abrasion — continued
genital organs, external
female S30.816 ☑
male S30.815 ☑
groin S30.811 ☑
gum S00.512 ☑
hand S60.51 ☑
head S00.91 ☑
ear — see Abrasion, ear
eyelid — see Abrasion, eyelid
lip S00.511 ☑
nose S00.31 ☑
oral cavity S00.512 ☑
scalp S00.01 ☑
specified site NEC S00.81 ☑
heel — see Abrasion, foot
hip S70.21 ☑
inguinal region S30.811 ☑
interscapular region S20.419 ☑
jaw S00.81 ☑
knee S80.21 ☑
labium (majus) (minus) S30.814 ☑
larynx S10.11 ☑
leg (lower) S80.81 ☑
knee — see Abrasion, knee
upper — see Abrasion, thigh
lip S00.511 ☑
lower back S30.810 ☑
lumbar region S30.810 ☑
malar region S00.81 ☑
mammary — see Abrasion, breast
mastoid region S00.81 ☑
mouth S00.512 ☑
nail
finger — see Abrasion, finger
toe — see Abrasion, toe
nape S10.81 ☑
nasal S00.31 ☑
neck S10.91 ☑
specified site NEC S10.81 ☑
throat S10.11 ☑
nose S00.31 ☑
occipital region S00.01 ☑
oral cavity S00.512 ☑
orbital region — see Abrasion, eyelid
palate S00.512 ☑
palm — see Abrasion, hand
parietal region S00.01 ☑
pelvis S30.810 ☑
penis S30.812 ☑
perineum
female S30.814 ☑
male S30.810 ☑
periocular area — see Abrasion, eyelid
phalanges
finger — see Abrasion, finger
toe — see Abrasion, toe
pharynx S10.11 ☑
pinna — see Abrasion, ear
popliteal space — see Abrasion, knee
prepuce S30.812 ☑
pubic region S30.810 ☑
pudendum
female S30.816 ☑
male S30.815 ☑
sacral region S30.810 ☑
scalp S00.01 ☑
scapular region — see Abrasion, shoulder
scrotum S30.813 ☑
shin — see Abrasion, leg
shoulder S40.21 ☑
skin NEC T14.8 ☑
sternal region S20.319 ☑
submaxillary region S00.81 ☑
submental region S00.81 ☑
subungual
finger (s) — see Abrasion, finger
toe (s) — see Abrasion, toe
supraclavicular fossa S10.81 ☑
supraorbital S00.81 ☑
temple S00.81 ☑
temporal region S00.81 ☑
testis S30.813 ☑
thigh S70.31 ☑
thorax, thoracic (wall) S20.91 ☑
back S20.41 ☑
front S20.31 ☑
throat S10.11 ☑
thumb S60.31 ☑
toe (s) (lesser) S90.416 ☑
great S90.41 ☑
tongue S00.512 ☑

Abrasion — continued
tooth, teeth (dentifrice) (habitual) (hard tissues) (occupational) (ritual) (traditional) K03.1
trachea S10.11 ☑
tunica vaginalis S30.813 ☑
tympanum, tympanic membrane — see Abrasion, ear
uvula S00.512 ☑
vagina S30.814 ☑
vocal cords S10.11 ☑
vulva S30.814 ☑
wrist S60.81 ☑
Abrism — see Poisoning, food, noxious, plant
Abruptio placentae O45.9 ☑
with
afibrinogenemia O45.01 ☑
coagulation defect O45.00 ☑
specified NEC O45.09 ☑
disseminated intravascular coagulation O45.02 ☑
hypofibrinogenemia O45.01 ☑
specified NEC O45.8 ☑
Abruption, placenta — see Abruptio placentae
Abscess (connective tissue) (embolic) (fistulous) (infective) (metastatic) (multiple) (pernicious) (pyogenic) (septic) L02.91
with
diverticular disease (intestine) K57.80
with bleeding K57.81
large intestine K57.20
with
bleeding K57.21
small intestine K57.40
with bleeding K57.41
small intestine K57.00
with
bleeding K57.01
large intestine K57.40
with bleeding K57.41
lymphangitis - code by site under Abscess
abdomen, abdominal
cavity K65.1
wall L02.211
abdominopelvic K65.1
accessory sinus — see Sinusitis
adrenal (capsule) (gland) E27.8
alveolar K04.7
with sinus K04.6
ambic A06.4
brain (and liver or lung abscess) A06.6
genitourinary tract A06.82
liver (without mention of brain or lung abscess) A06.4
lung (and liver) (without mention of brain abscess) A06.5
specified site NEC A06.89
spleen A06.89
anerobic A48.0
ankle — see Abscess, lower limb
anorectal K61.2
antecubital space — see Abscess, upper limb
antrum (chronic) (Highmore) — see Sinusitis, maxillary
anus K61.0
apical (tooth) K04.7
with sinus (alveolar) K04.6
appendix K35.3
areola (acute) (chronic) (nonpuerperal) N61.1
puerperal, postpartum or gestational — see Infection, nipple
arm (any part) — see Abscess, upper limb
artery (wall) I77.89
atheromatous I77.2
auricle, ear — see Abscess, ear, external
axilla (region) L02.41 ☑
lymph gland or node L04.2
back (any part, except buttock) L02.212
Bartholin's gland N75.1
with
abortion — see Abortion, by type complicated by, sepsis
ectopic or molar pregnancy O08.0
following ectopic or molar pregnancy O08.0
Bezold's — see Mastoiditis, acute
bilharziasis B65.1
bladder (wall) — see Cystitis, specified type NEC
bone (subperiosteal) (see also Osteomyelitis, specified type NEC)
accessory sinus (chronic) — see Sinusitis
chronic or old — see Osteomyelitis, chronic
jaw (lower) (upper) M27.2
mastoid — see Mastoiditis, acute, subperiosteal

Abscess — continued
bone — continued
petrous — see Petrositis
spinal (tuberculous) A18.01
nontuberculous — see Osteomyelitis, vertebra
bowel K63.0
brain (any part) (cystic) (otogenic) G06.0
amebic (with abscess of any other site) A06.6
gonococcal A54.82
pheomycotic (chromomycotic) B43.1
tuberculous A17.81
breast (acute) (chronic) (nonpuerperal) N61.1
newborn P39.0
puerperal, postpartum, gestational — see Mastitis, obstetric, purulent
broad ligament N73.2
acute N73.0
chronic N73.1
Brodie's (localized) (chronic) M86.8X ☑
bronchi J98.09
buccal cavity K12.2
bulbourethral gland N34.0
bursa M71.00
ankle M71.07 ☑
elbow M71.02 ☑
foot M71.07 ☑
hand M71.04 ☑
hip M71.05 ☑
knee M71.06 ☑
multiple sites M71.09
pharyngeal J39.1
shoulder M71.01 ☑
specified site NEC M71.08
wrist M71.03 ☑
buttock L02.31
canthus — see Blepharoconjunctivitis
cartilage — see Disorder, cartilage, specified type NEC
cecum K35.3
cerebellum, cerebellar G06.0
sequelae G09
cerebral (embolic) G06.0
sequelae G09
cervical (meaning neck) L02.11
lymph gland or node L04.0
cervix (stump) (uteri) — see Cervicitis
cheek (external) L02.01
inner K12.2
chest J86.9
with fistula J86.0
wall L02.213
chin L02.01
choroid — see Inflammation, chorioretinal
circumtonsillar J36
cold (lung) (tuberculous) (see also Tuberculosis, abscess, lung)
articular — see Tuberculosis, joint
colon (wall) K63.0
colostomy K94.02
conjunctiva — see Conjunctivitis, acute
cornea H16.31 ☑
corpus
cavernosum N48.21
luteum — see Oophoritis
Cowper's gland N34.0
cranium G06.0
cul-de-sac (Douglas') (posterior) — see Peritonitis, pelvic, female
cutaneous — see Abscess, by site
dental K04.7
with sinus (alveolar) K04.6
dentoalveolar K04.7
with sinus K04.6
diaphragm, diaphragmatic K65.1
Douglas' cul-de-sac or pouch — see Peritonitis, pelvic, female
Dubois A50.59
ear (middle) (see also Otitis, media, suppurative)
acute — see Otitis, media, suppurative, acute
external H60.0 ☑
entamebic — see Abscess, amebic
enterostomy K94.12
epididymis N45.4
epidural G06.2
brain G06.0
spinal cord G06.1
epiglottis J38.7
epiploon, epiploic K65.1
erysipelatous — see Erysipelas
esophagus K20.8
ethmoid (bone) (chronic) (sinus) J32.2

☑ Additional character required

Abscess — *continued*
external auditory canal — *see* Abscess, ear, external
extradural G06.2
  brain G06.0
    sequelae G09
  spinal cord G06.1
extraperitoneal K68.19
eye — *see* Endophthalmitis, purulent
eyelid H00.03 ☑
face (any part, except ear, eye and nose) L02.01
fallopian tube — *see* Salpingitis
fascia M72.8
fauces J39.1
fecal K63.0
femoral (region) — *see* Abscess, lower limb
filaria, filarial — *see* Infestation, filarial
finger (any) (*see also* Abscess, hand)
  nail — *see* Cellulitis, finger
foot L02.61 ☑
forehead L02.01
frontal sinus (chronic) J32.1
gallbladder K81.0
genital organ or tract
  female (external) N76.4
  male N49.9
    multiple sites N49.8
    specified NEC N49.8
gestational mammary O91.11 ☑
gestational subareolar O91.11 ☑
gingival — *see* Peridontitis, aggressive, localized
gland, glandular (lymph) (acute) — *see* Lymphadenitis, acute
gluteal (region) L02.31
gonorrheal — *see* Gonococcus
groin L02.214
gum — *see* Peridontitis, aggressive, localized
hand L02.51 ☑
head NEC L02.811
  face (any part, except ear, eye and nose) L02.01
heart — *see* Carditis
heel — *see* Abscess, foot
helminthic — *see* Infestation, helminth
hepatic (cholangitic) (hematogenic) (lymphogenic) (pylephlebitic) K75.0
  amebic A06.4
hip (region) — *see* Abscess, lower limb
ileocecal K35.3
ileostomy (bud) K94.12
iliac (region) L02.214
  fossa K35.3
infraclavicular (fossa) — *see* Abscess, upper limb
inguinal (region) L02.214
  lymph gland or node L04.1
intestine, intestinal NEC K63.0
  rectal K61.1
intra-abdominal (*see also* Abscess, peritoneum) K65.1
  postprocedural T81.4 ☑
  retroperitoneal K68.11
intracranial G06.0
intramammary — *see* Abscess, breast
intraorbital — *see* Abscess, orbit
intraperitoneal K65.1
intraspinal G06.1
intrasphincteric (anus) K61.4
intratonsillar J36
ischiorectal (fossa) K61.3
jaw (bone) (lower) (upper) M27.2
joint — *see* Arthritis, pyogenic or pyemic
  spine (tuberculous) A18.01
    nontuberculous — *see* Spondylopathy, infective
kidney N15.1
  with calculus N20.0
    with hydronephrosis N13.6
  puerperal (postpartum) O86.21
knee (*see also* Abscess, lower limb)
  joint M00.9
labium (majus) (minus) N76.4
lacrimal
  caruncle — *see* Inflammation, lacrimal, passages, acute
  gland — *see* Dacryoadenitis
  passages (duct) (sac) — *see* Inflammation, lacrimal, passages, acute
lacunar N34.0
larynx J38.7
lateral (alveolar) K04.7
  with sinus K04.6
leg (any part) — *see* Abscess, lower limb
lens H27.8

lingual K14.0
  tonsil J36
lip K13.0
Littre's gland N34.0
liver (cholangitic) (hematogenic) (lymphogenic) (pylephlebitic) (pyogenic) K75.0
  amebic (due to Entamoeba histolytica) (dysenteric) (tropical) A06.4
    with
      brain abscess (and liver or lung abscess) A06.6
      lung abscess A06.5
loin (region) L02.211
lower limb L02.41 ☑
lumbar (tuberculous) A18.01
  nontuberculous L02.212
lung (miliary) (putrid) J85.2
  with pneumonia J85.1
    due to specified organism (*see* Pneumonia, in (due to))
  amebic (with liver abscess) A06.5
    with
      brain abscess A06.6
      pneumonia A06.5
lymph, lymphatic, gland or node (acute) (*see also* Lymphadenitis, acute)
  mesentery I88.0
malar M27.2
mammary gland — *see* Abscess, breast
marginal, anus K61.0
mastoid — *see* Mastoiditis, acute
maxilla, maxillary M27.2
  molar (tooth) K04.7
    with sinus K04.6
  premolar K04.7
  sinus (chronic) J32.0
mediastinum J85.3
meibomian gland — *see* Hordeolum
meninges G06.2
mesentery, mesenteric K65.1
mesosalpinx — *see* Salpingitis
mons pubis L02.215
mouth (floor) K12.2
muscle — *see* Myositis, infective
myocardium I40.0
nabothian (follicle) — *see* Cervicitis
nasal J32.9
nasopharyngeal J39.1
navel L02.216
  newborn P38.9
    with mild hemorrhage P38.1
    without hemorrhage P38.9
neck (region) L02.11
  lymph gland or node L04.0
nephritic — *see* Abscess, kidney
nipple N61.1
  associated with
    lactation — *see* Pregnancy, complicated by
    pregnancy — *see* Pregnancy, complicated by
nose (external) (fossa) (septum) J34.0
  sinus (chronic) — *see* Sinusitis
omentum K65.1
operative wound T81.4 ☑
orbit, orbital — *see* Cellulitis, orbit
otogenic G06.0
ovary, ovarian (corpus luteum) — *see* Oophoritis
oviduct — *see* Oophoritis
palate (soft) K12.2
  hard M27.2
palmar (space) — *see* Abscess, hand
pancreas (duct) — *see* Pancreatitis, acute
parafrenal N48.21
parametric, parametrium N73.2
  acute N73.0
  chronic N73.1
paranephric N15.1
parapancreatic — *see* Pancreatitis, acute
parapharyngeal J39.0
pararectal K61.1
parasinus — *see* Sinusitis
parauterine (*see also* Disease, pelvis, inflammatory) N73.2
paravaginal — *see* Vaginitis
parietal region (scalp) L02.811
parodontal — *see* Peridontitis, aggressive, localized
parotid (duct) (gland) K11.3
  region K12.2
pectoral (region) L02.213
pelvis, pelvic
  female — *see* Disease, pelvis, inflammatory
  male, peritoneal K65.1

penis N48.21
  gonococcal (accessory gland) (periurethral) A54.1
perianal K61.0
periapical K04.7
  with sinus (alveolar) K04.6
periappendicular K35.3
pericardial I30.1
pericecal K35.3
pericemental — *see* Peridontitis, aggressive, localized
pericholecystic — *see* Cholecystitis, acute
pericoronal — *see* Peridontitis, aggressive, localized
peridental — *see* Peridontitis, aggressive, localized
perimetric (*see also* Disease, pelvis, inflammatory) N73.2
perinephric, perinephritic — *see* Abscess, kidney
perineum, perineal (superficial) L02.215
  urethra N34.0
periodontal (parietal) — *see* Peridontitis, aggressive, localized
  apical K04.7
periosteum, periosteal (*see also* Osteomyelitis, specified type NEC)
  with osteomyelitis (*see also* Osteomyelitis, specified type NEC)
    acute — *see* Osteomyelitis, acute
    chronic — *see* Osteomyelitis, chronic
peripharyngeal J39.0
peripleuritic J86.9
  with fistula J86.0
periprostatic N41.2
perirectal K61.1
perirenal (tissue) — *see* Abscess, kidney
perisinuous (nose) — *see* Sinusitis
peritoneum, peritoneal (perforated) (ruptured) K65.1
  with appendicitis K35.3
  pelvic
    female — *see* Peritonitis, pelvic, female
    male K65.1
  postoperative T81.4 ☑
  puerperal, postpartum, childbirth O85
  tuberculous A18.31
peritonsillar J36
perityphlic K35.3
periureteral N28.89
periurethral N34.0
  gonococcal (accessory gland) (periurethral) A54.1
periuterine (*see also* Disease, pelvis, inflammatory) N73.2
perivesical — *see* Cystitis, specified type NEC
petrous bone — *see* Petrositis
phagedenic NOS L02.91
  chancroid A57
pharynx, pharyngeal (lateral) J39.1
pilonidal L05.01
pituitary (gland) E23.6
pleura J86.9
  with fistula J86.0
popliteal — *see* Abscess, lower limb
postcecal K35.3
postlaryngeal J38.7
postnasal J34.0
postoperative (any site) T81.4 ☑
  retroperitoneal K68.11
postpharyngeal J39.0
posttonsillar J36
post-typhoid A01.09
pouch of Douglas — *see* Peritonitis, pelvic, female
premammary — *see* Abscess, breast
prepatellar — *see* Abscess, lower limb
prostate N41.2
  gonococcal (acute) (chronic) A54.22
psoas muscle K68.12
puerperal - code by site under Puerperal, abscess
pulmonary — *see* Abscess, lung
pulp, pulpal (dental) K04.01
  irreversible K04.02
  reversible K04.01
rectovaginal septum K63.0
rectovesical — *see* Cystitis, specified type NEC
rectum K61.1
renal — *see* Abscess, kidney
retina — *see* Inflammation, chorioretinal
retrobulbar — *see* Abscess, orbit
retrocecal K65.1
retrolaryngeal J38.7

Adenoma — continued
  tubular — continued
    female D27.9
    male D29.20
  tubulovillous (see also Neoplasm, benign, by site)
    adenocarcinoma in — see Neoplasm, malignant, by site
    adenocarcinoma in situ — see Neoplasm, in situ, by site
  villous — see Neoplasm, uncertain behavior, by site
    adenocarcinoma in — see Neoplasm, malignant, by site
    adenocarcinoma in situ — see Neoplasm, in situ, by site
  water-clear cell D35.1
Adenomatosis
  endocrine (multiple) E31.20
    single specified site — see Neoplasm, uncertain behavior, by site
  erosive of nipple D24 ☑
  pluriendocrine — see Adenomatosis, endocrine
  pulmonary D38.1
    malignant — see Neoplasm, lung, malignant
  specified site — see Neoplasm, benign, by site
  unspecified site D12.6
Adenomatous
  goiter (nontoxic) E04.9
    with hyperthyroidism — see Hyperthyroidism, with, goiter, nodular
    toxic — see Hyperthyroidism, with, goiter, nodular
Adenomyoma (see also Neoplasm, benign, by site)
  prostate — see Enlarged, prostate
Adenomyometritis N80.0
Adenomyosis N80.0
Adenopathy (lymph gland) R59.9
  generalized R59.1
  inguinal R59.0
  localized R59.0
  mediastinal R59.0
  mesentery R59.0
  syphilitic (secondary) A51.49
  tracheobronchial R59.0
    tuberculous A15.4
      primary (progressive) A15.7
  tuberculous (see also Tuberculosis, lymph gland) A18.2
    tracheobronchial A15.4
      primary (progressive) A15.7
Adenosalpingitis — see Salpingitis
Adenosarcoma — see Neoplasm, malignant, by site
Adenosclerosis I88.8
Adenosis (sclerosing) breast — see Fibroadenosis, breast
Adenovirus, as cause of disease classified elsewhere B97.0
Adentia (complete) (partial) — see Absence, teeth
Adherent (see also Adhesions)
  labia (minora) N90.89
  pericardium (nonrheumatic) I31.0
    rheumatic I09.2
  placenta (with hemorrhage) O72.0
    without hemorrhage O73.0
  prepuce, newborn N47.0
  scar (skin) L90.5
  tendon in scar L90.5
Adhesions, adhesive (postinfective) K66.0
  with intestinal obstruction K56.50
    complete K56.52
    incomplete K56.51
    partial K56.51
  abdominal (wall) — see Adhesions, peritoneum
  appendix K38.8
  bile duct (common) (hepatic) K83.8
  bladder (sphincter) N32.89
  bowel — see Adhesions, peritoneum
  cardiac I31.0
    rheumatic I09.2
  cecum — see Adhesions, peritoneum
  cervicovaginal N88.1
    congenital Q52.8
    postpartal O90.89
      old N88.1
  cervix N88.1
  ciliary body NEC — see Adhesions, iris
  clitoris N90.89
  colon — see Adhesions, peritoneum
  common duct K83.8
  congenital (see also Anomaly, by site)
    fingers — see Syndactylism, complex, fingers
    omental, anomalous Q43.3
    peritoneal Q43.3
    tongue (to gum or roof of mouth) Q38.3

Adhesions — continued
  conjunctiva (acquired) H11.21 ☑
    congenital Q15.8
  cystic duct K82.8
  diaphragm — see Adhesions, peritoneum
  due to foreign body — see Foreign body
  duodenum — see Adhesions, peritoneum
  ear
    middle H74.1 ☑
  epididymis N50.89
  epidural — see Adhesions, meninges
  epiglottis J38.7
  eyelid H02.59
  female pelvis N73.6
  gallbladder K82.8
  globe H44.89
  heart I31.0
    rheumatic I09.2
  ileocecal (coil) — see Adhesions, peritoneum
  ileum — see Adhesions, peritoneum
  intestine (see also Adhesions, peritoneum)
    with obstruction K56.50
      complete K56.52
      incomplete K56.51
      partial K56.51
  intra-abdominal — see Adhesions, peritoneum
  iris H21.50 ☑
    anterior H21.51 ☑
    goniosynechiae H21.52 ☑
    posterior H21.54 ☑
    to corneal graft T85.898 ☑
  joint — see Ankylosis
    knee M23.8X ☑
    temporomandibular M26.61 ☑
  labium (majus) (minus), congenital Q52.5
  liver — see Adhesions, peritoneum
  lung J98.4
  mediastinum J98.59
  meninges (cerebral) (spinal) G96.12
    congenital Q07.8
    tuberculous (cerebral) (spinal) A17.0
  mesenteric — see Adhesions, peritoneum
  nasal (septum) (to turbinates) J34.89
  ocular muscle — see Strabismus, mechanical
  omentum — see Adhesions, peritoneum
  ovary N73.6
    congenital (to cecum, kidney or omentum) Q50.39
  paraovarian N73.6
  pelvic (peritoneal)
    female N73.6
      postprocedural N99.4
    male — see Adhesions, peritoneum
    postpartal (old) N73.6
    tuberculous A18.17
  penis to scrotum (congenital) Q55.8
  periappendiceal (see also Adhesions, peritoneum)
  pericardium (nonrheumatic) I31.0
    focal I31.8
    rheumatic I09.2
    tuberculous A18.84
  pericholecystic K82.8
  perigastric — see Adhesions, peritoneum
  periovarian N73.6
  periprostatic N42.89
  perirectal — see Adhesions, peritoneum
  perirenal N28.89
  peritoneum, peritoneal (postinfective)
    with obstruction (intestinal) K56.50
      complete K56.52
      incomplete K56.51
      partial K56.51
    congenital Q43.3
    pelvic, female N73.6
      postprocedural N99.4
    postpartal, pelvic N73.6
    postprocedural K66.0
    to uterus N73.6
  peritubal N73.6
  periureteral N28.89
  periuterine N73.6
  perivesical N32.89
  perivesicular (seminal vesicle) N50.89
  pleura, pleuritic J94.8
    tuberculous NEC A15.6
  pleuropericardial J94.8
  postoperative (gastrointestinal tract) K66.0
    with obstruction (see also Obstruction, intestine, postoperative) K91.30
    due to foreign body accidentally left in wound — see Foreign body, accidentally left during a procedure

Adhesions — continued
  postoperative — continued
    pelvic peritoneal N99.4
    urethra — see Stricture, urethra, postprocedural
    vagina N99.2
  postpartal, old (vulva or perineum) N90.89
  preputial, prepuce N47.5
  pulmonary J98.4
  pylorus — see Adhesions, peritoneum
  sciatic nerve — see Lesion, nerve, sciatic
  seminal vesicle N50.89
  shoulder (joint) — see Capsulitis, adhesive
  sigmoid flexure — see Adhesions, peritoneum
  spermatic cord (acquired) N50.89
    congenital Q55.4
  spinal canal G96.12
  stomach — see Adhesions, peritoneum
  subscapular — see Capsulitis, adhesive
  temporomandibular M26.61 ☑
  tendinitis (see also Tenosynovitis, specified type NEC)
    shoulder — see Capsulitis, adhesive
  testis N44.8
  tongue, congenital (to gum or roof of mouth) Q38.3
    acquired K14.8
  trachea J39.8
  tubo-ovarian N73.6
  tunica vaginalis N44.8
  uterus N73.6
    internal N85.6
    to abdominal wall N73.6
  vagina (chronic) N89.5
    postoperative N99.2
  vitreomacular H43.82 ☑
  vitreous H43.89
  vulva N90.89
Adiaspiromycosis B48.8
Adie (-Holmes) pupil or syndrome — see Anomaly, pupil, function, tonic pupil
Adiponecrosis neonatorum P83.88
Adiposis (see also Obesity)
  cerebralis E23.6
  dolorosa E88.2
Adiposity (see also Obesity)
  heart — see Degeneration, myocardial
  localized E65
Adiposogenital dystrophy E23.6
Adjustment
  disorder — see Disorder, adjustment
  implanted device — see Encounter (for), adjustment (of)
  prosthesis, external — see Fitting
  reaction — see Disorder, adjustment
Administration of tPA (rtPA) in a different facility within the last 24 hours prior to admission to current facility Z92.82
Admission (for) (see also Encounter (for))
  adjustment (of)
    artificial
      arm Z44.00 ☑
        complete Z44.01 ☑
        partial Z44.02 ☑
      eye Z44.2 ☑
      leg Z44.10 ☑
        complete Z44.11 ☑
        partial Z44.12 ☑
    brain neuropacemaker Z46.2
    implanted Z45.42
    breast
      implant Z45.81 ☑
      prosthesis (external) Z44.3 ☑
    colostomy belt Z46.89
    contact lenses Z46.0
    cystostomy device Z46.6
    dental prosthesis Z46.3
    device NEC
      abdominal Z46.89
      implanted Z45.89
        cardiac Z45.09
          defibrillator (with synchronous cardiac pacemaker) Z45.02
          pacemaker (cardiac resynchronization therapy (CRT-P)) Z45.018
          pulse generator Z45.010
          resynchronization therapy defibrillator (CRT-D) Z45.02
      hearing device Z45.328
        bone conduction Z45.320
        cochlear Z45.321
      infusion pump Z45.1
      nervous system Z45.49

☑ **Additional character required**

Admission — *continued*
  adjustment — *continued*
        CSF drainage Z45.41
        hearing device — *see* Admission,
          adjustment, device, implanted,
          hearing device
        neuropacemaker Z45.42
        visual substitution Z45.31
      specified NEC Z45.89
      vascular access Z45.2
      visual substitution Z45.31
    nervous system Z46.2
      implanted — *see* Admission, adjustment,
        device, implanted, nervous system
    orthodontic Z46.4
    prosthetic Z44.9
      arm — *see* Admission, adjustment, artificial,
        arm
      breast Z44.3 ☑
      dental Z46.3
      eye Z44.2 ☑
      leg — *see* Admission, adjustment, artificial,
        leg
      specified type NEC Z44.8
    substitution
      auditory Z46.2
        implanted — *see* Admission, adjustment,
          device, implanted, hearing device
      nervous system Z46.2
        implanted — *see* Admission, adjustment,
          device, implanted, nervous system
      visual Z46.2
        implanted Z45.31
    urinary Z46.6
  hearing aid Z46.1
    implanted — *see* Admission, adjustment,
      device, implanted, hearing device
  ileostomy device Z46.89
  intestinal appliance or device NEC Z46.89
  neuropacemaker (brain) (peripheral nerve)
    (spinal cord) Z46.2
    implanted Z45.42
  orthodontic device Z46.4
  orthopedic (brace) (cast) (device)
    (shoes) Z46.89
  pacemaker (cardiac resynchronization therapy
    (CRT-P))
    cardiac Z45.018
      pulse generator Z45.010
    nervous system Z46.2
      implanted Z45.42
  portacath (port-a-cath) Z45.2
  prosthesis Z44.9
    arm — *see* Admission, adjustment, artificial,
      arm
    breast Z44.3 ☑
    dental Z46.3
    eye Z44.2 ☑
    leg — *see* Admission, adjustment, artificial,
      leg
    specified NEC Z44.8
  spectacles Z46.0
  aftercare (*see also* Aftercare) Z51.89
    postpartum
      immediately after delivery Z39.0
      routine follow-up Z39.2
    radiation therapy (antineoplastic) Z51.0
  attention to artificial opening (of) Z43.9
    artificial vagina Z43.7
    colostomy Z43.3
    cystostomy Z43.5
    enterostomy Z43.4
    gastrostomy Z43.1
    ileostomy Z43.2
    jejunostomy Z43.4
    nephrostomy Z43.6
    specified site NEC Z43.8
      intestinal tract Z43.4
      urinary tract Z43.6
    tracheostomy Z43.0
    ureterostomy Z43.6
    urethrostomy Z43.6
  breast augmentation or reduction Z41.1
  breast reconstruction following
    mastectomy Z42.1
  change of
    dressing (nonsurgical) Z48.00
    neuropacemaker device (brain) (peripheral
      nerve) (spinal cord) Z46.2
      implanted Z45.42
    surgical dressing Z48.01

Admission — *continued*
  circumcision, ritual or routine (in absence of
    diagnosis) Z41.2
  clinical research investigation (control) (normal
    comparison) (participant) Z00.6
  contraceptive management Z30.9
  cosmetic surgery NEC Z41.1
  counseling (*see also* Counseling)
    dietary Z71.3
    gestational carrier Z31.7
    HIV Z71.7
    human immunodeficiency virus Z71.7
    nonattending third party Z71.0
    procreative management NEC Z31.69
  delivery, full-term, uncomplicated O80
    cesarean, without indication O82
  desensitization to allergens Z51.6
  dietary surveillance and counseling Z71.3
  ear piercing Z41.3
  examination at health care facility (adult) (*see also*
    Examination) Z00.00
    with abnormal findings Z00.01
    clinical research investigation (control) (normal
      comparison) (participant) Z00.6
    dental Z01.20
      with abnormal findings Z01.21
    donor (potential) Z00.5
    ear Z01.10
      with abnormal findings NEC Z01.118
    eye Z01.00
      with abnormal findings Z01.01
    general, specified reason NEC Z00.8
    hearing Z01.10
      with abnormal findings NEC Z01.118
    postpartum checkup Z39.2
    psychiatric (general) Z00.8
      requested by authority Z04.6
    vision Z01.00
      with abnormal findings Z01.01
  fitting (of)
    artificial
      arm — *see* Admission, adjustment, artificial,
        arm
      eye Z44.2 ☑
      leg — *see* Admission, adjustment, artificial,
        leg
    brain neuropacemaker Z46.2
      implanted Z45.42
    breast prosthesis (external) Z44.3 ☑
    colostomy belt Z46.89
    contact lenses Z46.0
    cystostomy device Z46.6
    dental prosthesis Z46.3
    dentures Z46.3
    device NEC
      abdominal Z46.89
      nervous system Z46.2
        implanted — *see* Admission, adjustment,
          device, implanted, nervous system
      orthodontic Z46.4
      prosthetic Z44.9
        breast Z44.3 ☑
        dental Z46.3
        eye Z44.2 ☑
      substitution
        auditory Z46.2
          implanted — *see* Admission, adjustment,
            device, implanted, hearing device
        nervous system Z46.2
          implanted — *see* Admission, adjustment,
            device, implanted, nervous system
        visual Z46.2
          implanted Z45.31
    hearing aid Z46.1
    ileostomy device Z46.89
    intestinal appliance or device NEC Z46.89
    neuropacemaker (brain) (peripheral nerve)
      (spinal cord) Z46.2
      implanted Z45.42
    orthodontic device Z46.4
    orthopedic device (brace) (cast) (shoes) Z46.89
    prosthesis Z44.9
      arm — *see* Admission, adjustment, artificial,
        arm
      breast Z44.3 ☑
      dental Z46.3
      eye Z44.2 ☑
      leg — *see* Admission, adjustment, artificial,
        leg
      specified type NEC Z44.8
    spectacles Z46.0
  follow-up examination Z09

Admission — *continued*
  intrauterine device management Z30.431
    initial prescription Z30.014
  mental health evaluation Z00.8
    requested by authority Z04.6
  observation — *see* Observation
  Papanicolaou smear, cervix Z12.4
    for suspected malignant neoplasm Z12.4
  plastic and reconstructive surgery following
    medical procedure or healed injury
    NEC Z42.8
  plastic surgery, cosmetic NEC Z41.1
  postpartum observation
    immediately after delivery Z39.0
    routine follow-up Z39.2
  poststerilization (for restoration) Z31.0
    aftercare Z31.42
  procreative management Z31.9
  prophylactic (measure) (*see also* Encounter,
    prophylactic measures)
    organ removal Z40.00
      breast Z40.01
      fallopian tube (s) Z40.03
        with ovary (s) Z40.02
      ovary (s) Z40.02
      specified organ NEC Z40.09
      testes Z40.09
    vaccination Z23
  psychiatric examination (general) Z00.8
    requested by authority Z04.6
  radiation therapy (antineoplastic) Z51.0
  reconstructive surgery following medical
    procedure or healed injury NEC Z42.8
  removal of
    cystostomy catheter Z43.5
    drains Z48.03
    dressing (nonsurgical) Z48.00
    implantable subdermal contraceptive Z30.46
    intrauterine contraceptive device Z30.432
    neuropacemaker (brain) (peripheral nerve)
      (spinal cord) Z46.2
      implanted Z45.42
    staples Z48.02
    surgical dressing Z48.01
    sutures Z48.02
    ureteral stent Z46.6
  respirator [ventilator] use during power
    failure Z99.12
  restoration of organ continuity
    (poststerilization) Z31.0
    aftercare Z31.42
  sensitivity test (*see also* Test, skin)
    allergy NEC Z01.82
    Mantoux Z11.1
  tuboplasty following previous sterilization Z31.0
    aftercare Z31.42
  vasoplasty following previous sterilization Z31.0
    aftercare Z31.42
  vision examination Z01.00
    with abnormal findings Z01.01
  waiting period for admission to other
    facility Z75.1
Adnexitis (suppurative) — *see* Salpingo-oophoritis
Adolescent X-linked adrenoleukodystrophy E71.521
Adrenal (gland) — *see* condition
Adrenalism, tuberculous A18.7
Adrenalitis, adrenitis E27.8
  autoimmune E27.1
  meningococcal, hemorrhagic A39.1
Adrenarche, premature E27.0
Adrenocortical syndrome — *see* Cushing's,
  syndrome
Adrenogenital syndrome E25.9
  acquired E25.8
  congenital E25.0
  salt loss E25.0
Adrenogenitalism, congenital E25.0
Adrenoleukodystrophy E71.529
  neonatal E71.511
  X-linked E71.529
    Addison only phenotype E71.528
    Addison-Schilder E71.528
    adolescent E71.521
    adrenomyeloneuropathy E71.522
    childhood cerebral E71.520
    other specified E71.528
Adrenomyeloneuropathy E71.522
Adventitious bursa — *see* Bursopathy, specified
  type NEC
Adverse effect — *see* Table of Drugs and Chemicals,
  categories T36-T50, with 6th character 5
Advice — *see* Counseling

Adynamia - Agenesis

Adynamia (episodica) (hereditary) (periodic) G72.3
Aeration lung imperfect, newborn — *see* Atelectasis
Aerobullosis T70.3 ☑
Aerocele — *see* Embolism, air
Aerodermectasia
   subcutaneous (traumatic) T79.7 ☑
Aerodontalgia T70.29 ☑
Aeroembolism T70.3 ☑
Aerogenes capsulatus infection A48.0
Aero-otitis media T70.0 ☑
Aerophagy, aerophagia (psychogenic) F45.8
Aerophobia F40.228
Aerosinusitis T70.1 ☑
Aerotitis T70.0 ☑
Affection — *see* Disease
Afibrinogenemia (*see also* Defect, coagulation)
   D68.8
   acquired D65
   congenital D68.2
   following ectopic or molar pregnancy O08.1
   in abortion — *see* Abortion, by type, complicated
     by, afibrinogenemia
   puerperal O72.3
African
   sleeping sickness B56.9
   tick fever A68.1
   trypanosomiasis B56.9
     gambian B56.0
     rhodesian B56.1
Aftercare (*see also* Care) Z51.89
   following surgery (for) (on)
     amputation Z47.81
     attention to
       drains Z48.03
       dressings (nonsurgical) Z48.00
         surgical Z48.01
       sutures Z48.02
     circulatory system Z48.812
     delayed (planned) wound closure Z48.1
     digestive system Z48.815
     explantation of joint prosthesis (staged
       procedure)
       hip Z47.32
       knee Z47.33
       shoulder Z47.31
     genitourinary system Z48.816
     joint replacement Z47.1
     neoplasm Z48.3
     nervous system Z48.811
     oral cavity Z48.814
     organ transplant
       bone marrow Z48.290
       heart Z48.21
       heart-lung Z48.280
       kidney Z48.22
       liver Z48.23
       lung Z48.24
       multiple organs NEC Z48.288
       specified NEC Z48.298
     orthopedic NEC Z47.89
     planned wound closure Z48.1
     removal of internal fixation device Z47.2
     respiratory system Z48.813
     scoliosis Z47.82
     sense organs Z48.810
     skin and subcutaneous tissue Z48.817
     specified body system
       circulatory Z48.812
       digestive Z48.815
       genitourinary Z48.816
       nervous Z48.811
       oral cavity Z48.814
       respiratory Z48.813
       sense organs Z48.810
       skin and subcutaneous tissue Z48.817
       teeth Z48.814
     specified NEC Z48.89
     spinal Z47.89
     teeth Z48.814
   fracture - code to fracture with seventh character
     D
   involving
     removal of
       drains Z48.03
       dressings (nonsurgical) Z48.00
       staples Z48.02
       surgical dressings Z48.01
       sutures Z48.02
   neuropacemaker (brain) (peripheral nerve)
     (spinal cord) Z46.2
     implanted Z45.42
   orthopedic NEC Z47.89

Aftercare — *continued*
   postprocedural — *see* Aftercare, following
     surgery
After-cataract — *see* Cataract, secondary
Agalactia (primary) O92.3
   elective, secondary or therapeutic O92.5
Agammaglobulinemia (acquired (secondary))
   (nonfamilial) D80.1
   with
     immunoglobulin-bearing B-lymphocytes D80.1
     lymphopenia D81.9
   autosomal recessive (Swiss type) D80.0
   Bruton's X-linked D80.0
   common variable (CVAgamma) D80.1
   congenital sex-linked D80.0
   hereditary D80.0
   lymphopenic D81.9
   Swiss type (autosomal recessive) D80.0
   X-linked (with growth hormone deficiency)
     (Bruton) D80.0
Aganglionosis (bowel) (colon) Q43.1
Age (old) — *see* Senility
Agenesis
   adrenal (gland) Q89.1
   alimentary tract (complete) (partial) NEC Q45.8
     upper Q40.8
   anus, anal (canal) Q42.3
     with fistula Q42.2
   aorta Q25.41
   appendix Q42.8
   arm (complete) Q71.0 ☑
     with hand present Q71.1 ☑
   artery (peripheral) Q27.9
     brain Q28.3
     coronary Q24.5
     pulmonary Q25.79
     specified NEC Q27.8
     umbilical Q27.0
   auditory (canal) (external) Q16.1
   auricle (ear) Q16.0
   bile duct or passage Q44.5
   bladder Q64.5
   bone Q79.9
   brain Q00.0
     part of Q04.3
   breast (with nipple present) Q83.8
     with absent nipple Q83.0
   bronchus Q32.4
   canaliculus lacrimalis Q10.4
   carpus — *see* Agenesis, hand
   cartilage Q79.9
   cecum Q42.8
   cerebellum Q04.3
   cervix Q51.5
   chin Q18.8
   cilia Q10.3
   circulatory system, part NOS Q28.9
   clavicle Q74.0
   clitoris Q52.6
   coccyx Q76.49
   colon Q42.9
     specified NEC Q42.8
   corpus callosum Q04.0
   cricoid cartilage Q31.8
   diaphragm (with hernia) Q79.1
   digestive organ (s) or tract (complete) (partial)
     NEC Q45.8
     upper Q40.8
   ductus arteriosus Q28.8
   duodenum Q41.0
   ear Q16.9
     auricle Q16.0
     lobe Q17.8
   ejaculatory duct Q55.4
   endocrine (gland) NEC Q89.2
   epiglottis Q31.8
   esophagus Q39.8
   eustachian tube Q16.2
   eye Q11.1
     adnexa Q15.8
   eyelid (fold) Q10.3
   face
     bones NEC Q75.8
     specified part NEC Q18.8
   fallopian tube Q50.6
   femur — *see* Defect, reduction, lower limb,
     longitudinal, femur
   fibula — *see* Defect, reduction, lower limb,
     longitudinal, fibula
   finger (complete) (partial) — *see* Agenesis, hand
   foot (and toes) (complete) (partial) Q72.3 ☑

Agenesis — *continued*
   forearm (with hand present) — *see* Agenesis, arm,
     with hand present
     and hand Q71.2 ☑
   gallbladder Q44.0
   gastric Q40.2
   genitalia, genital (organ (s))
     female Q52.8
       external Q52.71
       internal NEC Q52.8
     male Q55.8
   glottis Q31.8
   hair Q84.0
   hand (and fingers) (complete) (partial) Q71.3 ☑
   heart Q24.8
     valve NEC Q24.8
       pulmonary Q22.0
   hepatic Q44.7
   humerus — *see* Defect, reduction, upper limb
   hymen Q52.4
   ileum Q41.2
   incus Q16.3
   intestine (small) Q41.9
     large Q42.9
       specified NEC Q42.8
   iris (dilator fibers) Q13.1
   jaw M26.09
   jejunum Q41.1
   kidney(s) (partial) Q60.2
     bilateral Q60.1
     unilateral Q60.0
   labium (majus) (minus) Q52.71
   labyrinth, membranous Q16.5
   lacrimal apparatus Q10.4
   larynx Q31.8
   leg (complete) Q72.0 ☑
     with foot present Q72.1 ☑
     lower leg (with foot present) — *see* Agenesis,
       leg, with foot present
       and foot Q72.2 ☑
   lens Q12.3
   limb (complete) Q73.0
     lower — *see* Agenesis, leg
     upper — *see* Agenesis, arm
   lip Q38.0
   liver Q44.7
   lung (fissure) (lobe) (bilateral) (unilateral) Q33.3
   mandible, maxilla M26.09
   metacarpus — *see* Agenesis, hand
   metatarsus — *see* Agenesis, foot
   muscle Q79.8
     eyelid Q10.3
     ocular Q15.8
   musculoskeletal system NEC Q79.8
   nail (s) Q84.3
   neck, part Q18.8
   nerve Q07.8
   nervous system, part NEC Q07.8
   nipple Q83.2
   nose Q30.1
   nuclear Q07.8
   organ
     of Corti Q16.5
     or site not listed — *see* Anomaly, by site
   osseous meatus (ear) Q16.1
   ovary
     bilateral Q50.02
     unilateral Q50.01
   oviduct Q50.6
   pancreas Q45.0
   parathyroid (gland) Q89.2
   parotid gland (s) Q38.4
   patella Q74.1
   pelvic girdle (complete) (partial) Q74.2
   penis Q55.5
   pericardium Q24.8
   pituitary (gland) Q89.2
   prostate Q55.4
   punctum lacrimale Q10.4
   radioulnar — *see* Defect, reduction, upper limb
   radius — *see* Defect, reduction, upper limb,
     longitudinal, radius
   rectum Q42.1
     with fistula Q42.0
   renal Q60.2
     bilateral Q60.1
     unilateral Q60.0
   respiratory organ NEC Q34.8
   rib Q76.6
   roof of orbit Q75.8
   round ligament Q52.8
   sacrum Q76.49

☑ **Additional character required**

Adynamia - Agenesis

ICD-10-CM INDEX TO DISEASES AND INJURIES

Agenesis — *continued*
salivary gland Q38.4
scapula Q74.0
scrotum Q55.29
seminal vesicles Q55.4
septum
  atrial Q21.1
  between aorta and pulmonary artery Q21.4
  ventricular Q20.4
shoulder girdle (complete) (partial) Q74.0
skull (bone) Q75.8
  with
    anencephaly Q00.0
    encephalocele — *see* Encephalocele
    hydrocephalus Q03.9
      with spina bifida — *see* Spina bifida, by site,
        with hydrocephalus
    microcephaly Q02
spermatic cord Q55.4
spinal cord Q06.0
spine Q76.49
spleen Q89.01
sternum Q76.7
stomach Q40.2
submaxillary gland (s) (congenital) Q38.4
tarsus — *see* Agenesis, foot
tendon Q79.8
testicle Q55.0
thymus (gland) Q89.2
thyroid (gland) E03.1
  cartilage Q31.8
tibia — *see* Defect, reduction, lower limb,
  longitudinal, tibia
tibiofibular — *see* Defect, reduction, lower limb,
  specified type NEC
toe (and foot) (complete) (partial) — *see*
  Agenesis, foot
tongue Q38.3
trachea (cartilage) Q32.1
ulna — *see* Defect, reduction, upper limb,
  longitudinal, ulna
upper limb — *see* Agenesis, arm
ureter Q62.4
urethra Q64.5
urinary tract NEC Q64.8
uterus Q51.0
uvula Q38.5
vagina Q52.0
vas deferens Q55.4
vein (s) (peripheral) Q27.9
  brain Q28.3
  great NEC Q26.8
  portal Q26.5
vena cava (inferior) (superior) Q26.8
vermis of cerebellum Q04.3
vertebra Q76.49
vulva Q52.71
Ageusia R43.2
Agitated — *see* condition
Agitation R45.1
Aglossia (congenital) Q38.3
Aglossia-adactylia syndrome Q87.0
Aglycogenosis E74.00
Agnosia (body image) (other senses) (tactile) R48.1
developmental F88
verbal R48.1
  auditory R48.1
    developmental F80.2
  developmental F80.2
visual (object) R48.3
Agoraphobia F40.00
with panic disorder F40.01
without panic disorder F40.02
Agrammatism R48.8
Agranulocytopenia — *see* Agranulocytosis
Agranulocytosis (chronic) (cyclical) (genetic)
  (infantile) (periodic) (pernicious) (*see also*
  Neutropenia) D70.9
congenital D70.0
cytoreductive cancer chemotherapy
  sequela D70.1
drug-induced D70.2
  due to cytoreductive cancer
    chemotherapy D70.1
due to infection D70.3
secondary D70.4
  drug-induced D70.2
  due to cytoreductive cancer
    chemotherapy D70.1
Agraphia (absolute) R48.8
with alexia R48.0
developmental F81.81

Ague (dumb) — *see* Malaria
Agyria Q04.3
Ahumada-del Castillo syndrome E23.0
Aichomophobia F40.298
AIDS (related complex) B20
Ailment heart — *see* Disease, heart
Ailurophobia F40.218
Ainhum (disease) L94.6
AIN — *see* Neoplasia, intraepithelial, anal
AIPHI (acute idiopathic pulmonary hemorrhage in
  infants (over 28 days old)) R04.81
Air
anterior mediastinum J98.2
compressed, disease T70.3 ☑
conditioner lung or pneumonitis J67.7
embolism (artery) (cerebral) (any site) T79.0 ☑
  with ectopic or molar pregnancy O08.2
  due to implanted device NEC — *see*
    Complications, by site and type, specified
    NEC
  following
    abortion — *see* Abortion by type,
      complicated by, embolism
    ectopic or molar pregnancy O08.2
    infusion, therapeutic injection or
      transfusion T80.0 ☑
  in pregnancy, childbirth or puerperium — *see*
    Embolism, obstetric
  traumatic T79.0 ☑
hunger, psychogenic F45.8
rarefied, effects of — *see* Effect, adverse, high
  altitude
sickness T75.3 ☑
Airplane sickness T75.3 ☑
Akathisia (drug-induced) (treatment-induced)
  G25.71
neuroleptic induced (acute) G25.71
tardive G25.71
Akinesia R29.898
Akinetic mutism R41.89
Akureyri's disease G93.3
Alactasia, congenital E73.0
Alagille's syndrome Q44.7
Alastrim B03
Albers-Schönberg syndrome Q78.2
Albert's syndrome — *see* Tendinitis, Achilles
Albinism, albino E70.30
with hematologic abnormality E70.339
  Chédiak-Higashi syndrome E70.330
  Hermansky-Pudlak syndrome E70.331
  other specified E70.338
I E70.320
II E70.321
ocular E70.319
  autosomal recessive E70.311
  other specified E70.318
  X-linked E70.310
oculocutaneous E70.329
  other specified E70.328
  tyrosinase (ty) negative E70.320
  tyrosinase (ty) positive E70.321
other specified E70.39
Albinismus E70.30
Albright (-McCune) (-Sternberg) syndrome Q78.1
Albuminous — *see* condition
Albuminuria, albuminuric (acute) (chronic)
  (subacute) (*see also* Proteinuria) R80.9
complicating pregnancy — *see* Proteinuria,
  gestational
with
  gestational hypertension — *see* Pre-
    eclampsia
  pre-existing hypertension — *see*
    Hypertension, complicating pregnancy,
    pre-existing, with, pre-eclampsia
gestational — *see* Proteinuria, gestational
with
  gestational hypertension — *see* Pre-eclampsia
  pre-existing hypertension — *see*
    Hypertension, complicating pregnancy,
    pre-existing, with, pre-eclampsia
orthostatic R80.2
postural R80.2
pre-eclamptic — *see* Pre-eclampsia
scarlatinal A38.8
Albuminurophobia F40.298
Alcaptonuria E70.29
Alcohol, alcoholic, alcohol-induced
addiction (without remission) F10.20
  with remission F10.21
amnestic disorder, persisting F10.96
  with dependence F10.26

Alcohol — *continued*
anxiety disorder F10.980
bipolar and related disorder F10.94
depressive disorder F10.94
major neurocognitive disorder, amnestic-
  confabulatory type F10.96
major neurocognitive disorder, nonamnestic-
  confabulatory type F10.97
mild neurocognitive disorder F10.988
psychotic disorder F10.959
sexual dysfunction F10.981
sleep disorder F10.982
brain syndrome, chronic F10.97
  with dependence F10.27
cardiopathy I42.6
counseling and surveillance Z71.41
  family member Z71.42
delirium (acute) (tremens) (withdrawal) F10.231
  with intoxication F10.921
  in
    abuse F10.121
    dependence F10.221
dementia F10.97
  with dependence F10.27
deterioration F10.97
  with dependence F10.27
hallucinosis (acute) F10.951
  in
    abuse F10.151
    dependence F10.251
insanity F10.959
intoxication (acute) (without
  dependence) F10.129
  with
    delirium F10.121
    dependence F10.229
      with delirium F10.221
      uncomplicated F10.220
    uncomplicated F10.120
jealousy F10.988
Korsakoff's, Korsakov's, Korsakow's F10.26
liver K70.9
  acute — *see* Disease, liver, alcoholic, hepatitis
mania (acute) (chronic) F10.959
paranoia, paranoid (type) psychosis F10.950
pellagra E52
poisoning, accidental (acute) NEC — *see* Table of
  Drugs and Chemicals, alcohol, poisoning
psychosis — *see* Psychosis, alcoholic
withdrawal (without convulsions) F10.239
  with delirium F10.231
Alcoholism (chronic) (without remission) F10.20
with
  psychosis — *see* Psychosis, alcoholic
  remission F10.21
Korsakov's F10.96
  with dependence F10.26
Alder (-Reilly) anomaly or syndrome (leukocyte
  granulation) D72.0
Aldosteronism E26.9
familial (type I) E26.02
glucocorticoid-remediable E26.02
primary (due to (bilateral) adrenal
  hyperplasia) E26.09
primary NEC E26.09
secondary E26.1
specified NEC E26.89
Aldosteronoma D44.10
Aldrich (-Wiskott) syndrome (eczema-
  thrombocytopenia) D82.0
Alektorophobia F40.218
Aleppo boil B55.1
Aleukemic — *see* condition
Aleukia
congenital D70.0
hemorrhagica D61.9
  congenital D61.09
splenica D73.1
Alexia R48.0
developmental F81.0
secondary to organic lesion R48.0
Algoneurodystrophy M89.00
ankle M89.07 ☑
foot M89.07 ☑
forearm M89.03 ☑
hand M89.04 ☑
lower leg M89.06 ☑
multiple sites M89.0 ☑
shoulder M89.01 ☑
specified site NEC M89.08
thigh M89.05 ☑
upper arm M89.02 ☑

Algophobia - Amnesia

Algophobia F40.298
Alienation, mental — *see* Psychosis
Alkalemia E87.3
Alkalosis E87.3
  metabolic E87.3
    with respiratory acidosis E87.4
  respiratory E87.3
Alkaptonuria E70.29
Allen-Masters syndrome N83.8
Allergy, allergic (reaction) (to) T78.40 ☑
  air-borne substance NEC (rhinitis) J30.89
  alveolitis (extrinsic) J67.9
    due to
      Aspergillus clavatus J67.4
      Cryptostroma corticale J67.6
      organisms (fungal, thermophilic
        actinomycete) growing in ventilation (air
        conditioning) systems J67.7
    specified type NEC J67.8
  anaphylactic reaction or shock T78.2 ☑
  angioneurotic edema T78.3 ☑
  animal (dander) (epidermal) (hair) (rhinitis) J30.81
  bee sting (anaphylactic shock) — *see* Toxicity,
    venom, arthropod, bee
  biological — *see* Allergy, drug
  colitis (*see also* Colitis, allergic) K52.29
  dander (animal) (rhinitis) J30.81
  dandruff (rhinitis) J30.81
  dental restorative material (existing) K08.55
  dermatitis — *see* Dermatitis, contact, allergic
  diathesis — *see* History, allergy
  drug, medicament & biological (any) (external)
    (internal) T78.40 ☑
    correct substance properly administered — *see*
      Table of Drugs and Chemicals, by drug,
      adverse effect
    wrong substance given or taken NEC (by
      accident) — *see* Table of Drugs and
      Chemicals, by drug, poisoning
  due to pollen J30.1
  dust (house) (stock) (rhinitis) J30.89
    with asthma — *see* Asthma, allergic extrinsic
  eczema — *see* Dermatitis, contact, allergic
  epidermal (animal) (rhinitis) J30.81
  feathers (rhinitis) J30.89
  food (any) (ingested) NEC T78.1 ☑
    anaphylactic shock — *see* Shock, anaphylactic,
      due to food
    dermatitis — *see* Dermatitis, due to, food
    dietary counseling and surveillance Z71.3
    in contact with skin L23.6
    rhinitis J30.5
    status (without reaction) Z91.018
      eggs Z91.012
      milk products Z91.011
      peanuts Z91.010
      seafood Z91.013
      specified NEC Z91.018
  gastrointestinal (*see also* specific type of allergic
    reaction)
    meaning colitis (*see also* Colitis, allergic) K52.29
    meaning gastroenteritis (*see also*
      Gastroenteritis, allergic) K52.29
    meaning other adverse food reaction not
      elsewhere classified T78.1 ☑
  grain J30.1
  grass (hay fever) (pollen) J30.1
    asthma — *see* Asthma, allergic extrinsic
  hair (animal) (rhinitis) J30.81
  history (of) — *see* History, allergy
  horse serum — *see* Allergy, serum
  inhalant (rhinitis) J30.89
    pollen J30.1
  kapok (rhinitis) J30.89
  medicine — *see* Allergy, drug
  milk protein (*see also* Allergy, food) Z91.011
    anaphylactic reaction T78.07 ☑
    dermatitis L27.2
    enterocolitis syndrome K52.21
    enteropathy K52.22
    gastroenteritis K52.29
    gastroesophageal reflux (*see also* Reaction,
      adverse, food) K21.9
      with esophagitis K21.0
    proctocolitis K52.82
  nasal, seasonal due to pollen J30.1
  pneumonia J82
  pollen (any) (hay fever) J30.1
    asthma — *see* Asthma, allergic extrinsic
  primrose J30.1
  primula J30.1
  proctocolitis K52.82

Allergy — *continued*
  purpura D69.0
  ragweed (hay fever) (pollen) J30.1
    asthma — *see* Asthma, allergic extrinsic
  rose (pollen) J30.1
  seasonal NEC J30.2
  Senecio jacobae (pollen) J30.1
  serum (*see also* Reaction, serum) T80.69 ☑
    anaphylactic shock T80.59 ☑
  shock (anaphylactic) T78.2 ☑
    due to
      administration of blood and blood
        products T80.51 ☑
      adverse effect of correct medicinal substance
        properly administered T88.6 ☑
      immunization T80.52 ☑
      serum NEC T80.59 ☑
      vaccination T80.52 ☑
  specific NEC T78.49 ☑
  tree (any) (hay fever) (pollen) J30.1
    asthma — *see* Asthma, allergic extrinsic
  upper respiratory J30.9
  urticaria L50.0
  vaccine — *see* Allergy, serum
  wheat — *see* Allergy, food
Allescheriasis B48.2
Alligator skin disease Q80.9
Allocheiria, allochiria R20.8
Almeida's disease — *see* Paracoccidioidomycosis
Alopecia (hereditaria) (seborrheica) L65.9
  androgenic L64.9
    drug-induced L64.0
    specified NEC L64.8
  areata L63.9
    ophiasis L63.2
    specified NEC L63.8
    totalis L63.0
    universalis L63.1
  cicatricial L66.9
    specified NEC L66.8
  circumscripta L63.9
  congenital, congenitalis Q84.0
  due to cytotoxic drugs NEC L65.8
  mucinosa L65.2
  postinfective NEC L65.8
  postpartum L65.0
  premature L64.8
  specific (syphilitic) A51.32
  specified NEC L65.8
  syphilitic (secondary) A51.32
  totalis (capitis) L63.0
  universalis (entire body) L63.1
  X-ray L58.1
Alpers' disease G31.81
Alpine sickness T70.29 ☑
Alport syndrome Q87.81
ALTE (apparent life threatening event) in newborn
  and infant R68.13
Alteration (of), Altered
  awareness
    transient R40.4
    unintended under general anesthesia, during
      procedure T88.53
  mental status R41.82
  pattern of family relationships affecting
    child Z62.898
  sensation
    following
      cerebrovascular disease I69.998
        cerebral infarction I69.398
        intracerebral hemorrhage I69.198
        nontraumatic intracranial hemorrhage
          NEC I69.298
        specified disease NEC I69.898
        subarachnoid hemorrhage I69.098
Alternating — *see* condition
Altitude, high (effects) — *see* Effect, adverse, high
  altitude
Aluminosis (of lung) J63.0
Alveolitis
  allergic (extrinsic) — *see* Pneumonitis,
    hypersensitivity
  due to
    Aspergillus clavatus J67.4
    Cryptostroma corticale J67.6
  fibrosing (cryptogenic) (idiopathic) J84.112
  jaw M27.3
  sicca dolorosa M27.3
Alveolus, alveolar — *see* condition
Alymphocytosis D72.810
  thymic (with immunodeficiency) D82.1
Alymphoplasia, thymic D82.1

Alzheimer's disease or sclerosis — *see* Disease,
  Alzheimer's
Amastia (with nipple present) Q83.8
  with absent nipple Q83.0
Amathophobia F40.228
Amaurosis (acquired) (congenital) (*see also*
  Blindness)
  fugax G45.3
  hysterical F44.6
  Leber's congenital H35.50
  uremic — *see* Uremia
Amaurotic idiocy (infantile) (juvenile) (late) E75.4
Amaxophobia F40.248
Ambiguous genitalia Q56.4
Amblyopia (congenital) (ex anopsia) (partial)
  (suppression) H53.00
  anisometropic — *see* Amblyopia, refractive
  deprivation H53.01 ☑
  hysterical F44.6
  nocturnal (*see also* Blindness, night)
    vitamin A deficiency E50.5
  refractive H53.02 ☑
  strabismic H53.03 ☑
  suspect H53.04 ☑
  tobacco H53.8
  toxic NEC H53.8
  uremic — *see* Uremia
Ameba, amebic (histolytica) (*see also* Amebiasis)
  abscess (liver) A06.4
Amebiasis A06.9
  with abscess — *see* Abscess, amebic
  acute A06.0
  chronic (intestine) A06.1
    with abscess — *see* Abscess, amebic
  cutaneous A06.7
  cutis A06.7
  cystitis A06.81
  genitourinary tract NEC A06.82
  hepatic — *see* Abscess, liver, amebic
  intestine A06.0
  nondysenteric colitis A06.2
  skin A06.7
  specified site NEC A06.89
Ameboma (of intestine) A06.3
Amelia Q73.0
  lower limb — *see* Agenesis, leg
  upper limb — *see* Agenesis, arm
Ameloblastoma (*see also* Cyst, calcifying
  odontogenic)
  long bones C40.9 ☑
    lower limb C40.2 ☑
    upper limb C40.0 ☑
  malignant C41.1
    jaw (bone) (lower) C41.1
      upper C41.0
  tibial C40.2 ☑
Amelogenesis imperfecta K00.5
  nonhereditaria (segmentalis) K00.4
Amenorrhea N91.2
  hyperhormonal E28.8
  primary N91.0
  secondary N91.1
Amentia — *see* Disability, intellectual
  Meynert's (nonalcoholic) F04
American
  leishmaniasis B55.2
  mountain tick fever A93.2
Ametropia — *see* Disorder, refraction
AMH (asymptomatic microscopic hematuria) R31.21
Amianthosis J61
Amimia R48.8
Amino-acid disorder E72.9
  anemia D53.0
Aminoacidopathy E72.9
Aminoaciduria E72.9
Amnes (t)ic syndrome (post-traumatic) F04
  induced by
    alcohol F10.96
      with dependence F10.26
    psychoactive NEC F19.96
      with
        abuse F19.16
        dependence F19.26
    sedative F13.96
      with dependence F13.26
Amnesia R41.3
  anterograde R41.1
  auditory R48.8
  dissociative F44.0
    with dissociative fugue F44.1
  hysterical F44.0
  postictal in epilepsy — *see* Epilepsy

☑ **Additional character required**

Amnesia — *continued*
  psychogenic F44.0
  retrograde R41.2
  transient global G45.4
Amnion, amniotic — *see* condition
Amnionitis — *see* Pregnancy, complicated by
Amok F68.8
Amoral traits F60.89
Amphetamine (or other stimulant)-induced
  anxiety disorder F15.980
  bipolar and related disorder F15.94
  delirium F15.921
  depressive disorder F15.94
  obsessive-compulsive and related
    disorder F15.988
  psychotic disorder F15.959
  sexual dysfunction F15.981
  sleep disorder F15.982
  stimulant withdrawal F15.23
Ampulla
  lower esophagus K22.8
  phrenic K22.8
Amputation (*see also* Absence, by site, acquired)
  neuroma (postoperative) (traumatic) — *see*
    Complications, amputation stump, neuroma
  stump (surgical)
    abnormal, painful, or with complication (late)
      — *see* Complications, amputation stump
    healed or old NOS Z89.9
  traumatic (complete) (partial)
    arm (upper) (complete) S48.91 ☑
      at
        elbow S58.01 ☑
          partial S58.02 ☑
        shoulder joint (complete) S48.01 ☑
          partial S48.02 ☑
      between
        elbow and wrist (complete) S58.11 ☑
          partial S58.12 ☑
        shoulder and elbow (complete) S48.11 ☑
          partial S48.12 ☑
      partial S48.92 ☑
    breast (complete) S28.21 ☑
      partial S28.22 ☑
    clitoris (complete) S38.211 ☑
      partial S38.212 ☑
    ear (complete) S08.11 ☑
      partial S08.12 ☑
    finger (complete) (metacarpophalangeal) S68.11 ☑
      index S68.11 ☑
      little S68.11 ☑
      middle S68.11 ☑
      partial S68.12 ☑
        index S68.12 ☑
        little S68.12 ☑
        middle S68.12 ☑
        ring S68.12 ☑
      ring S68.11 ☑
      thumb — *see* Amputation, traumatic, thumb
      transphalangeal (complete) S68.61 ☑
        index S68.61 ☑
        little S68.61 ☑
        middle S68.61 ☑
        partial S68.62 ☑
          index S68.62 ☑
          little S68.62 ☑
          middle S68.62 ☑
          ring S68.62 ☑
        ring S68.61 ☑
    foot (complete) S98.91 ☑
      at ankle level S98.01 ☑
        partial S98.02 ☑
      midfoot S98.31 ☑
        partial S98.32 ☑
      partial S98.92 ☑
    forearm (complete) S58.91 ☑
      at elbow level (complete) S58.01 ☑
        partial S58.02 ☑
      between elbow and wrist
        (complete) S58.11 ☑
        partial S58.12 ☑
      partial S58.92 ☑
    genital organ (s) (external)
      female (complete) S38.211 ☑
        partial S38.212 ☑
      male
        penis (complete) S38.221 ☑
          partial S38.222 ☑
        scrotum (complete) S38.231 ☑
          partial S38.232 ☑
        testes (complete) S38.231 ☑
          partial S38.232 ☑

Amputation — *continued*
  traumatic — *continued*
    hand (complete) (wrist level) S68.41 ☑
      finger (s) alone — *see* Amputation, traumatic,
        finger
      partial S68.42 ☑
      thumb alone — *see* Amputation, traumatic,
        thumb
      transmetacarpal (complete) S68.71 ☑
        partial S68.72 ☑
    head
      ear — *see* Amputation, traumatic, ear
      nose (partial) S08.812 ☑
        complete S08.811 ☑
      part S08.89 ☑
        scalp S08.0 ☑
    hip (and thigh) (complete) S78.91 ☑
      at hip joint (complete) S78.01 ☑
        partial S78.02 ☑
      between hip and knee (complete) S78.11 ☑
        partial S78.12 ☑
      partial S78.92 ☑
    labium (majus) (minus) (complete) S38.21 ☑
      partial S38.21 ☑
    leg (lower) S88.91 ☑
      at knee level S88.01 ☑
        partial S88.02 ☑
      between knee and ankle S88.11 ☑
        partial S88.12 ☑
      partial S88.92 ☑
    nose (partial) S08.812 ☑
      complete S08.811 ☑
    penis (complete) S38.221 ☑
      partial S38.222 ☑
    scrotum (complete) S38.231 ☑
      partial S38.232 ☑
    shoulder — *see* Amputation, traumatic, arm
      at shoulder joint — *see* Amputation,
        traumatic, arm, at shoulder joint
    testes (complete) S38.231 ☑
      partial S38.232 ☑
    thigh — *see* Amputation, traumatic, hip
    thorax, part of S28.1 ☑
      breast — *see* Amputation, traumatic, breast
    thumb (complete)
      (metacarpophalangeal) S68.01 ☑
      partial S68.02 ☑
      transphalangeal (complete) S68.51 ☑
        partial S68.52 ☑
    toe (lesser) S98.13 ☑
      great S98.11 ☑
        partial S98.12 ☑
      more than one S98.21 ☑
        partial S98.22 ☑
      partial S98.14 ☑
    vulva (complete) S38.211 ☑
      partial S38.212 ☑
Amputee (bilateral) (old) Z89.9
Amsterdam dwarfism Q87.1
Amusia R48.8
  developmental F80.89
Amyelencephalus, amyelencephaly Q00.0
Amyelia Q06.0
Amygdalitis — *see* Tonsillitis
Amygdalolith J35.8
Amyloid heart (disease) E85.4 [I43]
Amyloidosis (generalized) (primary) E85.9
  with lung involvement E85.4 [J99]
  familial E85.2
  genetic E85.2
  heart E85.4 [I43]
  hemodialysis-associated E85.3
  light chain (AL) E85.81
  liver E85.4 [K77]
  localized E85.4
  neuropathic heredofamilial E85.1
  non-neuropathic heredofamilial E85.0
  organ limited E85.4
  Portuguese E85.1
  pulmonary E85.4 [J99]
  secondary systemic E85.3
  senile systemic (SSA) E85.82
  skin (lichen) (macular) E85.4 [L99]
  specified NEC E85.89
  subglottic E85.4 [J99]
  wild-type transthyretin-related (ATTR) E85.82
Amylopectinosis (brancher enzyme deficiency)
  E74.03
Amylophagia — *see* Pica
Amyoplasia congenita Q79.8
Amyotonia M62.89
  congenita G70.2

Amyotrophia, amyotrophy, amyotrophic G71.8
  congenita Q79.8
  diabetic — *see* Diabetes, amyotrophy
  lateral sclerosis G12.21
  neuralgic G54.5
  spinal progressive G12.25
Anacidity, gastric K31.83
  psychogenic F45.8
Anaerosis of newborn P28.89
Analbuminemia E88.09
Analgesia — *see* Anesthesia
Analphalipoproteinemia E78.6
Anaphylactic
  purpura D69.0
  shock or reaction — *see* Shock, anaphylactic
Anaphylactoid shock or reaction — *see* Shock,
  anaphylactic
Anaphylactoid syndrome of pregnancy O88.01 ☑
Anaphylaxis — *see* Shock, anaphylactic
Anaplasia cervix (*see also* Dysplasia, cervix) N87.9
Anaplasmosis, human A77.49
Anarthria R47.1
Anasarca R60.1
  cardiac — *see* Failure, heart, congestive
  lung J18.2
  newborn P83.2
  nutritional E43
  pulmonary J18.2
  renal N04.9
Anastomosis
  aneurysmal — *see* Aneurysm
  arteriovenous ruptured brain I60.8
  intestinal K63.89
    complicated NEC K91.89
      involving urinary tract N99.89
  retinal and choroidal vessels (congenital) Q14.8
Anatomical narrow angle H40.03 ☑
Ancylostoma, ancylostomiasis (braziliense)
  (caninum) (ceylanicum) (duodenale) B76.0
  Necator americanus B76.1
Andersen's disease (glycogen storage) E74.09
Anderson-Fabry disease E75.21
Andes disease T70.29 ☑
Andrews' disease (bacterid) L08.89
Androblastoma
  benign
    specified site — *see* Neoplasm, benign, by site
    unspecified site
      female D27.9
      male D29.20
  malignant
    specified site — *see* Neoplasm, malignant, by
      site
    unspecified site
      female C56.9
      male C62.90
  specified site — *see* Neoplasm, uncertain
    behavior, by site
  tubular
    with lipid storage
      specified site — *see* Neoplasm, benign, by
        site
      unspecified site
        female D27.9
        male D29.20
    specified site — *see* Neoplasm, benign, by site
    unspecified site
      female D39.10
      male D40.10
Androgen insensitivity syndrome (*see also*
  Syndrome, androgen insensitivity) E34.50
Androgen resistance syndrome (*see also* Syndrome,
  androgen insensitivity) E34.50
Android pelvis Q74.2
  with disproportion (fetopelvic) O33.3 ☑
    causing obstructed labor O65.3
Androphobia F40.290
Anectasis, pulmonary (newborn) — *see* Atelectasis
Anemia (essential) (general) (hemoglobin
  deficiency) (infantile) (primary) (profound) D64.9
  with (due to) (in)
    disorder of
      anaerobic glycolysis D55.2
      pentose phosphate pathway D55.1
    koilonychia D50.9
  achlorhydric D50.8
  achrestic D53.1
  Addison (-Biermer) (pernicious) D51.0
  agranulocytic — *see* Agranulocytosis

Anemia

Anemia — *continued*
  amino-acid-deficiency D53.0
  aplastic D61.9
    congenital D61.09
    drug-induced D61.1
    due to
      drugs D61.1
      external agents NEC D61.2
      infection D61.2
      radiation D61.2
    idiopathic D61.3
    red cell (pure) D60.9
      chronic D60.0
      congenital D61.01
      specified type NEC D60.8
      transient D60.1
    specified type NEC D61.89
    toxic D61.2
  aregenerative
    congenital D61.09
  asiderotic D50.9
  atypical (primary) D64.9
  Baghdad spring D55.0
  Balantidium coli A07.0
  Biermer's (pernicious) D51.0
  blood loss (chronic) D50.0
    acute D62
  bothriocephalus B70.0 *[D63.8]*
  brickmaker's B76.9 *[D63.8]*
  cerebral I67.89
  childhood D58.9
  chlorotic D50.8
  chronic
    blood loss D50.0
    hemolytic D58.9
      idiopathic D59.9
    simple D53.9
  chronica congenita aregenerativa D61.09
  combined system disease NEC D51.0 *[G32.0]*
    due to dietary vitamin B12 deficiency D51.3
      [G32.0]
  complicating pregnancy, childbirth or
      puerperium — *see* Pregnancy, complicated
      by (management affected by), anemia
  congenital P61.4
    aplastic D61.09
    due to isoimmunization NOS P55.9
    dyserythropoietic, dyshematopoietic D64.4
    following fetal blood loss P61.3
    Heinz body D58.2
    hereditary hemolytic NOS D58.9
    pernicious D51.0
    spherocytic D58.0
  Cooley's (erythroblastic) D56.1
  cytogenic D51.0
  deficiency D53.9
    2, 3 diphosphoglycerate mutase D55.2
    2, 3 PG D55.2
    6 phosphogluconate dehydrogenase D55.1
    6-PGD D55.1
    amino-acid D53.0
    combined B12 and folate D53.1
    enzyme D55.9
      drug-induced (hemolytic) D59.2
      glucose-6-phosphate dehydrogenase
        (G6PD) D55.0
      glycolytic D55.2
      nucleotide metabolism D55.3
      related to hexose monophosphate (HMP)
        shunt pathway NEC D55.1
      specified type NEC D55.8
    erythrocytic glutathione D55.1
    folate D52.9
      dietary D52.0
      drug-induced D52.1
    folic acid D52.9
      dietary D52.0
      drug-induced D52.1
    G SH D55.1
    GGS-R D55.1
    glucose-6-phosphate dehydrogenase D55.0
    glutathione reductase D55.1
    glyceraldehyde phosphate
      dehydrogenase D55.2
    G6PD D55.0
    hexokinase D55.2
    iron D50.9
      secondary to blood loss (chronic) D50.0
    nutritional D53.9
      with
        poor iron absorption D50.8
        specified deficiency NEC D53.8

Anemia — *continued*
  deficiency — *continued*
    phosphofructo-aldolase D55.2
    phosphoglycerate kinase D55.2
    PK D55.2
    protein D53.0
    pyruvate kinase D55.2
    transcobalamin II D51.2
    triose-phosphate isomerase D55.2
    vitamin B12 NOS D51.9
      dietary D51.3
      due to
        intrinsic factor deficiency D51.0
        selective vitamin B12 malabsorption with
          proteinuria D51.1
      pernicious D51.0
      specified type NEC D51.8
  Diamond-Blackfan (congenital
      hypoplastic) D61.01
  dibothriocephalus B70.0 *[D63.8]*
  dimorphic D53.1
  diphasic D53.1
  Diphyllobothrium (Dibothriocephalus) B70.0
      [D63.8]
  due to (in) (with)
    antineoplastic chemotherapy D64.81
    blood loss (chronic) D50.0
      acute D62
    chemotherapy, antineoplastic D64.81
    chronic disease classified elsewhere NEC D63.8
    chronic kidney disease D63.1
    deficiency
      amino-acid D53.0
      copper D53.8
      folate (folic acid) D52.9
        dietary D52.0
        drug-induced D52.1
      molybdenum D53.8
      protein D53.0
      zinc D53.8
    dietary vitamin B12 deficiency D51.3
    disorder of
      glutathione metabolism D55.1
      nucleotide metabolism D55.3
    drug — *see* Anemia, by type (*see also* Table of
      Drugs and Chemicals)
    end stage renal disease D63.1
    enzyme disorder D55.9
    fetal blood loss P61.3
    fish tapeworm (D.latum) infestation B70.0
      [D63.8]
    hemorrhage (chronic) D50.0
      acute D62
    impaired absorption D50.9
    loss of blood (chronic) D50.0
      acute D62
    myxedema E03.9 *[D63.8]*
    Necator americanus B76.1 *[D63.8]*
    prematurity P61.2
    selective vitamin B12 malabsorption with
      proteinuria D51.1
    transcobalamin II deficiency D51.2
  Dyke-Young type (secondary)
      (symptomatic) D59.1
  dyserythropoietic (congenital) D64.4
  dyshematopoietic (congenital) D64.4
  Egyptian B76.9 *[D63.8]*
  elliptocytosis — *see* Elliptocytosis
  enzyme-deficiency, drug-induced D59.2
  epidemic (*see also* Ancylostomiasis) B76.9 *[D63.8]*
  erythroblastic
    familial D56.1
    newborn (*see also* Disease, hemolytic) P55.9
    of childhood D56.1
  erythrocytic glutathione deficiency D55.1
  erythropoietin-resistant anemia (EPO resistant
      anemia) D63.1
  Faber's (achlorhydric anemia) D50.9
  factitious (self-induced blood letting) D50.0
  familial erythroblastic D56.1
  Fanconi's (congenital pancytopenia) D61.09
  favism D55.0
  fish tapeworm (D. latum) infestation B70.0 *[D63.8]*
  folate (folic acid) deficiency D52.9
  glucose-6-phosphate dehydrogenase (G6PD)
      deficiency D55.0
  glutathione-reductase deficiency D55.1
  goat's milk D52.0
  granulocytic — *see* Agranulocytosis
  Heinz body, congenital D58.2
  hemolytic D58.9
    acquired D59.9

Anemia — *continued*
  hemolytic — *continued*
    with hemoglobinuria NEC D59.6
    autoimmune NEC D59.1
    infectious D59.4
    specified type NEC D59.8
    toxic D59.4
  acute D59.9
    due to enzyme deficiency specified type
      NEC D55.8
    Lederer's D59.1
  autoimmune D59.1
    drug-induced D59.0
  chronic D58.9
    idiopathic D59.9
  cold type (secondary) (symptomatic) D59.1
  congenital (spherocytic) — *see* Spherocytosis
  due to
    cardiac conditions D59.4
    drugs (nonautoimmune) D59.2
      autoimmune D59.0
    enzyme disorder D55.9
      drug-induced D59.2
    presence of shunt or other internal prosthetic
      device D59.4
  familial D58.9
  hereditary D58.9
    due to enzyme disorder D55.9
      specified type NEC D55.8
    specified type NEC D58.8
  idiopathic (chronic) D59.9
  mechanical D59.4
  microangiopathic D59.4
  nonautoimmune D59.4
    drug-induced D59.2
  nonspherocytic
    congenital or hereditary NEC D55.8
      glucose-6-phosphate dehydrogenase
        deficiency D55.0
      pyruvate kinase deficiency D55.2
      type
        I D55.1
        II D55.2
    type
      I D55.1
      II D55.2
  secondary D59.4
    autoimmune D59.1
  specified (hereditary) type NEC D58.8
  Stransky-Regala type (*see also*
      Hemoglobinopathy) D58.8
  symptomatic D59.4
    autoimmune D59.1
  toxic D59.4
  warm type (secondary) (symptomatic) D59.1
  hemorrhagic (chronic) D50.0
    acute D62
  Herrick's D57.1
  hexokinase deficiency D55.2
  hookworm B76.9 *[D63.8]*
  hypochromic (idiopathic) (microcytic)
      (normoblastic) D50.9
    due to blood loss (chronic) D50.0
      acute D62
    familial sex-linked D64.0
    pyridoxine-responsive D64.3
    sideroblastic, sex-linked D64.0
  hypoplasia, red blood cells D61.9
    congenital or familial D61.01
  hypoplastic (idiopathic) D61.9
    congenital or familial (of childhood) D61.01
  hypoproliferative (refractive) D61.9
  idiopathic D64.9
    aplastic D61.3
    hemolytic, chronic D59.9
  in (due to) (with)
    chronic kidney disease D63.1
    end stage renal disease D63.1
    failure, kidney (renal) D63.1
    neoplastic disease (*see also* Neoplasm) D63.0
  intertropical (*see also* Ancylostomiasis) D63.8
  iron deficiency D50.9
    secondary to blood loss (chronic) D50.0
      acute D62
    specified type NEC D50.8
  Joseph-Diamond-Blackfan (congenital
      hypoplastic) D61.01
  Lederer's (hemolytic) D59.1
  leukoerythroblastic D61.82
  macrocytic D53.9
    nutritional D52.0
    tropical D52.8

☑ **Additional character required**

Anemia — *continued*
  malarial (*see also* Malaria) B54 *[D63.8]*
  malignant (progressive) D51.0
  malnutrition D53.9
  marsh (*see also* Malaria) B54 *[D63.8]*
  Mediterranean (with other
      hemoglobinopathy) D56.9
  megaloblastic D53.1
    combined B12 and folate deficiency D53.1
    hereditary D51.1
    nutritional D52.0
    orotic aciduria D53.0
    refractory D53.1
    specified type NEC D53.1
  megalocytic D53.1
  microcytic (hypochromic) D50.9
    due to blood loss (chronic) D50.0
      acute D62
    familial D56.8
  microdrepanocytosis D57.40
  microelliptopoikilocytic (Rietti-Greppi-
      Micheli) D56.9
  miner's B76.9 *[D63.8]*
  myelodysplastic D46.9
  myelofibrosis D75.81
  myelogenous D64.89
  myelopathic D64.89
  myelophthisic D61.82
  myeloproliferative D47.Z9
  newborn P61.4
    due to
      ABO (antibodies, isoimmunization, maternal/
          fetal incompatibility) P55.1
      Rh (antibodies, isoimmunization, maternal/
          fetal incompatibility) P55.0
    following fetal blood loss P61.3
    posthemorrhagic (fetal) P61.3
  nonspherocytic hemolytic — *see* Anemia,
      hemolytic, nonspherocytic
  normocytic (infectional) D64.9
    due to blood loss (chronic) D50.0
      acute D62
    myelophthisic D61.82
  nutritional (deficiency) D53.9
    with
      poor iron absorption D50.8
      specified deficiency NEC D53.8
    megaloblastic D52.0
  of prematurity P61.2
  orotaciduric (congenital) (hereditary) D53.0
  osteosclerotic D64.89
  ovalocytosis (hereditary) — *see* Elliptocytosis
  paludal (*see also* Malaria) B54 *[D63.8]*
  pernicious (congenital) (malignant)
      (progressive) D51.0
  pleochromic D64.89
    of sprue D52.8
  posthemorrhagic (chronic) D50.0
    acute D62
    newborn P61.3
  postoperative (postprocedural)
    due to (acute) blood loss D62
      chronic blood loss D50.0
    specified NEC D64.9
  postpartum O90.81
  pressure D64.89
  progressive D64.9
    malignant D51.0
    pernicious D51.0
  protein-deficiency D53.0
  pseudoleukemica infantum D64.89
  pure red cell D60.9
    congenital D61.01
  pyridoxine-responsive D64.3
  pyruvate kinase deficiency D55.2
  refractory D46.4
    with
      excess of blasts D46.20
        1 (RAEB 1) D46.21
        2 (RAEB 2) D46.22
        in transformation (RAEB T) — *see* Leukemia,
            acute myeloblastic
      hemochromatosis D46.1
      sideroblasts (ring) (RARS) D46.1
    megaloblastic D53.1
    sideroblastic D46.1
    sideropenic D50.9
    without ring sideroblasts, so stated D46.0
    without sideroblasts without excess of
        blasts D46.0
  Rietti-Greppi-Micheli D56.9
  scorbutic D53.2

Anemia — *continued*
  secondary to
    blood loss (chronic) D50.0
      acute D62
    hemorrhage (chronic) D50.0
      acute D62
  semiplastic D61.89
  sickle-cell — *see* Disease, sickle-cell
  sideroblastic D64.3
    hereditary D64.0
    hypochromic, sex-linked D64.0
    pyridoxine-responsive NEC D64.3
    refractory D46.1
    secondary (due to)
      disease D64.1
      drugs and toxins D64.2
    specified type NEC D64.3
  sideropenic (refractory) D50.9
    due to blood loss (chronic) D50.0
      acute D62
  simple chronic D53.9
  specified type NEC D64.89
  spherocytic (hereditary) — *see* Spherocytosis
  splenic D64.89
  splenomegalic D64.89
  stomatocytosis D58.8
  syphilitic (acquired) (late) A52.79 *[D63.8]*
  target cell D64.89
  thalassemia D56.9
  thrombocytopenic — *see* Thrombocytopenia
  toxic D61.2
  tropical B76.9 *[D63.8]*
    macrocytic D52.8
  tuberculous A18.89 *[D63.8]*
  vegan D51.3
  vitamin
    B6-responsive D64.3
    B12 deficiency (dietary) pernicious D51.0
  von Jaksch's D64.89
  Witts' (achlorhydric anemia) D50.8
Anemophobia F40.228
Anencephalus, anencephaly Q00.0
Anergasia — *see* Psychosis, organic
Anesthesia, anesthetic R20.0
  complication or reaction NEC (*see also*
      Complications, anesthesia) T88.59 ☑
    due to
      correct substance properly administered
          — *see* Table of Drugs and Chemicals, by
          drug, adverse effect
      overdose or wrong substance given — *see*
          Table of Drugs and Chemicals, by drug,
          poisoning
    unintended awareness under general
        anesthesia during procedure T88.53 ☑
    personal history of Z92.84
  cornea H18.81 ☑
  dissociative F44.6
  functional (hysterical) F44.6
  hyperesthetic, thalamic G89.0
  hysterical F44.6
  local skin lesion R20.0
  sexual (psychogenic) F52.1
  shock (due to) T88.2 ☑
  skin R20.0
  testicular N50.9
Anetoderma (maculosum) (of) L90.8
  Jadassohn-Pellizzari L90.2
  Schweniger-Buzzi L90.1
Aneurin deficiency E51.9
Aneurysm (anastomotic) (artery) (cirsoid) (diffuse)
    (false) (fusiform) (multiple) (saccular) I72.9
  abdominal (aorta) I71.4
    ruptured I71.3
    syphilitic A52.01
  aorta, aortic (nonsyphilitic) I71.9
    abdominal I71.4
      ruptured I71.3
    arch I71.2
      ruptured I71.1
    arteriosclerotic I71.9
      ruptured I71.8
    ascending I71.2
      ruptured I71.1
    congenital Q25.43
    descending I71.9
      abdominal I71.4
        ruptured I71.3
      ruptured I71.8
      thoracic I71.2
        ruptured I71.1
    root Q25.43

Aneurysm — *continued*
  aorta, aortic — *continued*
    ruptured I71.8
    sinus, congenital Q25.43
    syphilitic A52.01
    thoracic I71.2
      ruptured I71.1
    thoracoabdominal I71.6
      ruptured I71.5
    thorax, thoracic (arch) I71.2
      ruptured I71.1
    transverse I71.2
      ruptured I71.1
    valve (heart) (*see also* Endocarditis, aortic) I35.8
  arteriosclerotic I72.9
    cerebral I67.1
      ruptured — *see* Hemorrhage, intracranial,
          subarachnoid
  arteriovenous (congenital) (*see also*
      Malformation, arteriovenous)
    acquired I77.0
      brain I67.1
      coronary I25.41
      pulmonary I28.0
    brain Q28.2
      ruptured I60.8
    peripheral — *see* Malformation, arteriovenous,
        peripheral
    precerebral vessels Q28.0
    specified site NEC (*see also* Malformation,
        arteriovenous)
      acquired I77.0
  basal — *see* Aneurysm, brain
  basilar (trunk) I72.5
  berry (congenital) (nonruptured) I67.1
    ruptured I60.7
  brain I67.1
    arteriosclerotic I67.1
      ruptured — *see* Hemorrhage, intracranial,
          subarachnoid
    arteriovenous (congenital)
        (nonruptured) Q28.2
      acquired I67.1
        ruptured I60.8
      ruptured I60.8
    berry (congenital) (nonruptured) I67.1
      ruptured (*see also* Hemorrhage, intracranial,
          subarachnoid) I60.7
    congenital Q28.3
      ruptured I60.7
    meninges I67.1
      ruptured I60.8
    miliary (congenital) (nonruptured) I67.1
      ruptured (*see also* Hemorrhage, intracranial,
          subarachnoid) I60.7
    mycotic I33.0
    ruptured — *see* Hemorrhage, intracranial,
        subarachnoid
    syphilitic (hemorrhage) A52.05
  cardiac (false) (*see also* Aneurysm, heart) I25.3
  carotid artery (common) (external) I72.0
    internal (intracranial) I67.1
      extracranial portion I72.0
      ruptured into brain I60.0 ☑
    syphilitic A52.09
      intracranial A52.05
  cavernous sinus I67.1
    arteriovenous (congenital)
        (nonruptured) Q28.3
      ruptured I60.8
  celiac I72.8
  central nervous system, syphilitic A52.05
  cerebral — *see* Aneurysm, brain
  chest — *see* Aneurysm, thorax
  circle of Willis I67.1
    congenital Q28.3
      ruptured I60.6
    ruptured I60.6
  common iliac artery I72.3
  congenital (peripheral) Q27.8
    aorta (root) (sinus) Q25.43
    brain Q28.3
      ruptured I60.7
    coronary Q24.5
    digestive system Q27.8
    lower limb Q27.8
    pulmonary Q25.79
    retina Q14.1
    specified site NEC Q27.8
    upper limb Q27.8
  conjunctiva — *see* Abnormality, conjunctiva,
      vascular

Aneurysm - Angiostrongyliasis

Aneurysm — *continued*
conus arteriosus — *see* Aneurysm, heart
coronary (arteriosclerotic) (artery) I25.41
arteriovenous, congenital Q24.5
congenital Q24.5
ruptured — *see* Infarct, myocardium
syphilitic A52.06
vein I25.89
cylindroid (aorta) I71.9
ruptured I71.8
syphilitic A52.01
ductus arteriosus Q25.0
endocardial, infective (any valve) I33.0
femoral (artery) (ruptured) I72.4
gastroduodenal I72.8
gastroepiploic I72.8
heart (wall) (chronic or with a stated duration of over 4 weeks) I25.3
valve — *see* Endocarditis
hepatic I72.8
iliac (common) (artery) (ruptured) I72.3
infective I72.9
endocardial (any valve) I33.0
innominate (nonsyphilitic) I72.8
syphilitic A52.09
interauricular septum — *see* Aneurysm, heart
interventricular septum — *see* Aneurysm, heart
intrathoracic (nonsyphilitic) I71.2
ruptured I71.1
syphilitic A52.01
lower limb I72.4
lung (pulmonary artery) I28.1
mediastinal (nonsyphilitic) I72.8
syphilitic A52.09
miliary (congenital) I67.1
ruptured — *see* Hemorrhage, intracerebral, subarachnoid, intracranial
mitral (heart) (valve) I34.8
mural — *see* Aneurysm, heart
mycotic I72.9
endocardial (any valve) I33.0
ruptured, brain — *see* Hemorrhage, intracerebral, subarachnoid
myocardium — *see* Aneurysm, heart
neck I72.0
pancreaticoduodenal I72.8
patent ductus arteriosus Q25.0
peripheral NEC I72.8
congenital Q27.8
digestive system Q27.8
lower limb Q27.8
specified site NEC Q27.8
upper limb Q27.8
popliteal (artery) (ruptured) I72.4
precerebral
congenital (nonruptured) Q28.1
specified site, NEC I72.5
pulmonary I28.1
arteriovenous Q25.72
acquired I28.0
syphilitic A52.09
valve (heart) — *see* Endocarditis, pulmonary
racemose (peripheral) I72.9
congenital — *see* Aneurysm, congenital
radial I72.1
Rasmussen NEC A15.0
renal (artery) I72.2
retina (*see also* Disorder, retina, microaneurysms)
congenital Q14.1
diabetic — *see* Diabetes, microaneurysms, retinal
sinus of Valsalva Q25.49
specified NEC I72.8
spinal (cord) I72.8
syphilitic (hemorrhage) A52.09
splenic I72.8
subclavian (artery) (ruptured) I72.8
syphilitic A52.09
superior mesenteric I72.8
syphilitic (aorta) A52.01
central nervous system A52.05
congenital (late) A50.54 [I79.0]
spine, spinal A52.09
thoracoabdominal (aorta) I71.6
ruptured I71.5
syphilitic A52.01
thorax, thoracic (aorta) (arch) (nonsyphilitic) I71.2
ruptured I71.1
syphilitic A52.01
traumatic (complication) (early), specified site — *see* Injury, blood vessel
tricuspid (heart) (valve) I07.8

Aneurysm — *continued*
ulnar I72.1
upper limb (ruptured) I72.1
valve, valvular — *see* Endocarditis
venous (*see also* Varix) I86.8
congenital Q27.8
digestive system Q27.8
lower limb Q27.8
specified site NEC Q27.8
upper limb Q27.8
ventricle — *see* Aneurysm, heart
vertebral artery I72.6
visceral NEC I72.8
Angelman syndrome Q93.5
Anger R45.4
Angiectasis, angiectopia I99.8
Angiitis I77.6
allergic granulomatous M30.1
hypersensitivity M31.0
necrotizing M31.9
specified NEC M31.8
nervous system, granulomatous I67.7
Angina (attack) (cardiac) (chest) (heart) (pectoris) (syndrome) (vasomotor) I20.9
with
atherosclerotic heart disease — *see* Arteriosclerosis, coronary (artery),
documented spasm I20.1
abdominal K55.1
accelerated — *see* Angina, unstable
agranulocytic — *see* Agranulocytosis
angiospastic — *see* Angina, with documented spasm
aphthous B08.5
crescendo — *see* Angina, unstable
croupous J05.0
cruris I73.9
de novo effort — *see* Angina, unstable
diphtheritic, membranous A36.0
equivalent — *see* Angina, unstable
exudative, chronic J37.0
following acute myocardial infarction I23.7
gangrenous diphtheritic A36.0
intestinal K55.1
Ludovici K12.2
Ludwig's K12.2
malignant diphtheritic A36.0
membranous J05.0
diphtheritic A36.0
Vincent's A69.1
mesenteric K55.1
monocytic — *see* Mononucleosis, infectious
of effort — *see* Angina, specified NEC
phlegmonous J36
diphtheritic A36.0
post-infarctional I23.7
pre-infarctional — *see* Angina, unstable
Prinzmetal — *see* Angina, with documented spasm
progressive — *see* Angina, unstable
pseudomembranous A69.1
pultaceous, diphtheritic A36.0
spasm-induced — *see* Angina, with documented spasm
specified NEC I20.8
stable I20.8
stenocardia — *see* Angina, specified NEC
stridulous, diphtheritic A36.2
tonsil J36
trachealis J05.0
unstable I20.0
variant — *see* Angina, with documented spasm
Vincent's A69.1
worsening effort — *see* Angina, unstable
Angioblastoma — *see* Neoplasm, connective tissue, uncertain behavior
Angiocholecystitis — *see* Cholecystitis, acute
Angiocholitis (*see also* Cholecystitis, acute) K83.0
Angiodysgenesis spinalis G95.19
Angiodysplasia (cecum) (colon) K55.20
with bleeding K55.21
duodenum (and stomach) K31.819
with bleeding K31.811
stomach (and duodenum) K31.819
with bleeding K31.811
Angioedema (allergic) (any site) (with urticaria) T78.3 ☑
hereditary D84.1
Angioendothelioma — *see* Neoplasm, uncertain behavior, by site
benign D18.00
intra-abdominal D18.03
intracranial D18.02

Angioendothelioma — *continued*
benign — *continued*
skin D18.01
specified site NEC D18.09
bone — *see* Neoplasm, bone, malignant
Ewing's — *see* Neoplasm, bone, malignant
Angioendotheliomatosis C85.8 ☑
Angiofibroma (*see also* Neoplasm, benign, by site)
juvenile
specified site — *see* Neoplasm, benign, by site
unspecified site D10.6
Angiohemophilia (A) (B) D68.0
Angioid streaks (choroid) (macula) (retina) H35.33
Angiokeratoma — *see* Neoplasm, skin, benign
corporis diffusum E75.21
Angioleiomyoma — *see* Neoplasm, connective tissue, benign
Angiolipoma (*see also* Lipoma)
infiltrating — *see* Lipoma
Angioma (*see also* Hemangioma, by site)
capillary I78.1
hemorrhagicum hereditaria I78.0
intra-abdominal D18.03
intracranial D18.02
malignant — *see* Neoplasm, connective tissue, malignant
plexiform D18.00
intra-abdominal D18.03
intracranial D18.02
skin D18.01
specified site NEC D18.09
senile I78.1
serpiginosum L81.7
skin D18.01
specified site NEC D18.09
spider I78.1
stellate I78.1
venous Q28.3
Angiomatosis Q82.8
bacillary A79.89
encephalotrigeminal Q85.8
hemorrhagic familial I78.0
hereditary familial I78.0
liver K76.4
Angiomyolipoma — *see* Lipoma
Angiomyoliposarcoma — *see* Neoplasm, connective tissue, malignant
Angiomyoma — *see* Neoplasm, connective tissue, benign
Angiomyosarcoma — *see* Neoplasm, connective tissue, malignant
Angiomyxoma — *see* Neoplasm, connective tissue, uncertain behavior
Angioneurosis F45.8
Angioneurotic edema (allergic) (any site) (with urticaria) T78.3 ☑
hereditary D84.1
Angiopathia, angiopathy I99.9
cerebral I67.9
amyloid E85.4 [I68.0]
diabetic (peripheral) — *see* Diabetes, angiopathy
peripheral I73.9
diabetic — *see* Diabetes, angiopathy
specified type NEC I73.89
retinae syphilitica A52.05
retinalis (juvenilis)
diabetic — *see* Diabetes, retinopathy
proliferative — *see* Retinopathy, proliferative
Angiosarcoma (*see also* Neoplasm, connective tissue, malignant)
liver C22.3
Angiosclerosis — *see* Arteriosclerosis
Angiospasm (peripheral) (traumatic) (vessel) I73.9
brachial plexus G54.0
cerebral G45.9
cervical plexus G54.2
nerve
arm — *see* Mononeuropathy, upper limb
axillary G54.0
median — *see* Lesion, nerve, median
ulnar — *see* Lesion, nerve, ulnar
axillary G54.0
leg — *see* Mononeuropathy, lower limb
median — *see* Lesion, nerve, median
plantar — *see* Lesion, nerve, plantar
ulnar — *see* Lesion, nerve, ulnar
Angiospastic disease or edema I73.9
Angiostrongyliasis
due to
Parastrongylus
cantonensis B83.2
costaricensis B81.3

Angiostrongyliasis — *continued*
  intestinal B81.3
Anguillulosis — *see* Strongyloidiasis
Angulation
  cecum — *see* Obstruction, intestine
  coccyx (acquired) (*see also* subcategory) M43.8 ☑
    congenital NEC Q76.49
  femur (acquired) (*see also* Deformity, limb,
    specified type NEC, thigh)
    congenital Q74.2
  intestine (large) (small) — *see* Obstruction,
    intestine
  sacrum (acquired) (*see also* subcategory) M43.8 ☑
    congenital NEC Q76.49
  sigmoid (flexure) — *see* Obstruction, intestine
  spine — *see* Dorsopathy, deforming, specified
    NEC
  tibia (acquired) (*see also* Deformity, limb,
    specified type NEC, lower leg)
    congenital Q74.2
  ureter N13.5
    with infection N13.6
  wrist (acquired) (*see also* Deformity, limb,
    specified type NEC, forearm)
    congenital Q74.0
Angulus infectiosus (lips) K13.0
Anhedonia R45.84
  sexual F52.0
Anhidrosis L74.4
Anhydration E86.0
Anhydremia E86.0
Anidrosis L74.4
Aniridia (congenital) Q13.1
Anisakiasis (infection) (infestation) B81.0
Anisakis larvae infestation B81.0
Aniseikonia H52.32
Anisocoria (pupil) H57.02
  congenital Q13.2
Anisocytosis R71.8
Anisometropia (congenital) H52.31
Ankle — *see* condition
Ankyloblepharon (eyelid) (acquired) (*see also*
  Blepharophimosis)
  filiforme (adnatum) (congenital) Q10.3
  total Q10.3
Ankyloglossia Q38.1
Ankylosis (fibrous) (osseous) (joint) M24.60
  ankle M24.67 ☑
  arthrodesis status Z98.1
  cricoarytenoid (cartilage) (joint) (larynx) J38.7
  dental K03.5
  ear ossicles H74.31 ☑
  elbow M24.62 ☑
  foot M24.67 ☑
  hand M24.64 ☑
  hip M24.65 ☑
  incostapedial joint (infectional) — *see* Ankylosis,
    ear ossicles
  jaw (temporomandibular) M26.61 ☑
  knee M24.66 ☑
  lumbosacral M43.27
  postoperative (status) Z98.1
  produced by surgical fusion, status Z98.1
  sacro-iliac (joint) M43.28
  shoulder M24.61 ☑
  spine (joint) (*see also* Fusion, spine)
    spondylitic — *see* Spondylitis, ankylosing
  surgical Z98.1
  temporomandibular M26.61 ☑
  tooth, teeth (hard tissues) K03.5
  wrist M24.63 ☑
Ankylostoma — *see* Ancylostoma
Ankylostomiasis — *see* Ancylostomiasis
Ankylurethria — *see* Stricture, urethra
Annular (*see also* condition)
  detachment, cervix N88.8
  organ or site, congenital NEC — *see* Distortion
  pancreas (congenital) Q45.1
Anodontia (complete) (partial) (vera) K00.0
  acquired K08.10 ☑
Anomaly, anomalous (congenital) (unspecified type)
  Q89.9
  abdominal wall NEC Q79.59
  acoustic nerve Q07.8
  adrenal (gland) Q89.1
  Alder (-Reilly) (leukocyte granulation) D72.0
  alimentary tract Q45.9
    upper Q40.9
  alveolar M26.70
    hyperplasia M26.79
      mandibular M26.72
      maxillary M26.71

Anomaly — *continued*
  alveolar — *continued*
    hypoplasia M26.79
      mandibular M26.74
      maxillary M26.73
    ridge (process) M26.79
    specified NEC M26.79
  ankle (joint) Q74.2
  anus Q43.9
  aorta (arch) NEC Q25.40
    coarctation (preductal) (postductal) Q25.1
  aortic cusp or valve Q23.9
  appendix Q43.8
  apple peel syndrome Q41.1
  aqueduct of Sylvius Q03.0
    with spina bifida — *see* Spina bifida, with
      hydrocephalus
  arm Q74.0
  arteriovenous NEC
    coronary Q24.5
    gastrointestinal Q27.33
      acquired — *see* Angiodysplasia
  artery (peripheral) Q27.9
    basilar NEC Q28.1
    cerebral Q28.3
    coronary Q24.5
    digestive system Q27.8
    eye Q15.8
    great Q25.9
      specified NEC Q25.8
    lower limb Q27.8
    peripheral Q27.9
      specified NEC Q27.8
    pulmonary NEC Q25.79
    renal Q27.2
    retina Q14.1
    specified site NEC Q27.8
    subclavian Q27.8
      origin Q25.48
    umbilical Q27.0
    upper limb Q27.8
    vertebral NEC Q28.1
  aryteno-epiglottic folds Q31.8
  atrial
    bands or folds Q20.8
    septa Q21.1
  atrioventricular
    excitation I45.6
    septum Q21.0
  auditory canal Q17.8
  auricle
    ear Q17.8
      causing impairment of hearing Q16.9
    heart Q20.8
  Axenfeld's Q15.0
  back Q89.9
  band
    atrial Q20.8
    heart Q24.8
    ventricular Q24.8
  Bartholin's duct Q38.4
  biliary duct or passage Q44.5
  bladder Q64.70
    absence Q64.5
    diverticulum Q64.6
    exstrophy Q64.10
      cloacal Q64.12
      extroversion Q64.19
      specified type NEC Q64.19
      supravesical fissure Q64.11
    neck obstruction Q64.31
    specified type NEC Q64.79
  bone Q79.9
    arm Q74.0
    face Q75.9
    leg Q74.2
    pelvic girdle Q74.2
    shoulder girdle Q74.0
    skull Q75.9
      with
        anencephaly Q00.0
        encephalocele — *see* Encephalocele
        hydrocephalus Q03.9
          with spina bifida — *see* Spina bifida, by
            site, with hydrocephalus
        microcephaly Q02
  brain (multiple) Q04.9
    vessel Q28.3
  breast Q83.9
  broad ligament Q50.6
  bronchus Q32.4
  bulbus cordis Q21.9

Anomaly — *continued*
  bursa Q79.9
  canal of Nuck Q52.4
  canthus Q10.3
  capillary Q27.9
  cardiac Q24.9
    chambers Q20.9
      specified NEC Q20.8
    septal closure Q21.9
      specified NEC Q21.8
    valve NEC Q24.8
      pulmonary Q22.3
  cardiovascular system Q28.8
  carpus Q74.0
  caruncle, lacrimal Q10.6
  cascade stomach Q40.2
  cauda equina Q06.3
  cecum Q43.9
  cerebral Q04.9
    vessels Q28.3
  cervix Q51.9
  Chédiak-Higashi (-Steinbrinck) (congenital
    gigantism of peroxidase granules) E70.330
  cheek Q18.9
  chest wall Q67.8
    bones Q76.9
  chin Q18.9
  chordae tendineae Q24.8
  choroid Q14.3
    plexus Q07.8
  chromosomes, chromosomal Q99.9
    D (1) — *see* condition, chromosome 13
    E (3) — *see* condition, chromosome 18
    G — *see* condition, chromosome 21
    sex
      female phenotype Q97.8
      gonadal dysgenesis (pure) Q99.1
      Klinefelter's Q98.4
      male phenotype Q98.9
      Turner's Q96.9
    specified NEC Q99.8
  cilia Q10.3
  circulatory system Q28.9
  clavicle Q74.0
  clitoris Q52.6
  coccyx Q76.49
  colon Q43.9
  common duct Q44.5
  communication
    coronary artery Q24.5
    left ventricle with right atrium Q21.0
  concha (ear) Q17.3
  connection
    portal vein Q26.5
    pulmonary venous Q26.4
      partial Q26.3
      total Q26.2
    renal artery with kidney Q27.2
  cornea (shape) Q13.4
  coronary artery or vein Q24.5
  cranium — *see* Anomaly, skull
  cricoid cartilage Q31.8
  cystic duct Q44.5
  dental
    alveolar — *see* Anomaly, alveolar
    arch relationship M26.20
      specified NEC M26.29
  dentofacial M26.9
    alveolar — *see* Anomaly, alveolar
    dental arch relationship M26.20
      specified NEC M26.29
    functional M26.50
      specified NEC M26.59
    jaw-cranial base relationship M26.10
      asymmetry M26.12
      maxillary M26.11
      specified type NEC M26.19
    jaw size M26.00
      macrogenia M26.05
      mandibular
        hyperplasia M26.03
        hypoplasia M26.04
      maxillary
        hyperplasia M26.01
        hypoplasia M26.02
      microgenia M26.06
      specified type NEC M26.09
    malocclusion M26.4
      dental arch relationship NEC M26.29
      jaw-cranial base relationship — *see* Anomaly,
        dentofacial, jaw-cranial base relationship
      jaw size — *see* Anomaly, dentofacial, jaw size

Anomaly

Anomaly — *continued*
- dentofacial — *continued*
  - specified type NEC M26.89
  - temporomandibular joint M26.60 ☑
    - adhesions M26.61 ☑
    - ankylosis M26.61 ☑
    - arthralgia M26.62 ☑
    - articular disc M26.63 ☑
    - specified type NEC M26.69
  - tooth position, fully erupted M26.30
    - specified NEC M26.39
- dermatoglyphic Q82.8
- diaphragm (apertures) NEC Q79.1
- digestive organ (s) or tract Q45.9
  - lower Q43.9
  - upper Q40.9
- distance, interarch (excessive) (inadequate) M26.25
- distribution, coronary artery Q24.5
- ductus
  - arteriosus Q25.0
  - botalli Q25.0
- duodenum Q43.9
- dura (brain) Q04.9
  - spinal cord Q06.9
- ear (external) Q17.9
  - causing impairment of hearing Q16.9
  - inner Q16.5
  - middle (causing impairment of hearing) Q16.4
    - ossicles Q16.3
- Ebstein's (heart) (tricuspid valve) Q22.5
- ectodermal Q82.9
- Eisenmenger's (ventricular septal defect) Q21.8
- ejaculatory duct Q55.4
- elbow Q74.0
- endocrine gland NEC Q89.2
- epididymis Q55.4
- epiglottis Q31.8
- esophagus Q39.9
- eustachian tube Q17.8
- eye Q15.9
  - anterior segment Q13.9
    - specified NEC Q13.89
  - posterior segment Q14.9
    - specified NEC Q14.8
  - ptosis (eyelid) Q10.0
  - specified NEC Q15.8
- eyebrow Q18.8
- eyelid Q10.3
  - ptosis Q10.0
- face Q18.9
  - bone (s) Q75.9
- fallopian tube Q50.6
- fascia Q79.9
- femur NEC Q74.2
- fibula NEC Q74.2
- finger Q74.0
- fixation, intestine Q43.3
- flexion (joint) NOS Q74.9
  - hip or thigh Q65.89
- foot NEC Q74.2
  - varus (congenital) Q66.3
- foramen
  - Botalli Q21.1
  - ovale Q21.1
- forearm Q74.0
- forehead Q75.8
- form, teeth K00.4
- fovea centralis Q14.1
- frontal bone — *see* Anomaly, skull
- gallbladder (position) (shape) (size) Q44.1
- Gartner's duct Q52.4
- gastrointestinal tract Q45.9
- genitalia, genital organ (s) or system
  - female Q52.9
    - external Q52.70
    - internal NOS Q52.9
  - male Q55.9
    - hydrocele P83.5
    - specified NEC Q55.8
- genitourinary NEC
  - female Q52.9
  - male Q55.9
- Gerbode Q21.0
- glottis Q31.8
- granulation or granulocyte, genetic (constitutional) (leukocyte) D72.0
- gum Q38.6
- gyri Q07.9
- hair Q84.2
- hand Q74.0
- hard tissue formation in pulp K04.3

Anomaly — *continued*
- head — *see* Anomaly, skull
- heart Q24.9
  - auricle Q20.8
  - bands or folds Q24.8
  - fibroelastosis cordis I42.4
  - obstructive NEC Q22.6
  - patent ductus arteriosus (Botalli) Q25.0
  - septum Q21.9
    - auricular Q21.1
    - interatrial Q21.1
    - interventricular Q21.0
      - with pulmonary stenosis or atresia, dextraposition of aorta and hypertrophy of right ventricle Q21.3
    - specified NEC Q21.8
    - ventricular Q21.0
      - with pulmonary stenosis or atresia, dextraposition of aorta and hypertrophy of right ventricle Q21.3
  - tetralogy of Fallot Q21.3
  - valve NEC Q24.8
    - aortic
      - bicuspid valve Q23.1
      - insufficiency Q23.1
      - stenosis Q23.0
        - subaortic Q24.4
    - mitral
      - insufficiency Q23.3
      - stenosis Q23.2
    - pulmonary Q22.3
      - atresia Q22.0
      - insufficiency Q22.2
      - stenosis Q22.1
        - infundibular Q24.3
        - subvalvular Q24.3
    - tricuspid
      - atresia Q22.4
      - stenosis Q22.4
  - ventricle Q20.8
- heel NEC Q74.2
- Hegglin's D72.0
- hemianencephaly Q00.0
- hemicephaly Q00.0
- hemicrania Q00.0
- hepatic duct Q44.5
- hip NEC Q74.2
- hourglass stomach Q40.2
- humerus Q74.0
- hydatid of Morgagni
  - female Q50.5
  - male (epididymal) Q55.4
    - testicular Q55.29
- hymen Q52.4
- hypersegmentation of neutrophils, hereditary D72.0
- hypophyseal Q89.2
- ileocecal (coil) (valve) Q43.9
- ileum Q43.9
- ilium NEC Q74.2
- integument Q84.9
  - specified NEC Q84.8
- interarch distance (excessive) (inadequate) M26.25
- intervertebral cartilage or disc Q76.49
- intestine (large) (small) Q43.9
  - with anomalous adhesions, fixation or malrotation Q43.3
- iris Q13.2
- ischium NEC Q74.2
- jaw — *see* Anomaly, dentofacial
  - alveolar — *see* Anomaly, alveolar
- jaw-cranial base relationship — *see* Anomaly, dentofacial, jaw-cranial base relationship
- jejunum Q43.8
- joint Q74.9
  - specified NEC Q74.8
- Jordan's D72.0
- kidney (s) (calyx) (pelvis) Q63.9
  - artery Q27.2
  - specified NEC Q63.8
- Klippel-Feil (brevicollis) Q76.1
- knee Q74.1
- labium (majus) (minus) Q52.70
- labyrinth, membranous Q16.5
- lacrimal apparatus or duct Q10.6
- larynx, laryngeal (muscle) Q31.9
  - web (bed) Q31.0
- lens Q12.9
- leukocytes, genetic D72.0
  - granulation (constitutional) D72.0
- lid (fold) Q10.3

Anomaly — *continued*
- ligament Q79.9
  - broad Q50.6
  - round Q52.8
- limb Q74.9
  - lower NEC Q74.2
    - reduction deformity — *see* Defect, reduction, lower limb
  - upper Q74.0
- lip Q38.0
- liver Q44.7
  - duct Q44.5
- lower limb NEC Q74.2
- lumbosacral (joint) (region) Q76.49
  - kyphosis — *see* Kyphosis, congenital
  - lordosis — *see* Lordosis, congenital
- lung (fissure) (lobe) Q33.9
- mandible — *see* Anomaly, dentofacial
- maxilla — *see* Anomaly, dentofacial
- May (-Hegglin) D72.0
- meatus urinarius NEC Q64.79
- meningeal bands or folds Q07.9
  - constriction of Q07.8
  - spinal Q06.9
- meninges Q07.9
  - cerebral Q04.8
  - spinal Q06.9
- meningocele Q05.9
- mesentery Q45.9
- metacarpus Q74.0
- metatarsus NEC Q74.2
- middle ear Q16.4
  - ossicles Q16.3
- mitral (leaflets) (valve) Q23.9
  - insufficiency Q23.3
  - specified NEC Q23.8
  - stenosis Q23.2
- mouth Q38.6
- Müllerian (*see also* Anomaly, by site)
  - uterus NEC Q51.818
- multiple NEC Q89.7
- muscle Q79.9
  - eyelid Q10.3
- musculoskeletal system, except limbs Q79.9
- myocardium Q24.8
- nail Q84.6
- narrowness, eyelid Q10.3
- nasal sinus (wall) Q30.8
- neck (any part) Q18.9
- nerve Q07.9
  - acoustic Q07.8
  - optic Q07.8
- nervous system (central) Q07.9
- nipple Q83.9
- nose, nasal (bones) (cartilage) (septum) (sinus) Q30.9
  - specified NEC Q30.8
- ocular muscle Q15.8
- omphalomesenteric duct Q43.0
- opening, pulmonary veins Q26.4
- optic
  - disc Q14.2
  - nerve Q07.8
- opticociliary vessels Q13.2
- orbit (eye) Q10.7
- organ Q89.9
  - of Corti Q16.5
- origin
  - artery
    - innominate Q25.8
    - pulmonary Q25.79
    - renal Q27.2
    - subclavian Q25.48
- osseous meatus (ear) Q16.1
- ovary Q50.39
- oviduct Q50.6
- palate (hard) (soft) NEC Q38.5
- pancreas or pancreatic duct Q45.3
- papillary muscles Q24.8
- parathyroid gland Q89.2
- paraurethral ducts Q64.79
- parotid (gland) Q38.4
- patella Q74.1
- Pelger-Huët (hereditary hyposegmentation) D72.0
- pelvic girdle NEC Q74.2
- pelvis (bony) NEC Q74.2
  - rachitic E64.3
- penis (glans) Q55.69
- pericardium Q24.8
- peripheral vascular system Q27.9
- Peter's Q13.4

☑ **Additional character required**

Anomaly — *continued*
  pharynx Q38.8
  pigmentation L81.9
    congenital Q82.8
  pituitary (gland) Q89.2
  pleural (folds) Q34.0
  portal vein Q26.5
    connection Q26.5
  position, tooth, teeth, fully erupted M26.30
    specified NEC M26.39
  precerebral vessel Q28.1
  prepuce Q55.69
  prostate Q55.4
  pulmonary Q33.9
    artery NEC Q25.79
    valve Q22.3
      atresia Q22.0
      insufficiency Q22.2
      specified type NEC Q22.3
      stenosis Q22.1
        infundibular Q24.3
        subvalvular Q24.3
    venous connection Q26.4
      partial Q26.3
      total Q26.2
  pupil Q13.2
    function H57.00
      anisocoria H57.02
      Argyll Robertson pupil H57.01
      miosis H57.03
      mydriasis H57.04
      specified type NEC H57.09
      tonic pupil H57.05 ☑
  pylorus Q40.3
  radius Q74.0
  rectum Q43.9
  reduction (extremity) (limb)
    femur (longitudinal) — *see* Defect, reduction,
      lower limb, longitudinal, femur
    fibula (longitudinal) — *see* Defect, reduction,
      lower limb, longitudinal, fibula
    lower limb — *see* Defect, reduction, lower limb
    radius (longitudinal) — *see* Defect, reduction,
      upper limb, longitudinal, radius
    tibia (longitudinal) — *see* Defect, reduction,
      lower limb, longitudinal, tibia
    ulna (longitudinal) — *see* Defect, reduction,
      upper limb, longitudinal, ulna
    upper limb — *see* Defect, reduction, upper limb
  refraction — *see* Disorder, refraction
  renal Q63.9
    artery Q27.2
    pelvis Q63.9
      specified NEC Q63.8
  respiratory system Q34.9
    specified NEC Q34.8
  retina Q14.1
  rib Q76.6
    cervical Q76.5
  Rieger's Q13.81
  rotation — *see* Malrotation
    hip or thigh Q65.89
  round ligament Q52.8
  sacroiliac (joint) NEC Q74.2
  sacrum NEC Q76.49
    kyphosis — *see* Kyphosis, congenital
    lordosis — *see* Lordosis, congenital
  saddle nose, syphilitic A50.57
  salivary duct or gland Q38.4
  scapula Q74.0
  scrotum — *see* Malformation, testis and scrotum
  sebaceous gland Q82.9
  seminal vesicles Q55.4
  sense organs NEC Q07.8
  sex chromosomes NEC (*see also* Anomaly,
    chromosomes)
    female phenotype Q97.8
    male phenotype Q98.9
  shoulder (girdle) (joint) Q74.0
  sigmoid (flexure) Q43.9
  simian crease Q82.8
  sinus of Valsalva Q25.49
  skeleton generalized Q78.9
  skin (appendage) Q82.9
  skull Q75.9
    with
      anencephaly Q00.0
      encephalocele — *see* Encephalocele
      hydrocephalus Q03.9
        with spina bifida — *see* Spina bifida, by site,
          with hydrocephalus
      microcephaly Q02

Anomaly — *continued*
  specified organ or site NEC Q89.8
  spermatic cord Q55.4
  spine, spinal NEC Q76.49
    column NEC Q76.49
      kyphosis — *see* Kyphosis, congenital
      lordosis — *see* Lordosis, congenital
    cord Q06.9
    nerve root Q07.8
  spleen Q89.09
    agenesis Q89.01
  stenonian duct Q38.4
  sternum NEC Q76.7
  stomach Q40.3
  submaxillary gland Q38.4
  tarsus NEC Q74.2
  tendon Q79.9
  testis — *see* Malformation, testis and scrotum
  thigh NEC Q74.2
  thorax (wall) Q67.8
    bony Q76.9
  throat Q38.8
  thumb Q74.0
  thymus gland Q89.2
  thyroid (gland) Q89.2
    cartilage Q31.8
  tibia NEC Q74.2
    saber A50.56
  toe Q74.2
  tongue Q38.3
  tooth, teeth K00.9
    eruption K00.6
    position, fully erupted M26.30
    spacing, fully erupted M26.30
  trachea (cartilage) Q32.1
  tragus Q17.9
  tricuspid (leaflet) (valve) Q22.9
    atresia or stenosis Q22.4
    Ebstein's Q22.5
  Uhl's (hypoplasia of myocardium, right
    ventricle) Q24.8
  ulna Q74.0
  umbilical artery Q27.0
  union
    cricoid cartilage and thyroid cartilage Q31.8
    thyroid cartilage and hyoid bone Q31.8
    trachea with larynx Q31.8
  upper limb Q74.0
  urachus Q64.4
  ureter Q62.8
    obstructive NEC Q62.39
      cecoureterocele Q62.32
      orthotopic ureterocele Q62.31
  urethra Q64.70
    absence Q64.5
    double Q64.74
    fistula to rectum Q64.73
    obstructive Q64.39
      stricture Q64.32
    prolapse Q64.71
    specified type NEC Q64.79
  urinary tract Q64.9
  uterus Q51.9
    with only one functioning horn Q51.4
  uvula Q38.5
  vagina Q52.4
  valleculae Q31.8
  valve (heart) NEC Q24.8
    coronary sinus Q24.5
    inferior vena cava Q24.8
    pulmonary Q22.3
    sinus coronario Q24.5
    venae cavae inferioris Q24.8
  vas deferens Q55.4
  vascular Q27.9
    brain Q28.3
    ring Q25.45
  vein (s) (peripheral) Q27.9
    brain Q28.3
    cerebral Q28.3
    coronary Q24.5
    developmental Q28.3
    great Q26.9
      specified NEC Q26.8
  vena cava (inferior) (superior) Q26.9
  venous — *see* Anomaly, vein (s)
  venous return Q26.8
  ventricular
    bands or folds Q24.8
    septa Q21.0
  vertebra Q76.49
    kyphosis — *see* Kyphosis, congenital
    lordosis — *see* Lordosis, congenital

Anomaly — *continued*
  vesicourethral orifice Q64.79
  vessel (s) Q27.9
    optic papilla Q14.2
    precerebral Q28.1
  vitelline duct Q43.0
  vitreous body or humor Q14.0
  vulva Q52.70
  wrist (joint) Q74.0
Anomia R48.8
Anonychia (congenital) Q84.3
  acquired L60.8
Anophthalmos, anophthalmus (congenital) (globe)
  Q11.1
  acquired Z90.01
Anopia, anopsia H53.46 ☑
  quadrant H53.46 ☑
Anorchia, anorchism, anorchidism Q55.0
Anorexia R63.0
  hysterical F44.89
  nervosa F50.00
    atypical F50.9
    binge-eating type F50.2
      with purging F50.02
    restricting type F50.01
Anorgasmy, psychogenic (female) F52.31
  male F52.32
Anosmia R43.0
  hysterical F44.6
  postinfectional J39.8
Anosognosia R41.89
Anosteoplasia Q78.9
Anovulatory cycle N97.0
Anoxemia R09.02
  newborn P84
Anoxia (pathological) R09.02
  altitude T70.29 ☑
  cerebral G93.1
    complicating
      anesthesia (general) (local) or other
        sedation T88.59 ☑
      in labor and delivery O74.3
      in pregnancy O29.21 ☑
      postpartum, puerperal O89.2
    delivery (cesarean) (instrumental) O75.4
    during a procedure G97.81
    newborn P84
    resulting from a procedure G97.82
  due to
    drowning T75.1 ☑
    high altitude T70.29 ☑
  heart — *see* Insufficiency, coronary
  intrauterine P84
  myocardial — *see* Insufficiency, coronary
  newborn P84
  spinal cord G95.11
  systemic (by suffocation) (low content in
    atmosphere) — *see* Asphyxia, traumatic
Anteflexion — *see* Anteversion
Antenatal
  care (normal pregnancy) Z34.90
  screening (encounter for) of mother (*see also*
    Encounter, antenatal screening) Z36.9
Antepartum — *see* condition
Anterior — *see* condition
Antero-occlusion M26.220
Anteversion
  cervix — *see* Anteversion, uterus
  femur (neck), congenital Q65.89
  uterus, uterine (cervix) (postinfectional)
    (postpartal, old) N85.4
    congenital Q51.818
    in pregnancy or childbirth — *see* Pregnancy,
      complicated by
Anthophobia F40.228
Anthracosilicosis J60
Anthracosis (lung) (occupational) J60
  lingua K14.3
Anthrax A22.9
  with pneumonia A22.1
  cerebral A22.8
  colitis A22.2
  cutaneous A22.0
  gastrointestinal A22.2
  inhalation A22.1
  intestinal A22.2
  meningitis A22.8
  pulmonary A22.1
  respiratory A22.1
  sepsis A22.7
  specified manifestation NEC A22.8

Anthropoid - Appendicitis

Anthropoid pelvis Q74.2
 with disproportion (fetopelvic) O33.0
Anthropophobia F40.10
 generalized F40.11
Antibodies, maternal (blood group) — *see*
 Isoimmunization, affecting management of
 pregnancy
  anti-D — *see* Isoimmunization, affecting
   management of pregnancy, Rh
  newborn P55.0
Antibody
 anticardiolipin R76.0
  with
   hemorrhagic disorder D68.312
   hypercoagulable state D68.61
 antiphosphatidylglycerol R76.0
  with
   hemorrhagic disorder D68.312
   hypercoagulable state D68.61
 antiphosphatidylinositol R76.0
  with
   hemorrhagic disorder D68.312
   hypercoagulable state D68.61
 antiphosphatidylserine R76.0
  with
   hemorrhagic disorder D68.312
   hypercoagulable state D68.61
 antiphospholipid R76.0
  with
   hemorrhagic disorder D68.312
   hypercoagulable state D68.61
Anticardiolipin syndrome D68.61
Anticoagulant, circulating (intrinsic) (*see also* -
 Disorder, hemorrhagic) D68.318
  drug-induced (extrinsic) (*see also* - Disorder,
   hemorrhagic) D68.32
  iatrogenic D68.32
Antidiuretic hormone syndrome E22.2
Antimonial cholera — *see* Poisoning, antimony
Antiphospholipid
 antibody
  with hemorrhagic disorder D68.312
  syndrome D68.61
Antisocial personality F60.2
Antithrombinemia — *see* Circulating anticoagulants
Antithromboplastinemia D68.318
Antithromboplastinogenemia D68.318
Antitoxin complication or reaction — *see*
 Complications, vaccination
Antlophobia F40.228
Antritis J32.0
 maxilla J32.0
  acute J01.00
   recurrent J01.01
 stomach K29.60
  with bleeding K29.61
Antrum, antral — *see* condition
Anuria R34
 calculous (impacted) (recurrent) (*see also*
  Calculus, urinary) N20.9
 following
  abortion — *see* Abortion by type complicated
   by, renal failure
  ectopic or molar pregnancy O08.4
 newborn P96.0
 postprocedural N99.0
 postrenal N13.8
 traumatic (following crushing) T79.5 ☑
Anus, anal — *see* condition
Anusitis K62.89
Anxiety F41.9
 depression F41.8
 episodic paroxysmal F41.0
 generalized F41.1
 hysteria F41.8
 neurosis F41.1
 panic type F41.0
 reaction F41.1
 separation, abnormal (of childhood) F93.0
 specified NEC F41.8
 state F41.1
Aorta, aortic — *see* condition
Aortectasia — *see* Ectasia, aorta
 with aneurysm — *see* Aneurysm, aorta
Aortitis (nonsyphilitic) (calcific) I77.6
 arteriosclerotic I70.0
 Doehle-Heller A52.02
 luetic A52.02
 rheumatic — *see* Endocarditis, acute, rheumatic
 specific (syphilitic) A52.02
 syphilitic A52.02
  congenital A50.54 [I79.1]

Apathetic thyroid storm — *see* Thyrotoxicosis
Apathy R45.3
Apeirophobia F40.228
Apepsia K30
 psychogenic F45.8
Aperistalsis, esophagus K22.0
Apertognathia M26.29
Apert's syndrome Q87.0
Aphagia R13.0
 psychogenic F50.9
Aphakia (acquired) (postoperative) H27.0 ☑
 congenital Q12.3
Aphasia (amnestic) (global) (nominal) (semantic)
 (syntactic) R47.01
 acquired, with epilepsy (Landau-Kleffner
  syndrome) — *see* Epilepsy, specified NEC
 auditory (developmental) F80.2
 developmental (receptive type) F80.2
  expressive type F80.1
  Wernicke's F80.2
 following
  cerebrovascular disease I69.920
   cerebral infarction I69.320
   intracerebral hemorrhage I69.120
   nontraumatic intracranial hemorrhage
    NEC I69.220
   specified disease NEC I69.820
   subarachnoid hemorrhage I69.020
 primary progressive G31.01 [F02.80]
  with behavioral disturbance G31.01 [F02.81]
 progressive isolated G31.01 [F02.80]
  with behavioral disturbance G31.01 [F02.81]
 sensory F80.2
 syphilis, tertiary A52.19
 Wernicke's (developmental) F80.2
Aphonia (organic) R49.1
 hysterical F44.4
 psychogenic F44.4
Aphthae, aphthous (*see also* condition)
 Bednar's K12.0
 cachectic K14.0
 epizootic B08.8
 fever B08.8
 oral (recurrent) K12.0
 stomatitis (major) (minor) K12.0
 thrush B37.0
 ulcer (oral) (recurrent) K12.0
  genital organ (s) NEC
   female N76.6
   male N50.89
  larynx J38.7
Apical — *see* condition
Apiphobia F40.218
Aplasia (*see also* Agenesis)
 abdominal muscle syndrome Q79.4
 alveolar process (acquired) — *see* Anomaly,
  alveolar
  congenital Q38.6
 aorta (congenital) Q25.41
 axialis extracorticalis (congenita) E75.29
 bone marrow (myeloid) D61.9
  congenital D61.01
 brain Q00.0
  part of Q04.3
 bronchus Q32.4
 cementum K00.4
 cerebellum Q04.3
 cervix (congenital) Q51.5
 congenital pure red cell D61.01
 corpus callosum Q04.0
 cutis congenita Q84.8
 erythrocyte congenital D61.01
 extracortical axial E75.29
 eye Q11.1
 fovea centralis (congenital) Q14.1
 gallbladder, congenital Q44.0
 iris Q13.1
 labyrinth, membranous Q16.5
 limb (congenital) Q73.8
  lower — *see* Defect, reduction, lower limb
  upper — *see* Agenesis, arm
 lung, congenital (bilateral) (unilateral) Q33.3
 pancreas Q45.0
 parathyroid-thymic D82.1
 Pelizaeus-Merzbacher E75.29
 penis Q55.5
 prostate Q55.4
 red cell (with thymoma) D60.9
  acquired D60.9
   due to drugs D60.9
  adult D60.9
  chronic D60.0

Aplasia — *continued*
 red cell — *continued*
  congenital D61.01
  constitutional D61.01
  due to drugs D60.9
  hereditary D61.01
  of infants D61.01
  primary D61.01
  pure D61.01
   due to drugs D60.9
  specified type NEC D60.8
  transient D60.1
 round ligament Q52.8
 skin Q84.8
 spermatic cord Q55.4
 spleen Q89.01
 testicle Q55.0
 thymic, with immunodeficiency D82.1
 thyroid (congenital) (with myxedema) E03.1
 uterus Q51.0
 ventral horn cell Q06.1
Apnea, apneic (of) (spells) R06.81
 newborn NEC P28.4
  obstructive P28.4
  sleep (central) (obstructive) (primary) P28.3
  prematurity P28.4
 sleep G47.30
  central (primary) G47.31
   idiopathic G47.31
   in conditions classified elsewhere G47.37
  obstructive (adult) (pediatric) G47.33
   hypopnea G47.33
  primary central G47.31
  specified NEC G47.39
Apneumatosis, newborn P28.0
Apocrine metaplasia (breast) — *see* Dysplasia,
 mammary, specified type NEC
Apophysitis (bone) (*see also* Osteochondropathy)
 calcaneus M92.8
 juvenile M92.9
Apoplectiform convulsions (cerebral ischemia)
 I67.82
Apoplexia, apoplexy, apoplectic
 adrenal A39.1
 heart (auricle) (ventricle) — *see* Infarct,
  myocardium
 heat T67.0 ☑
 hemorrhagic (stroke) — *see* Hemorrhage,
  intracranial
 meninges, hemorrhagic — *see* Hemorrhage,
  intracranial, subarachnoid
 uremic N18.9 [I68.8]
Appearance
 bizarre R46.1
 specified NEC R46.89
 very low level of personal hygiene R46.0
Appendage
 epididymal (organ of Morgagni) Q55.4
 intestine (epiploic) Q43.8
 preauricular Q17.0
 testicular (organ of Morgagni) Q55.29
Appendicitis (pneumococcal) (retrocecal) K37
 with
  perforation or rupture K35.2
  peritoneal abscess K35.3
  peritonitis NEC K35.3
   generalized (with perforation or
    rupture) K35.2
   localized (with perforation or rupture) K35.3
 acute (catarrhal) (fulminating)
  (gangrenous) (obstructive) (retrocecal)
  (suppurative) K35.80
  with
   peritoneal abscess K35.3
   peritonitis NEC K35.3
    generalized (with perforation or
     rupture) K35.2
    localized (with perforation or
     rupture) K35.3
   specified NEC K35.89
 amebic A06.89
 chronic (recurrent) K36
 exacerbation — *see* Appendicitis, acute
 gangrenous — *see* Appendicitis, acute
 healed (obliterative) K36
 interval K36
 neurogenic K36
 obstructive K36
 recurrent K36
 relapsing K36
 subacute (adhesive) K36
 subsiding K36

☑ **Additional character required**

Appendicitis — *continued*
  suppurative — *see* Appendicitis, acute
  tuberculous A18.32
Appendicopathia oxyurica B80
Appendix, appendicular (*see also* condition)
  epididymis Q55.4
  Morgagni
    female Q50.5
    male (epididymal) Q55.4
      testicular Q55.29
  testis Q55.29
Appetite
  depraved — *see* Pica
  excessive R63.2
  lack or loss (*see also* Anorexia) R63.0
    nonorganic origin F50.89
    psychogenic F50.89
  perverted (hysterical) — *see* Pica
Apple peel syndrome Q41.1
Apprehension state F41.1
Apprehensiveness, abnormal F41.9
Approximal wear K03.0
Apraxia (classic) (ideational) (ideokinetic)
  (ideomotor) (motor) (verbal) R48.2
  following
    cerebrovascular disease I69.990
      cerebral infarction I69.390
      intracerebral hemorrhage I69.190
      nontraumatic intracranial hemorrhage
        NEC I69.290
      specified disease NEC I69.890
      subarachnoid hemorrhage I69.090
  oculomotor, congenital H51.8
Aptyalism K11.7
Apudoma — *see* Neoplasm, uncertain behavior, by
  site
Aqueous misdirection H40.83 ☑
Arabicum elephantiasis — *see* Infestation, filarial
Arachnitis — *see* Meningitis
Arachnodactyly — *see* Syndrome, Marfan's
Arachnoiditis (acute) (adhesive) (basal) (brain)
  (cerebrospinal) — *see* Meningitis
Arachnophobia F40.210
Arboencephalitis, Australian A83.4
Arborization block (heart) I45.5
ARC (AIDS-related complex) B20
Arch
  aortic Q25.49
  bovine Q25.49
Arches — *see* condition
Arcuate uterus Q51.810
Arcuatus uterus Q51.810
Arcus (cornea) senilis — *see* Degeneration, cornea,
  senile
Arc-welder's lung J63.4
Areflexia R29.2
Areola — *see* condition
Argentaffinoma (*see also* Neoplasm, uncertain
  behavior, by site)
  malignant — *see* Neoplasm, malignant, by site
  syndrome E34.0
Argininemia E72.21
Arginosuccinic aciduria E72.22
Argyll Robertson phenomenon, pupil or syndrome
  (syphilitic) A52.19
  atypical H57.09
  nonsyphilitic H57.09
Argyria, argyriasis
  conjunctival H11.13 ☑
  from drug or medicament — *see* Table of Drugs
    and Chemicals, by substance
Argyrosis, conjunctival H11.13 ☑
Arhinencephaly Q04.1
Ariboflavinosis E53.0
Arm — *see* condition
Arnold-Chiari disease, obstruction or syndrome
  (type II) Q07.00
  with
    hydrocephalus Q07.02
      with spina bifida Q07.03
    spina bifida Q07.01
      with hydrocephalus Q07.03
  type III — *see* Encephalocele
  type IV Q04.8
Aromatic amino-acid metabolism disorder E70.9
  specified NEC E70.8
Arousals, confusional G47.51
Arrest, arrested
  cardiac I46.9
    complicating
      abortion — *see* Abortion, by type,
        complicated by, cardiac arrest

Arrest — *continued*
  cardiac — *continued*
    anesthesia (general) (local) or other sedation
      — *see* Table of Drugs and Chemicals, by
      drug,
      in labor and delivery O74.2
      in pregnancy O29.11 ☑
      postpartum, puerperal O89.1
    delivery (cesarean) (instrumental) O75.4
    due to
      cardiac condition I46.2
      specified condition NEC I46.8
    intraoperative I97.71 ☑
    newborn P29.81
    personal history, successfully
      resuscitated Z86.74
    postprocedural I97.12 ☑
      obstetric procedure O75.4
  cardiorespiratory — *see* Arrest, cardiac
  circulatory — *see* Arrest, cardiac
  deep transverse O64.0 ☑
  development or growth
    bone — *see* Disorder, bone, development or
      growth
    child R62.50
    tracheal rings Q32.1
  epiphyseal
    complete
      femur M89.15 ☑
      humerus M89.12 ☑
      tibia M89.16 ☑
      ulna M89.13 ☑
    forearm M89.13 ☑
      specified NEC M89.13 ☑
      ulna — *see* Arrest, epiphyseal, by type, ulna
    lower leg M89.16 ☑
      specified NEC M89.168
      tibia — *see* Arrest, epiphyseal, by type, tibia
    partial
      femur M89.15 ☑
      humerus M89.12 ☑
      tibia M89.16 ☑
      ulna M89.13 ☑
    specified NEC M89.18
  granulopoiesis — *see* Agranulocytosis
  growth plate — *see* Arrest, epiphyseal
  heart — *see* Arrest, cardiac
  legal, anxiety concerning Z65.3
  physeal — *see* Arrest, epiphyseal
  respiratory R09.2
    newborn P28.81
  sinus I45.5
  spermatogenesis (complete) — *see* Azoospermia
    incomplete — *see* Oligospermia
  transverse (deep) O64.0 ☑
Arrhenoblastoma
  benign
    specified site — *see* Neoplasm, benign, by site
    unspecified site
      female D27.9
      male D29.20
  malignant
    specified site — *see* Neoplasm, malignant, by
      site
    unspecified site
      female C56.9
      male C62.90
  specified site — *see* Neoplasm, uncertain
    behavior, by site
  unspecified site
    female D39.10
    male D40.10
Arrhythmia (auricle) (cardiac) (juvenile) (nodal) (reflex)
  (sinus) (supraventricular) (transitory) (ventricle) I49.9
  block I45.9
  extrasystolic I49.49
  newborn
    bradycardia P29.12
    occurring before birth P03.819
      before onset of labor P03.810
      during labor P03.811
    tachycardia P29.11
  psychogenic F45.8
  specified NEC I49.8
  vagal R55
  ventricular re-entry I47.0
Arrillaga-Ayerza syndrome (pulmonary sclerosis
  with pulmonary hypertension) I27.0
Arsenical pigmentation L81.8
  from drug or medicament — *see* Table of Drugs
    and Chemicals
Arsenism — *see* Poisoning, arsenic

Arterial — *see* condition
Arteriofibrosis — *see* Arteriosclerosis
Arteriolar sclerosis — *see* Arteriosclerosis
Arteriolith — *see* Arteriosclerosis
Arteriolitis I77.6
  necrotizing, kidney I77.5
  renal — *see* Hypertension, kidney
Arteriolosclerosis — *see* Arteriosclerosis
Arterionephrosclerosis — *see* Hypertension, kidney
Arteriopathy I77.9
Arteriosclerosis, arteriosclerotic (diffuse) (obliterans)
  (of) (senile) (with calcification) I70.90
  aorta I70.0
  arteries of extremities — *see* Arteriosclerosis,
    extremities
  brain I67.2
  bypass graft
    coronary — *see* Arteriosclerosis, coronary,
      bypass graft
    extremities — *see* Arteriosclerosis, extremities,
      bypass graft
  cardiac — *see* Disease, heart, ischemic,
    atherosclerotic
  cardiopathy — *see* Disease, heart, ischemic,
    atherosclerotic
  cardiorenal — *see* Hypertension, cardiorenal
  cardiovascular — *see* Disease, heart, ischemic,
    atherosclerotic
  carotid (*see also* Occlusion, artery, carotid) I65.2 ☑
  central nervous system I67.2
  cerebral I67.2
  cerebrovascular I67.2
  coronary (artery) I25.10
    due to
      calcified coronary lesion (severely) I25.84
      lipid rich plaque I25.83
    bypass graft I25.810
      with
        angina pectoris I25.709
          with documented spasm I25.701
          specified type NEC I25.708
          unstable I25.700
        ischemic chest pain I25.709
      autologous artery I25.810
        with
          angina pectoris I25.729
            with documented spasm I25.721
            specified type I25.728
            unstable I25.720
          ischemic chest pain I25.729
      autologous vein I25.810
        with
          angina pectoris I25.719
            with documented spasm I25.711
            specified type I25.718
            unstable I25.710
          ischemic chest pain I25.719
      nonautologous biological I25.810
        with
          angina pectoris I25.739
            with documented spasm I25.731
            specified type I25.738
            unstable I25.730
          ischemic chest pain I25.739
      specified type NEC I25.810
        with
          angina pectoris I25.799
            with documented spasm I25.791
            specified type I25.798
            unstable I25.790
          ischemic chest pain I25.799
    native vessel
      with
        angina pectoris I25.119
          with documented spasm I25.111
          specified type NEC I25.118
          unstable I25.110
        ischemic chest pain I25.119
    transplanted heart I25.811
      bypass graft I25.812
        with
          angina pectoris I25.769
            with documented spasm I25.761
            specified type I25.768
            unstable I25.760
          ischemic chest pain I25.769
      native coronary artery I25.811
        with
          angina pectoris I25.759
            with documented spasm I25.751
            specified type I25.758
            unstable I25.750
          ischemic chest pain I25.759

Arteriosclerosis

Arteriosclerosis — *continued*
　extremities (native arteries) I70.209
　　bypass graft I70.309
　　　autologous vein graft I70.409
　　　　leg I70.409
　　　　　with
　　　　　　gangrene (and intermittent
　　　　　　　claudication, rest pain and
　　　　　　　ulcer) I70.469
　　　　　　intermittent claudication I70.419
　　　　　　rest pain (and intermittent
　　　　　　　claudication) I70.429
　　　　　bilateral I70.403
　　　　　　with
　　　　　　　gangrene (and intermittent
　　　　　　　　claudication, rest pain and
　　　　　　　　ulcer) I70.463
　　　　　　　intermittent claudication I70.413
　　　　　　　rest pain (and intermittent
　　　　　　　　claudication) I70.423
　　　　　　specified type NEC I70.493
　　　　　left I70.402
　　　　　　with
　　　　　　　gangrene (and intermittent
　　　　　　　　claudication, rest pain and
　　　　　　　　ulcer) I70.462
　　　　　　　intermittent claudication I70.412
　　　　　　　rest pain (and intermittent
　　　　　　　　claudication) I70.422
　　　　　　　ulceration (and intermittent
　　　　　　　　claudication and rest
　　　　　　　　pain) I70.449
　　　　　　　ankle I70.443
　　　　　　　calf I70.442
　　　　　　　foot site NEC I70.445
　　　　　　　heel I70.444
　　　　　　　lower leg NEC I70.448
　　　　　　　midfoot I70.444
　　　　　　　thigh I70.441
　　　　　　specified type NEC I70.492
　　　　　right I70.401
　　　　　　with
　　　　　　　gangrene (and intermittent
　　　　　　　　claudication, rest pain and
　　　　　　　　ulcer) I70.461
　　　　　　　intermittent claudication I70.411
　　　　　　　rest pain (and intermittent
　　　　　　　　claudication) I70.421
　　　　　　　ulceration (and intermittent
　　　　　　　　claudication and rest
　　　　　　　　pain) I70.439
　　　　　　　ankle I70.433
　　　　　　　calf I70.432
　　　　　　　foot site NEC I70.435
　　　　　　　heel I70.434
　　　　　　　lower leg NEC I70.438
　　　　　　　midfoot I70.434
　　　　　　　thigh I70.431
　　　　　　specified type NEC I70.491
　　　　　specified type NEC I70.499
　　　　specified NEC I70.408
　　　　　with
　　　　　　gangrene (and intermittent
　　　　　　　claudication, rest pain and
　　　　　　　ulcer) I70.468
　　　　　　intermittent claudication I70.418
　　　　　　rest pain (and intermittent
　　　　　　　claudication) I70.428
　　　　　　ulceration (and intermittent
　　　　　　　claudication and rest pain) I70.45
　　　　　specified type NEC I70.498
　　　leg I70.309
　　　　with
　　　　　gangrene (and intermittent claudication,
　　　　　　rest pain and ulcer) I70.369
　　　　　intermittent claudication I70.319
　　　　　rest pain (and intermittent
　　　　　　claudication) I70.329
　　　　bilateral I70.303
　　　　　with
　　　　　　gangrene (and intermittent
　　　　　　　claudication, rest pain and
　　　　　　　ulcer) I70.363
　　　　　　intermittent claudication I70.313
　　　　　　rest pain (and intermittent
　　　　　　　claudication) I70.323
　　　　　specified type NEC I70.393
　　　　left I70.302
　　　　　with
　　　　　　gangrene (and intermittent
　　　　　　　claudication, rest pain and
　　　　　　　ulcer) I70.362

Arteriosclerosis — *continued*
　extremities — *continued*
　　　intermittent claudication I70.312
　　　rest pain (and intermittent
　　　　claudication) I70.322
　　　ulceration (and intermittent
　　　　claudication and rest pain) I70.349
　　　　ankle I70.343
　　　　calf I70.342
　　　　foot site NEC I70.345
　　　　heel I70.344
　　　　lower leg NEC I70.348
　　　　midfoot I70.344
　　　　thigh I70.341
　　　specified type NEC I70.392
　　right I70.301
　　　with
　　　　gangrene (and intermittent
　　　　　claudication, rest pain and
　　　　　ulcer) I70.361
　　　　intermittent claudication I70.311
　　　　rest pain (and intermittent
　　　　　claudication) I70.321
　　　　ulceration (and intermittent
　　　　　claudication and rest pain) I70.339
　　　　　ankle I70.333
　　　　　calf I70.332
　　　　　foot site NEC I70.335
　　　　　heel I70.334
　　　　　lower leg NEC I70.338
　　　　　midfoot I70.334
　　　　　thigh I70.331
　　　　specified type NEC I70.391
　　specified type NEC I70.399
　　nonautologous biological graft I70.509
　　　leg I70.509
　　　　with
　　　　　gangrene (and intermittent
　　　　　　claudication, rest pain and
　　　　　　ulcer) I70.569
　　　　　intermittent claudication I70.519
　　　　　rest pain (and intermittent
　　　　　　claudication) I70.529
　　　　bilateral I70.503
　　　　　with
　　　　　　gangrene (and intermittent
　　　　　　　claudication, rest pain and
　　　　　　　ulcer) I70.563
　　　　　　intermittent claudication I70.513
　　　　　　rest pain (and intermittent
　　　　　　　claudication) I70.523
　　　　　specified type NEC I70.593
　　　　left I70.502
　　　　　with
　　　　　　gangrene (and intermittent
　　　　　　　claudication, rest pain and
　　　　　　　ulcer) I70.562
　　　　　　intermittent claudication I70.512
　　　　　　rest pain (and intermittent
　　　　　　　claudication) I70.522
　　　　　　ulceration (and intermittent
　　　　　　　claudication and rest
　　　　　　　pain) I70.549
　　　　　　ankle I70.543
　　　　　　calf I70.542
　　　　　　foot site NEC I70.545
　　　　　　heel I70.544
　　　　　　lower leg NEC I70.548
　　　　　　midfoot I70.544
　　　　　　thigh I70.541
　　　　　specified type NEC I70.592
　　　　right I70.501
　　　　　with
　　　　　　gangrene (and intermittent
　　　　　　　claudication, rest pain and
　　　　　　　ulcer) I70.561
　　　　　　intermittent claudication I70.511
　　　　　　rest pain (and intermittent
　　　　　　　claudication) I70.521
　　　　　　ulceration (and intermittent
　　　　　　　claudication and rest
　　　　　　　pain) I70.539
　　　　　　ankle I70.533
　　　　　　calf I70.532
　　　　　　foot site NEC I70.535
　　　　　　heel I70.534
　　　　　　lower leg NEC I70.538
　　　　　　midfoot I70.534
　　　　　　thigh I70.531
　　　　　specified type NEC I70.591
　　　　specified type NEC I70.599
　　　specified NEC I70.508

Arteriosclerosis — *continued*
　extremities — *continued*
　　　with
　　　　gangrene (and intermittent
　　　　　claudication, rest pain and
　　　　　ulcer) I70.568
　　　　intermittent claudication I70.518
　　　　rest pain (and intermittent
　　　　　claudication) I70.528
　　　　ulceration (and intermittent
　　　　　claudication and rest pain) I70.55
　　　specified type NEC I70.598
　　nonbiological graft I70.609
　　　leg I70.609
　　　　with
　　　　　gangrene (and intermittent
　　　　　　claudication, rest pain and
　　　　　　ulcer) I70.669
　　　　　intermittent claudication I70.619
　　　　　rest pain (and intermittent
　　　　　　claudication) I70.629
　　　　bilateral I70.603
　　　　　with
　　　　　　gangrene (and intermittent
　　　　　　　claudication, rest pain and
　　　　　　　ulcer) I70.663
　　　　　　intermittent claudication I70.613
　　　　　　rest pain (and intermittent
　　　　　　　claudication) I70.623
　　　　　specified type NEC I70.693
　　　　left I70.602
　　　　　with
　　　　　　gangrene (and intermittent
　　　　　　　claudication, rest pain and
　　　　　　　ulcer) I70.662
　　　　　　intermittent claudication I70.612
　　　　　　rest pain (and intermittent
　　　　　　　claudication) I70.622
　　　　　　ulceration (and intermittent
　　　　　　　claudication and rest
　　　　　　　pain) I70.649
　　　　　　ankle I70.643
　　　　　　calf I70.642
　　　　　　foot site NEC I70.645
　　　　　　heel I70.644
　　　　　　lower leg NEC I70.648
　　　　　　midfoot I70.644
　　　　　　thigh I70.641
　　　　　specified type NEC I70.692
　　　　right I70.601
　　　　　with
　　　　　　gangrene (and intermittent
　　　　　　　claudication, rest pain and
　　　　　　　ulcer) I70.661
　　　　　　intermittent claudication I70.611
　　　　　　rest pain (and intermittent
　　　　　　　claudication) I70.621
　　　　　　ulceration (and intermittent
　　　　　　　claudication and rest
　　　　　　　pain) I70.639
　　　　　　ankle I70.633
　　　　　　calf I70.632
　　　　　　foot site NEC I70.635
　　　　　　heel I70.634
　　　　　　lower leg NEC I70.638
　　　　　　midfoot I70.634
　　　　　　thigh I70.631
　　　　　specified type NEC I70.691
　　　　specified type NEC I70.699
　　　specified NEC I70.608
　　　　with
　　　　　gangrene (and intermittent
　　　　　　claudication, rest pain and
　　　　　　ulcer) I70.668
　　　　　intermittent claudication I70.618
　　　　　rest pain (and intermittent
　　　　　　claudication) I70.628
　　　　　ulceration (and intermittent
　　　　　　claudication and rest pain) I70.65
　　　　specified type NEC I70.698
　　specified graft NEC I70.709
　　　leg I70.709
　　　　with
　　　　　gangrene (and intermittent
　　　　　　claudication, rest pain and
　　　　　　ulcer) I70.769
　　　　　intermittent claudication I70.719
　　　　　rest pain (and intermittent
　　　　　　claudication) I70.729
　　　　bilateral I70.703
　　　　　with

☑ **Additional character required**

Arteriosclerosis — *continued*
  extremities — *continued*
    gangrene (and intermittent claudication, rest pain and ulcer) I70.763
    intermittent claudication I70.713
    rest pain (and intermittent claudication) I70.723
    specified type NEC I70.793
    left I70.702
      with
        gangrene (and intermittent claudication, rest pain and ulcer) I70.762
        intermittent claudication I70.712
        rest pain (and intermittent claudication) I70.722
        ulceration (and intermittent claudication and rest pain) I70.749
        ankle I70.743
        calf I70.742
        foot site NEC I70.745
        heel I70.744
        lower leg NEC I70.748
        midfoot I70.744
        thigh I70.741
      specified type NEC I70.792
    right I70.701
      with
        gangrene (and intermittent claudication, rest pain and ulcer) I70.761
        intermittent claudication I70.711
        rest pain (and intermittent claudication) I70.721
        ulceration (and intermittent claudication and rest pain) I70.739
        ankle I70.733
        calf I70.732
        foot site NEC I70.735
        heel I70.734
        lower leg NEC I70.738
        midfoot I70.734
        thigh I70.731
      specified type NEC I70.791
    specified type NEC I70.799
    specified NEC I70.708
      with
        gangrene (and intermittent claudication, rest pain and ulcer) I70.768
        intermittent claudication I70.718
        rest pain (and intermittent claudication) I70.728
        ulceration (and intermittent claudication and rest pain) I70.75
      specified type NEC I70.798
    specified NEC I70.308
      with
        gangrene (and intermittent claudication, rest pain and ulcer) I70.368
        intermittent claudication I70.318
        rest pain (and intermittent claudication) I70.328
        ulceration (and intermittent claudication and rest pain) I70.35
      specified type NEC I70.398
  leg I70.209
    with
      gangrene (and intermittent claudication, rest pain and ulcer) I70.269
      intermittent claudication I70.219
      rest pain (and intermittent claudication) I70.229
    bilateral I70.203
      with
        gangrene (and intermittent claudication, rest pain and ulcer) I70.263
        intermittent claudication I70.213
        rest pain (and intermittent claudication) I70.223
      specified type NEC I70.293
    left I70.202
      with
        gangrene (and intermittent claudication, rest pain and ulcer) I70.262
        intermittent claudication I70.212
        rest pain (and intermittent claudication) I70.222

Arteriosclerosis — *continued*
  extremities — *continued*
      ulceration (and intermittent claudication and rest pain) I70.249
      ankle I70.243
      calf I70.242
      foot site NEC I70.245
      heel I70.244
      lower leg NEC I70.248
      midfoot I70.244
      thigh I70.241
    specified type NEC I70.292
    right I70.201
      with
        gangrene (and intermittent claudication, rest pain and ulcer) I70.261
        intermittent claudication I70.211
        rest pain (and intermittent claudication) I70.221
        ulceration (and intermittent claudication and rest pain) I70.239
        ankle I70.233
        calf I70.232
        foot site NEC I70.235
        heel I70.234
        lower leg NEC I70.238
        midfoot I70.234
        thigh I70.231
      specified type NEC I70.291
    specified site NEC I70.208
      with
        gangrene (and intermittent claudication, rest pain and ulcer) I70.268
        intermittent claudication I70.218
        rest pain (and intermittent claudication) I70.228
        ulceration (and intermittent claudication and rest pain) I70.25
      specified type NEC I70.298
  generalized I70.91
  heart (disease) — *see* Arteriosclerosis, coronary (artery),
  kidney — *see* Hypertension, kidney
  medial — *see* Arteriosclerosis, extremities
  mesenteric (artery) K55.1
  Mönckeberg's — *see* Arteriosclerosis, extremities
  myocarditis I51.4
  peripheral (of extremities) — *see* Arteriosclerosis, extremities
  pulmonary (idiopathic) I27.0
  renal (arterioles) (*see also* Hypertension, kidney)
    artery I70.1
  retina (vascular) I70.8 *[H35.0 ☑]*
  specified artery NEC I70.8
  spinal (cord) G95.19
  vertebral (artery) I67.2
Arteriospasm I73.9
Arteriovenous — *see* condition
Arteritis I77.6
  allergic M31.0
  aorta (nonsyphilitic) I77.6
    syphilitic A52.02
  aortic arch M31.4
  brachiocephalic M31.4
  brain I67.7
    syphilitic A52.04
  cerebral I67.7
    in
      diseases classified elsewhere I68.2
      systemic lupus erythematosus M32.19
    listerial A32.89
    syphilitic A52.04
    tuberculous A18.89
  coronary (artery) I25.89
    rheumatic I01.8
      chronic I09.89
    syphilitic A52.06
  cranial (left) (right), giant cell M31.6
  deformans — *see* Arteriosclerosis
  giant cell NEC M31.6
    with polymyalgia rheumatica M31.5
  necrosing or necrotizing M31.9
    specified NEC M31.8
  nodosa M30.0
  obliterans — *see* Arteriosclerosis
  pulmonary I28.8
  rheumatic — *see* Fever, rheumatic
  senile — *see* Arteriosclerosis
  suppurative I77.2
  syphilitic (general) A52.09
    brain A52.04

Arteritis — *continued*
  syphilitic — *continued*
    coronary A52.06
    spinal A52.09
  temporal, giant cell M31.6
  young female aortic arch syndrome M31.4
Artery, arterial (*see also* condition)
  abscess I77.89
  single umbilical Q27.0
Arthralgia (allergic) (*see also* Pain, joint)
  in caisson disease T70.3 ☑
  temporomandibular M26.62 ☑
Arthritis, arthritic (acute) (chronic) (nonpyogenic) (subacute) M19.90
  allergic — *see* Arthritis, specified form NEC
  ankylosing (crippling) (spine) (*see also* Spondylitis, ankylosing)
    sites other than spine — *see* Arthritis, specified form NEC
  atrophic — *see* Osteoarthritis
    spine — *see* Spondylitis, ankylosing
  back — *see* Spondylopathy, inflammatory
  blennorrhagic (gonococcal) A54.42
  Charcot's — *see* Arthropathy, neuropathic
    diabetic — *see* Diabetes, arthropathy, neuropathic
    syringomyelic G95.0
  chylous (filarial) (*see also* category M01) B74.9
  climacteric (any site) NEC — *see* Arthritis, specified form NEC
  crystal (-induced) — *see* Arthritis, in, crystals
  deformans — *see* Osteoarthritis
  degenerative — *see* Osteoarthritis
  due to or associated with
    acromegaly E22.0
    brucellosis — *see* Brucellosis
    caisson disease T70.3 ☑
    diabetes — *see* Diabetes, arthropathy
    dracontiasis (*see also* category M01) B72
    enteritis NEC
      regional — *see* Enteritis, regional
    erysipelas (*see also* category M01) A46
    erythema
      epidemic A25.1
      nodosum L52
    filariasis NOS B74.9
    glanders A24.0
    helminthiasis (*see also* category M01) B83.9
    hemophilia D66 *[M36.2]*
    Henoch- (Schönlein) purpura D69.0 *[M36.4]*
    human parvovirus (*see also* category M01) B97.6
    infectious disease NEC — *see* category M01
    leprosy (*see also* category M01) (*see also* Leprosy) A30.9
    Lyme disease A69.23
    mycobacteria (*see also* category M01) A31.8
    parasitic disease NEC (*see also* category M01) B89
    paratyphoid fever (*see also* category M01) (*see also* Fever, paratyphoid) A01.4
    rat bite fever (*see also* category M01) A25.1
    regional enteritis — *see* Enteritis, regional
    respiratory disorder NOS J98.9
    serum sickness (*see also* Reaction, serum) T80.69 ☑
    syringomyelia G95.0
    typhoid fever A01.04
  epidemic erythema A25.1
  febrile — *see* Fever, rheumatic
  gonococcal A54.42
  gouty (acute) — *see* Gout
  in (due to)
    acromegaly (*see also* subcategory M14.8 ☑) E22.0
    amyloidosis (*see also* subcategory M14.8 ☑) E85.4
    bacterial disease (*see also* subcategory M01) A49.9
    Behçet's syndrome M35.2
    caisson disease (*see also* subcategory M14.8 ☑) T70.3 ☑
    coliform bacilli (Escherichia coli) — *see* Arthritis, in, pyogenic organism NEC
    crystals M11.9
      dicalcium phosphate — *see* Arthritis, in, crystals, specified type NEC
      hydroxyapatite M11.0 ☑
      pyrophosphate — *see* Arthritis, in, crystals, specified type NEC
      specified type NEC M11.80
        ankle M11.87 ☑
        elbow M11.82 ☑
        foot joint M11.87 ☑

Arthritis

Arthritis — *continued*
  in — *continued*
    hand joint M11.84 ☑
    hip M11.85 ☑
    knee M11.86 ☑
    multiple sites M11.8 ☑
    shoulder M11.81 ☑
    vertebrae M11.88
    wrist M11.83 ☑
  dermatoarthritis, lipoid E78.81
  dracontiasis (dracunculiasis) (*see also* category M01) B72
  endocrine disorder NEC (*see also* subcategory M14.8 ☑) E34.9
  enteritis, infectious NEC (*see also* category M01) A09
    specified organism NEC (*see also* category M01) A08.8
  erythema
    multiforme (*see also* subcategory M14.8 ☑) L51.9
    nodosum (*see also* subcategory M14.8 ☑) L52
  gout — *see* Gout
  helminthiasis NEC (*see also* category M01) B83.9
  hemochromatosis (*see also* subcategory M14.8 ☑) E83.118
  hemoglobinopathy NEC D58.2 *[M36.3]*
  hemophilia NEC D66 *[M36.2]*
  Hemophilus influenzae M00.8 ☑ *[B96.3]*
  Henoch (-Schönlein) purpura D69.0 *[M36.4]*
  hyperparathyroidism NEC (*see also* subcategory M14.8 ☑) E21.3
  hypersensitivity reaction NEC T78.49 ☑ *[M36.4]*
  hypogammaglobulinemia (*see also* subcategory M14.8 ☑) D80.1
  hypothyroidism NEC (*see also* subcategory M14.8 ☑) E03.9
  infection — *see* Arthritis, pyogenic or pyemic
    spine — *see* Spondylopathy, infective
  infectious disease NEC — *see* category M01
  leprosy (*see also* category M01) A30.9
  leukemia NEC C95.9 ☑ *[M36.1]*
  lipoid dermatoarthritis E78.81
  Lyme disease A69.23
  Mediterranean fever, familial (*see also* subcategory M14.8 ☑) M04.1
  Meningococcus A39.83
  metabolic disorder NEC (*see also* subcategory M14.8 ☑) E88.9
  multiple myelomatosis C90.0 ☑ *[M36.1]*
  mumps B26.85
  mycosis NEC (*see also* category M01) B49
  myelomatosis (multiple) C90.0 ☑ *[M36.1]*
  neurological disorder NEC G98.0
  ochronosis (*see also* subcategory M14.8 ☑) E70.29
  O'nyong-nyong (*see also* category M01) A92.1
  parasitic disease NEC (*see also* category M01) B89
  paratyphoid fever (*see also* category M01) A01.4
  Pseudomonas — *see* Arthritis, pyogenic, bacterial NEC
  psoriasis L40.50
  pyogenic organism NEC — *see* Arthritis, pyogenic, bacterial NEC
  Reiter's disease — *see* Reiter's disease
  respiratory disorder NEC (*see also* subcategory M14.8 ☑) J98.9
  reticulosis, malignant (*see also* subcategory M14.8 ☑) C86.0
  rubella B06.82
  Salmonella (arizonae) (cholerae-suis) (enteritidis) (typhimurium) A02.23
  sarcoidosis D86.86
  specified bacteria NEC — *see* Arthritis, pyogenic, bacterial NEC
  sporotrichosis B42.82
  syringomyelia G95.0
  thalassemia NEC D56.9 *[M36.3]*
  tuberculosis — *see* Tuberculosis, arthritis
  typhoid fever A01.04
  urethritis, Reiter's — *see* Reiter's disease
  viral disease NEC (*see also* category M01) B34.9
  infectious or infective (*see also* Arthritis, pyogenic or pyemic)
    spine — *see* Spondylopathy, infective
  juvenile M08.90
    with systemic onset — *see* Still's disease
    ankle M08.97 ☑
    elbow M08.92 ☑

Arthritis — *continued*
  juvenile — *continued*
    foot joint M08.97 ☑
    hand joint M08.94 ☑
    hip M08.95 ☑
    knee M08.96 ☑
    multiple site M08.99
    pauciarticular M08.40
      ankle M08.47 ☑
      elbow M08.42 ☑
      foot joint M08.47 ☑
      hand joint M08.44 ☑
      hip M08.45 ☑
      knee M08.46 ☑
      shoulder M08.41 ☑
      vertebrae M08.48
      wrist M08.43 ☑
    psoriatic L40.54
    rheumatoid — *see* Arthritis, rheumatoid, juvenile
    shoulder M08.91 ☑
    vertebra M08.98
    specified type NEC M08.80
      ankle M08.87 ☑
      elbow M08.82 ☑
      foot joint M08.87 ☑
      hand joint M08.84 ☑
      hip M08.85 ☑
      knee M08.86 ☑
      multiple site M08.89
      shoulder M08.81 ☑
      specified joint NEC M08.88
      vertebrae M08.88
      wrist M08.83 ☑
    wrist M08.93 ☑
  meaning osteoarthritis — *see* Osteoarthritis
  meningococcal A39.83
  menopausal (any site) NEC — *see* Arthritis, specified form NEC
  mutilans (psoriatic) L40.52
  mycotic NEC (*see also* category M01) B49
  neuropathic (Charcot) — *see* Arthropathy, neuropathic
    diabetic — *see* Diabetes, arthropathy, neuropathic
    nonsyphilitic NEC G98.0
    syringomyelic G95.0
  ochronotic (*see also* subcategory M14.8 ☑) E70.29
  palindromic (any site) — *see* Rheumatism, palindromic
  pneumococcal M00.10
    ankle M00.17 ☑
    elbow M00.12 ☑
    foot joint — *see* Arthritis, pneumococcal, ankle
    hand joint M00.14 ☑
    hip M00.15 ☑
    knee M00.16 ☑
    multiple site M00.19
    shoulder M00.11 ☑
    vertebra M00.18
    wrist M00.13 ☑
  postdysenteric — *see* Arthropathy, postdysenteric
  postmeningococcal A39.84
  postrheumatic, chronic — *see* Arthropathy, postrheumatic, chronic
  primary progressive (*see also* Arthritis, specified form NEC)
    spine — *see* Spondylitis, ankylosing
  psoriatic L40.50
  purulent (any site except spine) — *see* Arthritis, pyogenic or pyemic
    spine — *see* Spondylopathy, infective
  pyogenic or pyemic (any site except spine) M00.9
    bacterial NEC M00.80
      ankle M00.87 ☑
      elbow M00.82 ☑
      foot joint — *see* Arthritis, pyogenic, bacterial NEC, ankle
      hand joint M00.84 ☑
      hip M00.85 ☑
      knee M00.86 ☑
      multiple site M00.89
      shoulder M00.81 ☑
      vertebra M00.88
      wrist M00.83 ☑
    pneumococcal — *see* Arthritis, pneumococcal
    spine — *see* Spondylopathy, infective
    staphylococcal — *see* Arthritis, staphylococcal
    streptococcal — *see* Arthritis, streptococcal NEC
      pneumococcal — *see* Arthritis, pneumococcal
  reactive — *see* Reiter's disease

Arthritis — *continued*
  rheumatic (*see also* Arthritis, rheumatoid)
    acute or subacute — *see* Fever, rheumatic
  rheumatoid M06.9
    with
      carditis — *see* Rheumatoid, carditis
      endocarditis — *see* Rheumatoid, carditis
      heart involvement NEC — *see* Rheumatoid, carditis
      lung involvement — *see* Rheumatoid, lung
      myocarditis — *see* Rheumatoid, carditis
      myopathy — *see* Rheumatoid, myopathy
      pericarditis — *see* Rheumatoid, carditis
      polyneuropathy — *see* Rheumatoid, polyneuropathy
      rheumatoid factor — *see* Arthritis, rheumatoid, seropositive
      splenoadenomegaly and leukopenia — *see* Felty's syndrome
      vasculitis — *see* Rheumatoid, vasculitis
      visceral involvement NEC — *see* Rheumatoid, arthritis, with involvement of organs NEC
    juvenile (with or without rheumatoid factor) M08.00
      ankle M08.07 ☑
      elbow M08.02 ☑
      foot joint M08.07 ☑
      hand joint M08.04 ☑
      hip M08.05 ☑
      knee M08.06 ☑
      multiple site M08.09
      shoulder M08.01 ☑
      vertebra M08.08
      wrist M08.03 ☑
    seronegative M06.00
      ankle M06.07 ☑
      elbow M06.02 ☑
      foot joint M06.07 ☑
      hand joint M06.04 ☑
      hip M06.05 ☑
      knee M06.06 ☑
      multiple site M06.09
      shoulder M06.01 ☑
      vertebra M06.08
      wrist M06.03 ☑
    seropositive M05.9
      specified NEC M05.80
        ankle M05.87 ☑
        elbow M05.82 ☑
        foot joint M05.87 ☑
        hand joint M05.84 ☑
        hip M05.85 ☑
        knee M05.86 ☑
        multiple sites M05.89
        shoulder M05.81 ☑
        vertebra — *see* Spondylitis, ankylosing
        wrist M05.83 ☑
      without organ involvement M05.70
        ankle M05.77 ☑
        elbow M05.72 ☑
        foot joint M05.77 ☑
        hand joint M05.74 ☑
        hip M05.75 ☑
        knee M05.76 ☑
        multiple sites M05.79
        shoulder M05.71 ☑
        vertebra — *see* Spondylitis, ankylosing
        wrist M05.73 ☑
    specified type NEC M06.80
      ankle M06.87 ☑
      elbow M06.82 ☑
      foot joint M06.87 ☑
      hand joint M06.84 ☑
      hip M06.85 ☑
      knee M06.86 ☑
      multiple site M06.89
      shoulder M06.81 ☑
      vertebra M06.88
      wrist M06.83 ☑
    spine — *see* Spondylitis, ankylosing
  rubella B06.82
  scorbutic (*see also* subcategory M14.8 ☑) E54
  senile or senescent — *see* Osteoarthritis
  septic (any site except spine) — *see* Arthritis, pyogenic or pyemic
    spine — *see* Spondylopathy, infective
  serum (nontherapeutic) (therapeutic) — *see* Arthropathy, postimmunization
  specified form NEC M13.80
    ankle M13.87 ☑
    elbow M13.82 ☑
    foot joint M13.87 ☑

Arthritis — *continued*
specified form NEC — *continued*
hand joint M13.84 ☑
hip M13.85 ☑
knee M13.86 ☑
multiple site M13.89
shoulder M13.81 ☑
specified joint NEC M13.88
wrist M13.83 ☑
spine (*see also* Spondylopathy, inflammatory)
infectious or infective NEC — *see*
Spondylopathy, infective
Marie-Strümpell — *see* Spondylitis, ankylosing
pyogenic — *see* Spondylopathy, infective
rheumatoid — *see* Spondylitis, ankylosing
traumatic (old) — *see* Spondylopathy, traumatic
tuberculous A18.01
staphylococcal M00.00
ankle M00.07 ☑
elbow M00.02 ☑
foot joint — *see* Arthritis, staphylococcal, ankle
hand joint M00.04 ☑
hip M00.05 ☑
knee M00.06 ☑
multiple site M00.09
shoulder M00.01 ☑
vertebra M00.08
wrist M00.03 ☑
streptococcal NEC M00.20
ankle M00.27 ☑
elbow M00.22 ☑
foot joint — *see* Arthritis, streptococcal, ankle
hand joint M00.24 ☑
hip M00.25 ☑
knee M00.26 ☑
multiple site M00.29
shoulder M00.21 ☑
vertebra M00.28
wrist M00.23 ☑
suppurative — *see* Arthritis, pyogenic or pyemic
syphilitic (late) A52.16
congenital A50.55 [M12.80]
syphilitica deformans (Charcot) A52.16
temporomandibular M26.69
toxic of menopause (any site) — *see* Arthritis, specified form NEC
transient — *see* Arthropathy, specified form NEC
traumatic (chronic) — *see* Arthropathy, traumatic
tuberculous A18.02
spine A18.01
uratic — *see* Gout
urethritica (Reiter's) — *see* Reiter's disease
vertebral — *see* Spondylopathy, inflammatory
villous (any site) — *see* Arthropathy, specified form NEC
Arthrocele — *see* Effusion, joint
Arthrodesis status Z98.1
Arthrodynia (*see also* Pain, joint)
Arthrodysplasia Q74.9
Arthrofibrosis, joint — *see* Ankylosis
Arthrogryposis (congenital) Q68.8
multiplex congenita Q74.3
Arthrokatadysis M24.7
Arthropathy (*see also* Arthritis) M12.9
Charcot's — *see* Arthropathy, neuropathic
diabetic — *see* Diabetes, arthropathy, neuropathic
syringomyelic G95.0
cricoarytenoid J38.7
crystal (-induced) — *see* Arthritis, in, crystals
diabetic NEC — *see* Diabetes, arthropathy
distal interphalangeal, psoriatic L40.51
enteropathic M07.60
ankle M07.67 ☑
elbow M07.62 ☑
foot joint M07.67 ☑
hand joint M07.64 ☑
hip M07.65 ☑
knee M07.66 ☑
multiple site M07.69
shoulder M07.61 ☑
vertebra M07.68
wrist M07.63 ☑
following intestinal bypass M02.00
ankle M02.07 ☑
elbow M02.02 ☑
foot joint M02.07 ☑
hand joint M02.04 ☑
hip M02.05 ☑
knee M02.06 ☑
multiple site M02.09
shoulder M02.01 ☑

Arthropathy — *continued*
following intestinal bypass — *continued*
vertebra M02.08
wrist M02.03 ☑
gouty (*see also* Gout)
in (due to)
Lesch-Nyhan syndrome E79.1 [M14.8 ☑]
sickle-cell disorders D57 [M14.8 ☑]
hemophilic NEC D66 [M36.2]
in (due to)
hyperparathyroidism NEC E21.3 [M14.8 ☑]
metabolic disease NOS E88.9 [M14.8 ☑]
in (due to)
acromegaly E22.0 [M14.8 ☑]
amyloidosis E85.4 [M14.8 ☑]
blood disorder NOS D75.9 [M36.3]
diabetes — *see* Diabetes, arthropathy
endocrine disease NOS E34.9 [M14.8 ☑]
erythema
multiforme L51.9 [M14.8 ☑]
nodosum L52 [M14.8 ☑]
hemochromatosis E83.118 [M14.8 ☑]
hemoglobinopathy NEC D58.2 [M36.3]
hemophilia NEC D66 [M36.2]
Henoch-Schönlein purpura D69.0 [M36.4]
hyperthyroidism E05.90 [M14.8 ☑]
hypothyroidism E03.9 [M14.8 ☑]
infective endocarditis I33.0 [M12.80]
leukemia NEC C95.9 ☑ [M36.1]
malignant histiocytosis C96.A [M36.1]
metabolic disease NOS E88.9 [M14.8 ☑]
multiple myeloma C90.0 ☑ [M36.1]
neoplastic disease NOS (*see also*
Neoplasm) D49.9 [M36.1]
nutritional deficiency (*see also* subcategory
M14.8 ☑) E63.9
psoriasis NOS L40.50
sarcoidosis D86.86
syphilis (late) A52.77
congenital A50.55 [M12.80]
thyrotoxicosis (*see also* subcategory M14.8 ☑)
E05.90
ulcerative colitis K51.90 [M07.60]
viral hepatitis (postinfective) NEC B19.9
[M12.80]
Whipple's disease (*see also* subcategory M14.8 ☑)
K90.81
Jaccoud — *see* Arthropathy, postrheumatic, chronic
juvenile — *see* Arthritis, juvenile
psoriatic L40.54
mutilans (psoriatic) L40.52
neuropathic (Charcot) M14.60
ankle M14.67 ☑
diabetic — *see* Diabetes, arthropathy, neuropathic
elbow M14.62 ☑
foot joint M14.67 ☑
hand joint M14.64 ☑
hip M14.65 ☑
knee M14.66 ☑
multiple site M14.69
nonsyphilitic NEC G98.0
shoulder M14.61 ☑
syringomyelic G95.0
vertebra M14.68
wrist M14.63 ☑
osteopulmonary — *see* Osteoarthropathy, hypertrophic, specified NEC
postdysenteric M02.10
ankle M02.17 ☑
elbow M02.12 ☑
foot joint M02.17 ☑
hand joint M02.14 ☑
hip M02.15 ☑
knee M02.16 ☑
multiple site M02.19
shoulder M02.11 ☑
vertebra M02.18
wrist M02.13 ☑
postimmunization M02.20
ankle M02.27 ☑
elbow M02.22 ☑
foot joint M02.27 ☑
hand joint M02.24 ☑
hip M02.25 ☑
knee M02.26 ☑
multiple site M02.29
shoulder M02.21 ☑
vertebra M02.28
wrist M02.23 ☑

Arthropathy — *continued*
postinfectious NEC B99 ☑ [M12.80]
in (due to)
enteritis due to Yersinia enterocolitica A04.6
[M12.80]
syphilis A52.77
viral hepatitis NEC B19.9 [M12.80]
postrheumatic, chronic (Jaccoud) M12.00
ankle M12.07 ☑
elbow M12.02 ☑
foot joint M12.07 ☑
hand joint M12.04 ☑
hip M12.05 ☑
knee M12.06 ☑
multiple site M12.09
shoulder M12.01 ☑
specified joint NEC M12.08
vertebrae M12.08
wrist M12.03 ☑
psoriatic NEC L40.59
interphalangeal, distal L40.51
reactive M02.9
in (due to)
infective endocarditis I33.0 [M02.9]
specified type NEC M02.80
ankle M02.87 ☑
elbow M02.82 ☑
foot joint M02.87 ☑
hand joint M02.84 ☑
hip M02.85 ☑
knee M02.86 ☑
multiple site M02.89
shoulder M02.81 ☑
vertebra M02.88
wrist M02.83 ☑
specified form NEC M12.80
ankle M12.87 ☑
elbow M12.82 ☑
foot joint M12.87 ☑
hand joint M12.84 ☑
hip M12.85 ☑
knee M12.86 ☑
multiple site M12.89
shoulder M12.81 ☑
specified joint NEC M12.88
vertebrae M12.88
wrist M12.83 ☑
syringomyelic G95.0
tabes dorsalis A52.16
tabetic A52.16
transient — *see* Arthropathy, specified form NEC
traumatic M12.50
ankle M12.57 ☑
elbow M12.52 ☑
foot joint M12.57 ☑
hand joint M12.54 ☑
hip M12.55 ☑
knee M12.56 ☑
multiple site M12.59
shoulder M12.51 ☑
specified joint NEC M12.58
vertebrae M12.58
wrist M12.53 ☑
Arthropyosis — *see* Arthritis, pyogenic or pyemic
Arthrosis (deformans) (degenerative) (localized) (*see
also* Osteoarthritis) M19.90
spine — *see* Spondylosis
Arthus' phenomenon or reaction T78.41 ☑
due to
drug — *see* Table of Drugs and Chemicals, by
drug
Articular — *see* condition
Articulation, reverse (teeth) M26.24
Artificial
insemination complication — *see* Complications,
artificial, fertilization
opening status (functioning) (without
complication) Z93.9
anus (colostomy) Z93.3
colostomy Z93.3
cystostomy Z93.50
appendico-vesicostomy Z93.52
cutaneous Z93.51
specified NEC Z93.59
enterostomy Z93.4
gastrostomy Z93.1
ileostomy Z93.2
intestinal tract NEC Z93.4
jejunostomy Z93.4
nephrostomy Z93.6
specified site NEC Z93.8
tracheostomy Z93.0

Artificial — *continued*
  opening status — *continued*
    ureterostomy Z93.6
    urethrostomy Z93.6
    urinary tract NEC Z93.6
    vagina Z93.8
    vagina status Z93.8
Arytenoid — *see* condition
Asbestosis (occupational) J61
ASC-H (atypical squamous cells cannot exclude high grade squamous intraepithelial lesion on cytologic smear)
    anus R85.611
    cervix R87.611
    vagina R87.621
ASC-US (atypical squamous cells of undetermined significance on cytologic smear)
    anus R85.610
    cervix R87.610
    vagina R87.620
Ascariasis B77.9
  with
    complications NEC B77.89
    intestinal complications B77.0
    pneumonia, pneumonitis B77.81
Ascaridosis, ascaridiasis — *see* Ascariasis
Ascaris (infection) (infestation) (lumbricoides) — *see* Ascariasis
Ascending — *see* condition
Aschoff's bodies — *see* Myocarditis, rheumatic
Ascites (abdominal) R18.8
    cardiac (*see also* Failure, heart, right) I50.810
    chylous (nonfilarial) I89.8
      filarial — *see* Infestation, filarial
    due to
      cirrhosis, alcoholic K70.31
      hepatitis
        alcoholic K70.11
        chronic active K71.51
      S. japonicum B65.2
    heart (*see also* Failure, heart, right) I50.810
    malignant R18.0
    pseudochylous R18.8
    syphilitic A52.74
    tuberculous A18.31
Aseptic — *see* condition
Asherman's syndrome N85.6
Asialia K11.7
Asiatic cholera — *see* Cholera
Asimultagnosia (simultanagnosia) R48.3
Askin's tumor — *see* Neoplasm, connective tissue, malignant
Asocial personality F60.2
Asomatognosia R41.4
Aspartylglucosaminuria E77.1
Asperger's disease or syndrome F84.5
Aspergilloma — *see* Aspergillosis
Aspergillosis (with pneumonia) B44.9
    bronchopulmonary, allergic B44.81
    disseminated B44.7
    generalized B44.7
    pulmonary NEC B44.1
      allergic B44.81
      invasive B44.0
    specified NEC B44.89
    tonsillar B44.2
Aspergillus (flavus) (fumigatus) (infection) (terreus) — *see* Aspergillosis
Aspermatogenesis — *see* Azoospermia
Aspermia (testis) — *see* Azoospermia
Asphyxia, asphyxiation (by) R09.01
    antenatal P84
    birth P84
    bunny bag — *see* Asphyxia, due to, mechanical threat to breathing, trapped in bed clothes
    crushing S28.0 ☑
    drowning T75.1 ☑
    gas, fumes, or vapor — *see* Table of Drugs and Chemicals
    inhalation — *see* Inhalation
    intrauterine P84
    local I73.00
      with gangrene I73.01
    mucus (*see also* Foreign body, respiratory tract, causing asphyxia)
    newborn P84
    pathological R09.01
    postnatal P84
      mechanical — *see* Asphyxia, due to, mechanical threat to breathing
    prenatal P84
    reticularis R23.1

Asphyxia — *continued*
    strangulation — *see* Asphyxia, due to, mechanical threat to breathing
    submersion T75.1 ☑
    traumatic T71.9 ☑
      due to
        crushed chest S28.0 ☑
        foreign body (in) — *see* Foreign body, respiratory tract, causing asphyxia
        low oxygen content of ambient air T71.20 ☑
          due to
            being trapped in
              low oxygen environment T71.29 ☑
                in car trunk T71.221 ☑
                  circumstances
                    undetermined T71.224 ☑
                  done with intent to harm by
                    another person T71.223 ☑
                    self T71.222 ☑
                in refrigerator T71.231 ☑
                  circumstances
                    undetermined T71.234 ☑
                  done with intent to harm by
                    another person T71.233 ☑
                    self T71.232 ☑
            cave-in T71.21 ☑
      mechanical threat to breathing (accidental) T71.191 ☑
        circumstances undetermined T71.194 ☑
        done with intent to harm by
          another person T71.193 ☑
          self T71.192 ☑
        hanging T71.161 ☑
          circumstances undetermined T71.164 ☑
          done with intent to harm by
            another person T71.163 ☑
            self T71.162 ☑
        plastic bag T71.121 ☑
          circumstances undetermined T71.124 ☑
          done with intent to harm by
            another person T71.123 ☑
            self T71.122 ☑
        smothering
          in furniture T71.151 ☑
            circumstances
              undetermined T71.154 ☑
            done with intent to harm by
              another person T71.153 ☑
              self T71.152 ☑
          under
            another person's body T71.141 ☑
              circumstances
                undetermined T71.144 ☑
              done with intent to harm T71.143 ☑
            pillow T71.111 ☑
              circumstances
                undetermined T71.114 ☑
              done with intent to harm by
                another person T71.113 ☑
                self T71.112 ☑
        trapped in bed clothes T71.131 ☑
          circumstances undetermined T71.134 ☑
          done with intent to harm by
            another person T71.133 ☑
            self T71.132 ☑
    vomiting, vomitus — *see* Foreign body, respiratory tract, causing asphyxia
Aspiration
    amniotic (clear) fluid (newborn) P24.10
      with
        pneumonia (pneumonitis) P24.11
        respiratory symptoms P24.11
    blood
      newborn (without respiratory symptoms) P24.20
        with
          pneumonia (pneumonitis) P24.21
          respiratory symptoms P24.21
      specified age NEC — *see* Foreign body, respiratory tract
    bronchitis J69.0
    food or foreign body (with asphyxiation) — *see* Asphyxia, food
    liquor (amnii) (newborn) P24.10
      with
        pneumonia (pneumonitis) P24.11
        respiratory symptoms P24.11
    meconium (newborn) (without respiratory symptoms) P24.00
      with
        pneumonitis (pneumonitis) P24.01
        respiratory symptoms P24.01

Aspiration — *continued*
    milk (newborn) (without respiratory symptoms) P24.30
      with
        pneumonia (pneumonitis) P24.31
        respiratory symptoms P24.31
      specified age NEC — *see* Foreign body, respiratory tract
    mucus (*see also* Foreign body, by site, causing asphyxia)
      newborn P24.10
        with
          pneumonia (pneumonitis) P24.11
          respiratory symptoms P24.11
    neonatal P24.9
      specific NEC (without respiratory symptoms) P24.80
        with
          pneumonia (pneumonitis) P24.81
          respiratory symptoms P24.81
    newborn P24.9
      specific NEC (without respiratory symptoms) P24.80
        with
          pneumonia (pneumonitis) P24.81
          respiratory symptoms P24.81
    pneumonia J69.0
    pneumonitis J69.0
    syndrome of newborn — *see* Aspiration, by substance, with pneumonia
    vernix caseosa (newborn) P24.80
      with
        pneumonia (pneumonitis) P24.81
        respiratory symptoms P24.81
    vomitus (*see also* Foreign body, respiratory tract)
      newborn (without respiratory symptoms) P24.30
        with
          pneumonia (pneumonitis) P24.31
          respiratory symptoms P24.31
Asplenia (congenital) Q89.01
    postsurgical Z90.81
Assam fever B55.0
Assault, sexual — *see* Maltreatment
Assmann's focus NEC A15.0
Astasia (-abasia) (hysterical) F44.4
Asteatosis cutis L85.3
Astereognosia, astereognosis R48.1
Asterixis R27.8
    in liver disease K71.3
Asteroid hyalitis — *see* Deposit, crystalline
Asthenia, asthenic R53.1
    cardiac (*see also* Failure, heart) I50.9
      psychogenic F45.8
    cardiovascular (*see also* Failure, heart) I50.9
      psychogenic F45.8
    heart (*see also* Failure, heart) I50.9
      psychogenic F45.8
    hysterical F44.4
    myocardial (*see also* Failure, heart) I50.9
      psychogenic F45.8
    nervous F48.8
    neurocirculatory F45.8
    neurotic F48.8
    psychogenic F48.8
    psychoneurotic F48.8
    psychophysiologic F48.8
    reaction (psychophysiologic) F48.8
    senile R54
Asthenopia (*see also* Discomfort, visual)
    hysterical F44.6
    psychogenic F44.6
Asthenospermia — *see* Abnormal, specimen, male genital organs
Asthma, asthmatic (bronchial) (catarrh) (spasmodic) J45.909
    with
      chronic obstructive bronchitis J44.9
        with
          acute lower respiratory infection J44.0
          exacerbation (acute) J44.1
      chronic obstructive pulmonary disease J44.9
        with
          acute lower respiratory infection J44.0
          exacerbation (acute) J44.1
      exacerbation (acute) J45.901
    hay fever — *see* Asthma, allergic extrinsic
    rhinitis, allergic — *see* Asthma, allergic extrinsic
    status asthmaticus J45.902
    allergic extrinsic J45.909
      with
        exacerbation (acute) J45.901
        status asthmaticus J45.902

☑ **Additional character required**

Asthma — *continued*
  atopic — *see* Asthma, allergic extrinsic
  cardiac — *see* Failure, ventricular, left
  cardiobronchial I50.1
  childhood J45.909
    with
      exacerbation (acute) J45.901
      status asthmaticus J45.902
  chronic obstructive J44.9
    with
      acute lower respiratory infection J44.0
      exacerbation (acute) J44.1
  collier's J60
  cough variant J45.991
  detergent J69.8
  due to
    detergent J69.8
    inhalation of fumes J68.3
  eosinophilic J82
  extrinsic, allergic — *see* Asthma, allergic extrinsic
  grinder's J62.8
  hay — *see* Asthma, allergic extrinsic
  heart I50.1
  idiosyncratic — *see* Asthma, nonallergic
  intermittent (mild) J45.20
    with
      exacerbation (acute) J45.21
      status asthmaticus J45.22
  intrinsic, nonallergic — *see* Asthma, nonallergic
  Kopp's E32.8
  late-onset J45.909
    with
      exacerbation (acute) J45.901
      status asthmaticus J45.902
  mild intermittent J45.20
    with
      exacerbation (acute) J45.21
      status asthmaticus J45.22
  mild persistent J45.30
    with
      exacerbation (acute) J45.31
      status asthmaticus J45.32
  Millar's (laryngismus stridulus) J38.5
  miner's J60
  mixed J45.909
    with
      exacerbation (acute) J45.901
      status asthmaticus J45.902
  moderate persistent J45.40
    with
      exacerbation (acute) J45.41
      status asthmaticus J45.42
  nervous — *see* Asthma, nonallergic
  nonallergic (intrinsic) J45.909
    with
      exacerbation (acute) J45.901
      status asthmaticus J45.902
  persistent
    mild J45.30
      with
        exacerbation (acute) J45.31
        status asthmaticus J45.32
    moderate J45.40
      with
        exacerbation (acute) J45.41
        status asthmaticus J45.42
    severe J45.50
      with
        exacerbation (acute) J45.51
        status asthmaticus J45.52
  platinum J45.998
  pneumoconiotic NEC J64
  potter's J62.8
  predominantly allergic J45.909
  psychogenic F54
  pulmonary eosinophilic J82
  red cedar J67.8
  Rostan's I50.1
  sandblaster's J62.8
  sequoiosis J67.8
  severe persistent J45.50
    with
      exacerbation (acute) J45.51
      status asthmaticus J45.52
  specified NEC J45.998
  stonemason's J62.8
  thymic E32.8
  tuberculous — *see* Tuberculosis, pulmonary
  Wichmann's (laryngismus stridulus) J38.5
  wood J67.8
Astigmatism (compound) (congenital) H52.20 ☑
  irregular H52.21 ☑
  regular H52.22 ☑

Astraphobia F40.220
Astroblastoma
  specified site — *see* Neoplasm, malignant, by site
  unspecified site C71.9
Astrocytoma (cystic)
  anaplastic
    specified site — *see* Neoplasm, malignant, by
      site
    unspecified site C71.9
  fibrillary
    specified site — *see* Neoplasm, malignant, by
      site
    unspecified site C71.9
  fibrous
    specified site — *see* Neoplasm, malignant, by
      site
    unspecified site C71.9
  gemistocytic
    specified site — *see* Neoplasm, malignant, by
      site
    unspecified site C71.9
  juvenile
    specified site — *see* Neoplasm, malignant, by
      site
    unspecified site C71.9
  pilocytic
    specified site — *see* Neoplasm, malignant, by
      site
    unspecified site C71.9
  piloid
    specified site — *see* Neoplasm, malignant, by
      site
    unspecified site C71.9
  protoplasmic
    specified site — *see* Neoplasm, malignant, by
      site
    unspecified site C71.9
  specified site NEC — *see* Neoplasm, malignant,
    by site
  subependymal D43.2
    giant cell
      specified site — *see* Neoplasm, uncertain
        behavior, by site
      unspecified site D43.2
    specified site — *see* Neoplasm, uncertain
      behavior, by site
    unspecified site D43.2
  unspecified site C71.9
Astroglioma
  specified site — *see* Neoplasm, malignant, by site
  unspecified site C71.9
Asymbolia R48.8
Asymmetry (*see also* Distortion)
  between native and reconstructed breast N65.1
  face Q67.0
  jaw (lower) — *see* Anomaly, dentofacial, jaw-
    cranial base relationship, asymmetry
Asynergia, asynergy R27.8
  ventricular I51.89
Asystole (heart) — *see* Arrest, cardiac
At risk
  for
    dental caries Z91.849
      high Z91.843
      low Z91.841
      moderate Z91.842
    falling Z91.81
Ataxia, ataxy, ataxic R27.0
  acute R27.8
  brain (hereditary) G11.9
  cerebellar (hereditary) G11.9
    with defective DNA repair G11.3
    alcoholic G31.2
    early-onset G11.1
    in
      alcoholism G31.2
      myxedema E03.9 *[G13.2]*
      neoplastic disease (*see also* Neoplasm) D49.9
        [G32.81]
      specified disease NEC G32.81
    late-onset (Marie's) G11.2
  cerebral (hereditary) G11.9
  congenital nonprogressive G11.0
  family, familial — *see* Ataxia, hereditary
  following
    cerebrovascular disease I69.993
      cerebral infarction I69.393
      intracerebral hemorrhage I69.193
      nontraumatic intracranial hemorrhage
        NEC I69.293
      specified disease NEC I69.893
      subarachnoid hemorrhage I69.093

Ataxia — *continued*
  Friedreich's (heredofamilial) (cerebellar)
    (spinal) G11.1
  gait R26.0
    hysterical F44.4
  general R27.8
  gluten M35.9 *[G32.81]*
    with celiac disease K90.0 *[G32.81]*
  hereditary G11.9
    with neuropathy G60.2
    cerebellar — *see* Ataxia, cerebellar
    spastic G11.4
    specified NEC G11.8
    spinal (Friedreich's) G11.1
  heredofamilial — *see* Ataxia, hereditary
  Hunt's G11.1
  hysterical F44.4
  locomotor (progressive) (syphilitic) (partial)
    (spastic) A52.11
    diabetic — *see* Diabetes, ataxia
  Marie's (cerebellar) (heredofamilial) (late-
    onset) G11.2
  nonorganic origin F44.4
  nonprogressive, congenital G11.0
  psychogenic F44.4
  Roussy-Lévy G60.0
  Sanger-Brown's (hereditary) G11.2
  spastic hereditary G11.4
  spinal
    hereditary (Friedreich's) G11.1
    progressive (syphilitic) A52.11
  spinocerebellar, X-linked recessive G11.1
  telangiectasia (Louis-Bar) G11.3
Ataxia-telangiectasia (Louis-Bar) G11.3
Atelectasis (massive) (partial) (pressure) (pulmonary)
  J98.11
  newborn P28.10
    due to resorption P28.11
    partial P28.19
    primary P28.0
    secondary P28.19
  primary (newborn) P28.0
  tuberculous — *see* Tuberculosis, pulmonary
Atelocardia Q24.9
Atelomyelia Q06.1
Atheroembolism
  of
    extremities
      lower I75.02 ☑
      upper I75.01 ☑
    kidney I75.81
    specified NEC I75.89
Atheroma, atheromatous (*see also* Arteriosclerosis)
  I70.90
  aorta, aortic I70.0
    valve (*see also* Endocarditis, aortic) I35.8
  aorto-iliac I70.0
  artery — *see* Arteriosclerosis
  basilar (artery) I67.2
  carotid (artery) (common) (internal) I67.2
  cerebral (arteries) I67.2
  coronary (artery) I25.10
    with angina pectoris — *see* Arteriosclerosis,
      coronary (artery),
    degeneration — *see* Arteriosclerosis
  heart, cardiac — *see* Disease, heart, ischemic,
    atherosclerotic
  mitral (valve) I34.8
  myocardium, myocardial — *see* Disease, heart,
    ischemic, atherosclerotic
  pulmonary valve (heart) (*see also* Endocarditis,
    pulmonary) I37.8
  tricuspid (heart) (valve) I36.8
  valve, valvular — *see* Endocarditis
  vertebral (artery) I67.2
Atheromatosis — *see* Arteriosclerosis
Atherosclerosis (*see also* Arteriosclerosis)
  coronary
    artery I25.10
      with angina pectoris — *see* Arteriosclerosis,
        coronary (artery),
      due to
        calcified coronary lesion (severely) I25.84
        lipid rich plaque I25.83
    transplanted heart I25.811
      bypass graft I25.812
        with angina pectoris — *see* Arteriosclerosis,
          coronary (artery),
      native coronary artery I25.811
        with angina pectoris — *see* Arteriosclerosis,
          coronary (artery),

Athetosis - Atrophy

Athetosis (acquired) R25.8
  bilateral (congenital) G80.3
  congenital (bilateral) (double) G80.3
  double (congenital) G80.3
  unilateral R25.8
Athlete's
  foot B35.3
  heart I51.7
Athrepsia E41
Athyrea (acquired) (*see also* Hypothyroidism)
  congenital E03.1
Atonia, atony, atonic
  bladder (sphincter) (neurogenic) N31.2
  capillary I78.8
  cecum K59.8
    psychogenic F45.8
  colon — *see* Atony, intestine
  congenital P94.2
  esophagus K22.8
  intestine K59.8
    psychogenic F45.8
  stomach K31.89
    neurotic or psychogenic F45.8
  uterus (during labor) O62.2
    with hemorrhage (postpartum) O72.1
    postpartum (with hemorrhage) O72.1
      without hemorrhage O75.89
Atopy — *see* History, allergy
Atransferrinemia, congenital E88.09
Atresia, atretic
  alimentary organ or tract NEC Q45.8
    upper Q40.8
  ani, anus, anal (canal) Q42.3
    with fistula Q42.2
  aorta (ring) Q25.29
  aortic (orifice) (valve) Q23.0
    arch Q25.21
    congenital with hypoplasia of ascending aorta
      and defective development of left ventricle
      (with mitral stenosis) Q23.4
    in hypoplastic left heart syndrome Q23.4
  aqueduct of Sylvius Q03.0
    with spina bifida — *see* Spina bifida, with
      hydrocephalus
  artery NEC Q27.8
    cerebral Q28.3
    coronary Q24.5
    digestive system Q27.8
    eye Q15.8
    lower limb Q27.8
    pulmonary Q25.5
    specified site NEC Q27.8
    umbilical Q27.0
    upper limb Q27.8
  auditory canal (external) Q16.1
  bile duct (common) (congenital) (hepatic) Q44.2
    acquired — *see* Obstruction, bile duct
  bladder (neck) Q64.39
    obstruction Q64.31
  bronchus Q32.4
  cecum Q42.8
  cervix (acquired) N88.2
    congenital Q51.828
    in pregnancy or childbirth — *see* Anomaly,
      cervix, in pregnancy or childbirth
    causing obstructed labor O65.5
  choana Q30.0
  colon Q42.9
    specified NEC Q42.8
  common duct Q44.2
  cricoid cartilage Q31.8
  cystic duct Q44.2
    acquired K82.8
      with obstruction K82.0
  digestive organs NEC Q45.8
  duodenum Q41.0
  ear canal Q16.1
  ejaculatory duct Q55.4
  epiglottis Q31.8
  esophagus Q39.0
    with tracheoesophageal fistula Q39.1
  eustachian tube Q17.8
  fallopian tube (congenital) Q50.6
    acquired N97.1
  follicular cyst N83.0 ☑
  foramen of
    Luschka Q03.1
      with spina bifida — *see* Spina bifida, with
        hydrocephalus
    Magendie Q03.1
      with spina bifida — *see* Spina bifida, with
        hydrocephalus

Atresia — *continued*
  gallbladder Q44.1
  genital organ
    external
      female Q52.79
      male Q55.8
    internal
      female Q52.8
      male Q55.8
  glottis Q31.8
  gullet Q39.0
    with tracheoesophageal fistula Q39.1
  heart valve NEC Q24.8
    pulmonary Q22.0
    tricuspid Q22.4
  hymen Q52.3
    acquired (postinfective) N89.6
  ileum Q41.2
  intestine (small) Q41.9
    large Q42.9
      specified NEC Q42.8
  iris, filtration angle Q15.0
  jejunum Q41.1
  lacrimal apparatus Q10.4
  larynx Q31.8
  meatus urinarius Q64.33
  mitral valve Q23.2
    in hypoplastic left heart syndrome Q23.4
  nares (anterior) (posterior) Q30.0
  nasopharynx Q34.8
  nose, nostril Q30.0
    acquired J34.89
  organ or site NEC Q89.8
  osseous meatus (ear) Q16.1
  oviduct (congenital) Q50.6
    acquired N97.1
  parotid duct Q38.4
    acquired K11.8
  pulmonary (artery) Q25.5
    valve Q22.0
  pulmonic Q22.0
  pupil Q13.2
  rectum Q42.1
    with fistula Q42.0
  salivary duct Q38.4
    acquired K11.8
  sublingual duct Q38.4
    acquired K11.8
  submandibular duct Q38.4
    acquired K11.8
  submaxillary duct Q38.4
    acquired K11.8
  thyroid cartilage Q31.8
  trachea Q32.1
  tricuspid valve Q22.4
  ureter Q62.10
    pelvic junction Q62.11
    vesical orifice Q62.12
  ureteropelvic junction Q62.11
  ureterovesical orifice Q62.12
  urethra (valvular) Q64.39
    stricture Q64.32
  urinary tract NEC Q64.8
  uterus Q51.818
    acquired N85.8
  vagina (congenital) Q52.4
    acquired (postinfectional) (senile) N89.5
  vas deferens Q55.5
  vascular NEC Q27.8
    cerebral Q28.3
    digestive system Q27.8
    lower limb Q27.8
    specified site NEC Q27.8
    upper limb Q27.8
  vein NEC Q27.8
    digestive system Q27.8
    great Q26.8
    lower limb Q27.8
    portal Q26.5
    pulmonary Q26.4
      partial Q26.3
      total Q26.2
    specified site NEC Q27.8
    upper limb Q27.8
  vena cava (inferior) (superior) Q26.8
  vesicourethral orifice Q64.31
  vulva Q52.79
    acquired N90.5
Atrichia, atrichosis — *see* Alopecia
Atrophia (*see also* Atrophy)
  cutis senilis L90.8
    due to radiation L57.8

Atrophia — *continued*
  gyrata of choroid and retina H31.23
  senilis R54
    dermatological L90.8
      due to radiation (nonionizing) (solar) L57.8
  unguium L60.3
    congenita Q84.6
Atrophie blanche (en plaque) (de Milian) L95.0
Atrophoderma, atrophodermia (of) L90.9
  diffusum (idiopathic) L90.4
  maculatum L90.8
    et striatum L90.8
      due to syphilis A52.79
    syphilitic A51.39
  neuriticum L90.8
  Pasini and Pierini L90.3
  pigmentosum Q82.1
  reticulatum symmetricum faciei L66.4
  senile L90.8
    due to radiation (nonionizing) (solar) L57.8
  vermiculata (cheeks) L66.4
Atrophy, atrophic (of)
  adrenal (capsule) (gland) E27.49
    primary (autoimmune) E27.1
  alveolar process or ridge (edentulous) K08.20
  anal sphincter (disuse) N81.84
  appendix K38.8
  arteriosclerotic — *see* Arteriosclerosis
  bile duct (common) (hepatic) K83.8
  bladder N32.89
    neurogenic N31.8
  blanche (en plaque) (of Milian) L95.0
  bone (senile) NEC (*see also* Disorder, bone,
      specified type NEC)
    due to
      tabes dorsalis (neurogenic) A52.11
  brain (cortex) (progressive) G31.9
    frontotemporal circumscribed G31.01 *[F02.80]*
      with behavioral disturbance G31.01 *[F02.81]*
    senile NEC G31.1
  breast N64.2
    obstetric — *see* Disorder, breast, specified type
      NEC
  buccal cavity K13.79
  cardiac — *see* Degeneration, myocardial
  cartilage (infectional) (joint) — *see* Disorder,
      cartilage, specified NEC
  cerebellar — *see* Atrophy, brain
  cerebral — *see* Atrophy, brain
  cervix (mucosa) (senile) (uteri) N88.8
    menopausal N95.8
  Charcot-Marie-Tooth G60.0
  choroid (central) (macular) (myopic)
      (retina) H31.10 ☑
    diffuse secondary H31.12 ☑
    gyrate H31.23
    senile H31.11 ☑
  ciliary body — *see* Atrophy, iris
  conjunctiva (senile) H11.89
  corpus cavernosum N48.89
  cortical — *see* Atrophy, brain
  cystic duct K82.8
  Déjérine-Thomas G23.8
  disuse NEC — *see* Atrophy, muscle
  Duchenne-Aran G12.21
  ear H93.8 ☑
  edentulous alveolar ridge K08.20
  endometrium (senile) N85.8
    cervix N88.8
  enteric K63.89
  epididymis N50.89
  eyeball — *see* Disorder, globe, degenerated
      condition, atrophy
  eyelid (senile) — *see* Disorder, eyelid,
      degenerative
  facial (skin) L90.9
  fallopian tube (senile) N83.32 ☑
    with ovary N83.33 ☑
  fascioscapulohumeral (Landouzy-
      Déjérine) G71.0
  fatty, thymus (gland) E32.8
  gallbladder K82.8
  gastric K29.40
    with bleeding K29.41
  gastrointestinal K63.89
  glandular I89.8
  globe H44.52 ☑
  gum — *see* Recession, gingival
  hair L67.8
  heart (brown) — *see* Degeneration, myocardial
  hemifacial Q67.4
    Romberg G51.8

☑ **Additional character required**

Atrophy — *continued*
  infantile E41
    paralysis, acute — *see* Poliomyelitis, paralytic
  intestine K63.89
  iris (essential) (progressive) H21.26 ☑
    specified NEC H21.29
  kidney (senile) (terminal) (*see also* Sclerosis, renal) N26.1
    congenital or infantile Q60.5
      bilateral Q60.4
      unilateral Q60.3
    hydronephrotic — *see* Hydronephrosis
  lacrimal gland (primary) H04.14 ☑
    secondary H04.15 ☑
  Landouzy-Déjérine G71.0
  laryngitis, infective J37.0
  larynx J38.7
  Leber's optic (hereditary) H47.22
  lip K13.0
  liver (yellow) K72.90
    with coma K72.91
    acute, subacute K72.00
      with coma K72.01
    chronic K72.10
      with coma K72.11
  lung (senile) J98.4
  macular (dermatological) L90.8
    syphilitic, skin A51.39
    striated A52.79
  mandible (edentulous) K08.20
    minimal K08.21
    moderate K08.22
    severe K08.23
  maxilla K08.20
    minimal K08.24
    moderate K08.25
    severe K08.26
  muscle, muscular (diffuse) (general) (idiopathic) (primary) M62.50
    ankle M62.57 ☑
    Duchenne-Aran G12.21
    foot M62.57 ☑
    forearm M62.53 ☑
    hand M62.54 ☑
    infantile spinal G12.0
    lower leg M62.56 ☑
    multiple sites M62.59
    myelopathic — *see* Atrophy, muscle, spinal
    myotonic G71.11
    neuritic G58.9
    neuropathic (peroneal) (progressive) G60.0
    pelvic (disuse) N81.84
    peroneal G60.0
    progressive (bulbar) G12.21
      adult G12.1
      infantile (spinal) G12.0
      spinal G12.25
        adult G12.1
        infantile G12.0
    pseudohypertrophic G71.0
    shoulder region M62.51 ☑
    specified site NEC M62.58
    spinal G12.9
      adult form G12.1
      Aran-Duchenne G12.21
      childhood form, type II G12.1
      distal G12.1
      hereditary NEC G12.1
      infantile, type I (Werdnig-Hoffmann) G12.0
      juvenile form, type III (Kugelberg-Welander) G12.1
      progressive G12.25
      scapuloperoneal form G12.1
      specified NEC G12.8
    syphilitic A52.78
    thigh M62.55 ☑
    upper arm M62.52 ☑
  myocardium — *see* Degeneration, myocardial
  myometrium (senile) N85.8
    cervix N88.8
  myopathic NEC — *see* Atrophy, muscle
  myotonia G71.11
  nail L60.3
  nasopharynx J31.1
  nerve (*see also* Disorder, nerve)
    abducens — *see* Strabismus, paralytic, sixth nerve
    accessory G52.8
    acoustic or auditory — *see* subcategory H93.3
    cranial G52.9
      eighth (auditory) — *see* subcategory H93.3
      eleventh (accessory) G52.8

Atrophy — *continued*
  nerve — *continued*
    fifth (trigeminal) G50.8
    first (olfactory) G52.0
    fourth (trochlear) — *see* Strabismus, paralytic, fourth nerve
    second (optic) H47.20
    sixth (abducens) — *see* Strabismus, paralytic, sixth nerve
    tenth (pneumogastric) (vagus) G52.2
    third (oculomotor) — *see* Strabismus, paralytic, third nerve
    twelfth (hypoglossal) G52.3
  hypoglossal G52.3
  oculomotor — *see* Strabismus, paralytic, third nerve
  olfactory G52.0
  optic (papillomacular bundle)
    syphilitic (late) A52.15
      congenital A50.44
  pneumogastric G52.2
  trigeminal G50.8
  trochlear — *see* Strabismus, paralytic, fourth nerve
  vagus (pneumogastric) G52.2
  neurogenic, bone, tabetic A52.11
  nutritional E41
  old age R54
  olivopontocerebellar G23.8
  optic (nerve) H47.20
    glaucomatous H47.23 ☑
    hereditary H47.22
    primary H47.21 ☑
    specified type NEC H47.29 ☑
    syphilitic (late) A52.15
      congenital A50.44
  orbit H05.31 ☑
  ovary (senile) N83.31 ☑
    with fallopian tube N83.33 ☑
  oviduct (senile) — *see* Atrophy, fallopian tube
  palsy, diffuse (progressive) G12.22
  pancreas (duct) (senile) K86.89
  parotid gland K11.0
  pelvic muscle N81.84
  penis N48.89
  pharynx J39.2
  pluriglandular E31.8
    autoimmune E31.0
  polyarthritis M15.9
  prostate N42.89
  pseudohypertrophic (muscle) G71.0
  renal (*see also* Sclerosis, renal) N26.1
  retina, retinal (postinfectional) H35.89
  rhinitis J31.0
  salivary gland K11.0
  scar L90.5
  sclerosis, lobar (of brain) G31.09 *[F02.80]*
    with behavioral disturbance G31.09 *[F02.81]*
  scrotum N50.89
  seminal vesicle N50.89
  senile R54
    due to radiation (nonionizing) (solar) L57.8
  skin (patches) (spots) L90.9
    degenerative (senile) L90.8
    due to radiation (nonionizing) (solar) L57.8
    senile L90.8
  spermatic cord N50.89
  spinal (acute) (cord) G95.89
    muscular — *see* Atrophy, muscle, spinal
    paralysis G12.20
      acute — *see* Poliomyelitis, paralytic
      meaning progressive muscular atrophy G12.21
  spine (column) — *see* Spondylopathy, specified NEC
  spleen (senile) D73.0
  stomach K29.40
    with bleeding K29.41
  striate (skin) L90.6
    syphilitic A52.79
  subcutaneous L90.9
  sublingual gland K11.0
  submandibular gland K11.0
  submaxillary gland K11.0
  Sudeck's — *see* Algoneurodystrophy
  suprarenal (capsule) (gland) E27.49
    primary E27.1
  systemic affecting central nervous system in
    myxedema E03.9 *[G13.2]*
    neoplastic disease (*see also* Neoplasm) D49.9 *[G13.1]*
    specified disease NEC G13.8

Atrophy — *continued*
  tarso-orbital fascia, congenital Q10.3
  testis N50.0
  thenar, partial — *see* Syndrome, carpal tunnel
  thymus (fatty) E32.8
  thyroid (gland) (acquired) E03.4
    with cretinism E03.1
    congenital (with myxedema) E03.1
  tongue (senile) K14.8
    papillae K14.4
  trachea J39.8
  tunica vaginalis N50.89
  turbinate J34.89
  tympanic membrane (nonflaccid) H73.82 ☑
    flaccid H73.81 ☑
  upper respiratory tract J39.8
  uterus, uterine (senile) N85.8
    cervix N88.8
    due to radiation (intended effect) N85.8
      adverse effect or misadventure N99.89
  vagina (senile) N95.2
  vas deferens N50.89
  vascular I99.8
  vertebra (senile) — *see* Spondylopathy, specified NEC
  vulva (senile) N90.5
  Werdnig-Hoffmann G12.0
  yellow — *see* Failure, hepatic
Attack, attacks
  with alteration of consciousness (with automatisms) — *see* Epilepsy, localization-related, symptomatic, with complexpartial seizures
  Adams-Stokes I45.9
  akinetic — *see* Epilepsy, generalized, specified NEC
  angina — *see* Angina
  atonic — *see* Epilepsy, generalized, specified NEC
  benign shuddering G25.83
  cataleptic — *see* Catalepsy
  coronary — *see* Infarct, myocardium
  cyanotic, newborn P28.2
  drop NEC R55
  epileptic — *see* Epilepsy
  heart — *see* infarct, myocardium
  hysterical F44.9
  jacksonian — *see* Epilepsy, localization-related, symptomatic, with simple partial seizures
  myocardium, myocardial — *see* Infarct, myocardium
  myoclonic — *see* Epilepsy, generalized, specified NEC
  panic F41.0
  psychomotor — *see* Epilepsy, localization-related, symptomatic, with complex partial seizures
  salaam — *see* Epilepsy, spasms
  schizophreniform, brief F23
  shuddering, benign G25.83
  Stokes-Adams I45.9
  syncope R55
  transient ischemic (TIA) G45.9
    specified NEC G45.8
  unconsciousness R55
    hysterical F44.89
  vasomotor R55
  vasovagal (paroxysmal) (idiopathic) R55
  without alteration of consciousness — *see* Epilepsy, localization-related, symptomatic, with simple partial seizures
Attention (to)
  artificial
    opening (of) Z43.9
      digestive tract NEC Z43.4
        colon Z43.3
        ilium Z43.2
        stomach Z43.1
      specified NEC Z43.8
      trachea Z43.0
      urinary tract NEC Z43.6
        cystostomy Z43.5
        nephrostomy Z43.6
        ureterostomy Z43.6
        urethrostomy Z43.6
      vagina Z43.7
  colostomy Z43.3
  cystostomy Z43.5
  deficit disorder or syndrome F98.8
    with hyperactivity — *see* Disorder, attention-deficit hyperactivity
  gastrostomy Z43.1
  ileostomy Z43.2
  jejunostomy Z43.4

Attention — *continued*
　nephrostomy Z43.6
　surgical dressings Z48.01
　sutures Z48.02
　tracheostomy Z43.0
　ureterostomy Z43.6
　urethrostomy Z43.6
Attrition
　gum — *see* Recession, gingival
　tooth, teeth (excessive) (hard tissues) K03.0
Atypical, atypism (*see also* condition)
　cells (on cytolgocial smear) (endocervical) (endometrial) (glandular)
　　cervix R87.619
　　vagina R87.629
　cervical N87.9
　endometrium N85.9
　　hyperplasia N85.00
　parenting situation Z62.9
Auditory — *see* condition
Aujeszky's disease B33.8
Aurantiasis, cutis E67.1
Auricle, auricular (*see also* condition)
　cervical Q18.2
Auriculotemporal syndrome G50.8
Austin Flint murmur (aortic insufficiency) I35.1
Australian
　Q fever A78
　X disease A83.4
Autism, autistic (childhood) (infantile) F84.0
　atypical F84.9
　spectrum disorder F84.0
Autodigestion R68.89
Autoerythrocyte sensitization (syndrome) D69.2
Autographism L50.3
Autoimmune
　disease (systemic) M35.9
　inhibitors to clotting factors D68.311
　lymphoproliferative syndrome [ALPS] D89.82
　thyroiditis E06.3
Autointoxication R68.89
Automatism G93.89
　with temporal sclerosis G93.81
　epileptic — *see* Epilepsy, localization-related, symptomatic, with complex partial seizures
　paroxysmal, idiopathic — *see* Epilepsy, localization-related, symptomatic, with complex partial seizures
Autonomic, autonomous
　bladder (neurogenic) N31.2
　hysteria seizure F44.5
Autosensitivity, erythrocyte D69.2
Autosensitization, cutaneous L30.2
Autosome — *see* condition by chromosome involved
Autotopagnosia R48.1
Autotoxemia R68.89
Autumn — *see* condition
Avellis' syndrome G46.8
Aversion
　oral R63.3
　　newborn P92. ☑
　　nonorganic origin F98.2 ☑
　sexual F52.1
Aviator's
　disease or sickness — *see* Effect, adverse, high altitude
　ear T70.0 ☑
Avitaminosis (multiple) (*see also* Deficiency, vitamin) E56.9
　B E53.9
　　with
　　　beriberi E51.11
　　　pellagra E52
　B2 E53.0
　B6 E53.1
　B12 E53.8
　D E55.9
　　with rickets E55.0
　G E53.0
　K E56.1
　nicotinic acid E52
AVNRT (atrioventricular nodal re-entrant tachycardia) I47.1
AVRT (atrioventricular nodal re-entrant tachycardia) I47.1
Avulsion (traumatic)
　blood vessel — *see* Injury, blood vessel
　bone — *see* Fracture, by site
　cartilage (*see also* Dislocation, by site)
　　symphyseal (inner), complicating delivery O71.6

Avulsion — *continued*
　external site other than limb — *see* Wound, open, by site
　eye S05.7 ☑
　head (intracranial)
　　external site NEC S08.89 ☑
　　scalp S08.0 ☑
　internal organ or site — *see* Injury, by site
　joint (*see also* Dislocation, by site)
　　capsule — *see* Sprain, by site
　kidney S37.06 ☑
　ligament — *see* Sprain, by site
　limb (*see also* Amputation, traumatic, by site)
　　skin and subcutaneous tissue — *see* Wound, open, by site
　muscle — *see* Injury, muscle
　nerve (root) — *see* Injury, nerve
　scalp S08.0 ☑
　skin and subcutaneous tissue — *see* Wound, open, by site
　spleen S36.032 ☑
　symphyseal cartilage (inner), complicating delivery O71.6
　tendon — *see* Injury, muscle
　tooth S03.2 ☑
Awareness of heart beat R00.2
Axenfeld's
　anomaly or syndrome Q15.0
　degeneration (calcareous) Q13.4
Axilla, axillary (*see also* condition)
　breast Q83.1
Axonotmesis — *see* Injury, nerve
Ayerza's disease or syndrome (pulmonary artery sclerosis with pulmonary hypertension) I27.0
Azoospermia (organic) N46.01
　due to
　　drug therapy N46.021
　　efferent duct obstruction N46.023
　　infection N46.022
　　radiation N46.024
　　specified cause NEC N46.029
　　systemic disease N46.025
Azotemia R79.89
　meaning uremia N19
Aztec ear Q17.3
Azygos
　continuation inferior vena cava Q26.8
　lobe (lung) Q33.1

B

Baastrup's disease — *see* Kissing spine
Babesiosis B60.0
Babington's disease (familial hemorrhagic telangiectasia) I78.0
Babinski's syndrome A52.79
Baby
　crying constantly R68.11
　floppy (syndrome) P94.2
Bacillary — *see* condition
Bacilluria R82.71
Bacillus (*see also* Infection, bacillus)
　abortus infection A23.1
　anthracis infection A22.9
　coli infection (*see also* Escherichia coli) B96.20
　Flexner's A03.1
　mallei infection A24.0
　Shiga's A03.0
　suipestifer infection — *see* Infection, salmonella
Back — *see* condition
Backache (postural) M54.9
　sacroiliac M53.3
　specified NEC M54.89
Backflow — *see* Reflux
Backward reading (dyslexia) F81.0
Bacteremia R78.81
　with sepsis — *see* Sepsis
Bactericholia — *see* Cholecystitis, acute
Bacterid, bacteride (pustular) L40.3
Bacterium, bacteria, bacterial
　agent NEC, as cause of disease classified elsewhere B96.89
　in blood — *see* Bacteremia
　in urine — *see* Bacteriuria
Bacteriuria, bacteruria R82.71
　asymptomatic R82.71
Bacteroides
　fragilis, as cause of disease classified elsewhere B96.6

Bad
　heart — *see* Disease, heart
　trip
　　due to drug abuse — *see* Abuse, drug, hallucinogen
　　due to drug dependence — *see* Dependence, drug, hallucinogen
Baelz's disease (cheilitis glandularis apostematosa) K13.0
Baerensprung's disease (eczema marginatum) B35.6
Bagasse disease or pneumonitis J67.1
Bagassosis J67.1
Baker's cyst — *see* Cyst, Baker's
Bakwin-Krida syndrome (metaphyseal dysplasia) Q78.5
Balancing side interference M26.56
Balanitis (circinata) (erosiva) (gangrenosa) (phagedenic) (vulgaris) N48.1
　amebic A06.82
　candidal B37.42
　due to Haemophilus ducreyi A57
　gonococcal (acute) (chronic) A54.09
　xerotica obliterans N48.0
Balanoposthitis N47.6
　gonococcal (acute) (chronic) A54.09
　ulcerative (specific) A63.8
Balanorrhagia — *see* Balanitis
Balantidiasis, balantidiosis A07.0
Bald tongue K14.4
Baldness (*see also* Alopecia)
　male-pattern — *see* Alopecia, androgenic
Balkan grippe A78
Balloon disease — *see* Effect, adverse, high altitude
Balo's disease (concentric sclerosis) G37.5
Bamberger-Marie disease — *see* Osteoarthropathy, hypertrophic, specified type NEC
Bancroft's filariasis B74.0
Band (s)
　adhesive — *see* Adhesions, peritoneum
　anomalous or congenital (*see also* Anomaly, by site)
　　heart (atrial) (ventricular) Q24.8
　　intestine Q43.3
　　omentum Q43.3
　cervix N88.1
　constricting, congenital Q79.8
　gallbladder (congenital) Q44.1
　intestinal (adhesive) — *see* Adhesions, peritoneum
　obstructive
　　intestine K56.50
　　　complete K56.52
　　　incomplete K56.51
　　　partial K56.51
　　peritoneum K56.50
　　　complete K56.52
　　　incomplete K56.51
　　　partial K56.51
　periappendiceal, congenital Q43.3
　peritoneal (adhesive) — *see* Adhesions, peritoneum
　uterus N73.6
　　internal N85.6
　vagina N89.5
Bandemia D72.825
Bandl's ring (contraction), complicating delivery O62.4
Bangkok hemorrhagic fever A91
Bang's disease (brucella abortus) A23.1
Bankruptcy, anxiety concerning Z59.8
Bannister's disease T78.3 ☑
　hereditary D84.1
Banti's disease or syndrome (with cirrhosis) (with portal hypertension) K76.6
Bar, median, prostate — *see* Enlargement, enlarged, prostate
Barcoo disease or rot — *see* Ulcer, skin
Barlow's disease E54
Barodontalgia T70.29 ☑
Baron Münchausen syndrome — *see* Disorder, factitious
Barosinusitis T70.1 ☑
Barotitis T70.0 ☑
Barotrauma T70.29 ☑
　odontalgia T70.29 ☑
　otitic T70.0 ☑
　sinus T70.1 ☑
Barraquer (-Simons) disease or syndrome (progressive lipodystrophy) E88.1
Barré-Guillain disease or syndrome G61.0
Barré-Liéou syndrome (posterior cervical sympathetic) M53.0

Barrel chest M95.4
Barrett's
  disease — *see* Barrett's, esophagus
  esophagus K22.70
    with dysplasia K22.719
      high grade K22.711
      low grade K22.710
    without dysplasia K22.70
  syndrome — *see* Barrett's, esophagus
  ulcer K22.10
    with bleeding K22.11
    without bleeding K22.10
Bársony (-Polgár) (-Teschendorf) syndrome (corkscrew esophagus) K22.4
Bartholinitis (suppurating) N75.8
  gonococcal (acute) (chronic) (with abscess) A54.1
Barth syndrome E78.71
Bartonellosis A44.9
  cutaneous A44.1
  mucocutaneous A44.1
  specified NEC A44.8
  systemic A44.0
Barton's fracture S52.56 ☑
Bartter's syndrome E26.81
Basal — *see* condition
Basan's (hidrotic) ectodermal dysplasia Q82.4
Baseball finger — *see* Dislocation, finger
Basedow's disease (exophthalmic goiter) — *see* Hyperthyroidism, with, goiter
Basic — *see* condition
Basilar — *see* condition
Bason's (hidrotic) ectodermal dysplasia Q82.4
Basopenia — *see* Agranulocytosis
Basophilia D72.824
Basophilism (cortico-adrenal) (Cushing's) (pituitary) E24.0
Bassen-Kornzweig disease or syndrome E78.6
Bat ear Q17.5
Bateman's
  disease B08.1
  purpura (senile) D69.2
Bathing cramp T75.1 ☑
Bathophobia F40.248
Batten (-Mayou) disease E75.4
  retina E75.4 [H36]
Batten-Steinert syndrome G71.11
Battered — *see* Maltreatment
Battey Mycobacterium infection A31.0
Battle exhaustion F43.0
Battledore placenta O43.19 ☑
Baumgarten-Cruveilhier cirrhosis, disease or syndrome K74.69
Bauxite fibrosis (of lung) J63.1
Bayle's disease (general paresis) A52.17
Bazin's disease (primary) (tuberculous) A18.4
Beach ear — *see* Swimmer's, ear
Beaded hair (congenital) Q84.1
Béal conjunctivitis or syndrome B30.2
Beard's disease (neurasthenia) F48.8
Beat (s)
  atrial, premature I49.1
  ectopic I49.49
  elbow — *see* Bursitis, elbow
  escaped, heart I49.49
  hand — *see* Bursitis, hand
  knee — *see* Bursitis, knee
  premature I49.40
    atrial I49.1
    auricular I49.1
    supraventricular I49.1
Beau's
  disease or syndrome — *see* Degeneration, myocardial
  lines (transverse furrows on fingernails) L60.4
Bechterev's syndrome — *see* Spondylitis, ankylosing
Beck's syndrome (anterior spinal artery occlusion) I65.8
Becker's
  cardiomyopathy I42.8
  disease
    idiopathic mural endomyocardial disease I42.3
    myotonia congenita, recessive form G71.12
  dystrophy G71.0
  pigmented hairy nevus D22.5
Beckwith-Wiedemann syndrome Q87.3
Bed confinement status Z74.01
Bed sore — *see* Ulcer, pressure, by site
Bedbug bite (s) — *see* Bite (s), by site, superficial, insect
Bedclothes, asphyxiation or suffocation by — *see* Asphyxia, traumatic, due to, mechanical, trapped

Bednar's
  aphthae K12.0
  tumor — *see* Neoplasm, malignant, by site
Bedridden Z74.01
Bedsore — *see* Ulcer, pressure, by site
Bedwetting — *see* Enuresis
Bee sting (with allergic or anaphylactic shock) — *see* Toxicity, venom, arthropod, bee
Beer drinker's heart (disease) I42.6
Begbie's disease (exophthalmic goiter) — *see* Hyperthyroidism, with, goiter
Behavior
  antisocial
    adult Z72.811
    child or adolescent Z72.810
  disorder, disturbance — *see* Disorder, conduct
  disruptive — *see* Disorder, conduct
  drug seeking Z76.5
  inexplicable R46.2
  marked evasiveness R46.5
  obsessive-compulsive R46.81
  overactivity R46.3
  poor responsiveness R46.4
  self-damaging (life-style) Z72.89
  sleep-incompatible Z72.821
  slowness R46.4
  specified NEC R46.89
  strange (and inexplicable) R46.2
  suspiciousness R46.5
  type A pattern Z73.1
  undue concern or preoccupation with stressful events R46.6
  verbosity and circumstantial detail obscuring reason for contact R46.7
Behçet's disease or syndrome M35.2
Behr's disease — *see* Degeneration, macula
Beigel's disease or morbus (white piedra) B36.2
Bejel A65
Bekhterev's syndrome — *see* Spondylitis, ankylosing
Belching — *see* Eructation
Bell's
  mania F30.8
  palsy, paralysis G51.0
    infant or newborn P11.3
  spasm G51.3
Bence Jones albuminuria or proteinuria NEC R80.3
Bends T70.3 ☑
Benedikt's paralysis or syndrome G46.3
Benign (*see also* condition)
  prostatic hyperplasia — *see* Hyperplasia, prostate
Bennett's fracture (displaced) S62.21 ☑
Benson's disease — *see* Deposit, crystalline
Bent
  back (hysterical) F44.4
  nose M95.0
    congenital Q67.4
Bereavement (uncomplicated) Z63.4
Bergeron's disease (hysterical chorea) F44.4
Berger's disease — *see* Nephropathy, IgA
Beriberi (dry) E51.11
  heart (disease) E51.12
  polyneuropathy E51.11
  wet E51.12
    involving circulatory system E51.11
Berlin's disease or edema (traumatic) S05.8X ☑
Berlock (berloque) dermatitis L56.2
Bernard-Horner syndrome G90.2
Bernard-Soulier disease or thrombopathia D69.1
Bernhardt (-Roth) disease — *see* Mononeuropathy, lower limb, meralgia paresthetica
Bernheim's syndrome — *see* Failure, heart, right
Bertielliasis B71.8
Berylliosis (lung) J63.2
Besnier-Boeck (-Schaumann) disease — *see* Sarcoidosis
Besnier's
  lupus pernio D86.3
  prurigo L20.0
Bestiality F65.89
Best's disease H35.50
Beta-mercaptolactate-cysteine disulfiduria E72.09
Betalipoproteinemia, broad or floating E78.2
Betting and gambling Z72.6
  pathological (compulsive) F63.0
Bezoar T18.9 ☑
  intestine T18.3 ☑
  stomach T18.2 ☑
Bezold's abscess — *see* Mastoiditis, acute
Bianchi's syndrome R48.8
Bicornate or bicornis uterus Q51.3
  in pregnancy or childbirth O34.00
    causing obstructed labor O65.5
Bicuspid aortic valve Q23.1

Biedl-Bardet syndrome Q87.89
Bielschowsky (-Jansky) disease E75.4
Biermer's (pernicious) anemia or disease D51.0
Biett's disease L93.0
Bifid (congenital)
  apex, heart Q24.8
  clitoris Q52.6
  kidney Q63.8
  nose Q30.2
  patella Q74.1
  scrotum Q55.29
  toe NEC Q74.2
  tongue Q38.3
  ureter Q62.8
  uterus Q51.3
  uvula Q35.7
Biforis uterus (suprasimplex) Q51.3
Bifurcation (congenital)
  gallbladder Q44.1
  kidney pelvis Q63.8
  renal pelvis Q63.8
  rib Q76.6
  tongue, congenital Q38.3
  trachea Q32.1
  ureter Q62.8
  urethra Q64.74
  vertebra Q76.49
Big spleen syndrome D73.1
Bigeminal pulse R00.8
Bilateral — *see* condition
Bile
  duct — *see* condition
  pigments in urine R82.2
Bilharziasis (*see also* Schistosomiasis)
  chyluria B65.0
  cutaneous B65.3
  galacturia B65.0
  hematochyluria B65.0
  intestinal B65.1
  lipemia B65.9
  lipuria B65.0
  oriental B65.2
  piarhemia B65.9
  pulmonary NOS B65.9 [J99]
    pneumonia B65.9 [J17]
  tropical hematuria B65.0
  vesical B65.0
Biliary — *see* condition
Bilirubin metabolism disorder E80.7
  specified NEC E80.6
Bilirubinemia, familial nonhemolytic E80.4
Bilirubinuria R82.2
Biliuria R82.2
Bilocular stomach K31.2
Binswanger's disease I67.3
Biparta, bipartite
  carpal scaphoid Q74.0
  patella Q74.1
  vagina Q52.10
Bird
  face Q75.8
  fancier's disease or lung J67.2
Birt-Hogg-Dube syndrome Q87.89
Birth
  complications in mother — *see* Delivery, complicated
  compression during NOS P15.9
  defect — *see* Anomaly
  immature (less than 37 completed weeks) — *see* Preterm, newborn
    extremely (less than 28 completed weeks) — *see* Immaturity, extreme
  inattention, at or after — *see* Maltreatment, child, neglect
  injury NOS P15.9
    basal ganglia P11.1
    brachial plexus NEC P14.3
    brain (compression) (pressure) P11.2
    central nervous system NOS P11.9
    cerebellum P11.1
    cerebral hemorrhage P10.1
    external genitalia P15.5
    eye P15.3
    face P15.4
    fracture
      bone P13.9
        specified NEC P13.8
      clavicle P13.4
      femur P13.2
      humerus P13.3
      long bone, except femur P13.3
      radius and ulna P13.3

Birth — *continued*
- injury NOS — *continued*
  - skull P13.0
  - spine P11.5
  - tibia and fibula P13.3
- intracranial P11.2
  - laceration or hemorrhage P10.9
    - specified NEC P10.8
- intraventricular hemorrhage P10.2
- laceration
  - brain P10.1
  - by scalpel P15.8
  - peripheral nerve P14.9
- liver P15.0
- meninges
  - brain P11.1
  - spinal cord P11.5
- nerve
  - brachial plexus P14.3
  - cranial NEC (except facial) P11.4
  - facial P11.3
  - peripheral P14.9
  - phrenic (paralysis) P14.2
- paralysis
  - facial nerve P11.3
  - spinal P11.5
- penis P15.5
- rupture
  - spinal cord P11.5
- scalp P12.9
- scalpel wound P15.8
- scrotum P15.5
- skull NEC P13.1
  - fracture P13.0
- specified type NEC P15.8
- spinal cord P11.5
- spine P11.5
- spleen P15.1
- sternomastoid (hematoma) P15.2
- subarachnoid hemorrhage P10.3
- subcutaneous fat necrosis P15.6
- subdural hemorrhage P10.0
- tentorial tear P10.4
- testes P15.5
- vulva P15.5
- lack of care, at or after — *see* Maltreatment, child, neglect
- neglect, at or after — *see* Maltreatment, child, neglect
- palsy or paralysis, newborn, NOS (birth injury) P14.9
- premature (infant) — *see* Preterm, newborn
- shock, newborn P96.89
- trauma — *see* Birth, injury
- weight
  - low (2499 grams or less) — *see* Low, birthweight
    - extremely (999 grams or less) — *see* Low, birthweight, extreme
  - 4000 grams to 4499 grams P08.1
  - 4500 grams or more P08.0

Birthmark Q82.5
Bisalbuminemia E88.09
Biskra's button B55.1
Bite (s) (animal) (human)
- abdomen, abdominal
  - wall S31.159 ☑
    - with penetration into peritoneal cavity S31.659 ☑
    - epigastric region S31.152 ☑
      - with penetration into peritoneal cavity S31.652 ☑
    - left
      - lower quadrant S31.154 ☑
        - with penetration into peritoneal cavity S31.654 ☑
      - upper quadrant S31.151 ☑
        - with penetration into peritoneal cavity S31.651 ☑
    - periumbilic region S31.155 ☑
      - with penetration into peritoneal cavity S31.655 ☑
    - right
      - lower quadrant S31.153 ☑
        - with penetration into peritoneal cavity S31.653 ☑
      - upper quadrant S31.150 ☑
        - with penetration into peritoneal cavity S31.650 ☑
    - superficial NEC S30.871 ☑
      - insect S30.861 ☑

Bite — *continued*
- alveolar (process) — *see* Bite, oral cavity
- amphibian (venomous) — *see* Venom, bite, amphibian
- animal (*see also* Bite, by site)
  - venomous — *see* Venom
- ankle S91.05 ☑
  - superficial NEC S90.57 ☑
    - insect S90.56 ☑
- antecubital space — *see* Bite, elbow
- anus S31.835 ☑
  - superficial NEC S30.877 ☑
    - insect S30.867 ☑
- arm (upper) S41.15 ☑
  - lower — *see* Bite, forearm
  - superficial NEC S40.87 ☑
    - insect S40.86 ☑
- arthropod NEC — *see* Venom, bite, arthropod
- auditory canal (external) (meatus) — *see* Bite, ear
- auricle, ear — *see* Bite, ear
- axilla — *see* Bite, arm
- back (*see also* Bite, thorax, back)
  - lower S31.050 ☑
    - with penetration into retroperitoneal space S31.051 ☑
  - superficial NEC S30.870 ☑
    - insect S30.860 ☑
- bedbug — *see* Bite (s), by site, superficial, insect
- breast S21.05 ☑
  - superficial NEC S20.17 ☑
    - insect S20.16 ☑
- brow — *see* Bite, head, specified site NEC
- buttock S31.805 ☑
  - left S31.825 ☑
  - right S31.815 ☑
  - superficial NEC S30.870 ☑
    - insect S30.860 ☑
- calf — *see* Bite, leg
- canaliculus lacrimalis — *see* Bite, eyelid
- canthus, eye — *see* Bite, eyelid
- centipede — *see* Toxicity, venom, arthropod, centipede
- cheek (external) S01.45 ☑
  - superficial NEC S00.87 ☑
    - insect S00.86 ☑
  - internal — *see* Bite, oral cavity
- chest wall — *see* Bite, thorax
- chigger B88.0
- chin — *see* Bite, head, specified site NEC
- clitoris — *see* Bite, vulva
- costal region — *see* Bite, thorax
- digit (s)
  - hand — *see* Bite, finger
  - toe — *see* Bite, toe
- ear (canal) (external) S01.35 ☑
  - superficial NEC S00.47 ☑
    - insect S00.46 ☑
- elbow S51.05 ☑
  - superficial NEC S50.37 ☑
    - insect S50.36 ☑
- epididymis — *see* Bite, testis
- epigastric region — *see* Bite, abdomen
- epiglottis — *see* Bite, neck, specified site NEC
- esophagus, cervical S11.25 ☑
  - superficial NEC S10.17 ☑
    - insect S10.16 ☑
- eyebrow — *see* Bite, eyelid
- eyelid S01.15 ☑
  - superficial NEC S00.27 ☑
    - insect S00.26 ☑
- face NEC — *see* Bite, head, specified site NEC
- finger (s) S61.259 ☑
  - with
    - damage to nail S61.359 ☑
  - index S61.258 ☑
    - with
      - damage to nail S61.358 ☑
    - left S61.251 ☑
      - with
        - damage to nail S61.351 ☑
    - right S61.250 ☑
      - with
        - damage to nail S61.350 ☑
    - superficial NEC S60.478 ☑
      - insect S60.46 ☑
  - little S61.25 ☑
    - with
      - damage to nail S61.35 ☑
    - superficial NEC S60.47 ☑
      - insect S60.46 ☑
  - middle S61.25 ☑
    - with

Bite — *continued*
- finger — *continued*
  - damage to nail S61.35 ☑
  - superficial NEC S60.47 ☑
    - insect S60.46 ☑
  - ring S61.25 ☑
    - with
      - damage to nail S61.35 ☑
    - superficial NEC S60.47 ☑
      - insect S60.46 ☑
  - superficial NEC S60.479 ☑
    - insect S60.469 ☑
  - thumb — *see* Bite, thumb
- flank — *see* Bite, abdomen, wall
- flea — *see* Bite, by site, superficial, insect
- foot (except toe (s) alone) S91.35 ☑
  - superficial NEC S90.87 ☑
    - insect S90.86 ☑
  - toe — *see* Bite, toe
- forearm S51.85 ☑
  - elbow only — *see* Bite, elbow
  - superficial NEC S50.87 ☑
    - insect S50.86 ☑
- forehead — *see* Bite, head, specified site NEC
- genital organs, external
  - female S31.552 ☑
    - superficial NEC S30.876 ☑
      - insect S30.866 ☑
    - vagina and vulva — *see* Bite, vulva
  - male S31.551 ☑
    - penis — *see* Bite, penis
    - scrotum — *see* Bite, scrotum
    - superficial NEC S30.875 ☑
      - insect S30.865 ☑
    - testes — *see* Bite, testis
- groin — *see* Bite, abdomen, wall
- gum — *see* Bite, oral cavity
- hand S61.45 ☑
  - finger — *see* Bite, finger
  - superficial NEC S60.57 ☑
    - insect S60.56 ☑
  - thumb — *see* Bite, thumb
- head S01.95 ☑
  - cheek — *see* Bite, cheek
  - ear — *see* Bite, ear
  - eyelid — *see* Bite, eyelid
  - lip — *see* Bite, lip
  - nose — *see* Bite, nose
  - oral cavity — *see* Bite, oral cavity
  - scalp — *see* Bite, scalp
  - specified site NEC S01.85 ☑
    - superficial NEC S00.87 ☑
      - insect S00.86 ☑
  - superficial NEC S00.97 ☑
    - insect S00.96 ☑
  - temporomandibular area — *see* Bite, cheek
- heel — *see* Bite, foot
- hip S71.05 ☑
  - superficial NEC S70.27 ☑
    - insect S70.26 ☑
- hymen S31.45 ☑
- hypochondrium — *see* Bite, abdomen, wall
- hypogastric region — *see* Bite, abdomen, wall
- inguinal region — *see* Bite, abdomen, wall
- insect — *see* Bite, by site, superficial, insect
- instep — *see* Bite, foot
- interscapular region — *see* Bite, thorax, back
- jaw — *see* Bite, head, specified site NEC
- knee S81.05 ☑
  - superficial NEC S80.27 ☑
    - insect S80.26 ☑
- labium (majus) (minus) — *see* Bite, vulva
- lacrimal duct — *see* Bite, eyelid
- larynx S11.015 ☑
  - superficial NEC S10.17 ☑
    - insect S10.16 ☑
- leg (lower) S81.85 ☑
  - ankle — *see* Bite, ankle
  - foot — *see* Bite, foot
  - knee — *see* Bite, knee
  - superficial NEC S80.87 ☑
    - insect S80.86 ☑
  - toe — *see* Bite, toe
  - upper — *see* Bite, thigh
- lip S01.551 ☑
  - superficial NEC S00.571 ☑
    - insect S00.561 ☑
- lizard (venomous) — *see* Venom, bite, reptile
- loin — *see* Bite, abdomen, wall
- lower back — *see* Bite, back, lower
- lumbar region — *see* Bite, back, lower
- malar region — *see* Bite, head, specified site NEC

☑ **Additional character required**

Bite — *continued*
  mammary — *see* Bite, breast
  marine animals (venomous) — *see* Toxicity,
    venom, marine animal
  mastoid region — *see* Bite, head, specified site
    NEC
  mouth — *see* Bite, oral cavity
  nail
    finger — *see* Bite, finger
    toe — *see* Bite, toe
  nape — *see* Bite, neck, specified site NEC
  nasal (septum) (sinus) — *see* Bite, nose
  nasopharynx — *see* Bite, head, specified site NEC
  neck S11.95 ☑
    involving
      cervical esophagus — *see* Bite, esophagus,
        cervical
      larynx — *see* Bite, larynx
      pharynx — *see* Bite, pharynx
      thyroid gland S11.15 ☑
      trachea — *see* Bite, trachea
    specified site NEC S11.85 ☑
      superficial NEC S10.87 ☑
        insect S10.86 ☑
    superficial NEC S10.97 ☑
      insect S10.96 ☑
    throat S11.85 ☑
      superficial NEC S10.17 ☑
        insect S10.16 ☑
  nose (septum) (sinus) S01.25 ☑
    superficial NEC S00.37 ☑
      insect S00.36 ☑
  occipital region — *see* Bite, scalp
  oral cavity S01.552 ☑
    superficial NEC S00.572 ☑
      insect S00.562 ☑
  orbital region — *see* Bite, eyelid
  palate — *see* Bite, oral cavity
  palm — *see* Bite, hand
  parietal region — *see* Bite, scalp
  pelvis S31.050 ☑
    with penetration into retroperitoneal
      space S31.051 ☑
    superficial NEC S30.870 ☑
      insect S30.860 ☑
  penis S31.25 ☑
    superficial NEC S30.872 ☑
      insect S30.862 ☑
  perineum
    female — *see* Bite, vulva
    male — *see* Bite, pelvis
  periocular area (with or without lacrimal
    passages) — *see* Bite, eyelid
  phalanges
    finger — *see* Bite, finger
    toe — *see* Bite, toe
  pharynx S11.25 ☑
    superficial NEC S10.17 ☑
      insect S10.16 ☑
  pinna — *see* Bite, ear
  poisonous — *see* Venom
  popliteal space — *see* Bite, knee
  prepuce — *see* Bite, penis
  pubic region — *see* Bite, abdomen, wall
  rectovaginal septum — *see* Bite, vulva
  red bug B88.0
  reptile NEC (*see also* Venom, bite, reptile)
    nonvenomous — *see* Bite, by site
    snake — *see* Venom, bite, snake
  sacral region — *see* Bite, back, lower
  sacroiliac region — *see* Bite, back, lower
  salivary gland — *see* Bite, oral cavity
  scalp S01.05 ☑
    superficial NEC S00.07 ☑
      insect S00.06 ☑
  scapular region — *see* Bite, shoulder
  scrotum S31.35 ☑
    superficial NEC S30.873 ☑
      insect S30.863 ☑
  sea-snake (venomous) — *see* Toxicity, venom,
    snake, sea snake
  shin — *see* Bite, leg
  shoulder S41.05 ☑
    superficial NEC S40.27 ☑
      insect S40.26 ☑
  snake (*see also* Venom, bite, snake)
    nonvenomous — *see* Bite, by site
  spermatic cord — *see* Bite, testis
  spider (venomous) — *see* Toxicity, venom, spider
    nonvenomous — *see* Bite, by site, superficial,
      insect
  sternal region — *see* Bite, thorax, front

Bite — *continued*
  submaxillary region — *see* Bite, head, specified
    site NEC
  submental region — *see* Bite, head, specified
    site NEC
  subungual
    finger (s) — *see* Bite, finger
    toe — *see* Bite, toe
  superficial — *see* Bite, by site, superficial
  supraclavicular fossa S11.85 ☑
  supraorbital — *see* Bite, head, specified site NEC
  temple, temporal region — *see* Bite, head,
    specified site NEC
  temporomandibular area — *see* Bite, cheek
  testis S31.35 ☑
    superficial NEC S30.873 ☑
      insect S30.863 ☑
  thigh S71.15 ☑
    superficial NEC S70.37 ☑
      insect S70.36 ☑
  thorax, thoracic (wall) S21.95 ☑
    back S21.25 ☑
      with penetration into thoracic
        cavity S21.45 ☑
    breast — *see* Bite, breast
    front S21.15 ☑
      with penetration into thoracic
        cavity S21.35 ☑
    superficial NEC S20.97 ☑
      back S20.47 ☑
      front S20.37 ☑
      insect S20.96 ☑
        back S20.46 ☑
        front S20.36 ☑
  throat — *see* Bite, neck, throat
  thumb S61.05 ☑
    with
      damage to nail S61.15 ☑
    superficial NEC S60.37 ☑
      insect S60.36 ☑
  thyroid S11.15 ☑
    superficial NEC S10.87 ☑
      insect S10.86 ☑
  toe (s) S91.15 ☑
    with
      damage to nail S91.25 ☑
    great S91.15 ☑
      with
        damage to nail S91.25 ☑
    lesser S91.15 ☑
      with
        damage to nail S91.25 ☑
    superficial NEC S90.47 ☑
      great S90.47 ☑
      insect S90.46 ☑
        great S90.46 ☑
  tongue S01.552 ☑
  trachea S11.025 ☑
    superficial NEC S10.17 ☑
      insect S10.16 ☑
  tunica vaginalis — *see* Bite, testis
  tympanum, tympanic membrane — *see* Bite, ear
  umbilical region S31.155 ☑
  uvula — *see* Bite, oral cavity
  vagina — *see* Bite, vulva
  venomous — *see* Venom
  vocal cords S11.035 ☑
    superficial NEC S10.17 ☑
      insect S10.16 ☑
  vulva S31.45 ☑
    superficial NEC S30.874 ☑
      insect S30.864 ☑
  wrist S61.55 ☑
    superficial NEC S60.87 ☑
      insect S60.86 ☑
Biting, cheek or lip K13.1
Biventricular failure (heart) I50.82
Björck (-Thorson) syndrome (malignant carcinoid)
  E34.0
Black
  death A20.9
  eye S00.1 ☑
  hairy tongue K14.3
  heel (foot) S90.3 ☑
  lung (disease) J60
  palm (hand) S60.22 ☑
Blackfan-Diamond anemia or syndrome (congenital
  hypoplastic anemia) D61.01
Blackhead L70.0
Blackout R55
Bladder — *see* condition

Blast (air) (hydraulic) (immersion) (underwater)
  blindness S05.8X ☑
  injury
    abdomen or thorax — *see* Injury, by site
    ear (acoustic nerve trauma) — *see* Injury, nerve,
      acoustic, specified type NEC
    syndrome NEC T70.8 ☑
Blastoma — *see* Neoplasm, malignant, by site
  pulmonary — *see* Neoplasm, lung, malignant
Blastomycosis, blastomycotic B40.9
  Brazilian — *see* Paracoccidioidomycosis
  cutaneous B40.3
  disseminated B40.7
  European — *see* Cryptococcosis
  generalized B40.7
  keloidal B48.0
  North American B40.9
  primary pulmonary B40.0
  pulmonary B40.2
    acute B40.0
    chronic B40.1
  skin B40.3
  South American — *see* Paracoccidioidomycosis
  specified NEC B40.89
Bleb (s) R23.8
  emphysematous (lung) (solitary) J43.9
  endophthalmitis H59.43
  filtering (vitreous), after glaucoma surgery Z98.83
  inflamed (infected), postprocedural H59.40
    stage 1 H59.41
    stage 2 H59.42
    stage 3 H59.43
  lung (ruptured) J43.9
    congenital — *see* Atelectasis
    newborn P25.8
  subpleural (emphysematous) J43.9
Blebitis, postprocedural H59.40
  stage 1 H59.41
  stage 2 H59.42
  stage 3 H59.43
Bleeder (familial) (hereditary) — *see* Hemophilia
Bleeding (*see also* Hemorrhage)
  anal K62.5
  anovulatory N97.0
  atonic, following delivery O72.1
  capillary I78.8
    puerperal O72.2
  contact (postcoital) N93.0
  due to uterine subinvolution N85.3
  ear — *see* Otorrhagia
  excessive, associated with menopausal
    onset N92.4
  familial — *see* Defect, coagulation
  following intercourse N93.0
  gastrointestinal K92.2
  hemorrhoids — *see* Hemorrhoids
  intermenstrual (regular) N92.3
    irregular N92.1
  intraoperative — *see* Complication,
    intraoperative, hemorrhage
  irregular N92.6
  menopausal N92.4
  newborn, intraventricular — *see* Newborn,
    affected by, hemorrhage, intraventricular
  nipple N64.59
  nose R04.0
  ovulation N92.3
  postclimacteric N95.0
  postcoital N93.0
  postmenopausal N95.0
  postoperative — *see* Complication,
    postprocedural, hemorrhage
  preclimacteric N92.4
  pre-pubertal vaginal N93.1
  puberty (excessive, with onset of menstrual
    periods) N92.2
  rectum, rectal K62.5
    newborn P54.2
  tendencies — *see* Defect, coagulation
  throat R04.1
  tooth socket (post-extraction) K91.840
  umbilical stump P51.9
  uterus, uterine NEC N93.9
    climacteric N92.4
    dysfunctional or functional N93.8
    menopausal N92.4
    preclimacteric or premenopausal N92.4
    unrelated to menstrual cycle N93.9
  vagina, vaginal (abnormal) N93.9
    dysfunctional or functional N93.8
    newborn P54.6
    pre-pubertal N93.1
  vicarious N94.89

Blennorrhagia - Block

Blennorrhagia, blennorrhagic — *see* Gonorrhea
Blennorrhea (acute) (chronic) (*see also* Gonorrhea)
   inclusion (neonatal) (newborn) P39.1
   lower genitourinary tract (gonococcal) A54.00
   neonatorum (gonococcal ophthalmia) A54.31
Blepharelosis — *see* Entropion
Blepharitis (angularis) (ciliaris) (eyelid) (marginal)
   (nonulcerative) H01.009
   herpes zoster B02.39
   left H01.006
     lower H01.005
     upper H01.004
   right H01.003
     lower H01.002
     upper H01.001
   squamous H01.029
     left H01.026
       lower H01.025
       upper H01.024
     right H01.023
       lower H01.022
       upper H01.021
   ulcerative H01.019
     left H01.016
       lower H01.015
       upper H01.014
     right H01.013
       lower H01.012
       upper H01.011
Blepharochalasis H02.30
   congenital Q10.0
   left H02.36
     lower H02.35
     upper H02.34
   right H02.33
     lower H02.32
     upper H02.31
Blepharoclonus H02.59
Blepharoconjunctivitis H10.50 ☑
   angular H10.52 ☑
   contact H10.53 ☑
   ligneous H10.51 ☑
Blepharophimosis (eyelid) H02.529
   congenital Q10.3
   left H02.526
     lower H02.525
     upper H02.524
   right H02.523
     lower H02.522
     upper H02.521
Blepharoptosis H02.40 ☑
   congenital Q10.0
   mechanical H02.41 ☑
   myogenic H02.42 ☑
   neurogenic H02.43 ☑
   paralytic H02.43 ☑
Blepharopyorrhea, gonococcal A54.39
Blepharospasm G24.5
   drug induced G24.01
Blighted ovum O02.0
Blind (*see also* Blindness)
   bronchus (congenital) Q32.4
   loop syndrome K90.2
     congenital Q43.8
   sac, fallopian tube (congenital) Q50.6
   spot, enlarged — *see* Defect, visual field,
     localized, scotoma, blind spot area
   tract or tube, congenital NEC — *see* Atresia, by site
Blindness (acquired) (congenital) (both eyes)
   H54.0X ☑
   blast S05.8X ☑
   color — *see* Deficiency, color vision
   concussion S05.8X ☑
   cortical H47.619
     left brain H47.612
     right brain H47.611
   day H53.11
   due to injury (current episode) S05.9 ☑
     sequelae - code to injury with seventh
       character S
   eclipse (total) — *see* Retinopathy, solar
   emotional (hysterical) F44.6
   face H53.16
   hysterical F44.6
   legal (both eyes) (USA definition) H54.8
   mind R48.8
   night H53.60
     abnormal dark adaptation curve H53.61
     acquired H53.62
     congenital H53.63
     specified type NEC H53.69
     vitamin A deficiency E50.5

Blindness — *continued*
   one eye (other eye normal) H54.40
     left (normal vision on right) H54.42 ☑
       low vision on right H54.12 ☑
     low vision, other eye H54.10
     right (normal vision on left) H54.41 ☑
       low vision on left H54.11 ☑
   psychic R48.8
   river B73.01
   snow — *see* Photokeratitis
   sun, solar — *see* Retinopathy, solar
   transient — *see* Disturbance, vision, subjective,
     loss, transient
   traumatic (current episode) S05.9 ☑
   word (developmental) F81.0
     acquired R48.0
     secondary to organic lesion R48.0
Blister (nonthermal)
   abdominal wall S30.821 ☑
   alveolar process S00.522 ☑
   ankle S90.52 ☑
   antecubital space — *see* Blister, elbow
   anus S30.827 ☑
   arm (upper) S40.82 ☑
   auditory canal — *see* Blister, ear
   auricle — *see* Blister, ear
   axilla — *see* Blister, arm
   back, lower S30.820 ☑
   beetle dermatitis L24.89
   breast S20.12 ☑
   brow S00.82 ☑
   calf — *see* Blister, leg
   canthus — *see* Blister, eyelid
   cheek S00.82 ☑
     internal S00.522 ☑
   chest wall — *see* Blister, thorax
   chin S00.82 ☑
   costal region — *see* Blister, thorax
   digit (s)
     foot — *see* Blister, toe
     hand — *see* Blister, finger
   due to burn — *see* Burn, by site, second degree
   ear S00.42 ☑
   elbow S50.32 ☑
   epiglottis S10.12 ☑
   esophagus, cervical S10.12 ☑
   eyebrow — *see* Blister, eyelid
   eyelid S00.22 ☑
   face S00.82 ☑
   fever B00.1
   finger (s) S60.429 ☑
     index S60.42 ☑
     little S60.42 ☑
     middle S60.42 ☑
     ring S60.42 ☑
   foot (except toe (s) alone) S90.82 ☑
     toe — *see* Blister, toe
   forearm S50.82 ☑
     elbow only — *see* Blister, elbow
   forehead S00.82 ☑
   fracture - omit code
   genital organ
     female S30.826 ☑
     male S30.825 ☑
   gum S00.522 ☑
   hand S60.52 ☑
   head S00.92 ☑
     ear — *see* Blister, ear
     eyelid — *see* Blister, eyelid
     lip S00.521 ☑
     nose S00.82 ☑
     oral cavity S00.522 ☑
     scalp S00.02 ☑
     specified site NEC S00.82 ☑
   heel — *see* Blister, foot
   hip S70.22 ☑
   interscapular region S20.429 ☑
   jaw S00.82 ☑
   knee S80.22 ☑
   larynx S10.12 ☑
   leg (lower) S80.82 ☑
     knee — *see* Blister, knee
     upper — *see* Blister, thigh
   lip S00.521 ☑
   malar region S00.82 ☑
   mammary — *see* Blister, breast
   mastoid region S00.82 ☑
   mouth S00.522 ☑
   multiple, skin, nontraumatic R23.8
   nail
     finger — *see* Blister, finger
     toe — *see* Blister, toe

Blister — *continued*
   nasal S00.32 ☑
   neck S10.92 ☑
     specified site NEC S10.82 ☑
     throat S10.12 ☑
   nose S00.32 ☑
   occipital region S00.02 ☑
   oral cavity S00.522 ☑
   orbital region — *see* Blister, eyelid
   palate S00.522 ☑
   palm — *see* Blister, hand
   parietal region S00.02 ☑
   pelvis S30.820 ☑
   penis S30.822 ☑
   periocular area — *see* Blister, eyelid
   phalanges
     finger — *see* Blister, finger
     toe — *see* Blister, toe
   pharynx S10.12 ☑
   pinna — *see* Blister, ear
   popliteal space — *see* Blister, knee
   scalp S00.02 ☑
   scapular region — *see* Blister, shoulder
   scrotum S30.823 ☑
   shin — *see* Blister, leg
   shoulder S40.22 ☑
   sternal region S20.329 ☑
   submaxillary region S00.82 ☑
   submental region S00.82 ☑
   subungual
     finger (s) — *see* Blister, finger
     toe (s) — *see* Blister, toe
   supraclavicular fossa S10.82 ☑
   supraorbital S00.82 ☑
   temple S00.82 ☑
   temporal region S00.82 ☑
   testis S30.823 ☑
   thermal — *see* Burn, second degree, by site
   thigh S70.32 ☑
   thorax, thoracic (wall) S20.92 ☑
     back S20.42 ☑
     front S20.32 ☑
   throat S10.12 ☑
   thumb S60.32 ☑
   toe (s) S90.42 ☑
     great S90.42 ☑
   tongue S00.522 ☑
   trachea S10.12 ☑
   tympanum, tympanic membrane — *see* Blister,
     ear
   upper arm — *see* Blister, arm (upper)
   uvula S00.522 ☑
   vagina S30.824 ☑
   vocal cords S10.12 ☑
   vulva S30.824 ☑
   wrist S60.82 ☑
Bloating R14.0
Bloch-Sulzberger disease or syndrome Q82.3
Block, blocked
   alveolocapillary J84.10
   arborization (heart) I45.5
   arrhythmic I45.9
   atrioventricular (incomplete) (partial) I44.30
     with atrioventricular dissociation I44.2
     complete I44.2
       congenital Q24.6
     congenital Q24.6
     first degree I44.0
     second degree (types I and II) I44.1
     specified NEC I44.39
     third degree I44.2
     types I and II I44.1
   auriculoventricular — *see* Block, atrioventricular
   bifascicular (cardiac) I45.2
   bundle-branch (complete) (false)
     (incomplete) I45.4
     bilateral I45.2
     left I44.7
       with right bundle branch block I45.2
       hemiblock I44.60
         anterior I44.4
         posterior I44.5
       incomplete I44.7
         with right bundle branch block I45.2
     right I45.10
       with
         left bundle branch block I45.2
         left fascicular block I45.2
       specified NEC I45.19
     Wilson's type I45.19
   cardiac I45.9
   conduction I45.9
     complete I44.2

Block — *continued*
  fascicular (left) I44.60
    anterior I44.4
    posterior I44.5
    right I45.0
    specified NEC I44.69
  foramen Magendie (acquired) G91.1
    congenital Q03.1
      with spina bifida — *see* Spina bifida, by site, with hydrocephalus
  heart I45.9
    bundle branch I45.4
      bilateral I45.2
    complete (atrioventricular) I44.2
    congenital Q24.6
    first degree (atrioventricular) I44.0
    second degree (atrioventricular) I44.1
    specified type NEC I45.5
    third degree (atrioventricular) I44.2
  hepatic vein I82.0
  intraventricular (nonspecific) I45.4
    bundle branch
      bilateral I45.2
  kidney N28.9
    postcystoscopic or postprocedural N99.0
  Mobitz (types I and II) I44.1
  myocardial — *see* Block, heart
  nodal I45.5
  organ or site, congenital NEC — *see* Atresia, by site
  portal (vein) I81
  second degree (types I and II) I44.1
  sinoatrial I45.5
  sinoauricular I45.5
  third degree I44.2
  trifascicular I45.3
  tubal N97.1
  vein NOS I82.90
  Wenckebach (types I and II) I44.1
Blockage — *see* Obstruction
Blocq's disease F44.4
Blood
  constituents, abnormal R78.9
  disease D75.9
  donor — *see* Donor, blood
  dyscrasia D75.9
    with
      abortion — *see* Abortion, by type, complicated by, hemorrhage
      ectopic pregnancy O08.1
      molar pregnancy O08.1
    following ectopic or molar pregnancy O08.1
    newborn P61.9
    puerperal, postpartum O72.3
  flukes NEC — *see* Schistosomiasis
  in
    feces K92.1
      occult R19.5
    urine — *see* Hematuria
  mole O02.0
  occult in feces R19.5
  pressure
    decreased, due to shock following injury T79.4 ☑
    examination only Z01.30
    fluctuating I99.8
    high — *see* Hypertension
      borderline R03.0
      incidental reading, without diagnosis of hypertension R03.0
    low (*see also* Hypotension)
      incidental reading, without diagnosis of hypotension R03.1
  spitting — *see* Hemoptysis
  staining cornea — *see* Pigmentation, cornea, stromal
  transfusion
    reaction or complication — *see* Complications, transfusion
  type
    A (Rh positive) Z67.10
      Rh negative Z67.11
    AB (Rh positive) Z67.30
      Rh negative Z67.31
    B (Rh positive) Z67.20
      Rh negative Z67.21
    O (Rh positive) Z67.40
      Rh negative Z67.41
    Rh (positive) Z67.90
      negative Z67.91
  vessel rupture — *see* Hemorrhage
  vomiting — *see* Hematemesis

Blood-forming organs, disease D75.9
Bloodgood's disease — *see* Mastopathy, cystic
Bloom (-Machacek) (-Torre) syndrome Q82.8
Blount's disease or osteochondrosis — *see* Osteochondrosis, juvenile, tibia
Blue
  baby Q24.9
  diaper syndrome E72.09
  dome cyst (breast) — *see* Cyst, breast
  dot cataract Q12.0
  nevus D22.9
  sclera Q13.5
    with fragility of bone and deafness Q78.0
  toe syndrome I75.02 ☑
Blueness — *see* Cyanosis
Blues, postpartal O90.6
  baby O90.6
Blurring, visual H53.8
Blushing (abnormal) (excessive) R23.2
BMI — *see* Body, mass index
Boarder, hospital NEC Z76.4
  accompanying sick person Z76.3
  healthy infant or child Z76.2
    foundling Z76.1
Bockhart's impetigo L01.02
Bodechtel-Guttman disease (subacute sclerosing panencephalitis) A81.1
Boder-Sedgwick syndrome (ataxia-telangiectasia) G11.3
Body, bodies
  Aschoff's — *see* Myocarditis, rheumatic
  asteroid, vitreous — *see* Deposit, crystalline
  cytoid (retina) — *see* Occlusion, artery, retina
  drusen (degenerative) (macula) (retinal) (*see also* Degeneration, macula, drusen)
    optic disc — *see* Drusen, optic disc
  foreign — *see* Foreign body
  loose
    joint, except knee — *see* Loose, body, joint
      knee M23.4 ☑
    sheath, tendon — *see* Disorder, tendon, specified type NEC
  mass index (BMI)
    adult
      19.9 or less Z68.1
      20.0-20.9 Z68.20
      21.0-21.9 Z68.21
      22.0-22.9 Z68.22
      23.0-23.9 Z68.23
      24.0-24.9 Z68.24
      25.0-25.9 Z68.25
      26.0-26.9 Z68.26
      27.0-27.9 Z68.27
      28.0-28.9 Z68.28
      29.0-29.9 Z68.29
      30.0-30.9 Z68.30
      31.0-31.9 Z68.31
      32.0-32.9 Z68.32
      33.0-33.9 Z68.33
      34.0-34.9 Z68.34
      35.0-35.9 Z68.35
      36.0-36.9 Z68.36
      37.0-37.9 Z68.37
      38.0-38.9 Z68.38
      39.0-39.9 Z68.39
      40.0-44.9 Z68.41
      45.0-49.9 Z68.42
      50.0-59.9 Z68.43
      60.0-69.9 Z68.44
      70 and over Z68.45
    pediatric
      5th percentile to less than 85th percentile for age Z68.52
      85th percentile to less than 95th percentile for age Z68.53
      greater than or equal to ninety-fifth percentile for age Z68.54
      less than fifth percentile for age Z68.51
  Mooser's A75.2
  rice (*see also* Loose, body, joint)
    knee M23.4 ☑
  rocking F98.4
Boeck's
  disease or sarcoid — *see* Sarcoidosis
  lupoid (miliary) D86.3
Boerhaave's syndrome (spontaneous esophageal rupture) K22.3
Boggy
  cervix N88.8
  uterus N85.8
Boil (*see also* Furuncle, by site)
  Aleppo B55.1

Boil — *continued*
  Baghdad B55.1
  Delhi B55.1
  lacrimal
    gland — *see* Dacryoadenitis
    passages (duct) (sac) — *see* Inflammation, lacrimal, passages, acute
  Natal B55.1
  orbit, orbital — *see* Abscess, orbit
  tropical B55.1
Bold hives — *see* Urticaria
Bombé, iris — *see* Membrane, pupillary
Bone — *see* condition
Bonnevie-Ullrich syndrome (*see also* Turner's syndrome) Q87.1
Bonnier's syndrome — *see* subcategory H81.8
Bonvale dam fever T73.3 ☑
Bony block of joint — *see* Ankylosis
BOOP (bronchiolitis obliterans organized pneumonia) J84.89
Borderline
  diabetes mellitus R73.03
  hypertension R03.0
  osteopenia M85.8 ☑
  pelvis, with obstruction during labor O65.1
  personality F60.3
Borna disease A83.9
Bornholm disease B33.0
Boston exanthem A88.0
Botalli, ductus (patent) (persistent) Q25.0
Bothriocephalus latus infestation B70.0
Botulism (foodborne intoxication) A05.1
  infant A48.51
  non-foodborne A48.52
  wound A48.52
Bouba — *see* Yaws
Bouchard's nodes (with arthropathy) M15.2
Bouffée délirante F23
Bouillaud's disease or syndrome (rheumatic heart disease) I01.9
Bourneville's disease Q85.1
Boutonniere deformity (finger) — *see* Deformity, finger, boutonniere
Bouveret (-Hoffmann) syndrome (paroxysmal tachycardia) I47.9
Bovine heart — *see* Hypertrophy, cardiac
Bowel — *see* condition
Bowen's
  dermatosis (precancerous) — *see* Neoplasm, skin, in situ
  disease — *see* Neoplasm, skin, in situ
  epithelioma — *see* Neoplasm, skin, in situ
  type
    epidermoid carcinoma-in-situ — *see* Neoplasm, skin, in situ
    intraepidermal squamous cell carcinoma — *see* Neoplasm, skin, in situ
Bowing
  femur (*see also* Deformity, limb, specified type NEC, thigh)
    congenital Q68.3
  fibula (*see also* Deformity, limb, specified type NEC, lower leg)
    congenital Q68.4
  forearm (*see also* Deformity, limb, specified type NEC, forearm)
  leg (s), long bones, congenital Q68.5
  radius — *see* Deformity, limb, specified type NEC, forearm
  tibia (*see also* Deformity, limb, specified type NEC, lower leg)
    congenital Q68.4
Bowleg (s) (acquired) M21.16 ☑
  congenital Q68.5
  rachitic E64.3
Boyd's dysentery A03.2
Brachial — *see* condition
Brachycardia R00.1
Brachycephaly Q75.0
Bradley's disease A08.19
Bradyarrhythmia, cardiac I49.8
Bradycardia (sinoatrial) (sinus) (vagal) R00.1
  neonatal P29.12
  reflex G90.09
  tachycardia syndrome I49.5
Bradykinesia R25.8
Bradypnea R06.89
Bradytachycardia I49.5
Brailsford's disease or osteochondrosis — *see* Osteochondrosis, juvenile, radius
Brain (*see also* condition)
  death G93.82
  syndrome — *see* Syndrome, brain

Branched-chain amino-acid disorder E71.2
Branchial — *see* condition
  cartilage, congenital Q18.2
Branchiogenic remnant (in neck) Q18.0
Brandt's syndrome (acrodermatitis enteropathica)
    E83.2
Brash (water) R12
Bravais-jacksonian epilepsy — *see* Epilepsy,
    localization-related, symptomatic, with simple
    partial seizures
Braxton Hicks contractions — *see* False, labor
Brazilian leishmaniasis B55.2
BRBPR K62.5
Break, retina (without detachment) H33.30 ☑
    with retinal detachment — *see* Detachment,
      retina
  horseshoe tear H33.31 ☑
  multiple H33.33 ☑
  round hole H33.32 ☑
Breakdown
  device, graft or implant (*see also* Complications,
    by site and type, mechanical) T85.618 ☑
    arterial graft NEC — *see* Complication,
      cardiovascular device, mechanical, vascular
    breast (implant) T85.41 ☑
    catheter NEC T85.618 ☑
      cystostomy T83.010 ☑
      Hopkins T83.018 ☑
      ileostomy T83.018 ☑
      dialysis (renal) T82.41 ☑
        intraperitoneal T85.611 ☑
      infusion NEC T82.514 ☑
        cranial T85.610 ☑
        epidural T85.610 ☑
        intrathecal T85.610 ☑
        spinal T85.610 ☑
        subarachnoid T85.610 ☑
        subdural T85.610 ☑
      nephrostomy T83.012 ☑
      urethral indwelling T83.011 ☑
      urinary NEC T83.018 ☑
      urostomy T83.018 ☑
    electronic (electrode) (pulse generator)
      (stimulator)
      bone T84.310 ☑
      cardiac T82.119 ☑
        electrode T82.110 ☑
        pulse generator T82.111 ☑
        specified type NEC T82.118 ☑
      nervous system — *see* Complication,
        prosthetic device, mechanical, electronic
        nervous system stimulator
      urinary — *see* Complication, genitourinary,
        device, urinary, mechanical
    fixation, internal (orthopedic) NEC — *see*
      Complication, fixation device, mechanical
    gastrointestinal — *see* Complications,
      prosthetic device, mechanical,
      gastrointestinal device
    genital NEC T83.418 ☑
      intrauterine contraceptive device T83.31 ☑
      penile prosthesis (cylinder) (implanted)
        (pump) (reservoir) T83.410 ☑
      testicular prosthesis T83.411 ☑
    heart NEC — *see* Complication, cardiovascular
      device, mechanical
    intrathecal infusion pump T85.615 ☑
    joint prosthesis — *see* Complications..., joint
      prosthesis, internal, mechanical, by site
    nervous system, specified device
      NEC T85.615 ☑
    ocular NEC — *see* Complications, prosthetic
      device, mechanical, ocular device
    orthopedic NEC — *see* Complication,
      orthopedic, device, mechanical
    specified NEC T85.618 ☑
    subcutaneous device pocket
      nervous system prosthetic device, implant, or
        graft T85.890 ☑
      other internal prosthetic device, implant, or
        graft T85.898 ☑
    sutures, permanent T85.612 ☑
      used in bone repair — *see* Complications,
        fixation device, internal (orthopedic),
        mechanical
    urinary NEC T83.118 ☑
      graft T83.21 ☑
      sphincter, implanted T83.111 ☑
      stent (ileal conduit)
        (nephroureteral) T83.113 ☑
      ureteral indwelling T83.112 ☑

Breakdown — *continued*
  device — *continued*
    vascular NEC — *see* Complication,
      cardiovascular device, mechanical
    ventricular intracranial shunt T85.01 ☑
  nervous F48.8
  perineum O90.1
  respirator J95.850
    specified NEC J95.859
  ventilator J95.850
    specified NEC J95.859
Breast (*see also* condition)
  buds E30.1
    in newborn P96.89
  dense R92.2
  nodule (*see also* Lump, breast) N63.0
Breath
  foul R19.6
  holder, child R06.89
  holding spell R06.89
  shortness R06.02
Breathing
  labored — *see* Hyperventilation
  mouth R06.5
    causing malocclusion M26.5 ☑
  periodic R06.3
    high altitude G47.32
Breathlessness R06.81
Breda's disease — *see* Yaws
Breech presentation (mother) O32.1 ☑
  causing obstructed labor O64.1 ☑
  footling O32.8 ☑
    causing obstructed labor O64.8 ☑
  incomplete O32.8 ☑
    causing obstructed labor O64.8 ☑
Breisky's disease N90.4
Brennemann's syndrome I88.0
Brenner
  tumor (benign) D27.9
    borderline malignancy D39.1 ☑
    malignant C56 ☑
    proliferating D39.1 ☑
Bretonneau's disease or angina A36.0
Breus' mole O02.0
Brevicollis Q76.49
Brickmakers' anemia B76.9 *[D63.8]*
Bridge, myocardial Q24.5
Bright red blood per rectum (BRBPR) K62.5
Bright's disease (*see also* Nephritis)
  arteriosclerotic — *see* Hypertension, kidney
Brill (-Zinsser) disease (recrudescent typhus) A75.1
  flea-borne A75.2
  louse-borne A75.1
Brill-Symmers' disease C82.90
Brion-Kayser disease — *see* Fever, parathyroid
Briquet's disorder or syndrome F45.0
Brissaud's
  infantilism or dwarfism E23.0
  motor-verbal tic F95.2
Brittle
  bones disease Q78.0
  nails L60.3
    congenital Q84.6
Broad (*see also* condition)
  beta disease E78.2
  ligament laceration syndrome N83.8
Broad- or floating-betalipoproteinemia E78.2
Brock's syndrome (atelectasis due to enlarged lymph
    nodes) J98.19
Brocq-Duhring disease (dermatitis herpetiformis)
    L13.0
Brodie's abscess or disease M86.8X ☑
Broken
  arches (*see also* Deformity, limb, flat foot)
  arm (meaning upper limb) — *see* Fracture, arm
  back — *see* Fracture, vertebra
  bone — *see* Fracture
  implant or internal device — *see* Complications,
    by site and type, mechanical
  leg (meaning lower limb) — *see* Fracture, leg
  nose S02.2 ☑
  tooth, teeth — *see* Fracture, tooth
Bromhidrosis, bromidrosis L75.0
Bromidism, bromism G92
  due to
    correct substance properly administered — *see*
      Table of Drugs and Chemicals, by drug,
      adverse effect
    overdose or wrong substance given or taken —
      see Table of Drugs and Chemicals, by drug,
      poisoning
  chronic (dependence) F13.20

Bromidrosiphobia F40.298
Bronchi, bronchial — *see* condition
Bronchiectasis (cylindrical) (diffuse) (fusiform)
    (localized) (saccular) J47.9
  with
    acute
      bronchitis J47.0
      lower respiratory infection J47.0
    exacerbation (acute) J47.1
  congenital Q33.4
  tuberculous NEC — *see* Tuberculosis, pulmonary
Bronchiolectasis — *see* Bronchiectasis
Bronchiolitis (acute) (infective) (subacute) J21.9
  with
    bronchospasm or obstruction J21.9
    influenza, flu or grippe — *see* Influenza, with,
      respiratory manifestations NEC
  chemical (chronic) J68.4
    acute J68.0
  chronic (fibrosing) (obliterative) J44.9
  due to
    external agent — *see* Bronchitis, acute, due to
    human metapneumovirus J21.1
    respiratory syncytial virus J21.0
    specified organism NEC J21.8
  fibrosa obliterans J44.9
  influenzal — *see* Influenza, with, respiratory
    manifestations NEC
  obliterans J42
    with organizing pneumonia (BOOP) J84.89
  obliterative (chronic) (subacute) J44.9
    due to fumes or vapors J68.4
    due to chemicals, gases, fumes or vapors
      (inhalation) J68.4
  respiratory, interstitial lung disease J84.115
Bronchitis (diffuse) (fibrinous) (hypostatic) (infective)
    (membranous) J40
  with
    influenza, flu or grippe — *see* Influenza, with,
      respiratory manifestations NEC
    obstruction (airway) (lung) J44.9
    tracheitis (I5 years of age and above) J40
      acute or subacute J20.9
      chronic J42
      under I5 years of age J20.9
  acute or subacute (with bronchospasm or
    obstruction) J20.9
    with
      bronchiectasis J47.0
      chronic obstructive pulmonary disease J44.0
    chemical (due to gases, fumes or vapors) J68.0
    due to
      fumes or vapors J68.0
      Haemophilus influenzae J20.1
      Mycoplasma pneumoniae J20.0
      radiation J70.0
      specified organism NEC J20.8
      Streptococcus J20.2
      virus
        coxsackie J20.3
        echovirus J20.7
        parainfluenzae J20.4
        respiratory syncytial J20.5
        rhinovirus J20.6
    viral NEC J20.8
  allergic (acute) J45.909
    with
      exacerbation (acute) J45.901
      status asthmaticus J45.902
  arachidic T17.528 ☑
  aspiration (due to fumes or vapors) J68.0
  asthmatic J45.9 ☑
    chronic J44.9
      with
        acute lower respiratory infection J44.0
        exacerbation (acute) J44.1
  capillary — *see* Pneumonia, broncho
  caseous (tuberculous) A15.5
  Castellani's A69.8
  catarrhal (I5 years of age and above) J40
    acute — *see* Bronchitis, acute
    chronic J41.0
    under I5 years of age J20.9
  chemical (acute) (subacute) J68.0
    chronic J68.4
    due to fumes or vapors J68.0
      chronic J68.4
  chronic J42
    with
      airways obstruction J44.9
      tracheitis (chronic) J42
    asthmatic (obstructive) J44.9

Bronchitis — *continued*
  chronic — *continued*
    catarrhal J41.0
    chemical (due to fumes or vapors) J68.4
    due to
      chemicals, gases, fumes or vapors
        (inhalation) J68.4
      radiation J70.1
      tobacco smoking J41.0
    emphysematous J44.9
    mucopurulent J41.1
    non-obstructive J41.0
    obliterans J44.9
    obstructive J44.9
    purulent J41.1
    simple J41.0
  croupous — *see* Bronchitis, acute
  due to gases, fumes or vapors (chemical) J68.0
  emphysematous (obstructive) J44.9
  exudative — *see* Bronchitis, acute
  fetid J41.1
  grippal — *see* Influenza, with, respiratory
    manifestations NEC
  in those under I5 years age — *see* Bronchitis,
    acute
    chronic — *see* Bronchitis, chronic
  influenzal — *see* Influenza, with, respiratory
    manifestations NEC
  mixed simple and mucopurulent J41.8
  moulder's J62.8
  mucopurulent (chronic) (recurrent) J41.1
    acute or subacute J20.9
    simple (mixed) J41.8
  obliterans (chronic) J44.9
  obstructive (chronic) (diffuse) J44.9
  pituitous J41.1
  pneumococcal, acute or subacute J20.2
  pseudomembranous, acute or subacute — *see*
    Bronchitis, acute
  purulent (chronic) (recurrent) J41.1
    acute or subacute — *see* Bronchitis, acute
  putrid J41.1
  senile (chronic) J42
  simple and mucopurulent (mixed) J41.8
  smokers' J41.0
  spirochetal NEC A69.8
  subacute — *see* Bronchitis, acute
  suppurative (chronic) J41.1
    acute or subacute — *see* Bronchitis, acute
  tuberculous A15.5
  under I5 years of age — *see* Bronchitis, acute
    chronic — *see* Bronchitis, chronic
  viral NEC, acute or subacute (*see also* Bronchitis,
    acute) J20.8
Bronchoalveolitis J18.0
Bronchoaspergillosis B44.1
Bronchocele meaning goiter E04.0
Broncholithiasis J98.09
  tuberculous NEC A15.5
Bronchomalacia J98.09
  congenital Q32.2
Bronchomycosis NOS B49 *[J99]*
  candidal B37.1
Bronchopleuropneumonia — *see* Pneumonia,
  broncho
Bronchopneumonia — *see* Pneumonia, broncho
Bronchopneumonitis — *see* Pneumonia, broncho
Bronchopulmonary — *see* condition
Bronchopulmonitis — *see* Pneumonia, broncho
Bronchorrhagia (*see* Hemoptysis)
Bronchorrhea J98.09
  acute J20.9
  chronic (infective) (purulent) J42
Bronchospasm (acute) J98.01
  with
    bronchiolitis, acute J21.9
    bronchitis, acute (conditions in J20) — *see*
      Bronchitis, acute
  due to external agent — *see* condition,
    respiratory, acute, due to
  exercise induced J45.990
Bronchospirochetosis A69.8
  Castellani A69.8
Bronchostenosis J98.09
Bronchus — *see* condition
Brontophobia F40.220
Bronze baby syndrome P83.88
Brooke's tumor — *see* Neoplasm, skin, benign
Brown enamel of teeth (hereditary) K00.5
Brown's sheath syndrome H50.61 ☑
Brown-Séquard disease, paralysis or syndrome
  G83.81

Bruce sepsis A23.0
Brucellosis (infection) A23.9
  abortus A23.1
  canis A23.3
  dermatitis A23.9
  melitensis A23.0
  mixed A23.8
  sepsis A23.9
    melitensis A23.0
    specified NEC A23.8
  suis A23.2
Bruck-de Lange disease Q87.1
Bruck's disease — *see* Deformity, limb
BRUE (brief resolved unexplained event) R68.13
Brugsch's syndrome Q82.8
Bruise (skin surface intact) (*see also* Contusion)
  with
    open wound — *see* Wound, ope
    internal organ — *see* Injury, by site
    newborn P54.5
  scalp, due to birth injury, newborn P12.3
  umbilical cord O69.5 ☑
Bruit (arterial) R09.89
  cardiac R01.1
Brush burn — *see* Abrasion, by site
Bruton's X-linked agammaglobulinemia D80.0
Bruxism
  psychogenic F45.8
  sleep related G47.63
Bubbly lung syndrome P27.0
Bubo I88.8
  blennorrhagic (gonococcal) A54.89
  chancroidal A57
  climatic A55
  due to Haemophilus ducreyi A57
  gonococcal A54.89
  indolent (nonspecific) I88.8
  inguinal (nonspecific) I88.8
    chancroidal A57
    climatic A55
    due to H. ducreyi A57
    infective I88.8
  scrofulous (tuberculous) A18.2
  soft chancre A57
  suppurating — *see* Lymphadenitis, acute
  syphilitic (primary) A51.0
    congenital A50.07
  tropical A55
  virulent (chancroidal) A57
Bubonic plague A20.0
Bubonocele — *see* Hernia, inguinal
Buccal — *see* condition
Buchanan's disease or osteochondrosis M91.0
Buchem's syndrome (hyperostosis corticalis) M85.2
Bucket-handle fracture or tear (semilunar cartilage)
  — *see* Tear, meniscus
Budd-Chiari syndrome (hepatic vein thrombosis)
  I82.0
Budgerigar fancier's disease or lung J67.2
Buds
  breast E30.1
    in newborn P96.89
Buerger's disease (thromboangiitis obliterans) I73.1
Bulbar — *see* condition
Bulbus cordis (left ventricle) (persistent) Q21.8
Bulimia (nervosa) F50.2
  atypical F50.9
  normal weight F50.9
Bulky
  stools R19.5
  uterus N85.2
Bulla (e) R23.8
  lung (emphysematous) (solitary) J43.9
    newborn P25.8
Bullet wound (*see also* Wound, open)
  fracture - code as Fracture, by site
  internal organ — *see* Injury, by site
Bundle
  branch block (complete) (false) (incomplete) —
    see Block, bundle-branch
  of His — *see* condition
Bunion M21.61 ☑
  tailor's M21.62 ☑
Bunionette M21.62 ☑
Buphthalmia, buphthalmos (congenital) Q15.0
Burdwan fever B55.0
Bürger-Grütz disease or syndrome E78.3
Buried
  penis (congenital) Q55.64
    acquired N48.83
  roots K08.3
Burke's syndrome K86.89

Burkitt
  cell leukemia C91.0 ☑
  lymphoma (malignant) C83.7 ☑
    small noncleaved, diffuse C83.7 ☑
    spleen C83.77
    undifferentiated C83.7 ☑
  tumor C83.7 ☑
  type
    acute lymphoblastic leukemia C91.0 ☑
    undifferentiated C83.7 ☑
Burn (electricity) (flame) (hot gas, liquid or hot
  object) (radiation) (steam) (thermal) T30.0
  abdomen, abdominal (muscle) (wall) T21.02 ☑
    first degree T21.12 ☑
    second degree T21.22 ☑
    third degree T21.32 ☑
  above elbow T22.039 ☑
    first degree T22.139 ☑
    left T22.032 ☑
      first degree T22.132 ☑
      second degree T22.232 ☑
      third degree T22.332 ☑
    right T22.031 ☑
      first degree T22.131 ☑
      second degree T22.231 ☑
      third degree T22.331 ☑
    second degree T22.239 ☑
    third degree T22.339 ☑
  acid (caustic) (external) (internal) — *see*
    Corrosion, by site
  alimentary tract NEC T28.2 ☑
    esophagus T28.1 ☑
    mouth T28.0 ☑
    pharynx T28.0 ☑
  alkaline (caustic) (external) (internal) — *see*
    Corrosion, by site
  ankle T25.019 ☑
    first degree T25.119 ☑
    left T25.012 ☑
      first degree T25.112 ☑
      second degree T25.212 ☑
      third degree T25.312 ☑
    multiple with foot — *see* Burn, lower, limb,
      multiple, ankle and foot
    right T25.011 ☑
      first degree T25.111 ☑
      second degree T25.211 ☑
      third degree T25.311 ☑
    second degree T25.219 ☑
    third degree T25.319 ☑
  anus — *see* Burn, buttock
  arm (lower) (upper) — *see* Burn, upper, limb
  axilla T22.049 ☑
    first degree T22.149 ☑
    left T22.042 ☑
      first degree T22.142 ☑
      second degree T22.242 ☑
      third degree T22.342 ☑
    right T22.041 ☑
      first degree T22.141 ☑
      second degree T22.241 ☑
      third degree T22.341 ☑
    second degree T22.249 ☑
    third degree T22.349 ☑
  back (lower) T21.04 ☑
    first degree T21.14 ☑
    second degree T21.24 ☑
    third degree T21.34 ☑
    upper T21.03 ☑
      first degree T21.13 ☑
      second degree T21.23 ☑
      third degree T21.33 ☑
  blisters - code as Burn, second degree, by site
  breast (s) — *see* Burn, chest wall
  buttock (s) T21.05 ☑
    first degree T21.15 ☑
    second degree T21.25 ☑
    third degree T21.35 ☑
  calf T24.039 ☑
    first degree T24.139 ☑
    left T24.032 ☑
      first degree T24.132 ☑
      second degree T24.232 ☑
      third degree T24.332 ☑
    right T24.031 ☑
      first degree T24.131 ☑
      second degree T24.231 ☑
      third degree T24.331 ☑
    second degree T24.239 ☑
    third degree T24.339 ☑
  canthus (eye) — *see* Burn, eyelid
  caustic acid or alkaline — *see* Corrosion, by site

Cell - Chandler's

Cell (s), cellular (*see also* condition)
  in urine R82.99
Cellulitis (diffuse) (phlegmonous) (septic)
  (suppurative) L03.90
    abdominal wall L03.311
    anaerobic A48.0
    ankle — *see* Cellulitis, lower limb
    anus K61.0
    arm — *see* Cellulitis, upper limb
    auricle (ear) — *see* Cellulitis, ear
    axilla L03.11 ☑
    back (any part) L03.312
    breast (acute) (nonpuerperal) (subacute) N61.0
      nipple N61.0
    broad ligament
      acute N73.0
    buttock L03.317
    cervical (meaning neck) L03.221
    cervix (uteri) — *see* Cervicitis
    cheek (external) L03.211
      internal K12.2
    chest wall L03.313
    chronic L03.90
    clostridial A48.0
    corpus cavernosum N48.22
    digit
      finger — *see* Cellulitis, finger
      toe — *see* Cellulitis, toe
    Douglas' cul-de-sac or pouch
      acute N73.0
    drainage site (following operation) T81.4 ☑
    ear (external) H60.1 ☑
    eosinophilic (granulomatous) L98.3
    erysipelatous — *see* Erysipelas
    external auditory canal — *see* Cellulitis, ear
    eyelid — *see* Abscess, eyelid
    face NEC L03.211
    finger (intrathecal) (periosteal) (subcutaneous)
      (subcuticular) L03.01 ☑
    foot — *see* Cellulitis, lower limb
    gangrenous — *see* Gangrene
    genital organ NEC
      female (external) N76.4
      male N49.9
        multiple sites N49.8
        specified NEC N49.8
    gluteal (region) L03.317
    gonococcal A54.89
    groin L03.314
    hand — *see* Cellulitis, upper limb
    head NEC L03.811
      face (any part, except ear, eye and
        nose) L03.211
    heel — *see* Cellulitis, lower limb
    hip — *see* Cellulitis, lower limb
    jaw (region) L03.211
    knee — *see* Cellulitis, lower limb
    labium (majus) (minus) — *see* Vulvitis
    lacrimal passages — *see* Inflammation, lacrimal,
      passages
    larynx J38.7
    leg — *see* Cellulitis, lower limb
    lip K13.0
    lower limb L03.11 ☑
      toe — *see* Cellulitis, toe
    mouth (floor) K12.2
    multiple sites, so stated L03.90
    nasopharynx J39.1
    navel L03.316
      newborn P38.9
        with mild hemorrhage P38.1
        without hemorrhage P38.9
    neck (region) L03.221
    nipple (acute) (nonpuerperal) (subacute) N61.0
    nose (septum) (external) J34.0
    orbit, orbital H05.01 ☑
    palate (soft) K12.2
    pectoral (region) L03.313
    pelvis, pelvic (chronic)
      female (*see also* Disease, pelvis,
        inflammatory) N73.2
        acute N73.0
      following ectopic or molar pregnancy O08.0
      male K65.0
    penis N48.22
    perineal, perineum L03.315
    periorbital L03.213
    perirectal K61.1
    peritonsillar J36
    periurethral N34.0
    periuterine (*see also* Disease, pelvis,
      inflammatory) N73.2
      acute N73.0

Cellulitis — *continued*
  pharynx J39.1
  preseptal L03.213
  rectum K61.1
  retroperitoneal K68.9
  round ligament
    acute N73.0
  scalp (any part) L03.811
  scrotum N49.2
  seminal vesicle N49.0
  shoulder — *see* Cellulitis, upper limb
  specified site NEC L03.818
  submandibular (region) (space) (triangle) K12.2
    gland K11.3
  submaxillary (region) K12.2
    gland K11.3
  thigh — *see* Cellulitis, lower limb
  thumb (intrathecal) (periosteal) (subcutaneous)
    (subcuticular) — *see* Cellulitis, finger
  toe (intrathecal) (periosteal) (subcutaneous)
    (subcuticular) L03.03 ☑
  tonsil J36
  trunk L03.319
    abdominal wall L03.311
    back (any part) L03.312
    buttock L03.317
    chest wall L03.313
    groin L03.314
    perineal, perineum L03.315
    umbilicus L03.316
  tuberculous (primary) A18.4
  umbilicus L03.316
  upper limb L03.11 ☑
    axilla — *see* Cellulitis, axilla
    finger — *see* Cellulitis, finger
    thumb — *see* Cellulitis, finger
  vaccinal T88.0 ☑
  vocal cord J38.3
  vulva — *see* Vulvitis
  wrist — *see* Cellulitis, upper limb
Cementoblastoma, benign — *see* Cyst, calcifying
  odontogenic
Cementoma — *see* Cyst, calcifying odontogenic
Cementoperiostitis — *see* Periodontitis
Cementosis K03.4
Central auditory processing disorder H93.25
Central pain syndrome G89.0
Cephalematocele, cephal (o) hematocele
    newborn P52.8
      birth injury P10.8
    traumatic — *see* Hematoma, brain
Cephalematoma, cephalhematoma (calcified)
    newborn (birth injury) P12.0
    traumatic — *see* Hematoma, brain
Cephalgia, cephalalgia (*see also* Headache)
    histamine G44.009
      intractable G44.001
      not intractable G44.009
    trigeminal autonomic (TAC) NEC G44.099
      intractable G44.091
      not intractable G44.099
Cephalic — *see* condition
Cephalitis — *see* Encephalitis
Cephalocele — *see* Encephalocele
Cephalomenia N94.89
Cephalopelvic — *see* condition
Cerclage (with cervical incompetence) in pregnancy
  — *see* Incompetence, cervix, in pregnancy
Cerebellitis — *see* Encephalitis
Cerebellum, cerebellar — *see* condition
Cerebral — *see* condition
Cerebritis — *see* Encephalitis
Cerebro-hepato-renal syndrome Q87.89
Cerebromalacia — *see* Softening, brain
    sequelae of cerebrovascular disease I69.398
Cerebroside lipidosis E75.22
Cerebrospasticity (congenital) G80.1
Cerebrospinal — *see* condition
Cerebrum — *see* condition
Ceroid-lipofuscinosis, neuronal E75.4
Cerumen (accumulation) (impacted) H61.2 ☑
Cervical (*see also* condition)
    auricle Q18.2
    dysplasia in pregnancy — *see* Abnormal, cervix,
      in pregnancy or childbirth
    erosion in pregnancy — *see* Abnormal, cervix, in
      pregnancy or childbirth
    fibrosis in pregnancy — *see* Abnormal, cervix, in
      pregnancy or childbirth
    fusion syndrome Q76.1
    rib Q76.5
    shortening (complicating pregnancy) O26.87 ☑

Cervicalgia M54.2
Cervicitis (acute) (chronic) (nonvenereal) (senile
  (atrophic)) (subacute) (with ulceration) N72
    with
      abortion — *see* Abortion, by type complicated
        by genital tract and pelvic infection
      ectopic pregnancy O08.0
      molar pregnancy O08.0
    chlamydial A56.09
    gonococcal A54.03
    herpesviral A60.03
    puerperal (postpartum) O86.11
    syphilitic A52.76
    trichomonal A59.09
    tuberculous A18.16
Cervicocolpitis (emphysematosa) (*see also* Cervicitis)
  N72
Cervix — *see* condition
Cesarean delivery, previous, affecting management
  of pregnancy O34.219
    classical (vertical) scar O34.212
    low transverse scar O34.211
Céstan (-Chenais) paralysis or syndrome G46.3
Céstan-Raymond syndrome I65.8
Cestode infestation B71.9
  specified type NEC B71.8
Cestodiasis B71.9
Chabert's disease A22.9
Chacaleh E53.8
Chafing L30.4
Chagas' (-Mazza) disease (chronic) B57.2
  with
    cardiovascular involvement NEC B57.2
    digestive system involvement B57.30
      megacolon B57.32
      megaesophagus B57.31
      other specified B57.39
    megacolon B57.32
    megaesophagus B57.31
    myocarditis B57.2
    nervous system involvement B57.40
      meningitis B57.41
      meningoencephalitis B57.42
      other specified B57.49
    specified organ involvement NEC B57.5
  acute (with) B57.1
    cardiovascular NEC B57.0
    myocarditis B57.0
Chagres fever B50.9
Chairridden Z74.09
Chalasia (cardiac sphincter) K21.9
Chalazion H00.19
    left H00.16
      lower H00.15
      upper H00.14
    right H00.13
      lower H00.12
      upper H00.11
Chalcosis (*see also* Disorder, globe, degenerative,
  chalcosis)
    cornea — *see* Deposit, cornea
    crystalline lens — *see* Cataract, complicated
    retina H35.89
Chalicosis (pulmonum) J62.8
Chancre (any genital site) (hard) (hunterian) (mixed)
  (primary) (seronegative) (seropositive) (syphilitic)
  A51.0
    congenital A50.07
    conjunctiva NEC A51.2
    Ducrey's A57
    extragenital A51.2
    eyelid A51.2
    lip A51.2
    nipple A51.2
    Nisbet's A57
    of
      carate A67.0
      pinta A67.0
      yaws A66.0
    palate, soft A51.2
    phagedenic A57
    simple A57
    soft A57
      bubo A57
      palate A51.2
    urethra A51.0
    yaws A66.0
Chancroid (anus) (genital) (penis) (perineum)
  (rectum) (urethra) (vulva) A57
Chandler's disease (osteochondritis dissecans, hip)
  — *see* Osteochondritis, dissecans, hip

☑ Additional character required

Change (s) (in) (of) (*see also* Removal)
  arteriosclerotic — *see* Arteriosclerosis
  bone (*see also* Disorder, bone)
    diabetic — *see* Diabetes, bone change
  bowel habit R19.4
  cardiorenal (vascular) — *see* Hypertension,
    cardiorenal
  cardiovascular — *see* Disease, cardiovascular
  circulatory I99.9
  cognitive (mild) (organic) R41.89
  color, tooth, teeth
    during formation K00.8
    posteruptive K03.7
  contraceptive device Z30.433
  corneal membrane H18.30
    Bowman's membrane fold or rupture H18.31 ☑
    Descemet's membrane
      fold H18.32 ☑
      rupture H18.33 ☑
  coronary — *see* Disease, heart, ischemic
  degenerative, spine or vertebra — *see*
    Spondylosis
  dental pulp, regressive K04.2
  dressing (nonsurgical) Z48.00
    surgical Z48.01
  heart — *see* Disease, heart
  hip joint — *see* Derangement, joint, hip
  hyperplastic larynx J38.7
  hypertrophic
    nasal sinus J34.89
    turbinate, nasal J34.3
    upper respiratory tract J39.8
  indwelling catheter Z46.6
  inflammatory (*see also* Inflammation)
    sacroiliac M46.1
  job, anxiety concerning Z56.1
  joint — *see* Derangement, joint
  life — *see* Menopause
  mental status R41.82
  minimal (glomerular) (*see also* N00-N07 with
    fourth character .0) N05.0
  myocardium, myocardial — *see* Degeneration,
    myocardial
  of life — *see* Menopause
  pacemaker Z45.018
    pulse generator Z45.010
  personality (enduring) F68.8
    due to (secondary to)
      general medical condition F07.0
    secondary (nonspecific) F60.89
  regressive, dental pulp K04.2
  renal — *see* Disease, renal
  retina H35.9
    myopic (*see also* Myopia,
      degenerative) H44.2 ☑
  sacroiliac joint M53.3
  senile (*see also* condition) R54
  sensory R20.8
  skin R23.9
    acute, due to ultraviolet radiation L56.9
      specified NEC L56.8
    chronic, due to nonionizing radiation L57.9
      specified NEC L57.8
    cyanosis R23.0
    flushing R23.2
    pallor R23.1
    petechiae R23.3
    specified change NEC R23.8
    swelling — *see* Mass, localized
    texture R23.4
  trophic
    arm — *see* Mononeuropathy, upper limb
    leg — *see* Mononeuropathy, lower limb
  vascular I99.9
  vasomotor I73.9
  voice R49.9
    psychogenic F44.4
    specified NEC R49.8
Changing sleep-work schedule, affecting sleep
  G47.26
Changuinola fever A93.1
Chapping skin T69.8 ☑
Charcot-Marie-Tooth disease, paralysis or syndrome
  G60.0
Charcot's
  arthropathy — *see* Arthropathy, neuropathic
  cirrhosis K74.3
  disease (tabetic arthropathy) A52.16
  joint (disease) (tabetic) A52.16
    diabetic — *see* Diabetes, with, arthropathy
    syringomyelic G95.0
  syndrome (intermittent claudication) I73.9

CHARGE association Q89.8
Charley-horse (quadriceps) M62.831
  traumatic (quadriceps) S76.11 ☑
Charlouis' disease — *see* Yaws
Cheadle's disease E54
Checking (of)
  cardiac pacemaker (battery)
    (electrode(s)) Z45.018
    pulse generator Z45.010
  implantable subdermal contraceptive Z30.46
  intrauterine contraceptive device Z30.431
  wound Z48.0 ☑
    due to injury - code to Injury, by site, using
      appropriate seventh character for
      subsequent encounter
Check-up — *see* Examination
Chédiak-Higashi (-Steinbrinck) syndrome
  (congenital gigantism of peroxidase granules)
  E70.330
Cheek — *see* condition
Cheese itch B88.0
Cheese-washer's lung J67.8
Cheese-worker's lung J67.8
Cheilitis (acute) (angular) (catarrhal) (chronic)
  (exfoliative) (gangrenous) (glandular) (infectional)
  (suppurative) (ulcerative) (vesicular) K13.0
    actinic (due to sun) L56.8
      other than from sun L59.8
    candidal B37.83
Cheilodynia K13.0
Cheiloschisis — *see* Cleft, lip
Cheilosis (angular) K13.0
  with pellagra E52
  due to
    vitamin B2 (riboflavin) deficiency E53.0
Cheiromegaly M79.89
Cheiropompholyx L30.1
Cheloid — *see* Keloid
Chemical burn — *see* Corrosion, by site
Chemodectoma — *see* Paraganglioma,
  nonchromaffin
Chemosis, conjunctiva — *see* Edema, conjunctiva
Chemotherapy (session) (for)
  cancer Z51.11
  neoplasm Z51.11
Cherubism M27.8
Chest — *see* condition
Cheyne-Stokes breathing (respiration) R06.3
Chiari's
  disease or syndrome (hepatic vein
    thrombosis) I82.0
  malformation
    type I G93.5
    type II — *see* Spina bifida
  net Q24.8
Chicago disease B40.9
Chickenpox — *see* Varicella
Chiclero ulcer or sore B55.1
Chigger (infestation) B88.0
Chignon (disease) B36.8
  newborn (from vacuum extraction) (birth
    injury) P12.1
Chilaiditi's syndrome (subphrenic displacement,
  colon) Q43.3
Chilblain (s) (lupus) T69.1 ☑
Child
  custody dispute Z65.3
Childbirth — *see* Delivery
Childhood
  cerebral X-linked adrenoleukodystrophy E71.520
  period of rapid growth Z00.2
Chill (s) R68.83
  with fever R50.9
  congestive in malarial regions B54
  without fever R68.83
Chilomastigiasis A07.8
Chimera 46,XX/46,XY Q99.0
Chin — *see* condition
Chinese dysentery A03.9
Chionophobia F40.228
Chitral fever A93.1
Chlamydia, chlamydial A74.9
  cervicitis A56.09
  conjunctivitis A74.0
  cystitis A56.01
  endometritis A56.11
  epididymitis A56.19
  female
    pelvic inflammatory disease A56.11
    pelviperitonitis A56.11
  orchitis A56.19
  peritonitis A74.81

Chlamydia — *continued*
  pharyngitis A56.4
  proctitis A56.3
  psittaci (infection) A70
  salpingitis A56.11
  sexually-transmitted infection NEC A56.8
  specified NEC A74.89
  urethritis A56.01
  vulvovaginitis A56.02
Chlamydiosis — *see* Chlamydia
Chloasma (skin) (idiopathic) (symptomatic) L81.1
  eyelid H02.719
    hyperthyroid E05.90 *[H02.719]*
      with thyroid storm E05.91 *[H02.719]*
    left H02.716
      lower H02.715
      upper H02.714
    right H02.713
      lower H02.712
      upper H02.711
Chloroma C92.3
Chlorosis D50.9
  Egyptian B76.9 *[D63.8]*
  miner's B76.9 *[D63.8]*
Chlorotic anemia D50.8
Chocolate cyst (ovary) N80.1
Choked
  disc or disk — *see* Papilledema
  on food, phlegm, or vomitus NOS — *see* Foreign
    body, by site
  while vomiting NOS — *see* Foreign body, by site
Chokes (resulting from bends) T70.3 ☑
Choking sensation R09.89
Cholangiectasis K83.8
Cholangiocarcinoma
  with hepatocellular carcinoma, combined C22.0
  liver C22.1
  specified site NEC — *see* Neoplasm, malignant,
    by site
  unspecified site C22.1
Cholangiohepatitis K83.8
  due to fluke infestation B66.1
Cholangiohepatoma C22.0
Cholangiolitis (acute) (chronic) (extrahepatic)
  (gangrenous) (intrahepatic) K83.0
  paratyphoidal — *see* Fever, paratyphoid
  typhoidal A01.09
Cholangioma D13.4
  malignant — *see* Cholangiocarcinoma
Cholangitis (ascending) (primary) (recurrent)
  (sclerosing) (secondary) (stenosing) (suppurative)
  K83.0
  with calculus, bile duct — *see* Calculus, bile duct,
    with cholangitis
  chronic nonsuppurative destructive K74.3
Cholecystectasia K82.8
Cholecystitis K81.9
  with
    calculus, stones in
      bile duct (common) (hepatic) — *see* Calculus,
        bile duct, with cholecystitis
      cystic duct — *see* Calculus, gallbladder, with
        cholecystitis
      gallbladder — *see* Calculus, gallbladder, with
        cholecystitis
      choledocholithiasis — *see* Calculus, bile duct,
        with cholecystitis
      cholelithiasis — *see* Calculus, gallbladder, with
        cholecystitis
  acute (emphysematous) (gangrenous)
    (suppurative) K81.0
    with
      calculus, stones in
        cystic duct — *see* Calculus, gallbladder, with
          cholecystitis, acute
        gallbladder — *see* Calculus, gallbladder,
          with cholecystitis, acute
        choledocholithiasis — *see* Calculus, bile duct,
          with cholecystitis, acute
        cholelithiasis — *see* Calculus, gallbladder,
          with cholecystitis, acute
      chronic cholecystitis K81.2
        with gallbladder calculus K80.12
          with obstruction K80.13
  chronic K81.1
    with acute cholecystitis K81.2
      with gallbladder calculus K80.12
        with obstruction K80.13
  emphysematous (acute) — *see* Cholecystitis,
    acute
  gangrenous — *see* Cholecystitis, acute
  paratyphoidal, current A01.4

Cholecystitis - Chronic

Cholecystitis — *continued*
  suppurative — *see* Cholecystitis, acute
  typhoidal A01.09
Cholecystolithiasis — *see* Calculus, gallbladder
Choledochitis (suppurative) K83.0
Choledocholith — *see* Calculus, bile duct
Choledocholithiasis (common duct) (hepatic duct)
  — *see* Calculus, bile duct
  cystic — *see* Calculus, gallbladder
  typhoidal A01.09
Cholelithiasis (cystic duct) (gallbladder) (impacted)
  (multiple) — *see* Calculus, gallbladder
  bile duct (common) (hepatic) — *see* Calculus,
    bile duct
  hepatic duct — *see* Calculus, bile duct
  specified NEC K80.80
    with obstruction K80.81
Cholemia (*see also* Jaundice)
  familial (simple) (congenital) E80.4
  Gilbert's E80.4
Choleperitoneum, choleperitonitis K65.3
Cholera (Asiatic) (epidemic) (malignant) A00.9
  antimonial — *see* Poisoning, antimony
  classical A00.0
  due to Vibrio cholerae 01 A00.9
    biovar cholerae A00.0
    biovar eltor A00.1
    el tor A00.1
    el tor A00.1
Cholerine — *see* Cholera
Cholestasis NEC K83.1
  with hepatocyte injury K71.0
  due to total parenteral nutrition (TPN) K76.89
  pure K71.0
Cholesteatoma (ear) (middle) (with reaction)
  H71.9 ☑
  attic H71.0 ☑
  external ear (canal) H60.4 ☑
  mastoid H71.2 ☑
  postmastoidectomy cavity (recurrent) — *see*
    Complications, postmastoidectomy,
    recurrent cholesteatoma
  recurrent (postmastoidectomy) — *see*
    Complications, postmastoidectomy,
    recurrent cholesteatoma
  tympanum H71.1 ☑
Cholesteatosis, diffuse H71.3 ☑
Cholesteremia E78.00
Cholesterin in vitreous — *see* Deposit, crystalline
Cholesterol
  deposit
    retina H35.89
    vitreous — *see* Deposit, crystalline
  elevated (high) E78.00
    with elevated (high) triglycerides E78.2
    screening for Z13.220
  imbibition of gallbladder K82.4
Cholesterolemia (essential) (pure) E78.00
  familial E78.01
  hereditary E78.01
Cholesterolosis, cholesterosis (gallbladder) K82.4
  cerebrotendinous E75.5
Cholocolic fistula K82.3
Choluria R82.2
Chondritis M94.8X9
  auricular H61.03 ☑
  costal (Tietze's) M94.0
  external ear H61.03 ☑
  patella, posttraumatic — *see* Chondromalacia,
    patella
  pinna H61.03 ☑
  purulent M94.8X ☑
  tuberculous NEC A18.02
    intervertebral A18.01
Chondroblastoma (*see also* Neoplasm, bone,
  benign)
  malignant — *see* Neoplasm, bone, malignant
Chondrocalcinosis M11.20
  ankle M11.27 ☑
  elbow M11.22 ☑
  familial M11.10
    ankle M11.17 ☑
    elbow M11.12 ☑
    foot joint M11.17 ☑
    hand joint M11.14 ☑
    hip M11.15 ☑
    knee M11.16 ☑
    multiple site M11.19
    shoulder M11.11 ☑
    vertebrae M11.18
    wrist M11.13 ☑
  foot joint M11.27 ☑

Chondrocalcinosis — *continued*
  hand joint M11.24 ☑
  hip M11.25 ☑
  knee M11.26 ☑
  multiple site M11.29
  shoulder M11.21 ☑
  vertebrae M11.28
  specified type NEC M11.20
    ankle M11.27 ☑
    elbow M11.22 ☑
    foot joint M11.27 ☑
    hand joint M11.24 ☑
    hip M11.25 ☑
    knee M11.26 ☑
    multiple site M11.29
    shoulder M11.21 ☑
    vertebrae M11.28
    wrist M11.23 ☑
  wrist M11.23 ☑
Chondrodermatitis nodularis helicis or anthelicis —
  see Perichondritis, ear
Chondrodysplasia Q78.9
  with hemangioma Q78.4
  calcificans congenita Q77.3
  fetalis Q77.4
  metaphyseal (Jansen's) (McKusick's)
    (Schmid's) Q78.8
  punctata Q77.3
Chondrodystrophy, chondrodystrophia (familial)
  (fetalis) (hypoplastic) Q78.9
  calcificans congenita Q77.3
  myotonic (congenital) G71.13
  punctata Q77.3
Chondroectodermal dysplasia Q77.6
Chondrogenesis imperfecta Q77.4
Chondrolysis M94.35 ☑
Chondroma (*see also* Neoplasm, cartilage, benign)
  juxtacortical — *see* Neoplasm, bone, benign
  periosteal — *see* Neoplasm, bone, benign
Chondromalacia (systemic) M94.20
  acromioclavicular joint M94.21 ☑
  ankle M94.27 ☑
  elbow M94.22 ☑
  foot joint M94.27 ☑
  glenohumeral joint M94.21 ☑
  hand joint M94.24 ☑
  hip M94.25 ☑
  knee M94.26 ☑
    patella M22.4 ☑
  multiple sites M94.29
  patella M22.4 ☑
  rib M94.28
  sacroiliac joint M94.259
  shoulder M94.21 ☑
  sternoclavicular joint M94.21 ☑
  vertebral joint M94.28
  wrist M94.23 ☑
Chondromatosis (*see also* Neoplasm, cartilage,
  uncertain behavior)
  internal Q78.4
Chondromyxosarcoma — *see* Neoplasm, cartilage,
  malignant
Chondro-osteodysplasia (Morquio-Brailsford type)
  E76.219
Chondro-osteodystrophy E76.29
Chondro-osteoma — *see* Neoplasm, bone, benign
Chondropathia tuberosa M94.0
Chondrosarcoma — *see* Neoplasm, cartilage,
  malignant
  juxtacortical — *see* Neoplasm, bone, malignant
  mesenchymal — *see* Neoplasm, connective
    tissue, malignant
  myxoid — *see* Neoplasm, cartilage, malignant
Chordee (nonvenereal) N48.89
  congenital Q54.4
  gonococcal A54.09
Chorditis (fibrinous) (nodosa) (tuberosa) J38.2
Chordoma — *see* Neoplasm, vertebral (column),
  malignant
Chorea (chronic) (gravis) (posthemiplegic) (senile)
  (spasmodic) G25.5
  with
    heart involvement I02.0
      active or acute (conditions in I01 ☑) I02.0
      rheumatic I02.9
        with valvular disorder I02.0
      rheumatic heart disease (chronic) (inactive)
        (quiescent) - code to rheumatic heart
        condition involved
  drug-induced G25.4
  habit F95.8
  hereditary G10

Chorea — *continued*
  Huntington's G10
  hysterical F44.4
  minor I02.9
    with heart involvement I02.0
  progressive G25.5
    hereditary G10
  rheumatic (chronic) I02.9
    with heart involvement I02.0
  Sydenham's I02.9
    with heart involvement — *see* Chorea, with
      rheumatic heart disease
    nonrheumatic G25.5
Choreoathetosis (paroxysmal) G25.5
Chorioadenoma (destruens) D39.2
Chorioamnionitis O41.12 ☑
Chorioangioma D26.7
Choriocarcinoma — *see* Neoplasm, malignant, by
  site
  combined with
    embryonal carcinoma — *see* Neoplasm,
      malignant, by site
    other germ cell elements — *see* Neoplasm,
      malignant, by site
    teratoma — *see* Neoplasm, malignant, by site
  specified site — *see* Neoplasm, malignant, by site
  unspecified site
    female C58
    male C62.90
Chorioencephalitis (acute) (lymphocytic) (serous)
  A87.2
Chorioepithelioma — *see* Choriocarcinoma
Choriomeningitis (acute) (lymphocytic) (serous)
  A87.2
Chorionepithelioma — *see* Choriocarcinoma
Chorioretinitis (*see also* Inflammation, chorioretinal)
  disseminated (*see also* Inflammation,
    chorioretinal, disseminated)
    in neurosyphilis A52.19
  Egyptian B76.9 *[D63.8]*
  focal (*see also* Inflammation, chorioretinal, focal)
  histoplasmic B39.9 *[H32]*
  in (due to)
    histoplasmosis B39.9 *[H32]*
    syphilis (secondary) A51.43
      late A52.71
    toxoplasmosis (acquired) B58.01
      congenital (active) P37.1 *[H32]*
    tuberculosis A18.53
  juxtapapillary, juxtapapillaris — *see* Inflammation,
    chorioretinal, focal, juxtapapillary
  leprous A30.9 *[H32]*
  miner's B76.9 *[D63.8]*
  progressive myopia (degeneration) (*see also*
    Myopia, degenerative) H44.2 ☑
  syphilitic (secondary) A51.43
    congenital (early) A50.01 *[H32]*
      late A50.32
    late A52.71
  tuberculous A18.53
Chorioretinopathy, central serous H35.71 ☑
Choroid — *see* condition
Choroideremia H31.21
Choroiditis — *see* Chorioretinitis
Choroidopathy — *see* Disorder, choroid
Choroidoretinitis — *see* Chorioretinitis
Choroidoretinopathy, central serous — *see*
  Chorioretinopathy, central serous
Christian-Weber disease M35.6
Christmas disease D67
Chromaffinoma (*see also* Neoplasm, benign, by site)
  malignant — *see* Neoplasm, malignant, by site
Chromatopsia — *see* Deficiency, color vision
Chromhidrosis, chromidrosis L75.1
Chromoblastomycosis — *see* Chromomycosis
Chromoconversion R82.91
Chromomycosis B43.9
  brain abscess B43.1
  cerebral B43.1
  cutaneous B43.0
  skin B43.0
  specified NEC B43.8
  subcutaneous abscess or cyst B43.2
Chromophytosis B36.0
Chromosome — *see* condition by chromosome
  involved
  D (1) — *see* condition, chromosome 13
  E (3) — *see* condition, chromosome 18
  G — *see* condition, chromosome 21
Chromotrichomycosis B36.8
Chronic — *see* condition
  fracture — *see* Fracture, pathological

☑ **Additional character required**

Churg-Strauss syndrome M30.1
Chyle cyst, mesentery I89.8
Chylocele (nonfilarial) I89.8
   filarial (*see also* Infestation, filarial) B74.9 *[N51]*
   tunica vaginalis N50.89
      filarial (*see also* Infestation, filarial) B74.9 *[N51]*
Chylomicronemia (fasting) (with
   hyperprebetalipoproteinemia) E78.3
Chylopericardium I31.3
   acute I30.9
Chylothorax (nonfilarial) I89.8
   filarial (*see also* Infestation, filarial) B74.9 *[J91.8]*
Chylous — *see* condition
Chyluria (nonfilarial) R82.0
   due to
      bilharziasis B65.0
      Brugia (malayi) B74.1
         timori B74.2
      schistosomiasis (bilharziasis) B65.0
      Wuchereria (bancrofti) B74.0
   filarial — *see* Infestation, filarial
Cicatricial (deformity) — *see* Cicatrix
Cicatrix (adherent) (contracted) (painful) (vicious)
   (*see also* Scar) L90.5
   adenoid (and tonsil) J35.8
   alveolar process M26.79
   anus K62.89
   auricle — *see* Disorder, pinna, specified type NEC
   bile duct (common) (hepatic) K83.8
   bladder N32.89
   bone — *see* Disorder, bone, specified type NEC
   brain G93.89
   cervix (postoperative) (postpartal) N88.1
   common duct K83.8
   cornea H17.9
      tuberculous A18.59
   duodenum (bulb), obstructive K31.5
   esophagus K22.2
   eyelid — *see* Disorder, eyelid function
   hypopharynx J39.2
   lacrimal passages — *see* Obstruction, lacrimal
   larynx J38.7
   lung J98.4
   middle ear — *see* subcategory H74.8
   mouth K13.79
   muscle M62.89
      with contracture — *see* Contraction, muscle NEC
   nasopharynx J39.2
   palate (soft) K13.79
   penis N48.89
   pharynx J39.2
   prostate N42.89
   rectum K62.89
   retina — *see* Scar, chorioretinal
   semilunar cartilage — *see* Derangement,
      meniscus
   seminal vesicle N50.89
   skin L90.5
      infected L08.89
      postinfective L90.5
      tuberculous B90.8
   specified site NEC L90.5
   throat J39.2
   tongue K14.8
   tonsil (and adenoid) J35.8
   trachea J39.8
   tuberculous NEC B90.9
   urethra N36.8
   uterus N85.8
   vagina N89.8
      postoperative N99.2
   vocal cord J38.3
   wrist, constricting (annular) L90.5
CIDP (chronic inflammatory demyelinating
   polyneuropathy) G61.81
CIN — *see* Neoplasia, intraepithelial, cervix
CINCA (chronic infantile neurological, cutaneous and
   articular syndrome) M04.2
Cinchonism — *see* Deafness, ototoxic
   correct substance properly administered — *see*
      Table of Drugs and Chemicals, by drug,
      adverse effect
   overdose or wrong substance given or taken —
      see Table of Drugs and Chemicals, by drug,
      poisoning
Circle of Willis — *see* condition
Circular — *see* condition
Circulating anticoagulants (*see also* - Disorder,
   hemorrhagic) D68.318
   due to drugs (*see also* - Disorder,
      hemorrhagic) D68.32
   following childbirth O72.3

Circulation
   collateral, any site I99.8
   defective (lower extremity) I99.9
      congenital Q28.9
   embryonic Q28.9
   failure (peripheral) R57.9
      newborn P29.89
   fetal, persistent P29.38
   heart, incomplete Q28.9
Circulatory system — *see* condition
Circulus senilis (cornea) — *see* Degeneration, cornea,
   senile
Circumcision (in absence of medical indication)
   (ritual) (routine) Z41.2
Circumscribed — *see* condition
Circumvallate placenta O43.11 ☑
Cirrhosis, cirrhotic (hepatic) (liver) K74.60
   alcoholic K70.30
      with ascites K70.31
   atrophic — *see* Cirrhosis, liver
   Baumgarten-Cruveilhier K74.69
   biliary (cholangiolitic) (cholangitic) (hypertrophic)
      (obstructive) (pericholangiolitic) K74.5
      due to
         Clonorchiasis B66.1
         flukes B66.3
      primary K74.3
      secondary K74.4
   cardiac (of liver) K76.1
   Charcot's K74.3
   cholangiolitic, cholangitic, cholostatic
      (primary) K74.3
   congestive K76.1
   Cruveilhier-Baumgarten K74.69
   cryptogenic (liver) K74.69
   due to
      hepatolenticular degeneration E83.01
      Wilson's disease E83.01
      xanthomatosis E78.2
   fatty K76.0
      alcoholic K70.0
   Hanot's (hypertrophic) K74.3
   hepatic — *see* Cirrhosis, liver
   hypertrophic K74.3
   Indian childhood K74.69
   kidney — *see* Sclerosis, renal
   Laennec's K70.30
      with ascites K70.31
      alcoholic K70.30
         with ascites K70.31
      nonalcoholic K74.69
   liver K74.60
      alcoholic K70.30
         with ascites K70.31
      fatty K70.0
      congenital P78.81
      syphilitic A52.74
   lung (chronic) J84.10
   macronodular K74.69
      alcoholic K70.30
         with ascites K70.31
   micronodular K74.69
      alcoholic K70.30
         with ascites K70.31
   mixed type K74.69
   monolobular K74.3
   nephritis — *see* Sclerosis, renal
   nutritional K74.69
      alcoholic K70.30
         with ascites K70.31
   obstructive — *see* Cirrhosis, biliary
   ovarian N83.8
   pancreas (duct) K86.89
   pigmentary E83.110
   portal K74.69
      alcoholic K70.30
         with ascites K70.31
   postnecrotic K74.69
      alcoholic K70.30
         with ascites K70.31
   pulmonary J84.10
   renal — *see* Sclerosis, renal
   spleen D73.2
   stasis K76.1
   Todd's K74.3
   unilobar K74.3
   xanthomatous (biliary) K74.5
      due to xanthomatosis (familial) (metabolic)
         (primary) E78.2
Cistern, subarachnoid R93.0
Citrullinemia E72.23
Citrullinuria E72.23

Civatte's disease or poikiloderma L57.3
Clam digger's itch B65.3
Clammy skin R23.1
Clap — *see* Gonorrhea
Clarke-Hadfield syndrome (pancreatic infantilism)
   K86.89
Clark's paralysis G80.9
Clastothrix L67.8
Claude Bernard-Horner syndrome G90.2
   traumatic — *see* Injury, nerve, cervical
      sympathetic
Claude's disease or syndrome G46.3
Claudication (intermittent) I73.9
   cerebral (artery) G45.9
   spinal cord (arteriosclerotic) G95.19
      syphilitic A52.09
   venous (axillary) I87.8
Claudicatio venosa intermittens I87.8
Claustrophobia F40.240
Clavus (infected) L84
Clawfoot (congenital) Q66.89
   acquired — *see* Deformity, limb, clawfoot
Clawhand (acquired) (*see also* Deformity, limb,
   clawhand)
   congenital Q68.1
Clawtoe (congenital) Q66.89
   acquired — *see* Deformity, toe, specified NEC
Clay eating — *see* Pica
Cleansing of artificial opening — *see* Attention to,
   artificial, opening
Cleft (congenital) (*see also* Imperfect, closure)
   alveolar process M26.79
   branchial (persistent) Q18.2
      cyst Q18.0
      fistula Q18.0
      sinus Q18.0
   cricoid cartilage, posterior Q31.8
   foot Q72.7 ☑
   hand Q71.6 ☑
   lip (unilateral) Q36.9
      with cleft palate Q37.9
         hard Q37.1
            with soft Q37.5
         soft Q37.3
            with hard Q37.5
      bilateral Q36.0
         with cleft palate Q37.8
            hard Q37.0
               with soft Q37.4
            soft Q37.2
               with hard Q37.4
      median Q36.1
   nose Q30.2
   palate Q35.9
      with cleft lip (unilateral) Q37.9
         bilateral Q37.8
      hard Q35.1
         with
            cleft lip (unilateral) Q37.1
               bilateral Q37.0
            soft Q35.5
               with cleft lip (unilateral) Q37.5
                  bilateral Q37.4
      medial Q35.5
      soft Q35.3
         with
            cleft lip (unilateral) Q37.3
               bilateral Q37.2
            hard Q35.5
               with cleft lip (unilateral) Q37.5
                  bilateral Q37.4
   penis Q55.69
   scrotum Q55.29
   thyroid cartilage Q31.8
   uvula Q35.7
Cleidocranial dysostosis Q74.0
Cleptomania F63.2
Clicking hip (newborn) R29.4
Climacteric (female) (*see also* Menopause)
   arthritis (any site) NEC — *see* Arthritis, specified
      form NEC
   depression (single episode) F32.89
      recurrent episode F33.8
   melancholia (single episode) F32.89
      recurrent episode F33.8
   male (symptoms) (syndrome) NEC N50.89
   paranoid state F22
   polyarthritis NEC — *see* Arthritis, specified form
      NEC
   symptoms (female) N95.1
Clinical research investigation (clinical trial) (control
   subject) (normal comparison) (participant) Z00.6

Deficiency - Deformity

Clitoris - Colitis

Deficiency - Deformity

ICD-10-CM INDEX TO DISEASES AND INJURIES

ICD-10-CM INDEX TO DISEASES AND INJURIES

Deficiency — *continued*
  vitamin — *continued*
    PP (pellagra-preventing) E52
    specified NEC E56.8
    thiamin E51.9
      beriberi — *see* Beriberi
  zinc, dietary E60
Deficit (*see also* Deficiency)
  attention and concentration R41.840
    following
      cerebral infarction I69.310
      cerebrovascular disease I69.910
        specified disease NEC I69.810
      nontraumatic
        intracerebral hemorrhage I69.110
        specified intracranial hemorrhage
          NEC I69.210
        subarachnoid hemorrhage I69.010
    disorder — *see* Attention, deficit
  cognitive
    communication R41.841
    emotional
      following
        cerebral infarction I69.315
        cerebrovascular disease I69.915
          specified disease NEC I69.815
        nontraumatic
          intracerebral hemorrhage I69.115
          specified intracranial hemorrhage
            NEC I69.215
          subarachnoid hemorrhage I69.015
    following
      cerebral infarction I69.319
      cerebrovascular disease I69.919
        specified disease NEC I69.819
      nontraumatic
        intracerebral hemorrhage I69.119
        specified intracranial hemorrhage
          NEC I69.219
        subarachnoid hemorrhage I69.019
    social
      following
        cerebral infarction I69.315
        cerebrovascular disease I69.915
          specified disease NEC I69.815
        nontraumatic
          intracerebral hemorrhage I69.115
          specified intracranial hemorrhage
            NEC I69.215
          subarachnoid hemorrhage I69.015
  cognitive NEC R41.89
    following
      cerebral infarction I69.318
      cerebrovascular disease I69.918
        specified disease NEC I69.818
      nontraumatic
        intracerebral hemorrhage I69.118
        specified intracranial hemorrhage
          NEC I69.218
        subarachnoid hemorrhage I69.018
  concentration R41.840
  executive function R41.844
    following
      cerebral infarction I69.314
      cerebrovascular disease I69.914
        specified disease NEC I69.814
      nontraumatic
        intracerebral hemorrhage I69.114
        specified intracranial hemorrhage
          NEC I69.214
        subarachnoid hemorrhage I69.014
  frontal lobe R41.844
    following
      cerebral infarction I69.314
      cerebrovascular disease I69.914
        specified disease NEC I69.814
      nontraumatic
        intracerebral hemorrhage I69.114
        specified intracranial hemorrhage
          NEC I69.214
        subarachnoid hemorrhage I69.014
  memory
    following
      cerebral infarction I69.311
      cerebrovascular disease I69.911
        specified disease NEC I69.811
      nontraumatic
        intracerebral hemorrhage I69.111
        specified intracranial hemorrhage
          NEC I69.211
        subarachnoid hemorrhage I69.011

Deficit — *continued*
  neurologic NEC R29.818
    ischemic
      reversible (RIND) I63.9
        prolonged (PRIND) I63.9
    oxygen R09.02
    prolonged reversible ischemic neurologic
      (PRIND) I63.9
  psychomotor R41.843
    following
      cerebral infarction I69.313
      cerebrovascular disease I69.913
        specified disease NEC I69.813
      nontraumatic
        intracerebral hemorrhage I69.113
        specified intracranial hemorrhage
          NEC I69.213
        subarachnoid hemorrhage I69.013
  visuospatial R41.842
    following
      cerebral infarction I69.312
      cerebrovascular disease I69.912
        specified disease NEC I69.812
      nontraumatic
        intracerebral hemorrhage I69.112
        specified intracranial hemorrhage
          NEC I69.212
        subarachnoid hemorrhage I69.012
Deflection
  radius — *see* Deformity, limb, specified type NEC,
    forearm
  septum (acquired) (nasal) (nose) J34.2
  spine — *see* Curvature, spine
  turbinate (nose) J34.2
Defluvium
  capillorum — *see* Alopecia
  ciliorum — *see* Madarosis
  unguium L60.8
Deformity Q89.9
  abdomen, congenital Q89.9
  abdominal wall
    acquired M95.8
    congenital Q79.59
  acquired (unspecified site) M95.9
  adrenal gland Q89.1
  alimentary tract, congenital Q45.9
    upper Q40.9
  ankle (joint) (acquired) (*see also* Deformity, limb,
    lower leg)
    abduction — *see* Contraction, joint, ankle
    congenital Q68.8
    contraction — *see* Contraction, joint, ankle
    specified type NEC — *see* Deformity, limb, foot,
      specified NEC
  anus (acquired) K62.89
    congenital Q43.9
  aorta (arch) (congenital) Q25.40
    acquired I77.89
  aortic
    arch, acquired I77.89
    cusp or valve (congenital) Q23.8
      acquired (*see also* Endocarditis, aortic) I35.8
  arm (acquired) (upper) (*see also* Deformity, limb,
    upper arm)
    congenital Q68.8
    forearm — *see* Deformity, limb, forearm
  artery (congenital) (peripheral) NOS Q27.9
    acquired I77.89
    coronary (acquired) I25.9
      congenital Q24.5
    umbilical Q27.0
  atrial septal Q21.1
  auditory canal (external) (congenital) (*see also*
    Malformation, ear, external)
    acquired — *see* Disorder, ear, external, specified
      type NEC
  auricle
    ear (congenital) (*see also* Malformation, ear,
      external)
      acquired — *see* Disorder, pinna, deformity
  back — *see* Dorsopathy, deforming
  bile duct (common) (congenital) (hepatic) Q44.5
    acquired K83.8
  biliary duct or passage (congenital) Q44.5
    acquired K83.8
  bladder (neck) (trigone) (sphincter)
    (acquired) N32.89
    congenital Q64.79
  bone (acquired) NOS M95.9
    congenital Q79.9
    turbinate M95.0

Deformity — *continued*
  brain (congenital) Q04.9
    acquired G93.89
    reduction Q04.3
  breast (acquired) N64.89
    congenital Q83.9
    reconstructed N65.0
  bronchus (congenital) Q32.4
    acquired NEC J98.09
  bursa, congenital Q79.9
  canaliculi (lacrimalis) (acquired) (*see also* Disorder,
    lacrimal system, changes)
    congenital Q10.6
  canthus, acquired — *see* Disorder, eyelid,
    specified type NEC
  capillary (acquired) I78.8
  cardiovascular system, congenital Q28.9
  caruncle, lacrimal (acquired) (*see also* Disorder,
    lacrimal system, changes)
    congenital Q10.6
  cascade, stomach K31.2
  cecum (congenital) Q43.9
    acquired K63.89
  cerebral, acquired G93.89
    congenital Q04.9
  cervix (uterus) (acquired) NEC N88.8
    congenital Q51.9
  cheek (acquired) M95.2
    congenital Q18.9
  chest (acquired) (wall) M95.4
    congenital Q67.8
    sequelae (late effect) of rickets E64.3
  chin (acquired) M95.2
    congenital Q18.9
  choroid (congenital) Q14.3
    acquired H31.8
    plexus Q07.8
      acquired G96.19
  cicatricial — *see* Cicatrix
  cilia, acquired — *see* Disorder, eyelid, specified
    type NEC
  clavicle (acquired) M95.8
    congenital Q68.8
  clitoris (congenital) Q52.6
    acquired N90.89
  clubfoot — *see* Clubfoot
  coccyx (acquired) — *see* subcategory M43.8
  colon (congenital) Q43.9
    acquired K63.89
  concha (ear), congenital (*see also* Malformation,
    ear, external)
    acquired — *see* Disorder, pinna, deformity
  cornea (acquired) H18.70
    congenital Q13.4
    descemetocele — *see* Descemetocele
    ectasia — *see* Ectasia, cornea
    specified NEC H18.79 ☑
    staphyloma — *see* Staphyloma, cornea
  coronary artery (acquired) I25.9
    congenital Q24.5
  cranium (acquired) — *see* Deformity, skull
  cricoid cartilage (congenital) Q31.8
    acquired J38.7
  cystic duct (congenital) Q44.5
    acquired K82.8
  Dandy-Walker Q03.1
    with spina bifida — *see* Spina bifida
  diaphragm (congenital) Q79.1
    acquired J98.6
  digestive organ NOS Q45.9
  ductus arteriosus Q25.0
  duodenal bulb K31.89
  duodenum (congenital) Q43.9
    acquired K31.89
  dura — *see* Deformity, meninges
  ear (acquired) (*see also* Disorder, pinna,
    deformity)
    congenital (external) Q17.9
      internal Q16.5
      middle Q16.4
        ossicles Q16.3
      ossicles Q16.3
  ectodermal (congenital) NEC Q84.9
  ejaculatory duct (congenital) Q55.4
    acquired N50.89
  elbow (joint) (acquired) (*see also* Deformity, limb,
    upper arm)
    congenital Q68.8
    contraction — *see* Contraction, joint, elbow
  endocrine gland NEC Q89.2
  epididymis (congenital) Q55.4
    acquired N50.89

☑ **Additional character required**

Deformity — *continued*
  epiglottis (congenital) Q31.8
    acquired J38.7
  esophagus (congenital) Q39.9
    acquired K22.8
  eustachian tube (congenital) NEC Q17.8
  eye, congenital Q15.9
  eyebrow (congenital) Q18.8
  eyelid (acquired) (*see also* Disorder, eyelid,
    specified type NEC)
    congenital Q10.3
  face (acquired) M95.2
    congenital Q18.9
  fallopian tube, acquired N83.8
  femur (acquired) — *see* Deformity, limb, specified
    type NEC, thigh
  fetal
    with fetopelvic disproportion O33.7 ☑
      causing obstructed labor O66.3
  finger (acquired) M20.00 ☑
    boutonniere M20.02 ☑
    congenital Q68.1
    flexion contracture — *see* Contraction, joint,
      hand
    mallet finger M20.01 ☑
    specified NEC M20.09 ☑
    swan-neck M20.03 ☑
  flexion (joint) (acquired) (*see also* Deformity, limb,
    flexion) M21.20
    congenital NOS Q74.9
      hip Q65.89
  foot (acquired) (*see also* Deformity, limb, lower
    leg)
    cavovarus (congenital) Q66.1
    congenital NOS Q66.9
      specified type NEC Q66.89
    specified type NEC — *see* Deformity, limb, foot,
      specified NEC
    valgus (congenital) Q66.6
      acquired — *see* Deformity, valgus, ankle
    varus (congenital) NEC Q66.3
      acquired — *see* Deformity, varus, ankle
  forearm (acquired) (*see also* Deformity, limb,
    forearm)
    congenital Q68.8
  forehead (acquired) M95.2
    congenital Q75.8
  frontal bone (acquired) M95.2
    congenital Q75.8
  gallbladder (congenital) Q44.1
    acquired K82.8
  gastrointestinal tract (congenital) NOS Q45.9
    acquired K63.89
  genitalia, genital organ (s) or system NEC
    female (congenital) Q52.9
      acquired N94.89
      external Q52.70
    male (congenital) Q55.9
      acquired N50.89
  globe (eye) (congenital) Q15.8
    acquired H44.89
  gum, acquired NEC K06.8
  hand (acquired) — *see* Deformity, limb, hand
    congenital Q68.1
  head (acquired) M95.2
    congenital Q75.8
  heart (congenital) Q24.9
    septum Q21.9
      auricular Q21.1
      ventricular Q21.0
    valve (congenital) NEC Q24.8
      acquired — *see* Endocarditis
  heel (acquired) — *see* Deformity, foot
  hepatic duct (congenital) Q44.5
    acquired K83.8
  hip (joint) (acquired) (*see also* Deformity, limb,
    thigh)
    congenital Q65.9
    due to (previous) juvenile osteochondrosis —
      see Coxa, plana
    flexion — *see* Contraction, joint, hip
  hourglass — *see* Contraction, hourglass
  humerus (acquired) M21.82 ☑
    congenital Q74.0
  hypophyseal (congenital) Q89.2
  ileocecal (coil) (valve) (acquired) K63.89
    congenital Q43.9
  ileum (congenital) Q43.9
    acquired K63.89
  ilium (acquired) M95.5
    congenital Q74.2
  integument (congenital) Q84.9

Deformity — *continued*
  intervertebral cartilage or disc (acquired) — *see*
    Disorder, disc, specified NEC
  intestine (large) (small) (congenital) NOS Q43.9
    acquired K63.89
  intrinsic minus or plus (hand) — *see* Deformity,
    limb, specified type NEC, forearm
  iris (acquired) H21.89
    congenital Q13.2
  ischium (acquired) M95.5
    congenital Q74.2
  jaw (acquired) (congenital) M26.9
  joint (acquired) NEC M21.90
    congenital Q68.8
    elbow M21.92 ☑
    hand M21.94 ☑
    hip M21.95 ☑
    knee M21.96 ☑
    shoulder M21.92 ☑
    wrist M21.93 ☑
  kidney (s) (calyx) (pelvis) (congenital) Q63.9
    acquired N28.89
    artery (congenital) Q27.2
      acquired I77.89
  Klippel-Feil (brevicollis) Q76.1
  knee (acquired) NEC (*see also* Deformity, limb,
    lower leg)
    congenital Q68.2
  labium (majus) (minus) (congenital) Q52.79
    acquired N90.89
  lacrimal passages or duct (congenital) NEC Q10.6
    acquired — *see* Disorder, lacrimal system,
      changes
  larynx (muscle) (congenital) Q31.8
    acquired J38.7
    web (glottic) Q31.0
  leg (upper) (acquired) NEC (*see also* Deformity,
    limb, thigh)
    congenital Q68.8
    lower leg — *see* Deformity, limb, lower leg
  lens (acquired) H27.8
    congenital Q12.9
  lid (fold) (acquired) (*see also* Disorder, eyelid,
    specified type NEC)
    congenital Q10.3
  ligament (acquired) — *see* Disorder, ligament
    congenital Q79.9
  limb (acquired) M21.90
    clawfoot M21.53 ☑
    clawhand M21.51 ☑
    clubfoot M21.54 ☑
    clubhand M21.52 ☑
    congenital, except reduction deformity Q74.9
    flat foot M21.4 ☑
    flexion M21.20
      ankle M21.27 ☑
      elbow M21.22 ☑
      finger M21.24 ☑
      hip M21.25 ☑
      knee M21.26 ☑
      shoulder M21.21 ☑
      toe M21.27 ☑
      wrist M21.23 ☑
    foot
      claw — *see* Deformity, limb, clawfoot
      club — *see* Deformity, limb, clubfoot
      drop M21.37 ☑
      flat — *see* Deformity, limb, flat foot
      specified NEC M21.6X ☑
    forearm M21.93 ☑
    hand M21.94 ☑
    lower leg M21.96 ☑
    specified type NEC M21.80
      forearm M21.83 ☑
      lower leg M21.86 ☑
      thigh M21.85 ☑
      upper arm M21.82 ☑
    thigh M21.95 ☑
    unequal length M21.70
      short site is
        femur M21.75 ☑
        fibula M21.76 ☑
        humerus M21.72 ☑
        radius M21.73 ☑
        tibia M21.76 ☑
        ulna M21.73 ☑
    upper arm M21.92 ☑
    valgus — *see* Deformity, valgus
    varus — *see* Deformity, varus
    wrist drop M21.33 ☑
  lip (acquired) NEC K13.0
    congenital Q38.0

Deformity — *continued*
  liver (congenital) Q44.7
    acquired K76.89
  lumbosacral (congenital) (joint) (region) Q76.49
    acquired — *see* subcategory M43.8
    kyphosis — *see* Kyphosis, congenital
    lordosis — *see* Lordosis, congenital
  lung (congenital) Q33.9
    acquired J98.4
  lymphatic system, congenital Q89.9
  Madelung's (radius) Q74.0
  mandible (acquired) (congenital) M26.9
  maxilla (acquired) (congenital) M26.9
  meninges or membrane (congenital) Q07.9
    cerebral Q04.8
      acquired G96.19
    spinal cord (congenital) G96.19
      acquired G96.19
  metacarpus (acquired) — *see* Deformity, limb,
    forearm
    congenital Q74.0
  metatarsus (acquired) — *see* Deformity, foot
    congenital Q66.9
  middle ear (congenital) Q16.4
    ossicles Q16.3
  mitral (leaflets) (valve) I05.8
    parachute Q23.2
    stenosis, congenital Q23.2
  mouth (acquired) K13.79
    congenital Q38.6
  multiple, congenital NEC Q89.7
  muscle (acquired) M62.89
    congenital Q79.9
      sternocleidomastoid Q68.0
  musculoskeletal system (acquired) M95.9
    congenital Q79.9
    specified NEC M95.8
  nail (acquired) L60.8
    congenital Q84.6
  nasal — *see* Deformity, nose
  neck (acquired) M95.3
    congenital Q18.9
    sternocleidomastoid Q68.0
  nervous system (congenital) Q07.9
  nipple (congenital) Q83.9
    acquired N64.89
  nose (acquired) (cartilage) M95.0
    bone (turbinate) M95.0
    congenital Q30.9
      bent or squashed Q67.4
    saddle M95.0
      syphilitic A50.57
    septum (acquired) J34.2
      congenital Q30.8
    sinus (wall) (congenital) Q30.8
      acquired M95.0
    syphilitic (congenital) A50.57
      late A52.73
  ocular muscle (congenital) Q10.3
    acquired — *see* Strabismus, mechanical
  opticociliary vessels (congenital) Q13.2
  orbit (eye) (acquired) H05.30
    atrophy — *see* Atrophy, orbit
    congenital Q10.7
    due to
      bone disease NEC H05.32 ☑
      trauma or surgery H05.33 ☑
    enlargement — *see* Enlargement, orbit
    exostosis — *see* Exostosis, orbit
  organ of Corti (congenital) Q16.5
  ovary (congenital) Q50.39
    acquired N83.8
  oviduct, acquired N83.8
  palate (congenital) Q38.5
    acquired M27.8
    cleft (congenital) — *see* Cleft, palate
  pancreas (congenital) Q45.3
    acquired K86.89
  parathyroid (gland) Q89.2
  parotid (gland) (congenital) Q38.4
    acquired K11.8
  patella (acquired) — *see* Disorder, patella,
    specified NEC
  pelvis, pelvic (acquired) (bony) M95.5
    with disproportion (fetopelvic) O33.0
      causing obstructed labor O65.0
    congenital Q74.2
    rachitic sequelae (late effect) E64.3
  penis (glans) (congenital) Q55.69
    acquired N48.89
  pericardium (congenital) Q24.8
    acquired — *see* Pericarditis

Deformity - Degeneration

Deformity — *continued*
  pharynx (congenital) Q38.8
    acquired J39.2
  pinna, acquired (*see also* Disorder, pinna, deformity)
    congenital Q17.9
  pituitary (congenital) Q89.2
  posture — *see* Dorsopathy, deforming
  prepuce (congenital) Q55.69
    acquired N47.8
  prostate (congenital) Q55.4
    acquired N42.89
  pupil (congenital) Q13.2
    acquired — *see* Abnormality, pupillary
  pylorus (congenital) Q40.3
    acquired K31.89
  rachitic (acquired), old or healed E64.3
  radius (acquired) (*see also* Deformity, limb, forearm)
    congenital Q68.8
  rectum (congenital) Q43.9
    acquired K62.89
  reduction (extremity) (limb), congenital (*see also* condition and site) Q73.8
    brain Q04.3
    lower — *see* Defect, reduction, lower limb
    upper — *see* Defect, reduction, upper limb
  renal — *see* Deformity, kidney
  respiratory system (congenital) Q34.9
  rib (acquired) M95.4
    congenital Q76.6
      cervical Q76.5
  rotation (joint) (acquired) — *see* Deformity, limb, specified site NEC
    congenital Q74.9
    hip — *see* Deformity, limb, specified type NEC, thigh
      congenital Q65.89
  sacroiliac joint (congenital) Q74.2
    acquired — *see* subcategory M43.8
  sacrum (acquired) — *see* subcategory M43.8
  saddle
    back — *see* Lordosis
    nose M95.0
      syphilitic A50.57
  salivary gland or duct (congenital) Q38.4
    acquired K11.8
  scapula (acquired) M95.8
    congenital Q68.8
  scrotum (congenital) (*see also* Malformation, testis and scrotum)
    acquired N50.89
  seminal vesicles (congenital) Q55.4
    acquired N50.89
  septum, nasal (acquired) J34.2
  shoulder (joint) (acquired) — *see* Deformity, limb, upper arm
    congenital Q74.0
    contraction — *see* Contraction, joint, shoulder
  sigmoid (flexure) (congenital) Q43.9
    acquired K63.89
  skin (congenital) Q82.9
  skull (acquired) M95.2
    congenital Q75.8
      with
        anencephaly Q00.0
        encephalocele — *see* Encephalocele
        hydrocephalus Q03.9
          with spina bifida — *see* Spina bifida, by site, with hydrocephalus
        microcephaly Q02
  soft parts, organs or tissues (of pelvis)
    in pregnancy or childbirth NEC O34.8 ☑
      causing obstructed labor O65.5
  spermatic cord (congenital) Q55.4
    acquired N50.89
    torsion — *see* Torsion, spermatic cord
  spinal — *see* Dorsopathy, deforming
    column (acquired) — *see* Dorsopathy, deforming
    congenital Q67.5
    cord (congenital) Q06.9
      acquired G95.89
    nerve root (congenital) Q07.9
  spine (acquired) (*see also* Dorsopathy, deforming)
    congenital Q67.5
    rachitic E64.3
    specified NEC — *see* Dorsopathy, deforming, specified NEC
  spleen
    acquired D73.89
    congenital Q89.09

Deformity — *continued*
  Sprengel's (congenital) Q74.0
  sternocleidomastoid (muscle), congenital Q68.0
  sternum (acquired) M95.4
    congenital NEC Q76.7
  stomach (congenital) Q40.3
    acquired K31.89
  submandibular gland (congenital) Q38.4
  submaxillary gland (congenital) Q38.4
    acquired K11.8
  talipes — *see* Talipes
  testis (congenital) (*see also* Malformation, testis and scrotum)
    acquired N44.8
    torsion — *see* Torsion, testis
  thigh (acquired) (*see also* Deformity, limb, thigh)
    congenital NEC Q68.8
  thorax (acquired) (wall) M95.4
    congenital Q67.8
    sequelae of rickets E64.3
  thumb (acquired) (*see also* Deformity, finger)
    congenital NEC Q68.1
  thymus (tissue) (congenital) Q89.2
  thyroid (gland) (congenital) Q89.2
    cartilage Q31.8
      acquired J38.7
  tibia (acquired) (*see also* Deformity, limb, specified type NEC, lower leg)
    congenital NEC Q68.8
    saber (syphilitic) A50.56
  toe (acquired) M20.6 ☑
    congenital Q66.9
    hallux rigidus M20.2 ☑
    hallux valgus M20.1 ☑
    hallux varus M20.3 ☑
    hammer toe M20.4 ☑
    specified NEC M20.5X ☑
  tongue (congenital) Q38.3
    acquired K14.8
  tooth, teeth K00.2
  trachea (rings) (congenital) Q32.1
    acquired J39.8
  transverse aortic arch (congenital) Q25.49
  tricuspid (leaflets) (valve) I07.8
    atresia or stenosis Q22.4
    Ebstein's Q22.5
  trunk (acquired) M95.8
    congenital Q89.9
  ulna (acquired) (*see also* Deformity, limb, forearm)
    congenital NEC Q68.8
  urachus, congenital Q64.4
  ureter (opening) (congenital) Q62.8
    acquired N28.89
  urethra (congenital) Q64.79
    acquired N36.8
  urinary tract (congenital) Q64.9
    urachus Q64.4
  uterus (congenital) Q51.9
    acquired N85.8
  uvula (congenital) Q38.5
  vagina (acquired) N89.8
    congenital Q52.4
  valgus NEC M21.00
    ankle M21.07 ☑
    elbow M21.02 ☑
    hip M21.05 ☑
    knee M21.06 ☑
  valve, valvular (congenital) (heart) Q24.8
    acquired — *see* Endocarditis
  varus NEC M21.10
    ankle M21.17 ☑
    elbow M21.12 ☑
    hip M21.15 ☑
    knee M21.16 ☑
    tibia — *see* Osteochondrosis, juvenile, tibia
  vas deferens (congenital) Q55.4
    acquired N50.89
  vein (congenital) Q27.9
    great Q26.9
  vertebra — *see* Dorsopathy, deforming
  vertical talus (congenital) Q66.80
    left foot Q66.82
    right foot Q66.81
  vesicourethral orifice (acquired) N32.89
    congenital NEC Q64.79
  vessels of optic papilla (congenital) Q14.2
  visual field (contraction) — *see* Defect, visual field
  vitreous body, acquired H43.89
  vulva (congenital) Q52.79
    acquired N90.89
  wrist (joint) (acquired) (*see also* Deformity, limb, forearm)

Deformity — *continued*
  wrist — *continued*
    congenital Q68.8
    contraction — *see* Contraction, joint, wrist
Degeneration, degenerative
  adrenal (capsule) (fatty) (gland) (hyaline) (infectional) E27.8
  amyloid (*see also* Amyloidosis) E85.9
  anterior cornua, spinal cord G12.29
  anterior labral S43.49 ☑
  aorta, aortic I70.0
    fatty I77.89
  aortic valve (heart) — *see* Endocarditis, aortic
  arteriovascular — *see* Arteriosclerosis
  artery, arterial (atheromatous) (calcareous) (*see also* Arteriosclerosis)
    cerebral, amyloid E85.4 *[I68.0]*
    medial — *see* Arteriosclerosis, extremities
  articular cartilage NEC — *see* Derangement, joint, articular cartilage, by site
  atheromatous — *see* Arteriosclerosis
  basal nuclei or ganglia G23.9
    specified NEC G23.8
  bone NEC — *see* Disorder, bone, specified type NEC
  brachial plexus G54.0
  brain (cortical) (progressive) G31.9
    alcoholic G31.2
    arteriosclerotic I67.2
    childhood G31.9
      specified NEC G31.89
    cystic G31.89
      congenital Q04.6
    in
      alcoholism G31.2
      beriberi E51.2
      cerebrovascular disease I67.9
      congenital hydrocephalus Q03.9
        with spina bifida (*see also* Spina bifida)
      Fabry-Anderson disease E75.21
      Gaucher's disease E75.22
      Hunter's syndrome E76.1
      lipidosis
        cerebral E75.4
        generalized E75.6
      mucopolysaccharidosis — *see* Mucopolysaccharidosis
      myxedema E03.9 *[G32.89]*
      neoplastic disease (*see also* Neoplasm) D49.6 *[G32.89]*
      Niemann-Pick disease E75.249 *[G32.89]*
      sphingolipidosis E75.3 *[G32.89]*
      vitamin B12 deficiency E53.8 *[G32.89]*
    senile NEC G31.1
  breast N64.89
  Bruch's membrane — *see* Degeneration, choroid
  capillaries (fatty) I78.8
    amyloid E85.89 *[I79.8]*
  cardiac (*see also* Degeneration, myocardial)
    valve, valvular — *see* Endocarditis
  cardiorenal — *see* Hypertension, cardiorenal
  cardiovascular (*see also* Disease, cardiovascular)
    renal — *see* Hypertension, cardiorenal
  cerebellar NOS G31.9
    alcoholic G31.2
    primary (hereditary) (sporadic) G11.9
  cerebral — *see* Degeneration, brain
  cerebrovascular I67.9
    due to hypertension I67.4
  cervical plexus G54.2
  cervix N88.8
    due to radiation (intended effect) N88.8
      adverse effect or misadventure N99.89
  chamber angle H21.21 ☑
  changes, spine or vertebra — *see* Spondylosis
  chorioretinal (*see also* Degeneration, choroid)
    hereditary H31.20
  choroid (colloid) (drusen) H31.10 ☑
    atrophy — *see* Atrophy, choroidal
    hereditary — *see* Dystrophy, choroidal, hereditary
  ciliary body H21.22 ☑
  cochlear — *see* subcategory H83.8
  combined (spinal cord) (subacute) E53.8 *[G32.0]*
    with anemia (pernicious) D51.0 *[G32.0]*
      due to dietary vitamin B12 deficiency D51.3 *[G32.0]*
    in (due to)
      vitamin B12 deficiency E53.8 *[G32.0]*
        anemia D51.9 *[G32.0]*
  conjunctiva H11.10
    concretions — *see* Concretion, conjunctiva

☑ **Additional character required**

Degeneration — *continued*
  conjunctiva — *continued*
    deposits — *see* Deposit, conjunctiva
    pigmentations — *see* Pigmentation, conjunctiva
    pinguecula — *see* Pinguecula
    xerosis — *see* Xerosis, conjunctiva
  cornea H18.40
    calcerous H18.43
      band keratopathy H18.42 ☑
    familial, hereditary — *see* Dystrophy, cornea
    hyaline (of old scars) H18.49
    keratomalacia — *see* Keratomalacia
    nodular H18.45 ☑
    peripheral H18.46 ☑
    senile H18.41 ☑
    specified type NEC H18.49
  cortical (cerebellar) (parenchymatous) G31.89
    alcoholic G31.2
    diffuse, due to arteriopathy I67.2
  corticobasal G31.85
  cutis L98.8
    amyloid E85.4 [L99]
  dental pulp K04.2
  disc disease — *see* Degeneration, intervertebral disc NEC
  dorsolateral (spinal cord) — *see* Degeneration, combined
  extrapyramidal G25.9
  eye, macular (*see also* Degeneration, macula)
    congenital or hereditary — *see* Dystrophy, retina
  facet joints — *see* Spondylosis
  fatty
    liver NEC K76.0
      alcoholic K70.0
  grey matter (brain) (Alpers') G31.81
  heart (*see also* Degeneration, myocardial)
    amyloid E85.4 [I43]
    atheromatous — *see* Disease, heart, ischemic, atherosclerotic
    ischemic — *see* Disease, heart, ischemic
  hepatolenticular (Wilson's) E83.01
  hepatorenal K76.7
  hyaline (diffuse) (generalized)
    localized — *see* Degeneration, by site
  infrapatellar fat pad M79.4
  intervertebral disc NOS
    with
      myelopathy — *see* Disorder, disc, with, myelopathy
      radiculitis or radiculopathy — *see* Disorder, disc, with, radiculopathy
    cervical, cervicothoracic — *see* Disorder, disc, cervical, degeneration
      with
        myelopathy — *see* Disorder, disc, cervical, with myelopathy
        neuritis, radiculitis or radiculopathy — *see* Disorder, disc, cervical, with neuritis
    lumbar region M51.36
      with
        myelopathy M51.06
        neuritis, radiculitis, radiculopathy or sciatica M51.16
    lumbosacral region M51.37
      with
        neuritis, radiculitis, radiculopathy or sciatica M51.17
    sacrococcygeal region M53.3
    thoracic region M51.34
      with
        myelopathy M51.04
        neuritis, radiculitis, radiculopathy M51.14
    thoracolumbar region M51.35
      with
        myelopathy M51.05
        neuritis, radiculitis, radiculopathy M51.15
  intestine, amyloid E85.4
  iris (pigmentary) H21.23 ☑
  ischemic — *see* Ischemia
  joint disease — *see* Osteoarthritis
  kidney N28.89
    amyloid E85.4 [N29]
    cystic, congenital Q61.9
    fatty N28.89
    polycystic Q61.3
      adult type (autosomal dominant) Q61.2
      infantile type (autosomal recessive) NEC Q61.19
        collecting duct dilatation Q61.11

Degeneration — *continued*
  Kuhnt-Junius (*see also* Degeneration, macula) H35.32 ☑
  lens — *see* Cataract
  lenticular (familial) (progressive) (Wilson's) (with cirrhosis of liver) E83.01
  liver (diffuse) NEC K76.89
    amyloid E85.4 [K77]
    cystic K76.89
      congenital Q44.6
    fatty NEC K76.0
      alcoholic K70.0
    hypertrophic K76.89
    parenchymatous, acute or subacute K72.00
      with coma K72.01
    pigmentary K76.89
    toxic (acute) K71.9
  lung J98.4
  lymph gland I89.8
    hyaline I89.8
  macula, macular (acquired) (age-related) (senile) H35.30
    angioid streaks H35.33
    atrophic age-related H35.31 ☑
    congenital or hereditary — *see* Dystrophy, retina
    cystoid H35.35 ☑
    drusen H35.36 ☑
    dry age-related H35.31 ☑
    exudative H35.32 ☑
    hole H35.34 ☑
    nonexudative H35.31 ☑
    puckering H35.37 ☑
    toxic H35.38 ☑
    wet age-related H35.32 ☑
  membranous labyrinth, congenital (causing impairment of hearing) Q16.5
  meniscus — *see* Derangement, meniscus
  mitral — *see* Insufficiency, mitral
  Mönckeberg's — *see* Arteriosclerosis, extremities
  motor centers, senile G31.1
  multi-system G90.3
  mural — *see* Degeneration, myocardial
  muscle (fatty) (fibrous) (hyaline) (progressive) M62.89
    heart — *see* Degeneration, myocardial
  myelin, central nervous system G37.9
  myocardial, myocardium (fatty) (hyaline) (senile) I51.5
    with rheumatic fever (conditions in I00) I09.0
      active, acute or subacute I01.2
        with chorea I02.0
      inactive or quiescent (with chorea) I09.0
    hypertensive — *see* Hypertension, heart
    rheumatic — *see* Degeneration, myocardial, with rheumatic fever
    syphilitic A52.06
  nasal sinus (mucosa) J32.9
    frontal J32.1
    maxillary J32.0
  nerve — *see* Disorder, nerve
  nervous system G31.9
    alcoholic G31.2
    amyloid E85.4 [G99.8]
    autonomic G90.9
    fatty G31.89
    specified NEC G31.89
  nipple N64.89
  olivopontocerebellar (hereditary) (familial) G23.8
  osseous labyrinth — *see* subcategory H83.8
  ovary N83.8
    cystic N83.20 ☑
    microcystic N83.20 ☑
  pallidal pigmentary (progressive) G23.0
  pancreas K86.89
    tuberculous A18.83
  penis N48.89
  pigmentary (diffuse) (general)
    localized — *see* Degeneration, by site
    pallidal (progressive) G23.0
  pineal gland E34.8
  pituitary (gland) E23.6
  popliteal fat pad M79.4
  posterolateral (spinal cord) — *see* Degeneration, combined
  pulmonary valve (heart) I37.8
  pulp (tooth) K04.2
  pupillary margin H21.24 ☑
  renal — *see* Degeneration, kidney

Degeneration — *continued*
  retina H35.9
    hereditary (cerebroretinal) (congenital) (juvenile) (macula) (peripheral) (pigmentary) — *see* Dystrophy, retina
    Kuhnt-Junius (*see also* Degeneration, macula) H35.32 ☑
    macula (cystic) (exudative) (hole) (nonexudative) (pseudohole) (senile) (toxic) — *see* Degeneration, macula
    peripheral H35.40
      lattice H35.41 ☑
      microcystoid H35.42 ☑
      paving stone H35.43 ☑
      secondary
        pigmentary H35.45 ☑
        vitreoretinal H35.46 ☑
      senile reticular H35.44 ☑
    pigmentary (primary) (*see also* Dystrophy, retina)
      secondary — *see* Degeneration, retina, peripheral, secondary
    posterior pole — *see* Degeneration, macula
  saccule, congenital (causing impairment of hearing) Q16.5
  senile R54
    brain G31.1
    cardiac, heart or myocardium — *see* Degeneration, myocardial
    motor centers G31.1
    vascular — *see* Arteriosclerosis
  sinus (cystic) (*see also* Sinusitis)
    polypoid J33.1
  skin L98.8
    amyloid E85.4 [L99]
    colloid L98.8
  spinal (cord) G31.89
    amyloid E85.4 [G32.89]
    combined (subacute) — *see* Degeneration, combined
    dorsolateral — *see* Degeneration, combined
    familial NEC G31.89
    fatty G31.89
    funicular — *see* Degeneration, combined
    posterolateral — *see* Degeneration, combined
    subacute combined — *see* Degeneration, combined
    tuberculous A17.81
  spleen D73.0
    amyloid E85.4 [D77]
  stomach K31.89
  striatonigral G23.2
  suprarenal (capsule) (gland) E27.8
  synovial membrane (pulpy) — *see* Disorder, synovium, specified type NEC
  tapetoretinal — *see* Dystrophy, retina
  thymus (gland) E32.8
    fatty E32.8
  thyroid (gland) E07.89
  tricuspid (heart) (valve) I07.9
  tuberculous NEC — *see* Tuberculosis
  turbinate J34.89
  uterus (cystic) N85.8
  vascular (senile) — *see* Arteriosclerosis
    hypertensive — *see* Hypertension
  vitreoretinal, secondary — *see* Degeneration, retina, peripheral, secondary, vitreoretinal
  vitreous (body) H43.81 ☑
  Wallerian — *see* Disorder, nerve
  Wilson's hepatolenticular E83.01
Deglutition
  paralysis R13.0
    hysterical F44.4
  pneumonia J69.0
Degos' disease I77.89
Dehiscence (of)
  amputation stump T87.81
  cesarean wound O90.0
  closure of
    cornea T81.31 ☑
    craniotomy T81.32 ☑
    fascia (muscular) (superficial) T81.32 ☑
    internal organ or tissue T81.32 ☑
    laceration (external) (internal) T81.33 ☑
    ligament T81.32 ☑
    mucosa T81.31 ☑
    muscle or muscle flap T81.32 ☑
    ribs or rib cage T81.32 ☑
    skin and subcutaneous tissue (full-thickness) (superficial) T81.31 ☑
    skull T81.32 ☑
    sternum (sternotomy) T81.32 ☑

Dehiscence - Delivery

Dehiscence — *continued*
  closure of — *continued*
    tendon T81.32 ☑
    traumatic laceration (external)
      (internal) T81.33 ☑
    episiotomy O90.1
    operation wound NEC T81.31 ☑
      external operation wound
        (superficial) T81.31 ☑
      internal operation wound (deep) T81.32 ☑
    perineal wound (postpartum) O90.1
    traumatic injury wound repair T81.33 ☑
    wound T81.30 ☑
      traumatic repair T81.33 ☑
Dehydration E86.0
  newborn P74.1
Déjérine-Roussy syndrome G89.0
Déjérine-Sottas disease or neuropathy
  (hypertrophic) G60.0
Déjérine-Thomas atrophy G23.8
Delay, delayed
  any plane in pelvis
    complicating delivery O66.9
  birth or delivery NOS O63.9
  closure, ductus arteriosus (Botalli) P29.38
  coagulation — *see* Defect, coagulation
  conduction (cardiac) (ventricular) I45.9
  delivery, second twin, triplet, etc O63.2
  development R62.50
    global F88
    intellectual (specific) F81.9
    language F80.9
      due to hearing loss F80.4
    learning F81.9
    pervasive F84.9
    physiological R62.50
      specified stage NEC R62.0
    reading F81.0
    sexual E30.0
    speech F80.9
      due to hearing loss F80.4
    spelling F81.81
  ejaculation F52.32
  gastric emptying K30
  menarche E30.0
  menstruation (cause unknown) N91.0
  milestone R62.0
  passage of meconium (newborn) P76.0
  primary respiration P28.9
  puberty (constitutional) E30.0
  separation of umbilical cord P96.82
  sexual maturation, female E30.0
  sleep phase syndrome G47.21
  union, fracture — *see* Fracture, by site
  vaccination Z28.9
Deletion (s)
  autosome Q93.9
    identified by fluorescence in situ hybridization
      (FISH) Q93.89
    identified by in situ hybridization (ISH) Q93.89
  chromosome
    with complex rearrangements NEC Q93.7
    part of NEC Q93.5
    seen only at prometaphase Q93.89
    short arm
      4 Q93.3
      5p Q93.4
      22q11.2 Q93.81
    specified NEC Q93.89
  long arm chromosome 18 or 21 Q93.89
    with complex rearrangements NEC Q93.7
  microdeletions NEC Q93.88
Delhi boil or button B55.1
Delinquency (juvenile) (neurotic) F91.8
  group Z72.810
Delinquent immunization status Z28.3
Delirium, delirious (acute or subacute) (not alcohol-
  or drug-induced) (with dementia) R41.0
  alcoholic (acute) (tremens) (withdrawal) F10.921
    with intoxication F10.921
      in
        abuse F10.121
        dependence F10.221
  due to (secondary to)
    alcohol
      intoxication F10.921
        in
          abuse F10.121
          dependence F10.221
      withdrawal F10.231
    amphetamine intoxication F15.921
      in

Delirium — *continued*
  due to — *continued*
      abuse F15.121
      dependence F15.221
    anxiolytic
      intoxication F13.921
        in
          abuse F13.121
          dependence F13.221
      withdrawal F13.231
    cannabis intoxication (acute) F12.921
      in
        abuse F12.121
        dependence F12.221
    cocaine intoxication (acute) F14.921
      in
        abuse F14.121
        dependence F14.221
    general medical condition F05
    hallucinogen intoxication F16.921
      in
        abuse F16.121
        dependence F16.221
    hypnotic
      intoxication F13.921
        in
          abuse F13.121
          dependence F13.221
      withdrawal F13.231
    inhalant intoxication (acute) F18.921
      in
        abuse F18.121
        dependence F18.221
    multiple etiologies F05
    opioid intoxication (acute) F11.921
      in
        abuse F11.121
        dependence F11.221
    other (or unknown) substance F19.921
    phencyclidine intoxication (acute) F16.921
      in
        abuse F16.121
        dependence F16.221
    psychoactive substance NEC intoxication
      (acute) F19.921
      in
        abuse F19.121
        dependence F19.221
    sedative
      intoxication F13.921
        in
          abuse F13.121
          dependence F13.221
      withdrawal F13.231
    unknown etiology F05
  exhaustion F43.0
  hysterical F44.89
  postprocedural (postoperative) F05
  puerperal F05
  thyroid — *see* Thyrotoxicosis with thyroid storm
  traumatic — *see* Injury, intracranial
  tremens (alcohol-induced) F10.231
    sedative-induced F13.231
Delivery (childbirth) (labor)
  arrested active phase O62.1
  cesarean (for)
    abnormal
      pelvis (bony) (deformity) (major) NEC with
        disproportion (fetopelvic) O33.0
        with obstructed labor O65.0
      presentation or position O32.9 ☑
    abruptio placentae (*see also* Abruptio
      placentae) O45.9 ☑
    acromion presentation O32.2 ☑
    atony, uterus O62.2
    breech presentation O32.1 ☑
      incomplete O32.8 ☑
    brow presentation O32.3 ☑
    cephalopelvic disproportion O33.9
    cerclage O34.3 ☑
    chin presentation O32.3 ☑
    cicatrix of cervix O34.4 ☑
    contracted pelvis (general)
      inlet O33.2
      outlet O33.3 ☑
    cord presentation or prolapse O69.0 ☑
    cystocele O34.8 ☑
    deformity (acquired) (congenital)
      pelvic organs or tissues NEC O34.8 ☑
      pelvis (bony) NEC O33.0
    disproportion NOS O33.9
    eclampsia — *see* Eclampsia

Delivery — *continued*
  cesarean — *continued*
    face presentation O32.3 ☑
    failed
      forceps O66.5
      induction of labor O61.9
        instrumental O61.1
        mechanical O61.1
        medical O61.0
        specified NEC O61.8
        surgical O61.1
      trial of labor NOS O66.40
        following previous cesarean
          delivery O66.41
      vacuum extraction O66.5
      ventouse O66.5
    fetal-maternal hemorrhage O43.01 ☑
    hemorrhage (intrapartum) O67.9
      with coagulation defect O67.0
      specified cause NEC O67.8
    high head at term O32.4 ☑
    hydrocephalic fetus O33.6 ☑
    incarceration of uterus O34.51 ☑
    incoordinate uterine action O62.4
    increased size, fetus O33.5 ☑
    inertia, uterus O62.2
      primary O62.0
      secondary O62.1
    lateroversion, uterus O34.59 ☑
    mal lie O32.9 ☑
    malposition
      fetus O32.9 ☑
      pelvic organs or tissues NEC O34.8 ☑
      uterus NEC O34.59 ☑
    malpresentation NOS O32.9 ☑
    oblique presentation O32.2 ☑
    occurring after 37 completed weeks of
      gestation but before 39 completed weeks
      gestation due to (spontaneous) onset of
      labor O75.82
    oversize fetus O33.5 ☑
    pelvic tumor NEC O34.8 ☑
    placenta previa O44.0 ☑
      complete O44.0 ☑
        with hemorrhage O44.1 ☑
    placental insufficiency O36.51 ☑
    planned, occurring after 37 completed weeks
      of gestation but before 39 completed
      weeks gestation due to (spontaneous)
      onset of labor O75.82
    polyp, cervix O34.4 ☑
      causing obstructed labor O65.5
    poor dilatation, cervix O62.0
    pre-eclampsia O14.94
      mild O14.04
      moderate O14.04
      severe O14.14
        with hemolysis, elevated liver enzymes and
          low platelet count (HELLP) O14.24
    previous
      cesarean delivery O34.219
        classical (vertical) scar O34.212
        low transverse scar O34.211
      surgery (to)
        cervix O34.4 ☑
        gynecological NEC O34.8 ☑
        rectum O34.7 ☑
        uterus O34.29
        vagina O34.6 ☑
    prolapse
      arm or hand O32.2 ☑
      uterus O34.52 ☑
    prolonged labor NOS O63.9
    rectocele O34.8 ☑
    retroversion
      uterus O34.53 ☑
    rigid
      cervix O34.4 ☑
      pelvic floor O34.8 ☑
      perineum O34.7 ☑
      vagina O34.6 ☑
      vulva O34.7 ☑
    sacculation, pregnant uterus O34.59 ☑
    scar (s)
      cervix O34.4 ☑
      cesarean delivery O34.219
        classical (vertical) O34.212
        low transverse O34.211
      transmural uterine O34.29
      uterus O34.29
    Shirodkar suture in situ O34.3 ☑
    shoulder presentation O32.2 ☑

☑ **Additional character required**

Delivery — *continued*
  cesarean — *continued*
    stenosis or stricture, cervix O34.4 ☑
    streptococcus group B (GBS) carrier
        state O99.824
    transmural uterine scar O34.29
    transverse presentation or lie O32.2 ☑
    tumor, pelvic organs or tissues NEC O34.8 ☑
        cervix O34.4 ☑
    umbilical cord presentation or
        prolapse O69.0 ☑
    without indication O82
  completely normal case O80
  complicated O75.9
    by
        abnormal, abnormality (of)
            forces of labor O62.9
                specified type NEC O62.8
            glucose O99.814
            uterine contractions NOS O62.9
        abruptio placentae (*see also* Abruptio
            placentae) O45.9 ☑
        abuse
            physical O9A.32
            psychological O9A.52
            sexual O9A.42
        adherent placenta O72.0
            without hemorrhage O73.0
        alcohol use O99.314
        anemia (pre-existing) O99.02
        anesthetic death O74.8
        annular detachment of cervix O71.3
        atony, uterus O62.2
        attempted vacuum extraction and
            forceps O66.5
        Bandl's ring O62.4
        bariatric surgery status O99.844
        biliary tract disorder O26.62
        bleeding — *see* Delivery, complicated by,
            hemorrhage
        blood disorder NEC O99.12
        cervical dystocia (hypotonic) O62.2
            primary O62.0
            secondary O62.1
        circulatory system disorder O99.42
        compression of cord (umbilical) NEC O69.2 ☑
        condition NEC O99.89
        contraction, contracted ring O62.4
        cord (umbilical)
            around neck
                with compression O69.1 ☑
                without compression O69.81 ☑
            bruising O69.5 ☑
            complication O69.9 ☑
                specified NEC O69.89 ☑
            compression NEC O69.2 ☑
            entanglement O69.2 ☑
                without compression O69.82 ☑
            hematoma O69.5 ☑
            presentation O69.0 ☑
            prolapse O69.0 ☑
            short O69.3 ☑
            thrombosis (vessels) O69.5 ☑
            vascular lesion O69.5 ☑
        Couvelaire uterus O45.8X ☑
        damage to (injury to) NEC
            perineum O71.82
            periurethral tissue O71.82
            vulva O71.82
        delay following rupture of membranes
            (spontaneous) — *see* Pregnancy,
            complicated by, premature rupture of
            membranes
        depressed fetal heart tones O76
        diabetes O24.92
            gestational O24.429
                diet controlled O24.420
                insulin controlled O24.424
                oral drug controlled (antidiabetic)
                    (hypoglycemic) O24.425
            pre-existing O24.32
                specified NEC O24.82
                type 1 O24.02
                type 2 O24.12
        diastasis recti (abdominis) O71.89
        dilatation
            bladder O66.8
            cervix incomplete, poor or slow O62.0
        disease NEC O99.89
        disruptio uteri — *see* Delivery, complicated
            by, rupture, uterus
        drug use O99.324

Delivery — *continued*
  complicated — *continued*
    dysfunction, uterus NOS O62.9
        hypertonic O62.4
        hypotonic O62.2
            primary O62.0
            secondary O62.1
        incoordinate O62.4
    eclampsia O15.1
    embolism (pulmonary) — *see* Embolism,
        obstetric
    endocrine, nutritional or metabolic disease
        NEC O99.284
    failed
        attempted vaginal birth after previous
            cesarean delivery O66.41
        induction of labor O61.9
            instrumental O61.1
            mechanical O61.1
            medical O61.0
            specified NEC O61.8
            surgical O61.1
        trial of labor O66.40
    female genital mutilation O65.5
    fetal
        abnormal acid-base balance O68
        acidemia O68
        acidosis O68
        alkalosis O68
        death, early O02.1
        deformity O66.3
        heart rate or rhythm (abnormal) (non-
            reassuring) O76
        hypoxia O77.8
        stress O77.9
            due to drug administration O77.1
            electrocardiographic evidence of O77.8
            specified NEC O77.8
            ultrasound evidence of O77.8
    fever during labor O75.2
    gastric banding status O99.844
    gastric bypass status O99.844
    gastrointestinal disease NEC O99.62
    gestational
        diabetes O24.429
            diet controlled O24.420
            insulin (and diet) controlled O24.424
            oral drug controlled (antidiabetic)
                (hypoglycemic) O24.425
        edema O12.04
            with proteinuria O12.24
        proteinuria O12.14
    gonorrhea O98.22
    hematoma O71.7
        ischial spine O71.7
        pelvic O71.7
        vagina O71.7
        vulva or perineum O71.7
    hemorrhage (uterine) O67.9
        associated with
            afibrinogenemia O67.0
            coagulation defect O67.0
            hyperfibrinolysis O67.0
            hypofibrinogenemia O67.0
        due to
            low implantation of placenta O44.5 ☑
            low lying placenta O44.5 ☑
            placenta previa O44.1 ☑
                marginal O44.3 ☑
                partial O44.3 ☑
            premature separation of placenta
                (normally implanted) (*see also*
                Abruptio placentae) O45.9 ☑
            retained placenta O72.0
            uterine leiomyoma O67.8
        placenta NEC O67.8
        postpartum NEC (atonic)
            (immediate) O72.1
            with retained or trapped placenta O72.0
            delayed O72.2
            secondary O72.2
            third stage O72.0
    hourglass contraction, uterus O62.4
    hypertension, hypertensive (pre-existing)
        — *see* Hypertension, complicated by,
        childbirth (labor)
    hypotension O26.5 ☑
    incomplete dilatation (cervix) O62.0
    incoordinate uterus contractions O62.4
    inertia, uterus O62.2
        during latent phase of labor O62.0
        primary O62.0

Delivery — *continued*
  complicated — *continued*
    secondary O62.1
    infection (maternal) O98.92
        carrier state NEC O99.834
        gonorrhea O98.22
        human immunodeficiency virus
            (HIV) O98.72
        sexually transmitted NEC O98.32
        specified NEC O98.82
        syphilis O98.12
        tuberculosis O98.02
        viral hepatitis O98.42
        viral NEC O98.52
    injury (to mother) (*see also* Delivery,
        complicated, by, damage to) O71.9
        nonobstetric O9A.22
            caused by abuse — *see* Delivery,
                complicated by, abuse
    intrauterine fetal death, early O02.1
    inversion, uterus O71.2
    laceration (perineal) O70.9
        anus (sphincter) O70.4
            with third degree laceration (*see also*
                Delivery, complicated, by, laceration,
                perineum, third degree) O70.20
            with mucosa O70.3
            without third degree laceration O70.4
        bladder (urinary) O71.5
        bowel O71.5
        cervix (uteri) O71.3
        fourchette O70.0
        hymen O70.0
        labia O70.0
        pelvic
            floor O70.1
            organ NEC O71.5
        perineum, perineal O70.9
            first degree O70.0
            fourth degree O70.3
            muscles O70.1
            second degree O70.1
            skin O70.0
            slight O70.0
            third degree O70.20
                with
                    both external anal sphincter (EAS)
                        and internal anal sphincter (IAS)
                        torn (IIIc) O70.23
                    less than 50% of external anal
                        sphincter (EAS) thickness torn
                        (IIIa) O70.21
                    more than 50% external anal
                        sphincter (EAS) thickness torn
                        (IIIb) O70.22
                IIIa O70.21
                IIIb O70.22
                IIIc O70.23
        peritoneum (pelvic) O71.5
        rectovaginal (septum) (without perineal
            laceration) O71.4
            with perineum (*see also* Delivery,
                complicated, by, laceration,
                perineum, third degree) O70.20
                with anal or rectal mucosa O70.3
        specified NEC O71.89
        sphincter ani — *see* Delivery, complicated,
            by, laceration, anus (sphincter)
        urethra O71.5
        uterus O71.81
            before labor O71.81
        vagina, vaginal (deep) (high) (without
            perineal laceration) O71.4
            with perineum O70.0
            muscles, with perineum O70.1
        vulva O70.0
    liver disorder O26.62
    malignancy O9A.12
    malnutrition O25.2
    malposition, malpresentation
        placenta O44.0 ☑
            with hemorrhage O44.1 ☑
        uterus or cervix O65.5
        without obstruction (*see also* Delivery,
            complicated by, obstruction) O32.9 ☑
            breech O32.1 ☑
            compound O32.6 ☑
            face (brow) (chin) O32.3 ☑
            footling O32.8 ☑
            high head O32.4 ☑
            oblique O32.2 ☑
            specified NEC O32.8 ☑

☑ **Additional character required**

Delivery — continued
  complicated — continued
    transverse O32.2 ☑
    unstable lie O32.0 ☑
  meconium in amniotic fluid O77.0
  mental disorder NEC O99.344
  metrorrhexis — see Delivery, complicated by, rupture, uterus
  nervous system disorder O99.354
  obesity (pre-existing) O99.214
  obesity surgery status O99.844
  obstetric trauma O71.9
    specified NEC O71.89
  obstructed labor
    due to
      breech (complete) (frank)
        presentation O64.1 ☑
        incomplete O64.8 ☑
      brow presenation O64.3 ☑
      buttock presentation O64.1 ☑
      chin presentation O64.2 ☑
      compound presentation O64.5 ☑
      contracted pelvis O65.1
      deep transverse arrest O64.0 ☑
      deformed pelvis O65.0
      dystocia (fetal) O66.9
        due to
          conjoined twins O66.3
          fetal
            abnormality NEC O66.3
            ascites O66.3
            hydrops O66.3
            meningomyelocele O66.3
            sacral teratoma O66.3
            tumor O66.3
          hydrocephalic fetus O66.3
      shoulder O66.0
      face presentation O64.2 ☑
      fetopelvic disproportion O65.4
      footling presentation O64.8 ☑
      impacted shoulders O66.0
      incomplete rotation of fetal
        head O64.0 ☑
      large fetus O66.2
      locked twins O66.1
      malposition O64.9 ☑
        specified NEC O64.8 ☑
      malpresentation O64.9 ☑
        specified NEC O64.8 ☑
      multiple fetuses NEC O66.6
      pelvic
        abnormality (maternal) O65.9
          organ O65.5
          specified NEC O65.8
        contraction
          inlet O65.2
          mid-cavity O65.3
          outlet O65.3
        persistent (position)
          occipitoiliac O64.0 ☑
          occipitoposterior O64.0 ☑
          occipitosacral O64.0 ☑
          occipitotransverse O64.0 ☑
      prolapsed arm O64.4 ☑
      shoulder presentation O64.4 ☑
    specified NEC O66.8
  pathological retraction ring, uterus O62.4
  penetration, pregnant uterus by instrument O71.1
  perforation — see Delivery, complicated by, laceration
  placenta, placental
    ablatio (see also Abruptio placentae) O45.9 ☑
    abnormality O43.9 ☑
      specified NEC O43.89 ☑
    abruptio (see also Abruptio placentae) O45.9 ☑
    accreta O43.21 ☑
    adherent (with hemorrhage) O72.0
      without hemorrhage O73.0
    detachment (premature) (see also Abruptio placentae) O45.9 ☑
    disorder O43.9 ☑
      specified NEC O43.89 ☑
    hemorrhage NEC O67.8
    increta O43.22 ☑
    low (implantation) (lying) O44.4 ☑
      with hemorrhage O44.5 ☑
    malformation O43.10 ☑
    malposition O44.0 ☑
      without hemorrhage O44.1 ☑

Delivery — continued
  complicated — continued
    percreta O43.23 ☑
    previa (central) (complete) (lateral) (total) O44.0 ☑
      with hemorrhage O44.1 ☑
      marginal O44.2 ☑
        with hemorrhage O44.3 ☑
      partial O44.2 ☑
        with hemorrhage O44.3 ☑
    retained (with hemorrhage) O72.0
      without hemorrhage O73.0
    separation (premature) O45.9 ☑
      specified NEC O45.8X ☑
    vicious insertion O44.1 ☑
  precipitate labor O62.3
  premature rupture, membranes (see also Pregnancy, complicated by, premature rupture of membranes) O42.90
  prolapse
    arm or hand O32.2 ☑
    cord (umbilical) O69.0 ☑
    foot or leg O32.8 ☑
    uterus O34.52 ☑
  prolonged labor O63.9
    first stage O63.0
    second stage O63.1
  protozoal disease (maternal) O98.62
  respiratory disease NEC O99.52
  retained membranes or portions of placenta O72.2
    without hemorrhage O73.1
  retarded birth O63.9
  retention of secundines (with hemorrhage) O72.0
    without hemorrhage O73.0
    partial O72.2
      without hemorrhage O73.1
  rupture
    bladder (urinary) O71.5
    cervix O71.3
    pelvic organ NEC O71.5
    urethra O71.5
    uterus (during or after labor) O71.1
      before labor O71.0 ☑
  separation, pubic bone (symphysis pubis) O71.6
  shock O75.1
  shoulder presentation O64.4 ☑
  skin disorder NEC O99.72
  spasm, cervix O62.4
  stenosis or stricture, cervix O65.5
  streptococcus group B (GBS) carrier state O99.824
  subluxation of symphysis (pubis) O26.72
  syphilis (maternal) O98.12
  tear — see Delivery, complicated by, laceration
  tetanic uterus O62.4
  trauma (obstetrical) (see also Delivery, complicated, by, damage to) O71.9
    non-obstetric O9A.22
    periurethral O71.82
    specified NEC O71.89
  tuberculosis (maternal) O98.02
  tumor, pelvic organs or tissues NEC O65.5
  umbilical cord around neck
    with compression O69.1 ☑
    without compression O69.81 ☑
  uterine inertia O62.2
    during latent phase of labor O62.0
    primary O62.0
    secondary O62.1
  vasa previa O69.4 ☑
  velamentous insertion of cord O43.12 ☑
  specified complication NEC O75.89
delayed NOS O63.9
  following rupture of membranes
    artificial O75.5
  second twin, triplet, etc. O63.2
forceps, low following failed vacuum extraction O66.5
missed (at or near term) O36.4 ☑
normal O80
obstructed — see Delivery, complicated by, obstructed labor
precipitate O62.3
preterm (see also Pregnancy, complicated by, preterm labor) O60.10 ☑
spontaneous O80
term pregnancy NOS O80
uncomplicated O80

Delivery — continued
  vaginal, following previous cesarean
    delivery O34.219
    classical (vertical) scar O34.212
    low transverse scar O34.211
Delusions (paranoid) — see Disorder, delusional
Dementia (degenerative (primary)) (old age) (persisting) F03.90
  with
    aggressive behavior F03.91
    behavioral disturbance F03.91
    combative behavior F03.91
    Lewy bodies G31.83 [F02.80]
      with behavioral disturbance G31.83 [F02.81]
    Parkinsonism G31.83 [F02.80]
      with behavioral disturbance G31.83 [F02.81]
    Parkinson's disease G20 [F02.80]
      with behavioral disturbance G20 [F02.81]
    violent behavior F03.91
  alcoholic F10.97
    with dependence F10.27
  Alzheimer's type — see Disease, Alzheimer's
  arteriosclerotic — see Dementia, vascular
  atypical, Alzheimer's type — see Disease, Alzheimer's, specified NEC
  congenital — see Disability, intellectual
  frontal (lobe) G31.09 [F02.80]
    with behavioral disturbance G31.09 [F02.81]
  frontotemporal G31.09 [F02.80]
    with behavioral disturbance G31.09 [F02.81]
    specified NEC G31.09 [F02.80]
      with behavioral disturbance G31.09 [F02.81]
  in (due to)
    alcohol F10.97
      with dependence F10.27
    Alzheimer's disease — see Disease, Alzheimer's
    arteriosclerotic brain disease — see Dementia, vascular
    cerebral lipidoses E75. ☑ [F02.80]
      with behavioral disturbance E75. ☑ [F02.81]
    Creutzfeldt-Jakob disease (see also Creutzfeldt-Jakob disease or syndrome (with dementia)) A81.00
    epilepsy G40. ☑ [F02.80]
      with behavioral disturbance G40. ☑ [F02.81]
    hepatolenticular degeneration E83.01 [F02.80]
      with behavioral disturbance E83.01 [F02.81]
    human immunodeficiency virus (HIV) disease B20 [F02.80]
      with behavioral disturbance B20 [F02.81]
    Huntington's disease or chorea G10 [F02.80]
      with behavioral disturbance G10 [F02.81]
    hypercalcemia E83.52 [F02.80]
      with behavioral disturbance E83.52 [F02.81]
    hypothyroidism, acquired E03.9 [F02.80]
      with behavioral disturbance E03.9 [F02.81]
      due to iodine deficiency E01.8 [F02.80]
        with behavioral disturbance E01.8 [F02.81]
    inhalants F18.97
      with dependence F18.27
    multiple
      etiologies F03 ☑
      sclerosis G35 [F02.80]
        with behavioral disturbance G35 [F02.81]
    neurosyphilis A52.17 [F02.80]
      with behavioral disturbance A52.17 [F02.81]
      juvenile A50.49 [F02.80]
        with behavioral disturbance A50.49 [F02.81]
    niacin deficiency E52 [F02.80]
      with behavioral disturbance E52 [F02.81]
    paralysis agitans G20 [F02.80]
      with behavioral disturbance G20 [F02.81]
    Parkinson's disease G20 [F02.80]
    pellagra E52 [F02.80]
      with behavioral disturbance E52 [F02.81]
    Pick's G31.01 [F02.80]
      with behavioral disturbance G31.01 [F02.81]
    polyarteritis nodosa M30.0 [F02.80]
      with behavioral disturbance M30.0 [F02.81]
    psychoactive drug F19.97
      with dependence F19.27
      inhalants F18.97
        with dependence F18.27
      sedatives, hypnotics or anxiolytics F13.97
        with dependence F13.27
    sedatives, hypnotics or anxiolytics F13.97
      with dependence F13.27
    systemic lupus erythematosus M32. ☑ [F02.80]
      with behavioral disturbance M32. ☑ [F02.81]
    trypanosomiasis
      African B56.9 [F02.80]

☑ Additional character required

Delivery - Dementia

ICD-10-CM INDEX TO DISEASES AND INJURIES

Dementia — *continued*
  in — *continued*
    with behavioral disturbance B56.9 *[F02.81]*
    unknown etiology F03 ☑
    vitamin B12 deficiency E53.8 *[F02.80]*
      with behavioral disturbance E53.8 *[F02.81]*
    volatile solvents F18.97
      with dependence F18.27
      with behavioral disturbance G31.83 *[F02.81]*
  infantile, infantilis F84.3
  Lewy body G31.83 *[F02.80]*
    with behavioral disturbance G31.83 *[F02.81]*
  multi-infarct — *see* Dementia, vascular
  paralytica, paralytic (syphilitic) A52.17 *[F02.80]*
    with behavioral disturbance A52.17 *[F02.81]*
    juvenilis A50.45
  paretic A52.17
  praecox — *see* Schizophrenia
  presenile F03 ☑
    Alzheimer's type — *see* Disease, Alzheimer's,
      early onset
    primary degenerative F03 ☑
  progressive, syphilitic A52.17
  senile F03 ☑
    with acute confusional state F05
    Alzheimer's type — *see* Disease, Alzheimer's,
      late onset
    depressed or paranoid type F03 ☑
  vascular (acute onset) (mixed) (multi-infarct)
    (subcortical) F01.50
    with behavioral disturbance F01.51
Demineralization, bone — *see* Osteoporosis
Demodex folliculorum (infestation) B88.0
Demophobia F40.248
Demoralization R45.3
Demyelination, demyelinization
  central nervous system G37.9
    specified NEC G37.8
  corpus callosum (central) G37.1
  disseminated, acute G36.9
    specified NEC G36.8
  global G35
  in optic neuritis G36.0
Dengue (classical) (fever) A90
  hemorrhagic A91
  sandfly A93.1
Dennie-Marfan syphilitic syndrome A50.45
Dens evaginatus, in dente or invaginatus K00.2
Dense breasts R92.2
Density
  increased, bone (disseminated) (generalized)
    (spotted) — *see* Disorder, bone, density and
    structure, specified type NEC
  lung (nodular) J98.4
Dental (*see also* condition)
  examination Z01.20
    with abnormal findings Z01.21
  restoration
    aesthetically inadequate or displeasing K08.56
    defective K08.50
      specified NEC K08.59
    failure of marginal integrity K08.51
    failure of periodontal anatomical
      integrity K08.54
Dentia praecox K00.6
Denticles (pulp) K04.2
Dentigerous cyst K09.0
Dentin
  irregular (in pulp) K04.3
  opalescent K00.5
  secondary (in pulp) K04.3
  sensitive K03.89
Dentinogenesis imperfecta K00.5
Dentinoma — *see* Cyst, calcifying odontogenic
Dentition (syndrome) K00.7
  delayed K00.6
  difficult K00.7
  precocious K00.6
  premature K00.6
  retarded K00.6
Dependence (on) (syndrome) F19.20
  with remission F19.21
  alcohol (ethyl) (methyl) (without
    remission) F10.20
    with
      amnestic disorder, persisting F10.26
      anxiety disorder F10.280
      dementia, persisting F10.27
      intoxication F10.229
        with delirium F10.221
        uncomplicated F10.220
      mood disorder F10.24

Dependence — *continued*
  alcohol — *continued*
    psychotic disorder F10.259
      with
        delusions F10.250
        hallucinations F10.251
    remission F10.21
    sexual dysfunction F10.281
    sleep disorder F10.282
    specified disorder NEC F10.288
    withdrawal F10.239
      with
        delirium F10.231
        perceptual disturbance F10.232
      uncomplicated F10.230
    counseling and surveillance Z71.41
  amobarbital — *see* Dependence, drug, sedative
  amphetamine (s) (type) — *see* Dependence, drug,
    stimulant NEC
  amytal (sodium) — *see* Dependence, drug,
    sedative
  analgesic NEC F55.8
  anesthetic (agent) (gas) (general) (local) NEC —
    see Dependence, drug, psychoactive NEC
  anxiolytic NEC — *see* Dependence, drug, sedative
  barbital (s) — *see* Dependence, drug, sedative
  barbiturate (s) (compounds) (drugs classifiable to
    T42) — *see* Dependence, drug, sedative
  benzedrine — *see* Dependence, drug, stimulant
    NEC
  bhang — *see* Dependence, drug, cannabis
  bromide (s) NEC — *see* Dependence, drug,
    sedative
  caffeine — *see* Dependence, drug, stimulant NEC
  cannabis (sativa) (indica) (resin) (derivatives)
    (type) — *see* Dependence, drug, cannabis
  chloral (betaine) (hydrate) — *see* Dependence,
    drug, sedative
  chlordiazepoxide — *see* Dependence, drug,
    sedative
  coca (leaf) (derivatives) — *see* Dependence, drug,
    cocaine
  cocaine — *see* Dependence, drug, cocaine
  codeine — *see* Dependence, drug, opioid
  combinations of drugs F19.20
  dagga — *see* Dependence, drug, cannabis
  demerol — *see* Dependence, drug, opioid
  dexamphetamine — *see* Dependence, drug,
    stimulant NEC
  dexedrine — *see* Dependence, drug, stimulant
    NEC
  dextromethorphan — *see* Dependence, drug,
    opioid
  dextromoramide — *see* Dependence, drug,
    opioid
  dextro-nor-pseudo-ephedrine — *see*
    Dependence, drug, stimulant NEC
  dextrorphan — *see* Dependence, drug, opioid
  diazepam — *see* Dependence, drug, sedative
  dilaudid — *see* Dependence, drug, opioid
  D-lysergic acid diethylamide — *see* Dependence,
    drug, hallucinogen
  drug NEC F19.20
    with sleep disorder F19.282
    cannabis F12.20
      with
        anxiety disorder F12.280
        intoxication F12.229
          with
            delirium F12.221
            perceptual disturbance F12.222
          uncomplicated F12.220
        other specified disorder F12.288
        psychosis F12.259
          delusions F12.250
          hallucinations F12.251
        unspecified disorder F12.29
      in remission F12.21
    cocaine F14.20
      with
        anxiety disorder F14.280
        intoxication F14.229
          with
            delirium F14.221
            perceptual disturbance F14.222
          uncomplicated F14.220
        mood disorder F14.24
        other specified disorder F14.288
        psychosis F14.259
          delusions F14.250
          hallucinations F14.251
        sexual dysfunction F14.281

Dependence — *continued*
  drug NEC — *continued*
    sleep disorder F14.282
    unspecified disorder F14.29
    withdrawal F14.23
    in remission F14.21
    withdrawal symptoms in newborn P96.1
    counseling and surveillance Z71.51
    hallucinogen F16.20
      with
        anxiety disorder F16.280
        flashbacks F16.283
        intoxication F16.229
          with delirium F16.221
          uncomplicated F16.220
        mood disorder F16.24
        other specified disorder F16.288
        perception disorder, persisting F16.283
        psychosis F16.259
          delusions F16.250
          hallucinations F16.251
        unspecified disorder F16.29
      in remission F16.21
    in remission F19.21
    inhalant F18.20
      with
        anxiety disorder F18.280
        dementia, persisting F18.27
        intoxication F18.229
          with delirium F18.221
          uncomplicated F18.220
        mood disorder F18.24
        other specified disorder F18.288
        psychosis F18.259
          delusions F18.250
          hallucinations F18.251
        unspecified disorder F18.29
      in remission F18.21
    nicotine F17.200
      with disorder F17.209
      in remission F17.201
      specified disorder NEC F17.208
      withdrawal F17.203
      chewing tobacco F17.220
        with disorder F17.229
        in remission F17.221
        specified disorder NEC F17.228
        withdrawal F17.223
      cigarettes F17.210
        with disorder F17.219
        in remission F17.211
        specified disorder NEC F17.218
        withdrawal F17.213
      specified product NEC F17.290
        with disorder F17.299
        remission F17.291
        specified disorder NEC F17.298
        withdrawal F17.293
    opioid F11.20
      with
        intoxication F11.229
          with
            delirium F11.221
            perceptual disturbance F11.222
          uncomplicated F11.220
        mood disorder F11.24
        other specified disorder F11.288
        psychosis F11.259
          delusions F11.250
          hallucinations F11.251
        sexual dysfunction F11.281
        sleep disorder F11.282
        unspecified disorder F11.29
        withdrawal F11.23
      in remission F11.21
    psychoactive NEC F19.20
      with
        amnestic disorder F19.26
        anxiety disorder F19.280
        dementia F19.27
        intoxication F19.229
          with
            delirium F19.221
            perceptual disturbance F19.222
          uncomplicated F19.220
        mood disorder F19.24
        other specified disorder F19.288
        psychosis F19.259
          delusions F19.250
          hallucinations F19.251
        sexual dysfunction F19.281
        sleep disorder F19.282

Dependence - Depression

Dependence — *continued*
 drug NEC — *continued*
  unspecified disorder F19.29
  withdrawal F19.239
   with
    delirium F19.231
    perceptual disturbance F19.232
   uncomplicated F19.230
  sedative, hypnotic or anxiolytic F13.20
   with
    amnestic disorder F13.26
    anxiety disorder F13.280
    dementia, persisting F13.27
    intoxication F13.229
     with delirium F13.221
     uncomplicated F13.220
    mood disorder F13.24
    other specified disorder F13.288
    psychosis F13.259
     delusions F13.250
     hallucinations F13.251
    sexual dysfunction F13.281
    sleep disorder F13.282
    unspecified disorder F13.29
    withdrawal F13.239
     with
      delirium F13.231
      perceptual disturbance F13.232
     uncomplicated F13.230
   in remission F13.21
  stimulant NEC F15.20
   with
    anxiety disorder F15.280
    intoxication F15.229
     with
      delirium F15.221
      perceptual disturbance F15.222
     uncomplicated F15.220
    mood disorder F15.24
    other specified disorder F15.288
    psychosis F15.259
     delusions F15.250
     hallucinations F15.251
    sexual dysfunction F15.281
    sleep disorder F15.282
    unspecified disorder F15.29
    withdrawal F15.23
   in remission F15.21
 ethyl
  alcohol (without remission) F10.20
   with remission F10.21
  bromide — *see* Dependence, drug, sedative
  carbamate F19.20
  chloride F19.20
  morphine — *see* Dependence, drug, opioid
 ganja — *see* Dependence, drug, cannabis
 glue (airplane) (sniffing) — *see* Dependence,
  drug, inhalant
 glutethimide — *see* Dependence, drug, sedative
 hallucinogenics — *see* Dependence, drug,
  hallucinogen
 hashish — *see* Dependence, drug, cannabis
 hemp — *see* Dependence, drug, cannabis
 heroin (salt) (any) — *see* Dependence, drug,
  opioid
 hypnotic NEC — *see* Dependence, drug, sedative
 Indian hemp — *see* Dependence, drug, cannabis
 inhalants — *see* Dependence, drug, inhalant
 khat — *see* Dependence, drug, stimulant NEC
 laudanum — *see* Dependence, drug, opioid
 LSD (-25) (derivatives) — *see* Dependence, drug,
  hallucinogen
 luminal — *see* Dependence, drug, sedative
 lysergic acid — *see* Dependence, drug,
  hallucinogen
 maconha — *see* Dependence, drug, cannabis
 marihuana — *see* Dependence, drug, cannabis
 meprobamate — *see* Dependence, drug, sedative
 mescaline — *see* Dependence, drug,
  hallucinogen
 methadone — *see* Dependence, drug, opioid
 methamphetamine (s) — *see* Dependence, drug,
  stimulant NEC
 methaqualone — *see* Dependence, drug, sedative
 methyl
  alcohol (without remission) F10.20
   with remission F10.21
  bromide — *see* Dependence, drug, sedative
  morphine — *see* Dependence, drug, opioid
  phenidate — *see* Dependence, drug, stimulant
   NEC
  sulfonal — *see* Dependence, drug, sedative

Dependence — *continued*
 morphine (sulfate) (sulfite) (type) — *see*
  Dependence, drug, opioid
 narcotic (drug) NEC — *see* Dependence, drug,
  opioid
 nembutal — *see* Dependence, drug, sedative
 neraval — *see* Dependence, drug, sedative
 neravan — *see* Dependence, drug, sedative
 neurobarb — *see* Dependence, drug, sedative
 nicotine — *see* Dependence, drug, nicotine
 nitrous oxide F19.20
 nonbarbiturate sedatives and tranquilizers with
  similar effect — *see* Dependence, drug,
  sedative
 on
  artificial heart (fully implantable)
   (mechanical) Z95.812
  aspirator Z99.0
  care provider (because of) Z74.9
   impaired mobility Z74.09
   need for
    assistance with personal care Z74.1
    continuous supervision Z74.3
   no other household member able to render
    care Z74.2
   specified reason NEC Z74.8
  machine Z99.89
   enabling NEC Z99.89
   specified type NEC Z99.89
  renal dialysis (hemodialysis) (peritoneal) Z99.2
  respirator Z99.11
  ventilator Z99.11
  wheelchair Z99.3
 opiate — *see* Dependence, drug, opioid
 opioids — *see* Dependence, drug, opioid
 opium (alkaloids) (derivatives) (tincture) — *see*
  Dependence, drug, opioid
 oxygen (long-term) (supplemental) Z99.81
 paraldehyde — *see* Dependence, drug, sedative
 paregoric — *see* Dependence, drug, opioid
 PCP (phencyclidine) (or related substance) — *see*
  Dependence, drug, hallucinogen
 pentobarbital — *see* Dependence, drug, sedative
 pentobarbitone (sodium) — *see* Dependence,
  drug, sedative
 pentothal — *see* Dependence, drug, sedative
 peyote — *see* Dependence, drug, hallucinogen
 phencyclidine (PCP) (or related substance) — *see*
  Dependence, drug, hallucinogen
 phenmetrazine — *see* Dependence, drug,
  stimulant NEC
 phenobarbital — *see* Dependence, drug, sedative
 polysubstance F19.20
 psilocibin, psilocin, psilocyn, psilocyline — *see*
  Dependence, drug, hallucinogen
 psychostimulant NEC — *see* Dependence, drug,
  stimulant NEC
 secobarbital — *see* Dependence, drug, sedative
 seconal — *see* Dependence, drug, sedative
 sedative NEC — *see* Dependence, drug, sedative
 specified drug NEC — *see* Dependence, drug
 stimulant NEC — *see* Dependence, drug,
  stimulant NEC
 substance NEC — *see* Dependence, drug
 supplemental oxygen Z99.81
 tobacco — *see* Dependence, drug, nicotine
  counseling and surveillance Z71.6
 tranquilizer NEC — *see* Dependence, drug,
  sedative
 vitamin B6 E53.1
 volatile solvents — *see* Dependence, drug,
  inhalant
Dependency
 care-provider Z74.9
 passive F60.7
 reactions (persistent) F60.7
Depersonalization (in neurotic state) (neurotic)
 (syndrome) F48.1
Depletion
 extracellular fluid E86.9
 plasma E86.1
 potassium E87.6
  nephropathy N25.89
 salt or sodium E87.1
  causing heat exhaustion or prostration T67.4 ☑
  nephropathy N28.9
 volume NOS E86.9
Deployment (current) (military) status Z56.82
 in theater or in support of military war,
  peacekeeping and humanitarian
  operations Z56.82

Deployment — *continued*
 personal history of Z91.82
  military war, peacekeeping and humanitarian
   deployment (current or past
    conflict) Z91.82
 returned from Z91.82
Depolarization, premature I49.40
 atrial I49.1
 junctional I49.2
 specified NEC I49.49
 ventricular I49.3
Deposit
 bone in Boeck's sarcoid D86.89
 calcareous, calcium — *see* Calcification
 cholesterol
  retina H35.89
  vitreous (body) (humor) — *see* Deposit,
   crystalline
 conjunctiva H11.11 ☑
 cornea H18.00 ☑
  argentous H18.02 ☑
  due to metabolic disorder H18.03 ☑
  Kayser-Fleischer ring H18.04 ☑
  pigmentation — *see* Pigmentation, cornea
 crystalline, vitreous (body) (humor) H43.2 ☑
 hemosiderin in old scars of cornea — *see*
  Pigmentation, cornea, stromal
 metallic in lens — *see* Cataract, specified NEC
 skin R23.8
 tooth, teeth (betel) (black) (green) (materia alba)
  (orange) (tobacco) K03.6
 urate, kidney — *see* Calculus, kidney
Depraved appetite — *see* Pica
Depressed
 HDL cholesterol E78.6
Depression (acute) (mental) F32.9
 agitated (single episode) F32.2
 anaclitic — *see* Disorder, adjustment
 anxiety F41.8
  persistent F34.1
 arches (*see also* Deformity, limb, flat foot)
 atypical (single episode) F32.89
  recurrent episode F33.8
 basal metabolic rate R94.8
 bone marrow D75.89
 central nervous system R09.2
 cerebral R29.818
  newborn P91.4
 cerebrovascular I67.9
 chest wall M95.4
 climacteric (single episode) F32.89
  recurrent episode F33.8
 endogenous (without psychotic symptoms) F33.2
  with psychotic symptoms F33.3
 functional activity R68.89
 hysterical F44.89
 involutional (single episode) F32.89
  recurrent episode F33.8
 major F32.9
  with psychotic symptoms F32.3
  recurrent — *see* Disorder, depressive, recurrent
 manic-depressive — *see* Disorder, depressive,
  recurrent
 masked (single episode) F32.89
 medullary G93.89
 menopausal (single episode) F32.89
  recurrent episode F33.8
 metatarsus — *see* Depression, arches
 monopolar F33.9
 nervous F34.1
 neurotic F34.1
 nose M95.0
 postnatal F53
 postpartum F53
 post-psychotic of schizophrenia F32.89
 post-schizophrenic F32.89
 psychogenic (reactive) (single episode) F32.9
 psychoneurotic F34.1
 psychotic (single episode) F32.3
  recurrent F33.3
 reactive (psychogenic) (single episode) F32.9
  psychotic (single episode) F32.3
 recurrent — *see* Disorder, depressive, recurrent
 respiratory center G93.89
 seasonal — *see* Disorder, depressive, recurrent
 senile F03 ☑
 severe, single episode F32.2
 situational F43.21
 skull Q67.4
 specified NEC (single episode) F32.89
 sternum M95.4
 visual field — *see* Defect, visual field

Depression — *continued*
vital (recurrent) (without psychotic
symptoms) F33.2
with psychotic symptoms F33.3
single episode F32.2
Deprivation
cultural Z60.3
effects NOS T73.9 ☑
specified NEC T73.8 ☑
emotional NEC Z65.8
affecting infant or child — *see* Maltreatment,
child, psychological
food T73.0 ☑
protein — *see* Malnutrition
sleep Z72.820
social Z60.4
affecting infant or child — *see* Maltreatment,
child, psychological
specified NEC T73.8 ☑
vitamins — *see* Deficiency, vitamin
water T73.1 ☑
Derangement
ankle (internal) — *see* Derangement, joint, ankle
cartilage (articular) NEC — *see* Derangement,
joint, articular cartilage, by site
recurrent — *see* Dislocation, recurrent
cruciate ligament, anterior, current injury — *see*
Sprain, knee, cruciate, anterior
elbow (internal) — *see* Derangement, joint, elbow
hip (joint) (internal) (old) — *see* Derangement,
joint, hip
joint (internal) M24.9
ankylosis — *see* Ankylosis
articular cartilage M24.10
ankle M24.17 ☑
elbow M24.12 ☑
foot M24.17 ☑
hand M24.14 ☑
hip M24.15 ☑
knee NEC M23.9 ☑
loose body — *see* Loose, body
shoulder M24.11 ☑
wrist M24.13 ☑
contracture — *see* Contraction, joint
current injury (*see also* Dislocation)
knee, meniscus or cartilage — *see* Tear,
meniscus
dislocation
pathological — *see* Dislocation, pathological
recurrent — *see* Dislocation, recurrent
knee — *see* Derangement, knee
ligament — *see* Disorder, ligament
loose body — *see* Loose, body
recurrent — *see* Dislocation, recurrent
specified type NEC M24.80
ankle M24.87 ☑
elbow M24.82 ☑
foot joint M24.87 ☑
hand joint M24.84 ☑
hip M24.85 ☑
shoulder M24.81 ☑
wrist M24.83 ☑
temporomandibular M26.69
knee (recurrent) M23.9 ☑
ligament disruption, spontaneous M23.60 ☑
anterior cruciate M23.61 ☑
capsular M23.67 ☑
instability, chronic M23.5 ☑
lateral collateral M23.64 ☑
medial collateral M23.63 ☑
posterior cruciate M23.62 ☑
loose body M23.4 ☑
meniscus M23.30 ☑
cystic M23.00 ☑
lateral M23.002
anterior horn M23.04 ☑
posterior horn M23.05 ☑
specified NEC M23.06 ☑
medial M23.005
anterior horn M23.01 ☑
posterior horn M23.02 ☑
specified NEC M23.03 ☑
degenerate — *see* Derangement, knee,
meniscus, specified NEC
detached — *see* Derangement, knee,
meniscus, specified NEC
due to old tear or injury M23.20 ☑
lateral M23.20 ☑
anterior horn M23.24 ☑
posterior horn M23.25 ☑
specified NEC M23.26 ☑
medial M23.20 ☑

Derangement — *continued*
knee — *continued*
anterior horn M23.21 ☑
posterior horn M23.22 ☑
specified NEC M23.23 ☑
retained — *see* Derangement, knee,
meniscus, specified NEC
specified NEC M23.30 ☑
lateral M23.30 ☑
anterior horn M23.34 ☑
posterior horn M23.35 ☑
specified NEC M23.36 ☑
medial M23.30 ☑
anterior horn M23.31 ☑
posterior horn M23.32 ☑
specified NEC M23.33 ☑
old M23.8X ☑
specified NEC — *see* subcategory M23.8
low back NEC — *see* Dorsopathy, specified NEC
meniscus — *see* Derangement, knee, meniscus
mental — *see* Psychosis
patella, specified NEC — *see* Disorder, patella,
derangement NEC
semilunar cartilage (knee) — *see* Derangement,
knee, meniscus, specified NEC
shoulder (internal) — *see* Derangement, joint,
shoulder
Dercum's disease E88.2
Derealization (neurotic) F48.1
Dermal — *see* condition
Dermaphytid — *see* Dermatophytosis
Dermatitis (eczematous) L30.9
ab igne L59.0
acarine B88.0
actinic (due to sun) L57.8
other than from sun L59.8
allergic — *see* Dermatitis, contact, allergic
ambustionis, due to burn or scald — *see* Burn
amebic A06.7
ammonia L22
arsenical (ingested) L27.8
artefacta L98.1
psychogenic F54
atopic L20.9
psychogenic F54
specified NEC L20.89
autoimmune progesterone L30.8
berlock, berloque L56.2
blastomycotic B40.3
blister beetle L24.89
bullous, bullosa L13.9
mucosynechial, atrophic L12.1
seasonal L30.8
specified NEC L13.8
calorica L59.0
due to burn or scald — *see* Burn
caterpillar L24.89
cercarial B65.3
combustionis L59.0
due to burn or scald — *see* Burn
congelationis T69.1 ☑
contact (occupational) L25.9
allergic L23.9
due to
adhesives L23.1
cement L23.5
chemical products NEC L23.5
chromium L23.0
cosmetics L23.2
dander (cat) (dog) L23.81
drugs in contact with skin L23.3
dyes L23.4
food in contact with skin L23.6
hair (cat) (dog) L23.81
insecticide L23.5
metals L23.0
nickel L23.0
plants, non-food L23.7
plastic L23.5
rubber L23.5
specified agent NEC L23.89
due to
cement L25.3
chemical products NEC L25.3
cosmetics L25.0
dander (cat) (dog) L23.81
drugs in contact with skin L25.1
dyes L25.2
food in contact with skin L25.4
hair (cat) (dog) L23.81
plants, non-food L25.5
specified agent NEC L25.8

Dermatitis — *continued*
contact — *continued*
irritant L24.9
due to
cement L24.5
chemical products NEC L24.5
cosmetics L24.3
detergents L24.0
drugs in contact with skin L24.4
food in contact with skin L24.6
oils and greases L24.1
plants, non-food L24.7
solvents L24.2
specified agent NEC L24.89
contusiformis L52
diabetic — *see* E08-E13 with .620
diaper L22
diphtheritica A36.3
dry skin L85.3
due to
acetone (contact) (irritant) L24.2
acids (contact) (irritant) L24.5
adhesive (s) (allergic) (contact) (plaster) L23.1
irritant L24.5
alcohol (irritant) (skin contact) (substances in
category T51) L24.2
taken internally L27.8
alkalis (contact) (irritant) L24.5
arsenic (ingested) L27.8
carbon disulfide (contact) (irritant) L24.2
caustics (contact) (irritant) L24.5
cement (contact) L25.3
cereal (ingested) L27.2
chemical (s) NEC L25.3
taken internally L27.8
chlorocompounds L24.2
chromium (contact) (irritant) L24.81
coffee (ingested) L27.2
cold weather L30.8
cosmetics (contact) L25.0
allergic L23.2
irritant L24.3
cyclohexanes L24.2
dander (cat) (dog) L23.81
Demodex species B88.0
Dermanyssus gallinae B88.0
detergents (contact) (irritant) L24.0
dichromate L24.81
drugs and medicaments (generalized) (internal
use) L27.0
external — *see* Dermatitis, due to, drugs, in
contact with skin
in contact with skin L25.1
allergic L23.3
irritant L24.4
localized skin eruption L27.1
specified substance — *see* Table of Drugs and
Chemicals
dyes (contact) L25.2
allergic L23.4
irritant L24.89
epidermophytosis — *see* Dermatophytosis
esters L24.2
external irritant NEC L24.9
fish (ingested) L27.2
flour (ingested) L27.2
food (ingested) L27.2
in contact with skin L25.4
fruit (ingested) L27.2
furs (allergic) (contact) L23.81
glues — *see* Dermatitis, due to, adhesives
glycols L24.2
greases NEC (contact) (irritant) L24.1
hair (cat) (dog) L23.81
hot
objects and materials — *see* Burn
weather or places L59.0
hydrocarbons L24.2
infrared rays L59.8
ingestion, ingested substance L27.9
chemical NEC L27.8
drugs and medicaments — *see* Dermatitis,
due to, drugs
food L27.2
specified NEC L27.8
insecticide in contact with skin L24.5
internal agent L27.9
drugs and medicaments (generalized) — *see*
Dermatitis, due to, drugs
food L27.2
irradiation — *see* Dermatitis, due to, radioactive
substance

Dermatitis - Dermatosis

Dermatitis — *continued*
  due to — *continued*
    ketones L24.2
    lacquer tree (allergic) (contact) L23.7
    light (sun) NEC L57.8
      acute L56.8
      other L59.8
    Liponyssoides sanguineus B88.0
    low temperature L30.8
    meat (ingested) L27.2
    metals, metal salts (contact) (irritant) L24.81
    milk (ingested) L27.2
    nickel (contact) (irritant) L24.81
    nylon (contact) (irritant) L24.5
    oils NEC (contact) (irritant) L24.1
    paint solvent (contact) (irritant) L24.2
    petroleum products (contact) (irritant)
        (substances in T52.0) L24.2
    plants NEC (contact) L25.5
      allergic L23.7
      irritant L24.7
    plasters (adhesive) (any) (allergic)
        (contact) L23.1
      irritant L24.5
    plastic (contact) L25.3
    preservatives (contact) — *see* Dermatitis, due
        to, chemical, in contact with skin
    primrose (allergic) (contact) L23.7
    primula (allergic) (contact) L23.7
    radiation L59.8
      nonionizing (chronic exposure) L57.8
      sun NEC L57.8
        acute L56.8
    radioactive substance L58.9
      acute L58.0
      chronic L58.1
    radium L58.9
      acute L58.0
      chronic L58.1
    ragweed (allergic) (contact) L23.7
    Rhus (allergic) (contact) (diversiloba)
        (radicans) (toxicodendron) (venenata)
        (verniciflua) L23.7
    rubber (contact) L24.5
    Senecio jacobaea (allergic) (contact) L23.7
    solvents (contact) (irritant) (substances in
        categories T52) L24.2
    specified agent NEC (contact) L25.8
      allergic L23.89
      irritant L24.89
    sunshine NEC L57.8
      acute L56.8
    tetrachlorethylene (contact) (irritant) L24.2
    toluene (contact) (irritant) L24.2
    turpentine (contact) L24.2
    ultraviolet rays (sun NEC) (chronic
        exposure) L57.8
      acute L56.8
    vaccine or vaccination L27.0
      specified substance — *see* Table of Drugs and
          Chemicals
    varicose veins — *see* Varix, leg, with, inflammation
    X-rays L58.9
      acute L58.0
      chronic L58.1
  dyshydrotic L30.1
  dysmenorrheica N94.6
  escharotica — *see* Burn
  exfoliative, exfoliating (generalized) L26
    neonatorum L00
  eyelid (*see also* Dermatosis, eyelid)
    allergic H01.119
      left H01.116
        lower H01.115
        upper H01.114
      right H01.113
        lower H01.112
        upper H01.111
    contact — *see* Dermatitis, eyelid, allergic
    due to
      Demodex species B88.0
      herpes (zoster) B02.39
        simplex B00.59
    eczematous H01.139
      left H01.136
        lower H01.135
        upper H01.134
      right H01.133
        lower H01.132
        upper H01.131
  facta, factitia, factitial L98.1
    psychogenic F54

Dermatitis — *continued*
  flexural NEC L20.82
  friction L30.4
  fungus B36.9
    specified type NEC B36.8
  gangrenosa, gangrenous infantum L08.0
  harvest mite B88.0
  heat L59.0
  herpesviral, vesicular (ear) (lip) B00.1
  herpetiformis (bullous) (erythematous) (pustular)
      (vesicular) L13.0
    juvenile L12.2
    senile L12.0
  hiemalis L30.8
  hypostatic, hypostatica — *see* Varix, leg, with,
      inflammation
  infectious eczematoid L30.3
  infective L30.3
  irritant — *see* Dermatitis, contact, irritant
  Jacquet's (diaper dermatitis) L22
  Leptus B88.0
  lichenified NEC L28.0
  medicamentosa (generalized) (internal use) —
      see Dermatitis, due to drugs
  mite B88.0
  multiformis L13.0
    juvenile L12.2
  napkin L22
  neurotica L13.0
  nummular L30.0
  papillaris capillitii L73.0
  pellagrous E52
  perioral L71.0
  photocontact L56.2
  polymorpha dolorosa L13.0
  pruriginosa L13.0
  pruritic NEC L30.8
  psychogenic F54
  purulent L08.0
  pustular
    contagious B08.02
    subcorneal L13.1
  pyococcal L08.0
  pyogenica L08.0
  repens L40.2
  Ritter's (exfoliativa) L00
  Schamberg's L81.7
  schistosome B65.3
  seasonal bullous L30.8
  seborrheic L21.9
    infantile L21.1
    specified NEC L21.8
  sensitization NOS L23.9
  septic L08.0
  solare L57.8
  specified NEC L30.8
  stasis I87.2
    with
      varicose ulcer — *see* Varix, leg, with ulcer,
          with inflammation
      varicose veins — *see* Varix, leg, with,
          inflammation
    due to postthrombotic syndrome — *see*
        Syndrome, postthrombotic
  suppurative L08.0
  traumatic NEC L30.4
  trophoneurotica L13.0
  ultraviolet (sun) (chronic exposure) L57.8
    acute L56.8
  varicose — *see* Varix, leg, with inflammation
  vegetans L10.1
  verrucosa B43.0
  vesicular, herpesviral B00.1
Dermatoarthritis, lipoid E78.81
Dermatochalasis, eyelid H02.839
  left H02.836
    lower H02.835
    upper H02.834
  right H02.833
    lower H02.832
    upper H02.831
Dermatofibroma (lenticulare) — *see* Neoplasm, skin,
  benign
    protuberans — *see* Neoplasm, skin, uncertain
        behavior
Dermatofibrosarcoma (pigmented) (protuberans)
  — *see* Neoplasm, skin, malignant
Dermatographia L50.3
Dermatolysis (exfoliativa) (congenital) Q82.8
  acquired L57.4
  eyelids — *see* Blepharochalasis
  palpebrarum — *see* Blepharochalasis
  senile L57.4

Dermatomegaly NEC Q82.8
Dermatomucosomyositis M33.10
  with
    myopathy M33.12
    respiratory involvement M33.11
    specified organ involvement NEC M33.19
Dermatomycosis B36.9
  furfuracea B36.0
  specified type NEC B36.8
Dermatomyositis (acute) (chronic) — *see also*
  Dermatopolymyositis
    adult (*see also* Dermatomyositis, specified
        NEC) M33.10
    in (due to) neoplastic disease (*see also*
        Neoplasm) D49.9 *[M36.0]*
    juvenile M33.00
      with
        myopathy M33.02
        respiratory involvement M33.01
        specified organ involvement NEC M33.09
      without myopathy M33.03
    specified NEC M33.10
      with
        myopathy M33.12
        respiratory involvement M33.11
        specified organ involvement NEC M33.19
      without myopathy M33.13
Dermatoneuritis of children — *see* Poisoning,
  mercury
Dermatophilosis A48.8
Dermatophytid L30.2
Dermatophytide — *see* Dermatophytosis
Dermatophytosis (epidermophyton) (infection)
  (Microsporum) (tinea) (Trichophyton) B35.9
    beard B35.0
    body B35.4
    capitis B35.0
    corporis B35.4
    deep-seated B35.8
    disseminated B35.8
    foot B35.3
    granulomatous B35.8
    groin B35.6
    hand B35.2
    nail B35.1
    perianal (area) B35.6
    scalp B35.0
    specified NEC B35.8
Dermatopolymyositis M33.90
  with
    myopathy M33.92
    respiratory involvement M33.91
    specified organ involvement NEC M33.99
  in neoplastic disease (*see also* Neoplasm) D49.9
      [M36.0]
  juvenile M33.00
    with
      myopathy M33.02
      respiratory involvement M33.01
      specified organ involvement NEC M33.09
    specified NEC M33.10
      myopathy M33.12
      respiratory involvement M33.11
      specified organ involvement NEC M33.19
    without myopathy M33.93
Dermatopolyneuritis — *see* Poisoning, mercury
Dermatorrhexis Q79.6
  acquired L57.4
Dermatosclerosis (*see also* Scleroderma)
  localized L94.0
Dermatosis L98.9
  Andrews' L08.89
  Bowen's — *see* Neoplasm, skin, in situ
  bullous L13.9
    specified NEC L13.8
  exfoliativa L26
  eyelid (noninfectious)
    dermatitis — *see* Dermatitis, eyelid
    discoid lupus erythematosus — *see* Lupus,
        erythematosus, eyelid
    xeroderma — *see* Xeroderma, acquired, eyelid
  factitial L98.1
  febrile neutrophilic L98.2
  gonococcal A54.89
  herpetiformis L13.0
    juvenile L12.2
  linear IgA L13.8
  menstrual NEC L98.8
  neutrophilic, febrile L98.2
  occupational — *see* Dermatitis, contact
  papulosa nigra L82.1

☑ **Additional character required**

Dermatosis — *continued*
pigmentary L81.9
progressive L81.7
Schamberg's L81.7
psychogenic F54
purpuric, pigmented L81.7
pustular, subcorneal L13.1
transient acantholytic L11.1
Dermographia, dermographism L50.3
Dermoid (cyst) (*see also* Neoplasm, benign, by site)
with malignant transformation C56 ☑
due to radiation (nonionizing) L57.8
Dermopathy
infiltrative with thyrotoxicosis — *see*
Thyrotoxicosis
nephrogenic fibrosing L90.8
Dermophytosis — *see* Dermatophytosis
Descemetocele H18.73 ☑
Descemet's membrane — *see* condition
Descending — *see* condition
Descensus uteri — *see* Prolapse, uterus
Desert
rheumatism B38.0
sore — *see* Ulcer, skin
Desertion (newborn) — *see* Maltreatment
Desmoid (extra-abdominal) (tumor) — *see*
Neoplasm, connective tissue, uncertain behavior
abdominal D48.1
Despondency F32.9
Desquamation, skin R23.4
Destruction, destructive (*see also* Damage)
articular facet (*see also* Derangement, joint, specified type NEC)
knee M23.8X ☑
vertebra — *see* Spondylosis
bone (*see also* Disorder, bone, specified type NEC)
syphilitic A52.77
joint (*see also* Derangement, joint, specified type NEC)
sacroiliac M53.3
rectal sphincter K62.89
septum (nasal) J34.89
tuberculous NEC — *see* Tuberculosis
tympanum, tympanic membrane (nontraumatic)
— *see* Disorder, tympanic membrane, specified NEC
vertebral disc — *see* Degeneration, intervertebral disc
Destructiveness (*see also* Disorder, conduct)
adjustment reaction — *see* Disorder, adjustment
Desultory labor O62.2
Detachment
cartilage — *see* Sprain
cervix, annular N88.8
complicating delivery O71.3
choroid (old) (postinfectional) (simple) (spontaneous) H31.40 ☑
hemorrhagic H31.41 ☑
serous H31.42 ☑
ligament — *see* Sprain
meniscus (knee) (*see also* Derangement, knee, meniscus, specified NEC)
current injury — *see* Tear, meniscus
due to old tear or injury — *see* Derangement, knee, meniscus, due to old tear
retina (without retinal break) (serous) H33.2 ☑
with retinal:
break H33.00 ☑
giant H33.03 ☑
multiple H33.02 ☑
single H33.01 ☑
dialysis H33.04 ☑
pigment epithelium — *see* Degeneration, retina, separation of layers, pigment epithelium detachment
rhegmatogenous — *see* Detachment, retina, with retinal, break
specified NEC H33.8
total H33.05 ☑
traction H33.4 ☑
vitreous (body) H43.81 ☑
Detergent asthma J69.8
Deterioration
epileptic F06.8
general physical R53.81
heart, cardiac — *see* Degeneration, myocardial
mental — *see* Psychosis
myocardial, myocardium — *see* Degeneration, myocardial
senile (simple) R54
Deuteranomaly (anomalous trichromat) H53.53
Deuteranopia (complete) (incomplete) H53.53

Development
abnormal, bone Q79.9
arrested R62.50
bone — *see* Arrest, development or growth, bone
child R62.50
due to malnutrition E45
defective, congenital (*see also* Anomaly, by site)
cauda equina Q06.3
left ventricle Q24.8
in hypoplastic left heart syndrome Q23.4
valve Q24.8
pulmonary Q22.3
delayed (*see also* Delay, development) R62.50
arithmetical skills F81.2
language (skills) (expressive) F80.1
learning skill F81.9
mixed skills F88
motor coordination F82
reading F81.0
specified learning skill NEC F81.89
speech F80.9
spelling F81.81
written expression F81.81
imperfect, congenital (*see also* Anomaly, by site)
heart Q24.9
lungs Q33.6
incomplete
bronchial tree Q32.4
organ or site not listed — *see* Hypoplasia, by site
respiratory system Q34.9
sexual, precocious NEC E30.1
tardy, mental (*see also* Disability, intellectual) F79
Developmental — *see* condition
testing, infant or child — *see* Examination, child
Devergie's disease (pityriasis rubra pilaris) L44.0
Deviation (in)
conjugate palsy (eye) (spastic) H51.0
esophagus (acquired) K22.8
eye, skew H51.8
midline (jaw) (teeth) (dental arch) M26.29
specified site NEC — *see* Malposition
nasal septum J34.2
congenital Q67.4
opening and closing of the mandible M26.53
organ or site, congenital NEC — *see* Malposition, congenital
septum (nasal) (acquired) J34.2
congenital Q67.4
sexual F65.9
bestiality F65.89
erotomania F52.8
exhibitionism F65.2
fetishism, fetishistic F65.0
transvestism F65.1
frotteurism F65.81
masochism F65.51
multiple F65.89
necrophilia F65.89
nymphomania F52.8
pederosis F65.4
pedophilia F65.4
sadism, sadomasochism F65.52
satyriasis F52.8
specified type NEC F65.89
transvestism F64.1
voyeurism F65.3
teeth, midline M26.29
trachea J39.8
ureter, congenital Q62.61
Device
cerebral ventricle (communicating) in situ Z98.2
contraceptive — *see* Contraceptive, device
drainage, cerebrospinal fluid, in situ Z98.2
Devic's disease G36.0
Devil's
grip B33.0
pinches (purpura simplex) D69.2
Devitalized tooth K04.99
Devonshire colic — *see* Poisoning, lead
Dextraposition, aorta Q20.3
in tetralogy of Fallot Q21.3
Dextrinosis, limit (debrancher enzyme deficiency) E74.03
Dextrocardia (true) Q24.0
with
complete transposition of viscera Q89.3
situs inversus Q89.3
Dextrotransposition, aorta Q20.3
d-glycericacidemia E72.59
Dhat syndrome F48.8

Dhobi itch B35.6
Di George's syndrome D82.1
Di Guglielmo's disease C94.0 ☑
Diabetes, diabetic (mellitus) (sugar) E11.9
with
amyotrophy E11.44
arthropathy NEC E11.618
autonomic (poly) neuropathy E11.43
cataract E11.36
Charcot's joints E11.610
chronic kidney disease E11.22
circulatory complication NEC E11.59
complication E11.8
specified NEC E11.69
dermatitis E11.620
foot ulcer E11.621
gangrene E11.52
gastroparalysis E11.43
gastroparesis E11.43
glomerulonephrosis, intracapillary E11.21
glomerulosclerosis, intercapillary E11.21
hyperglycemia E11.65
hyperosmolarity E11.00
with coma E11.01
hypoglycemia E11.649
with coma E11.641
ketoacidosis E11.10
with coma E11.11
kidney complications NEC E11.29
Kimmelstiel-Wilson disease E11.21
loss of protective sensation (LOPS) — *see*
Diabetes, by type, with neuropathy
mononeuropathy E11.41
myasthenia E11.44
necrobiosis lipoidica E11.620
nephropathy E11.21
neuralgia E11.42
neurologic complication NEC E11.49
neuropathic arthropathy E11.610
neuropathy E11.40
ophthalmic complication NEC E11.39
oral complication NEC E11.638
osteomyelitis E11.69
periodontal disease E11.630
peripheral angiopathy E11.51
with gangrene E11.52
polyneuropathy E11.42
renal complication NEC E11.29
renal tubular degeneration E11.29
retinopathy E11.319
with macular edema E11.311
resolved following treatment E11.37 ☑
nonproliferative E11.329 ☑
with macular edema E11.321 ☑
mild E11.329 ☑
with macular edema E11.321 ☑
moderate E11.339 ☑
with macular edema E11.331 ☑
severe E11.349 ☑
with macular edema E11.341 ☑
proliferative E11.359 ☑
with
combined traction retinal detachment and rhegmatogenous retinal detachment E11.354 ☑
macular edema E11.351 ☑
stable proliferative diabetic retinopathy E11.355 ☑
traction retinal detachment involving the macula E11.352 ☑
traction retinal detachment not involving the macula E11.353 ☑
skin complication NEC E11.628
skin ulcer NEC E11.622
brittle — *see* Diabetes, type 1
bronzed E83.110
complicating pregnancy — *see* Pregnancy, complicated by, diabetes
dietary counseling and surveillance Z71.3
due to
autoimmune process — *see* Diabetes, type 1
immune mediated pancreatic islet beta-cell destruction — *see* Diabetes, type 1
due to drug or chemical E09.9
with
amyotrophy E09.44
arthropathy NEC E09.618
autonomic (poly) neuropathy E09.43
cataract E09.36
Charcot's joints E09.610
chronic kidney disease E09.22
circulatory complication NEC E09.59

Diabetes

Diabetes — *continued*
  due to drug or chemical — *continued*
    complication E09.8
      specified NEC E09.69
    dermatitis E09.620
    foot ulcer E09.621
    gangrene E09.52
    gastroparalysis E09.43
    gastroparesis E09.43
    glomerulonephrosis, intracapillary E09.21
    glomerulosclerosis, intercapillary E09.21
    hyperglycemia E09.65
    hyperosmolarity E09.00
      with coma E09.01
    hypoglycemia E09.649
      with coma E09.641
    ketoacidosis E09.10
      with coma E09.11
    kidney complications NEC E09.29
    Kimmelsteil-Wilson disease E09.21
    mononeuropathy E09.41
    myasthenia E09.44
    necrobiosis lipoidica E09.620
    nephropathy E09.21
    neuralgia E09.42
    neurologic complication NEC E09.49
    neuropathic arthropathy E09.610
    neuropathy E09.40
    ophthalmic complication NEC E09.39
    oral complication NEC E09.638
    periodontal disease E09.630
    peripheral angiopathy E09.51
      with gangrene E09.52
    polyneuropathy E09.42
    renal complication NEC E09.29
    renal tubular degeneration E09.29
    retinopathy E09.319
      with macular edema E09.311
      resolved following treatment E09.37 ☑
      nonproliferative E09.329 ☑
        with macular edema E09.321 ☑
        mild E09.329 ☑
          with macular edema E09.321 ☑
        moderate E09.339 ☑
          with macular edema E09.331 ☑
        severe E09.349 ☑
          with macular edema E09.341 ☑
      proliferative E09.359 ☑
        with
          combined traction retinal detachment
            and rhegmatogenous retinal
            detachment E09.354 ☑
          macular edema E09.351 ☑
          stable proliferative diabetic
            retinopathy E09.355 ☑
          traction retinal detachment involving
            the macula E09.352 ☑
          traction retinal detachment not
            involving the macula E09.353 ☑
    skin complication NEC E09.628
    skin ulcer NEC E09.622
  due to underlying condition E08.9
    with
      amyotrophy E08.44
      arthropathy NEC E08.618
      autonomic (poly) neuropathy E08.43
      cataract E08.36
      Charcot's joints E08.610
      chronic kidney disease E08.22
      circulatory complication NEC E08.59
      complication E08.8
        specified NEC E08.69
      dermatitis E08.620
      foot ulcer E08.621
      gangrene E08.52
      gastroparalysis E08.43
      gastroparesis E08.43
      glomerulonephrosis, intracapillary E08.21
      glomerulosclerosis, intercapillary E08.21
      hyperglycemia E08.65
      hyperosmolarity E08.00
        with coma E08.01
      hypoglycemia E08.649
        with coma E08.641
      ketoacidosis E08.10
        with coma E08.11
      kidney complications NEC E08.29
      Kimmelsteil-WIlson disease E08.21
      mononeuropathy E08.41
      myasthenia E08.44
      necrobiosis lipoidica E08.620
      nephropathy E08.21

Diabetes — *continued*
  due to underlying condition — *continued*
    neuralgia E08.42
    neurologic complication NEC E08.49
    neuropathic arthropathy E08.610
    neuropathy E08.42
    ophthalmic complication NEC E08.39
    oral complication NEC E08.638
    periodontal disease E08.630
    peripheral angiopathy E08.51
      with gangrene E08.52
    polyneuropathy E08.42
    renal complication NEC E08.29
    renal tubular degeneration E08.29
    retinopathy E08.319
      with macular edema E08.311
      resolved following treatment E08.37 ☑
      nonproliferative E08.329 ☑
        with macular edema E08.321 ☑
        mild E08.329 ☑
          with macular edema E08.321 ☑
        moderate E08.339 ☑
          with macular edema E08.331 ☑
        severe E08.349 ☑
          with macular edema E08.341 ☑
      proliferative E08.359 ☑
        with
          combined traction retinal detachment
            and rhegmatogenous retinal
            detachment E08.354 ☑
          macular edema E08.351 ☑
          stable proliferative diabetic
            retinopathy E08.355 ☑
          traction retinal detachment involving
            the macula E08.352 ☑
          traction retinal detachment not
            involving the macula E08.353 ☑
    skin complication NEC E08.628
    skin ulcer NEC E08.622
  gestational (in pregnancy) O24.419
    affecting newborn P70.0
    diet controlled O24.410
    in childbirth O24.429
      diet controlled O24.420
      insulin (and diet) controlled O24.424
      oral drug controlled (antidiabetic)
        (hypoglycemic) O24.425
    insulin (and diet) controlled O24.414
    oral drug controlled (antidiabetic)
      (hypoglycemic) O24.415
    puerperal O24.439
      diet controlled O24.430
      insulin (and diet) controlled O24.434
      oral drug controlled (antidiabetic)
        (hypoglycemic) O24.435
  hepatogenous E13.9
  idiopathic — *see* Diabetes, type 1
  inadequately controlled - code to Diabetes, by
    type, with hyperglycemia
  insipidus E23.2
    nephrogenic N25.1
    pituitary E23.2
    vasopressin resistant N25.1
  insulin dependent - code to type of diabetes
  juvenile-onset — *see* Diabetes, type 1
  ketosis-prone — *see* Diabetes, type 1
  latent R73.03
  neonatal (transient) P70.2
  non-insulin dependent - code to type of diabetes
  out of control - code to Diabetes, by type, with
    hyperglycemia
  phosphate E83.39
  poorly controlled - code to Diabetes, by type,
    with hyperglycemia
  postpancreatectomy — *see* Diabetes, specified
    type NEC
  postprocedural — *see* Diabetes, specified type
    NEC
  secondary diabetes mellitus NEC — *see* Diabetes,
    specified type NEC
  specified type NEC E13.9
    with
      amyotrophy E13.44
      arthropathy NEC E13.618
      autonomic (poly) neuropathy E13.43
      cataract E13.36
      Charcot's joints E13.610
      chronic kidney disease E13.22
      circulatory complication NEC E13.59
      complication E13.8
        specified NEC E13.69
      dermatitis E13.620

Diabetes — *continued*
  specified type NEC — *continued*
    foot ulcer E13.621
    gangrene E13.52
    gastroparalysis E13.43
    gastroparesis E13.43
    glomerulonephrosis, intracapillary E13.21
    glomerulosclerosis, intercapillary E13.21
    hyperglycemia E13.65
    hyperosmolarity E13.00
      with coma E13.01
    hypoglycemia E13.649
      with coma E13.641
    ketoacidosis E13.10
      with coma E13.11
    kidney complications NEC E13.29
    Kimmelsteil-Wilson disease E13.21
    mononeuropathy E13.41
    myasthenia E13.44
    necrobiosis lipoidica E13.620
    nephropathy E13.21
    neuralgia E13.42
    neurologic complication NEC E13.49
    neuropathic arthropathy E13.610
    neuropathy E13.40
    ophthalmic complication NEC E13.39
    oral complication NEC E13.638
    periodontal disease E13.630
    peripheral angiopathy E13.51
      with gangrene E13.52
    polyneuropathy E13.42
    renal complication NEC E13.29
    renal tubular degeneration E13.29
    retinopathy E13.319
      with macular edema E13.311
      resolved following treatment E13.37 ☑
      nonproliferative E13.329 ☑
        with macular edema E13.321 ☑
        mild E13.329 ☑
          with macular edema E13.321 ☑
        moderate E13.339 ☑
          with macular edema E13.331 ☑
        severe E13.349 ☑
          with macular edema E13.341 ☑
      proliferative E13.359 ☑
        with
          combined traction retinal detachment
            and rhegmatogenous retinal
            detachment E13.354 ☑
          macular edema E13.351 ☑
          stable proliferative diabetic
            retinopathy E13.355 ☑
          traction retinal detachment involving
            the macula E13.352 ☑
          traction retinal detachment not
            involving the macula E13.353 ☑
    skin complication NEC E13.628
    skin ulcer NEC E13.622
  steroid-induced — *see* Diabetes, due to, drug or
    chemical
  type 1 E10.9
    with
      amyotrophy E10.44
      arthropathy NEC E10.618
      autonomic (poly) neuropathy E10.43
      cataract E10.36
      Charcot's joints E10.610
      chronic kidney disease E10.22
      circulatory complication NEC E10.59
      complication E10.8
        specified NEC E10.69
      dermatitis E10.620
      foot ulcer E10.621
      gangrene E10.52
      gastroparalysis E10.43
      gastroparesis E10.43
      glomerulonephrosis, intracapillary E10.21
      glomerulosclerosis, intercapillary E10.21
      hyperglycemia E10.65
      hypoglycemia E10.649
        with coma E10.641
      ketoacidosis E10.10
        with coma E10.11
      kidney complications NEC E10.29
      Kimmelsteil-Wilson disease E10.21
      mononeuropathy E10.41
      myasthenia E10.44
      necrobiosis lipoidica E10.620
      nephropathy E10.21
      neuralgia E10.42
      neurologic complication NEC E10.49
      neuropathic arthropathy E10.610

☑ **Additional character required**

Diabetes — *continued*
  type 1 — *continued*
    neuropathy E10.40
    ophthalmic complication NEC E10.39
    oral complication NEC E10.638
    osteomyelitis E10.69
    periodontal disease E10.630
    peripheral angiopathy E10.51
      with gangrene E10.52
    polyneuropathy E10.42
    renal complication NEC E10.29
    renal tubular degeneration E10.29
    retinopathy E10.319
      with macular edema E10.311
      resolved following treatment E10.37 ☑
      nonproliferative E10.329 ☑
        with macular edema E10.321 ☑
        mild E10.329 ☑
          with macular edema E10.321 ☑
        moderate E10.339 ☑
          with macular edema E10.331 ☑
        severe E10.349 ☑
          with macular edema E10.341 ☑
      proliferative E10.359 ☑
        with
          combined traction retinal detachment
            and rhegmatogenous retinal
            detachment E10.354 ☑
          macular edema E10.351 ☑
          stable proliferative diabetic
            retinopathy E10.355 ☑
          traction retinal detachment involving
            the macula E10.352 ☑
          traction retinal detachment not
            involving the macula E10.353 ☑
    skin complication NEC E10.628
    skin ulcer NEC E10.622
  type 2 E11.9
    with
      amyotrophy E11.44
      arthropathy NEC E11.618
      autonomic (poly) neuropathy E11.43
      cataract E11.36
      Charcot's joints E11.610
      chronic kidney disease E11.22
      circulatory complication NEC E11.59
      complication E11.8
        specified NEC E11.69
      dermatitis E11.620
      foot ulcer E11.621
      gangrene E11.52
      gastroparalysis E11.43
      gastroparesis E11.43
      glomerulonephrosis, intracapillary E11.21
      glomerulosclerosis, intercapillary E11.21
      hyperglycemia E11.65
      hyperosmolarity E11.00
        with coma E11.01
      hypoglycemia E11.649
        with coma E11.641
      ketoacidosis E11.10
        with coma E11.11
      kidney complications NEC E11.29
      Kimmelstiel-Wilson disease E11.21
      mononeuropathy E11.41
      myasthenia E11.44
      necrobiosis lipoidica E11.620
      nephropathy E11.21
      neuralgia E11.42
      neurologic complication NEC E11.49
      neuropathic arthropathy E11.610
      neuropathy E11.40
      ophthalmic complication NEC E11.39
      oral complication NEC E11.638
      osteomyelitis E11.69
      periodontal disease E11.630
      peripheral angiopathy E11.51
        with gangrene E11.52
      polyneuropathy E11.42
      renal complication NEC E11.29
      renal tubular degeneration E11.29
      retinopathy E11.319
        with macular edema E11.311
        resolved following treatment E11.37 ☑
        nonproliferative E11.329 ☑
          with macular edema E11.321 ☑
          mild E11.329 ☑
            with macular edema E11.321 ☑
          moderate E11.339 ☑
            with macular edema E11.331 ☑
          severe E11.349 ☑
            with macular edema E11.341 ☑

Diabetes — *continued*
  type 2 — *continued*
      proliferative E11.359 ☑
        with
          combined traction retinal detachment
            and rhegmatogenous retinal
            detachment E11.354 ☑
          macular edema E11.351 ☑
          stable proliferative diabetic
            retinopathy E11.355 ☑
          traction retinal detachment involving
            the macula E11.352 ☑
          traction retinal detachment not
            involving the macula E11.353 ☑
    skin complication NEC E11.628
    skin ulcer NEC E11.622
  uncontrolled
    meaning
      hyperglycemia — *see* Diabetes, by type, with,
        hyperglycemia
      hypoglycemia — *see* Diabetes, by type, with,
        hypoglycemia
Diacyclothrombopathia D69.1
Diagnosis deferred R69
Dialysis (intermittent) (treatment)
  noncompliance (with) Z91.15
  renal (hemodialysis) (peritoneal), status Z99.2
  retina, retinal — *see* Detachment, retina, with
    retinal, dialysis
Diamond-Blackfan anemia (congenital hypoplastic)
  D61.01
Diamond-Gardener syndrome (autoerythrocyte
  sensitization) D69.2
Diaper rash L22
Diaphoresis (excessive) R61
Diaphragm — *see* condition
Diaphragmalgia R07.1
Diaphragmatitis, diaphragmitis J98.6
Diaphysial aclasis Q78.6
Diaphysitis — *see* Osteomyelitis, specified type NEC
Diarrhea, diarrheal (disease) (infantile)
  (inflammatory) R19.7
  achlorhydric K31.83
  allergic K52.29
    due to
      colitis — *see* Colitis, allergic
      enteritis — *see* Enteritis, allergic
  amebic (*see also* Amebiasis) A06.0
    with abscess — *see* Abscess, amebic
    acute A06.0
    chronic A06.1
    nondysenteric A06.2
  bacillary — *see* Dysentery, bacillary
  balantidial A07.0
  cachectic NEC K52.89
  Chilomastix A07.8
  choleriformis A00.1
  chronic (noninfectious) K52.9
  coccidial A07.3
  Cochin-China K90.1
    strongyloidiasis B78.0
  Dientamoeba A07.8
  dietetic (*see also* Diarrhea, allergic) K52.29
  drug-induced K52.1
  due to
    bacteria A04.9
      specified NEC A04.8
    Campylobacter A04.5
    Capillaria philippinensis B81.1
    Clostridium difficile
      not specified as recurrent A04.72
      recurrent A04.71
    Clostridium perfringens (C) (F) A04.8
    Cryptosporidium A07.2
    drugs K52.1
    Escherichia coli A04.4
      enteroaggregative A04.4
      enterohemorrhagic A04.3
      enteroinvasive A04.2
      enteropathogenic A04.0
      enterotoxigenic A04.1
      specified NEC A04.4
    food hypersensitivity (*see also* Diarrhea,
      allergic) K52.29
    Necator americanus B76.1
    S. japonicum B65.2
    specified organism NEC A08.8
      bacterial A04.8
      viral A08.39
    Staphylococcus A04.8
    Trichuris trichiuria B79
    virus — *see* Enteritis, viral
    Yersinia enterocolitica A04.6

Diarrhea — *continued*
  dysenteric A09
  endemic A09
  epidemic A09
  flagellate A07.9
  Flexner's (ulcerative) A03.1
  functional K59.1
    following gastrointestinal surgery K91.89
    psychogenic F45.8
  Giardia lamblia A07.1
  giardial A07.1
  hill K90.1
  infectious A09
  malarial — *see* Malaria
  mite B88.0
  mycotic NEC B49
  neonatal (noninfectious) P78.3
  nervous F45.8
  neurogenic K59.1
  noninfectious K52.9
  postgastrectomy K91.1
  postvagotomy K91.1
  protozoal A07.9
    specified NEC A07.8
  psychogenic F45.8
  specified
    bacterium NEC A04.8
    virus NEC A08.39
  strongyloidiasis B78.0
  toxic K52.1
  trichomonal A07.8
  tropical K90.1
  tuberculous A18.32
  viral — *see* Enteritis, viral
Diastasis
  cranial bones M84.88
    congenital NEC Q75.8
  joint (traumatic) — *see* Dislocation
  muscle M62.00
    ankle M62.07 ☑
    congenital Q79.8
    foot M62.07 ☑
    forearm M62.03 ☑
    hand M62.04 ☑
    lower leg M62.06 ☑
    pelvic region M62.05 ☑
    shoulder region M62.01 ☑
    specified site NEC M62.08
    thigh M62.05 ☑
    upper arm M62.02 ☑
  recti (abdomen)
    complicating delivery O71.89
    congenital Q79.59
Diastema, tooth, teeth, fully erupted M26.32
Diastematomyelia Q06.2
Diataxia, cerebral G80.4
Diathesis
  allergic — *see* History, allergy
  bleeding (familial) D69.9
  cystine (familial) E72.00
  gouty — *see* Gout
  hemorrhagic (familial) D69.9
    newborn NEC P53
  spasmophilic R29.0
Diaz's disease or osteochondrosis (juvenile) (talus)
  — *see* Osteochondrosis, juvenile, tarsus
Dibothriocephalus, dibothriocephaliasis (latus)
  (infection) (infestation) B70.0
    larval B70.1
Dicephalus, dicephaly Q89.4
Dichotomy, teeth K00.2
Dichromat, dichromatopsia (congenital) — *see*
  Deficiency, color vision
Dichuchwa A65
Dicroceliasis B66.2
Didelphia, didelphys — *see* Double uterus
Didymytis N45.1
  with orchitis N45.3
Dietary
  inadequacy or deficiency E63.9
  surveillance and counseling Z71.3
Dietl's crisis N13.8
Dieulafoy lesion (hemorrhagic)
  duodenum K31.82
  esophagus K22.8
  intestine (colon) K63.81
  stomach K31.82
Difficult, difficulty (in)
  acculturation Z60.3
  feeding R63.3
    newborn P92.9
      breast P92.5

Difficult — continued
  feeding — continued
    specified NEC P92.8
   nonorganic (infant or child) F98.29
  intubation, in anesthesia T88.4 ☑
  mechanical, gastroduodenal stoma K91.89
   causing obstruction (see also Obstruction,
    intestine, postoperative) K91.30
  micturition
   need to immediately re-void R39.191
   position dependent R39.192
   specified NEC R39.198
  reading (developmental) F81.0
   secondary to emotional disorders F93.9
  spelling (specific) F81.81
   with reading disorder F81.89
   due to inadequate teaching Z55.8
  swallowing — see Dysphagia
  walking R26.2
  work
   conditions NEC Z56.5
   schedule Z56.3
Diffuse — see condition
DiGeorge's syndrome (thymic hypoplasia) D82.1
Digestive — see condition
Dihydropyrimidine dehydrogenase disease (DPD)
  E88.89
Diktyoma — see Neoplasm, malignant, by site
Dilaceration, tooth K00.4
Dilatation
  anus K59.8
   venule — see Hemorrhoids
  aorta (focal) (general) — see Ectasia, aorta
   with aneurysm — see Aneurysm, aorta
   congenital Q25.44
  artery — see Aneurysm
  bladder (sphincter) N32.89
   congenital Q64.79
  blood vessel I99.8
  bronchial J47.9
   with
    exacerbation (acute) J47.1
    lower respiratory infection J47.0
  calyx (due to obstruction) — see Hydronephrosis
  capillaries I78.8
  cardiac (acute) (chronic) (see also Hypertrophy,
   cardiac)
   congenital Q24.8
   valve NEC Q24.8
    pulmonary Q22.3
   valve — see Endocarditis
  cavum septi pellucidi Q06.8
  cervix (uteri) (see also Incompetency, cervix)
   incomplete, poor, slow complicating
    delivery O62.0
  colon K59.39
   congenital Q43.1
   psychogenic F45.8
   toxic K59.31
  common duct (acquired) K83.8
   congenital Q44.5
  cystic duct (acquired) K82.8
   congenital Q44.5
  duct, mammary — see Ectasia, mammary duct
  duodenum K59.8
  esophagus K22.8
   congenital Q39.5
   due to achalasia K22.0
  eustachian tube, congenital Q17.8
  gallbladder K82.8
  gastric — see Dilatation, stomach
  heart (acute) (chronic) (see also Hypertrophy,
   cardiac)
   congenital Q24.8
   valve — see Endocarditis
  ileum K59.8
   psychogenic F45.8
  jejunum K59.8
   psychogenic F45.8
  kidney (calyx) (collecting structures) (cystic)
   (parenchyma) (pelvis) (idiopathic) N28.89
  lacrimal passages or duct — see Disorder, lacrimal
   system, changes
  lymphatic vessel I89.0
  mammary duct — see Ectasia, mammary duct
  Meckel's diverticulum (congenital) Q43.0
   malignant — see Table of Neoplasms, small
    intestine, malignant
  myocardium (acute) (chronic) — see Hypertrophy,
   cardiac
  organ or site, congenital NEC — see Distortion
  pancreatic duct K86.89

Dilatation — continued
  pericardium — see Pericarditis
  pharynx J39.2
  prostate N42.89
  pulmonary
   artery (idiopathic) I28.8
   valve, congenital Q22.3
  pupil H57.04
  rectum K59.39
  saccule, congenital Q16.5
  salivary gland (duct) K11.8
  sphincter ani K62.89
  stomach K31.89
   acute K31.0
   psychogenic F45.8
  submaxillary duct K11.8
  trachea, congenital Q32.1
  ureter (idiopathic) N28.82
   congenital Q62.2
   due to obstruction N13.4
  urethra (acquired) N36.8
  vasomotor I73.9
  vein I86.8
  ventricular, ventricle (acute) (chronic) (see also
   Hypertrophy, cardiac)
   cerebral, congenital Q04.8
  venule NEC I86.8
  vesical orifice N32.89
Dilated, dilation — see Dilatation
Diminished, diminution
  hearing (acuity) — see Deafness
  sense or sensation (cold) (heat) (tactile)
   (vibratory) R20.8
  vision NEC H54.7
  vital capacity R94.2
Diminuta taenia B71.0
Dimitri-Sturge-Weber disease Q85.8
Dimple
  congenital sacral Q82.6
  parasacral Q82.6
  pilonidal or postanal — see Cyst, pilonidal
Dioctophyme renalis (infection) (infestation) B83.8
Dipetalonemiasis B74.4
Diphallus Q55.69
Diphtheria, diphtheritic (gangrenous) (hemorrhagic)
  A36.9
  carrier (suspected) Z22.2
  cutaneous A36.3
  faucial A36.0
  infection of wound A36.3
  laryngeal A36.2
  myocarditis A36.81
  nasal, anterior A36.89
  nasopharyngeal A36.1
  neurological complication A36.89
  pharyngeal A36.0
  specified site NEC A36.89
  tonsillar A36.0
Diphyllobothriasis (intestine) B70.0
  larval B70.1
Diplacusis H93.22 ☑
Diplegia (upper limbs) G83.0
  congenital (cerebral) G80.8
  facial G51.0
  lower limbs G82.20
  spastic G80.1
Diplococcus, diplococcal — see condition
Diplopia H53.2
Dipsomania F10.20
  with
   psychosis — see Psychosis, alcoholic
   remission F10.21
Dipylidiasis B71.1
DIRA (deficiency of interleukin 1 receptor
  antagonist) M04.8
Direction, teeth, abnormal, fully erupted M26.30
Dirofilariasis B74.8
Dirt-eating child F98.3
Disability, disabilities
  heart — see Disease, heart
  intellectual F79
   with
    autistic features F84.9
   mild (I.Q.50-69) F70
   moderate (I.Q.35-49) F71
   profound (I.Q. under 20) F73
   severe (I.Q.20-34) F72
   specified level NEC F78
  knowledge acquisition F81.9
  learning F81.9
  limiting activities Z73.6
  spelling, specific F81.81

Disappearance of family member Z63.4
Disarticulation — see Amputation
  meaning traumatic amputation — see
   Amputation, traumatic
Discharge (from)
  abnormal finding in — see Abnormal, specimen
  breast (female) (male) N64.52
  diencephalic autonomic idiopathic — see
   Epilepsy, specified NEC
  ear (see also Otorrhea)
   blood — see Otorrhagia
  excessive urine R35.8
  nipple N64.52
  penile R36.9
  postnasal R09.82
  prison, anxiety concerning Z65.2
  urethral R36.9
   without blood R36.0
   hematospermia R36.1
  vaginal N89.8
Discitis, diskitis M46.40
  cervical region M46.42
  cervicothoracic region M46.43
  lumbar region M46.46
  lumbosacral region M46.47
  multiple sites M46.49
  occipito-atlanto-axial region M46.41
  pyogenic — see Infection, intervertebral disc,
   pyogenic
  sacrococcygeal region M46.48
  thoracic region M46.44
  thoracolumbar region M46.45
Discoid
  meniscus (congenital) Q68.6
  semilunar cartilage (congenital) — see
   Derangement, knee, meniscus, specified NEC
Discoloration
  nails L60.8
  teeth (posteruptive) K03.7
   during formation K00.8
Discomfort
  chest R07.89
  visual H53.14 ☑
Discontinuity, ossicles, ear H74.2 ☑
Discord (with)
  boss Z56.4
  classmates Z55.4
  counselor Z64.4
  employer Z56.4
  family Z63.8
  fellow employees Z56.4
  in-laws Z63.1
  landlord Z59.2
  lodgers Z59.2
  neighbors Z59.2
  probation officer Z64.4
  social worker Z64.4
  teachers Z55.4
  workmates Z56.4
Discordant connection
  atrioventricular (congenital) Q20.5
  ventriculoarterial Q20.3
Discrepancy
  centric occlusion maximum
   intercuspation M26.55
  leg length (acquired) — see Deformity, limb,
   unequal length
   congenital — see Defect, reduction, lower limb
  uterine size date O26.84 ☑
Discrimination
  ethnic Z60.5
  political Z60.5
  racial Z60.5
  religious Z60.5
  sex Z60.5
Disease, diseased (see also Syndrome)
  absorbent system I87.8
  acid-peptic K30
  Acosta's T70.29 ☑
  Adams-Stokes (-Morgagni) (syncope with heart
   block) I45.9
  Addison's anemia (pernicious) D51.0
  adenoids (and tonsils) J35.9
  adrenal (capsule) (cortex) (gland)
   (medullary) E27.9
   hyperfunction E27.0
   specified NEC E27.8
  ainhum L94.6
  airway
   obstructive, chronic J44.9
    due to
     cotton dust J66.0

☑ **Additional character required**

Disease — *continued*
  airway — *continued*
    specific organic dusts NEC J66.8
    reactive — *see* Asthma
  akamushi (scrub typhus) A75.3
  Albers-Schönberg (marble bones) Q78.2
  Albert's — *see* Tendinitis, Achilles
  alimentary canal K63.9
  alligator-skin Q80.9
    acquired L85.0
  alpha heavy chain C88.3
  alpine T70.29 ☑
  altitude T70.20 ☑
  alveolar ridge
    edentulous K06.9
      specified NEC K06.8
  alveoli, teeth K08.9
  Alzheimer's G30.9 *[F02.80]*
    with behavioral disturbance G30.9 *[F02.81]*
    early onset G30.0 *[F02.80]*
      with behavioral disturbance G30.0 *[F02.81]*
    late onset G30.1 *[F02.80]*
      with behavioral disturbance G30.1 *[F02.81]*
    specified NEC G30.8 *[F02.80]*
      with behavioral disturbance G30.8 *[F02.81]*
  amyloid — *see* Amyloidosis
  Andersen's (glycogenosis IV) E74.09
  Andes T70.29 ☑
  Andrews' (bacterid) L08.89
  angiospastic I73.9
    cerebral G45.9
    vein I87.8
  anterior
    chamber H21.9
    horn cell G12.29
  antiglomerular basement membrane (anti- GBM)
      antibody M31.0
    tubulo-interstitial nephritis N12
  antral — *see* Sinusitis, maxillary
  anus K62.9
    specified NEC K62.89
  aorta (nonsyphilitic) I77.9
    syphilitic NEC A52.02
  aortic (heart) (valve) I35.9
    rheumatic I06.9
  Apollo B30.3
  aponeuroses — *see* Enthesopathy
  appendix K38.9
    specified NEC K38.8
  aqueous (chamber) H21.9
  Arnold-Chiari — *see* Arnold-Chiari disease
  arterial I77.9
    occlusive — *see* Occlusion, by site
    due to stricture or stenosis I77.1
  arteriocardiorenal — *see* Hypertension, cardiorenal
  arteriolar (generalized) (obliterative) I77.9
  arteriorenal — *see* Hypertension, kidney
  arteriosclerotic (*see also* Arteriosclerosis)
    cardiovascular — *see* Disease, heart, ischemic, atherosclerotic
    coronary (artery) — *see* Disease, heart, ischemic, atherosclerotic
    heart — *see* Disease, heart, ischemic, atherosclerotic
  artery I77.9
    cerebral I67.9
    coronary I25.10
      with angina pectoris — *see* Arteriosclerosis, coronary (artery),
  arthropod-borne NOS (viral) A94
    specified type NEC A93.8
  atticoantral, chronic H66.20
    left H66.22
      with right H66.23
    right H66.21
      with left H66.23
  auditory canal — *see* Disorder, ear, external
  auricle, ear NEC — *see* Disorder, pinna
  Australian X A83.4
  autoimmune (systemic) NOS M35.9
    hemolytic (cold type) (warm type) D59.1
      drug-induced D59.0
    thyroid E06.3
  aviator's — *see* Effect, adverse, high altitude
  Ayerza's (pulmonary artery sclerosis with pulmonary hypertension) I27.0
  Babington's (familial hemorrhagic telangiectasia) I78.0
  bacterial A49.9
    specified NEC A48.8
    zoonotic A28.9
      specified type NEC A28.8

Disease — *continued*
  Baelz's (cheilitis glandularis apostematosa) K13.0
  bagasse J67.1
  balloon — *see* Effect, adverse, high altitude
  Bang's (brucella abortus) A23.1
  Bannister's T78.3 ☑
  barometer makers' — *see* Poisoning, mercury
  Barraquer (-Simons') (progressive lipodystrophy) E88.1
  Barrett's — *see* Barrett's, esophagus
  Bartholin's gland N75.9
  basal ganglia G25.9
    degenerative G23.9
      specified NEC G23.8
    specified NEC G25.89
  Basedow's (exophthalmic goiter) — *see* Hyperthyroidism, with, goiter (diffuse)
  Bateman's B08.1
  Batten-Steinert G71.11
  Battey A31.0
  Beard's (neurasthenia) F48.8
  Becker
    idiopathic mural endomyocardial I42.3
    myotonia congenita G71.12
  Begbie's (exophthalmic goiter) — *see* Hyperthyroidism, with, goiter (diffuse)
  behavioral, organic F07.9
  Beigel's (white piedra) B36.2
  Benson's — *see* Deposit, crystalline
  Bernard-Soulier (thrombopathy) D69.1
  Bernhardt (-Roth) — *see* Mononeuropathy, lower limb, meralgia paresthetica
  Biermer's (pernicious anemia) D51.0
  bile duct (common) (hepatic) K83.9
    with calculus, stones — *see* Calculus, bile duct
    specified NEC K83.8
  biliary (tract) K83.9
    specified NEC K83.8
  Billroth's — *see* Spina bifida
  bird fancier's J67.2
  black lung J60
  bladder N32.9
    in (due to)
      schistosomiasis (bilharziasis) B65.0 *[N33]*
    specified NEC N32.89
  bleeder's D66
  blood D75.9
    forming organs D75.9
    vessel I99.9
  Bloodgood's — *see* Mastopathy, cystic
  Bodechtel-Guttmann (subacute sclerosing panencephalitis) A81.1
  bone (*see also* Disorder, bone)
    aluminum M83.4
    fibrocystic NEC
      jaw M27.49
  bone-marrow D75.9
  Borna A83.9
  Bornholm (epidemic pleurodynia) B33.0
  Bouchard's (myopathic dilatation of the stomach) K31.0
  Bouillaud's (rheumatic heart disease) I01.9
  Bourneville (-Brissaud) (tuberous sclerosis) Q85.1
  Bouveret (-Hoffmann) (paroxysmal tachycardia) I47.9
  bowel K63.9
    functional K59.9
      psychogenic F45.8
  brain G93.9
    arterial, artery I67.9
    arteriosclerotic I67.2
    congenital Q04.9
    degenerative — *see* Degeneration, brain
    inflammatory — *see* Encephalitis
    organic G93.9
      arteriosclerotic I67.2
    parasitic NEC B71.9 *[G94]*
    senile NEC G31.1
    specified NEC G93.89
  breast (*see also* Disorder, breast) N64.9
    cystic (chronic) — *see* Mastopathy, cystic
    fibrocystic — *see* Mastopathy, cystic
    Paget's
      female, unspecified side C50.91 ☑
      male, unspecified side C50.92 ☑
    specified NEC N64.89
  Breda's — *see* Yaws
  Bretonneau's (diphtheritic malignant angina) A36.0
  Bright's — *see* Nephritis
    arteriosclerotic — *see* Hypertension, kidney
  Brill's (recrudescent typhus) A75.1

Disease — *continued*
  Brill-Zinsser (recrudescent typhus) A75.1
  Brion-Kayser — *see* Fever, paratyphoid
  broad
    beta E78.2
    ligament (noninflammatory) N83.9
      inflammatory — *see* Disease, pelvis, inflammatory
      specified NEC N83.8
  Brocq-Duhring (dermatitis herpetiformis) L13.0
  Brocq's
    meaning
      dermatitis herpetiformis L13.0
      prurigo L28.2
  bronchopulmonary J98.4
  bronchus NEC J98.09
  bronze Addison's E27.1
    tuberculous A18.7
  budgerigar fancier's J67.2
  bullous L13.9
    chronic of childhood L12.2
    specified NEC L13.8
  Buerger's (thromboangiitis obliterans) I73.1
  Bürger-Grütz (essential familial hyperlipemia) E78.3
  bursa — *see* Bursopathy
  caisson T70.3 ☑
  California — *see* Coccidioidomycosis
  capillaries I78.9
    specified NEC I78.8
  Carapata A68.0
  cardiac — *see* Disease, heart
  cardiopulmonary, chronic I27.9
  cardiorenal (hepatic) (hypertensive) (vascular) — *see* Hypertension, cardiorenal
  cardiovascular (atherosclerotic) I25.10
    with angina pectoris — *see* Arteriosclerosis, coronary (artery),
    congenital Q28.9
    newborn P29.9
      specified NEC P29.89
    hypertensive — *see* Hypertension, heart
    renal (hypertensive) — *see* Hypertension, cardiorenal
    syphilitic (asymptomatic) A52.00
  cartilage — *see* Disorder, cartilage
  Castellani's A69.8
  Castleman (unicentric) (multicentric) D47.Z2
    HHV-8-associated (*see also* Herpesvirus, human, 8) D47.Z2
  cat-scratch A28.1
  Cavare's (familial periodic paralysis) G72.3
  cecum K63.9
  celiac (adult) (infantile) (with steatorrhea) K90.0
  cellular tissue L98.9
  central core G71.2
  cerebellar, cerebellum — *see* Disease, brain
  cerebral (*see also* Disease, brain)
    degenerative — *see* Degeneration, brain
  cerebrospinal G96.9
  cerebrovascular I67.9
    acute I67.89
      embolic I63.4 ☑
      thrombotic I63.3 ☑
    arteriosclerotic I67.2
    specified NEC I67.89
  cervix (uteri) (noninflammatory) N88.9
    inflammatory — *see* Cervicitis
    specified NEC N88.8
  Chabert's A22.9
  Chandler's (osteochondritis dissecans, hip) — *see* Osteochondritis, dissecans, hip
  Charlouis — *see* Yaws
  Chédiak-Steinbrinck (-Higashi) (congenital gigantism of peroxidase granules) E70.330
  chest J98.9
  Chiari's (hepatic vein thrombosis) I82.0
  Chicago B40.9
  Chignon B36.8
  chigo, chigoe B88.1
  childhood granulomatous D71
  Chinese liver fluke B66.1
  chlamydial A74.9
    specified NEC A74.89
  cholecystic K82.9
  choroid H31.9
    specified NEC H31.8
  Christmas D67
  chronic bullous of childhood L12.2
  chylomicron retention E78.3
  ciliary body H21.9
    specified NEC H21.89

Disease

Disease — *continued*

circulatory (system) NEC I99.8
  newborn P29.9
  syphilitic A52.00
    congenital A50.54
coagulation factor deficiency (congenital) — *see* Defect, coagulation
coccidioidal — *see* Coccidioidomycosis
cold
  agglutinin or hemoglobinuria D59.1
    paroxysmal D59.6
  hemagglutinin (chronic) D59.1
collagen NOS (nonvascular) (vascular) M35.9
  specified NEC M35.8
colon K63.9
  functional K59.9
    congenital Q43.2
  ischemic (*see also* Ischemia, intestine, acute) K55.039
colonic inflammatory bowel, unclassified (IBDU) K52.3
combined system — *see* Degeneration, combined
compressed air T70.3 ☑
Concato's (pericardial polyserositis) A19.9
  nontubercular I31.1
  pleural — *see* Pleurisy, with effusion
conjunctiva H11.9
  chlamydial A74.0
  specified NEC H11.89
  viral B30.9
    specified NEC B30.8
connective tissue, systemic (diffuse) M35.9
  in (due to)
    hypogammaglobulinemia D80.1 *[M36.8]*
    ochronosis E70.29 *[M36.8]*
  specified NEC M35.8
Conor and Bruch's (boutonneuse fever) A77.1
Cooper's — *see* Mastopathy, cystic
Cori's (glycogenosis III) E74.03
corkhandler's or corkworker's J67.3
cornea H18.9
  specified NEC H18.89 ☑
coronary (artery) — *see* Disease, heart, ischemic, atherosclerotic
  congenital Q24.5
  ostial, syphilitic (aortic) (mitral) (pulmonary) A52.03
corpus cavernosum N48.9
  specified NEC N48.89
Cotugno's — *see* Sciatica
coxsackie (virus) NEC B34.1
cranial nerve NOS G52.9
Creutzfeldt-Jakob — *see* Creutzfeldt-Jakob disease or syndrome
Crocq's (acrocyanosis) I73.89
Crohn's — *see* Enteritis, regional
Curschmann G71.11
cystic
  breast (chronic) — *see* Mastopathy, cystic
  kidney, congenital Q61.9
  liver, congenital Q44.6
  lung J98.4
    congenital Q33.0
cytomegalic inclusion (generalized) B25.9
  with pneumonia B25.0
  congenital P35.1
cytomegaloviral B25.9
  specified NEC B25.8
Czerny's (periodic hydrarthrosis of the knee) — *see* Effusion, joint, knee
Daae (-Finsen) (epidemic pleurodynia) B33.0
Darling's — *see* Histoplasmosis capsulati
Débove's (splenomegaly) R16.1
deer fly — *see* Tularemia
Degos' I77.89
demyelinating, demyelinizing (nervous system) G37.9
  multiple sclerosis G35
  specified NEC G37.8
dense deposit (*see also* N00-N07 with fourth character .6) N05.6
deposition, hydroxyapatite — *see* Disease, hydroxyapatite deposition
de Quervain's (tendon sheath) M65.4
  thyroid (subacute granulomatous thyroiditis) E06.1
Devergie's (pityriasis rubra pilaris) L44.0
Devic's G36.0
diaphorase deficiency D74.0
diaphragm J98.6
diarrheal, infectious NEC A09

Disease — *continued*

digestive system K92.9
  specified NEC K92.89
disc, degenerative — *see* Degeneration, intervertebral disc
discogenic (*see also* Displacement, intervertebral disc NEC)
  with myelopathy — *see* Disorder, disc, with, myelopathy
diverticular — *see* Diverticula
Dubois (thymus) A50.59 *[E35]*
Duchenne-Griesinger G71.0
Duchenne's
  muscular dystrophy G71.0
  pseudohypertrophy, muscles G71.0
ductless glands E34.9
Duhring's (dermatitis herpetiformis) L13.0
duodenum K31.9
  specified NEC K31.89
Dupré's (meningism) R29.1
Dupuytren's (muscle contracture) M72.0
Durand-Nicholas-Favre (climatic bubo) A55
Duroziez's (congenital mitral stenosis) Q23.2
ear — *see* Disorder, ear
Eberth's — *see* Fever, typhoid
Ebola (virus) A98.4
Ebstein's heart Q22.5
Echinococcus — *see* Echinococcus
echovirus NEC B34.1
Eddowes' (brittle bones and blue sclera) Q78.0
edentulous (alveolar) ridge K06.9
  specified NEC K06.8
Edsall's T67.2 ☑
Eichstedt's (pityriasis versicolor) B36.0
Eisenmenger's (irreversible) I27.83
Ellis-van Creveld (chondroectodermal dysplasia) Q77.6
end stage renal (ESRD) N18.6
  due to hypertension I12.0
endocrine glands or system NEC E34.9
endomyocardial (eosinophilic) I42.3
English (rickets) E55.0
enteroviral, enterovirus NEC B34.1
  central nervous system NEC A88.8
epidemic B99.9
  specified NEC B99.8
epididymis N50.9
Erb (-Landouzy) G71.0
Erdheim-Chester (ECD) E88.89
esophagus K22.9
  functional K22.4
  psychogenic F45.8
  specified NEC K22.8
Eulenburg's (congenital paramyotonia) G71.19
eustachian tube — *see* Disorder, eustachian tube
external
  auditory canal — *see* Disorder, ear, external
  ear — *see* Disorder, ear, external
extrapyramidal G25.9
  specified NEC G25.89
eye H57.9
  anterior chamber H21.9
  inflammatory NEC H57.8
  muscle (external) — *see* Strabismus
  specified NEC H57.8
  syphilitic — *see* Oculopathy, syphilitic
eyeball H44.9
  specified NEC H44.89
eyelid — *see* Disorder, eyelid
  specified NEC — *see* Disorder, eyelid, specified type NEC
eyeworm of Africa B74.3
facial nerve (seventh) G51.9
  newborn (birth injury) P11.3
Fahr (of brain) G23.8
Fahr Volhard (of kidney) I12. ☑
fallopian tube (noninflammatory) N83.9
  inflammatory — *see* Salpingo-oophoritis
  specified NEC N83.8
familial periodic paralysis G72.3
Fanconi's (congenital pancytopenia) D61.09
fascia NEC (*see also* Disorder, muscle)
  inflammatory — *see* Myositis
  specified NEC M62.89
Fauchard's (periodontitis) — *see* Periodontitis
Favre-Durand-Nicolas (climatic bubo) A55
Fede's K14.0
Feer's — *see* Poisoning, mercury
female pelvic inflammatory (*see also* Disease, pelvis, inflammatory) N73.9
  syphilitic (secondary) A51.42
  tuberculous A18.17

Disease — *continued*

Fernels' (aortic aneurysm) I71.9
fibrocaseous of lung — *see* Tuberculosis, pulmonary
fibrocystic — *see* Fibrocystic disease
Fiedler's (leptospiral jaundice) A27.0
fifth B08.3
file-cutter's — *see* Poisoning, lead
fish-skin Q80.9
  acquired L85.0
Flajani (-Basedow) (exophthalmic goiter) — *see* Hyperthyroidism, with, goiter (diffuse)
flax-dresser's J66.1
fluke — *see* Infestation, fluke
foot and mouth B08.8
foot process N04.9
Forbes' (glycogenosis III) E74.03
Fordyce-Fox (apocrine miliaria) L75.2
Fordyce's (ectopic sebaceous glands) (mouth) Q38.6
Forestier's (rhizomelic pseudopolyarthritis) M35.3
  meaning ankylosing hyperostosis — *see* Hyperostosis, ankylosing
Fothergill's
  neuralgia — *see* Neuralgia, trigeminal
  scarlatina anginosa A38.9
Fournier (gangrene) N49.3
  female N76.89
fourth B08.8
Fox (-Fordyce) (apocrine miliaria) L75.2
Francis' — *see* Tularemia
Franklin C88.2
Frei's (climatic bubo) A55
Friedreich's
  combined systemic or ataxia G11.1
  myoclonia G25.3
frontal sinus — *see* Sinusitis, frontal
fungus NEC B49
Gaisböck's (polycythemia hypertonica) D75.1
gallbladder K82.9
  calculus — *see* Calculus, gallbladder
  cholecystitis — *see* Cholecystitis
  cholesterolosis K82.4
  fistula — *see* Fistula, gallbladder
  hydrops K82.1
  obstruction — *see* Obstruction, gallbladder
  perforation K82.2
  specified NEC K82.8
gamma heavy chain C88.2
Gamna's (siderotic splenomegaly) D73.2
Gamstorp's (adynamia episodica hereditaria) G72.3
Gandy-Nanta (siderotic splenomegaly) D73.2
ganister J62.8
gastric — *see* Disease, stomach
gastroesophageal reflux (GERD) K21.9
  with esophagitis K21.0
gastrointestinal (tract) K92.9
  amyloid E85.4
  functional K59.9
    psychogenic F45.8
  specified NEC K92.89
Gee (-Herter) (-Heubner) (-Thaysen) (nontropical sprue) K90.0
genital organs
  female N94.9
  male N50.9
Gerhardt's (erythromelalgia) I73.81
Gibert's (pityriasis rosea) L42
Gierke's (glycogenosis I) E74.01
Gilles de la Tourette's (motor-verbal tic) F95.2
gingiva K06.9
  plaque induced K05.00
  specified NEC K06.8
gland (lymph) I89.9
Glanzmann's (hereditary hemorrhagic thrombasthenia) D69.1
glass-blower's (cataract) — *see* Cataract, specified NEC
  salivary gland hypertrophy K11.1
Glisson's — *see* Rickets
globe H44.9
  specified NEC H44.89
glomerular (*see also* Glomerulonephritis)
  with edema — *see* Nephrosis
  acute — *see* Nephritis, acute
  chronic — *see* Nephritis, chronic
  minimal change N05.0
  rapidly progressive N01.9
glycogen storage E74.00
  Andersen's E74.09
  Cori's E74.03

☑ **Additional character required**

Disease — *continued*
  glycogen storage — *continued*
    Forbes' E74.03
    generalized E74.00
    glucose-6-phosphatase deficiency E74.01
    heart E74.02 *[143]*
    hepatorenal E74.09
    Hers' E74.09
    liver and kidney E74.09
    McArdle's E74.04
    muscle phosphofructokinase E74.09
    myocardium E74.02 *[143]*
    Pompe's E74.02
    Tauri's E74.09
    type 0 E74.09
    type I E74.01
    type II E74.02
    type III E74.03
    type IV E74.09
    type V E74.04
    type VI-XI E74.09
    Von Gierke's E74.01
  Goldstein's (familial hemorrhagic
      telangiectasia) I78.0
  gonococcal NOS A54.9
  graft-versus-host (GVH) D89.813
    acute D89.810
    acute on chronic D89.812
    chronic D89.811
  grainhandler's J67.8
  granulomatous (childhood) (chronic) D71
  Graves' (exophthalmic goiter) — *see*
      Hyperthyroidism, with, goiter (diffuse)
  Griesinger's — *see* Ancylostomiasis
  Grisel's M43.6
  Gruby's (tinea tonsurans) B35.0
  Guillain-Barré G61.0
  Guinon's (motor-verbal tic) F95.2
  gum K06.9
  gynecological N94.9
  H (Hartnup's) E72.02
  Haff — *see* Poisoning, mercury
  Hageman (congenital factor XII deficiency) D68.2
  hair (color) (shaft) L67.9
    follicles L73.9
      specified NEC L73.8
  Hamman's (spontaneous mediastinal
      emphysema) J98.2
  hand, foot and mouth B08.4
  Hansen's — *see* Leprosy
  Hantavirus, with pulmonary manifestations B33.4
    with renal manifestations A98.5
  Harada's H30.81 ☑
  Hartnup (pellagra-cerebellar ataxia-renal
      aminoaciduria) E72.02
  Hart's (pellagra-cerebellar ataxia-renal
      aminoaciduria) E72.02
  Hashimoto's (struma lymphomatosa) E06.3
  Hb — *see* Disease, hemoglobin
  heart (organic) I51.9
    with
      pulmonary edema (acute) (*see also* Failure,
          ventricular, left) I50.1
      rheumatic fever (conditions in I00)
        active I01.9
          with chorea I02.0
          specified NEC I01.8
        inactive or quiescent (with chorea) I09.9
          specified NEC I09.89
    amyloid E85.4 *[143]*
    aortic (valve) I35.9
    arteriosclerotic or sclerotic (senile) — *see*
        Disease, heart, ischemic, atherosclerotic
    artery, arterial — *see* Disease, heart, ischemic,
        atherosclerotic
    beer drinkers' I42.6
    beriberi (wet) E51.12
    black I27.0
    congenital Q24.9
      cyanotic Q24.9
      specified NEC Q24.8
    coronary — *see* Disease, heart, ischemic
    cryptogenic I51.9
    fibroid — *see* Myocarditis
    functional I51.89
      psychogenic F45.8
    glycogen storage E74.02 *[143]*
    gonococcal A54.83
    hypertensive — *see* Hypertension, heart
    hyperthyroid (*see also* Hyperthyroidism) E05.90
        [143]
      with thyroid storm E05.91 *[143]*

Disease — *continued*
  heart — *continued*
    ischemic (chronic or with a stated duration of
        over 4 weeks) I25.9
      atherosclerotic (of) I25.10
        with angina pectoris — *see* Arteriosclerosis,
            coronary (artery)
        coronary artery bypass graft — *see*
            Arteriosclerosis, coronary (artery),
            cardiomyopathy I25.5
        diagnosed on ECG or other special
            investigation, but currently presenting
            no symptoms I25.6
      silent I25.6
      specified form NEC I25.89
    kyphoscoliotic I27.1
    meningococcal A39.50
      endocarditis A39.51
      myocarditis A39.52
      pericarditis A39.53
    mitral I05.9
      specified NEC I05.8
    muscular — *see* Degeneration, myocardial
    psychogenic (functional) F45.8
    pulmonary (chronic) I27.9
      in schistosomiasis B65.9 *[152]*
      specified NEC I27.89
    rheumatic (chronic) (inactive) (old) (quiescent)
        (with chorea) I09.9
      active or acute I01.9
        with chorea (acute) (rheumatic)
            (Sydenham's) I02.0
      specified NEC I09.89
    senile — *see* Myocarditis
    syphilitic A52.06
      aortic A52.03
        aneurysm A52.01
      congenital A50.54 *[152]*
    thyrotoxic (*see also* Thyrotoxicosis) E05.90 *[143]*
      with thyroid storm E05.91 *[143]*
    valve, valvular (obstructive) (regurgitant) (*see
        also* Endocarditis)
      congenital NEC Q24.8
      pulmonary Q22.3
    vascular — *see* Disease, cardiovascular
  heavy chain NEC C88.2
    alpha C88.3
    gamma C88.2
    mu C88.2
  Hebra's
    pityriasis
      maculata et circinata L42
      rubra pilaris L44.0
    prurigo L28.2
  hematopoietic organs D75.9
  hemoglobin or Hb
    abnormal (mixed) NEC D58.2
      with thalassemia D56.9
    AS genotype D57.3
    Bart's D56.0
    C (Hb-C) D58.2
      with other abnormal hemoglobin NEC D58.2
      elliptocytosis D58.1
      Hb-S D57.2 ☑
      sickle-cell D57.2 ☑
      thalassemia D56.8
    Constant Spring D58.2
    D (Hb-D) D58.2
    E (Hb-E) D58.2
    E-beta thalassemia D56.5
    elliptocytosis D58.1
    H (Hb-H) (thalassemia) D56.0
      with other abnormal hemoglobin NEC D56.9
      Constant Spring D56.0
    I thalassemia D56.9
    M D74.0
    S or SS D57.1
    SC D57.2 ☑
    SD D57.8 ☑
    SE D57.8 ☑
    spherocytosis D58.0
    unstable, hemolytic D58.2
  hemolytic (newborn) P55.9
    autoimmune (cold type) (warm type) D59.1
    drug-induced D59.0
    due to or with
      incompatibility
        ABO (blood group) P55.1
        blood (group) (Duffy) (K(ell)) (Kidd) (Lewis)
            (M) (S) NEC P55.8
        Rh (blood group) (factor) P55.0
      Rh negative mother P55.0

Disease — *continued*
  hemolytic — *continued*
    specified type NEC P55.8
    unstable hemoglobin D58.2
  hemorrhagic D69.9
    newborn P53
  Henoch (-Schönlein) (purpura nervosa) D69.0
  hepatic — *see* Disease, liver
  hepatobiliary K83.9
    toxic K71.9
  hepatolenticular E83.01
  heredodegenerative NEC
    spinal cord G95.89
  herpesviral, disseminated B00.7
  Hers' (glycogenosis VI) E74.09
  Herter (-Gee) (-Heubner) (nontropical
      sprue) K90.0
  Heubner-Herter (nontropical sprue) K90.0
  high fetal gene or hemoglobin thalassemia D56.9
  Hildenbrand's — *see* Typhus
  hip (joint) M25.9
    congenital Q65.89
    suppurative M00.9
    tuberculous A18.02
  His (-Werner) (trench fever) A79.0
  Hodgson's I71.2
    ruptured I71.1
  Holla — *see* Spherocytosis
  hookworm B76.9
    specified NEC B76.8
  host-versus-graft D89.813
    acute D89.810
    acute on chronic D89.812
    chronic D89.811
  human immunodeficiency virus (HIV) B20
  Huntington's G10
    with dementia G10 *[F02.80]*
  Hutchinson's (cheiropompholyx) — *see*
      Hutchinson's disease
  hyaline (diffuse) (generalized)
    membrane (lung) (newborn) P22.0
      adult J80
  hydatid — *see* Echinococcus
  hydroxyapatite deposition M11.00
    ankle M11.07 ☑
    elbow M11.02 ☑
    foot joint M11.07 ☑
    hand joint M11.04 ☑
    hip M11.05 ☑
    knee M11.06 ☑
    multiple site M11.09
    shoulder M11.01 ☑
    vertebra M11.08
    wrist M11.03 ☑
  hyperkinetic — *see* Hyperkinesia
  hypertensive — *see* Hypertension
  hypophysis E23.7
  Iceland G93.3
  I-cell E77.0
  immune D89.9
  immunoproliferative (malignant) C88.9
    small intestinal C88.3
    specified NEC C88.8
  inclusion B25.9
    salivary gland B25.9
  infectious, infective B99.9
    congenital P37.9
      specified NEC P37.8
      viral P35.9
        specified type NEC P35.8
    specified NEC B99.8
  inflammatory
    penis N48.29
      abscess N48.21
      cellulitis N48.22
    prepuce N47.7
      balanoposthitis N47.6
    tubo-ovarian — *see* Salpingo-oophoritis
  intervertebral disc (*see also* Disorder, disc)
    with myelopathy — *see* Disorder, disc, with,
        myelopathy
    cervical, cervicothoracic — *see* Disorder, disc,
        cervical
    with
      myelopathy — *see* Disorder, disc, cervical,
          with myelopathy
      neuritis, radiculitis or radiculopathy — *see*
          Disorder, disc, cervical, with neuritis
      specified NEC — *see* Disorder, disc, cervical,
          specified type NEC
    lumbar (with)
      myelopathy M51.06

Disease

Disease — *continued*
    intervertebral disc — *continued*
      neuritis, radiculitis, radiculopathy or
        sciatica M51.16
      specified NEC M51.86
      lumbosacral (with)
        neuritis, radiculitis, radiculopathy or
          sciatica M51.17
        specified NEC M51.87
      specified NEC — *see* Disorder, disc, specified
        NEC
      thoracic (with)
        myelopathy M51.04
        neuritis, radiculitis or radiculopathy M51.14
        specified NEC M51.84
      thoracolumbar (with)
        myelopathy M51.05
        neuritis, radiculitis or radiculopathy M51.15
        specified NEC M51.85
    intestine K63.9
      functional K59.9
        psychogenic F45.8
        specified NEC K59.8
      organic K63.9
      protozoal A07.9
      specified NEC K63.89
    iris H21.9
      specified NEC H21.89
    iron metabolism or storage E83.10
    island (scrub typhus) A75.3
    itai-itai — *see* Poisoning, cadmium
    Jakob-Creutzfeldt — *see* Creutzfeldt-Jakob
      disease or syndrome
    jaw M27.9
      fibrocystic M27.49
      specified NEC M27.8
    jigger B88.1
    joint (*see also* Disorder, joint)
      Charcot's — *see* Arthropathy, neuropathic
        (Charcot)
      degenerative — *see* Osteoarthritis
        multiple M15.9
        spine — *see* Spondylosis
      hypertrophic — *see* Osteoarthritis
      sacroiliac M53.3
      specified NEC — *see* Disorder, joint, specified
        type NEC
      spine NEC — *see* Dorsopathy
      suppurative — *see* Arthritis, pyogenic or
        pyemic
    Jourdain's (acute gingivitis) K05.00
      nonplaque induced K05.01
      plaque induced K05.00
    Kaschin-Beck (endemic polyarthritis) M12.10
      ankle M12.17 ☑
      elbow M12.12 ☑
      foot joint M12.17 ☑
      hand joint M12.14 ☑
      hip M12.15 ☑
      knee M12.16 ☑
      multiple site M12.19
      shoulder M12.11 ☑
      vertebra M12.18
      wrist M12.13 ☑
    Katayama B65.2
    Kedani (scrub typhus) A75.3
    Keshan E59
    kidney (functional) (pelvis) N28.9
      chronic N18.9
        hypertensive — *see* Hypertension, kidney
        stage 1 N18.1
        stage 2 (mild) N18.2
        stage 3 (moderate) N18.3
        stage 4 (severe) N18.4
        stage 5 N18.5
      complicating pregnancy — *see* Pregnancy,
        complicated by, renal disease
      cystic (congenital) Q61.9
      diabetic — *see* E08-E13 with .22
      fibrocystic (congenital) Q61.8
      hypertensive — *see* Hypertension, kidney
      in (due to)
        schistosomiasis (bilharziasis) B65.9 *[N29]*
      multicystic Q61.4
      polycystic Q61.3
        adult type Q61.2
        childhood type NEC Q61.19
          collecting duct dilatation Q61.11
      Kimmelstiel (-Wilson) (intercapillary polycystic
        (congenital) glomerulosclerosis) — *see*
        E08-E13 with .21

Disease — *continued*
    Kimura D21.9
      specified site (*see* Neoplasm, connective tissue
        benign)
    Kinnier Wilson's (hepatolenticular
      degeneration) E83.01
    kissing — *see* Mononucleosis, infectious
    Klebs' (*see also* Glomerulonephritis) N05. ☑
    Klippel-Feil (brevicollis) Q76.1
    Köhler-Pellegrini-Stieda (calcification, knee joint)
      — *see* Bursitis, tibial collateral
    Kok Q89.8
    König's (osteochondritis dissecans) — *see*
      Osteochondritis, dissecans
    Korsakoff's (nonalcoholic) F04
      alcoholic F10.96
        with dependence F10.26
    Kostmann's (infantile genetic
      agranulocytosis) D70.0
    kuru A81.81
    Kyasanur Forest A98.2
    labyrinth, ear — *see* Disorder, ear, inner
    lacrimal system — *see* Disorder, lacrimal system
    Lafora's — *see* Epilepsy, generalized, idiopathic
    Lancereaux-Mathieu (leptospiral jaundice) A27.0
    Landry's G61.0
    Larrey-Weil (leptospiral jaundice) A27.0
    larynx J38.7
    legionnaires' A48.1
      nonpneumonic A48.2
    Lenegre's I44.2
    lens H27.9
      specified NEC H27.8
    Lev's (acquired complete heart block) I44.2
    Lewy body (dementia) G31.83 *[F02.80]*
      with behavioral disturbance G31.83 *[F02.81]*
    Lichtheim's (subacute combined sclerosis with
      pernicious anemia) D51.0
    Lightwood's (renal tubular acidosis) N25.89
    Lignac's (cystinosis) E72.04
    lip K13.0
    lipid-storage E75.6
      specified NEC E75.5
    Lipschütz's N76.6
    liver (chronic) (organic) K76.9
      alcoholic (chronic) K70.9
        acute — *see* Disease, liver, alcoholic, hepatitis
        cirrhosis K70.30
          with ascites K70.31
        failure K70.40
          with coma K70.41
        fatty liver K70.0
        fibrosis K70.2
        hepatitis K70.10
          with ascites K70.11
        sclerosis K70.2
      cystic, congenital Q44.6
      drug-induced (idiosyncratic) (toxic)
        (predictable) (unpredictable) — *see*
        Disease, liver, toxic
      end stage K72.90
        due to hepatitis — *see* Hepatitis
      fatty, nonalcoholic (NAFLD) K76.0
        alcoholic K70.0
      fibrocystic (congenital) Q44.6
      fluke
        Chinese B66.1
        oriental B66.1
        sheep B66.3
      gestational alloimmune (GALD) P78.84
      glycogen storage E74.09 *[K77]*
      in (due to)
        schistosomiasis (bilharziasis) B65.9 *[K77]*
      inflammatory K75.9
        alcoholic K70.1 ☑
        specified NEC K75.89
      polycystic (congenital) Q44.6
      toxic K71.9
        with
          cholestasis K71.0
          cirrhosis (liver) K71.7
          fibrosis (liver) K71.7
          focal nodular hyperplasia K71.8
          hepatic granuloma K71.8
          hepatic necrosis K71.10
            with coma K71.11
          hepatitis NEC K71.6
            acute K71.2
            chronic
              active K71.50
                with ascites K71.51
              lobular K71.4

Disease — *continued*
    liver — *continued*
          persistent K71.3
        lupoid K71.50
          with ascites K71.51
        peliosis hepatis K71.8
        veno-occlusive disease (VOD) of liver K71.8
      veno-occlusive K76.5
    Lobo's (keloid blastomycosis) B48.0
    Lobstein's (brittle bones and blue sclera) Q78.0
    Ludwig's (submaxillary cellulitis) K12.2
    lumbosacral region M53.87
    lung J98.4
      black J60
      congenital Q33.9
      cystic J98.4
        congenital Q33.0
      fibroid (chronic) — *see* Fibrosis, lung
      fluke B66.4
        oriental B66.4
      in
        amyloidosis E85.4 *[J99]*
        sarcoidosis D86.0
        Sjögren's syndrome M35.02
        systemic
          lupus erythematosus M32.13
          sclerosis M34.81
      interstitial J84.9
        of childhood, specified NEC J84.848
        respiratory bronchiolitis J84.115
        specified NEC J84.89
      obstructive (chronic) J44.9
        with
          acute
            bronchitis J44.0
            exacerbation NEC J44.1
            lower respiratory infection J44.0
          alveolitis, allergic J67.9
          asthma J44.9
          bronchiectasis J47.9
            with
              exacerbation (acute) J47.1
              lower respiratory infection J47.0
          bronchitis J44.9
            with
              exacerbation (acute) J44.1
              lower respiratory infection J44.0
          emphysema J43.9
          hypersensitivity pneumonitis J67.9
        decompensated J44.1
          with
            exacerbation (acute) J44.1
      polycystic J98.4
        congenital Q33.0
      rheumatoid (diffuse) (interstitial) — *see*
        Rheumatoid, lung
    Lutembacher's (atrial septal defect with mitral
      stenosis) Q21.1
    Lyme A69.20
    lymphatic (gland) (system) (channel) (vessel) I89.9
    lymphoproliferative D47.9
      specified NEC D47.Z9
      T-gamma D47.Z9
      X-linked D82.3
    Magitot's M27.2
    malarial — *see* Malaria
    malignant (*see also* Neoplasm, malignant, by site)
    Manson's B65.1
    maple bark J67.6
    maple-syrup-urine E71.0
    Marburg (virus) A98.3
    Marion's (bladder neck obstruction) N32.0
    Marsh's (exophthalmic goiter) — *see*
      Hyperthyroidism, with, goiter (diffuse)
    mastoid (process) — *see* Disorder, ear, middle
    Mathieu's (leptospiral jaundice) A27.0
    Maxcy's A75.2
    McArdle (-Schmid-Pearson) (glycogenosis
      V) E74.04
    mediastinum J98.59
    medullary center (idiopathic) (respiratory) G93.89
    Meige's (chronic hereditary edema) Q82.0
    meningococcal — *see* Infection, meningococcal
    mental F99
      organic F09
    mesenchymal M35.9
    mesenteric embolic (*see also* Ischemia, intestine,
      acute) K55.039
    metabolic, metabolism E88.9
      bilirubin E80.7
    metal-polisher's J62.8

Disease — *continued*
  metastatic (*see also* Neoplasm, secondary, by site) C79.9
  microvascular - code to condition
  microvillus
    atrophy Q43.8
    inclusion (MVD) Q43.8
  middle ear — *see* Disorder, ear, middle
  Mikulicz' (dryness of mouth, absent or decreased lacrimation) K11.8
  Milroy's (chronic hereditary edema) Q82.0
  Minamata — *see* Poisoning, mercury
  minicore G71.2
  Minor's G95.19
  Minot's (hemorrhagic disease, newborn) P53
  Minot-von Willebrand-Jürgens (angiohemophilia) D68.0
  Mitchell's (erythromelalgia) I73.81
  mitral (valve) I05.9
    nonrheumatic I34.9
  mixed connective tissue M35.1
  moldy hay J67.0
  Monge's T70.29 ☑
  Morgagni-Adams-Stokes (syncope with heart block) I45.9
  Morgagni's (syndrome) (hyperostosis frontalis interna) M85.2
  Morton's (with metatarsalgia) — *see* Lesion, nerve, plantar
  Morvan's G60.8
  motor neuron (bulbar) (mixed type) (spinal) G12.20
    amyotrophic lateral sclerosis G12.21
    familial G12.24
    progressive bulbar palsy G12.22
    specified NEC G12.29
  moyamoya I67.5
  mu heavy chain disease C88.2
  multicore G71.2
  muscle (*see also* Disorder, muscle)
    inflammatory — *see* Myositis
    ocular (external) — *see* Strabismus
  musculoskeletal system, soft tissue — *see also* Disorder, soft tissue
    specified NEC — *see* Disorder, soft tissue, specified type NEC
  mushroom workers' J67.5
  mycotic B49
  myelodysplastic, not classified C94.6
  myeloproliferative, not classified C94.6
    chronic D47.1
  myocardium, myocardial (*see also* Degeneration, myocardial) I51.5
    primary (idiopathic) I42.9
  myoneural G70.9
  Naegeli's D69.1
  nails L60.9
    specified NEC L60.8
  Nairobi (sheep virus) A93.8
  nasal J34.9
  nemaline body G71.2
  nerve — *see* Disorder, nerve
  nervous system G98.8
    autonomic G90.9
    central G96.9
      specified NEC G96.8
    congenital Q07.9
    parasympathetic G90.9
    specified NEC G98.8
    sympathetic G90.9
    vegetative G90.9
  neuromuscular system G70.9
  Newcastle B30.8
  Nicolas (-Durand)-Favre (climatic bubo) A55
  nipple N64.9
    Paget's C50.01 ☑
      female C50.01 ☑
      male C50.02 ☑
  Nishimoto (-Takeuchi) I67.5
  nonarthropod-borne NOS (viral) B34.9
    enterovirus NEC B34.1
  nonautoimmune hemolytic D59.4
    drug-induced D59.2
  Nonne-Milroy-Meige (chronic hereditary edema) Q82.0
  nose J34.9
  nucleus pulposus — *see* Disorder, disc
  nutritional E63.9
  oast-house-urine E72.19
    ocular
      herpesviral B00.50
      zoster B02.30

Disease — *continued*
  obliterative vascular I77.1
  Ohara's — *see* Tularemia
  Opitz's (congestive splenomegaly) D73.2
  Oppenheim-Urbach (necrobiosis lipoidica diabeticorum) — *see* E08-E13 with .620
  optic nerve NEC — *see* Disorder, nerve, optic
  orbit — *see* Disorder, orbit
  Oriental liver fluke B66.1
  Oriental lung fluke B66.4
  Ormond's N13.5
  Oropouche virus A93.0
  Osler-Rendu (familial hemorrhagic telangiectasia) I78.0
  osteofibrocystic E21.0
  Otto's M24.7
  outer ear — *see* Disorder, ear, external
  ovary (noninflammatory) N83.9
    cystic N83.20 ☑
    inflammatory — *see* Salpingo-oophoritis
    polycystic E28.2
    specified NEC N83.8
  Owren's (congenital) — *see* Defect, coagulation
  pancreas K86.9
    cystic K86.2
    fibrocystic E84.9
    specified NEC K86.89
  panvalvular I08.9
    specified NEC I08.8
  parametrium (noninflammatory) N83.9
  parasitic B89
    cerebral NEC B71.9 *[G94]*
    intestinal NOS B82.9
    mouth B37.0
    skin NOS B88.9
    specified type — *see* Infestation
    tongue B37.0
  parathyroid (gland) E21.5
    specified NEC E21.4
  Parkinson's G20
  parodontal K05.6
  Parrot's (syphilitic osteochondritis) A50.02
  Parry's (exophthalmic goiter) — *see* Hyperthyroidism, with, goiter (diffuse)
  Parson's (exophthalmic goiter) — *see* Hyperthyroidism, with, goiter (diffuse)
  Paxton's (white piedra) B36.2
  pearl-worker's — *see* Osteomyelitis, specified type NEC
  Pellegrini-Stieda (calcification, knee joint) — *see* Bursitis, tibial collateral
  pelvis, pelvic
    female NOS N94.9
      specified NEC N94.89
    gonococcal (acute) (chronic) A54.24
    inflammatory (female) N73.9
      acute N73.0
      chlamydial A56.11
      chronic N73.1
      specified NEC N73.8
      syphilitic (secondary) A51.42
        late A52.76
      tuberculous A18.17
    organ, female NEC N94.9
    peritoneum, female NEC N94.89
  penis N48.9
    inflammatory N48.29
      abscess N48.21
      cellulitis N48.22
    specified NEC N48.89
  periapical tissues NOS K04.90
  periodontal K05.6
    specified NEC K05.5
  periosteum — *see* Disorder, bone, specified type NEC
  peripheral
    arterial I73.9
    autonomic nervous system G90.9
    nerves — *see* Polyneuropathy
    vascular NOS I73.9
  peritoneum K66.9
    pelvic, female NEC N94.89
    specified NEC K66.8
  persistent mucosal (middle ear) H66.20
    left H66.22
      with right H66.23
    right H66.21
      with left H66.23
  Petit's — *see* Hernia, abdomen, specified site NEC
  pharynx J39.2
    specified NEC J39.2
  Phocas' — *see* Mastopathy, cystic

Disease — *continued*
  photochromogenic (acid-fast bacilli) (pulmonary) A31.0
    nonpulmonary A31.9
  Pick's G31.01 *[F02.80]*
    with behavioral disturbance G31.01 *[F02.81]*
    brain G31.01 *[F02.80]*
      with behavioral disturbance G31.01 *[F02.81]*
    of pericardium (pericardial pseudocirrhosis of liver) I31.1
  pigeon fancier's J67.2
  pineal gland E34.8
  pink — *see* Poisoning, mercury
  Pinkus' (lichen nitidus) L44.1
  pinworm B80
  Piry virus A93.8
  pituitary (gland) E23.7
  pituitary-snuff-taker's J67.8
  pleura (cavity) J94.9
    specified NEC J94.8
  pneumatic drill (hammer) T75.21 ☑
  Pollitzer's (hidradenitis suppurativa) L73.2
  polycystic
    kidney or renal Q61.3
      adult type Q61.2
      childhood type NEC Q61.19
        collecting duct dilatation Q61.11
    liver or hepatic Q44.6
    lung or pulmonary J98.4
      congenital Q33.0
    ovary, ovaries E28.2
    spleen Q89.09
  polyethylene T84.05 ☑
  Pompe's (glycogenosis II) E74.02
  Posadas-Wernicke B38.9
  Potain's (pulmonary edema) — *see* Edema, lung
  prepuce N47.8
    inflammatory N47.7
    balanoposthitis N47.6
  Pringle's (tuberous sclerosis) Q85.1
  prion, central nervous system A81.9
    specified NEC A81.89
  prostate N42.9
    specified NEC N42.89
  protozoal B64
    acanthamebiasis — *see* Acanthamebiasis
    African trypanosomiasis — *see* African trypanosomiasis
    babesiosis B60.0
    Chagas disease — *see* Chagas disease
    intestine, intestinal A07.9
    leishmaniasis — *see* Leishmaniasis
    malaria — *see* Malaria
    naegleriasis B60.2
    pneumocystosis B59
    specified organism NEC B60.8
    toxoplasmosis — *see* Toxoplasmosis
  pseudo-Hurler's E77.0
  psychiatric F99
  psychotic — *see* Psychosis
  Puente's (simple glandular cheilitis) K13.0
  puerperal (*see also* Puerperal) O90.89
  pulmonary (*see also* Disease, lung)
    artery I28.9
    chronic obstructive J44.9
      with
        acute bronchitis J44.0
          exacerbation (acute) J44.1
        lower respiratory infection (acute) J44.0
        decompensated J44.1
          with
            exacerbation (acute) J44.1
    heart I27.9
      specified NEC I27.89
    hypertensive (vascular) (*see also* Hypertension, pulmonary) I27.20
      primary (idiopathic) I27.0
    valve I37.9
      rheumatic I09.89
  pulp (dental) NOS K04.90
  pulseless M31.4
  Putnam's (subacute combined sclerosis with pernicious anemia) D51.0
  Pyle (-Cohn) (metaphyseal dysplasia) Q78.5
  ragpicker's or ragsorter's A22.1
  Raynaud's — *see* Raynaud's disease
  reactive airway — *see* Asthma
  Reclus' (cystic) — *see* Mastopathy, cystic
  rectum K62.9
    specified NEC K62.89
  Refsum's (heredopathia atactica polyneuritiformis) G60.1

Disease

Disease — *continued*
renal (functional) (pelvis) (*see also* Disease, kidney) N28.9
  with
    edema — *see* Nephrosis
    glomerular lesion — *see* Glomerulonephritis
      with edema — *see* Nephrosis
    interstitial nephritis N12
  acute N28.9
  chronic (*see also* Disease, kidney, chronic) N18.9
  cystic, congenital Q61.9
  diabetic — *see* E08-E13 with .22
  end-stage (failure) N18.6
    due to hypertension I12.0
  fibrocystic (congenital) Q61.8
  hypertensive — *see* Hypertension, kidney
  lupus M32.14
  phosphate-losing (tubular) N25.0
  polycystic (congenital) Q61.3
    adult type Q61.2
    childhood type NEC Q61.19
      collecting duct dilatation Q61.11
  rapidly progressive N01.9
  subacute N01.9
Rendu-Osler-Weber (familial hemorrhagic telangiectasia) I78.0
renovascular (arteriosclerotic) — *see* Hypertension, kidney
respiratory (tract) J98.9
  acute or subacute NOS J06.9
    due to
      chemicals, gases, fumes or vapors (inhalation) J68.3
      external agent J70.9
        specified NEC J70.8
      radiation J70.0
      smoke inhalation J70.5
    noninfectious J39.8
  chronic NOS J98.9
    due to
      chemicals, gases, fumes or vapors J68.4
      external agent J70.9
        specified NEC J70.8
      radiation J70.1
  newborn P27.9
    specified NEC P27.8
  due to
    chemicals, gases, fumes or vapors J68.9
      acute or subacute NEC J68.3
      chronic J68.4
    external agent J70.9
      specified NEC J70.8
  newborn P28.9
    specified type NEC P28.89
  upper J39.9
    acute or subacute J06.9
    noninfectious NEC J39.8
    specified NEC J39.8
    streptococcal J06.9
retina, retinal H35.9
  Batten's or Batten-Mayou E75.4 *[H36]*
  specified NEC H35.89
rheumatoid — *see* Arthritis, rheumatoid
rickettsial NOS A79.9
  specified type NEC A79.89
Riga (-Fede) (cachectic aphthae) K14.0
Riggs' (compound periodontitis) — *see* Periodontitis
Ritter's L00
Rivalta's (cervicofacial actinomycosis) A42.2
Robles' (onchocerciasis) B73.01
Roger's (congenital interventricular septal defect) Q21.0
Rosenthal's (factor XI deficiency) D68.1
Rossbach's (hyperchlorhydria) K30
Ross River B33.1
Rotes Quérol — *see* Hyperostosis, ankylosing
Roth (-Bernhardt) — *see* Mononeuropathy, lower limb, meralgia paresthetica
Runeberg's (progressive pernicious anemia) D51.0
sacroiliac NEC M53.3
salivary gland or duct K11.9
  inclusion B25.9
  specified NEC K11.8
  virus B25.9
sandworm B76.9
Schimmelbusch's — *see* Mastopathy, cystic
Schmorl's — *see* Schmorl's disease or nodes
Schönlein (-Henoch) (purpura rheumatica) D69.0
Schottmüller's — *see* Fever, paratyphoid

Disease — *continued*
Schultz's (agranulocytosis) — *see* Agranulocytosis
Schwalbe-Ziehen-Oppenheim G24.1
Schwartz-Jampel G71.13
sclera H15.9
  specified NEC H15.89
scrofulous (tuberculous) A18.2
scrotum N50.9
sebaceous glands L73.9
semilunar cartilage, cystic (*see also* Derangement, knee, meniscus, cystic)
seminal vesicle N50.9
serum NEC (*see also* Reaction, serum) T80.69 ☑
sexually transmitted A64
  anogenital
    herpesviral infection — *see* Herpes, anogenital
    warts A63.0
  chancroid A57
  chlamydial infection — *see* Chlamydia
  gonorrhea — *see* Gonorrhea
  granuloma inguinale A58
  specified organism NEC A63.8
  syphilis — *see* Syphilis
  trichomoniasis — *see* Trichomoniasis
Sézary C84.1 ☑
shimamushi (scrub typhus) A75.3
shipyard B30.0
sickle-cell D57.1
  with crisis (vasoocclusive pain) D57.00
    with
      acute chest syndrome D57.01
      splenic sequestration D57.02
  elliptocytosis D57.8 ☑
  Hb-C D57.20
    with crisis (vasoocclusive pain) D57.219
      with
        acute chest syndrome D57.211
        splenic sequestration D57.212
    without crisis D57.20
  Hb-SD D57.80
    with crisis D57.819
      with
        acute chest syndrome D57.811
        splenic sequestration D57.812
  Hb-SE D57.80
    with crisis D57.819
      with
        acute chest syndrome D57.811
        splenic sequestration D57.812
  specified NEC D57.80
    with crisis D57.819
      with
        acute chest syndrome D57.811
        splenic sequestration D57.812
  spherocytosis D57.80
    with crisis D57.819
      with
        acute chest syndrome D57.811
        splenic sequestration D57.812
  thalassemia D57.40
    with crisis (vasoocclusive pain) D57.419
      with
        acute chest syndrome D57.411
        splenic sequestration D57.412
    without crisis D57.40
silo-filler's J68.8
  bronchitis J68.0
  pneumonitis J68.0
  pulmonary edema J68.1
simian B B00.4
Simons' (progressive lipodystrophy) E88.1
sin nombre virus B33.4
sinus — *see* Sinusitis
Sirkari's B55.0
sixth B08.20
  due to human herpesvirus 6 B08.21
  due to human herpesvirus 7 B08.22
skin L98.9
  due to metabolic disorder NEC E88.9 *[L99]*
  specified NEC L98.8
slim (HIV) B20
small vessel I73.9
Sneddon-Wilkinson (subcorneal pustular dermatosis) L13.1
South African creeping B88.0
spinal (cord) G95.9
  congenital Q06.9
  specified NEC G95.89
spine (*see also* Spondylopathy)
  joint — *see* Dorsopathy
  tuberculous A18.01

Disease — *continued*
spinocerebellar (hereditary) G11.9
  specified NEC G11.8
spleen D73.9
  amyloid E85.4 *[D77]*
  organic D73.9
  polycystic Q89.09
  postinfectional D73.89
sponge-diver's — *see* Toxicity, venom, marine animal, sea anemone
Startle Q89.8
Steinert's G71.11
Sticker's (erythema infectiosum) B08.3
Stieda's (calcification, knee joint) — *see* Bursitis, tibial collateral
Stokes' (exophthalmic goiter) — *see* Hyperthyroidism, with, goiter (diffuse)
Stokes-Adams (syncope with heart block) I45.9
stomach K31.9
  functional, psychogenic F45.8
  specified NEC K31.89
stonemason's J62.8
storage
  glycogen — *see* Disease, glycogen storage
  mucopolysaccharide — *see* Mucopolysaccharidosis
striatopallidal system NEC G25.89
Stuart-Prower (congenital factor X deficiency) D68.2
Stuart's (congenital factor X deficiency) D68.2
subcutaneous tissue — *see* Disease, skin
supporting structures of teeth K08.9
  specified NEC K08.89
suprarenal (capsule) (gland) E27.9
  hyperfunction E27.0
  specified NEC E27.8
sweat glands L74.9
  specified NEC L74.8
Sweeley-Klionsky E75.21
Swift (-Feer) — *see* Poisoning, mercury
swimming-pool granuloma A31.1
Sylvest's (epidemic pleurodynia) B33.0
sympathetic nervous system G90.9
synovium — *see* Disorder, synovium
syphilitic — *see* Syphilis
systemic tissue mast cell C96.20
tanapox (virus) B08.71
Tangier E78.6
Tarral-Besnier (pityriasis rubra pilaris) L44.0
Tauri's E74.09
tear duct — *see* Disorder, lacrimal system
tendon, tendinous (*see also* Disorder, tendon)
  nodular — *see* Trigger finger
terminal vessel I73.9
testis N50.9
thalassemia Hb-S — *see* Disease, sickle-cell, thalassemia
Thaysen-Gee (nontropical sprue) K90.0
Thomsen G71.12
throat J39.2
  septic J02.0
thromboembolic — *see* Embolism
thymus (gland) E32.9
  specified NEC E32.8
thyroid (gland) E07.9
  heart (*see also* Hyperthyroidism) E05.90 *[I43]*
    with thyroid storm E05.91 *[I43]*
  specified NEC E07.89
Tietze's M94.0
tongue K14.9
  specified NEC K14.8
tonsils, tonsillar (and adenoids) J35.9
tooth, teeth K08.9
  hard tissues K03.9
    specified NEC K03.89
  pulp NEC K04.99
  specified NEC K08.89
Tourette's F95.2
trachea NEC J39.8
tricuspid I07.9
  nonrheumatic I36.9
triglyceride-storage E75.5
trophoblastic — *see* Mole, hydatidiform
tsutsugamushi A75.3
tube (fallopian) (noninflammatory) N83.9
  inflammatory — *see* Salpingitis
  specified NEC N83.8
tuberculous NEC — *see* Tuberculosis
tubo-ovarian (noninflammatory) N83.9
  inflammatory — *see* Salpingo-oophoritis
  specified NEC N83.8

☑ **Additional character required**

Disease — *continued*

tubotympanic, chronic — *see* Otitis, media, suppurative, chronic, tubotympanic
tubulo-interstitial N15.9
  specified NEC N15.8
tympanum — *see* Disorder, tympanic membrane
Uhl's Q24.8
Underwood's (sclerema neonatorum) P83.0
Unverricht (-Lundborg) — *see* Epilepsy, generalized, idiopathic
Urbach-Oppenheim (necrobiosis lipoidica diabeticorum) — *see* E08-E13 with .620
ureter N28.9
  in (due to)
    schistosomiasis (bilharziasis) B65.0 *[N29]*
urethra N36.9
  specified NEC N36.8
urinary (tract) N39.9
  bladder N32.9
    specified NEC N32.89
  specified NEC N39.8
uterus (noninflammatory) N85.9
  infective — *see* Endometritis
  inflammatory — *see* Endometritis
  specified NEC N85.8
uveal tract (anterior) H21.9
  posterior H31.9
vagabond's B85.1
vagina, vaginal (noninflammatory) N89.9
  inflammatory NEC N76.89
  specified NEC N89.8
valve, valvular I38
  multiple I08.9
    specified NEC I08.8
van Creveld-von Gierke (glycogenosis I) E74.01
vas deferens N50.9
vascular I99.9
  arteriosclerotic — *see* Arteriosclerosis
  ciliary body NEC — *see* Disorder, iris, vascular
  hypertensive — *see* Hypertension
  iris NEC — *see* Disorder, iris, vascular
  obliterative I77.1
    peripheral I73.9
  occlusive I99.8
  peripheral (occlusive) I73.9
    in diabetes mellitus — *see* E08-E13 with .51
vasomotor I73.9
vasospastic I73.9
vein I87.9
venereal (*see also* Disease, sexually transmitted) A64
  chlamydial NEC A56.8
    anus A56.3
    genitourinary NOS A56.2
    pharynx A56.4
    rectum A56.3
  fifth A55
  sixth A55
  specified nature or type NEC A63.8
vertebra, vertebral (*see also* Spondylopathy)
  disc — *see* Disorder, disc
vibration — *see* Vibration, adverse effects
viral, virus (*see also* Disease, by type of virus) B34.9
  arbovirus NOS A94
  arthropod-borne NOS A94
  congenital P35.9
    specified NEC P35.8
  Hanta (with renal manifestations) (Dobrava) (Puumala) (Seoul) A98.5
    with pulmonary manifestations (Andes) (Bayou) (Bermejo) (Black Creek Canal) (Choclo) (Juquitiba) (Laguna negra) (Lechiguanas) (New York) (Oran) (Sin nombre) B33.4
  Hantaan (Korean hemorrhagic fever) A98.5
  human immunodeficiency (HIV) B20
  Kunjin A83.4
  nonarthropod-borne NOS B34.9
  Powassan A84.8
  Rocio (encephalitis) A83.6
  Sin nombre (Hantavirus) (cardio)-pulmonary syndrome B33.4
  Tahyna B33.8
  vesicular stomatitis A93.8
vitreous H43.9
  specified NEC H43.89
vocal cord J38.3
Volkmann's, acquired T79.6 ☑
von Eulenburg's (congenital paramyotonia) G71.19
von Gierke's (glycogenosis I) E74.01

Disease — *continued*

von Graefe's — *see* Strabismus, paralytic, ophthalmoplegia, progressive
von Willebrand (-Jürgens) (angiohemophilia) D68.0
Vrolik's (osteogenesis imperfecta) Q78.0
vulva (noninflammatory) N90.9
  inflammatory NEC N76.89
  specified NEC N90.89
Wallgren's (obstruction of splenic vein with collateral circulation) I87.8
Wassilieff's (leptospiral jaundice) A27.0
wasting NEC R64
  due to malnutrition E41
Waterhouse-Friderichsen A39.1
Wegner's (syphilitic osteochondritis) A50.02
Weil's (leptospiral jaundice of lung) A27.0
Weir Mitchell's (erythromelalgia) I73.81
Werdnig-Hoffmann G12.0
Wermer's E31.21
Werner-His (trench fever) A79.0
Werner-Schultz (neutropenic splenomegaly) D73.81
Wernicke-Posadas B38.9
whipworm B79
white blood cells D72.9
  specified NEC D72.89
white matter R90.82
white-spot, meaning lichen sclerosus et atrophicus L90.0
  penis N48.0
  vulva N90.4
Wilkie's K55.1
Wilkinson-Sneddon (subcorneal pustular dermatosis) L13.1
Willis' — *see* Diabetes
Wilson's (hepatolenticular degeneration) E83.01
woolsorter's A22.1
yaba monkey tumor B08.72
yaba pox (virus) B08.72
Zika virus A92.5
zoonotic, bacterial A28.9
  specified type NEC A28.8
Disfigurement (due to scar) L90.5
Disgerminoma — *see* Dysgerminoma
DISH (diffuse idiopathic skeletal hyperostosis) — *see* Hyperostosis, ankylosing
Disinsertion, retina — *see* Detachment, retina
Dislocatable hip, congenital Q65.6
Dislocation (articular)
  with fracture — *see* Fracture
  acromioclavicular (joint) S43.10 ☑
    with displacement
      100%-200% S43.12 ☑
      more than 200% S43.13 ☑
    inferior S43.14 ☑
    posterior S43.15 ☑
  ankle S93.0 ☑
  astragalus — *see* Dislocation, ankle
  atlantoaxial S13.121 ☑
  atlantooccipital S13.111 ☑
  atloidooccipital S13.111 ☑
  breast bone S23.29 ☑
  capsule, joint - code by site under Dislocation
  carpal (bone) — *see* Dislocation, wrist
  carpometacarpal (joint) NEC S63.05 ☑
    thumb S63.04 ☑
  cartilage (joint) - code by site under Dislocation
  cervical spine (vertebra) — *see* Dislocation, vertebra, cervical
  chronic — *see* Dislocation, recurrent
  clavicle — *see* Dislocation, acromioclavicular joint
  coccyx S33.2 ☑
  congenital NEC Q68.8
  coracoid — *see* Dislocation, shoulder
  costal cartilage S23.29 ☑
  costochondral S23.29 ☑
  cricoarytenoid articulation S13.29 ☑
  cricothyroid articulation S13.29 ☑
  dorsal vertebra — *see* Dislocation, vertebra, thoracic
  ear ossicle — *see* Discontinuity, ossicles, ear
  elbow S53.10 ☑
    congenital Q68.8
    pathological — *see* Dislocation, pathological NEC, elbow
    radial head alone — *see* Dislocation, radial head
    recurrent — *see* Dislocation, recurrent, elbow
    traumatic S53.10 ☑
      anterior S53.11 ☑
      lateral S53.14 ☑
      medial S53.13 ☑

Dislocation — *continued*

  elbow — *continued*
    posterior S53.12 ☑
    specified type NEC S53.19 ☑
  eye, nontraumatic — *see* Luxation, globe
  eyeball, nontraumatic — *see* Luxation, globe
  femur
    distal end — *see* Dislocation, knee
    proximal end — *see* Dislocation, hip
  fibula
    distal end — *see* Dislocation, ankle
    proximal end — *see* Dislocation, knee
  finger S63.25 ☑
    index S63.25 ☑
    interphalangeal S63.27 ☑
      distal S63.29 ☑
        index S63.29 ☑
        little S63.29 ☑
        middle S63.29 ☑
        ring S63.29 ☑
      index S63.27 ☑
      little S63.27 ☑
      middle S63.27 ☑
      proximal S63.28 ☑
        index S63.28 ☑
        little S63.28 ☑
        middle S63.28 ☑
        ring S63.28 ☑
      ring S63.27 ☑
    little S63.25 ☑
    metacarpophalangeal S63.26 ☑
      index S63.26 ☑
      little S63.26 ☑
      middle S63.26 ☑
      ring S63.26 ☑
    middle S63.25 ☑
    recurrent — *see* Dislocation, recurrent, finger
    ring S63.25 ☑
    thumb — *see* Dislocation, thumb
  foot S93.30 ☑
    recurrent — *see* Dislocation, recurrent, foot
    specified site NEC S93.33 ☑
    tarsal joint S93.31 ☑
    tarsometatarsal joint S93.32 ☑
    toe — *see* Dislocation, toe
  fracture — *see* Fracture
  glenohumeral (joint) — *see* Dislocation, shoulder
  glenoid — *see* Dislocation, shoulder
  habitual — *see* Dislocation, recurrent
  hip S73.00 ☑
    anterior S73.03 ☑
      obturator S73.02 ☑
    central S73.04 ☑
    congenital (total) Q65.2
      bilateral Q65.1
      partial Q65.5
        bilateral Q65.4
        unilateral Q65.3 ☑
      unilateral Q65.0 ☑
    developmental M24.85 ☑
    pathological — *see* Dislocation, pathological NEC, hip
    posterior S73.01 ☑
    recurrent — *see* Dislocation, recurrent, hip
  humerus, proximal end — *see* Dislocation, shoulder
  incomplete — *see* Subluxation, by site
  incus — *see* Discontinuity, ossicles, ear
  infracoracoid — *see* Dislocation, shoulder
  innominate (pubic junction) (sacral junction) S33.39 ☑
    acetabulum — *see* Dislocation, hip
  interphalangeal (joint (s))
    finger S63.279 ☑
      distal S63.29 ☑
        index S63.29 ☑
        little S63.29 ☑
        middle S63.29 ☑
        ring S63.29 ☑
      index S63.27 ☑
      little S63.27 ☑
      middle S63.27 ☑
      proximal S63.28 ☑
        index S63.28 ☑
        little S63.28 ☑
        middle S63.28 ☑
        ring S63.28 ☑
      ring S63.27 ☑
    foot or toe — *see* Dislocation, toe
    thumb S63.12 ☑
  jaw (cartilage) (meniscus) S03.0 ☑

Dislocation — *continued*
  joint prosthesis — *see* Complications, joint
      prosthesis, mechanical, displacement, by site
  knee S83.106 ☑
      cap — *see* Dislocation, patella
      congenital Q68.2
      old M23.8X ☑
      patella — *see* Dislocation, patella
      pathological — *see* Dislocation, pathological
          NEC, knee
      proximal tibia
          anteriorly S83.11 ☑
          laterally S83.14 ☑
          medially S83.13 ☑
          posteriorly S83.12 ☑
      recurrent (*see also* Derangement, knee,
          specified NEC)
      specified type NEC S83.19 ☑
  lacrimal gland H04.16 ☑
  lens (complete) H27.10
      anterior H27.12 ☑
      congenital Q12.1
      ocular implant — *see* Complications,
          intraocular lens
      partial H27.11 ☑
      posterior H27.13 ☑
      traumatic S05.8X ☑
  ligament - code by site under Dislocation
  lumbar (vertebra) — *see* Dislocation, vertebra,
      lumbar
  lumbosacral (vertebra) (*see also* Dislocation,
      vertebra, lumbar)
      congenital Q76.49
  mandible S03.0 ☑
  meniscus (knee) — *see* Tear, meniscus
      other sites - code by site under Dislocation
  metacarpal (bone)
      distal end — *see* Dislocation, finger
      proximal end S63.06 ☑
  metacarpophalangeal (joint)
      finger S63.26 ☑
          index S63.26 ☑
          little S63.26 ☑
          middle S63.26 ☑
          ring S63.26 ☑
          thumb S63.11 ☑
  metatarsal (bone) — *see* Dislocation, foot
  metatarsophalangeal (joint (s)) — *see* Dislocation,
      toe
  midcarpal (joint) S63.03 ☑
  midtarsal (joint) — *see* Dislocation, foot
  neck S13.20 ☑
      specified site NEC S13.29 ☑
      vertebra — *see* Dislocation, vertebra, cervical
  nose (septal cartilage) S03.1 ☑
  occipitoatloid S13.111 ☑
  old — *see* Derangement, joint, specified type NEC
  ossicles, ear — *see* Discontinuity, ossicles, ear
  partial — *see* Subluxation, by site
  patella S83.006 ☑
      congenital Q74.1
      lateral S83.01 ☑
      recurrent (nontraumatic) M22.0 ☑
          incomplete M22.1 ☑
      specified type NEC S83.09 ☑
  pathological NEC M24.30
      ankle M24.37 ☑
      elbow M24.32 ☑
      foot joint M24.37 ☑
      hand joint M24.34 ☑
      hip M24.35 ☑
      knee M24.36 ☑
      lumbosacral joint — *see* subcategory M53.2
      pelvic region — *see* Dislocation, pathological,
          hip
      sacroiliac — *see* subcategory M53.2
      shoulder M24.31 ☑
      wrist M24.33 ☑
  pelvis NEC S33.30 ☑
      specified NEC S33.39 ☑
  phalanx
      finger or hand — *see* Dislocation, finger
      foot or toe — *see* Dislocation, toe
  prosthesis, internal — *see* Complications,
      prosthetic device, by site, mechanical
  radial head S53.006 ☑
      anterior S53.01 ☑
      posterior S53.02 ☑
      specified type NEC S53.09 ☑
  radiocarpal (joint) S63.02 ☑
  radiohumeral (joint) — *see* Dislocation, radial
      head

Dislocation — *continued*
  radioulnar (joint)
      distal S63.01 ☑
      proximal — *see* Dislocation, elbow
  radius
      distal end — *see* Dislocation, wrist
      proximal end — *see* Dislocation, radial head
  recurrent M24.40
      ankle M24.47 ☑
      elbow M24.42 ☑
      finger M24.44 ☑
      foot joint M24.47 ☑
      hand joint M24.44 ☑
      hip M24.45 ☑
      knee M24.46 ☑
          patella — *see* Dislocation, patella, recurrent
      patella — *see* Dislocation, patella, recurrent
      sacroiliac — *see* subcategory M53.2
      shoulder M24.41 ☑
      toe M24.47 ☑
      vertebra (*see also* subcategory) M43.5 ☑
          atlantoaxial M43.4
              with myelopathy M43.3
      wrist M24.43 ☑
  rib (cartilage) S23.29 ☑
  sacrococcygeal S33.2 ☑
  sacroiliac (joint) (ligament) S33.2 ☑
      congenital Q74.2
      recurrent — *see* subcategory M53.2
  sacrum S33.2 ☑
  scaphoid (bone) (hand) (wrist) — *see* Dislocation,
      wrist
      foot — *see* Dislocation, foot
  scapula — *see* Dislocation, shoulder, girdle,
      scapula
  semilunar cartilage, knee — *see* Tear, meniscus
  septal cartilage (nose) S03.1 ☑
  septum (nasal) (old) J34.2
  sesamoid bone - code by site under Dislocation
  shoulder (blade) (ligament) (joint)
      (traumatic) S43.006 ☑
      acromioclavicular — *see* Dislocation,
          acromioclavicular
      chronic — *see* Dislocation, recurrent, shoulder
      congenital Q68.8
      girdle S43.30 ☑
          scapula S43.31 ☑
          specified site NEC S43.39 ☑
      humerus S43.00 ☑
          anterior S43.01 ☑
          inferior S43.03 ☑
          posterior S43.02 ☑
      pathological — *see* Dislocation, pathological
          NEC, shoulder
      recurrent — *see* Dislocation, recurrent, shoulder
      specified type NEC S43.08 ☑
  spine
      cervical — *see* Dislocation, vertebra, cervical
      congenital Q76.49
      due to birth trauma P11.5
      lumbar — *see* Dislocation, vertebra, lumbar
      thoracic — *see* Dislocation, vertebra, thoracic
  spontaneous — *see* Dislocation, pathological
  sternoclavicular (joint) S43.206 ☑
      anterior S43.21 ☑
      posterior S43.22 ☑
  sternum S23.29 ☑
  subglenoid — *see* Dislocation, shoulder
  symphysis pubis S33.4 ☑
  talus — *see* Dislocation, ankle
  tarsal (bone) (joint (s)) — *see* Dislocation, foot
  tarsometatarsal (joint (s)) — *see* Dislocation, foot
  temporomandibular (joint) S03.0 ☑
  thigh, proximal end — *see* Dislocation, hip
  thorax S23.20 ☑
      specified site NEC S23.29 ☑
      vertebra — *see* Dislocation, vertebra
  thumb S63.10 ☑
      interphalangeal joint — *see* Dislocation,
          interphalangeal (joint), thumb
      metacarpophalangeal joint — *see* Dislocation,
          metacarpophalangeal (joint), thumb
  thyroid cartilage S13.29 ☑
  tibia
      distal end — *see* Dislocation, ankle
      proximal end — *see* Dislocation, knee
  tibiofibular (joint)
      distal — *see* Dislocation, ankle
      superior — *see* Dislocation, knee
  toe (s) S93.106 ☑
      great S93.10 ☑
          interphalangeal joint S93.11 ☑

Dislocation — *continued*
  toe — *continued*
      metatarsophalangeal joint S93.12 ☑
      interphalangeal joint S93.119 ☑
      lesser S93.106 ☑
          interphalangeal joint S93.11 ☑
          metatarsophalangeal joint S93.12 ☑
      metatarsophalangeal joint S93.12 ☑
  tooth S03.2 ☑
  trachea S23.29 ☑
  ulna
      distal end S63.07 ☑
      proximal end — *see* Dislocation, elbow
  ulnohumeral (joint) — *see* Dislocation, elbow
  vertebra (articular process) (body) (traumatic)
      cervical S13.101 ☑
          atlantoaxial joint S13.121 ☑
          atlantooccipital joint S13.111 ☑
          atloidooccipital joint S13.111 ☑
          joint between
              C0 and C1 S13.111 ☑
              C1 and C2 S13.121 ☑
              C2 and C3 S13.131 ☑
              C3 and C4 S13.141 ☑
              C4 and C5 S13.151 ☑
              C5and C6 S13.161 ☑
              C6and C7 S13.171 ☑
              C7and T1 S13.181 ☑
          occipitoatloid joint S13.111 ☑
      congenital Q76.49
      lumbar S33.101 ☑
          joint between
              L1and L2 S33.111 ☑
              L2and L3 S33.121 ☑
              L3 and L4 S33.131 ☑
              L4and L5 S33.141 ☑
      nontraumatic — *see* Displacement,
          intervertebral disc
      partial — *see* Subluxation, by site
      recurrent NEC — *see* subcategory M43.5
      thoracic S23.101 ☑
          joint between
              T1 and T2 S23.111 ☑
              T2 and T3 S23.121 ☑
              T3 and T4 S23.123 ☑
              T4 and T5 S23.131 ☑
              T5 and T6 S23.133 ☑
              T6 and T7 S23.141 ☑
              T7 and T8 S23.143 ☑
              T8 and T9 S23.151 ☑
              T9 and T10 S23.153 ☑
              T10 and T11 S23.161 ☑
              T11 and T12 S23.163 ☑
              T12 and L1 S23.171 ☑
  wrist (carpal bone) S63.006 ☑
      carpometacarpal joint — *see* Dislocation,
          carpometacarpal (joint)
      distal radioulnar joint — *see* Dislocation,
          radioulnar (joint), distal
      metacarpal bone, proximal — *see* Dislocation,
          metacarpal (bone), proximal end
      midcarpal — *see* Dislocation, midcarpal (joint)
      radiocarpal joint — *see* Dislocation, radiocarpal
          (joint)
      recurrent — *see* Dislocation, recurrent, wrist
      specified site NEC S63.09 ☑
      ulna — *see* Dislocation, ulna, distal end
  xiphoid cartilage S23.29 ☑
Disorder (of) (*see also* Disease)
  acantholytic L11.9
      specified NEC L11.8
  acute
      psychotic — *see* Psychosis, acute
      stress F43.0
  adjustment (grief) F43.20
      with
          anxiety F43.22
              with depressed mood F43.23
          conduct disturbance F43.24
              with emotional disturbance F43.25
          depressed mood F43.21
              with anxiety F43.23
          other specified symptom F43.29
  adrenal (capsule) (gland) (medullary) E27.9
      specified NEC E27.8
  adrenogenital E25.9
      drug-induced E25.8
      iatrogenic E25.8
      idiopathic E25.8
  adult personality (and behavior) F69
      specified NEC F68.8
  affective (mood) — *see* Disorder, mood

ICD-10-CM INDEX TO DISEASES AND INJURIES

Dislocation - Disorder

Disorder — *continued*
- aggressive, unsocialized F91.1
- alcohol-related F10.99
  - with
    - amnestic disorder, persisting F10.96
    - anxiety disorder F10.980
    - dementia, persisting F10.97
    - intoxication F10.929
      - with delirium F10.921
      - uncomplicated F10.920
    - mood disorder F10.94
    - other specified F10.988
    - psychotic disorder F10.959
      - with
        - delusions F10.950
        - hallucinations F10.951
    - sexual dysfunction F10.981
    - sleep disorder F10.982
- alcohol use
  - mild F10.10
    - with
      - alcohol-induced
        - anxiety disorder F10.180
        - bipolar and related disorder F10.14
        - depressive disorder F10.14
        - psychotic disorder F10.159
        - sexual dysfunction F10.181
        - sleep disorder F10.182
      - alcohol intoxication F10.129
        - delirium F10.121
    - in remission (early) (sustained) F10.11
  - moderate or severe F10.20
    - with
      - alcohol-induced
        - anxiety disorder F10.280
        - bipolar and related disorder F10.24
        - depressive disorder F10.24
        - major neurocognitive disorder, amnestic-confabulatory type F10.26
        - major neurocognitive disorder, nonamnestic-confabulatory type F10.27
        - mild neurocognitive disorder F10.288
        - psychotic disorder F10.259
        - sexual dysfunction F10.281
        - sleep disorder F10.282
      - alcohol intoxication F10.229
        - delirium F10.221
    - in remission (early) (sustained) F10.21
- allergic — *see* Allergy
- alveolar NEC J84.09
- amino-acid
  - cystathioninuria E72.19
  - cystinosis E72.04
  - cystinuria E72.01
  - glycinuria E72.09
  - homocystinuria E72.11
  - metabolism — *see* Disturbance, metabolism, amino-acid
  - specified NEC E72.8
  - neonatal, transitory P74.8
  - renal transport NEC E72.09
  - transport NEC E72.09
- amnesic, amnestic
  - alcohol-induced F10.96
    - with dependence F10.26
  - due to (secondary to) general medical condition F04
  - psychoactive NEC-induced F19.96
    - with
      - abuse F19.16
      - dependence F19.26
  - sedative, hypnotic or anxiolytic-induced F13.96
    - with dependence F13.26
- amphetamine-type substance use
  - mild F15.10
    - in remission (early) (sustained) F15.11
  - moderate F15.20
    - in remission (early) (sustained) F15.21
  - severe F15.20
    - in remission (early) (sustained) F15.21
- amphetamine (or other stimulant) use
  - mild
    - with
      - amphetamine (or other stimulant)-induced
        - anxiety disorder F15.180
        - bipolar and related disorder F15.14
        - depressive disorder F15.14
        - obsessive-compulsive and related disorder F15.188
        - psychotic disorder F15.159
        - sexual dysfunction F15.181

Disorder — *continued*
- amphetamine — *continued*
  - amphetamine, cocaine, or other stimulant intoxication
    - with perceptual disturbances F15.122
    - without perceptual disturbances F15.129
    - intoxication delirium F15.121
  - moderate or severe
    - with
      - amphetamine (or other stimulant)-induced
        - anxiety disorder F15.280
        - obsessive-compulsive and related disorder F15.288
        - sexual dysfunction F15.281
        - bipolar and related disorder F15.24
        - depressive disorder F15.24
        - psychotic disorder F15.259
      - amphetamine, cocaine, or other stimulant intoxication
        - with perceptual disturbances F15.222
        - without perceptual disturbances F15.229
        - intoxication delirium F15.221
- anaerobic glycolysis with anemia D55.2
- anxiety F41.9
  - due to (secondary to)
    - alcohol F10.980
      - in
        - abuse F10.180
        - dependence F10.280
    - amphetamine F15.980
      - in
        - abuse F15.180
        - dependence F15.280
    - anxiolytic F13.980
      - in
        - abuse F13.180
        - dependence F13.280
    - caffeine F15.980
      - in
        - abuse F15.180
        - dependence F15.280
    - cannabis F12.980
      - in
        - abuse F12.180
        - dependence F12.280
    - cocaine F14.980
      - in
        - abuse F14.180
        - dependence F14.180
    - general medical condition F06.4
    - hallucinogen F16.980
      - in
        - abuse F16.180
        - dependence F16.280
    - hypnotic F13.980
      - in
        - abuse F13.180
        - dependence F13.280
    - inhalant F18.980
      - in
        - abuse F18.180
        - dependence F18.280
    - phencyclidine F16.980
      - in
        - abuse F16.180
        - dependence F16.280
    - psychoactive substance NEC F19.980
      - in
        - abuse F19.180
        - dependence F19.280
    - sedative F13.980
      - in
        - abuse F13.180
        - dependence F13.280
    - volatile solvents F18.980
      - in
        - abuse F18.180
        - dependence F18.280
  - generalized F41.1
  - illness F45.21
  - mixed
    - with depression (mild) F41.8
    - specified NEC F41.3
  - organic F06.4
  - phobic F40.9
    - of childhood F40.8
  - specified NEC F41.8
- aortic valve — *see* Endocarditis, aortic
- aromatic amino-acid metabolism E70.9
  - specified NEC E70.8
- arteriole NEC I77.89
- artery NEC I77.89

Disorder — *continued*
- articulation — *see* Disorder, joint
- attachment (childhood)
  - disinhibited F94.2
  - reactive F94.1
- attention-deficit hyperactivity (adolescent) (adult) (child) F90.9
  - combined
    - presentation F90.2
    - type F90.2
  - hyperactive
    - impulsive presentation F90.1
    - type F90.1
  - inattentive
    - presentation F90.0
    - type F90.0
  - specified type NEC F90.8
- attention-deficit without hyperactivity (adolescent) (adult) (child) F98.8
- auditory processing (central) H93.25
- autistic F84.0
- autism spectrum F84.0
- autoimmune D89.89
- autonomic nervous system G90.9
  - specified NEC G90.8
- avoidant
  - child or adolescent F40.10
  - restrictive food intake F50.82
- balance
  - acid-base E87.8
    - mixed E87.4
  - electrolyte E87.8
  - fluid NEC E87.8
- behavioral (disruptive) — *see* Disorder, conduct
- beta-amino-acid metabolism E72.8
- bile acid and cholesterol metabolism E78.70
  - Barth syndrome E78.71
  - other specified E78.79
  - Smith-Lemli-Opitz syndrome E78.72
- bilirubin excretion E80.6
- binge eating F50.81
- binocular
  - movement H51.9
    - convergence
      - excess H51.12
      - insufficiency H51.11
    - internuclear ophthalmoplegia — *see* Ophthalmoplegia, internuclear
    - palsy of conjugate gaze H51.0
    - specified type NEC H51.8
  - vision NEC — *see* Disorder, vision, binocular
- bipolar (I) (type 1) F31.9
  - and related due to a known physiological condition
    - with
      - manic features F06.33
      - manic- or hypomanic-like episodes F06.33
      - mixed features F06.34
  - current (or most recent) episode
    - depressed F31.9
      - with psychotic features F31.5
      - without psychotic features F31.30
        - mild F31.31
        - moderate F31.32
        - severe (without psychotic features) F31.4
          - with psychotic features F31.5
    - hypomanic F31.0
    - manic F31.9
      - with psychotic features F31.2
      - without psychotic features F31.10
        - mild F31.11
        - moderate F31.12
        - severe (without psychotic features) F31.13
          - with psychotic features F31.2
    - mixed F31.60
      - mild F31.61
      - moderate F31.62
      - severe (without psychotic features) F31.63
        - with psychotic features F31.64
      - severe depression (without psychotic features) F31.4
        - with psychotic features F31.5
  - in remission (currently) F31.70
    - in full remission
      - most recent episode
        - depressed F31.76
        - hypomanic F31.72
        - manic F31.74
        - mixed F31.78
    - in partial remission
      - most recent episode

Disorder — *continued*
  bipolar — *continued*
      depressed F31.75
      hypomanic F31.71
      manic F31.73
      mixed F31.77
    specified NEC F31.89
    II (type 2) F31.81
    organic F06.30
    single manic episode F30.9
      mild F30.11
      moderate F30.12
      severe (without psychotic symptoms) F30.13
        with psychotic symptoms F30.2
  bladder N32.9
    functional NEC N31.9
    in schistosomiasis B65.0 *[N33]*
    specified NEC N32.89
  bleeding D68.9
  blood D75.9
    in congenital early syphilis A50.09 *[D77]*
  body dysmorphic F45.22
  bone M89.9
    continuity M84.9
      specified type NEC M84.80
        ankle M84.87 ☑
        fibula M84.86 ☑
        foot M84.87 ☑
        hand M84.84 ☑
        humerus M84.82 ☑
        neck M84.88
        pelvis M84.859
        radius M84.83 ☑
        rib M84.88
        shoulder M84.81 ☑
        skull M84.88
        thigh M84.85 ☑
        tibia M84.86 ☑
        ulna M84.83 ☑
        vertebra M84.88
    density and structure M85.9
      cyst (*see also* Cyst, bone, specified type NEC)
        aneurysmal — *see* Cyst, bone, aneurysmal
        solitary — *see* Cyst, bone, solitary
      diffuse idiopathic skeletal hyperostosis — *see*
        Hyperostosis, ankylosing
      fibrous dysplasia (monostotic) — *see*
        Dysplasia, fibrous, bone
      fluorosis — *see* Fluorosis, skeletal
      hyperostosis of skull M85.2
      osteitis condensans — *see* Osteitis,
        condensans
      specified type NEC M85.8 ☑
        ankle M85.87 ☑
        foot M85.87 ☑
        forearm M85.83 ☑
        hand M85.84 ☑
        lower leg M85.86 ☑
        multiple sites M85.89
        neck M85.88
        rib M85.88
        shoulder M85.81 ☑
        skull M85.88
        thigh M85.85 ☑
        upper arm M85.82 ☑
        vertebra M85.88
    development and growth NEC M89.20
      carpus M89.24 ☑
      clavicle M89.21 ☑
      femur M89.25 ☑
      fibula M89.26 ☑
      finger M89.24 ☑
      humerus M89.22 ☑
      ilium M89.259
      ischium M89.259
      metacarpus M89.24 ☑
      metatarsus M89.27 ☑
      multiple sites M89.29
      neck M89.28
      radius M89.23 ☑
      rib M89.28
      scapula M89.21 ☑
      skull M89.28
      tarsus M89.27 ☑
      tibia M89.26 ☑
      toe M89.27 ☑
      ulna M89.23 ☑
      vertebra M89.28
      specified type NEC M89.8X ☑
  brachial plexus G54.0
  branched-chain amino-acid metabolism E71.2
    specified NEC E71.19

Disorder — *continued*
  breast N64.9
    agalactia — *see* Agalactia
    associated with
      lactation O92.70
        specified NEC O92.79
      pregnancy O92.20
        specified NEC O92.29
      puerperium O92.20
        specified NEC O92.29
    cracked nipple — *see* Cracked nipple
    galactorrhea — *see* Galactorrhea
    hypogalactia O92.4
    lactation disorder NEC O92.79
    mastitis — *see* Mastitis
    nipple infection — *see* Infection, nipple
    retracted nipple — *see* Retraction, nipple
    specified type NEC N64.89
  Briquet's F45.0
  bullous, in diseases classified elsewhere L14
  caffeine use
    mild
      with
        caffeine-induced
          anxiety disorder F15.180
          sleep disorder F15.182
    moderate or severe
      with
        caffeine-induced
          anxiety disorder F15.280
          sleep disorder F15.282
  cannabis use
    mild F12.10
      with
        cannabis-induced
          anxiety disorder F12.180
          psychotic disorder F12.159
          sleep disorder F12.188
        cannabis intoxication delirium F12.121
          with perceptual disturbances F12.122
          without perceptual disturbances F12.129
      in remission (early) (sustained) F12.11
    moderate or severe F12.20
      with
        cannabis-induced
          anxiety disorder F12.280
          psychotic disorder F12.259
          sleep disorder F12.288
        cannabis intoxication
          with perceptual disturbances F12.222
          without perceptual disturbances F12.229
        delirium F12.221
      in remission (early) (sustained) F12.21
  carbohydrate
    absorption, intestinal NEC E74.39
    metabolism (congenital) E74.9
      specified NEC E74.8
  cardiac, functional I51.89
  carnitine metabolism E71.40
  cartilage M94.9
    articular NEC — *see* Derangement, joint,
      articular cartilage
    chondrocalcinosis — *see* Chondrocalcinosis
    specified type NEC M94.8X ☑
      articular — *see* Derangement, joint, articular
        cartilage
      multiple sites M94.8X0
  catatonia (due to known physiological condition)
    (with another mental disorder) F06.1
  catatonic
    due to (secondary to) known physiological
      condition F06.1
    organic F06.1
  central auditory processing H93.25
  cervical
    region NEC M53.82
    root (nerve) NEC G54.2
  character NOS F60.9
  childhood disintegrative NEC F84.3
  cholesterol and bile acid metabolism E78.70
    Barth syndrome E78.71
    other specified E78.79
    Smith-Lemli-Opitz syndrome E78.72
  choroid H31.9
    atrophy — *see* Atrophy, choroid
    degeneration — *see* Degeneration, choroid
    detachment — *see* Detachment, choroid
    dystrophy — *see* Dystrophy, choroid
    hemorrhage — *see* Hemorrhage, choroid
    rupture — *see* Rupture, choroid
    scar — *see* Scar, chorioretinal
    solar retinopathy — *see* Retinopathy, solar
    specified type NEC H31.8

Disorder — *continued*
  ciliary body — *see* Disorder, iris
    degeneration — *see* Degeneration, ciliary body
  coagulation (factor) (*see also* Defect,
    coagulation) D68.9
    newborn, transient P61.6
  cocaine use
    mild F14.10
      with
        amphetamine, cocaine, or other stimulant
          intoxication
          with perceptual disturbances F14.122
          without perceptual disturbances F14.129
        cocaine-induced
          anxiety disorder F14.180
          bipolar and related disorder F14.14
          depressive disorder F14.14
          obsessive-compulsive and related
            disorder F14.188
          psychotic disorder F14.159
          sexual dysfunction F14.181
          sleep disorder F14.182
        cocaine intoxication delirium F14.121
      in remission (early) (sustained) F14.11
    moderate or severe F14.20
      with
        amphetamine, cocaine, or other stimulant
          intoxication
          with perceptual disturbances F14.222
          without perceptual disturbances F14.229
        cocaine-induced
          anxiety disorder F14.280
          bipolar and related disorder F14.24
          depressive disorder F14.24
          obsessive-compulsive and related
            disorder F14.288
          psychotic disorder F14.259
          sexual dysfunction F14.281
          sleep disorder F14.282
        cocaine intoxication delirium F14.221
      in remission (early) (sustained) F14.21
  coccyx NEC M53.3
  cognitive F09
    due to (secondary to) general medical
      condition F09
    persisting R41.89
      due to
        alcohol F10.97
          with dependence F10.27
        anxiolytics F13.97
          with dependence F13.27
        hypnotics F13.97
          with dependence F13.27
        sedatives F13.97
          with dependence F13.27
        specified substance NEC F19.97
          with
            abuse F19.17
            dependence F19.27
  communication F80.9
    social pragmatic F80.82
  conduct (childhood) F91.9
    adjustment reaction — *see* Disorder,
      adjustment
    adolescent onset type F91.2
    childhood onset type F91.1
    compulsive F63.9
    confined to family context F91.0
    depressive F91.8
    group type F91.2
    hyperkinetic — *see* Disorder, attention-deficit
      hyperactivity
    oppositional defiance F91.3
    socialized F91.2
    solitary aggressive type F91.1
    specified NEC F91.8
    unsocialized (aggressive) F91.1
  conduction, heart I45.9
  congenital glycosylation (CDG) E74.8
  conjunctiva H11.9
    infection — *see* Conjunctivitis
  connective tissue, localized L94.9
    specified NEC L94.8
  conversion (functional neurological symptom
    disorder)
    with
      abnormal movement F44.4
      anesthesia or sensory loss F44.6
      attacks or seizures F44.5
      mixed symptoms F44.7
      special sensory symptoms F44.6
      speech symptoms F44.4

Disorder — continued
  conversion — continued
    swallowing symptoms F44.4
    weakness or paralysis F44.4
  convulsive (secondary) — see Convulsions
  cornea H18.9
    deformity — see Deformity, cornea
    degeneration — see Degeneration, cornea
    deposits — see Deposit, cornea
    due to contact lens H18.82 ☑
      specified as edema — see Edema, cornea
    edema — see Edema, cornea
    keratitis — see Keratitis
    keratoconjunctivitis — see Keratoconjunctivitis
    membrane change — see Change, corneal
      membrane
    neovascularization — see Neovascularization,
      cornea
    scar — see Opacity, cornea
    specified type NEC H18.89 ☑
    ulcer — see Ulcer, cornea
  corpus cavernosum N48.9
  cranial nerve — see Disorder, nerve, cranial
  cyclothymic F34.0
  defiant oppositional F91.3
  delusional (persistent) (systematized) F22
    induced F24
  depersonalization F48.1
  depressive F32.9
    due to known physiological condition
      with
        depressive features F06.31
        major depressive-like episode F06.32
        mixed features F06.34
    major F32.9
      with psychotic symptoms F32.3
      in remission (full) F32.5
        partial F32.4
      recurrent F33.9
        with psychotic features F33.3
      single episode F32.9
        mild F32.0
        moderate F32.1
        severe (without psychotic symptoms) F32.2
          with psychotic symptoms F32.3
    organic F06.31
    persistent F34.1
    recurrent F33.9
      current episode
        mild F33.0
        moderate F33.1
        severe (without psychotic symptoms) F33.2
          with psychotic symptoms F33.3
      in remission F33.40
        full F33.42
        partial F33.41
      specified NEC F33.8
    single episode — see Episode, depressive
    specified NEC F32.89
  developmental F89
    arithmetical skills F81.2
    coordination (motor) F82
    expressive writing F81.81
    language F80.9
      expressive F80.1
      mixed receptive and expressive F80.2
      receptive type F80.2
      specified NEC F80.89
    learning F81.9
      arithmetical F81.2
      reading F81.0
    mixed F88
    motor coordination or function F82
    pervasive F84.9
      specified NEC F84.8
    phonological F80.0
    reading F81.0
    scholastic skills (see also Disorder, learning)
      mixed F81.89
    specified NEC F88
    speech F80.9
      articulation F80.0
      specified NEC F80.89
    written expression F81.81
  diaphragm J98.6
  digestive (system) K92.9
    newborn P78.9
      specified NEC P78.89
    postprocedural — see Complication,
      gastrointestinal
    psychogenic F45.8

Disorder — continued
  disc (intervertebral) M51.9
    with
      myelopathy
        cervical region M50.00
        cervicothoracic region M50.03
        high cervical region M50.01
        lumbar region M51.06
        mid-cervical region M50.020
        sacrococcygeal region M53.3
        thoracic region M51.04
        thoracolumbar region M51.05
      radiculopathy
        cervical region M50.10
        cervicothoracic region M50.13
        high cervical region M50.11
        lumbar region M51.16
        lumbosacral region M51.17
        mid-cervical region M50.120
        sacrococcygeal region M53.3
        thoracic region M51.14
        thoracolumbar region M51.15
    cervical M50.90
      with
        myelopathy M50.00
          C2-C3 M50.01
          C3-C4 M50.01
          C4-C5 M50.021
          C5-C6 M50.022
          C6-C7 M50.023
          C7-T1 M50.03
          cervicothoracic region M50.03
          high cervical region M50.01
          mid-cervical region M50.020
        neuritis, radiculitis or radiculopathy M50.10
          C2-C3 M50.11
          C3-C4 M50.11
          C4-C5 M50.121
          C5-C6 M50.122
          C6-C7 M50.123
          C7-T1 M50.13
          cervicothoracic region M50.13
          high cervical region M50.11
          mid-cervical region M50.120
      C2-C3 M50.91
      C3-C4 M50.91
      C4-C5 M50.921
      C5-C6 M50.922
      C6-C7 M50.923
      C7-T1 M50.93
      cervicothoracic region M50.93
      degeneration M50.30
        C2-C3 M50.31
        C3-C4 M50.31
        C4-C5 M50.321
        C5-C6 M50.322
        C6-C7 M50.323
        C7-T1 M50.33
        cervicothoracic region M50.33
        high cervical region M50.31
        mid-cervical region M50.320
      displacement M50.20
        C2-C3 M50.21
        C3-C4 M50.21
        C4-C5 M50.221
        C5-C6 M50.222
        C6-C7 M50.223
        C7-T1 M50.23
        cervicothoracic region M50.23
        high cervical region M50.21
        mid-cervical region M50.220
      high cervical region M50.91
      mid-cervical region M50.920
      specified type NEC M50.80
        C2-C3 M50.81
        C3-C4 M50.81
        C4-C5 M50.821
        C5-C6 M50.822
        C6-C7 M50.823
        C7-T1 M50.83
        cervicothoracic region M50.83
        high cervical region M50.81
        mid-cervical region M50.820
    specified NEC
      lumbar region M51.86
      lumbosacral region M51.87
      sacrococcygeal region M53.3
      thoracic region M51.84
      thoracolumbar region M51.85
  disinhibited attachment (childhood) F94.2
  disintegrative, childhood NEC F84.3

Disorder — continued
  disruptive F91.9
    mood dysregulation F34.81
    specified NEC F91.8
  disruptive behavior — see Disorder, conduct
  dissocial personality F60.2
  dissociative F44.9
    affecting
      motor function F44.4
        and sensation F44.7
      sensation F44.6
        and motor function F44.7
    brief reactive F43.0
    due to (secondary to) general medical
      condition F06.8
    mixed F44.7
    organic F06.8
    other specified NEC F44.89
  double heterozygous sickling — see Disease,
    sickle-cell
  dream anxiety F51.5
  drug induced hemorrhagic D68.32
  drug related F19.99
    abuse — see Abuse, drug
    dependence — see Dependence, drug
  dysmorphic body F45.22
  dysthymic F34.1
  ear H93.9 ☑
    bleeding — see Otorrhagia
    deafness — see Deafness
    degenerative H93.09 ☑
    discharge — see Otorrhea
    external H61.9 ☑
      auditory canal stenosis — see Stenosis,
        external ear canal
      exostosis — see Exostosis, external ear canal
      impacted cerumen — see Impaction,
        cerumen
      otitis — see Otitis, externa
      perichondritis — see Perichondritis, ear
      pinna — see Disorder, pinna
      specified type NEC H61.89 ☑
        in diseases classified elsewhere H62.8X ☑
    inner H83.9 ☑
      vestibular dysfunction — see Disorder,
        vestibular function
    middle H74.9 ☑
      adhesive H74.1 ☑
      ossicle — see Abnormal, ear ossicles
      polyp — see Polyp, ear (middle)
      specified NEC, in diseases classified
        elsewhere H75.8 ☑
      postprocedural — see Complications, ear,
        procedure
      specified NEC, in diseases classified
        elsewhere H94.8 ☑
  eating (adult) (psychogenic) F50.9
    anorexia — see Anorexia
    binge F50.81
    bulimia F50.2
    child F98.29
      pica F98.3
      rumination disorder F98.21
    pica F50.89
      childhood F98.3
  electrolyte (balance) NEC E87.8
    with
      abortion — see Abortion by type
        complicated by specified condition NEC
      ectopic pregnancy O08.5
      molar pregnancy O08.5
    acidosis (metabolic) (respiratory) E87.2
    alkalosis (metabolic) (respiratory) E87.3
  elimination, transepidermal L87.9
    specified NEC L87.8
  emotional (persistent) F34.9
    of childhood F93.9
      specified NEC F93.8
  endocrine E34.9
    postprocedural E89.89
    specified NEC E89.89
  erectile (male) (organic) (see also Dysfunction,
    sexual, male, erectile) N52.9
    nonorganic F52.21
  erythematous — see Erythema
  esophagus K22.9
    functional K22.4
    psychogenic F45.8
  eustachian tube H69.9 ☑
    infection — see Salpingitis, eustachian
    obstruction — see Obstruction, eustachian tube
    patulous — see Patulous, eustachian tube

Disorder

Disorder — *continued*
- eustachian tube — *continued*
  - specified NEC H69.8 ☑
- exhibitionistic F65.2
- extrapyramidal G25.9
  - in diseases classified elsewhere — *see* category G26
  - specified type NEC G25.89
- eye H57.9
  - postprocedural — *see* Complication, postprocedural, eye
- eyelid H02.9
  - cyst — *see* Cyst, eyelid
  - degenerative H02.70
    - chloasma — *see* Chloasma, eyelid
    - madarosis — *see* Madarosis
    - specified type NEC H02.79
    - vitiligo — *see* Vitiligo, eyelid
    - xanthelasma — *see* Xanthelasma
  - dermatochalasis — *see* Dermatochalasis
  - edema — *see* Edema, eyelid
  - elephantiasis — *see* Elephantiasis, eyelid
  - foreign body, retained — *see* Foreign body, retained, eyelid
  - function H02.59
    - abnormal innervation syndrome — *see* Syndrome, abnormal innervation
    - blepharochalasis — *see* Blepharochalasis
    - blepharoclonus — *see* Blepharoclonus
    - blepharophimosis — *see* Blepharophimosis
    - blepharoptosis — *see* Blepharoptosis
    - lagophthalmos — *see* Lagophthalmos
    - lid retraction — *see* Retraction, lid
  - hypertrichosis — *see* Hypertrichosis, eyelid
  - specified type NEC H02.89
  - vascular H02.879
    - left H02.876
      - lower H02.875
      - upper H02.874
    - right H02.873
      - lower H02.872
      - upper H02.871
- factitious F68.10
  - with predominantly
    - psychological symptoms F68.11
      - with physical symptoms F68.13
    - physical symptoms F68.12
      - with psychological symptoms F68.13
- factor, coagulation — *see* Defect, coagulation
- fatty acid
  - metabolism E71.30
    - specified NEC E71.39
  - oxidation
    - LCAD E71.310
    - MCAD E71.311
    - SCAD E71.312
    - specified deficiency NEC E71.318
- feeding (infant or child) (*see also* Disorder, eating) R63.3
  - or eating disorder F50.9
  - specified NEC F50.9
- feigned (with obvious motivation) Z76.5
  - without obvious motivation — *see* Disorder, factitious
- female
  - hypoactive sexual desire F52.0
  - orgasmic F52.31
  - sexual interest/arousal F52.22
- fetishistic F65.0
- fibroblastic M72.9
  - specified NEC M72.8
- fluency
  - adult onset F98.5
  - childhood onset F80.81
  - following
    - cerebral infarction I69.323
    - cerebrovascular disease I69.923
      - specified disease NEC I69.823
    - intracerebral hemorrhage I69.123
    - nontraumatic intracranial hemorrhage NEC I69.223
    - subarachnoid hemorrhage I69.023
  - in conditions classified elsewhere R47.82
- fluid balance E87.8
- follicular (skin) L73.9
  - specified NEC L73.8
- frotteuristic F65.81
- fructose metabolism E74.10
  - essential fructosuria E74.11
  - fructokinase deficiency E74.11
  - fructose-1, 6-diphosphatase deficiency E74.19
  - hereditary fructose intolerance E74.12
  - other specified E74.19

Disorder — *continued*
- functional polymorphonuclear neutrophils D71
- gallbladder, biliary tract and pancreas in diseases classified elsewhere K87
- gambling F63.0
- gamma-glutamyl cycle E72.8
- gastric (functional) K31.9
  - motility K30
  - psychogenic F45.8
  - secretion K30
- gastrointestinal (functional) NOS K92.9
  - newborn P78.9
  - psychogenic F45.8
- gender-identity or -role F64.9
  - childhood F64.2
  - effect on relationship F66
  - of adolescence or adulthood F64.0
    - nontranssexual F64.8
  - specified NEC F64.8
  - uncertainty F66
- genito-pelvic pain penetration F52.6
- genitourinary system
  - female N94.9
  - male N50.9
  - psychogenic F45.8
- globe H44.9
  - degenerated condition H44.50
    - absolute glaucoma H44.51 ☑
    - atrophy H44.52 ☑
    - leucocoria H44.53 ☑
  - degenerative H44.30
    - chalcosis H44.31 ☑
    - myopia (*see also* Myopia, degenerative) H44.2 ☑
    - siderosis H44.32 ☑
    - specified type NEC H44.39 ☑
  - endophthalmitis — *see* Endophthalmitis
  - foreign body, retained — *see* Foreign body, intraocular, old, retained
  - hemophthalmos — *see* Hemophthalmos
  - hypotony H44.40
    - due to
      - ocular fistula H44.42 ☑
      - specified disorder NEC H44.43 ☑
    - flat anterior chamber H44.41 ☑
    - primary H44.44 ☑
  - luxation — *see* Luxation, globe
  - specified type NEC H44.89
- glomerular (in) N05.9
  - amyloidosis E85.4 [N08]
  - cryoglobulinemia D89.1 [N08]
  - disseminated intravascular coagulation D65 [N08]
  - Fabry's disease E75.21 [N08]
  - familial lecithin cholesterol acyltransferase deficiency E78.6 [N08]
  - Goodpasture's syndrome M31.0
  - hemolytic-uremic syndrome D59.3
  - Henoch (-Schönlein) purpura D69.0 [N08]
  - malariae malaria B52.0
  - microscopic polyangiitis M31.7 [N08]
  - multiple myeloma C90.0 ☑ [N08]
  - mumps B26.83
  - schistosomiasis B65.9 [N08]
  - sepsis NEC A41. ☑ [N08]
    - streptococcal A40. ☑ [N08]
  - sickle-cell disorders D57. ☑ [N08]
  - strongyloidiasis B78.9 [N08]
  - subacute bacterial endocarditis I33.0 [N08]
  - syphilis A52.75
  - systemic lupus erythematosus M32.14
  - thrombotic thrombocytopenic purpura M31.1 [N08]
  - Waldenström macroglobulinemia C88.0 [N08]
  - Wegener's granulomatosis M31.31
- gluconeogenesis E74.4
- glucosaminoglycan metabolism — *see* Disorder, metabolism, glucosaminoglycan
- glycine metabolism E72.50
  - d-glycericacidemia E72.59
  - hyperhydroxyprolinemia E72.59
  - hyperoxaluria E72.53
  - hyperprolinemia E72.59
  - non-ketotic hyperglycinemia E72.51
  - oxalosis E72.53
  - oxaluria E72.53
  - sarcosinemia E72.59
  - trimethylaminuria E72.52
- glycoprotein metabolism E77.9
  - specified NEC E77.8
- habit (and impulse) F63.9
  - involving sexual behavior NEC F65.9
  - specified NEC F63.89
- hallucinogen use
  - mild F16.10

Disorder — *continued*
- hallucinogen use — *continued*
  - with
    - hallucinogen-induced
      - anxiety disorder F16.180
      - bipolar and related disorder F16.14
      - depressive disorder F16.14
      - psychotic disorder F16.159
    - hallucinogen intoxication delirium F16.121
    - other hallucinogen intoxication F16.129
  - in remission (early) (sustained) F16.11
  - moderate or severe F16.20
    - with
      - hallucinogen-induced
        - anxiety disorder F16.280
        - bipolar and related disorder F16.24
        - depressive disorder F16.24
        - psychotic disorder F16.259
      - hallucinogen intoxication delirium F16.221
      - other hallucinogen intoxication F16.229
    - in remission (early) (sustained) F16.21
- heart action I49.9
- hematological D75.9
  - newborn (transient) P61.9
  - specified NEC P61.8
- hematopoietic organs D75.9
- hemorrhagic NEC D69.9
  - drug-induced D68.32
  - due to
    - extrinsic circulating anticoagulants D68.32
      - increase in
        - anti-IIa D68.32
        - anti-Xa D68.32
    - intrinsic
      - circulating anticoagulants D68.318
        - increase in
          - antithrombin D68.318
          - anti-VIIIa D68.318
          - anti-IXa D68.318
          - anti-XIa D68.318
  - following childbirth O72.3
- hemostasis — *see* Defect, coagulation
- histidine metabolism E70.40
  - histidinemia E70.41
  - other specified E70.49
- hoarding F42.3
- hyperkinetic — *see* Disorder, attention-deficit hyperactivity
- hyperleucine-isoleucinemia E71.19
- hypervalinemia E71.19
- hypoactive sexual desire F52.0
- hypochondriacal F45.20
  - body dysmorphic F45.22
  - neurosis F45.21
  - other specified F45.29
- identity
  - dissociative F44.81
  - of childhood F93.8
  - illness anxiety F45.21
- immune mechanism (immunity) D89.9
  - specified type NEC D89.89
- impaired renal tubular function N25.9
  - specified NEC N25.89
- impulse (control) F63.9
- inflammatory
  - pelvic, in diseases classified elsewhere — *see* category N74
  - penis N48.29
    - abscess N48.21
    - cellulitis N48.22
- inhalant use
  - mild F18.10
    - with
      - inhalant-induced
        - anxiety disorder F18.180
        - depressive disorder F18.14
        - major neurocognitive disorder F18.17
        - mild neurocognitive disorder F18.188
        - psychotic disorder F18.159
      - inhalant intoxication F18.129
      - inhalant intoxication delirium F18.121
    - in remission (early) (sustained) F18.11
  - moderate or severe F18.20
    - with
      - inhalant-induced
        - anxiety disorder F18.280
        - depressive disorder F18.24
        - major neurocognitive disorder F18.27
        - mild neurocognitive disorder F18.288
        - psychotic disorder F18.259
      - inhalant intoxication F18.229
      - inhalant intoxication delirium F18.221
    - in remission (early) (sustained) F18.21

☑ **Additional character required**

Disorder — *continued*
  integument, newborn P83.9
    specified NEC P83.88
  intermittent explosive F63.81
  internal secretion pancreas — *see* Increased,
      secretion, pancreas, endocrine
  intestine, intestinal
    carbohydrate absorption NEC E74.39
      postoperative K91.2
    functional NEC K59.9
      postoperative K91.89
    psychogenic F45.8
    vascular K55.9
      chronic K55.1
      specified NEC K55.8
  intraoperative (intraprocedural) — *see*
      Complications, intraoperative
  involuntary emotional expression (IEED) F48.2
  iris H21.9
    adhesions — *see* Adhesions, iris
    atrophy — *see* Atrophy, iris
    chamber angle recession — *see* Recession,
        chamber angle
    cyst — *see* Cyst, iris
    degeneration — *see* Degeneration, iris
    in diseases classified elsewhere H22
    iridodialysis — *see* Iridodialysis
    iridoschisis — *see* Iridoschisis
    miotic pupillary cyst — *see* Cyst, pupillary
    pupillary
      abnormality — *see* Abnormality, pupillary
      membrane — *see* Membrane, pupillary
    specified type NEC H21.89
    vascular NEC H21.1X ☑
  iron metabolism E83.10
    specified NEC E83.19
  isovaleric acidemia E71.110
  jaw, developmental M27.0
    temporomandibular (*see also* Anomaly,
        dentofacial, temporomandibular
        joint) M26.60 ☑
  joint M25.9
    derangement — *see* Derangement, joint
    effusion — *see* Effusion, joint
    fistula — *see* Fistula, joint
    hemarthrosis — *see* Hemarthrosis
    instability — *see* Instability, joint
    osteophyte — *see* Osteophyte
    pain — *see* Pain, joint
    psychogenic F45.8
    specified type NEC M25.80
      ankle M25.87 ☑
      elbow M25.82 ☑
      foot joint M25.87 ☑
      hand joint M25.84 ☑
      hip M25.85 ☑
      knee M25.86 ☑
      shoulder M25.81 ☑
      wrist M25.83 ☑
    stiffness — *see* Stiffness, joint
  ketone metabolism E71.32
  kidney N28.9
    functional (tubular) N25.9
    in
      schistosomiasis B65.9 *[N29]*
    tubular function N25.9
      specified NEC N25.89
  lacrimal system H04.9
    changes H04.69
    fistula — *see* Fistula, lacrimal
    gland H04.19
      atrophy — *see* Atrophy, lacrimal gland
      cyst — *see* Cyst, lacrimal, gland
      dacryops — *see* Dacryops
      dislocation — *see* Dislocation, lacrimal gland
      dry eye syndrome — *see* Syndrome, dry eye
      infection — *see* Dacryoadenitis
      granuloma — *see* Granuloma, lacrimal
      inflammation — *see* Inflammation, lacrimal
      obstruction — *see* Obstruction, lacrimal
    specified NEC H04.89
  lactation NEC O92.79
  language (developmental) F80.9
    expressive F80.1
    mixed receptive and expressive F80.2
    receptive F80.2
  late luteal phase dysphoric N94.89
  learning (specific) F81.9
    acalculia R48.8
    alexia R48.0
    mathematics F81.2
    reading F81.0

Disorder — *continued*
  learning — *continued*
    specified
      with impairment in
        mathematics F81.2
        reading F81.0
        written expression F81.81
    specified NEC F81.89
    spelling F81.81
    written expression F81.81
  lens H27.9
    aphakia — *see* Aphakia
    cataract — *see* Cataract
    dislocation — *see* Dislocation, lens
    specified type NEC H27.8
  ligament M24.20
    ankle M24.27 ☑
    attachment, spine — *see* Enthesopathy, spinal
    elbow M24.22 ☑
    foot joint M24.27 ☑
    hand joint M24.24 ☑
    hip M24.25 ☑
    knee — *see* Derangement, knee, specified NEC
    shoulder M24.21 ☑
    vertebra M24.28
    wrist M24.23 ☑
  ligamentous attachments (*see also*
      Enthesopathy)
    spine — *see* Enthesopathy, spinal
  lipid
    metabolism, congenital E78.9
    storage E75.6
      specified NEC E75.5
  lipoprotein
    deficiency (familial) E78.6
    metabolism E78.9
      specified NEC E78.89
  liver K76.9
    malarial B54 *[K77]*
  low back (*see also* Dorsopathy, specified NEC)
  lumbosacral
    plexus G54.1
    root (nerve) NEC G54.4
  lung, interstitial, drug-induced J70.4
    acute J70.2
    chronic J70.3
  lymphoproliferative, post-transplant (PTLD) D47.
      Z1
  lysine and hydroxylysine metabolism E72.3
  major neurocognitive — *see* Dementia, in (due to)
  male
    erectile (organic) (*see also* Dysfunction, sexual,
        male, erectile) N52.9
      nonorganic F52.21
    hypoactive sexual desire F52.0
    orgasmic F52.32
  manic F30.9
    organic F06.33
  mast cell activation — *see* Activation, mast cell
  mastoid (*see also* Disorder, ear, middle)
    postprocedural — *see* Complications, ear,
        procedure
  meniscus — *see* Derangement, knee, meniscus
  menopausal N95.9
    specified NEC N95.8
  menstrual N92.6
    psychogenic F45.8
    specified NEC N92.5
  mental (or behavioral) (nonpsychotic) F99
    due to (secondary to)
      amphetamine
        due to drug abuse — *see* Abuse, drug,
            stimulant
        due to drug dependence — *see*
            Dependence, drug, stimulant
      brain disease, damage and dysfunction F09
      caffeine use
        due to drug abuse — *see* Abuse, drug,
            stimulant
        due to drug dependence — *see*
            Dependence, drug, stimulant
      cannabis use
        due to drug abuse — *see* Abuse, drug,
            cannabis
        due to drug dependence — *see*
            Dependence, drug, cannabis
      general medical condition F09
      sedative or hypnotic use
        due to drug abuse — *see* Abuse, drug,
            sedative
        due to drug dependence — *see*
            Dependence, drug, sedative

Disorder — *continued*
  mental — *continued*
    tobacco (nicotine) use — *see* Dependence,
        drug, nicotine
    following organic brain damage F07.9
      frontal lobe syndrome F07.0
      personality change F07.0
      postconcussional syndrome F07.81
      specified NEC F07.89
    infancy, childhood or adolescence F98.9
    neurotic — *see* Neurosis
    organic or symptomatic F09
    presenile, psychotic F03 ☑
    problem NEC
    psychoneurotic — *see* Neurosis
    psychotic — *see* Psychosis
    puerperal F53
    senile, psychotic NEC F03 ☑
  metabolic, amino acid, transitory, newborn P74.8
  metabolism NOS E88.9
    amino-acid E72.9
      aromatic E70.9
        albinism — *see* Albinism
        histidine E70.40
          histidinemia E70.41
          other specified E70.49
        hyperphenylalaninemia E70.1
          classical phenylketonuria E70.0
        other specified E70.8
        tryptophan E70.5
        tyrosine E70.20
          hypertyrosinemia E70.21
          other specified E70.29
      branched chain E71.2
        3-methylglutaconic aciduria E71.111
        hyperleucine-isoleucinemia E71.19
        hypervalinemia E71.19
        isovaleric acidemia E71.110
        maple syrup urine disease E71.0
        methylmalonic acidemia E71.120
        organic aciduria NEC E71.118
        other specified E71.19
        proprionate NEC E71.128
        proprionic acidemia E71.121
      glycine E72.9
        d-glycericacidemia E72.59
        hyperhydroxyprolinemia E72.59
        hyperoxaluria E72.53
        hyperprolinemia E72.59
        non-ketotic hyperglycinemia E72.51
        other specified E72.59
        sarcosinemia E72.59
        trimethylaminuria E72.52
      hydroxylysine E72.3
      lysine E72.3
      ornithine E72.4
      other specified E72.8
        beta-amino acid E72.8
        gamma-glutamyl cycle E72.8
      straight-chain E72.8
      sulfur-bearing E72.10
        homocystinuria E72.11
        methylenetetrahydrofolate reductase
            deficiency E72.12
        other specified E72.19
    bile acid and cholesterol metabolism E78.70
    bilirubin E80.7
      specified NEC E80.6
    calcium E83.50
      hypercalcemia E83.52
      hypocalcemia E83.51
      other specified E83.59
    carbohydrate E74.9
      specified NEC E74.8
    cholesterol and bile acid metabolism E78.70
    congenital E88.9
    copper E83.00
      Wilson's disease E83.01
      specified type NEC E83.09
    cystinuria E72.01
    fructose E74.10
    galactose E74.20
    glucosaminoglycan E76.9
      mucopolysaccharidosis — *see*
          Mucopolysaccharidosis
      specified NEC E76.8
    glutamine E72.8
    glycine E72.50
    glycogen storage (hepatorenal) E74.09
    glycoprotein E77.9
      specified NEC E77.8
    glycosaminoglycan E76.9

Disorder

Disorder — *continued*
  metabolism — *continued*
    specified NEC E76.8
    in labor and delivery O75.89
    iron E83.10
    isoleucine E71.19
    leucine E71.19
    lipoid E78.9
    lipoprotein E78.9
      specified NEC E78.89
    magnesium E83.40
      hypermagnesemia E83.41
      hypomagnesemia E83.42
      other specified E83.49
    mineral E83.9
      specified NEC E83.89
    mitochondrial E88.40
      MELAS syndrome E88.41
      MERRF syndrome (myoclonic epilepsy
        associated with ragged-red fibers) E88.42
      other specified E88.49
    ornithine E72.4
    phosphatases E83.30
    phosphorus E83.30
      acid phosphatase deficiency E83.39
      hypophosphatasia E83.39
      hypophosphatemia E83.39
        familial E83.31
      other specified E83.39
      pseudovitamin D deficiency E83.32
    plasma protein NEC E88.09
    porphyrin — *see* Porphyria
    postprocedural E89.89
      specified NEC E89.89
    purine E79.9
      specified NEC E79.8
    pyrimidine E79.9
      specified NEC E79.8
    pyruvate E74.4
    serine E72.8
    sodium E87.8
    specified NEC E88.89
    threonine E72.8
    valine E71.19
    zinc E83.2
  methylmalonic acidemia E71.120
  micturition NEC (*see also* Difficulty,
    micturition) R39.198
    feeling of incomplete emptying R39.14
    hesitancy R39.11
    poor stream R39.12
    psychogenic F45.8
    split stream R39.13
    straining R39.16
    urgency R39.15
  mild neurocognitive G31.84
  mitochondrial metabolism E88.40
  mitral (valve) — *see* Endocarditis, mitral
  mixed
    anxiety and depressive F41.8
    of scholastic skills (developmental) F81.89
    receptive expressive language F80.2
  mood F39
    bipolar — *see* Disorder, bipolar
    depressive — *see* Disorder, depressive
    due to (secondary to)
      alcohol F10.94
      amphetamine F15.94
        in
          abuse F15.14
          dependence F15.24
      anxiolytic F13.94
        in
          abuse F13.14
          dependence F13.24
      cocaine F14.94
        in
          abuse F14.14
          dependence F14.24
      general medical condition F06.30
      hallucinogen F16.94
        in
          abuse F16.14
          dependence F16.24
      hypnotic F13.94
        in
          abuse F13.14
          dependence F13.24
      inhalant F18.94
        in
          abuse F18.14
          dependence F18.24

Disorder — *continued*
  mood — *continued*
    opioid F11.94
      in
        abuse F11.14
        dependence F11.24
    phencyclidine (PCP) F16.94
      in
        abuse F16.14
        dependence F16.24
    physiological condition F06.30
      with
        depressive features F06.31
        major depressive-like episode F06.32
        manic features F06.33
        mixed features F06.34
    psychoactive substance NEC F19.94
      in
        abuse F19.14
        dependence F19.24
    sedative F13.94
      in
        abuse F13.14
        dependence F13.24
    volatile solvents F18.94
      in
        abuse F18.14
        dependence F18.24
    manic episode F30.9
      with psychotic symptoms F30.2
      in remission (full) F30.4
      partial F30.3
      specified type NEC F30.8
      without psychotic symptoms F30.10
        mild F30.11
        moderate F30.12
        severe F30.13
    organic F06.30
      right hemisphere F07.89
    persistent F34.9
      cyclothymia F34.0
      dysthymia F34.1
      specified type NEC F34.89
    recurrent F39
    right hemisphere organic F07.89
  movement G25.9
    drug-induced G25.70
      akathisia G25.71
      specified NEC G25.79
    hysterical F44.4
    in diseases classified elsewhere — *see* category
      G26
    periodic limb G47.61
      sleep related G47.61
    specified NEC G25.89
    sleep related NEC G47.69
    stereotyped F98.4
    treatment-induced G25.9
  multiple personality F44.81
  muscle M62.9
    attachment, spine — *see* Enthesopathy, spinal
    in trichinellosis — *see* Trichinellosis, with
      muscle disorder
    psychogenic F45.8
    specified type NEC M62.89
    tone, newborn P94.9
      specified NEC P94.8
  muscular
    attachments (*see also* Enthesopathy)
      spine — *see* Enthesopathy, spinal
    urethra N36.44
  musculoskeletal system, soft tissue — *see*
    Disorder, soft tissue
    postprocedural M96.89
    psychogenic F45.8
  myoneural G70.9
    due to lead G70.1
    specified NEC G70.89
    toxic G70.1
  myotonic NEC G71.19
  nail, in diseases classified elsewhere L62
  neck region NEC — *see* Dorsopathy, specified NEC
  neonatal onset multisystemic inflammatory
    (NOMID) M04.2
  nerve G58.9
    abducent NEC — *see* Strabismus, paralytic,
      sixth nerve
    accessory G52.8
    acoustic — *see* subcategory H93.3
    auditory — *see* subcategory H93.3
    auriculotemporal G50.8
    axillary G54.0

Disorder — *continued*
  nerve — *continued*
    cerebral — *see* Disorder, nerve, cranial
    cranial G52.9
      eighth — *see* subcategory H93.3
      eleventh G52.8
      fifth G50.9
      first G52.0
      fourth NEC — *see* Strabismus, paralytic,
        fourth nerve
      multiple G52.7
      ninth G52.1
      second NEC — *see* Disorder, nerve, optic
      seventh NEC G51.8
      sixth NEC — *see* Strabismus, paralytic, sixth nerve
      specified NEC G52.8
      tenth G52.2
      third NEC — *see* Strabismus, paralytic, third
        nerve
      twelfth G52.3
    entrapment — *see* Neuropathy, entrapment
    facial G51.9
      specified NEC G51.8
    femoral — *see* Lesion, nerve, femoral
    glossopharyngeal NEC G52.1
    hypoglossal G52.3
    intercostal G58.0
    lateral
      cutaneous of thigh — *see* Mononeuropathy,
        lower limb, meralgia paresthetica
      popliteal — *see* Lesion, nerve, popliteal
    lower limb — *see* Mononeuropathy, lower limb
    medial popliteal — *see* Lesion, nerve, popliteal,
      medial
    median NEC — *see* Lesion, nerve, median
    multiple G58.7
    oculomotor NEC — *see* Strabismus, paralytic,
      third nerve
    olfactory G52.0
    optic NEC H47.09 ☑
      hemorrhage into sheath — *see* Hemorrhage,
        optic nerve
      ischemic H47.01 ☑
    peroneal — *see* Lesion, nerve, popliteal
    phrenic G58.8
    plantar — *see* Lesion, nerve, plantar
    pneumogastric G52.2
    posterior tibial — *see* Syndrome, tarsal tunnel
    radial — *see* Lesion, nerve, radial
    recurrent laryngeal G52.2
    root G54.9
      cervical G54.2
      lumbosacral G54.1
      specified NEC G54.8
      thoracic G54.3
    sciatic NEC — *see* Lesion, nerve, sciatic
    specified NEC G58.8
      lower limb — *see* Mononeuropathy, lower
        limb, specified NEC
      upper limb — *see* Mononeuropathy, upper
        limb, specified NEC
    sympathetic G90.9
    tibial — *see* Lesion, nerve, popliteal, medial
    trigeminal G50.9
      specified NEC G50.8
    trochlear NEC — *see* Strabismus, paralytic,
      fourth nerve
    ulnar — *see* Lesion, nerve, ulnar
    upper limb — *see* Mononeuropathy, upper limb
    vagus G52.2
  nervous system G98.8
    autonomic (peripheral) G90.9
      specified NEC G90.8
    central G96.9
      specified NEC G96.8
    parasympathetic G90.9
    specified NEC G98.8
    sympathetic G90.9
    vegetative G90.9
  neurocognitive R41.9
    major
      with
        aggressive behavior F01.51
        combative behavior F01.51
        violent behavior F01.51
      due to vascular disease, with behavioral
        disturbance F01.51
      in (due to) (other diseases classified
        elsewhere) (*see also* Dementia, in (due
        to)) F02.80
        with
          aggressive behavior F02.81

☑ **Additional character required**

Disorder — *continued*
   neurocognitive — *continued*
      combative behavior F02.81
      violent behavior F02.81
     without behavioral disturbance F01.50
    mild G31.84
   neurodevelopmental F89
    specified NEC F88
   neurohypophysis NEC E23.3
   neurological NEC R29.818
   neuromuscular G70.9
    hereditary NEC G71.9
    specified NEC G70.89
    toxic G70.1
   neurotic F48.9
    specified NEC F48.8
   neutrophil, polymorphonuclear D71
   nicotine use — *see* Dependence, drug, nicotine
   nightmare F51.5
   non-rapid eye movement sleep arousal
    sleep terror type F51.4
    sleepwalking type F51.3
   nose J34.9
    specified NEC J34.89
   obsessive-compulsive F42.9
    and related disorder due to a known
      physiological condition F06.8
   odontogenesis NOS K00.9
   opioid use
    with
     opioid-induced psychotic disorder F11.959
      with
       delusions F11.950
       hallucinations F11.951
    due to drug abuse — *see* Abuse, drug, opioid
    due to drug dependence — *see* Dependence,
     drug, opioid
    mild F11.10
     with
      opioid-induced
       anxiety disorder F11.188
       depressive disorder F11.14
       sexual dysfunction F11.181
      opioid intoxication
       with perceptual disturbances F11.122
       delirium F11.121
       without perceptual disturbances F11.129
     in remission (early) (sustained) F11.11
    moderate or severe F11.20
     with
      opioid-induced
       anxiety disorder F11.288
       anxiety disorder F11.988
       depressive disorder F11.24
       depressive disorder F11.94
       sexual dysfunction F11.281
       sexual dysfunction F11.981
      opioid intoxication
       with perceptual disturbances F11.222
       delirium F11.221
       without perceptual disturbances F11.229
     in remission (early) (sustained) F11.21
   oppositional defiant F91.3
   optic
    chiasm H47.49
     due to
      inflammatory disorder H47.41
      neoplasm H47.42
      vascular disorder H47.43
    disc H47.39 ☑
     coloboma — *see* Coloboma, optic disc
     drusen — *see* Drusen, optic disc
     pseudopapilledema — *see*
      Pseudopapilledema
    radiations — *see* Disorder, visual, pathway
    tracts — *see* Disorder, visual, pathway
   orbit H05.9
    cyst — *see* Cyst, orbit
    deformity — *see* Deformity, orbit
    edema — *see* Edema, orbit
    enophthalmos — *see* Enophthalmos
    exophthalmos — *see* Exophthalmos
    hemorrhage — *see* Hemorrhage, orbit
    inflammation — *see* Inflammation, orbit
    myopathy — *see* Myopathy, extraocular
     muscles
    retained foreign body — *see* Foreign body,
     orbit, old
    specified type NEC H05.89
   organic
    anxiety F06.4
    catatonic F06.1

Disorder — *continued*
   organic — *continued*
    delusional F06.2
    dissociative F06.8
    emotionally labile (asthenic) F06.8
    mood (affective) F06.30
    schizophrenia-like F06.2
   orgasmic (female) F52.31
    male F52.32
   ornithine metabolism E72.4
   overanxious F41.1
    of childhood F93.8
   pain
    with related psychological factors F45.42
    exclusively related to psychological
     factors F45.41
    genito-pelvic penetration disorder F52.6
   pancreatic internal secretion E16.9
    specified NEC E16.8
   panic F41.0
    with agoraphobia F40.01
   papulosquamous L44.9
    in diseases classified elsewhere L45
    specified NEC L44.8
   paranoid F22
    induced F24
    shared F24
   paraphilic F65.9
    specified NEC F65.89
   parathyroid (gland) E21.5
    specified NEC E21.4
   parietoalveolar NEC J84.09
   paroxysmal, mixed R56.9
   patella M22.9 ☑
    chondromalacia — *see* Chondromalacia, patella
    derangement NEC M22.3X ☑
    recurrent
     dislocation — *see* Dislocation, patella,
      recurrent
     subluxation — *see* Dislocation, patella,
      recurrent, incomplete
    specified NEC M22.8X ☑
   patellofemoral M22.2X ☑
   pedophilic F65.4
   pentose phosphate pathway with anemia D55.1
   perception, due to hallucinogens F16.983
    in
     abuse F16.183
     dependence F16.283
   peripheral nervous system NEC G64
   peroxisomal E71.50
    biogenesis
     neonatal adrenoleukodystrophy E71.511
     specified disorder NEC E71.518
     Zellweger syndrome E71.510
    rhizomelic chondrodysplasia punctata E71.540
    specified form NEC E71.548
     group 1 E71.518
     group 2 E71.53
     group 3 E71.542
    X-linked adrenoleukodystrophy E71.529
     adolescent E71.521
     adrenomyeloneuropathy E71.522
     childhood E71.520
     specified form NEC E71.528
    Zellweger-like syndrome E71.541
   persistent
    (somatoform) pain F45.41
    affective (mood) F34.9
   personality (*see also* Personality) F60.9
    affective F34.0
    aggressive F60.3
    amoral F60.2
    anankastic F60.5
    antisocial F60.2
    anxious F60.6
    asocial F60.2
    asthenic F60.7
    avoidant F60.6
    borderline F60.3
    change (secondary) due to general medical
     condition F07.0
    compulsive F60.5
    cyclothymic F34.0
    dependent (passive) F60.7
    depressive F34.1
    dissocial F60.2
    emotional instability F60.3
    expansive paranoid F60.0
    explosive F60.3
    following organic brain damage F07.9
    histrionic F60.4

Disorder — *continued*
   personality — *continued*
    hyperthymic F34.0
    hypothymic F34.1
    hysterical F60.4
    immature F60.89
    inadequate F60.7
    labile F60.3
    mixed (nonspecific) F60.89
    moral deficiency F60.2
    narcissistic F60.81
    negativistic F60.89
    obsessional F60.5
    obsessive (-compulsive) F60.5
    organic F07.9
    overconscientious F60.5
    paranoid F60.0
    passive (-dependent) F60.7
    passive-aggressive F60.89
    pathological NEC F60.9
    pseudosocial F60.2
    psychopathic F60.2
    schizoid F60.1
    schizotypal F21
    self-defeating F60.7
    specified NEC F60.89
    type A F60.5
    unstable (emotional) F60.3
   pervasive, developmental F84.9
   phencyclidine use
    mild F16.10
     with
      phencyclidine-induced
       anxiety disorder F16.180
       bipolar and related disorder F16.14
       depressive disorder F16.14
       psychotic disorder F16.159
      phencyclidine intoxication F16.129
      phencyclidine intoxication
       delirium F16.121
     in remission (early) (sustained) F16.11
    moderate or severe F16.20
     with
      phencyclidine-induced
       anxiety disorder F16.280
       bipolar and related disorder F16.24
       depressive disorder F16.24
       psychotic disorder F16.259
      phencyclidine intoxication F16.229
      phencyclidine intoxication
       delirium F16.221
     in remission (early) (sustained) F16.21
   phobic anxiety, childhood F40.8
   phosphate-losing tubular N25.0
   pigmentation L81.9
    choroid, congenital Q14.3
    diminished melanin formation L81.6
    iron L81.8
    specified NEC L81.8
   pinna (noninfective) H61.10 ☑
    deformity, acquired H61.11 ☑
    hematoma H61.12 ☑
    perichondritis — *see* Perichondritis, ear
    specified type NEC H61.19 ☑
   pituitary gland E23.7
    iatrogenic (postprocedural) E89.3
    specified NEC E23.6
   platelets D69.1
   plexus G54.9
    specified NEC G54.8
   polymorphonuclear neutrophils D71
   porphyrin metabolism — *see* Porphyria
   postconcussional F07.81
   posthallucinogen perception F16.983
    in
     abuse F16.183
     dependence F16.283
   postmenopausal N95.9
    specified NEC N95.8
   postprocedural (postoperative) — *see*
    Complications, postprocedural
   post-transplant lymphoproliferative D47.Z1
   post-traumatic stress (PTSD) F43.10
    acute F43.11
    chronic F43.12
   premenstrual dysphoric (PMDD) F32.81
   prepuce N47.8
   propionic acidemia E71.121
   prostate N42.9
    specified NEC N42.89
   psychogenic NOS (*see also* condition) F45.9
    anxiety F41.8

Disorder

Disorder — continued

psychogenic NOS — continued
  appetite F50.9
  asthenic F48.8
  cardiovascular (system) F45.8
  compulsive F42.8
  cutaneous F54
  depressive F32.9
  digestive (system) F45.8
  dysmenorrheic F45.8
  dyspneic F45.8
  endocrine (system) F54
  eye NEC F45.8
  feeding — see Disorder, eating
  functional NEC F45.8
  gastric F45.8
  gastrointestinal (system) F45.8
  genitourinary (system) F45.8
  heart (function) (rhythm) F45.8
  hyperventilatory F45.8
  hypochondriacal — see Disorder, hypochondriacal
  intestinal F45.8
  joint F45.8
  learning F81.9
  limb F45.8
  lymphatic (system) F45.8
  menstrual F45.8
  micturition F45.8
  monoplegic NEC F44.4
  motor F44.4
  muscle F45.8
  musculoskeletal F45.8
  neurocirculatory F45.8
  obsessive F42.8
  occupational F48.8
  organ or part of body NEC F45.8
  paralytic NEC F44.4
  phobic F40.9
  physical NEC F45.8
  rectal F45.8
  respiratory (system) F45.8
  rheumatic F45.8
  sexual (function) F52.9
  skin (allergic) (eczematous) F54
  sleep F51.9
  specified part of body NEC F45.8
  stomach F45.8
psychological F99
  associated with
    disease classified elsewhere F54
    sexual
      development F66
      relationship F66
    uncertainty about gender identity F64.9
psychomotor NEC F44.4
  hysterical F44.4
psychoneurotic (see also Neurosis)
  mixed NEC F48.8
psychophysiologic — see Disorder, somatoform
psychosexual F65.9
  development F66
  identity of childhood F64.2
psychosomatic NOS — see Disorder, somatoform
  multiple F45.0
  undifferentiated F45.1
psychotic — see Psychosis
  transient (acute) F23
puberty E30.9
  specified NEC E30.8
pulmonary (valve) — see Endocarditis, pulmonary
purine metabolism E79.9
pyrimidine metabolism E79.9
pyruvate metabolism E74.4
reactive attachment (childhood) F94.1
reading R48.0
  developmental (specific) F81.0
receptive language F80.2
receptor, hormonal, peripheral (see also Syndrome, androgen insensitivity) E34.50
recurrent brief depressive F33.8
reflex R29.2
refraction H52.7
  aniseikonia H52.32
  anisometropia H52.31
  astigmatism — see Astigmatism
  hypermetropia — see Hypermetropia
  myopia — see Myopia
  presbyopia H52.4
  specified NEC H52.6
relationship F68.8
  due to sexual orientation F66

Disorder — continued

REM sleep behavior G47.52
renal function, impaired (tubular) N25.9
resonance R49.9
  specified NEC R49.8
respiratory function, impaired (see also Failure, respiration)
  postprocedural — see Complication, postoperative, respiratory system
  psychogenic F45.8
retina H35.9
  angioid streaks H35.33
  changes in vascular appearance H35.01 ☑
  degeneration — see Degeneration, retina
  dystrophy (hereditary) — see Dystrophy, retina
  edema H35.81
  hemorrhage — see Hemorrhage, retina
  ischemia H35.82
  macular degeneration — see Degeneration, macula
  microaneurysms H35.04 ☑
  microvascular abnormality NEC H35.09
  neovascularization — see Neovascularization, retina
  retinopathy — see Retinopathy
  separation of layers H35.70
    central serous chorioretinopathy H35.71 ☑
    pigment epithelium detachment (serous) H35.72 ☑
    hemorrhagic H35.73 ☑
  specified type NEC H35.89
  telangiectasis — see Telangiectasis, retina
  vasculitis — see Vasculitis, retina
retroperitoneal K68.9
right hemisphere organic affective F07.89
rumination (infant or child) F98.21
sacrum, sacrococcygeal NEC M53.3
schizoaffective F25.9
  bipolar type F25.0
  depressive type F25.1
  manic type F25.0
  mixed type F25.0
  specified NEC F25.8
schizoid of childhood F84.5
schizophrenia spectrum and other psychotic disorder F29
  specified NEC F28
schizophreniform F20.81
  brief F23
schizotypal (personality) F21
secretion, thyrocalcitonin E07.0
sedative, hypnotic, or anxiolytic use
  mild F13.10
    with
      sedative, hypnotic, or anxiolytic-induced
        anxiety disorder F13.180
        bipolar and related disorder F13.14
        depressive disorder F13.14
        psychotic disorder F13.159
        sexual dysfunction F13.181
      sedative, hypnotic, or anxiolytic intoxication F13.129
      sedative, hypnotic, or anxiolytic intoxication delirium F13.121
    in remission (early) (sustained) F13.11
  moderate or severe F13.20
    with
      sedative, hypnotic, or anxiolytic-induced
        anxiety disorder F13.280
        bipolar and related disorder F13.24
        depressive disorder F13.24
        major neurocognitive disorder F13.27
        mild neurocognitive disorder F13.288
        psychotic disorder F13.259
        sexual dysfunction F13.281
      sedative, hypnotic, or anxiolytic intoxication F13.229
      sedative, hypnotic, or anxiolytic intoxication delirium F13.221
    in remission (early) (sustained) F13.21
seizure (see also Epilepsy) G40.909
  intractable G40.919
    with status epilepticus G40.911
semantic pragmatic F80.89
  with autism F84.0
sense of smell R43.1
  psychogenic F45.8
separation anxiety, of childhood F93.0
sexual
  arousal, female F52.22
  aversion F52.1
  function, psychogenic F52.9

Disorder — continued

sexual — continued
  interest/arousal, female F52.22
  masochism F65.51
  maturation F66
  nonorganic F52.9
  preference (see also Deviation, sexual) F65.9
    fetishistic transvestism F65.1
  relationship F66
  sadism F65.52
shyness, of childhood and adolescence F40.10
sibling rivalry F93.8
sickle-cell (sickling) (homozygous) — see Disease, sickle-cell
  heterozygous D57.3
  specified type NEC D57.8 ☑
  trait D57.3
sinus (nasal) J34.9
  specified NEC J34.89
skin L98.9
  atrophic L90.9
    specified NEC L90.8
  granulomatous L92.9
    specified NEC L92.8
  hypertrophic L91.9
    specified NEC L91.8
  infiltrative NEC L98.6
  newborn P83.9
    specified NEC P83.88
  picking F42.4
  psychogenic (allergic) (eczematous) F54
sleep G47.9
  breathing-related — see Apnea, sleep
  circadian rhythm G47.20
    advance sleep phase type G47.22
    delayed sleep phase type G47.21
    due to
      alcohol
        abuse F10.182
        dependence F10.282
        use F10.982
      amphetamines
        abuse F15.182
        dependence F15.282
        use F15.982
      caffeine
        abuse F15.182
        dependence F15.282
        use F15.982
      cocaine
        abuse F14.182
        dependence F14.282
        use F14.982
      drug NEC
        abuse F19.182
        dependence F19.282
        use F19.982
      opioid
        abuse F11.182
        dependence F11.282
        use F11.982
      psychoactive substance NEC
        abuse F19.182
        dependence F19.282
        use F19.982
      sedative, hypnotic, or anxiolytic
        abuse F13.182
        dependence F13.282
        use F13.982
      stimulant NEC
        abuse F15.182
        dependence F15.282
        use F15.982
    free running type G47.24
    in conditions classified elsewhere G47.27
    irregular sleep wake type G47.23
    jet lag type G47.25
    non-24-hour sleep-wake type G47.24
    shift work type G47.26
    specified NEC G47.29
  due to
    alcohol
      abuse F10.182
      dependence F10.282
      use F10.982
    amphetamine
      abuse F15.182
      dependence F15.282
      use F15.982
    anxiolytic
      abuse F13.182
      dependence F13.282

☑ **Additional character required**

Disorder — *continued*
  sleep — *continued*
    use F13.982
    caffeine
      abuse F15.182
      dependence F15.282
      use F15.982
    cocaine
      abuse F14.182
      dependence F14.282
      use F14.982
    drug NEC
      abuse F19.182
      dependence F19.282
      use F19.982
    hypnotic
      abuse F13.182
      dependence F13.282
      use F13.982
    opioid
      abuse F11.182
      dependence F11.282
      use F11.982
    psychoactive substance NEC
      abuse F19.182
      dependence F19.282
      use F19.982
    sedative
      abuse F13.182
      dependence F13.282
      use F13.982
    stimulant NEC
      abuse F15.182
      dependence F15.282
      use F15.982
  emotional F51.9
  excessive somnolence — *see* Hypersomnia
  hypersomnia type — *see* Hypersomnia
  initiating or maintaining — *see* Insomnia
  nightmares F51.5
  nonorganic F51.9
    specified NEC F51.8
  parasomnia type G47.50
  specified NEC G47.8
  terrors F51.4
  walking F51.3
  sleep-wake pattern or schedule (*see also* Disorder, sleep, circadian rhythm) G47.9
    specified NEC G47.8
  social
    anxiety (of childhood) F40.10
      generalized F40.11
    functioning in childhood F94.9
      specified NEC F94.8
    pragmatic F80.82
  soft tissue M79.9
    ankle M79.9
    due to use, overuse and pressure M70.90
      ankle M70.97 ☑
      bursitis — *see* Bursitis
      foot M70.97 ☑
      forearm M70.93 ☑
      hand M70.94 ☑
      lower leg M70.96 ☑
      multiple sites M70.99
      pelvic region M70.95 ☑
      shoulder region M70.91 ☑
      specified site NEC M70.98
      specified type NEC M70.80
        ankle M70.87 ☑
        foot M70.87 ☑
        forearm M70.83 ☑
        hand M70.84 ☑
        lower leg M70.86 ☑
        multiple sites M70.89
        pelvic region M70.85 ☑
        shoulder region M70.81 ☑
        specified site NEC M70.88
        thigh M70.85 ☑
        upper arm M70.82 ☑
      thigh M70.95 ☑
      upper arm M70.92 ☑
    foot M79.9
    forearm M79.9
    hand M79.9
    lower leg M79.9
    multiple sites M79.9
    occupational — *see* Disorder, soft tissue, due to use, overuse and pressure
    pelvic region M79.9
    shoulder region M79.9
    specified type NEC M79.89

Disorder — *continued*
  soft tissue — *continued*
    thigh M79.9
    upper arm M79.9
  somatic symptom F45.1
  somatization F45.0
  somatoform F45.9
    pain (persistent) F45.41
    somatization (multiple) (long-lasting) F45.0
    specified NEC F45.8
    undifferentiated F45.1
  somnolence, excessive — *see* Hypersomnia
  specific
    arithmetical F81.2
    developmental, of motor F82
    reading F81.0
    speech and language F80.9
    spelling F81.81
    written expression F81.81
  speech R47.9
    articulation (functional) (specific) F80.0
    developmental F80.9
    specified NEC R47.89
  speech-sound F80.0
  spelling (specific) F81.81
  spine (*see also* Dorsopathy)
    ligamentous or muscular attachments, peripheral — *see* Enthesopathy, spinal
    specified NEC — *see* Dorsopathy, specified NEC
  stereotyped, habit or movement F98.4
  stimulant use (other) (unspecified)
    mild F15.10
      in remission (early) (sustained) F15.11
    moderate or severe F15.20
      in remission (early) (sustained) F15.21
  stomach (functional) — *see* Disorder, gastric
  stress F43.9
    acute F43.0
    post-traumatic F43.10
      acute F43.11
      chronic F43.12
  substance use (other) (unknown)
    mild F19.10
      with substance-induced
        anxiety disorder F19.180
        bipolar and related disorder F19.14
        depressive disorder F19.14
        major neurocognitive disorder F19.17
        mild neurocognitive disorder F19.188
        obsessive-compulsive and related disorder F19.188
        sexual dysfunction F19.181
      substance intoxication F19.129
      substance intoxication delirium F19.121
    moderate or severe F19.20
      with substance-induced
        anxiety disorder F19.280
        bipolar and related disorder F19.24
        depressive disorder F19.24
        major neurocognitive disorder F19.27
        mild neurocognitive disorder F19.288
        obsessive-compulsive and related disorder F19.288
        sexual dysfunction F19.281
      in remission (early) (sustained) F19.21
      substance intoxication F19.229
      substance intoxication delirium F19.221
  sulfur-bearing amino-acid metabolism E72.10
  sweat gland (eccrine) L74.9
    apocrine L75.9
      specified NEC L75.8
    specified NEC L74.8
  synovium M67.90
    acromioclavicular M67.91 ☑
    ankle M67.97 ☑
    elbow M67.92 ☑
    foot M67.97 ☑
    forearm M67.93 ☑
    hand M67.94 ☑
    hip M67.95 ☑
    knee M67.96 ☑
    multiple sites M67.99
    rupture — *see* Rupture, synovium
    shoulder M67.91 ☑
    specified type NEC M67.80
      acromioclavicular M67.81 ☑
      ankle M67.87 ☑
      elbow M67.82 ☑
      foot M67.87 ☑
      hand M67.84 ☑
      hip M67.85 ☑
      knee M67.86 ☑

Disorder — *continued*
  synovium — *continued*
    multiple sites M67.89
    wrist M67.83 ☑
  synovitis — *see* Synovitis
  upper arm M67.92 ☑
  wrist M67.93 ☑
  temperature regulation, newborn P81.9
    specified NEC P81.8
  temporomandibular joint M26.60 ☑
  tendon M67.90
    acromioclavicular M67.91 ☑
    ankle M67.97 ☑
    contracture — *see* Contracture, tendon
    elbow M67.92 ☑
    foot M67.97 ☑
    forearm M67.93 ☑
    hand M67.94 ☑
    hip M67.95 ☑
    knee M67.96 ☑
    multiple sites M67.99
    rupture — *see* Rupture, tendon
    shoulder M67.91 ☑
    specified type NEC M67.80
      acromioclavicular M67.81 ☑
      ankle M67.87 ☑
      elbow M67.82 ☑
      foot M67.87 ☑
      hand M67.84 ☑
      hip M67.85 ☑
      knee M67.86 ☑
      multiple sites M67.89
      trunk M67.88
      wrist M67.83 ☑
    synovitis — *see* Synovitis
    tendinitis — *see* Tendinitis
    tenosynovitis — *see* Tenosynovitis
    trunk M67.98
    upper arm M67.92 ☑
    wrist M67.93 ☑
  thoracic root (nerve) NEC G54.3
  thyrocalcitonin hypersecretion E07.0
  thyroid (gland) E07.9
    function NEC, neonatal, transitory P72.2
    iodine-deficiency related E01.8
    specified NEC E07.89
  tic — *see* Tic
  tobacco use
    chewing tobacco (mild) (moderate) (severe)
      in remission (early) (sustained) F17.221
    cigarettes (mild) (moderate) (severe)
      in remission (early) (sustained) F17.211
    mild Z72.0
      in remission (early) (sustained) F17.201
    moderate F17.200
      in remission (early) (sustained) F17.201
    severe F17.200
      in remission (early) (sustained) F17.201
    specified product NEC (mild) (moderate) (severe)
      in remission (early) (sustained) F17.291
  tooth K08.9
    development K00.9
      specified NEC K00.8
    eruption K00.6
  Tourette's F95.2
  trance and possession F44.89
  transvestic F65.1
  trauma and stressor-related F43.9
    other specified F43.8
  tricuspid (valve) — *see* Endocarditis, tricuspid
  tryptophan metabolism E70.5
  tubular, phosphate-losing N25.0
  tubulo-interstitial (in)
    brucellosis A23.9 *[N16]*
    cystinosis E72.04
    diphtheria A36.84
    glycogen storage disease E74.00 *[N16]*
    leukemia NEC C95.9 ☑ *[N16]*
    lymphoma NEC C85.9 ☑ *[N16]*
    mixed cryoglobulinemia D89.1 *[N16]*
    multiple myeloma C90.0 ☑ *[N16]*
    Salmonella infection A02.25
    sarcoidosis D86.84
    sepsis A41.9 *[N16]*
      streptococcal A40.9 *[N16]*
    systemic lupus erythematosus M32.15
    toxoplasmosis B58.83
    transplant rejection T86.91 *[N16]*
    Wilson's disease E83.01 *[N16]*
  tubulo-renal function, impaired N25.9
    specified NEC N25.89

Disorder — *continued*
  tympanic membrane H73.9 ☑
    atrophy — *see* Atrophy, tympanic membrane
    infection — *see* Myringitis
    perforation — *see* Perforation, tympanum
    specified NEC H73.89 ☑
  unsocialized aggressive F91.1
  urea cycle metabolism E72.20
    argininemia E72.21
    arginosuccinic aciduria E72.22
    citrullinemia E72.23
    ornithine transcarbamylase deficiency E72.4
    other specified E72.29
  ureter (in) N28.9
    schistosomiasis B65.0 *[N29]*
    tuberculosis A18.11
  urethra N36.9
    specified NEC N36.8
  urinary system N39.9
    specified NEC N39.8
  valve, heart
    aortic — *see* Endocarditis, aortic
    mitral — *see* Endocarditis, mitral
    pulmonary — *see* Endocarditis, pulmonary
    rheumatic
      aortic — *see* Endocarditis, aortic, rheumatic
      mitral — *see* Endocarditis, mitral
      pulmonary — *see* Endocarditis, pulmonary, rheumatic
      tricuspid — *see* Endocarditis, tricuspid
    tricuspid — *see* Endocarditis, tricuspid
  vestibular function H81.9 ☑
    specified NEC — *see* subcategory H81.8
    in diseases classified elsewhere H82. ☑
    vertigo — *see* Vertigo
  vision, binocular H53.30
    abnormal retinal correspondence H53.31
    diplopia H53.2
    fusion with defective stereopsis H53.32
    simultaneous perception H53.33
    suppression H53.34
  visual
    cortex
      blindness H47.619
        left brain H47.612
        right brain H47.611
      due to
        inflammatory disorder H47.629
          left brain H47.622
          right brain H47.621
        neoplasm H47.639
          left brain H47.632
          right brain H47.631
        vascular disorder H47.649
          left brain H47.642
          right brain H47.641
    pathway H47.9
      due to
        inflammatory disorder H47.51 ☑
        neoplasm H47.52 ☑
        vascular disorder H47.53 ☑
      optic chiasm — *see* Disorder, optic, chiasm
  vitreous body H43.9
    crystalline deposits — *see* Deposit, crystalline
    degeneration — *see* Degeneration, vitreous
    hemorrhage — *see* Hemorrhage, vitreous
    opacities — *see* Opacity, vitreous
    prolapse — *see* Prolapse, vitreous
    specified type NEC H43.89
  voice R49.9
    specified type NEC R49.8
  volatile solvent use
    due to drug abuse — *see* Abuse, drug, inhalant
    due to drug dependence — *see* Dependence, drug, inhalant
  voyeuristic F65.3
  white blood cells D72.9
    specified NEC D72.89
  withdrawing, child or adolescent F40.10
Disorientation R41.0
Displacement, displaced
  acquired traumatic of bone, cartilage, joint, tendon NEC — *see* Dislocation
  adrenal gland (congenital) Q89.1
  appendix, retrocecal (congenital) Q43.8
  auricle (congenital) Q17.4
  bladder (acquired) N32.89
    congenital Q64.19
  brachial plexus (congenital) Q07.8
  brain stem, caudal (congenital) Q04.8
  canaliculus (lacrimalis), congenital Q10.6

Displacement — *continued*
  cardia through esophageal hiatus (congenital) Q40.1
  cerebellum, caudal (congenital) Q04.8
  cervix — *see* Malposition, uterus
  colon (congenital) Q43.3
  device, implant or graft (*see also* Complications, by site and type, mechanical) T85.628 ☑
    arterial graft NEC — *see* Complication, cardiovascular device, mechanical, vascular
    breast (implant) T85.42 ☑
    catheter NEC T85.628 ☑
      dialysis (renal) T82.42 ☑
        intraperitoneal T85.621 ☑
      infusion NEC T82.524 ☑
        spinal (epidural) (subdural) T85.620 ☑
      urinary
        cystostomy T83.020 ☑
        Hopkins T83.028 ☑
        ileostomy T83.028 ☑
        indwelling T83.021 ☑
        nephrostomy T83.022 ☑
        specified NEC T83.028 ☑
        urostomy T83.028 ☑
    electronic (electrode) (pulse generator) (stimulator) — *see* Complication, electronic stimulator
    fixation, internal (orthopedic) NEC — *see* Complication, fixation device, mechanical
    gastrointestinal — *see* Complications, prosthetic device, mechanical, gastrointestinal device
    genital NEC T83.428 ☑
      intrauterine contraceptive device (string) T83.32 ☑
      penile prosthesis (cylinder) (implanted) (pump) (reservoir) T83.420 ☑
      testicular prosthesis T83.421 ☑
    heart NEC — *see* Complication, cardiovascular device, mechanical
    joint prosthesis — *see* Complications, joint prosthesis, mechanical
    ocular — *see* Complications, prosthetic device, mechanical, ocular device
    orthopedic NEC — *see* Complication, orthopedic, device or graft, mechanical
    specified NEC T85.628 ☑
    urinary NEC T83.128 ☑
      graft T83.22 ☑
      sphincter, implanted T83.121 ☑
      stent (ileal conduit) (nephroureteral) T83.123 ☑
      ureteral indwelling T83.122 ☑
    vascular NEC — *see* Complication, cardiovascular device, mechanical
    ventricular intracranial shunt T85.02 ☑
  electronic stimulator
    bone T84.320 ☑
    cardiac — *see* Complications, cardiac device, electronic
    nervous system — *see* Complication, prosthetic device, mechanical, electronic nervous system stimulator
    urinary — *see* Complications, electronic stimulator, urinary
  esophageal mucosa into cardia of stomach, congenital Q39.8
  esophagus (acquired) K22.8
    congenital Q39.8
  eyeball (acquired) (lateral) (old) — *see* Displacement, globe
    congenital Q15.8
    current — *see* Avulsion, eye
  fallopian tube (acquired) N83.4 ☑
    congenital Q50.6
    opening (congenital) Q50.6
  gallbladder (congenital) Q44.1
  gastric mucosa (congenital) Q40.2
  globe (acquired) (old) (lateral) H05.21 ☑
    current — *see* Avulsion, eye
  heart (congenital) Q24.8
    acquired I51.89
  hymen (upward) (congenital) Q52.4
  intervertebral disc NEC
    with myelopathy — *see* Disorder, disc, with, myelopathy
    cervical, cervicothoracic (with) M50.20
      myelopathy — *see* Disorder, disc, cervical, with myelopathy
      neuritis, radiculitis or radiculopathy — *see* Disorder, disc, cervical, with neuritis
    due to trauma — *see* Dislocation, vertebra

Displacement — *continued*
  intervertebral disc NEC — *continued*
    lumbar region M51.26
      with
        myelopathy M51.06
        neuritis, radiculitis, radiculopathy or sciatica M51.16
    lumbosacral region M51.27
      with
        neuritis, radiculitis, radiculopathy or sciatica M51.17
    sacrococcygeal region M53.3
    thoracic region M51.24
      with
        myelopathy M51.04
        neuritis, radiculitis, radiculopathy M51.14
    thoracolumbar region M51.25
      with
        myelopathy M51.05
        neuritis, radiculitis, radiculopathy M51.15
  intrauterine device (string) T83.32 ☑
  kidney (acquired) N28.83
    congenital Q63.2
  lachrymal, lacrimal apparatus or duct (congenital) Q10.6
  lens, congenital Q12.1
  macula (congenital) Q14.1
  Meckel's diverticulum Q43.0
    malignant — *see* Table of Neoplasms, small intestine, malignant
  nail (congenital) Q84.6
    acquired L60.8
  opening of Wharton's duct in mouth Q38.4
  organ or site, congenital NEC — *see* Malposition, congenital
  ovary (acquired) N83.4 ☑
    congenital Q50.39
    free in peritoneal cavity (congenital) Q50.39
    into hernial sac N83.4 ☑
  oviduct (acquired) N83.4 ☑
    congenital Q50.6
  parathyroid (gland) E21.4
  parotid gland (congenital) Q38.4
  punctum lacrimale (congenital) Q10.6
  sacro-iliac (joint) (congenital) Q74.2
    current injury S33.2 ☑
    old — *see* subcategory M53.2
  salivary gland (any) (congenital) Q38.4
  spleen (congenital) Q89.09
  stomach, congenital Q40.2
  sublingual duct Q38.4
  tongue (downward) (congenital) Q38.3
  tooth, teeth, fully erupted M26.30
    horizontal M26.33
    vertical M26.34
  trachea (congenital) Q32.1
  ureter or ureteric opening or orifice (congenital) Q62.62
  uterine opening of oviducts or fallopian tubes Q50.6
  uterus, uterine — *see* Malposition, uterus
  ventricular septum Q21.0
    with rudimentary ventricle Q20.4
Disproportion
  between native and reconstructed breast N65.1
  fiber-type G71.2
Disruptio uteri — *see* Rupture, uterus
Disruption (of)
  ciliary body NEC H21.89
  closure of
    cornea T81.31 ☑
    craniotomy T81.32 ☑
    fascia (muscular) (superficial) T81.32 ☑
    internal organ or tissue T81.32 ☑
    laceration (external) (internal) T81.33 ☑
    ligament T81.32 ☑
    mucosa T81.31 ☑
    muscle or muscle flap T81.32 ☑
    ribs or rib cage T81.32 ☑
    skin and subcutaneous tissue (full-thickness) (superficial) T81.31 ☑
    skull T81.32 ☑
    sternum (sternotomy) T81.32 ☑
    tendon T81.32 ☑
    traumatic laceration (external) (internal) T81.33 ☑
  family Z63.8
    due to
      absence of family member due to military deployment Z63.31
      absence of family member NEC Z63.32

☑ **Additional character required**

Disruption — *continued*
  family — *continued*
    alcoholism and drug addiction in
      family Z63.72
    bereavement Z63.4
    death (assumed) or disappearance of family
      member Z63.4
    divorce or separation Z63.5
    drug addiction in family Z63.72
    return of family member from military
      deployment (current or past
      conflict) Z63.71
    stressful life events NEC Z63.79
  iris NEC H21.89
  ligament (s) (*see also* Sprain)
    knee
      current injury — *see* Dislocation, knee
      old (chronic) — *see* Derangement, knee,
        ligament, instability, chronic
      spontaneous NEC — *see* Derangement, knee,
        disruption ligament
  ossicular chain — *see* Discontinuity, ossicles, ear
  pelvic ring (stable) S32.810 ☑
    unstable S32.811 ☑
  wound T81.30 ☑
    episiotomy O90.1
    operation T81.31 ☑
      cesarean O90.0
      external operation wound
        (superficial) T81.31 ☑
      internal operation wound (deep) T81.32 ☑
    perineal (obstetric) O90.1
    traumatic injury repair T81.33 ☑
    traumatic injury wound repair T81.33 ☑
Dissatisfaction with
  employment Z56.9
  school environment Z55.4
Dissecting — *see* condition
Dissection
  aorta I71.00
    abdominal I71.02
    thoracic I71.01
    thoracoabdominal I71.03
  artery I77.70
    basilar (trunk) I77.75
    carotid I77.71
    cerebral (nonruptured) I67.0
      ruptured — *see* Hemorrhage, intracranial,
        subarachnoid
    coronary I25.42
    extremity
      lower I77.77
      upper I77.76
    iliac I77.72
    precerebral
      congenital (nonruptured) Q28.1
      specified site NEC I77.75
    renal I77.73
    specified NEC I77.79
    vertebral I77.74
  precerbral artery, congential (nonruptured) Q28.1
  Heartland A93.8
  traumatic — *see* Wound, open, by site
  vascular I99.8
  wound — *see* Wound, open
Disseminated — *see* condition
Dissociation
  auriculoventricular or atrioventricular (AV) (any
    degree) (isorhythmic) I45.89
    with heart block I44.2
  interference I45.89
Dissociative reaction, state F44.9
Dissolution, vertebra — *see* Osteoporosis
Distension, distention
  abdomen R14.0
  bladder N32.89
  cecum K63.89
  colon K63.89
  gallbladder K82.8
  intestine K63.89
  kidney N28.89
  liver K76.89
  seminal vesicle N50.89
  stomach K31.89
    acute K31.0
    psychogenic F45.8
  ureter — *see* Dilatation, ureter
  uterus N85.8
Distoma hepaticum infestation B66.3
Distomiasis B66.9
  bile passages B66.3
  hemic B65.9

Distomiasis — *continued*
  hepatic B66.3
    due to Clonorchis sinensis B66.1
  intestinal B66.5
  liver B66.3
    due to Clonorchis sinensis B66.1
  lung B66.4
  pulmonary B66.4
Distomolar (fourth molar) K00.1
Disto-occlusion (Division I) (Division II) M26.212
Distortion (s) (congenital)
  adrenal (gland) Q89.1
  arm NEC Q68.8
  bile duct or passage Q44.5
  bladder Q64.79
  brain Q04.9
  cervix (uteri) Q51.9
  chest (wall) Q67.8
    bones Q76.8
  clavicle Q74.0
  clitoris Q52.6
  coccyx Q76.49
  common duct Q44.5
  coronary Q24.5
  cystic duct Q44.5
  ear (auricle) (external) Q17.3
    inner Q16.5
    middle Q16.4
      ossicles Q16.3
  endocrine NEC Q89.2
  eustachian tube Q17.8
  eye (adnexa) Q15.8
  face bone (s) NEC Q75.8
  fallopian tube Q50.6
  femur NEC Q68.8
  fibula NEC Q68.8
  finger (s) Q68.1
  foot Q66.9
  genitalia, genital organ (s)
    female Q52.8
      external Q52.79
      internal NEC Q52.8
  gyri Q04.8
  hand bone (s) Q68.1
  heart (auricle) (ventricle) Q24.8
    valve (cusp) Q24.8
  hepatic duct Q44.5
  humerus NEC Q68.8
  hymen Q52.4
  intrafamilial communications Z63.8
  jaw NEC M26.89
  labium (majus) (minus) Q52.79
  leg NEC Q68.8
  lens Q12.8
  liver Q44.7
  lumbar spine Q76.49
    with disproportion O33.8
      causing obstructed labor O65.0
  lumbosacral (joint) (region) Q76.49
    kyphosis — *see* Kyphosis, congenital
    lordosis — *see* Lordosis, congenital
  nerve Q07.8
  nose Q30.8
  organ
    of Corti Q16.5
    or site not listed — *see* Anomaly, by site
  ossicles, ear Q16.3
  oviduct Q50.6
  pancreas Q45.3
  parathyroid (gland) Q89.2
  pituitary (gland) Q89.2
  radius NEC Q68.8
  sacroiliac joint Q74.2
  sacrum Q76.49
  scapula Q74.0
  shoulder girdle Q74.0
  skull bone (s) NEC Q75.8
    with
      anencephalus Q00.0
      encephalocele — *see* Encephalocele
      hydrocephalus Q03.9
        with spina bifida — *see* Spina bifida, with
          hydrocephalus
      microcephaly Q02
  spinal cord Q06.8
  spine Q76.49
    kyphosis — *see* Kyphosis, congenital
    lordosis — *see* Lordosis, congenital
  spleen Q89.09
  sternum NEC Q76.7
  thorax (wall) Q67.8
    bony Q76.8
  thymus (gland) Q89.2

Distortion — *continued*
  thyroid (gland) Q89.2
  tibia NEC Q68.8
  toe (s) Q66.9
  tongue Q38.3
  trachea (cartilage) Q32.1
  ulna NEC Q68.8
  ureter Q62.8
  urethra Q64.79
    causing obstruction Q64.39
  uterus Q51.9
  vagina Q52.4
  vertebra Q76.49
    kyphosis — *see* Kyphosis, congenital
    lordosis — *see* Lordosis, congenital
  visual (*see also* Disturbance, vision)
    shape and size H53.15
  vulva Q52.79
  wrist (bones) (joint) Q68.8
Distress
  abdomen — *see* Pain, abdominal
  acute respiratory R06.03
    syndrome (adult) (child) J80
  epigastric R10.13
  fetal P84
    complicating pregnancy — *see* Stress, fetal
  gastrointestinal (functional) K30
    psychogenic F45.8
  intestinal (functional) NOS K59.9
    psychogenic F45.8
  maternal, during labor and delivery O75.0
  relationship, with spouse or intimate partner Z63.0
  respiratory (adult) (child) R06.03
    newborn P22.9
      specified NEC P22.8
    orthopnea R06.01
    psychogenic F45.8
    shortness of breath R06.02
    specified type NEC R06.09
Distribution vessel, atypical Q27.9
  coronary artery Q24.5
  precerebral Q28.1
Districhiasis L68.8
Disturbance (s) (*see also* Disease)
  absorption K90.9
    calcium E58
    carbohydrate K90.49
    fat K90.49
      pancreatic K90.3
    protein K90.49
    starch K90.49
    vitamin — *see* Deficiency, vitamin
  acid-base equilibrium E87.8
    mixed E87.4
  activity and attention (with hyperkinesis) — *see*
    Disorder, attention-deficit hyperactivity
  amino acid transport E72.00
  assimilation, food K90.9
  auditory nerve, except deafness — *see*
    subcategory H93.3
  behavior — *see* Disorder, conduct
  blood clotting (mechanism) (*see also* Defect,
    coagulation) D68.9
  cerebral
    nerve — *see* Disorder, nerve, cranial
    status, newborn P91.9
      specified NEC P91.88
  circulatory I99.9
  conduct (*see also* Disorder, conduct) F91.9
    adjustment reaction — *see* Disorder,
      adjustment
    compulsive F63.9
    disruptive F91.9
    hyperkinetic — *see* Disorder, attention-deficit
      hyperactivity
    socialized F91.2
    specified NEC F91.8
    unsocialized F91.1
  coordination R27.8
  cranial nerve — *see* Disorder, nerve, cranial
  deep sensibility — *see* Disturbance, sensation
  digestive K30
    psychogenic F45.8
  electrolyte (*see also* Imbalance, electrolyte)
    newborn, transitory P74.4
      hyperammonemia P74.6
      potassium balance P74.3
      sodium balance P74.2
      specified type NEC P74.4
  emotions specific to childhood and
    adolescence F93.9
    with

Disturbance — *continued*
- emotions specific — *continued*
  - anxiety and fearfulness NEC F93.8
  - elective mutism F94.0
  - oppositional disorder F91.3
  - sensitivity (withdrawal) F40.10
  - shyness F40.10
  - social withdrawal F40.10
  - involving relationship problems F93.8
  - mixed F93.8
  - specified NEC F93.8
- endocrine (gland) E34.9
  - neonatal, transitory P72.9
  - specified NEC P72.8
- equilibrium R42
- fructose metabolism E74.10
- gait — *see* Gait
  - hysterical F44.4
  - psychogenic F44.4
- gastrointestinal (functional) K30
  - psychogenic F45.8
- habit, child F98.9
- hearing, except deafness and tinnitus — *see* Abnormal, auditory perception
- heart, functional (conditions in I44-I50)
  - due to presence of (cardiac) prosthesis I97.19 ☑
  - postoperative I97.89
    - cardiac surgery (*see also* Infarct, myocardium, associated with revascularization procedure) I97.19 ☑
- hormones E34.9
- innervation uterus (parasympathetic) (sympathetic) N85.8
- keratinization NEC
  - gingiva K05.10
    - nonplaque induced K05.11
    - plaque induced K05.10
  - lip K13.0
  - oral (mucosa) (soft tissue) K13.29
  - tongue K13.29
- learning (specific) — *see* Disorder, learning
- memory — *see* Amnesia
  - mild, following organic brain damage F06.8
- mental F99
  - associated with diseases classified elsewhere F54
- metabolism E88.9
  - with
    - abortion — *see* Abortion, by type with other specified complication
    - ectopic pregnancy O08.5
    - molar pregnancy O08.5
  - amino-acid E72.9
    - aromatic E70.9
    - branched-chain E71.2
    - straight-chain E72.8
    - sulfur-bearing E72.10
  - ammonia E72.20
  - arginine E72.21
  - arginosuccinic acid E72.22
  - carbohydrate E74.9
  - cholesterol E78.9
  - citrulline E72.23
  - cystathionine E72.19
  - general E88.9
  - glutamine E72.8
  - histidine E70.40
  - homocystine E72.19
  - hydroxylysine E72.3
  - in labor or delivery O75.89
  - iron E83.10
  - lipoid E78.9
  - lysine E72.3
  - methionine E72.19
  - neonatal, transitory P74.9
    - calcium and magnesium P71.9
      - specified type NEC P71.8
    - carbohydrate metabolism P70.9
      - specified type NEC P70.8
    - specified NEC P74.8
  - ornithine E72.4
  - phosphate E83.39
  - sodium NEC E87.8
  - threonine E72.8
  - tryptophan E70.5
  - tyrosine E70.20
  - urea cycle E72.20
- motor R29.2
- nervous, functional R45.0
- neuromuscular mechanism (eye), due to syphilis A52.15
- nutritional E63.9
  - nail L60.3

Disturbance — *continued*
- ocular motion H51.9
  - psychogenic F45.8
- oculogyric H51.8
  - psychogenic F45.8
- oculomotor H51.9
  - psychogenic F45.8
- olfactory nerve R43.1
- optic nerve NEC — *see* Disorder, nerve, optic
- oral epithelium, including tongue NEC K13.29
- perceptual due to
  - alcohol withdrawal F10.232
  - amphetamine intoxication F15.922
    - in
      - abuse F15.122
      - dependence F15.222
  - anxiolytic withdrawal F13.232
  - cannabis intoxication (acute) F12.922
    - in
      - abuse F12.122
      - dependence F12.222
  - cocaine intoxication (acute) F14.922
    - in
      - abuse F14.122
      - dependence F14.222
  - hypnotic withdrawal F13.232
  - opioid intoxication (acute) F11.922
    - in
      - abuse F11.122
      - dependence F11.222
  - phencyclidine intoxication (acute) F16.122
  - sedative withdrawal F13.232
- personality (pattern) (trait) (*see also* Disorder, personality) F60.9
  - following organic brain damage F07.9
- polyglandular E31.9
  - specified NEC E31.8
- potassium balance, newborn P74.3
- psychogenic F45.9
- psychomotor F44.4
- psychophysical visual H53.16
- pupillary — *see* Anomaly, pupil, function
- reflex R29.2
- rhythm, heart I49.9
- salivary secretion K11.7
- sensation (cold) (heat) (localization) (tactile discrimination) (texture) (vibratory) NEC R20.9
  - hysterical F44.6
  - skin R20.9
    - anesthesia R20.0
    - hyperesthesia R20.3
    - hypoesthesia R20.1
    - paresthesia R20.2
    - specified type NEC R20.8
  - smell R43.9
    - and taste (mixed) R43.8
    - anosmia R43.0
    - parosmia R43.1
    - specified NEC R43.8
  - taste R43.9
    - and smell (mixed) R43.8
    - parageusia R43.2
    - specified NEC R43.8
- sensory — *see* Disturbance, sensation
- situational (transient) (*see also* Disorder, adjustment)
  - acute F43.0
- sleep G47.9
  - nonorganic origin F51.9
- smell — *see* Disturbance, sensation, smell
- sociopathic F60.2
- sodium balance, newborn P74.2
- speech R47.9
  - developmental F80.9
  - specified NEC R47.89
- stomach (functional) K31.9
- sympathetic (nerve) G90.9
- taste — *see* Disturbance, sensation, taste
- temperature
  - regulation, newborn P81.9
    - specified NEC P81.8
  - sense R20.8
    - hysterical F44.6
- tooth
  - eruption K00.6
  - formation K00.4
  - structure, hereditary NEC K00.5
- touch — *see* Disturbance, sensation
- vascular I99.9
  - arteriosclerotic — *see* Arteriosclerosis
- vasomotor I73.9

Disturbance — *continued*
- vasospastic I73.9
- vision, visual H53.9
  - following
    - cerebral infarction I69.398
    - cerebrovascular disease I69.998
      - specified NEC I69.898
    - intracerebral hemorrhage I69.198
    - nontraumatic intracranial hemorrhage NEC I69.098
    - specified disease NEC I69.898
    - subarachnoid hemorrhage I69.098
  - psychophysical H53.16
  - specified NEC H53.8
  - subjective H53.10
    - day blindness H53.11
    - discomfort H53.14 ☑
    - distortions of shape and size H53.15
    - loss
      - sudden H53.13 ☑
      - transient H53.12 ☑
    - specified type NEC H53.19
- voice R49.9
  - psychogenic F44.4
  - specified NEC R49.8

Diuresis R35.8
Diver's palsy, paralysis or squeeze T70.3 ☑
Diverticulitis (acute) K57.92
- bladder — *see* Cystitis
- ileum — *see* Diverticulitis, intestine, small
- intestine K57.92
  - with
    - abscess, perforation or peritonitis K57.80
      - with bleeding K57.81
    - bleeding K57.93
  - congenital Q43.8
  - large K57.32
    - with
      - abscess, perforation or peritonitis K57.20
        - with bleeding K57.21
      - bleeding K57.33
      - small intestine K57.52
        - with
          - abscess, perforation or peritonitis K57.40
            - with bleeding K57.41
          - bleeding K57.53
  - small K57.12
    - with
      - abscess, perforation or peritonitis K57.00
        - with bleeding K57.01
      - bleeding K57.13
      - large intestine K57.52
        - with
          - abscess, perforation or peritonitis K57.40
            - with bleeding K57.41
          - bleeding K57.53

Diverticulosis K57.90
- with bleeding K57.91
- large intestine K57.30
  - with
    - bleeding K57.31
    - small intestine K57.50
      - with bleeding K57.51
- small intestine K57.10
  - with
    - bleeding K57.11
    - large intestine K57.50
      - with bleeding K57.51

Diverticulum, diverticula (multiple) K57.90
- appendix (noninflammatory) K38.2
- bladder (sphincter) N32.3
  - congenital Q64.6
- bronchus (congenital) Q32.4
  - acquired J98.09
- calyx, calyceal (kidney) N28.89
- cardia (stomach) K31.4
- cecum — *see* Diverticulosis, intestine, large
  - congenital Q43.8
- colon — *see* Diverticulosis, intestine, large
  - congenital Q43.8
- duodenum — *see* Diverticulosis, intestine, small
  - congenital Q43.8
- epiphrenic (esophagus) K22.5
- esophagus (congenital) Q39.6
  - acquired (epiphrenic) (pulsion) (traction) K22.5
- eustachian tube — *see* Disorder, eustachian tube, specified NEC
- fallopian tube N83.8
- gastric K31.4
- heart (congenital) Q24.8

Disturbance - Diverticulum

ICD-10-CM INDEX TO DISEASES AND INJURIES

Diverticulum — *continued*
ileum — *see* Diverticulosis, intestine, small
jejunum — *see* Diverticulosis, intestine, small
kidney (pelvis) (calyces) N28.89
with calculus — *see* Calculus, kidney
Meckel's (displaced) (hypertrophic) Q43.0
malignant — *see* Table of Neoplasms, small
intestine, malignant
midthoracic K22.5
organ or site, congenital NEC — *see* Distortion
pericardium (congenital) (cyst) Q24.8
acquired I31.8
pharyngoesophageal (congenital) Q39.6
acquired K22.5
pharynx (congenital) Q38.7
rectosigmoid — *see* Diverticulosis, intestine, large
congenital Q43.8
rectum — *see* Diverticulosis, intestine, large
Rokitansky's K22.5
seminal vesicle N50.89
sigmoid — *see* Diverticulosis, intestine, large
congenital Q43.8
stomach (acquired) K31.4
congenital Q40.2
trachea (acquired) J39.8
ureter (acquired) N28.89
congenital Q62.8
ureterovesical orifice N28.89
urethra (acquired) N36.1
congenital Q64.79
ventricle, left (congenital) Q24.8
vesical N32.3
congenital Q64.6
Zenker's (esophagus) K22.5
Division
cervix uteri (acquired) N88.8
glans penis Q55.69
labia minora (congenital) Q52.79
ligament (partial or complete) (current) (*see also*
Sprain)
with open wound — *see* Wound, open
muscle (partial or complete) (current) (*see also*
Injury, muscle)
with open wound — *see* Wound, open
nerve (traumatic) — *see* Injury, nerve
spinal cord — *see* Injury, spinal cord, by region
vein I87.8
Divorce, causing family disruption Z63.5
Dix-Hallpike neurolabyrinthitis — *see* Neuronitis,
vestibular
Dizziness R42
hysterical F44.89
psychogenic F45.8
DMAC (disseminated mycobacterium avium-
intracellulare complex) A31.2
DNR (do not resuscitate) Z66
Doan-Wiseman syndrome (primary splenic
neutropenia) — *see* Agranulocytosis
Doehle-Heller aortitis A52.02
Dog bite — *see* Bite
Dohle body panmyelopathic syndrome D72.0
Dolichocephaly Q67.2
Dolichocolon Q43.8
Dolichostenomelia — *see* Syndrome, Marfan's
Donohue's syndrome E34.8
Donor (organ or tissue) Z52.9
blood (whole) Z52.000
autologous Z52.010
specified component (lymphocytes) (platelets)
NEC Z52.008
autologous Z52.018
specified donor NEC Z52.098
specified donor NEC Z52.090
stem cells Z52.001
autologous Z52.011
specified donor NEC Z52.091
bone Z52.20
autologous Z52.21
marrow Z52.3
specified type NEC Z52.29
cornea Z52.5
egg (Oocyte) Z52.819
age 35 and over Z52.812
anonymous recipient Z52.812
designated recipient Z52.813
under age 35 Z52.810
anonymous recipient Z52.810
designated recipient Z52.811
kidney Z52.4
liver Z52.6
lung Z52.89

Donor — *continued*
lymphocyte — *see* Donor, blood, specified
components NEC
Oocyte — *see* Donor, egg
platelets Z52.008
potential, examination of Z00.5
semen Z52.89
skin Z52.10
autologous Z52.11
specified type NEC Z52.19
specified organ or tissue NEC Z52.89
sperm Z52.89
Donovanosis A58
Dorsalgia M54.9
psychogenic F45.41
specified NEC M54.89
Dorsopathy M53.9
deforming M43.9
specified NEC — *see* subcategory M43.8
specified NEC M53.80
cervical region M53.82
cervicothoracic region M53.83
lumbar region M53.86
lumbosacral region M53.87
occipito-atlanto-axial region M53.81
sacrococcygeal region M53.88
thoracic region M53.84
thoracolumbar region M53.85
Double
albumin E88.09
aortic arch Q25.45
auditory canal Q17.8
auricle (heart) Q20.8
bladder Q64.79
cervix Q51.820
with doubling of uterus (and vagina) Q51.10
with obstruction Q51.11
inlet ventricle Q20.4
kidney with double pelvis (renal) Q63.0
meatus urinarius Q64.75
monster Q89.4
outlet
left ventricle Q20.2
right ventricle Q20.1
pelvis (renal) with double ureter Q62.5
tongue Q38.3
ureter (one or both sides) Q62.5
with double pelvis (renal) Q62.5
urethra Q64.74
urinary meatus Q64.75
uterus Q51.2
with
doubling of cervix (and vagina) Q51.10
with obstruction Q51.11
in pregnancy or childbirth O34.59 ☑
causing obstructed labor O65.5
vagina Q52.10
with doubling of uterus (and cervix) Q51.10
with obstruction Q51.11
vision H53.2
vulva Q52.79
Douglas' pouch, cul-de-sac — *see* condition
Down syndrome Q90.9
meiotic nondisjunction Q90.0
mitotic nondisjunction Q90.1
mosaicism Q90.1
translocation Q90.2
DPD (dihydropyrimidine dehydrogenase deficiency)
E88.89
Dracontiasis B72
Dracunculiasis, dracunculosis B72
Dream state, hysterical F44.89
Dreschlera (hawaiiensis) (infection) B43.8
Drepanocytic anemia — *see* Disease, sickle-cell
Dresbach's syndrome (elliptocytosis) D58.1
Dressler's syndrome I24.1
Drift, ulnar — *see* Deformity, limb, specified type
NEC, forearm
Drinking (alcohol)
excessive, to excess NEC (without
dependence) F10.10
habitual (continual) (without remission) F10.20
with remission F10.21
Drip, postnasal (chronic) R09.82
due to
allergic rhinitis — *see* Rhinitis, allergic
common cold J00
gastroesophageal reflux — *see* Reflux,
gastroesophageal
nasopharyngitis — *see* Nasopharyngitis
other know condition - code to condition
sinusitis — *see* Sinusitis

Droop
facial R29.810
cerebrovascular disease I69.992
cerebral infarction I69.392
intracerebral hemorrhage I69.192
nontraumatic intracranial hemorrhage
NEC I69.292
specified disease NEC I69.892
subarachnoid hemorrhage I69.092
Drop (in)
attack NEC R55
finger — *see* Deformity, finger
foot — *see* Deformity, limb, foot, drop
hematocrit (precipitous) R71.0
hemoglobin R71.0
toe — *see* Deformity, toe, specified NEC
wrist — *see* Deformity, limb, wrist drop
Dropped heart beats I45.9
Dropsy, dropsical (*see also* Hydrops)
abdomen R18.8
brain — *see* Hydrocephalus
cardiac, heart — *see* Failure, heart, congestive
gangrenous — *see* Gangrene
heart — *see* Failure, heart, congestive
kidney — *see* Nephrosis
lung — *see* Edema, lung
newborn due to isoimmunization P56.0
pericardium — *see* Pericarditis
Drowned, drowning (near) T75.1 ☑
Drowsiness R40.0
Drug
abuse counseling and surveillance Z71.51
addiction — *see* Dependence
dependence — *see* Dependence
habit — *see* Dependence
harmful use — *see* Abuse, drug
induced fever R50.2
overdose — *see* Table of Drugs and Chemicals, by
drug, poisoning
poisoning — *see* Table of Drugs and Chemicals,
by drug, poisoning
resistant organism infection (*see also* Resistant,
organism, to, drug) Z16.30
therapy
long term (current) (prophylactic) — *see*
Therapy, drug long-term (current)
(prophylactic)
short term - omit code
wrong substance given or taken in error — *see*
Table of Drugs and Chemicals, by drug,
poisoning
Drunkenness (without dependence) F10.129
acute in alcoholism F10.229
chronic (without remission) F10.20
with remission F10.21
pathological (without dependence) F10.129
with dependence F10.229
sleep F51.9
Drusen
macula (degenerative) (retina) — *see*
Degeneration, macula, drusen
optic disc H47.32 ☑
Dry, dryness (*see also* condition)
larynx J38.7
mouth R68.2
due to dehydration E86.0
nose J34.89
socket (teeth) M27.3
throat J39.2
DSAP L56.5
Duane's syndrome H50.81 ☑
Dubin-Johnson disease or syndrome E80.6
Dubois' disease (thymus gland) A50.59 *[E35]*
Dubowitz' syndrome Q87.1
Duchenne-Aran muscular atrophy G12.21
Duchenne-Griesinger disease G71.0
Duchenne's
disease or syndrome
motor neuron disease G12.22
muscular dystrophy G71.0
locomotor ataxia (syphilitic) A52.11
paralysis
birth injury P14.0
due to or associated with
motor neuron disease G12.22
muscular dystrophy G71.0
Ducrey's chancre A57
Duct, ductus — *see* condition
Duhring's disease (dermatitis herpetiformis) L13.0
Dullness, cardiac (decreased) (increased) R01.2
Dumb ague — *see* Malaria
Dumbness — *see* Aphasia

Dumdum - Dysfunction

Dumdum fever B55.0
Dumping syndrome (postgastrectomy) K91.1
Duodenitis (nonspecific) (peptic) K29.80
   with bleeding K29.81
Duodenocholangitis — see Cholangitis
Duodenum, duodenal — see condition
Duplay's bursitis or periarthritis — see Tendinitis, calcific, shoulder
Duplication, duplex (see also Accessory)
   alimentary tract Q45.8
   anus Q43.4
   appendix (and cecum) Q43.4
   biliary duct (any) Q44.5
   bladder Q64.79
   cecum (and appendix) Q43.4
   cervix Q51.820
   chromosome NEC
     with complex rearrangements NEC Q92.5
     seen only at prometaphase Q92.8
   cystic duct Q44.5
   digestive organs Q45.8
   esophagus Q39.8
   frontonasal process Q75.8
   intestine (large) (small) Q43.4
   kidney Q63.0
   liver Q44.7
   pancreas Q45.3
   penis Q55.69
   respiratory organs NEC Q34.8
   salivary duct Q38.4
   spinal cord (incomplete) Q06.2
   stomach Q40.2
Dupré's disease (meningism) R29.1
Dupuytren's contraction or disease M72.0
Durand-Nicolas-Favre disease A55
Durotomy (inadvertent) (incidental) G97.41
Duroziez's disease (congenital mitral stenosis) Q23.2
Dutton's relapsing fever (West African) A68.1
Dwarfism E34.3
   achondroplastic Q77.4
   congenital E34.3
   constitutional E34.3
   hypochondroplastic Q77.4
   hypophyseal E23.0
   infantile E34.3
   Laron-type E34.3
   Lorain (-Levi) type E23.0
   metatropic Q77.8
   nephrotic-glycosuric (with hypophosphatemic rickets) E72.09
   nutritional E45
   pancreatic K86.89
   pituitary E23.0
   renal N25.0
   thanatophoric Q77.1
Dyke-Young anemia (secondary) (symptomatic) D59.1
Dysacusis — see Abnormal, auditory perception
Dysadrenocortism E27.9
   hyperfunction E27.0
Dysarthria R47.1
   following
     cerebral infarction I69.322
     cerebrovascular disease I69.922
       specified disease NEC I69.822
     intracerebral hemorrhage I69.122
     nontraumatic intracranial hemorrhage NEC I69.222
     subarachnoid hemorrhage I69.022
Dysautonomia (familial) G90.1
Dysbarism T70.3 ☑
Dysbasia R26.2
   angiosclerotica intermittens I73.9
   hysterical F44.4
   lordotica (progressiva) G24.1
   nonorganic origin F44.4
   psychogenic F44.4
Dysbetalipoproteinemia (familial) E78.2
Dyscalculia R48.8
   developmental F81.2
Dyschezia K59.00
Dyschondroplasia (with hemangiomata) Q78.4
Dyschromia (skin) L81.9
Dyscollagenosis M35.9
Dyscranio-pygo-phalangy Q87.0
Dyscrasia
   blood (with) D75.9
     antepartum hemorrhage — see Hemorrhage, antepartum, with coagulation defect
     newborn P61.9
       specified type NEC P61.8
     intrapartum hemorrhage O67.0

Dyscrasia — continued
   blood — continued
     puerperal, postpartum O72.3
     polyglandular, pluriglandular E31.9
Dysendocrinism E34.9
Dysentery, dysenteric (catarrhal) (diarrhea) (epidemic) (hemorrhagic) (infectious) (sporadic) (tropical) A09
   abscess, liver A06.4
   amebic (see also Amebiasis) A06.0
     with abscess — see Abscess, amebic
     acute A06.0
     chronic A06.1
   arthritis (see also category M01) A09
     bacillary (see also category M01) A03.9
   bacillary A03.9
     arthritis (see also category M01) A03.9
     Boyd A03.2
     Flexner A03.1
     Schmitz (-Stutzer) A03.0
     Shiga (-Kruse) A03.0
     Shigella A03.9
       boydii A03.2
       dysenteriae A03.0
       flexneri A03.1
       group A A03.0
       group B A03.1
       group C A03.2
       group D A03.3
       sonnei A03.3
       specified type NEC A03.8
     Sonne A03.3
     specified type NEC A03.8
   balantidial A07.0
   Balantidium coli A07.0
   Boyd's A03.2
   candidal B37.82
   Chilomastix A07.8
   Chinese A03.9
   coccidial A07.3
   Dientamoeba (fragilis) A07.8
   Embadomonas A07.8
   Entamoeba, entamebic — see Dysentery, amebic
   Flexner-Boyd A03.2
   Flexner's A03.1
   Giardia lamblia A07.1
   Hiss-Russell A03.1
   Lamblia A07.1
   leishmanial B55.0
   malarial — see Malaria
   metazoal B82.0
   monilial B37.82
   protozoal A07.9
   Salmonella A02.0
   schistosomal B65.1
   Schmitz (-Stutzer) A03.0
   Shiga (-Kruse) A03.0
   Shigella NOS — see Dysentery, bacillary
   Sonne A03.3
   strongyloidiasis B78.0
   trichomonal A07.8
   viral (see also Enteritis, viral) A08.4
Dysequilibrium R42
Dysesthesia R20.8
   hysterical F44.6
Dysfibrinogenemia (congenital) D68.2
Dysfunction
   adrenal E27.9
     hyperfunction E27.0
   autonomic
     due to alcohol G31.2
     somatoform F45.8
   bladder N31.9
     neurogenic NOS — see Dysfunction, bladder, neuromuscular
     neuromuscular NOS N31.9
       atonic (motor) (sensory) N31.2
       autonomous N31.2
       flaccid N31.2
       nonreflex N31.2
       reflex N31.1
       specified NEC N31.8
       uninhibited N31.0
   bleeding, uterus N93.8
   cerebral G93.89
   colon K59.9
     psychogenic F45.8
   colostomy K94.03
   cystic duct K82.8
   cystostomy (stoma) — see Complications, cystostomy

Dysfunction — continued
   ejaculatory N53.19
     anejaculatory orgasm N53.13
     painful N53.12
     premature F52.4
     retarded N53.11
   endocrine NOS E34.9
   endometrium N85.8
   enterostomy K94.13
   erectile — see Dysfunction, sexual, male, erectile
   gallbladder K82.8
   gastrostomy (stoma) K94.23
   gland, glandular NOS E34.9
   heart I51.89
   hemoglobin D75.89
   hepatic K76.89
   hypophysis E23.7
   hypothalamic NEC E23.3
   ileostomy (stoma) K94.13
   jejunostomy (stoma) K94.13
   kidney — see Disease, renal
   labyrinthine — see subcategory H83.2
   left ventricular, following sudden emotional stress I51.81
   liver K76.89
   male — see Dysfunction, sexual, male
   orgasmic (female) F52.31
     male F52.32
   ovary E28.9
     specified NEC E28.8
   papillary muscle I51.89
   parathyroid E21.4
   physiological NEC R68.89
     psychogenic F59
   pineal gland E34.8
   pituitary (gland) E23.3
   platelets D69.1
   polyglandular E31.9
     specified NEC E31.8
   psychophysiologic F59
   psychosexual F52.9
     with
       dyspareunia F52.6
       premature ejaculation F52.4
       vaginismus F52.5
   pylorus K31.9
   rectum K59.9
     psychogenic F45.8
   reflex (sympathetic) — see Syndrome, pain, complex regional I
   segmental — see Dysfunction, somatic
   senile R54
   sexual (due to) R37
     alcohol F10.981
     amphetamine F15.981
       in
         abuse F15.181
         dependence F15.281
     anxiolytic F13.981
       in
         abuse F13.181
         dependence F13.281
     cocaine F14.981
       in
         abuse F14.181
         dependence F14.281
     excessive sexual drive F52.8
     failure of genital response (male) F52.21
       female F52.22
     female N94.9
       aversion F52.1
       dyspareunia N94.10
         psychogenic F52.6
       frigidity F52.22
       nymphomania F52.8
       orgasmic F52.31
       psychogenic F52.9
         aversion F52.1
         dyspareunia F52.6
         frigidity F52.22
         nymphomania F52.8
         orgasmic F52.31
         vaginismus F52.5
       vaginismus N94.2
         psychogenic F52.5
     hypnotic F13.981
       in
         abuse F13.181
         dependence F13.281
     inhibited orgasm (female) F52.31
       male F52.32
     lack

☑ Additional character required

Dysfunction — *continued*
  sexual — *continued*
    of sexual enjoyment F52.1
    or loss of sexual desire F52.0
    male N53.9
      anejaculatory orgasm N53.13
      ejaculatory N53.19
        painful N53.12
        premature F52.4
        retarded N53.11
      erectile N52.9
        drug induced N52.2
        due to
          disease classified elsewhere N52.1
          drug N52.2
        postoperative (postprocedural) N52.39
          following
            cryotherapy N52.37
            interstitial seed therapy N52.36
            prostate ablative therapy N52.37
            prostatectomy N52.34
              radical N52.31
            radiation therapy N52.35
            radical cystectomy N52.32
            ultrasound ablative therapy N52.37
            urethral surgery N52.33
        psychogenic F52.21
        specified cause NEC N52.8
        vasculogenic
          arterial insufficiency N52.01
            with corporo-venous occlusive N52.03
          corporo-venous occlusive N52.02
            with arterial insufficiency N52.03
      impotence — *see* Dysfunction, sexual, male, erectile
      psychogenic F52.9
        aversion F52.1
        erectile F52.21
        orgasmic F52.32
        premature ejaculation F52.4
        satyriasis F52.8
        specified type NEC F52.8
      specified type NEC N53.8
    nonorganic F52.9
      specified NEC F52.8
    opioid F11.981
      in
        abuse F11.181
        dependence F11.281
    orgasmic dysfunction (female) F52.31
      male F52.32
    premature ejaculation F52.4
    psychoactive substances NEC F19.981
      in
        abuse F19.181
        dependence F19.281
    psychogenic F52.9
    sedative F13.981
      in
        abuse F13.181
        dependence F13.281
    sexual aversion F52.1
    vaginismus (nonorganic) (psychogenic) F52.5
  sinoatrial node I49.5
  somatic M99.09
    abdomen M99.09
    acromioclavicular M99.07
    cervical region M99.01
    cervicothoracic M99.01
    costochondral M99.08
    costovertebral M99.08
    head region M99.00
    hip M99.05
    lower extremity M99.06
    lumbar region M99.03
    lumbosacral M99.03
    occipitocervical M99.00
    pelvic region M99.05
    pubic M99.05
    rib cage M99.08
    sacral region M99.04
    sacrococcygeal M99.04
    sacroiliac M99.04
    specified NEC M99.09
    sternochondral M99.08
    sternoclavicular M99.07
    thoracic region M99.02
    thoracolumbar M99.02
    upper extremity M99.07
  somatoform autonomic F45.8
  stomach K31.89
    psychogenic F45.8

Dysfunction — *continued*
  suprarenal E27.9
    hyperfunction E27.0
  symbolic R48.9
    specified type NEC R48.8
  temporomandibular (joint) M26.69
    joint-pain syndrome M26.62 ☑
  testicular (endocrine) E29.9
    specified NEC E29.8
  thymus E32.9
  thyroid E07.9
  ureterostomy (stoma) — *see* Complications, stoma, urinary tract
  urethrostomy (stoma) — *see* Complications, stoma, urinary tract
  uterus, complicating delivery O62.9
    hypertonic O62.4
    hypotonic O62.2
      primary O62.0
      secondary O62.1
  ventricular I51.9
    with congestive heart failure (*see also* Failure, heart) I50.9
    left, reversible, following sudden emotional stress I51.81
Dysgenesis
  gonadal (due to chromosomal anomaly) Q96.9
    pure Q99.1
  renal Q60.5
    bilateral Q60.4
    unilateral Q60.3
  reticular D72.0
  tidal platelet D69.3
Dysgerminoma
  specified site — *see* Neoplasm, malignant, by site
  unspecified site
    female C56.9
    male C62.90
Dysgeusia R43.2
Dysgraphia R27.8
Dyshidrosis, dysidrosis L30.1
Dyskaryotic cervical smear R87.619
Dyskeratosis L85.8
  cervix — *see* Dysplasia, cervix
  congenital Q82.8
  uterus NEC N85.8
Dyskinesia G24.9
  biliary (cystic duct or gallbladder) K82.8
  drug induced
    orofacial G24.01
  esophagus K22.4
  hysterical F44.4
  intestinal K59.8
  nonorganic origin F44.4
  orofacial (idiopathic) G24.4
    drug induced G24.01
  psychogenic F44.4
  subacute, drug induced G24.01
  tardive G24.01
    neuroleptic induced G24.01
  trachea J39.8
  tracheobronchial J98.09
Dyslalia (developmental) F80.0
Dyslexia R48.0
  developmental F81.0
Dyslipidemia E78.5
  depressed HDL cholesterol E78.6
  elevated fasting triglycerides E78.1
Dysmaturity (*see also* Light for dates)
  pulmonary (newborn) (Wilson-Mikity) P27.0
Dysmenorrhea (essential) (exfoliative) N94.6
  congestive (syndrome) N94.6
  primary N94.4
  psychogenic F45.8
  secondary N94.5
Dysmetabolic syndrome X E88.81
Dysmetria R27.8
Dysmorphism (due to)
  alcohol Q86.0
  exogenous cause NEC Q86.8
  hydantoin Q86.1
  warfarin Q86.2
Dysmorphophobia (nondelusional) F45.22
  delusional F22
Dysnomia R47.01
Dysorexia R63.0
  psychogenic F50.89
Dysostosis
  cleidocranial, cleidocranialis Q74.0
  craniofacial Q75.1
  Fairbank's (idiopathic familial generalized osteophytosis) Q78.9

Dysostosis — *continued*
  mandibulofacial (incomplete) Q75.4
  multiplex E76.01
  oculomandibular Q75.5
Dyspareunia (female) N94.10
  deep N94.12
  male N53.12
  nonorganic F52.6
  psychogenic F52.6
  secondary N94.19
  specified NEC N94.19
  superficial (introital) N94.11
Dyspepsia R10.13
  atonic K30
  functional (allergic) (congenital) (gastrointestinal) (occupational) (reflex) K30
  intestinal K59.8
  nervous F45.8
  neurotic F45.8
  psychogenic F45.8
Dysphagia R13.10
  cervical R13.19
  following
    cerebral infarction I69.391
    cerebrovascular disease I69.991
      specified NEC I69.891
    intracerebral hemorrhage I69.191
    nontraumatic intracranial hemorrhage NEC I69.291
    specified disease NEC I69.891
    subarachnoid hemorrhage I69.091
  functional (hysterical) F45.8
  hysterical F45.8
  nervous (hysterical) F45.8
  neurogenic R13.19
  oral phase R13.11
  oropharyngeal phase R13.12
  pharyngeal phase R13.13
  pharyngoesophageal phase R13.14
  psychogenic F45.8
  sideropenic D50.1
  spastica K22.4
  specified NEC R13.19
Dysphagocytosis, congenital D71
Dysphasia R47.02
  developmental
    expressive type F80.1
    receptive type F80.2
  following
    cerebrovascular disease I69.921
      cerebral infarction I69.321
      intracerebral hemorrhage I69.121
      nontraumatic intracranial hemorrhage NEC I69.221
      specified disease NEC I69.821
      subarachnoid hemorrhage I69.021
Dysphonia R49.0
  functional F44.4
  hysterical F44.4
  psychogenic F44.4
  spastica J38.3
Dysphoria
  gender F64.9
    in
      adolescence and adulthood F64.0
      children F64.2
    specified NEC F64.8
  postpartal O90.6
Dyspituitarism E23.3
Dysplasia (*see also* Anomaly)
  acetabular, acetabulum, congenital Q65.89
  alveolar capillary, with vein misalignment J84.843
  anus (histologically confirmed) (mild) (moderate) K62.82
    severe D01.3
  arrhythmogenic right ventricular I42.8
  arterial, fibromuscular I77.3
  asphyxiating thoracic (congenital) Q77.2
  brain Q07.9
  bronchopulmonary, perinatal P27.1
  cervix (uteri) N87.9
    mild N87.0
    moderate N87.1
    severe D06.9
  chondroectodermal Q77.6
  colon D12.6
  craniometaphyseal Q78.8
  dentinal K00.5
  diaphyseal, progressive Q78.3
  dystrophic Q77.5
  ectodermal (anhidrotic) (congenital) (hereditary) Q82.4
    hydrotic Q82.8

Dysplasia - Echinococcus

Dysplasia — *continued*
    epithelial, uterine cervix — *see* Dysplasia, cervix
    eye (congenital) Q11.2
    fibrous
        bone NEC (monostotic) M85.00
            ankle M85.07 ☑
            foot M85.07 ☑
            forearm M85.03 ☑
            hand M85.04 ☑
            lower leg M85.06 ☑
            multiple site M85.09
            neck M85.08
            rib M85.08
            shoulder M85.01 ☑
            skull M85.08
            specified site NEC M85.08
            thigh M85.05 ☑
            toe M85.07 ☑
            upper arm M85.02 ☑
            vertebra M85.08
        diaphyseal, progressive Q78.3
        jaw M27.8
        polyostotic Q78.1
    florid osseous (*see also* Cyst, calcifying
        odontogenic)
    high grade, focal D12.6
    hip, congenital Q65.89
    joint, congenital Q74.8
    kidney Q61.4
        multicystic Q61.4
    leg Q74.2
    lung, congenital (not associated with short
        gestation) Q33.6
    mammary (gland) (benign) N60.9 ☑
        cyst (solitary) — *see* Cyst, breast
        cystic — *see* Mastopathy, cystic
        duct ectasia — *see* Ectasia, mammary duct
        fibroadenosis — *see* Fibroadenosis, breast
        fibrosclerosis — *see* Fibrosclerosis, breast
        specified type NEC N60.8 ☑
    metaphyseal Q78.5
    muscle Q79.8
    oculodentodigital Q87.0
    periapical (cemental) (cemento-osseous) — *see*
        Cyst, calcifying odontogenic
    periosteum — *see* Disorder, bone, specified type
        NEC
    polyostotic fibrous Q78.1
    prostate (*see also* Neoplasia, intraepithelial,
        prostate) N42.30
        severe D07.5
        specified NEC N42.39
    renal Q61.4
        multicystic Q61.4
    retinal, congenital Q14.1
    right ventricular, arrhythmogenic I42.8
    septo-optic Q04.4
    skin L98.8
    spinal cord Q06.1
    spondyloepiphyseal Q77.7
    thymic, with immunodeficiency D82.1
    vagina N89.3
        mild N89.0
        moderate N89.1
        severe NEC D07.2
    vulva N90.3
        mild N90.0
        moderate N90.1
        severe NEC D07.1
Dyspnea (nocturnal) (paroxysmal) R06.00
    asthmatic (bronchial) J45.909
        with
            exacerbation (acute) J45.901
            bronchitis J45.909
                with
                    exacerbation (acute) J45.901
                    status asthmaticus J45.902
            chronic J44.9
            status asthmaticus J45.902
    cardiac — *see* Failure, ventricular, left
    cardiac — *see* Failure, ventricular, left
    functional F45.8
    hyperventilation R06.4
    hysterical F45.8
    newborn P28.89
    orthopnea R06.01
    psychogenic F45.8
    shortness of breath R06.02
    specified type NEC R06.09
Dyspraxia R27.8
    developmental (syndrome) F82
Dysproteinemia E88.09

Dysreflexia, autonomic G90.4
Dysrhythmia
    cardiac I49.9
        newborn
            bradycardia P29.12
                occurring before birth P03.819
                    before onset of labor P03.810
                    during labor P03.811
            tachycardia P29.11
        postoperative I97.89
    cerebral or cortical — *see* Epilepsy
Dyssomnia — *see* Disorder, sleep
Dyssynergia
    biliary K83.8
    bladder sphincter N36.44
    cerebellaris myoclonica (Hunt's ataxia) G11.1
Dysthymia F34.1
Dysthyroidism E07.9
Dystocia O66.9
    affecting newborn P03.1
    cervical (hypotonic) O62.2
        affecting newborn P03.6
        primary O62.0
        secondary O62.1
    contraction ring O62.4
    fetal O66.9
        abnormality NEC O66.3
        conjoined twins O66.3
        oversize O66.2
    maternal O66.9
    positional O64.9 ☑
    shoulder (girdle) O66.0
        causing obstructed labor O66.0
    uterine NEC O62.4
Dystonia G24.9
    deformans progressiva G24.1
    drug induced NEC G24.09
        acute G24.02
        specified NEC G24.09
    familial G24.1
    idiopathic G24.1
        familial G24.1
        nonfamilial G24.2
        orofacial G24.4
    lenticularis G24.8
    musculorum deformans G24.1
    neuroleptic induced (acute) G24.02
    orofacial (idiopathic) G24.4
    oromandibular G24.4
        due to drug G24.01
    specified NEC G24.8
    torsion (familial) (idiopathic) G24.1
        acquired G24.8
        genetic G24.1
        symptomatic (nonfamilial) G24.2
Dystonic movements R25.8
Dystrophy, dystrophia
    adiposogenital E23.6
    Becker's type G71.0
    cervical sympathetic G90.2
    choroid (hereditary) H31.20
        central areolar H31.22
        choroideremia H31.21
        gyrate atrophy H31.23
        specified type NEC H31.29
    cornea (hereditary) H18.50
        endothelial H18.51
        epithelial H18.52
        granular H18.53
        lattice H18.54
        macular H18.55
        specified type NEC H18.59
    Duchenne's type G71.0
    due to malnutrition E45
    Erb's G71.0
    Fuchs' H18.51
    Gower's muscular G71.0
    hair L67.8
    infantile neuraxonal G31.89
    Landouzy-Déjérine type G71.0
    Leyden-Möbius G71.0
    muscular G71.0
        benign (Becker type) G71.0
        congenital (hereditary) (progressive) (with
            specific morphological abnormalities of
            the muscle fiber) G71.0
            myotonic G71.11
        distal G71.0
        Duchenne type G71.0
        Emery-Dreifuss G71.0
        Erb type G71.0
        facioscapulohumeral G71.0

Dystrophy — *continued*
    muscular — *continued*
        Gower's G71.0
        hereditary (progressive) G71.0
        Landouzy-Déjérine type G71.0
        limb-girdle G71.0
        myotonic G71.11
        progressive (hereditary) G71.0
            Charcot-Marie (-Tooth) type G60.0
        pseudohypertrophic (infantile) G71.0
        severe (Duchenne type) G71.0
    myocardium, myocardial — *see* Degeneration,
        myocardial
    myotonic, myotonica G71.11
    nail L60.3
        congenital Q84.6
    nutritional E45
    ocular G71.0
    oculocerebrorenal E72.03
    oculopharyngeal G71.0
    ovarian N83.8
    polyglandular E31.8
    reflex (neuromuscular) (sympathetic) — *see*
        Syndrome, pain, complex regional I
    retinal (hereditary) H35.50
        in
            lipid storage disorders E75.6 [H36]
            systemic lipidoses E75.6 [H36]
        involving
            pigment epithelium H35.54
            sensory area H35.53
        pigmentary H35.52
        vitreoretinal H35.51
    Salzmann's nodular — *see* Degeneration, cornea,
        nodular
    scapuloperoneal G71.0
    skin NEC L98.8
    sympathetic (reflex) — *see* Syndrome, pain,
        complex regional I
        cervical G90.2
    tapetoretinal H35.54
    thoracic, asphyxiating Q77.2
    unguium L60.3
        congenital Q84.6
    vitreoretinal H35.51
    vulva N90.4
    yellow (liver) — *see* Failure, hepatic
Dysuria R30.0
    psychogenic F45.8

E

Eales' disease H35.06 ☑
Ear (*see also* condition)
    piercing Z41.3
    tropical NEC B36.9 [H62.40]
        in
            aspergillosis B44.89
            candidiasis B37.84
            moniliasis B37.84
    wax (impacted) H61.20
        left H61.22
            with right H61.23
        right H61.21
            with left H61.23
Earache — *see* subcategory H92.0
Early satiety R68.81
Eaton-Lambert syndrome — *see* Syndrome,
    Lambert-Eaton
Eberth's disease (typhoid fever) A01.00
Ebola virus disease A98.4
Ebstein's anomaly or syndrome (heart) Q22.5
Eccentro-osteochondrodysplasia E76.29
Ecchondroma — *see* Neoplasm, bone, benign
Ecchondrosis D48.0
Ecchymosis R58
    conjunctiva — *see* Hemorrhage, conjunctiva
    eye (traumatic) — *see* Contusion, eyeball
    eyelid (traumatic) — *see* Contusion, eyelid
    newborn P54.5
    spontaneous R23.3
    traumatic — *see* Contusion
Echinococciasis — *see* Echinococcus
Echinococcosis — *see* Echinococcus
Echinococcus (infection) B67.90
    granulosus B67.4
        bone B67.2
        liver B67.0
        lung B67.1
        multiple sites B67.32

☑ **Additional character required**

Echinococcus — *continued*
granulosus — *continued*
specified site NEC B67.39
thyroid B67.31
liver NOS B67.8
granulosus B67.0
multilocularis B67.5
lung NEC B67.99
granulosus B67.1
multilocularis B67.69
multilocularis B67.7
liver B67.5
multiple sites B67.61
specified site NEC B67.69
specified site NEC B67.99
granulosus B67.39
multilocularis B67.69
thyroid NEC B67.99
granulosus B67.31
multilocularis B67.69 *[E35]*
Echinorhynchiasis B83.8
Echinostomiasis B66.8
Echolalia R48.8
Echovirus, as cause of disease classified elsewhere B97.12
Eclampsia, eclamptic (coma) (convulsions) (delirium) (with hypertension) NEC O15.9
complicating
labor and delivery O15.1
postpartum O15.2
pregnancy O15.0 ☑
puerperium O15.2
Economic circumstances affecting care Z59.9
Economo's disease A85.8
Ectasia, ectasis
annuloaortic I35.8
aorta I77.819
with aneurysm — *see* Aneurysm, aorta
abdominal I77.811
thoracic I77.810
thoracoabdominal I77.812
breast — *see* Ectasia, mammary duct
capillary I78.8
cornea H18.71 ☑
gastric antral vascular (GAVE) K31.819
with hemorrhage K31.811
without hemorrhage K31.819
mammary duct N60.4 ☑
salivary gland (duct) K11.8
sclera — *see* Sclerectasia
Ecthyma L08.0
contagiosum B08.02
gangrenosum L08.0
infectiosum B08.02
Ectocardia Q24.8
Ectodermal dysplasia (anhidrotic) Q82.4
Ectodermosis erosiva pluriorificialis L51.1
Ectopic, ectopia (congenital)
abdominal viscera Q45.8
due to defect in anterior abdominal wall Q79.59
ACTH syndrome E24.3
adrenal gland Q89.1
anus Q43.5
atrial beats I49.1
beats I49.49
atrial I49.1
ventricular I49.3
bladder Q64.10
bone and cartilage in lung Q33.5
brain Q04.8
breast tissue Q83.8
cardiac Q24.8
cerebral Q04.8
cordis Q24.8
endometrium — *see* Endometriosis
gastric mucosa Q40.2
gestation — *see* Pregnancy, by site
heart Q24.8
hormone secretion NEC E34.2
kidney (crossed) (pelvis) Q63.2
lens, lentis Q12.1
mole — *see* Pregnancy, by site
organ or site NEC — *see* Malposition, congenital
pancreas Q45.3
pregnancy — *see* Pregnancy, ectopic
pupil — *see* Abnormality, pupillary
renal Q63.2
sebaceous glands of mouth Q38.6
spleen Q89.09
testis Q53.00
bilateral Q53.02
unilateral Q53.01

Ectopic — *continued*
thyroid Q89.2
tissue in lung Q33.5
ureter Q62.63
ventricular beats I49.3
vesicae Q64.10
Ectromelia Q73.8
lower limb — *see* Defect, reduction, limb, lower, specified type NEC
upper limb — *see* Defect, reduction, limb, upper, specified type NEC
Ectropion H02.109
cervix N86
with cervicitis N72
congenital Q10.1
eyelid (paralytic) H02.109
cicatricial H02.119
left H02.116
lower H02.115
upper H02.114
right H02.113
lower H02.112
upper H02.111
congenital Q10.1
left H02.106
lower H02.105
upper H02.104
mechanical H02.129
left H02.126
lower H02.125
upper H02.124
right H02.123
lower H02.122
upper H02.121
right H02.103
lower H02.102
upper H02.101
senile H02.139
left H02.136
lower H02.135
upper H02.134
right H02.133
lower H02.132
upper H02.131
spastic H02.149
left H02.146
lower H02.145
upper H02.144
right H02.143
lower H02.142
upper H02.141
iris H21.89
lip (acquired) K13.0
congenital Q38.0
urethra N36.8
uvea H21.89
Eczema (acute) (chronic) (erythematous) (fissum) (rubrum) (squamous) (*see also* Dermatitis) L30.9
contact — *see* Dermatitis, contact
dyshydrotic L30.1
external ear — *see* Otitis, externa, acute, eczematoid
flexural L20.82
herpeticum B00.0
hypertrophicum L28.0
hypostatic — *see* Varix, leg, with, inflammation
impetiginous L01.1
infantile (due to any substance) L20.83
intertriginous L21.1
seborrheic L21.1
intertriginous NEC L30.4
infantile L21.1
intrinsic (allergic) L20.84
lichenified NEC L28.0
marginatum (hebrae) B35.6
pustular L30.3
stasis I87.2
with varicose veins — *see* Varix, leg, with, inflammation
vaccination, vaccinatum T88.1 ☑
varicose — *see* Varix, leg, with, inflammation
Eczematid L30.2
Eddowes (-Spurway) syndrome Q78.0
Edema, edematous (infectious) (pitting) (toxic) R60.9
with nephritis — *see* Nephrosis
allergic T78.3 ☑
amputation stump (surgical) (sequelae (late effect)) T87.89
angioneurotic (allergic) (any site) (with urticaria) T78.3 ☑
hereditary D84.1
angiospastic I73.9

Edema — *continued*
Berlin's (traumatic) S05.8X ☑
brain (cytotoxic) (vasogenic) G93.6
due to birth injury P11.0
newborn (anoxia or hypoxia) P52.4
birth injury P11.0
traumatic — *see* Injury, intracranial, cerebral edema
cardiac — *see* Failure, heart, congestive
cardiovascular — *see* Failure, heart, congestive
cerebral — *see* Edema, brain
cerebrospinal — *see* Edema, brain
cervix (uteri) (acute) N88.8
puerperal, postpartum O90.89
chronic hereditary Q82.0
circumscribed, acute T78.3 ☑
hereditary D84.1
conjunctiva H11.42 ☑
cornea H18.2 ☑
idiopathic H18.22 ☑
secondary H18.23 ☑
due to contact lens H18.21 ☑
due to
lymphatic obstruction I89.0
salt retention E87.0
epiglottis — *see* Edema, glottis
essential, acute T78.3 ☑
hereditary D84.1
extremities, lower — *see* Edema, legs
eyelid NEC H02.849
left H02.846
lower H02.845
upper H02.844
right H02.843
lower H02.842
upper H02.841
familial, hereditary Q82.0
famine — *see* Malnutrition, severe
generalized R60.1
glottis, glottic, glottidis (obstructive) (passive) J38.4
allergic T78.3 ☑
hereditary D84.1
heart — *see* Failure, heart, congestive
heat T67.7 ☑
hereditary Q82.0
inanition — *see* Malnutrition, severe
intracranial G93.6
iris H21.89
joint — *see* Effusion, joint
larynx — *see* Edema, glottis
legs R60.0
due to venous obstruction I87.1
hereditary Q82.0
localized R60.0
due to venous obstruction I87.1
lower limbs — *see* Edema, legs
lung J81.1
with heart condition or failure — *see* Failure, ventricular, left
acute J81.0
chemical (acute) J68.1
chronic J68.1
chronic J81.1
due to
chemicals, gases, fumes or vapors (inhalation) J68.1
external agent J70.9
specified NEC J70.8
radiation J70.1
due to
chemicals, fumes or vapors (inhalation) J68.1
external agent J70.9
specified NEC J70.8
high altitude T70.29 ☑
near drowning T75.1 ☑
radiation J70.0
meaning failure, left ventricle I50.1
lymphatic I89.0
due to mastectomy I97.2
macula H35.81
cystoid, following cataract surgery — *see* Complications, postprocedural, following cataract surgery
diabetic — *see* Diabetes, by type, with, retinopathy, with macular edema
malignant — *see* Gangrene, gas
Milroy's Q82.0
nasopharynx J39.2
newborn P83.30
hydrops fetalis — *see* Hydrops, fetalis
specified NEC P83.39

Edema - Elephantiasis

ICD-10-CM INDEX TO DISEASES AND INJURIES

Edema — *continued*
  nutritional (*see also* Malnutrition, severe)
    with dyspigmentation, skin and hair E40
  optic disc or nerve — *see* Papilledema
  orbit H05.22 ☑
  pancreas K86.89
  papilla, optic — *see* Papilledema
  penis N48.89
  periodic T78.3 ☑
    hereditary D84.1
  pharynx J39.2
  pulmonary — *see* Edema, lung
  Quincke's T78.3 ☑
    hereditary D84.1
  renal — *see* Nephrosis
  retina H35.81
    diabetic — *see* Diabetes, by type, with,
      retinopathy, with macular edema
  salt E87.0
  scrotum N50.89
  seminal vesicle N50.89
  spermatic cord N50.89
  spinal (cord) (vascular) (nontraumatic) G95.19
  starvation — *see* Malnutrition, severe
  stasis — *see* Hypertension, venous, (chronic)
  subglottic — *see* Edema, glottis
  supraglottic — *see* Edema, glottis
  testis N44.8
  tunica vaginalis N50.89
  vas deferens N50.89
  vulva (acute) N90.89
Edentulism — *see* Absence, teeth, acquired
Edsall's disease T67.2 ☑
Educational handicap Z55.9
  specified NEC Z55.8
Edward's syndrome — *see* Trisomy, 18
Effect, adverse
  abnormal gravitational (G) forces or
    states T75.81 ☑
  abuse — *see* Maltreatment
  air pressure T70.9 ☑
    specified NEC T70.8 ☑
  altitude (high) — *see* Effect, adverse, high altitude
  anesthesia (*see also* Anesthesia) T88.59 ☑
    in labor and delivery O74.9
    local, toxic
      in labor and delivery O74.4
      in pregnancy NEC O29.3 ☑
      postpartum, puerperal O89.3
    postpartum, puerperal O89.9
    specified NEC T88.59 ☑
      in labor and delivery O74.8
      postpartum, puerperal O89.8
    spinal and epidural T88.59 ☑
      headache T88.59 ☑
        in labor and delivery O74.5
        postpartum, puerperal O89.4
      specified NEC
        in labor and delivery O74.6
        postpartum, puerperal O89.5
  antitoxin — *see* Complications, vaccination
  atmospheric pressure T70.9 ☑
    due to explosion T70.8 ☑
    high T70.3 ☑
    low — *see* Effect, adverse, high altitude
    specified effect NEC T70.8 ☑
  biological, correct substance properly
    administered — *see* Effect, adverse, drug
  blood (derivatives) (serum) (transfusion) — *see*
    Complications, transfusion
  chemical substance — *see* Table of Drugs and
    Chemicals
  cold (temperature) (weather) T69.9 ☑
    chilblains T69.1 ☑
    frostbite — *see* Frostbite
    specified effect NEC T69.8 ☑
  drugs and medicaments T88.7 ☑
    specified drug — *see* Table of Drugs and
      Chemicals, by drug, adverse effect
    specified effect - code to condition
  electric current, electricity (shock) T75.4 ☑
    burn — *see* Burn
  exertion (excessive) T73.3 ☑
  exposure — *see* Exposure
  external cause NEC T75.89 ☑
  foodstuffs T78.1 ☑
    allergic reaction — *see* Allergy, food
      causing anaphylaxis — *see* Shock,
        anaphylactic, due to food
    noxious — *see* Poisoning, food, noxious
  gases, fumes, or vapors T59.9 ☑

Effect — *continued*
  gases — *continued*
    specified agent — *see* Table of Drugs and
      Chemicals
  glue (airplane) sniffing
    due to drug abuse — *see* Abuse, drug, inhalant
    due to drug dependence — *see* Dependence,
      drug, inhalant
  heat — *see* Heat
  high altitude NEC T70.29 ☑
    anoxia T70.29 ☑
    on
      ears T70.0 ☑
      sinuses T70.1 ☑
    polycythemia D75.1
  high pressure fluids T70.4 ☑
  hot weather — *see* Heat
  hunger T73.0 ☑
  immersion, foot — *see* Immersion
  immunization — *see* Complications, vaccination
  immunological agents — *see* Complications,
    vaccination
  infrared (radiation) (rays) NOS T66 ☑
    dermatitis or eczema L59.8
  infusion — *see* Complications, infusion
  lack of care of infants — *see* Maltreatment, child
  lightning — *see* Lightning
  medical care T88.9 ☑
    specified NEC T88.8 ☑
  medicinal substance, correct, properly
    administered — *see* Effect, adverse, drug
  motion T75.3 ☑
  noise, on inner ear — *see* subcategory H83.3
  overheated places — *see* Heat
  psychosocial, of work environment Z56.5
  radiation (diagnostic) (infrared) (natural source)
    (therapeutic) (ultraviolet) (X-ray) NOS T66 ☑
    dermatitis or eczema — *see* Dermatitis, due to,
      radiation
    fibrosis of lung J70.1
    pneumonitis J70.0
    pulmonary manifestations
      acute J70.0
      chronic J70.1
    skin L59.9
  radioactive substance NOS
    dermatitis or eczema — *see* Radiodermatitis
  reduced temperature T69.9 ☑
    immersion foot or hand — *see* Immersion
    specified effect NEC T69.8 ☑
  serum NEC (*see also* Reaction, serum) T80.69 ☑
  specified NEC T78.8 ☑
    external cause NEC T75.89 ☑
  strangulation — *see* Asphyxia, traumatic
  submersion T75.1 ☑
  thirst T73.1 ☑
  toxic — *see* Toxicity
  transfusion — *see* Complications, transfusion
  ultraviolet (radiation) (rays) NOS T66 ☑
    burn — *see* Burn
    dermatitis or eczema — *see* Dermatitis, due to,
      ultraviolet rays
      acute L56.8
  vaccine (any) — *see* Complications, vaccination
  vibration — *see* Vibration, adverse effects
  water pressure NEC T70.9 ☑
    specified NEC T70.8 ☑
  weightlessness T75.82 ☑
  whole blood — *see* Complications, transfusion
  work environment Z56.5
Effect (s) (of) (from) — *see* Effect, adverse NEC
Effects, late — *see* Sequelae
Effluvium
  anagen L65.1
  telogen L65.0
Effort syndrome (psychogenic) F45.8
Effusion
  amniotic fluid — *see* Pregnancy, complicated by,
    premature rupture of membranes
  brain (serous) G93.6
  bronchial — *see* Bronchitis
  cerebral G93.6
  cerebrospinal (*see also* Meningitis)
    vessel G93.6
  chest — *see* Effusion, pleura
  chylous, chyliform (pleura) J94.0
  intracranial G93.6
  joint M25.40
    ankle M25.47 ☑
    elbow M25.42 ☑
    foot joint M25.47 ☑
    hand joint M25.44 ☑

Effusion — *continued*
  joint — *continued*
    hip M25.45 ☑
    knee M25.46 ☑
    shoulder M25.41 ☑
    specified joint NEC M25.48
    wrist M25.43 ☑
  malignant pleural J91.0
  meninges — *see* Meningitis
  pericardium, pericardial (noninflammatory) I31.3
    acute — *see* Pericarditis, acute
  peritoneal (chronic) R18.8
  pleura, pleurisy, pleuritic, pleuropericardial J90
    chylous, chyliform J94.0
    due to systemic lupus erythematosis M32.13
    in conditions classified elsewhere J91.8
    influenzal — *see* Influenza, with, respiratory
      manifestations NEC
    malignant J91.0
    newborn P28.89
    tuberculous NEC A15.6
      primary (progressive) A15.7
  spinal — *see* Meningitis
  thorax, thoracic — *see* Effusion, pleura
Egg shell nails L60.3
  congenital Q84.6
Egyptian splenomegaly B65.1
Ehrlichiosis A77.40
  due to
    E. chafeensis A77.41
    E. sennetsu A79.81
    specified organism NEC A77.49
Ehlers-Danlos syndrome Q79.6
Eichstedt's disease B36.0
Eisenmenger's
  complex or syndrome I27.83
  defect Q21.8
Ejaculation
  delayed F52.32
  painful N53.12
  premature F52.4
  retarded N53.11
  retrograde N53.14
  semen, painful N53.12
    psychogenic F52.6
Ekbom's syndrome (restless legs) G25.81
Ekman's syndrome (brittle bones and blue sclera)
  Q78.0
Elastic skin Q82.8
  acquired L57.4
Elastofibroma — *see* Neoplasm, connective tissue,
  benign
Elastoma (juvenile) Q82.8
  Miescher's L87.2
Elastomyofibrosis I42.4
Elastosis
  actinic, solar L57.8
  atrophicans (senile) L57.4
  perforans serpiginosa L87.2
  senilis L57.4
Elbow — *see* condition
Electric current, electricity, effects (concussion)
  (fatal) (nonfatal) (shock) T75.4 ☑
  burn — *see* Burn
Electric feet syndrome E53.8
Electrocution T75.4 ☑
  from electroshock gun (taser) T75.4 ☑
Electrolyte imbalance E87.8
  with
    abortion — *see* Abortion by type, complicated
      by, electrolyte imbalance
    ectopic pregnancy O08.5
    molar pregnancy O08.5
Elephantiasis (nonfilarial) I89.0
  arabicum — *see* Infestation, filarial
  bancroftian B74.0
  congenital (any site) (hereditary) Q82.0
  due to
    Brugia (malayi) B74.1
      timori B74.2
    mastectomy I97.2
    Wuchereria (bancrofti) B74.0
  eyelid H02.859
    left H02.856
      lower H02.855
      upper H02.854
    right H02.853
      lower H02.852
      upper H02.851
  filarial, filariensis — *see* Infestation, filarial
  glandular I89.0
  graecorum A30.9

☑ **Additional character required**

Elephantiasis — *continued*
  lymphangiectatic I89.0
  lymphatic vessel I89.0
    due to mastectomy I97.2
  scrotum (nonfilarial) I89.0
  streptococcal I89.0
  surgical I97.89
    postmastectomy I97.2
  telangiectodes I89.0
  vulva (nonfilarial) N90.89
Elevated, elevation
  antibody titer R76.0
  basal metabolic rate R94.8
  blood pressure (*see also* Hypertension)
    reading (incidental) (isolated) (nonspecific), no
      diagnosis of hypertension R03.0
  blood sugar R73.9
  body temperature (of unknown origin) R50.9
  C-reactive protein (CRP) R79.82
  cancer antigen 125 [CA 125] R97.1
  carcinoembryonic antigen [CEA] R97.0
  cholesterol E78.00
    with high triglycerides E78.2
  conjugate, eye H51.0
  diaphragm, congenital Q79.1
  erythrocyte sedimentation rate R70.0
  fasting glucose R73.01
  fasting triglycerides E78.1
  finding on laboratory examination — *see*
    Findings, abnormal, inconclusive, without
    diagnosis, by type of exam
  GFR (glomerular filtration rate) — *see* Findings,
    abnormal, inconclusive, without diagnosis,
    by type of exam
  glucose tolerance (oral) R73.02
  immunoglobulin level R76.8
  indoleacetic acid R82.5
  lactic acid dehydrogenase (LDH) level R74.0
  leukocytes D72.829
  lipoprotein a level E78.8 ☑
  liver function
    study R94.5
    test R79.89
      alkaline phosphatase R74.8
      aminotransferase R74.0
      bilirubin R17
      hepatic enzyme R74.8
      lactate dehydrogenase R74.0
  lymphocytes D72.820
  prostate specific antigen [PSA] R97.20
  Rh titer — *see* Complication (s), transfusion,
    incompatibility reaction, Rh (factor)
  scapula, congenital Q74.0
  sedimentation rate R70.0
  SGOT R74.0
  SGPT R74.0
  transaminase level R74.0
  triglycerides E78.1
    with high cholesterol E78.2
  tumor associated antigens [TAA] NEC R97.8
  tumor specific antigens [TSA] NEC R97.8
  urine level of
    catecholamine R82.5
    indoleacetic acid R82.5
    17-ketosteroids R82.5
    steroids R82.5
    vanillylmandelic acid (VMA) R82.5
  venous pressure I87.8
  white blood cell count D72.829
    specified NEC D72.828
Elliptocytosis (congenital) (hereditary) D58.1
  Hb C (disease) D58.1
  hemoglobin disease D58.1
  sickle-cell (disease) D57.8 ☑
    trait D57.3
Ellison-Zollinger syndrome E16.4
Ellis-van Creveld syndrome (chondroectodermal
  dysplasia) Q77.6
Elongated, elongation (congenital) (*see also*
  Distortion)
  bone Q79.9
  cervix (uteri) Q51.828
    acquired N88.4
    hypertrophic N88.4
  colon Q43.8
  common bile duct Q44.5
  cystic duct Q44.5
  frenulum, penis Q55.69
  labia minora (acquired) N90.69
  ligamentum patellae Q74.1
  petiolus (epiglottidis) Q31.8
  tooth, teeth K00.2
  uvula Q38.6

Eltor cholera A00.1
Emaciation (due to malnutrition) E41
Embadomoniasis A07.8
Embedded tooth, teeth K01.0
  root only K08.3
Embolic — *see* condition
Embolism (multiple) (paradoxical) I74.9
  air (any site) (traumatic) T79.0 ☑
    following
      abortion — *see* Abortion by type
        complicated by embolism
      ectopic pregnancy O08.2
      infusion, therapeutic injection or
        transfusion T80.0 ☑
      molar pregnancy O08.2
      procedure NEC
        artery T81.719 ☑
          mesenteric T81.710 ☑
          renal T81.711 ☑
          specified NEC T81.718 ☑
        vein T81.72 ☑
    in pregnancy, childbirth or puerperium — *see*
      Embolism, obstetric
  amniotic fluid (pulmonary) (*see also* Embolism,
    obstetric)
    following
      abortion — *see* Abortion by type
        complicated by embolism
      ectopic pregnancy O08.2
      molar pregnancy O08.2
  aorta, aortic I74.10
    abdominal I74.09
      saddle I74.01
    bifurcation I74.09
    saddle I74.01
    thoracic I74.11
  artery I74.9
    auditory, internal I65.8
    basilar — *see* Occlusion, artery, basilar
    carotid (common) (internal) — *see* Occlusion,
      artery, carotid
    cerebellar (anterior inferior) (posterior inferior)
      (superior) I66.3
    cerebral — *see* Occlusion, artery, cerebral
    choroidal (anterior) I65.8
    communicating posterior I65.8
    coronary (*see also* Infarct, myocardium)
      not resulting in infarction I24.0
    extremity I74.4
      lower I74.3
      upper I74.2
    hypophyseal I65.8
    iliac I74.5
    limb I74.4
      lower I74.3
      upper I74.2
    mesenteric (with gangrene) (*see also* Ischemia,
      intestine, acute) K55.059
    ophthalmic — *see* Occlusion, artery, retina
    peripheral I74.4
    pontine I65.8
    precerebral — *see* Occlusion, artery, precerebral
    pulmonary — *see* Embolism, pulmonary
    renal N28.0
    retinal — *see* Occlusion, artery, retina
    septic I76
    specified NEC I74.8
    vertebral — *see* Occlusion, artery, vertebral
  basilar (artery) I65.1
  blood clot
    following
      abortion — *see* Abortion by type
        complicated by embolism
      ectopic or molar pregnancy O08.2
    in pregnancy, childbirth or puerperium — *see*
      Embolism, obstetric
  brain (*see also* Occlusion, artery, cerebral)
    following
      abortion — *see* Abortion by type
        complicated by embolism
      ectopic or molar pregnancy O08.2
    puerperal, postpartum, childbirth — *see*
      Embolism, obstetric
  capillary I78.8
  cardiac (*see also* Infarct, myocardium)
    not resulting in infarction I51.3
  carotid (artery) (common) (internal) — *see*
    Occlusion, artery, carotid
  cavernous sinus (venous) — *see* Embolism,
    intracranial venous sinus
  cerebral — *see* Occlusion, artery, cerebral
  cholesterol — *see* Atheroembolism

Embolism — *continued*
  coronary (artery or vein) (systemic) — *see*
    Occlusion, coronary
  due to device, implant or graft (*see also*
    Complications, by site and type, specified
    NEC)
    arterial graft NEC T82.818 ☑
    breast (implant) T85.818 ☑
    catheter NEC T85.818 ☑
      dialysis (renal) T82.818 ☑
        intraperitoneal T85.818 ☑
      infusion NEC T82.818 ☑
        spinal (epidural) (subdural) T85.810 ☑
      urinary (indwelling) T83.81 ☑
    electronic (electrode) (pulse generator)
      (stimulator)
      bone T84.81 ☑
      cardiac T82.817 ☑
      nervous system (brain) (peripheral nerve)
        (spinal) T85.810 ☑
      urinary T83.81 ☑
    fixation, internal (orthopedic) NEC T84.81 ☑
    gastrointestinal (bile duct)
      (esophagus) T85.818 ☑
    genital NEC T83.81 ☑
    heart (graft) (valve) T82.817 ☑
    joint prosthesis T84.81 ☑
    ocular (corneal graft) (orbital
      implant) T85.818 ☑
    orthopedic (bone graft) NEC T86.838
    specified NEC T85.818 ☑
    urinary (graft) NEC T83.81 ☑
    vascular NEC T82.818 ☑
    ventricular intracranial shunt T85.810 ☑
  extremities
    lower — *see* Embolism, vein, lower extremity
      arterial I74.3
    upper I74.2
  eye H34.9
  fat (cerebral) (pulmonary) (systemic) T79.1 ☑
    following
      abortion — *see* Abortion by type
        complicated by embolism
      ectopic or molar pregnancy O08.2
    complicating delivery — *see* Embolism,
      obstetric
    following
      abortion — *see* Abortion by type complicated
        by embolism
      ectopic or molar pregnancy O08.2
      infusion, therapeutic injection or transfusion
        air T80.0 ☑
  heart (fatty) (*see also* Infarct, myocardium)
    not resulting in infarction I51.3
  hepatic (vein) I82.0
  in pregnancy, childbirth or puerperium — *see*
    Embolism, obstetric
  intestine (artery) (vein) (with gangrene) (*see also*
    Ischemia, intestine, acute) K55.039
  intracranial (*see also* Occlusion, artery, cerebral)
    venous sinus (any) G08
      nonpyogenic I67.6
  intraspinal venous sinuses or veins G08
    nonpyogenic G95.19
  kidney (artery) N28.0
  lateral sinus (venous) — *see* Embolism,
    intracranial, venous sinus
  leg — *see* Embolism, vein, lower extremity
    arterial I74.3
  longitudinal sinus (venous) — *see* Embolism,
    intracranial, venous sinus
  lung (massive) — *see* Embolism, pulmonary
  meninges I66.8
  mesenteric (artery) (vein) (with gangrene) (*see
    also* Ischemia, intestine, acute) K55.059
  obstetric (in) (pulmonary)
    childbirth O88.22
      air O88.02
      amniotic fluid O88.12
      blood clot O88.22
      fat O88.82
      pyemic O88.32
      septic O88.32
      specified type NEC O88.82
    pregnancy O88.21 ☑
      air O88.01 ☑
      amniotic fluid O88.11 ☑
      blood clot O88.21 ☑
      fat O88.81 ☑
      pyemic O88.31 ☑
      septic O88.31 ☑
      specified type NEC O88.81 ☑

Elephantiasis - Embolism

ICD-10-CM INDEX TO DISEASES AND INJURIES

Embolism - Encephalitis

Embolism — *continued*
  obstetric — *continued*
    puerperal O88.23
      air O88.03
      amniotic fluid O88.13
      blood clot O88.23
      fat O88.83
      pyemic O88.33
      septic O88.33
      specified type NEC O88.83
  ophthalmic — *see* Occlusion, artery, retina
  penis N48.81
  peripheral artery NOS I74.4
  pituitary E23.6
  popliteal (artery) I74.3
  portal (vein) I81
  postoperative, postrpocedural
    artery T81.719 ☑
      mesenteric T81.710 ☑
      renal T81.711 ☑
      specified NEC T81.718 ☑
    vein T81.72 ☑
  precerebral artery — *see* Occlusion, artery, precerebral
  puerperal — *see* Embolism, obstetric
  pulmonary (acute) (artery) (vein) I26.99
    with acute cor pulmonale I26.09
    chronic I27.82
    following
      abortion — *see* Abortion by type complicated by embolism
      ectopic or molar pregnancy O08.2
    healed or old Z86.711
    in pregnancy, childbirth or puerperium — *see* Embolism, obstetric
    personal history of Z86.711
    saddle I26.92
      with acute cor pulmonale I26.02
    septic I26.90
      with acute cor pulmonale I26.01
  pyemic (multiple) I76
    following
      abortion — *see* Abortion by type complicated by embolism
      ectopic or molar pregnancy O08.2
    Hemophilus influenzae A41.3
    pneumococcal A40.3
      with pneumonia J13
    puerperal, postpartum, childbirth (any organism) — *see* Embolism, obstetric
    specified organism NEC A41.89
    staphylococcal A41.2
    streptococcal A40.9
  renal (artery) N28.0
    vein I82.3
  retina, retinal — *see* Occlusion, artery, retina
  saddle
    abdominal aorta I74.01
    pulmonary artery I26.92
      with acute cor pulmonale I26.02
  septic (arterial) I76
    complicating abortion — *see* Abortion, by type, complicated by, embolism
  sinus — *see* Embolism, intracranial, venous sinus
  soap complicating abortion — *see* Abortion, by type, complicated by, embolism
  spinal cord G95.19
    pyogenic origin G06.1
  spleen, splenic (artery) I74.8
  upper extremity I74.2
  vein (acute) I82.90
    antecubital I82.61 ☑
      chronic I82.71 ☑
    axillary I82.A1 ☑
      chronic I82.A2 ☑
    basilic I82.61 ☑
      chronic I82.71 ☑
    brachial I82.62 ☑
      chronic I82.72 ☑
    brachiocephalic (innominate) I82.290
      chronic I82.291
    cephalic I82.61 ☑
      chronic I82.71 ☑
    chronic I82.91
    deep (DVT) I82.40 ☑
      calf I82.4Z ☑
        chronic I82.5Z ☑
      lower leg I82.4Z ☑
        chronic I82.5Z ☑
      thigh I82.4Y ☑
        chronic I82.5Y ☑
      upper leg I82.4Y ☑

Embolism — *continued*
  vein — *continued*
      chronic I82.5Y ☑
    femoral I82.41 ☑
      chronic I82.51 ☑
    iliac (iliofemoral) I82.42 ☑
      chronic I82.52 ☑
    innominate I82.290
      chronic I82.291
    internal jugular I82.C1 ☑
      chronic I82.C2 ☑
    lower extremity
      deep I82.40 ☑
        chronic I82.50 ☑
        specified NEC I82.49 ☑
          chronic NEC I82.59 ☑
      distal
        deep I82.4Z ☑
      proximal
        deep I82.4Y ☑
          chronic I82.5Y ☑
      superficial I82.81 ☑
    popliteal I82.43 ☑
      chronic I82.53 ☑
    radial I82.62 ☑
      chronic I82.72 ☑
    renal I82.3
    saphenous (greater) (lesser) I82.81 ☑
    specified NEC I82.890
      chronic NEC I82.891
    subclavian I82.B1 ☑
      chronic I82.B2 ☑
    thoracic NEC I82.290
      chronic I82.291
    tibial I82.44 ☑
      chronic I82.54 ☑
    ulnar I82.62 ☑
      chronic I82.72 ☑
    upper extremity I82.60 ☑
      chronic I82.70 ☑
      deep I82.62 ☑
        chronic I82.72 ☑
      superficial I82.61 ☑
        chronic I82.71 ☑
    vena cava
      inferior (acute) I82.220
        chronic I82.221
      superior (acute) I82.210
        chronic I82.211
    venous sinus G08
    vessels of brain — *see* Occlusion, artery, cerebral
Embolus — *see* Embolism
Embryoma (*see also* Neoplasm, uncertain behavior, by site)
  benign — *see* Neoplasm, benign, by site
  kidney C64. ☑
  liver C22.0
  malignant (*see also* Neoplasm, malignant, by site)
    kidney C64. ☑
    liver C22.0
    testis C62.9 ☑
      descended (scrotal) C62.1 ☑
      undescended C62.0 ☑
  testis C62.9 ☑
    descended (scrotal) C62.1 ☑
    undescended C62.0 ☑
Embryonic
  circulation Q28.9
  heart Q28.9
  vas deferens Q55.4
Embryopathia NOS Q89.9
Embryotoxon Q13.4
Emesis — *see* Vomiting
Emotional lability R45.86
Emotionality, pathological F60.3
Emotogenic disease — *see* Disorder, psychogenic
Emphysema (atrophic) (bullous) (chronic) (interlobular) (lung) (obstructive) (pulmonary) (senile) (vesicular) J43.9
  cellular tissue (traumatic) T79.7 ☑
    surgical T81.82 ☑
  centrilobular J43.2
  compensatory J98.3
  congenital (interstitial) P25.0
  conjunctiva H11.89
  connective tissue (traumatic) T79.7 ☑
    surgical T81.82 ☑
  due to chemicals, gases, fumes or vapors J68.4
  eyelid (s) — *see* Disorder, eyelid, specified type NEC
    surgical T81.82 ☑
    traumatic T79.7 ☑

Emphysema — *continued*
  interstitial J98.2
    congenital P25.0
    perinatal period P25.0
  laminated tissue T79.7 ☑
    surgical T81.82 ☑
  mediastinal J98.2
    newborn P25.2
  orbit, orbital — *see* Disorder, orbit, specified type NEC
  panacinar J43.1
  panlobular J43.1
  specified NEC J43.8
  subcutaneous (traumatic) T79.7 ☑
    nontraumatic J98.2
    postprocedural T81.82 ☑
    surgical T81.82 ☑
  surgical T81.82 ☑
  thymus (gland) (congenital) E32.8
  traumatic (subcutaneous) T79.7 ☑
  unilateral J43.0
Empty nest syndrome Z60.0
Empyema (acute) (chest) (double) (pleura) (supradiaphragmatic) (thorax) J86.9
  with fistula J86.0
  accessory sinus (chronic) — *see* Sinusitis
  antrum (chronic) — *see* Sinusitis, maxillary
  brain (any part) — *see* Abscess, brain
  ethmoidal (chronic) (sinus) — *see* Sinusitis, ethmoidal
  extradural — *see* Abscess, extradural
  frontal (chronic) (sinus) — *see* Sinusitis, frontal
  gallbladder K81.0
  mastoid (process) (acute) — *see* Mastoiditis, acute
  maxilla, maxillary M27.2
    sinus (chronic) — *see* Sinusitis, maxillary
  nasal sinus (chronic) — *see* Sinusitis
  sinus (accessory) (chronic) (nasal) — *see* Sinusitis
  sphenoidal (sinus) (chronic) — *see* Sinusitis, sphenoidal
  subarachnoid — *see* Abscess, extradural
  subdural — *see* Abscess, subdural
  tuberculous A15.6
  ureter — *see* Ureteritis
  ventricular — *see* Abscess, brain
En coup de sabre lesion L94.1
Enamel pearls K00.2
Enameloma K00.2
Enanthema, viral B09
Encephalitis (chronic) (hemorrhagic) (idiopathic) (nonepidemic) (spurious) (subacute) G04.90
  acute (*see also* Encephalitis, viral) A86
    disseminated G04.00
      infectious G04.01
      noninfectious G04.81
      postimmunization (postvaccination) G04.02
      postinfectious G04.01
    inclusion body A85.8
    necrotizing hemorrhagic G04.30
      postimmunization G04.32
      postinfectious G04.31
      specified NEC G04.39
  arboviral, arbovirus NEC A85.2
  arthropod-borne NEC (viral) A85.2
  Australian A83.4
  California (virus) A83.5
  Central European (tick-borne) A84.1
  Czechoslovakian A84.1
  Dawson's (inclusion body) A81.1
  diffuse sclerosing A81.1
  disseminated, acute G04.00
  due to
    cat scratch disease A28.1
    human immunodeficiency virus (HIV) disease B20 *[G05.3]*
    malaria — *see* Malaria
    rickettsiosis — *see* Rickettsiosis
    smallpox inoculation G04.02
    typhus — *see* Typhus
  Eastern equine A83.2
  endemic (viral) A86
  epidemic NEC (viral) A86
  equine (acute) (infectious) (viral) A83.9
    Eastern A83.2
    Venezuelan A92.2
    Western A83.1
  Far Eastern (tick-borne) A84.0
  following vaccination or other immunization procedure G04.02
  herpes zoster B02.0
  herpesviral B00.4
    due to herpesvirus 6 B10.01

Encephalitis — *continued*
 herpesviral — *continued*
  due to herpesvirus 7 B10.09
  specified NEC B10.09
 Ilheus (virus) A83.8
 inclusion body A81.1
 in (due to)
  actinomycosis A42.82
  adenovirus A85.1
  African trypanosomiasis B56.9 *[G05.3]*
  Chagas' disease (chronic) B57.42
  cytomegalovirus B25.8
  enterovirus A85.0
  herpes (simplex) virus B00.4
   due to herpesvirus 6 B10.01
   due to herpesvirus 7 B10.09
   specified NEC B10.09
  infectious disease NEC B99 ☑ *[G05.3]*
  influenza — *see* Influenza, with,
   encephalopathy
  listeriosis A32.12
  measles B05.0
  mumps B26.2
  naegleriasis B60.2
  parasitic disease NEC B89 *[G05.3]*
  poliovirus A80.9 *[G05.3]*
  rubella B06.01
  syphilis
   congenital A50.42
   late A52.14
  systemic lupus erythematosus M32.19
  toxoplasmosis (acquired) B58.2
   congenital P37.1
  tuberculosis A17.82
  zoster B02.0
 infectious (acute) (virus) NEC A86
 Japanese (B type) A83.0
 La Crosse A83.5
 lead — *see* Poisoning, lead
 lethargica (acute) (infectious) A85.8
 louping ill A84.8
 lupus erythematosus, systemic M32.19
 lymphatica A87.2
 Mengo A85.8
 meningococcal A39.81
 Murray Valley A83.4
 otitic NEC H66.40 *[G05.3]*
 parasitic NOS B71.9
 periaxial G37.0
 periaxialis (concentrica) (diffuse) G37.5
 postchickenpox B01.11
 postexanthematous NEC B09
 postimmunization G04.02
 postinfectious NEC G04.01
 postmeasles B05.0
 postvaccinal G04.02
 postvaricella B01.11
 postviral NEC A86
 Powassan A84.8
 Rasmussen G04.81
 Rio Bravo A85.8
 Russian
  autumnal A83.0
  spring-summer (taiga) A84.0
 saturnine — *see* Poisoning, lead
 specified NEC G04.81
 St. Louis A83.3
 subacute sclerosing A81.1
 summer A83.0
 suppurative G04.81
 tick-borne A84.9
 Torula, torular (cryptococcal) B45.1
 toxic NEC G92
 trichinosis B75 *[G05.3]*
 type
  B A83.0
  C A83.3
 van Bogaert's A81.1
 Venezuelan equine A92.2
 Vienna A85.8
 viral, virus A86
  arthropod-borne NEC A85.2
   mosquito-borne A83.9
    Australian X disease A83.4
    California virus A83.5
    Eastern equine A83.2
    Japanese (B type) A83.0
    Murray Valley A83.4
    specified NEC A83.8
    St. Louis A83.3
    type B A83.0
    type C A83.3

Encephalitis — *continued*
 viral — *continued*
   Western equine A83.1
  tick-borne A84.9
   biundulant A84.1
   central European A84.1
   Czechoslovakian A84.1
   diphasic meningoencephalitis A84.1
   Far Eastern A84.0
   Russian spring-summer (taiga) A84.0
   specified NEC A84.8
  specified type NEC A85.8
 Western equine A83.1
Encephalocele (Q01.9)
 frontal Q01.0
 nasofrontal Q01.1
 occipital Q01.2
 specified NEC Q01.8
Encephalocystocele — *see* Encephalocele
Encephaloduroarteriomyosynangiosis (EDAMS) I67.5
Encephalomalacia (brain) (cerebellar) (cerebral) — *see* Softening, brain
Encephalomeningitis — *see* Meningoencephalitis
Encephalomeningocele — *see* Encephalocele
Encephalomeningomyelitis — *see* Meningoencephalitis
Encephalomyelitis (*see also* Encephalitis) G04.90
 acute disseminated G04.00
  infectious G04.01
  noninfectious G04.81
  postimmunization G04.02
  postinfectious G04.01
 acute necrotizing hemorrhagic G04.30
  postimmunization G04.32
  postinfectious G04.31
  specified NEC G04.39
 benign myalgic G93.3
 equine A83.9
  Eastern A83.2
  Venezuelan A92.2
  Western A83.1
 in diseases classified elsewhere G05.3
 myalgic, benign G93.3
 postchickenpox B01.11
 postinfectious NEC G04.01
 postmeasles B05.0
 postvaccinal G04.02
 postvaricella B01.11
 rubella B06.01
 specified NEC G04.81
 Venezuelan equine A92.2
Encephalomyelocele — *see* Encephalocele
Encephalomyelomeningitis — *see* Meningoencephalitis
Encephalomyelopathy G96.9
Encephalomyeloradiculitis (acute) G61.0
Encephalomyeloradiculoneuritis (acute) (Guillain-Barré) G61.0
Encephalomyeloradiculopathy G96.9
Encephalopathia hyperbilirubinemica, newborn P57.9
 due to isoimmunization (conditions in P55) P57.0
Encephalopathy (acute) G93.40
 acute necrotizing hemorrhagic G04.30
  postimmunization G04.32
  postinfectious G04.31
  specified NEC G04.39
 alcoholic G31.2
 anoxic — *see* Damage, brain, anoxic
 arteriosclerotic I67.2
 centrolobar progressive (Schilder) G37.0
 congenital Q07.9
 degenerative, in specified disease NEC G32.89
 demyelinating callosal G37.1
 due to
  drugs - (*see also* Table of Drugs and Chemicals) G92
 hepatic — *see* Failure, hepatic
 hyperbilirubinemic, newborn P57.9
  due to isoimmunization (conditions in P55) P57.0
 hypertensive I67.4
 hypoglycemic E16.2
 hypoxic — *see* Damage, brain, anoxic
 hypoxic ischemic P91.60
  mild P91.61
  moderate P91.62
  severe P91.63
 in (due to) (with)
  birth injury P11.1
  hyperinsulinism E16.1 *[G94]*

Encephalopathy — *continued*
 in — *continued*
  influenza — *see* Influenza, with, encephalopathy
  lack of vitamin (*see also* Deficiency, vitamin) E56.9 *[G32.89]*
  neoplastic disease (*see also* Neoplasm) D49.9 *[G13.1]*
  serum (*see also* Reaction, serum) T80.69 ☑
  syphilis A52.17
  trauma (postconcussional) F07.81
   current injury — *see* Injury, intracranial
  vaccination G04.02
 lead — *see* Poisoning, lead
 metabolic G93.41
  drug induced G92
  toxic G92
 myoclonic, early, symptomatic — *see* Epilepsy, generalized, specified NEC
 necrotizing, subacute (Leigh) G31.82
 neonatal P91.819
  in diseases classified elsewhere P91.811
 pellagrous E52 *[G32.89]*
 portosystemic — *see* Failure, hepatic
 postcontusional F07.81
  current injury — *see* Injury, intracranial, diffuse
 posthypoglycemic (coma) E16.1 *[G94]*
 postradiation G93.89
 saturnine — *see* Poisoning, lead
 septic G93.41
 specified NEC G93.49
 spongiform, subacute (viral) A81.09
 toxic G92
  metabolic G92
 traumatic (postconcussional) F07.81
  current injury — *see* Injury, intracranial
 vitamin B deficiency NEC E53.9 *[G32.89]*
  vitamin B1 E51.2
 Wernicke's E51.2
Encephalorrhagia — *see* Hemorrhage, intracranial, intracerebral
Encephalosis, posttraumatic F07.81
Enchondroma (*see also* Neoplasm, bone, benign)
Enchondromatosis (cartilaginous) (multiple) Q78.4
Encopresis R15.9
 functional F98.1
 nonorganic origin F98.1
 psychogenic F98.1
Encounter (with health service) (for) Z76.89
 adjustment and management (of)
  breast implant Z45.81 ☑
  implanted device NEC Z45.89
  myringotomy device (stent) (tube) Z45.82
 administrative purpose only Z02.9
  examination for
   adoption Z02.82
   armed forces Z02.3
   disability determination Z02.71
   driving license Z02.4
   employment Z02.1
   insurance Z02.6
   medical certificate NEC Z02.79
   paternity testing Z02.81
   residential institution admission Z02.2
   school admission Z02.0
   sports Z02.5
  specified reason NEC Z02.89
 aftercare — *see* Aftercare
 antenatal screening Z36.9
  cervical length Z36.86
  chromosomal anomalies Z36.0
  congenital cardiac abnormalities Z36.83
  elevated maternal serum alphafetoprotein level Z36.1
  fetal growth retardation Z36.4
  fetal lung maturity Z36.84
  fetal macrosomia Z36.88
  hydrops fetalis Z36.81
  intrauterine growth restriction (IUGR)/small-for-dates Z36.4
  isoimmunization Z36.5
  large-for-dates Z36.88
  malformations Z36.3
  non-visualized anatomy on a previous scan Z36.2
  nuchal translucency Z36.82
  raised alphafetoprotein level Z36.1
  risk of pre-term labor Z36.86
  specified type NEC Z36.89
  specified follow-up NEC Z36.2
  specified genetic defects NEC Z36.8A
  Streptococcus B Z36.85

Encounter - Endocarditis

ICD-10-CM INDEX TO DISEASES AND INJURIES

Encounter — *continued*
- antenatal screening — *continued*
  - suspected anomaly Z36.3
  - uncertain dates Z36.87
- assisted reproductive fertility procedure
  - cycle Z31.83
- blood typing Z01.83
  - Rh typing Z01.83
- breast augmentation or reduction Z41.1
- breast implant exchange (different material) (different size) Z45.81 ☑
- breast reconstruction following mastectomy Z42.1
- check-up — *see* Examination
- chemotherapy for neoplasm Z51.11
- colonoscopy, screening Z12.11
- counseling — *see* Counseling
- delivery, full-term, uncomplicated O80
  - cesarean, without indication O82
- desensitization to allergens Z51.6
- ear piercing Z41.3
- examination — *see* Examination
- expectant parent (s) (adoptive) pre-birth pediatrician visit Z76.81
- fertility preservation procedure (prior to cancer therapy) (prior to removal of gonads) Z31.84
- fitting (of) — *see* Fitting (and adjustment) (of)
- genetic
  - counseling
    - nonprocreative Z71.83
    - procreative Z31.5
  - testing — *see* Test, genetic
- hearing conservation and treatment Z01.12
- immunotherapy for neoplasm Z51.12
- in vitro fertilization cycle Z31.83
- instruction (in)
  - childbirth Z32.2
  - child care (postpartal) (prenatal) Z32.3
  - natural family planning
    - procreative Z31.61
    - to avoid pregnancy Z30.02
- insulin pump titration Z46.81
- joint prosthesis insertion following prior explantation of joint prosthesis (staged procedure)
  - hip Z47.32
  - knee Z47.33
  - shoulder Z47.31
- laboratory (as part of a general medical examination) Z00.00
  - with abnormal findings Z00.01
- mental health services (for)
  - abuse NEC
    - perpetrator Z69.82
    - victim Z69.81
  - child abuse
    - nonparental
      - perpetrator Z69.021
      - victim Z69.020
    - parental
      - perpetrator Z69.011
      - victim Z69.010
  - child neglect
    - nonparental
      - perpetrator Z69.021
      - victim Z69.020
    - parental
      - perpetrator Z69.011
      - victim Z69.010
  - child psychological abuse
    - nonparental
      - perpetrator Z69.021
      - victim Z69.020
    - parental
      - perpetrator Z69.011
      - victim Z69.010
  - child sexual abuse
    - nonparental
      - perpetrator Z69.021
      - victim Z69.020
    - parental
      - perpetrator Z69.011
      - victim Z69.010
  - non-spousal adult abuse (perpetrator) (victim) Z69.81
  - spousal or partner
    - abuse
      - perpetrator Z69.12
      - victim Z69.11
    - neglect
      - perpetrator Z69.12
      - victim Z69.11

Encounter — *continued*
- mental health services — *continued*
  - psychological abuse
    - perpetrator Z69.12
    - victim Z69.11
  - violence
    - perpetrator (physical) (sexual) Z69.12
    - victim (physical) Z69.11
      - sexual Z69.81
- observation (for) (ruled out)
  - exposure to (suspected)
    - anthrax Z03.810
    - biological agent NEC Z03.818
- pediatrician visit, by expectant parent (s) (adoptive) Z76.81
- placental sample (taken vaginally) (*see also* Encounter, antenatal screening) Z36.9
- plastic and reconstructive surgery following medical procedure or healed injury NEC Z42.8
- pregnancy
  - supervision of — *see* Pregnancy, supervision of
  - test Z32.00
    - result negative Z32.02
    - result positive Z32.01
- procreative management and counseling for gestational carrier Z31.7
- prophylactic measures Z29.9
  - antivenin Z29.12
  - fluoride administration Z29.3
  - immunotherapy for respiratory syncytial virus (RSV) Z29.11
  - rabies immune globin Z29.14
  - Rho (D) immune globulin Z29.13
  - specified NEC Z29.8
- radiation therapy (antineoplastic) Z51.0
- radiological (as part of a general medical examination) Z00.00
  - with abnormal findings Z00.01
- reconstructive surgery following medical procedure or healed injury NEC Z42.8
- removal (of) (*see also* Removal)
  - artificial
    - arm Z44.00 ☑
      - complete Z44.01 ☑
      - partial Z44.02 ☑
    - eye Z44.2 ☑
    - leg Z44.10 ☑
      - complete Z44.11 ☑
      - partial Z44.12 ☑
  - breast implant Z45.81 ☑
    - tissue expander (without synchronous insertion of permanent implant) Z45.81 ☑
  - device Z46.9
    - specified NEC Z46.89
  - external
    - fixation device - code to fracture with seventh character D
    - prosthesis, prosthetic device Z44.9
      - breast Z44.3 ☑
      - specified NEC Z44.8
  - implanted device NEC Z45.89
  - insulin pump Z46.81
  - internal fixation device Z47.2
  - myringotomy device (stent) (tube) Z45.82
  - nervous system device NEC Z46.2
    - brain neuropacemaker Z46.2
    - visual substitution device Z46.2
      - implanted Z45.31
  - non-vascular catheter Z46.82
  - orthodontic device Z46.4
  - stent
    - ureteral Z46.6
  - urinary device Z46.6
- repeat cervical smear to confirm findings of recent normal smear following initial abnormal smear Z01.42
- respirator [ventilator] use during power failure Z99.12
- Rh typing Z01.83
- screening — *see* Screening
- specified NEC Z76.89
- sterilization Z30.2
- suspected condition, ruled out
  - amniotic cavity and membrane Z03.71
  - cervical shortening Z03.75
  - fetal anomaly Z03.73
  - fetal growth Z03.74
  - maternal and fetal conditions NEC Z03.79
  - oligohydramnios Z03.71
  - placental problem Z03.72
  - polyhydramnios Z03.71

Encounter — *continued*
- suspected exposure (to), ruled out
  - anthrax Z03.810
  - biological agents NEC Z03.818
- termination of pregnancy, elective Z33.2
- testing — *see* Test
- therapeutic drug level monitoring Z51.81
- titration, insulin pump Z46.81
- to determine fetal viability of pregnancy O36.80 ☑
- training
  - insulin pump Z46.81
- X-ray of chest (as part of a general medical examination) Z00.00
  - with abnormal findings Z00.01

Encystment — *see* Cyst

Endarteritis (bacterial, subacute) (infective) I77.6
- brain I67.7
- cerebral or cerebrospinal I67.7
- deformans — *see* Arteriosclerosis
- embolic — *see* Embolism
- obliterans (*see also* Arteriosclerosis)
  - pulmonary I28.8
- pulmonary I28.8
- retina — *see* Vasculitis, retina
- senile — *see* Arteriosclerosis
- syphilitic A52.09
  - brain or cerebral A52.04
  - congenital A50.54 [I79.8]
- tuberculous A18.89

Endemic — *see* condition

Endocarditis (chronic) (marantic) (nonbacterial) (thrombotic) (valvular) I38
- with rheumatic fever (conditions in I00)
  - active — *see* Endocarditis, acute, rheumatic
  - inactive or quiescent (with chorea) I09.1
- acute or subacute I33.9
  - infective I33.0
  - rheumatic (aortic) (mitral) (pulmonary) (tricuspid) I01.1
    - with chorea (acute) (rheumatic) (Sydenham's) I02.0
- aortic (heart) (nonrheumatic) (valve) I35.8
  - with
    - mitral disease I08.0
      - with tricuspid (valve) disease I08.3
        - active or acute I01.1
          - with chorea (acute) (rheumatic) (Sydenham's) I02.0
    - rheumatic fever (conditions in I00)
      - active — *see* Endocarditis, acute, rheumatic
      - inactive or quiescent (with chorea) I06.9
    - tricuspid (valve) disease I08.2
      - with mitral (valve) disease I08.3
  - acute or subacute I33.9
  - arteriosclerotic I35.8
  - rheumatic I06.9
    - with mitral disease I08.0
      - with tricuspid (valve) disease I08.3
        - active or acute I01.1
          - with chorea (acute) (rheumatic) (Sydenham's) I02.0
    - active or acute I01.1
      - with chorea (acute) (rheumatic) (Sydenham's) I02.0
    - specified NEC I06.8
  - specified cause NEC I35.8
  - syphilitic A52.03
- arteriosclerotic I38
- atypical verrucous (Libman-Sacks) M32.11
- bacterial (acute) (any valve) (subacute) I33.0
- candidal B37.6
- congenital Q24.8
- constrictive I33.0
- Coxiella burnetii A78 [I39]
- Coxsackie B33.21
- due to
  - prosthetic cardiac valve T82.6 ☑
  - Q fever A78 [I39]
  - Serratia marcescens I33.0
  - typhoid (fever) A01.02
- gonococcal A54.83
- infectious or infective (acute) (any valve) (subacute) I33.0
- lenta (acute) (any valve) (subacute) I33.0
- Libman-Sacks M32.11
- listerial A32.82
- Löffler's I42.3
- malignant (acute) (any valve) (subacute) I33.0
- meningococcal A39.51
- mitral (chronic) (double) (fibroid) (heart) (inactive) (valve) (with chorea) I05.9

☑ **Additional character required**

Endocarditis — *continued*
  mitral — *continued*
    with
      aortic (valve) disease I08.0
        with tricuspid (valve) disease I08.3
          active or acute I01.1
            with chorea (acute) (rheumatic)
              (Sydenham's) I02.0
        rheumatic fever (conditions in I00)
          active — *see* Endocarditis, acute, rheumatic
          inactive or quiescent (with chorea) I05.9
        tricuspid (valve) disease I08.1
          with aortic (valve) disease I08.3
      active or acute I01.1
        with chorea (acute) (rheumatic)
          (Sydenham's) I02.0
      bacterial I33.0
      arteriosclerotic I34.8
      nonrheumatic I34.8
        acute or subacute I33.9
      specified NEC I05.8
    monilial B37.6
    multiple valves I08.9
      specified disorders I08.8
    mycotic (acute) (any valve) (subacute) I33.0
    pneumococcal (acute) (any valve)
      (subacute) I33.0
    pulmonary (chronic) (heart) (valve) I37.8
      with rheumatic fever (conditions in I00)
        active — *see* Endocarditis, acute, rheumatic
        inactive or quiescent (with chorea) I09.89
          with aortic, mitral or tricuspid disease I08.8
      acute or subacute I33.9
        rheumatic I01.1
          with chorea (acute) (rheumatic)
            (Sydenham's) I02.0
      arteriosclerotic I37.8
      congenital Q22.2
      rheumatic (chronic) (inactive) (with
        chorea) I09.89
        active or acute I01.1
          with chorea (acute) (rheumatic)
            (Sydenham's) I02.0
      syphilitic A52.03
    purulent (acute) (any valve) (subacute) I33.0
    Q fever A78 *[I39]*
    rheumatic (chronic) (inactive) (with chorea) I09.1
      active or acute (aortic) (mitral) (pulmonary)
        (tricuspid) I01.1
        with chorea (acute) (rheumatic)
          (Sydenham's) I02.0
    rheumatoid — *see* Rheumatoid, carditis
    septic (acute) (any valve) (subacute) I33.0
    streptococcal (acute) (any valve) (subacute) I33.0
    subacute — *see* Endocarditis, acute
    suppurative (acute) (any valve) (subacute) I33.0
    syphilitic A52.03
    toxic I33.9
    tricuspid (chronic) (heart) (inactive) (rheumatic)
      (valve) (with chorea) I07.9
      with
        aortic (valve) disease I08.2
          mitral (valve) disease I08.3
        mitral (valve) disease I08.1
          aortic (valve) disease I08.3
        rheumatic fever (conditions in I00)
          active — *see* Endocarditis, acute, rheumatic
          inactive or quiescent (with chorea) I07.8
      active or acute I01.1
        with chorea (acute) (rheumatic)
          (Sydenham's) I02.0
      arteriosclerotic I36.8
      nonrheumatic I36.8
        acute or subacute I33.9
      specified cause, except rheumatic I36.8
    tuberculous — *see* Tuberculosis, endocarditis
    typhoid A01.02
    ulcerative (acute) (any valve) (subacute) I33.0
    vegetative (acute) (any valve) (subacute) I33.0
    verrucous (atypical) (nonbacterial)
      (nonrheumatic) M32.11
Endocardium, endocardial (*see also* condition)
  cushion defect Q21.2
Endocervicitis (*see also* Cervicitis)
  due to intrauterine (contraceptive)
    device T83.69 ☑
  hyperplastic N72
Endocrine — *see* condition
Endocrinopathy, pluriglandular E31.9
Endodontic
  overfill M27.52
  underfill M27.53

Endodontitis K04.01
  irreversible K04.02
  reversible K04.01
Endomastoiditis — *see* Mastoiditis
Endometrioma N80.9
Endometriosis N80.9
  appendix N80.5
  bladder N80.8
  bowel N80.5
  broad ligament N80.3
  cervix N80.0
  colon N80.5
  cul-de-sac (Douglas') N80.3
  exocervix N80.0
  fallopian tube N80.2
  female genital organ NEC N80.8
  gallbladder N80.8
  in scar of skin N80.6
  internal N80.0
  intestine N80.5
  lung N80.8
  myometrium N80.0
  ovary N80.1
  parametrium N80.3
  pelvic peritoneum N80.3
  peritoneal (pelvic) N80.3
  rectovaginal septum N80.4
  rectum N80.5
  round ligament N80.3
  skin (scar) N80.6
  specified site NEC N80.8
  stromal D39.0
  thorax N80.8
  umbilicus N80.8
  uterus (internal) N80.0
  vagina N80.4
  vulva N80.8
Endometritis (decidual) (nonspecific) (purulent)
  (senile) (atrophic) (suppurative) N71.9
  with ectopic pregnancy O08.0
  acute N71.0
  blenorrhagic (gonococcal) (acute)
    (chronic) A54.24
  cervix, cervical (with erosion or ectropion) (*see*
    also Cervicitis)
    hyperplastic N72
  chlamydial A56.11
  chronic N71.1
  following
    abortion — *see* Abortion by type complicated
      by genital infection
    ectopic or molar pregnancy O08.0
  gonococcal, gonorrheal (acute) (chronic) A54.24
  hyperplastic (*see also* Hyperplasia,
    endometrial) N85.00
    cervix N72
  puerperal, postpartum, childbirth O86.12
  subacute N71.0
  tuberculous A18.17
Endometrium — *see* condition
Endomyocardiopathy, South African I42.3
Endomyocarditis — *see* Endocarditis
Endomyofibrosis I42.3
Endomyometritis — *see* Endometritis
Endopericarditis — *see* Endocarditis
Endoperineuritis — *see* Disorder, nerve
Endophlebitis — *see* Phlebitis
Endophthalmia — *see* Endophthalmitis, purulent
Endophthalmitis (acute) (infective) (metastatic)
  (subacute) H44.009
  bleb associated H59.4 — (*see also* Bleb,
    inflamed (infected), postprocedural)
  gonorrheal A54.39
  in (due to)
    cysticercosis B69.1
    onchocerciasis B73.01
    toxocariasis B83.0
  panuveitis — *see* Panuveitis
  parasitic H44.12 ☑
  purulent H44.00 ☑
    panophthalmitis — *see* Panophthalmitis
    vitreous abscess H44.02 ☑
  specified NEC H44.19
  sympathetic — *see* Uveitis, sympathetic
Endosalpingioma D28.2
Endosalpingiosis N94.89
Endosteitis — *see* Osteomyelitis
Endothelioma, bone — *see* Neoplasm, bone,
  malignant
Endotheliosis (hemorrhagic infectional) D69.8
Endotoxemia - code to condition
Endotrachelitis — *see* Cervicitis

Engelmann (-Camurati) syndrome Q78.3
English disease — *see* Rickets
Engman's disease L30.3
Engorgement
  breast N64.59
    newborn P83.4
    puerperal, postpartum O92.79
  lung (passive) — *see* Edema, lung
  pulmonary (passive) — *see* Edema, lung
  stomach K31.89
  venous, retina — *see* Occlusion, retina, vein,
    engorgement
Enlargement, enlarged (*see also* Hypertrophy)
  adenoids J35.2
    with tonsils J35.3
  alveolar ridge K08.89
    congenital — *see* Anomaly, alveolar
  apertures of diaphragm (congenital) Q79.1
  gingival K06.1
  heart, cardiac — *see* Hypertrophy, cardiac
  labium majus, childhood asymmetric
    (CALME) N90.61
  lacrimal gland, chronic H04.03 ☑
  liver — *see* Hypertrophy, liver
  lymph gland or node R59.9
    generalized R59.1
    localized R59.0
  orbit H05.34 ☑
  organ or site, congenital NEC — *see* Anomaly,
    by site
  parathyroid (gland) E21.0
  pituitary fossa R93.0
  prostate N40.0
    with lower urinary tract symptoms
      (LUTS) N40.1
    without lower urinary tract symptoms
      (LUTS) N40.0
  sella turcica R93.0
  spleen — *see* Splenomegaly
  thymus (gland) (congenital) E32.0
  thyroid (gland) — *see* Goiter
  tongue K14.8
  tonsils J35.1
    with adenoids J35.3
  uterus N85.2
  vestibular aqueduct Q16.5
Enophthalmos H05.40 ☑
  due to
    orbital tissue atrophy H05.41 ☑
    trauma or surgery H05.42 ☑
Enostosis M27.8
Entamebic, entamebiasis — *see* Amebiasis
Entanglement
  umbilical cord (s) O69.82 ☑
    with compression O69.2 ☑
    around neck (with compression) O69.81 ☑
      with compression O69.1 ☑
      without compression O69.81 ☑
    of twins in monoamniotic sac O69.2 ☑
    without compression O69.82 ☑
Enteralgia — *see* Pain, abdominal
Enteric — *see* condition
Enteritis (acute) (diarrheal) (hemorrhagic)
  (noninfective) K52.9
  adenovirus A08.2
  aertrycke infection A02.0
  allergic K52.29
    with
      eosinophilic gastritis or gastroenteritis K52.81
      food protein-induced enterocolitis
        syndrome K52.21
      food protein-induced enteropathy K52.22
  amebic (acute) A06.0
    with abscess — *see* Abscess, amebic
    chronic A06.1
      with abscess — *see* Abscess, amebic
      nondysenteric A06.2
    nondysenteric A06.2
  astrovirus A08.32
  bacillary NOS A03.9
  bacterial A04.9
    specified NEC A04.8
  calicivirus A08.31
  candidal B37.82
  Chilomastix A07.8
  choleriformis A00.1
  chronic (noninfectious) K52.9
    ulcerative — *see* Colitis, ulcerative
  cicatrizing (chronic) — *see* Enteritis, regional,
    small intestine
  Clostridium
    botulinum (food poisoning) A05.1

Enteritis — *continued*
- Clostridium — *continued*
  - difficile
    - not specified as recurrent A04.72
    - recurrent A04.71
- coccidial A07.3
- coxsackie virus A08.39
- dietetic (*see also* Enteritis, allergic) K52.29
- drug-induced K52.1
- due to
  - astrovirus A08.32
  - calicivirus A08.31
  - coxsackie virus A08.39
  - drugs K52.1
  - echovirus A08.39
  - enterovirus NEC A08.39
  - food hypersensitivity (*see also* Enteritis, allergic) K52.29
  - infectious organism (bacterial) (viral) — *see* Enteritis, infectious
  - torovirus A08.39
  - Yersinia enterocolitica A04.6
- echovirus A08.39
- eltor A00.1
- enterovirus NEC A08.39
- eosinophilic K52.81
- epidemic (infectious) A09
- fulminant (*see also* Ischemia, intestine, acute) K55.019
- gangrenous — *see* Enteritis, infectious
- giardial A07.1
- infectious NOS A09
  - due to
    - adenovirus A08.2
    - Aerobacter aerogenes A04.8
    - Arizona (bacillus) A02.0
    - bacteria NOS A04.9
      - specified NEC A04.8
    - Campylobacter A04.5
    - Clostridium difficile
      - not specified as recurrent A04.72
      - recurrent A04.71
    - Clostridium perfringens A04.8
    - Enterobacter aerogenes A04.8
    - enterovirus A08.39
    - Escherichia coli A04.4
      - enteroaggregative A04.4
      - enterohemorrhagic A04.3
      - enteroinvasive A04.2
      - enteropathogenic A04.0
      - enterotoxigenic A04.1
      - specified NEC A04.4
    - specified
      - bacteria NEC A04.8
      - virus NEC A08.39
    - Staphylococcus A04.8
    - virus NEC A08.4
      - specified type NEC A08.39
    - Yersinia enterocolitica A04.6
  - specified organism NEC A08.8
- influenzal — *see* Influenza, with, digestive manifestations
- ischemic K55.9
  - acute (*see also* Ischemia, intestine, acute) K55.019
  - chronic K55.1
- microsporidial A07.8
- mucomembranous, myxomembranous — *see* Syndrome, irritable bowel
- mucous — *see* Syndrome, irritable bowel
- necroticans A05.2
- necrotizing of newborn — *see* Enterocolitis, necrotizing, in newborn
- neurogenic — *see* Syndrome, irritable bowel
- newborn necrotizing — *see* Enterocolitis, necrotizing, in newborn
- noninfectious K52.9
- norovirus A08.11
- parasitic NEC B82.9
- paratyphoid (fever) — *see* Fever, paratyphoid
- protozoal A07.9
  - specified NEC A07.8
- radiation K52.0
- regional (of) K50.90
  - with
    - complication K50.919
      - abscess K50.914
      - fistula K50.913
      - intestinal obstruction K50.912
      - rectal bleeding K50.911
      - specified complication NEC K50.918
  - colon — *see* Enteritis, regional, large intestine

Enteritis — *continued*
- regional — *continued*
  - duodenum — *see* Enteritis, regional, small intestine
  - ileum — *see* Enteritis, regional, small intestine
  - jejunum — *see* Enteritis, regional, small intestine
  - large bowel — *see* Enteritis, regional, large intestine
  - large intestine (colon) (rectum) K50.10
    - with
      - complication K50.119
        - abscess K50.114
        - fistula K50.113
        - intestinal obstruction K50.112
        - rectal bleeding K50.111
        - small intestine (duodenum) (ileum) (jejunum) involvement K50.80
          - with
            - complication K50.819
              - abscess K50.814
              - fistula K50.813
              - intestinal obstruction K50.812
              - rectal bleeding K50.811
              - specified complication NEC K50.818
        - specified complication NEC K50.118
  - rectum — *see* Enteritis, regional, large intestine
  - small intestine (duodenum) (ileum) (jejunum) K50.00
    - with
      - complication K50.019
        - abscess K50.014
        - fistula K50.013
        - intestinal obstruction K50.012
        - large intestine (colon) (rectum) involvement K50.80
          - with
            - complication K50.819
              - abscess K50.814
              - fistula K50.813
              - intestinal obstruction K50.812
              - rectal bleeding K50.811
              - specified complication NEC K50.818
        - rectal bleeding K50.011
        - specified complication NEC K50.018
- rotaviral A08.0
- Salmonella, salmonellosis (arizonae) (choleraesuis) (enteritidis) (typhimurium) A02.0
- segmental — *see* Enteritis, regional
- septic A09
- Shigella — *see* Infection, Shigella
- small round structured NEC A08.19
- spasmodic, spastic — *see* Syndrome, irritable bowel
- staphylococcal A04.8
  - due to food A05.0
- torovirus A08.39
- toxic NEC K52.1
  - due to Clostridium difficile
    - not specified as recurrent A04.72
    - recurrent A04.71
- trichomonal A07.8
- tuberculous A18.32
- typhosa A01.00
- ulcerative (chronic) — *see* Colitis, ulcerative
- viral A08.4
  - adenovirus A08.2
  - enterovirus A08.39
  - Rotavirus A08.0
  - small round structured NEC A08.19
  - specified NEC A08.39
  - virus specified NEC A08.39

Enterobiasis B80
Enterobius vermicularis (infection) (infestation) B80
Enterocele (*see also* Hernia, abdomen)
- pelvic, pelvis (acquired) (congenital) N81.5
- vagina, vaginal (acquired) (congenital) NEC N81.5
Enterocolitis (*see also* Enteritis) K52.9
- due to Clostridium difficile
  - not specified as recurrent A04.72
  - recurrent A04.71
- fulminant ischemic (*see also* Ischemia, intestine, acute) K55.059
- granulomatous — *see* Enteritis, regional
- hemorrhagic (acute) (*see also* Ischemia, intestine, acute) K55.059
  - chronic K55.1
- infectious NEC A09
- ischemic K55.9

Enterocolitis — *continued*
- necrotizing K55.30
  - with
    - perforation K55.33
    - pneumatosis K55.32
      - and perforation K55.33
  - due to Clostridium difficile
    - not specified as recurrent A04.72
    - recurrent A04.71
  - in non-newborn K55.30
    - stage 1 (without pneumatosis, without perforation) K55.31
    - stage 2 (with pneumatosis, without perforation) K55.32
    - stage 3 (with pneumatosis, with perforation) K55.33
  - in newborn P77.9
    - stage 1 (without pneumatosis, without perforation) P77.1
    - stage 2 (with pneumatosis, without perforation) P77.2
    - stage 3 (with pneumatosis, with perforation) P77.3
  - without pneumatosis or perforation K55.31
- noninfectious K52.9
  - newborn — *see* Enterocolitis, necrotizing, in newborn
- pseudomembranous (newborn)
  - not specified as recurrent A04.72 ☑
  - recurrent A04.71
- radiation K52.0
  - newborn — *see* Enterocolitis, necrotizing, in newborn
- ulcerative (chronic) — *see* Pancolitis, ulcerative (chronic)
Enterogastritis — *see* Enteritis
Enteropathy K63.9
- food protein-induced enterocolitis K52.22
- celiac-gluten-sensitive K90.0
  - non-celiac K90.41
- hemorrhagic, terminal (*see also* Ischemia, intestine, acute) K55.059
- protein-losing K90.49
Enteroperitonitis — *see* Peritonitis
Enteroptosis K63.4
Enterorrhagia K92.2
Enterospasm (*see also* Syndrome, irritable, bowel)
- psychogenic F45.8
Enterostenosis (*see also* Obstruction, intestine, specified NEC) K56.699
Enterostomy
- complication — *see* Complication, enterostomy
- status Z93.4
Enterovirus, as cause of disease classified elsewhere B97.10
- coxsackievirus B97.11
- echovirus B97.12
- other specified B97.19
Enthesopathy (peripheral) M77.9
- Achilles tendinitis — *see* Tendinitis, Achilles
- ankle and tarsus M77.9
  - specified type NEC — *see* Enthesopathy, foot, specified type NEC
- anterior tibial syndrome M76.81 ☑
- calcaneal spur — *see* Spur, bone, calcaneal
- elbow region M77.8
  - lateral epicondylitis — *see* Epicondylitis, lateral
  - medial epicondylitis — *see* Epicondylitis, medial
- foot NEC M77.9
  - metatarsalgia — *see* Metatarsalgia
  - specified type NEC M77.5 ☑
- forearm M77.9
- gluteal tendinitis — *see* Tendinitis, gluteal
- hand M77.9
- hip — *see* Enthesopathy, lower limb, specified type NEC
- iliac crest spur — *see* Spur, bone, iliac crest
- iliotibial band syndrome — *see* Syndrome, iliotibial band
- knee — *see* Enthesopathy, lower limb, lower leg, specified type NEC
- lateral epicondylitis — *see* Epicondylitis, lateral
- lower limb (excluding foot) M76.9
  - Achilles tendinitis — *see* Tendinitis, Achilles
  - anterior tibial syndrome M76.81 ☑
  - gluteal tendinitis — *see* Tendinitis, gluteal
  - iliac crest spur — *see* Spur, bone, iliac crest
  - iliotibial band syndrome — *see* Syndrome, iliotibial band
  - patellar tendinitis — *see* Tendinitis, patellar

☑ **Additional character required**

Enthesopathy — *continued*
  lower limb — *continued*
    pelvic region — *see* Enthesopathy, lower limb,
      specified type NEC
    peroneal tendinitis — *see* Tendinitis, peroneal
    posterior tibial syndrome M76.82 ☑
    psoas tendinitis — *see* Tendinitis, psoas
    shoulder M77.9
    specified type NEC M76.89 ☑
    tibial collateral bursitis — *see* Bursitis, tibial
      collateral
  medial epicondylitis — *see* Epicondylitis, medial
  metatarsalgia — *see* Metatarsalgia
  multiple sites M77.9
  patellar tendinitis — *see* Tendinitis, patellar
  pelvis M77.9
  periarthritis of wrist — *see* Periarthritis, wrist
  peroneal tendinitis — *see* Tendinitis, peroneal
  posterior tibial syndrome M76.82 ☑
  psoas tendinitis — *see* Tendinitis, psoas
  shoulder region — *see* Lesion, shoulder
  specified site NEC M77.9
  specified type NEC M77.8
  spinal M46.00
    cervical region M46.02
    cervicothoracic region M46.03
    lumbar region M46.06
    lumbosacral region M46.07
    multiple sites M46.09
    occipito-atlanto-axial region M46.01
    sacrococcygeal region M46.08
    thoracic region M46.04
    thoracolumbar region M46.05
  tibial collateral bursitis — *see* Bursitis, tibial
    collateral
  upper arm M77.9
  wrist and carpus NEC M77.8
    calcaneal spur — *see* Spur, bone, calcaneal
    periarthritis of wrist — *see* Periarthritis, wrist
Entomophobia F40.218
Entomophthoromycosis B46.8
Entrance, air into vein — *see* Embolism, air
Entrapment, nerve — *see* Neuropathy, entrapment
Entropion (eyelid) (paralytic) H02.009
  cicatricial H02.019
    left H02.016
      lower H02.015
      upper H02.014
    right H02.013
      lower H02.012
      upper H02.011
  congenital Q10.2
  left H02.006
    lower H02.005
    upper H02.004
  mechanical H02.029
    left H02.026
      lower H02.025
      upper H02.024
    right H02.023
      lower H02.022
      upper H02.021
  right H02.003
    lower H02.002
    upper H02.001
  senile H02.039
    left H02.036
      lower H02.035
      upper H02.034
    right H02.033
      lower H02.032
      upper H02.031
  spastic H02.049
    left H02.046
      lower H02.045
      upper H02.044
    right H02.043
      lower H02.042
      upper H02.041
Enucleated eye (traumatic, current) S05.7 ☑
Enuresis R32
  functional F98.0
  habit disturbance F98.0
  nocturnal N39.44
    psychogenic F98.0
  nonorganic origin F98.0
  psychogenic F98.0
Eosinopenia — *see* Agranulocytosis
Eosinophilia (allergic) (hereditary) (idiopathic)
  (secondary) D72.1
  with
    angiolymphoid hyperplasia (ALHE) D18.01

Eosinophilia — *continued*
  infiltrative J82
  Löffler's J82
  peritoneal — *see* Peritonitis, eosinophilic
  pulmonary NEC J82
  tropical (pulmonary) J82
Eosinophilia-myalgia syndrome M35.8
Ependymitis (acute) (cerebral) (chronic) (granular) —
  see Encephalomyelitis
Ependymoblastoma
  specified site — *see* Neoplasm, malignant, by site
  unspecified site C71.9
Ependymoma (epithelial) (malignant)
  anaplastic
    specified site — *see* Neoplasm, malignant, by
      site
    unspecified site C71.9
  benign
    specified site — *see* Neoplasm, benign, by site
    unspecified site D33.2
  myxopapillary D43.2
    specified site — *see* Neoplasm, uncertain
      behavior, by site
    unspecified site D43.2
  papillary D43.2
    specified site — *see* Neoplasm, uncertain
      behavior, by site
    unspecified site D43.2
  specified site — *see* Neoplasm, malignant, by site
  unspecified site C71.9
Ependymopathy G93.89
Ephelis, ephelides L81.2
Epiblepharon (congenital) Q10.3
Epicanthus, epicanthic fold (eyelid) (congenital)
  Q10.3
Epicondylitis (elbow)
  lateral M77.1 ☑
  medial M77.0 ☑
Epicystitis — *see* Cystitis
Epidemic — *see* condition
Epidermidalization, cervix — *see* Dysplasia, cervix
Epidermis, epidermal — *see* condition
Epidermodysplasia verruciformis B07.8
Epidermolysis
  bullosa (congenital) Q81.9
    acquired L12.30
      drug-induced L12.31
      specified cause NEC L12.35
    dystrophica Q81.2
    letalis Q81.1
    simplex Q81.0
    specified NEC Q81.8
  necroticans combustiformis L51.2
    due to drug — *see* Table of Drugs and
      Chemicals, by drug
Epidermophytid — *see* Dermatophytosis
Epidermophytosis (infected) — *see*
  Dermatophytosis
Epididymis — *see* condition
Epididymitis (acute) (nonvenereal) (recurrent)
  (residual) N45.1
  with orchitis N45.3
  blennorrhagic (gonococcal) A54.23
  caseous (tuberculous) A18.15
  chlamydial A56.19
  filarial (*see also* Infestation, filarial) B74.9 *[N51]*
  gonococcal A54.23
  syphilitic A52.76
  tuberculous A18.15
Epididymo-orchitis (*see also* Epididymitis) N45.3
Epidural — *see* condition
Epigastrium, epigastric — *see* condition
Epigastrocele — *see* Hernia, ventral
Epiglottis — *see* condition
Epiglottitis, epiglottiditis (acute) J05.10
  with obstruction J05.11
  chronic J37.0
Epignathus Q89.4
Epilepsia partialis continua (*see also* Kozhevnikof's
  epilepsy) G40.1 ☑
Epilepsy, epileptic, epilepsia (attack) (cerebral)
  (convulsion) (fit) (seizure) G40.909
  Note: the following terms are to be considered
    equivalent to intractable: pharmacoresistant
    (pharmacologically resistant), treatment
    resistant, refractory (medically) and poorly
    controlled
  with
    complex partial seizures — *see* Epilepsy,
      localization-related, symptomatic, with
      complex partial seizures

Epilepsy — *continued*
  with — *continued*
    grand mal seizures on awakening — *see*
      Epilepsy, generalized, specified NEC
    myoclonic absences — *see* Epilepsy,
      generalized, specified NEC
    myoclonic-astatic seizures — *see* Epilepsy,
      generalized, specified NEC
    simple partial seizures — *see* Epilepsy,
      localization-related, symptomatic, with
      simple partial seizures
  akinetic — *see* Epilepsy, generalized, specified
    NEC
  benign childhood with centrotemporal EEG
    spikes — *see* Epilepsy, localization-related,
      idiopathic
  benign myoclonic in infancy G40.80 ☑
  Bravais-jacksonian — *see* Epilepsy, localization-
    related, symptomatic, with simple partial
    seizures
  childhood
    with occipital EEG paroxysms — *see* Epilepsy,
      localization-related, idiopathic
    absence G40.A09
      intractable G40.A19
        with status epilepticus G40.A11
        without status epilepticus G40.A19
      not intractable G40.A09
        with status epilepticus G40.A01
        without status epilepticus G40.A09
  climacteric — *see* Epilepsy, specified NEC
  cysticercosis B69.0
  deterioration (mental) F06.8
  due to syphilis A52.19
  focal — *see* Epilepsy, localization-related,
    symptomatic, with simple partial seizures
  generalized
    idiopathic G40.309
      intractable G40.319
        with status epilepticus G40.311
        without status epilepticus G40.319
      not intractable G40.309
        with status epilepticus G40.301
        without status epilepticus G40.309
    specified NEC G40.409
      intractable G40.419
        with status epilepticus G40.411
        without status epilepticus G40.419
      not intractable G40.409
        with status epilepticus G40.401
        without status epilepticus G40.409
  impulsive petit mal — *see* Epilepsy, juvenile
    myoclonic
  intractable G40.919
    with status epilepticus G40.911
    without status epilepticus G40.919
  juvenile absence G40.A09
    intractable G40.A19
      with status epilepticus G40.A11
      without status epilepticus G40.A19
    not intractable G40.A09
      with status epilepticus G40.A01
      without status epilepticus G40.A09
  juvenile myoclonic G40.B09
    intractable G40.B19
      with status epilepticus G40.B11
      without status epilepticus G40.B19
    not intractable G40.B09
      with status epilepticus G40.B01
      without status epilepticus G40.B09
  localization-related (focal) (partial)
    idiopathic G40.009
      with seizures of localized onset G40.009
        intractable G40.019
          with status epilepticus G40.011
          without status epilepticus G40.019
        not intractable G40.009
          with status epilepticus G40.001
          without status epilepticus G40.009
    symptomatic
      with complex partial seizures G40.209
        intractable G40.219
          with status epilepticus G40.211
          without status epilepticus G40.219
        not intractable G40.209
          with status epilepticus G40.201
          without status epilepticus G40.209
      with simple partial seizures G40.109
        intractable G40.119
          with status epilepticus G40.111
          without status epilepticus G40.119
        not intractable G40.109

Epilepsy — *continued*
  localization-related — *continued*
      with status epilepticus G40.101
       without status epilepticus G40.109
  myoclonus, myoclonic — *see* Epilepsy,
    generalized, specified NEC
    progressive — *see* Epilepsy, generalized,
     idiopathic
  not intractable G40.909
    with status epilepticus G40.901
    without status epilepticus G40.909
  on awakening — *see* Epilepsy, generalized,
    specified NEC
  parasitic NOS B71.9 *[G94]*
  partialis continua (see also Kozhevnikof's
    epilepsy) G40.1 ☑
  peripheral — *see* Epilepsy, specified NEC
  procursiva — *see* Epilepsy, localization-related,
    symptomatic, with simple partial seizures
  progressive (familial) myoclonic — *see* Epilepsy,
    generalized, idiopathic
  reflex — *see* Epilepsy, specified NEC
  related to
    alcohol G40.509
      not intractable G40.509
        with status epilepticus G40.501
        without status epliepticus G40.509
    drugs G40.509
      not intractable G40.509
        with status epilepticus G40.501
        without status epliepticus G40.509
    external causes G40.509
      not intractable G40.509
        with status epilepticus G40.501
        without status epliepticus G40.509
    hormonal changes G40.509
      not intractable G40.509
        with status epilepticus G40.501
        without status epliepticus G40.509
    sleep deprivation G40.509
      not intractable G40.509
        with status epilepticus G40.501
        without status epliepticus G40.509
    stress G40.509
      not intractable G40.509
        with status epilepticus G40.501
        without status epliepticus G40.509
  somatomotor — *see* Epilepsy, localization-related,
    symptomatic, with simple partial seizures
  somatosensory — *see* Epilepsy, localization-
    related, symptomatic, with simple partial
    seizures
  spasms G40.822
    intractable G40.824
      with status epilepticus G40.823
      without status epilepticus G40.824
    not intractable G40.822
      with status epilepticus G40.821
      without status epilepticus G40.822
  specified NEC G40.802
    intractable G40.804
      with status epilepticus G40.803
      without status epilepticus G40.804
    not intractable G40.802
      with status epilepticus G40.801
      without status epilepticus G40.802
  syndromes
    generalized
      idiopathic G40.309
        intractable G40.319
          with status epilepticus G40.311
          without status epilepticus G40.319
        not intractable G40.309
          with status epilepticus G40.301
          without status epilepticus G40.309
      specified NEC G40.409
        intractable G40.419
          with status epilepticus G40.411
          without status epilepticus G40.419
        not intractable G40.409
          with status epilepticus G40.401
          without status epilepticus G40.409
    localization-related (focal) (partial)
      idiopathic G40.009
        with seizures of localized onset G40.009
          intractable G40.019
            with status epilepticus G40.011
            without status epilepticus G40.019
          not intractable G40.009
            with status epilepticus G40.001
            without status epilepticus G40.009
    symptomatic

Epilepsy — *continued*
  syndromes — *continued*
      with complex partial seizures G40.209
        intractable G40.219
          with status epilepticus G40.211
          without status epilepticus G40.219
        not intractable G40.209
          with status epilepticus G40.201
          without status epilepticus G40.209
      with simple partial seizures G40.109
        intractable G40.119
          with status epilepticus G40.111
          without status epilepticus G40.119
        not intractable G40.109
          with status epilepticus G40.101
          without status epilepticus G40.109
      specified NEC G40.802
        intractable G40.804
          with status epilepticus G40.803
          without status epilepticus G40.804
        not intractable G40.802
          with status epilepticus G40.801
          without status epilepticus G40.802
    tonic (-clonic) — *see* Epilepsy, generalized,
      specified NEC
    twilight F05
    uncinate (gyrus) — *see* Epilepsy, localization-
      related, symptomatic, with complex partial
      seizures
    Unverricht (-Lundborg) (familial myoclonic) — *see*
      Epilepsy, generalized, idiopathic
    visceral — *see* Epilepsy, specified NEC
    visual — *see* Epilepsy, specified NEC
Epiloia Q85.1
Epimenorrhea N92.0
Epipharyngitis — *see* Nasopharyngitis
Epiphora H04.20 ☑
  due to
    excess lacrimation H04.21 ☑
    insufficient drainage H04.22 ☑
Epiphyseal arrest — *see* Arrest, epiphyseal
Epiphyseolysis, epiphysiolysis — *see*
  Osteochondropathy
Epiphysitis (see also Osteochondropathy)
  juvenile M92.9
  syphilitic (congenital) A50.02
Epiplocele — *see* Hernia, abdomen
Epiploitis — *see* Peritonitis
Epiplosarcomphalocele — *see* Hernia, umbilicus
Episcleritis (suppurative) H15.10 ☑
  in (due to)
    syphilis A52.71
    tuberculosis A18.51
  nodular H15.12 ☑
  periodica fugax H15.11 ☑
    angioneurotic — *see* Edema, angioneurotic
  syphilitic (late) A52.71
  tuberculous A18.51
Episode
  affective, mixed F39
  depersonalization (in neurotic state) F48.1
  depressive F32.9
    major F32.9
      mild F32.0
      moderate F32.1
      severe (without psychotic symptoms) F32.2
        with psychotic symptoms F32.3
    recurrent F33.9
      brief F33.8
    specified NEC F32.89
  hypomanic F30.8
  manic F30.9
    with
      psychotic symptoms F30.2
      remission (full) F30.4
        partial F30.3
    other specified F30.8
    recurrent F31.89
    without psychotic symptoms F30.10
      mild F30.11
      moderate F30.12
      severe (without psychotic symptoms) F30.13
        with psychotic symptoms F30.2
  psychotic F23
    organic F06.8
  schizophrenic (acute) NEC, brief F23
Epispadias (female) (male) Q64.0
Episplenitis D73.89
Epistaxis (multiple) R04.0
  hereditary I78.0
  vicarious menstruation N94.89

Epithelioma (malignant) — *(see also* Neoplasm,
  malignant, by site)
  adenoides cysticum — *see* Neoplasm, skin, benign
  basal cell — *see* Neoplasm, skin, malignant
  benign — *see* Neoplasm, benign, by site
  Bowen's — *see* Neoplasm, skin, in situ
  calcifying, of Malherbe — *see* Neoplasm, skin,
    benign
  external site — *see* Neoplasm, skin, malignant
  intraepidermal, Jadassohn — *see* Neoplasm, skin,
    benign
  squamous cell — *see* Neoplasm, malignant, by
    site
Epitheliomatosis pigmented Q82.1
Epitheliopathy, multifocal placoid pigment
  H30.14 ☑
Epithelium, epithelial — *see* condition
Epituberculosis (with atelectasis) (allergic) A15.7
Eponychia Q84.6
Epstein's
  nephrosis or syndrome — *see* Nephrosis
  pearl K09.8
Epulis (gingiva) (fibrous) (giant cell) K06.8
Equinia A24.0
Equinovarus (congenital) (talipes) Q66.0
  acquired — *see* Deformity, limb, clubfoot
Equivalent
  convulsive (abdominal) — *see* Epilepsy, specified
    NEC
  epileptic (psychic) — *see* Epilepsy, localization-
    related, symptomatic, with complex partial
    seizures
Erb (-Duchenne) paralysis (birth injury) (newborn)
  P14.0
Erb-Goldflam disease or syndrome G70.00
  with exacerbation (acute) G70.01
  in crisis G70.01
Erb's
  disease G71.0
  palsy, paralysis (brachial) (birth) (newborn) P14.0
    spinal (spastic) syphilitic A52.17
  pseudohypertrophic muscular dystrophy G71.0
Erdheim's syndrome (acromegalic macrospondylitis)
  E22.0
Erection, painful (persistent) — *see* Priapism
Ergosterol deficiency (vitamin D) E55.9
  with
    adult osteomalacia M83.8
    rickets — *see* Rickets
Ergotism (see also Poisoning, food, noxious, plant)
  from ergot used as drug (migraine therapy) — *see*
    Table of Drugs and Chemicals
Erosio interdigitalis blastomycetica B37.2
Erosion
  artery I77.2
    without rupture I77.89
  bone — *see* Disorder, bone, density and structure,
    specified NEC
  bronchus J98.09
  cartilage (joint) — *see* Disorder, cartilage,
    specified type NEC
  cervix (uteri) (acquired) (chronic) (congenital) N86
    with cervicitis N72
  cornea (nontraumatic) — *see* Ulcer, cornea
    recurrent H18.83 ☑
    traumatic — *see* Abrasion, cornea
  dental (idiopathic) (occupational) (due to diet,
    drugs or vomiting) K03.2
  duodenum, postpyloric — *see* Ulcer, duodenum
  esophagus K22.10
    with bleeding K22.11
  gastric — *see* Ulcer, stomach
  gastrojejunal — *see* Ulcer, gastrojejunal
  implanted mesh — *see* Complications, mesh
  intestine K63.3
  lymphatic vessel I89.8
  pylorus, pyloric (ulcer) — *see* Ulcer, stomach
  spine, aneurysmal A52.09
  stomach — *see* Ulcer, stomach
  subcutaneous device pocket
    nervous system prosthetic device, implant, or
      graft T85.890 ☑
    other internal prosthetic device, implant, or
      graft T85.898 ☑
  teeth (idiopathic) (occupational) (due to diet,
    drugs or vomiting) K03.2
  urethra N36.8
  uterus N85.8
Erotomania F52.8
Error
  metabolism, inborn — *see* Disorder, metabolism
  refractive — *see* Disorder, refraction

☑ **Additional character required**

Epilepsy - Error

ICD-10-CM INDEX TO DISEASES AND INJURIES

Eructation R14.2
  nervous or psychogenic F45.8
Eruption
  creeping B76.9
  drug (generalized) (taken internally) L27.0
    fixed L27.1
    in contact with skin — see Dermatitis, due to
      drugs
    localized L27.1
  Hutchinson, summer L56.4
  Kaposi's varicelliform B00.0
  napkin L22
  polymorphous light (sun) L56.4
  recalcitrant pustular L13.8
  ringed R23.8
  skin (nonspecific) R21
    creeping (meaning hookworm) B76.9
    due to inoculation/vaccination (generalized)
      (see also Dermatitis, due to, vaccine) L27.0
      localized L27.1
    erysipeloid A26.0
    feigned L98.1
    Kaposi's varicelliform B00.0
    lichenoid L28.0
    meaning dermatitis — see Dermatitis
    toxic NEC L53.0
  tooth, teeth, abnormal (incomplete) (late)
    (premature) (sequence) K00.6
  vesicular R23.8
Erysipelas (gangrenous) (infantile) (newborn)
  (phlegmonous) (suppurative) A46
  external ear A46 [H62.40]
  puerperal, postpartum O86.89
Erysipeloid A26.9
  cutaneous (Rosenbach's) A26.0
  disseminated A26.8
  sepsis A26.7
  specified NEC A26.8
Erythema, erythematous (infectional)
  (inflammation) L53.9
  ab igne L59.0
  annulare (centrifugum) (rheumaticum) L53.1
  arthriticum epidemicum A25.1
  brucellum — see Brucellosis
  chronic figurate NEC L53.3
  chronicum migrans (Borrelia burgdorferi) A69.20
  diaper L22
  due to
    chemical NEC L53.0
      in contact with skin L24.5
    drug (internal use) — see Dermatitis, due to,
      drugs
  elevatum diutinum L95.1
  endemic E52
  epidemic, arthritic A25.1
  figuratum perstans L53.3
  gluteal L22
  heat - code by site under Burn, first degree
  ichthyosiforme congenitum bullous Q80.3
  in diseases classified elsewhere L54
  induratum (nontuberculous) L52
    tuberculous A18.4
  infectiosum B08.3
  intertrigo L30.4
  iris L51.9
  marginatum L53.2
    in (due to) acute rheumatic fever I00
  medicamentosum — see Dermatitis, due to,
    drugs
  migrans A26.0
    chronicum A69.20
    tongue K14.1
  multiforme (major) (minor) L51.9
    bullous, bullosum L51.1
    conjunctiva L51.1
    nonbullous L51.0
    pemphigoides L12.0
    specified NEC L51.8
  napkin L22
  neonatorum P83.88
    toxic P83.1
  nodosum L52
    tuberculous A18.4
  palmar L53.8
  pernio T69.1 ☑
  rash, newborn P83.88
  scarlatiniform (recurrent) (exfoliative) L53.8
  solare L55.0
  specified NEC L53.8
  toxic, toxicum NEC L53.0
    newborn P83.1
  tuberculous (primary) A18.4

Erythematous, erythematosus — see condition
Erythermalgia (primary) I73.81
Erythralgia I73.81
Erythrasma L08.1
Erythredema (polyneuropathy) — see Poisoning,
  mercury
Erythremia (acute) C94.0 ☑
  chronic D45
  secondary D75.1
Erythroblastopenia (see also Aplasia, red cell) D60.9
  congenital D61.01
Erythroblastophthisis D61.09
Erythroblastosis (fetalis) (newborn) P55.9
  due to
    ABO (antibodies) (incompatibility)
      (isoimmunization) P55.1
    Rh (antibodies) (incompatibility)
      (isoimmunization) P55.0
Erythrocyanosis (crurum) I73.89
Erythrocythemia — see Erythremia
Erythrocytosis (megalosplenic) (secondary) D75.1
  familial D75.0
  oval, hereditary — see Elliptocytosis
  secondary D75.1
  stress D75.1
Erythroderma (secondary) (see also Erythema) L53.9
  bullous ichthyosiform, congenital Q80.3
  desquamativum L21.1
  ichthyosiform, congenital (bullous) Q80.3
  neonatorum P83.88
  psoriaticum L40.8
Erythrodysesthesia, palmar plantar (PPE) L27.1
Erythrogenesis imperfecta D61.09
Erythroleukemia C94.0 ☑
Erythromelalgia I73.81
Erythrophagocytosis D75.89
Erythrophobia F40.298
Erythroplakia, oral epithelium, and tongue K13.29
Erythroplasia (Queyrat) D07.4
  specified site — see Neoplasm, skin, in situ
  unspecified site D07.4
Escherichia coli (E. coli), as cause of disease classified
  elsewhere B96.20
  non-O157 Shiga toxin-producing (with known O
    group) B96.22
  non-Shiga toxin-producing B96.29
  O157 with confirmation of Shiga toxin when H
    antigen is unknown, or is not H7 B96.21
  O157:H- (nonmotile) with confirmation of Shiga
    toxin B96.21
  Shiga toxin-producing (with unspecified O
    group) (STEC) B96.23
  O157 B96.21
  O157:H7 with or without confirmation of Shiga
    toxin-production B96.21
  specified NEC B96.29
Esophagismus K22.4
Esophagitis (acute) (alkaline) (chemical) (chronic)
  (infectional) (necrotic) (peptic) (postoperative)
  K20.9
  candidal B37.81
  due to gastrointestinal reflux disease K21.0
  eosinophilic K20.0
  reflux K21.0
  specified NEC K20.8
  tuberculous A18.83
  ulcerative K22.10
    with bleeding K22.11
Esophagocele K22.5
Esophagomalacia K22.8
Esophagospasm K22.4
Esophagostenosis K22.2
Esophagostomiasis B81.8
Esophagotracheal — see condition
Esophagus — see condition
Esophoria H50.51
  convergence, excess H51.12
  divergence, insufficiency H51.8
Esotropia — see Strabismus, convergent
  concomitant
Espundia B55.2
Essential — see condition
Esthesioneuroblastoma C30.0
Esthesioneurocytoma C30.0
Esthesioneuroepithelioma C30.0
Esthiomene A55
Estivo-autumnal malaria (fever) B50.9
Estrangement (marital) Z63.5
  parent-child NEC Z62.890

Estriasis — see Myiasis
Ethanolism — see Alcoholism
Etherism — see Dependence, drug, inhalant
Ethmoid, ethmoidal — see condition
Ethmoiditis (chronic) (nonpurulent) (purulent) (see
  also Sinusitis, ethmoidal)
  influenzal — see Influenza, with, respiratory
    manifestations NEC
  Woakes' J33.1
Ethylism — see Alcoholism
Eulenburg's disease (congenital paramyotonia)
  G71.19
Eumycetoma B47.0
Eunuchoidism E29.1
  hypogonadotropic E23.0
European blastomycosis — see Cryptococcosis
Eustachian — see condition
Evaluation (for) (of)
  development state
    adolescent Z00.3
    period of
      delayed growth in childhood Z00.70
        with abnormal findings Z00.71
      rapid growth in childhood Z00.2
    puberty Z00.3
  growth and developmental state (period of rapid
    growth) Z00.2
    delayed growth Z00.70
      with abnormal findings Z00.71
  mental health (status) Z00.8
    requested by authority Z04.6
  period of
    delayed growth in childhood Z00.70
      with abnormal findings Z00.71
    rapid growth in childhood Z00.2
  suspected condition — see Observation
Evans syndrome D69.41
Event
  apparent life threatening in newborn and infant
    (ALTE) R68.13
  brief resolved unexplained event (BRUE) R68.13
Eventration (see also Hernia, ventral)
  colon into chest — see Hernia, diaphragm
  diaphragm (congenital) Q79.1
Eversion
  bladder N32.89
  cervix (uteri) N86
    with cervicitis N72
  foot NEC (see also Deformity, valgus, ankle)
    congenital Q66.6
  punctum lacrimale (postinfectional)
    (senile) H04.52 ☑
  ureter (meatus) N28.89
  urethra (meatus) N36.8
  uterus N81.4
Evidence
  cytologic
    of malignancy on anal smear R85.614
    of malignancy on cervical smear R87.614
    of malignancy on vaginal smear R87.624
Evisceration
  birth injury P15.8
  traumatic NEC
    eye — see Enucleated eye
Evulsion — see Avulsion
Ewing's sarcoma or tumor — see Neoplasm, bone,
  malignant
Examination (for) (following) (general) (of) (routine)
  Z00.00
  with abnormal findings Z00.01
  abuse, physical (alleged), ruled out
    adult Z04.71
    child Z04.72
  adolescent (development state) Z00.3
  alleged rape or sexual assault (victim), ruled out
    adult Z04.41
    child Z04.42
  allergy Z01.82
  annual (adult) (periodic) (physical) Z00.00
    with abnormal findings Z00.01
    gynecological Z01.419
      with abnormal findings Z01.411
  antibody response Z01.84
  blood — see Examination, laboratory
  blood pressure Z01.30
    with abnormal findings Z01.31
  cancer staging — see Neoplasm, malignant, by
    site
  cervical Papanicolaou smear Z12.4
    as part of routine gynecological
      examination Z01.419
      with abnormal findings Z01.411

Examination — *continued*
  child (over 28 days old) Z00.129
    with abnormal findings Z00.121
    under 28 days old — *see* Newborn, examination
  clinical research control or normal comparison
      (control) (participant) Z00.6
  contraceptive (drug) maintenance (routine) Z30.8
    device (intrauterine) Z30.431
  dental Z01.20
    with abnormal findings Z01.21
  developmental — *see* Examination, child
  donor (potential) Z00.5
  ear Z01.10
    with abnormal findings NEC Z01.118
  eye Z01.00
    with abnormal findings Z01.01
  following
    accident NEC Z04.3
      transport Z04.1
      work Z04.2
    assault, alleged, ruled out
      adult Z04.71
      child Z04.72
    motor vehicle accident Z04.1
    treatment (for) Z09
      combined NEC Z09
        fracture Z09
        malignant neoplasm Z08
      malignant neoplasm Z08
      mental disorder Z09
      specified condition NEC Z09
  follow-up (routine) (following) Z09
    chemotherapy NEC Z09
      malignant neoplasm Z08
    fracture Z09
    malignant neoplasm Z08
    postpartum Z39.2
    psychotherapy Z09
    radiotherapy NEC Z09
      malignant neoplasm Z08
    surgery NEC Z09
      malignant neoplasm Z08
  gynecological Z01.419
    with abnormal findings Z01.411
    for contraceptive maintenance Z30.8
  health — *see* Examination, medical
  hearing Z01.10
    with abnormal findings NEC Z01.118
    following failed hearing screening Z01.110
  immunity status testing Z01.84
  laboratory (as part of a general medical
      examination) Z00.00
    with abnormal findings Z00.01
    preprocedural Z01.812
  lactating mother Z39.1
  medical (adult) (for) (of) Z00.00
    with abnormal findings Z00.01
    administrative purpose only Z02.9
      specified NEC Z02.89
    admission to
      armed forces Z02.3
      old age home Z02.2
      prison Z02.89
      residential institution Z02.2
      school Z02.0
        following illness or medical
            treatment Z02.0
      summer camp Z02.89
    adoption Z02.82
    blood alcohol or drug level Z02.83
    camp (summer) Z02.89
    clinical research, normal subject (control)
        (participant) Z00.6
    control subject in clinical research (normal
        comparison) (participant) Z00.6
    donor (potential) Z00.5
    driving license Z02.4
    general (adult) Z00.00
      with abnormal findings Z00.01
    immigration Z02.89
    insurance purposes Z02.6
    marriage Z02.89
    medicolegal reasons NEC Z04.8
    naturalization Z02.89
    participation in sport Z02.5
    paternity testing Z02.81
    population survey Z00.8
    pre-employment Z02.1
    pre-operative — *see* Examination, pre-
        procedural
    pre-procedural
      cardiovascular Z01.810

Examination — *continued*
  medical — *continued*
    respiratory Z01.811
    specified NEC Z01.818
    preschool children
      for admission to school Z02.0
    prisoners
      for entrance into prison Z02.89
    recruitment for armed forces Z02.3
    specified NEC Z00.8
    sport competition Z02.5
  medicolegal reason NEC Z04.8
  newborn — *see* Newborn, examination
  pelvic (annual) (periodic) Z01.419
    with abnormal findings Z01.411
  period of rapid growth in childhood Z00.2
  periodic (adult) (annual) (routine) Z00.00
    with abnormal findings Z00.01
  physical (adult) (*see also* Examination, medical
      Z00.00)
    sports Z02.5
  postpartum
    immediately after delivery Z39.0
    routine follow-up Z39.2
  prenatal (normal pregnancy) (*see also* Pregnancy,
      normal) Z34.9 ☑
  pre-chemotherapy (antineoplastic) Z01.818
  pre-procedural (pre-operative)
    cardiovascular Z01.810
    laboratory Z01.812
    respiratory Z01.811
    specified NEC Z01.818
  prior to chemotherapy (antineoplastic) Z01.818
  psychiatric NEC Z00.8
    follow-up not needing further care Z09
    requested by authority Z04.6
  radiological (as part of a general medical
      examination) Z00.00
    with abnormal findings Z00.01
  repeat cervical smear to confirm findings
      of recent normal smear following initial
      abnormal smear Z01.42
  skin (hypersensitivity) Z01.82
  special (*see also* Examination, by type) Z01.89
    specified type NEC Z01.89
  specified type or reason NEC Z04.8
  teeth Z01.20
    with abnormal findings Z01.21
  urine — *see* Examination, laboratory
  vision Z01.00
    with abnormal findings Z01.01
Exanthem, exanthema (*see also* Rash)
  with enteroviral vesicular stomatitis B08.4
  Boston A88.0
  epidemic with meningitis A88.0 *[G02]*
  subitum B08.20
    due to human herpesvirus 6 B08.21
    due to human herpesvirus 7 B08.22
  viral, virus B09
    specified type NEC B08.8
Excess, excessive, excessively
  alcohol level in blood R78.0
  androgen (ovarian) E28.1
  attrition, tooth, teeth K03.0
  carotene, carotin (dietary) E67.1
  cold, effects of T69.9 ☑
    specified effect NEC T69.8 ☑
  convergence H51.12
  crying
    in child, adolescent, or adult R45.83
    in infant R68.11
  development, breast N62
  divergence H51.8
  drinking (alcohol) NEC (without
      dependence) F10.10
    habitual (continual) (without remission) F10.20
  eating R63.2
  estrogen E28.0
  fat (*see also* Obesity)
    in heart — *see* Degeneration, myocardial
    localized E65
  foreskin N47.8
  gas R14.0
  glucagon E16.3
  heat — *see* Heat
  intermaxillary vertical dimension of fully erupted
      teeth M26.37
  interocclusal distance of fully erupted
      teeth M26.37
  kalium E87.5
  large
    colon K59.39

Excess — *continued*
  large — *continued*
    congenital Q43.8
    infant P08.0
    organ or site, congenital NEC — *see* Anomaly,
        by site
  long
    organ or site, congenital NEC — *see* Anomaly,
        by site
  menstruation (with regular cycle) N92.0
    with irregular cycle N92.1
  napping Z72.821
  natrium E87.0
  number of teeth K00.1
  nutrient (dietary) NEC R63.2
  potassium (K) E87.5
  salivation K11.7
  secretion (*see also* Hypersecretion)
    milk O92.6
    sputum R09.3
    sweat R61
  sexual drive F52.8
  short
    organ or site, congenital NEC — *see* Anomaly,
        by site
    umbilical cord in labor or delivery O69.3 ☑
  skin L98.7
    and subcutaneous tissue L98.7
    eyelid (acquired) — *see* Blepharochalasis
      congenital Q10.3
  sodium (Na) E87.0
  spacing of fully erupted teeth M26.32
  sputum R09.3
  sweating R61
  thirst R63.1
    due to deprivation of water T73.1 ☑
  tuberosity of jaw M26.07
  vitamin
    A (dietary) E67.0
      administered as drug (prolonged intake)
          — *see* Table of Drugs and Chemicals,
          vitamins, adverse effect
      overdose or wrong substance given or taken
          — *see* Table of Drugs and Chemicals,
          vitamins, poisoning
    D (dietary) E67.3
      administered as drug (prolonged intake)
          — *see* Table of Drugs and Chemicals,
          vitamins, adverse effect
      overdose or wrong substance given or taken
          — *see* Table of Drugs and Chemicals,
          vitamins, poisoning
  weight
    gain R63.5
    loss R63.4
Excitability, abnormal, under minor stress
(personality disorder) F60.3
Excitation
  anomalous atrioventricular I45.6
  psychogenic F30.8
  reactive (from emotional stress, psychological
      trauma) F30.8
Excitement
  hypomanic F30.8
  manic F30.9
  mental, reactive (from emotional stress,
      psychological trauma) F30.8
  state, reactive (from emotional stress,
      psychological trauma) F30.8
Excoriation (traumatic) (*see also* Abrasion)
  neurotic L98.1
  skin picking disorder F42.4
Exfoliation
  due to erythematous conditions according to
      extent of body surface involved L49.0
    10-19 percent of body surface L49.1
    20-29 percent of body surface L49.2
    30-39 percent of body surface L49.3
    40-49 percent of body surface L49.4
    50-59 percent of body surface L49.5
    60-69 percent of body surface L49.6
    70-79 percent of body surface L49.7
    80-89 percent of body surface L49.8
    90-99 percent of body surface L49.9
    less than 10 percent of body surface L49.0
  teeth, due to systemic causes K08.0
Exfoliative — *see* condition
Exhaustion, exhaustive (physical NEC) R53.83
  battle F43.0
  cardiac — *see* Failure, heart
  delirium F43.0

☑ **Additional character required**

Exhaustion — *continued*
due to
cold T69.8 ☑
excessive exertion T73.3 ☑
exposure T73.2 ☑
neurasthenia F48.8
heart — *see* Failure, heart
heat (*see also* Heat, exhaustion) T67.5 ☑
due to
salt depletion T67.4 ☑
water depletion T67.3 ☑
maternal, complicating delivery O75.81
mental F48.8
myocardium, myocardial — *see* Failure, heart
nervous F48.8
old age R54
psychogenic F48.8
psychosis F43.0
senile R54
vital NEC Z73.0
Exhibitionism F65.2
Exocervicitis — *see* Cervicitis
Exomphalos Q79.2
meaning hernia — *see* Hernia, umbilicus
Exophoria H50.52
convergence, insufficiency H51.11
divergence, excess H51.8
Exophthalmos H05.2 ☑
congenital Q15.8
constant NEC H05.24 ☑
displacement, globe — *see* Displacement, globe
due to thyrotoxicosis (hyperthyroidism) — *see* Hyperthyroidism, with, goiter (diffuse)
dysthyroid — *see* Hyperthyroidism, with, goiter (diffuse)
goiter — *see* Hyperthyroidism, with, goiter (diffuse)
intermittent NEC H05.25 ☑
malignant — *see* Hyperthyroidism, with, goiter (diffuse)
orbital
edema — *see* Edema, orbit
hemorrhage — *see* Hemorrhage, orbit
pulsating NEC H05.26 ☑
thyrotoxic, thyrotropic — *see* Hyperthyroidism, with, goiter (diffuse)
Exostosis (*see also* Disorder, bone)
cartilaginous — *see* Neoplasm, bone, benign
congenital (multiple) Q78.6
external ear canal H61.81 ☑
gonococcal A54.49
jaw (bone) M27.8
multiple, congenital Q78.6
orbit H05.35 ☑
osteocartilaginous — *see* Neoplasm, bone, benign
syphilitic A52.77
Exotropia — *see* Strabismus, divergent concomitant
Explanation of
investigation finding Z71.2
medication Z71.89
Exposure (to) (*see also* Contact, with) T75.89 ☑
acariasis Z20.7
AIDS virus Z20.6
air pollution Z77.110
algae and algae toxins Z77.121
algae bloom Z77.121
anthrax Z20.810
aromatic amines Z77.020
aromatic (hazardous) compounds NEC Z77.028
aromatic dyes NOS Z77.028
arsenic Z77.012
asbestos Z77.090
bacterial disease NEC Z20.818
benzene Z77.021
blue-green algae bloom Z77.121
body fluids (potentially hazardous) Z77.21
brown tide Z77.121
chemicals (chiefly nonmedicinal) (hazardous) NEC Z77.098
cholera Z20.09
chromium compounds Z77.018
cold, effects of T69.9 ☑
specified effect NEC T69.8 ☑
communicable disease Z20.9
bacterial NEC Z20.818
specified NEC Z20.89
viral NEC Z20.828
cyanobacteria bloom Z77.121
disaster Z65.5
discrimination Z60.5
dyes Z77.098

Exposure — *continued*
effects of T73.9 ☑
environmental tobacco smoke (acute) (chronic) Z77.22
Escherichia coli (E. coli) Z20.01
exhaustion due to T73.2 ☑
fiberglass — *see* Table of Drugs and Chemicals, fiberglass
German measles Z20.4
gonorrhea Z20.2
hazardous metals NEC Z77.018
hazardous substances NEC Z77.29
hazards in the physical environment NEC Z77.128
hazards to health NEC Z77.9
human immunodeficiency virus (HIV) Z20.6
human T-lymphotropic virus type-1 (HTLV-1) Z20.89
implanted
mesh — *see* Complications, mesh
prosthetic materials NEC — *see* Complications, prosthetic materials NEC
infestation (parasitic) NEC Z20.7
intestinal infectious disease NEC Z20.09
Escherichia coli (E. coli) Z20.01
lead Z77.011
meningococcus Z20.811
mold (toxic) Z77.120
nickel dust Z77.018
noise Z77.122
occupational
air contaminants NEC Z57.39
dust Z57.2
environmental tobacco smoke Z57.31
extreme temperature Z57.6
noise Z57.0
radiation Z57.1
risk factors Z57.9
specified NEC Z57.8
toxic agents (gases) (liquids) (solids) (vapors) in agriculture Z57.4
toxic agents (gases) (liquids) (solids) (vapors) in industry NEC Z57.5
vibration Z57.7
parasitic disease NEC Z20.7
pediculosis Z20.7
persecution Z60.5
pfiesteria piscicida Z77.121
poliomyelitis Z20.89
polycyclic aromatic hydrocarbons Z77.028
pollution
air Z77.110
environmental NEC Z77.118
soil Z77.112
water Z77.111
prenatal (drugs) (toxic chemicals) — *see* Newborn, affected by, noxious substances transmitted via placenta or breast milk
rabies Z20.3
radiation, naturally occurring NEC Z77.123
radon Z77.123
red tide (Florida) Z77.121
rubella Z20.4
second hand tobacco smoke (acute) (chronic) Z77.22
in the perinatal period P96.81
sexually-transmitted disease Z20.2
smallpox (laboratory) Z20.89
syphilis Z20.2
terrorism Z65.4
torture Z65.4
tuberculosis Z20.1
uranium Z77.012
varicella Z20.820
venereal disease Z20.2
viral disease NEC Z20.828
war Z65.5
water pollution Z77.111
Exsanguination — *see* Hemorrhage
Exstrophy
abdominal contents Q45.8
bladder Q64.10
cloacal Q64.12
specified type NEC Q64.19
supravesical fissure Q64.11
Extensive — *see* condition
Extra (*see also* Accessory)
marker chromosomes (normal individual) Q92.61
in abnormal individual Q92.62
rib Q76.6
cervical Q76.5
Extrasystoles (supraventricular) I49.49
atrial I49.1

Extrasystoles — *continued*
auricular I49.1
junctional I49.2
ventricular I49.3
Extrauterine gestation or pregnancy — *see* Pregnancy, by site
Extravasation
blood R58
chyle into mesentery I89.8
pelvicalyceal N13.8
pyelosinus N13.8
urine (from ureter) R39.0
vesicant agent
antineoplastic chemotherapy T80.810 ☑
other agent NEC T80.818 ☑
Extremity — *see* condition, limb
Extrophy — *see* Exstrophy
Extroversion
bladder Q64.19
uterus N81.4
complicating delivery O71.2
postpartal (old) N81.4
Extruded tooth (teeth) M26.34
Extrusion
breast implant (prosthetic) T85.42 ☑
eye implant (globe) (ball) T85.328 ☑
intervertebral disc — *see* Displacement, intervertebral disc
ocular lens implant (prosthetic) — *see* Complications, intraocular lens
vitreous — *see* Prolapse, vitreous
Exudate
pleural — *see* Effusion, pleura
retina H35.89
Exudative — *see* condition
Eye, eyeball, eyelid — *see* condition
Eyestrain — *see* Disturbance, vision, subjective
Eyeworm disease of Africa B74.3

F

Faber's syndrome (achlorhydric anemia) D50.9
Fabry (-Anderson) disease E75.21
Faciocephalalgia, autonomic (*see also* Neuropathy, peripheral, autonomic) G90.09
Factor (s)
psychic, associated with diseases classified elsewhere F54
psychological
affecting physical conditions F54
or behavioral
affecting general medical condition F54
associated with disorders or diseases classified elsewhere F54
Fahr disease (of brain) G23.8
Fahr Volhard disease (of kidney) I12. ☑
Failure, failed
abortion — *see* Abortion, attempted
aortic (valve) I35.8
rheumatic I06.8
attempted abortion — *see* Abortion, attempted
biventricular I50.82
due to left heart failure I50.814
bone marrow — *see* Anemia, aplastic
cardiac — *see* Failure, heart
cardiorenal (chronic) (*see also* Failure, renal, and Failure, heart) I50.9
hypertensive I13.2
cardiorespiratory (*see also* Failure, heart) R09.2
cardiovascular (chronic) — *see* Failure, heart
cerebrovascular I67.9
cervical dilatation in labor O62.0
circulation, circulatory (peripheral) R57.9
newborn P29.89
compensation — *see* Disease, heart
compliance with medical treatment or regimen — *see* Noncompliance
congestive — *see* Failure, heart, congestive
dental implant (endosseous) M27.69
due to
failure of dental prosthesis M27.63
lack of attached gingiva M27.62
occlusal trauma (poor prosthetic design) M27.62
parafunctional habits M27.62
periodontal infection (peri-implantitis) M27.62
poor oral hygiene M27.62
osseointegration M27.61
due to

Failure — *continued*
  dental implant — *continued*
    complications of systemic disease M27.61
    poor bone quality M27.61
   iatrogenic M27.61
   post-osseointegration
    biological M27.62
    due to complications of systemic
     disease M27.62
    iatrogenic M27.62
    mechanical M27.63
   pre-integration M27.61
   pre-osseointegration M27.61
   specified NEC M27.69
  descent of head (at term) of pregnancy
   (mother) O32.4 ☑
  endosseous dental implant — *see* Failure, dental
   implant
  engagement of head (term of pregnancy)
   (mother) O32.4 ☑
  erection (penile) (*see also* Dysfunction, sexual,
   male, erectile) N52.9
   nonorganic F52.21
  examination (s), anxiety concerning Z55.2
  expansion terminal respiratory units (newborn)
   (primary) P28.0
  forceps NOS (with subsequent cesarean
   delivery) O66.5
  gain weight (child over 28 days old) R62.51
   adult R62.7
   newborn P92.6
  genital response (male) F52.21
   female F52.22
  heart (acute) (senile) (sudden) I50.9
   with
    acute pulmonary edema — *see* Failure,
     ventricular, left
    decompensation (*see also* Failure, heart, by
     type as diastolic or systolic, acute and
     chronic) I50.9
    dilatation — *see* Disease, heart
    normal ejection fraction — *see* Failure, heart,
     diastolic
    preserved ejection fraction — *see* Failure,
     heart, diastolic
    reduced ejection fraction — *see* Failure,
     heart, systolic
   arteriosclerotic I70.90
   biventricular I50.82
    due to left heart failure I50.814
   combined left-right sided I50.82
    due to left heart failure I50.814
   compensated (*see also* Failure, heart, by type as
    diastolic or systolic, chronic) I50.9
   complicating
    anesthesia (general) (local) or other sedation
     in labor and delivery O74.2
     in pregnancy O29.12 ☑
     postpartum, puerperal O89.1
    delivery (cesarean) (instrumental) O75.4
   congestive I50.9
    with rheumatic fever (conditions in I00)
     active I01.8
     inactive or quiescent (with chorea) I09.81
    newborn P29.0
    rheumatic (chronic) (inactive) (with
     chorea) I09.81
     active or acute I01.8
      with chorea I02.0
   decompensated (*see also* Failure, heart, by
    type as diastolic or systolic, acute and
    chronic) I50.9
   degenerative — *see* Degeneration, myocardial
   diastolic (congestive) (left ventricular) I50.30
    acute (congestive) I50.31
     and (on) chronic (congestive) I50.33
    chronic (congestive) I50.32
     and (on) acute (congestive) I50.33
    combined with systolic (congestive) I50.40
     acute (congestive) I50.41
      and (on) chronic (congestive) I50.43
     chronic (congestive) I50.42
      and (on) acute (congestive) I50.43
    due to presence of cardiac prosthesis I97.13 ☑
   end stage (*see also* Failure, heart, by type as
    diastolic or systolic, chronic) I50.84
   following cardiac surgery I97.13 ☑
   high output NOS I50.83
   hypertensive — *see* Hypertension, heart
   left (ventricular) (*see also* Failure, ventricular,
    left)

Failure — *continued*
  heart — *continued*
   combined diastolic and systolic — *see* Failure,
    heart, diastolic, combined with systolic
   diastolic — *see* Failure, heart, diastolic
   systolic — *see* Failure, heart, systolic
   low output (syndrome) NOS I50.9
   newborn P29.0
   organic — *see* Disease, heart
   peripartum O90.3
   postprocedural I97.13 ☑
   rheumatic (chronic) (inactive) I09.9
   right (isolated) (ventricular) I50.810
    acute I50.811
     and (on) chronic I50.813
    chronic I50.812
     and acute I50.813
    secondary to left heart failure I50.814
   specified NEC I50.89
  Note: heart failure stages A, B, C, and D are based
   on the American College of Cardiology and
   American Heart Association stages of heart
   failure, which complement and should
   not be confused with the New York Heart
   Association Classification of Heart Failure,
   into Class I, Class II, Class III, and Class IV
   stage A Z91.89
   stage B (*see also* Failure, heart, by type as
    diastolic or systolic) I50.9
   stage C (*see also* Failure, heart, by type as
    diastolic or systolic) I50.9
   stage D (*see also* Failure, heart, by type as
    diastolic or systolic, chronic) I50.84
   systolic (congestive) (left ventricular) I50.20
    acute (congestive) I50.21
     and (on) chronic (congestive) I50.23
    chronic (congestive) I50.22
     and (on) acute (congestive) I50.23
    combined with diastolic (congestive) I50.40
     acute (congestive) I50.41
      and (on) chronic (congestive) I50.43
     chronic (congestive) I50.42
      and (on) acute (congestive) I50.43
   thyrotoxic (*see also* Thyrotoxicosis) E05.90 *[I43]*
    with
     high output (*see also* Thyrotoxicosis) I50.83
    thyroid storm E05.91 *[I43]*
     high output (*see also*
      Thyrotoxicosis) I50.83
   valvular — *see* Endocarditis
  hepatic K72.90
   with coma K72.91
   acute or subacute K72.00
    with coma K72.01
    due to drugs K71.10
     with coma K71.11
   alcoholic (acute) (chronic) (subacute) K70.40
    with coma K70.41
   chronic K72.10
    with coma K72.11
    due to drugs (acute) (subacute)
     (chronic) K71.10
     with coma K71.11
    due to drugs (acute) (subacute)
     (chronic) K71.10
     with coma K71.11
   postprocedural K91.82
  hepatorenal K76.7
  induction (of labor) O61.9
   abortion — *see* Abortion, attempted
   by
    oxytocic drugs O61.0
    prostaglandins O61.0
   instrumental O61.1
   mechanical O61.1
   medical O61.0
   specified NEC O61.8
   surgical O61.1
  intubation during anesthesia T88.4 ☑
   in pregnancy O29.6 ☑
   labor and delivery O74.7
   postpartum, puerperal O89.6
  involution, thymus (gland) E32.0
  kidney (*see also* Disease, kidney, chronic) N19
   acute (*see also* Failure, renal, acute) N17.9
   diabetic — *see* E08-E13 with .22
  lactation (complete) O92.3
   partial O92.4
  Leydig's cell, adult E29.1
  liver — *see* Failure, hepatic
  menstruation at puberty N91.0
  mitral I05.8

Failure — *continued*
  myocardial, myocardium (*see also* Failure,
   heart) I50.9
   chronic (*see also* Failure, heart, congestive) I50.9
   congestive (*see also* Failure, heart,
    congestive) I50.9
  orgasm (female) (psychogenic) F52.31
   male F52.32
  ovarian (primary) E28.39
   iatrogenic E89.40
    asymptomatic E89.40
    symptomatic E89.41
   postprocedural (postablative) (postirradiation)
    (postsurgical) E89.40
    asymptomatic E89.40
    symptomatic E89.41
  ovulation causing infertility N97.0
  polyglandular, autoimmune E31.0
  prosthetic joint implant — *see* Complications,
   joint prosthesis, mechanical, breakdown,
   by site
  renal N19
   with
    tubular necrosis (acute) N17.0
   acute N17.9
    with
     cortical necrosis N17.1
     medullary necrosis N17.2
     tubular necrosis N17.0
    specified NEC N17.8
   chronic N18.9
    hypertensive — *see* Hypertension, kidney
   congenital P96.0
   end stage (chronic) N18.6
    due to hypertension I12.0
   following
    abortion — *see* Abortion by type
     complicated by specified condition NEC
    crushing T79.5 ☑
    ectopic or molar pregnancy O08.4
    labor and delivery (acute) O90.4
   hypertensive — *see* Hypertension, kidney
   postprocedural N99.0
  respiration, respiratory J96.90
   with
    hypercapnia J96.92
    hypercarbia J96.02
    hypoxia J96.91
   acute J96.00
    with
     hypercapnia J96.02
     hypercarbia J96.02
     hypoxia J96.01
   center G93.89
   acute and (on) chronic J96.20
    with
     hypercapnia J96.22
     hypercarbia J96.22
     hypoxia J96.21
   chronic J96.10
    with
     hypercapnia J96.12
     hypercarbia J96.12
     hypoxia J96.11
   newborn P28.5
   postprocedural (acute) J95.821
    acute and chronic J95.822
  rotation
   cecum Q43.3
   colon Q43.3
   intestine Q43.3
   kidney Q63.2
  sedation (conscious) (moderate) during
   procedure T88.52 ☑
   history of Z92.83
  segmentation (*see also* Fusion)
   fingers — *see* Syndactylism, complex, fingers
   vertebra Q76.49
    with scoliosis Q76.3
  seminiferous tubule, adult E29.1
  senile (general) R54
  sexual arousal (male) F52.21
   female F52.22
  testicular endocrine function E29.1
  to thrive (child over 28 days old) R62.51
   adult R62.7
   newborn P92.6
  transplant T86.92
   bone T86.831
    marrow T86.02
   cornea T86.841
   heart T86.22

☑ **Additional character required**

Failure

ICD-10-CM INDEX TO DISEASES AND INJURIES

Failure — *continued*
 transplant — *continued*
  with lung (s) T86.32
  intestine T86.851
  kidney T86.12
  liver T86.42
  lung (s) T86.811
   with heart T86.32
  pancreas T86.891
  skin (allograft) (autograft) T86.821
  specified organ or tissue NEC T86.891
  stem cell (peripheral blood) (umbilical cord) T86.5
 trial of labor (with subsequent cesarean delivery) O66.40
  following previous cesarean delivery O66.41
 tubal ligation N99.89
 urinary — *see* Disease, kidney, chronic
 vacuum extraction NOS (with subsequent cesarean delivery) O66.5
 vasectomy N99.89
 ventouse NOS (with subsequent cesarean delivery) O66.5
 ventricular (*see also* Failure, heart) I50.9
  left (*see also* Failure, heart, left) I50.1
   with rheumatic fever (conditions in I00)
    active I01.8
     with chorea I02.0
    inactive or quiescent (with chorea) I09.81
    rheumatic (chronic) (inactive) (with chorea) I09.81
     active or acute I01.8
      with chorea I02.0
  right — *see* Failure, heart, right
 vital centers, newborn P91.88
Fainting (fit) R55
Fallen arches — *see* Deformity, limb, flat foot
Falling, falls (repeated) R29.6
 any organ or part — *see* Prolapse
Fallopian
 insufflation Z31.41
 tube — *see* condition
Fallot's
 pentalogy Q21.8
 tetrad or tetralogy Q21.3
 triad or trilogy Q22.3
False (*see also* condition)
 croup J38.5
 joint — *see* Nonunion, fracture
 labor (pains) O47.9
  at or after 37 completed weeks of gestation O47.1
  before 37 completed weeks of gestation O47.0 ☑
 passage, urethra (prostatic) N36.5
 pregnancy F45.8
Family, familial (*see also* condition)
 disruption Z63.8
  involving divorce or separation Z63.5
 Li-Fraumeni (syndrome) Z15.01
 planning advice Z30.09
 problem Z63.9
  specified NEC Z63.8
 retinoblastoma C69.2 ☑
Famine (effects of) T73.0 ☑
 edema — *see* Malnutrition, severe
Fanconi (-de Toni) (-Debré) syndrome E72.09
 with cystinosis E72.04
Fanconi's anemia (congenital pancytopenia) D61.09
Farber's disease or syndrome E75.29
Farcy A24.0
Farmer's
 lung J67.0
 skin L57.8
Farsightedness — *see* Hypermetropia
Fascia — *see* condition
Fasciculation R25.3
Fasciitis M72.9
 diffuse (eosinophilic) M35.4
 infective M72.8
  necrotizing M72.6
 necrotizing M72.6
 nodular M72.4
 perirenal (with ureteral obstruction) N13.5
  with infection N13.6
 plantar M72.2
 specified NEC M72.8
 traumatic (old) M72.8
  current - code by site under Sprain
Fascioliasis B66.3
Fasciolopsis, fasciolopsiasis (intestinal) B66.5
Fascioscapulohumeral myopathy G71.0

Fast pulse R00.0
Fat
 embolism — *see* Embolism, fat
 excessive (*see also* Obesity)
  in heart — *see* Degeneration, myocardial
 in stool R19.5
 localized (pad) E65
  heart — *see* Degeneration, myocardial
  knee M79.4
  retropatellar M79.4
 necrosis
  breast N64.1
  mesentery K65.4
  omentum K65.4
 pad E65
  knee M79.4
Fatigue R53.83
 auditory deafness — *see* Deafness
 chronic R53.82
 combat F43.0
 general R53.83
  psychogenic F48.8
 heat (transient) T67.6 ☑
 muscle M62.89
 myocardium — *see* Failure, heart
 neoplasm-related R53.0
 nervous, neurosis F48.8
 operational F48.8
 psychogenic (general) F48.8
 senile R54
 voice R49.8
Fatness — *see* Obesity
Fatty (*see also* condition)
 apron E65
 degeneration — *see* Degeneration, fatty
 heart (enlarged) — *see* Degeneration, myocardial
 liver NEC K76.0
  alcoholic K70.0
  nonalcoholic K76.0
 necrosis — *see* Degeneration, fatty
Fauces — *see* condition
Fauchard's disease (periodontitis) — *see* Periodontitis
Faucitis J02.9
Favism (anemia) D55.0
Favus — *see* Dermatophytosis
Fazio-Londe disease or syndrome G12.1
Fear complex or reaction F40.9
Fear of — *see* Phobia
Feared complaint unfounded Z71.1
Febris, febrile (*see also* Fever)
 flava (*see also* Fever, yellow) A95.9
 melitensis A23.0
 pestis — *see* Plague
 recurrens — *see* Fever, relapsing
 rubra A38.9
Fecal
 incontinence R15.9
 smearing R15.1
 soiling R15.1
 urgency R15.2
Fecalith (impaction) K56.41
 appendix K38.1
 congenital P76.8
Fede's disease K14.0
Feeble rapid pulse due to shock following injury T79.4 ☑
Feeble-minded F70
Feeding
 difficulties R63.3
 problem R63.3
  newborn P92.9
   specified NEC P92.8
  nonorganic (adult) — *see* Disorder, eating
Feeling (of)
 foreign body in throat R09.89
Feer's disease — *see* Poisoning, mercury
Feet — *see* condition
Feigned illness Z76.5
Feil-Klippel syndrome (brevicollis) Q76.1
Feinmesser's (hidrotic) ectodermal dysplasia Q82.4
Felinophobia F40.218
Felon (*see also* Cellulitis, digit)
 with lymphangitis — *see* Lymphangitis, acute, digit
Felty's syndrome M05.00
 ankle M05.07 ☑
 elbow M05.02 ☑
 foot joint M05.07 ☑
 hand joint M05.04 ☑
 hip M05.05 ☑
 knee M05.06 ☑

Felty's — *continued*
 multiple site M05.09
 shoulder M05.01 ☑
 vertebra — *see* Spondylitis, ankylosing
 wrist M05.03 ☑
Female genital cutting status — *see* Female genital mutilation status (FGM)
Female genital mutilation status (FGM) N90.810
 specified NEC N90.818
 type I (clitorectomy status) N90.811
 type II (clitorectomy with excision of labia minora status) N90.812
 type III (infibulation status) N90.813
 type IV N90.818
Femur, femoral — *see* condition
Fenestration, fenestrated (*see also* Imperfect, closure)
 aortico-pulmonary Q21.4
 cusps, heart valve NEC Q24.8
  pulmonary Q22.3
 pulmonic cusps Q22.3
Fernell's disease (aortic aneurysm) I71.9
Fertile eunuch syndrome E23.0
Fetid
 breath R19.6
 sweat L75.0
Fetishism F65.0
 transvestic F65.1
Fetus, fetal (*see also* condition)
 alcohol syndrome (dysmorphic) Q86.0
 compressus O31.0 ☑
 hydantoin syndrome Q86.1
 lung tissue P28.0
 papyraceous O31.0 ☑
Fever (inanition) (of unknown origin) (persistent) (with chills) (with rigor) R50.9
 abortus A23.1
 Aden (dengue) A90
 African tick-borne A68.1
 American
  mountain (tick) A93.2
  spotted A77.0
 aphthous B08.8
 arbovirus, arboviral A94
  hemorrhagic A94
  specified NEC A93.8
 Argentinian hemorrhagic A96.0
 Assam B55.0
 Australian Q A78
 Bangkok hemorrhagic A91
 Barmah forest A92.8
 Bartonella A44.0
 bilious, hemoglobinuric B50.8
 blackwater B50.8
 blister B00.1
 Bolivian hemorrhagic A96.1
 Bonvale dam T73.3 ☑
 boutonneuse A77.1
 brain — *see* Encephalitis
 Brazilian purpuric A48.4
 breakbone A90
 Bullis A77.0
 Bunyamwera A92.8
 Burdwan B55.0
 Bwamba A92.8
 Cameroon — *see* Malaria
 Canton A75.9
 catarrhal (acute) J00
  chronic J31.0
 cat-scratch A28.1
 Central Asian hemorrhagic A98.0
 cerebral — *see* Encephalitis
 cerebrospinal meningococcal A39.0
 Chagres B50.9
 Chandipura A92.8
 Changuinola A93.1
 Charcot's (biliary) (hepatic) (intermittent) — *see* Calculus, bile duct
 Chikungunya (viral) (hemorrhagic) A92.0
 Chitral A93.1
 Colombo — *see* Fever, paratyphoid
 Colorado tick (virus) A93.2
 congestive (remittent) — *see* Malaria
 Congo virus A98.0
 continued malarial B50.9
 Corsican — *see* Malaria
 Crimean-Congo hemorrhagic A98.0
 Cyprus — *see* Brucellosis
 dandy A90
 deer fly — *see* Tularemia
 dengue (viral) A90
  hemorrhagic A91
  sandfly A93.1

Fracture

Fracture, traumatic — *continued*
  thorax — *continued*
    wedge compression S22.050 ☑
    first S22.019 ☑
      burst (stable) S22.011 ☑
        unstable S22.012 ☑
      specified type NEC S22.018 ☑
      wedge compression S22.010 ☑
    fourth S22.049 ☑
      burst (stable) S22.041 ☑
        unstable S22.042 ☑
      specified type NEC S22.048 ☑
      wedge compression S22.040 ☑
    ninth S22.079 ☑
      burst (stable) S22.071 ☑
        unstable S22.072 ☑
      specified type NEC S22.078 ☑
      wedge compression S22.070 ☑
    nondisplaced S22.001 ☑
    second S22.029 ☑
      burst (stable) S22.021 ☑
        unstable S22.022 ☑
      specified type NEC S22.028 ☑
      wedge compression S22.020 ☑
    seventh S22.069 ☑
      burst (stable) S22.061 ☑
        unstable S22.062 ☑
      specified type NEC S22.068 ☑
      wedge compression S22.060 ☑
    sixth S22.059 ☑
      burst (stable) S22.051 ☑
        unstable S22.052 ☑
      specified type NEC S22.058 ☑
      wedge compression S22.050 ☑
    specified type NEC S22.008 ☑
    tenth S22.079 ☑
      burst (stable) S22.071 ☑
        unstable S22.072 ☑
      specified type NEC S22.078 ☑
      wedge compression S22.070 ☑
    third S22.039 ☑
      burst (stable) S22.031 ☑
        unstable S22.032 ☑
      specified type NEC S22.038 ☑
      wedge compression S22.030 ☑
    twelfth S22.089 ☑
      burst (stable) S22.081 ☑
        unstable S22.082 ☑
      specified type NEC S22.088 ☑
      wedge compression S22.080 ☑
    wedge compression S22.000 ☑
  thumb S62.50 ☑
    distal phalanx (displaced) S62.52 ☑
      nondisplaced S62.52 ☑
    proximal phalanx (displaced) S62.51 ☑
      nondisplaced S62.51 ☑
  thyroid cartilage S12.8 ☑
  tibia (shaft) S82.20 ☑
    comminuted (displaced) S82.25 ☑
      nondisplaced S82.25 ☑
    condyles — *see* Fracture, tibia, upper end
    distal end — *see* Fracture, tibia, lower end
    epiphysis
      lower — *see* Fracture, tibia, lower end
      upper — *see* Fracture, tibia, upper end
    following insertion of implant, prosthesis or
      plate M96.67 ☑
    head (involving knee joint) — *see* Fracture,
      tibia, upper end
    intercondyloid eminence — *see* Fracture, tibia,
      upper end
    involving ankle or malleolus — *see* Fracture,
      ankle, medial malleolus
    lower end S82.30 ☑
      physeal S89.10 ☑
        Salter-Harris
          Type I S89.11 ☑
          Type II S89.12 ☑
          Type III S89.13 ☑
          Type IV S89.14 ☑
        specified NEC S89.19 ☑
      pilon (displaced) S82.87 ☑
        nondisplaced S82.87 ☑
      specified NEC S82.39 ☑
      torus S82.31 ☑
    malleolus — *see* Fracture, ankle, medial
      malleolus
    oblique (displaced) S82.23 ☑
      nondisplaced S82.23 ☑
    pilon — *see* Fracture, tibia, lower end, pilon
    proximal end — *see* Fracture, tibia, upper end
    segmental (displaced) S82.26 ☑

Fracture, traumatic — *continued*
  tibia — *continued*
    nondisplaced S82.26 ☑
    specified NEC S82.29 ☑
    spine — *see* Fracture, tibia, upper end, spine
    spiral (displaced) S82.24 ☑
      nondisplaced S82.24 ☑
    transverse (displaced) S82.22 ☑
      nondisplaced S82.22 ☑
    tuberosity — *see* Fracture, tibia, upper end,
      tuberosity
    upper end S82.10 ☑
      bicondylar (displaced) S82.14 ☑
        nondisplaced S82.14 ☑
      lateral condyle (displaced) S82.12 ☑
        nondisplaced S82.12 ☑
      medial condyle (displaced) S82.13 ☑
        nondisplaced S82.13 ☑
      physeal S89.00 ☑
        Salter-Harris
          Type I S89.01 ☑
          Type II S89.02 ☑
          Type III S89.03 ☑
          Type IV S89.04 ☑
        specified NEC S89.09 ☑
      plateau — *see* Fracture, tibia, upper end,
        bicondylar
      spine (displaced) S82.11 ☑
        nondisplaced S82.11 ☑
      torus S82.16 ☑
      specified NEC S82.19 ☑
      tuberosity (displaced) S82.15 ☑
        nondisplaced S82.15 ☑
  toe S92.91 ☑
    great (displaced) S92.40 ☑
      distal phalanx (displaced) S92.42 ☑
        nondisplaced S92.42 ☑
      nondisplaced S92.40 ☑
      proximal phalanx (displaced) S92.41 ☑
        nondisplaced S92.41 ☑
      specified NEC S92.49 ☑
    lesser (displaced) S92.50 ☑
      distal phalanx (displaced) S92.53 ☑
        nondisplaced S92.53 ☑
      medial phalanx (displaced) S92.52 ☑
        nondisplaced S92.52 ☑
      nondisplaced S92.50 ☑
      proximal phalanx (displaced) S92.51 ☑
        nondisplaced S92.51 ☑
      specified NEC S92.59 ☑
    physeal
      phalanx S99.20 ☑
        Salter-Harris
          Type I S99.21 ☑
          Type II S99.22 ☑
          Type III S99.23 ☑
          Type IV S99.24 ☑
        specified NEC S99.29 ☑
  tooth (root) S02.5 ☑
  trachea (cartilage) S12.8 ☑
  transverse process — *see* Fracture, vertebra
  trapezium or trapezoid bone — *see* Fracture,
    carpal
  trimalleolar — *see* Fracture, ankle, trimalleolar
  triquetrum (cuneiform of carpus) — *see* Fracture,
    carpal, triquetrum
  trochanter — *see* Fracture, femur, trochanteric
  tuberosity (external) — *see* Fracture, traumatic,
    by site
  ulna (shaft) S52.20 ☑
    bent bone S52.28 ☑
    coronoid process — *see* Fracture, ulna, upper
      end, coronoid process
    distal end — *see* Fracture, ulna, lower end
    following insertion of implant, prosthesis or
      plate M96.63 ☑
    head S52.60 ☑
    lower end S52.60 ☑
      physeal S59.00 ☑
        Salter-Harris
          Type I S59.01 ☑
          Type II S59.02 ☑
          Type III S59.03 ☑
          Type IV S59.04 ☑
        specified NEC S59.09 ☑
      specified NEC S52.69 ☑
      styloid process (displaced) S52.61 ☑
        nondisplaced S52.61 ☑
      torus S52.62 ☑
    proximal end — *see* Fracture, ulna, upper end
    shaft S52.20 ☑
      comminuted (displaced) S52.25 ☑

Fracture, traumatic — *continued*
  ulna — *continued*
    nondisplaced S52.25 ☑
    greenstick S52.21 ☑
    Monteggia's — *see* Monteggia's fracture
    oblique (displaced) S52.23 ☑
      nondisplaced S52.23 ☑
    segmental (displaced) S52.26 ☑
      nondisplaced S52.26 ☑
    specified NEC S52.29 ☑
    spiral (displaced) S52.24 ☑
      nondisplaced S52.24 ☑
    transverse (displaced) S52.22 ☑
      nondisplaced S52.22 ☑
    upper end S52.00 ☑
      coronoid process (displaced) S52.04 ☑
        nondisplaced S52.04 ☑
      olecranon process (displaced) S52.02 ☑
        with intraarticular extension S52.03 ☑
        nondisplaced S52.02 ☑
          with intraarticular extension S52.03 ☑
      specified NEC S52.09 ☑
      torus S52.01 ☑
  unciform — *see* Fracture, carpal, hamate
  vault of skull S02.0 ☑
  vertebra, vertebral (arch) (body) (column) (neural
    arch) (pedicle) (spinous process) (transverse
    process)
    atlas — *see* Fracture, neck, cervical vertebra,
      first
    axis — *see* Fracture, neck, cervical vertebra,
      second
    cervical (teardrop) S12.9 ☑
      axis — *see* Fracture, neck, cervical vertebra,
        second
      first (atlas) — *see* Fracture, neck, cervical
        vertebra, first
      second (axis) — *see* Fracture, neck, cervical
        vertebra, second
    chronic M84.48 ☑
    coccyx S32.2 ☑
    dorsal — *see* Fracture, thorax, vertebra
    lumbar S32.009 ☑
      burst (stable) S32.001 ☑
        unstable S32.002 ☑
      fifth S32.059 ☑
        burst (stable) S32.051 ☑
          unstable S32.052 ☑
        specified type NEC S32.058 ☑
        wedge compression S32.050 ☑
      first S32.019 ☑
        burst (stable) S32.011 ☑
          unstable S32.012 ☑
        specified type NEC S32.018 ☑
        wedge compression S32.010 ☑
      fourth S32.049 ☑
        burst (stable) S32.041 ☑
          unstable S32.042 ☑
        specified type NEC S32.048 ☑
        wedge compression S32.040 ☑
      second S32.029 ☑
        burst (stable) S32.021 ☑
          unstable S32.022 ☑
        specified type NEC S32.028 ☑
        wedge compression S32.020 ☑
      specified type NEC S32.008 ☑
      third S32.039 ☑
        burst (stable) S32.031 ☑
          unstable S32.032 ☑
        specified type NEC S32.038 ☑
        wedge compression S32.030 ☑
      wedge compression S32.000 ☑
    metastatic — *see* Collapse, vertebra, in,
      specified disease NEC (*see also* Neoplasm)
    newborn (birth injury) P11.5
    sacrum S32.10 ☑
      specified NEC S32.19 ☑
      Type
        1 S32.14 ☑
        2 S32.15 ☑
        3 S32.16 ☑
        4 S32.17 ☑
      Zone
        I S32.119 ☑
          displaced (minimally) S32.111 ☑
            severely S32.112 ☑
          nondisplaced S32.110 ☑
        II S32.129 ☑
          displaced (minimally) S32.121 ☑
            severely S32.122 ☑
          nondisplaced S32.120 ☑
        III S32.139 ☑

☑ **Additional character required**

Fracture, traumatic — *continued*
  vertebra — *continued*
       displaced (minimally) S32.131 ☑
        severely S32.132 ☑
       nondisplaced S32.130 ☑
    thoracic — *see* Fracture, thorax, vertebra
  vertex S02.0 ☑
  vomer (bone) S02.2 ☑
  wrist S62.10 ☑
    carpal — *see* Fracture, carpal bone
    navicular (scaphoid) (hand) — *see* Fracture,
      carpal, navicular
  xiphisternum, xiphoid (process) S22.24 ☑
  zygoma S02.402 ☑
    left side S02.40F ☑
    right side S02.40E ☑
Fragile, fragility
  autosomal site Q95.5
  bone, congenital (with blue sclera) Q78.0
  capillary (hereditary) D69.8
  hair L67.8
  nails L60.3
  non-sex chromosome site Q95.5
  X chromosome Q99.2
Fragilitas
  crinium L67.8
  ossium (with blue sclerae) (hereditary) Q78.0
  unguium L60.3
    congenital Q84.6
Fragments, cataract (lens), following cataract
  surgery H59.02 ☑
    retained foreign body — *see* Retained, foreign
      body fragments (type of)
Frailty (frail) R54
  mental R41.81
Frambesia, frambesial (tropica) (*see also* Yaws)
  initial lesion or ulcer A66.0
  primary A66.0
Frambeside
  gummatous A66.4
  of early yaws A66.2
Frambesioma A66.1
Franceschetti-Klein (-Wildervanck) disease or
  syndrome Q75.4
Francis' disease — *see* Tularemia
Franklin disease C88.2
Frank's essential thrombocytopenia D69.3
Fraser's syndrome Q87.0
Freckle (s) L81.2
  malignant melanoma in — *see* Melanoma
  melanotic (Hutchinson's) — *see*
    Melanoma, in situ
  retinal D49.81
Frederickson's hyperlipoproteinemia, type
  I and V E78.3
  IIA E78.00
  IIB and III E78.2
  IV E78.1
Freeman Sheldon syndrome Q87.0
Freezing (*see also* Effect, adverse, cold) T69.9 ☑
Freiberg's disease (infraction of metatarsal head or
  osteochondrosis) — *see* Osteochondrosis, juvenile,
  metatarsus
Frei's disease A55
Fremitus, friction, cardiac R01.2
Frenum, frenulum
  external os Q51.828
  tongue (shortening) (congenital) Q38.1
Frequency micturition (nocturnal) R35.0
  psychogenic F45.8
Frey's syndrome
  auriculotemporal G50.8
  hyperhidrosis L74.52
Friction
  burn — *see* Burn, by site
  fremitus, cardiac R01.2
  precordial R01.2
  sounds, chest R09.89
Friderichsen-Waterhouse syndrome or disease
  A39.1
Friedländer's B (bacillus) NEC (*see also* condition)
  A49.8
Friedreich's
  ataxia G11.1
  combined systemic disease G11.1
  facial hemihypertrophy Q67.4
  sclerosis (cerebellum) (spinal cord) G11.1
Frigidity F52.22
Fröhlich's syndrome E23.6
Frontal (*see also* condition)
  lobe syndrome F07.0

Frostbite (superficial) T33.90 ☑
  with
    partial thickness skin loss — *see* Frostbite
      (superficial), by site
    tissue necrosis T34.90 ☑
  abdominal wall T33.3 ☑
    with tissue necrosis T34.3 ☑
  ankle T33.81 ☑
    with tissue necrosis T34.81 ☑
  arm T33.4 ☑
    with tissue necrosis T34.4 ☑
    finger (s) — *see* Frostbite, finger
    hand — *see* Frostbite, hand
    wrist — *see* Frostbite, wrist
  ear T33.01 ☑
    with tissue necrosis T34.01 ☑
  face T33.09 ☑
    with tissue necrosis T34.09 ☑
  finger T33.53 ☑
    with tissue necrosis T34.53 ☑
  foot T33.82 ☑
    with tissue necrosis T34.82 ☑
  hand T33.52 ☑
    with tissue necrosis T34.52 ☑
  head T33.09 ☑
    with tissue necrosis T34.09 ☑
    ear — *see* Frostbite, ear
    nose — *see* Frostbite, nose
  hip (and thigh) T33.6 ☑
    with tissue necrosis T34.6 ☑
  knee T33.7 ☑
    with tissue necrosis T34.7 ☑
  leg T33.9 ☑
    with tissue necrosis T34.9 ☑
    ankle — *see* Frostbite, ankle
    foot — *see* Frostbite, foot
    knee — *see* Frostbite, knee
    lower T33.7 ☑
      with tissue necrosis T34.7 ☑
    thigh — *see* Frostbite, hip
    toe — *see* Frostbite, toe
  limb
    lower T33.99 ☑
      with tissue necrosis T34.99 ☑
    upper — *see* Frostbite, arm
  neck T33.1 ☑
    with tissue necrosis T34.1 ☑
  nose T33.02 ☑
    with tissue necrosis T34.02 ☑
  pelvis T33.3 ☑
    with tissue necrosis T34.3 ☑
  specified site NEC T33.99 ☑
    with tissue necrosis T34.99 ☑
  thigh — *see* Frostbite, hip
  thorax T33.2 ☑
    with tissue necrosis T34.2 ☑
  toes T33.83 ☑
    with tissue necrosis T34.83 ☑
  trunk T33.99 ☑
    with tissue necrosis T34.99 ☑
  wrist T33.51 ☑
    with tissue necrosis T34.51 ☑
Frotteurism F65.81
Frozen (*see also* Effect, adverse, cold) T69.9 ☑
  pelvis (female) N94.89
    male K66.8
  shoulder — *see* Capsulitis, adhesive
Fructokinase deficiency E74.11
Fructose 1,6 diphosphatase deficiency E74.19
Fructosemia (benign) (essential) E74.12
Fructosuria (benign) (essential) E74.11
Fuchs'
  black spot (myopic) (*see also* Myopia,
    degenerative) H44.2 ☑
  dystrophy (corneal endothelium) H18.51
  heterochromic cyclitis — *see* Cyclitis, Fuchs'
    heterochromic
Fucosidosis E77.1
Fugue R68.89
  dissociative F44.1
  hysterical (dissociative) F44.1
  postictal in epilepsy — *see* Epilepsy
  reaction to exceptional stress (transient) F43.0
Fulminant, fulminating — *see* condition
Functional (*see also* condition)
  bleeding (uterus) N93.8
Functioning, intellectual, borderline R41.83
Fundus — *see* condition
Fungemia NOS B49
Fungus, fungous
  cerebral G93.89
  disease NOS B49
  infection — *see* Infection, fungus

Funiculitis (acute) (chronic) (endemic) N49.1
  gonococcal (acute) (chronic) A54.23
  tuberculous A18.15
Funnel
  breast (acquired) M95.4
    congenital Q67.6
    sequelae (late effect) of rickets E64.3
  chest (acquired) M95.4
    congenital Q67.6
    sequelae (late effect) of rickets E64.3
  pelvis (acquired) M95.5
    with disproportion (fetopelvic) O33.3 ☑
      causing obstructed labor O65.3
    congenital Q74.2
FUO (fever of unknown origin) R50.9
Furfur L21.0
  microsporon B36.0
Furrier's lung J67.8
Furrowed K14.5
  nail (s) (transverse) L60.4
    congenital Q84.6
  tongue K14.5
    congenital Q38.3
Furuncle L02.92
  abdominal wall L02.221
  ankle — *see* Furuncle, lower limb
  anus K61.0
  antecubital space — *see* Furuncle, upper limb
  arm — *see* Furuncle, upper limb
  auditory canal, external — *see* Abscess, ear,
    external
  auricle (ear) — *see* Abscess, ear, external
  axilla (region) L02.42 ☑
  back (any part) L02.222
  breast N61.1
  buttock L02.32
  cheek (external) L02.02
  chest wall L02.223
  chin L02.02
  corpus cavernosum N48.21
  ear, external — *see* Abscess, ear, external
  external auditory canal — *see* Abscess, ear,
    external
  eyelid — *see* Abscess, eyelid
  face L02.02
  femoral (region) — *see* Furuncle, lower limb
  finger — *see* Furuncle, hand
  flank L02.221
  foot L02.62 ☑
  forehead L02.02
  gluteal (region) L02.32
  groin L02.224
  hand L02.52 ☑
  head L02.821
    face L02.02
  hip — *see* Furuncle, lower limb
  kidney — *see* Abscess, kidney
  knee — *see* Furuncle, lower limb
  labium (majus) (minus) N76.4
  lacrimal
    gland — *see* Dacryoadenitis
    passages (duct) (sac) — *see* Inflammation,
      lacrimal, passages, acute
  leg (any part) — *see* Furuncle, lower limb
  lower limb L02.42 ☑
  malignant A22.0
  mouth K12.2
  navel L02.226
  neck L02.12
  nose J34.0
  orbit, orbital — *see* Abscess, orbit
  palmar (space) — *see* Furuncle, hand
  partes posteriores L02.32
  pectoral region L02.223
  penis N48.21
  perineum L02.225
  pinna — *see* Abscess, ear, external
  popliteal — *see* Furuncle, lower limb
  prepatellar — *see* Furuncle, lower limb
  scalp L02.821
  seminal vesicle N49.0
  shoulder — *see* Furuncle, upper limb
  specified site NEC L02.828
  submandibular K12.2
  temple (region) L02.02
  thumb — *see* Furuncle, hand
  toe — *see* Furuncle, foot
  trunk L02.229
    abdominal wall L02.221
    back L02.222
    chest wall L02.223
    groin L02.224

Hemorrhage — *continued*
  tracheobronchial R04.89
    newborn P26.0
  traumatic - code to specific injury
    cerebellar — *see* Hemorrhage, brain
    intracranial — *see* Hemorrhage, brain
    recurring or secondary (following initial
        hemorrhage at time of injury) T79.2 ☑
  tuberculous NEC (*see also* Tuberculosis,
      pulmonary) A15.0
  tunica vaginalis N50.1
  ulcer - code by site under Ulcer, with
      hemorrhage K27.4
  umbilicus, umbilical
    cord
      after birth, newborn P51.9
      complicating delivery O69.5 ☑
    newborn P51.9
      massive P51.0
      slipped ligature P51.8
    stump P51.9
  urethra (idiopathic) N36.8
  uterus, uterine (abnormal) N93.9
    climacteric N92.4
    complicating delivery — *see* Hemorrhage,
        complicating, delivery
    dysfunctional or functional N93.8
    intermenstrual (regular) N92.3
      irregular N92.1
    postmenopausal N95.0
    postpartum — *see* Hemorrhage, postpartum
    preclimacteric or premenopausal N92.4
    prepubertal N93.8
    pubertal N92.2
  vagina (abnormal) N93.9
    newborn P54.6
  vas deferens N50.1
  vasa previa O69.4 ☑
  ventricular I61.5
  vesical N32.89
  viscera NEC R58
    newborn P54.8
  vitreous (humor) (intraocular) H43.1 ☑
  vulva N90.89
Hemorrhoids (bleeding) (without mention of
    degree) K64.9
  1st degree (grade/stage I) (without prolapse
      outside of anal canal) K64.0
  2nd degree (grade/stage II) (that prolapse with
      straining but retract spontaneously) K64.1
  3rd degree (grade/stage III) (that prolapse with
      straining and require manual replacement
      back inside anal canal) K64.2
  4th degree (grade/stage IV) (with prolapsed
      tissue that cannot be manually
      replaced) K64.3
  complicating
    pregnancy O22.4 ☑
    puerperium O87.2
  external K64.4
    with
      thrombosis K64.5
  internal (without mention of degree) K64.8
  prolapsed K64.8
  skin tags
    anus K64.4
    residual K64.4
  specified NEC K64.8
  strangulated (*see also* Hemorrhoids, by
      degree) K64.8
  thrombosed (*see also* Hemorrhoids, by
      degree) K64.5
  ulcerated (*see also* Hemorrhoids, by degree) K64.8
Hemosalpinx N83.6
  with
    hematocolpos N89.7
    hematometra N85.7
      with hematocolpos N89.7
Hemosiderosis (dietary) E83.19
  pulmonary, idiopathic E83.1 ☑ *[J84.03]*
  transfusion T80.89 ☑
Hemothorax (bacterial) (nontuberculous) J94.2
  newborn P54.8
  traumatic S27.1 ☑
    with pneumothorax S27.2 ☑
  tuberculous NEC A15.6
Henoch (-Schönlein) disease or syndrome (purpura)
    D69.0
Henpue, henpuye A66.6
Hepar lobatum (syphilitic) A52.74
Hepatalgia K76.89

Hepatitis K75.9
  acute B17.9
    with coma K72.01
    with hepatic failure — *see* Failure, hepatic
    alcoholic — *see* Hepatitis, alcoholic
    infectious B17.9
    non-viral K72.0 ☑
    viral B17.9
  alcoholic (acute) (chronic) K70.10
    with ascites K70.11
  amebic — *see* Abscess, liver, amebic
  anicteric, (viral) — *see* Hepatitis, viral
  antigen-associated (HAA) — *see* Hepatitis, B
  Australia-antigen (positive) — *see* Hepatitis, B
  autoimmune K75.4
  B B19.10
    with hepatic coma B19.11
    acute B16.9
      with
        delta-agent (coinfection) (without hepatic
            coma) B16.1
          with hepatic coma B16.0
        hepatic coma (without delta-agent
            coinfection) B16.2
    chronic B18.1
      with delta-agent B18.0
  bacterial NEC K75.89
  C (viral) B19.20
    with hepatic coma B19.21
    acute B17.10
      with hepatic coma B17.11
    chronic B18.2
  catarrhal (acute) B15.9
    with hepatic coma B15.0
  cholangiolitic K75.89
  cholestatic K75.89
  chronic K73.9
    active NEC K73.2
    lobular NEC K73.1
    persistent NEC K73.0
    specified NEC K73.8
  cytomegaloviral B25.1
  due to ethanol (acute) (chronic) — *see* Hepatitis,
      alcoholic
  epidemic B15.9
    with hepatic coma B15.0
  fulminant NEC (viral) — *see* Hepatitis, viral
  neonatal giant cell P59.29
  granulomatous NEC K75.3
  herpesviral B00.81
  history of
    B Z86.19
    C Z86.19
  homologous serum — *see* Hepatitis, viral, type B
  in (due to)
    mumps B26.81
    toxoplasmosis (acquired) B58.1
      congenital (active) P37.1 *[K77]*
  infectious, infective B15.9
    acute (subacute) B17.9
    chronic B18.9
  inoculation — *see* Hepatitis, viral, type B
  interstitial (chronic) K74.69
  lupoid NEC K75.4
  malignant NEC (with hepatic failure) K72.90
    with coma K72.91
  neonatal (idiopathic) (toxic) P59.29
  newborn P59.29
  postimmunization — *see* Hepatitis, viral, type B
  post-transfusion — *see* Hepatitis, viral, type B
  reactive, nonspecific K75.2
  serum — *see* Hepatitis, viral, type B
  specified type NEC
    with hepatic failure — *see* Failure, hepatic
  syphilitic (late) A52.74
    congenital (early) A50.08 *[K77]*
      late A50.59 *[K77]*
    secondary A51.45
  toxic (*see also* Disease, liver, toxic) K71.6
  tuberculous A18.83
  viral, virus B19.9
    with hepatic coma B19.0
    acute B17.9
    chronic B18.9
      specified NEC B18.8
    type
      B B18.1
        with delta-agent B18.0
      C B18.2
  congenital P35.3
  coxsackie B33.8 *[K77]*
  cytomegalic inclusion B25.1

Hepatitis — *continued*
  viral — *continued*
    in remission, any type - code to Hepatitis,
        chronic, by type
    non-A, non-B B17.8
    specified type NEC (with or without
        coma) B17.8
    type
      A B15.9
        with hepatic coma B15.0
      B B19.10
        with hepatic coma B19.11
        acute B16.9
          with
            delta-agent (coinfection) (without
                hepatic coma) B16.1
              with hepatic coma B16.0
            hepatic coma (without delta-agent
                coinfection) B16.2
        chronic B18.1
          with delta-agent B18.0
      C B19.20
        with hepatic coma B19.21
        acute B17.10
          with hepatic coma B17.11
        chronic B18.2
      E B17.2
    non-A, non-B B17.8
Hepatization lung (acute) — *see* Pneumonia, lobar
Hepatoblastoma C22.2
Hepatocarcinoma C22.0
Hepatocholangiocarcinoma C22.0
Hepatocholangioma, benign D13.4
Hepatocholangitis K75.89
Hepatolenticular degeneration E83.01
Hepatoma (malignant) C22.0
  benign D13.4
  embryonal C22.0
Hepatomegaly (*see also* Hypertrophy, liver)
  with splenomegaly R16.2
  congenital Q44.7
  in mononucleosis
    gammaherpesviral B27.09
    infectious specified NEC B27.89
Hepatoptosis K76.89
Hepatorenal syndrome following labor and delivery
    O90.4
Hepatosis K76.89
Hepatosplenomegaly R16.2
  hyperlipemic (Bürger-Grütz type) E78.3 *[K77]*
Hereditary — *see* condition
Heredodegeneration, macular — *see* Dystrophy,
    retina
Heredopathia atactica polyneuritiformis G60.1
Heredosyphilis — *see* Syphilis, congenital
Herlitz' syndrome Q81.1
Hermansky-Pudlak syndrome E70.331
Hermaphrodite, hermaphroditism (true) Q56.0
  46,XX with streak gonads Q99.1
  46,XX/46,XY Q99.0
  46,XY with streak gonads Q99.1
  chimera 46,XX/46,XY Q99.0
Hernia, hernial (acquired) (recurrent) K46.9
  with
    gangrene — *see* Hernia, by site, with, gangrene
    incarceration — *see* Hernia, by site, with,
        obstruction
    irreducible — *see* Hernia, by site, with,
        obstruction
    obstruction — *see* Hernia, by site, with,
        obstruction
    strangulation — *see* Hernia, by site, with,
        obstruction
  abdomen, abdominal K46.9
    with
      gangrene (and obstruction) K46.1
      obstruction K46.0
    femoral — *see* Hernia, femoral
    incisional — *see* Hernia, incisional
    inguinal — *see* Hernia, inguinal
    specified site NEC K45.8
      with
        gangrene (and obstruction) K45.1
        obstruction K45.0
    umbilical — *see* Hernia, umbilical
    wall — *see* Hernia, ventral
  appendix — *see* Hernia, abdomen
  bladder (mucosa) (sphincter)
    congenital (female) (male) Q79.51
    female — *see* Cystocele
    male N32.89
  brain, congenital — *see* Encephalocele

☑ **Additional character required**

Hernia — *continued*
  cartilage, vertebra — *see* Displacement, intervertebral disc
  cerebral, congenital (*see also* Encephalocele)
    endaural Q01.8
  ciliary body (traumatic) S05.2 ☑
  colon — *see* Hernia, abdomen
  Cooper's — *see* Hernia, abdomen, specified site NEC
  crural — *see* Hernia, femoral
  diaphragm, diaphragmatic K44.9
    with
      gangrene (and obstruction) K44.1
      obstruction K44.0
    congenital Q79.0
  direct (inguinal) — *see* Hernia, inguinal
  diverticulum, intestine — *see* Hernia, abdomen
  double (inguinal) — *see* Hernia, inguinal, bilateral
  due to adhesions (with obstruction) K56.50
  epigastric (*see also* Hernia, ventral) K43.9
  esophageal hiatus — *see* Hernia, hiatal
  external (inguinal) — *see* Hernia, inguinal
  fallopian tube N83.4 ☑
  fascia M62.89
  femoral K41.90
    with
      gangrene (and obstruction) K41.40
        not specified as recurrent K41.40
        recurrent K41.41
      obstruction K41.30
        not specified as recurrent K41.30
        recurrent K41.31
    bilateral K41.20
      with
        gangrene (and obstruction) K41.10
          not specified as recurrent K41.10
          recurrent K41.11
        obstruction K41.00
          not specified as recurrent K41.00
          recurrent K41.01
      not specified as recurrent K41.20
      recurrent K41.21
    unilateral K41.90
      with
        gangrene (and obstruction) K41.40
          not specified as recurrent K41.40
          recurrent K41.41
        obstruction K41.30
          not specified as recurrent K41.30
          recurrent K41.31
      not specified as recurrent K41.90
      recurrent K41.91
    not specified as recurrent K41.90
    recurrent K41.91
  foramen magnum G93.5
    congenital Q01.8
  funicular (umbilical) (*see also* Hernia, umbilicus)
    spermatic (cord) — *see* Hernia, inguinal
  gastrointestinal tract — *see* Hernia, abdomen
  Hesselbach's — *see* Hernia, femoral, specified site NEC
  hiatal (esophageal) (sliding) K44.9
    with
      gangrene (and obstruction) K44.1
      obstruction K44.0
    congenital Q40.1
  hypogastric — *see* Hernia, ventral
  incarcerated (*see also* Hernia, by site, with obstruction)
    with gangrene — *see* Hernia, by site, with gangrene
  incisional K43.2
    with
      gangrene (and obstruction) K43.1
      obstruction K43.0
  indirect (inguinal) — *see* Hernia, inguinal
  inguinal (direct) (external) (funicular) (indirect) (internal) (oblique) (scrotal) (sliding) K40.90
    with
      gangrene (and obstruction) K40.40
        not specified as recurrent K40.40
        recurrent K40.41
      obstruction K40.30
        not specified as recurrent K40.30
        recurrent K40.31
    not specified as recurrent K40.90
    recurrent K40.91
    bilateral K40.20
      with
        gangrene (and obstruction) K40.10
          not specified as recurrent K40.10
          recurrent K40.11

Hernia — *continued*
  inguinal — *continued*
      obstruction K40.00
        not specified as recurrent K40.00
        recurrent K40.01
      not specified as recurrent K40.20
      recurrent K40.21
    unilateral K40.90
      with
        gangrene (and obstruction) K40.40
          not specified as recurrent K40.40
          recurrent K40.41
        obstruction K40.30
          not specified as recurrent K40.30
          recurrent K40.31
      not specified as recurrent K40.90
      recurrent K40.91
  internal (*see also* Hernia, abdomen)
    inguinal — *see* Hernia, inguinal
  interstitial — *see* Hernia, abdomen
  intervertebral cartilage or disc — *see* Displacement, intervertebral disc
  intestine, intestinal — *see* Hernia, by site
  intra-abdominal — *see* Hernia, abdomen
  iris (traumatic) S05.2 ☑
  irreducible (*see also* Hernia, by site, with obstruction)
    with gangrene — *see* Hernia, by site, with gangrene
  ischiatic — *see* Hernia, abdomen, specified site NEC
  ischiorectal — *see* Hernia, abdomen, specified site NEC
  lens (traumatic) S05.2 ☑
  linea (alba) (semilunaris) — *see* Hernia, ventral
  Littre's — *see* Hernia, abdomen
  lumbar — *see* Hernia, abdomen, specified site NEC
  lung (subcutaneous) J98.4
  mediastinum J98.59
  mesenteric (internal) — *see* Hernia, abdomen
  midline — *see* Hernia, ventral
  muscle (sheath) M62.89
  nucleus pulposus — *see* Displacement, intervertebral disc
  oblique (inguinal) — *see* Hernia, inguinal
  obstructive (*see also* Hernia, by site, with obstruction)
    with gangrene — *see* Hernia, by site, with gangrene
  obturator — *see* Hernia, abdomen, specified site NEC
  omental — *see* Hernia, abdomen
  ovary N83.4 ☑
  oviduct N83.4 ☑
  paraesophageal (*see also* Hernia, diaphragm)
    congenital Q40.1
  parastomal K43.5
    with
      gangrene (and obstruction) K43.4
      obstruction K43.3
  paraumbilical — *see* Hernia, umbilicus
  perineal — *see* Hernia, abdomen, specified site NEC
  Petit's — *see* Hernia, abdomen, specified site NEC
  postoperative — *see* Hernia, incisional
  pregnant uterus — *see* Abnormal, uterus in pregnancy or childbirth
  prevesical N32.89
  properitoneal — *see* Hernia, abdomen, specified site NEC
  pudendal — *see* Hernia, abdomen, specified site NEC
  rectovaginal N81.6
  retroperitoneal — *see* Hernia, abdomen, specified site NEC
  Richter's — *see* Hernia, abdomen, with obstruction
  Rieux's, Riex's — *see* Hernia, abdomen, specified site NEC
  sac condition (adhesion) (dropsy) (inflammation) (laceration) (suppuration) - code by site under Hernia
  sciatic — *see* Hernia, abdomen, specified site NEC
  scrotum, scrotal — *see* Hernia, inguinal
  sliding (inguinal) (*see also* Hernia, inguinal)
    hiatus — *see* Hernia, hiatal
  spigelian — *see* Hernia, ventral
  spinal — *see* Spina bifida
  strangulated (*see also* Hernia, by site, with obstruction)

Hernia — *continued*
  strangulated — *continued*
    with gangrene — *see* Hernia, by site, with gangrene
  subxiphoid — *see* Hernia, ventral
  supra-umbilicus — *see* Hernia, ventral
  tendon — *see* Disorder, tendon, specified type NEC
  Treitz's (fossa) — *see* Hernia, abdomen, specified site NEC
  tunica vaginalis Q55.29
  umbilicus, umbilical K42.9
    with
      gangrene (and obstruction) K42.1
      obstruction K42.0
  ureter N28.89
  urethra, congenital Q64.79
  urinary meatus, congenital Q64.79
  uterus N81.4
    pregnant — *see* Abnormal, uterus in pregnancy or childbirth
  vaginal (anterior) (wall) — *see* Cystocele
  Velpeau's — *see* Hernia, femoral
  ventral K43.9
    with
      gangrene (and obstruction) K43.7
      obstruction K43.6
    recurrent — *see* Hernia, incisional
    incisional K43.2
      with
        gangrene (and obstruction) K43.1
        obstruction K43.0
    specified NEC K43.9
      with
        gangrene (and obstruction) K43.7
        obstruction K43.6
  vesical
    congenital (female) (male) Q79.51
    female — *see* Cystocele
    male N32.89
  vitreous (into wound) S05.2 ☑
    into anterior chamber — *see* Prolapse, vitreous
Herniation (*see also* Hernia)
  brain (stem) G93.5
  cerebral G93.5
  mediastinum J98.59
  nucleus pulposus — *see* Displacement, intervertebral disc
Herpangina B08.5
Herpes, herpesvirus, herpetic B00.9
  anogenital A60.9
    perianal skin A60.1
    rectum A60.1
    urogenital tract A60.00
      cervix A60.03
      male genital organ NEC A60.02
      penis A60.01
      specified site NEC A60.09
      vagina A60.04
      vulva A60.04
  blepharitis (zoster) B02.39
    simplex B00.59
  circinatus B35.4
    bullosus L12.0
  conjunctivitis (simplex) B00.53
    zoster B02.31
  cornea B02.33
  encephalitis B00.4
    due to herpesvirus 6 B10.01
    due to herpesvirus 7 B10.09
    specified NEC B10.09
  eye (zoster) B02.30
    simplex B00.50
  eyelid (zoster) B02.39
    simplex B00.59
  facialis B00.1
  febrilis B00.1
  geniculate ganglionitis B02.21
  genital, genitalis A60.00
    female A60.09
    male A60.02
  gestational, gestationis O26.4 ☑
  gingivostomatitis B00.2
  human B00.9
    1 — *see* Herpes, simplex
    2 — *see* Herpes, simplex
    3 — *see* Varicella
    4 — *see* Mononucleosis, Epstein-Barr (virus)
    5 — *see* Disease, cytomegalic inclusion (generalized)
    6
      encephalitis B10.01

☑ **Additional character required**

Herpes — continued
  human — continued
    specified NEC B10.81
      7
        encephalitis B10.09
        specified NEC B10.82
      8 B10.89
    infection NEC B10.89
      Kaposi's sarcoma associated B10.89
  iridocyclitis (simplex) B00.51
    zoster B02.32
  iris (vesicular erythema multiforme) L51.9
  iritis (simplex) B00.51
  Kaposi's sarcoma associated B10.89
  keratitis (simplex) (dendritic) (disciform)
    (interstitial) B00.52
    zoster (interstitial) B02.33
  keratoconjunctivitis (simplex) B00.52
    zoster B02.33
  labialis B00.1
  lip B00.1
  meningitis (simplex) B00.3
    zoster B02.1
  ophthalmicus (zoster) NEC B02.30
    simplex B00.50
  penis A60.01
  perianal skin A60.1
  pharyngitis, pharyngotonsillitis B00.2
  rectum A60.1
  scrotum A60.02
  sepsis B00.7
  simplex B00.9
    complicated NEC B00.89
    congenital P35.2
    conjunctivitis B00.53
    external ear B00.1
    eyelid B00.59
    hepatitis B00.81
    keratitis (interstitial) B00.52
    myleitis B00.82
    specified complication NEC B00.89
    visceral B00.89
  stomatitis B00.2
  tonsurans B35.0
  visceral B00.89
  vulva A60.04
  whitlow B00.89
  zoster (see also condition) B02.9
    auricularis B02.21
    complicated NEC B02.8
    conjunctivitis B02.31
    disseminated B02.7
    encephalitis B02.0
    eye (lid) B02.39
    geniculate ganglionitis B02.21
    keratitis (interstitial) B02.33
    meningitis B02.1
    myelitis B02.24
    neuritis, neuralgia B02.29
    ophthalmicus NEC B02.30
    oticus B02.21
    polyneuropathy B02.23
    specified complication NEC B02.8
    trigeminal neuralgia B02.22
Herpesvirus (human) — see Herpes
Herpetophobia F40.218
Herrick's anemia — see Disease, sickle-cell
Hers' disease E74.09
Herter-Gee syndrome K90.0
Herxheimer's reaction R68.89
Hesitancy
  of micturition R39.11
  urinary R39.11
Hesselbach's hernia — see Hernia, femoral, specified
  site NEC
Heterochromia (congenital) Q13.2
  cataract — see Cataract, complicated
  cyclitis (Fuchs) — see Cyclitis, Fuchs'
    heterochromic
  hair L67.1
  iritis — see Cyclitis, Fuchs' heterochromic
  retained metallic foreign body (nonmagnetic) —
    see Foreign body, intraocular, old, retained
    magnetic — see Foreign body, intraocular, old,
      retained, magnetic
  uveitis — see Cyclitis, Fuchs' heterochromic
Heterophoria — see Strabismus, heterophoria
Heterophyes, heterophyiasis (small intestine) B66.8
Heterotopia, heterotopic (see also Malposition,
  congenital)
  cerebralis Q04.8
Heterotropia — see Strabismus

Heubner-Herter disease K90.0
Hexadactylism Q69.9
HGSIL (cytology finding) (high grade squamous
  intraepithelial lesion on cytologic smear) (Pap
  smear finding)
  anus R85.613
  cervix R87.613
    biopsy (histology) finding — see Neoplasia,
      intraepithelial, cervix, grade II or grade III
  vagina R87.623
    biopsy (histology) finding — see Neoplasia,
      intraepithelial, vagina, grade II or grade III
Hibernoma — see Lipoma
Hiccup, hiccough R06.6
  epidemic B33.0
  psychogenic F45.8
Hidden penis (congenital) Q55.64
  acquired N48.83
Hidradenitis (axillaris) (suppurative) L73.2
Hidradenoma (nodular) (see also Neoplasm, skin,
  benign)
  clear cell — see Neoplasm, skin, benign
  papillary — see Neoplasm, skin, benign
Hidrocystoma — see Neoplasm, skin, benign
High
  altitude effects T70.20 ☑
    anoxia T70.29 ☑
    on
      ears T70.0 ☑
      sinuses T70.1 ☑
    polycythemia D75.1
  arch
    foot Q66.7
    palate, congenital Q38.5
  arterial tension — see Hypertension
  basal metabolic rate R94.8
  blood pressure (see also Hypertension)
    borderline R03.0
    reading (incidental) (isolated) (nonspecific),
      without diagnosis of hypertension R03.0
  cholesterol E78.00
    with high triglycerides E78.2
  diaphragm (congenital) Q79.1
  expressed emotional level within family Z63.8
  head at term O32.4 ☑
  palate, congenital Q38.5
  risk
    infant NEC Z76.2
    sexual behavior (heterosexual) Z72.51
      bisexual Z72.53
      homosexual Z72.52
  scrotal testis, testes
    bilateral Q53.23
    unilateral Q53.13
  temperature (of unknown origin) R50.9
  thoracic rib Q76.6
  triglycerides E78.1
    with high cholesterol E78.2
Hildenbrand's disease A75.0
Hilum — see condition
Hip — see condition
Hippel's disease Q85.8
Hippophobia F40.218
Hippus H57.09
Hirschsprung's disease or megacolon Q43.1
Hirsutism, hirsuties L68.0
Hirudiniasis
  external B88.3
  internal B83.4
Hiss-Russell dysentery A03.1
Histidinemia, histidinuria E70.41
Histiocytoma (see also Neoplasm, skin, benign)
  fibrous (see also Neoplasm, skin, benign)
    atypical — see Neoplasm, connective tissue,
      uncertain behavior
    malignant — see Neoplasm, connective tissue,
      malignant
Histiocytosis D76.3
  acute differentiated progressive C96.0
  Langerhans' cell NEC C96.6
    multifocal X
      multisystemic (disseminated) C96.0
      unisystemic C96.5
    pulmonary, adult (adult PLCH) J84.82
    unifocal (X) C96.6
  lipid, lipoid D76.3
    essential E75.29
  malignant C96.A
  mononuclear phagocytes NEC D76.1
    Langerhans' cells C96.6
  non-Langerhans cell D76.3
  polyostotic sclerosing D76.3

Histiocytosis — continued
  sinus, with massive lymphadenopathy D76.3
  syndrome NEC D76.3
  X NEC C96.6
    acute (progressive) C96.0
    chronic C96.6
    multifocal C96.5
    multisystemic C96.0
    unifocal C96.6
Histoplasmosis B39.9
  with pneumonia NEC B39.2
  African B39.5
  American — see Histoplasmosis, capsulati
  capsulati B39.4
    disseminated B39.3
    generalized B39.3
    pulmonary B39.2
      acute B39.0
      chronic B39.1
  Darling's B39.4
  duboisii B39.5
  lung NEC B39.2
History
  family (of) (see also History, personal (of))
    alcohol abuse Z81.1
    allergy NEC Z84.89
    anemia Z83.2
    arthritis Z82.61
    asthma Z82.5
    blindness Z82.1
    cardiac death (sudden) Z82.41
    carrier of genetic disease Z84.81
    chromosomal anomaly Z82.79
    chronic
      disabling disease NEC Z82.8
      lower respiratory disease Z82.5
    colonic polyps Z83.71
    congenital malformations and
      deformations Z82.79
      polycystic kidney Z82.71
    consanguinity Z84.3
    deafness Z82.2
    diabetes mellitus Z83.3
    disability NEC Z82.8
    disease or disorder (of)
      allergic NEC Z84.89
      behavioral NEC Z81.8
      blood and blood-forming organs Z83.2
      cardiovascular NEC Z82.49
      chronic disabling NEC Z82.8
      digestive Z83.79
      ear NEC Z83.52
      endocrine NEC Z83.49
      eye NEC Z83.518
        glaucoma Z83.511
      familial hypercholesterolemia Z83.42
      genitourinary NEC Z84.2
      glaucoma Z83.511
      hematological Z83.2
      immune mechanism Z83.2
      infectious NEC Z83.1
      ischemic heart Z82.49
      kidney Z84.1
      mental NEC Z81.8
      metabolic Z83.49
      musculoskeletal NEC Z82.69
      neurological NEC Z82.0
      nutritional Z83.49
      parasitic NEC Z83.1
      psychiatric NEC Z81.8
      respiratory NEC Z83.6
      skin and subcutaneous tissue NEC Z84.0
      specified NEC Z84.89
    drug abuse NEC Z81.3
    epilepsy Z82.0
    familial hypercholesterolemia Z83.42
    genetic disease carrier Z84.81
    glaucoma Z83.511
    hearing loss Z82.2
    human immunodeficiency virus (HIV)
      infection Z83.0
    Huntington's chorea Z82.0
    intellectual disability Z81.0
    leukemia Z80.6
    malignant neoplasm (of) NOS Z80.9
      bladder Z80.52
      breast Z80.3
      bronchus Z80.1
      digestive organ Z80.0
      gastrointestinal tract Z80.0
      genital organ Z80.49
        ovary Z80.41

☑ **Additional character required**

Herpes - History

ICD-10-CM INDEX TO DISEASES AND INJURIES

History — *continued*
   family — *continued*
      prostate Z80.42
      specified organ NEC Z80.49
      testis Z80.43
    hematopoietic NEC Z80.7
    intrathoracic organ NEC Z80.2
    kidney Z80.51
    lung Z80.1
    lymphatic NEC Z80.7
    ovary Z80.41
    prostate Z80.42
    respiratory organ NEC Z80.2
    specified site NEC Z80.8
    testis Z80.43
    trachea Z80.1
    urinary organ or tract Z80.59
      bladder Z80.52
      kidney Z80.51
   mental
    disorder NEC Z81.8
   multiple endocrine neoplasia (MEN)
    syndrome Z83.41
   osteoporosis Z82.62
   polycystic kidney Z82.71
   polyps (colon) Z83.71
   psychiatric disorder Z81.8
   psychoactive substance abuse NEC Z81.3
   respiratory condition NEC Z83.6
    asthma and other lower respiratory
      conditions Z82.5
   self-harmful behavior Z81.8
   SIDS (sudden infant death syndrome) Z84.82
   skin condition Z84.0
   specified condition NEC Z84.89
   stroke (cerebrovascular) Z82.3
   substance abuse NEC Z81.4
    alcohol Z81.1
    drug NEC Z81.3
    psychoactive NEC Z81.3
    tobacco Z81.2
   sudden
    cardiac death Z82.41
    infant death syndrome (SIDS) Z84.82
   tobacco abuse Z81.2
   violence, violent behavior Z81.8
   visual loss Z82.1
  personal (of) (*see also* History, family (of))
   abuse
    childhood Z62.819
      physical Z62.810
      psychological Z62.811
      sexual Z62.810
    adult Z91.419
      physical and sexual Z91.410
      psychological Z91.411
   alcohol dependence F10.21
   allergy (to) Z88.9
    analgesic agent NEC Z88.6
    anesthetic Z88.4
    antibiotic agent NEC Z88.1
    anti-infective agent NEC Z88.3
    contrast media Z91.041
    drugs, medicaments and biological
      substances Z88.9
      specified NEC Z88.8
    food Z91.018
      additives Z91.02
      eggs Z91.012
      milk products Z91.011
      peanuts Z91.010
      seafood Z91.013
      specified food NEC Z91.018
    insect Z91.038
      bee Z91.030
    latex Z91.040
    medicinal agents Z88.9
      specified NEC Z88.8
    narcotic agent NEC Z88.5
    nonmedicinal agents Z91.048
    penicillin Z88.0
    serum Z88.7
    specified NEC Z91.09
    sulfonamides Z88.2
    vaccine Z88.7
   anaphylactic shock Z87.892
   anaphylaxis Z87.892
   behavioral disorders Z86.59
   benign carcinoid tumor Z86.012
   benign neoplasm Z86.018
    carcinoid Z86.012
    brain Z86.011

History — *continued*
  personal — *continued*
    colonic polyps Z86.010
   brain injury (traumatic) Z87.820
   breast implant removal Z98.86
   calculi, renal Z87.442
   cancer — *see* History, personal (of), malignant
    neoplasm (of)
   cardiac arrest (death), successfully
    resuscitated Z86.74
   cerebral infarction without residual
    deficit Z86.73
   cervical dysplasia Z87.410
   chemotherapy for neoplastic condition Z92.21
   childhood abuse — *see* History, personal (of),
    abuse
   cleft lip (corrected) Z87.730
   cleft palate (corrected) Z87.730
   collapsed vertebra (healed) Z87.311
    due to osteoporosis Z87.310
   combat and operational stress reaction Z86.51
   congenital malformation (corrected) Z87.798
    circulatory system (corrected) Z87.74
    digestive system (corrected) NEC Z87.738
    ear (corrected) Z87.721
    eye (corrected) Z87.720
    face and neck (corrected) Z87.790
    genitourinary system (corrected)
      NEC Z87.718
    heart (corrected) Z87.74
    integument (corrected) Z87.76
    limb (s) (corrected) Z87.76
    musculoskeletal system (corrected) Z87.76
    neck (corrected) Z87.790
    nervous system (corrected) NEC Z87.728
    respiratory system (corrected) Z87.75
    sense organs (corrected) NEC Z87.728
    specified NEC Z87.798
   contraception Z92.0
   deployment (military) Z91.82
   diabetic foot ulcer Z86.31
   disease or disorder (of) Z87.898
    blood and blood-forming organs Z86.2
    circulatory system Z86.79
      specified condition NEC Z86.79
    connective tissue NEC Z87.39
    digestive system Z87.19
      colonic polyp Z86.010
      peptic ulcer disease Z87.11
      specified condition NEC Z87.19
    ear Z86.69
    endocrine Z86.39
      diabetic foot ulcer Z86.31
      gestational diabetes Z86.32
      specified type NEC Z86.39
    eye Z86.69
    genital (track) system NEC
      female Z87.42
      male Z87.438
    hematological Z86.2
    Hodgkin Z85.71
    immune mechanism Z86.2
    infectious Z86.19
      malaria Z86.13
      Methicillin resistant Staphylococcus aureus
        (MRSA) Z86.14
      poliomyelitis Z86.12
      specified NEC Z86.19
      tuberculosis Z86.11
    mental NEC Z86.59
    metabolic Z86.39
      diabetic foot ulcer Z86.31
      gestational diabetes Z86.32
      specified type NEC Z86.39
    musculoskeletal NEC Z87.39
    nervous system Z86.69
    nutritional Z86.39
    parasitic Z86.19
    respiratory system NEC Z87.09
    sense organs Z86.69
    skin Z87.2
    specified site or type NEC Z87.898
    subcutaneous tissue Z87.2
    trophoblastic Z87.59
    urinary system NEC Z87.448
   drug dependence — *see* Dependence, drug, by
    type, in remission
   drug therapy
    antineoplastic chemotherapy Z92.21
    estrogen Z92.23
    immunosuppression Z92.25
    inhaled steroids Z92.240

History — *continued*
  personal — *continued*
    monoclonal drug Z92.22
    specified NEC Z92.29
    steroid Z92.241
    systemic steroids Z92.241
   dysplasia
    cervical (mild) (moderate) Z87.410
      severe (grade III) Z86.001
    prostatic Z87.430
    vaginal (mild) (moderate) Z87.411
      severe (grade III) Z86.008
    vulvar (mild) (moderate) Z87.412
      severe (grade III) Z86.008
   embolism (venous) Z86.718
    pulmonary Z86.711
   encephalitis Z86.61
   estrogen therapy Z92.23
   extracorporeal membrane oxygenation
    (ECMO) Z92.81
   failed moderate sedation Z92.83
   failed conscious sedation Z92.83
   fall, falling Z91.81
   fracture (healed)
    fatigue Z87.312
    fragility Z87.310
    osteoporosis Z87.310
    pathological NEC Z87.311
    stress Z87.312
    traumatic Z87.81
   gestational diabetes Z86.32
   hepatitis
    B Z86.19
    C Z86.19
   Hodgkin disease Z85.71
   hyperthermia, malignant Z88.4
   hypospadias (corrected) Z87.710
   hysterectomy Z90.710
   immunosuppression therapy Z92.25
   in situ neoplasm
    breast Z86.000
    cervix uteri Z86.001
    specified NEC Z86.008
   infection NEC Z86.19
    central nervous system Z86.61
    Methicillin resistant Staphylococcus aureus
      (MRSA) Z86.14
    urinary (recurrent) (tract) Z87.440
   injury NEC Z87.828
   in utero procedure during pregnancy Z98.870
   in utero procedure while a fetus Z98.871
   irradiation Z92.3
   kidney stones Z87.442
   leukemia Z85.6
   lymphoma (non-Hodgkin) Z85.72
   malignant melanoma (skin) Z85.820
   malignant neoplasm (of) Z85.9
    accessory sinuses Z85.22
    anus NEC Z85.048
      carcinoid Z85.040
    bladder Z85.51
    bone Z85.830
    brain Z85.841
    breast Z85.3
    bronchus NEC Z85.118
      carcinoid Z85.110
    carcinoid — *see* History, personal (of),
      malignant neoplasm, by site, carcinoid
    cervix Z85.41
    colon NEC Z85.038
      carcinoid Z85.030
    digestive organ Z85.00
      specified NEC Z85.09
    endocrine gland NEC Z85.858
    epididymis Z85.48
    esophagus Z85.01
    eye Z85.840
    gastrointestinal tract — *see* History,
      malignant neoplasm, digestive organ
    genital organ
      female Z85.40
        specified NEC Z85.44
      male Z85.45
        specified NEC Z85.49
    hematopoietic NEC Z85.79
    intrathoracic organ Z85.20
    kidney NEC Z85.528
      carcinoid Z85.520
    large intestine NEC Z85.038
      carcinoid Z85.030
    larynx Z85.21
    liver Z85.05

☑ **Additional character required**

History — *continued*
  personal — *continued*
    lung NEC Z85.118
      carcinoid Z85.110
    mediastinum Z85.29
    Merkel cell Z85.821
    middle ear Z85.22
    nasal cavities Z85.22
    nervous system NEC Z85.848
    oral cavity Z85.819
      specified site NEC Z85.818
    ovary Z85.43
    pancreas Z85.07
    pharynx Z85.819
      specified site NEC Z85.818
    pelvis Z85.53
    pleura Z85.29
    prostate Z85.46
    rectosigmoid junction NEC Z85.048
      carcinoid Z85.040
    rectum NEC Z85.048
      carcinoid Z85.040
    respiratory organ Z85.20
    sinuses, accessory Z85.22
    skin NEC Z85.828
      melanoma Z85.820
      Merkel cell Z85.821
    small intestine NEC Z85.068
      carcinoid Z85.060
    soft tissue Z85.831
    specified site NEC Z85.89
    stomach NEC Z85.028
      carcinoid Z85.020
    testis Z85.47
    thymus NEC Z85.238
      carcinoid Z85.230
    thyroid Z85.850
    tongue Z85.810
    trachea Z85.12
    ureter Z85.54
    urinary organ or tract Z85.50
      specified NEC Z85.59
    uterus Z85.42
  maltreatment Z91.89
  medical treatment NEC Z92.89
  melanoma (malignant) (skin) Z85.820
  meningitis Z86.61
  mental disorder Z86.59
  Merkel cell carcinoma (skin) Z85.821
  Methicillin resistant Staphylococcus aureus
      (MRSA) Z86.14
  military deployment Z91.82
  military war, peacekeeping and humanitarian
      deployment (current or past
      conflict) Z91.82
  myocardial infarction (old) I25.2
  neglect (in)
    adult Z91.412
    childhood Z62.812
  neoplasm
    benign Z86.018
      brain Z86.011
      colon polyp Z86.010
    in situ
      breast Z86.000
      cervix uteri Z86.001
      specified NEC Z86.008
    malignant — *see* History of, malignant
      neoplasm
    uncertain behavior Z86.03
  nephrotic syndrome Z87.441
  nicotine dependence Z87.891
  noncompliance with medical treatment or
      regimen — *see* Noncompliance
  nutritional deficiency Z86.39
  obstetric complications Z87.59
    childbirth Z87.59
    pregnancy Z87.59
    pre-term labor Z87.51
    puerperium Z87.59
  osteoporosis fractures Z87.31 ☑
  parasuicide (attempt) Z91.5
  physical trauma NEC Z87.828
    self-harm or suicide attempt Z91.5
  poisoning NEC Z91.89
    self-harm or suicide attempt Z91.5
  poor personal hygiene Z91.89
  pneumonia (recurrent) Z87.01
  preterm labor Z87.51
  prolonged reversible ischemic neurologic
      deficit (PRIND) Z86.73
  procedure during pregnancy Z98.870

History — *continued*
  personal — *continued*
    procedure while a fetus Z98.871
    prostatic dysplasia Z87.430
    psychological
      abuse
        adult Z91.411
        child Z62.811
      trauma, specified NEC Z91.49
    radiation therapy Z92.3
    removal
      implant
        breast Z98.86
    renal calculi Z87.442
    respiratory condition NEC Z87.09
    retained foreign body fully removed Z87.821
    risk factors NEC Z91.89
    self-harm Z91.5
    self-poisoning attempt Z91.5
    sex reassignment Z87.890
    sleep-wake cycle problem Z72.821
    specified NEC Z87.898
    steroid therapy (systemic) Z92.241
      inhaled Z92.240
    stroke without residual deficits Z86.73
    substance abuse NEC F10-F19
    sudden cardiac arrest Z86.74
    sudden cardiac death successfully
        resuscitated Z86.74
    suicide attempt Z91.5
    surgery NEC Z98.890
      with uterine scar Z98.891
      sex reassignment Z87.890
      transplant — *see* Transplant
    thrombophlebitis Z86.72
    thrombosis (venous) Z86.718
      pulmonary Z86.711
    tobacco dependence Z87.891
    transient ischemic attack (TIA) without residual
        deficits Z86.73
    trauma (physical) NEC Z87.828
      psychological NEC Z91.49
      self-harm Z91.5
    traumatic brain injury Z87.820
    unhealthy sleep-wake cycle Z72.821
    unintended awareness under general
        anesthesia Z92.84
    urinary calculi Z87.442
    urinary (recurrent) (tract) infection (s) Z87.440
    uterine scar from previous surgery Z98.891
    vaginal dysplasia Z87.411
    venous thrombosis or embolism Z86.718
      pulmonary Z86.711
    vulvar dysplasia Z87.412
His-Werner disease A79.0
HIV (*see also* Human, immunodeficiency virus) B20
  laboratory evidence (nonconclusive) R75
  positive, seropositive Z21
  nonconclusive test (in infants) R75
Hives (bold) — *see* Urticaria
Hoarseness R49.0
Hobo Z59.0
Hodgkin disease — *see* Lymphoma, Hodgkin
Hodgson's disease I71.2
  ruptured I71.1
Hoffa-Kastert disease E88.89
Hoffa's disease E88.89
Hoffmann-Bouveret syndrome I47.9
Hoffmann's syndrome E03.9 *[G73.7]*
Hole (round)
  macula H35.34 ☑
  retina (without detachment) — *see* Break, retina,
      round hole
  with detachment — *see* Detachment, retina,
      with retinal, break
Holiday relief care Z75.5
Hollenhorst's plaque — *see* Occlusion, artery, retina
Hollow foot (congenital) Q66.7
  acquired — *see* Deformity, limb, foot, specified NEC
Holoprosencephaly Q04.2
Holt-Oram syndrome Q87.2
Homelessness Z59.0
Homesickness — *see* Disorder, adjustment
Homocystinemia, homocystinuria E72.11
Homogentisate 1,2-dioxygenase deficiency E70.29
Homologous serum hepatitis (prophylactic)
  (therapeutic) — *see* Hepatitis, viral, type B
Honeycomb lung J98.4
  congenital Q33.0
Hooded
  clitoris Q52.6
  penis Q55.69

Hookworm (anemia) (disease) (infection)
  (infestation) B76.9
  specified NEC B76.8
Hordeolum (eyelid) (externum) (recurrent) H00.019
  internum H00.029
    left H00.026
      lower H00.025
      upper H00.024
    right H00.023
      lower H00.022
      upper H00.021
  left H00.016
    lower H00.015
    upper H00.014
  right H00.013
    lower H00.012
    upper H00.011
Horn
  cutaneous L85.8
  nail L60.2
    congenital Q84.6
Horner (-Claude Bernard) syndrome G90.2
  traumatic — *see* Injury, nerve, cervical
    sympathetic
Horseshoe kidney (congenital) Q63.1
Horton's headache or neuralgia G44.099
  intractable G44.091
  not intractable G44.099
Hospital hopper syndrome — *see* Disorder, factitious
Hospitalism in children — *see* Disorder, adjustment
Hostility R45.5
  towards child Z62.3
Hot flashes
  menopausal N95.1
Hourglass (contracture) (*see also* Contraction,
  hourglass)
  stomach K31.89
    congenital Q40.2
    stricture K31.2
Household, housing circumstance affecting care
  Z59.9
  specified NEC Z59.8
Housemaid's knee — *see* Bursitis, prepatellar
Hudson (-Ståhli) line (cornea) — *see* Pigmentation,
  cornea, anterior
Human
  bite (open wound) (*see also* Bite)
    intact skin surface — *see* Bite, superficial
  herpesvirus — *see* Herpes
  immunodeficiency virus (HIV) disease
      (infection) B20
    asymptomatic status Z21
    contact Z20.6
    counseling Z71.7
    dementia B20 *[F02.80]*
      with behavioral disturbance B20 *[F02.81]*
    exposure to Z20.6
    laboratory evidence R75
    type-2 (HIV 2) as cause of disease classified
        elsewhere B97.35
  papillomavirus (HPV)
    DNA test positive
      high risk
        cervix R87.810
        vagina R87.811
      low risk
        cervix R87.820
        vagina R87.821
    screening for Z11.51
  T-cell lymphotropic virus
    type-1 (HTLV-I) infection B33.3
      as cause of disease classified
          elsewhere B97.33
    carrier Z22.6
    type-2 (HTLV-II) as cause of disease classified
        elsewhere B97.34
Humidifier lung or pneumonitis J67.7
Humiliation (experience) in childhood Z62.898
Humpback (acquired) — *see* Kyphosis
Hunchback (acquired) — *see* Kyphosis
Hunger T73.0 ☑
  air, psychogenic F45.8
Hungry bone syndrome E83.81
Hunner's ulcer — *see* Cystitis, chronic, interstitial
Hunter's
  glossitis D51.0
  syndrome E76.1
Huntington's disease or chorea G10
  with dementia G10 *[F02.80]*
    with behavioral disturbance G10 *[F02.81]*

☑ **Additional character required**

Hunt's
  disease or syndrome (herpetic geniculate ganglionitis) B02.21
    dyssynergia cerebellaris myoclonica G11.1
  neuralgia B02.21
Hurler (-Scheie) disease or syndrome E76.02
Hurst's disease G36.1
Hurthle cell
  adenocarcinoma C73
  adenoma D34
  carcinoma C73
  tumor D34
Hutchinson-Boeck disease or syndrome — see Sarcoidosis
Hutchinson-Gilford disease or syndrome E34.8
Hutchinson's
  disease, meaning
    angioma serpiginosum L81.7
    pompholyx (cheiropompholyx) L30.1
    prurigo estivalis L56.4
    summer eruption or summer prurigo L56.4
  melanotic freckle — see Melanoma, in situ
    malignant melanoma in — see Melanoma
  teeth or incisors (congenital syphilis) A50.52
  triad (congenital syphilis) A50.53
Hyalin plaque, sclera, senile H15.89
Hyaline membrane (disease) (lung) (pulmonary) (newborn) P22.0
Hyalinosis
  cutis (et mucosae) E78.89
  focal and segmental (glomerular) (see also N00-N07 with fourth character .1) N05.1
Hyalitis, hyalosis, asteroid (see also Deposit, crystalline)
  syphilitic (late) A52.71
Hydatid
  cyst or tumor — see Echinococcus
  mole — see Hydatidiform mole
  Morgagni
    female Q50.5
    male (epididymal) Q55.4
    testicular Q55.29
Hydatidiform mole (benign) (complicating pregnancy) (delivered) (undelivered) O01.9
  classical O01.0
  complete O01.0
  incomplete O01.1
  invasive D39.2
  malignant D39.2
  partial O01.1
Hydatidosis — see Echinococcus
Hydradenitis (axillaris) (suppurative) L73.2
Hydradenoma — see Hidradenoma
Hydramnios O40. ☑
Hydrancephaly, hydranencephaly Q04.3
  with spina bifida — see Spina bifida, with hydrocephalus
Hydrargyrism NEC — see Poisoning, mercury
Hydrarthrosis (see also Effusion, joint)
  gonococcal A54.42
  intermittent M12.40
    ankle M12.47 ☑
    elbow M12.42 ☑
    foot joint M12.47 ☑
    hand joint M12.44 ☑
    hip M12.45 ☑
    knee M12.46 ☑
    multiple site M12.49
    shoulder M12.41 ☑
    specified joint NEC M12.48
    wrist M12.43 ☑
  of yaws (early) (late) (see also subcategory M14.8 ☑) A66.6
  syphilitic (late) A52.77
    congenital A50.55 [M12.80]
Hydremia D64.89
Hydrencephalocele (congenital) — see Encephalocele
Hydrencephalomeningocele (congenital) — see Encephalocele
Hydroa R23.8
  aestivale L56.4
  vacciniforme L56.4
Hydroadenitis (axillaris) (suppurative) L73.2
Hydrocalycosis — see Hydronephrosis
Hydrocele (spermatic cord) (testis) (tunica vaginalis) N43.3
  canal of Nuck N94.89
  communicating N43.2
    congenital P83.5
  congenital P83.5
  encysted N43.0

Hydrocele — continued
  female NEC N94.89
  infected N43.1
  newborn P83.5
  round ligament N94.89
  specified NEC N43.2
  spinalis — see Spina bifida
  vulva N90.89
Hydrocephalus (acquired) (external) (internal) (malignant) (recurrent) G91.9
  aqueduct Sylvius stricture Q03.0
  causing disproportion O33.6 ☑
    with obstructed labor O66.3
  communicating G91.0
  congenital (external) (internal) Q03.9
    with spina bifida Q05.4
      cervical Q05.0
      dorsal Q05.1
      lumbar Q05.2
      lumbosacral Q05.2
      sacral Q05.3
      thoracic Q05.1
      thoracolumbar Q05.1
    specified NEC Q03.8
  due to toxoplasmosis (congenital) P37.1
  foramen Magendie block (acquired) G91.1
    congenital (see also Hydrocephalus, congenital) Q03.1
  in (due to)
    infectious disease NEC B89 [G91.4]
    neoplastic disease NEC (see also Neoplasm) G91.4
    parasitic disease B89 [G91.4]
  newborn Q03.9
    with spina bifida — see Spina bifida, with hydrocephalus
  noncommunicating G91.1
  normal pressure G91.2
    secondary G91.0
  obstructive G91.1
  otitic G93.2
  post-traumatic NEC G91.3
  secondary G91.4
    post-traumatic G91.3
  specified NEC G91.8
  syphilitic, congenital A50.49
Hydrocolpos (congenital) N89.8
Hydrocystoma — see Neoplasm, skin, benign
Hydroencephalocele (congenital) — see Encephalocele
Hydroencephalomeningocele (congenital) — see Encephalocele
Hydrohematopneumothorax — see Hemothorax
Hydromeningitis — see Meningitis
Hydromeningocele (spinal) (see also Spina bifida)
  cranial — see Encephalocele
Hydrometra N85.8
Hydrometrocolpos N89.8
Hydromicrocephaly Q02
Hydromphalos (since birth) Q45.8
Hydromyelia Q06.4
Hydromyelocele — see Spina bifida
Hydronephrosis (atrophic) (early) (functionless) (intermittent) (primary) (secondary) NEC N13.30
  with
    infection N13.6
    obstruction (by) (of)
      renal calculus N13.2
        with infection N13.6
      ureteral NEC N13.1
        with infection N13.6
        calculus N13.2
          with infection N13.6
      ureteropelvic junction (congenital) Q62.11
        acquired N13.0
          with infection N13.6
      ureteral stricture NEC N13.1
        with infection N13.6
  congenital Q62.0
    due to acquired occlusion of ureteropelvic junction N13.0
  specified type NEC N13.39
  tuberculous A18.11
Hydropericarditis — see Pericarditis
Hydropericardium — see Pericarditis
Hydroperitoneum R18.8
Hydrophobia — see Rabies
Hydrophthalmos Q15.0
Hydropneumohemothorax — see Hemothorax
Hydropneumopericarditis — see Pericarditis
Hydropneumopericardium — see Pericarditis

Hydropneumothorax J94.8
  traumatic — see Injury, intrathoracic, lung
  tuberculous NEC A15.6
Hydrops R60.9
  abdominis R18.8
  articulorum intermittens — see Hydrarthrosis, intermittent
  cardiac — see Failure, heart, congestive
  causing obstructed labor (mother) O66.3
  endolymphatic H81.0 ☑
  fetal — see Pregnancy, complicated by, hydrops, fetalis
  fetalis P83.2
    due to
      ABO isoimmunization P56.0
      alpha thalassemia D56.0
      hemolytic disease P56.90
        specified NEC P56.99
      isoimmunization (ABO) (Rh) P56.0
      other specified nonhemolytic disease NEC P83.2
      Rh incompatibility P56.0
    during pregnancy — see Pregnancy, complicated by, hydrops, fetalis
  gallbladder K82.1
  joint — see Effusion, joint
  labyrinth H81.0 ☑
  newborn (idiopathic) P83.2
    due to
      ABO isoimmunization P56.0
      alpha thalassemia D56.0
      hemolytic disease P56.90
        specified NEC P56.99
      isoimmunization (ABO) (Rh) P56.0
      Rh incompatibility P56.0
  nutritional — see Malnutrition, severe
  pericardium — see Pericarditis
  pleura — see Hydrothorax
  spermatic cord — see Hydrocele
Hydropyonephrosis N13.6
Hydrorachis Q06.4
Hydrorrhea (nasal) J34.89
  pregnancy — see Rupture, membranes, premature
Hydrosadenitis (axillaris) (suppurative) L73.2
Hydrosalpinx (fallopian tube) (follicularis) N70.11
Hydrothorax (double) (pleura) J94.8
  chylous (nonfilarial) I89.8
  filarial (see also Infestation, filarial) B74.9 [J91.8]
  traumatic — see Injury, intrathoracic
  tuberculous NEC (non primary) A15.6
Hydroureter (see also Hydronephrosis) N13.4
  with infection N13.6
  congenital Q62.39
Hydroureteronephrosis — see Hydronephrosis
Hydrourethra N36.8
Hydroxykynureninuria E70.8
Hydroxylysinemia E72.3
Hydroxyprolinemia E72.59
Hygiene, sleep
  abuse Z72.821
  inadequate Z72.821
  poor Z72.821
Hygroma (congenital) (cystic) D18.1
  praepatellare, prepatellar — see Bursitis, prepatellar
Hymen — see condition
Hymenolepis, hymenolepiasis (diminuta) (infection) (infestation) (nana) B71.0
Hypalgesia R20.8
Hyperacidity (gastric) K31.89
  psychogenic F45.8
Hyperactive, hyperactivity F90.9
  basal cell, uterine cervix — see Dysplasia, cervix
  bowel sounds R19.12
  cervix epithelial (basal) — see Dysplasia, cervix
  child F90.9
    attention deficit — see Disorder, attention-deficit hyperactivity
  detrusor muscle N32.81
  gastrointestinal K31.89
    psychogenic F45.8
  nasal mucous membrane J34.3
  stomach K31.89
  thyroid (gland) — see Hyperthyroidism
Hyperacusis H93.23 ☑
Hyperadrenalism E27.5
Hyperadrenocorticism E24.9
  congenital E25.0
  iatrogenic E24.2
    correct substance properly administered — see Table of Drugs and Chemicals, by drug, adverse effect

Infection

Infection — *continued*
  Oidium albicans B37.9
  Onchocerca (volvulus) — *see* Onchocerciasis
  oncovirus, as cause of disease classified
    elsewhere B97.32
  operation wound T81.4 ☑
  Opisthorchis (felineus) (viverrini) B66.0
  orbit, orbital — *see* Inflammation, orbit
  orthopoxvirus NEC B08.09
  ovary — *see* Salpingo-oophoritis
  Oxyuris vermicularis B80
  pancreas (acute) — *see* Pancreatitis, acute
    abscess — *see* Pancreatitis, acute
    specified NEC (*see also* Pancreatitis,
      acute) K85.80
  papillomavirus, as cause of disease classified
    elsewhere B97.7
  papovavirus NEC B34.4
  Paracoccidioides brasiliensis — *see*
    Paracoccidioidomycosis
  Paragonimus (westermani) B66.4
  parainfluenza virus B34.8
  parameningococcus NOS A39.9
  parapoxvirus B08.60
    specified NEC B08.69
  parasitic B89
  Parastrongylus
    cantonensis B83.2
    costaricensis B81.3
    paratyphoid A01.4
      Type A A01.1
      Type B A01.2
      Type C A01.3
  paraurethral ducts N34.2
  parotid gland — *see* Sialoadenitis
  parvovirus NEC B34.3
    as cause of disease classified elsewhere B97.6
  Pasteurella NEC A28.0
    multocida A28.0
    pestis — *see* Plague
    pseudotuberculosis A28.0
    septica (cat bite) (dog bite) A28.0
    tularensis — *see* Tularemia
  pelvic, female — *see* Disease, pelvis, inflammatory
  Penicillium (marneffei) B48.4
  penis (glans) (retention) NEC N48.29
  periapical K04.5
  peridental, periodontal K05.20
    generalized — *see* Peridontitis, aggressive,
      generalized
    localized — *see* Peridontitis, aggressive,
      localized
  perinatal period P39.9
    specified type NEC P39.8
  perineal repair (puerperal) O86.0
  periorbital — *see* Inflammation, orbit
  perirectal K62.89
  perirenal — *see* Infection, kidney
  peritoneal — *see* Peritonitis
  periureteral N28.89
  Petriellidium boydii B48.2
  pharynx (*see also* Pharyngitis)
    coxsackievirus B08.5
    posterior, lymphoid (chronic) J35.03
  Phialophora
    gougerotii (subcutaneous abscess or
      cyst) B43.2
    jeanselmei (subcutaneous abscess or
      cyst) B43.2
    verrucosa (skin) B43.0
  Piedraia hortae B36.3
  pinta A67.9
    intermediate A67.1
    late A67.2
    mixed A67.3
    primary A67.0
  pinworm B80
  pityrosporum furfur B36.0
  pleuro-pneumonia-like organism (PPLO)
    NEC A49.3
    as cause of disease classified elsewhere B96.0
  pneumococcus, pneumococcal NEC A49.1
    as cause of disease classified elsewhere B95.3
    generalized (purulent) A40.3
      with pneumonia J13
  Pneumocystis carinii (pneumonia) B59
  Pneumocystis jiroveci (pneumonia) B59
  port or reservoir T80.212 ☑
  postoperative T81.4 ☑
  postoperative wound T81.4 ☑
  postprocedural T81.4 ☑
  postvaccinal T88.0 ☑

Infection — *continued*
  prepuce NEC N47.7
    with penile inflammation N47.6
  prion — *see* Disease, prion, central nervous
    system
  prostate (capsule) — *see* Prostatitis
  Proteus (mirabilis) (morganii) (vulgaris) NEC A49.8
    as cause of disease classified elsewhere B96.4
  protozoal NEC B64
    intestinal A07.9
      specified NEC A07.8
    specified NEC B60.8
  Pseudallescheria boydii B48.2
  Pseudomonas NEC A49.8
    as cause of disease classified elsewhere B96.5
    mallei A24.0
    pneumonia J15.1
    pseudomallei — *see* Melioidosis
  puerperal O86.4
    genitourinary tract NEC O86.89
    major or generalized O85
    minor O86.4
    specified NEC O86.89
  pulmonary — *see* Infection, lung
  purulent — *see* Abscess
  Pyrenochaeta romeroi B47.0
  Q fever A78
  rectum (sphincter) K62.89
  renal (*see also* Infection, kidney)
    pelvis and ureter (cystic) N28.85
  reovirus, as cause of disease classified
    elsewhere B97.5
  respiratory (tract) NEC J98.8
    acute J22
    chronic J98.8
    influenzal (upper) (acute) — *see* Influenza, with,
      respiratory manifestations NEC
    lower (acute) J22
      chronic — *see* Bronchitis, chronic
    rhinovirus J00
    syncytial virus, as cause of disease classified
      elsewhere B97.4
    upper (acute) NOS J06.9
      chronic J39.8
      streptococcal J06.9
      viral NOS J06.9
  resulting from
    presence of internal prosthesis, implant, graft
      — *see* Complications, by site and type,
      infection
  retortamoniasis A07.8
  retroperitoneal NEC K68.9
  retrovirus B33.3
    as cause of disease classified elsewhere B97.30
      human
        immunodeficiency, type 2 (HIV 2) B97.35
        T-cell lymphotropic
          type I (HTLV-I) B97.33
          type II (HTLV-II) B97.34
      lentivirus B97.31
      oncovirus B97.32
      specified NEC B97.39
  Rhinosporidium (seeberi) B48.1
  rhinovirus
    as cause of disease classified elsewhere B97.89
    unspecified nature or site B34.8
  Rhizopus — *see* Mucormycosis
  rickettsial NOS A79.9
  roundworm (large) NEC B82.0
    Ascariasis (*see also* Ascariasis) B77.9
  rubella — *see* Rubella
  Saccharomyces — *see* Candidiasis
  salivary duct or gland (any) — *see* Sialoadenitis
  Salmonella (aertrycke) (arizonae) (callinarum)
    (cholerae-suis) (enteritidis) (suipestifer)
    (typhimurium) A02.9
    with
      (gastro)enteritis A02.0
      sepsis A02.1
      specified manifestation NEC A02.8
    due to food (poisoning) A02.9
    hirschfeldii A01.3
    localized A02.20
      arthritis A02.23
      meningitis A02.21
      osteomyelitis A02.24
      pneumonia A02.22
      pyelonephritis A02.25
      specified NEC A02.29
    paratyphi A01.4
      A A01.1
      B A01.2

Infection — *continued*
  Salmonella — *continued*
    C A01.3
    schottmuelleri A01.2
    typhi, typhosa — *see* Typhoid
  Sarcocystis A07.8
  scabies B86
  Schistosoma — *see* Infestation, Schistosoma
  scrotum (acute) NEC N49.2
  seminal vesicle — *see* Vesiculitis
  septic
    localized, skin — *see* Abscess
  sheep liver fluke B66.3
  Shigella A03.9
    boydii A03.2
    dysenteriae A03.0
    flexneri A03.1
    group
      A A03.0
      B A03.1
      C A03.2
      D A03.3
    Schmitz (-Stutzer) A03.0
    schmitzii A03.0
    shigae A03.0
    sonnei A03.3
    specified NEC A03.8
  shoulder (joint) NEC M00.9
    due to internal joint prosthesis T84.59 ☑
    skin NEC L08.9
  sinus (accessory) (chronic) (nasal) (*see also*
    Sinusitis)
    pilonidal — *see* Sinus, pilonidal
    skin NEC L08.89
  Skene's duct or gland — *see* Urethritis
  skin (local) (staphylococcal) (streptococcal) L08.9
    abscess - code by site under Abscess
    cellulitis - code by site under Cellulitis
    due to fungus B36.9
      specified type NEC B36.8
    mycotic B36.9
      specified type NEC B36.8
    newborn P39.4
    ulcer — *see* Ulcer, skin
  slow virus A81.9
    specified NEC A81.89
  Sparganum (mansoni) (proliferum) (baxteri) B70.1
  specific (*see also* Syphilis)
    to perinatal period — *see* Infection, congenital
  specified NEC B99.8
  spermatic cord NEC N49.1
  sphenoidal (sinus) — *see* Sinusitis, sphenoidal
  spinal cord NOS (*see also* Myelitis) G04.91
    abscess G06.1
    meninges — *see* Meningitis
    streptococcal G04.89
  Spirillum A25.0
  spirochetal NOS A69.9
    lung A69.8
    specified NEC A69.8
  Spirometra larvae B70.1
  spleen D73.89
  Sporotrichum, Sporothrix (schenckii) — *see*
    Sporotrichosis
  staphylococcal, unspecified site
    aureus (methicillin susceptible) (MSSA) A49.01
      methicillin resistant (MRSA) A49.02
    as cause of disease classified elsewhere B95.8
      aureus (methicillin susceptible)
        (MSSA) B95.61
        methicillin resistant (MRSA) B95.62
      specified NEC B95.7
    food poisoning A05.0
    generalized (purulent) A41.2
    pneumonia — *see* Pneumonia, staphylococcal
  Stellantchasmus falcatus B66.8
  streptobacillus moniliformis A25.1
  streptococcal NEC A49.1
    as cause of disease classified elsewhere B95.5
    B genitourinary complicating
      childbirth O98.82
      pregnancy O98.81 ☑
      puerperium O98.83
    congenital
      sepsis P36.10
        group B P36.0
        specified NEC P36.19
    generalized (purulent) A40.9
  Streptomyces B47.1
  Strongyloides (stercoralis) — *see* Strongyloidiasis
  stump (amputation) (surgical) — *see*
    Complication, amputation stump, infection

Infection — *continued*
  subcutaneous tissue, local L08.9
  suipestifer — *see* Infection, salmonella
  swimming pool bacillus A31.1
  Taenia — *see* Infestation, Taenia
  Taeniarhynchus saginatus B68.1
  tapeworm — *see* Infestation, tapeworm
  tendon (sheath) — *see* Tenosynovitis, infective
    NEC
  Ternidens diminutus B81.8
  testis — *see* Orchitis
  threadworm B80
  throat — *see* Pharyngitis
  thyroglossal duct K14.8
  toe (skin) L08.9
    cellulitis L03.03 ☑
      fungus B35.1
    nail L03.03 ☑
      fungus B35.1
  tongue NEC K14.0
    parasitic B37.0
  tonsil (and adenoid) (faucial) (lingual)
    (pharyngeal) — *see* Tonsillitis
  tooth, teeth K04.7
    periapical K04.7
    peridental, periodontal K05.20
      generalized — *see* Peridontitis, aggressive,
        generalized
      localized — *see* Peridontitis, aggressive,
        localized
    pulp K04.01
      irreversible K04.02
      reversible K04.01
    socket M27.3
  TORCH — *see* Infection, congenital
    without active infection P00.2
  Torula histolytica — *see* Cryptococcosis
  Toxocara (canis) (cati) (felis) B83.0
  Toxoplasma gondii — *see* Toxoplasma
  trachea, chronic J42
  trematode NEC — *see* Infestation, fluke
  trench fever A79.0
  Treponema pallidum — *see* Syphilis
  Trichinella (spiralis) B75
  Trichomonas A59.9
    cervix A59.09
    intestine A07.8
    prostate A59.02
    specified site NEC A59.8
    urethra A59.03
    urogenitalis A59.00
    vagina A59.01
    vulva A59.01
  Trichophyton, trichophytic — *see*
    Dermatophytosis
  Trichosporon (beigelii) cutaneum B36.2
  Trichostrongylus B81.2
  Trichuris (trichiura) B79
  Trombicula (irritans) B88.0
  Trypanosoma
    brucei
      gambiense B56.0
      rhodesiense B56.1
    cruzi — *see* Chagas' disease
  tubal — *see* Salpingo-oophoritis
  tuberculous NEC — *see* Tuberculosis
  tubo-ovarian — *see* Salpingo-oophoritis
  tunnel T80.212 ☑
  tunica vaginalis N49.1
  tympanic membrane NEC — *see* Myringitis
  typhoid (abortive) (ambulant) (bacillus) — *see*
    Typhoid
  typhus A75.9
    flea-borne A75.2
    mite-borne A75.3
    recrudescent A75.1
    tick-borne A77.9
      African A77.1
      North Asian A77.2
  umbilicus L08.82
  ureter N28.86
  urethra — *see* Urethritis
  urinary (tract) N39.0
    bladder — *see* Cystitis
    complicating
      pregnancy O23.4 ☑
        specified type NEC O23.3 ☑
    kidney — *see* Infection, kidney
    newborn P39.3
    puerperal (postpartum) O86.20
    tuberculous A18.13
    urethra — *see* Urethritis

Infection — *continued*
  uterus, uterine — *see* Endometritis
  vaccination T88.0 ☑
  vaccinia not from vaccination B08.011
  vagina (acute) — *see* Vaginitis
  varicella B01.9
  varicose veins — *see* Varix
  vas deferens NEC N49.1
  vesical — *see* Cystitis
  Vibrio
    cholerae A00.0
      El Tor A00.1
    parahaemolyticus (food poisoning) A05.3
    vulnificus
      as cause of disease classified
        elsewhere B96.82
      foodborne intoxication A05.5
  Vincent's (gum) (mouth) (tonsil) A69.1
  virus, viral NOS B34.9
    adenovirus
      as cause of disease classified elsewhere B97.0
      unspecified nature or site B34.0
    arborvirus, arbovirus arthropod-borne A94
    as cause of disease classified elsewhere B97.89
      adenovirus B97.0
      coronavirus B97.29
        SARS-associated B97.21
      coxsackievirus B97.11
      echovirus B97.12
      enterovirus B97.10
        coxsackievirus B97.11
        echovirus B97.12
        specified NEC B97.19
      human
        immunodeficiency, type 2 (HIV 2) B97.35
        T-cell lymphotropic,
          type I (HTLV-I) B97.33
          type II (HTLV-II) B97.34
        metapneumovirus B97.81
      papillomavirus B97.7
      parvovirus B97.6
      reovirus B97.5
      respiratory syncytial B97.4
      retrovirus B97.30
        human
          immunodeficiency, type 2 (HIV 2) B97.35
          T-cell lymphotropic,
            type I (HTLV-I) B97.33
            type II (HTLV-II) B97.34
        lentivirus B97.31
        oncovirus B97.32
        specified NEC B97.39
      specified NEC B97.89
    central nervous system A89
      atypical A81.9
        specified NEC A81.89
      enterovirus NEC A88.8
        meningitis A87.0
      slow virus A81.9
        specified NEC A81.89
      specified NEC A88.8
    chest J98.8
    cotia B08.8
    coxsackie (*see also* Infection, coxsackie) B34.1
      as cause of disease classified
        elsewhere B97.11
    ECHO
      as cause of disease classified
        elsewhere B97.12
      unspecified nature or site B34.1
    encephalitis, tick-borne A84.9
    enterovirus, as cause of disease classified
      elsewhere B97.10
      coxsackievirus B97.11
      echovirus B97.12
      specified NEC B97.19
    exanthem NOS B09
    human papilloma as cause of disease classified
      elsewhere B97.7
    human metapneumovirus as cause of disease
      classified elsewhere B97.81
    intestine — *see* Enteritis, viral
    respiratory syncytial
      as cause of disease classified elsewhere B97.4
      bronchopneumonia J12.1
      common cold syndrome J00
      nasopharyngitis (acute) J00
    rhinovirus
      as cause of disease classified
        elsewhere B97.89
      unspecified nature or site B34.8
    slow A81.9

Infection — *continued*
  virus — *continued*
    specified NEC A81.89
    specified type NEC B33.8
      as cause of disease classified
        elsewhere B97.89
      unspecified nature or site B34.8
    unspecified nature or site B34.9
    West Nile — *see* Virus, West Nile
  vulva (acute) — *see* Vulvitis
  West Nile — *see* Virus, West Nile
  whipworm B79
  worms B83.9
    specified type NEC B83.8
  Wuchereria (bancrofti) B74.0
    malayi B74.1
  yatapoxvirus B08.70
    specified NEC B08.79
  yeast (*see also* Candidiasis) B37.9
  yellow fever — *see* Fever, yellow
  Yersinia
    enterocolitica (intestinal) A04.6
    pestis — *see* Plague
    pseudotuberculosis A28.2
  Zeis' gland — *see* Hordeolum
  Zika virus A92.5
  zoonotic bacterial NOS A28.9
  Zopfia senegalensis B47.0
Infective, infectious — *see* condition
Infertility
  female N97.9
    age-related N97.8
    associated with
      anovulation N97.0
      cervical (mucus) disease or anomaly N88.3
      congenital anomaly
        cervix N88.3
        fallopian tube N97.1
        uterus N97.2
        vagina N97.8
      dysmucorrhea N88.3
      fallopian tube disease or anomaly N97.1
      pituitary-hypothalamic origin E23.0
      specified origin NEC N97.8
      Stein-Leventhal syndrome E28.2
      uterine disease or anomaly N97.2
      vaginal disease or anomaly N97.8
    due to
      cervical anomaly N88.3
      fallopian tube anomaly N97.1
      ovarian failure E28.39
      Stein-Leventhal syndrome E28.2
      uterine anomaly N97.2
      vaginal anomaly N97.8
    nonimplantation N97.2
    origin
      cervical N88.3
      tubal (block) (occlusion) (stenosis) N97.1
      uterine N97.2
      vaginal N97.8
  male N46.9
    azoospermia N46.01
      extratesticular cause N46.029
        drug therapy N46.021
        efferent duct obstruction N46.023
        infection N46.022
        radiation N46.024
        specified cause NEC N46.029
        systemic disease N46.025
    oligospermia N46.11
      extratesticular cause N46.129
        drug therapy N46.121
        efferent duct obstruction N46.123
        infection N46.122
        radiation N46.124
        specified cause NEC N46.129
        systemic disease N46.125
    specified type NEC N46.8
Infestation B88.9
  Acanthocheilonema (perstans)
    (streptocerca) B74.4
  Acariasis B88.0
    demodex folliculorum B88.0
    sarcoptes scabiei B86
    trombiculae B88.0
  Agamofilaria streptocerca B74.4
  Ancylostoma, ankylostoma (braziliense)
    (caninum) (ceylanicum) (duodenale) B76.0
    americanum B76.1
    new world B76.1
  Anisakis larvae, anisakiasis B81.0
  arthropod NEC B88.2

Infestation

Infestation — *continued*
  Ascaris lumbricoides — *see* Ascariasis
  Balantidium coli A07.0
  beef tapeworm B68.1
  Bothriocephalus (latus) B70.0
    larval B70.1
  broad tapeworm B70.0
    larval B70.1
  Brugia (malayi) B74.1
    timori B74.2
  candiru B88.8
  Capillaria
    hepatica B83.8
    philippinensis B81.1
  cat liver fluke B66.0
  cestodes B71.9
    diphyllobothrium — *see* Infestation, diphyllobothrium
    dipylidiasis B71.1
    hymenolepiasis B71.0
    specified type NEC B71.8
  chigger B88.0
  chigo, chigoe B88.1
  Clonorchis (sinensis) (liver) B66.1
  coccidial A07.3
  crab-lice B85.3
  Cysticercus cellulosae — *see* Cysticercosis
  Demodex (folliculorum) B88.0
  Dermanyssus gallinae B88.0
  Dermatobia (hominis) — *see* Myiasis
  Dibothriocephalus (latus) B70.0
    larval B70.1
  Dicrocoelium dendriticum B66.2
  Diphyllobothrium (adult) (latum) (intestinal) (pacificum) B70.0
    larval B70.1
  Diplogonoporus (grandis) B71.8
  Dipylidium caninum B67.4
  Distoma hepaticum B66.3
  dog tapeworm B67.4
  Dracunculus medinensis B72
  dragon worm B72
  dwarf tapeworm B71.0
  Echinococcus — *see* Echinococcus
  Echinostomum ilocanum B66.8
  Entamoeba (histolytica) — *see* Infection, Ameba
  Enterobius vermicularis B80
  eyelid
    in (due to)
      leishmaniasis B55.1
      loiasis B74.3
      onchocerciasis B73.09
      phthiriasis B85.3
      parasitic NOS B89
  eyeworm B74.3
  Fasciola (gigantica) (hepatica) (indica) B66.3
  Fasciolopsis (buski) (intestine) B66.5
  filarial B74.9
    bancroftian B74.0
    conjunctiva B74.9
    due to
      Acanthocheilonema (perstans) (streptocerca) B74.4
      Brugia (malayi) B74.1
        timori B74.2
      Dracunculus medinensis B72
      guinea worm B72
      loa loa B74.3
      Mansonella (ozzardi) (perstans) (streptocerca) B74.4
      Onchocerca volvulus B73.00
        eye B73.00
        eyelid B73.09
      Wuchereria (bancrofti) B74.0
    Malayan B74.1
    ozzardi B74.4
    specified type NEC B74.8
  fish tapeworm B70.0
    larval B70.1
  fluke B66.9
    blood NOS — *see* Schistosomiasis
    cat liver B66.0
    intestinal B66.5
    liver (sheep) B66.3
      cat B66.0
      Chinese B66.1
      due to clonorchiasis B66.1
      oriental B66.1
    lancet B66.2
    lung (oriental) B66.4
    sheep liver B66.3
    specified type NEC B66.8

Infestation — *continued*
  fly larvae — *see* Myiasis
  Gasterophilus (intestinalis) — *see* Myiasis
  Gastrodiscoides hominis B66.8
  Giardia lamblia A07.1
  Gnathostoma (spinigerum) B83.1
  Gongylonema B83.8
  guinea worm B72
  helminth B83.9
    angiostrongyliasis B83.2
      intestinal B81.3
    gnathostomiasis B83.1
    hirudiniasis, internal B83.4
    intestinal B82.0
      angiostrongyliasis B81.3
      anisakiasis B81.0
      ascariasis — *see* Ascariasis
      capillariasis B81.1
      cysticercosis — *see* Cysticercosis
      diphyllobothriasis — *see* Infestation, diphyllobothriasis
      dracunculiasis B72
      echinococcus — *see* Echinococcus
      enterobiasis B80
      filariasis — *see* Infestation, filarial
      fluke — *see* Infestation, fluke
      hookworm — *see* Infestation, hookworm
      mixed (types classifiable to more than one of the titles B65.0-B81.3 and B81.8) B81.4
      onchocerciasis — *see* Onchocerciasis
      schistosomiasis — *see* Infestation, schistosoma
      specified
        cestode NEC — *see* Infestation, cestode
        type NEC B81.8
      strongyloidiasis — *see* Strongyloidiasis
      taenia — *see* Infestation, taenia
      trichinellosis B75
      trichostrongyliasis B81.2
      trichuriasis B79
    specified type NEC B83.8
    syngamiasis B83.3
    visceral larva migrans B83.0
  Heterophyes (heterophyes) B66.8
  hookworm B76.9
    ancylostomiasis B76.0
    necatoriasis B76.1
    specified type NEC B76.8
  Hymenolepis (diminuta) (nana) B71.0
  intestinal NEC B82.9
  leeches (aquatic) (land) — *see* Hirudiniasis
  Leishmania — *see* Leishmaniasis
  lice, louse — *see* Infestation, Pediculus
  Linguatula B88.8
  Liponyssoides sanguineus B88.0
  Loa loa B74.3
    conjunctival B74.3
    eyelid B74.3
  louse — *see* Infestation, Pediculus
  maggots — *see* Myiasis
  Mansonella (ozzardi) (perstans) (streptocerca) B74.4
  Medina (worm) B72
  Metagonimus (yokogawai) B66.8
  microfilaria streptocerca — *see* Onchocerciasis
    eye B73.00
    eyelid B73.09
  mites B88.9
    scabic B86
  Monilia (albicans) — *see* Candidiasis
  mouth B37.0
  Necator americanus B76.1
  nematode NEC (intestinal) B82.0
    Ancylostoma B76.0
    conjunctiva NEC B83.9
    Enterobius vermicularis B80
    Gnathostoma spinigerum B83.1
    physaloptera B80
    specified NEC B81.8
    trichostrongylus B81.2
    trichuris (trichuria) B79
  Oesophagostomum (apiostomum) B81.8
  Oestrus ovis (*see also* Myiasis) B87.9
  Onchocerca (volvulus) — *see* Onchocerciasis
  Opisthorchis (felineus) (viverrini) B66.0
  orbit, parasitic NOS B89
  Oxyuris vermicularis B80
  Paragonimus (westermani) B66.4
  parasite, parasitic B89
    eyelid B89
    intestinal NOS B82.9
    mouth B37.0

Infestation — *continued*
  parasite — *continued*
    skin B88.9
    tongue B37.0
  Parastrongylus
    cantonensis B83.2
    costaricensis B81.3
  Pediculus B85.2
    body B85.1
    capitis (humanus) (any site) B85.0
    corporis (humanus) (any site) B85.1
    head B85.0
    mixed (classifiable to more than one of the titles B85.0-B85.3) B85.4
    pubis (any site) B85.3
  Pentastoma B88.8
  Phthirus (pubis) (any site) B85.3
    with any infestation classifiable to B85.0-B85.2 B85.4
  pinworm B80
  pork tapeworm (adult) B68.0
  protozoal NEC B64
    intestinal A07.9
      specified NEC A07.8
    specified NEC B60.8
  pubic, louse B85.3
  rat tapeworm B71.0
  red bug B88.0
  roundworm (large) NEC B82.0
    Ascariasis (*see also* Ascariasis) B77.9
  sandflea B88.1
  Sarcoptes scabiei B86
  scabies B86
  Schistosoma B65.9
    bovis B65.8
    cercariae B65.3
    haematobium B65.0
    intercalatum B65.8
    japonicum B65.2
    mansoni B65.1
    mattheei B65.8
    mekongi B65.8
    specified type NEC B65.8
    spindale B65.8
  screw worms — *see* Myiasis
  skin NOS B88.9
  Sparganum (mansoni) (proliferum) (baxteri) B70.1
    larval B70.1
  specified type NEC B88.8
  Spirometra larvae B70.1
  Stellantchasmus falcatus B66.8
  Strongyloides stercoralis — *see* Strongyloidiasis
  Taenia B68.9
    diminuta B71.0
    echinococcus — *see* Echinococcus
    mediocanellata B68.1
    nana B71.0
    saginata B68.1
    solium (intestinal form) B68.0
      larval form — *see* Cysticercosis
  Taeniarhynchus saginatus B68.1
  tapeworm B71.9
    beef B68.1
    broad B70.0
      larval B70.1
    dog B67.4
    dwarf B71.0
    fish B70.0
      larval B70.1
    pork B68.0
    rat B71.0
  Ternidens diminutus B81.8
  Tetranychus molestissimus B88.0
  threadworm B80
  tongue B37.0
  Toxocara (canis) (cati) (felis) B83.0
  trematode (s) NEC — *see* Infestation, fluke
  Trichinella (spiralis) B75
  Trichocephalus B79
  Trichomonas — *see* Trichomoniasis
  Trichostrongylus B81.2
  Trichuris (trichiura) B79
  Trombicula (irritans) B88.0
  Tunga penetrans B88.1
  Uncinaria americana B76.1
  Vandellia cirrhosa B88.8
  whipworm B79
  worms B83.9
    intestinal B82.0
  Wuchereria (bancrofti) B74.0

☑ **Additional character required**

Infiltrate, infiltration
  amyloid (generalized) (localized) — see
    Amyloidosis
  calcareous NEC R89.7
    localized — see Degeneration, by site
  calcium salt R89.7
  cardiac
    fatty — see Degeneration, myocardial
    glycogenic E74.02 *[143]*
  corneal — see Edema, cornea
  eyelid — see Inflammation, eyelid
  glycogen, glycogenic — see Disease, glycogen
    storage
  heart, cardiac
    fatty — see Degeneration, myocardial
    glycogenic E74.02 *[143]*
  inflammatory in vitreous H43.89
  kidney N28.89
  leukemic — see Leukemia
  liver K76.89
    fatty — see Fatty, liver NEC
    glycogen (see also Disease, glycogen
      storage) E74.03 *[K77]*
  lung R91.8
    eosinophilic J82
  lymphatic (see also Leukemia, lymphatic) C91.9 ☑
    gland I88.9
  muscle, fatty M62.89
  myocardium, myocardial
    fatty — see Degeneration, myocardial
    glycogenic E74.02 *[143]*
  on chest x-ray R91.8
  pulmonary R91.8
    with eosinophilia J82
  skin (lymphocytic) L98.6
  thymus (gland) (fatty) E32.8
  urine R39.0
  vesicant agent
    antineoplastic chemotherapy T80.810 ☑
    other agent NEC T80.818 ☑
  vitreous body H43.89
Infirmity R68.89
  senile R54
Inflammation, inflamed, inflammatory (with exudation)
  abducent (nerve) — see Strabismus, paralytic,
    sixth nerve
  accessory sinus (chronic) — see Sinusitis
  adrenal (gland) E27.8
  alveoli, teeth M27.3
    scorbutic E54
  anal canal, anus K62.89
  antrum (chronic) — see Sinusitis, maxillary
  appendix — see Appendicitis
  arachnoid — see Meningitis
  areola N61.0
    puerperal, postpartum or gestational — see
      Infection, nipple
  areolar tissue NOS L08.9
  artery — see Arteritis
  auditory meatus (external) — see Otitis, externa
  Bartholin's gland N75.8
  bile duct (common) (hepatic) or passage — see
    Cholangitis
  bladder — see Cystitis
  bone — see Osteomyelitis
  brain (see also Encephalitis)
    membrane — see Meningitis
  breast N61.0
    puerperal, postpartum, gestational — see
      Mastitis, obstetric
  broad ligament — see Disease, pelvis,
    inflammatory
  bronchi — see Bronchitis
  catarrhal J00
  cecum — see Appendicitis
  cerebral (see also Encephalitis)
    membrane — see Meningitis
  cerebrospinal
    meningococcal A39.0
  cervix (uteri) — see Cervicitis
  chest J98.8
  chorioretinal H30.9 ☑
    cyclitis — see Cyclitis
    disseminated H30.10 ☑
      generalized H30.13 ☑
      peripheral H30.12 ☑
      posterior pole H30.11 ☑
    epitheliopathy — see Epitheliopathy
    focal H30.00 ☑
      juxtapapillary H30.01 ☑
      macular H30.04 ☑

Inflammation — continued
  chorioretinal — continued
    paramacular — see Inflammation,
      chorioretinal, focal, macular
    peripheral H30.03 ☑
    posterior pole H30.02 ☑
    specified type NEC H30.89 ☑
  choroid — see Inflammation, chorioretinal
  chronic, postmastoidectomy cavity — see
    Complications, postmastoidectomy,
    inflammation
  colon — see Enteritis
  connective tissue (diffuse) NEC — see Disorder,
    soft tissue, specified type NEC
  cornea — see Keratitis
  corpora cavernosa N48.29
  cranial nerve — see Disorder, nerve, cranial
  Douglas' cul-de-sac or pouch (chronic) N73.0
  due to device, implant or graft (see also
    Complications, by site and type, infection or
    inflammation)
    arterial graft T82.7 ☑
    breast (implant) T85.79 ☑
    catheter T85.79 ☑
      dialysis (renal) T82.7 ☑
        intraperitoneal T85.71 ☑
      infusion T82.7 ☑
        cranial T85.735 ☑
        intrathecal T85.735 ☑
        spinal (epidural) (subdural) T85.735 ☑
        subarachnoid T85.735 ☑
      urinary T83.518 ☑
        cystostomy T83.510 ☑
        Hopkins T83.518 ☑
        ileostomy T83.518 ☑
        nephrostomy T83.512 ☑
        specified NEC T83.518 ☑
        urethral indwelling T83.511 ☑
        urostomy T83.518 ☑
    electronic (electrode) (pulse generator)
      (stimulator)
      bone T84.7 ☑
      cardiac T82.7 ☑
      nervous system T85.738 ☑
        brain T85.731 ☑
        cranial nerve T85.732 ☑
        gastric nerve T85.732 ☑
        neurostimulator generator T85.734 ☑
        peripheral nerve T85.732 ☑
        sacral nerve T85.732 ☑
        spinal cord T85.733 ☑
        vagal nerve T85.732 ☑
      urinary T83.590 ☑
    fixation, internal (orthopedic) NEC — see
      Complication, fixation device, infection
    gastrointestinal (bile duct)
      (esophagus) T85.79 ☑
      neurostimulator electrode (lead) T85.732 ☑
    genital NEC T83.69 ☑
    heart NEC T82.7 ☑
      valve (prosthesis) T82.6 ☑
        graft T82.7 ☑
    joint prosthesis — see Complication, joint
      prosthesis, infection
    ocular (corneal graft) (orbital implant)
      NEC T85.79 ☑
    orthopedic NEC T84.7 ☑
    penile (cylinder) (pump) (reservoir) T83.61 ☑
    specified NEC T85.79 ☑
    testicular T83.62 ☑
    urinary NEC T83.598 ☑
      ileal conduit stent T83.593 ☑
      implanted neurostimulation T83.590 ☑
      implanted sphincter T83.591 ☑
      indwelling ureteral stent T83.592 ☑
      nephroureteral stent T83.593 ☑
      specified stent NEC T83.593 ☑
    vascular NEC T82.7 ☑
    ventricular intracranial (communicating)
      shunt T85.730 ☑
  duodenum K29.80
    with bleeding K29.81
  dura mater — see Meningitis
  ear (middle) (see also Otitis, media)
    external — see Otitis, externa
    inner — see subcategory H83.0
  epididymis — see Epididymitis
  esophagus K20.9
  ethmoidal (sinus) (chronic) — see Sinusitis,
    ethmoidal
  eustachian tube (catarrhal) — see Salpingitis,
    eustachian

Inflammation — continued
  eyelid H01.9
    abscess — see Abscess, eyelid
    blepharitis — see Blepharitis
    chalazion — see Chalazion
    dermatosis (noninfectious) — see Dermatosis,
      eyelid
    hordeolum — see Hordeolum
    specified NEC H01.8
  fallopian tube — see Salpingo-oophoritis
  fascia — see Myositis
  follicular, pharynx J31.2
  frontal (sinus) (chronic) — see Sinusitis, frontal
  gallbladder — see Cholecystitis
  gastric — see Gastritis
  gastrointestinal — see Enteritis
  genital organ (internal) (diffuse)
    female — see Disease, pelvis, inflammatory
    male N49.9
      multiple sites N49.8
      specified NEC N49.8
  gland (lymph) — see Lymphadenitis
  glottis — see Laryngitis
  granular, pharynx J31.2
  gum K05.10
    nonplaque induced K05.11
    plaque induced K05.10
  heart — see Carditis
  hepatic duct — see Cholangitis
  ileoanal (internal) pouch K91.850
  ileum (see also Enteritis)
    regional or terminal — see Enteritis, regional
  intestine (any part) — see Enteritis
  intestinal pouch K91.850
  jaw (acute) (bone) (chronic) (lower) (suppurative)
    (upper) M27.2
  joint NEC — see Arthritis
    sacroiliac M46.1
  kidney — see Nephritis
  knee (joint) M13.169
    tuberculous A18.02
  labium (majus) (minus) — see Vulvitis
  lacrimal
    gland — see Dacryoadenitis
    passages (duct) (sac) (see also Dacryocystitis)
      canaliculitis — see Canaliculitis, lacrimal
  larynx — see Laryngitis
  leg NOS L08.9
  lip K13.0
  liver (capsule) (see also Hepatitis)
    chronic K73.9
    suppurative K75.0
  lung (acute) (see also Pneumonia)
    chronic J98.4
  lymph gland or node — see Lymphadenitis
  lymphatic vessel — see Lymphangitis
  maxilla, maxillary M27.2
    sinus (chronic) — see Sinusitis, maxillary
  membranes of brain or spinal cord — see
    Meningitis
  meninges — see Meningitis
  mouth K12.1
  muscle — see Myositis
  myocardium — see Myocarditis
  nasal sinus (chronic) — see Sinusitis
  nasopharynx — see Nasopharyngitis
  navel L08.82
  nerve NEC — see Neuralgia
  nipple N61.0
    puerperal, postpartum or gestational — see
      Infection, nipple
  nose — see Rhinitis
  oculomotor (nerve) — see Strabismus, paralytic,
    third nerve
  optic nerve — see Neuritis, optic
  orbit (chronic) H05.10
    acute H05.00
      abscess — see Abscess, orbit
      cellulitis — see Cellulitis, orbit
      osteomyelitis — see Osteomyelitis, orbit
      periostitis — see Periostitis, orbital
      tenonitis — see Tenonitis, eye
    granuloma — see Granuloma, orbit
    myositis — see Myositis, orbital
  ovary — see Salpingo-oophoritis
  oviduct — see Salpingo-oophoritis
  pancreas (acute) — see Pancreatitis
  parametrium N73.0
  parotid region L08.9
  pelvis, female — see Disease, pelvis, inflammatory
  penis (corpora cavernosa) N48.29
  perianal K62.89

Inflammation - Injury

Inflammation — *continued*
   pericardium — *see* Pericarditis
   perineum (female) (male) L08.9
   perirectal K62.89
   peritoneum — *see* Peritonitis
   periuterine — *see* Disease, pelvis, inflammatory
   perivesical — *see* Cystitis
   petrous bone (acute) (chronic) — *see* Petrositis
   pharynx (acute) — *see* Pharyngitis
   pia mater — *see* Meningitis
   pleura — *see* Pleurisy
   polyp, colon (*see also* Polyp, colon, inflammatory) K51.40
   prostate (*see also* Prostatitis)
      specified type NEC N41.8
   rectosigmoid — *see* Rectosigmoiditis
   rectum (*see also* Proctitis) K62.89
   respiratory, upper (*see also* Infection, respiratory, upper) J06.9
      acute, due to radiation J70.0
      chronic, due to external agent — *see* condition, respiratory, chronic, due to
      due to
         chemicals, gases, fumes or vapors (inhalation) J68.2
         radiation J70.1
   retina — *see* Chorioretinitis
   retrocecal — *see* Appendicitis
   retroperitoneal — *see* Peritonitis
   salivary duct or gland (any) (suppurative) — *see* Sialoadenitis
   scorbutic, alveoli, teeth E54
   scrotum N49.2
   seminal vesicle — *see* Vesiculitis
   sigmoid — *see* Enteritis
   sinus — *see* Sinusitis
   Skene's duct or gland — *see* Urethritis
   skin L08.9
   spermatic cord N49.1
   sphenoidal (sinus) — *see* Sinusitis, sphenoidal
   spinal
      cord — *see* Encephalitis
      membrane — *see* Meningitis
      nerve — *see* Disorder, nerve
   spine — *see* Spondylopathy, inflammatory
   spleen (capsule) D73.89
   stomach — *see* Gastritis
   subcutaneous tissue L08.9
   suprarenal (gland) E27.8
   synovial — *see* Tenosynovitis
   tendon (sheath) NEC — *see* Tenosynovitis
   testis — *see* Orchitis
   throat (acute) — *see* Pharyngitis
   thymus (gland) E32.8
   thyroid (gland) — *see* Thyroiditis
   tongue K14.0
   tonsil — *see* Tonsillitis
   trachea — *see* Tracheitis
   trochlear (nerve) — *see* Strabismus, paralytic, fourth nerve
   tubal — *see* Salpingo-oophoritis
   tuberculous NEC — *see* Tuberculosis
   tubo-ovarian — *see* Salpingo-oophoritis
   tunica vaginalis N49.1
   tympanic membrane — *see* Tympanitis
   umbilicus, umbilical L08.82
   uterine ligament — *see* Disease, pelvis, inflammatory
   uterus (catarrhal) — *see* Endometritis
   uveal tract (anterior) NOS (*see also* Iridocyclitis)
      posterior — *see* Chorioretinitis
   vagina — *see* Vaginitis
   vas deferens N49.1
   vein (*see also* Phlebitis)
      intracranial or intraspinal (septic) G08
      thrombotic I80.9
         leg — *see* Phlebitis, leg
         lower extremity — *see* Phlebitis, leg
   vocal cord J38.3
   vulva — *see* Vulvitis
   Wharton's duct (suppurative) — *see* Sialoadenitis
Inflation, lung, imperfect (newborn) — *see* Atelectasis
Influenza (bronchial) (epidemic) (respiratory (upper)) (unidentified influenza virus) J11.1
   with
      digestive manifestations J11.2
      encephalopathy J11.81
      enteritis J11.2
      gastroenteritis J11.2
      gastrointestinal manifestations J11.2
      laryngitis J11.1

Influenza — *continued*
   with — *continued*
      myocarditis J11.82
      otitis media J11.83
      pharyngitis J11.1
      pneumonia J11.00
         specified type J11.08
      respiratory manifestations NEC J11.1
      specified manifestation NEC J11.89
   A/H5N1 (*see also* Influenza, due to, identified novel influenza A virus) J09.X2
   avian (*see also* Influenza, due to, identified novel influenza A virus) J09.X2
   bird (*see also* Influenza, due to, identified novel influenza A virus) J09.X2
   novel (2009) H1N1 influenza (*see also* Influenza, due to, identified influenza virus NEC) J10.1
   novel influenza A/H1N1 (*see also* Influenza, due to, identified influenza virus NEC) J10.1
   due to
      avian (*see also* Influenza, due to, identified novel influenza A virus) J09.X2
      identified influenza virus NEC J10.1
         with
            digestive manifestations J10.2
            encephalopathy J10.81
            enteritis J10.2
            gastroenteritis J10.2
            gastrointestinal manifestations J10.2
            laryngitis J10.1
            myocarditis J10.82
            otitis media J10.83
            pharyngitis J10.1
            pneumonia (unspecified type) J10.00
               with same identified influenza virus J10.01
               specified type NEC J10.08
            respiratory manifestations NEC J10.1
            specified manifestation NEC J10.89
      identified novel influenza A virus J09.X2
         with
            digestive manifestations J09.X3
            encephalopathy J09.X9
            enteritis J09.X3
            gastroenteritis J09.X3
            gastrointestinal manifestations J09.X3
            laryngitis J09.X9
            myocarditis J09.X9
            otitis media J09.X9
            pharyngitis J09.X9
            pneumonia J09.X1
            respiratory manifestations NEC J09.X2
            specified manifestation NEC J09.X9
            upper respiratory symptoms J09.X2
      of other animal origin, not bird or swine (*see also* Influenza, due to, identified novel influenza A virus) J09.X2
      swine (viruses that normally cause infections in pigs) (*see also* Influenza, due to, identified novel influenza A virus) J09.X2
Influenza-like disease — *see* Influenza
Influenzal — *see* Influenza
Infraction, Freiberg's (metatarsal head) — *see* Osteochondrosis, juvenile, metatarsus
Infraeruption of tooth (teeth) M26.34
Infusion complication, misadventure, or reaction — *see* Complications, infusion
Ingestion
   chemical — *see* Table of Drugs and Chemicals, by substance, poisoning
   drug or medicament
      correct substance properly administered — *see* Table of Drugs and Chemicals, by drug, adverse effect
      overdose or wrong substance given or taken — *see* Table of Drugs and Chemicals, by drug, poisoning
   foreign body — *see* Foreign body, alimentary tract
   tularemia A21.3
Ingrowing
   hair (beard) L73.1
   nail (finger) (toe) L60.0
Inguinal (*see also* condition)
   testicle Q53.9
      bilateral Q53.212
      unilateral Q53.112
Inhalant-induced
   anxiety disorder F18.980
   depressive disorder F18.94
   major neurocognitive disorder F18.97
   mild neurocognitive disorder F18.988
   psychotic disorder F18.959

Inhalation
   anthrax A22.1
   flame T27.3 ☑
   food or foreign body — *see* Foreign body, by site
   gases, fumes, or vapors NEC T59.9 ☑
      specified agent — *see* Table of Drugs and Chemicals, by substance
   liquid or vomitus — *see* Asphyxia
   meconium (newborn) P24.00
      with
         pneumonia (pneumonitis) P24.01
         with respiratory symptoms P24.01
   mucus — *see* Asphyxia, mucus
   oil or gasoline (causing suffocation) — *see* Foreign body, by site
   smoke J70.5
      due to chemicals, gases, fumes and vapors J68.9
   steam — *see* Toxicity, vapors
   stomach contents or secretions — *see* Foreign body, by site
      due to anesthesia (general) (local) or other sedation T88.59 ☑
      in labor and delivery O74.0
      in pregnancy O29.01 ☑
      postpartum, puerperal O89.01
Inhibition, orgasm
   female F52.31
   male F52.32
Inhibitor, systemic lupus erythematosus (presence of) D68.62
Iniencephalus, iniencephaly Q00.2
Injection, traumatic jet (air) (industrial) (water) (paint or dye) T70.4 ☑
Injury (*see also* specified injury type) T14.90 ☑
   abdomen, abdominal S39.91 ☑
      blood vessel — *see* Injury, blood vessel, abdomen
      cavity — *see* Injury, intra-abdominal
      contusion S30.1 ☑
      internal — *see* Injury, intra-abdominal
      intra-abdominal organ — *see* Injury, intra-abdominal
      nerve — *see* Injury, nerve, abdomen
      open — *see* Wound, open, abdomen
      specified NEC S39.81 ☑
      superficial — *see* Injury, superficial, abdomen
   Achilles tendon S86.00 ☑
      laceration S86.02 ☑
      specified type NEC S86.09 ☑
      strain S86.01 ☑
   acoustic, resulting in deafness — *see* Injury, nerve, acoustic
   adrenal (gland) S37.819 ☑
      contusion S37.812 ☑
      laceration S37.813 ☑
      specified type NEC S37.818 ☑
   alveolar (process) S09.93 ☑
   ankle S99.91 ☑
      contusion — *see* Contusion, ankle
      dislocation — *see* Dislocation, ankle
      fracture — *see* Fracture, ankle
      nerve — *see* Injury, nerve, ankle
      open — *see* Wound, open, ankle
      specified type NEC S99.81 ☑
      sprain — *see* Sprain, ankle
      superficial — *see* Injury, superficial, ankle
   anterior chamber, eye — *see* Injury, eye, specified site NEC
   anus — *see* Injury, abdomen
   aorta (thoracic) S25.00 ☑
      abdominal S35.00 ☑
         laceration (minor) (superficial) S35.01 ☑
            major S35.02 ☑
         specified type NEC S35.09 ☑
      laceration (minor) (superficial) S25.01 ☑
         major S25.02 ☑
      specified type NEC S25.09 ☑
   arm (upper) S49.9 ☑
      blood vessel — *see* Injury, blood vessel, arm
      contusion — *see* Contusion, arm, upper
      fracture — *see* Fracture, humerus
      lower — *see* Injury, forearm
      muscle — *see* Injury, muscle, shoulder
      nerve — *see* Injury, nerve, arm
      open — *see* Wound, open, arm
      specified type NEC S49.8 ☑
      superficial — *see* Injury, superficial, arm
   artery (complicating trauma) (*see also* Injury, blood vessel, by site)
      cerebral or meningeal — *see* Injury, intracranial
      auditory canal (external) (meatus) S09.91 ☑

☑ **Additional character required**

Injury — continued
auricle, auris, ear S09.91 ☑
axilla — see Injury, shoulder
back — see Injury, back, lower
bile duct S36.13 ☑
birth (see also Birth, injury) P15.9
bladder (sphincter) S37.20 ☑
 at delivery O71.5
 contusion S37.22 ☑
 laceration S37.23 ☑
 obstetrical trauma O71.5
 specified type NEC S37.29 ☑
blast (air) (hydraulic) (immersion) (underwater)
  NEC T14.8 ☑
 acoustic nerve trauma — see Injury, nerve,
  acoustic
 bladder — see Injury, bladder
 brain — see Concussion
 colon — see Injury, intestine, large, blast injury
 ear (primary) S09.31 ☑
  secondary S09.39 ☑
 generalized T70.8 ☑
 lung — see Injury, intrathoracic, lung, blast
  injury
 multiple body organs T70.8 ☑
 peritoneum S36.81 ☑
 rectum S36.61 ☑
 retroperitoneum S36.898 ☑
 small intestine S36.419 ☑
  duodenum S36.410 ☑
  specified site NEC S36.418 ☑
 specified
  intra-abdominal organ NEC S36.898 ☑
  pelvic organ NEC S37.899 ☑
blood vessel NEC T14.8 ☑
 abdomen S35.9 ☑
  aorta — see Injury, aorta, abdominal
  celiac artery — see Injury, blood vessel, celiac
   artery
  iliac vessel — see Injury, blood vessel, iliac
  laceration S35.91 ☑
  mesenteric vessel — see Injury, mesenteric
  portal vein — see Injury, blood vessel, portal
   vein
  renal vessel — see Injury, blood vessel, renal
  specified vessel NEC S35.8X ☑
  splenic vessel — see Injury, blood vessel,
   splenic
  vena cava — see Injury, vena cava, inferior
 ankle — see Injury, blood vessel, foot
 aorta (abdominal) (thoracic) — see Injury, aorta
 arm (upper) NEC S45.90 ☑
  forearm — see Injury, blood vessel, forearm
  laceration S45.91 ☑
  specified
   site NEC S45.80 ☑
    laceration S45.81 ☑
    specified type NEC S45.89 ☑
   type NEC S45.99 ☑
  superficial vein S45.30 ☑
   laceration S45.31 ☑
   specified type NEC S45.39 ☑
 axillary
  artery S45.00 ☑
   laceration S45.01 ☑
   specified type NEC S45.09 ☑
  vein S45.20 ☑
   laceration S45.21 ☑
   specified type NEC S45.29 ☑
 azygos vein — see Injury, blood vessel, thoracic,
  specified site NEC
 brachial
  artery S45.10 ☑
   laceration S45.11 ☑
   specified type NEC S45.19 ☑
  vein S45.20 ☑
   laceration S45.219 ☑
   specified type NEC S45.29 ☑
 carotid artery (common) (external) (internal,
  extracranial) S15.00 ☑
  internal, intracranial S06.8 ☑
  laceration (minor) (superficial) S15.01 ☑
   major S15.02 ☑
  specified type NEC S15.09 ☑
 celiac artery S35.219 ☑
  branch S35.299 ☑
   laceration (minor) (superficial) S35.291 ☑
    major S35.292 ☑
   specified NEC S35.298 ☑
  laceration (minor) (superficial) S35.211 ☑
   major S35.212 ☑
  specified type NEC S35.218 ☑

Injury — continued
 blood vessel NEC — continued
  cerebral — see Injury, intracranial
  deep plantar — see Injury, blood vessel, plantar
   artery
  digital (hand) — see Injury, blood vessel, finger
  dorsal
   artery (foot) S95.00 ☑
    laceration S95.01 ☑
    specified type NEC S95.09 ☑
   vein (foot) S95.20 ☑
    laceration S95.21 ☑
    specified type NEC S95.29 ☑
  due to accidental laceration during procedure
   — see Laceration, accidental complicating
   surgery
  extremity — see Injury, blood vessel, limb
  femoral
   artery (common) (superficial) S75.00 ☑
    laceration (minor) (superficial) S75.01 ☑
     major S75.02 ☑
    specified type NEC S75.09 ☑
   vein (hip level) (thigh level) S75.10 ☑
    laceration (minor) (superficial) S75.11 ☑
     major S75.12 ☑
    specified type NEC S75.19 ☑
  finger S65.50 ☑
   index S65.50 ☑
    laceration S65.51 ☑
    specified type NEC S65.59 ☑
   laceration S65.51 ☑
   little S65.50 ☑
    laceration S65.51 ☑
    specified type NEC S65.59 ☑
   middle S65.50 ☑
    laceration S65.51 ☑
    specified type NEC S65.59 ☑
   specified type NEC S65.59 ☑
   thumb — see Injury, blood vessel, thumb
  foot S95.90 ☑
   dorsal
    artery — see Injury, blood vessel, dorsal,
     artery
    vein — see Injury, blood vessel, dorsal, vein
   laceration S95.91 ☑
   plantar artery — see Injury, blood vessel,
    plantar artery
   specified
    site NEC S95.80 ☑
     laceration S95.81 ☑
     specified type NEC S95.89 ☑
    specified type NEC S95.99 ☑
  forearm S55.90 ☑
   laceration S55.91 ☑
   radial artery — see Injury, blood vessel, radial
    artery
   specified
    site NEC S55.80 ☑
     laceration S55.81 ☑
     specified type NEC S55.89 ☑
    type NEC S55.99 ☑
   ulnar artery — see Injury, blood vessel, ulnar
    artery
   vein S55.20 ☑
    laceration S55.21 ☑
    specified type NEC S55.29 ☑
  gastric
   artery — see Injury, mesenteric, artery,
    branch
   vein — see Injury, blood vessel, abdomen
  gastroduodenal artery — see Injury,
   mesenteric, artery, branch
  greater saphenous vein (lower leg
   level) S85.30 ☑
  hip (and thigh) level S75.20 ☑
   laceration (minor) (superficial) S75.21 ☑
    major S75.22 ☑
   specified type NEC S75.29 ☑
  laceration S85.31 ☑
  specified type NEC S85.39 ☑
  hand (level) S65.90 ☑
   finger — see Injury, blood vessel, finger
   laceration S65.91 ☑
   palmar arch — see Injury, blood vessel,
    palmar arch
   radial artery — see Injury, blood vessel, radial
    artery, hand
   specified
    site NEC S65.80 ☑
     laceration S65.81 ☑
     specified type NEC S65.89 ☑
    type NEC S65.99 ☑

Injury — continued
 blood vessel NEC — continued
  thumb — see Injury, blood vessel, thumb
  ulnar artery — see Injury, blood vessel, ulnar
   artery, hand
  head S09.0 ☑
   intracranial — see Injury, intracranial
   multiple S09.0 ☑
  hepatic
   artery — see Injury, mesenteric, artery
   vein — see Injury, vena cava, inferior
  hip S75.90 ☑
   femoral artery — see Injury, blood vessel,
    femoral, artery
   femoral vein — see Injury, blood vessel,
    femoral, vein
   greater saphenous vein — see Injury, blood
    vessel, greater saphenous, hip level
   laceration S75.91 ☑
   specified
    site NEC S75.80 ☑
     laceration S75.81 ☑
     specified type NEC S75.89 ☑
    type NEC S75.99 ☑
  hypogastric (artery) (vein) — see Injury, blood
   vessel, iliac
  iliac S35.5 ☑
   artery S35.51 ☑
   specified vessel NEC S35.5 ☑
   uterine vessel — see Injury, blood vessel,
    uterine
   vein S35.51 ☑
  innominate — see Injury, blood vessel, thoracic,
   innominate
  intercostal (artery) (vein) — see Injury, blood
   vessel, thoracic, intercostal
  jugular vein (external) S15.20 ☑
   internal S15.30 ☑
    laceration (minor) (superficial) S15.31 ☑
     major S15.32 ☑
    specified type NEC S15.39 ☑
   laceration (minor) (superficial) S15.21 ☑
    major S15.22 ☑
   specified type NEC S15.29 ☑
  leg (level) (lower) S85.90 ☑
   greater saphenous — see Injury, blood vessel,
    greater saphenous
   laceration S85.91 ☑
   lesser saphenous — see Injury, blood vessel,
    lesser saphenous
   peroneal artery — see Injury, blood vessel,
    peroneal artery
   popliteal
    artery — see Injury, blood vessel, popliteal,
     artery
    vein — see Injury, blood vessel, popliteal,
     vein
   specified
    site NEC S85.80 ☑
     laceration S85.81 ☑
     specified type NEC S85.89 ☑
    type NEC S85.99 ☑
   thigh — see Injury, blood vessel, hip
   tibial artery — see Injury, blood vessel, tibial
    artery
  lesser saphenous vein (lower leg
   level) S85.40 ☑
   laceration S85.41 ☑
   specified type NEC S85.49 ☑
  limb
   lower — see Injury, blood vessel, leg
   upper — see Injury, blood vessel, arm
  lower back — see Injury, blood vessel,
   abdomen
   specified NEC — see Injury, blood vessel,
    abdomen, specified, site NEC
  mammary (artery) (vein) — see Injury, blood
   vessel, thoracic, specified site NEC
  mesenteric (inferior) (superior)
   artery — see Injury, mesenteric, artery
   vein — see Injury, mesenteric, vein
  neck S15.9 ☑
   specified site NEC S15.8 ☑
  ovarian (artery) (vein) — see subcategory S35.8
  palmar arch (superficial) S65.20 ☑
   deep S65.30 ☑
    laceration S65.31 ☑
    specified type NEC S65.39 ☑
   laceration S65.21 ☑
   specified type NEC S65.29 ☑
  pelvis — see Injury, blood vessel, abdomen

Injury

Injury — *continued*
    blood vessel NEC — *continued*
        specified NEC — *see* Injury, blood vessel,
            abdomen, specified, site NEC
        peroneal artery S85.20 ☑
           laceration S85.21 ☑
           specified type NEC S85.29 ☑
        plantar artery (deep) (foot) S95.10 ☑
           laceration S95.11 ☑
           specified type NEC S95.19 ☑
        popliteal
           artery S85.00 ☑
              laceration S85.01 ☑
              specified type NEC S85.09 ☑
           vein S85.50 ☑
              laceration S85.51 ☑
              specified type NEC S85.59 ☑
        portal vein S35.319 ☑
           laceration S35.311 ☑
           specified type NEC S35.318 ☑
        precerebral — *see* Injury, blood vessel, neck
        pulmonary (artery) (vein) — *see* Injury, blood
           vessel, thoracic, pulmonary
        radial artery (forearm level) S55.10 ☑
           hand and wrist (level) S65.10 ☑
              laceration S65.11 ☑
              specified type NEC S65.19 ☑
           laceration S55.11 ☑
           specified type NEC S55.19 ☑
        renal
           artery S35.40 ☑
              laceration S35.41 ☑
              specified NEC S35.49 ☑
           vein S35.40 ☑
              laceration S35.41 ☑
              specified NEC S35.49 ☑
        saphenous vein (greater) (lower leg level) — *see*
           Injury, blood vessel, greater saphenous
           hip and thigh level — *see* Injury, blood vessel,
              greater saphenous, hip level
           lesser — *see* Injury, blood vessel, lesser
              saphenous
        shoulder
           specified NEC — *see* Injury, blood vessel, arm,
              specified site NEC
           superficial vein — *see* Injury, blood vessel,
              arm, superficial vein
        specified NEC T14.8 ☑
        splenic
           artery — *see* Injury, blood vessel, celiac
              artery, branch
           vein S35.329 ☑
              laceration S35.321 ☑
              specified NEC S35.328 ☑
        subclavian — *see* Injury, blood vessel, thoracic,
           innominate
        thigh — *see* Injury, blood vessel, hip
        thoracic S25.90 ☑
           aorta S25.00 ☑
              laceration (minor) (superficial) S25.01 ☑
                 major S25.02 ☑
              specified type NEC S25.09 ☑
           azygos vein — *see* Injury, blood vessel,
              thoracic, specified, site NEC
           innominate
              artery S25.10 ☑
                laceration (minor) (superficial) S25.11 ☑
                 major S25.12 ☑
                specified type NEC S25.19 ☑
             vein S25.30 ☑
               laceration (minor) (superficial) S25.31 ☑
                major S25.32 ☑
               specified type NEC S25.39 ☑
           intercostal S25.50 ☑
              laceration S25.51 ☑
              specified type NEC S25.59 ☑
           laceration S25.91 ☑
           mammary vessel — *see* Injury, blood vessel,
              thoracic, specified, site NEC
           pulmonary S25.40 ☑
              laceration (minor) (superficial) S25.41 ☑
                 major S25.42 ☑
              specified type NEC S25.49 ☑
           specified
              site NEC S25.80 ☑
                laceration S25.81 ☑
                specified type NEC S25.89 ☑
             type NEC S25.99 ☑
           subclavian — *see* Injury, blood vessel,
             thoracic, innominate
           vena cava (superior) S25.20 ☑
             laceration (minor) (superficial) S25.21 ☑

Injury — *continued*
    blood vessel NEC — *continued*
           major S25.22 ☑
           specified type NEC S25.29 ☑
        thumb S65.40 ☑
           laceration S65.41 ☑
           specified type NEC S65.49 ☑
        tibial artery S85.10 ☑
           anterior S85.13 ☑
              laceration S85.14 ☑
              specified injury NEC S85.15 ☑
           laceration S85.11 ☑
           posterior S85.16 ☑
              laceration S85.17 ☑
              specified injury NEC S85.18 ☑
           specified injury NEC S85.12 ☑
        ulnar artery (forearm level) S55.00 ☑
           hand and wrist (level) S65.00 ☑
              laceration S65.01 ☑
              specified type NEC S65.09 ☑
           laceration S55.01 ☑
           specified type NEC S55.09 ☑
        upper arm (level) — *see* Injury, blood vessel,
           arm
        superficial vein — *see* Injury, blood vessel,
           arm, superficial vein
        uterine S35.5 ☑
           artery S35.53 ☑
           vein S35.53 ☑
        vena cava — *see* Injury, vena cava
        vertebral artery S15.10 ☑
           laceration (minor) (superficial) S15.11 ☑
              major S15.12 ☑
           specified type NEC S15.19 ☑
        wrist (level) — *see* Injury, blood vessel, hand
    brachial plexus S14.3 ☑
        newborn P14.3
    brain (traumatic) S06.9 ☑
        diffuse (axonal) S06.2X ☑
        focal S06.30 ☑
    brainstem S06.38 ☑
    breast NOS S29.9 ☑
    broad ligament — *see* Injury, pelvic organ,
        specified site NEC
    bronchus, bronchi — *see* Injury, intrathoracic,
        bronchus
    brow S09.90 ☑
    buttock S39.92 ☑
    canthus, eye S05.90 ☑
    cardiac plexus — *see* Injury, nerve, thorax,
        sympathetic
    cauda equina S34.3 ☑
    cavernous sinus — *see* Injury, intracranial
    cecum — *see* Injury, colon
    celiac ganglion or plexus — *see* Injury, nerve,
        lumbosacral, sympathetic
    cerebellum — *see* Injury, intracranial
    cerebral — *see* Injury, intracranial
    cervix (uteri) — *see* Injury, uterus
    cheek (wall) S09.93 ☑
    chest — *see* Injury, thorax
    childbirth (newborn) (*see also* Birth, injury)
        maternal NEC O71.9
    chin S09.93 ☑
    choroid (eye) — *see* Injury, eye, specified site NEC
    clitoris S39.94 ☑
    coccyx (*see also* Injury, back, lower)
        complicating delivery O71.6
    colon — *see* Injury, intestine, large
    common bile duct — *see* Injury, liver
    conjunctiva (superficial) — *see* Injury, eye,
        conjunctiva
    conus medullaris — *see* Injury, spinal, sacral
    cord
        spermatic (pelvic region) S37.898 ☑
           scrotal region S39.848 ☑
        spinal — *see* Injury, spinal cord, by region
    cornea — *see* Injury, eye, specified site NEC
        abrasion — *see* Injury, eye, cornea, abrasion
    cortex (cerebral) (*see also* Injury, intracranial)
        visual — *see* Injury, nerve, optic
    costal region NEC S29.9 ☑
    costochondral NEC S29.9 ☑
    cranial
        cavity — *see* Injury, intracranial
        nerve — *see* Injury, nerve, cranial
    crushing — *see* Crush
    cutaneous sensory nerve
    cystic duct — *see* Injury, liver
    deep tissue — *see* Contusion, by site
        meaning pressure ulcer — *see* Ulcer, pressure,
           unstageable, by site

Injury — *continued*
    delivery (newborn) P15.9
        maternal NEC O71.9
    Descemet's membrane — *see* Injury, eyeball,
        penetrating
    diaphragm — *see* Injury, intrathoracic, diaphragm
    duodenum — *see* Injury, intestine, small,
        duodenum
    ear (auricle) (external) (canal) S09.91 ☑
        abrasion — *see* Abrasion, ear
        bite — *see* Bite, ear
        blister — *see* Blister, ear
        bruise — *see* Contusion, ear
        contusion — *see* Contusion, ear
        external constriction — *see* Constriction,
           external, ear
        hematoma — *see* Hematoma, ear
        inner — *see* Injury, ear, middle
        laceration — *see* Laceration, ear
        middle S09.30 ☑
           blast — *see* Injury, blast, ear
           specified NEC S09.39 ☑
        puncture — *see* Puncture, ear
        superficial — *see* Injury, superficial, ear
    eighth cranial nerve (acoustic or auditory) — *see*
        Injury, nerve, acoustic
    elbow S59.90 ☑
        contusion — *see* Contusion, elbow
        dislocation — *see* Dislocation, elbow
        fracture — *see* Fracture, ulna, upper end
        open — *see* Wound, open, elbow
        specified NEC S59.80 ☑
        sprain — *see* Sprain, elbow
        superficial — *see* Injury, superficial, elbow
    eleventh cranial nerve (accessory) — *see* Injury,
        nerve, accessory
    epididymis S39.94 ☑
    epigastric region S39.91 ☑
    epiglottis NEC S19.89 ☑
    esophageal plexus — *see* Injury, nerve, thorax,
        sympathetic
    esophagus (thoracic part) (*see also* Injury,
        intrathoracic, esophagus)
        cervical NEC S19.85 ☑
    eustachian tube S09.30 ☑
    eye S05.9 ☑
        avulsion S05.7 ☑
        ball — *see* Injury, eyeball
        conjunctiva S05.0 ☑
        cornea
           abrasion S05.0 ☑
           laceration S05.3 ☑
              with prolapse S05.2 ☑
        lacrimal apparatus S05.8X ☑
        orbit penetration S05.4 ☑
        specified site NEC S05.8X ☑
    eyeball S05.8X ☑
        contusion S05.1 ☑
        penetrating S05.6 ☑
           with
              foreign body S05.5 ☑
              prolapse or loss of intraocular
                 tissue S05.2 ☑
              without prolapse or loss of intraocular
                 tissue S05.3 ☑
        specified type NEC S05.8 ☑
    eyebrow S09.93 ☑
    eyelid S09.93 ☑
        abrasion — *see* Abrasion, eyelid
        contusion — *see* Contusion, eyelid
        open — *see* Wound, open, eyelid
    face S09.93 ☑
    fallopian tube S37.509 ☑
        bilateral S37.502 ☑
           blast injury S37.512 ☑
           contusion S37.522 ☑
           laceration S37.532 ☑
           specified type NEC S37.592 ☑
        blast injury (primary) S37.519 ☑
           bilateral S37.512 ☑
           secondary — *see* Injury, fallopian tube,
              specified type NEC
           unilateral S37.511 ☑
        contusion S37.529 ☑
           bilateral S37.522 ☑
           unilateral S37.521 ☑
        laceration S37.539 ☑
           bilateral S37.532 ☑
           unilateral S37.531 ☑
        specified type NEC S37.599 ☑
           bilateral S37.592 ☑
           unilateral S37.591 ☑

☑ **Additional character required**

Injury — *continued*
  fallopian tube — *continued*
    unilateral S37.501 ☑
      blast injury S37.511 ☑
      contusion S37.521 ☑
      laceration S37.531 ☑
      specified type NEC S37.591 ☑
  fascia — *see* Injury, muscle
  fifth cranial nerve (trigeminal) — *see* Injury, nerve, trigeminal
  finger (nail) S69.9 ☑
    blood vessel — *see* Injury, blood vessel, finger
    contusion — *see* Contusion, finger
    dislocation — *see* Dislocation, finger
    fracture — *see* Fracture, finger
    muscle — *see* Injury, muscle, finger
    nerve — *see* Injury, nerve, digital, finger
    open — *see* Wound, open, finger
    specified NEC S69.8 ☑
    sprain — *see* Sprain, finger
    superficial — *see* Injury, superficial, finger
  first cranial nerve (olfactory) — *see* Injury, nerve, olfactory
  flank — *see* Injury, abdomen
  foot S99.92 ☑
    blood vessel — *see* Injury, blood vessel, foot
    contusion — *see* Contusion, foot
    dislocation — *see* Dislocation, foot
    fracture — *see* Fracture, foot
    muscle — *see* Injury, muscle, foot
    open — *see* Wound, open, foot
    specified type NEC S99.82 ☑
    sprain — *see* Sprain, foot
    superficial — *see* Injury, superficial, foot
  forceps NOS P15.9
  forearm S59.91 ☑
    blood vessel — *see* Injury, blood vessel, forearm
    contusion — *see* Contusion, forearm
    fracture — *see* Fracture, forearm
    muscle — *see* Injury, muscle, forearm
    nerve — *see* Injury, nerve, forearm
    open — *see* Wound, open, forearm
    specified NEC S59.81 ☑
    superficial — *see* Injury, superficial, forearm
  forehead S09.90 ☑
  fourth cranial nerve (trochlear) — *see* Injury, nerve, trochlear
  gallbladder S36.129 ☑
    contusion S36.122 ☑
    laceration S36.123 ☑
    specified NEC S36.128 ☑
  ganglion
    celiac, coeliac — *see* Injury, nerve, lumbosacral, sympathetic
    gasserian — *see* Injury, nerve, trigeminal
    stellate — *see* Injury, nerve, thorax, sympathetic
    thoracic sympathetic — *see* Injury, nerve, thorax, sympathetic
  gasserian ganglion — *see* Injury, nerve, trigeminal
  gastric artery — *see* Injury, blood vessel, celiac artery, branch
  gastroduodenal artery — *see* Injury, blood vessel, celiac artery, branch
  gastrointestinal tract — *see* Injury, intra-abdominal
    with open wound into abdominal cavity — *see* Wound, open, with penetration into peritoneal cavity
    colon — *see* Injury, intestine, large
    rectum — *see* Injury, intestine, large, rectum
      with open wound into abdominal cavity S36.61 ☑
    specified site NEC — *see* Injury, intra-abdominal, specified, site NEC
    stomach — *see* Injury, stomach
    small intestine — *see* Injury, intestine, small
  genital organ (s)
    external S39.94 ☑
      specified NEC S39.848 ☑
    internal S37.90 ☑
      fallopian tube — *see* Injury, fallopian tube
      ovary — *see* Injury, ovary
      prostate — *see* Injury, prostate
      seminal vesicle — *see* Injury, pelvis, organ, specified site NEC
      uterus — *see* Injury, uterus
      vas deferens — *see* Injury, pelvis, organ, specified site NEC
      obstetrical trauma O71.9
  gland
    lacrimal laceration — *see* Injury, eye, specified site NEC

Injury — *continued*
  gland — *continued*
    salivary S09.93 ☑
    thyroid NEC S19.84 ☑
  globe (eye) S05.90 ☑
    specified NEC S05.8X ☑
  groin — *see* Injury, abdomen
  gum S09.90 ☑
  hand S69.9 ☑
    blood vessel — *see* Injury, blood vessel, hand
    contusion — *see* Contusion, hand
    fracture — *see* Fracture, hand
    muscle — *see* Injury, muscle, hand
    nerve — *see* Injury, nerve, hand
    open — *see* Wound, open, hand
    specified NEC S69.8 ☑
    sprain — *see* Sprain, hand
    superficial — *see* Injury, superficial, hand
  head S09.90 ☑
    with loss of consciousness S06.9 ☑
    specified NEC S09.8 ☑
  heart S26.90 ☑
    with hemopericardium S26.00 ☑
      contusion S26.01 ☑
      laceration (mild) S26.020 ☑
        moderate S26.021 ☑
        major S26.022 ☑
      specified type NEC S26.09 ☑
    contusion S26.91 ☑
    laceration S26.92 ☑
    specified type NEC S26.99 ☑
    without hemopericardium S26.10 ☑
      contusion S26.11 ☑
      laceration S26.12 ☑
      specified type NEC S26.19 ☑
  heel — *see* Injury, foot
  hepatic
    artery — *see* Injury, blood vessel, celiac artery, branch
    duct — *see* Injury, liver
    vein — *see* Injury, vena cava, inferior
  hip S79.91 ☑
    blood vessel — *see* Injury, blood vessel, hip
    contusion — *see* Contusion, hip
    dislocation — *see* Dislocation, hip
    fracture — *see* Fracture, femur, neck
    muscle — *see* Injury, muscle, hip
    nerve — *see* Injury, nerve, hip
    open — *see* Wound, open, hip
    sprain — *see* Sprain, hip
    superficial — *see* Injury, superficial, hip
    specified NEC S79.81 ☑
  hymen S39.94 ☑
  hypogastric
    blood vessel — *see* Injury, blood vessel, iliac
    plexus — *see* Injury, nerve, lumbosacral, sympathetic
  ileum — *see* Injury, intestine, small
  iliac region S39.91 ☑
  instrumental (during surgery) — *see* Laceration, accidental complicating surgery
    birth injury — *see* Birth, injury
    nonsurgical — *see* Injury, by site
    obstetrical O71.9
      bladder O71.5
      cervix O71.3
      high vaginal O71.4
      perineal NOS O70.9
      urethra O71.5
      uterus O71.5
        with rupture or perforation O71.1
  internal T14.8 ☑
    aorta — *see* Injury, aorta
    bladder (sphincter) — *see* Injury, bladder
      with
        ectopic or molar pregnancy O08.6
        following ectopic or molar pregnancy O08.6
        obstetrical trauma O71.5
    bronchus, bronchi — *see* Injury, intrathoracic, bronchus
    cecum — *see* Injury, intestine, large
    cervix (uteri) (*see also* Injury, uterus)
      with ectopic or molar pregnancy O08.6
      following ectopic or molar pregnancy O08.6
      obstetrical trauma O71.3
    chest — *see* Injury, intrathoracic
    gastrointestinal tract — *see* Injury, intra-abdominal
    heart — *see* Injury, heart
    intestine NEC — *see* Injury, intestine
    intrauterine — *see* Injury, uterus

Injury — *continued*
  internal — *continued*
    mesentery — *see* Injury, intra-abdominal, specified, site NEC
    pelvis, pelvic (organ) S37.90 ☑
      following ectopic or molar pregnancy (subsequent episode) O08.6
      obstetrical trauma NEC O71.5
        rupture or perforation O71.1
      specified NEC S39.83 ☑
    rectum — *see* Injury, intestine, large, rectum
    stomach — *see* Injury, stomach
    ureter — *see* Injury, ureter
    urethra (sphincter) following ectopic or molar pregnancy O08.6
    uterus — *see* Injury, uterus
  interscapular area — *see* Injury, thorax
  intestine
    large S36.509 ☑
      ascending (right) S36.500 ☑
        blast injury (primary) S36.510 ☑
          secondary S36.590 ☑
        contusion S36.520 ☑
        laceration S36.530 ☑
        specified type NEC S36.590 ☑
      blast injury (primary) S36.519 ☑
        ascending (right) S36.510 ☑
        descending (left) S36.512 ☑
        rectum S36.61 ☑
        sigmoid S36.513 ☑
        specified site NEC S36.518 ☑
        transverse S36.511 ☑
      contusion S36.529 ☑
        ascending (right) S36.520 ☑
        descending (left) S36.522 ☑
        rectum S36.62 ☑
        sigmoid S36.523 ☑
        specified site NEC S36.528 ☑
        transverse S36.521 ☑
      descending (left) S36.502 ☑
        blast injury (primary) S36.512 ☑
          secondary S36.592 ☑
        contusion S36.522 ☑
        laceration S36.532 ☑
        specified type NEC S36.592 ☑
      laceration S36.539 ☑
        ascending (right) S36.530 ☑
        descending (left) S36.532 ☑
        rectum S36.63 ☑
        sigmoid S36.533 ☑
        specified site NEC S36.538 ☑
        transverse S36.531 ☑
      rectum S36.60 ☑
        blast injury (primary) S36.61 ☑
          secondary S36.69 ☑
        contusion S36.62 ☑
        laceration S36.63 ☑
        specified type NEC S36.69 ☑
      sigmoid S36.503 ☑
        blast injury (primary) S36.513 ☑
          secondary S36.593 ☑
        contusion S36.523 ☑
        laceration S36.533 ☑
        specified type NEC S36.593 ☑
      specified
        site NEC S36.508 ☑
          blast injury (primary) S36.518 ☑
            secondary S36.598 ☑
          contusion S36.528 ☑
          laceration S36.538 ☑
          specified type NEC S36.598 ☑
        type NEC S36.599 ☑
          ascending (right) S36.590 ☑
          descending (left) S36.592 ☑
          rectum S36.69 ☑
          sigmoid S36.593 ☑
          specified site NEC S36.598 ☑
          transverse S36.591 ☑
      transverse S36.501 ☑
        blast injury (primary) S36.511 ☑
          secondary S36.591 ☑
        contusion S36.521 ☑
        laceration S36.531 ☑
        specified type NEC S36.591 ☑
    small S36.409 ☑
      blast injury (primary) S36.419 ☑
        duodenum S36.410 ☑
        secondary S36.499 ☑
          duodenum S36.490 ☑
          specified site NEC S36.498 ☑
        specified site NEC S36.418 ☑
      contusion S36.429 ☑

Injury

Injury — *continued*
  intestine — *continued*
    duodenum S36.420 ☑
      specified site NEC S36.428 ☑
    duodenum S36.400 ☑
      blast injury (primary) S36.410 ☑
        secondary S36.490 ☑
      contusion S36.420 ☑
      laceration S36.430 ☑
      specified NEC S36.490 ☑
    laceration S36.439 ☑
      duodenum S36.430 ☑
      specified site NEC S36.438 ☑
    specified
      type NEC S36.499 ☑
        duodenum S36.490 ☑
        specified site NEC S36.498 ☑
      site NEC S36.408 ☑
  intra-abdominal S36.90 ☑
    adrenal gland — *see* Injury, adrenal gland
    bladder — *see* Injury, bladder
    colon — *see* Injury, intestine, large
    contusion S36.92 ☑
    fallopian tube — *see* Injury, fallopian tube
    gallbladder — *see* Injury, gallbladder
    intestine — *see* Injury, intestine
    laceration S36.93 ☑
    liver — *see* Injury, liver
    kidney — *see* Injury, kidney
    ovary — *see* Injury, ovary
    pancreas — *see* Injury, pancreas
    pelvic NOS S37.90 ☑
    peritoneum — *see* Injury, intra-abdominal, specified, site NEC
    prostate — *see* Injury, prostate
    rectum — *see* Injury, intestine, large, rectum
    retroperitoneum — *see* Injury, intra-abdominal, specified, site NEC
    seminal vesicle — *see* Injury, pelvis, organ, specified site NEC
    small intestine — *see* Injury, intestine, small
    specified
      site NEC S36.899 ☑
        contusion S36.892 ☑
        laceration S36.893 ☑
        specified type NEC S36.898 ☑
      type NEC S36.99 ☑
      pelvic S37.90 ☑
        specified
          site NEC S37.899 ☑
            specified type NEC S37.898 ☑
          type NEC S37.99 ☑
    spleen — *see* Injury, spleen
    stomach — *see* Injury, stomach
    ureter — *see* Injury, ureter
    urethra — *see* Injury, urethra
    uterus — *see* Injury, uterus
    vas deferens — *see* Injury, pelvis, organ, specified site NEC
  intracranial (traumatic) S06.9 ☑
    cerebellar hemorrhage, traumatic — *see* Injury, intracranial, focal
    cerebral edema, traumatic S06.1X ☑
      diffuse S06.1X ☑
      focal S06.1X ☑
    diffuse (axonal) S06.2X ☑
    epidural hemorrhage (traumatic) S06.4X ☑
    focal brain injury S06.30 ☑
      contusion — *see* Contusion, cerebral
      laceration — *see* Laceration, cerebral
    intracerebral hemorrhage, traumatic S06.36 ☑
      left side S06.35 ☑
      right side S06.34 ☑
    subarachnoid hemorrhage, traumatic S06.6X ☑
    subdural hemorrhage, traumatic S06.5X ☑
  intraocular — *see* Injury, eyeball, penetrating
  intrathoracic S27.9 ☑
    bronchus S27.409 ☑
      bilateral S27.402 ☑
      blast injury (primary) S27.419 ☑
        bilateral S27.412 ☑
        secondary — *see* Injury, intrathoracic, bronchus, specified type NEC
        unilateral S27.411 ☑
      contusion S27.429 ☑
        bilateral S27.422 ☑
        unilateral S27.421 ☑
      laceration S27.439 ☑
        bilateral S27.432 ☑
        unilateral S27.431 ☑
      specified type NEC S27.499 ☑
        bilateral S27.492 ☑

Injury — *continued*
  intrathoracic — *continued*
      unilateral S27.491 ☑
    unilateral S27.401 ☑
    diaphragm S27.809 ☑
      contusion S27.802 ☑
      laceration S27.803 ☑
      specified type NEC S27.808 ☑
    esophagus (thoracic) S27.819 ☑
      contusion S27.812 ☑
      laceration S27.813 ☑
      specified type NEC S27.818 ☑
    heart — *see* Injury, heart
    hemopneumothorax S27.2 ☑
    hemothorax S27.1 ☑
    lung S27.309 ☑
      aspiration J69.0
      bilateral S27.302 ☑
      blast injury (primary) S27.319 ☑
        bilateral S27.312 ☑
        secondary — *see* Injury, intrathoracic, lung, specified type NEC
        unilateral S27.311 ☑
      contusion S27.329 ☑
        bilateral S27.322 ☑
        unilateral S27.321 ☑
      laceration S27.339 ☑
        bilateral S27.332 ☑
        unilateral S27.331 ☑
      specified type NEC S27.399 ☑
        bilateral S27.392 ☑
        unilateral S27.391 ☑
      unilateral S27.301 ☑
    pleura S27.60 ☑
      laceration S27.63 ☑
      specified type NEC S27.69 ☑
    pneumothorax S27.0 ☑
    specified organ NEC S27.899 ☑
      contusion S27.892 ☑
      laceration S27.893 ☑
      specified type NEC S27.898 ☑
    thoracic duct — *see* Injury, intrathoracic, specified organ NEC
    thymus gland — *see* Injury, intrathoracic, specified organ NEC
    trachea, thoracic S27.50 ☑
      blast (primary) S27.51 ☑
      contusion S27.52 ☑
      laceration S27.53 ☑
      specified type NEC S27.59 ☑
  iris — *see* Injury, eye, specified site NEC
    penetrating — *see* Injury, eyeball, penetrating
  jaw S09.93 ☑
  jejunum — *see* Injury, intestine, small
  joint NOS T14.8 ☑
    old or residual — *see* Disorder, joint, specified type NEC
  kidney S37.00 ☑
    acute (nontraumatic) N17.9
    contusion — *see* Contusion, kidney
    laceration — *see* Laceration, kidney
    specified NEC S37.09 ☑
  knee S89.9 ☑
    contusion — *see* Contusion, knee
    dislocation — *see* Dislocation, knee
    meniscus (lateral) (medial) — *see* Sprain, knee, specified site NEC
      old injury or tear — *see* Derangement, knee, meniscus, due to old injury
    open — *see* Wound, open, knee
    specified NEC S89.8 ☑
    sprain — *see* Sprain, knee
    superficial — *see* Injury, superficial, knee
  labium (majus) (minus) S39.94 ☑
  labyrinth, ear S09.30 ☑
  lacrimal apparatus, duct, gland, or sac — *see* Injury, eye, specified site NEC
  larynx NEC S19.81 ☑
  leg (lower) S89.9 ☑
    blood vessel — *see* Injury, blood vessel, leg
    contusion — *see* Contusion, leg
    fracture — *see* Fracture, leg
    muscle — *see* Injury, muscle, leg
    nerve — *see* Injury, nerve, leg
    open — *see* Wound, open, leg
    specified NEC S89.8 ☑
    superficial — *see* Injury, superficial, leg
  lens, eye — *see* Injury, eye, specified site NEC
    penetrating — *see* Injury, eyeball, penetrating
  limb NEC T14.8 ☑
  lip S09.93 ☑

Injury — *continued*
  liver S36.119 ☑
    contusion S36.112 ☑
    laceration S36.113 ☑
      major (stellate) S36.116 ☑
      minor S36.114 ☑
      moderate S36.115 ☑
      specified NEC S36.118 ☑
  lower back S39.92 ☑
    specified NEC S39.82 ☑
  lumbar, lumbosacral (region) S39.92 ☑
    plexus — *see* Injury, lumbosacral plexus
  lumbosacral plexus S34.4 ☑
  lung (*see also* Injury, intrathoracic, lung)
    aspiration J69.0
    transfusion-related (TRALI) J95.84
  lymphatic thoracic duct — *see* Injury, intrathoracic, specified organ NEC
  malar region S09.93 ☑
  mastoid region S09.90 ☑
  maxilla S09.93 ☑
  mediastinum — *see* Injury, intrathoracic, specified organ NEC
  membrane, brain — *see* Injury, intracranial
  meningeal artery — *see* Injury, intracranial, subdural hemorrhage
  meninges (cerebral) — *see* Injury, intracranial
  mesenteric
    artery
      branch S35.299 ☑
        laceration (minor) (superficial) S35.291 ☑
          major S35.292 ☑
          specified NEC S35.298 ☑
      inferior S35.239 ☑
        laceration (minor) (superficial) S35.231 ☑
          major S35.232 ☑
          specified NEC S35.238 ☑
      superior S35.229 ☑
        laceration (minor) (superficial) S35.221 ☑
          major S35.222 ☑
          specified NEC S35.228 ☑
    plexus (inferior) (superior) — *see* Injury, nerve, lumbosacral, sympathetic
    vein
      inferior S35.349 ☑
        laceration S35.341 ☑
        specified NEC S35.348 ☑
      superior S35.339 ☑
        laceration S35.331 ☑
        specified NEC S35.338 ☑
  mesentery — *see* Injury, intra-abdominal, specified site NEC
  mesosalpinx — *see* Injury, pelvic organ, specified site NEC
  middle ear S09.30 ☑
  midthoracic region NOS S29.9 ☑
  mouth S09.93 ☑
  multiple NOS T07 ☑
  muscle (and fascia) (and tendon)
    abdomen S39.001 ☑
      laceration S39.021 ☑
      specified type NEC S39.091 ☑
      strain S39.011 ☑
    abductor
      thumb, forearm level — *see* Injury, muscle, thumb, abductor
    adductor
      thigh S76.20 ☑
        laceration S76.22 ☑
        specified type NEC S76.29 ☑
        strain S76.21 ☑
    ankle — *see* Injury, muscle, foot
    anterior muscle group, at leg level (lower) S86.20 ☑
      laceration S86.22 ☑
      specified type NEC S86.29 ☑
      strain S86.21 ☑
    arm (upper) — *see* Injury, muscle, shoulder
    biceps (parts NEC) S46.20 ☑
      laceration S46.22 ☑
      long head S46.10 ☑
        laceration S46.12 ☑
        strain S46.11 ☑
        specified type NEC S46.19 ☑
      specified type NEC S46.29 ☑
      strain S46.21 ☑
    extensor
      finger (s) (other than thumb) — *see* Injury, muscle, finger by site, extensor
      forearm level, specified NEC — *see* Injury, muscle, forearm, extensor
      thumb — *see* Injury, muscle, thumb, extensor

☑ **Additional character required**

Injury — *continued*
    muscle — *continued*
        toe (large) (ankle level) (foot level) — *see* Injury, muscle, toe, extensor
        finger
            extensor (forearm level) S56.40 ☑
                hand level S66.309 ☑
                    laceration S66.329 ☑
                    specified type NEC S66.399 ☑
                    strain S66.319 ☑
                laceration S56.429 ☑
                specified type NEC S56.499 ☑
                strain S56.419 ☑
            flexor (forearm level) S56.10 ☑
                hand level S66.109 ☑
                    laceration S66.129 ☑
                    specified type NEC S66.199 ☑
                    strain S66.119 ☑
                laceration S56.129 ☑
                specified type NEC S56.199 ☑
                strain S56.119 ☑
            intrinsic S66.509 ☑
                laceration S66.529 ☑
                specified type NEC S66.599 ☑
                strain S66.519 ☑
        index
            extensor (forearm level)
                hand level S66.308 ☑
                    laceration S66.32 ☑
                    specified type NEC S66.39 ☑
                    strain S66.31 ☑
                specified type NEC S56.492 ☑
            flexor (forearm level)
                hand level S66.108 ☑
                    laceration S66.12 ☑
                    specified type NEC S66.19 ☑
                    strain S66.11 ☑
                specified type NEC S56.19 ☑
                strain S56.11 ☑
            intrinsic S66.50 ☑
                laceration S66.52 ☑
                specified type NEC S66.59 ☑
                strain S66.51 ☑
        little
            extensor (forearm level)
                hand level S66.30 ☑
                    laceration S66.32 ☑
                    specified type NEC S66.39 ☑
                    strain S66.31 ☑
                laceration S56.42 ☑
                specified type NEC S56.49 ☑
                strain S56.41 ☑
            flexor (forearm level)
                hand level S66.10 ☑
                    laceration S66.12 ☑
                    specified type NEC S66.19 ☑
                    strain S66.11 ☑
                laceration S56.12 ☑
                specified type NEC S56.19 ☑
                strain S56.11 ☑
            intrinsic S66.50 ☑
                laceration S66.52 ☑
                specified type NEC S66.59 ☑
                strain S66.51 ☑
        middle
            extensor (forearm level)
                hand level S66.30 ☑
                    laceration S66.32 ☑
                    specified type NEC S66.39 ☑
                    strain S66.31 ☑
                laceration S56.42 ☑
                specified type NEC S56.49 ☑
                strain S56.41 ☑
            flexor (forearm level)
                hand level S66.10 ☑
                    laceration S66.12 ☑
                    specified type NEC S66.19 ☑
                    strain S66.11 ☑
                laceration S56.12 ☑
                specified type NEC S56.19 ☑
                strain S56.11 ☑
            intrinsic S66.50 ☑
                laceration S66.52 ☑
                specified type NEC S66.59 ☑
                strain S66.51 ☑
        ring
            extensor (forearm level)
                hand level S66.30 ☑
                    laceration S66.32 ☑
                    specified type NEC S66.39 ☑
                    strain S66.31 ☑
                laceration S56.42 ☑

Injury — *continued*
    muscle — *continued*
        specified type NEC S56.49 ☑
        strain S56.41 ☑
        flexor (forearm level)
            hand level S66.10 ☑
                laceration S66.12 ☑
                specified type NEC S66.19 ☑
                strain S66.11 ☑
            laceration S56.12 ☑
            specified type NEC S56.19 ☑
            strain S56.11 ☑
        intrinsic S66.50 ☑
            laceration S66.52 ☑
            specified type NEC S66.59 ☑
            strain S66.51 ☑
    flexor
        finger (s) (other than thumb) — *see* Injury, muscle, finger
        forearm level, specified NEC — *see* Injury, muscle, forearm, flexor
        thumb — *see* Injury, muscle, thumb, flexor
        toe (long) (ankle level) (foot level) — *see* Injury, muscle, toe, flexor
    foot S96.90 ☑
        intrinsic S96.20 ☑
            laceration S96.22 ☑
            specified type NEC S96.29 ☑
            strain S96.21 ☑
        laceration S96.92 ☑
        long extensor, toe — *see* Injury, muscle, toe, extensor
        long flexor, toe — *see* Injury, muscle, toe, flexor
        specified
            site NEC S96.80 ☑
                laceration S96.82 ☑
                specified type NEC S96.89 ☑
                strain S96.81 ☑
            type NEC S96.99 ☑
        strain S96.91 ☑
    forearm (level) S56.90 ☑
        extensor S56.50 ☑
            laceration S56.52 ☑
            specified type NEC S56.59 ☑
            strain S56.51 ☑
        flexor S56.20 ☑
            laceration S56.22 ☑
            specified type NEC S56.29 ☑
            strain S56.21 ☑
        laceration S56.92 ☑
        specified S56.99 ☑
            site NEC S56.80 ☑
                laceration S56.82 ☑
                strain S56.81 ☑
                type NEC S56.89 ☑
        strain S56.91 ☑
    hand (level) S66.90 ☑
        laceration S66.92 ☑
        specified
            site NEC S66.80 ☑
                laceration S66.82 ☑
                specified type NEC S66.89 ☑
                strain S66.81 ☑
            type NEC S66.99 ☑
        strain S66.91 ☑
    head S09.10 ☑
        laceration S09.12 ☑
        specified type NEC S09.19 ☑
        strain S09.11 ☑
    hip NEC S76.00 ☑
        laceration S76.02 ☑
        specified type NEC S76.09 ☑
        strain S76.01 ☑
    intrinsic
        ankle and foot level — *see* Injury, muscle, foot, intrinsic
        finger (other than thumb) — *see* Injury, muscle, finger by site, intrinsic
        foot (level) — *see* Injury, muscle, foot, intrinsic
        thumb — *see* Injury, muscle, thumb, intrinsic
    leg (level) (lower) S86.90 ☑
        Achilles tendon — *see* Injury, Achilles tendon
        anterior muscle group — *see* Injury, muscle, anterior muscle group
        laceration S86.92 ☑
        peroneal muscle group — *see* Injury, muscle, peroneal muscle group
        posterior muscle group — *see* Injury, muscle, posterior muscle group, leg level
        specified
            site NEC S86.80 ☑

Injury — *continued*
    muscle — *continued*
        laceration S86.82 ☑
        specified type NEC S86.89 ☑
        type NEC S86.99 ☑
    strain S86.91 ☑
    long
        extensor toe, at ankle and foot level — *see* Injury, muscle, toe, extensor
        flexor, toe, at ankle and foot level — *see* Injury, muscle, toe, flexor
        head, biceps — *see* Injury, muscle, biceps, long head
    lower back S39.002 ☑
        laceration S39.022 ☑
        specified type NEC S39.092 ☑
        strain S39.012 ☑
    neck (level) S16.9 ☑
        laceration S16.2 ☑
        specified type NEC S16.8 ☑
        strain S16.1 ☑
    pelvis S39.003 ☑
        laceration S39.023 ☑
        specified type NEC S39.093 ☑
        strain S39.013 ☑
    peroneal muscle group, at leg level (lower) S86.30 ☑
        laceration S86.32 ☑
        specified type NEC S86.39 ☑
        strain S86.31 ☑
    posterior muscle (group)
        leg level (lower) S86.10 ☑
            laceration S86.12 ☑
            specified type NEC S86.19 ☑
            strain S86.11 ☑
        thigh level S76.30 ☑
            laceration S76.32 ☑
            specified type NEC S76.39 ☑
            strain S76.31 ☑
    quadriceps (thigh) S76.10 ☑
        laceration S76.12 ☑
        specified type NEC S76.19 ☑
        strain S76.11 ☑
    shoulder S46.90 ☑
        laceration S46.92 ☑
        rotator cuff — *see* Injury, rotator cuff
        specified site NEC S46.80 ☑
            laceration S46.82 ☑
            strain S46.81 ☑
            specified type NEC S46.89 ☑
        strain S46.91 ☑
        specified type NEC S46.99 ☑
    thigh NEC (level) S76.90 ☑
        adductor — *see* Injury, muscle, adductor, thigh
        laceration S76.92 ☑
        posterior muscle (group) — *see* Injury, muscle, posterior muscle, thigh level
        quadriceps — *see* Injury, muscle, quadriceps
        specified
            site NEC S76.80 ☑
                laceration S76.82 ☑
                specified type NEC S76.89 ☑
                strain S76.81 ☑
            type NEC S76.99 ☑
        strain S76.91 ☑
    thorax (level) S29.009 ☑
        back wall S29.002 ☑
        front wall S29.001 ☑
        laceration S29.029 ☑
            back wall S29.022 ☑
            front wall S29.021 ☑
        specified type NEC S29.099 ☑
            back wall S29.092 ☑
            front wall S29.091 ☑
        strain S29.019 ☑
            back wall S29.012 ☑
            front wall S29.011 ☑
    thumb
        abductor (forearm level) S56.30 ☑
            laceration S56.32 ☑
            specified type NEC S56.39 ☑
            strain S56.31 ☑
        extensor (forearm level) S56.30 ☑
            hand level S66.20 ☑
                laceration S66.22 ☑
                specified type NEC S66.29 ☑
                strain S66.21 ☑
            laceration S56.32 ☑
            specified type NEC S56.39 ☑
            strain S56.31 ☑

Injury

Injury — *continued*
  muscle — *continued*
    flexor (forearm level) S56.00 ☑
      hand level S66.00 ☑
        laceration S66.02 ☑
        specified type NEC S66.09 ☑
        strain S66.01 ☑
      laceration S56.02 ☑
      specified type NEC S56.09 ☑
      strain S56.01 ☑
      wrist level — *see* Injury, muscle, thumb, flexor, hand level
    intrinsic S66.40 ☑
      laceration S66.42 ☑
      specified type NEC S66.49 ☑
      strain S66.41 ☑
    toe (*see also* Injury, muscle, foot)
      extensor, long S96.10 ☑
        laceration S96.12 ☑
        specified type NEC S96.19 ☑
        strain S96.11 ☑
      flexor, long S96.00 ☑
        laceration S96.02 ☑
        specified type NEC S96.09 ☑
        strain S96.01 ☑
    triceps S46.30 ☑
      laceration S46.32 ☑
      specified type NEC S46.39 ☑
      strain S46.31 ☑
    wrist (and hand) level — *see* Injury, muscle, hand
  musculocutaneous nerve — *see* Injury, nerve, musculocutaneous
  myocardium — *see* Injury, heart
  nape — *see* Injury, neck
  nasal (septum) (sinus) S09.92 ☑
  nasopharynx S09.92 ☑
  neck S19.9 ☑
    specified NEC S19.80 ☑
    specified site NEC S19.89 ☑
  nerve NEC T14.8 ☑
    abdomen S34.9 ☑
      peripheral S34.6 ☑
      specified site NEC S34.8 ☑
    abducens S04.4 ☑
      contusion S04.4 ☑
      laceration S04.4 ☑
      specified type NEC S04.4 ☑
    abducent — *see* Injury, nerve, abducens
    accessory S04.7 ☑
      contusion S04.7 ☑
      laceration S04.7 ☑
      specified type NEC S04.7 ☑
    acoustic S04.6 ☑
      contusion S04.6 ☑
      laceration S04.6 ☑
      specified type NEC S04.6 ☑
    ankle S94.9 ☑
      cutaneous sensory S94.3 ☑
      specified site NEC — *see* subcategory S94.8
    anterior crural, femoral — *see* Injury, nerve, femoral
    arm (upper) S44.9 ☑
      axillary — *see* Injury, nerve, axillary
      cutaneous — *see* Injury, nerve, cutaneous, arm
      median — *see* Injury, nerve, median, upper arm
      musculocutaneous — *see* Injury, nerve, musculocutaneous
      radial — *see* Injury, nerve, radial, upper arm
      specified site NEC — *see* subcategory S44.8
      ulnar — *see* Injury, nerve, ulnar, arm
    auditory — *see* Injury, nerve, acoustic
    axillary S44.3 ☑
    brachial plexus — *see* Injury, brachial plexus
    cervical sympathetic S14.5 ☑
    cranial S04.9 ☑
      contusion S04.9 ☑
      eighth (acoustic or auditory) — *see* Injury, nerve, acoustic
      eleventh (accessory) — *see* Injury, nerve, accessory
      fifth (trigeminal) — *see* Injury, nerve, trigeminal
      first (olfactory) — *see* Injury, nerve, olfactory
      fourth (trochlear) — *see* Injury, nerve, trochlear
      laceration S04.9 ☑
      ninth (glossopharyngeal) — *see* Injury, nerve, glossopharyngeal
      second (optic) — *see* Injury, nerve, optic

Injury — *continued*
  nerve NEC — *continued*
    seventh (facial) — *see* Injury, nerve, facial
    sixth (abducent) — *see* Injury, nerve, abducens
    specified
      nerve NEC S04.89 ☑
        contusion S04.89 ☑
        laceration S04.89 ☑
        specified type NEC S04.89 ☑
      type NEC S04.9 ☑
    tenth (pneumogastric or vagus) — *see* Injury, nerve, vagus
    third (oculomotor) — *see* Injury, nerve, oculomotor
    twelfth (hypoglossal) — *see* Injury, nerve, hypoglossal
    cutaneous sensory
      ankle (level) S94.3 ☑
      arm (upper) (level) S44.5 ☑
      foot (level) — *see* Injury, nerve, cutaneous sensory, ankle
      forearm (level) S54.3 ☑
      hip (level) S74.2 ☑
      leg (lower level) S84.2 ☑
      shoulder (level) — *see* Injury, nerve, cutaneous sensory, arm
      thigh (level) — *see* Injury, nerve, cutaneous sensory, hip
    deep peroneal — *see* Injury, nerve, peroneal, foot
    digital
      finger S64.4 ☑
        index S64.49 ☑
        little S64.49 ☑
        middle S64.49 ☑
        ring S64.49 ☑
      thumb S64.3 ☑
      toe — *see* Injury, nerve, ankle, specified site NEC
    eighth cranial (acoustic or auditory) — *see* Injury, nerve, acoustic
    eleventh cranial (accessory) — *see* Injury, nerve, accessory
    facial S04.5 ☑
      contusion S04.5 ☑
      laceration S04.5 ☑
      newborn P11.3
      specified type NEC S04.5 ☑
    femoral (hip level) (thigh level) S74.1 ☑
    fifth cranial (trigeminal) — *see* Injury, nerve, trigeminal
    finger (digital) — *see* Injury, nerve, digital, finger
    first cranial (olfactory) — *see* Injury, nerve, olfactory
    foot S94.9 ☑
      cutaneous sensory S94.3 ☑
      deep peroneal S94.2 ☑
      lateral plantar S94.0 ☑
      medial plantar S94.1 ☑
      specified site NEC — *see* subcategory S94.8
    forearm (level) S54.9 ☑
      cutaneous sensory — *see* Injury, nerve, cutaneous sensory, forearm
      median — *see* Injury, nerve, median
      radial — *see* Injury, nerve, radial
      specified site NEC — *see* subcategory S54.8
      ulnar — *see* Injury, nerve, ulnar
    fourth cranial (trochlear) — *see* Injury, nerve, trochlear
    glossopharyngeal S04.89 ☑
      specified type NEC S04.89 ☑
    hand S64.9 ☑
      median — *see* Injury, nerve, median, hand
      radial — *see* Injury, nerve, radial, hand
      specified NEC — *see* subcategory S64.8
      ulnar — *see* Injury, nerve, ulnar, hand
    hip (level) S74.9 ☑
      cutaneous sensory — *see* Injury, nerve, cutaneous sensory, hip
      femoral — *see* Injury, nerve, femoral
      sciatic — *see* Injury, nerve, sciatic
      specified site NEC — *see* subcategory S74.8
    hypoglossal S04.89 ☑
      specified type NEC S04.89 ☑
    lateral plantar S94.0 ☑
    leg (lower) S84.9 ☑
      cutaneous sensory — *see* Injury, nerve, cutaneous sensory, leg
      peroneal — *see* Injury, nerve, peroneal
      specified site NEC — *see* subcategory S84.8

Injury — *continued*
  nerve NEC — *continued*
    tibial — *see* Injury, nerve, tibial
    upper — *see* Injury, nerve, thigh
    lower
      back — *see* Injury, nerve, abdomen, specified site NEC
        peripheral — *see* Injury, nerve, abdomen, peripheral
      limb — *see* Injury, nerve, leg
    lumbar spinal — *see* Injury, nerve, spinal, lumbar
    lumbar plexus — *see* Injury, nerve, lumbosacral, sympathetic
    lumbosacral
      plexus — *see* Injury, nerve, lumbosacral, sympathetic
      sympathetic S34.5 ☑
    medial plantar S94.1 ☑
    median (forearm level) S54.1 ☑
      hand (level) S64.1 ☑
      upper arm (level) S44.1 ☑
      wrist (level) — *see* Injury, nerve, median, hand
    musculocutaneous S44.4 ☑
    musculospiral (upper arm level) — *see* Injury, nerve, radial, upper arm
    neck S14.9 ☑
      peripheral S14.4 ☑
      specified site NEC S14.8 ☑
      sympathetic S14.5 ☑
    ninth cranial (glossopharyngeal) — *see* Injury, nerve, glossopharyngeal
    oculomotor S04.1 ☑
      contusion S04.1 ☑
      laceration S04.1 ☑
      specified type NEC S04.1 ☑
    olfactory S04.81 ☑
      specified type NEC S04.81 ☑
    optic S04.01 ☑
      contusion S04.01 ☑
      laceration S04.01 ☑
      specified type NEC S04.01 ☑
    pelvic girdle — *see* Injury, nerve, hip
    pelvis — *see* Injury, nerve, abdomen, specified site NEC
      peripheral — *see* Injury, nerve, abdomen, peripheral
    peripheral NEC T14.8 ☑
      abdomen — *see* Injury, nerve, abdomen, peripheral
      lower back — *see* Injury, nerve, abdomen, peripheral
      neck — *see* Injury, nerve, neck, peripheral
      pelvis — *see* Injury, nerve, abdomen, peripheral
      specified NEC T14.8 ☑
    peroneal (lower leg level) S84.1 ☑
      foot S94.2 ☑
    plexus
      brachial — *see* Injury, brachial plexus
      celiac, coeliac — *see* Injury, nerve, lumbosacral, sympathetic
      mesenteric, inferior — *see* Injury, nerve, lumbosacral, sympathetic
      sacral — *see* Injury, lumbosacral plexus
      spinal
        brachial — *see* Injury, brachial plexus
        lumbosacral — *see* Injury, lumbosacral plexus
    pneumogastric — *see* Injury, nerve, vagus
    radial (forearm level) S54.2 ☑
      hand (level) S64.2 ☑
      upper arm (level) S44.2 ☑
      wrist (level) — *see* Injury, nerve, radial, hand
    root — *see* Injury, nerve, spinal, root
    sacral plexus — *see* Injury, lumbosacral plexus
    sacral spinal — *see* Injury, nerve, spinal, sacral
    sciatic (hip level) (thigh level) S74.0 ☑
    second cranial (optic) — *see* Injury, nerve, optic
    seventh cranial (facial) — *see* Injury, nerve, facial
    shoulder — *see* Injury, nerve, arm
    sixth cranial (abducent) — *see* Injury, nerve, abducens
    spinal
      plexus — *see* Injury, nerve, plexus, spinal
      root
        cervical S14.2 ☑
        dorsal S24.2 ☑
        lumbar S34.21 ☑
        sacral S34.22 ☑

☑ **Additional character required**

ICD-10-CM INDEX TO DISEASES AND INJURIES

Injury

Injury — *continued*
  nerve NEC — *continued*
    thoracic — *see* Injury, nerve, spinal, root, dorsal
    splanchnic — *see* Injury, nerve, lumbosacral, sympathetic
    sympathetic NEC — *see* Injury, nerve, lumbosacral, sympathetic
      cervical — *see* Injury, nerve, cervical sympathetic
    tenth cranial (pneumogastric or vagus) — *see* Injury, nerve, vagus
    thigh (level) — *see* Injury, nerve, hip
      cutaneous sensory — *see* Injury, nerve, cutaneous sensory, hip
      femoral — *see* Injury, nerve, femoral
      sciatic — *see* Injury, nerve, sciatic
      specified NEC — *see* Injury, nerve, hip
    third cranial (oculomotor) — *see* Injury, nerve, oculomotor
    thorax S24.9 ☑
      peripheral S24.3 ☑
      specified site NEC S24.8 ☑
      sympathetic S24.4 ☑
    thumb, digital — *see* Injury, nerve, digital, thumb
    tibial (lower leg level) (posterior) S84.0 ☑
    toe — *see* Injury, nerve, ankle
    trigeminal S04.3 ☑
      contusion S04.3 ☑
      laceration S04.3 ☑
      specified type NEC S04.3 ☑
    trochlear S04.2 ☑
      contusion S04.2 ☑
      laceration S04.2 ☑
      specified type NEC S04.2 ☑
    twelfth cranial (hypoglossal) — *see* Injury, nerve, hypoglossal
    ulnar (forearm level) S54.0 ☑
      arm (upper) (level) S44.0 ☑
      hand (level) S64.0 ☑
      wrist (level) — *see* Injury, nerve, ulnar, hand
    vagus S04.89 ☑
      specified type NEC S04.89 ☑
    wrist (level) — *see* Injury, nerve, hand
    ninth cranial nerve (glossopharyngeal) — *see* Injury, nerve, glossopharyngeal
  nose (septum) S09.92 ☑
  obstetrical O71.9
    specified NEC O71.89
  occipital (region) (scalp) S09.90 ☑
    lobe — *see* Injury, intracranial
  optic chiasm S04.02 ☑
  optic radiation S04.03 ☑
  optic tract and pathways S04.03 ☑
  orbit, orbital (region) — *see* Injury, eye
    penetrating (with foreign body) — *see* Injury, eye, orbit, penetrating
    specified NEC — *see* Injury, eye, specified site NEC
  ovary, ovarian S37.409 ☑
    bilateral S37.402 ☑
      contusion S37.422 ☑
      laceration S37.432 ☑
      specified type NEC S37.492 ☑
    blood vessel — *see* Injury, blood vessel, ovarian
    contusion S37.429 ☑
      bilateral S37.422 ☑
      unilateral S37.421 ☑
    laceration S37.439 ☑
      bilateral S37.432 ☑
      unilateral S37.431 ☑
    specified type NEC S37.499 ☑
      bilateral S37.492 ☑
      unilateral S37.491 ☑
    unilateral S37.401 ☑
      contusion S37.421 ☑
      laceration S37.431 ☑
      specified type NEC S37.491 ☑
  palate (hard) (soft) S09.93 ☑
  pancreas S36.209 ☑
    body S36.201 ☑
      contusion S36.221 ☑
      laceration S36.231 ☑
        major S36.261 ☑
        minor S36.241 ☑
        moderate S36.251 ☑
      specified type NEC S36.291 ☑
    contusion S36.229 ☑
    head S36.200 ☑
      contusion S36.220 ☑
      laceration S36.230 ☑

Injury — *continued*
  pancreas — *continued*
      major S36.260 ☑
      minor S36.240 ☑
      moderate S36.250 ☑
    specified type NEC S36.290 ☑
    laceration S36.239 ☑
      major S36.269 ☑
      minor S36.249 ☑
      moderate S36.259 ☑
    specified type NEC S36.299 ☑
    tail S36.202 ☑
      contusion S36.222 ☑
      laceration S36.232 ☑
        major S36.262 ☑
        minor S36.242 ☑
        moderate S36.252 ☑
      specified type NEC S36.292 ☑
  parietal (region) (scalp) S09.90 ☑
    lobe — *see* Injury, intracranial
  patellar ligament (tendon) S76.10 ☑
    laceration S76.12 ☑
    specified NEC S76.19 ☑
    strain S76.11 ☑
  pelvis, pelvic (floor) S39.93 ☑
    complicating delivery O70.1
    joint or ligament, complicating delivery O71.6
    organ S37.90 ☑
      with ectopic or molar pregnancy O08.6
      complication of abortion — *see* Abortion
      contusion S37.92 ☑
      following ectopic or molar pregnancy O08.6
      laceration S37.93 ☑
      obstetrical trauma NEC O71.5
      specified
        site NEC S37.899 ☑
          contusion S37.892 ☑
          laceration S37.893 ☑
          specified type NEC S37.898 ☑
        type NEC S37.99 ☑
    specified NEC S39.83 ☑
  penis S39.94 ☑
  perineum S39.94 ☑
  peritoneum S36.81 ☑
    laceration S36.893 ☑
  periurethral tissue — *see* Injury, urethra
    complicating delivery O71.82
  phalanges
    foot — *see* Injury, foot
    hand — *see* Injury, hand
  pharynx NEC S19.85 ☑
  pleura — *see* Injury, intrathoracic, pleura
  plexus
    brachial — *see* Injury, brachial plexus
    cardiac — *see* Injury, nerve, thorax, sympathetic
    celiac, coeliac — *see* Injury, nerve, lumbosacral, sympathetic
    esophageal — *see* Injury, nerve, thorax, sympathetic
    hypogastric — *see* Injury, nerve, lumbosacral, sympathetic
    lumbar, lumbosacral — *see* Injury, lumbosacral plexus
    mesenteric — *see* Injury, nerve, lumbosacral, sympathetic
    pulmonary — *see* Injury, nerve, thorax, sympathetic
  postcardiac surgery (syndrome) I97.0
  prepuce S39.94 ☑
  prostate S37.829 ☑
    contusion S37.822 ☑
    laceration S37.823 ☑
    specified type NEC S37.828 ☑
  pubic region S39.94 ☑
  pudendum S39.94 ☑
  pulmonary plexus — *see* Injury, nerve, thorax, sympathetic
  rectovaginal septum NEC S39.83 ☑
  rectum — *see* Injury, intestine, large, rectum
  retina — *see* Injury, eye, specified site NEC
    penetrating — *see* Injury, eyeball, penetrating
  retroperitoneal — *see* Injury, intra-abdominal, specified site NEC
  rotator cuff (muscle (s)) (tendon (s)) S46.00 ☑
    laceration S46.02 ☑
    specified type NEC S46.09 ☑
    strain S46.01 ☑
  round ligament — *see* Injury, pelvic organ, specified site NEC
  sacral plexus — *see* Injury, lumbosacral plexus
  salivary duct or gland S09.93 ☑

Injury — *continued*
  scalp S09.90 ☑
    newborn (birth injury) P12.9
      due to monitoring (electrode) (sampling incision) P12.4
      specified NEC P12.89
        caput succedaneum P12.81
  scapular region — *see* Injury, shoulder
  sclera — *see* Injury, eye, specified site NEC
    penetrating — *see* Injury, eyeball, penetrating
  scrotum S39.94 ☑
  second cranial nerve (optic) — *see* Injury, nerve, optic
  seminal vesicle — *see* Injury, pelvic organ, specified site NEC
  seventh cranial nerve (facial) — *see* Injury, nerve, facial
  shoulder S49.9 ☑
    blood vessel — *see* Injury, blood vessel, arm
    contusion — *see* Contusion, shoulder
    dislocation — *see* Dislocation, shoulder
    fracture — *see* Fracture, shoulder
    muscle — *see* Injury, muscle, shoulder
    nerve — *see* Injury, nerve, shoulder
    open — *see* Wound, open, shoulder
    specified type NEC S49.8 ☑
    sprain — *see* Sprain, shoulder girdle
    superficial — *see* Injury, superficial, shoulder
  sinus
    cavernous — *see* Injury, intracranial
    nasal S09.92 ☑
  sixth cranial nerve (abducent) — *see* Injury, nerve, abducens
  skeleton, birth injury P13.9
    specified part NEC P13.8
  skin NEC T14.8 ☑
    surface intact — *see* Injury, superficial
  skull NEC S09.90 ☑
  specified NEC T14.8 ☑
  spermatic cord (pelvic region) S37.898 ☑
    scrotal region S39.848 ☑
  spinal (cord)
    cervical (neck) S14.109 ☑
      anterior cord syndrome S14.139 ☑
        C1 level S14.131 ☑
        C2 level S14.132 ☑
        C3 level S14.133 ☑
        C4 level S14.134 ☑
        C5 level S14.135 ☑
        C6 level S14.136 ☑
        C7 level S14.137 ☑
        C8 level S14.138 ☑
      Brown-Séquard syndrome S14.149 ☑
        C1 level S14.141 ☑
        C2 level S14.142 ☑
        C3 level S14.143 ☑
        C4 level S14.144 ☑
        C5 level S14.145 ☑
        C6 level S14.146 ☑
        C7 level S14.147 ☑
        C8 level S14.148 ☑
      C1 level S14.101 ☑
      C2 level S14.102 ☑
      C3 level S14.103 ☑
      C4 level S14.104 ☑
      C5 level S14.105 ☑
      C6 level S14.106 ☑
      C7 level S14.107 ☑
      C8 level S14.108 ☑
      central cord syndrome S14.129 ☑
        C1 level S14.121 ☑
        C2 level S14.122 ☑
        C3 level S14.123 ☑
        C4 level S14.124 ☑
        C5 level S14.125 ☑
        C6 level S14.126 ☑
        C7 level S14.127 ☑
        C8 level S14.128 ☑
      complete lesion S14.119 ☑
        C1 level S14.111 ☑
        C2 level S14.112 ☑
        C3 level S14.113 ☑
        C4 level S14.114 ☑
        C5 level S14.115 ☑
        C6 level S14.116 ☑
        C7 level S14.117 ☑
        C8 level S14.118 ☑
      concussion S14.0 ☑
      edema S14.0 ☑
      incomplete lesion specified NEC S14.159 ☑
        C1 level S14.151 ☑
        C2 level S14.152 ☑

Injury

Injury — *continued*
  spinal — *continued*
    C3 level S14.153 ☑
    C4 level S14.154 ☑
    C5 level S14.155 ☑
    C6 level S14.156 ☑
    C7 level S14.157 ☑
    C8 level S14.158 ☑
    posterior cord syndrome S14.159 ☑
    C1 level S14.151 ☑
    C2 level S14.152 ☑
    C3 level S14.153 ☑
    C4 level S14.154 ☑
    C5 level S14.155 ☑
    C6 level S14.156 ☑
    C7 level S14.157 ☑
    C8 level S14.158 ☑
   dorsal — *see* Injury, spinal, thoracic
   lumbar S34.109 ☑
    complete lesion S34.119 ☑
     L1 level S34.111 ☑
     L2 level S34.112 ☑
     L3 level S34.113 ☑
     L4 level S34.114 ☑
     L5 level S34.115 ☑
    concussion S34.01 ☑
    edema S34.01 ☑
    incomplete lesion S34.129 ☑
     L1 level S34.121 ☑
     L2 level S34.122 ☑
     L3 level S34.123 ☑
     L4 level S34.124 ☑
     L5 level S34.125 ☑
    L1 level S34.101 ☑
    L2 level S34.102 ☑
    L3 level S34.103 ☑
    L4 level S34.104 ☑
    L5 level S34.105 ☑
   nerve root NEC
    cervical — *see* Injury, nerve, spinal, root, cervical
    dorsal — *see* Injury, nerve, spinal, root, dorsal
    lumbar S34.21 ☑
    sacral S34.22 ☑
    thoracic — *see* Injury, nerve, spinal, root, dorsal
   plexus
    brachial — *see* Injury, brachial plexus
    lumbosacral — *see* Injury, lumbosacral plexus
   sacral S34.139 ☑
    complete lesion S34.131 ☑
    incomplete lesion S34.132 ☑
   thoracic S24.109 ☑
    anterior cord syndrome S24.139 ☑
     T1 level S24.131 ☑
     T2-T6 level S24.132 ☑
     T7-T10 level S24.133 ☑
     T11-T12 level S24.134 ☑
    Brown-Séquard syndrome S24.149 ☑
     T1 level S24.141 ☑
     T2-T6 level S24.142 ☑
     T7-T10 level S24.143 ☑
     T11-T12 level S24.144 ☑
    complete lesion S24.119 ☑
     T1 level S24.111 ☑
     T2-T6 level S24.112 ☑
     T7-T10 level S24.113 ☑
     T11-T12 level S24.114 ☑
    concussion S24.0 ☑
    edema S24.0 ☑
    incomplete lesion specified NEC S24.159 ☑
     T1 level S24.151 ☑
     T2-T6 level S24.152 ☑
     T7-T10 level S24.153 ☑
     T11-T12 level S24.154 ☑
    posterior cord syndrome S24.159 ☑
     T1 level S24.151 ☑
     T2-T6 level S24.152 ☑
     T7-T10 level S24.153 ☑
     T11-T12 level S24.154 ☑
    T1 level S24.101 ☑
    T2-T6 level S24.102 ☑
    T7-T10 level S24.103 ☑
    T11-T12 level S24.104 ☑
  splanchnic nerve — *see* Injury, nerve, lumbosacral, sympathetic
  spleen S36.00 ☑
   contusion S36.029 ☑
    major S36.021 ☑
    minor S36.020 ☑
   laceration S36.039 ☑
    major (massive) (stellate) S36.032 ☑

Injury — *continued*
  spleen — *continued*
    moderate S36.031 ☑
    superficial (capsular) (minor) S36.030 ☑
   specified type NEC S36.09 ☑
  splenic artery — *see* Injury, blood vessel, celiac artery, branch
  stellate ganglion — *see* Injury, nerve, thorax, sympathetic
  sternal region S29.9 ☑
  stomach S36.30 ☑
   contusion S36.32 ☑
   laceration S36.33 ☑
   specified type NEC S36.39 ☑
  subconjunctival — *see* Injury, eye, conjunctiva
  subcutaneous NEC T14.8 ☑
  submaxillary region S09.93 ☑
  submental region S09.93 ☑
  subungual
   fingers — *see* Injury, hand
   toes — *see* Injury, foot
  superficial NEC T14.8 ☑
   abdomen, abdominal (wall) S30.92 ☑
    abrasion S30.811 ☑
    bite S30.871 ☑
     insect S30.861 ☑
    contusion S30.1 ☑
    external constriction S30.841 ☑
    foreign body S30.851 ☑
   abrasion — *see* Abrasion, by site
   adnexa, eye NEC — *see* Injury, eye, specified site NEC
   alveolar process — *see* Injury, superficial, oral cavity
   ankle S90.91 ☑
    abrasion — *see* Abrasion, ankle
    blister — *see* Blister, ankle
    bite — *see* Bite, ankle
    contusion — *see* Contusion, ankle
    external constriction — *see* Constriction, external, ankle
    foreign body — *see* Foreign body, superficial, ankle
   anus S30.98 ☑
   arm (upper) S40.92 ☑
    abrasion — *see* Abrasion, arm
    bite — *see* Bite, superficial, arm
    blister — *see* Blister, arm (upper)
    contusion — *see* Contusion, arm
    external constriction — *see* Constriction, external, arm
    foreign body — *see* Foreign body, superficial, arm
   auditory canal (external) (meatus) — *see* Injury, superficial, ear
   auricle — *see* Injury, superficial, ear
   axilla — *see* Injury, superficial, arm
   back (*see also* Injury, superficial, thorax, back)
    lower S30.91 ☑
     abrasion S30.810 ☑
     contusion S30.0 ☑
     external constriction S30.840 ☑
     superficial
      bite NEC S30.870 ☑
       insect S30.860 ☑
      foreign body S30.850 ☑
   bite NEC — *see* Bite, superficial NEC, by site
   blister — *see* Blister, by site
   breast S20.10 ☑
    abrasion — *see* Abrasion, breast
    bite — *see* Bite, superficial, breast
    contusion — *see* Contusion, breast
    external constriction — *see* Constriction, external, breast
    foreign body — *see* Foreign body, superficial, breast
   brow — *see* Injury, superficial, head, specified NEC
   buttock S30.91 ☑
   calf — *see* Injury, superficial, leg
   canthus, eye — *see* Injury, superficial, periocular area
   cheek (external) — *see* Injury, superficial, head, specified NEC
    internal — *see* Injury, superficial, oral cavity
   chest wall — *see* Injury, superficial, thorax
   chin — *see* Injury, superficial, head NEC
   clitoris S30.95 ☑
   conjunctiva — *see* Injury, eye, conjunctiva
    with foreign body (in conjunctival sac) — *see* Foreign body, conjunctival sac
   contusion — *see* Contusion, by site

Injury — *continued*
  superficial NEC — *continued*
   costal region — *see* Injury, superficial, thorax
   digit (s)
    hand — *see* Injury, superficial, finger
   ear (auricle) (canal) (external) S00.40 ☑
    abrasion — *see* Abrasion, ear
    bite — *see* Bite, superficial, ear
    contusion — *see* Contusion, ear
    external constriction — *see* Constriction, external, ear
    foreign body — *see* Foreign body, superficial, ear
   elbow S50.90 ☑
    abrasion — *see* Abrasion, elbow
    bite — *see* Bite, superficial, elbow
    blister — *see* Blister, elbow
    contusion — *see* Contusion, elbow
    external constriction — *see* Constriction, external, elbow
    foreign body — *see* Foreign body, superficial, elbow
   epididymis S30.94 ☑
   epigastric region S30.92 ☑
   epiglottis — *see* Injury, superficial, throat
   esophagus
    cervical — *see* Injury, superficial, throat
   external constriction — *see* Constriction, external, by site
   extremity NEC T14.8 ☑
   eyeball NEC — *see* Injury, eye, specified site NEC
   eyebrow — *see* Injury, superficial, periocular area
   eyelid S00.20 ☑
    abrasion — *see* Abrasion, eyelid
    bite — *see* Bite, superficial, eyelid
    contusion — *see* Contusion, eyelid
    external constriction — *see* Constriction, external, eyelid
    foreign body — *see* Foreign body, superficial, eyelid
   face NEC — *see* Injury, superficial, head, specified NEC
   finger (s) S60.949 ☑
    abrasion — *see* Abrasion, finger
    bite — *see* Bite, superficial, finger
    blister — *see* Blister, finger
    contusion — *see* Contusion, finger
    external constriction — *see* Constriction, external, finger
    foreign body — *see* Foreign body, superficial, finger
    insect bite — *see* Bite, by site, superficial, insect
    index S60.94 ☑
    little S60.94 ☑
    middle S60.94 ☑
    ring S60.94 ☑
   flank S30.92 ☑
   foot S90.92 ☑
    abrasion — *see* Abrasion, foot
    bite — *see* Bite, foot
    blister — *see* Blister, foot
    contusion — *see* Contusion, foot
    external constriction — *see* Constriction, external, foot
    foreign body — *see* Foreign body, superficial, foot
   forearm S50.91 ☑
    abrasion — *see* Abrasion, forearm
    bite — *see* Bite, forearm, superficial
    blister — *see* Blister, forearm
    contusion — *see* Contusion, forearm
    elbow only — *see* Injury, superficial, elbow
    external constriction — *see* Constriction, external, forearm
    foreign body — *see* Foreign body, superficial, forearm
   forehead — *see* Injury, superficial, head NEC
   foreign body — *see* Foreign body, superficial
   genital organs, external
    female S30.97 ☑
    male S30.96 ☑
   globe (eye) — *see* Injury, eye, specified site NEC
   groin S30.92 ☑
   gum — *see* Injury, superficial, oral cavity
   hand S60.92 ☑
    abrasion — *see* Abrasion, hand
    bite — *see* Bite, superficial, hand
    contusion — *see* Contusion, hand

☑ **Additional character required**

Injury — continued
  superficial NEC — continued
    external constriction — see Constriction, external, hand
    foreign body — see Foreign body, superficial, hand
    head S00.90 ☑
      ear — see Injury, superficial, ear
      eyelid — see Injury, superficial, eyelid
      nose S00.30 ☑
      oral cavity S00.502 ☑
      scalp S00.00 ☑
      specified site NEC S00.80 ☑
    heel — see Injury, superficial, foot
    hip S70.91 ☑
      abrasion — see Abrasion, hip
      bite — see Bite, superficial, hip
      blister — see Blister, hip
      contusion — see Contusion, hip
      external constriction — see Constriction, external, hip
      foreign body — see Foreign body, superficial, hip
    iliac region — see Injury, superficial, abdomen
    inguinal region — see Injury, superficial, abdomen
    insect bite — see Bite, by site, superficial, insect
    interscapular region — see Injury, superficial, thorax, back
    jaw — see Injury, superficial, head, specified NEC
    knee S80.91 ☑
      abrasion — see Abrasion, knee
      bite — see Bite, superficial, knee
      blister — see Blister, knee
      contusion — see Contusion, knee
      external constriction — see Constriction, external, knee
      foreign body — see Foreign body, superficial, knee
    labium (majus) (minus) S30.95 ☑
    lacrimal (apparatus) (gland) (sac) — see Injury, eye, specified site NEC
    larynx — see Injury, superficial, throat
    leg (lower) S80.92 ☑
      abrasion — see Abrasion, leg
      bite — see Bite, superficial, leg
      contusion — see Contusion, leg
      external constriction — see Constriction, external, leg
      foreign body — see Foreign body, superficial, leg
      knee — see Injury, superficial, knee
    limb NEC T14.8 ☑
    lip S00.501 ☑
    lower back S30.91 ☑
    lumbar region S30.91 ☑
    malar region — see Injury, superficial, head, specified NEC
    mammary — see Injury, superficial, breast
    mastoid region — see Injury, superficial, head, specified NEC
    mouth — see Injury, superficial, oral cavity
    muscle NEC T14.8 ☑
    nail NEC T14.8 ☑
      finger — see Injury, superficial, finger
      toe — see Injury, superficial, toe
    nasal (septum) — see Injury, superficial, nose
    neck S10.90 ☑
      specified site NEC S10.80 ☑
    nose (septum) S00.30 ☑
    occipital region — see Injury, superficial, scalp
    oral cavity S00.502 ☑
    orbital region — see Injury, superficial, periocular area
    palate — see Injury, superficial, oral cavity
    palm — see Injury, superficial, hand
    parietal region — see Injury, superficial, scalp
    pelvis S30.91 ☑
      girdle — see Injury, superficial, hip
    penis S30.93 ☑
    perineum
      female S30.95 ☑
      male S30.91 ☑
    periocular area S00.20 ☑
      abrasion — see Abrasion, eyelid
      bite — see Bite, superficial, eyelid
      contusion — see Contusion, eyelid
      external constriction — see Constriction, external, eyelid
      foreign body — see Foreign body, superficial, eyelid

Injury — continued
  superficial NEC — continued
    phalanges
      finger — see Injury, superficial, finger
      toe — see Injury, superficial, toe
    pharynx — see Injury, superficial, throat
    pinna — see Injury, superficial, ear
    popliteal space — see Injury, superficial, knee
    prepuce S30.93 ☑
    pubic region S30.91 ☑
    pudendum
      female S30.97 ☑
      male S30.96 ☑
    sacral region S30.91 ☑
    scalp S00.00 ☑
    scapular region — see Injury, superficial, shoulder
    sclera — see Injury, eye, specified site NEC
    scrotum S30.94 ☑
    shin — see Injury, superficial, leg
    shoulder S40.91 ☑
      abrasion — see Abrasion, shoulder
      bite — see Bite, superficial, shoulder
      blister — see Blister, shoulder
      contusion — see Contusion, shoulder
      external constriction — see Constriction, external, shoulder
      foreign body — see Foreign body, superficial, shoulder
    skin NEC T14.8 ☑
    sternal region — see Injury, superficial, thorax, front
    subconjunctival — see Injury, eye, specified site NEC
    subcutaneous NEC T14.8 ☑
    submaxillary region — see Injury, superficial, head, specified NEC
    submental region — see Injury, superficial, head, specified NEC
    subungual
      finger (s) — see Injury, superficial, finger
      toe (s) — see Injury, superficial, toe
    supraclavicular fossa — see Injury, superficial, neck
    supraorbital — see Injury, superficial, head, specified NEC
    temple — see Injury, superficial, head, specified NEC
    temporal region — see Injury, superficial, head, specified NEC
    testis S30.94 ☑
    thigh S70.92 ☑
      abrasion — see Abrasion, thigh
      bite — see Bite, superficial, thigh
      blister — see Blister, thigh
      contusion — see Contusion, thigh
      external constriction — see Constriction, external, thigh
      foreign body — see Foreign body, superficial, thigh
    thorax, thoracic (wall) S20.90 ☑
      abrasion — see Abrasion, thorax
      back S20.40 ☑
      bite — see Bite, thorax, superficial
      blister — see Blister, thorax
      contusion — see Contusion, thorax
      external constriction — see Constriction, external, thorax
      foreign body — see Foreign body, superficial, thorax
      front S20.30 ☑
    throat S10.10 ☑
      abrasion S10.11 ☑
      bite S10.17 ☑
        insect S10.16 ☑
      blister S10.12 ☑
      contusion S10.0 ☑
      external constriction S10.14 ☑
      foreign body S10.15 ☑
    thumb S60.93 ☑
      abrasion — see Abrasion, thumb
      bite — see Bite, superficial, thumb
      blister — see Blister, thumb
      contusion — see Contusion, thumb
      external constriction — see Constriction, external, thumb
      foreign body — see Foreign body, superficial, thumb
      insect bite — see Bite, by site, superficial, insect
      specified type NEC S60.39 ☑
    toe (s) S90.93 ☑

Injury — continued
  superficial NEC — continued
    abrasion — see Abrasion, toe
    bite — see Bite, toe
    blister — see Blister, toe
    contusion — see Contusion, toe
    external constriction — see Constriction, external, toe
    foreign body — see Foreign body, superficial, toe
    great S90.93 ☑
    tongue — see Injury, superficial, oral cavity
    tooth, teeth — see Injury, superficial, oral cavity
    trachea S10.10 ☑
    tunica vaginalis S30.94 ☑
    tympanum, tympanic membrane — see Injury, superficial, ear
    uvula — see Injury, superficial, oral cavity
    vagina S30.95 ☑
    vocal cords — see Injury, superficial, throat
    vulva S30.95 ☑
    wrist S60.91 ☑
  supraclavicular region — see Injury, neck
  supraorbital S09.93 ☑
  suprarenal gland (multiple) — see Injury, adrenal
  surgical complication (external or internal site) — see Laceration, accidental complicating surgery
  temple S09.90 ☑
  temporal region S09.90 ☑
  tendon (see also Injury, muscle, by site)
    abdomen — see Injury, muscle, abdomen
    Achilles — see Injury, Achilles tendon
    lower back — see Injury, muscle, lower back
    pelvic organs — see Injury, muscle, pelvis
  tenth cranial nerve (pneumogastric or vagus) — see Injury, nerve, vagus
  testis S39.94 ☑
  thigh S79.92 ☑
    blood vessel — see Injury, blood vessel, hip
    contusion — see Contusion, thigh
    fracture — see Fracture, femur
    muscle — see Injury, muscle, thigh
    nerve — see Injury, nerve, thigh
    open — see Wound, open, thigh
    specified NEC S79.82 ☑
    superficial — see Injury, superficial, thigh
  third cranial nerve (oculomotor) — see Injury, nerve, oculomotor
  thorax, thoracic S29.9 ☑
    blood vessel — see Injury, blood vessel, thorax
    cavity — see Injury, intrathoracic
    dislocation — see Dislocation, thorax
    external (wall) S29.9 ☑
      contusion — see Contusion, thorax
      nerve — see Injury, nerve, thorax
      open — see Wound, open, thorax
      specified NEC S29.8 ☑
      sprain — see Sprain, thorax
      superficial — see Injury, superficial, thorax
    fracture — see Fracture, thorax
    internal — see Injury, intrathoracic
    intrathoracic organ — see Injury, intrathoracic
    sympathetic ganglion — see Injury, nerve, thorax, sympathetic
  throat (see also Injury, neck) S19.9 ☑
  thumb S69.9 ☑
    blood vessel — see Injury, blood vessel, thumb
    contusion — see Contusion, thumb
    dislocation — see Dislocation, thumb
    fracture — see Fracture, thumb
    muscle — see Injury, muscle, thumb
    nerve — see Injury, nerve, digital, thumb
    open — see Wound, open, thumb
    specified NEC S69.8 ☑
    sprain — see Sprain, thumb
    superficial — see Injury, superficial, thumb
  thymus (gland) — see Injury, intrathoracic, specified organ NEC
  thyroid (gland) NEC S19.84 ☑
  toe S99.92 ☑
    contusion — see Contusion, toe
    dislocation — see Dislocation, toe
    fracture — see Fracture, toe
    muscle — see Injury, muscle, toe
    open — see Wound, open, toe
    specified type NEC S99.82 ☑
    sprain — see Sprain, toe
    superficial — see Injury, superficial, toe
  tongue S09.93 ☑
  tonsil S09.93 ☑
  tooth S09.93 ☑

Injury - Insufficiency

Injury — *continued*
- trachea (cervical) NEC S19.82 ☑
  - thoracic — *see* Injury, intrathoracic, trachea, thoracic
- transfusion-related acute lung (TRALI) J95.84
- tunica vaginalis S39.94 ☑
- twelfth cranial nerve (hypoglossal) — *see* Injury, nerve, hypoglossal
- ureter S37.10 ☑
  - contusion S37.12 ☑
  - laceration S37.13 ☑
  - specified type NEC S37.19 ☑
- urethra (sphincter) S37.30 ☑
  - at delivery O71.5
  - contusion S37.32 ☑
  - laceration S37.33 ☑
  - specified type NEC S37.39 ☑
- urinary organ S37.90 ☑
  - contusion S37.92 ☑
  - laceration S37.93 ☑
  - specified
    - site NEC S37.899 ☑
      - contusion S37.892 ☑
      - laceration S37.893 ☑
      - specified type NEC S37.898 ☑
    - type NEC S37.99 ☑
- uterus, uterine S37.60 ☑
  - with ectopic or molar pregnancy O08.6
  - blood vessel — *see* Injury, blood vessel, iliac
  - contusion S37.62 ☑
  - laceration S37.63 ☑
    - cervix at delivery O71.3
  - rupture associated with obstetrics — *see* Rupture, uterus
  - specified type NEC S37.69 ☑
- uvula S09.93 ☑
- vagina S39.93 ☑
  - abrasion S30.814 ☑
  - bite S31.45 ☑
    - insect S30.864 ☑
    - superficial NEC S30.874 ☑
  - contusion S30.23 ☑
  - crush S38.03 ☑
  - during delivery — *see* Laceration, vagina, during delivery
  - external constriction S30.844 ☑
  - insect bite S30.864 ☑
  - laceration S31.41 ☑
    - with foreign body S31.42 ☑
  - open wound S31.40 ☑
  - puncture S31.43 ☑
    - with foreign body S31.44 ☑
  - superficial S30.95 ☑
    - foreign body S30.854 ☑
- vas deferens — *see* Injury, pelvic organ, specified site NEC
- vascular NEC T14.8 ☑
- vein — *see* Injury, blood vessel
- vena cava (superior) S25.20 ☑
  - inferior S35.10 ☑
    - laceration (minor) (superficial) S35.11 ☑
      - major S35.12 ☑
    - specified type NEC S35.19 ☑
  - laceration (minor) (superficial) S25.21 ☑
    - major S25.22 ☑
  - specified type NEC S25.29 ☑
- vesical (sphincter) — *see* Injury, bladder
- visual cortex S04.04 ☑
- vitreous (humor) S05.90 ☑
  - specified NEC S05.8X ☑
- vocal cord NEC S19.83 ☑
- vulva S39.94 ☑
  - abrasion S30.814 ☑
  - bite S31.45 ☑
    - insect S30.864 ☑
    - superficial NEC S30.874 ☑
  - contusion S30.23 ☑
  - crush S38.03 ☑
  - during delivery — *see* Laceration, perineum, female, during delivery
  - external constriction S30.844 ☑
  - insect bite S30.864 ☑
  - laceration S31.41 ☑
    - with foreign body S31.42 ☑
  - open wound S31.40 ☑
  - puncture S31.43 ☑
    - with foreign body S31.44 ☑
  - superficial S30.95 ☑
    - foreign body S30.854 ☑
- whiplash (cervical spine) S13.4 ☑
- wrist S69.9 ☑
  - blood vessel — *see* Injury, blood vessel, hand

Injury — *continued*
- wrist — *continued*
  - contusion — *see* Contusion, wrist
  - dislocation — *see* Dislocation, wrist
  - fracture — *see* Fracture, wrist
  - muscle — *see* Injury, muscle, hand
  - nerve — *see* Injury, nerve, hand
  - open — *see* Wound, open, wrist
  - specified NEC S69.8 ☑
  - sprain — *see* Sprain, wrist
  - superficial — *see* Injury, superficial, wrist
Inoculation (*see also* Vaccination)
- complication or reaction — *see* Complications, vaccination
Insanity, insane (*see also* Psychosis)
- adolescent — *see* Schizophrenia
- confusional F28
  - acute or subacute F05
- delusional F22
- senile F03 ☑
Insect
- bite — *see* Bite, by site, superficial, insect
- venomous, poisoning NEC (by) — *see* Venom, arthropod
Insensitivity
- adrenocorticotropin hormone (ACTH) E27.49
- androgen E34.50
  - complete E34.51
  - partial E34.52
Insertion
- cord (umbilical) lateral or velamentous O43.12 ☑
- intrauterine contraceptive device (encounter for) — *see* Intrauterine contraceptive device
Insolation (sunstroke) T67.0 ☑
Insomnia (organic) G47.00
- adjustment F51.02
- adjustment disorder F51.02
- behavioral, of childhood Z73.819
  - combined type Z73.812
  - limit setting type Z73.811
  - sleep-onset association type Z73.810
- childhood Z73.819
- chronic F51.04
  - somatized tension F51.04
- conditioned F51.04
- due to
  - alcohol
    - abuse F10.182
    - dependence F10.282
    - use F10.982
  - amphetamines
    - abuse F15.182
    - dependence F15.282
    - use F15.982
  - anxiety disorder F51.05
  - caffeine
    - abuse F15.182
    - dependence F15.282
    - use F15.982
  - cocaine
    - abuse F14.182
    - dependence F14.282
    - use F14.982
  - depression F51.05
  - drug NEC
    - abuse F19.182
    - dependence F19.282
    - use F19.982
  - medical condition G47.01
  - mental disorder NEC F51.05
  - opioid
    - abuse F11.182
    - dependence F11.282
    - use F11.982
  - psychoactive substance NEC
    - abuse F19.182
    - dependence F19.282
    - use F19.982
  - sedative, hypnotic, or anxiolytic
    - abuse F13.182
    - dependence F13.282
    - use F13.982
  - stimulant NEC
    - abuse F15.182
    - dependence F15.282
    - use F15.982
- fatal familial (FFI) A81.83
- idiopathic F51.01
- learned F51.3
- nonorganic origin F51.01
- not due to a substance or known physiological condition F51.01
- specified NEC F51.09

Insomnia — *continued*
- paradoxical F51.03
- primary F51.01
- psychiatric F51.05
- psychophysiologic F51.04
- related to psychopathology F51.05
- short-term F51.02
- specified NEC G47.09
- stress-related F51.02
- transient F51.02
- without objective findings F51.02
Inspiration
- food or foreign body — *see* Foreign body, by site
- mucus — *see* Asphyxia, mucus
Inspissated bile syndrome (newborn) P59.1
Instability
- emotional (excessive) F60.3
- joint (post-traumatic) M25.30
  - ankle M25.37 ☑
  - due to old ligament injury — *see* Disorder, ligament
  - elbow M25.32 ☑
  - flail — *see* Flail, joint
  - foot M25.37 ☑
  - hand M25.34 ☑
  - hip M25.35 ☑
  - knee M25.36 ☑
  - lumbosacral — *see* subcategory M53.2
  - prosthesis — *see* Complications, joint prosthesis, mechanical, displacement, by site
  - sacroiliac — *see* subcategory M53.2
  - secondary to
    - old ligament injury — *see* Disorder, ligament
    - removal of joint prosthesis M96.89
  - shoulder (region) M25.31 ☑
  - spine — *see* subcategory M53.2
  - wrist M25.33 ☑
- knee (chronic) M23.5 ☑
- lumbosacral — *see* subcategory M53.2
- nervous F48.8
- personality (emotional) F60.3
- spine — *see* Instability, joint, spine
- vasomotor R55
Institutional syndrome (childhood) F94.2
Institutionalization, affecting child Z62.22
- disinhibited attachment F94.2
Insufficiency, insufficient
- accommodation, old age H52.4
- adrenal (gland) E27.40
  - primary E27.1
- adrenocortical E27.40
  - drug-induced E27.3
  - iatrogenic E27.3
  - primary E27.1
- anatomic crown height K08.89
- anterior (occlusal) guidance M26.54
- anus K62.89
- aortic (valve) I35.1
  - with
    - mitral (valve) disease I08.0
      - with tricuspid (valve) disease I08.3
    - stenosis I35.2
    - tricuspid (valve) disease I08.2
      - with mitral (valve) disease I08.3
  - congenital Q23.1
  - rheumatic I06.1
    - with
      - mitral (valve) disease I08.0
        - with tricuspid (valve) disease I08.3
      - stenosis I06.2
        - with mitral (valve) disease I08.0
          - with tricuspid (valve) disease I08.3
        - tricuspid (valve) disease I08.2
          - with mitral (valve) disease I08.3
  - specified cause NEC I35.1
  - syphilitic A52.03
- arterial I77.1
  - basilar G45.0
  - carotid (hemispheric) G45.1
  - cerebral I67.81
  - coronary (acute or subacute) I24.8
  - mesenteric K55.1
  - peripheral I73.9
  - precerebral (multiple) (bilateral) G45.2
  - vertebral G45.0
- arteriovenous I99.8
- biliary K83.8
- cardiac (*see also* Insufficiency, myocardial)
  - due to presence of (cardiac) prosthesis I97.11 ☑
  - postprocedural I97.11 ☑

☑ **Additional character required**

Insufficiency — *continued*
 cardiorenal, hypertensive I13.2
 cardiovascular — *see* Disease, cardiovascular
 cerebrovascular (acute) I67.81
  with transient focal neurological signs and
   symptoms G45.8
 circulatory NEC I99.8
  newborn P29.89
 clinical crown length K08.89
 convergence H51.11
 coronary (acute or subacute) I24.8
  chronic or with a stated duration of over 4
   weeks I25.89
 corticoadrenal E27.40
  primary E27.1
 dietary E63.9
 divergence H51.8
 food T73.0 ☑
 gastroesophageal K22.8
 gonadal
  ovary E28.39
  testis E29.1
 heart (*see also* Insufficiency, myocardial)
  newborn P29.0
  valve — *see* Endocarditis
 hepatic — *see* Failure, hepatic
 idiopathic autonomic G90.09
 interocclusal distance of fully erupted teeth
  (ridge) M26.36
 kidney N28.9
  acute N28.9
  chronic N18.9
 lacrimal (secretion) H04.12 ☑
  passages — *see* Stenosis, lacrimal
 liver — *see* Failure, hepatic
 lung — *see* Insufficiency, pulmonary
 mental (congenital) — *see* Disability, intellectual
 mesenteric K55.1
 mitral (valve) I34.0
  with
   aortic valve disease I08.0
    with tricuspid (valve) disease I08.3
   obstruction or stenosis I05.2
    with aortic valve disease I08.0
   tricuspid (valve) disease I08.1
    with aortic (valve) disease I08.3
  congenital Q23.3
  rheumatic I05.1
   with
    aortic valve disease I08.0
     with tricuspid (valve) disease I08.3
    obstruction or stenosis I05.2
     with aortic valve disease I08.0
      with tricuspid (valve) disease I08.3
    tricuspid (valve) disease I08.1
     with aortic (valve) disease I08.3
   active or acute I01.1
    with chorea, rheumatic (Sydenham's) I02.0
  specified cause, except rheumatic I34.0
 muscle (*see also* Disease, muscle)
  heart — *see* Insufficiency, myocardial
  ocular NEC H50.9
 myocardial, myocardium (with arteriosclerosis)
  (*see also* Failure, heart) I50.9
  with
   rheumatic fever (conditions in I00) I09.0
    active, acute or subacute I01.2
     with chorea I02.0
    inactive or quiescent (with chorea) I09.0
  congenital Q24.8
  hypertensive — *see* Hypertension, heart
  newborn P29.0
  rheumatic I09.0
   active, acute, or subacute I01.2
  syphilitic A52.06
 nourishment T73.0 ☑
 pancreatic K86.89
  exocrine K86.81
 parathyroid (gland) E20.9
 peripheral vascular (arterial) I73.9
 pituitary E23.0
 placental (mother) O36.51 ☑
 platelets D69.6
 prenatal care affecting management of
  pregnancy O09.3 ☑
 progressive pluriglandular E31.0
 pulmonary J98.4
  acute, following surgery (nonthoracic) J95.2
   thoracic J95.1
  chronic, following surgery J95.3
  following
   shock J98.4

Insufficiency — *continued*
 pulmonary — *continued*
  trauma J98.4
  newborn P28.5
  valve I37.1
   with stenosis I37.2
   congenital Q22.2
   rheumatic I09.89
    with aortic, mitral or tricuspid (valve)
     disease I08.8
 pyloric K31.89
 renal (acute) N28.9
  chronic N18.9
 respiratory R06.89
  newborn P28.5
 rotation — *see* Malrotation
 sleep syndrome F51.12
 social insurance Z59.7
 suprarenal E27.40
  primary E27.1
 tarso-orbital fascia, congenital Q10.3
 testis E29.1
 thyroid (gland) (acquired) E03.9
  congenital E03.1
 tricuspid (valve) (rheumatic) I07.1
  with
   aortic (valve) disease I08.2
    with mitral (valve) disease I08.3
   mitral (valve) disease I08.1
    with aortic (valve) disease I08.3
   obstruction or stenosis I07.2
    with aortic (valve) disease I08.2
     with mitral (valve) disease I08.3
  congenital Q22.8
  nonrheumatic I36.1
   with stenosis I36.2
 urethral sphincter R32
 valve, valvular (heart) I38
  aortic — *see* Insufficiency, aortic (valve)
  mitral — *see* Insufficiency, mitral (valve)
  pulmonary — *see* Insufficiency, pulmonary,
   valve
  tricuspid — *see* Insufficiency, tricuspid (valve)
  congenital Q24.8
 vascular I99.8
  intestine K55.9
   acute (*see also* Ischemia, intestine,
    acute) K55.059
   mesenteric K55.1
   peripheral I73.9
   renal — *see* Hypertension, kidney
 velopharyngeal
  acquired K13.79
  congenital Q38.8
 venous (chronic) (peripheral) I87.2
 ventricular — *see* Insufficiency, myocardial
 welfare support Z59.7
Insufflation, fallopian Z31.41
Insular — *see* condition
Insulinoma
 pancreas
  benign D13.7
  malignant C25.4
  uncertain behavior D37.8
 specified site
  benign — *see* Neoplasm, by site, benign
  malignant — *see* Neoplasm, by site, malignant
  uncertain behavior — *see* Neoplasm, by site,
   uncertain behavior
 unspecified site
  benign D13.7
  malignant C25.4
  uncertain behavior D37.8
Insuloma — *see* Insulinoma
Interference
 balancing side M26.56
 non-working side M26.56
Intermenstrual — *see* condition
Intermittent — *see* condition
Internal — *see* condition
Interrogation
 cardiac defibrillator (automatic)
  (implantable) Z45.02
 cardiac pacemaker Z45.018
 cardiac (event) (loop) recorder Z45.09
 infusion pump (implanted) (intrathecal) Z45.1
 neurostimulator Z46.2
Interruption
 aortic arch Q25.21
 bundle of His I44.30
 phase-shift, sleep cycle — *see* Disorder, sleep,
  circadian rhythm

Interruption — *continued*
 sleep phase-shift, or 24 hour sleep-wake cycle —
  see Disorder, sleep, circadian rhythm
Interstitial — *see* condition
Intertrigo L30.4
 labialis K13.0
Intervertebral disc — *see* condition
Intestine, intestinal — *see* condition
Intolerance
 carbohydrate K90.49
 disaccharide, hereditary E73.0
 fat NEC K90.49
  pancreatic K90.3
 food K90.49
  dietary counseling and surveillance Z71.3
 fructose E74.10
  hereditary E74.12
 glucose (-galactose) E74.39
 gluten K90.41
 lactose E73.9
  specified NEC E73.8
 lysine E72.3
 milk NEC K90.49
  lactose E73.9
 protein K90.49
 starch NEC K90.49
 sucrose (-isomaltose) E74.31
Intoxicated NEC (without dependence) — *see*
 Alcohol, intoxication
Intoxication
 acid E87.2
 alcoholic (acute) (without dependence) — *see*
  Alcohol, intoxication
 alimentary canal K52.1
 amphetamine (without dependence) — *see*
  Abuse, drug, stimulant, with intoxication
  with dependence — *see* Dependence, drug,
   stimulant, with intoxication
 anxiolytic (acute) (without dependence) — *see*
  Abuse, drug, sedative, with intoxication
  with dependence — *see* Dependence, drug,
   sedative, with intoxication
 caffeine F15.929
  with dependence — *see* Dependence, drug,
   stimulant, with intoxication
 cannabinoids (acute) (without dependence) —
  see Use, cannabis, with intoxication
  with
   abuse — *see* Abuse, drug, cannabis, with
    intoxication
   dependence — *see* Dependence, drug,
    cannabis, with intoxication
 chemical — *see* Table of Drugs and Chemicals
  via placenta or breast milk — *see* Absorption,
   chemical, through placenta
 cocaine (acute) (without dependence) — *see*
  Abuse, drug, cocaine, with intoxication
  with dependence — *see* Dependence, drug,
   cocaine, with intoxication
 drug
  acute (without dependence) — *see* Abuse,
   drug, by type with intoxication
   with dependence — *see* Dependence, drug,
    by type with intoxication
  addictive
   via placenta or breast milk — *see* Absorption,
    drug, addictive, through placenta
  newborn P93.8
   gray baby syndrome P93.0
  overdose or wrong substance given or taken —
   see Table of Drugs and Chemicals, by drug,
   poisoning
 enteric K52.1
 foodborne A05.9
  bacterial A05.9
  classical (Clostridium botulinum) A05.1
  due to
   Bacillus cereus A05.4
   bacterium A05.9
    specified NEC A05.8
   Clostridium
    botulinum A05.1
    perfringens A05.2
    welchii A05.2
   Salmonella A02.9
    with
     (gastro) enteritis A02.0
     localized infection (s) A02.20
      arthritis A02.23
      meningitis A02.21
      osteomyelitis A02.24
      pneumonia A02.22

Intoxication - Irritation

Intoxication — *continued*
  foodborne — *continued*
      pyelonephritis A02.25
      specified NEC A02.29
      sepsis A02.1
      specified manifestation NEC A02.8
    Staphylococcus A05.0
    Vibrio
      parahaemolyticus A05.3
      vulnificus A05.5
   enterotoxin, staphylococcal A05.0
   noxious — *see* Poisoning, food, noxious
  gastrointestinal K52.1
  hallucinogenic (without dependence) — *see*
    Abuse, drug, hallucinogen, with intoxication
   with dependence — *see* Dependence, drug,
    hallucinogen, with intoxication
  hypnotic (acute) (without dependence) — *see*
    Abuse, drug, sedative, with intoxication
   with dependence — *see* Dependence, drug,
    sedative, with intoxication
  inhalant (acute) (without dependence) — *see*
    Abuse, drug, inhalant, with intoxication
   with dependence — *see* Dependence, drug,
    inhalant, with intoxication
  meaning
   inebriation — *see* category F10
   poisoning — *see* Table of Drugs and Chemicals
  methyl alcohol (acute) (without dependence) —
    see Alcohol, intoxication
  opioid (acute) (without dependence) — *see*
    Abuse, drug, opioid, with intoxication
   with dependence — *see* Dependence, drug,
    opioid, with intoxication
  pathologic NEC (without dependence) — *see*
    Alcohol, intoxication
  phencyclidine (without dependence) — *see*
    Abuse, drug, hallucinogen, with intoxication
   with dependence - — *see* Dependence, drug,
    hallucinogen, with intoxication
  potassium (K) E87.5
  psychoactive substance NEC (without
    dependence) — *see* Abuse, drug,
    psychoactive NEC, with intoxication
   with dependence — *see* Dependence, drug,
    psychoactive NEC, with intoxication
  sedative (acute) (without dependence) — *see*
    Abuse, drug, sedative, with intoxication
   with dependence — *see* Dependence, drug,
    sedative, with intoxication
  serum (*see also* Reaction, serum) T80.69 ☑
  uremic — *see* Uremia
  volatile solvents (acute) (without dependence) —
    see Abuse, drug, inhalant, with intoxication
   with dependence — *see* Dependence, drug,
    inhalant, with intoxication
  water E87.79
Intraabdominal testis, testes
  bilateral Q53.211
  unilateral Q53.111
Intracranial — *see* condition
Intrahepatic gallbladder Q44.1
Intraligamentous — *see* condition
Intrathoracic (*see also* condition)
  kidney Q63.2
Intrauterine contraceptive device
  checking Z30.431
  insertion Z30.430
   immediately following removal Z30.433
  in situ Z97.5
  management Z30.431
  reinsertion Z30.433
  removal Z30.432
  replacement Z30.433
  retention in pregnancy O26.3 ☑
Intraventricular — *see* condition
Intrinsic deformity — *see* Deformity
Intubation, difficult or failed T88.4 ☑
Intumescence, lens (eye) (cataract) — *see* Cataract
Intussusception (bowel) (colon) (enteric) (ileocecal)
  (ileocolic) (intestine) (rectum) K56.1
  appendix K38.8
  congenital Q43.8
  ureter (with obstruction) N13.5
Invagination (bowel, colon, intestine or rectum)
  K56.1
Inversion
  albumin-globulin (A-G) ratio E88.09
  bladder N32.89
  cecum — *see* Intussusception
  cervix N88.8
  chromosome in normal individual Q95.1

Inversion — *continued*
  circadian rhythm — *see* Disorder, sleep, circadian
    rhythm
  nipple N64.59
   congenital Q83.8
   gestational — *see* Retraction, nipple
   puerperal, postpartum — *see* Retraction, nipple
  nyctohemeral rhythm — *see* Disorder, sleep,
    circadian rhythm
  optic papilla Q14.2
  organ or site, congenital NEC — *see* Anomaly,
    by site
  sleep rhythm — *see* Disorder, sleep, circadian rhythm
  testis (congenital) Q55.29
  uterus (chronic) (postinfectional) (postpartal,
    old) N85.5
   postpartum O71.2
  vagina (posthysterectomy) N99.3
  ventricular Q20.5
Investigation (*see also* Examination) Z04.9
  clinical research subject (control) (normal
    comparison) (participant) Z00.6
Involuntary movement, abnormal R25.9
Involution, involutional (*see also* condition)
  breast, cystic — *see* Dysplasia, mammary,
    specified type NEC
  depression (single episode) F32.89
   recurrent episode F33.9
  melancholia (single episode) F32.89
   recurrent episode F33.8
  ovary, senile — *see* Atrophy, ovary
  thymus failure E32.8
I.Q.
  under 20 F73
  20-34 F72
  35-49 F71
  50-69 F70
IRDS (type I) P22.0
  type II P22.1
Irideremia Q13.1
Iridis rubeosis — *see* Disorder, iris, vascular
Iridochoroiditis (panuveitis) — *see* Panuveitis
Iridocyclitis H20.9
  acute H20.0 ☑
   hypopyon H20.05 ☑
   primary H20.01 ☑
   recurrent H20.02 ☑
   secondary (noninfectious) H20.04 ☑
    infectious H20.03 ☑
  chronic H20.1 ☑
  due to allergy — *see* Iridocyclitis, acute,
    secondary
  endogenous — *see* Iridocyclitis, acute, primary
  Fuchs' — *see* Cyclitis, Fuchs' heterochromic
  gonococcal A54.32
  granulomatous — *see* Iridocyclitis, chronic
  herpes, herpetic (simplex) B00.51
   zoster B02.32
  hypopyon — *see* Iridocyclitis, acute, hypopyon
  in (due to)
   ankylosing spondylitis M45.9
   gonococcal infection A54.32
   herpes (simplex) virus B00.51
    zoster B02.32
   infectious disease NOS B99 ☑
   parasitic disease NOS B89 *[H22]*
   sarcoidosis D86.83
   syphilis A51.43
   tuberculosis A18.54
   zoster B02.32
  lens-induced H20.2 ☑
  nongranulomatous — *see* Iridocyclitis, acute
  recurrent — *see* Iridocyclitis, acute, recurrent
  rheumatic — *see* Iridocyclitis, chronic
  subacute — *see* Iridocyclitis, acute
  sympathetic — *see* Uveitis, sympathetic
  syphilitic (secondary) A51.43
  tuberculous (chronic) A18.54
  Vogt-Koyanagi H20.82 ☑
Iridocyclochoroiditis (panuveitis) — *see* Panuveitis
Iridodialysis H21.53 ☑
Iridodonesis H21.89
Iridoplegia (complete) (partial) (reflex) H57.09
Iridoschisis H21.25 ☑
Iris (*see also* condition)
  bombé — *see* Membrane, pupillary
Iritis (*see also* Iridocyclitis)
  chronic — *see* Iridocyclitis, chronic
  diabetic — *see* E08-E13 with .39
  due to
   herpes simplex B00.51
   leprosy A30.9 *[H22]*

Iritis — *continued*
  gonococcal A54.32
  gouty (*see also* Gout, by type) M10.9 *[H22]*
  granulomatous — *see* Iridocyclitis, chronic
  lens induced — *see* Iridocyclitis, lens-induced
  papulosa (syphilitic) A52.71
  rheumatic — *see* Iridocyclitis, chronic
  syphilitic (secondary) A51.43
   congenital (early) A50.01
   late A52.71
  tuberculous A18.54
Iron — *see* condition
Iron-miner's lung J63.4
Irradiated enamel (tooth, teeth) K03.89
Irradiation effects, adverse T66 ☑
Irreducible, irreducibility — *see* condition
Irregular, irregularity
  action, heart I49.9
  alveolar process K08.89
  bleeding N92.6
  breathing R06.89
  contour of cornea (acquired) — *see* Deformity,
    cornea
   congenital Q13.4
  contour, reconstructed breast N65.0
  dentin (in pulp) K04.3
  eye movements H55.89
   nystagmus — *see* Nystagmus
   saccadic H55.81
  labor O62.2
  menstruation (cause unknown) N92.6
  periods N92.6
  prostate N42.9
  pupil — *see* Abnormality, pupillary
  reconstructed breast N65.0
  respiratory R06.89
  septum (nasal) J34.2
  shape, organ or site, congenital NEC — *see*
    Distortion
  sleep-wake pattern (rhythm) G47.23
Irritable, irritability R45.4
  bladder N32.89
  bowel (syndrome) K58.9
   with
    constipation K58.1
    diarrhea K58.0
   mixed K58.2
   psychogenic F45.8
   specified NEC K58.8
  bronchial — *see* Bronchitis
  cerebral, in newborn P91.3
  colon (*see also* Irritable, bowel) K58.9
   with diarrhea K58.0
   psychogenic F45.8
  duodenum K59.8
  heart (psychogenic) F45.8
  hip — *see* Derangement, joint, specified type
    NEC, hip
  ileum K59.8
  infant R68.12
  jejunum K59.8
  rectum K59.8
  stomach K31.89
   psychogenic F45.8
  sympathetic G90.8
  urethra N36.8
Irritation
  anus K62.89
  axillary nerve G54.0
  bladder N32.89
  brachial plexus G54.0
  bronchial — *see* Bronchitis
  cervical plexus G54.2
  cervix — *see* Cervicitis
  choroid, sympathetic — *see* Endophthalmitis
  cranial nerve — *see* Disorder, nerve, cranial
  gastric K31.89
   psychogenic F45.8
  globe, sympathetic — *see* Uveitis, sympathetic
  labyrinth — *see* subcategory H83.2
  lumbosacral plexus G54.1
  meninges (traumatic) — *see* Injury, intracranial
   nontraumatic — *see* Meningismus
  nerve — *see* Disorder, nerve
  nervous R45.0
  penis N48.89
  perineum NEC L29.3
  peripheral autonomic nervous system G90.8
  peritoneum — *see* Peritonitis
  pharynx J39.2
  plantar nerve — *see* Lesion, nerve, plantar

☑ **Additional character required**

Irritation — *continued*
  spinal (cord) (traumatic) (*see also* Injury, spinal
      cord, by region)
    nerve G58.9
      root NEC — *see* Radiculopathy
      nontraumatic — *see* Myelopathy
    stomach K31.89
      psychogenic F45.8
    sympathetic nerve NEC G90.8
    ulnar nerve — *see* Lesion, nerve, ulnar
    vagina N89.8
Ischemia, ischemic I99.8
  brain — *see* Ischemia, cerebral
  bowel (transient)
    acute (*see also* Ischemia, intestine,
        acute) K55.059
    chronic K55.1
    due to mesenteric artery insufficiency K55.1
  cardiac (*see* Disease, heart, ischemic)
  cardiomyopathy I25.5
  cerebral (chronic) (generalized) I67.82
    arteriosclerotic I67.2
    intermittent G45.9
    newborn P91.0
    recurrent focal G45.8
    transient G45.9
  colon chronic (due to mesenteric artery
      insufficiency) K55.1
  coronary — *see* Disease, heart, ischemic
  demand (coronary) (*see also* Angina) I24.8
    with myocardial infarction I21.A1
    resulting in myocardial infarction I21.A1
  heart (chronic or with a stated duration of over 4
      weeks) I25.9
    acute or with a stated duration of 4 weeks or
        less I24.9
    subacute I24.9
  infarction, muscle — *see* Infarct, muscle
  intestine (large) (small) (transient) K55.9
    acute K55.059
      diffuse K55.052
      focal K55.051
      large K55.039
        diffuse K55.032
        focal K55.031
      small K55.019
        diffuse K55.012
        focal K55.011
    chronic K55.1
    due to mesenteric artery insufficiency K55.1
  kidney N28.0
  mesenteric, acute (*see also* Ischemia, intestine,
      acute) K55.059
  muscle, traumatic T79.6 ☑
  myocardium, myocardial (chronic or with a stated
      duration of over 4 weeks) I25.9
    acute, without myocardial infarction I51.3
    silent (asymptomatic) I25.6
    transient of newborn P29.4
  renal N28.0
  retina, retinal — *see* Occlusion, artery, retina
  small bowel
    acute K55.019
      diffuse K55.012
      focal K55.011
    chronic K55.1
    due to mesenteric artery insufficiency K55.1
  spinal cord G95.11
  subendocardial — *see* Insufficiency, coronary
  supply (coronary) (*see also* Angina) I25.9
    due to vasospasm I20.1
Ischial spine — *see* condition
Ischialgia — *see* Sciatica
Ischiopagus Q89.4
Ischium, ischial — *see* condition
Ischuria R34
Iselin's disease or osteochondrosis — *see*
    Osteochondrosis, juvenile, metatarsus
Islands of
  parotid tissue in
    lymph nodes Q38.6
    neck structures Q38.6
  submaxillary glands in
    fascia Q38.6
    lymph nodes Q38.6
    neck muscles Q38.6
Islet cell tumor, pancreas D13.7
Isoimmunization NEC (*see also* Incompatibility)
  affecting management of pregnancy (ABO) (with
      hydrops fetalis) O36.11 ☑
    anti-A sensitization O36.11 ☑
    anti-B sensitization O36.19 ☑

Isoimmunization — *continued*
  affecting management of pregnancy — *continued*
    anti-c sensitization O36.09 ☑
    anti-C sensitization O36.09 ☑
    anti-e sensitization O36.09 ☑
    anti-E sensitization O36.09 ☑
    Rh NEC O36.09 ☑
      anti-D antibody O36.01 ☑
    specified NEC O36.19 ☑
  newborn P55.9
    with
      hydrops fetalis P56.0
      kernicterus P57.0
    ABO (blood groups) P55.1
    Rhesus (Rh) factor P55.0
    specified type NEC P55.8
Isolation, isolated
  dwelling Z59.8
  family Z63.79
  social Z60.4
Isoleucinosis E71.19
Isomerism atrial appendages (with asplenia or
    polysplenia) Q20.6
Isosporiasis, isosporosis A07.3
Isovaleric acidemia E71.110
Issue of
  medical certificate Z02.79
    for disability determination Z02.71
  repeat prescription (appliance) (glasses)
      (medicinal substance, medicament,
      medicine) Z76.0
    contraception — *see* Contraception
Itch, itching (*see also* Pruritus)
  baker's L23.6
  barber's B35.0
  bricklayer's L24.5
  cheese B88.0
  clam digger's B65.3
  coolie B76.9
  copra B88.0
  dew B76.9
  dhobi B35.6
  filarial — *see* Infestation, filarial
  grain B88.0
  grocer's B88.0
  ground B76.9
  harvest B88.0
  jock B35.6
  Malabar B35.5
    beard B35.0
    foot B35.3
    scalp B35.0
  meaning scabies B86
  Norwegian B86
  perianal L29.0
  poultrymen's B88.0
  sarcoptic B86
  scabies B86
  scrub B88.0
  straw B88.0
  swimmer's B65.3
  water B76.9
  winter L29.8
Ivemark's syndrome (asplenia with congenital heart
    disease) Q89.01
Ivory bones Q78.2
Ixodiasis NEC B88.8

J

Jaccoud's syndrome — *see* Arthropathy,
    postrheumatic, chronic
Jackson's
  membrane Q43.3
  paralysis or syndrome G83.89
  veil Q43.3
Jacquet's dermatitis (diaper dermatitis) L22
Jadassohn-Pellizari's disease or anetoderma L90.2
Jadassohn's
  blue nevus — *see* Nevus
  intraepidermal epithelioma — *see* Neoplasm,
      skin, benign
Jaffe-Lichtenstein (-Uehlinger) syndrome — *see*
    Dysplasia, fibrous, bone NEC
Jakob-Creutzfeldt disease or syndrome — *see*
    Creutzfeldt-Jakob disease or syndrome
Jaksch-Luzet disease D64.89
Jamaican
  neuropathy G92
  paraplegic tropical ataxic-spastic syndrome G92

Janet's disease F48.8
Janiceps Q89.4
Jansky-Bielschowsky amaurotic idiocy E75.4
Japanese
  B-type encephalitis A83.0
  river fever A75.3
Jaundice (yellow) R17
  acholuric (familial) (splenomegalic) (*see also*
      Spherocytosis)
    acquired D59.8
  breast-milk (inhibitor) P59.3
  catarrhal (acute) B15.9
    with hepatic coma B15.0
  cholestatic (benign) R17
  due to or associated with
    delayed conjugation P59.8
      associated with (due to) preterm
          delivery P59.0
    preterm delivery P59.0
  epidemic (catarrhal) B15.9
    with hepatic coma B15.0
    leptospiral A27.0
    spirochetal A27.0
  familial nonhemolytic (congenital) (Gilbert) E80.4
    Crigler-Najjar E80.5
  febrile (acute) B15.9
    with hepatic coma B15.0
    leptospiral A27.0
    spirochetal A27.0
  hematogenous D59.9
  hemolytic (acquired) D59.9
    congenital — *see* Spherocytosis
  hemorrhagic (acute) (leptospiral)
      (spirochetal) A27.0
  infectious (acute) (subacute) B15.9
    with hepatic coma B15.0
    leptospiral A27.0
    spirochetal A27.0
  leptospiral (hemorrhagic) A27.0
  malignant (without coma) K72.90
    with coma K72.91
  newborn P59.9
    due to or associated with
      ABO
        antibodies P55.1
        incompatibility, maternal/fetal P55.1
        isoimmunization P55.1
      absence or deficiency of enzyme system for
          bilirubin conjugation (congenital) P59.8
      bleeding P58.1
      breast milk inhibitors to conjugation P59.3
        associated with preterm delivery P59.0
      bruising P58.0
      Crigler-Najjar syndrome E80.5
      delayed conjugation P59.8
        associated with preterm delivery P59.0
      drugs or toxins
        given to newborn P58.42
        transmitted from mother P58.41
      excessive hemolysis P58.9
        due to
          bleeding P58.1
          bruising P58.0
          drugs or toxins
            given to newborn P58.42
            transmitted from mother P58.41
          infection P58.2
          polycythemia P58.3
          swallowed maternal blood P58.5
          specified type NEC P58.8
      galactosemia E74.21
      Gilbert syndrome E80.4
      hemolytic disease P55.9
        ABO isoimmunization P55.1
        Rh isoimmunization P55.0
        specified NEC P55.8
      hepatocellular damage P59.20
        specified NEC P59.29
      hereditary hemolytic anemia P58.8
      hypothyroidism, congenital E03.1
      incompatibility, maternal/fetal NOS P55.9
      infection P58.2
      inspissated bile syndrome P59.1
      isoimmunization NOS P55.9
      mucoviscidosis E84.9
      polycythemia P58.3
      preterm delivery P59.0
      Rh
        antibodies P55.0
        incompatibility, maternal/fetal P55.0
        isoimmunization P55.0
      specified cause NEC P59.8

Jaundice - Kerion

Jaundice — *continued*
  newborn — *continued*
    swallowed maternal blood P58.5
    spherocytosis (congenital) D58.0
  neonatal — *see* Jaundice, newborn
  nonhemolytic congenital familial (Gilbert) E80.4
  nuclear, newborn (*see also* Kernicterus of newborn) P57.9
  obstructive (*see also* Obstruction, bile duct) K83.1
  post-immunization — *see* Hepatitis, viral, type, B
  post-transfusion — *see* Hepatitis, viral, type, B
  regurgitation (*see also* Obstruction, bile duct) K83.1
  serum (homologous) (prophylactic) (therapeutic) — *see* Hepatitis, viral, type, B
  spirochetal (hemorrhagic) A27.0
  symptomatic R17
    newborn P59.9
Jaw — *see* condition
Jaw-winking phenomenon or syndrome Q07.8
Jealousy
  alcoholic F10.988
  childhood F93.8
  sibling F93.8
Jejunitis — *see* Enteritis
Jejunostomy status Z93.4
Jejunum, jejunal — *see* condition
Jensen's disease — *see* Inflammation, chorioretinal, focal, juxtapapillary
Jerks, myoclonic G25.3
Jervell-Lange-Nielsen syndrome I45.81
Jeune's disease Q77.2
Jigger disease B88.1
Job's syndrome (chronic granulomatous disease) D71
Joint (*see also* condition)
  mice — *see* Loose, body, joint
    knee M23.4 ☑
Jordan's anomaly or syndrome D72.0
Joseph-Diamond-Blackfan anemia (congenital hypoplastic) D61.01
Jungle yellow fever A95.0
Jüngling's disease — *see* Sarcoidosis
Juvenile — *see* condition

K

Kahler's disease C90.0 ☑
Kakke E51.11
Kala-azar B55.0
Kallmann's syndrome E23.0
Kanner's syndrome (autism) — *see* Psychosis, childhood
Kaposi's
  dermatosis (xeroderma pigmentosum) Q82.1
  lichen ruber L44.0
    acuminatus L44.0
  sarcoma
    colon C46.4
    connective tissue C46.1
    gastrointestinal organ C46.4
    lung C46.5 ☑
    lymph node (multiple) C46.3
    palate (hard) (soft) C46.2
    rectum C46.4
    skin (multiple sites) C46.0
    specified site NEC C46.7
    stomach C46.4
    unspecified site C46.9
  varicelliform eruption B00.0
    vaccinia T88.1 ☑
Kartagener's syndrome or triad (sinusitis, bronchiectasis, situs inversus) Q89.3
Karyotype
  with abnormality except iso (Xq) Q96.2
  45,X Q96.0
  46,X
    iso (Xq) Q96.1
  46,XX Q98.3
    with streak gonads Q50.32
    hermaphrodite (true) Q99.1
    male Q98.3
  46,XY
    with streak gonads Q56.1
    female Q97.3
    hermaphrodite (true) Q99.1
  47,XXX Q97.0
  47,XXY Q98.0
  47,XYY Q98.5
Kaschin-Beck disease — *see* Disease, Kaschin-Beck

Katayama's disease or fever B65.2
Kawasaki's syndrome M30.3
Kayser-Fleischer ring (cornea) (pseudosclerosis) H18.04 ☑
Kaznelson's syndrome (congenital hypoplastic anemia) D61.01
Kearns-Sayre syndrome H49.81 ☑
Kedani fever A75.3
Kelis L91.0
Kelly (-Patterson) syndrome (sideropenic dysphagia) D50.1
Keloid, cheloid L91.0
  acne L73.0
  Addison's L94.0
  cornea — *see* Opacity, cornea
  Hawkin's L91.0
  scar L91.0
Keloma L91.0
Kenya fever A77.1
Keratectasia (*see also* Ectasia, cornea)
  congenital Q13.4
Keratinization of alveolar ridge mucosa
  excessive K13.23
  minimal K13.22
Keratinized residual ridge mucosa
  excessive K13.23
  minimal K13.22
Keratitis (nodular) (nonulcerative) (simple) (zonular) H16.9
  with ulceration (central) (marginal) (perforated) (ring) — *see* Ulcer, cornea
  actinic — *see* Photokeratitis
  arborescens (herpes simplex) B00.52
  areolar H16.11 ☑
  bullosa H16.8
  deep H16.309
    specified type NEC H16.399
  dendritic (a) (herpes simplex) B00.52
  disciform (is) (herpes simplex) B00.52
    varicella B01.81
  filamentary H16.12 ☑
  gonococcal (congenital or prenatal) A54.33
  herpes, herpetic (simplex) B00.52
    zoster B02.33
  in (due to)
    acanthamebiasis B60.13
    adenovirus B30.0
    exanthema (*see also* Exanthem) B09
    herpes (simplex) virus B00.52
    measles B05.81
    syphilis A50.31
    tuberculosis A18.52
    zoster B02.33
  interstitial (nonsyphilitic) H16.30 ☑
    diffuse H16.32 ☑
    herpes, herpetic (simplex) B00.52
      zoster B02.33
    sclerosing H16.33 ☑
    specified type NEC H16.39 ☑
    syphilitic (congenital) (late) A50.31
    tuberculous A18.52
  macular H16.11 ☑
  nummular H16.11 ☑
  oyster shuckers' H16.8
  parenchymatous — *see* Keratitis, interstitial
  petrificans H16.8
  postmeasles B05.81
  punctata
    leprosa A30.9 [*H16.14* ☑]
    syphilitic (profunda) A50.31
  punctate H16.14 ☑
  purulent H16.8
  rosacea L71.8
  sclerosing H16.33 ☑
  specified type NEC H16.8
  stellate H16.11 ☑
  striate H16.11 ☑
  superficial H16.10 ☑
    with conjunctivitis — *see* Keratoconjunctivitis
    due to light — *see* Photokeratitis
  suppurative H16.8
  syphilitic (congenital) (prenatal) A50.31
  trachomatous A71.1
    sequelae B94.0
  tuberculous A18.52
  vesicular H16.8
  xerotic (*see also* Keratomalacia) H16.8
    vitamin A deficiency E50.4
Keratoacanthoma L85.8
Keratocele — *see* Descemetocele
Keratoconjunctivitis H16.20 ☑
  Acanthamoeba B60.13

Keratoconjunctivitis — *continued*
  adenoviral B30.0
  epidemic B30.0
  exposure H16.21 ☑
  herpes, herpetic (simplex) B00.52
    zoster B02.33
  in exanthema (*see also* Exanthem) B09
  infectious B30.0
  lagophthalmic — *see* Keratoconjunctivitis, specified type NEC
  neurotrophic H16.23 ☑
  phlyctenular H16.25 ☑
  postmeasles B05.81
  shipyard B30.0
  sicca (Sjogren's) M35.0 ☑
    not Sjogren's H16.22 ☑
  specified type NEC H16.29 ☑
  tuberculous (phlyctenular) A18.52
  vernal H16.26 ☑
Keratoconus H18.60 ☑
  congenital Q13.4
  stable H18.61 ☑
  unstable H18.62 ☑
Keratocyst (dental) (odontogenic) — *see* Cyst, calcifying odontogenic
Keratoderma, keratodermia (congenital) (palmaris et plantaris) (symmetrical) Q82.8
  acquired L85.1
    in diseases classified elsewhere L86
  climactericum L85.1
  gonococcal A54.89
  gonorrheal A54.89
  punctata L85.2
  Reiter's — *see* Reiter's disease
Keratodermatocele — *see* Descemetocele
Keratoglobus H18.79 ☑
  congenital Q15.8
    with glaucoma Q15.0
Keratohemia — *see* Pigmentation, cornea, stromal
Keratoiritis (*see also* Iridocyclitis)
  syphilitic A50.39
  tuberculous A18.54
Keratoma L57.0
  palmaris and plantaris hereditarium Q82.8
  senile L57.0
Keratomalacia H18.44 ☑
  vitamin A deficiency E50.4
Keratomegaly Q13.4
Keratomycosis B49
  nigrans, nigricans (palmaris) B36.1
Keratopathy H18.9
  band H18.42 ☑
  bullous H18.1 ☑
  bullous (aphakic), following cataract surgery H59.01 ☑
Keratoscleritis, tuberculous A18.52
Keratosis L57.0
  actinic L57.0
  arsenical L85.8
  congenital, specified NEC Q80.8
  female genital NEC N94.89
  follicularis Q82.8
    acquired L11.0
    congenita Q82.8
    et parafollicularis in cutem penetrans L87.0
    spinulosa (decalvans) Q82.8
    vitamin A deficiency E50.8
  gonococcal A54.89
  male genital (external) N50.89
  nigricans L83
  obturans, external ear (canal) — *see* Cholesteatoma, external ear
  palmaris et plantaris (inherited) (symmetrical) Q82.8
    acquired L85.1
  penile N48.89
  pharynx J39.2
  pilaris, acquired L85.8
  punctata (palmaris et plantaris) L85.2
  scrotal N50.89
  seborrheic L82.1
    inflamed L82.0
  senile L57.0
  solar L57.0
  tonsillaris J35.8
  vagina N89.4
  vegetans Q82.8
  vitamin A deficiency E50.8
  vocal cord J38.3
Kerato-uveitis — *see* Iridocyclitis
Kerunoparalysis T75.09 ☑
Kerion (celsi) B35.0

☑ **Additional character required**

Kernicterus of newborn (not due to isoimmunization) P57.9
  due to isoimmunization (conditions in P55.0-P55.9) P57.0
  specified type NEC P57.8
Keshan disease E59
Ketoacidosis E87.2
  diabetic — see Diabetes, by type, with ketoacidosis
Ketonuria R82.4
Ketosis NEC E88.89
  diabetic — see Diabetes, by type, with with ketoacidosis
Kew Garden fever A79.1
Kidney — see condition
Kienböck's disease (see also Osteochondrosis, juvenile, hand, carpal lunate)
  adult M93.1
Kimmelstiel (-Wilson) disease — see Diabetes, Kimmelstiel (-Wilson) disease
Kimura disease D21.9
  specified site (see Neoplasm, connective tissue benign)
Kink, kinking
  artery I77.1
  hair (acquired) L67.8
  ileum or intestine — see Obstruction, intestine
  Lane's — see Obstruction, intestine
  organ or site, congenital NEC — see Anomaly, by site
  ureter (pelvic junction) N13.5
    with
      hydronephrosis N13.1
        with infection N13.6
      pyelonephritis (chronic) N11.1
    congenital Q62.39
  vein (s) I87.8
    caval I87.1
    peripheral I87.1
Kinnier Wilson's disease (hepatolenticular degeneration) E83.01
Kissing spine M48.20
  cervical region M48.22
  cervicothoracic region M48.23
  lumbar region M48.26
  lumbosacral region M48.27
  occipito-atlanto-axial region M48.21
  thoracic region M48.24
  thoracolumbar region M48.25
Klatskin's tumor C24.0
Klauder's disease A26.8
Klebs' disease (see also Glomerulonephritis) N05. ☑
Klebsiella (K.) pneumoniae, as cause of disease classified elsewhere B96.1
Klein (e)-Levin syndrome G47.13
Kleptomania F63.2
Klinefelter's syndrome Q98.4
  karyotype 47,XXY Q98.0
  male with more than two X chromosomes Q98.1
Klippel-Feil deficiency, disease, or syndrome (brevicollis) Q76.1
Klippel's disease I67.2
Klippel-Trenaunay (-Weber) syndrome Q87.2
Klumpke (-Déjerine) palsy, paralysis (birth) (newborn) P14.1
Knee — see condition
Knock knee (acquired) M21.06 ☑
  congenital Q74.1
Knot (s)
  intestinal, syndrome (volvulus) K56.2
  surfer S89.8 ☑
  umbilical cord (true) O69.2 ☑
Knotting (of)
  hair L67.8
  intestine K56.2
Knuckle pad (Garrod's) M72.1
Koch's
  infection — see Tuberculosis
  relapsing fever A68.9
Koch-Weeks' conjunctivitis — see Conjunctivitis, acute, mucopurulent
Köebner's syndrome Q81.8
Köenig's disease (osteochondritis dissecans) — see Osteochondritis, dissecans
Köhler-Pellegrini-Steida disease or syndrome (calcification, knee joint) — see Bursitis, tibial collateral
Köhler's disease
  patellar — see Osteochondrosis, juvenile, patella
  tarsal navicular — see Osteochondrosis, juvenile, tarsus
Koilonychia L60.3
  congenital Q84.6

Kojevnikov's, epilepsy — see Kozhevnikof's epilepsy
Koplik's spots B05.9
Kopp's asthma E32.8
Korsakoff's (Wernicke) disease, psychosis or syndrome (alcoholic) F10.96
  with dependence F10.26
  drug-induced
    due to drug abuse — see Abuse, drug, by type, with amnestic disorder
    due to drug dependence — see Dependence, drug, by type, with amnestic disorder
  nonalcoholic F04
Korsakov's disease, psychosis or syndrome — see Korsakoff's disease
Korsakow's disease, psychosis or syndrome — see Korsakoff's disease
Kostmann's disease or syndrome (infantile genetic agranulocytosis) — see Agranulocytosis
Kozhevnikof's epilepsy G40.109
  intractable G40.119
    with status epilepticus G40.111
    without status epilepticus G40.119
  not intractable G40.109
    with status epilepticus G40.101
    without status epilepticus G40.109
Krabbe's
  disease E75.23
  syndrome, congenital muscle hypoplasia Q79.8
Kraepelin-Morel disease — see Schizophrenia
Kraft-Weber-Dimitri disease Q85.8
Kraurosis
  ani K62.89
  penis N48.0
  vagina N89.8
  vulva N90.4
Kreotoxism A05.9
Krukenberg's
  spindle — see Pigmentation, cornea, posterior
  tumor C79.6 ☑
Kufs' disease E75.4
Kugelberg-Welander disease G12.1
Kuhnt-Junius degeneration (see also Degeneration, macula) H35.32 ☑
Kümmell's disease or spondylitis — see Spondylopathy, traumatic
Kupffer cell sarcoma C22.3
Kuru A81.81
Kussmaul's
  disease M30.0
  respiration E87.2
    in diabetic acidosis — see Diabetes, by type, with ketoacidosis
Kwashiorkor E40
  marasmic, marasmus type E42
Kyasanur Forest disease A98.2
Kyphoscoliosis, kyphoscoliotic (acquired) (see also Scoliosis) M41.9
  congenital Q67.5
  heart (disease) I27.1
  sequelae of rickets E64.3
  tuberculous A18.01
Kyphosis, kyphotic (acquired) M40.209
  cervical region M40.202
  cervicothoracic region M40.203
  congenital Q76.419
    cervical region Q76.412
    cervicothoracic region Q76.413
    occipito-atlanto-axial region Q76.411
    thoracic region Q76.414
    thoracolumbar region Q76.415
  Morquio-Brailsford type (spinal) (see also subcategory M49.8) E76.219
  postlaminectomy M96.3
  postradiation therapy M96.2
  postural (adolescent) M40.00
    cervicothoracic region M40.03
    thoracic region M40.04
    thoracolumbar region M40.05
  secondary NEC M40.10
    cervical region M40.12
    cervicothoracic region M40.13
    thoracic region M40.14
    thoracolumbar region M40.15
  sequelae of rickets E64.3
  specified type NEC M40.299
    cervical region M40.292
    cervicothoracic region M40.293
    thoracic region M40.294
    thoracolumbar region M40.295
  syphilitic, congenital A50.56
  thoracic region M40.204
  thoracolumbar region M40.205
  tuberculous A18.01

Kyrle disease L87.0

L

Labia, labium — see condition
Labile
  blood pressure R09.89
  vasomotor system I73.9
Labioglossal paralysis G12.29
Labioglossal paralysis G12.29
Labium leporinum — see Cleft, lip
Labor — see Delivery
Labored breathing — see Hyperventilation
Labyrinthitis (circumscribed) (destructive) (diffuse) (inner ear) (latent) (purulent) (suppurative) (see also subcategory) H83.0 ☑
  syphilitic A52.79
Laceration
  with abortion — see Abortion, by type, complicated by laceration of pelvic organs
  abdomen, abdominal
    wall S31.119 ☑
      with
        foreign body S31.129 ☑
        penetration into peritoneal cavity S31.619 ☑
          with foreign body S31.629 ☑
      epigastric region S31.112 ☑
        with
          foreign body S31.122 ☑
          penetration into peritoneal cavity S31.612 ☑
            with foreign body S31.622 ☑
      left
        lower quadrant S31.114 ☑
          with
            foreign body S31.124 ☑
            penetration into peritoneal cavity S31.614 ☑
              with foreign body S31.624 ☑
        upper quadrant S31.111 ☑
          with
            foreign body S31.121 ☑
            penetration into peritoneal cavity S31.611 ☑
              with foreign body S31.621 ☑
      periumbilic region S31.115 ☑
        with
          foreign body S31.125 ☑
          penetration into peritoneal cavity S31.615 ☑
            with foreign body S31.625 ☑
      right
        lower quadrant S31.113 ☑
          with
            foreign body S31.123 ☑
            penetration into peritoneal cavity S31.613 ☑
              with foreign body S31.623 ☑
        upper quadrant S31.110 ☑
          with
            foreign body S31.120 ☑
            penetration into peritoneal cavity S31.610 ☑
              with foreign body S31.620 ☑
  accidental, complicating surgery — see Complications, surgical, accidental puncture or laceration
  Achilles tendon S86.02 ☑
  adrenal gland S37.813 ☑
  alveolar (process) — see Laceration, oral cavity
  ankle S91.01 ☑
    with
      foreign body S91.02 ☑
  antecubital space — see Laceration, elbow
  anus (sphincter) S31.831 ☑
    with
      ectopic or molar pregnancy O08.6
      foreign body S31.832 ☑
    complicating delivery — see Delivery, complicated, by, laceration, anus (sphincter)
    following ectopic or molar pregnancy O08.6
    nontraumatic, nonpuerperal — see Fissure, anus
  arm (upper) S41.11 ☑
    with foreign body S41.12 ☑
    lower — see Laceration, forearm
  auditory canal (external) (meatus) — see Laceration, ear
  auricle, ear — see Laceration, ear

Laceration

Laceration — *continued*
- axilla — *see* Laceration, arm
- back (*see also* Laceration, thorax, back)
  - lower S31.010 ☑
    - with
      - foreign body S31.020 ☑
        - with penetration into retroperitoneal space S31.021 ☑
        - penetration into retroperitoneal space S31.011 ☑
- bile duct S36.13 ☑
- bladder S37.23 ☑
  - with ectopic or molar pregnancy O08.6
  - following ectopic or molar pregnancy O08.6
  - obstetrical trauma O71.5
- blood vessel — *see* Injury, blood vessel
- bowel (*see also* Laceration, intestine)
  - with ectopic or molar pregnancy O08.6
  - complicating abortion — *see* Abortion, by type, complicated by, specified condition NEC
  - following ectopic or molar pregnancy O08.6
  - obstetrical trauma O71.5
- brain (any part) (cortex) (diffuse) (membrane) (*see also* Injury, intracranial, diffuse)
  - during birth P10.8
    - with hemorrhage P10.1
  - focal — *see* Injury, intracranial, focal brain injury
- brainstem S06.38 ☑
- breast S21.01 ☑
  - with foreign body S21.02 ☑
- broad ligament S37.893 ☑
  - with ectopic or molar pregnancy O08.6
  - following ectopic or molar pregnancy O08.6
  - laceration syndrome N83.8
  - obstetrical trauma O71.6
  - syndrome (laceration) N83.8
- buttock S31.801 ☑
  - with foreign body S31.802 ☑
  - left S31.821 ☑
    - with foreign body S31.822 ☑
  - right S31.811 ☑
    - with foreign body S31.812 ☑
- calf — *see* Laceration, leg
- canaliculus lacrimalis — *see* Laceration, eyelid
- canthus, eye — *see* Laceration, eyelid
- capsule, joint — *see* Sprain
- causing eversion of cervix uteri (old) N86
- central (perineal), complicating delivery O70.9
- cerebellum, traumatic S06.37 ☑
- cerebral S06.33 ☑
  - left side S06.32 ☑
  - during birth P10.8
    - with hemorrhage P10.1
  - right side S06.31 ☑
- cervix (uteri)
  - with ectopic or molar pregnancy O08.6
  - following ectopic or molar pregnancy O08.6
  - nonpuerperal, nontraumatic N88.1
  - obstetrical trauma (current) O71.3
  - old (postpartal) N88.1
  - traumatic S37.63 ☑
- cheek (external) S01.41 ☑
  - with foreign body S01.42 ☑
  - internal — *see* Laceration, oral cavity
- chest wall — *see* Laceration, thorax
- chin — *see* Laceration, head, specified site NEC
- chordae tendinae NEC I51.1
  - concurrent with acute myocardial infarction — *see* Infarct, myocardium
  - following acute myocardial infarction (current complication) I23.4
- clitoris — *see* Laceration, vulva
- colon — *see* Laceration, intestine, large, colon
- common bile duct S36.13 ☑
- cortex (cerebral) — *see* Injury, intracranial, diffuse
- costal region — *see* Laceration, thorax
- cystic duct S36.13 ☑
- diaphragm S27.803 ☑
- digit (s)
  - hand — *see* Laceration, finger
  - foot — *see* Laceration, toe
- duodenum S36.430 ☑
- ear (canal) (external) S01.31 ☑
  - with foreign body S01.32 ☑
  - drum S09.2 ☑
- elbow S51.01 ☑
  - with
    - foreign body S51.02 ☑
- epididymis — *see* Laceration, testis
- epigastric region — *see* Laceration, abdomen, wall, epigastric region

Laceration — *continued*
- esophagus K22.8
  - traumatic
    - cervical S11.21 ☑
      - with foreign body S11.22 ☑
    - thoracic S27.813 ☑
- eye (ball) S05.3 ☑
  - with prolapse or loss of intraocular tissue S05.2 ☑
  - penetrating S05.6 ☑
- eyebrow — *see* Laceration, eyelid
- eyelid S01.11 ☑
  - with foreign body S01.12 ☑
- face NEC — *see* Laceration, head, specified site NEC
- fallopian tube S37.539 ☑
  - bilateral S37.532 ☑
  - unilateral S37.531 ☑
- finger (s) S61.219 ☑
  - with
    - damage to nail S61.319 ☑
      - with
        - foreign body S61.329 ☑
    - foreign body S61.229 ☑
  - index S61.218 ☑
    - with
      - damage to nail S61.318 ☑
        - with
          - foreign body S61.328 ☑
      - foreign body S61.228 ☑
    - left S61.211 ☑
      - with
        - damage to nail S61.311 ☑
          - with
            - foreign body S61.321 ☑
        - foreign body S61.221 ☑
    - right S61.210 ☑
      - with
        - damage to nail S61.310 ☑
          - with
            - foreign body S61.320 ☑
        - foreign body S61.220 ☑
  - little S61.218 ☑
    - with
      - damage to nail S61.318 ☑
        - with
          - foreign body S61.328 ☑
      - foreign body S61.228 ☑
    - left S61.217 ☑
      - with
        - damage to nail S61.317 ☑
          - with
            - foreign body S61.327 ☑
        - foreign body S61.227 ☑
    - right S61.216 ☑
      - with
        - damage to nail S61.316 ☑
          - with
            - foreign body S61.326 ☑
        - foreign body S61.226 ☑
  - middle S61.218 ☑
    - with
      - damage to nail S61.318 ☑
        - with
          - foreign body S61.328 ☑
      - foreign body S61.228 ☑
    - left S61.213 ☑
      - with
        - damage to nail S61.313 ☑
          - with
            - foreign body S61.323 ☑
        - foreign body S61.223 ☑
    - right S61.212 ☑
      - with
        - damage to nail S61.312 ☑
          - with
            - foreign body S61.322 ☑
        - foreign body S61.222 ☑
  - ring S61.218 ☑
    - with
      - damage to nail S61.318 ☑
        - with
          - foreign body S61.328 ☑
      - foreign body S61.228 ☑
    - left S61.215 ☑
      - with
        - damage to nail S61.315 ☑
          - with
            - foreign body S61.325 ☑
        - foreign body S61.225 ☑
    - right S61.214 ☑
      - with

Laceration — *continued*
- finger (s) — *continued*
  - damage to nail S61.314 ☑
    - with
      - foreign body S61.324 ☑
  - foreign body S61.224 ☑
- flank S31.119 ☑
  - with foreign body S31.129 ☑
- foot (except toe (s) alone) S91.319 ☑
  - with foreign body S91.329 ☑
  - left S91.312 ☑
    - with foreign body S91.322 ☑
  - right S91.311 ☑
    - with foreign body S91.321 ☑
  - toe — *see* Laceration, toe
- forearm S51.819 ☑
  - with
    - foreign body S51.829 ☑
  - elbow only — *see* Laceration, elbow
  - left S51.812 ☑
    - with
      - foreign body S51.822 ☑
  - right S51.811 ☑
    - with
      - foreign body S51.821 ☑
- forehead S01.81 ☑
  - with foreign body S01.82 ☑
- fourchette O70.0
  - with ectopic or molar pregnancy O08.6
  - complicating delivery O70.0
  - following ectopic or molar pregnancy O08.6
- gallbladder S36.123 ☑
- genital organs, external
  - female S31.512 ☑
    - with foreign body S31.522 ☑
    - vagina — *see* Laceration, vagina
    - vulva — *see* Laceration, vulva
  - male S31.511 ☑
    - with foreign body S31.521 ☑
    - penis — *see* Laceration, penis
    - scrotum — *see* Laceration, scrotum
    - testis — *see* Laceration, testis
- groin — *see* Laceration, abdomen, wall
- gum — *see* Laceration, oral cavity
- hand S61.419 ☑
  - with
    - foreign body S61.429 ☑
  - finger — *see* Laceration, finger
  - left S61.412 ☑
    - with
      - foreign body S61.422 ☑
  - right S61.411 ☑
    - with
      - foreign body S61.421 ☑
  - thumb — *see* Laceration, thumb
- head S01.91 ☑
  - with foreign body S01.92 ☑
  - cheek — *see* Laceration, cheek
  - ear — *see* Laceration, ear
  - eyelid — *see* Laceration, eyelid
  - lip — *see* Laceration, lip
  - nose — *see* Laceration, nose
  - oral cavity — *see* Laceration, oral cavity
  - scalp S01.01 ☑
    - with foreign body S01.02 ☑
  - specified site NEC S01.81 ☑
    - with foreign body S01.82 ☑
  - temporomandibular area — *see* Laceration, cheek
- heart — *see* Injury, heart, laceration
- heel — *see* Laceration, foot
- hepatic duct S36.13 ☑
- hip S71.019 ☑
  - with foreign body S71.029 ☑
  - left S71.012 ☑
    - with foreign body S71.022 ☑
  - right S71.011 ☑
    - with foreign body S71.021 ☑
- hymen — *see* Laceration, vagina
- hypochondrium — *see* Laceration, abdomen, wall
- hypogastric region — *see* Laceration, abdomen, wall
- ileum S36.438 ☑
- inguinal region — *see* Laceration, abdomen, wall
- instep — *see* Laceration, foot
- internal organ — *see* Injury, by site
- interscapular region — *see* Laceration, thorax, back
- intestine
  - large
    - colon S36.539 ☑
      - ascending S36.530 ☑

☑ **Additional character required**

Laceration — continued
  intestine — continued
        descending S36.532 ☑
        sigmoid S36.533 ☑
        specified site NEC S36.538 ☑
        rectum S36.63 ☑
        transverse S36.531 ☑
     small S36.439 ☑
        duodenum S36.430 ☑
        specified site NEC S36.438 ☑
  intra-abdominal organ S36.93 ☑
     intestine — see Laceration, intestine
     liver — see Laceration, liver
     pancreas — see Laceration, pancreas
     peritoneum S36.81 ☑
     specified site NEC S36.893 ☑
     spleen — see Laceration, spleen
     stomach — see Laceration, stomach
  intracranial NEC (see also Injury, intracranial, diffuse)
     birth injury P10.9
  jaw — see Laceration, head, specified site NEC
  jejunum S36.438 ☑
  joint capsule — see Sprain, by site
  kidney S37.03 ☑
     major (greater than 3 cm) (massive) (stellate) S37.06 ☑
     minor (less than 1 cm) S37.04 ☑
     moderate (1 to 3 cm) S37.05 ☑
     multiple S37.06 ☑
  knee S81.01 ☑
     with foreign body S81.02 ☑
  labium (majus) (minus) — see Laceration, vulva
  lacrimal duct — see Laceration, eyelid
  large intestine — see Laceration, intestine, large
  larynx S11.011 ☑
     with foreign body S11.012 ☑
  leg (lower) S81.819 ☑
     with foreign body S81.829 ☑
     foot — see Laceration, foot
     knee — see Laceration, knee
     left S81.812 ☑
        with foreign body S81.822 ☑
     right S81.811 ☑
        with foreign body S81.821 ☑
     upper — see Laceration, thigh
  ligament — see Sprain
  lip S01.511 ☑
     with foreign body S01.521 ☑
  liver S36.113 ☑
     major (stellate) S36.116 ☑
     minor S36.114 ☑
     moderate S36.115 ☑
  loin — see Laceration, abdomen, wall
  lower back — see Laceration, back, lower
  lumbar region — see Laceration, back, lower
  lung S27.339 ☑
     bilateral S27.332 ☑
     unilateral S27.331 ☑
  malar region — see Laceration, head, specified site NEC
  mammary — see Laceration, breast
  mastoid region — see Laceration, head, specified site NEC
  meninges — see Injury, intracranial, diffuse
  meniscus — see Tear, meniscus
  mesentery S36.893 ☑
  mesosalpinx S37.893 ☑
  mouth — see Laceration, oral cavity
  muscle — see Injury, muscle, by site, laceration
  nail
     finger — see Laceration, finger, with damage to nail
     toe — see Laceration, toe, with damage to nail
  nasal (septum) (sinus) — see Laceration, nose
  nasopharynx — see Laceration, head, specified site NEC
  neck S11.91 ☑
     with foreign body S11.92 ☑
     involving
        cervical esophagus S11.21 ☑
           with foreign body S11.22 ☑
        larynx — see Laceration, larynx
        pharynx — see Laceration, pharynx
        thyroid gland — see Laceration, thyroid gland
        trachea — see Laceration, trachea
     specified site NEC S11.81 ☑
        with foreign body S11.82 ☑
  nerve — see Injury, nerve
  nose (septum) (sinus) S01.21 ☑
     with foreign body S01.22 ☑

Laceration — continued
  ocular NOS S05.3 ☑
     adnexa NOS S01.11 ☑
  oral cavity S01.512 ☑
     with foreign body S01.522 ☑
  orbit (eye) — see Wound, open, ocular, orbit
  ovary S37.439 ☑
     bilateral S37.432 ☑
     unilateral S37.431 ☑
  palate — see Laceration, oral cavity
  palm — see Laceration, hand
  pancreas S36.239 ☑
     body S36.231 ☑
        major S36.261 ☑
        minor S36.241 ☑
        moderate S36.251 ☑
     head S36.230 ☑
        major S36.260 ☑
        minor S36.240 ☑
        moderate S36.250 ☑
     major S36.269 ☑
     minor S36.249 ☑
     moderate S36.259 ☑
     tail S36.232 ☑
        major S36.262 ☑
        minor S36.242 ☑
        moderate S36.252 ☑
  pelvic S31.010 ☑
     with
        foreign body S31.020 ☑
           penetration into retroperitoneal cavity S31.021 ☑
        penetration into retroperitoneal cavity S31.011 ☑
     floor (see also Laceration, back, lower)
        with ectopic or molar pregnancy O08.6
        complicating delivery O70.1
        following ectopic or molar pregnancy O08.6
        old (postpartal) N81.89
     organ S37.93 ☑
        with ectopic or molar pregnancy O08.6
        adrenal gland S37.813 ☑
        bladder S37.23 ☑
        fallopian tube — see Laceration, fallopian tube
        following ectopic or molar pregnancy O08.6
        kidney — see Laceration, kidney
        obstetrical trauma O71.5
        ovary — see Laceration, ovary
        prostate S37.823 ☑
        specified site NEC S37.893 ☑
        ureter S37.13 ☑
        urethra S37.33 ☑
        uterus S37.63 ☑
  penis S31.21 ☑
     with foreign body S31.22 ☑
  perineum
     female S31.41 ☑
        with
           ectopic or molar pregnancy O08.6
           foreign body S31.42 ☑
        during delivery O70.9
           first degree O70.0
           fourth degree O70.3
           second degree O70.1
           third degree (see also Delivery, complicated, by, laceration, perineum, third degree) O70.20
        old (postpartal) N81.89
        postpartal N81.89
        secondary (postpartal) O90.1
     male S31.119 ☑
        with foreign body S31.129 ☑
  periocular area (with or without lacrimal passages) — see Laceration, eyelid
  peritoneum S36.893 ☑
  periumbilic region — see Laceration, abdomen, wall, periumbilic
  periurethral tissue — see Laceration, urethra
  phalanges
     finger — see Laceration, finger
     toe — see Laceration, toe
  pharynx S11.21 ☑
     with foreign body S11.22 ☑
  pinna — see Laceration, ear
  popliteal space — see Laceration, knee
  prepuce — see Laceration, penis
  prostate S37.823 ☑
  pubic region S31.119 ☑
     with foreign body S31.129 ☑
  pudendum — see Laceration, genital organs, external

Laceration — continued
  rectovaginal septum — see Laceration, vagina
  rectum S36.63 ☑
  retroperitoneum S36.893 ☑
  round ligament S37.893 ☑
  sacral region — see Laceration, back, lower
  sacroiliac region — see Laceration, back, lower
  salivary gland — see Laceration, oral cavity
  scalp S01.01 ☑
     with foreign body S01.02 ☑
  scapular region — see Laceration, shoulder
  scrotum S31.31 ☑
     with foreign body S31.32 ☑
  seminal vesicle S37.893 ☑
  shin — see Laceration, leg
  shoulder S41.019 ☑
     with foreign body S41.029 ☑
     left S41.012 ☑
        with foreign body S41.022 ☑
     right S41.011 ☑
        with foreign body S41.021 ☑
  small intestine — see Laceration, intestine, small
  spermatic cord — see Laceration, testis
  spinal cord (meninges) (see also Injury, spinal cord, by region)
     due to injury at birth P11.5
     newborn (birth injury) P11.5
  spleen S36.039 ☑
     major (massive) (stellate) S36.032 ☑
     moderate S36.031 ☑
     superficial (minor) S36.030 ☑
  sternal region — see Laceration, thorax, front
  stomach S36.33 ☑
  submaxillary region — see Laceration, head, specified site NEC
  submental region — see Laceration, head, specified site NEC
  subungual
     finger (s) — see Laceration, finger, with damage to nail
     toe (s) — see Laceration, toe, with damage to nail
  suprarenal gland — see Laceration, adrenal gland
  temple, temporal region — see Laceration, head, specified site NEC
  temporomandibular area — see Laceration, cheek
  tendon — see Injury, muscle, by site, laceration
     Achilles S86.02 ☑
  tentorium cerebelli — see Injury, intracranial, diffuse
  testis S31.31 ☑
     with foreign body S31.32 ☑
  thigh S71.11 ☑
     with foreign body S71.12 ☑
  thorax, thoracic (wall) S21.91 ☑
     with foreign body S21.92 ☑
        back S21.22 ☑
           with penetration into thoracic cavity S21.42 ☑
        front S21.12 ☑
           with penetration into thoracic cavity S21.32 ☑
     back S21.21 ☑
        with
           foreign body S21.22 ☑
              with penetration into thoracic cavity S21.42 ☑
           penetration into thoracic cavity S21.41 ☑
     breast — see Laceration, breast
     front S21.11 ☑
        with
           foreign body S21.12 ☑
              with penetration into thoracic cavity S21.32 ☑
           penetration into thoracic cavity S21.31 ☑
  thumb S61.019 ☑
     with
        damage to nail S61.119 ☑
           with
              foreign body S61.129 ☑
        foreign body S61.029 ☑
     left S61.012 ☑
        with
           damage to nail S61.112 ☑
              with
                 foreign body S61.122 ☑
           foreign body S61.022 ☑
     right S61.011 ☑
        with
           damage to nail S61.111 ☑
              with
                 foreign body S61.121 ☑

Laceration — *continued*
  thumb — *continued*
      foreign body S61.021 ☑
  thyroid gland S11.11 ☑
    with foreign body S11.12 ☑
  toe (s) S91.119 ☑
    with
      damage to nail S91.219 ☑
        with
          foreign body S91.229 ☑
      foreign body S91.129 ☑
    great S91.113 ☑
      with
        damage to nail S91.213 ☑
          with
            foreign body S91.223 ☑
        foreign body S91.123 ☑
    left S91.112 ☑
      with
        damage to nail S91.212 ☑
          with
            foreign body S91.222 ☑
        foreign body S91.122 ☑
    right S91.111 ☑
      with
        damage to nail S91.211 ☑
          with
            foreign body S91.221 ☑
        foreign body S91.121 ☑
    lesser S91.116 ☑
      with
        damage to nail S91.216 ☑
          with
            foreign body S91.226 ☑
        foreign body S91.126 ☑
    left S91.115 ☑
      with
        damage to nail S91.215 ☑
          with
            foreign body S91.225 ☑
        foreign body S91.125 ☑
    right S91.114 ☑
      with
        damage to nail S91.214 ☑
          with
            foreign body S91.224 ☑
        foreign body S91.124 ☑
  tongue — *see* Laceration, oral cavity
  trachea S11.021 ☑
    with foreign body S11.022 ☑
  tunica vaginalis — *see* Laceration, testis
  tympanum, tympanic membrane — *see*
    Laceration, ear, drum
  umbilical region S31.115 ☑
    with foreign body S31.125 ☑
  ureter S37.13 ☑
  urethra S37.33 ☑
    with or following ectopic or molar
      pregnancy O08.6
    obstetrical trauma O71.5
  urinary organ NEC S37.893 ☑
  uterus S37.63 ☑
    with ectopic or molar pregnancy O08.6
    following ectopic or molar pregnancy O08.6
    nonpuerperal, nontraumatic N85.8
    obstetrical trauma NEC O71.81
    old (postpartal) N85.8
  uvula — *see* Laceration, oral cavity
  vagina S31.41 ☑
    with
      ectopic or molar pregnancy O08.6
      foreign body S31.42 ☑
    during delivery O71.4
      with perineal laceration — *see* Laceration,
        perineum, female, during delivery
    following ectopic or molar pregnancy O08.6
    nonpuerperal, nontraumatic N89.8
    old (postpartal) N89.8
  vas deferens S37.893 ☑
  vesical — *see* Laceration, bladder
  vocal cords S11.031 ☑
    with foreign body S11.032 ☑
  vulva S31.41 ☑
    with
      ectopic or molar pregnancy O08.6
      foreign body S31.42 ☑
    complicating delivery O70.0
    following ectopic or molar pregnancy O08.6
    nonpuerperal, nontraumatic N90.89
    old (postpartal) N90.89
  wrist S61.519 ☑
    with

Laceration — *continued*
  wrist — *continued*
      foreign body S61.529 ☑
    left S61.512 ☑
      with
        foreign body S61.522 ☑
    right S61.511 ☑
      with
        foreign body S61.521 ☑
Lack of
  achievement in school Z55.3
  adequate
    food Z59.4
    intermaxillary vertical dimension of fully
      erupted teeth M26.36
    sleep Z72.820
  appetite (*see* Anorexia) R63.0
  awareness R41.9
  care
    in home Z74.2
    of infant (at or after birth) T76.02 ☑
      confirmed T74.02 ☑
  cognitive functions R41.9
  coordination R27.9
    ataxia R27.0
    specified type NEC R27.8
  development (physiological) R62.50
    failure to thrive (child over 28 days old) R62.51
      adult R62.7
      newborn P92.6
    short stature R62.52
    specified type NEC R62.59
  energy R53.83
  financial resources Z59.6
  food T73.0 ☑
  growth R62.52
  heating Z59.1
  housing (permanent) (temporary) Z59.0
    adequate Z59.1
  learning experiences in childhood Z62.898
  leisure time (affecting life-style) Z73.2
  material resources Z59.9
  memory (*see also* Amnesia)
    mild, following organic brain damage F06.8
  ovulation N97.0
  parental supervision or control of child Z62.0
  person able to render necessary care Z74.2
  physical exercise Z72.3
  play experience in childhood Z62.898
  posterior occlusal support M26.57
  relaxation (affecting life-style) Z73.2
  sexual
    desire F52.0
    enjoyment F52.1
  shelter Z59.0
  sleep (adequate) Z72.820
  supervision of child by parent Z62.0
  support, posterior occlusal M26.57
  water T73.1 ☑
Lacrimal — *see* condition
Lacrimation, abnormal — *see* Epiphora
Lacrimonasal duct — *see* condition
Lactation, lactating (breast) (puerperal, postpartum)
  associated
    cracked nipple O92.13
    retracted nipple O92.03
  defective O92.4
  disorder NEC O92.79
  excessive O92.6
  failed (complete) O92.3
    partial O92.4
  mastitis NEC — *see* Mastitis, obstetric
  mother (care and/or examination) Z39.1
  nonpuerperal N64.3
Lacticemia, excessive E87.2
Lacunar skull Q75.8
Laennec's cirrhosis K70.30
  with ascites K70.31
  nonalcoholic K74.69
Lafora's disease — *see* Epilepsy, generalized,
  idiopathic
Lag, lid (nervous) — *see* Retraction, lid
Lagophthalmos (eyelid) (nervous) H02.209
  cicatricial H02.219
    left H02.216
      lower H02.215
      upper H02.214
    right H02.213
      lower H02.212
      upper H02.211
  keratoconjunctivitis — *see* Keratoconjunctivitis

Lagophthalmos — *continued*
  left H02.206
    lower H02.205
    upper H02.204
  mechanical H02.229
    left H02.226
      lower H02.225
      upper H02.224
    right H02.223
      lower H02.222
      upper H02.221
  paralytic H02.239
    left H02.236
      lower H02.235
      upper H02.234
    right H02.233
      lower H02.232
      upper H02.231
  right H02.203
    lower H02.202
    upper H02.201
Laki-Lorand factor deficiency — *see* Defect,
  coagulation, specified type NEC
Lalling F80.0
Lambert-Eaton syndrome — *see* Syndrome,
  Lambert-Eaton
Lambliasis, lambliosis A07.1
Landau-Kleffner syndrome — *see* Epilepsy, specified
  NEC
Landouzy-Déjérine dystrophy or
  facioscapulohumeral atrophy G71.0
Landouzy's disease (icterohemorrhagic
  leptospirosis) A27.0
Landry-Guillain-Barré, syndrome or paralysis G61.0
Landry's disease or paralysis G61.0
Lane's
  band Q43.3
  kink — *see* Obstruction, intestine
  syndrome K90.2
Langdon Down syndrome — *see* Trisomy, 21
Lapsed immunization schedule status Z28.3
Large
  baby (regardless of gestational age) (4000g to
    4499g) P08.1
  ear, congenital Q17.1
  physiological cup Q14.2
  stature R68.89
Large-for-dates NEC (infant) (4000g to 4499g) P08.1
  affecting management of pregnancy O36.6 ☑
  exceptionally (4500g or more) P08.0
Larsen-Johansson disease orosteochondrosis — *see*
  Osteochondrosis, juvenile, patella
Larsen's syndrome (flattened facies and multiple
  congenital dislocations) Q74.8
Larva migrans
  cutaneous B76.9
    Ancylostoma B76.0
  visceral B83.0
Laryngeal — *see* condition
Laryngismus (stridulus) J38.5
  congenital P28.89
  diphtheritic A36.2
Laryngitis (acute) (edematous) (fibrinous)
  (infective) (infiltrative) (malignant)
  (membranous) (phlegmonous) (pneumococcal)
  (pseudomembranous) (septic) (subglottic)
  (suppurative) (ulcerative) J04.0
  with
    influenza, flu, or grippe — *see* Influenza, with,
      laryngitis
    tracheitis (acute) — *see* Laryngotracheitis
  atrophic J37.0
  catarrhal J37.0
  chronic J37.0
    with tracheitis (chronic) J37.1
  diphtheritic A36.2
  due to external agent — *see* Inflammation,
    respiratory, upper, due to
  Hemophilus influenzae J04.0
  H. influenzae J04.0
  hypertrophic J37.0
  influenzal — *see* Influenza, with, respiratory
    manifestations NEC
  obstructive J05.0
  sicca J37.0
  spasmodic J05.0
    acute J04.0
  streptococcal J04.0
  stridulous J05.0
  syphilitic (late) A52.73
    congenital A50.59 *[J99]*
    early A50.03 *[J99]*

☑ **Additional character required**

Laryngitis — *continued*
 tuberculous A15.5
 Vincent's A69.1
Laryngocele (congenital) (ventricular) Q31.3
Laryngofissure J38.7
 congenital Q31.8
Laryngomalacia (congenital) Q31.5
Laryngopharyngitis (acute) J06.0
 chronic J37.0
 due to external agent — *see* Inflammation,
  respiratory, upper, due to
Laryngoplegia J38.00
 bilateral J38.02
 unilateral J38.01
Laryngoptosis J38.7
Laryngospasm J38.5
Laryngostenosis J38.6
Laryngotracheitis (acute) (Infectional) (infective)
 (viral) J04.2
 atrophic J37.1
 catarrhal J37.1
 chronic J37.1
 diphtheritic A36.2
 due to external agent — *see* Inflammation,
  respiratory, upper, due to
 Hemophilus influenzae J04.2
 hypertrophic J37.1
 influenzal — *see* Influenza, with, respiratory
  manifestations NEC
 pachydermic J38.7
 sicca J37.1
 spasmodic J38.5
  acute J05.0
 streptococcal J04.2
 stridulous J38.5
 syphilitic (late) A52.73
  congenital A50.59 [J99]
   early A50.03 [J99]
 tuberculous A15.5
 Vincent's A69.1
Laryngotracheobronchitis — *see* Bronchitis
Larynx, laryngeal — *see* condition
Lassa fever A96.2
Lassitude — *see* Weakness
Late
 talker R62.0
 walker R62.0
Late effect (s) — *see* Sequelae
Latent — *see* condition
Laterocession — *see* Lateroversion
Lateroflexion — *see* Lateroversion
Lateroversion
 cervix — *see* Lateroversion, uterus
 uterus, uterine (cervix) (postinfectional)
  (postpartal, old) N85.4
  congenital Q51.818
  in pregnancy or childbirth O34.59 ☑
Lathyrism — *see* Poisoning, food, noxious, plant
Launois' syndrome (pituitary gigantism) E22.0
Launois-Bensaude adenolipomatosis E88.89
Laurence-Moon (-Bardet)-Biedl syndrome Q87.89
Lax, laxity (*see also* Relaxation)
 ligament (ous) (*see also* Disorder, ligament)
  familial M35.7
  knee — *see* Derangement, knee
 skin (acquired) L57.4
  congenital Q82.8
Laxative habit F55.2
Lazy leukocyte syndrome D70.8
Lead miner's lung J63.6
Leak, leakage
 air NEC J93.82
  postprocedural J95.812
 amniotic fluid — *see* Rupture, membranes,
  premature
 blood (microscopic), fetal, into maternal
  circulation affecting management of
  pregnancy — *see* Pregnancy, complicated by
 cerebrospinal fluid G96.0
  from spinal (lumbar) puncture G97.0
 device, implant or graft (*see also* Complications,
  by site and type, mechanical)
  arterial graft NEC — *see* Complication,
   cardiovascular device, mechanical, vascular
  breast (implant) T85.43 ☑
  catheter NEC T85.638 ☑
   urinary T83.038 ☑
    cystostomy T83.030 ☑
    Hopkins T83.038 ☑
    ileostomy T83.038 ☑
    indwelling T83.031 ☑
    nephrostomy T83.032 ☑

Leak — *continued*
 device — *continued*
   specified NEC T83.038 ☑
   urostomy T83.038 ☑
  dialysis (renal) T82.43 ☑
   intraperitoneal T85.631 ☑
  infusion NEC T82.534 ☑
   spinal (epidural) (subdural) T85.630 ☑
  gastrointestinal — *see* Complications,
   prosthetic device, mechanical,
   gastrointestinal device
  genital NEC T83.498 ☑
   penile prosthesis (cylinder) (implanted)
    (pump) (reservoir) T83.490 ☑
   testicular prosthesis T83.491 ☑
  heart NEC — *see* Complication, cardiovascular
   device, mechanical
  joint prosthesis — *see* Complications, joint
   prosthesis, mechanical, specified NEC, by
   site
  ocular NEC — *see* Complications, prosthetic
   device, mechanical, ocular device
  orthopedic NEC — *see* Complication,
   orthopedic, device, mechanical
  persistent air J93.82
  specified NEC T85.638 ☑
  urinary NEC (*see also* Complication,
   genitourinary, device, urinary, mechanical)
   graft T83.23 ☑
  vascular NEC — *see* Complication,
   cardiovascular device, mechanical
  ventricular intracranial shunt T85.03 ☑
 urine — *see* Incontinence
Leaky heart — *see* Endocarditis
Learning defect (specific) F81.9
Leather bottle stomach C16.9
Leber's
 congenital amaurosis H35.50
 optic atrophy (hereditary) H47.22
Lederer's anemia D59.1
Leeches (external) — *see* Hirudiniasis
Leg — *see* condition
Legg (-Calvé)-Perthes disease, syndrome or
 osteochondrosis M91.1 ☑
Legionellosis A48.1
 nonpneumonic A48.2
Legionnaires'
 disease A48.1
  nonpneumonic A48.2
 pneumonia A48.1
Leigh's disease G31.82
Leiner's disease L21.1
Leiofibromyoma — *see* Leiomyoma
Leiomyoblastoma — *see* Neoplasm, connective
 tissue, benign
Leiomyofibroma (*see also* Neoplasm, connective
 tissue, benign)
 uterus (cervix) (corpus) D25.9
Leiomyoma (*see also* Neoplasm, connective tissue,
 benign)
 bizarre — *see* Neoplasm, connective tissue,
  benign
 cellular — *see* Neoplasm, connective tissue,
  benign
 epithelioid — *see* Neoplasm, connective tissue,
  benign
 uterus (cervix) (corpus) D25.9
  intramural D25.1
  submucous D25.0
  subserosal D25.2
 vascular — *see* Neoplasm, connective tissue,
  benign
Leiomyoma, leiomyomatosis (intravascular) — *see*
 Neoplasm, connective tissue, uncertain behavior
Leiomyosarcoma (*see also* Neoplasm, connective
 tissue, malignant)
 epithelioid — *see* Neoplasm, connective tissue,
  malignant
 myxoid — *see* Neoplasm, connective tissue,
  malignant
Leishmaniasis B55.9
 American (mucocutaneous) B55.2
  cutaneous B55.1
 Asian Desert B55.1
 Brazilian B55.2
 cutaneous (any type) B55.1
 dermal (*see also* Leishmaniasis, cutaneous)
  post-kala-azar B55.0
 eyelid B55.1
 infantile B55.0
 Mediterranean B55.0
 mucocutaneous (American) (New World) B55.2

Leishmaniasis — *continued*
 naso-oral B55.2
 nasopharyngeal B55.2
 old world B55.1
 tegumentaria diffusa B55.1
 visceral B55.0
Leishmanoid, dermal (*see also* Leishmaniasis,
 cutaneous)
 post-kala-azar B55.0
Lenegre's disease I44.2
Lengthening, leg — *see* Deformity, limb, unequal
 length
Lennert's lymphoma — *see* Lymphoma, Lennert's
Lennox-Gastaut syndrome G40.812
 intractable G40.814
  with status epilepticus G40.813
  without status epilepticus G40.814
 not intractable G40.812
  with status epilepticus G40.811
  without status epilepticus G40.812
Lens — *see* condition
Lenticonus (anterior) (posterior) (congenital) Q12.8
Lenticular degeneration, progressive E83.01
Lentiglobus (posterior) (congenital) Q12.8
Lentigo (congenital) L81.4
 maligna (*see also* Melanoma, in situ)
  melanoma — *see* Melanoma
Lentivirus, as cause of disease classified elsewhere
 B97.31
Leontiasis
 ossium M85.2
 syphilitic (late) A52.78
  congenital A50.59
Lepothrix A48.8
Lepra — *see* Leprosy
Leprechaunism E34.8
Leprosy A30. ☑
 with muscle disorder A30.9 [M63.80]
  ankle A30.9 [M63.87 ☑]
  foot A30.9 [M63.87 ☑]
  forearm A30.9 [M63.83 ☑]
  hand A30.9 [M63.84 ☑]
  lower leg A30.9 [M63.86 ☑]
  multiple sites A30.9 [M63.89]
  pelvic region A30.9 [M63.85 ☑]
  shoulder region A30.9 [M63.81 ☑]
  specified site NEC A30.9 [M63.88]
  thigh A30.9 [M63.85 ☑]
  upper arm A30.9 [M63.82 ☑]
 anesthetic A30.9
 BB A30.3
 BL A30.4
 borderline (infiltrated) (neuritic) A30.3
  lepromatous A30.4
  tuberculoid A30.2
 BT A30.2
 dimorphous (infiltrated) (neuritic) A30.3
 I A30.0
 indeterminate (macular) (neuritic) A30.0
 lepromatous (diffuse) (infiltrated) (macular)
  (neuritic) (nodular) A30.5
 LL A30.5
 macular (early) (neuritic) (simple) A30.9
 maculoanesthetic A30.9
 mixed A30.3
 neural A30.9
 nodular A30.5
 primary neuritic A30.3
 specified type NEC A30.8
 TT A30.1
 tuberculoid (major) (minor) A30.1
Leptocytosis, hereditary D56.9
Leptomeningitis (chronic) (circumscribed)
 (hemorrhagic) (nonsuppurative) — *see* Meningitis
Leptomeningopathy G96.19
Leptospiral — *see* condition
Leptospirochetal — *see* condition
Leptospirosis A27.9
 canicola A27.89
 due to Leptospira interrogans serovar
  icterohaemorrhagiae A27.0
 icterohemorrhagica A27.0
 pomona A27.89
 Weil's disease A27.0
Leptus dermatitis B88.0
Leriche's syndrome (aortic bifurcation occlusion)
 I74.09
Leri's pleonosteosis Q78.8
Leri-Weill syndrome Q77.8
Lermoyez' syndrome — *see* Vertigo, peripheral NEC
Lesch-Nyhan syndrome E79.1
Leser-Trélat disease L82.1
 inflamed L82.0

Lesion (s) (nontraumatic)
 abducens nerve — *see* Strabismus, paralytic, sixth
  nerve
 alveolar process K08.9
 angiocentric immunoproliferative D47.Z9
 anorectal K62.9
 aortic (valve) I35.9
 auditory nerve — *see* subcategory H93.3
 basal ganglion G25.9
 bile duct — *see* Disease, bile duct
 biomechanical M99.9
  specified type NEC M99.89
   abdomen M99.89
   acromioclavicular M99.87
   cervical region M99.81
   cervicothoracic M99.81
   costochondral M99.88
   costovertebral M99.88
   head region M99.80
   hip M99.85
   lower extremity M99.86
   lumbar region M99.83
   lumbosacral M99.83
   occipitocervical M99.80
   pelvic region M99.85
   pubic M99.85
   rib cage M99.88
   sacral region M99.84
   sacrococcygeal M99.84
   sacroiliac M99.84
   specified NEC M99.89
   sternochondral M99.88
   sternoclavicular M99.87
   thoracic region M99.82
   thoracolumbar M99.82
   upper extremity M99.87
 bladder N32.9
 bone — *see* Disorder, bone
 brachial plexus G54.0
 brain G93.9
  congenital Q04.9
  vascular I67.9
   degenerative I67.9
   hypertensive I67.4
 buccal cavity K13.79
 calcified — *see* Calcification
 canthus — *see* Disorder, eyelid
 carate — *see* Pinta, lesions
 cardia K31.9
 cardiac (*see also* Disease, heart) I51.9
  congenital Q24.9
  valvular — *see* Endocarditis
 cauda equina G83.4
 cecum K63.9
 cerebral — *see* Lesion, brain
 cerebrovascular I67.9
  degenerative I67.9
  hypertensive I67.4
 cervical (nerve) root NEC G54.2
 chiasmal — *see* Disorder, optic, chiasm
 chorda tympani G51.8
 coin, lung R91.1
 colon K63.9
 combined periodontic - endodontic K05.5
 congenital — *see* Anomaly, by site
 conjunctiva H11.9
 conus medullaris — *see* Injury, conus medullaris
 coronary artery — *see* Ischemia, heart
 cranial nerve G52.9
  eighth — *see* Disorder, ear
  eleventh G52.8
  fifth G50.9
  first G52.0
  fourth — *see* Strabismus, paralytic, fourth nerve
  seventh G51.9
  sixth — *see* Strabismus, paralytic, sixth nerve
  tenth G52.2
  twelfth G52.3
 cystic — *see* Cyst
 degenerative — *see* Degeneration
 duodenum K31.9
 edentulous (alveolar) ridge, associated with
  trauma, due to traumatic occlusion K06.2
 en coup de sabre L94.1
 eyelid — *see* Disorder, eyelid
 gasserian ganglion G50.8
 gastric K31.9
 gastroduodenal K31.9
 gastrointestinal K63.9
 gingiva, associated with trauma K06.2
 glomerular
  focal and segmental (*see also* N00-N07 with
   fourth character .1) N05.1

Lesion (s) — *continued*
 glomerular — *continued*
  minimal change (*see also* N00-N07 with fourth
   character .0) N05.0
 heart (organic) — *see* Disease, heart
 hyperchromic, due to pinta (carate) A67.1
 hyperkeratotic — *see* Hyperkeratosis
 hypothalamic E23.7
 ileocecal K63.9
 ileum K63.9
 iliohypogastric nerve G57.8 ☑
 inflammatory — *see* Inflammation
 intestine K63.9
 intracerebral — *see* Lesion, brain
 intrachiasmal (optic) — *see* Disorder, optic,
  chiasm
 intracranial, space-occupying R90.0
 joint — *see* Disorder, joint
  sacroiliac (old) M53.3
 keratotic — *see* Keratosis
 kidney — *see* Disease, renal
 laryngeal nerve (recurrent) G52.2
 lip K13.0
 liver K76.9
 lumbosacral
  plexus G54.1
  root (nerve) NEC G54.4
 lung (coin) R91.1
 maxillary sinus J32.0
 mitral I05.9
 Morel-Lavallée — *see* Hematoma, by site
 motor cortex NEC G93.89
 mouth K13.79
 nerve G58.9
  femoral G57.2 ☑
  median G56.1 ☑
   carpal tunnel syndrome — *see* Syndrome,
    carpal tunnel
  plantar G57.6 ☑
  popliteal (lateral) G57.3 ☑
   medial G57.4 ☑
  radial G56.3 ☑
  sciatic G57.0 ☑
  spinal — *see* Injury, nerve, spinal
  ulnar G56.2 ☑
 nervous system, congenital Q07.9
 nonallopathic — *see* Lesion, biomechanical
 nose (internal) J34.89
 obstructive — *see* Obstruction
 obturator nerve G57.8 ☑
 oral mucosa K13.70
 organ or site NEC — *see* Disease, by site
 osteolytic — *see* Osteolysis
 peptic K27.9
 periodontal, due to traumatic occlusion K05.5
 pharynx J39.2
 pigment, pigmented (skin) L81.9
 pinta — *see* Pinta, lesions
 polypoid — *see* Polyp
 prechiasmal (optic) — *see* Disorder, optic, chiasm
 primary (*see also* Syphilis, primary) A51.0
  carate A67.0
  pinta A67.0
  yaws A66.0
 pulmonary J98.4
  valve I37.9
 pylorus K31.9
 rectosigmoid K63.9
 retina, retinal H35.9
 sacroiliac (joint) (old) M53.3
 salivary gland K11.9
  benign lymphoepithelial K11.8
 saphenous nerve G57.8 ☑
 sciatic nerve G57.0 ☑
 secondary — *see* Syphilis, secondary
 shoulder (region) M75.9 ☑
  specified NEC M75.8 ☑
 sigmoid K63.9
 sinus (accessory) (nasal) J34.89
 skin L98.9
  suppurative L08.0
 SLAP S43.43 ☑
 spinal cord G95.9
  congenital Q06.9
 spleen D73.89
 stomach K31.9
 superior glenoid labrum S43.43 ☑
 syphilitic — *see* Syphilis

Lesion (s) — *continued*
 tertiary — *see* Syphilis, tertiary
 thoracic root (nerve) NEC G54.3
 tonsillar fossa J35.9
 tooth, teeth K08.9
  white spot
   chewing surface K02.51
   pit and fissure surface K02.51
   smooth surface K02.61
 traumatic — *see* specific type of injury by site
 tricuspid (valve) I07.9
  nonrheumatic I36.9
 trigeminal nerve G50.9
 ulcerated or ulcerative — *see* Ulcer, skin
 uterus N85.9
 vagus nerve G52.2
 valvular — *see* Endocarditis
 vascular I99.9
  affecting central nervous system I67.9
  following trauma NEC T14.8 ☑
  umbilical cord, complicating delivery O69.5 ☑
 warty — *see* Verruca
 white spot (tooth)
  chewing surface K02.51
  pit and fissure surface K02.51
  smooth surface K02.61
Lethargic — *see* condition
Lethargy R53.83
Letterer-Siwe's disease C96.0
Leukemia, leukemic C95.9 ☑
 acute basophilic C94.8 ☑
 acute bilineal C95.0 ☑
 acute erythroid C94.0 ☑
 acute lymphoblastic C91.0 ☑
 acute megakaryoblastic C94.2 ☑
 acute megakaryocytic C94.2 ☑
 acute mixed lineage C95.0 ☑
 acute monoblastic (monoblastic/
  monocytic) C93.0 ☑
 acute monocytic (monoblastic/
  monocytic) C93.0 ☑
 acute myeloblastic (minimal differentiation) (with
  maturation) C92.0 ☑
 acute myeloid
  with
   11q23-abnormality C92.6 ☑
   dysplasia of remaining hematopoesis
    and/or myelodysplastic disease in its
    history C92.A ☑
   multilineage dysplasia C92.A ☑
   variation of MLL-gene C92.6 ☑
  M6 (a) (b) C94.0 ☑
  M7 C94.2 ☑
 acute myelomonocytic C92.5 ☑
 acute promyelocytic C92.4 ☑
 adult T-cell (HTLV-1-associated) (acute variant)
  (chronic variant) (lymphomatoid variant)
  (smouldering variant) C91.5 ☑
 aggressive NK-cell C94.8 ☑
 AML (1/ETO) (M0) (M1) (M2) (without a FAB
  classification) C92.0 ☑
 AML M3 C92.4 ☑
 AML M4 (Eo with inv(16) or t(16;16)) C92.5 ☑
 AML M5 C93.0 ☑
 AML M5a C93.0 ☑
 AML M5b C93.0 ☑
 AML Me with t (15;17) and variants C92.4 ☑
 atypical chronic myeloid, BCR/ABL-
  negative C92.2 ☑
 biphenotypic acute C95.0 ☑
 blast cell C95.0 ☑
 Burkitt-type, mature B-cell C91.A ☑
 chronic lymphocytic, of B-cell type C91.1 ☑
 chronic monocytic C93.1 ☑
 chronic myelogenous (Philadelphia chromosome
  (Ph1) positive) (t(9;22)) (q34;q11) (with crisis
  of blast cells) C92.1 ☑
 chronic myeloid, BCR/ABL-positive C92.1 ☑
  atypical, BCR/ABL-negative C92.2 ☑
 chronic myelomonocytic C93.1 ☑
 chronic neutrophilic D47.1
 CMML (-1) (-2) (with eosinophilia) C93.1 ☑
 granulocytic (*see also* Category C92) C92.9 ☑
 hairy cell C91.4 ☑
 juvenile myelomonocytic C93.3 ☑
 lymphoid C91.9 ☑
  specified NEC C91.Z ☑
 mast cell C94.3 ☑
 mature B-cell, Burkitt-type C91.A ☑
 monocytic (subacute) C93.9 ☑
  specified NEC C93.Z ☑
 myelogenous (*see also* Category C92) C92.9 ☑

☑ **Additional character required**

Leukemia — *continued*
  myeloid C92.9 ☑
    specified NEC C92.Z ☑
  plasma cell C90.1 ☑
  plasmacytic C90.1 ☑
  prolymphocytic
    of B-cell type C91.3 ☑
    of T-cell type C91.6 ☑
  specified NEC C94.8 ☑
  stem cell, of unclear lineage C95.0 ☑
  subacute lymphocytic C91.9 ☑
  T-cell large granular lymphocytic C91.Z ☑
  unspecified cell type C95.9 ☑
    acute C95.0 ☑
    chronic C95.1 ☑
Leukemoid reaction (*see also* Reaction, leukemoid)
    D72.823
Leukoaraiosis (hypertensive) I67.81
Leukoariosis — *see* Leukoaraiosis
Leukocoria — *see* Disorder, globe, degenerated
    condition, leucocoria
Leukocytopenia D72.819
Leukocytosis D72.829
    eosinophilic D72.1
Leukoderma, leukodermia NEC L81.5
    syphilitic A51.39
      late A52.79
Leukodystrophy E75.29
Leukoedema, oral epithelium K13.29
Leukoencephalitis G04.81
    acute (subacute) hemorrhagic G36.1
      postimmunization or postvaccinal G04.02
    postinfectious G04.01
    subacute sclerosing A81.1
    van Bogaert's (sclerosing) A81.1
Leukoencephalopathy (*see also* Encephalopathy)
    G93.49
    Binswanger's I67.3
    heroin vapor G92
    metachromatic E75.25
    multifocal (progressive) A81.2
    postimmunization and postvaccinal G04.02
    progressive multifocal A81.2
    reversible, posterior G93.6
    van Bogaert's (sclerosing) A81.1
    vascular, progressive I67.3
Leukoerythroblastosis D75.9
Leukokeratosis (*see also* Leukoplakia)
    mouth K13.21
    nicotina palati K13.24
    oral mucosa K13.21
    tongue K13.21
    vocal cord J38.3
Leukokraurosis vulva (e) N90.4
Leukoma (cornea) (*see also* Opacity, cornea)
    adherent H17.0 ☑
    interfering with central vision — *see* Opacity,
      cornea, central
Leukomalacia, cerebral, newborn P91.2
    periventricular P91.2
Leukomelanopathy, hereditary D72.0
Leukonychia (punctata) (striata) L60.8
    congenital Q84.4
Leukopathia unguium L60.8
    congenital Q84.4
Leukopenia D72.819
    basophilic D72.818
    chemotherapy (cancer) induced D70.1
    congenital D70.0
    cyclic D70.0
    drug induced NEC D70.2
      due to cytoreductive cancer
        chemotherapy D70.1
    eosinophilic D72.818
    familial D70.0
    infantile genetic D70.0
    malignant D70.9
    periodic D70.0
    transitory neonatal P61.5
Leukopenic — *see* condition
Leukoplakia
    anus K62.89
    bladder (postinfectional) N32.89
    buccal K13.21
    cervix (uteri) N88.0
    esophagus K22.8
    gingiva K13.21
    hairy (oral mucosa) (tongue) K13.3
    kidney (pelvis) N28.89
    larynx J38.7
    lip K13.21
    mouth K13.21

Leukoplakia — *continued*
  oral epithelium, including tongue
      (mucosa) K13.21
    palate K13.21
    pelvis (kidney) N28.89
    penis (infectional) N48.0
    rectum K62.89
    syphilitic (late) A52.79
    tongue K13.21
    ureter (postinfectional) N28.89
    urethra (postinfectional) N36.8
    uterus N85.8
    vagina N89.4
    vocal cord J38.3
    vulva N90.4
Leukorrhea N89.8
    due to Trichomonas (vaginalis) A59.00
    trichomonal A59.00
Leukosarcoma C85.9 ☑
Levocardia (isolated) Q24.1
    with situs inversus Q89.3
Levotransposition Q20.5
Lev's disease or syndrome (acquired complete heart
    block) I44.2
Levulosuria — *see* Fructosuria
Levurid L30.2
Lewy body (ies) (dementia) (disease) G31.83
Leyden-Moebius dystrophy G71.0
Leydig cell
  carcinoma
    specified site — *see* Neoplasm, malignant, by
      site
    unspecified site
      female C56.9
      male C62.9 ☑
  tumor
    benign
      specified site — *see* Neoplasm, benign, by
        site
      unspecified site
        female D27. ☑
        male D29.2 ☑
    malignant
      specified site — *see* Neoplasm, malignant,
        by site
      unspecified site
        female C56. ☑
        male C62.9 ☑
      specified site — *see* Neoplasm, uncertain
        behavior, by site
      unspecified site
        female D39.1 ☑
        male D40.1 ☑
Leydig-Sertoli cell tumor
    specified site — *see* Neoplasm, benign, by site
    unspecified site
      female D27. ☑
      male D29.2 ☑
LGSIL (Low grade squamous intraepithelial lesion on
    cytologic smear of)
    anus R85.612
    cervix R87.612
    vagina R87.622
Liar, pathologic F60.2
Libido
    decreased R68.82
Libman-Sacks disease M32.11
Lice (infestation) B85.2
    body (Pediculus corporis) B85.1
    crab B85.3
    head (Pediculus capitis) B85.0
    mixed (classifiable to more than one of the titles
      B85.0-B85.3) B85.4
    pubic (Phthirus pubis) B85.3
Lichen L28.0
    albus L90.0
      penis N48.0
      vulva N90.4
    amyloidosis E85.4 *[L99]*
    atrophicus L90.0
      penis N48.0
      vulva N90.4
    congenital Q82.8
    myxedematosus L98.5
    nitidus L44.1
    pilaris Q82.8
      acquired L85.8
    planopilaris L66.1
    planus (chronicus) L43.9
      annularis L43.8
      bullous L43.1
      follicular L66.1

Lichen — *continued*
  planus — *continued*
    hypertrophic L43.0
    moniliformis L44.3
    of Wilson L43.9
    specified NEC L43.8
    subacute (active) L43.3
    tropicus L43.3
  ruber
    acuminatus L44.0
    moniliformis L44.3
    planus L43.9
  sclerosus (et atrophicus) L90.0
    penis N48.0
    vulva N90.4
  scrofulosus (primary) (tuberculous) A18.4
  simplex (chronicus) (circumscriptus) L28.0
  striatus L44.2
  urticatus L28.2
Lichenification L28.0
Lichenoides tuberculosis (primary) A18.4
Lichtheim's disease or syndrome — *see*
    Degeneration, combined
Lien migrans D73.89
Ligament — *see* condition
Light
  for gestational age — *see* Light for dates
  headedness R42
Light-for-dates (infant) P05.00
  with weight of
    499 grams or less P05.01
    500-749 grams P05.02
    750-999 grams P05.03
    1000-1249 grams P05.04
    1250-1499 grams P05.05
    1500-1749 grams P05.06
    1750-1999 grams P05.07
    2000-2499 grams P05.08
    2500 grams and over P05.09
  specified NEC P05.09
  and small-for-dates — *see* Small for dates
  affecting management of pregnancy O36.59 ☑
Lightning (effects) (stroke) (struck by) T75.00 ☑
  burn — *see* Burn
  foot E53.8
  shock T75.01 ☑
  specified effect NEC T75.09 ☑
Lightwood-Albright syndrome N25.89
Lightwood's disease or syndrome (renal tubular
    acidosis) N25.89
Lignac (-de Toni) (-Fanconi) (-Debré) disease or
    syndrome E72.09
  with cystinosis E72.04
Ligneous thyroiditis E06.5
Likoff's syndrome I20.8
Limb — *see* condition
Limbic epilepsy personality syndrome F07.0
Limitation, limited
  activities due to disability Z73.6
  cardiac reserve — *see* Disease, heart
  eye muscle duction, traumatic — *see* Strabismus,
    mechanical
  mandibular range of motion M26.52
Lindau (-von Hippel) disease Q85.8
Line (s)
  Beau's L60.4
  Harris' — *see* Arrest, epiphyseal
  Hudson's (cornea) — *see* Pigmentation, cornea,
    anterior
  Stähli's (cornea) — *see* Pigmentation, cornea,
    anterior
Linea corneae senilis — *see* Change, cornea, senile
Lingua
  geographica K14.1
  nigra (villosa) K14.3
  plicata K14.5
  tylosis K13.29
Lingual — *see* condition
Linguatulosis B88.8
Linitis (gastric) plastica C16.9
Lip — *see* condition
Lipedema — *see* Edema
Lipemia (*see also* Hyperlipidemia)
  retina, retinalis E78.3
Lipidosis E75.6
  cerebral (infantile) (juvenile) (late) E75.4
  cerebroretinal E75.4
  cerebroside E75.22
  cholesterol (cerebral) E75.5
  glycolipid E75.21
  hepatosplenomegalic E78.3

ICD-10-CM INDEX TO DISEASES AND INJURIES

Lipidosis — *continued*
  sphingomyelin — *see* Niemann-Pick disease or syndrome
  sulfatide E75.29
Lipoadenoma — *see* Neoplasm, benign, by site
Lipoblastoma — *see* Lipoma
Lipoblastomatosis — *see* Lipoma
Lipochondrodystrophy E76.01
Lipodermatosclerosis — *see* Varix, leg, with, inflammation
  ulcerated — *see* Varix, leg, with, ulcer, with inflammation by site
Lipochrome histiocytosis (familial) D71
Lipodystrophia progressiva E88.1
Lipodystrophy (progressive) E88.1
  insulin E88.1
  intestinal K90.81
  mesenteric K65.4
Lipofibroma — *see* Lipoma
Lipofuscinosis, neuronal (with ceroidosis) E75.4
Lipogranuloma, sclerosing L92.8
Lipogranulomatosis E78.89
Lipoid (*see also* condition)
  histiocytosis D76.3
    essential E75.29
  nephrosis N04.9
  proteinosis of Urbach E78.89
Lipoidemia — *see* Hyperlipidemia
Lipoidosis — *see* Lipidosis
Lipoma D17.9
  fetal D17.9
    fat cell D17.9
  infiltrating D17.9
  intramuscular D17.9
  pleomorphic D17.9
  site classification
    arms (skin) (subcutaneous) D17.2 ☑
    connective tissue D17.30
      intra-abdominal D17.5
      intrathoracic D17.4
      peritoneum D17.79
      retroperitoneum D17.79
      specified site NEC D17.39
      spermatic cord D17.6
    face (skin) (subcutaneous) D17.0
    genitourinary organ NEC D17.72
    head (skin) (subcutaneous) D17.0
    intra-abdominal D17.5
    intrathoracic D17.4
    kidney D17.71
    legs (skin) (subcutaneous) D17.2 ☑
    neck (skin) (subcutaneous) D17.0
    peritoneum D17.79
    retroperitoneum D17.79
    skin D17.30
      specified site NEC D17.39
    specified site NEC D17.79
    spermatic cord D17.6
    subcutaneous D17.30
      specified site NEC D17.39
    trunk (skin) (subcutaneous) D17.1
    unspecified D17.9
  spindle cell D17.9
Lipomatosis E88.2
  dolorosa (Dercum) E88.2
  fetal — *see* Lipoma
  Launois-Bensaude E88.89
Lipomyoma — *see* Lipoma
Lipomyxoma — *see* Lipoma
Lipomyxosarcoma — *see* Neoplasm, connective tissue, malignant
Lipoprotein metabolism disorder E78.9
Lipoproteinemia E78.5
  broad-beta E78.2
  floating-beta E78.2
  hyper-pre-beta E78.1
Liposarcoma (*see also* Neoplasm, connective tissue, malignant)
  dedifferentiated — *see* Neoplasm, connective tissue, malignant
  differentiated type — *see* Neoplasm, connective tissue, malignant
  embryonal — *see* Neoplasm, connective tissue, malignant
  mixed type — *see* Neoplasm, connective tissue, malignant
  myxoid — *see* Neoplasm, connective tissue, malignant
  pleomorphic — *see* Neoplasm, connective tissue, malignant
  round cell — *see* Neoplasm, connective tissue, malignant

Liposarcoma — *continued*
  well differentiated type — *see* Neoplasm, connective tissue, malignant
Liposynovitis prepatellaris E88.89
Lipping, cervix N86
Lipschütz disease or ulcer N76.6
Lipuria R82.0
  schistosomiasis (bilharziasis) B65.0
Lisping F80.0
Lissauer's paralysis A52.17
Lissencephalia, lissencephaly Q04.3
Listeriosis, listerellosis A32.9
  congenital (disseminated) P37.2
  cutaneous A32.0
  neonatal, newborn (disseminated) P37.2
  oculoglandular A32.81
  specified NEC A32.89
Lithemia E79.0
Lithiasis — *see* Calculus
Lithosis J62.8
Lithuria R82.99
Litigation, anxiety concerning Z65.3
Little leaguer's elbow — *see* Epicondylitis, medial
Little's disease G80.9
Littre's
  gland — *see* condition
  hernia — *see* Hernia, abdomen
Littritis — *see* Urethritis
Livedo (annularis) (racemosa) (reticularis) R23.1
Liver — *see* condition
Living alone (problems with) Z60.2
  with handicapped person Z74.2
Lloyd's syndrome — *see* Adenomatosis, endocrine
Loa loa, loaiasis, loasis B74.3
Lobar — *see* condition
Lobomycosis B48.0
Lobo's disease B48.0
Lobotomy syndrome F07.0
Lobstein (-Ekman) disease or syndrome Q78.0
Lobster-claw hand Q71.6 ☑
Lobulation (congenital) (*see also* Anomaly, by site)
  kidney, Q63.1
  liver, abnormal Q44.7
  spleen Q89.09
Lobule, lobular — *see* condition
Local, localized — *see* condition
Locked-in state G83.5
Locked twins causing obstructed labor O66.1
Locking
  joint — *see* Derangement, joint, specified type NEC
    knee — *see* Derangement, knee
Lockjaw — *see* Tetanus
Löffler's
  endocarditis I42.3
  eosinophilia J82
  pneumonia J82
  syndrome (eosinophilic pneumonitis) J82
Loiasis (with conjunctival infestation) (eyelid) B74.3
Lone Star fever A77.0
Long
  labor O63.9
    first stage O63.0
    second stage O63.1
  QT syndrome I45.81
Long-term (current) (prophylactic) drug therapy (use of)
  agents affecting estrogen receptors and estrogen levels NEC Z79.818
  anastrozole (Arimidex) Z79.811
  antibiotics Z79.2
    short-term use - omit code
  anticoagulants Z79.01
  anti-inflammatory, non-steroidal (NSAID) Z79.1
  antiplatelet Z79.02
  antithrombotics Z79.02
  aromatase inhibitors Z79.811
  aspirin Z79.82
  birth control pill or patch Z79.3
  bisphosphonates Z79.83
  contraceptive, oral Z79.3
  drug, specified NEC Z79.899
  estrogen receptor downregulators Z79.818
  Evista Z79.810
  exemestane (Aromasin) Z79.811
  Fareston Z79.810
  fulvestrant (Faslodex) Z79.818
  gonadotropin-releasing hormone (GnRH) agonist Z79.818
  goserelin acetate (Zoladex) Z79.818
  hormone replacement Z79.890
  insulin Z79.4

Long-term — *continued*
  letrozole (Femara) Z79.811
  leuprolide acetate (leuprorelin) (Lupron) Z79.818
  megestrol acetate (Megace) Z79.818
  methadone for pain management Z79.891
  Nolvadex Z79.810
  non-steroidal anti-inflammatories (NSAID) Z79.1
  opiate analgesic Z79.891
  oral
    antidiabetic Z79.84
    contraceptive Z79.3
    hypoglycemic Z79.84
  raloxifene (Evista) Z79.810
  selective estrogen receptor modulators (SERMs) Z79.810
  steroids
    inhaled Z79.51
    systemic Z79.52
  tamoxifen (Nolvadex) Z79.810
  toremifene (Fareston) Z79.810
Longitudinal stripes or grooves, nails L60.8
  congenital Q84.6
Loop
  intestine — *see* Volvulus
  vascular on papilla (optic) Q14.2
Loose (*see also* condition)
  body
    joint M24.00
      ankle M24.07 ☑
      elbow M24.02 ☑
      hand M24.04 ☑
      hip M24.05 ☑
      knee M23.4 ☑
      shoulder (region) M24.01 ☑
      specified site NEC M24.08
      vertebra M24.08
      toe M24.07 ☑
      wrist M24.03 ☑
      knee M23.4 ☑
    sheath, tendon — *see* Disorder, tendon, specified type NEC
  cartilage — *see* Loose, body, joint
  skin and subcutaneous tissue (following bariatric surgery weight loss) (following dietary weight loss) L98.7
  tooth, teeth K08.89
Loosening
  aseptic
    joint prosthesis — *see* Complications, joint prosthesis, mechanical, loosening, by site
    epiphysis — *see* Osteochondropathy
  mechanical
    joint prosthesis — *see* Complications, joint prosthesis, mechanical, loosening, by site
Looser-Milkman (-Debray) syndrome M83.8
Lop ear (deformity) Q17.3
Lorain (-Levi) short stature syndrome E23.0
Lordosis M40.50
  acquired — *see* Lordosis, specified type NEC
  congenital Q76.429
    lumbar region Q76.426
    lumbosacral region Q76.427
    sacral region Q76.428
    sacrococcygeal region Q76.428
    thoracolumbar region Q76.425
  lumbar region M40.56
  lumbosacral region M40.57
  postsurgical M96.4
  postural — *see* Lordosis, specified type NEC
  rachitic (late effect) (sequelae) E64.3
  sequelae of rickets E64.3
  specified type NEC M40.40
    lumbar region M40.46
    lumbosacral region M40.47
    thoracolumbar region M40.45
  thoracolumbar region M40.55
  tuberculous A18.01
Loss (of)
  appetite (*see* Anorexia) R63.0
    hysterical F50.89
    nonorganic origin F50.89
    psychogenic F50.89
  blood — *see* Hemorrhage
  bone — *see* Loss, substance of, bone
  control, sphincter, rectum R15.9
    nonorganic origin F98.1
  consciousness, transient R55
    traumatic — *see* Injury, intracranial
  elasticity, skin R23.4
  family (member) in childhood Z62.898
  fluid (acute) E86.9
  function of labyrinth — *see* subcategory H83.2

☑ **Additional character required**

Loss — *continued*
- hair, nonscarring — *see* Alopecia
- hearing (*see also* Deafness)
  - central NOS H90.5
  - conductive H90.2
    - bilateral H90.0
    - unilateral
      - with
        - restricted hearing on the contralateral side H90.A1 ☑
        - unrestricted hearing on the contralateral side H90.1 ☑
  - mixed conductive and sensorineural hearing loss H90.8
    - bilateral H90.6
    - unilateral
      - with
        - restricted hearing on the contralateral side H90.A3 ☑
        - unrestricted hearing on the contralateral side H90.7 ☑
  - neural NOS H90.5
  - perceptive NOS H90.5
  - sensorineural NOS H90.5
    - bilateral H90.3
    - unilateral
      - with
        - restricted hearing on the contralateral side H90.A2 ☑
        - unrestricted hearing on the contralateral side H90.4 ☑
  - sensory NOS H90.5
- height R29.890
- limb or member, traumatic, current — *see* Amputation, traumatic
- love relationship in childhood Z62.898
- memory (*see also* Amnesia)
  - mild, following organic brain damage F06.8
- mind — *see* Psychosis
- occlusal vertical dimension of fully erupted teeth M26.37
- organ or part — *see* Absence, by site, acquired
- ossicles, ear (partial) H74.32 ☑
- parent in childhood Z63.4
- pregnancy, recurrent N96
  - care in current pregnancy O26.2 ☑
  - without current pregnancy N96
- recurrent pregnancy — *see* Loss, pregnancy, recurrent
- self-esteem, in childhood Z62.898
- sense of
  - smell — *see* Disturbance, sensation, smell
  - taste — *see* Disturbance, sensation, taste
  - touch R20.8
- sensory R44.9
  - dissociative F44.6
- sexual desire F52.0
- sight (acquired) (complete) (congenital) — *see* Blindness
- substance of
  - bone — *see* Disorder, bone, density and structure, specified NEC
    - horizontal alveolar K06.3
  - cartilage — *see* Disorder, cartilage, specified type NEC
    - auricle (ear) — *see* Disorder, pinna, specified type NEC
  - vitreous (humor) H15.89
- tooth, teeth — *see* Absence, teeth, acquired
- vision, visual H54.7
  - both eyes H54.3
  - one eye H54.60
    - left (normal vision on right) H54.62
    - right (normal vision on left) H54.61
  - specified as blindness — *see* Blindness
  - subjective
    - sudden H53.13 ☑
    - transient H53.12 ☑
- vitreous — *see* Prolapse, vitreous
- voice — *see* Aphonia
- weight (abnormal) (cause unknown) R63.4

Louis-Bar syndrome (ataxia-telangiectasia) G11.3
Louping ill (encephalitis) A84.8
Louse, lousiness — *see* Lice
Low
- achiever, school Z55.3
- back syndrome M54.5
- basal metabolic rate R94.8
- birthweight (2499 grams or less) P07.10
  - with weight of
    - 1000-1249 grams P07.14
    - 1250-1499 grams P07.15

Low — *continued*
- birthweight — *continued*
  - 1500-1749 grams P07.16
  - 1750-1999 grams P07.17
  - 2000-2499 grams P07.18
  - extreme (999 grams or less) P07.00
    - with weight of
      - 499 grams or less P07.01
      - 500-749 grams P07.02
      - 750-999 grams P07.03
  - for gestational age — *see* Light for dates
- blood pressure (*see also* Hypotension)
  - reading (incidental) (isolated) (nonspecific) R03.1
- cardiac reserve — *see* Disease, heart
- function (*see also* Hypofunction)
  - kidney N28.9
- hematocrit D64.9
- hemoglobin D64.9
- income Z59.6
- level of literacy Z55.0
- lying
  - kidney N28.89
  - organ or site, congenital — *see* Malposition, congenital
- output syndrome (cardiac) — *see* Failure, heart
- platelets (blood) — *see* Thrombocytopenia
- reserve, kidney N28.89
- salt syndrome E87.1
- self esteem R45.81
- set ears Q17.4
- vision H54.2X ☑
  - one eye (other eye normal) H54.50
    - left (normal vision on right) H54.52A ☑
    - other eye blind — *see* Blindness
    - right (normal vision on left) H54.511 ☑

Low-density-lipoprotein-type (LDL)
- hyperlipoproteinemia E78.00
Lowe's syndrome E72.03
Lown-Ganong-Levine syndrome I45.6
LSD reaction (acute) (without dependence) F16.90
- with dependence F16.20
L-shaped kidney Q63.8
Ludwig's angina or disease K12.2
Lues (venerea), luetic — *see* Syphilis
Luetscher's syndrome (dehydration) E86.0
Lumbago, lumbalgia M54.5
- with sciatica M54.4 ☑
  - due to intervertebral disc disorder M51.17
- due to displacement, intervertebral disc M51.27
  - with sciatica M51.17
Lumbar — *see* condition
Lumbarization, vertebra, congenital Q76.49
Lumbermen's itch B88.0
Lump (*see also* Mass)
- breast N63.0
  - axillary tail
    - left N63.32
    - right N63.31
  - left
    - lower inner quadrant N63.24
    - lower outer quadrant N63.23
    - unspecified quadrant N63.20
    - upper inner quadrant N63.22
    - upper outer quadrant N63.21
  - right
    - lower inner quadrant N63.14
    - lower outer quadrant N63.13
    - unspecified quadrant N63.10
    - upper inner quadrant N63.12
    - upper outer quadrant N63.11
  - subareolar
    - left N63.42
    - right N63.41
Lunacy — *see* Psychosis
Lung — *see* condition
Lupoid (miliary) of Boeck D86.3
Lupus
- anticoagulant D68.62
  - with
    - hemorrhagic disorder D68.312
    - hypercoagulable state D68.62
  - finding without diagnosis R76.0
- discoid (local) L93.0
- erythematosus (discoid) (local) L93.0
  - disseminated — *see* Lupus, erythematosus, systemic
  - eyelid H01.129
    - left H01.126
      - lower H01.125
      - upper H01.124
    - right H01.123

Lupus — *continued*
- erythematosus — *continued*
  - lower H01.122
  - upper H01.121
  - profundus L93.2
  - specified NEC L93.2
  - subacute cutaneous L93.1
  - systemic M32.9
    - with organ or system involvement M32.10
      - endocarditis M32.11
      - lung M32.13
      - pericarditis M32.12
      - renal (glomerular) M32.14
        - tubulo-interstitial M32.15
      - specified organ or system NEC M32.19
    - drug-induced M32.0
    - inhibitor (presence of) D68.62
      - with
        - hemorrhagic disorder D68.312
        - hypercoagulable state D68.62
      - finding without diagnosis R76.0
    - specified NEC M32.8
- exedens A18.4
- hydralazine M32.0
  - correct substance properly administered — *see* Table of Drugs and Chemicals, by drug, adverse effect
  - overdose or wrong substance given or taken — *see* Table of Drugs and Chemicals, by drug, poisoning
- nephritis (chronic) M32.14
- nontuberculous, not disseminated L93.0
- panniculitis L93.2
- pernio (Besnier) D86.3
- systemic — *see* Lupus, erythematosus, systemic
- tuberculous A18.4
  - eyelid L93.2
  - vulgaris A18.4
    - eyelid A18.4
Luteinoma D27. ☑
Lutembacher's disease or syndrome (atrial septal defect with mitral stenosis) Q21.1
Luteoma D27. ☑
Lutz (-Splendore-de Almeida) disease — *see* Paracoccidioidomycosis
Luxation (*see also* Dislocation)
- eyeball (nontraumatic) — *see* Luxation, globe
  - birth injury P15.3
- globe, nontraumatic H44.82 ☑
- lacrimal gland — *see* Dislocation, lacrimal gland
- lens (old) (partial) (spontaneous)
  - congenital Q12.1
  - syphilitic A50.39
Lycanthropy F22
Lyell's syndrome L51.2
- due to drug L51.2
  - correct substance properly administered — *see* Table of Drugs and Chemicals, by drug, adverse effect
  - overdose or wrong substance given or taken — *see* Table of Drugs and Chemicals, by drug, poisoning
Lyme disease A69.20
Lymph
- gland or node — *see* condition
- scrotum — *see* Infestation, filarial
Lymphadenitis I88.9
- with ectopic or molar pregnancy O08.0
- acute L04.9
  - axilla L04.2
  - face L04.0
  - head L04.0
  - hip L04.3
  - limb
    - lower L04.3
    - upper L04.2
  - neck L04.0
  - shoulder L04.2
  - specified site NEC L04.8
  - trunk L04.1
- anthracosis (occupational) J60
- any site, except mesenteric I88.9
  - chronic I88.1
  - subacute I88.1
- breast
  - gestational — *see* Mastitis, obstetric
  - puerperal, postpartum (nonpurulent) O91.22
- chancroidal (congenital) A57
- chronic I88.1
  - mesenteric I88.0
- due to
  - Brugia (malayi) B74.1

Melanoma — *continued*
  skin — *continued*
    eyebrow C43.39
    eyelid (lower) (upper) C43.1 ☑
    face C43.30
      specified NEC C43.39
    female genital organ (external) NEC C51.9
    finger C43.6 ☑
    flank C43.59
    foot C43.7 ☑
    forearm C43.6 ☑
    forehead C43.39
    foreskin C60.0
    glabella C43.39
    gluteal region C43.59
    groin C43.59
    hand C43.6 ☑
    heel C43.7 ☑
    helix C43.2 ☑
    hip C43.7 ☑
    interscapular region C43.59
    jaw (external) C43.39
    knee C43.7 ☑
    labium C51.9
      majus C51.0
      minus C51.1
    leg C43.7 ☑
    lip (lower) (upper) C43.0
    lower limb NEC C43.7 ☑
    male genital organ (external) NEC C63.9
    nail
      finger C43.6 ☑
      toe C43.7 ☑
    nasolabial groove C43.39
    nates C43.59
    neck C43.4
    nose (external) C43.31
    overlapping site C43.8
    palpebra C43.1 ☑
    penis C60.9
    perianal skin C43.51
    perineum C43.51
    pinna C43.2 ☑
    popliteal fossa or space C43.7 ☑
    prepuce C60.0
    pudendum C51.9
    scalp C43.4
    scrotum C63.2
    shoulder C43.6 ☑
    skin NEC C43.9
    submammary fold C43.52
    temple C43.39
    thigh C43.7 ☑
    toe C43.7 ☑
    trunk NEC C43.59
    umbilicus C43.59
    upper limb NEC C43.6 ☑
    vulva C51.9
      overlapping sites C51.8
  spindle cell
    with epithelioid, mixed — *see* Melanoma, skin, by site
    type A C69.4 ☑
    type B C69.4 ☑
  superficial spreading — *see* Melanoma, skin, by site
Melanosarcoma (*see also* Melanoma)
  epithelioid cell — *see* Melanoma
Melanosis L81.4
  addisonian E27.1
    tuberculous A18.7
  adrenal E27.1
  colon K63.89
  conjunctiva — *see* Pigmentation, conjunctiva
    congenital Q13.89
  cornea (presenile) (senile) (*see also* Pigmentation, cornea)
    congenital Q13.4
  eye NEC H57.8
    congenital Q15.8
  lenticularis progressiva Q82.1
  liver K76.89
  precancerous (*see also* Melanoma, in situ)
    malignant melanoma in — *see* Melanoma
  Riehl's L81.4
  sclera H15.89
    congenital Q13.89
  suprarenal E27.1
  tar L81.4
  toxic L81.4
Melanuria R82.99
MELAS syndrome E88.41

Melasma L81.1
  adrenal (gland) E27.1
  suprarenal (gland) E27.1
Melena K92.1
  with ulcer - code by site under Ulcer, with hemorrhage K27.4
  due to swallowed maternal blood P78.2
  newborn, neonatal P54.1
    due to swallowed maternal blood P78.2
Meleney's
  gangrene (cutaneous) — *see* Ulcer, skin
  ulcer (chronic undermining) — *see* Ulcer, skin
Melioidosis A24.9
  acute A24.1
  chronic A24.2
  fulminating A24.1
  pneumonia A24.1
  pulmonary (chronic) A24.2
    acute A24.1
    subacute A24.2
  sepsis A24.1
  specified NEC A24.3
  subacute A24.2
Melitensis, febris A23.0
Melkersson (-Rosenthal) syndrome G51.2
Mellitus, diabetes — *see* Diabetes
Melorheostosis (bone) — *see* Disorder, bone, density and structure, specified NEC
Meloschisis Q18.4
Melotia Q17.4
Membrana
  capsularis lentis posterior Q13.89
  epipapillaris Q14.2
Membranacea placenta O43.19 ☑
Membranaceous uterus N85.8
Membrane (s), membranous (*see also* condition)
  cyclitic — *see* Membrane, pupillary
  folds, congenital — *see* Web
  Jackson's Q43.3
  over face of newborn P28.9
  premature rupture — *see* Rupture, membranes, premature
  pupillary H21.4 ☑
    persistent Q13.89
  retained (with hemorrhage) (complicating delivery) O72.2
    without hemorrhage O73.1
  secondary cataract — *see* Cataract, secondary
  unruptured (causing asphyxia) — *see* Asphyxia, newborn
  vitreous — *see* Opacity, vitreous, membranes and strands
Membranitis — *see* Chorioamnionitis
Memory disturbance, lack or loss (*see also* Amnesia)
  mild, following organic brain damage F06.8
Menadione deficiency E56.1
Menarche
  delayed E30.0
  precocious E30.1
Mendacity, pathologic F60.2
Mendelson's syndrome (due to anesthesia) J95.4
  in labor and delivery O74.0
  in pregnancy O29.01 ☑
  obstetric O74.0
  postpartum, puerperal O89.01
Ménétrier's disease or syndrome K29.60
  with bleeding K29.61
Ménière's disease, syndrome or vertigo H81.0 ☑
Meninges, meningeal — *see* condition
Meningioma (*see also* Neoplasm, meninges, benign)
  angioblastic — *see* Neoplasm, meninges, benign
  angiomatous — *see* Neoplasm, meninges, benign
  endotheliomatous — *see* Neoplasm, meninges, benign
  fibroblastic — *see* Neoplasm, meninges, benign
  fibrous — *see* Neoplasm, meninges, benign
  hemangioblastic — *see* Neoplasm, meninges, benign
  hemangiopericytic — *see* Neoplasm, meninges, benign
  malignant — *see* Neoplasm, meninges, malignant
  meningiothelial — *see* Neoplasm, meninges, benign
  meningotheliomatous — *see* Neoplasm, meninges, benign
  mixed — *see* Neoplasm, meninges, benign
  multiple — *see* Neoplasm, meninges, uncertain behavior
  papillary — *see* Neoplasm, meninges, uncertain behavior
  psammomatous — *see* Neoplasm, meninges, benign

Meningioma — *continued*
  syncytial — *see* Neoplasm, meninges, benign
  transitional — *see* Neoplasm, meninges, benign
Meningiomatosis (diffuse) — *see* Neoplasm, meninges, uncertain behavior
Meningism — *see* Meningismus
Meningismus (infectional) (pneumococcal) R29.1
  due to serum or vaccine R29.1
  influenzal — *see* Influenza, with, manifestations NEC
Meningitis (basal) (basic) (brain) (cerebral) (cervical) (congestive) (diffuse) (hemorrhagic) (infantile) (membranous) (metastatic) (nonspecific) (pontine) (progressive) (simple) (spinal) (subacute) (sympathetic) (toxic) G03.9
  abacterial G03.0
  actinomycotic A42.81
  adenoviral A87.1
  arbovirus A87.8
  aseptic (acute) G03.0
  bacterial G00.9
    Escherichia coli (E. coli) G00.8
    Friedländer (bacillus) G00.8
    gram-negative G00.9
    H. influenzae G00.0
    Klebsiella G00.8
    pneumococcal G00.1
    specified organism NEC G00.8
    staphylococcal G00.3
    streptococcal (acute) G00.2
  benign recurrent (Mollaret) G03.2
  candidal B37.5
  caseous (tuberculous) A17.0
  cerebrospinal A39.0
  chronic NEC G03.1
  clear cerebrospinal fluid NEC G03.0
  coxsackievirus A87.0
  cryptococcal B45.1
  diplococcal (gram positive) A39.0
  echovirus A87.0
  enteroviral A87.0
  eosinophilic B83.2
  epidemic NEC A39.0
  Escherichia coli (E. coli) G00.8
  fibrinopurulent G00.9
    specified organism NEC G00.8
  Friedländer (bacillus) G00.8
  gonococcal A54.81
  gram-negative cocci G00.9
  gram-positive cocci G00.9
  Haemophilus (influenzae) G00.0
  H. influenzae G00.0
  in (due to)
    adenovirus A87.1
    African trypanosomiasis B56.9 *[G02]*
    anthrax A22.8
    bacterial disease NEC A48.8 *[G01]*
    Chagas' disease (chronic) B57.41
    chickenpox B01.0
    coccidioidomycosis B38.4
    Diplococcus pneumoniae G00.1
    enterovirus A87.0
    herpes (simplex) virus B00.3
      zoster B02.1
    infectious mononucleosis B27.92
    leptospirosis A27.81
    Listeria monocytogenes A32.11
    Lyme disease A69.21
    measles B05.1
    mumps (virus) B26.1
    neurosyphilis (late) A52.13
    parasitic disease NEC B89 *[G02]*
    poliovirus A80.9 *[G02]*
    preventive immunization, inoculation or vaccination G03.8
    rubella B06.02
    Salmonella infection A02.21
    specified cause NEC G03.8
    Streptococcal pneumoniae G00.1
    typhoid fever A01.01
    varicella B01.0
    viral disease NEC A87.8
    whooping cough A37.90
    zoster B02.1
  infectious G00.9
  influenzal (H. influenzae) G00.0
  Klebsiella G00.8
  leptospiral (aseptic) A27.81
  lymphocytic (acute) (benign) (serous) A87.2
  meningococcal A39.0
  Mima polymorpha G00.8
  Mollaret (benign recurrent) G03.2

☑ **Additional character required**

Meningitis — *continued*
  monilial B37.5
  mycotic NEC B49 *[G02]*
  Neisseria A39.0
  nonbacterial G03.0
  nonpyogenic NEC G03.0
  ossificans G96.19
  pneumococcal streptococcus pneumoniae G00.1
  poliovirus A80.9 *[G02]*
  postmeasles B05.1
  purulent G00.9
    specified organism NEC G00.8
  pyogenic G00.9
    specified organism NEC G00.8
  Salmonella (arizonae) (Cholerae-Suis) (enteritidis) (typhimurium) A02.21
  septic G00.9
    specified organism NEC G00.8
  serosa circumscripta NEC G03.0
  serous NEC G93.2
  specified organism NEC G00.8
  sporotrichosis B42.81
  staphylococcal G00.3
  sterile G03.0
  Streptococcal (acute) G00.2
    pneumoniae G00.1
  suppurative G00.9
    specified organism NEC G00.8
  syphilitic (late) (tertiary) A52.13
    acute A51.41
    congenital A50.41
    secondary A51.41
  Torula histolytica (cryptococcal) B45.1
  traumatic (complication of injury) T79.8 ☑
  tuberculous A17.0
  typhoid A01.01
  viral NEC A87.9
  Yersinia pestis A20.3
Meningocele (spinal) (*see also* Spina bifida)
  with hydrocephalus — *see* Spina bifida, by site, with hydrocephalus
  acquired (traumatic) G96.19
  cerebral — *see* Encephalocele
Meningocerebritis — *see* Meningoencephalitis
Meningococcemia A39.4
  acute A39.2
  chronic A39.3
Meningococcus, meningococcal (*see also* condition) A39.9
  adrenalitis, hemorrhagic A39.1
  carrier (suspected) of Z22.31
  meningitis (cerebrospinal) A39.0
Meningoencephalitis (*see also* Encephalitis) G04.90
  acute NEC (*see also* Encephalitis, viral) A86
  bacterial NEC G04.2
  California A83.5
  diphasic A84.1
  eosinophilic B83.2
  epidemic A39.81
  herpesviral, herpetic B00.4
    due to herpesvirus 6 B10.01
    due to herpesvirus 7 B10.09
    specified NEC B10.09
  in (due to)
    blastomycosis NEC B40.81
    diseases classified elsewhere G05.3
    free-living amebae B60.2
    Hemophilus influenzae (H .influenzae) G00.0
    herpes B00.4
      due to herpesvirus 6 B10.01
      due to herpesvirus 7 B10.09
      specified NEC B10.09
    H. influenzae G00.0
    Lyme disease A69.22
    mercury — *see* subcategory T56.1
    mumps B26.2
    Naegleria (amebae) (organisms) (fowleri) B60.2
    Parastrongylus cantonensis B83.2
    toxoplasmosis (acquired) B58.2
      congenital P37.1
  infectious (acute) (viral) A86
  influenzal (H. influenzae) G00.0
  Listeria monocytogenes A32.12
  lymphocytic (serous) A87.2
  mumps B26.2
  parasitic NEC B89 *[G05.3]*
  pneumococcal G04.2
  primary amebic B60.2
  specific (syphilitic) A52.14
  specified organism NEC G04.81
  staphylococcal G04.2
  streptococcal G04.2

Meningoencephalitis — *continued*
  syphilitic A52.14
  toxic NEC G92
    due to mercury — *see* subcategory T56.1
  tuberculous A17.82
  virus NEC A86
Meningoencephalocele (*see also* Encephalocele)
  syphilitic A52.19
  congenital A50.49
Meningoencephalomyelitis (*see also* Meningoencephalitis)
  acute NEC (viral) A86
    disseminated G04.00
      postimmunization or postvaccination G04.02
      postinfectious G04.01
    due to
      actinomycosis A42.82
      Torula B45.1
      Toxoplasma or toxoplasmosis (acquired) B58.2
        congenital P37.1
    postimmunization or postvaccination G04.02
Meningoencephalomyelopathy G96.9
Meningoencephalopathy G96.9
Meningomyelitis (*see also* Meningoencephalitis)
  bacterial NEC G04.2
  blastomycotic NEC B40.81
  cryptococcal B45.1
  in diseases classified elsewhere G05.4
  meningococcal A39.81
  syphilitic A52.14
  tuberculous A17.82
Meningomyelocele (*see also* Spina bifida)
  syphilitic A52.19
Meningomyeloneuritis — *see* Meningoencephalitis
Meningoradiculitis — *see* Meningitis
Meningovascular — *see* condition
Menkes' disease or syndrome E83.09
  meaning maple-syrup-urine disease E71.0
Menometrorrhagia N92.1
Menopause, menopausal (asymptomatic) (state) Z78.0
  arthritis (any site) NEC — *see* Arthritis, specified form NEC
  bleeding N92.4
  depression (single episode) F32.89
    agitated (single episode) F32.2
      recurrent episode F33.9
    psychotic (single episode) F32.89
      recurrent episode F33.9
    recurrent episode F33.8
  melancholia (single episode) F32.89
    recurrent episode F33.8
  paranoid state F22
  premature E28.319
    asymptomatic E28.319
      postirradiation E89.40
      postsurgical E89.40
    symptomatic E28.310
      postirradiation E89.41
      postsurgical E89.41
  psychosis NEC F28
  symptomatic N95.1
  toxic polyarthritis NEC — *see* Arthritis, specified form NEC
Menorrhagia (primary) N92.0
  climacteric N92.4
    menopausal N92.4
  menopausal N92.4
  postclimacteric N95.0
  postmenopausal N95.0
  preclimacteric or premenopausal N92.4
  pubertal (menses retained) N92.2
Menostaxis N92.0
Menses, retention N94.89
Menstrual — *see* Menstruation
Menstruation
  absent — *see* Amenorrhea
  anovulatory N97.0
  cycle, irregular N92.6
  delayed N91.0
  disorder N93.9
    psychogenic F45.8
  during pregnancy O20.8
  excessive (with regular cycle) N92.0
    with irregular cycle N92.1
    at puberty N92.2
  frequent N92.0
  infrequent — *see* Oligomenorrhea
  irregular N92.6
    specified NEC N92.5
  latent N92.5
  membranous N92.5

Menstruation — *continued*
  painful (*see also* Dysmenorrhea) N94.6
    primary N94.4
    psychogenic F45.8
    secondary N94.5
  passage of clots N92.0
  precocious E30.1
  protracted N92.5
  rare — *see* Oligomenorrhea
  retained N94.89
  retrograde N92.5
  scanty — *see* Oligomenorrhea
  suppression N94.89
  vicarious (nasal) N94.89
Mental (*see also* condition)
  deficiency — *see* Disability, intellectual
  deterioration — *see* Psychosis
  disorder — *see* Disorder, mental
  exhaustion F48.8
  insufficiency (congenital) — *see* Disability, intellectual
  observation without need for further medical care Z03.89
  retardation — *see* Disability, intellectual
  subnormality — *see* Disability, intellectual
  upset — *see* Disorder, mental
Meralgia paresthetica G57.1 ☑
Mercurial — *see* condition
Mercurialism — *see* subcategory T56.1
MERRF syndrome (myoclonic epilepsy associated with ragged-red fiber) E88.42
Merkel cell tumor — *see* Carcinoma, Merkel cell
Merocele — *see* Hernia, femoral
Meromelia
  lower limb — *see* Defect, reduction, lower limb
    intercalary
      femur — *see* Defect, reduction, lower limb, specified type NEC
      tibiofibular (complete) (incomplete) — *see* Defect, reduction, lower limb
  upper limb — *see* Defect, reduction, upper limb
    intercalary, humeral, radioulnar — *see* Agenesis, arm, with hand present
Merzbacher-Pelizaeus disease E75.29
Mesaortitis — *see* Aortitis
Mesarteritis — *see* Arteritis
Mesencephalitis — *see* Encephalitis
Mesenchymoma (*see also* Neoplasm, connective tissue, uncertain behavior)
  benign — *see* Neoplasm, connective tissue, benign
  malignant — *see* Neoplasm, connective tissue, malignant
Mesenteritis
  retractile K65.4
  sclerosing K65.4
Mesentery, mesenteric — *see* condition
Mesiodens, mesiodentes K00.1
Mesio-occlusion M26.213
Mesocolon — *see* condition
Mesonephroma (malignant) — *see* Neoplasm, malignant, by site
  benign — *see* Neoplasm, benign, by site
Mesophlebitis — *see* Phlebitis
Mesostromal dysgenesia Q13.89
Mesothelioma (malignant) C45.9
  benign
    mesentery D19.1
    mesocolon D19.1
    omentum D19.1
    peritoneum D19.1
    pleura D19.0
    specified site NEC D19.7
    unspecified site D19.9
  biphasic C45.9
    benign
      mesentery D19.1
      mesocolon D19.1
      omentum D19.1
      peritoneum D19.1
      pleura D19.0
      specified site NEC D19.7
      unspecified site D19.9
  cystic D48.4
  epithelioid C45.9
    benign
      mesentery D19.1
      mesocolon D19.1
      omentum D19.1
      peritoneum D19.1
      pleura D19.0
      specified site NEC D19.7
      unspecified site D19.9

Personality — *continued*
  inadequate F60.7
  labile (emotional) F60.3
  mixed (nonspecific) F60.89
  morally defective F60.2
  multiple F44.81
  narcissistic F60.81
  obsessional F60.5
  obsessive (-compulsive) F60.5
  organic F07.0
  overconscientious F60.5
  paranoid F60.0
  passive (-dependent) F60.7
  passive-aggressive F60.89
  pathologic F60.9
  pattern defect or disturbance F60.9
  pseudopsychopathic (organic) F07.0
  pseudoretarded (organic) F07.0
  psychoinfantile F60.4
  psychoneurotic NEC F60.89
  psychopathic F60.2
  querulant F60.0
  sadistic F60.89
  schizoid F60.1
  self-defeating F60.7
  sensitive paranoid F60.0
  sociopathic (amoral) (antisocial) (asocial)
    (dissocial) F60.2
  specified NEC F60.89
  type A Z73.1
  unstable (emotional) F60.3
Perthes' disease — *see* Legg-Calvé-Perthes disease
Pertussis (*see also* Whooping cough) A37.90
Perversion, perverted
  appetite F50.89
    psychogenic F50.89
  function
    pituitary gland E23.2
      posterior lobe E22.2
  sense of smell and taste R43.8
    psychogenic F45.8
  sexual — *see* Deviation, sexual
Pervious, congenital (*see also* Imperfect, closure)
  ductus arteriosus Q25.0
Pes (congenital) (*see also* Talipes)
  acquired (*see also* Deformity, limb, foot, specified
    NEC)
    planus — *see* Deformity, limb, flat foot
  adductus Q66.89
  cavus Q66.7
  deformity NEC, acquired — *see* Deformity, limb,
    foot, specified NEC
  planus (acquired) (any degree) (*see also*
    Deformity, limb, flat foot)
    rachitic sequelae (late effect) E64.3
  valgus Q66.6
Pest, pestis — *see* Plague
Petechia, petechiae R23.3
  newborn P54.5
Petechial typhus A75.9
Peter's anomaly Q13.4
Petit mal seizure — *see* Epilepsy, generalized,
  specified NEC
Petit's hernia — *see* Hernia, abdomen, specified site
  NEC
Petrellidosis B48.2
Petrositis H70.20 ☑
  acute H70.21 ☑
  chronic H70.22 ☑
Peutz-Jeghers disease or syndrome Q85.8
Peyronie's disease N48.6
PFAPA (periodic fever, aphthous stomatitis,
  pharyngitis, and adenopathy syndrome) M04.8
Pfeiffer's disease — *see* Mononucleosis, infectious
Phagedena (dry) (moist) (sloughing) (*see also*
  Gangrene)
  geometric L88
  penis N48.29
  tropical — *see* Ulcer, skin
  vulva N76.6
Phagedenic — *see* condition
Phakoma H35.89
Phakomatosis (*see also* specific eponymous
  syndromes) Q85.9
  Bourneville's Q85.1
  specified NEC Q85.8
Phantom limb syndrome (without pain) G54.7
  with pain G54.6
Pharyngeal pouch syndrome D82.1
Pharyngitis (acute) (catarrhal) (gangrenous)
  (infective) (malignant) (membranous)
  (phlegmonous) (pseudomembranous) (simple)
  (subacute) (suppurative) (ulcerative) (viral) J02.9

Pharyngitis — *continued*
  with influenza, flu, or grippe — *see* Influenza,
    with, pharyngitis
  aphthous B08.5
  atrophic J31.2
  chlamydial A56.4
  chronic (atrophic) (granular) (hypertrophic) J31.2
  coxsackievirus B08.5
  diphtheritic A36.0
  enteroviral vesicular B08.5
  follicular (chronic) J31.2
  fusospirochetal A69.1
  gonococcal A54.5
  granular (chronic) J31.2
  herpesviral B00.2
  hypertrophic J31.2
  infectional, chronic J31.2
  influenzal — *see* Influenza, with, respiratory
    manifestations NEC
  lymphonodular, acute (enteroviral) B08.8
  pneumococcal J02.8
  purulent J02.9
  putrid J02.9
  septic J02.0
  sicca J31.2
  specified organism NEC J02.8
  staphylococcal J02.8
  streptococcal J02.0
  syphilitic, congenital (early) A50.03
  tuberculous A15.8
  vesicular, enteroviral B08.5
  viral NEC J02.8
Pharyngoconjunctivitis, viral B30.2
Pharyngolaryngitis (acute) J06.0
  chronic J37.0
Pharyngoplegia J39.2
Pharyngotonsillitis, herpesviral B00.2
Pharyngotracheitis, chronic J42
Pharynx, pharyngeal — *see* condition
Phencyclidine-induced
  anxiety disorder F16.980
  bipolar and related disorder F16.94
  depressive disorder F16.94
  psychotic disorder F16.959
Phenomenon
  Arthus' — *see* Arthus' phenomenon
  jaw-winking Q07.8
  lupus erythematosus (LE) cell M32.9
  Raynaud's (secondary) I73.00
    with gangrene I73.01
  vasomotor R55
  vasospastic I73.9
  vasovagal R55
  Wenckebach's I44.1
Phenylketonuria E70.1
  classical E70.0
  maternal E70.1
Pheochromoblastoma
  specified site — *see* Neoplasm, malignant, by site
  unspecified site C74.10
Pheochromocytoma
  malignant
    specified site — *see* Neoplasm, malignant, by
      site
    unspecified site C74.10
  specified site — *see* Neoplasm, benign, by site
  unspecified site D35.00
Pheohyphomycosis — *see* Chromomycosis
Pheomycosis — *see* Chromomycosis
Phimosis (congenital) (due to infection) N47.1
  chancroidal A57
Phlebectasia (*see also* Varix)
  congenital Q27.4
Phlebitis (infective) (pyemic) (septic) (suppurative)
  I80.9
  antepartum — *see* Thrombophlebitis,
    antepartum
  blue — *see* Phlebitis, leg, deep
  breast, superficial I80.8
  cavernous (venous) sinus — *see* Phlebitis,
    intracranial (venous) sinus
  cerebral (venous) sinus — *see* Phlebitis,
    intracranial (venous) sinus
  chest wall, superficial I80.8
  cranial (venous) sinus — *see* Phlebitis, intracranial
    (venous) sinus
  deep (vessels) — *see* Phlebitis, leg, deep
  due to implanted device — *see* Complications, by
    site and type, specified NEC
  during or resulting from a procedure T81.72 ☑
  femoral vein (superficial) I80.1 ☑
  femoropopliteal vein I80.0 ☑

Phlebitis — *continued*
  gestational — *see* Phlebopathy, gestational
  hepatic veins I80.8
  iliofemoral — *see* Phlebitis, femoral vein
  intracranial (venous) sinus (any) G08
    nonpyogenic I67.6
  intraspinal venous sinuses and veins G08
    nonpyogenic G95.19
  lateral (venous) sinus — *see* Phlebitis, intracranial
    (venous) sinus
  leg I80.3
    antepartum — *see* Thrombophlebitis,
      antepartum
    deep (vessels) NEC I80.20 ☑
      iliac I80.21 ☑
      popliteal vein I80.22 ☑
      specified vessel NEC I80.29 ☑
      tibial vein I80.23 ☑
    femoral vein (superficial) I80.1 ☑
    superficial (vessels) I80.0 ☑
  longitudinal sinus — *see* Phlebitis, intracranial
    (venous) sinus
  lower limb — *see* Phlebitis, leg
  migrans, migrating (superficial) I82.1
  pelvic
    with ectopic or molar pregnancy O08.0
    following ectopic or molar pregnancy O08.0
    puerperal, postpartum O87.1
  popliteal vein — *see* Phlebitis, leg, deep, popliteal
  portal (vein) K75.1
  postoperative T81.72 ☑
  pregnancy — *see* Thrombophlebitis, antepartum
  puerperal, postpartum, childbirth O87.0
    deep O87.1
    pelvic O87.1
    superficial O87.0
  retina — *see* Vasculitis, retina
  saphenous (accessory) (great) (long) (small) —
    see Phlebitis, leg, superficial
  sinus (meninges) — *see* Phlebitis, intracranial
    (venous) sinus
  specified site NEC I80.8
  syphilitic A52.09
  tibial vein — *see* Phlebitis, leg, deep, tibial
  ulcerative I80.9
    leg — *see* Phlebitis, leg
  umbilicus I80.8
  uterus (septic) — *see* Endometritis
  varicose (leg) (lower limb) — *see* Varix, leg, with,
    inflammation
Phlebofibrosis I87.8
Phleboliths I87.8
Phlebopathy,
  gestational O22.9 ☑
  puerperal O87.9
Phlebosclerosis I87.8
Phlebothrombosis (*see also* Thrombosis)
  antepartum — *see* Thrombophlebitis,
    antepartum
  pregnancy — *see* Thrombophlebitis, antepartum
  puerperal — *see* Thrombophlebitis, puerperal
Phlebotomus fever A93.1
Phlegmasia
  alba dolens O87.1
    nonpuerperal — *see* Phlebitis, femoral vein
  cerulea dolens — *see* Phlebitis, leg, deep
Phlegmon — *see* Abscess
Phlegmonous — *see* condition
Phlyctenulosis (allergic) (keratoconjunctivitis)
  (nontuberculous) (*see also* Keratoconjunctivitis)
  cornea — *see* Keratoconjunctivitis
  tuberculous A18.52
Phobia, phobic F40.9
  animal F40.218
    spiders F40.210
  examination F40.298
  reaction F40.9
  simple F40.298
  social F40.10
    generalized F40.11
  specific (isolated) F40.298
    animal F40.218
      spiders F40.210
    blood F40.230
    injection F40.231
    injury F40.233
    men F40.290
    natural environment F40.228
      thunderstorms F40.220
    situational F40.248
      bridges F40.242
      closed in spaces F40.240

Phobia — *continued*
  specific — *continued*
    flying F40.243
    heights F40.241
   specified focus NEC F40.298
   transfusion F40.231
   women F40.291
  specified NEC F40.8
   medical care NEC F40.232
  state F40.9
Phocas' disease — *see* Mastopathy, cystic
Phocomelia Q73.1
  lower limb — *see* Agenesis, leg, with foot present
  upper limb — *see* Agenesis, arm, with hand present
Phoria H50.50
Phosphate-losing tubular disorder N25.0
Phosphatemia E83.39
Phosphaturia E83.39
Photodermatitis (sun) L56.8
  chronic L57.8
  due to drug L56.8
  light other than sun L59.8
Photokeratitis H16.13 ☑
Photophobia H53.14 ☑
Photophthalmia — *see* Photokeratitis
Photopsia H53.19
Photoretinitis — *see* Retinopathy, solar
Photosensitivity, photosensitization (sun) skin L56.8
  light other than sun L59.8
Phrenitis — *see* Encephalitis
Phrynoderma (vitamin A deficiency) E50.8
Phthiriasis (pubis) B85.3
  with any infestation classifiable to B85.0-B85.2 B85.4
Phthirus infestation — *see* Phthiriasis
Phthisis (*see also* Tuberculosis)
  bulbi (infectional) — *see* Disorder, globe, degenerated condition, atrophy
  eyeball (due to infection) — *see* Disorder, globe, degenerated condition, atrophy
Phycomycosis — *see* Zygomycosis
Physalopteriasis B81.8
Physical restraint status Z78.1
Phytobezoar T18.9 ☑
  intestine T18.3 ☑
  stomach T18.2 ☑
Pian — *see* Yaws
Pianoma A66.1
Pica F50.89
  in adults F50.89
  infant or child F98.3
Picking, nose F98.8
Pick-Niemann disease — *see* Niemann-Pick disease or syndrome
Pick's
  cerebral atrophy G31.01 *[F02.80]*
   with behavioral disturbance G31.01 *[F02.81]*
  disease or syndrome (brain) G31.01 *[F02.80]*
   with behavioral disturbance G31.01 *[F02.81]*
   brain G31.01 *[F02.80]*
    with behavioral disturbance G31.01 *[F02.81]*
   pericardium (pericardial pseudocirrhosis of liver) I31.1
  syndrome
   brain G31.01 *[F02.80]*
    with behavioral disturbance G31.01 *[F02.81]*
   of heart (pericardial pseudocirrhosis of liver) I31.1
Pickwickian syndrome E66.2
Piebaldism E70.39
Piedra (beard) (scalp) B36.8
  black B36.3
  white B36.2
Pierre Robin deformity or syndrome Q87.0
Pierson's disease or osteochondrosis M91.0
Pig-bel A05.2
Pigeon
  breast or chest (acquired) M95.4
   congenital Q67.7
   rachitic sequelae (late effect) E64.3
  breeder's disease or lung J67.2
  fancier's disease or lung J67.2
  toe — *see* Deformity, toe, specified NEC
Pigmentation (abnormal) (anomaly) L81.9
  conjunctiva H11.13 ☑
  cornea (anterior) H18.01 ☑
   posterior H18.05 ☑
   stromal H18.06 ☑
  diminished melanin formation NEC L81.6
  iron L81.8
  lids, congenital Q82.8
  limbus corneae — *see* Pigmentation, cornea

Pigmentation — *continued*
  metals L81.8
  optic papilla, congenital Q14.2
  retina, congenital (grouped) (nevoid) Q14.1
  scrotum, congenital Q82.8
  tattoo L81.8
Piles (*see also* Hemorrhoids) K64.9
Pili
  annulati or torti (congenital) Q84.1
  incarnati L73.1
Pill roller hand (intrinsic) — *see* Parkinsonism
Pilomatrixoma — *see* Neoplasm, skin, benign
  malignant — *see* Neoplasm, skin, malignant
Pilonidal — *see* condition
Pimple R23.8
PIN — *see* Neoplasia, intraepithelial, prostate
Pinched nerve — *see* Neuropathy, entrapment
Pindborg tumor — *see* Cyst, calcifying odontogenic
Pineal body or gland — *see* condition
Pinealoblastoma C75.3
Pinealoma D44.5
  malignant C75.3
Pineoblastoma C75.3
Pineocytoma D44.5
Pinguecula H11.15 ☑
Pingueculitis H10.81 ☑
Pinhole meatus (*see also* Stricture, urethra) N35.9
Pink
  disease — *see* subcategory T56.1
  eye — *see* Conjunctivitis, acute, mucopurulent
Pinkus' disease (lichen nitidus) L44.1
Pinpoint
  meatus — *see* Stricture, urethra
  os (uteri) — *see* Stricture, cervix
Pins and needles R20.2
Pinta A67.9
  cardiovascular lesions A67.2
  chancre (primary) A67.0
  erythematous plaques A67.1
  hyperchromic lesions A67.1
  hyperkeratosis A67.1
  lesions A67.9
   cardiovascular A67.2
   hyperchromic A67.1
   intermediate A67.1
   late A67.2
   mixed A67.3
   primary A67.0
   skin (achromic) (cicatricial) (dyschromic) A67.2
    hyperchromic A67.1
    mixed (achromic and hyperchromic) A67.3
  papule (primary) A67.0
  skin lesions (achromic) (cicatricial) (dyschromic) A67.2
   hyperchromic A67.1
   mixed (achromic and hyperchromic) A67.3
  vitiligo A67.2
Pintids A67.1
Pinworm (disease) (infection) (infestation) B80
Piroplasmosis B60.0
Pistol wound — *see* Gunshot wound
Pitchers' elbow — *see* Derangement, joint, specified type NEC, elbow
Pithecoid pelvis Q74.2
  with disproportion (fetopelvic) O33.0
   causing obstructed labor O65.0
Pithiatism F48.8
Pitted — *see* Pitting
Pitting (*see also* Edema) R60.9
  lip R60.0
  nail L60.8
  teeth K00.4
Pituitary gland — *see* condition
Pituitary-snuff-taker's disease J67.8
Pityriasis (capitis) L21.0
  alba L30.5
  circinata (et maculata) L42
  furfuracea L21.0
  Hebra's L26
  lichenoides L41.0
   chronica L41.1
   et varioliformis (acuta) L41.0
  maculata (et circinata) L30.5
  nigra B36.1
  pilaris, Hebra's L44.0
  rosea L42
  rotunda L44.8
  rubra (Hebra) pilaris L44.0
  simplex L30.5
  specified type NEC L30.5
  streptogenes L30.5
  versicolor (scrotal) B36.0

Placenta, placental — *see* Pregnancy, complicated by (care of) (management affected by), specified condition
Placentitis O41.14 ☑
Plagiocephaly Q67.3
Plague A20.9
  abortive A20.8
  ambulatory A20.8
  asymptomatic A20.8
  bubonic A20.0
  cellulocutaneous A20.1
  cutaneobubonic A20.1
  lymphatic gland A20.0
  meningitis A20.3
  pharyngeal A20.8
  pneumonic (primary) (secondary) A20.2
  pulmonary, pulmonic A20.2
  septicemic A20.7
  tonsillar A20.8
   septicemic A20.7
Planning, family
  contraception Z30.9
  procreation Z31.69
Plaque (s)
  artery, arterial — *see* Arteriosclerosis
  calcareous — *see* Calcification
  coronary, lipid rich I25.83
  epicardial I31.8
  erythematous, of pinta A67.1
  Hollenhorst's — *see* Occlusion, artery, retina
  lipid rich, coronary I25.83
  pleural (without asbestos) J92.9
   with asbestos J92.0
  tongue K13.29
Plasmacytoma C90.3 ☑
  extramedullary C90.2 ☑
  medullary C90.0 ☑
  solitary C90.3 ☑
Plasmacytopenia D72.818
Plasmacytosis D72.822
Plaster ulcer — *see* Ulcer, pressure, by site
Plateau iris syndrome (post-iridectomy) (postprocedural) (without glaucoma) H21.82
  with glaucoma H40.22 ☑
Platybasia Q75.8
Platyonychia (congenital) Q84.6
  acquired L60.8
Platypelloid pelvis M95.5
  with disproportion (fetopelvic) O33.0
   causing obstructed labor O65.0
  congenital Q74.2
Platyspondylisis Q76.49
Plaut (-Vincent) disease (*see also* Vincent's) A69.1
Plethora R23.2
  newborn P61.1
Pleura, pleural — *see* condition
Pleuralgia R07.81
Pleurisy (acute) (adhesive) (chronic) (costal) (diaphragmatic) (double) (dry) (fibrinous) (fibrous) (interlobar) (latent) (plastic) (primary) (residual) (sicca) (sterile) (subacute) (unresolved) R09.1
  with
   adherent pleura J86.0
   effusion J90
    chylous, chyliform J94.0
    tuberculous (non primary) A15.6
     primary (progressive) A15.7
    tuberculosis — *see* Pleurisy, tuberculous (non primary)
  encysted — *see* Pleurisy, with effusion
  exudative — *see* Pleurisy, with effusion
  fibrinopurulent, fibropurulent — *see* Pyothorax
  hemorrhagic — *see* Hemothorax
  pneumococcal J90
  purulent — *see* Pyothorax
  septic — *see* Pyothorax
  serofibrinous — *see* Pleurisy, with effusion
  seropurulent — *see* Pyothorax
  serous — *see* Pleurisy, with effusion
  staphylococcal J86.9
  streptococcal J90
  suppurative — *see* Pyothorax
  traumatic (post) (current) — *see* Injury, intrathoracic, pleura
  tuberculous (with effusion) (non primary) A15.6
   primary (progressive) A15.7
Pleuritis sicca — *see* Pleurisy
Pleurobronchopneumonia — *see* Pneumonia, broncho-
Pleurodynia R07.81
  epidemic B33.0
  viral B33.0

Pleuropericarditis - Pneumonia

Pleuropericarditis (see also Pericarditis)
  acute I30.9
Pleuropneumonia (acute) (bilateral) (double)
  (septic) (see also Pneumonia) J18.8
  chronic — see Fibrosis, lung
Pleuro-pneumonia-like-organism (PPLO), as cause
  of disease classified elsewhere B96.0
Pleurorrhea — see Pleurisy, with effusion
Plexitis, brachial G54.0
Plica
  polonica B85.0
  syndrome, knee M67.5 ☑
  tonsil J35.8
Plicated tongue K14.5
Plug
  bronchus NEC J98.09
  meconium (newborn) NEC syndrome P76.0
  mucus — see Asphyxia, mucus
Plumbism — see subcategory T56.0
Plummer's disease E05.20
  with thyroid storm E05.21
Plummer-Vinson syndrome D50.1
Pluricarential syndrome of infancy E40
Plus (and minus) hand (intrinsic) — see Deformity,
  limb, specified type NEC, forearm
Pneumathemia — see Air, embolism
Pneumatic hammer (drill) syndrome T75.21 ☑
Pneumatocele (lung) J98.4
  intracranial G93.89
  tension J44.9
Pneumatosis
  cystoides intestinalis K63.89
  intestinalis K63.89
  peritonei K66.8
Pneumaturia R39.89
Pneumoblastoma — see Neoplasm, lung, malignant
Pneumocephalus G93.89
Pneumococcemia A40.3
Pneumococcus, pneumococcal — see condition
Pneumoconiosis (due to) (inhalation of) J64
  with tuberculosis (any type in A15) J65
  aluminum J63.0
  asbestos J61
  bagasse, bagassosis J67.1
  bauxite J63.1
  beryllium J63.2
  coal miners' (simple) J60
  coalworkers' (simple) J60
  collier's J60
  cotton dust J66.0
  diatomite (diatomaceous earth) J62.8
  dust
    inorganic NEC J63.6
    lime J62.8
    marble J62.8
    organic NEC J66.8
  fumes or vapors (from silo) J68.9
  graphite J63.3
  grinder's J62.8
  kaolin J62.8
  mica J62.8
  millstone maker's J62.8
  mineral fibers NEC J61
  miner's J60
  moldy hay J67.0
  potter's J62.8
  rheumatoid — see Rheumatoid, lung
  sandblaster's J62.8
  silica, silicate NEC J62.8
    with carbon J60
  stonemason's J62.8
  talc (dust) J62.0
Pneumocystis carinii pneumonia B59
Pneumocystis jiroveci (pneumonia) B59
Pneumocystosis (with pneumonia) B59
Pneumohemopericardium I31.2
Pneumohemothorax J94.2
  traumatic S27.2 ☑
Pneumohydropericardium — see Pericarditis
Pneumohydrothorax — see Hydrothorax
Pneumomediastinum J98.2
  congenital or perinatal P25.2
Pneumomycosis B49 [J99]
Pneumonia (acute) (double) (migratory) (purulent)
  (septic) (unresolved) J18.9
  with
    lung abscess J85.1
      due to specified organism — see Pneumonia,
        in (due to)
    influenza — see Influenza, with, pneumonia
  adenoviral J12.0
  adynamic J18.2

Pneumonia — continued
  alba A50.04
  allergic (eosinophilic) J82
  alveolar — see Pneumonia, lobar
  anaerobes J15.8
  anthrax A22.1
  apex, apical — see Pneumonia, lobar
  Ascaris B77.81
  aspiration J69.0
    due to
      aspiration of microorganisms
        bacterial J15.9
        viral J12.9
      food (regurgitated) J69.0
      gastric secretions J69.0
      milk (regurgitated) J69.0
      oils, essences J69.1
      solids, liquids NEC J69.8
      vomitus J69.0
    newborn P24.81
      amniotic fluid (clear) P24.11
      blood P24.21
      liquor (amnii) P24.11
      meconium P24.01
      milk P24.31
      mucus P24.11
      food (regurgitated) P24.31
      specified NEC P24.81
      stomach contents P24.31
    postprocedural J95.4
  atypical NEC J18.9
  bacillus J15.9
    specified NEC J15.8
  bacterial J15.9
    specified NEC J15.8
  Bacteroides (fragilis) (oralis)
    (melaninogenicus) J15.8
  basal, basic, basilar — see Pneumonia, by type
  bronchiolitis obliterans organized (BOOP) J84.89
  broncho-, bronchial (confluent) (croupous)
    (diffuse) (disseminated) (hemorrhagic)
    (involving lobes) (lobar) (terminal) J18.0
    allergic (eosinophilic) J82
    aspiration — see Pneumonia, aspiration
    bacterial J15.9
      specified NEC J15.8
    chronic — see Fibrosis, lung
    diplococcal J13
    Eaton's agent J15.7
    Escherichia coli (E. coli) J15.5
    Friedländer's bacillus J15.0
    Hemophilus influenzae J14
    hypostatic J18.2
    inhalation (see also Pneumonia, aspiration)
      due to fumes or vapors (chemical) J68.0
      of oils or essences J69.1
    Klebsiella (pneumoniae) J15.0
    lipid, lipoid J69.1
      endogenous J84.89
    Mycoplasma (pneumoniae) J15.7
    pleuro-pneumonia-like-organisms (PPLO) J15.7
    pneumococcal J13
    Proteus J15.6
    Pseudomonas J15.1
    Serratia marcescens J15.6
    specified organism NEC J16.8
    staphylococcal — see Pneumonia,
      staphylococcal
    streptococcal NEC J15.4
      group B J15.3
      pneumoniae J13
    viral, virus — see Pneumonia, viral
  Butyrivibrio (fibriosolvens) J15.8
  Candida B37.1
  caseous — see Tuberculosis, pulmonary
  catarrhal — see Pneumonia, broncho
  chlamydial J16.0
    congenital P23.1
  cholesterol J84.89
  cirrhotic (chronic) — see Fibrosis, lung
  Clostridium (haemolyticum) (novyi) J15.8
  confluent — see Pneumonia, broncho
  congenital (infective) P23.9
    due to
      bacterium NEC P23.6
      Chlamydia P23.1
      Escherichia coli P23.4
      Haemophilus influenzae P23.6
      infective organism NEC P23.8
      Klebsiella pneumoniae P23.6
      Mycoplasma P23.6
      Pseudomonas P23.5

Pneumonia — continued
  congenital — continued
    Staphylococcus P23.6
    Streptococcus (except group B) P23.6
      group B P23.3
    viral agent P23.0
    specified NEC P23.8
  croupous — see Pneumonia, lobar
  cryptogenic organizing J84.116
  cytomegalic inclusion B25.0
  cytomegaloviral B25.0
  deglutition — see Pneumonia, aspiration
  desquamative interstitial J84.117
  diffuse — see Pneumonia, broncho
  diplococcal, diplococcus (broncho-) (lobar) J13
  disseminated (focal) — see Pneumonia, broncho
  Eaton's agent J15.7
  embolic, embolism — see Embolism, pulmonary
  Enterobacter J15.6
  eosinophilic J82
  Escherichia coli (E. coli) J15.5
  Eubacterium J15.8
  fibrinous — see Pneumonia, lobar
  fibroid, fibrous (chronic) — see Fibrosis, lung
  Friedländer's bacillus J15.0
  Fusobacterium (nucleatum) J15.8
  gangrenous J85.0
  giant cell (measles) B05.2
  gonococcal A54.84
  gram-negative bacteria NEC J15.6
    anaerobic J15.8
  Hemophilus influenzae (broncho) (lobar) J14
  human metapneumovirus J12.3
  hypostatic (broncho) (lobar) J18.2
  in (due to)
    actinomycosis A42.0
    adenovirus J12.0
    anthrax A22.1
    ascariasis B77.81
    aspergillosis B44.9
    Bacillus anthracis A22.1
    Bacterium anitratum J15.6
    candidiasis B37.1
    chickenpox B01.2
    Chlamydia J16.0
      neonatal P23.1
    coccidioidomycosis B38.2
      acute B38.0
      chronic B38.1
    cytomegalovirus disease B25.0
    Diplococcus (pneumoniae) J13
    Eaton's agent J15.7
    Enterobacter J15.6
    Escherichia coli (E. coli) J15.5
    Friedländer's bacillus J15.0
    fumes and vapors (chemical) (inhalation) J68.0
    gonorrhea A54.84
    Hemophilus influenzae (H. influenzae) J14
    Herellea J15.6
    histoplasmosis B39.2
      acute B39.0
      chronic B39.1
    human metapneumovirus J12.3
    Klebsiella (pneumoniae) J15.0
    measles B05.2
    Mycoplasma (pneumoniae) J15.7
    nocardiasis, nocardiosis A43.0
    ornithosis A70
    parainfluenza virus J12.2
    pleuro-pneumonia-like-organism (PPLO) J15.7
    pneumococcus J13
    pneumocystosis (Pneumocystis carinii)
      (Pneumocystis jiroveci) B59
    Proteus J15.6
    Pseudomonas NEC J15.1
      pseudomallei A24.1
    psittacosis A70
    Q fever A78
    respiratory syncytial virus J12.1
    rheumatic fever I00 [J17]
    rubella B06.81
    Salmonella (infection) A02.22
      typhi A01.03
    schistosomiasis B65.9 [J17]
    Serratia marcescens J15.6
    specified
      bacterium NEC J15.8
      organism NEC J16.8
    spirochetal NEC A69.8
    Staphylococcus J15.20
      aureus (methicillin susceptible)
        (MSSA) J15.211

☑ **Additional character required**

Pneumonia — continued
in — continued
methicillin resistant (MRSA) J15.212
specified NEC J15.29
Streptococcus J15.4
group B J15.3
pneumoniae J13
specified NEC J15.4
toxoplasmosis B58.3
tularemia A21.2
typhoid (fever) A01.03
varicella B01.2
virus — see Pneumonia, viral
whooping cough A37.91
due to
Bordetella parapertussis A37.11
Bordetella pertussis A37.01
specified NEC A37.81
Yersinia pestis A20.2
inhalation of food or vomit — see Pneumonia,
aspiration
interstitial J84.9
chronic J84.111
desquamative J84.117
due to
collagen vascular disease J84.17
known underlying cause J84.17
idiopathic NOS J84.111
in disease classified elsewhere J84.17
lymphocytic (due to collagen vascular disease)
(in diseases classified elsewhere) J84.17
lymphoid J84.2
non-specific J84.89
due to
collagen vascular disease J84.17
known underlying cause J84.17
idiopathic J84.113
in diseases classified elsewhere J84.17
plasma cell B59
pseudomonas J15.1
usual J84.112
due to collagen vascular disease J84.17
idiopathic J84.112
in diseases classified elsewhere J84.17
Klebsiella (pneumoniae) J15.0
lipid, lipoid (exogenous) J69.1
endogenous J84.89
lobar (disseminated) (double) (interstitial) J18.1
bacterial J15.9
specified NEC J15.8
chronic — see Fibrosis, lung
Escherichia coli (E. coli) J15.5
Friedländer's bacillus J15.0
Hemophilus influenzae J14
hypostatic J18.2
Klebsiella (pneumoniae) J15.0
pneumococcal J13
Proteus J15.6
Pseudomonas J15.1
specified organism NEC J16.8
staphylococcal — see Pneumonia,
staphylococcal
streptococcal NEC J15.4
Streptococcus pneumoniae J13
viral, virus — see Pneumonia, viral
lobular — see Pneumonia, broncho
Löffler's J82
lymphoid interstitial J84.2
massive — see Pneumonia, lobar
meconium P24.01
MRSA (Methicillin resistant Staphylococcus
aureus) J15.212
MSSA (methicillin susceptible Staphylococcus
aureus) J15.211
multilobar — see Pneumonia, by type
Mycoplasma (pneumoniae) J15.7
necrotic J85.0
neonatal P23.9
aspiration — see Aspiration, by substance, with
pneumonia
nitrogen dioxide J68.0
organizing J84.89
due to
collagen vascular disease J84.17
known underlying cause J84.17
in diseases classified elsewhere J84.17
orthostatic J18.2
parainfluenza virus J12.2
parenchymatous — see Fibrosis, lung
passive J18.2
patchy — see Pneumonia, broncho
Peptococcus J15.8

Pneumonia — continued
Peptostreptococcus J15.8
plasma cell (of infants) B59
pleurolobar — see Pneumonia, lobar
pleuro-pneumonia-like organism (PPLO) J15.7
pneumococcal (broncho) (lobar) J13
Pneumocystis (carinii) (jiroveci) B59
postinfectional NEC B99 ☑ [J17]
postmeasles B05.2
Proteus J15.6
Pseudomonas J15.1
psittacosis A70
radiation J70.0
respiratory syncytial virus J12.1
resulting from a procedure J95.89
rheumatic I00 [J17]
Salmonella (arizonae) (cholerae-suis) (enteritidis)
(typhimurium) A02.22
typhi A01.03
typhoid fever A01.03
SARS-associated coronavirus J12.81
segmented, segmental — see Pneumonia,
broncho-
Serratia marcescens J15.6
specified NEC J18.8
bacterium NEC J15.8
organism NEC J16.8
virus NEC J12.89
spirochetal NEC A69.8
staphylococcal (broncho) (lobar) J15.20
aureus (methicillin susceptible) (MSSA) J15.211
methicillin resistant (MRSA) J15.212
specified NEC J15.29
static, stasis J18.2
streptococcal NEC (broncho) (lobar) J15.4
group
A J15.4
B J15.3
specified NEC J15.4
Streptococcus pneumoniae J13
syphilitic, congenital (early) A50.04
traumatic (complication) (early)
(secondary) T79.8 ☑
tuberculous (any) — see Tuberculosis, pulmonary
tularemic A21.2
varicella B01.2
Veillonella J15.8
ventilator associated J95.851
viral, virus (broncho) (interstitial) (lobar) J12.9
adenoviral J12.0
congenital P23.0
human metapneumovirus J12.3
parainfluenza J12.2
respiratory syncytial J12.1
SARS-associated coronavirus J12.81
specified NEC J12.89
white (congenital) A50.04
Pneumonic — see condition
Pneumonitis (acute) (primary) (see also Pneumonia)
air-conditioner J67.7
allergic (due to) J67.9
organic dust NEC J67.8
red cedar dust J67.8
sequoiosis J67.8
wood dust J67.8
aspiration J69.0
due to
anesthesia J95.4
during
labor and delivery O74.0
pregnancy O29.01 ☑
puerperium O89.01
fumes or gases J68.0
obstetric O74.0
chemical (due to gases, fumes or vapors)
(inhalation) J68.0
due to anesthesia J95.4
cholesterol J84.89
crack (cocaine) J68.0
chronic — see Fibrosis, lung
congenital rubella P35.0
due to
beryllium J68.0
cadmium J68.0
crack (cocaine) J68.0
detergent J69.8
fluorocarbon-polymer J68.0
food, vomit (aspiration) J69.0
fumes or vapors J68.0
gases, fumes or vapors (inhalation) J68.0
inhalation
blood J69.8

Pneumonitis — continued
due to — continued
essences J69.1
food (regurgitated), milk, vomit J69.0
oils, essences J69.1
saliva J69.0
solids, liquids NEC J69.8
manganese J68.0
nitrogen dioxide J68.0
oils, essences J69.1
solids, liquids NEC J69.8
toxoplasmosis (acquired) B58.3
congenital P37.1
vanadium J68.0
ventilator J95.851
eosinophilic J82
hypersensitivity J67.9
air conditioner lung J67.7
bagassosis J67.1
bird fancier's lung J67.2
farmer's lung J67.0
maltworker's lung J67.4
maple bark-stripper's lung J67.6
mushroom worker's lung J67.5
specified organic dust NEC J67.8
suberosis J67.3
interstitial (chronic) J84.89
acute J84.114
lymphoid J84.2
non-specific J84.89
idiopathic J84.113
lymphoid, interstitial J84.2
meconium P24.01
postanesthetic J95.4
correct substance properly administered — see
Table of Drugs and Chemicals, by drug,
adverse effect
in labor and delivery O74.0
in pregnancy O29.01 ☑
obstetric O74.0
overdose or wrong substance given or taken
(by accident) — see Table of Drugs and
Chemicals, by drug, poisoning
postpartum, puerperal O89.01
postoperative J95.4
obstetric O74.0
radiation J70.0
rubella, congenital P35.0
ventilation (air-conditioning) J67.7
ventilator associated J95.851
wood-dust J67.8
Pneumonoconiosis — see Pneumoconiosis
Pneumoparotid K11.8
Pneumopathy NEC J98.4
alveolar J84.09
due to organic dust NEC J66.8
parietoalveolar J84.09
Pneumopericarditis (see also Pericarditis)
acute I30.9
Pneumopericardium (see also Pericarditis)
congenital P25.3
newborn P25.3
traumatic (post) — see Injury, heart
Pneumophagia (psychogenic) F45.8
Pneumopleurisy, pneumopleuritis (see also
Pneumonia) J18.8
Pneumopyopericardium I30.1
Pneumopyothorax — see Pyopneumothorax
with fistula J86.0
Pneumorrhagia (see also Hemorrhage, lung)
tuberculous — see Tuberculosis, pulmonary
Pneumothorax NOS J93.9
acute J93.83
chronic J93.81
congenital P25.1
perinatal period P25.1
postprocedural J95.811
specified NEC J93.83
spontaneous NOS J93.83
newborn P25.1
primary J93.11
secondary J93.12
tension J93.0
tense valvular, infectional J93.0
tension (spontaneous) J93.0
traumatic S27.0 ☑
with hemothorax S27.2 ☑
tuberculous — see Tuberculosis, pulmonary
Podagra (see also Gout) M10.9
Podencephalus Q01.9
Poikilocytosis R71.8

Poikiloderma - Polyneuropathy

Poikiloderma L81.6
  Civatte's L57.3
  congenital Q82.8
  vasculare atrophicans L94.5
Poikilodermatomyositis M33.10
  with
    myopathy M33.12
    respiratory involvement M33.11
    specified organ involvement NEC M33.19
Pointed ear (congenital) Q17.3
Poison ivy, oak, sumac or other plant dermatitis
    (allergic) (contact) L23.7
Poisoning (acute) (see also Table of Drugs and
    Chemicals)
  algae and toxins T65.82 ☑
  Bacillus B (aertrycke) (cholerae (suis))
    (paratyphosus) (suipestifer) A02.9
    botulinus A05.1
  bacterial toxins A05.9
  berries, noxious — see Poisoning, food, noxious,
    berries
  botulism A05.1
  ciguatera fish T61.0 ☑
  Clostridium botulinum A05.1
  death-cap (Amanita phalloides) (Amanita verna)
    — see Poisoning, food, noxious, mushrooms
  drug — see Table of Drugs and Chemicals, by
    drug, poisoning
  epidemic, fish (noxious) — see Poisoning, seafood
    bacterial A05.9
  fava bean D55.0
  fish (noxious) T61.9 ☑
    bacterial — see Intoxication, foodborne, by
      agent
    ciguatera fish — see Poisoning, ciguatera fish
    scombroid fish — see Poisoning, scombroid fish
    specified type NEC T61.77 ☑
  food (acute) (diseased) (infected) (noxious)
      NEC T62.9 ☑
    bacterial — see Intoxication, foodborne, by
      agent
    due to
      Bacillus (aertrycke) (choleraesuis)
        (paratyphosus) (suipestifer) A02.9
        botulinus A05.1
      Clostridium (perfringens) (Welchii) A05.2
      salmonella (aertrycke) (callinarum)
        (choleraesuis) (enteritidis) (paratyphi)
        (suipestifer) A02.9
        with
          gastroenteritis A02.0
          sepsis A02.1
      staphylococcus A05.0
      Vibrio
        parahaemolyticus A05.3
        vulnificus A05.5
    noxious or naturally toxic T62.9 ☑
      berries — see subcategory T62.1
      fish — see Poisoning, seafood
      mushrooms — see subcategory T62.0X
      plants NEC — see subcategory T62.2X
      seafood — see Poisoning, seafood
      specified NEC — see subcategory T62.8X
  ichthyotoxism — see Poisoning, seafood
  kreotoxism, food A05.9
  latex T65.81 ☑
  lead T56.0 ☑
  mushroom — see Poisoning, food, noxious,
    mushroom
  mussels (see also Poisoning, shellfish)
    bacterial — see Intoxication, foodborne, by
      agent
  nicotine (tobacco) T65.2 ☑
  noxious foodstuffs — see Poisoning, food,
    noxious
  plants, noxious — see Poisoning, food, noxious,
    plants NEC
  ptomaine — see Poisoning, food
  radiation J70.0
  Salmonella (arizonae) (cholerae-suis) (enteritidis)
    (typhimurium) A02.9
  scombroid fish T61.1 ☑
  seafood (noxious) T61.9 ☑
    bacterial — see Intoxication, foodborne, by
      agent
    fish — see Poisoning, fish
    shellfish — see Poisoning, shellfish
    specified NEC — see subcategory T61.8X
  shellfish (amnesic) (azaspiracid) (diarrheic)
    (neurotoxic) (noxious) (paralytic) T61.78 ☑
    bacterial — see Intoxication, foodborne, by
      agent

Poisoning — continued
  shellfish — continued
    ciguatera mollusk — see Poisoning, ciguatera
      fish
  specified substance NEC T65.891 ☑
  Staphylococcus, food A05.0
  tobacco (nicotine) T65.2 ☑
  water E87.79
Poker spine — see Spondylitis, ankylosing
Poland syndrome Q79.8
Polioencephalitis (acute) (bulbar) A80.9
  inferior G12.22
  influenzal — see Influenza, with, encephalopathy
  superior hemorrhagic (acute) (Wernicke's) E51.2
  Wernicke's E51.2
Polioencephalomyelitis (acute) (anterior) A80.9
  with beriberi E51.2
Polioencephalopathy, superior hemorrhagic E51.2
  with
    beriberi E51.11
    pellagra E52
Poliomeningoencephalitis — see
  Meningoencephalitis
Poliomyelitis (acute) (anterior) (epidemic) A80.9
  with paralysis (bulbar) — see Poliomyelitis, paralytic
  abortive A80.4
  ascending (progressive) — see Poliomyelitis,
    paralytic
  bulbar (paralytic) — see Poliomyelitis, paralytic
  congenital P35.8
  nonepidemic A80.9
  nonparalytic A80.4
  paralytic A80.30
    specified NEC A80.39
    vaccine-associated A80.0
    wild virus
      imported A80.1
      indigenous A80.2
  spinal, acute A80.9
Poliosis (eyebrow) (eyelashes) L67.1
  circumscripta, acquired L67.1
Pollakiuria R35.0
  psychogenic F45.8
Pollinosis J30.1
Pollitzer's disease L73.2
Polyadenitis (see also Lymphadenitis)
  malignant A20.0
Polyalgia M79.89
Polyangiitis M30.0
  microscopic M31.7
  overlap syndrome M30.8
Polyarteritis
  microscopic M31.7
  nodosa M30.0
    with lung involvement M30.1
    juvenile M30.2
    related condition NEC M30.8
Polyarthralgia — see Pain, joint
Polyarthritis, polyarthropathy (see also Arthritis)
    M13.0
  due to or associated with other specified
    conditions — see Arthritis
  epidemic (Australian) (with exanthema) B33.1
  infective — see Arthritis, pyogenic or pyemic
  inflammatory M06.4
  juvenile (chronic) (seronegative) M08.3
  migratory — see Fever, rheumatic
  rheumatic, acute — see Fever, rheumatic
Polyarthrosis M15.9
  post-traumatic M15.3
  primary M15.0
  specified NEC M15.8
Polycarential syndrome of infancy E40
Polychondritis (atrophic) (chronic) (see also Disorder,
    cartilage, specified type NEC)
  relapsing M94.1
Polycoria Q13.2
Polycystic (disease)
  degeneration, kidney Q61.3
    autosomal dominant (adult type) Q61.2
    autosomal recessive (infantile type) NEC Q61.19
  kidney Q61.3
    autosomal
      dominant Q61.2
      recessive NEC Q61.19
    autosomal dominant (adult type) Q61.2
    autosomal recessive (childhood type)
      NEC Q61.19
    infantile type NEC Q61.19
  liver Q44.6
  lung J98.4
    congenital Q33.0

Polycystic — continued
  ovary, ovaries E28.2
  spleen Q89.09
Polycythemia (secondary) D75.1
  acquired D75.1
  benign (familial) D75.0
  due to
    donor twin P61.1
    erythropoietin D75.1
    fall in plasma volume D75.1
    high altitude D75.1
    maternal-fetal transfusion P61.1
    stress D75.1
  emotional D75.1
  erythropoietin D75.1
  familial (benign) D75.0
  Gaisböck's (hypertonica) D75.1
  high altitude D75.1
  hypertonica D75.1
  hypoxemic D75.1
  neonatorum P61.1
  nephrogenous D75.1
  relative D75.1
  secondary D75.1
  spurious D75.1
  stress D75.1
  vera D45
Polycytosis cryptogenica D75.1
Polydactylism, polydactyly Q69.9
  toes Q69.2
Polydipsia R63.1
Polydystrophy, pseudo-Hurler E77.0
Polyembryoma — see Neoplasm, malignant, by site
Polyglandular
  deficiency E31.0
  dyscrasia E31.9
  dysfunction E31.9
  syndrome E31.8
Polyhydramnios O40. ☑
Polymastia Q83.1
Polymenorrhea N92.0
Polymyalgia M35.3
  arteritica, giant cell M31.5
  rheumatica M35.3
    with giant cell arteritis M31.5
Polymyositis (acute) (chronic) (hemorrhagic) M33.20
  with
    myopathy M33.22
    respiratory involvement M33.21
    skin involvement — see Dermatopolymyositis
    specified organ involvement NEC M33.29
  ossificans (generalisata) (progressiva) — see
    Myositis, ossificans, progressiva
Polyneuritis, polyneuritic (see also Polyneuropathy)
  acute (post-) infective G61.0
  alcoholic G62.1
  cranialis G52.7
  demyelinating, chronic inflammatory
    (CIDP) G61.81
  diabetic — see Diabetes, polyneuropathy
  diphtheritic A36.83
  due to lack of vitamin NEC E56.9 [G63]
  endemic E51.11
  erythredema — see subcategory T56.1
  febrile, acute G61.0
  hereditary ataxic G60.1
  idiopathic, acute G61.0
  infective (acute) G61.0
  inflammatory, chronic demyelinating
    (CIDP) G61.81
  nutritional E63.9 [G63]
  postinfective (acute) G61.0
  specified NEC G62.89
Polyneuropathy (peripheral) G62.9
  alcoholic G62.1
  amyloid (Portuguese) E85.1 [G63]
    transthyretin-related (ATTR) familial E85.1
  arsenical G62.2
  critical illness G62.81
  demyelinating, chronic inflammatory
    (CIDP) G61.81
  diabetic — see Diabetes, polyneuropathy
  drug-induced G62.0
  hereditary G60.9
    specified NEC G60.8
  idiopathic G60.9
    progressive G60.3
  in (due to)
    alcohol G62.1
      sequelae G65.2
    amyloidosis, familial (Portuguese) E85.1 [G63]
    antitetanus serum G61.1

☑ **Additional character required**

Polyneuropathy — continued
  in — continued
    arsenic G62.2
      sequelae G65.2
    avitaminosis NEC E56.9 [G63]
    beriberi E51.11
    collagen vascular disease NEC M35.9 [G63]
    deficiency (of)
      B (-complex) vitamins E53.9 [G63]
      vitamin B6 E53.1 [G63]
    diabetes — see Diabetes, polyneuropathy
    diphtheria A36.83
    drug or medicament G62.0
      correct substance properly administered — see Table of Drugs and Chemicals, by drug, adverse effect
      overdose or wrong substance given or taken — see Table of Drugs and Chemicals, by drug, poisoning
    endocrine disease NEC E34.9 [G63]
    herpes zoster B02.23
    hypoglycemia E16.2 [G63]
    infectious
      disease NEC B99 ☑ [G63]
      mononucleosis B27.91
    lack of vitamin NEC E56.9 [G63]
    lead G62.2
      sequelae G65.2
    leprosy A30.9 [G63]
    Lyme disease A69.22
    metabolic disease NEC E88.9 [G63]
    microscopic polyangiitis M31.7 [G63]
    mumps B26.84
    neoplastic disease (see also Neoplasm) D49.9 [G63]
    nutritional deficiency NEC E63.9 [G63]
    organophosphate compounds G62.2
      sequelae G65.2
    parasitic disease NEC B89 [G63]
    pellagra E52 [G63]
    polyarteritis nodosa M30.0
    porphyria E80.20 [G63]
    radiation G62.82
    rheumatoid arthritis — see Rheumatoid, polyneuropathy
    sarcoidosis D86.89
    serum G61.1
    syphilis (late) A52.15
      congenital A50.43
    systemic
      connective tissue disorder M35.9 [G63]
      lupus erythematosus M32.19
    toxic agent NEC G62.2
      sequelae G65.2
    transthyretin-related (ATTR) familial amyloid E85.1
    triorthocresyl phosphate G62.2
      sequelae G65.2
    tuberculosis A17.89
    uremia N18.9 [G63]
    vitamin B12 deficiency E53.8 [G63]
      with anemia (pernicious) D51.0 [G63]
        due to dietary deficiency D51.3 [G63]
    zoster B02.23
  inflammatory G61.9
    chronic demyelinating (CIDP) G61.81
    sequelae G65.1
    specified NEC G61.89
  lead G62.2
    sequelae G65.2
  nutritional NEC E63.9 [G63]
  postherpetic (zoster) B02.23
  progressive G60.3
  radiation-induced G62.82
  sensory (hereditary) (idiopathic) G60.8
  specified NEC G62.89
  syphilitic (late) A52.15
    congenital A50.43
Polyopia H53.8
Polyorchism, polyorchidism Q55.21
Polyosteoarthritis (see also Osteoarthritis, generalized) M15.9
  post-traumatic M15.3
  specified NEC M15.8
Polyostotic fibrous dysplasia Q78.1
Polyotia Q17.0
Polyp, polypus
  accessory sinus J33.8
  adenocarcinoma in — see Neoplasm, malignant, by site
  adenocarcinoma in situ in — see Neoplasm, in situ, by site

Polyp, polypus — continued
  adenoid tissue J33.0
  adenomatous (see also Neoplasm, benign, by site)
    adenocarcinoma in — see Neoplasm, malignant, by site
    adenocarcinoma in situ in — see Neoplasm, in situ, by site
    carcinoma in — see Neoplasm, malignant, by site
    carcinoma in situ in — see Neoplasm, in situ, by site
    multiple — see Neoplasm, benign
      adenocarcinoma in — see Neoplasm, malignant, by site
      adenocarcinoma in situ in — see Neoplasm, in situ, by site
  antrum J33.8
  anus, anal (canal) K62.0
  Bartholin's gland N84.3
  bladder D41.4
  carcinoma in — see Neoplasm, malignant, by site
  carcinoma in situ in — see Neoplasm, in situ, by site
  cecum D12.0
  cervix (uteri) N84.1
    in pregnancy or childbirth — see Pregnancy, complicated by, abnormal, cervix
    mucous N84.1
    nonneoplastic N84.1
  choanal J33.0
  cholesterol K82.4
  clitoris N84.3
  colon K63.5
    adenomatous D12.6
    ascending D12.2
    cecum D12.0
    descending D12.4
    inflammatory K51.40
      with
        abscess K51.414
        complication K51.419
          specified NEC K51.418
        fistula K51.413
        intestinal obstruction K51.412
        rectal bleeding K51.411
    sigmoid D12.5
    transverse D12.3
  corpus uteri N84.0
  dental K04.01
    irreversible K04.02
    reversible K04.01
  duodenum K31.7
  ear (middle) H74.4 ☑
  endometrium N84.0
  ethmoidal (sinus) J33.8
  fallopian tube N84.8
  female genital tract N84.9
    specified NEC N84.8
  frontal (sinus) J33.8
  gallbladder K82.4
  gingiva, gum K06.8
  labia, labium (majus) (minus) N84.3
  larynx (mucous) J38.1
    adenomatous D14.1
  malignant — see Neoplasm, malignant, by site
  maxillary (sinus) J33.8
  middle ear — see Polyp, ear (middle)
  myometrium N84.0
  nares
    anterior J33.9
    posterior J33.0
  nasal (mucous) J33.9
    cavity J33.0
    septum J33.0
  nasopharyngeal J33.0
  nose (mucous) J33.9
  oviduct N84.8
  pharynx J39.2
  placenta O90.89
  prostate — see Enlargement, enlarged, prostate
  pudenda, pudendum N84.3
  pulpal (dental) K04.01
    irreversible K04.02
    reversible K04.01
  rectum (nonadenomatous) K62.1
    adenomatous — see Polyp, adenomatous
  septum (nasal) J33.0
  sinus (accessory) (ethmoidal) (frontal) (maxillary) (sphenoidal) J33.8
  sphenoidal (sinus) J33.8
  stomach K31.7
    adenomatous D13.1

Polyp, polypus — continued
  tube, fallopian N84.8
  turbinate, mucous membrane J33.8
  umbilical, newborn P83.6
  ureter N28.89
  urethra N36.2
  uterus (body) (corpus) (mucous) N84.0
    cervix N84.1
    in pregnancy or childbirth — see Pregnancy, complicated by, tumor, uterus
  vagina N84.2
  vocal cord (mucous) J38.1
  vulva N84.3
Polyphagia R63.2
Polyploidy Q92.7
Polypoid — see condition
Polyposis (see also Polyp)
  coli (adenomatous) D12.6
    adenocarcinoma in C18.9
    adenocarcinoma in situ in — see Neoplasm, in situ, by site
    carcinoma in C18.9
  colon (adenomatous) D12.6
  familial D12.6
    adenocarcinoma in situ in — see Neoplasm, in situ, by site
  intestinal (adenomatous) D12.6
  malignant lymphomatous C83.1 ☑
  multiple, adenomatous (see also Neoplasm, benign) D36.9
Polyradiculitis — see Polyneuropathy
Polyradiculoneuropathy (acute) (postinfective) (segmentally demyelinating) G61.0
Polyserositis
  due to pericarditis I31.1
  pericardial I31.1
  periodic, familial E85.0
  tuberculous A19.9
    acute A19.1
    chronic A19.8
Polysplenia syndrome Q89.09
Polysyndactyly (see also Syndactylism, syndactyly) Q70.4
Polytrichia L68.3
Polyunguia Q84.6
Polyuria R35.8
  nocturnal R35.1
  psychogenic F45.8
Pompe's disease (glycogen storage) E74.02
Pompholyx L30.1
Poncet's disease (tuberculous rheumatism) A18.09
Pond fracture — see Fracture, skull
Ponos B55.0
Pons, pontine — see condition
Poor
  aesthetic of existing restoration of tooth K08.56
  contractions, labor O62.2
  gingival margin to tooth restoration K08.51
  personal hygiene R46.0
  prenatal care, affecting management of pregnancy — see Pregnancy, complicated by, insufficient, prenatal care
  sucking reflex (newborn) R29.2
  urinary stream R39.12
  vision NEC H54.7
Poradenitis, nostras inguinalis or venerea A55
Porencephaly (congenital) (developmental) (true) Q04.6
  acquired G93.0
  nondevelopmental G93.0
  traumatic (post) F07.89
Porocephaliasis B88.8
Porokeratosis Q82.8
Poroma, eccrine — see Neoplasm, skin, benign
Porphyria (South African) E80.20
  acquired E80.20
  acute intermittent (hepatic) (Swedish) E80.21
  cutanea tarda (hereditary) (symptomatic) E80.1
  due to drugs E80.20
    correct substance properly administered — see Table of Drugs and Chemicals, by drug, adverse effect
    overdose or wrong substance given or taken — see Table of Drugs and Chemicals, by drug, poisoning
  erythropoietic (congenital) (hereditary) E80.0
  hepatocutaneous type E80.1
  secondary E80.20
  toxic NEC E80.20
  variegata E80.20
Porphyrinuria — see Porphyria
Porphyruria — see Porphyria

Portal — *see* condition
Port wine nevus, mark, or stain Q82.5
Posadas-Wernicke disease B38.9
Positive
  culture (nonspecific)
    blood R78.81
    bronchial washings R84.5
    cerebrospinal fluid R83.5
    cervix uteri R87.5
    nasal secretions R84.5
    nipple discharge R89.5
    nose R84.5
      staphylococcus (Methicillin
        susceptible) Z22.321
        Methicillin resistant Z22.322
    peritoneal fluid R85.5
    pleural fluid R84.5
    prostatic secretions R86.5
    saliva R85.5
    seminal fluid R86.5
    sputum R84.5
    synovial fluid R89.5
    throat scrapings R84.5
    urine R82.79
    vagina R87.5
    vulva R87.5
    wound secretions R89.5
  PPD (skin test) R76.11
  serology for syphilis A53.0
    false R76.8
    with signs or symptoms - code as Syphilis, by
      site and stage
  skin test, tuberculin (without active
    tuberculosis) R76.11
  test, human immunodeficiency virus (HIV) R75
  VDRL A53.0
    with signs or symptoms - code by site and
      stage under Syphilis A53.9
  Wassermann reaction A53.0
Postcardiotomy syndrome I97.0
Postcaval ureter Q62.62
Postcholecystectomy syndrome K91.5
Postclimacteric bleeding N95.0
Postcommissurotomy syndrome I97.0
Postconcussional syndrome F07.81
Postcontusional syndrome F07.81
Postcricoid region — *see* condition
Post-dates (40-42 weeks) (pregnancy) (mother) O48.0
  more than 42 weeks gestation O48.1
Postencephalitic syndrome F07.89
Posterior — *see* condition
Posterolateral sclerosis (spinal cord) — *see*
  Degeneration, combined
Postexanthematous — *see* condition
Postfebrile — *see* condition
Postgastrectomy dumping syndrome K91.1
Posthemiplegic chorea — *see* Monoplegia
Posthemorrhagic anemia (chronic) D50.0
  acute D62
  newborn P61.3
Postherpetic neuralgia (zoster) B02.29
  trigeminal B02.22
Posthitis N47.7
Postimmunization complication or reaction — *see*
  Complications, vaccination
Postinfectious — *see* condition
Postlaminectomy syndrome NEC M96.1
Postleukotomy syndrome F07.0
Postmastectomy lymphedema (syndrome) I97.2
Postmaturity, postmature (over 42 weeks)
  maternal (over 42 weeks gestation) O48.1
  newborn P08.22
Postmeasles complication NEC (*see also* condition)
  B05.89
Postmenopausal
  endometrium (atrophic) N95.8
    suppurative (*see also* Endometritis) N71.9
  osteoporosis — *see* Osteoporosis, postmenopausal
Postnasal drip R09.82
  due to
    allergic rhinitis — *see* Rhinitis, allergic
    common cold J00
    gastroesophageal reflux — *see* Reflux,
      gastroesophageal
    nasopharyngitis — *see* Nasopharyngitis
    other know condition - code to condition
    sinusitis — *see* Sinusitis
Postnatal — *see* condition
Postoperative (postprocedural) — *see* Complication,
  postoperative
  pneumothorax, therapeutic Z98.3
  state NEC Z98.890

Postpancreatectomy hyperglycemia E89.1
Postpartum — *see* Puerperal
Postphlebitic syndrome — *see* Syndrome,
  postthrombotic
Postpoliomyelitic (*see also* condition)
  osteopathy — *see* Osteopathy, after poliomyelitis
Postpolio (myelitic) syndrome G14
Postprocedural (*see also* Postoperative)
  hypoinsulinemia E89.1
Postschizophrenic depression F32.89
Postsurgery status (*see also* Status (post))
  pneumothorax, therapeutic Z98.3
Post-term (40-42 weeks) (pregnancy) (mother) O48.0
  infant P08.21
  more than 42 weeks gestation (mother) O48.1
Post-traumatic brain syndrome, nonpsychotic
  F07.81
Post-typhoid abscess A01.09
Postures, hysterical F44.2
Postvaccinal reaction or complication — *see*
  Complications, vaccination
Postvalvulotomy syndrome I97.0
Potain's
  disease (pulmonary edema) — *see* Edema, lung
  syndrome (gastrectasis with dyspepsia) K31.0
Potter's
  asthma J62.8
  facies Q60.6
  lung J62.8
  syndrome (with renal agenesis) Q60.6
Pott's
  curvature (spinal) A18.01
  disease or paraplegia A18.01
  spinal curvature A18.01
  tumor, puffy — *see* Osteomyelitis, specified type
    NEC
Pouch
  bronchus Q32.4
  Douglas' — *see* condition
  esophagus, esophageal, congenital Q39.6
    acquired K22.5
  gastric K31.4
  Hartmann's K82.8
  pharynx, pharyngeal (congenital) Q38.7
Pouchitis K91.850
Poultrymen's itch B88.0
Poverty NEC Z59.6
  extreme Z59.5
Poxvirus NEC B08.8
Prader-Willi syndrome Q87.1
Preauricular appendage or tag Q17.0
Prebetalipoproteinemia (acquired) (essential)
  (familial) (hereditary) (primary) (secondary) E78.1
  with chylomicronemia E78.3
Precipitate labor or delivery O62.3
Preclimacteric bleeding (menorrhagia) N92.4
Precocious
  adrenarche E30.1
  menarche E30.1
  menstruation E30.1
  pubarche E30.1
  puberty E30.1
    central E22.8
  sexual development NEC E30.1
  thelarche E30.8
Precocity, sexual (constitutional) (cryptogenic)
  (female) (idiopathic) (male) E30.1
  with adrenal hyperplasia E25.9
    congenital E25.0
Precordial pain R07.2
Predeciduous teeth K00.2
Prediabetes, prediabetic R73.03
  complicating
    pregnancy — *see* Pregnancy, complicated by,
      diseases of, specified type or system NEC
    puerperium O99.89
Predislocation status of hip at birth Q65.6
Pre-eclampsia O14.9 ☑
  with pre-existing hypertension — *see*
    Hypertension, complicating pregnancy, pre-
    existing, with, pre-eclampsia
  complicating
    childbirth O14.94
    puerperium O14.95
  mild O14.0 ☑
    complicating
      childbirth O14.04
      puerperium O14.05
  moderate O14.0 ☑
    complicating
      childbirth O14.04
      puerperium O14.05

Pre-eclampsia — *continued*
  severe O14.1 ☑
    with hemolysis, elevated liver enzymes and low
      platelet count (HELLP) O14.2 ☑
    complicating
      childbirth O14.24
      puerperium O14.25
    complicating
      childbirth O14.14
      puerperium O14.15
Pre-eruptive color change, teeth, tooth K00.8
Pre-excitation atrioventricular conduction I45.6
Preglaucoma H40.00 ☑
Pregnancy (single) (uterine) (*see also* Delivery and
  Puerperal)
  Note: The Tabular must be reviewed for
    assignment of the appropriate character
    indicating the trimester of the pregnancy
  Note: The Tabular must be reviewed for
    assignment of appropriate seventh character
    for multiple gestation codes in Chapter 15
  abdominal (ectopic) O00.00
    with intrauterine pregnancy O00.01
    with viable fetus O36.7 ☑
  ampullar O00.10 ☑
    with intrauterine pregnancy O00.11 ☑
  biochemical O02.81
  broad ligament O00.80
    with intrauterine pregnancy O00.81
  cervical O00.80
    with intrauterine pregnancy O00.81
  chemical O02.81
  complicated NOS O26.9 ☑
  complicated by (care of) (management affected
    by)
    abnormal, abnormality
      cervix O34.4 ☑
        causing obstructed labor O65.5
      cord (umbilical) O69.9 ☑
      fetal heart rate or rhythm O36.83 ☑
      findings on antenatal screening of
        mother O28.9
        biochemical O28.1
        cytological O28.2
        chromosomal O28.5
        genetic O28.5
        hematological O28.0
        radiological O28.4
        specified NEC O28.8
        ultrasonic O28.3
      glucose (tolerance) NEC O99.810
      pelvic organs O34.9 ☑
        specified NEC O34.8 ☑
          causing obstructed labor O65.5
      pelvis (bony) (major) NEC O33.0
      perineum O34.7 ☑
      position
        placenta O44.0 ☑
          with hemorrhage O44.1 ☑
        uterus O34.59 ☑
      uterus O34.59 ☑
        causing obstructed labor O65.5
        congenital O34.0 ☑
      vagina O34.6 ☑
        causing obstructed labor O65.5
      vulva O34.7 ☑
        causing obstructed labor O65.5
    abruptio placentae — *see* Abruptio placentae
    abscess or cellulitis
      bladder O23.1 ☑
      breast O91.11 ☑
      genital organ or tract O23.9 ☑
    abuse
      physical O9A.31 ☑
      psychological O9A.51 ☑
      sexual O9A.41 ☑
    adverse effect anesthesia O29.9 ☑
      aspiration pneumonitis O29.01 ☑
      cardiac arrest O29.11 ☑
      cardiac complication NEC O29.19 ☑
      cardiac failure O29.12 ☑
      central nervous system complication
        NEC O29.29 ☑
      cerebral anoxia O29.21 ☑
      failed or difficult intubation O29.6 ☑
      inhalation of stomach contents or secretions
        NOS O29.01 ☑
      local, toxic reaction O29.3X ☑
      Mendelson's syndrome O29.01 ☑
      pressure collapse of lung O29.02 ☑
      pulmonary complications NEC O29.09 ☑
      specified NEC O29.8X ☑

Pregnancy — *continued*
   complicated by — *continued*
      spinal and epidural type NEC O29.5X ☑
         induced headache O29.4 ☑
      albuminuria (*see also* Proteinuria, gestational) O12.1 ☑
      alcohol use O99.31 ☑
      amnionitis O41.12 ☑
      anaphylactoid syndrome of pregnancy O88.01 ☑
      anemia (conditions in D50-D64) (pre-existing) O99.01 ☑
         complicating the puerperium O99.03
      antepartum hemorrhage O46.9 ☑
         with coagulation defect — *see* Hemorrhage, antepartum, with coagulation defect
         specified NEC O46.8X ☑
      appendicitis O99.61 ☑
      atrophy (yellow) (acute) liver (subacute) O26.61 ☑
      bariatric surgery status O99.84 ☑
      bicornis or bicornuate uterus O34.0 ☑
      biliary tract problems O26.61 ☑
      breech presentation O32.1 ☑
      cardiovascular diseases (conditions in I00-I09, I20-I52, I70-I99) O99.41 ☑
      cerebrovascular disorders (conditions in I60-I69) O99.41 ☑
      cervical shortening O26.87 ☑
      cervicitis O23.51 ☑
      chloasma (gravidarum) O26.89 ☑
      cholestasis (intrahepatic) O26.61 ☑
      cholecystitis O99.61 ☑
      chorioamnionitis O41.12 ☑
      circulatory system disorder (conditions in I00-I09, I20-I99, O99.41) ☑
      compound presentation O32.6 ☑
      conjoined twins O30.02 ☑
      connective system disorders (conditions in M00-M99) O99.89
      contracted pelvis (general) O33.1
         inlet O33.2
         outlet O33.3 ☑
      convulsions (eclamptic) (uremic) (*see also* Eclampsia) O15.9
      cracked nipple O92.11 ☑
      cystitis O23.1 ☑
      cystocele O34.8 ☑
      death of fetus (near term) O36.4 ☑
         early pregnancy O02.1
         of one fetus or more in multiple gestation O31.2 ☑
      deciduitis O41.14 ☑
      decreased fetal movement O36.81 ☑
      dental problems O99.61 ☑
      diabetes (mellitus) O24.91 ☑
         gestational (pregnancy induced) — *see* Diabetes, gestational
         pre-existing O24.31 ☑
            specified NEC O24.81 ☑
            type 1 O24.01 ☑
            type 2 O24.11 ☑
      digestive system disorders (conditions in K00-K93) O99.61 ☑
      diseases of — *see* Pregnancy, complicated by, specified body system disease
         biliary tract O26.61 ☑
         blood NEC (conditions in D65-D77) O99.11 ☑
         liver O26.61 ☑
         specified NEC O99.89
      disorders of — *see* Pregnancy, complicated by, specified body system disorder
         amniotic fluid and membranes O41.9 ☑
            specified NEC O41.8X ☑
         biliary tract O26.61 ☑
         ear and mastoid process (conditions in H60-H95) O99.89
         eye and adnexa (conditions in H00-H59) O99.89
         liver O26.61 ☑
         skin (conditions in L00-L99) O99.71 ☑
         specified NEC O99.89
      displacement, uterus NEC O34.59 ☑
         causing obstructed labor O65.5
      disproportion (due to) O33.9
         fetal (ascites) (hydrops) (meningomyelocele) (sacral teratoma) (tumor) deformities NEC O33.7 ☑
         generally contracted pelvis O33.1
         hydrocephalic fetus O33.6 ☑
         inlet contraction of pelvis O33.2
         mixed maternal and fetal origin O33.4 ☑

Pregnancy — *continued*
   complicated by — *continued*
      specified NEC O33.8
      double uterus O34.0 ☑
         causing obstructed labor O65.5
      drug use (conditions in F11-F19) O99.32 ☑
      eclampsia, eclamptic (coma) (convulsions) (delirium) (nephritis) (uremia) (*see also* Eclampsia) O15. ☑
      ectopic pregnancy — *see* Pregnancy, ectopic
      edema O12.0 ☑
         with
            gestational hypertension, mild (*see also* Pre-eclampsia) O14.0 ☑
            proteinuria O12.2 ☑
      effusion, amniotic fluid — *see* Pregnancy, complicated by, premature rupture of membranes
      elderly
         multigravida O09.52 ☑
         primigravida O09.51 ☑
      embolism (*see also* Embolism, obstetric, pregnancy) O88.
      endocrine diseases NEC O99.28 ☑
      endometritis O86.12
      excessive weight gain O26.0 ☑
      exhaustion O26.81 ☑
         during labor and delivery O75.81
      face presentation O32.3 ☑
      failed induction of labor O61.9
         instrumental O61.1
         mechanical O61.1
         medical O61.0
         specified NEC O61.8
         surgical O61.1
      failed or difficult intubation for anesthesia O29.6 ☑
      false labor (pains) O47.9
         at or after 37 completed weeks of pregnancy O47.1
         before 37 completed weeks of pregnancy O47.0 ☑
      fatigue O26.81 ☑
         during labor and delivery O75.81
      fatty metamorphosis of liver O26.61 ☑
      female genital mutilation O34.8 ☑ [N90.81 ☑]
      fetal (maternal care for)
         abnormality or damage O35.9 ☑
            acid-base balance O68
            specified type NEC O35.8 ☑
         acidemia O68
         acidosis O68
         alkalosis O68
         anemia and thrombocytopenia O36.82 ☑
         anencephaly O35.0 ☑
         chromosomal abnormality (conditions in Q90-Q99) O35.1 ☑
         conjoined twins O30.02 ☑
         damage from
            amniocentesis O35.7 ☑
            biopsy procedures O35.7 ☑
            drug addiction O35.5 ☑
            hematological investigation O35.7 ☑
            intrauterine contraceptive device O35.7 ☑
            maternal
               alcohol addiction O35.4 ☑
               cytomegalovirus infection O35.3 ☑
               disease NEC O35.8 ☑
               drug addiction O35.5 ☑
               listeriosis O35.8 ☑
               rubella O35.3 ☑
               toxoplasmosis O35.8 ☑
               viral infection O35.3 ☑
            medical procedure NEC O35.7 ☑
            radiation O35.6 ☑
         death (near term) O36.4 ☑
            early pregnancy O02.1
         decreased movement O36.81 ☑
         disproportion due to deformity (fetal) O33.7 ☑
         excessive growth (large for dates) O36.6 ☑
         growth retardation O36.59 ☑
            light for dates O36.59 ☑
            small for dates O36.59 ☑
         heart rate irregularity (bradycardia) (decelerations) (tachycardia) O76
         hereditary disease O35.2 ☑
         hydrocephalus O35.0 ☑
         intrauterine death O36.4 ☑
         poor growth O36.59 ☑
            light for dates O36.59 ☑
            small for dates O36.59 ☑

Pregnancy — *continued*
   complicated by — *continued*
      problem O36.9 ☑
         specified NEC O36.89 ☑
      reduction (elective) O31.3 ☑
      selective termination O31.3 ☑
      spina bifida O35.0 ☑
      thrombocytopenia O36.82 ☑
      fibroid (tumor) (uterus) O34.1 ☑
      fissure of nipple O92.11 ☑
      gallstones O99.61 ☑
      gastric banding status O99.84 ☑
      gastric bypass status O99.84 ☑
      genital herpes (asymptomatic) (history of) (inactive) O98.3 ☑
      genital tract infection O23.9 ☑
      glomerular diseases (conditions in N00-N07) O26.83 ☑
         with hypertension, pre-existing — *see* Hypertension, complicating, pregnancy, pre-existing, with, renal disease
      gonorrhea O98.21 ☑
      grand multiparity O09.4 ☑
      habitual aborter — *see* Pregnancy, complicated by, recurrent pregnancy loss
      HELLP syndrome (hemolysis, elevated liver enzymes and low platelet count) O14.2 ☑
      hemorrhage
         antepartum — *see* Hemorrhage, antepartum
         before 20 completed weeks gestation O20.9
            specified NEC O20.8
         due to premature separation, placenta (*see also* Abruptio placentae) O45.9 ☑
         early O20.9
            specified NEC O20.8
         threatened abortion O20.0
      hemorrhoids O22.4 ☑
      hepatitis (viral) O98.41 ☑
      herniation of uterus O34.59 ☑
      high
         head at term O32.4 ☑
         risk — *see* Supervision (of) (for), high-risk
      history of in utero procedure during previous pregnancy O09.82 ☑
      HIV O98.71 ☑
      human immunodeficiency virus (HIV) disease O98.71 ☑
      hydatidiform mole (*see also* Mole, hydatidiform) O01.9
      hydramnios O40. ☑
      hydrocephalic fetus (disproportion) O33.6 ☑
      hydrops
         amnii O40. ☑
         fetalis O36.2 ☑
            associated with isoimmunization (*see also* Pregnancy, complicated by, isoimmunization) O36.11 ☑
      hydrorrhea O42.90
      hyperemesis (gravidarum) (mild) (*see also* Hyperemesis, gravidarum) O21.0
      hypertension — *see* Hypertension, complicating pregnancy
      hypertensive
         heart and renal disease, pre-existing — *see* Hypertension, complicating, pregnancy, pre-existing, with, heart disease, with renal disease
         heart disease, pre-existing — *see* Hypertension, complicating, pregnancy, pre-existing, with, heart disease
         renal disease, pre-existing — *see* Hypertension, complicating, pregnancy, pre-existing, with, renal disease
      hypotension O26.5 ☑
      immune disorders NEC (conditions in D80-D89) O99.11 ☑
      incarceration, uterus O34.51 ☑
      incompetent cervix O34.3 ☑
      inconclusive fetal viability O36.80 ☑
      infection (s) O98.91 ☑
         amniotic fluid or sac O41.10 ☑
         bladder O23.1 ☑
         carrier state NEC O99.830
            streptococcus B O99.820
         genital organ or tract O23.9 ☑
            specified NEC O23.59 ☑
         genitourinary tract O23.9 ☑
         gonorrhea O98.21 ☑
         hepatitis (viral) O98.41 ☑
         HIV O98.71 ☑
         human immunodeficiency virus (HIV) O98.71 ☑

Pregnancy

Pregnancy — *continued*
  complicated by — *continued*
    kidney O23.0 ☑
    nipple O91.01 ☑
    parasitic disease O98.91 ☑
      specified NEC O98.81 ☑
    protozoal disease O98.61 ☑
    sexually transmitted NEC O98.31 ☑
    specified type NEC O98.81 ☑
    syphilis O98.11 ☑
    tuberculosis O98.01 ☑
    urethra O23.2 ☑
    urinary (tract) O23.4 ☑
      specified NEC O23.3 ☑
    viral disease O98.51 ☑
  injury or poisoning (conditions in S00-T88) O9A.21 ☑
    due to abuse
      physical O9A.31 ☑
      psychological O9A.51 ☑
      sexual O9A.41 ☑
  insufficient
    prenatal care O09.3 ☑
    weight gain O26.1 ☑
  insulin resistance O26.89 ☑
  intrauterine fetal death (near term) O36.4 ☑
    early pregnancy O02.1
    multiple gestation (one fetus or more) O31.2 ☑
  isoimmunization O36.11 ☑
    anti-A sensitization O36.11 ☑
    anti-B sensitization O36.19 ☑
    Rh O36.09 ☑
      anti-D antibody O36.01 ☑
    specified NEC O36.19 ☑
  laceration of uterus NEC O71.81
  malformation
    placenta, placental (vessel) O43.10 ☑
      specified NEC O43.19 ☑
    uterus (congenital) O34.0 ☑
  malnutrition (conditions in E40-E46) O25.1 ☑
  maternal hypotension syndrome O26.5 ☑
  mental disorders (conditions in F01-F09, F20-F99) O99.34 ☑
    alcohol use O99.31 ☑
    drug use O99.32 ☑
    smoking O99.33 ☑
  mentum presentation O32.3 ☑
  metabolic disorders O99.28 ☑
  missed
    abortion O02.1
    delivery O36.4 ☑
  multiple gestations O30.9 ☑
    conjoined twins O30.02 ☑
    specified number of multiples NEC — *see* Pregnancy, multiple (gestation), specified NEC
    quadruplet — *see* Pregnancy, quadruplet
    specified complication NEC O31.8X ☑
    triplet — *see* Pregnancy, triplet
    twin — *see* Pregnancy, twin
  musculoskeletal condition (conditions is M00-M99) O99.89
  necrosis, liver (conditions in K72) O26.61 ☑
  neoplasm
    benign
      cervix O34.4 ☑
      corpus uteri O34.1 ☑
      uterus O34.1 ☑
    malignant O9A.11 ☑
  nephropathy NEC O26.83 ☑
  nervous system condition (conditions in G00-G99) O99.35 ☑
  nutritional diseases NEC O99.28 ☑
  obesity (pre-existing) O99.21 ☑
  obesity surgery status O99.84 ☑
  oblique lie or presentation O32.2 ☑
  older mother — *see* Pregnancy, complicated by, elderly
  oligohydramnios O41.0 ☑
    with premature rupture of membranes (*see also* Pregnancy, complicated by, premature rupture of membranes) O42. ☑
  onset (spontaneous) of labor after 37 completed weeks of gestation but before 39 completed weeks gestation, with delivery by (planned) cesarean section O75.82
  oophoritis O23.52 ☑
  overdose, drug (*see also* Table of Drugs and Chemicals, by drug, poisoning) O9A.21 ☑

Pregnancy — *continued*
  complicated by — *continued*
    oversize fetus O33.5 ☑
    papyraceous fetus O31.0 ☑
    pelvic inflammatory disease O99.89
    periodontal disease O99.61 ☑
    peripheral neuritis O26.82 ☑
    peritoneal (pelvic) adhesions O99.89
    phlebitis O22.9 ☑
    phlebopathy O22.9 ☑
    phlebothrombosis (superficial) O22.2 ☑
      deep O22.3 ☑
    placenta accreta O43.21 ☑
    placenta increta O43.22 ☑
    placenta percreta O43.23 ☑
    placenta previa O44.0 ☑
      complete O44.0 ☑
        with hemorrhage O44.1 ☑
      marginal O44.2 ☑
        with hemorrhage O44.3 ☑
      partial O44.2 ☑
        with hemorrhage O44.3 ☑
    placental disorder O43.9 ☑
      specified NEC O43.89 ☑
    placental dysfunction O43.89 ☑
    placental infarction O43.81 ☑
    placental insufficiency O36.51 ☑
    placental transfusion syndromes
      fetomaternal O43.01 ☑
      fetus to fetus O43.02 ☑
      maternofetal O43.01 ☑
    placentitis O41.14 ☑
    pneumonia O99.51 ☑
    poisoning (*see also* Table of Drugs and Chemicals) O9A.21 ☑
    polyhydramnios O40 ☑
    polymorphic eruption of pregnancy O26.86
    poor obstetric history NEC O09.29 ☑
    postmaturity (post-term) (40 to 42 weeks) O48.0
    more than 42 completed weeks gestation (prolonged) O48.1
    pre-eclampsia O14.9 ☑
      mild O14.0 ☑
      moderate O14.0 ☑
      severe O14.1 ☑
        with hemolysis, elevated liver enzymes and low platelet count (HELLP) O14.2 ☑
    premature labor — *see* Pregnancy, complicated by, preterm labor
    premature rupture of membranes O42.90
      full-term, unspecified as to length of time between rupture and onset of labor O42.92
      with onset of labor
        within 24 hours O42.00
          at or after 37 weeks gestation, onset of labor within 24 hours of rupture O42.02
          pre-term (before 37 completed weeks of gestation) O42.01 ☑
        after 24 hours O42.10
          at or after 37 weeks gestation, onset of labor more than 24 hours following rupture O42.12
          pre-term (before 37 completed weeks of gestation) O42.11 ☑
      at or after 37 weeks gestation, unspecified as to length of time between rupture and onset of labor O42.92
      pre-term (before 37 completed weeks of gestation) O42.91 ☑
    premature separation of placenta (*see also* Abruptio placentae) O45.9 ☑
    presentation, fetal — *see* Delivery, complicated by, malposition
    preterm delivery O60.10 ☑
    preterm labor
      with delivery O60.10 ☑
        preterm O60.10 ☑
        term O60.20 ☑
      second trimester
        with term delivery O60.22 ☑
        without delivery O60.02
        with preterm delivery
          second trimester O60.12 ☑
          third trimester O60.13 ☑
      third trimester
        with term delivery O60.23 ☑
        without delivery O60.03
        with third trimester preterm delivery O60.14 ☑

Pregnancy — *continued*
  complicated by — *continued*
    without delivery O60.00
      second trimester O60.02
      third trimester O60.03
    previous history of — *see* Pregnancy, supervision of, high-risk
    prolapse, uterus O34.52 ☑
    proteinuria (gestational) (*see also* Proteinuria, gestational) O12.1 ☑
    with edema O12.2 ☑
    pruritic urticarial papules and plaques of pregnancy (PUPPP) O26.86
    pruritus (neurogenic) O26.89 ☑
    psychosis or psychoneurosis (puerperal) F53
    ptyalism O26.89 ☑
    PUPPP (pruritic urticarial papules and plaques of pregnancy) O26.86
    pyelitis O23.0 ☑
    recurrent pregnancy loss O26.2 ☑
    renal disease or failure NEC O26.83 ☑
      with secondary hypertension, pre-existing — *see* Hypertension, complicating, pregnancy, pre-existing, secondary
      hypertensive, pre-existing — *see* Hypertension, complicating, pregnancy, pre-existing, with, renal disease
    respiratory condition (conditions in J00-J99) O99.51 ☑
    retained, retention
      dead ovum O02.0
      intrauterine contraceptive device O26.3 ☑
    retroversion, uterus O34.53 ☑
    Rh immunization, incompatibility or sensitization NEC O36.09 ☑
      anti-D antibody O36.01 ☑
    rupture
      amnion (premature) (*see also* Pregnancy, complicated by, premature rupture of membranes) O42 ☑
      membranes (premature) (*see also* Pregnancy, complicated by, premature rupture of membranes) O42 ☑
      uterus (during labor) O71.1
        before onset of labor O71.0 ☑
    salivation (excessive) O26.89 ☑
    salpingitis O23.52 ☑
    salpingo-oophoritis O23.52 ☑
    sepsis (conditions in A40, A41) O98.81 ☑
    size date discrepancy (uterine) O26.84 ☑
    skin condition (conditions in L00-L99) O99.71 ☑
    smoking (tobacco) O99.33 ☑
    social problem O09.7 ☑
    specified condition NEC O26.89 ☑
    spotting O26.85 ☑
    streptococcus group B (GBS) carrier state O99.820
    subluxation of symphysis (pubis) O26.71 ☑
    syphilis (conditions in A50-A53) O98.11 ☑
    threatened
      abortion O20.0
      labor O47.9
        at or after 37 completed weeks of gestation O47.1
        before 37 completed weeks of gestation O47.0 ☑
    thrombophlebitis (superficial) O22.2 ☑
    thrombosis O22.9 ☑
      cerebral venous O22.5 ☑
      cerebrovenous sinus O22.5 ☑
      deep O22.3 ☑
    tobacco use disorder (smoking) O99.33 ☑
    torsion of uterus O34.59 ☑
    toxemia O14.9 ☑
    transverse lie or presentation O32.2 ☑
    tuberculosis (conditions in A15-A19) O98.01 ☑
    tumor (benign)
      cervix O34.4 ☑
      malignant O9A.11 ☑
      uterus O34.1 ☑
    unstable lie O32.0 ☑
    upper respiratory infection O99.51 ☑
    urethritis O23.2 ☑
    uterine size date discrepancy O26.84 ☑
    vaginitis or vulvitis O23.59 ☑
    varicose veins (lower extremities) O22.0 ☑
      genitals O22.1 ☑
      legs O22.0 ☑
      perineal O22.1 ☑
      vaginal or vulval O22.1 ☑

☑ **Additional character required**

Pregnancy   ICD-10-CM INDEX TO DISEASES AND INJURIES

Pregnancy — continued
  complicated by — continued
    venereal disease NEC (conditions in
      A63.8) O98.31 ☑
    venous disorders O22.9 ☑
      specified NEC O22.8X ☑
    viral diseases (conditions in A80-B09,
      B25-B34) O98.51 ☑
    very young mother — see Pregnancy,
      complicated by, young mother
    vomiting O21.9
      due to diseases classified elsewhere O21.8
      hyperemesis gravidarum (mild) (see also
        Hyperemesis, gravidarum) O21.0
      late (occurring after 20 weeks of
        gestation) O21.2
    young mother
      multigravida O09.62 ☑
      primigravida O09.61 ☑
  concealed O09.3 ☑
  continuing following
    elective fetal reduction of one or more
      fetus O31.3 ☑
    intrauterine death of one or more
      fetus O31.2 ☑
    spontaneous abortion of one or more
      fetus O31.1 ☑
  cornual O00.80
    with intrauterine pregnancy O00.81
  ectopic (ruptured) O00.90
    with intrauterine pregnancy O00.91
    abdominal O00.00
      with
        intrauterine pregnancy O00.01
        viable fetus O36.7 ☑
    cervical O00.80
      with intrauterine pregnancy O00.81
    complicated (by) O08.9
      afibrinogenemia O08.1
      cardiac arrest O08.81
      chemical damage of pelvic organ (s) O08.6
      circulatory collapse O08.3
      defibrination syndrome O08.1
      electrolyte imbalance O08.5
      embolism (amniotic fluid) (blood clot)
        (pulmonary) (septic) O08.2
      endometritis O08.0
      genital tract and pelvic infection O08.0
      hemorrhage (delayed) (excessive) O08.1
      infection
        genital tract or pelvic O08.0
        kidney 008.83
        urinary tract O08.83
      intravascular coagulation O08.1
      laceration of pelvic organ (s) O08.6
      metabolic disorder O08.5
      oliguria O08.4
      oophoritis O08.0
      parametritis O08.0
      pelvic peritonitis O08.0
      perforation of pelvic organ (s) O08.6
      renal failure or shutdown O08.4
      salpingitis or salpingo-oophoritis O08.0
      sepsis O08.82
      shock O08.83
        septic O08.82
      specified condition NEC O08.89
      tubular necrosis (renal) O08.4
      uremia O08.4
      urinary infection O08.83
      venous complication NEC O08.7
        embolism O08.2
    cornual O00.80
      with intrauterine pregnancy O00.81
    intraligamentous O00.80
      with intrauterine pregnancy O00.81
    mural O00.80
      with intrauterine pregnancy O00.81
    ovarian O00.20 ☑
      with intrauterine pregnancy O00.21 ☑
    specified site NEC O00.80
      with intrauterine pregnancy O00.81
    tubal (ruptured) O00.10 ☑
      with intrauterine pregnancy O00.11 ☑
  examination (normal) Z34.9 ☑
    high-risk — see Pregnancy, supervision of,
      high-risk
    first Z34.0 ☑
    specified Z34.8 ☑
  extrauterine — see Pregnancy, ectopic
  fallopian O00.10 ☑
    with intrauterine pregnancy O00.11 ☑

Pregnancy — continued
  false F45.8
  gestational carrier Z33.3
  hidden O09.3 ☑
  high-risk — see Pregnancy, supervision of,
    high-risk
  incidental finding Z33.1
  interstitial O00.80
    with intrauterine pregnancy O00.81
  intraligamentous O00.80
    with intrauterine pregnancy O00.81
  intramural O00.80
    with intrauterine pregnancy O00.81
  intraperitoneal O00.00
    with intrauterine pregnancy O00.01
  isthmian O00.10 ☑
    with intrauterine pregnancy O00.11 ☑
  mesometric (mural) O00.80
    with intrauterine pregnancy O00.81
  molar NEC O02.0
    complicated (by) O08.9
      afibrinogenemia O08.1
      cardiac arrest O08.81
      chemical damage of pelvic organ (s) O08.6
      circulatory collapse O08.3
      defibrination syndrome O08.1
      electrolyte imbalance O08.5
      embolism (amniotic fluid) (blood clot)
        (pulmonary) (septic) O08.2
      endometritis O08.0
      genital tract and pelvic infection O08.0
      hemorrhage (delayed) (excessive) O08.1
      infection
        genital tract or pelvic O08.0
        kidney O08.83
        urinary tract O08.83
      intravascular coagulation O08.1
      laceration of pelvic organ (s) O08.6
      metabolic disorder O08.5
      oliguria O08.4
      oophoritis O08.0
      parametritis O08.0
      pelvic peritonitis O08.0
      perforation of pelvic organ (s) O08.6
      renal failure or shutdown O08.4
      salpingitis or salpingo-oophoritis O08.0
      sepsis O08.82
      shock O08.3
        septic O08.82
      specified condition NEC O08.89
      tubular necrosis (renal) O08.4
      uremia O08.4
      urinary infection O08.83
      venous complication NEC O08.7
        embolism O08.2
    hydatidiform (see also Mole,
      hydatidiform) O01.9
  multiple (gestation) O30.9 ☑
    greater than quadruplets — see Pregnancy,
      multiple (gestation), specified NEC
    specified NEC O30.80 ☑
      with
        two or more monoamniotic
          fetuses O30.82 ☑
        two or more monochorionic
          fetuses O30.81 ☑
      two or more monoamniotic fetuses O30.82 ☑
      two or more monochorionic
        fetuses O30.81 ☑
      unable to determine number of placenta and
        number of amniotic sacs O30.89 ☑
      unspecified number of placenta and
        unspecified number of amniotic
        sacs O30.80 ☑
  mural O00.80
    with intrauterine pregnancy O00.81
  normal (supervision of) Z34.9 ☑
    high-risk — see Pregnancy, supervision of,
      high-risk
    first Z34.0 ☑
    specified Z34.8 ☑
  ovarian O00.20 ☑
    with intrauterine pregnancy O00.21 ☑
  postmature (40 to 42 weeks) O48.0
    more than 42 weeks gestation O48.1
  post-term (40 to 42 weeks) O48.0
  prenatal care only Z34.9 ☑
    high-risk — see Pregnancy, supervision of,
      high-risk
    first Z34.0 ☑
    specified Z34.8 ☑
  prolonged (more than 42 weeks gestation) O48.1

Pregnancy — continued
  quadruplet O30.20 ☑
    with
      two or more monoamniotic fetuses O30.22 ☑
      two or more monochorionic
        fetuses O30.21 ☑
    two or more monoamniotic fetuses O30.22 ☑
    two or more monochorionic fetuses O30.21 ☑
    unable to determine number of placenta and
      number of amniotic sacs O30.29 ☑
    unspecified number of placenta and
      unspecified number of amniotic
      sacs O30.20 ☑
  quintuplet — see Pregnancy, multiple (gestation),
    specified NEC
  sextuplet — see Pregnancy, multiple (gestation),
    specified NEC
  supervision of
    concealed pregnancy O09.3 ☑
    elderly mother
      multigravida O09.52 ☑
      primigravida O09.51 ☑
    hidden pregnancy O09.3 ☑
    high-risk O09.9 ☑
      due to (history of)
        ectopic pregnancy O09.1 ☑
        elderly — see Pregnancy, supervision,
          elderly mother
        grand multiparity O09.4 ☑
        infertility O09.0 ☑
        insufficient prenatal care O09.3 ☑
        in utero procedure during previous
          pregnancy O09.82 ☑
        in vitro fertilization O09.81 ☑
        molar pregnancy O09.A ☑
        multiple previous pregnancies O09.4 ☑
        older mother — see Pregnancy, supervision
          of, elderly mother
        poor reproductive or obstetric history
          NEC O09.29 ☑
        pre-term labor O09.21 ☑
        previous
          neonatal death O09.29 ☑
        social problems O09.7 ☑
        specified NEC O09.89 ☑
        very young mother — see Pregnancy,
          supervision, young mother
      resulting from in vitro fertilization O09.81 ☑
    normal Z34.9 ☑
      first Z34.0 ☑
      specified NEC Z34.8 ☑
    young mother
      multigravida O09.62 ☑
      primigravida O09.61 ☑
  triplet O30.10 ☑
    with
      two or more monoamniotic fetuses O30.12 ☑
      two or more monochorionic
        fetuses O30.11 ☑
    two or more monoamniotic fetuses O30.12 ☑
    two or more monochorionic fetuses O30.11 ☑
    unable to determine number of placenta and
      number of amniotic sacs O30.19 ☑
    unspecified number of placenta and
      unspecified number of amniotic
      sacs O30.10 ☑
  tubal (with abortion) (with rupture) O00.10 ☑
    with intrauterine pregnancy O00.11 ☑
  twin O30.00 ☑
    conjoined O30.02 ☑
    dichorionic/diamniotic (two placenta, two
      amniotic sacs) O30.04 ☑
    monochorionic/diamniotic (one placenta, two
      amniotic sacs) O30.03 ☑
    monochorionic/monoamniotic (one placenta,
      one amniotic sac) O30.01 ☑
    unable to determine number of placenta and
      number of amniotic sacs O30.09 ☑
    unspecified number of placenta and
      unspecified number of amniotic
      sacs O30.00 ☑
  unwanted Z64.0
  weeks of gestation
    8 weeks Z3A.08
    9 weeks Z3A.09
    10 weeks Z3A.10
    11 weeks Z3A.11
    12 weeks Z3A.12
    13 weeks Z3A.13
    14 weeks Z3A.14
    15 weeks Z3A.15
    16 weeks Z3A.16

Pregnancy — *continued*
  weeks of gestation — *continued*
    17 weeks Z3A.17
    18 weeks Z3A.18
    19 weeks Z3A.19
    20 weeks Z3A.20
    21 weeks Z3A.21
    22 weeks Z3A.22
    23 weeks Z3A.23
    24 weeks Z3A.24
    25 weeks Z3A.25
    26 weeks Z3A.26
    27 weeks Z3A.27
    28 weeks Z3A.28
    29 weeks Z3A.29
    30 weeks Z3A.30
    31 weeks Z3A.31
    32 weeks Z3A.32
    33 weeks Z3A.33
    34 weeks Z3A.34
    35 weeks Z3A.35
    36 weeks Z3A.36
    37 weeks Z3A.37
    38 weeks Z3A.38
    39 weeks Z3A.39
    40 weeks Z3A.40
    41 weeks Z3A.41
    42 weeks Z3A.42
    greater than 42 weeks Z3A.49
    less than 8 weeks Z3A.01
    not specified Z3A.00
  Preiser's disease — *see* Osteonecrosis, secondary, due to, trauma, metacarpus
  Pre-kwashiorkor — *see* Malnutrition, severe
  Preleukemia (syndrome) D46.9
  Preluxation, hip, congenital Q65.6
  Premature (*see also* condition)
    adrenarche E27.0
    aging E34.8
    beats I49.40
      atrial I49.1
      auricular I49.1
      supraventricular I49.1
    birth NEC — *see* Preterm, newborn
    closure, foramen ovale Q21.8
    contraction
      atrial I49.1
      atrioventricular I49.2
      auricular I49.1
      auriculoventricular I49.49
      heart (extrasystole) I49.49
      junctional I49.2
      ventricular I49.3
    delivery (*see also* Pregnancy, complicated by, preterm labor) O60.10 ☑
    ejaculation F52.4
    infant NEC — *see* Preterm, newborn
    light-for-dates — *see* Light for dates
    labor — *see* Pregnancy, complicated by, preterm labor
    lungs P28.0
    menopause E28.319
      asymptomatic E28.319
      symptomatic E28.310
    newborn
      extreme (less than 28 completed weeks) — *see* Immaturity, extreme
      less than 37 completed weeks — *see* Preterm, newborn
    puberty E30.1
    rupture membranes or amnion — *see* Pregnancy, complicated by, premature rupture of membranes
    senility E34.8
    thelarche E30.8
    ventricular systole I49.3
  Prematurity NEC (less than 37 completed weeks) — *see* Preterm, newborn
    extreme (less than 28 completed weeks) — *see* Immaturity, extreme
  Premenstrual
    dysphoric disorder (PMDD) F32.81
    tension (syndrome) N94.3
  Premolarization, cuspids K00.2
  Prenatal
    care, normal pregnancy — *see* Pregnancy, normal
    screening of mother (*see also* Encounter, antenatal screening) Z36.9
    teeth K00.6
  Preparatory care for subsequent treatment NEC
    for dialysis Z49.01
      peritoneal Z49.02

Prepartum — *see* condition
Preponderance, left or right ventricular I51.7
Prepuce — *see* condition
PRES (posterior reversible encephalopathy syndrome) I67.83
Presbycardia R54
Presbycusis, presbyacusia H91.1 ☑
Presbyesophagus K22.8
Presbyophrenia F03 ☑
Presbyopia H52.4
Prescription of contraceptives (initial) Z30.019
  barrier Z30.018
  diaphragm Z30.018
  emergency (postcoital) Z30.012
  implantable subdermal Z30.017
  injectable Z30.013
  intrauterine contraceptive device Z30.014
  pills Z30.011
  postcoital (emergency) Z30.012
  repeat Z30.40
    barrier Z30.49
    diaphragm Z30.49
    implantable subdermal Z30.46
    injectable Z30.42
    pills Z30.41
    specified type NEC Z30.49
    transdermal patch hormonal Z30.45
    vaginal ring hormonal Z30.44
  specified type NEC Z30.018
    transdermal patch hormonal Z30.016
    vaginal ring hormonal Z30.015
Presence (of)
  ankle-joint implant (functional) (prosthesis) Z96.66 ☑
  aortocoronary (bypass) graft Z95.1
  arterial-venous shunt (dialysis) Z99.2
  artificial
    eye (globe) Z97.0
    heart (fully implantable) (mechanical) Z95.812
      valve Z95.2
    larynx Z96.3
    lens (intraocular) Z96.1
    limb (complete) (partial) Z97.1 ☑
      arm Z97.1 ☑
        bilateral Z97.15
      leg Z97.1 ☑
        bilateral Z97.16
  audiological implant (functional) Z96.29
  bladder implant (functional) Z96.0
  bone
    conduction hearing device Z96.29
    implant (functional) NEC Z96.7
    joint (prosthesis) — *see* Presence, joint implant
  cardiac
    defibrillator (functional) (with synchronous cardiac pacemaker) Z95.810
    implant or graft Z95.9
      specified type NEC Z95.818
    pacemaker Z95.0
    resynchronization therapy
      defibrillator Z95.810
      pacemaker Z95.0
  cerebrospinal fluid drainage device Z98.2
  cochlear implant (functional) Z96.21
  contact lens (es) Z97.3
  coronary artery graft or prosthesis Z95.5
  CRT-D (cardiac resynchronization therapy defibrillator) Z95.810
  CRT-P (cardiac resynchronization therapy pacemaker) Z95.0
  cardioverter-defibrillator (ICD) Z95.810
  CSF shunt Z98.2
  dental prosthesis device Z97.2
  dentures Z97.2
  device (external) NEC Z97.8
    cardiac NEC Z95.818
    heart assist Z95.811
    implanted (functional) Z96.9
      specified NEC Z96.89
    prosthetic Z97.8
  ear implant Z96.20
    cochlear implant Z96.21
    myringotomy tube Z96.22
    specified type NEC Z96.29
  elbow-joint implant (functional) (prosthesis) Z96.62 ☑
  endocrine implant (functional) NEC Z96.49
  eustachian tube stent or device (functional) Z96.29
  external hearing-aid or device Z97.4
  finger-joint implant (functional) (prosthetic) Z96.69 ☑

Presence — *continued*
  functional implant Z96.9
    specified NEC Z96.89
  graft
    cardiac NEC Z95.818
    vascular NEC Z95.828
  hearing-aid or device (external) Z97.4
    implant (bone) (cochlear) (functional) Z96.21
  heart assist device Z95.811
  heart valve implant (functional) Z95.2
    prosthetic Z95.2
    specified type NEC Z95.4
    xenogenic Z95.3
  hip-joint implant (functional) (prosthesis) Z96.64 ☑
  ICD (cardioverter-defibrillator) Z95.810
  implanted device (artificial) (functional) (prosthetic) Z96.9
    automatic cardiac defibrillator (with synchronous cardiac pacemaker) Z95.810
    cardiac pacemaker Z95.0
    cochlear Z96.21
    dental Z96.5
    heart Z95.812
    heart valve Z95.2
      prosthetic Z95.2
      specified NEC Z95.4
      xenogenic Z95.3
    insulin pump Z96.41
    intraocular lens Z96.1
    joint Z96.60
      ankle Z96.66 ☑
      elbow Z96.62 ☑
      finger Z96.69 ☑
      hip Z96.64 ☑
      knee Z96.65 ☑
      shoulder Z96.61 ☑
      specified NEC Z96.698
      wrist Z96.63 ☑
    larynx Z96.3
    myringotomy tube Z96.22
    otological Z96.20
      cochlear Z96.21
      eustachian stent Z96.29
      myringotomy Z96.22
      specified NEC Z96.29
      stapes Z96.29
    skin Z96.81
    skull plate Z96.7
    specified NEC Z96.89
    urogenital Z96.0
  insulin pump (functional) Z96.41
  intestinal bypass or anastomosis Z98.0
  intraocular lens (functional) Z96.1
  intrauterine contraceptive device (IUD) Z97.5
  intravascular implant (functional) (prosthetic) NEC Z95.9
    coronary artery Z95.5
    defibrillator (with synchronous cardiac pacemaker) Z95.810
    peripheral vessel (with angioplasty) Z95.820
  joint implant (prosthetic) (any) Z96.60
    ankle — *see* Presence, ankle joint implant
    elbow — *see* Presence, elbow joint implant
    finger — *see* Presence, finger joint implant
    hip — *see* Presence, hip joint implant
    knee — *see* Presence, knee joint implant
    shoulder — *see* Presence, shoulder joint implant
    specified joint NEC Z96.698
    wrist — *see* Presence, wrist joint implant
  knee-joint implant (functional) (prosthesis) Z96.65 ☑
  laryngeal implant (functional) Z96.3
  mandibular implant (dental) Z96.5
  myringotomy tube (s) Z96.22
  orthopedic-joint implant (prosthetic) (any) — *see* Presence, joint implant
  otological implant (functional) Z96.29
  shoulder-joint implant (functional) (prosthesis) Z96.61 ☑
  skull-plate implant Z96.7
  spectacles Z97.3
  stapes implant (functional) Z96.29
  systemic lupus erythematosus [SLE] inhibitor D68.62
  tendon implant (functional) (graft) Z96.7
  tooth root (s) implant Z96.5
  ureteral stent Z96.0
  urethral stent Z96.0
  urogenital implant (functional) Z96.0
  vascular implant or device Z95.9
    access port device Z95.828

☑ **Additional character required**

Presence — *continued*
    vascular implant or device — *continued*
        specified type NEC Z95.828
        wrist-joint implant (functional)
            (prosthesis) Z96.63 ☑
Presenile (*see also* condition)
    dementia F03 ☑
    premature aging E34.8
Presentation, fetal — *see* Delivery, complicated by, malposition
Prespondylolisthesis (congenital) Q76.2
Pressure
    area, skin — *see* Ulcer, pressure, by site
    brachial plexus G54.0
    brain G93.5
        injury at birth NEC P11.1
    cerebral — *see* Pressure, brain
    chest R07.89
    cone, tentorial G93.5
    hyposystolic (*see also* Hypotension)
        incidental reading, without diagnosis of hypotension R03.1
    increased
        intracranial (benign) G93.2
            injury at birth P11.0
        intraocular H40.05 ☑
    lumbosacral plexus G54.1
    mediastinum J98.59
    necrosis (chronic) — *see* Ulcer, pressure, by site
    parental, inappropriate (excessive) Z62.6
    sore (chronic) — *see* Ulcer, pressure, by site
    spinal cord G95.20
    ulcer (chronic) — *see* Ulcer, pressure, by site
    venous, increased I87.8
Pre-syncope R55
Preterm
    delivery (*see also* Pregnancy, complicated by, preterm labor) O60.10 ☑
    labor — *see* Pregnancy, complicated by, preterm labor
    newborn (infant) P07.30
        gestational age
            28 completed weeks (28 weeks, 0 days through 28 weeks, 6 days) P07.31
            29 completed weeks (29 weeks, 0 days through 29 weeks, 6 days) P07.32
            30 completed weeks (30 weeks, 0 days through 30 weeks, 6 days) P07.33
            31 completed weeks (31 weeks, 0 days through 31 weeks, 6 days) P07.34
            32 completed weeks (32 weeks, 0 days through 32 weeks, 6 days) P07.35
            33 completed weeks (33 weeks, 0 days through 33 weeks, 6 days) P07.36
            34 completed weeks (34 weeks, 0 days through 34 weeks, 6 days) P07.37
            35 completed weeks (35 weeks, 0 days through 35 weeks, 6 days) P07.38
            36 completed weeks (36 weeks, 0 days through 36 weeks, 6 days) P07.39
Previa
    placenta (total) (without hemorrhage) O44.0 ☑
        with hemorrhage O44.1 ☑
        complete O44.0 ☑
            with hemorrhage O44.1 ☑
        low (*see also* Delivery, complicated, by, placenta, low) O44.4 ☑
            with hemorrhage O44.5 ☑
        marginal O44.2 ☑
            with hemorrhage O44.3 ☑
        partial O44.2 ☑
            with hemorrhage O44.3 ☑
    vasa O69.4 ☑
Priapism N48.30
    due to
        disease classified elsewhere N48.32
        drug N48.33
        specified cause NEC N48.39
        trauma N48.31
Prickling sensation (skin) R20.2
Prickly heat L74.0
Primary — *see* condition
Primigravida
    elderly, affecting management of pregnancy, labor and delivery (supervision only) — *see* Pregnancy, complicated by, elderly, primigravida
    older, affecting management of pregnancy, labor and delivery (supervision only) — *see* Pregnancy, complicated by, elderly, primigravida

Primigravida — *continued*
    very young, affecting management of pregnancy, labor and delivery (supervision only) — *see* Pregnancy, complicated by, young mother, primigravida
Primipara
    elderly, affecting management of pregnancy, labor and delivery (supervision only) — *see* Pregnancy, complicated by, elderly, primigravida
    older, affecting management of pregnancy, labor and delivery (supervision only) — *see* Pregnancy, complicated by, elderly, primigravida
    very young, affecting management of pregnancy, labor and delivery (supervision only) — *see* Pregnancy, complicated by, young mother, primigravida
Primus varus (bilateral) Q66.2 ☑
PRIND (Prolonged reversible ischemic neurologic deficit) I63.9
Pringle's disease (tuberous sclerosis) Q85.1
Prinzmetal angina I20.1
Prizefighter ear — *see* Cauliflower ear
Problem (with) (related to)
    academic Z55.8
    acculturation Z60.3
    adjustment (to)
        change of job Z56.1
        life-cycle transition Z60.0
        pension Z60.0
        retirement Z60.0
    adopted child Z62.821
    alcoholism in family Z63.72
    atypical parenting situation Z62.9
    bankruptcy Z59.8
    behavioral (adult) F69
        drug seeking Z76.5
    birth of sibling affecting child Z62.898
    care (of)
        provider dependency Z74.9
            specified NEC Z74.8
        sick or handicapped person in family or household Z63.6
    child
        abuse (affecting the child) — *see* Maltreatment, child
        custody or support proceedings Z65.3
        in welfare custody Z62.21
        in care of non-parental family member Z62.21
        in foster care Z62.21
        living in orphanage or group home Z62.22
    child-rearing Z62.9
        specified NEC Z62.898
    communication (developmental) F80.9
    conflict or discord (with)
        boss Z56.4
        classmates Z55.4
        counselor Z64.4
        employer Z56.4
        family Z63.9
            specified NEC Z63.8
        probation officer Z64.4
        social worker Z64.4
        teachers Z55.4
        workmates Z56.4
    conviction in legal proceedings Z65.0
        with imprisonment Z65.1
    counselor Z64.4
    creditors Z59.8
    digestive K92.9
    drug addict in family Z63.72
    ear — *see* Disorder, ear
    economic Z59.9
        affecting care Z59.9
        specified NEC Z59.8
    education Z55.9
        specified NEC Z55.8
    employment Z56.9
        change of job Z56.1
        discord Z56.4
        environment Z56.5
        sexual harassment Z56.81
        specified NEC Z56.89
        stress NEC Z56.6
        stressful schedule Z56.3
        threat of job loss Z56.2
        unemployment Z56.0
    enuresis, child F98.0
    eye H57.9
    failed examinations (school) Z55.2
    falling Z91.81

Problem — *continued*
    family (*see also* Disruption, family) Z63.9
        specified NEC Z63.8
    feeding (elderly) (infant) R63.3
        newborn P92.9
            breast P92.5
            overfeeding P92.4
            slow P92.2
            specified NEC P92.8
            underfeeding P92.3
        nonorganic F50.89
    finance Z59.9
        specified NEC Z59.8
    foreclosure on loan Z59.8
    foster child Z62.822
    frightening experience (s) in childhood Z62.898
    genital NEC
        female N94.9
        male N50.9
    health care Z75.9
        specified NEC Z75.8
    hearing — *see* Deafness
    homelessness Z59.0
    housing Z59.9
        inadequate Z59.1
        isolated Z59.8
        specified NEC Z59.8
    identity (of childhood) F93.8
    illegitimate pregnancy (unwanted) Z64.0
    illiteracy Z55.0
    impaired mobility Z74.09
    imprisonment or incarceration Z65.1
    inadequate teaching affecting education Z55.8
    inappropriate (excessive) parental pressure Z62.6
    influencing health status NEC Z78.9
    in-law Z63.1
    institutionalization, affecting child Z62.22
    intrafamilial communication Z63.8
    jealousy, child F93.8
    landlord Z59.2
    language (developmental) F80.9
    learning (developmental) F81.9
    legal Z65.3
        conviction without imprisonment Z65.0
        imprisonment Z65.1
        release from prison Z65.2
    life-management Z73.9
        specified NEC Z73.89
    life-style Z72.9
        gambling Z72.6
        high-risk sexual behavior (heterosexual) Z72.51
            bisexual Z72.53
            homosexual Z72.52
        inappropriate eating habits Z72.4
        self-damaging behavior NEC Z72.89
        specified NEC Z72.89
        tobacco use Z72.0
    literacy Z55.9
        low level Z55.0
        specified NEC Z55.8
    living alone Z60.2
    lodgers Z59.2
    loss of love relationship in childhood Z62.898
    marital Z63.0
        involving
            divorce Z63.5
            estrangement Z63.5
            gender identity F66
    mastication K08.89
    medical
        care, within family Z63.6
        facilities Z75.9
            specified NEC Z75.8
    mental F48.9
    multiparity Z64.1
    negative life events in childhood Z62.9
        altered pattern of family relationships Z62.898
        frightening experience Z62.898
        loss of
            love relationship Z62.898
            self-esteem Z62.898
        physical abuse (alleged) — *see* Maltreatment, child
        removal from home Z62.29
        specified event NEC Z62.898
    neighbor Z59.2
    neurological NEC R29.818
    new step-parent affecting child Z62.898
    none (feared complaint unfounded) Z71.1
    occupational NEC Z56.89
    parent-child — *see* Conflict, parent-child
    personal hygiene Z91.89

Problem — *continued*
  personality F69
  phase-of-life transition, adjustment Z60.0
  presence of sick or disabled person in family or
    household Z63.79
    needing care Z63.6
  primary support group (family) Z63.9
    specified NEC Z63.8
  probation officer Z64.4
  psychiatric F99
  psychosexual (development) F66
  psychosocial Z65.9
    religious or spiritual Z65.8
    specified NEC Z65.8
  relationship Z63.9
    childhood F93.8
  release from prison Z65.2
    religious or spiritual Z65.8
  removal from home affecting child Z62.29
  seeking and accepting known hazardous and
    harmful
    behavioral or psychological interventions Z65.8
    chemical, nutritional or physical
      interventions Z65.8
  sexual function (nonorganic) F52.9
  sight H54.7
  sleep disorder, child F51.9
  smell — *see* Disturbance, sensation, smell
  social
    environment Z60.9
      specified NEC Z60.8
    exclusion and rejection Z60.4
    worker Z64.4
  speech R47.9
    developmental F80.9
    specified NEC R47.89
  swallowing — *see* Dysphagia
  taste — *see* Disturbance, sensation, taste
  tic, child F95.0
  underachievement in school Z55.3
  unemployment Z56.0
    threatened Z56.2
  unwanted pregnancy Z64.0
  upbringing Z62.9
    specified NEC Z62.898
  urinary N39.9
  voice production R47.89
  work schedule (stressful) Z56.3
Procedure (surgical)
  converted
    arthroscopic to open Z53.33
    laparoscopic to open Z53.31
    specified procedure NEC to open Z53.39
    thoracoscopic to open Z53.32
  for purpose other than remedying health
    state Z41.9
    specified NEC Z41.8
  not done Z53.9
    because of
      administrative reasons Z53.8
      contraindication Z53.09
        smoking Z53.01
      patient's decision Z53.20
        for reasons of belief or group
          pressure Z53.1
        left against medical advice (AMA) Z53.21
        specified reason NEC Z53.29
      specified reason NEC Z53.8
Procidentia (uteri) N81.3
Proctalgia K62.89
  fugax K59.4
  spasmodic K59.4
Proctitis K62.89
  amebic (acute) A06.0
  chlamydial A56.3
  gonococcal A54.6
  granulomatous — *see* Enteritis, regional, large
    intestine
  herpetic A60.1
  radiation K62.7
  tuberculous A18.32
  ulcerative (chronic) K51.20
    with
      complication K51.219
        abscess K51.214
        fistula K51.213
        obstruction K51.212
        rectal bleeding K51.211
        specified NEC K51.218
Proctocele
  female (without uterine prolapse) N81.6
    with uterine prolapse N81.2

Proctocele — *continued*
  female — *continued*
    complete N81.3
  male K62.3
Proctocolitis
  food-induced eosinophilic K52.82
  food protein-induced K52.82
  milk protein-induced K52.82
  mucosal — *see* Rectosigmoiditis, ulcerative
Proctoptosis K62.3
Proctorrhagia K62.5
Proctosigmoiditis K63.89
  ulcerative (chronic) — *see* Rectosigmoiditis,
    ulcerative
Proctospasm K59.4
  psychogenic F45.8
Profichet's disease — *see* Disorder, soft tissue,
  specified type NEC
Progeria E34.8
Prognathism (mandibular) (maxillary) M26.19
Progonoma (melanotic) — *see* Neoplasm, benign,
  by site
Progressive — *see* condition
Prolactinoma
  specified site — *see* Neoplasm, benign, by site
  unspecified site D35.2
Prolapse, prolapsed
  anus, anal (canal) (sphincter) K62.2
  arm or hand O32.2 ☑
    causing obstructed labor O64.4 ☑
  bladder (mucosa) (sphincter) (acquired)
    congenital Q79.4
    female — *see* Cystocele
    male N32.89
  breast implant (prosthetic) T85.49 ☑
  cecostomy K94.09
  cecum K63.4
  cervix, cervical (hypertrophied) N81.2
    anterior lip, obstructing labor O65.5
    congenital Q51.828
    postpartal, old N81.2
    stump N81.85
  ciliary body (traumatic) — *see* Laceration,
    eye(ball), with prolapse or loss of interocular
    tissue
  colon (pedunculated) K63.4
  colostomy K94.09
  disc (intervertebral) — *see* Displacement,
    intervertebral disc
  eye implant (orbital) T85.398 ☑
    lens (ocular) — *see* Complications, intraocular
      lens
  fallopian tube N83.4 ☑
  gastric (mucosa) K31.89
  genital, female N81.9
    specified NEC N81.89
  globe, nontraumatic — *see* Luxation, globe
  ileostomy bud K94.19
  intervertebral disc — *see* Displacement,
    intervertebral disc
  intestine (small) K63.4
  iris (traumatic) — *see* Laceration, eye(ball), with
    prolapse or loss of interocular tissue
    nontraumatic H21.89
  kidney N28.83
    congenital Q63.2
  laryngeal muscles or ventricle J38.7
  liver K76.89
  meatus urinarius N36.8
  mitral (valve) I34.1
  ocular lens implant — *see* Complications,
    intraocular lens
  organ or site, congenital NEC — *see* Malposition,
    congenital
  ovary N83.4 ☑
  pelvic floor, female N81.89
  perineum, female N81.89
  rectum (mucosa) (sphincter) K62.3
    due to trichuris trichuria B79
  spleen D73.89
  stomach K31.89
  umbilical cord
    complicating delivery O69.0 ☑
  urachus, congenital Q64.4
  ureter N28.89
    with obstruction N13.5
      with infection N13.6
  ureterovesical orifice N28.89
  urethra (acquired) (infected) (mucosa) N36.8
    congenital Q64.71
  urinary meatus N36.8
    congenital Q64.72

Prolapse — *continued*
  uterovaginal N81.4
    complete N81.3
    incomplete N81.2
  uterus (with prolapse of vagina) N81.4
    complete N81.3
    congenital Q51.818
    first degree N81.2
    in pregnancy or childbirth — *see* Pregnancy,
      complicated by, abnormal, uterus
    incomplete N81.2
    postpartal (old) N81.4
    second degree N81.2
    third degree N81.3
  uveal (traumatic) — *see* Laceration, eye(ball), with
    prolapse or loss of interocular tissue
  vagina (anterior) (wall) — *see* Cystocele
    with prolapse of uterus N81.4
      complete N81.3
      incomplete N81.2
    posterior wall N81.6
    posthysterectomy N99.3
  vitreous (humor) H43.0 ☑
    in wound — *see* Laceration, eye(ball), with
      prolapse or loss of interocular tissue
  womb — *see* Prolapse, uterus
Prolapsus, female N81.9
  specified NEC N81.89
Proliferation (s)
  prostate, atypical small acinar N42.32
  primary cutaneous CD30-positive large
    T-cell C86.6
Proliferative — *see* condition
Prolonged, prolongation (of)
  bleeding (time) (idiopathic) R79.1
  coagulation (time) R79.1
  gestation (over 42 completed weeks)
    mother O48.1
    newborn P08.22
  interval I44.0
  labor O63.9
    first stage O63.0
    second stage O63.1
  partial thromboplastin time (PTT) R79.1
  pregnancy (more than 42 weeks gestation) O48.1
  prothrombin time R79.1
  QT interval I45.81
  uterine contractions in labor O62.4
Prominence, prominent
  auricle (congenital) (ear) Q17.5
  ischial spine or sacral promontory
    with disproportion (fetopelvic) O33.0
      causing obstructed labor O65.0
  nose (congenital) acquired M95.0
Promiscuity — *see* High, risk, sexual behavior
Pronation
  ankle — *see* Deformity, limb, foot, specified NEC
  foot (*see also* Deformity, limb, foot, specified NEC)
    congenital Q74.2
Prophylactic
  administration of
    antibiotics, long-term Z79.2
      short-term use - omit code
    drug (*see also* Long-term (current) drug therapy
      (use of)) Z79.899
    medication Z79.899
  organ removal (for neoplasia
    management) Z40.00
    breast Z40.01
    fallopian tube (s) Z40.03
      with ovary (s) Z40.02
    ovary (s) Z40.02
    specified site NEC Z40.09
  surgery Z40.9
    for risk factors related to malignant neoplasm
      — *see* Prophylactic, organ removal
    specified NEC Z40.8
  vaccination Z23
Propionic acidemia E71.121
Proptosis (ocular) (*see also* Exophthalmos)
  thyroid — *see* Hyperthyroidism, with goiter
Prosecution, anxiety concerning Z65.3
Prosopagnosia R48.3
Prostadynia N42.81
Prostate, prostatic — *see* condition
Prostatism — *see* Hyperplasia, prostate
Prostatitis (congestive) (suppurative) (with cystitis)
  N41.9
  acute N41.0
  cavitary N41.8
  chronic N41.1
  diverticular N41.8

Prostatitis — *continued*
  due to Trichomonas (vaginalis) A59.02
  fibrous N41.1
  gonococcal (acute) (chronic) A54.22
  granulomatous N41.4
  hypertrophic N41.1
  subacute N41.1
  trichomonal A59.02
  tuberculous A18.14
Prostatocystitis N41.3
Prostatorrhea N42.89
Prostatosis N42.82
Prostration R53.83
  heat (*see also* Heat, exhaustion)
    anhydrotic T67.3 ☑
    due to
      salt (and water) depletion T67.4 ☑
      water depletion T67.3 ☑
  nervous F48.8
  senile R54
Protanomaly (anomalous trichromat) H53.54
Protanopia (complete) (incomplete) H53.54
Protection (against) (from) — *see* Prophylactic
Protein
  deficiency NEC — *see* Malnutrition
  malnutrition — *see* Malnutrition
  sickness (*see also* Reaction, serum) T80.69 ☑
Proteinemia R77.9
Proteinosis
  alveolar (pulmonary) J84.01
  lipid or lipoid (of Urbach) E78.89
Proteinuria R80.9
  Bence Jones R80.3
  complicating pregnancy — *see* Proteinuria, gestational
  gestational
    complicating
      childbirth O12.14
      pregnancy O12.1 ☑
        with edema O12.2 ☑
      puerperium O12.15
  idiopathic R80.0
  isolated R80.0
    with glomerular lesion N06.9
      dense deposit disease N06.6
      diffuse
        crescentic glomerulonephritis N06.7
        endocapillary proliferative glomerulonephritis N06.4
        mesangiocapillary glomerulonephritis N06.5
        focal and segmental hyalinosis or sclerosis N06.1
        membranous (diffuse) N06.2
        mesangial proliferative (diffuse) N06.3
        minimal change N06.0
      specified pathology NEC N06.8
  orthostatic R80.2
    with glomerular lesion — *see* Proteinuria, isolated, with glomerular lesion
  persistent R80.1
    with glomerular lesion — *see* Proteinuria, isolated, with glomerular lesion
  postural R80.2
    with glomerular lesion — *see* Proteinuria, isolated, with glomerular lesion
  pre-eclamptic — *see* Pre-eclampsia
  puerperal O12.15
  specified type NEC R80.8
Proteolysis, pathologic D65
Proteus (mirabilis) (morganii), as cause of disease classified elsewhere B96.4
Prothrombin gene mutation D68.52
Protoporphyria, erythropoietic E80.0
Protozoal (*see also* condition)
  disease B64
    specified NEC B60.8
Protrusion, protrusio
  acetabuli M24.7
  acetabulum (into pelvis) M24.7
  device, implant or graft (*see also* Complications, by site and type, mechanical) T85.698 ☑
    arterial graft NEC — *see* Complication, cardiovascular device, mechanical, vascular
    breast (implant) T85.49 ☑
    catheter NEC T85.698 ☑
      cystostomy T83.090 ☑
      dialysis (renal) T82.49 ☑
        intraperitoneal T85.691 ☑
      infusion NEC T82.594 ☑
        spinal (epidural) (subdural) T85.690 ☑

Protrusion — *continued*
  device — *continued*
    urinary (*see also* Complications, catheter, urinary) T83.098 ☑
    electronic (electrode) (pulse generator) (stimulator)
      bone T84.390 ☑
      nervous system — *see* Complication, prosthetic device, mechanical, electronic nervous system stimulator
    fixation, internal (orthopedic) NEC — *see* Complication, fixation device, mechanical
    gastrointestinal — *see* Complications, prosthetic device, mechanical, gastrointestinal device
    genital NEC T83.498 ☑
      intrauterine contraceptive device T83.39 ☑
      penile prosthesis (cylinder) (implanted) (pump) (reservoir) T83.490 ☑
      testicular prosthesis T83.491 ☑
    heart NEC — *see* Complication, cardiovascular device, mechanical
    joint prosthesis — *see* Complications, joint prosthesis, mechanical, specified NEC, by site
    ocular NEC — *see* Complications, prosthetic device, mechanical, ocular device
    orthopedic NEC — *see* Complication, orthopedic, device, mechanical
    specified NEC T85.628 ☑
    urinary NEC (*see also* Complication, genitourinary, device, urinary, mechanical)
      graft T83.29 ☑
    vascular NEC — *see* Complication, cardiovascular device, mechanical
    ventricular intracranial shunt T85.09 ☑
    intervertebral disc — *see* Displacement, intervertebral disc
    joint prosthesis — *see* Complications, joint prosthesis, mechanical, specified NEC, by site
    nucleus pulposus — *see* Displacement, intervertebral disc
Prune belly (syndrome) Q79.4
Prurigo (ferox) (gravis) (Hebrae) (Hebra's) (mitis) (simplex) L28.2
  Besnier's L20.0
  estivalis L56.4
  nodularis L28.1
  psychogenic F45.8
Pruritus, pruritic (essential) L29.9
  ani, anus L29.0
    psychogenic F45.8
  anogenital L29.3
    psychogenic F45.8
  due to onchocerca volvulus B73.1
  gravidarum — *see* Pregnancy, complicated by, specified pregnancy-related condition NEC
  hiemalis L29.8
  neurogenic (any site) F45.8
  perianal L29.0
  psychogenic (any site) F45.8
  scroti, scrotum L29.1
    psychogenic F45.8
  senile, senilis L29.8
  specified NEC L29.8
    psychogenic F45.8
  Trichomonas A59.9
  vulva, vulvae L29.2
    psychogenic F45.8
Pseudarthrosis, pseudoarthrosis (bone) — *see* Nonunion, fracture
  clavicle, congenital Q74.0
  joint, following fusion or arthrodesis M96.0
Pseudoaneurysm — *see* Aneurysm
Pseudoangioma I81
Pseudoangina (pectoris) — *see* Angina
Pseudoarteriosus Q28.8
Pseudoarthrosis — *see* Pseudarthrosis
Pseudobulbar affect (PBA) F48.2
Pseudochromhidrosis L67.8
Pseudocirrhosis, liver, pericardial I31.1
Pseudocowpox B08.03
Pseudocoxalgia M91.3 ☑
Pseudocroup J38.5
Pseudo-Cushing's syndrome, alcohol-induced E24.4
Pseudocyesis F45.8
Pseudocyst
  lung J98.4
  pancreas K86.3
  retina — *see* Cyst, retina
Pseudoelephantiasis neuroarthritica Q82.0

Pseudoexfoliation, capsule (lens) — *see* Cataract, specified NEC
Pseudofolliculitis barbae L73.1
Pseudoglioma H44.89
Pseudohemophilia (Bernuth's) (hereditary) (type B) D68.0
  Type A D69.8
  vascular D69.8
Pseudohermaphroditism Q56.3
  adrenal E25.8
  female Q56.2
    with adrenocortical disorder E25.8
    without adrenocortical disorder Q56.2
    adrenal (congenital) E25.0
    unspecified E25.9
  male Q56.1
    with
      adrenocortical disorder E25.8
      androgen resistance E34.51
      cleft scrotum Q56.1
      feminizing testis E34.51
      5-alpha-reductase deficiency E29.1
    without gonadal disorder Q56.1
    adrenal E25.8
    unspecified E25.9
Pseudo-Hurler's polydystrophy E77.0
Pseudohydrocephalus G93.2
Pseudohypertrophic muscular dystrophy (Erb's) G71.0
Pseudohypertrophy, muscle G71.0
Pseudohypoparathyroidism E20.1
Pseudoinsomnia F51.03
Pseudoleukemia, infantile D64.89
Pseudomembranous — *see* condition
Pseudomenses (newborn) P54.6
Pseudomenstruation (newborn) P54.6
Pseudomeningocele (cerebral) (infective) (post-traumatic) G96.19
  postprocedural (spinal) G97.82
Pseudomonas
  aeruginosa, as cause of disease classified elsewhere B96.5
  mallei infection A24.0
    as cause of disease classified elsewhere B96.5
  pseudomallei, as cause of disease classified elsewhere B96.5
Pseudomyotonia G71.19
Pseudomyxoma peritonei C78.6
Pseudoneuritis, optic (nerve) (disc) (papilla), congenital Q14.2
Pseudo-obstruction intestine (acute) (chronic) (idiopathic) (intermittent secondary) (primary) K59.8
Pseudopapilledema H47.33 ☑
  congenital Q14.2
Pseudoparalysis
  arm or leg R29.818
  atonic, congenital P94.2
Pseudopelade L66.0
Pseudophakia Z96.1
Pseudopolyarthritis, rhizomelic M35.3
Pseudopolycythemia D75.1
Pseudopseudohypoparathyroidism E20.1
Pseudopterygium H11.81 ☑
Pseudoptosis (eyelid) — *see* Blepharochalasis
Pseudopuberty, precocious
  female heterosexual E25.8
  male isosexual E25.8
Pseudorickets (renal) N25.0
Pseudorubella B08.20
Pseudoscterema, newborn P83.88
Pseudosclerosis (brain)
  of Westphal (Strümpell) E83.01
  Jakob's — *see* Creutzfeldt-Jakob disease or syndrome
  spastic — *see* Creutzfeldt-Jakob disease or syndrome
Pseudotetanus — *see* Convulsions
Pseudotetany R29.0
  hysterical F44.5
Pseudotruncus arteriosus Q25.49
Pseudotuberculosis A28.2
  enterocolitis A04.8
  pasteurella (infection) A28.0
Pseudotumor
  cerebri G93.2
  orbital H05.11 ☑
Pseudoxanthoma elasticum Q82.8
Psilosis (sprue) (tropical) K90.1
  nontropical K90.0
Psittacosis A70
Psoitis M60.88

Psoriasis - Puberty

Psoriasis L40.9
    arthropathic L40.50
        arthritis mutilans L40.52
        distal interphalangeal L40.51
        juvenile L40.54
        other specified L40.59
        spondylitis L40.53
    buccal K13.29
    flexural L40.8
    guttate L40.4
    mouth K13.29
    nummular L40.0
    plaque L40.0
    psychogenic F54
    pustular (generalized) L40.1
        palmaris et plantaris L40.3
    specified NEC L40.8
    vulgaris L40.0
Psychasthenia F48.8
Psychiatric disorder or problem F99
Psychogenic (see also condition)
    factors associated with physical conditions F54
Psychological and behavioral factors affecting
    medical condition F59
Psychoneurosis, psychoneurotic (see also Neurosis)
    anxiety (state) F41.1
    depersonalization F48.1
    hypochondriacal F45.21
    hysteria F44.9
    neurasthenic F48.8
    personality NEC F60.89
Psychopathy, psychopathic
    affectionless F94.2
    autistic F84.5
    constitution, post-traumatic F07.81
    personality — see Disorder, personality
    sexual — see Deviation, sexual
    state F60.2
Psychosexual identity disorder of childhood F64.2
Psychosis, psychotic F29
    acute (transient) F23
        hysterical F44.9
    affective — see Disorder, mood
    alcoholic F10.959
        with
            abuse F10.159
            anxiety disorder F10.980
                with
                    abuse F10.180
                    dependence F10.280
            delirium tremens F10.231
            delusions F10.950
                with
                    abuse F10.150
                    dependence F10.250
            dementia F10.97
                with dependence F10.27
            dependence F10.259
            hallucinosis F10.951
                with
                    abuse F10.151
                    dependence F10.251
            mood disorder F10.94
                with
                    abuse F10.14
                    dependence F10.24
            paranoia F10.950
                with
                    abuse F10.150
                    dependence F10.250
            persisting amnesia F10.96
                with dependence F10.26
        amnestic confabulatory F10.96
            with dependence F10.26
        delirium tremens F10.231
        Korsakoff's, Korsakov's, Korsakow's F10.26
        paranoid type F10.950
            with
                abuse F10.150
                dependence F10.250
    anergastic — see Psychosis, organic
    arteriosclerotic (simple type)
        (uncomplicated) F01.50
        with behavioral disturbance F01.51
    childhood F84.0
        atypical F84.8
    climacteric — see Psychosis, involutional
    confusional F29
        acute or subacute F05
        reactive F23
    cycloid F23
    depressive — see Disorder, depressive

Psychosis — continued
    disintegrative (childhood) F84.3
    drug-induced — see F11-F19 with .x59
        paranoid and hallucinatory states — see
            F11-F19 with .x50 or .x51
    due to or associated with
        addiction, drug — see F11-F19 with .x59
        dependence
            alcohol F10.259
            drug — see F11-F19 with .x59
        epilepsy F06.8
        Huntington's chorea F06.8
        ischemia, cerebrovascular (generalized) F06.8
        multiple sclerosis F06.8
        physical disease F06.8
        presenile dementia F03 ☑
        senile dementia F03 ☑
        vascular disease (arteriosclerotic)
            (cerebral) F01.50
            with behavioral disturbance F01.51
    epileptic F06.8
    episode F23
        due to or associated with physical
            condition F06.8
    exhaustive F43.0
    hallucinatory, chronic F28
    hypomanic F30.8
    hysterical (acute) F44.9
    induced F24
    infantile F84.0
        atypical F84.8
    infective (acute) (subacute) F05
    involutional F28
        depressive — see Disorder, depressive
        melancholic — see Disorder, depressive
        paranoid (state) F22
    Korsakoff's, Korsakov's, Korsakow's
        (nonalcoholic) F04
        alcoholic F10.96
            in dependence F10.26
        induced by other psychoactive substance —
            see categories F11-F19 with .x5x
    mania, manic (single episode) F30.2
        recurrent type F31.89
    manic-depressive — see Disorder, bipolar
    menopausal — see Psychosis, involutional
    mixed schizophrenic and affective F25.8
    multi-infarct (cerebrovascular) F01.50
        with behavioral disturbance F01.51
    nonorganic F29
        specified NEC F28
    organic F09
        due to or associated with
            arteriosclerosis (cerebral) — see Psychosis,
                arteriosclerotic
            cerebrovascular disease, arteriosclerotic —
                see Psychosis, arteriosclerotic
            childbirth — see Psychosis, puerperal
            Creutzfeldt-Jakob disease or syndrome — see
                Creutzfeldt-Jakob disease or syndrome
            dependence, alcohol F10.259
            disease
                alcoholic liver F10.259
                brain, arteriosclerotic — see Psychosis,
                    arteriosclerotic
                cerebrovascular F01.50
                    with behavioral disturbance F01.51
                Creutzfeldt-Jakob — see Creutzfeldt-Jakob
                    disease or syndrome
            endocrine or metabolic F06.8
                acute or subacute F05
            liver, alcoholic F10.259
            epilepsy transient (acute) F05
            infection
                brain (intracranial) F06.8
                    acute or subacute F05
            intoxication
                alcoholic (acute) F10.259
                drug F19 with .x59 F11 ☑
            ischemia, cerebrovascular (generalized) —
                see Psychosis, arteriosclerotic
            puerperium — see Psychosis, puerperal
            trauma, brain (birth) (from electric current)
                (surgical) F06.8
                acute or subacute F05
        infective F06.8
            acute or subacute F05
        post-traumatic F06.8
            acute or subacute F05
    paranoiac F22
    paranoid (climacteric) (involutional)
        (menopausal) F22

Psychosis — continued
    paranoid — continued
        psychogenic (acute) F23
        schizophrenic F20.0
        senile F03 ☑
    postpartum F53
    presbyophrenic (type) F03 ☑
    presenile F03 ☑
    psychogenic (paranoid) F23
        depressive F32.3
    puerperal F53
        specified type — see Psychosis, by type
    reactive (brief) (transient) (emotional stress)
        (psychological trauma) F23
        depressive F32.3
            recurrent F33.3
        excitative type F30.8
    schizoaffective F25.9
        depressive type F25.1
        manic type F25.0
    schizophrenia, schizophrenic — see
        Schizophrenia
    schizophrenia-like, in epilepsy F06.2
    schizophreniform F20.81
        affective type F25.9
        brief F23
        confusional type F23
        mixed type F25.0
    senile NEC F03 ☑
        depressed or paranoid type F03 ☑
        simple deterioration F03 ☑
        specified type - code to condition
    shared F24
    situational (reactive) F23
    symbiotic (childhood) F84.3
    symptomatic F09
Psychosomatic — see Disorder, psychosomatic
Psychosyndrome, organic F07.9
Psychotic episode due to or associated with physical
    condition F06.8
Pterygium (eye) H11.00 ☑
    amyloid H11.01 ☑
    central H11.02 ☑
    colli Q18.3
    double H11.03 ☑
    peripheral
        progressive H11.05 ☑
        stationary H11.04 ☑
    recurrent H11.06 ☑
Ptilosis (eyelid) — see Madarosis
Ptomaine (poisoning) — see Poisoning, food
Ptosis (see also Blepharoptosis)
    adiposa (false) — see Blepharoptosis
    breast N64.81
    cecum K63.4
    colon K63.4
    congenital (eyelid) Q10.0
        specified site NEC — see Anomaly, by site
    eyelid — see Blepharoptosis
        congenital Q10.0
    gastric K31.89
    intestine K63.4
    kidney N28.83
    liver K76.89
    renal N28.83
    splanchnic K63.4
    spleen D73.89
    stomach K31.89
    viscera K63.4
PTP D69.51
Ptyalism (periodic) K11.7
    hysterical F45.8
    pregnancy — see Pregnancy, complicated by,
        specified pregnancy-related condition NEC
    psychogenic F45.8
Ptyalolithiasis K11.5
Pubarche, precocious E30.1
Pubertas praecox E30.1
Puberty (development state) Z00.3
    bleeding (excessive) N92.2
    delayed E30.0
    precocious (constitutional) (cryptogenic)
        (idiopathic) E30.1
        central E22.8
        due to
            ovarian hyperfunction E28.1
                estrogen E28.0
            testicular hyperfunction E29.0
    premature E30.1
        due to
            adrenal cortical hyperfunction E25.8
            pineal tumor E34.8
            pituitary (anterior) hyperfunction E22.8

☑ Additional character required

Puckering, macula — *see* Degeneration, macula, puckering
Pudenda, pudendum — *see* condition
Puente's disease (simple glandular cheilitis) K13.0
Puerperal, puerperium (complicated by, complications)
  abnormal glucose (tolerance test) O99.815
  abscess
    areola O91.02
      associated with lactation O91.03
    Bartholin's gland O86.19
    breast O91.12
      associated with lactation O91.13
    cervix (uteri) O86.11
    genital organ NEC O86.19
    kidney O86.21
    mammary O91.12
      associated with lactation O91.13
    nipple O91.02
      associated with lactation O91.03
    peritoneum O85
    subareolar O91.12
      associated with lactation O91.13
    urinary tract — *see* Puerperal, infection, urinary
    uterus O86.12
    vagina (wall) O86.13
    vaginorectal O86.13
    vulvovaginal gland O86.13
  adnexitis O86.19
  afibrinogenemia, or other coagulation
    defect O72.3
  albuminuria (acute) (subacute) — *see* Proteinuria, gestational
  alcohol use O99.315
  anemia O90.81
    pre-existing (pre-pregnancy) O99.03
  anesthetic death O89.8
  apoplexy O99.43
  bariatric surgery status O99.845
  blood disorder NEC O99.13
  blood dyscrasia O72.3
  cardiomyopathy O90.3
  cerebrovascular disorder (conditions in
    I60-I69) O99.43
  cervicitis O86.11
  circulatory system disorder O99.43
  coagulopathy (any) O99.13
    with hemorrhage O72.3
  complications O90.9
    specified NEC O90.89
  convulsions — *see* Eclampsia
  cystitis O86.22
  cystopyelitis O86.29
  delirium NEC F05
  diabetes O24.93
    gestational — *see* Puerperal, gestational diabetes
    pre-existing O24.33
      specified NEC O24.83
      type 1 O24.03
      type 2 O24.13
  digestive system disorder O99.63
  disease O90.9
    breast NEC O92.29
    cerebrovascular (acute) O99.43
    nonobstetric NEC O99.89
    tubo-ovarian O86.19
    Valsuani's O99.03
  disorder O90.9
    biliary tract O26.63
    lactation O92.70
    liver O26.63
    nonobstetric NEC O99.89
  disruption
    cesarean wound O90.0
    episiotomy wound O90.1
    perineal laceration wound O90.1
  drug use O99.325
  eclampsia (with pre-existing hypertension) O15.2
  embolism (pulmonary) (blood clot) — *see*
    Embolism, obstetric, puerperal
  endocrine, nutritional or metabolic disease
    NEC O99.285
  endophlebitis — *see* Puerperal, phlebitis
  endotrachelitis O86.11
  failure
    lactation (complete) O92.3
      partial O92.4
    renal, acute O90.4
  fever (of unknown origin) O86.4
    septic O85
  fissure, nipple O92.12
    associated with lactation O92.13

Puerperal — *continued*
  fistula
    breast (due to mastitis) O91.12
      associated with lactation O91.13
    nipple O91.02
      associated with lactation O91.03
  galactophoritis O91.22
    associated with lactation O91.23
  galactorrhea O92.6
  gastric banding status O99.845
  gastric bypass status O99.845
  gastrointestinal disease NEC O99.63
  gestational
    diabetes O24.439
      diet controlled O24.430
      insulin (and diet) controlled O24.434
      oral drug controlled (antidiabetic)
        (hypoglycemic) O24.435
    edema O12.05
      with proteinuria O12.25
    proteinuria O12.15
  gonorrhea O98.23
  hematoma, subdural O99.43
  hemiplegia, cerebral O99.355
    due to cerebrovascular disorder O99.43
  hemorrhage O72.1
    brain O99.43
    bulbar O99.43
    cerebellar O99.43
    cerebral O99.43
    cortical O99.43
    delayed or secondary O72.2
    extradural O99.43
    internal capsule O99.43
    intracranial O99.43
    intrapontine O99.43
    meningeal O99.43
    pontine O99.43
    retained placenta O72.0
    subarachnoid O99.43
    subcortical O99.43
    subdural O99.43
    third stage O72.0
    uterine, delayed O72.2
    ventricular O99.43
  hemorrhoids O87.2
  hepatorenal syndrome O90.4
  hypertension — *see* Hypertension, complicating,
    puerperium
  hypertrophy, breast O92.29
  induration breast (fibrous) O92.29
  infection O86.4
    cervix O86.11
    generalized O85
    genital tract NEC O86.19
      obstetric surgical wound O86.0
    kidney (bacillus coli) O86.21
    maternal O98.93
      carrier state NEC O99.835
      gonorrhea O98.23
      human immunodeficiency virus (HIV) O98.73
      protozoal O98.63
      sexually transmitted NEC O98.33
      specified NEC O98.83
      streptococcus group B (GBS) carrier
        state O99.825
      syphilis O98.13
      tuberculosis O98.03
      viral hepatitis O98.43
      viral NEC O98.53
    nipple O91.02
      associated with lactation O91.03
    peritoneum O85
    renal O86.21
    specified NEC O86.89
    urinary (asymptomatic) (tract) NEC O86.20
      bladder O86.22
      kidney O86.21
      specified site NEC O86.29
      urethra O86.22
    vagina O86.13
    vein — *see* Puerperal, phlebitis
  ischemia, cerebral O99.43
  lymphangitis O86.89
    breast O91.22
      associated with lactation O91.23
  malignancy O9A.13
  malnutrition O25.3
  mammillitis O91.02
    associated with lactation O91.03
  mammitis O91.22
    associated with lactation O91.23

Puerperal — *continued*
  mania F30.8
  mastitis O91.22
    associated with lactation O91.23
    purulent O91.12
      associated with lactation O91.13
  melancholia — *see* Disorder, depressive
  mental disorder NEC O99.345
  metroperitonitis O85
  metrorrhagia — *see* Hemorrhage, postpartum
  metrosalpingitis O86.19
  metrovaginitis O86.13
  milk leg O87.1
  monoplegia, cerebral O99.43
  mood disturbance O90.6
  necrosis, liver (acute) (subacute) (conditions in
    subcategory K72.0) O26.63
    with renal failure O90.4
  nervous system disorder O99.355
  neuritis O90.89
  obesity (pre-existing prior to pregnancy) O99.215
  obesity surgery status O99.845
  occlusion, precerebral artery O99.43
  paralysis
    bladder (sphincter) O90.89
    cerebral O99.43
  paralytic stroke O99.43
  parametritis O85
  paravaginitis O86.13
  pelviperitonitis O85
  perimetritis O86.12
  perimetrosalpingitis O86.19
  perinephritis O86.21
  periphlebitis — *see* Puerperal phlebitis
  peritoneal infection O85
  peritonitis (pelvic) O85
  perivaginitis O86.13
  phlebitis O87.0
    deep O87.1
    pelvic O87.1
    superficial O87.0
  phlebothrombosis, deep O87.1
  phlegmasia alba dolens O87.1
  placental polyp O90.89
  pneumonia, embolic — *see* Embolism, obstetric,
    puerperal
  pre-eclampsia — *see* Pre-eclampsia
  psychosis F53
  pyelitis O86.21
  pyelocystitis O86.29
  pyelonephritis O86.21
  pyelonephrosis O86.21
  pyemia O85
  pyocystitis O86.29
  pyohemia O85
  pyometra O86.12
  pyonephritis O86.21
  pyosalpingitis O86.19
  pyrexia (of unknown origin) O86.4
  renal
    disease NEC O90.89
    failure O90.4
  respiratory disease NEC O99.53
  retention
    decidua — *see* Retention, decidua
    placenta O72.0
    secundines — *see* Retention, secundines
  retracted nipple O92.02
  salpingo-ovaritis O86.19
  salpingoperitonitis O85
  secondary perineal tear O90.1
  sepsis (pelvic) O85
  sepsis O85
  septic thrombophlebitis O86.81
  skin disorder NEC O99.73
  specified condition NEC O99.89
  stroke O99.43
  subinvolution (uterus) O90.89
  subluxation of symphysis (pubis) O26.73
  suppuration — *see* Puerperal, abscess
  tetanus A34
  thelitis O91.02
    associated with lactation O91.03
  thrombocytopenia O72.3
  thrombophlebitis (superficial) O87.0
    deep O87.1
    pelvic O87.1
    septic O86.81
  thrombosis (venous) — *see* Thrombosis,
    puerperal
  thyroiditis O90.5

Puerperal — *continued*
  toxemia (eclamptic) (pre-eclamptic) (with convulsions) O15.2
  trauma, non-obstetric O9A.23
    caused by abuse (physical) (suspected) O9A.33
      confirmed O9A.33
      psychological (suspected) O9A.53
        confirmed O9A.53
      sexual (suspected) O9A.43
        confirmed O9A.43
  uremia (due to renal failure) O90.4
  urethritis O86.22
  vaginitis O86.13
  varicose veins (legs) O87.4
    vulva or perineum O87.8
  venous O87.9
  vulvitis O86.19
  vulvovaginitis O86.13
  white leg O87.1
Puerperium — *see* Puerperal
Pulmolithiasis J98.4
Pulmonary — *see* condition
Pulpitis (acute) (anachoretic) (chronic) (hyperplastic) (putrescent) (suppurative) (ulcerative) K04.01
  irreversible K04.02
  reversible K04.01
Pulpless tooth K04.99
Pulse
  alternating R00.8
  bigeminal R00.8
  fast R00.0
  feeble, rapid due to shock following injury T79.4 ☑
  rapid R00.0
  weak R09.89
Pulsus alternans or trigeminus R00.8
Punch drunk F07.81
Punctum lacrimale occlusion — *see* Obstruction, lacrimal
Puncture
  abdomen, abdominal
    wall S31.139 ☑
      with
        foreign body S31.149 ☑
        penetration into peritoneal cavity S31.639 ☑
          with foreign body S31.649 ☑
      epigastric region S31.132 ☑
        with
          foreign body S31.142 ☑
          penetration into peritoneal cavity S31.632 ☑
            with foreign body S31.642 ☑
      left
        lower quadrant S31.134 ☑
          with
            foreign body S31.144 ☑
            penetration into peritoneal cavity S31.634 ☑
              with foreign body S31.644 ☑
        upper quadrant S31.131 ☑
          with
            foreign body S31.141 ☑
            penetration into peritoneal cavity S31.631 ☑
              with foreign body S31.641 ☑
      periumbilic region S31.135 ☑
        with
          foreign body S31.145 ☑
          penetration into peritoneal cavity S31.635 ☑
            with foreign body S31.645 ☑
      right
        lower quadrant S31.133 ☑
          with
            foreign body S31.143 ☑
            penetration into peritoneal cavity S31.633 ☑
              with foreign body S31.643 ☑
        upper quadrant S31.130 ☑
          with
            foreign body S31.140 ☑
            penetration into peritoneal cavity S31.630 ☑
              with foreign body S31.640 ☑
  accidental, complicating surgery — *see* Complication, accidental puncture or laceration
  alveolar (process) — *see* Puncture, oral cavity
  ankle S91.039 ☑
    with
      foreign body S91.049 ☑

Puncture — *continued*
  ankle — *continued*
    left S91.032 ☑
      with
        foreign body S91.042 ☑
    right S91.031 ☑
      with
        foreign body S91.041 ☑
  anus S31.833 ☑
    with foreign body S31.834 ☑
  arm (upper) S41.139 ☑
    with foreign body S41.149 ☑
    left S41.132 ☑
      with foreign body S41.142 ☑
    lower — *see* Puncture, forearm
    right S41.131 ☑
      with foreign body S41.141 ☑
  auditory canal (external) (meatus) — *see* Puncture, ear
  auricle, ear — *see* Puncture, ear
  axilla — *see* Puncture, arm
  back (*see also* Puncture, thorax, back)
    lower S31.030 ☑
      with
        foreign body S31.040 ☑
          with penetration into retroperitoneal space S31.041 ☑
        penetration into retroperitoneal space S31.031 ☑
  bladder (traumatic) S37.29 ☑
    nontraumatic N32.89
  breast S21.039 ☑
    with foreign body S21.049 ☑
    left S21.032 ☑
      with foreign body S21.042 ☑
    right S21.031 ☑
      with foreign body S21.041 ☑
  buttock S31.803 ☑
    with foreign body S31.804 ☑
    left S31.823 ☑
      with foreign body S31.824 ☑
    right S31.813 ☑
      with foreign body S31.814 ☑
  by
    device, implant or graft — *see* Complications, by site and type, mechanical
    foreign body left accidentally in operative wound T81.539 ☑
    instrument (any) during a procedure, accidental — *see* Puncture, accidental complicating surgery
  calf — *see* Puncture, leg
  canaliculus lacrimalis — *see* Puncture, eyelid
  canthus, eye — *see* Puncture, eyelid
  cervical esophagus S11.23 ☑
    with foreign body S11.24 ☑
  cheek (external) S01.439 ☑
    with foreign body S01.449 ☑
    left S01.432 ☑
      with foreign body S01.442 ☑
    right S01.431 ☑
      with foreign body S01.441 ☑
    internal — *see* Puncture, oral cavity
  chest wall — *see* Puncture, thorax
  chin — *see* Puncture, head, specified site NEC
  clitoris — *see* Puncture, vulva
  costal region — *see* Puncture, thorax
  digit (s)
    hand — *see* Puncture, finger
    foot — *see* Puncture, toe
  ear (canal) (external) S01.339 ☑
    with foreign body S01.349 ☑
    left S01.332 ☑
      with foreign body S01.342 ☑
    right S01.331 ☑
      with foreign body S01.341 ☑
    drum S09.2 ☑
  elbow S51.039 ☑
    with
      foreign body S51.049 ☑
    left S51.032 ☑
      with
        foreign body S51.042 ☑
    right S51.031 ☑
      with
        foreign body S51.041 ☑
  epididymis — *see* Puncture, testis
  epigastric region — *see* Puncture, abdomen, wall, epigastric
  epiglottis S11.83 ☑
    with foreign body S11.84 ☑

Puncture — *continued*
  esophagus
    cervical S11.23 ☑
      with foreign body S11.24 ☑
    thoracic S27.818 ☑
  eyeball S05.6 ☑
    with foreign body S05.5 ☑
  eyebrow — *see* Puncture, eyelid
  eyelid S01.13 ☑
    with foreign body S01.14 ☑
    left S01.132 ☑
      with foreign body S01.142 ☑
    right S01.131 ☑
      with foreign body S01.141 ☑
  face NEC — *see* Puncture, head, specified site NEC
  finger (s) S61.239 ☑
    with
      damage to nail S61.339 ☑
        with
          foreign body S61.349 ☑
      foreign body S61.249 ☑
    index S61.238 ☑
      with
        damage to nail S61.338 ☑
          with
            foreign body S61.348 ☑
        foreign body S61.248 ☑
      left S61.231 ☑
        with
          damage to nail S61.331 ☑
            with
              foreign body S61.341 ☑
          foreign body S61.241 ☑
      right S61.230 ☑
        with
          damage to nail S61.330 ☑
            with
              foreign body S61.340 ☑
          foreign body S61.240 ☑
    little S61.238 ☑
      with
        damage to nail S61.338 ☑
          with
            foreign body S61.348 ☑
        foreign body S61.248 ☑
      left S61.237 ☑
        with
          damage to nail S61.337 ☑
            with
              foreign body S61.347 ☑
          foreign body S61.247 ☑
      right S61.236 ☑
        with
          damage to nail S61.336 ☑
            with
              foreign body S61.346 ☑
          foreign body S61.246 ☑
    middle S61.238 ☑
      with
        damage to nail S61.338 ☑
          with
            foreign body S61.348 ☑
        foreign body S61.248 ☑
      left S61.233 ☑
        with
          damage to nail S61.333 ☑
            with
              foreign body S61.343 ☑
          foreign body S61.243 ☑
      right S61.232 ☑
        with
          damage to nail S61.332 ☑
            with
              foreign body S61.342 ☑
          foreign body S61.242 ☑
    ring S61.238 ☑
      with
        damage to nail S61.338 ☑
          with
            foreign body S61.348 ☑
        foreign body S61.248 ☑
      left S61.235 ☑
        with
          damage to nail S61.335 ☑
            with
              foreign body S61.345 ☑
          foreign body S61.245 ☑
      right S61.234 ☑
        with
          damage to nail S61.334 ☑
            with
              foreign body S61.344 ☑
          foreign body S61.244 ☑

☑ **Additional character required**

Puerperal - Puncture

ICD-10-CM INDEX TO DISEASES AND INJURIES

Puncture — *continued*
- flank S31.139 ☑
  - with foreign body S31.149 ☑
- foot (except toe (s) alone) S91.339 ☑
  - with foreign body S91.349 ☑
  - left S91.332 ☑
    - with foreign body S91.342 ☑
  - right S91.331 ☑
    - with foreign body S91.341 ☑
  - toe — *see* Puncture, toe
- forearm S51.839 ☑
  - with
    - foreign body S51.849 ☑
  - elbow only — *see* Puncture, elbow
  - left S51.832 ☑
    - with
      - foreign body S51.842 ☑
  - right S51.831 ☑
    - with
      - foreign body S51.841 ☑
- forehead — *see* Puncture, head, specified site NEC
- genital organs, external
  - female S31.532 ☑
    - with foreign body S31.542 ☑
    - vagina — *see* Puncture, vagina
    - vulva — *see* Puncture, vulva
  - male S31.531 ☑
    - with foreign body S31.541 ☑
    - penis — *see* Puncture, penis
    - scrotum — *see* Puncture, scrotum
    - testis — *see* Puncture, testis
- groin — *see* Puncture, abdomen, wall
- gum — *see* Puncture, oral cavity
- hand S61.439 ☑
  - with
    - foreign body S61.449 ☑
  - finger — *see* Puncture, finger
  - left S61.432 ☑
    - with
      - foreign body S61.442 ☑
  - right S61.431 ☑
    - with
      - foreign body S61.441 ☑
  - thumb — *see* Puncture, thumb
- head S01.93 ☑
  - with foreign body S01.94 ☑
  - cheek — *see* Puncture, cheek
  - ear — *see* Puncture, ear
  - eyelid — *see* Puncture, eyelid
  - lip — *see* Puncture, oral cavity
  - nose — *see* Puncture, nose
  - oral cavity — *see* Puncture, oral cavity
  - scalp S01.03 ☑
    - with foreign body S01.04 ☑
  - specified site NEC S01.83 ☑
    - with foreign body S01.84 ☑
  - temporomandibular area — *see* Puncture, cheek
- heart S26.99 ☑
  - with hemopericardium S26.09 ☑
  - without hemopericardium S26.19 ☑
- heel — *see* Puncture, foot
- hip S71.039 ☑
  - with foreign body S71.049 ☑
  - left S71.032 ☑
    - with foreign body S71.042 ☑
  - right S71.031 ☑
    - with foreign body S71.041 ☑
- hymen — *see* Puncture, vagina
- hypochondrium — *see* Puncture, abdomen, wall
- hypogastric region — *see* Puncture, abdomen, wall
- inguinal region — *see* Puncture, abdomen, wall
- instep — *see* Puncture, foot
- internal organs — *see* Injury, by site
- interscapular region — *see* Puncture, thorax, back
- intestine
  - large
    - colon S36.599 ☑
      - ascending S36.590 ☑
      - descending S36.592 ☑
      - sigmoid S36.593 ☑
      - specified site NEC S36.598 ☑
      - transverse S36.591 ☑
    - rectum S36.69 ☑
  - small S36.499 ☑
    - duodenum S36.490 ☑
    - specified site NEC S36.498 ☑
- intra-abdominal organ S36.99 ☑
  - gallbladder S36.128 ☑
  - intestine — *see* Puncture, intestine

Puncture — *continued*
- intra-abdominal organ — *continued*
  - liver S36.118 ☑
  - pancreas — *see* Puncture, pancreas
  - peritoneum S36.81 ☑
  - specified site NEC S36.898 ☑
  - spleen S36.09 ☑
  - stomach S36.39 ☑
- jaw — *see* Puncture, head, specified site NEC
- knee S81.039 ☑
  - with foreign body S81.049 ☑
  - left S81.032 ☑
    - with foreign body S81.042 ☑
  - right S81.031 ☑
    - with foreign body S81.041 ☑
- labium (majus) (minus) — *see* Puncture, vulva
- lacrimal duct — *see* Puncture, eyelid
- larynx S11.013 ☑
  - with foreign body S11.014 ☑
- leg (lower) S81.839 ☑
  - with foreign body S81.849 ☑
  - foot — *see* Puncture, foot
  - knee — *see* Puncture, knee
  - left S81.832 ☑
    - with foreign body S81.842 ☑
  - right S81.831 ☑
    - with foreign body S81.841 ☑
  - upper — *see* Puncture, thigh
- lip S01.531 ☑
  - with foreign body S01.541 ☑
- loin — *see* Puncture, abdomen, wall
- lower back — *see* Puncture, back, lower
- lumbar region — *see* Puncture, back, lower
- malar region — *see* Puncture, head, specified site NEC
- mammary — *see* Puncture, breast
- mastoid region — *see* Puncture, head, specified site NEC
- mouth — *see* Puncture, oral cavity
- nail
  - finger — *see* Puncture, finger, with damage to nail
  - toe — *see* Puncture, toe, with damage to nail
- nasal (septum) (sinus) — *see* Puncture, nose
- nasopharynx — *see* Puncture, head, specified site NEC
- neck S11.93 ☑
  - with foreign body S11.94 ☑
  - involving
    - cervical esophagus — *see* Puncture, cervical esophagus
    - larynx — *see* Puncture, larynx
    - pharynx — *see* Puncture, pharynx
    - thyroid gland — *see* Puncture, thyroid gland
    - trachea — *see* Puncture, trachea
  - specified site NEC S11.83 ☑
    - with foreign body S11.84 ☑
- nose (septum) (sinus) S01.23 ☑
  - with foreign body S01.24 ☑
- ocular — *see* Puncture, eyeball
- oral cavity S01.532 ☑
  - with foreign body S01.542 ☑
- orbit S05.4 ☑
- palate — *see* Puncture, oral cavity
- palm — *see* Puncture, hand
- pancreas S36.299 ☑
  - body S36.291 ☑
  - head S36.290 ☑
  - tail S36.292 ☑
- pelvis — *see* Puncture, back, lower
- penis S31.23 ☑
  - with foreign body S31.24 ☑
- perineum
  - female S31.43 ☑
    - with foreign body S31.44 ☑
  - male S31.139 ☑
    - with foreign body S31.149 ☑
- periocular area (with or without lacrimal passages) — *see* Puncture, eyelid
- phalanges
  - finger — *see* Puncture, finger
  - toe — *see* Puncture, toe
- pharynx S11.23 ☑
  - with foreign body S11.24 ☑
- pinna — *see* Puncture, ear
- popliteal space — *see* Puncture, knee
- prepuce — *see* Puncture, penis
- pubic region S31.139 ☑
  - with foreign body S31.149 ☑
- pudendum — *see* Puncture, genital organs, external
- rectovaginal septum — *see* Puncture, vagina

Puncture — *continued*
- sacral region — *see* Puncture, back, lower
- sacroiliac region — *see* Puncture, back, lower
- salivary gland — *see* Puncture, oral cavity
- scalp S01.03 ☑
  - with foreign body S01.04 ☑
- scapular region — *see* Puncture, shoulder
- scrotum S31.33 ☑
  - with foreign body S31.34 ☑
- shin — *see* Puncture, leg
- shoulder S41.039 ☑
  - with foreign body S41.049 ☑
  - left S41.032 ☑
    - with foreign body S41.042 ☑
  - right S41.031 ☑
    - with foreign body S41.041 ☑
- spermatic cord — *see* Puncture, testis
- sternal region — *see* Puncture, thorax, front
- submaxillary region — *see* Puncture, head, specified site NEC
- submental region — *see* Puncture, head, specified site NEC
- subungual
  - finger (s) — *see* Puncture, finger, with damage to nail
  - toe — *see* Puncture, toe, with damage to nail
- supraclavicular fossa — *see* Puncture, neck, specified site NEC
- temple, temporal region — *see* Puncture, head, specified site NEC
- temporomandibular area — *see* Puncture, cheek
- testis S31.33 ☑
  - with foreign body S31.34 ☑
- thigh S71.139 ☑
  - with foreign body S71.149 ☑
  - left S71.132 ☑
    - with foreign body S71.142 ☑
  - right S71.131 ☑
    - with foreign body S71.141 ☑
- thorax, thoracic (wall) S21.93 ☑
  - with foreign body S21.94 ☑
  - back S21.23 ☑
    - with
      - foreign body S21.24 ☑
        - with penetration S21.44 ☑
      - penetration S21.43 ☑
  - breast — *see* Puncture, breast
  - front S21.13 ☑
    - with
      - foreign body S21.14 ☑
        - with penetration S21.34 ☑
      - penetration S21.33 ☑
- throat — *see* Puncture, neck
- thumb S61.039 ☑
  - with
    - damage to nail S61.139 ☑
      - with
        - foreign body S61.149 ☑
    - foreign body S61.049 ☑
  - left S61.032 ☑
    - with
      - damage to nail S61.132 ☑
        - with
          - foreign body S61.142 ☑
      - foreign body S61.042 ☑
  - right S61.031 ☑
    - with
      - damage to nail S61.131 ☑
        - with
          - foreign body S61.141 ☑
      - foreign body S61.041 ☑
- thyroid gland S11.13 ☑
  - with foreign body S11.14 ☑
- toe (s) S91.139 ☑
  - with
    - damage to nail S91.239 ☑
      - with
        - foreign body S91.249 ☑
    - foreign body S91.149 ☑
  - great S91.133 ☑
    - with
      - damage to nail S91.233 ☑
        - with
          - foreign body S91.243 ☑
      - foreign body S91.143 ☑
    - left S91.132 ☑
      - with
        - damage to nail S91.232 ☑
          - with
            - foreign body S91.242 ☑
        - foreign body S91.142 ☑
    - right S91.131 ☑

Puncture - Quadricuspid

Puncture — *continued*
  toe (s) — *continued*
    with
      damage to nail S91.231 ☑
        with
          foreign body S91.241 ☑
        foreign body S91.141 ☑
    lesser S91.136 ☑
      with
        damage to nail S91.236 ☑
          with
            foreign body S91.246 ☑
        foreign body S91.146 ☑
    left S91.135 ☑
      with
        damage to nail S91.235 ☑
          with
            foreign body S91.245 ☑
        foreign body S91.145 ☑
    right S91.134 ☑
      with
        damage to nail S91.234 ☑
          with
            foreign body S91.244 ☑
        foreign body S91.144 ☑
  tongue — *see* Puncture, oral cavity
  trachea S11.023 ☑
    with foreign body S11.024 ☑
  tunica vaginalis — *see* Puncture, testis
  tympanum, tympanic membrane S09.2 ☑
  umbilical region S31.135 ☑
    with foreign body S31.145 ☑
  uvula — *see* Puncture, oral cavity
  vagina S31.43 ☑
    with foreign body S31.44 ☑
  vocal cords S11.033 ☑
    with foreign body S11.034 ☑
  vulva S31.43 ☑
    with foreign body S31.44 ☑
  wrist S61.539 ☑
    with
      foreign body S61.549 ☑
    left S61.532 ☑
      with
        foreign body S61.542 ☑
    right S61.531 ☑
      with
        foreign body S61.541 ☑
PUO (pyrexia of unknown origin) R50.9
Pupillary membrane (persistent) Q13.89
Pupillotonia — *see* Anomaly, pupil, function, tonic pupil
Purpura D69.2
  abdominal D69.0
  allergic D69.0
  anaphylactoid D69.0
  annularis telangiectodes L81.7
  arthritic D69.0
  autoerythrocyte sensitization D69.2
  autoimmune D69.0
  bacterial D69.0
  Bateman's (senile) D69.2
  capillary fragility (hereditary) (idiopathic) D69.8
  cryoglobulinemic D89.1
  Devil's pinches D69.2
  fibrinolytic — *see* Fibrinolysis
  fulminans, fulminous D65
  gangrenous D65
  hemorrhagic, hemorrhagica D69.3
    not due to thrombocytopenia D69.0
  Henoch (-Schönlein) (allergic) D69.0
  hypergammaglobulinemic (benign) (Waldenström) D89.0
  idiopathic (thrombocytopenic) D69.3
    nonthrombocytopenic D69.0
  immune thrombocytopenic D69.3
  infectious D69.0
  malignant D69.0
  neonatorum P54.5
  nervosa D69.0
  newborn P54.5
  nonthrombocytopenic D69.2
    hemorrhagic D69.0
    idiopathic D69.0
  nonthrombopenic D69.2
  peliosis rheumatica D69.0
  posttransfusion (post-transfusion) (from (fresh) whole blood or blood products) D69.51
  primary D69.49
  red cell membrane sensitivity D69.2
  rheumatica D69.0
  Schönlein (-Henoch) (allergic) D69.0

Purpura — *continued*
  scorbutic E54 *[D77]*
  senile D69.2
  simplex D69.2
  symptomatica D69.0
  telangiectasia annularis L81.7
  thrombocytopenic D69.49
    congenital D69.42
    hemorrhagic D69.3
    hereditary D69.42
    idiopathic D69.3
    immune D69.3
    neonatal, transitory P61.0
    thrombotic M31.1
  thrombohemolytic — *see* Fibrinolysis
  thrombolytic — *see* Fibrinolysis
  thrombopenic D69.49
  thrombotic, thrombocytopenic M31.1
  toxic D69.0
  vascular D69.0
  visceral symptoms D69.0
Purpuric spots R23.3
Purulent — *see* condition
Pus
  in
    stool R19.5
    urine N39.0
  tube (rupture) — *see* Salpingo-oophoritis
Pustular rash L08.0
Pustule (nonmalignant) L08.9
  malignant A22.0
Pustulosis palmaris et plantaris L40.3
Putnam (-Dana) disease or syndrome — *see* Degeneration, combined
Putrescent pulp (dental) K04.1
Pyarthritis, pyarthrosis — *see* Arthritis, pyogenic or pyemic
  tuberculous — *see* Tuberculosis, joint
Pyelectasis — *see* Hydronephrosis
Pyelitis (congenital) (uremic) (*see also* Pyelonephritis)
  with
    calculus — *see* category N20
      with hydronephrosis N13.2
    contracted kidney N11.9
  acute N10
  chronic N11.9
    with calculus — *see* category N20
      with hydronephrosis N13.2
  cystica N28.84
  puerperal (postpartum) O86.21
  tuberculous A18.11
Pyelocystitis — *see* Pyelonephritis
Pyelonephritis (*see also* Nephritis, tubulo-interstitial)
  with
    calculus — *see* category N20
      with hydronephrosis N13.2
    contracted kidney N11.9
  acute N10
  calculus — *see* category N20
    with hydronephrosis N13.2
  chronic N11.9
    with calculus — *see* category N20
      with hydronephrosis N13.2
    associated with ureteral obstruction or stricture N11.1
    nonobstructive N11.8
      with reflux (vesicoureteral) N11.0
    obstructive N11.1
    specified NEC N11.8
  in (due to)
    brucellosis A23.9 *[N16]*
    cryoglobulinemia (mixed) D89.1 *[N16]*
    cystinosis E72.04
    diphtheria A36.84
    glycogen storage disease E74.09 *[N16]*
    leukemia NEC C95.9 ☑ *[N16]*
    lymphoma NEC C85.90 *[N16]*
    multiple myeloma C90.0 ☑ *[N16]*
    obstruction N11.1
    Salmonella infection A02.25
    sarcoidosis D86.84
    sepsis A41.9 *[N16]*
    Sjögren's disease M35.04
    toxoplasmosis B58.83
    transplant rejection T86.91 *[N16]*
    Wilson's disease E83.01 *[N16]*
  nonobstructive N12
    with reflux (vesicoureteral) N11.0
    chronic N11.8
  syphilitic A52.75
Pyelonephrosis (obstructive) N11.1
  chronic N11.9

Pyelophlebitis I80.8
Pyeloureteritis cystica N28.85
Pyemia, pyemic (fever) (infection) (purulent) (*see also* Sepsis)
  joint — *see* Arthritis, pyogenic or pyemic
  liver K75.1
  pneumococcal A40.3
  portal K75.1
  postvaccinal T88.0 ☑
  puerperal, postpartum, childbirth O85
  specified organism NEC A41.89
  tuberculous — *see* Tuberculosis, miliary
Pygopagus Q89.4
Pyknoepilepsy (idiopathic) — *see* Pyknolepsy
Pyknolepsy G40.A09
  intractable G40.A19
    with status epilepticus G40.A11
    without status epilepticus G40.A19
  not intractable G40.A09
    with status epilepticus G40.A01
    without status epilepticus G40.A09
Pylephlebitis K75.1
Pyle's syndrome Q78.5
Pylethrombophlebitis K75.1
Pylethrombosis K75.1
Pyloritis K29.90
  with bleeding K29.91
Pylorospasm (reflex) NEC K31.3
  congenital or infantile Q40.0
  newborn Q40.0
  neurotic F45.8
  psychogenic F45.8
Pylorus, pyloric — *see* condition
Pyoarthrosis — *see* Arthritis, pyogenic or pyemic
Pyocele
  mastoid — *see* Mastoiditis, acute
  sinus (accessory) — *see* Sinusitis
  turbinate (bone) J32.9
  urethra (*see also* Urethritis) N34.0
Pyocolpos — *see* Vaginitis
Pyocystitis N30.80
  with hematuria N30.81
Pyoderma, pyodermia L08.0
  gangrenosum L88
  newborn P39.4
  phagedenic L88
  vegetans L08.81
Pyodermatitis L08.0
  vegetans L08.81
Pyogenic — *see* condition
Pyohydronephrosis N13.6
Pyometra, pyometrium, pyometritis — *see* Endometritis
Pyomyositis (tropical) — *see* Myositis, infective
Pyonephritis N12
Pyonephrosis N13.6
  tuberculous A18.11
Pyo-oophoritis — *see* Salpingo-oophoritis
Pyo-ovarium — *see* Salpingo-oophoritis
Pyopericarditis, pyopericardium I30.1
Pyophlebitis — *see* Phlebitis
Pyopneumopericardium I30.1
Pyopneumothorax (infective) J86.9
  with fistula J86.0
  tuberculous NEC A15.6
Pyosalpinx, pyosalpingitis (*see also* Salpingo-oophoritis)
Pyothorax J86.9
  with fistula J86.0
  tuberculous NEC A15.6
Pyoureter N28.89
  tuberculous A18.11
Pyramidopallidonigral syndrome G20
Pyrexia (of unknown origin) R50.9
  atmospheric T67.0 ☑
  during labor NEC O75.2
  heat T67.0 ☑
  newborn P81.9
    environmentally-induced P81.0
  persistent R50.9
  puerperal O86.4
Pyroglobulinemia NEC E88.09
Pyromania F63.1
Pyrosis R12
Pyuria (bacterial) N39.0

Q

Q fever A78
  with pneumonia A78
Quadricuspid aortic valve Q23.8

☑ **Additional character required**

Quadrilateral fever A78
Quadriparesis — *see* Quadriplegia
    meaning muscle weakness M62.81
Quadriplegia G82.50
    complete
        C1-C4 level G82.51
        C5-C7 level G82.53
    congenital (cerebral) (spinal) G80.8
        spastic G80.0
    embolic (current episode) I63.4 ☑
    functional R53.2
    incomplete
        C1-C4 level G82.52
        C5-C7 level G82.54
    thrombotic (current episode) I63.3 ☑
    traumatic - code to injury with seventh character S
        current episode — *see* Injury, spinal (cord),
            cervical
Quadruplet, pregnancy — *see* Pregnancy,
    quadruplet
Quarrelsomeness F60.3
Queensland fever A77.3
Quervain's disease M65.4
    thyroid E06.1
Queyrat's erythroplasia D07.4
    penis D07.4
    specified site — *see* Neoplasm, skin, in situ
    unspecified site D07.4
Quincke's disease or edema T78.3 ☑
    hereditary D84.1
Quinsy (gangrenous) J36
Quintan fever A79.0
Quintuplet, pregnancy — *see* Pregnancy, quintuplet

R

Rabbit fever — *see* Tularemia
Rabies A82.9
    contact Z20.3
    exposure to Z20.3
    inoculation reaction — *see* Complications,
        vaccination
    sylvatic A82.0
    urban A82.1
Rachischisis — *see* Spina bifida
Rachitic (*see also* condition)
    deformities of spine (late effect) (sequelae) E64.3
    pelvis (late effect) (sequelae) E64.3
        with disproportion (fetopelvic) O33.0
            causing obstructed labor O65.0
Rachitis, rachitism (acute) (tarda) (*see also* Rickets)
    renalis N25.0
    sequelae E64.3
Radial nerve — *see* condition
Radiation
    burn — *see* Burn
    effects NOS T66 ☑
    sickness NOS T66 ☑
    therapy, encounter for Z51.0
Radiculitis (pressure) (vertebrogenic) — *see*
    Radiculopathy
Radiculomyelitis (*see also* Encephalitis)
    toxic, due to
        Clostridium tetani A35
        Corynebacterium diphtheriae A36.82
Radiculopathy M54.10
    cervical region M54.12
    cervicothoracic region M54.13
    due to
        disc disorder
            C3 M50.11
            C4 M50.11
            C5 M50.121
            C6 M50.122
            C7 M50.123
            C8 M50.13
        displacement of intervertebral disc — *see*
            Disorder, disc, with, radiculopathy
    leg M54.1 ☑
    lumbar region M54.16
    lumbosacral region M54.17
    occipito-atlanto-axial region M54.11
    postherpetic B02.29
    sacrococcygeal region M54.18
    syphilitic A52.11
    thoracic region (with visceral pain) M54.14
    thoracolumbar region M54.15
Radiodermal burns (acute, chronic, or occupational)
    — *see* Burn

Radiodermatitis L58.9
    acute L58.0
    chronic L58.1
Radiotherapy session Z51.0
RAEB (refractory anemia with excess blasts) D46.2 ☑
Rage, meaning rabies — *see* Rabies
Ragpicker's disease A22.1
Ragsorter's disease A22.1
Raillietiniasis B71.8
Railroad neurosis F48.8
Railway spine F48.8
Raised (*see also* Elevated)
    antibody titer R76.0
Rake teeth, tooth M26.39
Rales R09.89
Ramifying renal pelvis Q63.8
Ramsay-Hunt disease or syndrome (*see also* Hunt's
    disease) B02.21
    meaning dyssynergia cerebellaris
        myoclonica G11.1
Ranula K11.6
    congenital Q38.4
Rape
    adult
        confirmed T74.21 ☑
        suspected T76.21 ☑
    alleged, observation or examination, ruled out
        adult Z04.41
        child Z04.42
    child
        confirmed T74.22 ☑
        suspected T76.22 ☑
Rapid
    feeble pulse, due to shock, following
        injury T79.4 ☑
    heart (beat) R00.0
        psychogenic F45.8
    second stage (delivery) O62.3
    time-zone change syndrome — *see* Disorder,
        sleep, circadian rhythm, psychogenic
Rarefaction, bone — *see* Disorder, bone, density and
    structure, specified NEC
Rash (toxic) R21
    canker A38.9
    diaper L22
    drug (internal use) L27.0
        contact (*see also* Dermatitis, due to, drugs,
            external) L25.1
    following immunization T88.1 ☑
    food — *see* Dermatitis, due to, food
    heat L74.0
    napkin (psoriasiform) L22
    nettle — *see* Urticaria
    pustular L08.0
    rose R21
        epidemic B06.9
    scarlet A38.9
    serum (*see also* Reaction, serum) T80.69 ☑
    wandering tongue K14.1
Rasmussen aneurysm — *see* Tuberculosis,
    pulmonary
Rasmussen encephalitis G04.81
Rat-bite fever A25.9
    due to Streptobacillus moniliformis A25.1
    spirochetal (morsus muris) A25.0
Rathke's pouch tumor D44.3
Raymond (-Céstan) syndrome I65.8
Raynaud's disease, phenomenon or syndrome
    (secondary) I73.00
    with gangrene (symmetric) I73.01
RDS (newborn) (type I) P22.0
    type II P22.1
Reaction (*see also* Disorder)
    adaptation — *see* Disorder, adjustment
    adjustment (anxiety) (conduct disorder)
        (depressiveness) (distress) — *see* Disorder,
        adjustment
        with
            mutism, elective (child) (adolescent) F94.0
    adverse
        food (any) (ingested) NEC T78.1 ☑
            anaphylactic — *see* Shock, anaphylactic, due
                to food
    affective — *see* Disorder, mood
    allergic — *see* Allergy
    anaphylactic — *see* Shock, anaphylactic
    anaphylactoid — *see* Shock, anaphylactic
    anesthesia — *see* Anesthesia, complication
    antitoxin (prophylactic) (therapeutic) — *see*
        Complications, vaccination
    anxiety F41.1
    Arthus — *see* Arthus' phenomenon

Reaction — *continued*
    asthenic F48.8
    combat and operational stress F43.0
    compulsive F42.8
    conversion F44.9
    crisis, acute F43.0
    deoxyribonuclease (DNA) (DNase)
        hypersensitivity D69.2
    depressive (single episode) F32.9
        affective (single episode) F31.4
            recurrent episode F33.9
        neurotic F34.1
        psychoneurotic F34.1
        psychotic F32.3
        recurrent — *see* Disorder, depressive, recurrent
    dissociative F44.9
    drug NEC T88.7 ☑
        addictive — *see* Dependence, drug
            transmitted via placenta or breast milk — *see*
                Absorption, drug, addictive, through
                placenta
        allergic — *see* Allergy, drug
        lichenoid L43.2
        newborn P93.8
            gray baby syndrome P93.0
        overdose or poisoning (by accident) — *see* Table
            of Drugs and Chemicals, by drug, poisoning
        photoallergic L56.1
        phototoxic L56.0
        withdrawal — *see* Dependence, by drug, with,
            withdrawal
            infant of dependent mother P96.1
            newborn P96.1
        wrong substance given or taken (by accident)
            — *see* Table of Drugs and Chemicals, by
            drug, poisoning
    fear F40.9
        child (abnormal) F93.8
    febrile nonhemolytic transfusion (FNHTR) R50.84
    fluid loss, cerebrospinal G97.1
    foreign
        body NEC — *see* Granuloma, foreign body
            in operative wound (inadvertently left) — *see*
                Foreign body, accidentally left during a
                procedure
        substance accidentally left during a procedure
            (chemical) (powder) (talc) T81.60 ☑
            aseptic peritonitis T81.61 ☑
            body or object (instrument) (sponge) (swab)
                — *see* Foreign body, accidentally left
                during a procedure
            specified reaction NEC T81.69 ☑
    grief — *see* Disorder, adjustment
    Herxheimer's R68.89
    hyperkinetic — *see* Hyperkinesia
    hypochondriacal F45.20
    hypoglycemic, due to insulin E16.0
        with coma (diabetic) — *see* Diabetes, coma
            nondiabetic E15
        therapeutic misadventure — *see* subcategory
            T38.3
    hypomanic F30.8
    hysterical F44.9
    immunization — *see* Complications, vaccination
    incompatibility
        ABO blood group (infusion) (transfusion)
            — *see* Complication (s), transfusion,
            incompatibility reaction, ABO
            delayed serologic T80.39 ☑
        minor blood group (Duffy) (E) (K(ell)) (Kidd)
            (Lewis) (M) (N) (P) (S) T80.89 ☑
        Rh (factor) (infusion) (transfusion) —
            see Complication (s), transfusion,
            incompatibility reaction, Rh (factor)
    inflammatory — *see* Infection
    infusion — *see* Complications, infusion
    inoculation (immune serum) — *see*
        Complications, vaccination
    insulin T38.3 ☑
    involutional psychotic — *see* Disorder, depressive
    leukemoid D72.823
        basophilic D72.823
        lymphocytic D72.823
        monocytic D72.823
        myelocytic D72.823
        neutrophilic D72.823
    LSD (acute)
        due to drug abuse — *see* Abuse, drug,
            hallucinogen
        due to drug dependence — *see* Dependence,
            drug, hallucinogen
    lumbar puncture G97.1

Retained — *continued*
　fragments — *continued*
　　metal Z18.10
　　nonmagnetic metal Z18.12
　　nontherapeutic radioactive Z18.09
　　organic NEC Z18.39
　　plastic Z18.2
　　quill (s) (animal) Z18.31
　　radioactive (nontherapeutic) NEC Z18.09
　　specified NEC Z18.89
　　spine (s) (animal) Z18.31
　　stone Z18.83
　　tooth (teeth) Z18.32
　　wood Z18.33
　gallstones, following cholecystectomy K91.86
Retardation
　development, developmental, specific — *see* Disorder, developmental
　endochondral bone growth — *see* Disorder, bone, development or growth
　growth R62.50
　　due to malnutrition E45
　mental — *see* Disability, intellectual
　motor function, specific F82
　physical (child) R62.52
　　due to malnutrition E45
　reading (specific) F81.0
　spelling (specific) (without reading disorder) F81.81
Retching — *see* Vomiting
Retention (*see also* Retained)
　bladder — *see* Retention, urine
　carbon dioxide E87.2
　cholelithiasis following cholecystectomy K91.86
　cyst — *see* Cyst
　dead
　　fetus (at or near term) (mother) O36.4 ☑
　　　early fetal death O02.1
　　ovum O02.0
　decidua (fragments) (following delivery) (with hemorrhage) O72.2
　　without hemorrhage O73.1
　deciduous tooth K00.6
　dental root K08.3
　fecal — *see* Constipation
　fetus
　　dead O36.4 ☑
　　　early O02.1
　fluid R60.9
　foreign body (*see also* Foreign body, retained)
　　current trauma - code as Foreign body, by site or type
　gallstones, following cholecystectomy K91.86
　gastric K31.89
　intrauterine contraceptive device, in pregnancy — *see* Pregnancy, complicated by, retention, intrauterine device
　membranes (complicating delivery) (with hemorrhage) O72.2
　　with abortion — *see* Abortion, by type
　　without hemorrhage O73.1
　meniscus — *see* Derangement, meniscus
　menses N94.89
　milk (puerperal, postpartum) O92.79
　nitrogen, extrarenal R39.2
　ovary syndrome N99.83
　placenta (total) (with hemorrhage) O72.0
　　without hemorrhage O73.0
　　portions or fragments (with hemorrhage) O72.2
　　　without hemorrhage O73.1
　products of conception
　　early pregnancy (dead fetus) O02.1
　　following
　　　delivery (with hemorrhage) O72.2
　　　　without hemorrhage O73.1
　secundines (following delivery) (with hemorrhage) O72.0
　　without hemorrhage O73.0
　　complicating puerperium (delayed hemorrhage) O72.2
　　partial O72.2
　　　without hemorrhage O73.1
　smegma, clitoris N90.89
　urine R33.9
　　due to hyperplasia (hypertrophy) of prostate — *see* Hyperplasia, prostate
　　drug-induced R33.0
　　organic R33.8
　　　drug-induced R33.0
　　psychogenic F45.8
　　specified NEC R33.8
　water (in tissues) — *see* Edema

Reticular erythematous mucinosis L98.5
Reticulation, dust — *see* Pneumoconiosis
Reticulocytosis R70.1
Reticuloendotheliosis
　acute infantile C96.0
　leukemic C91.4 ☑
　nonlipid C96.0
Reticulohistiocytoma (giant-cell) D76.3
Reticuloid, actinic L57.1
Reticulosis (skin)
　acute of infancy C96.0
　hemophagocytic, familial D76.1
　histiocytic medullary C96.A
　lipomelanotic I89.8
　malignant (midline) C86.0
　polymorphic C86.0
　Sézary — *see* Sézary disease
Retina, retinal (*see also* condition)
　dark area D49.81
Retinitis (*see also* Inflammation, chorioretinal)
　albuminurica N18.9 *[H32]*
　diabetic — *see* Diabetes, retinitis
　disciformis — *see* Degeneration, macula
　focal — *see* Inflammation, chorioretinal, focal
　gravidarum — *see* Pregnancy, complicated by, specified pregnancy-related condition NEC
　juxtapapillaris — *see* Inflammation, chorioretinal, focal, juxtapapillary
　luetic — *see* Retinitis, syphilitic
　pigmentosa H35.52
　proliferans — *see* Disorder, globe, degenerative, specified type NEC
　proliferating — *see* Disorder, globe, degenerative, specified type NEC
　renal N18.9 *[H32]*
　syphilitic (early) (secondary) A51.43
　　central, recurrent A52.71
　　congenital (early) A50.01 *[H32]*
　　late A52.71
　tuberculous A18.53
Retinoblastoma C69.2 ☑
　differentiated C69.2 ☑
　undifferentiated C69.2 ☑
Retinochoroiditis (*see also* Inflammation, chorioretinal)
　disseminated — *see* Inflammation, chorioretinal, disseminated
　　syphilitic A52.71
　focal — *see* Inflammation, chorioretinal
　juxtapapillaris — *see* Inflammation, chorioretinal, focal, juxtapapillary
Retinopathy (background) H35.00
　arteriosclerotic I70.8 *[H35.0 ☑]*
　atherosclerotic I70.8 *[H35.0 ☑]*
　central serous — *see* Chorioretinopathy, central serous
　Coats H35.02 ☑
　diabetic — *see* Diabetes, retinopathy
　exudative H35.02 ☑
　hypertensive H35.03 ☑
　in (due to)
　　diabetes — *see* Diabetes, retinopathy
　　sickle-cell disorders D57. ☑ *[H36]*
　of prematurity H35.10 ☑
　　stage 0 H35.11 ☑
　　stage 1 H35.12 ☑
　　stage 2 H35.13 ☑
　　stage 3 H35.14 ☑
　　stage 4 H35.15 ☑
　　stage 5 H35.16 ☑
　pigmentary, congenital — *see* Dystrophy, retina
　proliferative NEC H35.2 ☑
　　diabetic — *see* Diabetes, retinopathy, proliferative
　　sickle-cell D57. ☑ *[H36]*
　solar H31.02 ☑
Retinoschisis H33.10 ☑
　congenital Q14.1
　specified type NEC H33.19 ☑
Retortamoniasis A07.8
Retractile testis Q55.22
Retraction
　cervix — *see* Retroversion, uterus
　drum (membrane) — *see* Disorder, tympanic membrane, specified NEC
　finger — *see* Deformity, finger
　lid H02.539
　　left H02.536
　　　lower H02.535
　　　upper H02.534
　　right H02.533
　　　lower H02.532
　　　upper H02.531

Retraction — *continued*
　lung J98.4
　mediastinum J98.59
　nipple N64.53
　　associated with
　　　lactation O92.03
　　　pregnancy O92.01 ☑
　　　puerperium O92.02
　　congenital Q83.8
　palmar fascia M72.0
　pleura — *see* Pleurisy
　ring, uterus (Bandl's) (pathological) O62.4
　sternum (congenital) Q76.7
　　acquired M95.4
　uterus — *see* Retroversion, uterus
　valve (heart) — *see* Endocarditis
Retrobulbar — *see* condition
Retrocecal — *see* condition
Retrocession — *see* Retroversion
Retrodisplacement — *see* Retroversion
Retroflection, retroflexion — *see* Retroversion
Retrognathia, retrognathism (mandibular) (maxillary) M26.19
Retrograde menstruation N92.5
Retroperineal — *see* condition
Retroperitoneal — *see* condition
Retroperitonitis K68.9
Retropharyngeal — *see* condition
Retroplacental — *see* condition
Retroposition — *see* Retroversion
Retroprosthetic membrane T85.398 ☑
Retrosternal thyroid (congenital) Q89.2
Retroversion, retroverted
　cervix — *see* Retroversion, uterus
　female NEC — *see* Retroversion, uterus
　iris H21.89
　testis (congenital) Q55.29
　uterus (acquired) (acute) (any degree) (asymptomatic) (cervix) (postinfectional) (postpartal, old) N85.4
　　congenital Q51.818
　　in pregnancy O34.53 ☑
Retrovirus, as cause of disease classified elsewhere B97.30
　human
　　immunodeficiency, type 2 (HIV 2) B97.35
　　T-cell lymphotropic
　　　type I (HTLV-I) B97.33
　　　type II (HTLV-II) B97.34
　lentivirus B97.31
　oncovirus B97.32
　specified NEC B97.39
Retrusion, premaxilla (developmental) M26.09
Rett's disease or syndrome F84.2
Reverse peristalsis R19.2
Reye's syndrome G93.7
Rh (factor)
　hemolytic disease (newborn) P55.0
　incompatibility, immunization or sensitization
　　affecting management of pregnancy NEC O36.09 ☑
　　　anti-D antibody O36.01 ☑
　　newborn P55.0
　　transfusion reaction — *see* Complication (s), transfusion, incompatibility reaction, Rh (factor)
　negative mother affecting newborn P55.0
　titer elevated — *see* Complication (s), transfusion, incompatibility reaction, Rh (factor)
　transfusion reaction — *see* Complication (s), transfusion, incompatibility reaction, Rh (factor)
Rhabdomyolysis (idiopathic) NEC M62.82
　traumatic T79.6 ☑
Rhabdomyoma (*see also* Neoplasm, connective tissue, benign)
　adult — *see* Neoplasm, connective tissue, benign
　fetal — *see* Neoplasm, connective tissue, benign
　glycogenic — *see* Neoplasm, connective tissue, benign
Rhabdomyosarcoma (any type) — *see* Neoplasm, connective tissue, malignant
Rhabdosarcoma — *see* Rhabdomyosarcoma
Rhesus (factor) incompatibility — *see* Rh, incompatibility
Rheumatic (acute) (subacute) (chronic)
　adherent pericardium I09.2
　coronary arteritis I01.9
　degeneration, myocardium I09.0
　fever (acute) — *see* Fever, rheumatic
　heart — *see* Disease, heart, rheumatic

☑ **Additional character required**

Rheumatic — *continued*
  myocardial degeneration — *see* Degeneration,
    myocardium
  myocarditis (chronic) (inactive) (with
    chorea) I09.0
    active or acute I01.2
    with chorea (acute) (rheumatic)
      (Sydenham's) I02.0
  pancarditis, acute I01.8
    with chorea (acute (rheumatic)
      Sydenham's) I02.0
  pericarditis (active) (acute) (with effusion) (with
    pneumonia) I01.0
    with chorea (acute) (rheumatic)
      (Sydenham's) I02.0
    chronic or inactive I09.2
  pneumonia I00 [J17]
  torticollis M43.6
  typhoid fever A01.09
Rheumatism (articular) (neuralgic) (nonarticular)
  M79.0
  gout — *see* Arthritis, rheumatoid
  intercostal, meaning Tietze's disease M94.0
  palindromic (any site) M12.30
    ankle M12.37 ☑
    elbow M12.32 ☑
    foot joint M12.37 ☑
    hand joint M12.34 ☑
    hip M12.35 ☑
    knee M12.36 ☑
    multiple site M12.39
    shoulder M12.31 ☑
    specified joint NEC M12.38
    vertebrae M12.38
    wrist M12.33 ☑
  sciatic M54.4 ☑
Rheumatoid (*see also* condition)
  arthritis (*see also* Arthritis, rheumatoid)
    with involvement of organs NEC M05.60
      ankle M05.67 ☑
      elbow M05.62 ☑
      foot joint M05.67 ☑
      hand joint M05.64 ☑
      hip M05.65 ☑
      knee M05.66 ☑
      multiple site M05.69
      shoulder M05.61 ☑
      vertebra — *see* Spondylitis, ankylosing
      wrist M05.63 ☑
    seronegative — *see* Arthritis, rheumatoid,
      seronegative
    seropositive — *see* Arthritis, rheumatoid,
      seropositive
  carditis M05.30
    ankle M05.37 ☑
    elbow M05.32 ☑
    foot joint M05.37 ☑
    hand joint M05.34 ☑
    hip M05.35 ☑
    knee M05.36 ☑
    multiple site M05.39
    shoulder M05.31 ☑
    vertebra — *see* Spondylitis, ankylosing
    wrist M05.33 ☑
  endocarditis — *see* Rheumatoid, carditis
  lung (disease) M05.10
    ankle M05.17 ☑
    elbow M05.12 ☑
    foot joint M05.17 ☑
    hand joint M05.14 ☑
    hip M05.15 ☑
    knee M05.16 ☑
    multiple site M05.19
    shoulder M05.11 ☑
    vertebra — *see* Spondylitis, ankylosing
    wrist M05.13 ☑
  myocarditis — *see* Rheumatoid, carditis
  myopathy M05.40
    ankle M05.47 ☑
    elbow M05.42 ☑
    foot joint M05.47 ☑
    hand joint M05.44 ☑
    hip M05.45 ☑
    knee M05.46 ☑
    multiple site M05.49
    shoulder M05.41 ☑
    vertebra — *see* Spondylitis, ankylosing
    wrist M05.43 ☑
  pericarditis — *see* Rheumatoid, carditis
  polyarthritis — *see* Arthritis, rheumatoid
  polyneuropathy M05.50
    ankle M05.57 ☑

Rheumatoid — *continued*
  polyneuropathy — *continued*
    elbow M05.52 ☑
    foot joint M05.57 ☑
    hand joint M05.54 ☑
    hip M05.55 ☑
    knee M05.56 ☑
    multiple site M05.59
    shoulder M05.51 ☑
    vertebra — *see* Spondylitis, ankylosing
    wrist M05.53 ☑
  vasculitis M05.20
    ankle M05.27 ☑
    elbow M05.22 ☑
    foot joint M05.27 ☑
    hand joint M05.24 ☑
    hip M05.25 ☑
    knee M05.26 ☑
    multiple site M05.29
    shoulder M05.21 ☑
    vertebra — *see* Spondylitis, ankylosing
    wrist M05.23 ☑
Rhinitis (atrophic) (catarrhal) (chronic) (croupous)
  (fibrinous) (granulomatous) (hyperplastic)
  (hypertrophic) (membranous) (obstructive)
  (purulent) (suppurative) (ulcerative) J31.0
  with
    sore throat — *see* Nasopharyngitis
  acute J00
  allergic J30.9
    with asthma J45.909
      with
        exacerbation (acute) J45.901
        status asthmaticus J45.902
    due to
      food J30.5
      pollen J30.1
    nonseasonal J30.89
    perennial J30.89
    seasonal NEC J30.2
    specified NEC J30.89
  infective J00
  pneumococcal J00
  syphilitic A52.73
    congenital A50.05 [J99]
  tuberculous A15.8
  vasomotor J30.0
Rhinoantritis (chronic) — *see* Sinusitis, maxillary
Rhinodacryolith — *see* Dacryolith
Rhinolith (nasal sinus) J34.89
Rhinomegaly J34.89
Rhinopharyngitis (acute) (subacute) (*see also*
  Nasopharyngitis)
  chronic J31.1
  destructive ulcerating A66.5
  mutilans A66.5
Rhinophyma L71.1
Rhinorrhea J34.89
  cerebrospinal (fluid) G96.0
  paroxysmal — *see* Rhinitis, allergic
  spasmodic — *see* Rhinitis, allergic
Rhinosalpingitis — *see* Salpingitis, eustachian
Rhinoscleroma A48.8
Rhinosporidiosis B48.1
Rhinovirus infection NEC B34.8
Rhizomelic chondrodysplasia punctata E71.540
Rhythm
  atrioventricular nodal I49.8
  disorder I49.9
    coronary sinus I49.8
    ectopic I49.8
    nodal I49.8
  escape I49.9
  heart, abnormal I49.9
  idioventricular I44.2
  nodal I49.8
  sleep, inversion G47.2 ☑
    nonorganic origin — *see* Disorder, sleep,
      circadian rhythm, psychogenic
Rhytidosis facialis L98.8
Rib (*see also* condition)
  cervical Q76.5
Riboflavin deficiency E53.0
Rice bodies (*see also* Loose, body, joint)
  knee M23.4 ☑
Richter syndrome — *see* Leukemia, chronic
  lymphocytic, B-cell type
Richter's hernia — *see* Hernia, abdomen, with
  obstruction
Ricinism — *see* Poisoning, food, noxious, plant
Rickets (active) (acute) (adolescent) (chest wall)
  (congenital) (current) (infantile) (intestinal) E55.0

Rickets — *continued*
  adult — *see* Osteomalacia
  celiac K90.0
  hypophosphatemic with nephrotic-glycosuric
    dwarfism E72.09
  inactive E64.3
  kidney N25.0
  renal N25.0
  sequelae, any E64.3
  vitamin-D-resistant E83.31 [M90.80]
Rickettsial disease A79.9
  specified type NEC A79.89
Rickettsialpox (Rickettsia akari) A79.1
Rickettsiosis A79.9
  due to
    Ehrlichia sennetsu A79.81
    Rickettsia akari (rickettsialpox) A79.1
  specified type NEC A79.89
  tick-borne A77.9
  vesicular A79.1
Rider's bone — *see* Ossification, muscle, specified
  NEC
Ridge, alveolus (*see also* condition)
  flabby K06.8
Ridged ear, congenital Q17.3
Riedel's
  lobe, liver Q44.7
  struma, thyroiditis or disease E06.5
Rieger's anomaly or syndrome Q13.81
Riehl's melanosis L81.4
Rietti-Greppi-Micheli anemia D56.9
Rieux's hernia — *see* Hernia, abdomen, specified
  site NEC
Riga (-Fede) disease K14.0
Riggs' disease — *see* Periodontitis
Right aortic arch Q25.47
Right middle lobe syndrome J98.11
Rigid, rigidity (*see also* condition)
  abdominal R19.30
    with severe abdominal pain R10.0
    epigastric R19.36
    generalized R19.37
    left lower quadrant R19.34
    left upper quadrant R19.32
    periumbilic R19.35
    right lower quadrant R19.33
    right upper quadrant R19.31
  articular, multiple, congenital Q68.8
  cervix (uteri) in pregnancy — *see* Pregnancy,
    complicated by, abnormal, cervix
  hymen (acquired) (congenital) N89.6
  nuchal R29.1
  pelvic floor in pregnancy — *see* Pregnancy,
    complicated by, abnormal, pelvic organs or
    tissues NEC
  perineum or vulva in pregnancy — *see*
    Pregnancy, complicated by, abnormal, vulva
  spine — *see* Dorsopathy, specified NEC
  vagina in pregnancy — *see* Pregnancy,
    complicated by, abnormal, vagina
Rigors R68.89
  with fever R50.9
Riley-Day syndrome G90.1
RIND (reversible ischemic neurologic deficit) I63.9
Ring (s)
  aorta (vascular) Q25.45
  Bandl's O62.4
  contraction, complicating delivery O62.4
  esophageal, lower (muscular) K22.2
  Fleischer's (cornea) H18.04 ☑
  hymenal, tight (acquired) (congenital) N89.6
  Kayser-Fleischer (cornea) H18.04 ☑
  retraction, uterus, pathological O62.4
  Schatzki's (esophagus) (lower) K22.2
    congenital Q39.3
  Soemmerring's — *see* Cataract, secondary
  vascular (congenital) Q25.8
    aorta Q25.45
Ringed hair (congenital) Q84.1
Ringworm B35.9
  beard B35.0
  black dot B35.0
  body B35.4
  Burmese B35.5
  corporeal B35.4
  foot B35.3
  groin B35.6
  hand B35.2
  honeycomb B35.0
  nails B35.1
  perianal (area) B35.6
  scalp B35.0

☑ **Additional character required**

Ringworm - Rupture

Ringworm — *continued*
  specified NEC B35.8
  Tokelau B35.5
Rise, venous pressure I87.8
Rising, PSA following treatment for malignant neoplasm of prostate R97.21
Risk
  for
    dental caries Z91.849
      high Z91.843
      low Z91.841
      moderate Z91.842
    suicidal
      meaning personal history of attempted suicide Z91.5
      meaning suicidal ideation — *see* Ideation, suicidal
Ritter's disease L00
Rivalry, sibling Z62.891
Rivalta's disease A42.2
River blindness B73.01
Robert's pelvis Q74.2
  with disproportion (fetopelvic) O33.0
    causing obstructed labor O65.0
Robin (-Pierre) syndrome Q87.0
Robinow-Silvermann-Smith syndrome Q87.1
Robinson's (hidrotic) ectodermal dysplasia or syndrome Q82.4
Robles' disease B73.01
Rocky Mountain (spotted) fever A77.0
Roetheln — *see* Rubella
Roger's disease Q21.0
Rokitansky-Aschoff sinuses (gallbladder) K82.8
Rolando's fracture (displaced) S62.22 ☑
  nondisplaced S62.22 ☑
Romano-Ward (prolonged QT interval) syndrome I45.81
Romberg's disease or syndrome G51.8
Roof, mouth — *see* condition
Rosacea L71.9
  acne L71.9
  keratitis L71.8
  specified NEC L71.8
Rosary, rachitic E55.0
Rose
  cold J30.1
  fever J30.1
  rash R21
    epidemic B06.9
Rosenbach's erysipeloid A26.0
Rosenthal's disease or syndrome D68.1
Roseola B09
  infantum B08.20
    due to human herpesvirus 6 B08.21
    due to human herpesvirus 7 B08.22
Rossbach's disease K31.89
  psychogenic F45.8
Ross River disease or fever B33.1
Rostan's asthma (cardiac) — *see* Failure, ventricular, left
Rotation
  anomalous, incomplete or insufficient, intestine Q43.3
  cecum (congenital) Q43.3
  colon (congenital) Q43.3
  spine, incomplete or insufficient — *see* Dorsopathy, deforming, specified NEC
  tooth, teeth, fully erupted M26.35
  vertebra, incomplete or insufficient — *see* Dorsopathy, deforming, specified NEC
Rotes Quérol disease or syndrome — *see* Hyperostosis, ankylosing
Roth (-Bernhardt) disease or syndrome — *see* Meralgia paraesthetica
Rothmund (-Thomson) syndrome Q82.8
Rotor's disease or syndrome E80.6
Round
  back (with wedging of vertebrae) — *see* Kyphosis
    sequelae (late effect) of rickets E64.3
  worms (large) (infestation) NEC B82.0
    Ascariasis (*see also* Ascariasis) B77.9
Roussy-Lévy syndrome G60.0
Rubella (German measles) B06.9
  complication NEC B06.09
    neurological B06.00
  congenital P35.0
  contact Z20.4
  exposure to Z20.4
  maternal
    manifest rubella in infant P35.0
    care for (suspected) damage to fetus O35.3 ☑

Rubella — *continued*
  maternal — *continued*
    suspected damage to fetus affecting management of pregnancy O35.3 ☑
    specified complications NEC B06.89
Rubeola (meaning measles) — *see* Measles
  meaning rubella — *see* Rubella
Rubeosis, iris — *see* Disorder, iris, vascular
Rubinstein-Taybi syndrome Q87.2
Rudimentary (congenital) (*see also* Agenesis)
  arm — *see* Defect, reduction, upper limb
  bone Q79.9
  cervix uteri Q51.828
  eye Q11.2
  lobule of ear Q17.3
  patella Q74.1
  respiratory organs in thoracopagus Q89.4
  tracheal bronchus Q32.4
  uterus Q51.818
    in male Q56.1
  vagina Q52.0
Ruled out condition — *see* Observation, suspected
Rumination R11.10
  with nausea R11.2
  disorder of infancy F98.21
  neurotic F42.8
  newborn P92.1
  obsessional F42.8
  psychogenic F42.8
Runeberg's disease D51.0
Runny nose R09.89
Rupia (syphilitic) A51.39
  congenital A50.06
  tertiary A52.79
Rupture, ruptured
  abscess (spontaneous) - code by site under Abscess
  aneurysm — *see* Aneurysm
  anus (sphincter) — *see* Laceration, anus
  aorta, aortic I71.8
    abdominal I71.3
    arch I71.1
    ascending I71.1
    descending I71.8
      abdominal I71.3
      thoracic I71.1
    syphilitic A52.01
    thoracoabdominal I71.5
    thorax, thoracic I71.1
    transverse I71.1
    traumatic — *see* Injury, aorta, laceration, major
    valve or cusp (*see also* Endocarditis, aortic) I35.8
  appendix (with peritonitis) K35.2
    with localized peritonitis K35.3
  arteriovenous fistula, brain I60.8
  artery I77.2
    brain — *see* Hemorrhage, intracranial, intracerebral
    coronary — *see* Infarct, myocardium
    heart — *see* Infarct, myocardium
    pulmonary I28.8
    traumatic (complication) — *see* Injury, blood vessel
  bile duct (common) (hepatic) K83.2
    cystic K82.2
  bladder (sphincter) (nontraumatic) (spontaneous) N32.89
    following ectopic or molar pregnancy O08.6
    obstetrical trauma O71.5
    traumatic S37.29 ☑
  blood vessel (*see also* Hemorrhage)
    brain — *see* Hemorrhage, intracranial, intracerebral
    heart — *see* Infarct, myocardium
    traumatic (complication) — *see* Injury, blood vessel, laceration, major, by site
  bone — *see* Fracture
  bowel (nontraumatic) K63.1
  brain
    aneurysm (congenital) (*see also* Hemorrhage, intracranial, subarachnoid)
      syphilitic A52.05
    hemorrhagic — *see* Hemorrhage, intracranial, intracerebral
  capillaries I78.8
  cardiac (auricle) (ventricle) (wall) I23.3
    with hemopericardium I23.0
    infectional I40.9
    traumatic — *see* Injury, heart
  cartilage (articular) (current) (*see also* Sprain)
    knee S83.3 ☑
    semilunar — *see* Tear, meniscus

Rupture — *continued*
  cecum (with peritonitis) K65.0
    with peritoneal abscess K35.3
    traumatic S36.598 ☑
  celiac artery, traumatic — *see* Injury, blood vessel, celiac artery, laceration, major
  cerebral aneurysm (congenital) (*see* Hemorrhage, intracranial, subarachnoid)
  cervix (uteri)
    with ectopic or molar pregnancy O08.6
    following ectopic or molar pregnancy O08.6
    obstetrical trauma O71.3
    traumatic S37.69 ☑
  chordae tendineae NEC I51.1
    concurrent with acute myocardial infarction — *see* Infarct, myocardium
    following acute myocardial infarction (current complication) I23.4
  choroid (direct) (indirect) (traumatic) H31.32 ☑
  circle of Willis I60.6
  colon (nontraumatic) K63.1
    traumatic — *see* Injury, intestine, large
  cornea (traumatic) — *see* Injury, eye, laceration
  coronary (artery) (thrombotic) — *see* Infarct, myocardium
  corpus luteum (infected) (ovary) N83.1 ☑
  cyst — *see* Cyst
  cystic duct K82.2
  Descemet's membrane — *see* Change, corneal membrane, Descemet's, rupture
    traumatic — *see* Injury, eye, laceration
  diaphragm, traumatic — *see* Injury, intrathoracic, diaphragm
  disc — *see* Rupture, intervertebral disc
  diverticulum (intestine) K57.80
    with bleeding K57.81
    bladder N32.3
    large intestine K57.20
      with
        bleeding K57.21
        small intestine K57.40
          with bleeding K57.41
      small intestine K57.00
      with
        bleeding K57.01
        large intestine K57.40
          with bleeding K57.41
  duodenal stump K31.89
  ear drum (nontraumatic) (*see also* Perforation, tympanum)
    traumatic S09.2 ☑
    due to blast injury — *see* Injury, blast, ear
  esophagus K22.3
  eye (without prolapse or loss of intraocular tissue) — *see* Injury, eye, laceration
  fallopian tube NEC (nonobstetric) (nontraumatic) N83.8
    due to pregnancy O00.10 ☑
      with intrauterine pregnancy O00.11 ☑
  fontanel P13.1
  gallbladder K82.2
    traumatic S36.128 ☑
  gastric (*see also* Rupture, stomach)
    vessel K92.2
  globe (eye) (traumatic) — *see* Injury, eye, laceration
  graafian follicle (hematoma) N83.0 ☑
  heart — *see* Rupture, cardiac
  hymen (nontraumatic) (nonintentional) N89.8
  internal organ, traumatic — *see* Injury, by site
  intervertebral disc — *see* Displacement, intervertebral disc
    traumatic — *see* Rupture, traumatic, intervertebral disc
  intestine NEC (nontraumatic) K63.1
    traumatic — *see* Injury, intestine
  iris (*see also* Abnormality, pupillary)
    traumatic — *see* Injury, eye, laceration
  joint capsule, traumatic — *see* Sprain
  kidney (traumatic) S37.06 ☑
    birth injury P15.8
    nontraumatic N28.89
  lacrimal duct (traumatic) — *see* Injury, eye, specified site NEC
  lens (cataract) (traumatic) — *see* Cataract, traumatic
  ligament, traumatic — *see* Rupture, traumatic, ligament, by site
  liver S36.116 ☑
    birth injury P15.0
  lymphatic vessel I89.8

☑ **Additional character required**

Rupture

Rupture — *continued*
  marginal sinus (placental) (with hemorrhage)
      — *see* Hemorrhage, antepartum, specified
      cause NEC
  membrana tympani (nontraumatic) — *see*
      Perforation, tympanum
  membranes (spontaneous)
    artificial
      delayed delivery following O75.5
      delayed delivery following — *see* Pregnancy,
        complicated by, premature rupture of
        membranes
  meningeal artery I60.8
  meniscus (knee) (*see also* Tear, meniscus)
    old — *see* Derangement, meniscus
    site other than knee - code as Sprain
  mesenteric artery, traumatic — *see* Injury,
      mesenteric, artery, laceration, major
  mesentery (nontraumatic) K66.8
    traumatic — *see* Injury, intra-abdominal,
      specified, site NEC
  mitral (valve) I34.8
  muscle (traumatic) (*see also* Strain)
    diastasis — *see* Diastasis, muscle
    nontraumatic M62.10
      ankle M62.17 ☑
      foot M62.17 ☑
      forearm M62.13 ☑
      hand M62.14 ☑
      lower leg M62.16 ☑
      pelvic region M62.15 ☑
      shoulder region M62.11 ☑
      specified site NEC M62.18
      thigh M62.15 ☑
      upper arm M62.12 ☑
    traumatic — *see* Strain, by site
  musculotendinous junction NEC, nontraumatic
      — *see* Rupture, tendon, spontaneous
  mycotic aneurysm causing cerebral hemorrhage
      — *see* Hemorrhage, intracranial,
      subarachnoid
  myocardium, myocardial — *see* Rupture, cardiac
    traumatic — *see* Injury, heart
  nontraumatic, meaning hernia — *see* Hernia
  obstructed — *see* Hernia, by site, obstructed
  operation wound — *see* Disruption, wound,
      operation
  ovary, ovarian N83.8
    corpus luteum cyst N83.1 ☑
    follicle (graafian) N83.0 ☑
  oviduct (nonobstetric) (nontraumatic) N83.8
    due to pregnancy O00.10 ☑
      with intrauterine pregnancy O00.11 ☑
  pancreas (nontraumatic) K86.89
    traumatic S36.299 ☑
  papillary muscle NEC I51.2
    following acute myocardial infarction (current
      complication) I23.5
  pelvic
    floor, complicating delivery O70.1
    organ NEC, obstetrical trauma O71.5
  perineum (nonobstetric) (nontraumatic) N90.89
    complicating delivery — *see* Delivery,
      complicated, by, laceration, anus
      (sphincter)
  postoperative wound — *see* Disruption, wound,
      operation
  prostate (traumatic) S37.828 ☑
  pulmonary
    artery I28.8
    valve (heart) I37.8
    vein I28.8
    vessel I28.8
  pus tube — *see* Salpingitis
  pyosalpinx — *see* Salpingitis
  rectum (nontraumatic) K63.1
    traumatic S36.69 ☑
  retina, retinal (traumatic) (without detachment)
      (*see also* Break, retina)
    with detachment — *see* Detachment, retina,
      with retinal, break
  rotator cuff (nontraumatic) M75.10 ☑
    complete M75.12 ☑
    incomplete M75.11 ☑
  sclera — *see* Injury, eye, laceration
  sigmoid (nontraumatic) K63.1
    traumatic S36.593 ☑
  spinal cord (*see also* Injury, spinal cord, by region)
    due to injury at birth P11.5
    newborn (birth injury) P11.5
  spleen (traumatic) S36.09 ☑
    birth injury P15.1

Rupture — *continued*
  spleen — *continued*
    congenital (birth injury) P15.1
    due to P. vivax malaria B51.0
    nontraumatic D73.5
    spontaneous D73.5
  splenic vein R58
    traumatic — *see* Injury, blood vessel, splenic
      vein
  stomach (nontraumatic) (spontaneous) K31.89
    traumatic S36.39 ☑
  supraspinatus (complete) (incomplete)
      (nontraumatic) — *see* Tear, rotator cuff
  symphysis pubis
    obstetric O71.6
    traumatic S33.4 ☑
  synovium (cyst) M66.10
    ankle M66.17 ☑
    elbow M66.12 ☑
    finger M66.14 ☑
    foot M66.17 ☑
    forearm M66.13 ☑
    hand M66.14 ☑
    pelvic region M66.15 ☑
    shoulder region M66.11 ☑
    specified site NEC M66.18
    thigh M66.15 ☑
    toe M66.17 ☑
    upper arm M66.12 ☑
    wrist M66.13 ☑
  tendon (traumatic) — *see* Strain
    nontraumatic (spontaneous) M66.9
      ankle M66.87 ☑
      extensor M66.20
        ankle M66.27 ☑
        foot M66.27 ☑
        forearm M66.23 ☑
        hand M66.24 ☑
        lower leg M66.26 ☑
        multiple sites M66.29
        pelvic region M66.25 ☑
        shoulder region M66.21 ☑
        specified site NEC M66.28
        thigh M66.25 ☑
        upper arm M66.22 ☑
      flexor M66.30
        ankle M66.37 ☑
        foot M66.37 ☑
        forearm M66.33 ☑
        hand M66.34 ☑
        lower leg M66.36 ☑
        multiple sites M66.39
        pelvic region M66.35 ☑
        shoulder region M66.31 ☑
        specified site NEC M66.38
        thigh M66.35 ☑
        upper arm M66.32 ☑
      foot M66.87 ☑
      forearm M66.83 ☑
      hand M66.84 ☑
      lower leg M66.86 ☑
      multiple sites M66.89
      pelvic region M66.85 ☑
      shoulder region M66.81 ☑
      specified
        site NEC M66.88
        tendon M66.80
      thigh M66.85 ☑
      upper arm M66.82 ☑
  thoracic duct I89.8
  tonsil J35.8
  traumatic
    aorta — *see* Injury, aorta, laceration, major
    diaphragm — *see* Injury, intrathoracic,
      diaphragm
    external site — *see* Wound, open, by site
    eye — *see* Injury, eye, laceration
    internal organ — *see* Injury, by site
    intervertebral disc
      cervical S13.0 ☑
      lumbar S33.0 ☑
      thoracic S23.0 ☑
    kidney S37.06 ☑
    ligament (*see also* Sprain)
      ankle — *see* Sprain, ankle
      carpus — *see* Rupture, traumatic, ligament,
        wrist
      collateral (hand) — *see* Rupture, traumatic,
        ligament, finger, collateral
      finger (metacarpophalangeal)
        (interphalangeal) S63.40 ☑
        collateral S63.41 ☑

Rupture — *continued*
  traumatic — *continued*
        index S63.41 ☑
        little S63.41 ☑
        middle S63.41 ☑
        ring S63.41 ☑
      index S63.40 ☑
      little S63.40 ☑
      middle S63.40 ☑
      palmar S63.42 ☑
        index S63.42 ☑
        little S63.42 ☑
        middle S63.42 ☑
        ring S63.42 ☑
      ring S63.40 ☑
      specified site NEC S63.499 ☑
        index S63.49 ☑
        little S63.49 ☑
        middle S63.49 ☑
        ring S63.49 ☑
      volar plate S63.43 ☑
        index S63.43 ☑
        little S63.43 ☑
        middle S63.43 ☑
        ring S63.43 ☑
    foot — *see* Sprain, foot
    radial collateral S53.2 ☑
    radiocarpal — *see* Rupture, traumatic,
      ligament, wrist, radiocarpal
    ulnar collateral S53.3 ☑
    ulnocarpal — *see* Rupture, traumatic,
      ligament, wrist, ulnocarpal
    wrist S63.30 ☑
      collateral S63.31 ☑
      radiocarpal S63.32 ☑
      specified site NEC S63.39 ☑
      ulnocarpal (palmar) S63.33 ☑
    liver S36.116 ☑
    membrana tympani — *see* Rupture, ear drum,
      traumatic
    muscle or tendon — *see* Strain
    myocardium — *see* Injury, heart
    pancreas S36.299 ☑
    rectum S36.69 ☑
    sigmoid S36.593 ☑
    spleen S36.09 ☑
    stomach S36.39 ☑
    symphysis pubis S33.4 ☑
    tympanum, tympanic (membrane) — *see*
      Rupture, ear drum, traumatic
    ureter S37.19 ☑
    uterus S37.69 ☑
    vagina — *see* Injury, vagina
    vena cava — *see* Injury, vena cava, laceration,
      major
  tricuspid (heart) (valve) I07.8
  tube, tubal (nonobstetric) (nontraumatic) N83.8
    abscess — *see* Salpingitis
    due to pregnancy O00.10 ☑
      with intrauterine pregnancy O00.11 ☑
  tympanum, tympanic (membrane)
      (nontraumatic) (*see also* Perforation,
      tympanic membrane) H72.9 ☑
    traumatic — *see* Rupture, ear drum, traumatic
  umbilical cord, complicating delivery O69.89 ☑
  ureter (traumatic) S37.19 ☑
    nontraumatic N28.89
  urethra (nontraumatic) N36.8
    with ectopic or molar pregnancy O08.6
    following ectopic or molar pregnancy O08.6
    obstetrical trauma O71.5
    traumatic S37.39 ☑
  uterosacral ligament (nonobstetric)
      (nontraumatic) N83.8
  uterus (traumatic) S37.69 ☑
    before labor O71.0 ☑
    during or after labor O71.1
    nonpuerperal, nontraumatic N85.8
    pregnant (during labor) O71.1
      before labor O71.0 ☑
  vagina — *see* Injury, vagina
  valve, valvular (heart) — *see* Endocarditis
  varicose vein — *see* Varix
  varix — *see* Varix
  vena cava R58
    traumatic — *see* Injury, vena cava, laceration, major
  vesical (urinary) N32.89
  vessel (blood) R58
    pulmonary I28.8
    traumatic — *see* Injury, blood vessel
  viscus R19.8
  vulva complicating delivery O70.0

Seizure - Septum

Seizure — *continued*
  partial — *continued*
    simple — *see* Epilepsy, localization-related,
      symptomatic, with simple partial seizures
  petit mal G40.409
    intractable G40.419
      with status epilepticus G40.411
      without status epilepticus G40.419
    not intractable G40.409
      with status epilepticus G40.401
      without status epilepticus G40.409
  post traumatic R56.1
  recurrent G40.909
  specified NEC G40.89
  uncinate — *see* Epilepsy, localization-related,
    symptomatic, with complex partial seizures
Selenium deficiency, dietary E59
Self-damaging behavior (life-style) Z72.89
Self-harm (attempted)
  history (personal) Z91.5
    in family Z81.8
Self-mutilation (attempted)
  history (personal) Z91.5
    in family Z81.8
Self-poisoning
  history (personal) Z91.5
    in family Z81.8
  observation following (alleged) attempt Z03.6
Semicoma R40.1
Seminal vesiculitis N49.0
Seminoma C62.9 ☑
  specified site — *see* Neoplasm, malignant, by site
Senear-Usher disease or syndrome L10.4
Senectus R54
Senescence (without mention of psychosis) R54
Senile, senility (*see also* condition) R41.81
  with
    acute confusional state F05
    mental changes NOS F03 ☑
    psychosis NEC — *see* Psychosis, senile
  asthenia R54
  cervix (atrophic) N88.8
  debility R54
  endometrium (atrophic) N85.8
  fallopian tube (atrophic) — *see* Atrophy, fallopian
    tube
  heart (failure) R54
  ovary (atrophic) — *see* Atrophy, ovary
  premature E34.8
  vagina, vaginitis (atrophic) N95.2
  wart L82.1
Sensation
  burning (skin) R20.8
    tongue K14.6
  loss of R20.8
  prickling (skin) R20.2
  tingling (skin) R20.2
Sense loss
  smell — *see* Disturbance, sensation, smell
  taste — *see* Disturbance, sensation, taste
  touch R20.8
Sensibility disturbance (cortical) (deep) (vibratory)
  R20.9
Sensitive, sensitivity (*see also* Allergy)
  carotid sinus G90.01
  child (excessive) F93.8
  cold, autoimmune D59.1
  dentin K03.89
  gluten (non-celiac) K90.41
  latex Z91.040
  methemoglobin D74.8
  tuberculin, without clinical or radiological
    symptoms R76.11
  visual
    glare H53.71
    impaired contrast H53.72
Sensitiver Beziehungswahn F22
Sensitization, auto-erythrocytic D69.2
Separation
  anxiety, abnormal (of childhood) F93.0
  apophysis, traumatic - code as Fracture, by site
  choroid — *see* Detachment, choroid
  epiphysis, epiphyseal
    nontraumatic (*see also* Osteochondropathy,
      specified type NEC)
      upper femoral — *see* Slipped, epiphysis,
        upper femoral
    traumatic - code as Fracture, by site
  fracture — *see* Fracture
  infundibulum cardiac from right ventricle by a
    partition Q24.3

Separation — *continued*
  joint (traumatic) (current) - code by site under
    Dislocation
  pubic bone, obstetrical trauma O71.6
  retina, retinal — *see* Detachment, retina
  symphysis pubis, obstetrical trauma O71.6
  tracheal ring, incomplete, congenital Q32.1
Sepsis (generalized) (unspecified organism) A41.9
  with
    organ dysfunction (acute) (multiple) R65.20
      with septic shock R65.21
  actinomycotic A42.7
  adrenal hemorrhage syndrome
    (meningococcal) A39.1
  anaerobic A41.4
  Bacillus anthracis A22.7
  Brucella (*see also* Brucellosis) A23.9
  candidal B37.7
  cryptogenic A41.9
  due to device, implant or graft T85.79 ☑
    arterial graft NEC T82.7 ☑
    breast (implant) T85.79 ☑
    catheter NEC T85.79 ☑
      dialysis (renal) T82.7 ☑
        intraperitoneal T85.71 ☑
      infusion NEC T82.7 ☑
        spinal (cranial) (epidural) (intrathecal)
          (spinal) (subarachnoid)
          (subdural) T85.735 ☑
      urethral indwelling T83.511 ☑
      urinary T83.518 ☑
    ectopic or molar pregnancy O08.82
    electronic (electrode) (pulse generator)
      (stimulator)
      bone T84.7 ☑
      cardiac T82.7 ☑
      nervous system T85.738 ☑
        brain T85.731 ☑
        neurostimulator generator T85.734 ☑
        peripheral nerve T85.732 ☑
        spinal cord T85.733 ☑
      urinary T83.590 ☑
    fixation, internal (orthopedic) — *see*
      Complication, fixation device, infection
    gastrointestinal (bile duct)
      (esophagus) T85.79 ☑
      neurostimulator electrode (lead) T85.732 ☑
    genital T83.69 ☑
    heart NEC T82.7 ☑
      valve (prosthesis) T82.6 ☑
        graft T82.7 ☑
    joint prosthesis — *see* Complication, joint
      prosthesis, infection
    ocular (corneal graft) (orbital implant) T85.79 ☑
    orthopedic NEC T84.7 ☑
      fixation device, internal — *see* Complication,
        fixation device, infection
    specified NEC T85.79 ☑
    vascular T82.7 ☑
    ventricular intracranial (communicating)
      shunt T85.730 ☑
  during labor O75.3
  Enterococcus A41.81
  Erysipelothrix (rhusiopathiae) (erysipeloid) A26.7
  Escherichia coli (E. coli) A41.5 ☑
  extraintestinal yersiniosis A28.2
  following
    abortion (subsequent episode) O08.0
      current episode — *see* Abortion
    ectopic or molar pregnancy O08.82
    immunization T88.0 ☑
    infusion, therapeutic injection or transfusion
      NEC T80.29 ☑
  gangrenous A41.9
  gonococcal A54.86
  Gram-negative (organism) A41.5 ☑
    anaerobic A41.4
  Haemophilus influenzae A41.3
  herpesviral B00.7
  intra-abdominal K65.1
  intraocular — *see* Endophthalmitis, purulent
  Listeria monocytogenes A32.7
  localized - code to specific localized infection
    in operation wound T81.4 ☑
    skin — *see* Abscess
  malleus A24.0
  melioidosis A24.1
  meningeal — *see* Meningitis
  meningococcal A39.4
    acute A39.2
    chronic A39.3

Sepsis — *continued*
  MSSA (Methicillin susceptible Staphylococcus
    aureus) A41.01
  newborn P36.9
    due to
      anaerobes NEC P36.5
      Escherichia coli P36.4
      Staphylococcus P36.30
        aureus P36.2
        specified NEC P36.39
      Streptococcus P36.10
        group B P36.0
        specified NEC P36.19
    specified NEC P36.8
  Pasteurella multocida A28.0
  pelvic, puerperal, postpartum, childbirth O85
  postprocedural T81.4 ☑
  pneumococcal A40.3
  puerperal, postpartum, childbirth (pelvic) O85
  Salmonella (arizonae) (cholerae-suis) (enteritidis)
    (typhimurium) A02.1
  severe R65.20
    with septic shock R65.21
  skin, localized — *see* Abscess
  Shigella (*see also* Dysentery, bacillary) A03.9
  specified organism NEC A41.89
  Staphylococcus, staphylococcal A41.2
    aureus (methicillin susceptible) (MSSA) A41.01
      methicillin resistant (MRSA) A41.02
    coagulase-negative A41.1
    specified NEC A41.1
  Streptococcus, streptococcal A40.9
    agalactiae A40.1
    group
      A A40.0
      B A40.1
      D A41.81
    neonatal P36.10
      group B P36.0
      specified NEC P36.19
    pneumoniae A40.3
    pyogenes A40.0
    specified NEC A40.8
  tracheostomy stoma J95.02
  tularemic A21.7
  umbilical, umbilical cord (newborn) — *see* Sepsis,
    newborn
  Yersinia pestis A20.7
Septate — *see* Septum
Septic — *see* condition
  arm — *see* Cellulitis, upper limb
    with lymphangitis — *see* Lymphangitis, acute,
      upper limb
  embolus — *see* Embolism
  finger — *see* Cellulitis, digit
    with lymphangitis — *see* Lymphangitis, acute,
      digit
  foot — *see* Cellulitis, lower limb
    with lymphangitis — *see* Lymphangitis, acute,
      lower limb
  gallbladder (acute) K81.0
  hand — *see* Cellulitis, upper limb
    with lymphangitis — *see* Lymphangitis, acute,
      upper limb
  joint — *see* Arthritis, pyogenic or pyemic
  leg — *see* Cellulitis, lower limb
    with lymphangitis — *see* Lymphangitis, acute,
      lower limb
  nail (*see also* Cellulitis, digit)
    with lymphangitis — *see* Lymphangitis, acute, digit
  sore (*see also* Abscess)
    throat J02.0
      streptococcal J02.0
  spleen (acute) D73.89
  teeth, tooth (pulpal origin) K04.4
  throat — *see* Pharyngitis
  thrombus — *see* Thrombosis
  toe — *see* Cellulitis, digit
    with lymphangitis — *see* Lymphangitis, acute,
      digit
  tonsils, chronic J35.01
    with adenoiditis J35.03
  uterus — *see* Endometritis
Septicemia A41.9
  meaning sepsis — *see* Sepsis
Septum, septate (congenital) (*see also* Anomaly, by
  site)
  anal Q42.3
    with fistula Q42.2
  aqueduct of Sylvius Q03.0
    with spina bifida — *see* Spina bifida, by site,
      with hydrocephalus

☑ **Additional character required**

Septum — *continued*
- uterus (complete) (partial) Q51.2
- vagina Q52.10
  - in pregnancy — *see* Pregnancy, complicated by, abnormal vagina
    - causing obstructed labor O65.5
  - longitudinal Q52.129
    - microperforate
      - left side Q52.124
      - right side Q52.123
    - nonobstruction Q52.120
    - obstructing Q52.129
      - left side Q52.122
      - right side Q52.121
  - transverse Q52.11
Sequelae (of) (*see also* condition)
- abscess, intracranial or intraspinal (conditions in G06) G09
- amputation - code to injury with seventh character S
- burn and corrosion - code to injury with seventh character S
- calcium deficiency E64.8
- cerebrovascular disease — *see* Sequelae, disease, cerebrovascular
- childbirth O94
- contusion - code to injury with seventh character S
- corrosion — *see* Sequelae, burn and corrosion
- crushing injury - code to injury with seventh character S
- disease
  - cerebrovascular I69.90
    - alteration of sensation I69.998
    - aphasia I69.920
    - apraxia I69.990
    - ataxia I69.993
    - cognitive deficits I69.91 ☑
    - disturbance of vision I69.998
    - dysarthria I69.922
    - dysphagia I69.991
    - dysphasia I69.921
    - facial droop I69.992
    - facial weakness I69.992
    - fluency disorder I69.923
    - hemiplegia I69.95 ☑
    - hemorrhage
      - intracerebral — *see* Sequelae, hemorrhage, intracerebral
      - intracranial, nontraumatic NEC — *see* Sequelae, hemorrhage, intracranial, nontraumatic
      - subarachnoid — *see* Sequelae, hemorrhage, subarachnoid
    - language deficit I69.928
    - monoplegia
      - lower limb I69.94 ☑
      - upper limb I69.93 ☑
    - paralytic syndrome I69.96 ☑
    - specified effect NEC I69.998
  - specified type NEC I69.80
    - alteration of sensation I69.898
    - aphasia I69.820
    - apraxia I69.890
    - ataxia I69.893
    - cognitive deficits I69.81 ☑
    - disturbance of vision I69.898
    - dysarthria I69.822
    - dysphagia I69.891
    - dysphasia I69.821
    - facial droop I69.892
    - facial weakness I69.892
    - fluency disorder I69.823
    - hemiplegia I69.85 ☑
    - language deficit I69.828
    - monoplegia
      - lower limb I69.84 ☑
      - upper limb I69.83 ☑
    - paralytic syndrome I69.86 ☑
    - specified effect NEC I69.898
    - speech deficit I69.928
    - speech deficit I69.828
  - stroke NOS — *see* Sequelae, stroke NOS
- dislocation - code to injury with seventh character S
- encephalitis or encephalomyelitis (conditions in G04) G09
  - in infectious disease NEC B94.8
  - viral B94.1
- external cause - code to injury with seventh character S

Sequelae — *continued*
- foreign body entering natural orifice - code to injury with seventh character S
- fracture - code to injury with seventh character S
- frostbite - code to injury with seventh character S
- Hansen's disease B92
- hemorrhage
  - intracerebral I69.10
    - alteration of sensation I69.198
    - aphasia I69.120
    - apraxia I69.190
    - ataxia I69.193
    - cognitive deficits I69.11 ☑
    - disturbance of vision I69.198
    - dysarthria I69.122
    - dysphagia I69.191
    - dysphasia I69.121
    - facial droop I69.192
    - facial weakness I69.192
    - fluency disorder I69.123
    - hemiplegia I69.15 ☑
    - language deficit NEC I69.128
    - monoplegia
      - lower limb I69.14 ☑
      - upper limb I69.13 ☑
    - paralytic syndrome I69.16 ☑
    - specified effect NEC I69.198
    - speech deficit NEC I69.128
  - intracranial, nontraumatic NEC I69.20
    - alteration of sensation I69.298
    - aphasia I69.220
    - apraxia I69.290
    - ataxia I69.293
    - cognitive deficits I69.21 ☑
    - disturbance of vision I69.298
    - dysarthria I69.222
    - dysphagia I69.291
    - dysphasia I69.221
    - facial droop I69.292
    - facial weakness I69.292
    - fluency disorder I69.223
    - hemiplegia I69.25 ☑
    - language deficit NEC I69.228
    - monoplegia
      - lower limb I69.24 ☑
      - upper limb I69.23 ☑
    - paralytic syndrome I69.26 ☑
    - specified effect NEC I69.298
    - speech deficit NEC I69.228
  - subarachnoid I69.00
    - alteration of sensation I69.098
    - aphasia I69.020
    - apraxia I69.090
    - ataxia I69.093
    - cognitive deficits — *see* subcategory I69.01
    - disturbance of vision I69.098
    - dysarthria I69.022
    - dysphagia I69.091
    - dysphasia I69.021
    - facial droop I69.092
    - facial weakness I69.092
    - fluency disorder I69.023
    - hemiplegia I69.05 ☑
    - language deficit NEC I69.028
    - monoplegia
      - lower limb I69.04 ☑
      - upper limb I69.03 ☑
    - paralytic syndrome I69.06 ☑
    - specified effect NEC I69.098
    - speech deficit NEC I69.028
- hepatitis, viral B94.2
- hyperalimentation E68
- infarction
  - cerebral I69.30
    - alteration of sensation I69.398
    - aphasia I69.320
    - apraxia I69.390
    - ataxia I69.393
    - cognitive deficits I69.31 ☑
    - disturbance of vision I69.398
    - dysarthria I69.322
    - dysphagia I69.391
    - dysphasia I69.321
    - facial droop I69.392
    - facial weakness I69.392
    - fluency disorder I69.323
    - hemiplegia I69.35 ☑
    - language deficit NEC I69.328
    - monoplegia
      - lower limb I69.34 ☑
      - upper limb I69.33 ☑

Sequelae — *continued*
- infarction — *continued*
  - paralytic syndrome I69.36 ☑
  - specified effect NEC I69.398
  - speech deficit NEC I69.328
- infection, pyogenic, intracranial or intraspinal G09
- infectious disease B94.9
  - specified NEC B94.8
- injury - code to injury with seventh character S
- leprosy B92
- meningitis
  - bacterial (conditions in G00) G09
  - other or unspecified cause (conditions in G03) G09
- muscle (and tendon) injury - code to injury with seventh character S
- myelitis — *see* Sequelae, encephalitis
- niacin deficiency E64.8
- nutritional deficiency E64.9
  - specified NEC E64.8
- obstetrical condition O94
- parasitic disease B94.9
- phlebitis or thrombophlebitis of intracranial or intraspinal venous sinuses and veins (conditions in G08) G09
- poisoning - code to poisoning with seventh character S
  - nonmedicinal substance — *see* Sequelae, toxic effect, nonmedicinal substance
- poliomyelitis (acute) B91
- pregnancy O94
- protein-energy malnutrition E64.0
- puerperium O94
- rickets E64.3
- selenium deficiency E64.8
- sprain and strain - code to injury with seventh character S
- stroke NOS I69.30
  - alteration in sensation I69.398
  - aphasia I69.320
  - apraxia I69.390
  - ataxia I69.393
  - cognitive deficits I69.31 ☑
  - disturbance of vision I69.398
  - dysarthria I69.322
  - dysphagia I69.391
  - dysphasia I69.321
  - facial droop I69.392
  - facial weakness I69.392
  - hemiplegia I69.35 ☑
  - language deficit NEC I69.328
  - monoplegia
    - lower limb I69.34 ☑
    - upper limb I69.33 ☑
  - paralytic syndrome I69.36 ☑
  - specified effect NEC I69.398
  - speech deficit NEC I69.328
- tendon and muscle injury - code to injury with seventh character S
- thiamine deficiency E64.8
- trachoma B94.0
- tuberculosis B90.9
  - bones and joints B90.2
  - central nervous system B90.0
  - genitourinary B90.1
  - pulmonary (respiratory) B90.9
  - specified organs NEC B90.8
- viral
  - encephalitis B94.1
  - hepatitis B94.2
- vitamin deficiency NEC E64.8
  - A E64.1
  - B E64.8
  - C E64.2
- wound, open - code to injury with seventh character S
Sequestration (*see also* Sequestrum)
- disk — *see* Displacement, intervertebral disk
- lung, congenital Q33.2
Sequestrum
- bone — *see* Osteomyelitis, chronic
- dental M27.2
- jaw bone M27.2
- orbit — *see* Osteomyelitis, orbit
- sinus (accessory) (nasal) — *see* Sinusitis
Sequoiosis lung or pneumonitis J67.8
Serology for syphilis
- doubtful
  - with signs or symptoms - code by site and stage under Syphilis

Serology — *continued*
  doubtful — *continued*
    follow-up of latent syphilis — *see* Syphilis, latent
    negative, with signs or symptoms - code by site and stage under Syphilis
    positive A53.0
      with signs or symptoms - code by site and stage under Syphilis
    reactivated A53.0
Seroma (*see also* Hematoma)
  postprocedural — *see* Complication, postprocedural, seroma
  traumatic, secondary and recurrent T79.2 ☑
Seropurulent — *see* condition
Serositis, multiple K65.8
  pericardial I31.1
  peritoneal K65.8
Serous — *see* condition
Sertoli cell
  adenoma
    specified site — *see* Neoplasm, benign, by site
    unspecified site
      female D27.9
      male D29.20
  carcinoma
    specified site — *see* Neoplasm, malignant, by site
    unspecified site (male) C62.9 ☑
      female C56.9
  tumor
    with lipid storage
      specified site — *see* Neoplasm, benign, by site
      unspecified site
        female D27.9
        male D29.20
    specified site — *see* Neoplasm, benign, by site
    unspecified site
      female D27.9
      male D29.20
Sertoli-Leydig cell tumor — *see* Neoplasm, benign, by site
  specified site — *see* Neoplasm, benign, by site
  unspecified site
    female D27.9
    male D29.20
Serum
  allergy, allergic reaction (*see also* Reaction, serum) T80.69 ☑
    shock (*see also* Shock, anaphylactic) T80.59 ☑
  arthritis (*see also* Reaction, serum) T80.69 ☑
  complication or reaction NEC (*see also* Reaction, serum) T80.69 ☑
  disease NEC (*see also* Reaction, serum) T80.69 ☑
  hepatitis (*see also* Hepatitis, viral, type B)
    carrier (suspected) of B18.1
  intoxication (*see also* Reaction, serum) T80.69 ☑
  neuritis (*see also* Reaction, serum) T80.69 ☑
  neuropathy G61.1
  poisoning NEC (*see also* Reaction, serum) T80.69 ☑
  rash NEC (*see also* Reaction, serum) T80.69 ☑
  reaction NEC (*see also* Reaction, serum) T80.69 ☑
  sickness NEC (*see also* Reaction, serum) T80.69 ☑
  urticaria (*see also* Reaction, serum) T80.69 ☑
Sesamoiditis M25.8 ☑
Sever's disease or osteochondrosis — *see* Osteochondrosis, juvenile, tarsus
Severe sepsis R65.20
  with septic shock R65.21
Sex
  chromosome mosaics Q97.8
    lines with various numbers of X chromosomes Q97.2
  education Z70.8
  reassignment surgery status Z87.890
Sextuplet pregnancy — *see* Pregnancy, sextuplet
Sexual
  function, disorder of (psychogenic) F52.9
  immaturity (female) (male) E30.0
  impotence (psychogenic) organic origin NEC — *see* Dysfunction, sexual, male
  precocity (constitutional) (cryptogenic) (female) (idiopathic) (male) E30.1
Sexuality, pathologic — *see* Deviation, sexual
Sézary disease C84.1 ☑
Shadow, lung R91.8
Shaking palsy or paralysis — *see* Parkinsonism
Shallowness, acetabulum — *see* Derangement, joint, specified type NEC, hip
Shaver's disease J63.1

Sheath (tendon) — *see* condition
Sheathing, retinal vessels H35.01 ☑
Shedding
  nail L60.8
  premature, primary (deciduous) teeth K00.6
Sheehan's disease or syndrome E23.0
Shelf, rectal K62.89
Shell teeth K00.5
Shellshock (current) F43.0
  lasting state — *see* Disorder, post-traumatic stress
Shield kidney Q63.1
Shift
  auditory threshold (temporary) H93.24 ☑
  mediastinal R93.8
Shifting sleep-work schedule (affecting sleep) G47.26
Shiga (-Kruse) dysentery A03.0
Shiga's bacillus A03.0
Shigella (dysentery) — *see* Dysentery, bacillary
Shigellosis A03.9
  Group A A03.0
  Group B A03.1
  Group C A03.2
  Group D A03.3
Shin splints S86.89 ☑
Shingles — *see* Herpes, zoster
Shipyard disease or eye B30.0
Shirodkar suture, in pregnancy — *see* Pregnancy, complicated by, incompetent cervix
Shock R57.9
  with ectopic or molar pregnancy O08.3
  adrenal (cortical) (Addisonian) E27.2
  adverse food reaction (anaphylactic) — *see* Shock, anaphylactic, due to food
  allergic — *see* Shock, anaphylactic
  anaphylactic T78.2 ☑
    chemical — *see* Table of Drugs and Chemicals
    due to drug or medicinal substance
      correct substance properly administered T88.6 ☑
      overdose or wrong substance given or taken (by accident) — *see* Table of Drugs and Chemicals, by drug, poisoning
    due to food (nonpoisonous) T78.00 ☑
      additives T78.06 ☑
      dairy products T78.07 ☑
      eggs T78.08 ☑
      fish T78.03 ☑
        shellfish T78.02 ☑
      fruit T78.04 ☑
      milk T78.07 ☑
      nuts T78.05 ☑
        multiple types T78.05 ☑
        peanuts T78.01 ☑
      peanuts T78.01 ☑
      seeds T78.05 ☑
      specified type NEC T78.09 ☑
      vegetable T78.04 ☑
    following sting (s) — *see* Venom
    immunization T80.52 ☑
    serum T80.59 ☑
      blood and blood products T80.51 ☑
      immunization T80.52 ☑
      specified NEC T80.59 ☑
      vaccination T80.52 ☑
  anaphylactoid — *see* Shock, anaphylactic
  anesthetic
    correct substance properly administered T88.2 ☑
    overdose or wrong substance given or taken — *see* Table of Drugs and Chemicals, by drug, poisoning
    specified anesthetic — *see* Table of Drugs and Chemicals, by drug, poisoning
  cardiogenic R57.0
  chemical substance — *see* Table of Drugs and Chemicals
  complicating ectopic or molar pregnancy O08.3
  culture — *see* Disorder, adjustment
  drug
    due to correct substance properly administered T88.6 ☑
    overdose or wrong substance given or taken (by accident) — *see* Table of Drugs and Chemicals, by drug, poisoning
  during or after labor and delivery O75.1
  electric T75.4 ☑
    (taser) T75.4 ☑
  endotoxic R65.21
    postprocedural (resulting from a procedure, not elsewhere classified) T81.12 ☑

Shock — *continued*
  following
    ectopic or molar pregnancy O08.3
    injury (immediate) (delayed) T79.4 ☑
    labor and delivery O75.1
  food (anaphylactic) — *see* Shock, anaphylactic, due to food
  from electroshock gun (taser) T75.4 ☑
  gram-negative R65.21
    postprocedural (resulting from a procedure, not elsewhere classified) T81.12 ☑
  hematologic R57.8
  hemorrhagic R57.8
    surgery (intraoperative) (postoperative) T81.19 ☑
    trauma T79.4 ☑
  hypovolemic R57.1
    surgical T81.19 ☑
    traumatic T79.4 ☑
  insulin E15
    therapeutic misadventure — *see* subcategory T38.3
  kidney N17.0
    traumatic (following crushing) T79.5 ☑
  liver K72.00
  lightning T75.01 ☑
  lung J80
  obstetric O75.1
    with ectopic or molar pregnancy O08.3
    following ectopic or molar pregnancy O08.3
  pleural (surgical) T81.19 ☑
    due to trauma T79.4 ☑
  postprocedural (postoperative) T81.10 ☑
    with ectopic or molar pregnancy O08.3
    cardiogenic T81.11 ☑
    endotoxic T81.12 ☑
    following ectopic or molar pregnancy O08.3
    gram-negative T81.12 ☑
    hypovolemic T81.19 ☑
    septic T81.12 ☑
    specified type NEC T81.19 ☑
  psychic F43.0
  septic (due to severe sepsis) R65.21
  specified NEC R57.8
  surgical T81.10 ☑
  taser gun (taser) T75.4 ☑
  therapeutic misadventure NEC T81.10 ☑
  thyroxin
    overdose or wrong substance given or taken — *see* Table of Drugs and Chemicals, by drug, poisoning
  toxic, syndrome A48.3
  transfusion — *see* Complications, transfusion
  traumatic (immediate) (delayed) T79.4 ☑
Shoemaker's chest M95.4
Short, shortening, shortness
  arm (acquired) (*see also* Deformity, limb, unequal length)
    congenital Q71.81 ☑
    forearm — *see* Deformity, limb, unequal length
  bowel syndrome K91.2
  breath R06.02
  cervical (complicating pregnancy) O26.87 ☑
    non-gravid uterus N88.3
  common bile duct, congenital Q44.5
  cord (umbilical), complicating delivery O69.3 ☑
  cystic duct, congenital Q44.5
  esophagus (congenital) Q39.8
  femur (acquired) — *see* Deformity, limb, unequal length, femur
    congenital — *see* Defect, reduction, lower limb, longitudinal, femur
  frenum, frenulum, linguae (congenital) Q38.1
  hip (acquired) (*see also* Deformity, limb, unequal length)
    congenital Q65.89
  leg (acquired) (*see also* Deformity, limb, unequal length)
    congenital Q72.81 ☑
    lower leg (*see also* Deformity, limb, unequal length)
  limbed stature, with immunodeficiency D82.2
  lower limb (acquired) (*see also* Deformity, limb, unequal length)
    congenital Q72.81 ☑
  organ or site, congenital NEC — *see* Distortion
  palate, congenital Q38.5
  radius (acquired) (*see also* Deformity, limb, unequal length)
    congenital — *see* Defect, reduction, upper limb, longitudinal, radius
  rib syndrome Q77.2

☑ **Additional character required**

Short — *continued*
- stature (child) (hereditary) (idiopathic) NEC R62.52
  - constitutional E34.3
  - due to endocrine disorder E34.3
  - Laron-type E34.3
- tendon (*see also* Contraction, tendon)
  - with contracture of joint — *see* Contraction, joint
  - Achilles (acquired) M67.0 ☑
    - congenital Q66.89
    - congenital Q79.8
- thigh (acquired) (*see also* Deformity, limb, unequal length, femur)
  - congenital — *see* Defect, reduction, lower limb, longitudinal, femur
- tibialis anterior (tendon) — *see* Contraction, tendon
- umbilical cord
  - complicating delivery O69.3 ☑
- upper limb, congenital — *see* Defect, reduction, upper limb, specified type NEC
- urethra N36.8
- uvula, congenital Q38.5
- vagina (congenital) Q52.4

Shortsightedness — *see* Myopia
Shoshin (acute fulminating beriberi) E51.11
Shoulder — *see* condition
Shovel-shaped incisors K00.2
Shower, thromboembolic — *see* Embolism
Shunt
- arterial-venous (dialysis) Z99.2
- arteriovenous, pulmonary (acquired) I28.0
  - congenital Q25.72
- cerebral ventricle (communicating) in situ Z98.2
- surgical, prosthetic, with complications — *see* Complications, cardiovascular, device or implant
Shutdown, renal N28.9
Shy-Drager syndrome G90.3
Sialadenitis, sialadenosis (any gland) (chronic) (periodic) (suppurative) — *see* Sialoadenitis
Sialectasia K11.8
Sialidosis E77.1
Sialitis, silitis (any gland) (chronic) (suppurative) — *see* Sialoadenitis
Sialoadenitis (any gland) (periodic) (suppurative) K11.20
- acute K11.21
  - recurrent K11.22
- chronic K11.23
Sialoadenopathy K11.9
Sialoangitis — *see* Sialoadenitis
Sialodochitis (fibrinosa) — *see* Sialoadenitis
Sialodocholithiasis K11.5
Sialolithiasis K11.5
Sialometaplasia, necrotizing K11.8
Sialorrhea (*see also* Ptyalism)
- periodic — *see* Sialoadenitis
Sialosis K11.7
Siamese twin Q89.4
Sibling rivalry Z62.891
Sicard's syndrome G52.7
Sicca syndrome M35.00
- with
  - keratoconjunctivitis M35.01
  - lung involvement M35.02
  - myopathy M35.03
  - renal tubulo-interstitial disorders M35.04
  - specified organ involvement NEC M35.09
Sick R69
- or handicapped person in family Z63.79
  - needing care at home Z63.6
- sinus (syndrome) I49.5
Sick-euthyroid syndrome E07.81
Sickle-cell
- anemia — *see* Disease, sickle-cell
- trait D57.3
Sicklemia (*see also* Disease, sickle-cell)
- trait D57.3
Sickness
- air (travel) T75.3 ☑
- airplane T75.3 ☑
- alpine T70.29 ☑
- altitude T70.20 ☑
- Andes T70.29 ☑
- aviator's T70.29 ☑
- balloon T70.29 ☑
- car T75.3 ☑
- compressed air T70.3 ☑
- decompression T70.3 ☑
- green D50.8

Sickness — *continued*
- milk — *see* Poisoning, food, noxious
- motion T75.3 ☑
- mountain T70.29 ☑
  - acute D75.1
- protein (*see also* Reaction, serum) T80.69 ☑
- radiation T66 ☑
- roundabout (motion) T75.3 ☑
- sea T75.3 ☑
- serum NEC (*see also* Reaction, serum) T80.69 ☑
- sleeping (African) B56.9
  - by Trypanosoma B56.9
    - brucei
      - gambiense B56.0
      - rhodesiense B56.1
  - East African B56.1
  - Gambian B56.0
  - Rhodesian B56.1
  - West African B56.0
- swing (motion) T75.3 ☑
- train (railway) (travel) T75.3 ☑
- travel (any vehicle) T75.3 ☑
Sideropenia — *see* Anemia, iron deficiency
Siderosilicosis J62.8
Siderosis (lung) J63.4
- eye (globe) — *see* Disorder, globe, degenerative, siderosis
Siemens' syndrome (ectodermal dysplasia) Q82.8
Sighing R06.89
- psychogenic F45.8
Sigmoid (*see also* condition)
- flexure — *see* condition
- kidney Q63.1
Sigmoiditis (*see also* Enteritis) K52.9
- infectious A09
- noninfectious K52.9
Silfverskiöld's syndrome Q78.9
Silicosiderosis J62.8
Silicosis, silicotic (simple) (complicated) J62.8
- with tuberculosis J65
Silicotuberculosis J65
Silo-fillers' disease J68.8
- bronchitis J68.0
- pneumonitis J68.0
- pulmonary edema J68.1
Silver's syndrome Q87.1
Simian malaria B53.1
Simmonds' cachexia or disease E23.0
Simons' disease or syndrome (progressive lipodystrophy) E88.1
Simple, simplex — *see* condition
Simulation, conscious (of illness) Z76.5
Simultanagnosia (asimultagnosia) R48.3
Sin Nombre virus disease (Hantavirus) (cardio)-pulmonary syndrome B33.4
Sinding-Larsen disease or osteochondrosis — *see* Osteochondrosis, juvenile, patella
Singapore hemorrhagic fever A91
Singer's node or nodule J38.2
Single
- atrium Q21.2
- coronary artery Q24.5
- umbilical artery Q27.0
- ventricle Q20.4
Singultus R06.6
- epidemicus B33.0
Sinus (*see also* Fistula)
- abdominal K63.89
- arrest I45.5
- arrhythmia I49.8
- bradycardia R00.1
- branchial cleft (internal) (external) Q18.0
- coccygeal — *see* Sinus, pilonidal
- dental K04.6
- dermal (congenital) Q06.8
  - with abscess Q06.8
  - coccygeal, pilonidal — *see* Sinus, coccygeal
- infected, skin NEC L08.89
- marginal, ruptured or bleeding — *see* Hemorrhage, antepartum, specified cause NEC
- medial, face and neck Q18.8
- pause I45.5
- pericranii Q01.9
- pilonidal (infected) (rectum) L05.92
  - with abscess L05.02
- preauricular Q18.1
- rectovaginal N82.3
- Rokitansky-Aschoff (gallbladder) K82.8
- sacrococcygeal (dermoid) (infected) — *see* Sinus, pilonidal
- tachycardia R00.0
  - paroxysmal I47.1

Sinus — *continued*
- tarsi syndrome M25.57 ☑
- testis N50.89
- tract (postinfective) — *see* Fistula
- urachus Q64.4
Sinusitis (accessory) (chronic) (hyperplastic) (nasal) (nonpurulent) (purulent) J32.9
- acute J01.90
  - ethmoidal J01.20
    - recurrent J01.21
  - frontal J01.10
    - recurrent J01.11
  - involving more than one sinus, other than pansinusitis J01.80
    - recurrent J01.81
  - maxillary J01.00
    - recurrent J01.01
  - pansinusitis J01.40
    - recurrent J01.41
  - recurrent J01.91
  - specified NEC J01.80
    - recurrent J01.81
  - sphenoidal J01.30
    - recurrent J01.31
- allergic — *see* Rhinitis, allergic
- due to high altitude T70.1 ☑
- ethmoidal J32.2
  - acute J01.20
    - recurrent J01.21
- frontal J32.1
  - acute J01.10
    - recurrent J01.11
- influenzal — *see* Influenza, with, respiratory manifestations NEC
- involving more than one sinus but not pansinusitis J32.8
  - acute J01.80
    - recurrent J01.81
- maxillary J32.0
  - acute J01.00
    - recurrent J01.01
- sphenoidal J32.3
  - acute J01.30
    - recurrent J01.31
- tuberculous, any sinus A15.8
Sinusitis-bronchiectasis-situs inversus (syndrome) (triad) Q89.3
Sipple's syndrome E31.22
Sirenomelia (syndrome) Q87.2
Siriasis T67.0 ☑
Sirkari's disease B55.0
Siti A65
Situation, psychiatric F99
Situational
- disturbance (transient) — *see* Disorder, adjustment
  - acute F43.0
- maladjustment — *see* Disorder, adjustment
- reaction — *see* Disorder, adjustment
  - acute F43.0
Situs inversus or transversus (abdominalis) (thoracis) Q89.3
Sixth disease B08.20
- due to human herpesvirus 6 B08.21
- due to human herpesvirus 7 B08.22
Sjögren-Larsson syndrome Q87.1
Sjögren's syndrome or disease — *see* Sicca syndrome
Skeletal — *see* condition
Skene's gland — *see* condition
Skenitis — *see* Urethritis
Skerljevo A65
Skevas-Zerfus disease — *see* Toxicity, venom, marine animal, sea anemone
Skin (*see also* condition)
- clammy R23.1
- donor — *see* Donor, skin
- hidebound M35.9
Slate-dressers' or slate-miners' lung J62.8
Sleep
- apnea — *see* Apnea, sleep
- deprivation Z72.820
- disorder or disturbance G47.9
  - child F51.9
    - nonorganic origin F51.9
    - specified NEC G47.8
- disturbance G47.9
  - nonorganic origin F51.9
- drunkenness F51.9
- rhythm inversion G47.2 ☑
- terrors F51.4
- walking F51.3
  - hysterical F44.89

Sleep hygiene
    abuse Z72.821
    inadequate Z72.821
    poor Z72.821
Sleeping sickness — *see* Sickness, sleeping
Sleeplessness — *see* Insomnia
    menopausal N95.1
Sleep-wake schedule disorder G47.20
Slim disease (in HIV infection) B20
Slipped, slipping
    epiphysis (traumatic) (*see also*
        Osteochondropathy, specified type NEC)
        capital femoral (traumatic)
            acute (on chronic) S79.01 ☑
        current traumatic - code as Fracture, by site
        upper femoral (nontraumatic) M93.00 ☑
            acute M93.01 ☑
                on chronic M93.03 ☑
            chronic M93.02 ☑
    intervertebral disc — *see* Displacement,
        intervertebral disc
    ligature, umbilical P51.8
    patella — *see* Disorder, patella, derangement NEC
    rib M89.8X8
    sacroiliac joint — *see* subcategory M53.2
    tendon — *see* Disorder, tendon
    ulnar nerve, nontraumatic — *see* Lesion, nerve,
        ulnar
    vertebra NEC — *see* Spondylolisthesis
Slocumb's syndrome E27.0
Sloughing (multiple) (phagedena) (skin) (*see also*
    Gangrene)
    abscess — *see* Abscess
    appendix K38.8
    fascia — *see* Disorder, soft tissue, specified type
        NEC
    scrotum N50.89
    tendon — *see* Disorder, tendon
    transplanted organ — *see* Rejection, transplant
    ulcer — *see* Ulcer, skin
Slow
    feeding, newborn P92.2
    flow syndrome, coronary I20.8
    heart (beat) R00.1
Slowing, urinary stream R39.198
Sluder's neuralgia (syndrome) G44.89
Slurred, slurring speech R47.81
Small (ness)
    for gestational age — *see* Small for dates
    introitus, vagina N89.6
    kidney (unknown cause) N27.9
        bilateral N27.1
        unilateral N27.0
    ovary (congenital) Q50.39
    pelvis
        with disproportion (fetopelvic) O33.1
            causing obstructed labor O65.1
    uterus N85.8
    white kidney N03.9
Small-and-light-for-dates — *see* Small for dates
Small-for-dates (infant) P05.10
    with weight of
        499 grams or less P05.11
        500-749 grams P05.12
        750-999 grams P05.13
        1000-1249 grams P05.14
        1250-1499 grams P05.15
        1500-1749 grams P05.16
        1750-1999 grams P05.17
        2000-2499 grams P05.18
        2500 grams and over P05.19
    specified NEC P05.19
Smallpox B03
Smearing, fecal R15.1
Smith-Lemli-Opitz syndrome E78.72
Smith's fracture S52.54 ☑
Smoker — *see* Dependence, drug, nicotine
Smoker's
    bronchitis J41.0
    cough J41.0
    palate K13.24
    throat J31.2
    tongue K13.24
Smoking
    passive Z77.22
Smothering spells R06.81
Snaggle teeth, tooth M26.39
Snapping
    finger — *see* Trigger finger
    hip — *see* Derangement, joint, specified type
        NEC, hip
        involving the iliotibial band M76.3 ☑

Snapping — *continued*
    knee — *see* Derangement, knee
        involving the iliotibial band M76.3 ☑
Sneddon-Wilkinson disease or syndrome (sub-
    corneal pustular dermatosis) L13.1
Sneezing (intractable) R06.7
Sniffing
    cocaine
        abuse — *see* Abuse, drug, cocaine
        dependence — *see* Dependence, drug, cocaine
    gasoline
        abuse — *see* Abuse, drug, inhalant
        dependence — *see* Dependence, drug, inhalant
    glue (airplane)
        abuse — *see* Abuse, drug, inhalant
        drug dependence — *see* Dependence, drug,
            inhalant
Sniffles
    newborn P28.89
Snoring R06.83
Snow blindness — *see* Photokeratitis
Snuffles (non-syphilitic) R06.5
    newborn P28.89
    syphilitic (infant) A50.05 *[J99]*
Social
    exclusion Z60.4
        due to discrimination or persecution
            (perceived) Z60.5
    migrant Z59.0
        acculturation difficulty Z60.3
    rejection Z60.4
        due to discrimination or persecution Z60.5
    role conflict NEC Z73.5
    skills inadequacy NEC Z73.4
    transplantation Z60.3
Sodoku A25.0
Soemmerring's ring — *see* Cataract, secondary
Soft (*see also* condition)
    nails L60.3
Softening
    bone — *see* Osteomalacia
    brain (necrotic) (progressive) G93.89
        congenital Q04.8
        embolic I63.4 ☑
        hemorrhagic — *see* Hemorrhage, intracranial,
            intracerebral
        occlusive I63.5 ☑
        thrombotic I63.3 ☑
    cartilage M94.2 ☑
        patella M22.4 ☑
    cerebellar — *see* Softening, brain
    cerebral — *see* Softening, brain
    cerebrospinal — *see* Softening, brain
    myocardial, heart — *see* Degeneration,
        myocardial
    spinal cord G95.89
    stomach K31.89
Soldier's
    heart F45.8
    patches I31.0
Solitary
    cyst, kidney N28.1
    kidney, congenital Q60.0
Solvent abuse — *see* Abuse, drug, inhalant
    dependence — *see* Dependence, drug, inhalant
Somatization reaction, somatic reaction — *see*
    Disorder, somatoform
Somnambulism F51.3
    hysterical F44.89
Somnolence R40.0
    nonorganic origin F51.11
Sonne dysentery A03.3
Soor B37.0
Sore
    bed — *see* Ulcer, pressure, by site
    chiclero B55.1
    Delhi B55.1
    desert — *see* Ulcer, skin
    eye H57.1 ☑
    Lahore B55.1
    mouth K13.79
        canker K12.0
    muscle M79.1
    Naga — *see* Ulcer, skin
    of skin — *see* Ulcer, skin
    oriental B55.1
    pressure — *see* Ulcer, pressure, by site
    skin L98.9
    soft A57
    throat (acute) (*see also* Pharyngitis)
        with influenza, flu, or grippe — *see* Influenza,
            with, respiratory manifestations NEC

Sore — *continued*
    throat — *continued*
        chronic J31.2
        coxsackie (virus) B08.5
        diphtheritic A36.0
        herpesviral B00.2
        influenzal — *see* Influenza, with, respiratory
            manifestations NEC
        septic J02.0
        streptococcal (ulcerative) J02.0
        viral NEC J02.8
            coxsackie B08.5
        tropical — *see* Ulcer, skin
        veldt — *see* Ulcer, skin
Soto's syndrome (cerebral gigantism) Q87.3
South African cardiomyopathy syndrome I42.8
Southeast Asian hemorrhagic fever A91
Spacing
    abnormal, tooth, teeth, fully erupted M26.30
    excessive, tooth, fully erupted M26.32
Spade-like hand (congenital) Q68.1
Spading nail L60.8
    congenital Q84.6
Spanish collar N47.1
Sparganosis B70.1
Spasm (s), spastic, spasticity (*see also* condition)
    R25.2
    accommodation — *see* Spasm, of
        accommodation
    ampulla of Vater K83.4
    anus, ani (sphincter) (reflex) K59.4
        psychogenic F45.8
    artery I73.9
        cerebral G45.9
    Bell's G51.3
    bladder (sphincter, external or internal) N32.89
        psychogenic F45.8
    bronchus, bronchiole J98.01
    cardia K22.0
    cardiac I20.1
    carpopedal — *see* Tetany
    cerebral (arteries) (vascular) G45.9
    cervix, complicating delivery O62.4
    ciliary body (of accommodation) — *see* Spasm, of
        accommodation
    colon (*see also* Irritable, bowel) K58.9
        with diarrhea K58.0
        psychogenic F45.8
    common duct K83.8
    compulsive — *see* Tic
    conjugate H51.8
    coronary (artery) I20.1
    diaphragm (reflex) R06.6
        epidemic B33.0
        psychogenic F45.8
    duodenum K59.8
    epidemic diaphragmatic (transient) B33.0
    esophagus (diffuse) K22.4
        psychogenic F45.8
    facial G51.3
    fallopian tube N83.8
    gastrointestinal (tract) K31.89
        psychogenic F45.8
    glottis J38.5
        hysterical F44.4
        psychogenic F45.8
            conversion reaction F44.4
        reflex through recurrent laryngeal nerve J38.5
    habit — *see* Tic
    heart I20.1
    hemifacial (clonic) G51.3
    hourglass — *see* Contraction, hourglass
    hysterical F44.4
    infantile — *see* Epilepsy, spasms
    inferior oblique, eye H51.8
    intestinal (*see also* Syndrome, irritable
        bowel) K58.9
        psychogenic F45.8
    larynx, laryngeal J38.5
        hysterical F44.4
        psychogenic F45.8
            conversion reaction F44.4
    levator palpebrae superioris — *see* Disorder,
        eyelid function
    muscle NEC M62.838
        back M62.830
    nerve, trigeminal G51.0
    nervous F45.8
    nodding F98.4
    occupational F48.8
    oculogyric H51.8
        psychogenic F45.8

☑ **Additional character required**

Sleep - Spasm

ICD-10-CM INDEX TO DISEASES AND INJURIES

Spasm — *continued*
  of accommodation H52.53 ☑
  ophthalmic artery — *see* Occlusion, artery, retina
  perineal, female N94.89
  peroneo-extensor (*see also* Deformity, limb, flat
    foot)
  pharynx (reflex) J39.2
    hysterical F45.8
    psychogenic F45.8
  psychogenic F45.8
  pylorus NEC K31.3
    adult hypertrophic K31.89
    congenital or infantile Q40.0
    psychogenic F45.8
  rectum (sphincter) K59.4
    psychogenic F45.8
  retinal (artery) — *see* Occlusion, artery, retina
  sigmoid (*see also* Syndrome, irritable
    bowel) K58.9
    psychogenic F45.8
  sphincter of Oddi K83.4
  stomach K31.89
    neurotic F45.8
  throat J39.2
    hysterical F45.8
    psychogenic F45.8
  tic F95.9
    chronic F95.1
    transient of childhood F95.0
  tongue K14.8
  torsion (progressive) G24.1
  trigeminal nerve — *see* Neuralgia, trigeminal
  ureter N13.5
  urethra (sphincter) N35.9
  uterus N85.8
    complicating labor O62.4
  vagina N94.2
    psychogenic F52.5
  vascular I73.9
  vasomotor I73.9
  vein NEC I87.8
  viscera — *see* Pain, abdominal
Spasmodic — *see* condition
Spasmophilia — *see* Tetany
Spasmus nutans F98.4
Spastic, spasticity (*see also* Spasm)
  child (cerebral) (congenital) (paralysis) G80.1
Speaker's throat R49.8
Specific, specified — *see* condition
Speech
  defect, disorder, disturbance, impediment R47.9
    psychogenic, in childhood and
      adolescence F98.8
    slurring R47.81
    specified NEC R47.89
Spencer's disease A08.19
Spens' syndrome (syncope with heart block) I45.9
Sperm counts (fertility testing) Z31.41
  postvasectomy Z30.8
    reversal Z31.42
Spermatic cord — *see* condition
Spermatocele N43.40
  congenital Q55.4
  multiple N43.42
  single N43.41
Spermatocystitis N49.0
Spermatocytoma C62.9 ☑
  specified site — *see* Neoplasm, malignant, by site
Spermatorrhea N50.89
Sphacelus — *see* Gangrene
Sphenoidal — *see* condition
Sphenoiditis (chronic) — *see* Sinusitis, sphenoidal
Sphenopalatine ganglion neuralgia G90.09
Sphericity, increased, lens (congenital) Q12.4
Spherocytosis (congenital) (familial) (hereditary)
  D58.0
  hemoglobin disease D58.0
  sickle-cell (disease) D57.8 ☑
Spherophakia Q12.4
Sphincter — *see* condition
Sphincteritis, sphincter of Oddi — *see* Cholangitis
Sphingolipidosis E75.3
  specified NEC E75.29
Sphingomyelinosis E75.3
Spicule tooth K00.2
Spider
  bite — *see* Toxicity, venom, spider
  fingers — *see* Syndrome, Marfan's
  nevus I78.1
  toes — *see* Syndrome, Marfan's
  vascular I78.1

Spiegler-Fendt
  benign lymphocytoma L98.8
  sarcoid L08.89
Spielmeyer-Vogt disease E75.4
Spina bifida (aperta) Q05.9
  with hydrocephalus NEC Q05.4
  cervical Q05.5
    with hydrocephalus Q05.0
  dorsal Q05.6
    with hydrocephalus Q05.1
  lumbar Q05.7
    with hydrocephalus Q05.2
  lumbosacral Q05.7
    with hydrocephalus Q05.2
  occulta Q76.0
  sacral Q05.8
    with hydrocephalus Q05.3
  thoracic Q05.6
    with hydrocephalus Q05.1
  thoracolumbar Q05.6
    with hydrocephalus Q05.1
Spindle, Krukenberg's — *see* Pigmentation, cornea,
  posterior
Spine, spinal — *see* condition
Spiradenoma (eccrine) — *see* Neoplasm, skin,
  benign
Spirillosis A25.0
Spirillum
  minus A25.0
  obermeieri infection A68.0
Spirochetal — *see* condition
Spirochetosis A69.9
  arthritic, arthritica A69.9
  bronchopulmonary A69.8
  icterohemorrhagic A27.0
  lung A69.8
Spirometrosis B70.1
Spitting blood — *see* Hemoptysis
Splanchnoptosis K63.4
Spleen, splenic — *see* condition
Splenectasis — *see* Splenomegaly
Splenitis (interstitial) (malignant) (nonspecific)
  D73.89
  malarial (*see also* Malaria) B54 [D77]
  tuberculous A18.85
Splenocele D73.89
Splenomegaly, splenomegalia (Bengal)
  (cryptogenic) (idiopathic) (tropical) R16.1
  with hepatomegaly R16.2
  cirrhotic D73.2
  congenital Q89.09
  congestive, chronic D73.2
  Egyptian B65.1
  Gaucher's E75.22
  malarial (*see also* Malaria) B54 [D77]
  neutropenic D73.81
  Niemann-Pick — *see* Niemann-Pick disease or
    syndrome
  siderotic D73.2
  syphilitic A52.79
    congenital (early) A50.08 [D77]
Splenopathy D73.9
Splenoptosis D73.89
Splenosis D73.89
Splinter — *see* Foreign body, superficial, by site
Split, splitting
  foot Q72.7 ☑
  hand Q71.6 ☑
  heart sounds R01.2
  lip, congenital — *see* Cleft, lip
  nails L60.3
  urinary stream R39.13
Spondylarthrosis — *see* Spondylosis
Spondylitis (chronic) (*see also* Spondylopathy,
  inflammatory)
  ankylopoietica — *see* Spondylitis, ankylosing
  ankylosing (chronic) M45.9
    with lung involvement M45.9 [J99]
    cervical region M45.2
    cervicothoracic region M45.3
    juvenile M08.1
    lumbar region M45.6
    lumbosacral region M45.7
    multiple sites M45.0
    occipito-atlanto-axial region M45.1
    sacrococcygeal region M45.8
    thoracic region M45.4
    thoracolumbar region M45.5
  atrophic (ligamentous) — *see* Spondylitis,
    ankylosing
  deformans (chronic) — *see* Spondylosis
  gonococcal A54.41

Spondylitis — *continued*
  gouty (*see also* Gout, by type, vertebrae) M10.08
  in (due to)
    brucellosis A23.9 [M49.80]
      cervical region A23.9 [M49.82]
      cervicothoracic region A23.9 [M49.83]
      lumbar region A23.9 [M49.86]
      lumbosacral region A23.9 [M49.87]
      multiple sites A23.9 [M49.89]
      occipito-atlanto-axial region A23.9 [M49.81]
      sacrococcygeal region A23.9 [M49.88]
      thoracic region A23.9 [M49.84]
      thoracolumbar region A23.9 [M49.85]
    enterobacteria (*see also* subcategory
      M49.8) A04.9
    tuberculosis A18.01
  infectious NEC — *see* Spondylopathy, infective
  juvenile ankylosing (chronic) M08.1
  Kümmell's — *see* Spondylopathy, traumatic
  Marie-Strümpell — *see* Spondylitis, ankylosing
  muscularis — *see* Spondylopathy, specified NEC
  psoriatic L40.53
  rheumatoid — *see* Spondylitis, ankylosing
  rhizomelica — *see* Spondylitis, ankylosing
  sacroiliac NEC M46.1
  senescent, senile — *see* Spondylosis
  traumatic (chronic) or post-traumatic — *see*
    Spondylopathy, traumatic
  tuberculous A18.01
  typhosa A01.05
Spondylolisthesis (acquired) (degenerative) M43.10
  with disproportion (fetopelvic) O33.0
    causing obstructed labor O65.0
  cervical region M43.12
  cervicothoracic region M43.13
  congenital Q76.2
  lumbar region M43.16
  lumbosacral region M43.17
  multiple sites M43.19
  occipito-atlanto-axial region M43.11
  sacrococcygeal region M43.18
  thoracic region M43.14
  thoracolumbar region M43.15
  traumatic (old) M43.10
    acute
      fifth cervical (displaced) S12.430 ☑
        nondisplaced S12.431 ☑
        specified type NEC (displaced) S12.450 ☑
          nondisplaced S12.451 ☑
        type III S12.44 ☑
      fourth cervical (displaced) S12.330 ☑
        nondisplaced S12.331 ☑
        specified type NEC (displaced) S12.350 ☑
          nondisplaced S12.351 ☑
        type III S12.34 ☑
      second cervical (displaced) S12.130 ☑
        nondisplaced S12.131 ☑
        specified type NEC (displaced) S12.150 ☑
          nondisplaced S12.151 ☑
        type III S12.14 ☑
      seventh cervical (displaced) S12.630 ☑
        nondisplaced S12.631 ☑
        specified type NEC (displaced) S12.650 ☑
          nondisplaced S12.651 ☑
        type III S12.64 ☑
      sixth cervical (displaced) S12.530 ☑
        nondisplaced S12.531 ☑
        specified type NEC (displaced) S12.550 ☑
          nondisplaced S12.551 ☑
        type III S12.54 ☑
      third cervical (displaced) S12.230 ☑
        nondisplaced S12.231 ☑
        specified type NEC (displaced) S12.250 ☑
          nondisplaced S12.251 ☑
        type III S12.24 ☑
Spondylolysis (acquired) M43.00
  cervical region M43.02
  cervicothoracic region M43.03
  congenital Q76.2
  lumbar region M43.06
  lumbosacral region M43.07
    with disproportion (fetopelvic) O33.0
      causing obstructed labor O65.8
  multiple sites M43.09
  occipito-atlanto-axial region M43.01
  sacrococcygeal region M43.08
  thoracic region M43.04
  thoracolumbar region M43.05
Spondylopathy M48.9
  infective NEC M46.50
    cervical region M46.52
    cervicothoracic region M46.53

Spondylopathy - Sprain

Spondylopathy — *continued*
  infective NEC — *continued*
    lumbar region M46.56
    lumbosacral region M46.57
    multiple sites M46.59
    occipito-atlanto-axial region M46.51
    sacrococcygeal region M46.58
    thoracic region M46.54
    thoracolumbar region M46.55
  inflammatory M46.90
    cervical region M46.92
    cervicothoracic region M46.93
    lumbar region M46.96
    lumbosacral region M46.97
    multiple sites M46.99
    occipito-atlanto-axial region M46.91
    sacrococcygeal region M46.98
    specified type NEC M46.80
      cervical region M46.82
      cervicothoracic region M46.83
      lumbar region M46.86
      lumbosacral region M46.87
      multiple sites M46.89
      occipito-atlanto-axial region M46.81
      sacrococcygeal region M46.88
      thoracic region M46.84
      thoracolumbar region M46.85
    thoracic region M46.94
    thoracolumbar region M46.95
  neuropathic, in
    syringomyelia and syringobulbia G95.0
    tabes dorsalis A52.11
  specified NEC — *see* subcategory M48.8
  traumatic M48.30
    cervical region M48.32
    cervicothoracic region M48.33
    lumbar region M48.36
    lumbosacral region M48.37
    occipito-atlanto-axial region M48.31
    sacrococcygeal region M48.38
    thoracic region M48.34
    thoracolumbar region M48.35
Spondylosis M47.9
  with
    disproportion (fetopelvic) O33.0
      causing obstructed labor O65.0
    myelopathy NEC M47.10
      cervical region M47.12
      cervicothoracic region M47.13
      lumbar region M47.16
      occipito-atlanto-axial region M47.11
      thoracic region M47.14
      thoracolumbar region M47.15
    radiculopathy M47.20
      cervical region M47.22
      cervicothoracic region M47.23
      lumbar region M47.26
      lumbosacral region M47.27
      occipito-atlanto-axial region M47.21
      sacrococcygeal region M47.28
      thoracic region M47.24
      thoracolumbar region M47.25
  specified NEC M47.899
    cervical region M47.892
    cervicothoracic region M47.893
    lumbar region M47.896
    lumbosacral region M47.897
    occipito-atlanto-axial region M47.891
    sacrococcygeal region M47.898
    thoracic region M47.894
    thoracolumbar region M47.895
  traumatic — *see* Spondylopathy, traumatic
  without myelopathy or radiculopathy M47.819
    cervical region M47.812
    cervicothoracic region M47.813
    lumbar region M47.816
    lumbosacral region M47.817
    occipito-atlanto-axial region M47.811
    sacrococcygeal region M47.818
    thoracic region M47.814
    thoracolumbar region M47.815
Sponge
  inadvertently left in operation wound — *see*
    Foreign body, accidentally left during a
    procedure
  kidney (medullary) Q61.5
Sponge-diver's disease — *see* Toxicity, venom,
  marine animal, sea anemone
Spongioblastoma (any type) — *see* Neoplasm,
  malignant, by site
  specified site — *see* Neoplasm, malignant, by site
  unspecified site C71.9

Spongioneuroblastoma — *see* Neoplasm,
  malignant, by site
Spontaneous (*see also* condition)
  fracture (cause unknown) — *see* Fracture,
    pathological
Spoon nail L60.3
  congenital Q84.6
Sporadic — *see* condition
Sporothrix schenckii infection — *see* Sporotrichosis
Sporotrichosis B42.9
  arthritis B42.82
  disseminated B42.7
  generalized B42.7
  lymphocutaneous (fixed) (progressive) B42.1
  pulmonary B42.0
  specified NEC B42.89
Spots, spotting (in) (of)
  Bitot's (*see also* Pigmentation, conjunctiva)
    in the young child E50.1
    vitamin A deficiency E50.1
  café, au lait L81.3
  Cayenne pepper I78.1
  cotton wool, retina — *see* Occlusion, artery, retina
  de Morgan's (senile angiomas) I78.1
  Fuchs' black (myopic) (*see also* Myopia,
    degenerative) H44.2 ☑
  intermenstrual (regular) N92.0
    irregular N92.1
  Koplik's B05.9
  liver L81.4
  pregnancy O26.85 ☑
  purpuric R23.3
  ruby I78.1
Spotted fever — *see* Fever, spotted N92.3
Sprain (joint) (ligament)
  acromioclavicular joint or ligament S43.5 ☑
  ankle S93.40 ☑
    calcaneofibular ligament S93.41 ☑
    deltoid ligament S93.42 ☑
    internal collateral ligament — *see* Sprain, ankle,
      specified ligament NEC
    specified ligament NEC S93.49 ☑
    talofibular ligament — *see* Sprain, ankle,
      specified ligament NEC
    tibiofibular ligament S93.43 ☑
  anterior longitudinal, cervical S13.4 ☑
  atlas, atlanto-axial, atlanto-occipital S13.4 ☑
  breast bone — *see* Sprain, sternum
  calcaneofibular — *see* Sprain, ankle
  carpal — *see* Sprain, wrist
  carpometacarpal — *see* Sprain, hand, specified
    site NEC
  cartilage
    costal S23.41 ☑
    semilunar (knee) — *see* Sprain, knee, specified
      site NEC
      with current tear — *see* Tear, meniscus
    thyroid region S13.5 ☑
    xiphoid — *see* Sprain, sternum
  cervical, cervicodorsal, cervicothoracic S13.4 ☑
  chondrosternal S23.421 ☑
  coracoclavicular S43.8 ☑
  coracohumeral S43.41 ☑
  coronary, knee — *see* Sprain, knee, specified site
    NEC
  costal cartilage S23.41 ☑
  cricoarytenoid articulation or ligament S13.5 ☑
  cricothyroid articulation S13.5 ☑
  cruciate, knee — *see* Sprain, knee, cruciate
  deltoid, ankle — *see* Sprain, ankle
  dorsal (spine) S23.3 ☑
  elbow S53.40 ☑
    radial collateral ligament S53.43 ☑
    radiohumeral S53.41 ☑
    rupture
      radial collateral ligament — *see* Rupture,
        traumatic, ligament, radial collateral
      ulnar collateral ligament — *see* Rupture,
        traumatic, ligament, ulnar collateral
    specified type NEC S53.49 ☑
    ulnar collateral ligament S53.44 ☑
    ulnohumeral S53.42 ☑
  femur, head — *see* Sprain, hip
  fibular collateral, knee — *see* Sprain, knee,
    collateral
  fibulocalcaneal — *see* Sprain, ankle
  finger (s) S63.61 ☑
    index S63.61 ☑
    interphalangeal (joint) S63.63 ☑
      index S63.63 ☑
      little S63.63 ☑
      middle S63.63 ☑

Sprain — *continued*
  finger — *continued*
    ring S63.63 ☑
    little S63.61 ☑
    middle S63.61 ☑
    ring S63.61 ☑
    metacarpophalangeal (joint) S63.65 ☑
    specified site NEC S63.69 ☑
      index S63.69 ☑
      little S63.69 ☑
      middle S63.69 ☑
      ring S63.69 ☑
  foot S93.60 ☑
    specified ligament NEC S93.69 ☑
    tarsal ligament S93.61 ☑
    tarsometatarsal ligament S93.62 ☑
    toe — *see* Sprain, toe
  hand S63.9 ☑
    finger — *see* Sprain, finger
    specified site NEC — *see* subcategory S63.8
    thumb — *see* Sprain, thumb
  head S03.9 ☑
  hip S73.10 ☑
    iliofemoral ligament S73.11 ☑
    ischiocapsular (ligament) S73.12 ☑
    specified NEC S73.19 ☑
  iliofemoral — *see* Sprain, hip
  innominate
    acetabulum — *see* Sprain, hip
    sacral junction S33.6 ☑
  internal
    collateral, ankle — *see* Sprain, ankle
    semilunar cartilage — *see* Sprain, knee,
      specified site NEC
  interphalangeal
    finger — *see* Sprain, finger, interphalangeal
      (joint)
    toe — *see* Sprain, toe, interphalangeal joint
  ischiocapsular — *see* Sprain, hip
  ischiofemoral — *see* Sprain, hip
  jaw (articular disc) (cartilage) (meniscus) S03.4 ☑
    old M26.69
  knee S83.9 ☑
    collateral ligament S83.40 ☑
      lateral (fibular) S83.42 ☑
      medial (tibial) S83.41 ☑
    cruciate ligament S83.50 ☑
      anterior S83.51 ☑
      posterior S83.52 ☑
    lateral (fibular) collateral ligament S83.42 ☑
    medial (tibial) collateral ligament S83.41 ☑
    patellar ligament S76.11 ☑
    specified site NEC S83.8X ☑
    superior tibiofibular joint (ligament) S83.6 ☑
  lateral collateral, knee — *see* Sprain, knee,
    collateral
  lumbar (spine) S33.5 ☑
  lumbosacral S33.9 ☑
  mandible (articular disc) S03.4 ☑
    old M26.69
  medial collateral, knee — *see* Sprain, knee,
    collateral
  meniscus
    jaw S03.4 ☑
      old M26.69
    knee — *see* Sprain, knee, specified site NEC
      with current tear — *see* Tear, meniscus
        old — *see* Derangement, knee, meniscus,
          due to old tear
    mandible S03.4 ☑
      old M26.69
  metacarpal (distal) (proximal) — *see* Sprain, hand,
    specified site NEC
  metacarpophalangeal — *see* Sprain, finger,
    metacarpophalangeal (joint)
  metatarsophalangeal — *see* Sprain, toe,
    metatarsophalangeal joint
  midcarpal — *see* Sprain, hand, specified site NEC
  midtarsal — *see* Sprain, foot, specified site NEC
  neck S13.9 ☑
    anterior longitudinal cervical ligament S13.4 ☑
    atlanto-axial joint S13.4 ☑
    atlanto-occipital joint S13.4 ☑
    cervical spine S13.4 ☑
    cricoarytenoid ligament S13.5 ☑
    cricothyroid ligament S13.5 ☑
    specified site NEC S13.8 ☑
    thyroid region (cartilage) S13.5 ☑
  nose S03.8 ☑
  orbicular, hip — *see* Sprain, hip
  patella — *see* Sprain, knee, specified site NEC
  patellar ligament S76.11 ☑

☑ **Additional character required**

Sprain — *continued*
  pelvis NEC S33.8 ☑
  phalanx
    finger — *see* Sprain, finger
    toe — *see* Sprain, toe
  pubofemoral — *see* Sprain, hip
  radiocarpal — *see* Sprain, wrist
  radiohumeral — *see* Sprain, elbow
  radius, collateral — *see* Rupture, traumatic,
    ligament, radial collateral
  rib (cage) S23.41 ☑
  rotator cuff (capsule) S43.42 ☑
  sacroiliac (region)
    chronic or old — *see* subcategory M53.2
    joint S33.6 ☑
  scaphoid (hand) — *see* Sprain, hand, specified
    site NEC
  scapula (r) — *see* Sprain, shoulder girdle,
    specified site NEC
  semilunar cartilage (knee) — *see* Sprain, knee,
    specified site NEC
    with current tear — *see* Tear, meniscus
      old — *see* Derangement, knee, meniscus, due
        to old tear
  shoulder joint S43.40 ☑
    acromioclavicular joint (ligament) — *see* Sprain,
      acromioclavicular joint
    blade — *see* Sprain, shoulder, girdle, specified
      site NEC
    coracoclavicular joint (ligament) — *see* Sprain,
      coracoclavicular joint
    coracohumeral ligament — *see* Sprain,
      coracohumeral joint
    girdle S43.9 ☑
      specified site NEC S43.8 ☑
    rotator cuff — *see* Sprain, rotator cuff
    specified site NEC S43.49 ☑
    sternoclavicular joint (ligament) — *see* Sprain,
      sternoclavicular joint
  spine
    cervical S13.4 ☑
    lumbar S33.5 ☑
    thoracic S23.3 ☑
  sternoclavicular joint S43.6 ☑
  sternum S23.429 ☑
    chondrosternal joint S23.421 ☑
    specified site NEC S23.428 ☑
    sternoclavicular (joint) (ligament) S23.420 ☑
  symphysis
    jaw S03.4 ☑
      old M26.69
    mandibular S03.4 ☑
      old M26.69
  talofibular — *see* Sprain, ankle
  tarsal — *see* Sprain, foot, specified site NEC
  tarsometatarsal — *see* Sprain, foot, specified site
    NEC
  temporomandibular S03.4 ☑
    old M26.69
  thorax S23.9 ☑
    ribs S23.41 ☑
    specified site NEC S23.8 ☑
    spine S23.3 ☑
    sternum — *see* Sprain, sternum
  thumb S63.60 ☑
    interphalangeal (joint) S63.62 ☑
    metacarpophalangeal (joint) S63.64 ☑
    specified site NEC S63.68 ☑
  thyroid cartilage or region S13.5 ☑
  tibia (proximal end) — *see* Sprain, knee, specified
    site NEC
  tibial collateral, knee — *see* Sprain, knee, collateral
  tibiofibular
    distal — *see* Sprain, ankle
    superior — *see* Sprain, knee, specified site NEC
  toe (s) S93.50 ☑
    great S93.50 ☑
    interphalangeal joint S93.51 ☑
      great S93.51 ☑
      lesser S93.51 ☑
    lesser S93.50 ☑
    metatarsophalangeal joint S93.52 ☑
      great S93.52 ☑
      lesser S93.52 ☑
  ulna, collateral — *see* Rupture, traumatic,
    ligament, ulnar collateral
  ulnohumeral — *see* Sprain, elbow
  wrist S63.50 ☑
    carpal S63.51 ☑
    radiocarpal S63.52 ☑
    specified site NEC S63.59 ☑
  xiphoid cartilage — *see* Sprain, sternum

Sprengel's deformity (congenital) Q74.0
Sprue (tropical) K90.1
  celiac K90.0
  idiopathic K90.49
  meaning thrush B37.0
  nontropical K90.0
Spur, bone (*see also* Enthesopathy)
  calcaneal M77.3 ☑
  iliac crest M76.2 ☑
  nose (septum) J34.89
Spurway's syndrome Q78.0
Sputum
  abnormal (amount) (color) (odor)
    (purulent) R09.3
  blood-stained R04.2
  excessive (cause unknown) R09.3
Squamous (*see also* condition)
  epithelium in
    cervical canal (congenital) Q51.828
    uterine mucosa (congenital) Q51.818
Squashed nose M95.0
  congenital Q67.4
Squeeze, diver's T70.3 ☑
Squint (*see also* Strabismus)
  accommodative — *see* Strabismus, convergent
    concomitant
St. Hubert's disease A82.9
Stab (*see also* Laceration)
  internal organs — *see* Injury, by site
Stafne's cyst or cavity M27.0
Staggering gait R26.0
  hysterical F44.4
Staghorn calculus — *see* Calculus, kidney
Stähli's line (cornea) (pigment) — *see* Pigmentation,
  cornea, anterior
Stain, staining
  meconium (newborn) P96.83
  port wine Q82.5
  tooth, teeth (hard tissues) (extrinsic) K03.6
    due to
      accretions K03.6
      deposits (betel) (black) (green) (materia alba)
        (orange) (soft) (tobacco) K03.6
      metals (copper) (silver) K03.7
      nicotine K03.6
      pulpal bleeding K03.7
      tobacco K03.6
    intrinsic K00.8
Stammering (*see also* Disorder, fluency) F80.81
Standstill
  auricular I45.5
  cardiac — *see* Arrest, cardiac
  sinoatrial I45.5
  ventricular — *see* Arrest, cardiac
Stannosis J63.5
Stanton's disease — *see* Melioidosis
Staphylitis (acute) (catarrhal) (chronic) (gangrenous)
  (membranous) (suppurative) (ulcerative) K12.2
Staphylococcal scalded skin syndrome L00
Staphylococcemia A41.2
Staphylococcus, staphylococcal (*see also* condition)
  as cause of disease classified elsewhere B95.8
    aureus (methicillin susceptible) (MSSA) B95.61
      methicillin resistant (MRSA) B95.62
    specified NEC, as cause of disease classified
      elsewhere B95.7
Staphyloma (sclera)
  cornea H18.72 ☑
  equatorial H15.81 ☑
  localized (anterior) H15.82 ☑
  posticum H15.83 ☑
  ring H15.85 ☑
Stargardt's disease — *see* Dystrophy, retina
Starvation (inanition) (due to lack of food) T73.0 ☑
  edema — *see* Malnutrition, severe
Stasis
  bile (noncalculous) K83.1
  bronchus J98.09
    with infection — *see* Bronchitis
  cardiac — *see* Failure, heart, congestive
  cecum K59.8
  colon K59.8
  dermatitis I87.2
    with
      varicose ulcer — *see* Varix, leg, with ulcer,
        with inflammation
      varicose veins — *see* Varix, leg, with,
        inflammation
    due to postthrombotic syndrome — *see*
      Syndrome, postthrombotic
  duodenal K31.5
  eczema — *see* Varix, leg, with, inflammation

Stasis — *continued*
  edema — *see* Hypertension, venous (chronic),
    idiopathic
  foot T69.0 ☑
  ileocecal coil K59.8
  ileum K59.8
  intestinal K59.8
  jejunum K59.8
  kidney N19
  liver (cirrhotic) K76.1
  lymphatic I89.8
  pneumonia J18.2
  pulmonary — *see* Edema, lung
  rectal K59.8
  renal N19
    tubular N17.0
  ulcer — *see* Varix, leg, with, ulcer
    without varicose veins I87.2
  urine — *see* Retention, urine
  venous I87.8
State (of)
  affective and paranoid, mixed, organic
    psychotic F06.8
  agitated R45.1
    acute reaction to stress F43.0
  anxiety (neurotic) F41.1
  apprehension F41.1
  burn-out Z73.0
  climacteric, female Z78.0
    symptomatic N95.1
  compulsive F42.8
    mixed with obsessional thoughts F42.2
  confusional (psychogenic) F44.89
    acute (*see also* Delirium)
      with
        arteriosclerotic dementia F01.50
          with behavioral disturbance F01.51
        senility or dementia F05
      alcoholic F10.231
    epileptic F05
    reactive (from emotional stress, psychological
      trauma) F44.89
    subacute — *see* Delirium
  convulsive — *see* Convulsions
  crisis F43.0
  depressive F32.9
    neurotic F34.1
  dissociative F44.9
  emotional shock (stress) R45.7
  hypercoagulation — *see* Hypercoagulable
  locked-in G83.5
  menopausal Z78.0
    symptomatic N95.1
  neurotic F48.9
    with depersonalization F48.1
  obsessional F42.8
  oneiroid (schizophrenia-like) F23
  organic
    hallucinatory (nonalcoholic) F06.0
    paranoid (-hallucinatory) F06.2
  panic F41.0
  paranoid F22
    climacteric F22
    involutional F22
    menopausal F22
    organic F06.2
    senile F03 ☑
    simple F22
  persistent vegetative R40.3
  phobic F40.9
  postleukotomy F07.0
  pregnant
    gestational carrier Z33.3
    incidental Z33.1
  psychogenic, twilight F44.89
  psychopathic (constitutional) F60.2
  psychotic, organic (*see also* Psychosis, organic)
    mixed paranoid and affective F06.8
    senile or presenile F03 ☑
    transient NEC F06.8
      with
        hallucinations F06.0
        depression F06.31
  residual schizophrenic F20.5
  restlessness R45.1
  stress (emotional) R45.7
  tension (mental) F48.9
    specified NEC F48.8
  transient organic psychotic NEC F06.8
    depressive type F06.31
    hallucinatory type F06.0

State — *continued*
- twilight
  - epileptic F05
  - psychogenic F44.89
- vegetative, persistent R40.3
- vital exhaustion Z73.0
- withdrawal, — *see* Withdrawal, state

Status (post) (*see also* Presence (of))
- absence, epileptic — *see* Epilepsy, by type, with status epilepticus
- administration of tPA (rtPA) in a different facility within the last 24 hours prior to admission to current facility Z92.82
- adrenalectomy (unilateral) (bilateral) E89.6
- anastomosis Z98.0
- angioplasty (peripheral) Z98.62
  - with implant Z95.820
  - coronary artery Z98.61
    - with implant Z95.5
- anginosus I20.9
- aortocoronary bypass Z95.1
- arthrodesis Z98.1
- artificial opening (of) Z93.9
  - gastrointestinal tract Z93.4
  - specified NEC Z93.8
  - urinary tract Z93.6
  - vagina Z93.8
- asthmaticus — *see* Asthma, by type, with status asthmaticus
- awaiting organ transplant Z76.82
- bariatric surgery Z98.84
- bed confinement Z74.01
- bleb, filtering (vitreous), after glaucoma surgery Z98.83
- breast implant Z98.82
  - removal Z98.86
- cataract extraction Z98.4 ☑
- cholecystectomy Z90.49
- clitorectomy N90.811
  - with excision of labia minora N90.812
- colectomy (complete) (partial) Z90.49
- colonization — *see* Carrier (suspected) of
- colostomy Z93.3
- convulsivus idiopathicus — *see* Epilepsy, by type, with status epilepticus
- coronary artery angioplasty — *see* Status, angioplasty, coronary artery
- coronary artery bypass graft Z95.1
- cystectomy (urinary bladder) Z90.6
- cystostomy Z93.50
  - appendico-vesicostomy Z93.52
  - cutaneous Z93.51
  - specified NEC Z93.59
- delinquent immunization Z28.3
- dental Z98.818
  - crown Z98.811
  - fillings Z98.811
  - restoration Z98.811
  - sealant Z98.810
  - specified NEC Z98.818
- deployment (current) (military) Z56.82
- dialysis (hemodialysis) (peritoneal) Z99.2
- do not resuscitate (DNR) Z66
- donor — *see* Donor
- embedded fragments — *see* Retained, foreign body fragments (type of)
- embedded splinter — *see* Retained, foreign body fragments (type of)
- enterostomy Z93.4
- epileptic, epilepticus (*see also* Epilepsy, by type, with status epilepticus) G40.901
- estrogen receptor
  - negative Z17.1
  - positive Z17.0
- female genital cutting — *see* Female genital mutilation status
- female genital mutilation — *see* Female genital mutilation status
- filtering (vitreous) bleb after glaucoma surgery Z98.83
- gastrectomy (complete) (partial) Z90.3
- gastric banding Z98.84
- gastric bypass for obesity Z98.84
- gastrostomy Z93.1
- human immunodeficiency virus (HIV) infection, asymptomatic Z21
- hysterectomy (complete) (total) Z90.710
  - partial (with remaining cervical stump) Z90.711
- ileostomy Z93.2
- implant
  - breast Z98.82
  - infibulation N90.813

Status — *continued*
- intestinal bypass Z98.0
- jejunostomy Z93.4
- laryngectomy Z90.02
- lapsed immunization schedule Z28.3
- lymphaticus E32.8
- malignancy
  - castrate resistant prostate Z19.2
  - hormone resistant Z19.2
  - hormone sensitive Z19.1
- marmoratus G80.3
- mastectomy (unilateral) (bilateral) Z90.1 ☑
- military deployment status (current) Z56.82
  - in theater or in support of military war, peacekeeping and humanitarian operations Z56.82
- nephrectomy (unilateral) (bilateral) Z90.5
- nephrostomy Z93.6
- obesity surgery Z98.84
- oophorectomy
  - bilateral Z90.722
  - unilateral Z90.721
- organ replacement
  - by artificial or mechanical device or prosthesis of
    - artery Z95.828
    - bladder Z96.0
    - blood vessel Z95.828
    - breast Z97.8
    - eye globe Z97.0
    - heart Z95.812
      - valve Z95.2
    - intestine Z97.8
    - joint Z96.60
      - hip — *see* Presence, hip joint implant
      - knee — *see* Presence, knee joint implant
      - specified site NEC Z96.698
    - kidney Z97.8
    - larynx Z96.3
    - lens Z96.1
    - limbs — *see* Presence, artificial, limb
    - liver Z97.8
    - lung Z97.8
    - pancreas Z97.8
  - by organ transplant (heterologous) (homologous) — *see* Transplant
- pacemaker
  - brain Z96.89
  - cardiac Z95.0
  - specified NEC Z96.89
- pancreatectomy Z90.410
  - complete Z90.410
  - partial Z90.411
  - total Z90.410
- physical restraint Z78.1
- pneumonectomy (complete) (partial) Z90.2
- pneumothorax, therapeutic Z98.3
- postcommotio cerebri F07.81
- postoperative (postprocedural) NEC Z98.890
  - breast implant Z98.82
  - dental Z98.818
    - crown Z98.811
    - fillings Z98.811
    - restoration Z98.811
    - sealant Z98.810
    - specified NEC Z98.818
  - uterine scar Z98.891
  - pneumothorax, therapeutic Z98.3
- postpartum (routine follow-up) Z39.2
  - care immediately after delivery Z39.0
- postsurgical (postprocedural) NEC Z98.890
  - pneumothorax, therapeutic Z98.3
- pregnancy, incidental Z33.1
- prosthesis coronary angioplasty Z95.5
- pseudophakia Z96.1
- renal dialysis (hemodialysis) (peritoneal) Z99.2
- retained foreign body — *see* Retained, foreign body fragments (type of)
- reversed jejunal transposition (for bypass) Z98.0
- salpingo-oophorectomy
  - bilateral Z90.722
  - unilateral Z90.721
- sex reassignment surgery status Z87.890
- shunt
  - arteriovenous (for dialysis) Z99.2
  - cerebrospinal fluid Z98.2
  - ventricular (communicating) (for drainage) Z98.2
- splenectomy Z90.81
- thymicolymphaticus E32.8
- thymicus E32.8
- thymolymphaticus E32.8

Status — *continued*
- thyroidectomy (hypothyroidism) E89.0
- tooth (teeth) extraction (*see also* Absence, teeth, acquired) K08.409
- tPA (rtPA) administration in a different facility within the last 24 hours prior to admission to current facility Z92.82
- tracheostomy Z93.0
- transplant — *see* Transplant
  - organ removed Z98.85
- tubal ligation Z98.51
- underimmunization Z28.3
- ureterostomy Z93.6
- urethrostomy Z93.6
- vagina, artificial Z93.8
- vasectomy Z98.52
- wheelchair confinement Z99.3

Stealing
- child problem F91.8
  - in company with others Z72.810
- pathological (compulsive) F63.2

Steam burn — *see* Burn

Steatocystoma multiplex L72.2

Steatohepatitis (nonalcoholic) (NASH) K75.81

Steatoma L72.3
- eyelid (cystic) — *see* Dermatosis, eyelid
  - infected — *see* Hordeolum

Steatorrhea (chronic) K90.9
- with lacteal obstruction K90.2
- idiopathic (adult) (infantile) K90.9
- pancreatic K90.3
- primary K90.0
- tropical K90.1

Steatosis E88.89
- heart — *see* Degeneration, myocardial
- kidney N28.89
- liver NEC K76.0

Steele-Richardson-Olszewski disease or syndrome G23.1

Steinbrocker's syndrome G90.8

Steinert's disease G71.11

Stein-Leventhal syndrome E28.2

Stein's syndrome E28.2

STEMI (*see also* - Infarct, myocardium, ST elevation) I21.3

Stenocardia I20.8

Stenocephaly Q75.8

Stenosis, stenotic (cicatricial) (*see also* Stricture)
- ampulla of Vater K83.1
- anus, anal (canal) (sphincter) K62.4
  - and rectum K62.4
  - congenital Q42.3
    - with fistula Q42.2
- aorta (ascending) (supraventricular) (congenital) Q25.1
  - arteriosclerotic I70.0
  - calcified I70.0
  - supravalvular Q25.3
- aortic (valve) I35.0
  - with insufficiency I35.2
  - congenital Q23.0
  - rheumatic I06.0
    - with
      - incompetency, insufficiency or regurgitation I06.2
        - with mitral (valve) disease I08.0
          - with tricuspid (valve) disease I08.3
      - mitral (valve) disease I08.0
        - with tricuspid (valve) disease I08.3
      - tricuspid (valve) disease I08.2
        - with mitral (valve) disease I08.3
  - specified cause NEC I35.0
  - syphilitic A52.03
- aqueduct of Sylvius (congenital) Q03.0
  - with spina bifida — *see* Spina bifida, by site, with hydrocephalus
  - acquired G91.1
- artery NEC (*see also* Arteriosclerosis) I77.1
  - celiac I77.4
  - cerebral — *see* Occlusion, artery, cerebral
  - extremities — *see* Arteriosclerosis, extremities
  - precerebral — *see* Occlusion, artery, precerebral
  - pulmonary (congenital) Q25.6
    - acquired I28.8
  - renal I70.1
  - stent
    - coronary T82.855 ☑
    - peripheral T82.856 ☑
- bile duct (common) (hepatic) K83.1
  - congenital Q44.3
- bladder-neck (acquired) N32.0
  - congenital Q64.31

☑ **Additional character required**

Stenosis — *continued*
  brain G93.89
  bronchus J98.09
    congenital Q32.3
    syphilitic A52.72
  cardia (stomach) K22.2
    congenital Q39.3
  cardiovascular — *see* Disease, cardiovascular
  caudal M48.08
  cervix, cervical (canal) N88.2
    congenital Q51.828
    in pregnancy or childbirth — *see* Pregnancy,
        complicated by, abnormal cervix
  colon (*see also* Obstruction, intestine)
    congenital Q42.9
      specified NEC Q42.8
  colostomy K94.03
  common (bile) duct K83.1
    congenital Q44.3
  coronary (artery) — *see* Disease, heart, ischemic,
      atherosclerotic
  cystic duct — *see* Obstruction, gallbladder
  due to presence of device, implant or graft
      (*see also* Complications, by site and type,
      specified NEC) T85.858 ☑
    arterial graft NEC T82.858 ☑
    breast (implant) T85.858 ☑
    catheter T85.858 ☑
      dialysis (renal) T82.858 ☑
        intraperitoneal T85.858 ☑
      infusion NEC T82.858 ☑
        spinal (epidural) (subdural) T85.850 ☑
      urinary (indwelling) T83.85 ☑
    fixation, internal (orthopedic) NEC T84.85 ☑
    gastrointestinal (bile duct)
        (esophagus) T85.858 ☑
    genital NEC T83.85 ☑
    heart NEC T82.857 ☑
    joint prosthesis T84.85 ☑
    ocular (corneal graft) (orbital implant)
        NEC T85.858 ☑
    orthopedic NEC T84.85 ☑
    specified NEC T85.858 ☑
    urinary NEC T83.85 ☑
    vascular NEC T82.858 ☑
    ventricular intracranial shunt T85.850 ☑
  duodenum K31.5
    congenital Q41.0
  ejaculatory duct NEC N50.89
  endocervical os — *see* Stenosis, cervix
  enterostomy K94.13
  esophagus K22.2
    congenital Q39.3
    syphilitic A52.79
      congenital A50.59 *[K23]*
  eustachian tube — *see* Obstruction, eustachian
      tube
  external ear canal (acquired) H61.30 ☑
    congenital Q16.1
    due to
      inflammation H61.32 ☑
      trauma H61.31 ☑
    postprocedural H95.81 ☑
    specified cause NEC H61.39 ☑
  gallbladder — *see* Obstruction, gallbladder
  glottis J38.6
  heart valve (congenital) Q24.8
    aortic Q23.0
    mitral Q23.2
    pulmonary Q22.1
    tricuspid Q22.4
  hepatic duct K83.1
  hymen N89.6
  hypertrophic subaortic (idiopathic) I42.1
  ileum (*see also* Obstruction, intestine, specified
      NEC) K56.699
    congenital Q41.2
  infundibulum cardia Q24.3
  intervertebral foramina (*see also* Lesion,
      biomechanical, specified NEC)
    connective tissue M99.79
      abdomen M99.79
      cervical region M99.71
      cervicothoracic M99.71
      head region M99.70
      lumbar region M99.73
      lumbosacral M99.73
      occipitocervical M99.70
      sacral region M99.74
      sacrococcygeal M99.74
      sacroiliac M99.74
      specified NEC M99.79

Stenosis — *continued*
  intervertebral foramina — *continued*
      thoracic region M99.72
      thoracolumbar M99.72
    disc M99.79
      abdomen M99.79
      cervical region M99.71
      cervicothoracic M99.71
      head region M99.70
      lower extremity M99.76
      lumbar region M99.73
      lumbosacral M99.73
      occipitocervical M99.70
      pelvic M99.75
      rib cage M99.78
      sacral region M99.74
      sacrococcygeal M99.74
      sacroiliac M99.74
      specified NEC M99.79
      thoracic region M99.72
      thoracolumbar M99.72
      upper extremity M99.77
    osseous M99.69
      abdomen M99.69
      cervical region M99.61
      cervicothoracic M99.61
      head region M99.60
      lower extremity M99.66
      lumbar region M99.63
      lumbosacral M99.63
      occipitocervical M99.60
      pelvic M99.65
      rib cage M99.68
      sacral region M99.64
      sacrococcygeal M99.64
      sacroiliac M99.64
      specified NEC M99.69
      thoracic region M99.62
      thoracolumbar M99.62
      upper extremity M99.67
    subluxation — *see* Stenosis, intervertebral
        foramina, osseous
  intestine (*see also* Obstruction, intestine)
    congenital (small) Q41.9
      large Q42.9
        specified NEC Q42.8
      specified NEC Q41.8
  jejunum (*see also* Obstruction, intestine, specified
      NEC) K56.699
    congenital Q41.1
  lacrimal (passage)
    canaliculi H04.54 ☑
    congenital Q10.5
    duct H04.55 ☑
    punctum H04.56 ☑
    sac H04.57 ☑
  lacrimonasal duct — *see* Stenosis, lacrimal, duct
    congenital Q10.5
  larynx J38.6
    congenital NEC Q31.8
      subglottic Q31.1
    syphilitic A52.73
      congenital A50.59 *[J99]*
  mitral (chronic) (inactive) (valve) I05.0
    with
      aortic valve disease I08.0
      incompetency, insufficiency or
          regurgitation I05.2
    active or acute I01.1
      with rheumatic or Sydenham's chorea I02.0
    congenital Q23.2
    specified cause, except rheumatic I34.2
    syphilitic A52.03
  myocardium, myocardial (*see also* Degeneration,
      myocardial)
    hypertrophic subaortic (idiopathic) I42.1
  nares (anterior) (posterior) J34.89
    congenital Q30.0
  nasal duct (*see also* Stenosis, lacrimal, duct)
    congenital Q10.5
  nasolacrimal duct (*see also* Stenosis, lacrimal,
      duct)
    congenital Q10.5
  neural canal (*see also* Lesion, biomechanical,
      specified NEC)
    connective tissue M99.49
      abdomen M99.49
      cervical region M99.41
      cervicothoracic M99.41
      head region M99.40
      lower extremity M99.46
      lumbar region M99.43

Stenosis — *continued*
  neural canal — *continued*
      lumbosacral M99.43
      occipitocervical M99.40
      pelvic M99.45
      rib cage M99.48
      sacral region M99.44
      sacrococcygeal M99.44
      sacroiliac M99.44
      specified NEC M99.49
      thoracic region M99.42
      thoracolumbar M99.42
      upper extremity M99.47
    intervertebral disc M99.59
      abdomen M99.59
      cervical region M99.51
      cervicothoracic M99.51
      head region M99.50
      lower extremity M99.56
      lumbar region M99.53
      lumbosacral M99.53
      occipitocervical M99.50
      pelvic M99.55
      rib cage M99.58
      sacral region M99.54
      sacrococcygeal M99.54
      sacroiliac M99.54
      specified NEC M99.59
      thoracic region M99.52
      thoracolumbar M99.52
      upper extremity M99.57
    osseous M99.39
      abdomen M99.39
      cervical region M99.31
      cervicothoracic M99.31
      head region M99.30
      lower extremity M99.36
      lumbar region M99.33
      lumbosacral M99.33
      pelvic M99.35
      rib cage M99.38
      occipitocervical M99.30
      sacral region M99.34
      sacrococcygeal M99.34
      sacroiliac M99.34
      specified NEC M99.39
      thoracic region M99.32
      thoracolumbar M99.32
      upper extremity M99.37
    subluxation M99.29
      cervical region M99.21
      cervicothoracic M99.21
      head region M99.20
      lower extremity M99.26
      lumbar region M99.23
      lumbosacral M99.23
      occipitocervical M99.20
      pelvic M99.25
      rib cage M99.28
      sacral region M99.24
      sacrococcygeal M99.24
      sacroiliac M99.24
      specified NEC M99.29
      thoracic region M99.22
      thoracolumbar M99.22
      upper extremity M99.27
  organ or site, congenital NEC — *see* Atresia, by site
  papilla of Vater K83.1
  pulmonary (artery) (congenital) Q25.6
    with ventricular septal defect, transposition
        of aorta, and hypertrophy of right
        ventricle Q21.3
    acquired I28.8
    in tetralogy of Fallot Q21.3
    infundibular Q24.3
    subvalvular Q24.3
    supravalvular Q25.6
    valve I37.0
      with insufficiency I37.2
      congenital Q22.1
      rheumatic I09.89
        with aortic, mitral or tricuspid (valve)
            disease I08.8
    vein, acquired I28.8
    vessel NEC I28.8
  pulmonic (congenital) Q22.1
    infundibular Q24.3
    subvalvular Q24.3
  pylorus (hypertrophic) (acquired) K31.1
    adult K31.1
    congenital Q40.0
    infantile Q40.0

Stricture — *continued*
  pylorus (hypertrophic) K31.1
    adult K31.1
    congenital Q40.0
    infantile Q40.0
  rectosigmoid (*see also* Obstruction, intestine, specified NEC) K56.699
  rectum (sphincter) K62.4
    congenital Q42.1
      with fistula Q42.0
    due to
      chlamydial lymphogranuloma A55
      irradiation K91.89
      lymphogranuloma venereum A55
    gonococcal A54.6
    inflammatory (chlamydial) A55
    syphilitic A52.74
    tuberculous A18.32
  renal artery I70.1
    congenital Q27.1
  salivary duct or gland (any) K11.8
  sigmoid (flexure) — *see* Obstruction, intestine
  spermatic cord N50.89
  stoma (following) (of)
    colostomy K94.03
    enterostomy K94.13
    gastrostomy K94.23
    ileostomy K94.13
    tracheostomy J95.03
  stomach K31.89
    congenital Q40.2
    hourglass K31.2
  subaortic Q24.4
    hypertrophic (acquired) (idiopathic) I42.1
  subglottic J38.6
  syphilitic NEC A52.79
  trachea J39.8
    congenital Q32.1
    syphilitic A52.73
    tuberculous NEC A15.5
  tracheostomy J95.03
  tricuspid (valve) — *see* Stenosis, tricuspid
  tunica vaginalis N50.89
  ureter (postoperative) N13.5
    with
      hydronephrosis N13.1
        with infection N13.6
      pyelonephritis (chronic) N11.1
    congenital — *see* Atresia, ureter
    tuberculous A18.11
  ureteropelvic junction (congenital) Q62.11
    acquired, with hydronephrosis N13.0
  ureterovesical orifice N13.5
    with infection N13.6
  urethra (organic) (spasmodic) N35.9
    associated with schistosomiasis B65.0 *[N37]*
    congenital Q64.39
      valvular (posterior) Q64.2
    due to
      infection — *see* Stricture, urethra, postinfective
      trauma — *see* Stricture, urethra, post-traumatic
    gonococcal, gonorrheal A54.01
    infective NEC — *see* Stricture, urethra, postinfective
    late effect (sequelae) of injury — *see* Stricture, urethra, post-traumatic
    postcatheterization — *see* Stricture, urethra, postprocedural
    postinfective NEC
      female N35.12
      male N35.119
        anterior urethra N35.114
        bulbous urethra N35.112
        meatal N35.111
        membranous urethra N35.113
    postobstetric N35.021
    postoperative — *see* Stricture, urethra, postprocedural
    postprocedural
      female N99.12
      male N99.114
        anterior bulbous urethra N99.113
        bulbous urethra N99.111
        fossa navicularis N99.115
        meatal N99.110
        membranous urethra N99.112
    post-traumatic
      female N35.028
        due to childbirth N35.021
      male N35.014

Stricture — *continued*
  urethra — *continued*
    anterior urethra N35.013
    bulbous urethra N35.011
    meatal N35.010
    membranous urethra N35.012
    sequela (late effect) of
      childbirth N35.021
      injury — *see* Stricture, urethra, post-traumatic
    specified cause NEC N35.8
    syphilitic A52.76
    traumatic — *see* Stricture, urethra, post-traumatic
    valvular (posterior), congenital Q64.2
  urinary meatus — *see* Stricture, urethra
  uterus, uterine (synechiae) N85.6
    os (external) (internal) — *see* Stricture, cervix
  vagina (outlet) — *see* Stenosis, vagina
  valve (cardiac) (heart) (*see also* Endocarditis)
    congenital
      aortic Q23.0
      mitral Q23.2
      pulmonary Q22.1
      tricuspid Q22.4
  vas deferens N50.89
    congenital Q55.4
  vein I87.1
  vena cava (inferior) (superior) NEC I87.1
    congenital Q26.0
  vesicourethral orifice N32.0
    congenital Q64.31
  vulva (acquired) N90.5
Stridor R06.1
  congenital (larynx) P28.89
Stridulous — *see* condition
Stroke (apoplectic) (brain) (embolic) (ischemic) (paralytic) (thrombotic) I63.9
  cryptogenic (*see also* infarction, cerebral) I63.9
  epileptic — *see* Epilepsy
  heat T67.0 ☑
  in evolution I63.9
  intraoperative
    during cardiac surgery I97.810
    during other surgery I97.811
  lightning — *see* Lightning
  meaning
    cerebral hemorrhage - code to Hemorrhage, intracranial
    cerebral infarction - code to Infarction, cerebral
  postprocedural
    following cardiac surgery I97.820
    following other surgery I97.821
  unspecified (NOS) I63.9
Stromatosis, endometrial D39.0
Strongyloidiasis, strongyloidosis B78.9
  cutaneous B78.1
  disseminated B78.7
  intestinal B78.0
Strophulus pruriginosus L28.2
Struck by lightning — *see* Lightning
Struma (*see also* Goiter)
  Hashimoto E06.3
  lymphomatosa E06.3
  nodosa (simplex) E04.9
    endemic E01.2
      multinodular E01.1
    multinodular E04.2
      iodine-deficiency related E01.1
    toxic or with hyperthyroidism E05.20
      with thyroid storm E05.21
      multinodular E05.20
        with thyroid storm E05.21
      uninodular E05.10
        with thyroid storm E05.11
    toxicosa E05.20
      with thyroid storm E05.21
      multinodular E05.20
        with thyroid storm E05.21
      uninodular E05.10
        with thyroid storm E05.11
    uninodular E04.1
  ovarii D27. ☑
  Riedel's E06.5
Strumipriva cachexia E03.4
Strümpell-Marie spine — *see* Spondylitis, ankylosing
Strümpell-Westphal pseudosclerosis E83.01
Stuart deficiency disease (factor X) D68.2
Stuart-Prower factor deficiency (factor X) D68.2
Student's elbow — *see* Bursitis, elbow, olecranon
Stump — *see* Amputation
Stunting, nutritional E45

Stupor (catatonic) R40.1
  depressive (single episode) F32.89
    recurrent episode F33.8
  dissociative F44.2
  manic F30.2
  manic-depressive F31.89
  psychogenic (anergic) F44.2
  reaction to exceptional stress (transient) F43.0
Sturge (-Weber) (-Dimitri) (-Kalischer) disease or syndrome Q85.8
Stuttering F80.81
  adult onset F98.5
  childhood onset F80.81
  following cerebrovascular disease — *see* Disorder, fluency. following cerebrovascular disease
  in conditions classified elsewhere R47.82
Sty, stye (external) (internal) (meibomian) (zeisian) — *see* Hordeolum
Subacidity, gastric K31.89
  psychogenic F45.8
Subacute — *see* condition
Subarachnoid — *see* condition
Subcortical — *see* condition
Subcostal syndrome, nerve compression — *see* Mononeuropathy, upper limb, specified site NEC
Subcutaneous, subcuticular — *see* condition
Subdural — *see* condition
Subendocardium — *see* condition
Subependymoma
  specified site — *see* Neoplasm, uncertain behavior, by site
  unspecified site D43.2
Suberosis J67.3
Subglossitis — *see* Glossitis
Subhemophilia D66
Subinvolution
  breast (postlactational) (postpuerperal) N64.89
  puerperal O90.89
  uterus (chronic) (nonpuerperal) N85.3
  puerperal O90.89
Sublingual — *see* condition
Sublinguitis — *see* Sialoadenitis
Subluxatable hip Q65.6
Subluxation (*see also* Dislocation)
  acromioclavicular S43.11 ☑
  ankle S93.0 ☑
  atlantoaxial, recurrent M43.4
    with myelopathy M43.3
  carpometacarpal (joint) NEC S63.05 ☑
    thumb S63.04 ☑
  complex, vertebral — *see* Complex, subluxation
  congenital (*see also* Malposition, congenital)
    hip — *see* Dislocation, hip, congenital, partial
    joint (excluding hip)
      lower limb Q68.8
      shoulder Q68.8
      upper limb Q68.8
  elbow (traumatic) S53.10 ☑
    anterior S53.11 ☑
    lateral S53.14 ☑
    medial S53.13 ☑
    posterior S53.12 ☑
    specified type NEC S53.19 ☑
  finger S63.20 ☑
    index S63.20 ☑
    interphalangeal S63.22 ☑
      distal S63.24 ☑
        index S63.24 ☑
        little S63.24 ☑
        middle S63.24 ☑
        ring S63.24 ☑
      index S63.22 ☑
      little S63.22 ☑
      middle S63.22 ☑
      proximal S63.23 ☑
        index S63.23 ☑
        little S63.23 ☑
        middle S63.23 ☑
        ring S63.23 ☑
      ring S63.22 ☑
    little S63.20 ☑
    metacarpophalangeal S63.21 ☑
      index S63.21 ☑
      little S63.21 ☑
      middle S63.21 ☑
      ring S63.21 ☑
    middle S63.20 ☑
    ring S63.20 ☑
  foot S93.30 ☑
    specified site NEC S93.33 ☑
    tarsal joint S93.31 ☑
    tarsometatarsal joint S93.32 ☑
    toe — *see* Subluxation, toe

☑ **Additional character required**

Subluxation — *continued*
hip S73.00 ☑
  anterior S73.03 ☑
    obturator S73.02 ☑
  central S73.04 ☑
  posterior S73.01 ☑
interphalangeal (joint)
  finger S63.22 ☑
    distal joint S63.24 ☑
      index S63.24 ☑
      little S63.24 ☑
      middle S63.24 ☑
      ring S63.24 ☑
    index S63.22 ☑
    little S63.22 ☑
    middle S63.22 ☑
    proximal joint S63.23 ☑
      index S63.23 ☑
      little S63.23 ☑
      middle S63.23 ☑
      ring S63.23 ☑
    ring S63.22 ☑
  thumb S63.12 ☑
  toe S93.13 ☑
    great S93.13 ☑
    lesser S93.13 ☑
joint prosthesis — *see* Complications, joint
  prosthesis, mechanical, displacement, by site
knee S83.10 ☑
  cap — *see* Subluxation, patella
  patella — *see* Subluxation, patella
  proximal tibia
    anteriorly S83.11 ☑
    laterally S83.14 ☑
    medially S83.13 ☑
    posteriorly S83.12 ☑
  specified type NEC S83.19 ☑
lens — *see* Dislocation, lens, partial
ligament, traumatic — *see* Sprain, by site
metacarpal (bone)
  proximal end S63.06 ☑
metacarpophalangeal (joint)
  finger S63.21 ☑
    index S63.21 ☑
    little S63.21 ☑
    middle S63.21 ☑
    ring S63.21 ☑
  thumb S63.11 ☑
metatarsophalangeal joint S93.14 ☑
  great toe S93.14 ☑
  lesser toe S93.14 ☑
midcarpal (joint) S63.03 ☑
patella S83.00 ☑
  lateral S83.01 ☑
  recurrent (nontraumatic) — *see* Dislocation,
    patella, recurrent, incomplete
  specified type NEC S83.09 ☑
pathological — *see* Dislocation, pathological
radial head S53.00 ☑
  anterior S53.01 ☑
  nursemaid's elbow S53.03 ☑
  posterior S53.02 ☑
  specified type NEC S53.09 ☑
radiocarpal (joint) S63.02 ☑
radioulnar (joint)
  distal S63.01 ☑
  proximal — *see* Subluxation, elbow
shoulder
  congenital Q68.8
  girdle S43.30 ☑
    scapula S43.31 ☑
    specified site NEC S43.39 ☑
  traumatic S43.00 ☑
    anterior S43.01 ☑
    inferior S43.03 ☑
    posterior S43.02 ☑
    specified type NEC S43.08 ☑
sternoclavicular (joint) S43.20 ☑
  anterior S43.21 ☑
  posterior S43.22 ☑
symphysis (pubis)
thumb S63.103 ☑
  interphalangeal joint — *see* Subluxation,
    interphalangeal (joint), thumb
  metacarpophalangeal joint — *see* Subluxation,
    metacarpophalangeal (joint), thumb
toe (s) S93.10 ☑
  great S93.10 ☑
    interphalangeal joint S93.13 ☑
    metatarsophalangeal joint S93.14 ☑
  interphalangeal joint S93.13 ☑
  lesser S93.10 ☑

Subluxation — *continued*
toe — *continued*
    interphalangeal joint S93.13 ☑
    metatarsophalangeal joint S93.14 ☑
  metatarsophalangeal joint S93.149 ☑
ulnohumeral joint — *see* Subluxation, elbow
vertebral
  recurrent NEC — *see* subcategory M43.5
  traumatic
    cervical S13.100 ☑
      atlantoaxial joint S13.120 ☑
      atlantooccipital joint S13.110 ☑
      atloidooccipital joint S13.110 ☑
      joint between
        C0 and C1 S13.110 ☑
        C1 and C2 S13.120 ☑
        C2 and C3 S13.130 ☑
        C3 and C4 S13.140 ☑
        C4 and C5 S13.150 ☑
        C5and C6 S13.160 ☑
        C6and C7 S13.170 ☑
        C7and T1 S13.180 ☑
      occipitoatloid joint S13.110 ☑
    lumbar S33.100 ☑
      joint between
        L1and L2 S33.110 ☑
        L2and L3 S33.120 ☑
        L3 and L4 S33.130 ☑
        L4and L5 S33.140 ☑
    thoracic S23.100 ☑
      joint between
        T1and T2 S23.110 ☑
        T2and T3 S23.120 ☑
        T3 and T4 S23.122 ☑
        T4 and T5 S23.130 ☑
        T5 and T6 S23.132 ☑
        T6 and T7 S23.140 ☑
        T7 and T8 S23.142 ☑
        T8 and T9 S23.150 ☑
        T9 and T10 S23.152 ☑
        T10 and T11 S23.160 ☑
        T11 and T12 S23.162 ☑
        T12 and L1 S23.170 ☑
ulna
  distal end S63.07 ☑
  proximal end — *see* Subluxation, elbow
wrist (carpal bone) S63.00 ☑
  carpometacarpal joint — *see* Subluxation,
    carpometacarpal (joint)
  distal radioulnar joint — *see* Subluxation,
    radioulnar (joint), distal
  metacarpal bone, proximal — *see* Subluxation,
    metacarpal (bone), proximal end
  midcarpal — *see* Subluxation, midcarpal (joint)
  radiocarpal joint — *see* Subluxation,
    radiocarpal (joint)
  recurrent — *see* Dislocation, recurrent, wrist
  specified site NEC S63.09 ☑
  ulna — *see* Subluxation, ulna, distal end
Submaxillary — *see* condition
Submersion (fatal) (nonfatal) T75.1 ☑
Submucous — *see* condition
Subnormal, subnormality
  accommodation (old age) H52.4
  mental — *see* Disability, intellectual
  temperature (accidental) T68 ☑
Subphrenic — *see* condition
Subscapular nerve — *see* condition
Subseptus uterus Q51.2
Subsiding appendicitis K36
Substance (other psychoactive)-induced
  anxiety disorder F19.980
  bipolar and related disorder F19.94
  delirium F19.921
  depressive disorder F19.94
  major neurocognitive disorder F19.97
  mild neurocognitive disorder F19.988
  obsessive-compulsive and related
    disorder F19.988
  psychotic disorder F19.959
  sexual dysfunction F19.981
  sleep disorder F19.982
Substernal thyroid E04.9
  congenital Q89.2
Substitution disorder F44.9
Subtentorial — *see* condition
Subthyroidism (acquired) (*see also* Hypothyroidism)
  congenital E03.1
Succenturiate placenta O43.19 ☑
Sucking thumb, child (excessive) F98.8
Sudamen, sudamina L74.1
Sudanese kala-azar B55.0

Sudden
  heart failure — *see* Failure, heart
  hearing loss — *see* Deafness, sudden
Sudeck's atrophy, disease, or syndrome — *see*
  Algoneurodystrophy
Suffocation — *see* Asphyxia, traumatic
Sugar
  blood
    high (transient) R73.9
    low (transient) E16.2
  in urine R81
Suicide, suicidal (attempted) T14.91 ☑
  by poisoning — *see* Table of Drugs and Chemicals
  history of (personal) Z91.5
    in family Z81.8
  ideation — *see* Ideation, suicidal
  risk
    meaning personal history of attempted
      suicide Z91.5
    meaning suicidal ideation — *see* Ideation,
      suicidal
  tendencies
    meaning personal history of attempted
      suicide Z91.5
    meaning suicidal ideation — *see* Ideation,
      suicidal
  trauma — *see* nature of injury by site
Suipestifer infection — *see* Infection, salmonella
Sulfhemoglobinemia, sulphemoglobinemia
  (acquired) (with methemoglobinemia) D74.8
Sumatran mite fever A75.3
Summer — *see* condition
Sunburn L55.9
  due to
    tanning bed (acute) L56.8
      chronic L57.8
    ultraviolet radiation (acute) L56.8
      chronic L57.8
  first degree L55.0
  second degree L55.1
  third degree L55.2
SUNCT (short lasting unilateral neuralgiform
  headache with conjunctival injection and tearing)
  G44.059
  intractable G44.051
  not intractable G44.059
Sundowning F05
Sunken acetabulum — *see* Derangement, joint,
  specified type NEC, hip
Sunstroke T67.0 ☑
Superfecundation — *see* Pregnancy, multiple
Superfetation — *see* Pregnancy, multiple
Superinvolution (uterus) N85.8
Supernumerary (congenital)
  aortic cusps Q23.8
  auditory ossicles Q16.3
  bone Q79.8
  breast Q83.1
  carpal bones Q74.0
  cusps, heart valve NEC Q24.8
    aortic Q23.8
    mitral Q23.2
    pulmonary Q22.3
  digit (s) Q69.9
  ear (lobule) Q17.0
  fallopian tube Q50.6
  finger Q69.0
  hymen Q52.4
  kidney Q63.0
  lacrimonasal duct Q10.6
  lobule (ear) Q17.0
  mitral cusps Q23.2
  muscle Q79.8
  nipple (s) Q83.3
  organ or site not listed — *see* Accessory
  ossicles, auditory Q16.3
  ovary Q50.31
  oviduct Q50.6
  pulmonary, pulmonic cusps Q22.3
  rib Q76.6
    cervical or first (syndrome) Q76.5
  roots (of teeth) K00.2
  spleen Q89.09
  tarsal bones Q74.2
  teeth K00.1
  testis Q55.29
  thumb Q69.1
  toe Q69.2
  uterus Q51.2
  vagina Q52.1 ☑
  vertebra Q76.49

Syndrome

Syndrome — *continued*
Clarke-Hadfield K86.89
Clerambault's automatism G93.89
Clouston's (hidrotic ectodermal dysplasia) Q82.4
clumsiness, clumsy child F82
cluster headache G44.009
  intractable G44.001
  not intractable G44.009
Coffin-Lowry Q89.8
cold injury (newborn) P80.0
combined immunity deficiency D81.9
compartment (deep) (posterior) (traumatic) T79.A0 ☑
  abdomen T79.A3 ☑
  lower extremity (hip, buttock, thigh, leg, foot, toes) T79.A2 ☑
  nontraumatic
    abdomen M79.A3
    lower extremity (hip, buttock, thigh, leg, foot, toes) M79.A2 ☑
    specified site NEC M79.A9
    upper extremity (shoulder, arm, forearm, wrist, hand, fingers) M79.A1 ☑
  postprocedural — *see* Syndrome, compartment, nontraumatic
  specified site NEC T79.A9 ☑
  upper extremity (shoulder, arm, forearm, wrist, hand, fingers) T79.A1 ☑
complex regional pain — *see* Syndrome, pain, complex regional
compression T79.5 ☑
  anterior spinal — *see* Syndrome, anterior, spinal artery, compression
  cauda equina G83.4
  celiac artery I77.4
  vertebral artery M47.029
    occipito-atlanto-axial region M47.021
    cervical region M47.022
concussion F07.81
congenital
  affecting multiple systems NEC Q87.89
  central alveolar hypoventilation G47.35
  facial diplegia Q87.0
  muscular hypertrophy-cerebral Q87.89
  oculo-auriculovertebral Q87.0
  oculofacial diplegia (Moebius) Q87.0
  rubella (manifest) P35.0
congestion-fibrosis (pelvic), female N94.89
congestive dysmenorrhea N94.6
Conn's E26.01
connective tissue M35.9
  overlap NEC M35.1
conus medullaris G95.81
cord
  anterior G83.82
  posterior G83.83
coronary
  acute NEC I24.9
  insufficiency or intermediate I20.0
  slow flow I20.8
Costen's (complex) M26.69
costochondral junction M94.0
costoclavicular G54.0
costovertebral E22.0
Cowden Q85.8
craniovertebral M53.0
Creutzfeldt-Jakob — *see* Creutzfeldt-Jakob disease or syndrome
cri-du-chat Q93.4
crib death R99
cricopharyngeal — *see* Dysphagia
croup J05.0
CRPS I — *see* Syndrome, pain, complex regional I
crush T79.5 ☑
cubital tunnel — *see* Lesion, nerve, ulnar
Curschmann (-Batten) (-Steinert) G71.11
Cushing's E24.9
  alcohol-induced E24.4
  due to
    alcohol
    drugs E24.2
    ectopic ACTH E24.3
    overproduction of pituitary ACTH E24.0
  drug-induced E24.2
  overdose or wrong substance given or taken — *see* Table of Drugs and Chemicals, by drug, poisoning
  pituitary-dependent E24.0
  specified type NEC E24.8
cryopyrin-associated periodic M04.2
cryptophthalmos Q87.0
cystic duct stump K91.5

Syndrome — *continued*
Dana-Putnam D51.0
Danbolt (-Cross) (acrodermatitis enteropathica) E83.2
Dandy-Walker Q03.1
  with spina bifida Q07.01
Danlos' Q79.6
defibrination (*see also* Fibrinolysis)
  with
    antepartum hemorrhage — *see* Hemorrhage, antepartum, with coagulation defect
    intrapartum hemorrhage — *see* Hemorrhage, complicating, delivery
  newborn P60
  postpartum O72.3
Degos' I77.89
Déjérine-Roussy G89.0
delayed sleep phase G47.21
demyelinating G37.9
dependence — *see* F10-F19 with fourth character .2
depersonalization (-derealization) F48.1
De Quervain E34.51
de Toni-Fanconi (-Debré) E72.09
  with cystinosis E72.04
diabetes mellitus-hypertension-nephrosis — *see* Diabetes, nephrosis
diabetes mellitus in newborn infant P70.2
diabetes-nephrosis — *see* Diabetes, nephrosis
diabetic amyotrophy — *see* Diabetes, amyotrophy
dialysis associated steal T82.898 ☑
Diamond-Blackfan D61.01
Diamond-Gardener D69.2
DIC (diffuse or disseminated intravascular coagulopathy) D65
di George's D82.1
Dighton's Q78.0
disequilibrium E87.8
Döhle body-panmyelopathic D72.0
dorsolateral medullary G46.4
double athetosis G80.3
Down (*see also* Down syndrome) Q90.9
Dresbach's (elliptocytosis) D58.1
Dressler's (postmyocardial infarction) I24.1
  postcardiotomy I97.0
drug withdrawal, infant of dependent mother P96.1
dry eye H04.12 ☑
due to abnormality
  chromosomal Q99.9
    sex
      female phenotype Q97.9
      male phenotype Q98.9
    specified NEC Q99.8
dumping (postgastrectomy) K91.1
  nonsurgical K31.89
Dupré's (meningism) R29.1
dysmetabolic X E88.81
dyspraxia, developmental F82
Eagle-Barrett Q79.4
Eaton-Lambert — *see* Syndrome, Lambert-Eaton
Ebstein's Q22.5
ectopic ACTH E24.3
eczema-thrombocytopenia D82.0
Eddowes' Q78.0
effort (psychogenic) F45.8
Eisenmenger's I27.83
Ehlers-Danlos Q79.6
Ekman's Q78.0
electric feet E53.8
Ellis-van Creveld Q77.6
empty nest Z60.0
endocrine-hypertensive E27.0
entrapment — *see* Neuropathy, entrapment
eosinophilia-myalgia M35.8
epileptic (*see also* Epilepsy, by type)
  absence G40.A09
    intractable G40.A19
      with status epilepticus G40.A11
      without status epilepticus G40.A19
    not intractable G40.A09
      with status epilepticus G40.A01
      without status epilepticus G40.A09
Erdheim-Chester (ECD) E88.89
Erdheim's E22.0
erythrocyte fragmentation D59.4
Evans D69.41
exhaustion F48.8
extrapyramidal G25.9
  specified NEC G25.89
eye retraction — *see* Strabismus

Syndrome — *continued*
eyelid-malar-mandible Q87.0
Faber's D50.9
facial pain, paroxysmal G50.0
Fallot's Q21.3
familial cold autoinflammatory M04.2
familial eczema-thrombocytopenia (Wiskott-Aldrich) D82.0
Fanconi (-de Toni) (-Debré) E72.09
  with cystinosis E72.04
Fanconi's (anemia) (congenital pancytopenia) D61.09
fatigue
  chronic R53.82
  psychogenic F48.8
faulty bowel habit K59.39
Feil-Klippel (brevicollis) Q76.1
Felty's — *see* Felty's syndrome
fertile eunuch E23.0
fetal
  alcohol (dysmorphic) Q86.0
  hydantoin Q86.1
Fiedler's I40.1
first arch Q87.0
fish odor E72.8
Fisher's G61.0
Fitzhugh-Curtis
  due to
    Chlamydia trachomatis A74.81
    Neisseria gonorrhoea (gonococcal peritonitis) A54.85
Fitz's (*see also* Pancreatitis, acute) K85.80
Flajani (-Basedow) E05.00
  with thyroid storm E05.01
flatback — *see* Flatback syndrome
floppy
  baby P94.2
  iris (intraoeprative) (IFIS) H21.81
  mitral valve I34.1
flush E34.0
Foix-Alajouanine G95.19
Fong's Q87.2
food protein-induced enterocolitis K52.21
foramen magnum G93.5
Foster-Kennedy H47.14 ☑
Foville's (peduncular) G46.3
fragile X Q99.2
Franceschetti Q75.4
Frey's
  auriculotemporal G50.8
  hyperhidrosis L74.52
Friderichsen-Waterhouse A39.1
Froin's G95.89
frontal lobe F07.0
Fukuhara E88.49
functional
  bowel K59.9
  prepubertal castrate E29.1
Gaisböck's D75.1
ganglion (basal ganglia brain) G25.9
  geniculi G51.1
Gardner-Diamond D69.2
gastroesophageal
  junction K22.0
  laceration-hemorrhage K22.6
gastrojejunal loop obstruction K91.89
Gee-Herter-Heubner K90.0
Gelineau's G47.419
  with cataplexy G47.411
genito-anorectal A55
Gerstmann-Sträussler-Scheinker (GSS) A81.82
Gianotti-Crosti L44.4
giant platelet (Bernard-Soulier) D69.1
Gilles de la Tourette's F95.2
goiter-deafness E07.1
Goldberg Q89.8
Goldberg-Maxwell E34.51
Good's D83.8
Gopalan' (burning feet) E53.8
Gorlin's Q87.89
Gougerot-Blum L81.7
Gouley's I31.1
Gower's R55
gray or grey (newborn) P93.0
  platelet D69.1
Gubler-Millard G46.3
Guillain-Barré (-Strohl) G61.0
gustatory sweating G50.8
Hadfield-Clarke K86.89
hair tourniquet — *see* Constriction, external, by site
Hamman's J98.19

☑ **Additional character required**

Syndrome — *continued*
  hand-foot L27.1
  hand-shoulder G90.8
  hantavirus (cardio)-pulmonary (HPS)
    (HCPS) B33.4
  happy puppet Q93.5
  Harada's H30.81 ☑
  Hayem-Faber D50.9
  headache NEC G44.89
    complicated NEC G44.59
  Heberden's I20.8
  Hedinger's E34.0
  Hegglin's D72.0
  HELLP (hemolysis, elevated liver enzymes and
    low platelet count) O14.2 ☑
    complicating
      childbirth O14.24
      puerperium O14.25
  hemolytic-uremic D59.3
  hemophagocytic, infection-associated D76.2
  Henoch-Schönlein D69.0
  hepatic flexure K59.8
  hepatopulmonary K76.81
  hepatorenal K76.7
    following delivery O90.4
    postoperative or postprocedural K91.83
    postpartum, puerperal O90.4
  hepatourologic K76.7
  Herter (-Gee) (nontropical sprue) K90.0
  Heubner-Herter K90.0
  Heyd's K76.7
  Hilger's G90.09
  histamine-like (fish poisoning) — *see* Poisoning,
    fish
  histiocytic D76.3
  histiocytosis NEC D76.3
  HIV infection, acute B20
  Hoffmann-Werdnig G12.0
  Hollander-Simons E88.1
  Hoppe-Goldflam G70.00
    with exacerbation (acute) G70.01
    in crisis G70.01
  Horner's G90.2
  hungry bone E83.81
  hunterian glossitis D51.0
  Hutchinson's triad A50.53
  hyperabduction G54.0
  hyperammonemia-hyperornithinemia-
    homocitrullinemia E72.4
  hypereosinophilic (idiopathic) D72.1
  hyperimmunoglobulin D M04.1
  hyperimmunoglobulin E (IgE) D82.4
  hyperkalemic E87.5
  hyperkinetic — *see* Hyperkinesia
  hypermobility M35.7
  hypernatremia E87.0
  hyperosmolarity E87.0
  hyperperfusion G97.82
  hypersplenic D73.1
  hypertransfusion, newborn P61.1
  hyperventilation F45.8
  hyperviscosity (of serum)
    polycythemic D75.1
    sclerothymic D58.8
  hypoglycemic (familial) (neonatal) E16.2
  hypokalemic E87.6
  hyponatremic E87.1
  hypopituitarism E23.0
  hypoplastic left-heart Q23.4
  hypopotassemia E87.6
  hyposmolality E87.1
  hypotension, maternal O26.5 ☑
  hypothenar hammer I73.89
  hypoventilation, obesity (OHS) E66.2
  ICF (intravascular coagulation-fibrinolysis) D65
  idiopathic
    cardiorespiratory distress, newborn P22.0
    nephrotic (infantile) N04.9
  iliotibial band M76.3 ☑
  immobility, immobilization (paraplegic) M62.3
  immune reconstitution D89.3
  immune reconstitution inflammatory [IRIS] D89.3
  immunity deficiency, combined D81.9
  immunodeficiency
    acquired — *see* Human, immunodeficiency
      virus (HIV) disease
    combined D81.9
  impending coronary I20.0
  impingement, shoulder M75.4 ☑
  inappropriate secretion of antidiuretic
    hormone E22.2

Syndrome — *continued*
  infant
    of diabetic mother P70.1
      gestational diabetes P70.0
  infantilism (pituitary) E23.0
  inferior vena cava I87.1
  inspissated bile (newborn) P59.1
  institutional (childhood) F94.2
  insufficient sleep F51.12
  intermediate coronary (artery) I20.0
  interspinous ligament — *see* Spondylopathy,
    specified NEC
  intestinal
    carcinoid E34.0
    knot K56.2
  intravascular coagulation-fibrinolysis (ICF) D65
  iodine-deficiency, congenital E00.9
    type
      mixed E00.2
      myxedematous E00.1
      neurological E00.0
  IRDS (idiopathic respiratory distress,
    newborn) P22.0
  irritable
    bowel K58.9
      with
        constipation K58.1
        diarrhea K58.0
      mixed K58.2
      psychogenic F45.8
      specified NEC K58.8
    heart (psychogenic) F45.8
    weakness F48.8
  ischemic
    bowel (transient) K55.9
      chronic K55.1
      due to mesenteric artery insufficiency K55.1
    steal T82.898 ☑
  IVC (intravascular coagulopathy) D65
  Ivemark's Q89.01
  Jaccoud's — *see* Arthropathy, postrheumatic,
    chronic
  Jackson's G83.89
  Jakob-Creutzfeldt — *see* Creutzfeldt-Jakob
    disease or syndrome
  jaw-winking Q07.8
  Jervell-Lange-Nielsen I45.81
  jet lag G47.25
  Job's D71
  Joseph-Diamond-Blackfan D61.01
  jugular foramen G52.7
  Kabuki Q89.8
  Kanner's (autism) F84.0
  Kartagener's Q89.3
  Kelly's D50.1
  Kimmelstiel-Wilson — *see* Diabetes, specified
    type, with Kimmelstiel-Wilson disease
  Klein (e)-Levine G47.13
  Klippel-Feil (brevicollis) Q76.1
  Köhler-Pellegrini-Steida — *see* Bursitis, tibial
    collateral
  König's K59.8
  Korsakoff (-Wernicke) (nonalcoholic) F04
    alcoholic F10.26
  Kostmann's D70.0
  Krabbe's congenital muscle hypoplasia Q79.8
  labyrinthine — *see* subcategory H83.2
  lacunar NEC G46.7
  Lambert-Eaton G70.80
    in
      neoplastic disease G73.1
      specified disease NEC G70.81
  Landau-Kleffner — *see* Epilepsy, specified NEC
  Larsen's Q74.8
  lateral
    cutaneous nerve of thigh G57.1 ☑
    medullary G46.4
  Launois' E22.0
  lazy
    leukocyte D70.8
    posture M62.3
  Lemiere I80.8
  Lennox-Gastaut G40.812
    intractable G40.814
      with status epilepticus G40.813
      without status epilepticus G40.814
    not intractable G40.812
      with status epilepticus G40.811
      without status epilepticus G40.812
  lenticular, progressive E83.01
  Leopold-Levi's E05.90
  Lev's I44.2

Syndrome — *continued*
  Li-Fraumeni Z15.01
  Lichtheim's D51.0
  Lightwood's N25.89
  Lignac (de Toni) (-Fanconi) (-Debré) E72.09
    with cystinosis E72.04
  Likoff's I20.8
  limbic epilepsy personality F07.0
  liver-kidney K76.7
  lobotomy F07.0
  Loffler's J82
  long arm 18 or 21 deletion Q93.89
  long QT I45.81
  Louis-Barré G11.3
  low
    atmospheric pressure T70.29 ☑
    back M54.5
    output (cardiac) I50.9
  lower radicular, newborn (birth injury) P14.8
  Luetscher's (dehydration) E86.0
  Lupus anticoagulant D68.62
  Lutembacher's Q21.1
  macrophage activation D76.1
    due to infection D76.2
  magnesium-deficiency R29.0
  Majeed M04.8
  Mal de Debarquement R42
  malabsorption K90.9
    postsurgical K91.2
  malformation, congenital, due to
    alcohol Q86.0
    exogenous cause NEC Q86.8
    hydantoin Q86.1
    warfarin Q86.2
  malignant
    carcinoid E34.0
    neuroleptic G21.0
  Mallory-Weiss K22.6
  mandibulofacial dysostosis Q75.4
  manic-depressive — *see* Disorder, bipolar
  maple-syrup-urine E71.0
  Marable's I77.4
  Marfan's Q87.40
    with
      cardiovascular manifestations Q87.418
        aortic dilation Q87.410
      ocular manifestations Q87.42
      skeletal manifestations Q87.43
  Marie's (acromegaly) E22.0
  mast cell activation — *see* Activation, mast cell
  maternal hypotension — *see* Syndrome,
    hypotension, maternal
  May (-Hegglin) D72.0
  McArdle (-Schmidt) (-Pearson) E74.04
  McQuarrie's E16.2
  meconium plug (newborn) P76.0
  median arcuate ligament I77.4
  Meekeren-Ehlers-Danlos Q79.6
  megavitamin-B6 E67.2
  Meige G24.4
  MELAS E88.41
  Mendelson's O74.0
  MERRF (myoclonic epilepsy associated with
    ragged-red fibers) E88.42
  mesenteric
    artery (superior) K55.1
    vascular insufficiency K55.1
  metabolic E88.81
  metastatic carcinoid E34.0
  micrognathia-glossoptosis Q87.0
  midbrain NEC G93.89
  middle lobe (lung) J98.19
  middle radicular G54.0
  migraine (*see also* Migraine) G43.909
  Mikulicz' K11.8
  milk-alkali E83.52
  Millard-Gubler G46.3
  Miller-Dieker Q93.88
  Miller-Fisher G61.0
  Minkowski-Chauffard D58.0
  Mirizzi's K83.1
  MNGIE (Mitochondrial Neurogastrointestinal
    Encephalopathy) E88.49
  Möbius, ophthalmoplegic migraine — *see*
    Migraine, ophthalmoplegic
  monofixation H50.42
  Morel-Moore M85.2
  Morel-Morgagni M85.2
  Morgagni (-Morel) (-Stewart) M85.2
  Morgagni-Adams-Stokes I45.9
  Muckle-Wells M04.2

Syndrome — *continued*
    mucocutaneous lymph node (acute febrile) (MCLS) M30.3
    multiple endocrine neoplasia (MEN) — *see* Neoplasia, endocrine, multiple (MEN)
    multiple operations — *see* Disorder, factitious
    Mounier-Kuhn Q32.4
        with bronchiectasis J47.9
            with
                exacerbation (acute) J47.1
                lower respiratory infection J47.0
        acquired J98.09
            with bronchiectasis J47.9
                with
                    exacerbation (acute) J47.1
                    lower respiratory infection J47.0
    myasthenic G70.9
        in
            diabetes mellitus — *see* Diabetes, amyotrophy
            endocrine disease NEC E34.9 *[G73.3]*
            neoplastic disease (*see also* Neoplasm) D49.9 *[G73.3]*
            thyrotoxicosis (hyperthyroidism) E05.90 *[G73.3]*
                with thyroid storm E05.91 *[G73.3]*
    myelodysplastic D46.9
        with
            5q deletion D46.C
            isolated del (5q) chromosomal abnormality D46.C
        lesions, low grade D46.20
        specified NEC D46.Z
    myelopathic pain G89.0
    myeloproliferative (chronic) D47.1
    myofascial pain M79.1
    Naffziger's G54.0
    nail patella Q87.2
    NARP (Neuropathy, Ataxia and Retinitis pigmentosa) E88.49
    neonatal abstinence P96.1
    nephritic (*see also* Nephritis)
        with edema — *see* Nephrosis
        acute N00.9
        chronic N03.9
        rapidly progressive N01.9
    nephrotic (congenital) (*see also* Nephrosis) N04.9
        with
            dense deposit disease N04.6
            diffuse
                crescentic glomerulonephritis N04.7
                endocapillary proliferative glomerulonephritis N04.4
                membranous glomerulonephritis N04.2
                mesangial proliferative glomerulonephritis N04.3
                mesangiocapillary glomerulonephritis N04.5
            focal and segmental glomerular lesions N04.1
            minor glomerular abnormality N04.0
            specified morphological changes NEC N04.8
        diabetic — *see* Diabetes, nephrosis
    neurologic neglect R41.4
    Nezelof's D81.4
    Nonne-Milroy-Meige Q82.0
    Nothnagel's vasomotor acroparesthesia I73.89
    obesity hypoventilation (OHS) E66.2
    oculomotor H51.9
    ophthalmoplegia-cerebellar ataxia — *see* Strabismus, paralytic, third nerve
    oral allergy T78.1 ☑
    oral-facial-digital Q87.0
    organic
        affective F06.30
        amnesic (not alcohol- or drug-induced) F04
        brain F09
        depressive F06.31
        hallucinosis F06.0
        personality F07.0
    Ormond's N13.5
    oro-facial-digital Q87.0
    os trigonum Q68.8
    Osler-Weber-Rendu I78.0
    osteoporosis-osteomalacia M83.8
    Osterreicher-Turner Q87.2
    otolith — *see* subcategory H81.8
    oto-palatal-digital Q87.0
    outlet (thoracic) G54.0
    ovary
        polycystic E28.2
        resistant E28.39
        sclerocystic E28.2

Syndrome — *continued*
    Owren's D68.2
    Paget-Schroetter I82.890
    pain (*see also* Pain)
        complex regional I G90.50
            lower limb G90.52 ☑
            specified site NEC G90.59
            upper limb G90.51 ☑
        complex regional II — *see* Causalgia
    painful
        bruising D69.2
        feet E53.8
        prostate N42.81
    paralysis agitans — *see* Parkinsonism
    paralytic G83.9
        specified NEC G83.89
    Parinaud's H51.0
    parkinsonian — *see* Parkinsonism
    Parkinson's — *see* Parkinsonism
    paroxysmal facial pain G50.0
    Parry's E05.00
        with thyroid storm E05.01
    Parsonage (-Aldren)-Turner G54.5
    patella clunk M25.86 ☑
    Paterson (-Brown) (-Kelly) D50.1
    pectoral girdle I77.89
    pectoralis minor I77.89
    pediatric autoimmune neuropsychiatric disorders associated with streptococcal infections (PANDAS) D89.89
    Pelger-Huet D72.0
    pellagra-cerebellar ataxia-renal aminoaciduria E72.02
    pellagroid E52
    Pellegrini-Stieda — *see* Bursitis, tibial collateral
    pelvic congestion-fibrosis, female N94.89
    penta X Q97.1
    peptic ulcer — *see* Ulcer, peptic
    perabduction I77.89
    periodic fever M04.1
    periodic fever, aphthous stomatitis, pharyngitis, and adenopathy [PFAPA] M04.8
    periodic headache, in adults and children — *see* Headache, periodic syndromes in adults and children
    periurethral fibrosis N13.5
    phantom limb (without pain) G54.7
        with pain G54.6
    pharyngeal pouch D82.1
    Pick's — *see* Disease, Pick's
    Pickwickian E66.2
    PIE (pulmonary infiltration with eosinophilia) J82
    pigmentary pallidal degeneration (progressive) G23.0
    pineal E34.8
    pituitary E22.0
    plantar fascia M72.2
    placental transfusion — *see* Pregnancy, complicated by, placental transfusion syndromes
    plateau iris (post-iridectomy) (postprocedural) H21.82
    Plummer-Vinson D50.1
    pluricarential of infancy E40
    plurideficiency E40
    pluriglandular (compensatory) E31.8
        autoimmune E31.0
    pneumatic hammer T75.21 ☑
    polyangiitis overlap M30.8
    polycarential of infancy E40
    polyglandular E31.8
        autoimmune E31.0
    polysplenia Q89.09
    pontine NEC G93.89
    popliteal
        artery entrapment I77.89
        web Q87.89
    postcardiac injury
        postcardiotomy I97.0
        postmyocardial infarction I24.1
    postcardiotomy I97.0
    post chemoembolization - code to associated conditions
    postcholecystectomy K91.5
    postcommissurotomy I97.0
    postconcussional F07.81
    postcontusional F07.81
    postencephalitic F07.89
    posterior
        cervical sympathetic M53.0
        cord G83.83
        fossa compression G93.5
        reversible encephalopathy (PRES) I67.83

Syndrome — *continued*
    postgastrectomy (dumping) K91.1
    postgastric surgery K91.1
    postinfarction I24.1
    postlaminectomy NEC M96.1
    postleukotomy F07.0
    postmastectomy lymphedema I97.2
    postmyocardial infarction I24.1
    postoperative NEC T81.9 ☑
        blind loop K90.2
    postpartum panhypopituitary (Sheehan) E23.0
    postpolio (myelitic) G14
    postthrombotic I87.009
        with
            inflammation I87.02 ☑
                with ulcer I87.03 ☑
            specified complication NEC I87.09 ☑
            ulcer I87.01 ☑
                with inflammation I87.03 ☑
        asymptomatic I87.00 ☑
    postvagotomy K91.1
    postvalvulotomy I97.0
    postviral NEC G93.3
        fatigue G93.3
    Potain's K31.0
    potassium intoxication E87.5
    precerebral artery (multiple) (bilateral) G45.2
    preinfarction I20.0
    preleukemic D46.9
    premature senility E34.8
    premenstrual dysphoric F32.89
    premenstrual tension N94.3
    Prinzmetal-Massumi R07.1
    prune belly Q79.4
    pseudocarpal tunnel (sublimis) — *see* Syndrome, carpal tunnel
    pseudoparalytica G70.00
        with exacerbation (acute) G70.01
        in crisis G70.01
    pseudo -Turner's Q87.1
    psycho-organic (nonpsychotic severity) F07.9
        acute or subacute F05
        depressive type F06.31
        hallucinatory type F06.0
        nonpsychotic severity F07.0
        specified NEC F07.89
    pulmonary
        arteriosclerosis I27.0
        dysmaturity (Wilson-Mikity) P27.0
        hypoperfusion (idiopathic) P22.0
        renal (hemorrhagic) (Goodpasture's) M31.0
    pure
        motor lacunar G46.5
        sensory lacunar G46.6
    Putnam-Dana D51.0
    pyogenic arthritis, pyoderma gangrenosum, and acne [PAPA] M04.8
    pyramidopallidonigral G20
    pyriformis — *see* Lesion, nerve, sciatic
    QT interval prolongation I45.81
    radicular NEC — *see* Radiculopathy
        upper limbs, newborn (birth injury) P14.3
    rapid time-zone change G47.25
    Rasmussen G04.81
    Raymond (-Céstan) I65.8
    Raynaud's I73.00
        with gangrene I73.01
    RDS (respiratory distress syndrome, newborn) P22.0
    reactive airways dysfunction J68.3
    Refsum's G60.1
    Reifenstein E34.52
    renal glomerulohyalinosis-diabetic — *see* Diabetes, nephrosis
    Rendu-Osler-Weber I78.0
    residual ovary N99.83
    resistant ovary E28.39
    respiratory
        distress
            acute J80
                adult J80
                child J80
                idiopathic J84.114
            newborn (idiopathic) (type I) P22.0
                type II P22.1
    restless legs G25.81
    retinoblastoma (familial) C69.2 ☑
    retroperitoneal fibrosis N13.5
    retroviral seroconversion (acute) Z21
    Reye's G93.7
    Richter — *see* Leukemia, chronic lymphocytic, B-cell type

☑ **Additional character required**

ICD-10-CM INDEX TO DISEASES AND INJURIES

Syndrome

Syndrome — *continued*
  Ridley's I50.1
  right
    heart, hypoplastic Q22.6
    ventricular obstruction — *see* Failure, heart,
      congestive
  Romano-Ward (prolonged QT interval) I45.81
  rotator cuff, shoulder (*see also* Tear, rotator
    cuff) M75.10 ☑
  Rotes Quérol — *see* Hyperostosis, ankylosing
  Roth — *see* Meralgia paresthetica
  rubella (congenital) P35.0
  Ruvalcaba-Myhre-Smith E71.440
  Rytand-Lipsitch I44.2
  salt
    depletion E87.1
      due to heat NEC T67.8 ☑
        causing heat exhaustion or
          prostration T67.4 ☑
    low E87.1
  salt-losing N28.89
  Scaglietti-Dagnini E22.0
  scalenus anticus (anterior) G54.0
  scapulocostal — *see* Mononeuropathy, upper
    limb, specified site NEC
  scapuloperoneal G71.0
  schizophrenic, of childhood NEC F84.5
  Schnitzler D47.2
  Scholte's E34.0
  Schroeder's E27.0
  Schüller-Christian C96.5
  Schwachman's — *see* Syndrome, Shwachman's
  Schwartz (-Jampel) G71.13
  Schwartz-Bartter E22.2
  scimitar Q26.8
  sclerocystic ovary E28.2
  Seitelberger's G31.89
  septicemic adrenal hemorrhage A39.1
  seroconversion, retroviral (acute) Z21
  serous meningitis G93.2
  severe acute respiratory (SARS) J12.81
  shaken infant T74.4 ☑
  shock (traumatic) T79.4 ☑
    kidney N17.0
      following crush injury T79.5 ☑
    toxic A48.3
  shock-lung J80
  Shone's - code to specific anomalies
  short
    bowel K91.2
    rib Q77.2
  shoulder-hand — *see* Algoneurodystrophy
  Shwachman's D70.4
  sicca — *see* Sicca syndrome
  sick
    cell E87.1
    sinus I49.5
  sick-euthyroid E07.81
  sideropenic D50.1
  Siemens' ectodermal dysplasia Q82.4
  Silfversköld's Q78.9
  Simons' E88.1
  sinus tarsi M25.57 ☑
  sinusitis-bronchiectasis-situs inversus Q89.3
  Sipple's E31.22
  sirenomelia Q87.2
  Slocumb's E27.0
  slow flow, coronary I20.8
  Sluder's G44.89
  Smith-Magenis Q93.88
  Sneddon-Wilkinson L13.1
  Soto's Q87.3
  South African cardiomyopathy I42.8
  spasmodic
    upward movement, eyes H51.8
    winking F95.8
  Spen's I45.9
  splenic
    agenesis Q89.01
    flexure K59.8
    neutropenia D73.81
  Spurway's Q78.0
  staphylococcal scalded skin L00
  steal
    arteriovenous T82.898 ☑
    ischemic T82.898 ☑
    subclavian G45.8
  Stein-Leventhal E28.2
  Stein's E28.2
  Stevens-Johnson syndrome L51.1
    toxic epidermal necrolysis overlap L51.3
  Stewart-Morel M85.2

Syndrome — *continued*
  Stickler Q89.8
  stiff baby Q89.8
  stiff man G25.82
  Still-Felty — *see* Felty's syndrome
  Stokes (-Adams) I45.9
  stone heart I50.1
  straight back, congenital Q76.49
  subclavian steal G45.8
  subcoracoid-pectoralis minor G54.0
  subcostal nerve compression I77.89
  subphrenic interposition Q43.3
  superior
    cerebellar artery I63.8
    mesenteric artery K55.1
    semi-circular canal dehiscence H83.8X ☑
    vena cava I87.1
  supine hypotensive (maternal) — *see* Syndrome,
    hypotension, maternal
  suprarenal cortical E27.0
  supraspinatus (*see also* Tear, rotator
    cuff) M75.10 ☑
  Susac G93.49
  swallowed blood P78.2
  sweat retention L74.0
  Swyer Q99.1
  Symond's G93.2
  sympathetic
    cervical paralysis G90.2
    pelvic, female N94.89
  systemic inflammatory response (SIRS), of
    non-infectious origin (without organ
    dysfunction) R65.10
    with acute organ dysfunction R65.11
  tachycardia-bradycardia I49.5
  takotsubo I51.81
  TAR (thrombocytopenia with absent
    radius) Q87.2
  tarsal tunnel G57.5 ☑
  teething K00.7
  tegmental G93.89
  telangiectasic-pigmentation-cataract Q82.8
  temporal pyramidal apex — *see* Otitis, media,
    suppurative, acute
  temporomandibular joint-pain-
    dysfunction M26.62 ☑
  Terry's (*see also* Myopia, degenerative) H44.2 ☑
  testicular feminization (*see also* Syndrome,
    androgen insensitivity) E34.51
  thalamic pain (hyperesthetic) G89.0
  thoracic outlet (compression) G54.0
  Thorson-Björck E34.0
  thrombocytopenia with absent radius
    (TAR) Q87.2
  thyroid-adrenocortical insufficiency E31.0
  tibial
    anterior M76.81 ☑
    posterior M76.82 ☑
  Tietze's M94.0
  time-zone (rapid) G47.25
  Toni-Fanconi E72.09
    with cystinosis E72.04
  Touraine's Q79.8
  tourniquet — *see* Constriction, external, by site
  toxic shock A48.3
  transient left ventricular apical balloning I51.81
  traumatic vasospastic T75.22 ☑
  Treacher Collins Q75.4
  triple X, female Q97.0
  trisomy Q92.9
    13 Q91.7
      meiotic nondisjunction Q91.4
      mitotic nondisjunction Q91.5
      mosaicism Q91.5
      translocation Q91.6
    18 Q91.3
      meiotic nondisjunction Q91.0
      mitotic nondisjunction Q91.1
      mosaicism Q91.1
      translocation Q91.2
    20 (q) (p) Q92.8
    21 Q90.9
      meiotic nondisjunction Q90.0
      mitotic nondisjunction Q90.1
      mosaicism Q90.1
      translocation Q90.2
    22 Q92.8
  tropical wet feet T69.0 ☑
  Trousseau's I82.1
  tumor lysis (following antineoplastic
    chemotherapy) (spontaneous) NEC E88.3

Syndrome — *continued*
  tumor necrosis factor receptor associated
    periodic (TRAPS) M04.1
  Twiddler's (due to)
    automatic implantable defibrillator T82.198 ☑
    cardiac pacemaker T82.198 ☑
  Unverricht (-Lundborg) — *see* Epilepsy,
    generalized, idiopathic
  upward gaze H51.8
  uremia, chronic (*see also* Disease, kidney,
    chronic) N18.9
  urethral N34.3
  urethro-oculo-articular — *see* Reiter's disease
  urohepatic K76.7
  vago-hypoglossal G52.7
  vascular NEC in cerebrovascular disease G46.8
  vasoconstriction, reversible
    cerebrovascular I67.841
  vasomotor I73.9
  vasospastic (traumatic) T75.22 ☑
  vasovagal R55
  van Buchem's M85.2
  van der Hoeve's Q78.0
  VATER Q87.2
  velo-cardio-facial Q93.81
  vena cava (inferior) (superior) (obstruction) I87.1
  vertebral
    artery G45.0
      compression — *see* Syndrome, anterior,
        spinal artery, compression
    steal G45.0
  vertebro-basilar artery G45.0
  vertebrogenic (pain) M54.89
  vertiginous — *see* Disorder, vestibular function
  Vinson-Plummer D50.1
  virus B34.9
  visceral larva migrans B83.0
  visual disorientation H53.8
  vitamin B6 deficiency E53.1
  vitreal corneal H59.01 ☑
  vitreous (touch) H59.01 ☑
  Vogt-Koyanagi H20.82 ☑
  Volkmann's T79.6 ☑
  von Schroetter's I82.890
  von Willebrand (-Jürgen) D68.0
  Waldenström-Kjellberg D50.1
  Wallenberg's G46.3
  water retention E87.79
  Waterhouse (-Friderichsen) A39.1
  Weber-Gubler G46.3
  Weber-Leyden G46.3
  Weber's G46.3
  Wegener's M31.30
    with
      kidney involvement M31.31
      lung involvement M31.30
        with kidney involvement M31.31
  Weingarten's (tropical eosinophilia) J82
  Weiss-Baker G90.09
  Werdnig-Hoffman G12.0
  Wermer's E31.21
  Werner's E34.8
  Wernicke-Korsakoff (nonalcoholic) F04
    alcoholic F10.26
  West's — *see* Epilepsy, spasms
  Westphal-Strümpell E83.01
  wet
    feet (maceration) (tropical) T69.0 ☑
    lung, newborn P22.1
  whiplash S13.4 ☑
  whistling face Q87.0
  Wilkie's K55.1
  Wilkinson-Sneddon L13.1
  Willebrand (-Jürgens) D68.0
  Wilson's (hepatolenticular degeneration) E83.01
  Wiskott-Aldrich D82.0
  withdrawal — *see* Withdrawal, state
    drug
      infant of dependent mother P96.1
      therapeutic use, newborn P96.2
  Woakes' (ethmoiditis) J33.1
  Wright's (hyperabduction) G54.0
  X I20.9
  XXXX Q97.1
  XXXXX Q97.1
  XXXXY Q98.1
  XXY Q98.0
  yellow nail L60.5
  Zahorsky's B08.5
  Zellweger syndrome E71.510
  Zellweger-like syndrome E71.541

Synechia (anterior) (iris) (posterior) (pupil) (*see also* Adhesions, iris)
  intra-uterine (traumatic) N85.6
Synesthesia R20.8
Syngamiasis, syngamosis B83.3
Synodontia K00.2
Synorchidism, synorchism Q55.1
Synostosis (congenital) Q78.8
  astragalo-scaphoid Q74.2
  radioulnar Q74.0
Synovial sarcoma — *see* Neoplasm, connective tissue, malignant
Synovioma (malignant) (*see also* Neoplasm, connective tissue, malignant)
  benign — *see* Neoplasm, connective tissue, benign
Synoviosarcoma — *see* Neoplasm, connective tissue, malignant
Synovitis (*see also* Tenosynovitis) M65.9
  crepitant
    hand M70.0 ☑
    wrist M70.03 ☑
  gonococcal A54.49
  gouty — *see* Gout
  in (due to)
    crystals M65.8 ☑
    gonorrhea A54.49
    syphilis (late) A52.78
    use, overuse, pressure — *see* Disorder, soft tissue, due to use
  infective NEC — *see* Tenosynovitis, infective NEC
  specified NEC — *see* Tenosynovitis, specified type NEC
  syphilitic A52.78
    congenital (early) A50.02
  toxic — *see* Synovitis, transient
  transient M67.3 ☑
    ankle M67.37 ☑
    elbow M67.32 ☑
    foot joint M67.37 ☑
    hand joint M67.34 ☑
    hip M67.35 ☑
    knee M67.36 ☑
    multiple site M67.39
    pelvic region M67.35 ☑
    shoulder M67.31 ☑
    specified joint NEC M67.38
    wrist M67.33 ☑
  traumatic, current — *see* Sprain
  tuberculous — *see* Tuberculosis, synovitis
  villonodular (pigmented) M12.2 ☑
    ankle M12.27 ☑
    elbow M12.22 ☑
    foot joint M12.27 ☑
    hand joint M12.24 ☑
    hip M12.25 ☑
    knee M12.26 ☑
    multiple site M12.29
    pelvic region M12.25 ☑
    shoulder M12.21 ☑
    specified joint NEC M12.28
    vertebrae M12.28
    wrist M12.23 ☑
Syphilid A51.39
  congenital A50.06
  newborn A50.06
  tubercular (late) A52.79
Syphilis, syphilitic (acquired) A53.9
  abdomen (late) A52.79
  acoustic nerve A52.15
  adenopathy (secondary) A51.49
  adrenal (gland) (with cortical hypofunction) A52.79
  age under 2 years NOS (*see also* Syphilis, congenital, early)
    acquired A51.9
  alopecia (secondary) A51.32
  anemia (late) A52.79 [D63.8]
  aneurysm (aorta) (ruptured) A52.01
    central nervous system A52.05
    congenital A50.54 [I79.0]
  anus (late) A52.74
    primary A51.1
    secondary A51.39
  aorta (arch) (abdominal) (thoracic) A52.02
    aneurysm A52.01
  aortic (insufficiency) (regurgitation) (stenosis) A52.03
    aneurysm A52.01
  arachnoid (adhesive) (cerebral) (spinal) A52.13
  asymptomatic — *see* Syphilis, latent
  ataxia (locomotor) A52.11

Syphilis, syphilitic — *continued*
  atrophoderma maculatum A51.39
  auricular fibrillation A52.06
  bladder (late) A52.76
  bone A52.77
    secondary A51.46
  brain A52.17
  breast (late) A52.79
  bronchus (late) A52.72
  bubo (primary) A51.0
  bulbar palsy A52.19
  bursa (late) A52.78
  cardiac decompensation A52.06
  cardiovascular A52.00
  central nervous system (late) (recurrent) (relapse) (tertiary) A52.3
    with
      ataxia A52.11
      general paralysis A52.17
        juvenile A50.45
      paresis (general) A52.17
        juvenile A50.45
      tabes (dorsalis) A52.11
        juvenile A50.45
      taboparesis A52.17
        juvenile A50.45
    aneurysm A52.05
    congenital A50.40
    juvenile A50.40
    remission in (sustained) A52.3
    serology doubtful, negative, or positive A52.3
    specified nature or site NEC A52.19
    vascular A52.05
  cerebral A52.17
    meningovascular A52.13
    nerves (multiple palsies) A52.15
    sclerosis A52.17
    thrombosis A52.05
  cerebrospinal (tabetic type) A52.12
  cerebrovascular A52.05
  cervix (late) A52.76
  chancre (multiple) A51.0
    extragenital A51.2
    Rollet's A51.0
  Charcot's joint A52.16
  chorioretinitis A51.43
    congenital A50.01
    late A52.71
    prenatal A50.01
  choroiditis — *see* Syphilitic chorioretinitis
  choroidoretinitis — *see* Syphilitic chorioretinitis
  ciliary body (secondary) A51.43
    late A52.71
  colon (late) A52.74
  combined spinal sclerosis A52.11
  condyloma (latum) A51.31
  congenital A50.9
    with
      paresis (general) A50.45
      tabes (dorsalis) A50.45
      taboparesis A50.45
    chorioretinitis, choroiditis A50.01 [H32]
    early, or less than 2 years after birth NEC A50.2
      with manifestations — *see* Syphilis, congenital, early, symptomatic
      latent (without manifestations) A50.1
        negative spinal fluid test A50.1
        serology positive A50.1
      symptomatic A50.09
        cutaneous A50.06
        mucocutaneous A50.07
        oculopathy A50.01
        osteochondropathy A50.02
        pharyngitis A50.03
        pneumonia A50.04
        rhinitis A50.05
        visceral A50.08
    interstitial keratitis A50.31
    juvenile neurosyphilis A50.45
    late, or 2 years or more after birth NEC A50.7
      chorioretinitis, choroiditis A50.32
      interstitial keratitis A50.31
      juvenile neurosyphilis A50.45
      latent (without manifestations) A50.6
        negative spinal fluid test A50.6
        serology positive A50.6
      symptomatic or with manifestations NEC A50.59
        arthropathy A50.55
        cardiovascular A50.54
        Clutton's joints A50.51
        Hutchinson's teeth A50.52

Syphilis, syphilitic — *continued*
  congenital — *continued*
        Hutchinson's triad A50.53
        osteochondropathy A50.56
        saddle nose A50.57
  conjugal A53.9
    tabes A52.11
  conjunctiva (late) A52.71
  contact Z20.2
  cord bladder A52.19
  cornea, late A52.71
  coronary (artery) (sclerosis) A52.06
  coryza, congenital A50.05
  cranial nerve A52.15
    multiple palsies A52.15
  cutaneous — *see* Syphilis, skin
  dacryocystitis (late) A52.71
  degeneration, spinal cord A52.12
  dementia paralytica A52.17
    juvenilis A50.45
  destruction of bone A52.77
  dilatation, aorta A52.01
  due to blood transfusion A53.9
  dura mater A52.13
  ear A52.79
    inner A52.79
      nerve (eighth) A52.15
      neurorecurrence A52.15
  early A51.9
    cardiovascular A52.00
    central nervous system A52.3
    latent (without manifestations) (less than 2 years after infection) A51.5
      negative spinal fluid test A51.5
      serological relapse after treatment A51.5
      serology positive A51.5
    relapse (treated, untreated) A51.9
    skin A51.39
    symptomatic A51.9
      extragenital chancre A51.2
      primary, except extragenital chancre A51.0
      secondary (*see also* Syphilis, secondary) A51.39
        relapse (treated, untreated) A51.49
    ulcer A51.39
  eighth nerve (neuritis) A52.15
  endemic A65
  endocarditis A52.03
    aortic A52.03
    pulmonary A52.03
  epididymis (late) A52.76
  epiglottis (late) A52.73
  epiphysitis (congenital) (early) A50.02
  episcleritis (late) A52.71
  esophagus A52.79
  eustachian tube A52.73
  exposure to Z20.2
  eye A52.71
  eyelid (late) (with gumma) A52.71
  fallopian tube (late) A52.76
  fracture A52.77
  gallbladder (late) A52.74
  gastric (polyposis) (late) A52.74
  general A53.9
    paralysis A52.17
      juvenile A50.45
  genital (primary) A51.0
  glaucoma A52.71
  gumma NEC A52.79
    cardiovascular system A52.00
    central nervous system A52.3
    congenital A50.59
  heart (block) (decompensation) (disease) (failure) A52.06 [I52]
    valve NEC A52.03
  hemianesthesia A52.19
  hemianopsia A52.71
  hemiparesis A52.17
  hemiplegia A52.17
  hepatic artery A52.09
  hepatis A52.74
  hepatomegaly, congenital A50.08
  hereditaria tarda — *see* Syphilis, congenital, late
  hereditary — *see* Syphilis, congenital
  Hutchinson's teeth A50.52
  hyalitis A52.71
  inactive — *see* Syphilis, latent
  infantum — *see* Syphilis, congenital
  inherited — *see* Syphilis, congenital
  internal ear A52.79
  intestine (late) A52.74
  iris, iritis (secondary) A51.43
    late A52.71

Syphilis, syphilitic — *continued*
  joint (late) A52.77
  keratitis (congenital) (interstitial) (late) A50.31
  kidney (late) A52.75
  lacrimal passages (late) A52.71
  larynx (late) A52.73
  late A52.9
    cardiovascular A52.00
    central nervous system A52.3
    kidney A52.75
    latent or 2 years or more after infection
      (without manifestations) A52.8
      negative spinal fluid test A52.8
      serology positive A52.8
    paresis A52.17
    specified site NEC A52.79
    symptomatic or with manifestations A52.79
    tabes A52.11
  latent A53.0
    with signs or symptoms - code by site and
      stage under Syphilis
    central nervous system A52.2
    date of infection unspecified A53.0
    early, or less than 2 years after infection A51.5
    follow-up of latent syphilis A53.0
      date of infection unspecified A53.0
      late, or 2 years or more after infection A52.8
    late, or 2 years or more after infection A52.8
    positive serology (only finding) A53.0
      date of infection unspecified A53.0
      early, or less than 2 years after infection A51.5
      late, or 2 years or more after infection A52.8
  lens (late) A52.71
  leukoderma A51.39
    late A52.79
  lienitis A52.79
  lip A51.39
    chancre (primary) A51.2
    late A52.79
  Lissauer's paralysis A52.17
  liver A52.74
  locomotor ataxia A52.11
  lung A52.72
  lymph gland (early) (secondary) A51.49
    late A52.79
  lymphadenitis (secondary) A51.49
  macular atrophy of skin A51.39
    striated A52.79
  mediastinum (late) A52.73
  meninges (adhesive) (brain) (spinal cord) A52.13
  meningitis A52.13
    acute (secondary) A51.41
    congenital A50.41
  meningoencephalitis A52.14
  meningovascular A52.13
    congenital A50.41
  mesarteritis A52.09
    brain A52.04
  middle ear A52.77
  mitral stenosis A52.03
  monoplegia A52.17
  mouth (secondary) A51.39
    late A52.79
  mucocutaneous (secondary) A51.39
    late A52.79
  mucous
    membrane (secondary) A51.39
      late A52.79
    patches A51.39
      congenital A50.07
  mulberry molars A50.52
  muscle A52.78
  myocardium A52.06
  nasal sinus (late) A52.73
  neonatorum — *see* Syphilis, congenital
  nephrotic syndrome (secondary) A51.44
  nerve palsy (any cranial nerve) A52.15
    multiple A52.15
  nervous system, central A52.3
  neuritis A52.15
    acoustic A52.15
  neurorecidive of retina A52.19
  neuroretinitis A52.19
  newborn — *see* Syphilis, congenital
  nodular superficial (late) A52.79
  nonvenereal A65
  nose (late) A52.73
    saddle back deformity A50.57
  occlusive arterial disease A52.09
  oculopathy A52.71
  ophthalmic (late) A52.71
  optic nerve (atrophy) (neuritis) (papilla) A52.15

Syphilis, syphilitic — *continued*
  orbit (late) A52.71
  organic A53.9
  osseous (late) A52.77
  osteochondritis (congenital) (early) A50.02 *[M90.80]*
  osteoporosis A52.77
  ovary (late) A52.76
  oviduct (late) A52.76
  palate (late) A52.79
  pancreas (late) A52.74
  paralysis A52.17
    general A52.17
      juvenile A50.45
  paresis (general) A52.17
    juvenile A50.45
  paresthesia A52.19
  Parkinson's disease or syndrome A52.19
  paroxysmal tachycardia A52.06
  pemphigus (congenital) A50.06
  penis (chancre) A51.0
    late A52.76
  pericardium A52.06
  perichondritis, larynx (late) A52.73
  periosteum (late) A52.77
    congenital (early) A50.02 *[M90.80]*
    early (secondary) A51.46
  peripheral nerve A52.79
  petrous bone (late) A52.77
  pharynx (late) A52.73
    secondary A51.39
  pituitary (gland) A52.79
  pleura (late) A52.73
  pneumonia, white A50.04
  pontine lesion A52.17
  portal vein A52.09
  primary A51.0
    anal A51.1
    and secondary — *see* Syphilis, secondary
    central nervous system A52.3
    extragenital chancre NEC A51.2
    fingers A51.2
    genital A51.0
    lip A51.2
    specified site NEC A51.2
    tonsils A51.2
  prostate (late) A52.76
  ptosis (eyelid) A52.71
  pulmonary (late) A52.72
    artery A52.09
  pyelonephritis (late) A52.75
  recently acquired, symptomatic A51.9
  rectum (late) A52.74
  respiratory tract (late) A52.73
  retina, late A52.71
  retrobulbar neuritis A52.15
  salpingitis A52.76
  sclera (late) A52.71
  sclerosis
    cerebral A52.17
    coronary A52.06
    multiple A52.11
  scotoma (central) A52.71
  scrotum (late) A52.76
  secondary (and primary) A51.49
    adenopathy A51.49
    anus A51.39
    bone A51.46
    chorioretinitis, choroiditis A51.43
    hepatitis A51.45
    liver A51.45
    lymphadenitis A51.49
    meningitis (acute) A51.41
    mouth A51.39
    mucous membranes A51.39
    periosteum, periostitis A51.46
    pharynx A51.39
    relapse (treated, untreated) A51.49
    skin A51.39
    specified form NEC A51.49
    tonsil A51.39
    ulcer A51.39
    viscera NEC A51.49
    vulva A51.39
  seminal vesicle (late) A52.76
  seronegative with signs or symptoms - code by
    site and stage under Syphilis
  seropositive
    with signs or symptoms - code by site and
      stage under Syphilis
    follow-up of latent syphilis — *see* Syphilis,
      latent
    only finding — *see* Syphilis, latent

Syphilis, syphilitic — *continued*
  seventh nerve (paralysis) A52.15
  sinus, sinusitis (late) A52.73
  skeletal system A52.77
  skin (with ulceration) (early) (secondary) A51.39
    late or tertiary A52.79
  small intestine A52.74
  spastic spinal paralysis A52.17
  spermatic cord (late) A52.76
  spinal (cord) A52.12
  spleen A52.79
  splenomegaly A52.79
  spondylitis A52.77
  staphyloma A52.71
  stigmata (congenital) A50.59
  stomach A52.74
  synovium A52.78
  tabes dorsalis (late) A52.11
    juvenile A50.45
  tabetic type A52.11
    juvenile A50.45
  taboparesis A52.17
    juvenile A50.45
  tachycardia A52.06
  tendon (late) A52.78
  tertiary A52.9
    with symptoms NEC A52.79
    cardiovascular A52.00
    central nervous system A52.3
    multiple NEC A52.79
    specified site NEC A52.79
  testis A52.76
  thorax A52.73
  throat A52.73
  thymus (gland) (late) A52.79
  thyroid (late) A52.79
  tongue (late) A52.79
  tonsil (lingual) (late) A52.73
    primary A51.2
    secondary A51.39
  trachea (late) A52.73
  tunica vaginalis (late) A52.76
  ulcer (any site) (early) (secondary) A51.39
    late A52.79
    perforating A52.79
      foot A52.11
  urethra (late) A52.76
  urogenital (late) A52.76
  uterus (late) A52.76
  uveal tract (secondary) A51.43
    late A52.71
  uveitis (secondary) A51.43
    late A52.71
  uvula (late) (perforated) A52.79
  vagina A51.0
    late A52.76
  valvulitis NEC A52.03
  vascular A52.00
    brain (cerebral) A52.05
  ventriculi A52.74
  vesicae urinariae (late) A52.76
  viscera (abdominal) (late) A52.74
    secondary A51.49
  vitreous (opacities) (late) A52.71
    hemorrhage A52.71
  vulva A51.0
    late A52.76
    secondary A51.39
Syphiloma A52.79
  cardiovascular system A52.00
  central nervous system A52.3
  circulatory system A52.00
  congenital A50.59
Syphilophobia F45.29
Syringadenoma (*see also* Neoplasm, skin, benign)
  papillary — *see* Neoplasm, skin, benign
Syringobulbia G95.0
Syringocystadenoma — *see* Neoplasm, skin, benign
  papillary — *see* Neoplasm, skin, benign
Syringoma (*see also* Neoplasm, skin, benign)
  chondroid — *see* Neoplasm, skin, benign
Syringomyelia G95.0
Syringomyelitis — *see* Encephalitis
Syringomyelocele — *see* Spina bifida
Syringopontia G95.0
System, systemic (*see also* condition)
  disease, combined — *see* Degeneration,
    combined
  inflammatory response syndrome (SIRS) of
    non-infectious origin (without organ
    dysfunction) R65.10
    with acute organ dysfunction R65.11

Ulcer

Ulcer, ulcerated, ulcerating, ulceration, ulcerative
— continued
  lower limb — continued
    with
      bone involvement without evidence of
        necrosis L97.906
      bone necrosis L97.904
      exposed fat layer L97.902
      muscle involvement without evidence of
        necrosis L97.905
      muscle necrosis L97.903
      skin breakdown only L97.901
      specified severity NEC L97.908
    ankle L97.309
      with
        bone involvement without evidence of
          necrosis L97.306
        bone necrosis L97.304
        exposed fat layer L97.302
        muscle involvement without evidence of
          necrosis L97.305
        muscle necrosis L97.303
        skin breakdown only L97.301
        specified severity NEC L97.308
      left L97.329
        with
          bone involvement without evidence of
            necrosis L97.326
          bone necrosis L97.324
          exposed fat layer L97.322
          muscle involvement without evidence of
            necrosis L97.325
          muscle necrosis L97.323
          skin breakdown only L97.321
          specified severity NEC L97.328
      right L97.319
        with
          bone involvement without evidence of
            necrosis L97.316
          bone necrosis L97.314
          exposed fat layer L97.312
          muscle involvement without evidence of
            necrosis L97.315
          muscle necrosis L97.313
          skin breakdown only L97.311
          specified severity NEC L97.318
    calf L97.209
      with
        bone involvement without evidence of
          necrosis L97.206
        bone necrosis L97.204
        exposed fat layer L97.202
        muscle involvement without evidence of
          necrosis L97.205
        muscle necrosis L97.203
        skin breakdown only L97.201
        specified severity NEC L97.208
      left L97.229
        with
          bone involvement without evidence of
            necrosis L97.226
          bone necrosis L97.224
          exposed fat layer L97.222
          muscle involvement without evidence of
            necrosis L97.225
          muscle necrosis L97.223
          skin breakdown only L97.221
          specified severity NEC L97.228
      right L97.219
        with
          bone involvement without evidence of
            necrosis L97.216
          bone necrosis L97.214
          exposed fat layer L97.212
          muscle involvement without evidence of
            necrosis L97.215
          muscle necrosis L97.213
          skin breakdown only L97.211
          specified severity NEC L97.218
    decubitus — see Ulcer, pressure, by site
    foot specified NEC L97.509
      with
        bone involvement without evidence of
          necrosis L97.506
        bone necrosis L97.504
        exposed fat layer L97.502
        muscle involvement without evidence of
          necrosis L97.505
        muscle necrosis L97.503
        skin breakdown only L97.501
        specified severity NEC L97.508
      left L97.529

Ulcer, ulcerated, ulcerating, ulceration, ulcerative
— continued
  lower limb — continued
    with
      bone involvement without evidence of
        necrosis L97.526
      bone necrosis L97.524
      exposed fat layer L97.522
      muscle involvement without evidence of
        necrosis L97.525
      muscle necrosis L97.523
      skin breakdown only L97.521
      specified severity NEC L97.528
    right L97.519
      with
        bone involvement without evidence of
          necrosis L97.516
        bone necrosis L97.514
        exposed fat layer L97.512
        muscle involvement without evidence of
          necrosis L97.515
        muscle necrosis L97.513
        skin breakdown only L97.511
        specified severity NEC L97.518
    heel L97.409
      with
        bone involvement without evidence of
          necrosis L97.406
        bone necrosis L97.404
        exposed fat layer L97.402
        muscle involvement without evidence of
          necrosis L97.405
        muscle necrosis L97.403
        skin breakdown only L97.401
        specified severity NEC L97.408
      left L97.429
        with
          bone involvement without evidence of
            necrosis L97.426
          bone necrosis L97.424
          exposed fat layer L97.422
          muscle involvement without evidence of
            necrosis L97.425
          muscle necrosis L97.423
          skin breakdown only L97.421
          specified severity NEC L97.428
      right L97.419
        with
          bone involvement without evidence of
            necrosis L97.416
          bone necrosis L97.414
          exposed fat layer L97.412
          muscle involvement without evidence of
            necrosis L97.415
          muscle necrosis L97.413
          skin breakdown only L97.411
          specified severity NEC L97.418
    left L97.929
      with
        bone involvement without evidence of
          necrosis L97.926
        bone necrosis L97.924
        exposed fat layer L97.922
        muscle involvement without evidence of
          necrosis L97.925
        muscle necrosis L97.923
        skin breakdown only L97.921
        specified severity NEC L97.928
    lower leg NOS L97.909
      with
        bone involvement without evidence of
          necrosis L97.906
        bone necrosis L97.904
        exposed fat layer L97.902
        muscle involvement without evidence of
          necrosis L97.905
        muscle necrosis L97.903
        skin breakdown only L97.901
        specified severity NEC L97.908
    left L97.929
      with
        bone involvement without evidence of
          necrosis L97.926
        bone necrosis L97.924
        exposed fat layer L97.922
        muscle involvement without evidence of
          necrosis L97.925
        muscle necrosis L97.923
        skin breakdown only L97.921
        specified severity NEC L97.928
    right L97.919
      with

Ulcer, ulcerated, ulcerating, ulceration, ulcerative
— continued
  lower limb — continued
      bone involvement without evidence of
        necrosis L97.916
      bone necrosis L97.914
      exposed fat layer L97.912
      muscle involvement without evidence of
        necrosis L97.915
      muscle necrosis L97.913
      skin breakdown only L97.911
      specified severity NEC L97.918
    specified site NEC L97.809
      with
        bone involvement without evidence of
          necrosis L97.806
        bone necrosis L97.804
        exposed fat layer L97.802
        muscle involvement without evidence of
          necrosis L97.805
        muscle necrosis L97.803
        skin breakdown only L97.801
        specified severity NEC L97.808
      left L97.829
        with
          bone involvement without evidence of
            necrosis L97.826
          bone necrosis L97.824
          exposed fat layer L97.822
          muscle involvement without evidence
            of necrosis L97.825
          muscle necrosis L97.823
          skin breakdown only L97.821
          specified severity NEC L97.828
      right L97.819
        with
          bone involvement without evidence of
            necrosis L97.816
          bone necrosis L97.814
          exposed fat layer L97.812
          muscle involvement without evidence
            of necrosis L97.815
          muscle necrosis L97.813
          skin breakdown only L97.811
          specified severity NEC L97.818
    midfoot L97.409
      with
        bone involvement without evidence of
          necrosis L97.406
        bone necrosis L97.404
        exposed fat layer L97.402
        muscle involvement without evidence of
          necrosis L97.405
        muscle necrosis L97.403
        skin breakdown only L97.401
        specified severity NEC L97.408
    left L97.429
      with
        bone involvement without evidence of
          necrosis L97.426
        bone necrosis L97.424
        exposed fat layer L97.422
        muscle involvement without evidence of
          necrosis L97.425
        muscle necrosis L97.423
        skin breakdown only L97.421
        specified severity NEC L97.428
    right L97.419
      with
        bone involvement without evidence of
          necrosis L97.416
        bone necrosis L97.414
        exposed fat layer L97.412
        muscle involvement without evidence of
          necrosis L97.415
        muscle necrosis L97.413
        skin breakdown only L97.411
        specified severity NEC L97.418
    right L97.919
      with
        bone involvement without evidence of
          necrosis L97.916
        bone necrosis L97.914
        exposed fat layer L97.912
        muscle involvement without evidence of
          necrosis L97.915
        muscle necrosis L97.913
        skin breakdown only L97.911
        specified severity NEC L97.918
    thigh L97.109
      with

☑ **Additional character required**

Ulcer, ulcerated, ulcerating, ulceration, ulcerative
— *continued*
  lower limb — *continued*
    bone involvement without evidence of
      necrosis L97.106
    bone necrosis L97.104
    muscle involvement without evidence of
      necrosis L97.105
    exposed fat layer L97.102
    muscle necrosis L97.103
    skin breakdown only L97.101
    specified severity NEC L97.108
   left L97.129
    with
      bone involvement without evidence of
        necrosis L97.126
      bone necrosis L97.124
      exposed fat layer L97.122
      muscle involvement without evidence of
        necrosis L97.125
      muscle necrosis L97.123
      skin breakdown only L97.121
      specified severity NEC L97.128
   right L97.119
    with
      bone involvement without evidence of
        necrosis L97.116
      bone necrosis L97.114
      exposed fat layer L97.112
      muscle involvement without evidence of
        necrosis L97.115
      muscle necrosis L97.113
      skin breakdown only L97.111
      specified severity NEC L97.118
   toe L97.509
    with
      bone involvement without evidence of
        necrosis L97.506
      bone necrosis L97.504
      exposed fat layer L97.502
      muscle involvement without evidence of
        necrosis L97.505
      muscle necrosis L97.503
      skin breakdown only L97.501
      specified severity NEC L97.508
    left L97.529
      with
        bone involvement without evidence of
          necrosis L97.526
        bone necrosis L97.524
        exposed fat layer L97.522
        muscle involvement without evidence of
          necrosis L97.525
        muscle necrosis L97.523
        skin breakdown only L97.521
        specified severity NEC L97.528
    right L97.519
      with
        bone involvement without evidence of
          necrosis L97.516
        bone necrosis L97.514
        exposed fat layer L97.512
        muscle involvement without evidence of
          necrosis L97.515
        muscle necrosis L97.513
        skin breakdown only L97.511
        specified severity NEC L97.518
  leprous A30.1
  syphilitic A52.19
  varicose — *see* Varix, leg, with, ulcer
  luetic — *see* Ulcer, syphilitic
  lung J98.4
   tuberculous — *see* Tuberculosis, pulmonary
  malignant — *see* Neoplasm, malignant, by site
  marginal NEC — *see* Ulcer, gastrojejunal
  meatus (urinarius) N34.2
  Meckel's diverticulum Q43.0
   malignant — *see* Table of Neoplasms, small
    intestine, malignant
  Meleney's (chronic undermining) — *see* Ulcer,
   skin
  Mooren's (cornea) — *see* Ulcer, cornea, Mooren's
  mycobacterial (skin) A31.1
  nasopharynx J39.2
  neck, uterus N86
  neurogenic NEC — *see* Ulcer, skin
  nose, nasal (passage) (infective) (septum) J34.0
   skin — *see* Ulcer, skin
   spirochetal A69.8
   varicose (bleeding) I86.8
  oral mucosa (traumatic) K12.1
  palate (soft) K12.1

Ulcer, ulcerated, ulcerating, ulceration, ulcerative
— *continued*
  penis (chronic) N48.5
  peptic (site unspecified) K27.9
   with
    hemorrhage K27.4
     and perforation K27.6
    perforation K27.5
   acute K27.3
    with
     hemorrhage K27.0
      and perforation K27.2
     perforation K27.1
   chronic K27.7
    with
     hemorrhage K27.4
      and perforation K27.6
     perforation K27.5
   esophagus K22.10
    with bleeding K22.11
   newborn P78.82
  perforating K27.5
   skin — *see* Ulcer, skin
  peritonsillar J35.8
  phagedenic (tropical) — *see* Ulcer, skin
  pharynx J39.2
  phlebitis — *see* Phlebitis
  plaster — *see* Ulcer, pressure, by site
  popliteal space — *see* Ulcer, lower limb
  postpyloric — *see* Ulcer, duodenum
  prepuce N47.7
  prepyloric — *see* Ulcer, stomach
  pressure (pressure area) L89.9 ☑
   ankle L89.5 ☑
   back L89.1 ☑
   buttock L89.3 ☑
   coccyx L89.15 ☑
   contiguous site of back, buttock, hip L89.4 ☑
   elbow L89.0 ☑
   face L89.81 ☑
   head L89.81 ☑
   heel L89.6 ☑
   hip L89.2 ☑
   sacral region (tailbone) L89.15 ☑
   specified site NEC L89.89 ☑
   stage 1 (healing) (pre-ulcer skin changes
    limited to persistent focal edema)
    ankle L89.5 ☑
    back L89.1 ☑
    buttock L89.3 ☑
    coccyx L89.15 ☑
    contiguous site of back, buttock, hip L89.4 ☑
    elbow L89.0 ☑
    face L89.81 ☑
    head L89.81 ☑
    heel L89.6 ☑
    hip L89.2 ☑
    sacral region (tailbone) L89.15 ☑
    specified site NEC L89.89 ☑
   stage 2 (healing) (abrasion, blister, partial
    thickness skin loss involving epidermis
    and/or dermis)
    ankle L89.5 ☑
    back L89.1 ☑
    buttock L89.3 ☑
    coccyx L89.15 ☑
    contiguous site of back, buttock, hip L89.4 ☑
    elbow L89.0 ☑
    face L89.81 ☑
    head L89.81 ☑
    heel L89.6 ☑
    hip L89.2 ☑
    sacral region (tailbone) L89.15 ☑
    specified site NEC L89.89 ☑
   stage 3 (healing) (full thickness skin loss
    involving damage or necrosis of
    subcutaneous tissue)
    ankle L89.5 ☑
    back L89.1 ☑
    buttock L89.3 ☑
    coccyx L89.15 ☑
    contiguous site of back, buttock, hip L89.4 ☑
    elbow L89.0 ☑
    face L89.81 ☑
    head L89.81 ☑
    heel L89.6 ☑
    hip L89.2 ☑
    sacral region (tailbone) L89.15 ☑
    specified site NEC L89.89 ☑
   stage 4 (healing) (necrosis of soft tissues
    through to underlying muscle, tendon, or
    bone)

Ulcer, ulcerated, ulcerating, ulceration, ulcerative
— *continued*
  pressure — *continued*
   ankle L89.5 ☑
   back L89.1 ☑
   buttock L89.3 ☑
   coccyx L89.15 ☑
   contiguous site of back, buttock, hip L89.4 ☑
   elbow L89.0 ☑
   face L89.81 ☑
   head L89.81 ☑
   heel L89.6 ☑
   hip L89.2 ☑
   sacral region (tailbone) L89.15 ☑
   specified site NEC L89.89 ☑
   unspecified stage
    ankle L89.5 ☑
    back L89.1 ☑
    buttock L89.3 ☑
    coccyx L89.15 ☑
    contiguous site of back, buttock, hip L89.4 ☑
    elbow L89.0 ☑
    face L89.81 ☑
    head L89.81 ☑
    heel L89.6 ☑
    hip L89.2 ☑
    sacral region (tailbone) L89.15 ☑
    specified site NEC L89.89 ☑
   unstageable
    ankle L89.5 ☑
    back L89.1 ☑
    buttock L89.3 ☑
    coccyx L89.15 ☑
    contiguous site of back, buttock, hip L89.4 ☑
    elbow L89.0 ☑
    face L89.81 ☑
    head L89.81 ☑
    heel L89.6 ☑
    hip L89.2 ☑
    sacral region (tailbone) L89.15 ☑
    specified site NEC L89.89 ☑
  primary of intestine K63.3
   with perforation K63.1
  prostate N41.9
  pyloric — *see* Ulcer, stomach
  rectosigmoid K63.3
   with perforation K63.1
  rectum (sphincter) (solitary) K62.6
   stercoraceous, stercoral K62.6
  retina — *see* Inflammation, chorioretinal
  rodent (*see also* Neoplasm, skin, malignant)
  sclera — *see* Scleritis
  scrofulous (tuberculous) A18.2
  scrotum N50.89
   tuberculous A18.15
   varicose I86.1
  seminal vesicle N50.89
  sigmoid — *see* Ulcer, intestine
  skin (atrophic) (chronic) (neurogenic) (non-
   healing) (perforating) (pyogenic) (trophic)
   (tropical) L98.499
   with gangrene — *see* Gangrene
   amebic A06.7
   back — *see* Ulcer, back
   buttock — *see* Ulcer, buttock
   decubitus — *see* Ulcer, pressure
   lower limb — *see* Ulcer, lower limb
   mycobacterial A31.1
   specified site NEC L98.499
    with
     bone involvement without evidence of
      necrosis L98.496
     bone necrosis L98.494
     exposed fat layer L98.492
     muscle involvement without evidence of
      necrosis L98.495
     muscle necrosis L98.493
     skin breakdown only L98.491
     specified severity NEC L98.498
   tuberculous (primary) A18.4
   varicose — *see* Ulcer, varicose
  sloughing — *see* Ulcer, skin
  solitary, anus or rectum (sphincter) K62.6
  sore throat J02.9
   streptococcal J02.0
  spermatic cord N50.89
  spine (tuberculous) A18.01
  stasis (venous) — *see* Varix, leg, with, ulcer
   without varicose veins I87.2
  stercoraceous, stercoral K63.3
   with perforation K63.1
   anus or rectum K62.6

Ulcer - Urethritis

Ulcer, ulcerated, ulcerating, ulceration, ulcerative — *continued*
  stoma, stomal — *see* Ulcer, gastrojejunal
  stomach (eroded) (peptic) (round) K25.9
    with
      hemorrhage K25.4
        and perforation K25.6
      perforation K25.5
    acute K25.3
      with
        hemorrhage K25.0
          and perforation K25.2
        perforation K25.1
    chronic K25.7
      with
        hemorrhage K25.4
          and perforation K25.6
        perforation K25.5
  stomal — *see* Ulcer, gastrojejunal
  stomatitis K12.1
  stress — *see* Ulcer, peptic
  strumous (tuberculous) A18.2
  submucosal, bladder — *see* Cystitis, interstitial
  syphilitic (any site) (early) (secondary) A51.39
    late A52.79
    perforating A52.79
      foot A52.11
  testis N50.89
  thigh — *see* Ulcer, lower limb
  throat J39.2
    diphtheritic A36.0
  toe — *see* Ulcer, lower limb
  tongue (traumatic) K14.0
  tonsil J35.8
    diphtheritic A36.0
  trachea J39.8
  trophic — *see* Ulcer, skin
  tropical — *see* Ulcer, skin
  tuberculous — *see* Tuberculosis, ulcer
  tunica vaginalis N50.89
  turbinate J34.89
  typhoid (perforating) — *see* Typhoid
  unspecified site — *see* Ulcer, skin
  urethra (meatus) — *see* Urethritis
  uterus N85.8
    cervix N86
      with cervicitis N72
    neck N86
      with cervicitis N72
  vagina N76.5
    in Behçet's disease M35.2 [N77.0]
    pessary N89.8
  valve, heart I33.0
  varicose (lower limb, any part) (*see also* Varix, leg, with, ulcer)
    broad ligament I86.2
    esophagus — *see* Varix, esophagus
    inflamed or infected — *see* Varix, leg, with ulcer, with inflammation
    nasal septum I86.8
    perineum I86.3
    scrotum I86.1
    specified site NEC I86.8
    sublingual I86.0
    vulva I86.3
  vas deferens N50.89
  vulva (acute) (infectional) N76.6
    in (due to)
      Behçet's disease M35.2 [N77.0]
      herpesviral (herpes simplex) infection A60.04
      tuberculosis A18.18
  vulvobuccal, recurring N76.6
  X-ray L58.1
  yaws A66.4
Ulcerosa scarlatina A38.8
Ulcus (*see also* Ulcer)
  cutis tuberculosum A18.4
  duodeni — *see* Ulcer, duodenum
  durum (syphilitic) A51.0
    extragenital A51.2
  gastrojejunale — *see* Ulcer, gastrojejunal
  hypostaticum — *see* Ulcer, varicose
  molle (cutis) (skin) A57
  serpens corneae — *see* Ulcer, cornea, central
  ventriculi — *see* Ulcer, stomach
Ulegyria Q04.8
Ulerythema
  ophryogenes, congenital Q84.2
  sycosiforme L73.8
Ullrich (-Bonnevie) (-Turner) syndrome (*see also* Turner's syndrome) Q87.1
Ullrich-Feichtiger syndrome Q87.0

Ulnar — *see* condition
Ulorrhagia, ulorrhea K06.8
Umbilicus, umbilical — *see* condition
Unacceptable
  contours of tooth K08.54
  morphology of tooth K08.54
Unavailability (of)
  bed at medical facility Z75.1
  health service-related agencies Z75.4
  medical facilities (at) Z75.3
    due to
      investigation by social service agency Z75.2
      lack of services at home Z75.0
      remoteness from facility Z75.3
      waiting list Z75.1
    home Z75.0
    outpatient clinic Z75.3
  schooling Z55.1
  social service agencies Z75.4
Uncinaria americana infestation B76.1
Uncinariasis B76.9
Uncongenial work Z56.5
Unconscious (ness) — *see* Coma
Under observation — *see* Observation
Underachievement in school Z55.3
Underdevelopment (*see also* Undeveloped)
  nose Q30.1
  sexual E30.0
Underdosing (*see also* Table of Drugs and Chemicals, categories T36-T50, with final character 6) Z91.14
  intentional NEC Z91.128
    due to financial hardship of patient Z91.120
  unintentional NEC Z91.138
    due to patient's age related debility Z91.130
Underfeeding, newborn P92.3
Underfill, endodontic M27.53
Underimmunization status Z28.3
Undernourishment — *see* Malnutrition
Undernutrition — *see* Malnutrition
Underweight R63.6
  for gestational age — *see* Light for dates
Underwood's disease P83.0
Undescended (*see also* Malposition, congenital)
  cecum Q43.3
  colon Q43.3
  testicle — *see* Cryptorchid
Undeveloped, undevelopment (*see also* Hypoplasia)
  brain (congenital) Q02
  cerebral (congenital) Q02
  heart Q24.8
  lung Q33.6
  testis E29.1
  uterus E30.0
Undiagnosed (disease) R69
Undulant fever — *see* Brucellosis
Unemployment, anxiety concerning Z56.0
  threatened Z56.2
Unequal length (acquired) (limb) (*see also* Deformity, limb, unequal length)
  leg (*see also* Deformity, limb, unequal length)
    congenital Q72.9 ☑
Unextracted dental root K08.3
Unguis incarnatus L60.0
Unhappiness R45.2
Unicornate uterus Q51.4
  in pregnancy or childbirth O34.00
Unilateral (*see also* condition)
  development, breast N64.89
  organ or site, congenital NEC — *see* Agenesis, by site
Unilocular heart Q20.8
Union, abnormal (*see also* Fusion)
  larynx and trachea Q34.8
Universal mesentery Q43.3
Unrepairable overhanging of dental restorative materials K08.52
Unsatisfactory
  restoration of tooth K08.50
    specified NEC K08.59
  sample of cytologic smear
    anus R85.615
    cervix R87.615
    vagina R87.625
  surroundings Z59.1
  work Z56.5
Unsoundness of mind — *see* Psychosis
Unstable
  back NEC — *see* Instability, joint, spine
  hip (congenital) Q65.6
    acquired — *see* Derangement, joint, specified type NEC, hip

Unstable — *continued*
  joint — *see* Instability, joint
    secondary to removal of joint prosthesis M96.89
  lie (mother) O32.0 ☑
  lumbosacral joint (congenital)
    acquired — *see* subcategory M53.2
  sacroiliac — *see* subcategory M53.2
  spine NEC — *see* Instability, joint, spine
Unsteadiness on feet R26.81
Untruthfulness, child problem F91.8
Unverricht (-Lundborg) disease or epilepsy — *see* Epilepsy, generalized, idiopathic
Unwanted pregnancy Z64.0
Upbringing, institutional Z62.22
  away from parents NEC Z62.29
  in care of non-parental family member Z62.21
  in foster care Z62.21
  in orphanage or group home Z62.22
  in welfare custody Z62.21
Upper respiratory — *see* condition
Upset
  gastric K30
  gastrointestinal K30
    psychogenic F45.8
  intestinal (large) (small) K59.9
    psychogenic F45.8
  menstruation N93.9
  mental F48.9
  stomach K30
    psychogenic F45.8
Urachus (*see also* condition)
  patent or persistent Q64.4
Urbach-Oppenheim disease (necrobiosis lipoidica diabeticorum) — *see* E08-E13 with .620
Urbach's lipoid proteinosis E78.89
Urbach-Wiethe disease E78.89
Urban yellow fever A95.1
Urea
  blood, high — *see* Uremia
  cycle metabolism disorder — *see* Disorder, urea cycle metabolism
Uremia, uremic N19
  with
    ectopic or molar pregnancy O08.4
    polyneuropathy N18.9 *[G63]*
  chronic NOS (*see also* Disease, kidney, chronic) N18.9
    due to hypertension — *see* Hypertensive, kidney
  complicating
    ectopic or molar pregnancy O08.4
  congenital P96.0
  extrarenal R39.2
  following ectopic or molar pregnancy O08.4
  newborn P96.0
  prerenal R39.2
Ureter, ureteral — *see* condition
Ureteralgia N23
Ureterectasis — *see* Hydroureter
Ureteritis N28.89
  cystica N28.86
  due to calculus N20.1
    with calculus, kidney N20.2
      with hydronephrosis N13.2
  gonococcal (acute) (chronic) A54.21
  nonspecific N28.89
Ureterocele N28.89
  congenital (orthotopic) Q62.31
    ectopic Q62.32
Ureterolith, ureterolithiasis — *see* Calculus, ureter
Ureterostomy
  attention to Z43.6
  status Z93.6
Urethra, urethral — *see* condition
Urethralgia R39.89
Urethritis (anterior) (posterior) N34.2
  calculous N21.1
  candidal B37.41
  chlamydial A56.01
  diplococcal (gonococcal) A54.01
    with abscess (accessory gland) (periurethral) A54.1
  gonococcal A54.01
    with abscess (accessory gland) (periurethral) A54.1
  nongonococcal N34.1
    Reiter's — *see* Reiter's disease
  nonspecific N34.1
  nonvenereal N34.1
  postmenopausal N34.2
  puerperal O86.22

☑ **Additional character required**

Urethritis — *continued*
Reiter's — *see* Reiter's disease
specified NEC N34.2
trichomonal or due to Trichomonas
(vaginalis) A59.03
Urethrocele N81.0
with
cystocele — *see* Cystocele
prolapse of uterus — *see* Prolapse, uterus
Urethrolithiasis (with colic or infection) N21.1
Urethrorectal — *see* condition
Urethrorrhagia N36.8
Urethrorrhea R36.9
Urethrostomy
attention to Z43.6
status Z93.6
Urethrotrigonitis — *see* Trigonitis
Urethrovaginal — *see* condition
Urgency
fecal R15.2
hypertensive — *see* Hypertension
urinary R39.15
Urhidrosis, uridrosis L74.8
Uric acid in blood (increased) E79.0
Uricacidemia (asymptomatic) E79.0
Uricemia (asymptomatic) E79.0
Uricosuria R82.99
Urinary — *see* condition
Urination
frequent R35.0
painful R30.9
Urine
blood in — *see* Hematuria
discharge, excessive R35.8
enuresis, nonorganic origin F98.0
extravasation R39.0
frequency R35.0
incontinence R32
nonorganic origin F98.0
intermittent stream R39.198
pus in N39.0
retention or stasis R33.9
organic R33.8
drug-induced R33.0
psychogenic F45.8
secretion
deficient R34
excessive R35.8
frequency R35.0
stream
intermittent R39.198
slowing R39.198
splitting R39.13
weak R39.12
Urinemia — *see* Uremia
Urinoma, urethra N36.8
Uroarthritis, infectious (Reiter's) — *see* Reiter's
disease
Urodialysis R34
Urolithiasis — *see* Calculus, urinary
Uronephrosis — *see* Hydronephrosis
Uropathy N39.9
obstructive N13.9
specified NEC N13.8
reflux N13.9
specified NEC N13.8
vesicoureteral reflux-associated — *see* Reflux,
vesicoureteral
Urosepsis - code to condition
Urticaria L50.9
with angioneurotic edema T78.3 ☑
hereditary D84.1
allergic L50.0
cholinergic L50.5
chronic L50.8
cold, familial L50.2
contact L50.6
dermatographic L50.3
due to
cold or heat L50.2
drugs L50.0
food L50.0
inhalants L50.0
plants L50.6
serum (*see also* Reaction, serum) T80.69 ☑
factitial L50.3
familial cold M04.2
giant T78.3 ☑
hereditary D84.1
gigantea T78.3 ☑
idiopathic L50.1

Urticaria — *continued*
larynx T78.3 ☑
hereditary D84.1
neonatorum P83.88
nonallergic L50.1
papulosa (Hebra) L28.2
pigmentosa D47.01
congenital Q82.2
of neonatal onset Q82.2
of newborn onset Q82.2
recurrent periodic L50.8
serum (*see also* Reaction, serum) T80.69 ☑
solar L56.3
specified type NEC L50.8
thermal (cold) (heat) L50.2
vibratory L50.4
xanthelasmoidea — *see* Urticaria pigmentosa
Use (of)
alcohol Z72.89
with
intoxication F10.929
sleep disorder F10.982
harmful — *see* Abuse, alcohol
amphetamines — *see* Use, stimulant NEC
caffeine — *see* Use, stimulant NEC
cannabis F12.90
with
anxiety disorder F12.980
intoxication F12.929
with
delirium F12.921
perceptual disturbance F12.922
uncomplicated F12.920
other specified disorder F12.988
psychosis F12.959
delusions F12.950
hallucinations F12.951
unspecified disorder F12.99
cocaine F14.90
with
anxiety disorder F14.980
intoxication F14.929
with
delirium F14.921
perceptual disturbance F14.922
uncomplicated F14.920
other specified disorder F14.988
psychosis F14.959
delusions F14.950
hallucinations F14.951
sexual dysfunction F14.981
sleep disorder F14.982
unspecified disorder F14.99
harmful — *see* Abuse, drug, cocaine
drug (s) NEC F19.90
with sleep disorder F19.982
harmful — *see* Abuse, drug, by type
hallucinogen NEC F16.90
with
anxiety disorder F16.980
intoxication F16.929
with
delirium F16.921
uncomplicated F16.920
mood disorder F16.94
other specified disorder F16.988
perception disorder (flashbacks) F16.983
psychosis F16.959
delusions F16.950
hallucinations F16.951
unspecified disorder F16.99
harmful — *see* Abuse, drug, hallucinogen NEC
inhalants F18.90
with
anxiety disorder F18.980
intoxication F18.929
with delirium F18.921
uncomplicated F18.920
mood disorder F18.94
other specified disorder F18.988
persisting dementia F18.97
psychosis F18.959
delusions F18.950
hallucinations F18.951
unspecified disorder F18.99
harmful — *see* Abuse, drug, inhalant
methadone — *see* Use, opioid
nonprescribed drugs F19.90
harmful — *see* Abuse, non-psychoactive
substance
opioid F11.90
with

Use — *continued*
opioid — *continued*
disorder F11.99
mood F11.94
sleep F11.982
specified type NEC F11.988
intoxication F11.929
with
delirium F11.921
perceptual disturbance F11.922
uncomplicated F11.920
withdrawal F11.93
harmful — *see* Abuse, drug, opioid
patent medicines F19.90
harmful — *see* Abuse, non-psychoactive
substance
psychoactive drug NEC F19.90
with
anxiety disorder F19.980
intoxication F19.929
with
delirium F19.921
perceptual disturbance F19.922
uncomplicated F19.920
mood disorder F19.94
other specified disorder F19.988
persisting
amnestic disorder F19.96
dementia F19.97
psychosis F19.959
delusions F19.950
hallucinations F19.951
sexual dysfunction F19.981
sleep disorder F19.982
unspecified disorder F19.99
withdrawal F19.939
with
delirium F19.931
perceptual disturbance F19.932
uncomplicated F19.930
harmful — *see* Abuse, drug NEC, psychoactive
NEC
sedative, hypnotic, or anxiolytic F13.90
with
anxiety disorder F13.980
intoxication F13.929
with
delirium F13.921
uncomplicated F13.920
other specified disorder F13.988
persisting
amnestic disorder F13.96
dementia F13.97
psychosis F13.959
delusions F13.950
hallucinations F13.951
sexual dysfunction F13.981
sleep disorder F13.982
unspecified disorder F13.99
harmful — *see* Abuse, drug, sedative, hypnotic,
or anxiolytic
stimulant NEC F15.90
with
anxiety disorder F15.980
intoxication F15.929
with
delirium F15.921
perceptual disturbance F15.922
uncomplicated F15.920
mood disorder F15.94
other specified disorder F15.988
psychosis F15.959
delusions F15.950
hallucinations F15.951
sexual dysfunction F15.981
sleep disorder F15.982
unspecified disorder F15.99
withdrawal F15.93
harmful — *see* Abuse, drug, stimulant NEC
tobacco Z72.0
with dependence — *see* Dependence, drug,
nicotine
volatile solvents (*see also* Use, inhalant) F18.90
harmful — *see* Abuse, drug, inhalant
Usher-Senear disease or syndrome L10.4
Uta B55.1
Uteromegaly N85.2
Uterovaginal — *see* condition
Uterovesical — *see* condition
Uveal — *see* condition
Uveitis (anterior) (*see also* Iridocyclitis)
acute — *see* Iridocyclitis, acute

Uveitis — *continued*
　chronic — *see* Iridocyclitis, chronic
　due to toxoplasmosis (acquired) B58.09
　　congenital P37.1
　granulomatous — *see* Iridocyclitis, chronic
　heterochromic — *see* Cyclitis, Fuchs'
　　heterochromic
　lens-induced — *see* Iridocyclitis, lens-induced
　posterior — *see* Chorioretinitis
　sympathetic H44.13 ☑
　syphilitic (secondary) A51.43
　　congenital (early) A50.01
　　late A52.71
　tuberculous A18.54
Uveoencephalitis — *see* Inflammation, chorioretinal
Uveokeratitis — *see* Iridocyclitis
Uveoparotitis D86.89
Uvula — *see* condition
Uvulitis (acute) (catarrhal) (chronic) (membranous)
　(suppurative) (ulcerative) K12.2

V

Vaccination (prophylactic)
　complication or reaction — *see* Complications,
　　vaccination
　delayed Z28.9
　encounter for Z23
　not done — *see* Immunization, not done, because
　　(of)
Vaccinia (generalized) (localized) T88.1 ☑
　congenital P35.8
　without vaccination B08.011
Vacuum, in sinus (accessory) (nasal) J34.89
Vagabond, vagabondage Z59.0
Vagabond's disease B85.1
Vagina, vaginal — *see* condition
Vaginalitis (tunica) (testis) N49.1
Vaginismus (reflex) N94.2
　functional F52.5
　nonorganic F52.5
　psychogenic F52.5
　secondary N94.2
Vaginitis (acute) (circumscribed) (diffuse)
　(emphysematous) (nonvenereal) (ulcerative) N76.0
　with ectopic or molar pregnancy O08.0
　amebic A06.82
　atrophic, postmenopausal N95.2
　bacterial N76.0
　blennorrhagic (gonococcal) A54.02
　candidal B37.3
　chlamydial A56.02
　chronic N76.1
　due to Trichomonas (vaginalis) A59.01
　following ectopic or molar pregnancy O08.0
　gonococcal A54.02
　　with abscess (accessory gland)
　　　(periurethral) A54.1
　granuloma A58
　in (due to)
　　candidiasis B37.3
　　herpesviral (herpes simplex) infection A60.04
　　pinworm infection B80 [N77.1]
　monilial B37.3
　mycotic (candidal) B37.3
　postmenopausal atrophic N95.2
　puerperal (postpartum) O86.13
　senile (atrophic) N95.2
　subacute or chronic N76.1
　syphilitic (early) A51.0
　　late A52.76
　trichomonal A59.01
　tuberculous A18.18
Vaginosis — *see* Vaginitis
Vagotonia G52.2
Vagrancy Z59.0
VAIN — *see* Neoplasia, intraepithelial, vagina
Vallecula — *see* condition
Valley fever B38.0
Valsuani's disease — *see* Anemia, obstetric
Valve, valvular (formation) (*see also* condition)
　cerebral ventricle (communicating) in situ Z98.2
　cervix, internal os Q51.828
　congenital NEC — *see* Atresia, by site
　ureter (pelvic junction) (vesical orifice) Q62.39
　urethra (congenital) (posterior) Q64.2
Valvulitis (chronic) — *see* Endocarditis
Valvulopathy — *see* Endocarditis
Van Bogaert's leukoencephalopathy (sclerosing)
　(subacute) A81.1

Van Bogaert-Scherer-Epstein disease or syndrome
　E75.5
Van Buchem's syndrome M85.2
Van Creveld-von Gierke disease E74.01
Van der Hoeve (-de Kleyn) syndrome Q78.0
Van der Woude's syndrome Q38.0
Van Neck's disease or osteochondrosis M91.0
Vanishing lung J44.9
Vapor asphyxia or suffocation T59.9 ☑
　specified agent — *see* Table of Drugs and Chemicals
Variance, lethal ball, prosthetic heart valve T82.09 ☑
Variants, thalassemic D56.8
Variations in hair color L67.1
Varicella B01.9
　with
　　complications NEC B01.89
　　encephalitis B01.11
　　encephalomyelitis B01.11
　　meningitis B01.0
　　myelitis B01.12
　　pneumonia B01.2
　congenital P35.8
Varices — *see* Varix
Varicocele (scrotum) (thrombosed) I86.1
　ovary I86.2
　perineum I86.3
　spermatic cord (ulcerated) I86.1
Varicose
　aneurysm (ruptured) I77.0
　dermatitis — *see* Varix, leg, with, inflammation
　eczema — *see* Varix, leg, with, inflammation
　phlebitis — *see* Varix, with, inflammation
　tumor — *see* Varix
　ulcer (lower limb, any part) (*see also* Varix, leg,
　　with, ulcer)
　　anus (*see also* Hemorrhoids) K64.8
　　esophagus — *see* Varix, esophagus
　　inflamed or infected — *see* Varix, leg, with ulcer,
　　　with inflammation
　　nasal septum I86.8
　　perineum I86.3
　　scrotum I86.1
　　specified site NEC I86.8
　vein — *see* Varix
　vessel — *see* Varix, leg
Varicosis, varicosities, varicosity — *see* Varix
Variola (major) (minor) B03
Varioloid B03
Varix (lower limb) (ruptured) I83.90
　with
　　edema I83.899
　　inflammation I83.10
　　　with ulcer (venous) I83.209
　　pain I83.819
　　specified complication NEC I83.899
　　stasis dermatitis I83.10
　　　with ulcer (venous) I83.209
　　swelling I83.899
　　ulcer I83.009
　　　with inflammation I83.209
　aneurysmal I77.0
　asymptomatic I83.9 ☑
　bladder I86.2
　broad ligament I86.2
　complicating
　　childbirth (lower extremity) O87.4
　　　anus or rectum O87.2
　　　genital (vagina, vulva or perineum) O87.8
　　pregnancy (lower extremity) O22.0 ☑
　　　anus or rectum O22.4 ☑
　　　genital (vagina, vulva or perineum) O22.1 ☑
　　puerperium (lower extremity) O87.4
　　　anus or rectum O87.2
　　　genital (vagina, vulva, perineum) O87.8
　congenital (any site) Q27.8
　esophagus (idiopathic) (primary)
　　(ulcerated) I85.00
　　bleeding I85.01
　　congenital Q27.8
　　in (due to)
　　　alcoholic liver disease I85.10
　　　　bleeding I85.11
　　　cirrhosis of liver I85.10
　　　　bleeding I85.11
　　　portal hypertension I85.10
　　　　bleeding I85.11
　　　schistosomiasis I85.10
　　　　bleeding I85.11
　　　toxic liver disease I85.10
　　　　bleeding I85.11
　　secondary I85.10
　　　bleeding I85.11

Varix — *continued*
　gastric I86.4
　inflamed or infected I83.10
　　ulcerated I83.209
　labia (majora) I86.3
　leg (asymptomatic) I83.90
　　with
　　　edema I83.899
　　　inflammation I83.10
　　　　with ulcer — *see* Varix, leg, with, ulcer, with
　　　　　inflammation by site
　　　pain I83.819
　　　specified complication NEC I83.899
　　　swelling I83.899
　　　ulcer I83.009
　　　　with inflammation I83.209
　　　　ankle I83.003
　　　　　with inflammation I83.203
　　　　calf I83.002
　　　　　with inflammation I83.202
　　　　foot NEC I83.005
　　　　　with inflammation I83.205
　　　　heel I83.004
　　　　　with inflammation I83.204
　　　　lower leg NEC I83.008
　　　　　with inflammation I83.208
　　　　midfoot I83.004
　　　　　with inflammation I83.204
　　　　thigh I83.001
　　　　　with inflammation I83.201
　　bilateral (asymptomatic) I83.93
　　　with
　　　　edema I83.893
　　　　pain I83.813
　　　　specified complication NEC I83.893
　　　　swelling I83.893
　　　　ulcer I83.0 ☑
　　　　　with inflammation I83.209
　　left (asymptomatic) I83.92
　　　with
　　　　edema I83.892
　　　　pain I83.812
　　　　specified complication NEC I83.892
　　　　swelling I83.892
　　　　inflammation I83.12
　　　　　with ulcer — *see* Varix, leg, with, ulcer,
　　　　　　with inflammation by site
　　　　ulcer I83.029
　　　　　with inflammation I83.229
　　　　　ankle I83.023
　　　　　　with inflammation I83.223
　　　　　calf I83.022
　　　　　　with inflammation I83.222
　　　　　foot NEC I83.025
　　　　　　with inflammation I83.225
　　　　　heel I83.024
　　　　　　with inflammation I83.224
　　　　　lower leg NEC I83.028
　　　　　　with inflammation I83.228
　　　　　midfoot I83.024
　　　　　　with inflammation I83.224
　　　　　thigh I83.021
　　　　　　with inflammation I83.221
　　right (asymptomatic) I83.91
　　　with
　　　　edema I83.891
　　　　pain I83.811
　　　　specified complication NEC I83.891
　　　　swelling I83.891
　　　　inflammation I83.11
　　　　　with ulcer — *see* Varix, leg, with, ulcer,
　　　　　　with inflammation by site
　　　　ulcer I83.019
　　　　　with inflammation I83.219
　　　　　ankle I83.013
　　　　　　with inflammation I83.213
　　　　　calf I83.012
　　　　　　with inflammation I83.212
　　　　　foot NEC I83.015
　　　　　　with inflammation I83.215
　　　　　heel I83.014
　　　　　　with inflammation I83.214
　　　　　lower leg NEC I83.018
　　　　　　with inflammation I83.218
　　　　　midfoot I83.014
　　　　　　with inflammation I83.214
　　　　　thigh I83.011
　　　　　　with inflammation I83.211
　nasal septum I86.8
　orbit I86.8
　　congenital Q27.8
　ovary I86.2

Varix — *continued*
 papillary I78.1
 pelvis I86.2
 perineum I86.3
 pharynx I86.8
 placenta O43.89 ☑
 renal papilla I86.8
 retina H35.09
 scrotum (ulcerated) I86.1
 sigmoid colon I86.8
 specified site NEC I86.8
 spinal (cord) (vessels) I86.8
 spleen, splenic (vein) (with phlebolith) I86.8
 stomach I86.4
 sublingual I86.0
 ulcerated I83.009
  inflamed or infected I83.209
 uterine ligament I86.2
 vagina I86.8
 vocal cord I86.8
 vulva I86.3
Vas deferens — *see* condition
Vas deferentitis N49.1
Vasa previa O69.4 ☑
 hemorrhage from, affecting newborn P50.0
Vascular (*see also* condition)
 loop on optic papilla Q14.2
 spasm I73.9
 spider I78.1
Vascularization, cornea — *see* Neovascularization, cornea
Vasculitis I77.6
 allergic D69.0
 cryoglobulinemic D89.1
 disseminated I77.6
 hypocomplementemic M31.8
 kidney I77.89
 livedoid L95.0
 nodular L95.8
 retina H35.06 ☑
 rheumatic — *see* Fever, rheumatic
 rheumatoid — *see* Rheumatoid, vasculitis
 skin (limited to) L95.9
  specified NEC L95.8
 systemic M31.8
Vasculopathy, necrotizing M31.9
 cardiac allograft T86.290
 specified NEC M31.8
Vasitis (nodosa) N49.1
 tuberculous A18.15
Vasodilation I73.9
Vasomotor — *see* condition
Vasoplasty, after previous sterilization Z31.0
 aftercare Z31.42
Vasospasm (vasoconstriction) I73.9
 cerebral (cerebrovascular) (artery) I67.848
  reversible I67.841
 coronary I20.1
 nerve
  arm — *see* Mononeuropathy, upper limb
  brachial plexus G54.0
  cervical plexus G54.2
  leg — *see* Mononeuropathy, lower limb
 peripheral NOS I73.9
 retina (artery) — *see* Occlusion, artery, retina
Vasospastic — *see* condition
Vasovagal attack (paroxysmal) R55
 psychogenic F45.8
VATER syndrome Q87.2
Vater's ampulla — *see* condition
Vegetation, vegetative
 adenoid (nasal fossa) J35.8
 endocarditis (acute) (any valve) (subacute) I33.0
 heart (mycotic) (valve) I33.0
Veil
 Jackson's Q43.3
Vein, venous — *see* condition
Veldt sore — *see* Ulcer, skin
Velpeau's hernia — *see* Hernia, femoral
Venereal
 bubo A55
 disease A64
 granuloma inguinale A58
 lymphogranuloma (Durand-Nicolas-Favre) A55
Venofibrosis I87.8
Venom, venomous — *see* Table of Drugs and Chemicals, by animal or substance, poisoning
Venous — *see* condition
Ventilator lung, newborn P27.8
Ventral — *see* condition
Ventricle, ventricular (*see also* condition)
 escape I49.3

Ventricle — *continued*
 inversion Q20.5
Ventriculitis (cerebral) (*see also* Encephalitis) G04.90
Ventriculostomy status Z98.2
Vernet's syndrome G52.7
Verneuil's disease (syphilitic bursitis) A52.78
Verruca (due to HPV) (filiformis) (simplex) (viral) (vulgaris) B07.9
 acuminata A63.0
 necrogenica (primary) (tuberculosa) A18.4
 plana B07.8
 plantaris B07.0
 seborrheica L82.1
  inflamed L82.0
 senile (seborrheic) L82.1
  inflamed L82.0
 tuberculosa (primary) A18.4
 venereal A63.0
Verrucosities — *see* Verruca
Verruga peruana, peruviana A44.1
Version
 with extraction
 cervix — *see* Malposition, uterus
 uterus (postinfectional) (postpartal, old) — *see* Malposition, uterus
Vertebra, vertebral — *see* condition
Vertical talus (congenital) Q66.80
 left foot Q66.82
 right foot Q66.81
Vertigo R42
 auditory — *see* Vertigo, aural
 aural H81.31 ☑
 benign paroxysmal (positional) H81.1 ☑
 central (origin) H81.4 ☑
 cerebral H81.4 ☑
 Dix and Hallpike (epidemic) — *see* Neuronitis, vestibular
 due to infrasound T75.23 ☑
 epidemic A88.1
  Dix and Hallpike — *see* Neuronitis, vestibular
  Pedersen's — *see* Neuronitis, vestibular
  vestibular neuronitis — *see* Neuronitis, vestibular
 hysterical F44.89
 infrasound T75.23 ☑
 labyrinthine — *see* subcategory H81.0
 laryngeal R05
 malignant positional H81.4 ☑
 Ménière's — *see* subcategory H81.0
 menopausal N95.1
 otogenic — *see* Vertigo, aural
 paroxysmal positional, benign — *see* Vertigo, benign paroxysmal
 Pedersen's (epidemic) — *see* Neuronitis, vestibular
 peripheral NEC H81.39 ☑
 positional
  benign paroxysmal — *see* Vertigo, benign paroxysmal
  malignant H81.4 ☑
Very-low-density-lipoprotein-type (VLDL)
 hyperlipoproteinemia E78.1
Vesania — *see* Psychosis
Vesical — *see* condition
Vesicle
 cutaneous R23.8
 seminal — *see* condition
 skin R23.8
Vesicocolic — *see* condition
Vesicoperineal — *see* condition
Vesicorectal — *see* condition
Vesicourethrorectal — *see* condition
Vesicovaginal — *see* condition
Vesicular — *see* condition
Vesiculitis (seminal) N49.0
 amebic A06.82
 gonorrheal (acute) (chronic) A54.23
 trichomonal A59.09
 tuberculous A18.15
Vestibulitis (ear) (*see also* subcategory) H83.0 ☑
 nose (external) J34.89
 vulvar N94.810
Vestibulopathy, acute peripheral (recurrent) — *see* Neuronitis, vestibular
Vestige, vestigial (*see also* Persistence)
 branchial Q18.0
 structures in vitreous Q14.0
Vibration
 adverse effects T75.20 ☑
  pneumatic hammer syndrome T75.21 ☑
  specified effect NEC T75.29 ☑

Vibration — *continued*
 adverse effects — *continued*
  vasospastic syndrome T75.22 ☑
  vertigo from infrasound T75.23 ☑
 exposure (occupational) Z57.7
 vertigo T75.23 ☑
Vibriosis A28.9
Victim (of)
 crime Z65.4
 disaster Z65.5
 terrorism Z65.4
 torture Z65.4
 war Z65.5
Vidal's disease L28.0
Villaret's syndrome G52.7
Villous — *see* condition
VIN — *see* Neoplasia, intraepithelial, vulva
Vincent's infection (angina) (gingivitis) A69.1
 stomatitis NEC A69.1
Vinson-Plummer syndrome D50.1
Violence, physical R45.6
Viosterol deficiency — *see* Deficiency, calciferol
Vipoma — *see* Neoplasm, malignant, by site
Viremia B34.9
Virilism (adrenal) E25.9
 congenital E25.0
Virilization (female) (suprarenal) E25.9
 congenital E25.0
 isosexual E28.2
Virulent bubo A57
Virus, viral (*see also* condition)
 as cause of disease classified elsewhere B97.89
 cytomegalovirus B25.9
 human immunodeficiency (HIV) — *see* Human, immunodeficiency virus (HIV) disease
 infection — *see* Infection, virus
 specified NEC B34.8
 swine influenza (viruses that normally cause infections in pigs) (*see also* Influenza, due to, identified novel influenza A virus) J09.X2
 West Nile (fever) A92.30
  with
   complications NEC A92.39
   cranial nerve disorders A92.32
   encephalitis A92.31
   encephalomyelitis A92.31
   neurologic manifestation NEC A92.32
   optic neuritis A92.32
   polyradiculitis A92.32
Viscera, visceral — *see* condition
Visceroptosis K63.4
Visible peristalsis R19.2
Vision, visual
 binocular, suppression H53.34
 blurred, blurring H53.8
  hysterical F44.6
 defect, defective NEC H54.7
 disorientation (syndrome) H53.8
 disturbance H53.9
  hysterical F44.6
 double H53.2
 examination Z01.00
  with abnormal findings Z01.01
 field, limitation (defect) — *see* Defect, visual field
 hallucinations R44.1
 halos H53.19
 loss — *see* Loss, vision
  sudden — *see* Disturbance, vision, subjective, loss, sudden
 low (both eyes) — *see* Low, vision
 perception, simultaneous without fusion H53.33
Vitality, lack or want of R53.83
 newborn P96.89
Vitamin deficiency — *see* Deficiency, vitamin
Vitelline duct, persistent Q43.0
Vitiligo L80
 eyelid H02.739
  left H02.736
   lower H02.735
   upper H02.734
  right H02.733
   lower H02.732
   upper H02.731
 pinta A67.2
 vulva N90.89
Vitreal corneal syndrome H59.01 ☑
Vitreoretinopathy, proliferative (*see also* Retinopathy, proliferative)
 with retinal detachment — *see* Detachment, retina, traction

Vitreous - Wernicke-Korsakoff's

Vitreous (see also condition)
  touch syndrome — see Complication, postprocedural, following cataract surgery
Vocal cord — see condition
Vogt-Koyanagi syndrome H20.82 ☑
Vogt's disease or syndrome G80.3
Vogt-Spielmeyer amaurotic idiocy or disease E75.4
Voice
  change R49.9
    specified NEC R49.8
  loss — see Aphonia
Volhynian fever A79.0
Volkmann's ischemic contracture or paralysis (complicating trauma) T79.6 ☑
Volvulus (bowel) (colon) (intestine) K56.2
  with perforation K56.2
  congenital Q43.8
  duodenum K31.5
  fallopian tube — see Torsion, fallopian tube
  oviduct — see Torsion, fallopian tube
  stomach (due to absence of gastrocolic ligament) K31.89
Vomiting R11.10
  with nausea R11.2
  asphyxia — see Foreign body, by site, causing asphyxia, gastric contents
  bilious (cause unknown) R11.14
    in newborn P92.01
    following gastro-intestinal surgery K91.0
  blood — see Hematemesis
  causing asphyxia, choking, or suffocation — see Foreign body, by site
  cyclical G43.A0
    with refractory migraine G43.A1
    intractable G43.A1
    not intractable G43.A0
    psychogenic F50.89
    without refractory migraine G43.A0
  fecal mater R11.13
  following gastrointestinal surgery K91.0
    psychogenic F50.89
  functional K31.89
  hysterical F50.89
  nervous F50.89
  neurotic F50.89
  newborn NEC P92.09
    bilious P92.01
  periodic R11.10
    psychogenic F50.89
  projectile R11.12
  psychogenic F50.89
  uremic — see Uremia
  without nausea R11.11
Vomito negro — see Fever, yellow
Von Bezold's abscess — see Mastoiditis, acute
Von Economo-Cruchet disease A85.8
Von Eulenburg's disease G71.19
Von Gierke's disease E74.01
Von Hippel (-Lindau) disease or syndrome Q85.8
Von Jaksch's anemia or disease D64.89
Von Recklinghausen
  disease (neurofibromatosis) Q85.01
    bones E21.0
Von Schroetter's syndrome I82.890
Von Willebrand (-Jurgens) (-Minot) disease or syndrome D68.0
Von Zumbusch's disease L40.1
Voyeurism F65.3
Vrolik's disease Q78.0
Vulva — see condition
Vulvismus N94.2
Vulvitis (acute) (allergic) (atrophic) (hypertrophic) (intertriginous) (senile) N76.2
  with ectopic or molar pregnancy O08.0
  adhesive, congenital Q52.79
  blennorrhagic (gonococcal) A54.02
  candidal B37.3
  chlamydial A56.02
  due to Haemophilus ducreyi A57
  following ectopic or molar pregnancy O08.0
  gonococcal A54.02
    with abscess (accessory gland) (periurethral) A54.1
  herpesviral A60.04
  leukoplakic N90.4
  monilial B37.3
  puerperal (postpartum) O86.19
  subacute or chronic N76.3
  syphilitic (early) A51.0
    late A52.76
  trichomonal A59.01
  tuberculous A18.18

Vulvodynia N94.819
  specified NEC N94.818
Vulvorectal — see condition
Vulvovaginitis (acute) — see Vaginitis

W

Waiting list, person on Z75.1
  for organ transplant Z76.82
  undergoing social agency investigation Z75.2
Waldenström-Kjellberg syndrome D50.1
Waldenström
  hypergammaglobulinemia D89.0
  syndrome or macroglobulinemia C88.0
Walking
  difficulty R26.2
    psychogenic F44.4
  sleep F51.3
    hysterical F44.89
Wall, abdominal — see condition
Wallenberg's disease or syndrome G46.3
Wallgren's disease I87.8
Wandering
  gallbladder, congenital Q44.1
  in diseases classified elsewhere Z91.83
  kidney, congenital Q63.8
  organ or site, congenital NEC — see Malposition, congenital, by site
  pacemaker (heart) I49.8
  spleen D73.89
War neurosis F48.8
Wart (due to HPV) (filiform) (infectious) (viral) B07.9
  anogenital region (venereal) A63.0
  common B07.8
  external genital organs (venereal) A63.0
  flat B07.8
  Hassal-Henle's (of cornea) H18.49
  Peruvian A44.1
  plantar B07.0
  prosector (tuberculous) A18.4
  seborrheic L82.1
    inflamed L82.0
  senile (seborrheic) L82.1
    inflamed L82.0
  tuberculous A18.4
  venereal A63.0
Warthin's tumor — see Neoplasm, salivary gland, benign
Wassilieff's disease A27.0
Wasting
  disease R64
    due to malnutrition E41
  extreme (due to malnutrition) E41
  muscle NEC — see Atrophy, muscle
Water
  clefts (senile cataract) — see Cataract, senile, incipient
  deprivation of T73.1 ☑
  intoxication E87.79
  itch B76.9
  lack of T73.1 ☑
  loading E87.70
  on
    brain — see Hydrocephalus
    chest J94.8
  poisoning E87.79
Waterbrash R12
Waterhouse (-Friderichsen) syndrome or disease (meningococcal) A39.1
Water-losing nephritis N25.89
Watermelon stomach K31.819
  with hemorrhage K31.811
  without hemorrhage K31.819
Watsoniasis B66.8
Wax in ear — see Impaction, cerumen
Weak, weakening, weakness (generalized) R53.1
  arches (acquired) (see also Deformity, limb, flat foot)
  bladder (sphincter) R32
  facial R29.810
    following
      cerebrovascular disease I69.992
        cerebral infarction I69.392
        intracerebral hemorrhage I69.192
        nontraumatic intracranial hemorrhage NEC I69.292
        specified disease NEC I69.892
        stroke I69.392
        subarachnoid hemorrhage I69.092
  foot (double) — see Weak, arches

Weak — continued
  heart, cardiac — see Failure, heart
  mind F70
  muscle M62.81
  myocardium — see Failure, heart
  newborn P96.89
  pelvic fundus N81.89
  pubocervical tissue N81.82
  senile R54
  rectovaginal tissue N81.83
  urinary stream R39.12
  valvular — see Endocarditis
Wear, worn (with normal or routine use)
  articular bearing surface of internal joint prosthesis — see Complications, joint prosthesis, mechanical, wear of articular bearing surfaces, by site
  device, implant or graft — see Complications, by site, mechanical complication
  tooth, teeth (approximal) (hard tissues) (interproximal) (occlusal) K03.0
Weather, weathered
  effects of
    cold T69.9 ☑
      specified effect NEC T69.8 ☑
    hot — see Heat
  skin L57.8
Weaver's syndrome Q87.3
Web, webbed (congenital)
  duodenal Q43.8
  esophagus Q39.4
  fingers Q70.1 ☑
  larynx (glottic) (subglottic) Q31.0
  neck (pterygium colli) Q18.3
  Paterson-Kelly D50.1
  popliteal syndrome Q87.89
  toes Q70.3 ☑
Weber-Christian disease M35.6
Weber-Cockayne syndrome (epidermolysis bullosa) Q81.8
Weber-Gubler syndrome G46.3
Weber-Leyden syndrome G46.3
Weber-Osler syndrome I78.0
Weber's paralysis or syndrome G46.3
Wedge-shaped or wedging vertebra — see Collapse, vertebra NEC
Wegener's granulomatosis or syndrome M31.30
  with
    kidney involvement M31.31
    lung involvement M31.30
      with kidney involvement M31.31
Wegner's disease A50.02
Weight
  1000-2499 grams at birth (low) — see Low, birthweight
  999 grams or less at birth (extremely low) — see Low, birthweight, extreme
  and length below 10th percentile for gestational age P05.1 ☑
  below but length above 10th percentile for gestational age P05.0 ☑
  gain (abnormal) (excessive) R63.5
    in pregnancy — see Pregnancy, complicated by, excessive weight gain
    low — see Pregnancy, complicated by, insufficient, weight gain
  loss (abnormal) (cause unknown) R63.4
Weightlessness (effect of) T75.82 ☑
Weil (l)-Marchesani syndrome Q87.1
Weil's disease A27.0
Weingarten's syndrome J82
Weir Mitchell's disease I73.81
Weiss-Baker syndrome G90.09
Wells' disease L98.3
Wen — see Cyst, sebaceous
Wenckebach's block or phenomenon I44.1
Werdnig-Hoffmann syndrome (muscular atrophy) G12.0
Werlhof's disease D69.3
Wermer's disease or syndrome E31.21
Werner-His disease A79.0
Werner's disease or syndrome E34.8
Wernicke-Korsakoff's syndrome or psychosis (alcoholic) F10.96
  with dependence F10.26
  drug-induced
    due to drug abuse — see Abuse, drug, by type, with amnestic disorder
    due to drug dependence — see Dependence, drug, by type, with amnestic disorder
  nonalcoholic F04

Wernicke-Posadas disease B38.9
Wernicke's
   developmental aphasia F80.2
   disease or syndrome E51.2
   encephalopathy E51.2
   polioencephalitis, superior E51.2
West African fever B50.8
Westphal-Strümpell syndrome E83.01
West's syndrome — see Epilepsy, spasms
Wet
   feet, tropical (maceration) (syndrome) — see
      Immersion, foot
   lung (syndrome), newborn P22.1
Wharton's duct — see condition
Wheal — see Urticaria
Wheezing R06.2
Whiplash injury S13.4 ☑
Whipple's disease (see also subcategory M14.8 ☑)
   K90.81
Whipworm (disease) (infection) (infestation) B79
Whistling face Q87.0
White (see also condition)
   kidney, small N03.9
   leg, puerperal, postpartum, childbirth O87.1
   mouth B37.0
   patches of mouth K13.29
   spot lesions, teeth
      chewing surface K02.51
      pit and fissure surface K02.51
      smooth surface K02.61
Whitehead L70.0
Whitlow (see also Cellulitis, digit)
   with lymphangitis — see Lymphangitis, acute, digit
   herpesviral B00.89
Whitmore's disease or fever — see Melioidosis
Whooping cough A37.90
   with pneumonia A37.91
      due to Bordetella
         bronchiseptica A37.81
         parapertussis A37.11
         pertussis A37.01
         specified organism NEC A37.81
   due to
      Bordetella
         bronchiseptica A37.80
            with pneumonia A37.81
         parapertussis A37.10
            with pneumonia A37.11
         pertussis A37.00
            with pneumonia A37.01
         specified NEC A37.80
            with pneumonia A37.81
Wichman's asthma J38.5
Wide cranial sutures, newborn P96.3
Widening aorta — see Ectasia, aorta
   with aneurysm — see Aneurysm, aorta
Wilkie's disease or syndrome K55.1
Wilkinson-Sneddon disease or syndrome L13.1
Willebrand (-Jürgens) thrombopathy D68.0
Willige-Hunt disease or syndrome G23.1
Wilms' tumor C64 ☑
Wilson-Mikity syndrome P27.0
Wilson's
   disease or syndrome E83.01
   hepatolenticular degeneration E83.01
   lichen ruber L43.9
Window (see also Imperfect, closure)
   aorticopulmonary Q21.4
Winter — see condition
Wiskott-Aldrich syndrome D82.0
Withdrawal state (see also Dependence, drug by
   type, with withdrawal)
   alcohol
      with perceptual disturbances F10.232
      without perceptual disturbances F10.239
   caffeine F15.93
   cannabis F12.288
   newborn
      correct therapeutic substance properly
         administered P96.2
      infant of dependent mother P96.1
   therapeutic substance, neonatal P96.2
Witts' anemia D50.8
Witzelsucht F07.0
Woakes' ethmoiditis or syndrome J33.1
Wolff-Hirschorn syndrome Q93.3
Wolff-Parkinson-White syndrome I45.6
Wolhynian fever A79.0
Wolman's disease E75.5
Wood lung or pneumonitis J67.8
Woolly, wooly hair (congenital) (nevus) Q84.1
Woolsorter's disease A22.1

Word
   blindness (congenital) (developmental) F81.0
   deafness (congenital) (developmental) H93.25
Worm (s) (infection) (infestation) (see also Infestation,
   helminth)
   guinea B72
   in intestine NEC B82.0
Worm-eaten soles A66.3
Worn out — see Exhaustion
   cardiac
      defibrillator (with synchronous cardiac
         pacemaker) Z45.02
      pacemaker
         battery Z45.010
         lead Z45.018
      device, implant or graft — see Complications, by
         site, mechanical
Worried well Z71.1
Worries R45.82
Wound check Z48.0 ☑
   due to injury - code to Injury, by site, using
      appropriate seventh character for
      subsequent encounter
Wound, open T14.8 ☑
   abdomen, abdominal
      wall S31.109 ☑
         with penetration into peritoneal
            cavity S31.609 ☑
         bite — see Bite, abdomen, wall
         epigastric region S31.102 ☑
            with penetration into peritoneal
               cavity S31.602 ☑
            bite — see Bite, abdomen, wall, epigastric
               region
            laceration — see Laceration, abdomen,
               wall, epigastric region
            puncture — see Puncture, abdomen, wall,
               epigastric region
         laceration — see Laceration, abdomen, wall
         left
            lower quadrant S31.104 ☑
               with penetration into peritoneal
                  cavity S31.604 ☑
               bite — see Bite, abdomen, wall, left, lower
                  quadrant
               laceration — see Laceration, abdomen,
                  wall, left, lower quadrant
               puncture — see Puncture, abdomen,
                  wall, left, lower quadrant
            upper quadrant S31.101 ☑
               with penetration into peritoneal
                  cavity S31.601 ☑
               bite — see Bite, abdomen, wall, left,
                  upper quadrant
               laceration — see Laceration, abdomen,
                  wall, left, upper quadrant
               puncture — see Puncture, abdomen,
                  wall, left, upper quadrant
         periumbilic region S31.105 ☑
            with penetration into peritoneal
               cavity S31.605 ☑
            bite — see Bite, abdomen, wall, periumbilic
               region
            laceration — see Laceration, abdomen,
               wall, periumbilic region
            puncture — see Puncture, abdomen, wall,
               periumbilic region
         puncture — see Puncture, abdomen, wall
         right
            lower quadrant S31.103 ☑
               with penetration into peritoneal
                  cavity S31.603 ☑
               bite — see Bite, abdomen, wall, right,
                  lower quadrant
               laceration — see Laceration, abdomen,
                  wall, right, lower quadrant
               puncture — see Puncture, abdomen,
                  wall, right, lower quadrant
            upper quadrant S31.100 ☑
               with penetration into peritoneal
                  cavity S31.600 ☑
               bite — see Bite, abdomen, wall, right,
                  upper quadrant
               laceration — see Laceration, abdomen,
                  wall, right, upper quadrant
               puncture — see Puncture, abdomen,
                  wall, right, upper quadrant
   alveolar (process) — see Wound, open, oral cavity
   ankle S91.00 ☑
      bite — see Bite, ankle
      laceration — see Laceration, ankle
      puncture — see Puncture, ankle

Wound, open — continued
   antecubital space — see Wound, open, elbow
   anterior chamber, eye — see Wound, open, ocular
   anus S31.839 ☑
      bite S31.835 ☑
      laceration — see Laceration, anus
      puncture — see Puncture, anus
   arm (upper) S41.10 ☑
      with amputation — see Amputation, traumatic,
         arm
      bite — see Bite, arm
      forearm — see Wound, open, forearm
      laceration — see Laceration, arm
      puncture — see Puncture, arm
   auditory canal (external) (meatus) — see Wound,
      open, ear
   auricle, ear — see Wound, open, ear
   axilla — see Wound, open, arm
   back (see also Wound, open, thorax, back)
      lower S31.000 ☑
         with penetration into retroperitoneal
            space S31.001 ☑
         bite — see Bite, back, lower
         laceration — see Laceration, back, lower
         puncture — see Puncture, back, lower
   bite — see Bite
   blood vessel — see Injury, blood vessel
   breast S21.00 ☑
      with amputation — see Amputation, traumatic,
         breast
      bite — see Bite, breast
      laceration — see Laceration, breast
      puncture — see Puncture, breast
   buttock S31.809 ☑
      bite — see Bite, buttock
      laceration — see Laceration, buttock
      left S31.829 ☑
      puncture — see Puncture, buttock
      right S31.819 ☑
   calf — see Wound, open, leg
   canaliculus lacrimalis — see Wound, open, eyelid
   canthus, eye — see Wound, open, eyelid
   cervical esophagus S11.20 ☑
      bite S11.25 ☑
      laceration — see Laceration, esophagus,
         traumatic, cervical
      puncture — see Puncture, cervical esophagus
   cheek (external) S01.40 ☑
      bite — see Bite, cheek
      laceration — see Laceration, cheek
      puncture — see Puncture, cheek
      internal — see Wound, open, oral cavity
   chest wall — see Wound, open, thorax
   chin — see Wound, open, head, specified site NEC
   choroid — see Wound, open, ocular
   ciliary body (eye) — see Wound, open, ocular
   clitoris S31.40 ☑
      with amputation — see Amputation, traumatic,
         clitoris
      bite S31.45 ☑
      laceration — see Laceration, vulva
      puncture — see Puncture, vulva
   conjunctiva — see Wound, open, ocular
   cornea — see Wound, open, ocular
   costal region — see Wound, open, thorax
   Descemet's membrane — see Wound, open,
      ocular
   digit (s)
      foot — see Wound, open, toe
      hand — see Wound, open, finger
   ear (canal) (external) S01.30 ☑
      with amputation — see Amputation, traumatic,
         ear
      bite — see Bite, ear
      laceration — see Laceration, ear
      puncture — see Puncture, ear
      drum S09.2 ☑
   elbow S51.00 ☑
      bite — see Bite, elbow
      laceration — see Laceration, elbow
      puncture — see Puncture, elbow
   epididymis — see Wound, open, testis
   epigastric region S31.102 ☑
      with penetration into peritoneal
         cavity S31.602 ☑
      bite — see Bite, abdomen, wall, epigastric
         region
      laceration — see Laceration, abdomen, wall,
         epigastric region
      puncture — see Puncture, abdomen, wall,
         epigastric region

Wound

Wound, open — *continued*
  epiglottis — *see* Wound, open, neck, specified
    site NEC
  esophagus (thoracic) S27.819 ☑
    cervical — *see* Wound, open, cervical
      esophagus
      laceration S27.813 ☑
      specified type NEC S27.818 ☑
  eye — *see* Wound, open, ocular
  eyeball — *see* Wound, open, ocular
  eyebrow — *see* Wound, open, eyelid
  eyelid S01.10 ☑
    bite — *see* Bite, eyelid
    laceration — *see* Laceration, eyelid
    puncture — *see* Puncture, eyelid
  face NEC — *see* Wound, open, head, specified
    site NEC
  finger (s) S61.209 ☑
    with
      amputation — *see* Amputation, traumatic,
        finger
      damage to nail S61.309 ☑
    bite — *see* Bite, finger
    index S61.208 ☑
      with
        damage to nail S61.308 ☑
      left S61.201 ☑
        with
          damage to nail S61.301 ☑
      right S61.200 ☑
        with
          damage to nail S61.300 ☑
    laceration — *see* Laceration, finger
    little S61.208 ☑
      with
        damage to nail S61.308 ☑
      left S61.207 ☑
        with damage to nail S61.307 ☑
      right S61.206 ☑
        with damage to nail S61.306 ☑
    middle S61.208 ☑
      with
        damage to nail S61.308 ☑
      left S61.203 ☑
        with damage to nail S61.303 ☑
      right S61.202 ☑
        with damage to nail S61.302 ☑
    puncture — *see* Puncture, finger
    ring S61.208 ☑
      with
        damage to nail S61.308 ☑
      left S61.205 ☑
        with damage to nail S61.305 ☑
      right S61.204 ☑
        with damage to nail S61.304 ☑
  flank — *see* Wound, open, abdomen, wall
  foot (except toe (s) alone) S91.30 ☑
    with amputation — *see* Amputation, traumatic,
      foot
    bite — *see* Bite, foot
    laceration — *see* Laceration, foot
    puncture — *see* Puncture, foot
    toe — *see* Wound, open, toe
  forearm S51.80 ☑
    with
      amputation — *see* Amputation, traumatic,
        forearm
    bite — *see* Bite, forearm
    elbow only — *see* Wound, open, elbow
    laceration — *see* Laceration, forearm
    puncture — *see* Puncture, forearm
  forehead — *see* Wound, open, head, specified
    site NEC
  genital organs, external
    with amputation — *see* Amputation, traumatic,
      genital organs
    bite — *see* Bite, genital organ
    female S31.502 ☑
      vagina S31.40 ☑
      vulva S31.40 ☑
    laceration — *see* Laceration, genital organ
    male S31.501 ☑
      penis S31.20 ☑
      scrotum S31.30 ☑
      testes S31.30 ☑
    puncture — *see* Puncture, genital organ
  globe (eye) — *see* Wound, open, ocular
  groin — *see* Wound, open, abdomen, wall
  gum — *see* Wound, open, oral cavity
  hand S61.40 ☑
    with

Wound, open — *continued*
  hand — *continued*
      amputation — *see* Amputation, traumatic,
        hand
    bite — *see* Bite, hand
    finger (s) — *see* Wound, open, finger
    laceration — *see* Laceration, hand
    puncture — *see* Puncture, hand
    thumb — *see* Wound, open, thumb
  head S01.90 ☑
    bite — *see* Bite, head
    cheek — *see* Wound, open, cheek
    ear — *see* Wound, open, ear
    eyelid — *see* Wound, open, eyelid
    laceration — *see* Laceration, head
    lip — *see* Wound, open, lip
    nose S01.20 ☑
    oral cavity — *see* Wound, open, oral cavity
    puncture — *see* Puncture, head
    scalp — *see* Wound, open, scalp
    specified site NEC S01.80 ☑
    temporomandibular area — *see* Wound, open,
      cheek
  heel — *see* Wound, open, foot
  hip S71.00 ☑
    with amputation — *see* Amputation, traumatic,
      hip
    bite — *see* Bite, hip
    laceration — *see* Laceration, hip
    puncture — *see* Puncture, hip
  hymen S31.40 ☑
    bite — *see* Bite, vulva
    laceration — *see* Laceration, vagina
    puncture — *see* Puncture, vagina
  hypochondrium S31.109 ☑
    bite — *see* Bite, hypochondrium
    laceration — *see* Laceration, hypochondrium
    puncture — *see* Puncture, hypochondrium
  hypogastric region S31.109 ☑
    bite — *see* Bite, hypogastric region
    laceration — *see* Laceration, hypogastric region
    puncture — *see* Puncture, hypogastric region
  iliac (region) — *see* Wound, open, inguinal region
  inguinal region S31.109 ☑
    bite — *see* Bite, abdomen, wall, lower quadrant
    laceration — *see* Laceration, inguinal region
    puncture — *see* Puncture, inguinal region
  instep — *see* Wound, open, foot
  interscapular region — *see* Wound, open, thorax,
    back
  intraocular — *see* Wound, open, ocular
  iris — *see* Wound, open, ocular
  jaw — *see* Wound, open, head, specified site NEC
  knee S81.00 ☑
    bite — *see* Bite, knee
    laceration — *see* Laceration, knee
    puncture — *see* Puncture, knee
  labium (majus) (minus) — *see* Wound, open,
    vulva
  laceration — *see* Laceration, by site
  lacrimal duct — *see* Wound, open, eyelid
  larynx S11.019 ☑
    bite — *see* Bite, larynx
    laceration — *see* Laceration, larynx
    puncture — *see* Puncture, larynx
  left
    lower quadrant S31.104 ☑
      with penetration into peritoneal
        cavity S31.604 ☑
      bite — *see* Bite, abdomen, wall, left, lower
        quadrant
      laceration — *see* Laceration, abdomen, wall,
        left, lower quadrant
      puncture — *see* Puncture, abdomen, wall,
        left, lower quadrant
    upper quadrant S31.101 ☑
      with penetration into peritoneal
        cavity S31.601 ☑
      bite — *see* Bite, abdomen, wall, left, upper
        quadrant
      laceration — *see* Laceration, abdomen, wall,
        left, upper quadrant
      puncture — *see* Puncture, abdomen, wall,
        left, upper quadrant
  leg (lower) S81.80 ☑
    with amputation — *see* Amputation, traumatic,
      leg
    ankle — *see* Wound, open, ankle
    bite — *see* Bite, leg
    foot — *see* Wound, open, foot
    knee — *see* Wound, open, knee

Wound, open — *continued*
  leg — *continued*
    laceration — *see* Laceration, leg
    puncture — *see* Puncture, leg
    toe — *see* Wound, open, toe
    upper — *see* Wound, open, thigh
  lip S01.501 ☑
    bite — *see* Bite, lip
    laceration — *see* Laceration, lip
    puncture — *see* Puncture, lip
  loin S31.109 ☑
    bite — *see* Bite, abdomen, wall
    laceration — *see* Laceration, loin
    puncture — *see* Puncture, loin
  lower back — *see* Wound, open, back, lower
  lumbar region — *see* Wound, open, back, lower
  malar region — *see* Wound, open, head, specified
    site NEC
  mammary — *see* Wound, open, breast
  mastoid region — *see* Wound, open, head,
    specified site NEC
  mouth — *see* Wound, open, oral cavity
  nail
    finger — *see* Wound, open, finger, with damage
      to nail
    toe — *see* Wound, open, toe, with damage to nail
  nape (neck) — *see* Wound, open, neck
  nasal (septum) (sinus) — *see* Wound, open, nose
  nasopharynx — *see* Wound, open, head, specified
    site NEC
  neck S11.90 ☑
    bite — *see* Bite, neck
    involving
      cervical esophagus S11.20 ☑
      larynx — *see* Wound, open, larynx
      pharynx S11.20 ☑
      thyroid S11.10 ☑
      trachea (cervical) S11.029 ☑
        bite — *see* Bite, trachea
        laceration S11.021 ☑
          with foreign body S11.022 ☑
        puncture S11.023 ☑
          with foreign body S11.024 ☑
    laceration — *see* Laceration, neck
    puncture — *see* Puncture, neck
    specified site NEC S11.80 ☑
      specified type NEC S11.89 ☑
  nose (septum) (sinus) S01.20 ☑
    with amputation — *see* Amputation, traumatic,
      nose
    bite — *see* Bite, nose
    laceration — *see* Laceration, nose
    puncture — *see* Puncture, nose
  ocular S05.90 ☑
    avulsion (traumatic enucleation) S05.7 ☑
    eyeball S05.6 ☑
      with foreign body S05.5 ☑
    eyelid — *see* Wound, open, eyelid
    laceration and rupture S05.3 ☑
      with prolapse or loss of intraocular
        tissue S05.2 ☑
    orbit (penetrating) (with or without foreign
      body) S05.4 ☑
    periocular area — *see* Wound, open, eyelid
    specified NEC S05.8X ☑
  oral cavity S01.502 ☑
    bite S01.552 ☑
    laceration — *see* Laceration, oral cavity
    puncture — *see* Puncture, oral cavity
  orbit — *see* Wound, open, ocular, orbit
  palate — *see* Wound, open, oral cavity
  palm — *see* Wound, open, hand
  pelvis, pelvic (*see also* Wound, open, back, lower)
    girdle — *see* Wound, open, hip
  penetrating — *see* Puncture, by site
  penis S31.20 ☑
    with amputation — *see* Amputation, traumatic,
      penis
    bite S31.25 ☑
    laceration — *see* Laceration, penis
    puncture — *see* Puncture, penis
  perineum
    bite — *see* Bite, perineum
    female S31.502 ☑
    laceration — *see* Laceration, perineum
    male S31.501 ☑
    puncture — *see* Puncture, perineum
  periocular area (with or without lacrimal
    passages) — *see* Wound, open, eyelid
  periumbilic region S31.105 ☑
    with penetration into peritoneal
      cavity S31.605 ☑

☑ **Additional character required**

Wound, open — *continued*
  periumbilic region — *continued*
    bite — *see* Bite, abdomen, wall, periumbilic region
    laceration — *see* Laceration, abdomen, wall, periumbilic region
    puncture — *see* Puncture, abdomen, wall, periumbilic region
  phalanges
    finger — *see* Wound, open, finger
    toe — *see* Wound, open, toe
  pharynx S11.20 ☑
  pinna — *see* Wound, open, ear
  popliteal space — *see* Wound, open, knee
  prepuce — *see* Wound, open, penis
  pubic region — *see* Wound, open, back, lower
  pudendum — *see* Wound, open, genital organs, external
  puncture wound — *see* Puncture
  rectovaginal septum — *see* Wound, open, vagina
  right
    lower quadrant S31.103 ☑
      with penetration into peritoneal cavity S31.603 ☑
      bite — *see* Bite, abdomen, wall, right, lower quadrant
      laceration — *see* Laceration, abdomen, wall, right, lower quadrant
      puncture — *see* Puncture, abdomen, wall, right, lower quadrant
    upper quadrant S31.100 ☑
      with penetration into peritoneal cavity S31.600 ☑
      bite — *see* Bite, abdomen, wall, right, upper quadrant
      laceration — *see* Laceration, abdomen, wall, right, upper quadrant
      puncture — *see* Puncture, abdomen, wall, right, upper quadrant
  sacral region — *see* Wound, open, back, lower
  sacroiliac region — *see* Wound, open, back, lower
  salivary gland — *see* Wound, open, oral cavity
  scalp S01.00 ☑
    bite S01.05 ☑
    laceration — *see* Laceration, scalp
    puncture — *see* Puncture, scalp
  scalpel, newborn (birth injury) P15.8
  scapular region — *see* Wound, open, shoulder
  sclera — *see* Wound, open, ocular
  scrotum S31.30 ☑
    with amputation — *see* Amputation, traumatic, scrotum
    bite S31.35 ☑
    laceration — *see* Laceration, scrotum
    puncture — *see* Puncture, scrotum
  shin — *see* Wound, open, leg
  shoulder S41.00 ☑
    with amputation — *see* Amputation, traumatic, arm
    bite — *see* Bite, shoulder
    laceration — *see* Laceration, shoulder
    puncture — *see* Puncture, shoulder
  skin NOS T14.8 ☑
  spermatic cord — *see* Wound, open, testis
  sternal region — *see* Wound, open, thorax, front wall
  submaxillary region — *see* Wound, open, head, specified site NEC
  submental region — *see* Wound, open, head, specified site NEC
  subungual
    finger (s) — *see* Wound, open, finger
    toe (s) — *see* Wound, open, toe
  supraclavicular region — *see* Wound, open, neck, specified site NEC
  temple, temporal region — *see* Wound, open, head, specified site NEC
  temporomandibular area — *see* Wound, open, head, specified site NEC
  testis S31.30 ☑
    with amputation — *see* Amputation, traumatic, testes
    bite S31.35 ☑
    laceration — *see* Laceration, testis
    puncture — *see* Puncture, testis
  thigh S71.10 ☑
    with amputation — *see* Amputation, traumatic, hip
    bite — *see* Bite, thigh
    laceration — *see* Laceration, thigh
    puncture — *see* Puncture, thigh

Wound, open — *continued*
  thorax, thoracic (wall) S21.90 ☑
    back S21.20 ☑
      with penetration S21.40 ☑
    bite — *see* Bite, thorax
    breast — *see* Wound, open, breast
    front S21.10 ☑
      with penetration S21.30 ☑
    laceration — *see* Laceration, thorax
    puncture — *see* Puncture, thorax
  throat — *see* Wound, open, neck
  thumb S61.009 ☑
    with
      amputation — *see* Amputation, traumatic, thumb
      damage to nail S61.109 ☑
    bite — *see* Bite, thumb
    laceration — *see* Laceration, thumb
    left S61.002 ☑
      with
        damage to nail S61.102 ☑
    puncture — *see* Puncture, thumb
    right S61.001 ☑
      with
        damage to nail S61.101 ☑
  thyroid (gland) — *see* Wound, open, neck, thyroid
  toe (s) S91.109 ☑
    with
      amputation — *see* Amputation, traumatic, toe
      damage to nail S91.209 ☑
    bite — *see* Bite, toe
    great S91.103 ☑
      with
        damage to nail S91.203 ☑
      left S91.102 ☑
        with
          damage to nail S91.202 ☑
      right S91.101 ☑
        with
          damage to nail S91.201 ☑
    laceration — *see* Laceration, toe
    lesser S91.106 ☑
      with
        damage to nail S91.206 ☑
      left S91.105 ☑
        with
          damage to nail S91.205 ☑
      right S91.104 ☑
        with
          damage to nail S91.204 ☑
    puncture — *see* Puncture, toe
  tongue — *see* Wound, open, oral cavity
  trachea (cervical region) — *see* Wound, open, neck, trachea
  tunica vaginalis — *see* Wound, open, testis
  tympanum, tympanic membrane S09.2 ☑
    laceration — *see* Laceration, ear, drum
    puncture — *see* Puncture, tympanum
  umbilical region — *see* Wound, open, abdomen, wall, periumbilic region
  uvula — *see* Wound, open, oral cavity
  vagina S31.40 ☑
    bite S31.45 ☑
    laceration — *see* Laceration, vagina
    puncture — *see* Puncture, vagina
  vocal cord S11.039 ☑
    bite — *see* Bite, vocal cord
    laceration S11.031 ☑
      with foreign body S11.032 ☑
    puncture S11.033 ☑
      with foreign body S11.034 ☑
  vitreous (humor) — *see* Wound, open, ocular
  vulva S31.40 ☑
    with amputation — *see* Amputation, traumatic, vulva
    bite S31.45 ☑
    laceration — *see* Laceration, vulva
    puncture — *see* Puncture, vulva
  wrist S61.50 ☑
    bite — *see* Bite, wrist
    laceration — *see* Laceration, wrist
    puncture — *see* Puncture, wrist
Wound, superficial — *see* Injury (*see also* specified injury type)
Wright's syndrome G54.0
Wrist — *see* condition
Wrong drug (by accident) (given in error) — *see* Table of Drugs and Chemicals, by drug, poisoning
Wry neck — *see* Torticollis
Wuchereria (bancrofti) infestation B74.0
Wuchereriasis B74.0
Wuchernde Struma Langhans C73

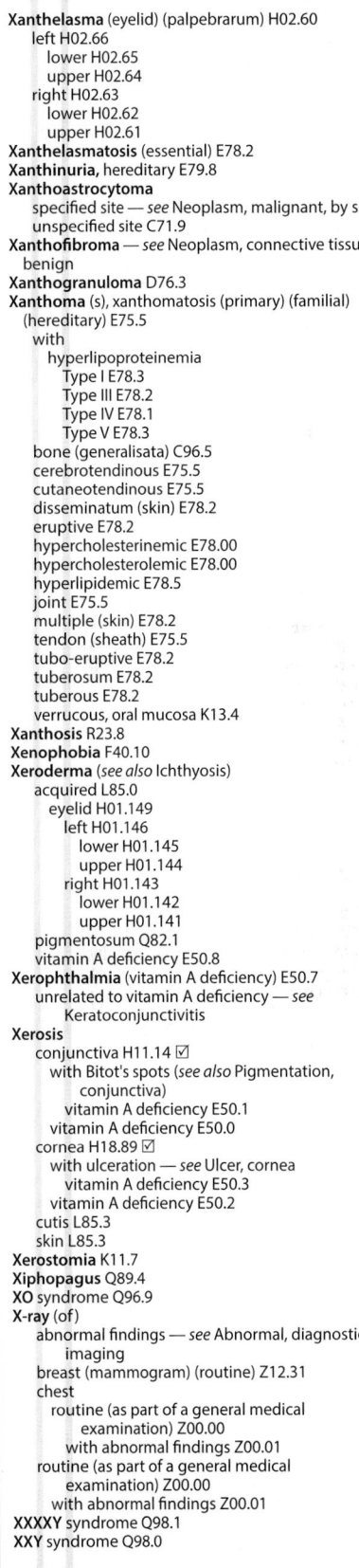

X

Xanthelasma (eyelid) (palpebrarum) H02.60
  left H02.66
    lower H02.65
    upper H02.64
  right H02.63
    lower H02.62
    upper H02.61
Xanthelasmatosis (essential) E78.2
Xanthinuria, hereditary E79.8
Xanthoastrocytoma
  specified site — *see* Neoplasm, malignant, by site
  unspecified site C71.9
Xanthofibroma — *see* Neoplasm, connective tissue, benign
Xanthogranuloma D76.3
Xanthoma (s), xanthomatosis (primary) (familial) (hereditary) E75.5
  with
    hyperlipoproteinemia
      Type I E78.3
      Type III E78.2
      Type IV E78.1
      Type V E78.3
  bone (generalisata) C96.5
  cerebrotendinous E75.5
  cutaneotendinous E75.5
  disseminatum (skin) E78.2
  eruptive E78.2
  hypercholesterinemic E78.00
  hypercholesterolemic E78.00
  hyperlipidemic E78.5
  joint E75.5
  multiple (skin) E78.2
  tendon (sheath) E75.5
  tubo-eruptive E78.2
  tuberosum E78.2
  tuberous E78.2
  verrucous, oral mucosa K13.4
Xanthosis R23.8
Xenophobia F40.10
Xeroderma (*see also* Ichthyosis)
  acquired L85.0
  eyelid H01.149
    left H01.146
      lower H01.145
      upper H01.144
    right H01.143
      lower H01.142
      upper H01.141
  pigmentosum Q82.1
  vitamin A deficiency E50.8
Xerophthalmia (vitamin A deficiency) E50.7
  unrelated to vitamin A deficiency — *see* Keratoconjunctivitis
Xerosis
  conjunctiva H11.14 ☑
    with Bitot's spots (*see also* Pigmentation, conjunctiva)
      vitamin A deficiency E50.1
    vitamin A deficiency E50.0
  cornea H18.89 ☑
    with ulceration — *see* Ulcer, cornea
      vitamin A deficiency E50.3
    vitamin A deficiency E50.2
  cutis L85.3
  skin L85.3
Xerostomia K11.7
Xiphopagus Q89.4
XO syndrome Q96.9
X-ray (of)
  abnormal findings — *see* Abnormal, diagnostic imaging
  breast (mammogram) (routine) Z12.31
  chest
    routine (as part of a general medical examination) Z00.00
      with abnormal findings Z00.01
    routine (as part of a general medical examination) Z00.00
      with abnormal findings Z00.01
XXXXY syndrome Q98.1
XXY syndrome Q98.0

Y

Yaba pox (virus disease) B08.72
Yatapoxvirus B08.70
  specified NEC B08.79

Yawning - Zymotic

Yawning R06.89
  psychogenic F45.8
Yaws A66.9
  bone lesions A66.6
  butter A66.1
  chancre A66.0
  cutaneous, less than five years after
     infection A66.2
  early (cutaneous) (macular) (maculopapular)
     (micropapular) (papular) A66.2
    frambeside A66.2
    skin lesions NEC A66.2
  eyelid A66.2
  ganglion A66.6
  gangosis, gangosa A66.5
  gumma, gummata A66.4
    bone A66.6
  gummatous
    frambeside A66.4
    osteitis A66.6
    periostitis A66.6
  hydrarthrosis (*see also* subcategory M14.8 ☑) A66.6
  hyperkeratosis (early) (late) A66.3
  initial lesions A66.0
  joint lesions (*see also* subcategory M14.8 ☑) A66.6
  juxta-articular nodules A66.7
  late nodular (ulcerated) A66.4
  latent (without clinical manifestations) (with
     positive serology) A66.8
  mother A66.0
  mucosal A66.7
  multiple papillomata A66.1
  nodular, late (ulcerated) A66.4
  osteitis A66.6
  papilloma, plantar or palmar A66.1
  periostitis (hypertrophic) A66.6
  specified NEC A66.7
  ulcers A66.4
  wet crab A66.1
Yeast infection (*see also* Candidiasis) B37.9
Yellow
  atrophy (liver) — *see* Failure, hepatic
  fever — *see* Fever, yellow
  jack — *see* Fever, yellow
  jaundice — *see* Jaundice
  nail syndrome L60.5
Yersiniosis (*see also* Infection, Yersinia)
  extraintestinal A28.2
  intestinal A04.6

Z

Zahorsky's syndrome (herpangina) B08.5
Zellweger's syndrome Q87.89
Zenker's diverticulum (esophagus) K22.5
Ziehen-Oppenheim disease G24.1
Zieve's syndrome K70.0
Zika NOS A92.5
Zinc
  deficiency, dietary E60
  metabolism disorder E83.2
Zollinger-Ellison syndrome E16.4
Zona — *see* Herpes, zoster
Zoophobia F40.218
Zoster (herpes) — *see* Herpes, zoster
Zygomycosis B46.9
  specified NEC B46.8
Zymotic — *see* condition

☑ **Additional character required**

ICD-10-CM Table of Neoplasms

The list below gives the code numbers for neoplasms by anatomical site. For each site there are six possible code numbers according to whether the neoplasm in question is malignant, benign, in situ, of uncertain behavior, or of unspecified nature. The description of the neoplasm will often indicate which of the six columns is appropriate; e.g., malignant melanoma of skin, benign fibroadenoma of breast, carcinoma in situ of cervix uteri.

Where such descriptors are not present, the remainder of the Index should be consulted where guidance is given to the appropriate column for each morphological (histological) variety listed; e.g., Mesonephroma—see Neoplasm, malignant; Embryoma—see also Neoplasm, uncertain behavior; Disease, Bowen's—see Neoplasm, skin, in situ. However, the guidance in the Index can be overridden if one of the descriptors mentioned above is present; e.g., malignant adenoma of colon is coded to C18.9 and not to D12.6 as the adjective 'malignant' overrides the Index entry 'Adenoma—see also Neoplasm, benign.'

Codes listed with a dash (-) following the code have a required additional character for laterality. The Tabular must be reviewed for the complete code.

Neoplasm	Malignant Primary	Malignant Secondary	Ca in situ	Benign	Uncertain Behavior	Unspecified Behavior
Neoplasm, neoplastic	C80.1	C79.9	D09.9	D36.9	D48.9	D49.9
abdomen, abdominal	C76.2	C79.8-	D09.8	D36.7	D48.7	D49.89
cavity	C76.2	C79.8-	D09.8	D36.7	D48.7	D49.89
organ	C76.2	C79.8-	D09.8	D36.7	D48.7	D49.89
viscera	C76.2	C79.8-	D09.8	D36.7	D48.7	D49.89
wall (see also Neoplasm, abdomen, wall, skin)	C44.509	C79.2-	D04.5	D23.5	D48.5	D49.2
connective tissue	C49.4	C79.8-	-	D21.4	D48.1	D49.2
skin	C44.509	-	-	-	-	-
basal cell carcinoma	C44.519	-	-	-	-	-
specified type NEC	C44.599	-	-	-	-	-
squamous cell carcinoma	C44.529	-	-	-	-	-
abdominopelvic	C76.8	C79.8-	-	D36.7	D48.7	D49.89
accessory sinus — see Neoplasm, sinus						
acoustic nerve	C72.4-	C79.49	-	D33.3	D43.3	D49.7
adenoid (pharynx) (tissue)	C11.1	C79.89	D00.08	D10.6	D37.05	D49.0
adipose tissue (see also Neoplasm, connective tissue)	C49.4	C79.89	-	D21.9	D48.1	D49.2
adnexa (uterine)	C57.4	C79.89	D07.39	D28.7	D39.8	D49.59
adrenal	C74.9-	C79.7-	D09.3	D35.0-	D44.1-	D49.7
capsule	C74.9-	C79.7-	D09.3	D35.0-	D44.1-	D49.7
cortex	C74.0-	C79.7-	D09.3	D35.0-	D44.1-	D49.7
gland	C74.9-	C79.7-	D09.3	D35.0-	D44.1-	D49.7
medulla	C74.1-	C79.7-	D09.3	D35.0-	D44.1-	D49.7
ala nasi (external) (see also Neoplasm, skin, nose)	C44.301	C79.2	D04.39	D23.39	D48.5	D49.2
alimentary canal or tract NEC	C26.9	C78.80	D01.9	D13.9	D37.9	D49.0
alveolar	C03.9	C79.89	D00.03	D10.39	D37.09	D49.0
mucosa	C03.9	C79.89	D00.03	D10.39	D37.09	D49.0
lower	C03.1	C79.89	D00.03	D10.39	D37.09	D49.0
upper	C03.0	C79.89	D00.03	D10.39	D37.09	D49.0
ridge or process	C41.1	C79.51	-	D16.5-	D48.0	D49.2
carcinoma	C03.9	C79.8-	-	-	-	-
lower	C03.1	C79.8-	-	-	-	-
upper	C03.0	C79.8-	-	-	-	-
lower	C41.1	C79.51	-	D16.5-	D48.0	D49.2
mucosa	C03.9	C79.89	D00.03	D10.39	D37.09	D49.0
lower	C03.1	C79.89	D00.03	D10.39	D37.09	D49.0
upper	C03.0	C79.89	D00.03	D10.39	D37.09	D49.0
upper	C41.0	C79.51	-	D16.4-	D48.0	D49.2
sulcus	C06.1	C79.89	D00.02	D10.39	D37.09	D49.0
alveolus	C03.9	C79.89	D00.03	D10.39	D37.09	D49.0
lower	C03.1	C79.89	D00.03	D10.39	D37.09	D49.0
upper	C03.0	C79.89	D00.03	D10.39	D37.09	D49.0
ampulla of Vater	C24.1	C78.89	D01.5	D13.5	D37.6	D49.0
ankle NEC	C76.5-	C79.89	D04.7-	D36.7	D48.7	D49.89
anorectum, anorectal (junction)	C21.8	C78.5	D01.3	D12.9	D37.8	D49.0
antecubital fossa or space	C76.4-	C79.89	D04.6-	D36.7	D48.7	D49.89
antrum (Highmore) (maxillary)	C31.0	C78.39	D02.3	D14.0	D38.5	D49.1
pyloric	C16.3	C78.89	D00.2	D13.1	D37.1	D49.0
tympanicum	C30.1	C78.39	D02.3	D14.0	D38.5	D49.1
anus, anal	C21.0	C78.5	D01.3	D12.9	D37.8	D49.0
canal	C21.1	C78.5	D01.3	D12.9	D37.8	D49.0
cloacogenic zone	C21.2	C78.5	D01.3	D12.9	D37.8	D49.0
margin (see also Neoplasm, anus, skin)	C44.500	C79.2	D04.5	D23.5	D48.5	D49.2
overlapping lesion with rectosigmoid junction or rectum	C21.8	-	-	-	-	-
skin	C44.500	C79.2	D04.5	D23.5	D48.5	D49.2
basal cell carcinoma	C44.510	-	-	-	-	-
specified type NEC	C44.590	-	-	-	-	-
squamous cell carcinoma	C44.520	-	-	-	-	-
sphincter	C21.1	C78.5	D01.3	D12.9	D37.8	D49.0
aorta (thoracic)	C49.3	C79.89	-	D21.3	D48.1	D49.2
abdominal	C49.4	C79.89	-	D21.4	D48.1	D49.2
aortic body	C75.5	C79.89	-	D35.6	D44.7	D49.7

Neoplasm	Malignant Primary	Malignant Secondary	Ca in situ	Benign	Uncertain Behavior	Unspecified Behavior
aponeurosis	C49.9	C79.89	-	D21.9	D48.1	D49.2
palmar	C49.1-	C79.89	-	D21.1-	D48.1	D49.2
plantar	C49.2-	C79.89	-	D21.2-	D48.1	D49.2
appendix	C18.1	C78.5	D01.0	D12.1	D37.3	D49.0
arachnoid	C70.9	C79.49	-	D32.9	D42.9	D49.7
cerebral	C70.0	C79.32	-	D32.0	D42.0	D49.7
spinal	C70.1	C79.49	-	D32.1	D42.1	D49.7
areola	C50.0-	C79.81	D05.-	D24.-	D48.6-	D49.3
arm NEC	C76.4-	C79.89	D04.6-	D36.7	D48.7	D49.89
artery — see Neoplasm, connective tissue						
aryepiglottic fold	C13.1	C79.89	D00.08	D10.7	D37.05	D49.0
hypopharyngeal aspect	C13.1	C79.89	D00.08	D10.7	D37.05	D49.0
laryngeal aspect	C32.1	C78.39	D02.0	D14.1	D38.0	D49.1
marginal zone	C13.1	C79.89	D00.08	D10.7	D37.05	D49.0
arytenoid (cartilage)	C32.3	C78.39	D02.0	D14.1	D38.0	D49.1
fold — see Neoplasm, aryepiglottic						
associated with transplanted organ	C80.2	-	-	-	-	-
atlas	C41.2	C79.51	-	D16.6	D48.0	D49.2
atrium, cardiac	C38.0	C79.89	-	D15.1	D48.7	D49.89
auditory						
canal (external) (skin)	C44.20-	C79.2	D04.2-	D23.2-	D48.5	D49.2
internal	C30.1	C78.39	D02.3	D14.0	D38.5	D49.1
nerve	C72.4-	C79.49	-	D33.3	D43.3	D49.7
tube	C30.1	C78.39	D02.3	D14.0	D38.5	D49.1
opening	C11.2	C79.89	D00.08	D10.6	D37.05	D49.0
auricle, ear (see also Neoplasm, skin, ear)	C44.20-	C79.2	D04.2-	D23.2-	D48.5	D49.2
auricular canal (external) (see also Neoplasm, skin, ear)	C44.20-	C79.2	D04.2-	D23.2-	D48.5	D49.2
internal	C30.1	C78.39	D02.3	D14.0	D38.5	D49.2
autonomic nerve or nervous system NEC (see Neoplasm, nerve, peripheral)						
axilla, axillary	C76.1	C79.89	D09.8	D36.7	D48.7	D49.89
fold (see also Neoplasm, skin, trunk)	C44.509	C79.2	D04.5	D23.5	D48.5	D49.2
back NEC	C76.8	C79.89	D04.5	D36.7	D48.7	D49.89
Bartholin's gland	C51.0	C79.82	D07.1	D28.0	D39.8	D49.59
basal ganglia	C71.0	C79.31	-	D33.0	D43.0	D49.6
basis pedunculi	C71.7	C79.31	-	D33.1	D43.1	D49.6
bile or biliary (tract)	C24.9	C78.89	D01.5	D13.5	D37.6	D49.0
canaliculi (biliferi) (intrahepatic)	C22.1	C78.7	D01.5	D13.4	D37.6	D49.0
canals, interlobular	C22.1	C78.89	D01.5	D13.4	D37.6	D49.0
duct or passage (common) (cystic) (extrahepatic)	C24.0	C78.89	D01.5	D13.5	D37.6	D49.0
interlobular	C22.1	C78.89	D01.5	D13.4	D37.6	D49.0
intrahepatic	C22.1	C78.7	D01.5	D13.4	D37.6	D49.0
and extrahepatic	C24.8	C78.89	D01.5	D13.5	D37.6	D49.0
bladder (urinary)	C67.9	C79.11	D09.0	D30.3	D41.4	D49.4
dome	C67.1	C79.11	D09.0	D30.3	D41.4	D49.4
neck	C67.5	C79.11	D09.0	D30.3	D41.4	D49.4
orifice	C67.9	C79.11	D09.0	D30.3	D41.4	D49.4
ureteric	C67.6	C79.11	D09.0	D30.3	D41.4	D49.4
urethral	C67.5	C79.11	D09.0	D30.3	D41.4	D49.4
overlapping lesion	C67.8					
sphincter	C67.8	C79.11	D09.0	D30.3	D41.4	D49.4
trigone	C67.0	C79.11	D09.0	D30.3	D41.4	D49.4
urachus	C67.7	C79.11	D09.0	D30.3	D41.4	D49.4
wall	C67.9	C79.11	D09.0	D30.3	D41.4	D49.4
anterior	C67.3	C79.11	D09.0	D30.3	D41.4	D49.4
lateral	C67.2	C79.11	D09.0	D30.3	D41.4	D49.4
posterior	C67.4	C79.11	D09.0	D30.3	D41.4	D49.4
blood vessel — see Neoplasm, connective tissue						
bone (periosteum)	C41.9	C79.51	-	D16.9-	D48.0	D49.2
acetabulum	C41.4	C79.51	-	D16.8-	D48.0	D49.2
ankle	C40.3-	C79.51	-	D16.3-	-	-
arm NEC	C40.0-	C79.51	-	D16.0-	-	-
astragalus	C40.3-	C79.51	-	D16.3-	-	-
atlas	C41.2	C79.51	-	D16.6-	D48.0	D49.2
axis	C41.2	C79.51	-	D16.6-	D48.0	D49.2
back NEC	C41.2	C79.51	-	D16.6-	D48.0	D49.2
calcaneus	C40.3-	C79.51	-	D16.3-	-	-
calvarium	C41.0	C79.51	-	D16.4-	D48.0	D49.2
carpus (any)	C40.1-	C79.51	-	D16.1-	-	-
cartilage NEC	C41.9	C79.51	-	D16.9-	D48.0	D49.2
clavicle	C41.3	C79.51	-	D16.7-	D48.0	D49.2
clivus	C41.0	C79.51	-	D16.4-	D48.0	D49.2
coccygeal vertebra	C41.4	C79.51	-	D16.8-	D48.0	D49.2
coccyx	C41.4	C79.51	-	D16.8-	D48.0	D49.2
costal cartilage	C41.3	C79.51	-	D16.7-	D48.0	D49.2
costovertebral joint	C41.3	C79.51	-	D16.7-	D48.0	D49.2
cranial	C41.0	C79.51	-	D16.4-	D48.0	D49.2
cuboid	C40.3-	C79.51	-	D16.3-	-	-
cuneiform	C41.9	C79.51	-	D16.9-	D48.0	D49.2
elbow	C40.0-	C79.51	-	D16.0-	-	-

Neoplasm	Malignant Primary	Malignant Secondary	Ca in situ	Benign	Uncertain Behavior	Unspecified Behavior
bone — *continued*						
ethmoid (labyrinth)	C41.0	C79.51	-	D16.4-	D48.0	D49.2
face	C41.0	C79.51	-	D16.4-	D48.0	D49.2
femur (any part)	C40.2-	C79.51	-	D16.2-	-	-
fibula (any part)	C40.2-	C79.51	-	D16.2-	-	-
finger (any)	C40.1-	C79.51	-	D16.1-	-	-
foot	C40.3-	C79.51	-	D16.3-	-	-
forearm	C40.0-	C79.51	-	D16.0-	-	-
frontal	C41.0	C79.51	-	D16.4-	D48.0	D49.2
hand	C40.1-	C79.51	-	D16.1-	-	-
heel	C40.3-	C79.51	-	D16.3-	-	-
hip	C41.4	C79.51	-	D16.8-	D48.0	D49.2
humerus (any part)	C40.0-	C79.51	-	D16.0-	-	-
hyoid	C41.0	C79.51	-	D16.4-	D48.0	D49.2
ilium	C41.4	C79.51	-	D16.8-	D48.0	D49.2
innominate	C41.4	C79.51	-	D16.8-	D48.0	D49.2
intervertebral cartilage or disc	C41.2	C79.51	-	D16.6-	D48.0	D49.2
ischium	C41.4	C79.51	-	D16.8-	D48.0	D49.2
jaw (lower)	C41.1	C79.51	-	D16.5-	D48.0	D49.2
knee	C40.2-	C79.51	-	D16.2-	-	-
leg NEC	C40.2-	C79.51	-	D16.2-	-	-
limb NEC	C40.9-	C79.51	-	D16.9-	-	-
lower (long bones)	C40.2-	C79.51	-	D16.2-	-	-
short bones	C40.3-	C79.51	-	D16.3-	-	-
upper (long bones)	C40.0-	C79.51	-	D16.0-	-	-
short bones	C40.1-	C79.51	-	D16.1-	-	-
malar	C41.0	C79.51	-	D16.4-	D48.0	D49.2
mandible	C41.1	C79.51	-	D16.5-	D48.0	D49.2
marrow NEC (any bone)	C96.9	C79.52	-	-	D47.9	D49.89
mastoid	C41.0	C79.51	-	D16.4-	D48.0	D49.2
maxilla, maxillary (superior)	C41.0	C79.51	-	D16.4-	D48.0	D49.2
inferior	C41.1	C79.51	-	D16.5-	D48.0	D49.2
metacarpus (any)	C40.1-	C79.51	-	D16.1-	-	-
metatarsus (any)	C40.3-	C79.51	-	D16.3-	-	-
overlapping sites	C40.8-	-	-	-	-	-
navicular						
ankle	C40.3-	C79.51	-	-	-	-
hand	C40.1-	C79.51	-	-	-	-
nose, nasal	C41.0	C79.51	-	D16.4-	D48.0	D49.2
occipital	C41.0	C79.51	-	D16.4-	D48.0	D49.2
orbit	C41.0	C79.51	-	D16.4-	D48.0	D49.2
parietal	C41.0	C79.51	-	D16.4-	D48.0	D49.2
patella	C40.2-	C79.51	-	-	-	-
pelvic	C41.4	C79.51	-	D16.8	D48.0	D49.2
phalanges						
foot	C40.3-	C79.51	-	-	-	-
hand	C40.1-	C79.51	-	-	-	-
pubic	C41.4	C79.51	-	D16.8	D48.0	D49.2
radius (any part)	C40.0-	C79.51	-	D16.0-	-	-
rib	C41.3	C79.51	-	D16.7	D48.0	D49.2
sacral vertebra	C41.4	C79.51	-	D16.8	D48.0	D49.2
sacrum	C41.4	C79.51	-	D16.8	D48.0	D49.2
scaphoid						
of ankle	C40.3-	C79.51	-	-	-	-
of hand	C40.1-	C79.51	-	-	-	-
scapula (any part)	C40.0-	C79.51	-	D16.0-	-	-
sella turcica	C41.0	C79.51	-	D16.4-	D48.0	D49.2
shoulder	C40.0-	C79.51	-	D16.0-	-	-
skull	C41.0	C79.51	-	D16.4-	D48.0	D49.2
sphenoid	C41.0	C79.51	-	D16.4-	D48.0	D49.2
spine, spinal (column)	C41.2	C79.51	-	D16.6	D48.0	D49.2
coccyx	C41.4	C79.51	-	D16.8	D48.0	D49.2
sacrum	C41.4	C79.51	-	D16.8	D48.0	D49.2
sternum	C41.3	C79.51	-	D16.7	D48.0	D49.2
tarsus (any)	C40.3-	C79.51	-	-	-	-
temporal	C41.0	C79.51	-	D16.4-	D48.0	D49.2
thumb	C40.1-	C79.51	-	-	-	-
tibia (any part)	C40.2-	C79.51	-	-	-	-
toe (any)	C40.3-	C79.51	-	-	-	-
trapezium	C40.1-	C79.51	-	-	-	-
trapezoid	C40.1-	C79.51	-	-	-	-
turbinate	C41.0	C79.51	-	D16.4-	D48.0	D49.2
ulna (any part)	C40.0-	C79.51	-	D16.0-	-	-
unciform	C40.1-	C79.51	-	-	-	-
vertebra (column)	C41.2	C79.51	-	D16.6	D48.0	D49.2
coccyx	C41.4	C79.51	-	D16.8	D48.0	D49.2
sacrum	C41.4	C79.51	-	D16.8	D48.0	D49.2
vomer	C41.0	C79.51	-	D16.4-	D48.0	D49.2
wrist	C40.1-	C79.51	-	-	-	-
xiphoid process	C41.3	C79.51	-	D16.7	D48.0	D49.2
zygomatic	C41.0	C79.51	-	D16.4-	D48.0	D49.2
book-leaf (mouth) *ventral surface of tongue and floor of mouth*	C06.89	C79.89	D00.00	D10.39	D37.09	D49.0
bowel — *see* Neoplasm, intestine						
brachial plexus	C47.1-	C79.89	-	D36.12	D48.2	D49.2
brain NEC	C71.9	C79.31	-	D33.2	D43.2	D49.6
basal ganglia	C71.0	C79.31	-	D33.0	D43.0	D49.6
cerebellopontine angle	C71.6	C79.31	-	D33.1	D43.1	D49.6

Neoplasm	Malignant Primary	Malignant Secondary	Ca in situ	Benign	Uncertain Behavior	Unspecified Behavior
brain NEC — *continued*						
cerebellum NOS	C71.6	C79.31	-	D33.1	D43.1	D49.6
cerebrum	C71.0	C79.31	-	D33.0	D43.0	D49.6
choroid plexus	C71.7	C79.31	-	D33.1	D43.1	D49.6
corpus callosum	C71.8	C79.31	-	D33.2	D43.2	D49.6
corpus striatum	C71.0	C79.31	-	D33.0	D43.0	D49.6
cortex (cerebral)	C71.0	C79.31	-	D33.0	D43.0	D49.6
frontal lobe	C71.1	C79.31	-	D33.0	D43.0	D49.6
globus pallidus	C71.0	C79.31	-	D33.0	D43.0	D49.6
hippocampus	C71.2	C79.31	-	D33.0	D43.0	D49.6
hypothalamus	C71.0	C79.31	-	D33.0	D43.0	D49.6
internal capsule	C71.0	C79.31	-	D33.0	D43.0	D49.6
medulla oblongata	C71.7	C79.31	-	D33.1	D43.1	D49.6
meninges	C70.0	C79.32	-	D32.0	D42.0	D49.7
midbrain	C71.7	C79.31	-	D33.1	D43.1	D49.6
occipital lobe	C71.4	C79.31	-	D33.0	D43.0	D49.6
overlapping lesion	C71.8	C79.31	-	-	-	-
parietal lobe	C71.3	C79.31	-	D33.0	D43.0	D49.6
peduncle	C71.7	C79.31	-	D33.1	D43.1	D49.6
pons	C71.7	C79.31	-	D33.1	D43.1	D49.6
stem	C71.7	C79.31	-	D33.1	D43.1	D49.6
tapetum	C71.8	C79.31	-	D33.2	D43.2	D49.6
temporal lobe	C71.2	C79.31	-	D33.0	D43.0	D49.6
thalamus	C71.0	C79.31	-	D33.0	D43.0	D49.6
uncus	C71.2	C79.31	-	D33.0	D43.0	D49.6
ventricle (floor)	C71.5	C79.31	-	D33.0	D43.0	D49.6
fourth	C71.7	C79.31	-	D33.1	D43.1	D49.6
branchial (cleft) (cyst) (vestiges)	C10.4	C79.89	D00.08	D10.5	D37.05	D49.0
breast (connective tissue) (glandular tissue) (soft parts)	C50.9-	C79.81	D05.-	D24.-	D48.6-	D49.3
areola	C50.0-	C79.81	D05.-	D24.-	D48.6-	D49.3
axillary tail	C50.6-	C79.81	D05.-	D24.-	D48.6-	D49.3
central portion	C50.1-	C79.81	D05.-	D24.-	D48.6-	D49.3
inner	C50.8-	C79.81	D05.-	D24.-	D48.6-	D49.3
lower	C50.8-	C79.81	D05.-	D24.-	D48.6-	D49.3
lower-inner quadrant	C50.3-	C79.81	D05.-	D24.-	D48.6-	D49.3
lower-outer quadrant	C50.5-	C79.81	D05.-	D24.-	D48.6-	D49.3
mastectomy site (skin) (*see also* Neoplasm, breast, skin)	C44.501	C79.2	-	-	-	-
specified as breast tissue	C50.8-	C79.81	-	-	-	-
midline	C50.8-	C79.81	D05.-	D24.-	D48.6-	D49.3
nipple	C50.0-	C79.81	D05.-	D24.-	D48.6-	D49.3
outer	C50.8-	C79.81	D05.-	D24.-	D48.6-	D49.3
overlapping lesion	C50.8-	-	-	-	-	-
skin	C44.501	C79.2	D04.5	D23.5	D48.5	D49.2
basal cell carcinoma	C44.511	-	-	-	-	-
specified type NEC	C44.591	-	-	-	-	-
squamous cell carcinoma	C44.521	-	-	-	-	-
tail (axillary)	C50.6-	C79.81	D05.-	D24.-	D48.6-	D49.3
upper	C50.8-	C79.81	D05.-	D24.-	D48.6-	D49.3
upper-inner quadrant	C50.2-	C79.81	D05.-	D24.-	D48.6-	D49.3
upper-outer quadrant	C50.4-	C79.81	D05.-	D24.-	D48.6-	D49.3
broad ligament	C57.1	C79.82	D07.39	D28.2	D39.8	D49.59
bronchiogenic, bronchogenic (lung)	C34.9-	C78.0-	D02.2-	D14.3-	D38.1	D49.1
bronchiole	C34.9-	C78.0-	D02.2-	D14.3-	D38.1	D49.1
bronchus	C34.9-	C78.0-	D02.2-	D14.3-	D38.1	D49.1
carina	C34.0-	C78.0-	D02.2-	D14.3-	D38.1	D49.1
lower lobe of lung	C34.3-	C78.0-	D02.2-	D14.3-	D38.1	D49.1
main	C34.0-	C78.0-	D02.2-	D14.3-	D38.1	D49.1
middle lobe of lung	C34.2	C78.0-	D02.21	D14.31	D38.1	D49.1
overlapping lesion	C34.8-	-	-	-	-	-
upper lobe of lung	C34.1-	C78.0-	D02.2-	D14.3-	D38.1	D49.1
brow	C44.309	C79.2	D04.39	D23.39	D48.5	D49.2
basal cell carcinoma	C44.319	-	-	-	-	-
specified type NEC	C44.399	-	-	-	-	-
squamous cell carcinoma	C44.329	-	-	-	-	-
buccal (cavity)	C06.9	C79.89	D00.00	D10.39	D37.09	D49.0
commissure	C06.0	C79.89	D00.02	D10.39	D37.09	D49.0
groove (lower) (upper)	C06.1	C79.89	D00.02	D10.39	D37.09	D49.0
mucosa	C06.0	C79.89	D00.02	D10.39	D37.09	D49.0
sulcus (lower) (upper)	C06.1	C79.89	D00.02	D10.39	D37.09	D49.0
bulbourethral gland	C68.0	C79.19	D09.19	D30.4	D41.3	D49.59
bursa — *see* Neoplasm, connective tissue						
buttock NEC	C76.3	C79.89	D04.5	D36.7	D48.7	D49.89
calf	C76.5-	C79.89	D04.7-	D36.7	D48.7	D49.89
calvarium	C41.0	C79.51	-	D16.4-	D48.0	D49.2
calyx, renal	C65.-	C79.0-	D09.19	D30.1-	D41.1-	D49.51-
canal						
anal	C21.1	C78.5	D01.3	D12.9	D37.8	D49.0
auditory (external) (*see also* Neoplasm, skin, ear)	C44.20-	C79.2	D04.2-	D23.2-	D48.5	D49.2
auricular (external) (*see also* Neoplasm, skin, ear)	C44.20-	C79.2	D04.2-	D23.2-	D48.5	D49.2
canaliculi, biliary (biliferi) (intrahepatic)	C22.1	C78.7	D01.5	D13.4	D37.6	D49.0
canthus (eye) (inner) (outer)	C44.10-	C79.2	D04.1-	D23.1-	D48.5	D49.2
basal cell carcinoma	C44.11-	-	-	-	-	-
specified type NEC	C44.19-	-	-	-	-	-
squamous cell carcinoma	C44.12-	-	-	-	-	-

Neoplasm	Malignant Primary	Malignant Secondary	Ca in situ	Benign	Uncertain Behavior	Unspecified Behavior
capillary — see Neoplasm, connective tissue						
caput coli	C18.0	C78.5	D01.0	D12.0	D37.4	D49.0
carcinoid — see Tumor, carcinoid						
cardia (gastric)	C16.0	C78.89	D00.2	D13.1	D37.1	D49.0
cardiac orifice (stomach)	C16.0	C78.89	D00.2	D13.1	D37.1	D49.0
cardio-esophageal junction	C16.0	C78.89	D00.2	D13.1	D37.1	D49.0
cardio-esophagus	C16.0	C78.89	D00.2	D13.1	D37.1	D49.0
carina (bronchus)	C34.0-	C78.0-	D02.2-	D14.3-	D38.1	D49.1
carotid (artery)	C49.0	C79.89	-	D21.0	D48.1	D49.2
body	C75.4	C79.89	-	D35.5	D44.6	D49.7
carpus (any bone)	C40.1-	C79.51	-	D16.1-	-	-
cartilage (articular) (joint) NEC (see also Neoplasm, bone)	C41.9	C79.51	-	D16.9-	D48.0	D49.2
arytenoid	C32.3	C78.39	D02.0	D14.1	D38.0	D49.1
auricular	C49.0	C79.89	-	D21.0	D48.1	D49.2
bronchi	C34.0-	C78.39	-	D14.3-	D38.1	D49.1
costal	C41.3	C79.51	-	D16.7	D48.0	D49.2
cricoid	C32.3	C78.39	D02.0	D14.1	D38.0	D49.1
cuneiform	C32.3	C78.39	D02.0	D14.1	D38.0	D49.1
ear (external)	C49.0	C79.89	-	D21.0	D48.1	D49.2
ensiform	C41.3	C79.51	-	D16.7	D48.0	D49.2
epiglottis	C32.1	C78.39	D02.0	D14.1	D38.0	D49.1
anterior surface	C10.1	C79.89	D00.08	D10.5	D37.05	D49.0
eyelid	C49.0	C79.89	-	D21.0	D48.1	D49.2
intervertebral	C41.2	C79.51	-	D16.6	D48.0	D49.2
larynx, laryngeal	C32.3	C78.39	D02.0	D14.1	D38.0	D49.1
nose, nasal	C30.0	C78.39	D02.3	D14.0	D38.5	D49.1
pinna	C49.0	C79.89	-	D21.0	D48.1	D49.2
rib	C41.3	C79.51	-	D16.7	D48.0	D49.2
semilunar (knee)	C40.2-	C79.51	-	D16.2-	D48.0	D49.2
thyroid	C32.3	C78.39	D02.0	D14.1	D38.0	D49.1
trachea	C33	C78.39	D02.1	D14.2	D38.1	D49.1
cauda equina	C72.1	C79.49	-	D33.4	D43.4	D49.7
cavity						
buccal	C06.9	C79.89	D00.00	D10.30	D37.09	D49.0
nasal	C30.0	C78.39	D02.3	D14.0	D38.5	D49.1
oral	C06.9	C79.89	D00.00	D10.30	D37.09	D49.0
peritoneal	C48.2	C78.6	-	D20.1	D48.4	D49.0
tympanic	C30.1	C78.39	D02.3	D14.0	D38.5	D49.1
cecum	C18.0	C78.5	D01.0	D12.0	D37.4	D49.0
central nervous system	C72.9	C79.40	-	-	-	-
cerebellopontine (angle)	C71.6	C79.31	-	D33.1	D43.1	D49.6
cerebellum, cerebellar	C71.6	C79.31	-	D33.1	D43.1	D49.6
cerebrum, cerebral (cortex) (hemisphere) (white matter)	C71.0	C79.31	-	D33.0	D43.0	D49.6
meninges	C70.0	C79.32	-	D32.0	D42.0	D49.7
peduncle	C71.7	C79.31	-	D33.1	D43.1	D49.6
ventricle	C71.5	C79.31	-	D33.0	D43.0	D49.6
fourth	C71.7	C79.31	-	D33.1	D43.1	D49.6
cervical region	C76.0	C79.89	D09.8	D36.7	D48.7	D49.89
cervix (cervical) (uteri) (uterus)	C53.9	C79.82	D06.9	D26.0	D39.0	D49.59
canal	C53.0	C79.82	D06.0	D26.0	D39.0	D49.59
endocervix (canal) (gland)	C53.0	C79.82	D06.0	D26.0	D39.0	D49.59
exocervix	C53.1	C79.82	D06.1	D26.0	D39.0	D49.59
external os	C53.1	C79.82	D06.1	D26.0	D39.0	D49.59
internal os	C53.0	C79.82	D06.0	D26.0	D39.0	D49.59
nabothian gland	C53.0	C79.82	D06.0	D26.0	D39.0	D49.59
overlapping lesion	C53.8	-	-	-	-	-
squamocolumnar junction	C53.8	C79.82	D06.7	D26.0	D39.0	D49.59
stump	C53.8	C79.82	D06.7	D26.0	D39.0	D49.59
cheek	C76.0	C79.89	D09.8	D36.7	D48.7	D49.89
external	C44.309	C79.2	D04.39	D23.39	D48.5	D49.2
basal cell carcinoma	C44.319	-	-	-	-	-
specified type NEC	C44.399	-	-	-	-	-
squamous cell carcinoma	C44.329	-	-	-	-	-
inner aspect	C06.0	C79.89	D00.02	D10.39	D37.09	D49.0
internal	C06.0	C79.89	D00.02	D10.39	D37.09	D49.0
mucosa	C06.0	C79.89	D00.02	D10.39	D37.09	D49.0
chest (wall) NEC	C76.1	C79.89	D09.8	D36.7	D48.7	D49.89
chiasma opticum	C72.3-	C79.49	-	D33.3	D43.3	D49.7
chin	C44.309	C79.2	D04.39	D23.39	D48.5	D49.2
basal cell carcinoma	C44.319	-	-	-	-	-
specified type NEC	C44.399	-	-	-	-	-
squamous cell carcinoma	C44.329	-	-	-	-	-
choana	C11.3	C79.89	D00.08	D10.6	D37.05	D49.0
cholangiole	C22.1	C78.89	D01.5	D13.4	D37.6	D49.0
choledochal duct	C24.0	C78.89	D01.5	D13.5	D37.6	D49.0
choroid	C69.3-	C79.49	D09.2-	D31.3-	D48.7	D49.81
plexus	C71.5	C79.31	-	D33.0	D43.0	D49.6
ciliary body	C69.4-	C79.49	D09.2-	D31.4-	D48.7	D49.89
clavicle	C41.3	C79.51	-	D16.7	D48.0	D49.2
clitoris	C51.2	C79.82	D07.1	D28.0	D39.8	D49.59
clivus	C41.0	C79.51	-	D16.4-	D48.0	D49.2
cloacogenic zone	C21.2	C78.5	D01.3	D12.9	D37.8	D49.0
coccygeal						
body or glomus	C49.5	C79.8º	-	D21.5	D48.1	D49.2
vertebra	C41.4	C79.51	-	D16.8	D48.0	D49.2

Neoplasm	Malignant Primary	Malignant Secondary	Ca in situ	Benign	Uncertain Behavior	Unspecified Behavior
coccyx	C41.4	C79.51	-	D16.8	D48.0	D49.2
colon (see also Neoplasm, intestine, large)	C18.9	C78.5	-	-	-	-
with rectum	C19	C78.5	D01.1	D12.7	D37.5	D49.0
column, spinal — see Neoplasm, spine						
columnella (see also Neoplasm, skin, face)	C44.390	C79.2	D04.39	D23.39	D48.5	D49.2
commissure						
labial, lip	C00.6	C79.89	D00.01	D10.39	D37.01	D49.0
laryngeal	C32.0	C78.39	D02.0	D14.1	D38.0	D49.1
common (bile) duct	C24.0	C78.89	D01.5	D13.5	D37.6	D49.0
concha (see also Neoplasm, skin, ear)	C44.20-	C79.2	D04.2-	D23.2-	D48.5	D49.2
nose	C30.0	C78.39	D02.3	D14.0	D38.5	D49.1
conjunctiva	C69.0-	C79.49	D09.2-	D31.0-	D48.7	D49.89
connective tissue NEC	C49.9	C79.89	-	D21.9	D48.1	D49.2

Note: For neoplasms of connective tissue (blood vessel, bursa, fascia, ligament, muscle, peripheral nerves, sympathetic and parasympathetic nerves and ganglia, synovia, tendon, etc.) or of morphological types that indicate connective tissue, code according to the list under "Neoplasm, connective tissue". For sites that do not appear in this list, code to neoplasm of that site; e.g., fibrosarcoma, pancreas (C25.9).

Note: Morphological types that indicate connective tissue appear in their proper place in the alphabetic index with the instruction "see Neoplasm, connective tissue ...."

Neoplasm	Malignant Primary	Malignant Secondary	Ca in situ	Benign	Uncertain Behavior	Unspecified Behavior
abdomen	C49.4	C79.89	-	D21.4	D48.1	D49.2
abdominal wall	C49.4	C79.89	-	D21.4	D48.1	D49.2
ankle	C49.2-	C79.89	-	D21.2-	D48.1	D49.2
antecubital fossa or space	C49.1-	C79.89	-	D21.1-	D48.1	D49.2
arm	C49.1-	C79.89	-	D21.1-	D48.1	D49.2
auricle (ear)	C49.0	C79.89	-	D21.0	D48.1	D49.2
axilla	C49.3	C79.89	-	D21.3	D48.1	D49.2
back	C49.6	C79.89	-	D21.6	D48.1	D49.2
breast — see Neoplasm, breast						
buttock	C49.5	C79.89	-	D21.5	D48.1	D49.2
calf	C49.2-	C79.89	-	D21.2-	D48.1	D49.2
cervical region	C49.0	C79.89	-	D21.0	D48.1	D49.2
cheek	C49.0	C79.89	-	D21.0	D48.1	D49.2
chest (wall)	C49.3	C79.89	-	D21.3	D48.1	D49.2
chin	C49.0	C79.89	-	D21.0	D48.1	D49.2
diaphragm	C49.3	C79.89	-	D21.3	D48.1	D49.2
ear (external)	C49.0	C79.89	-	D21.0	D48.1	D49.2
elbow	C49.1-	C79.89	-	D21.1-	D48.1	D49.2
extrarectal	C49.5	C79.89	-	D21.5	D48.1	D49.2
extremity	C49.9	C79.89	-	D21.9	D48.1	D49.2
lower	C49.2-	C79.89	-	D21.2-	D48.1	D49.2
upper	C49.1-	C79.89	-	D21.1-	D48.1	D49.2
eyelid	C49.0	C79.89	-	D21.0	D48.1	D49.2
face	C49.0	C79.89	-	D21.0	D48.1	D49.2
finger	C49.1-	C79.89	-	D21.1-	D48.1	D49.2
flank	C49.6	C79.89	-	D21.6	D48.1	D49.2
foot	C49.2-	C79.89	-	D21.2-	D48.1	D49.2
forearm	C49.1-	C79.89	-	D21.1-	D48.1	D49.2
forehead	C49.0	C79.89	-	D21.0	D48.1	D49.2
gastric	C49.4	C79.89	-	D21.4	D48.1	D49.2
gastrointestinal	C49.4	C79.89	-	D21.4	D48.1	D49.2
gluteal region	C49.5	C79.89	-	D21.5	D48.1	D49.2
great vessels NEC	C49.3	C79.89	-	D21.3	D48.1	D49.2
groin	C49.5	C79.89	-	D21.5	D48.1	D49.2
hand	C49.1-	C79.89	-	D21.1-	D48.1	D49.2
head	C49.0	C79.89	-	D21.0	D48.1	D49.2
heel	C49.2-	C79.89	-	D21.2-	D48.1	D49.2
hip	C49.2-	C79.89	-	D21.2-	D48.1	D49.2
hypochondrium	C49.4	C79.89	-	D21.4	D48.1	D49.2
iliopsoas muscle	C49.5	C79.89	-	D21.5	D48.1	D49.2
infraclavicular region	C49.3	C79.89	-	D21.3	D48.1	D49.2
inguinal (canal) (region)	C49.5	C79.89	-	D21.5	D48.1	D49.2
intestinal	C49.4	C79.89	-	D21.4	D48.1	D49.2
intrathoracic	C49.3	C79.89	-	D21.3	D48.1	D49.2
ischiorectal fossa	C49.5	C79.89	-	D21.5	D48.1	D49.2
jaw	C03.9	C79.89	D00.03	D10.39	D37.09	D49.0
knee	C49.2-	C79.89	-	D21.2-	D48.1	D49.2
leg	C49.2-	C79.89	-	D21.2-	D48.1	D49.2
limb NEC	C49.9	C79.89	-	D21.9	D48.1	D49.2
lower	C49.2-	C79.89	-	D21.2-	D48.1	D49.2
upper	C49.1-	C79.89	-	D21.1-	D48.1	D49.2
nates	C49.5	C79.89	-	D21.5	D48.1	D49.2
neck	C49.0	C79.89	-	D21.0	D48.1	D49.2
orbit	C69.6-	C79.49	D09.2-	D31.6-	D48.1	D49.89
overlapping lesion	C49.8	-	-	-	-	-
pararectal	C49.5	C79.89	-	D21.5	D48.1	D49.2
para-urethral	C49.5	C79.89	-	D21.5	D48.1	D49.2
paravaginal	C49.5	C79.89	-	D21.5	D48.1	D49.2
pelvis (floor)	C49.5	C79.89	-	D21.5	D48.1	D49.2
pelvo-abdominal	C49.8	C79.89	-	D21.6	D48.1	D49.2
perineum	C49.5	C79.89	-	D21.5	D48.1	D49.2
perirectal (tissue)	C49.5	C79.89	-	D21.5	D48.1	D49.2
periurethral (tissue)	C49.5	C79.89	-	D21.5	D48.1	D49.2
popliteal fossa or space	C49.2-	C79.89	-	D21.2-	D48.1	D49.2
presacral	C49.5	C79.89	-	D21.5	D48.1	D49.2

connective - fibula

ICD-10-CM TABLE OF NEOPLASMS

Neoplasm	Malignant Primary	Malignant Secondary	Ca in situ	Benign	Uncertain Behavior	Unspecified Behavior
connective tissue NEC — *continued*						
psoas muscle	C49.4	C79.89	-	D21.4	D48.1	D49.2
pterygoid fossa	C49.0	C79.89	-	D21.0	D48.1	D49.2
rectovaginal septum or wall	C49.5	C79.89	-	D21.5	D48.1	D49.2
rectovesical	C49.5	C79.89	-	D21.5	D48.1	D49.2
retroperitoneum	C48.0	C78.6	-	D20.0	D48.3	D49.0
sacrococcygeal region	C49.5	C79.89	-	D21.5	D48.1	D49.2
scalp	C49.0	C79.89	-	D21.0	D48.1	D49.2
scapular region	C49.3	C79.89	-	D21.3	D48.1	D49.2
shoulder	C49.1-	C79.89	-	D21.1-	D48.1	D49.2
skin (dermis) NEC (*see also* Neoplasm, skin, by site)	C44.90	C79.2	D04.9	D23.9	D48.5	D49.2
stomach	C49.4	C79.89	-	D21.4	D48.1	D49.2
submental	C49.0	C79.89	-	D21.0	D48.1	D49.2
supraclavicular region	C49.0	C79.89	-	D21.0	D48.1	D49.2
temple	C49.0	C79.89	-	D21.0	D48.1	D49.2
temporal region	C49.0	C79.89	-	D21.0	D48.1	D49.2
thigh	C49.2-	C79.89	-	D21.2-	D48.1	D49.2
thoracic (duct) (wall)	C49.3	C79.89	-	D21.3	D48.1	D49.2
thorax	C49.3	C79.89	-	D21.3	D48.1	D49.2
thumb	C49.1-	C79.89	-	D21.1-	D48.1	D49.2
toe	C49.2-	C79.89	-	D21.2-	D48.1	D49.2
trunk	C49.6	C79.89	-	D21.6	D48.1	D49.2
umbilicus	C49.4	C79.89	-	D21.4	D48.1	D49.2
vesicorectal	C49.5	C79.89	-	D21.5	D48.1	D49.2
wrist	C49.1-	C79.89	-	D21.1-	D48.1	D49.2
conus medullaris	C72.0	C79.49	-	D33.4	D43.4	D49.7
cord (true) (vocal)	C32.0	C78.39	D02.0	D14.1	D38.0	D49.1
false	C32.1	C78.39	D02.0	D14.1	D38.0	D49.1
spermatic	C63.1-	C79.82	D07.69	D29.8	D40.8	D49.59
spinal (cervical) (lumbar) (thoracic)	C72.0	C79.49	-	D33.4	D43.4	D49.7
cornea (limbus)	C69.1-	C79.49	D09.2-	D31.1-	D48.7	D49.89
corpus						
albicans	C56.-	C79.6-	D07.39	D27.-	D39.1-	D49.59
callosum, brain	C71.0	C79.31	-	D33.2	D43.2	D49.6
cavernosum	C60.2	C79.82	D07.4	D29.0	D40.8	D49.59
gastric	C16.2	C78.89	D00.2	D13.1	D37.1	D49.0
overlapping sites	C54.8	-	-	-	-	-
penis	C60.2	C79.82	D07.4	D29.0	D40.8	D49.59
striatum, cerebrum	C71.0	C79.31	-	D33.0	D43.0	D49.6
uteri	C54.9	C79.82	D07.0	D26.1	D39.0	D49.59
isthmus	C54.0	C79.82	D07.0	D26.1	D39.0	D49.59
cortex						
adrenal	C74.0-	C79.7-	D09.3	D35.0-	D44.1-	D49.7
cerebral	C71.0	C79.31	-	D33.0	D43.0	D49.6
costal cartilage	C41.3	C79.51	-	D16.7	D48.0	D49.2
costovertebral joint	C41.3	C79.51	-	D16.7	D48.0	D49.2
Cowper's gland	C68.0	C79.19	D09.19	D30.4	D41.3	D49.59
cranial (fossa, any)	C71.9	C79.31	-	D33.2	D43.2	D49.6
meninges	C70.0	C79.32	-	D32.0	D42.0	D49.7
nerve	C72.50	C79.49	-	D33.3	D43.3	D49.7
specified NEC	C72.59	C79.49	-	D33.3	D43.3	D49.7
craniobuccal pouch	C75.2	C79.89	D09.3	D35.2	D44.3	D49.7
craniopharyngeal (duct) (pouch)	C75.2	C79.89	D09.3	D35.3	D44.4	D49.7
cricoid	C13.0	C79.89	D00.08	D10.7	D37.05	D49.0
cartilage	C32.3	C78.39	D02.0	D14.1	D38.0	D49.1
cricopharynx	C13.0	C79.89	D00.08	D10.7	D37.05	D49.0
crypt of Morgagni	C21.8	C78.5	D01.3	D12.9	D37.8	D49.0
crystalline lens	C69.4-	C79.49	D09.2-	D31.4-	D48.7	D49.89
cul-de-sac (Douglas')	C48.1	C78.6	-	D20.1	D48.4	D49.0
cuneiform cartilage	C32.3	C78.39	D02.0	D14.1	D38.0	D49.1
cutaneous — *see* Neoplasm, skin						
cutis — *see* Neoplasm, skin						
cystic (bile) duct (common)	C24.0	C78.89	D01.5	D13.5	D37.6	D49.0
dermis — *see* Neoplasm, skin						
diaphragm	C49.3	C79.89	-	D21.3	D48.1	D49.2
digestive organs, system, tube, or tract NEC	C26.9	C78.89	D01.9	D13.9	D37.9	D49.0
disc, intervertebral	C41.2	C79.51	-	D16.6	D48.0	D49.2
disease, generalized	C80.0	-	-	-	-	-
disseminated	C80.0	-	-	-	-	-
Douglas' cul-de-sac or pouch	C48.1	C78.6	-	D20.1	D48.4	D49.0
duodenojejunal junction	C17.8	C78.4	D01.49	D13.39	D37.2	D49.0
duodenum	C17.0	C78.4	D01.49	D13.2	D37.2	D49.0
dura (cranial) (mater)	C70.9	C79.49	-	D32.9	D42.9	D49.7
cerebral	C70.0	C79.32	-	D32.0	D42.0	D49.7
spinal	C70.1	C79.49	-	D32.1	D42.1	D49.7
ear (external) (*see also* Neoplasm, skin, ear)	C44.20-	C79.2	D04.2-	D23.2-	D48.5	D49.2
auricle or auris (*see also* Neoplasm, skin, ear)	C44.20-	C79.2	D04.2-	D23.2-	D48.5	D49.2
canal, external (*see also* Neoplasm, skin, ear)	C44.20-	C79.2	D04.2-	D23.2-	D48.5	D49.2
cartilage	C49.0	C79.89	-	D21.0	D48.1	D49.2
external meatus (*see also* Neoplasm, skin, ear)	C44.20-	C79.2	D04.2-	D23.2-	D48.5	D49.2
inner	C30.1	C78.39	D02.3	D14.0	D38.5	D49.1
lobule (*see also* Neoplasm, skin, ear)	C44.20-	C79.2	D04.2-	D23.2-	D48.5	D49.2

Neoplasm	Malignant Primary	Malignant Secondary	Ca in situ	Benign	Uncertain Behavior	Unspecified Behavior
ear — *continued*						
middle	C30.1	C78.39	D02.3	D14.0	D38.5	D49.1
overlapping lesion with accessory sinuses	C31.8					
skin	C44.20-	C79.2	D04.2-	D23.2-	D48.5	D49.2
basal cell carcinoma	C44.21-	-	-	-	-	-
specified type NEC	C44.29-	-	-	-	-	-
squamous cell carcinoma	C44.22-	-	-	-	-	-
earlobe	C44.20-	C79.2	D04.2-	D23.2-	D48.5	D49.2
basal cell carcinoma	C44.21-	-	-	-	-	-
specified type NEC	C44.29-	-	-	-	-	-
squamous cell carcinoma	C44.22-	-	-	-	-	-
ejaculatory duct	C63.7	C79.82	D07.69	D29.8	D40.8	D49.59
elbow NEC	C76.4-	C79.89	D04.6-	D36.7	D48.7	D49.89
endocardium	C38.0	C79.89	-	D15.1	D48.7	D49.89
endocervix (canal) (gland)	C53.0	C79.82	D06.0	D26.0	D39.0	D49.59
endocrine gland NEC	C75.9	C79.89	D09.3	D35.9	D44.9	D49.7
pluriglandular	C75.8	C79.89	D09.3	D35.7	D44.9	D49.7
endometrium (gland) (stroma)	C54.1	C79.82	D07.0	D26.1	D39.0	D49.59
ensiform cartilage	C41.3	C79.51	-	D16.7	D48.0	D49.2
enteric — *see* Neoplasm, intestine						
ependyma (brain)	C71.5	C79.31	-	D33.0	D43.0	D49.6
fourth ventricle	C71.7	C79.31	-	D33.1	D43.1	D49.6
epicardium	C38.0	C79.89	-	D15.1	D48.7	D49.89
epididymis	C63.0-	C79.82	D07.69	D29.3-	D40.8	D49.59
epidural	C72.9	C79.49	-	D33.9	D43.9	D49.7
epiglottis	C32.1	C78.39	D02.0	D14.1	D38.0	D49.1
anterior aspect or surface	C10.1	C79.89	D00.08	D10.5	D37.05	D49.0
cartilage	C32.3	C78.39	D02.0	D14.1	D38.0	D49.1
free border (margin)	C10.1	C79.89	D00.08	D10.5	D37.05	D49.0
junctional region	C10.8	C79.89	D00.08	D10.5	D37.05	D49.0
posterior (laryngeal) surface	C32.1	C78.39	D02.0	D14.1	D38.0	D49.1
suprahyoid portion	C32.1	C78.39	D02.0	D14.1	D38.0	D49.1
esophagogastric junction	C16.0	C78.89	D00.2	D13.1	D37.1	D49.0
esophagus	C15.9	C78.89	D00.1	D13.0	D37.8	D49.0
abdominal	C15.5	C78.89	D00.1	D13.0	D37.8	D49.0
cervical	C15.3	C78.89	D00.1	D13.0	D37.8	D49.0
distal (third)	C15.5	C78.89	D00.1	D13.0	D37.8	D49.0
lower (third)	C15.5	C78.89	D00.1	D13.0	D37.8	D49.0
middle (third)	C15.4	C78.89	D00.1	D13.0	D37.8	D49.0
overlapping lesion	C15.8	-	-	-	-	-
proximal (third)	C15.3	C78.89	D00.1	D13.0	D37.8	D49.0
thoracic	C15.4	C78.89	D00.1	D13.0	D37.8	D49.0
upper (third)	C15.3	C78.89	D00.1	D13.0	D37.8	D49.0
ethmoid (sinus)	C31.1	C78.39	D02.3	D14.0	D38.5	D49.1
bone or labyrinth	C41.0	C79.51	-	D16.4-	D48.0	D49.2
eustachian tube	C30.1	C78.39	D02.3	D14.0	D38.5	D49.1
exocervix	C53.1	C79.82	D06.1	D26.0	D39.0	D49.59
external						
meatus (ear) (*see also* Neoplasm, skin, ear)	C44.20-	C79.2	D04.2-	D23.2-	D48.5	D49.2
os, cervix uteri	C53.1	C79.82	D06.1	D26.0	D39.0	D49.59
extradural	C72.9	C79.49	-	D33.9	D43.9	D49.7
extrahepatic (bile) duct	C24.0	C78.89	D01.5	D13.5	D37.6	D49.0
overlapping lesion with gallbladder	C24.8					
extraocular muscle	C69.6-	C79.49	D09.2-	D31.6-	D48.7	D49.89
extrarectal	C76.3	C79.89	D09.8	D36.7	D48.7	D49.89
extremity	C76.8	C79.89	D04.8	D36.7	D48.7	D49.89
lower	C76.5-	C79.89	D04.7-	D36.7	D48.7	D49.89
upper	C76.4-	C79.89	D04.6-	D36.7	D48.7	D49.89
eye NEC	C69.9-	C79.49	D09.2	D31.9	D48.7	D49.89
overlapping sites	C69.8	-	-	-	-	-
eyeball	C69.9-	C79.49	D09.2-	D31.9-	D48.7	D49.89
eyebrow	C44.309	C79.2	D04.39	D23.39	D48.5	D49.2
basal cell carcinoma	C44.319	-	-	-	-	-
specified type NEC	C44.399	-	-	-	-	-
squamous cell carcinoma	C44.329	-	-	-	-	-
eyelid (lower) (skin) (upper)	C44.10-	-	-	-	-	-
basal cell carcinoma	C44.11-	-	-	-	-	-
specified type NEC	C44.19-	-	-	-	-	-
squamous cell carcinoma	C44.12-	-	-	-	-	-
cartilage	C49.0	C79.89	-	D21.0	D48.1	D49.2
face NEC	C76.0	C79.89	D04.39	D36.7	D48.7	D49.89
fallopian tube (accessory)	C57.0-	C79.82	D07.39	D28.2	D39.8	D49.59
falx (cerebella) (cerebri)	C70.0	C79.32	-	D32.0	D42.0	D49.7
fascia (*see also* Neoplasm, connective tissue)						
palmar	C49.1-	C79.89	-	D21.1-	D48.1	D49.2
plantar	C49.2-	C79.89	-	D21.2-	D48.1	D49.2
fatty tissue — *see* Neoplasm, connective tissue						
fauces, faucial NEC	C10.9	C79.89	D00.08	D10.5	D37.05	D49.0
pillars	C09.1	C79.89	D00.08	D10.5	D37.05	D49.0
tonsil	C09.9	C79.89	D00.08	D10.4	D37.05	D49.0
femur (any part)	C40.2-	-	-	D16.2-	-	-
fetal membrane	C58	C79.82	D07.0	D26.7	D39.2	D49.59
fibrous tissue — *see* Neoplasm, connective tissue						
fibula (any part)	C40.2-	C79.51	-	D16.2-	-	-

Neoplasm	Malignant Primary	Malignant Secondary	Ca in situ	Benign	Uncertain Behavior	Unspecified Behavior
filum terminale	C72.0	C79.49	-	D33.4	D43.4	D49.7
finger NEC	C76.4-	C79.89	D04.6-	D36.7	D48.7	D49.89
flank NEC	C76.8	C79.89	D04.5	D36.7	D48.7	D49.89
follicle, nabothian	C53.0	C79.82	D06.0	D26.0	D39.0	D49.59
foot NEC	C76.5-	C79.89	D04.7-	D36.7	D48.7	D49.89
forearm NEC	C76.4-	C79.89	D04.6-	D36.7	D48.7	D49.89
forehead (skin)	C44.309	C79.2	D04.39	D23.39	D48.5	D49.2
basal cell carcinoma	C44.319	-	-	-	-	-
specified type NEC	C44.399	-	-	-	-	-
squamous cell carcinoma	C44.329	-	-	-	-	-
foreskin	C60.0	C79.82	D07.4	D29.0	D40.8	D49.59
fornix						
pharyngeal	C11.3	C79.89	D00.08	D10.6	D37.05	D49.0
vagina	C52	C79.82	D07.2	D28.1	D39.8	D49.59
fossa (of)						
anterior (cranial)	C71.9	C79.31	-	D33.2	D43.2	D49.6
cranial	C71.9	C79.31	-	D33.2	D43.2	D49.6
ischiorectal	C76.3	C79.89	D09.8	D36.7	D48.7	D49.89
middle (cranial)	C71.9	C79.31	-	D33.2	D43.2	D49.6
piriform	C12	C79.89	D00.08	D10.7	D37.05	D49.0
pituitary	C75.1	C79.89	D09.3	D35.2	D44.3	D49.7
posterior (cranial)	C71.9	C79.31	-	D33.2	D43.2	D49.6
pterygoid	C49.0	C79.89	-	D21.0	D48.1	D49.2
pyriform	C12	C79.89	D00.08	D10.7	D37.05	D49.0
Rosenmuller	C11.2	C79.89	D00.08	D10.6	D37.05	D49.0
tonsillar	C09.0	C79.89	D00.08	D10.5	D37.05	D49.0
fourchette	C51.9	C79.82	D07.1	D28.0	D39.8	D49.59
frenulum						
labii — see Neoplasm, lip, internal						
linguae	C02.2	C79.89	D00.07	D10.1	D37.02	D49.0
frontal						
bone	C41.0	C79.51	-	D16.4-	D48.0	D49.2
lobe, brain	C71.1	C79.31	-	D33.0	D43.0	D49.6
pole	C71.1	C79.31	-	D33.0	D43.0	D49.6
sinus	C31.2	C78.39	D02.3	D14.0	D38.5	D49.1
fundus						
stomach	C16.1	C78.89	D00.2	D13.1	D37.1	D49.0
uterus	C54.3	C79.82	D07.0	D26.1	D39.0	D49.59
gall duct (extrahepatic)	C24.0	C78.89	D01.5	D13.5	D37.6	D49.0
intrahepatic	C22.1	C78.7	D01.5	D13.4	D37.6	D49.0
gallbladder	C23	C78.89	D01.5	D13.5	D37.6	D49.0
overlapping lesion with extrahepatic bile ducts	C24.8	-	-	-	-	-
ganglia (see also Neoplasm, nerve, peripheral)	C47.9	C79.89	-	D36.10	D48.2	D49.2
basal	C71.0	C79.31	-	D33.0	D43.0	D49.6
cranial nerve	C72.50	C79.49	-	D33.3	D43.3	D49.7
Gartner's duct	C52	C79.82	D07.2	D28.1	D39.8	D49.59
gastric — see Neoplasm, stomach						
gastrocolic	C26.9	C78.89	D01.9	D13.9	D37.9	D49.0
gastroesophageal junction	C16.0	C78.89	D00.2	D13.1	D37.1	D49.0
gastrointestinal (tract) NEC	C26.9	C78.89	D01.9	D13.9	D37.9	D49.0
generalized	C80.0	-	-	-	-	-
genital organ or tract						
female NEC	C57.9	C79.82	D07.30	D28.9	D39.9	D49.59
overlapping lesion	C57.8	-	-	-	-	-
specified site NEC	C57.7	C79.82	D07.39	D28.7	D39.8	D49.59
male NEC	C63.9	C79.82	D07.60	D29.9	D40.9	D49.59
overlapping lesion	C63.8	-	-	-	-	-
specified site NEC	C63.7	C79.82	D07.69	D29.8	D40.8	D49.59
genitourinary tract						
female	C57.9	C79.82	D07.30	D28.9	D39.9	D49.59
male	C63.9	C79.82	D07.60	D29.9	D40.9	D49.59
gingiva (alveolar) (marginal)	C03.9	C79.89	D00.03	D10.39	D37.09	D49.0
lower	C03.1	C79.89	D00.03	D10.39	D37.09	D49.0
mandibular	C03.1	C79.89	D00.03	D10.39	D37.09	D49.0
maxillary	C03.0	C79.89	D00.03	D10.39	D37.09	D49.0
upper	C03.0	C79.89	D00.03	D10.39	D37.09	D49.0
gland, glandular (lymphatic) (system) (see also Neoplasm, lymph gland)						
endocrine NEC	C75.9	C79.89	D09.3	D35.9	D44.9	D49.7
salivary — see Neoplasm, salivary gland						
glans penis	C60.1	C79.82	D07.4	D29.0	D40.8	D49.59
globus pallidus	C71.0	C79.31	-	D33.0	D43.0	D49.6
glomus						
coccygeal	C49.5	C79.89	-	D21.5	D48.1	D49.2
jugularis	C75.5	C79.89	-	D35.6	D44.7	D49.7
glosso-epiglottic fold(s)	C10.1	C79.89	D00.08	D10.5	D37.05	D49.0
glossopalatine fold	C09.1	C79.89	D00.08	D10.5	D37.05	D49.0
glossopharyngeal sulcus	C09.0	C79.89	D00.08	D10.5	D37.05	D49.0
glottis	C32.0	C78.39	D02.0	D14.1	D38.0	D49.1
gluteal region	C76.3	C79.89	D04.5	D36.7	D48.7	D49.89
great vessels NEC	C49.3	C79.89	-	D21.3	D48.1	D49.2
groin NEC	C76.3	C79.89	D04.5	D36.7	D48.7	D49.89
gum	C03.9	C79.89	D00.03	D10.39	D37.09	D49.0
lower	C03.1	C79.89	D00.03	D10.39	D37.09	D49.0
upper	C03.0	C79.89	D00.03	D10.39	D37.09	D49.0
hand NEC	C76.4-	C79.89	D04.6-	D36.7	D48.7	D49.89

Neoplasm	Malignant Primary	Malignant Secondary	Ca in situ	Benign	Uncertain Behavior	Unspecified Behavior
head NEC	C76.0	C79.89	D04.4	D36.7	D48.7	D49.89
heart	C38.0	C79.89	-	D15.1	D48.7	D49.89
heel NEC	C76.5-	C79.89	D04.7-	D36.7	D48.7	D49.89
helix (see also Neoplasm, skin, ear)	C44.20-	C79.2	D04.2-	D23.2-	D48.5	D49.2
hematopoietic, hemopoietic tissue NEC	C96.9	-	-	-	-	-
specified NEC	C96.Z	-	-	-	-	-
hemisphere, cerebral	C71.0	C79.31	-	D33.0	D43.0	D49.6
hemorrhoidal zone	C21.1	C78.5	D01.3	D12.9	D37.8	D49.0
hepatic (see also Index to disease, by histology)	C22.9	C78.7	D01.5	D13.4	D37.6	D49.0
duct (bile)	C24.0	C78.89	D01.5	D13.5	D37.6	D49.0
flexure (colon)	C18.3	C78.5	D01.0	D12.3	D37.4	D49.0
primary	C22.8	C78.7	D01.5	D13.4	D37.6	D49.0
hepatobiliary	C24.9	C78.89	D01.5	D13.5	D37.6	D49.0
hepatoblastoma	C22.2	C78.7	D01.5	D13.4	D37.6	D49.0
hepatoma	C22.0	C78.7	D01.5	D13.4	D37.6	D49.0
hilus of lung	C34.0-	C78.0-	D02.2-	D14.3-	D38.1	D49.1
hip NEC	C76.5-	C79.89	D04.7-	D36.7	D48.7	D49.89
hippocampus, brain	C71.2	C79.31	-	D33.0	D43.0	D49.6
humerus (any part)	C40.0-	C79.51	-	D16.0-		
hymen	C52	C79.82	D07.2	D28.1	D39.8	D49.59
hypopharynx, hypopharyngeal NEC	C13.9	C79.89	D00.08	D10.7	D37.05	D49.0
overlapping lesion	C13.8	-	-	-	-	-
postcricoid region	C13.0	C79.89	D00.08	D10.7	D37.05	D49.0
posterior wall	C13.2	C79.89	D00.08	D10.7	D37.05	D49.0
pyriform fossa (sinus)	C12	C79.89	D00.08	D10.7	D37.05	D49.0
hypophysis	C75.1	C79.89	D09.3	D35.2	D44.3	D49.7
hypothalamus	C71.0	C79.31	-	D33.0	D43.0	D49.6
ileocecum, ileocecal (coil) (junction) (valve)	C18.0	C78.5	D01.0	D12.0	D37.4	D49.0
ileum	C17.2	C78.4	D01.49	D13.39	D37.2	D49.0
ilium	C41.4	C79.51	-	D16.8	D48.0	D49.2
immunoproliferative NEC	C88.9	-	-	-	-	-
infraclavicular (region)	C76.1	C79.89	D04.5	D36.7	D48.7	D49.89
inguinal (region)	C76.3	C79.89	D04.5	D36.7	D48.7	D49.89
insula	C71.0	C79.31	-	D33.0	D43.0	D49.6
insular tissue (pancreas)	C25.4	C78.89	D01.7	D13.7	D37.8	D49.0
brain	C71.0	C79.31	-	D33.0	D43.0	D49.6
interarytenoid fold	C13.1	C79.89	D00.08	D10.7	D37.05	D49.0
hypopharyngeal aspect	C13.1	C79.89	D00.08	D10.7	D37.05	D49.0
laryngeal aspect	C32.1	C78.39	D02.0	D14.1	D38.0	D49.1
marginal zone	C13.1	C79.89	D00.08	D10.7	D37.05	D49.0
interdental papillae	C03.9	C79.89	D00.03	D10.39	D37.09	D49.0
lower	C03.1	C79.89	D00.03	D10.39	D37.09	D49.0
upper	C03.0	C79.89	D00.03	D10.39	D37.09	D49.0
internal						
capsule	C71.0	C79.31	-	D33.0	D43.0	D49.6
os (cervix)	C53.0	C79.82	D06.0	D26.0	D39.0	D49.59
intervertebral cartilage or disc	C41.2	C79.51	-	D16.6	D48.0	D49.2
intestine, intestinal	C26.0	C78.80	D01.40	D13.9	D37.8	D49.0
large	C18.9	C78.5	D01.0	D12.6	D37.4	D49.0
appendix	C18.1	C78.5	D01.0	D12.1	D37.3	D49.0
caput coli	C18.0	C78.5	D01.0	D12.0	D37.4	D49.0
cecum	C18.0	C78.5	D01.0	D12.0	D37.4	D49.0
colon	C18.9	C78.5	D01.0	D12.6	D37.4	D49.0
and rectum	C19	C78.5	D01.1	D12.7	D37.5	D49.0
ascending	C18.2	C78.5	D01.0	D12.2	D37.4	D49.0
caput	C18.0	C78.5	D01.0	D12.0	D37.4	D49.0
descending	C18.6	C78.5	D01.0	D12.4	D37.4	D49.0
distal	C18.6	C78.5	D01.0	D12.4	D37.4	D49.0
left	C18.6	C78.5	D01.0	D12.4	D37.4	D49.0
overlapping lesion	C18.8	-	-	-	-	-
pelvic	C18.7	C78.5	D01.0	D12.5	D37.4	D49.0
right	C18.2	C78.5	D01.0	D12.2	D37.4	D49.0
sigmoid (flexure)	C18.7	C78.5	D01.0	D12.5	D37.4	D49.0
transverse	C18.4	C78.5	D01.0	D12.3	D37.4	D49.0
hepatic flexure	C18.3	C78.5	D01.0	D12.3	D37.4	D49.0
ileocecum, ileocecal (coil) (valve)	C18.0	C78.5	D01.0	D12.0	D37.4	D49.0
overlapping lesion	C18.8	-	-	-	-	-
sigmoid flexure (lower) (upper)	C18.7	C78.5	D01.0	D12.5	D37.4	D49.0
splenic flexure	C18.5	C78.5	D01.0	D12.3	D37.4	D49.0
small	C17.9	C78.4	D01.40	D13.30	D37.2	D49.0
duodenum	C17.0	C78.4	D01.49	D13.2	D37.2	D49.0
ileum	C17.2	C78.4	D01.49	D13.39	D37.2	D49.0
jejunum	C17.1	C78.4	D01.49	D13.39	D37.2	D49.0
overlapping lesion	C17.8	-	-	-	-	-
tract NEC	C26.0	C78.89	D01.40	D13.9	D37.8	D49.0
intra-abdominal	C76.2	C79.89	D09.8	D36.7	D48.7	D49.89
intracranial NEC	C71.9	C79.31	-	D33.2	D43.2	D49.6
intrahepatic (bile) duct	C22.1	C78.7	D01.5	D13.4	D37.6	D49.0
intraocular	C69.9-	C79.49	D09.2-	D31.9-	D48.7	D49.89
intraorbital	C69.6-	C79.49	D09.2-	D31.6-	D48.7	D49.89
intrasellar	C75.1	C79.89	D09.3	D35.2	D44.3	D49.7
intrathoracic (cavity) (organs)	C76.1	C79.89	D09.8	D15.7	D48.7	D49.89
specified NEC	C76.1	C79.89	D09.8	D15.7	-	-
iris	C69.4-	C79.49	D09.2-	D31.4-	D48.7	D49.89
ischiorectal (fossa)	C76.3	C79.89	D09.8	D36.7	D48.7	D49.89
ischium	C41.4	C79.51	-	D16.8	D48.0	D49.2

Neoplasm	Malignant Primary	Malignant Secondary	Ca in situ	Benign	Uncertain Behavior	Unspecified Behavior
nasopharynx, nasopharyngeal—*continued*						
wall—*continued*						
lateral	C11.2	C79.89	D00.08	D10.6	D37.05	D49.0
posterior	C11.1	C79.89	D00.08	D10.6	D37.05	D49.0
superior	C11.0	C79.89	D00.08	D10.6	D37.05	D49.0
nates (*see also* Neoplasm, skin, trunk)	C44.509	C79.2	D04.5	D23.5	D48.5	D49.2
neck NEC	C76.0	C79.89	D09.8	D36.7	D48.7	D49.89
skin	C44.40	-	-	-	-	-
basal cell carcinoma	C44.41	-	-	-	-	-
specified type NEC	C44.49	-	-	-	-	-
squamous cell carcinoma	C44.42	-	-	-	-	-
nerve (ganglion)	C47.9	C79.89	-	D36.10	D48.2	D49.2
abducens	C72.59	C79.49	-	D33.3	D43.3	D49.7
accessory (spinal)	C72.59	C79.49	-	D33.3	D43.3	D49.7
acoustic	C72.4-	C79.49	-	D33.3	D43.3	D49.7
auditory	C72.4-	C79.49	-	D33.3	D43.3	D49.7
autonomic NEC (*see also* Neoplasm, nerve, peripheral)	C47.9	C79.89	-	D36.10	D48.2	D49.2
brachial	C47.1-	C79.89	-	D36.12	D48.2	D49.2
cranial	C72.50	C79.49	-	D33.3	D43.3	D49.7
specified NEC	C72.59	C79.49	-	D33.3	D43.3	D49.7
facial	C72.59	C79.49	-	D33.3	D43.3	D49.7
femoral	C47.2-	C79.89	-	D36.13	D48.2	D49.2
ganglion NEC (*see also* Neoplasm, nerve, peripheral)	C47.9	C79.89	-	D36.10	D48.2	D49.2
glossopharyngeal	C72.59	C79.49	-	D33.3	D43.3	D49.7
hypoglossal	C72.59	C79.49	-	D33.3	D43.3	D49.7
intercostal	C47.3	C79.89	-	D36.14	D48.2	D49.2
lumbar	C47.6	C79.89	-	D36.17	D48.2	D49.2
median	C47.1-	C79.89	-	D36.12	D48.2	D49.2
obturator	C47.2-	C79.89	-	D36.13	D48.2	D49.2
oculomotor	C72.59	C79.49	-	D33.3	D43.3	D49.7
olfactory	C47.2-	C79.49	-	D33.3	D43.3	D49.7
optic	C72.3-	C79.49	-	D33.3	D43.3	D49.7
parasympathetic NEC	C47.9	C79.89	-	D36.10	D48.2	D49.2
peripheral NEC	C47.9	C79.89	-	D36.10	D48.2	D49.2
abdomen	C47.4	C79.89	-	D36.15	D48.2	D49.2
abdominal wall	C47.4	C79.89	-	D36.15	D48.2	D49.2
ankle	C47.2-	C79.89	-	D36.13	D48.2	D49.2
antecubital fossa or space	C47.1-	C79.89	-	D36.12	D48.2	D49.2
arm	C47.1-	C79.89	-	D36.12	D48.2	D49.2
auricle (ear)	C47.0	C79.89	-	D36.11	D48.2	D49.2
axilla	C47.3	C79.89	-	D36.12	D48.2	D49.2
back	C47.6	C79.89	-	D36.17	D48.2	D49.2
buttock	C47.5	C79.89	-	D36.16	D48.2	D49.2
calf	C47.2-	C79.89	-	D36.13	D48.2	D49.2
cervical region	C47.0	C79.89	-	D36.11	D48.2	D49.2
cheek	C47.0	C79.89	-	D36.11	D48.2	D49.2
chest (wall)	C47.3	C79.89	-	D36.14	D48.2	D49.2
chin	C47.0	C79.89	-	D36.11	D48.2	D49.2
ear (external)	C47.0	C79.89	-	D36.11	D48.2	D49.2
elbow	C47.1-	C79.89	-	D36.12	D48.2	D49.2
extrarectal	C47.5	C79.89	-	D36.16	D48.2	D49.2
extremity	C47.9	C79.89	-	D36.10	D48.2	D49.2
lower	C47.2-	C79.89	-	D36.13	D48.2	D49.2
upper	C47.1-	C79.89	-	D36.12	D48.2	D49.2
eyelid	C47.0	C79.89	-	D36.11	D48.2	D49.2
face	C47.0	C79.89	-	D36.11	D48.2	D49.2
finger	C47.1-	C79.89	-	D36.12	D48.2	D49.2
flank	C47.6	C79.89	-	D36.17	D48.2	D49.2
foot	C47.2-	C79.89	-	D36.13	D48.2	D49.2
forearm	C47.1-	C79.89	-	D36.12	D48.2	D49.2
forehead	C47.0	C79.89	-	D36.11	D48.2	D49.2
gluteal region	C47.5	C79.89	-	D36.16	D48.2	D49.2
groin	C47.5	C79.89	-	D36.16	D48.2	D49.2
hand	C47.1-	C79.89	-	D36.12	D48.2	D49.2
head	C47.0	C79.89	-	D36.11	D48.2	D49.2
heel	C47.2-	C79.89	-	D36.13	D48.2	D49.2
hip	C47.2-	C79.89	-	D36.13	D48.2	D49.2
infraclavicular region	C47.3	C79.89	-	D36.14	D48.2	D49.2
inguinal (canal) (region)	C47.5	C79.89	-	D36.16	D48.2	D49.2
intrathoracic	C47.3	C79.89	-	D36.14	D48.2	D49.2
ischiorectal fossa	C47.5	C79.89	-	D36.16	D48.2	D49.2
knee	C47.2-	C79.89	-	D36.13	D48.2	D49.2
leg	C72.2-	C79.89	-	D36.13	D48.2	D49.2
limb NEC	C47.9	C79.89	-	D36.10	D48.2	D49.2
lower	C47.2-	C79.89	-	D36.13	D48.2	D49.2
upper	C47.1-	C79.89	-	D36.12	D48.2	D49.2
nates	C47.5	C79.89	-	D36.16	D48.2	D49.2
neck	C47.0	C79.89	-	D36.11	D48.2	D49.2
orbit	C69.6-	C79.49	-	D31.6-	D48.7	D49.2
pararectal	C47.5	C79.89	-	D36.16	D48.2	D49.2
paraurethral	C47.5	C79.89	-	D36.16	D48.2	D49.2
paravaginal	C47.5	C79.89	-	D36.16	D48.2	D49.2
pelvis (floor)	C47.5	C79.89	-	D36.16	D48.2	D49.2
pelvoabdominal	C47.8	C79.89	-	D36.17	D48.2	D49.2
perineum	C47.5	C79.89	-	D36.16	D48.2	D49.2
perirectal (tissue)	C47.5	C79.89	-	D36.16	D48.2	D49.2

Neoplasm	Malignant Primary	Malignant Secondary	Ca in situ	Benign	Uncertain Behavior	Unspecified Behavior
nerve—*continued*						
peripheral NEC—*continued*						
periurethral (tissue)	C47.5	C79.89	-	D36.16	D48.2	D49.2
popliteal fossa or space	C47.2-	C79.89	-	D36.13	D48.2	D49.2
presacral	C47.5	C79.89	-	D36.16	D48.2	D49.2
pterygoid fossa	C47.0	C79.89	-	D36.11	D48.2	D49.2
rectovaginal septum or wall	C47.5	C79.89	-	D36.16	D48.2	D49.2
rectovesical	C47.5	C79.89	-	D36.16	D48.2	D49.2
sacrococcygeal region	C47.5	C79.89	-	D36.16	D48.2	D49.2
scalp	C47.0	C79.89	-	D36.11	D48.2	D49.2
scapular region	C47.3	C79.89	-	D36.14	D48.2	D49.2
shoulder	C47.1-	C79.89	-	D36.12	D48.2	D49.2
submental	C47.0	C79.89	-	D36.11	D48.2	D49.2
supraclavicular region	C47.0	C79.89	-	D36.11	D48.2	D49.2
temple	C47.0	C79.89	-	D36.11	D48.2	D49.2
temporal region	C47.0	C79.89	-	D36.11	D48.2	D49.2
thigh	C47.2-	C79.89	-	D36.13	D48.2	D49.2
thoracic (duct) (wall)	C47.3	C79.89	-	D36.14	D48.2	D49.2
thorax	C47.3	C79.89	-	D36.14	D48.2	D49.2
thumb	C47.1-	C79.89	-	D36.12	D48.2	D49.2
toe	C47.2-	C79.89	-	D36.13	D48.2	D49.2
trunk	C47.6	C79.89	-	D36.17	D48.2	D49.2
umbilicus	C47.4	C79.89	-	D36.15	D48.2	D49.2
vesicorectal	C47.5	C79.89	-	D36.16	D48.2	D49.2
wrist	C47.1-	C79.89	-	D36.12	D48.2	D49.2
radial	C47.1-	C79.89	-	D36.12	D48.2	D49.2
sacral	C47.5	C79.89	-	D36.16	D48.2	D49.2
sciatic	C47.2-	C79.89	-	D36.13	D48.2	D49.2
spinal NEC	C47.9	C79.89	-	D36.10	D48.2	D49.2
accessory	C72.59	C79.49	-	D33.3	D43.3	D49.7
sympathetic NEC (*see also* Neoplasm, nerve, peripheral)	C47.9	C79.89	-	D36.10	D48.2	D49.2
trigeminal	C72.59	C79.49	-	D33.3	D43.3	D49.7
trochlear	C72.59	C79.49	-	D33.3	D43.3	D49.7
ulnar	C47.1-	C79.89	-	D36.12	D48.2	D49.2
vagus	C72.59	C79.49	-	D33.3	D43.3	D49.7
nervous system (central)	C72.9	C79.40	-	D33.9	D43.9	D49.7
autonomic — *see* Neoplasm, nerve, peripheral						
parasympathetic — *see* Neoplasm, nerve, peripheral						
specified site NEC	-	C79.49	-	D33.7	D43.8	-
sympathetic — *see* Neoplasm, nerve, peripheral						
nevus — *see* Nevus						
nipple	C50.0-	C79.81	D05.-	D24.-	-	-
nose, nasal	C76.0	C79.89	D09.8	D36.7	D48.7	D49.89
ala (external) (nasi) (*see also* Neoplasm, nose, skin)	C44.301	C79.2	D04.39	D23.39	D48.5	D49.2
bone	C41.0	C79.51	-	D16.4-	D48.0	D49.2
cartilage	C30.0	C78.39	D02.3	D14.0	D38.5	D49.1
cavity	C30.0	C78.39	D02.3	D14.0	D38.5	D49.1
choana	C11.3	C79.89	D00.08	D10.6	D37.05	D49.0
external (skin) (*see also* Neoplasm, nose, skin)	C44.301	C79.2	D04.39	D23.39	D48.5	D49.2
fossa	C30.0	C78.39	D02.3	D14.0	D38.5	D49.1
internal	C30.0	C78.39	D02.3	D14.0	D38.5	D49.1
mucosa	C30.0	C78.39	D02.3	D14.0	D38.5	D49.1
septum	C30.0	C78.39	D02.3	D14.0	D38.5	D49.1
posterior margin	C11.3	C79.89	D00.08	D10.6	D37.05	D49.0
sinus — *see* Neoplasm, sinus						
skin	C44.301	C79.2	D04.39	D23.39	D48.5	D49.2
basal cell carcinoma	C44.311	-	-	-	-	-
specified type NEC	C44.391	-	-	-	-	-
squamous cell carcinoma	C44.321	-	-	-	-	-
turbinate (mucosa)	C30.0	C78.39	D02.3	D14.0	D38.5	D49.1
bone	C41.0	C79.51	-	D16.4-	D48.0	D49.2
vestibule	C30.0	C78.39	D02.3	D14.0	D38.5	D49.1
nostril	C30.0	C78.39	D02.3	D14.0	D38.5	D49.1
nucleus pulposus	C41.2	C79.51	-	D16.6	D48.0	D49.2
occipital						
bone	C41.0	C79.51	-	D16.4-	D48.0	D49.2
lobe or pole, brain	C71.4	C79.31	-	D33.0	D43.0	D49.6
odontogenic — *see* Neoplasm, jaw bone						
olfactory nerve or bulb	C72.2-	C79.49	-	D33.3	D43.3	D49.7
olive (brain)	C71.7	C79.31	-	D33.1	D43.1	D49.6
omentum	C48.1	C78.6	-	D20.1	D48.4	D49.0
operculum (brain)	C71.0	C79.31	-	D33.0	D43.0	D49.6
optic nerve, chiasm, or tract	C72.3-	C79.49	-	D33.3	D43.3	D49.7
oral (cavity)	C06.9	C79.89	D00.00	D10.30	D37.09	D49.0
ill-defined	C14.8	C79.89	D00.00	D10.30	D37.09	D49.0
mucosa	C06.0	C79.89	D00.02	D10.39	D37.09	D49.0
orbit	C69.6-	C79.49	D09.2-	D31.6-	D48.7	D49.89
autonomic nerve	C69.6-	C79.49	-	D31.6-	D48.7	D49.2
bone	C41.0	C79.51	-	D16.4-	D48.0	D49.2
eye	C69.6-	C79.49	D09.2-	D31.6-	D48.7	D49.89
peripheral nerves	C69.6-	C79.49	-	D31.6-	D48.7	D49.2
soft parts	C69.6-	C79.49	D09.2-	D31.6-	D48.7	D49.89

Neoplasm	Malignant Primary	Malignant Secondary	Ca in situ	Benign	Uncertain Behavior	Unspecified Behavior
organ of Zuckerkandl	C75.5	C79.89	-	D35.6	D44.7	D49.7
oropharynx	C10.9	C79.89	D00.08	D10.5	D37.05	D49.0
branchial cleft (vestige)	C10.4	C79.89	D00.08	D10.5	D37.05	D49.0
junctional region	C10.8	C79.89	D00.08	D10.5	D37.05	D49.0
lateral wall	C10.2	C79.89	D00.08	D10.5	D37.05	D49.0
overlapping lesion	C10.8	-	-	-	-	-
pillars or fauces	C09.1	C79.89	D00.08	D10.5	D37.05	D49.0
posterior wall	C10.3	C79.89	D00.08	D10.5	D37.05	D49.0
vallecula	C10.0	C79.89	D00.08	D10.5	D37.05	D49.0
os						
external	C53.1	C79.82	D06.1	D26.0	D39.0	D49.59
internal	C53.0	C79.82	D06.0	D26.0	D39.0	D49.59
ovary	C56.-	C79.6-	D07.39	D27.-	D39.1-	D49.59
oviduct	C57.0-	C79.82	D07.39	D28.2	D39.8	D49.59
palate	C05.9	C79.89	D00.00	D10.39	D37.09	D49.0
hard	C05.0	C79.89	D00.05	D10.39	D37.09	D49.0
junction of hard and soft palate	C05.9	C79.89	D00.00	D10.39	D37.09	D49.0
overlapping lesions	C05.8	-	-	-	-	-
soft	C05.1	C79.89	D00.04	D10.39	D37.09	D49.0
nasopharyngeal surface	C11.3	C79.89	D00.08	D10.6	D37.05	D49.0
posterior surface	C11.3	C79.89	D00.08	D10.6	D37.05	D49.0
superior surface	C11.3	C79.89	D00.08	D10.6	D37.05	D49.0
palatoglossal arch	C09.1	C79.89	D00.00	D10.5	D37.09	D49.0
palatopharyngeal arch	C09.1	C79.89	D00.00	D10.5	D37.09	D49.0
pallium	C71.0	C79.31	-	D33.0	D43.0	D49.6
palpebra	C44.10-	C79.2	D04.1-	D23.1-	D48.5	D49.2
basal cell carcinoma	C44.11-	-	-	-	-	-
specified type NEC	C44.19-	-	-	-	-	-
squamous cell carcinoma	C44.12-	-	-	-	-	-
pancreas	C25.9	C78.89	D01.7	D13.6	D37.8	D49.0
body	C25.1	C78.89	D01.7	D13.6	D37.8	D49.0
duct (of Santorini) (of Wirsung)	C25.3	C78.89	D01.7	D13.6	D37.8	D49.0
ectopic tissue	C25.7	C78.89	-	D13.6	D37.8	D49.0
head	C25.0	C78.89	D01.7	D13.6	D37.8	D49.0
islet cells	C25.4	C78.89	D01.7	D13.7	D37.8	D49.0
neck	C25.7	C78.89	D01.7	D13.6	D37.8	D49.0
overlapping lesion	C25.8	-	-	-	-	-
tail	C25.2	C78.89	D01.7	D13.6	D37.8	D49.0
para-aortic body	C75.5	C79.89	-	D35.6	D44.7	D49.7
paraganglion NEC	C75.5	C79.89	-	D35.6	D44.7	D49.7
parametrium	C57.3	C79.82	-	D28.2	D39.8	D49.59
paranephric	C48.0	C78.6	-	D20.0	D48.3	D49.0
pararectal	C76.3	C79.89	-	D36.7	D48.7	D49.89
parasagittal (region)	C76.0	C79.89	D09.8	D36.7	D48.7	D49.89
parasellar	C72.9	C79.49	-	D33.9	D43.8	D49.7
parathyroid (gland)	C75.0	C79.89	D09.3	D35.1	D44.2	D49.7
paraurethral	C76.3	C79.89	-	D36.7	D48.7	D49.89
gland	C68.1	C79.19	D09.19	D30.8	D41.8	D49.59
paravaginal	C76.3	C79.89	-	D36.7	D48.7	D49.89
parenchyma, kidney	C64.-	C79.0-	D09.19	D30.0-	D41.0-	D49.51-
parietal						
bone	C41.0	C79.51	-	D16.4-	D48.0	D49.2
lobe, brain	C71.3	C79.31	-	D33.0	D43.0	D49.6
paroophoron	C57.1	C79.82	D07.39	D28.2	D39.8	D49.59
parotid (duct) (gland)	C07	C79.89	D00.00	D11.0	D37.030	D49.0
parovarium	C57.1	C79.82	D07.39	D28.2	D39.8	D49.59
patella	C40.20	C79.51	-	-	-	-
peduncle, cerebral	C71.7	C79.31	-	D33.1	D43.1	D49.6
pelvirectal junction	C19	C78.5	D01.1	D12.7	D37.5	D49.0
pelvis, pelvic	C76.3	C79.89	D09.8	D36.7	D48.7	D49.89
bone	C41.4	C79.51	-	D16.8	D48.0	D49.2
floor	C76.3	C79.89	D09.8	D36.7	D48.7	D49.89
renal	C65.-	C79.0-	D09.19	D30.1-	D41.1-	D49.51-
viscera	C76.3	C79.89	D09.8	D36.7	D48.7	D49.89
wall	C76.3	C79.89	D09.8	D36.7	D48.7	D49.89
pelvo-abdominal	C76.8	C79.89	D09.8	D36.7	D48.7	D49.89
penis	C60.9	C79.82	D07.4	D29.0	D40.8	D49.59
body	C60.2	C79.82	D07.4	D29.0	D40.8	D49.59
corpus (cavernosum)	C60.2	C79.82	D07.4	D29.0	D40.8	D49.59
glans	C60.1	C79.82	D07.4	D29.0	D40.8	D49.59
overlapping sites	C60.8	-	-	-	-	-
skin NEC	C60.9	C79.82	D07.4	D29.0	D40.8	D49.59
periadrenal (tissue)	C48.0	C78.6	-	D20.0	D48.3	D49.0
perianal (skin) (see also Neoplasm, anus, skin)	C44.500	C79.2	D04.5	D23.5	D48.5	D49.2
pericardium	C38.0	C79.89	-	D15.1	D48.7	D49.89
perinephric	C48.0	C78.6	-	D20.0	D48.3	D49.0
perineum	C76.3	C79.89	D09.8	D36.7	D48.7	D49.89
periodontal tissue NEC	C03.9	C79.89	D00.03	D10.39	D37.09	D49.0
periosteum — see Neoplasm, bone						
peripancreatic	C48.0	C78.6	-	D20.0	D48.3	D49.0
peripheral nerve NEC	C47.9	C79.89	-	D36.10	D48.2	D49.2
perirectal (tissue)	C76.3	C79.89	-	D36.7	D48.7	D49.89
perirenal (tissue)	C48.0	C78.6	-	D20.0	D48.3	D49.0
peritoneum, peritoneal (cavity)	C48.2	C78.6	-	D20.1	D48.4	D49.0
benign mesothelial tissue — see Mesothelioma, benign						
overlapping lesion	C48.8	-	-	-	-	-
with digestive organs	C26.9	-	-	-	-	-

Neoplasm	Malignant Primary	Malignant Secondary	Ca in situ	Benign	Uncertain Behavior	Unspecified Behavior
peritoneum — *continued*						
parietal	C48.1	C78.6	-	D20.1	D48.4	D49.0
pelvic	C48.1	C78.6	-	D20.1	D48.4	D49.0
specified part NEC	C48.1	C78.6	-	D20.1	D48.4	D49.0
peritonsillar (tissue)	C76.0	C79.89	D09.8	D36.7	D48.7	D49.89
periurethral tissue	C76.3	C79.89	-	D36.7	D48.7	D49.89
phalanges						
foot	C40.3-	C79.51	-	D16.3-	-	-
hand	C40.1-	C79.51	-	D16.1-	-	-
pharynx, pharyngeal	C14.0	C79.89	D00.08	D10.9	D37.05	D49.0
bursa	C11.1	C79.89	D00.08	D10.6	D37.05	D49.0
fornix	C11.3	C79.89	D00.08	D10.6	D37.05	D49.0
recess	C11.2	C79.89	D00.08	D10.6	D37.05	D49.0
region	C14.0	C79.89	D00.08	D10.9	D37.05	D49.0
tonsil	C11.1	C79.89	D00.08	D10.6	D37.05	D49.0
wall (lateral) (posterior)	C14.0	C79.89	D00.08	D10.9	D37.05	D49.0
pia mater	C70.9	C79.40	-	D32.9	D42.9	D49.7
cerebral	C70.0	C79.32	-	D32.0	D42.0	D49.7
cranial	C70.0	C79.32	-	D32.0	D42.0	D49.7
spinal	C70.1	C79.49	-	D32.1	D42.1	D49.7
pillars of fauces	C09.1	C79.89	D00.08	D10.5	D37.05	D49.0
pineal (body) (gland)	C75.3	C79.89	D09.3	D35.4	D44.5	D49.7
pinna (ear) NEC (*see also* Neoplasm, skin, ear)	C44.20-	C79.2	D04.2-	D23.2-	D48.5	D49.2
piriform fossa or sinus	C12	C79.89	D00.08	D10.7	D37.05	D49.0
pituitary (body) (fossa) (gland) (lobe)	C75.1	C79.89	D09.3	D35.2	D44.3	D49.7
placenta	C58	C79.82	D07.0	D26.7	D39.2	D49.59
pleura, pleural (cavity)	C38.4	C78.2	-	D19.0	D38.2	D49.1
overlapping lesion with heart or mediastinum	C38.8	-	-	-	-	-
parietal	C38.4	C78.2	-	D19.0	D38.2	D49.1
visceral	C38.4	C78.2	-	D19.0	D38.2	D49.1
plexus						
brachial	C47.1-	C79.89	-	D36.12	D48.2	D49.2
cervical	C47.0	C79.89	-	D36.11	D48.2	D49.2
choroid	C71.5	C79.31	-	D33.0	D43.0	D49.6
lumbosacral	C47.5	C79.89	-	D36.16	D48.2	D49.2
sacral	C47.5	C79.89	-	D36.16	D48.2	D49.2
pluriendocrine	C75.8	C79.89	D09.3	D35.7	D44.9	D49.7
pole						
frontal	C71.1	C79.31	-	D33.0	D43.0	D49.6
occipital	C71.4	C79.31	-	D33.0	D43.0	D49.6
pons (varolii)	C71.7	C79.31	-	D33.1	D43.1	D49.6
popliteal fossa or space	C76.5-	C79.89	D04.7-	D36.7	D48.7	D49.89
postcricoid (region)	C13.0	C79.89	D00.08	D10.7	D37.05	D49.0
posterior fossa (cranial)	C71.9	C79.31	-	D33.2	D43.2	D49.6
postnasal space	C11.9	C79.89	D00.08	D10.6	D37.05	D49.0
prepuce	C60.0	C79.82	D07.4	D29.0	D40.8	D49.59
prepylorus	C16.4	C78.89	D00.2	D13.1	D37.1	D49.0
presacral (region)	C76.3	C79.89	-	D36.7	D48.7	D49.89
prostate (gland)	C61	C79.82	D07.5	D29.1	D40.0	D49.59
utricle	C68.0	C79.19	D09.19	D30.4	D41.3	D49.59
pterygoid fossa	C49.0	C79.89	-	D21.0	D48.1	D49.2
pubic bone	C41.4	C79.51	-	D16.8	D48.0	D49.2
pudenda, pudendum (female)	C51.9	C79.82	D07.1	D28.0	D39.8	D49.59
pulmonary (*see also* Neoplasm, lung)	C34.9-	C78.0-	D02.2-	D14.3-	D38.1	D49.1
putamen	C71.0	C79.31	-	D33.0	D43.0	D49.6
pyloric						
antrum	C16.3	C78.89	D00.2	D13.1	D37.1	D49.0
canal	C16.4	C78.89	D00.2	D13.1	D37.1	D49.0
pylorus	C16.4	C78.89	D00.2	D13.1	D37.1	D49.0
pyramid (brain)	C71.7	C79.31	-	D33.1	D43.1	D49.6
pyriform fossa or sinus	C12	C79.89	D00.08	D10.7	D37.05	D49.0
radius (any part)	C40.0-	C79.51	-	D16.0-	-	-
Rathke's pouch	C75.1	C79.89	D09.3	D35.2	D44.3	D49.7
rectosigmoid (junction)	C19	C78.5	D01.1	D12.7	D37.5	D49.0
overlapping lesion with anus or rectum	C21.8	-	-	-	-	-
rectouterine pouch	C48.1	C78.6	-	D20.1	D48.4	D49.0
rectovaginal septum or wall	C76.3	C79.89	D09.8	D36.7	D48.7	D49.89
rectovesical septum	C76.3	C79.89	D09.8	D36.7	D48.7	D49.89
rectum (ampulla)	C20	C78.5	D01.2	D12.8	D37.5	D49.0
and colon	C19	C78.5	D01.1	D12.7	D37.5	D49.0
overlapping lesion with anus or rectosigmoid junction	C21.8	-	-	-	-	-
renal	C64.-	C79.0-	D09.19	D30.0-	D41.0-	D49.51-
calyx	C65.-	C79.0-	D09.19	D30.1-	D41.1-	D49.51-
hilus	C65.-	C79.0-	D09.19	D30.1-	D41.1-	D49.51-
parenchyma	C64.-	C79.0-	D09.19	D30.0-	D41.0-	D49.51-
pelvis	C65.-	C79.0-	D09.19	D30.1-	D41.1-	D49.51-
respiratory						
organs or system NEC	C39.9	C78.30	D02.4	D14.4	D38.6	D49.1
tract NEC	C39.9	C78.30	D02.4	D14.4	D38.5	D49.1
upper	C39.0	C78.30	D02.4	D14.0	D38.5	D49.1
retina	C69.2-	C79.49	D09.2-	D31.2-	D48.7	D49.81
retrobulbar	C69.6-	C79.49	-	D31.6-	D48.7	D49.89
retrocecal	C48.0	C78.6	-	D20.0	D48.3	D49.0
retromolar (area) (triangle) (trigone)	C06.2	C79.89	D00.00	D10.39	D37.09	D49.0
retro-orbital	C76.0	C79.89	D09.8	D36.7	D48.7	D49.89

Substance	Poisoning, Accidental unintentional	Poisoning, Intentional self-harm	Poisoning, Assault	Poisoning, Undetermined	Adverse effect	Underdosing
Anesthetic NEC — *continued*						
local NEC	T41.3X1	T41.3X2	T41.3X3	T41.3X4	T41.3X5	T41.3X6
rectal	T41.201	T41.202	T41.203	T41.204	T41.205	T41.206
general	T41.201	T41.202	T41.203	T41.204	T41.205	T41.206
local	T41.3X1	T41.3X2	T41.3X3	T41.3X4	T41.3X5	T41.3X6
regional NEC	T41.3X1	T41.3X2	T41.3X3	T41.3X4	T41.3X5	T41.3X6
spinal NEC	T41.3X1	T41.3X2	T41.3X3	T41.3X4	T41.3X5	T41.3X6
thiobarbiturate	T41.1X1	T41.1X2	T41.1X3	T41.1X4	T41.1X5	T41.1X6
topical	T41.3X1	T41.3X2	T41.3X3	T41.3X4	T41.3X5	T41.3X6
Aneurine	T45.2X1	T45.2X2	T45.2X3	T45.2X4	T45.2X5	T45.2X6
Angio-Conray	T50.8X1	T50.8X2	T50.8X3	T50.8X4	T50.8X5	T50.8X6
Angiotensin	T44.5X1	T44.5X2	T44.5X3	T44.5X4	T44.5X5	T44.5X6
Angiotensinamide	T44.991	T44.992	T44.993	T44.994	T44.995	T44.996
Anhydrohydroxy-progesterone	T38.5X1	T38.5X2	T38.5X3	T38.5X4	T38.5X5	T38.5X6
Anhydron	T50.2X1	T50.2X2	T50.2X3	T50.2X4	T50.2X5	T50.2X6
Anileridine	T40.4X1	T40.4X2	T40.4X3	T40.4X4	T40.4X5	T40.4X6
Aniline (dye) (liquid)	T65.3X1	T65.3X2	T65.3X3	T65.3X4	--	--
analgesic	T39.1X1	T39.1X2	T39.1X3	T39.1X4	T39.1X5	T39.1X6
derivatives, therapeutic NEC	T39.1X1	T39.1X2	T39.1X3	T39.1X4	T39.1X5	T39.1X6
vapor	T65.3X1	T65.3X2	T65.3X3	T65.3X4	--	--
Aniscoropine	T44.3X1	T44.3X2	T44.3X3	T44.3X4	T44.3X5	T44.3X6
Anise oil	T47.5X1	T47.5X2	T47.5X3	T47.5X4	T47.5X5	T47.5X6
Anisidine	T65.3X1	T65.3X2	T65.3X3	T65.3X4	--	--
Anisindione	T45.511	T45.512	T45.513	T45.514	T45.515	T45.516
Anisotropine methyl-bromide	T44.3X1	T44.3X2	T44.3X3	T44.3X4	T44.3X5	T44.3X6
Anistreplase	T45.611	T45.612	T45.613	T45.614	T45.615	T45.616
Anorexiant (central)	T50.5X1	T50.5X2	T50.5X3	T50.5X4	T50.5X5	T50.5X6
Anorexic agents	T50.5X1	T50.5X2	T50.5X3	T50.5X4	T50.5X5	T50.5X6
Ansamycin	T36.6X1	T36.6X2	T36.6X3	T36.6X4	T36.6X5	T36.6X6
Ant (bite) (sting)	T63.421	T63.422	T63.423	T63.424	--	--
Ant poison — *see* Insecticide						
Antabuse	T50.6X1	T50.6X2	T50.6X3	T50.6X4	T50.6X5	T50.6X6
Antacid NEC	T47.1X1	T47.1X2	T47.1X3	T47.1X4	T47.1X5	T47.1X6
Antagonist						
Aldosterone	T50.0X1	T50.0X2	T50.0X3	T50.0X4	T50.0X5	T50.0X6
alpha-adrenoreceptor	T44.6X1	T44.6X2	T44.6X3	T44.6X4	T44.6X5	T44.6X6
anticoagulant	T45.7X1	T45.7X2	T45.7X3	T45.7X4	T45.7X5	T45.7X6
beta-adrenoreceptor	T44.7X1	T44.7X2	T44.7X3	T44.7X4	T44.7X5	T44.7X6
extrapyramidal NEC	T44.3X1	T44.3X2	T44.3X3	T44.3X4	T44.3X5	T44.3X6
folic acid	T45.1X1	T45.1X2	T45.1X3	T45.1X4	T45.1X5	T45.1X6
H2 receptor	T47.0X1	T47.0X2	T47.0X3	T47.0X4	T47.0X5	T47.0X6
heavy metal	T45.8X1	T45.8X2	T45.8X3	T45.8X4	T45.8X5	T45.8X6
narcotic analgesic	T50.7X1	T50.7X2	T50.7X3	T50.7X4	T50.7X5	T50.7X6
opiate	T50.7X1	T50.7X2	T50.7X3	T50.7X4	T50.7X5	T50.7X6
pyrimidine	T45.1X1	T45.1X2	T45.1X3	T45.1X4	T45.1X5	T45.1X6
serotonin	T46.5X1	T46.5X2	T46.5X3	T46.5X4	T46.5X5	T46.5X6
Antazolin (e)	T45.0X1	T45.0X2	T45.0X3	T45.0X4	T45.0X5	T45.0X6
Anterior pituitary hormone NEC	T38.811	T38.812	T38.813	T38.814	T38.815	T38.816
Anthelmintic NEC	T37.4X1	T37.4X2	T37.4X3	T37.4X4	T37.4X5	T37.4X6
Anthiolimine	T37.4X1	T37.4X2	T37.4X3	T37.4X4	T37.4X5	T37.4X6
Anthralin	T49.4X1	T49.4X2	T49.4X3	T49.4X4	T49.4X5	T49.4X6
Anthramycin	T45.1X1	T45.1X2	T45.1X3	T45.1X4	T45.1X5	T45.1X6
Antiadrenergic NEC	T44.8X1	T44.8X2	T44.8X3	T44.8X4	T44.8X5	T44.8X6
Antiallergic NEC	T45.0X1	T45.0X2	T45.0X3	T45.0X4	T45.0X5	T45.0X6
Anti-anemic (drug) (preparation)	T45.8X1	T45.8X2	T45.8X3	T45.8X4	T45.8X5	T45.8X6
Antiandrogen NEC	T38.6X1	T38.6X2	T38.6X3	T38.6X4	T38.6X5	T38.6X6
Antianxiety drug NEC	T43.501	T43.502	T43.503	T43.504	T43.505	T43.506
Antiaris toxicaria	T65.891	T65.892	T65.893	T65.894	--	--
Antiarteriosclerotic drug	T46.6X1	T46.6X2	T46.6X3	T46.6X4	T46.6X5	T46.6X6
Antiasthmatic drug NEC	T48.6X1	T48.6X2	T48.6X3	T48.6X4	T48.6X5	T48.6X6
Antibiotic NEC	T36.91	T36.92	T36.93	T36.94	T36.95	T36.96
aminoglycoside	T36.5X1	T36.5X2	T36.5X3	T36.5X4	T36.5X5	T36.5X6
anticancer	T45.1X1	T45.1X2	T45.1X3	T45.1X4	T45.1X5	T45.1X6
antifungal	T36.7X1	T36.7X2	T36.7X3	T36.7X4	T36.7X5	T36.7X6
antimycobacterial	T36.5X1	T36.5X2	T36.5X3	T36.5X4	T36.5X5	T36.5X6
antineoplastic	T45.1X1	T45.1X2	T45.1X3	T45.1X4	T45.1X5	T45.1X6
cephalosporin (group)	T36.1X1	T36.1X2	T36.1X3	T36.1X4	T36.1X5	T36.1X6
chloramphenicol (group)	T36.2X1	T36.2X2	T36.2X3	T36.2X4	T36.2X5	T36.2X6
ENT	T49.6X1	T49.6X2	T49.6X3	T49.6X4	T49.6X5	T49.6X6
eye	T49.5X1	T49.5X2	T49.5X3	T49.5X4	T49.5X5	T49.5X6
fungicidal (local)	T49.0X1	T49.0X2	T49.0X3	T49.0X4	T49.0X5	T49.0X6
intestinal	T36.8X1	T36.8X2	T36.8X3	T36.8X4	T36.8X5	T36.8X6
b-lactam NEC	T36.1X1	T36.1X2	T36.1X3	T36.1X4	T36.1X5	T36.1X6
local	T49.0X1	T49.0X2	T49.0X3	T49.0X4	T49.0X5	T49.0X6
macrolides	T36.3X1	T36.3X2	T36.3X3	T36.3X4	T36.3X5	T36.3X6
polypeptide	T36.8X1	T36.8X2	T36.8X3	T36.8X4	T36.8X5	T36.8X6
specified NEC	T36.8X1	T36.8X2	T36.8X3	T36.8X4	T36.8X5	T36.8X6
tetracycline (group)	T36.4X1	T36.4X2	T36.4X3	T36.4X4	T36.4X5	T36.4X6
throat	T49.6X1	T49.6X2	T49.6X3	T49.6X4	T49.6X5	T49.6X6
Anticancer agents NEC	T45.1X1	T45.1X2	T45.1X3	T45.1X4	T45.1X5	T45.1X6
Anticholesterolemic drug NEC	T46.6X1	T46.6X2	T46.6X3	T46.6X4	T46.6X5	T46.6X6
Anticholinergic NEC	T44.3X1	T44.3X2	T44.3X3	T44.3X4	T44.3X5	T44.3X6
Anticholinesterase	T44.0X1	T44.0X2	T44.0X3	T44.0X4	T44.0X5	T44.0X6
organophosphorus	T44.0X1	T44.0X2	T44.0X3	T44.0X4	T44.0X5	T44.0X6
insecticide	T60.0X1	T60.0X2	T60.0X3	T60.0X4	--	--
nerve gas	T59.891	T59.892	T59.893	T59.894	--	--
reversible	T44.0X1	T44.0X2	T44.0X3	T44.0X4	T44.0X5	T44.0X6
ophthalmological	T49.5X1	T49.5X2	T49.5X3	T49.5X4	T49.5X5	T49.5X6
Anticoagulant NEC	T45.511	T45.512	T45.513	T45.514	T45.515	T45.516
Antagonist	T45.7X1	T45.7X2	T45.7X3	T45.7X4	T45.7X5	T45.7X6
Anti-common-cold drug NEC	T48.5X1	T48.5X2	T48.5X3	T48.5X4	T48.5X5	T48.5X6
Anticonvulsant	T42.71	T42.72	T42.73	T42.74	T42.75	T42.76
barbiturate	T42.3X1	T42.3X2	T42.3X3	T42.3X4	T42.3X5	T42.3X6
combination (with barbiturate)	T42.3X1	T42.3X2	T42.3X3	T42.3X4	T42.3X5	T42.3X6
hydantoin	T42.0X1	T42.0X2	T42.0X3	T42.0X4	T42.0X5	T42.0X6
hypnotic NEC	T42.6X1	T42.6X2	T42.6X3	T42.6X4	T42.6X5	T42.6X6
oxazolidinedione	T42.2X1	T42.2X2	T42.2X3	T42.2X4	T42.2X5	T42.2X6
pyrimidinedione	T42.6X1	T42.6X2	T42.6X3	T42.6X4	T42.6X5	T42.6X6
specified NEC	T42.6X1	T42.6X2	T42.6X3	T42.6X4	T42.6X5	T42.6X6
succinimide	T42.2X1	T42.2X2	T42.2X3	T42.2X4	T42.2X5	T42.2X6
Anti-D immunoglobulin (human)	T50.Z11	T50.Z12	T50.Z13	T50.Z14	T50.Z15	T50.Z16
Antidepressant	T43.201	T43.202	T43.203	T43.204	T43.205	T43.206
monoamine oxidase inhibitor	T43.1X1	T43.1X2	T43.1X3	T43.1X4	T43.1X5	T43.1X6
selective serotonin norepinephrine reuptake inhibitor	T43.211	T43.212	T43.213	T43.214	T43.215	T43.216
selective serotonin reuptake inhibitor	T43.221	T43.222	T43.223	T43.224	T43.225	T43.226
specified NEC	T43.291	T43.292	T43.293	T43.294	T43.295	T43.296
tetracyclic	T43.021	T43.022	T43.023	T43.024	T43.025	T43.026
triazolopyridine	T43.211	T43.212	T43.213	T43.214	T43.215	T43.216
tricyclic	T43.011	T43.012	T43.013	T43.014	T43.015	T43.016
Antidiabetic NEC	T38.3X1	T38.3X2	T38.3X3	T38.3X4	T38.3X5	T38.3X6
biguanide	T38.3X1	T38.3X2	T38.3X3	T38.3X4	T38.3X5	T38.3X6
and sulfonyl combined	T38.3X1	T38.3X2	T38.3X3	T38.3X4	T38.3X5	T38.3X6
combined	T38.3X1	T38.3X2	T38.3X3	T38.3X4	T38.3X5	T38.3X6
sulfonylurea	T38.3X1	T38.3X2	T38.3X3	T38.3X4	T38.3X5	T38.3X6
Antidiarrheal drug NEC	T47.6X1	T47.6X2	T47.6X3	T47.6X4	T47.6X5	T47.6X6
absorbent	T47.6X1	T47.6X2	T47.6X3	T47.6X4	T47.6X5	T47.6X6
Antidiphtheria serum	T50.Z11	T50.Z12	T50.Z13	T50.Z14	T50.Z15	T50.Z16
Antidiuretic hormone	T38.891	T38.892	T38.893	T38.894	T38.895	T38.896
Antidote NEC	T50.6X1	T50.6X2	T50.6X3	T50.6X4	T50.6X5	T50.6X6
heavy metal	T45.8X1	T45.8X2	T45.8X3	T45.8X4	T45.8X5	T45.8X6
Antidysrhythmic NEC	T46.2X1	T46.2X2	T46.2X3	T46.2X4	T46.2X5	T46.2X6
Antiemetic drug	T45.0X1	T45.0X2	T45.0X3	T45.0X4	T45.0X5	T45.0X6
Antiepilepsy agent	T42.71	T42.72	T42.73	T42.74	T42.75	T42.76
combination	T42.5X1	T42.5X2	T42.5X3	T42.5X4	T42.5X5	T42.5X6
mixed	T42.5X1	T42.5X2	T42.5X3	T42.5X4	T42.5X5	T42.5X6
specified, NEC	T42.6X1	T42.6X2	T42.6X3	T42.6X4	T42.6X5	T42.6X6
Antiestrogen NEC	T38.6X1	T38.6X2	T38.6X3	T38.6X4	T38.6X5	T38.6X6
Antifertility pill	T38.4X1	T38.4X2	T38.4X3	T38.4X4	T38.4X5	T38.4X6
Antifibrinolytic drug	T45.621	T45.622	T45.623	T45.624	T45.625	T45.626
Antifilarial drug	T37.4X1	T37.4X2	T37.4X3	T37.4X4	T37.4X5	T37.4X6
Antiflatulent	T47.5X1	T47.5X2	T47.5X3	T47.5X4	T47.5X5	T47.5X6
Antifreeze	T65.91	T65.92	T65.93	T65.94	--	--
alcohol	T51.1X1	T51.1X2	T51.1X3	T51.1X4	--	--
ethylene glycol	T51.8X1	T51.8X2	T51.8X3	T51.8X4	--	--
Antifungal						
antibiotic (systemic)	T36.7X1	T36.7X2	T36.7X3	T36.7X4	T36.7X5	T36.7X6
anti-infective NEC	T37.91	T37.92	T37.93	T37.94	T37.95	T37.96
disinfectant, local	T49.0X1	T49.0X2	T49.0X3	T49.0X4	T49.0X5	T49.0X6
nonmedicinal (spray)	T60.3X1	T60.3X2	T60.3X3	T60.3X4	--	--
topical	T49.0X1	T49.0X2	T49.0X3	T49.0X4	T49.0X5	T49.0X6
Anti-gastric-secretion drug NEC	T47.1X1	T47.1X2	T47.1X3	T47.1X4	T47.1X5	T47.1X6
Antigonadotrophin NEC	T38.6X1	T38.6X2	T38.6X3	T38.6X4	T38.6X5	T38.6X6
Antihallucinogen	T43.501	T43.502	T43.503	T43.504	T43.505	T43.506
Antihelmintics	T37.4X1	T37.4X2	T37.4X3	T37.4X4	T37.4X5	T37.4X6
Antihemophilic						
factor	T45.8X1	T45.8X2	T45.8X3	T45.8X4	T45.8X5	T45.8X6
fraction	T45.8X1	T45.8X2	T45.8X3	T45.8X4	T45.8X5	T45.8X6
globulin concentrate	T45.7X1	T45.7X2	T45.7X3	T45.7X4	T45.7X5	T45.7X6
human plasma	T45.8X1	T45.8X2	T45.8X3	T45.8X4	T45.8X5	T45.8X6
plasma, dried	T45.7X1	T45.7X2	T45.7X3	T45.7X4	T45.7X5	T45.7X6
Antihemorrhoidal preparation	T49.2X1	T49.2X2	T49.2X3	T49.2X4	T49.2X5	T49.2X6
Antiheparin drug	T45.7X1	T45.7X2	T45.7X3	T45.7X4	T45.7X5	T45.7X6
Antihistamine	T45.0X1	T45.0X2	T45.0X3	T45.0X4	T45.0X5	T45.0X6
Antihookworm drug	T37.4X1	T37.4X2	T37.4X3	T37.4X4	T37.4X5	T37.4X6

Substance	Poisoning, Accidental unintentional	Poisoning, Intentional self-harm	Poisoning, Assault	Poisoning, Undetermined	Adverse effect	Underdosing
Anti-human lymphocytic globulin	T50.Z11	T50.Z12	T50.Z13	T50.Z14	T50.Z15	T50.Z16
Antihyperlipidemic drug	T46.6X1	T46.6X2	T46.6X3	T46.6X4	T46.6X5	T46.6X6
Antihypertensive drug NEC	T46.5X1	T46.5X2	T46.5X3	T46.5X4	T46.5X5	T46.5X6
Anti-infective NEC	T37.91	T37.92	T37.93	T37.94	T37.95	T37.96
anthelmintic	T37.4X1	T37.4X2	T37.4X3	T37.4X4	T37.4X5	T37.4X6
antibiotics	T36.91	T36.92	T36.93	T36.94	T36.95	T36.96
specified NEC	T36.8X1	T36.8X2	T36.8X3	T36.8X4	T36.8X5	T36.8X6
antimalarial	T37.2X1	T37.2X2	T37.2X3	T37.2X4	T37.2X5	T37.2X6
antimycobacterial NEC	T37.1X1	T37.1X2	T37.1X3	T37.1X4	T37.1X5	T37.1X6
antibiotics	T36.5X1	T36.5X2	T36.5X3	T36.5X4	T36.5X5	T36.5X6
antiprotozoal NEC	T37.3X1	T37.3X2	T37.3X3	T37.3X4	T37.3X5	T37.3X6
blood	T37.2X1	T37.2X2	T37.2X3	T37.2X4	T37.2X5	T37.2X6
antiviral	T37.5X1	T37.5X2	T37.5X3	T37.5X4	T37.5X5	T37.5X6
arsenical	T37.8X1	T37.8X2	T37.8X3	T37.8X4	T37.8X5	T37.8X6
bismuth, local	T49.0X1	T49.0X2	T49.0X3	T49.0X4	T49.0X5	T49.0X6
ENT	T49.6X1	T49.6X2	T49.6X3	T49.6X4	T49.6X5	T49.6X6
eye NEC	T49.5X1	T49.5X2	T49.5X3	T49.5X4	T49.5X5	T49.5X6
heavy metals NEC	T37.8X1	T37.8X2	T37.8X3	T37.8X4	T37.8X5	T37.8X6
local NEC	T49.0X1	T49.0X2	T49.0X3	T49.0X4	T49.0X5	T49.0X6
specified NEC	T49.0X1	T49.0X2	T49.0X3	T49.0X4	T49.0X5	T49.0X6
mixed	T37.91	T37.92	T37.93	T37.94	T37.95	T37.96
ophthalmic preparation	T49.5X1	T49.5X2	T49.5X3	T49.5X4	T49.5X5	T49.5X6
topical NEC	T49.0X1	T49.0X2	T49.0X3	T49.0X4	T49.0X5	T49.0X6
Anti-inflammatory drug NEC	T39.391	T39.392	T39.393	T39.394	T39.395	T39.396
local	T49.0X1	T49.0X2	T49.0X3	T49.0X4	T49.0X5	T49.0X6
nonsteroidal NEC	T39.391	T39.392	T39.393	T39.394	T39.395	T39.396
propionic acid derivative	T39.311	T39.312	T39.313	T39.314	T39.315	T39.316
specified NEC	T39.391	T39.392	T39.393	T39.394	T39.395	T39.396
Antikaluretic	T50.3X1	T50.3X2	T50.3X3	T50.3X4	T50.3X5	T50.3X6
Antiknock (tetraethyl lead)	T56.0X1	T56.0X2	T56.0X3	T56.0X4	--	--
Antilipemic drug NEC	T46.6X1	T46.6X2	T46.6X3	T46.6X4	T46.6X5	T46.6X6
Antimalarial	T37.2X1	T37.2X2	T37.2X3	T37.2X4	T37.2X5	T37.2X6
prophylactic NEC	T37.2X1	T37.2X2	T37.2X3	T37.2X4	T37.2X5	T37.2X6
pyrimidine derivative	T37.2X1	T37.2X2	T37.2X3	T37.2X4	T37.2X5	T37.2X6
Antimetabolite	T45.1X1	T45.1X2	T45.1X3	T45.1X4	T45.1X5	T45.1X6
Antimitotic agent	T45.1X1	T45.1X2	T45.1X3	T45.1X4	T45.1X5	T45.1X6
Antimony (compounds) (vapor) NEC	T56.891	T56.892	T56.893	T56.894	--	--
anti-infectives	T37.8X1	T37.8X2	T37.8X3	T37.8X4	T37.8X5	T37.8X6
dimercaptosuccinate	T37.3X1	T37.3X2	T37.3X3	T37.3X4	T37.3X5	T37.3X6
hydride	T56.891	T56.892	T56.893	T56.894	--	--
pesticide (vapor)	T60.8X1	T60.8X2	T60.8X3	T60.8X4	--	--
potassium (sodium) tartrate	T37.8X1	T37.8X2	T37.8X3	T37.8X4	T37.8X5	T37.8X6
sodium dimercaptosuccinate	T37.3X1	T37.3X2	T37.3X3	T37.3X4	T37.3X5	T37.3X6
tartrated	T37.8X1	T37.8X2	T37.8X3	T37.8X4	T37.8X5	T37.8X6
Antimuscarinic NEC	T44.3X1	T44.3X2	T44.3X3	T44.3X4	T44.3X5	T44.3X6
Antimycobacterial drug NEC	T37.1X1	T37.1X2	T37.1X3	T37.1X4	T37.1X5	T37.1X6
antibiotics	T36.5X1	T36.5X2	T36.5X3	T36.5X4	T36.5X5	T36.5X6
combination	T37.1X1	T37.1X2	T37.1X3	T37.1X4	T37.1X5	T37.1X6
Antinausea drug	T45.0X1	T45.0X2	T45.0X3	T45.0X4	T45.0X5	T45.0X6
Antinematode drug	T37.4X1	T37.4X2	T37.4X3	T37.4X4	T37.4X5	T37.4X6
Antineoplastic NEC	T45.1X1	T45.1X2	T45.1X3	T45.1X4	T45.1X5	T45.1X6
alkaloidal	T45.1X1	T45.1X2	T45.1X3	T45.1X4	T45.1X5	T45.1X6
antibiotics	T45.1X1	T45.1X2	T45.1X3	T45.1X4	T45.1X5	T45.1X6
combination	T45.1X1	T45.1X2	T45.1X3	T45.1X4	T45.1X5	T45.1X6
estrogen	T38.5X1	T38.5X2	T38.5X3	T38.5X4	T38.5X5	T38.5X6
steroid	T38.7X1	T38.7X2	T38.7X3	T38.7X4	T38.7X5	T38.7X6
Antiparasitic drug (systemic)	T37.91	T37.92	T37.93	T37.94	T37.95	T37.96
local	T49.0X1	T49.0X2	T49.0X3	T49.0X4	T49.0X5	T49.0X6
specified NEC	T37.8X1	T37.8X2	T37.8X3	T37.8X4	T37.8X5	T37.8X6
Antiparkinsonism drug NEC	T42.8X1	T42.8X2	T42.8X3	T42.8X4	T42.8X5	T42.8X6
Antiperspirant NEC	T49.2X1	T49.2X2	T49.2X3	T49.2X4	T49.2X5	T49.2X6
Antiphlogistic NEC	T39.4X1	T39.4X2	T39.4X3	T39.4X4	T39.4X5	T39.4X6
Antiplatyhelmintic drug	T37.4X1	T37.4X2	T37.4X3	T37.4X4	T37.4X5	T37.4X6
Antiprotozoal drug NEC	T37.3X1	T37.3X2	T37.3X3	T37.3X4	T37.3X5	T37.3X6
blood	T37.2X1	T37.2X2	T37.2X3	T37.2X4	T37.2X5	T37.2X6
local	T49.0X1	T49.0X2	T49.0X3	T49.0X4	T49.0X5	T49.0X6
Antipruritic drug NEC	T49.1X1	T49.1X2	T49.1X3	T49.1X4	T49.1X5	T49.1X6
Antipsychotic drug	T43.501	T43.502	T43.503	T43.504	T43.505	T43.506
specified NEC	T43.591	T43.592	T43.593	T43.594	T43.595	T43.596
Antipyretic	T39.91	T39.92	T39.93	T39.94	T39.95	T39.96
specified NEC	T39.8X1	T39.8X2	T39.8X3	T39.8X4	T39.8X5	T39.8X6
Antipyrine	T39.2X1	T39.2X2	T39.2X3	T39.2X4	T39.2X5	T39.2X6
Antirabies hyperimmune serum	T50.Z11	T50.Z12	T50.Z13	T50.Z14	T50.Z15	T50.Z16
Antirheumatic NEC	T39.4X1	T39.4X2	T39.4X3	T39.4X4	T39.4X5	T39.4X6
Antirigidity drug NEC	T42.8X1	T42.8X2	T42.8X3	T42.8X4	T42.8X5	T42.8X6
Antischistosomal drug	T37.4X1	T37.4X2	T37.4X3	T37.4X4	T37.4X5	T37.4X6
Antiscorpion sera	T50.Z11	T50.Z12	T50.Z13	T50.Z14	T50.Z15	T50.Z16
Antiseborrheics	T49.4X1	T49.4X2	T49.4X3	T49.4X4	T49.4X5	T49.4X6
Antiseptics (external) (medicinal)	T49.0X1	T49.0X2	T49.0X3	T49.0X4	T49.0X5	T49.0X6
Antistine	T45.0X1	T45.0X2	T45.0X3	T45.0X4	T45.0X5	T45.0X6
Antitapeworm drug	T37.4X1	T37.4X2	T37.4X3	T37.4X4	T37.4X5	T37.4X6
Antitetanus immunoglobulin	T50.Z11	T50.Z12	T50.Z13	T50.Z14	T50.Z15	T50.Z16
Antithrombotic	T45.521	T45.522	T45.523	T45.524	T45.525	T45.526
Antithyroid drug NEC	T38.2X1	T38.2X2	T38.2X3	T38.2X4	T38.2X5	T38.2X6
Antitoxin	T50.Z11	T50.Z12	T50.Z13	T50.Z14	T50.Z15	T50.Z16
diphtheria	T50.Z11	T50.Z12	T50.Z13	T50.Z14	T50.Z15	T50.Z16
gas gangrene	T50.Z11	T50.Z12	T50.Z13	T50.Z14	T50.Z15	T50.Z16
tetanus	T50.Z11	T50.Z12	T50.Z13	T50.Z14	T50.Z15	T50.Z16
Antitrichomonal drug	T37.3X1	T37.3X2	T37.3X3	T37.3X4	T37.3X5	T37.3X6
Antituberculars	T37.1X1	T37.1X2	T37.1X3	T37.1X4	T37.1X5	T37.1X6
antibiotics	T36.5X1	T36.5X2	T36.5X3	T36.5X4	T36.5X5	T36.5X6
Antitussive NEC	T48.3X1	T48.3X2	T48.3X3	T48.3X4	T48.3X5	T48.3X6
codeine mixture	T40.2X1	T40.2X2	T40.2X3	T40.2X4	T40.2X5	T40.2X6
opiate	T40.2X1	T40.2X2	T40.2X3	T40.2X4	T40.2X5	T40.2X6
Antivaricose drug	T46.8X1	T46.8X2	T46.8X3	T46.8X4	T46.8X5	T46.8X6
Antivenin, antivenom (sera)	T50.Z11	T50.Z12	T50.Z13	T50.Z14	T50.Z15	T50.Z16
crotaline	T50.Z11	T50.Z12	T50.Z13	T50.Z14	T50.Z15	T50.Z16
spider bite	T50.Z11	T50.Z12	T50.Z13	T50.Z14	T50.Z15	T50.Z16
Antivertigo drug	T45.0X1	T45.0X2	T45.0X3	T45.0X4	T45.0X5	T45.0X6
Antiviral drug NEC	T37.5X1	T37.5X2	T37.5X3	T37.5X4	T37.5X5	T37.5X6
eye	T49.5X1	T49.5X2	T49.5X3	T49.5X4	T49.5X5	T49.5X6
Antiwhipworm drug	T37.4X1	T37.4X2	T37.4X3	T37.4X4	T37.4X5	T37.4X6
Antrol (*see also* by specific chemical substance)	T60.91	T60.92	T60.93	T60.94	--	--
fungicide	T60.91	T60.92	T60.93	T60.94	--	--
ANTU (alpha naphthylthiourea)	T60.4X1	T60.4X2	T60.4X3	T60.4X4	--	--
Apalcillin	T36.0X1	T36.0X2	T36.0X3	T36.0X4	T36.0X5	T36.0X6
APC	T48.5X1	T48.5X2	T48.5X3	T48.5X4	T48.5X5	T48.5X6
Aplonidine	T44.4X1	T44.4X2	T44.4X3	T44.4X4	T44.4X5	T44.4X6
Apomorphine	T47.7X1	T47.7X2	T47.7X3	T47.7X4	T47.7X5	T47.7X6
Appetite depressants, central	T50.5X1	T50.5X2	T50.5X3	T50.5X4	T50.5X5	T50.5X6
Apraclonidine (hydrochloride)	T44.4X1	T44.4X2	T44.4X3	T44.4X4	T44.4X5	T44.4X6
Apresoline	T46.5X1	T46.5X2	T46.5X3	T46.5X4	T46.5X5	T46.5X6
Aprindine	T46.2X1	T46.2X2	T46.2X3	T46.2X4	T46.2X5	T46.2X6
Aprobarbital	T42.3X1	T42.3X2	T42.3X3	T42.3X4	T42.3X5	T42.3X6
Apronalide	T42.6X1	T42.6X2	T42.6X3	T42.6X4	T42.6X5	T42.6X6
Aprotinin	T45.621	T45.622	T45.623	T45.624	T45.625	T45.626
Aptocaine	T41.3X1	T41.3X2	T41.3X3	T41.3X4	T41.3X5	T41.3X6
Aqua fortis	T54.2X1	T54.2X2	T54.2X3	T54.2X4	--	--
Ara-A	T37.5X1	T37.5X2	T37.5X3	T37.5X4	T37.5X5	T37.5X6
Ara-C	T45.1X1	T45.1X2	T45.1X3	T45.1X4	T45.1X5	T45.1X6
Arachis oil	T49.3X1	T49.3X2	T49.3X3	T49.3X4	T49.3X5	T49.3X6
cathartic	T47.4X1	T47.4X2	T47.4X3	T47.4X4	T47.4X5	T47.4X6
Aralen	T37.2X1	T37.2X2	T37.2X3	T37.2X4	T37.2X5	T37.2X6
Arecoline	T44.1X1	T44.1X2	T44.1X3	T44.1X4	T44.1X5	T44.1X6
Arginine	T50.991	T50.992	T50.993	T50.994	T50.995	T50.996
glutamate	T50.991	T50.992	T50.993	T50.994	T50.995	T50.996
Argyrol	T49.0X1	T49.0X2	T49.0X3	T49.0X4	T49.0X5	T49.0X6
ENT agent	T49.6X1	T49.6X2	T49.6X3	T49.6X4	T49.6X5	T49.6X6
ophthalmic preparation	T49.5X1	T49.5X2	T49.5X3	T49.5X4	T49.5X5	T49.5X6
Aristocort	T38.0X1	T38.0X2	T38.0X3	T38.0X4	T38.0X5	T38.0X6
ENT agent	T49.6X1	T49.6X2	T49.6X3	T49.6X4	T49.6X5	T49.6X6
ophthalmic preparation	T49.5X1	T49.5X2	T49.5X3	T49.5X4	T49.5X5	T49.5X6
topical NEC	T49.0X1	T49.0X2	T49.0X3	T49.0X4	T49.0X5	T49.0X6
Aromatics, corrosive	T54.1X1	T54.1X2	T54.1X3	T54.1X4	--	--
disinfectants	T54.1X1	T54.1X2	T54.1X3	T54.1X4	--	--
Arsenate of lead	T57.0X1	T57.0X2	T57.0X3	T57.0X4	--	--
herbicide	T57.0X1	T57.0X2	T57.0X3	T57.0X4	--	--
Arsenic, arsenicals (compounds) (dust) (vapor) **NEC**	T57.0X1	T57.0X2	T57.0X3	T57.0X4	--	--
anti-infectives	T37.8X1	T37.8X2	T37.8X3	T37.8X4	T37.8X5	T37.8X6
pesticide (dust) (fumes)	T57.0X1	T57.0X2	T57.0X3	T57.0X4	--	--
Arsine (gas)	T57.0X1	T57.0X2	T57.0X3	T57.0X4	--	--
Arsphenamine (silver)	T37.8X1	T37.8X2	T37.8X3	T37.8X4	T37.8X5	T37.8X6
Arsthinol	T37.3X1	T37.3X2	T37.3X3	T37.3X4	T37.3X5	T37.3X6
Artane	T44.3X1	T44.3X2	T44.3X3	T44.3X4	T44.3X5	T44.3X6
Arthropod (venomous) **NEC**	T63.481	T63.482	T63.483	T63.484	--	--
Articaine	T41.3X1	T41.3X2	T41.3X3	T41.3X4	T41.3X5	T41.3X6
Asbestos	T57.8X1	T57.8X2	T57.8X3	T57.8X4	--	--
Ascaridole	T37.4X1	T37.4X2	T37.4X3	T37.4X4	T37.4X5	T37.4X6
Ascorbic acid	T45.2X1	T45.2X2	T45.2X3	T45.2X4	T45.2X5	T45.2X6
Asiaticoside	T49.0X1	T49.0X2	T49.0X3	T49.0X4	T49.0X5	T49.0X6
Asparaginase	T45.1X1	T45.1X2	T45.1X3	T45.1X4	T45.1X5	T45.1X6
Aspidium (oleoresin)	T37.4X1	T37.4X2	T37.4X3	T37.4X4	T37.4X5	T37.4X6
Aspirin (aluminum) (soluble)	T39.011	T39.012	T39.013	T39.014	T39.015	T39.016
Aspoxicillin	T36.0X1	T36.0X2	T36.0X3	T36.0X4	T36.0X5	T36.0X6
Astemizole	T45.0X1	T45.0X2	T45.0X3	T45.0X4	T45.0X5	T45.0X6
Astringent (local)	T49.2X1	T49.2X2	T49.2X3	T49.2X4	T49.2X5	T49.2X6
specified NEC	T49.2X1	T49.2X2	T49.2X3	T49.2X4	T49.2X5	T49.2X6
Astromicin	T36.5X1	T36.5X2	T36.5X3	T36.5X4	T36.5X5	T36.5X6
Ataractic drug NEC	T43.501	T43.502	T43.503	T43.504	T43.505	T43.506
Atenolol	T44.7X1	T44.7X2	T44.7X3	T44.7X4	T44.7X5	T44.7X6
Atonia drug, intestinal	T47.4X1	T47.4X2	T47.4X3	T47.4X4	T47.4X5	T47.4X6

Atophan - Benzothiadiazides

Substance	Poisoning, Accidental unintentional	Poisoning, Intentional self-harm	Poisoning, Assault	Poisoning, Undetermined	Adverse effect	Underdosing
Atophan	T50.4X1	T50.4X2	T50.4X3	T50.4X4	T50.4X5	T50.4X6
Atracurium besilate	T48.1X1	T48.1X2	T48.1X3	T48.1X4	T48.1X5	T48.1X6
Atropine	T44.3X1	T44.3X2	T44.3X3	T44.3X4	T44.3X5	T44.3X6
derivative	T44.3X1	T44.3X2	T44.3X3	T44.3X4	T44.3X5	T44.3X6
methonitrate	T44.3X1	T44.3X2	T44.3X3	T44.3X4	T44.3X5	T44.3X6
Attapulgite	T47.6X1	T47.6X2	T47.6X3	T47.6X4	T47.6X5	T47.6X6
Auramine	T65.891	T65.892	T65.893	T65.894	--	--
dye	T65.6X1	T65.6X2	T65.6X3	T65.6X4	--	--
fungicide	T60.3X1	T60.3X2	T60.3X3	T60.3X4	--	--
Auranofin	T39.4X1	T39.4X2	T39.4X3	T39.4X4	T39.4X5	T39.4X6
Aurantiin	T46.991	T46.992	T46.993	T46.994	T46.995	T46.996
Aureomycin	T36.4X1	T36.4X2	T36.4X3	T36.4X4	T36.4X5	T36.4X6
ophthalmic preparation	T49.5X1	T49.5X2	T49.5X3	T49.5X4	T49.5X5	T49.5X6
topical NEC	T49.0X1	T49.0X2	T49.0X3	T49.0X4	T49.0X5	T49.0X6
Aurothioglucose	T39.4X1	T39.4X2	T39.4X3	T39.4X4	T39.4X5	T39.4X6
Aurothioglycanide	T39.4X1	T39.4X2	T39.4X3	T39.4X4	T39.4X5	T39.4X6
Aurothiomalate sodium	T39.4X1	T39.4X2	T39.4X3	T39.4X4	T39.4X5	T39.4X6
Aurotioprol	T39.4X1	T39.4X2	T39.4X3	T39.4X4	T39.4X5	T39.4X6
Automobile fuel	T52.0X1	T52.0X2	T52.0X3	T52.0X4	--	--
Autonomic nervous system agent NEC	T44.901	T44.902	T44.903	T44.904	T44.905	T44.906
Avlosulfon	T37.1X1	T37.1X2	T37.1X3	T37.1X4	T37.1X5	T37.1X6
Avomine	T42.6X1	T42.6X2	T42.6X3	T42.6X4	T42.6X5	T42.6X6
Axerophthol	T45.2X1	T45.2X2	T45.2X3	T45.2X4	T45.2X5	T45.2X6
Azacitidine	T45.1X1	T45.1X2	T45.1X3	T45.1X4	T45.1X5	T45.1X6
Azacyclonol	T43.591	T43.592	T43.593	T43.594	T43.595	T43.596
Azadirachta	T60.2X1	T60.2X2	T60.2X3	T60.2X4	--	--
Azanidazole	T37.3X1	T37.3X2	T37.3X3	T37.3X4	T37.3X5	T37.3X6
Azapetine	T46.7X1	T46.7X2	T46.7X3	T46.7X4	T46.7X5	T46.7X6
Azapropazone	T39.2X1	T39.2X2	T39.2X3	T39.2X4	T39.2X5	T39.2X6
Azaribine	T45.1X1	T45.1X2	T45.1X3	T45.1X4	T45.1X5	T45.1X6
Azaserine	T45.1X1	T45.1X2	T45.1X3	T45.1X4	T45.1X5	T45.1X6
Azatadine	T45.0X1	T45.0X2	T45.0X3	T45.0X4	T45.0X5	T45.0X6
Azatepa	T45.1X1	T45.1X2	T45.1X3	T45.1X4	T45.1X5	T45.1X6
Azathioprine	T45.1X1	T45.1X2	T45.1X3	T45.1X4	T45.1X5	T45.1X6
Azelaic acid	T49.0X1	T49.0X2	T49.0X3	T49.0X4	T49.0X5	T49.0X6
Azelastine	T45.0X1	T45.0X2	T45.0X3	T45.0X4	T45.0X5	T45.0X6
Azidocillin	T36.0X1	T36.0X2	T36.0X3	T36.0X4	T36.0X5	T36.0X6
Azidothymidine	T37.5X1	T37.5X2	T37.5X3	T37.5X4	T37.5X5	T37.5X6
Azinphos (ethyl) (methyl)	T60.0X1	T60.0X2	T60.0X3	T60.0X4	--	--
Aziridine (chelating)	T54.1X1	T54.1X2	T54.1X3	T54.1X4	--	--
Azithromycin	T36.3X1	T36.3X2	T36.3X3	T36.3X4	T36.3X5	T36.3X6
Azlocillin	T36.0X1	T36.0X2	T36.0X3	T36.0X4	T36.0X5	T36.0X6
Azobenzene smoke	T65.3X1	T65.3X2	T65.3X3	T65.3X4	--	--
acaricide	T60.8X1	T60.8X2	T60.8X3	T60.8X4	--	--
Azosulfamide	T37.0X1	T37.0X2	T37.0X3	T37.0X4	T37.0X5	T37.0X6
AZT	T37.5X1	T37.5X2	T37.5X3	T37.5X4	T37.5X5	T37.5X6
Aztreonam	T36.1X1	T36.1X2	T36.1X3	T36.1X4	T36.1X5	T36.1X6
Azulfidine	T37.0X1	T37.0X2	T37.0X3	T37.0X4	T37.0X5	T37.0X6
Azuresin	T50.8X1	T50.8X2	T50.8X3	T50.8X4	T50.8X5	T50.8X6
B						
Bacampicillin	T36.0X1	T36.0X2	T36.0X3	T36.0X4	T36.0X5	T36.0X6
Bacillus						
lactobacillus	T47.8X1	T47.8X2	T47.8X3	T47.8X4	T47.8X5	T47.8X6
subtilis	T47.6X1	T47.6X2	T47.6X3	T47.6X4	T47.6X5	T47.6X6
Bacimycin	T49.0X1	T49.0X2	T49.0X3	T49.0X4	T49.0X5	T49.0X6
ophthalmic preparation	T49.5X1	T49.5X2	T49.5X3	T49.5X4	T49.5X5	T49.5X6
Bacitracin zinc	T49.0X1	T49.0X2	T49.0X3	T49.0X4	T49.0X5	T49.0X6
with neomycin	T49.0X1	T49.0X2	T49.0X3	T49.0X4	T49.0X5	T49.0X6
ENT agent	T49.6X1	T49.6X2	T49.6X3	T49.6X4	T49.6X5	T49.6X6
ophthalmic preparation	T49.5X1	T49.5X2	T49.5X3	T49.5X4	T49.5X5	T49.5X6
topical NEC	T49.0X1	T49.0X2	T49.0X3	T49.0X4	T49.0X5	T49.0X6
Baclofen	T42.8X1	T42.8X2	T42.8X3	T42.8X4	T42.8X5	T42.8X6
Baking soda	T50.991	T50.992	T50.993	T50.994	T50.995	T50.996
BAL	T45.8X1	T45.8X2	T45.8X3	T45.8X4	T45.8X5	T45.8X6
Bambuterol	T48.6X1	T48.6X2	T48.6X3	T48.6X4	T48.6X5	T48.6X6
Bamethan (sulfate)	T46.7X1	T46.7X2	T46.7X3	T46.7X4	T46.7X5	T46.7X6
Bamifylline	T48.6X1	T48.6X2	T48.6X3	T48.6X4	T48.6X5	T48.6X6
Bamipine	T45.0X1	T45.0X2	T45.0X3	T45.0X4	T45.0X5	T45.0X6
Baneberry — *see* Actaea spicata						
Banewort — *see* Belladonna						
Barbenyl	T42.3X1	T42.3X2	T42.3X3	T42.3X4	T42.3X5	T42.3X6
Barbexaclone	T42.6X1	T42.6X2	T42.6X3	T42.6X4	T42.6X5	T42.6X6
Barbital	T42.3X1	T42.3X2	T42.3X3	T42.3X4	T42.3X5	T42.3X6
sodium	T42.3X1	T42.3X2	T42.3X3	T42.3X4	T42.3X5	T42.3X6
Barbitone	T42.3X1	T42.3X2	T42.3X3	T42.3X4	T42.3X5	T42.3X6
Barbiturate NEC	T42.3X1	T42.3X2	T42.3X3	T42.3X4	T42.3X5	T42.3X6
with tranquilizer	T42.3X1	T42.3X2	T42.3X3	T42.3X4	T42.3X5	T42.3X6
anesthetic (intravenous)	T41.1X1	T41.1X2	T41.1X3	T41.1X4	T41.1X5	T41.1X6
Barium (carbonate) (chloride) (sulfite)	T57.8X1	T57.8X2	T57.8X3	T57.8X4	--	--
diagnostic agent	T50.8X1	T50.8X2	T50.8X3	T50.8X4	T50.8X5	T50.8X6
pesticide	T60.4X1	T60.4X2	T60.4X3	T60.4X4	--	--
rodenticide	T60.4X1	T60.4X2	T60.4X3	T60.4X4	--	--
sulfate (medicinal)	T50.8X1	T50.8X2	T50.8X3	T50.8X4	T50.8X5	T50.8X6

Substance	Poisoning, Accidental unintentional	Poisoning, Intentional self-harm	Poisoning, Assault	Poisoning, Undetermined	Adverse effect	Underdosing
Barrier cream	T49.3X1	T49.3X2	T49.3X3	T49.3X4	T49.3X5	T49.3X6
Basic fuchsin	T49.0X1	T49.0X2	T49.0X3	T49.0X4	T49.0X5	T49.0X6
Battery acid or fluid	T54.2X1	T54.2X2	T54.2X3	T54.2X4	--	--
Bay rum	T51.8X1	T51.8X2	T51.8X3	T51.8X4	--	--
BCG (vaccine)	T50.A91	T50.A92	T50.A93	T50.A94	T50.A95	T50.A96
BCNU	T45.1X1	T45.1X2	T45.1X3	T45.1X4	T45.1X5	T45.1X6
Bearsfoot	T62.2X1	T62.2X2	T62.2X3	T62.2X4	--	--
Beclamide	T42.6X1	T42.6X2	T42.6X3	T42.6X4	T42.6X5	T42.6X6
Beclomethasone	T44.5X1	T44.5X2	T44.5X3	T44.5X4	T44.5X5	T44.5X6
Bee (sting) (venom)	T63.441	T63.442	T63.443	T63.444	--	--
Befunolol	T49.5X1	T49.5X2	T49.5X3	T49.5X4	T49.5X5	T49.5X6
Bekanamycin	T36.5X1	T36.5X2	T36.5X3	T36.5X4	T36.5X5	T36.5X6
Belladonna (*see also* Nightshade)						
alkaloids	T44.3X1	T44.3X2	T44.3X3	T44.3X4	T44.3X5	T44.3X6
extract	T44.3X1	T44.3X2	T44.3X3	T44.3X4	T44.3X5	T44.3X6
herb	T44.3X1	T44.3X2	T44.3X3	T44.3X4	T44.3X5	T44.3X6
Bemegride	T50.7X1	T50.7X2	T50.7X3	T50.7X4	T50.7X5	T50.7X6
Benactyzine	T44.3X1	T44.3X2	T44.3X3	T44.3X4	T44.3X5	T44.3X6
Benadryl	T45.0X1	T45.0X2	T45.0X3	T45.0X4	T45.0X5	T45.0X6
Benaprizine	T44.3X1	T44.3X2	T44.3X3	T44.3X4	T44.3X5	T44.3X6
Benazepril	T46.4X1	T46.4X2	T46.4X3	T46.4X4	T46.4X5	T46.4X6
Bencyclane	T46.7X1	T46.7X2	T46.7X3	T46.7X4	T46.7X5	T46.7X6
Bendazol	T46.3X1	T46.3X2	T46.3X3	T46.3X4	T46.3X5	T46.3X6
Bendrofluazide	T50.2X1	T50.2X2	T50.2X3	T50.2X4	T50.2X5	T50.2X6
Bendroflumethiazide	T50.2X1	T50.2X2	T50.2X3	T50.2X4	T50.2X5	T50.2X6
Benemid	T50.4X1	T50.4X2	T50.4X3	T50.4X4	T50.4X5	T50.4X6
Benethamine penicillin	T36.0X1	T36.0X2	T36.0X3	T36.0X4	T36.0X5	T36.0X6
Benexate	T47.1X1	T47.1X2	T47.1X3	T47.1X4	T47.1X5	T47.1X6
Benfluorex	T46.6X1	T46.6X2	T46.6X3	T46.6X4	T46.6X5	T46.6X6
Benfotiamine	T45.2X1	T45.2X2	T45.2X3	T45.2X4	T45.2X5	T45.2X6
Benisone	T49.0X1	T49.0X2	T49.0X3	T49.0X4	T49.0X5	T49.0X6
Benomyl	T60.0X1	T60.0X2	T60.0X3	T60.0X4	--	--
Benoquin	T49.8X1	T49.8X2	T49.8X3	T49.8X4	T49.8X5	T49.8X6
Benoxinate	T41.3X1	T41.3X2	T41.3X3	T41.3X4	T41.3X5	T41.3X6
Benperidol	T43.4X1	T43.4X2	T43.4X3	T43.4X4	T43.4X5	T43.4X6
Benproperine	T48.3X1	T48.3X2	T48.3X3	T48.3X4	T48.3X5	T48.3X6
Benserazide	T42.8X1	T42.8X2	T42.8X3	T42.8X4	T42.8X5	T42.8X6
Bentazepam	T42.4X1	T42.4X2	T42.4X3	T42.4X4	T42.4X5	T42.4X6
Bentiromide	T50.8X1	T50.8X2	T50.8X3	T50.8X4	T50.8X5	T50.8X6
Bentonite	T49.3X1	T49.3X2	T49.3X3	T49.3X4	T49.3X5	T49.3X6
Benzalbutyramide	T46.6X1	T46.6X2	T46.6X3	T46.6X4	T46.6X5	T46.6X6
Benzalkonium (chloride)	T49.0X1	T49.0X2	T49.0X3	T49.0X4	T49.0X5	T49.0X6
ophthalmic preparation	T49.5X1	T49.5X2	T49.5X3	T49.5X4	T49.5X5	T49.5X6
Benzamidosalicylate (calcium)	T37.1X1	T37.1X2	T37.1X3	T37.1X4	T37.1X5	T37.1X6
Benzamine	T41.3X1	T41.3X2	T41.3X3	T41.3X4	T41.3X5	T41.3X6
lactate	T49.1X1	T49.1X2	T49.1X3	T49.1X4	T49.1X5	T49.1X6
Benzamphetamine	T50.5X1	T50.5X2	T50.5X3	T50.5X4	T50.5X5	T50.5X6
Benzapril hydrochloride	T46.5X1	T46.5X2	T46.5X3	T46.5X4	T46.5X5	T46.5X6
Benzathine benzylpenicillin	T36.0X1	T36.0X2	T36.0X3	T36.0X4	T36.0X5	T36.0X6
Benzathine penicillin	T36.0X1	T36.0X2	T36.0X3	T36.0X4	T36.0X5	T36.0X6
Benzatropine	T42.8X1	T42.8X2	T42.8X3	T42.8X4	T42.8X5	T42.8X6
Benzbromarone	T50.4X1	T50.4X2	T50.4X3	T50.4X4	T50.4X5	T50.4X6
Benzcarbimine	T45.1X1	T45.1X2	T45.1X3	T45.1X4	T45.1X5	T45.1X6
Benzedrex	T44.991	T44.992	T44.993	T44.994	T44.995	T44.996
Benzedrine (amphetamine)	T43.621	T43.622	T43.623	T43.624	T43.625	T43.626
Benzenamine	T65.3X1	T65.3X2	T65.3X3	T65.3X4	--	--
Benzene	T52.1X1	T52.1X2	T52.1X3	T52.1X4	--	--
homologues (acetyl) (dimethyl)(methyl) (solvent)	T52.2X1	T52.2X2	T52.2X3	T52.2X4	--	--
Benzethonium (chloride)	T49.0X1	T49.0X2	T49.0X3	T49.0X4	T49.0X5	T49.0X6
Benzfetamine	T50.5X1	T50.5X2	T50.5X3	T50.5X4	T50.5X5	T50.5X6
Benzhexol	T44.3X1	T44.3X2	T44.3X3	T44.3X4	T44.3X5	T44.3X6
Benzhydramine (chloride)	T45.0X1	T45.0X2	T45.0X3	T45.0X4	T45.0X5	T45.0X6
Benzidine	T65.891	T65.892	T65.893	T65.894	--	--
Benzilonium bromide	T44.3X1	T44.3X2	T44.3X3	T44.3X4	T44.3X5	T44.3X6
Benzimidazole	T60.3X1	T60.3X2	T60.3X3	T60.3X4	--	--
Benzin (e) — *see* Ligroin						
Benziodarone	T46.3X1	T46.3X2	T46.3X3	T46.3X4	T46.3X5	T46.3X6
Benznidazole	T37.3X1	T37.3X2	T37.3X3	T37.3X4	T37.3X5	T37.3X6
Benzocaine	T41.3X1	T41.3X2	T41.3X3	T41.3X4	T41.3X5	T41.3X6
Benzodiapin	T42.4X1	T42.4X2	T42.4X3	T42.4X4	T42.4X5	T42.4X6
Benzodiazepine NEC	T42.4X1	T42.4X2	T42.4X3	T42.4X4	T42.4X5	T42.4X6
Benzoic acid	T49.0X1	T49.0X2	T49.0X3	T49.0X4	T49.0X5	T49.0X6
with salicylic acid	T49.0X1	T49.0X2	T49.0X3	T49.0X4	T49.0X5	T49.0X6
Benzoin (tincture)	T48.5X1	T48.5X2	T48.5X3	T48.5X4	T48.5X5	T48.5X6
Benzol (benzene)	T52.1X1	T52.1X2	T52.1X3	T52.1X4	--	--
vapor	T52.0X1	T52.0X2	T52.0X3	T52.0X4	--	--
Benzomorphan	T40.2X1	T40.2X2	T40.2X3	T40.2X4	T40.2X5	T40.2X6
Benzonatate	T48.3X1	T48.3X2	T48.3X3	T48.3X4	T48.3X5	T48.3X6
Benzophenones	T49.3X1	T49.3X2	T49.3X3	T49.3X4	T49.3X5	T49.3X6
Benzopyrone	T46.991	T46.992	T46.993	T46.994	T46.995	T46.996
Benzothiadiazides	T50.2X1	T50.2X2	T50.2X3	T50.2X4	T50.2X5	T50.2X6

Substance	Poisoning, Accidental unintentional	Poisoning, Intentional self-harm	Poisoning, Assault	Poisoning, Undetermined	Adverse effect	Underdosing
Benzoxonium chloride	T49.0X1	T49.0X2	T49.0X3	T49.0X4	T49.0X5	T49.0X6
Benzoyl peroxide	T49.0X1	T49.0X2	T49.0X3	T49.0X4	T49.0X5	T49.0X6
Benzoylpas calcium	T37.1X1	T37.1X2	T37.1X3	T37.1X4	T37.1X5	T37.1X6
Benzperidin	T43.591	T43.592	T43.593	T43.594	T43.595	T43.596
Benzperidol	T43.591	T43.592	T43.593	T43.594	T43.595	T43.596
Benzphetamine	T50.5X1	T50.5X2	T50.5X3	T50.5X4	T50.5X5	T50.5X6
Benzpyrinium bromide	T44.1X1	T44.1X2	T44.1X3	T44.1X4	T44.1X5	T44.1X6
Benzquinamide	T45.0X1	T45.0X2	T45.0X3	T45.0X4	T45.0X5	T45.0X6
Benzthiazide	T50.2X1	T50.2X2	T50.2X3	T50.2X4	T50.2X5	T50.2X6
Benztropine						
anticholinergic	T44.3X1	T44.3X2	T44.3X3	T44.3X4	T44.3X5	T44.3X6
antiparkinson	T42.8X1	T42.8X2	T42.8X3	T42.8X4	T42.8X5	T42.8X6
Benzydamine	T49.0X1	T49.0X2	T49.0X3	T49.0X4	T49.0X5	T49.0X6
Benzyl						
acetate	T52.8X1	T52.8X2	T52.8X3	T52.8X4	--	--
alcohol	T49.0X1	T49.0X2	T49.0X3	T49.0X4	T49.0X5	T49.0X6
benzoate	T49.0X1	T49.0X2	T49.0X3	T49.0X4	T49.0X5	T49.0X6
Benzoic acid	T49.0X1	T49.0X2	T49.0X3	T49.0X4	T49.0X5	T49.0X6
morphine	T40.2X1	T40.2X2	T40.2X3	T40.2X4	--	--
nicotinate	T46.6X1	T46.6X2	T46.6X3	T46.6X4	T46.6X5	T46.6X6
penicillin	T36.0X1	T36.0X2	T36.0X3	T36.0X4	T36.0X5	T36.0X6
Benzylhydrochlorthia-zide	T50.2X1	T50.2X2	T50.2X3	T50.2X4	T50.2X5	T50.2X6
Benzylpenicillin	T36.0X1	T36.0X2	T36.0X3	T36.0X4	T36.0X5	T36.0X6
Benzylthiouracil	T38.2X1	T38.2X2	T38.2X3	T38.2X4	T38.2X5	T38.2X6
Bephenium hydroxy-naphthoate	T37.4X1	T37.4X2	T37.4X3	T37.4X4	T37.4X5	T37.4X6
Bepridil	T46.1X1	T46.1X2	T46.1X3	T46.1X4	T46.1X5	T46.1X6
Bergamot oil	T65.891	T65.892	T65.893	T65.894	--	--
Bergapten	T50.991	T50.992	T50.993	T50.994	T50.995	T50.996
Berries, poisonous	T62.1X1	T62.1X2	T62.1X3	T62.1X4	--	--
Beryllium (compounds)	T56.7X1	T56.7X2	T56.7X3	T56.7X4	--	--
b-acetyldigoxin	T46.0X1	T46.0X2	T46.0X3	T46.0X4	T46.0X5	T46.0X6
beta adrenergic blocking agent, heart	T44.7X1	T44.7X2	T44.7X3	T44.7X4	T44.7X5	T44.7X6
b-benzalbutyramide	T46.6X1	T46.6X2	T46.6X3	T46.6X4	T46.6X5	T46.6X6
Betacarotene	T45.2X1	T45.2X2	T45.2X3	T45.2X4	T45.2X5	T45.2X6
b-eucaine	T49.1X1	T49.1X2	T49.1X3	T49.1X4	T49.1X5	T49.1X6
Beta-Chlor	T42.6X1	T42.6X2	T42.6X3	T42.6X4	T42.6X5	T42.6X6
b-galactosidase	T47.5X1	T47.5X2	T47.5X3	T47.5X4	T47.5X5	T47.5X6
Betahistine	T46.7X1	T46.7X2	T46.7X3	T46.7X4	T46.7X5	T46.7X6
Betaine	T47.5X1	T47.5X2	T47.5X3	T47.5X4	T47.5X5	T47.5X6
Betamethasone	T49.0X1	T49.0X2	T49.0X3	T49.0X4	T49.0X5	T49.0X6
topical	T49.0X1	T49.0X2	T49.0X3	T49.0X4	T49.0X5	T49.0X6
Betamicin	T36.8X1	T36.8X2	T36.8X3	T36.8X4	T36.8X5	T36.8X6
Betanidine	T46.5X1	T46.5X2	T46.5X3	T46.5X4	T46.5X5	T46.5X6
b-sitosterol(s)	T46.6X1	T46.6X2	T46.6X3	T46.6X4	T46.6X5	T46.6X6
Betaxolol	T44.7X1	T44.7X2	T44.7X3	T44.7X4	T44.7X5	T44.7X6
Betazole	T50.8X1	T50.8X2	T50.8X3	T50.8X4	T50.8X5	T50.8X6
Bethanechol	T44.1X1	T44.1X2	T44.1X3	T44.1X4	T44.1X5	T44.1X6
chloride	T44.1X1	T44.1X2	T44.1X3	T44.1X4	T44.1X5	T44.1X6
Bethanidine	T46.5X1	T46.5X2	T46.5X3	T46.5X4	T46.5X5	T46.5X6
Betoxycaine	T41.3X1	T41.3X2	T41.3X3	T41.3X4	T41.3X5	T41.3X6
Betula oil	T49.3X1	T49.3X2	T49.3X3	T49.3X4	T49.3X5	T49.3X6
Bevantolol	T44.7X1	T44.7X2	T44.7X3	T44.7X4	T44.7X5	T44.7X6
Bevonium metilsulfate	T44.3X1	T44.3X2	T44.3X3	T44.3X4	T44.3X5	T44.3X6
Bezafibrate	T46.6X1	T46.6X2	T46.6X3	T46.6X4	T46.6X5	T46.6X6
Bezitramide	T40.4X1	T40.4X2	T40.4X3	T40.4X4	T40.4X5	T40.4X6
BHA	T50.991	T50.992	T50.993	T50.994	T50.995	T50.996
Bhang	T40.7X1	T40.7X2	T40.7X3	T40.7X4	T40.7X5	T40.7X6
BHC (medicinal)	T49.0X1	T49.0X2	T49.0X3	T49.0X4	T49.0X5	T49.0X6
nonmedicinal (vapor)	T53.6X1	T53.6X2	T53.6X3	T53.6X4	--	--
Bialamicol	T37.3X1	T37.3X2	T37.3X3	T37.3X4	T37.3X5	T37.3X6
Bibenzonium bromide	T48.3X1	T48.3X2	T48.3X3	T48.3X4	T48.3X5	T48.3X6
Bibrocathol	T49.5X1	T49.5X2	T49.5X3	T49.5X4	T49.5X5	T49.5X6
Bichloride of mercury — *see* Mercury, chloride						
Bichromates (calcium) (potassium)(sodium) (crystals)	T57.8X1	T57.8X2	T57.8X3	T57.8X4	--	--
fumes	T56.2X1	T56.2X2	T56.2X3	T56.2X4	--	--
Biclotymol	T49.6X1	T49.6X2	T49.6X3	T49.6X4	T49.6X5	T49.6X6
Bicucculine	T50.7X1	T50.7X2	T50.7X3	T50.7X4	T50.7X5	T50.7X6
Bifemelane	T43.291	T43.292	T43.293	T43.294	T43.295	T43.296
Biguanide derivatives, oral	T38.3X1	T38.3X2	T38.3X3	T38.3X4	T38.3X5	T38.3X6
Bile salts	T47.5X1	T47.5X2	T47.5X3	T47.5X4	T47.5X5	T47.5X6
Biligrafin	T50.8X1	T50.8X2	T50.8X3	T50.8X4	T50.8X5	T50.8X6
Bilopaque	T50.8X1	T50.8X2	T50.8X3	T50.8X4	T50.8X5	T50.8X6
Binifibrate	T46.6X1	T46.6X2	T46.6X3	T46.6X4	T46.6X5	T46.6X6
Binitrobenzol	T65.3X1	T65.3X2	T65.3X3	T65.3X4	--	--
Bioflavonoid(s)	T46.991	T46.992	T46.993	T46.994	T46.995	T46.996
Biological substance NEC	T50.901	T50.902	T50.903	T50.904	T50.905	T50.906
Biotin	T45.2X1	T45.2X2	T45.2X3	T45.2X4	T45.2X5	T45.2X6
Biperiden	T44.3X1	T44.3X2	T44.3X3	T44.3X4	T44.3X5	T44.3X6
Bisacodyl	T47.2X1	T47.2X2	T47.2X3	T47.2X4	T47.2X5	T47.2X6
Bisbentiamine	T45.2X1	T45.2X2	T45.2X3	T45.2X4	T45.2X5	T45.2X6
Bisbutiamine	T45.2X1	T45.2X2	T45.2X3	T45.2X4	T45.2X5	T45.2X6
Bisdequalinium (salts) (diacetate)	T49.6X1	T49.6X2	T49.6X3	T49.6X4	T49.6X5	T49.6X6
Bishydroxycoumarin	T45.511	T45.512	T45.513	T45.514	T45.515	T45.516
Bismarsen	T37.8X1	T37.8X2	T37.8X3	T37.8X4	T37.8X5	T37.8X6
Bismuth salts	T47.6X1	T47.6X2	T47.6X3	T47.6X4	T47.6X5	T47.6X6
aluminate	T47.1X1	T47.1X2	T47.1X3	T47.1X4	T47.1X5	T47.1X6
anti-infectives	T37.8X1	T37.8X2	T37.8X3	T37.8X4	T37.8X5	T37.8X6
formic iodide	T49.0X1	T49.0X2	T49.0X3	T49.0X4	T49.0X5	T49.0X6
glycolylarsenate	T49.0X1	T49.0X2	T49.0X3	T49.0X4	T49.0X5	T49.0X6
nonmedicinal (compounds) NEC	T65.91	T65.92	T65.93	T65.94	--	--
subcarbonate	T47.6X1	T47.6X2	T47.6X3	T47.6X4	T47.6X5	T47.6X6
subsalicylate	T37.8X1	T37.8X2	T37.8X3	T37.8X4	T37.8X5	T37.8X6
sulfarsphenamine	T37.8X1	T37.8X2	T37.8X3	T37.8X4	T37.8X5	T37.8X6
Bisoprolol	T44.7X1	T44.7X2	T44.7X3	T44.7X4	T44.7X5	T44.7X6
Bisoxatin	T47.2X1	T47.2X2	T47.2X3	T47.2X4	T47.2X5	T47.2X6
Bisulepin (hydrochloride)	T45.0X1	T45.0X2	T45.0X3	T45.0X4	T45.0X5	T45.0X6
Bithionol	T37.8X1	T37.8X2	T37.8X3	T37.8X4	T37.8X5	T37.8X6
anthelminthic	T37.4X1	T37.4X2	T37.4X3	T37.4X4	T37.4X5	T37.4X6
Bitolterol	T48.6X1	T48.6X2	T48.6X3	T48.6X4	T48.6X5	T48.6X6
Bitoscanate	T37.4X1	T37.4X2	T37.4X3	T37.4X4	T37.4X5	T37.4X6
Bitter almond oil	T62.8X1	T62.8X2	T62.8X3	T62.8X4	--	--
Bittersweet	T62.2X1	T62.2X2	T62.2X3	T62.2X4	--	--
Black						
flag	T60.91	T60.92	T60.93	T60.94	--	--
henbane	T62.2X1	T62.2X2	T62.2X3	T62.2X4	--	--
leaf (40)	T60.91	T60.92	T60.93	T60.94	--	--
widow spider (bite)	T63.311	T63.312	T63.313	T63.314	--	--
antivenin	T50.Z11	T50.Z12	T50.Z13	T50.Z14	T50.Z15	T50.Z16
Blast furnace gas (carbon monoxide from)	T58.8X1	T58.8X2	T58.8X3	T58.8X4	--	--
Bleach	T54.91	T54.92	T54.93	T54.94	--	--
Bleaching agent (medicinal)	T49.4X1	T49.4X2	T49.4X3	T49.4X4	T49.4X5	T49.4X6
Bleomycin	T45.1X1	T45.1X2	T45.1X3	T45.1X4	T45.1X5	T45.1X6
Blockain	T41.3X1	T41.3X2	T41.3X3	T41.3X4	T41.3X5	T41.3X6
infiltration (subcutaneous)	T41.3X1	T41.3X2	T41.3X3	T41.3X4	T41.3X5	T41.3X6
nerve block (peripheral) (plexus)	T41.3X1	T41.3X2	T41.3X3	T41.3X4	T41.3X5	T41.3X6
topical (surface)	T41.3X1	T41.3X2	T41.3X3	T41.3X4	T41.3X5	T41.3X6
Blockers, calcium channel	T46.1X1	T46.1X2	T46.1X3	T46.1X4	T46.1X5	T46.1X6
Blood (derivatives) (natural) (plasma) (whole)	T45.8X1	T45.8X2	T45.8X3	T45.8X4	T45.8X5	T45.8X6
dried	T45.8X1	T45.8X2	T45.8X3	T45.8X4	T45.8X5	T45.8X6
drug affecting NEC	T45.91	T45.92	T45.93	T45.94	T45.95	T45.96
expander NEC	T45.8X1	T45.8X2	T45.8X3	T45.8X4	T45.8X5	T45.8X6
fraction NEC	T45.8X1	T45.8X2	T45.8X3	T45.8X4	T45.8X5	T45.8X6
substitute (macromolecular)	T45.8X1	T45.8X2	T45.8X3	T45.8X4	T45.8X5	T45.8X6
Blue velvet	T40.2X1	T40.2X2	T40.2X3	T40.2X4	--	--
Bone meal	T62.8X1	T62.8X2	T62.8X3	T62.8X4	--	--
Bonine	T45.0X1	T45.0X2	T45.0X3	T45.0X4	T45.0X5	T45.0X6
Bopindolol	T44.7X1	T44.7X2	T44.7X3	T44.7X4	T44.7X5	T44.7X6
Boracic acid	T49.0X1	T49.0X2	T49.0X3	T49.0X4	T49.0X5	T49.0X6
ENT agent	T49.6X1	T49.6X2	T49.6X3	T49.6X4	T49.6X5	T49.6X6
ophthalmic preparation	T49.5X1	T49.5X2	T49.5X3	T49.5X4	T49.5X5	T49.5X6
Borane complex	T57.8X1	T57.8X2	T57.8X3	T57.8X4	--	--
Borate(s)	T57.8X1	T57.8X2	T57.8X3	T57.8X4	--	--
buffer	T50.991	T50.992	T50.993	T50.994	T50.995	T50.996
cleanser	T54.91	T54.92	T54.93	T54.94	--	--
sodium	T57.8X1	T57.8X2	T57.8X3	T57.8X4	--	--
Borax (cleanser)	T54.91	T54.92	T54.93	T54.94	--	--
Bordeaux mixture	T60.3X1	T60.3X2	T60.3X3	T60.3X4	--	--
Boric acid	T49.0X1	T49.0X2	T49.0X3	T49.0X4	T49.0X5	T49.0X6
ENT agent	T49.6X1	T49.6X2	T49.6X3	T49.6X4	T49.6X5	T49.6X6
ophthalmic preparation	T49.5X1	T49.5X2	T49.5X3	T49.5X4	T49.5X5	T49.5X6
Bornaprine	T44.3X1	T44.3X2	T44.3X3	T44.3X4	T44.3X5	T44.3X6
Boron	T57.8X1	T57.8X2	T57.8X3	T57.8X4	--	--
hydride NEC	T57.8X1	T57.8X2	T57.8X3	T57.8X4	--	--
fumes or gas	T57.8X1	T57.8X2	T57.8X3	T57.8X4	--	--
trifluoride	T59.891	T59.892	T59.893	T59.894	--	--
Botox	T48.291	T48.292	T48.293	T48.294	T48.295	T48.296
Botulinus anti-toxin (type A, B)	T50.Z11	T50.Z12	T50.Z13	T50.Z14	T50.Z15	T50.Z16
Brake fluid vapor	T59.891	T59.892	T59.893	T59.894	--	--
Brallobarbital	T42.3X1	T42.3X2	T42.3X3	T42.3X4	T42.3X5	T42.3X6
Bran (wheat)	T47.4X1	T47.4X2	T47.4X3	T47.4X4	T47.4X5	T47.4X6
Brass (fumes)	T56.891	T56.892	T56.893	T56.894	--	--
Brasso	T52.0X1	T52.0X2	T52.0X3	T52.0X4	--	--
Bretylium tosilate	T46.2X1	T46.2X2	T46.2X3	T46.2X4	T46.2X5	T46.2X6
Brevital (sodium)	T41.1X1	T41.1X2	T41.1X3	T41.1X4	T41.1X5	T41.1X6
Brinase	T45.3X1	T45.3X2	T45.3X3	T45.3X4	T45.3X5	T45.3X6
British antilewisite	T45.8X1	T45.8X2	T45.8X3	T45.8X4	T45.8X5	T45.8X6

Brodifacoum - Calcium

Substance	Poisoning, Accidental unintentional	Poisoning, Intentional self-harm	Poisoning, Assault	Poisoning, Undetermined	Adverse effect	Underdosing
Brodifacoum	T60.4X1	T60.4X2	T60.4X3	T60.4X4	--	--
Bromal (hydrate)	T42.6X1	T42.6X2	T42.6X3	T42.6X4	T42.6X5	T42.6X6
Bromazepam	T42.4X1	T42.4X2	T42.4X3	T42.4X4	T42.4X5	T42.4X6
Bromazine	T45.0X1	T45.0X2	T45.0X3	T45.0X4	T45.0X5	T45.0X6
Brombenzylcyanide	T59.3X1	T59.3X2	T59.3X3	T59.3X4	--	--
Bromelains	T45.3X1	T45.3X2	T45.3X3	T45.3X4	T45.3X5	T45.3X6
Bromethalin	T60.4X1	T60.4X2	T60.4X3	T60.4X4	--	--
Bromhexine	T48.4X1	T48.4X2	T48.4X3	T48.4X4	T48.4X5	T48.4X6
Bromide salts	T42.6X1	T42.6X2	T42.6X3	T42.6X4	T42.6X5	T42.6X6
Bromindione	T45.511	T45.512	T45.513	T45.514	T45.515	T45.516
Bromine						
compounds (medicinal)	T42.6X1	T42.6X2	T42.6X3	T42.6X4	T42.6X5	T42.6X6
sedative	T42.6X1	T42.6X2	T42.6X3	T42.6X4	T42.6X5	T42.6X6
vapor	T59.891	T59.892	T59.893	T59.894	--	--
Bromisoval	T42.6X1	T42.6X2	T42.6X3	T42.6X4	T42.6X5	T42.6X6
Bromisovalum	T42.6X1	T42.6X2	T42.6X3	T42.6X4	T42.6X5	T42.6X6
Bromobenzylcyanide	T59.3X1	T59.3X2	T59.3X3	T59.3X4	--	--
Bromochlorosalicylani-lide	T49.0X1	T49.0X2	T49.0X3	T49.0X4	T49.0X5	T49.0X6
Bromocriptine	T42.8X1	T42.8X2	T42.8X3	T42.8X4	T42.8X5	T42.8X6
Bromodiphenhydramine	T45.0X1	T45.0X2	T45.0X3	T45.0X4	T45.0X5	T45.0X6
Bromoform	T42.6X1	T42.6X2	T42.6X3	T42.6X4	T42.6X5	T42.6X6
Bromophenol blue reagent	T50.991	T50.992	T50.993	T50.994	T50.995	T50.996
Bromopride	T47.8X1	T47.8X2	T47.8X3	T47.8X4	T47.8X5	T47.8X6
Bromosalicylchloranitide	T49.0X1	T49.0X2	T49.0X3	T49.0X4	T49.0X5	T49.0X6
Bromosalicylhydroxamic acid	T37.1X1	T37.1X2	T37.1X3	T37.1X4	T37.1X5	T37.1X6
Bromo-seltzer	T39.1X1	T39.1X2	T39.1X3	T39.1X4	T39.1X5	T39.1X6
Bromoxynil	T60.3X1	T60.3X2	T60.3X3	T60.3X4	--	--
Bromperidol	T43.4X1	T43.4X2	T43.4X3	T43.4X4	T43.4X5	T43.4X6
Brompheniramine	T45.0X1	T45.0X2	T45.0X3	T45.0X4	T45.0X5	T45.0X6
Bromsulfophthalein	T50.8X1	T50.8X2	T50.8X3	T50.8X4	T50.8X5	T50.8X6
Bromural	T42.6X1	T42.6X2	T42.6X3	T42.6X4	T42.6X5	T42.6X6
Bromvaletone	T42.6X1	T42.6X2	T42.6X3	T42.6X4	T42.6X5	T42.6X6
Bronchodilator NEC	T48.6X1	T48.6X2	T48.6X3	T48.6X4	T48.6X5	T48.6X6
Brotizolam	T42.4X1	T42.4X2	T42.4X3	T42.4X4	T42.4X5	T42.4X6
Brovincamine	T46.7X1	T46.7X2	T46.7X3	T46.7X4	T46.7X5	T46.7X6
Brown recluse spider (bite) (venom)	T63.331	T63.332	T63.333	T63.334	--	--
Brown spider (bite) (venom)	T63.391	T63.392	T63.393	T63.394	--	--
Broxaterol	T48.6X1	T48.6X2	T48.6X3	T48.6X4	T48.6X5	T48.6X6
Broxuridine	T45.1X1	T45.1X2	T45.1X3	T45.1X4	T45.1X5	T45.1X6
Broxyquinoline	T37.8X1	T37.8X2	T37.8X3	T37.8X4	T37.8X5	T37.8X6
Bruceine	T48.291	T48.292	T48.293	T48.294	T48.295	T48.296
Brucia	T62.2X1	T62.2X2	T62.2X3	T62.2X4	--	--
Brucine	T65.1X1	T65.1X2	T65.1X3	T65.1X4	--	--
Brunswick green — *see* Copper						
Bruten — *see* Ibuprofen						
Bryonia	T47.2X1	T47.2X2	T47.2X3	T47.2X4	T47.2X5	T47.2X6
Buclizine	T45.0X1	T45.0X2	T45.0X3	T45.0X4	T45.0X5	T45.0X6
Buclosamide	T49.0X1	T49.0X2	T49.0X3	T49.0X4	T49.0X5	T49.0X6
Budesonide	T44.5X1	T44.5X2	T44.5X3	T44.5X4	T44.5X5	T44.5X6
Budralazine	T46.5X1	T46.5X2	T46.5X3	T46.5X4	T46.5X5	T46.5X6
Bufferin	T39.011	T39.012	T39.013	T39.014	T39.015	T39.016
Buflomedil	T46.7X1	T46.7X2	T46.7X3	T46.7X4	T46.7X5	T46.7X6
Buformin	T38.3X1	T38.3X2	T38.3X3	T38.3X4	T38.3X5	T38.3X6
Bufotenine	T40.991	T40.992	T40.993	T40.994	--	--
Bufrolin	T48.6X1	T48.6X2	T48.6X3	T48.6X4	T48.6X5	T48.6X6
Bufylline	T48.6X1	T48.6X2	T48.6X3	T48.6X4	T48.6X5	T48.6X6
Bulk filler	T50.5X1	T50.5X2	T50.5X3	T50.5X4	T50.5X5	T50.5X6
cathartic	T47.4X1	T47.4X2	T47.4X3	T47.4X4	T47.4X5	T47.4X6
Bumetanide	T50.1X1	T50.1X2	T50.1X3	T50.1X4	T50.1X5	T50.1X6
Bunaftine	T46.2X1	T46.2X2	T46.2X3	T46.2X4	T46.2X5	T46.2X6
Bunamiodyl	T50.8X1	T50.8X2	T50.8X3	T50.8X4	T50.8X5	T50.8X6
Bunazosin	T44.6X1	T44.6X2	T44.6X3	T44.6X4	T44.6X5	T44.6X6
Bunitrolol	T44.7X1	T44.7X2	T44.7X3	T44.7X4	T44.7X5	T44.7X6
Buphenine	T46.7X1	T46.7X2	T46.7X3	T46.7X4	T46.7X5	T46.7X6
Bupivacaine	T41.3X1	T41.3X2	T41.3X3	T41.3X4	T41.3X5	T41.3X6
infiltration (subcutaneous)	T41.3X1	T41.3X2	T41.3X3	T41.3X4	T41.3X5	T41.3X6
nerve block (peripheral) (plexus)	T41.3X1	T41.3X2	T41.3X3	T41.3X4	T41.3X5	T41.3X6
spinal	T41.3X1	T41.3X2	T41.3X3	T41.3X4	T41.3X5	T41.3X6
Bupranolol	T44.7X1	T44.7X2	T44.7X3	T44.7X4	T44.7X5	T44.7X6
Buprenorphine	T40.4X1	T40.4X2	T40.4X3	T40.4X4	T40.4X5	T40.4X6
Bupropion	T43.291	T43.292	T43.293	T43.294	T43.295	T43.296
Burimamide	T47.1X1	T47.1X2	T47.1X3	T47.1X4	T47.1X5	T47.1X6
Buserelin	T38.891	T38.892	T38.893	T38.894	T38.895	T38.896
Buspirone	T43.591	T43.592	T43.593	T43.594	T43.595	T43.596
Busulfan, busulphan	T45.1X1	T45.1X2	T45.1X3	T45.1X4	T45.1X5	T45.1X6
Butabarbital (sodium)	T42.3X1	T42.3X2	T42.3X3	T42.3X4	T42.3X5	T42.3X6
Butabarbitone	T42.3X1	T42.3X2	T42.3X3	T42.3X4	T42.3X5	T42.3X6
Butabarpal	T42.3X1	T42.3X2	T42.3X3	T42.3X4	T42.3X5	T42.3X6
Butacaine	T41.3X1	T41.3X2	T41.3X3	T41.3X4	T41.3X5	T41.3X6
Butalamine	T46.7X1	T46.7X2	T46.7X3	T46.7X4	T46.7X5	T46.7X6
Butalbital	T42.3X1	T42.3X2	T42.3X3	T42.3X4	T42.3X5	T42.3X6
Butallylonal	T42.3X1	T42.3X2	T42.3X3	T42.3X4	T42.3X5	T42.3X6

Substance	Poisoning, Accidental unintentional	Poisoning, Intentional self-harm	Poisoning, Assault	Poisoning, Undetermined	Adverse effect	Underdosing
Butamben	T41.3X1	T41.3X2	T41.3X3	T41.3X4	T41.3X5	T41.3X6
Butamirate	T48.3X1	T48.3X2	T48.3X3	T48.3X4	T48.3X5	T48.3X6
Butane (distributed in mobile container)	T59.891	T59.892	T59.893	T59.894	--	--
distributed through pipes	T59.891	T59.892	T59.893	T59.894	--	--
incomplete combustion	T58.11	T58.12	T58.13	T58.14	--	--
Butanilicaine	T41.3X1	T41.3X2	T41.3X3	T41.3X4	T41.3X5	T41.3X6
Butanol	T51.3X1	T51.3X2	T51.3X3	T51.3X4	--	--
Butanone, 2-butanone	T52.4X1	T52.4X2	T52.4X3	T52.4X4	--	--
Butantrone	T49.4X1	T49.4X2	T49.4X3	T49.4X4	T49.4X5	T49.4X6
Butaperazine	T43.3X1	T43.3X2	T43.3X3	T43.3X4	T43.3X5	T43.3X6
Butazolidin	T39.2X1	T39.2X2	T39.2X3	T39.2X4	T39.2X5	T39.2X6
Butetamate	T48.6X1	T48.6X2	T48.6X3	T48.6X4	T48.6X5	T48.6X6
Butethal	T42.3X1	T42.3X2	T42.3X3	T42.3X4	T42.3X5	T42.3X6
Butethamate	T44.3X1	T44.3X2	T44.3X3	T44.3X4	T44.3X5	T44.3X6
Buthalitone (sodium)	T41.1X1	T41.1X2	T41.1X3	T41.1X4	T41.1X5	T41.1X6
Butisol (sodium)	T42.3X1	T42.3X2	T42.3X3	T42.3X4	T42.3X5	T42.3X6
Butizide	T50.2X1	T50.2X2	T50.2X3	T50.2X4	T50.2X5	T50.2X6
Butobarbital	T42.3X1	T42.3X2	T42.3X3	T42.3X4	T42.3X5	T42.3X6
sodium	T42.3X1	T42.3X2	T42.3X3	T42.3X4	T42.3X5	T42.3X6
Butobarbitone	T42.3X1	T42.3X2	T42.3X3	T42.3X4	T42.3X5	T42.3X6
Butoconazole (nitrate)	T49.0X1	T49.0X2	T49.0X3	T49.0X4	T49.0X5	T49.0X6
Butorphanol	T40.4X1	T40.4X2	T40.4X3	T40.4X4	T40.4X5	T40.4X6
Butriptyline	T43.011	T43.012	T43.013	T43.014	T43.015	T43.016
Butropium bromide	T44.3X1	T44.3X2	T44.3X3	T44.3X4	T44.3X5	T44.3X6
Butter of antimony — *see* Antimony						
Buttercups	T62.2X1	T62.2X2	T62.2X3	T62.2X4	--	--
Butyl						
acetate (secondary)	T52.8X1	T52.8X2	T52.8X3	T52.8X4	--	--
alcohol	T51.3X1	T51.3X2	T51.3X3	T51.3X4	--	--
aminobenzoate	T41.3X1	T41.3X2	T41.3X3	T41.3X4	T41.3X5	T41.3X6
butyrate	T52.8X1	T52.8X2	T52.8X3	T52.8X4	--	--
carbinol	T51.3X1	T51.3X2	T51.3X3	T51.3X4	--	--
carbitol	T52.3X1	T52.3X2	T52.3X3	T52.3X4	--	--
cellosolve	T52.3X1	T52.3X2	T52.3X3	T52.3X4	--	--
chloral (hydrate)	T42.6X1	T42.6X2	T42.6X3	T42.6X4	T42.6X5	T42.6X6
formate	T52.8X1	T52.8X2	T52.8X3	T52.8X4	--	--
lactate	T52.8X1	T52.8X2	T52.8X3	T52.8X4	--	--
propionate	T52.8X1	T52.8X2	T52.8X3	T52.8X4	--	--
scopolamine bromide	T44.3X1	T44.3X2	T44.3X3	T44.3X4	T44.3X5	T44.3X6
thiobarbital sodium	T41.1X1	T41.1X2	T41.1X3	T41.1X4	T41.1X5	T41.1X6
Butylated hydroxy-anisole	T50.991	T50.992	T50.993	T50.994	T50.995	T50.996
Butylchloral hydrate	T42.6X1	T42.6X2	T42.6X3	T42.6X4	T42.6X5	T42.6X6
Butyltoluene	T52.2X1	T52.2X2	T52.2X3	T52.2X4	--	--
Butyn	T41.3X1	T41.3X2	T41.3X3	T41.3X4	T41.3X5	T41.3X6
Butyrophenone (-based tranquilizers)	T43.4X1	T43.4X2	T43.4X3	T43.4X4	T43.4X5	T43.4X6
C						
Cabergoline	T42.8X1	T42.8X2	T42.8X3	T42.8X4	T42.8X5	T42.8X6
Cacodyl, cacodylic acid	T57.0X1	T57.0X2	T57.0X3	T57.0X4	--	--
Cactinomycin	T45.1X1	T45.1X2	T45.1X3	T45.1X4	T45.1X5	T45.1X6
Cade oil	T49.4X1	T49.4X2	T49.4X3	T49.4X4	T49.4X5	T49.4X6
Cadexomer iodine	T49.0X1	T49.0X2	T49.0X3	T49.0X4	T49.0X5	T49.0X6
Cadmium (chloride) (fumes) (oxide)	T56.3X1	T56.3X2	T56.3X3	T56.3X4	--	--
sulfide (medicinal) NEC	T49.4X1	T49.4X2	T49.4X3	T49.4X4	T49.4X5	T49.4X6
Cadralazine	T46.5X1	T46.5X2	T46.5X3	T46.5X4	T46.5X5	T46.5X6
Caffeine	T43.611	T43.612	T43.613	T43.614	T43.615	T43.616
Calabar bean	T62.2X1	T62.2X2	T62.2X3	T62.2X4	--	--
Caladium seguinum	T62.2X1	T62.2X2	T62.2X3	T62.2X4	--	--
Calamine (lotion)	T49.3X1	T49.3X2	T49.3X3	T49.3X4	T49.3X5	T49.3X6
Calcifediol	T45.2X1	T45.2X2	T45.2X3	T45.2X4	T45.2X5	T45.2X6
Calciferol	T45.2X1	T45.2X2	T45.2X3	T45.2X4	T45.2X5	T45.2X6
Calcitonin	T50.991	T50.992	T50.993	T50.994	T50.995	T50.996
Calcitriol	T45.2X1	T45.2X2	T45.2X3	T45.2X4	T45.2X5	T45.2X6
Calcium	T50.3X1	T50.3X2	T50.3X3	T50.3X4	T50.3X5	T50.3X6
actylsalicylate	T39.011	T39.012	T39.013	T39.014	T39.015	T39.016
benzamidosalicylate	T37.1X1	T37.1X2	T37.1X3	T37.1X4	T37.1X5	T37.1X6
bromide	T42.6X1	T42.6X2	T42.6X3	T42.6X4	T42.6X5	T42.6X6
bromolactobionate	T42.6X1	T42.6X2	T42.6X3	T42.6X4	T42.6X5	T42.6X6
carbaspirin	T39.011	T39.012	T39.013	T39.014	T39.015	T39.016
carbimide	T50.6X1	T50.6X2	T50.6X3	T50.6X4	T50.6X5	T50.6X6
carbonate	T47.1X1	T47.1X2	T47.1X3	T47.1X4	T47.1X5	T47.1X6
chloride	T50.991	T50.992	T50.993	T50.994	T50.995	T50.996
anhydrous	T50.991	T50.992	T50.993	T50.994	T50.995	T50.996
cyanide	T57.8X1	T57.8X2	T57.8X3	T57.8X4	--	--
dioctyl sulfosuccinate	T47.4X1	T47.4X2	T47.4X3	T47.4X4	T47.4X5	T47.4X6
disodium edathamil	T45.8X1	T45.8X2	T45.8X3	T45.8X4	T45.8X5	T45.8X6
disodium edetate	T45.8X1	T45.8X2	T45.8X3	T45.8X4	T45.8X5	T45.8X6
dobesilate	T46.991	T46.992	T46.993	T46.994	T46.995	T46.996
EDTA	T45.8X1	T45.8X2	T45.8X3	T45.8X4	T45.8X5	T45.8X6
ferrous citrate	T45.4X1	T45.4X2	T45.4X3	T45.4X4	T45.4X5	T45.4X6
folinate	T45.8X1	T45.8X2	T45.8X3	T45.8X4	T45.8X5	T45.8X6

Substance	Poisoning, Accidental unintentional	Poisoning, Intentional self-harm	Poisoning, Assault	Poisoning, Undetermined	Adverse effect	Underdosing
Calcium — *continued*						
glubionate	T50.3X1	T50.3X2	T50.3X3	T50.3X4	T50.3X5	T50.3X6
gluconate	T50.3X1	T50.3X2	T50.3X3	T50.3X4	T50.3X5	T50.3X6
gluconogalactogluc-onate	T50.3X1	T50.3X2	T50.3X3	T50.3X4	T50.3X5	T50.3X6
hydrate, hydroxide	T54.3X1	T54.3X2	T54.3X3	T54.3X4	--	--
hypochlorite	T54.3X1	T54.3X2	T54.3X3	T54.3X4		
iodide	T48.4X1	T48.4X2	T48.4X3	T48.4X4	T48.4X5	T48.4X6
ipodate	T50.8X1	T50.8X2	T50.8X3	T50.8X4	T50.8X5	T50.8X6
lactate	T50.3X1	T50.3X2	T50.3X3	T50.3X4	T50.3X5	T50.3X6
leucovorin	T45.8X1	T45.8X2	T45.8X3	T45.8X4	T45.8X5	T45.8X6
mandelate	T37.91	T37.92	T37.93	T37.94	T37.95	T37.96
oxide	T54.3X1	T54.3X2	T54.3X3	T54.3X4	--	--
pantothenate	T45.2X1	T45.2X2	T45.2X3	T45.2X4	T45.2X5	T45.2X6
phosphate	T50.3X1	T50.3X2	T50.3X3	T50.3X4	T50.3X5	T50.3X6
salicylate	T39.091	T39.092	T39.093	T39.094	T39.095	T39.096
salts	T50.3X1	T50.3X2	T50.3X3	T50.3X4	T50.3X5	T50.3X6
Calculus-dissolving drug	T50.991	T50.992	T50.993	T50.994	T50.995	T50.996
Calomel	T49.0X1	T49.0X2	T49.0X3	T49.0X4	T49.0X5	T49.0X6
Caloric agent	T50.3X1	T50.3X2	T50.3X3	T50.3X4	T50.3X5	T50.3X6
Calusterone	T38.7X1	T38.7X2	T38.7X3	T38.7X4	T38.7X5	T38.7X6
Camazepam	T42.4X1	T42.4X2	T42.4X3	T42.4X4	T42.4X5	T42.4X6
Camomile	T49.0X1	T49.0X2	T49.0X3	T49.0X4	T49.0X5	T49.0X6
Camoquin	T37.2X1	T37.2X2	T37.2X3	T37.2X4	T37.2X5	T37.2X6
Camphor						
insecticide	T60.2X1	T60.2X2	T60.2X3	T60.2X4	--	--
medicinal	T49.8X1	T49.8X2	T49.8X3	T49.8X4	T49.8X5	T49.8X6
Camylofin	T44.3X1	T44.3X2	T44.3X3	T44.3X4	T44.3X5	T44.3X6
Cancer chemotherapy drug regimen	T45.1X1	T45.1X2	T45.1X3	T45.1X4	T45.1X5	T45.1X6
Candeptin	T49.0X1	T49.0X2	T49.0X3	T49.0X4	T49.0X5	T49.0X6
Candicidin	T49.0X1	T49.0X2	T49.0X3	T49.0X4	T49.0X5	T49.0X6
Cannabinol	T40.7X1	T40.7X2	T40.7X3	T40.7X4	T40.7X5	T40.7X6
Cannabis (derivatives)	T40.7X1	T40.7X2	T40.7X3	T40.7X4	T40.7X5	T40.7X6
Canned heat	T51.1X1	T51.1X2	T51.1X3	T51.1X4	--	--
Canrenoic acid	T50.0X1	T50.0X2	T50.0X3	T50.0X4	T50.0X5	T50.0X6
Canrenone	T50.0X1	T50.0X2	T50.0X3	T50.0X4	T50.0X5	T50.0X6
Cantharides, cantharidin, cantharis	T49.8X1	T49.8X2	T49.8X3	T49.8X4	T49.8X5	T49.8X6
Canthaxanthin	T50.991	T50.992	T50.993	T50.994	T50.995	T50.996
Capillary-active drug NEC	T46.901	T46.902	T46.903	T46.904	T46.905	T46.906
Capreomycin	T36.8X1	T36.8X2	T36.8X3	T36.8X4	T36.8X5	T36.8X6
Capsicum	T49.4X1	T49.4X2	T49.4X3	T49.4X4	T49.4X5	T49.4X6
Captafol	T60.3X1	T60.3X2	T60.3X3	T60.3X4	--	--
Captan	T60.3X1	T60.3X2	T60.3X3	T60.3X4	--	--
Captodiame, captodiamine	T43.591	T43.592	T43.593	T43.594	T43.595	T43.596
Captopril	T46.4X1	T46.4X2	T46.4X3	T46.4X4	T46.4X5	T46.4X6
Caramiphen	T44.3X1	T44.3X2	T44.3X3	T44.3X4	T44.3X5	T44.3X6
Carazolol	T44.7X1	T44.7X2	T44.7X3	T44.7X4	T44.7X5	T44.7X6
Carbachol	T44.1X1	T44.1X2	T44.1X3	T44.1X4	T44.1X5	T44.1X6
Carbacrylamine (resin)	T50.3X1	T50.3X2	T50.3X3	T50.3X4	T50.3X5	T50.3X6
Carbamate (insecticide)	T60.0X1	T60.0X2	T60.0X3	T60.0X4	--	--
Carbamate (sedative)	T42.6X1	T42.6X2	T42.6X3	T42.6X4	T42.6X5	T42.6X6
herbicide	T60.0X1	T60.0X2	T60.0X3	T60.0X4	--	--
insecticide	T60.0X1	T60.0X2	T60.0X3	T60.0X4	--	--
Carbamazepine	T42.1X1	T42.1X2	T42.1X3	T42.1X4	T42.1X5	T42.1X6
Carbamide	T47.3X1	T47.3X2	T47.3X3	T47.3X4	T47.3X5	T47.3X6
peroxide	T49.0X1	T49.0X2	T49.0X3	T49.0X4	T49.0X5	T49.0X6
topical	T49.8X1	T49.8X2	T49.8X3	T49.8X4	T49.8X5	T49.8X6
Carbamylcholine chloride	T44.1X1	T44.1X2	T44.1X3	T44.1X4	T44.1X5	T44.1X6
Carbaril	T60.0X1	T60.0X2	T60.0X3	T60.0X4	--	--
Carbarsone	T37.3X1	T37.3X2	T37.3X3	T37.3X4	T37.3X5	T37.3X6
Carbaryl	T60.0X1	T60.0X2	T60.0X3	T60.0X4	--	--
Carbaspirin	T39.011	T39.012	T39.013	T39.014	T39.015	T39.016
Carbazochrome (salicylate) (sodium sulfonate)	T49.4X1	T49.4X2	T49.4X3	T49.4X4	T49.4X5	T49.4X6
Carbenicillin	T36.0X1	T36.0X2	T36.0X3	T36.0X4	T36.0X5	T36.0X6
Carbenoxolone	T47.1X1	T47.1X2	T47.1X3	T47.1X4	T47.1X5	T47.1X6
Carbetapentane	T48.3X1	T48.3X2	T48.3X3	T48.3X4	T48.3X5	T48.3X6
Carbethyl salicylate	T39.091	T39.092	T39.093	T39.094	T39.095	T39.096
Carbidopa (with levodopa)	T42.8X1	T42.8X2	T42.8X3	T42.8X4	T42.8X5	T42.8X6
Carbimazole	T38.2X1	T38.2X2	T38.2X3	T38.2X4	T38.2X5	T38.2X6
Carbinol	T51.1X1	T51.1X2	T51.1X3	T51.1X4	--	--
Carbinoxamine	T45.0X1	T45.0X2	T45.0X3	T45.0X4	T45.0X5	T45.0X6
Carbiphene	T39.8X1	T39.8X2	T39.8X3	T39.8X4	T39.8X5	T39.8X6
Carbitol	T52.3X1	T52.3X2	T52.3X3	T52.3X4	--	--
Carbo medicinalis	T47.6X1	T47.6X2	T47.6X3	T47.6X4	T47.6X5	T47.6X6
Carbocaine	T41.3X1	T41.3X2	T41.3X3	T41.3X4	T41.3X5	T41.3X6
infiltration (subcutaneous)	T41.3X1	T41.3X2	T41.3X3	T41.3X4	T41.3X5	T41.3X6
nerve block (peripheral) (plexus)	T41.3X1	T41.3X2	T41.3X3	T41.3X4	T41.3X5	T41.3X6
topical (surface)	T41.3X1	T41.3X2	T41.3X3	T41.3X4	T41.3X5	T41.3X6
Carbocisteine	T48.4X1	T48.4X2	T48.4X3	T48.4X4	T48.4X5	T48.4X6
Carbocromen	T46.3X1	T46.3X2	T46.3X3	T46.3X4	T46.3X5	T46.3X6
Carbol fuchsin	T49.0X1	T49.0X2	T49.0X3	T49.0X4	T49.0X5	T49.0X6

Substance	Poisoning, Accidental unintentional	Poisoning, Intentional self-harm	Poisoning, Assault	Poisoning, Undetermined	Adverse effect	Underdosing
Carbolic acid (*see also* Phenol)	T54.0X1	T54.0X2	T54.0X3	T54.0X4	--	--
Carbolonium (bromide)	T48.1X1	T48.1X2	T48.1X3	T48.1X4	T48.1X5	T48.1X6
Carbomycin	T36.8X1	T36.8X2	T36.8X3	T36.8X4	T36.8X5	T36.8X6
Carbon						
bisulfide (liquid)	T65.4X1	T65.4X2	T65.4X3	T65.4X4	--	--
vapor	T65.4X1	T65.4X2	T65.4X3	T65.4X4	--	--
dioxide (gas)	T59.7X1	T59.7X2	T59.7X3	T59.7X4	--	--
medicinal	T41.5X1	T41.5X2	T41.5X3	T41.5X4	T41.5X5	T41.5X6
nonmedicinal	T59.7X1	T59.7X2	T59.7X3	T59.7X4	--	--
snow	T49.4X1	T49.4X2	T49.4X3	T49.4X4	T49.4X5	T49.4X6
disulfide (liquid)	T65.4X1	T65.4X2	T65.4X3	T65.4X4	--	--
vapor	T65.4X1	T65.4X2	T65.4X3	T65.4X4	--	--
monoxide (from incomplete combustion)	T58.91	T58.92	T58.93	T58.94	--	--
blast furnace gas	T58.8X1	T58.8X2	T58.8X3	T58.8X4	--	--
butane (distributed in mobile container)	T58.11	T58.12	T58.13	T58.14	--	--
distributed through pipes	T58.11	T58.12	T58.13	T58.14	--	--
charcoal fumes	T58.2X1	T58.2X2	T58.2X3	T58.2X4	--	--
coal	T58.2X1	T58.2X2	T58.2X3	T58.2X4	--	--
coke (in domestic stoves, fireplaces)	T58.2X1	T58.2X2	T58.2X3	T58.2X4	--	--
gas (piped)	T58.11	T58.12	T58.13	T58.14	--	--
solid (in domestic stoves, fireplaces)	T58.2X1	T58.2X2	T58.2X3	T58.2X4	--	--
exhaust gas (motor) not in transit	T58.01	T58.02	T58.03	T58.04	--	--
combustion engine, any not in watercraft	T58.01	T58.02	T58.03	T58.04	--	--
farm tractor, not in transit	T58.01	T58.02	T58.03	T58.04	--	--
gas engine	T58.01	T58.02	T58.03	T58.04	--	--
motor pump	T58.01	T58.02	T58.03	T58.04	--	--
motor vehicle, not in transit	T58.01	T58.02	T58.03	T58.04	--	--
fuel (in domestic use)	T58.2X1	T58.2X2	T58.2X3	T58.2X4	--	--
gas (piped)	T58.11	T58.12	T58.13	T58.14	--	--
in mobile container	T58.11	T58.12	T58.13	T58.14	--	--
piped (natural)	T58.11	T58.12	T58.13	T58.14	--	--
utility	T58.11	T58.12	T58.13	T58.14	--	--
in mobile container	T58.11	T58.12	T58.13	T58.14	--	--
illuminating gas	T58.11	T58.12	T58.13	T58.14	--	--
industrial fuels or gases, any	T58.8X1	T58.8X2	T58.8X3	T58.8X4	--	--
kerosene (in domestic stoves, fireplaces)	T58.2X1	T58.2X2	T58.2X3	T58.2X4	--	--
kiln gas or vapor	T58.8X1	T58.8X2	T58.8X3	T58.8X4	--	--
motor exhaust gas, not in transit	T58.01	T58.02	T58.03	T58.04	--	--
piped gas (manufactured) (natural)	T58.11	T58.12	T58.13	T58.14	--	--
producer gas	T58.8X1	T58.8X2	T58.8X3	T58.8X4	--	--
propane (distributed in mobile container)	T58.11	T58.12	T58.13	T58.14	--	--
distributed through pipes	T58.11	T58.12	T58.13	T58.14	--	--
specified source NEC	T58.8X1	T58.8X2	T58.8X3	T58.8X4	--	--
stove gas	T58.11	T58.12	T58.13	T58.14	--	--
piped	T58.11	T58.12	T58.13	T58.14	--	--
utility gas	T58.11	T58.12	T58.13	T58.14	--	--
piped	T58.11	T58.12	T58.13	T58.14	--	--
water gas	T58.11	T58.12	T58.13	T58.14	--	--
wood (in domestic stoves, fireplaces)	T58.2X1	T58.2X2	T58.2X3	T58.2X4	--	--
tetrachloride (vapor) NEC	T53.0X1	T53.0X2	T53.0X3	T53.0X4	--	--
liquid (cleansing agent) NEC	T53.0X1	T53.0X2	T53.0X3	T53.0X4	--	--
solvent	T53.0X1	T53.0X2	T53.0X3	T53.0X4	--	--
Carbonic acid gas	T59.7X1	T59.7X2	T59.7X3	T59.7X4	--	--
anhydrase inhibitor NEC	T50.2X1	T50.2X2	T50.2X3	T50.2X4	T50.2X5	T50.2X6
Carbophenothion	T60.0X1	T60.0X2	T60.0X3	T60.0X4	--	--
Carboplatin	T45.1X1	T45.1X2	T45.1X3	T45.1X4	T45.1X5	T45.1X6
Carboprost	T48.0X1	T48.0X2	T48.0X3	T48.0X4	T48.0X5	T48.0X6
Carboquone	T45.1X1	T45.1X2	T45.1X3	T45.1X4	T45.1X5	T45.1X6
Carbowax	T49.3X1	T49.3X2	T49.3X3	T49.3X4	T49.3X5	T49.3X6
Carboxymethyl-cellulose	T47.4X1	T47.4X2	T47.4X3	T47.4X4	T47.4X5	T47.4X6
S-Carboxymethyl-cysteine	T48.4X1	T48.4X2	T48.4X3	T48.4X4	T48.4X5	T48.4X6
Carbrital	T42.3X1	T42.3X2	T42.3X3	T42.3X4	T42.3X5	T42.3X6
Carbromal	T42.6X1	T42.6X2	T42.6X3	T42.6X4	T42.6X5	T42.6X6

2018 ICD-10-CM

ICD-10-CM TABLE OF DRUGS AND CHEMICALS

Chlorzoxazone - Cocaine

Chlorzoxazone - Cocaine

ICD-10-CM TABLE OF DRUGS AND CHEMICALS

Substance	Poisoning, Accidental unintentional	Poisoning, Intentional self-harm	Poisoning, Assault	Poisoning, Undetermined	Adverse effect	Underdosing
Chlorzoxazone	T42.8X1	T42.8X2	T42.8X3	T42.8X4	T42.8X5	T42.8X6
Choke damp	T59.7X1	T59.7X2	T59.7X3	T59.7X4	--	--
Cholagogues	T47.5X1	T47.5X2	T47.5X3	T47.5X4	T47.5X5	T47.5X6
Cholebrine	T50.8X1	T50.8X2	T50.8X3	T50.8X4	T50.8X5	T50.8X6
Cholecalciferol	T45.2X1	T45.2X2	T45.2X3	T45.2X4	T45.2X5	T45.2X6
Cholecystokinin	T50.8X1	T50.8X2	T50.8X3	T50.8X4	T50.8X5	T50.8X6
Cholera vaccine	T50.A91	T50.A92	T50.A93	T50.A94	T50.A95	T50.A96
Choleretic	T47.5X1	T47.5X2	T47.5X3	T47.5X4	T47.5X5	T47.5X6
Cholesterol-lowering agents	T46.6X1	T46.6X2	T46.6X3	T46.6X4	T46.6X5	T46.6X6
Cholestyramine (resin)	T46.6X1	T46.6X2	T46.6X3	T46.6X4	T46.6X5	T46.6X6
Cholic acid	T47.5X1	T47.5X2	T47.5X3	T47.5X4	T47.5X5	T47.5X6
Choline	T48.6X1	T48.6X2	T48.6X3	T48.6X4	T48.6X5	T48.6X6
chloride	T50.991	T50.992	T50.993	T50.994	T50.995	T50.996
dihydrogen citrate	T50.991	T50.992	T50.993	T50.994	T50.995	T50.996
salicylate	T39.091	T39.092	T39.093	T39.094	T39.095	T39.096
theophyllinate	T48.6X1	T48.6X2	T48.6X3	T48.6X4	T48.6X5	T48.6X6
Cholinergic (drug) **NEC**	T44.1X1	T44.1X2	T44.1X3	T44.1X4	T44.1X5	T44.1X6
muscle tone enhancer	T44.1X1	T44.1X2	T44.1X3	T44.1X4	T44.1X5	T44.1X6
organophosphorus	T44.0X1	T44.0X2	T44.0X3	T44.0X4	T44.0X5	T44.0X6
insecticide	T60.0X1	T60.0X2	T60.0X3	T60.0X4	--	--
nerve gas	T59.891	T59.892	T59.893	T59.894	--	--
trimethyl ammonium propanediol	T44.1X1	T44.1X2	T44.1X3	T44.1X4	T44.1X5	T44.1X6
Cholinesterase reactivator	T50.6X1	T50.6X2	T50.6X3	T50.6X4	T50.6X5	T50.6X6
Cholografin	T50.8X1	T50.8X2	T50.8X3	T50.8X4	T50.8X5	T50.8X6
Chorionic gonadotropin	T38.891	T38.892	T38.893	T38.894	T38.895	T38.896
Chromate	T56.2X1	T56.2X2	T56.2X3	T56.2X4	--	--
dust or mist	T56.2X1	T56.2X2	T56.2X3	T56.2X4	--	--
lead (*see also* lead)	T56.0X1	T56.0X2	T56.0X3	T56.0X4	--	--
paint	T56.0X1	T56.0X2	T56.0X3	T56.0X4	--	--
Chromic						
acid	T56.2X1	T56.2X2	T56.2X3	T56.2X4	--	--
dust or mist	T56.2X1	T56.2X2	T56.2X3	T56.2X4	--	--
phosphate 32P	T45.1X1	T45.1X2	T45.1X3	T45.1X4	T45.1X5	T45.1X6
Chromium	T56.2X1	T56.2X2	T56.2X3	T56.2X4	--	--
compounds — *see* Chromate						
sesquioxide	T50.8X1	T50.8X2	T50.8X3	T50.8X4	T50.8X5	T50.8X6
Chromomycin A3	T45.1X1	T45.1X2	T45.1X3	T45.1X4	T45.1X5	T45.1X6
Chromonar	T46.3X1	T46.3X2	T46.3X3	T46.3X4	T46.3X5	T46.3X6
Chromyl chloride	T56.2X1	T56.2X2	T56.2X3	T56.2X4	--	--
Chrysarobin	T49.4X1	T49.4X2	T49.4X3	T49.4X4	T49.4X5	T49.4X6
Chrysazin	T47.2X1	T47.2X2	T47.2X3	T47.2X4	T47.2X5	T47.2X6
Chymar	T45.3X1	T45.3X2	T45.3X3	T45.3X4	T45.3X5	T45.3X6
ophthalmic preparation	T49.5X1	T49.5X2	T49.5X3	T49.5X4	T49.5X5	T49.5X6
Chymopapain	T45.3X1	T45.3X2	T45.3X3	T45.3X4	T45.3X5	T45.3X6
Chymotrypsin	T45.3X1	T45.3X2	T45.3X3	T45.3X4	T45.3X5	T45.3X6
ophthalmic preparation	T49.5X1	T49.5X2	T49.5X3	T49.5X4	T49.5X5	T49.5X6
Cianidanol	T50.991	T50.992	T50.993	T50.994	T50.995	T50.996
Cianopramine	T43.011	T43.012	T43.013	T43.014	T43.015	T43.016
Cibenzoline	T46.2X1	T46.2X2	T46.2X3	T46.2X4	T46.2X5	T46.2X6
Ciclacillin	T36.0X1	T36.0X2	T36.0X3	T36.0X4	T36.0X5	T36.0X6
Ciclobarbital — *see* Hexobarbital						
Ciclonicate	T46.7X1	T46.7X2	T46.7X3	T46.7X4	T46.7X5	T46.7X6
Ciclopirox (olamine)	T49.0X1	T49.0X2	T49.0X3	T49.0X4	T49.0X5	T49.0X6
Ciclosporin	T45.1X1	T45.1X2	T45.1X3	T45.1X4	T45.1X5	T45.1X6
Cicuta maculata or virosa	T62.2X1	T62.2X2	T62.2X3	T62.2X4	--	--
Cicutoxin	T62.2X1	T62.2X2	T62.2X3	T62.2X4	--	--
Cigarette lighter fluid	T52.0X1	T52.0X2	T52.0X3	T52.0X4	--	--
Cigarettes (tobacco)	T65.221	T65.222	T65.223	T65.224	--	--
Ciguatoxin	T61.01	T61.02	T61.03	T61.04	--	--
Cilazapril	T46.4X1	T46.4X2	T46.4X3	T46.4X4	T46.4X5	T46.4X6
Cimetidine	T47.0X1	T47.0X2	T47.0X3	T47.0X4	T47.0X5	T47.0X6
Cimetropium bromide	T44.3X1	T44.3X2	T44.3X3	T44.3X4	T44.3X5	T44.3X6
Cinchocaine	T41.3X1	T41.3X2	T41.3X3	T41.3X4	T41.3X5	T41.3X6
topical (surface)	T41.3X1	T41.3X2	T41.3X3	T41.3X4	T41.3X5	T41.3X6
Cinchona	T37.2X1	T37.2X2	T37.2X3	T37.2X4	T37.2X5	T37.2X6
Cinchonine alkaloids	T37.2X1	T37.2X2	T37.2X3	T37.2X4	T37.2X5	T37.2X6
Cinchophen	T50.4X1	T50.4X2	T50.4X3	T50.4X4	T50.4X5	T50.4X6
Cinepazide	T46.7X1	T46.7X2	T46.7X3	T46.7X4	T46.7X5	T46.7X6
Cinnamedrine	T48.5X1	T48.5X2	T48.5X3	T48.5X4	T48.5X5	T48.5X6
Cinnarizine	T45.0X1	T45.0X2	T45.0X3	T45.0X4	T45.0X5	T45.0X6
Cinoxacin	T37.8X1	T37.8X2	T37.8X3	T37.8X4	T37.8X5	T37.8X6
Ciprofibrate	T46.6X1	T46.6X2	T46.6X3	T46.6X4	T46.6X5	T46.6X6
Ciprofloxacin	T36.8X1	T36.8X2	T36.8X3	T36.8X4	T36.8X5	T36.8X6
Cisapride	T47.8X1	T47.8X2	T47.8X3	T47.8X4	T47.8X5	T47.8X6
Cisplatin	T45.1X1	T45.1X2	T45.1X3	T45.1X4	T45.1X5	T45.1X6
Citalopram	T43.221	T43.222	T43.223	T43.224	T43.225	T43.226
Citanest	T41.3X1	T41.3X2	T41.3X3	T41.3X4	T41.3X5	T41.3X6
infiltration (subcutaneous)	T41.3X1	T41.3X2	T41.3X3	T41.3X4	T41.3X5	T41.3X6
nerve block (peripheral) (plexus)	T41.3X1	T41.3X2	T41.3X3	T41.3X4	T41.3X5	T41.3X6
Citric acid	T47.5X1	T47.5X2	T47.5X3	T47.5X4	T47.5X5	T47.5X6
Citrovorum (factor)	T45.8X1	T45.8X2	T45.8X3	T45.8X4	T45.8X5	T45.8X6
Claviceps purpurea	T62.2X1	T62.2X2	T62.2X3	T62.2X4	--	--

Substance	Poisoning, Accidental unintentional	Poisoning, Intentional self-harm	Poisoning, Assault	Poisoning, Undetermined	Adverse effect	Underdosing
Clavulanic acid	T36.1X1	T36.1X2	T36.1X3	T36.1X4	T36.1X5	T36.1X6
Cleaner, cleansing agent, type not specified	T65.891	T65.892	T65.893	T65.894	--	--
of paint or varnish	T52.91	T52.92	T52.93	T52.94	--	--
specified type NEC	T65.891	T65.892	T65.893	T65.894	--	--
Clebopride	T47.8X1	T47.8X2	T47.8X3	T47.8X4	T47.8X5	T47.8X6
Clefamide	T37.3X1	T37.3X2	T37.3X3	T37.3X4	T37.3X5	T37.3X6
Clemastine	T45.0X1	T45.0X2	T45.0X3	T45.0X4	T45.0X5	T45.0X6
Clematis vitalba	T62.2X1	T62.2X2	T62.2X3	T62.2X4	--	--
Clemizole	T45.0X1	T45.0X2	T45.0X3	T45.0X4	T45.0X5	T45.0X6
penicillin	T36.0X1	T36.0X2	T36.0X3	T36.0X4	T36.0X5	T36.0X6
Clenbuterol	T48.6X1	T48.6X2	T48.6X3	T48.6X4	T48.6X5	T48.6X6
Clidinium bromide	T44.3X1	T44.3X2	T44.3X3	T44.3X4	T44.3X5	T44.3X6
Clindamycin	T36.8X1	T36.8X2	T36.8X3	T36.8X4	T36.8X5	T36.8X6
Clinofibrate	T46.6X1	T46.6X2	T46.6X3	T46.6X4	T46.6X5	T46.6X6
Clioquinol	T37.8X1	T37.8X2	T37.8X3	T37.8X4	T37.8X5	T37.8X6
Cliradon	T40.2X1	T40.2X2	T40.2X3	T40.2X4	--	--
Clobazam	T42.4X1	T42.4X2	T42.4X3	T42.4X4	T42.4X5	T42.4X6
Clobenzorex	T50.5X1	T50.5X2	T50.5X3	T50.5X4	T50.5X5	T50.5X6
Clobetasol	T49.0X1	T49.0X2	T49.0X3	T49.0X4	T49.0X5	T49.0X6
Clobetasone	T49.0X1	T49.0X2	T49.0X3	T49.0X4	T49.0X5	T49.0X6
Clobutinol	T48.3X1	T48.3X2	T48.3X3	T48.3X4	T48.3X5	T48.3X6
Clocortolone	T38.0X1	T38.0X2	T38.0X3	T38.0X4	T38.0X5	T38.0X6
Clodantoin	T49.0X1	T49.0X2	T49.0X3	T49.0X4	T49.0X5	T49.0X6
Clodronic acid	T50.991	T50.992	T50.993	T50.994	T50.995	T50.996
Clofazimine	T37.1X1	T37.1X2	T37.1X3	T37.1X4	T37.1X5	T37.1X6
Clofedanol	T48.3X1	T48.3X2	T48.3X3	T48.3X4	T48.3X5	T48.3X6
Clofenamide	T50.2X1	T50.2X2	T50.2X3	T50.2X4	T50.2X5	T50.2X6
Clofenotane	T49.0X1	T49.0X2	T49.0X3	T49.0X4	T49.0X5	T49.0X6
Clofezone	T39.2X1	T39.2X2	T39.2X3	T39.2X4	T39.2X5	T39.2X6
Clofibrate	T46.6X1	T46.6X2	T46.6X3	T46.6X4	T46.6X5	T46.6X6
Clofibride	T46.6X1	T46.6X2	T46.6X3	T46.6X4	T46.6X5	T46.6X6
Cloforex	T50.5X1	T50.5X2	T50.5X3	T50.5X4	T50.5X5	T50.5X6
Clomethiazole	T42.6X1	T42.6X2	T42.6X3	T42.6X4	T42.6X5	T42.6X6
Clometocillin	T36.0X1	T36.0X2	T36.0X3	T36.0X4	T36.0X5	T36.0X6
Clomifene	T38.5X1	T38.5X2	T38.5X3	T38.5X4	T38.5X5	T38.5X6
Clomiphene	T38.5X1	T38.5X2	T38.5X3	T38.5X4	T38.5X5	T38.5X6
Clomipramine	T43.011	T43.012	T43.013	T43.014	T43.015	T43.016
Clomocycline	T36.4X1	T36.4X2	T36.4X3	T36.4X4	T36.4X5	T36.4X6
Clonazepam	T42.4X1	T42.4X2	T42.4X3	T42.4X4	T42.4X5	T42.4X6
Clonidine	T46.5X1	T46.5X2	T46.5X3	T46.5X4	T46.5X5	T46.5X6
Clonixin	T39.8X1	T39.8X2	T39.8X3	T39.8X4	T39.8X5	T39.8X6
Clopamide	T50.2X1	T50.2X2	T50.2X3	T50.2X4	T50.2X5	T50.2X6
Clopenthixol	T43.4X1	T43.4X2	T43.4X3	T43.4X4	T43.4X5	T43.4X6
Cloperastine	T48.3X1	T48.3X2	T48.3X3	T48.3X4	T48.3X5	T48.3X6
Clophedianol	T48.3X1	T48.3X2	T48.3X3	T48.3X4	T48.3X5	T48.3X6
Cloponone	T36.2X1	T36.2X2	T36.2X3	T36.2X4	T36.2X5	T36.2X6
Cloprednol	T38.0X1	T38.0X2	T38.0X3	T38.0X4	T38.0X5	T38.0X6
Cloral betaine	T42.6X1	T42.6X2	T42.6X3	T42.6X4	T42.6X5	T42.6X6
Cloramfenicol	T36.2X1	T36.2X2	T36.2X3	T36.2X4	T36.2X5	T36.2X6
Clorazepate (dipotassium)	T42.4X1	T42.4X2	T42.4X3	T42.4X4	T42.4X5	T42.4X6
Clorexolone	T50.2X1	T50.2X2	T50.2X3	T50.2X4	T50.2X5	T50.2X6
Clorfenamine	T45.0X1	T45.0X2	T45.0X3	T45.0X4	T45.0X5	T45.0X6
Clorgiline	T43.1X1	T43.1X2	T43.1X3	T43.1X4	T43.1X5	T43.1X6
Clorotepine	T44.3X1	T44.3X2	T44.3X3	T44.3X4	T44.3X5	T44.3X6
Clorox (bleach)	T54.91	T54.92	T54.93	T54.94	--	--
Clorprenaline	T48.6X1	T48.6X2	T48.6X3	T48.6X4	T48.6X5	T48.6X6
Clortermine	T50.5X1	T50.5X2	T50.5X3	T50.5X4	T50.5X5	T50.5X6
Clotiapine	T43.591	T43.592	T43.593	T43.594	T43.595	T43.596
Clotiazepam	T42.4X1	T42.4X2	T42.4X3	T42.4X4	T42.4X5	T42.4X6
Clotibric acid	T46.6X1	T46.6X2	T46.6X3	T46.6X4	T46.6X5	T46.6X6
Clotrimazole	T49.0X1	T49.0X2	T49.0X3	T49.0X4	T49.0X5	T49.0X6
Cloxacillin	T36.0X1	T36.0X2	T36.0X3	T36.0X4	T36.0X5	T36.0X6
Cloxazolam	T42.4X1	T42.4X2	T42.4X3	T42.4X4	T42.4X5	T42.4X6
Cloxiquine	T49.0X1	T49.0X2	T49.0X3	T49.0X4	T49.0X5	T49.0X6
Clozapine	T42.4X1	T42.4X2	T42.4X3	T42.4X4	T42.4X5	T42.4X6
Coagulant NEC	T45.7X1	T45.7X2	T45.7X3	T45.7X4	T45.7X5	T45.7X6
Coal (carbon monoxide from) (*see also* Carbon, monoxide, coal)	T58.2X1	T58.2X2	T58.2X3	T58.2X4	--	--
oil — *see* Kerosene						
tar	T49.1X1	T49.1X2	T49.1X3	T49.1X4	T49.1X5	T49.1X6
fumes	T59.891	T59.892	T59.893	T59.894	--	--
medicinal (ointment)	T49.4X1	T49.4X2	T49.4X3	T49.4X4	T49.4X5	T49.4X6
analgesics NEC	T39.2X1	T39.2X2	T39.2X3	T39.2X4	T39.2X5	T39.2X6
naphtha (solvent)	T52.0X1	T52.0X2	T52.0X3	T52.0X4	--	--
Cobalamine	T45.2X1	T45.2X2	T45.2X3	T45.2X4	T45.2X5	T45.2X6
Cobalt (nonmedicinal) (fumes) (industrial)	T56.891	T56.892	T56.893	T56.894	--	--
medicinal (trace) (chloride)	T45.8X1	T45.8X2	T45.8X3	T45.8X4	T45.8X5	T45.8X6
Cobra (venom)	T63.041	T63.042	T63.043	T63.044	--	--
Coca (leaf)	T40.5X1	T40.5X2	T40.5X3	T40.5X4	T40.5X5	T40.5X6
Cocaine	T40.5X1	T40.5X2	T40.5X3	T40.5X4	T40.5X5	T40.5X6
topical anesthetic	T41.3X1	T41.3X2	T41.3X3	T41.3X4	T41.3X5	T41.3X6

Substance	Poisoning, Accidental unintentional	Poisoning, Intentional self-harm	Poisoning, Assault	Poisoning, Undetermined	Adverse effect	Underdosing
Cocarboxylase	T45.3X1	T45.3X2	T45.3X3	T45.3X4	T45.3X5	T45.3X6
Coccidioidin	T50.8X1	T50.8X2	T50.8X3	T50.8X4	T50.8X5	T50.8X6
Cocculus indicus	T62.1X1	T62.1X2	T62.1X3	T62.1X4	--	--
Cochineal	T65.6X1	T65.6X2	T65.6X3	T65.6X4	--	--
medicinal products	T50.991	T50.992	T50.993	T50.994	T50.995	T50.996
Codeine	T40.2X1	T40.2X2	T40.2X3	T40.2X4	T40.2X5	T40.2X6
Cod-liver oil	T45.2X1	T45.2X2	T45.2X3	T45.2X4	T45.2X5	T45.2X6
Coenzyme A	T50.991	T50.992	T50.993	T50.994	T50.995	T50.996
Coffee	T62.8X1	T62.8X2	T62.8X3	T62.8X4	--	--
Cogalactoiso-merase	T50.991	T50.992	T50.993	T50.994	T50.995	T50.996
Cogentin	T44.3X1	T44.3X2	T44.3X3	T44.3X4	T44.3X5	T44.3X6
Coke fumes or gas (carbon monoxide)	T58.2X1	T58.2X2	T58.2X3	T58.2X4	--	--
industrial use	T58.8X1	T58.8X2	T58.8X3	T58.8X4	--	--
Colace	T47.4X1	T47.4X2	T47.4X3	T47.4X4	T47.4X5	T47.4X6
Colaspase	T45.1X1	T45.1X2	T45.1X3	T45.1X4	T45.1X5	T45.1X6
Colchicine	T50.4X1	T50.4X2	T50.4X3	T50.4X4	T50.4X5	T50.4X6
Colchicum	T62.2X1	T62.2X2	T62.2X3	T62.2X4	--	--
Cold cream	T49.3X1	T49.3X2	T49.3X3	T49.3X4	T49.3X5	T49.3X6
Colecalciferol	T45.2X1	T45.2X2	T45.2X3	T45.2X4	T45.2X5	T45.2X6
Colestipol	T46.6X1	T46.6X2	T46.6X3	T46.6X4	T46.6X5	T46.6X6
Colestyramine	T46.6X1	T46.6X2	T46.6X3	T46.6X4	T46.6X5	T46.6X6
Colimycin	T36.8X1	T36.8X2	T36.8X3	T36.8X4	T36.8X5	T36.8X6
Colistimethate	T36.8X1	T36.8X2	T36.8X3	T36.8X4	T36.8X5	T36.8X6
Colistin	T36.8X1	T36.8X2	T36.8X3	T36.8X4	T36.8X5	T36.8X6
sulfate (eye preparation)	T49.5X1	T49.5X2	T49.5X3	T49.5X4	T49.5X5	T49.5X6
Collagen	T50.991	T50.992	T50.993	T50.994	T50.995	T50.996
Collagenase	T49.4X1	T49.4X2	T49.4X3	T49.4X4	T49.4X5	T49.4X6
Collodion	T49.3X1	T49.3X2	T49.3X3	T49.3X4	T49.3X5	T49.3X6
Colocynth	T47.2X1	T47.2X2	T47.2X3	T47.2X4	T47.2X5	T47.2X6
Colophony adhesive	T49.3X1	T49.3X2	T49.3X3	T49.3X4	T49.3X5	T49.3X6
Colorant (see also Dye)	T50.991	T50.992	T50.993	T50.994	T50.995	T50.996
Coloring matter — see Dye(s)						
Combustion gas (after combustion) — see Carbon, monoxide						
prior to combustion	T59.891	T59.892	T59.893	T59.894	--	--
Compazine	T43.3X1	T43.3X2	T43.3X3	T43.3X4	T43.3X5	T43.3X6
Compound						
42 (warfarin)	T60.4X1	T60.4X2	T60.4X3	T60.4X4	--	--
269 (endrin)	T60.1X1	T60.1X2	T60.1X3	T60.1X4	--	--
497 (dieldrin)	T60.1X1	T60.1X2	T60.1X3	T60.1X4	--	--
1080 (sodium fluoroacetate)	T60.4X1	T60.4X2	T60.4X3	T60.4X4	--	--
3422 (parathion)	T60.0X1	T60.0X2	T60.0X3	T60.0X4	--	--
3911 (phorate)	T60.0X1	T60.0X2	T60.0X3	T60.0X4	--	--
3956 (toxaphene)	T60.1X1	T60.1X2	T60.1X3	T60.1X4	--	--
4049 (malathion)	T60.0X1	T60.0X2	T60.0X3	T60.0X4	--	--
4069 (malathion)	T60.0X1	T60.0X2	T60.0X3	T60.0X4	--	--
4124 (dicapthon)	T60.0X1	T60.0X2	T60.0X3	T60.0X4	--	--
E (cortisone)	T38.0X1	T38.0X2	T38.0X3	T38.0X4	T38.0X5	T38.0X6
F (hydrocortisone)	T38.0X1	T38.0X2	T38.0X3	T38.0X4	T38.0X5	T38.0X6
Congener, anabolic	T38.7X1	T38.7X2	T38.7X3	T38.7X4	T38.7X5	T38.7X6
Congo red	T50.8X1	T50.8X2	T50.8X3	T50.8X4	T50.8X5	T50.8X6
Coniine, conine	T62.2X1	T62.2X2	T62.2X3	T62.2X4	--	--
Conium (maculatum)	T62.2X1	T62.2X2	T62.2X3	T62.2X4	--	--
Conjugated estrogenic substances	T38.5X1	T38.5X2	T38.5X3	T38.5X4	T38.5X5	T38.5X6
Contac	T48.5X1	T48.5X2	T48.5X3	T48.5X4	T48.5X5	T48.5X6
Contact lens solution	T49.5X1	T49.5X2	T49.5X3	T49.5X4	T49.5X5	T49.5X6
Contraceptive (oral)	T38.4X1	T38.4X2	T38.4X3	T38.4X4	T38.4X5	T38.4X6
vaginal	T49.8X1	T49.8X2	T49.8X3	T49.8X4	T49.8X5	T49.8X6
Contrast medium, radiography	T50.8X1	T50.8X2	T50.8X3	T50.8X4	T50.8X5	T50.8X6
Convallaria glycosides	T46.0X1	T46.0X2	T46.0X3	T46.0X4	T46.0X5	T46.0X6
Convallaria majalis	T62.2X1	T62.2X2	T62.2X3	T62.2X4	--	--
berry	T62.1X1	T62.1X2	T62.1X3	T62.1X4	--	--
Copper (dust) (fumes) (nonmedicinal) NEC	T56.4X1	T56.4X2	T56.4X3	T56.4X4	--	--
arsenate, arsenite	T57.0X1	T57.0X2	T57.0X3	T57.0X4	--	--
insecticide	T60.2X1	T60.2X2	T60.2X3	T60.2X4	--	--
emetic	T47.7X1	T47.7X2	T47.7X3	T47.7X4	T47.7X5	T47.7X6
fungicide	T60.3X1	T60.3X2	T60.3X3	T60.3X4	--	--
gluconate	T49.0X1	T49.0X2	T49.0X3	T49.0X4	T49.0X5	T49.0X6
insecticide	T60.2X1	T60.2X2	T60.2X3	T60.2X4	--	--
medicinal (trace)	T45.8X1	T45.8X2	T45.8X3	T45.8X4	T45.8X5	T45.8X6
oleate	T49.0X1	T49.0X2	T49.0X3	T49.0X4	T49.0X5	T49.0X6
sulfate	T56.4X1	T56.4X2	T56.4X3	T56.4X4	--	--
cupric	T56.4X1	T56.4X2	T56.4X3	T56.4X4	--	--
fungicide	T60.3X1	T60.3X2	T60.3X3	T60.3X4	--	--
medicinal						
ear	T49.6X1	T49.6X2	T49.6X3	T49.6X4	T49.6X5	T49.6X6

Substance	Poisoning, Accidental unintentional	Poisoning, Intentional self-harm	Poisoning, Assault	Poisoning, Undetermined	Adverse effect	Underdosing
Copper — continued						
sulfate — continued						
emetic	T47.7X1	T47.7X2	T47.7X3	T47.7X4	T47.7X5	T47.7X6
eye	T49.5X1	T49.5X2	T49.5X3	T49.5X4	T49.5X5	T49.5X6
cuprous	T56.4X1	T56.4X2	T56.4X3	T56.4X4	--	--
fungicide	T60.3X1	T60.3X2	T60.3X3	T60.3X4	--	--
medicinal						
ear	T49.6X1	T49.6X2	T49.6X3	T49.6X4	T49.6X5	T49.6X6
emetic	T47.7X1	T47.7X2	T47.7X3	T47.7X4	T47.7X5	T47.7X6
eye	T49.5X1	T49.5X2	T49.5X3	T49.5X4	T49.5X5	T49.5X6
Copperhead snake (bite) (venom)	T63.061	T63.062	T63.063	T63.064	--	--
Coral (sting)	T63.691	T63.692	T63.693	T63.694	--	--
snake (bite) (venom)	T63.021	T63.022	T63.023	T63.024	--	--
Corbadrine	T49.6X1	T49.6X2	T49.6X3	T49.6X4	T49.6X5	T49.6X6
Cordite	T65.891	T65.892	T65.893	T65.894	--	--
vapor	T59.891	T59.892	T59.893	T59.894	--	--
Cordran	T49.0X1	T49.0X2	T49.0X3	T49.0X4	T49.0X5	T49.0X6
Corn cures	T49.4X1	T49.4X2	T49.4X3	T49.4X4	T49.4X5	T49.4X6
Corn starch	T49.3X1	T49.3X2	T49.3X3	T49.3X4	T49.3X5	T49.3X6
Cornhusker's lotion	T49.3X1	T49.3X2	T49.3X3	T49.3X4	T49.3X5	T49.3X6
Coronary vasodilator NEC	T46.3X1	T46.3X2	T46.3X3	T46.3X4	T46.3X5	T46.3X6
Corrosive NEC	T54.91	T54.92	T54.93	T54.94	--	--
acid NEC	T54.2X1	T54.2X2	T54.2X3	T54.2X4	--	--
aromatics	T54.1X1	T54.1X2	T54.1X3	T54.1X4	--	--
disinfectant	T54.1X1	T54.1X2	T54.1X3	T54.1X4	--	--
fumes NEC	T54.91	T54.92	T54.93	T54.94	--	--
specified NEC	T54.91	T54.92	T54.93	T54.94	--	--
sublimate	T56.1X1	T56.1X2	T56.1X3	T56.1X4	--	--
Cortate	T38.0X1	T38.0X2	T38.0X3	T38.0X4	T38.0X5	T38.0X6
Cort-Dome	T38.0X1	T38.0X2	T38.0X3	T38.0X4	T38.0X5	T38.0X6
ENT agent	T49.6X1	T49.6X2	T49.6X3	T49.6X4	T49.6X5	T49.6X6
ophthalmic preparation	T49.5X1	T49.5X2	T49.5X3	T49.5X4	T49.5X5	T49.5X6
topical NEC	T49.0X1	T49.0X2	T49.0X3	T49.0X4	T49.0X5	T49.0X6
Cortef	T38.0X1	T38.0X2	T38.0X3	T38.0X4	T38.0X5	T38.0X6
ENT agent	T49.6X1	T49.6X2	T49.6X3	T49.6X4	T49.6X5	T49.6X6
ophthalmic preparation	T49.5X1	T49.5X2	T49.5X3	T49.5X4	T49.5X5	T49.5X6
topical NEC	T49.0X1	T49.0X2	T49.0X3	T49.0X4	T49.0X5	T49.0X6
Corticosteroid	T38.0X1	T38.0X2	T38.0X3	T38.0X4	T38.0X5	T38.0X6
ENT agent	T49.6X1	T49.6X2	T49.6X3	T49.6X4	T49.6X5	T49.6X6
mineral	T50.0X1	T50.0X2	T50.0X3	T50.0X4	T50.0X5	T50.0X6
ophthalmic	T49.5X1	T49.5X2	T49.5X3	T49.5X4	T49.5X5	T49.5X6
topical NEC	T49.0X1	T49.0X2	T49.0X3	T49.0X4	T49.0X5	T49.0X6
Corticotropin	T38.811	T38.812	T38.813	T38.814	T38.815	T38.816
Cortisol	T49.0X1	T49.0X2	T49.0X3	T49.0X4	T49.0X5	T49.0X6
ENT agent	T49.6X1	T49.6X2	T49.6X3	T49.6X4	T49.6X5	T49.6X6
ophthalmic preparation	T49.5X1	T49.5X2	T49.5X3	T49.5X4	T49.5X5	T49.5X6
topical NEC	T49.0X1	T49.0X2	T49.0X3	T49.0X4	T49.0X5	T49.0X6
Cortisone (acetate)	T38.0X1	T38.0X2	T38.0X3	T38.0X4	T38.0X5	T38.0X6
ENT agent	T49.6X1	T49.6X2	T49.6X3	T49.6X4	T49.6X5	T49.6X6
ophthalmic preparation	T49.5X1	T49.5X2	T49.5X3	T49.5X4	T49.5X5	T49.5X6
topical NEC	T49.0X1	T49.0X2	T49.0X3	T49.0X4	T49.0X5	T49.0X6
Cortivazol	T38.0X1	T38.0X2	T38.0X3	T38.0X4	T38.0X5	T38.0X6
Cortogen	T38.0X1	T38.0X2	T38.0X3	T38.0X4	T38.0X5	T38.0X6
ENT agent	T49.6X1	T49.6X2	T49.6X3	T49.6X4	T49.6X5	T49.6X6
ophthalmic preparation	T49.5X1	T49.5X2	T49.5X3	T49.5X4	T49.5X5	T49.5X6
Cortone	T38.0X1	T38.0X2	T38.0X3	T38.0X4	T38.0X5	T38.0X6
ENT agent	T49.6X1	T49.6X2	T49.6X3	T49.6X4	T49.6X5	T49.6X6
ophthalmic preparation	T49.5X1	T49.5X2	T49.5X3	T49.5X4	T49.5X5	T49.5X6
Cortril	T38.0X1	T38.0X2	T38.0X3	T38.0X4	T38.0X5	T38.0X6
ENT agent	T49.6X1	T49.6X2	T49.6X3	T49.6X4	T49.6X5	T49.6X6
ophthalmic preparation	T49.5X1	T49.5X2	T49.5X3	T49.5X4	T49.5X5	T49.5X6
topical NEC	T49.0X1	T49.0X2	T49.0X3	T49.0X4	T49.0X5	T49.0X6
Corynebacterium parvum	T45.1X1	T45.1X2	T45.1X3	T45.1X4	T45.1X5	T45.1X6
Cosmetic preparation	T49.8X1	T49.8X2	T49.8X3	T49.8X4	T49.8X5	T49.8X6
Cosmetics	T49.8X1	T49.8X2	T49.8X3	T49.8X4	T49.8X5	T49.8X6
Cosyntropin	T38.811	T38.812	T38.813	T38.814	T38.815	T38.816
Cotarnine	T45.7X1	T45.7X2	T45.7X3	T45.7X4	T45.7X5	T45.7X6
Co-trimoxazole	T36.8X1	T36.8X2	T36.8X3	T36.8X4	T36.8X5	T36.8X6
Cottonseed oil	T49.3X1	T49.3X2	T49.3X3	T49.3X4	T49.3X5	T49.3X6
Cough mixture (syrup)	T48.4X1	T48.4X2	T48.4X3	T48.4X4	T48.4X5	T48.4X6
containing opiates	T40.2X1	T40.2X2	T40.2X3	T40.2X4	T40.2X5	T40.2X6
expectorants	T48.4X1	T48.4X2	T48.4X3	T48.4X4	T48.4X5	T48.4X6
Coumadin	T45.511	T45.512	T45.513	T45.514	T45.515	T45.516
rodenticide	T60.4X1	T60.4X2	T60.4X3	T60.4X4	--	--
Coumaphos	T60.0X1	T60.0X2	T60.0X3	T60.0X4	--	--
Coumarin	T45.511	T45.512	T45.513	T45.514	T45.515	T45.516
Coumetarol	T45.511	T45.512	T45.513	T45.514	T45.515	T45.516
Cowbane	T62.2X1	T62.2X2	T62.2X3	T62.2X4	--	--
Cozyme	T45.2X1	T45.2X2	T45.2X3	T45.2X4	T45.2X5	T45.2X6
Crack	T40.5X1	T40.5X2	T40.5X3	T40.5X4	--	--
Crataegus extract	T46.0X1	T46.0X2	T46.0X3	T46.0X4	T46.0X5	T46.0X6
Creolin	T54.1X1	T54.1X2	T54.1X3	T54.1X4	--	--
disinfectant	T54.1X1	T54.1X2	T54.1X3	T54.1X4	--	--

Substance	Poisoning, Accidental unintentional	Poisoning, Intentional self-harm	Poisoning, Assault	Poisoning, Undetermined	Adverse effect	Underdosing
Fenofibrate	T46.6X1	T46.6X2	T46.6X3	T46.6X4	T46.6X5	T46.6X6
Fenoprofen	T39.311	T39.312	T39.313	T39.314	T39.315	T39.316
Fenoterol	T48.6X1	T48.6X2	T48.6X3	T48.6X4	T48.6X5	T48.6X6
Fenoverine	T44.3X1	T44.3X2	T44.3X3	T44.3X4	T44.3X5	T44.3X6
Fenoxazoline	T48.5X1	T48.5X2	T48.5X3	T48.5X4	T48.5X5	T48.5X6
Fenproporex	T50.5X1	T50.5X2	T50.5X3	T50.5X4	T50.5X5	T50.5X6
Fenquizone	T50.2X1	T50.2X2	T50.2X3	T50.2X4	T50.2X5	T50.2X6
Fentanyl	T40.4X1	T40.4X2	T40.4X3	T40.4X4	T40.4X5	T40.4X6
Fentazin	T43.3X1	T43.3X2	T43.3X3	T43.3X4	T43.3X5	T43.3X6
Fenthion	T60.0X1	T60.0X2	T60.0X3	T60.0X4	--	--
Fenticlor	T49.0X1	T49.0X2	T49.0X3	T49.0X4	T49.0X5	T49.0X6
Fenylbutazone	T39.2X1	T39.2X2	T39.2X3	T39.2X4	T39.2X5	T39.2X6
Feprazone	T39.2X1	T39.2X2	T39.2X3	T39.2X4	T39.2X5	T39.2X6
Fer de lance (bite) (venom)	T63.061	T63.062	T63.063	T63.064	--	--
Ferric (*see also* Iron)						
chloride	T45.4X1	T45.4X2	T45.4X3	T45.4X4	T45.4X5	T45.4X6
citrate	T45.4X1	T45.4X2	T45.4X3	T45.4X4	T45.4X5	T45.4X6
hydroxide						
colloidal	T45.4X1	T45.4X2	T45.4X3	T45.4X4	T45.4X5	T45.4X6
polymaltose	T45.4X1	T45.4X2	T45.4X3	T45.4X4	T45.4X5	T45.4X6
pyrophosphate	T45.4X1	T45.4X2	T45.4X3	T45.4X4	T45.4X5	T45.4X6
Ferritin	T45.4X1	T45.4X2	T45.4X3	T45.4X4	T45.4X5	T45.4X6
Ferrocholinate	T45.4X1	T45.4X2	T45.4X3	T45.4X4	T45.4X5	T45.4X6
Ferrodextrane	T45.4X1	T45.4X2	T45.4X3	T45.4X4	T45.4X5	T45.4X6
Ferropolimaler	T45.4X1	T45.4X2	T45.4X3	T45.4X4	T45.4X5	T45.4X6
Ferrous (*see also* Iron)						
phosphate	T45.4X1	T45.4X2	T45.4X3	T45.4X4	T45.4X5	T45.4X6
salt	T45.4X1	T45.4X2	T45.4X3	T45.4X4	T45.4X5	T45.4X6
with folic acid	T45.4X1	T45.4X2	T45.4X3	T45.4X4	T45.4X5	T45.4X6
Ferrous fumerate, gluconate, lactate, salt NEC, sulfate (medicinal)	T45.4X1	T45.4X2	T45.4X3	T45.4X4	T45.4X5	T45.4X6
Ferrovanadium (fumes)	T59.891	T59.892	T59.893	T59.894	--	--
Ferrum — *see* Iron						
Fertilizers NEC	T65.891	T65.892	T65.893	T65.894	--	--
with herbicide mixture	T60.3X1	T60.3X2	T60.3X3	T60.3X4	--	--
Fetoxilate	T47.6X1	T47.6X2	T47.6X3	T47.6X4	T47.6X5	T47.6X6
Fiber, dietary	T47.4X1	T47.4X2	T47.4X3	T47.4X4	T47.4X5	T47.4X6
Fiberglass	T65.831	T65.832	T65.833	T65.834	--	--
Fibrinogen (human)	T45.8X1	T45.8X2	T45.8X3	T45.8X4	T45.8X5	T45.8X6
Fibrinolysin (human)	T45.691	T45.692	T45.693	T45.694	T45.695	T45.696
Fibrinolysis						
affecting drug	T45.601	T45.602	T45.603	T45.604	T45.605	T45.606
inhibitor NEC	T45.621	T45.622	T45.623	T45.624	T45.625	T45.626
Fibrinolytic drug	T45.611	T45.612	T45.613	T45.614	T45.615	T45.616
Filix mas	T37.4X1	T37.4X2	T37.4X3	T37.4X4	T37.4X5	T37.4X6
Filtering cream	T49.3X1	T49.3X2	T49.3X3	T49.3X4	T49.3X5	T49.3X6
Fiorinal	T39.011	T39.012	T39.013	T39.014	T39.015	T39.016
Firedamp	T59.891	T59.892	T59.893	T59.894	--	--
Fish, noxious, nonbacterial	T61.91	T61.92	T61.93	T61.94	--	--
ciguatera	T61.01	T61.02	T61.03	T61.04	--	--
scombroid	T61.11	T61.12	T61.13	T61.14	--	--
shell	T61.781	T61.782	T61.783	T61.784	--	--
specified NEC	T61.771	T61.772	T61.773	T61.774	--	--
Flagyl	T37.3X1	T37.3X2	T37.3X3	T37.3X4	T37.3X5	T37.3X6
Flavine adenine dinucleotide	T45.2X1	T45.2X2	T45.2X3	T45.2X4	T45.2X5	T45.2X6
Flavodic acid	T46.991	T46.992	T46.993	T46.994	T46.995	T46.996
Flavoxate	T44.3X1	T44.3X2	T44.3X3	T44.3X4	T44.3X5	T44.3X6
Flaxedil	T48.1X1	T48.1X2	T48.1X3	T48.1X4	T48.1X5	T48.1X6
Flaxseed (medicinal)	T49.3X1	T49.3X2	T49.3X3	T49.3X4	T49.3X5	T49.3X6
Flecainide	T46.2X1	T46.2X2	T46.2X3	T46.2X4	T46.2X5	T46.2X6
Fleroxacin	T36.8X1	T36.8X2	T36.8X3	T36.8X4	T36.8X5	T36.8X6
Floctafenine	T39.8X1	T39.8X2	T39.8X3	T39.8X4	T39.8X5	T39.8X6
Flomax	T44.6X1	T44.6X2	T44.6X3	T44.6X4	T44.6X5	T44.6X6
Flomoxef	T36.1X1	T36.1X2	T36.1X3	T36.1X4	T36.1X5	T36.1X6
Flopropione	T44.3X1	T44.3X2	T44.3X3	T44.3X4	T44.3X5	T44.3X6
Florantyrone	T47.5X1	T47.5X2	T47.5X3	T47.5X4	T47.5X5	T47.5X6
Floraquin	T37.8X1	T37.8X2	T37.8X3	T37.8X4	T37.8X5	T37.8X6
Florinef	T38.0X1	T38.0X2	T38.0X3	T38.0X4	T38.0X5	T38.0X6
ENT agent	T49.6X1	T49.6X2	T49.6X3	T49.6X4	T49.6X5	T49.6X6
ophthalmic preparation	T49.5X1	T49.5X2	T49.5X3	T49.5X4	T49.5X5	T49.5X6
topical NEC	T49.0X1	T49.0X2	T49.0X3	T49.0X4	T49.0X5	T49.0X6
Flowers of sulfur	T49.4X1	T49.4X2	T49.4X3	T49.4X4	T49.4X5	T49.4X6
Floxuridine	T45.1X1	T45.1X2	T45.1X3	T45.1X4	T45.1X5	T45.1X6
Fluanisone	T43.4X1	T43.4X2	T43.4X3	T43.4X4	T43.4X5	T43.4X6
Flubendazole	T37.4X1	T37.4X2	T37.4X3	T37.4X4	T37.4X5	T37.4X6
Fluclorolone acetonide	T49.0X1	T49.0X2	T49.0X3	T49.0X4	T49.0X5	T49.0X6
Flucloxacillin	T36.0X1	T36.0X2	T36.0X3	T36.0X4	T36.0X5	T36.0X6
Fluconazole	T37.8X1	T37.8X2	T37.8X3	T37.8X4	T37.8X5	T37.8X6
Flucytosine	T37.8X1	T37.8X2	T37.8X3	T37.8X4	T37.8X5	T37.8X6
Fludeoxyglucose (18F)	T50.8X1	T50.8X2	T50.8X3	T50.8X4	T50.8X5	T50.8X6
Fludiazepam	T42.4X1	T42.4X2	T42.4X3	T42.4X4	T42.4X5	T42.4X6
Fludrocortisone	T50.0X1	T50.0X2	T50.0X3	T50.0X4	T50.0X5	T50.0X6
ENT agent	T49.6X1	T49.6X2	T49.6X3	T49.6X4	T49.6X5	T49.6X6
ophthalmic preparation	T49.5X1	T49.5X2	T49.5X3	T49.5X4	T49.5X5	T49.5X6
topical NEC	T49.0X1	T49.0X2	T49.0X3	T49.0X4	T49.0X5	T49.0X6
Fludroxycortide	T49.0X1	T49.0X2	T49.0X3	T49.0X4	T49.0X5	T49.0X6
Flufenamic acid	T39.391	T39.392	T39.393	T39.394	T39.395	T39.396
Fluindione	T45.511	T45.512	T45.513	T45.514	T45.515	T45.516
Flumequine	T37.8X1	T37.8X2	T37.8X3	T37.8X4	T37.8X5	T37.8X6
Flumethasone	T49.0X1	T49.0X2	T49.0X3	T49.0X4	T49.0X5	T49.0X6
Flumethiazide	T50.2X1	T50.2X2	T50.2X3	T50.2X4	T50.2X5	T50.2X6
Flumidin	T37.5X1	T37.5X2	T37.5X3	T37.5X4	T37.5X5	T37.5X6
Flunarizine	T46.7X1	T46.7X2	T46.7X3	T46.7X4	T46.7X5	T46.7X6
Flunidazole	T37.8X1	T37.8X2	T37.8X3	T37.8X4	T37.8X5	T37.8X6
Flunisolide	T48.6X1	T48.6X2	T48.6X3	T48.6X4	T48.6X5	T48.6X6
Flunitrazepam	T42.4X1	T42.4X2	T42.4X3	T42.4X4	T42.4X5	T42.4X6
Fluocinolone (acetonide)	T49.0X1	T49.0X2	T49.0X3	T49.0X4	T49.0X5	T49.0X6
Fluocinonide	T49.0X1	T49.0X2	T49.0X3	T49.0X4	T49.0X5	T49.0X6
Fluocortin (butyl)	T49.0X1	T49.0X2	T49.0X3	T49.0X4	T49.0X5	T49.0X6
Fluocortolone	T49.0X1	T49.0X2	T49.0X3	T49.0X4	T49.0X5	T49.0X6
Fluohydrocortisone	T38.0X1	T38.0X2	T38.0X3	T38.0X4	T38.0X5	T38.0X6
ENT agent	T49.6X1	T49.6X2	T49.6X3	T49.6X4	T49.6X5	T49.6X6
ophthalmic preparation	T49.5X1	T49.5X2	T49.5X3	T49.5X4	T49.5X5	T49.5X6
topical NEC	T49.0X1	T49.0X2	T49.0X3	T49.0X4	T49.0X5	T49.0X6
Fluonid	T49.0X1	T49.0X2	T49.0X3	T49.0X4	T49.0X5	T49.0X6
Fluopromazine	T43.3X1	T43.3X2	T43.3X3	T43.3X4	T43.3X5	T43.3X6
Fluoracetate	T60.8X1	T60.8X2	T60.8X3	T60.8X4	--	--
Fluorescein	T50.8X1	T50.8X2	T50.8X3	T50.8X4	T50.8X5	T50.8X6
Fluorhydrocortisone	T50.0X1	T50.0X2	T50.0X3	T50.0X4	T50.0X5	T50.0X6
Fluoride (nonmedicinal) (pesticide) (sodium) NEC	T60.8X1	T60.8X2	T60.8X3	T60.8X4	--	--
hydrogen — *see* Hydrofluoric acid						
medicinal NEC	T50.991	T50.992	T50.993	T50.994	T50.995	T50.996
dental use	T49.7X1	T49.7X2	T49.7X3	T49.7X4	T49.7X5	T49.7X6
not pesticide NEC	T54.91	T54.92	T54.93	T54.94	--	--
stannous	T49.7X1	T49.7X2	T49.7X3	T49.7X4	T49.7X5	T49.7X6
Fluorinated corticosteroids	T38.0X1	T38.0X2	T38.0X3	T38.0X4	T38.0X5	T38.0X6
Fluorine (gas)	T59.5X1	T59.5X2	T59.5X3	T59.5X4	--	--
salt — *see* Fluoride(s)						
Fluoristan	T49.7X1	T49.7X2	T49.7X3	T49.7X4	T49.7X5	T49.7X6
Fluormetholone	T49.0X1	T49.0X2	T49.0X3	T49.0X4	T49.0X5	T49.0X6
Fluoroacetate	T60.8X1	T60.8X2	T60.8X3	T60.8X4	--	--
Fluorocarbon monomer	T53.6X1	T53.6X2	T53.6X3	T53.6X4	--	--
Fluorocytosine	T37.8X1	T37.8X2	T37.8X3	T37.8X4	T37.8X5	T37.8X6
Fluorodeoxyuridine	T45.1X1	T45.1X2	T45.1X3	T45.1X4	T45.1X5	T45.1X6
Fluorometholone	T49.0X1	T49.0X2	T49.0X3	T49.0X4	T49.0X5	T49.0X6
ophthalmic preparation	T49.5X1	T49.5X2	T49.5X3	T49.5X4	T49.5X5	T49.5X6
Fluorophosphate insecticide	T60.0X1	T60.0X2	T60.0X3	T60.0X4	--	--
Fluorosol	T46.3X1	T46.3X2	T46.3X3	T46.3X4	T46.3X5	T46.3X6
Fluorouracil	T45.1X1	T45.1X2	T45.1X3	T45.1X4	T45.1X5	T45.1X6
Fluorphenylalanine	T49.5X1	T49.5X2	T49.5X3	T49.5X4	T49.5X5	T49.5X6
Fluothane	T41.0X1	T41.0X2	T41.0X3	T41.0X4	T41.0X5	T41.0X6
Fluoxetine	T43.221	T43.222	T43.223	T43.224	T43.225	T43.226
Fluoxymesterone	T38.7X1	T38.7X2	T38.7X3	T38.7X4	T38.7X5	T38.7X6
Flupenthixol	T43.4X1	T43.4X2	T43.4X3	T43.4X4	T43.4X5	T43.4X6
Flupentixol	T43.4X1	T43.4X2	T43.4X3	T43.4X4	T43.4X5	T43.4X6
Fluphenazine	T43.3X1	T43.3X2	T43.3X3	T43.3X4	T43.3X5	T43.3X6
Fluprednidene	T49.0X1	T49.0X2	T49.0X3	T49.0X4	T49.0X5	T49.0X6
Fluprednisolone	T38.0X1	T38.0X2	T38.0X3	T38.0X4	T38.0X5	T38.0X6
Fluradoline	T39.8X1	T39.8X2	T39.8X3	T39.8X4	T39.8X5	T39.8X6
Flurandrenolide	T49.0X1	T49.0X2	T49.0X3	T49.0X4	T49.0X5	T49.0X6
Flurandrenolone	T49.0X1	T49.0X2	T49.0X3	T49.0X4	T49.0X5	T49.0X6
Flurazepam	T42.4X1	T42.4X2	T42.4X3	T42.4X4	T42.4X5	T42.4X6
Flurbiprofen	T39.311	T39.312	T39.313	T39.314	T39.315	T39.316
Flurobate	T49.0X1	T49.0X2	T49.0X3	T49.0X4	T49.0X5	T49.0X6
Fluroxene	T41.0X1	T41.0X2	T41.0X3	T41.0X4	T41.0X5	T41.0X6
Fluspirilene	T43.591	T43.592	T43.593	T43.594	T43.595	T43.596
Flutamide	T38.6X1	T38.6X2	T38.6X3	T38.6X4	T38.6X5	T38.6X6
Flutazolam	T42.4X1	T42.4X2	T42.4X3	T42.4X4	T42.4X5	T42.4X6
Fluticasone propionate	T38.0X1	T38.0X2	T38.0X3	T38.0X4	T38.0X5	T38.0X6
Flutoprazepam	T42.4X1	T42.4X2	T42.4X3	T42.4X4	T42.4X5	T42.4X6
Flutropium bromide	T48.6X1	T48.6X2	T48.6X3	T48.6X4	T48.6X5	T48.6X6
Fluvoxamine	T43.221	T43.222	T43.223	T43.224	T43.225	T43.226
Folacin	T45.8X1	T45.8X2	T45.8X3	T45.8X4	T45.8X5	T45.8X6
Folic acid	T45.8X1	T45.8X2	T45.8X3	T45.8X4	T45.8X5	T45.8X6
with ferrous salt	T45.2X1	T45.2X2	T45.2X3	T45.2X4	T45.2X5	T45.2X6
antagonist	T45.1X1	T45.1X2	T45.1X3	T45.1X4	T45.1X5	T45.1X6
Folinic acid	T45.8X1	T45.8X2	T45.8X3	T45.8X4	T45.8X5	T45.8X6
Folium stramoniae	T48.6X1	T48.6X2	T48.6X3	T48.6X4	T48.6X5	T48.6X6
Follicle-stimulating hormone, human	T38.811	T38.812	T38.813	T38.814	T38.815	T38.816
Folpet	T60.3X1	T60.3X2	T60.3X3	T60.3X4	--	--
Fominoben	T48.3X1	T48.3X2	T48.3X3	T48.3X4	T48.3X5	T48.3X6

Food, foodstuffs, noxious, nonbacterial, NEC - Gas NEC

Substance	Poisoning, Accidental unintentional	Poisoning, Intentional self-harm	Poisoning, Assault	Poisoning, Undetermined	Adverse effect	Underdosing
Food, foodstuffs, noxious, nonbacterial, NEC	T62.91	T62.92	T62.93	T62.94	--	--
berries	T62.1X1	T62.1X2	T62.1X3	T62.1X4	--	--
fish (*see also* Fish)	T61.91	T61.92	T61.93	T61.94	--	--
mushrooms	T62.0X1	T62.0X2	T62.0X3	T62.0X4	--	--
plants	T62.2X1	T62.2X2	T62.2X3	T62.2X4	--	--
seafood	T61.91	T61.92	T61.93	T61.94	--	--
specified NEC	T61.8X1	T61.8X2	T61.8X3	T61.8X4	--	--
seeds	T62.2X1	T62.2X2	T62.2X3	T62.2X4	--	--
shellfish	T61.781	T61.782	T61.783	T61.784	--	--
specified NEC	T62.8X1	T62.8X2	T62.8X3	T62.8X4	--	--
Fool's parsley	T62.2X1	T62.2X2	T62.2X3	T62.2X4	--	--
Formaldehyde (solution), gas or vapor	T59.2X1	T59.2X2	T59.2X3	T59.2X4	--	--
fungicide	T60.3X1	T60.3X2	T60.3X3	T60.3X4	--	--
Formalin	T59.2X1	T59.2X2	T59.2X3	T59.2X4	--	--
fungicide	T60.3X1	T60.3X2	T60.3X3	T60.3X4	--	--
vapor	T59.2X1	T59.2X2	T59.2X3	T59.2X4	--	--
Formic acid	T54.2X1	T54.2X2	T54.2X3	T54.2X4	--	--
vapor	T59.891	T59.892	T59.893	T59.894	--	--
Foscarnet sodium	T37.5X1	T37.5X2	T37.5X3	T37.5X4	T37.5X5	T37.5X6
Fosfestrol	T38.5X1	T38.5X2	T38.5X3	T38.5X4	T38.5X5	T38.5X6
Fosfomycin	T36.8X1	T36.8X2	T36.8X3	T36.8X4	T36.8X5	T36.8X6
Fosfonet sodium	T37.5X1	T37.5X2	T37.5X3	T37.5X4	T37.5X5	T37.5X6
Fosinopril	T46.4X1	T46.4X2	T46.4X3	T46.4X4	T46.4X5	T46.4X6
sodium	T46.4X1	T46.4X2	T46.4X3	T46.4X4	T46.4X5	T46.4X6
Fowler's solution	T57.0X1	T57.0X2	T57.0X3	T57.0X4	--	--
Foxglove	T62.2X1	T62.2X2	T62.2X3	T62.2X4	--	--
Framycetin	T36.5X1	T36.5X2	T36.5X3	T36.5X4	T36.5X5	T36.5X6
Frangula	T47.2X1	T47.2X2	T47.2X3	T47.2X4	T47.2X5	T47.2X6
extract	T47.2X1	T47.2X2	T47.2X3	T47.2X4	T47.2X5	T47.2X6
Frei antigen	T50.8X1	T50.8X2	T50.8X3	T50.8X4	T50.8X5	T50.8X6
Freon	T53.5X1	T53.5X2	T53.5X3	T53.5X4	--	--
Fructose	T50.3X1	T50.3X2	T50.3X3	T50.3X4	T50.3X5	T50.3X6
Frusemide	T50.1X1	T50.1X2	T50.1X3	T50.1X4	T50.1X5	T50.1X6
FSH	T38.811	T38.812	T38.813	T38.814	T38.815	T38.816
Ftorafur	T45.1X1	T45.1X2	T45.1X3	T45.1X4	T45.1X5	T45.1X6
Fuel						
automobile	T52.0X1	T52.0X2	T52.0X3	T52.0X4	--	--
exhaust gas, not in transit	T58.01	T58.02	T58.03	T58.04	--	--
vapor NEC	T52.0X1	T52.0X2	T52.0X3	T52.0X4	--	--
gas (domestic use) (*see also* Carbon, monoxide, fuel, utility)	T59.891	T59.892	T59.893	T59.894	--	--
utility	T59.891	T59.892	T59.893	T59.894	--	--
in mobile container	T59.891	T59.892	T59.893	T59.894	--	--
incomplete combustion of — *see* Carbon, monoxide, fuel, utility						
piped (natural)	T59.891	T59.892	T59.893	T59.894	--	--
industrial, incomplete combustion	T58.8X1	T58.8X2	T58.8X3	T58.8X4	--	--
Fugillin	T36.8X1	T36.8X2	T36.8X3	T36.8X4	T36.8X5	T36.8X6
Fulminate of mercury	T56.1X1	T56.1X2	T56.1X3	T56.1X4	--	--
Fulvicin	T36.7X1	T36.7X2	T36.7X3	T36.7X4	T36.7X5	T36.7X6
Fumadil	T36.8X1	T36.8X2	T36.8X3	T36.8X4	T36.8X5	T36.8X6
Fumagillin	T36.8X1	T36.8X2	T36.8X3	T36.8X4	T36.8X5	T36.8X6
Fumaric acid	T49.4X1	T49.4X2	T49.4X3	T49.4X4	T49.4X5	T49.4X6
Fumes (from)	T59.91	T59.92	T59.93	T59.94		
carbon monoxide — *see* Carbon, monoxide						
charcoal (domestic use) — *see* Charcoal, fumes						
chloroform — *see* Chloroform						
coke (in domestic stoves, fireplaces) — *see* Coke fumes						
corrosive NEC	T54.91	T54.92	T54.93	T54.94		
ether — *see* ether						
freons	T53.5X1	T53.5X2	T53.5X3	T53.5X4	--	--
hydrocarbons	T59.891	T59.892	T59.893	T59.894	--	--
petroleum (liquefied)	T59.891	T59.892	T59.893	T59.894	--	--
distributed through pipes (pure or mixed with air)	T59.891	T59.892	T59.893	T59.894	--	--
lead — *see* lead						
metal — *see* Metals, or the specified metal						
nitrogen dioxide	T59.0X1	T59.0X2	T59.0X3	T59.0X4	--	--
pesticides — *see* Pesticides						

Substance	Poisoning, Accidental unintentional	Poisoning, Intentional self-harm	Poisoning, Assault	Poisoning, Undetermined	Adverse effect	Underdosing
Fumes — *continued*						
petroleum (liquefied)	T59.891	T59.892	T59.893	T59.894	--	--
distributed through pipes (pure or mixed with air)	T59.891	T59.892	T59.893	T59.894	--	--
polyester	T59.891	T59.892	T59.893	T59.894	--	--
specified source NEC (*see also* substance specified)	T59.891	T59.892	T59.893	T59.894	--	--
sulfur dioxide	T59.1X1	T59.1X2	T59.1X3	T59.1X4	--	--
Fumigant NEC	T60.91	T60.92	T60.93	T60.94	--	--
Fungi, noxious, used as food	T62.0X1	T62.0X2	T62.0X3	T62.0X4	--	--
Fungicide NEC (nonmedicinal)	T60.3X1	T60.3X2	T60.3X3	T60.3X4	--	--
Fungizone	T36.7X1	T36.7X2	T36.7X3	T36.7X4	T36.7X5	T36.7X6
topical	T49.0X1	T49.0X2	T49.0X3	T49.0X4	T49.0X5	T49.0X6
Furacin	T49.0X1	T49.0X2	T49.0X3	T49.0X4	T49.0X5	T49.0X6
Furadantin	T37.91	T37.92	T37.93	T37.94	T37.95	T37.96
Furazolidone	T37.8X1	T37.8X2	T37.8X3	T37.8X4	T37.8X5	T37.8X6
Furazolium chloride	T49.0X1	T49.0X2	T49.0X3	T49.0X4	T49.0X5	T49.0X6
Furfural	T52.8X1	T52.8X2	T52.8X3	T52.8X4	--	--
Furnace (coal burning) (domestic), **gas from**	T58.2X1	T58.2X2	T58.2X3	T58.2X4	--	--
industrial	T58.8X1	T58.8X2	T58.8X3	T58.8X4	--	--
Furniture polish	T65.891	T65.892	T65.893	T65.894	--	--
Furosemide	T50.1X1	T50.1X2	T50.1X3	T50.1X4	T50.1X5	T50.1X6
Furoxone	T37.91	T37.92	T37.93	T37.94	T37.95	T37.96
Fursultiamine	T45.2X1	T45.2X2	T45.2X3	T45.2X4	T45.2X5	T45.2X6
Fusafungine	T36.8X1	T36.8X2	T36.8X3	T36.8X4	T36.8X5	T36.8X6
Fusel oil (any) (amyl) (butyl) (propyl), vapor	T51.3X1	T51.3X2	T51.3X3	T51.3X4	--	--
Fusidate (ethanolamine) (sodium)	T36.8X1	T36.8X2	T36.8X3	T36.8X4	T36.8X5	T36.8X6
Fusidic acid	T36.8X1	T36.8X2	T36.8X3	T36.8X4	T36.8X5	T36.8X6
Fytic acid, nonasodium	T50.6X1	T50.6X2	T50.6X3	T50.6X4	T50.6X5	T50.6X6
G						
GABA	T43.8X1	T43.8X2	T43.8X3	T43.8X4	T43.8X5	T43.8X6
Gadopentetic acid	T50.8X1	T50.8X2	T50.8X3	T50.8X4	T50.8X5	T50.8X6
Galactose	T50.3X1	T50.3X2	T50.3X3	T50.3X4	T50.3X5	T50.3X6
b-Galactosidase	T47.5X1	T47.5X2	T47.5X3	T47.5X4	T47.5X5	T47.5X6
Galantamine	T44.0X1	T44.0X2	T44.0X3	T44.0X4	T44.0X5	T44.0X6
Gallamine (triethiodide)	T48.1X1	T48.1X2	T48.1X3	T48.1X4	T48.1X5	T48.1X6
Gallium citrate	T50.991	T50.992	T50.993	T50.994	T50.995	T50.996
Gallopamil	T46.1X1	T46.1X2	T46.1X3	T46.1X4	T46.1X5	T46.1X6
Gamboge	T47.2X1	T47.2X2	T47.2X3	T47.2X4	T47.2X5	T47.2X6
Gamimune	T50.Z11	T50.Z12	T50.Z13	T50.Z14	T50.Z15	T50.Z16
Gamma globulin	T50.Z11	T50.Z12	T50.Z13	T50.Z14	T50.Z15	T50.Z16
Gamma-aminobutyric acid	T43.8X1	T43.8X2	T43.8X3	T43.8X4	T43.8X5	T43.8X6
Gamma-benzene hexachloride (medicinal)	T49.0X1	T49.0X2	T49.0X3	T49.0X4	T49.0X5	T49.0X6
nonmedicinal, vapor	T53.6X1	T53.6X2	T53.6X3	T53.6X4	--	--
Gamma-BHC (medicinal) (*see also* Gammabenzene hexachloride)	T49.0X1	T49.0X2	T49.0X3	T49.0X4	T49.0X5	T49.0X6
Gamulin	T50.Z11	T50.Z12	T50.Z13	T50.Z14	T50.Z15	T50.Z16
Ganciclovir (sodium)	T37.5X1	T37.5X2	T37.5X3	T37.5X4	T37.5X5	T37.5X6
Ganglionic blocking drug NEC	T44.2X1	T44.2X2	T44.2X3	T44.2X4	T44.2X5	T44.2X6
specified NEC	T44.2X1	T44.2X2	T44.2X3	T44.2X4	T44.2X5	T44.2X6
Ganja	T40.7X1	T40.7X2	T40.7X3	T40.7X4	T40.7X5	T40.7X6
Garamycin	T36.5X1	T36.5X2	T36.5X3	T36.5X4	T36.5X5	T36.5X6
ophthalmic preparation	T49.5X1	T49.5X2	T49.5X3	T49.5X4	T49.5X5	T49.5X6
topical NEC	T49.0X1	T49.0X2	T49.0X3	T49.0X4	T49.0X5	T49.0X6
Gardenal	T42.3X1	T42.3X2	T42.3X3	T42.3X4	T42.3X5	T42.3X6
Gardepanyl	T42.3X1	T42.3X2	T42.3X3	T42.3X4	T42.3X5	T42.3X6
Gas NEC	T59.91	T59.92	T59.93	T59.94	--	--
acetylene	T59.891	T59.892	T59.893	T59.894	--	--
incomplete combustion of	T58.11	T58.12	T58.13	T58.14		
air contaminants, source or type not specified	T59.91	T59.92	T59.93	T59.94	--	--
anesthetic	T41.0X1	T41.0X2	T41.0X3	T41.0X4	T41.0X5	T41.0X6
blast furnace	T58.8X1	T58.8X2	T58.8X3	T58.8X4	--	--
butane — *see* butane						
carbon monoxide — *see* Carbon, monoxide						
chlorine	T59.4X1	T59.4X2	T59.4X3	T59.4X4	--	--
coal	T58.2X1	T58.2X2	T58.2X3	T58.2X4	--	--
cyanide	T57.3X1	T57.3X2	T57.3X3	T57.3X4	--	--
dicyanogen	T65.0X1	T65.0X2	T65.0X3	T65.0X4	--	--
domestic — *see* Domestic gas						

Ipodate, calcium - Lauryl sulfoacetate

Substance	Poisoning, Accidental unintentional	Poisoning, Intentional self-harm	Poisoning, Assault	Poisoning, Undetermined	Adverse effect	Underdosing
Ipodate, calcium	T50.8X1	T50.8X2	T50.8X3	T50.8X4	T50.8X5	T50.8X6
Ipral	T42.3X1	T42.3X2	T42.3X3	T42.3X4	T42.3X5	T42.3X6
Ipratropium (bromide)	T48.6X1	T48.6X2	T48.6X3	T48.6X4	T48.6X5	T48.6X6
Ipriflavone	T46.3X1	T46.3X2	T46.3X3	T46.3X4	T46.3X5	T46.3X6
Iprindole	T43.011	T43.012	T43.013	T43.014	T43.015	T43.016
Iproclozide	T43.1X1	T43.1X2	T43.1X3	T43.1X4	T43.1X5	T43.1X6
Iprofenin	T50.8X1	T50.8X2	T50.8X3	T50.8X4	T50.8X5	T50.8X6
Iproheptine	T49.2X1	T49.2X2	T49.2X3	T49.2X4	T49.2X5	T49.2X6
Iproniazid	T43.1X1	T43.1X2	T43.1X3	T43.1X4	T43.1X5	T43.1X6
Iproplatin	T45.1X1	T45.1X2	T45.1X3	T45.1X4	T45.1X5	T45.1X6
Iproveratril	T46.1X1	T46.1X2	T46.1X3	T46.1X4	T46.1X5	T46.1X6
Iron (compounds) (medicinal) NEC	T45.4X1	T45.4X2	T45.4X3	T45.4X4	T45.4X5	T45.4X6
ammonium	T45.4X1	T45.4X2	T45.4X3	T45.4X4	T45.4X5	T45.4X6
dextran injection	T45.4X1	T45.4X2	T45.4X3	T45.4X4	T45.4X5	T45.4X6
nonmedicinal	T56.891	T56.892	T56.893	T56.894	--	--
salts	T45.4X1	T45.4X2	T45.4X3	T45.4X4	T45.4X5	T45.4X6
sorbitex	T45.4X1	T45.4X2	T45.4X3	T45.4X4	T45.4X5	T45.4X6
sorbitol citric acid complex	T45.4X1	T45.4X2	T45.4X3	T45.4X4	T45.4X5	T45.4X6
Irrigating fluid (vaginal)	T49.8X1	T49.8X2	T49.8X3	T49.8X4	T49.8X5	T49.8X6
eye	T49.5X1	T49.5X2	T49.5X3	T49.5X4	T49.5X5	T49.5X6
Isepamicin	T36.5X1	T36.5X2	T36.5X3	T36.5X4	T36.5X5	T36.5X6
Isoaminile (citrate)	T48.3X1	T48.3X2	T48.3X3	T48.3X4	T48.3X5	T48.3X6
Isoamyl nitrite	T46.3X1	T46.3X2	T46.3X3	T46.3X4	T46.3X5	T46.3X6
Isobenzan	T60.1X1	T60.1X2	T60.1X3	T60.1X4	--	--
Isobutyl acetate	T52.8X1	T52.8X2	T52.8X3	T52.8X4	--	--
Isocarboxazid	T43.1X1	T43.1X2	T43.1X3	T43.1X4	T43.1X5	T43.1X6
Isoconazole	T49.0X1	T49.0X2	T49.0X3	T49.0X4	T49.0X5	T49.0X6
Isocyanate	T65.0X1	T65.0X2	T65.0X3	T65.0X4	--	--
Isoephedrine	T44.991	T44.992	T44.993	T44.994	T44.995	T44.996
Isoetarine	T48.6X1	T48.6X2	T48.6X3	T48.6X4	T48.6X5	T48.6X6
Isoethadione	T42.2X1	T42.2X2	T42.2X3	T42.2X4	T42.2X5	T42.2X6
Isoetharine	T44.5X1	T44.5X2	T44.5X3	T44.5X4	T44.5X5	T44.5X6
Isoflurane	T41.0X1	T41.0X2	T41.0X3	T41.0X4	T41.0X5	T41.0X6
Isoflurophate	T44.0X1	T44.0X2	T44.0X3	T44.0X4	T44.0X5	T44.0X6
Isomaltose, ferric complex	T45.4X1	T45.4X2	T45.4X3	T45.4X4	T45.4X5	T45.4X6
Isometheptene	T44.3X1	T44.3X2	T44.3X3	T44.3X4	T44.3X5	T44.3X6
Isoniazid	T37.1X1	T37.1X2	T37.1X3	T37.1X4	T37.1X5	T37.1X6
with						
rifampicin	T36.6X1	T36.6X2	T36.6X3	T36.6X4	T36.6X5	T36.6X6
thioacetazone	T37.1X1	T37.1X2	T37.1X3	T37.1X4	T37.1X5	T37.1X6
Isonicotinic acid hydrazide	T37.1X1	T37.1X2	T37.1X3	T37.1X4	T37.1X5	T37.1X6
Isonipecaine	T40.4X1	T40.4X2	T40.4X3	T40.4X4	T40.4X5	T40.4X6
Isopentaquine	T37.2X1	T37.2X2	T37.2X3	T37.2X4	T37.2X5	T37.2X6
Isophane insulin	T38.3X1	T38.3X2	T38.3X3	T38.3X4	T38.3X5	T38.3X6
Isophorone	T65.891	T65.892	T65.893	T65.894	--	--
Isophosphamide	T45.1X1	T45.1X2	T45.1X3	T45.1X4	T45.1X5	T45.1X6
Isopregnenone	T38.5X1	T38.5X2	T38.5X3	T38.5X4	T38.5X5	T38.5X6
Isoprenaline	T48.6X1	T48.6X2	T48.6X3	T48.6X4	T48.6X5	T48.6X6
Isopromethazine	T43.3X1	T43.3X2	T43.3X3	T43.3X4	T43.3X5	T43.3X6
Isopropamide	T44.3X1	T44.3X2	T44.3X3	T44.3X4	T44.3X5	T44.3X6
iodide	T44.3X1	T44.3X2	T44.3X3	T44.3X4	T44.3X5	T44.3X6
Isopropanol	T51.2X1	T51.2X2	T51.2X3	T51.2X4	--	--
Isopropyl						
acetate	T52.8X1	T52.8X2	T52.8X3	T52.8X4	--	--
alcohol	T51.2X1	T51.2X2	T51.2X3	T51.2X4	--	--
medicinal	T49.4X1	T49.4X2	T49.4X3	T49.4X4	T49.4X5	T49.4X6
ether	T52.8X1	T52.8X2	T52.8X3	T52.8X4	--	--
Isopropylaminophenazone	T39.2X1	T39.2X2	T39.2X3	T39.2X4	T39.2X5	T39.2X6
Isoproterenol	T48.6X1	T48.6X2	T48.6X3	T48.6X4	T48.6X5	T48.6X6
Isosorbide dinitrate	T46.3X1	T46.3X2	T46.3X3	T46.3X4	T46.3X5	T46.3X6
Isothipendyl	T45.0X1	T45.0X2	T45.0X3	T45.0X4	T45.0X5	T45.0X6
Isotretinoin	T50.991	T50.992	T50.993	T50.994	T50.995	T50.996
Isoxazolyl penicillin	T36.0X1	T36.0X2	T36.0X3	T36.0X4	T36.0X5	T36.0X6
Isoxicam	T39.391	T39.392	T39.393	T39.394	T39.395	T39.396
Isoxsuprine	T46.7X1	T46.7X2	T46.7X3	T46.7X4	T46.7X5	T46.7X6
Ispagula	T47.4X1	T47.4X2	T47.4X3	T47.4X4	T47.4X5	T47.4X6
husk	T47.4X1	T47.4X2	T47.4X3	T47.4X4	T47.4X5	T47.4X6
Isradipine	T46.1X1	T46.1X2	T46.1X3	T46.1X4	T46.1X5	T46.1X6
I-thyroxine sodium	T38.1X1	T38.1X2	T38.1X3	T38.1X4	T38.1X5	T38.1X6
Itraconazole	T37.8X1	T37.8X2	T37.8X3	T37.8X4	T37.8X5	T37.8X6
Itramin tosilate	T46.3X1	T46.3X2	T46.3X3	T46.3X4	T46.3X5	T46.3X6
Ivermectin	T37.4X1	T37.4X2	T37.4X3	T37.4X4	T37.4X5	T37.4X6
Izoniazid	T37.1X1	T37.1X2	T37.1X3	T37.1X4	T37.1X5	T37.1X6
with thioacetazone	T37.1X1	T37.1X2	T37.1X3	T37.1X4	T37.1X5	T37.1X6
J						
Jalap	T47.2X1	T47.2X2	T47.2X3	T47.2X4	T47.2X5	T47.2X6
Jamaica						
dogwood (bark)	T39.8X1	T39.8X2	T39.8X3	T39.8X4	T39.8X5	T39.8X6
ginger	T65.891	T65.892	T65.893	T65.894	--	--
root	T62.2X1	T62.2X2	T62.2X3	T62.2X4	--	--
Jatropha	T62.2X1	T62.2X2	T62.2X3	T62.2X4	--	--
curcas	T62.2X1	T62.2X2	T62.2X3	T62.2X4	--	--
Jectofer	T45.4X1	T45.4X2	T45.4X3	T45.4X4	T45.4X5	T45.4X6

Substance	Poisoning, Accidental unintentional	Poisoning, Intentional self-harm	Poisoning, Assault	Poisoning, Undetermined	Adverse effect	Underdosing
Jellyfish (sting)	T63.621	T63.622	T63.623	T63.624	--	--
Jequirity (bean)	T62.2X1	T62.2X2	T62.2X3	T62.2X4	--	--
Jimson weed (stramonium)	T62.2X1	T62.2X2	T62.2X3	T62.2X4	--	--
seeds	T62.2X1	T62.2X2	T62.2X3	T62.2X4	--	--
Josamycin	T36.3X1	T36.3X2	T36.3X3	T36.3X4	T36.3X5	T36.3X6
Juniper tar	T49.1X1	T49.1X2	T49.1X3	T49.1X4	T49.1X5	T49.1X6
K						
Kallidinogenase	T46.7X1	T46.7X2	T46.7X3	T46.7X4	T46.7X5	T46.7X6
Kallikrein	T46.7X1	T46.7X2	T46.7X3	T46.7X4	T46.7X5	T46.7X6
Kanamycin	T36.5X1	T36.5X2	T36.5X3	T36.5X4	T36.5X5	T36.5X6
Kantrex	T36.5X1	T36.5X2	T36.5X3	T36.5X4	T36.5X5	T36.5X6
Kaolin	T47.6X1	T47.6X2	T47.6X3	T47.6X4	T47.6X5	T47.6X6
light	T47.6X1	T47.6X2	T47.6X3	T47.6X4	T47.6X5	T47.6X6
Karaya (gum)	T47.4X1	T47.4X2	T47.4X3	T47.4X4	T47.4X5	T47.4X6
Kebuzone	T39.2X1	T39.2X2	T39.2X3	T39.2X4	T39.2X5	T39.2X6
Kelevan	T60.1X1	T60.1X2	T60.1X3	T60.1X4	--	--
Kemithal	T41.1X1	T41.1X2	T41.1X3	T41.1X4	T41.1X5	T41.1X6
Kenacort	T38.0X1	T38.0X2	T38.0X3	T38.0X4	T38.0X5	T38.0X6
Keratolytic drug NEC	T49.4X1	T49.4X2	T49.4X3	T49.4X4	T49.4X5	T49.4X6
anthracene	T49.4X1	T49.4X2	T49.4X3	T49.4X4	T49.4X5	T49.4X6
Keratoplastic NEC	T49.4X1	T49.4X2	T49.4X3	T49.4X4	T49.4X5	T49.4X6
Kerosene, kerosine (fuel) (solvent) NEC	T52.0X1	T52.0X2	T52.0X3	T52.0X4	--	--
insecticide	T52.0X1	T52.0X2	T52.0X3	T52.0X4	--	--
vapor	T52.0X1	T52.0X2	T52.0X3	T52.0X4	--	--
Ketamine	T41.291	T41.292	T41.293	T41.294	T41.295	T41.296
Ketazolam	T42.4X1	T42.4X2	T42.4X3	T42.4X4	T42.4X5	T42.4X6
Ketazon	T39.2X1	T39.2X2	T39.2X3	T39.2X4	T39.2X5	T39.2X6
Ketobemidone	T40.4X1	T40.4X2	T40.4X3	T40.4X4	--	--
Ketoconazole	T49.0X1	T49.0X2	T49.0X3	T49.0X4	T49.0X5	T49.0X6
Ketols	T52.4X1	T52.4X2	T52.4X3	T52.4X4	--	--
Ketone oils	T52.4X1	T52.4X2	T52.4X3	T52.4X4	--	--
Ketoprofen	T39.311	T39.312	T39.313	T39.314	T39.315	T39.316
Ketorolac	T39.8X1	T39.8X2	T39.8X3	T39.8X4	T39.8X5	T39.8X6
Ketotifen	T45.0X1	T45.0X2	T45.0X3	T45.0X4	T45.0X5	T45.0X6
Khat	T43.691	T43.692	T43.693	T43.694	--	--
Khellin	T46.3X1	T46.3X2	T46.3X3	T46.3X4	T46.3X5	T46.3X6
Khelloside	T46.3X1	T46.3X2	T46.3X3	T46.3X4	T46.3X5	T46.3X6
Kiln gas or vapor (carbon monoxide)	T58.8X1	T58.8X2	T58.8X3	T58.8X4	--	--
Kitasamycin	T36.3X1	T36.3X2	T36.3X3	T36.3X4	T36.3X5	T36.3X6
Konsyl	T47.4X1	T47.4X2	T47.4X3	T47.4X4	T47.4X5	T47.4X6
Kosam seed	T62.2X1	T62.2X2	T62.2X3	T62.2X4	--	--
Krait (venom)	T63.091	T63.092	T63.093	T63.094	--	--
Kwell (insecticide)	T60.1X1	T60.1X2	T60.1X3	T60.1X4	--	--
anti-infective (topical)	T49.0X1	T49.0X2	T49.0X3	T49.0X4	T49.0X5	T49.0X6
L						
Labetalol	T44.8X1	T44.8X2	T44.8X3	T44.8X4	T44.8X5	T44.8X6
Laburnum (seeds)	T62.2X1	T62.2X2	T62.2X3	T62.2X4	--	--
leaves	T62.2X1	T62.2X2	T62.2X3	T62.2X4	--	--
Lachesine	T49.5X1	T49.5X2	T49.5X3	T49.5X4	T49.5X5	T49.5X6
Lacidipine	T46.5X1	T46.5X2	T46.5X3	T46.5X4	T46.5X5	T46.5X6
Lacquer	T65.6X1	T65.6X2	T65.6X3	T65.6X4	--	--
Lacrimogenic gas	T59.3X1	T59.3X2	T59.3X3	T59.3X4	--	--
Lactated potassic saline	T50.3X1	T50.3X2	T50.3X3	T50.3X4	T50.3X5	T50.3X6
Lactic acid	T49.8X1	T49.8X2	T49.8X3	T49.8X4	T49.8X5	T49.8X6
Lactobacillus						
acidophilus	T47.6X1	T47.6X2	T47.6X3	T47.6X4	T47.6X5	T47.6X6
compound	T47.6X1	T47.6X2	T47.6X3	T47.6X4	T47.6X5	T47.6X6
bifidus, lyophilized	T47.6X1	T47.6X2	T47.6X3	T47.6X4	T47.6X5	T47.6X6
bulgaricus	T47.6X1	T47.6X2	T47.6X3	T47.6X4	T47.6X5	T47.6X6
sporogenes	T47.6X1	T47.6X2	T47.6X3	T47.6X4	T47.6X5	T47.6X6
Lactoflavin	T45.2X1	T45.2X2	T45.2X3	T45.2X4	T45.2X5	T45.2X6
Lactose (as excipient)	T50.901	T50.902	T50.903	T50.904	T50.905	T50.906
Lactuca (virosa) (extract)	T42.6X1	T42.6X2	T42.6X3	T42.6X4	T42.6X5	T42.6X6
Lactucarium	T42.6X1	T42.6X2	T42.6X3	T42.6X4	T42.6X5	T42.6X6
Lactulose	T47.3X1	T47.3X2	T47.3X3	T47.3X4	T47.3X5	T47.3X6
Laevo — see Levo-						
Lanatosides	T46.0X1	T46.0X2	T46.0X3	T46.0X4	T46.0X5	T46.0X6
Lanolin	T49.3X1	T49.3X2	T49.3X3	T49.3X4	T49.3X5	T49.3X6
Largactil	T43.3X1	T43.3X2	T43.3X3	T43.3X4	T43.3X5	T43.3X6
Larkspur	T62.2X1	T62.2X2	T62.2X3	T62.2X4	--	--
Laroxyl	T43.011	T43.012	T43.013	T43.014	T43.015	T43.016
Lasix	T50.1X1	T50.1X2	T50.1X3	T50.1X4	T50.1X5	T50.1X6
Lassar's paste	T49.4X1	T49.4X2	T49.4X3	T49.4X4	T49.4X5	T49.4X6
Latamoxef	T36.1X1	T36.1X2	T36.1X3	T36.1X4	T36.1X5	T36.1X6
Latex	T65.811	T65.812	T65.813	T65.814	--	--
Lathyrus (seed)	T62.2X1	T62.2X2	T62.2X3	T62.2X4	--	--
Laudanum	T40.0X1	T40.0X2	T40.0X3	T40.0X4	T40.0X5	T40.0X6
Laudexium	T48.1X1	T48.1X2	T48.1X3	T48.1X4	T48.1X5	T48.1X6
Laughing gas	T41.0X1	T41.0X2	T41.0X3	T41.0X4	T41.0X5	T41.0X6
Laurel, black or cherry	T62.2X1	T62.2X2	T62.2X3	T62.2X4	--	--
Laurolinium	T49.0X1	T49.0X2	T49.0X3	T49.0X4	T49.0X5	T49.0X6
Lauryl sulfoacetate	T49.2X1	T49.2X2	T49.2X3	T49.2X4	T49.2X5	T49.2X6

Substance	Poisoning, Accidental unintentional	Poisoning, Intentional self-harm	Poisoning, Assault	Poisoning, Undetermined	Adverse effect	Underdosing
Laxative NEC	T47.4X1	T47.4X2	T47.4X3	T47.4X4	T47.4X5	T47.4X6
osmotic	T47.3X1	T47.3X2	T47.3X3	T47.3X4	T47.3X5	T47.3X6
saline	T47.3X1	T47.3X2	T47.3X3	T47.3X4	T47.3X5	T47.3X6
stimulant	T47.2X1	T47.2X2	T47.2X3	T47.2X4	T47.2X5	T47.2X6
L-dopa	T42.8X1	T42.8X2	T42.8X3	T42.8X4	T42.8X5	T42.8X6
Lead (dust) (fumes) (vapor) NEC	T56.0X1	T56.0X2	T56.0X3	T56.0X4	--	--
acetate	T49.2X1	T49.2X2	T49.2X3	T49.2X4	T49.2X5	T49.2X6
alkyl (fuel additive)	T56.0X1	T56.0X2	T56.0X3	T56.0X4	--	--
anti-infectives	T37.8X1	T37.8X2	T37.8X3	T37.8X4	T37.8X5	T37.8X6
antiknock compound (tetraethyl)	T56.0X1	T56.0X2	T56.0X3	T56.0X4	--	--
arsenate, arsenite (dust) (herbicide) (insecticide) (vapor)	T57.0X1	T57.0X2	T57.0X3	T57.0X4	--	--
carbonate	T56.0X1	T56.0X2	T56.0X3	T56.0X4	--	--
paint	T56.0X1	T56.0X2	T56.0X3	T56.0X4	--	--
chromate	T56.0X1	T56.0X2	T56.0X3	T56.0X4	--	--
paint	T56.0X1	T56.0X2	T56.0X3	T56.0X4	--	--
dioxide	T56.0X1	T56.0X2	T56.0X3	T56.0X4	--	--
inorganic	T56.0X1	T56.0X2	T56.0X3	T56.0X4	--	--
iodide	T56.0X1	T56.0X2	T56.0X3	T56.0X4	--	--
pigment (paint)	T56.0X1	T56.0X2	T56.0X3	T56.0X4	--	--
monoxide (dust)	T56.0X1	T56.0X2	T56.0X3	T56.0X4	--	--
paint	T56.0X1	T56.0X2	T56.0X3	T56.0X4	--	--
organic	T56.0X1	T56.0X2	T56.0X3	T56.0X4	--	--
oxide	T56.0X1	T56.0X2	T56.0X3	T56.0X4	--	--
paint	T56.0X1	T56.0X2	T56.0X3	T56.0X4	--	--
paint	T56.0X1	T56.0X2	T56.0X3	T56.0X4	--	--
salts	T56.0X1	T56.0X2	T56.0X3	T56.0X4	--	--
specified compound NEC	T56.0X1	T56.0X2	T56.0X3	T56.0X4	--	--
tetra-ethyl	T56.0X1	T56.0X2	T56.0X3	T56.0X4	--	--
Lebanese red	T40.7X1	T40.7X2	T40.7X3	T40.7X4	T40.7X5	T40.7X6
Lefetamine	T39.8X1	T39.8X2	T39.8X3	T39.8X4	T39.8X5	T39.8X6
Lenperone	T43.4X1	T43.4X2	T43.4X3	T43.4X4	T43.4X5	T43.4X6
Lente lietin (insulin)	T38.3X1	T38.3X2	T38.3X3	T38.3X4	T38.3X5	T38.3X6
Leptazol	T50.7X1	T50.7X2	T50.7X3	T50.7X4	T50.7X5	T50.7X6
Leptophos	T60.0X1	T60.0X2	T60.0X3	T60.0X4	--	--
Leritine	T40.2X1	T40.2X2	T40.2X3	T40.2X4	T40.2X5	T40.2X6
Letosteine	T48.4X1	T48.4X2	T48.4X3	T48.4X4	T48.4X5	T48.4X6
Letter	T38.1X1	T38.1X2	T38.1X3	T38.1X4	T38.1X5	T38.1X6
Lettuce opium	T42.6X1	T42.6X2	T42.6X3	T42.6X4	T42.6X5	T42.6X6
Leucinocaine	T41.3X1	T41.3X2	T41.3X3	T41.3X4	T41.3X5	T41.3X6
Leucocianidol	T46.991	T46.992	T46.993	T46.994	T46.995	T46.996
Leucovorin (factor)	T45.8X1	T45.8X2	T45.8X3	T45.8X4	T45.8X5	T45.8X6
Leukeran	T45.1X1	T45.1X2	T45.1X3	T45.1X4	T45.1X5	T45.1X6
Leuprolide	T38.891	T38.892	T38.893	T38.894	T38.895	T38.896
Levalbuterol	T48.6X1	T48.6X2	T48.6X3	T48.6X4	T48.6X5	T48.6X6
Levallorphan	T50.7X1	T50.7X2	T50.7X3	T50.7X4	T50.7X5	T50.7X6
Levamisole	T37.4X1	T37.4X2	T37.4X3	T37.4X4	T37.4X5	T37.4X6
Levanil	T42.6X1	T42.6X2	T42.6X3	T42.6X4	T42.6X5	T42.6X6
Levarterenol	T44.4X1	T44.4X2	T44.4X3	T44.4X4	T44.4X5	T44.4X6
Levdropropizine	T48.3X1	T48.3X2	T48.3X3	T48.3X4	T48.3X5	T48.3X6
Levobunolol	T49.5X1	T49.5X2	T49.5X3	T49.5X4	T49.5X5	T49.5X6
Levocabastine (hydrochloride)	T45.0X1	T45.0X2	T45.0X3	T45.0X4	T45.0X5	T45.0X6
Levocarnitine	T50.991	T50.992	T50.993	T50.994	T50.995	T50.996
Levodopa	T42.8X1	T42.8X2	T42.8X3	T42.8X4	T42.8X5	T42.8X6
with carbidopa	T42.8X1	T42.8X2	T42.8X3	T42.8X4	T42.8X5	T42.8X6
Levo-dromoran	T40.2X1	T40.2X2	T40.2X3	T40.2X4	T40.2X5	T40.2X6
Levoglutamide	T50.991	T50.992	T50.993	T50.994	T50.995	T50.996
Levoid	T38.1X1	T38.1X2	T38.1X3	T38.1X4	T38.1X5	T38.1X6
Levo-iso-methadone	T40.3X1	T40.3X2	T40.3X3	T40.3X4	T40.3X5	T40.3X6
Levomepromazine	T43.3X1	T43.3X2	T43.3X3	T43.3X4	T43.3X5	T43.3X6
Levonordefrin	T49.6X1	T49.6X2	T49.6X3	T49.6X4	T49.6X5	T49.6X6
Levonorgestrel	T38.4X1	T38.4X2	T38.4X3	T38.4X4	T38.4X5	T38.4X6
with ethinylestradiol	T38.5X1	T38.5X2	T38.5X3	T38.5X4	T38.5X5	T38.5X6
Levopromazine	T43.3X1	T43.3X2	T43.3X3	T43.3X4	T43.3X5	T43.3X6
Levoprome	T42.6X1	T42.6X2	T42.6X3	T42.6X4	T42.6X5	T42.6X6
Levopropoxyphene	T40.4X1	T40.4X2	T40.4X3	T40.4X4	T40.4X5	T40.4X6
Levopropylhexedrine	T50.5X1	T50.5X2	T50.5X3	T50.5X4	T50.5X5	T50.5X6
Levoproxyphylline	T48.6X1	T48.6X2	T48.6X3	T48.6X4	T48.6X5	T48.6X6
Levorphanol	T40.4X1	T40.4X2	T40.4X3	T40.4X4	T40.4X5	T40.4X6
Levothyroxine	T38.1X1	T38.1X2	T38.1X3	T38.1X4	T38.1X5	T38.1X6
sodium	T38.1X1	T38.1X2	T38.1X3	T38.1X4	T38.1X5	T38.1X6
Levsin	T44.3X1	T44.3X2	T44.3X3	T44.3X4	T44.3X5	T44.3X6
Levulose	T50.3X1	T50.3X2	T50.3X3	T50.3X4	T50.3X5	T50.3X6
Lewisite (gas), **not in war**	T57.0X1	T57.0X2	T57.0X3	T57.0X4	--	--
Librium	T42.4X1	T42.4X2	T42.4X3	T42.4X4	T42.4X5	T42.4X6
Lidex	T49.0X1	T49.0X2	T49.0X3	T49.0X4	T49.0X5	T49.0X6
Lidocaine	T41.3X1	T41.3X2	T41.3X3	T41.3X4	T41.3X5	T41.3X6
regional	T41.3X1	T41.3X2	T41.3X3	T41.3X4	T41.3X5	T41.3X6
spinal	T41.3X1	T41.3X2	T41.3X3	T41.3X4	T41.3X5	T41.3X6
Lidofenin	T50.8X1	T50.8X2	T50.8X3	T50.8X4	T50.8X5	T50.8X6
Lidoflazine	T46.1X1	T46.1X2	T46.1X3	T46.1X4	T46.1X5	T46.1X6
Lighter fluid	T52.0X1	T52.0X2	T52.0X3	T52.0X4	--	--
Lignin hemicellulose	T47.6X1	T47.6X2	T47.6X3	T47.6X4	T47.6X5	T47.6X6
Lignocaine	T41.3X1	T41.3X2	T41.3X3	T41.3X4	T41.3X5	T41.3X6
regional	T41.3X1	T41.3X2	T41.3X3	T41.3X4	T41.3X5	T41.3X6
spinal	T41.3X1	T41.3X2	T41.3X3	T41.3X4	T41.3X5	T41.3X6
Ligroin (e) (solvent)	T52.0X1	T52.0X2	T52.0X3	T52.0X4	--	--
vapor	T59.891	T59.892	T59.893	T59.894	--	--
Ligustrum vulgare	T62.2X1	T62.2X2	T62.2X3	T62.2X4	--	--
Lily of the valley	T62.2X1	T62.2X2	T62.2X3	T62.2X4	--	--
Lime (chloride)	T54.3X1	T54.3X2	T54.3X3	T54.3X4	--	--
Limonene	T52.8X1	T52.8X2	T52.8X3	T52.8X4	--	--
Lincomycin	T36.8X1	T36.8X2	T36.8X3	T36.8X4	T36.8X5	T36.8X6
Lindane (insecticide) (nonmedicinal) (vapor)	T53.6X1	T53.6X2	T53.6X3	T53.6X4	--	--
medicinal	T49.0X1	T49.0X2	T49.0X3	T49.0X4	T49.0X5	T49.0X6
Liniments NEC	T49.91	T49.92	T49.93	T49.94	T49.95	T49.96
Linoleic acid	T46.6X1	T46.6X2	T46.6X3	T46.6X4	T46.6X5	T46.6X6
Linolenic acid	T46.6X1	T46.6X2	T46.6X3	T46.6X4	T46.6X5	T46.6X6
Linseed	T47.4X1	T47.4X2	T47.4X3	T47.4X4	T47.4X5	T47.4X6
Liothyronine	T38.1X1	T38.1X2	T38.1X3	T38.1X4	T38.1X5	T38.1X6
Liotrix	T38.1X1	T38.1X2	T38.1X3	T38.1X4	T38.1X5	T38.1X6
Lipancreatin	T47.5X1	T47.5X2	T47.5X3	T47.5X4	T47.5X5	T47.5X6
Lipo-alprostadil	T46.7X1	T46.7X2	T46.7X3	T46.7X4	T46.7X5	T46.7X6
Lipo-Lutin	T38.5X1	T38.5X2	T38.5X3	T38.5X4	T38.5X5	T38.5X6
Lipotropic drug NEC	T50.901	T50.902	T50.903	T50.904	T50.905	T50.906
Liquefied petroleum gases	T59.891	T59.892	T59.893	T59.894	--	--
piped (pure or mixed with air)	T59.891	T59.892	T59.893	T59.894	--	--
Liquid						
paraffin	T47.4X1	T47.4X2	T47.4X3	T47.4X4	T47.4X5	T47.4X6
petrolatum	T47.4X1	T47.4X2	T47.4X3	T47.4X4	T47.4X5	T47.4X6
topical	T49.3X1	T49.3X2	T49.3X3	T49.3X4	T49.3X5	T49.3X6
specified NEC	T65.891	T65.892	T65.893	T65.894	--	--
substance	T65.91	T65.92	T65.93	T65.94	--	--
Liquor creosolis compositus	T65.891	T65.892	T65.893	T65.894	--	--
Liquorice	T48.4X1	T48.4X2	T48.4X3	T48.4X4	T48.4X5	T48.4X6
extract	T47.8X1	T47.8X2	T47.8X3	T47.8X4	T47.8X5	T47.8X6
Lisinopril	T46.4X1	T46.4X2	T46.4X3	T46.4X4	T46.4X5	T46.4X6
Lisuride	T42.8X1	T42.8X2	T42.8X3	T42.8X4	T42.8X5	T42.8X6
Lithane	T43.8X1	T43.8X2	T43.8X3	T43.8X4	T43.8X5	T43.8X6
Lithium	T56.891	T56.892	T56.893	T56.894	--	--
gluconate	T43.591	T43.592	T43.593	T43.594	T43.595	T43.596
salts (carbonate)	T43.591	T43.592	T43.593	T43.594	T43.595	T43.596
Lithonate	T43.8X1	T43.8X2	T43.8X3	T43.8X4	T43.8X5	T43.8X6
Liver						
extract	T45.8X1	T45.8X2	T45.8X3	T45.8X4	T45.8X5	T45.8X6
for parenteral use	T45.8X1	T45.8X2	T45.8X3	T45.8X4	T45.8X5	T45.8X6
fraction 1	T45.8X1	T45.8X2	T45.8X3	T45.8X4	T45.8X5	T45.8X6
hydrolysate	T45.8X1	T45.8X2	T45.8X3	T45.8X4	T45.8X5	T45.8X6
Lizard (bite) (venom)	T63.121	T63.122	T63.123	T63.124	--	--
LMD	T45.8X1	T45.8X2	T45.8X3	T45.8X4	T45.8X5	T45.8X6
Lobelia	T62.2X1	T62.2X2	T62.2X3	T62.2X4	--	--
Lobeline	T50.7X1	T50.7X2	T50.7X3	T50.7X4	T50.7X5	T50.7X6
Local action drug NEC	T49.8X1	T49.8X2	T49.8X3	T49.8X4	T49.8X5	T49.8X6
Locorten	T49.0X1	T49.0X2	T49.0X3	T49.0X4	T49.0X5	T49.0X6
Lofepramine	T43.011	T43.012	T43.013	T43.014	T43.015	T43.016
Lolium temulentum	T62.2X1	T62.2X2	T62.2X3	T62.2X4	--	--
Lomotil	T47.6X1	T47.6X2	T47.6X3	T47.6X4	T47.6X5	T47.6X6
Lomustine	T45.1X1	T45.1X2	T45.1X3	T45.1X4	T45.1X5	T45.1X6
Lonidamine	T45.1X1	T45.1X2	T45.1X3	T45.1X4	T45.1X5	T45.1X6
Loperamide	T47.6X1	T47.6X2	T47.6X3	T47.6X4	T47.6X5	T47.6X6
Loprazolam	T42.4X1	T42.4X2	T42.4X3	T42.4X4	T42.4X5	T42.4X6
Lorajmine	T46.2X1	T46.2X2	T46.2X3	T46.2X4	T46.2X5	T46.2X6
Loratidine	T45.0X1	T45.0X2	T45.0X3	T45.0X4	T45.0X5	T45.0X6
Lorazepam	T42.4X1	T42.4X2	T42.4X3	T42.4X4	T42.4X5	T42.4X6
Lorcainide	T46.2X1	T46.2X2	T46.2X3	T46.2X4	T46.2X5	T46.2X6
Lormetazepam	T42.4X1	T42.4X2	T42.4X3	T42.4X4	T42.4X5	T42.4X6
Lotions NEC	T49.91	T49.92	T49.93	T49.94	T49.95	T49.96
Lotusate	T42.3X1	T42.3X2	T42.3X3	T42.3X4	T42.3X5	T42.3X6
Lovastatin	T46.6X1	T46.6X2	T46.6X3	T46.6X4	T46.6X5	T46.6X6
Lowila	T49.2X1	T49.2X2	T49.2X3	T49.2X4	T49.2X5	T49.2X6
Loxapine	T43.591	T43.592	T43.593	T43.594	T43.595	T43.596
Lozenges (throat)	T49.6X1	T49.6X2	T49.6X3	T49.6X4	T49.6X5	T49.6X6
LSD	T40.8X1	T40.8X2	T40.8X3	T40.8X4	--	--
L-Tryptophan — *see* amino acid						
Lubricant, eye	T49.5X1	T49.5X2	T49.5X3	T49.5X4	T49.5X5	T49.5X6
Lubricating oil NEC	T52.0X1	T52.0X2	T52.0X3	T52.0X4	--	--
Lucanthone	T37.4X1	T37.4X2	T37.4X3	T37.4X4	T37.4X5	T37.4X6
Luminal	T42.3X1	T42.3X2	T42.3X3	T42.3X4	T42.3X5	T42.3X6
Lung irritant (gas) NEC	T59.91	T59.92	T59.93	T59.94	--	--
Luteinizing hormone	T38.811	T38.812	T38.813	T38.814	T38.815	T38.816
Lutocylol	T38.5X1	T38.5X2	T38.5X3	T38.5X4	T38.5X5	T38.5X6

Substance	Poisoning, Accidental unintentional	Poisoning, Intentional self-harm	Poisoning, Assault	Poisoning, Undetermined	Adverse effect	Underdosing
Lutromone	T38.5X1	T38.5X2	T38.5X3	T38.5X4	T38.5X5	T38.5X6
Lututrin	T48.291	T48.292	T48.293	T48.294	T48.295	T48.296
Lye (concentrated)	T54.3X1	T54.3X2	T54.3X3	T54.3X4	--	--
Lygranum (skin test)	T50.8X1	T50.8X2	T50.8X3	T50.8X4	T50.8X5	T50.8X6
Lymecycline	T36.4X1	T36.4X2	T36.4X3	T36.4X4	T36.4X5	T36.4X6
Lymphogranuloma venereum antigen	T50.8X1	T50.8X2	T50.8X3	T50.8X4	T50.8X5	T50.8X6
Lynestrenol	T38.4X1	T38.4X2	T38.4X3	T38.4X4	T38.4X5	T38.4X6
Lyovac Sodium Edecrin	T50.1X1	T50.1X2	T50.1X3	T50.1X4	T50.1X5	T50.1X6
Lypressin	T38.891	T38.892	T38.893	T38.894	T38.895	T38.896
Lysergic acid diethylamide	T40.8X1	T40.8X2	T40.8X3	T40.8X4	--	--
Lysergide	T40.8X1	T40.8X2	T40.8X3	T40.8X4	--	--
Lysine vasopressin	T38.891	T38.892	T38.893	T38.894	T38.895	T38.896
Lysol	T54.1X1	T54.1X2	T54.1X3	T54.1X4	--	--
Lysozyme	T49.0X1	T49.0X2	T49.0X3	T49.0X4	T49.0X5	T49.0X6
Lytta (vitatta)	T49.8X1	T49.8X2	T49.8X3	T49.8X4	T49.8X5	T49.8X6
M						
Mace	T59.3X1	T59.3X2	T59.3X3	T59.3X4	--	--
Macrogol	T50.991	T50.992	T50.993	T50.994	T50.995	T50.996
Macrolide						
anabolic drug	T38.7X1	T38.7X2	T38.7X3	T38.7X4	T38.7X5	T38.7X6
antibiotic	T36.3X1	T36.3X2	T36.3X3	T36.3X4	T36.3X5	T36.3X6
Mafenide	T49.0X1	T49.0X2	T49.0X3	T49.0X4	T49.0X5	T49.0X6
Magaldrate	T47.1X1	T47.1X2	T47.1X3	T47.1X4	T47.1X5	T47.1X6
Magic mushroom	T40.991	T40.992	T40.993	T40.994	--	--
Magnamycin	T36.8X1	T36.8X2	T36.8X3	T36.8X4	T36.8X5	T36.8X6
Magnesia magma	T47.1X1	T47.1X2	T47.1X3	T47.1X4	T47.1X5	T47.1X6
Magnesium NEC	T56.891	T56.892	T56.893	T56.894	--	--
carbonate	T47.1X1	T47.1X2	T47.1X3	T47.1X4	T47.1X5	T47.1X6
citrate	T47.4X1	T47.4X2	T47.4X3	T47.4X4	T47.4X5	T47.4X6
hydroxide	T47.1X1	T47.1X2	T47.1X3	T47.1X4	T47.1X5	T47.1X6
oxide	T47.1X1	T47.1X2	T47.1X3	T47.1X4	T47.1X5	T47.1X6
peroxide	T49.0X1	T49.0X2	T49.0X3	T49.0X4	T49.0X5	T49.0X6
salicylate	T39.091	T39.092	T39.093	T39.094	T39.095	T39.096
silicofluoride	T50.3X1	T50.3X2	T50.3X3	T50.3X4	T50.3X5	T50.3X6
sulfate	T47.4X1	T47.4X2	T47.4X3	T47.4X4	T47.4X5	T47.4X6
thiosulfate	T45.0X1	T45.0X2	T45.0X3	T45.0X4	T45.0X5	T45.0X6
trisilicate	T47.1X1	T47.1X2	T47.1X3	T47.1X4	T47.1X5	T47.1X6
Malathion (medicinal)	T49.0X1	T49.0X2	T49.0X3	T49.0X4	T49.0X5	T49.0X6
insecticide	T60.0X1	T60.0X2	T60.0X3	T60.0X4	--	--
Male fern extract	T37.4X1	T37.4X2	T37.4X3	T37.4X4	T37.4X5	T37.4X6
M-AMSA	T45.1X1	T45.1X2	T45.1X3	T45.1X4	T45.1X5	T45.1X6
Mandelic acid	T37.8X1	T37.8X2	T37.8X3	T37.8X4	T37.8X5	T37.8X6
Manganese (dioxide) (salts)	T57.2X1	T57.2X2	T57.2X3	T57.2X4	--	--
medicinal	T50.991	T50.992	T50.993	T50.994	T50.995	T50.996
Mannitol	T47.3X1	T47.3X2	T47.3X3	T47.3X4	T47.3X5	T47.3X6
hexanitrate	T46.3X1	T46.3X2	T46.3X3	T46.3X4	T46.3X5	T46.3X6
Mannomustine	T45.1X1	T45.1X2	T45.1X3	T45.1X4	T45.1X5	T45.1X6
MAO inhibitors	T43.1X1	T43.1X2	T43.1X3	T43.1X4	T43.1X5	T43.1X6
Mapharsen	T37.8X1	T37.8X2	T37.8X3	T37.8X4	T37.8X5	T37.8X6
Maphenide	T49.0X1	T49.0X2	T49.0X3	T49.0X4	T49.0X5	T49.0X6
Maprotiline	T43.021	T43.022	T43.023	T43.024	T43.025	T43.026
Marcaine	T41.3X1	T41.3X2	T41.3X3	T41.3X4	T41.3X5	T41.3X6
infiltration (subcutaneous)	T41.3X1	T41.3X2	T41.3X3	T41.3X4	T41.3X5	T41.3X6
nerve block (peripheral) (plexus)	T41.3X1	T41.3X2	T41.3X3	T41.3X4	T41.3X5	T41.3X6
Marezine	T45.0X1	T45.0X2	T45.0X3	T45.0X4	T45.0X5	T45.0X6
Marihuana	T40.7X1	T40.7X2	T40.7X3	T40.7X4	T40.7X5	T40.7X6
Marijuana	T40.7X1	T40.7X2	T40.7X3	T40.7X4	T40.7X5	T40.7X6
Marine (sting)	T63.691	T63.692	T63.693	T63.694	--	--
animals (sting)	T63.691	T63.692	T63.693	T63.694	--	--
plants (sting)	T63.711	T63.712	T63.713	T63.714	--	--
Marplan	T43.1X1	T43.1X2	T43.1X3	T43.1X4	T43.1X5	T43.1X6
Marsh gas	T59.891	T59.892	T59.893	T59.894	--	--
Marsilid	T43.1X1	T43.1X2	T43.1X3	T43.1X4	T43.1X5	T43.1X6
Matulane	T45.1X1	T45.1X2	T45.1X3	T45.1X4	T45.1X5	T45.1X6
Mazindol	T50.5X1	T50.5X2	T50.5X3	T50.5X4	T50.5X5	T50.5X6
MCPA	T60.3X1	T60.3X2	T60.3X3	T60.3X4	--	--
MDMA	T43.621	T43.622	T43.623	T43.624	T43.625	T43.626
Meadow saffron	T62.2X1	T62.2X2	T62.2X3	T62.2X4	--	--
Measles virus vaccine (attenuated)	T50.B91	T50.B92	T50.B93	T50.B94	T50.B95	T50.B96
Meat, noxious	T62.8X1	T62.8X2	T62.8X3	T62.8X4	--	--
Meballymal	T42.3X1	T42.3X2	T42.3X3	T42.3X4	T42.3X5	T42.3X6
Mebanazine	T43.1X1	T43.1X2	T43.1X3	T43.1X4	T43.1X5	T43.1X6
Mebaral	T42.3X1	T42.3X2	T42.3X3	T42.3X4	T42.3X5	T42.3X6
Mebendazole	T37.4X1	T37.4X2	T37.4X3	T37.4X4	T37.4X5	T37.4X6
Mebeverine	T44.3X1	T44.3X2	T44.3X3	T44.3X4	T44.3X5	T44.3X6
Mebhydrolin	T45.0X1	T45.0X2	T45.0X3	T45.0X4	T45.0X5	T45.0X6
Mebumal	T42.3X1	T42.3X2	T42.3X3	T42.3X4	T42.3X5	T42.3X6
Mebutamate	T43.591	T43.592	T43.593	T43.594	T43.595	T43.596
Mecamylamine	T44.2X1	T44.2X2	T44.2X3	T44.2X4	T44.2X5	T44.2X6
Mechlorethamine	T45.1X1	T45.1X2	T45.1X3	T45.1X4	T45.1X5	T45.1X6
Mecillinam	T36.0X1	T36.0X2	T36.0X3	T36.0X4	T36.0X5	T36.0X6
Meclizine (hydrochloride)	T45.0X1	T45.0X2	T45.0X3	T45.0X4	T45.0X5	T45.0X6
Meclocycline	T36.4X1	T36.4X2	T36.4X3	T36.4X4	T36.4X5	T36.4X6
Meclofenamate	T39.391	T39.392	T39.393	T39.394	T39.395	T39.396
Meclofenamic acid	T39.391	T39.392	T39.393	T39.394	T39.395	T39.396
Meclofenoxate	T43.691	T43.692	T43.693	T43.694	T43.695	T43.696
Meclozine	T45.0X1	T45.0X2	T45.0X3	T45.0X4	T45.0X5	T45.0X6
Mecobalamin	T45.8X1	T45.8X2	T45.8X3	T45.8X4	T45.8X5	T45.8X6
Mecoprop	T60.3X1	T60.3X2	T60.3X3	T60.3X4	--	--
Mecrilate	T49.3X1	T49.3X2	T49.3X3	T49.3X4	T49.3X5	T49.3X6
Mecysteine	T48.4X1	T48.4X2	T48.4X3	T48.4X4	T48.4X5	T48.4X6
Medazepam	T42.4X1	T42.4X2	T42.4X3	T42.4X4	T42.4X5	T42.4X6
Medicament NEC	T50.901	T50.902	T50.903	T50.904	T50.905	T50.906
Medinal	T42.3X1	T42.3X2	T42.3X3	T42.3X4	T42.3X5	T42.3X6
Medomin	T42.3X1	T42.3X2	T42.3X3	T42.3X4	T42.3X5	T42.3X6
Medrogestone	T38.5X1	T38.5X2	T38.5X3	T38.5X4	T38.5X5	T38.5X6
Medroxalol	T44.8X1	T44.8X2	T44.8X3	T44.8X4	T44.8X5	T44.8X6
Medroxyprogesterone acetate (depot)	T38.5X1	T38.5X2	T38.5X3	T38.5X4	T38.5X5	T38.5X6
Medrysone	T49.0X1	T49.0X2	T49.0X3	T49.0X4	T49.0X5	T49.0X6
Mefenamic acid	T39.391	T39.392	T39.393	T39.394	T39.395	T39.396
Mefenorex	T50.5X1	T50.5X2	T50.5X3	T50.5X4	T50.5X5	T50.5X6
Mefloquine	T37.2X1	T37.2X2	T37.2X3	T37.2X4	T37.2X5	T37.2X6
Mefruside	T50.2X1	T50.2X2	T50.2X3	T50.2X4	T50.2X5	T50.2X6
Megahallucinogen	T40.901	T40.902	T40.903	T40.904	T40.905	T40.906
Megestrol	T38.5X1	T38.5X2	T38.5X3	T38.5X4	T38.5X5	T38.5X6
Meglumine						
antimoniate	T37.8X1	T37.8X2	T37.8X3	T37.8X4	T37.8X5	T37.8X6
diatrizoate	T50.8X1	T50.8X2	T50.8X3	T50.8X4	T50.8X5	T50.8X6
iodipamide	T50.8X1	T50.8X2	T50.8X3	T50.8X4	T50.8X5	T50.8X6
iotroxate	T50.8X1	T50.8X2	T50.8X3	T50.8X4	T50.8X5	T50.8X6
MEK (methyl ethyl ketone)	T52.4X1	T52.4X2	T52.4X3	T52.4X4	--	--
Meladinin	T49.3X1	T49.3X2	T49.3X3	T49.3X4	T49.3X5	T49.3X6
Meladrazine	T44.3X1	T44.3X2	T44.3X3	T44.3X4	T44.3X5	T44.3X6
Melaleuca alternifolia oil	T49.0X1	T49.0X2	T49.0X3	T49.0X4	T49.0X5	T49.0X6
Melanizing agents	T49.3X1	T49.3X2	T49.3X3	T49.3X4	T49.3X5	T49.3X6
Melanocyte-stimulating hormone	T38.891	T38.892	T38.893	T38.894	T38.895	T38.896
Melarsonyl potassium	T37.3X1	T37.3X2	T37.3X3	T37.3X4	T37.3X5	T37.3X6
Melarsoprol	T37.3X1	T37.3X2	T37.3X3	T37.3X4	T37.3X5	T37.3X6
Melia azedarach	T62.2X1	T62.2X2	T62.2X3	T62.2X4	--	--
Melitracen	T43.011	T43.012	T43.013	T43.014	T43.015	T43.016
Mellaril	T43.3X1	T43.3X2	T43.3X3	T43.3X4	T43.3X5	T43.3X6
Meloxine	T49.3X1	T49.3X2	T49.3X3	T49.3X4	T49.3X5	T49.3X6
Melperone	T43.4X1	T43.4X2	T43.4X3	T43.4X4	T43.4X5	T43.4X6
Melphalan	T45.1X1	T45.1X2	T45.1X3	T45.1X4	T45.1X5	T45.1X6
Memantine	T43.8X1	T43.8X2	T43.8X3	T43.8X4	T43.8X5	T43.8X6
Menadiol	T45.7X1	T45.7X2	T45.7X3	T45.7X4	T45.7X5	T45.7X6
sodium sulfate	T45.7X1	T45.7X2	T45.7X3	T45.7X4	T45.7X5	T45.7X6
Menadione	T45.7X1	T45.7X2	T45.7X3	T45.7X4	T45.7X5	T45.7X6
sodium bisulfite	T45.7X1	T45.7X2	T45.7X3	T45.7X4	T45.7X5	T45.7X6
Menaphthone	T45.7X1	T45.7X2	T45.7X3	T45.7X4	T45.7X5	T45.7X6
Menaquinone	T45.7X1	T45.7X2	T45.7X3	T45.7X4	T45.7X5	T45.7X6
Menatetrenone	T45.7X1	T45.7X2	T45.7X3	T45.7X4	T45.7X5	T45.7X6
Meningococcal vaccine	T50.A91	T50.A92	T50.A93	T50.A94	T50.A95	T50.A96
Menningovax (-AC) (-C)	T50.A91	T50.A92	T50.A93	T50.A94	T50.A95	T50.A96
Menotropins	T38.811	T38.812	T38.813	T38.814	T38.815	T38.816
Menthol	T48.5X1	T48.5X2	T48.5X3	T48.5X4	T48.5X5	T48.5X6
Mepacrine	T37.2X1	T37.2X2	T37.2X3	T37.2X4	T37.2X5	T37.2X6
Meparfynol	T42.6X1	T42.6X2	T42.6X3	T42.6X4	T42.6X5	T42.6X6
Mepartricin	T36.7X1	T36.7X2	T36.7X3	T36.7X4	T36.7X5	T36.7X6
Mepazine	T43.3X1	T43.3X2	T43.3X3	T43.3X4	T43.3X5	T43.3X6
Mepenzolate	T44.3X1	T44.3X2	T44.3X3	T44.3X4	T44.3X5	T44.3X6
bromide	T44.3X1	T44.3X2	T44.3X3	T44.3X4	T44.3X5	T44.3X6
Meperidine	T40.4X1	T40.4X2	T40.4X3	T40.4X4	T40.4X5	T40.4X6
Mephebarbital	T42.3X1	T42.3X2	T42.3X3	T42.3X4	T42.3X5	T42.3X6
Mephenamin (e)	T42.8X1	T42.8X2	T42.8X3	T42.8X4	T42.8X5	T42.8X6
Mephenesin	T42.8X1	T42.8X2	T42.8X3	T42.8X4	T42.8X5	T42.8X6
Mephenhydramine	T45.0X1	T45.0X2	T45.0X3	T45.0X4	T45.0X5	T45.0X6
Mephenoxalone	T42.8X1	T42.8X2	T42.8X3	T42.8X4	T42.8X5	T42.8X6
Mephentermine	T44.991	T44.992	T44.993	T44.994	T44.995	T44.996
Mephenytoin	T42.0X1	T42.0X2	T42.0X3	T42.0X4	T42.0X5	T42.0X6
with phenobarbital	T42.3X1	T42.3X2	T42.3X3	T42.3X4	T42.3X5	T42.3X6
Mephobarbital	T42.3X1	T42.3X2	T42.3X3	T42.3X4	T42.3X5	T42.3X6
Mephosfolan	T60.0X1	T60.0X2	T60.0X3	T60.0X4	--	--
Mepindolol	T44.7X1	T44.7X2	T44.7X3	T44.7X4	T44.7X5	T44.7X6
Mepiperphenidol	T44.3X1	T44.3X2	T44.3X3	T44.3X4	T44.3X5	T44.3X6
Mepitiostane	T38.7X1	T38.7X2	T38.7X3	T38.7X4	T38.7X5	T38.7X6
Mepivacaine	T41.3X1	T41.3X2	T41.3X3	T41.3X4	T41.3X5	T41.3X6
epidural	T41.3X1	T41.3X2	T41.3X3	T41.3X4	T41.3X5	T41.3X6
Meprednisone	T38.0X1	T38.0X2	T38.0X3	T38.0X4	T38.0X5	T38.0X6
Meprobam	T43.591	T43.592	T43.593	T43.594	T43.595	T43.596
Meprobamate	T43.591	T43.592	T43.593	T43.594	T43.595	T43.596
Meproscillarin	T46.0X1	T46.0X2	T46.0X3	T46.0X4	T46.0X5	T46.0X6
Meprylcaine	T41.3X1	T41.3X2	T41.3X3	T41.3X4	T41.3X5	T41.3X6

Substance	Poisoning, Accidental unintentional	Poisoning, Intentional self-harm	Poisoning, Assault	Poisoning, Undetermined	Adverse effect	Underdosing
Meptazinol	T39.8X1	T39.8X2	T39.8X3	T39.8X4	T39.8X5	T39.8X6
Mepyramine	T45.0X1	T45.0X2	T45.0X3	T45.0X4	T45.0X5	T45.0X6
Mequitazine	T43.3X1	T43.3X2	T43.3X3	T43.3X4	T43.3X5	T43.3X6
Meralluride	T50.2X1	T50.2X2	T50.2X3	T50.2X4	T50.2X5	T50.2X6
Merbaphen	T50.2X1	T50.2X2	T50.2X3	T50.2X4	T50.2X5	T50.2X6
Merbromin	T49.0X1	T49.0X2	T49.0X3	T49.0X4	T49.0X5	T49.0X6
Mercaptobenzothiazole salts	T49.0X1	T49.0X2	T49.0X3	T49.0X4	T49.0X5	T49.0X6
Mercaptomerin	T50.2X1	T50.2X2	T50.2X3	T50.2X4	T50.2X5	T50.2X6
Mercaptopurine	T45.1X1	T45.1X2	T45.1X3	T45.1X4	T45.1X5	T45.1X6
Mercumatilin	T50.2X1	T50.2X2	T50.2X3	T50.2X4	T50.2X5	T50.2X6
Mercuramide	T50.2X1	T50.2X2	T50.2X3	T50.2X4	T50.2X5	T50.2X6
Mercurochrome	T49.0X1	T49.0X2	T49.0X3	T49.0X4	T49.0X5	T49.0X6
Mercurophylline	T50.2X1	T50.2X2	T50.2X3	T50.2X4	T50.2X5	T50.2X6
Mercury, mercurial, mercuric, mercurous (compounds) (cyanide) (fumes) (nonmedicinal) (vapor) **NEC**	T56.1X1	T56.1X2	T56.1X3	T56.1X4	--	--
ammoniated	T49.0X1	T49.0X2	T49.0X3	T49.0X4	T49.0X5	T49.0X6
anti-infective						
local	T49.0X1	T49.0X2	T49.0X3	T49.0X4	T49.0X5	T49.0X6
systemic	T37.8X1	T37.8X2	T37.8X3	T37.8X4	T37.8X5	T37.8X6
topical	T49.0X1	T49.0X2	T49.0X3	T49.0X4	T49.0X5	T49.0X6
chloride (ammoniated)	T49.0X1	T49.0X2	T49.0X3	T49.0X4	T49.0X5	T49.0X6
fungicide	T56.1X1	T56.1X2	T56.1X3	T56.1X4	--	--
diuretic NEC	T50.2X1	T50.2X2	T50.2X3	T50.2X4	T50.2X5	T50.2X6
fungicide	T56.1X1	T56.1X2	T56.1X3	T56.1X4	--	--
organic (fungicide)	T56.1X1	T56.1X2	T56.1X3	T56.1X4	--	--
oxide, yellow	T49.0X1	T49.0X2	T49.0X3	T49.0X4	T49.0X5	T49.0X6
Mersalyl	T50.2X1	T50.2X2	T50.2X3	T50.2X4	T50.2X5	T50.2X6
Merthiolate	T49.0X1	T49.0X2	T49.0X3	T49.0X4	T49.0X5	T49.0X6
ophthalmic preparation	T49.5X1	T49.5X2	T49.5X3	T49.5X4	T49.5X5	T49.5X6
Meruvax	T50.B91	T50.B92	T50.B93	T50.B94	T50.B95	T50.B96
Mesalazine	T47.8X1	T47.8X2	T47.8X3	T47.8X4	T47.8X5	T47.8X6
Mescal buttons	T40.991	T40.992	T40.993	T40.994	--	--
Mescaline	T40.991	T40.992	T40.993	T40.994	--	--
Mesna	T48.4X1	T48.4X2	T48.4X3	T48.4X4	T48.4X5	T48.4X6
Mesoglycan	T46.6X1	T46.6X2	T46.6X3	T46.6X4	T46.6X5	T46.6X6
Mesoridazine	T43.3X1	T43.3X2	T43.3X3	T43.3X4	T43.3X5	T43.3X6
Mestanolone	T38.7X1	T38.7X2	T38.7X3	T38.7X4	T38.7X5	T38.7X6
Mesterolone	T38.7X1	T38.7X2	T38.7X3	T38.7X4	T38.7X5	T38.7X6
Mestranol	T38.5X1	T38.5X2	T38.5X3	T38.5X4	T38.5X5	T38.5X6
Mesulergine	T42.8X1	T42.8X2	T42.8X3	T42.8X4	T42.8X5	T42.8X6
Mesulfen	T49.0X1	T49.0X2	T49.0X3	T49.0X4	T49.0X5	T49.0X6
Mesuximide	T42.2X1	T42.2X2	T42.2X3	T42.2X4	T42.2X5	T42.2X6
Metabutethamine	T41.3X1	T41.3X2	T41.3X3	T41.3X4	T41.3X5	T41.3X6
Metactesylacetate	T49.0X1	T49.0X2	T49.0X3	T49.0X4	T49.0X5	T49.0X6
Metacycline	T36.4X1	T36.4X2	T36.4X3	T36.4X4	T36.4X5	T36.4X6
Metaldehyde (snail killer) **NEC**	T60.8X1	T60.8X2	T60.8X3	T60.8X4	--	--
Metals (heavy) (nonmedicinal)	T56.91	T56.92	T56.93	T56.94	--	--
dust, fumes, or vapor NEC	T56.91	T56.92	T56.93	T56.94	--	--
light NEC	T56.91	T56.92	T56.93	T56.94	--	--
dust, fumes, or vapor NEC	T56.91	T56.92	T56.93	T56.94	--	--
specified NEC	T56.891	T56.892	T56.893	T56.894	--	--
thallium	T56.811	T56.812	T56.813	T56.814	--	--
Metamfetamine	T43.621	T43.622	T43.623	T43.624	T43.625	T43.626
Metamizole sodium	T39.2X1	T39.2X2	T39.2X3	T39.2X4	T39.2X5	T39.2X6
Metampicillin	T36.0X1	T36.0X2	T36.0X3	T36.0X4	T36.0X5	T36.0X6
Metamucil	T47.4X1	T47.4X2	T47.4X3	T47.4X4	T47.4X5	T47.4X6
Metandienone	T38.7X1	T38.7X2	T38.7X3	T38.7X4	T38.7X5	T38.7X6
Metandrostenolone	T38.7X1	T38.7X2	T38.7X3	T38.7X4	T38.7X5	T38.7X6
Metaphen	T49.0X1	T49.0X2	T49.0X3	T49.0X4	T49.0X5	T49.0X6
Metaphos	T60.0X1	T60.0X2	T60.0X3	T60.0X4	--	--
Metapramine	T43.011	T43.012	T43.013	T43.014	T43.015	T43.016
Metaproterenol	T48.291	T48.292	T48.293	T48.294	T48.295	T48.296
Metaraminol	T44.4X1	T44.4X2	T44.4X3	T44.4X4	T44.4X5	T44.4X6
Metaxalone	T42.8X1	T42.8X2	T42.8X3	T42.8X4	T42.8X5	T42.8X6
Metenolone	T38.7X1	T38.7X2	T38.7X3	T38.7X4	T38.7X5	T38.7X6
Metergoline	T42.8X1	T42.8X2	T42.8X3	T42.8X4	T42.8X5	T42.8X6
Metescufylline	T46.991	T46.992	T46.993	T46.994	T46.995	T46.996
Metetoin	T42.0X1	T42.0X2	T42.0X3	T42.0X4	T42.0X5	T42.0X6
Metformin	T38.3X1	T38.3X2	T38.3X3	T38.3X4	T38.3X5	T38.3X6
Methacholine	T44.1X1	T44.1X2	T44.1X3	T44.1X4	T44.1X5	T44.1X6
Methacycline	T36.4X1	T36.4X2	T36.4X3	T36.4X4	T36.4X5	T36.4X6
Methadone	T40.3X1	T40.3X2	T40.3X3	T40.3X4	T40.3X5	T40.3X6
Methallenestril	T38.5X1	T38.5X2	T38.5X3	T38.5X4	T38.5X5	T38.5X6
Methallenoestril	T38.5X1	T38.5X2	T38.5X3	T38.5X4	T38.5X5	T38.5X6
Methamphetamine	T43.621	T43.622	T43.623	T43.624	T43.625	T43.626
Methampyrone	T39.2X1	T39.2X2	T39.2X3	T39.2X4	T39.2X5	T39.2X6
Methandienone	T38.7X1	T38.7X2	T38.7X3	T38.7X4	T38.7X5	T38.7X6
Methandriol	T38.7X1	T38.7X2	T38.7X3	T38.7X4	T38.7X5	T38.7X6
Methandrostenolone	T38.7X1	T38.7X2	T38.7X3	T38.7X4	T38.7X5	T38.7X6
Methane	T59.891	T59.892	T59.893	T59.894	--	--
Methanethiol	T59.891	T59.892	T59.893	T59.894	--	--

Substance	Poisoning, Accidental unintentional	Poisoning, Intentional self-harm	Poisoning, Assault	Poisoning, Undetermined	Adverse effect	Underdosing
Methaniazide	T37.1X1	T37.1X2	T37.1X3	T37.1X4	T37.1X5	T37.1X6
Methanol (vapor)	T51.1X1	T51.1X2	T51.1X3	T51.1X4	--	--
Methantheline	T44.3X1	T44.3X2	T44.3X3	T44.3X4	T44.3X5	T44.3X6
Methanthelinium bromide	T44.3X1	T44.3X2	T44.3X3	T44.3X4	T44.3X5	T44.3X6
Methaphenilene	T45.0X1	T45.0X2	T45.0X3	T45.0X4	T45.0X5	T45.0X6
Methapyrilene	T45.0X1	T45.0X2	T45.0X3	T45.0X4	T45.0X5	T45.0X6
Methaqualone (compound)	T42.6X1	T42.6X2	T42.6X3	T42.6X4	T42.6X5	T42.6X6
Metharbital	T42.3X1	T42.3X2	T42.3X3	T42.3X4	T42.3X5	T42.3X6
Methazolamide	T50.2X1	T50.2X2	T50.2X3	T50.2X4	T50.2X5	T50.2X6
Methdilazine	T43.3X1	T43.3X2	T43.3X3	T43.3X4	T43.3X5	T43.3X6
Methedrine	T43.621	T43.622	T43.623	T43.624	T43.625	T43.626
Methenamine (mandelate)	T37.8X1	T37.8X2	T37.8X3	T37.8X4	T37.8X5	T37.8X6
Methenolone	T38.7X1	T38.7X2	T38.7X3	T38.7X4	T38.7X5	T38.7X6
Methergine	T48.0X1	T48.0X2	T48.0X3	T48.0X4	T48.0X5	T48.0X6
Methetoin	T42.0X1	T42.0X2	T42.0X3	T42.0X4	T42.0X5	T42.0X6
Methiacil	T38.2X1	T38.2X2	T38.2X3	T38.2X4	T38.2X5	T38.2X6
Methicillin	T36.0X1	T36.0X2	T36.0X3	T36.0X4	T36.0X5	T36.0X6
Methimazole	T38.2X1	T38.2X2	T38.2X3	T38.2X4	T38.2X5	T38.2X6
Methiodal sodium	T50.8X1	T50.8X2	T50.8X3	T50.8X4	T50.8X5	T50.8X6
Methionine	T50.991	T50.992	T50.993	T50.994	T50.995	T50.996
Methisazone	T37.5X1	T37.5X2	T37.5X3	T37.5X4	T37.5X5	T37.5X6
Methisoprinol	T37.5X1	T37.5X2	T37.5X3	T37.5X4	T37.5X5	T37.5X6
Methitural	T42.3X1	T42.3X2	T42.3X3	T42.3X4	T42.3X5	T42.3X6
Methixene	T44.3X1	T44.3X2	T44.3X3	T44.3X4	T44.3X5	T44.3X6
Methobarbital, methobarbitone	T42.3X1	T42.3X2	T42.3X3	T42.3X4	T42.3X5	T42.3X6
Methocarbamol	T42.8X1	T42.8X2	T42.8X3	T42.8X4	T42.8X5	T42.8X6
skeletal muscle relaxant	T48.1X1	T48.1X2	T48.1X3	T48.1X4	T48.1X5	T48.1X6
Methohexital	T41.1X1	T41.1X2	T41.1X3	T41.1X4	T41.1X5	T41.1X6
Methohexitone	T41.1X1	T41.1X2	T41.1X3	T41.1X4	T41.1X5	T41.1X6
Methoin	T42.0X1	T42.0X2	T42.0X3	T42.0X4	T42.0X5	T42.0X6
Methopholine	T39.8X1	T39.8X2	T39.8X3	T39.8X4	T39.8X5	T39.8X6
Methopromazine	T43.3X1	T43.3X2	T43.3X3	T43.3X4	T43.3X5	T43.3X6
Methorate	T48.3X1	T48.3X2	T48.3X3	T48.3X4	T48.3X5	T48.3X6
Methoserpidine	T46.5X1	T46.5X2	T46.5X3	T46.5X4	T46.5X5	T46.5X6
Methotrexate	T45.1X1	T45.1X2	T45.1X3	T45.1X4	T45.1X5	T45.1X6
Methotrimeprazine	T43.3X1	T43.3X2	T43.3X3	T43.3X4	T43.3X5	T43.3X6
Methoxa-Dome	T49.3X1	T49.3X2	T49.3X3	T49.3X4	T49.3X5	T49.3X6
Methoxamine	T44.4X1	T44.4X2	T44.4X3	T44.4X4	T44.4X5	T44.4X6
Methoxsalen	T50.991	T50.992	T50.993	T50.994	T50.995	T50.996
Methoxyaniline	T65.3X1	T65.3X2	T65.3X3	T65.3X4	--	--
Methoxybenzyl penicillin	T36.0X1	T36.0X2	T36.0X3	T36.0X4	T36.0X5	T36.0X6
Methoxychlor	T53.7X1	T53.7X2	T53.7X3	T53.7X4	--	--
Methoxy-DDT	T53.7X1	T53.7X2	T53.7X3	T53.7X4	--	--
2-Methoxyethanol	T52.3X1	T52.3X2	T52.3X3	T52.3X4	--	--
Methoxyflurane	T41.0X1	T41.0X2	T41.0X3	T41.0X4	T41.0X5	T41.0X6
Methoxyphenamine	T48.6X1	T48.6X2	T48.6X3	T48.6X4	T48.6X5	T48.6X6
Methoxypromazine	T43.3X1	T43.3X2	T43.3X3	T43.3X4	T43.3X5	T43.3X6
5-Methoxypsoralen (5-MOP)	T50.991	T50.992	T50.993	T50.994	T50.995	T50.996
8-Methoxypsoralen (8-MOP)	T50.991	T50.992	T50.993	T50.994	T50.995	T50.996
Methscopolamine bromide	T44.3X1	T44.3X2	T44.3X3	T44.3X4	T44.3X5	T44.3X6
Methsuximide	T42.2X1	T42.2X2	T42.2X3	T42.2X4	T42.2X5	T42.2X6
Methyclothiazide	T50.2X1	T50.2X2	T50.2X3	T50.2X4	T50.2X5	T50.2X6
Methyl						
acetate	T52.4X1	T52.4X2	T52.4X3	T52.4X4	--	--
acetone	T52.4X1	T52.4X2	T52.4X3	T52.4X4	--	--
acrylate	T65.891	T65.892	T65.893	T65.894	--	--
alcohol	T51.1X1	T51.1X2	T51.1X3	T51.1X4	--	--
aminophenol	T65.3X1	T65.3X2	T65.3X3	T65.3X4	--	--
amphetamine	T43.621	T43.622	T43.623	T43.624	T43.625	T43.626
androstanolone	T38.7X1	T38.7X2	T38.7X3	T38.7X4	T38.7X5	T38.7X6
atropine	T44.3X1	T44.3X2	T44.3X3	T44.3X4	T44.3X5	T44.3X6
benzene	T52.2X1	T52.2X2	T52.2X3	T52.2X4	--	--
benzoate	T52.8X1	T52.8X2	T52.8X3	T52.8X4	--	--
benzol	T52.2X1	T52.2X2	T52.2X3	T52.2X4	--	--
bromide (gas)	T59.891	T59.892	T59.893	T59.894	--	--
fumigant	T60.8X1	T60.8X2	T60.8X3	T60.8X4	--	--
butanol	T51.3X1	T51.3X2	T51.3X3	T51.3X4	--	--
carbinol	T51.1X1	T51.1X2	T51.1X3	T51.1X4	--	--
carbonate	T52.8X1	T52.8X2	T52.8X3	T52.8X4	--	--
CCNU	T45.1X1	T45.1X2	T45.1X3	T45.1X4	T45.1X5	T45.1X6
cellosolve	T52.91	T52.92	T52.93	T52.94	--	--
cellulose	T47.4X1	T47.4X2	T47.4X3	T47.4X4	T47.4X5	T47.4X6
chloride (gas)	T59.891	T59.892	T59.893	T59.894	--	--
chloroformate	T59.3X1	T59.3X2	T59.3X3	T59.3X4	--	--
cyclohexane	T52.8X1	T52.8X2	T52.8X3	T52.8X4	--	--
cyclohexanol	T51.8X1	T51.8X2	T51.8X3	T51.8X4	--	--
cyclohexanone	T52.8X1	T52.8X2	T52.8X3	T52.8X4	--	--
cyclohexyl acetate	T52.8X1	T52.8X2	T52.8X3	T52.8X4	--	--
demeton	T60.0X1	T60.0X2	T60.0X3	T60.0X4	--	--
dihydromorphinone	T40.2X1	T40.2X2	T40.2X3	T40.2X4	T40.2X5	T40.2X6
ergometrine	T48.0X1	T48.0X2	T48.0X3	T48.0X4	T48.0X5	T48.0X6
ergonovine	T48.0X1	T48.0X2	T48.0X3	T48.0X4	T48.0X5	T48.0X6
ethyl ketone	T52.4X1	T52.4X2	T52.4X3	T52.4X4	--	--

Methyl - Monoxidine hydrochloride

Substance	Poisoning, Accidental unintentional	Poisoning, Intentional self-harm	Poisoning, Assault	Poisoning, Undetermined	Adverse effect	Underdosing
Methyl — *continued*						
glucamine antimonate	T37.8X1	T37.8X2	T37.8X3	T37.8X4	T37.8X5	T37.8X6
hydrazine	T65.891	T65.892	T65.893	T65.894	--	--
iodide	T65.891	T65.892	T65.893	T65.894	--	--
isobutyl ketone	T52.4X1	T52.4X2	T52.4X3	T52.4X4	--	--
isothiocyanate	T60.3X1	T60.3X2	T60.3X3	T60.3X4	--	--
mercaptan	T59.891	T59.892	T59.893	T59.894	--	--
morphine NEC	T40.2X1	T40.2X2	T40.2X3	T40.2X4	T40.2X5	T40.2X6
nicotinate	T49.4X1	T49.4X2	T49.4X3	T49.4X4	T49.4X5	T49.4X6
paraben	T49.0X1	T49.0X2	T49.0X3	T49.0X4	T49.0X5	T49.0X6
parafynol	T42.6X1	T42.6X2	T42.6X3	T42.6X4	T42.6X5	T42.6X6
parathion	T60.0X1	T60.0X2	T60.0X3	T60.0X4	--	--
peridol	T43.4X1	T43.4X2	T43.4X3	T43.4X4	T43.4X5	T43.4X6
phenidate	T43.631	T43.632	T43.633	T43.634	T43.635	T43.636
prednisolone	T38.0X1	T38.0X2	T38.0X3	T38.0X4	T38.0X5	T38.0X6
ENT agent	T49.6X1	T49.6X2	T49.6X3	T49.6X4	T49.6X5	T49.6X6
ophthalmic preparation	T49.5X1	T49.5X2	T49.5X3	T49.5X4	T49.5X5	T49.5X6
topical NEC	T49.0X1	T49.0X2	T49.0X3	T49.0X4	T49.0X5	T49.0X6
propylcarbinol	T51.3X1	T51.3X2	T51.3X3	T51.3X4	--	--
rosaniline NEC	T49.0X1	T49.0X2	T49.0X3	T49.0X4	T49.0X5	T49.0X6
salicylate	T49.2X1	T49.2X2	T49.2X3	T49.2X4	T49.2X5	T49.2X6
sulfate (fumes)	T59.891	T59.892	T59.893	T59.894	--	--
liquid	T52.8X1	T52.8X2	T52.8X3	T52.8X4	--	--
sulfonal	T42.6X1	T42.6X2	T42.6X3	T42.6X4	T42.6X5	T42.6X6
testosterone	T38.7X1	T38.7X2	T38.7X3	T38.7X4	T38.7X5	T38.7X6
thiouracil	T38.2X1	T38.2X2	T38.2X3	T38.2X4	T38.2X5	T38.2X6
Methylamphetamine	T43.621	T43.622	T43.623	T43.624	T43.625	T43.626
Methylated spirit	T51.1X1	T51.1X2	T51.1X3	T51.1X4	--	--
Methylatropine nitrate	T44.3X1	T44.3X2	T44.3X3	T44.3X4	T44.3X5	T44.3X6
Methylbenactyzium bromide	T44.3X1	T44.3X2	T44.3X3	T44.3X4	T44.3X5	T44.3X6
Methylbenzethonium chloride	T49.0X1	T49.0X2	T49.0X3	T49.0X4	T49.0X5	T49.0X6
Methylcellulose	T47.4X1	T47.4X2	T47.4X3	T47.4X4	T47.4X5	T47.4X6
laxative	T47.4X1	T47.4X2	T47.4X3	T47.4X4	T47.4X5	T47.4X6
Methylchlorophenoxy-acetic acid	T60.3X1	T60.3X2	T60.3X3	T60.3X4	--	--
Methyldopa	T46.5X1	T46.5X2	T46.5X3	T46.5X4	T46.5X5	T46.5X6
Methyldopate	T46.5X1	T46.5X2	T46.5X3	T46.5X4	T46.5X5	T46.5X6
Methylene						
blue	T50.6X1	T50.6X2	T50.6X3	T50.6X4	T50.6X5	T50.6X6
chloride or dichloride (solvent) NEC	T53.4X1	T53.4X2	T53.4X3	T53.4X4	--	--
Methylenedioxyamphet-amine	T43.621	T43.622	T43.623	T43.624	T43.625	T43.626
Methylenedioxymetham-phetamine	T43.621	T43.622	T43.623	T43.624	T43.625	T43.626
Methylergometrine	T48.0X1	T48.0X2	T48.0X3	T48.0X4	T48.0X5	T48.0X6
Methylergonovine	T48.0X1	T48.0X2	T48.0X3	T48.0X4	T48.0X5	T48.0X6
Methylestrenolone	T38.5X1	T38.5X2	T38.5X3	T38.5X4	T38.5X5	T38.5X6
Methylethyl cellulose	T50.991	T50.992	T50.993	T50.994	T50.995	T50.996
Methylhexabital	T42.3X1	T42.3X2	T42.3X3	T42.3X4	T42.3X5	T42.3X6
Methylmorphine	T40.2X1	T40.2X2	T40.2X3	T40.2X4	T40.2X5	T40.2X6
Methylparaben (ophthalmic)	T49.5X1	T49.5X2	T49.5X3	T49.5X4	T49.5X5	T49.5X6
Methylparafynol	T42.6X1	T42.6X2	T42.6X3	T42.6X4	T42.6X5	T42.6X6
Methylpentynol, methylpenthynol	T42.6X1	T42.6X2	T42.6X3	T42.6X4	T42.6X5	T42.6X6
Methylphenidate	T43.631	T43.632	T43.633	T43.634	T43.635	T43.636
Methylphenobarbital	T42.3X1	T42.3X2	T42.3X3	T42.3X4	T42.3X5	T42.3X6
Methylpolysiloxane	T47.1X1	T47.1X2	T47.1X3	T47.1X4	T47.1X5	T47.1X6
Methylprednisolone — *see* Methyl, prednisolone						
Methylrosaniline	T49.0X1	T49.0X2	T49.0X3	T49.0X4	T49.0X5	T49.0X6
Methylrosanilinium chloride	T49.0X1	T49.0X2	T49.0X3	T49.0X4	T49.0X5	T49.0X6
Methyltestosterone	T38.7X1	T38.7X2	T38.7X3	T38.7X4	T38.7X5	T38.7X6
Methylthionine chloride	T50.6X1	T50.6X2	T50.6X3	T50.6X4	T50.6X5	T50.6X6
Methylthioninium chloride	T50.6X1	T50.6X2	T50.6X3	T50.6X4	T50.6X5	T50.6X6
Methylthiouracil	T38.2X1	T38.2X2	T38.2X3	T38.2X4	T38.2X5	T38.2X6
Methyprylon	T42.6X1	T42.6X2	T42.6X3	T42.6X4	T42.6X5	T42.6X6
Methysergide	T46.5X1	T46.5X2	T46.5X3	T46.5X4	T46.5X5	T46.5X6
Metiamide	T47.1X1	T47.1X2	T47.1X3	T47.1X4	T47.1X5	T47.1X6
Meticillin	T36.0X1	T36.0X2	T36.0X3	T36.0X4	T36.0X5	T36.0X6
Meticrane	T50.2X1	T50.2X2	T50.2X3	T50.2X4	T50.2X5	T50.2X6
Metildigoxin	T46.0X1	T46.0X2	T46.0X3	T46.0X4	T46.0X5	T46.0X6
Metipranolol	T49.5X1	T49.5X2	T49.5X3	T49.5X4	T49.5X5	T49.5X6
Metirosine	T46.5X1	T46.5X2	T46.5X3	T46.5X4	T46.5X5	T46.5X6
Metisazone	T37.5X1	T37.5X2	T37.5X3	T37.5X4	T37.5X5	T37.5X6
Metixene	T44.3X1	T44.3X2	T44.3X3	T44.3X4	T44.3X5	T44.3X6
Metizoline	T48.5X1	T48.5X2	T48.5X3	T48.5X4	T48.5X5	T48.5X6
Metoclopramide	T45.0X1	T45.0X2	T45.0X3	T45.0X4	T45.0X5	T45.0X6
Metofenazate	T43.3X1	T43.3X2	T43.3X3	T43.3X4	T43.3X5	T43.3X6
Metofoline	T39.8X1	T39.8X2	T39.8X3	T39.8X4	T39.8X5	T39.8X6
Metolazone	T50.2X1	T50.2X2	T50.2X3	T50.2X4	T50.2X5	T50.2X6
Metopon	T40.2X1	T40.2X2	T40.2X3	T40.2X4	T40.2X5	T40.2X6
Metoprine	T45.1X1	T45.1X2	T45.1X3	T45.1X4	T45.1X5	T45.1X6

Substance	Poisoning, Accidental unintentional	Poisoning, Intentional self-harm	Poisoning, Assault	Poisoning, Undetermined	Adverse effect	Underdosing
Metoprolol	T44.7X1	T44.7X2	T44.7X3	T44.7X4	T44.7X5	T44.7X6
Metrifonate	T60.0X1	T60.0X2	T60.0X3	T60.0X4	--	--
Metrizamide	T50.8X1	T50.8X2	T50.8X3	T50.8X4	T50.8X5	T50.8X6
Metrizoic acid	T50.8X1	T50.8X2	T50.8X3	T50.8X4	T50.8X5	T50.8X6
Metronidazole	T37.8X1	T37.8X2	T37.8X3	T37.8X4	T37.8X5	T37.8X6
Metycaine	T41.3X1	T41.3X2	T41.3X3	T41.3X4	T41.3X5	T41.3X6
infiltration (subcutaneous)	T41.3X1	T41.3X2	T41.3X3	T41.3X4	T41.3X5	T41.3X6
nerve block (peripheral) (plexus)	T41.3X1	T41.3X2	T41.3X3	T41.3X4	T41.3X5	T41.3X6
topical (surface)	T41.3X1	T41.3X2	T41.3X3	T41.3X4	T41.3X5	T41.3X6
Metyrapone	T50.8X1	T50.8X2	T50.8X3	T50.8X4	T50.8X5	T50.8X6
Mevinphos	T60.0X1	T60.0X2	T60.0X3	T60.0X4	--	--
Mexazolam	T42.4X1	T42.4X2	T42.4X3	T42.4X4	T42.4X5	T42.4X6
Mexenone	T49.3X1	T49.3X2	T49.3X3	T49.3X4	T49.3X5	T49.3X6
Mexiletine	T46.2X1	T46.2X2	T46.2X3	T46.2X4	T46.2X5	T46.2X6
Mezereon	T62.2X1	T62.2X2	T62.2X3	T62.2X4	--	--
berries	T62.1X1	T62.1X2	T62.1X3	T62.1X4	--	--
Mezlocillin	T36.0X1	T36.0X2	T36.0X3	T36.0X4	T36.0X5	T36.0X6
Mianserin	T43.021	T43.022	T43.023	T43.024	T43.025	T43.026
Micatin	T49.0X1	T49.0X2	T49.0X3	T49.0X4	T49.0X5	T49.0X6
Miconazole	T49.0X1	T49.0X2	T49.0X3	T49.0X4	T49.0X5	T49.0X6
Micronomicin	T36.5X1	T36.5X2	T36.5X3	T36.5X4	T36.5X5	T36.5X6
Midazolam	T42.4X1	T42.4X2	T42.4X3	T42.4X4	T42.4X5	T42.4X6
Midecamycin	T36.3X1	T36.3X2	T36.3X3	T36.3X4	T36.3X5	T36.3X6
Mifepristone	T38.6X1	T38.6X2	T38.6X3	T38.6X4	T38.6X5	T38.6X6
Milk of magnesia	T47.1X1	T47.1X2	T47.1X3	T47.1X4	T47.1X5	T47.1X6
Millipede (tropical) (venomous)	T63.411	T63.412	T63.413	T63.414	--	--
Miltown	T43.591	T43.592	T43.593	T43.594	T43.595	T43.596
Milverine	T44.3X1	T44.3X2	T44.3X3	T44.3X4	T44.3X5	T44.3X6
Minaprine	T43.291	T43.292	T43.293	T43.294	T43.295	T43.296
Minaxolone	T41.291	T41.292	T41.293	T41.294	T41.295	T41.296
Mineral						
acids	T54.2X1	T54.2X2	T54.2X3	T54.2X4	--	--
oil (laxative)(medicinal)	T47.4X1	T47.4X2	T47.4X3	T47.4X4	T47.4X5	T47.4X6
emulsion	T47.2X1	T47.2X2	T47.2X3	T47.2X4	T47.2X5	T47.2X6
nonmedicinal	T52.0X1	T52.0X2	T52.0X3	T52.0X4	--	--
topical	T49.3X1	T49.3X2	T49.3X3	T49.3X4	T49.3X5	T49.3X6
salt NEC	T50.3X1	T50.3X2	T50.3X3	T50.3X4	T50.3X5	T50.3X6
spirits	T52.0X1	T52.0X2	T52.0X3	T52.0X4	--	--
Mineralocorticosteroid	T50.0X1	T50.0X2	T50.0X3	T50.0X4	T50.0X5	T50.0X6
Minocycline	T36.4X1	T36.4X2	T36.4X3	T36.4X4	T36.4X5	T36.4X6
Minoxidil	T46.7X1	T46.7X2	T46.7X3	T46.7X4	T46.7X5	T46.7X6
Miokamycin	T36.3X1	T36.3X2	T36.3X3	T36.3X4	T36.3X5	T36.3X6
Miotic drug	T49.5X1	T49.5X2	T49.5X3	T49.5X4	T49.5X5	T49.5X6
Mipafox	T60.0X1	T60.0X2	T60.0X3	T60.0X4	--	--
Mirex	T60.1X1	T60.1X2	T60.1X3	T60.1X4	--	--
Mirtazapine	T43.021	T43.022	T43.023	T43.024	T43.025	T43.026
Misonidazole	T37.3X1	T37.3X2	T37.3X3	T37.3X4	T37.3X5	T37.3X6
Misoprostol	T47.1X1	T47.1X2	T47.1X3	T47.1X4	T47.1X5	T47.1X6
Mithramycin	T45.1X1	T45.1X2	T45.1X3	T45.1X4	T45.1X5	T45.1X6
Mitobronitol	T45.1X1	T45.1X2	T45.1X3	T45.1X4	T45.1X5	T45.1X6
Mitoguazone	T45.1X1	T45.1X2	T45.1X3	T45.1X4	T45.1X5	T45.1X6
Mitolactol	T45.1X1	T45.1X2	T45.1X3	T45.1X4	T45.1X5	T45.1X6
Mitomycin	T45.1X1	T45.1X2	T45.1X3	T45.1X4	T45.1X5	T45.1X6
Mitopodozide	T45.1X1	T45.1X2	T45.1X3	T45.1X4	T45.1X5	T45.1X6
Mitotane	T45.1X1	T45.1X2	T45.1X3	T45.1X4	T45.1X5	T45.1X6
Mitoxantrone	T45.1X1	T45.1X2	T45.1X3	T45.1X4	T45.1X5	T45.1X6
Mivacurium chloride	T48.1X1	T48.1X2	T48.1X3	T48.1X4	T48.1X5	T48.1X6
Miyari bacteria	T47.6X1	T47.6X2	T47.6X3	T47.6X4	T47.6X5	T47.6X6
Moclobemide	T43.1X1	T43.1X2	T43.1X3	T43.1X4	T43.1X5	T43.1X6
Moderil	T46.5X1	T46.5X2	T46.5X3	T46.5X4	T46.5X5	T46.5X6
Mofebutazone	T39.2X1	T39.2X2	T39.2X3	T39.2X4	T39.2X5	T39.2X6
Mogadon — *see* Nitrazepam						
Molindone	T43.591	T43.592	T43.593	T43.594	T43.595	T43.596
Molsidomine	T46.3X1	T46.3X2	T46.3X3	T46.3X4	T46.3X5	T46.3X6
Mometasone	T49.0X1	T49.0X2	T49.0X3	T49.0X4	T49.0X5	T49.0X6
Monistat	T49.0X1	T49.0X2	T49.0X3	T49.0X4	T49.0X5	T49.0X6
Monkshood	T62.2X1	T62.2X2	T62.2X3	T62.2X4	--	--
Monoamine oxidase inhibitor NEC	T43.1X1	T43.1X2	T43.1X3	T43.1X4	T43.1X5	T43.1X6
hydrazine	T43.1X1	T43.1X2	T43.1X3	T43.1X4	T43.1X5	T43.1X6
Monobenzone	T49.4X1	T49.4X2	T49.4X3	T49.4X4	T49.4X5	T49.4X6
Monochloroacetic acid	T60.3X1	T60.3X2	T60.3X3	T60.3X4	--	--
Monochlorobenzene	T53.7X1	T53.7X2	T53.7X3	T53.7X4	--	--
Monoethanolamine	T46.8X1	T46.8X2	T46.8X3	T46.8X4	T46.8X5	T46.8X6
oleate	T46.8X1	T46.8X2	T46.8X3	T46.8X4	T46.8X5	T46.8X6
Monooctanoin	T50.991	T50.992	T50.993	T50.994	T50.995	T50.996
Monophenylbutazone	T39.2X1	T39.2X2	T39.2X3	T39.2X4	T39.2X5	T39.2X6
Monosodium glutamate	T65.891	T65.892	T65.893	T65.894	--	--
Monosulfiram	T49.0X1	T49.0X2	T49.0X3	T49.0X4	T49.0X5	T49.0X6
Monoxide, carbon — *see* Carbon, monoxide						
Monoxidine hydrochloride	T46.1X1	T46.1X2	T46.1X3	T46.1X4	T46.1X5	T46.1X6

Substance	Poisoning, Accidental unintentional	Poisoning, Intentional self-harm	Poisoning, Assault	Poisoning, Undetermined	Adverse effect	Underdosing
Monuron	T60.3X1	T60.3X2	T60.3X3	T60.3X4	--	--
Moperone	T43.4X1	T43.4X2	T43.4X3	T43.4X4	T43.4X5	T43.4X6
Mopidamol	T45.1X1	T45.1X2	T45.1X3	T45.1X4	T45.1X5	T45.1X6
MOPP (mechloreth-amine + vincristine + prednisone + procarba-zine)	T45.1X1	T45.1X2	T45.1X3	T45.1X4	T45.1X5	T45.1X6
Morfin	T40.2X1	T40.2X2	T40.2X3	T40.2X4	T40.2X5	T40.2X6
Morinamide	T37.1X1	T37.1X2	T37.1X3	T37.1X4	T37.1X5	T37.1X6
Morning glory seeds	T40.991	T40.992	T40.993	T40.994	--	--
Moroxydine	T37.5X1	T37.5X2	T37.5X3	T37.5X4	T37.5X5	T37.5X6
Morphazinamide	T37.1X1	T37.1X2	T37.1X3	T37.1X4	T37.1X5	T37.1X6
Morphine	T40.2X1	T40.2X2	T40.2X3	T40.2X4	T40.2X5	T40.2X6
antagonist	T50.7X1	T50.7X2	T50.7X3	T50.7X4	T50.7X5	T50.7X6
Morpholinylethylmorphine	T40.2X1	T40.2X2	T40.2X3	T40.2X4		
Morsuximide	T42.2X1	T42.2X2	T42.2X3	T42.2X4	T42.2X5	T42.2X6
Mosapramine	T43.591	T43.592	T43.593	T43.594	T43.595	T43.596
Moth balls (see also Pesticides)	T60.2X1	T60.2X2	T60.2X3	T60.2X4	--	--
naphthalene	T60.2X1	T60.2X2	T60.2X3	T60.2X4	--	--
paradichlorobenzene	T60.1X1	T60.1X2	T60.1X3	T60.1X4	--	--
Motor exhaust gas	T58.01	T58.02	T58.03	T58.04	--	--
Mouthwash (antiseptic) (zinc chloride)	T49.6X1	T49.6X2	T49.6X3	T49.6X4	T49.6X5	T49.6X6
Moxastine	T45.0X1	T45.0X2	T45.0X3	T45.0X4	T45.0X5	T45.0X6
Moxaverine	T44.3X1	T44.3X2	T44.3X3	T44.3X4	T44.3X5	T44.3X6
Moxisylyte	T46.7X1	T46.7X2	T46.7X3	T46.7X4	T46.7X5	T46.7X6
Mucilage, plant	T47.4X1	T47.4X2	T47.4X3	T47.4X4	T47.4X5	T47.4X6
Mucolytic drug	T48.4X1	T48.4X2	T48.4X3	T48.4X4	T48.4X5	T48.4X6
Mucomyst	T48.4X1	T48.4X2	T48.4X3	T48.4X4	T48.4X5	T48.4X6
Mucous membrane agents (external)	T49.91	T49.92	T49.93	T49.94	T49.95	T49.96
specified NEC	T49.8X1	T49.8X2	T49.8X3	T49.8X4	T49.8X5	T49.8X6
Mumps						
immune globulin (human)	T50.Z11	T50.Z12	T50.Z13	T50.Z14	T50.Z15	T50.Z16
skin test antigen	T50.8X1	T50.8X2	T50.8X3	T50.8X4	T50.8X5	T50.8X6
vaccine	T50.B91	T50.B92	T50.B93	T50.B94	T50.B95	T50.B96
Mumpsvax	T50.B91	T50.B92	T50.B93	T50.B94	T50.B95	T50.B96
Mupirocin	T49.0X1	T49.0X2	T49.0X3	T49.0X4	T49.0X5	T49.0X6
Muriatic acid — see Hydrochloric acid						
Muromonab-CD3	T45.1X1	T45.1X2	T45.1X3	T45.1X4	T45.1X5	T45.1X6
Muscle-action drug NEC	T48.201	T48.202	T48.203	T48.204	T48.205	T48.206
Muscle affecting agents NEC	T48.201	T48.202	T48.203	T48.204	T48.205	T48.206
oxytocic	T48.0X1	T48.0X2	T48.0X3	T48.0X4	T48.0X5	T48.0X6
relaxants	T48.201	T48.202	T48.203	T48.204	T48.205	T48.206
central nervous system	T42.8X1	T42.8X2	T42.8X3	T42.8X4	T42.8X5	T42.8X6
skeletal	T48.1X1	T48.1X2	T48.1X3	T48.1X4	T48.1X5	T48.1X6
smooth	T44.3X1	T44.3X2	T44.3X3	T44.3X4	T44.3X5	T44.3X6
Muscle relaxant — see Relaxant, muscle						
Muscle-tone depressant, central NEC	T42.8X1	T42.8X2	T42.8X3	T42.8X4	T42.8X5	T42.8X6
specified NEC	T42.8X1	T42.8X2	T42.8X3	T42.8X4	T42.8X5	T42.8X6
Mushroom, noxious	T62.0X1	T62.0X2	T62.0X3	T62.0X4	--	--
Mussel, noxious	T61.781	T61.782	T61.783	T61.784	--	--
Mustard (emetic)	T47.7X1	T47.7X2	T47.7X3	T47.7X4	T47.7X5	T47.7X6
black	T47.7X1	T47.7X2	T47.7X3	T47.7X4	T47.7X5	T47.7X6
gas, not in war	T59.91	T59.92	T59.93	T59.94	--	--
nitrogen	T45.1X1	T45.1X2	T45.1X3	T45.1X4	T45.1X5	T45.1X6
Mustine	T45.1X1	T45.1X2	T45.1X3	T45.1X4	T45.1X5	T45.1X6
M-vac	T45.1X1	T45.1X2	T45.1X3	T45.1X4	T45.1X5	T45.1X6
Mycifradin	T36.5X1	T36.5X2	T36.5X3	T36.5X4	T36.5X5	T36.5X6
topical	T49.0X1	T49.0X2	T49.0X3	T49.0X4	T49.0X5	T49.0X6
Mycitracin	T36.8X1	T36.8X2	T36.8X3	T36.8X4	T36.8X5	T36.8X6
ophthalmic preparation	T49.5X1	T49.5X2	T49.5X3	T49.5X4	T49.5X5	T49.5X6
Mycostatin	T36.7X1	T36.7X2	T36.7X3	T36.7X4	T36.7X5	T36.7X6
topical	T49.0X1	T49.0X2	T49.0X3	T49.0X4	T49.0X5	T49.0X6
Mycotoxins	T64.81	T64.82	T64.83	T64.84	--	--
aflatoxin	T64.01	T64.02	T64.03	T64.04	--	--
specified NEC	T64.81	T64.82	T64.83	T64.84	--	--
Mydriacyl	T44.3X1	T44.3X2	T44.3X3	T44.3X4	T44.3X5	T44.3X6
Mydriatic drug	T49.5X1	T49.5X2	T49.5X3	T49.5X4	T49.5X5	T49.5X6
Myelobromal	T45.1X1	T45.1X2	T45.1X3	T45.1X4	T45.1X5	T45.1X6
Myleran	T45.1X1	T45.1X2	T45.1X3	T45.1X4	T45.1X5	T45.1X6
Myochrysin (e)	T39.2X1	T39.2X2	T39.2X3	T39.2X4	T39.2X5	T39.2X6
Myoneural blocking agents	T48.1X1	T48.1X2	T48.1X3	T48.1X4	T48.1X5	T48.1X6
Myralact	T49.0X1	T49.0X2	T49.0X3	T49.0X4	T49.0X5	T49.0X6
Myristica fragrans	T62.2X1	T62.2X2	T62.2X3	T62.2X4	--	--
Myristicin	T65.891	T65.892	T65.893	T65.894	--	--
Mysoline	T42.3X1	T42.3X2	T42.3X3	T42.3X4	T42.3X5	T42.3X6
N						
Nabilone	T40.7X1	T40.7X2	T40.7X3	T40.7X4	T40.7X5	T40.7X6
Nabumetone	T39.391	T39.392	T39.393	T39.394	T39.395	T39.396

Substance	Poisoning, Accidental unintentional	Poisoning, Intentional self-harm	Poisoning, Assault	Poisoning, Undetermined	Adverse effect	Underdosing
Nadolol	T44.7X1	T44.7X2	T44.7X3	T44.7X4	T44.7X5	T44.7X6
Nafcillin	T36.0X1	T36.0X2	T36.0X3	T36.0X4	T36.0X5	T36.0X6
Nafoxidine	T38.6X1	T38.6X2	T38.6X3	T38.6X4	T38.6X5	T38.6X6
Naftazone	T46.991	T46.992	T46.993	T46.994	T46.995	T46.996
Naftidrofuryl (oxalate)	T46.7X1	T46.7X2	T46.7X3	T46.7X4	T46.7X5	T46.7X6
Naftifine	T49.0X1	T49.0X2	T49.0X3	T49.0X4	T49.0X5	T49.0X6
Nail polish remover	T52.91	T52.92	T52.93	T52.94	--	--
Nalbuphine	T40.4X1	T40.4X2	T40.4X3	T40.4X4	T40.4X5	T40.4X6
Naled	T60.0X1	T60.0X2	T60.0X3	T60.0X4	--	--
Nalidixic acid	T37.8X1	T37.8X2	T37.8X3	T37.8X4	T37.8X5	T37.8X6
Nalorphine	T50.7X1	T50.7X2	T50.7X3	T50.7X4	T50.7X5	T50.7X6
Naloxone	T50.7X1	T50.7X2	T50.7X3	T50.7X4	T50.7X5	T50.7X6
Naltrexone	T50.7X1	T50.7X2	T50.7X3	T50.7X4	T50.7X5	T50.7X6
Namenda	T43.8X1	T43.8X2	T43.8X3	T43.8X4	T43.8X5	T43.8X6
Nandrolone	T38.7X1	T38.7X2	T38.7X3	T38.7X4	T38.7X5	T38.7X6
Naphazoline	T48.5X1	T48.5X2	T48.5X3	T48.5X4	T48.5X5	T48.5X6
Naphtha (painters') (petroleum)	T52.0X1	T52.0X2	T52.0X3	T52.0X4	--	--
solvent	T52.0X1	T52.0X2	T52.0X3	T52.0X4	--	--
vapor	T52.0X1	T52.0X2	T52.0X3	T52.0X4	--	--
Naphthalene (non-chlorinated)	T60.2X1	T60.2X2	T60.2X3	T60.2X4	--	--
chlorinated	T60.1X1	T60.1X2	T60.1X3	T60.1X4	--	--
vapor	T60.1X1	T60.1X2	T60.1X3	T60.1X4	--	--
insecticide or moth repellent	T60.2X1	T60.2X2	T60.2X3	T60.2X4	--	--
chlorinated	T60.1X1	T60.1X2	T60.1X3	T60.1X4	--	--
vapor	T60.2X1	T60.2X2	T60.2X3	T60.2X4	--	--
chlorinated	T60.1X1	T60.1X2	T60.1X3	T60.1X4	--	--
Naphthol	T65.891	T65.892	T65.893	T65.894	--	--
Naphthylamine	T65.891	T65.892	T65.893	T65.894	--	--
Naphthylthiourea (ANTU)	T60.4X1	T60.4X2	T60.4X3	T60.4X4	--	--
Naprosyn — see Naproxen						
Naproxen	T39.311	T39.312	T39.313	T39.314	T39.315	T39.316
Narcotic (drug)	T40.601	T40.602	T40.603	T40.604	T40.605	T40.606
analgesic NEC	T40.601	T40.602	T40.603	T40.604	T40.605	T40.606
antagonist	T50.7X1	T50.7X2	T50.7X3	T50.7X4	T50.7X5	T50.7X6
specified NEC	T40.691	T40.692	T40.693	T40.694	T40.695	T40.696
synthetic	T40.4X1	T40.4X2	T40.4X3	T40.4X4	T40.4X5	T40.4X6
Narcotine	T48.3X1	T48.3X2	T48.3X3	T48.3X4	T48.3X5	T48.3X6
Nardil	T43.1X1	T43.1X2	T43.1X3	T43.1X4	T43.1X5	T43.1X6
Nasal drug NEC	T49.6X1	T49.6X2	T49.6X3	T49.6X4	T49.6X5	T49.6X6
Natamycin	T49.0X1	T49.0X2	T49.0X3	T49.0X4	T49.0X5	T49.0X6
Natrium cyanide — see Cyanide(s)						
Natural						
blood (product)	T45.8X1	T45.8X2	T45.8X3	T45.8X4	T45.8X5	T45.8X6
gas (piped)	T59.891	T59.892	T59.893	T59.894	--	--
incomplete combustion	T58.11	T58.12	T58.13	T58.14	--	--
Nealbarbital	T42.3X1	T42.3X2	T42.3X3	T42.3X4	T42.3X5	T42.3X6
Nectadon	T48.3X1	T48.3X2	T48.3X3	T48.3X4	T48.3X5	T48.3X6
Nedocromil	T48.6X1	T48.6X2	T48.6X3	T48.6X4	T48.6X5	T48.6X6
Nefopam	T39.8X1	T39.8X2	T39.8X3	T39.8X4	T39.8X5	T39.8X6
Nematocyst (sting)	T63.691	T63.692	T63.693	T63.694	--	--
Nembutal	T42.3X1	T42.3X2	T42.3X3	T42.3X4	T42.3X5	T42.3X6
Nemonapride	T43.591	T43.592	T43.593	T43.594	T43.595	T43.596
Neoarsphenamine	T37.8X1	T37.8X2	T37.8X3	T37.8X4	T37.8X5	T37.8X6
Neocinchophen	T50.4X1	T50.4X2	T50.4X3	T50.4X4	T50.4X5	T50.4X6
Neomycin (derivatives)	T36.5X1	T36.5X2	T36.5X3	T36.5X4	T36.5X5	T36.5X6
with						
bacitracin	T49.0X1	T49.0X2	T49.0X3	T49.0X4	T49.0X5	T49.0X6
neostigmine	T44.0X1	T44.0X2	T44.0X3	T44.0X4	T44.0X5	T44.0X6
ENT agent	T49.6X1	T49.6X2	T49.6X3	T49.6X4	T49.6X5	T49.6X6
ophthalmic preparation	T49.5X1	T49.5X2	T49.5X3	T49.5X4	T49.5X5	T49.5X6
topical NEC	T49.0X1	T49.0X2	T49.0X3	T49.0X4	T49.0X5	T49.0X6
Neonal	T42.3X1	T42.3X2	T42.3X3	T42.3X4	T42.3X5	T42.3X6
Neoprontosil	T37.0X1	T37.0X2	T37.0X3	T37.0X4	T37.0X5	T37.0X6
Neosalvarsan	T37.8X1	T37.8X2	T37.8X3	T37.8X4	T37.8X5	T37.8X6
Neosilversalvarsan	T37.8X1	T37.8X2	T37.8X3	T37.8X4	T37.8X5	T37.8X6
Neosporin	T36.8X1	T36.8X2	T36.8X3	T36.8X4	T36.8X5	T36.8X6
ENT agent	T49.6X1	T49.6X2	T49.6X3	T49.6X4	T49.6X5	T49.6X6
ophthalmic preparation	T49.5X1	T49.5X2	T49.5X3	T49.5X4	T49.5X5	T49.5X6
topical NEC	T49.0X1	T49.0X2	T49.0X3	T49.0X4	T49.0X5	T49.0X6
Neostigmine bromide	T44.0X1	T44.0X2	T44.0X3	T44.0X4	T44.0X5	T44.0X6
Neraval	T42.3X1	T42.3X2	T42.3X3	T42.3X4	T42.3X5	T42.3X6
Neravan	T42.3X1	T42.3X2	T42.3X3	T42.3X4	T42.3X5	T42.3X6
Nerium oleander	T62.2X1	T62.2X2	T62.2X3	T62.2X4	--	--
Nerve gas, not in war	T59.91	T59.92	T59.93	T59.94	--	--
Nesacaine	T41.3X1	T41.3X2	T41.3X3	T41.3X4	T41.3X5	T41.3X6
infiltration (subcutaneous)	T41.3X1	T41.3X2	T41.3X3	T41.3X4	T41.3X5	T41.3X6
nerve block (peripheral) (plexus)	T41.3X1	T41.3X2	T41.3X3	T41.3X4	T41.3X5	T41.3X6
Netilmicin	T36.5X1	T36.5X2	T36.5X3	T36.5X4	T36.5X5	T36.5X6
Neurobarb	T42.3X1	T42.3X2	T42.3X3	T42.3X4	T42.3X5	T42.3X6
Neuroleptic drug NEC	T43.501	T43.502	T43.503	T43.504	T43.505	T43.506

Neuromuscular blocking drug - Octotiamine

Substance	Poisoning, Accidental unintentional	Poisoning, Intentional self-harm	Poisoning, Assault	Poisoning, Undetermined	Adverse effect	Underdosing
Neuromuscular blocking drug	T48.1X1	T48.1X2	T48.1X3	T48.1X4	T48.1X5	T48.1X6
Neutral insulin injection	T38.3X1	T38.3X2	T38.3X3	T38.3X4	T38.3X5	T38.3X6
Neutral spirits	T51.0X1	T51.0X2	T51.0X3	T51.0X4	--	--
beverage	T51.0X1	T51.0X2	T51.0X3	T51.0X4	--	--
Niacin	T46.7X1	T46.7X2	T46.7X3	T46.7X4	T46.7X5	T46.7X6
Niacinamide	T45.2X1	T45.2X2	T45.2X3	T45.2X4	T45.2X5	T45.2X6
Nialamide	T43.1X1	T43.1X2	T43.1X3	T43.1X4	T43.1X5	T43.1X6
Niaprazine	T42.6X1	T42.6X2	T42.6X3	T42.6X4	T42.6X5	T42.6X6
Nicametate	T46.7X1	T46.7X2	T46.7X3	T46.7X4	T46.7X5	T46.7X6
Nicardipine	T46.1X1	T46.1X2	T46.1X3	T46.1X4	T46.1X5	T46.1X6
Nicergoline	T46.7X1	T46.7X2	T46.7X3	T46.7X4	T46.7X5	T46.7X6
Nickel (carbonyl) (tetra-carbonyl)(fumes) (vapor)	T56.891	T56.892	T56.893	T56.894	--	--
Nickelocene	T56.891	T56.892	T56.893	T56.894	--	--
Niclosamide	T37.4X1	T37.4X2	T37.4X3	T37.4X4	T37.4X5	T37.4X6
Nicofuranose	T46.7X1	T46.7X2	T46.7X3	T46.7X4	T46.7X5	T46.7X6
Nicomorphine	T40.2X1	T40.2X2	T40.2X3	T40.2X4	--	--
Nicorandil	T46.3X1	T46.3X2	T46.3X3	T46.3X4	T46.3X5	T46.3X6
Nicotiana (plant)	T62.2X1	T62.2X2	T62.2X3	T62.2X4	--	--
Nicotinamide	T45.2X1	T45.2X2	T45.2X3	T45.2X4	T45.2X5	T45.2X6
Nicotine (insecticide) (spray) (sulfate) NEC	T60.2X1	T60.2X2	T60.2X3	T60.2X4	--	--
from tobacco	T65.291	T65.292	T65.293	T65.294	--	--
cigarettes	T65.221	T65.222	T65.223	T65.224	--	--
not insecticide	T65.291	T65.292	T65.293	T65.294	--	--
Nicotinic acid	T46.7X1	T46.7X2	T46.7X3	T46.7X4	T46.7X5	T46.7X6
Nicotinyl alcohol	T46.7X1	T46.7X2	T46.7X3	T46.7X4	T46.7X5	T46.7X6
Nicoumalone	T45.511	T45.512	T45.513	T45.514	T45.515	T45.516
Nifedipine	T46.1X1	T46.1X2	T46.1X3	T46.1X4	T46.1X5	T46.1X6
Nifenazone	T39.2X1	T39.2X2	T39.2X3	T39.2X4	T39.2X5	T39.2X6
Nifuraldezone	T37.91	T37.92	T37.93	T37.94	T37.95	T37.96
Nifuratel	T37.8X1	T37.8X2	T37.8X3	T37.8X4	T37.8X5	T37.8X6
Nifurtimox	T37.3X1	T37.3X2	T37.3X3	T37.3X4	T37.3X5	T37.3X6
Nifurtoinol	T37.8X1	T37.8X2	T37.8X3	T37.8X4	T37.8X5	T37.8X6
Nightshade, deadly (solanum) (see also Belladonna)	T62.2X1	T62.2X2	T62.2X3	T62.2X4	--	--
berry	T62.1X1	T62.1X2	T62.1X3	T62.1X4	--	--
Nikethamide	T50.7X1	T50.7X2	T50.7X3	T50.7X4	T50.7X5	T50.7X6
Nilstat	T36.7X1	T36.7X2	T36.7X3	T36.7X4	T36.7X5	T36.7X6
topical	T49.0X1	T49.0X2	T49.0X3	T49.0X4	T49.0X5	T49.0X6
Nilutamide	T38.6X1	T38.6X2	T38.6X3	T38.6X4	T38.6X5	T38.6X6
Nimesulide	T39.391	T39.392	T39.393	T39.394	T39.395	T39.396
Nimetazepam	T42.4X1	T42.4X2	T42.4X3	T42.4X4	T42.4X5	T42.4X6
Nimodipine	T46.1X1	T46.1X2	T46.1X3	T46.1X4	T46.1X5	T46.1X6
Nimorazole	T37.3X1	T37.3X2	T37.3X3	T37.3X4	T37.3X5	T37.3X6
Nimustine	T45.1X1	T45.1X2	T45.1X3	T45.1X4	T45.1X5	T45.1X6
Niridazole	T37.4X1	T37.4X2	T37.4X3	T37.4X4	T37.4X5	T37.4X6
Nisentil	T40.2X1	T40.2X2	T40.2X3	T40.2X4	T40.2X5	T40.2X6
Nisoldipine	T46.1X1	T46.1X2	T46.1X3	T46.1X4	T46.1X5	T46.1X6
Nitramine	T65.3X1	T65.3X2	T65.3X3	T65.3X4	--	--
Nitrate, organic	T46.3X1	T46.3X2	T46.3X3	T46.3X4	T46.3X5	T46.3X6
Nitrazepam	T42.4X1	T42.4X2	T42.4X3	T42.4X4	T42.4X5	T42.4X6
Nitrefazole	T50.6X1	T50.6X2	T50.6X3	T50.6X4	T50.6X5	T50.6X6
Nitrendipine	T46.1X1	T46.1X2	T46.1X3	T46.1X4	T46.1X5	T46.1X6
Nitric						
acid (liquid)	T54.2X1	T54.2X2	T54.2X3	T54.2X4	--	--
vapor	T59.891	T59.892	T59.893	T59.894	--	--
oxide (gas)	T59.0X1	T59.0X2	T59.0X3	T59.0X4	--	--
Nitrimidazine	T37.3X1	T37.3X2	T37.3X3	T37.3X4	T37.3X5	T37.3X6
Nitrite, amyl (medicinal) (vapor)	T46.3X1	T46.3X2	T46.3X3	T46.3X4	T46.3X5	T46.3X6
Nitroaniline	T65.3X1	T65.3X2	T65.3X3	T65.3X4	--	--
vapor	T59.891	T59.892	T59.893	T59.894	--	--
Nitrobenzene, nitrobenzol	T65.3X1	T65.3X2	T65.3X3	T65.3X4	--	--
vapor	T65.3X1	T65.3X2	T65.3X3	T65.3X4	--	--
Nitrocellulose	T65.891	T65.892	T65.893	T65.894	--	--
lacquer	T65.891	T65.892	T65.893	T65.894	--	--
Nitrodiphenyl	T65.3X1	T65.3X2	T65.3X3	T65.3X4	--	--
Nitrofural	T49.0X1	T49.0X2	T49.0X3	T49.0X4	T49.0X5	T49.0X6
Nitrofurantoin	T37.8X1	T37.8X2	T37.8X3	T37.8X4	T37.8X5	T37.8X6
Nitrofurazone	T49.0X1	T49.0X2	T49.0X3	T49.0X4	T49.0X5	T49.0X6
Nitrogen	T59.0X1	T59.0X2	T59.0X3	T59.0X4	--	--
mustard	T45.1X1	T45.1X2	T45.1X3	T45.1X4	T45.1X5	T45.1X6
Nitroglycerin, nitro-glycerol (medicinal)	T46.3X1	T46.3X2	T46.3X3	T46.3X4	T46.3X5	T46.3X6
nonmedicinal	T65.5X1	T65.5X2	T65.5X3	T65.5X4	--	--
fumes	T65.5X1	T65.5X2	T65.5X3	T65.5X4	--	--
Nitroglycol	T52.3X1	T52.3X2	T52.3X3	T52.3X4	--	--
Nitrohydrochloric acid	T54.2X1	T54.2X2	T54.2X3	T54.2X4	--	--
Nitromersol	T49.0X1	T49.0X2	T49.0X3	T49.0X4	T49.0X5	T49.0X6
Nitronaphthalene	T65.891	T65.892	T65.893	T65.894	--	--
Nitrophenol	T54.0X1	T54.0X2	T54.0X3	T54.0X4	--	--

Substance	Poisoning, Accidental unintentional	Poisoning, Intentional self-harm	Poisoning, Assault	Poisoning, Undetermined	Adverse effect	Underdosing
Nitropropane	T52.8X1	T52.8X2	T52.8X3	T52.8X4	--	--
Nitroprusside	T46.5X1	T46.5X2	T46.5X3	T46.5X4	T46.5X5	T46.5X6
Nitrosodimethylamine	T65.3X1	T65.3X2	T65.3X3	T65.3X4	--	--
Nitrothiazol	T37.4X1	T37.4X2	T37.4X3	T37.4X4	T37.4X5	T37.4X6
Nitrotoluene, nitrotoluol	T65.3X1	T65.3X2	T65.3X3	T65.3X4	--	--
vapor	T65.3X1	T65.3X2	T65.3X3	T65.3X4	--	--
Nitrous						
acid (liquid)	T54.2X1	T54.2X2	T54.2X3	T54.2X4	--	--
fumes	T59.891	T59.892	T59.893	T59.894	--	--
ether spirit	T46.3X1	T46.3X2	T46.3X3	T46.3X4	T46.3X5	T46.3X6
oxide	T41.0X1	T41.0X2	T41.0X3	T41.0X4	T41.0X5	T41.0X6
Nitroxoline	T37.8X1	T37.8X2	T37.8X3	T37.8X4	T37.8X5	T37.8X6
Nitrozone	T49.0X1	T49.0X2	T49.0X3	T49.0X4	T49.0X5	T49.0X6
Nizatidine	T47.0X1	T47.0X2	T47.0X3	T47.0X4	T47.0X5	T47.0X6
Nizofenone	T43.8X1	T43.8X2	T43.8X3	T43.8X4	T43.8X5	T43.8X6
Noctec	T42.6X1	T42.6X2	T42.6X3	T42.6X4	T42.6X5	T42.6X6
Noludar	T42.6X1	T42.6X2	T42.6X3	T42.6X4	T42.6X5	T42.6X6
Nomegestrol	T38.5X1	T38.5X2	T38.5X3	T38.5X4	T38.5X5	T38.5X6
Nomifensine	T43.291	T43.292	T43.293	T43.294	T43.295	T43.296
Nonoxinol	T49.8X1	T49.8X2	T49.8X3	T49.8X4	T49.8X5	T49.8X6
Nonylphenoxy (polyethoxy-ethanol)	T49.8X1	T49.8X2	T49.8X3	T49.8X4	T49.8X5	T49.8X6
Noptil	T42.3X1	T42.3X2	T42.3X3	T42.3X4	T42.3X5	T42.3X6
Noradrenaline	T44.4X1	T44.4X2	T44.4X3	T44.4X4	T44.4X5	T44.4X6
Noramidopyrine	T39.2X1	T39.2X2	T39.2X3	T39.2X4	T39.2X5	T39.2X6
methanesulfonate sodium	T39.2X1	T39.2X2	T39.2X3	T39.2X4	T39.2X5	T39.2X6
Norbormide	T60.4X1	T60.4X2	T60.4X3	T60.4X4	--	--
Nordazepam	T42.4X1	T42.4X2	T42.4X3	T42.4X4	T42.4X5	T42.4X6
Norepinephrine	T44.4X1	T44.4X2	T44.4X3	T44.4X4	T44.4X5	T44.4X6
Norethandrolone	T38.7X1	T38.7X2	T38.7X3	T38.7X4	T38.7X5	T38.7X6
Norethindrone	T38.4X1	T38.4X2	T38.4X3	T38.4X4	T38.4X5	T38.4X6
Norethisterone (acetate) (enantate)	T38.4X1	T38.4X2	T38.4X3	T38.4X4	T38.4X5	T38.4X6
with ethinylestradiol	T38.5X1	T38.5X2	T38.5X3	T38.5X4	T38.5X5	T38.5X6
Noretynodrel	T38.5X1	T38.5X2	T38.5X3	T38.5X4	T38.5X5	T38.5X6
Norfenefrine	T44.4X1	T44.4X2	T44.4X3	T44.4X4	T44.4X5	T44.4X6
Norfloxacin	T36.8X1	T36.8X2	T36.8X3	T36.8X4	T36.8X5	T36.8X6
Norgestrel	T38.4X1	T38.4X2	T38.4X3	T38.4X4	T38.4X5	T38.4X6
Norgestrienone	T38.4X1	T38.4X2	T38.4X3	T38.4X4	T38.4X5	T38.4X6
Norlestrin	T38.4X1	T38.4X2	T38.4X3	T38.4X4	T38.4X5	T38.4X6
Norlutin	T38.4X1	T38.4X2	T38.4X3	T38.4X4	T38.4X5	T38.4X6
Normal serum albumin (human), salt-poor	T45.8X1	T45.8X2	T45.8X3	T45.8X4	T45.8X5	T45.8X6
Normethandrone	T38.5X1	T38.5X2	T38.5X3	T38.5X4	T38.5X5	T38.5X6
Normison — see Benzodiazepines						
Normorphine	T40.2X1	T40.2X2	T40.2X3	T40.2X4	--	--
Norpseudoephedrine	T50.5X1	T50.5X2	T50.5X3	T50.5X4	T50.5X5	T50.5X6
Nortestosterone (furanpropionate)	T38.7X1	T38.7X2	T38.7X3	T38.7X4	T38.7X5	T38.7X6
Nortriptyline	T43.011	T43.012	T43.013	T43.014	T43.015	T43.016
Noscapine	T48.3X1	T48.3X2	T48.3X3	T48.3X4	T48.3X5	T48.3X6
Nose preparations	T49.6X1	T49.6X2	T49.6X3	T49.6X4	T49.6X5	T49.6X6
Novobiocin	T36.5X1	T36.5X2	T36.5X3	T36.5X4	T36.5X5	T36.5X6
Novocain (infiltration) (topical)	T41.3X1	T41.3X2	T41.3X3	T41.3X4	T41.3X5	T41.3X6
nerve block (peripheral) (plexus)	T41.3X1	T41.3X2	T41.3X3	T41.3X4	T41.3X5	T41.3X6
spinal	T41.3X1	T41.3X2	T41.3X3	T41.3X4	T41.3X5	T41.3X6
Noxious foodstuff	T62.91	T62.92	T62.93	T62.94	--	--
specified NEC	T62.8X1	T62.8X2	T62.8X3	T62.8X4	--	--
Noxiptiline	T43.011	T43.012	T43.013	T43.014	T43.015	T43.016
Noxytiolin	T49.0X1	T49.0X2	T49.0X3	T49.0X4	T49.0X5	T49.0X6
NPH Iletin (insulin)	T38.3X1	T38.3X2	T38.3X3	T38.3X4	T38.3X5	T38.3X6
Numorphan	T40.2X1	T40.2X2	T40.2X3	T40.2X4	T40.2X5	T40.2X6
Nunol	T42.3X1	T42.3X2	T42.3X3	T42.3X4	T42.3X5	T42.3X6
Nupercaine (spinal anesthetic)	T41.3X1	T41.3X2	T41.3X3	T41.3X4	T41.3X5	T41.3X6
topical (surface)	T41.3X1	T41.3X2	T41.3X3	T41.3X4	T41.3X5	T41.3X6
Nutmeg oil (liniment)	T49.3X1	T49.3X2	T49.3X3	T49.3X4	T49.3X5	T49.3X6
Nutritional supplement	T50.901	T50.902	T50.903	T50.904	T50.905	T50.906
Nux vomica	T65.1X1	T65.1X2	T65.1X3	T65.1X4	--	--
Nydrazid	T37.1X1	T37.1X2	T37.1X3	T37.1X4	T37.1X5	T37.1X6
Nylidrin	T46.7X1	T46.7X2	T46.7X3	T46.7X4	T46.7X5	T46.7X6
Nystatin	T36.7X1	T36.7X2	T36.7X3	T36.7X4	T36.7X5	T36.7X6
topical	T49.0X1	T49.0X2	T49.0X3	T49.0X4	T49.0X5	T49.0X6
Nytol	T45.0X1	T45.0X2	T45.0X3	T45.0X4	T45.0X5	T45.0X6
O						
Obidoxime chloride	T50.6X1	T50.6X2	T50.6X3	T50.6X4	T50.6X5	T50.6X6
Octafonium (chloride)	T49.3X1	T49.3X2	T49.3X3	T49.3X4	T49.3X5	T49.3X6
Octamethyl pyrophos-phoramide	T60.0X1	T60.0X2	T60.0X3	T60.0X4	--	--
Octanoin	T50.991	T50.992	T50.993	T50.994	T50.995	T50.996
Octatropine methyl-bromide	T44.3X1	T44.3X2	T44.3X3	T44.3X4	T44.3X5	T44.3X6
Octotiamine	T45.2X1	T45.2X2	T45.2X3	T45.2X4	T45.2X5	T45.2X6

Neuromuscular blocking drug - Octotiamine

ICD-10-CM TABLE OF DRUGS AND CHEMICALS

Substance	Poisoning, Accidental unintentional	Poisoning, Intentional self-harm	Poisoning, Assault	Poisoning, Undetermined	Adverse effect	Underdosing
Octoxinol (9)	T49.8X1	T49.8X2	T49.8X3	T49.8X4	T49.8X5	T49.8X6
Octreotide	T38.991	T38.992	T38.993	T38.994	T38.995	T38.996
Octyl nitrite	T46.3X1	T46.3X2	T46.3X3	T46.3X4	T46.3X5	T46.3X6
Oestradiol	T38.5X1	T38.5X2	T38.5X3	T38.5X4	T38.5X5	T38.5X6
Oestriol	T38.5X1	T38.5X2	T38.5X3	T38.5X4	T38.5X5	T38.5X6
Oestrogen	T38.5X1	T38.5X2	T38.5X3	T38.5X4	T38.5X5	T38.5X6
Oestrone	T38.5X1	T38.5X2	T38.5X3	T38.5X4	T38.5X5	T38.5X6
Ofloxacin	T36.8X1	T36.8X2	T36.8X3	T36.8X4	T36.8X5	T36.8X6
Oil (of)	T65.891	T65.892	T65.893	T65.894	--	--
bitter almond	T62.8X1	T62.8X2	T62.8X3	T62.8X4	--	--
cloves	T49.7X1	T49.7X2	T49.7X3	T49.7X4	T49.7X5	T49.7X6
colors	T65.6X1	T65.6X2	T65.6X3	T65.6X4	--	--
fumes	T59.891	T59.892	T59.893	T59.894	--	--
lubricating	T52.0X1	T52.0X2	T52.0X3	T52.0X4	--	--
Niobe	T52.8X1	T52.8X2	T52.8X3	T52.8X4	--	--
vitriol (liquid)	T54.2X1	T54.2X2	T54.2X3	T54.2X4	--	--
fumes	T54.2X1	T54.2X2	T54.2X3	T54.2X4	--	--
wintergreen (bitter) NEC	T49.3X1	T49.3X2	T49.3X3	T49.3X4	T49.3X5	T49.3X6
Oily preparation (for skin)	T49.3X1	T49.3X2	T49.3X3	T49.3X4	T49.3X5	T49.3X6
Ointment NEC	T49.3X1	T49.3X2	T49.3X3	T49.3X4	T49.3X5	T49.3X6
Olanzapine	T43.591	T43.592	T43.593	T43.594	T43.595	T43.596
Oleander	T62.2X1	T62.2X2	T62.2X3	T62.2X4	--	--
Oleandomycin	T36.3X1	T36.3X2	T36.3X3	T36.3X4	T36.3X5	T36.3X6
Oleandrin	T46.0X1	T46.0X2	T46.0X3	T46.0X4	T46.0X5	T46.0X6
Oleic acid	T46.6X1	T46.6X2	T46.6X3	T46.6X4	T46.6X5	T46.6X6
Oleovitamin A	T45.2X1	T45.2X2	T45.2X3	T45.2X4	T45.2X5	T45.2X6
Oleum ricini	T47.2X1	T47.2X2	T47.2X3	T47.2X4	T47.2X5	T47.2X6
Olive oil (medicinal) NEC	T47.4X1	T47.4X2	T47.4X3	T47.4X4	T47.4X5	T47.4X6
Olivomycin	T45.1X1	T45.1X2	T45.1X3	T45.1X4	T45.1X5	T45.1X6
Olsalazine	T47.8X1	T47.8X2	T47.8X3	T47.8X4	T47.8X5	T47.8X6
Omeprazole	T47.1X1	T47.1X2	T47.1X3	T47.1X4	T47.1X5	T47.1X6
OMPA	T60.0X1	T60.0X2	T60.0X3	T60.0X4	--	--
Oncovin	T45.1X1	T45.1X2	T45.1X3	T45.1X4	T45.1X5	T45.1X6
Ondansetron	T45.0X1	T45.0X2	T45.0X3	T45.0X4	T45.0X5	T45.0X6
Ophthaine	T41.3X1	T41.3X2	T41.3X3	T41.3X4	T41.3X5	T41.3X6
Ophthetic	T41.3X1	T41.3X2	T41.3X3	T41.3X4	T41.3X5	T41.3X6
Opiate NEC	T40.601	T40.602	T40.603	T40.604	T40.605	T40.606
antagonists	T50.7X1	T50.7X2	T50.7X3	T50.7X4	T50.7X5	T50.7X6
Opioid NEC	T40.2X1	T40.2X2	T40.2X3	T40.2X4	T40.2X5	T40.2X6
Opipramol	T43.011	T43.012	T43.013	T43.014	T43.015	T43.016
Opium alkaloids (total)	T40.0X1	T40.0X2	T40.0X3	T40.0X4	T40.0X5	T40.0X6
standardized powdered	T40.0X1	T40.0X2	T40.0X3	T40.0X4	T40.0X5	T40.0X6
tincture (camphorated)	T40.0X1	T40.0X2	T40.0X3	T40.0X4	T40.0X5	T40.0X6
Oracon	T38.4X1	T38.4X2	T38.4X3	T38.4X4	T38.4X5	T38.4X6
Oragrafin	T50.8X1	T50.8X2	T50.8X3	T50.8X4	T50.8X5	T50.8X6
Oral contraceptives	T38.4X1	T38.4X2	T38.4X3	T38.4X4	T38.4X5	T38.4X6
Oral rehydration salts	T50.3X1	T50.3X2	T50.3X3	T50.3X4	T50.3X5	T50.3X6
Orazamide	T50.991	T50.992	T50.993	T50.994	T50.995	T50.996
Orciprenaline	T48.291	T48.292	T48.293	T48.294	T48.295	T48.296
Organidin	T48.4X1	T48.4X2	T48.4X3	T48.4X4	T48.4X5	T48.4X6
Organonitrate NEC	T46.3X1	T46.3X2	T46.3X3	T46.3X4	T46.3X5	T46.3X6
Organophosphates	T60.0X1	T60.0X2	T60.0X3	T60.0X4	--	--
Orimune	T50.B91	T50.B92	T50.B93	T50.B94	T50.B95	T50.B96
Orinase	T38.3X1	T38.3X2	T38.3X3	T38.3X4	T38.3X5	T38.3X6
Ormeloxifene	T38.6X1	T38.6X2	T38.6X3	T38.6X4	T38.6X5	T38.6X6
Ornidazole	T37.3X1	T37.3X2	T37.3X3	T37.3X4	T37.3X5	T37.3X6
Ornithine aspartate	T50.991	T50.992	T50.993	T50.994	T50.995	T50.996
Ornoprostil	T47.1X1	T47.1X2	T47.1X3	T47.1X4	T47.1X5	T47.1X6
Orphenadrine (hydrochloride)	T42.8X1	T42.8X2	T42.8X3	T42.8X4	T42.8X5	T42.8X6
Ortal (sodium)	T42.3X1	T42.3X2	T42.3X3	T42.3X4	T42.3X5	T42.3X6
Orthoboric acid	T49.0X1	T49.0X2	T49.0X3	T49.0X4	T49.0X5	T49.0X6
ENT agent	T49.6X1	T49.6X2	T49.6X3	T49.6X4	T49.6X5	T49.6X6
ophthalmic preparation	T49.5X1	T49.5X2	T49.5X3	T49.5X4	T49.5X5	T49.5X6
Orthocaine	T41.3X1	T41.3X2	T41.3X3	T41.3X4	T41.3X5	T41.3X6
Orthodichlorobenzene	T53.7X1	T53.7X2	T53.7X3	T53.7X4	--	--
Ortho-Novum	T38.4X1	T38.4X2	T38.4X3	T38.4X4	T38.4X5	T38.4X6
Orthotolidine (reagent)	T54.2X1	T54.2X2	T54.2X3	T54.2X4	--	--
Osmic acid (liquid)	T54.2X1	T54.2X2	T54.2X3	T54.2X4	--	--
fumes	T54.2X1	T54.2X2	T54.2X3	T54.2X4	--	--
Osmotic diuretics	T50.2X1	T50.2X2	T50.2X3	T50.2X4	T50.2X5	T50.2X6
Otilonium bromide	T44.3X1	T44.3X2	T44.3X3	T44.3X4	T44.3X5	T44.3X6
Otorhinolaryngological drug NEC	T49.6X1	T49.6X2	T49.6X3	T49.6X4	T49.6X5	T49.6X6
Ouabain (e)	T46.0X1	T46.0X2	T46.0X3	T46.0X4	T46.0X5	T46.0X6
Ovarian						
hormone	T38.5X1	T38.5X2	T38.5X3	T38.5X4	T38.5X5	T38.5X6
stimulant	T38.5X1	T38.5X2	T38.5X3	T38.5X4	T38.5X5	T38.5X6
Ovral	T38.4X1	T38.4X2	T38.4X3	T38.4X4	T38.4X5	T38.4X6
Ovulen	T38.4X1	T38.4X2	T38.4X3	T38.4X4	T38.4X5	T38.4X6
Oxacillin	T36.0X1	T36.0X2	T36.0X3	T36.0X4	T36.0X5	T36.0X6
Oxalic acid	T54.2X1	T54.2X2	T54.2X3	T54.2X4	--	--
ammonium salt	T50.991	T50.992	T50.993	T50.994	T50.995	T50.996
Oxamniquine	T37.4X1	T37.4X2	T37.4X3	T37.4X4	T37.4X5	T37.4X6
Oxanamide	T43.591	T43.592	T43.593	T43.594	T43.595	T43.596

Substance	Poisoning, Accidental unintentional	Poisoning, Intentional self-harm	Poisoning, Assault	Poisoning, Undetermined	Adverse effect	Underdosing
Oxandrolone	T38.7X1	T38.7X2	T38.7X3	T38.7X4	T38.7X5	T38.7X6
Oxantel	T37.4X1	T37.4X2	T37.4X3	T37.4X4	T37.4X5	T37.4X6
Oxapium iodide	T44.3X1	T44.3X2	T44.3X3	T44.3X4	T44.3X5	T44.3X6
Oxaprotiline	T43.021	T43.022	T43.023	T43.024	T43.025	T43.026
Oxaprozin	T39.311	T39.312	T39.313	T39.314	T39.315	T39.316
Oxatomide	T45.0X1	T45.0X2	T45.0X3	T45.0X4	T45.0X5	T45.0X6
Oxazepam	T42.4X1	T42.4X2	T42.4X3	T42.4X4	T42.4X5	T42.4X6
Oxazimedrine	T50.5X1	T50.5X2	T50.5X3	T50.5X4	T50.5X5	T50.5X6
Oxazolam	T42.4X1	T42.4X2	T42.4X3	T42.4X4	T42.4X5	T42.4X6
Oxazolidine derivatives	T42.2X1	T42.2X2	T42.2X3	T42.2X4	T42.2X5	T42.2X6
Oxazolidinedione (derivative)	T42.2X1	T42.2X2	T42.2X3	T42.2X4	T42.2X5	T42.2X6
Ox bile extract	T47.5X1	T47.5X2	T47.5X3	T47.5X4	T47.5X5	T47.5X6
Oxcarbazepine	T42.1X1	T42.1X2	T42.1X3	T42.1X4	T42.1X5	T42.1X6
Oxedrine	T44.4X1	T44.4X2	T44.4X3	T44.4X4	T44.4X5	T44.4X6
Oxeladin (citrate)	T48.3X1	T48.3X2	T48.3X3	T48.3X4	T48.3X5	T48.3X6
Oxendolone	T38.5X1	T38.5X2	T38.5X3	T38.5X4	T38.5X5	T38.5X6
Oxetacaine	T41.3X1	T41.3X2	T41.3X3	T41.3X4	T41.3X5	T41.3X6
Oxethazine	T41.3X1	T41.3X2	T41.3X3	T41.3X4	T41.3X5	T41.3X6
Oxetorone	T39.8X1	T39.8X2	T39.8X3	T39.8X4	T39.8X5	T39.8X6
Oxiconazole	T49.0X1	T49.0X2	T49.0X3	T49.0X4	T49.0X5	T49.0X6
Oxidizing agent NEC	T54.91	T54.92	T54.93	T54.94	--	--
Oxipurinol	T50.4X1	T50.4X2	T50.4X3	T50.4X4	T50.4X5	T50.4X6
Oxitriptan	T43.291	T43.292	T43.293	T43.294	T43.295	T43.296
Oxitropium bromide	T48.6X1	T48.6X2	T48.6X3	T48.6X4	T48.6X5	T48.6X6
Oxodipine	T46.1X1	T46.1X2	T46.1X3	T46.1X4	T46.1X5	T46.1X6
Oxolamine	T48.3X1	T48.3X2	T48.3X3	T48.3X4	T48.3X5	T48.3X6
Oxolinic acid	T37.8X1	T37.8X2	T37.8X3	T37.8X4	T37.8X5	T37.8X6
Oxomemazine	T43.3X1	T43.3X2	T43.3X3	T43.3X4	T43.3X5	T43.3X6
Oxophenarsine	T37.3X1	T37.3X2	T37.3X3	T37.3X4	T37.3X5	T37.3X6
Oxprenolol	T44.7X1	T44.7X2	T44.7X3	T44.7X4	T44.7X5	T44.7X6
Oxsoralen	T49.3X1	T49.3X2	T49.3X3	T49.3X4	T49.3X5	T49.3X6
Oxtriphylline	T48.6X1	T48.6X2	T48.6X3	T48.6X4	T48.6X5	T48.6X6
Oxybate sodium	T41.291	T41.292	T41.293	T41.294	T41.295	T41.296
Oxybuprocaine	T41.3X1	T41.3X2	T41.3X3	T41.3X4	T41.3X5	T41.3X6
Oxybutynin	T44.3X1	T44.3X2	T44.3X3	T44.3X4	T44.3X5	T44.3X6
Oxychlorosene	T49.0X1	T49.0X2	T49.0X3	T49.0X4	T49.0X5	T49.0X6
Oxycodone	T40.2X1	T40.2X2	T40.2X3	T40.2X4	T40.2X5	T40.2X6
Oxyfedrine	T46.3X1	T46.3X2	T46.3X3	T46.3X4	T46.3X5	T46.3X6
Oxygen	T41.5X1	T41.5X2	T41.5X3	T41.5X4	T41.5X5	T41.5X6
Oxylone	T49.0X1	T49.0X2	T49.0X3	T49.0X4	T49.0X5	T49.0X6
ophthalmic preparation	T49.5X1	T49.5X2	T49.5X3	T49.5X4	T49.5X5	T49.5X6
Oxymesterone	T38.7X1	T38.7X2	T38.7X3	T38.7X4	T38.7X5	T38.7X6
Oxymetazoline	T48.5X1	T48.5X2	T48.5X3	T48.5X4	T48.5X5	T48.5X6
Oxymetholone	T38.7X1	T38.7X2	T38.7X3	T38.7X4	T38.7X5	T38.7X6
Oxymorphone	T40.2X1	T40.2X2	T40.2X3	T40.2X4	T40.2X5	T40.2X6
Oxypertine	T43.591	T43.592	T43.593	T43.594	T43.595	T43.596
Oxyphenbutazone	T39.2X1	T39.2X2	T39.2X3	T39.2X4	T39.2X5	T39.2X6
Oxyphencyclimine	T44.3X1	T44.3X2	T44.3X3	T44.3X4	T44.3X5	T44.3X6
Oxyphenisatine	T47.2X1	T47.2X2	T47.2X3	T47.2X4	T47.2X5	T47.2X6
Oxyphenonium bromide	T44.3X1	T44.3X2	T44.3X3	T44.3X4	T44.3X5	T44.3X6
Oxypolygelatin	T45.8X1	T45.8X2	T45.8X3	T45.8X4	T45.8X5	T45.8X6
Oxyquinoline (derivatives)	T37.8X1	T37.8X2	T37.8X3	T37.8X4	T37.8X5	T37.8X6
Oxytetracycline	T36.4X1	T36.4X2	T36.4X3	T36.4X4	T36.4X5	T36.4X6
Oxytocic drug NEC	T48.0X1	T48.0X2	T48.0X3	T48.0X4	T48.0X5	T48.0X6
Oxytocin (synthetic)	T48.0X1	T48.0X2	T48.0X3	T48.0X4	T48.0X5	T48.0X6
Ozone	T59.891	T59.892	T59.893	T59.894	--	--
P						
PABA	T49.3X1	T49.3X2	T49.3X3	T49.3X4	T49.3X5	T49.3X6
Packed red cells	T45.8X1	T45.8X2	T45.8X3	T45.8X4	T45.8X5	T45.8X6
Padimate	T49.3X1	T49.3X2	T49.3X3	T49.3X4	T49.3X5	T49.3X6
Paint NEC	T65.6X1	T65.6X2	T65.6X3	T65.6X4	--	--
cleaner	T52.91	T52.92	T52.93	T52.94	--	--
fumes NEC	T59.891	T59.892	T59.893	T59.894	--	--
lead (fumes)	T56.0X1	T56.0X2	T56.0X3	T56.0X4	--	--
solvent NEC	T52.8X1	T52.8X2	T52.8X3	T52.8X4	--	--
stripper	T52.8X1	T52.8X2	T52.8X3	T52.8X4	--	--
Palfium	T40.2X1	T40.2X2	T40.2X3	T40.2X4	--	--
Palm kernel oil	T50.991	T50.992	T50.993	T50.994	T50.995	T50.996
Paludrine	T37.2X1	T37.2X2	T37.2X3	T37.2X4	T37.2X5	T37.2X6
PAM (pralidoxime)	T50.6X1	T50.6X2	T50.6X3	T50.6X4	T50.6X5	T50.6X6
Pamaquine (naphthoute)	T37.2X1	T37.2X2	T37.2X3	T37.2X4	T37.2X5	T37.2X6
Panadol	T39.1X1	T39.1X2	T39.1X3	T39.1X4	T39.1X5	T39.1X6
Pancreatic						
digestive secretion stimulant	T47.8X1	T47.8X2	T47.8X3	T47.8X4	T47.8X5	T47.8X6
dornase	T45.3X1	T45.3X2	T45.3X3	T45.3X4	T45.3X5	T45.3X6
Pancreatin	T47.5X1	T47.5X2	T47.5X3	T47.5X4	T47.5X5	T47.5X6
Pancrelipase	T47.5X1	T47.5X2	T47.5X3	T47.5X4	T47.5X5	T47.5X6
Pancuronium (bromide)	T48.1X1	T48.1X2	T48.1X3	T48.1X4	T48.1X5	T48.1X6
Pangamic acid	T45.2X1	T45.2X2	T45.2X3	T45.2X4	T45.2X5	T45.2X6
Panthenol	T45.2X1	T45.2X2	T45.2X3	T45.2X4	T45.2X5	T45.2X6
topical	T49.8X1	T49.8X2	T49.8X3	T49.8X4	T49.8X5	T49.8X6
Pantopon	T40.0X1	T40.0X2	T40.0X3	T40.0X4	T40.0X5	T40.0X6
Pantothenic acid	T45.2X1	T45.2X2	T45.2X3	T45.2X4	T45.2X5	T45.2X6

Panwarfin - Pesticide

Substance	Poisoning, Accidental unintentional	Poisoning, Intentional self-harm	Poisoning, Assault	Poisoning, Undetermined	Adverse effect	Underdosing
Panwarfin	T45.511	T45.512	T45.513	T45.514	T45.515	T45.516
Papain	T47.5X1	T47.5X2	T47.5X3	T47.5X4	T47.5X5	T47.5X6
– digestant	T47.5X1	T47.5X2	T47.5X3	T47.5X4	T47.5X5	T47.5X6
Papaveretum	T40.0X1	T40.0X2	T40.0X3	T40.0X4	T40.0X5	T40.0X6
Papaverine	T44.3X1	T44.3X2	T44.3X3	T44.3X4	T44.3X5	T44.3X6
Para-acetamidophenol	T39.1X1	T39.1X2	T39.1X3	T39.1X4	T39.1X5	T39.1X6
Para-aminobenzoic acid	T49.3X1	T49.3X2	T49.3X3	T49.3X4	T49.3X5	T49.3X6
Para-aminophenol derivatives	T39.1X1	T39.1X2	T39.1X3	T39.1X4	T39.1X5	T39.1X6
Para-aminosalicylic acid	T37.1X1	T37.1X2	T37.1X3	T37.1X4	T37.1X5	T37.1X6
Paracetaldehyde	T42.6X1	T42.6X2	T42.6X3	T42.6X4	T42.6X5	T42.6X6
Paracetamol	T39.1X1	T39.1X2	T39.1X3	T39.1X4	T39.1X5	T39.1X6
Parachlorophenol (camphorated)	T49.0X1	T49.0X2	T49.0X3	T49.0X4	T49.0X5	T49.0X6
Paracodin	T40.2X1	T40.2X2	T40.2X3	T40.2X4	T40.2X5	T40.2X6
Paradione	T42.2X1	T42.2X2	T42.2X3	T42.2X4	T42.2X5	T42.2X6
Paraffin(s) (wax)	T52.0X1	T52.0X2	T52.0X3	T52.0X4	--	--
– liquid (medicinal)	T47.4X1	T47.4X2	T47.4X3	T47.4X4	T47.4X5	T47.4X6
– – nonmedicinal	T52.0X1	T52.0X2	T52.0X3	T52.0X4	--	--
Paraformaldehyde	T60.3X1	T60.3X2	T60.3X3	T60.3X4	--	--
Paraldehyde	T42.6X1	T42.6X2	T42.6X3	T42.6X4	T42.6X5	T42.6X6
Paramethadione	T42.2X1	T42.2X2	T42.2X3	T42.2X4	T42.2X5	T42.2X6
Paramethasone	T38.0X1	T38.0X2	T38.0X3	T38.0X4	T38.0X5	T38.0X6
– acetate	T49.0X1	T49.0X2	T49.0X3	T49.0X4	T49.0X5	T49.0X6
Paraoxon	T60.0X1	T60.0X2	T60.0X3	T60.0X4	--	--
Paraquat	T60.3X1	T60.3X2	T60.3X3	T60.3X4	--	--
Parasympatholytic NEC	T44.3X1	T44.3X2	T44.3X3	T44.3X4	T44.3X5	T44.3X6
Parasympathomimetic drug NEC	T44.1X1	T44.1X2	T44.1X3	T44.1X4	T44.1X5	T44.1X6
Parathion	T60.0X1	T60.0X2	T60.0X3	T60.0X4	--	--
Parathormone	T50.991	T50.992	T50.993	T50.994	T50.995	T50.996
Parathyroid extract	T50.991	T50.992	T50.993	T50.994	T50.995	T50.996
Paratyphoid vaccine	T50.A91	T50.A92	T50.A93	T50.A94	T50.A95	T50.A96
Paredrine	T44.4X1	T44.4X2	T44.4X3	T44.4X4	T44.4X5	T44.4X6
Paregoric	T40.0X1	T40.0X2	T40.0X3	T40.0X4	T40.0X5	T40.0X6
Pargyline	T46.5X1	T46.5X2	T46.5X3	T46.5X4	T46.5X5	T46.5X6
Paris green	T57.0X1	T57.0X2	T57.0X3	T57.0X4	--	--
– insecticide	T57.0X1	T57.0X2	T57.0X3	T57.0X4	--	--
Parnate	T43.1X1	T43.1X2	T43.1X3	T43.1X4	T43.1X5	T43.1X6
Paromomycin	T36.5X1	T36.5X2	T36.5X3	T36.5X4	T36.5X5	T36.5X6
Paroxypropione	T45.1X1	T45.1X2	T45.1X3	T45.1X4	T45.1X5	T45.1X6
Parzone	T40.2X1	T40.2X2	T40.2X3	T40.2X4	T40.2X5	T40.2X6
PAS	T37.1X1	T37.1X2	T37.1X3	T37.1X4	T37.1X5	T37.1X6
Pasiniazid	T37.1X1	T37.1X2	T37.1X3	T37.1X4	T37.1X5	T37.1X6
PBB (polybrominated biphenyls)	T65.891	T65.892	T65.893	T65.894	--	--
PCB	T65.891	T65.892	T65.893	T65.894	--	--
PCP						
– meaning pentachlorophenol	T60.1X1	T60.1X2	T60.1X3	T60.1X4	--	--
– – fungicide	T60.3X1	T60.3X2	T60.3X3	T60.3X4	--	--
– – herbicide	T60.3X1	T60.3X2	T60.3X3	T60.3X4	--	--
– – insecticide	T60.1X1	T60.1X2	T60.1X3	T60.1X4	--	--
– meaning phencyclidine	T40.991	T40.992	T40.993	T40.994	--	--
Peach kernel oil (emulsion)	T47.4X1	T47.4X2	T47.4X3	T47.4X4	T47.4X5	T47.4X6
Peanut oil (emulsion) **NEC**	T47.4X1	T47.4X2	T47.4X3	T47.4X4	T47.4X5	T47.4X6
– topical	T49.3X1	T49.3X2	T49.3X3	T49.3X4	T49.3X5	T49.3X6
Pearly Gates (morning glory seeds)	T40.991	T40.992	T40.993	T40.994	--	--
Pecazine	T43.3X1	T43.3X2	T43.3X3	T43.3X4	T43.3X5	T43.3X6
Pectin	T47.6X1	T47.6X2	T47.6X3	T47.6X4	T47.6X5	T47.6X6
Pefloxacin	T37.8X1	T37.8X2	T37.8X3	T37.8X4	T37.8X5	T37.8X6
Pegademase, bovine	T50.Z91	T50.Z92	T50.Z93	T50.Z94	T50.Z95	T50.Z96
Pelletierine tannate	T37.4X1	T37.4X2	T37.4X3	T37.4X4	T37.4X5	T37.4X6
Pemirolast (potassium)	T48.6X1	T48.6X2	T48.6X3	T48.6X4	T48.6X5	T48.6X6
Pemoline	T50.7X1	T50.7X2	T50.7X3	T50.7X4	T50.7X5	T50.7X6
Pempidine	T44.2X1	T44.2X2	T44.2X3	T44.2X4	T44.2X5	T44.2X6
Penamecillin	T36.0X1	T36.0X2	T36.0X3	T36.0X4	T36.0X5	T36.0X6
Penbutolol	T44.7X1	T44.7X2	T44.7X3	T44.7X4	T44.7X5	T44.7X6
Penethamate	T36.0X1	T36.0X2	T36.0X3	T36.0X4	T36.0X5	T36.0X6
Penfluridol	T43.591	T43.592	T43.593	T43.594	T43.595	T43.596
Penflutizide	T50.2X1	T50.2X2	T50.2X3	T50.2X4	T50.2X5	T50.2X6
Pengitoxin	T46.0X1	T46.0X2	T46.0X3	T46.0X4	T46.0X5	T46.0X6
Penicillamine	T50.6X1	T50.6X2	T50.6X3	T50.6X4	T50.6X5	T50.6X6
Penicillin (any)	T36.0X1	T36.0X2	T36.0X3	T36.0X4	T36.0X5	T36.0X6
Penicillinase	T45.3X1	T45.3X2	T45.3X3	T45.3X4	T45.3X5	T45.3X6
Penicilloyl polylysine	T50.8X1	T50.8X2	T50.8X3	T50.8X4	T50.8X5	T50.8X6
Penimepicycline	T36.4X1	T36.4X2	T36.4X3	T36.4X4	T36.4X5	T36.4X6
Pentachloroethane	T53.6X1	T53.6X2	T53.6X3	T53.6X4	--	--
Pentachloronaphthalene	T53.7X1	T53.7X2	T53.7X3	T53.7X4	--	--
Pentachlorophenol (pesticide)	T60.1X1	T60.1X2	T60.1X3	T60.1X4	--	--
– fungicide	T60.3X1	T60.3X2	T60.3X3	T60.3X4	--	--
– herbicide	T60.3X1	T60.3X2	T60.3X3	T60.3X4	--	--
– insecticide	T60.1X1	T60.1X2	T60.1X3	T60.1X4	--	--
Pentaerythritol	T46.3X1	T46.3X2	T46.3X3	T46.3X4	T46.3X5	T46.3X6
– chloral	T42.6X1	T42.6X2	T42.6X3	T42.6X4	T42.6X5	T42.6X6
– tetranitrate NEC	T46.3X1	T46.3X2	T46.3X3	T46.3X4	T46.3X5	T46.3X6
Pentaerythrityl tetranitrate	T46.3X1	T46.3X2	T46.3X3	T46.3X4	T46.3X5	T46.3X6
Pentagastrin	T50.8X1	T50.8X2	T50.8X3	T50.8X4	T50.8X5	T50.8X6
Pentalin	T53.6X1	T53.6X2	T53.6X3	T53.6X4	--	--
Pentamethonium bromide	T44.2X1	T44.2X2	T44.2X3	T44.2X4	T44.2X5	T44.2X6
Pentamidine	T37.3X1	T37.3X2	T37.3X3	T37.3X4	T37.3X5	T37.3X6
Pentanol	T51.3X1	T51.3X2	T51.3X3	T51.3X4	--	--
Pentapyrrolinium (bitartrate)	T44.2X1	T44.2X2	T44.2X3	T44.2X4	T44.2X5	T44.2X6
Pentaquine	T37.2X1	T37.2X2	T37.2X3	T37.2X4	T37.2X5	T37.2X6
Pentazocine	T40.4X1	T40.4X2	T40.4X3	T40.4X4	T40.4X5	T40.4X6
Pentetrazole	T50.7X1	T50.7X2	T50.7X3	T50.7X4	T50.7X5	T50.7X6
Penthienate bromide	T44.3X1	T44.3X2	T44.3X3	T44.3X4	T44.3X5	T44.3X6
Pentifylline	T46.7X1	T46.7X2	T46.7X3	T46.7X4	T46.7X5	T46.7X6
Pentobarbital	T42.3X1	T42.3X2	T42.3X3	T42.3X4	T42.3X5	T42.3X6
– sodium	T42.3X1	T42.3X2	T42.3X3	T42.3X4	T42.3X5	T42.3X6
Pentobarbitone	T42.3X1	T42.3X2	T42.3X3	T42.3X4	T42.3X5	T42.3X6
Pentolonium tartrate	T44.2X1	T44.2X2	T44.2X3	T44.2X4	T44.2X5	T44.2X6
Pentosan polysulfate (sodium)	T39.8X1	T39.8X2	T39.8X3	T39.8X4	T39.8X5	T39.8X6
Pentostatin	T45.1X1	T45.1X2	T45.1X3	T45.1X4	T45.1X5	T45.1X6
Pentothal	T41.1X1	T41.1X2	T41.1X3	T41.1X4	T41.1X5	T41.1X6
Pentoxifylline	T46.7X1	T46.7X2	T46.7X3	T46.7X4	T46.7X5	T46.7X6
Pentoxyverine	T48.3X1	T48.3X2	T48.3X3	T48.3X4	T48.3X5	T48.3X6
Pentrinat	T46.3X1	T46.3X2	T46.3X3	T46.3X4	T46.3X5	T46.3X6
Pentylenetetrazole	T50.7X1	T50.7X2	T50.7X3	T50.7X4	T50.7X5	T50.7X6
Pentylsalicylamide	T37.1X1	T37.1X2	T37.1X3	T37.1X4	T37.1X5	T37.1X6
Pentymal	T42.3X1	T42.3X2	T42.3X3	T42.3X4	T42.3X5	T42.3X6
Peplomycin	T45.1X1	T45.1X2	T45.1X3	T45.1X4	T45.1X5	T45.1X6
Peppermint (oil)	T47.5X1	T47.5X2	T47.5X3	T47.5X4	T47.5X5	T47.5X6
Pepsin	T47.5X1	T47.5X2	T47.5X3	T47.5X4	T47.5X5	T47.5X6
– digestant	T47.5X1	T47.5X2	T47.5X3	T47.5X4	T47.5X5	T47.5X6
Pepstatin	T47.1X1	T47.1X2	T47.1X3	T47.1X4	T47.1X5	T47.1X6
Peptavlon	T50.8X1	T50.8X2	T50.8X3	T50.8X4	T50.8X5	T50.8X6
Perazine	T43.3X1	T43.3X2	T43.3X3	T43.3X4	T43.3X5	T43.3X6
Percaine (spinal)	T41.3X1	T41.3X2	T41.3X3	T41.3X4	T41.3X5	T41.3X6
– topical (surface)	T41.3X1	T41.3X2	T41.3X3	T41.3X4	T41.3X5	T41.3X6
Perchloroethylene	T53.3X1	T53.3X2	T53.3X3	T53.3X4	--	--
– medicinal	T37.4X1	T37.4X2	T37.4X3	T37.4X4	T37.4X5	T37.4X6
– vapor	T53.3X1	T53.3X2	T53.3X3	T53.3X4	--	--
Percodan	T40.2X1	T40.2X2	T40.2X3	T40.2X4	T40.2X5	T40.2X6
Percogesic (*see also* acetaminophen)	T45.0X1	T45.0X2	T45.0X3	T45.0X4	T45.0X5	T45.0X6
Percorten	T38.0X1	T38.0X2	T38.0X3	T38.0X4	T38.0X5	T38.0X6
Pergolide	T42.8X1	T42.8X2	T42.8X3	T42.8X4	T42.8X5	T42.8X6
Pergonal	T38.811	T38.812	T38.813	T38.814	T38.815	T38.816
Perhexilene	T46.3X1	T46.3X2	T46.3X3	T46.3X4	T46.3X5	T46.3X6
Perhexiline (maleate)	T46.3X1	T46.3X2	T46.3X3	T46.3X4	T46.3X5	T46.3X6
Periactin	T45.0X1	T45.0X2	T45.0X3	T45.0X4	T45.0X5	T45.0X6
Periciazine	T43.3X1	T43.3X2	T43.3X3	T43.3X4	T43.3X5	T43.3X6
Periclor	T42.6X1	T42.6X2	T42.6X3	T42.6X4	T42.6X5	T42.6X6
Perindopril	T46.4X1	T46.4X2	T46.4X3	T46.4X4	T46.4X5	T46.4X6
Perisoxal	T39.8X1	T39.8X2	T39.8X3	T39.8X4	T39.8X5	T39.8X6
Peritoneal dialysis solution	T50.3X1	T50.3X2	T50.3X3	T50.3X4	T50.3X5	T50.3X6
Peritrate	T46.3X1	T46.3X2	T46.3X3	T46.3X4	T46.3X5	T46.3X6
Perlapine	T42.4X1	T42.4X2	T42.4X3	T42.4X4	T42.4X5	T42.4X6
Permanganate	T65.891	T65.892	T65.893	T65.894	--	--
Permethrin	T60.1X1	T60.1X2	T60.1X3	T60.1X4	--	--
Pernocton	T42.3X1	T42.3X2	T42.3X3	T42.3X4	T42.3X5	T42.3X6
Pernoston	T42.3X1	T42.3X2	T42.3X3	T42.3X4	T42.3X5	T42.3X6
Peronine	T40.2X1	T40.2X2	T40.2X3	T40.2X4	--	--
Perphenazine	T43.3X1	T43.3X2	T43.3X3	T43.3X4	T43.3X5	T43.3X6
Pertofrane	T43.011	T43.012	T43.013	T43.014	T43.015	T43.016
Pertussis						
– immune serum (human)	T50.Z11	T50.Z12	T50.Z13	T50.Z14	T50.Z15	T50.Z16
– vaccine (with diphtheria toxoid) (with tetanus toxoid)	T50.A11	T50.A12	T50.A13	T50.A14	T50.A15	T50.A16
Peruvian balsam	T49.0X1	T49.0X2	T49.0X3	T49.0X4	T49.0X5	T49.0X6
Peruvoside	T46.0X1	T46.0X2	T46.0X3	T46.0X4	T46.0X5	T46.0X6
Pesticide (dust) (fumes) (vapor) **NEC**	T60.91	T60.92	T60.93	T60.94	--	--
– arsenic	T57.0X1	T57.0X2	T57.0X3	T57.0X4	--	--
– chlorinated	T60.1X1	T60.1X2	T60.1X3	T60.1X4	--	--
– cyanide	T65.0X1	T65.0X2	T65.0X3	T65.0X4	--	--
– kerosene	T52.0X1	T52.0X2	T52.0X3	T52.0X4	--	--
– mixture (of compounds)	T60.91	T60.92	T60.93	T60.94	--	--
– naphthalene	T60.2X1	T60.2X2	T60.2X3	T60.2X4	--	--
– organochlorine (compounds)	T60.1X1	T60.1X2	T60.1X3	T60.1X4	--	--
– petroleum (distillate) (products) NEC	T60.8X1	T60.8X2	T60.8X3	T60.8X4	--	--
– specified ingredient NEC	T60.8X1	T60.8X2	T60.8X3	T60.8X4	--	--
– strychnine	T65.1X1	T65.1X2	T65.1X3	T65.1X4	--	--
– thallium	T60.4X1	T60.4X2	T60.4X3	T60.4X4	--	--

Substance	Poisoning, Accidental unintentional	Poisoning, Intentional self-harm	Poisoning, Assault	Poisoning, Undetermined	Adverse effect	Underdosing
Pethidine	T40.4X1	T40.4X2	T40.4X3	T40.4X4	T40.4X5	T40.4X6
Petrichloral	T42.6X1	T42.6X2	T42.6X3	T42.6X4	T42.6X5	T42.6X6
Petrol	T52.0X1	T52.0X2	T52.0X3	T52.0X4	--	--
vapor	T52.0X1	T52.0X2	T52.0X3	T52.0X4	--	--
Petrolatum	T49.3X1	T49.3X2	T49.3X3	T49.3X4	T49.3X5	T49.3X6
hydrophilic	T49.3X1	T49.3X2	T49.3X3	T49.3X4	T49.3X5	T49.3X6
liquid	T47.4X1	T47.4X2	T47.4X3	T47.4X4	T47.4X5	T47.4X6
topical	T49.3X1	T49.3X2	T49.3X3	T49.3X4	T49.3X5	T49.3X6
nonmedicinal	T52.0X1	T52.0X2	T52.0X3	T52.0X4	--	--
red veterinary	T49.3X1	T49.3X2	T49.3X3	T49.3X4	T49.3X5	T49.3X6
white	T49.3X1	T49.3X2	T49.3X3	T49.3X4	T49.3X5	T49.3X6
Petroleum (products) NEC	T52.0X1	T52.0X2	T52.0X3	T52.0X4	--	--
benzine(s) — see Ligroin						
ether — see Ligroin						
jelly — see Petrolatum						
naphtha — see Ligroin						
pesticide	T60.8X1	T60.8X2	T60.8X3	T60.8X4	--	--
solids	T52.0X1	T52.0X2	T52.0X3	T52.0X4	--	--
solvents	T52.0X1	T52.0X2	T52.0X3	T52.0X4	--	--
vapor	T52.0X1	T52.0X2	T52.0X3	T52.0X4	--	--
Peyote	T40.991	T40.992	T40.993	T40.994		
Phanodorm, phanodorn	T42.3X1	T42.3X2	T42.3X3	T42.3X4	T42.3X5	T42.3X6
Phanquinone	T37.3X1	T37.3X2	T37.3X3	T37.3X4	T37.3X5	T37.3X6
Phanquone	T37.3X1	T37.3X2	T37.3X3	T37.3X4	T37.3X5	T37.3X6
Pharmaceutical						
adjunct NEC	T50.901	T50.902	T50.903	T50.904	T50.905	T50.906
excipient NEC	T50.901	T50.902	T50.903	T50.904	T50.905	T50.906
sweetener	T50.901	T50.902	T50.903	T50.904	T50.905	T50.906
viscous agent	T50.901	T50.902	T50.903	T50.904	T50.905	T50.906
Phemitone	T42.3X1	T42.3X2	T42.3X3	T42.3X4	T42.3X5	T42.3X6
Phenacaine	T41.3X1	T41.3X2	T41.3X3	T41.3X4	T41.3X5	T41.3X6
Phenacemide	T42.6X1	T42.6X2	T42.6X3	T42.6X4	T42.6X5	T42.6X6
Phenacetin	T39.1X1	T39.1X2	T39.1X3	T39.1X4	T39.1X5	T39.1X6
Phenadoxone	T40.2X1	T40.2X2	T40.2X3	T40.2X4	--	--
Phenaglycodol	T43.591	T43.592	T43.593	T43.594	T43.595	T43.596
Phenantoin	T42.0X1	T42.0X2	T42.0X3	T42.0X4	T42.0X5	T42.0X6
Phenaphthazine reagent	T50.991	T50.992	T50.993	T50.994	T50.995	T50.996
Phenazocine	T40.4X1	T40.4X2	T40.4X3	T40.4X4	T40.4X5	T40.4X6
Phenazone	T39.2X1	T39.2X2	T39.2X3	T39.2X4	T39.2X5	T39.2X6
Phenazopyridine	T39.8X1	T39.8X2	T39.8X3	T39.8X4	T39.8X5	T39.8X6
Phenbenicillin	T36.0X1	T36.0X2	T36.0X3	T36.0X4	T36.0X5	T36.0X6
Phenbutrazate	T50.5X1	T50.5X2	T50.5X3	T50.5X4	T50.5X5	T50.5X6
Phencyclidine	T40.991	T40.992	T40.993	T40.994	T40.995	T40.996
Phendimetrazine	T50.5X1	T50.5X2	T50.5X3	T50.5X4	T50.5X5	T50.5X6
Phenelzine	T43.1X1	T43.1X2	T43.1X3	T43.1X4	T43.1X5	T43.1X6
Phenemal	T42.3X1	T42.3X2	T42.3X3	T42.3X4	T42.3X5	T42.3X6
Phenergan	T42.6X1	T42.6X2	T42.6X3	T42.6X4	T42.6X5	T42.6X6
Pheneticillin	T36.0X1	T36.0X2	T36.0X3	T36.0X4	T36.0X5	T36.0X6
Pheneturide	T42.6X1	T42.6X2	T42.6X3	T42.6X4	T42.6X5	T42.6X6
Phenformin	T38.3X1	T38.3X2	T38.3X3	T38.3X4	T38.3X5	T38.3X6
Phenglutarimide	T44.3X1	T44.3X2	T44.3X3	T44.3X4	T44.3X5	T44.3X6
Phenicarbazide	T39.8X1	T39.8X2	T39.8X3	T39.8X4	T39.8X5	T39.8X6
Phenindamine	T45.0X1	T45.0X2	T45.0X3	T45.0X4	T45.0X5	T45.0X6
Phenindione	T45.511	T45.512	T45.513	T45.514	T45.515	T45.516
Pheniprazine	T43.1X1	T43.1X2	T43.1X3	T43.1X4	T43.1X5	T43.1X6
Pheniramine	T45.0X1	T45.0X2	T45.0X3	T45.0X4	T45.0X5	T45.0X6
Phenisatin	T47.2X1	T47.2X2	T47.2X3	T47.2X4	T47.2X5	T47.2X6
Phenmetrazine	T50.5X1	T50.5X2	T50.5X3	T50.5X4	T50.5X5	T50.5X6
Phenobal	T42.3X1	T42.3X2	T42.3X3	T42.3X4	T42.3X5	T42.3X6
Phenobarbital	T42.3X1	T42.3X2	T42.3X3	T42.3X4	T42.3X5	T42.3X6
with						
mephenytoin	T42.3X1	T42.3X2	T42.3X3	T42.3X4	T42.3X5	T42.3X6
phenytoin	T42.3X1	T42.3X2	T42.3X3	T42.3X4	T42.3X5	T42.3X6
sodium	T42.3X1	T42.3X2	T42.3X3	T42.3X4	T42.3X5	T42.3X6
Phenobarbitone	T42.3X1	T42.3X2	T42.3X3	T42.3X4	T42.3X5	T42.3X6
Phenobutiodil	T50.8X1	T50.8X2	T50.8X3	T50.8X4	T50.8X5	T50.8X6
Phenoctide	T49.0X1	T49.0X2	T49.0X3	T49.0X4	T49.0X5	T49.0X6
Phenol	T49.0X1	T49.0X2	T49.0X3	T49.0X4	T49.0X5	T49.0X6
disinfectant	T54.0X1	T54.0X2	T54.0X3	T54.0X4	--	--
in oil injection	T46.8X1	T46.8X2	T46.8X3	T46.8X4	T46.8X5	T46.8X6
medicinal	T49.1X1	T49.1X2	T49.1X3	T49.1X4	T49.1X5	T49.1X6
nonmedicinal NEC	T54.0X1	T54.0X2	T54.0X3	T54.0X4	--	--
pesticide	T60.8X1	T60.8X2	T60.8X3	T60.8X4	--	--
red	T50.8X1	T50.8X2	T50.8X3	T50.8X4	T50.8X5	T50.8X6
Phenolic preparation	T49.1X1	T49.1X2	T49.1X3	T49.1X4	T49.1X5	T49.1X6
Phenolphthalein	T47.2X1	T47.2X2	T47.2X3	T47.2X4	T47.2X5	T47.2X6
Phenolsulfonphthalein	T50.8X1	T50.8X2	T50.8X3	T50.8X4	T50.8X5	T50.8X6
Phenomorphan	T40.2X1	T40.2X2	T40.2X3	T40.2X4	--	--
Phenonyl	T42.3X1	T42.3X2	T42.3X3	T42.3X4	T42.3X5	T42.3X6
Phenoperidine	T40.4X1	T40.4X2	T40.4X3	T40.4X4	--	--
Phenopyrazone	T46.991	T46.992	T46.993	T46.994	T46.995	T46.996
Phenoquin	T50.4X1	T50.4X2	T50.4X3	T50.4X4	T50.4X5	T50.4X6
Phenothiazine (psychotropic) NEC	T43.3X1	T43.3X2	T43.3X3	T43.3X4	T43.3X5	T43.3X6
insecticide	T60.2X1	T60.2X2	T60.2X3	T60.2X4	--	--

Substance	Poisoning, Accidental unintentional	Poisoning, Intentional self-harm	Poisoning, Assault	Poisoning, Undetermined	Adverse effect	Underdosing
Phenothrin	T49.0X1	T49.0X2	T49.0X3	T49.0X4	T49.0X5	T49.0X6
Phenoxybenzamine	T46.7X1	T46.7X2	T46.7X3	T46.7X4	T46.7X5	T46.7X6
Phenoxyethanol	T49.0X1	T49.0X2	T49.0X3	T49.0X4	T49.0X5	T49.0X6
Phenoxymethyl penicillin	T36.0X1	T36.0X2	T36.0X3	T36.0X4	T36.0X5	T36.0X6
Phenprobamate	T42.8X1	T42.8X2	T42.8X3	T42.8X4	T42.8X5	T42.8X6
Phenprocoumon	T45.511	T45.512	T45.513	T45.514	T45.515	T45.516
Phensuximide	T42.2X1	T42.2X2	T42.2X3	T42.2X4	T42.2X5	T42.2X6
Phentermine	T50.5X1	T50.5X2	T50.5X3	T50.5X4	T50.5X5	T50.5X6
Phenthicillin	T36.0X1	T36.0X2	T36.0X3	T36.0X4	T36.0X5	T36.0X6
Phentolamine	T46.7X1	T46.7X2	T46.7X3	T46.7X4	T46.7X5	T46.7X6
Phenyl						
butazone	T39.2X1	T39.2X2	T39.2X3	T39.2X4	T39.2X5	T39.2X6
enediamine	T65.3X1	T65.3X2	T65.3X3	T65.3X4	--	--
hydrazine	T65.3X1	T65.3X2	T65.3X3	T65.3X4	--	--
antineoplastic	T45.1X1	T45.1X2	T45.1X3	T45.1X4	T45.1X5	T45.1X6
mercuric compounds — see Mercury						
salicylate	T49.3X1	T49.3X2	T49.3X3	T49.3X4	T49.3X5	T49.3X6
Phenylalanine mustard	T45.1X1	T45.1X2	T45.1X3	T45.1X4	T45.1X5	T45.1X6
Phenylbutazone	T39.2X1	T39.2X2	T39.2X3	T39.2X4	T39.2X5	T39.2X6
Phenylenediamine	T65.3X1	T65.3X2	T65.3X3	T65.3X4	--	--
Phenylephrine	T44.4X1	T44.4X2	T44.4X3	T44.4X4	T44.4X5	T44.4X6
Phenylethylbiguanide	T38.3X1	T38.3X2	T38.3X3	T38.3X4	T38.3X5	T38.3X6
Phenylmercuric						
acetate	T49.0X1	T49.0X2	T49.0X3	T49.0X4	T49.0X5	T49.0X6
borate	T49.0X1	T49.0X2	T49.0X3	T49.0X4	T49.0X5	T49.0X6
nitrate	T49.0X1	T49.0X2	T49.0X3	T49.0X4	T49.0X5	T49.0X6
Phenylmethylbarbitone	T42.3X1	T42.3X2	T42.3X3	T42.3X4	T42.3X5	T42.3X6
Phenylpropanol	T47.5X1	T47.5X2	T47.5X3	T47.5X4	T47.5X5	T47.5X6
Phenylpropanolamine	T44.991	T44.992	T44.993	T44.994	T44.995	T44.996
Phenylsulfthion	T60.0X1	T60.0X2	T60.0X3	T60.0X4	--	--
Phenyltoloxamine	T45.0X1	T45.0X2	T45.0X3	T45.0X4	T45.0X5	T45.0X6
Phenyramidol, phenyramidon	T39.8X1	T39.8X2	T39.8X3	T39.8X4	T39.8X5	T39.8X6
Phenytoin	T42.0X1	T42.0X2	T42.0X3	T42.0X4	T42.0X5	T42.0X6
with Phenobarbital	T42.3X1	T42.3X2	T42.3X3	T42.3X4	T42.3X5	T42.3X6
pHisoHex	T49.2X1	T49.2X2	T49.2X3	T49.2X4	T49.2X5	T49.2X6
Pholcodine	T48.3X1	T48.3X2	T48.3X3	T48.3X4	T48.3X5	T48.3X6
Pholedrine	T46.991	T46.992	T46.993	T46.994	T46.995	T46.996
Phorate	T60.0X1	T60.0X2	T60.0X3	T60.0X4	--	--
Phosdrin	T60.0X1	T60.0X2	T60.0X3	T60.0X4	--	--
Phosfolan	T60.0X1	T60.0X2	T60.0X3	T60.0X4	--	--
Phosgene (gas)	T59.891	T59.892	T59.893	T59.894		
Phosphamidon	T60.0X1	T60.0X2	T60.0X3	T60.0X4	--	--
Phosphate	T65.891	T65.892	T65.893	T65.894		
laxative	T47.4X1	T47.4X2	T47.4X3	T47.4X4	T47.4X5	T47.4X6
organic	T60.0X1	T60.0X2	T60.0X3	T60.0X4	--	--
solvent	T52.91	T52.92	T52.93	T52.94		
tricresyl	T65.891	T65.892	T65.893	T65.894		
Phosphine	T57.1X1	T57.1X2	T57.1X3	T57.1X4		
fumigant	T57.1X1	T57.1X2	T57.1X3	T57.1X4	--	--
Phospholine	T49.5X1	T49.5X2	T49.5X3	T49.5X4	T49.5X5	T49.5X6
Phosphoric acid	T54.2X1	T54.2X2	T54.2X3	T54.2X4	--	--
Phosphorus (compound) NEC	T57.1X1	T57.1X2	T57.1X3	T57.1X4		
pesticide	T60.0X1	T60.0X2	T60.0X3	T60.0X4	--	--
Phthalates	T65.891	T65.892	T65.893	T65.894		
Phthalic anhydride	T65.891	T65.892	T65.893	T65.894		
Phthalimidoglutarimide	T42.6X1	T42.6X2	T42.6X3	T42.6X4	T42.6X5	T42.6X6
Phthalylsulfathiazole	T37.0X1	T37.0X2	T37.0X3	T37.0X4	T37.0X5	T37.0X6
Phylloquinone	T45.7X1	T45.7X2	T45.7X3	T45.7X4	T45.7X5	T45.7X6
Physeptone	T40.3X1	T40.3X2	T40.3X3	T40.3X4	T40.3X5	T40.3X6
Physostigma venenosum	T62.2X1	T62.2X2	T62.2X3	T62.2X4		
Physostigmine	T49.5X1	T49.5X2	T49.5X3	T49.5X4	T49.5X5	T49.5X6
Phytolacca decandra	T62.2X1	T62.2X2	T62.2X3	T62.2X4		
berries	T62.1X1	T62.1X2	T62.1X3	T62.1X4		
Phytomenadione	T45.7X1	T45.7X2	T45.7X3	T45.7X4	T45.7X5	T45.7X6
Phytonadione	T45.7X1	T45.7X2	T45.7X3	T45.7X4	T45.7X5	T45.7X6
Picoperine	T48.3X1	T48.3X2	T48.3X3	T48.3X4	T48.3X5	T48.3X6
Picosulfate (sodium)	T47.2X1	T47.2X2	T47.2X3	T47.2X4	T47.2X5	T47.2X6
Picric (acid)	T54.2X1	T54.2X2	T54.2X3	T54.2X4	--	--
Picrotoxin	T50.7X1	T50.7X2	T50.7X3	T50.7X4	T50.7X5	T50.7X6
Piketoprofen	T49.0X1	T49.0X2	T49.0X3	T49.0X4	T49.0X5	T49.0X6
Pilocarpine	T44.1X1	T44.1X2	T44.1X3	T44.1X4	T44.1X5	T44.1X6
Pilocarpus (jaborandi) extract	T44.1X1	T44.1X2	T44.1X3	T44.1X4	T44.1X5	T44.1X6
Pilsicainide (hydrochloride)	T46.2X1	T46.2X2	T46.2X3	T46.2X4	T46.2X5	T46.2X6
Pimaricin	T36.7X1	T36.7X2	T36.7X3	T36.7X4	T36.7X5	T36.7X6
Pimeclone	T50.7X1	T50.7X2	T50.7X3	T50.7X4	T50.7X5	T50.7X6
Pimelic ketone	T52.8X1	T52.8X2	T52.8X3	T52.8X4	--	--
Pimethixene	T45.0X1	T45.0X2	T45.0X3	T45.0X4	T45.0X5	T45.0X6
Piminodine	T40.2X1	T40.2X2	T40.2X3	T40.2X4	T40.2X5	T40.2X6
Pimozide	T43.591	T43.592	T43.593	T43.594	T43.595	T43.596
Pinacidil	T46.5X1	T46.5X2	T46.5X3	T46.5X4	T46.5X5	T46.5X6
Pinaverium bromide	T44.3X1	T44.3X2	T44.3X3	T44.3X4	T44.3X5	T44.3X6
Pinazepam	T42.4X1	T42.4X2	T42.4X3	T42.4X4	T42.4X5	T42.4X6
Pindolol	T44.7X1	T44.7X2	T44.7X3	T44.7X4	T44.7X5	T44.7X6

Substance	Poisoning, Accidental unintentional	Poisoning, Intentional self-harm	Poisoning, Assault	Poisoning, Undetermined	Adverse effect	Underdosing
Pindone	T60.4X1	T60.4X2	T60.4X3	T60.4X4	--	--
Pine oil (disinfectant)	T65.891	T65.892	T65.893	T65.894	--	--
Pinkroot	T37.4X1	T37.4X2	T37.4X3	T37.4X4	T37.4X5	T37.4X6
Pipadone	T40.2X1	T40.2X2	T40.2X3	T40.2X4	--	--
Pipamazine	T45.0X1	T45.0X2	T45.0X3	T45.0X4	T45.0X5	T45.0X6
Pipamperone	T43.4X1	T43.4X2	T43.4X3	T43.4X4	T43.4X5	T43.4X6
Pipazetate	T48.3X1	T48.3X2	T48.3X3	T48.3X4	T48.3X5	T48.3X6
Pipemidic acid	T37.8X1	T37.8X2	T37.8X3	T37.8X4	T37.8X5	T37.8X6
Pipenzolate bromide	T44.3X1	T44.3X2	T44.3X3	T44.3X4	T44.3X5	T44.3X6
Piperacetazine	T43.3X1	T43.3X2	T43.3X3	T43.3X4	T43.3X5	T43.3X6
Piperacillin	T36.0X1	T36.0X2	T36.0X3	T36.0X4	T36.0X5	T36.0X6
Piperazine	T37.4X1	T37.4X2	T37.4X3	T37.4X4	T37.4X5	T37.4X6
estrone sulfate	T38.5X1	T38.5X2	T38.5X3	T38.5X4	T38.5X5	T38.5X6
Piper cubeba	T62.2X1	T62.2X2	T62.2X3	T62.2X4	--	--
Piperidione	T48.3X1	T48.3X2	T48.3X3	T48.3X4	T48.3X5	T48.3X6
Piperidolate	T44.3X1	T44.3X2	T44.3X3	T44.3X4	T44.3X5	T44.3X6
Piperocaine	T41.3X1	T41.3X2	T41.3X3	T41.3X4	T41.3X5	T41.3X6
infiltration (subcutaneous)	T41.3X1	T41.3X2	T41.3X3	T41.3X4	T41.3X5	T41.3X6
nerve block (peripheral) (plexus)	T41.3X1	T41.3X2	T41.3X3	T41.3X4	T41.3X5	T41.3X6
topical (surface)	T41.3X1	T41.3X2	T41.3X3	T41.3X4	T41.3X5	T41.3X6
Piperonyl butoxide	T60.8X1	T60.8X2	T60.8X3	T60.8X4	--	--
Pipethanate	T44.3X1	T44.3X2	T44.3X3	T44.3X4	T44.3X5	T44.3X6
Pipobroman	T45.1X1	T45.1X2	T45.1X3	T45.1X4	T45.1X5	T45.1X6
Pipotiazine	T43.3X1	T43.3X2	T43.3X3	T43.3X4	T43.3X5	T43.3X6
Pipoxizine	T45.0X1	T45.0X2	T45.0X3	T45.0X4	T45.0X5	T45.0X6
Pipradrol	T43.691	T43.692	T43.693	T43.694	T43.695	T43.696
Piprinhydrinate	T45.0X1	T45.0X2	T45.0X3	T45.0X4	T45.0X5	T45.0X6
Pirarubicin	T45.1X1	T45.1X2	T45.1X3	T45.1X4	T45.1X5	T45.1X6
Pirazinamide	T37.1X1	T37.1X2	T37.1X3	T37.1X4	T37.1X5	T37.1X6
Pirbuterol	T48.6X1	T48.6X2	T48.6X3	T48.6X4	T48.6X5	T48.6X6
Pirenzepine	T47.1X1	T47.1X2	T47.1X3	T47.1X4	T47.1X5	T47.1X6
Piretanide	T50.1X1	T50.1X2	T50.1X3	T50.1X4	T50.1X5	T50.1X6
Piribedil	T42.8X1	T42.8X2	T42.8X3	T42.8X4	T42.8X5	T42.8X6
Piridoxilate	T46.3X1	T46.3X2	T46.3X3	T46.3X4	T46.3X5	T46.3X6
Piritramide	T40.4X1	T40.4X2	T40.4X3	T40.4X4	--	--
Piromidic acid	T37.8X1	T37.8X2	T37.8X3	T37.8X4	T37.8X5	T37.8X6
Piroxicam	T39.391	T39.392	T39.393	T39.394	T39.395	T39.396
beta-cyclodextrin complex	T39.8X1	T39.8X2	T39.8X3	T39.8X4	T39.8X5	T39.8X6
Pirozadil	T46.6X1	T46.6X2	T46.6X3	T46.6X4	T46.6X5	T46.6X6
Piscidia (bark) (erythrina)	T39.8X1	T39.8X2	T39.8X3	T39.8X4	T39.8X5	T39.8X6
Pitch	T65.891	T65.892	T65.893	T65.894	--	--
Pitkin's solution	T41.3X1	T41.3X2	T41.3X3	T41.3X4	T41.3X5	T41.3X6
Pitocin	T48.0X1	T48.0X2	T48.0X3	T48.0X4	T48.0X5	T48.0X6
Pitressin (tannate)	T38.891	T38.892	T38.893	T38.894	T38.895	T38.896
Pituitary extracts (posterior)	T38.891	T38.892	T38.893	T38.894	T38.895	T38.896
anterior	T38.811	T38.812	T38.813	T38.814	T38.815	T38.816
Pituitrin	T38.891	T38.892	T38.893	T38.894	T38.895	T38.896
Pivampicillin	T36.0X1	T36.0X2	T36.0X3	T36.0X4	T36.0X5	T36.0X6
Pivmecillinam	T36.0X1	T36.0X2	T36.0X3	T36.0X4	T36.0X5	T36.0X6
Placental hormone	T38.891	T38.892	T38.893	T38.894	T38.895	T38.896
Placidyl	T42.6X1	T42.6X2	T42.6X3	T42.6X4	T42.6X5	T42.6X6
Plague vaccine	T50.A91	T50.A92	T50.A93	T50.A94	T50.A95	T50.A96
Plant						
food or fertilizer NEC	T65.891	T65.892	T65.893	T65.894	--	--
containing herbicide	T60.3X1	T60.3X2	T60.3X3	T60.3X4	--	--
noxious, used as food	T62.2X1	T62.2X2	T62.2X3	T62.2X4	--	--
berries	T62.1X1	T62.1X2	T62.1X3	T62.1X4	--	--
seeds	T62.2X1	T62.2X2	T62.2X3	T62.2X4	--	--
specified type NEC	T62.2X1	T62.2X2	T62.2X3	T62.2X4	--	--
Plasma	T45.8X1	T45.8X2	T45.8X3	T45.8X4	T45.8X5	T45.8X6
expander NEC	T45.8X1	T45.8X2	T45.8X3	T45.8X4	T45.8X5	T45.8X6
protein fraction (human)	T45.8X1	T45.8X2	T45.8X3	T45.8X4	T45.8X5	T45.8X6
Plasmanate	T45.8X1	T45.8X2	T45.8X3	T45.8X4	T45.8X5	T45.8X6
Plasminogen (tissue) **activator**	T45.611	T45.612	T45.613	T45.614	T45.615	T45.616
Plaster dressing	T49.3X1	T49.3X2	T49.3X3	T49.3X4	T49.3X5	T49.3X6
Plastic dressing	T49.3X1	T49.3X2	T49.3X3	T49.3X4	T49.3X5	T49.3X6
Plegicil	T43.3X1	T43.3X2	T43.3X3	T43.3X4	T43.3X5	T43.3X6
Plicamycin	T45.1X1	T45.1X2	T45.1X3	T45.1X4	T45.1X5	T45.1X6
Podophyllotoxin	T49.8X1	T49.8X2	T49.8X3	T49.8X4	T49.8X5	T49.8X6
Podophyllum (resin)	T49.4X1	T49.4X2	T49.4X3	T49.4X4	T49.4X5	T49.4X6
Poison NEC	T65.91	T65.92	T65.93	T65.94	--	--
Poisonous berries	T62.1X1	T62.1X2	T62.1X3	T62.1X4	--	--
Pokeweed (any part)	T62.2X1	T62.2X2	T62.2X3	T62.2X4	--	--
Poldine metilsulfate	T44.3X1	T44.3X2	T44.3X3	T44.3X4	T44.3X5	T44.3X6
Polidexide (sulfate)	T46.6X1	T46.6X2	T46.6X3	T46.6X4	T46.6X5	T46.6X6
Polidocanol	T46.8X1	T46.8X2	T46.8X3	T46.8X4	T46.8X5	T46.8X6
Poliomyelitis vaccine	T50.B91	T50.B92	T50.B93	T50.B94	T50.B95	T50.B96
Polish (car) (floor) (furni-ture) (metal) (porcelain) (silver)	T65.891	T65.892	T65.893	T65.894	--	--
abrasive	T65.891	T65.892	T65.893	T65.894	--	--
porcelain	T65.891	T65.892	T65.893	T65.894	--	--
Poloxalkol	T47.4X1	T47.4X2	T47.4X3	T47.4X4	T47.4X5	T47.4X6
Poloxamer	T47.4X1	T47.4X2	T47.4X3	T47.4X4	T47.4X5	T47.4X6
Polyaminostyrene resins	T50.3X1	T50.3X2	T50.3X3	T50.3X4	T50.3X5	T50.3X6
Polycarbophil	T47.4X1	T47.4X2	T47.4X3	T47.4X4	T47.4X5	T47.4X6
Polychlorinated biphenyl	T65.891	T65.892	T65.893	T65.894	--	--
Polycycline	T36.4X1	T36.4X2	T36.4X3	T36.4X4	T36.4X5	T36.4X6
Polyester fumes	T59.891	T59.892	T59.893	T59.894	--	--
Polyester resin hardener	T52.91	T52.92	T52.93	T52.94	--	--
fumes	T59.891	T59.892	T59.893	T59.894	--	--
Polyestradiol phosphate	T38.5X1	T38.5X2	T38.5X3	T38.5X4	T38.5X5	T38.5X6
Polyethanolamine alkyl sulfate	T49.2X1	T49.2X2	T49.2X3	T49.2X4	T49.2X5	T49.2X6
Polyethylene adhesive	T49.3X1	T49.3X2	T49.3X3	T49.3X4	T49.3X5	T49.3X6
Polyferose	T45.4X1	T45.4X2	T45.4X3	T45.4X4	T45.4X5	T45.4X6
Polygeline	T45.8X1	T45.8X2	T45.8X3	T45.8X4	T45.8X5	T45.8X6
Polymyxin	T36.8X1	T36.8X2	T36.8X3	T36.8X4	T36.8X5	T36.8X6
B	T36.8X1	T36.8X2	T36.8X3	T36.8X4	T36.8X5	T36.8X6
ENT agent	T49.6X1	T49.6X2	T49.6X3	T49.6X4	T49.6X5	T49.6X6
ophthalmic preparation	T49.5X1	T49.5X2	T49.5X3	T49.5X4	T49.5X5	T49.5X6
topical NEC	T49.0X1	T49.0X2	T49.0X3	T49.0X4	T49.0X5	T49.0X6
E sulfate (eye preparation)	T49.5X1	T49.5X2	T49.5X3	T49.5X4	T49.5X5	T49.5X6
Polynoxylin	T49.0X1	T49.0X2	T49.0X3	T49.0X4	T49.0X5	T49.0X6
Polyoestradiol phosphate	T38.5X1	T38.5X2	T38.5X3	T38.5X4	T38.5X5	T38.5X6
Polyoxymethyleneurea	T49.0X1	T49.0X2	T49.0X3	T49.0X4	T49.0X5	T49.0X6
Polysilane	T47.8X1	T47.8X2	T47.8X3	T47.8X4	T47.8X5	T47.8X6
Polytetrafluoroethylene (inhaled)	T59.891	T59.892	T59.893	T59.894	--	--
Polythiazide	T50.2X1	T50.2X2	T50.2X3	T50.2X4	T50.2X5	T50.2X6
Polyvidone	T45.8X1	T45.8X2	T45.8X3	T45.8X4	T45.8X5	T45.8X6
Polyvinylpyrrolidone	T45.8X1	T45.8X2	T45.8X3	T45.8X4	T45.8X5	T45.8X6
Pontocaine (hydrochloride) (infiltration) (topical)	T41.3X1	T41.3X2	T41.3X3	T41.3X4	T41.3X5	T41.3X6
nerve block (peripheral) (plexus)	T41.3X1	T41.3X2	T41.3X3	T41.3X4	T41.3X5	T41.3X6
spinal	T41.3X1	T41.3X2	T41.3X3	T41.3X4	T41.3X5	T41.3X6
Porfiromycin	T45.1X1	T45.1X2	T45.1X3	T45.1X4	T45.1X5	T45.1X6
Posterior pituitary hormone NEC	T38.891	T38.892	T38.893	T38.894	T38.895	T38.896
Pot	T40.7X1	T40.7X2	T40.7X3	T40.7X4	T40.7X5	T40.7X6
Potash (caustic)	T54.3X1	T54.3X2	T54.3X3	T54.3X4	--	--
Potassic saline injection (lactated)	T50.3X1	T50.3X2	T50.3X3	T50.3X4	T50.3X5	T50.3X6
Potassium (salts) **NEC**	T50.3X1	T50.3X2	T50.3X3	T50.3X4	T50.3X5	T50.3X6
aminobenzoate	T45.8X1	T45.8X2	T45.8X3	T45.8X4	T45.8X5	T45.8X6
aminosalicylate	T37.1X1	T37.1X2	T37.1X3	T37.1X4	T37.1X5	T37.1X6
antimony 'tartrate'	T37.8X1	T37.8X2	T37.8X3	T37.8X4	T37.8X5	T37.8X6
arsenite (solution)	T57.0X1	T57.0X2	T57.0X3	T57.0X4	--	--
bichromate	T56.2X1	T56.2X2	T56.2X3	T56.2X4	--	--
bisulfate	T47.3X1	T47.3X2	T47.3X3	T47.3X4	T47.3X5	T47.3X6
bromide	T42.6X1	T42.6X2	T42.6X3	T42.6X4	T42.6X5	T42.6X6
canrenoate	T50.0X1	T50.0X2	T50.0X3	T50.0X4	T50.0X5	T50.0X6
carbonate	T54.3X1	T54.3X2	T54.3X3	T54.3X4	--	--
chlorate NEC	T65.891	T65.892	T65.893	T65.894	--	--
chloride	T50.3X1	T50.3X2	T50.3X3	T50.3X4	T50.3X5	T50.3X6
citrate	T50.991	T50.992	T50.993	T50.994	T50.995	T50.996
cyanide	T65.0X1	T65.0X2	T65.0X3	T65.0X4	--	--
ferric hexacyanoferrate (medicinal)	T50.6X1	T50.6X2	T50.6X3	T50.6X4	T50.6X5	T50.6X6
nonmedicinal	T65.891	T65.892	T65.893	T65.894	--	--
Fluoride	T57.8X1	T57.8X2	T57.8X3	T57.8X4	--	--
glucaldrate	T47.1X1	T47.1X2	T47.1X3	T47.1X4	T47.1X5	T47.1X6
hydroxide	T54.3X1	T54.3X2	T54.3X3	T54.3X4	--	--
iodate	T49.0X1	T49.0X2	T49.0X3	T49.0X4	T49.0X5	T49.0X6
iodide	T48.4X1	T48.4X2	T48.4X3	T48.4X4	T48.4X5	T48.4X6
nitrate	T57.8X1	T57.8X2	T57.8X3	T57.8X4	--	--
oxalate	T65.891	T65.892	T65.893	T65.894	--	--
perchlorate (nonmedicinal) NEC	T65.891	T65.892	T65.893	T65.894	--	--
antithyroid	T38.2X1	T38.2X2	T38.2X3	T38.2X4	T38.2X5	T38.2X6
medicinal	T38.2X1	T38.2X2	T38.2X3	T38.2X4	T38.2X5	T38.2X6
Permanganate (nonmedicinal)	T65.891	T65.892	T65.893	T65.894	--	--
medicinal	T49.0X1	T49.0X2	T49.0X3	T49.0X4	T49.0X5	T49.0X6
sulfate	T47.2X1	T47.2X2	T47.2X3	T47.2X4	T47.2X5	T47.2X6
Potassium-removing resin	T50.3X1	T50.3X2	T50.3X3	T50.3X4	T50.3X5	T50.3X6
Potassium-retaining drug	T50.3X1	T50.3X2	T50.3X3	T50.3X4	T50.3X5	T50.3X6
Povidone	T45.8X1	T45.8X2	T45.8X3	T45.8X4	T45.8X5	T45.8X6
iodine	T49.0X1	T49.0X2	T49.0X3	T49.0X4	T49.0X5	T49.0X6
Practolol	T44.7X1	T44.7X2	T44.7X3	T44.7X4	T44.7X5	T44.7X6
Prajmalium bitartrate	T46.2X1	T46.2X2	T46.2X3	T46.2X4	T46.2X5	T46.2X6
Pralidoxime (iodide)	T50.6X1	T50.6X2	T50.6X3	T50.6X4	T50.6X5	T50.6X6
chloride	T50.6X1	T50.6X2	T50.6X3	T50.6X4	T50.6X5	T50.6X6
Pramiverine	T44.3X1	T44.3X2	T44.3X3	T44.3X4	T44.3X5	T44.3X6
Pramocaine	T49.1X1	T49.1X2	T49.1X3	T49.1X4	T49.1X5	T49.1X6
Pramoxine	T49.1X1	T49.1X2	T49.1X3	T49.1X4	T49.1X5	T49.1X6

Substance	Poisoning, Accidental unintentional	Poisoning, Intentional self-harm	Poisoning, Assault	Poisoning, Undetermined	Adverse effect	Underdosing
Prasterone	T38.7X1	T38.7X2	T38.7X3	T38.7X4	T38.7X5	T38.7X6
Pravastatin	T46.6X1	T46.6X2	T46.6X3	T46.6X4	T46.6X5	T46.6X6
Prazepam	T42.4X1	T42.4X2	T42.4X3	T42.4X4	T42.4X5	T42.4X6
Praziquantel	T37.4X1	T37.4X2	T37.4X3	T37.4X4	T37.4X5	T37.4X6
Prazitone	T43.291	T43.292	T43.293	T43.294	T43.295	T43.296
Prazosin	T44.6X1	T44.6X2	T44.6X3	T44.6X4	T44.6X5	T44.6X6
Prednicarbate	T49.0X1	T49.0X2	T49.0X3	T49.0X4	T49.0X5	T49.0X6
Prednimustine	T45.1X1	T45.1X2	T45.1X3	T45.1X4	T45.1X5	T45.1X6
Prednisolone	T38.0X1	T38.0X2	T38.0X3	T38.0X4	T38.0X5	T38.0X6
ENT agent	T49.6X1	T49.6X2	T49.6X3	T49.6X4	T49.6X5	T49.6X6
ophthalmic preparation	T49.5X1	T49.5X2	T49.5X3	T49.5X4	T49.5X5	T49.5X6
steaglate	T49.0X1	T49.0X2	T49.0X3	T49.0X4	T49.0X5	T49.0X6
topical NEC	T49.0X1	T49.0X2	T49.0X3	T49.0X4	T49.0X5	T49.0X6
Prednisone	T38.0X1	T38.0X2	T38.0X3	T38.0X4	T38.0X5	T38.0X6
Prednylidene	T38.0X1	T38.0X2	T38.0X3	T38.0X4	T38.0X5	T38.0X6
Pregnandiol	T38.5X1	T38.5X2	T38.5X3	T38.5X4	T38.5X5	T38.5X6
Pregneninolone	T38.5X1	T38.5X2	T38.5X3	T38.5X4	T38.5X5	T38.5X6
Preludin	T43.691	T43.692	T43.693	T43.694	T43.695	T43.696
Premarin	T38.5X1	T38.5X2	T38.5X3	T38.5X4	T38.5X5	T38.5X6
Premedication anesthetic	T41.201	T41.202	T41.203	T41.204	T41.205	T41.206
Prenalterol	T44.5X1	T44.5X2	T44.5X3	T44.5X4	T44.5X5	T44.5X6
Prenoxdiazine	T48.3X1	T48.3X2	T48.3X3	T48.3X4	T48.3X5	T48.3X6
Prenylamine	T46.3X1	T46.3X2	T46.3X3	T46.3X4	T46.3X5	T46.3X6
Preparation H	T49.8X1	T49.8X2	T49.8X3	T49.8X4	T49.8X5	T49.8X6
Preparation, local	T49.4X1	T49.4X2	T49.4X3	T49.4X4	T49.4X5	T49.4X6
Preservative (nonmedicinal)	T65.891	T65.892	T65.893	T65.894	--	--
medicinal	T50.901	T50.902	T50.903	T50.904	T50.905	T50.906
wood	T60.91	T60.92	T60.93	T60.94	--	--
Prethcamide	T50.7X1	T50.7X2	T50.7X3	T50.7X4	T50.7X5	T50.7X6
Pride of China	T62.2X1	T62.2X2	T62.2X3	T62.2X4	--	--
Pridinol	T44.3X1	T44.3X2	T44.3X3	T44.3X4	T44.3X5	T44.3X6
Prifinium bromide	T44.3X1	T44.3X2	T44.3X3	T44.3X4	T44.3X5	T44.3X6
Prilocaine	T41.3X1	T41.3X2	T41.3X3	T41.3X4	T41.3X5	T41.3X6
infiltration (subcutaneous)	T41.3X1	T41.3X2	T41.3X3	T41.3X4	T41.3X5	T41.3X6
nerve block (peripheral) (plexus)	T41.3X1	T41.3X2	T41.3X3	T41.3X4	T41.3X5	T41.3X6
regional	T41.3X1	T41.3X2	T41.3X3	T41.3X4	T41.3X5	T41.3X6
Primaquine	T37.2X1	T37.2X2	T37.2X3	T37.2X4	T37.2X5	T37.2X6
Primidone	T42.6X1	T42.6X2	T42.6X3	T42.6X4	T42.6X5	T42.6X6
Primula (veris)	T62.2X1	T62.2X2	T62.2X3	T62.2X4	--	--
Prinadol	T40.2X1	T40.2X2	T40.2X3	T40.2X4	T40.2X5	T40.2X6
Priscol, Priscoline	T44.6X1	T44.6X2	T44.6X3	T44.6X4	T44.6X5	T44.6X6
Pristinamycin	T36.3X1	T36.3X2	T36.3X3	T36.3X4	T36.3X5	T36.3X6
Privet	T62.2X1	T62.2X2	T62.2X3	T62.2X4	--	--
berries	T62.1X1	T62.1X2	T62.1X3	T62.1X4	--	--
Privine	T44.4X1	T44.4X2	T44.4X3	T44.4X4	T44.4X5	T44.4X6
Pro-Banthine	T44.3X1	T44.3X2	T44.3X3	T44.3X4	T44.3X5	T44.3X6
Probarbital	T42.3X1	T42.3X2	T42.3X3	T42.3X4	T42.3X5	T42.3X6
Probenecid	T50.4X1	T50.4X2	T50.4X3	T50.4X4	T50.4X5	T50.4X6
Probucol	T46.6X1	T46.6X2	T46.6X3	T46.6X4	T46.6X5	T46.6X6
Procainamide	T46.2X1	T46.2X2	T46.2X3	T46.2X4	T46.2X5	T46.2X6
Procaine	T41.3X1	T41.3X2	T41.3X3	T41.3X4	T41.3X5	T41.3X6
benzylpenicillin	T36.0X1	T36.0X2	T36.0X3	T36.0X4	T36.0X5	T36.0X6
nerve block (periphreal) (plexus)	T41.3X1	T41.3X2	T41.3X3	T41.3X4	T41.3X5	T41.3X6
penicillin G	T36.0X1	T36.0X2	T36.0X3	T36.0X4	T36.0X5	T36.0X6
regional	T41.3X1	T41.3X2	T41.3X3	T41.3X4	T41.3X5	T41.3X6
spinal	T41.3X1	T41.3X2	T41.3X3	T41.3X4	T41.3X5	T41.3X6
Procalmidol	T43.591	T43.592	T43.593	T43.594	T43.595	T43.596
Procarbazine	T45.1X1	T45.1X2	T45.1X3	T45.1X4	T45.1X5	T45.1X6
Procaterol	T44.5X1	T44.5X2	T44.5X3	T44.5X4	T44.5X5	T44.5X6
Prochlorperazine	T43.3X1	T43.3X2	T43.3X3	T43.3X4	T43.3X5	T43.3X6
Procyclidine	T44.3X1	T44.3X2	T44.3X3	T44.3X4	T44.3X5	T44.3X6
Producer gas	T58.8X1	T58.8X2	T58.8X3	T58.8X4	--	--
Profadol	T40.4X1	T40.4X2	T40.4X3	T40.4X4	T40.4X5	T40.4X6
Profenamine	T44.3X1	T44.3X2	T44.3X3	T44.3X4	T44.3X5	T44.3X6
Profenil	T44.3X1	T44.3X2	T44.3X3	T44.3X4	T44.3X5	T44.3X6
Proflavine	T49.0X1	T49.0X2	T49.0X3	T49.0X4	T49.0X5	T49.0X6
Progabide	T42.6X1	T42.6X2	T42.6X3	T42.6X4	T42.6X5	T42.6X6
Progesterone	T38.5X1	T38.5X2	T38.5X3	T38.5X4	T38.5X5	T38.5X6
Progestin	T38.5X1	T38.5X2	T38.5X3	T38.5X4	T38.5X5	T38.5X6
oral contraceptive	T38.4X1	T38.4X2	T38.4X3	T38.4X4	T38.4X5	T38.4X6
Progestogen NEC	T38.5X1	T38.5X2	T38.5X3	T38.5X4	T38.5X5	T38.5X6
Progestone	T38.5X1	T38.5X2	T38.5X3	T38.5X4	T38.5X5	T38.5X6
Proglumide	T47.1X1	T47.1X2	T47.1X3	T47.1X4	T47.1X5	T47.1X6
Proguanil	T37.2X1	T37.2X2	T37.2X3	T37.2X4	T37.2X5	T37.2X6
Prolactin	T38.811	T38.812	T38.813	T38.814	T38.815	T38.816
Prolintane	T43.691	T43.692	T43.693	T43.694	T43.695	T43.696
Proloid	T38.1X1	T38.1X2	T38.1X3	T38.1X4	T38.1X5	T38.1X6
Proluton	T38.5X1	T38.5X2	T38.5X3	T38.5X4	T38.5X5	T38.5X6
Promacetin	T37.1X1	T37.1X2	T37.1X3	T37.1X4	T37.1X5	T37.1X6
Promazine	T43.3X1	T43.3X2	T43.3X3	T43.3X4	T43.3X5	T43.3X6
Promedol	T40.2X1	T40.2X2	T40.2X3	T40.2X4	--	--
Promegestone	T38.5X1	T38.5X2	T38.5X3	T38.5X4	T38.5X5	T38.5X6

Substance	Poisoning, Accidental unintentional	Poisoning, Intentional self-harm	Poisoning, Assault	Poisoning, Undetermined	Adverse effect	Underdosing
Promethazine (teoclate)	T43.3X1	T43.3X2	T43.3X3	T43.3X4	T43.3X5	T43.3X6
Promin	T37.1X1	T37.1X2	T37.1X3	T37.1X4	T37.1X5	T37.1X6
Pronase	T45.3X1	T45.3X2	T45.3X3	T45.3X4	T45.3X5	T45.3X6
Pronestyl (hydrochloride)	T46.2X1	T46.2X2	T46.2X3	T46.2X4	T46.2X5	T46.2X6
Pronetalol	T44.7X1	T44.7X2	T44.7X3	T44.7X4	T44.7X5	T44.7X6
Prontosil	T37.0X1	T37.0X2	T37.0X3	T37.0X4	T37.0X5	T37.0X6
Propachlor	T60.3X1	T60.3X2	T60.3X3	T60.3X4	--	--
Propafenone	T46.2X1	T46.2X2	T46.2X3	T46.2X4	T46.2X5	T46.2X6
Propallylonal	T42.3X1	T42.3X2	T42.3X3	T42.3X4	T42.3X5	T42.3X6
Propamidine	T49.0X1	T49.0X2	T49.0X3	T49.0X4	T49.0X5	T49.0X6
Propane (distributed in mobile container)	T59.891	T59.892	T59.893	T59.894	--	--
distributed through pipes	T59.891	T59.892	T59.893	T59.894	--	--
incomplete combustion	T58.11	T58.12	T58.13	T58.14	--	--
Propanidid	T41.291	T41.292	T41.293	T41.294	T41.295	T41.296
Propanil	T60.3X1	T60.3X2	T60.3X3	T60.3X4	--	--
1-Propanol	T51.3X1	T51.3X2	T51.3X3	T51.3X4	--	--
2-Propanol	T51.2X1	T51.2X2	T51.2X3	T51.2X4	--	--
Propantheline	T44.3X1	T44.3X2	T44.3X3	T44.3X4	T44.3X5	T44.3X6
bromide	T44.3X1	T44.3X2	T44.3X3	T44.3X4	T44.3X5	T44.3X6
Proparacaine	T41.3X1	T41.3X2	T41.3X3	T41.3X4	T41.3X5	T41.3X6
Propatylnitrate	T46.3X1	T46.3X2	T46.3X3	T46.3X4	T46.3X5	T46.3X6
Propicillin	T36.0X1	T36.0X2	T36.0X3	T36.0X4	T36.0X5	T36.0X6
Propiolactone	T49.0X1	T49.0X2	T49.0X3	T49.0X4	T49.0X5	T49.0X6
Propiomazine	T45.0X1	T45.0X2	T45.0X3	T45.0X4	T45.0X5	T45.0X6
Propionaldehyde (medicinal)	T42.6X1	T42.6X2	T42.6X3	T42.6X4	T42.6X5	T42.6X6
Propionate (calcium) (sodium)	T49.0X1	T49.0X2	T49.0X3	T49.0X4	T49.0X5	T49.0X6
Propion gel	T49.0X1	T49.0X2	T49.0X3	T49.0X4	T49.0X5	T49.0X6
Propitocaine	T41.3X1	T41.3X2	T41.3X3	T41.3X4	T41.3X5	T41.3X6
infiltration (subcutaneous)	T41.3X1	T41.3X2	T41.3X3	T41.3X4	T41.3X5	T41.3X6
nerve block (peripheral) (plexus)	T41.3X1	T41.3X2	T41.3X3	T41.3X4	T41.3X5	T41.3X6
Propofol	T41.291	T41.292	T41.293	T41.294	T41.295	T41.296
Propoxur	T60.0X1	T60.0X2	T60.0X3	T60.0X4	--	--
Propoxycaine	T41.3X1	T41.3X2	T41.3X3	T41.3X4	T41.3X5	T41.3X6
infiltration (subcutaneous)	T41.3X1	T41.3X2	T41.3X3	T41.3X4	T41.3X5	T41.3X6
nerve block (peripheral) (plexus)	T41.3X1	T41.3X2	T41.3X3	T41.3X4	T41.3X5	T41.3X6
topical (surface)	T41.3X1	T41.3X2	T41.3X3	T41.3X4	T41.3X5	T41.3X6
Propoxyphene	T40.4X1	T40.4X2	T40.4X3	T40.4X4	T40.4X5	T40.4X6
Propranolol	T44.7X1	T44.7X2	T44.7X3	T44.7X4	T44.7X5	T44.7X6
Propyl						
alcohol	T51.3X1	T51.3X2	T51.3X3	T51.3X4	--	--
carbinol	T51.3X1	T51.3X2	T51.3X3	T51.3X4	--	--
hexadrine	T44.4X1	T44.4X2	T44.4X3	T44.4X4	T44.4X5	T44.4X6
iodone	T50.8X1	T50.8X2	T50.8X3	T50.8X4	T50.8X5	T50.8X6
thiouracil	T38.2X1	T38.2X2	T38.2X3	T38.2X4	T38.2X5	T38.2X6
Propylaminopheno-thiazine	T43.3X1	T43.3X2	T43.3X3	T43.3X4	T43.3X5	T43.3X6
Propylene	T59.891	T59.892	T59.893	T59.894	--	--
Propylhexedrine	T48.5X1	T48.5X2	T48.5X3	T48.5X4	T48.5X5	T48.5X6
Propyliodone	T50.8X1	T50.8X2	T50.8X3	T50.8X4	T50.8X5	T50.8X6
Propylparaben (ophthalmic)	T49.5X1	T49.5X2	T49.5X3	T49.5X4	T49.5X5	T49.5X6
Propylthiouracil	T38.2X1	T38.2X2	T38.2X3	T38.2X4	T38.2X5	T38.2X6
Propyphenazone	T39.2X1	T39.2X2	T39.2X3	T39.2X4	T39.2X5	T39.2X6
Proquazone	T39.391	T39.392	T39.393	T39.394	T39.395	T39.396
Proscillaridin	T46.0X1	T46.0X2	T46.0X3	T46.0X4	T46.0X5	T46.0X6
Prostacyclin	T45.521	T45.522	T45.523	T45.524	T45.525	T45.526
Prostaglandin (I2)	T45.521	T45.522	T45.523	T45.524	T45.525	T45.526
E1	T46.7X1	T46.7X2	T46.7X3	T46.7X4	T46.7X5	T46.7X6
E2	T48.0X1	T48.0X2	T48.0X3	T48.0X4	T48.0X5	T48.0X6
F2 alpha	T48.0X1	T48.0X2	T48.0X3	T48.0X4	T48.0X5	T48.0X6
Prostigmin	T44.0X1	T44.0X2	T44.0X3	T44.0X4	T44.0X5	T44.0X6
Prosultiamine	T45.2X1	T45.2X2	T45.2X3	T45.2X4	T45.2X5	T45.2X6
Protamine sulfate	T45.7X1	T45.7X2	T45.7X3	T45.7X4	T45.7X5	T45.7X6
zinc insulin	T38.3X1	T38.3X2	T38.3X3	T38.3X4	T38.3X5	T38.3X6
Protease	T47.5X1	T47.5X2	T47.5X3	T47.5X4	T47.5X5	T47.5X6
Protectant, skin NEC	T49.3X1	T49.3X2	T49.3X3	T49.3X4	T49.3X5	T49.3X6
Protein hydrolysate	T50.991	T50.992	T50.993	T50.994	T50.995	T50.996
Prothiaden — *see* Dothiepin hydrochloride						
Prothionamide	T37.1X1	T37.1X2	T37.1X3	T37.1X4	T37.1X5	T37.1X6
Prothipendyl	T43.591	T43.592	T43.593	T43.594	T43.595	T43.596
Prothoate	T60.0X1	T60.0X2	T60.0X3	T60.0X4	--	--
Prothrombin						
activator	T45.7X1	T45.7X2	T45.7X3	T45.7X4	T45.7X5	T45.7X6
synthesis inhibitor	T45.511	T45.512	T45.513	T45.514	T45.515	T45.516
Protionamide	T37.1X1	T37.1X2	T37.1X3	T37.1X4	T37.1X5	T37.1X6
Protirelin	T38.891	T38.892	T38.893	T38.894	T38.895	T38.896
Protokylol	T48.6X1	T48.6X2	T48.6X3	T48.6X4	T48.6X5	T48.6X6
Protopam	T50.6X1	T50.6X2	T50.6X3	T50.6X4	T50.6X5	T50.6X6
Protoveratrine(s) (A) (B)	T46.5X1	T46.5X2	T46.5X3	T46.5X4	T46.5X5	T46.5X6
Protriptyline	T43.011	T43.012	T43.013	T43.014	T43.015	T43.016
Provera	T38.5X1	T38.5X2	T38.5X3	T38.5X4	T38.5X5	T38.5X6
Provitamin A	T45.2X1	T45.2X2	T45.2X3	T45.2X4	T45.2X5	T45.2X6

Substance	Poisoning, Accidental unintentional	Poisoning, Intentional self-harm	Poisoning, Assault	Poisoning, Undetermined	Adverse effect	Underdosing
Proxibarbal	T42.3X1	T42.3X2	T42.3X3	T42.3X4	T42.3X5	T42.3X6
Proxymetacaine	T41.3X1	T41.3X2	T41.3X3	T41.3X4	T41.3X5	T41.3X6
Proxyphylline	T48.6X1	T48.6X2	T48.6X3	T48.6X4	T48.6X5	T48.6X6
Prozac — *see* Fluoxetine hydrochloride						
Prunus						
laurocerasus	T62.2X1	T62.2X2	T62.2X3	T62.2X4	--	--
virginiana	T62.2X1	T62.2X2	T62.2X3	T62.2X4	--	--
Prussian blue						
commercial	T65.891	T65.892	T65.893	T65.894	--	--
therapeutic	T50.6X1	T50.6X2	T50.6X3	T50.6X4	T50.6X5	T50.6X6
Prussic acid	T65.0X1	T65.0X2	T65.0X3	T65.0X4	--	--
vapor	T57.3X1	T57.3X2	T57.3X3	T57.3X4	--	--
Pseudoephedrine	T44.991	T44.992	T44.993	T44.994	T44.995	T44.996
Psilocin	T40.991	T40.992	T40.993	T40.994	--	--
Psilocybin	T40.991	T40.992	T40.993	T40.994	--	--
Psilocybine	T40.991	T40.992	T40.993	T40.994	--	--
Psoralene (nonmedicinal)	T65.891	T65.892	T65.893	T65.894	--	--
Psoralens (medicinal)	T50.991	T50.992	T50.993	T50.994	T50.995	T50.996
PSP (phenolsulfonphthalein)	T50.8X1	T50.8X2	T50.8X3	T50.8X4	T50.8X5	T50.8X6
Psychodysleptic drug NEC	T40.901	T40.902	T40.903	T40.904	T40.905	T40.906
Psychostimulant	T43.601	T43.602	T43.603	T43.604	T43.605	T43.606
amphetamine	T43.621	T43.622	T43.623	T43.624	T43.625	T43.626
caffeine	T43.611	T43.612	T43.613	T43.614	T43.615	T43.616
methylphenidate	T43.631	T43.632	T43.633	T43.634	T43.635	T43.636
specified NEC	T43.691	T43.692	T43.693	T43.694	T43.695	T43.696
Psychotherapeutic drug NEC	T43.91	T43.92	T43.93	T43.94	T43.95	T43.96
antidepressants (*see also* Antidepressant)	T43.201	T43.202	T43.203	T43.204	T43.205	T43.206
specified NEC	T43.8X1	T43.8X2	T43.8X3	T43.8X4	T43.8X5	T43.8X6
tranquilizers NEC	T43.501	T43.502	T43.503	T43.504	T43.505	T43.506
Psychotomimetic agents	T40.901	T40.902	T40.903	T40.904	T40.905	T40.906
Psychotropic drug NEC	T43.91	T43.92	T43.93	T43.94	T43.95	T43.96
specified NEC	T43.8X1	T43.8X2	T43.8X3	T43.8X4	T43.8X5	T43.8X6
Psyllium hydrophilic mucilloid	T47.4X1	T47.4X2	T47.4X3	T47.4X4	T47.4X5	T47.4X6
Pteroylglutamic acid	T45.8X1	T45.8X2	T45.8X3	T45.8X4	T45.8X5	T45.8X6
Pteroyltriglutamate	T45.1X1	T45.1X2	T45.1X3	T45.1X4	T45.1X5	T45.1X6
PTFE — *see* Polytetrafluoroethylene						
Pulp						
devitalizing paste	T49.7X1	T49.7X2	T49.7X3	T49.7X4	T49.7X5	T49.7X6
dressing	T49.7X1	T49.7X2	T49.7X3	T49.7X4	T49.7X5	T49.7X6
Pulsatilla	T62.2X1	T62.2X2	T62.2X3	T62.2X4	--	--
Pumpkin seed extract	T37.4X1	T37.4X2	T37.4X3	T37.4X4	T37.4X5	T37.4X6
Purex (bleach)	T54.91	T54.92	T54.93	T54.94	--	--
Purgative NEC (*see also* Cathartic)	T47.4X1	T47.4X2	T47.4X3	T47.4X4	T47.4X5	T47.4X6
Purine analogue (antineoplastic)	T45.1X1	T45.1X2	T45.1X3	T45.1X4	T45.1X5	T45.1X6
Purine diuretics	T50.2X1	T50.2X2	T50.2X3	T50.2X4	T50.2X5	T50.2X6
Purinethol	T45.1X1	T45.1X2	T45.1X3	T45.1X4	T45.1X5	T45.1X6
PVP	T45.8X1	T45.8X2	T45.8X3	T45.8X4	T45.8X5	T45.8X6
Pyrabital	T39.8X1	T39.8X2	T39.8X3	T39.8X4	T39.8X5	T39.8X6
Pyramidon	T39.2X1	T39.2X2	T39.2X3	T39.2X4	T39.2X5	T39.2X6
Pyrantel	T37.4X1	T37.4X2	T37.4X3	T37.4X4	T37.4X5	T37.4X6
Pyrathiazine	T45.0X1	T45.0X2	T45.0X3	T45.0X4	T45.0X5	T45.0X6
Pyrazinamide	T37.1X1	T37.1X2	T37.1X3	T37.1X4	T37.1X5	T37.1X6
Pyrazinoic acid (amide)	T37.1X1	T37.1X2	T37.1X3	T37.1X4	T37.1X5	T37.1X6
Pyrazole (derivatives)	T39.2X1	T39.2X2	T39.2X3	T39.2X4	T39.2X5	T39.2X6
Pyrazolone analgesic NEC	T39.2X1	T39.2X2	T39.2X3	T39.2X4	T39.2X5	T39.2X6
Pyrethrin, pyrethrum (nonmedicinal)	T60.2X1	T60.2X2	T60.2X3	T60.2X4	--	--
Pyrethrum extract	T49.0X1	T49.0X2	T49.0X3	T49.0X4	T49.0X5	T49.0X6
Pyribenzamine	T45.0X1	T45.0X2	T45.0X3	T45.0X4	T45.0X5	T45.0X6
Pyridine	T52.8X1	T52.8X2	T52.8X3	T52.8X4	--	--
aldoxime methiodide	T50.6X1	T50.6X2	T50.6X3	T50.6X4	T50.6X5	T50.6X6
aldoxime methyl chloride	T50.6X1	T50.6X2	T50.6X3	T50.6X4	T50.6X5	T50.6X6
vapor	T59.891	T59.892	T59.893	T59.894	--	--
Pyridium	T39.8X1	T39.8X2	T39.8X3	T39.8X4	T39.8X5	T39.8X6
Pyridostigmine bromide	T44.0X1	T44.0X2	T44.0X3	T44.0X4	T44.0X5	T44.0X6
Pyridoxal phosphate	T45.2X1	T45.2X2	T45.2X3	T45.2X4	T45.2X5	T45.2X6
Pyridoxine	T45.2X1	T45.2X2	T45.2X3	T45.2X4	T45.2X5	T45.2X6
Pyrilamine	T45.0X1	T45.0X2	T45.0X3	T45.0X4	T45.0X5	T45.0X6
Pyrimethamine	T37.2X1	T37.2X2	T37.2X3	T37.2X4	T37.2X5	T37.2X6
with sulfadoxine	T37.2X1	T37.2X2	T37.2X3	T37.2X4	T37.2X5	T37.2X6
Pyrimidine antagonist	T45.1X1	T45.1X2	T45.1X3	T45.1X4	T45.1X5	T45.1X6
Pyriminil	T60.4X1	T60.4X2	T60.4X3	T60.4X4	--	--
Pyrithione zinc	T49.4X1	T49.4X2	T49.4X3	T49.4X4	T49.4X5	T49.4X6
Pyrithyldione	T42.6X1	T42.6X2	T42.6X3	T42.6X4	T42.6X5	T42.6X6
Pyrogallic acid	T49.0X1	T49.0X2	T49.0X3	T49.0X4	T49.0X5	T49.0X6
Pyrogallol	T49.0X1	T49.0X2	T49.0X3	T49.0X4	T49.0X5	T49.0X6
Pyroxylin	T49.3X1	T49.3X2	T49.3X3	T49.3X4	T49.3X5	T49.3X6

Substance	Poisoning, Accidental unintentional	Poisoning, Intentional self-harm	Poisoning, Assault	Poisoning, Undetermined	Adverse effect	Underdosing
Pyrrobutamine	T45.0X1	T45.0X2	T45.0X3	T45.0X4	T45.0X5	T45.0X6
Pyrrolizidine alkaloids	T62.8X1	T62.8X2	T62.8X3	T62.8X4	--	--
Pyrvinium chloride	T37.4X1	T37.4X2	T37.4X3	T37.4X4	T37.4X5	T37.4X6
PZI	T38.3X1	T38.3X2	T38.3X3	T38.3X4	T38.3X5	T38.3X6
Q						
Quaalude	T42.6X1	T42.6X2	T42.6X3	T42.6X4	T42.6X5	T42.6X6
Quarternary ammonium						
anti-infective	T49.0X1	T49.0X2	T49.0X3	T49.0X4	T49.0X5	T49.0X6
ganglion blocking	T44.2X1	T44.2X2	T44.2X3	T44.2X4	T44.2X5	T44.2X6
parasympatholytic	T44.3X1	T44.3X2	T44.3X3	T44.3X4	T44.3X5	T44.3X6
Quazepam	T42.4X1	T42.4X2	T42.4X3	T42.4X4	T42.4X5	T42.4X6
Quicklime	T54.3X1	T54.3X2	T54.3X3	T54.3X4	--	--
Quillaja extract	T48.4X1	T48.4X2	T48.4X3	T48.4X4	T48.4X5	T48.4X6
Quinacrine	T37.2X1	T37.2X2	T37.2X3	T37.2X4	T37.2X5	T37.2X6
Quinaglute	T46.2X1	T46.2X2	T46.2X3	T46.2X4	T46.2X5	T46.2X6
Quinalbarbital	T42.3X1	T42.3X2	T42.3X3	T42.3X4	T42.3X5	T42.3X6
Quinalbarbitone sodium	T42.3X1	T42.3X2	T42.3X3	T42.3X4	T42.3X5	T42.3X6
Quinalphos	T60.0X1	T60.0X2	T60.0X3	T60.0X4	--	--
Quinapril	T46.4X1	T46.4X2	T46.4X3	T46.4X4	T46.4X5	T46.4X6
Quinestradiol	T38.5X1	T38.5X2	T38.5X3	T38.5X4	T38.5X5	T38.5X6
Quinestradol	T38.5X1	T38.5X2	T38.5X3	T38.5X4	T38.5X5	T38.5X6
Quinestrol	T38.5X1	T38.5X2	T38.5X3	T38.5X4	T38.5X5	T38.5X6
Quinethazone	T50.2X1	T50.2X2	T50.2X3	T50.2X4	T50.2X5	T50.2X6
Quingestanol	T38.4X1	T38.4X2	T38.4X3	T38.4X4	T38.4X5	T38.4X6
Quinidine	T46.2X1	T46.2X2	T46.2X3	T46.2X4	T46.2X5	T46.2X6
Quinine	T37.2X1	T37.2X2	T37.2X3	T37.2X4	T37.2X5	T37.2X6
Quiniobine	T37.8X1	T37.8X2	T37.8X3	T37.8X4	T37.8X5	T37.8X6
Quinisocaine	T49.1X1	T49.1X2	T49.1X3	T49.1X4	T49.1X5	T49.1X6
Quinocide	T37.2X1	T37.2X2	T37.2X3	T37.2X4	T37.2X5	T37.2X6
Quinoline (derivatives) **NEC**	T37.8X1	T37.8X2	T37.8X3	T37.8X4	T37.8X5	T37.8X6
Quinupramine	T43.011	T43.012	T43.013	T43.014	T43.015	T43.016
Quotane	T41.3X1	T41.3X2	T41.3X3	T41.3X4	T41.3X5	T41.3X6
R						
Rabies						
immune globulin (human)	T50.Z11	T50.Z12	T50.Z13	T50.Z14	T50.Z15	T50.Z16
vaccine	T50.B91	T50.B92	T50.B93	T50.B94	T50.B95	T50.B96
Racemoramide	T40.2X1	T40.2X2	T40.2X3	T40.2X4	--	--
Racemorphan	T40.2X1	T40.2X2	T40.2X3	T40.2X4	T40.2X5	T40.2X6
Racepinefrin	T44.5X1	T44.5X2	T44.5X3	T44.5X4	T44.5X5	T44.5X6
Raclopride	T43.591	T43.592	T43.593	T43.594	T43.595	T43.596
Radiator alcohol	T51.1X1	T51.1X2	T51.1X3	T51.1X4	--	--
Radioactive drug NEC	T50.8X1	T50.8X2	T50.8X3	T50.8X4	T50.8X5	T50.8X6
Radio-opaque (drugs) (materials)	T50.8X1	T50.8X2	T50.8X3	T50.8X4	T50.8X5	T50.8X6
Ramifenazone	T39.2X1	T39.2X2	T39.2X3	T39.2X4	T39.2X5	T39.2X6
Ramipril	T46.4X1	T46.4X2	T46.4X3	T46.4X4	T46.4X5	T46.4X6
Ranitidine	T47.0X1	T47.0X2	T47.0X3	T47.0X4	T47.0X5	T47.0X6
Ranunculus	T62.2X1	T62.2X2	T62.2X3	T62.2X4	--	--
Rat poison NEC	T60.4X1	T60.4X2	T60.4X3	T60.4X4	--	--
Rattlesnake (venom)	T63.011	T63.012	T63.013	T63.014	--	--
Raubasine	T46.7X1	T46.7X2	T46.7X3	T46.7X4	T46.7X5	T46.7X6
Raudixin	T46.5X1	T46.5X2	T46.5X3	T46.5X4	T46.5X5	T46.5X6
Rautensin	T46.5X1	T46.5X2	T46.5X3	T46.5X4	T46.5X5	T46.5X6
Rautina	T46.5X1	T46.5X2	T46.5X3	T46.5X4	T46.5X5	T46.5X6
Rautotal	T46.5X1	T46.5X2	T46.5X3	T46.5X4	T46.5X5	T46.5X6
Rauwiloid	T46.5X1	T46.5X2	T46.5X3	T46.5X4	T46.5X5	T46.5X6
Rauwoldin	T46.5X1	T46.5X2	T46.5X3	T46.5X4	T46.5X5	T46.5X6
Rauwolfia (alkaloids)	T46.5X1	T46.5X2	T46.5X3	T46.5X4	T46.5X5	T46.5X6
Razoxane	T45.1X1	T45.1X2	T45.1X3	T45.1X4	T45.1X5	T45.1X6
Realgar	T57.0X1	T57.0X2	T57.0X3	T57.0X4	--	--
Recombinant (R) — *see* specific protein						
Red blood cells, packed	T45.8X1	T45.8X2	T45.8X3	T45.8X4	T45.8X5	T45.8X6
Red squill (scilliroside)	T60.4X1	T60.4X2	T60.4X3	T60.4X4	--	--
Reducing agent, industrial NEC	T65.891	T65.892	T65.893	T65.894	--	--
Refrigerant gas (chlorofluoro-carbon)	T53.5X1	T53.5X2	T53.5X3	T53.5X4	--	--
not chlorofluoro-carbon	T59.891	T59.892	T59.893	T59.894	--	--
Regroton	T50.2X1	T50.2X2	T50.2X3	T50.2X4	T50.2X5	T50.2X6
Rehydration salts (oral)	T50.3X1	T50.3X2	T50.3X3	T50.3X4	T50.3X5	T50.3X6
Rela	T42.8X1	T42.8X2	T42.8X3	T42.8X4	T42.8X5	T42.8X6
Relaxant, muscle						
anesthetic	T48.1X1	T48.1X2	T48.1X3	T48.1X4	T48.1X5	T48.1X6
central nervous system	T42.8X1	T42.8X2	T42.8X3	T42.8X4	T42.8X5	T42.8X6
skeletal NEC	T48.1X1	T48.1X2	T48.1X3	T48.1X4	T48.1X5	T48.1X6
smooth NEC	T44.3X1	T44.3X2	T44.3X3	T44.3X4	T44.3X5	T44.3X6
Remoxipride	T43.591	T43.592	T43.593	T43.594	T43.595	T43.596
Renese	T50.2X1	T50.2X2	T50.2X3	T50.2X4	T50.2X5	T50.2X6
Renografin	T50.8X1	T50.8X2	T50.8X3	T50.8X4	T50.8X5	T50.8X6
Replacement solution	T50.3X1	T50.3X2	T50.3X3	T50.3X4	T50.3X5	T50.3X6
Reproterol	T48.6X1	T48.6X2	T48.6X3	T48.6X4	T48.6X5	T48.6X6
Rescinnamine	T46.5X1	T46.5X2	T46.5X3	T46.5X4	T46.5X5	T46.5X6
Reserpin (e)	T46.5X1	T46.5X2	T46.5X3	T46.5X4	T46.5X5	T46.5X6

Substance	Poisoning, Accidental unintentional	Poisoning, Intentional self-harm	Poisoning, Assault	Poisoning, Undetermined	Adverse effect	Underdosing
Resorcin, resorcinol (nonmedicinal)	T65.891	T65.892	T65.893	T65.894	--	--
medicinal	T49.4X1	T49.4X2	T49.4X3	T49.4X4	T49.4X5	T49.4X6
Respaire	T48.4X1	T48.4X2	T48.4X3	T48.4X4	T48.4X5	T48.4X6
Respiratory drug NEC	T48.901	T48.902	T48.903	T48.904	T48.905	T48.906
antiasthmatic NEC	T48.6X1	T48.6X2	T48.6X3	T48.6X4	T48.6X5	T48.6X6
anti-common-cold NEC	T48.5X1	T48.5X2	T48.5X3	T48.5X4	T48.5X5	T48.5X6
expectorant NEC	T48.4X1	T48.4X2	T48.4X3	T48.4X4	T48.4X5	T48.4X6
stimulant	T48.901	T48.902	T48.903	T48.904	T48.905	T48.906
Retinoic acid	T49.0X1	T49.0X2	T49.0X3	T49.0X4	T49.0X5	T49.0X6
Retinol	T45.2X1	T45.2X2	T45.2X3	T45.2X4	T45.2X5	T45.2X6
Rh (D) immune globulin (human)	T50.Z11	T50.Z12	T50.Z13	T50.Z14	T50.Z15	T50.Z16
Rhodine	T39.011	T39.012	T39.013	T39.014	T39.015	T39.016
RhoGAM	T50.Z11	T50.Z12	T50.Z13	T50.Z14	T50.Z15	T50.Z16
Rhubarb						
dry extract	T47.2X1	T47.2X2	T47.2X3	T47.2X4	T47.2X5	T47.2X6
tincture, compound	T47.2X1	T47.2X2	T47.2X3	T47.2X4	T47.2X5	T47.2X6
Ribavirin	T37.5X1	T37.5X2	T37.5X3	T37.5X4	T37.5X5	T37.5X6
Riboflavin	T45.2X1	T45.2X2	T45.2X3	T45.2X4	T45.2X5	T45.2X6
Ribostamycin	T36.5X1	T36.5X2	T36.5X3	T36.5X4	T36.5X5	T36.5X6
Ricin	T62.2X1	T62.2X2	T62.2X3	T62.2X4	--	--
Ricinus communis	T62.2X1	T62.2X2	T62.2X3	T62.2X4	--	--
Rickettsial vaccine NEC	T50.A91	T50.A92	T50.A93	T50.A94	T50.A95	T50.A96
Rifabutin	T36.6X1	T36.6X2	T36.6X3	T36.6X4	T36.6X5	T36.6X6
Rifamide	T36.6X1	T36.6X2	T36.6X3	T36.6X4	T36.6X5	T36.6X6
Rifampicin	T36.6X1	T36.6X2	T36.6X3	T36.6X4	T36.6X5	T36.6X6
with isoniazid	T37.1X1	T37.1X2	T37.1X3	T37.1X4	T37.1X5	T37.1X6
Rifampin	T36.6X1	T36.6X2	T36.6X3	T36.6X4	T36.6X5	T36.6X6
Rifamycin	T36.6X1	T36.6X2	T36.6X3	T36.6X4	T36.6X5	T36.6X6
Rifaximin	T36.6X1	T36.6X2	T36.6X3	T36.6X4	T36.6X5	T36.6X6
Rimantadine	T37.5X1	T37.5X2	T37.5X3	T37.5X4	T37.5X5	T37.5X6
Rimazolium metilsulfate	T39.8X1	T39.8X2	T39.8X3	T39.8X4	T39.8X5	T39.8X6
Rimifon	T37.1X1	T37.1X2	T37.1X3	T37.1X4	T37.1X5	T37.1X6
Rimiterol	T48.6X1	T48.6X2	T48.6X3	T48.6X4	T48.6X5	T48.6X6
Ringer (lactate) solution	T50.3X1	T50.3X2	T50.3X3	T50.3X4	T50.3X5	T50.3X6
Ristocetin	T36.8X1	T36.8X2	T36.8X3	T36.8X4	T36.8X5	T36.8X6
Ritalin	T43.631	T43.632	T43.633	T43.634	T43.635	T43.636
Ritodrine	T44.5X1	T44.5X2	T44.5X3	T44.5X4	T44.5X5	T44.5X6
Roach killer — *see* Insecticide						
Rociverine	T44.3X1	T44.3X2	T44.3X3	T44.3X4	T44.3X5	T44.3X6
Rocky Mountain spotted fever vaccine	T50.A91	T50.A92	T50.A93	T50.A94	T50.A95	T50.A96
Rodenticide NEC	T60.4X1	T60.4X2	T60.4X3	T60.4X4	--	--
Rohypnol	T42.4X1	T42.4X2	T42.4X3	T42.4X4	T42.4X5	T42.4X6
Rokitamycin	T36.3X1	T36.3X2	T36.3X3	T36.3X4	T36.3X5	T36.3X6
Rolaids	T47.1X1	T47.1X2	T47.1X3	T47.1X4	T47.1X5	T47.1X6
Rolitetracycline	T36.4X1	T36.4X2	T36.4X3	T36.4X4	T36.4X5	T36.4X6
Romilar	T48.3X1	T48.3X2	T48.3X3	T48.3X4	T48.3X5	T48.3X6
Ronifibrate	T46.6X1	T46.6X2	T46.6X3	T46.6X4	T46.6X5	T46.6X6
Rosaprostol	T47.1X1	T47.1X2	T47.1X3	T47.1X4	T47.1X5	T47.1X6
Rose bengal sodium (131I)	T50.8X1	T50.8X2	T50.8X3	T50.8X4	T50.8X5	T50.8X6
Rose water ointment	T49.3X1	T49.3X2	T49.3X3	T49.3X4	T49.3X5	T49.3X6
Rosoxacin	T37.8X1	T37.8X2	T37.8X3	T37.8X4	T37.8X5	T37.8X6
Rotenone	T60.2X1	T60.2X2	T60.2X3	T60.2X4	--	--
Rotoxamine	T45.0X1	T45.0X2	T45.0X3	T45.0X4	T45.0X5	T45.0X6
Rough-on-rats	T60.4X1	T60.4X2	T60.4X3	T60.4X4	--	--
Roxatidine	T47.0X1	T47.0X2	T47.0X3	T47.0X4	T47.0X5	T47.0X6
Roxithromycin	T36.3X1	T36.3X2	T36.3X3	T36.3X4	T36.3X5	T36.3X6
Rt-PA	T45.611	T45.612	T45.613	T45.614	T45.615	T45.616
Rubbing alcohol	T51.2X1	T51.2X2	T51.2X3	T51.2X4	--	--
Rubefacient	T49.4X1	T49.4X2	T49.4X3	T49.4X4	T49.4X5	T49.4X6
Rubella vaccine	T50.B91	T50.B92	T50.B93	T50.B94	T50.B95	T50.B96
Rubeola vaccine	T50.B91	T50.B92	T50.B93	T50.B94	T50.B95	T50.B96
Rubidium chloride Rb82	T50.8X1	T50.8X2	T50.8X3	T50.8X4	T50.8X5	T50.8X6
Rubidomycin	T45.1X1	T45.1X2	T45.1X3	T45.1X4	T45.1X5	T45.1X6
Rue	T62.2X1	T62.2X2	T62.2X3	T62.2X4	--	--
Rufocromomycin	T45.1X1	T45.1X2	T45.1X3	T45.1X4	T45.1X5	T45.1X6
Russel's viper venin	T45.7X1	T45.7X2	T45.7X3	T45.7X4	T45.7X5	T45.7X6
Ruta (graveolens)	T62.2X1	T62.2X2	T62.2X3	T62.2X4	--	--
Rutinum	T46.991	T46.992	T46.993	T46.994	T46.995	T46.996
Rutoside	T46.991	T46.992	T46.993	T46.994	T46.995	T46.996
S						
Sabadilla (plant)	T62.2X1	T62.2X2	T62.2X3	T62.2X4	--	--
pesticide	T60.2X1	T60.2X2	T60.2X3	T60.2X4	--	--
Saccharated iron oxide	T45.8X1	T45.8X2	T45.8X3	T45.8X4	T45.8X5	T45.8X6
Saccharin	T50.901	T50.902	T50.903	T50.904	T50.905	T50.906
Saccharomyces boulardii	T47.6X1	T47.6X2	T47.6X3	T47.6X4	T47.6X5	T47.6X6
Safflower oil	T46.6X1	T46.6X2	T46.6X3	T46.6X4	T46.6X5	T46.6X6
Safrazine	T43.1X1	T43.1X2	T43.1X3	T43.1X4	T43.1X5	T43.1X6
Salazosulfapyridine	T37.0X1	T37.0X2	T37.0X3	T37.0X4	T37.0X5	T37.0X6
Salbutamol	T48.6X1	T48.6X2	T48.6X3	T48.6X4	T48.6X5	T48.6X6
Salicylamide	T39.091	T39.092	T39.093	T39.094	T39.095	T39.096
Salicylate NEC	T39.091	T39.092	T39.093	T39.094	T39.095	T39.096
methyl	T49.3X1	T49.3X2	T49.3X3	T49.3X4	T49.3X5	T49.3X6
theobromine calcium	T50.2X1	T50.2X2	T50.2X3	T50.2X4	T50.2X5	T50.2X6
Salicylazosulfapyridine	T37.0X1	T37.0X2	T37.0X3	T37.0X4	T37.0X5	T37.0X6
Salicylhydroxamic acid	T49.0X1	T49.0X2	T49.0X3	T49.0X4	T49.0X5	T49.0X6
Salicylic acid	T49.4X1	T49.4X2	T49.4X3	T49.4X4	T49.4X5	T49.4X6
with benzoic acid	T49.4X1	T49.4X2	T49.4X3	T49.4X4	T49.4X5	T49.4X6
congeners	T39.091	T39.092	T39.093	T39.094	T39.095	T39.096
derivative	T39.091	T39.092	T39.093	T39.094	T39.095	T39.096
salts	T39.091	T39.092	T39.093	T39.094	T39.095	T39.096
Salinazid	T37.1X1	T37.1X2	T37.1X3	T37.1X4	T37.1X5	T37.1X6
Salmeterol	T48.6X1	T48.6X2	T48.6X3	T48.6X4	T48.6X5	T48.6X6
Salol	T49.3X1	T49.3X2	T49.3X3	T49.3X4	T49.3X5	T49.3X6
Salsalate	T39.091	T39.092	T39.093	T39.094	T39.095	T39.096
Salt substitute	T50.901	T50.902	T50.903	T50.904	T50.905	T50.906
Salt-replacing drug	T50.901	T50.902	T50.903	T50.904	T50.905	T50.906
Salt-retaining mineralocorticoid	T50.0X1	T50.0X2	T50.0X3	T50.0X4	T50.0X5	T50.0X6
Saluretic NEC	T50.2X1	T50.2X2	T50.2X3	T50.2X4	T50.2X5	T50.2X6
Saluron	T50.2X1	T50.2X2	T50.2X3	T50.2X4	T50.2X5	T50.2X6
Salvarsan 606 (neosilver) (silver)	T37.8X1	T37.8X2	T37.8X3	T37.8X4	T37.8X5	T37.8X6
Sambucus canadensis	T62.2X1	T62.2X2	T62.2X3	T62.2X4	--	--
berry	T62.1X1	T62.1X2	T62.1X3	T62.1X4	--	--
Sandril	T46.5X1	T46.5X2	T46.5X3	T46.5X4	T46.5X5	T46.5X6
Sanguinaria canadensis	T62.2X1	T62.2X2	T62.2X3	T62.2X4	--	--
Saniflush (cleaner)	T54.2X1	T54.2X2	T54.2X3	T54.2X4	--	--
Santonin	T37.4X1	T37.4X2	T37.4X3	T37.4X4	T37.4X5	T37.4X6
Santyl	T49.8X1	T49.8X2	T49.8X3	T49.8X4	T49.8X5	T49.8X6
Saralasin	T46.5X1	T46.5X2	T46.5X3	T46.5X4	T46.5X5	T46.5X6
Sarcolysin	T45.1X1	T45.1X2	T45.1X3	T45.1X4	T45.1X5	T45.1X6
Sarkomycin	T45.1X1	T45.1X2	T45.1X3	T45.1X4	T45.1X5	T45.1X6
Saroten	T43.011	T43.012	T43.013	T43.014	T43.015	T43.016
Saturnine — *see* Lead						
Savin (oil)	T49.4X1	T49.4X2	T49.4X3	T49.4X4	T49.4X5	T49.4X6
Scammony	T47.2X1	T47.2X2	T47.2X3	T47.2X4	T47.2X5	T47.2X6
Scarlet red	T49.8X1	T49.8X2	T49.8X3	T49.8X4	T49.8X5	T49.8X6
Scheele's green	T57.0X1	T57.0X2	T57.0X3	T57.0X4	--	--
insecticide	T57.0X1	T57.0X2	T57.0X3	T57.0X4	--	--
Schizontozide (blood) (tissue)	T37.2X1	T37.2X2	T37.2X3	T37.2X4	T37.2X5	T37.2X6
Schradan	T60.0X1	T60.0X2	T60.0X3	T60.0X4	--	--
Schweinfurth green	T57.0X1	T57.0X2	T57.0X3	T57.0X4	--	--
insecticide	T57.0X1	T57.0X2	T57.0X3	T57.0X4	--	--
Scilla, rat poison	T60.4X1	T60.4X2	T60.4X3	T60.4X4	--	--
Scillaren	T60.4X1	T60.4X2	T60.4X3	T60.4X4	--	--
Sclerosing agent	T46.8X1	T46.8X2	T46.8X3	T46.8X4	T46.8X5	T46.8X6
Scombrotoxin	T61.11	T61.12	T61.13	T61.14	--	--
Scopolamine	T44.3X1	T44.3X2	T44.3X3	T44.3X4	T44.3X5	T44.3X6
Scopolia extract	T44.3X1	T44.3X2	T44.3X3	T44.3X4	T44.3X5	T44.3X6
Scouring powder	T65.891	T65.892	T65.893	T65.894	--	--
Sea						
anemone (sting)	T63.631	T63.632	T63.633	T63.634	--	--
cucumber (sting)	T63.691	T63.692	T63.693	T63.694	--	--
snake (bite) (venom)	T63.091	T63.092	T63.093	T63.094	--	--
urchin spine (puncture)	T63.691	T63.692	T63.693	T63.694	--	--
Seafood	T61.91	T61.92	T61.93	T61.94	--	--
specified NEC	T61.8X1	T61.8X2	T61.8X3	T61.8X4	--	--
Secbutabarbital	T42.3X1	T42.3X2	T42.3X3	T42.3X4	T42.3X5	T42.3X6
Secbutabarbitone	T42.3X1	T42.3X2	T42.3X3	T42.3X4	T42.3X5	T42.3X6
Secnidazole	T37.3X1	T37.3X2	T37.3X3	T37.3X4	T37.3X5	T37.3X6
Secobarbital	T42.3X1	T42.3X2	T42.3X3	T42.3X4	T42.3X5	T42.3X6
Seconal	T42.3X1	T42.3X2	T42.3X3	T42.3X4	T42.3X5	T42.3X6
Secretin	T50.8X1	T50.8X2	T50.8X3	T50.8X4	T50.8X5	T50.8X6
Sedative NEC	T42.71	T42.72	T42.73	T42.74	T42.75	T42.76
mixed NEC	T42.6X1	T42.6X2	T42.6X3	T42.6X4	T42.6X5	T42.6X6
Sedormid	T42.6X1	T42.6X2	T42.6X3	T42.6X4	T42.6X5	T42.6X6
Seed disinfectant or dressing	T60.8X1	T60.8X2	T60.8X3	T60.8X4	--	--
Seeds (poisonous)	T62.2X1	T62.2X2	T62.2X3	T62.2X4	--	--
Selegiline	T42.8X1	T42.8X2	T42.8X3	T42.8X4	T42.8X5	T42.8X6
Selenium NEC	T56.891	T56.892	T56.893	T56.894	--	--
disulfide or sulfide	T49.4X1	T49.4X2	T49.4X3	T49.4X4	T49.4X5	T49.4X6
fumes	T59.891	T59.892	T59.893	T59.894	--	--
sulfide	T49.4X1	T49.4X2	T49.4X3	T49.4X4	T49.4X5	T49.4X6
Selenomethionine (75Se)	T50.8X1	T50.8X2	T50.8X3	T50.8X4	T50.8X5	T50.8X6
Selsun	T49.4X1	T49.4X2	T49.4X3	T49.4X4	T49.4X5	T49.4X6
Semustine	T45.1X1	T45.1X2	T45.1X3	T45.1X4	T45.1X5	T45.1X6
Senega syrup	T48.4X1	T48.4X2	T48.4X3	T48.4X4	T48.4X5	T48.4X6
Senna	T47.2X1	T47.2X2	T47.2X3	T47.2X4	T47.2X5	T47.2X6
Sennoside A+B	T47.2X1	T47.2X2	T47.2X3	T47.2X4	T47.2X5	T47.2X6
Septisol	T49.2X1	T49.2X2	T49.2X3	T49.2X4	T49.2X5	T49.2X6
Seractide	T38.811	T38.812	T38.813	T38.814	T38.815	T38.816
Serax	T42.4X1	T42.4X2	T42.4X3	T42.4X4	T42.4X5	T42.4X6
Serenesil	T42.6X1	T42.6X2	T42.6X3	T42.6X4	T42.6X5	T42.6X6
Serenium (hydrochloride)	T37.91	T37.92	T37.93	T37.94	T37.95	T37.96
Serepax — *see* Oxazepam						
Sermorelin	T38.891	T38.892	T38.893	T38.894	T38.895	T38.896
Sernyl	T41.1X1	T41.1X2	T41.1X3	T41.1X4	T41.1X5	T41.1X6

2018 ICD-10-CM ICD-10-CM TABLE OF DRUGS AND CHEMICALS

Serotonin - Sodium

Substance	Poisoning, Accidental unintentional	Poisoning, Intentional self-harm	Poisoning, Assault	Poisoning, Undetermined	Adverse effect	Underdosing
Serotonin	T50.991	T50.992	T50.993	T50.994	T50.995	T50.996
Serpasil	T46.5X1	T46.5X2	T46.5X3	T46.5X4	T46.5X5	T46.5X6
Serrapeptase	T45.3X1	T45.3X2	T45.3X3	T45.3X4	T45.3X5	T45.3X6
Serum						
antibotulinus	T50.Z11	T50.Z12	T50.Z13	T50.Z14	T50.Z15	T50.Z16
anticytotoxic	T50.Z11	T50.Z12	T50.Z13	T50.Z14	T50.Z15	T50.Z16
antidiphtheria	T50.Z11	T50.Z12	T50.Z13	T50.Z14	T50.Z15	T50.Z16
antimeningococcus	T50.Z11	T50.Z12	T50.Z13	T50.Z14	T50.Z15	T50.Z16
anti-Rh	T50.Z11	T50.Z12	T50.Z13	T50.Z14	T50.Z15	T50.Z16
anti-snake-bite	T50.Z11	T50.Z12	T50.Z13	T50.Z14	T50.Z15	T50.Z16
antitetanic	T50.Z11	T50.Z12	T50.Z13	T50.Z14	T50.Z15	T50.Z16
antitoxic	T50.Z11	T50.Z12	T50.Z13	T50.Z14	T50.Z15	T50.Z16
complement (inhibitor)	T45.8X1	T45.8X2	T45.8X3	T45.8X4	T45.8X5	T45.8X6
convalescent	T50.Z11	T50.Z12	T50.Z13	T50.Z14	T50.Z15	T50.Z16
hemolytic complement	T45.8X1	T45.8X2	T45.8X3	T45.8X4	T45.8X5	T45.8X6
immune (human)	T50.Z11	T50.Z12	T50.Z13	T50.Z14	T50.Z15	T50.Z16
protective NEC	T50.Z11	T50.Z12	T50.Z13	T50.Z14	T50.Z15	T50.Z16
Setastine	T45.0X1	T45.0X2	T45.0X3	T45.0X4	T45.0X5	T45.0X6
Setoperone	T43.591	T43.592	T43.593	T43.594	T43.595	T43.596
Sewer gas	T59.91	T59.92	T59.93	T59.94	--	--
Shampoo	T55.0X1	T55.0X2	T55.0X3	T55.0X4	--	--
Shellfish, noxious, nonbacterial	T61.781	T61.782	T61.783	T61.784	--	--
Sildenafil	T46.7X1	T46.7X2	T46.7X3	T46.7X4	T46.7X5	T46.7X6
Silibinin	T50.991	T50.992	T50.993	T50.994	T50.995	T50.996
Silicone NEC	T65.891	T65.892	T65.893	T65.894	--	--
medicinal	T49.3X1	T49.3X2	T49.3X3	T49.3X4	T49.3X5	T49.3X6
Silvadene	T49.0X1	T49.0X2	T49.0X3	T49.0X4	T49.0X5	T49.0X6
Silver	T49.0X1	T49.0X2	T49.0X3	T49.0X4	T49.0X5	T49.0X6
anti-infectives	T49.0X1	T49.0X2	T49.0X3	T49.0X4	T49.0X5	T49.0X6
arsphenamine	T37.8X1	T37.8X2	T37.8X3	T37.8X4	T37.8X5	T37.8X6
colloidal	T49.0X1	T49.0X2	T49.0X3	T49.0X4	T49.0X5	T49.0X6
nitrate	T49.0X1	T49.0X2	T49.0X3	T49.0X4	T49.0X5	T49.0X6
ophthalmic preparation	T49.5X1	T49.5X2	T49.5X3	T49.5X4	T49.5X5	T49.5X6
toughened (keratolytic)	T49.4X1	T49.4X2	T49.4X3	T49.4X4	T49.4X5	T49.4X6
nonmedicinal (dust)	T56.891	T56.892	T56.893	T56.894	--	--
protein	T49.5X1	T49.5X2	T49.5X3	T49.5X4	T49.5X5	T49.5X6
salvarsan	T37.8X1	T37.8X2	T37.8X3	T37.8X4	T37.8X5	T37.8X6
sulfadiazine	T49.4X1	T49.4X2	T49.4X3	T49.4X4	T49.4X5	T49.4X6
Silymarin	T50.991	T50.992	T50.993	T50.994	T50.995	T50.996
Simaldrate	T47.1X1	T47.1X2	T47.1X3	T47.1X4	T47.1X5	T47.1X6
Simazine	T60.3X1	T60.3X2	T60.3X3	T60.3X4	--	--
Simethicone	T47.1X1	T47.1X2	T47.1X3	T47.1X4	T47.1X5	T47.1X6
Simfibrate	T46.6X1	T46.6X2	T46.6X3	T46.6X4	T46.6X5	T46.6X6
Simvastatin	T46.6X1	T46.6X2	T46.6X3	T46.6X4	T46.6X5	T46.6X6
Sincalide	T50.8X1	T50.8X2	T50.8X3	T50.8X4	T50.8X5	T50.8X6
Sinequan	T43.011	T43.012	T43.013	T43.014	T43.015	T43.016
Singoserp	T46.5X1	T46.5X2	T46.5X3	T46.5X4	T46.5X5	T46.5X6
Sintrom	T45.511	T45.512	T45.513	T45.514	T45.515	T45.516
Sisomicin	T36.5X1	T36.5X2	T36.5X3	T36.5X4	T36.5X5	T36.5X6
Sitosterols	T46.6X1	T46.6X2	T46.6X3	T46.6X4	T46.6X5	T46.6X6
Skeletal muscle relaxants	T48.1X1	T48.1X2	T48.1X3	T48.1X4	T48.1X5	T48.1X6
Skin						
agents (external)	T49.91	T49.92	T49.93	T49.94	T49.95	T49.96
specified NEC	T49.8X1	T49.8X2	T49.8X3	T49.8X4	T49.8X5	T49.8X6
test antigen	T50.8X1	T50.8X2	T50.8X3	T50.8X4	T50.8X5	T50.8X6
Sleep-eze	T45.0X1	T45.0X2	T45.0X3	T45.0X4	T45.0X5	T45.0X6
Sleeping draught, pill	T42.71	T42.72	T42.73	T42.74	T42.75	T42.76
Smallpox vaccine	T50.B11	T50.B12	T50.B13	T50.B14	T50.B15	T50.B16
Smelter fumes NEC	T56.91	T56.92	T56.93	T56.94	--	--
Smog	T59.1X1	T59.1X2	T59.1X3	T59.1X4	--	--
Smoke NEC	T59.811	T59.812	T59.813	T59.814	--	--
Smooth muscle relaxant	T44.3X1	T44.3X2	T44.3X3	T44.3X4	T44.3X5	T44.3X6
Snail killer NEC	T60.8X1	T60.8X2	T60.8X3	T60.8X4	--	--
Snake venom or bite	T63.001	T63.002	T63.003	T63.004	--	--
hemocoagulase	T45.7X1	T45.7X2	T45.7X3	T45.7X4	T45.7X5	T45.7X6
Snuff	T65.211	T65.212	T65.213	T65.214	--	--
Soap (powder) (product)	T55.0X1	T55.0X2	T55.0X3	T55.0X4	--	--
enema	T47.4X1	T47.4X2	T47.4X3	T47.4X4	T47.4X5	T47.4X6
medicinal, soft	T49.2X1	T49.2X2	T49.2X3	T49.2X4	T49.2X5	T49.2X6
superfatted	T49.2X1	T49.2X2	T49.2X3	T49.2X4	T49.2X5	T49.2X6
Sobrerol	T48.4X1	T48.4X2	T48.4X3	T48.4X4	T48.4X5	T48.4X6
Soda (caustic)	T54.3X1	T54.3X2	T54.3X3	T54.3X4	--	--
bicarb	T47.1X1	T47.1X2	T47.1X3	T47.1X4	T47.1X5	T47.1X6
chlorinated — *see* Sodium, hypochlorite						
Sodium						
acetosulfone	T37.1X1	T37.1X2	T37.1X3	T37.1X4	T37.1X5	T37.1X6
acetrizoate	T50.8X1	T50.8X2	T50.8X3	T50.8X4	T50.8X5	T50.8X6
acid phosphate	T50.3X1	T50.3X2	T50.3X3	T50.3X4	T50.3X5	T50.3X6
alginate	T47.8X1	T47.8X2	T47.8X3	T47.8X4	T47.8X5	T47.8X6
amidotrizoate	T50.8X1	T50.8X2	T50.8X3	T50.8X4	T50.8X5	T50.8X6
aminopterin	T45.1X1	T45.1X2	T45.1X3	T45.1X4	T45.1X5	T45.1X6
amylosulfate	T47.8X1	T47.8X2	T47.8X3	T47.8X4	T47.8X5	T47.8X6
Sodium — *continued*						
amytal	T42.3X1	T42.3X2	T42.3X3	T42.3X4	T42.3X5	T42.3X6
antimony gluconate	T37.3X1	T37.3X2	T37.3X3	T37.3X4	T37.3X5	T37.3X6
arsenate	T57.0X1	T57.0X2	T57.0X3	T57.0X4	--	--
aurothiomalate	T39.4X1	T39.4X2	T39.4X3	T39.4X4	T39.4X5	T39.4X6
aurothiosulfate	T39.4X1	T39.4X2	T39.4X3	T39.4X4	T39.4X5	T39.4X6
barbiturate	T42.3X1	T42.3X2	T42.3X3	T42.3X4	T42.3X5	T42.3X6
basic phosphate	T47.4X1	T47.4X2	T47.4X3	T47.4X4	T47.4X5	T47.4X6
bicarbonate	T47.1X1	T47.1X2	T47.1X3	T47.1X4	T47.1X5	T47.1X6
bichromate	T57.8X1	T57.8X2	T57.8X3	T57.8X4	--	--
biphosphate	T50.3X1	T50.3X2	T50.3X3	T50.3X4	T50.3X5	T50.3X6
bisulfate	T65.891	T65.892	T65.893	T65.894	--	--
borate						
cleanser	T57.8X1	T57.8X2	T57.8X3	T57.8X4	--	--
eye	T49.5X1	T49.5X2	T49.5X3	T49.5X4	T49.5X5	T49.5X6
therapeutic	T49.8X1	T49.8X2	T49.8X3	T49.8X4	T49.8X5	T49.8X6
bromide	T42.6X1	T42.6X2	T42.6X3	T42.6X4	T42.6X5	T42.6X6
cacodylate (nonmedicinal) NEC	T50.8X1	T50.8X2	T50.8X3	T50.8X4	T50.8X5	T50.8X6
anti-infective	T37.8X1	T37.8X2	T37.8X3	T37.8X4	T37.8X5	T37.8X6
herbicide	T60.3X1	T60.3X2	T60.3X3	T60.3X4	--	--
calcium edetate	T45.8X1	T45.8X2	T45.8X3	T45.8X4	T45.8X5	T45.8X6
carbonate NEC	T54.3X1	T54.3X2	T54.3X3	T54.3X4	--	--
chlorate NEC	T65.891	T65.892	T65.893	T65.894	--	--
herbicide	T54.91	T54.92	T54.93	T54.94	--	--
chloride	T50.3X1	T50.3X2	T50.3X3	T50.3X4	T50.3X5	T50.3X6
with glucose	T50.3X1	T50.3X2	T50.3X3	T50.3X4	T50.3X5	T50.3X6
chromate	T65.891	T65.892	T65.893	T65.894	--	--
citrate	T50.991	T50.992	T50.993	T50.994	T50.995	T50.996
cromoglicate	T48.6X1	T48.6X2	T48.6X3	T48.6X4	T48.6X5	T48.6X6
cyanide	T65.0X1	T65.0X2	T65.0X3	T65.0X4	--	--
cyclamate	T50.3X1	T50.3X2	T50.3X3	T50.3X4	T50.3X5	T50.3X6
dehydrocholate	T45.8X1	T45.8X2	T45.8X3	T45.8X4	T45.8X5	T45.8X6
diatrizoate	T50.8X1	T50.8X2	T50.8X3	T50.8X4	T50.8X5	T50.8X6
dibunate	T48.4X1	T48.4X2	T48.4X3	T48.4X4	T48.4X5	T48.4X6
dioctyl sulfosuccinate	T47.4X1	T47.4X2	T47.4X3	T47.4X4	T47.4X5	T47.4X6
dipantoyl ferrate	T45.8X1	T45.8X2	T45.8X3	T45.8X4	T45.8X5	T45.8X6
edetate	T45.8X1	T45.8X2	T45.8X3	T45.8X4	T45.8X5	T45.8X6
ethacrynate	T50.1X1	T50.1X2	T50.1X3	T50.1X4	T50.1X5	T50.1X6
feredetate	T45.8X1	T45.8X2	T45.8X3	T45.8X4	T45.8X5	T45.8X6
Fluoride — *see* Fluoride						
fluoroacetate (dust) (pesticide)	T60.4X1	T60.4X2	T60.4X3	T60.4X4	--	--
free salt	T50.3X1	T50.3X2	T50.3X3	T50.3X4	T50.3X5	T50.3X6
fusidate	T36.8X1	T36.8X2	T36.8X3	T36.8X4	T36.8X5	T36.8X6
glucaldrate	T47.1X1	T47.1X2	T47.1X3	T47.1X4	T47.1X5	T47.1X6
glucosulfone	T37.1X1	T37.1X2	T37.1X3	T37.1X4	T37.1X5	T37.1X6
glutamate	T45.8X1	T45.8X2	T45.8X3	T45.8X4	T45.8X5	T45.8X6
hydrogen carbonate	T50.3X1	T50.3X2	T50.3X3	T50.3X4	T50.3X5	T50.3X6
hydroxide	T54.3X1	T54.3X2	T54.3X3	T54.3X4	--	--
hypochlorite (bleach) NEC	T54.3X1	T54.3X2	T54.3X3	T54.3X4	--	--
disinfectant	T54.3X1	T54.3X2	T54.3X3	T54.3X4	--	--
medicinal (anti-infective) (external)	T49.0X1	T49.0X2	T49.0X3	T49.0X4	T49.0X5	T49.0X6
vapor	T54.3X1	T54.3X2	T54.3X3	T54.3X4	--	--
hyposulfite	T49.0X1	T49.0X2	T49.0X3	T49.0X4	T49.0X5	T49.0X6
indigotin disulfonate	T50.8X1	T50.8X2	T50.8X3	T50.8X4	T50.8X5	T50.8X6
iodide	T50.991	T50.992	T50.993	T50.994	T50.995	T50.996
I-131	T50.8X1	T50.8X2	T50.8X3	T50.8X4	T50.8X5	T50.8X6
therapeutic	T38.2X1	T38.2X2	T38.2X3	T38.2X4	T38.2X5	T38.2X6
iodohippurate (131I)	T50.8X1	T50.8X2	T50.8X3	T50.8X4	T50.8X5	T50.8X6
iopodate	T50.8X1	T50.8X2	T50.8X3	T50.8X4	T50.8X5	T50.8X6
iothalamate	T50.8X1	T50.8X2	T50.8X3	T50.8X4	T50.8X5	T50.8X6
iron edetate	T45.4X1	T45.4X2	T45.4X3	T45.4X4	T45.4X5	T45.4X6
lactate (compound solution)	T45.8X1	T45.8X2	T45.8X3	T45.8X4	T45.8X5	T45.8X6
lauryl (sulfate)	T49.2X1	T49.2X2	T49.2X3	T49.2X4	T49.2X5	T49.2X6
L-triiodothyronine	T38.1X1	T38.1X2	T38.1X3	T38.1X4	T38.1X5	T38.1X6
magnesium citrate	T50.991	T50.992	T50.993	T50.994	T50.995	T50.996
mersalate	T50.2X1	T50.2X2	T50.2X3	T50.2X4	T50.2X5	T50.2X6
metasilicate	T65.891	T65.892	T65.893	T65.894	--	--
metrizoate	T50.8X1	T50.8X2	T50.8X3	T50.8X4	T50.8X5	T50.8X6
monofluoroacetate (pesticide)	T60.1X1	T60.1X2	T60.1X3	T60.1X4	--	--
morrhuate	T46.8X1	T46.8X2	T46.8X3	T46.8X4	T46.8X5	T46.8X6
nafcillin	T36.0X1	T36.0X2	T36.0X3	T36.0X4	T36.0X5	T36.0X6
nitrate (oxidizing agent)	T65.891	T65.892	T65.893	T65.894	--	--
nitrite	T50.6X1	T50.6X2	T50.6X3	T50.6X4	T50.6X5	T50.6X6
nitroferricyanide	T46.5X1	T46.5X2	T46.5X3	T46.5X4	T46.5X5	T46.5X6
nitroprusside	T46.5X1	T46.5X2	T46.5X3	T46.5X4	T46.5X5	T46.5X6
oxalate	T65.891	T65.892	T65.893	T65.894	--	--
oxide/peroxide	T65.891	T65.892	T65.893	T65.894	--	--
oxybate	T41.291	T41.292	T41.293	T41.294	T41.295	T41.296
para-aminohippurate	T50.8X1	T50.8X2	T50.8X3	T50.8X4	T50.8X5	T50.8X6

Serotonin - Sodium

ICD-10-CM TABLE OF DRUGS AND CHEMICALS

Substance	Poisoning, Accidental unintentional	Poisoning, Intentional self-harm	Poisoning, Assault	Poisoning, Undetermined	Adverse effect	Underdosing
Sodium — *continued*						
perborate (nonmedicinal) NEC	T65.891	T65.892	T65.893	T65.894	--	--
medicinal	T49.0X1	T49.0X2	T49.0X3	T49.0X4	T49.0X5	T49.0X6
soap	T55.0X1	T55.0X2	T55.0X3	T55.0X4	--	--
percarbonate — *see* Sodium, perborate						
pertechnetate Tc99m	T50.8X1	T50.8X2	T50.8X3	T50.8X4	T50.8X5	T50.8X6
phosphate						
cellulose	T45.8X1	T45.8X2	T45.8X3	T45.8X4	T45.8X5	T45.8X6
dibasic	T47.2X1	T47.2X2	T47.2X3	T47.2X4	T47.2X5	T47.2X6
monobasic	T47.2X1	T47.2X2	T47.2X3	T47.2X4	T47.2X5	T47.2X6
phytate	T50.6X1	T50.6X2	T50.6X3	T50.6X4	T50.6X5	T50.6X6
picosulfate	T47.2X1	T47.2X2	T47.2X3	T47.2X4	T47.2X5	T47.2X6
polyhydroxyaluminium monocarbonate	T47.1X1	T47.1X2	T47.1X3	T47.1X4	T47.1X5	T47.1X6
polystyrene sulfonate	T50.3X1	T50.3X2	T50.3X3	T50.3X4	T50.3X5	T50.3X6
propionate	T49.0X1	T49.0X2	T49.0X3	T49.0X4	T49.0X5	T49.0X6
propyl hydroxybenzoate	T50.991	T50.992	T50.993	T50.994	T50.995	T50.996
psylliate	T46.8X1	T46.8X2	T46.8X3	T46.8X4	T46.8X5	T46.8X6
removing resins	T50.3X1	T50.3X2	T50.3X3	T50.3X4	T50.3X5	T50.3X6
salicylate	T39.091	T39.092	T39.093	T39.094	T39.095	T39.096
salt NEC	T50.3X1	T50.3X2	T50.3X3	T50.3X4	T50.3X5	T50.3X6
selenate	T60.2X1	T60.2X2	T60.2X3	T60.2X4	--	--
stibogluconate	T37.3X1	T37.3X2	T37.3X3	T37.3X4	T37.3X5	T37.3X6
sulfate	T47.4X1	T47.4X2	T47.4X3	T47.4X4	T47.4X5	T47.4X6
sulfoxone	T37.1X1	T37.1X2	T37.1X3	T37.1X4	T37.1X5	T37.1X6
tetradecyl sulfate	T46.8X1	T46.8X2	T46.8X3	T46.8X4	T46.8X5	T46.8X6
thiopental	T41.1X1	T41.1X2	T41.1X3	T41.1X4	T41.1X5	T41.1X6
thiosalicylate	T39.091	T39.092	T39.093	T39.094	T39.095	T39.096
thiosulfate	T50.6X1	T50.6X2	T50.6X3	T50.6X4	T50.6X5	T50.6X6
tolbutamide	T38.3X1	T38.3X2	T38.3X3	T38.3X4	T38.3X5	T38.3X6
(L) -triiodothyronine	T38.1X1	T38.1X2	T38.1X3	T38.1X4	T38.1X5	T38.1X6
tyropanoate	T50.8X1	T50.8X2	T50.8X3	T50.8X4	T50.8X5	T50.8X6
valproate	T42.6X1	T42.6X2	T42.6X3	T42.6X4	T42.6X5	T42.6X6
versenate	T50.6X1	T50.6X2	T50.6X3	T50.6X4	T50.6X5	T50.6X6
Sodium-free salt	T50.901	T50.902	T50.903	T50.904	T50.905	T50.906
Sodium-removing resin	T50.3X1	T50.3X2	T50.3X3	T50.3X4	T50.3X5	T50.3X6
Soft soap	T55.0X1	T55.0X2	T55.0X3	T55.0X4	--	--
Solanine	T62.2X1	T62.2X2	T62.2X3	T62.2X4	--	--
berries	T62.1X1	T62.1X2	T62.1X3	T62.1X4	--	--
Solanum dulcamara	T62.2X1	T62.2X2	T62.2X3	T62.2X4	--	--
berries	T62.1X1	T62.1X2	T62.1X3	T62.1X4	--	--
Solapsone	T37.1X1	T37.1X2	T37.1X3	T37.1X4	T37.1X5	T37.1X6
Solar lotion	T49.3X1	T49.3X2	T49.3X3	T49.3X4	T49.3X5	T49.3X6
Solasulfone	T37.1X1	T37.1X2	T37.1X3	T37.1X4	T37.1X5	T37.1X6
Soldering fluid	T65.891	T65.892	T65.893	T65.894	--	--
Solid substance	T65.91	T65.92	T65.93	T65.94	--	--
specified NEC	T65.891	T65.892	T65.893	T65.894	--	--
Solvent, industrial NEC	T52.91	T52.92	T52.93	T52.94	--	--
naphtha	T52.0X1	T52.0X2	T52.0X3	T52.0X4	--	--
petroleum	T52.0X1	T52.0X2	T52.0X3	T52.0X4	--	--
specified NEC	T52.8X1	T52.8X2	T52.8X3	T52.8X4	--	--
Soma	T42.8X1	T42.8X2	T42.8X3	T42.8X4	T42.8X5	T42.8X6
Somatorelin	T38.891	T38.892	T38.893	T38.894	T38.895	T38.896
Somatostatin	T38.991	T38.992	T38.993	T38.994	T38.995	T38.996
Somatotropin	T38.811	T38.812	T38.813	T38.814	T38.815	T38.816
Somatrem	T38.811	T38.812	T38.813	T38.814	T38.815	T38.816
Somatropin	T38.811	T38.812	T38.813	T38.814	T38.815	T38.816
Sominex	T45.0X1	T45.0X2	T45.0X3	T45.0X4	T45.0X5	T45.0X6
Somnos	T42.6X1	T42.6X2	T42.6X3	T42.6X4	T42.6X5	T42.6X6
Somonal	T42.3X1	T42.3X2	T42.3X3	T42.3X4	T42.3X5	T42.3X6
Soneryl	T42.3X1	T42.3X2	T42.3X3	T42.3X4	T42.3X5	T42.3X6
Soothing syrup	T50.901	T50.902	T50.903	T50.904	T50.905	T50.906
Sopor	T42.6X1	T42.6X2	T42.6X3	T42.6X4	T42.6X5	T42.6X6
Soporific	T42.71	T42.72	T42.73	T42.74	T42.75	T42.76
Soporific drug	T42.71	T42.72	T42.73	T42.74	T42.75	T42.76
specified type NEC	T42.6X1	T42.6X2	T42.6X3	T42.6X4	T42.6X5	T42.6X6
Sorbide nitrate	T46.3X1	T46.3X2	T46.3X3	T46.3X4	T46.3X5	T46.3X6
Sorbitol	T47.4X1	T47.4X2	T47.4X3	T47.4X4	T47.4X5	T47.4X6
Sotalol	T44.7X1	T44.7X2	T44.7X3	T44.7X4	T44.7X5	T44.7X6
Sotradecol	T46.8X1	T46.8X2	T46.8X3	T46.8X4	T46.8X5	T46.8X6
Soysterol	T46.6X1	T46.6X2	T46.6X3	T46.6X4	T46.6X5	T46.6X6
Spacoline	T44.3X1	T44.3X2	T44.3X3	T44.3X4	T44.3X5	T44.3X6
Spanish fly	T49.8X1	T49.8X2	T49.8X3	T49.8X4	T49.8X5	T49.8X6
Sparine	T43.3X1	T43.3X2	T43.3X3	T43.3X4	T43.3X5	T43.3X6
Sparteine	T48.0X1	T48.0X2	T48.0X3	T48.0X4	T48.0X5	T48.0X6
Spasmolytic						
anticholinergics	T44.3X1	T44.3X2	T44.3X3	T44.3X4	T44.3X5	T44.3X6
autonomic	T44.3X1	T44.3X2	T44.3X3	T44.3X4	T44.3X5	T44.3X6
bronchial NEC	T48.6X1	T48.6X2	T48.6X3	T48.6X4	T48.6X5	T48.6X6
quaternary ammonium	T44.3X1	T44.3X2	T44.3X3	T44.3X4	T44.3X5	T44.3X6
skeletal muscle NEC	T48.1X1	T48.1X2	T48.1X3	T48.1X4	T48.1X5	T48.1X6
Spectinomycin	T36.5X1	T36.5X2	T36.5X3	T36.5X4	T36.5X5	T36.5X6

Substance	Poisoning, Accidental unintentional	Poisoning, Intentional self-harm	Poisoning, Assault	Poisoning, Undetermined	Adverse effect	Underdosing
Speed	T43.621	T43.622	T43.623	T43.624	T43.625	T43.626
Spermicide	T49.8X1	T49.8X2	T49.8X3	T49.8X4	T49.8X5	T49.8X6
Spider (bite) (venom)	T63.391	T63.392	T63.393	T63.394	--	--
antivenin	T50.Z11	T50.Z12	T50.Z13	T50.Z14	T50.Z15	T50.Z16
Spigelia (root)	T37.4X1	T37.4X2	T37.4X3	T37.4X4	T37.4X5	T37.4X6
Spindle inactivator	T50.4X1	T50.4X2	T50.4X3	T50.4X4	T50.4X5	T50.4X6
Spiperone	T43.4X1	T43.4X2	T43.4X3	T43.4X4	T43.4X5	T43.4X6
Spiramycin	T36.3X1	T36.3X2	T36.3X3	T36.3X4	T36.3X5	T36.3X6
Spirapril	T46.4X1	T46.4X2	T46.4X3	T46.4X4	T46.4X5	T46.4X6
Spirilene	T43.591	T43.592	T43.593	T43.594	T43.595	T43.596
Spirit(s) (neutral) **NEC**	T51.0X1	T51.0X2	T51.0X3	T51.0X4	--	--
beverage	T51.0X1	T51.0X2	T51.0X3	T51.0X4	--	--
industrial	T51.0X1	T51.0X2	T51.0X3	T51.0X4	--	--
mineral	T52.0X1	T52.0X2	T52.0X3	T52.0X4	--	--
of salt — *see* Hydrochloric acid						
surgical	T51.0X1	T51.0X2	T51.0X3	T51.0X4	--	--
Spironolactone	T50.0X1	T50.0X2	T50.0X3	T50.0X4	T50.0X5	T50.0X6
Spiroperidol	T43.4X1	T43.4X2	T43.4X3	T43.4X4	T43.4X5	T43.4X6
Sponge, absorbable (gelatin)	T45.7X1	T45.7X2	T45.7X3	T45.7X4	T45.7X5	T45.7X6
Sporostacin	T49.0X1	T49.0X2	T49.0X3	T49.0X4	T49.0X5	T49.0X6
Spray (aerosol)	T65.91	T65.92	T65.93	T65.94	--	--
cosmetic	T65.891	T65.892	T65.893	T65.894	--	--
medicinal NEC	T50.901	T50.902	T50.903	T50.904	T50.905	T50.906
pesticides — *see* Pesticides						
specified content — *see* specific substance						
Spurge flax	T62.2X1	T62.2X2	T62.2X3	T62.2X4	--	--
Spurges	T62.2X1	T62.2X2	T62.2X3	T62.2X4	--	--
Sputum viscosity-lowering drug	T48.4X1	T48.4X2	T48.4X3	T48.4X4	T48.4X5	T48.4X6
Squill	T46.0X1	T46.0X2	T46.0X3	T46.0X4	T46.0X5	T46.0X6
rat poison	T60.4X1	T60.4X2	T60.4X3	T60.4X4	--	--
Squirting cucumber (cathartic)	T47.2X1	T47.2X2	T47.2X3	T47.2X4	T47.2X5	T47.2X6
Stains	T65.6X1	T65.6X2	T65.6X3	T65.6X4	--	--
Stannous fluoride	T49.7X1	T49.7X2	T49.7X3	T49.7X4	T49.7X5	T49.7X6
Stanolone	T38.7X1	T38.7X2	T38.7X3	T38.7X4	T38.7X5	T38.7X6
Stanozolol	T38.7X1	T38.7X2	T38.7X3	T38.7X4	T38.7X5	T38.7X6
Staphisagria or stavesacre (pediculicide)	T49.0X1	T49.0X2	T49.0X3	T49.0X4	T49.0X5	T49.0X6
Starch	T50.901	T50.902	T50.903	T50.904	T50.905	T50.906
Stelazine	T43.3X1	T43.3X2	T43.3X3	T43.3X4	T43.3X5	T43.3X6
Stemetil	T43.3X1	T43.3X2	T43.3X3	T43.3X4	T43.3X5	T43.3X6
Stepronin	T48.4X1	T48.4X2	T48.4X3	T48.4X4	T48.4X5	T48.4X6
Sterculia	T47.4X1	T47.4X2	T47.4X3	T47.4X4	T47.4X5	T47.4X6
Sternutator gas	T59.891	T59.892	T59.893	T59.894	--	--
Steroid	T38.0X1	T38.0X2	T38.0X3	T38.0X4	T38.0X5	T38.0X6
anabolic	T38.7X1	T38.7X2	T38.7X3	T38.7X4	T38.7X5	T38.7X6
androgenic	T38.7X1	T38.7X2	T38.7X3	T38.7X4	T38.7X5	T38.7X6
antineoplastic, hormone	T38.7X1	T38.7X2	T38.7X3	T38.7X4	T38.7X5	T38.7X6
estrogen	T38.5X1	T38.5X2	T38.5X3	T38.5X4	T38.5X5	T38.5X6
ENT agent	T49.6X1	T49.6X2	T49.6X3	T49.6X4	T49.6X5	T49.6X6
ophthalmic preparation	T49.5X1	T49.5X2	T49.5X3	T49.5X4	T49.5X5	T49.5X6
topical NEC	T49.0X1	T49.0X2	T49.0X3	T49.0X4	T49.0X5	T49.0X6
Stibine	T56.891	T56.892	T56.893	T56.894	--	--
Stibogluconate	T37.3X1	T37.3X2	T37.3X3	T37.3X4	T37.3X5	T37.3X6
Stibophen	T37.4X1	T37.4X2	T37.4X3	T37.4X4	T37.4X5	T37.4X6
Stilbamidine (isetionate)	T37.3X1	T37.3X2	T37.3X3	T37.3X4	T37.3X5	T37.3X6
Stilbestrol	T38.5X1	T38.5X2	T38.5X3	T38.5X4	T38.5X5	T38.5X6
Stilboestrol	T38.5X1	T38.5X2	T38.5X3	T38.5X4	T38.5X5	T38.5X6
Stimulant						
central nervous system (*see also* Psychostimulant)	T43.601	T43.602	T43.603	T43.604	T43.605	T43.606
analeptics	T50.7X1	T50.7X2	T50.7X3	T50.7X4	T50.7X5	T50.7X6
opiate antagonist	T50.7X1	T50.7X2	T50.7X3	T50.7X4	T50.7X5	T50.7X6
psychotherapeutic NEC (*see also* Psychotherapeutic drug)	T43.601	T43.602	T43.603	T43.604	T43.605	T43.606
specified NEC	T43.691	T43.692	T43.693	T43.694	T43.695	T43.696
respiratory	T48.901	T48.902	T48.903	T48.904	T48.905	T48.906
Stone-dissolving drug	T50.901	T50.902	T50.903	T50.904	T50.905	T50.906
Storage battery (cells) (acid)	T54.2X1	T54.2X2	T54.2X3	T54.2X4	--	--
Stovaine	T41.3X1	T41.3X2	T41.3X3	T41.3X4	T41.3X5	T41.3X6
infiltration (subcutaneous)	T41.3X1	T41.3X2	T41.3X3	T41.3X4	T41.3X5	T41.3X6
nerve block (peripheral) (plexus)	T41.3X1	T41.3X2	T41.3X3	T41.3X4	T41.3X5	T41.3X6
spinal	T41.3X1	T41.3X2	T41.3X3	T41.3X4	T41.3X5	T41.3X6
topical (surface)	T41.3X1	T41.3X2	T41.3X3	T41.3X4	T41.3X5	T41.3X6
Stovarsal	T37.8X1	T37.8X2	T37.8X3	T37.8X4	T37.8X5	T37.8X6
Stove gas — *see* Gas, stove						
Stoxil	T49.5X1	T49.5X2	T49.5X3	T49.5X4	T49.5X5	T49.5X6

Stramonium - Syrosingopine

Substance	Poisoning, Accidental unintentional	Poisoning, Intentional self-harm	Poisoning, Assault	Poisoning, Undetermined	Adverse effect	Underdosing
Stramonium	T48.6X1	T48.6X2	T48.6X3	T48.6X4	T48.6X5	T48.6X6
natural state	T62.2X1	T62.2X2	T62.2X3	T62.2X4	--	--
Streptodornase	T45.3X1	T45.3X2	T45.3X3	T45.3X4	T45.3X5	T45.3X6
Streptoduocin	T36.5X1	T36.5X2	T36.5X3	T36.5X4	T36.5X5	T36.5X6
Streptokinase	T45.611	T45.612	T45.613	T45.614	T45.615	T45.616
Streptomycin (derivative)	T36.5X1	T36.5X2	T36.5X3	T36.5X4	T36.5X5	T36.5X6
Streptonivicin	T36.5X1	T36.5X2	T36.5X3	T36.5X4	T36.5X5	T36.5X6
Streptovarycin	T36.5X1	T36.5X2	T36.5X3	T36.5X4	T36.5X5	T36.5X6
Streptozocin	T45.1X1	T45.1X2	T45.1X3	T45.1X4	T45.1X5	T45.1X6
Streptozotocin	T45.1X1	T45.1X2	T45.1X3	T45.1X4	T45.1X5	T45.1X6
Stripper (paint) (solvent)	T52.8X1	T52.8X2	T52.8X3	T52.8X4	--	--
Strobane	T60.1X1	T60.1X2	T60.1X3	T60.1X4	--	--
Strofantina	T46.0X1	T46.0X2	T46.0X3	T46.0X4	T46.0X5	T46.0X6
Strophanthin (g) (k)	T46.0X1	T46.0X2	T46.0X3	T46.0X4	T46.0X5	T46.0X6
Strophanthus	T46.0X1	T46.0X2	T46.0X3	T46.0X4	T46.0X5	T46.0X6
Strophantin	T46.0X1	T46.0X2	T46.0X3	T46.0X4	T46.0X5	T46.0X6
Strophantin-g	T46.0X1	T46.0X2	T46.0X3	T46.0X4	T46.0X5	T46.0X6
Strychnine (nonmedicinal) (pesticide) (salts)	T65.1X1	T65.1X2	T65.1X3	T65.1X4	--	--
medicinal	T48.291	T48.292	T48.293	T48.294	T48.295	T48.296
Strychnos (ignatii) — *see* Strychnine						
Styramate	T42.8X1	T42.8X2	T42.8X3	T42.8X4	T42.8X5	T42.8X6
Styrene	T65.891	T65.892	T65.893	T65.894	--	--
Succinimide, antiepileptic or anticonvulsant	T42.2X1	T42.2X2	T42.2X3	T42.2X4	T42.2X5	T42.2X6
mercuric — *see* Mercury						
Succinylcholine	T48.1X1	T48.1X2	T48.1X3	T48.1X4	T48.1X5	T48.1X6
Succinylsulfathiazole	T37.0X1	T37.0X2	T37.0X3	T37.0X4	T37.0X5	T37.0X6
Sucralfate	T47.1X1	T47.1X2	T47.1X3	T47.1X4	T47.1X5	T47.1X6
Sucrose	T50.3X1	T50.3X2	T50.3X3	T50.3X4	T50.3X5	T50.3X6
Sufentanil	T40.4X1	T40.4X2	T40.4X3	T40.4X4	T40.4X5	T40.4X6
Sulbactam	T36.0X1	T36.0X2	T36.0X3	T36.0X4	T36.0X5	T36.0X6
Sulbenicillin	T36.0X1	T36.0X2	T36.0X3	T36.0X4	T36.0X5	T36.0X6
Sulbentine	T49.0X1	T49.0X2	T49.0X3	T49.0X4	T49.0X5	T49.0X6
Sulfacetamide	T49.0X1	T49.0X2	T49.0X3	T49.0X4	T49.0X5	T49.0X6
ophthalmic preparation	T49.5X1	T49.5X2	T49.5X3	T49.5X4	T49.5X5	T49.5X6
Sulfachlorpyridazine	T37.0X1	T37.0X2	T37.0X3	T37.0X4	T37.0X5	T37.0X6
Sulfacitine	T37.0X1	T37.0X2	T37.0X3	T37.0X4	T37.0X5	T37.0X6
Sulfadiasulfone sodium	T37.0X1	T37.0X2	T37.0X3	T37.0X4	T37.0X5	T37.0X6
Sulfadiazine	T37.0X1	T37.0X2	T37.0X3	T37.0X4	T37.0X5	T37.0X6
silver (topical)	T49.0X1	T49.0X2	T49.0X3	T49.0X4	T49.0X5	T49.0X6
Sulfadimethoxine	T37.0X1	T37.0X2	T37.0X3	T37.0X4	T37.0X5	T37.0X6
Sulfadimidine	T37.0X1	T37.0X2	T37.0X3	T37.0X4	T37.0X5	T37.0X6
Sulfadoxine	T37.0X1	T37.0X2	T37.0X3	T37.0X4	T37.0X5	T37.0X6
with pyrimethamine	T37.2X1	T37.2X2	T37.2X3	T37.2X4	T37.2X5	T37.2X6
Sulfaethidole	T37.0X1	T37.0X2	T37.0X3	T37.0X4	T37.0X5	T37.0X6
Sulfafurazole	T37.0X1	T37.0X2	T37.0X3	T37.0X4	T37.0X5	T37.0X6
Sulfaguanidine	T37.0X1	T37.0X2	T37.0X3	T37.0X4	T37.0X5	T37.0X6
Sulfalene	T37.0X1	T37.0X2	T37.0X3	T37.0X4	T37.0X5	T37.0X6
Sulfaloxate	T37.0X1	T37.0X2	T37.0X3	T37.0X4	T37.0X5	T37.0X6
Sulfaloxic acid	T37.0X1	T37.0X2	T37.0X3	T37.0X4	T37.0X5	T37.0X6
Sulfamazone	T39.2X1	T39.2X2	T39.2X3	T39.2X4	T39.2X5	T39.2X6
Sulfamerazine	T37.0X1	T37.0X2	T37.0X3	T37.0X4	T37.0X5	T37.0X6
Sulfameter	T37.0X1	T37.0X2	T37.0X3	T37.0X4	T37.0X5	T37.0X6
Sulfamethazine	T37.0X1	T37.0X2	T37.0X3	T37.0X4	T37.0X5	T37.0X6
Sulfamethizole	T37.0X1	T37.0X2	T37.0X3	T37.0X4	T37.0X5	T37.0X6
Sulfamethoxazole	T37.0X1	T37.0X2	T37.0X3	T37.0X4	T37.0X5	T37.0X6
with trimethoprim	T36.8X1	T36.8X2	T36.8X3	T36.8X4	T36.8X5	T36.8X6
Sulfamethoxydiazine	T37.0X1	T37.0X2	T37.0X3	T37.0X4	T37.0X5	T37.0X6
Sulfamethoxypyridazine	T37.0X1	T37.0X2	T37.0X3	T37.0X4	T37.0X5	T37.0X6
Sulfamethylthiazole	T37.0X1	T37.0X2	T37.0X3	T37.0X4	T37.0X5	T37.0X6
Sulfametoxydiazine	T37.0X1	T37.0X2	T37.0X3	T37.0X4	T37.0X5	T37.0X6
Sulfamidopyrine	T39.2X1	T39.2X2	T39.2X3	T39.2X4	T39.2X5	T39.2X6
Sulfamonomethoxine	T37.0X1	T37.0X2	T37.0X3	T37.0X4	T37.0X5	T37.0X6
Sulfamoxole	T37.0X1	T37.0X2	T37.0X3	T37.0X4	T37.0X5	T37.0X6
Sulfamylon	T49.0X1	T49.0X2	T49.0X3	T49.0X4	T49.0X5	T49.0X6
Sulfan blue (diagnostic dye)	T50.8X1	T50.8X2	T50.8X3	T50.8X4	T50.8X5	T50.8X6
Sulfanilamide	T37.0X1	T37.0X2	T37.0X3	T37.0X4	T37.0X5	T37.0X6
Sulfanilylguanidine	T37.0X1	T37.0X2	T37.0X3	T37.0X4	T37.0X5	T37.0X6
Sulfaperin	T37.0X1	T37.0X2	T37.0X3	T37.0X4	T37.0X5	T37.0X6
Sulfaphenazole	T37.0X1	T37.0X2	T37.0X3	T37.0X4	T37.0X5	T37.0X6
Sulfaphenylthiazole	T37.0X1	T37.0X2	T37.0X3	T37.0X4	T37.0X5	T37.0X6
Sulfaproxyline	T37.0X1	T37.0X2	T37.0X3	T37.0X4	T37.0X5	T37.0X6
Sulfapyridine	T37.0X1	T37.0X2	T37.0X3	T37.0X4	T37.0X5	T37.0X6
Sulfapyrimidine	T37.0X1	T37.0X2	T37.0X3	T37.0X4	T37.0X5	T37.0X6
Sulfarsphenamine	T37.8X1	T37.8X2	T37.8X3	T37.8X4	T37.8X5	T37.8X6
Sulfasalazine	T37.0X1	T37.0X2	T37.0X3	T37.0X4	T37.0X5	T37.0X6
Sulfasuxidine	T37.0X1	T37.0X2	T37.0X3	T37.0X4	T37.0X5	T37.0X6
Sulfasymazine	T37.0X1	T37.0X2	T37.0X3	T37.0X4	T37.0X5	T37.0X6
Sulfated amylopectin	T47.8X1	T47.8X2	T47.8X3	T47.8X4	T47.8X5	T47.8X6
Sulfathiazole	T37.0X1	T37.0X2	T37.0X3	T37.0X4	T37.0X5	T37.0X6
Sulfatostearate	T49.2X1	T49.2X2	T49.2X3	T49.2X4	T49.2X5	T49.2X6
Sulfinpyrazone	T50.4X1	T50.4X2	T50.4X3	T50.4X4	T50.4X5	T50.4X6
Sulfiram	T49.0X1	T49.0X2	T49.0X3	T49.0X4	T49.0X5	T49.0X6
Sulfisomidine	T37.0X1	T37.0X2	T37.0X3	T37.0X4	T37.0X5	T37.0X6
Sulfisoxazole	T37.0X1	T37.0X2	T37.0X3	T37.0X4	T37.0X5	T37.0X6
ophthalmic preparation	T49.5X1	T49.5X2	T49.5X3	T49.5X4	T49.5X5	T49.5X6
Sulfobromophthalein (sodium)	T50.8X1	T50.8X2	T50.8X3	T50.8X4	T50.8X5	T50.8X6
Sulfobromphthalein	T50.8X1	T50.8X2	T50.8X3	T50.8X4	T50.8X5	T50.8X6
Sulfogaiacol	T48.4X1	T48.4X2	T48.4X3	T48.4X4	T48.4X5	T48.4X6
Sulfomyxin	T36.8X1	T36.8X2	T36.8X3	T36.8X4	T36.8X5	T36.8X6
Sulfonal	T42.6X1	T42.6X2	T42.6X3	T42.6X4	T42.6X5	T42.6X6
Sulfonamide NEC	T37.0X1	T37.0X2	T37.0X3	T37.0X4	T37.0X5	T37.0X6
eye	T49.5X1	T49.5X2	T49.5X3	T49.5X4	T49.5X5	T49.5X6
Sulfonazide	T37.1X1	T37.1X2	T37.1X3	T37.1X4	T37.1X5	T37.1X6
Sulfones	T37.1X1	T37.1X2	T37.1X3	T37.1X4	T37.1X5	T37.1X6
Sulfonethylmethane	T42.6X1	T42.6X2	T42.6X3	T42.6X4	T42.6X5	T42.6X6
Sulfonmethane	T42.6X1	T42.6X2	T42.6X3	T42.6X4	T42.6X5	T42.6X6
Sulfonphthal, sulfonphthol	T50.8X1	T50.8X2	T50.8X3	T50.8X4	T50.8X5	T50.8X6
Sulfonylurea derivatives, oral	T38.3X1	T38.3X2	T38.3X3	T38.3X4	T38.3X5	T38.3X6
Sulforidazine	T43.3X1	T43.3X2	T43.3X3	T43.3X4	T43.3X5	T43.3X6
Sulfoxone	T37.1X1	T37.1X2	T37.1X3	T37.1X4	T37.1X5	T37.1X6
Sulfur, sulfurated, sulfuric, sulfurous, sulfuryl (compounds NEC) (medicinal)	T49.4X1	T49.4X2	T49.4X3	T49.4X4	T49.4X5	T49.4X6
acid	T54.2X1	T54.2X2	T54.2X3	T54.2X4	--	--
dioxide (gas)	T59.1X1	T59.1X2	T59.1X3	T59.1X4	--	--
ether — *see* Ether(s)						
hydrogen	T59.6X1	T59.6X2	T59.6X3	T59.6X4	--	--
medicinal (keratolytic) (ointment) NEC	T49.4X1	T49.4X2	T49.4X3	T49.4X4	T49.4X5	T49.4X6
ointment	T49.0X1	T49.0X2	T49.0X3	T49.0X4	T49.0X5	T49.0X6
pesticide (vapor)	T60.91	T60.92	T60.93	T60.94	--	--
vapor NEC	T59.891	T59.892	T59.893	T59.894	--	--
Sulfuric acid	T54.2X1	T54.2X2	T54.2X3	T54.2X4	--	--
Sulglicotide	T47.1X1	T47.1X2	T47.1X3	T47.1X4	T47.1X5	T47.1X6
Sulindac	T39.391	T39.392	T39.393	T39.394	T39.395	T39.396
Sulisatin	T47.2X1	T47.2X2	T47.2X3	T47.2X4	T47.2X5	T47.2X6
Sulisobenzone	T49.3X1	T49.3X2	T49.3X3	T49.3X4	T49.3X5	T49.3X6
Sulkowitch's reagent	T50.8X1	T50.8X2	T50.8X3	T50.8X4	T50.8X5	T50.8X6
Sulmetozine	T44.3X1	T44.3X2	T44.3X3	T44.3X4	T44.3X5	T44.3X6
Suloctidil	T46.7X1	T46.7X2	T46.7X3	T46.7X4	T46.7X5	T46.7X6
Sulph-see also Sulf-						
Sulphadiazine	T37.0X1	T37.0X2	T37.0X3	T37.0X4	T37.0X5	T37.0X6
Sulphadimethoxine	T37.0X1	T37.0X2	T37.0X3	T37.0X4	T37.0X5	T37.0X6
Sulphadimidine	T37.0X1	T37.0X2	T37.0X3	T37.0X4	T37.0X5	T37.0X6
Sulphadione	T37.1X1	T37.1X2	T37.1X3	T37.1X4	T37.1X5	T37.1X6
Sulphafurazole	T37.0X1	T37.0X2	T37.0X3	T37.0X4	T37.0X5	T37.0X6
Sulphamethizole	T37.0X1	T37.0X2	T37.0X3	T37.0X4	T37.0X5	T37.0X6
Sulphamethoxazole	T37.0X1	T37.0X2	T37.0X3	T37.0X4	T37.0X5	T37.0X6
Sulphan blue	T50.8X1	T50.8X2	T50.8X3	T50.8X4	T50.8X5	T50.8X6
Sulphaphenazole	T37.0X1	T37.0X2	T37.0X3	T37.0X4	T37.0X5	T37.0X6
Sulphapyridine	T37.0X1	T37.0X2	T37.0X3	T37.0X4	T37.0X5	T37.0X6
Sulphasalazine	T37.0X1	T37.0X2	T37.0X3	T37.0X4	T37.0X5	T37.0X6
Sulphinpyrazone	T50.4X1	T50.4X2	T50.4X3	T50.4X4	T50.4X5	T50.4X6
Sulpiride	T43.591	T43.592	T43.593	T43.594	T43.595	T43.596
Sulprostone	T48.0X1	T48.0X2	T48.0X3	T48.0X4	T48.0X5	T48.0X6
Sulpyrine	T39.2X1	T39.2X2	T39.2X3	T39.2X4	T39.2X5	T39.2X6
Sultamicillin	T36.0X1	T36.0X2	T36.0X3	T36.0X4	T36.0X5	T36.0X6
Sulthiame	T42.6X1	T42.6X2	T42.6X3	T42.6X4	T42.6X5	T42.6X6
Sultiame	T42.6X1	T42.6X2	T42.6X3	T42.6X4	T42.6X5	T42.6X6
Sultopride	T43.591	T43.592	T43.593	T43.594	T43.595	T43.596
Sumatriptan	T39.8X1	T39.8X2	T39.8X3	T39.8X4	T39.8X5	T39.8X6
Sunflower seed oil	T46.6X1	T46.6X2	T46.6X3	T46.6X4	T46.6X5	T46.6X6
Superinone	T48.4X1	T48.4X2	T48.4X3	T48.4X4	T48.4X5	T48.4X6
Suprofen	T39.311	T39.312	T39.313	T39.314	T39.315	T39.316
Suramin (sodium)	T37.4X1	T37.4X2	T37.4X3	T37.4X4	T37.4X5	T37.4X6
Surfacaine	T41.3X1	T41.3X2	T41.3X3	T41.3X4	T41.3X5	T41.3X6
Surital	T41.1X1	T41.1X2	T41.1X3	T41.1X4	T41.1X5	T41.1X6
Sutilains	T45.3X1	T45.3X2	T45.3X3	T45.3X4	T45.3X5	T45.3X6
Suxamethonium (chloride)	T48.1X1	T48.1X2	T48.1X3	T48.1X4	T48.1X5	T48.1X6
Suxethonium (chloride)	T48.1X1	T48.1X2	T48.1X3	T48.1X4	T48.1X5	T48.1X6
Suxibuzone	T39.2X1	T39.2X2	T39.2X3	T39.2X4	T39.2X5	T39.2X6
Sweet niter spirit	T46.3X1	T46.3X2	T46.3X3	T46.3X4	T46.3X5	T46.3X6
Sweet oil (birch)	T49.3X1	T49.3X2	T49.3X3	T49.3X4	T49.3X5	T49.3X6
Sweetener	T50.901	T50.902	T50.903	T50.904	T50.905	T50.906
Sym-dichloroethyl ether	T53.6X1	T53.6X2	T53.6X3	T53.6X4	--	--
Sympatholytic NEC	T44.8X1	T44.8X2	T44.8X3	T44.8X4	T44.8X5	T44.8X6
haloalkylamine	T44.8X1	T44.8X2	T44.8X3	T44.8X4	T44.8X5	T44.8X6
Sympathomimetic NEC	T44.901	T44.902	T44.903	T44.904	T44.905	T44.906
anti-common-cold	T48.5X1	T48.5X2	T48.5X3	T48.5X4	T48.5X5	T48.5X6
bronchodilator	T48.6X1	T48.6X2	T48.6X3	T48.6X4	T48.6X5	T48.6X6
specified NEC	T44.991	T44.992	T44.993	T44.994	T44.995	T44.996
Synagis	T50.B91	T50.B92	T50.B93	T50.B94	T50.B95	T50.B96
Synalar	T49.0X1	T49.0X2	T49.0X3	T49.0X4	T49.0X5	T49.0X6
Synthroid	T38.1X1	T38.1X2	T38.1X3	T38.1X4	T38.1X5	T38.1X6
Syntocinon	T48.0X1	T48.0X2	T48.0X3	T48.0X4	T48.0X5	T48.0X6
Syrosingopine	T46.5X1	T46.5X2	T46.5X3	T46.5X4	T46.5X5	T46.5X6

Substance	Poisoning, Accidental unintentional	Poisoning, Intentional self-harm	Poisoning, Assault	Poisoning, Undetermined	Adverse effect	Underdosing
Systemic drug	T45.91	T45.92	T45.93	T45.94	T45.95	T45.96
specified NEC	T45.8X1	T45.8X2	T45.8X3	T45.8X4	T45.8X5	T45.8X6
2,4,5-T	T60.3X1	T60.3X2	T60.3X3	T60.3X4	--	--
T						
Tablets (see also specified substance)	T50.901	T50.902	T50.903	T50.904	T50.905	T50.906
Tace	T38.5X1	T38.5X2	T38.5X3	T38.5X4	T38.5X5	T38.5X6
Tacrine	T44.0X1	T44.0X2	T44.0X3	T44.0X4	T44.0X5	T44.0X6
Tadalafil	T46.7X1	T46.7X2	T46.7X3	T46.7X4	T46.7X5	T46.7X6
Talampicillin	T36.0X1	T36.0X2	T36.0X3	T36.0X4	T36.0X5	T36.0X6
Talbutal	T42.3X1	T42.3X2	T42.3X3	T42.3X4	T42.3X5	T42.3X6
Talc powder	T49.3X1	T49.3X2	T49.3X3	T49.3X4	T49.3X5	T49.3X6
Talcum	T49.3X1	T49.3X2	T49.3X3	T49.3X4	T49.3X5	T49.3X6
Taleranol	T38.6X1	T38.6X2	T38.6X3	T38.6X4	T38.6X5	T38.6X6
Tamoxifen	T38.6X1	T38.6X2	T38.6X3	T38.6X4	T38.6X5	T38.6X6
Tamsulosin	T44.6X1	T44.6X2	T44.6X3	T44.6X4	T44.6X5	T44.6X6
Tandearil, tanderil	T39.2X1	T39.2X2	T39.2X3	T39.2X4	T39.2X5	T39.2X6
Tannic acid	T49.2X1	T49.2X2	T49.2X3	T49.2X4	T49.2X5	T49.2X6
medicinal (astringent)	T49.2X1	T49.2X2	T49.2X3	T49.2X4	T49.2X5	T49.2X6
Tannin — see Tannic acid						
Tansy	T62.2X1	T62.2X2	T62.2X3	T62.2X4	--	--
TAO	T36.3X1	T36.3X2	T36.3X3	T36.3X4	T36.3X5	T36.3X6
Tapazole	T38.2X1	T38.2X2	T38.2X3	T38.2X4	T38.2X5	T38.2X6
Tar NEC	T52.0X1	T52.0X2	T52.0X3	T52.0X4	--	--
camphor	T60.1X1	T60.1X2	T60.1X3	T60.1X4	--	--
distillate	T49.1X1	T49.1X2	T49.1X3	T49.1X4	T49.1X5	T49.1X6
fumes	T59.891	T59.892	T59.893	T59.894	--	--
medicinal	T49.1X1	T49.1X2	T49.1X3	T49.1X4	T49.1X5	T49.1X6
ointment	T49.1X1	T49.1X2	T49.1X3	T49.1X4	T49.1X5	T49.1X6
Taractan	T43.591	T43.592	T43.593	T43.594	T43.595	T43.596
Tarantula (venomous)	T63.321	T63.322	T63.323	T63.324	--	--
Tartar emetic	T37.8X1	T37.8X2	T37.8X3	T37.8X4	T37.8X5	T37.8X6
Tartaric acid	T65.891	T65.892	T65.893	T65.894	--	--
Tartrate, laxative	T47.4X1	T47.4X2	T47.4X3	T47.4X4	T47.4X5	T47.4X6
Tartrated antimony (anti-infective)	T37.8X1	T37.8X2	T37.8X3	T37.8X4	T37.8X5	T37.8X6
Tauromustine	T45.1X1	T45.1X2	T45.1X3	T45.1X4	T45.1X5	T45.1X6
TCA — see Trichloroacetic acid						
TCDD	T53.7X1	T53.7X2	T53.7X3	T53.7X4	--	--
TDI (vapor)	T65.0X1	T65.0X2	T65.0X3	T65.0X4	--	--
Tear						
gas	T59.3X1	T59.3X2	T59.3X3	T59.3X4	--	--
solution	T49.5X1	T49.5X2	T49.5X3	T49.5X4	T49.5X5	T49.5X6
Teclothiazide	T50.2X1	T50.2X2	T50.2X3	T50.2X4	T50.2X5	T50.2X6
Teclozan	T37.3X1	T37.3X2	T37.3X3	T37.3X4	T37.3X5	T37.3X6
Tegafur	T45.1X1	T45.1X2	T45.1X3	T45.1X4	T45.1X5	T45.1X6
Tegretol	T42.1X1	T42.1X2	T42.1X3	T42.1X4	T42.1X5	T42.1X6
Teicoplanin	T36.8X1	T36.8X2	T36.8X3	T36.8X4	T36.8X5	T36.8X6
Telepaque	T50.8X1	T50.8X2	T50.8X3	T50.8X4	T50.8X5	T50.8X6
Tellurium	T56.891	T56.892	T56.893	T56.894	--	--
fumes	T56.891	T56.892	T56.893	T56.894	--	--
TEM	T45.1X1	T45.1X2	T45.1X3	T45.1X4	T45.1X5	T45.1X6
Temazepam	T42.4X1	T42.4X2	T42.4X3	T42.4X4	T42.4X5	T42.4X6
Temocillin	T36.0X1	T36.0X2	T36.0X3	T36.0X4	T36.0X5	T36.0X6
Tenamfetamine	T43.621	T43.622	T43.623	T43.624	T43.625	T43.626
Teniposide	T45.1X1	T45.1X2	T45.1X3	T45.1X4	T45.1X5	T45.1X6
Tenitramine	T46.3X1	T46.3X2	T46.3X3	T46.3X4	T46.3X5	T46.3X6
Tenoglicin	T48.4X1	T48.4X2	T48.4X3	T48.4X4	T48.4X5	T48.4X6
Tenonitrozole	T37.3X1	T37.3X2	T37.3X3	T37.3X4	T37.3X5	T37.3X6
Tenoxicam	T39.391	T39.392	T39.393	T39.394	T39.395	T39.396
TEPA	T45.1X1	T45.1X2	T45.1X3	T45.1X4	T45.1X5	T45.1X6
TEPP	T60.0X1	T60.0X2	T60.0X3	T60.0X4	--	--
Teprotide	T46.5X1	T46.5X2	T46.5X3	T46.5X4	T46.5X5	T46.5X6
Terazosin	T44.6X1	T44.6X2	T44.6X3	T44.6X4	T44.6X5	T44.6X6
Terbufos	T60.0X1	T60.0X2	T60.0X3	T60.0X4	--	--
Terbutaline	T48.6X1	T48.6X2	T48.6X3	T48.6X4	T48.6X5	T48.6X6
Terconazole	T49.0X1	T49.0X2	T49.0X3	T49.0X4	T49.0X5	T49.0X6
Terfenadine	T45.0X1	T45.0X2	T45.0X3	T45.0X4	T45.0X5	T45.0X6
Teriparatide (acetate)	T50.991	T50.992	T50.993	T50.994	T50.995	T50.996
Terizidone	T37.1X1	T37.1X2	T37.1X3	T37.1X4	T37.1X5	T37.1X6
Terlipressin	T38.891	T38.892	T38.893	T38.894	T38.895	T38.896
Terodiline	T46.3X1	T46.3X2	T46.3X3	T46.3X4	T46.3X5	T46.3X6
Teroxalene	T37.4X1	T37.4X2	T37.4X3	T37.4X4	T37.4X5	T37.4X6
Terpin (cis) hydrate	T48.4X1	T48.4X2	T48.4X3	T48.4X4	T48.4X5	T48.4X6
Terramycin	T36.4X1	T36.4X2	T36.4X3	T36.4X4	T36.4X5	T36.4X6
Tertatolol	T44.7X1	T44.7X2	T44.7X3	T44.7X4	T44.7X5	T44.7X6
Tessalon	T48.3X1	T48.3X2	T48.3X3	T48.3X4	T48.3X5	T48.3X6
Testolactone	T38.7X1	T38.7X2	T38.7X3	T38.7X4	T38.7X5	T38.7X6
Testosterone	T38.7X1	T38.7X2	T38.7X3	T38.7X4	T38.7X5	T38.7X6
Tetanus toxoid or vaccine	T50.A91	T50.A92	T50.A93	T50.A94	T50.A95	T50.A96
antitoxin	T50.Z11	T50.Z12	T50.Z13	T50.Z14	T50.Z15	T50.Z16
immune globulin (human)	T50.Z11	T50.Z12	T50.Z13	T50.Z14	T50.Z15	T50.Z16
toxoid	T50.A91	T50.A92	T50.A93	T50.A94	T50.A95	T50.A96
with diphtheria toxoid	T50.A21	T50.A22	T50.A23	T50.A24	T50.A25	T50.A26
with pertussis	T50.A11	T50.A12	T50.A13	T50.A14	T50.A15	T50.A16
Tetrabenazine	T43.591	T43.592	T43.593	T43.594	T43.595	T43.596
Tetracaine	T41.3X1	T41.3X2	T41.3X3	T41.3X4	T41.3X5	T41.3X6
nerve block (peripheral) (plexus)	T41.3X1	T41.3X2	T41.3X3	T41.3X4	T41.3X5	T41.3X6
regional	T41.3X1	T41.3X2	T41.3X3	T41.3X4	T41.3X5	T41.3X6
spinal	T41.3X1	T41.3X2	T41.3X3	T41.3X4	T41.3X5	T41.3X6
Tetrachlorethylene — see Tetrachloroethylene						
Tetrachlormethiazide	T50.2X1	T50.2X2	T50.2X3	T50.2X4	T50.2X5	T50.2X6
2,3,7,8-Tetrachlorodibenzo-p-dioxin	T53.7X1	T53.7X2	T53.7X3	T53.7X4	--	--
Tetrachloroethane	T53.6X1	T53.6X2	T53.6X3	T53.6X4	--	--
vapor	T53.6X1	T53.6X2	T53.6X3	T53.6X4	--	--
paint or varnish	T53.6X1	T53.6X2	T53.6X3	T53.6X4	--	--
Tetrachloroethylene (liquid)	T53.3X1	T53.3X2	T53.3X3	T53.3X4	--	--
medicinal	T37.4X1	T37.4X2	T37.4X3	T37.4X4	T37.4X5	T37.4X6
vapor	T53.3X1	T53.3X2	T53.3X3	T53.3X4	--	--
Tetrachloromethane — see Carbon tetrachloride						
Tetracosactide	T38.811	T38.812	T38.813	T38.814	T38.815	T38.816
Tetracosactrin	T38.811	T38.812	T38.813	T38.814	T38.815	T38.816
Tetracycline	T36.4X1	T36.4X2	T36.4X3	T36.4X4	T36.4X5	T36.4X6
ophthalmic preparation	T49.5X1	T49.5X2	T49.5X3	T49.5X4	T49.5X5	T49.5X6
topical NEC	T49.0X1	T49.0X2	T49.0X3	T49.0X4	T49.0X5	T49.0X6
Tetradifon	T60.8X1	T60.8X2	T60.8X3	T60.8X4	--	--
Tetradotoxin	T61.771	T61.772	T61.773	T61.774	--	--
Tetraethyl						
lead	T56.0X1	T56.0X2	T56.0X3	T56.0X4	--	--
pyrophosphate	T60.0X1	T60.0X2	T60.0X3	T60.0X4	--	--
Tetraethylammonium chloride	T44.2X1	T44.2X2	T44.2X3	T44.2X4	T44.2X5	T44.2X6
Tetraethylthiuram disulfide	T50.6X1	T50.6X2	T50.6X3	T50.6X4	T50.6X5	T50.6X6
Tetrahydroaminoacridine	T44.0X1	T44.0X2	T44.0X3	T44.0X4	T44.0X5	T44.0X6
Tetrahydrocannabinol	T40.7X1	T40.7X2	T40.7X3	T40.7X4	T40.7X5	T40.7X6
Tetrahydrofuran	T52.8X1	T52.8X2	T52.8X3	T52.8X4	--	--
Tetrahydronaphthalene	T52.8X1	T52.8X2	T52.8X3	T52.8X4	--	--
Tetrahydrozoline	T49.5X1	T49.5X2	T49.5X3	T49.5X4	T49.5X5	T49.5X6
Tetralin	T52.8X1	T52.8X2	T52.8X3	T52.8X4	--	--
Tetramethrin	T60.2X1	T60.2X2	T60.2X3	T60.2X4	--	--
Tetramethylthiuram (disulfide) NEC	T60.3X1	T60.3X2	T60.3X3	T60.3X4	--	--
medicinal	T49.0X1	T49.0X2	T49.0X3	T49.0X4	T49.0X5	T49.0X6
Tetramisole	T37.4X1	T37.4X2	T37.4X3	T37.4X4	T37.4X5	T37.4X6
Tetranicotinoyl fructose	T46.7X1	T46.7X2	T46.7X3	T46.7X4	T46.7X5	T46.7X6
Tetrazepam	T42.4X1	T42.4X2	T42.4X3	T42.4X4	T42.4X5	T42.4X6
Tetronal	T42.6X1	T42.6X2	T42.6X3	T42.6X4	T42.6X5	T42.6X6
Tetryl	T65.3X1	T65.3X2	T65.3X3	T65.3X4	--	--
Tetrylammonium chloride	T44.2X1	T44.2X2	T44.2X3	T44.2X4	T44.2X5	T44.2X6
Tetryzoline	T49.5X1	T49.5X2	T49.5X3	T49.5X4	T49.5X5	T49.5X6
Thalidomide	T45.1X1	T45.1X2	T45.1X3	T45.1X4	T45.1X5	T45.1X6
Thallium (compounds) (dust) NEC	T56.811	T56.812	T56.813	T56.814	--	--
pesticide	T60.4X1	T60.4X2	T60.4X3	T60.4X4	--	--
THC	T40.7X1	T40.7X2	T40.7X3	T40.7X4	T40.7X5	T40.7X6
Thebacon	T48.3X1	T48.3X2	T48.3X3	T48.3X4	T48.3X5	T48.3X6
Thebaine	T40.2X1	T40.2X2	T40.2X3	T40.2X4	T40.2X5	T40.2X6
Thenoic acid	T49.6X1	T49.6X2	T49.6X3	T49.6X4	T49.6X5	T49.6X6
Thenyldiamine	T45.0X1	T45.0X2	T45.0X3	T45.0X4	T45.0X5	T45.0X6
Theobromine (calcium salicylate)	T48.6X1	T48.6X2	T48.6X3	T48.6X4	T48.6X5	T48.6X6
sodium salicylate	T48.6X1	T48.6X2	T48.6X3	T48.6X4	T48.6X5	T48.6X6
Theophyllamine	T48.6X1	T48.6X2	T48.6X3	T48.6X4	T48.6X5	T48.6X6
Theophylline	T48.6X1	T48.6X2	T48.6X3	T48.6X4	T48.6X5	T48.6X6
aminobenzoic acid	T48.6X1	T48.6X2	T48.6X3	T48.6X4	T48.6X5	T48.6X6
ethylenediamine	T48.6X1	T48.6X2	T48.6X3	T48.6X4	T48.6X5	T48.6X6
piperazine p-amino-benzoate	T48.6X1	T48.6X2	T48.6X3	T48.6X4	T48.6X5	T48.6X6
Thiabendazole	T37.4X1	T37.4X2	T37.4X3	T37.4X4	T37.4X5	T37.4X6
Thialbarbital	T41.1X1	T41.1X2	T41.1X3	T41.1X4	T41.1X5	T41.1X6
Thiamazole	T38.2X1	T38.2X2	T38.2X3	T38.2X4	T38.2X5	T38.2X6
Thiambutosine	T37.1X1	T37.1X2	T37.1X3	T37.1X4	T37.1X5	T37.1X6
Thiamine	T45.2X1	T45.2X2	T45.2X3	T45.2X4	T45.2X5	T45.2X6
Thiamphenicol	T36.2X1	T36.2X2	T36.2X3	T36.2X4	T36.2X5	T36.2X6
Thiamylal	T41.1X1	T41.1X2	T41.1X3	T41.1X4	T41.1X5	T41.1X6
sodium	T41.1X1	T41.1X2	T41.1X3	T41.1X4	T41.1X5	T41.1X6
Thiazesim	T43.291	T43.292	T43.293	T43.294	T43.295	T43.296
Thiazides (diuretics)	T50.2X1	T50.2X2	T50.2X3	T50.2X4	T50.2X5	T50.2X6
Thiazinamium metilsulfate	T43.3X1	T43.3X2	T43.3X3	T43.3X4	T43.3X5	T43.3X6
Thiethylperazine	T43.3X1	T43.3X2	T43.3X3	T43.3X4	T43.3X5	T43.3X6
Thimerosal	T49.0X1	T49.0X2	T49.0X3	T49.0X4	T49.0X5	T49.0X6
ophthalmic preparation	T49.5X1	T49.5X2	T49.5X3	T49.5X4	T49.5X5	T49.5X6
Thioacetazone	T37.1X1	T37.1X2	T37.1X3	T37.1X4	T37.1X5	T37.1X6
with isoniazid	T37.1X1	T37.1X2	T37.1X3	T37.1X4	T37.1X5	T37.1X6

Substance	Poisoning, Accidental unintentional	Poisoning, Intentional self-harm	Poisoning, Assault	Poisoning, Undetermined	Adverse effect	Underdosing
Thiobarbital sodium	T41.1X1	T41.1X2	T41.1X3	T41.1X4	T41.1X5	T41.1X6
Thiobarbiturate anesthetic	T41.1X1	T41.1X2	T41.1X3	T41.1X4	T41.1X5	T41.1X6
Thiobismol	T37.8X1	T37.8X2	T37.8X3	T37.8X4	T37.8X5	T37.8X6
Thiobutabarbital sodium	T41.1X1	T41.1X2	T41.1X3	T41.1X4	T41.1X5	T41.1X6
Thiocarbamate (insecticide)	T60.0X1	T60.0X2	T60.0X3	T60.0X4	--	--
Thiocarbamide	T38.2X1	T38.2X2	T38.2X3	T38.2X4	T38.2X5	T38.2X6
Thiocarbarsone	T37.8X1	T37.8X2	T37.8X3	T37.8X4	T37.8X5	T37.8X6
Thiocarlide	T37.1X1	T37.1X2	T37.1X3	T37.1X4	T37.1X5	T37.1X6
Thioctamide	T50.991	T50.992	T50.993	T50.994	T50.995	T50.996
Thioctic acid	T50.991	T50.992	T50.993	T50.994	T50.995	T50.996
Thiofos	T60.0X1	T60.0X2	T60.0X3	T60.0X4	--	--
Thioglycolate	T49.4X1	T49.4X2	T49.4X3	T49.4X4	T49.4X5	T49.4X6
Thioglycolic acid	T65.891	T65.892	T65.893	T65.894	--	--
Thioguanine	T45.1X1	T45.1X2	T45.1X3	T45.1X4	T45.1X5	T45.1X6
Thiomercaptomerin	T50.2X1	T50.2X2	T50.2X3	T50.2X4	T50.2X5	T50.2X6
Thiomerin	T50.2X1	T50.2X2	T50.2X3	T50.2X4	T50.2X5	T50.2X6
Thiomersal	T49.0X1	T49.0X2	T49.0X3	T49.0X4	T49.0X5	T49.0X6
Thionazin	T60.0X1	T60.0X2	T60.0X3	T60.0X4	--	--
Thiopental (sodium)	T41.1X1	T41.1X2	T41.1X3	T41.1X4	T41.1X5	T41.1X6
Thiopentone (sodium)	T41.1X1	T41.1X2	T41.1X3	T41.1X4	T41.1X5	T41.1X6
Thiopropazate	T43.3X1	T43.3X2	T43.3X3	T43.3X4	T43.3X5	T43.3X6
Thioproperazine	T43.3X1	T43.3X2	T43.3X3	T43.3X4	T43.3X5	T43.3X6
Thioridazine	T43.3X1	T43.3X2	T43.3X3	T43.3X4	T43.3X5	T43.3X6
Thiosinamine	T49.3X1	T49.3X2	T49.3X3	T49.3X4	T49.3X5	T49.3X6
Thiotepa	T45.1X1	T45.1X2	T45.1X3	T45.1X4	T45.1X5	T45.1X6
Thiothixene	T43.4X1	T43.4X2	T43.4X3	T43.4X4	T43.4X5	T43.4X6
Thiouracil (benzyl) (methyl) (propyl)	T38.2X1	T38.2X2	T38.2X3	T38.2X4	T38.2X5	T38.2X6
Thiourea	T38.2X1	T38.2X2	T38.2X3	T38.2X4	T38.2X5	T38.2X6
Thiphenamil	T44.3X1	T44.3X2	T44.3X3	T44.3X4	T44.3X5	T44.3X6
Thiram	T60.3X1	T60.3X2	T60.3X3	T60.3X4	--	--
medicinal	T49.2X1	T49.2X2	T49.2X3	T49.2X4	T49.2X5	T49.2X6
Thonzylamine (systemic)	T45.0X1	T45.0X2	T45.0X3	T45.0X4	T45.0X5	T45.0X6
mucosal decongestant	T48.5X1	T48.5X2	T48.5X3	T48.5X4	T48.5X5	T48.5X6
Thorazine	T43.3X1	T43.3X2	T43.3X3	T43.3X4	T43.3X5	T43.3X6
Thorium dioxide suspension	T50.8X1	T50.8X2	T50.8X3	T50.8X4	T50.8X5	T50.8X6
Thornapple	T62.2X1	T62.2X2	T62.2X3	T62.2X4	--	--
Throat drug NEC	T49.6X1	T49.6X2	T49.6X3	T49.6X4	T49.6X5	T49.6X6
Thrombin	T45.7X1	T45.7X2	T45.7X3	T45.7X4	T45.7X5	T45.7X6
Thrombolysin	T45.611	T45.612	T45.613	T45.614	T45.615	T45.616
Thromboplastin	T45.7X1	T45.7X2	T45.7X3	T45.7X4	T45.7X5	T45.7X6
Thurfyl nicotinate	T46.7X1	T46.7X2	T46.7X3	T46.7X4	T46.7X5	T46.7X6
Thymol	T49.0X1	T49.0X2	T49.0X3	T49.0X4	T49.0X5	T49.0X6
Thymopentin	T37.5X1	T37.5X2	T37.5X3	T37.5X4	T37.5X5	T37.5X6
Thymoxamine	T46.7X1	T46.7X2	T46.7X3	T46.7X4	T46.7X5	T46.7X6
Thymus extract	T38.891	T38.892	T38.893	T38.894	T38.895	T38.896
Thyreotrophic hormone	T38.811	T38.812	T38.813	T38.814	T38.815	T38.816
Thyroglobulin	T38.1X1	T38.1X2	T38.1X3	T38.1X4	T38.1X5	T38.1X6
Thyroid (hormone)	T38.1X1	T38.1X2	T38.1X3	T38.1X4	T38.1X5	T38.1X6
Thyrolar	T38.1X1	T38.1X2	T38.1X3	T38.1X4	T38.1X5	T38.1X6
Thyrotrophin	T38.811	T38.812	T38.813	T38.814	T38.815	T38.816
Thyrotropic hormone	T38.811	T38.812	T38.813	T38.814	T38.815	T38.816
Thyroxine	T38.1X1	T38.1X2	T38.1X3	T38.1X4	T38.1X5	T38.1X6
Tiabendazole	T37.4X1	T37.4X2	T37.4X3	T37.4X4	T37.4X5	T37.4X6
Tiamizide	T50.2X1	T50.2X2	T50.2X3	T50.2X4	T50.2X5	T50.2X6
Tianeptine	T43.291	T43.292	T43.293	T43.294	T43.295	T43.296
Tiapamil	T46.1X1	T46.1X2	T46.1X3	T46.1X4	T46.1X5	T46.1X6
Tiapride	T43.591	T43.592	T43.593	T43.594	T43.595	T43.596
Tiaprofenic acid	T39.311	T39.312	T39.313	T39.314	T39.315	T39.316
Tiaramide	T39.8X1	T39.8X2	T39.8X3	T39.8X4	T39.8X5	T39.8X6
Ticarcillin	T36.0X1	T36.0X2	T36.0X3	T36.0X4	T36.0X5	T36.0X6
Ticlatone	T49.0X1	T49.0X2	T49.0X3	T49.0X4	T49.0X5	T49.0X6
Ticlopidine	T45.521	T45.522	T45.523	T45.524	T45.525	T45.526
Ticrynafen	T50.1X1	T50.1X2	T50.1X3	T50.1X4	T50.1X5	T50.1X6
Tidiacic	T50.991	T50.992	T50.993	T50.994	T50.995	T50.996
Tiemonium	T44.3X1	T44.3X2	T44.3X3	T44.3X4	T44.3X5	T44.3X6
iodide	T44.3X1	T44.3X2	T44.3X3	T44.3X4	T44.3X5	T44.3X6
Tienilic acid	T50.1X1	T50.1X2	T50.1X3	T50.1X4	T50.1X5	T50.1X6
Tifenamil	T44.3X1	T44.3X2	T44.3X3	T44.3X4	T44.3X5	T44.3X6
Tigan	T45.0X1	T45.0X2	T45.0X3	T45.0X4	T45.0X5	T45.0X6
Tigloidine	T44.3X1	T44.3X2	T44.3X3	T44.3X4	T44.3X5	T44.3X6
Tilactase	T47.5X1	T47.5X2	T47.5X3	T47.5X4	T47.5X5	T47.5X6
Tiletamine	T41.291	T41.292	T41.293	T41.294	T41.295	T41.296
Tilidine	T40.4X1	T40.4X2	T40.4X3	T40.4X4	--	--
Timepidium bromide	T44.3X1	T44.3X2	T44.3X3	T44.3X4	T44.3X5	T44.3X6
Timiperone	T43.4X1	T43.4X2	T43.4X3	T43.4X4	T43.4X5	T43.4X6
Timolol	T44.7X1	T44.7X2	T44.7X3	T44.7X4	T44.7X5	T44.7X6
Tin (chloride) (dust) (oxide) NEC	T56.6X1	T56.6X2	T56.6X3	T56.6X4	--	--
anti-infectives	T37.8X1	T37.8X2	T37.8X3	T37.8X4	T37.8X5	T37.8X6
Tincture, iodine — *see* Iodine						
Tindal	T43.3X1	T43.3X2	T43.3X3	T43.3X4	T43.3X5	T43.3X6
Tinidazole	T37.3X1	T37.3X2	T37.3X3	T37.3X4	T37.3X5	T37.3X6
Tinoridine	T39.8X1	T39.8X2	T39.8X3	T39.8X4	T39.8X5	T39.8X6

Substance	Poisoning, Accidental unintentional	Poisoning, Intentional self-harm	Poisoning, Assault	Poisoning, Undetermined	Adverse effect	Underdosing
Tiocarlide	T37.1X1	T37.1X2	T37.1X3	T37.1X4	T37.1X5	T37.1X6
Tioclomarol	T45.511	T45.512	T45.513	T45.514	T45.515	T45.516
Tioconazole	T49.0X1	T49.0X2	T49.0X3	T49.0X4	T49.0X5	T49.0X6
Tioguanine	T45.1X1	T45.1X2	T45.1X3	T45.1X4	T45.1X5	T45.1X6
Tiopronin	T50.991	T50.992	T50.993	T50.994	T50.995	T50.996
Tiotixene	T43.4X1	T43.4X2	T43.4X3	T43.4X4	T43.4X5	T43.4X6
Tioxolone	T49.4X1	T49.4X2	T49.4X3	T49.4X4	T49.4X5	T49.4X6
Tipepidine	T48.3X1	T48.3X2	T48.3X3	T48.3X4	T48.3X5	T48.3X6
Tiquizium bromide	T44.3X1	T44.3X2	T44.3X3	T44.3X4	T44.3X5	T44.3X6
Tiratricol	T38.1X1	T38.1X2	T38.1X3	T38.1X4	T38.1X5	T38.1X6
Tisopurine	T50.4X1	T50.4X2	T50.4X3	T50.4X4	T50.4X5	T50.4X6
Titanium (compounds) (vapor)	T56.891	T56.892	T56.893	T56.894	--	--
dioxide	T49.3X1	T49.3X2	T49.3X3	T49.3X4	T49.3X5	T49.3X6
ointment	T49.3X1	T49.3X2	T49.3X3	T49.3X4	T49.3X5	T49.3X6
oxide	T49.3X1	T49.3X2	T49.3X3	T49.3X4	T49.3X5	T49.3X6
tetrachloride	T56.891	T56.892	T56.893	T56.894	--	--
Titanocene	T56.891	T56.892	T56.893	T56.894	--	--
Titroid	T38.1X1	T38.1X2	T38.1X3	T38.1X4	T38.1X5	T38.1X6
Tizanidine	T42.8X1	T42.8X2	T42.8X3	T42.8X4	T42.8X5	T42.8X6
TMTD	T60.3X1	T60.3X2	T60.3X3	T60.3X4	--	--
TNT (fumes)	T65.3X1	T65.3X2	T65.3X3	T65.3X4	--	--
Toadstool	T62.0X1	T62.0X2	T62.0X3	T62.0X4	--	--
Tobacco NEC	T65.291	T65.292	T65.293	T65.294	--	--
cigarettes	T65.221	T65.222	T65.223	T65.224	--	--
Indian	T62.2X1	T62.2X2	T62.2X3	T62.2X4	--	--
smoke, second-hand	T65.221	T65.222	T65.223	T65.224	--	--
Tobramycin	T36.5X1	T36.5X2	T36.5X3	T36.5X4	T36.5X5	T36.5X6
Tocainide	T46.2X1	T46.2X2	T46.2X3	T46.2X4	T46.2X5	T46.2X6
Tocoferol	T45.2X1	T45.2X2	T45.2X3	T45.2X4	T45.2X5	T45.2X6
Tocopherol	T45.2X1	T45.2X2	T45.2X3	T45.2X4	T45.2X5	T45.2X6
acetate	T45.2X1	T45.2X2	T45.2X3	T45.2X4	T45.2X5	T45.2X6
Tocosamine	T48.0X1	T48.0X2	T48.0X3	T48.0X4	T48.0X5	T48.0X6
Todralazine	T46.5X1	T46.5X2	T46.5X3	T46.5X4	T46.5X5	T46.5X6
Tofisopam	T42.4X1	T42.4X2	T42.4X3	T42.4X4	T42.4X5	T42.4X6
Tofranil	T43.011	T43.012	T43.013	T43.014	T43.015	T43.016
Toilet deodorizer	T65.891	T65.892	T65.893	T65.894	--	--
Tolamolol	T44.7X1	T44.7X2	T44.7X3	T44.7X4	T44.7X5	T44.7X6
Tolazamide	T38.3X1	T38.3X2	T38.3X3	T38.3X4	T38.3X5	T38.3X6
Tolazoline	T46.7X1	T46.7X2	T46.7X3	T46.7X4	T46.7X5	T46.7X6
Tolbutamide (sodium)	T38.3X1	T38.3X2	T38.3X3	T38.3X4	T38.3X5	T38.3X6
Tolciclate	T49.0X1	T49.0X2	T49.0X3	T49.0X4	T49.0X5	T49.0X6
Tolmetin	T39.391	T39.392	T39.393	T39.394	T39.395	T39.396
Tolnaftate	T49.0X1	T49.0X2	T49.0X3	T49.0X4	T49.0X5	T49.0X6
Tolonidine	T46.5X1	T46.5X2	T46.5X3	T46.5X4	T46.5X5	T46.5X6
Toloxatone	T42.6X1	T42.6X2	T42.6X3	T42.6X4	T42.6X5	T42.6X6
Tolperisone	T44.3X1	T44.3X2	T44.3X3	T44.3X4	T44.3X5	T44.3X6
Tolserol	T42.8X1	T42.8X2	T42.8X3	T42.8X4	T42.8X5	T42.8X6
Toluene (liquid)	T52.2X1	T52.2X2	T52.2X3	T52.2X4	--	--
diisocyanate	T65.0X1	T65.0X2	T65.0X3	T65.0X4	--	--
Toluidine	T65.891	T65.892	T65.893	T65.894	--	--
vapor	T59.891	T59.892	T59.893	T59.894	--	--
Toluol (liquid)	T52.2X1	T52.2X2	T52.2X3	T52.2X4	--	--
vapor	T52.2X1	T52.2X2	T52.2X3	T52.2X4	--	--
Toluylenediamine	T65.3X1	T65.3X2	T65.3X3	T65.3X4	--	--
Tolylene-2,4-diisocyanate	T65.0X1	T65.0X2	T65.0X3	T65.0X4	--	--
Tonic NEC	T50.901	T50.902	T50.903	T50.904	T50.905	T50.906
Topical action drug NEC	T49.91	T49.92	T49.93	T49.94	T49.95	T49.96
ear, nose or throat	T49.6X1	T49.6X2	T49.6X3	T49.6X4	T49.6X5	T49.6X6
eye	T49.5X1	T49.5X2	T49.5X3	T49.5X4	T49.5X5	T49.5X6
skin	T49.91	T49.92	T49.93	T49.94	T49.95	T49.96
specified NEC	T49.8X1	T49.8X2	T49.8X3	T49.8X4	T49.8X5	T49.8X6
Toquizine	T44.3X1	T44.3X2	T44.3X3	T44.3X4	T44.3X5	T44.3X6
Toremifene	T38.6X1	T38.6X2	T38.6X3	T38.6X4	T38.6X5	T38.6X6
Tosylchloramide sodium	T49.8X1	T49.8X2	T49.8X3	T49.8X4	T49.8X5	T49.8X6
Toxaphene (dust) (spray)	T60.1X1	T60.1X2	T60.1X3	T60.1X4	--	--
Toxin, diphtheria (Schick Test)	T50.8X1	T50.8X2	T50.8X3	T50.8X4	T50.8X5	T50.8X6
Toxoid						
combined	T50.A21	T50.A22	T50.A23	T50.A24	T50.A25	T50.A26
diphtheria	T50.A91	T50.A92	T50.A93	T50.A94	T50.A95	T50.A96
tetanus	T50.A91	T50.A92	T50.A93	T50.A94	T50.A95	T50.A96
Trace element NEC	T45.8X1	T45.8X2	T45.8X3	T45.8X4	T45.8X5	T45.8X6
Tractor fuel NEC	T52.0X1	T52.0X2	T52.0X3	T52.0X4	--	--
Tragacanth	T50.991	T50.992	T50.993	T50.994	T50.995	T50.996
Tramadol	T40.4X1	T40.4X2	T40.4X3	T40.4X4	T40.4X5	T40.4X6
Tramazoline	T48.5X1	T48.5X2	T48.5X3	T48.5X4	T48.5X5	T48.5X6
Tranexamic acid	T45.621	T45.622	T45.623	T45.624	T45.625	T45.626
Tranilast	T45.0X1	T45.0X2	T45.0X3	T45.0X4	T45.0X5	T45.0X6
Tranquilizer NEC	T43.501	T43.502	T43.503	T43.504	T43.505	T43.506
with hypnotic or sedative	T42.6X1	T42.6X2	T42.6X3	T42.6X4	T42.6X5	T42.6X6
benzodiazepine NEC	T42.4X1	T42.4X2	T42.4X3	T42.4X4	T42.4X5	T42.4X6
butyrophenone NEC	T43.4X1	T43.4X2	T43.4X3	T43.4X4	T43.4X5	T43.4X6
carbamate	T43.591	T43.592	T43.593	T43.594	T43.595	T43.596
dimethylamine	T43.3X1	T43.3X2	T43.3X3	T43.3X4	T43.3X5	T43.3X6
ethylamine	T43.3X1	T43.3X2	T43.3X3	T43.3X4	T43.3X5	T43.3X6

Substance	Poisoning, Accidental unintentional	Poisoning, Intentional self-harm	Poisoning, Assault	Poisoning, Undetermined	Adverse effect	Underdosing
Tranquilizer NEC — *continued*						
hydroxyzine	T43.591	T43.592	T43.593	T43.594	T43.595	T43.596
major NEC	T43.501	T43.502	T43.503	T43.504	T43.505	T43.506
penothiazine NEC	T43.3X1	T43.3X2	T43.3X3	T43.3X4	T43.3X5	T43.3X6
phenothiazine-based	T43.3X1	T43.3X2	T43.3X3	T43.3X4	T43.3X5	T43.3X6
piperazine NEC	T43.3X1	T43.3X2	T43.3X3	T43.3X4	T43.3X5	T43.3X6
piperidine	T43.3X1	T43.3X2	T43.3X3	T43.3X4	T43.3X5	T43.3X6
propylamine	T43.3X1	T43.3X2	T43.3X3	T43.3X4	T43.3X5	T43.3X6
specified NEC	T43.591	T43.592	T43.593	T43.594	T43.595	T43.596
thioxanthene NEC	T43.591	T43.592	T43.593	T43.594	T43.595	T43.596
Tranxene	T42.4X1	T42.4X2	T42.4X3	T42.4X4	T42.4X5	T42.4X6
Tranylcypromine	T43.1X1	T43.1X2	T43.1X3	T43.1X4	T43.1X5	T43.1X6
Trapidil	T46.3X1	T46.3X2	T46.3X3	T46.3X4	T46.3X5	T46.3X6
Trasentine	T44.3X1	T44.3X2	T44.3X3	T44.3X4	T44.3X5	T44.3X6
Travert	T50.3X1	T50.3X2	T50.3X3	T50.3X4	T50.3X5	T50.3X6
Trazodone	T43.211	T43.212	T43.213	T43.214	T43.215	T43.216
Trecator	T37.1X1	T37.1X2	T37.1X3	T37.1X4	T37.1X5	T37.1X6
Treosulfan	T45.1X1	T45.1X2	T45.1X3	T45.1X4	T45.1X5	T45.1X6
Tretamine	T45.1X1	T45.1X2	T45.1X3	T45.1X4	T45.1X5	T45.1X6
Tretinoin	T49.0X1	T49.0X2	T49.0X3	T49.0X4	T49.0X5	T49.0X6
Tretoquinol	T48.6X1	T48.6X2	T48.6X3	T48.6X4	T48.6X5	T48.6X6
Triacetin	T49.0X1	T49.0X2	T49.0X3	T49.0X4	T49.0X5	T49.0X6
Triacetoxyanthracene	T49.4X1	T49.4X2	T49.4X3	T49.4X4	T49.4X5	T49.4X6
Triacetyloleandomycin	T36.3X1	T36.3X2	T36.3X3	T36.3X4	T36.3X5	T36.3X6
Triamcinolone	T38.0X1	T38.0X2	T38.0X3	T38.0X4	T38.0X5	T38.0X6
ENT agent	T49.6X1	T49.6X2	T49.6X3	T49.6X4	T49.6X5	T49.6X6
hexacetonide	T49.0X1	T49.0X2	T49.0X3	T49.0X4	T49.0X5	T49.0X6
ophthalmic preparation	T49.5X1	T49.5X2	T49.5X3	T49.5X4	T49.5X5	T49.5X6
topical NEC	T49.0X1	T49.0X2	T49.0X3	T49.0X4	T49.0X5	T49.0X6
Triampyzine	T44.3X1	T44.3X2	T44.3X3	T44.3X4	T44.3X5	T44.3X6
Triamterene	T50.2X1	T50.2X2	T50.2X3	T50.2X4	T50.2X5	T50.2X6
Triazine (herbicide)	T60.3X1	T60.3X2	T60.3X3	T60.3X4	--	--
Triaziquone	T45.1X1	T45.1X2	T45.1X3	T45.1X4	T45.1X5	T45.1X6
Triazolam	T42.4X1	T42.4X2	T42.4X3	T42.4X4	T42.4X5	T42.4X6
Triazole (herbicide)	T60.3X1	T60.3X2	T60.3X3	T60.3X4	--	--
Tribenoside	T46.991	T46.992	T46.993	T46.994	T46.995	T46.996
Tribromacetaldehyde	T42.6X1	T42.6X2	T42.6X3	T42.6X4	T42.6X5	T42.6X6
Tribromoethanol, rectal	T41.291	T41.292	T41.293	T41.294	T41.295	T41.296
Tribromomethane	T42.6X1	T42.6X2	T42.6X3	T42.6X4	T42.6X5	T42.6X6
Trichlorethane	T53.2X1	T53.2X2	T53.2X3	T53.2X4	--	--
Trichlorethylene	T53.2X1	T53.2X2	T53.2X3	T53.2X4	--	--
Trichlorfon	T60.0X1	T60.0X2	T60.0X3	T60.0X4	--	--
Trichlormethiazide	T50.2X1	T50.2X2	T50.2X3	T50.2X4	T50.2X5	T50.2X6
Trichlormethine	T45.1X1	T45.1X2	T45.1X3	T45.1X4	T45.1X5	T45.1X6
Trichloroacetic acid, Trichloracetic acid	T54.2X1	T54.2X2	T54.2X3	T54.2X4	--	--
medicinal	T49.4X1	T49.4X2	T49.4X3	T49.4X4	T49.4X5	T49.4X6
Trichloroethane	T53.2X1	T53.2X2	T53.2X3	T53.2X4	--	--
Trichloroethanol	T42.6X1	T42.6X2	T42.6X3	T42.6X4	T42.6X5	T42.6X6
Trichloroethyl phosphate	T42.6X1	T42.6X2	T42.6X3	T42.6X4	T42.6X5	T42.6X6
Trichloroethylene (liquid) (vapor)	T53.2X1	T53.2X2	T53.2X3	T53.2X4	--	--
anesthetic (gas)	T41.0X1	T41.0X2	T41.0X3	T41.0X4	T41.0X5	T41.0X6
vapor NEC	T53.2X1	T53.2X2	T53.2X3	T53.2X4	--	--
Trichlorofluoromethane NEC	T53.5X1	T53.5X2	T53.5X3	T53.5X4	--	--
Trichloronate	T60.0X1	T60.0X2	T60.0X3	T60.0X4	--	--
2,4,5-Trichlorophen-oxyacetic acid	T60.3X1	T60.3X2	T60.3X3	T60.3X4	--	--
Trichloropropane	T53.6X1	T53.6X2	T53.6X3	T53.6X4	--	--
Trichlorotriethylamine	T45.1X1	T45.1X2	T45.1X3	T45.1X4	T45.1X5	T45.1X6
Trichomonacides NEC	T37.3X1	T37.3X2	T37.3X3	T37.3X4	T37.3X5	T37.3X6
Trichomycin	T36.7X1	T36.7X2	T36.7X3	T36.7X4	T36.7X5	T36.7X6
Triclobisonium chloride	T49.0X1	T49.0X2	T49.0X3	T49.0X4	T49.0X5	T49.0X6
Triclocarban	T49.0X1	T49.0X2	T49.0X3	T49.0X4	T49.0X5	T49.0X6
Triclofos	T42.6X1	T42.6X2	T42.6X3	T42.6X4	T42.6X5	T42.6X6
Triclosan	T49.0X1	T49.0X2	T49.0X3	T49.0X4	T49.0X5	T49.0X6
Tricresyl phosphate	T65.891	T65.892	T65.893	T65.894	--	--
solvent	T52.91	T52.92	T52.93	T52.94	--	--
Tricyclamol chloride	T44.3X1	T44.3X2	T44.3X3	T44.3X4	T44.3X5	T44.3X6
Tridesilon	T49.0X1	T49.0X2	T49.0X3	T49.0X4	T49.0X5	T49.0X6
Tridihexethyl iodide	T44.3X1	T44.3X2	T44.3X3	T44.3X4	T44.3X5	T44.3X6
Tridione	T42.2X1	T42.2X2	T42.2X3	T42.2X4	T42.2X5	T42.2X6
Trientine	T45.8X1	T45.8X2	T45.8X3	T45.8X4	T45.8X5	T45.8X6
Triethanolamine NEC	T54.3X1	T54.3X2	T54.3X3	T54.3X4	--	--
detergent	T54.3X1	T54.3X2	T54.3X3	T54.3X4	--	--
trinitrate (biphosphate)	T46.3X1	T46.3X2	T46.3X3	T46.3X4	T46.3X5	T46.3X6
Triethanomelamine	T45.1X1	T45.1X2	T45.1X3	T45.1X4	T45.1X5	T45.1X6
Triethylenemelamine	T45.1X1	T45.1X2	T45.1X3	T45.1X4	T45.1X5	T45.1X6
Triethylenephosphoramide	T45.1X1	T45.1X2	T45.1X3	T45.1X4	T45.1X5	T45.1X6
Triethylenethiophosphoramide	T45.1X1	T45.1X2	T45.1X3	T45.1X4	T45.1X5	T45.1X6
Trifluoperazine	T43.3X1	T43.3X2	T43.3X3	T43.3X4	T43.3X5	T43.3X6
Trifluoroethyl vinyl ether	T41.0X1	T41.0X2	T41.0X3	T41.0X4	T41.0X5	T41.0X6
Trifluperidol	T43.4X1	T43.4X2	T43.4X3	T43.4X4	T43.4X5	T43.4X6
Triflupromazine	T43.3X1	T43.3X2	T43.3X3	T43.3X4	T43.3X5	T43.3X6
Trifluridine	T37.5X1	T37.5X2	T37.5X3	T37.5X4	T37.5X5	T37.5X6
Triflusal	T45.521	T45.522	T45.523	T45.524	T45.525	T45.526
Trihexyphenidyl	T44.3X1	T44.3X2	T44.3X3	T44.3X4	T44.3X5	T44.3X6
Triiodothyronine	T38.1X1	T38.1X2	T38.1X3	T38.1X4	T38.1X5	T38.1X6
Trilene	T41.0X1	T41.0X2	T41.0X3	T41.0X4	T41.0X5	T41.0X6
Trilostane	T38.991	T38.992	T38.993	T38.994	T38.995	T38.996
Trimebutine	T44.3X1	T44.3X2	T44.3X3	T44.3X4	T44.3X5	T44.3X6
Trimecaine	T41.3X1	T41.3X2	T41.3X3	T41.3X4	T41.3X5	T41.3X6
Trimeprazine (tartrate)	T44.3X1	T44.3X2	T44.3X3	T44.3X4	T44.3X5	T44.3X6
Trimetaphan camsilate	T44.2X1	T44.2X2	T44.2X3	T44.2X4	T44.2X5	T44.2X6
Trimetazidine	T46.7X1	T46.7X2	T46.7X3	T46.7X4	T46.7X5	T46.7X6
Trimethadione	T42.2X1	T42.2X2	T42.2X3	T42.2X4	T42.2X5	T42.2X6
Trimethaphan	T44.2X1	T44.2X2	T44.2X3	T44.2X4	T44.2X5	T44.2X6
Trimethidinium	T44.2X1	T44.2X2	T44.2X3	T44.2X4	T44.2X5	T44.2X6
Trimethobenzamide	T45.0X1	T45.0X2	T45.0X3	T45.0X4	T45.0X5	T45.0X6
Trimethoprim	T37.8X1	T37.8X2	T37.8X3	T37.8X4	T37.8X5	T37.8X6
with sulfamethoxazole	T36.8X1	T36.8X2	T36.8X3	T36.8X4	T36.8X5	T36.8X6
Trimethylcarbinol	T51.3X1	T51.3X2	T51.3X3	T51.3X4	--	--
Trimethylpsoralen	T49.3X1	T49.3X2	T49.3X3	T49.3X4	T49.3X5	T49.3X6
Trimeton	T45.0X1	T45.0X2	T45.0X3	T45.0X4	T45.0X5	T45.0X6
Trimetrexate	T45.1X1	T45.1X2	T45.1X3	T45.1X4	T45.1X5	T45.1X6
Trimipramine	T43.011	T43.012	T43.013	T43.014	T43.015	T43.016
Trimustine	T45.1X1	T45.1X2	T45.1X3	T45.1X4	T45.1X5	T45.1X6
Trinitrine	T46.3X1	T46.3X2	T46.3X3	T46.3X4	T46.3X5	T46.3X6
Trinitrobenzol	T65.3X1	T65.3X2	T65.3X3	T65.3X4	--	--
Trinitrophenol	T65.3X1	T65.3X2	T65.3X3	T65.3X4	--	--
Trinitrotoluene (fumes)	T65.3X1	T65.3X2	T65.3X3	T65.3X4	--	--
Trional	T42.6X1	T42.6X2	T42.6X3	T42.6X4	T42.6X5	T42.6X6
Triorthocresyl phosphate	T65.891	T65.892	T65.893	T65.894	--	--
Trioxide of arsenic	T57.0X1	T57.0X2	T57.0X3	T57.0X4	--	--
Trioxysalen	T49.4X1	T49.4X2	T49.4X3	T49.4X4	T49.4X5	T49.4X6
Tripamide	T50.2X1	T50.2X2	T50.2X3	T50.2X4	T50.2X5	T50.2X6
Triparanol	T46.6X1	T46.6X2	T46.6X3	T46.6X4	T46.6X5	T46.6X6
Tripelennamine	T45.0X1	T45.0X2	T45.0X3	T45.0X4	T45.0X5	T45.0X6
Triperiden	T44.3X1	T44.3X2	T44.3X3	T44.3X4	T44.3X5	T44.3X6
Triperidol	T43.4X1	T43.4X2	T43.4X3	T43.4X4	T43.4X5	T43.4X6
Triphenylphosphate	T65.891	T65.892	T65.893	T65.894	--	--
Triple						
bromides	T42.6X1	T42.6X2	T42.6X3	T42.6X4	T42.6X5	T42.6X6
carbonate	T47.1X1	T47.1X2	T47.1X3	T47.1X4	T47.1X5	T47.1X6
vaccine						
DPT	T50.A11	T50.A12	T50.A13	T50.A14	T50.A15	T50.A16
including pertussis	T50.A11	T50.A12	T50.A13	T50.A14	T50.A15	T50.A16
MMR	T50.B91	T50.B92	T50.B93	T50.B94	T50.B95	T50.B96
Triprolidine	T45.0X1	T45.0X2	T45.0X3	T45.0X4	T45.0X5	T45.0X6
Trisodium hydrogen edetate	T50.6X1	T50.6X2	T50.6X3	T50.6X4	T50.6X5	T50.6X6
Trisoralen	T49.3X1	T49.3X2	T49.3X3	T49.3X4	T49.3X5	T49.3X6
Trisulfapyrimidines	T37.0X1	T37.0X2	T37.0X3	T37.0X4	T37.0X5	T37.0X6
Trithiozine	T44.3X1	T44.3X2	T44.3X3	T44.3X4	T44.3X5	T44.3X6
Tritiozine	T44.3X1	T44.3X2	T44.3X3	T44.3X4	T44.3X5	T44.3X6
Tritoqualine	T45.0X1	T45.0X2	T45.0X3	T45.0X4	T45.0X5	T45.0X6
Trofosfamide	T45.1X1	T45.1X2	T45.1X3	T45.1X4	T45.1X5	T45.1X6
Troleandomycin	T36.3X1	T36.3X2	T36.3X3	T36.3X4	T36.3X5	T36.3X6
Trolnitrate (phosphate)	T46.3X1	T46.3X2	T46.3X3	T46.3X4	T46.3X5	T46.3X6
Tromantadine	T37.5X1	T37.5X2	T37.5X3	T37.5X4	T37.5X5	T37.5X6
Trometamol	T50.2X1	T50.2X2	T50.2X3	T50.2X4	T50.2X5	T50.2X6
Tromethamine	T50.2X1	T50.2X2	T50.2X3	T50.2X4	T50.2X5	T50.2X6
Tronothane	T41.3X1	T41.3X2	T41.3X3	T41.3X4	T41.3X5	T41.3X6
Tropacine	T44.3X1	T44.3X2	T44.3X3	T44.3X4	T44.3X5	T44.3X6
Tropatepine	T44.3X1	T44.3X2	T44.3X3	T44.3X4	T44.3X5	T44.3X6
Tropicamide	T44.3X1	T44.3X2	T44.3X3	T44.3X4	T44.3X5	T44.3X6
Trospium chloride	T44.3X1	T44.3X2	T44.3X3	T44.3X4	T44.3X5	T44.3X6
Troxerutin	T46.991	T46.992	T46.993	T46.994	T46.995	T46.996
Troxidone	T42.2X1	T42.2X2	T42.2X3	T42.2X4	T42.2X5	T42.2X6
Tryparsamide	T37.3X1	T37.3X2	T37.3X3	T37.3X4	T37.3X5	T37.3X6
Trypsin	T45.3X1	T45.3X2	T45.3X3	T45.3X4	T45.3X5	T45.3X6
Tryptizol	T43.011	T43.012	T43.013	T43.014	T43.015	T43.016
TSH	T38.811	T38.812	T38.813	T38.814	T38.815	T38.816
Tuaminoheptane	T48.5X1	T48.5X2	T48.5X3	T48.5X4	T48.5X5	T48.5X6
Tuberculin, purified protein derivative (PPD)	T50.8X1	T50.8X2	T50.8X3	T50.8X4	T50.8X5	T50.8X6
Tubocurare	T48.1X1	T48.1X2	T48.1X3	T48.1X4	T48.1X5	T48.1X6
Tubocurarine (chloride)	T48.1X1	T48.1X2	T48.1X3	T48.1X4	T48.1X5	T48.1X6
Tulobuterol	T48.6X1	T48.6X2	T48.6X3	T48.6X4	T48.6X5	T48.6X6
Turpentine (spirits of)	T52.8X1	T52.8X2	T52.8X3	T52.8X4	--	--
vapor	T52.8X1	T52.8X2	T52.8X3	T52.8X4	--	--
Tybamate	T43.591	T43.592	T43.593	T43.594	T43.595	T43.596
Tyloxapol	T48.4X1	T48.4X2	T48.4X3	T48.4X4	T48.4X5	T48.4X6
Tymazoline	T48.5X1	T48.5X2	T48.5X3	T48.5X4	T48.5X5	T48.5X6
Typhoid-paratyphoid vaccine	T50.A91	T50.A92	T50.A93	T50.A94	T50.A95	T50.A96
Typhus vaccine	T50.A91	T50.A92	T50.A93	T50.A94	T50.A95	T50.A96
Tyropanoate	T50.8X1	T50.8X2	T50.8X3	T50.8X4	T50.8X5	T50.8X6
Tyrothricin	T49.6X1	T49.6X2	T49.6X3	T49.6X4	T49.6X5	T49.6X6
ENT agent	T49.6X1	T49.6X2	T49.6X3	T49.6X4	T49.6X5	T49.6X6
ophthalmic preparation	T49.5X1	T49.5X2	T49.5X3	T49.5X4	T49.5X5	T49.5X6

Ufenamate - Veratrum

Substance	Poisoning, Accidental unintentional	Poisoning, Intentional self-harm	Poisoning, Assault	Poisoning, Undetermined	Adverse effect	Underdosing
U						
Ufenamate	T39.391	T39.392	T39.393	T39.394	T39.395	T39.396
Ultraviolet light protectant	T49.3X1	T49.3X2	T49.3X3	T49.3X4	T49.3X5	T49.3X6
Undecenoic acid	T49.0X1	T49.0X2	T49.0X3	T49.0X4	T49.0X5	T49.0X6
Undecoylium	T49.0X1	T49.0X2	T49.0X3	T49.0X4	T49.0X5	T49.0X6
Undecylenic acid (derivatives)	T49.0X1	T49.0X2	T49.0X3	T49.0X4	T49.0X5	T49.0X6
Unna's boot	T49.3X1	T49.3X2	T49.3X3	T49.3X4	T49.3X5	T49.3X6
Unsaturated fatty acid	T46.6X1	T46.6X2	T46.6X3	T46.6X4	T46.6X5	T46.6X6
Uracil mustard	T45.1X1	T45.1X2	T45.1X3	T45.1X4	T45.1X5	T45.1X6
Uramustine	T45.1X1	T45.1X2	T45.1X3	T45.1X4	T45.1X5	T45.1X6
Urapidil	T46.5X1	T46.5X2	T46.5X3	T46.5X4	T46.5X5	T46.5X6
Urari	T48.1X1	T48.1X2	T48.1X3	T48.1X4	T48.1X5	T48.1X6
Urate oxidase	T50.4X1	T50.4X2	T50.4X3	T50.4X4	T50.4X5	T50.4X6
Urea	T47.3X1	T47.3X2	T47.3X3	T47.3X4	T47.3X5	T47.3X6
peroxide	T49.0X1	T49.0X2	T49.0X3	T49.0X4	T49.0X5	T49.0X6
stibamine	T37.4X1	T37.4X2	T37.4X3	T37.4X4	T37.4X5	T37.4X6
topical	T49.8X1	T49.8X2	T49.8X3	T49.8X4	T49.8X5	T49.8X6
Urethane	T45.1X1	T45.1X2	T45.1X3	T45.1X4	T45.1X5	T45.1X6
Urginea (maritima) (scilla) — see Squill						
Uric acid metabolism drug NEC	T50.4X1	T50.4X2	T50.4X3	T50.4X4	T50.4X5	T50.4X6
Uricosuric agent	T50.4X1	T50.4X2	T50.4X3	T50.4X4	T50.4X5	T50.4X6
Urinary anti-infective	T37.8X1	T37.8X2	T37.8X3	T37.8X4	T37.8X5	T37.8X6
Urofollitropin	T38.812	T38.812	T38.813	T38.814	T38.815	T38.816
Urokinase	T45.611	T45.612	T45.613	T45.614	T45.615	T45.616
Urokon	T50.8X1	T50.8X2	T50.8X3	T50.8X4	T50.8X5	T50.8X6
Ursodeoxycholic acid	T50.991	T50.992	T50.993	T50.994	T50.995	T50.996
Ursodiol	T50.991	T50.992	T50.993	T50.994	T50.995	T50.996
Urtica	T62.2X1	T62.2X2	T62.2X3	T62.2X4	--	--
Utility gas — see Gas, utility						
V						
Vaccine NEC	T50.Z91	T50.Z92	T50.Z93	T50.Z94	T50.Z95	T50.Z96
antineoplastic	T50.Z91	T50.Z92	T50.Z93	T50.Z94	T50.Z95	T50.Z96
bacterial NEC	T50.A91	T50.A92	T50.A93	T50.A94	T50.A95	T50.A96
with						
other bacterial component	T50.A21	T50.A22	T50.A23	T50.A24	T50.A25	T50.A26
pertussis component	T50.A11	T50.A12	T50.A13	T50.A14	T50.A15	T50.A16
viral-rickettsial component	T50.A21	T50.A22	T50.A23	T50.A24	T50.A25	T50.A26
mixed NEC	T50.A21	T50.A22	T50.A23	T50.A24	T50.A25	T50.A26
BCG	T50.A91	T50.A92	T50.A93	T50.A94	T50.A95	T50.A96
cholera	T50.A91	T50.A92	T50.A93	T50.A94	T50.A95	T50.A96
diphtheria	T50.A91	T50.A92	T50.A93	T50.A94	T50.A95	T50.A96
with tetanus	T50.A21	T50.A22	T50.A23	T50.A24	T50.A25	T50.A26
and pertussis	T50.A11	T50.A12	T50.A13	T50.A14	T50.A15	T50.A16
influenza	T50.B91	T50.B92	T50.B93	T50.B94	T50.B95	T50.B96
measles	T50.B91	T50.B92	T50.B93	T50.B94	T50.B95	T50.B96
with mumps and rubella	T50.B91	T50.B92	T50.B93	T50.B94	T50.B95	T50.B96
meningococcal	T50.A91	T50.A92	T50.A93	T50.A94	T50.A95	T50.A96
mumps	T50.B91	T50.B92	T50.B93	T50.B94	T50.B95	T50.B96
paratyphoid	T50.A91	T50.A92	T50.A93	T50.A94	T50.A95	T50.A96
pertussis	T50.A11	T50.A12	T50.A13	T50.A14	T50.A15	T50.A16
with diphtheria	T50.A11	T50.A12	T50.A13	T50.A14	T50.A15	T50.A16
and tetanus	T50.A11	T50.A12	T50.A13	T50.A14	T50.A15	T50.A16
with other component	T50.A11	T50.A12	T50.A13	T50.A14	T50.A15	T50.A16
plague	T50.A91	T50.A92	T50.A93	T50.A94	T50.A95	T50.A96
poliomyelitis	T50.B91	T50.B92	T50.B93	T50.B94	T50.B95	T50.B96
poliovirus	T50.B91	T50.B92	T50.B93	T50.B94	T50.B95	T50.B96
rabies	T50.B91	T50.B92	T50.B93	T50.B94	T50.B95	T50.B96
respiratory syncytial virus	T50.B91	T50.B92	T50.B93	T50.B94	T50.B95	T50.B96
rickettsial NEC	T50.A91	T50.A92	T50.A93	T50.A94	T50.A95	T50.A96
with						
bacterial component	T50.A21	T50.A22	T50.A23	T50.A24	T50.A25	T50.A26
Rocky Mountain spotted fever	T50.A91	T50.A92	T50.A93	T50.A94	T50.A95	T50.A96
rubella	T50.B91	T50.B92	T50.B93	T50.B94	T50.B95	T50.B96
sabin oral	T50.B91	T50.B92	T50.B93	T50.B94	T50.B95	T50.B96
smallpox	T50.B11	T50.B12	T50.B13	T50.B14	T50.B15	T50.B16
TAB	T50.A91	T50.A92	T50.A93	T50.A94	T50.A95	T50.A96
tetanus	T50.A91	T50.A92	T50.A93	T50.A94	T50.A95	T50.A96
typhoid	T50.A91	T50.A92	T50.A93	T50.A94	T50.A95	T50.A96
typhus	T50.A91	T50.A92	T50.A93	T50.A94	T50.A95	T50.A96
viral NEC	T50.B91	T50.B92	T50.B93	T50.B94	T50.B95	T50.B96
yellow fever	T50.B91	T50.B92	T50.B93	T50.B94	T50.B95	T50.B96
Vaccinia immune globulin	T50.Z11	T50.Z12	T50.Z13	T50.Z14	T50.Z15	T50.Z16
Vaginal contraceptives	T49.8X1	T49.8X2	T49.8X3	T49.8X4	T49.8X5	T49.8X6
Valerian						
root	T42.6X1	T42.6X2	T42.6X3	T42.6X4	T42.6X5	T42.6X6
tincture	T42.6X1	T42.6X2	T42.6X3	T42.6X4	T42.6X5	T42.6X6
Valethamate bromide	T44.3X1	T44.3X2	T44.3X3	T44.3X4	T44.3X5	T44.3X6
Valisone	T49.0X1	T49.0X2	T49.0X3	T49.0X4	T49.0X5	T49.0X6
Valium	T42.4X1	T42.4X2	T42.4X3	T42.4X4	T42.4X5	T42.4X6

Substance	Poisoning, Accidental unintentional	Poisoning, Intentional self-harm	Poisoning, Assault	Poisoning, Undetermined	Adverse effect	Underdosing
Valmid	T42.6X1	T42.6X2	T42.6X3	T42.6X4	T42.6X5	T42.6X6
Valnoctamide	T42.6X1	T42.6X2	T42.6X3	T42.6X4	T42.6X5	T42.6X6
Valproate (sodium)	T42.6X1	T42.6X2	T42.6X3	T42.6X4	T42.6X5	T42.6X6
Valproic acid	T42.6X1	T42.6X2	T42.6X3	T42.6X4	T42.6X5	T42.6X6
Valpromide	T42.6X1	T42.6X2	T42.6X3	T42.6X4	T42.6X5	T42.6X6
Vanadium	T56.891	T56.892	T56.893	T56.894	--	--
Vancomycin	T36.8X1	T36.8X2	T36.8X3	T36.8X4	T36.8X5	T36.8X6
Vapor (see also Gas)	T59.91	T59.92	T59.93	T59.94		
kiln (carbon monoxide)	T58.8X1	T58.8X2	T58.8X3	T58.8X4		
lead — see lead						
specified source NEC	T59.891	T59.892	T59.893	T59.894	--	--
Vardenafil	T46.7X1	T46.7X2	T46.7X3	T46.7X4	T46.7X5	T46.7X6
Varicose reduction drug	T46.8X1	T46.8X2	T46.8X3	T46.8X4	T46.8X5	T46.8X6
Varnish	T65.4X1	T65.4X2	T65.4X3	T65.4X4	--	--
cleaner	T52.91	T52.92	T52.93	T52.94	--	--
Vaseline	T49.3X1	T49.3X2	T49.3X3	T49.3X4	T49.3X5	T49.3X6
Vasodilan	T46.7X1	T46.7X2	T46.7X3	T46.7X4	T46.7X5	T46.7X6
Vasodilator						
coronary NEC	T46.3X1	T46.3X2	T46.3X3	T46.3X4	T46.3X5	T46.3X6
peripheral NEC	T46.7X1	T46.7X2	T46.7X3	T46.7X4	T46.7X5	T46.7X6
Vasopressin	T38.891	T38.892	T38.893	T38.894	T38.895	T38.896
Vasopressor drugs	T38.891	T38.892	T38.893	T38.894	T38.895	T38.896
Vecuronium bromide	T48.1X1	T48.1X2	T48.1X3	T48.1X4	T48.1X5	T48.1X6
Vegetable extract, astringent	T49.2X1	T49.2X2	T49.2X3	T49.2X4	T49.2X5	T49.2X6
Venlafaxine	T43.211	T43.212	T43.213	T43.214	T43.215	T43.216
Venom, venomous (bite) (sting)	T63.91	T63.92	T63.93	T63.94	--	--
amphibian NEC	T63.831	T63.832	T63.833	T63.834	--	--
animal NEC	T63.891	T63.892	T63.893	T63.894	--	--
ant	T63.421	T63.422	T63.423	T63.424	--	--
arthropod NEC	T63.481	T63.482	T63.483	T63.484	--	--
bee	T63.441	T63.442	T63.443	T63.444	--	--
centipede	T63.411	T63.412	T63.413	T63.414	--	--
fish	T63.591	T63.592	T63.593	T63.594	--	--
frog	T63.811	T63.812	T63.813	T63.814	--	--
hornet	T63.451	T63.452	T63.453	T63.454	--	--
insect NEC	T63.481	T63.482	T63.483	T63.484	--	--
lizard	T63.121	T63.122	T63.123	T63.124	--	--
marine						
animals	T63.691	T63.692	T63.693	T63.694	--	--
bluebottle	T63.611	T63.612	T63.613	T63.614	--	--
jellyfish NEC	T63.621	T63.622	T63.623	T63.624	--	--
Portugese Man-o-war	T63.611	T63.612	T63.613	T63.614	--	--
sea anemone	T63.631	T63.632	T63.633	T63.634	--	--
specified NEC	T63.691	T63.692	T63.693	T63.694	--	--
fish	T63.591	T63.592	T63.593	T63.594	--	--
plants	T63.711	T63.712	T63.713	T63.714	--	--
sting ray	T63.511	T63.512	T63.513	T63.514	--	--
millipede (tropical)	T63.411	T63.412	T63.413	T63.414	--	--
plant NEC	T63.791	T63.792	T63.793	T63.794	--	--
marine	T63.711	T63.712	T63.713	T63.714	--	--
reptile	T63.191	T63.192	T63.193	T63.194	--	--
gila monster	T63.111	T63.112	T63.113	T63.114	--	--
lizard NEC	T63.121	T63.122	T63.123	T63.124	--	--
scorpion	T63.2X1	T63.2X2	T63.2X3	T63.2X4	--	--
snake	T63.001	T63.002	T63.003	T63.004	--	--
African NEC	T63.081	T63.082	T63.083	T63.084	--	--
American (North) (South) NEC	T63.061	T63.062	T63.063	T63.064	--	--
Asian	T63.081	T63.082	T63.083	T63.084	--	--
Australian	T63.071	T63.072	T63.073	T63.074	--	--
cobra	T63.041	T63.042	T63.043	T63.044	--	--
coral snake	T63.021	T63.022	T63.023	T63.024	--	--
rattlesnake	T63.011	T63.012	T63.013	T63.014	--	--
specified NEC	T63.091	T63.092	T63.093	T63.094	--	--
taipan	T63.031	T63.032	T63.033	T63.034	--	--
specified NEC	T63.891	T63.892	T63.893	T63.894	--	--
spider	T63.301	T63.302	T63.303	T63.304	--	--
black widow	T63.311	T63.312	T63.313	T63.314	--	--
brown recluse	T63.331	T63.332	T63.333	T63.334	--	--
specified NEC	T63.391	T63.392	T63.393	T63.394	--	--
tarantula	T63.321	T63.322	T63.323	T63.324	--	--
sting ray	T63.511	T63.512	T63.513	T63.514	--	--
toad	T63.821	T63.822	T63.823	T63.824	--	--
wasp	T63.461	T63.462	T63.463	T63.464	--	--
Venous sclerosing drug NEC	T46.8X1	T46.8X2	T46.8X3	T46.8X4	T46.8X5	T46.8X6
Ventolin — see Albuterol						
Veramon	T42.3X1	T42.3X2	T42.3X3	T42.3X4	T42.3X5	T42.3X6
Verapamil	T46.1X1	T46.1X2	T46.1X3	T46.1X4	T46.1X5	T46.1X6
Veratrine	T46.5X1	T46.5X2	T46.5X3	T46.5X4	T46.5X5	T46.5X6
Veratrum						
album	T62.2X1	T62.2X2	T62.2X3	T62.2X4	--	--
alkaloids	T46.5X1	T46.5X2	T46.5X3	T46.5X4	T46.5X5	T46.5X6
viride	T62.2X1	T62.2X2	T62.2X3	T62.2X4	--	--

Ufenamate - Veratrum · ICD-10-CM TABLE OF DRUGS AND CHEMICALS

Substance	Poisoning, Accidental unintentional	Poisoning, Intentional self-harm	Poisoning, Assault	Poisoning, Undetermined	Adverse effect	Underdosing
Verdigris	T60.3X1	T60.3X2	T60.3X3	T60.3X4	--	--
Veronal	T42.3X1	T42.3X2	T42.3X3	T42.3X4	T42.3X5	T42.3X6
Veroxil	T37.4X1	T37.4X2	T37.4X3	T37.4X4	T37.4X5	T37.4X6
Versenate	T50.6X1	T50.6X2	T50.6X3	T50.6X4	T50.6X5	T50.6X6
Versidyne	T39.8X1	T39.8X2	T39.8X3	T39.8X4	T39.8X5	T39.8X6
Vetrabutine	T48.0X1	T48.0X2	T48.0X3	T48.0X4	T48.0X5	T48.0X6
Vidarabine	T37.5X1	T37.5X2	T37.5X3	T37.5X4	T37.5X5	T37.5X6
Vienna						
green	T57.0X1	T57.0X2	T57.0X3	T57.0X4	--	--
insecticide	T60.2X1	T60.2X2	T60.2X3	T60.2X4	--	--
red	T57.0X1	T57.0X2	T57.0X3	T57.0X4	--	--
pharmaceutical dye	T50.991	T50.992	T50.993	T50.994	T50.995	T50.996
Vigabatrin	T42.6X1	T42.6X2	T42.6X3	T42.6X4	T42.6X5	T42.6X6
Viloxazine	T43.291	T43.292	T43.293	T43.294	T43.295	T43.296
Viminol	T39.8X1	T39.8X2	T39.8X3	T39.8X4	T39.8X5	T39.8X6
Vinbarbital, vinbarbitone	T42.3X1	T42.3X2	T42.3X3	T42.3X4	T42.3X5	T42.3X6
Vinblastine	T45.1X1	T45.1X2	T45.1X3	T45.1X4	T45.1X5	T45.1X6
Vinburnine	T46.7X1	T46.7X2	T46.7X3	T46.7X4	T46.7X5	T46.7X6
Vincamine	T45.1X1	T45.1X2	T45.1X3	T45.1X4	T45.1X5	T45.1X6
Vincristine	T45.1X1	T45.1X2	T45.1X3	T45.1X4	T45.1X5	T45.1X6
Vindesine	T45.1X1	T45.1X2	T45.1X3	T45.1X4	T45.1X5	T45.1X6
Vinesthene, vinethene	T41.0X1	T41.0X2	T41.0X3	T41.0X4	T41.0X5	T41.0X6
Vinorelbine tartrate	T45.1X1	T45.1X2	T45.1X3	T45.1X4	T45.1X5	T45.1X6
Vinpocetine	T46.7X1	T46.7X2	T46.7X3	T46.7X4	T46.7X5	T46.7X6
Vinyl						
acetate	T65.891	T65.892	T65.893	T65.894	--	--
bital	T42.3X1	T42.3X2	T42.3X3	T42.3X4	T42.3X5	T42.3X6
bromide	T65.891	T65.892	T65.893	T65.894	--	--
chloride	T59.891	T59.892	T59.893	T59.894	--	--
ether	T41.0X1	T41.0X2	T41.0X3	T41.0X4	T41.0X5	T41.0X6
Vinylbital	T42.3X1	T42.3X2	T42.3X3	T42.3X4	T42.3X5	T42.3X6
Vinylidene chloride	T65.891	T65.892	T65.893	T65.894	--	--
Vioform	T37.8X1	T37.8X2	T37.8X3	T37.8X4	T37.8X5	T37.8X6
topical	T49.0X1	T49.0X2	T49.0X3	T49.0X4	T49.0X5	T49.0X6
Viomycin	T36.8X1	T36.8X2	T36.8X3	T36.8X4	T36.8X5	T36.8X6
Viosterol	T45.2X1	T45.2X2	T45.2X3	T45.2X4	T45.2X5	T45.2X6
Viper (venom)	T63.091	T63.092	T63.093	T63.094	--	--
Viprynium	T37.4X1	T37.4X2	T37.4X3	T37.4X4	T37.4X5	T37.4X6
Viquidil	T46.7X1	T46.7X2	T46.7X3	T46.7X4	T46.7X5	T46.7X6
Viral vaccine NEC	T50.B91	T50.B92	T50.B93	T50.B94	T50.B95	T50.B96
Virginiamycin	T36.8X1	T36.8X2	T36.8X3	T36.8X4	T36.8X5	T36.8X6
Virugon	T37.5X1	T37.5X2	T37.5X3	T37.5X4	T37.5X5	T37.5X6
Viscous agent	T50.901	T50.902	T50.903	T50.904	T50.905	T50.906
Visine	T49.5X1	T49.5X2	T49.5X3	T49.5X4	T49.5X5	T49.5X6
Visnadine	T46.3X1	T46.3X2	T46.3X3	T46.3X4	T46.3X5	T46.3X6
Vitamin NEC	T45.2X1	T45.2X2	T45.2X3	T45.2X4	T45.2X5	T45.2X6
A	T45.2X1	T45.2X2	T45.2X3	T45.2X4	T45.2X5	T45.2X6
B NEC	T45.2X1	T45.2X2	T45.2X3	T45.2X4	T45.2X5	T45.2X6
nicotinic acid	T46.7X1	T46.7X2	T46.7X3	T46.7X4	T46.7X5	T46.7X6
B1	T45.2X1	T45.2X2	T45.2X3	T45.2X4	T45.2X5	T45.2X6
B2	T45.2X1	T45.2X2	T45.2X3	T45.2X4	T45.2X5	T45.2X6
B6	T45.2X1	T45.2X2	T45.2X3	T45.2X4	T45.2X5	T45.2X6
B12	T45.2X1	T45.2X2	T45.2X3	T45.2X4	T45.2X5	T45.2X6
B15	T45.2X1	T45.2X2	T45.2X3	T45.2X4	T45.2X5	T45.2X6
C	T45.2X1	T45.2X2	T45.2X3	T45.2X4	T45.2X5	T45.2X6
D	T45.2X1	T45.2X2	T45.2X3	T45.2X4	T45.2X5	T45.2X6
D2	T45.2X1	T45.2X2	T45.2X3	T45.2X4	T45.2X5	T45.2X6
D3	T45.2X1	T45.2X2	T45.2X3	T45.2X4	T45.2X5	T45.2X6
E	T45.2X1	T45.2X2	T45.2X3	T45.2X4	T45.2X5	T45.2X6
E acetate	T45.2X1	T45.2X2	T45.2X3	T45.2X4	T45.2X5	T45.2X6
hematopoietic	T45.8X1	T45.8X2	T45.8X3	T45.8X4	T45.8X5	T45.8X6
K NEC	T45.7X1	T45.7X2	T45.7X3	T45.7X4	T45.7X5	T45.7X6
K1	T45.7X1	T45.7X2	T45.7X3	T45.7X4	T45.7X5	T45.7X6
K2	T45.7X1	T45.7X2	T45.7X3	T45.7X4	T45.7X5	T45.7X6
PP	T45.2X1	T45.2X2	T45.2X3	T45.2X4	T45.2X5	T45.2X6
ulceroprotectant	T47.1X1	T47.1X2	T47.1X3	T47.1X4	T47.1X5	T47.1X6
Vleminckx's solution	T49.4X1	T49.4X2	T49.4X3	T49.4X4	T49.4X5	T49.4X6
Voltaren — see Diclofenac sodium						
W						
Warfarin	T45.511	T45.512	T45.513	T45.514	T45.515	T45.516
rodenticide	T60.4X1	T60.4X2	T60.4X3	T60.4X4	--	--
sodium	T45.511	T45.512	T45.513	T45.514	T45.515	T45.516
Wasp (sting)	T63.461	T63.462	T63.463	T63.464	--	--
Water						
balance drug	T50.3X1	T50.3X2	T50.3X3	T50.3X4	T50.3X5	T50.3X6
distilled	T50.3X1	T50.3X2	T50.3X3	T50.3X4	T50.3X5	T50.3X6
gas — see Gas, water						
incomplete combustion of — see Carbon, monoxide, fuel, utility						
hemlock	T62.2X1	T62.2X2	T62.2X3	T62.2X4	--	--
moccasin (venom)	T63.061	T63.062	T63.063	T63.064	--	--
purified	T50.3X1	T50.3X2	T50.3X3	T50.3X4	T50.3X5	T50.3X6

Substance	Poisoning, Accidental unintentional	Poisoning, Intentional self-harm	Poisoning, Assault	Poisoning, Undetermined	Adverse effect	Underdosing
Wax (paraffin) (petroleum)	T52.0X1	T52.0X2	T52.0X3	T52.0X4	--	--
automobile	T65.891	T65.892	T65.893	T65.894	--	--
floor	T52.0X1	T52.0X2	T52.0X3	T52.0X4	--	--
Weed killers NEC	T60.3X1	T60.3X2	T60.3X3	T60.3X4	--	--
Welldorm	T42.6X1	T42.6X2	T42.6X3	T42.6X4	T42.6X5	T42.6X6
White						
arsenic	T57.0X1	T57.0X2	T57.0X3	T57.0X4	--	--
hellebore	T62.2X1	T62.2X2	T62.2X3	T62.2X4	--	--
lotion (keratolytic)	T49.4X1	T49.4X2	T49.4X3	T49.4X4	T49.4X5	T49.4X6
spirit	T52.0X1	T52.0X2	T52.0X3	T52.0X4	--	--
Whitewash	T65.891	T65.892	T65.893	T65.894	--	--
Whole blood (human)	T45.8X1	T45.8X2	T45.8X3	T45.8X4	T45.8X5	T45.8X6
Wild						
black cherry	T62.2X1	T62.2X2	T62.2X3	T62.2X4	--	--
poisonous plants NEC	T62.2X1	T62.2X2	T62.2X3	T62.2X4	--	--
Window cleaning fluid	T65.891	T65.892	T65.893	T65.894	--	--
Wintergreen (oil)	T49.3X1	T49.3X2	T49.3X3	T49.3X4	T49.3X5	T49.3X6
Wisterine	T62.2X1	T62.2X2	T62.2X3	T62.2X4	--	--
Witch hazel	T49.2X1	T49.2X2	T49.2X3	T49.2X4	T49.2X5	T49.2X6
Wood alcohol or spirit	T51.1X1	T51.1X2	T51.1X3	T51.1X4	--	--
Wool fat (hydrous)	T49.3X1	T49.3X2	T49.3X3	T49.3X4	T49.3X5	T49.3X6
Woorali	T48.1X1	T48.1X2	T48.1X3	T48.1X4	T48.1X5	T48.1X6
Wormseed, American	T37.4X1	T37.4X2	T37.4X3	T37.4X4	T37.4X5	T37.4X6
X						
Xamoterol	T44.5X1	T44.5X2	T44.5X3	T44.5X4	T44.5X5	T44.5X6
Xanthine diuretics	T50.2X1	T50.2X2	T50.2X3	T50.2X4	T50.2X5	T50.2X6
Xanthinol nicotinate	T46.7X1	T46.7X2	T46.7X3	T46.7X4	T46.7X5	T46.7X6
Xanthotoxin	T49.3X1	T49.3X2	T49.3X3	T49.3X4	T49.3X5	T49.3X6
Xantinol nicotinate	T46.7X1	T46.7X2	T46.7X3	T46.7X4	T46.7X5	T46.7X6
Xantocillin	T36.0X1	T36.0X2	T36.0X3	T36.0X4	T36.0X5	T36.0X6
Xenon (127Xe) (133Xe)	T50.8X1	T50.8X2	T50.8X3	T50.8X4	T50.8X5	T50.8X6
Xenysalate	T49.4X1	T49.4X2	T49.4X3	T49.4X4	T49.4X5	T49.4X6
Xibornol	T37.8X1	T37.8X2	T37.8X3	T37.8X4	T37.8X5	T37.8X6
Xigris	T45.511	T45.512	T45.513	T45.514	T45.515	T45.516
Xipamide	T50.2X1	T50.2X2	T50.2X3	T50.2X4	T50.2X5	T50.2X6
Xylene (vapor)	T52.2X1	T52.2X2	T52.2X3	T52.2X4	--	--
Xylocaine (infiltration) (topical)	T41.3X1	T41.3X2	T41.3X3	T41.3X4	T41.3X5	T41.3X6
nerve block (peripheral) (plexus)	T41.3X1	T41.3X2	T41.3X3	T41.3X4	T41.3X5	T41.3X6
spinal	T41.3X1	T41.3X2	T41.3X3	T41.3X4	T41.3X5	T41.3X6
Xylol (vapor)	T52.2X1	T52.2X2	T52.2X3	T52.2X4	--	--
Xylometazoline	T48.5X1	T48.5X2	T48.5X3	T48.5X4	T48.5X5	T48.5X6
Y						
Yeast	T45.2X1	T45.2X2	T45.2X3	T45.2X4	T45.2X5	T45.2X6
dried	T45.2X1	T45.2X2	T45.2X3	T45.2X4	T45.2X5	T45.2X6
Yellow						
fever vaccine	T50.B91	T50.B92	T50.B93	T50.B94	T50.B95	T50.B96
jasmine	T62.2X1	T62.2X2	T62.2X3	T62.2X4	--	--
phenolphthalein	T47.2X1	T47.2X2	T47.2X3	T47.2X4	T47.2X5	T47.2X6
Yew	T62.2X1	T62.2X2	T62.2X3	T62.2X4	--	--
Yohimbic acid	T40.991	T40.992	T40.993	T40.994	T40.995	T40.996
Z						
Zactane	T39.8X1	T39.8X2	T39.8X3	T39.8X4	T39.8X5	T39.8X6
Zalcitabine	T37.5X1	T37.5X2	T37.5X3	T37.5X4	T37.5X5	T37.5X6
Zaroxolyn	T50.2X1	T50.2X2	T50.2X3	T50.2X4	T50.2X5	T50.2X6
Zephiran (topical)	T49.0X1	T49.0X2	T49.0X3	T49.0X4	T49.0X5	T49.0X6
ophthalmic preparation	T49.5X1	T49.5X2	T49.5X3	T49.5X4	T49.5X5	T49.5X6
Zeranol	T38.7X1	T38.7X2	T38.7X3	T38.7X4	T38.7X5	T38.7X6
Zerone	T51.1X1	T51.1X2	T51.1X3	T51.1X4	--	--
Zidovudine	T37.5X1	T37.5X2	T37.5X3	T37.5X4	T37.5X5	T37.5X6
Zimeldine	T43.221	T43.222	T43.223	T43.224	T43.225	T43.226
Zinc (compounds) (fumes) (vapor) NEC	T56.5X1	T56.5X2	T56.5X3	T56.5X4	--	--
anti-infectives	T49.0X1	T49.0X2	T49.0X3	T49.0X4	T49.0X5	T49.0X6
antivaricose	T46.8X1	T46.8X2	T46.8X3	T46.8X4	T46.8X5	T46.8X6
bacitracin	T49.0X1	T49.0X2	T49.0X3	T49.0X4	T49.0X5	T49.0X6
chloride (mouthwash)	T49.6X1	T49.6X2	T49.6X3	T49.6X4	T49.6X5	T49.6X6
chromate	T56.5X1	T56.5X2	T56.5X3	T56.5X4	--	--
gelatin	T49.3X1	T49.3X2	T49.3X3	T49.3X4	T49.3X5	T49.3X6
oxide	T49.3X1	T49.3X2	T49.3X3	T49.3X4	T49.3X5	T49.3X6
plaster	T49.3X1	T49.3X2	T49.3X3	T49.3X4	T49.3X5	T49.3X6
peroxide	T49.0X1	T49.0X2	T49.0X3	T49.0X4	T49.0X5	T49.0X6
pesticides	T56.5X1	T56.5X2	T56.5X3	T56.5X4	--	--
phosphide	T60.4X1	T60.4X2	T60.4X3	T60.4X4	--	--
pyrithionate	T49.4X1	T49.4X2	T49.4X3	T49.4X4	T49.4X5	T49.4X6
stearate	T49.3X1	T49.3X2	T49.3X3	T49.3X4	T49.3X5	T49.3X6
sulfate	T49.5X1	T49.5X2	T49.5X3	T49.5X4	T49.5X5	T49.5X6
ENT agent	T49.6X1	T49.6X2	T49.6X3	T49.6X4	T49.6X5	T49.6X6
ophthalmic solution	T49.5X1	T49.5X2	T49.5X3	T49.5X4	T49.5X5	T49.5X6
topical NEC	T49.0X1	T49.0X2	T49.0X3	T49.0X4	T49.0X5	T49.0X6
undecylenate	T49.0X1	T49.0X2	T49.0X3	T49.0X4	T49.0X5	T49.0X6
Zineb	T60.0X1	T60.0X2	T60.0X3	T60.0X4	--	--
Zinostatin	T45.1X1	T45.1X2	T45.1X3	T45.1X4	T45.1X5	T45.1X6

Zipeprol - Zyprexa

Substance	Poisoning, Accidental unintentional	Poisoning, Intentional self-harm	Poisoning, Assault	Poisoning, Undetermined	Adverse effect	Underdosing
Zipeprol	T48.3X1	T48.3X2	T48.3X3	T48.3X4	T48.3X5	T48.3X6
Zofenopril	T46.4X1	T46.4X2	T46.4X3	T46.4X4	T46.4X5	T46.4X6
Zolpidem	T42.6X1	T42.6X2	T42.6X3	T42.6X4	T42.6X5	T42.6X6
Zomepirac	T39.391	T39.392	T39.393	T39.394	T39.395	T39.396
Zopiclone	T42.6X1	T42.6X2	T42.6X3	T42.6X4	T42.6X5	T42.6X6
Zorubicin	T45.1X1	T45.1X2	T45.1X3	T45.1X4	T45.1X5	T45.1X6

Substance	Poisoning, Accidental unintentional	Poisoning, Intentional self-harm	Poisoning, Assault	Poisoning, Undetermined	Adverse effect	Underdosing
Zotepine	T43.591	T43.592	T43.593	T43.594	T43.595	T43.596
Zovant	T45.511	T45.512	T45.513	T45.514	T45.515	T45.516
Zoxazolamine	T42.8X1	T42.8X2	T42.8X3	T42.8X4	T42.8X5	T42.8X6
Zuclopenthixol	T43.4X1	T43.4X2	T43.4X3	T43.4X4	T43.4X5	T43.4X6
Zygadenus (venenosus)	T62.2X1	T62.2X2	T62.2X3	T62.2X4	--	--
Zyprexa	T43.591	T43.592	T43.593	T43.594	T43.595	T43.596

ICD-10-CM Index to External Causes of Injuries

The vertical yellow line appears at the 2nd and 4th indentations throughout the index.

A

Abandonment (causing exposure to weather conditions) (with intent to injure or kill) NEC X58 ☑
Abuse (adult) (child) (mental) (physical) (sexual) X58 ☑
Accident (to) X58 ☑
  aircraft (in transit) (powered) (*see also* Accident, transport, aircraft)
    due to, caused by cataclysm — *see* Forces of nature, by type
  animal-rider — *see* Accident, transport, animal-rider
  animal-drawn vehicle — *see* Accident, transport, animal-drawn vehicle occupant
  automobile — *see* Accident, transport, car occupant
  bare foot water skier V94.4 ☑
  boat, boating (*see also* Accident, watercraft)
    striking swimmer
      powered V94.11 ☑
      unpowered V94.12 ☑
  bus — *see* Accident, transport, bus occupant
  cable car, not on rails V98.0 ☑
    on rails — *see* Accident, transport, streetcar occupant
  car — *see* Accident, transport, car occupant
  caused by, due to
    animal NEC W64 ☑
    chain hoist W24.0 ☑
    cold (excessive) — *see* Exposure, cold
    corrosive liquid, substance — *see* Table of Drugs and Chemicals
    cutting or piercing instrument — *see* Contact, with, by type of instrument
    drive belt W24.0 ☑
    electric
      current — *see* Exposure, electric current
      motor (*see also* Contact, with, by type of machine) W31.3 ☑
      current (of) W86.8 ☑
    environmental factor NEC X58 ☑
    explosive material — *see* Explosion
    fire, flames — *see* Exposure, fire
    firearm missile — *see* Discharge, firearm by type
    heat (excessive) — *see* Heat
    hot — *see* Contact, with, hot
    ignition — *see* Ignition
    lifting device W24.0 ☑
    lightning — *see* subcategory T75.0
      causing fire — *see* Exposure, fire
    machine, machinery — *see* Contact, with, by type of machine
    natural factor NEC X58 ☑
    pulley (block) W24.0 ☑
    radiation — *see* Radiation
    steam X13.1 ☑
      inhalation X13.0 ☑
      pipe X16 ☑
    thunderbolt — *see* subcategory T75.0
      causing fire — *see* Exposure, fire
    transmission device W24.1 ☑
  coach — *see* Accident, transport, bus occupant
  coal car — *see* Accident, transport, industrial vehicle occupant
  diving (*see also* Fall, into, water)
    with
      drowning or submersion — *see* Drowning
  forklift — *see* Accident, transport, industrial vehicle occupant
  heavy transport vehicle NOS — *see* Accident, transport, truck occupant
  ice yacht V98.2 ☑
  in
    medical, surgical procedure
      as, or due to misadventure — *see* Misadventure
      causing an abnormal reaction or later complication without mention of misadventure (*see also* Complication of or following, by type of procedure) Y84.9
  land yacht V98.1 ☑
  late effect of — *see* W00-X58 with 7th character S
  logging car — *see* Accident, transport, industrial vehicle occupant

Accident — *continued*
  machine, machinery (*see also* Contact, with, by type of machine)
  on board watercraft V93.69 ☑
    explosion — *see* Explosion, in, watercraft
    fire — *see* Burn, on board watercraft
    powered craft V93.63 ☑
      ferry boat V93.61 ☑
      fishing boat V93.62 ☑
      jet skis V93.63 ☑
      liner V93.61 ☑
      merchant ship V93.60 ☑
      passenger ship V93.61 ☑
      sailboat V93.64 ☑
  mine tram — *see* Accident, transport, industrial vehicle occupant
  mobility scooter (motorized) — *see* Accident, transport, pedestrian, conveyance, specified type NEC
  motor scooter — *see* Accident, transport, motorcyclist
  motor vehicle NOS (traffic) (*see also* Accident, transport) V89.2 ☑
    nontraffic V89.0 ☑
    three-wheeled NOS — *see* Accident, transport, three-wheeled motor vehicle occupant
  motorcycle NOS — *see* Accident, transport, motorcyclist
  nonmotor vehicle NOS (nontraffic) (*see also* Accident, transport) V89.1 ☑
    traffic NOS V89.3 ☑
  nontraffic (victim's mode of transport NOS) V88.9 ☑
    collision (between) V88.7 ☑
      bus and truck V88.5 ☑
      car and:
        bus V88.3 ☑
        pickup V88.2 ☑
        three-wheeled motor vehicle V88.0 ☑
        train V88.6 ☑
        truck V88.4 ☑
        two-wheeled motor vehicle V88.0 ☑
        van V88.2 ☑
      specified vehicle NEC and:
        three-wheeled motor vehicle V88.1 ☑
        two-wheeled motor vehicle V88.1 ☑
    known mode of transport — *see* Accident, transport, by type of vehicle
    noncollision V88.8 ☑
  on board watercraft V93.89 ☑
    powered craft V93.83 ☑
      ferry boat V93.81 ☑
      fishing boat V93.82 ☑
      jet skis V93.83 ☑
      liner V93.81 ☑
      merchant ship V93.80 ☑
      passenger ship V93.81 ☑
    unpowered craft V93.88 ☑
      canoe V93.85 ☑
      inflatable V93.86 ☑
        in tow
          recreational V94.31 ☑
          specified NEC V94.32 ☑
      kayak V93.85 ☑
      sailboat V93.84 ☑
      surf-board V93.88 ☑
      water skis V93.87 ☑
      windsurfer V93.88 ☑
  parachutist V97.29 ☑
    entangled in object V97.21 ☑
    injured on landing V97.22 ☑
  pedal cycle — *see* Accident, transport, pedal cyclist
  pedestrian (on foot)
    with
      another pedestrian W51 ☑
        with fall W03 ☑
          due to ice or snow W00.0 ☑
        on pedestrian conveyance NEC V00.09 ☑
      roller skater (in-line) V00.01 ☑
      skate boarder V00.02 ☑
      transport vehicle — *see* Accident, transport
    on pedestrian conveyance — *see* Accident, transport, pedestrian, conveyance
  pick-up truck or van — *see* Accident, transport, pickup truck occupant
  quarry truck — *see* Accident, transport, industrial vehicle occupant

Accident — *continued*
  railway vehicle (any) (in motion) — *see* Accident, transport, railway vehicle occupant
    due to cataclysm — *see* Forces of nature, by type
  scooter (non-motorized) — *see* Accident, transport, pedestrian, conveyance, scooter
  sequelae of — *see* W00-X58 with 7th character S
  skateboard — *see* Accident, transport, pedestrian, conveyance, skateboard
  ski (ing) — *see* Accident, transport, pedestrian, conveyance
    lift V98.3 ☑
  specified cause NEC X58 ☑
  streetcar — *see* Accident, transport, streetcar occupant
  traffic (victim's mode of transport NOS) V87.9 ☑
    collision (between) V87.7 ☑
      bus and truck V87.5 ☑
      car and:
        bus V87.3 ☑
        pickup V87.2 ☑
        three-wheeled motor vehicle V87.0 ☑
        train V87.6 ☑
        truck V87.4 ☑
        two-wheeled motor vehicle V87.0 ☑
        van V87.2 ☑
      specified vehicle NEC and:
        three-wheeled motor vehicle V87.1 ☑
        two-wheeled motor vehicle V87.1 ☑
    known mode of transport — *see* Accident, transport, by type of vehicle
    noncollision V87.8 ☑
  transport (involving injury to) V99 ☑
    18 wheeler — *see* Accident, transport, truck occupant
    agricultural vehicle occupant (nontraffic) V84.9 ☑
      driver V84.5 ☑
      hanger-on V84.7 ☑
      passenger V84.6 ☑
      traffic V84.3 ☑
        driver V84.0 ☑
        hanger-on V84.2 ☑
        passenger V84.1 ☑
      while boarding or alighting V84.4 ☑
    aircraft NEC V97.89 ☑
      military NEC V97.818 ☑
        with civilian aircraft V97.810 ☑
        civilian injured by V97.811 ☑
      occupant injured (in)
        nonpowered craft accident V96.9 ☑
          balloon V96.00 ☑
            collision V96.03 ☑
            crash V96.01 ☑
            explosion V96.05 ☑
            fire V96.04 ☑
            forced landing V96.02 ☑
            specified type NEC V96.09 ☑
          glider V96.20 ☑
            collision V96.23 ☑
            crash V96.21 ☑
            explosion V96.25 ☑
            fire V96.24 ☑
            forced landing V96.22 ☑
            specified type NEC V96.29 ☑
          hang glider V96.10 ☑
            collision V96.13 ☑
            crash V96.11 ☑
            explosion V96.15 ☑
            fire V96.14 ☑
            forced landing V96.12 ☑
            specified type NEC V96.19 ☑
          specified craft NEC V96.8 ☑
        powered craft accident V95.9 ☑
          fixed wing NEC
            commercial V95.30 ☑
              collision V95.33 ☑
              crash V95.31 ☑
              explosion V95.35 ☑
              fire V95.34 ☑
              forced landing V95.32 ☑
              specified type NEC V95.39 ☑
            private V95.20 ☑
              collision V95.23 ☑
              crash V95.21 ☑
              explosion V95.25 ☑
              fire V95.24 ☑

Accident

☑ **Additional character required**

Accident — *continued*
  transport — *continued*
    nontraffic V71.1 ☑
    pickup truck (traffic) V73.6 ☑
      nontraffic V73.1 ☑
    railway vehicle (traffic) V75.6 ☑
      nontraffic V75.1 ☑
    specified vehicle NEC (traffic) V76.6 ☑
      nontraffic V76.1 ☑
    stationary object (traffic) V77.6 ☑
      nontraffic V77.1 ☑
    streetcar (traffic) V76.6 ☑
      nontraffic V76.1 ☑
    three wheeled motor vehicle
      (traffic) V72.6 ☑
      nontraffic V72.1 ☑
    truck (traffic) V74.6 ☑
      nontraffic V74.1 ☑
    two wheeled motor vehicle
      (traffic) V72.6 ☑
      nontraffic V72.1 ☑
    van (traffic) V73.6 ☑
      nontraffic V73.1 ☑
    noncollision accident (traffic) V78.6 ☑
      nontraffic V78.1 ☑
   specified type NEC V79.88 ☑
    military vehicle V79.81 ☑
  cable car, not on rails V98.0 ☑
   on rails — *see* Accident, transport, streetcar
    occupant
  car occupant V49.9 ☑
   ambulance occupant — *see* Accident,
    transport, ambulance occupant
   collision (with)
    animal (traffic) V40.9 ☑
     being ridden (traffic) V46.9 ☑
      nontraffic V46.3 ☑
      while boarding or alighting V46.4 ☑
     nontraffic V40.3 ☑
      while boarding or alighting V40.4 ☑
    animal-drawn vehicle (traffic) V46.9 ☑
     nontraffic V46.3 ☑
     while boarding or alighting V46.4 ☑
    bus (traffic) V44.9 ☑
     nontraffic V44.3 ☑
     while boarding or alighting V44.4 ☑
    car (traffic) V43.92 ☑
     nontraffic V43.32 ☑
     while boarding or alighting V43.42 ☑
    motor vehicle NOS (traffic) V49.60 ☑
     nontraffic V49.20 ☑
     specified type NEC (traffic) V49.69 ☑
      nontraffic V49.29 ☑
    pedal cycle (traffic) V41.9 ☑
     nontraffic V41.3 ☑
     while boarding or alighting V41.4 ☑
    pickup truck (traffic) V43.93 ☑
     nontraffic V43.33 ☑
     while boarding or alighting V43.43 ☑
    railway vehicle (traffic) V45.9 ☑
     nontraffic V45.3 ☑
     while boarding or alighting V45.4 ☑
    specified vehicle NEC (traffic) V46.9 ☑
     nontraffic V46.3 ☑
     while boarding or alighting V46.4 ☑
    sport utility vehicle (traffic) V43.91 ☑
     nontraffic V43.31 ☑
     while boarding or alighting V43.41 ☑
    stationary object (traffic) V47.9 ☑
     nontraffic V47.3 ☑
     while boarding or alighting V47.4 ☑
    streetcar (traffic) V46.9 ☑
     nontraffic V46.3 ☑
     while boarding or alighting V46.4 ☑
    three wheeled motor vehicle
     (traffic) V42.9 ☑
     nontraffic V42.3 ☑
     while boarding or alighting V42.4 ☑
    truck (traffic) V44.9 ☑
     nontraffic V44.3 ☑
     while boarding or alighting V44.4 ☑
    two wheeled motor vehicle
     (traffic) V42.9 ☑
     nontraffic V42.3 ☑
     while boarding or alighting V42.4 ☑
    van (traffic) V43.94 ☑
     nontraffic V43.34 ☑
     while boarding or alighting V43.44 ☑
   driver
    collision (with)
     animal (traffic) V40.5 ☑
      being ridden (traffic) V46.5 ☑

      nontraffic V46.0 ☑
     nontraffic V40.0 ☑
    animal-drawn vehicle (traffic) V46.5 ☑
     nontraffic V46.0 ☑
    bus (traffic) V44.5 ☑
     nontraffic V44.0 ☑
    car (traffic) V43.52 ☑
     nontraffic V43.02 ☑
    motor vehicle NOS (traffic) V49.40 ☑
     nontraffic V49.00 ☑
     specified type NEC (traffic) V49.49 ☑
      nontraffic V49.09 ☑
    pedal cycle (traffic) V41.5 ☑
     nontraffic V41.0 ☑
    pickup truck (traffic) V43.53 ☑
     nontraffic V43.03 ☑
    railway vehicle (traffic) V45.5 ☑
     nontraffic V45.0 ☑
    specified vehicle NEC (traffic) V46.5 ☑
     nontraffic V46.0 ☑
    sport utility vehicle (traffic) V43.51 ☑
     nontraffic V43.01 ☑
    stationary object (traffic) V47.5 ☑
     nontraffic V47.0 ☑
    streetcar (traffic) V46.5 ☑
     nontraffic V46.0 ☑
    three wheeled motor vehicle
     (traffic) V42.5 ☑
     nontraffic V42.0 ☑
    truck (traffic) V44.5 ☑
     nontraffic V44.0 ☑
    two wheeled motor vehicle
     (traffic) V42.5 ☑
     nontraffic V42.0 ☑
    van (traffic) V43.54 ☑
     nontraffic V43.04 ☑
    noncollision accident (traffic) V48.5 ☑
     nontraffic V48.0 ☑
   noncollision accident (traffic) V48.9 ☑
    nontraffic V48.3 ☑
    while boarding or alighting V48.4 ☑
   nontraffic V49.3 ☑
   hanger-on
    collision (with)
     animal (traffic) V40.7 ☑
      being ridden (traffic) V46.7 ☑
       nontraffic V46.2 ☑
      nontraffic V40.2 ☑
     animal-drawn vehicle (traffic) V46.7 ☑
      nontraffic V46.2 ☑
     bus (traffic) V44.7 ☑
      nontraffic V44.2 ☑
     car (traffic) V43.72 ☑
      nontraffic V43.22 ☑
     pedal cycle (traffic) V41.7 ☑
      nontraffic V41.2 ☑
     pickup truck (traffic) V43.73 ☑
      nontraffic V43.23 ☑
     railway vehicle (traffic) V45.7 ☑
      nontraffic V45.2 ☑
     specified vehicle NEC (traffic) V46.7 ☑
      nontraffic V46.2 ☑
     sport utility vehicle (traffic) V43.71 ☑
      nontraffic V43.21 ☑
     stationary object (traffic) V47.7 ☑
      nontraffic V47.2 ☑
     streetcar (traffic) V46.7 ☑
      nontraffic V46.2 ☑
     three wheeled motor vehicle
      (traffic) V42.7 ☑
      nontraffic V42.2 ☑
     truck (traffic) V44.7 ☑
      nontraffic V44.2 ☑
     two wheeled motor vehicle
      (traffic) V42.7 ☑
      nontraffic V42.2 ☑
     van (traffic) V43.74 ☑
      nontraffic V43.24 ☑
    noncollision accident (traffic) V48.7 ☑
     nontraffic V48.2 ☑
   passenger
    collision (with)
     animal (traffic) V40.6 ☑
      being ridden (traffic) V46.6 ☑
       nontraffic V46.1 ☑
      nontraffic V40.1 ☑
     animal-drawn vehicle (traffic) V46.6 ☑
      nontraffic V46.1 ☑
     bus (traffic) V44.6 ☑
      nontraffic V44.1 ☑

    car (traffic) V43.62 ☑
     nontraffic V43.12 ☑
    motor vehicle NOS (traffic) V49.50 ☑
     nontraffic V49.10 ☑
     specified type NEC (traffic) V49.59 ☑
      nontraffic V49.19 ☑
    pedal cycle (traffic) V41.6 ☑
     nontraffic V41.1 ☑
    pickup truck (traffic) V43.63 ☑
     nontraffic V43.13 ☑
    railway vehicle (traffic) V45.6 ☑
     nontraffic V45.1 ☑
    specified vehicle NEC (traffic) V46.6 ☑
     nontraffic V46.1 ☑
    sport utility vehicle (traffic) V43.61 ☑
     nontraffic V43.11 ☑
    stationary object (traffic) V47.6 ☑
     nontraffic V47.1 ☑
    streetcar (traffic) V46.6 ☑
     nontraffic V46.1 ☑
    three wheeled motor vehicle
     (traffic) V42.6 ☑
     nontraffic V42.1 ☑
    truck (traffic) V44.6 ☑
     nontraffic V44.1 ☑
    two wheeled motor vehicle
     (traffic) V42.6 ☑
     nontraffic V42.1 ☑
    van (traffic) V43.64 ☑
     nontraffic V43.14 ☑
    noncollision accident (traffic) V48.6 ☑
     nontraffic V48.1 ☑
   specified type NEC V49.88 ☑
    military vehicle V49.81 ☑
  coal car — *see* Accident, transport, industrial
   vehicle occupant
  construction vehicle occupant
   (nontraffic) V85.9 ☑
   driver V85.5 ☑
   hanger-on V85.7 ☑
   passenger V85.6 ☑
   traffic V85.3 ☑
    driver V85.0 ☑
    hanger-on V85.2 ☑
    passenger V85.1 ☑
   while boarding or alighting V85.4 ☑
  dirt bike rider (nontraffic) V86.96 ☑
   driver V86.56 ☑
   hanger-on V86.76 ☑
   passenger V86.66 ☑
   traffic V86.36 ☑
    driver V86.06 ☑
    hanger-on V86.26 ☑
    passenger V86.16 ☑
   while boarding or alighting V86.46 ☑
  due to cataclysm — *see* Forces of nature,
   by type
  dune buggy occupant (nontraffic) V86.93 ☑
   driver V86.53 ☑
   hanger-on V86.73 ☑
   passenger V86.63 ☑
   traffic V86.33 ☑
    driver V86.03 ☑
    hanger-on V86.23 ☑
    passenger V86.13 ☑
   while boarding or alighting V86.43 ☑
  forklift — *see* Accident, transport, industrial
   vehicle occupant
  go cart — *see* Accident, transport, all-terrain
   vehicle occupant
  golf cart — *see* Accident, transport, all-terrain
   vehicle occupant
  heavy transport vehicle occupant — *see*
   Accident, transport, truck occupant
  ice yacht V98.2 ☑
  industrial vehicle occupant (nontraffic) V83.9 ☑
   driver V83.5 ☑
   hanger-on V83.7 ☑
   passenger V83.6 ☑
   traffic V83.3 ☑
    driver V83.0 ☑
    hanger-on V83.2 ☑
    passenger V83.1 ☑
   while boarding or alighting V83.4 ☑
  interurban electric car — *see* Accident,
   transport, streetcar
  land yacht V98.1 ☑
  logging car — *see* Accident, transport,
   industrial vehicle occupant
  military vehicle occupant (traffic) V86.34 ☑

☑ **Additional character required**

415

Accident

Accident — *continued*
  transport — *continued*
    driver V86.04 ☑
    hanger-on V86.24 ☑
    nontraffic V86.94 ☑
      driver V86.54 ☑
      hanger-on V86.74 ☑
      passenger V86.64 ☑
    passenger V86.14 ☑
    while boarding or alighting V86.44 ☑
    mine tram — *see* Accident, transport, industrial vehicle occupant
    motorcoach — *see* Accident, transport, bus occupant
    motor/cross bike rider (*see also* Accident, transport, dirt bike rider) V86.96 ☑
    motorcyclist V29.9 ☑
      collision (with)
        animal (traffic) V20.9 ☑
          being ridden (traffic) V26.9 ☑
            nontraffic V26.2 ☑
              while boarding or alighting V26.3 ☑
          nontraffic V20.2 ☑
          while boarding or alighting V20.3 ☑
        animal-drawn vehicle (traffic) V26.9 ☑
          nontraffic V26.2 ☑
          while boarding or alighting V26.3 ☑
        bus (traffic) V24.9 ☑
          nontraffic V24.2 ☑
          while boarding or alighting V24.3 ☑
        car (traffic) V23.9 ☑
          nontraffic V23.2 ☑
          while boarding or alighting V23.3 ☑
        motor vehicle NOS (traffic) V29.60 ☑
          nontraffic V29.20 ☑
          specified type NEC (traffic) V29.69 ☑
            nontraffic V29.29 ☑
        pedal cycle (traffic) V21.9 ☑
          nontraffic V21.2 ☑
          while boarding or alighting V21.3 ☑
        pickup truck (traffic) V23.9 ☑
          nontraffic V23.2 ☑
          while boarding or alighting V23.3 ☑
        railway vehicle (traffic) V25.9 ☑
          nontraffic V25.2 ☑
          while boarding or alighting V25.3 ☑
        specified vehicle NEC (traffic) V26.9 ☑
          nontraffic V26.2 ☑
          while boarding or alighting V26.3 ☑
        stationary object (traffic) V27.9 ☑
          nontraffic V27.2 ☑
          while boarding or alighting V27.3 ☑
        streetcar (traffic) V26.9 ☑
          nontraffic V26.2 ☑
          while boarding or alighting V26.3 ☑
        three wheeled motor vehicle (traffic) V22.9 ☑
          nontraffic V22.2 ☑
          while boarding or alighting V22.3 ☑
        truck (traffic) V24.9 ☑
          nontraffic V24.2 ☑
          while boarding or alighting V24.3 ☑
        two wheeled motor vehicle (traffic) V22.9 ☑
          nontraffic V22.2 ☑
          while boarding or alighting V22.3 ☑
        van (traffic) V23.9 ☑
          nontraffic V23.2 ☑
          while boarding or alighting V23.3 ☑
      driver
        collision (with)
          animal (traffic) V20.4 ☑
            being ridden (traffic) V26.4 ☑
              nontraffic V26.0 ☑
            nontraffic V20.0 ☑
          animal-drawn vehicle (traffic) V26.4 ☑
            nontraffic V26.0 ☑
          bus (traffic) V24.4 ☑
            nontraffic V24.0 ☑
          car (traffic) V23.4 ☑
            nontraffic V23.0 ☑
          motor vehicle NOS (traffic) V29.40 ☑
            nontraffic V29.00 ☑
            specified type NEC (traffic) V29.49 ☑
              nontraffic V29.09 ☑
          pedal cycle (traffic) V21.4 ☑
            nontraffic V21.0 ☑
          pickup truck (traffic) V23.4 ☑
            nontraffic V23.0 ☑
          railway vehicle (traffic) V25.4 ☑
            nontraffic V25.0 ☑
          specified vehicle NEC (traffic) V26.4 ☑

Accident — *continued*
  transport — *continued*
          nontraffic V26.0 ☑
        stationary object (traffic) V27.4 ☑
          nontraffic V27.0 ☑
        streetcar (traffic) V26.4 ☑
          nontraffic V26.0 ☑
        three wheeled motor vehicle (traffic) V22.4 ☑
          nontraffic V22.0 ☑
        truck (traffic) V24.4 ☑
          nontraffic V24.0 ☑
        two wheeled motor vehicle (traffic) V22.4 ☑
          nontraffic V22.0 ☑
        van (traffic) V23.4 ☑
          nontraffic V23.0 ☑
      noncollision accident (traffic) V28.4 ☑
        nontraffic V28.0 ☑
      noncollision accident (traffic) V28.9 ☑
        nontraffic V28.2 ☑
        while boarding or alighting V28.3 ☑
      nontraffic V29.3 ☑
      passenger
        collision (with)
          animal (traffic) V20.5 ☑
            being ridden (traffic) V26.5 ☑
              nontraffic V26.1 ☑
            nontraffic V20.1 ☑
          animal-drawn vehicle (traffic) V26.5 ☑
            nontraffic V26.1 ☑
          bus (traffic) V24.5 ☑
            nontraffic V24.1 ☑
          car (traffic) V23.5 ☑
            nontraffic V23.1 ☑
          motor vehicle NOS (traffic) V29.50 ☑
            nontraffic V29.10 ☑
            specified type NEC (traffic) V29.59 ☑
              nontraffic V29.19 ☑
          pedal cycle (traffic) V21.5 ☑
            nontraffic V21.1 ☑
          pickup truck (traffic) V23.5 ☑
            nontraffic V23.1 ☑
          railway vehicle (traffic) V25.5 ☑
            nontraffic V25.1 ☑
          specified vehicle NEC (traffic) V26.5 ☑
            nontraffic V26.1 ☑
          stationary object (traffic) V27.5 ☑
            nontraffic V27.1 ☑
          streetcar (traffic) V26.5 ☑
            nontraffic V26.1 ☑
          three wheeled motor vehicle (traffic) V22.5 ☑
            nontraffic V22.1 ☑
          truck (traffic) V24.5 ☑
            nontraffic V24.1 ☑
          two wheeled motor vehicle (traffic) V22.5 ☑
            nontraffic V22.1 ☑
          van (traffic) V23.5 ☑
            nontraffic V23.1 ☑
        noncollision accident (traffic) V28.5 ☑
          nontraffic V28.1 ☑
      specified type NEC V29.88 ☑
        military vehicle V29.81 ☑
    motor vehicle NEC occupant (traffic) V89.2 ☑
    occupant (of)
      aircraft (powered) V95.9 ☑
        fixed wing
          commercial — *see* Accident, transport, aircraft, occupant, powered, fixed wing, commercial
          private — *see* Accident, transport, aircraft, occupant, powered, fixed wing, private
        nonpowered V96.9 ☑
        specified NEC V95.8 ☑
      airport battery-powered vehicle — *see* Accident, transport, industrial vehicle occupant
      all-terrain vehicle (ATV) — *see* Accident, transport, all-terrain vehicle occupant
      animal-drawn vehicle — *see* Accident, transport, animal-drawn vehicle occupant
      automobile — *see* Accident, transport, car occupant
      balloon V96.00 ☑
      battery-powered vehicle — *see* Accident, transport, industrial vehicle occupant
      bicycle — *see* Accident, transport, pedal cyclist

Accident — *continued*
  transport — *continued*
      motorized — *see* Accident, transport, motorcycle rider
      boat NEC — *see* Accident, watercraft
      bulldozer — *see* Accident, transport, construction vehicle occupant
      bus — *see* Accident, transport, bus occupant
      cable car (on rails) (*see also* Accident, transport, streetcar occupant)
        not on rails V98.0 ☑
      car (*see also* Accident, transport, car occupant)
        cable (on rails) (*see also* Accident, transport, streetcar occupant)
        not on rails V98.0 ☑
      coach — *see* Accident, transport, bus occupant
      coal-car — *see* Accident, transport, industrial vehicle occupant
      digger — *see* Accident, transport, construction vehicle occupant
      dump truck — *see* Accident, transport, construction vehicle occupant
      earth-leveler — *see* Accident, transport, construction vehicle occupant
      farm machinery (self-propelled) — *see* Accident, transport, agricultural vehicle occupant
      forklift — *see* Accident, transport, industrial vehicle occupant
      glider (unpowered) V96.20 ☑
        hang V96.10 ☑
        powered (microlight) (ultralight) — *see* Accident, transport, aircraft, occupant, powered, glider
      glider (unpowered) NEC V96.20 ☑
      hang-glider V96.10 ☑
      harvester — *see* Accident, transport, agricultural vehicle occupant
      heavy (transport) vehicle — *see* Accident, transport, truck occupant
      helicopter — *see* Accident, transport, aircraft, occupant, helicopter
      ice-yacht V98.2 ☑
      kite (carrying person) V96.8 ☑
      land-yacht V98.1 ☑
      logging car — *see* Accident, transport, industrial vehicle occupant
      mechanical shovel — *see* Accident, transport, construction vehicle occupant
      microlight — *see* Accident, transport, aircraft, occupant, powered, glider
      minibus — *see* Accident, transport, pickup truck occupant
      minivan — *see* Accident, transport, pickup truck occupant
      moped — *see* Accident, transport, motorcycle
      motor scooter — *see* Accident, transport, motorcycle
      motorcycle (with sidecar) — *see* Accident, transport, motorcycle
      off-road motor-vehicle (*see also* Accident, transport, all-terrain vehicle occupant) V86.99 ☑
      pedal cycle (*see also* Accident, transport, pedal cyclist)
      pick-up (truck) — *see* Accident, transport, pickup truck occupant
      railway (train) (vehicle) (subterranean) (elevated) — *see* Accident, transport, railway vehicle occupant
      rickshaw — *see* Accident, transport, pedal cycle
        motorized — *see* Accident, transport, three-wheeled motor vehicle
        pedal driven — *see* Accident, transport, pedal cyclist
      road-roller — *see* Accident, transport, construction vehicle occupant
      ship NOS V94.9 ☑
      ski-lift (chair) (gondola) V98.3 ☑
      snowmobile — *see* Accident, transport, snowmobile occupant
      spacecraft, spaceship — *see* Accident, transport, aircraft, occupant, spacecraft
      sport utility vehicle — *see* Accident, transport, pickup truck occupant
      streetcar (interurban) (operating on public street or highway) — *see* Accident, transport, streetcar occupant

☑ **Additional character required**

Accident — *continued*
  transport — *continued*
    SUV — *see* Accident, transport, pickup truck occupant
    téléférique V98.0 ☑
    three-wheeled vehicle (motorized) (*see also* Accident, transport, three-wheeled motor vehicle occupant)
      nonmotorized — *see* Accident, transport, pedal cycle
    tractor (farm) (and trailer) — *see* Accident, transport, agricultural vehicle occupant
    train — *see* Accident, transport, railway vehicle occupant
    tram — *see* Accident, transport, streetcar occupant
      in mine or quarry — *see* Accident, transport, industrial vehicle occupant
    tricycle — *see* Accident, transport, pedal cycle
      motorized — *see* Accident, transport, three-wheeled motor vehicle
    trolley — *see* Accident, transport, streetcar occupant
      in mine or quarry — *see* Accident, transport, industrial vehicle occupant
    tub, in mine or quarry — *see* Accident, transport, industrial vehicle occupant
    ultralight — *see* Accident, transport, aircraft, occupant, powered, glider
    van — *see* Accident, transport, van occupant
    vehicle NEC V89.9 ☑
      heavy transport — *see* Accident, transport, truck occupant
      motor (traffic) NEC V89.2 ☑
      nontraffic NEC V89.0 ☑
    watercraft NOS V94.9 ☑
      causing drowning — *see* Drowning, resulting from accident to boat
  off-road motor-vehicle (*see also* Accident, transport, all-terrain vehicle occupant) V86.99 ☑
  parachutist V97.29 ☑
    after accident to aircraft — *see* Accident, transport, aircraft
    entangled in object V97.21 ☑
    injured on landing V97.22 ☑
  pedal cyclist V19.9 ☑
    collision (with)
      animal (traffic) V10.9 ☑
        being ridden (traffic) V16.9 ☑
          nontraffic V16.2 ☑
          while boarding or alighting V16.3 ☑
        nontraffic V10.2 ☑
        while boarding or alighting V10.3 ☑
      animal-drawn vehicle (traffic) V16.9 ☑
        nontraffic V16.2 ☑
        while boarding or alighting V16.3 ☑
      bus (traffic) V14.9 ☑
        nontraffic V14.2 ☑
        while boarding or alighting V14.3 ☑
      car (traffic) V13.9 ☑
        nontraffic V13.2 ☑
        while boarding or alighting V13.3 ☑
      motor vehicle NOS (traffic) V19.60 ☑
        nontraffic V19.20 ☑
        specified type NEC (traffic) V19.69 ☑
          nontraffic V19.29 ☑
      pedal cycle (traffic) V11.9 ☑
        nontraffic V11.2 ☑
        while boarding or alighting V11.3 ☑
      pickup truck (traffic) V13.9 ☑
        nontraffic V13.2 ☑
        while boarding or alighting V13.3 ☑
      railway vehicle (traffic) V15.9 ☑
        nontraffic V15.2 ☑
        while boarding or alighting V15.3 ☑
      specified vehicle NEC (traffic) V16.9 ☑
        nontraffic V16.2 ☑
        while boarding or alighting V16.3 ☑
      stationary object (traffic) V17.9 ☑
        nontraffic V17.2 ☑
        while boarding or alighting V17.3 ☑
      streetcar (traffic) V16.9 ☑
        nontraffic V16.2 ☑
        while boarding or alighting V16.3 ☑
      three wheeled motor vehicle (traffic) V12.9 ☑
        nontraffic V12.2 ☑
        while boarding or alighting V12.3 ☑
      truck (traffic) V14.9 ☑
        nontraffic V14.2 ☑

Accident — *continued*
  transport — *continued*
        while boarding or alighting V14.3 ☑
      two wheeled motor vehicle (traffic) V12.9 ☑
        nontraffic V12.2 ☑
        while boarding or alighting V12.3 ☑
      van (traffic) V13.9 ☑
        nontraffic V13.2 ☑
        while boarding or alighting V13.3 ☑
    driver
      collision (with)
        animal (traffic) V10.4 ☑
          being ridden (traffic) V16.4 ☑
            nontraffic V16.0 ☑
          nontraffic V10.0 ☑
        animal-drawn vehicle (traffic) V16.4 ☑
          nontraffic V16.0 ☑
        bus (traffic) V14.4 ☑
          nontraffic V14.0 ☑
        car (traffic) V13.4 ☑
          nontraffic V13.0 ☑
        motor vehicle NOS (traffic) V19.40 ☑
          nontraffic V19.00 ☑
          specified type NEC (traffic) V19.49 ☑
            nontraffic V19.09 ☑
        pedal cycle (traffic) V11.4 ☑
          nontraffic V11.0 ☑
        pickup truck (traffic) V13.4 ☑
          nontraffic V13.0 ☑
        railway vehicle (traffic) V15.4 ☑
          nontraffic V15.0 ☑
        specified vehicle NEC (traffic) V16.4 ☑
          nontraffic V16.0 ☑
        stationary object (traffic) V17.4 ☑
          nontraffic V17.0 ☑
        streetcar (traffic) V16.4 ☑
          nontraffic V16.0 ☑
        three wheeled motor vehicle (traffic) V12.4 ☑
          nontraffic V12.0 ☑
        truck (traffic) V14.4 ☑
          nontraffic V14.0 ☑
        two wheeled motor vehicle (traffic) V12.4 ☑
          nontraffic V12.0 ☑
        van (traffic) V13.4 ☑
          nontraffic V13.0 ☑
      noncollision accident (traffic) V18.4 ☑
        nontraffic V18.0 ☑
    noncollision accident (traffic) V18.9 ☑
      nontraffic V18.2 ☑
      while boarding or alighting V18.3 ☑
    nontraffic V19.3 ☑
    passenger
      collision (with)
        animal (traffic) V10.5 ☑
          being ridden (traffic) V16.5 ☑
            nontraffic V16.1 ☑
          nontraffic V10.1 ☑
        animal-drawn vehicle (traffic) V16.5 ☑
          nontraffic V16.1 ☑
        bus (traffic) V14.5 ☑
          nontraffic V14.1 ☑
        car (traffic) V13.5 ☑
          nontraffic V13.1 ☑
        motor vehicle NOS (traffic) V19.50 ☑
          nontraffic V19.10 ☑
          specified type NEC (traffic) V19.59 ☑
            nontraffic V19.19 ☑
        pedal cycle (traffic) V11.5 ☑
          nontraffic V11.1 ☑
        pickup truck (traffic) V13.5 ☑
          nontraffic V13.1 ☑
        railway vehicle (traffic) V15.5 ☑
          nontraffic V15.1 ☑
        specified vehicle NEC (traffic) V16.5 ☑
          nontraffic V16.1 ☑
        stationary object (traffic) V17.5 ☑
          nontraffic V17.1 ☑
        streetcar (traffic) V16.5 ☑
          nontraffic V16.1 ☑
        three wheeled motor vehicle (traffic) V12.5 ☑
          nontraffic V12.1 ☑
        truck (traffic) V14.5 ☑
          nontraffic V14.1 ☑
        two wheeled motor vehicle (traffic) V12.5 ☑
          nontraffic V12.1 ☑
        van (traffic) V13.5 ☑
          nontraffic V13.1 ☑

Accident — *continued*
  transport — *continued*
      noncollision accident (traffic) V18.5 ☑
      nontraffic V18.1 ☑
    specified type NEC V19.88 ☑
      military vehicle V19.81 ☑
  pedestrian
    conveyance (occupant) V09.9 ☑
      baby stroller V00.828 ☑
        collision (with) V09.9 ☑
          animal being ridden or animal drawn vehicle V06.99 ☑
            nontraffic V06.09 ☑
            traffic V06.19 ☑
          bus or heavy transport V04.99 ☑
            nontraffic V04.09 ☑
            traffic V04.19 ☑
          car V03.99 ☑
            nontraffic V03.09 ☑
            traffic V03.19 ☑
          pedal cycle V01.99 ☑
            nontraffic V01.09 ☑
            traffic V01.19 ☑
          pick-up truck or van V03.99 ☑
            nontraffic V03.09 ☑
            traffic V03.19 ☑
          railway (train) (vehicle) V05.99 ☑
            nontraffic V05.09 ☑
            traffic V05.19 ☑
          streetcar V06.99 ☑
            nontraffic V06.09 ☑
            traffic V06.19 ☑
          stationary object V00.822 ☑
          two- or three-wheeled motor vehicle V02.99 ☑
            nontraffic V02.09 ☑
            traffic V02.19 ☑
          vehicle V09.9 ☑
            animal-drawn V06.99 ☑
              nontraffic V06.09 ☑
              traffic V06.19 ☑
            motor
              nontraffic V09.00 ☑
              traffic V09.20 ☑
        fall V00.821 ☑
        nontraffic V09.1 ☑
          involving motor vehicle NEC V09.00 ☑
        traffic V09.3 ☑
          involving motor vehicle NEC V09.20 ☑
      flat-bottomed NEC V00.388 ☑
        collision (with) V09.9 ☑
          animal being ridden or animal drawn vehicle V06.99 ☑
            nontraffic V06.09 ☑
            traffic V06.19 ☑
          bus or heavy transport V04.99 ☑
            nontraffic V04.09 ☑
            traffic V04.19 ☑
          car V03.99 ☑
            nontraffic V03.09 ☑
            traffic V03.19 ☑
          pedal cycle V01.99 ☑
            nontraffic V01.09 ☑
            traffic V01.19 ☑
          pick-up truck or van V03.99 ☑
            nontraffic V03.09 ☑
            traffic V03.19 ☑
          railway (train) (vehicle) V05.99 ☑
            nontraffic V05.09 ☑
            traffic V05.19 ☑
          stationary object V00.382 ☑
          streetcar V06.99 ☑
            nontraffic V06.09 ☑
            traffic V06.19 ☑
          two- or three-wheeled motor vehicle V02.99 ☑
            nontraffic V02.09 ☑
            traffic V02.19 ☑
          vehicle V09.9 ☑
            animal-drawn V06.99 ☑
              nontraffic V06.09 ☑
              traffic V06.19 ☑
            motor
              nontraffic V09.00 ☑
              traffic V09.20 ☑
        fall V00.381 ☑
        nontraffic V09.1 ☑
          involving motor vehicle NEC V09.00 ☑
      snow
        board — *see* Accident, transport, pedestrian, conveyance, snow board

Accident

Accident — *continued*
  transport — *continued*
          ski — *see* Accident, transport,
            pedestrian, conveyance, skis
            (snow)
        traffic V09.3 ☑
          involving motor vehicle NEC V09.20 ☑
      gliding type NEC V00.288 ☑
        collision (with) V09.9 ☑
          animal being ridden or animal drawn
            vehicle V06.99 ☑
              nontraffic V06.09 ☑
              traffic V06.19 ☑
          bus or heavy transport V04.99 ☑
            nontraffic V04.09 ☑
            traffic V04.19 ☑
          car V03.99 ☑
            nontraffic V03.09 ☑
            traffic V03.19 ☑
          pedal cycle V01.99 ☑
            nontraffic V01.09 ☑
            traffic V01.19 ☑
          pick-up truck or van V03.99 ☑
            nontraffic V03.09 ☑
            traffic V03.19 ☑
          railway (train) (vehicle) V05.99 ☑
            nontraffic V05.09 ☑
            traffic V05.19 ☑
          stationary object V00.282 ☑
          streetcar V06.99 ☑
            nontraffic V06.09 ☑
            traffic V06.19 ☑
          two- or three-wheeled motor
            vehicle V02.99 ☑
              nontraffic V02.09 ☑
              traffic V02.19 ☑
          vehicle V09.9 ☑
            animal-drawn V06.99 ☑
              nontraffic V06.09 ☑
              traffic V06.19 ☑
            motor
              nontraffic V09.00 ☑
              traffic V09.20 ☑
        fall V00.281 ☑
        heelies — *see* Accident, transport,
          pedestrian, conveyance, heelies
        ice skate — *see* Accident, transport,
          pedestrian, conveyance, ice skate
        nontraffic V09.1 ☑
          involving motor vehicle NEC V09.00 ☑
        sled — *see* Accident, transport,
          pedestrian, conveyance, sled
        traffic V09.3 ☑
          involving motor vehicle NEC V09.20 ☑
        wheelies — *see* Accident, transport,
          pedestrian, conveyance, heelies
      heelies V00.158 ☑
        colliding with stationary
          object V00.152 ☑
        fall V00.151 ☑
      ice skates V00.218 ☑
        collision (with) V09.9 ☑
          animal being ridden or animal drawn
            vehicle V06.99 ☑
              nontraffic V06.09 ☑
              traffic V06.19 ☑
          bus or heavy transport V04.99 ☑
            nontraffic V04.09 ☑
            traffic V04.19 ☑
          car V03.99 ☑
            nontraffic V03.09 ☑
            traffic V03.19 ☑
          pedal cycle V01.99 ☑
            nontraffic V01.09 ☑
            traffic V01.19 ☑
          pick-up truck or van V03.99 ☑
            nontraffic V03.09 ☑
            traffic V03.19 ☑
          railway (train) (vehicle) V05.99 ☑
            nontraffic V05.09 ☑
            traffic V05.19 ☑
          streetcar V06.99 ☑
            nontraffic V06.09 ☑
            traffic V06.19 ☑
          stationary object V00.212 ☑
          two- or three-wheeled motor
            vehicle V02.99 ☑
              nontraffic V02.09 ☑
              traffic V02.19 ☑
          vehicle V09.9 ☑
            animal-drawn V06.99 ☑
              nontraffic V06.09 ☑

Accident — *continued*
  transport — *continued*
          traffic V06.19 ☑
        motor
          nontraffic V09.00 ☑
          traffic V09.20 ☑
      fall V00.211 ☑
      nontraffic V09.1 ☑
        involving motor vehicle NEC V09.00 ☑
      traffic V09.3 ☑
        involving motor vehicle NEC V09.20 ☑
      motorized mobility scooter V00.838 ☑
        collision with stationary
          object V00.832 ☑
        fall from V00.831 ☑
      nontraffic V09.1 ☑
        involving motor vehicle V09.00 ☑
          military V09.01 ☑
          specified type NEC V09.09 ☑
      roller skates (non in-line) V00.128 ☑
        collision (with) V09.9 ☑
          animal being ridden or animal drawn
            vehicle V06.91 ☑
              nontraffic V06.01 ☑
              traffic V06.11 ☑
          bus or heavy transport V04.91 ☑
            nontraffic V04.01 ☑
            traffic V04.11 ☑
          car V03.91 ☑
            nontraffic V03.01 ☑
            traffic V03.11 ☑
          pedal cycle V01.91 ☑
            nontraffic V01.01 ☑
            traffic V01.11 ☑
          pick-up truck or van V03.91 ☑
            nontraffic V03.01 ☑
            traffic V03.11 ☑
          railway (train) (vehicle) V05.91 ☑
            nontraffic V05.01 ☑
            traffic V05.11 ☑
          streetcar V06.91 ☑
            nontraffic V06.01 ☑
            traffic V06.11 ☑
          stationary object V00.122 ☑
          two- or three-wheeled motor
            vehicle V02.91 ☑
              nontraffic V02.01 ☑
              traffic V02.11 ☑
          vehicle V09.9 ☑
            animal-drawn V06.91 ☑
              nontraffic V06.01 ☑
              traffic V06.11 ☑
            motor
              nontraffic V09.00 ☑
              traffic V09.20 ☑
        fall V00.121 ☑
      in-line V00.118 ☑
        collision — *see also* Accident, transport,
          pedestrian, conveyance occupant,
          roller skates, collision
          with stationary object V00.112 ☑
        fall V00.111 ☑
      nontraffic V09.1 ☑
        involving motor vehicle NEC V09.00 ☑
      traffic V09.3 ☑
        involving motor vehicle NEC V09.20 ☑
      rolling shoes V00.158 ☑
        colliding with stationary
          object V00.152 ☑
        fall V00.151 ☑
      rolling type NEC V00.188 ☑
        collision (with) V09.9 ☑
          animal being ridden or animal drawn
            vehicle V06.99 ☑
              nontraffic V06.09 ☑
              traffic V06.19 ☑
          bus or heavy transport V04.99 ☑
            nontraffic V04.09 ☑
            traffic V04.19 ☑
          car V03.99 ☑
            nontraffic V03.09 ☑
            traffic V03.19 ☑
          pedal cycle V01.99 ☑
            nontraffic V01.09 ☑
            traffic V01.19 ☑
          pick-up truck or van V03.99 ☑
            nontraffic V03.09 ☑
            traffic V03.19 ☑
          railway (train) (vehicle) V05.99 ☑
            nontraffic V05.09 ☑
            traffic V05.19 ☑
          stationary object V00.182 ☑

Accident — *continued*
  transport — *continued*
          streetcar V06.99 ☑
            nontraffic V06.09 ☑
            traffic V06.19 ☑
          two- or three-wheeled motor
            vehicle V02.99 ☑
              nontraffic V02.09 ☑
              traffic V02.19 ☑
          vehicle V09.9 ☑
            animal-drawn V06.99 ☑
              nontraffic V06.09 ☑
              traffic V06.19 ☑
            motor
              nontraffic V09.00 ☑
              traffic V09.20 ☑
        fall V00.181 ☑
        in-line roller skate — *see* Accident,
          transport, pedestrian, conveyance,
          roller skate, in-line
        nontraffic V09.1 ☑
          involving motor vehicle NEC V09.00 ☑
        roller skate — *see* Accident, transport,
          pedestrian, conveyance, roller skate
        scooter (non-motorized) — *see* Accident,
          transport, pedestrian, conveyance,
          scooter
        skateboard — *see* Accident, transport,
          pedestrian, conveyance, skateboard
        traffic V09.3 ☑
          involving motor vehicle NEC V09.20 ☑
      scooter (non-motorized) V00.148 ☑
        collision (with) V09.9 ☑
          animal being ridden or animal drawn
            vehicle V06.99 ☑
              nontraffic V06.09 ☑
              traffic V06.19 ☑
          bus or heavy transport V04.99 ☑
            nontraffic V04.09 ☑
            traffic V04.19 ☑
          car V03.99 ☑
            nontraffic V03.09 ☑
            traffic V03.19 ☑
          pedal cycle V01.99 ☑
            nontraffic V01.09 ☑
            traffic V01.19 ☑
          pick-up truck or van V03.99 ☑
            nontraffic V03.09 ☑
            traffic V03.19 ☑
          railway (train) (vehicle) V05.99 ☑
            nontraffic V05.09 ☑
            traffic V05.19 ☑
          streetcar V06.99 ☑
            nontraffic V06.09 ☑
            traffic V06.19 ☑
          stationary object V00.142 ☑
          two- or three-wheeled motor
            vehicle V02.99 ☑
              nontraffic V02.09 ☑
              traffic V02.19 ☑
          vehicle V09.9 ☑
            animal-drawn V06.99 ☑
              nontraffic V06.09 ☑
              traffic V06.19 ☑
            motor
              nontraffic V09.00 ☑
              traffic V09.20 ☑
        fall V00.141 ☑
        nontraffic V09.1 ☑
          involving motor vehicle NEC V09.00 ☑
        traffic V09.3 ☑
          involving motor vehicle NEC V09.20 ☑
      skate board V00.138 ☑
        collision (with) V09.9 ☑
          animal being ridden or animal drawn
            vehicle V06.92 ☑
              nontraffic V06.02 ☑
              traffic V06.12 ☑
          bus or heavy transport V04.92 ☑
            nontraffic V04.02 ☑
            traffic V04.12 ☑
          car V03.92 ☑
            nontraffic V03.02 ☑
            traffic V03.12 ☑
          pedal cycle V01.92 ☑
            nontraffic V01.02 ☑
            traffic V01.12 ☑
          pick-up truck or van V03.92 ☑
            nontraffic V03.02 ☑
            traffic V03.12 ☑
          railway (train) (vehicle) V05.92 ☑
            nontraffic V05.02 ☑

☑ **Additional character required**

Accident — *continued*
  transport — *continued*
    traffic V05.12 ☑
    streetcar V06.92 ☑
      nontraffic V06.02 ☑
      traffic V06.12 ☑
    stationary object V00.132 ☑
    two- or three-wheeled motor
      vehicle V02.92 ☑
      nontraffic V02.02 ☑
      traffic V02.12 ☑
    vehicle V09.9 ☑
      animal-drawn V06.92 ☑
        nontraffic V06.02 ☑
        traffic V06.12 ☑
      motor
        nontraffic V09.00 ☑
        traffic V09.20 ☑
    fall V00.131 ☑
    nontraffic V09.1 ☑
      involving motor vehicle NEC V09.00 ☑
    traffic V09.3 ☑
      involving motor vehicle NEC V09.20 ☑
  sled V00.228 ☑
    collision (with) V09.9 ☑
      animal being ridden or animal drawn
        vehicle V06.99 ☑
        nontraffic V06.09 ☑
        traffic V06.19 ☑
      bus or heavy transport V04.99 ☑
        nontraffic V04.09 ☑
        traffic V04.19 ☑
      car V03.99 ☑
        nontraffic V03.09 ☑
        traffic V03.19 ☑
      pedal cycle V01.99 ☑
        nontraffic V01.09 ☑
        traffic V01.19 ☑
      pick-up truck or van V03.99 ☑
        nontraffic V03.09 ☑
        traffic V03.19 ☑
      railway (train) (vehicle) V05.99 ☑
        nontraffic V05.09 ☑
        traffic V05.19 ☑
      streetcar V06.99 ☑
        nontraffic V06.09 ☑
        traffic V06.19 ☑
      stationary object V00.222 ☑
      two- or three-wheeled motor
        vehicle V02.99 ☑
        nontraffic V02.09 ☑
        traffic V02.19 ☑
      vehicle V09.9 ☑
        animal-drawn V06.99 ☑
          nontraffic V06.09 ☑
          traffic V06.19 ☑
        motor
          nontraffic V09.00 ☑
          traffic V09.20 ☑
    fall V00.221 ☑
    nontraffic V09.1 ☑
      involving motor vehicle NEC V09.00 ☑
    traffic V09.3 ☑
      involving motor vehicle NEC V09.20 ☑
  skis (snow) V00.328 ☑
    collision (with) V09.9 ☑
      animal being ridden or animal drawn
        vehicle V06.99 ☑
        nontraffic V06.09 ☑
        traffic V06.19 ☑
      bus or heavy transport V04.99 ☑
        nontraffic V04.09 ☑
        traffic V04.19 ☑
      car V03.99 ☑
        nontraffic V03.09 ☑
        traffic V03.19 ☑
      pedal cycle V01.99 ☑
        nontraffic V01.09 ☑
        traffic V01.19 ☑
      pick-up truck or van V03.99 ☑
        nontraffic V03.09 ☑
        traffic V03.19 ☑
      railway (train) (vehicle) V05.99 ☑
        nontraffic V05.09 ☑
        traffic V05.19 ☑
      streetcar V06.99 ☑
        nontraffic V06.09 ☑
        traffic V06.19 ☑
      stationary object V00.322 ☑
      two- or three-wheeled motor
        vehicle V02.99 ☑
        nontraffic V02.09 ☑

Accident — *continued*
  transport — *continued*
    traffic V02.19 ☑
    vehicle V09.9 ☑
      animal-drawn V06.99 ☑
        nontraffic V06.09 ☑
        traffic V06.19 ☑
      motor
        nontraffic V09.00 ☑
        traffic V09.20 ☑
    fall V00.321 ☑
    nontraffic V09.1 ☑
      involving motor vehicle NEC V09.00 ☑
    traffic V09.3 ☑
      involving motor vehicle NEC V09.20 ☑
  snow board V00.318 ☑
    collision (with) V09.9 ☑
      animal being ridden or animal drawn
        vehicle V06.99 ☑
        nontraffic V06.09 ☑
        traffic V06.19 ☑
      bus or heavy transport V04.99 ☑
        nontraffic V04.09 ☑
        traffic V04.19 ☑
      car V03.99 ☑
        nontraffic V03.09 ☑
        traffic V03.19 ☑
      pedal cycle V01.99 ☑
        nontraffic V01.09 ☑
        traffic V01.19 ☑
      pick-up truck or van V03.99 ☑
        nontraffic V03.09 ☑
        traffic V03.19 ☑
      railway (train) (vehicle) V05.99 ☑
        nontraffic V05.09 ☑
        traffic V05.19 ☑
      streetcar V06.99 ☑
        nontraffic V06.09 ☑
        traffic V06.19 ☑
      stationary object V00.312 ☑
      two- or three-wheeled motor
        vehicle V02.99 ☑
        nontraffic V02.09 ☑
      vehicle V09.9 ☑
        animal-drawn V06.99 ☑
          nontraffic V06.09 ☑
          traffic V06.19 ☑
        motor
          nontraffic V09.00 ☑
          traffic V09.20 ☑
    fall V00.311 ☑
    nontraffic V09.1 ☑
      involving motor vehicle NEC V09.00 ☑
    traffic V09.3 ☑
      involving motor vehicle NEC V09.20 ☑
  specified type NEC V00.898 ☑
    collision (with) V09.9 ☑
      animal being ridden or animal drawn
        vehicle V06.99 ☑
        nontraffic V06.09 ☑
        traffic V06.19 ☑
      bus or heavy transport V04.99 ☑
        nontraffic V04.09 ☑
        traffic V04.19 ☑
      car V03.99 ☑
        nontraffic V03.09 ☑
        traffic V03.19 ☑
      pedal cycle V01.99 ☑
        nontraffic V01.09 ☑
        traffic V01.19 ☑
      pick-up truck or van V03.99 ☑
        nontraffic V03.09 ☑
        traffic V03.19 ☑
      railway (train) (vehicle) V05.99 ☑
        nontraffic V05.09 ☑
        traffic V05.19 ☑
      streetcar V06.99 ☑
        nontraffic V06.09 ☑
        traffic V06.19 ☑
      stationary object V00.892 ☑
      two- or three-wheeled motor
        vehicle V02.99 ☑
        nontraffic V02.09 ☑
        traffic V02.19 ☑
      vehicle V09.9 ☑
        animal-drawn V06.99 ☑
          nontraffic V06.09 ☑
          traffic V06.19 ☑
        motor
          nontraffic V09.00 ☑
          traffic V09.20 ☑

Accident — *continued*
  transport — *continued*
    fall V00.891 ☑
    nontraffic V09.1 ☑
      involving motor vehicle NEC V09.00 ☑
    traffic V09.3 ☑
      involving motor vehicle NEC V09.20 ☑
    traffic V09.3 ☑
      involving motor vehicle V09.20 ☑
        military V09.21 ☑
        specified type NEC V09.29 ☑
  wheelchair (powered) V00.818 ☑
    collision (with) V09.9 ☑
      animal being ridden or animal drawn
        vehicle V06.99 ☑
        nontraffic V06.09 ☑
        traffic V06.19 ☑
      bus or heavy transport V04.99 ☑
        nontraffic V04.09 ☑
        traffic V04.19 ☑
      car V03.99 ☑
        nontraffic V03.09 ☑
        traffic V03.19 ☑
      pedal cycle V01.99 ☑
        nontraffic V01.09 ☑
        traffic V01.19 ☑
      pick-up truck or van V03.99 ☑
        nontraffic V03.09 ☑
        traffic V03.19 ☑
      railway (train) (vehicle) V05.99 ☑
        nontraffic V05.09 ☑
        traffic V05.19 ☑
      streetcar V06.99 ☑
        nontraffic V06.09 ☑
        traffic V06.19 ☑
      stationary object V00.812 ☑
      two- or three-wheeled motor
        vehicle V02.99 ☑
        nontraffic V02.09 ☑
        traffic V02.19 ☑
      vehicle V09.9 ☑
        animal-drawn V06.99 ☑
          nontraffic V06.09 ☑
          traffic V06.19 ☑
        motor
          nontraffic V09.00 ☑
          traffic V09.20 ☑
    fall V00.811 ☑
    nontraffic V09.1 ☑
      involving motor vehicle NEC V09.00 ☑
    traffic V09.3 ☑
      involving motor vehicle NEC V09.20 ☑
  wheeled shoe V00.158 ☑
    colliding with stationary
      object V00.152 ☑
    fall V00.151 ☑
  on foot (*see also* Accident, pedestrian)
    collision (with)
      animal being ridden or animal drawn
        vehicle V06.90 ☑
        nontraffic V06.00 ☑
        traffic V06.10 ☑
      bus or heavy transport V04.90 ☑
        nontraffic V04.00 ☑
        traffic V04.10 ☑
      car V03.90 ☑
        nontraffic V03.00 ☑
        traffic V03.10 ☑
      pedal cycle V01.90 ☑
        nontraffic V01.00 ☑
        traffic V01.10 ☑
      pick-up truck or van V03.90 ☑
        nontraffic V03.00 ☑
        traffic V03.10 ☑
      railway (train) (vehicle) V05.90 ☑
        nontraffic V05.00 ☑
        traffic V05.10 ☑
      streetcar V06.90 ☑
        nontraffic V06.00 ☑
        traffic V06.10 ☑
      two- or three-wheeled motor
        vehicle V02.90 ☑
        nontraffic V02.00 ☑
        traffic V02.10 ☑
      vehicle V09.9 ☑
        animal-drawn V06.90 ☑
          nontraffic V06.00 ☑
          traffic V06.10 ☑
        motor
          nontraffic V09.00 ☑
          traffic V09.20 ☑
    nontraffic V09.1 ☑

☑ **Additional character required**

Accident

Accident *— continued*
　transport *— continued*
　　involving motor vehicle V09.00 ☑
　　　military V09.01 ☑
　　　specified type NEC V09.09 ☑
　　traffic V09.3 ☑
　　　involving motor vehicle V09.20 ☑
　　　　military V09.21 ☑
　　　　specified type NEC V09.29 ☑
　　person NEC (unknown way or
　　　transportation) V99 ☑
　　collision (between)
　　　bus (with)
　　　　heavy transport vehicle (traffic) V87.5 ☑
　　　　　nontraffic V88.5 ☑
　　　car (with)
　　　　nontraffic V88.5 ☑
　　　　bus (traffic) V87.3 ☑
　　　　　nontraffic V88.3 ☑
　　　　heavy transport vehicle (traffic) V87.4 ☑
　　　　　nontraffic V88.4 ☑
　　　　pick-up truck or van (traffic) V87.2 ☑
　　　　　nontraffic V88.2 ☑
　　　　train or railway vehicle (traffic) V87.6 ☑
　　　　　nontraffic V88.6 ☑
　　　　two-or three-wheeled motor vehicle
　　　　　(traffic) V87.0 ☑
　　　　　nontraffic V88.0 ☑
　　　　motor vehicle (traffic) NEC V87.7 ☑
　　　　　nontraffic V88.7 ☑
　　　　two-or three-wheeled vehicle (with)
　　　　　(traffic)
　　　　　motor vehicle NEC V87.1 ☑
　　　　　　nontraffic V88.1 ☑
　　　nonmotor vehicle (collision) (noncollision)
　　　　(traffic) V87.9 ☑
　　　　nontraffic V88.9 ☑
　　pickup truck occupant V59.9 ☑
　　　collision (with)
　　　　animal (traffic) V50.9 ☑
　　　　　being ridden (traffic) V56.9 ☑
　　　　　　nontraffic V56.3 ☑
　　　　　　while boarding or alighting V56.4 ☑
　　　　　nontraffic V50.3 ☑
　　　　　while boarding or alighting V50.4 ☑
　　　　animal-drawn vehicle (traffic) V56.9 ☑
　　　　　nontraffic V56.3 ☑
　　　　　while boarding or alighting V56.4 ☑
　　　　bus (traffic) V54.9 ☑
　　　　　nontraffic V54.3 ☑
　　　　　while boarding or alighting V54.4 ☑
　　　　car (traffic) V53.9 ☑
　　　　　nontraffic V53.3 ☑
　　　　　while boarding or alighting V53.4 ☑
　　　　motor vehicle NOS (traffic) V59.60 ☑
　　　　　nontraffic V59.20 ☑
　　　　　specified type NEC (traffic) V59.69 ☑
　　　　　　nontraffic V59.29 ☑
　　　　pedal cycle (traffic) V51.9 ☑
　　　　　nontraffic V51.3 ☑
　　　　　while boarding or alighting V51.4 ☑
　　　　pickup truck (traffic) V53.9 ☑
　　　　　nontraffic V53.3 ☑
　　　　　while boarding or alighting V53.4 ☑
　　　　railway vehicle (traffic) V55.9 ☑
　　　　　nontraffic V55.3 ☑
　　　　　while boarding or alighting V55.4 ☑
　　　　specified vehicle NEC (traffic) V56.9 ☑
　　　　　nontraffic V56.3 ☑
　　　　　while boarding or alighting V56.4 ☑
　　　　stationary object (traffic) V57.9 ☑
　　　　　nontraffic V57.3 ☑
　　　　　while boarding or alighting V57.4 ☑
　　　　streetcar (traffic) V56.9 ☑
　　　　　nontraffic V56.3 ☑
　　　　　while boarding or alighting V56.4 ☑
　　　　three wheeled motor vehicle
　　　　　(traffic) V52.9 ☑
　　　　　nontraffic V52.3 ☑
　　　　　while boarding or alighting V52.4 ☑
　　　　truck (traffic) V54.9 ☑
　　　　　nontraffic V54.3 ☑
　　　　　while boarding or alighting V54.4 ☑
　　　　two wheeled motor vehicle
　　　　　(traffic) V52.9 ☑
　　　　　nontraffic V52.3 ☑
　　　　　while boarding or alighting V52.4 ☑
　　　　van (traffic) V53.9 ☑
　　　　　nontraffic V53.3 ☑
　　　　　while boarding or alighting V53.4 ☑
　　　driver
　　　　collision (with)

Accident *— continued*
　transport *— continued*
　　animal (traffic) V50.5 ☑
　　　being ridden (traffic) V56.5 ☑
　　　　nontraffic V56.0 ☑
　　　nontraffic V50.0 ☑
　　animal-drawn vehicle (traffic) V56.5 ☑
　　　nontraffic V56.0 ☑
　　bus (traffic) V54.5 ☑
　　　nontraffic V54.0 ☑
　　car (traffic) V53.5 ☑
　　　nontraffic V53.0 ☑
　　motor vehicle NOS (traffic) V59.40 ☑
　　　nontraffic V59.00 ☑
　　　specified type NEC (traffic) V59.49 ☑
　　　　nontraffic V59.09 ☑
　　pedal cycle (traffic) V51.5 ☑
　　　nontraffic V51.0 ☑
　　pickup truck (traffic) V53.5 ☑
　　　nontraffic V53.0 ☑
　　railway vehicle (traffic) V55.5 ☑
　　　nontraffic V55.0 ☑
　　specified vehicle NEC (traffic) V56.5 ☑
　　　nontraffic V56.0 ☑
　　stationary object (traffic) V57.5 ☑
　　　nontraffic V57.0 ☑
　　streetcar (traffic) V56.5 ☑
　　　nontraffic V56.0 ☑
　　three wheeled motor vehicle
　　　(traffic) V52.5 ☑
　　　nontraffic V52.0 ☑
　　truck (traffic) V54.5 ☑
　　　nontraffic V54.0 ☑
　　two wheeled motor vehicle
　　　(traffic) V52.5 ☑
　　　nontraffic V52.0 ☑
　　van (traffic) V53.5 ☑
　　　nontraffic V53.0 ☑
　　noncollision accident (traffic) V58.5 ☑
　　　nontraffic V58.0 ☑
　noncollision accident (traffic) V58.9 ☑
　　nontraffic V58.3 ☑
　　while boarding or alighting V58.4 ☑
　nontraffic V59.3 ☑
　hanger-on
　　collision (with)
　　　animal (traffic) V50.7 ☑
　　　　being ridden (traffic) V56.7 ☑
　　　　　nontraffic V56.2 ☑
　　　　nontraffic V50.2 ☑
　　　animal-drawn vehicle (traffic) V56.7 ☑
　　　　nontraffic V56.2 ☑
　　　bus (traffic) V54.7 ☑
　　　　nontraffic V54.2 ☑
　　　car (traffic) V53.7 ☑
　　　　nontraffic V53.2 ☑
　　　pedal cycle (traffic) V51.7 ☑
　　　　nontraffic V51.2 ☑
　　　pickup truck (traffic) V53.7 ☑
　　　　nontraffic V53.2 ☑
　　　railway vehicle (traffic) V55.7 ☑
　　　　nontraffic V55.2 ☑
　　　specified vehicle NEC (traffic) V56.7 ☑
　　　　nontraffic V56.2 ☑
　　　stationary object (traffic) V57.7 ☑
　　　　nontraffic V57.2 ☑
　　　streetcar (traffic) V56.7 ☑
　　　　nontraffic V56.2 ☑
　　　three wheeled motor vehicle
　　　　(traffic) V52.7 ☑
　　　　nontraffic V52.2 ☑
　　　truck (traffic) V54.7 ☑
　　　　nontraffic V54.2 ☑
　　　two wheeled motor vehicle
　　　　(traffic) V52.7 ☑
　　　　nontraffic V52.2 ☑
　　　van (traffic) V53.7 ☑
　　　　nontraffic V53.2 ☑
　　　noncollision accident (traffic) V58.7 ☑
　　　　nontraffic V58.2 ☑
　passenger
　　collision (with)
　　　animal (traffic) V50.6 ☑
　　　　being ridden (traffic) V56.6 ☑
　　　　　nontraffic V56.1 ☑
　　　　nontraffic V50.1 ☑
　　　animal-drawn vehicle (traffic) V56.6 ☑
　　　　nontraffic V56.1 ☑
　　　bus (traffic) V54.6 ☑
　　　　nontraffic V54.1 ☑
　　　car (traffic) V53.6 ☑
　　　　nontraffic V53.1 ☑

Accident *— continued*
　transport *— continued*
　　motor vehicle NOS (traffic) V59.50 ☑
　　　nontraffic V59.10 ☑
　　　specified type NEC (traffic) V59.59 ☑
　　　　nontraffic V59.19 ☑
　　pedal cycle (traffic) V51.6 ☑
　　　nontraffic V51.1 ☑
　　pickup truck (traffic) V53.6 ☑
　　　nontraffic V53.1 ☑
　　railway vehicle (traffic) V55.6 ☑
　　　nontraffic V55.1 ☑
　　specified vehicle NEC (traffic) V56.6 ☑
　　　nontraffic V56.1 ☑
　　stationary object (traffic) V57.6 ☑
　　　nontraffic V57.1 ☑
　　streetcar (traffic) V56.6 ☑
　　　nontraffic V56.1 ☑
　　three wheeled motor vehicle
　　　(traffic) V52.6 ☑
　　　nontraffic V52.1 ☑
　　truck (traffic) V54.6 ☑
　　　nontraffic V54.1 ☑
　　two wheeled motor vehicle
　　　(traffic) V52.6 ☑
　　　nontraffic V52.1 ☑
　　van (traffic) V53.6 ☑
　　　nontraffic V53.1 ☑
　　noncollision accident (traffic) V58.6 ☑
　　　nontraffic V58.1 ☑
　specified type NEC V59.88 ☑
　　military vehicle V59.81 ☑
　quarry truck — *see* Accident, transport,
　　industrial vehicle occupant
　race car — *see* Accident, transport, motor
　　vehicle NEC occupant
　railway vehicle occupant V81.9 ☑
　　collision (with) V81.3 ☑
　　　motor vehicle (non-military)
　　　　(traffic) V81.1 ☑
　　　　military V81.83 ☑
　　　　nontraffic V81.0 ☑
　　　rolling stock V81.2 ☑
　　　specified object NEC V81.3 ☑
　　during derailment V81.7 ☑
　　　with antecedent collision — *see* Accident,
　　　　transport, railway vehicle occupant,
　　　　collision
　　explosion V81.81 ☑
　　fall (in railway vehicle) V81.5 ☑
　　　during derailment V81.7 ☑
　　　　with antecedent collision — *see* Accident,
　　　　　transport, railway vehicle occupant,
　　　　　collision
　　　from railway vehicle V81.6 ☑
　　　　during derailment V81.7 ☑
　　　　　with antecedent collision — *see*
　　　　　　Accident, transport, railway vehicle
　　　　　　occupant, collision
　　　while boarding or alighting V81.4 ☑
　　fire V81.81 ☑
　　object falling onto train V81.82 ☑
　　specified type NEC V81.89 ☑
　　while boarding or alighting V81.4 ☑
　ski lift V98.3 ☑
　snowmobile occupant (nontraffic) V86.92 ☑
　　driver V86.52 ☑
　　hanger-on V86.72 ☑
　　passenger V86.62 ☑
　　traffic V86.32 ☑
　　　driver V86.02 ☑
　　　hanger-on V86.22 ☑
　　　passenger V86.12 ☑
　　while boarding or alighting V86.42 ☑
　specified NEC V98.8 ☑
　sport utility vehicle occupant (*see also* Accident,
　　transport, pickup truck occupant)
　streetcar occupant V82.9 ☑
　　collision (with) V82.3 ☑
　　　motor vehicle (traffic) V82.1 ☑
　　　　nontraffic V82.0 ☑
　　　rolling stock V82.2 ☑
　　during derailment V82.7 ☑
　　　with antecedent collision — *see* Accident,
　　　　transport, streetcar occupant, collision
　　fall (in streetcar) V82.5 ☑
　　　during derailment V82.7 ☑
　　　　with antecedent collision — *see* Accident,
　　　　　transport, streetcar occupant,
　　　　　collision
　　　from streetcar V82.6 ☑
　　　　during derailment V82.7 ☑

☑ **Additional character required**

Accident — *continued*
  transport — *continued*
        with antecedent collision — *see*
          Accident, transport, streetcar
          occupant, collision
        while boarding or alighting V82.4 ☑
      while boarding or alighting V82.4 ☑
      specified type NEC V82.8 ☑
      while boarding or alighting V82.4 ☑
    three-wheeled motor vehicle
      occupant V39.9 ☑
      collision (with)
        animal (traffic) V30.9 ☑
          being ridden (traffic) V36.9 ☑
            nontraffic V36.3 ☑
            while boarding or alighting V36.4 ☑
          nontraffic V30.3 ☑
          while boarding or alighting V30.4 ☑
        animal-drawn vehicle (traffic) V36.9 ☑
          nontraffic V36.3 ☑
          while boarding or alighting V36.4 ☑
        bus (traffic) V34.9 ☑
          nontraffic V34.3 ☑
          while boarding or alighting V34.4 ☑
        car (traffic) V33.9 ☑
          nontraffic V33.3 ☑
          while boarding or alighting V33.4 ☑
        motor vehicle NOS (traffic) V39.60 ☑
          nontraffic V39.20 ☑
          specified type NEC (traffic) V39.69 ☑
            nontraffic V39.29 ☑
        pedal cycle (traffic) V31.9 ☑
          nontraffic V31.3 ☑
          while boarding or alighting V31.4 ☑
        pickup truck (traffic) V33.9 ☑
          nontraffic V33.3 ☑
          while boarding or alighting V33.4 ☑
        railway vehicle (traffic) V35.9 ☑
          nontraffic V35.3 ☑
          while boarding or alighting V35.4 ☑
        specified vehicle NEC (traffic) V36.9 ☑
          nontraffic V36.3 ☑
          while boarding or alighting V36.4 ☑
        stationary object (traffic) V37.9 ☑
          nontraffic V37.3 ☑
          while boarding or alighting V37.4 ☑
        streetcar (traffic) V36.9 ☑
          nontraffic V36.3 ☑
          while boarding or alighting V36.4 ☑
        three wheeled motor vehicle
          (traffic) V32.9 ☑
          nontraffic V32.3 ☑
          while boarding or alighting V32.4 ☑
        truck (traffic) V34.9 ☑
          nontraffic V34.3 ☑
          while boarding or alighting V34.4 ☑
        two wheeled motor vehicle
          (traffic) V32.9 ☑
          nontraffic V32.3 ☑
          while boarding or alighting V32.4 ☑
        van (traffic) V33.9 ☑
          nontraffic V33.3 ☑
          while boarding or alighting V33.4 ☑
      driver
        collision (with)
          animal (traffic) V30.5 ☑
            being ridden (traffic) V36.5 ☑
              nontraffic V36.0 ☑
            nontraffic V30.0 ☑
          animal-drawn vehicle (traffic) V36.5 ☑
            nontraffic V36.0 ☑
          bus (traffic) V34.5 ☑
            nontraffic V34.0 ☑
          car (traffic) V33.5 ☑
            nontraffic V33.0 ☑
          motor vehicle NOS (traffic) V39.40 ☑
            nontraffic V39.00 ☑
            specified type NEC (traffic) V39.49 ☑
              nontraffic V39.09 ☑
          pedal cycle (traffic) V31.5 ☑
            nontraffic V31.0 ☑
          pickup truck (traffic) V33.5 ☑
            nontraffic V33.0 ☑
          railway vehicle (traffic) V35.5 ☑
            nontraffic V35.0 ☑
          specified vehicle NEC (traffic) V36.5 ☑
            nontraffic V36.0 ☑
          stationary object (traffic) V37.5 ☑
            nontraffic V37.0 ☑
          streetcar (traffic) V36.5 ☑
            nontraffic V36.0 ☑

Accident — *continued*
  transport — *continued*
        three wheeled motor vehicle
          (traffic) V32.5 ☑
          nontraffic V32.0 ☑
        truck (traffic) V34.5 ☑
          nontraffic V34.0 ☑
        two wheeled motor vehicle
          (traffic) V32.5 ☑
          nontraffic V32.0 ☑
        van (traffic) V33.5 ☑
          nontraffic V33.0 ☑
      noncollision accident (traffic) V38.5 ☑
        nontraffic V38.0 ☑
    noncollision accident (traffic) V38.9 ☑
      nontraffic V38.3 ☑
      while boarding or alighting V38.4 ☑
    nontraffic V39.3 ☑
    hanger-on
      collision (with)
        animal (traffic) V30.7 ☑
          being ridden (traffic) V36.7 ☑
            nontraffic V36.2 ☑
          nontraffic V30.2 ☑
        animal-drawn vehicle (traffic) V36.7 ☑
          nontraffic V36.2 ☑
        bus (traffic) V34.7 ☑
          nontraffic V34.2 ☑
        car (traffic) V33.7 ☑
          nontraffic V33.2 ☑
        pedal cycle (traffic) V31.7 ☑
          nontraffic V31.2 ☑
        pickup truck (traffic) V33.7 ☑
          nontraffic V33.2 ☑
        railway vehicle (traffic) V35.7 ☑
          nontraffic V35.2 ☑
        specified vehicle NEC (traffic) V36.7 ☑
          nontraffic V36.2 ☑
        stationary object (traffic) V37.7 ☑
          nontraffic V37.2 ☑
        streetcar (traffic) V36.7 ☑
          nontraffic V36.2 ☑
        three wheeled motor vehicle
          (traffic) V32.7 ☑
          nontraffic V32.2 ☑
        truck (traffic) V34.7 ☑
          nontraffic V34.2 ☑
        two wheeled motor vehicle
          (traffic) V32.7 ☑
          nontraffic V32.2 ☑
        van (traffic) V33.7 ☑
          nontraffic V33.2 ☑
      noncollision accident (traffic) V38.7 ☑
        nontraffic V38.2 ☑
    passenger
      collision (with)
        animal (traffic) V30.6 ☑
          being ridden (traffic) V36.6 ☑
            nontraffic V36.1 ☑
          nontraffic V30.1 ☑
        animal-drawn vehicle (traffic) V36.6 ☑
          nontraffic V36.1 ☑
        bus (traffic) V34.6 ☑
          nontraffic V34.1 ☑
        car (traffic) V33.6 ☑
          nontraffic V33.1 ☑
        motor vehicle NOS (traffic) V39.50 ☑
          nontraffic V39.10 ☑
          specified type NEC (traffic) V39.59 ☑
            nontraffic V39.19 ☑
        pedal cycle (traffic) V31.6 ☑
          nontraffic V31.1 ☑
        pickup truck (traffic) V33.6 ☑
          nontraffic V33.1 ☑
        railway vehicle (traffic) V35.6 ☑
          nontraffic V35.1 ☑
        specified vehicle NEC (traffic) V36.6 ☑
          nontraffic V36.1 ☑
        stationary object (traffic) V37.6 ☑
          nontraffic V37.1 ☑
        streetcar (traffic) V36.6 ☑
          nontraffic V36.1 ☑
        three wheeled motor vehicle
          (traffic) V32.6 ☑
          nontraffic V32.1 ☑
        truck (traffic) V34.6 ☑
          nontraffic V34.1 ☑
        two wheeled motor vehicle
          (traffic) V32.6 ☑
          nontraffic V32.1 ☑
        van (traffic) V33.6 ☑
          nontraffic V33.1 ☑

Accident — *continued*
  transport — *continued*
      noncollision accident (traffic) V38.6 ☑
        nontraffic V38.1 ☑
    specified type NEC V39.89 ☑
      military vehicle V39.81 ☑
    tractor (farm) (and trailer) — *see* Accident,
      transport, agricultural vehicle occupant
    tram — *see* Accident, transport, streetcar
      in mine or quarry — *see* Accident, transport,
        industrial vehicle occupant
    trolley — *see* Accident, transport, streetcar
      in mine or quarry — *see* Accident, transport,
        industrial vehicle occupant
    truck (heavy) occupant V69.9 ☑
      collision (with)
        animal (traffic) V60.9 ☑
          being ridden (traffic) V66.9 ☑
            nontraffic V66.3 ☑
            while boarding or alighting V66.4 ☑
          nontraffic V60.3 ☑
          while boarding or alighting V60.4 ☑
        animal-drawn vehicle (traffic) V66.9 ☑
          nontraffic V66.3 ☑
          while boarding or alighting V66.4 ☑
        bus (traffic) V64.9 ☑
          nontraffic V64.3 ☑
          while boarding or alighting V64.4 ☑
        car (traffic) V63.9 ☑
          nontraffic V63.3 ☑
          while boarding or alighting V63.4 ☑
        motor vehicle NOS (traffic) V69.60 ☑
          nontraffic V69.20 ☑
          specified type NEC (traffic) V69.69 ☑
            nontraffic V69.29 ☑
        pedal cycle (traffic) V61.9 ☑
          nontraffic V61.3 ☑
          while boarding or alighting V61.4 ☑
        pickup truck (traffic) V63.9 ☑
          nontraffic V63.3 ☑
          while boarding or alighting V63.4 ☑
        railway vehicle (traffic) V65.9 ☑
          nontraffic V65.3 ☑
          while boarding or alighting V65.4 ☑
        specified vehicle NEC (traffic) V66.9 ☑
          nontraffic V66.3 ☑
          while boarding or alighting V66.4 ☑
        stationary object (traffic) V67.9 ☑
          nontraffic V67.3 ☑
          while boarding or alighting V67.4 ☑
        streetcar (traffic) V66.9 ☑
          nontraffic V66.3 ☑
          while boarding or alighting V66.4 ☑
        three wheeled motor vehicle
          (traffic) V62.9 ☑
          nontraffic V62.3 ☑
          while boarding or alighting V62.4 ☑
        truck (traffic) V64.9 ☑
          nontraffic V64.3 ☑
          while boarding or alighting V64.4 ☑
        two wheeled motor vehicle
          (traffic) V62.9 ☑
          nontraffic V62.3 ☑
          while boarding or alighting V62.4 ☑
        van (traffic) V63.9 ☑
          nontraffic V63.3 ☑
          while boarding or alighting V63.4 ☑
      driver
        collision (with)
          animal (traffic) V60.5 ☑
            being ridden (traffic) V66.5 ☑
              nontraffic V66.0 ☑
            nontraffic V60.0 ☑
          animal-drawn vehicle (traffic) V66.5 ☑
            nontraffic V66.0 ☑
          bus (traffic) V64.5 ☑
            nontraffic V64.0 ☑
          car (traffic) V63.5 ☑
            nontraffic V63.0 ☑
          motor vehicle NOS (traffic) V69.40 ☑
            nontraffic V69.00 ☑
            specified type NEC (traffic) V69.49 ☑
              nontraffic V69.09 ☑
          pedal cycle (traffic) V61.5 ☑
            nontraffic V61.0 ☑
          pickup truck (traffic) V63.5 ☑
            nontraffic V63.0 ☑
          railway vehicle (traffic) V65.5 ☑
            nontraffic V65.0 ☑
          specified vehicle NEC (traffic) V66.5 ☑
            nontraffic V66.0 ☑
          stationary object (traffic) V67.5 ☑

Accident

Accident — *continued*
  transport — *continued*
      nontraffic V67.0 ☑
      streetcar (traffic) V66.5 ☑
        nontraffic V66.0 ☑
      three wheeled motor vehicle
        (traffic) V62.5 ☑
        nontraffic V62.0 ☑
      truck (traffic) V64.5 ☑
        nontraffic V64.0 ☑
      two wheeled motor vehicle
        (traffic) V62.5 ☑
        nontraffic V62.0 ☑
      van (traffic) V63.5 ☑
        nontraffic V63.0 ☑
     noncollision accident (traffic) V68.5 ☑
      nontraffic V68.0 ☑
    dump — *see* Accident, transport,
      construction vehicle occupant
    hanger-on
     collision (with)
      animal (traffic) V60.7 ☑
       being ridden (traffic) V66.7 ☑
        nontraffic V66.2 ☑
       nontraffic V60.2 ☑
      animal-drawn vehicle (traffic) V66.7 ☑
       nontraffic V66.2 ☑
      bus (traffic) V64.7 ☑
       nontraffic V64.2 ☑
      car (traffic) V63.7 ☑
       nontraffic V63.2 ☑
      pedal cycle (traffic) V61.7 ☑
       nontraffic V61.2 ☑
      pickup truck (traffic) V63.7 ☑
       nontraffic V63.2 ☑
      railway vehicle (traffic) V65.7 ☑
       nontraffic V65.2 ☑
      specified vehicle NEC (traffic) V66.7 ☑
       nontraffic V66.2 ☑
      stationary object (traffic) V67.7 ☑
       nontraffic V67.2 ☑
      streetcar (traffic) V66.7 ☑
       nontraffic V66.2 ☑
      three wheeled motor vehicle
       (traffic) V62.7 ☑
       nontraffic V62.2 ☑
      truck (traffic) V64.7 ☑
       nontraffic V64.2 ☑
      two wheeled motor vehicle
       (traffic) V62.7 ☑
       nontraffic V62.2 ☑
      van (traffic) V63.7 ☑
       nontraffic V63.2 ☑
     noncollision accident (traffic) V68.7 ☑
      nontraffic V68.2 ☑
    noncollision accident (traffic) V68.9 ☑
     nontraffic V68.3 ☑
     while boarding or alighting V68.4 ☑
    nontraffic V69.3 ☑
    passenger
     collision (with)
      animal (traffic) V60.6 ☑
       being ridden (traffic) V66.6 ☑
        nontraffic V66.1 ☑
       nontraffic V60.1 ☑
      animal-drawn vehicle (traffic) V66.6 ☑
       nontraffic V66.1 ☑
      bus (traffic) V64.6 ☑
       nontraffic V64.1 ☑
      car (traffic) V63.6 ☑
       nontraffic V63.1 ☑
      motor vehicle NOS (traffic) V69.50 ☑
       nontraffic V69.10 ☑
       specified type NEC (traffic) V69.59 ☑
        nontraffic V69.19 ☑
      pedal cycle (traffic) V61.6 ☑
       nontraffic V61.1 ☑
      pickup truck (traffic) V63.6 ☑
       nontraffic V63.1 ☑
      railway vehicle (traffic) V65.6 ☑
       nontraffic V65.1 ☑
      specified vehicle NEC (traffic) V66.6 ☑
       nontraffic V66.1 ☑
      stationary object (traffic) V67.6 ☑
       nontraffic V67.1 ☑
      streetcar (traffic) V66.6 ☑
       nontraffic V66.1 ☑
      three wheeled motor vehicle
       (traffic) V62.6 ☑
       nontraffic V62.1 ☑
      truck (traffic) V64.6 ☑
       nontraffic V64.1 ☑

Accident — *continued*
  transport — *continued*
      two wheeled motor vehicle
       (traffic) V62.6 ☑
       nontraffic V62.1 ☑
      van (traffic) V63.6 ☑
       nontraffic V63.1 ☑
     noncollision accident (traffic) V68.6 ☑
      nontraffic V68.1 ☑
    pickup — *see* Accident, transport, pickup
     truck occupant
    specified type NEC V69.88 ☑
     military vehicle V69.81 ☑
   van occupant V59.9 ☑
    collision (with)
     animal (traffic) V50.9 ☑
      being ridden (traffic) V56.9 ☑
       nontraffic V56.3 ☑
       while boarding or alighting V56.4 ☑
      nontraffic V50.3 ☑
      while boarding or alighting V50.4 ☑
     animal-drawn vehicle (traffic) V56.9 ☑
      nontraffic V56.3 ☑
      while boarding or alighting V56.4 ☑
     bus (traffic) V54.9 ☑
      nontraffic V54.3 ☑
      while boarding or alighting V54.4 ☑
     car (traffic) V53.9 ☑
      nontraffic V53.3 ☑
      while boarding or alighting V53.4 ☑
     motor vehicle NOS (traffic) V59.60 ☑
      nontraffic V59.20 ☑
      specified type NEC (traffic) V59.69 ☑
       nontraffic V59.29 ☑
     pedal cycle (traffic) V51.9 ☑
      nontraffic V51.3 ☑
      while boarding or alighting V51.4 ☑
     pickup truck (traffic) V53.9 ☑
      nontraffic V53.3 ☑
      while boarding or alighting V53.4 ☑
     railway vehicle (traffic) V55.9 ☑
      nontraffic V55.3 ☑
      while boarding or alighting V55.4 ☑
     specified vehicle NEC (traffic) V56.9 ☑
      nontraffic V56.3 ☑
      while boarding or alighting V56.4 ☑
     stationary object (traffic) V57.9 ☑
      nontraffic V57.3 ☑
      while boarding or alighting V57.4 ☑
     streetcar (traffic) V56.9 ☑
      nontraffic V56.3 ☑
      while boarding or alighting V56.4 ☑
     three wheeled motor vehicle
      (traffic) V52.9 ☑
      nontraffic V52.3 ☑
      while boarding or alighting V52.4 ☑
     truck (traffic) V54.9 ☑
      nontraffic V54.3 ☑
      while boarding or alighting V54.4 ☑
     two wheeled motor vehicle
      (traffic) V52.9 ☑
      nontraffic V52.3 ☑
      while boarding or alighting V52.4 ☑
     van (traffic) V53.9 ☑
      nontraffic V53.3 ☑
      while boarding or alighting V53.4 ☑
    driver
     collision (with)
      animal (traffic) V50.5 ☑
       being ridden (traffic) V56.5 ☑
        nontraffic V56.0 ☑
       nontraffic V50.0 ☑
      animal-drawn vehicle (traffic) V56.5 ☑
       nontraffic V56.0 ☑
      bus (traffic) V54.5 ☑
       nontraffic V54.0 ☑
      car (traffic) V53.5 ☑
       nontraffic V53.0 ☑
      motor vehicle NOS (traffic) V59.40 ☑
       nontraffic V59.00 ☑
       specified type NEC (traffic) V59.49 ☑
        nontraffic V59.09 ☑
      pedal cycle (traffic) V51.5 ☑
       nontraffic V51.0 ☑
      pickup truck (traffic) V53.5 ☑
       nontraffic V53.0 ☑
      railway vehicle (traffic) V55.5 ☑
       nontraffic V55.0 ☑
      specified vehicle NEC (traffic) V56.5 ☑
       nontraffic V56.0 ☑
      stationary object (traffic) V57.5 ☑
       nontraffic V57.0 ☑

Accident — *continued*
  transport — *continued*
      streetcar (traffic) V56.5 ☑
       nontraffic V56.0 ☑
     three wheeled motor vehicle
      (traffic) V52.5 ☑
      nontraffic V52.0 ☑
     truck (traffic) V54.5 ☑
      nontraffic V54.0 ☑
     two wheeled motor vehicle
      (traffic) V52.5 ☑
      nontraffic V52.0 ☑
     van (traffic) V53.5 ☑
      nontraffic V53.0 ☑
     noncollision accident (traffic) V58.5 ☑
      nontraffic V58.0 ☑
    noncollision accident (traffic) V58.9 ☑
     nontraffic V58.3 ☑
     while boarding or alighting V58.4 ☑
    nontraffic V59.3 ☑
    hanger-on
     collision (with)
      animal (traffic) V50.7 ☑
       being ridden (traffic) V56.7 ☑
        nontraffic V56.2 ☑
       nontraffic V50.2 ☑
      animal-drawn vehicle (traffic) V56.7 ☑
       nontraffic V56.2 ☑
      bus (traffic) V54.7 ☑
       nontraffic V54.2 ☑
      car (traffic) V53.7 ☑
       nontraffic V53.2 ☑
      pedal cycle (traffic) V51.7 ☑
       nontraffic V51.2 ☑
      pickup truck (traffic) V53.7 ☑
       nontraffic V53.2 ☑
      railway vehicle (traffic) V55.7 ☑
       nontraffic V55.2 ☑
      specified vehicle NEC (traffic) V56.7 ☑
       nontraffic V56.2 ☑
      stationary object (traffic) V57.7 ☑
       nontraffic V57.2 ☑
      streetcar (traffic) V56.7 ☑
       nontraffic V56.2 ☑
      three wheeled motor vehicle
       (traffic) V52.7 ☑
       nontraffic V52.2 ☑
      truck (traffic) V54.7 ☑
       nontraffic V54.2 ☑
      two wheeled motor vehicle
       (traffic) V52.7 ☑
       nontraffic V52.2 ☑
      van (traffic) V53.7 ☑
       nontraffic V53.2 ☑
     noncollision accident (traffic) V58.7 ☑
      nontraffic V58.2 ☑
    passenger
     collision (with)
      animal (traffic) V50.6 ☑
       being ridden (traffic) V56.6 ☑
        nontraffic V56.1 ☑
       nontraffic V50.1 ☑
      animal-drawn vehicle (traffic) V56.6 ☑
       nontraffic V56.1 ☑
      bus (traffic) V54.6 ☑
       nontraffic V54.1 ☑
      car (traffic) V53.6 ☑
       nontraffic V53.1 ☑
      motor vehicle NOS (traffic) V59.50 ☑
       nontraffic V59.10 ☑
       specified type NEC (traffic) V59.59 ☑
        nontraffic V59.19 ☑
      pedal cycle (traffic) V51.6 ☑
       nontraffic V51.1 ☑
      pickup truck (traffic) V53.6 ☑
       nontraffic V53.1 ☑
      railway vehicle (traffic) V55.6 ☑
       nontraffic V55.1 ☑
      specified vehicle NEC (traffic) V56.6 ☑
       nontraffic V56.1 ☑
      stationary object (traffic) V57.6 ☑
       nontraffic V57.1 ☑
      streetcar (traffic) V56.6 ☑
       nontraffic V56.1 ☑
      three wheeled motor vehicle
       (traffic) V52.6 ☑
       nontraffic V52.1 ☑
      truck (traffic) V54.6 ☑
       nontraffic V54.1 ☑
      two wheeled motor vehicle
       (traffic) V52.6 ☑
       nontraffic V52.1 ☑

☑ **Additional character required**

Accident — *continued*
  transport — *continued*
    van (traffic) V53.6 ☑
      nontraffic V53.1 ☑
    noncollision accident (traffic) V58.6 ☑
      nontraffic V58.1 ☑
    specified type NEC V59.88 ☑
      military vehicle V59.81 ☑
    watercraft occupant — *see* Accident, watercraft
  vehicle NEC V89.9 ☑
    animal-drawn NEC — *see* Accident, transport, animal-drawn vehicle occupant
  special
    agricultural — *see* Accident, transport, agricultural vehicle occupant
    construction — *see* Accident, transport, construction vehicle occupant
    industrial — *see* Accident, transport, industrial vehicle occupant
    three-wheeled NEC (motorized) — *see* Accident, transport, three-wheeled motor vehicle occupant
  watercraft V94.9 ☑
    causing
      drowning — *see* Drowning, due to, accident to, watercraft
      injury NEC V91.89 ☑
        crushed between craft and object V91.19 ☑
        powered craft V91.13 ☑
          ferry boat V91.11 ☑
          fishing boat V91.12 ☑
          jet skis V91.13 ☑
          liner V91.11 ☑
          merchant ship V91.10 ☑
          passenger ship V91.11 ☑
        unpowered craft V91.18 ☑
          canoe V91.15 ☑
          inflatable V91.16 ☑
          kayak V91.15 ☑
          sailboat V91.14 ☑
          surf-board V91.18 ☑
          windsurfer V91.18 ☑
      fall on board V91.29 ☑
        powered craft V91.23 ☑
          ferry boat V91.21 ☑
          fishing boat V91.22 ☑
          jet skis V91.23 ☑
          liner V91.21 ☑
          merchant ship V91.20 ☑
          passenger ship V91.21 ☑
        unpowered craft
          canoe V91.25 ☑
          inflatable V91.26 ☑
          kayak V91.25 ☑
          sailboat V91.24 ☑
      fire on board causing burn V91.09 ☑
        powered craft V91.03 ☑
          ferry boat V91.01 ☑
          fishing boat V91.02 ☑
          jet skis V91.03 ☑
          liner V91.01 ☑
          merchant ship V91.00 ☑
          passenger ship V91.01 ☑
        unpowered craft V91.08 ☑
          canoe V91.05 ☑
          inflatable V91.06 ☑
          kayak V91.05 ☑
          sailboat V91.04 ☑
          surf-board V91.08 ☑
          water skis V91.07 ☑
          windsurfer V91.08 ☑
      hit by falling object V91.39 ☑
        powered craft V91.33 ☑
          ferry boat V91.31 ☑
          fishing boat V91.32 ☑
          jet skis V91.33 ☑
          liner V91.31 ☑
          merchant ship V91.30 ☑
          passenger ship V91.31 ☑
        unpowered craft V91.38 ☑
          canoe V91.35 ☑
          inflatable V91.36 ☑
          kayak V91.35 ☑
          sailboat V91.34 ☑
          surf-board V91.38 ☑
          water skis V91.37 ☑
          windsurfer V91.38 ☑
      specified type NEC V91.89 ☑
        powered craft V91.83 ☑
          ferry boat V91.81 ☑
          fishing boat V91.82 ☑

Accident — *continued*
  watercraft — *continued*
          jet skis V91.83 ☑
          liner V91.81 ☑
          merchant ship V91.80 ☑
          passenger ship V91.81 ☑
        unpowered craft V91.88 ☑
          canoe V91.85 ☑
          inflatable V91.86 ☑
          kayak V91.85 ☑
          sailboat V91.84 ☑
          surf-board V91.88 ☑
          water skis V91.87 ☑
          windsurfer V91.88 ☑
    due to, caused by cataclysm — *see* Forces of nature, by type
    military NEC V94.818 ☑
      with civilian watercraft V94.810 ☑
      civilian in water injured by V94.811 ☑
    nonpowered, struck by
      nonpowered vessel V94.22 ☑
      powered vessel V94.21 ☑
    specified type NEC V94.89 ☑
    striking swimmer
      powered V94.11 ☑
      unpowered V94.12 ☑
Acid throwing (assault) Y08.89 ☑
Activity (involving) (of victim at time of event) Y93.9
  aerobic and step exercise (class) Y93.A3
  alpine skiing Y93.23
  animal care NEC Y93.K9
  arts and handcrafts NEC Y93.D9
  athletics NEC Y93.79
  athletics played as a team or group NEC Y93.69
  athletics played individually NEC Y93.59
  baking Y93.G3
  ballet Y93.41
  barbells Y93.B3
  BASE (Building, Antenna, Span, Earth) jumping Y93.33
  baseball Y93.64
  basketball Y93.67
  bathing (personal) Y93.E1
  beach volleyball Y93.68
  bike riding Y93.55
  blackout game Y93.85
  boogie boarding Y93.18
  bowling Y93.54
  boxing Y93.71
  brass instrument playing Y93.J4
  building construction Y93.H3
  bungee jumping Y93.34
  calisthenics Y93.A2
  canoeing (in calm and turbulent water) Y93.16
  capture the flag Y93.6A
  cardiorespiratory exercise NEC Y93.A9
  caregiving (providing) NEC Y93.F9
    bathing Y93.F1
    lifting Y93.F2
  cellular
    communication device Y93.C2
    telephone Y93.C2
  challenge course Y93.A5
  cheerleading Y93.45
  choking game Y93.85
  circuit training Y93.A4
  cleaning
    floor Y93.E5
  climbing NEC Y93.39
    mountain Y93.31
    rock Y93.31
    wall Y93.31
  clothing care and maintenance NEC Y93.E9
  combatives Y93.75
  computer
    keyboarding Y93.C1
    technology NEC Y93.C9
  confidence course Y93.A5
  construction (building) Y93.H3
  cooking and baking Y93.G3
  cool down exercises Y93.A2
  cricket Y93.69
  crocheting Y93.D1
  cross country skiing Y93.24
  dancing (all types) Y93.41
  digging
    dirt Y93.H1
  dirt digging Y93.H1
  dishwashing Y93.G1
  diving (platform) (springboard) Y93.12
    underwater Y93.15
  dodge ball Y93.6A

Activity — *continued*
  downhill skiing Y93.23
  drum playing Y93.J2
  dumbbells Y93.B3
  electronic
    devices NEC Y93.C9
      hand held interactive Y93.C2
    game playing (using) (with)
      interactive device Y93.C2
      keyboard or other stationary device Y93.C1
  elliptical machine Y93.A1
  exercise (s)
    machines ((primarily) for)
      cardiorespiratory conditioning Y93.A1
      muscle strengthening Y93.B1
    muscle strengthening (non-machine) NEC Y93.B9
  external motion NEC Y93.I9
    rollercoaster Y93.I1
  fainting game Y93.85
  field hockey Y93.65
  figure skating (pairs) (singles) Y93.21
  flag football Y93.62
  floor mopping and cleaning Y93.E5
  food preparation and clean up Y93.G1
  football (American) NOS Y93.61
    flag Y93.62
    tackle Y93.61
    touch Y93.62
  four square Y93.6A
  free weights Y93.B3
  frisbee (ultimate) Y93.74
  furniture
    building Y93.D3
    finishing Y93.D3
    repair Y93.D3
  game playing (electronic)
    using keyboard or other stationary device Y93.C1
    using interactive device Y93.C2
  gardening Y93.H2
  golf Y93.53
  grass drills Y93.A6
  grilling and smoking food Y93.G2
  grooming and shearing an animal Y93.K3
  guerilla drills Y93.A6
  gymnastics (rhythmic) Y93.43
  handball Y93.73
  handcrafts NEC Y93.D9
  hand held interactive electronic device Y93.C2
  hang gliding Y93.35
  hiking (on level or elevated terrain) Y93.01
  hockey (ice) Y93.22
    field Y93.65
  horseback riding Y93.52
  household (interior) maintenance NEC Y93.E9
  ice NEC Y93.29
    dancing Y93.21
    hockey Y93.22
    skating Y93.21
  inline roller skating Y93.51
  ironing Y93.E4
  judo Y93.75
  jumping (off) NEC Y93.39
    BASE (Building, Antenna, Span, Earth) Y93.33
    bungee Y93.34
    jacks Y93.A2
    rope Y93.56
  jumping jacks Y93.A2
  jumping rope Y93.56
  karate Y93.75
  kayaking (in calm and turbulent water) Y93.16
  keyboarding (computer) Y93.C1
  kickball Y93.6A
  knitting Y93.D1
  lacrosse Y93.65
  land maintenance NEC Y93.H9
  landscaping Y93.H2
  laundry Y93.E2
  machines (exercise)
    primarily for cardiorespiratory conditioning Y93.A1
    primarily for muscle strengthening Y93.B1
  maintenance
    exterior building NEC Y93.H9
    household (interior) NEC Y93.E9
    land Y93.H9
    property Y93.H9
  marching (on level or elevated terrain) Y93.01
  martial arts Y93.75
  microwave oven Y93.G3
  milking an animal Y93.K2

Activity - Assault

Activity — *continued*
- mopping (floor) Y93.E5
- mountain climbing Y93.31
- muscle strengthening
  - exercises (non-machine) NEC Y93.B9
  - machines Y93.B1
- musical keyboard (electronic) playing Y93.J1
- Nordic skiing Y93.24
- obstacle course Y93.A5
- oven (microwave) Y93.G3
- packing up and unpacking in moving to a new residence Y93.E6
- parasailing Y93.19
- pass out game Y93.85
- percussion instrument playing NEC Y93.J2
- personal
  - bathing and showering Y93.E1
  - hygiene NEC Y93.E8
  - showering Y93.E1
- physical games generally associated with school recess, summer camp and children Y93.6A
- physical training NEC Y93.A9
- piano playing Y93.J1
- Pilates Y93.B4
- platform diving Y93.12
- playing musical instrument
  - brass instrument Y93.J4
  - drum Y93.J2
  - musical keyboard (electronic) Y93.J1
  - percussion instrument NEC Y93.J2
  - piano Y93.J1
  - string instrument Y93.J3
  - winds instrument Y93.J4
- property maintenance
  - exterior NEC Y93.H9
  - interior NEC Y93.E9
- pruning (garden and lawn) Y93.H2
- pull-ups Y93.B2
- push-ups Y93.B2
- racquetball Y93.73
- rafting (in calm and turbulent water) Y93.16
- raking (leaves) Y93.H1
- rappelling Y93.32
- refereeing a sports activity Y93.81
- residential relocation Y93.E6
- rhythmic gymnastics Y93.43
- rhythmic movement NEC Y93.49
- riding
  - horseback Y93.52
  - rollercoaster Y93.I1
- rock climbing Y93.31
- rollercoaster riding Y93.I1
- roller skating (inline) Y93.51
- rough housing and horseplay Y93.83
- rowing (in calm and turbulent water) Y93.16
- rugby Y93.63
- running Y93.02
- SCUBA diving Y93.15
- sewing Y93.D2
- shoveling Y93.H1
  - dirt Y93.H1
  - snow Y93.H1
- showering (personal) Y93.E1
- sit-ups Y93.B2
- skateboarding Y93.51
- skating (ice) Y93.21
  - roller Y93.51
- skiing (alpine) (downhill) Y93.23
  - cross country Y93.24
  - nordic Y93.24
  - water Y93.17
- sledding (snow) Y93.23
- sleeping (sleep) Y93.84
- smoking and grilling food Y93.G2
- snorkeling Y93.15
- snow NEC Y93.29
  - boarding Y93.23
  - shoveling Y93.H1
  - sledding Y93.23
  - tubing Y93.23
- soccer Y93.66
- softball Y93.64
- specified NEC Y93.89
- spectator at an event Y93.82
- sports NEC Y93.79
  - sports played as a team or group NEC Y93.69
  - sports played individually NEC Y93.59
- springboard diving Y93.12
- squash Y93.73
- stationary bike Y93.A1
- step (stepping) exercise (class) Y93.A3
- stepper machine Y93.A1

Activity — *continued*
- stove Y93.G3
- string instrument playing Y93.J3
- surfing Y93.18
  - wind Y93.18
- swimming Y93.11
- tackle football Y93.61
- tap dancing Y93.41
- tennis Y93.73
- tobogganing Y93.23
- touch football Y93.62
- track and field events (non-running) Y93.57
  - running Y93.02
- trampoline Y93.44
- treadmill Y93.A1
- trimming shrubs Y93.H2
- tubing (in calm and turbulent water) Y93.16
  - snow Y93.23
- ultimate frisbee Y93.74
- underwater diving Y93.15
- unpacking in moving to a new residence Y93.E6
- use of stove, oven and microwave oven Y93.G3
- vacuuming Y93.E3
- volleyball (beach) (court) Y93.68
- wake boarding Y93.17
- walking an animal Y93.K1
- walking (on level or elevated terrain) Y93.01
  - an animal Y93.K1
- wall climbing Y93.31
- warm up and cool down exercises Y93.A2
- water NEC Y93.19
  - aerobics Y93.14
  - craft NEC Y93.19
  - exercise Y93.14
  - polo Y93.13
  - skiing Y93.17
  - sliding Y93.18
  - survival training and testing Y93.19
- weeding (garden and lawn) Y93.H2
- wind instrument playing Y93.J4
- windsurfing Y93.18
- wrestling Y93.72
- yoga Y93.42

Adverse effect of drugs — *see* Table of Drugs and Chemicals
Aerosinusitis — *see* Air, pressure
After-effect, late — *see* Sequelae
Air
- blast in war operations — *see* War operations, air blast
- pressure
  - change, rapid
    - during
      - ascent W94.29 ☑
        - while (in) (surfacing from)
          - aircraft W94.23 ☑
          - deep water diving W94.21 ☑
          - underground W94.22 ☑
      - descent W94.39 ☑
        - in
          - aircraft W94.31 ☑
          - water W94.32 ☑
  - high, prolonged W94.0 ☑
  - low, prolonged W94.12 ☑
    - due to residence or long visit at high altitude W94.11 ☑
Alpine sickness W94.11 ☑
Altitude sickness W94.11 ☑
Anaphylactic shock, anaphylaxis — *see* Table of Drugs and Chemicals
Andes disease W94.11 ☑
Arachnidism, arachnoidism X58 ☑
Arson (with intent to injure or kill) X97 ☑
Asphyxia, asphyxiation
- by
  - food (bone) (seed) — *see* categories T17 and T18 ☑
  - gas (*see also* Table of Drugs and Chemicals)
    - legal
      - execution — *see* Legal, intervention, gas
      - intervention — *see* Legal, intervention, gas
  - from
    - fire (*see also* Exposure, fire)
      - in war operations — *see* War operations, fire
    - ignition — *see* Ignition
    - vomitus T17.81 ☑
  - in war operations — *see* War operations, restriction of airway
Aspiration
- food (any type) (into respiratory tract) (with asphyxia, obstruction respiratory tract, suffocation) — *see* categories T17 and T18 ☑

Aspiration — *continued*
- foreign body — *see* Foreign body, aspiration
- vomitus (with asphyxia, obstruction respiratory tract, suffocation) T17.81 ☑
Assassination (attempt) — *see* Assault
Assault (homicidal) (by) (in) Y09
- arson X97 ☑
- bite (of human being) Y04.1 ☑
- bodily force Y04.8 ☑
  - bite Y04.1 ☑
  - bumping into Y04.2 ☑
    - sexual — *see* subcategories T74.0, T76.0 ☑
  - unarmed fight Y04.0 ☑
- bomb X96.9 ☑
  - antipersonnel X96.0 ☑
  - fertilizer X96.3 ☑
  - gasoline X96.1 ☑
  - letter X96.2 ☑
  - petrol X96.1 ☑
  - pipe X96.3 ☑
  - specified NEC X96.8 ☑
- brawl (hand) (fists) (foot) (unarmed) Y04.0 ☑
- burning, burns (by fire) NEC X97 ☑
  - acid Y08.89 ☑
  - caustic, corrosive substance Y08.89 ☑
  - chemical from swallowing caustic, corrosive substance — *see* Table of Drugs and Chemicals
  - cigarette (s) X97 ☑
  - hot object X98.9 ☑
    - fluid NEC X98.2 ☑
    - household appliance X98.3 ☑
    - specified NEC X98.8 ☑
    - steam X98.0 ☑
    - tap water X98.1 ☑
    - vapors X98.0 ☑
  - scalding — *see* Assault, burning
  - steam X98.0 ☑
  - vitriol Y08.89 ☑
- caustic, corrosive substance (gas) Y08.89 ☑
- crashing of
  - aircraft Y08.81 ☑
  - motor vehicle Y03.8 ☑
    - pushed in front of Y02.0 ☑
    - run over Y03.0 ☑
    - specified NEC Y03.8 ☑
- cutting or piercing instrument X99.9 ☑
  - dagger X99.2 ☑
  - glass X99.0 ☑
  - knife X99.1 ☑
  - specified NEC X99.8 ☑
  - sword X99.2 ☑
- dagger X99.2 ☑
- drowning (in) X92.9 ☑
  - bathtub X92.0 ☑
  - natural water X92.3 ☑
  - specified NEC X92.8 ☑
  - swimming pool X92.1 ☑
    - following fall X92.2 ☑
- dynamite X96.8 ☑
- explosive (s) (material) X96.9 ☑
- fight (hand) (fists) (foot) (unarmed) Y04.0 ☑
  - with weapon — *see* Assault, by type of weapon
- fire X97 ☑
- firearm X95.9 ☑
  - airgun X95.01 ☑
  - handgun X93 ☑
  - hunting rifle X94.1 ☑
  - larger X94.9 ☑
    - specified NEC X94.8 ☑
  - machine gun X94.2 ☑
  - shotgun X94.0 ☑
  - specified NEC X95.8 ☑
- gunshot (wound) NEC — *see* Assault, firearm, by type
- incendiary device X97 ☑
- injury Y09
  - to child due to criminal abortion attempt NEC Y08.89 ☑
- knife X99.1 ☑
- late effect of — *see* X92-Y08 with 7th character S
- placing before moving object NEC Y02.8 ☑
  - motor vehicle Y02.0 ☑
- poisoning — *see* categories T36-T65 with 7th character S
- puncture, any part of body — *see* Assault, cutting or piercing instrument
- pushing
  - before moving object NEC Y02.8 ☑
    - motor vehicle Y02.0 ☑
    - subway train Y02.1 ☑
    - train Y02.1 ☑

☑ **Additional character required**

Assault — *continued*
  from high place Y01 ☑
  rape T74.2 ☑
  scalding — *see* Assault, burning
  sequelae of — *see* X92-Y08 with 7th character S
  sexual (by bodily force) T74.2 ☑
  shooting — *see* Assault, firearm
  specified means NEC Y08.89 ☑
  stab, any part of body — *see* Assault, cutting or
      piercing instrument
  steam X98.0 ☑
  striking against
    other person Y04.2 ☑
    sports equipment Y08.09 ☑
      baseball bat Y08.02 ☑
      hockey stick Y08.01 ☑
  struck by
    sports equipment Y08.09 ☑
      baseball bat Y08.02 ☑
      hockey stick Y08.01 ☑
  submersion — *see* Assault, drowning
  violence Y09
  weapon Y09
    blunt Y00 ☑
    cutting or piercing — *see* Assault, cutting or
        piercing instrument
    firearm — *see* Assault, firearm
  wound Y09
    cutting — *see* Assault, cutting or piercing
        instrument
    gunshot — *see* Assault, firearm
    knife X99.1 ☑
    piercing — *see* Assault, cutting or piercing
        instrument
    puncture — *see* Assault, cutting or piercing
        instrument
    stab — *see* Assault, cutting or piercing
        instrument
Attack by mammals NEC W55.89 ☑
Avalanche — *see* Landslide
Aviator's disease — *see* Air, pressure

B

Barotitis, barodontalgia, barosinusitis, barotrauma
    (otitic) (sinus) — *see* Air, pressure
Battered (baby) (child) (person) (syndrome) X58 ☑
Bayonet wound W26.1 ☑
  in
    legal intervention — *see* Legal, intervention,
        sharp object, bayonet
    war operations — *see* War operations, combat
    stated as undetermined whether accidental or
        intentional Y28.8 ☑
    suicide (attempt) X78.2 ☑
Bean in nose — *see* categories T17 and T18 ☑
Bed set on fire NEC — *see* Exposure, fire,
    uncontrolled, building, bed
Beheading (by guillotine)
  homicide X99.9 ☑
  legal execution — *see* Legal, intervention
Bending, injury in (prolonged) (static) X50.1 ☑
Bends — *see* Air, pressure, change
Bite, bitten by
  alligator W58.01 ☑
  arthropod (nonvenomous) NEC W57 ☑
  bull W55.21 ☑
  cat W55.01 ☑
  cow W55.21 ☑
  crocodile W58.11 ☑
  dog W54.0 ☑
  goat W55.31 ☑
  hoof stock NEC W55.31 ☑
  horse W55.11 ☑
  human being (accidentally) W50.3 ☑
    with intent to injure or kill Y04.1 ☑
    as, or caused by, a crowd or human stampede
        (with fall) W52 ☑
    assault Y04.1 ☑
    homicide (attempt) Y04.1 ☑
    in
      fight Y04.1 ☑
  insect (nonvenomous) W57 ☑
  lizard (nonvenomous) W59.01 ☑
  mammal NEC W55.81 ☑
    marine W56.31 ☑
  marine animal (nonvenomous) W56.81 ☑
  millipede W57 ☑
  moray eel W56.51 ☑
  mouse W53.01 ☑

Bite, bitten by — *continued*
  person (s) (accidentally) W50.3 ☑
    with intent to injure or kill Y04.1 ☑
    as, or caused by, a crowd or human stampede
        (with fall) W52 ☑
    assault Y04.1 ☑
    homicide (attempt) Y04.1 ☑
    in
      fight Y04.1 ☑
  pig W55.41 ☑
  raccoon W55.51 ☑
  rat W53.11 ☑
  reptile W59.81 ☑
    lizard W59.01 ☑
    snake W59.11 ☑
    turtle W59.21 ☑
      terrestrial W59.81 ☑
  rodent W53.81 ☑
    mouse W53.01 ☑
    rat W53.11 ☑
    specified NEC W53.81 ☑
    squirrel W53.21 ☑
  shark W56.41 ☑
  sheep W55.31 ☑
  snake (nonvenomous) W59.11 ☑
  spider (nonvenomous) W57 ☑
  squirrel W53.21 ☑
Blast (air) in war operations — *see* War operations,
    blast
Blizzard X37.2 ☑
Blood alcohol level Y90.9
  less than 20mg/100ml Y90.0
  presence in blood, level not specified Y90.9
  20-39mg/100ml Y90.1
  40-59mg/100ml Y90.2
  60-79mg/100ml Y90.3
  80-99mg/100ml Y90.4
  100-119mg/100ml Y90.5
  120-199mg/100ml Y90.6
  200-239mg/100ml Y90.7
Blow X58 ☑
  by law-enforcing agent, police (on duty) — *see*
      Legal, intervention, manhandling
    blunt object — *see* Legal, intervention, blunt
        object
Blowing up — *see* Explosion
Brawl (hand) (fists) (foot) Y04.0 ☑
Breakage (accidental) (part of)
  ladder (causing fall) W11 ☑
  scaffolding (causing fall) W12 ☑
Broken
  glass, contact with — *see* Contact, with, glass
  power line (causing electric shock) W85 ☑
Bumping against, into (accidentally)
  object NEC W22.8 ☑
    with fall — *see* Fall, due to, bumping against,
        object
    caused by crowd or human stampede (with
        fall) W52 ☑
    sports equipment W21.9 ☑
  person (s) W51 ☑
    with fall W03 ☑
      due to ice or snow W00.0 ☑
    assault Y04.2 ☑
    caused by, a crowd or human stampede (with
        fall) W52 ☑
    homicide (attempt) Y04.2 ☑
  sports equipment W21.9 ☑
Burn, burned, burning (accidental) (by) (from) (on)
  acid NEC — *see* Table of Drugs and Chemicals
  bed linen — *see* Exposure, fire, uncontrolled, in
      building, bed
  blowtorch X08.8 ☑
    with ignition of clothing NEC X06.2 ☑
      nightwear X05 ☑
  bonfire, campfire (controlled) (*see also* Exposure,
      fire, controlled, not in building)
    uncontrolled — *see* Exposure, fire,
        uncontrolled, not in building
  candle X08.8 ☑
    with ignition of clothing NEC X06.2 ☑
      nightwear X05 ☑
  caustic liquid, substance (external) (internal) NEC
      — *see* Table of Drugs and Chemicals
  chemical (external) (internal) (*see also* Table of
      Drugs and Chemicals)
    in war operations — *see* War operations. fire
  cigar (s) or cigarette (s) X08.8 ☑
    with ignition of clothing NEC X06.2 ☑
      nightwear X05 ☑
  clothes, clothing NEC (from controlled
      fire) X06.2 ☑

Burn, burned, burning — *continued*
  clothes, clothing NEC — *continued*
    with conflagration — *see* Exposure, fire,
        uncontrolled, building
      not in building or structure — *see* Exposure,
          fire, uncontrolled, not in building
  cooker (hot) X15.8 ☑
    stated as undetermined whether accidental or
        intentional Y27.3 ☑
    suicide (attempt) X77.3 ☑
  electric blanket X16 ☑
  engine (hot) X17 ☑
  fire, flames — *see* Exposure, fire
  flare, Very pistol — *see* Discharge, firearm NEC
  heat
    from appliance (electrical) (household) X15.8 ☑
      cooker X15.8 ☑
      hotplate X15.2 ☑
      kettle X15.8 ☑
      light bulb X15.8 ☑
      saucepan X15.3 ☑
      skillet X15.3 ☑
      stove X15.0 ☑
    stated as undetermined whether accidental
        or intentional Y27.3 ☑
    suicide (attempt) X77.3 ☑
      toaster X15.1 ☑
  in local application or packing during medical
      or surgical procedure Y63.5
  heating
    appliance, radiator or pipe X16 ☑
  homicide (attempt) — *see* Assault, burning
  hot
    air X14.1 ☑
    cooker X15.8 ☑
    drink X10.0 ☑
    engine X17 ☑
    fat X10.2 ☑
    fluid NEC X12 ☑
    food X10.1 ☑
    gases X14.1 ☑
    heating appliance X16 ☑
    household appliance NEC X15.8 ☑
    kettle X15.8 ☑
    liquid NEC X12 ☑
    machinery X17 ☑
    metal (molten) (liquid) NEC X18 ☑
    object (not producing fire or flames)
        NEC X19 ☑
    oil (cooking) X10.2 ☑
    pipe (s) X16 ☑
    radiator X16 ☑
    saucepan (glass) (metal) X15.3 ☑
    stove (kitchen) X15.0 ☑
    substance NEC X19 ☑
      caustic or corrosive NEC — *see* Table of Drugs
          and Chemicals
    toaster X15.1 ☑
    tool X17 ☑
    vapor X13.1 ☑
    water (tap) — *see* Contact, with, hot, tap water
  hotplate X15.2 ☑
    suicide (attempt) X77.3 ☑
  ignition — *see* Ignition
  in war operations — *see* War operations, fire
  inflicted by other person X97 ☑
    by hot objects, hot vapor, and steam — *see*
        Assault, burning, hot object
  internal, from swallowed caustic, corrosive
      liquid, substance — *see* Table of Drugs and
      Chemicals
  iron (hot) X15.8 ☑
    stated as undetermined whether accidental or
        intentional Y27.3 ☑
    suicide (attempt) X77.3 ☑
  kettle (hot) X15.8 ☑
    stated as undetermined whether accidental or
        intentional Y27.3 ☑
    suicide (attempt) X77.3 ☑
  lamp (flame) X08.8 ☑
    with ignition of clothing NEC X06.2 ☑
      nightwear X05 ☑
  lighter (cigar) (cigarette) X08.8 ☑
    with ignition of clothing NEC X06.2 ☑
      nightwear X05 ☑
  lightning — *see* subcategory T75.0
    causing fire — *see* Exposure, fire
  liquid (boiling) (hot) NEC X12 ☑
    stated as undetermined whether accidental or
        intentional Y27.2 ☑
    suicide (attempt) X77.2 ☑

Contact

Contact — *continued*
  with — *continued*
        suicide (attempt) X77.2 ☑
      in bathtub X11.0 ☑
      running X11.1 ☑
      stated as undetermined whether
        accidental or intentional Y27.1 ☑
      suicide (attempt) X77.1 ☑
    toaster X15.1 ☑
    tool X17 ☑
    vapors X13.1 ☑
      inhalation X13.0 ☑
    water (tap) X11.8 ☑
      boiling X12 ☑
        stated as undetermined whether
          accidental or intentional Y27.2 ☑
        suicide (attempt) X77.2 ☑
      heated on stove X12 ☑
        stated as undetermined whether
          accidental or intentional Y27.2 ☑
        suicide (attempt) X77.2 ☑
      in bathtub X11.0 ☑
      running X11.1 ☑
      stated as undetermined whether
        accidental or intentional Y27.1 ☑
      suicide (attempt) X77.1 ☑
    hotplate X15.2 ☑
    ice-pick W27.4 ☑
    insect (nonvenomous) NEC W57 ☑
    kettle (hot) X15.8 ☑
    knife W26.0 ☑
      assault X99.1 ☑
      electric W29.1 ☑
      stated as undetermined whether accidental
        or intentional Y28.1 ☑
      suicide (attempt) X78.1 ☑
    lathe (metalworking) W31.1 ☑
      turnings W45.8 ☑
      woodworking W31.2 ☑
    lawnmower (powered) (ridden) W28 ☑
      causing electrocution W86.8 ☑
        suicide (attempt) X83.1 ☑
      unpowered W27.1 ☑
    lift, lifting (devices) W24.0 ☑
      agricultural operations W30.89 ☑
      shaft W24.0 ☑
    liquefied gas — *see* Exposure, cold, man-made
    liquid air, hydrogen, nitrogen — *see* Exposure,
      cold, man-made
    lizard (nonvenomous) W59.09 ☑
      bite W59.01 ☑
      strike W59.02 ☑
    llama — *see* Contact, with, hoof stock NEC
    macaw W61.19 ☑
      bite W61.11 ☑
      strike W61.12 ☑
    machine, machinery W31.9 ☑
      abrasive wheel W31.1 ☑
      agricultural including animal-
        powered W30.9 ☑
        combine harvester W30.0 ☑
        grain storage elevator W30.3 ☑
        hay derrick W30.2 ☑
        power take-off device W30.1 ☑
        reaper W30.0 ☑
        specified NEC W30.89 ☑
        thresher W30.0 ☑
        transport vehicle, stationary W30.81 ☑
      band saw W31.2 ☑
      bench saw W31.2 ☑
      circular saw W31.2 ☑
      commercial NEC W31.82 ☑
      drilling, metal (industrial) W31.1 ☑
      earth-drilling W31.0 ☑
      earthmoving or scraping W31.89 ☑
      excavating W31.89 ☑
      forging machine W31.1 ☑
      gas turbine W31.3 ☑
      hot X17 ☑
      internal combustion engine W31.3 ☑
      land drill W31.0 ☑
      lathe W31.1 ☑
      lifting (devices) W24.0 ☑
      metal drill W31.1 ☑
      metalworking (industrial) W31.1 ☑
      milling, metal W31.1 ☑
      mining W31.0 ☑
      molding W31.2 ☑
      overhead plane W31.2 ☑
      power press, metal W31.1 ☑
      prime mover W31.3 ☑
      printing W31.89 ☑

Contact — *continued*
  with — *continued*
      radial saw W31.2 ☑
      recreational W31.81 ☑
      roller-coaster W31.81 ☑
      rolling mill, metal W31.1 ☑
      sander W31.2 ☑
      seabed drill W31.0 ☑
      shaft
        hoist W31.0 ☑
        lift W31.0 ☑
      specified NEC W31.89 ☑
      spinning W31.89 ☑
      steam engine W31.3 ☑
      transmission W24.1 ☑
      undercutter W31.0 ☑
      water driven turbine W31.3 ☑
      weaving W31.89 ☑
      woodworking or forming
        (industrial) W31.2 ☑
    mammal (feces) (urine) W55.89 ☑
      bull — *see* Contact, with, bull
      cat — *see* Contact, with, cat
      cow — *see* Contact, with, cow
      goat — *see* Contact, with, goat
      hoof stock — *see* Contact, with, hoof stock
      horse — *see* Contact, with, horse
      marine W56.39 ☑
        dolphin — *see* Contact, with, dolphin
        orca — *see* Contact, with, orca
        sea lion — *see* Contact, with, sea lion
        specified NEC W56.39 ☑
          bite W56.31 ☑
          strike W56.32 ☑
      pig — *see* Contact, with, pig
      raccoon — *see* Contact, with, raccoon
      rodent — *see* Contact, with, rodent
      sheep — *see* Contact, with, sheep
      specified NEC W55.89 ☑
        bite W55.81 ☑
        strike W55.82 ☑
    marine
      animal W56.89 ☑
        bite W56.81 ☑
        dolphin — *see* Contact, with, dolphin
        fish NEC — *see* Contact, with, fish
        mammal — *see* Contact, with, mammal,
          marine
        orca — *see* Contact, with, orca
        sea lion — *see* Contact, with, sea lion
        shark — *see* Contact, with, shark
        strike W56.82 ☑
    meat
      grinder (domestic) W29.0 ☑
        industrial W31.82 ☑
        nonpowered W27.4 ☑
      slicer (domestic) W29.0 ☑
        industrial W31.82 ☑
    merry go round W31.81 ☑
    metal, hot (liquid) (molten) NEC X18 ☑
    millipede W57 ☑
    nail W45.0 ☑
      gun W29.4 ☑
    needle (sewing) W27.3 ☑
      hypodermic W46.0 ☑
        contaminated W46.1 ☑
    object (blunt) NEC
      hot NEC X19 ☑
      legal intervention — *see* Legal, intervention,
        blunt object
      sharp NEC W45.8 ☑
        inflicted by other person NEC W45.8 ☑
          stated as
            intentional homicide (attempt) —
              see Assault, cutting or piercing
              instrument
            legal intervention — *see* Legal,
              intervention, sharp object
            self-inflicted X78.9 ☑
    orca W56.29 ☑
      bite W56.21 ☑
      strike W56.22 ☑
    overhead plane W31.2 ☑
    paper (as sharp object) W26.2 ☑
    paper-cutter W27.5 ☑
    parrot W61.09 ☑
      bite W61.01 ☑
      strike W61.02 ☑
    pig W55.49 ☑
      bite W55.41 ☑
      strike W55.42 ☑
    pipe, hot X16 ☑

Contact — *continued*
  with — *continued*
    pitchfork W27.1 ☑
    plane (metal) (wood) W27.0 ☑
      overhead W31.2 ☑
    plant thorns, spines, sharp leaves or other
      mechanisms W60 ☑
    powered
      garden cultivator W29.3 ☑
      household appliance, implement, or
        machine W29.8 ☑
      saw (industrial) W31.2 ☑
        hand W29.8 ☑
    printing machine W31.89 ☑
    psittacine bird W61.29 ☑
      bite W61.21 ☑
      macaw — *see* Contact, with, macaw
      parrot — *see* Contact, with, parrot
      strike W61.22 ☑
    pulley (block) (transmission) W24.0 ☑
      agricultural operations W30.89 ☑
    raccoon W55.59 ☑
      bite W55.51 ☑
      strike W55.52 ☑
    radial-saw (industrial) W31.2 ☑
    radiator (hot) X16 ☑
    rake W27.1 ☑
    rattlesnake X58 ☑
    reaper W30.0 ☑
    reptile W59.89 ☑
      lizard — *see* Contact, with, lizard
      snake — *see* Contact, with, snake
      specified NEC W59.89 ☑
        bite W59.81 ☑
        crushing W59.83 ☑
        strike W59.82 ☑
      turtle — *see* Contact, with, turtle
    rivet gun (powered) W29.4 ☑
    road scraper — *see* Accident, transport,
      construction vehicle
    rodent (feces) (urine) W53.89 ☑
      bite W53.81 ☑
      mouse W53.09 ☑
        bite W53.01 ☑
      rat W53.19 ☑
        bite W53.11 ☑
      specified NEC W53.89 ☑
        bite W53.81 ☑
      squirrel W53.29 ☑
        bite W53.21 ☑
    roller coaster W31.81 ☑
    rope NEC W24.0 ☑
      agricultural operations W30.89 ☑
    saliva — *see* Contact, with, by type of animal
    sander W29.8 ☑
      industrial W31.2 ☑
    saucepan (hot) (glass) (metal) X15.3 ☑
    saw W27.0 ☑
      band (industrial) W31.2 ☑
      bench (industrial) W31.2 ☑
      chain W29.3 ☑
      hand W27.0 ☑
    sawing machine, metal W31.1 ☑
    scissors W27.2 ☑
    scorpion X58 ☑
    screwdriver W27.0 ☑
      powered W29.8 ☑
    sea
      anemone, cucumber or urchin (spine) X58 ☑
      lion W56.19 ☑
        bite W56.11 ☑
        strike W56.12 ☑
    serpent — *see* Contact, with, snake, by type
    sewing-machine (electric) (powered) W29.2 ☑
      not powered W27.8 ☑
    shaft (hoist) (lift) (transmission) NEC W24.0 ☑
      agricultural W30.89 ☑
    shark W56.49 ☑
      bite W56.41 ☑
      strike W56.42 ☑
    sharp object (s) W26.9 ☑
      specified NEC W26.8 ☑
    shears (hand) W27.2 ☑
      powered (industrial) W31.1 ☑
        domestic W29.2 ☑
    sheep W55.39 ☑
      bite W55.31 ☑
      strike W55.32 ☑
    shovel W27.8 ☑
      steam — *see* Accident, transport,
        construction vehicle
    snake (nonvenomous) W59.19 ☑

☑ **Additional character required**

Contact — ICD-10-CM INDEX TO EXTERNAL CAUSES OF INJURIES

Contact — continued
  with — continued
    bite W59.11 ☑
    crushing W59.13 ☑
    strike W59.12 ☑
  spade W27.1 ☑
  spider (venomous) X58 ☑
  spin-drier W29.2 ☑
  spinning machine W31.89 ☑
  splinter W45.8 ☑
  sports equipment W21.9 ☑
  staple gun (powered) W29.8 ☑
  steam X13.1 ☑
    engine W31.3 ☑
    inhalation X13.0 ☑
    pipe X16 ☑
    shovel W31.89 ☑
  stove (hot) (kitchen) X15.0 ☑
  substance, hot NEC X19 ☑
    molten (metal) X18 ☑
  sword W26.1 ☑
    assault X99.2 ☑
    stated as undetermined whether accidental
      or intentional Y28.2 ☑
    suicide (attempt) X78.2 ☑
  tarantula X58 ☑
  thresher W30.0 ☑
  tin can lid W26.8 ☑
  toad W62.1 ☑
  toaster (hot) X15.1 ☑
  tool W27.8 ☑
    hand (not powered) W27.8 ☑
      auger W27.0 ☑
      axe W27.0 ☑
      can opener W27.4 ☑
      chisel W27.0 ☑
      fork W27.4 ☑
      garden W27.1 ☑
      handsaw W27.0 ☑
      hoe W27.1 ☑
      ice-pick W27.4 ☑
      kitchen utensil W27.4 ☑
      manual
        lawn mower W27.1 ☑
        sewing machine W27.8 ☑
      meat grinder W27.4 ☑
      needle (sewing) W27.3 ☑
        hypodermic W46.0 ☑
          contaminated W46.1 ☑
      paper cutter W27.5 ☑
      pitchfork W27.1 ☑
      rake W27.1 ☑
      scissors W27.2 ☑
      screwdriver W27.0 ☑
      specified NEC W27.8 ☑
      workbench W27.0 ☑
    hot X17 ☑
    powered W29.8 ☑
      blender W29.0 ☑
        commercial W31.82 ☑
      can opener W29.0 ☑
        commercial W31.82 ☑
      chainsaw W29.3 ☑
      clothes dryer W29.2 ☑
        commercial W31.82 ☑
      dishwasher W29.2 ☑
        commercial W31.82 ☑
      edger W29.3 ☑
      electric fan W29.2 ☑
        commercial W31.82 ☑
      electric knife W29.1 ☑
      food processor W29.0 ☑
        commercial W31.82 ☑
      garbage disposal W29.0 ☑
        commercial W31.82 ☑
      garden tool W29.3 ☑
      hedge trimmer W29.3 ☑
      ice maker W29.0 ☑
        commercial W31.82 ☑
      kitchen appliance W29.0 ☑
        commercial W31.82 ☑
      lawn mower W28 ☑
      meat grinder W29.0 ☑
        commercial W31.82 ☑
      mixer W29.0 ☑
        commercial W31.82 ☑
      rototiller® W29.3 ☑
      sewing machine W29.2 ☑
        commercial W31.82 ☑
      washing machine W29.2 ☑
        commercial W31.82 ☑

Contact — continued
  with — continued
    transmission device (belt, cable, chain, gear,
      pinion, shaft) W24.1 ☑
      agricultural operations W30.89 ☑
    turbine (gas) (water-driven) W31.3 ☑
    turkey W61.49 ☑
      peck W61.43 ☑
      strike W61.42 ☑
    turtle (nonvenomous) W59.29 ☑
      bite W59.21 ☑
      strike W59.22 ☑
    terrestrial W59.89 ☑
      bite W59.81 ☑
      crushing W59.83 ☑
      strike W59.82 ☑
    under-cutter W31.0 ☑
    urine — see Contact, with, by type of animal
    vehicle
      agricultural use (transport) — see Accident,
        transport, agricultural vehicle
        not on public highway W30.81 ☑
      industrial use (transport) — see Accident,
        transport, industrial vehicle
        not on public highway W31.83 ☑
      off-road use (transport) — see Accident,
        transport, all-terrain or off-road vehicle
        not on public highway W31.83 ☑
      special construction use (transport) — see
        Accident, transport, construction vehicle
        not on public highway W31.83 ☑
    venomous
      animal X58 ☑
      arthropods X58 ☑
      lizard X58 ☑
      marine animal NEC X58 ☑
      marine plant NEC X58 ☑
      millipedes (tropical) X58 ☑
      plant (s) X58 ☑
      snake X58 ☑
      spider X58 ☑
    viper X58 ☑
    washing-machine (powered) W29.2 ☑
    wasp X58 ☑
    weaving-machine W31.89 ☑
    winch W24.0 ☑
      agricultural operations W30.89 ☑
    wire NEC W24.0 ☑
      agricultural operations W30.89 ☑
    wood slivers W45.8 ☑
    yellow jacket X58 ☑
    zebra — see Contact, with, hoof stock NEC
  pressure X50.9 ☑
  stress X50.9 ☑
Coup de soleil X32 ☑
Crash
  aircraft (in transit) (powered) V95.9 ☑
    balloon V96.01 ☑
    fixed wing NEC (private) V95.21 ☑
      commercial V95.31 ☑
    glider V96.21 ☑
      hang V96.11 ☑
      powered V95.11 ☑
    helicopter V95.01 ☑
    in war operations — see War operations,
      destruction of aircraft
    microlight V95.11 ☑
    nonpowered V96.9 ☑
      specified NEC V96.8 ☑
    powered NEC V95.8 ☑
    stated as
      homicide (attempt) Y08.81 ☑
      suicide (attempt) X83.0 ☑
    ultralight V95.11 ☑
  spacecraft V95.41 ☑
  transport vehicle NEC (see also Accident,
    transport) V89.9 ☑
    homicide (attempt) Y03.8 ☑
    motor NEC (traffic) V89.2 ☑
      homicide (attempt) Y03.8 ☑
      suicide (attempt) — see Suicide, collision
Cruelty (mental) (physical) (sexual) X58 ☑
Crushed (accidentally) X58 ☑
  between objects (moving) (stationary and
    moving) W23.0 ☑
    stationary W23.1 ☑
  by
    alligator W58.03 ☑
    avalanche NEC — see Landslide
    cave-in W20.0 ☑
      caused by cataclysmic earth surface
        movement — see Landslide

Crushed — continued
  by — continued
    crocodile W58.13 ☑
    crowd or human stampede W52 ☑
    falling
      aircraft V97.39 ☑
        in war operations — see War operations,
          destruction of aircraft
      earth, material W20.0 ☑
        caused by cataclysmic earth surface
          movement — see Landslide
      object NEC W20.8 ☑
    landslide NEC — see Landslide
    lizard (nonvenomous) W59.09 ☑
    machinery — see Contact, with, by type of
      machine
    reptile NEC W59.89 ☑
    snake (nonvenomous) W59.13 ☑
  in
    machinery — see Contact, with, by type of
      machine
Cut, cutting (any part of body) (accidental) (see also
  Contact, with, by object or machine)
  during medical or surgical treatment as
    misadventure — see Index to Diseases and
    Injuries, Complications
  homicide (attempt) — see Assault, cutting or
    piercing instrument
  inflicted by other person — see Assault, cutting or
    piercing instrument
  legal
    execution — see Legal, intervention
    intervention — see Legal, intervention, sharp
      object
  machine NEC (see also Contact, with, by type of
    machine) W31.9 ☑
  self-inflicted — see Suicide, cutting or piercing
    instrument
  suicide (attempt) — see Suicide, cutting or
    piercing instrument
Cyclone (any injury) X37.1 ☑

D

Decapitation (accidental circumstances) NEC X58 ☑
  homicide X99.9 ☑
  legal execution — see Legal, intervention
Dehydration from lack of water X58 ☑
Deprivation X58 ☑
Derailment (accidental)
  railway (rolling stock) (train) (vehicle) (without
    antecedent collision) V81.7 ☑
    with antecedent collision — see Accident,
      transport, railway vehicle occupant
  streetcar (without antecedent collision) V82.7 ☑
    with antecedent collision — see Accident,
      transport, streetcar occupant
Descent
  parachute (voluntary) (without accident to
    aircraft) V97.29 ☑
    due to accident to aircraft — see Accident,
      transport, aircraft
Desertion X58 ☑
Destitution X58 ☑
Disability, late effect or sequela of injury — see
  Sequelae
Discharge (accidental)
  airgun W34.010 ☑
    assault X95.01 ☑
    homicide (attempt) X95.01 ☑
    stated as undetermined whether accidental or
      intentional Y24.0 ☑
    suicide (attempt) X74.01 ☑
  BB gun — see Discharge, airgun
  firearm (accidental) W34.00 ☑
    assault X95.9 ☑
    handgun (pistol) (revolver) W32.0 ☑
      assault X93 ☑
      homicide (attempt) X93 ☑
      legal intervention — see Legal, intervention,
        firearm, handgun
      stated as undetermined whether accidental
        or intentional Y22 ☑
      suicide (attempt) X72 ☑
    homicide (attempt) X95.9 ☑
    hunting rifle W33.02 ☑
      assault X94.1 ☑
      homicide (attempt) X94.1 ☑
    legal intervention
      injuring

Explosion - Exposure

Explosion — *continued*
  homicide (attempt) X96.9 ☑
    antipersonnel bomb — *see* Explosion, antipersonnel bomb
    fertilizer bomb — *see* Explosion, fertilizer bomb
    gasoline bomb — *see* Explosion, gasoline bomb
    letter bomb — *see* Explosion, letter bomb
    pipe bomb — *see* Explosion, pipe bomb
    specified NEC X96.8 ☑
  hose, pressurized W37.8 ☑
  hot water heater, tank (in machinery) W35 ☑
    on watercraft — *see* Explosion, in, watercraft
  in, on
    dump W40.8 ☑
    factory W40.8 ☑
    mine (of explosive gases) NEC W40.1 ☑
    watercraft V93.59 ☑
      powered craft V93.53 ☑
        ferry boat V93.51 ☑
        fishing boat V93.52 ☑
        jet skis V93.53 ☑
        liner V93.51 ☑
        merchant ship V93.50 ☑
        passenger ship V93.51 ☑
        sailboat V93.54 ☑
  letter bomb W40.8 ☑
    assault X96.2 ☑
    homicide (attempt) X96.2 ☑
    suicide (attempt) X75 ☑
  machinery (*see also* Contact, with, by type of machine)
    on board watercraft — *see* Explosion, in, watercraft
    pressure vessel — *see* Explosion, by type of vessel
  methane W40.1 ☑
  mine W40.1 ☑
  missile NEC W40.8 ☑
  mortar bomb W40.8 ☑
    in
      assault X96.8 ☑
      homicide (attempt) X96.8 ☑
      legal intervention
        injuring
          bystander Y35.192 ☑
          law enforcement personnel Y35.191 ☑
          suspect Y35.193 ☑
      suicide (attempt) X75 ☑
  munitions (dump) (factory) W40.8 ☑
  pipe, pressurized W37.8 ☑
    bomb W40.8 ☑
      assault X96.4 ☑
      homicide (attempt) X96.4 ☑
      suicide (attempt) X75 ☑
  pressure, pressurized
    cooker W38 ☑
    gas tank (in machinery) W36.3 ☑
    hose W37.8 ☑
    pipe W37.8 ☑
    specified device NEC W38 ☑
    tire W37.8 ☑
      bicycle W37.0 ☑
    vessel (in machinery) W38 ☑
  propane W40.1 ☑
  self-inflicted X75 ☑
  shell (artillery) NEC W40.8 ☑
    during war operations — *see* War operations, explosion
    in
      legal intervention
        injuring
          bystander Y35.122 ☑
          law enforcement personnel Y35.121 ☑
          suspect Y35.123 ☑
    war — *see* War operations, explosion
  spacecraft V95.45 ☑
  steam or water lines (in machinery) W37.8 ☑
  stove W40.9 ☑
  stated as undetermined whether accidental or intentional Y25 ☑
  suicide (attempt) X75 ☑
  tire, pressurized W37.8 ☑
    bicycle W37.0 ☑
  undetermined whether accidental or intentional Y25 ☑
  vehicle tire NEC W37.8 ☑
    bicycle W37.0 ☑
  war operations — *see* War operations, explosion
Exposure (to) X58 ☑
  air pressure change — *see* Air, pressure

Exposure — *continued*
  cold (accidental) (excessive) (extreme) (natural) (place) X31 ☑
    assault Y08.89 ☑
    due to
      man-made conditions W93.8 ☑
        dry ice (contact) W93.01 ☑
          inhalation W93.02 ☑
        liquid air (contact) (hydrogen) (nitrogen) W93.11 ☑
          inhalation W93.12 ☑
        refrigeration unit (deep freeze) W93.2 ☑
      suicide (attempt) X83.2 ☑
      weather (conditions) X31 ☑
    homicide (attempt) Y08.89 ☑
    self-inflicted X83.2 ☑
  due to abandonment or neglect X58 ☑
  electric current W86.8 ☑
    appliance (faulty) W86.8 ☑
      domestic W86.0 ☑
    caused by other person Y08.89 ☑
    conductor (faulty) W86.1 ☑
    control apparatus (faulty) W86.1 ☑
    electric power generating plant, distribution station W86.1 ☑
    electroshock gun — *see* Exposure, electric current, taser
    high-voltage cable W85 ☑
    homicide (attempt) Y08.89 ☑
    legal execution — *see* Legal, intervention, specified means NEC
    lightning — *see* subcategory T75.0
    live rail W86.8 ☑
    misadventure in medical or surgical procedure in electroshock therapy Y63.4
    motor (electric) (faulty) W86.8 ☑
      domestic W86.0 ☑
    self-inflicted X83.1 ☑
    specified NEC W86.8 ☑
      domestic W86.0 ☑
    stun gun — *see* Exposure, electric current, taser
    suicide (attempt) X83.1 ☑
    taser W86.8 ☑
      assault Y08.89 ☑
      legal intervention Y35
      self-harm (intentional) X83.8 ☑
      undetermined intent Y33 ☑
    third rail W86.8 ☑
    transformer (faulty) W86.1 ☑
    transmission lines W85 ☑
  environmental tobacco smoke X58 ☑
  excessive
    cold — *see* Exposure, cold
    heat (natural) NEC X30 ☑
      man-made W92 ☑
  factor (s) NOS X58 ☑
    environmental NEC X58 ☑
    man-made NEC W99 ☑
    natural NEC — *see* Forces of nature
    specified NEC X58 ☑
  fire, flames (accidental) X08.8 ☑
    assault X97 ☑
    campfire — *see* Exposure, fire, controlled, not in building
    controlled (in)
      with ignition (of) clothing (*see also* Ignition, clothes) X06.2 ☑
        nightwear X05 ☑
      bonfire — *see* Exposure, fire, controlled, not in building
      brazier (in building or structure) (*see also* Exposure, fire, controlled, building)
        not in building or structure — *see* Exposure, fire, controlled, not in building
      building or structure X02.0 ☑
        with
          fall from building X02.3 ☑
          injury due to building collapse X02.2 ☑
          from building X02.5 ☑
          smoke inhalation X02.1 ☑
        hit by object from building X02.4 ☑
        specified mode of injury NEC X02.8 ☑
      fireplace, furnace or stove — *see* Exposure, fire, controlled, building
      not in building or structure X03.0 ☑
        with
          fall X03.3 ☑
          smoke inhalation X03.1 ☑
        hit by object X03.4 ☑
        specified mode of injury NEC X03.8 ☑

Exposure — *continued*
  fire, flames — *continued*
    trash — *see* Exposure, fire, controlled, not in building
    fireplace — *see* Exposure, fire, controlled, building
    fittings or furniture (in building or structure) (uncontrolled) — *see* Exposure, fire, uncontrolled, building
    forest (uncontrolled) — *see* Exposure, fire, uncontrolled, not in building
    grass (uncontrolled) — *see* Exposure, fire, uncontrolled, not in building
    hay (uncontrolled) — *see* Exposure, fire, uncontrolled, not in building
    homicide (attempt) X97 ☑
    ignition of highly flammable material X04 ☑
    in, of, on, starting in
      machinery — *see* Contact, with, by type of machine
      motor vehicle (in motion) (*see also* Accident, transport, occupant by type of vehicle) V87.8 ☑
        with collision — *see* Collision
      railway rolling stock, train, vehicle V81.81 ☑
        with collision — *see* Accident, transport, railway vehicle occupant
      street car (in motion) V82.8 ☑
        with collision — *see* Accident, transport, streetcar occupant
      transport vehicle NEC (*see also* Accident, transport)
        with collision — *see* Collision
      war operations (*see also* War operations, fire)
        from nuclear explosion — *see* War operations, nuclear weapons
      watercraft (in transit) (not in transit) V91.09 ☑
        localized — *see* Burn, on board watercraft, due to, fire on board
        powered craft V91.03 ☑
          ferry boat V91.01 ☑
          fishing boat V91.02 ☑
          jet skis V91.03 ☑
          liner V91.01 ☑
          merchant ship V91.00 ☑
          passenger ship V91.01 ☑
        unpowered craft V91.08 ☑
          canoe V91.05 ☑
          inflatable V91.06 ☑
          kayak V91.05 ☑
          sailboat V91.04 ☑
          surf-board V91.08 ☑
          water skis V91.07 ☑
          windsurfer V91.08 ☑
    lumber (uncontrolled) — *see* Exposure, fire, uncontrolled, not in building
    mine (uncontrolled) — *see* Exposure, fire, uncontrolled, not in building
    prairie (uncontrolled) — *see* Exposure, fire, uncontrolled, not in building
    resulting from
      explosion — *see* Explosion
      lightning X08.8 ☑
    self-inflicted X76 ☑
    specified NEC X08.8 ☑
    started by other person X97 ☑
    stove — *see* Exposure, fire, controlled, building
    stated as undetermined whether accidental or intentional Y26 ☑
    suicide (attempt) X76 ☑
    tunnel (uncontrolled) — *see* Exposure, fire, uncontrolled, not in building
    uncontrolled
      in building or structure X00.0 ☑
        with
          fall from building X00.3 ☑
          injury due to building collapse X00.2 ☑
          jump from building X00.5 ☑
          smoke inhalation X00.1 ☑
        bed X08.00 ☑
          due to
            cigarette X08.01 ☑
            specified material NEC X08.09 ☑
        furniture NEC X08.20 ☑
          due to
            cigarette X08.21 ☑
            specified material NEC X08.29 ☑
        hit by object from building X00.4 ☑
        sofa X08.10 ☑
          due to
            cigarette X08.11 ☑
            specified material NEC X08.19 ☑

☑ **Additional character required**

Exposure — *continued*
  fire, flames — *continued*
      specified mode of injury NEC X00.8 ☑
      not in building or structure (any) X01.0 ☑
        with
          fall X01.3 ☑
          smoke inhalation X01.1 ☑
        hit by object X01.4 ☑
        specified mode of injury NEC X01.8 ☑
      undetermined whether accidental or
        intentional Y26 ☑
  forces of nature NEC — *see* Forces of nature
  G-forces (abnormal) W49.9 ☑
  gravitational forces (abnormal) W49.9 ☑
  heat (natural) NEC — *see* Heat
  high-pressure jet (hydraulic)
    (pneumatic) W49.9 ☑
  hydraulic jet W49.9 ☑
  inanimate mechanical force W49.9 ☑
  jet, high-pressure (hydraulic)
    (pneumatic) W49.9 ☑
  lightning — *see* subcategory T75.0
    causing fire — *see* Exposure, fire
  mechanical forces NEC W49.9 ☑
    animate NEC W64 ☑
    inanimate NEC W49.9 ☑
  noise W42.9 ☑
    supersonic W42.0 ☑
  noxious substance — *see* Table of Drugs and
    Chemicals
  pneumatic jet W49.9 ☑
  prolonged in deep-freeze unit or
    refrigerator W93.2 ☑
  radiation — *see* Radiation
  smoke (*see also* Exposure, fire)
    tobacco, second hand Z77.22
  specified factors NEC X58 ☑
  sunlight X32 ☑
    man-made (sun lamp) W89.8 ☑
    tanning bed W89.1 ☑
  supersonic waves W42.0 ☑
  transmission line (s), electric W85 ☑
  vibration W49.9 ☑
  waves
    infrasound W49.9 ☑
    sound W42.9 ☑
    supersonic W42.0 ☑
  weather NEC — *see* Forces of nature
External cause status Y99.9
  child assisting in compensated work for
    family Y99.8
  civilian activity done for financial or other
    compensation Y99.0
  civilian activity done for income or pay Y99.0
  family member assisting in compensated work
    for other family member Y99.8
  hobby not done for income Y99.8
  leisure activity Y99.8
  military activity Y99.1
  off-duty activity of military personnel Y99.8
  recreation or sport not for income or while a
    student Y99.8
  specified NEC Y99.8
  student activity Y99.8
  volunteer activity Y99.2

F

Factors, supplemental
  alcohol
    blood level
      less than 20mg/100ml Y90.0
      presence in blood, level not specified Y90.9
      20-39mg/100ml Y90.1
      40-59mg/100ml Y90.2
      60-79mg/100ml Y90.3
      80-99mg/100ml Y90.4
      100-119mg/100ml Y90.5
      120-199mg/100ml Y90.6
      200-239mg/100ml Y90.7
      240mg/100ml or more Y90.8
      presence in blood, but level not specified Y90.9
  environmental-pollution-related condition —
    see Z57 ☑
  nosocomial condition Y95
  work-related condition Y99.0
Failure
  in suture or ligature during surgical
    procedure Y65.2

Failure — *continued*
  mechanical, of instrument or apparatus
    (any) (during any medical or surgical
    procedure) Y65.8
  sterile precautions (during medical and surgical
    care) — *see* Misadventure, failure, sterile
    precautions, by type of procedure
  to
    introduce tube or instrument Y65.4
      endotracheal tube during anesthesia Y65.3
    make curve (transport vehicle) NEC — *see*
      Accident, transport
    remove tube or instrument Y65.4
Fall, falling (accidental) W19 ☑
  building W20.1 ☑
    burning (uncontrolled fire) X00.3 ☑
  down
    embankment W17.81 ☑
    escalator W10.0 ☑
    hill W17.81 ☑
    ladder W11 ☑
    ramp W10.2 ☑
    stairs, steps W10.9 ☑
  due to
    bumping against
      object W18.00 ☑
        sharp glass W18.02 ☑
        specified NEC W18.09 ☑
        sports equipment W18.01 ☑
      person W03 ☑
        due to ice or snow W00.0 ☑
        on pedestrian conveyance — *see* Accident,
          transport, pedestrian, conveyance
    collision with another person W03 ☑
      due to ice or snow W00.0 ☑
      involving pedestrian conveyance — *see*
        Accident, transport, pedestrian,
        conveyance
    grocery cart tipping over W17.82 ☑
    ice or snow W00.9 ☑
      from one level to another W00.2 ☑
      on stairs or steps W00.1 ☑
      involving pedestrian conveyance — *see*
        Accident, transport, pedestrian,
        conveyance
      on same level W00.0 ☑
    slipping (on moving sidewalk) W01.0 ☑
      with subsequent striking against
        object W01.10 ☑
        furniture W01.190 ☑
        sharp object W01.119 ☑
          glass W01.110 ☑
          power tool or machine W01.111 ☑
          specified NEC W01.118 ☑
        specified NEC W01.198 ☑
    striking against
      object W18.00 ☑
        sharp glass W18.02 ☑
        specified NEC W18.09 ☑
        sports equipment W18.01 ☑
      person W03 ☑
        due to ice or snow W00.0 ☑
        on pedestrian conveyance — *see* Accident,
          transport, pedestrian, conveyance
  earth (with asphyxia or suffocation (by pressure))
    — *see* Earth, falling
  from, off, out of
    aircraft NEC (with accident to aircraft
      NEC) V97.0 ☑
      while boarding or alighting V97.1 ☑
    balcony W13.0 ☑
    bed W06 ☑
    boat, ship, watercraft NEC (with drowning or
      submersion) — *see* Drowning, due to, fall
      overboard
      with hitting bottom or object V94.0 ☑
    bridge W13.1 ☑
    building W13.9 ☑
      burning (uncontrolled fire) X00.3 ☑
    cavity W17.2 ☑
    chair W07 ☑
    cherry picker W17.89 ☑
    cliff W15 ☑
    dock W17.4 ☑
    embankment W17.81 ☑
    escalator W10.0 ☑
    flagpole W13.8 ☑
    furniture NEC W08 ☑
    grocery cart W17.82 ☑
    haystack W17.89 ☑
    high place NEC W17.89 ☑

Fall, falling — *continued*
  from, off, out of — *continued*
    stated as undetermined whether accidental
      or intentional Y30 ☑
    hole W17.2 ☑
    incline W10.2 ☑
    ladder W11 ☑
    lifting device W17.89 ☑
    machine, machinery (*see also* Contact, with, by
      type of machine)
      not in operation W17.89 ☑
    manhole W17.1 ☑
    mobile elevated work platform
      [MEWP] W17.89 ☑
    motorized mobility scooter W05.2 ☑
    one level to another NEC W17.89 ☑
      intentional, purposeful, suicide
        (attempt) X80 ☑
      stated as undetermined whether accidental
        or intentional Y30 ☑
    pit W17.2 ☑
    playground equipment W09.8 ☑
      jungle gym W09.2 ☑
      slide W09.0 ☑
      swing W09.1 ☑
    quarry W17.89 ☑
    railing W13.9 ☑
    ramp W10.2 ☑
    roof W13.2 ☑
    scaffolding W12 ☑
    scooter (nonmotorized) W05.1 ☑
      motorized mobility W05.2 ☑
    sky lift W17.89 ☑
    stairs, steps W10.9 ☑
      curb W10.1 ☑
      due to ice or snow W00.1 ☑
      escalator W10.0 ☑
      incline W10.2 ☑
      ramp W10.2 ☑
      sidewalk curb W10.1 ☑
      specified NEC W10.8 ☑
    stepladder W11 ☑
    storm drain W17.1 ☑
    streetcar NEC V82.6 ☑
      with antecedent collision — *see* Accident,
        transport, streetcar occupant
      while boarding or alighting V82.4 ☑
    structure NEC W13.8 ☑
      burning (uncontrolled fire) X00.3 ☑
    table W08 ☑
    toilet W18.11 ☑
      with subsequent striking against
        object W18.12 ☑
    train NEC V81.6 ☑
      during derailment (without antecedent
        collision) V81.7 ☑
        with antecedent collision — *see* Accident,
          transport, railway vehicle occupant
      while boarding or alighting V81.4 ☑
    transport vehicle after collision — *see* Accident,
      transport, by type of vehicle, collision
    tree W14 ☑
    vehicle (in motion) NEC (*see also* Accident,
      transport) V89.9 ☑
      motor NEC (*see also* Accident, transport,
        occupant, by type of vehicle) V87.8 ☑
      stationary W17.89 ☑
      while boarding or alighting — *see*
        Accident, transport, by type of vehicle,
        while boarding or alighting
    viaduct W13.8 ☑
    wall W13.8 ☑
    watercraft (*see also* Drowning, due to, fall
      overboard)
      with hitting bottom or object V94.0 ☑
    well W17.0 ☑
    wheelchair, non-moving W05.0 ☑
      powered — *see* Accident, transport,
        pedestrian, conveyance occupant,
        specified type NEC
    window W13.4 ☑
  in, on
    aircraft NEC V97.0 ☑
      with accident to aircraft V97.0 ☑
      while boarding or alighting V97.1 ☑
    bathtub (empty) W18.2 ☑
      filled W16.212 ☑
        causing drowning W16.211 ☑
    escalator W10.0 ☑
    incline W10.2 ☑
    ladder W11 ☑

Incident - Legal

Incident, adverse — *continued*
  device — *continued*
    prosthetic Y78.2
    rehabilitative Y78.1
    surgical Y78.3
    therapeutic Y78.1
  urology Y73.8
    accessory Y73.2
    diagnostic Y73.0
    miscellaneous Y73.8
    monitoring Y73.0
    prosthetic Y73.2
    rehabilitative Y73.1
    surgical Y73.3
    therapeutic Y73.1
Incineration (accidental) — *see* Exposure, fire
Infanticide — *see* Assault
Infrasound waves (causing injury) W49.9 ☑
Ingestion
  foreign body (causing injury) (with obstruction) — *see* Foreign body, alimentary canal
  poisonous
    plant (s) X58 ☑
    substance NEC — *see* Table of Drugs and Chemicals
Inhalation
  excessively cold substance, man-made — *see* Exposure, cold, man-made
  food (any type) (into respiratory tract) (with asphyxia, obstruction respiratory tract, suffocation) — *see* categories T17 and T18 ☑
  foreign body — *see* Foreign body, aspiration
  gastric contents (with asphyxia, obstruction respiratory passage, suffocation) T17.81 ☑
  hot air or gases X14.0 ☑
  liquid air, hydrogen, nitrogen W93.12 ☑
    suicide (attempt) X83.2 ☑
  steam X13.0 ☑
    assault X98.0 ☑
    stated as undetermined whether accidental or intentional Y27.0 ☑
    suicide (attempt) X77.0 ☑
  toxic gas — *see* Table of Drugs and Chemicals
  vomitus (with asphyxia, obstruction respiratory passage, suffocation) T17.81 ☑
Injury, injured (accidental(ly)) NOS X58 ☑
  by, caused by, from
    assault — *see* Assault
    law-enforcing agent, police, in course of legal intervention — *see* Legal intervention
    suicide (attempt) X83.8 ☑
  due to, in
    civil insurrection — *see* War operations
    fight (*see also* Assault, fight) Y04.0 ☑
    war operations — *see* War operations
  homicide (*see also* Assault) Y09
  inflicted (by)
    in course of arrest (attempted), suppression of disturbance, maintenance of order, by law-enforcing agents — *see* Legal intervention
    other person
      stated as
        accidental X58 ☑
        intentional, homicide (attempt) — *see* Assault
        undetermined whether accidental or intentional Y33 ☑
    purposely (inflicted) by other person (s) — *see* Assault
  self-inflicted X83.8 ☑
    stated as accidental X58 ☑
  specified cause NEC X58 ☑
  undetermined whether accidental or intentional Y33 ☑
Insolation, effects X30 ☑
Insufficient nourishment X58 ☑
Interruption of respiration (by)
  food (lodged in esophagus) — *see* categories T17 and T18 ☑
  vomitus (lodged in esophagus) T17.81 ☑
Intervention, legal — *see* Legal intervention
Intoxication
  drug — *see* Table of Drugs and Chemicals
  poison — *see* Table of Drugs and Chemicals

J

Jammed (accidentally)
  between objects (moving) (stationary and moving) W23.0 ☑

Jammed — *continued*
  between objects — *continued*
    stationary W23.1 ☑
Jumped, jumping
  before moving object NEC X81.8 ☑
    motor vehicle X81.0 ☑
    subway train X81.1 ☑
    train X81.1 ☑
    undetermined whether accidental or intentional Y31 ☑
  from
    boat (into water) voluntarily, without accident (to or on boat) W16.712 ☑
      with
        accident to or on boat — *see* Accident, watercraft
        drowning or submersion W16.711 ☑
          suicide (attempt) X71.3 ☑
        striking bottom W16.722 ☑
          causing drowning W16.721 ☑
    building (*see also* Jumped, from, high place) W13.9 ☑
      burning (uncontrolled fire) X00.5 ☑
    high place NEC W17.89 ☑
      suicide (attempt) X80 ☑
      undetermined whether accidental or intentional Y30 ☑
    structure (*see also* Jumped, from, high place) W13.9 ☑
      burning (uncontrolled fire) X00.5 ☑
  into water W16.92 ☑
    causing drowning W16.91 ☑
    from, off watercraft — *see* Jumped, from, boat
    in
      natural body W16.612 ☑
        causing drowning W16.611 ☑
        striking bottom W16.622 ☑
          causing drowning W16.621 ☑
      specified place NEC W16.812 ☑
        causing drowning W16.811 ☑
        striking
          bottom W16.822 ☑
            causing drowning W16.821 ☑
          wall W16.832 ☑
            causing drowning W16.831 ☑
      swimming pool W16.512 ☑
        causing drowning W16.511 ☑
        striking
          bottom W16.522 ☑
            causing drowning W16.521 ☑
          wall W16.532 ☑
            causing drowning W16.531 ☑
    suicide (attempt) X71.3 ☑

K

Kicked by
  animal NEC W55.82 ☑
  person (s) (accidentally) W50.1 ☑
    with intent to injure or kill Y04.0 ☑
    as, or caused by, a crowd or human stampede (with fall) W52 ☑
    assault Y04.0 ☑
    homicide (attempt) Y04.0 ☑
    in
      fight Y04.0 ☑
      legal intervention
        injuring
          bystander Y35.812 ☑
          law enforcement personnel Y35.811 ☑
          suspect Y35.813 ☑
Kicking
  against
    object W22.8 ☑
      sports equipment W21.9 ☑
    stationary W22.09 ☑
      sports equipment W21.89 ☑
    person — *see* Striking against, person
    sports equipment W21.9 ☑
  carpet stretcher with knee X50.3 ☑
Killed, killing (accidentally) NOS (*see also* Injury) X58 ☑
  in
    action — *see* War operations
    brawl, fight (hand) (fists) (foot) Y04.0 ☑
    by weapon (*see also* Assault)
      cutting, piercing — *see* Assault, cutting or piercing instrument
      firearm — *see* Discharge, firearm, by type, homicide

Killed, killing — *continued*
  self
    stated as
      accident NOS X58 ☑
      suicide — *see* Suicide
      undetermined whether accidental or intentional Y33 ☑
Kneeling (prolonged) (static) X50.1 ☑
Knocked down (accidentally) (by) NOS X58 ☑
  animal (not being ridden) NEC (*see also* Struck by, by type of animal)
  crowd or human stampede W52 ☑
  person W51 ☑
    in brawl, fight Y04.0 ☑
  transport vehicle NEC (*see also* Accident, transport) V09.9 ☑

L

Laceration NEC — *see* Injury
Lack of
  care (helpless person) (infant) (newborn) X58 ☑
  food except as result of abandonment or neglect X58 ☑
    due to abandonment or neglect X58 ☑
  water except as result of transport accident X58 ☑
    due to transport accident — *see* Accident, transport, by type
  helpless person, infant, newborn X58 ☑
Landslide (falling on transport vehicle) X36.1 ☑
  caused by collapse of man-made structure X36.0 ☑
Late effect — *see* Sequelae
Legal
  execution (any method) — *see* Legal, intervention
  intervention (by)
    baton — *see* Legal, intervention, blunt object, baton
    bayonet — *see* Legal, intervention, sharp object, bayonet
    blow — *see* Legal, intervention, manhandling
    blunt object
      baton
        injuring
          bystander Y35.312 ☑
          law enforcement personnel Y35.311 ☑
          suspect Y35.313 ☑
        injuring
          bystander Y35.302 ☑
          law enforcement personnel Y35.301 ☑
          suspect Y35.303 ☑
      specified NEC
        injuring
          bystander Y35.392 ☑
          law enforcement personnel Y35.391 ☑
          suspect Y35.393 ☑
      stave
        injuring
          bystander Y35.392 ☑
          law enforcement personnel Y35.391 ☑
          suspect Y35.393 ☑
    bomb — *see* Legal, intervention, explosive
    cutting or piercing instrument — *see* Legal, intervention, sharp object
    dynamite — *see* Legal, intervention, explosive, dynamite
    explosive (s)
      dynamite
        injuring
          bystander Y35.112 ☑
          law enforcement personnel Y35.111 ☑
          suspect Y35.113 ☑
      grenade
        injuring
          bystander Y35.192 ☑
          law enforcement personnel Y35.191 ☑
          suspect Y35.193 ☑
      injuring
        bystander Y35.102 ☑
        law enforcement personnel Y35.101 ☑
        suspect Y35.103 ☑
      mortar bomb
        injuring
          bystander Y35.192 ☑
          law enforcement personnel Y35.191 ☑
          suspect Y35.193 ☑
      shell
        injuring
          bystander Y35.122 ☑

☑ **Additional character required**

Legal — *continued*
  intervention — *continued*
      law enforcement personnel Y35.121 ☑
      suspect Y35.123 ☑
    specified NEC
      injuring
        bystander Y35.192 ☑
        law enforcement personnel Y35.191 ☑
        suspect Y35.193 ☑
    firearm (s) (discharge)
      handgun
        injuring
          bystander Y35.022 ☑
          law enforcement personnel Y35.021 ☑
          suspect Y35.023 ☑
      injuring
        bystander Y35.002 ☑
        law enforcement personnel Y35.001 ☑
        suspect Y35.003 ☑
      machine gun
        injuring
          bystander Y35.012 ☑
          law enforcement personnel Y35.011 ☑
          suspect Y35.013 ☑
      rifle pellet
        injuring
          bystander Y35.032 ☑
          law enforcement personnel Y35.031 ☑
          suspect Y35.033 ☑
      rubber bullet
        injuring
          bystander Y35.042 ☑
          law enforcement personnel Y35.041 ☑
          suspect Y35.043 ☑
      shotgun — *see* Legal, intervention, firearm, specified NEC
      specified NEC
        injuring
          bystander Y35.092 ☑
          law enforcement personnel Y35.091 ☑
          suspect Y35.093 ☑
    gas (asphyxiation) (poisoning)
      injuring
        bystander Y35.202 ☑
        law enforcement personnel Y35.201 ☑
        suspect Y35.203 ☑
      specified NEC
        injuring
          bystander Y35.292 ☑
          law enforcement personnel Y35.291 ☑
          suspect Y35.293 ☑
      tear gas
        injuring
          bystander Y35.212 ☑
          law enforcement personnel Y35.211 ☑
          suspect Y35.213 ☑
    grenade — *see* Legal, intervention, explosive, grenade
      injuring
        bystander Y35.92 ☑
        law enforcement personnel Y35.91 ☑
        suspect Y35.93 ☑
    late effect (of) — *see* with 7th character S Y35 ☑
    manhandling
      injuring
        bystander Y35.812 ☑
        law enforcement personnel Y35.811 ☑
        suspect Y35.813 ☑
    sequelae (of) — *see* with 7th character S Y35 ☑
    sharp objects
      bayonet
        injuring
          bystander Y35.412 ☑
          law enforcement personnel Y35.411 ☑
          suspect Y35.413 ☑
      injuring
        bystander Y35.402 ☑
        law enforcement personnel Y35.401 ☑
        suspect Y35.403 ☑
      specified NEC
        injuring
          bystander Y35.492 ☑
          law enforcement personnel Y35.491 ☑
          suspect Y35.493 ☑
    specified means NEC
      injuring
        bystander Y35.892 ☑
        law enforcement personnel Y35.891 ☑
        suspect Y35.893 ☑
    stabbing — *see* Legal, intervention, sharp object

Legal — *continued*
  intervention — *continued*
    stave — *see* Legal, intervention, blunt object, stave
    tear gas — *see* Legal, intervention, gas, tear gas
    truncheon — *see* Legal, intervention, blunt object, stave
Lifting (*see also* Overexertion)
  heavy objects X50.0 ☑
  weights X50.0 ☑
Lightning (shock) (stroke) (struck by) — *see* subcategory T75.0
  causing fire — *see* Exposure, fire
Loss of control (transport vehicle) NEC — *see* Accident, transport
Lost at sea NOS — *see* Drowning, due to, fall overboard
Low
  pressure (effects) — *see* Air, pressure, low
  temperature (effects) — *see* Exposure, cold
Lying before train, vehicle or other moving object X81.8 ☑
  subway train X81.1 ☑
  train X81.1 ☑
  undetermined whether accidental or intentional Y31 ☑
Lynching — *see* Assault

M

Malfunction (mechanism or component) (of)
  firearm W34.10 ☑
    airgun W34.110 ☑
    BB gun W34.110 ☑
    gas, air or spring-operated gun NEC W34.118 ☑
    handgun W32.1 ☑
    hunting rifle W33.12 ☑
    larger firearm W33.10 ☑
      specified NEC W33.19 ☑
    machine gun W33.13 ☑
    paintball gun W34.111 ☑
    pellet gun W34.110 ☑
    shotgun W33.11 ☑
    specified NEC W34.19 ☑
    Very pistol [flare] W34.19 ☑
  handgun — *see* Malfunction, firearm, handgun
Maltreatment — *see* Perpetrator
Mangled (accidentally) NOS X58 ☑
Manhandling (in brawl, fight) Y04.0 ☑
  legal intervention — *see* Legal, intervention, manhandling
Manslaughter (nonaccidental) — *see* Assault
Mauled by animal NEC W55.89 ☑
Medical procedure, complication of (delayed or as an abnormal reaction without mention of misadventure) — *see* Complication of or following, by specified type of procedure
  due to or as a result of misadventure — *see* Misadventure
Melting (due to fire) (*see also* Exposure, fire)
  apparel NEC X06.3 ☑
  clothes, clothing NEC X06.3 ☑
    nightwear X05 ☑
  fittings or furniture (burning building) (uncontrolled fire) X00.8 ☑
  nightwear X05 ☑
  plastic jewelry X06.1 ☑
Mental cruelty X58 ☑
Military operations (injuries to military and civilians occurring during peacetime on military property and during routine military exercises and operations) (by) (from) (involving) Y37.90 ☑
  air blast Y37.20 ☑
  aircraft
    destruction — *see* Military operations, destruction of aircraft
    airway restriction — *see* Military operations, restriction of airways
  asphyxiation — *see* Military operations, restriction of airways
  biological weapons Y37.6X ☑
  blast Y37.20 ☑
  blast fragments Y37.20 ☑
  blast wave Y37.20 ☑
  blast wind Y37.20 ☑
  bomb Y37.20 ☑
    dirty Y37.50 ☑
    gasoline Y37.31 ☑
    incendiary Y37.31 ☑
    petrol Y37.31 ☑

Military operations — *continued*
  bullet Y37.43 ☑
    incendiary Y37.32 ☑
    rubber Y37.41 ☑
  chemical weapons Y37.7X ☑
  combat
    hand to hand (unarmed) combat Y37.44 ☑
    using blunt or piercing object Y37.45 ☑
  conflagration — *see* Military operations, fire
  conventional warfare NEC Y37.49 ☑
  depth-charge Y37.01 ☑
  destruction of aircraft Y37.10 ☑
    due to
      air to air missile Y37.11 ☑
      collision with other aircraft Y37.12 ☑
      detonation (accidental) of onboard munitions and explosives Y37.14 ☑
      enemy fire or explosives Y37.11 ☑
      explosive placed on aircraft Y37.11 ☑
      onboard fire Y37.13 ☑
      rocket propelled grenade [RPG] Y37.11 ☑
      small arms fire Y37.11 ☑
      surface to air missile Y37.11 ☑
    specified NEC Y37.19 ☑
  detonation (accidental) of
    onboard marine weapons Y37.05 ☑
    own munitions or munitions launch device Y37.24 ☑
  dirty bomb Y37.50 ☑
  explosion (of) Y37.20 ☑
    aerial bomb Y37.21 ☑
    bomb NOS (*see also* Military operations, bomb (s)) Y37.20 ☑
    own munitions or munitions launch device (accidental) Y37.24 ☑
    fragments Y37.20 ☑
    grenade Y37.29 ☑
    guided missile Y37.22 ☑
    improvised explosive device [IED] (person-borne) (roadside) (vehicle-borne) Y37.23 ☑
    land mine Y37.29 ☑
    marine mine (at sea) (in harbor) Y37.02 ☑
    marine weapon Y37.00 ☑
      specified NEC Y37.09 ☑
    sea-based artillery shell Y37.03 ☑
    specified NEC Y37.29 ☑
    torpedo Y37.04 ☑
  fire Y37.30 ☑
    specified NEC Y37.39 ☑
  firearms
    discharge Y37.43 ☑
    pellets Y37.42 ☑
  flamethrower Y37.33 ☑
  fragments (from) (of)
    improvised explosive device [IED] (person-borne) (roadside) (vehicle-borne) Y37.26 ☑
    munitions Y37.25 ☑
    specified NEC Y37.29 ☑
    weapons Y37.27 ☑
  friendly fire Y37.92 ☑
  hand to hand (unarmed) combat Y37.44 ☑
  hot substances — *see* Military operations, fire
  incendiary bullet Y37.32 ☑
  nuclear weapon (effects of) Y37.50 ☑
    acute radiation exposure Y37.54 ☑
    blast pressure Y37.51 ☑
    direct blast Y37.51 ☑
    direct heat Y37.53 ☑
    fallout exposure Y37.54 ☑
    fireball Y37.53 ☑
    indirect blast (struck or crushed by blast debris) (being thrown by blast) Y37.52 ☑
    ionizing radiation (immediate exposure) Y37.54 ☑
    nuclear radiation Y37.54 ☑
    radiation
      ionizing (immediate exposure) Y37.54 ☑
      nuclear Y37.54 ☑
      thermal Y37.53 ☑
    specified NEC Y37.59 ☑
    secondary effects Y37.54 ☑
    thermal radiation Y37.53 ☑
  restriction of air (airway)
    intentional Y37.46 ☑
    unintentional Y37.47 ☑
  rubber bullets Y37.41 ☑
  shrapnel NOS Y37.29 ☑
  suffocation — *see* Military operations, restriction of airways
  unconventional warfare NEC Y37.7X ☑
  underwater blast NOS Y37.00 ☑
  warfare

Military operations — *continued*
  warfare — *continued*
    conventional NEC Y37.49 ☑
    unconventional NEC Y37.7X ☑
  weapons
    biological weapons Y37.6X ☑
    chemical Y37.7X ☑
    nuclear (effects of) Y37.50 ☑
      acute radiation exposure Y37.54 ☑
      blast pressure Y37.51 ☑
      direct blast Y37.51 ☑
      direct heat Y37.53 ☑
      fallout exposure Y37.54 ☑
      fireball Y37.53 ☑
      indirect blast (struck or crushed by blast debris) (being thrown by blast) Y37.52 ☑
      radiation
        ionizing (immediate exposure) Y37.54 ☑
          nuclear Y37.54 ☑
          thermal Y37.53 ☑
      secondary effects Y37.54 ☑
      specified NEC Y37.59 ☑
    of mass destruction [WMD] Y37.91 ☑
    weapon of mass destruction [WMD] Y37.91 ☑
Misadventure (s) to patient (s) during surgical or medical care Y69
  contaminated medical or biological substance (blood, drug, fluid) Y64.9
    administered (by) NEC Y64.9
      immunization Y64.1
      infusion Y64.0
      injection Y64.1
      specified means NEC Y64.8
      transfusion Y64.0
      vaccination Y64.1
  excessive amount of blood or other fluid during transfusion or infusion Y63.0
  failure
    in dosage Y63.9
      electroshock therapy Y63.4
      inappropriate temperature (too hot or too cold) in local application and packing Y63.5
      infusion
        excessive amount of fluid Y63.0
        incorrect dilution of fluid Y63.1
      insulin-shock therapy Y63.4
      nonadministration of necessary drug or biological substance Y63.6
      overdose — *see* Table of Drugs and Chemicals
        radiation, in therapy Y63.2
      radiation
        overdose Y63.2
      specified procedure NEC Y63.8
      transfusion
        excessive amount of blood Y63.0
    mechanical, of instrument or apparatus (any) (during any procedure) Y65.8
    sterile precautions (during procedure) Y62.9
      aspiration of fluid or tissue (by puncture or catheterization, except heart) Y62.6
      biopsy (except needle aspiration) Y62.8
        needle (aspirating) Y62.6
      blood sampling Y62.6
      catheterization Y62.6
        heart Y62.5
      dialysis (kidney) Y62.2
      endoscopic examination Y62.4
      enema Y62.8
      immunization Y62.3
      infusion Y62.1
      injection Y62.3
      needle biopsy Y62.6
      paracentesis (abdominal) (thoracic) Y62.6
      perfusion Y62.2
      puncture (lumbar) Y62.6
      removal of catheter or packing Y62.8
      specified procedure NEC Y62.8
      surgical operation Y62.0
      transfusion Y62.1
      vaccination Y62.3
    suture or ligature during surgical procedure Y65.2
    to introduce or to remove tube or instrument — *see* Failure, to
  hemorrhage — *see* Index to Diseases and Injuries, Complication (s)
  inadvertent exposure of patient to radiation Y63.3

Misadventure — *continued*
  inappropriate
    operation performed — *see* Inappropriate operation performed
    temperature (too hot or too cold) in local application or packing Y63.5
  infusion (*see also* Misadventure, by type, infusion) Y69
    excessive amount of fluid Y63.0
    incorrect dilution of fluid Y63.1
    wrong fluid Y65.1
  mismatched blood in transfusion Y65.0
  nonadministration of necessary drug or biological substance Y63.6
  overdose — *see* Table of Drugs and Chemicals
    radiation (in therapy) Y63.2
  perforation — *see* Index to Diseases and Injuries, Complication (s)
  performance of inappropriate operation — *see* Inappropriate operation performed
  puncture — *see* Index to Diseases and Injuries, Complication (s)
  specified type NEC Y65.8
    failure
      suture or ligature during surgical operation Y65.2
      to introduce or to remove tube or instrument — *see* Failure, to
    infusion of wrong fluid Y65.1
    performance of inappropriate operation — *see* Inappropriate operation performed
    transfusion of mismatched blood Y65.0
    wrong
      fluid in infusion Y65.1
      placement of endotracheal tube during anesthetic procedure Y65.3
  transfusion — *see* Misadventure, by type, transfusion
    excessive amount of blood Y63.0
    mismatched blood Y65.0
  wrong
    drug given in error — *see* Table of Drugs and Chemicals
    fluid in infusion Y65.1
    placement of endotracheal tube during anesthetic procedure Y65.3
Mismatched blood in transfusion Y65.0
Motion sickness T75.3 ☑
Mountain sickness W94.11 ☑
Mudslide (of cataclysmic nature) — *see* Landslide
Murder (attempt) — *see* Assault

N

Nail
  contact with W45.0 ☑
    gun W29.4 ☑
  embedded in skin W45.0 ☑
Neglect (criminal) (homicidal intent) X58 ☑
Noise (causing injury) (pollution) W42.9 ☑
  supersonic W42.0 ☑
Nonadministration (of)
  drug or biological substance (necessary) Y63.6
  surgical and medical care Y66
Nosocomial condition Y95

O

Object
  falling
    from, in, on, hitting
      machinery — *see* Contact, with, by type of machine
  set in motion by
    accidental explosion or rupture of pressure vessel W38 ☑
    firearm — *see* Discharge, firearm, by type
    machine (ry) — *see* Contact, with, by type of machine
Overdose (drug) — *see* Table of Drugs and Chemicals
  radiation Y63.2
Overexertion X50.9 ☑
  from
    prolonged static or awkward postures X50.1 ☑
    repetitive movements X50.3 ☑
    specified strenuous movements or postures NEC X50.9 ☑
    strenuous movement or load X50.0 ☑

Overexposure (accidental) (to)
  cold (*see also* Exposure, cold) X31 ☑
    due to man-made conditions — *see* Exposure, cold, man-made
  heat (*see also* Heat) X30 ☑
  radiation — *see* Radiation
  radioactivity W88.0 ☑
  sun (sunburn) X32 ☑
  weather NEC — *see* Forces of nature
  wind NEC — *see* Forces of nature
Overheated — *see* Heat
Overturning (accidental)
  machinery — *see* Contact, with, by type of machine
  transport vehicle NEC (*see also* Accident, transport) V89.9 ☑
  watercraft (causing drowning, submersion) (*see also* Drowning, due to, accident to, watercraft, overturning)
    causing injury except drowning or submersion — *see* Accident, watercraft, causing, injury NEC

P

Parachute descent (voluntary) (without accident to aircraft) V97.29 ☑
  due to accident to aircraft — *see* Accident, transport, aircraft
Pecked by bird W61.99 ☑
Perforation during medical or surgical treatment as misadventure — *see* Index to Diseases and Injuries, Complication (s)
Perpetrator, perpetration, of assault, maltreatment and neglect (by) Y07.9
  boyfriend Y07.03
  brother Y07.410
    stepbrother Y07.435
  coach Y07.53
  cousin
    female Y07.491
    male Y07.490
  daycare provider Y07.519
    at-home
      adult care Y07.512
      childcare Y07.510
    care center
      adult care Y07.513
      childcare Y07.511
  family member NEC Y07.499
  father Y07.11
    adoptive Y07.13
    foster Y07.420
    stepfather Y07.430
  foster father Y07.420
  foster mother Y07.421
  girl friend Y07.04
  healthcare provider Y07.529
    mental health Y07.521
    specified NEC Y07.528
  husband Y07.01
  instructor Y07.53
  mother Y07.12
    adoptive Y07.14
    foster Y07.421
    stepmother Y07.433
  nonfamily member Y07.50
    specified NEC Y07.59
  nurse Y07.528
  occupational therapist Y07.528
  partner of parent
    female Y07.434
    male Y07.432
  physical therapist Y07.528
  sister Y07.411
  speech therapist Y07.528
  stepbrother Y07.435
  stepfather Y07.430
  stepmother Y07.433
  stepsister Y07.436
  teacher Y07.53
  wife Y07.02
Piercing — *see* Contact, with, by type of object or machine
Pinched
  between objects (moving) (stationary and moving) W23.0 ☑
    stationary W23.1 ☑
Pinned under machine (ry) — *see* Contact, with, by type of machine

☑ **Additional character required**

Place of occurrence Y92.9
  abandoned house Y92.89
  airplane Y92.813
  airport Y92.520
  ambulatory health services establishment NEC Y92.538
  ambulatory surgery center Y92.530
  amusement park Y92.831
  apartment (co-op) — see Place of occurrence, residence, apartment
  assembly hall Y92.29
  bank Y92.510
  barn Y92.71
  baseball field Y92.320
  basketball court Y92.310
  beach Y92.832
  boarding house — see Place of occurrence, residence, boarding house
  boat Y92.814
  bowling alley Y92.39
  bridge Y92.89
  building under construction Y92.61
  bus Y92.811
    station Y92.521
  cafe Y92.511
  campsite Y92.833
  campus — see Place of occurrence, school
  canal Y92.89
  car Y92.810
  casino Y92.59
  children's home — see Place of occurrence, residence, institutional, orphanage
  church Y92.22
  cinema Y92.26
  clubhouse Y92.29
  coal pit Y92.64
  college (community) Y92.214
  condominium — see Place of occurrence, residence, apartment
  construction area — see Place of occurrence, industrial and construction area
  convalescent home — see Place of occurrence, residence, institutional, nursing home
  court-house Y92.240
  cricket ground Y92.328
  cultural building Y92.258
    art gallery Y92.250
    museum Y92.251
    music hall Y92.252
    opera house Y92.253
    specified NEC Y92.258
    theater Y92.254
  dancehall Y92.252
  day nursery Y92.210
  dentist office Y92.531
  derelict house Y92.89
  desert Y92.820
  dock NOS Y92.89
  dockyard Y92.62
  doctor's office Y92.531
  dormitory — see Place of occurrence, residence, institutional, school dormitory
  dry dock Y92.62
  factory (building) (premises) Y92.63
  farm (land under cultivation) (outbuildings) Y92.79
    barn Y92.71
    chicken coop Y92.72
    field Y92.73
    hen house Y92.72
    house — see Place of occurrence, residence, house
    orchard Y92.74
    specified NEC Y92.79
  football field Y92.321
  forest Y92.821
  freeway Y92.411
  gallery Y92.250
  garage (commercial) Y92.59
    boarding house Y92.044
    military base Y92.135
    mobile home Y92.025
    nursing home Y92.124
    orphanage Y92.114
    private house Y92.015
    reform school Y92.155
  gas station Y92.524
  gasworks Y92.69
  golf course Y92.39
  gravel pit Y92.64
  grocery Y92.512
  gymnasium Y92.39

Place of occurrence — continued
  handball court Y92.318
  harbor Y92.89
  harness racing course Y92.39
  healthcare provider office Y92.531
  highway (interstate) Y92.411
  hill Y92.828
  hockey rink Y92.330
  home — see Place of occurrence, residence
  hospice — see Place of occurrence, residence, institutional, nursing home
  hospital Y92.239
    cafeteria Y92.233
    corridor Y92.232
    operating room Y92.234
    patient
      bathroom Y92.231
      room Y92.230
    specified NEC Y92.238
  hotel Y92.59
  house (see also Place of occurrence, residence)
    abandoned Y92.89
    under construction Y92.61
  industrial and construction area (yard) Y92.69
    building under construction Y92.61
    dock Y92.62
    dry dock Y92.62
    factory Y92.63
    gasworks Y92.69
    mine Y92.64
    oil rig Y92.65
    pit Y92.64
    power station Y92.69
    shipyard Y92.62
    specified NEC Y92.69
    tunnel under construction Y92.69
    workshop Y92.69
  kindergarten Y92.211
  lacrosse field Y92.328
  lake Y92.828
  library Y92.241
  mall Y92.59
  market Y92.512
  marsh Y92.828
  military
    base — see Place of occurrence, residence, institutional, military base
    training ground Y92.84
  mine Y92.64
  mosque Y92.22
  motel Y92.59
  motorway (interstate) Y92.411
  mountain Y92.828
  movie-house Y92.26
  museum Y92.251
  music-hall Y92.252
  not applicable Y92.9
  nuclear power station Y92.69
  nursing home — see Place of occurrence, residence, institutional, nursing home
  office building Y92.59
  offshore installation Y92.65
  oil rig Y92.65
  old people's home — see Place of occurrence, residence, institutional, specified NEC
  opera-house Y92.253
  orphanage — see Place of occurrence, residence, institutional, orphanage
  outpatient surgery center Y92.530
  park (public) Y92.830
    amusement Y92.831
  parking garage Y92.89
    lot Y92.481
  pavement Y92.480
  physician office Y92.531
  polo field Y92.328
  pond Y92.828
  post office Y92.242
  power station Y92.69
  prairie Y92.828
  prison — see Place of occurrence, residence, institutional, prison
  public
    administration building Y92.248
      city hall Y92.243
      courthouse Y92.240
      library Y92.241
      post office Y92.242
      specified NEC Y92.248
    building NEC Y92.29
    hall Y92.29
    place NOS Y92.89

Place of occurrence — continued
  race course Y92.39
  radio station Y92.59
  railway line (bridge) Y92.85
  ranch (outbuildings) — see Place of occurrence, farm
  recreation area Y92.838
    amusement park Y92.831
    beach Y92.832
    campsite Y92.833
    park (public) Y92.830
    seashore Y92.832
    specified NEC Y92.838
  religious institution Y92.22
  reform school — see Place of occurrence, residence, institutional, reform school
  residence (non-institutional) (private) Y92.009
    apartment Y92.039
      bathroom Y92.031
      bedroom Y92.032
      kitchen Y92.030
      specified NEC Y92.038
    bathroom Y92.002
    bedroom Y92.003
    boarding house Y92.049
      bathroom Y92.041
      bedroom Y92.042
      driveway Y92.043
      garage Y92.044
      garden Y92.046
      kitchen Y92.040
      specified NEC Y92.048
      swimming pool Y92.045
      yard Y92.046
    dining room Y92.001
    garden Y92.007
    home Y92.009
    house, single family Y92.019
      bathroom Y92.012
      bedroom Y92.013
      dining room Y92.011
      driveway Y92.014
      garage Y92.015
      garden Y92.017
      kitchen Y92.010
      specified NEC Y92.018
      swimming pool Y92.016
      yard Y92.017
    institutional Y92.10
      children's home — see Place of occurrence, residence, institutional, orphanage
      hospice — see Place of occurrence, residence, institutional, nursing home
      military base Y92.139
        barracks Y92.133
        garage Y92.135
        garden Y92.137
        kitchen Y92.130
        mess hall Y92.131
        specified NEC Y92.138
        swimming pool Y92.136
        yard Y92.137
      nursing home Y92.129
        bathroom Y92.121
        bedroom Y92.122
        driveway Y92.123
        garage Y92.124
        garden Y92.126
        kitchen Y92.120
        specified NEC Y92.128
        swimming pool Y92.125
        yard Y92.126
      orphanage Y92.119
        bathroom Y92.111
        bedroom Y92.112
        driveway Y92.113
        garage Y92.114
        garden Y92.116
        kitchen Y92.110
        specified NEC Y92.118
        swimming pool Y92.115
        yard Y92.116
      prison Y92.149
        bathroom Y92.142
        cell Y92.143
        courtyard Y92.147
        dining room Y92.141
        kitchen Y92.140
        specified NEC Y92.148
        swimming pool Y92.146
      reform school Y92.159
        bathroom Y92.152

☑ **Additional character required**

Place of occurrence — *continued*
  residence — *continued*
    bedroom Y92.153
    dining room Y92.151
    driveway Y92.154
    garage Y92.155
    garden Y92.157
    kitchen Y92.150
    specified NEC Y92.158
    swimming pool Y92.156
    yard Y92.157
   school dormitory Y92.169
    bathroom Y92.162
    bedroom Y92.163
    dining room Y92.161
    kitchen Y92.160
    specified NEC Y92.168
   specified NEC Y92.199
    bathroom Y92.192
    bedroom Y92.193
    dining room Y92.191
    driveway Y92.194
    garage Y92.195
    garden Y92.197
    kitchen Y92.190
    specified NEC Y92.198
    swimming pool Y92.196
    yard Y92.197
  kitchen Y92.000
  mobile home Y92.029
   bathroom Y92.022
   bedroom Y92.023
   dining room Y92.021
   driveway Y92.024
   garage Y92.025
   garden Y92.027
   kitchen Y92.020
   specified NEC Y92.028
   swimming pool Y92.026
   yard Y92.027
  specified place in residence NEC Y92.008
  specified residence type NEC Y92.099
   bathroom Y92.091
   bedroom Y92.092
   driveway Y92.093
   garage Y92.094
   garden Y92.096
   kitchen Y92.090
   specified NEC Y92.098
   swimming pool Y92.095
   yard Y92.096
  restaurant Y92.511
  riding school Y92.39
  river Y92.828
  road Y92.488
  rodeo ring Y92.39
  rugby field Y92.328
  same day surgery center Y92.530
  sand pit Y92.64
  school (private) (public) (state) Y92.219
   college Y92.214
   daycare center Y92.210
   elementary school Y92.211
   high school Y92.213
   kindergarten Y92.211
   middle school Y92.212
   specified NEC Y92.218
   trace school Y92.215
   university Y92.214
   vocational school Y92.215
  sea (shore) Y92.832
  senior citizen center Y92.29
  service area
   airport Y92.520
   bus station Y92.521
   gas station Y92.524
   highway rest stop Y92.523
   railway station Y92.522
  shipyard Y92.62
  shop (commercial) Y92.513
  sidewalk Y92.480
  silo Y92.79
  skating rink (roller) Y92.331
   ice Y92.330
  slaughter house Y92.86
  soccer field Y92.322
  specified place NEC Y92.89
  sports area Y92.39
   athletic
    court Y92.318
     basketball Y92.310
     specified NEC Y92.318

Place of occurrence — *continued*
  sports area — *continued*
    squash Y92.311
    tennis Y92.312
   field Y92.328
    baseball Y92.320
    cricket ground Y92.328
    football Y92.321
    hockey Y92.328
    soccer Y92.322
    specified NEC Y92.328
   golf course Y92.39
   gymnasium Y92.39
   riding school Y92.39
   skating rink (roller) Y92.331
    ice Y92.330
   stadium Y92.39
   swimming pool Y92.34
  squash court Y92.311
  stadium Y92.39
  steeplechasing course Y92.39
  store Y92.512
  stream Y92.828
  street and highway Y92.410
   bike path Y92.482
   freeway Y92.411
   highway ramp Y92.415
   interstate highway Y92.411
   local residential or business street Y92.414
   motorway Y92.411
   parkway Y92.412
   parking lot Y92.481
   sidewalk Y92.480
   specified NEC Y92.488
   state road Y92.413
  subway car Y92.816
  supermarket Y92.512
  swamp Y92.828
  swimming pool (public) Y92.34
   private (at) Y92.095
    boarding house Y92.045
    military base Y92.136
    mobile home Y92.026
    nursing home Y92.125
    orphanage Y92.115
    prison Y92.146
    reform school Y92.156
    single family residence Y92.016
  synagogue Y92.22
  television station Y92.59
  tennis court Y92.312
  theater Y92.254
  trade area Y92.59
   bank Y92.510
   cafe Y92.511
   casino Y92.59
   garage Y92.59
   hotel Y92.59
   market Y92.512
   office building Y92.59
   radio station Y92.59
   restaurant Y92.511
   shop Y92.513
   shopping mall Y92.59
   store Y92.512
   supermarket Y92.512
   television station Y92.59
   warehouse Y92.59
  trailer park, residential — *see* Place of occurrence, residence, mobile home
  trailer site NOS Y92.89
  train Y92.815
   station Y92.522
  truck Y92.812
  tunnel under construction Y92.69
  urgent (health) care center Y92.532
  university Y92.214
  vehicle (transport) Y92.818
   airplane Y92.813
   boat Y92.814
   bus Y92.811
   car Y92.810
   specified NEC Y92.818
   subway car Y92.816
   train Y92.815
   truck Y92.812
  warehouse Y92.59
  water reservoir Y92.89
  wilderness area Y92.828
   desert Y92.820
   forest Y92.821
   marsh Y92.828

Place of occurrence — *continued*
  wilderness area — *continued*
   mountain Y92.828
   prairie Y92.828
   specified NEC Y92.828
   swamp Y92.828
  workshop Y92.69
  yard, private Y92.096
   boarding house Y92.046
   single family house Y92.017
   mobile home Y92.027
  youth center Y92.29
  zoo (zoological garden) Y92.834
Plumbism — *see* Table of Drugs and Chemicals, lead
Poisoning (accidental) (by) (*see also* Table of Drugs and Chemicals)
  by plant, thorns, spines, sharp leaves or other mechanisms NEC X58 ☑
  carbon monoxide
   generated by
    motor vehicle — *see* Accident, transport
    watercraft (in transit) (not in transit) V93.89 ☑
     ferry boat V93.81 ☑
     fishing boat V93.82 ☑
     jet skis V93.83 ☑
     liner V93.81 ☑
     merchant ship V93.80 ☑
     passenger ship V93.81 ☑
     powered craft NEC V93.83 ☑
  caused by injection of poisons into skin by plant thorns, spines, sharp leaves X58 ☑
   marine or sea plants (venomous) X58 ☑
  exhaust gas
   generated by
    motor vehicle — *see* Accident, transport
    watercraft (in transit) (not in transit) V93.89 ☑
     ferry boat V93.81 ☑
     fishing boat V93.82 ☑
     jet skis V93.83 ☑
     liner V93.81 ☑
     merchant ship V93.80 ☑
     passenger ship V93.81 ☑
     powered craft NEC V93.83 ☑
  fumes or smoke due to
   explosion (*see also* Explosion) W40.9 ☑
   fire — *see* Exposure, fire
   ignition — *see* Ignition
  gas
   in legal intervention — *see* Legal, intervention, gas
   legal execution — *see* Legal, intervention, gas
  in war operations — *see* War operations
  legal
   execution — *see* Legal, intervention, gas
   intervention
    by gas — *see* Legal, intervention, gas
    other specified means — *see* Legal, intervention, specified means NEC
Powder burn (by) (from)
  airgun W34.110 ☑
  BB gun W34.110 ☑
  firearm NEC W34.19 ☑
  gas, air or spring-operated gun NEC W34.118 ☑
  handgun W32.1 ☑
  hunting rifle W33.12 ☑
  larger firearm W33.10 ☑
   specified NEC W33.19 ☑
  machine gun W33.13 ☑
  paintball gun W34.111 ☑
  pellet gun W34.110 ☑
  shotgun W33.11 ☑
  Very pistol [flare] W34.19 ☑
Premature cessation (of) surgical and medical care Y66
Privation (food) (water) X58 ☑
Procedure (operation)
  correct, on wrong side or body part (wrong side) (wrong site) Y65.53
  intended for another patient done on wrong patient Y65.52
  performed on patient not scheduled for surgery Y65.52
  performed on wrong patient Y65.52
  wrong, performed on correct patient Y65.51
Prolonged
  sitting in transport vehicle — *see* Travel, by type of vehicle
  stay in
   high altitude as cause of anoxia, barodontalgia, barotitis or hypoxia W94.11 ☑
   weightless environment X52 ☑
Pulling, excessive (*see also* Overexertion) X50.9 ☑

☑ **Additional character required**

Puncture, puncturing (see also Contact, with, by type of object or machine)
 by
  plant thorns, spines, sharp leaves or other mechanisms NEC W60 ☑
  during medical or surgical treatment as misadventure — see Index to Diseases and Injuries, Complication (s)
Pushed, pushing (accidental) (injury in)
 by other person (s) (accidental) W51 ☑
  with fall W03 ☑
   due to ice or snow W00.0 ☑
  as, or caused by, a crowd or human stampede (with fall) W52 ☑
  before moving object NEC Y02.8 ☑
   motor vehicle Y02.0 ☑
   subway train Y02.1 ☑
   train Y02.1 ☑
  from
   high place NEC
    in accidental circumstances W17.89 ☑
    stated as
     intentional, homicide (attempt) Y01 ☑
     undetermined whether accidental or intentional Y30 ☑
   transport vehicle NEC (see also Accident, transport) V89.9 ☑
    stated as
     intentional, homicide (attempt) Y08.89 ☑
 overexertion X50.9 ☑

R

Radiation (exposure to)
 arc lamps W89.0 ☑
 atomic power plant (malfunction) NEC W88.1 ☑
 complication of or abnormal reaction to medical radiotherapy Y84.2
 electromagnetic, ionizing W88.0 ☑
 gamma rays W88.1 ☑
 in
  war operations (from or following nuclear explosion) — see War operations
 inadvertent exposure of patient (receiving test or therapy) Y63.3
 infrared (heaters and lamps) W90.1 ☑
  excessive heat from W92 ☑
 ionized, ionizing (particles, artificially accelerated)
  radioisotopes W88.1 ☑
  specified NEC W88.8 ☑
  x-rays W88.0 ☑
 isotopes, radioactive — see Radiation, radioactive isotopes
 laser (s) W90.2 ☑
  in war operations — see War operations
  misadventure in medical care Y63.2
 light sources (man-made visible and ultraviolet) W89.9 ☑
  natural X32 ☑
  specified NEC W89.8 ☑
  tanning bed W89.1 ☑
  welding light W89.0 ☑
 man-made visible light W89.9 ☑
  specified NEC W89.8 ☑
  tanning bed W89.1 ☑
  welding light W89.0 ☑
 microwave W90.8 ☑
 misadventure in medical or surgical procedure Y63.2
 natural NEC X39.08 ☑
  radon X39.01 ☑
 overdose (in medical or surgical procedure) Y63.2
 radar W90.0 ☑
 radioactive isotopes (any) W88.1 ☑
  atomic power plant malfunction W88.1 ☑
  misadventure in medical or surgical treatment Y63.2
 radiofrequency W90.0 ☑
 radium NEC W88.1 ☑
 sun X32 ☑
 ultraviolet (light) (man-made) W89.9 ☑
  natural X32 ☑
  specified NEC W89.8 ☑
  tanning bed W89.1 ☑
  welding light W89.0 ☑
 welding arc, torch, or light W89.0 ☑
  excessive heat from W92 ☑
 x-rays (hard) (soft) W88.0 ☑
Range disease W94.11 ☑
Rape (attempted) T74.2 ☑

Rat bite W53.11 ☑
Reaching (prolonged) (static) X50.1 ☑
Reaction, abnormal to medical procedure (see also Complication of or following, by type of procedure) Y84.9
 with misadventure — see Misadventure
 biologicals — see Table of Drugs and Chemicals
 drugs — see Table of Drugs and Chemicals
 vaccine — see Table of Drugs and Chemicals
Recoil
 airgun W34.110 ☑
 BB gun W34.110 ☑
 firearm NEC W34.19 ☑
 gas, air or spring-operated gun NEC W34.118 ☑
 handgun W32.1 ☑
 hunting rifle W33.12 ☑
 larger firearm W33.10 ☑
  specified NEC W33.19 ☑
 machine gun W33.13 ☑
 paintball gun W34.111 ☑
 pellet W34.110 ☑
 shotgun W33.11 ☑
 Very pistol [flare] W34.19 ☑
Reduction in
 atmospheric pressure — see Air, pressure, change
Rock falling on or hitting (accidentally) (person) W20.8 ☑
 in cave-in W20.0 ☑
Run over (accidentally) (by)
 animal (not being ridden) NEC W55.89 ☑
 machinery — see Contact, with, by specified type of machine
 transport vehicle NEC (see also Accident, transport) V09.9 ☑
  intentional homicide (attempt) Y03.0 ☑
  motor NEC V09.20 ☑
   intentional homicide (attempt) Y03.0 ☑
Running
 before moving object X81.8 ☑
  motor vehicle X81.0 ☑
Running off, away
 animal (being ridden) (see also Accident, transport) V80.918 ☑
  not being ridden W55.89 ☑
 animal-drawn vehicle NEC (see also Accident, transport) V80.928 ☑
 highway, road (way), street
  transport vehicle NEC (see also Accident, transport) V89.9 ☑
Rupture pressurized devices — see Explosion, by type of device

S

Saturnism — see Table of Drugs and Chemicals, lead
Scald, scalding (accidental) (by) (from) (in) X19 ☑
 air (hot) X14.1 ☑
 gases (hot) X14.1 ☑
 homicide (attempt) — see Assault, burning, hot object
 inflicted by other person
  stated as intentional, homicide (attempt) — see Assault, burning, hot object
 liquid (boiling) (hot) NEC X12 ☑
  stated as undetermined whether accidental or intentional Y27.2 ☑
  suicide (attempt) X77.2 ☑
 local application of externally applied substance in medical or surgical care Y63.5
 metal (molten) (liquid) (hot) NEC X18 ☑
 self-inflicted X77.9 ☑
 stated as undetermined whether accidental or intentional Y27.8 ☑
 steam X13.1 ☑
  assault X98.0 ☑
  stated as undetermined whether accidental or intentional Y27.0 ☑
  suicide (attempt) X77.0 ☑
 suicide (attempt) X77.9 ☑
 vapor (hot) X13.1 ☑
  assault X98.0 ☑
  stated as undetermined whether accidental or intentional Y27.0 ☑
  suicide (attempt) X77.0 ☑
Scratched by
 cat W55.03 ☑
 person (s) (accidentally) W50.4 ☑
  with intent to injure or kill Y04.0 ☑

Scratched by — continued
 person (s) — continued
  as, or caused by, a crowd or human stampede (with fall) W52 ☑
  assault Y04.0 ☑
  homicide (attempt) Y04.0 ☑
  in
   fight Y04.0 ☑
   legal intervention
    injuring
     bystander Y35.892 ☑
     law enforcement personnel Y35.891 ☑
     suspect Y35.893 ☑
Seasickness T75.3 ☑
Self-harm NEC (see also External cause by type, undetermined whether accidental or intentional)
 intentional — see Suicide
 poisoning NEC — see Table of drugs and biologicals, accident
Self-inflicted (injury) NEC (see also External cause by type, undetermined whether accidental or intentional)
 intentional — see Suicide
 poisoning NEC — see Table of drugs and biologicals, accident
Sequelae (of)
 accident NEC — see W00-X58 with 7th character S
 assault (homicidal) (any means) — see X92-Y08 with 7th character S
 homicide, attempt (any means) — see X92-Y08 with 7th character S
 injury undetermined whether accidentally or purposely inflicted — see Y21-Y33 with 7th character S
 intentional self-harm (classifiable to X71-X83) — see X71-X83 with 7th character S
 legal intervention — see with 7th character S Y35 ☑
 motor vehicle accident — see V00-V99 with 7th character S
 suicide, attempt (any means) — see X71-X83 with 7th character S
 transport accident — see V00-V99 with 7th character S
 war operations — see War operations
Shock
 electric — see Exposure, electric current
 from electric appliance (any) (faulty) W86.8 ☑
  domestic W86.0 ☑
  suicide (attempt) X83.1 ☑
Shooting, shot (accidental(ly)) (see also Discharge, firearm, by type)
 herself or himself — see Discharge, firearm by type, self-inflicted
 homicide (attempt) — see Discharge, firearm by type, homicide
 in war operations — see War operations
 inflicted by other person — see Discharge, firearm by type, homicide
  accidental — see Discharge, firearm, by type of firearm
 legal
  execution — see Legal, intervention, firearm
  intervention — see Legal, intervention, firearm
 self-inflicted — see Discharge, firearm by type, suicide
  accidental — see Discharge, firearm, by type of firearm
 suicide (attempt) — see Discharge, firearm by type, suicide
Shoving (accidentally) by other person — see Pushed, by other person
Sickness
 alpine W94.11 ☑
 motion — see Motion
 mountain W94.11 ☑
Sinking (accidental)
 watercraft (causing drowning, submersion) (see also Drowning, due to, accident to, watercraft, sinking)
  causing injury except drowning or submersion — see Accident, watercraft, causing, injury NEC
Siriasis X32 ☑
Sitting (prolonged) (static) X50.1 ☑
Slashed wrists — see Cut, self-inflicted
Slipping (accidental) (on same level)
 (with fall) W01.0 ☑
 on
  ice W00.0 ☑
   with skates — see Accident, transport, pedestrian, conveyance

Slipping - Struck

Slipping — *continued*
  on — *continued*
    mud W01.0 ☑
    oil W01.0 ☑
    snow W00.0 ☑
      with skis — *see* Accident, transport, pedestrian, conveyance
    surface (slippery) (wet) NEC W01.0 ☑
  without fall W18.40 ☑
    due to
      specified NEC W18.49 ☑
      stepping from one level to another W18.43 ☑
      stepping into hole or opening W18.42 ☑
      stepping on object W18.41 ☑
Sliver, wood, contact with W45.8 ☑
Smoldering (due to fire) — *see* Exposure, fire
Sodomy (attempted) by force T74.2 ☑
Sound waves (causing injury) W42.9 ☑
  supersonic W42.0 ☑
Splinter, contact with W45.8 ☑
Stab, stabbing — *see* Cut
Standing (prolonged) (static) X50.1 ☑
Starvation X58 ☑
Status of external cause Y99.9
  child assisting in compensated work for family Y99.8
  civilian activity done for financial or other compensation Y99.0
  civilian activity done for income or pay Y99.0
  family member assisting in compensated work for other family member Y99.8
  hobby not done for income Y99.8
  leisure activity Y99.8
  military activity Y99.1
  off-duty activity of military personnel Y99.8
  recreation or sport not for income or while a student Y99.8
  specified NEC Y99.8
  student activity Y99.8
  volunteer activity Y99.2
Stepped on
  by
    animal (not being ridden) NEC W55.89 ☑
    crowd or human stampede W52 ☑
    person W50.0 ☑
Stepping on
  object W22.8 ☑
    with fall W18.31 ☑
    sports equipment W21.9 ☑
    stationary W22.09 ☑
      sports equipment W21.89 ☑
  person W51 ☑
    by crowd or human stampede W52 ☑
  sports equipment W21.9 ☑
Sting
  arthropod, nonvenomous W57 ☑
  insect, nonvenomous W57 ☑
Storm (cataclysmic) — *see* Forces of nature, cataclysmic storm
Straining, excessive (*see also* Overexertion) X50.9 ☑
Strangling — *see* Strangulation
Strangulation (accidental) T71
Strenuous movements (*see also* Overexertion) X50.9 ☑
Striking against
  airbag (automobile) W22.10 ☑
    driver side W22.11 ☑
    front passenger side W22.12 ☑
    specified NEC W22.19 ☑
  bottom when
    diving or jumping into water (in) W16.822 ☑
      causing drowning W16.821 ☑
      from boat W16.722 ☑
        causing drowning W16.721 ☑
      natural body W16.622 ☑
        causing drowning W16.821 ☑
      swimming pool W16.522 ☑
        causing drowning W16.521 ☑
    falling into water (in) W16.322 ☑
      causing drowning W16.321 ☑
      fountain — *see* Striking against, bottom when, falling into water, specified NEC
      natural body W16.122 ☑
        causing drowning W16.121 ☑
      reservoir — *see* Striking against, bottom when, falling into water, specified NEC
      specified NEC W16.322 ☑
        causing drowning W16.321 ☑
      swimming pool W16.022 ☑
        causing drowning W16.021 ☑
  diving board (swimming-pool) W21.4 ☑
  object W22.8 ☑

Striking against — *continued*
  object — *continued*
    with
      drowning or submersion — *see* Drowning
      fall — *see* Fall, due to, bumping against, object
    caused by crowd or human stampede (with fall) W52 ☑
    furniture W22.03 ☑
    lamppost W22.02 ☑
    sports equipment W21.9 ☑
    stationary W22.09 ☑
      sports equipment W21.89 ☑
    wall W22.01 ☑
  person (s) W51 ☑
    with fall W03 ☑
      due to ice or snow W00.0 ☑
    as, or caused by, a crowd or human stampede (with fall) W52 ☑
    assault Y04.2 ☑
    homicide (attempt) Y04.2 ☑
  sports equipment W21.9 ☑
  wall (when) W22.01 ☑
    diving or jumping into water (in) W16.832 ☑
      causing drowning W16.831 ☑
      swimming pool W16.532 ☑
        causing drowning W16.531 ☑
    falling into water (in) W16.332 ☑
      causing drowning W16.331 ☑
    fountain — *see* Striking against, wall when, falling into water, specified NEC
    natural body W16.132 ☑
      causing drowning W16.131 ☑
    reservoir — *see* Striking against, wall when, falling into water, specified NEC
    specified NEC W16.332 ☑
      causing drowning W16.331 ☑
    swimming pool W16.032 ☑
      causing drowning W16.031 ☑
    swimming pool (when) W22.042 ☑
      causing drowning W22.041 ☑
      diving or jumping into water W16.532 ☑
        causing drowning W16.531 ☑
      falling into water W16.032 ☑
        causing drowning W16.031 ☑
Struck (accidentally) by
  airbag (automobile) W22.10 ☑
    driver side W22.11 ☑
    front passenger side W22.12 ☑
    specified NEC W22.19 ☑
  alligator W58.02 ☑
  animal (not being ridden) NEC W55.89 ☑
  avalanche — *see* Landslide
  ball (hit) (thrown) W21.00 ☑
    assault Y08.09 ☑
    baseball W21.03 ☑
    basketball W21.05 ☑
    golf ball W21.04 ☑
    football W21.01 ☑
    soccer W21.02 ☑
    softball W21.07 ☑
    specified NEC W21.09 ☑
    volleyball W21.06 ☑
  bat or racquet
    baseball bat W21.11 ☑
      assault Y08.02 ☑
    golf club W21.13 ☑
      assault Y08.09 ☑
    specified NEC W21.19 ☑
      assault Y08.09 ☑
    tennis racquet W21.12 ☑
      assault Y08.09 ☑
  bullet (*see also* Discharge, firearm by type)
    in war operations — *see* War operations
  crocodile W58.12 ☑
  dog W54.1 ☑
  flare, Very pistol — *see* Discharge, firearm NEC
  hailstones X39.8 ☑
  hockey (ice)
    field
      puck W21.221 ☑
      stick W21.211 ☑
    puck W21.220 ☑
    stick W21.210 ☑
      assault Y08.01 ☑
  landslide — *see* Landslide
  law-enforcement agent (on duty) — *see* Legal, intervention, manhandling
    with blunt object — *see* Legal, intervention, blunt object
  lightning — *see* subcategory T75.0
    causing fire — *see* Exposure, fire

Struck by — *continued*
  machine — *see* Contact, with, by type of machine
  mammal NEC W55.89 ☑
  marine W56.32 ☑
  marine animal W56.82 ☑
  missile
    firearm — *see* Discharge, firearm by type
    in war operations — *see* War operations, missile
  object W22.8 ☑
    blunt W22.8 ☑
      assault Y00 ☑
      suicide (attempt) X79 ☑
      undetermined whether accidental or intentional Y29 ☑
    falling W20.8 ☑
      from, in, on
        building W20.1 ☑
          burning (uncontrolled fire) X00.4 ☑
        cataclysmic
          earth surface movement NEC — *see* Landslide
          storm — *see* Forces of nature, cataclysmic storm
        cave-in W20.0 ☑
        earthquake X34 ☑
        machine (in operation) — *see* Contact, with, by type of machine
        structure W20.1 ☑
          burning X00.4 ☑
        transport vehicle (in motion) — *see* Accident, transport, by type of vehicle
    watercraft V93.49 ☑
      due to
        accident to craft V91.39 ☑
          powered craft V91.33 ☑
            ferry boat V91.31 ☑
            fishing boat V91.32 ☑
            jet skis V91.33 ☑
            liner V91.31 ☑
            merchant ship V91.30 ☑
            passenger ship V91.31 ☑
          unpowered craft V91.38 ☑
            canoe V91.35 ☑
            inflatable V91.36 ☑
            kayak V91.35 ☑
            sailboat V91.34 ☑
            surf-board V91.38 ☑
            windsurfer V91.38 ☑
        powered craft V93.43 ☑
          ferry boat V93.41 ☑
          fishing boat V93.42 ☑
          jet skis V93.43 ☑
          liner V93.41 ☑
          merchant ship V93.40 ☑
          passenger ship V93.41 ☑
        unpowered craft V93.48 ☑
          sailboat V93.44 ☑
          surf-board V93.48 ☑
          windsurfer V93.48 ☑
  moving NEC W20.8 ☑
  projected W20.8 ☑
    assault Y00 ☑
    in sports W21.9 ☑
      assault Y08.09 ☑
      ball W21.00 ☑
        baseball W21.03 ☑
        basketball W21.05 ☑
        football W21.01 ☑
        golf ball W21.04 ☑
        soccer W21.02 ☑
        softball W21.07 ☑
        specified NEC W21.09 ☑
        volleyball W21.06 ☑
      bat or racquet
        baseball bat W21.11 ☑
          assault Y08.02 ☑
        golf club W21.13 ☑
          assault Y08.09 ☑
        specified NEC W21.19 ☑
          assault Y08.09 ☑
        tennis racquet W21.12 ☑
          assault Y08.09 ☑
      hockey (ice)
        field
          puck W21.221 ☑
          stick W21.211 ☑
        puck W21.220 ☑
        stick W21.210 ☑
          assault Y08.01 ☑
      specified NEC W21.89 ☑
  set in motion by explosion — *see* Explosion
  thrown W20.8 ☑

☑ **Additional character required**

Struck by — *continued*
  object — *continued*
    assault Y00 ☑
    in sports W21.9 ☑
      assault Y08.09 ☑
      ball W21.00 ☑
        baseball W21.03 ☑
        basketball W21.05 ☑
        football W21.01 ☑
        golf ball W21.04 ☑
        soccer W21.02 ☑
        soft ball W21.07 ☑
        specified NEC W21.09 ☑
        volleyball W21.06 ☑
      bat or racquet
        baseball bat W21.11 ☑
          assault Y08.02 ☑
        golf club W21.13 ☑
          assault Y08.09 ☑
        specified NEC W21.19 ☑
          assault Y08.09 ☑
        tennis racquet W21.12 ☑
          assault Y08.09 ☑
      hockey (ice)
        field
          puck W21.221 ☑
          stick W21.211 ☑
        puck W21.220 ☑
        stick W21.210 ☑
          assault Y08.01 ☑
      specified NEC W21.89 ☑
  other person (s) W50.0 ☑
    with
      blunt object W22.8 ☑
        intentional, homicide (attempt) Y00 ☑
      sports equipment W21.9 ☑
      undetermined whether accidental or
        intentional Y29 ☑
    fall W03 ☑
      due to ice or snow W00.0 ☑
    as, or caused by, a crowd or human stampede
      (with fall) W52 ☑
    assault Y04.2 ☑
    homicide (attempt) Y04.2 ☑
    in legal intervention
      injuring
        bystander Y35.812 ☑
        law enforcement personnel Y35.811 ☑
        suspect Y35.813 ☑
    sports equipment W21.9 ☑
  police (on duty) — *see* Legal, intervention,
    manhandling
    with blunt object — *see* Legal, intervention,
      blunt object
  sports equipment W21.9 ☑
    assault Y08.09 ☑
    ball W21.00 ☑
      baseball W21.03 ☑
      basketball W21.05 ☑
      football W21.01 ☑
      golf ball W21.04 ☑
      soccer W21.02 ☑
      soft ball W21.07 ☑
      specified NEC W21.09 ☑
      volleyball W21.06 ☑
    bat or racquet
      baseball bat W21.11 ☑
        assault Y08.02 ☑
      golf club W21.13 ☑
        assault Y08.09 ☑
      specified NEC W21.19 ☑
      tennis racquet W21.12 ☑
        assault Y08.09 ☑
    cleats (shoe) W21.31 ☑
    foot wear NEC W21.39 ☑
    football helmet W21.81 ☑
    hockey (ice)
      field
        puck W21.221 ☑
        stick W21.211 ☑
      puck W21.220 ☑
      stick W21.210 ☑
        assault Y08.01 ☑
    skate blades W21.32 ☑
    specified NEC W21.89 ☑
      assault Y08.09 ☑
  thunderbolt — *see* subcategory T75.0
    causing fire — *see* Exposure, fire
  transport vehicle NEC (*see also* Accident,
    transport) V09.9 ☑
    intentional, homicide (attempt) Y03.0 ☑

Struck by — *continued*
  transport vehicle NEC — *continued*
    motor NEC (*see also* Accident,
      transport) V09.20 ☑
      homicide Y03.0 ☑
    vehicle (transport) NEC — *see* Accident, transport,
      by type of vehicle
    stationary (falling from jack, hydraulic lift,
      ramp) W20.8 ☑
Stumbling
  over
    animal NEC W01.0 ☑
      with fall W18.09 ☑
    carpet, rug or (small) object W22.8 ☑
      with fall W18.09 ☑
    person W51 ☑
      with fall W03 ☑
        due to ice or snow W00.0 ☑
  without fall W18.40 ☑
    due to
      specified NEC W18.49 ☑
      stepping from one level to another W18.43 ☑
      stepping into hole or opening W18.42 ☑
      stepping on object W18.41 ☑
Submersion (accidental) — *see* Drowning
Suffocation (accidental) (by external means) (by
  pressure) (mechanical) (*see also* category) T71 ☑
  due to, by
    avalanche — *see* Landslide
    explosion — *see* Explosion
    fire — *see* Exposure, fire
    food, any type (aspiration) (ingestion)
      (inhalation) — *see* categories T17
      and T18 ☑
    ignition — *see* Ignition
    landslide — *see* Landslide
    machine (ry) — *see* Contact, with, by type of
      machine
    vomitus (aspiration) (inhalation) T17.81 ☑
  in
    burning building X00.8 ☑
Suicide, suicidal (attempted) (by) X83.8 ☑
  blunt object X79 ☑
  burning, burns X76 ☑
    hot object X77.9 ☑
      fluid NEC X77.2 ☑
      household appliance X77.3 ☑
      specified NEC X77.8 ☑
      steam X77.0 ☑
      tap water X77.1 ☑
      vapors X77.0 ☑
  caustic substance — *see* Table of Drugs and
    Chemicals
  cold, extreme X83.2 ☑
  collision of motor vehicle with
    motor vehicle X82.0 ☑
    specified NEC X82.8 ☑
    train X82.1 ☑
    tree X82.2 ☑
  crashing of aircraft X83.0 ☑
  cut (any part of body) X78.9 ☑
  cutting or piercing instrument X78.9 ☑
    dagger X78.2 ☑
    glass X78.0 ☑
    knife X78.1 ☑
    specified NEC X78.8 ☑
    sword X78.2 ☑
  drowning (in) X71.9 ☑
    bathtub X71.0 ☑
    natural water X71.3 ☑
    specified NEC X71.8 ☑
    swimming pool X71.1 ☑
      following fall X71.2 ☑
  electrocution X83.1 ☑
  explosive (s) (material) X75 ☑
  fire, flames X76 ☑
  firearm X74.9 ☑
    airgun X74.01 ☑
    handgun X72 ☑
    hunting rifle X73.1 ☑
    larger X73.9 ☑
      specified NEC X73.8 ☑
    machine gun X73.2 ☑
    shotgun X73.0 ☑
    specified NEC X74.8 ☑
  hanging X83.8 ☑
  hot object — *see* Suicide, burning, hot object
  jumping
    before moving object X81.8 ☑
      motor vehicle X81.0 ☑
      subway train X81.1 ☑
      train X81.1 ☑

Suicide, suicidal — *continued*
  jumping — *continued*
    from high place X80 ☑
  late effect of attempt — *see* X71-X83 with 7th
    character S
  lying before moving object, train, vehicle X81.8 ☑
  poisoning — *see* Table of Drugs and Chemicals
  puncture (any part of body) — *see* Suicide,
    cutting or piercing instrument
  scald — *see* Suicide, burning, hot object
  sequelae of attempt — *see* X71-X83 with 7th
    character S
  sharp object (any) — *see* Suicide, cutting or
    piercing instrument
  shooting — *see* Suicide, firearm
  specified means NEC X83.8 ☑
  stab (any part of body) — *see* Suicide, cutting or
    piercing instrument
  steam, hot vapors X77.0 ☑
  strangulation X83.8 ☑
  submersion — *see* Suicide, drowning
  suffocation X83.8 ☑
  wound NEC X83.8 ☑
Sunstroke X32 ☑
Supersonic waves (causing injury) W42.0 ☑
Surgical procedure, complication of (delayed
  or as an abnormal reaction without mention
  of misadventure) (*see also* Complication of or
  following, by type of procedure)
  due to or as a result of misadventure — *see*
    Misadventure
Swallowed, swallowing
  foreign body — *see* Foreign body, alimentary
    canal
  poison — *see* Table of Drugs and Chemicals
  substance
    caustic or corrosive — *see* Table of Drugs and
      Chemicals
    poisonous — *see* Table of Drugs and Chemicals

T

Tackle in sport W03 ☑
Terrorism (involving) Y38.80 ☑
  biological weapons Y38.6X ☑
  chemical weapons Y38.7X ☑
  conflagration Y38.3X ☑
  drowning and submersion Y38.89 ☑
  explosion Y38.2X ☑
    destruction of aircraft Y38.1X ☑
    marine weapons Y38.0X ☑
  fire Y38.3X ☑
  firearms Y38.4X ☑
  hot substances Y38.3X ☑
  lasers Y38.89 ☑
  nuclear weapons Y38.5X ☑
  piercing or stabbing instruments Y38.89 ☑
  secondary effects Y38.9X ☑
  specified method NEC Y38.89 ☑
  suicide bomber Y38.81 ☑
Thirst X58 ☑
Threat to breathing
  aspiration — *see* Aspiration
  due to cave-in, falling earth or substance NEC T71
Thrown (accidentally)
  against part (any) of or object in transport vehicle
    (in motion) NEC (*see also* Accident, transport)
  from
    high place, homicide (attempt) Y01 ☑
    machinery — *see* Contact, with, by type of
      machine
    transport vehicle NEC (*see also* Accident,
      transport) V89.9 ☑
  off — *see* Thrown, from
Thunderbolt — *see* subcategory T75.0
  causing fire — *see* Exposure, fire
Tidal wave (any injury) NEC — *see* Forces of nature,
  tidal wave
Took
  overdose (drug) — *see* Table of Drugs and
    Chemicals
  poison — *see* Table of Drugs and Chemicals
Tornado (any injury) X37.1 ☑
Torrential rain (any injury) X37.8 ☑
Torture X58 ☑
Trampled by animal NEC W55.89 ☑
Trapped (accidentally)
  between objects (moving) (stationary and
    moving) — *see* Caught
  by part (any) of

A05.4 Foodborne Bacillus cereus intoxication · CC/MCC Exc

A05.5 Foodborne Vibrio vulnificus intoxication · CC/MCC Exc

A05.8 Other specified bacterial foodborne intoxications · CC/MCC Exc

A05.9 Bacterial foodborne intoxication, unspecified

A06 Amebiasis

INCLUDES infection due to Entamoeba histolytica

EXCLUDES1 other protozoal intestinal diseases (A07.-)

EXCLUDES2 acanthamebiasis (B60.1-)

Naegleriasis (B60.2)

A06.0 Acute amebic dysentery · CC/MCC Exc
Acute amebiasis
Intestinal amebiasis NOS

A06.1 Chronic intestinal amebiasis · CC/MCC Exc

A06.2 Amebic nondysenteric colitis · CC/MCC Exc

A06.3 Ameboma of intestine · CC/MCC Exc
Ameboma NOS

A06.4 Amebic liver abscess · MCC CC/MCC Exc
Hepatic amebiasis

A06.5 Amebic lung abscess · HCC MCC CC/MCC Exc
Amebic abscess of lung (and liver)

A06.6 Amebic brain abscess · MCC CC/MCC Exc
Amebic abscess of brain (and liver) (and lung)

A06.7 Cutaneous amebiasis

A06.8 Amebic infection of other sites

A06.81 Amebic cystitis · CC/MCC Exc

A06.82 Other amebic genitourinary infections · CC/MCC Exc
Amebic balanitis
Amebic vesiculitis
Amebic vulvovaginitis

A06.89 Other amebic infections · CC/MCC Exc
Amebic appendicitis
Amebic splenic abscess

A06.9 Amebiasis, unspecified

A07 Other protozoal intestinal diseases

A07.0 Balantidiasis
Balantidial dysentery

A07.1 Giardiasis [lambliasis] · HCC RHCC CC/MCC Exc

A07.2 Cryptosporidiosis · CC/MCC Exc

A07.3 Isosporiasis
Infection due to Isospora belli and Isospora hominis
Intestinal coccidiosis
Isosporosis

A07.4 Cyclosporiasis · CC/MCC Exc

A07.8 Other specified protozoal intestinal diseases · CC/MCC Exc
Intestinal microsporidiosis
Intestinal trichomoniasis
Sarcocystosis
Sarcosporidiosis

A07.9 Protozoal intestinal disease, unspecified · CC/MCC Exc
Flagellate diarrhea
Protozoal colitis
Protozoal diarrhea
Protozoal dysentery

A08 Viral and other specified intestinal infections

EXCLUDES1 influenza with involvement of gastrointestinal tract (J09.X3, J10.2, J11.2)

A08.0 Rotaviral enteritis · CC/MCC Exc

A08.1 Acute gastroenteropathy due to Norwalk agent and other small round viruses

A08.11 Acute gastroenteropathy due to Norwalk agent · CC/MCC Exc
Acute gastroenteropathy due to Norovirus
Acute gastroenteropathy due to Norwalk-like agent

A08.19 Acute gastroenteropathy due to other small round viruses · CC/MCC Exc
Acute gastroenteropathy due to small round virus [SRV] NOS

A08.2 Adenoviral enteritis · CC/MCC Exc

A08.3 Other viral enteritis

A08.31 Calicivirus enteritis · CC/MCC Exc

A08.32 Astrovirus enteritis · CC/MCC Exc

A08.39 Other viral enteritis · CC/MCC Exc
Coxsackie virus enteritis
Echovirus enteritis
Enterovirus enteritis NEC
Torovirus enteritis

A08.4 Viral intestinal infection, unspecified
AHA: Q3 2016
Viral enteritis NOS
Viral gastroenteritis NOS
Viral gastroenteropathy NOS

A08.8 Other specified intestinal infections

A09 Infectious gastroenteritis and colitis, unspecified · CC/MCC Exc
Infectious colitis NOS
Infectious enteritis NOS
Infectious gastroenteritis NOS
EXCLUDES1 colitis NOS (K52.9)
diarrhea NOS (R19.7)
enteritis NOS (K52.9)
gastroenteritis NOS (K52.9)
noninfective gastroenteritis and colitis, unspecified (K52.9)

Tuberculosis (A15-A19)

INCLUDES infections due to Mycobacterium tuberculosis and Mycobacterium bovis

EXCLUDES1 congenital tuberculosis (P37.0)
nonspecific reaction to test for tuberculosis without active tuberculosis (R76.1-)
pneumoconiosis associated with tuberculosis, any type in A15 (J65)
positive PPD (R76.11)
positive tuberculin skin test without active tuberculosis (R76.11)
sequelae of tuberculosis (B90.-)
silicotuberculosis (J65)

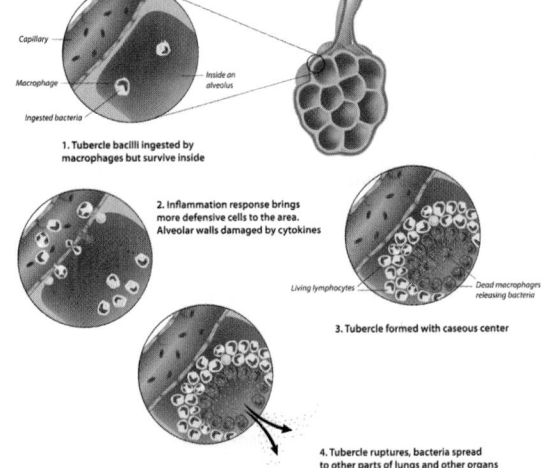

Figure 1.1 Progression of tuberculosis

A15 Respiratory tuberculosis

A15.0 Tuberculosis of lung · CC/MCC Exc
Tuberculous bronchiectasis
Tuberculous fibrosis of lung
Tuberculous pneumonia
Tuberculous pneumothorax

A15.4 Tuberculosis of intrathoracic lymph nodes · CC/MCC Exc
Tuberculosis of hilar lymph nodes
Tuberculosis of mediastinal lymph nodes
Tuberculosis of tracheobronchial lymph nodes
EXCLUDES1 tuberculosis specified as primary (A15.7)

A15.5 Tuberculosis of larynx, trachea **and** bronchus   cc CC/MCC Exc
  Tuberculosis of bronchus
  Tuberculosis of glottis
  Tuberculosis of larynx
  Tuberculosis of trachea
A15.6 Tuberculous pleurisy   cc CC/MCC Exc
  Tuberculosis of pleura Tuberculous empyema
  EXCLUDES1 *primary respiratory tuberculosis (A15.7)*
A15.7 Primary respiratory tuberculosis   cc CC/MCC Exc
A15.8 Other respiratory tuberculosis   cc CC/MCC Exc
  Mediastinal tuberculosis
  Nasopharyngeal tuberculosis
  Tuberculosis of nose
  Tuberculosis of sinus [any nasal]
A15.9 Respiratory tuberculosis unspecified   cc CC/MCC Exc
4ᵗʰ **A17 Tuberculosis of** nervous system
  A17.0 Tuberculosis meningitis   MCC CC/MCC Exc
    Tuberculosis of meninges (cerebral)(spinal)
    Tuberculous leptomeningitis
    EXCLUDES1 *tuberculous meningoencephalitis (A17.82)*
  A17.1 Meningeal tuberculoma   MCC CC/MCC Exc
    Tuberculoma of meninges (cerebral) (spinal)
    EXCLUDES2 *tuberculoma of brain and spinal cord (A17.81)*
  5ᵗʰ **A17.8 Other tuberculosis of** nervous system
    A17.81 Tuberculoma of brain and spinal cord   MCC CC/MCC Exc
      Tuberculous abscess of brain and spinal cord
    A17.82 Tuberculous meningoencephalitis   MCC CC/MCC Exc
      Tuberculous myelitis
    A17.83 Tuberculous neuritis   MCC
      Tuberculous mononeuropathy
    A17.89 Other tuberculosis of nervous system   MCC CC/MCC Exc
      Tuberculous polyneuropathy
  A17.9 Tuberculosis of nervous system, unspecified   cc CC/MCC Exc
4ᵗʰ **A18 Tuberculosis of** other organs
  5ᵗʰ **A18.0 Tuberculosis of** bones and joints
    A18.01 Tuberculosis of spine   cc CC/MCC Exc
      Pott's disease or curvature of spine
      Tuberculous arthritis
      Tuberculous osteomyelitis of spine
      Tuberculous spondylitis
    A18.02 Tuberculous arthritis of other joints   cc CC/MCC Exc
      Tuberculosis of hip (joint)
      Tuberculosis of knee (joint)
    A18.03 Tuberculosis of other bones   cc CC/MCC Exc
      Tuberculous mastoiditis
      Tuberculous osteomyelitis
    A18.09 Other musculoskeletal tuberculosis   cc CC/MCC Exc
      Tuberculous myositis
      Tuberculous synovitis
      Tuberculous tenosynovitis
  5ᵗʰ **A18.1 Tuberculosis of** genitourinary system
    A18.10 Tuberculosis of genitourinary system, unspecified   cc CC/MCC Exc
    A18.11 Tuberculosis of kidney and ureter   cc CC/MCC Exc
    A18.12 Tuberculosis of bladder   cc CC/MCC Exc
    A18.13 Tuberculosis of other urinary organs   cc CC/MCC Exc
      Tuberculous urethritis
    A18.14 Tuberculosis of prostate   A cc ♂ CC/MCC Exc
    A18.15 Tuberculosis of other male genital organs   cc ♂ CC/MCC Exc
    A18.16 Tuberculosis of cervix   cc ♀ CC/MCC Exc
    A18.17 Tuberculous female pelvic inflammatory disease   cc ♀ CC/MCC Exc
      Tuberculous endometritis
      Tuberculous oophoritis and salpingitis
    A18.18 Tuberculosis of other female genital organs   cc ♀ CC/MCC Exc
      Tuberculous ulceration of vulva
  A18.2 Tuberculous peripheral lymphadenopathy   cc CC/MCC Exc
    Tuberculous adenitis

    EXCLUDES2 *tuberculosis of bronchial and mediastinal lymph nodes*
      (A15.4)
      tuberculosis of mesenteric and retroperitoneal lymph
      nodes (A18.39)
      tuberculous tracheobronchial adenopathy (A15.4)
  5ᵗʰ **A18.3 Tuberculosis of** intestines, peritoneum and mesenteric glands
    A18.31 Tuberculous peritonitis   MCC CC/MCC Exc
      Tuberculous ascites
    A18.32 Tuberculous enteritis   cc CC/MCC Exc
      Tuberculosis of anus and rectum
      Tuberculosis of intestine (large) (small)
    A18.39 Retroperitoneal tuberculosis   cc CC/MCC Exc
      Tuberculosis of mesenteric glands
      Tuberculosis of retroperitoneal (lymph glands)
  A18.4 Tuberculosis of skin and subcutaneous tissue   cc CC/MCC Exc
    Erythema induratum, tuberculous
    Lupus excedens
    Lupus vulgaris NOS
    Lupus vulgaris of eyelid
    Scrofuloderma
    Tuberculosis of external ear
    EXCLUDES2 *lupus erythematosus (L93.-)*
      lupus NOS (M32.9)
      systemic (M32.-)
  5ᵗʰ **A18.5 Tuberculosis of** eye
    EXCLUDES2 *lupus vulgaris of eyelid (A18.4)*
    A18.50 Tuberculosis of eye, unspecified   cc CC/MCC Exc
    A18.51 Tuberculous episcleritis   cc CC/MCC Exc
    A18.52 Tuberculous keratitis   cc CC/MCC Exc
      Tuberculous interstitial keratitis
      Tuberculous keratoconjunctivitis (interstitial)
        (phlyctenular)
    A18.53 Tuberculous chorioretinitis   cc CC/MCC Exc
    A18.54 Tuberculous iridocyclitis   cc CC/MCC Exc
    A18.59 Other tuberculosis of eye   cc CC/MCC Exc
      Tuberculous conjunctivitis
  A18.6 Tuberculosis of (inner) (middle) ear   cc CC/MCC Exc
    Tuberculous otitis media
    EXCLUDES2 *tuberculosis of external ear (A18.4)*
      tuberculous mastoiditis (A18.03)
  A18.7 Tuberculosis of adrenal glands   cc CC/MCC Exc
    Tuberculous Addison's disease
  5ᵗʰ **A18.8 Tuberculosis of other** specified organs
    A18.81 Tuberculosis of thyroid gland   cc CC/MCC Exc
    A18.82 Tuberculosis of other endocrine glands   cc CC/MCC Exc
      Tuberculosis of pituitary gland
      Tuberculosis of thymus gland
    A18.83 Tuberculosis of digestive tract organs, not elsewhere classified   cc CC/MCC Exc
      EXCLUDES1 *tuberculosis of intestine (A18.32)*
    A18.84 Tuberculosis of heart   cc CC/MCC Exc
      Tuberculous cardiomyopathy
      Tuberculous endocarditis
      Tuberculous myocarditis
      Tuberculous pericarditis
    A18.85 Tuberculosis of spleen   cc CC/MCC Exc
    A18.89 Tuberculosis of other sites   cc CC/MCC Exc
      Tuberculosis of muscle
      Tuberculous cerebral arteritis
4ᵗʰ **A19 Miliary tuberculosis**
  INCLUDES *disseminated tuberculosis*
    generalized tuberculosis
    tuberculous polyserositis
  A19.0 Acute miliary tuberculosis of a single specified site   MCC CC/MCC Exc
  A19.1 Acute miliary tuberculosis of multiple sites   MCC CC/MCC Exc
  A19.2 Acute miliary tuberculosis, unspecified   MCC CC/MCC Exc
  A19.8 Other miliary tuberculosis   MCC CC/MCC Exc
  A19.9 Miliary tuberculosis, unspecified   MCC CC/MCC Exc

Unspecified Code   Other Specified Code   Manifestation Code   N Newborn   P Pediatric   M Maternity   A Adult   ♂ Male   ♀ Female
● New Code   ▲ Revised Code Title   ►◄ Revised Text   NOTES   *INCLUDES*   *EXCLUDES 1* Not coded here   *EXCLUDES 2* Not included here
4ᵗʰ 4ᵗʰ character required   5ᵗʰ 5ᵗʰ character required   6ᵗʰ 6ᵗʰ character required   7ᵗʰ 7ᵗʰ character required
7ˣ Extension 'X' Alert   HAC Hospital-acquired condition (HAC) alert   AHA AHA Coding Clinic©

Certain zoonotic bacterial diseases (A20-A28)

A20 Plague
- *INCLUDES* infection due to Yersinia pestis
  - **A20.0** Bubonic **plague** `MCC` `CC/MCC Exc`
  - **A20.1** Cellulocutaneous **plague** `MCC` `CC/MCC Exc`
  - **A20.2** Pneumonic **plague** `HCC` `MCC` `CC/MCC Exc`
  - **A20.3** **Plague** meningitis `MCC` `CC/MCC Exc`
  - **A20.7** Septicemic **plague** `HCC` `MCC` `CC/MCC Exc`
  - **A20.8** Other forms of plague `MCC` `CC/MCC Exc`
    Abortive plague
    Asymptomatic plague
    Pestis minor
  - **A20.9** **Plague, unspecified** `MCC` `CC/MCC Exc`

A21 Tularemia
- *INCLUDES* deer-fly fever
  - infection due to Francisella tularensis
  - rabbit fever
  - **A21.0** Ulceroglandular **tularemia** `CC` `CC/MCC Exc`
  - **A21.1** Oculoglandular **tularemia** `CC` `CC/MCC Exc`
    Ophthalmic tularemia
  - **A21.2** Pulmonary **tularemia** `CC` `HCC` `CC/MCC Exc`
  - **A21.3** Gastrointestinal **tularemia** `CC` `CC/MCC Exc`
    Abdominal tularemia
  - **A21.7** Generalized **tularemia** `CC` `CC/MCC Exc`
  - **A21.8** Other forms of tularemia `CC` `CC/MCC Exc`
  - **A21.9** **Tularemia, unspecified** `CC` `CC/MCC Exc`

A22 Anthrax
- *INCLUDES* infection due to Bacillus anthracis
  - **A22.0** Cutaneous **anthrax** `CC` `CC/MCC Exc`
    Malignant carbuncle
    Malignant pustule
  - **A22.1** Pulmonary **anthrax** `HCC` `MCC` `CC/MCC Exc`
    Inhalation anthrax
    Ragpicker's disease
    Woolsorter's disease
  - **A22.2** Gastrointestinal **anthrax** `CC` `CC/MCC Exc`
  - **A22.7** **Anthrax** sepsis `HCC` `MCC` `PDx MCC` `CC/MCC Exc`
  - **A22.8** Other forms of anthrax `CC` `CC/MCC Exc`
    Anthrax meningitis
  - **A22.9** **Anthrax, unspecified** `CC` `CC/MCC Exc`

A23 Brucellosis
- *INCLUDES* Malta fever
  - Mediterranean fever
  - undulant fever
  - **A23.0** **Brucellosis due to Brucella** melitensis
  - **A23.1** **Brucellosis due to Brucella** abortus
  - **A23.2** **Brucellosis due to Brucella** suis
  - **A23.3** **Brucellosis due to Brucella** canis
  - **A23.8** Other brucellosis `CC` `CC/MCC Exc`
  - **A23.9** **Brucellosis, unspecified** `CC` `CC/MCC Exc`

A24 Glanders and melioidosis
  - **A24.0** Glanders `CC` `CC/MCC Exc`
    Infection due to Pseudomonas mallei
    Malleus
  - **A24.1** Acute and fulminating **melioidosis** `CC` `CC/MCC Exc`
    Melioidosis pneumonia
    Melioidosis sepsis
  - **A24.2** Subacute and chronic **melioidosis** `CC` `CC/MCC Exc`
  - **A24.3** Other melioidosis `CC` `CC/MCC Exc`
  - **A24.9** **Melioidosis, unspecified** `CC` `CC/MCC Exc`
    Infection due to Pseudomonas pseudomallei NOS
    Whitmore's disease

A25 Rat-bite fevers
  - **A25.0** Spirillosis `CC` `CC/MCC Exc`
    Sodoku
  - **A25.1** Streptobacillosis `CC` `CC/MCC Exc`
    Epidemic arthritic erythema
    Haverhill fever
    Streptobacillary rat-bite fever

  - **A25.9** **Rat-bite fever, unspecified** `CC` `CC/MCC Exc`

A26 Erysipeloid
  - **A26.0** Cutaneous **erysipeloid**
    Erythema migrans
  - **A26.7** **Erysipelothrix** sepsis `HCC` `MCC` `PDx MCC` `CC/MCC Exc`
  - **A26.8** Other forms of erysipeloid
  - **A26.9** **Erysipeloid, unspecified**

A27 Leptospirosis
  - **A27.0** Leptospirosis icterohemorrhagica `CC` `CC/MCC Exc`
    Leptospiral or spirochetal jaundice (hemorrhagic)
    Weil's disease
  - **A27.8** Other forms of leptospirosis
    - **A27.81** Aseptic meningitis in leptospirosis `MCC` `CC/MCC Exc`
    - **A27.89** Other forms of leptospirosis `CC` `CC/MCC Exc`
  - **A27.9** **Leptospirosis, unspecified** `CC` `CC/MCC Exc`

A28 Other zoonotic bacterial diseases, not elsewhere classified
  - **A28.0** Pasteurellosis `CC` `CC/MCC Exc`
  - **A28.1** Cat-scratch disease `CC` `CC/MCC Exc`
    Cat-scratch fever
  - **A28.2** Extraintestinal yersiniosis `CC` `CC/MCC Exc`
    EXCLUDES1 enteritis due to Yersinia enterocolitica (A04.6)
    plague (A20.-)
  - **A28.8** Other specified zoonotic bacterial diseases, not elsewhere classified `CC` `CC/MCC Exc`
  - **A28.9** Zoonotic bacterial disease, unspecified `CC` `CC/MCC Exc`

Other bacterial diseases (A30-A49)

A30 Leprosy [Hansen's disease]
- *INCLUDES* infection due to Mycobacterium leprae
- *EXCLUDES1* sequelae of leprosy (B92)
  - **A30.0** Indeterminate **leprosy** `CC` `CC/MCC Exc`
    AHA: Q3 2016
    I leprosy
  - **A30.1** Tuberculoid **leprosy** `CC` `CC/MCC Exc`
    AHA: Q3 2016
    TT leprosy
  - **A30.2** Borderline tuberculoid **leprosy** `CC` `CC/MCC Exc`
    AHA: Q3 2016
    BT leprosy
  - **A30.3** Borderline **leprosy** `CC` `CC/MCC Exc`
    AHA: Q3 2016
    BB leprosy
  - **A30.4** Borderline lepromatous **leprosy** `CC` `CC/MCC Exc`
    AHA: Q3 2016
    BL leprosy
  - **A30.5** Lepromatous **leprosy** `CC` `CC/MCC Exc`
    AHA: Q3 2016
    LL leprosy
  - **A30.8** Other forms of leprosy `CC` `CC/MCC Exc`
    AHA: Q3 2016
  - **A30.9** **Leprosy, unspecified** `CC` `CC/MCC Exc`
    AHA: Q3 2016

A31 Infection due to other mycobacteria
- *EXCLUDES2* leprosy (A30.-)
  - tuberculosis (A15-A19)
  - **A31.0** Pulmonary mycobacterial infection `CC` `HCC` `RxHCC` `CC/MCC Exc`
    AHA: Q3 2016
    Infection due to Mycobacterium avium
    Infection due to Mycobacterium intracellulare [Battey bacillus]
    Infection due to Mycobacterium kansasii
  - **A31.1** Cutaneous mycobacterial infection `CC` `CC/MCC Exc`
    AHA: Q3 2016
    Buruli ulcer
    Infection due to Mycobacterium marinum
    Infection due to Mycobacterium ulcerans
  - **A31.2** Disseminated **mycobacterium avium-intracellulare complex (DMAC)** `CC` `HCC` `RxHCC` `CC/MCC Exc`
    AHA: Q3 2016
    MAC sepsis

`PDx` Unacceptable principal diagnosis symbol per Medicare code edits   `?` Code exempt from diagnosis present on admission requirement
`?` Questionable admission   `CC` Complication or comorbidity   `CC/MCC Exc` CC/MCC exclusion   `MCC` Major complication or comorbidity
`PDx CC` Principal diagnosis as its own CC   `PDx MCC` Principal diagnosis as its own MCC   `HCC` HCC diagnosis code   `RxHCC` RxHCC diagnosis code
MACRA code   `Z1` Z code as first-listed diagnosis

A31.8 Other mycobacterial infections   CC CC/MCC Exc
     AHA: Q3 2016
A31.9 **Mycobacterial infection, unspecified**   CC CC/MCC Exc
     AHA: Q3 2016
     Atypical mycobacterial infection NOS
     Mycobacteriosis NOS

A32 Listeriosis
    INCLUDES   listerial foodborne infection
    EXCLUDES1 neonatal (disseminated) listeriosis (P37.2)
   A32.0 **Cutaneous** listeriosis   CC CC/MCC Exc
      AHA: Q3 2016
   A32.1 **Listerial meningitis and meningoencephalitis**
      A32.11 **Listerial** meningitis   CC CC/MCC Exc
         AHA: Q3 2016
      A32.12 **Listerial** meningoencephalitis   CC CC/MCC Exc
         AHA: Q3 2016
   A32.7 **Listerial** sepsis   HCC MCC PDx MCC CC/MCC Exc
      AHA: Q3 2016
   A32.8 **Other forms of listeriosis**
      A32.81 **Oculoglandular** listeriosis   CC CC/MCC Exc
         AHA: Q3 2016
      A32.82 **Listerial** endocarditis   CC CC/MCC Exc
         AHA: Q3 2016
      A32.89 **Other forms of listeriosis**   CC CC/MCC Exc
         AHA: Q3 2016
         Listerial cerebral arteritis
   A32.9 **Listeriosis, unspecified**   CC CC/MCC Exc
      AHA: Q3 2016

A33 **Tetanus neonatorum**   N MCC CC/MCC Exc
     AHA: Q3 2016
A34 **Obstetrical tetanus**   M CC ♀ CC/MCC Exc
     AHA: Q3 2016
A35 **Other tetanus**   MCC CC/MCC Exc
     AHA: Q3 2016
     Tetanus NOS
     EXCLUDES1 obstetrical tetanus (A34)
         tetanus neonatorum (A33)

A36 Diphtheria
   A36.0 **Pharyngeal** diphtheria   CC CC/MCC Exc
      AHA: Q3 2016
      Diphtheritic membranous angina
      Tonsillar diphtheria
   A36.1 **Nasopharyngeal** diphtheria   CC CC/MCC Exc
      AHA: Q3 2016
   A36.2 **Laryngeal** diphtheria   CC CC/MCC Exc
      AHA: Q3 2016
      Diphtheritic laryngotracheitis
   A36.3 **Cutaneous** diphtheria   CC CC/MCC Exc
      AHA: Q3 2016
      EXCLUDES2 erythrasma (L08.1)
   A36.8 **Other diphtheria**
      A36.81 **Diphtheritic** cardiomyopathy   CC HCC RhHCC CC/MCC Exc
         AHA: Q3 2016
         Diphtheritic myocarditis
      A36.82 **Diphtheritic** radiculomyelitis   CC CC/MCC Exc
         AHA: Q3 2016
      A36.83 **Diphtheritic** polyneuritis   CC CC/MCC Exc
         AHA: Q3 2016
      A36.84 **Diphtheritic** tubulo-interstitial
         nephropathy   CC CC/MCC Exc
         AHA: Q3 2016
      A36.85 **Diphtheritic** cystitis   CC CC/MCC Exc
         AHA: Q3 2016
      A36.86 **Diphtheritic** conjunctivitis   CC CC/MCC Exc
         AHA: Q3 2016
      A36.89 **Other diphtheritic complications**   CC CC/MCC Exc
         AHA: Q3 2016
         Diphtheritic peritonitis
   A36.9 **Diphtheria, unspecified**   CC CC/MCC Exc
      AHA: Q3 2016

A37 Whooping cough
   A37.0 **Whooping cough due to** Bordetella pertussis
      A37.00 **Whooping cough due to Bordetella pertussis**
         without pneumonia   CC CC/MCC Exc
         AHA: Q3 2016
      A37.01 **Whooping cough due to Bordetella pertussis**
         with pneumonia   MCC PDx MCC CC/MCC Exc
         AHA: Q3 2016
   A37.1 **Whooping cough due to** Bordetella parapertussis
      A37.10 **Whooping cough due to Bordetella parapertussis**
         without pneumonia   CC CC/MCC Exc
         AHA: Q3 2016
      A37.11 **Whooping cough due to Bordetella parapertussis**
         with pneumonia   MCC PDx MCC CC/MCC Exc
         AHA: Q3 2016
   A37.8 **Whooping cough due to** other Bordetella species
      A37.80 **Whooping cough due to other Bordetella species**
         without pneumonia   CC CC/MCC Exc
         AHA: Q3 2016
      A37.81 **Whooping cough due to other Bordetella species**
         with pneumonia   MCC PDx MCC CC/MCC Exc
         AHA: Q3 2016
   A37.9 **Whooping cough, unspecified species**
      A37.90 **Whooping cough, unspecified species without**
         pneumonia   CC CC/MCC Exc
         AHA: Q3 2016
      A37.91 **Whooping cough, unspecified species with**
         pneumonia   MCC PDx MCC CC/MCC Exc
         AHA: Q3 2016

A38 Scarlet fever
    INCLUDES   scarlatina
    EXCLUDES2 streptococcal sore throat (J02.0)
   A38.0 **Scarlet fever** with otitis media   CC CC/MCC Exc
      AHA: Q3 2016
   A38.1 **Scarlet fever** with myocarditis   CC CC/MCC Exc
      AHA: Q3 2016
   A38.8 **Scarlet fever** with other complications   CC CC/MCC Exc
      AHA: Q3 2016
   A38.9 **Scarlet fever,** uncomplicated   CC CC/MCC Exc
      AHA: Q3 2016
      Scarlet fever, NOS

A39 Meningococcal infection
   A39.0 **Meningococcal** meningitis   MCC CC/MCC Exc
      AHA: Q3 2016
   A39.1 **Waterhouse-Friderichsen syndrome**   HCC MCC RhHCC CC/MCC Exc
      AHA: Q3 2016
      Meningococcal hemorrhagic adrenalitis
      Meningococcic adrenal syndrome
   A39.2 **Acute meningococcemia**   HCC MCC CC/MCC Exc
      AHA: Q3 2016
   A39.3 **Chronic meningococcemia**   HCC MCC CC/MCC Exc
      AHA: Q3 2016
   A39.4 **Meningococcemia, unspecified**   HCC CC CC/MCC Exc
      AHA: Q3 2016
   A39.5 **Meningococcal** heart disease
      A39.50 **Meningococcal carditis, unspecified**   MCC CC/MCC Exc
         AHA: Q3 2016
      A39.51 **Meningococcal** endocarditis   MCC CC/MCC Exc
         AHA: Q3 2016
      A39.52 **Meningococcal** myocarditis   MCC CC/MCC Exc
         AHA: Q3 2016
      A39.53 **Meningococcal** pericarditis   MCC CC/MCC Exc
         AHA: Q3 2016
   A39.8 **Other meningococcal infections**
      A39.81 **Meningococcal** encephalitis   MCC CC/MCC Exc
         AHA: Q3 2016
      A39.82 **Meningococcal** retrobulbar neuritis   CC CC/MCC Exc
         AHA: Q3 2016
      A39.83 **Meningococcal** arthritis   CC HCC CC/MCC Exc
         AHA: Q3 2016
      A39.84 **Postmeningococcal** arthritis   CC HCC CC/MCC Exc
         AHA: Q3 2016

Unspecified Code	Other Specified Code	Manifestation Code	N Newborn	P Pediatric	M Maternity	A Adult	♂ Male	♀ Female

● New Code   ▲ Revised Code Title   ▶◀ Revised Text   **NOTES**   *INCLUDES*   *EXCLUDES 1* Not coded here   *EXCLUDES 2* Not included here
④ 4th character required   ⑤ 5th character required   ⑥ 6th character required   ⑦ 7th character required
⑦ Extension 'X' Alert   **HAC** Hospital-acquired condition (HAC) alert   **AHA** AHA Coding Clinic©

A39.89 **Other meningococcal infections** cc CC/MCC Exc
  AHA: Q3 2016
  Meningococcal conjunctivitis

A39.9 **Meningococcal infection, unspecified** cc CC/MCC Exc
  AHA: Q3 2016
  Meningococcal disease NOS

A40 Streptococcal sepsis
  Code first postprocedural streptococcal sepsis (T81.4-)
  streptococcal sepsis during labor (O75.3)
  streptococcal sepsis following abortion or ectopic or molar pregnancy (O03-O07, O08.0)
  streptococcal sepsis following immunization (T88.0)
  streptococcal sepsis following infusion, transfusion or therapeutic injection (T80.2-)

  EXCLUDES1 neonatal (P36.0-P36.1)
      puerperal sepsis (O85)
      sepsis due to Streptococcus, group D (A41.81)

  A40.0 **Sepsis due to streptococcus, group A** HCC MCC CC/MCC Exc
    AHA: Q3 2016
  A40.1 **Sepsis due to streptococcus, group B** HCC MCC CC/MCC Exc
    AHA: Q3 2016
  A40.3 **Sepsis due to Streptococcus pneumoniae** HCC MCC
    AHA: Q3 2016
    Pneumococcal sepsis
  A40.8 **Other streptococcal sepsis** HCC MCC CC/MCC Exc
    AHA: Q3 2016
  A40.9 **Streptococcal sepsis, unspecified** HCC MCC CC/MCC Exc
    AHA: Q3 2016

A41 Other sepsis
  Code first postprocedural sepsis (T81.4-)
  sepsis during labor (O75.3)
  sepsis following abortion, ectopic or molar pregnancy (O03-O07, O08.0)
  sepsis following immunization (T88.0)
  sepsis following infusion, transfusion or therapeutic injection (T80.2-)

  EXCLUDES1 bacteremia NOS (R78.81)
      neonatal (P36.-)
      puerperal sepsis (O85)
      streptococcal sepsis (A40.-)

  EXCLUDES2 sepsis (due to) (in) actinomycotic (A42.7)
      sepsis (due to) (in) anthrax (A22.7)
      sepsis (due to) (in) candidal (B37.7)
      sepsis (due to) (in) Erysipelothrix (A26.7)
      sepsis (due to) (in) extraintestinal yersiniosis (A28.2)
      sepsis (due to) (in) gonococcal (A54.86)
      sepsis (due to) (in) herpesviral (B00.7)
      sepsis (due to) (in) listerial (A32.7)
      sepsis (due to) (in) melioidosis (A24.1)
      sepsis (due to) (in) meningococcal (A39.2-A39.4)
      sepsis (due to) (in) plague (A20.7)
      sepsis (due to) (in) tularemia (A21.7)
      toxic shock syndrome (A48.3)

  A41.0 **Sepsis due to Staphylococcus aureus**
    A41.01 **Sepsis due to Methicillin susceptible Staphylococcus aureus** HCC MCC CC/MCC Exc
      AHA: Q3 2016
      MSSA sepsis
      Staphylococcus aureus sepsis NOS
    A41.02 **Sepsis due to Methicillin resistant Staphylococcus aureus** HCC MCC CC/MCC Exc
      AHA: Q3 2016
  A41.1 **Sepsis due to other specified staphylococcus** HCC MCC CC/MCC Exc
    AHA: Q3 2016
    Coagulase negative staphylococcus sepsis
  A41.2 **Sepsis due to unspecified staphylococcus** HCC MCC CC/MCC Exc
    AHA: Q3 2016

A41.3 **Sepsis due to Hemophilus influenzae** HCC MCC CC/MCC Exc
  AHA: Q3 2016
A41.4 **Sepsis due to anaerobes** HCC MCC CC/MCC Exc
  AHA: Q3 2016
  EXCLUDES1 gas gangrene (A48.0)
A41.5 **Sepsis due to other Gram-negative organisms**
  A41.50 **Gram-negative sepsis, unspecified** HCC MCC CC/MCC Exc
    AHA: Q3 2016
    Gram-negative sepsis NOS
  A41.51 **Sepsis due to Escherichia coli [E. coli]** HCC MCC CC/MCC Exc
    AHA: Q3 2016
  A41.52 **Sepsis due to Pseudomonas** HCC MCC CC/MCC Exc
    AHA: Q3 2016
    Pseudomonas aeroginosa
  A41.53 **Sepsis due to Serratia** HCC MCC CC/MCC Exc
    AHA: Q3 2016
  A41.59 **Other Gram-negative sepsis** HCC MCC CC/MCC Exc
    AHA: Q3 2016
A41.8 **Other specified sepsis**
  A41.81 **Sepsis due to Enterococcus** HCC MCC CC/MCC Exc
    AHA: Q3 2016
  A41.89 **Other specified sepsis** HCC MCC CC/MCC Exc
    AHA: Q3 2016
A41.9 **Sepsis, unspecified organism** HCC MCC CC/MCC Exc
  AHA: Q3 2016
  Septicemia NOS

A42 Actinomycosis
  EXCLUDES1 actinomycetoma (B47.1)
  A42.0 **Pulmonary actinomycosis** cc HCC CC/MCC Exc
    AHA: Q3 2016
  A42.1 **Abdominal actinomycosis** cc CC/MCC Exc
    AHA: Q3 2016
  A42.2 **Cervicofacial actinomycosis** cc CC/MCC Exc
    AHA: Q3 2016
  A42.7 **Actinomycotic sepsis** HCC MCC CC/MCC Exc
    AHA: Q3 2016
  A42.8 **Other forms of actinomycosis**
    A42.81 **Actinomycotic meningitis** cc CC/MCC Exc
      AHA: Q3 2016
    A42.82 **Actinomycotic encephalitis** cc CC/MCC Exc
      AHA: Q3 2016
    A42.89 **Other forms of actinomycosis** cc CC/MCC Exc
      AHA: Q3 2016
  A42.9 **Actinomycosis, unspecified** cc CC/MCC Exc
    AHA: Q3 2016

A43 Nocardiosis
  A43.0 **Pulmonary nocardiosis** cc HCC CC/MCC Exc
    AHA: Q3 2016
  A43.1 **Cutaneous nocardiosis** cc CC/MCC Exc
    AHA: Q3 2016
  A43.8 **Other forms of nocardiosis** cc CC/MCC Exc
    AHA: Q3 2016
  A43.9 **Nocardiosis, unspecified** cc CC/MCC Exc
    AHA: Q3 2016

A44 Bartonellosis
  A44.0 **Systemic bartonellosis** cc CC/MCC Exc
    AHA: Q3 2016
    Oroya fever
  A44.1 **Cutaneous and mucocutaneous bartonellosis** cc CC/MCC Exc
    AHA: Q3 2016
    Verruga peruana
  A44.8 **Other forms of bartonellosis** cc CC/MCC Exc
    AHA: Q3 2016
  A44.9 **Bartonellosis, unspecified** cc CC/MCC Exc
    AHA: Q3 2016

A46 Erysipelas
  AHA: Q3 2016
  EXCLUDES1 postpartum or puerperal erysipelas (O86.89)

A48 Other bacterial diseases, not elsewhere classified
  EXCLUDES1 actinomycetoma (B47.1)

PDx Unacceptable principal diagnosis symbol per Medicare code edits   POA Code exempt from diagnosis present on admission requirement
? Questionable admission   cc Complication or comorbidity   CC/MCC Exc CC/MCC exclusion   MCC Major complication or comorbidity
Principal diagnosis as its own CC   Principal diagnosis as its own MCC   HCC HCC diagnosis code   RxHCC RxHCC diagnosis code
MACRA code   Z Z code as first-listed diagnosis

A48.0 Gas gangrene HCC MCC⊘ CC/MCC Exc
AHA: Q3 2016
Clostridial cellulitis
Clostridial myonecrosis

A48.1 Legionnaires' disease HCC MCC⊘ CC/MCC Exc
AHA: Q3 2016

A48.2 Nonpneumonic Legionnaires' disease [Pontiac fever]
AHA: Q3 2016

A48.3 Toxic shock syndrome HCC MCC⊘ CC/MCC Exc
AHA: Q3 2016
Use additional code to identify the organism (B95, B96)
EXCLUDES1 endotoxic shock NOS (R57.8)
sepsis NOS (A41.9)

A48.4 Brazilian purpuric fever
AHA: Q3 2016
Systemic Hemophilus aegyptius infection

5ᵗʰ **A48.5** Other specified botulism
Non-foodborne intoxication due to toxins of Clostridium botulinum [C. botulinum]
EXCLUDES1 food poisoning due to toxins of Clostridium botulinum (A05.1)

A48.51 Infant botulism P CC⊘ CC/MCC Exc
AHA: Q3 2016

A48.52 Wound botulism CC⊘ CC/MCC Exc
AHA: Q3 2016
Non-foodborne botulism NOS
Use additional code for associated wound

A48.8 Other specified bacterial diseases
AHA: Q3 2016

4ᵗʰ **A49** Bacterial infection of unspecified site
EXCLUDES1 bacterial agents as the cause of diseases classified elsewhere (B95-B96)
chlamydial infection NOS (A74.9)
meningococcal infection NOS (A39.9)
rickettsial infection NOS (A79.9)
spirochetal infection NOS (A69.9)

5ᵗʰ **A49.0** Staphylococcal infection, unspecified site

A49.01 Methicillin susceptible Staphylococcus aureus infection, unspecified site
AHA: Q3 2016
Methicillin susceptible Staphylococcus aureus (MSSA) infection
Staphylococcus aureus infection NOS

A49.02 Methicillin resistant Staphylococcus aureus infection, unspecified site
AHA: Q3 2016
Methicillin resistant Staphylococcus aureus (MRSA) infection

A49.1 Streptococcal infection, unspecified site
AHA: Q3 2016

A49.2 Hemophilus influenzae infection, unspecified site
AHA: Q3 2016

A49.3 Mycoplasma infection, unspecified site
AHA: Q3 2016

A49.8 Other bacterial infections of unspecified site
AHA: Q3 2016

A49.9 Bacterial infection, unspecified
AHA: Q3 2016
EXCLUDES1 bacteremia NOS (R78.81)

Infections with a predominantly sexual mode of transmission (A50-A64)

EXCLUDES1 human immunodeficiency virus [HIV] disease (B20)
nonspecific and nongonococcal urethritis (N34.1)
Reiter's disease (M02.3-)

4ᵗʰ **A50** Congenital syphilis

5ᵗʰ **A50.0** Early congenital syphilis, symptomatic
Any congenital syphilitic condition specified as early or manifest less than two years after birth.

A50.01 Early congenital syphilitic oculopathy CC⊘ CC/MCC Exc

A50.02 Early congenital syphilitic osteochondropathy CC⊘ CC/MCC Exc

A50.03 Early congenital syphilitic pharyngitis CC⊘ CC/MCC Exc
Early congenital syphilitic laryngitis

A50.04 Early congenital syphilitic pneumonia CC⊘ CC/MCC Exc

A50.05 Early congenital syphilitic rhinitis CC⊘ CC/MCC Exc

A50.06 Early cutaneous congenital syphilis CC⊘ CC/MCC Exc

A50.07 Early mucocutaneous congenital syphilis CC⊘ CC/MCC Exc

A50.08 Early visceral congenital syphilis CC⊘ CC/MCC Exc

A50.09 Other early congenital syphilis, symptomatic CC⊘ CC/MCC Exc

A50.1 Early congenital syphilis, latent
Congenital syphilis without clinical manifestations, with positive serological reaction and negative spinal fluid test, less than two years after birth.

A50.2 Early congenital syphilis, unspecified CC⊘ CC/MCC Exc
Congenital syphilis NOS less than two years after birth.

5ᵗʰ **A50.3** Late congenital syphilitic oculopathy
EXCLUDES1 Hutchinson's triad (A50.53)

A50.30 Late congenital syphilitic oculopathy, unspecified CC⊘ CC/MCC Exc

A50.31 Late congenital syphilitic interstitial keratitis CC⊘ CC/MCC Exc

A50.32 Late congenital syphilitic chorioretinitis CC⊘ CC/MCC Exc

A50.39 Other late congenital syphilitic oculopathy CC⊘ CC/MCC Exc

5ᵗʰ **A50.4** Late congenital neurosyphilis [juvenile neurosyphilis]
Use additional code to identify any associated mental disorder
EXCLUDES1 Hutchinson's triad (A50.53)

A50.40 Late congenital neurosyphilis, unspecified CC⊘ CC/MCC Exc
Juvenile neurosyphilis NOS

A50.41 Late congenital syphilitic meningitis MCC⊘ CC/MCC Exc

A50.42 Late congenital syphilitic encephalitis MCC⊘ CC/MCC Exc

A50.43 Late congenital syphilitic polyneuropathy CC⊘ CC/MCC Exc

A50.44 Late congenital syphilitic optic nerve atrophy CC⊘ CC/MCC Exc

A50.45 Juvenile general paresis CC⊘ CC/MCC Exc
Dementia paralytica juvenilis
Juvenile tabetoparetic neurosyphilis

A50.49 Other late congenital neurosyphilis CC⊘ CC/MCC Exc
Juvenile tabes dorsalis

5ᵗʰ **A50.5** Other late congenital syphilis, symptomatic
Any congenital syphilitic condition specified as late or manifest two years or more after birth.

A50.51 Clutton's joints CC⊘ CC/MCC Exc

A50.52 Hutchinson's teeth CC⊘ CC/MCC Exc

A50.53 Hutchinson's triad CC⊘ CC/MCC Exc

A50.54 Late congenital cardiovascular syphilis CC⊘ CC/MCC Exc

A50.55 Late congenital syphilitic arthropathy CC⊘ HCC CC/MCC Exc

A50.56 Late congenital syphilitic osteochondropathy CC⊘ CC/MCC Exc

A50.57 Syphilitic saddle nose CC⊘ CC/MCC Exc

A50.59 Other late congenital syphilis, symptomatic CC⊘ CC/MCC Exc

A50.6 Late congenital syphilis, latent
Congenital syphilis without clinical manifestations, with positive serological reaction and negative spinal fluid test, two years or more after birth.

A50.7 Late congenital syphilis, unspecified
Congenital syphilis NOS two years or more after birth.

A50.9 Congenital syphilis, unspecified

4ᵗʰ **A51** Early syphilis

A51.0 Primary genital syphilis
Syphilitic chancre NOS

A51.1 Primary anal syphilis

A51.2 Primary syphilis of other sites

5ᵗʰ **A51.3** Secondary syphilis of skin and mucous membranes

A51.31 Condyloma latum CC⊘ CC/MCC Exc

A51.32 Syphilitic alopecia CC⊘ CC/MCC Exc

Unspecified Code	Other Specified Code	Manifestation Code	N Newborn	P Pediatric	M Maternity	A Adult	♂ Male	♀ Female

● New Code ▲ Revised Code Title ►◄ Revised Text **NOTES** INCLUDES EXCLUDES 1 Not coded here EXCLUDES 2 Not included here
4ᵗʰ 4ᵗʰ character required 5ᵗʰ 5ᵗʰ character required 6ᵗʰ 6ᵗʰ character required 7ᵗʰ 7ᵗʰ character required
7ᵗʰ Extension 'X' Alert HAC Hospital-acquired condition (HAC) alert AHA AHA Coding Clinic©

2018 ICD-10-CM

When symbols appear on a code that requires a 7th character extension, refer to Appendix B to identify applicable 7th character codes.

453

A51.39 Other secondary syphilis of skin

Syphilitic leukoderma

Syphilitic mucous patch

EXCLUDES1 late syphilitic leukoderma (A52.79)

A51.4 Other secondary **syphilis**

A51.41 Secondary syphilitic meningitis

A51.42 Secondary syphilitic **female pelvic disease**

A51.43 Secondary syphilitic oculopathy

Secondary syphilitic chorioretinitis

Secondary syphilitic iridocyclitis, iritis

Secondary syphilitic uveitis

A51.44 Secondary syphilitic nephritis

A51.45 Secondary syphilitic hepatitis

A51.46 Secondary syphilitic osteopathy

A51.49 Other secondary syphilitic conditions

Secondary syphilitic lymphadenopathy

Secondary syphilitic myositis

A51.5 Early **syphilis**, latent

Syphilis (acquired) without clinical manifestations, with positive serological reaction and negative spinal fluid test, less than two years after infection.

A51.9 Early syphilis, unspecified

A52 Late **syphilis**

A52.0 Cardiovascular **and** cerebrovascular **syphilis**

A52.00 Cardiovascular syphilis, unspecified

A52.01 Syphilitic aneurysm of aorta

A52.02 Syphilitic aortitis

A52.03 Syphilitic endocarditis

Syphilitic aortic valve incompetence or stenosis

Syphilitic mitral valve stenosis

Syphilitic pulmonary valve regurgitation

A52.04 Syphilitic cerebral arteritis

A52.05 Other cerebrovascular syphilis

Syphilitic cerebral aneurysm (ruptured) (non-ruptured)

Syphilitic cerebral thrombosis

A52.06 Other syphilitic heart involvement

Syphilitic coronary artery disease

Syphilitic myocarditis

Syphilitic pericarditis

A52.09 Other cardiovascular syphilis

A52.1 Symptomatic **neurosyphilis**

A52.10 Symptomatic neurosyphilis, unspecified

A52.11 Tabes dorsalis

Locomotor ataxia (progressive)

Tabetic neurosyphilis

A52.12 Other cerebrospinal syphilis

A52.13 Late syphilitic meningitis

A52.14 Late syphilitic encephalitis

A52.15 Late syphilitic neuropathy

Late syphilitic acoustic neuritis

Late syphilitic optic (nerve) atrophy

Late syphilitic polyneuropathy

Late syphilitic retrobulbar neuritis

A52.16 Charcôt's arthropathy (tabetic)

A52.17 General paresis

Dementia paralytica

A52.19 Other symptomatic neurosyphilis

Syphilitic parkinsonism

A52.2 Asymptomatic **neurosyphilis**

A52.3 Neurosyphilis, unspecified

Gumma (syphilitic)

Syphilis (late)

Syphiloma

A52.7 Other symptomatic **late syphilis**

A52.71 Late syphilitic oculopathy

Late syphilitic chorioretinitis

Late syphilitic episcleritis

A52.72 Syphilis of lung and bronchus

A52.73 Symptomatic late syphilis of other respiratory organs

A52.74 Syphilis of liver and other viscera

Late syphilitic peritonitis

A52.75 Syphilis of kidney and ureter

Syphilitic glomerular disease

A52.76 Other genitourinary symptomatic late **syphilis**

Late syphilitic female pelvic inflammatory disease

A52.77 Syphilis of bone and joint

A52.78 Syphilis of other musculoskeletal tissue

Late syphilitic bursitis

Syphilis [stage unspecified] of bursa

Syphilis [stage unspecified] of muscle

Syphilis [stage unspecified] of synovium

Syphilis [stage unspecified] of tendon

A52.79 Other symptomatic late syphilis

Late syphilitic leukoderma

Syphilis of adrenal gland

Syphilis of pituitary gland

Syphilis of thyroid gland

Syphilitic splenomegaly

EXCLUDES1 syphilitic leukoderma (secondary) (A51.39)

A52.8 Late syphilis, latent

Syphilis (acquired) without clinical manifestations, with positive serological reaction and negative spinal fluid test, two years or more after infection.

A52.9 Late syphilis, unspecified

A53 Other and unspecified syphilis

A53.0 Latent syphilis, unspecified as early or late

Latent syphilis NOS

Positive serological reaction for syphilis

A53.9 Syphilis, unspecified

Infection due to Treponema pallidum NOS

Syphilis (acquired) NOS

EXCLUDES1 syphilis NOS under two years of age (A50.2)

A54 Gonococcal **infection**

A54.0 Gonococcal infection of lower genitourinary tract without periurethral or accessory gland abscess

EXCLUDES1 gonococcal infection with genitourinary gland abscess (A54.1)

gonococcal infection with periurethral abscess (A54.1)

A54.00 Gonococcal infection of lower genitourinary tract, unspecified

A54.01 Gonococcal cystitis and urethritis, unspecified

A54.02 Gonococcal vulvovaginitis, unspecified

A54.03 Gonococcal cervicitis, unspecified

A54.09 Other gonococcal infection of lower genitourinary tract

A54.1 Gonococcal infection of lower genitourinary tract with periurethral and accessory gland abscess

Gonococcal Bartholin's gland abscess

A54.2 Gonococcal pelviperitonitis and other gonococcal genitourinary **infection**

A54.21 Gonococcal infection of kidney and ureter

A54.22 Gonococcal prostatitis

A54.23 Gonococcal infection of other male genital organs

Gonococcal epididymitis

Gonococcal orchitis

A54.24 Gonococcal female pelvic inflammatory disease

Gonococcal pelviperitonitis

EXCLUDES1 gonococcal peritonitis (A54.85)

A54.29 Other gonococcal genitourinary infections

A54.3 Gonococcal infection of eye

A54.30 Gonococcal infection of eye, unspecified

A54.31 Gonococcal conjunctivitis

Ophthalmia neonatorum due to gonococcus

A54.32 Gonococcal iridocyclitis

A54.33 Gonococcal keratitis

PDx Unacceptable principal diagnosis symbol per Medicare code edits   Code exempt from diagnosis present on admission requirement

❓ Questionable admission   Complication or comorbidity   CC/MCC Exc CC/MCC exclusion   MCC Major complication or comorbidity

PDx/CC Principal diagnosis as its own CC   Principal diagnosis as its own MCC   HCC HCC diagnosis code   RxHCC RxHCC diagnosis code

MACRA code   Z1 Z code as first-listed diagnosis

A54.39 **Other gonococcal eye infection** `CC` `CC/MCC Exc`
Gonococcal endophthalmia

5ᵗʰ A54.4 **Gonococcal infection of** musculoskeletal system

A54.40 **Gonococcal infection of musculoskeletal system, unspecified** `CC` `HCC` `CC/MCC Exc`

A54.41 **Gonococcal** spondylopathy `CC` `HCC`

A54.42 **Gonococcal** arthritis `CC` `HCC`

EXCLUDES2 *gonococcal infection of spine (A54.41)*

A54.43 **Gonococcal** osteomyelitis `CC` `HCC` `CC/MCC Exc`

EXCLUDES2 *gonococcal infection of spine (A54.41)*

A54.49 **Gonococcal infection of other musculoskeletal tissue** `CC` `HCC` `CC/MCC Exc`
Gonococcal bursitis
Gonococcal myositis
Gonococcal synovitis
Gonococcal tenosynovitis

A54.5 **Gonococcal** pharyngitis

A54.6 **Gonococcal infection of** anus and rectum

5ᵗʰ A54.8 **Other gonococcal infections**

A54.81 **Gonococcal** meningitis `MCC` `CC/MCC Exc`

A54.82 **Gonococcal** brain abscess `CC` `CC/MCC Exc`

A54.83 **Gonococcal** heart infection `CC` `CC/MCC Exc`
Gonococcal endocarditis
Gonococcal myocarditis
Gonococcal pericarditis

A54.84 **Gonococcal** pneumonia `CC` `HCC` `CC/MCC Exc`

A54.85 **Gonococcal** peritonitis `CC` `HCC` `CC/MCC Exc`

EXCLUDES1 *gonococcal pelviperitonitis (A54.24)*

A54.86 **Gonococcal** sepsis `HCC` `MCC` `PDx MCC` `CC/MCC Exc`

A54.89 **Other gonococcal infections** `CC` `CC/MCC Exc`
Gonococcal keratoderma
Gonococcal lymphadenitis

A54.9 **Gonococcal infection, unspecified** `CC` `CC/MCC Exc`

A55 **Chlamydial lymphogranuloma (venereum)**
Climatic or tropical bubo
Durand-Nicolas-Favre disease
Esthiomene
Lymphogranuloma inguinale

4ᵗʰ A56 **Other sexually transmitted chlamydial diseases**

INCLUDES *sexually transmitted diseases due to Chlamydia trachomatis*

EXCLUDES1 *neonatal chlamydial conjunctivitis (P39.1)*
neonatal chlamydial pneumonia (P23.1)

EXCLUDES2 *chlamydial lymphogranuloma (A55)*
conditions classified to A74.-

5ᵗʰ A56.0 **Chlamydial infection of** lower genitourinary tract

A56.00 **Chlamydial infection of lower genitourinary tract, unspecified**

A56.01 **Chlamydial** cystitis and urethritis

A56.02 **Chlamydial** vulvovaginitis ♀

A56.09 **Other chlamydial infection of lower genitourinary tract**
Chlamydial cervicitis

5ᵗʰ A56.1 **Chlamydial infection of** pelviperitoneum and other genitourinary organs

A56.11 **Chlamydial female pelvic inflammatory disease** ♀

A56.19 **Other chlamydial genitourinary infection**
Chlamydial epididymitis
Chlamydial orchitis

A56.2 **Chlamydial infection of genitourinary tract, unspecified**

A56.3 **Chlamydial infection of** anus and rectum

A56.4 **Chlamydial infection of** pharynx

A56.8 **Sexually transmitted chlamydial infection of other sites**

A57 **Chancroid**
Ulcus molle

A58 **Granuloma inguinale**
Donovanosis

4ᵗʰ A59 **Trichomoniasis**

EXCLUDES2 *intestinal trichomoniasis (A07.8)*

5ᵗʰ A59.0 **Urogenital** trichomoniasis

A59.00 **Urogenital trichomoniasis, unspecified**
Fluor (vaginalis) due to Trichomonas
Leukorrhea (vaginalis) due to Trichomonas

A59.01 **Trichomonal** vulvovaginitis ♀

A59.02 **Trichomonal** prostatitis ♂

A59.03 **Trichomonal** cystitis and urethritis

A59.09 **Other urogenital trichomoniasis**
Trichomonas cervicitis

A59.8 **Trichomoniasis of other sites**

A59.9 **Trichomoniasis, unspecified**

4ᵗʰ A60 **Anogenital herpesviral [herpes simplex] infections**

5ᵗʰ A60.0 **Herpesviral infection of** genitalia and urogenital tract

A60.00 **Herpesviral infection of urogenital system, unspecified**

A60.01 **Herpesviral infection of** penis ♂

A60.02 **Herpesviral infection of other male genital organs** ♂

A60.03 **Herpesviral** cervicitis ♀

A60.04 **Herpesviral** vulvovaginitis ♀
Herpesviral [herpes simplex] ulceration
Herpesviral [herpes simplex] vaginitis
Herpesviral [herpes simplex] vulvitis

A60.09 **Herpesviral infection of other urogenital tract**

A60.1 **Herpesviral infection of** perianal skin and rectum

A60.9 **Anogenital herpesviral infection, unspecified**

4ᵗʰ A63 **Other predominantly sexually transmitted diseases, not elsewhere classified**

EXCLUDES2 *molluscum contagiosum (B08.1)*
papilloma of cervix (D26.0)

A63.0 **Anogenital (venereal) warts**
Anogenital warts due to (human) papillomavirus [HPV]
Condyloma acuminatum

A63.8 **Other specified predominantly sexually transmitted diseases**

A64 **Unspecified sexually transmitted disease**

Other spirochetal diseases (A65-A69)

EXCLUDES2 *leptospirosis (A27.-)*
syphilis (A50-A53)

A65 **Nonvenereal syphilis**
Bejel
Endemic syphilis
Njovera

4ᵗʰ A66 **Yaws**

INCLUDES *bouba*
frambesia (tropica)
pian

A66.0 **Initial lesions of yaws**
Chancre of yaws
Frambesia, initial or primary
Initial frambesial ulcer
Mother yaw

A66.1 **Multiple** papillomata and wet crab **yaws**
Frambesioma
Pianoma
Plantar or palmar papilloma of yaws

A66.2 **Other early skin lesions of yaws**
Cutaneous yaws, less than five years after infection
Early yaws (cutaneous)(macular)(maculopapular) (micropapular)(papular)
Frambeside of early yaws

A66.3 **Hyperkeratosis of yaws**
Ghoul hand
Hyperkeratosis, palmar or plantar (early) (late) due to yaws
Worm-eaten soles

A66.4 **Gummata and ulcers of yaws**
Gummatous frambeside
Nodular late yaws (ulcerated)

A66.5 **Gangosa**
Rhinopharyngitis mutilans

Unspecified Code	Other Specified Code	Manifestation Code

N Newborn P Pediatric M Maternity A Adult ♂ Male ♀ Female
● New Code ▲ Revised Code Title ►◄ Revised Text NOTES INCLUDES EXCLUDES 1 Not coded here EXCLUDES 2 Not included here
4ᵗʰ 4th character required 5ᵗʰ 5th character required 6ᵗʰ 6th character required 7ᵗʰ 7th character required
7ˣ Extension 'X' Alert HAC Hospital-acquired condition (HAC) alert **AHA** AHA Coding Clinic©

A66.6 Bone and joint lesions of yaws   HCC
    Yaws ganglion
    Yaws goundou
    Yaws gumma, bone
    Yaws gummatous osteitis or periostitis
    Yaws hydrarthrosis
    Yaws osteitis
    Yaws periostitis (hypertrophic)
A66.7 Other manifestations of yaws
    Juxta-articular nodules of yaws
    Mucosal yaws
A66.8 Latent yaws
    Yaws without clinical manifestations, with positive serology
A66.9 Yaws, unspecified

A67 Pinta [carate]
A67.0 Primary lesions of pinta
    Chancre (primary) of pinta
    Papule (primary) of pinta
A67.1 Intermediate lesions of pinta
    Erythematous plaques of pinta
    Hyperchromic lesions of pinta
    Hyperkeratosis of pinta
    Pintids
A67.2 Late lesions of pinta
    Achromic skin lesions of pinta
    Cicatricial skin lesions of pinta
    Dyschromic skin lesions of pinta
A67.3 Mixed lesions of pinta
    Achromic with hyperchromic skin lesions of pinta [carate]
A67.9 Pinta, unspecified

A68 Relapsing fevers
    INCLUDES recurrent fever
    EXCLUDES2 Lyme disease (A69.2-)
A68.0 Louse-borne relapsing fever   CC CC/MCC Exc
    Relapsing fever due to Borrelia recurrentis
A68.1 Tick-borne relapsing fever   CC CC/MCC Exc
    Relapsing fever due to any Borrelia species other than Borrelia recurrentis
A68.9 Relapsing fever, unspecified   CC CC/MCC Exc

A69 Other spirochetal infections
A69.0 Necrotizing ulcerative stomatitis
    Cancrum oris
    Fusospirochetal gangrene
    Noma
    Stomatitis gangrenosa
A69.1 Other Vincent's infections   CC CC/MCC Exc
    Fusospirochetal pharyngitis
    Necrotizing ulcerative (acute) gingivitis
    Necrotizing ulcerative (acute) gingivostomatitis
    Spirochetal stomatitis
    Trench mouth
    Vincent's angina
    Vincent's gingivitis
A69.2 Lyme disease
    Erythema chronicum migrans due to Borrelia burgdorferi
  A69.20 Lyme disease, unspecified   CC CC/MCC Exc
  A69.21 Meningitis due to Lyme disease   CC CC/MCC Exc
  A69.22 Other neurologic disorders in Lyme disease   CC CC/MCC Exc
     Cranial neuritis
     Meningoencephalitis
     Polyneuropathy
  A69.23 Arthritis due to Lyme disease   CC HCC CC/MCC Exc
  A69.29 Other conditions associated with Lyme disease   CC CC/MCC Exc
     AHA: Q3 2016
     Myopericarditis due to Lyme disease
A69.8 Other specified spirochetal infections
A69.9 Spirochetal infection, unspecified

Other diseases caused by chlamydiae (A70-A74)

    EXCLUDES1 sexually transmitted chlamydial diseases (A55-A56)
A70 Chlamydia psittaci infections   CC CC/MCC Exc
    Ornithosis
    Parrot fever
    Psittacosis
A71 Trachoma
    EXCLUDES1 sequelae of trachoma (B94.0)
A71.0 Initial stage of trachoma
    Trachoma dubium
A71.1 Active stage of trachoma
    Granular conjunctivitis (trachomatous)
    Trachomatous follicular conjunctivitis
    Trachomatous pannus
A71.9 Trachoma, unspecified
A74 Other diseases caused by chlamydiae
    EXCLUDES1 neonatal chlamydial conjunctivitis (P39.1)
          neonatal chlamydial pneumonia (P23.1)
          Reiter's disease (M02.3-)
          sexually transmitted chlamydial diseases (A55-A56)
    EXCLUDES2 chlamydial pneumonia (J16.0)
A74.0 Chlamydial conjunctivitis
    Paratrachoma
A74.8 Other chlamydial diseases
  A74.81 Chlamydial peritonitis
  A74.89 Other chlamydial diseases
A74.9 Chlamydial infection, unspecified
    Chlamydiosis NOS

Rickettsioses (A75-A79)

A75 Typhus fever
    EXCLUDES1 rickettsiosis due to Ehrlichia sennetsu (A79.81)
A75.0 Epidemic louse-borne typhus fever due to Rickettsia prowazekii   CC CC/MCC Exc
    Classical typhus (fever)
    Epidemic (louse-borne) typhus
A75.1 Recrudescent typhus [Brill's disease]   CC CC/MCC Exc
    Brill-Zinsser disease
A75.2 Typhus fever due to Rickettsia typhi   CC CC/MCC Exc
    Murine (flea-borne) typhus
A75.3 Typhus fever due to Rickettsia tsutsugamushi   CC CC/MCC Exc
    Scrub (mite-borne) typhus
    Tsutsugamushi fever
A75.9 Typhus fever, unspecified   CC CC/MCC Exc
    Typhus (fever) NOS
A77 Spotted fever [tick-borne rickettsioses]
A77.0 Spotted fever due to Rickettsia rickettsii   CC CC/MCC Exc
    Rocky Mountain spotted fever
    Sao Paulo fever
A77.1 Spotted fever due to Rickettsia conorii   CC CC/MCC Exc
    African tick typhus
    Boutonneuse fever
    India tick typhus
    Kenya tick typhus
    Marseilles fever
    Mediterranean tick fever
A77.2 Spotted fever due to Rickettsia siberica   CC CC/MCC Exc
    North Asian tick fever
    Siberian tick typhus
A77.3 Spotted fever due to Rickettsia australis   CC CC/MCC Exc
    Queensland tick typhus
A77.4 Ehrlichiosis
    EXCLUDES1 Rickettsiosis due to Ehrlichia sennetsu (A79.81)
  A77.40 Ehrlichiosis, unspecified   CC CC/MCC Exc
  A77.41 Ehrlichiosis chafeensis [E. chafeensis]   CC CC/MCC Exc
  A77.49 Other ehrlichiosis   CC CC/MCC Exc
A77.8 Other spotted fevers   CC CC/MCC Exc
A77.9 Spotted fever, unspecified   CC CC/MCC Exc
    Tick-borne typhus NOS

PDxM Unacceptable principal diagnosis symbol per Medicare code edits   PDx Code exempt from diagnosis present on admission requirement
? Questionable admission   CC Complication or comorbidity   CC/MCC CC/MCC exclusion   MCC Major complication or comorbidity
Principal diagnosis as its own CC   Principal diagnosis as its own MCC   HCC HCC diagnosis code   RxHCC RxHCC diagnosis code
MACRA code   Z1 Z code as first-listed diagnosis

456   When symbols appear on a code that requires a 7th character extension, refer to Appendix B to identify applicable 7th character codes.   **2018 ICD-10-CM**

A78 Q fever [CC] [CC/MCC Exc]
Infection due to Coxiella burnetii
Nine Mile fever
Quadrilateral fever

[4th] **A79 Other rickettsioses**
A79.0 Trench fever [CC] [CC/MCC Exc]
Quintan fever
Wolhynian fever
A79.1 Rickettsialpox due to Rickettsia akari [CC] [CC/MCC Exc]
Kew Garden fever
Vesicular rickettsiosis
[5th] **A79.8 Other specified rickettsioses**
A79.81 Rickettsiosis due to Ehrlichia sennetsu [CC] [CC/MCC Exc]
A79.89 Other specified rickettsioses [CC] [CC/MCC Exc]
A79.9 Rickettsiosis, unspecified [CC] [CC/MCC Exc]
Rickettsial infection NOS

Viral and prion infections of the central nervous system (A80-A89)

[EXCLUDES1] *postpolio syndrome (G14)*
sequelae of poliomyelitis (B91)
sequelae of viral encephalitis (B94.1)

[4th] **A80 Acute poliomyelitis**
A80.0 Acute paralytic poliomyelitis, vaccine-associated [MCC] [CC/MCC Exc]
A80.1 Acute paralytic poliomyelitis, wild virus, imported [MCC] [CC/MCC Exc]
A80.2 Acute paralytic poliomyelitis, wild virus, indigenous [MCC] [CC/MCC Exc]
[5th] **A80.3 Acute paralytic poliomyelitis, other and unspecified**
A80.30 Acute paralytic poliomyelitis, unspecified [MCC] [CC/MCC Exc]
A80.39 Other acute paralytic poliomyelitis [MCC] [CC/MCC Exc]
A80.4 Acute nonparalytic poliomyelitis
A80.9 Acute poliomyelitis, unspecified

[4th] **A81 Atypical virus infections of central nervous system**
[INCLUDES] *diseases of the central nervous system caused by prions*
Use additional code to identify:
dementia with behavioral disturbance (F02.81)
dementia without behavioral disturbance (F02.80)
[5th] **A81.0 Creutzfeldt-Jakob disease**
A81.00 Creutzfeldt-Jakob disease, unspecified [CC] [RxHCC] [CC/MCC Exc]
Jakob-Creutzfeldt disease, unspecified
A81.01 Variant Creutzfeldt-Jakob disease [CC] [RxHCC] [CC/MCC Exc]
vCJD
A81.09 Other Creutzfeldt-Jakob disease [CC] [RxHCC] [CC/MCC Exc]
CJD
Familial Creutzfeldt-Jakob disease
Iatrogenic Creutzfeldt-Jakob disease
Sporadic Creutzfeldt-Jakob disease
Subacute spongiform encephalopathy (with dementia)
A81.1 Subacute sclerosing panencephalitis [CC] [RxHCC] [CC/MCC Exc]
Dawson's inclusion body encephalitis
Van Bogaert's sclerosing leukoencephalopathy
A81.2 Progressive multifocal leukoencephalopathy [CC] [RxHCC] [CC/MCC Exc]
Multifocal leukoencephalopathy NOS
[5th] **A81.8 Other atypical virus infections of central nervous system**
A81.81 Kuru [CC] [RxHCC] [CC/MCC Exc]
A81.82 Gerstmann-Sträussler-Scheinker syndrome [CC] [RxHCC] [CC/MCC Exc]
GSS syndrome
A81.83 Fatal familial insomnia [CC] [RxHCC] [CC/MCC Exc]
FFI
A81.89 Other atypical virus infections of central nervous system [CC] [RxHCC] [CC/MCC Exc]
A81.9 Atypical virus infection of central nervous system, unspecified [CC] [RxHCC] [CC/MCC Exc]
Prion diseases of the central nervous system NOS

[4th] **A82 Rabies**
A82.0 Sylvatic rabies [CC] [CC/MCC Exc]
A82.1 Urban rabies [CC] [CC/MCC Exc]
A82.9 Rabies, unspecified [CC] [CC/MCC Exc]

[4th] **A83 Mosquito-borne viral encephalitis**
[INCLUDES] *mosquito-borne viral meningoencephalitis*
[EXCLUDES2] *Venezuelan equine encephalitis (A92.2)*
West Nile fever (A92.3-)
West Nile virus (A92.3-)
A83.0 Japanese encephalitis [MCC] [CC/MCC Exc]
A83.1 Western equine encephalitis [MCC] [CC/MCC Exc]
A83.2 Eastern equine encephalitis [MCC] [CC/MCC Exc]
A83.3 St Louis encephalitis [MCC] [CC/MCC Exc]
A83.4 Australian encephalitis [MCC] [CC/MCC Exc]
Kunjin virus disease
A83.5 California encephalitis [MCC] [CC/MCC Exc]
California meningoencephalitis
La Crosse encephalitis
A83.6 Rocio virus disease [MCC] [CC/MCC Exc]
A83.8 Other mosquito-borne viral encephalitis [MCC] [CC/MCC Exc]
A83.9 Mosquito-borne viral encephalitis, unspecified [MCC] [CC/MCC Exc]

[4th] **A84 Tick-borne viral encephalitis**
[INCLUDES] *tick-borne viral meningoencephalitis*
A84.0 Far Eastern tick-borne encephalitis [Russian spring-summer encephalitis] [MCC] [CC/MCC Exc]
A84.1 Central European tick-borne encephalitis [MCC] [CC/MCC Exc]
A84.8 Other tick-borne viral encephalitis [MCC] [CC/MCC Exc]
Louping ill
Powassan virus disease
A84.9 Tick-borne viral encephalitis, unspecified [MCC] [CC/MCC Exc]

[4th] **A85 Other viral encephalitis, not elsewhere classified**
[INCLUDES] *specified viral encephalomyelitis NEC*
specified viral meningoencephalitis NEC
[EXCLUDES1] *benign myalgic encephalomyelitis (G93.3)*
encephalitis due to cytomegalovirus (B25.8)
encephalitis due to herpesvirus NEC (B10.0-)
encephalitis due to herpesvirus [herpes simplex] (B00.4)
encephalitis due to measles virus (B05.0)
encephalitis due to mumps virus (B26.2)
encephalitis due to poliomyelitis virus (A80.-)
encephalitis due to zoster (B02.0)
lymphocytic choriomeningitis (A87.2)
A85.0 Enteroviral encephalitis [CC] [CC/MCC Exc]
Enteroviral encephalomyelitis
A85.1 Adenoviral encephalitis [CC] [CC/MCC Exc]
Adenoviral meningoencephalitis
A85.2 Arthropod-borne viral encephalitis, unspecified [MCC] [CC/MCC Exc]
[EXCLUDES1] *West nile virus with encephalitis (A92.31)*
A85.8 Other specified viral encephalitis [CC] [CC/MCC Exc]
Encephalitis lethargica
Von Economo-Cruchet disease

A86 Unspecified viral encephalitis [CC] [CC/MCC Exc]
Viral encephalomyelitis NOS
Viral meningoencephalitis NOS

[4th] **A87 Viral meningitis**
[EXCLUDES1] *meningitis due to herpesvirus [herpes simplex] (B00.3)*
meningitis due to herpesvirus [herpes simplex] (B00.3)
meningitis due to measles virus (B05.1)
meningitis due to mumps virus (B26.1)
meningitis due to poliomyelitis virus (A80.-)
meningitis due to zoster (B02.1)
A87.0 Enteroviral meningitis [CC] [CC/MCC Exc]
Coxsackievirus meningitis
Echovirus meningitis
A87.1 Adenoviral meningitis [CC] [CC/MCC Exc]
A87.2 Lymphocytic choriomeningitis [CC] [CC/MCC Exc]
Lymphocytic meningoencephalitis
A87.8 Other viral meningitis [CC] [CC/MCC Exc]
A87.9 Viral meningitis, unspecified [CC] [CC/MCC Exc]

Unspecified Code | Other Specified Code | Manifestation Code | [N] Newborn | [P] Pediatric | [M] Maternity | [A] Adult | ♂ Male | ♀ Female
● New Code | ▲ Revised Code Title | ►◄ Revised Text | [NOTES] | [INCLUDES] | [EXCLUDES1] Not coded here | [EXCLUDES2] Not included here
[4th] 4th character required | [5th] 5th character required | [6th] 6th character required | [7th] 7th character required
[X] Extension 'X' Alert | [HAC] Hospital-acquired condition (HAC) alert | AHA AHA Coding Clinic©

B08.22 **Exanthema subitum [sixth disease] due to human herpesvirus 7** [Q]
Roseola infantum due to human herpesvirus 7

B08.3 **Erythema infectiosum [fifth disease]** [CC] [CC/MCC Exc]

B08.4 **Enteroviral vesicular stomatitis with exanthem**
Hand, foot and mouth disease

B08.5 **Enteroviral vesicular pharyngitis**
Herpangina

[5th] B08.6 **Parapoxvirus infections**

B08.60 **Parapoxvirus infection, unspecified**

B08.61 **Bovine stomatitis**

B08.62 **Sealpox**

B08.69 **Other parapoxvirus infections**

[5th] B08.7 **Yatapoxvirus infections**

B08.70 **Yatapoxvirus infection, unspecified**

B08.71 **Tanapox virus disease** [CC] [CC/MCC Exc]

B08.72 **Yaba pox virus disease**
Yaba monkey tumor disease

B08.79 **Other yatapoxvirus infections**

B08.8 **Other specified viral infections characterized by skin and mucous membrane lesions**
Enteroviral lymphonodular pharyngitis
Foot-and-mouth disease
Poxvirus NEC

B09 **Unspecified viral infection characterized by skin and mucous membrane lesions**
Viral enanthema NOS
Viral exanthema NOS

Other human herpesviruses (B10)

[4th] B10 **Other human herpesviruses**

[EXCLUDES2] *cytomegalovirus (B25.9)*
Epstein-Barr virus (B27.0-)
herpes NOS (B00.9)
herpes simplex (B00.-)
herpes zoster (B02.-)
human herpesvirus NOS (B00.-)
human herpesvirus 1 and 2 (B00.-)
human herpesvirus 3 (B01.-, B02.-)
human herpesvirus 4 (B27.0-)
human herpesvirus 5 (B25.-)
varicella (B01.-)
zoster (B02.-)

[5th] B10.0 **Other human herpesvirus encephalitis**

[EXCLUDES2] *herpes encephalitis NOS (B00.4)*
herpes simplex encephalitis (B00.4)
human herpesvirus encephalitis (B00.4)
simian B herpes virus encephalitis (B00.4)

B10.01 **Human herpesvirus 6 encephalitis** [MCC] [CC/MCC Exc]

B10.09 **Other human herpesvirus encephalitis** [MCC] [CC/MCC Exc]
Human herpesvirus 7 encephalitis

[5th] B10.8 **Other human herpesvirus infection**

B10.81 **Human herpesvirus 6 infection**

B10.82 **Human herpesvirus 7 infection**

B10.89 **Other human herpesvirus infection**
Human herpesvirus 8 infection
Kaposi's sarcoma-associated herpesvirus infection

Viral hepatitis (B15-B19)

[EXCLUDES1] *sequelae of viral hepatitis (B94.2)*
[EXCLUDES2] *cytomegaloviral hepatitis (B25.1)*
herpesviral [herpes simplex] hepatitis (B00.81)

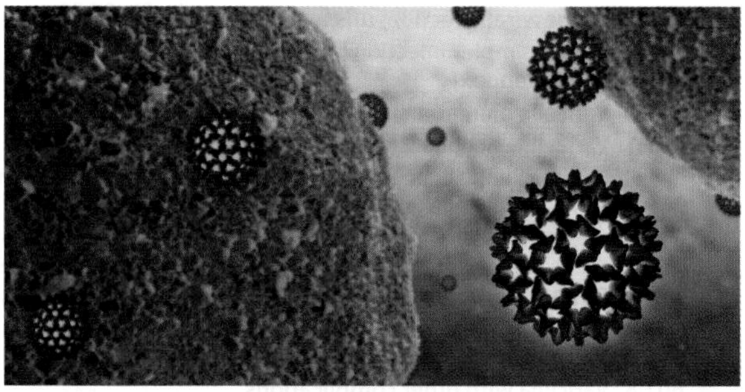

Figure 1.3 Hepatitis B virus

[4th] B15 **Acute hepatitis A**

B15.0 **Hepatitis A with hepatic coma** [MCC] [CC/MCC Exc]

B15.9 **Hepatitis A without hepatic coma** [CC] [CC/MCC Exc]
Hepatitis A (acute)(viral) NOS

[4th] B16 **Acute hepatitis B**

B16.0 **Acute hepatitis B with delta-agent with hepatic coma** [MCC] [CC/MCC Exc]

B16.1 **Acute hepatitis B with delta-agent without hepatic coma** [CC] [CC/MCC Exc]

B16.2 **Acute hepatitis B without delta-agent with hepatic coma** [MCC] [CC/MCC Exc]

B16.9 **Acute hepatitis B without delta-agent and without hepatic coma** [CC] [CC/MCC Exc]
AHA: Q3 2016
Hepatitis B (acute) (viral) NOS

[4th] B17 **Other acute viral hepatitis**

B17.0 **Acute delta-(super) infection of hepatitis B carrier** [CC] [CC/MCC Exc]

[5th] B17.1 **Acute hepatitis C**

B17.10 **Acute hepatitis C without hepatic coma** [CC] [CC/MCC Exc]
Acute hepatitis C NOS

B17.11 **Acute hepatitis C with hepatic coma** [MCC] [CC/MCC Exc]

B17.2 **Acute hepatitis E** [CC] [CC/MCC Exc]

B17.8 **Other specified acute viral hepatitis** [CC] [CC/MCC Exc]
Hepatitis non-A non-B (acute) (viral) NEC

B17.9 **Acute viral hepatitis, unspecified** [CC] [CC/MCC Exc]
Acute hepatitis NOS
Acute infectious hepatitis NOS

[4th] B18 **Chronic viral hepatitis**

[INCLUDES] *Carrier of viral hepatitis*

B18.0 **Chronic viral hepatitis B with delta-agent** [CC] [HCC] [RxHCC] [CC/MCC Exc]

B18.1 **Chronic viral hepatitis B without delta-agent** [CC] [HCC] [RxHCC] [CC/MCC Exc]
Carrier of viral hepatitis B
Chronic (viral) hepatitis B

B18.2 **Chronic viral hepatitis C** [HCC] [RxHCC]
AHA: Q1 2017
Carrier of viral hepatitis C

B18.8 **Other chronic viral hepatitis** [CC] [HCC] [RxHCC] [CC/MCC Exc]
Carrier of other viral hepatitis

B18.9 **Chronic viral hepatitis, unspecified** [CC] [HCC] [RxHCC] [CC/MCC Exc]
Carrier of unspecified viral hepatitis

[4th] B19 **Unspecified viral hepatitis**

B19.0 **Unspecified viral hepatitis with hepatic coma** [MCC] [CC/MCC Exc]

[5th] B19.1 **Unspecified viral hepatitis B**

B19.10 **Unspecified viral hepatitis B without hepatic coma** [CC] [CC/MCC Exc]
Unspecified viral hepatitis B NOS

B19.11 **Unspecified viral hepatitis B with hepatic coma** [MCC] [CC/MCC Exc]

[5th] B19.2 **Unspecified viral hepatitis C**

B19.20 **Unspecified viral hepatitis C without hepatic coma**
Viral hepatitis C NOS

B19.21 **Unspecified viral hepatitis C with hepatic coma** [MCC] [CC/MCC Exc]

B19.9 **Unspecified viral hepatitis without hepatic coma** [CC] [CC/MCC Exc]
Viral hepatitis NOS

[PDx] Unacceptable principal diagnosis symbol per Medicare code edits [POA] Code exempt from diagnosis present on admission requirement
[Q] Questionable admission [CC] Complication or comorbidity [CC/MCC Exc] CC/MCC exclusion [MCC] Major complication or comorbidity
[PDx CC] Principal diagnosis as its own CC [PDx MCC] Principal diagnosis as its own MCC [HCC] HCC diagnosis code [RxHCC] RxHCC diagnosis code
MACRA code [Z-1] Z code as first-listed diagnosis

 When symbols appear on a code that requires a 7th character extension, refer to Appendix B to identify applicable 7th character codes.

Human immunodeficiency virus [HIV] disease (B20)

B20 Human immunodeficiency virus [HIV] disease HCC MCC RxHCC CC/MCC Exc
- *INCLUDES* acquired immune deficiency syndrome [AIDS]
  - AIDS-related complex [ARC]
  - HIV infection, symptomatic

Code first Human immunodeficiency virus [HIV] disease complicating pregnancy, childbirth and the puerperium, if applicable (O98.7-)

Use additional code(s) to identify all manifestations of HIV infection

- *EXCLUDES1* asymptomatic human immunodeficiency virus [HIV] infection status (Z21)
  - exposure to HIV virus (Z20.6)
  - inconclusive serologic evidence of HIV (R75)

Other viral diseases (B25-B34)

4ᵗʰ **B25 Cytomegaloviral disease**
- *EXCLUDES1* congenital cytomegalovirus infection (P35.1)
  - cytomegaloviral mononucleosis (B27.1-)
- **B25.0 Cytomegaloviral** pneumonitis HCC MCC PDx MCC RxHCC CC/MCC Exc
- **B25.1 Cytomegaloviral** hepatitis CC HCC PDx CPG RxHCC
- **B25.2 Cytomegaloviral** pancreatitis HCC MCC PDx MCC RxHCC CC/MCC Exc
- **B25.8 Other cytomegaloviral diseases** CC HCC RxHCC CC/MCC Exc
  - Cytomegaloviral encephalitis
- **B25.9 Cytomegaloviral disease, unspecified** CC HCC RxHCC CC/MCC Exc

4ᵗʰ **B26 Mumps**
- *INCLUDES* epidemic parotitis
  - infectious parotitis
- **B26.0 Mumps** orchitis CC ♂ CC/MCC Exc
- **B26.1 Mumps** meningitis MCC CC/MCC Exc
- **B26.2 Mumps** encephalitis MCC CC/MCC Exc
- **B26.3 Mumps** pancreatitis CC CC/MCC Exc
- 5ᵗʰ **B26.8 Mumps with other complications**
  - **B26.81 Mumps** hepatitis CC CC/MCC Exc
  - **B26.82 Mumps** myocarditis CC CC/MCC Exc
  - **B26.83 Mumps** nephritis CC CC/MCC Exc
  - **B26.84 Mumps** polyneuropathy CC CC/MCC Exc
  - **B26.85 Mumps** arthritis CC HCC CC/MCC Exc
  - **B26.89 Other mumps complications** CC CC/MCC Exc
- **B26.9 Mumps** without complication
  - Mumps NOS
  - Mumps parotitis NOS

4ᵗʰ **B27 Infectious** mononucleosis
- *INCLUDES* glandular fever
  - monocytic angina
  - Pfeiffer's disease
- 5ᵗʰ **B27.0 Gammaherpesviral** mononucleosis
  - Mononucleosis due to Epstein-Barr virus
  - **B27.00 Gammaherpesviral mononucleosis** without complication
  - **B27.01 Gammaherpesviral mononucleosis** with polyneuropathy
  - **B27.02 Gammaherpesviral mononucleosis** with meningitis
  - **B27.09 Gammaherpesviral mononucleosis with other complications**
    - Hepatomegaly in gammaherpesviral mononucleosis
- 5ᵗʰ **B27.1 Cytomegaloviral** mononucleosis
  - **B27.10 Cytomegaloviral mononucleosis** without complications
  - **B27.11 Cytomegaloviral mononucleosis** with polyneuropathy
  - **B27.12 Cytomegaloviral mononucleosis** with meningitis
  - **B27.19 Cytomegaloviral mononucleosis** with other complication
    - Hepatomegaly in cytomegaloviral mononucleosis
- 5ᵗʰ **B27.8 Other** infectious mononucleosis
  - **B27.80 Other infectious mononucleosis** without complication
  - **B27.81 Other infectious mononucleosis** with polyneuropathy
  - **B27.82 Other infectious mononucleosis** with meningitis
  - **B27.89 Other infectious mononucleosis with other complication**
    - Hepatomegaly in other infectious mononucleosis

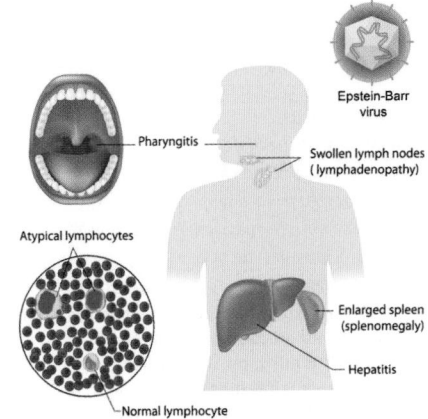

Figure 1.4 Infectious mononucleosis

- 5ᵗʰ **B27.9 Infectious mononucleosis,** unspecified
  - **B27.90 Infectious mononucleosis, unspecified** without complication
  - **B27.91 Infectious mononucleosis, unspecified** with polyneuropathy
  - **B27.92 Infectious mononucleosis, unspecified** with meningitis
  - **B27.99 Infectious mononucleosis, unspecified** with other complication
    - Hepatomegaly in unspecified infectious mononucleosis

4ᵗʰ **B30 Viral conjunctivitis**
- *EXCLUDES1* herpesviral [herpes simplex] ocular disease (B00.5)
  - ocular zoster (B02.3)
- **B30.0 Keratoconjunctivitis due to adenovirus**
  - Epidemic keratoconjunctivitis
  - Shipyard eye
- **B30.1 Conjunctivitis due to adenovirus**
  - Acute adenoviral follicular conjunctivitis
  - Swimming-pool conjunctivitis
- **B30.2 Viral** pharyngoconjunctivitis
- **B30.3 Acute epidemic hemorrhagic conjunctivitis (enteroviral)**
  - Conjunctivitis due to coxsackievirus 24
  - Conjunctivitis due to enterovirus 70
  - Hemorrhagic conjunctivitis (acute)(epidemic)
- **B30.8 Other viral conjunctivitis**
  - Newcastle conjunctivitis
- **B30.9 Viral conjunctivitis, unspecified**

4ᵗʰ **B33 Other viral diseases, not elsewhere classified**
- **B33.0 Epidemic myalgia**
  - Bornholm disease
- **B33.1 Ross River disease** CC CC/MCC Exc
  - Epidemic polyarthritis and exanthema
  - Ross River fever
- 5ᵗʰ **B33.2 Viral** carditis
  - Coxsackie (virus) carditis
  - **B33.20 Viral carditis, unspecified** CC CC/MCC Exc
  - **B33.21 Viral** endocarditis CC CC/MCC Exc
  - **B33.22 Viral** myocarditis CC CC/MCC Exc
  - **B33.23 Viral** pericarditis CC CC/MCC Exc
  - **B33.24 Viral** cardiomyopathy HCC RxHCC
- **B33.3 Retrovirus infections, not elsewhere classified**
  - Retrovirus infection NOS

Unspecified Code   Other Specified Code   Manifestation Code   Ⓝ Newborn   Ⓟ Pediatric   Ⓜ Maternity   Ⓐ Adult   ♂ Male   ♀ Female
● New Code   ▲ Revised Code Title   ►◄ Revised Text   *NOTES*   *INCLUDES*   *EXCLUDES 1* Not coded here   *EXCLUDES 2* Not included here
4ᵗʰ 4ᵗʰ character required   5ᵗʰ 5ᵗʰ character required   6ᵗʰ 6ᵗʰ character required   7ᵗʰ 7ᵗʰ character required
Ⓧ Extension 'X' Alert   HAC Hospital-acquired condition (HAC) alert   AHA AHA Coding Clinic©

2018 ICD-10-CM   When symbols appear on a code that requires a 7th character extension, refer to Appendix B to identify applicable 7th character codes.   **461**

B33.4 Hantavirus (cardio)-pulmonary syndrome [HPS] [HCPS] cc CC/MCC Exc
Hantavirus disease with pulmonary manifestations
Sin nombre virus disease
Use additional code to identify any associated acute kidney failure (N17.9)
EXCLUDES1 *hantavirus disease with renal manifestations (A98.5)*
hemorrhagic fever with renal manifestations (A98.5)

B33.8 Other specified viral diseases
EXCLUDES1 *anogenital human papillomavirus infection (A63.0)*
viral warts due to human papillomavirus infection (B07)

B34 Viral infection of unspecified site
EXCLUDES1 *anogenital human papillomavirus infection (A63.0)*
cytomegaloviral disease NOS (B25.9)
herpesvirus [herpes simplex] infection NOS (B00.9)
retrovirus infection NOS (B33.3)
viral agents as the cause of diseases classified elsewhere (B97.-)
viral warts due to human papillomavirus infection (B07)

B34.0 Adenovirus infection, unspecified
B34.1 Enterovirus infection, unspecified
Coxsackievirus infection NOS
Echovirus infection NOS
B34.2 Coronavirus infection, unspecified
EXCLUDES1 *pneumonia due to SARS-associated coronavirus (J12.81)*
B34.3 Parvovirus infection, unspecified cc CC/MCC Exc
B34.4 Papovavirus infection, unspecified
B34.8 Other viral infections of unspecified site
B34.9 Viral infection, unspecified
AHA: Q3 2016
Viremia NOS

Mycoses (B35-B49)

EXCLUDES2 *hypersensitivity pneumonitis due to organic dust (J67.-)*
mycosis fungoides (C84.0-)

B35 Dermatophytosis
INCLUDES *favus*
infections due to species of Epidermophyton, Micro-sporum and Trichophyton
tinea, any type except those in B36.-

B35.0 Tinea barbae and tinea capitis
Beard ringworm
Kerion
Scalp ringworm
Sycosis, mycotic
B35.1 Tinea unguium
Dermatophytic onychia
Dermatophytosis of nail
Onychomycosis
Ringworm of nails
B35.2 Tinea manuum
Dermatophytosis of hand
Hand ringworm
B35.3 Tinea pedis
Athlete's foot
Dermatophytosis of foot
Foot ringworm
B35.4 Tinea corporis
Ringworm of the body
B35.5 Tinea imbricata
Tokelau
B35.6 Tinea cruris
Dhobi itch
Groin ringworm
Jock itch
B35.8 Other dermatophytoses
Disseminated dermatophytosis
Granulomatous dermatophytosis

B35.9 Dermatophytosis, unspecified
Ringworm NOS

B36 Other superficial mycoses
B36.0 Pityriasis versicolor
Tinea flava
Tinea versicolor
B36.1 Tinea nigra
Keratomycosis nigricans palmaris
Microsporosis nigra
Pityriasis nigra
B36.2 White piedra
Tinea blanca
B36.3 Black piedra
B36.8 Other specified superficial mycoses
B36.9 Superficial mycosis, unspecified

B37 Candidiasis
INCLUDES *candidosis*
moniliasis
EXCLUDES1 *neonatal candidiasis (P37.5)*
B37.0 Candidal stomatitis cc CC/MCC Exc
Oral thrush
B37.1 Pulmonary candidiasis HCC MCC RxHCC CC/MCC Exc
Candidal bronchitis
Candidal pneumonia
B37.2 Candidiasis of skin and nail
Candidal onychia
Candidal paronychia
EXCLUDES2 *diaper dermatitis (L22)*
B37.3 Candidiasis of vulva and vagina ♀
Candidal vulvovaginitis
Monilial vulvovaginitis
Vaginal thrush
B37.4 Candidiasis of other urogenital sites
B37.41 Candidal cystitis and urethritis cc HAC CC/MCC Exc
B37.42 Candidal balanitis
B37.49 Other urogenital candidiasis cc HAC CC/MCC Exc
Candidal pyelonephritis
B37.5 Candidal meningitis MCC CC/MCC Exc
B37.6 Candidal endocarditis MCC CC/MCC Exc
B37.7 Candidal sepsis HCC MCC PDx/MCC RxHCC CC/MCC Exc
Disseminated candidiasis
Systemic candidiasis
B37.8 Candidiasis of other sites
B37.81 Candidal esophagitis cc HCC RxHCC CC/MCC Exc
B37.82 Candidal enteritis cc CC/MCC Exc
Candidal proctitis
B37.83 Candidal cheilitis cc CC/MCC Exc
B37.84 Candidal otitis externa cc CC/MCC Exc
B37.89 Other sites of candidiasis cc CC/MCC Exc
Candidal osteomyelitis
B37.9 Candidiasis, unspecified
Thrush NOS

B38 Coccidioidomycosis
B38.0 Acute pulmonary coccidioidomycosis cc HCC CC/MCC Exc
B38.1 Chronic pulmonary coccidioidomycosis cc HCC CC/MCC Exc
B38.2 Pulmonary coccidioidomycosis, unspecified cc HCC CC/MCC Exc
B38.3 Cutaneous coccidioidomycosis cc CC/MCC Exc
B38.4 Coccidioidomycosis meningitis MCC CC/MCC Exc
B38.7 Disseminated coccidioidomycosis cc CC/MCC Exc
Generalized coccidioidomycosis
B38.8 Other forms of coccidioidomycosis
B38.81 Prostatic coccidioidomycosis cc ♂ CC/MCC Exc
B38.89 Other forms of coccidioidomycosis cc CC/MCC Exc
B38.9 Coccidioidomycosis, unspecified cc CC/MCC Exc

B39 Histoplasmosis
Code first associated AIDS (B20)
Use additional code for any associated manifestations, such as:
endocarditis (I39)
meningitis (G02)
pericarditis (I32)
retinitis (H32)

PDx Unacceptable principal diagnosis symbol per Medicare code edits   PDx Code exempt from diagnosis present on admission requirement
? Questionable admission   cc Complication or comorbidity   CC/MCC Exc CC/MCC exclusion   MCC Major complication or comorbidity
PDx/CC Principal diagnosis as its own CC   PDx/MCC Principal diagnosis as its own MCC   HCC HCC diagnosis code   RxHCC RxHCC diagnosis code
MACRA code   Z code as first-listed diagnosis

462   When symbols appear on a code that requires a 7th character extension, refer to Appendix B to identify applicable 7th character codes.   2018 ICD-10-CM

B39.0   Acute pulmonary **histoplasmosis capsulati**   HCC MCC CC/MCC Exc

B39.1   Chronic pulmonary **histoplasmosis capsulati**   HCC MCC CC/MCC Exc

B39.2   Pulmonary **histoplasmosis capsulati,**
        unspecified   HCC MCC CC/MCC Exc

B39.3   Disseminated **histoplasmosis capsulati**   CC/MCC Exc
        Generalized histoplasmosis capsulati

B39.4   **Histoplasmosis capsulati, unspecified**
        American histoplasmosis

B39.5   **Histoplasmosis** duboisii
        African histoplasmosis

B39.9   **Histoplasmosis, unspecified**

B40   Blastomycosis

        EXCLUDES1 *Brazilian blastomycosis (B41.-)*
                   keloidal blastomycosis (B48.0)

B40.0   Acute pulmonary **blastomycosis**   HCC CC/MCC Exc

B40.1   Chronic pulmonary **blastomycosis**   HCC CC/MCC Exc

B40.2   Pulmonary **blastomycosis, unspecified**   HCC CC/MCC Exc

B40.3   Cutaneous **blastomycosis**   CC/MCC Exc

B40.7   Disseminated **blastomycosis**   CC/MCC Exc
        Generalized blastomycosis

B40.8   Other forms of blastomycosis

        B40.81   **Blastomycotic meningoencephalitis**   CC/MCC Exc
                 Meningomyelitis due to blastomycosis

        B40.89   Other forms of blastomycosis   CC/MCC Exc

B40.9   **Blastomycosis, unspecified**   CC/MCC Exc

B41   Paracoccidioidomycosis

        INCLUDES *Brazilian blastomycosis*
                  Lutz' disease

B41.0   Pulmonary **paracoccidioidomycosis**   HCC CC/MCC Exc

B41.7   Disseminated **paracoccidioidomycosis**   CC/MCC Exc
        Generalized paracoccidioidomycosis

B41.8   Other forms of **paracoccidioidomycosis**   CC/MCC Exc

B41.9   **Paracoccidioidomycosis, unspecified**   CC/MCC Exc

B42   Sporotrichosis

B42.0   Pulmonary **sporotrichosis**

B42.1   Lymphocutaneous **sporotrichosis**

B42.7   Disseminated **sporotrichosis**
        Generalized sporotrichosis

B42.8   Other forms of sporotrichosis

        B42.81   Cerebral **sporotrichosis**
                 Meningitis due to sporotrichosis

        B42.82   **Sporotrichosis** arthritis   HCC

        B42.89   Other forms of sporotrichosis

B42.9   **Sporotrichosis, unspecified**

B43   Chromomycosis and pheomycotic abscess

B43.0   Cutaneous **chromomycosis**
        Dermatitis verrucosa

B43.1   Pheomycotic **brain abscess**
        Cerebral chromomycosis

B43.2   Subcutaneous **pheomycotic abscess and cyst**

B43.8   Other forms of chromomycosis

B43.9   **Chromomycosis, unspecified**

B44   Aspergillosis

        INCLUDES *aspergilloma*

B44.0   Invasive **pulmonary aspergillosis**   HCC MCC PDx MCC RxHCC CC/MCC Exc

B44.1   Other **pulmonary aspergillosis**   HCC RxHCC CC/MCC Exc

B44.2   Tonsillar **aspergillosis**   HCC RxHCC CC/MCC Exc

B44.7   Disseminated **aspergillosis**   HCC RxHCC CC/MCC Exc
        Generalized aspergillosis

B44.8   Other forms of aspergillosis

        B44.81   **Allergic bronchopulmonary**
                 aspergillosis   HCC RxHCC CC/MCC Exc

        B44.89   Other forms of aspergillosis   HCC RxHCC CC/MCC Exc

B44.9   **Aspergillosis, unspecified**   HCC RxHCC CC/MCC Exc

B45   Cryptococcosis

B45.0   Pulmonary **cryptococcosis**   HCC RxHCC CC/MCC Exc

B45.1   Cerebral **cryptococcosis**   HCC MCC PDx MCC RxHCC CC/MCC Exc
        Cryptococcal meningitis
        Cryptococcosis meningocerebralis

B45.2   Cutaneous **cryptococcosis**   HCC RxHCC CC/MCC Exc

B45.3   Osseous **cryptococcosis**   HCC RxHCC CC/MCC Exc

B45.7   Disseminated **cryptococcosis**   HCC RxHCC CC/MCC Exc
        Generalized cryptococcosis

B45.8   **Other forms of cryptococcosis**   HCC RxHCC CC/MCC Exc

B45.9   **Cryptococcosis, unspecified**   HCC RxHCC CC/MCC Exc

B46   Zygomycosis

B46.0   Pulmonary **mucormycosis**   HCC MCC RxHCC CC/MCC Exc

B46.1   Rhinocerebral **mucormycosis**   HCC MCC RxHCC CC/MCC Exc

B46.2   Gastrointestinal **mucormycosis**   HCC MCC RxHCC CC/MCC Exc

B46.3   Cutaneous **mucormycosis**   HCC MCC RxHCC CC/MCC Exc
        Subcutaneous mucormycosis

B46.4   Disseminated **mucormycosis**   HCC MCC RxHCC CC/MCC Exc
        Generalized mucormycosis

B46.5   **Mucormycosis, unspecified**   HCC MCC RxHCC CC/MCC Exc

B46.8   Other zygomycoses
        Entomophthoromycosis

B46.9   **Zygomycosis, unspecified**   HCC MCC RxHCC CC/MCC Exc
        Phycomycosis NOS

B47   Mycetoma

B47.0   Eumycetoma   CC/MCC Exc
        Madura foot, mycotic
        Maduromycosis

B47.1   **Actinomycetoma**   CC/MCC Exc

B47.9   **Mycetoma, unspecified**   CC/MCC Exc
        Madura foot NOS

B48   Other mycoses, not elsewhere classified

B48.0   **Lobomycosis**
        Keloidal blastomycosis
        Lobo's disease

B48.1   **Rhinosporidiosis**

B48.2   **Allescheriasis**   CC/MCC Exc
        Infection due to Pseudallescheria boydii

        EXCLUDES1 *eumycetoma (B47.0)*

B48.3   **Geotrichosis**   CC/MCC Exc
        Geotrichum stomatitis

B48.4   **Penicillosis**   HCC RxHCC CC/MCC Exc

B48.8   Other specified mycoses   HCC RxHCC CC/MCC Exc
        Adiaspiromycosis
        Infection of tissue and organs by Alternaria
        Infection of tissue and organs by Drechslera
        Infection of tissue and organs by Fusarium
        Infection of tissue and organs by saprophytic fungi NEC

B49   Unspecified mycosis   CC/MCC Exc
        Fungemia NOS

Protozoal diseases (B50-B64)

        EXCLUDES1 *amebiasis (A06.-)*
                   other protozoal intestinal diseases (A07.-)

B50   Plasmodium falciparum malaria

        INCLUDES *mixed infections of Plasmodium falciparum with any other*
                  Plasmodium species

B50.0   **Plasmodium falciparum malaria** with cerebral
        complications   CC/MCC Exc
        Cerebral malaria NOS

B50.8   **Other severe and complicated Plasmodium**
        falciparum malaria   CC/MCC Exc
        Severe or complicated Plasmodium falciparum malaria NOS

B50.9   **Plasmodium falciparum malaria, unspecified**   MCC CC/MCC Exc

B51   Plasmodium vivax malaria

        INCLUDES *mixed infections of Plasmodium vivax with other Plasmodium*
                  species, except Plasmodium falciparum

        EXCLUDES1 *plasmodium vivax with Plasmodium falciparum (B50.-)*

B51.0   **Plasmodium vivax malaria** with rupture of spleen   CC/MCC Exc

B51.8   **Plasmodium vivax malaria** with other complications   CC/MCC Exc

B51.9   **Plasmodium vivax malaria** without complication   CC/MCC Exc
        Plasmodium vivax malaria NOS

Unspecified Code   Other Specified Code   Manifestation Code   N Newborn   P Pediatric   M Maternity   A Adult   ♂ Male   ♀ Female
● New Code   ▲ Revised Code Title   ▶◀ Revised Text   **NOTES**   INCLUDES   EXCLUDES 1   Not coded here   EXCLUDES 2   Not included here
4ᵗʰ character required   5ᵗʰ character required   6ᵗʰ character required   7ᵗʰ character required
Extension 'X' Alert   HAC Hospital-acquired condition (HAC) alert   **AHA** AHA Coding Clinic©

B52 **Plasmodium** malariae **malaria**

INCLUDES   mixed infections of Plasmodium malariae with other Plasmodium species, except Plasmodium falciparum and Plasmodium vivax

EXCLUDES1 Plasmodium falciparum (B50.-)

Plasmodium vivax (B51.-)

B52.0 **Plasmodium malariae malaria** with nephropathy

B52.8 **Plasmodium malariae malaria** with other complications

B52.9 **Plasmodium malariae malaria** without complication

Plasmodium malariae malaria NOS

B53 Other specified **malaria**

B53.0 **Plasmodium** ovale **malaria**

EXCLUDES1 Plasmodium ovale with Plasmodium falciparum (B50.-)

Plasmodium ovale with Plasmodium malariae (B52.-)

Plasmodium ovale with Plasmodium vivax (B51.-)

B53.1 **Malaria due to** simian plasmodia

EXCLUDES1 Malaria due to simian plasmodia with Plasmodium falciparum (B50.-)

Malaria due to simian plasmodia with Plasmodium malariae (B52.-)

Malaria due to simian plasmodia with Plasmodium ovale (B53.0)

Malaria due to simian plasmodia with Plasmodium vivax (B51.-)

B53.8 **Other malaria, not elsewhere classified**

B54 Unspecified **malaria**

B55 **Leishmaniasis**

B55.0 **Visceral leishmaniasis**

Kala-azar

Post-kala-azar dermal leishmaniasis

B55.1 Cutaneous **leishmaniasis**

B55.2 Mucocutaneous **leishmaniasis**

B55.9 **Leishmaniasis, unspecified**

B56 African **trypanosomiasis**

B56.0 Gambiense **trypanosomiasis**

Infection due to Trypanosoma brucei gambiense

West African sleeping sickness

B56.1 Rhodesiense **trypanosomiasis**

East African sleeping sickness

Infection due to Trypanosoma brucei rhodesiense

B56.9 **African trypanosomiasis, unspecified**

Sleeping sickness NOS

B57 Chagas' **disease**

INCLUDES   American trypanosomiasis

infection due to Trypanosoma cruzi

B57.0 **Acute** Chagas' disease with heart involvement

Acute Chagas' disease with myocarditis

B57.1 Acute **Chagas' disease** without heart involvement

Acute Chagas' disease NOS

B57.2 **Chagas' disease (chronic)** with heart involvement

American trypanosomiasis NOS

Chagas' disease (chronic) NOS

Chagas' disease (chronic) with myocarditis

Trypanosomiasis NOS

B57.3 **Chagas' disease (chronic)** with digestive system involvement

B57.30 **Chagas' disease with digestive system involvement, unspecified**

B57.31 Megaesophagus in Chagas' disease

B57.32 Megacolon in Chagas' disease

B57.39 **Other digestive system involvement in Chagas' disease**

B57.4 **Chagas' disease (chronic)** with nervous system involvement

B57.40 **Chagas' disease with nervous system involvement, unspecified**

B57.41 Meningitis in Chagas' disease

B57.42 Meningoencephalitis in Chagas' disease

B57.49 **Other nervous system involvement in Chagas' disease**

B57.5 Chagas' disease (chronic) with other organ involvement

B58 Toxoplasmosis

INCLUDES   infection due to Toxoplasma gondii

EXCLUDES1 congenital toxoplasmosis (P37.1)

B58.0 Toxoplasma oculopathy

B58.00 **Toxoplasma oculopathy, unspecified**

B58.01 **Toxoplasma** chorioretinitis

B58.09 Other **toxoplasma oculopathy**

Toxoplasma uveitis

B58.1 **Toxoplasma** hepatitis

B58.2 **Toxoplasma** meningoencephalitis

B58.3 **Pulmonary** toxoplasmosis

B58.8 **Toxoplasmosis** with other organ involvement

B58.81 **Toxoplasma** myocarditis

B58.82 **Toxoplasma** myositis

B58.83 **Toxoplasma** tubulo-interstitial nephropathy

Toxoplasma pyelonephritis

B58.89 **Toxoplasmosis with other organ involvement**

B58.9 **Toxoplasmosis, unspecified**

B59 Pneumocystosis

Pneumonia due to Pneumocystis carinii

Pneumonia due to Pneumocystis jiroveci

B60 Other protozoal diseases, not elsewhere classified

EXCLUDES1 cryptosporidiosis (A07.2)

intestinal microsporidiosis (A07.8)

isosporiasis (A07.3)

B60.0 **Babesiosis**

Piroplasmosis

B60.1 **Acanthamebiasis**

B60.10 **Acanthamebiasis, unspecified**

B60.11 Meningoencephalitis due to Acanthamoeba (culbertsoni)

B60.12 Conjunctivitis due to Acanthamoeba

B60.13 Keratoconjunctivitis due to Acanthamoeba

B60.19 **Other acanthamebic disease**

B60.2 **Naegleriasis**

Primary amebic meningoencephalitis

B60.8 Other specified protozoal diseases

Microsporidiosis

B64 Unspecified protozoal disease

Helminthiases (B65-B83)

B65 Schistosomiasis [bilharziasis]

INCLUDES   snail fever

B65.0 **Schistosomiasis due to Schistosoma** haematobium **[urinary schistosomiasis]**

B65.1 **Schistosomiasis due to Schistosoma** mansoni **[intestinal schistosomiasis]**

B65.2 **Schistosomiasis due to Schistosoma** japonicum

Asiatic schistosomiasis

B65.3 **Cercarial dermatitis**

Swimmer's itch

B65.8 **Other schistosomiasis**

Infection due to Schistosoma intercalatum

Infection due to Schistosoma mattheei

Infection due to Schistosoma mekongi

B65.9 Schistosomiasis, unspecified

B66 Other fluke infections

B66.0 **Opisthorchiasis**

Infection due to cat liver fluke

Infection due to Opisthorchis (felineus)(viverrini)

B66.1 **Clonorchiasis**

Chinese liver fluke disease

Infection due to Clonorchis sinensis

Oriental liver fluke disease

PDx Unacceptable principal diagnosis symbol per Medicare code edits   POA Code exempt from diagnosis present on admission requirement

? Questionable admission   CC Complication or comorbidity   CC/MCC Exc CC/MCC exclusion   MCC Major complication or comorbidity

CC Principal diagnosis as its own CC   MCC Principal diagnosis as its own MCC   HCC HCC diagnosis code   RxHCC RxHCC diagnosis code

MACRA code   Z1 Z code as first-listed diagnosis

B66.2 **Dicroceliasis** [CC] [CC/MCC Exc]
Infection due to Dicrocoelium dendriticum
Lancet fluke infection
B66.3 **Fascioliasis** [CC] [CC/MCC Exc]
Infection due to Fasciola gigantica
Infection due to Fasciola hepatica
Infection due to Fasciola indica
Sheep liver fluke disease
B66.4 **Paragonimiasis** [CC] [HCC] [CC/MCC Exc]
Infection due to Paragonimus species
Lung fluke disease
Pulmonary distomiasis
B66.5 **Fasciolopsiasis** [CC] [CC/MCC Exc]
Infection due to Fasciolopsis buski
Intestinal distomiasis
B66.8 **Other specified fluke infections** [CC] [CC/MCC Exc]
Echinostomiasis
Heterophyiasis
Metagonimiasis
Nanophyetiasis
Watsoniasis
B66.9 **Fluke infection, unspecified**

[4th] **B67 Echinococcosis**
[INCLUDES] *hydatidosis*
B67.0 **Echinococcus granulosus infection of liver** [CC] [CC/MCC Exc]
B67.1 **Echinococcus granulosus infection of lung** [CC] [HCC] [CC/MCC Exc]
B67.2 **Echinococcus granulosus infection of bone** [CC] [CC/MCC Exc]
[5th] B67.3 **Echinococcus granulosus infection, other and multiple sites**
B67.31 **Echinococcus granulosus infection, thyroid gland** [CC] [CC/MCC Exc]
B67.32 **Echinococcus granulosus infection, multiple sites** [CC] [CC/MCC Exc]
B67.39 **Echinococcus granulosus infection, other sites** [CC] [CC/MCC Exc]
B67.4 **Echinococcus granulosus infection, unspecified** [CC] [CC/MCC Exc]
Dog tapeworm (infection)
B67.5 **Echinococcus multilocularis infection of liver** [CC] [CC/MCC Exc]
[5th] B67.6 **Echinococcus multilocularis infection, other and multiple sites**
B67.61 **Echinococcus multilocularis infection, multiple sites** [CC] [CC/MCC Exc]
B67.69 **Echinococcus multilocularis infection, other sites** [CC] [CC/MCC Exc]
B67.7 **Echinococcus multilocularis infection, unspecified** [CC] [CC/MCC Exc]
B67.8 **Echinococcosis, unspecified, of liver** [CC] [CC/MCC Exc]
[5th] B67.9 **Echinococcosis, other and unspecified**
B67.90 **Echinococcosis, unspecified** [CC] [CC/MCC Exc]
Echinococcosis NOS
B67.99 **Other echinococcosis** [CC] [CC/MCC Exc]

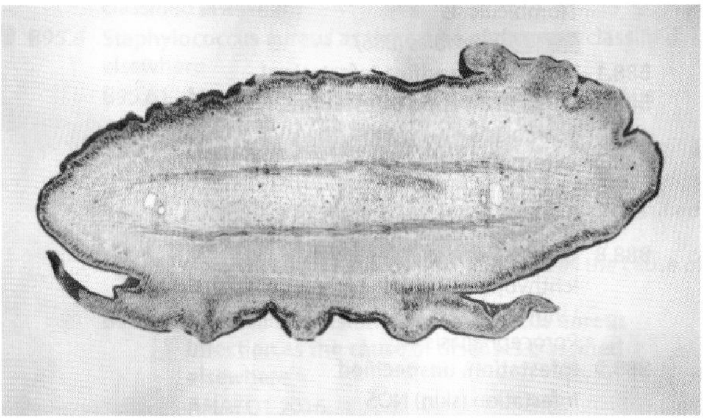

Figure 1.5 Taeniasis

[4th] **B68 Taeniasis**
[EXCLUDES1] *cysticercosis (B69.-)*
B68.0 **Taenia solium taeniasis** [CC] [CC/MCC Exc]
Pork tapeworm (infection)
B68.1 **Taenia saginata taeniasis** [CC] [CC/MCC Exc]
Beef tapeworm (infection)
Infection due to adult tapeworm Taenia saginata
B68.9 **Taeniasis, unspecified** [CC] [CC/MCC Exc]

[4th] **B69 Cysticercosis**
[INCLUDES] *cysticerciasis infection due to larval form of Taenia solium*
B69.0 **Cysticercosis of central nervous system** [CC] [CC/MCC Exc]
B69.1 **Cysticercosis of eye** [CC] [CC/MCC Exc]
[5th] B69.8 **Cysticercosis of other sites**
B69.81 **Myositis in cysticercosis** [CC] [CC/MCC Exc]
B69.89 **Cysticercosis of other sites** [CC] [CC/MCC Exc]
B69.9 **Cysticercosis, unspecified** [CC] [CC/MCC Exc]

[4th] **B70 Diphyllobothriasis and sparganosis**
B70.0 **Diphyllobothriasis** [CC] [CC/MCC Exc]
Diphyllobothrium (adult) (latum) (pacificum) infection
Fish tapeworm (infection)
[EXCLUDES2] *larval diphyllobothriasis (B70.1)*
B70.1 **Sparganosis** [CC] [CC/MCC Exc]
Infection due to Sparganum (mansoni) (proliferum)
Infection due to Spirometra larva
Larval diphyllobothriasis
Spirometrosis

[4th] **B71 Other cestode infections**
B71.0 **Hymenolepiasis** [CC] [CC/MCC Exc]
Dwarf tapeworm infection
Rat tapeworm (infection)
B71.1 **Dipylidiasis** [CC] [CC/MCC Exc]
B71.8 **Other specified cestode infections** [CC] [CC/MCC Exc]
Coenurosis
B71.9 **Cestode infection, unspecified**
Tapeworm (infection) NOS

B72 Dracunculiasis [CC] [CC/MCC Exc]
[INCLUDES] *guinea worm infection*
infection due to Dracunculus medinensis

[4th] **B73 Onchocerciasis**
[INCLUDES] *onchocerca volvulus infection*
onchocercosis
river blindness
[5th] B73.0 **Onchocerciasis with eye disease**
B73.00 **Onchocerciasis with eye involvement, unspecified** [CC] [CC/MCC Exc]
B73.01 **Onchocerciasis with endophthalmitis** [CC] [CC/MCC Exc]
B73.02 **Onchocerciasis with glaucoma** [CC] [CC/MCC Exc]
B73.09 **Onchocerciasis with other eye involvement** [CC] [CC/MCC Exc]
Infestation of eyelid due to onchocerciasis
B73.1 **Onchocerciasis without eye disease** [CC] [CC/MCC Exc]

[4th] **B74 Filariasis**
[EXCLUDES2] *onchocerciasis (B73)*
tropical (pulmonary) eosinophilia NOS (J82)
B74.0 **Filariasis due to Wuchereria bancrofti** [CC] [CC/MCC Exc]
Bancroftian elephantiasis
Bancroftian filariasis
B74.1 **Filariasis due to Brugia malayi** [CC] [CC/MCC Exc]
B74.2 **Filariasis due to Brugia timori** [CC] [CC/MCC Exc]
B74.3 **Loiasis** [CC] [CC/MCC Exc]
Calabar swelling
Eyeworm disease of Africa
Loa loa infection
B74.4 **Mansonelliasis** [CC] [CC/MCC Exc]
Infection due to Mansonella ozzardi
Infection due to Mansonella perstans
Infection due to Mansonella streptocerca
B74.8 **Other filariases** [CC] [CC/MCC Exc]
Dirofilariasis
B74.9 **Filariasis, unspecified** [CC] [CC/MCC Exc]

B75 Trichinellosis [CC] [CC/MCC Exc]
[INCLUDES] *infection due to Trichinella species*
trichiniasis

[4th] **B76 Hookworm diseases**
[INCLUDES] *uncinariasis*

Unspecified Code | Other Specified Code | Manifestation Code | [N] Newborn | [P] Pediatric | [M] Maternity | [A] Adult | ♂ Male | ♀ Female
● New Code | ▲ Revised Code Title | ►◄ Revised Text | [NOTES] | [INCLUDES] | [EXCLUDES1] Not coded here | [EXCLUDES2] Not included here
[4th] 4th character required | [5th] 5th character required | [6th] 6th character required | [7th] 7th character required
[X] Extension 'X' Alert | [HAC] Hospital-acquired condition (HAC) alert | AHA AHA Coding Clinic©

When symbols appear on a code that requires a 7th character extension, refer to Appendix B to identify applicable 7th character codes.

C02.9 **Malignant neoplasm of tongue, unspecified** [HCC]

C03 Malignant neoplasm of gum

INCLUDES *malignant neoplasm of alveolar (ridge) mucosa*
malignant neoplasm of gingiva

Use additional code to identify:

alcohol abuse and dependence (F10.-)

history of tobacco dependence (Z87.891)

tobacco dependence (F17.-)

tobacco use (Z72.0)

EXCLUDES2 *malignant odontogenic neoplasms (C41.0-C41.1)*

C03.0 **Malignant neoplasm of** upper gum [HCC]

C03.1 **Malignant neoplasm of** lower gum [HCC]

C03.9 **Malignant neoplasm of gum, unspecified** [HCC]

C04 Malignant neoplasm of floor of mouth

Use additional code to identify:

alcohol abuse and dependence (F10.-)

history of tobacco dependence (Z87.891)

tobacco dependence (F17.-)

tobacco use (Z72.0)

C04.0 **Malignant neoplasm of** anterior floor **of mouth** [HCC]

Malignant neoplasm of anterior to the premolar-canine junction

C04.1 **Malignant neoplasm of** lateral floor **of mouth** [HCC]

C04.8 **Malignant neoplasm of** overlapping sites **of floor of mouth** [HCC]

C04.9 **Malignant neoplasm of floor of mouth, unspecified** [HCC]

C05 Malignant neoplasm of palate

Use additional code to identify:

alcohol abuse and dependence (F10.-)

history of tobacco dependence (Z87.891)

tobacco dependence (F17.-)

tobacco use (Z72.0)

EXCLUDES1 *Kaposi's sarcoma of palate (C46.2)*

C05.0 **Malignant neoplasm of** hard **palate** [HCC]

C05.1 **Malignant neoplasm of** soft **palate** [HCC]

EXCLUDES2 *malignant neoplasm of nasopharyngeal surface of soft palate (C11.3)*

C05.2 **Malignant neoplasm of** uvula [HCC]

C05.8 **Malignant neoplasm of** overlapping sites **of palate** [HCC]

C05.9 **Malignant neoplasm of palate, unspecified** [HCC]

Malignant neoplasm of roof of mouth

C06 Malignant neoplasm of other and unspecified parts of mouth

Use additional code to identify:

alcohol abuse and dependence (F10.-)

history of tobacco dependence (Z87.891)

tobacco dependence (F17.-)

tobacco use (Z72.0)

C06.0 **Malignant neoplasm of** cheek mucosa [HCC]

Malignant neoplasm of buccal mucosa NOS
Malignant neoplasm of internal cheek

C06.1 **Malignant neoplasm of** vestibule **of mouth** [HCC]

Malignant neoplasm of buccal sulcus (upper) (lower)
Malignant neoplasm of labial sulcus (upper) (lower)

C06.2 **Malignant neoplasm of** retromolar area [HCC]

C06.8 **Malignant neoplasm of** overlapping sites **of other and unspecified parts of mouth**

C06.80 **Malignant neoplasm of overlapping sites of unspecified parts of mouth** [HCC]

C06.89 **Malignant neoplasm of overlapping sites of other parts of mouth** [HCC]

'book leaf' neoplasm [ventral surface of tongue and floor of mouth]

C06.9 **Malignant neoplasm of mouth, unspecified** [HCC]

Malignant neoplasm of minor salivary gland, unspecified site
Malignant neoplasm of oral cavity NOS

C07 Malignant neoplasm of parotid gland [HCC]

Use additional code to identify:

alcohol abuse and dependence (F10.-)

exposure to environmental tobacco smoke (Z77.22)

exposure to tobacco smoke in the perinatal period (P96.81)

history of tobacco dependence (Z87.891)

occupational exposure to environmental tobacco smoke (Z57.31)

tobacco dependence (F17.-)

tobacco use (Z72.0)

C08 Malignant neoplasm of other and unspecified major salivary glands

INCLUDES *malignant neoplasm of salivary ducts*

Use additional code to identify:

alcohol abuse and dependence (F10.-)

exposure to environmental tobacco smoke (Z77.22)

exposure to tobacco smoke in the perinatal period (P96.81)

history of tobacco dependence (Z87.891)

occupational exposure to environmental tobacco smoke (Z57.31)

tobacco dependence (F17.-)

tobacco use (Z72.0)

EXCLUDES1 *malignant neoplasms of specified minor salivary glands which are classified according to their anatomical location*

EXCLUDES2 *malignant neoplasms of minor salivary glands NOS (C06.9)*
malignant neoplasm of parotid gland (C07)

C08.0 **Malignant neoplasm of** submandibular gland [HCC]

Malignant neoplasm of submaxillary gland

C08.1 **Malignant neoplasm of** sublingual gland [HCC]

C08.9 **Malignant neoplasm of major salivary gland, unspecified** [HCC]

Malignant neoplasm of salivary gland (major) NOS

C09 Malignant neoplasm of tonsil

Use additional code to identify:

alcohol abuse and dependence (F10.-)

exposure to environmental tobacco smoke (Z77.22)

exposure to tobacco smoke in the perinatal period (P96.81)

history of tobacco dependence (Z87.891)

occupational exposure to environmental tobacco smoke (Z57.31)

tobacco dependence (F17.-)

tobacco use (Z72.0)

EXCLUDES2 *malignant neoplasm of lingual tonsil (C02.4)*
malignant neoplasm of pharyngeal tonsil (C11.1)

C09.0 **Malignant neoplasm of** tonsillar fossa [HCC]

C09.1 **Malignant neoplasm of** tonsillar pillar (anterior) (posterior) [HCC]

C09.8 **Malignant neoplasm of** overlapping sites **of tonsil** [HCC]

C09.9 **Malignant neoplasm of tonsil, unspecified** [HCC]

Malignant neoplasm of tonsil NOS
Malignant neoplasm of faucial tonsils
Malignant neoplasm of palatine tonsils

C10 Malignant neoplasm of oropharynx

Use additional code to identify:

alcohol abuse and dependence (F10.-)

exposure to environmental tobacco smoke (Z77.22)

exposure to tobacco smoke in the perinatal period (P96.81)

history of tobacco dependence (Z87.891)

occupational exposure to environmental tobacco smoke (Z57.31)

tobacco dependence (F17.-)

tobacco use (Z72.0)

EXCLUDES2 *malignant neoplasm of tonsil (C09.-)*

C10.0 **Malignant neoplasm of** vallecula [HCC]

C10.1 **Malignant neoplasm of** anterior surface of epiglottis [HCC]

Malignant neoplasm of epiglottis, free border [margin]
Malignant neoplasm of glossoepiglottic fold(s)

EXCLUDES2 *malignant neoplasm of epiglottis (suprahyoid portion) NOS (C32.1)*

C10.2 **Malignant neoplasm of** lateral wall **of oropharynx** [HCC]

C10.3 **Malignant neoplasm of** posterior wall **of oropharynx** [HCC]

C10.4 **Malignant neoplasm of** branchial cleft [HCC]

Malignant neoplasm of branchial cyst [site of neoplasm]

C10.8 **Malignant neoplasm of** overlapping sites **of oropharynx** [HCC]

Malignant neoplasm of junctional region of oropharynx

C10.9 **Malignant neoplasm of oropharynx, unspecified** [HCC]

C11 Malignant neoplasm of nasopharynx

Use additional code to identify:

exposure to environmental tobacco smoke (Z77.22)

PDx⃣ Unacceptable principal diagnosis symbol per Medicare code edits   PDx⃣ Code exempt from diagnosis present on admission requirement
❓ Questionable admission   ℅ Complication or comorbidity   CC-MCC EX CC/MCC exclusion   MCC Major complication or comorbidity
Principal diagnosis as its own CC   Principal diagnosis as its own MCC   HCC HCC diagnosis code   RxHCC RxHCC diagnosis code
MACRA code   Z1 Z code as first-listed diagnosis

When symbols appear on a code that requires a 7th character extension, refer to Appendix B to identify applicable 7th character codes.   **2018 ICD-10-CM**

exposure to tobacco smoke in the perinatal period (P96.81)

history of tobacco dependence (Z87.891)

occupational exposure to environmental tobacco smoke (Z57.31)

tobacco dependence (F17.-)

tobacco use (Z72.0)

C11.0 **Malignant neoplasm of** superior wall **of nasopharynx** `HCC`

Malignant neoplasm of roof of nasopharynx

C11.1 **Malignant neoplasm of** posterior wall **of nasopharynx** `HCC`

Malignant neoplasm of adenoid

Malignant neoplasm of pharyngeal tonsil

C11.2 **Malignant neoplasm of** lateral wall **of nasopharynx** `HCC`

Malignant neoplasm of fossa of Rosenmüller

Malignant neoplasm of opening of auditory tube

Malignant neoplasm of pharyngeal recess

C11.3 **Malignant neoplasm of** anterior wall **of nasopharynx** `HCC`

Malignant neoplasm of floor of nasopharynx

Malignant neoplasm of nasopharyngeal (anterior) (posterior) surface of soft palate

Malignant neoplasm of posterior margin of nasal choana

Malignant neoplasm of posterior margin of nasal septum

C11.8 **Malignant neoplasm of** overlapping sites **of nasopharynx** `HCC`

C11.9 **Malignant neoplasm of nasopharynx, unspecified** `HCC`

Malignant neoplasm of nasopharyngeal wall NOS

C12 **Malignant neoplasm of** pyriform sinus `HCC`

AHA: Q2 2002, Q4 2002

Malignant neoplasm of pyriform fossa

Use additional code to identify:

exposure to environmental tobacco smoke (Z77.22)

exposure to tobacco smoke in the perinatal period (P96.81)

history of tobacco dependence (Z87.891)

occupational exposure to environmental tobacco smoke (Z57.31)

tobacco dependence (F17.-)

tobacco use (Z72.0)

4ᵗʰ C13 **Malignant neoplasm of** hypopharynx

Use additional code to identify:

exposure to environmental tobacco smoke (Z77.22)

exposure to tobacco smoke in the perinatal period (P96.81)

history of tobacco dependence (Z87.891)

occupational exposure to environmental tobacco smoke (Z57.31)

tobacco dependence (F17.-)

tobacco use (Z72.0)

EXCLUDES2 _malignant neoplasm of pyriform sinus (C12)_

C13.0 **Malignant neoplasm of** postcricoid region `HCC`

C13.1 **Malignant neoplasm of** aryepiglottic fold, hypopharyngeal aspect `HCC`

Malignant neoplasm of aryepiglottic fold, marginal zone

Malignant neoplasm of aryepiglottic fold NOS

Malignant neoplasm of interarytenoid fold, marginal zone

Malignant neoplasm of interarytenoid fold NOS

EXCLUDES2 _malignant neoplasm of aryepiglottic fold or interarytenoid fold, laryngeal aspect (C32.1)_

C13.2 **Malignant neoplasm of** posterior wall **of hypopharynx** `HCC`

C13.8 **Malignant neoplasm of** overlapping sites **of hypopharynx** `HCC`

C13.9 **Malignant neoplasm of hypopharynx, unspecified** `HCC`

Malignant neoplasm of hypopharyngeal wall NOS

4ᵗʰ C14 **Malignant neoplasm of** other and ill-defined sites in the lip, oral cavity and pharynx

Use additional code to identify:

alcohol abuse and dependence (F10.-)

exposure to environmental tobacco smoke (Z77.22)

exposure to tobacco smoke in the perinatal period (P96.81)

history of tobacco dependence (Z87.891)

occupational exposure to environmental tobacco smoke (Z57.31)

tobacco dependence (F17.-)

tobacco use (Z72.0)

EXCLUDES1 _malignant neoplasm of oral cavity NOS (C06.9)_

C14.0 **Malignant neoplasm of pharynx, unspecified** `HCC`

C14.2 **Malignant neoplasm of** Waldeyer's ring `HCC`

C14.8 **Malignant neoplasm of** overlapping sites of lip, oral cavity and pharynx `HCC`

Primary malignant neoplasm of two or more contiguous sites of lip, oral cavity and pharynx

EXCLUDES1 _'book leaf' neoplasm [ventral surface of tongue and floor of mouth] (C06.89)_

Malignant neoplasms of digestive organs (C15-C26)

EXCLUDES1 _Kaposi's sarcoma of gastrointestinal sites (C46.4)_

EXCLUDES2 _gastrointestinal stromal tumors (C49.A-)_

4ᵗʰ C15 **Malignant neoplasm of** esophagus

Use additional code to identify:

alcohol abuse and dependence (F10.-)

C15.3 **Malignant neoplasm of** upper third of esophagus ⚥ `HCC` CC/MCC Exc

C15.4 **Malignant neoplasm of** middle third of esophagus ⚥ `HCC` CC/MCC Exc

C15.5 **Malignant neoplasm of** lower third of esophagus ⚥ `HCC` CC/MCC Exc

EXCLUDES1 _malignant neoplasm of cardio-esophageal junction (C16.0)_

C15.8 **Malignant neoplasm of** overlapping sites of esophagus ⚥ `HCC` CC/MCC Exc

C15.9 **Malignant neoplasm of esophagus, unspecified** ⚥ `HCC` CC/MCC Exc

4ᵗʰ C16 **Malignant neoplasm of** stomach

Use additional code to identify:

alcohol abuse and dependence (F10.-)

EXCLUDES2 _malignant carcinoid tumor of the stomach (C7A.092)_

C16.0 **Malignant neoplasm of** cardia ⚥ `HCC` `RxHCC` CC/MCC Exc

Malignant neoplasm of cardiac orifice

Malignant neoplasm of cardio-esophageal junction

Malignant neoplasm of esophagus and stomach

Malignant neoplasm of gastro-esophageal junction

C16.1 **Malignant neoplasm of** fundus **of stomach** ⚥ `HCC` `RxHCC` CC/MCC Exc

C16.2 **Malignant neoplasm of** body **of stomach** ⚥ `HCC` `RxHCC` CC/MCC Exc

C16.3 **Malignant neoplasm of** pyloric antrum ⚥ `HCC` `RxHCC` CC/MCC Exc

Malignant neoplasm of gastric antrum

C16.4 **Malignant neoplasm of** pylorus ⚥ `HCC` `RxHCC` CC/MCC Exc

Malignant neoplasm of prepylorus

Malignant neoplasm of pyloric canal

C16.5 **Malignant neoplasm of** lesser curvature **of stomach, unspecified** ⚥ `HCC` `RxHCC` CC/MCC Exc

Malignant neoplasm of lesser curvature of stomach, not classifiable to C16.1-C16.4

C16.6 **Malignant neoplasm of** greater curvature **of stomach, unspecified** ⚥ `HCC` `RxHCC` CC/MCC Exc

Malignant neoplasm of greater curvature of stomach, not classifiable to C16.0-C16.4

C16.8 **Malignant neoplasm of** overlapping sites **of stomach** ⚥ `HCC` `RxHCC` CC/MCC Exc

C16.9 **Malignant neoplasm of stomach, unspecified** ⚥ `HCC` `RxHCC` CC/MCC Exc

Gastric cancer NOS

4ᵗʰ C17 **Malignant neoplasm of** small intestine

EXCLUDES1 _malignant carcinoid tumors of the small intestine (C7A.01)_

C17.0 **Malignant neoplasm of** duodenum ⚥ `HCC` `RxHCC` CC/MCC Exc

C17.1 **Malignant neoplasm of** jejunum ⚥ `HCC` `RxHCC` CC/MCC Exc

C17.2 **Malignant neoplasm of** ileum ⚥ `HCC` `RxHCC` CC/MCC Exc

EXCLUDES1 _malignant neoplasm of ileocecal valve (C18.0)_

C17.3 Meckel's diverticulum, **malignant** ⚥ `HCC` `RxHCC` CC/MCC Exc

EXCLUDES1 _Meckel's diverticulum, congenital (Q43.0)_

C17.8 **Malignant neoplasm of** overlapping sites **of small intestine** ⚥ `HCC` `RxHCC` CC/MCC Exc

C17.9 **Malignant neoplasm of small intestine, unspecified** ⚥ `HCC` `RxHCC` CC/MCC Exc

4ᵗʰ C18 **Malignant neoplasm of** colon

EXCLUDES1 _malignant carcinoid tumors of the colon (C7A.02-)_

C18.0 **Malignant neoplasm of** cecum ⚥ `HCC` CC/MCC Exc

Malignant neoplasm of ileocecal valve

C18.1 **Malignant neoplasm of** appendix ⚥ `HCC` CC/MCC Exc

Unspecified Code   Other Specified Code   Manifestation Code   Ⓝ Newborn   Ⓟ Pediatric   Ⓜ Maternity   Ⓐ Adult   ♂ Male   ♀ Female

● New Code   ▲ Revised Code Title   ▶◀ Revised Text   **NOTES**   _INCLUDES_   _EXCLUDES 1_ Not coded here   _EXCLUDES 2_ Not included here

4ᵗʰ 4ᵗʰ character required   5ᵗʰ 5ᵗʰ character required   6ᵗʰ 6ᵗʰ character required   7ᵗʰ 7ᵗʰ character required

7ᵗʰ Extension 'X' Alert   `HAC` Hospital-acquired condition (HAC) alert   **AHA** AHA Coding Clinic©

C47.6 - C49.A9

CHAPTER 2: NEOPLASMS (C00-D49)

C69.12 - C74.92

CHAPTER 2: NEOPLASMS (C00-D49)

C76.50 - C80

CHAPTER 2: NEOPLASMS (C00-D49)

C76.50 Malignant neoplasm of unspecified lower limb `HCC`

C76.51 Malignant neoplasm of right lower limb `HCC`

C76.52 Malignant neoplasm of left lower limb `HCC`

C76.8 Malignant neoplasm of other specified ill-defined sites `HCC`

Malignant neoplasm of overlapping ill-defined sites

C77 Secondary and unspecified malignant neoplasm of lymph nodes

EXCLUDES1 *malignant neoplasm of lymph nodes, specified as primary (C81-C86, C88, C96.-)*

mesentary metastasis of carcinoid tumor (C7B.04)

secondary carcinoid tumors of distant lymph nodes (C7B.01)

C77.0 Secondary and unspecified malignant neoplasm of lymph nodes of head, face and neck `HCC RxHCC CC/MCC Exc`

Secondary and unspecified malignant neoplasm of supraclavicular lymph nodes

C77.1 Secondary and unspecified malignant neoplasm of intrathoracic lymph nodes `HCC RxHCC CC/MCC Exc`

C77.2 Secondary and unspecified malignant neoplasm of intra-abdominal lymph nodes `HCC RxHCC CC/MCC Exc`

C77.3 Secondary and unspecified malignant neoplasm of axilla and upper limb lymph nodes `HCC RxHCC CC/MCC Exc`

Secondary and unspecified malignant neoplasm of pectoral lymph nodes

C77.4 Secondary and unspecified malignant neoplasm of inguinal and lower limb lymph nodes `HCC RxHCC CC/MCC Exc`

C77.5 Secondary and unspecified malignant neoplasm of intrapelvic lymph nodes `HCC RxHCC CC/MCC Exc`

C77.8 Secondary and unspecified malignant neoplasm of lymph nodes of multiple regions

C77.9 Secondary and unspecified malignant neoplasm of lymph node, unspecified `HCC RxHCC CC/MCC Exc`

C78 Secondary malignant neoplasm of respiratory and digestive organs

EXCLUDES1 *secondary carcinoid tumors of liver (C7B.02)*

secondary carcinoid tumors of peritoneum (C7B.04)

EXCLUDES2 *lymph node metastases (C77.0)*

C78.0 Secondary malignant neoplasm of lung

C78.00 Secondary malignant neoplasm of unspecified lung `HCC RxHCC CC/MCC Exc`

C78.01 Secondary malignant neoplasm of right lung `HCC RxHCC CC/MCC Exc`

C78.02 Secondary malignant neoplasm of left lung `HCC RxHCC CC/MCC Exc`

C78.1 Secondary malignant neoplasm of mediastinum `HCC RxHCC CC/MCC Exc`

C78.2 Secondary malignant neoplasm of pleura `HCC RxHCC CC/MCC Exc`

C78.3 Secondary malignant neoplasm of other and unspecified respiratory organs

C78.30 Secondary malignant neoplasm of unspecified respiratory organ `HCC RxHCC CC/MCC Exc`

C78.39 Secondary malignant neoplasm of other respiratory organs `HCC RxHCC CC/MCC Exc`

C78.4 Secondary malignant neoplasm of small intestine `HCC RxHCC CC/MCC Exc`

C78.5 Secondary malignant neoplasm of large intestine and rectum `HCC RxHCC CC/MCC Exc`

C78.6 Secondary malignant neoplasm of retroperitoneum and peritoneum `HCC RxHCC CC/MCC Exc`

AHA: Q2 2017

C78.7 Secondary malignant neoplasm of liver and intrahepatic bile duct `HCC RxHCC CC/MCC Exc`

C78.8 Secondary malignant neoplasm of other and unspecified digestive organs

C78.80 Secondary malignant neoplasm of unspecified digestive organ `HCC RxHCC CC/MCC Exc`

C78.89 Secondary malignant neoplasm of other digestive organs `HCC RxHCC CC/MCC Exc`

Code also exocrine pancreatic insufficiency (K86.81)

C79 Secondary malignant neoplasm of other and unspecified sites

EXCLUDES1 *secondary carcinoid tumors (C7B.-)*

secondary neuroendocrine tumors (C7B.-)

C79.0 Secondary malignant neoplasm of kidney and renal pelvis

C79.00 Secondary malignant neoplasm of unspecified kidney and renal pelvis `HCC RxHCC CC/MCC Exc`

C79.01 Secondary malignant neoplasm of right kidney and renal pelvis `HCC RxHCC CC/MCC Exc`

C79.02 Secondary malignant neoplasm of left kidney and renal pelvis `HCC RxHCC CC/MCC Exc`

C79.1 Secondary malignant neoplasm of bladder and other and unspecified urinary organs

C79.10 Secondary malignant neoplasm of unspecified urinary organs `HCC RxHCC CC/MCC Exc`

C79.11 Secondary malignant neoplasm of bladder `HCC RxHCC CC/MCC Exc`

EXCLUDES2 *lymph node metastases (C77.0)*

C79.19 Secondary malignant neoplasm of other urinary organs `HCC RxHCC CC/MCC Exc`

C79.2 Secondary malignant neoplasm of skin `HCC RxHCC CC/MCC Exc`

EXCLUDES1 *secondary Merkel cell carcinoma (C7B.1)*

C79.3 Secondary malignant neoplasm of brain and cerebral meninges

C79.31 Secondary malignant neoplasm of brain `HCC RxHCC CC/MCC Exc`

C79.32 Secondary malignant neoplasm of cerebral meninges `HCC RxHCC CC/MCC Exc`

C79.4 Secondary malignant neoplasm of other and unspecified parts of nervous system

C79.40 Secondary malignant neoplasm of unspecified part of nervous system `HCC RxHCC CC/MCC Exc`

C79.49 Secondary malignant neoplasm of other parts of nervous system `HCC RxHCC CC/MCC Exc`

C79.5 Secondary malignant neoplasm of bone and bone marrow

EXCLUDES1 *secondary carcinoid tumors of bone (C7B.03)*

C79.51 Secondary malignant neoplasm of bone `HCC RxHCC CC/MCC Exc`

C79.52 Secondary malignant neoplasm of bone marrow `HCC RxHCC CC/MCC Exc`

C79.6 Secondary malignant neoplasm of ovary

C79.60 Secondary malignant neoplasm of unspecified ovary `HCC RxHCC ♀ CC/MCC Exc`

C79.61 Secondary malignant neoplasm of right ovary `HCC RxHCC ♀ CC/MCC Exc`

C79.62 Secondary malignant neoplasm of left ovary `HCC RxHCC ♀ CC/MCC Exc`

C79.7 Secondary malignant neoplasm of adrenal gland

C79.70 Secondary malignant neoplasm of unspecified adrenal gland `HCC RxHCC CC/MCC Exc`

C79.71 Secondary malignant neoplasm of right adrenal gland `HCC RxHCC CC/MCC Exc`

C79.72 Secondary malignant neoplasm of left adrenal gland `HCC RxHCC CC/MCC Exc`

C79.8 Secondary malignant neoplasm of other specified sites

C79.81 Secondary malignant neoplasm of breast `HCC RxHCC CC/MCC Exc`

C79.82 Secondary malignant neoplasm of genital organs `HCC RxHCC CC/MCC Exc`

C79.89 Secondary malignant neoplasm of other specified sites `HCC RxHCC CC/MCC Exc`

AHA: Q2 2017

C79.9 Secondary malignant neoplasm of unspecified site `HCC RxHCC CC/MCC Exc`

Metastatic cancer NOS

Metastatic disease NOS

EXCLUDES1 *carcinomatosis NOS (C80.0)*

generalized cancer NOS (C80.0)

malignant (primary) neoplasm of unspecified site (C80.1)

C80 Malignant neoplasm without specification of site

EXCLUDES1 *malignant carcinoid tumor of unspecified site (C7A.00)*

malignant neoplasm of specified multiple sites- code to each site

---

PDxEx Unacceptable principal diagnosis symbol per Medicare code edits   POA Code exempt from diagnosis present on admission requirement

? Questionable admission   c✓ Complication or comorbidity   CC/MCC Exc CC/MCC exclusion   MC✓ Major complication or comorbidity

PDx CC Principal diagnosis as its own CC   PDx MCC Principal diagnosis as its own MCC   HCC HCC diagnosis code   RxHCC RxHCC diagnosis code

MACRA code   Z1 Z code as first-listed diagnosis

480

484

486

When symbols appear on a code that requires a 7th character extension, refer to Appendix B to identify applicable 7th character codes.

2018 ICD-10-CM

C80.0 **Disseminated malignant neoplasm, unspecified** ♂♀ HCC RxHCC CC/MCC Exc
Carcinomatosis NOS
Generalized cancer, unspecified site (primary) (secondary)
Generalized malignancy, unspecified site (primary) (secondary)

C80.1 **Malignant (primary) neoplasm, unspecified** HCC
Cancer NOS
Cancer unspecified site (primary)
Carcinoma unspecified site (primary)
Malignancy unspecified site (primary)
EXCLUDES1 secondary malignant neoplasm of unspecified site (C79.9)

C80.2 **Malignant neoplasm associated with transplanted organ** ♂♀ HCC PDxIn CC/MCC Exc
Code first complication of transplanted organ (T86.-)
Use additional code to identify the specific malignancy

Malignant neoplasms of lymphoid, hematopoietic and related tissue (C81-C96)

EXCLUDES2 Kaposi's sarcoma of lymph nodes (C46.3)
secondary and unspecified neoplasm of lymph nodes (C77.-)
secondary neoplasm of bone marrow (C79.52)
secondary neoplasm of spleen (C78.89)

4ᵗʰ C81 **Hodgkin lymphoma**
EXCLUDES1 personal history of Hodgkin lymphoma (Z85.71)

5ᵗʰ C81.0 Nodular lymphocyte predominant **Hodgkin lymphoma**
C81.00 **Nodular lymphocyte predominant Hodgkin lymphoma, unspecified site**
C81.01 **Nodular lymphocyte predominant Hodgkin lymphoma, lymph nodes of** head, face, and neck ♂♀ HCC CC/MCC Exc
C81.02 **Nodular lymphocyte predominant Hodgkin lymphoma,** intrathoracic **lymph nodes** ♂♀ HCC CC/MCC Exc
C81.03 **Nodular lymphocyte predominant Hodgkin lymphoma,** intra-abdominal **lymph nodes** ♂♀ HCC CC/MCC Exc
C81.04 **Nodular lymphocyte predominant Hodgkin lymphoma, lymph nodes of** axilla and upper limb ♂♀ HCC CC/MCC Exc
C81.05 **Nodular lymphocyte predominant Hodgkin lymphoma, lymph nodes of** inguinal region and lower limb ♂♀ HCC CC/MCC Exc
C81.06 **Nodular lymphocyte predominant Hodgkin lymphoma,** intrapelvic **lymph nodes** ♂♀ HCC CC/MCC Exc
C81.07 **Nodular lymphocyte predominant Hodgkin lymphoma,** spleen ♂♀ HCC CC/MCC Exc
C81.08 **Nodular lymphocyte predominant Hodgkin lymphoma, lymph nodes of** multiple sites ♂♀ HCC CC/MCC Exc
C81.09 **Nodular lymphocyte predominant Hodgkin lymphoma, extranodal and solid organ sites** ♂♀ HCC CC/MCC Exc

5ᵗʰ C81.1 Nodular sclerosis Hodgkin **lymphoma**
Nodular sclerosis classical Hodgkin lymphoma
C81.10 **Nodular sclerosis Hodgkin lymphoma, unspecified site** ♂♀ HCC CC/MCC Exc
C81.11 **Nodular sclerosis Hodgkin lymphoma, lymph nodes of** head, face, and neck ♂♀ HCC CC/MCC Exc
C81.12 **Nodular sclerosis Hodgkin lymphoma,** intrathoracic **lymph nodes** ♂♀ HCC CC/MCC Exc
C81.13 **Nodular sclerosis Hodgkin lymphoma,** intra-abdominal **lymph nodes** ♂♀ HCC CC/MCC Exc
C81.14 **Nodular sclerosis Hodgkin lymphoma, lymph nodes of** axilla and upper limb ♂♀ HCC CC/MCC Exc
C81.15 **Nodular sclerosis Hodgkin lymphoma, lymph nodes of** inguinal region and lower limb ♂♀ HCC CC/MCC Exc
C81.16 **Nodular sclerosis Hodgkin lymphoma,** intrapelvic **lymph nodes** ♂♀ HCC CC/MCC Exc
C81.17 **Nodular sclerosis Hodgkin lymphoma,** spleen ♂♀ HCC CC/MCC Exc

C81.18 **Nodular sclerosis Hodgkin lymphoma, lymph nodes of** multiple sites ♂♀ HCC CC/MCC Exc
C81.19 **Nodular sclerosis Hodgkin lymphoma,** extranodal and solid organ sites ♂♀ HCC CC/MCC Exc

5ᵗʰ C81.2 Mixed cellularity **Hodgkin lymphoma**
Mixed cellularity classical Hodgkin lymphoma
C81.20 **Mixed cellularity Hodgkin lymphoma, unspecified site** ♂♀ HCC CC/MCC Exc
C81.21 **Mixed cellularity Hodgkin lymphoma, lymph nodes of** head, face, and neck ♂♀ HCC CC/MCC Exc
C81.22 **Mixed cellularity Hodgkin lymphoma,** intrathoracic **lymph nodes** ♂♀ HCC CC/MCC Exc
C81.23 **Mixed cellularity Hodgkin lymphoma,** intra-abdominal **lymph nodes** ♂♀ HCC CC/MCC Exc
C81.24 **Mixed cellularity Hodgkin lymphoma, lymph nodes of** axilla and upper limb ♂♀ HCC CC/MCC Exc
C81.25 **Mixed cellularity Hodgkin lymphoma, lymph nodes of** inguinal region and lower limb ♂♀ HCC CC/MCC Exc
C81.26 **Mixed cellularity Hodgkin lymphoma,** intrapelvic **lymph nodes** ♂♀ HCC CC/MCC Exc
C81.27 **Mixed cellularity Hodgkin lymphoma,** spleen ♂♀ HCC CC/MCC Exc
C81.28 **Mixed cellularity Hodgkin lymphoma, lymph nodes of** multiple sites ♂♀ HCC CC/MCC Exc
C81.29 **Mixed cellularity Hodgkin lymphoma,** extranodal and solid organ sites ♂♀ HCC CC/MCC Exc

5ᵗʰ C81.3 Lymphocyte depleted **Hodgkin lymphoma**
Lymphocyte depleted classical Hodgkin lymphoma
C81.30 **Lymphocyte depleted Hodgkin lymphoma, unspecified site** ♂♀ HCC CC/MCC Exc
C81.31 **Lymphocyte depleted Hodgkin lymphoma, lymph nodes of** head, face, and neck ♂♀ HCC CC/MCC Exc
C81.32 **Lymphocyte depleted Hodgkin lymphoma,** intrathoracic **lymph nodes** ♂♀ HCC CC/MCC Exc
C81.33 **Lymphocyte depleted Hodgkin lymphoma,** intra-abdominal **lymph nodes** ♂♀ HCC CC/MCC Exc
C81.34 **Lymphocyte depleted Hodgkin lymphoma, lymph nodes of** axilla and upper limb ♂♀ HCC CC/MCC Exc
C81.35 **Lymphocyte depleted Hodgkin lymphoma, lymph nodes of** inguinal region and lower limb ♂♀ HCC CC/MCC Exc
C81.36 **Lymphocyte depleted Hodgkin lymphoma,** intrapelvic **lymph nodes** ♂♀ HCC CC/MCC Exc
C81.37 **Lymphocyte depleted Hodgkin lymphoma,** spleen ♂♀ HCC CC/MCC Exc
C81.38 **Lymphocyte depleted Hodgkin lymphoma, lymph nodes of** multiple sites ♂♀ HCC CC/MCC Exc
C81.39 **Lymphocyte depleted Hodgkin lymphoma, extranodal and solid organ sites** ♂♀ HCC CC/MCC Exc

5ᵗʰ C81.4 Lymphocyte-rich Hodgkin **lymphoma**
Lymphocyte-rich classical Hodgkin lymphoma
EXCLUDES1 nodular lymphocyte predominant Hodgkin lymphoma (C81.0-)
C81.40 **Lymphocyte-rich Hodgkin lymphoma, unspecified site** ♂♀ HCC CC/MCC Exc
C81.41 **Lymphocyte-rich Hodgkin lymphoma, lymph nodes of** head, face, and neck ♂♀ HCC CC/MCC Exc
C81.42 **Lymphocyte-rich Hodgkin lymphoma,** intrathoracic **lymph nodes** ♂♀ HCC CC/MCC Exc
C81.43 **Lymphocyte-rich Hodgkin lymphoma,** intra-abdominal **lymph nodes** ♂♀ HCC CC/MCC Exc
C81.44 **Lymphocyte-rich Hodgkin lymphoma, lymph nodes of** axilla and upper limb ♂♀ HCC CC/MCC Exc
C81.45 **Lymphocyte-rich Hodgkin lymphoma, lymph nodes of** inguinal region and lower limb ♂♀ HCC CC/MCC Exc
C81.46 **Lymphocyte-rich Hodgkin lymphoma,** intrapelvic **lymph nodes** ♂♀ HCC CC/MCC Exc
C81.47 **Lymphocyte-rich Hodgkin lymphoma,** spleen ♂♀ HCC CC/MCC Exc
C81.48 **Lymphocyte-rich Hodgkin lymphoma, lymph nodes of** multiple sites ♂♀ HCC CC/MCC Exc
C81.49 **Lymphocyte-rich Hodgkin lymphoma,** extranodal and solid organ sites ♂♀ HCC CC/MCC Exc

---

Unspecified Code Other Specified Code Manifestation Code N Newborn P Pediatric M Maternity A Adult ♂ Male ♀ Female
● New Code ▲ Revised Code Title ►◄ Revised Text NOTES INCLUDES EXCLUDES1 Not coded here EXCLUDES2 Not included here
4ᵗʰ 4ᵗʰ character required 5ᵗʰ 5ᵗʰ character required 6ᵗʰ 6ᵗʰ character required 7ᵗʰ 7ᵗʰ character required
7ᵗʰ Extension 'X' Alert HAC Hospital-acquired condition (HAC) alert AHA AHA Coding Clinic©

C81.7 Other Hodgkin lymphoma
Classical Hodgkin lymphoma NOS
Other classical Hodgkin lymphoma

C81.70 **Other Hodgkin lymphoma, unspecified site**

C81.71 Other Hodgkin lymphoma, lymph nodes of head, face, and neck

C81.72 Other Hodgkin lymphoma, intrathoracic lymph nodes

C81.73 Other Hodgkin lymphoma, intra-abdominal lymph nodes

C81.74 Other Hodgkin lymphoma, lymph nodes of axilla and upper limb

C81.75 Other Hodgkin lymphoma, lymph nodes of inguinal region and lower limb

C81.76 Other Hodgkin lymphoma, intrapelvic lymph nodes

C81.77 Other Hodgkin lymphoma, spleen

C81.78 Other Hodgkin lymphoma, lymph nodes of multiple sites

C81.79 Other Hodgkin lymphoma, extranodal and solid organ sites

C81.9 Hodgkin lymphoma, unspecified

C81.90 **Hodgkin lymphoma, unspecified, unspecified site**

C81.91 Hodgkin lymphoma, unspecified, lymph nodes of head, face, and neck

C81.92 Hodgkin lymphoma, unspecified, intrathoracic lymph nodes

C81.93 Hodgkin lymphoma, unspecified, intra-abdominal lymph nodes

C81.94 Hodgkin lymphoma, unspecified, lymph nodes of axilla and upper limb

C81.95 Hodgkin lymphoma, unspecified, lymph nodes of inguinal region and lower limb

C81.96 Hodgkin lymphoma, unspecified, intrapelvic lymph nodes

C81.97 Hodgkin lymphoma, unspecified, spleen

C81.98 Hodgkin lymphoma, unspecified, lymph nodes of multiple sites

C81.99 Hodgkin lymphoma, unspecified, extranodal and solid organ sites

C82 Follicular lymphoma
INCLUDES follicular lymphoma with or without diffuse areas
EXCLUDES1 mature T/NK-cell lymphomas (C84.-)
　　　　　personal history of non-Hodgkin lymphoma (Z85.72)

C82.0 Follicular lymphoma grade I

C82.00 **Follicular lymphoma grade I, unspecified site**

C82.01 Follicular lymphoma grade I, lymph nodes of head, face, and neck

C82.02 Follicular lymphoma grade I, intrathoracic lymph nodes

C82.03 Follicular lymphoma grade I, intra-abdominal lymph nodes

C82.04 Follicular lymphoma grade I, lymph nodes of axilla and upper limb

C82.05 Follicular lymphoma grade I, lymph nodes of inguinal region and lower limb

C82.06 Follicular lymphoma grade I, intrapelvic lymph nodes

C82.07 Follicular lymphoma grade I, spleen

C82.08 Follicular lymphoma grade I, lymph nodes of multiple sites

C82.09 Follicular lymphoma grade I, extranodal and solid organ sites

C82.1 Follicular lymphoma grade II

C82.10 **Follicular lymphoma grade II, unspecified site**

C82.11 Follicular lymphoma grade II, lymph nodes of head, face, and neck

C82.12 Follicular lymphoma grade II, intrathoracic lymph nodes

C82.13 Follicular lymphoma grade II, intra-abdominal lymph nodes

C82.14 Follicular lymphoma grade II, lymph nodes of axilla and upper limb

C82.15 Follicular lymphoma grade II, lymph nodes of inguinal region and lower limb

C82.16 Follicular lymphoma grade II, intrapelvic lymph nodes

C82.17 Follicular lymphoma grade II, spleen

C82.18 Follicular lymphoma grade II, lymph nodes of multiple sites

C82.19 Follicular lymphoma grade II, extranodal and solid organ sites

C82.2 Follicular lymphoma grade III, unspecified

C82.20 **Follicular lymphoma grade III, unspecified, unspecified site**

C82.21 Follicular lymphoma grade III, unspecified, lymph nodes of head, face, and neck

C82.22 Follicular lymphoma grade III, unspecified, intrathoracic lymph nodes

C82.23 Follicular lymphoma grade III, unspecified, intra-abdominal lymph nodes

C82.24 Follicular lymphoma grade III, unspecified, lymph nodes of axilla and upper limb

C82.25 Follicular lymphoma grade III, unspecified, lymph nodes of inguinal region and lower limb

C82.26 Follicular lymphoma grade III, unspecified, intrapelvic lymph nodes

C82.27 Follicular lymphoma grade III, unspecified, spleen

C82.28 Follicular lymphoma grade III, unspecified, lymph nodes of multiple sites

C82.29 Follicular lymphoma grade III, unspecified, extranodal and solid organ sites

C82.3 Follicular lymphoma grade IIIa

C82.30 **Follicular lymphoma grade IIIa, unspecified site**

C82.31 Follicular lymphoma grade IIIa, lymph nodes of head, face, and neck

C82.32 Follicular lymphoma grade IIIa, intrathoracic lymph nodes

C82.33 Follicular lymphoma grade IIIa, intra-abdominal lymph nodes

C82.34 Follicular lymphoma grade IIIa, lymph nodes of axilla and upper limb

C82.35 Follicular lymphoma grade IIIa, lymph nodes of inguinal region and lower limb

C82.36 Follicular lymphoma grade IIIa, intrapelvic lymph nodes

C82.37 Follicular lymphoma grade IIIa, spleen

C82.38 Follicular lymphoma grade IIIa, lymph nodes of multiple sites

C82.39 Follicular lymphoma grade IIIa, extranodal and solid organ sites

C82.4 Follicular lymphoma grade IIIb

C82.40 **Follicular lymphoma grade IIIb, unspecified site**

C82.41 Follicular lymphoma grade IIIb, lymph nodes of head, face, and neck

C82.42 Follicular lymphoma grade IIIb, intrathoracic lymph nodes

C82.43 Follicular lymphoma grade IIIb, intra-abdominal lymph nodes

C82.44 Follicular lymphoma grade IIIb, lymph nodes of axilla and upper limb

C82.45 Follicular lymphoma grade IIIb, lymph nodes of inguinal region and lower limb

C82.46 Follicular lymphoma grade IIIb, intrapelvic lymph nodes

C82.47 Follicular lymphoma grade IIIb, spleen

PDx Unacceptable principal diagnosis symbol per Medicare code edits　　POA Code exempt from diagnosis present on admission requirement
? Questionable admission　　CC Complication or comorbidity　　CC/MCC Exc CC/MCC exclusion　　MCC Major complication or comorbidity
Principal diagnosis as its own CC　　Principal diagnosis as its own MCC　　HCC HCC diagnosis code　　RxHCC RxHCC diagnosis code
MACRA code　　Z1 Z code as first-listed diagnosis

C82.48 Follicular lymphoma grade IIIb, lymph nodes of multiple sites cc HCC CC/MCC Exc

C82.49 Follicular lymphoma grade IIIb, extranodal and solid organ sites cc HCC CC/MCC Exc

5ᵗʰ C82.5 Diffuse follicle center lymphoma

C82.50 Diffuse follicle center lymphoma, unspecified site cc HCC CC/MCC Exc

C82.51 Diffuse follicle center lymphoma, lymph nodes of head, face, and neck cc HCC CC/MCC Exc

C82.52 Diffuse follicle center lymphoma, intrathoracic lymph nodes cc HCC CC/MCC Exc

C82.53 Diffuse follicle center lymphoma, intra-abdominal lymph nodes cc HCC CC/MCC Exc

C82.54 Diffuse follicle center lymphoma, lymph nodes of axilla and upper limb cc HCC CC/MCC Exc

C82.55 Diffuse follicle center lymphoma, lymph nodes of inguinal region and lower limb cc HCC CC/MCC Exc

C82.56 Diffuse follicle center lymphoma, intrapelvic lymph nodes cc HCC CC/MCC Exc

C82.57 Diffuse follicle center lymphoma, spleen cc HCC CC/MCC Exc

C82.58 Diffuse follicle center lymphoma, lymph nodes of multiple sites cc HCC CC/MCC Exc

C82.59 Diffuse follicle center lymphoma, extranodal and solid organ sites cc HCC CC/MCC Exc

5ᵗʰ C82.6 Cutaneous follicle center lymphoma

C82.60 Cutaneous follicle center lymphoma, unspecified site cc HCC CC/MCC Exc

C82.61 Cutaneous follicle center lymphoma, lymph nodes of head, face, and neck cc HCC CC/MCC Exc

C82.62 Cutaneous follicle center lymphoma, intrathoracic lymph nodes cc HCC CC/MCC Exc

C82.63 Cutaneous follicle center lymphoma, intra-abdominal lymph nodes cc HCC CC/MCC Exc

C82.64 Cutaneous follicle center lymphoma, lymph nodes of axilla and upper limb cc HCC CC/MCC Exc

C82.65 Cutaneous follicle center lymphoma, lymph nodes of inguinal region and lower limb cc HCC CC/MCC Exc

C82.66 Cutaneous follicle center lymphoma, intrapelvic lymph nodes cc HCC CC/MCC Exc

C82.67 Cutaneous follicle center lymphoma, spleen cc HCC CC/MCC Exc

C82.68 Cutaneous follicle center lymphoma, lymph nodes of multiple sites cc HCC CC/MCC Exc

C82.69 Cutaneous follicle center lymphoma, extranodal and solid organ sites cc HCC CC/MCC Exc

5ᵗʰ C82.8 Other types of follicular lymphoma

C82.80 Other types of follicular lymphoma, unspecified site cc HCC CC/MCC Exc

C82.81 Other types of follicular lymphoma, lymph nodes of head, face, and neck cc HCC CC/MCC Exc

C82.82 Other types of follicular lymphoma, intrathoracic lymph nodes cc HCC CC/MCC Exc

C82.83 Other types of follicular lymphoma, intra-abdominal lymph nodes cc HCC CC/MCC Exc

C82.84 Other types of follicular lymphoma, lymph nodes of axilla and upper limb cc HCC CC/MCC Exc

C82.85 Other types of follicular lymphoma, lymph nodes of inguinal region and lower limb cc HCC CC/MCC Exc

C82.86 Other types of follicular lymphoma, intrapelvic lymph nodes cc HCC CC/MCC Exc

C82.87 Other types of follicular lymphoma, spleen cc HCC CC/MCC Exc

C82.88 Other types of follicular lymphoma, lymph nodes of multiple sites cc HCC CC/MCC Exc

C82.89 Other types of follicular lymphoma, extranodal and solid organ sites cc HCC CC/MCC Exc

5ᵗʰ C82.9 Follicular lymphoma, unspecified

C82.90 Follicular lymphoma, unspecified, unspecified site cc HCC CC/MCC Exc

C82.91 Follicular lymphoma, unspecified, lymph nodes of head, face, and neck cc HCC CC/MCC Exc

C82.92 Follicular lymphoma, unspecified, intrathoracic lymph nodes cc HCC CC/MCC Exc

C82.93 Follicular lymphoma, unspecified, intra-abdominal lymph nodes cc HCC CC/MCC Exc

C82.94 Follicular lymphoma, unspecified, lymph nodes of axilla and upper limb cc HCC CC/MCC Exc

C82.95 Follicular lymphoma, unspecified, lymph nodes of inguinal region and lower limb cc HCC CC/MCC Exc

C82.96 Follicular lymphoma, unspecified, intrapelvic lymph nodes cc HCC CC/MCC Exc

C82.97 Follicular lymphoma, unspecified, spleen cc HCC CC/MCC Exc

C82.98 Follicular lymphoma, unspecified, lymph nodes of multiple sites cc HCC CC/MCC Exc

C82.99 Follicular lymphoma, unspecified, extranodal and solid organ sites cc HCC CC/MCC Exc

4ᵗʰ C83 Non-follicular lymphoma

EXCLUDES1 personal history of non-Hodgkin lymphoma (Z85.72)

5ᵗʰ C83.0 Small cell B-cell lymphoma

Lymphoplasmacytic lymphoma
Nodal marginal zone lymphoma
Non-leukemic variant of B-CLL
Splenic marginal zone lymphoma

EXCLUDES1 chronic lymphocytic leukemia (C91.1)
mature T/NK-cell lymphomas (C84.-)
Waldenström macroglobulinemia (C88.0)

C83.00 Small cell B-cell lymphoma, unspecified site cc HCC CC/MCC Exc

C83.01 Small cell B-cell lymphoma, lymph nodes of head, face, and neck cc HCC CC/MCC Exc

C83.02 Small cell B-cell lymphoma, intrathoracic lymph nodes cc HCC CC/MCC Exc

C83.03 Small cell B-cell lymphoma, intra-abdominal lymph nodes cc HCC CC/MCC Exc

C83.04 Small cell B-cell lymphoma, lymph nodes of axilla and upper limb cc HCC CC/MCC Exc

C83.05 Small cell B-cell lymphoma, lymph nodes of inguinal region and lower limb cc HCC CC/MCC Exc

C83.06 Small cell B-cell lymphoma, intrapelvic lymph nodes cc HCC CC/MCC Exc

C83.07 Small cell B-cell lymphoma, spleen cc HCC CC/MCC Exc

C83.08 Small cell B-cell lymphoma, lymph nodes of multiple sites cc HCC CC/MCC Exc

C83.09 Small cell B-cell lymphoma, extranodal and solid organ sites cc HCC CC/MCC Exc

5ᵗʰ C83.1 Mantle cell lymphoma

Centrocytic lymphoma
Malignant lymphomatous polyposis

C83.10 Mantle cell lymphoma, unspecified site cc HCC CC/MCC Exc

C83.11 Mantle cell lymphoma, lymph nodes of head, face, and neck cc HCC CC/MCC Exc

C83.12 Mantle cell lymphoma, intrathoracic lymph nodes cc HCC CC/MCC Exc

C83.13 Mantle cell lymphoma, intra-abdominal lymph nodes cc HCC CC/MCC Exc

C83.14 Mantle cell lymphoma, lymph nodes of axilla and upper limb cc HCC CC/MCC Exc

C83.15 Mantle cell lymphoma, lymph nodes of inguinal region and lower limb cc HCC CC/MCC Exc

C83.16 Mantle cell lymphoma, intrapelvic lymph nodes cc HCC CC/MCC Exc

C83.17 Mantle cell lymphoma, spleen cc HCC CC/MCC Exc

C83.18 Mantle cell lymphoma, lymph nodes of multiple sites cc HCC CC/MCC Exc

C83.19 Mantle cell lymphoma, extranodal and solid organ sites cc HCC CC/MCC Exc

5ᵗʰ C83.3 Diffuse large B-cell lymphoma

Anaplastic diffuse large B-cell lymphoma
CD30-positive diffuse large B-cell lymphoma
Centroblastic diffuse large B-cell lymphoma
Diffuse large B-cell lymphoma, subtype not specified
Immunoblastic diffuse large B-cell lymphoma

Unspecified Code   Other Specified Code   Manifestation Code   N Newborn   P Pediatric   M Maternity   A Adult   ♂ Male   ♀ Female
● New Code   ▲ Revised Code Title   ▶◀ Revised Text   NOTES   INCLUDES   EXCLUDES 1 Not coded here   EXCLUDES 2 Not included here
4ᵗʰ 4ᵗʰ character required   5ᵗʰ 5ᵗʰ character required   6ᵗʰ 6ᵗʰ character required   7ᵗʰ 7ᵗʰ character required
7ˣ Extension 'X' Alert   HAC Hospital-acquired condition (HAC) alert   AHA AHA Coding Clinic©

Plasmablastic diffuse large B-cell lymphoma
Diffuse large B-cell lymphoma, subtype not specified
T-cell rich diffuse large B-cell lymphoma

EXCLUDES1 mediastinal (thymic) large B-cell lymphoma (C85.2-)

mature T/NK-cell lymphomas (C84.-)

C83.30 **Diffuse large B-cell lymphoma, unspecified site** cc HCC CC/MCC Exc

C83.31 **Diffuse large B-cell lymphoma, lymph nodes of** head, face, and neck cc HCC CC/MCC Exc

C83.32 **Diffuse large B-cell lymphoma, intrathoracic lymph nodes**

C83.33 **Diffuse large B-cell lymphoma, intra-abdominal lymph nodes**

C83.34 **Diffuse large B-cell lymphoma, lymph nodes of** axilla and upper limb

C83.35 **Diffuse large B-cell lymphoma, lymph nodes of** inguinal region and lower limb

C83.36 **Diffuse large B-cell lymphoma, intrapelvic lymph nodes**

C83.37 **Diffuse large B-cell lymphoma, spleen** cc HCC CC/MCC Exc

C83.38 **Diffuse large B-cell lymphoma, lymph nodes of** multiple sites cc HCC CC/MCC Exc

C83.39 **Diffuse large B-cell lymphoma, extranodal and solid organ sites** cc HCC CC/MCC Exc

5ᵗʰ **C83.5** Lymphoblastic (diffuse) lymphoma
B-precursor lymphoma
Lymphoblastic B-cell lymphoma
Lymphoblastic lymphoma NOS
Lymphoblastic T-cell lymphoma
T-precursor lymphoma

C83.50 **Lymphoblastic (diffuse) lymphoma, unspecified site** cc HCC CC/MCC Exc

C83.51 **Lymphoblastic (diffuse) lymphoma, lymph nodes of** head, face, and neck cc HCC CC/MCC Exc

C83.52 **Lymphoblastic (diffuse) lymphoma, intrathoracic lymph nodes** cc HCC CC/MCC Exc

C83.53 **Lymphoblastic (diffuse) lymphoma, intra-abdominal lymph nodes**

C83.54 **Lymphoblastic (diffuse) lymphoma, lymph nodes of** axilla and upper limb cc HCC CC/MCC Exc

C83.55 **Lymphoblastic (diffuse) lymphoma, lymph nodes of** inguinal region and lower limb cc HCC CC/MCC Exc

C83.56 **Lymphoblastic (diffuse) lymphoma, intrapelvic lymph nodes**

C83.57 **Lymphoblastic (diffuse) lymphoma, spleen** cc HCC CC/MCC Exc

C83.58 **Lymphoblastic (diffuse) lymphoma, lymph nodes of** multiple sites cc HCC CC/MCC Exc

C83.59 **Lymphoblastic (diffuse) lymphoma, extranodal and** solid organ sites cc HCC CC/MCC Exc

5ᵗʰ **C83.7** Burkitt lymphoma
Atypical Burkitt lymphoma
Burkitt-like lymphoma

EXCLUDES1 mature B-cell leukemia Burkitt type (C91.A-)

C83.70 **Burkitt lymphoma, unspecified site** cc HCC CC/MCC Exc

C83.71 **Burkitt lymphoma, lymph nodes of** head, face, and neck cc HCC CC/MCC Exc

C83.72 **Burkitt lymphoma, intrathoracic lymph nodes** cc HCC CC/MCC Exc

C83.73 **Burkitt lymphoma, intra-abdominal lymph nodes** cc HCC CC/MCC Exc

C83.74 **Burkitt lymphoma, lymph nodes of** axilla and upper limb cc HCC CC/MCC Exc

C83.75 **Burkitt lymphoma, lymph nodes of** inguinal region and lower limb cc HCC CC/MCC Exc

C83.76 **Burkitt lymphoma, intrapelvic lymph nodes** cc HCC CC/MCC Exc

C83.77 **Burkitt lymphoma, spleen** cc HCC CC/MCC Exc

C83.78 **Burkitt lymphoma, lymph nodes of** multiple sites cc HCC CC/MCC Exc

C83.79 **Burkitt lymphoma, extranodal and solid organ sites** cc HCC CC/MCC Exc

5ᵗʰ **C83.8** Other non-follicular lymphoma
Intravascular large B-cell lymphoma
Lymphoid granulomatosis
Primary effusion B-cell lymphoma

EXCLUDES1 mediastinal (thymic) large B-cell lymphoma (C85.2-)

T-cell rich B-cell lymphoma (C83.3-)

C83.80 **Other non-follicular lymphoma, unspecified site** cc HCC CC/MCC Exc

C83.81 **Other non-follicular lymphoma, lymph nodes of** head, face, and neck cc HCC CC/MCC Exc

C83.82 **Other non-follicular lymphoma, intrathoracic lymph nodes**

C83.83 **Other non-follicular lymphoma, intra-abdominal lymph nodes** cc HCC CC/MCC Exc

C83.84 **Other non-follicular lymphoma, lymph nodes of** axilla and upper limb cc HCC CC/MCC Exc

C83.85 **Other non-follicular lymphoma, lymph nodes of** inguinal region and lower limb cc HCC CC/MCC Exc

C83.86 **Other non-follicular lymphoma, intrapelvic lymph nodes**

C83.87 **Other non-follicular lymphoma, spleen** cc HCC CC/MCC Exc

C83.88 **Other non-follicular lymphoma, lymph nodes of** multiple sites cc HCC CC/MCC Exc

C83.89 **Other non-follicular lymphoma, extranodal and solid organ sites** cc HCC CC/MCC Exc

5ᵗʰ **C83.9** Non-follicular (diffuse) lymphoma, unspecified

C83.90 **Non-follicular (diffuse) lymphoma, unspecified, unspecified site** cc HCC CC/MCC Exc

C83.91 **Non-follicular (diffuse) lymphoma, unspecified, lymph nodes of** head, face, and neck cc HCC CC/MCC Exc

C83.92 **Non-follicular (diffuse) lymphoma, unspecified, intrathoracic lymph nodes** cc HCC CC/MCC Exc

C83.93 **Non-follicular (diffuse) lymphoma, unspecified, intra-abdominal lymph nodes** cc HCC CC/MCC Exc

C83.94 **Non-follicular (diffuse) lymphoma, unspecified, lymph nodes of** axilla and upper limb cc HCC

C83.95 **Non-follicular (diffuse) lymphoma, unspecified, lymph nodes of** inguinal region and lower limb cc HCC CC/MCC Exc

C83.96 **Non-follicular (diffuse) lymphoma, unspecified, intrapelvic lymph nodes** cc HCC CC/MCC Exc

C83.97 **Non-follicular (diffuse) lymphoma, unspecified, spleen** cc HCC CC/MCC Exc

C83.98 **Non-follicular (diffuse) lymphoma, unspecified, lymph nodes of** multiple sites cc HCC CC/MCC Exc

C83.99 **Non-follicular (diffuse) lymphoma, unspecified, extranodal and solid organ sites** cc HCC CC/MCC Exc

4ᵗʰ **C84** Mature T/NK-cell lymphomas

EXCLUDES1 personal history of non-Hodgkin lymphoma (Z85.72)

5ᵗʰ **C84.0** Mycosis fungoides

EXCLUDES1 peripheral T-cell lymphoma, not classified (C84.4-)

C84.00 **Mycosis fungoides, unspecified site** cc HCC RxHCC CC/MCC Exc

C84.01 **Mycosis fungoides, lymph nodes of** head, face, and neck cc HCC RxHCC CC/MCC Exc

C84.02 **Mycosis fungoides, intrathoracic lymph nodes** cc HCC RxHCC CC/MCC Exc

C84.03 **Mycosis fungoides, intra-abdominal lymph nodes** cc HCC RxHCC CC/MCC Exc

C84.04 **Mycosis fungoides, lymph nodes of** axilla and upper limb cc HCC RxHCC CC/MCC Exc

C84.05 **Mycosis fungoides, lymph nodes of** inguinal region and lower limb cc HCC RxHCC CC/MCC Exc

C84.06 **Mycosis fungoides, intrapelvic lymph nodes** cc HCC RxHCC CC/MCC Exc

C84.07 **Mycosis fungoides, spleen** cc HCC RxHCC CC/MCC Exc

C84.08 **Mycosis fungoides, lymph nodes of** multiple sites cc HCC RxHCC CC/MCC Exc

C84.09 **Mycosis fungoides, extranodal and solid organ sites** cc HCC RxHCC CC/MCC Exc

5ᵗʰ **C84.1** Sézary disease

C84.10 **Sézary disease, unspecified site** cc HCC RxHCC CC/MCC Exc

PDxⁿ Unacceptable principal diagnosis symbol per Medicare code edits   Pxₐ Code exempt from diagnosis present on admission requirement

? Questionable admission   cc Complication or comorbidity   CC/MCC Exc CC/MCC exclusion   MCC Major complication or comorbidity

PDₓ Principal diagnosis as its own CC   Mₓ Principal diagnosis as its own MCC   HCC HCC diagnosis code   RxHCC RxHCC diagnosis code

MACRA code   Z Z code as first-listed diagnosis

C84.11 Sézary disease, lymph nodes of head, face, and neck
C84.12 Sézary disease, intrathoracic lymph nodes
C84.13 Sézary disease, intra-abdominal lymph nodes
C84.14 Sézary disease, lymph nodes of axilla and upper limb
C84.15 Sézary disease, lymph nodes of inguinal region and lower limb
C84.16 Sézary disease, intrapelvic lymph nodes
C84.17 Sézary disease, spleen
C84.18 Sézary disease, lymph nodes of multiple sites
C84.19 Sézary disease, extranodal and solid organ sites

C84.4 Peripheral T-cell lymphoma, not classified
Lennert's lymphoma
Lymphoepithelioid lymphoma
Mature T-cell lymphoma, not elsewhere classified
  C84.40 Peripheral T-cell lymphoma, not classified, unspecified site
  C84.41 Peripheral T-cell lymphoma, not classified, lymph nodes of head, face, and neck
  C84.42 Peripheral T-cell lymphoma, not classified, intrathoracic lymph nodes
  C84.43 Peripheral T-cell lymphoma, not classified, intra-abdominal lymph nodes
  C84.44 Peripheral T-cell lymphoma, not classified, lymph nodes of axilla and upper limb
  C84.45 Peripheral T-cell lymphoma, not classified, lymph nodes of inguinal region and lower limb
  C84.46 Peripheral T-cell lymphoma, not classified, intrapelvic lymph nodes
  C84.47 Peripheral T-cell lymphoma, not classified, spleen
  C84.48 Peripheral T-cell lymphoma, not classified, lymph nodes of multiple sites
  C84.49 Peripheral T-cell lymphoma, not classified, extranodal and solid organ sites

C84.6 Anaplastic large cell lymphoma, ALK-positive
Anaplastic large cell lymphoma, CD30-positive
  C84.60 Anaplastic large cell lymphoma, ALK-positive, unspecified site
  C84.61 Anaplastic large cell lymphoma, ALK-positive, lymph nodes of head, face, and neck
  C84.62 Anaplastic large cell lymphoma, ALK-positive, intrathoracic lymph nodes
  C84.63 Anaplastic large cell lymphoma, ALK-positive, intra-abdominal lymph nodes
  C84.64 Anaplastic large cell lymphoma, ALK-positive, lymph nodes of axilla and upper limb
  C84.65 Anaplastic large cell lymphoma, ALK-positive, lymph nodes of inguinal region and lower limb
  C84.66 Anaplastic large cell lymphoma, ALK-positive, intrapelvic lymph nodes
  C84.67 Anaplastic large cell lymphoma, ALK-positive, spleen
  C84.68 Anaplastic large cell lymphoma, ALK-positive, lymph nodes of multiple sites
  C84.69 Anaplastic large cell lymphoma, ALK-positive, extranodal and solid organ sites

C84.7 Anaplastic large cell lymphoma, ALK-negative
  EXCLUDES1 primary cutaneous CD30-positive T-cell proliferations (C86.6-)
  C84.70 Anaplastic large cell lymphoma, ALK-negative, unspecified site
  C84.71 Anaplastic large cell lymphoma, ALK-negative, lymph nodes of head, face, and neck

C84.72 Anaplastic large cell lymphoma, ALK-negative, intrathoracic lymph nodes
C84.73 Anaplastic large cell lymphoma, ALK-negative, intra-abdominal lymph nodes
C84.74 Anaplastic large cell lymphoma, ALK-negative, lymph nodes of axilla and upper limb
C84.75 Anaplastic large cell lymphoma, ALK-negative, lymph nodes of inguinal region and lower limb
C84.76 Anaplastic large cell lymphoma, ALK-negative, intrapelvic lymph nodes
C84.77 Anaplastic large cell lymphoma, ALK-negative, spleen
C84.78 Anaplastic large cell lymphoma, ALK-negative, lymph nodes of multiple sites
C84.79 Anaplastic large cell lymphoma, ALK-negative, extranodal and solid organ sites

C84.A Cutaneous T-cell lymphoma, unspecified
  C84.A0 Cutaneous T-cell lymphoma, unspecified, unspecified site
  C84.A1 Cutaneous T-cell lymphoma, unspecified lymph nodes of head, face, and neck
  C84.A2 Cutaneous T-cell lymphoma, unspecified, intrathoracic lymph nodes
  C84.A3 Cutaneous T-cell lymphoma, unspecified, intra-abdominal lymph nodes
  C84.A4 Cutaneous T-cell lymphoma, unspecified, lymph nodes of axilla and upper limb
  C84.A5 Cutaneous T-cell lymphoma, unspecified, lymph nodes of inguinal region and lower limb
  C84.A6 Cutaneous T-cell lymphoma, unspecified, intrapelvic lymph nodes
  C84.A7 Cutaneous T-cell lymphoma, unspecified, spleen
  C84.A8 Cutaneous T-cell lymphoma, unspecified, lymph nodes of multiple sites
  C84.A9 Cutaneous T-cell lymphoma, unspecified, extranodal and solid organ sites

C84.Z Other mature T/NK-cell lymphomas
  NOTES If T-cell lineage or involvement is mentioned in conjunction with a specific lymphoma, code to the more specific description.
  EXCLUDES1 angioimmunoblastic T-cell lymphoma (C86.5)
    blastic NK-cell lymphoma (C86.4)
    enteropathy-type T-cell lymphoma (C86.2)
    extranodal NK-cell lymphoma, nasal type (C86.0)
    hepatosplenic T-cell lymphoma (C86.1)
    primary cutaneous CD30-positive T-cell proliferations (C86.6)
    subcutaneous panniculitis-like T-cell lymphoma (C86.3)
    T-cell leukemia (C91.1-)
  C84.Z0 Other mature T/NK-cell lymphomas, unspecified site
  C84.Z1 Other mature T/NK-cell lymphomas, lymph nodes of head, face, and neck
  C84.Z2 Other mature T/NK-cell lymphomas, intrathoracic lymph nodes
  C84.Z3 Other mature T/NK-cell lymphomas, intra-abdominal lymph nodes
  C84.Z4 Other mature T/NK-cell lymphomas, lymph nodes of axilla and upper limb
  C84.Z5 Other mature T/NK-cell lymphomas, lymph nodes of inguinal region and lower limb
  C84.Z6 Other mature T/NK-cell lymphomas, intrapelvic lymph nodes
  C84.Z7 Other mature T/NK-cell lymphomas, spleen
  C84.Z8 Other mature T/NK-cell lymphomas, lymph nodes of multiple sites

Unspecified Code   Other Specified Code   Manifestation Code   Ⓝ Newborn   Ⓟ Pediatric   Ⓜ Maternity   Ⓐ Adult   ♂ Male   ♀ Female
● New Code   ▲ Revised Code Title   ►◄ Revised Text   NOTES   INCLUDES   EXCLUDES 1 Not coded here   EXCLUDES 2 Not included here
4th character required   5th character required   6th character required   7th character required
Extension 'X' Alert   HAC Hospital-acquired condition (HAC) alert   AHA AHA Coding Clinic©

C84.Z9 **Other mature T/NK-cell lymphomas,** extranodal and solid organ sites

C84.9 **Mature T/NK-cell lymphomas,** unspecified
NK/T cell lymphoma NOS
EXCLUDES1 mature T-cell lymphoma, not elsewhere classified (C84.4-)

C84.90 **Mature T/NK-cell lymphomas, unspecified, unspecified site**

C84.91 **Mature T/NK-cell lymphomas, unspecified, lymph nodes of** head, face, and neck

C84.92 **Mature T/NK-cell lymphomas, unspecified,** intrathoracic **lymph nodes**

C84.93 **Mature T/NK-cell lymphomas, unspecified, intra-**abdominal **lymph nodes**

C84.94 **Mature T/NK-cell lymphomas, unspecified, lymph nodes of** axilla and upper limb

C84.95 **Mature T/NK-cell lymphomas, unspecified, lymph nodes of** inguinal region and lower limb

C84.96 **Mature T/NK-cell lymphomas, unspecified,** intrapelvic **lymph nodes**

C84.97 **Mature T/NK-cell lymphomas, unspecified,** spleen

C84.98 **Mature T/NK-cell lymphomas, unspecified, lymph nodes of** multiple sites

C84.99 **Mature T/NK-cell lymphomas, unspecified,** extranodal and solid organ sites

C85 **Other specified and unspecified types of non-Hodgkin lymphoma**
EXCLUDES1 other specified types of T/NK-cell lymphoma (C86.-)
personal history of non-Hodgkin lymphoma (Z85.72)

C85.1 Unspecified **B-cell lymphoma**
NOTES If B-cell lineage or involvement is mentioned in conjunction with a specific lymphoma, code to the more specific description.

C85.10 **Unspecified B-cell lymphoma, unspecified site**

C85.11 **Unspecified B-cell lymphoma, lymph nodes of** head, face, and neck

C85.12 **Unspecified B-cell lymphoma,** intrathoracic **lymph nodes**

C85.13 **Unspecified B-cell lymphoma,** intra-abdominal **lymph nodes**

C85.14 **Unspecified B-cell lymphoma, lymph nodes of** axilla and upper limb

C85.15 **Unspecified B-cell lymphoma, lymph nodes of** inguinal region and lower limb

C85.16 **Unspecified B-cell lymphoma,** intrapelvic **lymph nodes**

C85.17 **Unspecified B-cell lymphoma,** spleen

C85.18 **Unspecified B-cell lymphoma, lymph nodes of** multiple sites

C85.19 **Unspecified B-cell lymphoma,** extranodal and solid organ sites

C85.2 Mediastinal (thymic) **large B-cell lymphoma**

C85.20 **Mediastinal (thymic) large B-cell lymphoma, unspecified site**

C85.21 **Mediastinal (thymic) large B-cell lymphoma, lymph nodes of** head, face, and neck

C85.22 **Mediastinal (thymic) large B-cell lymphoma,** intrathoracic **lymph nodes**

C85.23 **Mediastinal (thymic) large B-cell lymphoma, intra-**abdominal **lymph nodes**

C85.24 **Mediastinal (thymic) large B-cell lymphoma, lymph nodes of** axilla and upper limb

C85.25 **Mediastinal (thymic) large B-cell lymphoma, lymph nodes of** inguinal region and lower limb

C85.26 **Mediastinal (thymic) large B-cell lymphoma,** intrapelvic **lymph nodes**

C85.27 **Mediastinal (thymic) large B-cell lymphoma,** spleen

C85.28 **Mediastinal (thymic) large B-cell lymphoma, lymph nodes of** multiple sites

C85.29 **Mediastinal (thymic) large B-cell lymphoma,** extranodal and solid organ sites

C85.8 **Other specified** types of non-Hodgkin lymphoma

C85.80 **Other specified types of non-Hodgkin lymphoma, unspecified site**

C85.81 **Other specified types of non-Hodgkin lymphoma, lymph nodes of** head, face, and neck

C85.82 **Other specified types of non-Hodgkin lymphoma,** intrathoracic **lymph nodes**

C85.83 **Other specified types of non-Hodgkin lymphoma,** intra-abdominal **lymph nodes**

C85.84 **Other specified types of non-Hodgkin lymphoma, lymph nodes of** axilla and upper limb

C85.85 **Other specified types of non-Hodgkin lymphoma, lymph nodes of** inguinal region and lower limb

C85.86 **Other specified types of non-Hodgkin lymphoma,** intrapelvic **lymph nodes**

C85.87 **Other specified types of non-Hodgkin lymphoma,** spleen

C85.88 **Other specified types of non-Hodgkin lymphoma, lymph nodes of** multiple sites

C85.89 **Other specified types of non-Hodgkin lymphoma,** extranodal and solid organ sites

C85.9 **Non-Hodgkin lymphoma,** unspecified
Lymphoma NOS
Malignant lymphoma NOS
Non-Hodgkin lymphoma NOS

C85.90 **Non-Hodgkin lymphoma, unspecified, unspecified site**

C85.91 **Non-Hodgkin lymphoma, unspecified, lymph nodes of** head, face, and neck

C85.92 **Non-Hodgkin lymphoma, unspecified,** intrathoracic **lymph nodes**

C85.93 **Non-Hodgkin lymphoma, unspecified,** intra-abdominal **lymph nodes**

C85.94 **Non-Hodgkin lymphoma, unspecified, lymph nodes of** axilla and upper limb

C85.95 **Non-Hodgkin lymphoma, unspecified, lymph nodes of** inguinal region and lower limb

C85.96 **Non-Hodgkin lymphoma, unspecified,** intrapelvic **lymph nodes**

C85.97 **Non-Hodgkin lymphoma, unspecified,** spleen

C85.98 **Non-Hodgkin lymphoma, unspecified, lymph nodes of** multiple sites

C85.99 **Non-Hodgkin lymphoma, unspecified,** extranodal and solid organ sites

C86 **Other specified** types of T/NK-cell lymphoma
EXCLUDES1 anaplastic large cell lymphoma, ALK negative (C84.7-)
anaplastic large cell lymphoma, ALK positive (C84.6-)
mature T/NK-cell lymphomas (C84.-)
other specified types of non-Hodgkin lymphoma (C85.8-)

C86.0 Extranodal **NK/T-cell lymphoma,** nasal type

C86.1 Hepatosplenic **T-cell lymphoma**
Alpha-beta and gamma delta types

C86.2 Enteropathy-type (intestinal) **T-cell lymphoma**
Enteropathy associated T-cell lymphoma

C86.3 Subcutaneous panniculitis-like **T-cell lymphoma**

C86.4 Blastic **NK-cell lymphoma**
Blastic plasmacytoid dendritic cell neoplasm (BPDCN)

C86.5 Angioimmunoblastic **T-cell lymphoma**
Angioimmunoblastic lymphadenopathy with dysproteinemia (AILD)

C86.6 Primary cutaneous CD30-positive **T-cell proliferations**
Lymphomatoid papulosis
Primary cutaneous anaplastic large cell lymphoma
Primary cutaneous CD30-positive large T-cell lymphoma

PDᵢₐ Unacceptable principal diagnosis symbol per Medicare code edits   POA Code exempt from diagnosis present on admission requirement
? Questionable admission   Complication or comorbidity   CC/MCC Exc CC/MCC exclusion   McC Major complication or comorbidity
PDx Principal diagnosis as its own CC   Principal diagnosis as its own MCC   HCC HCC diagnosis code   RxHCC RxHCC diagnosis code
MACRA code   Z1 Z code as first-listed diagnosis

C88 Malignant immunoproliferative diseases and certain other B-cell lymphomas
  EXCLUDES1 *B-cell lymphoma, unspecified (C85.1-)*
    personal history of other malignant neoplasms of lymphoid, hematopoietic and related tissues (Z85.79)

  C88.0 Waldenström macroglobulinemia   HCC
    Lymphoplasmacytic lymphoma with IgM-production
    Macroglobulinemia (idiopathic) (primary)
    EXCLUDES1 *small cell B-cell lymphoma (C83.0)*

  C88.2 Heavy chain disease   cc⊘ HCC CC/MCC Exc
    Franklin disease
    Gamma heavy chain disease
    Mu heavy chain disease

  C88.3 Immunoproliferative small intestinal disease   cc⊘ HCC CC/MCC Exc
    Alpha heavy chain disease
    Mediterranean lymphoma

  C88.4 Extranodal marginal zone B-cell lymphoma of mucosa-associated lymphoid tissue [MALT-lymphoma]   HCC CC/MCC Exc
    Lymphoma of skin-associated lymphoid tissue [SALT-lymphoma]
    Lymphoma of bronchial-associated lymphoid tissue [BALT-lymphoma]
    EXCLUDES1 *high malignant (diffuse large B-cell) lymphoma (C83.3-)*

  C88.8 Other malignant immunoproliferative diseases   cc⊘ HCC CC/MCC Exc

  C88.9 Malignant immunoproliferative disease, unspecified   cc⊘ HCC CC/MCC Exc
    Immunoproliferative disease NOS

C90 Multiple myeloma and malignant plasma cell neoplasms
  EXCLUDES1 *personal history of other malignant neoplasms of lymphoid, hematopoietic and related tissues (Z85.79)*

  C90.0 Multiple myeloma
    Kahler's disease
    Medullary plasmacytoma
    Myelomatosis
    Plasma cell myeloma
    EXCLUDES1 *solitary myeloma (C90.3-)*
             solitary plasmactyoma (C90.3-)

    C90.00 Multiple myeloma not having achieved remission   cc⊘ HCC RxHCC CC/MCC Exc
      Multiple myeloma with failed remission
      Multiple myeloma NOS
    C90.01 Multiple myeloma in remission   cc⊘ HCC RxHCC CC/MCC Exc
    C90.02 Multiple myeloma in relapse   cc⊘ HCC RxHCC CC/MCC Exc

  C90.1 Plasma cell leukemia
    Plasmacytic leukemia
    C90.10 Plasma cell leukemia not having achieved remission   cc⊘ HCC RxHCC CC/MCC Exc
      Plasma cell leukemia with failed remission
      Plasma cell leukemia NOS
    C90.11 Plasma cell leukemia in remission   cc⊘ HCC RxHCC CC/MCC Exc
    C90.12 Plasma cell leukemia in relapse   cc⊘ HCC RxHCC CC/MCC Exc

  C90.2 Extramedullary plasmacytoma
    C90.20 Extramedullary plasmacytoma not having achieved remission   cc⊘ HCC RxHCC CC/MCC Exc
      Extramedullary plasmacytoma with failed remission
      Extramedullary plasmacytoma NOS
    C90.21 Extramedullary plasmacytoma in remission   cc⊘ HCC RxHCC CC/MCC Exc
    C90.22 Extramedullary plasmacytoma in relapse   cc⊘ HCC RxHCC CC/MCC Exc

  C90.3 Solitary plasmacytoma
    Localized malignant plasma cell tumor NOS
    Plasmacytoma NOS
    Solitary myeloma
    C90.30 Solitary plasmacytoma not having achieved remission   cc⊘ HCC RxHCC CC/MCC Exc
      Solitary plasmacytoma with failed remission
      Solitary plasmacytoma NOS
    C90.31 Solitary plasmacytoma in remission   cc⊘ HCC RxHCC CC/MCC Exc
    C90.32 Solitary plasmacytoma in relapse   cc⊘ HCC RxHCC CC/MCC Exc

C91 Lymphoid leukemia
  EXCLUDES1 *personal history of leukemia (Z85.6)*

  C91.0 Acute lymphoblastic leukemia [ALL]
    NOTES   Code C91.0 should only be used for T-cell and B-cell precursor leukemia
    C91.00 Acute lymphoblastic leukemia not having achieved remission   cc⊘ HCC CC/MCC Exc
      Acute lymphoblastic leukemia with failed remission
      Acute lymphoblastic leukemia NOS
    C91.01 Acute lymphoblastic leukemia, in remission   cc⊘ HCC CC/MCC Exc
    C91.02 Acute lymphoblastic leukemia, in relapse   cc⊘ HCC CC/MCC Exc

  C91.1 Chronic lymphocytic leukemia of B-cell type
    Lymphoplasmacytic leukemia
    Richter syndrome
    EXCLUDES1 *lymphoplasmacytic lymphoma (C83.0-)*
    C91.10 Chronic lymphocytic leukemia of B-cell type not having achieved remission   cc⊘ HCC CC/MCC Exc
      Chronic lymphocytic leukemia of B-cell type with failed remission
      Chronic lymphocytic leukemia of B-cell type NOS
    C91.11 Chronic lymphocytic leukemia of B-cell type in remission   cc⊘ HCC CC/MCC Exc
    C91.12 Chronic lymphocytic leukemia of B-cell type in relapse   cc⊘ HCC CC/MCC Exc

  C91.3 Prolymphocytic leukemia of B-cell type
    C91.30 Prolymphocytic leukemia of B-cell type not having achieved remission   cc⊘ HCC CC/MCC Exc
      Prolymphocytic leukemia of B-cell type with failed remission
      Prolymphocytic leukemia of B-cell type NOS
    C91.31 Prolymphocytic leukemia of B-cell type, in remission   cc⊘ HCC CC/MCC Exc
    C91.32 Prolymphocytic leukemia of B-cell type, in relapse   cc⊘ HCC CC/MCC Exc

  C91.4 Hairy cell leukemia
    Leukemic reticuloendotheliosis
    C91.40 Hairy cell leukemia not having achieved remission   cc⊘ HCC CC/MCC Exc
      Hairy cell leukemia with failed remission
      Hairy cell leukemia NOS
    C91.41 Hairy cell leukemia, in remission   cc⊘ HCC CC/MCC Exc
    C91.42 Hairy cell leukemia, in relapse   cc⊘ HCC CC/MCC Exc

  C91.5 Adult T-cell lymphoma/leukemia (HTLV-1-associated)
    Acute variant of adult T-cell lymphoma/leukemia (HTLV-1-associated)
    Chronic variant of adult T-cell lymphoma/leukemia (HTLV-1-associated)
    Lymphomatoid variant of adult T-cell lymphoma/leukemia (HTLV-1-associated)
    Smouldering variant of adult T-cell lymphoma/leukemia (HTLV-1-associated)
    C91.50 Adult T-cell lymphoma/leukemia (HTLV-1-associated) not having achieved remission   A cc⊘ HCC CC/MCC Exc
      Adult T-cell lymphoma/leukemia (HTLV-1-associated) with failed remission
      Adult T-cell lymphoma/leukemia (HTLV-1-associated) NOS
    C91.51 Adult T-cell lymphoma/leukemia (HTLV-1-associated), in remission   A cc⊘ HCC CC/MCC Exc
    C91.52 Adult T-cell lymphoma/leukemia (HTLV-1-associated), in relapse   A cc⊘ HCC CC/MCC Exc

  C91.6 Prolymphocytic leukemia of T-cell type
    C91.60 Prolymphocytic leukemia of T-cell type not having achieved remission   cc⊘ HCC CC/MCC Exc
      Prolymphocytic leukemia of T-cell type with failed remission
      Prolymphocytic leukemia of T-cell type NOS
    C91.61 Prolymphocytic leukemia of T-cell type, in remission   cc⊘ HCC CC/MCC Exc

---

Unspecified Code   Other Specified Code   Manifestation Code   N Newborn   P Pediatric   M Maternity   A Adult   ♂ Male   ♀ Female
● New Code   ▲ Revised Code Title   ►◄ Revised Text   NOTES   INCLUDES   EXCLUDES1 Not coded here   EXCLUDES2 Not included here
4th character required   5th character required   6th character required   7th character required
Extension 'X' Alert   HAC Hospital-acquired condition (HAC) alert   AHA AHA Coding Clinic©

C91.62 **Prolymphocytic leukemia of T-cell type,** in relapse `CC` `HCC` `CC/MCC Exc`

🔟 C91.A Mature B-cell leukemia Burkitt-type

EXCLUDES1 *Burkitt lymphoma (C83.7-)*

C91.A0 **Mature B-cell leukemia Burkitt-type** not having achieved remission `CC` `HCC` `CC/MCC Exc`

Mature B-cell leukemia Burkitt-type with failed remission

Mature B-cell leukemia Burkitt-type NOS

C91.A1 **Mature B-cell leukemia Burkitt-type,** in remission `CC` `HCC` `CC/MCC Exc`

C91.A2 **Mature B-cell leukemia Burkitt-type,** in relapse `CC` `HCC` `CC/MCC Exc`

🔟 C91.Z Other lymphoid leukemia

T-cell large granular lymphocytic leukemia (associated with rheumatoid arthritis)

C91.Z0 **Other lymphoid leukemia** not having achieved remission `CC` `HCC` `CC/MCC Exc`

Other lymphoid leukemia with failed remission

Other lymphoid leukemia NOS

C91.Z1 **Other lymphoid leukemia, in remission** `CC` `HCC` `CC/MCC Exc`

C91.Z2 **Other lymphoid leukemia, in relapse** `CC` `HCC` `CC/MCC Exc`

🔟 C91.9 Lymphoid leukemia, unspecified

C91.90 **Lymphoid leukemia, unspecified** not having achieved remission `CC` `HCC` `CC/MCC Exc`

Lymphoid leukemia with failed remission

Lymphoid leukemia NOS

C91.91 **Lymphoid leukemia, unspecified, in remission** `CC` `HCC` `CC/MCC Exc`

C91.92 **Lymphoid leukemia, unspecified, in relapse** `CC` `HCC` `CC/MCC Exc`

🔘 C92 Myeloid leukemia

INCLUDES *granulocytic leukemia*

myelogenous leukemia

EXCLUDES1 *personal history of leukemia (Z85.6)*

🔟 C92.0 Acute myeloblastic leukemia

Acute myeloblastic leukemia, minimal differentiation

Acute myeloblastic leukemia (with maturation)

Acute myeloblastic leukemia 1/ETO

Acute myeloblastic leukemia M0

Acute myeloblastic leukemia M1

Acute myeloblastic leukemia M2

Acute myeloblastic leukemia with t(8;21)

Acute myeloblastic leukemia (without a FAB classification) NOS

Refractory anemia with excess blasts in transformation [RAEB T]

EXCLUDES1 *acute exacerbation of chronic myeloid leukemia (C92.10)*

refractory anemia with excess of blasts not in transformation (D46.2-)

C92.00 **Acute myeloblastic leukemia,** not having achieved remission `CC` `HCC` `CC/MCC Exc`

Acute myeloblastic leukemia with failed remission

Acute myeloblastic leukemia NOS

C92.01 **Acute myeloblastic leukemia,** in remission `CC` `HCC` `CC/MCC Exc`

C92.02 **Acute myeloblastic leukemia, in relapse** `CC` `HCC` `CC/MCC Exc`

🔟 C92.1 Chronic myeloid leukemia, BCR/ABL-positive

Chronic myelogenous leukemia, Philadelphia chromosome (Ph1) positive

Chronic myelogenous leukemia, t(9;22) (q34;q11)

Chronic myelogenous leukemia with crisis of blast cells

EXCLUDES1 *atypical chronic myeloid leukemia BCR/ABL-negative (C92.2-)*

chronic myelomonocytic leukemia (C93.1-)

chronic myeloproliferative disease (D47.1)

C92.10 **Chronic myeloid leukemia, BCR/ABL-positive,** not having achieved remission `CC` `HCC` `RxHCC` `CC/MCC Exc`

Chronic myeloid leukemia, BCR/ABL-positive with failed remission

Chronic myeloid leukemia, BCR/ABL-positive NOS

C92.11 **Chronic myeloid leukemia, BCR/ABL-positive,** in remission `CC` `HCC` `RxHCC` `CC/MCC Exc`

C92.12 **Chronic myeloid leukemia, BCR/ABL-positive,** in relapse `CC` `HCC` `RxHCC` `CC/MCC Exc`

🔟 C92.2 Atypical chronic myeloid leukemia, BCR/ABL-negative

C92.20 **Atypical chronic myeloid leukemia, BCR/ABL-negative,** not having achieved remission `CC` `HCC` `RxHCC` `CC/MCC Exc`

Atypical chronic myeloid leukemia, BCR/ABL-negative with failed remission

Atypical chronic myeloid leukemia, BCR/ABL-negative NOS

C92.21 **Atypical chronic myeloid leukemia, BCR/ABL-negative,** in remission `CC` `HCC` `RxHCC` `CC/MCC Exc`

C92.22 **Atypical chronic myeloid leukemia, BCR/ABL-negative,** in relapse `CC` `HCC` `RxHCC` `CC/MCC Exc`

🔟 C92.3 Myeloid sarcoma

A malignant tumor of immature myeloid cells

Chloroma

Granulocytic sarcoma

C92.30 **Myeloid sarcoma,** not having achieved remission `CC` `HCC` `RxHCC` `CC/MCC Exc`

Myeloid sarcoma with failed remission

Myeloid sarcoma NOS

C92.31 **Myeloid sarcoma, in remission** `CC` `HCC` `RxHCC` `CC/MCC Exc`

C92.32 **Myeloid sarcoma, in relapse** `CC` `HCC` `RxHCC` `CC/MCC Exc`

🔟 C92.4 Acute promyelocytic leukemia

AML M3

AML Me with t(15;17) and variants

C92.40 **Acute promyelocytic leukemia,** not having achieved remission `CC` `HCC` `CC/MCC Exc`

Acute promyelocytic leukemia with failed remission

Acute promyelocytic leukemia NOS

C92.41 **Acute promyelocytic leukemia, in remission** `CC` `HCC` `CC/MCC Exc`

C92.42 **Acute promyelocytic leukemia, in relapse** `CC` `HCC` `CC/MCC Exc`

🔟 C92.5 Acute myelomonocytic leukemia

AML M4

AML M4 Eo with inv(16) or t(16;16)

C92.50 **Acute myelomonocytic leukemia,** not having achieved remission `CC` `HCC` `CC/MCC Exc`

Acute myelomonocytic leukemia with failed remission

Acute myelomonocytic leukemia NOS

C92.51 **Acute myelomonocytic leukemia, in remission** `CC` `HCC` `CC/MCC Exc`

C92.52 **Acute myelomonocytic leukemia, in relapse** `CC` `HCC` `CC/MCC Exc`

🔟 C92.6 Acute myeloid leukemia with 11q23-abnormality

Acute myeloid leukemia with variation of MLL-gene

C92.60 **Acute myeloid leukemia with 11q23-abnormality** not having achieved remission `CC` `HCC` `CC/MCC Exc`

Acute myeloid leukemia with 11q23-abnormality with failed remission

Acute myeloid leukemia with 11q23-abnormality NOS

C92.61 **Acute myeloid leukemia with 11q23-abnormality** in remission `CC` `HCC` `CC/MCC Exc`

C92.62 **Acute myeloid leukemia with 11q23-abnormality** in relapse `CC` `HCC` `CC/MCC Exc`

🔟 C92.A Acute myeloid leukemia with multilineage dysplasia

Acute myeloid leukemia with dysplasia of remaining hematopoesis and/or myelodysplastic disease in its history

C92.A0 **Acute myeloid leukemia with multilineage dysplasia,** not having achieved remission `CC` `HCC` `CC/MCC Exc`

Acute myeloid leukemia with multilineage dysplasia with failed remission

Acute myeloid leukemia with multilineage dysplasia NOS

C92.A1 **Acute myeloid leukemia with multilineage dysplasia, in remission** `CC` `HCC` `CC/MCC Exc`

C92.A2 **Acute myeloid leukemia with multilineage dysplasia, in relapse** `CC` `HCC` `CC/MCC Exc`

PDxₙ Unacceptable principal diagnosis symbol per Medicare code edits   ₚₐ Code exempt from diagnosis present on admission requirement
❓ Questionable admission   `CC` Complication or comorbidity   `CC/MCC Exc` CC/MCC exclusion   `MCC` Major complication or comorbidity
Principal diagnosis as its own CC   Principal diagnosis as its own MCC   `HCC` HCC diagnosis code   `RxHCC` RxHCC diagnosis code
MACRA code   `Z1` Z code as first-listed diagnosis

5ᵗʰ C92.Z Other myeloid leukemia

C92.Z0 Other myeloid leukemia not having achieved remission ♂ⵎ HCC RxHCC CC/MCC Exc
Myeloid leukemia NEC with failed remission
Myeloid leukemia NEC

C92.Z1 Other myeloid leukemia, in remission ♂ⵎ HCC RxHCC CC/MCC Exc

C92.Z2 Other myeloid leukemia, in relapse ♂ⵎ HCC RxHCC CC/MCC Exc

5ᵗʰ C92.9 Myeloid leukemia, unspecified

C92.90 Myeloid leukemia, unspecified, not having achieved remission ♂ⵎ HCC RxHCC CC/MCC Exc
Myeloid leukemia, unspecified with failed remission
Myeloid leukemia, unspecified NOS

C92.91 Myeloid leukemia, unspecified in remission ♂ⵎ HCC RxHCC CC/MCC Exc

C92.92 Myeloid leukemia, unspecified in relapse ♂ⵎ HCC RxHCC CC/MCC Exc

4ᵗʰ C93 Monocytic leukemia

INCLUDES monocytoid leukemia

EXCLUDES1 personal history of leukemia (Z85.6)

5ᵗʰ C93.0 Acute monoblastic/monocytic leukemia
AML M5
AML M5a
AML M5b

C93.00 Acute monoblastic/monocytic leukemia, not having achieved remission ♂ⵎ HCC CC/MCC Exc
Acute monoblastic/monocytic leukemia with failed remission
Acute monoblastic/monocytic leukemia NOS

C93.01 Acute monoblastic/monocytic leukemia, in remission ♂ⵎ HCC CC/MCC Exc

C93.02 Acute monoblastic/monocytic leukemia, in relapse ♂ⵎ HCC CC/MCC Exc

5ᵗʰ C93.1 Chronic myelomonocytic leukemia
Chronic monocytic leukemia
CMML-1
CMML-2
CMML with eosinophilia

C93.10 Chronic myelomonocytic leukemia not having achieved remission ♂ⵎ HCC RxHCC CC/MCC Exc
Chronic myelomonocytic leukemia with failed remission
Chronic myelomonocytic leukemia NOS

C93.11 Chronic myelomonocytic leukemia, in remission ♂ⵎ HCC RxHCC CC/MCC Exc

C93.12 Chronic myelomonocytic leukemia, in relapse ♂ⵎ HCC RxHCC CC/MCC Exc

5ᵗʰ C93.3 Juvenile myelomonocytic leukemia

C93.30 Juvenile myelomonocytic leukemia, not having achieved remission P ♂ⵎ HCC RxHCC CC/MCC Exc
Juvenile myelomonocytic leukemia with failed remission
Juvenile myelomonocytic leukemia NOS

C93.31 Juvenile myelomonocytic leukemia, in remission P ♂ⵎ HCC RxHCC CC/MCC Exc

C93.32 Juvenile myelomonocytic leukemia, in relapse P ♂ⵎ HCC RxHCC CC/MCC Exc

5ᵗʰ C93.Z Other monocytic leukemia

C93.Z0 Other monocytic leukemia, not having achieved remission ♂ⵎ HCC RxHCC CC/MCC Exc
Other monocytic leukemia NOS

C93.Z1 Other monocytic leukemia, in remission ♂ⵎ HCC RxHCC CC/MCC Exc

C93.Z2 Other monocytic leukemia, in relapse ♂ⵎ HCC RxHCC CC/MCC Exc

5ᵗʰ C93.9 Monocytic leukemia, unspecified

C93.90 Monocytic leukemia, unspecified, not having achieved remission ♂ⵎ HCC RxHCC CC/MCC Exc
Monocytic leukemia, unspecified with failed remission
Monocytic leukemia, unspecified NOS

C93.91 Monocytic leukemia, unspecified in remission ♂ⵎ HCC RxHCC CC/MCC Exc

C93.92 Monocytic leukemia, unspecified in relapse ♂ⵎ HCC RxHCC CC/MCC Exc

4ᵗʰ C94 Other leukemias of specified cell type

EXCLUDES1 leukemic reticuloendotheliosis (C91.4-)
myelodysplastic syndromes (D46.-)
personal history of leukemia (Z85.6)
plasma cell leukemia (C90.1-)

5ᵗʰ C94.0 Acute erythroid leukemia
Acute myeloid leukemia M6(a)(b)
Erythroleukemia

C94.00 Acute erythroid leukemia, not having achieved remission ♂ⵎ HCC CC/MCC Exc
Acute erythroid leukemia with failed remission
Acute erythroid leukemia NOS

C94.01 Acute erythroid leukemia, in remission ♂ⵎ HCC CC/MCC Exc

C94.02 Acute erythroid leukemia, in relapse ♂ⵎ HCC CC/MCC Exc

5ᵗʰ C94.2 Acute megakaryoblastic leukemia
Acute myeloid leukemia M7
Acute megakaryocytic leukemia

C94.20 Acute megakaryoblastic leukemia not having achieved remission ♂ⵎ HCC CC/MCC Exc
Acute megakaryoblastic leukemia with failed remission
Acute megakaryoblastic leukemia NOS

C94.21 Acute megakaryoblastic leukemia, in remission ♂ⵎ HCC CC/MCC Exc

C94.22 Acute megakaryoblastic leukemia, in relapse ♂ⵎ HCC CC/MCC Exc

5ᵗʰ C94.3 Mast cell leukemia

C94.30 Mast cell leukemia not having achieved remission ♂ⵎ HCC RxHCC CC/MCC Exc
Mast cell leukemia with failed remission
Mast cell leukemia NOS

C94.31 Mast cell leukemia, in remission ♂ⵎ HCC RxHCC CC/MCC Exc

C94.32 Mast cell leukemia, in relapse ♂ⵎ HCC RxHCC CC/MCC Exc

5ᵗʰ C94.4 Acute panmyelosis with myelofibrosis
Acute myelofibrosis

EXCLUDES1 myelofibrosis NOS (D75.81)
secondary myelofibrosis NOS (D75.81)

C94.40 Acute panmyelosis with myelofibrosis not having achieved remission ♂ⵎ HCC CC/MCC Exc
Acute myelofibrosis NOS
Acute panmyelosis with myelofibrosis with failed remission
Acute panmyelosis NOS

C94.41 Acute panmyelosis with myelofibrosis, in remission ♂ⵎ HCC CC/MCC Exc

C94.42 Acute panmyelosis with myelofibrosis, in relapse ♂ⵎ HCC CC/MCC Exc

C94.6 Myelodysplastic disease, not classified ♂ⵎ HCC CC/MCC Exc
Myeloproliferative disease, not classified

5ᵗʰ C94.8 Other specified leukemias
Aggressive NK-cell leukemia
Acute basophilic leukemia

C94.80 Other specified leukemias not having achieved remission ♂ⵎ HCC RxHCC CC/MCC Exc
Other specified leukemia with failed remission
Other specified leukemias NOS

C94.81 Other specified leukemias, in remission ♂ⵎ HCC RxHCC CC/MCC Exc

C94.82 Other specified leukemias, in relapse ♂ⵎ HCC RxHCC CC/MCC Exc

4ᵗʰ C95 Leukemia of unspecified cell type

EXCLUDES1 personal history of leukemia (Z85.6)

5ᵗʰ C95.0 Acute leukemia of unspecified cell type
Acute bilineal leukemia
Acute mixed lineage leukemia
Biphenotypic acute leukemia
Stem cell leukemia of unclear lineage

EXCLUDES1 acute exacerbation of unspecified chronic leukemia (C95.10)

Unspecified Code Other Specified Code Manifestation Code Ⓝ Newborn Ⓟ Pediatric Ⓜ Maternity Ⓐ Adult ♂ Male ♀ Female
● New Code ▲ Revised Code Title ▶◀ Revised Text NOTES INCLUDES EXCLUDES 1 Not coded here EXCLUDES 2 Not included here
4ᵗʰ 4ᵗʰ character required 5ᵗʰ 5ᵗʰ character required 6ᵗʰ 6ᵗʰ character required 7ᵗʰ 7ᵗʰ character required
7ᵗʰ Extension 'X' Alert HAC Hospital-acquired condition (HAC) alert AHA AHA Coding Clinic©

C95.00 **Acute leukemia of unspecified cell type** not having achieved remission   cc HCC CC/MCC Exc
Acute leukemia of unspecified cell type with failed remission
Acute leukemia NOS

C95.01 **Acute leukemia of unspecified cell type, in remission**   cc HCC CC/MCC Exc

C95.02 **Acute leukemia of unspecified cell type, in relapse**   cc HCC CC/MCC Exc

5ᵗʰ C95.1 Chronic leukemia of unspecified cell type

C95.10 **Chronic leukemia of unspecified cell type not having achieved remission**   cc HCC CC/MCC Exc
Chronic leukemia of unspecified cell type with failed remission
Chronic leukemia NOS

C95.11 **Chronic leukemia of unspecified cell type, in remission**   cc HCC CC/MCC Exc

C95.12 **Chronic leukemia of unspecified cell type, in relapse**   cc HCC CC/MCC Exc

5ᵗʰ C95.9 Leukemia, unspecified

C95.90 **Leukemia, unspecified** not having achieved remission   cc HCC CC/MCC Exc
Leukemia, unspecified with failed remission
Leukemia NOS

C95.91 **Leukemia, unspecified, in remission**   cc HCC CC/MCC Exc

C95.92 **Leukemia, unspecified, in relapse**   cc HCC CC/MCC Exc

4ᵗʰ C96 **Other and unspecified malignant neoplasms of lymphoid, hematopoietic and related tissue**
EXCLUDES1 personal history of other malignant neoplasms of lymphoid, hematopoietic and related tissues (Z85.79)

C96.0 **Multifocal and multisystemic (disseminated) Langerhans-cell histiocytosis**   cc HCC CC/MCC Exc
Histiocytosis X, multisystemic
Letterer-Siwe disease
EXCLUDES1 adult pulmonary Langerhans cell histiocytosis (J84.82)
multifocal and unisystemic Langerhans-cell histiocytosis (C96.5)
unifocal Langerhans-cell histiocytosis (C96.6)

▲ 5ᵗʰ C96.2 **Malignant mast cell ►neoplasm◄**   HCC RxHCC
EXCLUDES1 indolent mastocytosis ►(D47.02)◄
mast cell leukemia (C94.30)
mastocytosis (congenital) (cutaneous) (Q82.2)

● C96.20 **Malignant** mast cell **neoplasm, unspecified**   cc CC/MCC Exc
● C96.21 **Aggressive systemic** mastocytosis   cc CC/MCC Exc
● C96.22 **Mast cell** sarcoma   cc CC/MCC Exc
● C96.29 **Other malignant** mast cell **neoplasm**   cc CC/MCC Exc

C96.4 **Sarcoma of dendritic cells (accessory cells)**   cc HCC CC/MCC Exc
Follicular dendritic cell sarcoma
Interdigitating dendritic cell sarcoma
Langerhans cell sarcoma

C96.5 **Multifocal and unisystemic Langerhans-cell histiocytosis**   cc HCC CC/MCC Exc
Hand-Schüller-Christian disease
Histiocytosis X, multifocal
EXCLUDES1 multifocal and multisystemic (disseminated) Langerhans-cell histiocytosis (C96.0)
unifocal Langerhans-cell histiocytosis (C96.6)

C96.6 **Unifocal Langerhans-cell histiocytosis**   cc HCC CC/MCC Exc
Eosinophilic granuloma
Histiocytosis X, unifocal
Histiocytosis X NOS
Langerhans-cell histiocytosis NOS
EXCLUDES1 multifocal and multisysemic (disseminated) Langerhans-cell histiocytosis (C96.0)
multifocal and unisystemic Langerhans-cell histiocytosis (C96.5)

C96.A **Histiocytic sarcoma**   cc HCC CC/MCC Exc
Malignant histiocytosis

C96.Z **Other specified malignant neoplasms of lymphoid, hematopoietic and related tissue**   cc HCC CC/MCC Exc

C96.9 **Malignant neoplasm of lymphoid, hematopoietic and related tissue, unspecified**   cc HCC CC/MCC Exc

In situ neoplasms (D00-D09)

INCLUDES   Bowen's disease
erythroplasia
grade III intraepithelial neoplasia
Queyrat's erythroplasia

4ᵗʰ D00 **Carcinoma in situ of** oral cavity, esophagus and stomach
EXCLUDES1 melanoma in situ (D03.-)

5ᵗʰ D00.0 **Carcinoma in situ of** lip, oral cavity and pharynx
Use additional code to identify:
exposure to environmental tobacco smoke (Z77.22)
exposure to tobacco smoke in the perinatal period (P96.81)
history of tobacco dependence (Z87.891)
occupational exposure to environmental tobacco smoke (Z57.31)
tobacco dependence (F17.-)
tobacco use (Z72.0)
EXCLUDES1 carcinoma in situ of aryepiglottic fold or interarytenoid fold, laryngeal aspect (D02.0)
carcinoma in situ of epiglottis NOS (D02.0)
carcinoma in situ of epiglottis suprahyoid portion (D02.0)
carcinoma in situ of skin of lip (D03.0, D04.0)

D00.00 **Carcinoma in situ of** oral cavity, unspecified site
D00.01 **Carcinoma in situ of** labial mucosa and vermilion border
D00.02 **Carcinoma in situ of** buccal mucosa
D00.03 **Carcinoma in situ of** gingiva and edentulous alveolar ridge
D00.04 **Carcinoma in situ of** soft palate
D00.05 **Carcinoma in situ of** hard palate
D00.06 **Carcinoma in situ of** floor of mouth
D00.07 **Carcinoma in situ of** tongue
D00.08 **Carcinoma in situ of** pharynx
Carcinoma in situ of aryepiglottic fold NOS
Carcinoma in situ of hypopharyngeal aspect of aryepiglottic fold
Carcinoma in situ of marginal zone of aryepiglottic fold

D00.1 **Carcinoma in situ of** esophagus
D00.2 **Carcinoma in situ of** stomach

4ᵗʰ D01 **Carcinoma in situ of** other and unspecified digestive organs
EXCLUDES1 melanoma in situ (D03.-)

D01.0 **Carcinoma in situ of** colon
EXCLUDES1 carcinoma in situ of rectosigmoid junction (D01.1)

D01.1 **Carcinoma in situ of** rectosigmoid junction
D01.2 **Carcinoma in situ of** rectum
D01.3 **Carcinoma in situ of** anus and anal canal
Anal intraepithelial neoplasia III [AIN III]
Severe dysplasia of anus
EXCLUDES1 anal intraepithelial neoplasia I and II [AIN I and AIN II] (K62.82)
carcinoma in situ of anal margin (D04.5)
carcinoma in situ of anal skin (D04.5)
carcinoma in situ of perianal skin (D04.5)

5ᵗʰ D01.4 **Carcinoma in situ of other and unspecified parts of** intestine
EXCLUDES1 carcinoma in situ of ampulla of Vater (D01.5)
D01.40 **Carcinoma in situ of unspecified part of intestine**
D01.49 **Carcinoma in situ of other parts of intestine**

D01.5 **Carcinoma in situ of** liver, gallbladder and bile ducts
Carcinoma in situ of ampulla of Vater

D01.7 **Carcinoma in situ of other specified digestive organs**
Carcinoma in situ of pancreas

D01.9 **Carcinoma in situ of digestive organ, unspecified**

PDxⓘ Unacceptable principal diagnosis symbol per Medicare code edits   POA Code exempt from diagnosis present on admission requirement
? Questionable admission   cc Complication or comorbidity   CC/MCC Exc CC/MCC exclusion   MCC Major complication or comorbidity
Principal diagnosis as its own CC   Principal diagnosis as its own MCC   HCC HCC diagnosis code   RxHCC RxHCC diagnosis code
MACRA code   Z1 Z code as first-listed diagnosis

CHAPTER 2: NEOPLASMS (C00-D49)

496   When symbols appear on a code that requires a 7th character extension, refer to Appendix B to identify applicable 7th character codes.   **2018 ICD-10-CM**

[4th] **D02 Carcinoma in situ of middle ear and respiratory system**
Use additional code to identify:
exposure to environmental tobacco smoke (Z77.22)
exposure to tobacco smoke in the perinatal period (P96.81)
history of tobacco dependence (Z87.891)
occupational exposure to environmental tobacco smoke (Z57.31)
tobacco dependence (F17.-)
tobacco use (Z72.0)
[EXCLUDES1] *melanoma in situ (D03.-)*

D02.0 Carcinoma in situ of larynx
Carcinoma in situ of aryepiglottic fold or interarytenoid fold, laryngeal aspect
Carcinoma in situ of epiglottis (suprahyoid portion)
[EXCLUDES1] *carcinoma in situ of aryepiglottic fold or interarytenoid fold NOS (D00.08)*
carcinoma in situ of hypopharyngeal aspect (D00.08)
carcinoma in situ of marginal zone (D00.08)

D02.1 Carcinoma in situ of trachea
[5th] **D02.2 Carcinoma in situ of bronchus and lung**
D02.20 Carcinoma in situ of unspecified bronchus and lung
D02.21 Carcinoma in situ of right bronchus and lung
D02.22 Carcinoma in situ of left bronchus and lung
D02.3 Carcinoma in situ of other parts of respiratory system
Carcinoma in situ of accessory sinuses
Carcinoma in situ of middle ear
Carcinoma in situ of nasal cavities
[EXCLUDES1] *carcinoma in situ of ear (external) (skin) (D04.2-)*
carcinoma in situ of nose NOS D09.8
carcinoma in situ of skin of nose (D04.3)
D02.4 Carcinoma in situ of respiratory system, unspecified

[4th] **D03 Melanoma in situ**
D03.0 Melanoma in situ of lip [HCC]
[5th] **D03.1 Melanoma in situ of eyelid, including canthus**
D03.10 Melanoma in situ of unspecified eyelid, including canthus [HCC]
D03.11 Melanoma in situ of right eyelid, including canthus [HCC]
D03.12 Melanoma in situ of left eyelid, including canthus [HCC]
[5th] **D03.2 Melanoma in situ of ear and external auricular canal**
D03.20 Melanoma in situ of unspecified ear and external auricular canal [HCC]
D03.21 Melanoma in situ of right ear and external auricular canal [HCC]
D03.22 Melanoma in situ of left ear and external auricular canal [HCC]
[5th] **D03.3 Melanoma in situ of other and unspecified parts of face**
D03.30 Melanoma in situ of unspecified part of face [HCC]
D03.39 Melanoma in situ of other parts of face [HCC]
D03.4 Melanoma in situ of scalp and neck [HCC]
[5th] **D03.5 Melanoma in situ of trunk**
D03.51 Melanoma in situ of anal skin [HCC]
Melanoma in situ of anal margin
Melanoma in situ of perianal skin
D03.52 Melanoma in situ of breast (skin) (soft tissue) [HCC]
D03.59 Melanoma in situ of other part of trunk [HCC]
[5th] **D03.6 Melanoma in situ of upper limb, including shoulder**
D03.60 Melanoma in situ of unspecified upper limb, including shoulder [HCC]
D03.61 Melanoma in situ of right upper limb, including shoulder [HCC]
D03.62 Melanoma in situ of left upper limb, including shoulder [HCC]
[5th] **D03.7 Melanoma in situ of lower limb, including hip**
D03.70 Melanoma in situ of unspecified lower limb, including hip [HCC]
D03.71 Melanoma in situ of right lower limb, including hip [HCC]
D03.72 Melanoma in situ of left lower limb, including hip [HCC]
D03.8 Melanoma in situ of other sites [HCC]
Melanoma in situ of scrotum
[EXCLUDES1] *carcinoma in situ of scrotum (D07.61)*
D03.9 Melanoma in situ, unspecified [HCC]

[4th] **D04 Carcinoma in situ of skin**
[EXCLUDES1] *erythroplasia of Queyrat (penis) NOS (D07.4)*
melanoma in situ (D03.-)
D04.0 Carcinoma in situ of skin of lip
[EXCLUDES1] *carcinoma in situ of vermilion border of lip (D00.01)*
[5th] **D04.1 Carcinoma in situ of skin of eyelid, including canthus**
D04.10 Carcinoma in situ of skin of unspecified eyelid, including canthus
D04.11 Carcinoma in situ of skin of right eyelid, including canthus
D04.12 Carcinoma in situ of skin of left eyelid, including canthus
[5th] **D04.2 Carcinoma in situ of skin of ear and external auricular canal**
D04.20 Carcinoma in situ of skin of unspecified ear and external auricular canal
D04.21 Carcinoma in situ of skin of right ear and external auricular canal
D04.22 Carcinoma in situ of skin of left ear and external auricular canal
[5th] **D04.3 Carcinoma in situ of skin of other and unspecified parts of face**
D04.30 Carcinoma in situ of skin of unspecified part of face
D04.39 Carcinoma in situ of skin of other parts of face
D04.4 Carcinoma in situ of skin of scalp and neck
D04.5 Carcinoma in situ of skin of trunk
Carcinoma in situ of anal margin
Carcinoma in situ of anal skin
Carcinoma in situ of perianal skin
Carcinoma in situ of skin of breast
[EXCLUDES1] *carcinoma in situ of anus NOS (D01.3)*
carcinoma in situ of scrotum (D07.61)
carcinoma in situ of skin of genital organs (D07.-)
[5th] **D04.6 Carcinoma in situ of skin of upper limb, including shoulder**
D04.60 Carcinoma in situ of skin of unspecified upper limb, including shoulder
D04.61 Carcinoma in situ of skin of right upper limb, including shoulder
D04.62 Carcinoma in situ of skin of left upper limb, including shoulder
[5th] **D04.7 Carcinoma in situ of skin of lower limb, including hip**
D04.70 Carcinoma in situ of skin of unspecified lower limb, including hip
D04.71 Carcinoma in situ of skin of right lower limb, including hip
D04.72 Carcinoma in situ of skin of left lower limb, including hip
D04.8 Carcinoma in situ of skin of other sites
D04.9 Carcinoma in situ of skin, unspecified

[4th] **D05 Carcinoma in situ of breast**
[EXCLUDES1] *carcinoma in situ of skin of breast (D04.5)*
melanoma in situ of breast (skin) (D03.5)
Paget's disease of breast or nipple (C50.-)
[5th] **D05.0 Lobular carcinoma in situ of breast**
D05.00 Lobular carcinoma in situ of unspecified breast
D05.01 Lobular carcinoma in situ of right breast
D05.02 Lobular carcinoma in situ of left breast
[5th] **D05.1 Intraductal carcinoma in situ of breast**
D05.10 Intraductal carcinoma in situ of unspecified breast
D05.11 Intraductal carcinoma in situ of right breast
D05.12 Intraductal carcinoma in situ of left breast
[5th] **D05.8 Other specified type of carcinoma in situ of breast**
D05.80 Other specified type of carcinoma in situ of unspecified breast
D05.81 Other specified type of carcinoma in situ of right breast

Unspecified Code Other Specified Code Manifestation Code [N] Newborn [P] Pediatric [M] Maternity [A] Adult ♂ Male ♀ Female
● New Code ▲ Revised Code Title ►◄ Revised Text [NOTES] INCLUDES [EXCLUDES1] Not coded here [EXCLUDES2] Not included here
[4th] 4th character required [5th] 5th character required [6th] 6th character required [7th] 7th character required
[X] Extension 'X' Alert [HAC] Hospital-acquired condition (HAC) alert AHA AHA Coding Clinic©

D05.82 **Other specified type of carcinoma in situ of** left **breast**

🔵 D05.9 Unspecified **type of carcinoma in situ of** breast

D05.90 **Unspecified type of carcinoma in situ of unspecified breast**

D05.91 **Unspecified type of carcinoma in situ of** right **breast**

D05.92 **Unspecified type of carcinoma in situ of** left **breast**

🔵 D06 **Carcinoma in situ of** cervix uteri

INCLUDES *cervical adenocarcinoma in situ*

cervical intraepithelial glandular neoplasia

cervical intraepithelial neoplasia III [CIN III]

severe dysplasia of cervix uteri

EXCLUDES1 *cervical intraepithelial neoplasia II [CIN II] (N87.1)*

cytologic evidence of malignancy of cervix without histologic confirmation (R87.614)

high grade squamous intraepithelial lesion (HGSIL) of cervix (R87.613)

melanoma in situ of cervix (D03.5)

moderate cervical dysplasia (N87.1)

D06.0 **Carcinoma in situ of** endocervix ♀

D06.1 **Carcinoma in situ of** exocervix ♀

D06.7 **Carcinoma in situ of** other parts **of cervix** ♀

D06.9 **Carcinoma in situ of cervix, unspecified** ♀

🔵 D07 **Carcinoma in situ of** other and unspecified genital organs

EXCLUDES1 *melanoma in situ of trunk (D03.5)*

D07.0 **Carcinoma in situ of** endometrium ♀

D07.1 **Carcinoma in situ of** vulva ♀

Severe dysplasia of vulva

Vulvar intraepithelial neoplasia III [VIN III]

EXCLUDES1 *moderate dysplasia of vulva (N90.1)*

vulvar intraepithelial neoplasia II [VIN II] (N90.1)

D07.2 **Carcinoma in situ of** vagina ♀

Severe dysplasia of vagina

Vaginal intraepithelial neoplasia III [VAIN III]

EXCLUDES1 *moderate dysplasia of vagina (N89.1)*

vaginal intraepithelial neoplasia II [VIN II] (N89.1)

🔵 D07.3 **Carcinoma in situ of** other and unspecified female genital organs

D07.30 **Carcinoma in situ of unspecified female genital organs** ♀

D07.39 **Carcinoma in situ of other female genital organs** ♀

D07.4 **Carcinoma in situ of** penis ♂

Erythroplasia of Queyrat NOS

D07.5 **Carcinoma in situ of** prostate ♂

Prostatic intraepithelial neoplasia III [PIN III]

Severe dysplasia of prostate

EXCLUDES1 *dysplasia (mild) (moderate) of prostate (N42.3-)*

prostatic intraepithelial neoplasia II [PIN II] (N42.3-)

🔵 D07.6 **Carcinoma in situ of** other and unspecified male genital organs

D07.60 **Carcinoma in situ of unspecified male genital organs** ♂

D07.61 **Carcinoma in situ of** scrotum ♂

D07.69 **Carcinoma in situ of other male genital organs** ♂

🔵 D09 **Carcinoma in situ of** other and unspecified sites

EXCLUDES1 *melanoma in situ (D03.-)*

D09.0 **Carcinoma in situ of** bladder

🔵 D09.1 **Carcinoma in situ of** other and unspecified urinary organs

D09.10 **Carcinoma in situ of unspecified urinary organ**

D09.19 **Carcinoma in situ of other urinary organs**

🔵 D09.2 **Carcinoma in situ of** eye

EXCLUDES1 *carcinoma in situ of skin of eyelid (D04.1-)*

D09.20 **Carcinoma in situ of unspecified eye**

D09.21 **Carcinoma in situ of** right **eye**

D09.22 **Carcinoma in situ of** left **eye**

D09.3 **Carcinoma in situ of** thyroid and other endocrine glands

EXCLUDES1 *carcinoma in situ of endocrine pancreas (D01.7)*

carcinoma in situ of ovary (D07.39)

carcinoma in situ of testis (D07.69)

D09.8 **Carcinoma in situ of** other specified sites

D09.9 **Carcinoma in situ, unspecified**

Benign neoplasms, except benign neuroendocrine tumors (D10-D36)

🔵 D10 **Benign neoplasm of** mouth and pharynx

D10.0 **Benign neoplasm of** lip

Benign neoplasm of lip (frenulum) (inner aspect) (mucosa) (vermilion border)

EXCLUDES1 *benign neoplasm of skin of lip (D22.0, D23.0)*

D10.1 **Benign neoplasm of** tongue

Benign neoplasm of lingual tonsil

D10.2 **Benign neoplasm of** floor of mouth

🔵 D10.3 **Benign neoplasm of other and unspecified parts of mouth**

D10.30 **Benign neoplasm of unspecified part of mouth**

D10.39 **Benign neoplasm of other parts of mouth**

Benign neoplasm of minor salivary gland NOS

EXCLUDES1 *benign odontogenic neoplasms (D16.4-D16.5)*

benign neoplasm of mucosa of lip (D10.0)

benign neoplasm of nasopharyngeal surface of soft palate (D10.6)

D10.4 **Benign neoplasm of** tonsil

Benign neoplasm of tonsil (faucial) (palatine)

EXCLUDES1 *benign neoplasm of lingual tonsil (D10.1)*

benign neoplasm of pharyngeal tonsil (D10.6)

benign neoplasm of tonsillar fossa (D10.5)

benign neoplasm of tonsillar pillars (D10.5)

D10.5 **Benign neoplasm of** other parts of oropharynx

Benign neoplasm of epiglottis, anterior aspect

Benign neoplasm of tonsillar fossa

Benign neoplasm of tonsillar pillars

Benign neoplasm of vallecula

EXCLUDES1 *benign neoplasm of epiglottis NOS (D14.1)*

benign neoplasm of epiglottis, suprahyoid portion (D14.1)

D10.6 **Benign neoplasm of** nasopharynx

Benign neoplasm of pharyngeal tonsil

Benign neoplasm of posterior margin of septum and choanae

D10.7 **Benign neoplasm of** hypopharynx

D10.9 **Benign neoplasm of pharynx, unspecified**

🔵 D11 **Benign neoplasm of** major salivary glands

EXCLUDES1 *benign neoplasms of specified minor salivary glands which are classified according to their anatomical location*

benign neoplasms of minor salivary glands NOS (D10.39)

D11.0 **Benign neoplasm of** parotid gland

D11.7 **Benign neoplasm of** other major salivary glands

Benign neoplasm of sublingual salivary gland

Benign neoplasm of submandibular salivary gland

D11.9 **Benign neoplasm of major salivary gland, unspecified**

🔵 D12 **Benign neoplasm of** colon, rectum, anus and anal canal

EXCLUDES1 *benign carcinoid tumors of the large intestine, and rectum (D3A.02-)*

D12.0 **Benign neoplasm of** cecum

Benign neoplasm of ileocecal valve

D12.1 **Benign neoplasm of** appendix

EXCLUDES1 *benign carcinoid tumor of the appendix (D3A.020)*

D12.2 **Benign neoplasm of** ascending colon

AHA: Q1 2017

D12.3 **Benign neoplasm of** transverse colon

AHA: Q1 2017

Benign neoplasm of hepatic flexure

Benign neoplasm of splenic flexure

D12.4 **Benign neoplasm of** descending colon

D12.5 **Benign neoplasm of** sigmoid colon

D12.6 **Benign neoplasm of colon, unspecified**

AHA: Q1 2017

Adenomatosis of colon

Benign neoplasm of large intestine NOS

Polyposis (hereditary) of colon

EXCLUDES1 *inflammatory polyp of colon (K51.4-)*

polyp of colon NOS (K63.5)

PDx🚫 Unacceptable principal diagnosis symbol per Medicare code edits   POA Code exempt from diagnosis present on admission requirement

❓ Questionable admission   🄲 Complication or comorbidity   CC/MCC EXC CC/MCC exclusion   MCC Major complication or comorbidity

🄲 Principal diagnosis as its own CC   🄼 Principal diagnosis as its own MCC   HCC HCC diagnosis code   RxHCC RxHCC diagnosis code

MACRA code   Z1 Z code as first-listed diagnosis

When symbols appear on a code that requires a 7th character extension, refer to Appendix B to identify applicable 7th character codes.

2018 ICD-10-CM

D12.7 Benign neoplasm of rectosigmoid junction
D12.8 Benign neoplasm of rectum
[EXCLUDES1] *benign carcinoid tumor of the rectum (D3A.026)*
D12.9 Benign neoplasm of anus and anal canal
Benign neoplasm of anus NOS
[EXCLUDES1] *benign neoplasm of anal margin (D22.5, D23.5)*
benign neoplasm of anal skin (D22.5, D23.5)
benign neoplasm of perianal skin (D22.5, D23.5)

[4th] **D13 Benign neoplasm of other and ill-defined parts of digestive system**
[EXCLUDES1] *benign stromal tumors of digestive system (D21.4)*
D13.0 Benign neoplasm of esophagus
D13.1 Benign neoplasm of stomach
[EXCLUDES1] *benign carcinoid tumor of the stomach (D3A.092)*
D13.2 Benign neoplasm of duodenum
[EXCLUDES1] *benign carcinoid tumor of the duodenum (D3A.010)*
[5th] D13.3 Benign neoplasm of other and unspecified parts of small intestine
[EXCLUDES1] *benign carcinoid tumors of the small intestine(D3A.01-)*
benign neoplasm of ileocecal valve (D12.0)
D13.30 Benign neoplasm of unspecified part of small intestine
D13.39 Benign neoplasm of other parts of small intestine
D13.4 Benign neoplasm of liver
Benign neoplasm of intrahepatic bile ducts
D13.5 Benign neoplasm of extrahepatic bile ducts
D13.6 Benign neoplasm of pancreas
[EXCLUDES1] *benign neoplasm of endocrine pancreas (D13.7)*
D13.7 Benign neoplasm of endocrine pancreas
Islet cell tumor
Benign neoplasm of islets of Langerhans
Use additional code to identify any functional activity.
D13.9 Benign neoplasm of ill-defined sites within the digestive system
Benign neoplasm of digestive system NOS
Benign neoplasm of intestine NOS
Benign neoplasm of spleen

[4th] **D14 Benign neoplasm of middle ear and respiratory system**
D14.0 Benign neoplasm of middle ear, nasal cavity and accessory sinuses
Benign neoplasm of cartilage of nose
[EXCLUDES1] *benign neoplasm of auricular canal (external) (D22.2-, D23.2-)*
benign neoplasm of bone of ear (D16.4)
benign neoplasm of bone of nose (D16.4)
benign neoplasm of cartilage of ear (D21.0)
benign neoplasm of ear (external)(skin) (D22.2-, D23.2-)
benign neoplasm of nose NOS (D36.7)
benign neoplasm of skin of nose (D22.39, D23.39)
benign neoplasm of olfactory bulb (D33.3)
benign neoplasm of posterior margin of septum and choanae (D10.6)
polyp of accessory sinus (J33.8)
polyp of ear (middle) (H74.4)
polyp of nasal (cavity) (J33.-)
D14.1 Benign neoplasm of larynx
Adenomatous polyp of larynx
Benign neoplasm of epiglottis (suprahyoid portion)
[EXCLUDES1] *benign neoplasm of epiglottis, anterior aspect (D10.5)*
polyp (nonadenomatous) of vocal cord or larynx (J38.1)
D14.2 Benign neoplasm of trachea
[5th] D14.3 Benign neoplasm of bronchus and lung
[EXCLUDES1] *benign carcinoid tumor of the bronchus and lung (D3A.090)*
D14.30 Benign neoplasm of unspecified bronchus and lung
D14.31 Benign neoplasm of right bronchus and lung
D14.32 Benign neoplasm of left bronchus and lung
D14.4 Benign neoplasm of respiratory system, unspecified

[4th] **D15 Benign neoplasm of other and unspecified intrathoracic organs**
[EXCLUDES1] *benign neoplasm of mesothelial tissue (D19.-)*
D15.0 Benign neoplasm of thymus
[EXCLUDES1] *benign carcinoid tumor of the thymus (D3A.091)*
D15.1 Benign neoplasm of heart
[EXCLUDES1] *benign neoplasm of great vessels (D21.3)*
D15.2 Benign neoplasm of mediastinum
D15.7 Benign neoplasm of other specified intrathoracic organs
D15.9 Benign neoplasm of intrathoracic organ, unspecified

[4th] **D16 Benign neoplasm of bone and articular cartilage**
[EXCLUDES1] *benign neoplasm of connective tissue of ear (D21.0)*
benign neoplasm of connective tissue of eyelid (D21.0)
benign neoplasm of connective tissue of larynx (D14.1)
benign neoplasm of connective tissue of nose (D14.0)
benign neoplasm of synovia (D21.-)
[5th] D16.0 Benign neoplasm of scapula and long bones of upper limb
D16.00 Benign neoplasm of scapula and long bones of unspecified upper limb
D16.01 Benign neoplasm of scapula and long bones of right upper limb
D16.02 Benign neoplasm of scapula and long bones of left upper limb
[5th] D16.1 Benign neoplasm of short bones of upper limb
D16.10 Benign neoplasm of short bones of unspecified upper limb
D16.11 Benign neoplasm of short bones of right upper limb
D16.12 Benign neoplasm of short bones of left upper limb
[5th] D16.2 Benign neoplasm of long bones of lower limb
D16.20 Benign neoplasm of long bones of unspecified lower limb
D16.21 Benign neoplasm of long bones of right lower limb
D16.22 Benign neoplasm of long bones of left lower limb
[5th] D16.3 Benign neoplasm of short bones of lower limb
D16.30 Benign neoplasm of short bones of unspecified lower limb
D16.31 Benign neoplasm of short bones of right lower limb
D16.32 Benign neoplasm of short bones of left lower limb
D16.4 Benign neoplasm of bones of skull and face
Benign neoplasm of maxilla (superior)
Benign neoplasm of orbital bone
Keratocyst of maxilla
Keratocystic odontogenic tumor of maxilla
[EXCLUDES2] *benign neoplasm of lower jaw bone (D16.5)*
D16.5 Benign neoplasm of lower jaw bone
Keratocyst of mandible
Keratocystic odontogenic tumor of mandible
D16.6 Benign neoplasm of vertebral column
[EXCLUDES1] *benign neoplasm of sacrum and coccyx (D16.8)*
D16.7 Benign neoplasm of ribs, sternum and clavicle
D16.8 Benign neoplasm of pelvic bones, sacrum and coccyx
D16.9 Benign neoplasm of bone and articular cartilage, unspecified

[4th] **D17 Benign lipomatous neoplasm**
D17.0 Benign lipomatous neoplasm of skin and subcutaneous tissue of head, face and neck
D17.1 Benign lipomatous neoplasm of skin and subcutaneous tissue of trunk
[5th] D17.2 Benign lipomatous neoplasm of skin and subcutaneous tissue of limb
D17.20 Benign lipomatous neoplasm of skin and subcutaneous tissue of unspecified limb
D17.21 Benign lipomatous neoplasm of skin and subcutaneous tissue of right arm
D17.22 Benign lipomatous neoplasm of skin and subcutaneous tissue of left arm
D17.23 Benign lipomatous neoplasm of skin and subcutaneous tissue of right leg

Unspecified Code Other Specified Code Manifestation Code [N] Newborn [P] Pediatric [M] Maternity [A] Adult ♂ Male ♀ Female
● New Code ▲ Revised Code Title ►◄ Revised Text [NOTES] [INCLUDES] [EXCLUDES1] Not coded here [EXCLUDES2] Not included here
[4th] 4th character required [5th] 5th character required [6th] 6th character required [7th] 7th character required
[7th] Extension 'X' Alert [HAC] Hospital-acquired condition (HAC) alert AHA AHA Coding Clinic©

D17.24   Benign lipomatous neoplasm of skin and subcutaneous tissue of left leg

(5ᵗʰ) D17.3   Benign lipomatous neoplasm of skin and subcutaneous tissue of other and unspecified sites

D17.30   Benign lipomatous neoplasm of skin and subcutaneous tissue of unspecified sites

D17.39   Benign lipomatous neoplasm of skin and subcutaneous tissue of other sites

D17.4   Benign lipomatous neoplasm of intrathoracic organs

D17.5   Benign lipomatous neoplasm of intra-abdominal organs

EXCLUDES1 *benign lipomatous neoplasm of peritoneum and retroperitoneum (D17.79)*

D17.6   Benign lipomatous neoplasm of spermatic cord   ♂

(5ᵗʰ) D17.7   Benign lipomatous neoplasm of other sites

D17.71   Benign lipomatous neoplasm of kidney

D17.72   Benign lipomatous neoplasm of other genitourinary organ

D17.79   Benign lipomatous neoplasm of other sites
Benign lipomatous neoplasm of peritoneum
Benign lipomatous neoplasm of retroperitoneum

D17.9   Benign lipomatous neoplasm, unspecified
Lipoma NOS

(4ᵗʰ) D18   Hemangioma and lymphangioma, any site

EXCLUDES1 *benign neoplasm of glomus jugulare (D35.6)*
blue or pigmented nevus (D22.-)
nevus NOS (D22.-)
vascular nevus (Q82.5)

(5ᵗʰ) D18.0   Hemangioma
Angioma NOS
Cavernous nevus

D18.00   Hemangioma unspecified site

D18.01   Hemangioma of skin and subcutaneous tissue

D18.02   Hemangioma of intracranial structures   HCC

D18.03   Hemangioma of intra-abdominal structures

D18.09   Hemangioma of other sites

D18.1   Lymphangioma, any site

(4ᵗʰ) D19   Benign neoplasm of mesothelial tissue

D19.0   Benign neoplasm of mesothelial tissue of pleura

D19.1   Benign neoplasm of mesothelial tissue of peritoneum

D19.7   Benign neoplasm of mesothelial tissue of other sites

D19.9   Benign neoplasm of mesothelial tissue, unspecified
Benign mesothelioma NOS

(4ᵗʰ) D20   Benign neoplasm of soft tissue of retroperitoneum and peritoneum

EXCLUDES1 *benign lipomatous neoplasm of peritoneum and retroperitoneum (D17.79)*
benign neoplasm of mesothelial tissue (D19.-)

D20.0   Benign neoplasm of soft tissue of retroperitoneum

D20.1   Benign neoplasm of soft tissue of peritoneum

(4ᵗʰ) D21   Other benign neoplasms of connective and other soft tissue

INCLUDES   *benign neoplasm of blood vessel*
benign neoplasm of bursa
benign neoplasm of cartilage
benign neoplasm of fascia
benign neoplasm of fat
benign neoplasm of ligament, except uterine
benign neoplasm of lymphatic channel
benign neoplasm of muscle
benign neoplasm of synovia
benign neoplasm of tendon (sheath)
benign stromal tumors

EXCLUDES1 *benign neoplasm of articular cartilage (D16.-)*
benign neoplasm of cartilage of larynx (D14.1)
benign neoplasm of cartilage of nose (D14.0)
benign neoplasm of connective tissue of breast (D24.-)
benign neoplasm of peripheral nerves and autonomic nervous system (D36.1-)
benign neoplasm of peritoneum (D20.1)

benign neoplasm of retroperitoneum (D20.0)
benign neoplasm of uterine ligament, any (D28.2)
benign neoplasm of vascular tissue (D18.-)
hemangioma (D18.0-)
lipomatous neoplasm (D17.-)
lymphangioma (D18.1)
uterine leiomyoma (D25.-)

D21.0   Benign neoplasm of connective and other soft tissue of head, face and neck
Benign neoplasm of connective tissue of ear
Benign neoplasm of connective tissue of eyelid

EXCLUDES1 *benign neoplasm of connective tissue of orbit (D31.6-)*

(5ᵗʰ) D21.1   Benign neoplasm of connective and other soft tissue of upper limb, including shoulder

D21.10   Benign neoplasm of connective and other soft tissue of unspecified upper limb, including shoulder

D21.11   Benign neoplasm of connective and other soft tissue of right upper limb, including shoulder

D21.12   Benign neoplasm of connective and other soft tissue of left upper limb, including shoulder

(5ᵗʰ) D21.2   Benign neoplasm of connective and other soft tissue of lower limb, including hip

D21.20   Benign neoplasm of connective and other soft tissue of unspecified lower limb, including hip

D21.21   Benign neoplasm of connective and other soft tissue of right lower limb, including hip

D21.22   Benign neoplasm of connective and other soft tissue of left lower limb, including hip

D21.3   Benign neoplasm of connective and other soft tissue of thorax
Benign neoplasm of axilla
Benign neoplasm of diaphragm
Benign neoplasm of great vessels

EXCLUDES1 *benign neoplasm of heart (D15.1)*
benign neoplasm of mediastinum (D15.2)
benign neoplasm of thymus (D15.0)

D21.4   Benign neoplasm of connective and other soft tissue of abdomen
Benign stromal tumors of abdomen

D21.5   Benign neoplasm of connective and other soft tissue of pelvis

EXCLUDES1 *benign neoplasm of any uterine ligament (D28.2)*
uterine leiomyoma (D25.-)

D21.6   Benign neoplasm of connective and other soft tissue of trunk, unspecified
Benign neoplasm of back NOS

D21.9   Benign neoplasm of connective and other soft tissue, unspecified

(4ᵗʰ) D22   Melanocytic nevi

INCLUDES   *atypical nevus*
blue hairy pigmented nevus
nevus NOS

D22.0   Melanocytic nevi of lip

(5ᵗʰ) D22.1   Melanocytic nevi of eyelid, including canthus

D22.10   Melanocytic nevi of unspecified eyelid, including canthus

D22.11   Melanocytic nevi of right eyelid, including canthus

D22.12   Melanocytic nevi of left eyelid, including canthus

(5ᵗʰ) D22.2   Melanocytic nevi of ear and external auricular canal

D22.20   Melanocytic nevi of unspecified ear and external auricular canal

D22.21   Melanocytic nevi of right ear and external auricular canal

D22.22   Melanocytic nevi of left ear and external auricular canal

(5ᵗʰ) D22.3   Melanocytic nevi of other and unspecified parts of face

D22.30   Melanocytic nevi of unspecified part of face

D22.39   Melanocytic nevi of other parts of face

D22.4   Melanocytic nevi of scalp and neck

POA Unacceptable principal diagnosis symbol per Medicare code edits   POA Code exempt from diagnosis present on admission requirement
？ Questionable admission   C Complication or comorbidity   CC/MCC Exc CC/MCC exclusion   MCC Major complication or comorbidity
Principal diagnosis as its own CC   Principal diagnosis as its own MCC   HCC HCC diagnosis code   RxHCC RxHCC diagnosis code
MACRA code   Z1 Z code as first-listed diagnosis

D22.5 Melanocytic nevi of trunk
Melanocytic nevi of anal margin
Melanocytic nevi of anal skin
Melanocytic nevi of perianal skin
Melanocytic nevi of skin of breast

5ᵗʰ D22.6 Melanocytic nevi of upper limb, including shoulder
D22.60 Melanocytic nevi of unspecified upper limb, including shoulder
D22.61 Melanocytic nevi of right upper limb, including shoulder
D22.62 Melanocytic nevi of left upper limb, including shoulder

5ᵗʰ D22.7 Melanocytic nevi of lower limb, including hip
D22.70 Melanocytic nevi of unspecified lower limb, including hip
D22.71 Melanocytic nevi of right lower limb, including hip
D22.72 Melanocytic nevi of left lower limb, including hip

D22.9 Melanocytic nevi, unspecified

4ᵗʰ D23 Other benign neoplasms of skin
INCLUDES benign neoplasm of hair follicles
benign neoplasm of sebaceous glands
benign neoplasm of sweat glands
EXCLUDES1 benign lipomatous neoplasms of skin (D17.0-D17.3)
melanocytic nevi (D22.-)

D23.0 Other benign neoplasm of skin of lip
EXCLUDES1 benign neoplasm of vermilion border of lip (D10.0)

5ᵗʰ D23.1 Other benign neoplasm of skin of eyelid, including canthus
D23.10 Other benign neoplasm of skin of unspecified eyelid, including canthus
D23.11 Other benign neoplasm of skin of right eyelid, including canthus
D23.12 Other benign neoplasm of skin of left eyelid, including canthus

5ᵗʰ D23.2 Other benign neoplasm of skin of ear and external auricular canal
D23.20 Other benign neoplasm of skin of unspecified ear and external auricular canal
D23.21 Other benign neoplasm of skin of right ear and external auricular canal
D23.22 Other benign neoplasm of skin of left ear and external auricular canal

5ᵗʰ D23.3 Other benign neoplasm of skin of other and unspecified parts of face
D23.30 Other benign neoplasm of skin of unspecified part of face
D23.39 Other benign neoplasm of skin of other parts of face

D23.4 Other benign neoplasm of skin of scalp and neck

D23.5 Other benign neoplasm of skin of trunk
Other benign neoplasm of anal margin
Other benign neoplasm of anal skin
Other benign neoplasm of perianal skin
Other benign neoplasm of skin of breast
EXCLUDES1 benign neoplasm of anus NOS (D12.9)

5ᵗʰ D23.6 Other benign neoplasm of skin of upper limb, including shoulder
D23.60 Other benign neoplasm of skin of unspecified upper limb, including shoulder
D23.61 Other benign neoplasm of skin of right upper limb, including shoulder
D23.62 Other benign neoplasm of skin of left upper limb, including shoulder

5ᵗʰ D23.7 Other benign neoplasm of skin of lower limb, including hip
D23.70 Other benign neoplasm of skin of unspecified lower limb, including hip
D23.71 Other benign neoplasm of skin of right lower limb, including hip
D23.72 Other benign neoplasm of skin of left lower limb, including hip

D23.9 Other benign neoplasm of skin, unspecified

4ᵗʰ D24 Benign neoplasm of breast
INCLUDES benign neoplasm of connective tissue of breast
benign neoplasm of soft parts of breast
fibroadenoma of breast
EXCLUDES2 adenofibrosis of breast (N60.2)
benign cyst of breast (N60.-)
benign mammary dysplasia (N60.-)
benign neoplasm of skin of breast (D22.5, D23.5)
fibrocystic disease of breast (N60.-)

D24.1 Benign neoplasm of right breast
D24.2 Benign neoplasm of left breast
D24.9 Benign neoplasm of unspecified breast

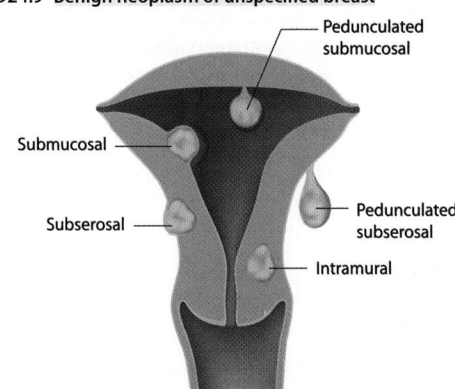

Figure 2.5 Uterine fibroids

4ᵗʰ D25 Leiomyoma of uterus
INCLUDES uterine fibroid
uterine fibromyoma
uterine myoma
D25.0 Submucous leiomyoma of uterus ♀
D25.1 Intramural leiomyoma of uterus ♀
Interstitial leiomyoma of uterus
D25.2 Subserosal leiomyoma of uterus ♀
Subperitoneal leiomyoma of uterus
D25.9 Leiomyoma of uterus, unspecified ♀

4ᵗʰ D26 Other benign neoplasms of uterus
D26.0 Other benign neoplasm of cervix uteri ♀
D26.1 Other benign neoplasm of corpus uteri ♀
D26.7 Other benign neoplasm of other parts of uterus ♀
D26.9 Other benign neoplasm of uterus, unspecified ♀

4ᵗʰ D27 Benign neoplasm of ovary
Use additional code to identify any functional activity.
EXCLUDES2 corpus albicans cyst (N83.2-)
corpus luteum cyst (N83.1-)
endometrial cyst (N80.1)
follicular (atretic) cyst (N83.0-)
graafian follicle cyst (N83.0-)
ovarian cyst NEC (N83.2-)
ovarian retention cyst (N83.2-)
D27.0 Benign neoplasm of right ovary ♀
D27.1 Benign neoplasm of left ovary ♀
D27.9 Benign neoplasm of unspecified ovary ♀

4ᵗʰ D28 Benign neoplasm of other and unspecified female genital organs
INCLUDES adenomatous polyp
benign neoplasm of skin of female genital organs
benign teratoma
EXCLUDES1 epoophoron cyst (Q50.5)
fimbrial cyst (Q50.4)
Gartner's duct cyst (Q52.4)
parovarian cyst (Q50.5)

| Unspecified Code | Other Specified Code | Manifestation Code | N Newborn | P Pediatric | M Maternity | A Adult | ♂ Male | ♀ Female |

● New Code ▲ Revised Code Title ►◄ Revised Text NOTES INCLUDES EXCLUDES1 Not coded here EXCLUDES2 Not included here
4ᵗʰ 4ᵗʰ character required 5ᵗʰ 5ᵗʰ character required 6ᵗʰ 6ᵗʰ character required 7ᵗʰ 7ᵗʰ character required
7ˣ Extension 'X' Alert HAC Hospital-acquired condition (HAC) alert AHA AHA Coding Clinic©

D28.0 Benign neoplasm of vulva ♀
D28.1 Benign neoplasm of vagina ♀
D28.2 Benign neoplasm of uterine tubes and ligaments ♀
Benign neoplasm of fallopian tube
Benign neoplasm of uterine ligament (broad) (round)
D28.7 **Benign neoplasm of other specified female genital organs** ♀
D28.9 **Benign neoplasm of female genital organ, unspecified** ♀

[4th] D29 Benign neoplasm of male genital organs
[INCLUDES] *benign neoplasm of skin of male genital organs*
D29.0 Benign neoplasm of penis ♂
D29.1 Benign neoplasm of prostate ♂
[EXCLUDES1] *enlarged prostate (N40.-)*
[5th] D29.2 Benign neoplasm of testis
Use additional code to identify any functional activity.
D29.20 **Benign neoplasm of unspecified testis** ♂
D29.21 Benign neoplasm of right testis ♂
D29.22 Benign neoplasm of left testis ♂
[5th] D29.3 Benign neoplasm of epididymis
D29.30 **Benign neoplasm of unspecified epididymis** ♂
D29.31 Benign neoplasm of right epididymis ♂
D29.32 Benign neoplasm of left epididymis ♂
D29.4 Benign neoplasm of scrotum ♂
Benign neoplasm of skin of scrotum
D29.8 **Benign neoplasm of other specified male genital organs** ♂
Benign neoplasm of seminal vesicle
Benign neoplasm of spermatic cord
Benign neoplasm of tunica vaginalis
D29.9 **Benign neoplasm of male genital organ, unspecified** ♂

[4th] D30 Benign neoplasm of urinary organs
[5th] D30.0 Benign neoplasm of kidney
[EXCLUDES1] *benign carcinoid tumor of the kidney (D3A.093)*
benign neoplasm of renal calyces (D30.1-)
benign neoplasm of renal pelvis (D30.1-)
D30.00 **Benign neoplasm of unspecified kidney**
D30.01 Benign neoplasm of right kidney
D30.02 Benign neoplasm of left kidney
[5th] D30.1 Benign neoplasm of renal pelvis
D30.10 **Benign neoplasm of unspecified renal pelvis**
D30.11 Benign neoplasm of right renal pelvis
D30.12 Benign neoplasm of left renal pelvis
[5th] D30.2 Benign neoplasm of ureter
[EXCLUDES1] *benign neoplasm of ureteric orifice of bladder (D30.3)*
D30.20 **Benign neoplasm of unspecified ureter**
D30.21 Benign neoplasm of right ureter
D30.22 Benign neoplasm of left ureter
D30.3 Benign neoplasm of bladder
Benign neoplasm of ureteric orifice of bladder
Benign neoplasm of urethral orifice of bladder
D30.4 Benign neoplasm of urethra
[EXCLUDES1] *benign neoplasm of urethral orifice of bladder (D30.3)*
D30.8 **Benign neoplasm of other specified urinary organs**
Benign neoplasm of paraurethral glands
D30.9 **Benign neoplasm of urinary organ, unspecified**
Benign neoplasm of urinary system NOS

[4th] D31 Benign neoplasm of eye and adnexa
[EXCLUDES1] *benign neoplasm of connective tissue of eyelid (D21.0)*
benign neoplasm of optic nerve (D33.3)
benign neoplasm of skin of eyelid (D22.1-, D23.1-)
[5th] D31.0 Benign neoplasm of conjunctiva
D31.00 **Benign neoplasm of unspecified conjunctiva**
D31.01 Benign neoplasm of right conjunctiva
D31.02 Benign neoplasm of left conjunctiva
[5th] D31.1 Benign neoplasm of cornea
D31.10 **Benign neoplasm of unspecified cornea**
D31.11 Benign neoplasm of right cornea
D31.12 Benign neoplasm of left cornea
[5th] D31.2 Benign neoplasm of retina
[EXCLUDES1] *dark area on retina (D49.81)*
hemangioma of retina (D49.81)
neoplasm of unspecified behavior of retina and choroid (D49.81)
retinal freckle (D49.81)
D31.20 **Benign neoplasm of unspecified retina**
D31.21 Benign neoplasm of right retina
D31.22 Benign neoplasm of left retina
[5th] D31.3 Benign neoplasm of choroid
D31.30 **Benign neoplasm of unspecified choroid**
D31.31 Benign neoplasm of right choroid
D31.32 Benign neoplasm of left choroid
[5th] D31.4 Benign neoplasm of ciliary body
D31.40 **Benign neoplasm of unspecified ciliary body**
D31.41 Benign neoplasm of right ciliary body
D31.42 Benign neoplasm of left ciliary body
[5th] D31.5 Benign neoplasm of lacrimal gland and duct
Benign neoplasm of lacrimal sac
Benign neoplasm of nasolacrimal duct
D31.50 **Benign neoplasm of unspecified lacrimal gland and duct**
D31.51 Benign neoplasm of right lacrimal gland and duct
D31.52 Benign neoplasm of left lacrimal gland and duct
[5th] D31.6 Benign neoplasm of unspecified site of orbit
Benign neoplasm of connective tissue of orbit
Benign neoplasm of extraocular muscle
Benign neoplasm of peripheral nerves of orbit
Benign neoplasm of retrobulbar tissue
Benign neoplasm of retro-ocular tissue
[EXCLUDES1] *benign neoplasm of orbital bone (D16.4)*
D31.60 **Benign neoplasm of unspecified site of unspecified orbit**
D31.61 Benign neoplasm of unspecified site of right orbit
D31.62 Benign neoplasm of unspecified site of left orbit
[5th] D31.9 Benign neoplasm of unspecified part of eye
Benign neoplasm of eyeball
D31.90 **Benign neoplasm of unspecified part of unspecified eye**
D31.91 Benign neoplasm of unspecified part of right eye
D31.92 Benign neoplasm of unspecified part of left eye

[4th] D32 Benign neoplasm of meninges
D32.0 Benign neoplasm of cerebral meninges [HCC]
D32.1 Benign neoplasm of spinal meninges [HCC]
D32.9 **Benign neoplasm of meninges, unspecified** [HCC]
Meningioma NOS

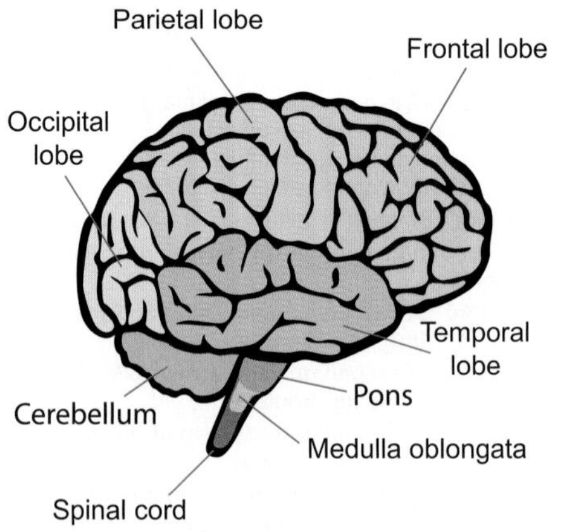
Parietal lobe
Frontal lobe
Occipital lobe
Temporal lobe
Pons
Cerebellum
Medulla oblongata
Spinal cord

Figure 2.6 Brain lobes

Unacceptable principal diagnosis symbol per Medicare code edits · Code exempt from diagnosis present on admission requirement · Questionable admission · Complication or comorbidity · CC/MCC exclusion · Major complication or comorbidity · Principal diagnosis as its own CC · Principal diagnosis as its own MCC · [HCC] HCC diagnosis code · [RxHCC] RxHCC diagnosis code · MACRA code · Z code as first-listed diagnosis

⁴ᵈ D33 Benign neoplasm of brain and other parts of central nervous system
 EXCLUDES1 *angioma (D18.0-)*
 benign neoplasm of meninges (D32.-)
 benign neoplasm of peripheral nerves and autonomic nervous system (D36.1-)
 hemangioma (D18.0-)
 neurofibromatosis (Q85.0-)
 retro-ocular benign neoplasm (D31.6-)

 D33.0 **Benign neoplasm of brain,** supratentorial   HCC
  Benign neoplasm of cerebral ventricle
  Benign neoplasm of cerebrum
  Benign neoplasm of frontal lobe
  Benign neoplasm of occipital lobe
  Benign neoplasm of parietal lobe
  Benign neoplasm of temporal lobe
  EXCLUDES1 *benign neoplasm of fourth ventricle (D33.1)*

 D33.1 **Benign neoplasm of brain,** infratentorial   HCC
  Benign neoplasm of brain stem
  Benign neoplasm of cerebellum
  Benign neoplasm of fourth ventricle

 D33.2 **Benign neoplasm of brain, unspecified**   HCC

 D33.3 **Benign neoplasm of** cranial nerves   HCC
  Benign neoplasm of olfactory bulb

 D33.4 **Benign neoplasm of** spinal cord   HCC

 D33.7 **Benign neoplasm of** other specified parts of central nervous system   HCC

 D33.9 **Benign neoplasm of central nervous system, unspecified**   HCC
  Benign neoplasm of nervous system (central) NOS

D34 **Benign neoplasm of** thyroid gland
 Use additional code to identify any functional activity

⁴ᵈ D35 **Benign neoplasm of** other and unspecified endocrine glands
 Use additional code to identify any functional activity
 EXCLUDES1 *benign neoplasm of endocrine pancreas (D13.7)*
  benign neoplasm of ovary (D27.-)
  benign neoplasm of testis (D29.2.-)
  benign neoplasm of thymus (D15.0)

 ⁵ᵈ D35.0 **Benign neoplasm of** adrenal gland
  D35.00 **Benign neoplasm of unspecified adrenal gland**
  D35.01 **Benign neoplasm of** right **adrenal gland**
  D35.02 **Benign neoplasm of** left **adrenal gland**

 D35.1 **Benign neoplasm of** parathyroid **gland**

 D35.2 **Benign neoplasm of** pituitary **gland**   HCC

 D35.3 **Benign neoplasm of** craniopharyngeal duct   HCC

 D35.4 **Benign neoplasm of** pineal **gland**   HCC

 D35.5 **Benign neoplasm of** carotid body

 D35.6 **Benign neoplasm of** aortic body and other paraganglia
  Benign tumor of glomus jugulare

 D35.7 **Benign neoplasm of** other specified **endocrine glands**

 D35.9 **Benign neoplasm of endocrine gland, unspecified**
  Benign neoplasm of unspecified endocrine gland

⁴ᵈ D36 **Benign neoplasm of** other and unspecified sites

 D36.0 **Benign neoplasm of** lymph nodes
  EXCLUDES1 *lymphangioma (D18.1)*

 ⁵ᵈ D36.1 **Benign neoplasm of** peripheral nerves and autonomic nervous system
  EXCLUDES1 *benign neoplasm of peripheral nerves of orbit (D31.6-)*
   neurofibromatosis (Q85.0-)

  D36.10 **Benign neoplasm of peripheral nerves and autonomic nervous system, unspecified**
  D36.11 **Benign neoplasm of peripheral nerves and autonomic nervous system of** face, head, and neck
  D36.12 **Benign neoplasm of peripheral nerves and autonomic nervous system,** upper limb, including shoulder
  D36.13 **Benign neoplasm of peripheral nerves and autonomic nervous system of** lower limb, including hip
  D36.14 **Benign neoplasm of peripheral nerves and autonomic nervous system of** thorax

  D36.15 **Benign neoplasm of peripheral nerves and autonomic nervous system of** abdomen
  D36.16 **Benign neoplasm of peripheral nerves and autonomic nervous system of** pelvis
  D36.17 **Benign neoplasm of peripheral nerves and autonomic nervous system of** trunk, unspecified

 D36.7 **Benign neoplasm of** other specified sites
  Benign neoplasm of nose NOS

 D36.9 **Benign neoplasm, unspecified site**

Benign neuroendocrine tumors (D3A)

⁴ᵈ D3A **Benign neuroendocrine tumors**
 Code also any associated multiple endocrine neoplasia [MEN] syndromes (E31.2-)
 Use additional code to identify any associated endocrine syndrome, such as:
 carcinoid syndrome (E34.0)
 EXCLUDES2 *benign pancreatic islet cell tumors (D13.7)*

 ⁵ᵈ D3A.0 **Benign carcinoid tumors**
  D3A.00 **Benign carcinoid tumor of unspecified site**
   Carcinoid tumor NOS

  ⁶ᵈ D3A.01 **Benign carcinoid tumors of the** small intestine
   D3A.010 **Benign carcinoid tumor of the** duodenum
   D3A.011 **Benign carcinoid tumor of the** jejunum
   D3A.012 **Benign carcinoid tumor of the** ileum
   D3A.019 **Benign carcinoid tumor of the small intestine, unspecified portion**

  ⁶ᵈ D3A.02 **Benign carcinoid tumors of the** appendix, large intestine, and rectum
   D3A.020 **Benign carcinoid tumor of the** appendix
   D3A.021 **Benign carcinoid tumor of the** cecum
   D3A.022 **Benign carcinoid tumor of the** ascending colon
   D3A.023 **Benign carcinoid tumor of the** transverse colon
   D3A.024 **Benign carcinoid tumor of the** descending colon
   D3A.025 **Benign carcinoid tumor of the** sigmoid colon
   D3A.026 **Benign carcinoid tumor of the** rectum
   D3A.029 **Benign carcinoid tumor of the large intestine, unspecified portion**
    Benign carcinoid tumor of the colon NOS

  ⁶ᵈ D3A.09 **Benign carcinoid tumors of** other sites
   D3A.090 **Benign carcinoid tumor of the** bronchus and lung
   D3A.091 **Benign carcinoid tumor of the** thymus
   D3A.092 **Benign carcinoid tumor of the** stomach
   D3A.093 **Benign carcinoid tumor of the** kidney
   D3A.094 **Benign carcinoid tumor of the** foregut, unspecified
   D3A.095 **Benign carcinoid tumor of the** midgut, unspecified
   D3A.096 **Benign carcinoid tumor of the** hindgut, unspecified
   D3A.098 **Benign carcinoid tumors of** other sites

 D3A.8 **Other benign neuroendocrine tumors**
  Neuroendocrine tumor NOS

Neoplasms of uncertain behavior, polycythemia vera and myelodysplastic syndromes (D37-D48)

 NOTES Categories D37-D44, and D48 classify by site neoplasms of uncertain behavior, i.e., histologic confirmation whether the neoplasm is malignant or benign cannot be made.
 EXCLUDES1 *neoplasms of unspecified behavior (D49.-)*

⁴ᵈ D37 **Neoplasm of uncertain behavior of** oral cavity and digestive organs
 EXCLUDES1 *stromal tumors of uncertain behavior of digestive system (D48.1)*

Unspecified Code   Other Specified Code   Manifestation Code   N Newborn   P Pediatric   M Maternity   A Adult   ♂ Male   ♀ Female
● New Code   ▲ Revised Code Title   ►◄ Revised Text   NOTES   *INCLUDES*   *EXCLUDES 1* Not coded here   *EXCLUDES 2* Not included here
⁴ᵈ 4ᵗʰ character required   ⁵ᵈ 5ᵗʰ character required   ⁶ᵈ 6ᵗʰ character required   ⁷ᵈ 7ᵗʰ character required
⁷ᵈ Extension 'X' Alert   HAC Hospital-acquired condition (HAC) alert   AHA AHA Coding Clinic©

2018 ICD-10-CM   When symbols appear on a code that requires a 7th character extension, refer to Appendix B to identify applicable 7th character codes.   **503**

Ⓢ D37.0 **Neoplasm of uncertain behavior of** lip, oral cavity and pharynx

EXCLUDES1 *neoplasm of uncertain behavior of aryepiglottic fold or interarytenoid fold, laryngeal aspect (D38.0)*

neoplasm of uncertain behavior of epiglottis NOS (D38.0)

neoplasm of uncertain behavior of skin of lip (D48.5)

neoplasm of uncertain behavior of suprahyoid portion of epiglottis (D38.0)

D37.01 **Neoplasm of uncertain behavior of** lip

Neoplasm of uncertain behavior of vermilion border of lip

D37.02 **Neoplasm of uncertain behavior of** tongue

Ⓢ D37.03 **Neoplasm of uncertain behavior of the** major salivary glands

D37.030 **Neoplasm of uncertain behavior of the** parotid **salivary glands**

D37.031 **Neoplasm of uncertain behavior of the** sublingual **salivary glands**

D37.032 **Neoplasm of uncertain behavior of the** submandibular **salivary glands**

D37.039 **Neoplasm of uncertain behavior of the major salivary glands, unspecified**

D37.04 **Neoplasm of uncertain behavior of the** minor salivary glands

Neoplasm of uncertain behavior of submucosal salivary glands of lip

Neoplasm of uncertain behavior of submucosal salivary glands of cheek

Neoplasm of uncertain behavior of submucosal salivary glands of hard palate

Neoplasm of uncertain behavior of submucosal salivary glands of soft palate

D37.05 **Neoplasm of uncertain behavior of** pharynx

Neoplasm of uncertain behavior of aryepiglottic fold of pharynx NOS

Neoplasm of uncertain behavior of hypopharyngeal aspect of aryepiglottic fold of pharynx

Neoplasm of uncertain behavior of marginal zone of aryepiglottic fold of pharynx

D37.09 **Neoplasm of uncertain behavior of** other specified **sites of the oral cavity**

D37.1 **Neoplasm of uncertain behavior of** stomach

D37.2 **Neoplasm of uncertain behavior of** small intestine

D37.3 **Neoplasm of uncertain behavior of** appendix

D37.4 **Neoplasm of uncertain behavior of** colon

D37.5 **Neoplasm of uncertain behavior of** rectum

Neoplasm of uncertain behavior of rectosigmoid junction

D37.6 **Neoplasm of uncertain behavior of** liver, gallbladder and bile ducts

Neoplasm of uncertain behavior of ampulla of Vater

D37.8 **Neoplasm of uncertain behavior of** other specified digestive organs

Neoplasm of uncertain behavior of anal canal

Neoplasm of uncertain behavior of anal sphincter

Neoplasm of uncertain behavior of anus NOS

Neoplasm of uncertain behavior of esophagus

Neoplasm of uncertain behavior of intestine NOS

Neoplasm of uncertain behavior of pancreas

EXCLUDES1 *neoplasm of uncertain behavior of anal margin (D48.5)*

neoplasm of uncertain behavior of anal skin (D48.5)

neoplasm of uncertain behavior of perianal skin (D48.5)

D37.9 **Neoplasm of uncertain behavior of digestive organ, unspecified**

Ⓐ D38 **Neoplasm of uncertain behavior of** middle ear and respiratory and intrathoracic organs

EXCLUDES1 *neoplasm of uncertain behavior of heart (D48.7)*

D38.0 **Neoplasm of uncertain behavior of** larynx

Neoplasm of uncertain behavior of aryepiglottic fold or interarytenoid fold, laryngeal aspect

Neoplasm of uncertain behavior of epiglottis (suprahyoid portion)

EXCLUDES1 *neoplasm of uncertain behavior of aryepiglottic fold or interarytenoid fold NOS (D37.05)*

neoplasm of uncertain behavior of hypopharyngeal aspect of aryepiglottic fold (D37.05)

neoplasm of uncertain behavior of marginal zone of aryepiglottic fold (D37.05)

D38.1 **Neoplasm of uncertain behavior of** trachea, bronchus and lung

D38.2 **Neoplasm of uncertain behavior of** pleura

D38.3 **Neoplasm of uncertain behavior of** mediastinum

D38.4 **Neoplasm of uncertain behavior of** thymus

D38.5 **Neoplasm of uncertain behavior of** other respiratory organs

Neoplasm of uncertain behavior of accessory sinuses

Neoplasm of uncertain behavior of cartilage of nose

Neoplasm of uncertain behavior of middle ear

Neoplasm of uncertain behavior of nasal cavities

EXCLUDES1 *neoplasm of uncertain behavior of ear (external) (skin) (D48.5)*

neoplasm of uncertain behavior of nose NOS (D48.7)

neoplasm of uncertain behavior of skin of nose (D48.5)

D38.6 **Neoplasm of uncertain behavior of respiratory organ, unspecified**

Ⓐ D39 **Neoplasm of uncertain behavior of** female genital organs

D39.0 **Neoplasm of uncertain behavior of** uterus ♀

Ⓢ D39.1 **Neoplasm of uncertain behavior of** ovary

Use additional code to identify any functional activity.

D39.10 **Neoplasm of uncertain behavior of unspecified ovary** ♀

D39.11 **Neoplasm of uncertain behavior of** right **ovary** ♀

D39.12 **Neoplasm of uncertain behavior of** left **ovary** ♀

D39.2 **Neoplasm of uncertain behavior of** placenta Ⓜ♀

Chorioadenoma destruens

Invasive hydatidiform mole

Malignant hydatidiform mole

EXCLUDES1 *hydatidiform mole NOS (O01.9)*

D39.8 **Neoplasm of uncertain behavior of** other specified **female genital organs** ♀

Neoplasm of uncertain behavior of skin of female genital organs

D39.9 **Neoplasm of uncertain behavior of female genital organ, unspecified** ♀

Ⓐ D40 **Neoplasm of uncertain behavior of** male genital organs

D40.0 **Neoplasm of uncertain behavior of** prostate ♂

Ⓢ D40.1 **Neoplasm of uncertain behavior of** testis

D40.10 **Neoplasm of uncertain behavior of unspecified testis** ♂

D40.11 **Neoplasm of uncertain behavior of** right **testis** ♂

D40.12 **Neoplasm of uncertain behavior of** left **testis** ♂

D40.8 **Neoplasm of uncertain behavior of** other specified **male genital organs** ♂

Neoplasm of uncertain behavior of skin of male genital organs

D40.9 **Neoplasm of uncertain behavior of male genital organ, unspecified** ♂

Ⓐ D41 **Neoplasm of uncertain behavior of** urinary organs

Ⓢ D41.0 **Neoplasm of uncertain behavior of** kidney

EXCLUDES1 *neoplasm of uncertain behavior of renal pelvis (D41.1-)*

D41.00 **Neoplasm of uncertain behavior of unspecified kidney**

D41.01 **Neoplasm of uncertain behavior of** right **kidney**

D41.02 **Neoplasm of uncertain behavior of** left **kidney**

Ⓢ D41.1 **Neoplasm of uncertain behavior of** renal pelvis

D41.10 **Neoplasm of uncertain behavior of unspecified renal pelvis**

D41.11 **Neoplasm of uncertain behavior of** right **renal pelvis**

D41.12 **Neoplasm of uncertain behavior of** left **renal pelvis**

Ⓢ D41.2 **Neoplasm of uncertain behavior of** ureter

D41.20 **Neoplasm of uncertain behavior of unspecified ureter**

ᴾᴰˣ Unacceptable principal diagnosis symbol per Medicare code edits   ᴾᴰˣ Code exempt from diagnosis present on admission requirement
🅀 Questionable admission   ©ᶜ Complication or comorbidity   ᶜᶜ/ᴹᶜᶜ CC/MCC exclusion   ᴹᶜᶜ Major complication or comorbidity
ℂℂ Principal diagnosis as its own CC   ℳℂ Principal diagnosis as its own MCC   HCC HCC diagnosis code   RxHCC RxHCC diagnosis code
MACRA code   🆉 Z code as first-listed diagnosis

When symbols appear on a code that requires a 7th character extension, refer to Appendix B to identify applicable 7th character codes.   **2018 ICD-10-CM**

D41.21 Neoplasm of uncertain behavior of right ureter
D41.22 Neoplasm of uncertain behavior of left ureter
D41.3 Neoplasm of uncertain behavior of urethra
D41.4 Neoplasm of uncertain behavior of bladder
D41.8 Neoplasm of uncertain behavior of other specified urinary organs
D41.9 Neoplasm of uncertain behavior of unspecified urinary organ

⁴ᵗʰ D42 Neoplasm of uncertain behavior of meninges
D42.0 Neoplasm of uncertain behavior of cerebral meninges   HCC
D42.1 Neoplasm of uncertain behavior of spinal meninges   HCC
D42.9 Neoplasm of uncertain behavior of meninges, unspecified   HCC

⁴ᵗʰ D43 Neoplasm of uncertain behavior of brain and central nervous system
EXCLUDES1 neoplasm of uncertain behavior of peripheral nerves and autonomic nervous system (D48.2)
D43.0 Neoplasm of uncertain behavior of brain, supratentorial   HCC
Neoplasm of uncertain behavior of cerebral ventricle
Neoplasm of uncertain behavior of cerebrum
Neoplasm of uncertain behavior of frontal lobe
Neoplasm of uncertain behavior of occipital lobe
Neoplasm of uncertain behavior of parietal lobe
Neoplasm of uncertain behavior of temporal lobe
EXCLUDES1 neoplasm of uncertain behavior of fourth ventricle (D43.1)
D43.1 Neoplasm of uncertain behavior of brain, infratentorial   HCC
Neoplasm of uncertain behavior of brain stem
Neoplasm of uncertain behavior of cerebellum
Neoplasm of uncertain behavior of fourth ventricle
D43.2 Neoplasm of uncertain behavior of brain, unspecified   HCC
D43.3 Neoplasm of uncertain behavior of cranial nerves   HCC
D43.4 Neoplasm of uncertain behavior of spinal cord   HCC
D43.8 Neoplasm of uncertain behavior of other specified parts of central nervous system   HCC
D43.9 Neoplasm of uncertain behavior of central nervous system, unspecified   HCC
Neoplasm of uncertain behavior of nervous system (central) NOS

⁴ᵗʰ D44 Neoplasm of uncertain behavior of endocrine glands
EXCLUDES1 multiple endocrine adenomatosis (E31.2-)
multiple endocrine neoplasia (E31.2-)
neoplasm of uncertain behavior of endocrine pancreas (D37.8)
neoplasm of uncertain behavior of ovary (D39.1-)
neoplasm of uncertain behavior of testis (D40.1-)
neoplasm of uncertain behavior of thymus (D38.4)
D44.0 Neoplasm of uncertain behavior of thyroid gland
⁵ᵗʰ D44.1 Neoplasm of uncertain behavior of adrenal gland
Use additional code to identify any functional activity.
D44.10 Neoplasm of uncertain behavior of unspecified adrenal gland
D44.11 Neoplasm of uncertain behavior of right adrenal gland
D44.12 Neoplasm of uncertain behavior of left adrenal gland
D44.2 Neoplasm of uncertain behavior of parathyroid gland
D44.3 Neoplasm of uncertain behavior of pituitary gland   HCC
Use additional code to identify any functional activity.
D44.4 Neoplasm of uncertain behavior of craniopharyngeal duct   HCC
D44.5 Neoplasm of uncertain behavior of pineal gland   HCC
D44.6 Neoplasm of uncertain behavior of carotid body   HCC
D44.7 Neoplasm of uncertain behavior of aortic body and other paraganglia   HCC
AHA: Q4 2016
D44.9 Neoplasm of uncertain behavior of unspecified endocrine gland
D45 Polycythemia vera   HCC
EXCLUDES1 familial polycythemia (D75.0)
secondary polycythemia (D75.1)

⁴ᵗʰ D46 Myelodysplastic syndromes
Use additional code for adverse effect, if applicable, to identify drug (T36-T50 with fifth or sixth character 5)
EXCLUDES2 drug-induced aplastic anemia (D61.1)
D46.0 Refractory anemia without ring sideroblasts, so stated   HCC RxHCC
Refractory anemia without sideroblasts, without excess of blasts
D46.1 Refractory anemia with ring sideroblasts   HCC RxHCC
RARS
⁵ᵗʰ D46.2 Refractory anemia with excess of blasts [RAEB]
D46.20 Refractory anemia with excess of blasts, unspecified   HCC RxHCC
RAEB NOS
D46.21 Refractory anemia with excess of blasts 1   HCC RxHCC
RAEB 1
D46.22 Refractory anemia with excess of blasts 2   CC HCC RxHCC CC/MCC Exc
RAEB 2
D46.A Refractory cytopenia with multilineage dysplasia   HCC RxHCC
D46.B Refractory cytopenia with multilineage dysplasia and ring sideroblasts   HCC RxHCC
RCMD RS
D46.C Myelodysplastic syndrome with isolated del(5q) chromosomal abnormality   CC HCC RxHCC CC/MCC Exc
Myelodysplastic syndrome with 5q deletion
5q minus syndrome NOS
D46.4 Refractory anemia, unspecified   HCC RxHCC
D46.Z Other myelodysplastic syndromes   HCC RxHCC
EXCLUDES1 chronic myelomonocytic leukemia (C93.1-)
D46.9 Myelodysplastic syndrome, unspecified   HCC RxHCC
Myelodysplasia NOS

⁴ᵗʰ D47 Other neoplasms of uncertain behavior of lymphoid, hematopoietic and related tissue
▲ ⁵ᵗʰ D47.0 ►Mast cell neoplasms◄ of uncertain behavior
EXCLUDES1 congenital cutaneous mastocytosis (Q82.2-)
histiocytic neoplasms of uncertain behavior (D47.Z9)
malignant mast cell neoplasm (C96.2-)
● D47.01 Cutaneous mastocytosis   CC CC/MCC Exc
Diffuse cutaneous mastocytosis
Maculopapular cutaneous mastocytosis
Solitary mastocytoma
Telangiectasia macularis eruptiva perstans
Urticaria pigmentosa
EXCLUDES1 congenital (diffuse) (maculopapular) cutaneous mastocytosis (Q82.2)
congenital urticaria pigmentosa (Q82.2)
extracutaneous mastocytoma (D47.09)
● D47.02 Systemic mastocytosis   CC CC/MCC Exc
Indolent systemic mastocytosis
Isolated bone marrow mastocytosis
Smoldering systemic mastocytosis
Systemic mastocytosis, with an associated hematological non-mast cell lineage disease (SM-AHNMD)
Code also, if applicable, any associated hematological non-mast cell lineage disease, such as:
acute myeloid leukemia (C92.6-, C92.A-)
chronic myelomonocytic leukemia (C93.1-)
essential thrombocytosis (D47.3)
hypereosinophilic syndrome (D72.1)
myelodysplastic syndrome (D46.9)
myeloproliferative syndrome (D47.1)
non-Hodgkin lymphoma (C82-C85)
plasma cell myeloma (C90.0-)
polycythemia vera (D45)
EXCLUDES1 aggressive systemic mastocytosis (C96.21)
mast cell leukemia (C94.3-)

Unspecified Code   Other Specified Code   Manifestation Code   N Newborn   P Pediatric   M Maternity   A Adult   ♂ Male   ♀ Female
● New Code   ▲ Revised Code Title   ►◄ Revised Text   NOTES   INCLUDES   EXCLUDES 1 Not coded here   EXCLUDES 2 Not included here
⁴ᵗʰ 4ᵗʰ character required   ⁵ᵗʰ 5ᵗʰ character required   ⁶ᵗʰ 6ᵗʰ character required   ⁷ᵗʰ 7ᵗʰ character required
⁷ˣ Extension 'X' Alert   HAC Hospital-acquired condition (HAC) alert   AHA AHA Coding Clinic©

● D47.09 **Other** mast cell **neoplasms of uncertain behavior** cc CC/MCC Exc
Extracutaneous mastocytoma
Mast cell tumor NOS
Mastocytoma NOS
Mastocytosis NOS

D47.1 **Chronic myeloproliferative disease** cc HCC CC/MCC Exc
Chronic neutrophilic leukemia
Myeloproliferative disease, unspecified
EXCLUDES1 *atypical chronic myeloid leukemia BCR/ABL-negative (C92.2-)*
chronic myeloid leukemia BCR/ABL-positive (C92.1-)
myelofibrosis NOS (D75.81)
myelophthisic anemia (D61.82)
myelophthisis (D61.82)
secondary myelofibrosis NOS (D75.81)

D47.2 **Monoclonal gammopathy**
Monoclonal gammopathy of undetermined significance [MGUS]

D47.3 **Essential (hemorrhagic) thrombocythemia** HCC
Essential thrombocytosis
Idiopathic hemorrhagic thrombocythemia

D47.4 **Osteomyelofibrosis** HCC RxHCC
Chronic idiopathic myelofibrosis
Myelofibrosis (idiopathic) (with myeloid metaplasia)
Myelosclerosis (megakaryocytic) with myeloid metaplasia
Secondary myelofibrosis in myeloproliferative disease
EXCLUDES1 *acute myelofibrosis (C94.4-)*

5ᵗʰ D47.Z **Other specified neoplasms of uncertain behavior of lymphoid, hematopoietic and related tissue**

D47.Z1 **Post-transplant lymphoproliferative disorder (PTLD)** cc HCC PDxIn CC/MCC Exc
Code first complications of transplanted organs and tissue (T86.-)

D47.Z2 **Castleman disease** cc HCC CC/MCC Exc
AHA: Q4 2016
Code also if applicable human herpesvirus 8 infection (B10.89)
EXCLUDES2 *Kaposi's sarcoma (C46-)*

D47.Z9 **Other specified neoplasms of uncertain behavior of lymphoid, hematopoietic and related tissue** cc HCC CC/MCC Exc
Histiocytic tumors of uncertain behavior

D47.9 **Neoplasm of uncertain behavior of lymphoid, hematopoietic and related tissue, unspecified** cc HCC CC/MCC Exc
Lymphoproliferative disease NOS

4ᵗʰ D48 **Neoplasm of uncertain behavior of other and unspecified sites**
EXCLUDES1 *neurofibromatosis (nonmalignant) (Q85.0-)*

D48.0 **Neoplasm of uncertain behavior of** bone and articular cartilage
EXCLUDES1 *neoplasm of uncertain behavior of cartilage of ear (D48.1)*
neoplasm of uncertain behavior of cartilage of larynx (D38.0)
neoplasm of uncertain behavior of cartilage of nose (D38.5)
neoplasm of uncertain behavior of connective tissue of eyelid (D48.1)
neoplasm of uncertain behavior of synovia (D48.1)

D48.1 **Neoplasm of uncertain behavior of** connective and other soft tissue
Neoplasm of uncertain behavior of connective tissue of ear
Neoplasm of uncertain behavior of connective tissue of eyelid
Stromal tumors of uncertain behavior of digestive system
EXCLUDES1 *neoplasm of uncertain behavior of articular cartilage (D48.0)*
neoplasm of uncertain behavior of cartilage of larynx (D38.0)
neoplasm of uncertain behavior of cartilage of nose (D38.5)

neoplasm of uncertain behavior of connective tissue of breast (D48.6-)

D48.2 **Neoplasm of uncertain behavior of** peripheral nerves and autonomic nervous system
EXCLUDES1 *neoplasm of uncertain behavior of peripheral nerves of orbit (D48.7)*

D48.3 **Neoplasm of uncertain behavior of** retroperitoneum

D48.4 **Neoplasm of uncertain behavior of** peritoneum

D48.5 **Neoplasm of uncertain behavior of** skin
Neoplasm of uncertain behavior of anal margin
Neoplasm of uncertain behavior of anal skin
Neoplasm of uncertain behavior of perianal skin
Neoplasm of uncertain behavior of skin of breast
EXCLUDES1 *neoplasm of uncertain behavior of anus NOS (D37.8)*
neoplasm of uncertain behavior of skin of genital organs (D39.8, D40.8)
neoplasm of uncertain behavior of vermilion border of lip (D37.0)

5ᵗʰ D48.6 **Neoplasm of uncertain behavior of** breast
Neoplasm of uncertain behavior of connective tissue of breast
Cystosarcoma phyllodes
EXCLUDES1 *neoplasm of uncertain behavior of skin of breast (D48.5)*

D48.60 **Neoplasm of uncertain behavior of unspecified breast**

D48.61 **Neoplasm of uncertain behavior of** right **breast**

D48.62 **Neoplasm of uncertain behavior of** left **breast**

D48.7 **Neoplasm of uncertain behavior of** other specified sites
Neoplasm of uncertain behavior of eye
Neoplasm of uncertain behavior of heart
Neoplasm of uncertain behavior of peripheral nerves of orbit
EXCLUDES1 *neoplasm of uncertain behavior of connective tissue (D48.1)*
neoplasm of uncertain behavior of skin of eyelid (D48.5)

D48.9 **Neoplasm of uncertain behavior, unspecified**

Neoplasms of unspecified behavior (D49)

4ᵗʰ D49 **Neoplasms of unspecified behavior**
NOTES Category D49 classifies by site neoplasms of unspecified morphology and behavior. The term 'mass', unless otherwise stated, is not to be regarded as a neoplastic growth.
INCLUDES *'growth' NOS*
neoplasm NOS
new growth NOS
tumor NOS
EXCLUDES1 *neoplasms of uncertain behavior (D37-D44, D48)*

D49.0 **Neoplasm of unspecified behavior of** digestive system
EXCLUDES1 *neoplasm of unspecified behavior of margin of anus (D49.2)*
neoplasm of unspecified behavior of perianal skin (D49.2)
neoplasm of unspecified behavior of skin of anus (D49.2)

D49.1 **Neoplasm of unspecified behavior of** respiratory system

D49.2 **Neoplasm of unspecified behavior of** bone, soft tissue, and skin
EXCLUDES1 *neoplasm of unspecified behavior of anal canal (D49.0)*
neoplasm of unspecified behavior of anus NOS (D49.0)
neoplasm of unspecified behavior of bone marrow (D49.89)
neoplasm of unspecified behavior of cartilage of larynx (D49.1)
neoplasm of unspecified behavior of cartilage of nose (D49.1)
neoplasm of unspecified behavior of connective tissue of breast (D49.3)

PDxIn Unacceptable principal diagnosis symbol per Medicare code edits   PDx Code exempt from diagnosis present on admission requirement
❓ Questionable admission   cc Complication or comorbidity   CC/MCC Exc CC/MCC exclusion   MCC Major complication or comorbidity
Principal diagnosis as its own CC   Principal diagnosis as its own MCC   HCC HCC diagnosis code   RxHCC RxHCC diagnosis code
MACRA code   Z1 Z code as first-listed diagnosis

neoplasm of unspecified behavior of skin of genital organs (D49.59)

neoplasm of unspecified behavior of vermilion border of lip (D49.0)

D49.3 Neoplasm of unspecified behavior of breast

  EXCLUDES1 neoplasm of unspecified behavior of skin of breast (D49.2)

D49.4 Neoplasm of unspecified behavior of bladder

D49.5 Neoplasm of unspecified behavior of other genitourinary organs

  D49.51 Neoplasm of **unspecified behavior** of kidney

    D49.511 Neoplasm of unspecified behavior of right **kidney**

      AHA: Q4 2016

    D49.512 Neoplasm of unspecified behavior of left **kidney**

      AHA: Q4 2016

    D49.519 Neoplasm of unspecified **behavior of** unspecified **kidney**

      AHA: Q4 2016

  D49.59 Neoplasm of unspecified behavior of other genitourinary organ

    AHA: Q4 2016

D49.6 Neoplasm of unspecified behavior of brain   HCC

  EXCLUDES1 neoplasm of unspecified behavior of cerebral meninges (D49.7)

  neoplasm of unspecified behavior of cranial nerves (D49.7)

D49.7 Neoplasm of unspecified behavior of endocrine glands and other parts of nervous system

  EXCLUDES1 neoplasm of unspecified behavior of peripheral, sympathetic, and parasympathetic nerves and ganglia (D49.2)

D49.8 Neoplasm of unspecified behavior of other specified sites

  EXCLUDES1 neoplasm of unspecified behavior of eyelid (skin) (D49.2)

  neoplasm of unspecified behavior of eyelid cartilage (D49.2)

  neoplasm of unspecified behavior of great vessels (D49.2)

  neoplasm of unspecified behavior of optic nerve (D49.7)

  D49.81 Neoplasm of unspecified behavior of retina and choroid

    Dark area on retina

    Retinal freckle

  D49.89 Neoplasm of unspecified behavior of other specified sites

D49.9 Neoplasm of unspecified behavior of unspecified site

Unspecified Code   Other-Specified Code   Manifestation Code   N Newborn   P Pediatric   M Maternity   A Adult   ♂ Male   ♀ Female

● New Code   ▲ Revised Code Title   ►◄ Revised Text   **NOTES**   *INCLUDES*   *EXCLUDES 1* Not coded here   *EXCLUDES 2* Not included here

4th character required   5th character required   6th character required   7th character required

Extension 'X' Alert   HAC Hospital-acquired condition (HAC) alert   **AHA** AHA Coding Clinic©

NOTES

Chapter 3: Diseases of the Blood and Blood-Forming Organs and Certain Disorders Involving the Immune Mechanism (D50-D89)

Diseases of the blood and blood-forming organs and certain disorders involving the immune mechanism (D50-D89)

EXCLUDES2 autoimmune disease (systemic) NOS (M35.9)

certain conditions originating in the perinatal period (P00-P96)

complications of pregnancy, childbirth and the puerperium (O00-O9A)

congenital malformations, deformations and chromosomal abnormalities (Q00-Q99)

endocrine, nutritional and metabolic diseases (E00-E88)

human immunodeficiency virus [HIV] disease (B20)

injury, poisoning and certain other consequences of external causes (S00-T88)

neoplasms (C00-D49)

symptoms, signs and abnormal clinical and laboratory findings, not elsewhere classified (R00-R94)

This chapter contains the following blocks:

D50-D53 Nutritional anemias
D55-D59 Hemolytic anemias
D60-D64 Aplastic and other anemias and other bone marrow failure syndromes
D65-D69 Coagulation defects, purpura and other hemorrhagic conditions
D70-D77 Other disorders of blood and blood-forming organs
D78 Intraoperative and postprocedural complications of the spleen
D80-D89 Certain disorders involving the immune mechanism

Nutritional anemias (D50-D53)

4ᵗʰ **D50** Iron deficiency anemia

INCLUDES asiderotic anemia
hypochromic anemia

D50.0 Iron deficiency anemia secondary to blood loss (chronic)
Posthemorrhagic anemia (chronic)
EXCLUDES1 acute posthemorrhagic anemia (D62)
congenital anemia from fetal blood loss (P61.3)

D50.1 Sideropenic dysphagia
Kelly-Paterson syndrome
Plummer-Vinson syndrome

D50.8 Other iron deficiency anemias
Iron deficiency anemia due to inadequate dietary iron intake

D50.9 Iron deficiency anemia, unspecified

4ᵗʰ **D51** Vitamin B12 deficiency anemia
EXCLUDES1 vitamin B12 deficiency (E53.8)

D51.0 Vitamin B12 deficiency anemia due to intrinsic factor deficiency
Addison anemia
Biermer anemia
Pernicious (congenital) anemia
Congenital intrinsic factor deficiency

D51.1 Vitamin B12 deficiency anemia due to selective vitamin B12 malabsorption with proteinuria
Imerslund (Gräsbeck) syndrome
Megaloblastic hereditary anemia

D51.2 Transcobalamin II deficiency

D51.3 Other dietary vitamin B12 deficiency anemia
Vegan anemia

D51.8 Other vitamin B12 deficiency anemias

D51.9 Vitamin B12 deficiency anemia, unspecified

4ᵗʰ **D52** Folate deficiency anemia
EXCLUDES1 folate deficiency without anemia (E53.8)

D52.0 Dietary folate deficiency anemia
Nutritional megaloblastic anemia

D52.1 Drug-induced folate deficiency anemia
Use additional code for adverse effect, if applicable, to identify drug (T36-T50 with fifth or sixth character 5)

D52.8 Other folate deficiency anemias

D52.9 Folate deficiency anemia, unspecified
Folic acid deficiency anemia NOS

4ᵗʰ **D53** Other nutritional anemias
INCLUDES megaloblastic anemia unresponsive to vitamin B12 or folate therapy

D53.0 Protein deficiency anemia
Amino-acid deficiency anemia
Orotaciduric anemia
EXCLUDES1 Lesch-Nyhan syndrome (E79.1)

D53.1 Other megaloblastic anemias, not elsewhere classified
Megaloblastic anemia NOS
EXCLUDES1 Di Guglielmo's disease (C94.0)

D53.2 Scorbutic anemia
EXCLUDES1 scurvy (E54)

D53.8 Other specified nutritional anemias
Anemia associated with deficiency of copper
Anemia associated with deficiency of molybdenum
Anemia associated with deficiency of zinc
EXCLUDES1 nutritional deficiencies without anemia, such as:
copper deficiency NOS (E61.0)
molybdenum deficiency NOS (E61.5)
zinc deficiency NOS (E60)

D53.9 Nutritional anemia, unspecified
Simple chronic anemia
EXCLUDES1 anemia NOS (D64.9)

Hemolytic anemias (D55-D59)

4ᵗʰ **D55** Anemia due to enzyme disorders
EXCLUDES1 drug-induced enzyme deficiency anemia (D59.2)

D55.0 Anemia due to glucose-6-phosphate dehydrogenase [G6PD] deficiency　HCC
Favism
G6PD deficiency anemia

D55.1 Anemia due to other disorders of glutathione metabolism　HCC
Anemia (due to) enzyme deficiencies, except G6PD, related to the hexose monophosphate [HMP] shunt pathway
Anemia (due to) hemolytic nonspherocytic (hereditary), type I

D55.2 Anemia due to disorders of glycolytic enzymes　HCC
Hemolytic nonspherocytic (hereditary) anemia, type II
Hexokinase deficiency anemia
Pyruvate kinase [PK] deficiency anemia
Triose-phosphate isomerase deficiency anemia
EXCLUDES1 disorders of glycolysis not associated with anemia (E74.8)

D55.3 Anemia due to disorders of nucleotide metabolism　HCC

D55.8 Other anemias due to enzyme disorders　HCC

D55.9 Anemia due to enzyme disorder, unspecified　HCC

4ᵗʰ **D56** Thalassemia
EXCLUDES1 sickle-cell thalassemia (D57.4-)

D56.0 Alpha thalassemia　HCC RxHCC
Alpha thalassemia major
Hemoglobin H Constant Spring
Hemoglobin H disease
Hydrops fetalis due to alpha thalassemia

Unspecified Code	Other Specified Code	Manifestation Code	N Newborn	P Pediatric	M Maternity	A Adult	♂ Male	♀ Female

● New Code　▲ Revised Code Title　►◄ Revised Text　NOTES　INCLUDES　EXCLUDES 1 Not coded here　EXCLUDES 2 Not included here
4ᵗʰ 4th character required　5ᵗʰ 5th character required　6ᵗʰ 6th character required　7ᵗʰ 7th character required
7ᵗʰ Extension 'X' Alert　HAC Hospital-acquired condition (HAC) alert　AHA AHA Coding Clinic©

2018 ICD-10-CM　　When symbols appear on a code that requires a 7th character extension, refer to Appendix B to identify applicable 7th character codes.　　**509**

Chapter 3: Diseases of the Blood and Blood-Forming Organs and Certain Disorders Involving the Immune Mechanism (D50-D89)

D56.1 - D58.2

Tabular List

Severe alpha thalassemia
Triple gene defect alpha thalassemia
Use additional code, if applicable, for hydrops fetalis due to alpha thalassemia (P56.99)
  EXCLUDES1 alpha thalassemia trait or minor (D56.3)
    asymptomatic alpha thalassemia (D56.3)
    hydrops fetalis due to isoimmunization (P56.0)
    hydrops fetalis not due to immune hemolysis (P83.2)

D56.1 Beta thalassemia HCC RxHCC
  Beta thalassemia major
  Cooley's anemia
  Homozygous beta thalassemia
  Severe beta thalassemia
  Thalassemia intermedia
  Thalassemia major
  EXCLUDES1 beta thalassemia minor (D56.3)
    beta thalassemia trait (D56.3)
    delta-beta thalassemia (D56.2)
    hemoglobin E-beta thalassemia (D56.5)
    sickle-cell beta thalassemia (D57.4-)

D56.2 Delta-beta thalassemia HCC
  Homozygous delta-beta thalassemia
  EXCLUDES1 delta-beta thalassemia minor (D56.3)
    delta-beta thalassemia trait (D56.3)

D56.3 Thalassemia minor
  Alpha thalassemia minor
  Alpha thalassemia silent carrier
  Alpha thalassemia trait
  Beta thalassemia minor
  Beta thalassemia trait
  Delta-beta thalassemia minor
  Delta-beta thalassemia trait
  Thalassemia trait NOS
  EXCLUDES1 alpha thalassemia (D56.0)
    beta thalassemia (D56.1)
    delta-beta thalassemia (D56.2)
    hemoglobin E-beta thalassemia (D56.5)
    sickle-cell trait (D57.3)

D56.4 Hereditary persistence of fetal hemoglobin [HPFH] HCC
D56.5 Hemoglobin E-beta thalassemia HCC RxHCC
  EXCLUDES1 beta thalassemia (D56.1)
    beta thalassemia minor (D56.3)
    beta thalassemia trait (D56.3)
    delta-beta thalassemia (D56.2)
    delta-beta thalassemia trait (D56.3)
    hemoglobin E disease (D58.2)
    other hemoglobinopathies (D58.2)
    sickle-cell beta thalassemia (D57.4-)

D56.8 Other thalassemias HCC
  Dominant thalassemia
  Hemoglobin C thalassemia
  Mixed thalassemia
  Thalassemia with other hemoglobinopathy
  EXCLUDES1 hemoglobin C disease (D58.2)
    hemoglobin E disease (D58.2)
    other hemoglobinopathies (D58.2)
    sickle-cell anemia (D57.-)
    sickle-cell thalassemia (D57.4)

D56.9 Thalassemia, unspecified
  Mediterranean anemia (with other hemoglobinopathy)

4ᵗʰ **D57 Sickle-cell disorders**
  Use additional code for any associated fever (R50.81)
  EXCLUDES1 other hemoglobinopathies (D58.-)

5ᵗʰ **D57.0 Hb-SS disease with crisis**
  Sickle-cell disease NOS with crisis
  Hb-SS disease with vasoocclusive pain
    D57.00 Hb-SS disease with crisis, unspecified HCC MCC RxHCC CC/MCC Exc

D57.01 Hb-SS disease with acute chest syndrome HCC MCC RxHCC CC/MCC Exc
D57.02 Hb-SS disease with splenic sequestration HCC MCC RxHCC CC/MCC Exc

D57.1 Sickle-cell disease without crisis HCC RxHCC
  Hb-SS disease without crisis
  Sickle-cell anemia NOS
  Sickle-cell disease NOS
  Sickle-cell disorder NOS

5ᵗʰ **D57.2 Sickle-cell/Hb-C disease**
  Hb-SC disease
  Hb-S/Hb-C disease
    D57.20 Sickle-cell/Hb-C disease without crisis HCC RxHCC
  6ᵗʰ **D57.21 Sickle-cell/Hb-C disease with crisis**
      D57.211 Sickle-cell/Hb-C disease with acute chest syndrome HCC MCC PDx CC RxHCC CC/MCC Exc
      D57.212 Sickle-cell/Hb-C disease with splenic sequestration HCC MCC RxHCC CC/MCC Exc
      D57.219 Sickle-cell/Hb-C disease with crisis, unspecified HCC MCC RxHCC CC/MCC Exc
        Sickle-cell/Hb-C disease with crisis NOS

D57.3 Sickle-cell trait HCC
  Hb-S trait
  Heterozygous hemoglobin S

5ᵗʰ **D57.4 Sickle-cell thalassemia**
  Sickle-cell beta thalassemia
  Thalassemia Hb-S disease
    D57.40 Sickle-cell thalassemia without crisis HCC RxHCC
      Microdrepanocytosis
      Sickle-cell thalassemia NOS
  6ᵗʰ **D57.41 Sickle-cell thalassemia with crisis**
      Sickle-cell thalassemia with vasoocclusive pain
      D57.411 Sickle-cell thalassemia with acute chest syndrome HCC MCC PDx CC RxHCC CC/MCC Exc
      D57.412 Sickle-cell thalassemia with splenic sequestration HCC MCC RxHCC CC/MCC Exc
      D57.419 Sickle-cell thalassemia with crisis, unspecified HCC MCC RxHCC CC/MCC Exc
        Sickle-cell thalassemia with crisis NOS

5ᵗʰ **D57.8 Other sickle-cell disorders**
  Hb-SD disease
  Hb-SE disease
    D57.80 Other sickle-cell disorders without crisis HCC RxHCC
  6ᵗʰ **D57.81 Other sickle-cell disorders with crisis**
      D57.811 Other sickle-cell disorders with acute chest syndrome HCC MCC RxHCC CC/MCC Exc
      D57.812 Other sickle-cell disorders with splenic sequestration HCC MCC RxHCC CC/MCC Exc
      D57.819 Other sickle-cell disorders with crisis, unspecified HCC MCC RxHCC CC/MCC Exc
        Other sickle-cell disorders with crisis NOS

4ᵗʰ **D58 Other hereditary hemolytic anemias**
  EXCLUDES1 hemolytic anemia of the newborn (P55.-)
D58.0 Hereditary spherocytosis HCC
  Acholuric (familial) jaundice
  Congenital (spherocytic) hemolytic icterus
  Minkowski-Chauffard syndrome
D58.1 Hereditary elliptocytosis HCC
  Elliptocytosis (congenital)
  Ovalocytosis (congenital) (hereditary)
D58.2 Other hemoglobinopathies HCC
  Abnormal hemoglobin NOS
  Congenital Heinz body anemia
  Hb-C disease
  Hb-D disease
  Hb-E disease
  Hemoglobinopathy NOS
  Unstable hemoglobin hemolytic disease
  EXCLUDES1 familial polycythemia (D75.0)
    Hb-M disease (D74.0)
    hemoglobin E-beta thalassemia (D56.5)

PDx Unacceptable principal diagnosis symbol per Medicare code edits   POA Code exempt from diagnosis present on admission requirement
? Questionable admission   CC Complication or comorbidity   CC/MCC Exc CC/MCC exclusion   MCC Major complication or comorbidity
CC Principal diagnosis as its own CC   MCC Principal diagnosis as its own MCC   HCC HCC diagnosis code   RxHCC RxHCC diagnosis code
MACRA code   Z1 Z code as first-listed diagnosis

D56.1 – D58.2

CHAPTER 3: DISEASES OF THE BLOOD AND BLOOD-FORMING ORGANS AND CERTAIN DISORDERS INVOLVING THE IMMUNE MECHANISM (D50-D89)

Chapter 3: Diseases of the Blood and Blood-Forming Organs and Certain Disorders Involving the Immune Mechanism (D50-D89)

Tabular List

D58.8 - D63.0

hereditary persistence of fetal hemoglobin [HPFH]
(D56.4)

high-altitude polycythemia (D75.1)

methemoglobinemia (D74.-)

other hemoglobinopathies with thalassemia (D56.8)

D58.8 Other specified hereditary hemolytic anemias cc⊕ HCC CC/MCC Exc
Stomatocytosis

D58.9 Hereditary hemolytic anemia, unspecified cc⊕ HCC CC/MCC Exc

4ᵗʰ **D59 Acquired hemolytic anemia**

D59.0 Drug-induced autoimmune hemolytic anemia cc⊕ HCC RxHCC CC/MCC Exc
Use additional code for adverse effect, if applicable, to identify drug (T36-T50 with fifth or sixth character 5)

D59.1 Other autoimmune hemolytic anemias
Autoimmune hemolytic disease (cold type) (warm type)
Chronic cold hemagglutinin disease
Cold agglutinin disease
Cold agglutinin hemoglobinuria
Cold type (secondary) (symptomatic) hemolytic anemia
Warm type (secondary) (symptomatic) hemolytic anemia
EXCLUDES1 Evans syndrome (D69.41)
  hemolytic disease of newborn (P55.-)
  paroxysmal cold hemoglobinuria (D59.6)

D59.2 Drug-induced nonautoimmune hemolytic anemia cc⊕ HCC RxHCC CC/MCC Exc
Drug-induced enzyme deficiency anemia
Use additional code for adverse effect, if applicable, to identify drug (T36-T50 with fifth or sixth character 5)

D59.3 Hemolytic-uremic syndrome HCC MCC⊕ RxHCC CC/MCC Exc
Use additional code to identify associated:
E. coli infection (B96.2-)
Pneumococcal pneumonia (J13)
Shigella dysenteriae (A03.9)

D59.4 Other nonautoimmune hemolytic anemias cc⊕ HCC RxHCC CC/MCC Exc
Mechanical hemolytic anemia
Microangiopathic hemolytic anemia
Toxic hemolytic anemia

D59.5 Paroxysmal nocturnal hemoglobinuria [Marchiafava-Micheli] HCC RxHCC
EXCLUDES1 hemoglobinuria NOS (R82.3)

D59.6 Hemoglobinuria due to hemolysis from other external causes HCC RxHCC
Hemoglobinuria from exertion
March hemoglobinuria
Paroxysmal cold hemoglobinuria
Use additional code (Chapter 20) to identify external cause
EXCLUDES1 hemoglobinuria NOS (R82.3)

D59.8 Other acquired hemolytic anemias HCC RxHCC

D59.9 Acquired hemolytic anemia, unspecified cc⊕ HCC RxHCC CC/MCC Exc
Idiopathic hemolytic anemia, chronic

Aplastic and other anemias and other bone marrow failure syndromes (D60-D64)

4ᵗʰ **D60 Acquired pure red cell aplasia [erythroblastopenia]**
INCLUDES red cell aplasia (acquired) (adult) (with thymoma)
EXCLUDES1 congenital red cell aplasia (D61.01)

D60.0 Chronic acquired pure red cell aplasia HCC MCC⊕ RxHCC CC/MCC Exc

D60.1 Transient acquired pure red cell aplasia HCC MCC⊕ RxHCC CC/MCC Exc

D60.8 Other acquired pure red cell aplasias HCC MCC⊕ RxHCC CC/MCC Exc

D60.9 Acquired pure red cell aplasia, unspecified HCC MCC⊕ RxHCC CC/MCC Exc

4ᵗʰ **D61 Other aplastic anemias and other bone marrow failure syndromes**
EXCLUDES1 neutropenia (D70.-)

5ᵗʰ **D61.0 Constitutional aplastic anemia**

D61.01 Constitutional (pure) red blood cell aplasia cc⊕ HCC RxHCC CC/MCC Exc
Blackfan-Diamond syndrome
Congenital (pure) red cell aplasia
Familial hypoplastic anemia
Primary (pure) red cell aplasia

Red cell (pure) aplasia of infants
EXCLUDES1 acquired red cell aplasia (D60.9)

D61.09 Other constitutional aplastic anemia cc⊕ HCC RxHCC CC/MCC Exc
Fanconi's anemia
Pancytopenia with malformations

D61.1 Drug-induced aplastic anemia HCC MCC⊕ RxHCC CC/MCC Exc
Use additional code for adverse effect, if applicable, to identify drug (T36-T50 with fifth or sixth character 5)

D61.2 Aplastic anemia due to other external agents HCC MCC⊕ RxHCC CC/MCC Exc
Code first, if applicable, toxic effects of substances chiefly nonmedicinal as to source (T51-T65)

D61.3 Idiopathic aplastic anemia HCC MCC⊕ RxHCC CC/MCC Exc

5ᵗʰ **D61.8 Other specified aplastic anemias and other bone marrow failure syndromes**

6ᵗʰ **D61.81 Pancytopenia**
EXCLUDES1 pancytopenia (due to) (with) aplastic anemia (D61.9)
  pancytopenia (due to) (with) bone marrow infiltration (D61.82)
  pancytopenia (due to) (with) congenital (pure) red cell aplasia (D61.01)
  pancytopenia (due to) (with) hairy cell leukemia (C91.4-)
  pancytopenia (due to) (with) human immunodeficiency virus disease (B20.-)
  pancytopenia (due to) (with) leukoerythroblastic anemia (D61.82)
  pancytopenia (due to) (with) myeloproliferative disease (D47.1)
EXCLUDES2 pancytopenia (due to) (with) myelodysplastic syndromes (D46.-)

D61.810 Antineoplastic chemotherapy induced pancytopenia HCC MCC⊕ CC/MCC Exc
EXCLUDES2 aplastic anemia due to antineoplastic chemotherapy (D61.1)

D61.811 Other drug-induced pancytopenia HCC MCC⊕ CC/MCC Exc
EXCLUDES2 aplastic anemia due to drugs (D61.1)

D61.818 Other pancytopenia cc⊕ HCC CC/MCC Exc

D61.82 Myelophthisis cc⊕ HCC RxHCC CC/MCC Exc
Leukoerythroblastic anemia
Myelophthisic anemia
Panmyelophthisis
Code also the underlying disorder, such as:
  malignant neoplasm of breast (C50.-)
  tuberculosis (A15.-)
EXCLUDES1 idiopathic myelofibrosis (D47.1)
  myelofibrosis NOS (D75.81)
  myelofibrosis with myeloid metaplasia (D47.4)
  primary myelofibrosis (D47.1)
  secondary myelofibrosis (D75.81)

D61.89 Other specified aplastic anemias and other bone marrow failure syndromes HCC MCC⊕ RxHCC CC/MCC Exc

D61.9 Aplastic anemia, unspecified cc⊕ HCC RxHCC CC/MCC Exc
Hypoplastic anemia NOS
Medullary hypoplasia

D62 Acute posthemorrhagic anemia cc⊕ CC/MCC Exc
EXCLUDES1 anemia due to chronic blood loss (D50.0)
  blood loss anemia NOS (D50.0)
  congenital anemia from fetal blood loss (P61.3)

4ᵗʰ **D63 Anemia in chronic diseases classified elsewhere**

D63.0 Anemia in neoplastic disease
Code first neoplasm (C00-D49)
EXCLUDES1 aplastic anemia due to antineoplastic chemotherapy (D61.1)
EXCLUDES2 anemia due to antineoplastic chemotherapy (D64.81)

Unspecified Code   Other Specified Code   Manifestation Code   N Newborn   P Pediatric   M Maternity   A Adult   ♂ Male   ♀ Female
● New Code   ▲ Revised Code Title   ►◄ Revised Text   NOTES   INCLUDES   EXCLUDES 1 Not coded here   EXCLUDES 2 Not included here
4ᵗʰ 4ᵗʰ character required   5ᵗʰ 5ᵗʰ character required   6ᵗʰ 6ᵗʰ character required   7ᵗʰ 7ᵗʰ character required
7ᵗʰ Extension 'X' Alert   HAC Hospital-acquired condition (HAC) alert   AHA AHA Coding Clinic©

D58.8 - D63.0

CHAPTER 3: DISEASES OF THE BLOOD AND BLOOD-FORMING ORGANS AND CERTAIN DISORDERS INVOLVING THE IMMUNE MECHANISM (D50-D89)

Chapter 3: Diseases of the Blood and Blood-Forming Organs and Certain Disorders Involving the Immune Mechanism (D50-D89)

D63.1 - D68.318

Tabular List

D63.1 - D68.318

CHAPTER 3: DISEASES OF THE BLOOD AND BLOOD-FORMING ORGANS AND CERTAIN DISORDERS INVOLVING THE IMMUNE MECHANISM (D50-D89)

D63.1 Anemia in chronic kidney disease
Erythropoietin resistant anemia (EPO resistant anemia)
Code first underlying chronic kidney disease (CKD) (N18.-)

D63.8 Anemia in other chronic diseases classified elsewhere
Code first underlying disease, such as:
diphyllobothriasis (B70.0)
hookworm disease (B76.0-B76.9)
hypothyroidism (E00.0-E03.9)
malaria (B50.0-B54)
symptomatic late syphilis (A52.79)
tuberculosis (A18.89)

D64 Other anemias
EXCLUDES1 refractory anemia (D46.-)
refractory anemia with excess blasts in transformation [RAEB T] (C92.0-)

D64.0 Hereditary sideroblastic anemia HCC RxHCC
Sex-linked hypochromic sideroblastic anemia

D64.1 Secondary sideroblastic anemia due to disease HCC RxHCC
Code first underlying disease

D64.2 Secondary sideroblastic anemia due to drugs and toxins HCC RxHCC
Code first poisoning due to drug or toxin, if applicable (T36-T65 with fifth or sixth character 1-4 or 6)
Use additional code for adverse effect, if applicable, to identify drug (T36-T50 with fifth or sixth character 5)

D64.3 Other sideroblastic anemias HCC RxHCC
Sideroblastic anemia NOS
Pyridoxine-responsive sideroblastic anemia NEC

D64.4 Congenital dyserythropoietic anemia
Dyshematopoietic anemia (congenital)
EXCLUDES1 Blackfan-Diamond syndrome (D61.01)
Di Guglielmo's disease (C94.0)

D64.8 Other specified anemias

D64.81 Anemia due to antineoplastic chemotherapy
Antineoplastic chemotherapy induced anemia
EXCLUDES1 aplastic anemia due to antineoplastic chemotherapy (D61.1)
EXCLUDES2 anemia in neoplastic disease (D63.0)

D64.89 Other specified anemias
Infantile pseudoleukemia

D64.9 Anemia, unspecified

Coagulation defects, purpura and other hemorrhagic conditions (D65-D69)

D65 Disseminated intravascular coagulation [defibrination syndrome] HCC MCC CC/MCC Exc
Afibrinogenemia, acquired
Consumption coagulopathy
Diffuse or disseminated intravascular coagulation [DIC]
Fibrinolytic hemorrhage, acquired
Fibrinolytic purpura
Purpura fulminans
EXCLUDES1 disseminated intravascular coagulation (complicating):
abortion or ectopic or molar pregnancy (O00-O07, O08.1)
in newborn (P60)
pregnancy, childbirth and the puerperium (O45.0, O46.0, O67.0, O72.3)

D66 Hereditary factor VIII deficiency HCC MCC CC/MCC Exc
Classical hemophilia
Deficiency factor VIII (with functional defect)
Hemophilia NOS
Hemophilia A
EXCLUDES1 factor VIII deficiency with vascular defect (D68.0)

D67 Hereditary factor IX deficiency HCC MCC CC/MCC Exc
Christmas disease
Factor IX deficiency (with functional defect)
Hemophilia B
Plasma thromboplastin component [PTC] deficiency

D68 Other coagulation defects
EXCLUDES1 abnormal coagulation profile (R79.1)
coagulation defects complicating abortion or ectopic or molar pregnancy (O00-O07, O08.1)
coagulation defects complicating pregnancy, childbirth and the puerperium (O45.0, O46.0, O67.0, O72.3)

D68.0 Von Willebrand's disease CC HCC CC/MCC Exc
Angiohemophilia
Factor VIII deficiency with vascular defect
Vascular hemophilia
EXCLUDES1 capillary fragility (hereditary) (D69.8)
factor VIII deficiency NOS (D66)
factor VIII deficiency with functional defect (D66)

D68.1 Hereditary factor XI deficiency CC HCC CC/MCC Exc
Hemophilia C
Plasma thromboplastin antecedent [PTA] deficiency
Rosenthal's disease

D68.2 Hereditary deficiency of other clotting factors CC HCC CC/MCC Exc
AC globulin deficiency
Congenital afibrinogenemia
Deficiency of factor I [fibrinogen]
Deficiency of factor II [prothrombin]
Deficiency of factor V [labile]
Deficiency of factor VII [stable]
Deficiency of factor X [Stuart-Prower]
Deficiency of factor XII [Hageman]
Deficiency of factor XIII [fibrin stabilizing]
Dysfibrinogenemia (congenital)
Hypoproconvertinemia
Owren's disease
Proaccelerin deficiency

D68.3 Hemorrhagic disorder due to circulating anticoagulants

D68.31 Hemorrhagic disorder due to intrinsic circulating anticoagulants, antibodies, or inhibitors

D68.311 Acquired hemophilia CC HCC CC/MCC Exc
Autoimmune hemophilia
Autoimmune inhibitors to clotting factors
Secondary hemophilia

D68.312 Antiphospholipid antibody with hemorrhagic disorder CC HCC CC/MCC Exc
Lupus anticoagulant (LAC) with hemorrhagic disorder
Systemic lupus erythematosus [SLE] inhibitor with hemorrhagic disorder
EXCLUDES1 antiphospholipid antibody, finding without diagnosis (R76.0)
antiphospholipid antibody syndrome (D68.61)
antiphospholipid antibody with hypercoagulable state (D68.61)
lupus anticoagulant (LAC) finding without diagnosis (R76.0)
lupus anticoagulant (LAC) with hypercoagulable state (D68.62)
systemic lupus erythematosus [SLE] inhibitor finding without diagnosis (R76.0)
systemic lupus erythematosus [SLE] inhibitor with hypercoagulable state (D68.62)

D68.318 Other hemorrhagic disorder due to intrinsic circulating anticoagulants, antibodies, or inhibitors CC HCC CC/MCC Exc
Antithromboplastinemia
Antithromboplastinogenemia
Hemorrhagic disorder due to intrinsic increase in antithrombin
Hemorrhagic disorder due to intrinsic increase in anti-VIIIa
Hemorrhagic disorder due to intrinsic increase in anti-IXa

PDx Unacceptable principal diagnosis symbol per Medicare code edits   POA Code exempt from diagnosis present on admission requirement
? Questionable admission   CC Complication or comorbidity   CC/MCC Exc CC/MCC exclusion   MCC Major complication or comorbidity
Principal diagnosis as its own CC   Principal diagnosis as its own MCC   HCC HCC diagnosis code   RxHCC RxHCC diagnosis code
MACRA code   Z1 Z code as first-listed diagnosis

512   When symbols appear on a code that requires a 7th character extension, refer to Appendix B to identify applicable 7th character codes.   2018 ICD-10-CM

Chapter 3: Diseases of the Blood and Blood-Forming Organs and Certain Disorders Involving the Immune Mechanism (D50-D89)

Tabular List

D68.32 - D69.9

Hemorrhagic disorder due to intrinsic increase in anti-XIa

D68.32 **Hemorrhagic disorder due to** extrinsic **circulating anticoagulants** ♂ⓔ HCC CC/MCC Exc

AHA: Q1 2016

Drug-induced hemorrhagic disorder
Hemorrhagic disorder due to increase in anti-IIa
Hemorrhagic disorder due to increase in anti-Xa
Hyperheparinemia
Use additional code for adverse effect, if applicable, to identify drug (T45.515, T45.525)

D68.4 **Acquired coagulation factor deficiency** ♂ⓔ HCC CC/MCC Exc

Deficiency of coagulation factor due to liver disease
Deficiency of coagulation factor due to vitamin K deficiency

EXCLUDES1 *vitamin K deficiency of newborn (P53)*

5ᵗʰ D68.5 **Primary thrombophilia**

Primary hypercoagulable states

EXCLUDES1 *antiphospholipid syndrome (D68.61)*

lupus anticoagulant (D68.62)

secondary activated protein C resistance (D68.69)

secondary antiphospholipid antibody syndrome (D68.69)

secondary lupus anticoagulant with hypercoagulable state (D68.69)

secondary systemic lupus erythematosus [SLE] inhibitor with hypercoagulable state (D68.69)

systemic lupus erythematosus [SLE] inhibitor finding without diagnosis (R76.0)

systemic lupus erythematosus [SLE] inhibitor with hemorrhagic disorder (D68.312)

thrombotic thrombocytopenic purpura (M31.1)

D68.51 **Activated protein C resistance** ♂ⓔ HCC RxHCC CC/MCC Exc

Factor V Leiden mutation

D68.52 **Prothrombin gene mutation** ♂ⓔ HCC RxHCC CC/MCC Exc

D68.59 **Other primary thrombophilia** ♂ⓔ HCC RxHCC CC/MCC Exc

Antithrombin III deficiency
Hypercoagulable state NOS
Primary hypercoagulable state NEC
Primary thrombophilia NEC
Protein C deficiency
Protein S deficiency
Thrombophilia NOS

5ᵗʰ D68.6 **Other thrombophilia**

Other hypercoagulable states

EXCLUDES1 *diffuse or disseminated intravascular coagulation [DIC] (D65)*

heparin induced thrombocytopenia (HIT) (D75.82)

hyperhomocysteinemia (E72.11)

D68.61 **Antiphospholipid syndrome** ♂ⓔ HCC RxHCC CC/MCC Exc

Anticardiolipin syndrome
Antiphospholipid antibody syndrome

EXCLUDES1 *anti-phospholipid antibody, finding without diagnosis (R76.0)*

anti-phospholipid antibody with hemorrhagic disorder (D68.312)

lupus anticoagulant syndrome (D68.62)

D68.62 **Lupus anticoagulant syndrome** ♂ⓔ HCC RxHCC CC/MCC Exc

Lupus anticoagulant
Presence of systemic lupus erythematosus [SLE] inhibitor

EXCLUDES1 *anticardiolipin syndrome (D68.61)*

antiphospholipid syndrome (D68.61)

lupus anticoagulant (LAC) finding without diagnosis (R76.0)

lupus anticoagulant (LAC) with hemorrhagic disorder (D68.312)

D68.69 **Other thrombophilia** ♂ⓔ HCC RxHCC CC/MCC Exc

Hypercoagulable states NEC
Secondary hypercoagulable state NOS

D68.8 **Other specified coagulation defects** ♂ⓔ HCC CC/MCC Exc

EXCLUDES1 *hemorrhagic disease of newborn (P53)*

D68.9 **Coagulation defect, unspecified** ♂ⓔ HCC CC/MCC Exc

4ᵗʰ D69 **Purpura and other hemorrhagic conditions**

EXCLUDES1 *benign hypergammaglobulinemic purpura (D89.0)*

cryoglobulinemic purpura (D89.1)

essential (hemorrhagic) thrombocythemia (D47.3)

hemorrhagic thrombocythemia (D47.3)

purpura fulminans (D65)

thrombotic thrombocytopenic purpura (M31.1)

Waldenström hypergammaglobulinemic purpura (D89.0)

D69.0 **Allergic purpura** ♂ⓔ HCC CC/MCC Exc

Allergic vasculitis
Nonthrombocytopenic hemorrhagic purpura
Nonthrombocytopenic idiopathic purpura
Purpura anaphylactoid
Purpura Henoch(-Schönlein)
Purpura rheumatica
Vascular purpura

EXCLUDES1 *thrombocytopenic hemorrhagic purpura (D69.3)*

D69.1 **Qualitative platelet defects** HCC

Bernard-Soulier [giant platelet] syndrome
Glanzmann's disease
Grey platelet syndrome
Thromboasthenia (hemorrhagic) (hereditary)
Thrombocytopathy

EXCLUDES1 *von Willebrand's disease (D68.0)*

D69.2 **Other nonthrombocytopenic purpura** HCC

Purpura NOS
Purpura simplex
Senile purpura

D69.3 **Immune thrombocytopenic purpura** ♂ⓔ HCC CC/MCC Exc

Hemorrhagic (thrombocytopenic) purpura
Idiopathic thrombocytopenic purpura
Tidal platelet dysgenesis

5ᵗʰ D69.4 **Other primary thrombocytopenia**

EXCLUDES1 *transient neonatal thrombocytopenia (P61.0)*

Wiskott-Aldrich syndrome (D82.0)

D69.41 **Evans syndrome** ♂ⓔ HCC CC/MCC Exc

D69.42 **Congenital and hereditary thrombocytopenia purpura** ♂ⓔ HCC CC/MCC Exc

Congenital thrombocytopenia
Hereditary thrombocytopenia
Code first congenital or hereditary disorder, such as:
thrombocytopenia with absent radius (TAR syndrome) (Q87.2)

D69.49 **Other primary thrombocytopenia** HCC

Megakaryocytic hypoplasia
Primary thrombocytopenia NOS

5ᵗʰ D69.5 **Secondary thrombocytopenia**

EXCLUDES1 *heparin induced thrombocytopenia (HIT) (D75.82)*

transient thrombocytopenia of newborn (P61.0)

D69.51 **Posttransfusion purpura**

Posttransfusion purpura from whole blood (fresh) or blood products
PTP

D69.59 **Other secondary thrombocytopenia**

D69.6 **Thrombocytopenia, unspecified** HCC

D69.8 **Other specified hemorrhagic conditions** HCC

Capillary fragility (hereditary)
Vascular pseudohemophilia

D69.9 **Hemorrhagic condition, unspecified** HCC

Unspecified Code   Other Specified Code   Manifestation Code   Ⓝ Newborn   Ⓟ Pediatric   Ⓜ Maternity   Ⓐ Adult   ♂ Male   ♀ Female
● New Code   ▲ Revised Code Title   ▶◀ Revised Text   **NOTES**   *INCLUDES*   *EXCLUDES 1* Not coded here   *EXCLUDES 2* Not included here
4ᵗʰ 4ᵗʰ character required   5ᵗʰ 5ᵗʰ character required   6ᵗʰ 6ᵗʰ character required   7ᵗʰ 7ᵗʰ character required
7ˣ Extension 'X' Alert   **HAC** Hospital-acquired condition (HAC) alert   **AHA** AHA Coding Clinic©

D68.32 – D69.9

CHAPTER 3: DISEASES OF THE BLOOD AND BLOOD-FORMING ORGANS AND CERTAIN DISORDERS INVOLVING THE IMMUNE MECHANISM (D50-D89)

Chapter 3: Diseases of the Blood and Blood-Forming Organs and Certain Disorders Involving the Immune Mechanism (D50-D89)

D80 - D89.1

Tabular List

D80 - D89.1

CHAPTER 3: DISEASES OF THE BLOOD AND BLOOD-FORMING ORGANS AND CERTAIN DISORDERS INVOLVING THE IMMUNE MECHANISM (D50-D89)

Certain disorders involving the immune mechanism (D80-D89)

INCLUDES defects in the complement system

immunodeficiency disorders, except human immunodeficiency virus [HIV] disease

sarcoidosis

EXCLUDES1 autoimmune disease (systemic) NOS (M35.9)

functional disorders of polymorphonuclear neutrophils (D71)

human immunodeficiency virus [HIV] disease (B20)

D80 Immunodeficiency with predominantly antibody defects

D80.0 **Hereditary** hypogammaglobulinemia

Autosomal recessive agammaglobulinemia (Swiss type)

X-linked agammaglobulinemia [Bruton] (with growth hormone deficiency)

D80.1 **Nonfamilial** hypogammaglobulinemia

Agammaglobulinemia with immunoglobulin-bearing B-lymphocytes

Common variable agammaglobulinemia [CVAgamma]

Hypogammaglobulinemia NOS

D80.2 **Selective deficiency of** immunoglobulin A [IgA]

D80.3 **Selective deficiency of** immunoglobulin G [IgG] subclasses

D80.4 **Selective deficiency of** immunoglobulin M [IgM]

D80.5 **Immunodeficiency with increased** immunoglobulin M [IgM]

D80.6 **Antibody deficiency with** near-normal immunoglobulins or with hyperimmunoglobulinemia

D80.7 **Transient hypogammaglobulinemia of** infancy

D80.8 **Other immunodeficiencies with predominantly** antibody defects

Kappa light chain deficiency

D80.9 **Immunodeficiency with predominantly antibody defects, unspecified**

D81 Combined immunodeficiencies

EXCLUDES1 autosomal recessive agammaglobulinemia (Swiss type) (D80.0)

D81.0 **Severe combined immunodeficiency [SCID] with** reticular dysgenesis

D81.1 **Severe combined immunodeficiency [SCID] with** low T- and B-cell numbers

D81.2 **Severe combined immunodeficiency [SCID] with** low or normal B-cell numbers

D81.3 **Adenosine deaminase [ADA] deficiency**

D81.4 **Nezelof's syndrome**

D81.5 **Purine nucleoside phosphorylase [PNP] deficiency**

D81.6 **Major histocompatibility complex class I deficiency**

Bare lymphocyte syndrome

D81.7 **Major histocompatibility complex class II deficiency**

D81.8 **Other combined immunodeficiencies**

D81.81 Biotin-dependent carboxylase **deficiency**

Multiple carboxylase deficiency

EXCLUDES1 biotin-dependent carboxylase deficiency due to dietary deficiency of biotin (E53.8)

D81.810 Biotinidase deficiency

D81.818 **Other biotin-dependent carboxylase deficiency**

Holocarboxylase synthetase deficiency

Other multiple carboxylase deficiency

D81.819 **Biotin-dependent carboxylase deficiency, unspecified**

Multiple carboxylase deficiency, unspecified

D81.89 **Other combined immunodeficiencies**

D81.9 **Combined immunodeficiency, unspecified**

Severe combined immunodeficiency disorder [SCID] NOS

D82 Immunodeficiency associated with other major defects

EXCLUDES1 ataxia telangiectasia [Louis-Bar] (G11.3)

D82.0 **Wiskott-Aldrich syndrome**

Immunodeficiency with thrombocytopenia and eczema

D82.1 **Di George's syndrome**

Pharyngeal pouch syndrome

Thymic alymphoplasia

Thymic aplasia or hypoplasia with immunodeficiency

D82.2 **Immunodeficiency with short-limbed stature**

D82.3 **Immunodeficiency following hereditary defective response to Epstein-Barr virus**

X-linked lymphoproliferative disease

D82.4 **Hyperimmunoglobulin E [IgE] syndrome**

D82.8 **Immunodeficiency associated with other specified major defects**

D82.9 **Immunodeficiency associated with major defect, unspecified**

D83 Common variable immunodeficiency

D83.0 **Common variable immunodeficiency with** predominant abnormalities of B-cell numbers and function

D83.1 **Common variable immunodeficiency with** predominant immunoregulatory T-cell disorders

D83.2 **Common variable immunodeficiency with** autoantibodies to B- or T-cells

D83.8 **Other common variable immunodeficiencies**

D83.9 **Common variable immunodeficiency, unspecified**

D84 Other immunodeficiencies

D84.0 **Lymphocyte function antigen-1 [LFA-1] defect**

D84.1 **Defects in the** complement system

C1 esterase inhibitor [C1-INH] deficiency

D84.8 **Other specified immunodeficiencies**

D84.9 **Immunodeficiency, unspecified**

D86 Sarcoidosis

D86.0 **Sarcoidosis of** lung

D86.1 **Sarcoidosis of** lymph nodes

D86.2 **Sarcoidosis of** lung with sarcoidosis of lymph nodes

D86.3 **Sarcoidosis of** skin

D86.8 **Sarcoidosis of** other sites

D86.81 **Sarcoid** meningitis

D86.82 **Multiple cranial nerve palsies in** sarcoidosis

D86.83 **Sarcoid** iridocyclitis

D86.84 **Sarcoid** pyelonephritis

Tubulo-interstitial nephropathy in sarcoidosis

D86.85 **Sarcoid** myocarditis

D86.86 **Sarcoid** arthropathy

Polyarthritis in sarcoidosis

D86.87 **Sarcoid** myositis

D86.89 **Sarcoidosis of** other sites

Hepatic granuloma

Uveoparotid fever [Heerfordt]

D86.9 **Sarcoidosis, unspecified**

D89 Other disorders involving the immune mechanism, not elsewhere classified

EXCLUDES1 hyperglobulinemia NOS (R77.1)

monoclonal gammopathy (of undetermined significance) (D47.2)

EXCLUDES2 transplant failure and rejection (T86.-)

D89.0 **Polyclonal hypergammaglobulinemia**

Benign hypergammaglobulinemic purpura

Polyclonal gammopathy NOS

D89.1 **Cryoglobulinemia**

Cryoglobulinemic purpura

Cryoglobulinemic vasculitis

Essential cryoglobulinemia

Idiopathic cryoglobulinemia

Mixed cryoglobulinemia

Primary cryoglobulinemia

Secondary cryoglobulinemia

PDx Unacceptable principal diagnosis symbol per Medicare code edits   Code exempt from diagnosis present on admission requirement

Questionable admission   Complication or comorbidity   CC/MCC exclusion   Major complication or comorbidity

Principal diagnosis as its own CC   Principal diagnosis as its own MCC   HCC HCC diagnosis code   RxHCC RxHCC diagnosis code

MACRA code   Z code as first-listed diagnosis

D89.2 **Hypergammaglobulinemia, unspecified**

D89.3 **Immune reconstitution syndrome** [HCC] [RxHCC]
Immune reconstitution inflammatory syndrome [IRIS]
Use additional code for adverse effect, if applicable, to identify drug (T36-T50 with fifth or sixth character 5)

[5th] D89.4 **Mast cell activation syndrome and related disorders**
[EXCLUDES1] *aggressive systemic mastocytosis ►(C96.21)◄*
►congenital◄ cutaneous mastocytosis (Q82.2)
(non-congenital) cutaneous mastocytosis (D47.01)
(indolent) systemic mastocytosis (D47.02)
malignant mast cell neoplasm (C96.2-)
malignant mastocytoma (C96.29)
mast cell leukemia (C94.3-)
mast cell sarcoma (C96.22)
mastocytoma NOS (D47.09)
other mast cell neoplasms of uncertain behavior (D47.09)
systemic mastocytosis associated with a clonal hematologic non-mast cell lineage disease (SM-AHNMD) (D47.02)

D89.40 **Mast cell activation, unspecified** [HCC] [RxHCC]
AHA: Q4 2016
Mast cell activation disorder, unspecified
Mast cell activation syndrome, NOS

D89.41 **Monoclonal mast cell activation syndrome** [HCC] [RxHCC]
AHA: Q4 2016

D89.42 **Idiopathic mast cell activation syndrome** [HCC] [RxHCC]
AHA: Q4 2016

D89.43 **Secondary mast cell activation** [HCC] [RxHCC]
AHA: Q4 2016
Secondary mast cell activation syndrome
Code also underlying etiology, if known

D89.49 **Other mast cell activation disorder** [HCC] [RxHCC]
AHA: Q4 2016
Other mast cell activation syndrome

[5th] D89.8 **Other specified disorders involving the immune mechanism, not elsewhere classified**

[6th] D89.81 **Graft-versus-host disease**
Code first underlying cause, such as:
complications of transplanted organs and tissue (T86.-)
complications of blood transfusion (T80.89)
Use additional code to identify associated manifestations, such as:
desquamative dermatitis (L30.8)
diarrhea (R19.7)
elevated bilirubin (R17)
hair loss (L65.9)

D89.810 **Acute graft-versus-host disease** [CC] [HCC] [RxHCC] [PDx] [CC/MCC Exc]

D89.811 **Chronic graft-versus-host disease** [CC] [HCC] [RxHCC] [PDx] [CC/MCC Exc]

D89.812 **Acute on chronic graft-versus-host disease** [CC] [HCC] [RxHCC] [PDx] [CC/MCC Exc]

D89.813 **Graft-versus-host disease, unspecified** [CC] [HCC] [RxHCC] [PDx] [CC/MCC Exc]

D89.82 **Autoimmune lymphoproliferative syndrome [ALPS]** [HCC] [RxHCC]

D89.89 **Other specified disorders involving the immune mechanism, not elsewhere classified** [HCC] [RxHCC]
[EXCLUDES1] *human immunodeficiency virus disease (B20)*

D89.9 **Disorder involving the immune mechanism, unspecified** [HCC] [RxHCC]
AHA: Q3 2015
Immune disease NOS

NOTES

Anatomy of the Endocrine System

1. **An Outline of the Endocrine System**
   a) The endocrine system is primarily responsible for maintaining the body's homeostasis through various hormones.
   b) The endocrine system is based on the ductless endocrine glands that secrete their hormones directly into the blood stream. These hormones are further carried to the target organs through the blood stream.
   c) The pituitary gland (or hypophysis) is regarded as the master gland of the endocrine system. This gland is monitored and controlled by the hypothalamus of the brain.

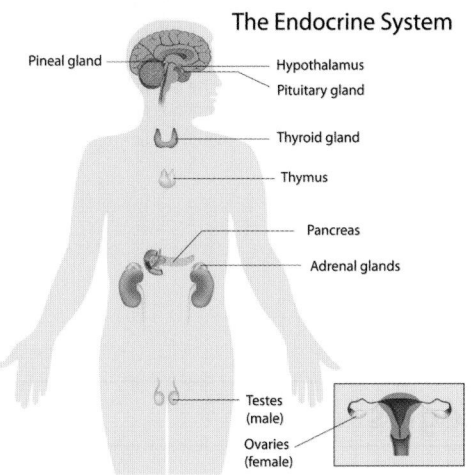

The Endocrine System

2. **The Endocrine Hormones**
   a) The names of various endocrine hormones of the body are as follows:
      i) epinephrine
      ii) norepinephrine
      iii) oxytocin
      iv) vasopressin
      v) insulin
      vi) growth hormone
      vii) cortisol
      viii) estrogen
      ix) testosterone
   b) The hormones monitor and control the processes of cellular respiration, growth, reproduction and electrolyte balances of the body. They also regulate the reproductive cycles, growth and the secretion of other hormones.

3. **The Hypothalamus (of the Brain)**
   a) The hypothalamus controls the secretions of the pituitary gland.
   b) The hypothalamus controls and monitors the secretions of the endocrine system.
   c) The endocrine system can influence the functions of the hypothalamus via negative feedback mechanisms.

4. **The Major Endocrine Glands**
   a) The names of the major endocrine glands are as follows:
      i) anterior pituitary gland
      ii) posterior pituitary gland
      iii) pineal gland
      iv) thyroid gland
      v) parathyroid gland
      vi) thymus
      vii) adrenal gland
      viii) pancreatic islets
      ix) ovaries
      x) testes

5. **The Anatomy of the Anterior Pituitary Gland**
   The anterior pituitary gland is constituted by the glandular epithelium and generates the following hormones, which are listed below:
   a) Growth Hormone

      The growth hormone stimulates cell metabolism and growth of bones and muscles.
   b) Thyroid Stimulating Hormone (TSH)

      The TSH stimulates the thyroid gland for the production of T3, T4 and calcitonin hormones.
   c) Adrenocorticotropic Hormone (ACTH)

      The ACTH stimulates the adrenal cortex for the secretion of the hormone cortisol.
   d) Melanocyte Stimulating Hormone (MSH)

      The MSH stimulates melanocytes for the production of melanin, which causes darkening of the skin.
   e) Luteinizing Hormone (LH)

      The LH stimulates the production of testosterone in males and progesterone in females.
   f) Prolactin

      The Prolactin provides stimulation for milk production in the mammary glands of female after child birth.

6. **The Anatomy of the Posterior Pituitary Gland**
   The posterior pituitary gland is also known as neurohypophysis. It is made up of the posterior lobe of the pituitary gland. The hormones of the posterior pituitary gland are listed below:
   a) Antidiuretic Hormone (ADH)/Vasopressin

      Function of vasopressin is to enhance water re-absorption in the kidney tubules. Deficiency of vasopressin can cause Diabetes insipidus.
   b) Oxytocin

      Oxytocin facilitates childbirth by causing the contraction of uterine smooth muscles. It also facilitates lactation by causing constriction of the mammary glands during breastfeeding.

7. **The Anatomy of the Thyroid Gland**
   a) The thyroid gland is located below the thyroid cartilage in the neck region. It is one of the largest endocrine glands in the body.
   b) The overactive thyroid gland causes excessive secretion of thyroid hormone or hyperthyroidism.
   c) The underactive thyroid gland causes a condition of lack of thyroid hormone, which is known as the hypothyroidism.
   d) The hormone calcitonin is secreted by the extrafollicular cells of the thyroid gland. It causes an increased excretion of the calcium and phosphate ions via the kidneys.

8. **The Anatomy of the Parathyroid Glands**
   a) The parathyroid glands are four in number and remain embedded in the posterior surface of the thyroid gland in the neck region. These glands secrete parathyroid hormone or parathormone (PTH).
   b) PTH stimulates the bone cells to release calcium and phosphate into the blood stream.
   c) A deficiency of PTH causes hypoparathyroidism.
   d) The high levels of PTH can result in the condition of hyperparathyroidism.

9. **The Anatomy of Adrenal Glands**
   a) The adrenal (or suprarenal) glands are located on top of each kidney.
   b) The adrenal gland is divided into the following components:
      i) adrenal medulla (or the inner portion)
      ii) adrenal cortex (or the outer portion)
   c) The hormones epinephrine (or adrenalin) and norepinephrine (or noradrenalin) are produced by the adrenal medulla.
   d) The adrenal cortex is divided into the following three layers:
      i) outer layer of adrenal cortex secretes aldosterone, which is a mineralocorticoid hormone and regulates sodium reabsorption and potassium excretion by the kidney.

ii)　hormone cortisol (or hydrocortisone) is secreted by the middle layer of adrenal cortex. It stimulates the liver to manufacture glucose from the circulating amino acids. The cortisol also possesses anti-inflammatory properties.

iii)　adrenal male sex hormones (or androgens) are produced by the inner layer of the adrenal cortex. These hormones enhance the male sex characteristics. The androgens are also the precursors of all estrogens (or the female sex hormones) and stimulate the female sex drive. Testosterone is the primary and most well-known androgen.

e)　A deficit of adrenal cortex hormones causes Addison's disease.

f)　An increased secretion of adrenal cortex causes Cushing's syndrome.

10. The Anatomy of the Pancreas

a)　The pancreas is a glandular organ of both digestive and endocrine systems.

b)　The islets of Langerhans of pancreas constitute its endocrine portion, and produce insulin and glucagon hormones for the regulation of blood glucose levels.

c)　The blood glucose concentration is regulated by the negative feedback mechanism.

d)　The clinical abnormality of diabetes mellitus is caused by the insufficient production of insulin.

11. The Anatomy of the Testes and Ovaries

a)　Each of the two testes is the component of the reproductive and endocrine systems and produces the male sex hormone, testosterone.

b)　Testosterone is responsible for the development of secondary male sex characteristics, which include facial and chest hairs, narrow hips, broad shoulders and deep voice.

c)　Each of the two ovaries is an ovum-producing reproductive organ and secretes estrogen and progesterone, which are the female sex hormones.

d)　Estrogen and progesterone are responsible for the development of the female reproductive organs and the development of secondary female sex characteristics, which include the fat deposition on thighs, hips and legs, high-pitched voice, broad hips and breast enlargement.

12. The Anatomy of the Thymus Gland

a)　The thymus gland is regarded as a specialized organ of the immune system that produces the hormone thymosin.

b)　Thymosin stimulates the production of the T-lymphocyte white blood cells (or T cells) that are critical cells of the adaptive immune system and protect the body against the invasion of foreign microbes.

13. The Anatomy of the Pineal Gland

a)　The pineal gland is also known as the pineal body, epiphysis cerebri or epiphysis. It is a small endocrine gland located near the thalamus inside the human brain.

b)　The pineal gland secretes the following hormones:

i)　melatonin, which regulates the body rhythms (wake and sleep patterns) and inhibits the functions of the reproductive system.

ii)　serotonin, which acts as a neurotransmitter and vasoconstrictor.

Common Pathologies

Adrenal Insufficiency
This is a condition in which the production of steroid hormones such as cortisol and aldosterone becomes low. Symptoms include fatigue, stomach upset, dehydration, and skin changes. Addison's disease is a type of adrenal insufficiency.

Cushing's Syndrome
This is a condition in which overproduction of a pituitary gland hormone (ACTH) leads to an overactive adrenal gland. A similar condition called Cushing's disease may occur in people, particularly children, who take high doses of corticosteroid medications.

Gigantism (acromegaly) and other growth hormone problems
This is a condition in which, if the pituitary gland produces too much growth hormone, a child's bones and body parts may grow abnormally fast. If growth hormone levels are too low, a child can stop growing in height.

Hyperthyroidism
This is a condition in which the thyroid gland produces too much thyroid hormone, leading to weight loss, fast heart rate, sweating, and nervousness. The most common cause for an overactive thyroid is an autoimmune disorder called Grave's disease.

Hypothyroidism
This is a condition in which, the thyroid gland does not produce enough thyroid hormone, leading to fatigue, constipation, dry skin, and depression. The underactive gland can cause slowed development in children. Some types of hypothyroidism are present at birth.

Hypopituitarism
This is a condition in which the pituitary gland releases little or no hormones. It may be caused by a number of different diseases. Women with this condition may stop getting their periods.

Polycystic Ovary Syndrome (PCOS)
This is a condition in which overproduction of androgens interfere with the development of eggs and their release from the female ovaries. PCOS is a leading cause of infertility.

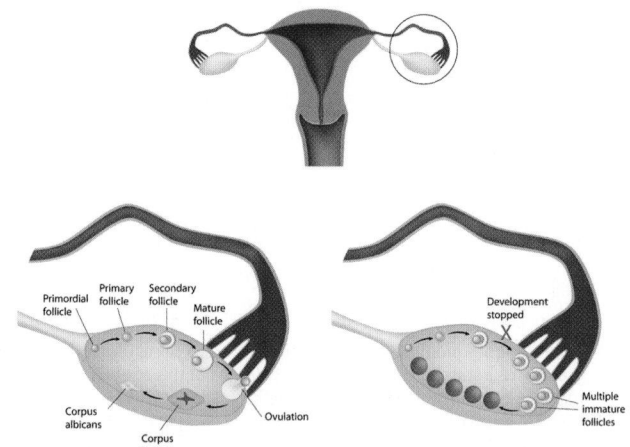

Normal Ovary　　　　*Polycystic Ovary*

Precocious Puberty
This is a condition in which abnormally early puberty occurs when glands tell the body to release sex hormones too soon in life.

Endocrine, nutritional and metabolic diseases (E00-E89)

NOTES All neoplasms, whether functionally active or not, are classified in Chapter 2. Appropriate codes in this chapter (i.e. E05.8, E07.0, E16-E31, E34.-) may be used as additional codes to indicate either functional activity by neoplasms and ectopic endocrine tissue or hyperfunction and hypofunction of endocrine glands associated with neoplasms and other conditions classified elsewhere.

EXCLUDES1 transitory endocrine and metabolic disorders specific to newborn (P70-P74)

This chapter contains the following blocks:

E00-E07   Disorders of thyroid gland
E08-E13   Diabetes mellitus
E15-E16   Other disorders of glucose regulation and pancreatic internal secretion
E20-E35   Disorders of other endocrine glands
E36   Intraoperative complications of endocrine system
E40-E46   Malnutrition
E50-E64   Other nutritional deficiencies
E65-E68   Overweight, obesity and other hyperalimentation
E70-E88   Metabolic disorders
E89   Postprocedural endocrine and metabolic complications and disorders, not elsewhere classified

Disorders of thyroid gland (E00-E07)

E00   Congenital iodine-deficiency syndrome

Use additional code (F70-F79) to identify associated intellectual disabilities.

EXCLUDES1 subclinical iodine-deficiency hypothyroidism (E02)

E00.0   Congenital iodine-deficiency syndrome, neurological type RxHCC

Endemic cretinism, neurological type

E00.1   Congenital iodine-deficiency syndrome, myxedematous type RxHCC

Endemic hypothyroid cretinism
Endemic cretinism, myxedematous type

E00.2   Congenital iodine-deficiency syndrome, mixed type RxHCC

Endemic cretinism, mixed type

E00.9   Congenital iodine-deficiency syndrome, unspecified RxHCC

Congenital iodine-deficiency hypothyroidism NOS
Endemic cretinism NOS

E01   Iodine-deficiency related thyroid disorders and allied conditions

EXCLUDES1 congenital iodine-deficiency syndrome (E00.-)
subclinical iodine-deficiency hypothyroidism (E02)

E01.0   Iodine-deficiency related diffuse (endemic) goiter RxHCC

E01.1   Iodine-deficiency related multinodular (endemic) goiter RxHCC

Iodine-deficiency related nodular goiter

E01.2   Iodine-deficiency related (endemic) goiter, unspecified RxHCC

Endemic goiter NOS

E01.8   Other iodine-deficiency related thyroid disorders and allied conditions RxHCC

Acquired iodine-deficiency hypothyroidism NOS

E02   Subclinical iodine-deficiency hypothyroidism RxHCC

E03   Other hypothyroidism

EXCLUDES1 iodine-deficiency related hypothyroidism (E00-E02)
postprocedural hypothyroidism (E89.0)

E03.0   Congenital hypothyroidism with diffuse goiter RxHCC

Congenital parenchymatous goiter (nontoxic)
Congenital goiter (nontoxic) NOS

EXCLUDES1 transitory congenital goiter with normal function (P72.0)

E03.1   Congenital hypothyroidism without goiter RxHCC

Aplasia of thyroid (with myxedema)
Congenital atrophy of thyroid
Congenital hypothyroidism NOS

E03.2   Hypothyroidism due to medicaments and other exogenous substances RxHCC

Code first poisoning due to drug or toxin, if applicable (T36-T65 with fifth or sixth character 1-4 or 6)
Use additional code for adverse effect, if applicable, to identify drug (T36-T50 with fifth or sixth character 5)

E03.3   Postinfectious hypothyroidism RxHCC

E03.4   Atrophy of thyroid (acquired) RxHCC

EXCLUDES1 congenital atrophy of thyroid (E03.1)

E03.5   Myxedema coma HCC MCC RxHCC CC/MCC Exc

E03.8   Other specified hypothyroidism RxHCC

E03.9   Hypothyroidism, unspecified RxHCC

Myxedema NOS

E04   Other nontoxic goiter

EXCLUDES1 congenital goiter (NOS) (diffuse) (parenchymatous) (E03.0)
iodine-deficiency related goiter (E00-E02)

E04.0   Nontoxic diffuse goiter RxHCC

Diffuse (colloid) nontoxic goiter
Simple nontoxic goiter

E04.1   Nontoxic single thyroid nodule RxHCC

Colloid nodule (cystic) (thyroid)
Nontoxic uninodular goiter
Thyroid (cystic) nodule NOS

E04.2   Nontoxic multinodular goiter RxHCC

Cystic goiter NOS
Multinodular (cystic) goiter NOS

E04.8   Other specified nontoxic goiter RxHCC

E04.9   Nontoxic goiter, unspecified RxHCC

Goiter NOS
Nodular goiter (nontoxic) NOS

E05   Thyrotoxicosis [hyperthyroidism]

EXCLUDES1 chronic thyroiditis with transient thyrotoxicosis (E06.2)
neonatal thyrotoxicosis (P72.1)

E05.0   Thyrotoxicosis with diffuse goiter

Exophthalmic or toxic goiter NOS
Graves' disease
Toxic diffuse goiter

E05.00   Thyrotoxicosis with diffuse goiter without thyrotoxic crisis or storm RxHCC

E05.01   Thyrotoxicosis with diffuse goiter with thyrotoxic crisis or storm MCC RxHCC CC/MCC Exc

E05.1   Thyrotoxicosis with toxic single thyroid nodule

Thyrotoxicosis with toxic uninodular goiter

E05.10   Thyrotoxicosis with toxic single thyroid nodule without thyrotoxic crisis or storm RxHCC

E05.11   Thyrotoxicosis with toxic single thyroid nodule with thyrotoxic crisis or storm MCC RxHCC CC/MCC Exc

E05.2   Thyrotoxicosis with toxic multinodular goiter

Toxic nodular goiter NOS

E05.20   Thyrotoxicosis with toxic multinodular goiter without thyrotoxic crisis or storm RxHCC

E05.21   Thyrotoxicosis with toxic multinodular goiter with thyrotoxic crisis or storm MCC RxHCC CC/MCC Exc

E05.3   Thyrotoxicosis from ectopic thyroid tissue

E05.30   Thyrotoxicosis from ectopic thyroid tissue without thyrotoxic crisis or storm RxHCC

E05.31   Thyrotoxicosis from ectopic thyroid tissue with thyrotoxic crisis or storm MCC RxHCC CC/MCC Exc

E05.4   Thyrotoxicosis factitia

E05.40   Thyrotoxicosis factitia without thyrotoxic crisis or storm RxHCC

E05.41   Thyrotoxicosis factitia with thyrotoxic crisis or storm MCC RxHCC CC/MCC Exc

E05.8   Other thyrotoxicosis

Overproduction of thyroid-stimulating hormone

E05.80   Other thyrotoxicosis without thyrotoxic crisis or storm RxHCC

E05.81   Other thyrotoxicosis with thyrotoxic crisis or storm MCC RxHCC CC/MCC Exc

E05.9   Thyrotoxicosis, unspecified

Hyperthyroidism NOS

E05.90   Thyrotoxicosis, unspecified without thyrotoxic crisis or storm RxHCC

Unspecified Code   Other Specified Code   Manifestation Code   N Newborn   P Pediatric   M Maternity   A Adult   ♂ Male   ♀ Female
● New Code   ▲ Revised Code Title   ▶◀ Revised Text   **NOTES**   *INCLUDES*   *EXCLUDES 1* Not coded here   *EXCLUDES 2* Not included here
④ 4th character required   ⑤ 5th character required   ⑥ 6th character required   ⑦ 7th character required
Ⓧ Extension 'X' Alert   HAC Hospital-acquired condition (HAC) alert   AHA AHA Coding Clinic©

E05.91   **Thyrotoxicosis, unspecified** with thyrotoxic crisis or
            storm   MCC° RxHCC CC/MCC Exc

E06   **Thyroiditis**
       EXCLUDES1 postpartum thyroiditis (O90.5)

       E06.0   **Acute thyroiditis**   CC° RxHCC CC/MCC Exc
                Abscess of thyroid
                Pyogenic thyroiditis
                Suppurative thyroiditis
                Use additional code (B95-B97) to identify infectious agent.

       E06.1   **Subacute thyroiditis**   RxHCC
                de Quervain thyroiditis
                Giant-cell thyroiditis
                Granulomatous thyroiditis
                Nonsuppurative thyroiditis
                Viral thyroiditis
                EXCLUDES1 autoimmune thyroiditis (E06.3)

       E06.2   **Chronic thyroiditis** with transient thyrotoxicosis   RxHCC
                EXCLUDES1 autoimmune thyroiditis (E06.3)

       E06.3   **Autoimmune thyroiditis**   RxHCC
                Hashimoto's thyroiditis
                Hashitoxicosis (transient)
                Lymphadenoid goiter
                Lymphocytic thyroiditis
                Struma lymphomatosa

       E06.4   **Drug-induced thyroiditis**   RxHCC
                Use additional code for adverse effect, if applicable, to
                identify drug (T36-T50 with fifth or sixth character 5)

       E06.5   **Other chronic thyroiditis**   RxHCC
                Chronic fibrous thyroiditis
                Chronic thyroiditis NOS
                Ligneous thyroiditis
                Riedel thyroiditis

       E06.9   **Thyroiditis, unspecified**   RxHCC

E07   **Other disorders of thyroid**

       E07.0   **Hypersecretion of calcitonin**   RxHCC
                C-cell hyperplasia of thyroid
                Hypersecretion of thyrocalcitonin

       E07.1   **Dyshormogenetic goiter**   RxHCC
                Familial dyshormogenetic goiter
                Pendred's syndrome
                EXCLUDES1 transitory congenital goiter with normal function
                (P72.0)

       E07.8   **Other specified disorders of thyroid**
                E07.81   **Sick-euthyroid syndrome**
                          Euthyroid sick-syndrome
                E07.89   **Other specified disorders of thyroid**   RxHCC
                          Abnormality of thyroid-binding globulin
                          Hemorrhage of thyroid
                          Infarction of thyroid

       E07.9   **Disorder of thyroid, unspecified**   RxHCC

Diabetes mellitus (E08-E13)

E08   **Diabetes mellitus** due to underlying condition
       Code first the underlying condition, such as:
       congenital rubella (P35.0)
       Cushing's syndrome (E24.-)
       cystic fibrosis (E84.-)
       malignant neoplasm (C00-C96)
       malnutrition (E40-E46)
       pancreatitis and other diseases of the pancreas (K85-K86.-)
       Use additional code to identify control using:
       insulin (Z79.4)
       oral antidiabetic drugs (Z79.84)
       oral hypoglycemic drugs (Z79.84)
       EXCLUDES1 drug or chemical induced diabetes mellitus (E09.-)
                   gestational diabetes (O24.4-)
                   neonatal diabetes mellitus (P70.2)
                   postpancreatectomy diabetes mellitus (E13.-)
                   postprocedural diabetes mellitus (E13.-)

                   secondary diabetes mellitus NEC (E13.-)
                   type 1 diabetes mellitus (E10.-)
                   type 2 diabetes mellitus (E11.-)

       E08.0   **Diabetes mellitus due to underlying condition with**
                hyperosmolarity
                E08.00   **Diabetes mellitus due to underlying condition with**
                          hyperosmolarity without nonketotic hyperglycemic-
                          hyperosmolar coma (NKHHC)   HAC HCC MCC° RxHCC CC/MCC Exc
                E08.01   **Diabetes mellitus due to underlying condition with**
                          hyperosmolarity with coma   HAC HCC MCC° RxHCC CC/MCC Exc

       E08.1   **Diabetes mellitus due to underlying condition with**
                ketoacidosis
                E08.10   **Diabetes mellitus due to underlying condition with**
                          ketoacidosis without coma   HAC HCC MCC° RxHCC CC/MCC Exc
                E08.11   **Diabetes mellitus due to underlying condition with**
                          ketoacidosis with coma   HCC MCC° RxHCC CC/MCC Exc

       E08.2   **Diabetes mellitus due to underlying condition with** kidney
                complications
                E08.21   **Diabetes mellitus due to underlying condition with**
                          diabetic nephropathy   HCC RxHCC
                          Diabetes mellitus due to underlying condition with
                             intercapillary glomerulosclerosis
                          Diabetes mellitus due to underlying condition with
                             intracapillary glomerulonephrosis
                          Diabetes mellitus due to underlying condition with
                             Kimmelstiel-Wilson disease
                E08.22   **Diabetes mellitus due to underlying condition with**
                          diabetic chronic kidney disease   HCC RxHCC
                          Use additional code to identify stage of chronic
                          kidney disease (N18.1-N18.6)
                E08.29   **Diabetes mellitus due to underlying condition with**
                          other diabetic kidney complication   HCC RxHCC
                          Renal tubular degeneration in diabetes mellitus due
                             to underlying condition

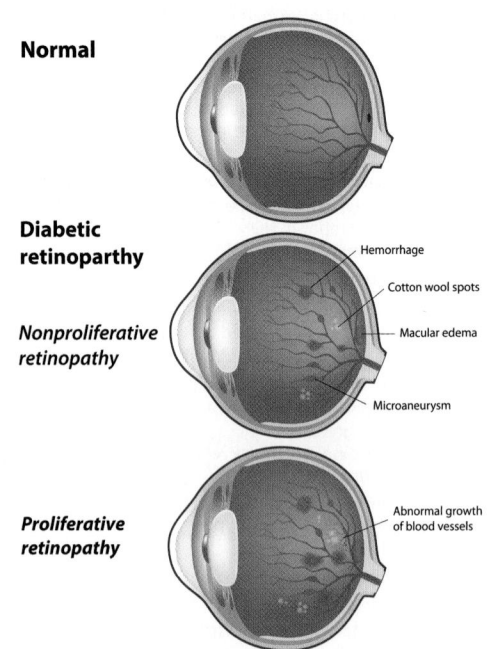

Normal

Diabetic retinoparthy

Nonproliferative retinopathy

Proliferative retinopathy

Hemorrhage
Cotton wool spots
Macular edema
Microaneurism
Abnormal growth of blood vessels

Figure 4.1 Diabetic retinopathy

       E08.3   **Diabetes mellitus due to underlying condition with**
                ophthalmic complications
                E08.31   **Diabetes mellitus due to underlying condition with**
                          unspecified diabetic retinopathy
                          E08.311   **Diabetes mellitus due to underlying**
                                     condition with unspecified diabetic
                                     retinopathy with macular edema   HCC RxHCC

PDx Unacceptable principal diagnosis symbol per Medicare code edits   POA Code exempt from diagnosis present on admission requirement
? Questionable admission   CC° Complication or comorbidity   CC/MCC Exc CC/MCC exclusion   MCC° Major complication or comorbidity
PDx Principal diagnosis as its own CC   PDx Principal diagnosis as its own MCC   HCC HCC diagnosis code   RxHCC RxHCC diagnosis code
MACRA code   Z1 Z code as first-listed diagnosis

E08.319 Diabetes mellitus due to underlying condition with unspecified diabetic retinopathy without macular edema HCC RxHCC

6th E08.32 Diabetes mellitus due to underlying condition with mild nonproliferative diabetic retinopathy

Diabetes mellitus due to underlying condition with nonproliferative diabetic retinopathy NOS

One of the following 7th characters is to be assigned to codes in subcategory E08.32 to designate laterality of the disease:

1 = right eye
2 = left eye
3 = bilateral
9 = unspecified eye

7th E08.321 Diabetes mellitus due to underlying condition with mild nonproliferative diabetic retinopathy with macular edema HCC RxHCC

7th E08.329 Diabetes mellitus due to underlying condition with mild nonproliferative diabetic retinopathy without macular edema HCC RxHCC

6th E08.33 Diabetes mellitus due to underlying condition with moderate nonproliferative diabetic retinopathy

One of the following 7th characters is to be assigned to codes in subcategory E08.33 to designate laterality of the disease:

1 = right eye
2 = left eye
3 = bilateral
9 = unspecified eye

7th E08.331 Diabetes mellitus due to underlying condition with moderate nonproliferative diabetic retinopathy with macular edema HCC RxHCC

7th E08.339 Diabetes mellitus due to underlying condition with moderate nonproliferative diabetic retinopathy without macular edema HCC RxHCC

6th E08.34 Diabetes mellitus due to underlying condition with severe nonproliferative diabetic retinopathy

One of the following 7th characters is to be assigned to codes in subcategory E08.34 to designate laterality of the disease:

1 = right eye
2 = left eye
3 = bilateral
9 = unspecified eye

7th E08.341 Diabetes mellitus due to underlying condition with severe nonproliferative diabetic retinopathy with macular edema HCC RxHCC

7th E08.349 Diabetes mellitus due to underlying condition with severe nonproliferative diabetic retinopathy without macular edema HCC RxHCC

6th E08.35 Diabetes mellitus due to underlying condition with proliferative diabetic retinopathy

One of the following 7th characters is to be assigned to codes in subcategory E08.35 to designate laterality of the disease:

1 = right eye
2 = left eye
3 = bilateral
9 = unspecified eye

7th E08.351 Diabetes mellitus due to underlying condition with proliferative diabetic retinopathy with macular edema HCC RxHCC

7th E08.352 Diabetes mellitus due to underlying condition with proliferative diabetic retinopathy with traction retinal detachment involving the macula HCC RxHCC

7th E08.353 Diabetes mellitus due to underlying condition with proliferative diabetic retinopathy with traction retinal detachment not involving the macula HCC RxHCC

7th E08.354 Diabetes mellitus due to underlying condition with proliferative diabetic retinopathy with combined traction retinal detachment and rhegmatogenous retinal detachment HCC RxHCC

7th E08.355 Diabetes mellitus due to underlying condition with stable proliferative diabetic retinopathy HCC RxHCC

7th E08.359 Diabetes mellitus due to underlying condition with proliferative diabetic retinopathy without macular edema HCC RxHCC

E08.36 Diabetes mellitus due to underlying condition with diabetic cataract HCC RxHCC

7th E08.37 Diabetes mellitus due to underlying condition with diabetic macular edema, resolved following treatment HCC RxHCC

One of the following 7th characters is to be assigned to code E08.37 to designate laterality of the disease:

1 = right eye
2 = left eye
3 = bilateral
9 = unspecified eye

E08.39 Diabetes mellitus due to underlying condition with other diabetic ophthalmic complication HCC RxHCC

Use additional code to identify manifestation, such as:

diabetic glaucoma (H40-H42)

5th E08.4 Diabetes mellitus due to underlying condition with neurological complications

E08.40 Diabetes mellitus due to underlying condition with diabetic neuropathy, unspecified HCC RxHCC

E08.41 Diabetes mellitus due to underlying condition with diabetic mononeuropathy HCC RxHCC

E08.42 Diabetes mellitus due to underlying condition with diabetic polyneuropathy HCC RxHCC

Diabetes mellitus due to underlying condition with diabetic neuralgia

E08.43 Diabetes mellitus due to underlying condition with diabetic autonomic (poly)neuropathy HCC RxHCC

AHA: Q4 2013

Diabetes mellitus due to underlying condition with diabetic gastroparesis

E08.44 Diabetes mellitus due to underlying condition with diabetic amyotrophy HCC RxHCC

E08.49 Diabetes mellitus due to underlying condition with other diabetic neurological complication HCC RxHCC

5th E08.5 Diabetes mellitus due to underlying condition with circulatory complications

E08.51 Diabetes mellitus due to underlying condition with diabetic peripheral angiopathy without gangrene HCC RxHCC

E08.52 Diabetes mellitus due to underlying condition with diabetic peripheral angiopathy with gangrene CC HCC PDx ⬆ RxHCC CC/MCC Exc

Diabetes mellitus due to underlying condition with diabetic gangrene

E08.59 Diabetes mellitus due to underlying condition with other circulatory complications HCC RxHCC

5th E08.6 Diabetes mellitus due to underlying condition with other specified complications

6th E08.61 Diabetes mellitus due to underlying condition with diabetic arthropathy

E08.610 Diabetes mellitus due to underlying condition with diabetic neuropathic arthropathy HCC RxHCC

Diabetes mellitus due to underlying condition with Charcôt's joints

Unspecified Code   Other Specified Code   Manifestation Code   N Newborn   P Pediatric   M Maternity   A Adult   ♂ Male   ♀ Female
● New Code   ▲ Revised Code Title   ►◄ Revised Text   NOTES   INCLUDES   EXCLUDES 1 Not coded here   EXCLUDES 2 Not included here
4th character required   5th character required   6th character required   7th character required
Extension 'X' Alert   HAC Hospital-acquired condition (HAC) alert   AHA AHA Coding Clinic©

CHAPTER 4: ENDOCRINE, NUTRITIONAL AND METABOLIC DISEASES (E00-E89)

E13.359 - E16.9

E13.359 Other specified diabetes mellitus with proliferative diabetic retinopathy without macular edema HCC RxHCC

E13.36 Other specified diabetes mellitus with diabetic cataract HCC RxHCC

E13.37 Other specified diabetes mellitus with diabetic macular edema, resolved following treatment HCC RxHCC
One of the following 7th characters is to be assigned to code E13.37 to designate laterality of the disease:
1 = right eye
2 = left eye
3 = bilateral
9 = unspecified eye

E13.39 Other specified diabetes mellitus with other diabetic ophthalmic complication HCC RxHCC
Use additional code to identify manifestation, such as:
diabetic glaucoma (H40-H42)

E13.4 Other specified diabetes mellitus with neurological complications

E13.40 Other specified diabetes mellitus with diabetic neuropathy, unspecified HCC RxHCC

E13.41 Other specified diabetes mellitus with diabetic mononeuropathy HCC RxHCC

E13.42 Other specified diabetes mellitus with diabetic polyneuropathy HCC RxHCC
Other specified diabetes mellitus with diabetic neuralgia

E13.43 Other specified diabetes mellitus with diabetic autonomic (poly)neuropathy HCC RxHCC
AHA: Q4 2013
Other specified diabetes mellitus with diabetic gastroparesis

E13.44 Other specified diabetes mellitus with diabetic amyotrophy HCC RxHCC

E13.49 Other specified diabetes mellitus with other diabetic neurological complication HCC RxHCC

E13.5 Other specified diabetes mellitus with circulatory complications

E13.51 Other specified diabetes mellitus with diabetic peripheral angiopathy without gangrene HCC RxHCC

E13.52 Other specified diabetes mellitus with diabetic peripheral angiopathy with gangrene PDx HCC PCC RxHCC CC/MCC Exc
Other specified diabetes mellitus with diabetic gangrene

E13.59 Other specified diabetes mellitus with other circulatory complications HCC RxHCC

E13.6 Other specified diabetes mellitus with other specified complications

E13.61 Other specified diabetes mellitus with diabetic arthropathy

E13.610 Other specified diabetes mellitus with diabetic neuropathic arthropathy HCC RxHCC
Other specified diabetes mellitus with Charcôt's joints

E13.618 Other specified diabetes mellitus with other diabetic arthropathy HCC RxHCC

E13.62 Other specified diabetes mellitus with skin complications

E13.620 Other specified diabetes mellitus with diabetic dermatitis HCC RxHCC
Other specified diabetes mellitus with diabetic necrobiosis lipoidica

E13.621 Other specified diabetes mellitus with foot ulcer HCC RxHCC
Use additional code to identify site of ulcer (L97.4-, L97.5-)

E13.622 Other specified diabetes mellitus with other skin ulcer HCC RxHCC
Use additional code to identify site of ulcer (L97.1-L97.9, L98.41-L98.49)

E13.628 Other specified diabetes mellitus with other skin complications HCC RxHCC

E13.63 Other specified diabetes mellitus with oral complications

E13.630 Other specified diabetes mellitus with periodontal disease HCC RxHCC

E13.638 Other specified diabetes mellitus with other oral complications HCC RxHCC

E13.64 Other specified diabetes mellitus with hypoglycemia

E13.641 Other specified diabetes mellitus with hypoglycemia with coma HCC MCC RxHCC CC/MCC Exc

E13.649 Other specified diabetes mellitus with hypoglycemia without coma HCC RxHCC

E13.65 Other specified diabetes mellitus with hyperglycemia HCC RxHCC

E13.69 Other specified diabetes mellitus with other specified complication HCC RxHCC
AHA: Q4 2016
Use additional code to identify complication

E13.8 Other specified diabetes mellitus with unspecified complications HCC RxHCC

E13.9 Other specified diabetes mellitus without complications HCC ? RxHCC

Other disorders of glucose regulation and pancreatic internal secretion (E15-E16)

E15 Nondiabetic hypoglycemic coma CC HAC HCC CC/MCC Exc
INCLUDES drug-induced insulin coma in nondiabetic
hyperinsulinism with hypoglycemic coma
hypoglycemic coma NOS

E16 Other disorders of pancreatic internal secretion

E16.0 Drug-induced hypoglycemia without coma
EXCLUDES1 diabetes with hypoglycemia without coma ▶(E09.649)◄
Use additional code for adverse effect, if applicable, to identify drug (T36-T50 with fifth or sixth character 5)

E16.1 Other hypoglycemia
Functional hyperinsulinism
Functional nonhyperinsulinemic hypoglycemia
Hyperinsulinism NOS
Hyperplasia of pancreatic islet beta cells NOS
EXCLUDES1 diabetes with hypoglycemia (E08.649, E10.649, E11.649, E13.649)
hypoglycemia in infant of diabetic mother (P70.1)
neonatal hypoglycemia (P70.4)

E16.2 Hypoglycemia, unspecified
AHA: Q3 2016
EXCLUDES1 diabetes with hypoglycemia (E08.649, E10.649, E11.649, E13.649)

E16.3 Increased secretion of glucagon RxHCC
Hyperplasia of pancreatic endocrine cells with glucagon excess

E16.4 Increased secretion of gastrin RxHCC
Hypergastrinemia
Hyperplasia of pancreatic endocrine cells with gastrin excess
Zollinger-Ellison syndrome

E16.8 Other specified disorders of pancreatic internal secretion RxHCC
Increased secretion from endocrine pancreas of growth hormone-releasing hormone
Increased secretion from endocrine pancreas of pancreatic polypeptide
Increased secretion from endocrine pancreas of somatostatin
Increased secretion from endocrine pancreas of vasoactive-intestinal polypeptide

E16.9 Disorder of pancreatic internal secretion, unspecified RxHCC
Islet-cell hyperplasia NOS
Pancreatic endocrine cell hyperplasia NOS

PDx Unacceptable principal diagnosis symbol per Medicare code edits   Code exempt from diagnosis present on admission requirement
? Questionable admission   CC Complication or comorbidity   CC/MCC Exc CC/MCC exclusion   MCC Major complication or comorbidity
PDx CC Principal diagnosis as its own CC   PDx MCC Principal diagnosis as its own MCC   HCC HCC diagnosis code   RxHCC RxHCC diagnosis code
MACRA code   Z code as first-listed diagnosis

Disorders of other endocrine glands (E20-E35)

EXCLUDES1 *galactorrhea (N64.3)*

gynecomastia (N62)

4ᵗʰ **E20 Hypoparathyroidism**

EXCLUDES1 *Di George's syndrome (D82.1)*

postprocedural hypoparathyroidism (E89.2)

tetany NOS (R29.0)

transitory neonatal hypoparathyroidism (P71.4)

E20.0 Idiopathic **hypoparathyroidism**   HCC RxHCC

E20.1 Pseudohypoparathyroidism

E20.8 **Other hypoparathyroidism**   HCC RxHCC

E20.9 **Hypoparathyroidism, unspecified**   HCC RxHCC

Parathyroid tetany

4ᵗʰ **E21 Hyperparathyroidism and other disorders of parathyroid gland**

EXCLUDES1 *adult osteomalacia (M83.-)*

ectopic hyperparathyroidism (E34.2)

familial hypocalciuric hypercalcemia (E83.52)

hungry bone syndrome (E83.81)

infantile and juvenile osteomalacia (E55.0)

E21.0 Primary **hyperparathyroidism**   HCC RxHCC

Hyperplasia of parathyroid

Osteitis fibrosa cystica generalisata [von Recklinghausen's disease of bone]

E21.1 Secondary **hyperparathyroidism, not elsewhere classified**   HCC RxHCC

EXCLUDES1 *secondary hyperparathyroidism of renal origin (N25.81)*

E21.2 **Other hyperparathyroidism**   HCC RxHCC

Tertiary hyperparathyroidism

EXCLUDES1 *familial hypocalciuric hypercalcemia (E83.52)*

E21.3 **Hyperparathyroidism, unspecified**   HCC RxHCC

E21.4 Other specified disorders of parathyroid gland   HCC RxHCC

E21.5 **Disorder of parathyroid gland, unspecified**   HCC RxHCC

4ᵗʰ **E22 Hyperfunction of pituitary gland**

EXCLUDES1 *Cushing's syndrome (E24.-)*

Nelson's syndrome (E24.1)

overproduction of ACTH not associated with Cushing's disease (E27.0)

overproduction of pituitary ACTH (E24.0)

overproduction of thyroid-stimulating hormone (E05.8-)

E22.0 **Acromegaly and pituitary gigantism**   HCC RxHCC

Overproduction of growth hormone

EXCLUDES1 *constitutional gigantism (E34.4)*

constitutional tall stature (E34.4)

increased secretion from endocrine pancreas of growth hormone-releasing hormone (E16.8)

E22.1 **Hyperprolactinemia**   cc⊘ HCC RxHCC CC/MCC Exc

Use additional code for adverse effect, if applicable, to identify drug (T36-T50 with fifth or sixth character 5)

E22.2 **Syndrome of inappropriate secretion of antidiuretic hormone**   cc⊘ HCC RxHCC CC/MCC Exc

E22.8 **Other hyperfunction of pituitary gland**   cc⊘ HCC RxHCC CC/MCC Exc

Central precocious puberty

E22.9 **Hyperfunction of pituitary gland, unspecified**   cc⊘ HCC RxHCC CC/MCC Exc

4ᵗʰ **E23 Hypofunction and other disorders of the pituitary gland**

INCLUDES   *the listed conditions whether the disorder is in the pituitary or the hypothalamus*

EXCLUDES1 *postprocedural hypopituitarism (E89.3)*

E23.0 **Hypopituitarism**   cc⊘ HCC RxHCC CC/MCC Exc

Fertile eunuch syndrome

Hypogonadotropic hypogonadism

Idiopathic growth hormone deficiency

Isolated deficiency of gonadotropin

Isolated deficiency of growth hormone

Isolated deficiency of pituitary hormone

Kallmann's syndrome

Lorain-Levi short stature

Necrosis of pituitary gland (postpartum)

Panhypopituitarism

Pituitary cachexia

Pituitary insufficiency NOS

Pituitary short stature

Sheehan's syndrome

Simmonds' disease

E23.1 **Drug-induced hypopituitarism**   HCC RxHCC

Use additional code for adverse effect, if applicable, to identify drug (T36-T50 with fifth or sixth character 5)

E23.2 **Diabetes insipidus**   cc⊘ HCC RxHCC CC/MCC Exc

EXCLUDES1 *nephrogenic diabetes insipidus (N25.1)*

E23.3 **Hypothalamic dysfunction, not elsewhere classified**   HCC RxHCC

EXCLUDES1 *Prader-Willi syndrome (Q87.1)*

Russell-Silver syndrome (Q87.1)

E23.6 **Other disorders of pituitary gland**   HCC RxHCC

Abscess of pituitary

Adiposogenital dystrophy

E23.7 **Disorder of pituitary gland, unspecified**   HCC RxHCC

4ᵗʰ **E24 Cushing's syndrome**

EXCLUDES1 *congenital adrenal hyperplasia (E25.0)*

E24.0 Pituitary-dependent **Cushing's disease**   cc⊘ HCC RxHCC CC/MCC Exc

Overproduction of pituitary ACTH

Pituitary-dependent hypercorticalism

E24.1 Nelson's syndrome   HCC RxHCC

E24.2 Drug-induced **Cushing's syndrome**   cc⊘ HCC RxHCC CC/MCC Exc

Use additional code for adverse effect, if applicable, to identify drug (T36-T50 with fifth or sixth character 5)

E24.3 Ectopic ACTH syndrome   cc⊘ HCC RxHCC CC/MCC Exc

E24.4 Alcohol-induced pseudo-**Cushing's syndrome**   cc⊘ HCC RxHCC CC/MCC Exc

E24.8 **Other Cushing's syndrome**   cc⊘ HCC RxHCC CC/MCC Exc

E24.9 **Cushing's syndrome, unspecified**   cc⊘ HCC RxHCC CC/MCC Exc

4ᵗʰ **E25 Adrenogenital disorders**

INCLUDES   *adrenogenital syndromes, virilizing or feminizing, whether acquired or due to adrenal hyperplasia consequent on inborn enzyme defects in hormone synthesis*

Female adrenal pseudohermaphroditism

Female heterosexual precocious pseudopuberty

Male isosexual precocious pseudopuberty

Male macrogenitosomia praecox

Male sexual precocity with adrenal hyperplasia

Male virilization (female)

EXCLUDES1 *indeterminate sex and pseudohermaphroditism (Q56)*

chromosomal abnormalities (Q90-Q99)

E25.0 Congenital **adrenogenital disorders** associated with enzyme deficiency   HCC RxHCC

Congenital adrenal hyperplasia

21-Hydroxylase deficiency

Salt-losing congenital adrenal hyperplasia

E25.8 **Other adrenogenital disorders**   HCC RxHCC

Idiopathic adrenogenital disorder

Use additional code for adverse effect, if applicable, to identify drug (T36-T50 with fifth or sixth character 5)

E25.9 **Adrenogenital disorder, unspecified**   HCC RxHCC

Adrenogenital syndrome NOS

4ᵗʰ **E26 Hyperaldosteronism**

5ᵗʰ E26.0 Primary **hyperaldosteronism**

E26.01 **Conn's syndrome**   HCC RxHCC

Code also adrenal adenoma (D35.0-)

E26.02 **Glucocorticoid-remediable aldosteronism**   HCC RxHCC

Familial aldosteronism type I

E26.09 **Other primary hyperaldosteronism**   HCC RxHCC

Primary aldosteronism due to adrenal hyperplasia (bilateral)

E26.1 Secondary **hyperaldosteronism**   HCC RxHCC

5ᵗʰ E26.8 **Other hyperaldosteronism**

E26.81 **Bartter's syndrome**   HCC RxHCC

E26.89 **Other hyperaldosteronism**   HCC RxHCC

Unspecified Code   Other Specified Code   Manifestation Code   Ⓝ Newborn   Ⓟ Pediatric   Ⓜ Maternity   Ⓐ Adult   ♂ Male   ♀ Female

● New Code   ▲ Revised Code Title   ▶◀ Revised Text   **NOTES**   *INCLUDES*   *EXCLUDES1* Not coded here   *EXCLUDES2* Not included here

4ᵗʰ 4ᵗʰ character required   5ᵗʰ 5ᵗʰ character required   6ᵗʰ 6ᵗʰ character required   7ᵗʰ 7ᵗʰ character required

Ⓧ Extension 'X' Alert   HAC Hospital-acquired condition (HAC) alert   **AHA** AHA Coding Clinic©

E26.9 **Hyperaldosteronism, unspecified** `HCC` `RxHCC`
 Aldosteronism NOS
 Hyperaldosteronism NOS

E27 **Other disorders of adrenal gland**
 E27.0 **Other adrenocortical overactivity** `c⊘` `HCC` `RxHCC` `cc/mcc Exc`
  Overproduction of ACTH, not associated with Cushing's
   disease
  Premature adrenarche
  EXCLUDES1 *Cushing's syndrome (E24.-)*

 E27.1 **Primary adrenocortical insufficiency** `c⊘` `HCC` `RxHCC` `cc/mcc Exc`
  Addison's disease
  Autoimmune adrenalitis
  EXCLUDES1 *Addison only phenotype adrenoleukodystrophy*
   (E71.528)
    amyloidosis (E85.-)
    tuberculous Addison's disease (A18.7)
    Waterhouse-Friderichsen syndrome (A39.1)

 E27.2 **Addisonian crisis** `c⊘` `HCC` `RxHCC` `cc/mcc Exc`
  Adrenal crisis
  Adrenocortical crisis

 E27.3 **Drug-induced adrenocortical insufficiency** `c⊘` `HCC` `RxHCC` `cc/mcc Exc`
  Use additional code for adverse effect, if applicable, to
   identify drug (T36-T50 with fifth or sixth character 5)

 E27.4 **Other and unspecified adrenocortical insufficiency**
  EXCLUDES1 *adrenoleukodystrophy [Addison-Schilder] (E71.528)*
    Waterhouse-Friderichsen syndrome (A39.1)
  E27.40 **Unspecified adrenocortical**
   insufficiency `c⊘` `HCC` `RxHCC` `cc/mcc Exc`
    Adrenocortical insufficiency NOS
    Hypoaldosteronism
  E27.49 **Other adrenocortical insufficiency** `c⊘` `HCC` `RxHCC` `cc/mcc Exc`
    Adrenal hemorrhage
    Adrenal infarction

 E27.5 **Adrenomedullary hyperfunction** `c⊘` `HCC` `RxHCC` `cc/mcc Exc`
  Adrenomedullary hyperplasia
  Catecholamine hypersecretion

 E27.8 **Other specified disorders of adrenal gland** `HCC` `RxHCC`
  Abnormality of cortisol-binding globulin

 E27.9 **Disorder of adrenal gland, unspecified** `HCC` `RxHCC`

E28 **Ovarian dysfunction**
 EXCLUDES1 *isolated gonadotropin deficiency (E23.0)*
    postprocedural ovarian failure (E89.4-)

 E28.0 **Estrogen excess** ♀
  Use additional code for adverse effect, if applicable, to
   identify drug (T36-T50 with fifth or sixth character 5)

 E28.1 **Androgen excess** ♀
  Hypersecretion of ovarian androgens
  Use additional code for adverse effect, if applicable, to
   identify drug (T36-T50 with fifth or sixth character 5)

 E28.2 **Polycystic ovarian syndrome** ♀
  Sclerocystic ovary syndrome
  Stein-Leventhal syndrome

 E28.3 **Primary ovarian failure**
  EXCLUDES1 *pure gonadal dysgenesis (Q99.1)*
    Turner's syndrome (Q96.-)
  E28.31 **Premature menopause**
   E28.310 **Symptomatic premature menopause** `A` ♀
    Symptoms such as flushing, sleeplessness,
     headache, lack of concentration,
     associated with premature menopause
   E28.319 **Asymptomatic premature menopause** `A` ♀
    Premature menopause NOS
  E28.39 **Other primary ovarian failure** ♀
    Decreased estrogen
    Resistant ovary syndrome

 E28.8 **Other ovarian dysfunction** ♀
  Ovarian hyperfunction NOS
  EXCLUDES1 *postprocedural ovarian failure (E89.4-)*

 E28.9 **Ovarian dysfunction, unspecified** ♀

E29 **Testicular dysfunction**
 EXCLUDES1 *androgen insensitivity syndrome (E34.5-)*
    azoospermia or oligospermia NOS (N46.0-N46.1)
    isolated gonadotropin deficiency (E23.0)
    Klinefelter's syndrome (Q98.0-Q98.1, Q98.4)

 E29.0 **Testicular hyperfunction** ♂
  Hypersecretion of testicular hormones

 E29.1 **Testicular hypofunction** ♂
  Defective biosynthesis of testicular androgen NOS
  5-delta-Reductase deficiency (with male
   pseudohermaphroditism)
  Testicular hypogonadism NOS
  Use additional code for adverse effect, if applicable, to
   identify drug (T36-T50 with fifth or sixth character 5)
  EXCLUDES1 *postprocedural testicular hypofunction (E89.5)*

 E29.8 **Other testicular dysfunction** ♂
 E29.9 **Testicular dysfunction, unspecified** ♂

E30 **Disorders of puberty, not elsewhere classified**
 E30.0 **Delayed puberty**
  Constitutional delay of puberty
  Delayed sexual development

 E30.1 **Precocious puberty** `P`
  Precocious menstruation
  EXCLUDES1 *Albright (-McCune) (-Sternberg) syndrome (Q78.1)*
    central precocious puberty (E22.8)
    congenital adrenal hyperplasia (E25.0)
    female heterosexual precocious pseudopuberty (E25.-)
    male isosexual precocious pseudopuberty (E25.-)

 E30.8 **Other disorders of puberty** `P`
  Premature thelarche

 E30.9 **Disorder of puberty, unspecified**

E31 **Polyglandular dysfunction**
 EXCLUDES1 *ataxia telangiectasia [Louis-Bar] (G11.3)*
    dystrophia myotonica [Steinert] (G71.11)
    pseudohypoparathyroidism (E20.1)

 E31.0 **Autoimmune polyglandular failure** `HCC` `RxHCC`
  Schmidt's syndrome

 E31.1 **Polyglandular hyperfunction** `HCC` `RxHCC`
  EXCLUDES1 *multiple endocrine adenomatosis (E31.2-)*
    multiple endocrine neoplasia (E31.2-)

 E31.2 **Multiple endocrine neoplasia [MEN] syndromes**
  Multiple endocrine adenomatosis
  Code also any associated malignancies and other conditions
   associated with the syndromes
  E31.20 **Multiple endocrine neoplasia [MEN] syndrome,**
   unspecified `HCC` `RxHCC`
    Multiple endocrine adenomatosis NOS
    Multiple endocrine neoplasia [MEN] syndrome NOS
  E31.21 **Multiple endocrine neoplasia [MEN] type I** `HCC` `RxHCC`
    Wermer's syndrome
  E31.22 **Multiple endocrine neoplasia [MEN] type IIA** `HCC` `RxHCC`
    Sipple's syndrome
  E31.23 **Multiple endocrine neoplasia [MEN] type IIB** `HCC` `RxHCC`
 E31.8 **Other polyglandular dysfunction** `HCC` `RxHCC`
 E31.9 **Polyglandular dysfunction, unspecified** `HCC` `RxHCC`

E32 **Diseases of thymus**
 EXCLUDES1 *aplasia or hypoplasia of thymus with immunodeficiency*
   (D82.1)
    myasthenia gravis (G70.0)

 E32.0 **Persistent hyperplasia of thymus** `HCC` `RxHCC`
  Hypertrophy of thymus

 E32.1 **Abscess of thymus** `c⊘` `HCC` `RxHCC` `cc/mcc Exc`

 E32.8 **Other diseases of thymus** `HCC` `RxHCC`
  EXCLUDES1 *aplasia or hypoplasia with immunodeficiency (D82.1)*
    thymoma (D15.0)

 E32.9 **Disease of thymus, unspecified** `HCC` `RxHCC`

E34 **Other endocrine disorders**
 EXCLUDES1 *pseudohypoparathyroidism (E20.1)*

`PDx` Unacceptable principal diagnosis symbol per Medicare code edits `PoA` Code exempt from diagnosis present on admission requirement
`?` Questionable admission `c⊘` Complication or comorbidity `cc/mcc Exc` CC/MCC exclusion `mcc⊘` Major complication or comorbidity
`CC` Principal diagnosis as its own CC `MCC` Principal diagnosis as its own MCC `HCC` HCC diagnosis code `RxHCC` RxHCC diagnosis code
MACRA code `Z1` Z code as first-listed diagnosis

E34.0 **Carcinoid syndrome** CC⊕ HCC RxHCC CC/MCC Exc⊕
    NOTES May be used as an additional code to identify functional activity associated with a carcinoid tumor.

E34.1 **Other hypersecretion of intestinal hormones**

E34.2 **Ectopic hormone secretion, not elsewhere classified**
    EXCLUDES1 ectopic ACTH syndrome (E24.3)

E34.3 **Short stature due to endocrine disorder**
    Constitutional short stature
    Laron-type short stature
    EXCLUDES1 achondroplastic short stature (Q77.4)
        hypochondroplastic short stature (Q77.4)
        nutritional short stature (E45)
        pituitary short stature (E23.0)
        progeria (E34.8)
        renal short stature (N25.0)
        Russell-Silver syndrome (Q87.1)
        short-limbed stature with immunodeficiency (D82.2)
        short stature in specific dysmorphic syndromes - code to syndrome - see Alphabetical Index
        short stature NOS (R62.52)

E34.4 **Constitutional tall stature** HCC RxHCC
    Constitutional gigantism

5ᵗʰ E34.5 **Androgen insensitivity syndrome**
    E34.50 **Androgen insensitivity syndrome, unspecified**
        Androgen insensitivity NOS
    E34.51 **Complete androgen insensitivity syndrome**
        Complete androgen insensitivity
        de Quervain syndrome
        Goldberg-Maxwell syndrome
    E34.52 **Partial androgen insensitivity syndrome**
        Partial androgen insensitivity
        Reifenstein syndrome

E34.8 **Other specified endocrine disorders**
    Pineal gland dysfunction
    Progeria
    EXCLUDES2 pseudohypoparathyroidism (E20.1)

E34.9 **Endocrine disorder, unspecified**
    Endocrine disturbance NOS
    Hormone disturbance NOS

E35 **Disorders of endocrine glands in diseases classified elsewhere**
    Code first underlying disease, such as:
    late congenital syphilis of thymus gland [Dubois disease] (A50.5)
    Use additional code, if applicable, to identify:
    sequelae of tuberculosis of other organs (B90.8)
    EXCLUDES1 Echinococcus granulosus infection of thyroid gland (B67.3)
        meningococcal hemorrhagic adrenalitis (A39.1)
        syphilis of endocrine gland (A52.79)
        tuberculosis of adrenal gland, except calcification (A18.7)
        tuberculosis of endocrine gland NEC (A18.82)
        tuberculosis of thyroid gland (A18.81)
        Waterhouse-Friderichsen syndrome (A39.1)

Intraoperative complications of endocrine system (E36)

4ᵗʰ E36 **Intraoperative complications of endocrine system**
    EXCLUDES2 postprocedural endocrine and metabolic complications and disorders, not elsewhere classified (E89.-)

5ᵗʰ E36.0 **Intraoperative hemorrhage and hematoma of an endocrine system organ or structure complicating a procedure**
    EXCLUDES1 intraoperative hemorrhage and hematoma of an endocrine system organ or structure due to accidental puncture or laceration during a procedure (E36.1-)
    E36.01 **Intraoperative hemorrhage and hematoma of an endocrine system organ or structure complicating an endocrine system procedure** CC⊕ CC/MCC Exc⊕
    E36.02 **Intraoperative hemorrhage and hematoma of an endocrine system organ or structure complicating other procedure** CC⊕ CC/MCC Exc⊕

5ᵗʰ E36.1 **Accidental puncture and laceration of an endocrine system organ or structure during a procedure**
    E36.11 **Accidental puncture and laceration of an endocrine system organ or structure during an endocrine system procedure** CC⊕ CC/MCC Exc⊕
    E36.12 **Accidental puncture and laceration of an endocrine system organ or structure during other procedure** CC⊕ CC/MCC Exc⊕

E36.8 **Other intraoperative complications of endocrine system**
    Use additional code, if applicable, to further specify disorder

Malnutrition (E40-E46)

    EXCLUDES1 intestinal malabsorption (K90.-)
        sequelae of protein-calorie malnutrition (E64.0)
    EXCLUDES2 nutritional anemias (D50-D53)
        starvation (T73.0)

E40 **Kwashiorkor** HCC MCC⊕ CC/MCC Exc⊕
    Severe malnutrition with nutritional edema with dyspigmentation of skin and hair
    EXCLUDES1 marasmic kwashiorkor (E42)

E41 **Nutritional marasmus** HCC MCC⊕ CC/MCC Exc⊕
    Severe malnutrition with marasmus
    EXCLUDES1 marasmic kwashiorkor (E42)

E42 **Marasmic kwashiorkor** HCC MCC⊕ CC/MCC Exc⊕
    Intermediate form severe protein-calorie malnutrition
    Severe protein-calorie malnutrition with signs of both kwashiorkor and marasmus

E43 **Unspecified severe protein-calorie malnutrition** HCC MCC⊕ CC/MCC Exc⊕
    Starvation edema

4ᵗʰ E44 **Protein-calorie malnutrition of moderate and mild degree**
    E44.0 **Moderate protein-calorie malnutrition** CC⊕ HCC CC/MCC Exc⊕
    E44.1 **Mild protein-calorie malnutrition** CC⊕ HCC CC/MCC Exc⊕

E45 **Retarded development following protein-calorie malnutrition** CC⊕ HCC CC/MCC Exc⊕
    Nutritional short stature
    Nutritional stunting
    Physical retardation due to malnutrition

E46 **Unspecified protein-calorie malnutrition** CC⊕ HCC CC/MCC Exc⊕
    Malnutrition NOS
    Protein-calorie imbalance NOS
    EXCLUDES1 nutritional deficiency NOS (E63.9)

Other nutritional deficiencies (E50-E64)

    EXCLUDES2 nutritional anemias (D50-D53)

4ᵗʰ E50 **Vitamin A deficiency**
    EXCLUDES1 sequelae of vitamin A deficiency (E64.1)
    E50.0 **Vitamin A deficiency with conjunctival xerosis**
    E50.1 **Vitamin A deficiency with Bitot's spot and conjunctival xerosis**
        Bitot's spot in the young child
    E50.2 **Vitamin A deficiency with corneal xerosis**
    E50.3 **Vitamin A deficiency with corneal ulceration and xerosis**
    E50.4 **Vitamin A deficiency with keratomalacia**
    E50.5 **Vitamin A deficiency with night blindness**
    E50.6 **Vitamin A deficiency with xerophthalmic scars of cornea**
    E50.7 **Other ocular manifestations of vitamin A deficiency**
        Xerophthalmia NOS
    E50.8 **Other manifestations of vitamin A deficiency**
        Follicular keratosis
        Xeroderma
    E50.9 **Vitamin A deficiency, unspecified**
        Hypovitaminosis A NOS

4ᵗʰ E51 **Thiamine deficiency**
    EXCLUDES1 sequelae of thiamine deficiency (E64.8)
    5ᵗʰ E51.1 **Beriberi**
        E51.11 **Dry beriberi** CC⊕ CC/MCC Exc⊕
            Beriberi NOS
            Beriberi with polyneuropathy

Unspecified Code   Other Specified Code   Manifestation Code Ⓝ Newborn Ⓟ Pediatric Ⓜ Maternity Ⓐ Adult ♂ Male ♀ Female
● New Code   ▲ Revised Code Title   ▶◀ Revised Text **NOTES** *INCLUDES* *EXCLUDES 1* Not coded here *EXCLUDES 2* Not included here
4ᵗʰ 4ᵗʰ character required 5ᵗʰ 5ᵗʰ character required 6ᵗʰ 6ᵗʰ character required 7ᵗʰ 7ᵗʰ character required
7ᵗʰ Extension 'X' Alert HAC Hospital-acquired condition (HAC) alert **AHA** AHA Coding Clinic©

E51.12 **Wet beriberi**   CC CC/MCC Exc
            Beriberi with cardiovascular manifestations
            Cardiovascular beriberi
            Shoshin disease
E51.2 **Wernicke's encephalopathy**   CC CC/MCC Exc
E51.8 **Other manifestations of thiamine deficiency** CC CC/MCC Exc
E51.9 **Thiamine deficiency, unspecified** CC CC/MCC Exc

E52 Niacin **deficiency [pellagra]**
        Niacin (-tryptophan) deficiency
        Nicotinamide deficiency
        Pellagra (alcoholic)
        EXCLUDES1 sequelae of niacin deficiency (E64.8)

E53 **Deficiency of** other B group vitamins
        EXCLUDES1 sequelae of vitamin B deficiency (E64.8)
    E53.0 Riboflavin **deficiency**   CC CC/MCC Exc
            Ariboflavinosis
            Vitamin B2 deficiency
    E53.1 Pyridoxine **deficiency**
            Vitamin B6 deficiency
            EXCLUDES1 pyridoxine-responsive sideroblastic anemia (D64.3)
    E53.8 **Deficiency of other** specified **B group vitamins**
            Biotin deficiency
            Cyanocobalamin deficiency
            Folate deficiency
            Folic acid deficiency
            Pantothenic acid deficiency
            Vitamin B12 deficiency
            EXCLUDES1 folate deficiency anemia (D52.-)
                      vitamin B12 deficiency anemia (D51.-)
    E53.9 **Vitamin B deficiency, unspecified**

E54 Ascorbic acid **deficiency**
        Deficiency of vitamin C
        Scurvy
        EXCLUDES1 scorbutic anemia (D53.2)
                  sequelae of vitamin C deficiency (E64.2)

E55 Vitamin D **deficiency**
        EXCLUDES1 adult osteomalacia (M83.-)
                  osteoporosis (M80.-)
                  sequelae of rickets (E64.3)
    E55.0 **Rickets, active**   CC RxHCC CC/MCC Exc
            Infantile osteomalacia
            Juvenile osteomalacia
            EXCLUDES1 celiac rickets (K90.0)
                      Crohn's rickets (K50.-)
                      hereditary vitamin D-dependent rickets (E83.32)
                      inactive rickets (E64.3)
                      renal rickets (N25.0)
                      sequelae of rickets (E64.3)
                      vitamin D-resistant rickets (E83.31)
    E55.9 **Vitamin D deficiency, unspecified**
            Avitaminosis D

E56 Other vitamin **deficiencies**
        EXCLUDES1 sequelae of other vitamin deficiencies (E64.8)
    E56.0 **Deficiency of** vitamin E
    E56.1 **Deficiency of** vitamin K
            EXCLUDES1 deficiency of coagulation factor due to vitamin K
                      deficiency (D68.4)
                      vitamin K deficiency of newborn (P53)
    E56.8 **Deficiency of other vitamins**
    E56.9 **Vitamin deficiency, unspecified**

E58 Dietary calcium **deficiency**
        EXCLUDES1 disorders of calcium metabolism (E83.5-)
                  sequelae of calcium deficiency (E64.8)

E59 Dietary selenium **deficiency**
        Keshan disease
        EXCLUDES1 sequelae of selenium deficiency (E64.8)

E60 Dietary zinc **deficiency**

E61 **Deficiency of other nutrient elements**
        Use additional code for adverse effect, if applicable, to identify drug
        (T36-T50 with fifth or sixth character 5)
        EXCLUDES1 disorders of mineral metabolism (E83.-)
                  iodine deficiency related thyroid disorders (E00-E02)
                  sequelae of malnutrition and other nutritional deficiencies
                  (E64.-)
    E61.0 Copper **deficiency**
    E61.1 Iron **deficiency**
            EXCLUDES1 iron deficiency anemia (D50.-)
    E61.2 Magnesium **deficiency**
    E61.3 Manganese **deficiency**
    E61.4 Chromium **deficiency**
    E61.5 Molybdenum **deficiency**
    E61.6 Vanadium **deficiency**
    E61.7 **Deficiency of** multiple nutrient elements
    E61.8 **Deficiency of other specified nutrient elements**
    E61.9 **Deficiency of nutrient element, unspecified**

E63 **Other nutritional deficiencies**
        EXCLUDES1 dehydration (E86.0)
                  failure to thrive, adult (R62.7)
                  failure to thrive, child (R62.51)
                  feeding problems in newborn (P92.-)
                  sequelae of malnutrition and other nutritional deficiencies
                  (E64.-)
    E63.0 Essential fatty acid [EFA] **deficiency**
    E63.1 Imbalance of constituents of food intake
    E63.8 **Other specified nutritional deficiencies**
    E63.9 **Nutritional deficiency, unspecified**

E64 **Sequelae of malnutrition and other nutritional deficiencies**
        NOTES   This category is to be used to indicate conditions in
                categories E43, E44, E46, E50-E63 as the cause of sequelae,
                which are themselves classified elsewhere. The 'sequelae'
                include conditions specified as such; they also include the
                late effects of diseases classifiable to the above categories if
                the disease itself is no longer present
        Code first condition resulting from (sequela) of malnutrition and
        other nutritional deficiencies
    E64.0 **Sequelae of** protein-calorie **malnutrition** CC POA HCC CC/MCC Exc
            EXCLUDES2 retarded development following protein-calorie
                      malnutrition (E45)
    E64.1 **Sequelae of** vitamin A **deficiency**   POA
    E64.2 **Sequelae of** vitamin C **deficiency**   POA
    E64.3 **Sequelae of** rickets   POA
    E64.8 **Sequelae of other nutritional deficiencies** POA
    E64.9 **Sequelae of unspecified nutritional deficiency** POA

Overweight, obesity and other hyperalimentation (E65-E68)

E65 **Localized adiposity**
        Fat pad

E66 **Overweight and obesity**
        Code first obesity complicating pregnancy, childbirth and the
        puerperium, if applicable (O99.21-)
        Use additional code to identify body mass index (BMI), if known (Z68.-)
        EXCLUDES1 adiposogenital dystrophy (E23.6)
                  lipomatosis NOS (E88.2)
                  lipomatosis dolorosa [Dercum] (E88.2)
                  Prader-Willi syndrome (Q87.1)
    E66.0 **Obesity** due to excess calories
        E66.01 Morbid (severe) **obesity due to excess
                calories**   HAC HCC RxHCC
                EXCLUDES1 morbid (severe) obesity with alveolar
                          hypoventilation (E66.2)
        E66.09 **Other obesity due to excess calories** ?
    E66.1 Drug-induced **obesity**   ?
            Use additional code for adverse effect, if applicable, to
            identify drug (T36-T50 with fifth or sixth character 5)

PDxⁿ Unacceptable principal diagnosis symbol per Medicare code edits   POA Code exempt from diagnosis present on admission requirement
? Questionable admission   CC Complication or comorbidity   CC/MCC Exc CC/MCC exclusion   MCC Major complication or comorbidity
PDx CC Principal diagnosis as its own CC   PDx MCC Principal diagnosis as its own MCC   HCC HCC diagnosis code   RxHCC RxHCC diagnosis code
MACRA code   Z Z code as first-listed diagnosis

E66.2 Morbid (severe) obesity with alveolar hypoventilation [CC] [HCC] [RxHCC] [CC/MCC Exc]
Obesity hypoventilation syndrome (OHS)
Pickwickian syndrome
E66.3 Overweight
E66.8 Other obesity [?]
E66.9 Obesity, unspecified [?]
AHA: Q4 2013
Obesity NOS
[4th] E67 Other hyperalimentation
[EXCLUDES1] hyperalimentation NOS (R63.2)
sequelae of hyperalimentation (E68)
E67.0 Hypervitaminosis A
E67.1 Hypercarotinemia
E67.2 Megavitamin-B6 syndrome
E67.3 Hypervitaminosis D
E67.8 Other specified hyperalimentation
E68 Sequelae of hyperalimentation
Code first condition resulting from (sequela) of hyperalimentation

Metabolic disorders (E70-E88)

[EXCLUDES1] androgen insensitivity syndrome (E34.5-)
congenital adrenal hyperplasia (E25.0)
Ehlers-Danlos syndrome (Q79.6)
hemolytic anemias attributable to enzyme disorders (D55.-)
Marfan's syndrome (Q87.4)
5-alpha-reductase deficiency (E29.1)

[4th] E70 Disorders of aromatic amino-acid metabolism
E70.0 Classical phenylketonuria [CC] [HCC] [RxHCC] [CC/MCC Exc]
E70.1 Other hyperphenylalaninemias [CC] [HCC] [RxHCC] [CC/MCC Exc]
[5th] E70.2 Disorders of tyrosine metabolism
[EXCLUDES1] transitory tyrosinemia of newborn (P74.5)
E70.20 Disorder of tyrosine metabolism, unspecified [CC] [HCC] [RxHCC] [CC/MCC Exc]
E70.21 Tyrosinemia [CC] [HCC] [RxHCC] [CC/MCC Exc]
Hypertyrosinemia
E70.29 Other disorders of tyrosine metabolism [CC] [HCC] [RxHCC] [CC/MCC Exc]
Alkaptonuria
Ochronosis
[5th] E70.3 Albinism
E70.30 Albinism, unspecified [CC] [HCC] [RxHCC] [CC/MCC Exc]
[6th] E70.31 Ocular albinism
E70.310 X-linked ocular albinism [CC] [HCC] [RxHCC] [CC/MCC Exc]
E70.311 Autosomal recessive ocular albinism [CC] [HCC] [RxHCC] [CC/MCC Exc]
E70.318 Other ocular albinism [CC] [HCC] [RxHCC] [CC/MCC Exc]
E70.319 Ocular albinism, unspecified [CC] [HCC] [RxHCC] [CC/MCC Exc]
[6th] E70.32 Oculocutaneous albinism
[EXCLUDES1] Chediak-Higashi syndrome (E70.330)
Hermansky-Pudlak syndrome (E70.331)
E70.320 Tyrosinase negative oculocutaneous albinism [CC] [HCC] [RxHCC] [CC/MCC Exc]
Albinism I
Oculocutaneous albinism ty-neg
E70.321 Tyrosinase positive oculocutaneous albinism [CC] [HCC] [RxHCC] [CC/MCC Exc]
Albinism II
Oculocutaneous albinism ty-pos
E70.328 Other oculocutaneous albinism [CC] [HCC] [RxHCC] [CC/MCC Exc]
Cross syndrome
E70.329 Oculocutaneous albinism, unspecified [CC] [HCC] [RxHCC] [CC/MCC Exc]
[6th] E70.33 Albinism with hematologic abnormality
E70.330 Chediak-Higashi syndrome [CC] [HCC] [RxHCC] [CC/MCC Exc]
E70.331 Hermansky-Pudlak syndrome [CC] [HCC] [RxHCC] [CC/MCC Exc]
E70.338 Other albinism with hematologic abnormality [CC] [HCC] [RxHCC] [CC/MCC Exc]
E70.339 Albinism with hematologic abnormality, unspecified [CC] [HCC] [RxHCC] [CC/MCC Exc]
E70.39 Other specified albinism [CC] [HCC] [RxHCC] [CC/MCC Exc]
Piebaldism
[5th] E70.4 Disorders of histidine metabolism
E70.40 Disorders of histidine metabolism, unspecified [CC] [HCC] [RxHCC] [CC/MCC Exc]
E70.41 Histidinemia [CC] [HCC] [RxHCC] [CC/MCC Exc]
E70.49 Other disorders of histidine metabolism [CC] [HCC] [RxHCC] [CC/MCC Exc]
E70.5 Disorders of tryptophan metabolism [CC] [HCC] [RxHCC] [CC/MCC Exc]
E70.8 Other disorders of aromatic amino-acid metabolism [CC] [HCC] [RxHCC] [CC/MCC Exc]
E70.9 Disorder of aromatic amino-acid metabolism, unspecified [CC] [HCC] [RxHCC] [CC/MCC Exc]

[4th] E71 Disorders of branched-chain amino-acid metabolism and fatty-acid metabolism
E71.0 Maple-syrup-urine disease [CC] [HCC] [RxHCC] [CC/MCC Exc]
[5th] E71.1 Other disorders of branched-chain amino-acid metabolism
[6th] E71.11 Branched-chain organic acidurias
E71.110 Isovaleric acidemia [CC] [HCC] [RxHCC] [CC/MCC Exc]
E71.111 3-methylglutaconic aciduria [CC] [HCC] [RxHCC] [CC/MCC Exc]
E71.118 Other branched-chain organic acidurias [CC] [HCC] [RxHCC] [CC/MCC Exc]
[6th] E71.12 Disorders of propionate metabolism
E71.120 Methylmalonic acidemia [CC] [HCC] [RxHCC] [CC/MCC Exc]
E71.121 Propionic acidemia [CC] [HCC] [RxHCC] [CC/MCC Exc]
E71.128 Other disorders of propionate metabolism [CC] [HCC] [RxHCC] [CC/MCC Exc]
E71.19 Other disorders of branched-chain amino-acid metabolism [CC] [HCC] [RxHCC] [CC/MCC Exc]
Hyperleucine-isoleucinemia
Hypervalinemia
E71.2 Disorder of branched-chain amino-acid metabolism, unspecified [CC] [HCC] [RxHCC] [CC/MCC Exc]
[5th] E71.3 Disorders of fatty-acid metabolism
[EXCLUDES1] peroxisomal disorders (E71.5)
Refsum's disease (G60.1)
Schilder's disease (G37.0)
[EXCLUDES2] carnitine deficiency due to inborn error of metabolism (E71.42)
E71.30 Disorder of fatty-acid metabolism, unspecified [RxHCC]
[6th] E71.31 Disorders of fatty-acid oxidation
E71.310 Long chain/very long chain acyl CoA dehydrogenase deficiency [CC] [HCC] [RxHCC] [CC/MCC Exc]
LCAD
VLCAD
E71.311 Medium chain acyl CoA dehydrogenase deficiency [CC] [HCC] [RxHCC] [CC/MCC Exc]
MCAD
E71.312 Short chain acyl CoA dehydrogenase deficiency [CC] [HCC] [RxHCC] [CC/MCC Exc]
SCAD
E71.313 Glutaric aciduria type II [CC] [HCC] [RxHCC] [CC/MCC Exc]
Glutaric aciduria type II A
Glutaric aciduria type II B
Glutaric aciduria type II C
[EXCLUDES1] glutaric aciduria (type 1) NOS (E72.3)
E71.314 Muscle carnitine palmitoyltransferase deficiency [CC] [HCC] [RxHCC] [CC/MCC Exc]
E71.318 Other disorders of fatty-acid oxidation [CC] [HCC] [RxHCC] [CC/MCC Exc]
E71.32 Disorders of ketone metabolism [CC] [HCC] [RxHCC] [CC/MCC Exc]
E71.39 Other disorders of fatty-acid metabolism [CC] [HCC] [RxHCC] [CC/MCC Exc]
[5th] E71.4 Disorders of carnitine metabolism
[EXCLUDES1] Muscle carnitine palmitoyltransferase deficiency (E71.314)

Unspecified Code Other Specified Code Manifestation Code [N] Newborn [P] Pediatric [M] Maternity [A] Adult ♂ Male ♀ Female
● New Code ▲ Revised Code Title ►◄ Revised Text [NOTES] [INCLUDES] [EXCLUDES1] Not coded here [EXCLUDES2] Not included here
[4th] 4th character required [5th] 5th character required [6th] 6th character required [7th] 7th character required
[7th] Extension 'X' Alert [HAC] Hospital-acquired condition (HAC) alert AHA AHA Coding Clinic©

E71.40 **Disorder of carnitine metabolism, unspecified** HCC RxHCC

E71.41 Primary **carnitine deficiency** HCC RxHCC

E71.42 **Carnitine deficiency due to** inborn errors of metabolism HCC RxHCC

Code also associated inborn error or metabolism

E71.43 Iatrogenic carnitine **deficiency** HCC RxHCC

Carnitine deficiency due to hemodialysis

Carnitine deficiency due to Valproic acid therapy

E71.44 Other secondary **carnitine deficiency**

E71.440 **Ruvalcaba-Myhre-Smith syndrome** HCC RxHCC

E71.448 **Other secondary carnitine deficiency** HCC RxHCC

E71.5 **Peroxisomal** disorders

EXCLUDES1 Schilder's disease (G37.0)

E71.50 **Peroxisomal disorder, unspecified** cc HCC RxHCC CC/MCC Exc

E71.51 **Disorders of peroxisome** biogenesis

Group 1 peroxisomal disorders

EXCLUDES1 Refsum's disease (G60.1)

E71.510 **Zellweger syndrome** cc HCC RxHCC CC/MCC Exc

E71.511 **Neonatal adrenoleukodystrophy** cc HCC RxHCC CC/MCC Exc

EXCLUDES1 X-linked adrenoleukodystrophy (E71.42-)

E71.518 **Other disorders of peroxisome biogenesis** cc HCC RxHCC CC/MCC Exc

E71.52 X-linked **adrenoleukodystrophy**

E71.520 Childhood cerebral X-linked **adrenoleukodystrophy** cc HCC RxHCC CC/MCC Exc

E71.521 Adolescent X-linked **adrenoleukodystrophy** cc HCC RxHCC CC/MCC Exc

E71.522 Adrenomyeloneuropathy cc HCC RxHCC CC/MCC Exc

E71.528 **Other X-linked adrenoleukodystrophy** cc HCC RxHCC CC/MCC Exc

Addison only phenotype adrenoleukodystrophy

Addison-Schilder adrenoleukodystrophy

E71.529 **X-linked adrenoleukodystrophy, unspecified type** cc HCC RxHCC CC/MCC Exc

E71.53 Other group 2 peroxisomal disorders cc HCC RxHCC CC/MCC Exc

E71.54 **Other peroxisomal disorders**

E71.540 **Rhizomelic chondrodysplasia punctata** cc HCC RxHCC CC/MCC Exc

EXCLUDES1 chondrodysplasia punctata NOS (Q77.3)

E71.541 **Zellweger-like syndrome** cc HCC RxHCC CC/MCC Exc

E71.542 **Other group 3 peroxisomal disorders** cc HCC RxHCC CC/MCC Exc

E71.548 **Other peroxisomal disorders** cc HCC RxHCC CC/MCC Exc

E72 **Other disorders of amino-acid metabolism**

EXCLUDES1 disorders of:

aromatic amino-acid metabolism (E70.-)

branched-chain amino-acid metabolism (E71.0-E71.2)

fatty-acid metabolism (E71.3)

purine and pyrimidine metabolism (E79.-)

gout (M1A.-, M10.-)

E72.0 **Disorders of amino-acid** transport

EXCLUDES1 disorders of tryptophan metabolism (E70.5)

E72.00 **Disorders of amino-acid transport, unspecified** cc HCC RxHCC CC/MCC Exc

E72.01 Cystinuria cc HCC RxHCC CC/MCC Exc

E72.02 **Hartnup's disease** cc HCC RxHCC CC/MCC Exc

E72.03 **Lowe's syndrome** cc HCC RxHCC

Use additional code for associated glaucoma (H42)

E72.04 Cystinosis cc HCC RxHCC CC/MCC Exc

Fanconi (-de Toni) (-Debré) syndrome with cystinosis

EXCLUDES1 Fanconi (-de Toni) (-Debré) syndrome without cystinosis (E72.09)

E72.09 **Other disorders of amino-acid transport** cc HCC RxHCC CC/MCC Exc

Fanconi (-de Toni) (-Debré) syndrome, unspecified

E72.1 **Disorders of** sulfur-bearing amino-acid metabolism

EXCLUDES1 cystinosis (E72.04)

cystinuria (E72.01)

transcobalamin II deficiency (D51.2)

E72.10 **Disorders of sulfur-bearing amino-acid metabolism, unspecified** cc HCC RxHCC CC/MCC Exc

E72.11 **Homocystinuria** cc HCC RxHCC CC/MCC Exc

Cystathionine synthase deficiency

E72.12 **Methylenetetrahydrofolate reductase deficiency** cc HCC RxHCC CC/MCC Exc

E72.19 **Other disorders of sulfur-bearing amino-acid metabolism** cc HCC RxHCC CC/MCC Exc

Cystathioninuria

Methioninemia

Sulfite oxidase deficiency

E72.2 **Disorders of** urea cycle metabolism

EXCLUDES1 disorders of ornithine metabolism (E72.4)

E72.20 **Disorder of urea cycle metabolism, unspecified** cc HCC RxHCC CC/MCC Exc

Hyperammonemia

EXCLUDES1 hyperammonemia-hyperornithinemia-homocitrullinemia syndrome E72.4

transient hyperammonemia of newborn (P74.6)

E72.21 **Argininemia** cc HCC RxHCC CC/MCC Exc

E72.22 **Arginosuccinic aciduria** cc HCC RxHCC CC/MCC Exc

E72.23 **Citrullinemia** cc HCC RxHCC CC/MCC Exc

E72.29 **Other disorders of urea cycle metabolism** cc HCC RxHCC CC/MCC Exc

E72.3 **Disorders of** lysine and hydroxylysine metabolism cc HCC RxHCC CC/MCC Exc

Glutaric aciduria NOS

Glutaric aciduria (type I)

Hydroxylysinemia

Hyperlysinemia

EXCLUDES1 glutaric aciduria type II (E71.313)

Refsum's disease (G60.1)

Zellweger syndrome (E71.510)

E72.4 **Disorders of** ornithine metabolism cc HCC RxHCC CC/MCC Exc

Hyperammonemia-Hyperornithinemia-Homocitrullinemia syndrome

Ornithinemia (types I, II)

Ornithine transcarbamylase deficiency

EXCLUDES1 hereditary choroidal dystrophy (H31.2-)

E72.5 **Disorders of** glycine metabolism

E72.50 **Disorder of glycine metabolism, unspecified** cc HCC RxHCC CC/MCC Exc

E72.51 Non-ketotic hyperglycinemia cc HCC RxHCC CC/MCC Exc

E72.52 Trimethylaminuria cc HCC RxHCC CC/MCC Exc

E72.53 Hyperoxaluria cc HCC RxHCC CC/MCC Exc

Oxalosis

Oxaluria

E72.59 **Other disorders of glycine metabolism** cc HCC RxHCC CC/MCC Exc

D-glycericacidemia

Hyperhydroxyprolinemia

Hyperprolinemia (types I, II)

Sarcosinemia

E72.8 **Other specified disorders of amino-acid metabolism** cc HCC RxHCC CC/MCC Exc

Disorders of beta-amino-acid metabolism

Disorders of gamma-glutamyl cycle

E72.9 **Disorder of amino-acid metabolism, unspecified** cc HCC RxHCC CC/MCC Exc

E73 **Lactose intolerance**

E73.0 Congenital **lactase deficiency**

E73.1 Secondary **lactase deficiency**

E73.8 **Other lactose intolerance**

E73.9 **Lactose intolerance, unspecified**

E74 **Other disorders of carbohydrate metabolism**

EXCLUDES1 diabetes mellitus (E08-E13)

hypoglycemia NOS (E16.2)

increased secretion of glucagon (E16.3)

mucopolysaccharidosis (E76.0-E76.3)

PDX Unacceptable principal diagnosis symbol per Medicare code edits   POA Code exempt from diagnosis present on admission requirement

? Questionable admission   cc Complication or comorbidity   CC/MCC Exc CC/MCC exclusion   MCC Major complication or comorbidity

Principal diagnosis as its own CC   Principal diagnosis as its own MCC   HCC HCC diagnosis code   RxHCC RxHCC diagnosis code

MACRA code   Z1 Z code as first-listed diagnosis

536   When symbols appear on a code that requires a 7th character extension, refer to Appendix B to identify applicable 7th character codes.   **2018 ICD-10-CM**

5ᵗʰ **E74.0** Glycogen storage **disease**

    E74.00 **Glycogen storage disease, unspecified** cᶜ⊘ HCC RxHCC CC/MCC Exc⊘

    E74.01 von Gierke **disease** cᶜ⊘ HCC RxHCC CC/MCC Exc⊘

        Type I glycogen storage disease

    E74.02 Pompe **disease** cᶜ⊘ HCC RxHCC CC/MCC Exc⊘

        Cardiac glycogenosis

        Type II glycogen storage disease

    E74.03 Cori **disease** cᶜ⊘ HCC RxHCC CC/MCC Exc⊘

        Forbes disease

        Type III glycogen storage disease

    E74.04 McArdle **disease** cᶜ⊘ HCC RxHCC CC/MCC Exc⊘

        Type V glycogen storage disease

    E74.09 **Other glycogen storage disease** cᶜ⊘ HCC RxHCC CC/MCC Exc⊘

        Andersen disease

        Hers disease

        Tauri disease

        Glycogen storage disease, types 0, IV, VI-XI

        Liver phosphorylase deficiency

        Muscle phosphofructokinase deficiency

5ᵗʰ **E74.1** **Disorders of** fructose **metabolism**

    EXCLUDES1 *muscle phosphofructokinase deficiency (E74.09)*

    E74.10 **Disorder of fructose metabolism, unspecified**

    E74.11 Essential fructosuria

        Fructokinase deficiency

    E74.12 Hereditary **fructose intolerance**

        Fructosemia

    E74.19 **Other disorders of fructose metabolism**

        Fructose-1, 6-diphosphatase deficiency

5ᵗʰ **E74.2** **Disorders of** galactose **metabolism**

    E74.20 **Disorders of galactose metabolism, unspecified** cᶜ⊘ HCC RxHCC CC/MCC Exc⊘

    E74.21 Galactosemia cᶜ⊘ HCC RxHCC CC/MCC Exc⊘

    E74.29 **Other disorders of galactose metabolism** cᶜ⊘ HCC RxHCC CC/MCC Exc⊘

        Galactokinase deficiency

5ᵗʰ **E74.3** **Other disorders of** intestinal carbohydrate absorption

    EXCLUDES2 *lactose intolerance (E73.-)*

    E74.31 **Sucrase-isomaltase deficiency**

    E74.39 **Other disorders of intestinal carbohydrate absorption**

        Disorder of intestinal carbohydrate absorption NOS

        Glucose-galactose malabsorption

        Sucrase deficiency

E74.4 **Disorders of** pyruvate metabolism and gluconeogenesis cᶜ⊘ HCC RxHCC CC/MCC Exc⊘

    Deficiency of phosphoenolpyruvate carboxykinase

    Deficiency of pyruvate carboxylase

    Deficiency of pyruvate dehydrogenase

    EXCLUDES1 *disorders of pyruvate metabolism and gluconeogenesis with anemia (D55.-)*

        Leigh's syndrome (G31.82)

E74.8 Other specified disorders of carbohydrate metabolism cᶜ⊘ HCC RxHCC CC/MCC Exc⊘

    Essential pentosuria

    Renal glycosuria

E74.9 **Disorder of carbohydrate metabolism, unspecified** HCC RxHCC

4ᵗʰ **E75** **Disorders of** sphingolipid **metabolism and** other lipid storage disorders

    EXCLUDES1 *mucolipidosis, types I-III (E77.0-E77.1)*

        Refsum's disease (G60.1)

5ᵗʰ **E75.0** GM2 gangliosidosis

    E75.00 **GM2 gangliosidosis, unspecified** cᶜ⊘ RxHCC CC/MCC Exc⊘

    E75.01 Sandhoff **disease** cᶜ⊘ RxHCC CC/MCC Exc⊘

    E75.02 Tay-Sachs **disease** cᶜ⊘ RxHCC CC/MCC Exc⊘

    E75.09 **Other GM2 gangliosidosis** cᶜ⊘ RxHCC CC/MCC Exc⊘

        Adult GM2 gangliosidosis

        Juvenile GM2 gangliosidosis

5ᵗʰ **E75.1** **Other and unspecified gangliosidosis**

    E75.10 Unspecified gangliosidosis cᶜ⊘ RxHCC CC/MCC Exc⊘

        Gangliosidosis NOS

    E75.11 Mucolipidosis IV cᶜ⊘ RxHCC CC/MCC Exc⊘

    E75.19 **Other gangliosidosis** cᶜ⊘ RxHCC CC/MCC Exc⊘

        GM1 gangliosidosis

        GM3 gangliosidosis

5ᵗʰ **E75.2** **Other sphingolipidosis**

    EXCLUDES1 *adrenoleukodystrophy [Addison-Schilder] (E71.528)*

    E75.21 Fabry (-Anderson) **disease** HCC RxHCC

    E75.22 Gaucher **disease** HCC RxHCC

    E75.23 Krabbe **disease** cᶜ⊘ HCC RxHCC CC/MCC Exc⊘

6ᵗʰ   **E75.24** **Niemann-Pick disease**

        E75.240 **Niemann-Pick disease** type A HCC RxHCC

        E75.241 **Niemann-Pick disease** type B HCC RxHCC

        E75.242 **Niemann-Pick disease** type C HCC RxHCC

        E75.243 **Niemann-Pick disease** type D HCC RxHCC

        E75.248 **Other Niemann-Pick disease** HCC RxHCC

        E75.249 Niemann-Pick disease, unspecified HCC RxHCC

    E75.25 **Metachromatic leukodystrophy** cᶜ⊘ RxHCC CC/MCC Exc⊘

    E75.29 **Other sphingolipidosis** cᶜ⊘ RxHCC CC/MCC Exc⊘

        Farber's syndrome

        Sulfatase deficiency

        Sulfatide lipidosis

E75.3 **Sphingolipidosis, unspecified** HCC RxHCC

E75.4 **Neuronal ceroid lipofuscinosis** cᶜ⊘ RxHCC CC/MCC Exc⊘

    Batten disease

    Bielschowsky-Jansky disease

    Kufs disease

    Spielmeyer-Vogt disease

E75.5 **Other lipid storage disorders** RxHCC

    Cerebrotendinous cholesterosis [van Bogaert-Scherer-Epstein]

    Wolman's disease

E75.6 **Lipid storage disorder, unspecified** RxHCC

4ᵗʰ **E76** **Disorders of** glycosaminoglycan **metabolism**

5ᵗʰ **E76.0** **Mucopolysaccharidosis,** type I

    E76.01 Hurler's **syndrome** cᶜ⊘ HCC RxHCC CC/MCC Exc⊘

    E76.02 Hurler-Scheie **syndrome** cᶜ⊘ HCC RxHCC CC/MCC Exc⊘

    E76.03 Scheie's **syndrome** cᶜ⊘ HCC RxHCC CC/MCC Exc⊘

E76.1 **Mucopolysaccharidosis,** type II cᶜ⊘ HCC RxHCC CC/MCC Exc⊘

    Hunter's syndrome

5ᵗʰ **E76.2** **Other mucopolysaccharidoses**

6ᵗʰ   **E76.21** Morquio **mucopolysaccharidoses**

        E76.210 **Morquio** A **mucopolysaccharidoses** cᶜ⊘ HCC RxHCC CC/MCC Exc⊘

            Classic Morquio syndrome

            Morquio syndrome A

            Mucopolysaccharidosis, type IVA

        E76.211 **Morquio** B **mucopolysaccharidoses** cᶜ⊘ HCC RxHCC CC/MCC Exc⊘

            Morquio-like mucopolysaccharidoses

            Morquio-like syndrome

            Morquio syndrome B

            Mucopolysaccharidosis, type IVB

        E76.219 **Morquio mucopolysaccharidoses, unspecified** cᶜ⊘ HCC RxHCC CC/MCC Exc⊘

            Morquio syndrome

            Mucopolysaccharidosis, type IV

    E76.22 Sanfilippo **mucopolysaccharidoses** cᶜ⊘ HCC RxHCC CC/MCC Exc⊘

        Mucopolysaccharidosis, type III (A) (B) (C) (D)

        Sanfilippo A syndrome

        Sanfilippo B syndrome

        Sanfilippo C syndrome

        Sanfilippo D syndrome

    E76.29 **Other mucopolysaccharidoses** cᶜ⊘ HCC RxHCC CC/MCC Exc⊘

        beta-Glucuronidase deficiency

        Maroteaux-Lamy (mild) (severe) syndrome

        Mucopolysaccharidosis, types VI, VII

E76.3 **Mucopolysaccharidosis, unspecified** cᶜ⊘ HCC RxHCC CC/MCC Exc⊘

E76.8 **Other disorders of glucosaminoglycan metabolism** cᶜ⊘ HCC RxHCC CC/MCC Exc⊘

E76.9 Glucosaminoglycan metabolism disorder, unspecified cᶜ⊘ HCC RxHCC CC/MCC Exc⊘

4ᵗʰ **E77** **Disorders of** glycoprotein **metabolism**

Unspecified Code Other Specified Code Manifestation Code Ⓝ Newborn Ⓟ Pediatric Ⓜ Maternity Ⓐ Adult ♂ Male ♀ Female
  ● New Code ▲ Revised Code Title ►◄ Revised Text **NOTES** *INCLUDES* EXCLUDES1 Not coded here EXCLUDES2 Not included here
  4ᵗʰ 4ᵗʰ character required 5ᵗʰ 5ᵗʰ character required 6ᵗʰ 6ᵗʰ character required 7ᵗʰ 7ᵗʰ character required
  ⊘ Extension 'X' Alert HAC Hospital-acquired condition (HAC) alert **AHA** AHA Coding Clinic©

2018 ICD-10-CM   When symbols appear on a code that requires a 7th character extension, refer to Appendix B to identify applicable 7th character codes.   **537**

E77.0 Defects in post-translational modification of lysosomal enzymes `HCC` `RxHCC`
- Mucolipidosis II [I-cell disease]
- Mucolipidosis III [pseudo-Hurler polydystrophy]

E77.1 Defects in glycoprotein degradation `HCC` `RxHCC`
- Aspartylglucosaminuria
- Fucosidosis
- Mannosidosis
- Sialidosis [mucolipidosis I]

E77.8 **Other disorders of glycoprotein metabolism** `HCC` `RxHCC`

E77.9 **Disorder of glycoprotein metabolism, unspecified** `HCC` `RxHCC`

E78 **Disorders of** lipoprotein metabolism and other lipidemias
> EXCLUDES1 sphingolipidosis (E75.0-E75.3)

E78.0 Pure hypercholesterolemia `RxHCC`

  E78.00 Pure hypercholesterolemia, unspecified `RxHCC`
> AHA: Q4 2016
- Fredrickson's hyperlipoproteinemia, type IIa
- Hyperbetalipoproteinemia
- Low-density-lipoprotein-type [LDL] hyperlipoproteinemia
- (Pure) hypercholesterolemia NOS

  E78.01 Familial hypercholesterolemia `RxHCC`
> AHA: Q4 2016

E78.1 Pure hyperglyceridemia `RxHCC`
- Elevated fasting triglycerides
- Endogenous hyperglyceridemia
- Fredrickson's hyperlipoproteinemia, type IV
- Hyperlipidemia, group B
- Hyperprebetalipoproteinemia
- Very-low-density-lipoprotein-type [VLDL] hyperlipoproteinemia

E78.2 Mixed hyperlipidemia `RxHCC`
- Broad- or floating-betalipoproteinemia
- Combined hyperlipidemia NOS
- Elevated cholesterol with elevated triglycerides NEC
- Fredrickson's hyperlipoproteinemia, type IIb or III
- Hyperbetalipoproteinemia with prebetalipoproteinemia
- Hypercholesteremia with endogenous hyperglyceridemia
- Hyperlipidemia, group C
- Tubo-eruptive xanthoma
- Xanthoma tuberosum
> EXCLUDES1 cerebrotendinous cholesterosis [van Bogaert-Scherer-Epstein] (E75.5)
> familial combined hyperlipidemia (E78.4)

E78.3 Hyperchylomicronemia `RxHCC`
- Chylomicron retention disease
- Fredrickson's hyperlipoproteinemia, type I or V
- Hyperlipidemia, group D
- Mixed hyperglyceridemia

E78.4 Other hyperlipidemia `RxHCC`
- Familial combined hyperlipidemia

E78.5 **Hyperlipidemia, unspecified** `RxHCC`

E78.6 Lipoprotein deficiency `RxHCC`
- Abetalipoproteinemia
- Depressed HDL cholesterol
- High-density lipoprotein deficiency
- Hypoalphalipoproteinemia
- Hypobetalipoproteinemia (familial)
- Lecithin cholesterol acyltransferase deficiency
- Tangier disease

E78.7 Disorders of bile acid and cholesterol metabolism
> EXCLUDES1 Niemann-Pick disease type C (E75.242)

  E78.70 **Disorder of bile acid and cholesterol metabolism, unspecified** `RxHCC`

  E78.71 Barth syndrome `CC` `CC/MCC Exc`

  E78.72 Smith-Lemli-Opitz syndrome `CC` `CC/MCC Exc`

  E78.79 Other disorders of bile acid and cholesterol metabolism `RxHCC`

E78.8 Other disorders of lipoprotein metabolism
  E78.81 Lipoid dermatoarthritis `RxHCC`
  E78.89 Other lipoprotein metabolism disorders `RxHCC`

E78.9 **Disorder of lipoprotein metabolism, unspecified** `RxHCC`

E79 **Disorders of** purine and pyrimidine metabolism
> EXCLUDES1 Ataxia-telangiectasia (Q87.1)
> Bloom's syndrome (Q82.8)
> Cockayne's syndrome (Q87.1)
> calculus of kidney (N20.0)
> combined immunodeficiency disorders (D81.-)
> Fanconi's anemia (D61.09)
> gout (M1A.-, M10.-)
> orotaciduric anemia (D53.0)
> progeria (E34.8)
> Werner's syndrome (E34.8)
> xeroderma pigmentosum (Q82.1)

E79.0 Hyperuricemia without signs of inflammatory arthritis and tophaceous disease
- Asymptomatic hyperuricemia

E79.1 Lesch-Nyhan syndrome `CC` `HCC` `RxHCC` `CC/MCC Exc`
- HGPRT deficiency

E79.2 Myoadenylate deaminase deficiency `CC` `HCC` `RxHCC` `CC/MCC Exc`

E79.8 Other disorders of purine and pyrimidine metabolism `CC` `HCC` `RxHCC` `CC/MCC Exc`
- Hereditary xanthinuria

E79.9 **Disorder of purine and pyrimidine metabolism, unspecified** `CC` `HCC` `RxHCC` `CC/MCC Exc`

E80 **Disorders of** porphyrin and bilirubin metabolism
> INCLUDES defects of catalase and peroxidase

E80.0 Hereditary erythropoietic porphyria `CC` `HCC` `RxHCC` `CC/MCC Exc`
- Congenital erythropoietic porphyria
- Erythropoietic protoporphyria

E80.1 Porphyria cutanea tarda `CC` `HCC` `RxHCC` `CC/MCC Exc`

E80.2 Other and unspecified porphyria
  E80.20 Unspecified porphyria `CC` `HCC` `RxHCC` `CC/MCC Exc`
- Porphyria NOS

  E80.21 Acute intermittent (hepatic) porphyria `CC` `HCC` `RxHCC` `CC/MCC Exc`

  E80.29 Other porphyria `CC` `HCC` `RxHCC` `CC/MCC Exc`
- Hereditary coproporphyria

E80.3 Defects of catalase and peroxidase `CC` `HCC` `RxHCC` `CC/MCC Exc`
- Acatalasia [Takahara]

E80.4 Gilbert syndrome

E80.5 Crigler-Najjar syndrome

E80.6 Other disorders of bilirubin metabolism
- Dubin-Johnson syndrome
- Rotor's syndrome

E80.7 **Disorder of bilirubin metabolism, unspecified**

E83 **Disorders of** mineral metabolism
> EXCLUDES1 dietary mineral deficiency (E58-E61)
> parathyroid disorders (E20-E21)
> vitamin D deficiency (E55.-)

E83.0 Disorders of copper metabolism
  E83.00 **Disorder of copper metabolism, unspecified** `RxHCC`
  E83.01 Wilson's disease `RxHCC`
> Code also associated Kayser Fleischer ring (H18.04-)
  E83.09 Other disorders of copper metabolism `RxHCC`
- Menkes' (kinky hair) (steely hair) disease

E83.1 Disorders of iron metabolism
> EXCLUDES1 iron deficiency anemia (D50.-)
> sideroblastic anemia (D64.0-D64.3)

  E83.10 **Disorder of iron metabolism, unspecified** `RxHCC`

  E83.11 Hemochromatosis
> EXCLUDES1 GALD (P78.84)
> Gestational alloimmune liver disease (P78.84)
> Neonatal hemochromatosis (P78.84)

    E83.110 Hereditary hemochromatosis `HCC` `RxHCC`
- Bronzed diabetes
- Pigmentary cirrhosis (of liver)
- Primary (hereditary) hemochromatosis

    E83.111 **Hemochromatosis** due to repeated red blood cell transfusions
- Iron overload due to repeated red blood cell transfusions

PDxn Unacceptable principal diagnosis symbol per Medicare code edits   POA Code exempt from diagnosis present on admission requirement
? Questionable admission   `CC` Complication or comorbidity   CC/MCC EXC CC/MCC exclusion   MCC Major complication or comorbidity
Principal diagnosis as its own CC   Principal diagnosis as its own MCC   `HCC` HCC diagnosis code   `RxHCC` RxHCC diagnosis code
MACRA code   Z1 Z code as first-listed diagnosis

538   When symbols appear on a code that requires a 7th character extension, refer to Appendix B to identify applicable 7th character codes.   **2018 ICD-10-CM**

Transfusion (red blood cell) associated hemochromatosis

E83.118 **Other hemochromatosis** [RxHCC]

E83.119 **Hemochromatosis, unspecified** [RxHCC]

E83.19 **Other disorders of iron metabolism** [RxHCC]

Use additional code, if applicable, for idiopathic pulmonary hemosiderosis (J84.03)

E83.2 **Disorders of zinc metabolism**

Acrodermatitis enteropathica

[5th] E83.3 **Disorders of phosphorus metabolism and phosphatases**

[EXCLUDES1] *adult osteomalacia (M83.-)*

osteoporosis (M80.-)

E83.30 **Disorder of phosphorus metabolism, unspecified** [RxHCC]

E83.31 **Familial hypophosphatemia** [RxHCC]

Vitamin D-resistant osteomalacia

Vitamin D-resistant rickets

[EXCLUDES1] *vitamin D-deficiency rickets (E55.0)*

E83.32 **Hereditary vitamin D-dependent rickets (type 1) (type 2)** [RxHCC]

25-hydroxyvitamin D 1-alpha-hydroxylase deficiency

Pseudovitamin D deficiency

Vitamin D receptor defect

E83.39 **Other disorders of phosphorus metabolism** [RxHCC]

Acid phosphatase deficiency

Hypophosphatasia

[5th] E83.4 **Disorders of magnesium metabolism**

E83.40 **Disorders of magnesium metabolism, unspecified**

E83.41 **Hypermagnesemia**

AHA: Q4 2016

E83.42 **Hypomagnesemia**

E83.49 **Other disorders of magnesium metabolism**

[5th] E83.5 **Disorders of calcium metabolism**

[EXCLUDES1] *chondrocalcinosis (M11.1-M11.2)*

hungry bone syndrome (E83.81)

hyperparathyroidism (E21.0-E21.3)

E83.50 **Unspecified disorder of calcium metabolism**

E83.51 **Hypocalcemia**

E83.52 **Hypercalcemia**

Familial hypocalciuric hypercalcemia

E83.59 **Other disorders of calcium metabolism**

Idiopathic hypercalciuria

[5th] E83.8 **Other disorders of mineral metabolism**

E83.81 **Hungry bone syndrome**

E83.89 **Other disorders of mineral metabolism**

E83.9 **Disorder of mineral metabolism, unspecified**

[4th] E84 **Cystic fibrosis**

[INCLUDES] *mucoviscidosis*

Code also exocrine pancreatic insufficiency (K86.81)

E84.0 **Cystic fibrosis with pulmonary manifestations** [HCC] [MCC] [RxHCC] [CC/MCC Exc]

Use additional code to identify any infectious organism present, such as:

Pseudomonas (B96.5)

[5th] E84.1 **Cystic fibrosis with intestinal manifestations**

E84.11 **Meconium ileus in cystic fibrosis** [N] [HCC] [MCC] [RxHCC] [CC/MCC Exc]

[EXCLUDES1] *meconium ileus not due to cystic fibrosis (P76.0)*

E84.19 **Cystic fibrosis with other intestinal manifestations** [CC] [HCC] [RxHCC] [CC/MCC Exc]

Distal intestinal obstruction syndrome

E84.8 **Cystic fibrosis with other manifestations** [CC] [HCC] [RxHCC] [CC/MCC Exc]

E84.9 **Cystic fibrosis, unspecified** [CC] [HCC] [RxHCC] [CC/MCC Exc]

[4th] E85 **Amyloidosis**

[EXCLUDES2] *Alzheimer's disease (G30.0-)*

E85.0 **Non-neuropathic heredofamilial amyloidosis** [CC] [HCC] [CC/MCC Exc]

Hereditary amyloid nephropathy

Code also associated disorders, such as:

autoinflammatory syndromes (M04.-)

[EXCLUDES2] *Transthyretin-related (ATTR) familial amyloid cardiomyopathy (E85.4)*

E85.1 **Neuropathic heredofamilial amyloidosis** [CC] [HCC] [CC/MCC Exc]

AHA: Q4 2012

Amyloid polyneuropathy (Portuguese)

Transthyretin-related (ATTR) familial amyloid polyneuropathy

E85.2 **Heredofamilial amyloidosis, unspecified** [CC] [HCC] [CC/MCC Exc]

E85.3 **Secondary systemic amyloidosis** [CC] [HCC] [CC/MCC Exc]

Hemodialysis-associated amyloidosis

E85.4 **Organ-limited amyloidosis** [CC] [HCC] [CC/MCC Exc]

Localized amyloidosis

Transthyretin-related (ATTR) familial amyloid cardiomyopathy

[5th] E85.8 **Other amyloidosis** [HCC]

● E85.81 **Light chain (AL) amyloidosis** [CC] [CC/MCC Exc]

● E85.82 **Wild-type transthyretin-related (ATTR) amyloidosis** [CC] [CC/MCC Exc]

Senile systemic amyloidosis (SSA)

● E85.89 **Other amyloidosis** [CC] [CC/MCC Exc]

E85.9 **Amyloidosis, unspecified** [CC] [HCC] [CC/MCC Exc]

[4th] E86 **Volume depletion**

Use additional code(s) for any associated disorders of electrolyte and acid-base balance (E87.-)

[EXCLUDES1] *dehydration of newborn (P74.1)*

hypovolemic shock NOS (R57.1)

postprocedural hypovolemic shock (T81.19)

traumatic hypovolemic shock (T79.4)

E86.0 **Dehydration**

E86.1 **Hypovolemia**

Depletion of volume of plasma

E86.9 **Volume depletion, unspecified**

[4th] E87 **Other disorders of fluid, electrolyte and acid-base balance**

[EXCLUDES1] *diabetes insipidus (E23.2)*

electrolyte imbalance associated with hyperemesis gravidarum (O21.1)

electrolyte imbalance following ectopic or molar pregnancy (O08.5)

familial periodic paralysis (G72.3)

E87.0 **Hyperosmolality and hypernatremia** [CC] [CC/MCC Exc]

Sodium [Na] excess

Sodium [Na] overload

E87.1 **Hypo-osmolality and hyponatremia** [CC] [CC/MCC Exc]

Sodium [Na] deficiency

[EXCLUDES1] *syndrome of inappropriate secretion of antidiuretic hormone (E22.2)*

E87.2 **Acidosis** [CC] [CC/MCC Exc]

Acidosis NOS

Lactic acidosis

Metabolic acidosis

Respiratory acidosis

[EXCLUDES1] *diabetic acidosis - see categories E08-E10, E13 with ketoacidosis*

E87.3 **Alkalosis** [CC] [CC/MCC Exc]

Alkalosis NOS

Metabolic alkalosis

Respiratory alkalosis

E87.4 **Mixed disorder of acid-base balance** [CC] [CC/MCC Exc]

E87.5 **Hyperkalemia**

Potassium [K] excess

Potassium [K] overload

E87.6 **Hypokalemia**

Potassium [K] deficiency

[5th] E87.7 **Fluid overload**

[EXCLUDES1] *edema NOS (R60.9)*

fluid retention (R60.9)

E87.70 **Fluid overload, unspecified**

E87.71 **Transfusion associated circulatory overload**

Fluid overload due to transfusion (blood) (blood components)

TACO

E87.79 **Other fluid overload**

E87.8   Other disorders of electrolyte and fluid balance, not elsewhere classified
Electrolyte imbalance NOS
Hyperchloremia
Hypochloremia

4ᵗʰ E88   Other and unspecified metabolic disorders
Use additional codes for associated conditions
EXCLUDES1 *histiocytosis X (chronic) (C96.6)*

5ᵗʰ E88.0   Disorders of plasma-protein metabolism, not elsewhere classified
EXCLUDES1 *disorder of lipoprotein metabolism (E78.-)*
monoclonal gammopathy (of undetermined significance) (D47.2)
polyclonal hypergammaglobulinemia (D89.0)
Waldenström macroglobulinemia (C88.0)

E88.01   Alpha-1-antitrypsin deficiency   HCC RxHCC
AAT deficiency

E88.09   Other disorders of plasma-protein metabolism, not elsewhere classified
Bisalbuminemia

E88.1   Lipodystrophy, not elsewhere classified
Lipodystrophy NOS
EXCLUDES1 *Whipple's disease (K90.81)*

E88.2   Lipomatosis, not elsewhere classified   RxHCC
Lipomatosis NOS
Lipomatosis (Check) dolorosa [Dercum]

E88.3   Tumor lysis syndrome   MCC CC/MCC Exc
Tumor lysis syndrome (spontaneous)
Tumor lysis syndrome following antineoplastic drug chemotherapy
Use additional code for adverse effect, if applicable, to identify drug (T45.1X5)

5ᵗʰ E88.4   Mitochondrial metabolism disorders
EXCLUDES1 *disorders of pyruvate metabolism (E74.4)*
Kearns-Sayre syndrome (H49.81)
Leber's disease (H47.22)
Leigh's encephalopathy (G31.82)
Mitochondrial myopathy, NEC (G71.3)
Reye's syndrome (G93.7)

E88.40   Mitochondrial metabolism disorder, unspecified   cc HCC RxHCC CC/MCC Exc

E88.41   MELAS syndrome   cc HCC RxHCC CC/MCC Exc
Mitochondrial myopathy, encephalopathy, lactic acidosis and stroke-like episodes

E88.42   MERRF syndrome   cc HCC RxHCC CC/MCC Exc
Myoclonic epilepsy associated with ragged-red fibers
Code also progressive myoclonic epilepsy (G40.3-)

E88.49   Other mitochondrial metabolism disorders   cc HCC RxHCC CC/MCC Exc

5ᵗʰ E88.8   Other specified metabolic disorders
E88.81   Metabolic syndrome
Dysmetabolic syndrome X
Use additional codes for associated manifestations, such as:
obesity (E66.-)

E88.89   Other specified metabolic disorders   HCC RxHCC
Launois-Bensaude adenolipomatosis
EXCLUDES1 *adult pulmonary Langerhans cell histiocytosis (J84.82)*

E88.9   Metabolic disorder, unspecified

Postprocedural endocrine and metabolic complications and disorders, not elsewhere classified (E89)

4ᵗʰ E89   Postprocedural endocrine and metabolic complications and disorders, not elsewhere classified
EXCLUDES2 *intraoperative complications of endocrine system organ or structure (E36.0-, E36.1-, E36.8)*

E89.0   Postprocedural hypothyroidism   RxHCC
Postirradiation hypothyroidism
Postsurgical hypothyroidism

E89.1   Postprocedural hypoinsulinemia   cc CC/MCC Exc
Postpancreatectomy hyperglycemia
Postsurgical hypoinsulinemia
Use additional code, if applicable, to identify:
acquired absence of pancreas (Z90.41-)
diabetes mellitus (postpancreatectomy) (postprocedural) (E13.-)
insulin use (Z79.4)
EXCLUDES1 *transient postprocedural hyperglycemia (R73.9)*
transient postprocedural hypoglycemia (E16.2)

E89.2   Postprocedural hypoparathyroidism   HCC RxHCC
Parathyroprival tetany

E89.3   Postprocedural hypopituitarism   HCC RxHCC
Postirradiation hypopituitarism

5ᵗʰ E89.4   Postprocedural ovarian failure
E89.40   Asymptomatic postprocedural ovarian failure   ♀
Postprocedural ovarian failure NOS

E89.41   Symptomatic postprocedural ovarian failure   ♀
Symptoms such as flushing, sleeplessness, headache, lack of concentration, associated with postprocedural menopause

E89.5   Postprocedural testicular hypofunction   ♂

E89.6   Postprocedural adrenocortical (-medullary) hypofunction   cc HCC RxHCC CC/MCC Exc

5ᵗʰ E89.8   Other postprocedural endocrine and metabolic complications and disorders
6ᵗʰ E89.81   Postprocedural hemorrhage of an endocrine system organ or structure following a procedure
E89.810   Postprocedural hemorrhage of an endocrine system organ or structure following an endocrine system procedure   cc CC/MCC Exc

E89.811   Postprocedural hemorrhage of an endocrine system organ or structure following other procedure   cc CC/MCC Exc

6ᵗʰ E89.82   Postprocedural hematoma and seroma of an endocrine system organ or structure
E89.820   Postprocedural hematoma of an endocrine system organ or structure following an endocrine system procedure   cc CC/MCC Exc

E89.821   Postprocedural hematoma of an endocrine system organ or structure following other procedure   cc CC/MCC Exc

E89.822   Postprocedural seroma of an endocrine system organ or structure following an endocrine system procedure   cc CC/MCC Exc

E89.823   Postprocedural seroma of an endocrine system organ or structure following other procedure   cc CC/MCC Exc

E89.89   Other postprocedural endocrine and metabolic complications and disorders   cc CC/MCC Exc
Use additional code, if applicable, to further specify disorder

---

PDxMₑ Unacceptable principal diagnosis symbol per Medicare code edits   PDx Code exempt from diagnosis present on admission requirement
❓ Questionable admission   cc Complication or comorbidity   CC/MCC Exc CC/MCC exclusion   MCC Major complication or comorbidity
PDx CC Principal diagnosis as its own CC   PDx MCC Principal diagnosis as its own MCC   HCC HCC diagnosis code   RxHCC RxHCC diagnosis code
MACRA code   Z Z code as first-listed diagnosis

NOTES

NOTES

Chapter 5: Mental, Behavioral and Neurodevelopmental Disorders (F01-F99)

Mental, Behavioral and Neurodevelopmental disorders (F01-F99)

INCLUDES *disorders of psychological development*

EXCLUDES2 *symptoms, signs and abnormal clinical laboratory findings, not elsewhere classified (R00-R99)*

This chapter contains the following blocks:

F01-F09	Mental disorders due to known physiological conditions
F10-F19	Mental and behavioral disorders due to psychoactive substance use
F20-F29	Schizophrenia, schizotypal, delusional, and other non-mood psychotic disorders
F30-F39	Mood [affective] disorders
F40-F48	Anxiety, dissociative, stress-related, somatoform and other nonpsychotic mental disorders
F50-F59	Behavioral syndromes associated with physiological disturbances and physical factors
F60-F69	Disorders of adult personality and behavior
F70-F79	Intellectual disabilities
F80-F89	Pervasive and specific developmental disorders
F90-F98	Behavioral and emotional disorders with onset usually occurring in childhood and adolescence
F99	Unspecified mental disorder

Mental disorders due to known physiological conditions (F01-F09)

NOTES This block comprises a range of mental disorders grouped together on the basis of their having in common a demonstrable etiology in cerebral disease, brain injury, or other insult leading to cerebral dysfunction. The dysfunction may be primary, as in diseases, injuries, and insults that affect the brain directly and selectively; or secondary, as in systemic diseases and disorders that attack the brain only as one of the multiple organs or systems of the body that are involved.

4ᵗʰ **F01 Vascular dementia**

Vascular dementia as a result of infarction of the brain due to vascular disease, including hypertensive cerebrovascular disease.

INCLUDES *arteriosclerotic dementia*

Code first the underlying physiological condition or sequelae of cerebrovascular disease.

5ᵗʰ **F01.5 Vascular dementia**

F01.50 Vascular dementia without behavioral disturbance   A RxHCC PDxIn

Major neurocognitive disorder without behavioral disturbance

F01.51 Vascular dementia with behavioral disturbance   A CC RxHCC PDxIn CC/MCC Exc

Major neurocognitive disorder due to vascular disease, with behavioral disturbance

Major neurocognitive disorder with aggressive behavior

Major neurocognitive disorder with combative behavior

Major neurocognitive disorder with violent behavior

Vascular dementia with aggressive behavior

Vascular dementia with combative behavior

Vascular dementia with violent behavior

Use additional code, if applicable, to identify wandering in vascular dementia (Z91.83)

4ᵗʰ **F02 Dementia in other diseases classified elsewhere**

INCLUDES *Major neurocognitive disorder in other diseases classified elsewhere*

Code first the underlying physiological condition, such as:

Alzheimer's (G30.-)

cerebral lipidosis (E75.4)

Creutzfeldt-Jakob disease (A81.0-)

dementia with Lewy bodies (G31.83)

dementia with Parkinsonism (G31.83)

epilepsy and recurrent seizures (G40.-)

frontotemporal dementia (G31.09)

hepatolenticular degeneration (E83.0)

human immunodeficiency virus [HIV] disease (B20)

Huntington's disease (G10)

hypercalcemia (E83.52)

hypothyroidism, acquired (E00-E03.-)

intoxications (T36-T65)

Jakob-Creutzfeldt disease (A81.0-)

multiple sclerosis (G35)

neurosyphilis (A52.17)

niacin deficiency [pellagra] (E52)

Parkinson's disease (G20)

Pick's disease (G31.01)

polyarteritis nodosa (M30.0)

prion disease (A81.9)

systemic lupus erythematosus (M32.-)

traumatic brain injury (S06.-)

trypanosomiasis (B56.-, B57.-)

vitamin B deficiency (E53.8)

EXCLUDES2 *dementia in alcohol and psychoactive substance disorders (F10-F19, with .17, .27, .97)*

vascular dementia (F01.5-)

5ᵗʰ **F02.8 Dementia in other diseases classified elsewhere**

F02.80 Dementia in other diseases classified elsewhere without behavioral disturbance   RxHCC

AHA: Q1 2017, Q2 2016, Q4 2016

Dementia in other diseases classified elsewhere NOS

Major neurocognitive disorder in other diseases classified elsewhere

F02.81 Dementia in other diseases classified elsewhere with behavioral disturbance   CC RxHCC CC/MCC Exc

AHA: Q1 2017, Q2 2017

Dementia in other diseases classified elsewhere with aggressive behavior

Dementia in other diseases classified elsewhere with combative behavior

Dementia in other diseases classified elsewhere with violent behavior

Major neurocognitive disorder in other diseases classified elsewhere with aggressive behavior

Major neurocognitive disorder in other diseases classified elsewhere with combative behavior

Major neurocognitive disorder in other diseases classified elsewhere with violent behavior

Use additional code, if applicable, to identify wandering in dementia in conditions classified elsewhere (Z91.83)

4ᵗʰ **F03 Unspecified dementia**

Presenile dementia NOS

Presenile psychosis NOS

Primary degenerative dementia NOS

Senile dementia NOS

Senile dementia depressed or paranoid type

Senile psychosis NOS

EXCLUDES1 *senility NOS (R41.81)*

EXCLUDES2 *mild memory disturbance due to known physiological condition (F06.8)*

senile dementia with delirium or acute confusional state (F05)

5ᵗʰ **F03.9 Unspecified dementia**

F03.90 Unspecified dementia without behavioral disturbance   A RxHCC

Dementia NOS

Unspecified Code   Other Specified Code   Manifestation Code   N Newborn   P Pediatric   M Maternity   A Adult   ♂ Male   ♀ Female
● New Code   ▲ Revised Code Title   ▶◀ Revised Text   NOTES   INCLUDES   EXCLUDES 1 Not coded here   EXCLUDES 2 Not included here
4ᵗʰ 4ᵗʰ character required   5ᵗʰ 5ᵗʰ character required   6ᵗʰ 6ᵗʰ character required   7ᵗʰ 7ᵗʰ character required
7ᵗʰ Extension 'X' Alert   HAC Hospital-acquired condition (HAC) alert   AHA AHA Coding Clinic©

F03.91   **Unspecified dementia with behavioral disturbance**   A cc RxHCC CC/MCC Exc
Unspecified dementia with aggressive behavior
Unspecified dementia with combative behavior
Unspecified dementia with violent behavior
Use additional code, if applicable, to identify wandering in unspecified dementia (Z91.83)

F04   **Amnestic disorder due to known physiological condition**   RxHCC PDxIn
Korsakov's psychosis or syndrome, nonalcoholic
Code first the underlying physiological condition
EXCLUDES1   *amnesia NOS (R41.3)*
anterograde amnesia (R41.1)
dissociative amnesia (F44.0)
retrograde amnesia (R41.2)
EXCLUDES2   *alcohol-induced or unspecified Korsakov's syndrome (F10.26, F10.96)*
Korsakov's syndrome induced by other psychoactive substances (F13.26, F13.96, F19.16, F19.26, F19.96)

F05   **Delirium due to known physiological condition**   cc PDxIn CC/MCC Exc
Acute or subacute brain syndrome
Acute or subacute confusional state (nonalcoholic)
Acute or subacute infective psychosis
Acute or subacute organic reaction
Acute or subacute psycho-organic syndrome
Delirium of mixed etiology
Delirium superimposed on dementia
Sundowning
Code first the underlying physiological condition
EXCLUDES1   *delirium NOS (R41.0)*
EXCLUDES2   *delirium tremens alcohol-induced or unspecified (F10.231, F10.921)*

F06   **Other mental disorders due to known physiological condition**
INCLUDES   *mental disorders due to endocrine disorder*
mental disorders due to exogenous hormone
mental disorders due to exogenous toxic substance
mental disorders due to primary cerebral disease
mental disorders due to somatic illness
mental disorders due to systemic disease affecting the brain
Code first the underlying physiological condition
EXCLUDES1   *unspecified dementia (F03)*
EXCLUDES2   *delirium due to known physiological condition (F05)*
dementia as classified in F01-F02
other mental disorders associated with alcohol and other psychoactive substances (F10-F19)

F06.0   **Psychotic disorder with hallucinations due to known physiological condition**   cc PDxIn CC/MCC Exc
Organic hallucinatory state (nonalcoholic)
EXCLUDES2   *hallucinations and perceptual disturbance induced by alcohol and other psychoactive substances (F10-F19 with .151, .251, .951)*
schizophrenia (F20.-)

F06.1   **Catatonic disorder due to known physiological condition**   PDxIn
Catatonia associated with another mental disorder
Catatonia NOS
EXCLUDES1   *catatonic stupor (R40.1)*
stupor NOS (R40.1)
EXCLUDES2   *catatonic schizophrenia (F20.2)*
dissociative stupor (F44.2)

F06.2   **Psychotic disorder with delusions due to known physiological condition**   PDxIn CC/MCC Exc
Paranoid and paranoid-hallucinatory organic states
Schizophrenia-like psychosis in epilepsy
EXCLUDES2   *alcohol and drug-induced psychotic disorder (F10-F19 with .150, .250, .950)*
brief psychotic disorder (F23)
delusional disorder (F22)
schizophrenia (F20.-)

F06.3   **Mood disorder due to known physiological condition**
EXCLUDES2   *mood disorders due to alcohol and other psychoactive substances (F10-F19 with .14, .24, .94)*
mood disorders, not due to known physiological condition or unspecified (F30-F39)

F06.30   **Mood disorder due to known physiological condition, unspecified**   PDxIn

F06.31   **Mood disorder due to known physiological condition with depressive features**   PDxIn
Depressive disorder due to known physiological condition, with depressive features

F06.32   **Mood disorder due to known physiological condition with major depressive-like episode**   PDxIn
Depressive disorder due to known physiological condition, with major depressive-like episode

F06.33   **Mood disorder due to known physiological condition with manic features**   PDxIn
Bipolar and related disorder due to a known physiological condition, with manic features
Bipolar and related disorder due to known physiological condition, with manic- or hypomanic-like episodes

F06.34   **Mood disorder due to known physiological condition with mixed features**   PDxIn
Bipolar and related disorder due to known physiological condition, with mixed features
Depressive disorder due to known physiological condition, with mixed features

F06.4   **Anxiety disorder due to known physiological condition**   PDxIn
EXCLUDES2   *anxiety disorders due to alcohol and other psychoactive substances (F10-F19 with .180, .280, .980)*
anxiety disorders, not due to known physiological condition or unspecified (F40.-, F41.-)

F06.8   **Other specified mental disorders due to known physiological condition**   PDxIn
Epileptic psychosis NOS
Obsessive-compulsive and related disorder due to a known physiological condition
Organic dissociative disorder
Organic emotionally labile [asthenic] disorder

F07   **Personality and behavioral disorders due to known physiological condition**
Code first the underlying physiological condition

F07.0   **Personality change due to known physiological condition**   PDxIn
Frontal lobe syndrome
Limbic epilepsy personality syndrome
Lobotomy syndrome
Organic personality disorder
Organic pseudopsychopathic personality
Organic pseudoretarded personality
Postleucotomy syndrome
Code first underlying physiological condition
EXCLUDES1   *mild cognitive impairment (G31.84)*
postconcussional syndrome (F07.81)
postencephalitic syndrome (F07.89)
signs and symptoms involving emotional state (R45.-)
EXCLUDES2   *specific personality disorder (F60.-)*

F07.8   **Other personality and behavioral disorders due to known physiological condition**

F07.81   **Postconcussional syndrome**   PDxIn
Postcontusional syndrome (encephalopathy)
Post-traumatic brain syndrome, nonpsychotic
Use additional code to identify associated post-traumatic headache, if applicable (G44.3-)
EXCLUDES1   *current concussion (brain) (S06.0-)*
postencephalitic syndrome (F07.89)

F07.89   **Other personality and behavioral disorders due to known physiological condition**   PDxIn
Postencephalitic syndrome
Right hemispheric organic affective disorder

PDxIn Unacceptable principal diagnosis symbol per Medicare code edits   POA Code exempt from diagnosis present on admission requirement
❓ Questionable admission   cc Complication or comorbidity   CC/MCC Exc CC/MCC exclusion   MCC Major complication or comorbidity
PCC Principal diagnosis as its own CC   PMCC Principal diagnosis as its own MCC   HCC HCC diagnosis code   RxHCC RxHCC diagnosis code
MACRA code   Z1 Z code as first-listed diagnosis

F07.9 **Unspecified personality and behavioral disorder due to known physiological condition** PDxIn

Organic psychosyndrome

F09 **Unspecified mental disorder due to known physiological condition** PDxIn

Mental disorder NOS due to known physiological condition
Organic brain syndrome NOS
Organic mental disorder NOS
Organic psychosis NOS
Symptomatic psychosis NOS
Code first the underlying physiological condition

EXCLUDES1 psychosis NOS (F29)

Mental and behavioral disorders due to psychoactive substance use (F10-F19)

4ᵗʰ F10 **Alcohol related disorders**

Use additional code for blood alcohol level, if applicable (Y90.-)

5ᵗʰ F10.1 **Alcohol** abuse

EXCLUDES1 alcohol dependence (F10.2-)
        alcohol use, unspecified (F10.9-)

F10.10 **Alcohol abuse,** uncomplicated
Alcohol use disorder, mild

● F10.11 **Alcohol** abuse, in remission
Alcohol use disorder, mild, in early remission
Alcohol use disorder, mild, in sustained remission

6ᵗʰ F10.12 **Alcohol abuse with** intoxication

F10.120 **Alcohol abuse with intoxication,** uncomplicated HCC

F10.121 **Alcohol abuse with intoxication** delirium cꞏ HCC CC/MCC Exc

F10.129 **Alcohol abuse with intoxication, unspecified** HCC

F10.14 **Alcohol abuse with alcohol-induced mood disorder** cꞏ HCC CC/MCC Exc
Alcohol use disorder, mild, with alcohol-induced bipolar or related disorder
Alcohol use disorder, mild, with alcohol-induced depressive disorder

6ᵗʰ F10.15 **Alcohol abuse with** alcohol-induced psychotic disorder

F10.150 **Alcohol abuse with alcohol-induced psychotic disorder with** delusions HCC

F10.151 **Alcohol abuse with alcohol-induced psychotic disorder with** hallucinations cꞏ HCC CC/MCC Exc

F10.159 **Alcohol abuse with alcohol-induced psychotic disorder, unspecified** cꞏ HCC CC/MCC Exc

6ᵗʰ F10.18 **Alcohol abuse with** other alcohol-induced disorders

F10.180 **Alcohol abuse with alcohol-induced** anxiety disorder cꞏ HCC CC/MCC Exc

F10.181 **Alcohol abuse with alcohol-induced** sexual dysfunction cꞏ HCC CC/MCC Exc

F10.182 **Alcohol abuse with alcohol-induced** sleep disorder HCC

F10.188 **Alcohol abuse with other alcohol-induced disorder** cꞏ HCC CC/MCC Exc

F10.19 **Alcohol abuse with unspecified alcohol-induced disorder** cꞏ HCC CC/MCC Exc

5ᵗʰ F10.2 **Alcohol** dependence

EXCLUDES1 alcohol abuse (F10.1-)
        alcohol use, unspecified (F10.9-)

EXCLUDES2 toxic effect of alcohol (T51.0-)

F10.20 **Alcohol dependence,** uncomplicated HCC
Alcohol use disorder, moderate
Alcohol use disorder, severe

F10.21 **Alcohol dependence,** in remission HCC
Alcohol use disorder, moderate, in early remission
Alcohol use disorder, moderate, in sustained remission

Alcohol use disorder, severe, in early remission
Alcohol use disorder, severe, in sustained remission

6ᵗʰ F10.22 **Alcohol dependence** with intoxication
Acute drunkenness (in alcoholism)

EXCLUDES2 alcohol dependence with withdrawal (F10.23-)

F10.220 **Alcohol dependence with intoxication,** uncomplicated HCC

F10.221 **Alcohol dependence with intoxication** delirium cꞏ HCC CC/MCC Exc

F10.229 **Alcohol dependence with intoxication, unspecified** HCC

6ᵗʰ F10.23 **Alcohol dependence with** withdrawal

EXCLUDES2 Alcohol dependence with intoxication (F10.22-)

F10.230 **Alcohol dependence with withdrawal,** uncomplicated cꞏ HCC CC/MCC Exc

F10.231 **Alcohol dependence with withdrawal** delirium cꞏ HCC CC/MCC Exc

F10.232 **Alcohol dependence with withdrawal** with perceptual disturbance cꞏ HCC CC/MCC Exc

F10.239 **Alcohol dependence with withdrawal, unspecified** cꞏ HCC CC/MCC Exc

F10.24 **Alcohol dependence with alcohol-induced** mood disorder cꞏ HCC CC/MCC Exc
Alcohol use disorder, moderate, with alcohol-induced bipolar or related disorder
Alcohol use disorder, moderate, with alcohol-induced depressive disorder
Alcohol use disorder, severe, with alcohol-induced bipolar or related disorder
Alcohol use disorder, severe, with alcohol-induced depressive disorder

6ᵗʰ F10.25 **Alcohol dependence with alcohol-induced** psychotic disorder

F10.250 **Alcohol dependence with alcohol-induced psychotic disorder** with delusions HCC

F10.251 **Alcohol dependence with alcohol-induced psychotic disorder** with hallucinations cꞏ HCC CC/MCC Exc

F10.259 **Alcohol dependence with alcohol-induced psychotic disorder, unspecified** cꞏ HCC CC/MCC Exc

F10.26 **Alcohol dependence with alcohol-induced** persisting amnestic disorder HCC
Alcohol use disorder, moderate, with alcohol-induced major neurocognitive disorder, amnestic-confabulatory type
Alcohol use disorder, severe, with alcohol-induced major neurocognitive disorder, amnestic-confabulatory type

F10.27 **Alcohol dependence with alcohol-induced** persisting dementia cꞏ HCC CC/MCC Exc
Alcohol use disorder, moderate, with alcohol-induced major neurocognitive disorder, nonamnestic-confabulatory type
Alcohol use disorder, severe, with alcohol-induced major neurocognitive disorder, nonamnestic-confabulatory type

6ᵗʰ F10.28 **Alcohol dependence with** other alcohol-induced disorders

F10.280 **Alcohol dependence with alcohol-induced** anxiety disorder cꞏ HCC CC/MCC Exc

F10.281 **Alcohol dependence with alcohol-induced** sexual dysfunction cꞏ HCC CC/MCC Exc

F10.282 **Alcohol dependence with alcohol-induced** sleep disorder HCC

F10.288 **Alcohol dependence with other alcohol-induced disorder** cꞏ HCC CC/MCC Exc
Alcohol use disorder, moderate, with alcohol-induced mild neurocognitive disorder
Alcohol use disorder, severe, with alcohol-induced mild neurocognitive disorder

---

Unspecified Code Other Specified Code Manifestation Code N Newborn P Pediatric M Maternity A Adult ♂ Male ♀ Female
● New Code ▲ Revised Code Title ►◄ Revised Text **NOTES** *INCLUDES* *EXCLUDES 1* Not coded here *EXCLUDES 2* Not included here
4ᵗʰ 4ᵗʰ character required 5ᵗʰ 5ᵗʰ character required 6ᵗʰ 6ᵗʰ character required 7ᵗʰ 7ᵗʰ character required
Extension 'X' Alert HAC Hospital-acquired condition (HAC) alert **AHA** AHA Coding Clinic©

F10.29 **Alcohol dependence with unspecified alcohol-induced disorder** cᶜ HCC cc/mcc Exc

5ᵗʰ F10.9 **Alcohol** use, unspecified

> EXCLUDES1 *alcohol abuse (F10.1-)*
>
> *alcohol dependence (F10.2-)*

6ᵗʰ F10.92 **Alcohol use, unspecified** with intoxication

F10.920 **Alcohol use, unspecified with intoxication, uncomplicated** HCC

F10.921 **Alcohol use, unspecified with intoxication delirium** cᶜ HCC cc/mcc Exc

F10.929 **Alcohol use,** unspecified **with intoxication, unspecified** HCC

F10.94 **Alcohol use, unspecified with alcohol-induced mood disorder** cᶜ HCC cc/mcc Exc

Alcohol induced bipolar or related disorder, without use disorder

Alcohol induced depressive disorder, without use disorder

6ᵗʰ F10.95 **Alcohol use, unspecified with** alcohol-induced psychotic disorder

F10.950 **Alcohol use, unspecified with alcohol-induced psychotic disorder with delusions** HCC

F10.951 **Alcohol use, unspecified with alcohol-induced psychotic disorder with hallucinations** cᶜ HCC cc/mcc Exc

F10.959 **Alcohol use,** unspecified **with alcohol-induced psychotic disorder, unspecified** cᶜ HCC cc/mcc Exc

Alcohol-induced psychotic disorder without use disorder

F10.96 **Alcohol use, unspecified with** alcohol-induced persisting amnestic disorder HCC

Alcohol-induced major neurocognitive disorder, amnestic-confabulatory type, without use disorder

F10.97 **Alcohol use, unspecified with** alcohol-induced persisting dementia HCC

Alcohol-induced major neurocognitive disorder, nonamnestic-confabulatory type, without use disorder

6ᵗʰ F10.98 **Alcohol use, unspecified with** other alcohol-induced disorders

F10.980 **Alcohol use, unspecified with alcohol-induced** anxiety disorder cᶜ HCC cc/mcc Exc

Alcohol induced anxiety disorder, without use disorder

F10.981 **Alcohol use, unspecified with alcohol-induced** sexual dysfunction cᶜ HCC cc/mcc Exc

Alcohol induced sexual dysfunction, without use disorder

F10.982 **Alcohol use, unspecified with alcohol-induced** sleep disorder HCC

Alcohol induced sleep disorder, without use disorder

F10.988 **Alcohol use, unspecified with** other alcohol-induced disorder cᶜ HCC cc/mcc Exc

Alcohol induced mild neurocognitive disorder, without use disorder

F10.99 **Alcohol use, unspecified with unspecified alcohol-induced disorder** cᶜ HCC cc/mcc Exc

4ᵗʰ F11 **Opioid** related disorders

5ᵗʰ F11.1 **Opioid** abuse

> EXCLUDES1 *opioid dependence (F11.2-)*
>
> *opioid use, unspecified (F11.9-)*

F11.10 **Opioid abuse,** uncomplicated

Opioid use disorder, mild

● F11.11 **Opioid** abuse, in remission

Opioid use disorder, mild, in early remission

Opioid use disorder, mild, in sustained remission

6ᵗʰ F11.12 **Opioid abuse** with intoxication

F11.120 **Opioid abuse with intoxication, uncomplicated** HCC

F11.121 **Opioid abuse with intoxication delirium** cᶜ HCC cc/mcc Exc

F11.122 **Opioid abuse with intoxication with perceptual disturbance** HCC

F11.129 **Opioid abuse with intoxication, unspecified** HCC

F11.14 **Opioid abuse with opioid-induced mood disorder** HCC

Opioid use disorder, mild, with opioid-induced depressive disorder

6ᵗʰ F11.15 **Opioid abuse with opioid-induced** psychotic disorder

F11.150 **Opioid abuse with opioid-induced psychotic disorder with delusions** cᶜ HCC cc/mcc Exc

F11.151 **Opioid abuse with opioid-induced psychotic disorder with hallucinations** cᶜ HCC cc/mcc Exc

F11.159 **Opioid abuse with opioid-induced psychotic disorder, unspecified** HCC

6ᵗʰ F11.18 **Opioid abuse with** other opioid-induced disorder

F11.181 **Opioid abuse with opioid-induced sexual dysfunction** HCC

F11.182 **Opioid abuse with opioid-induced sleep disorder** HCC

F11.188 **Opioid abuse with other opioid-induced disorder** HCC

F11.19 **Opioid abuse with unspecified opioid-induced disorder** HCC

5ᵗʰ F11.2 **Opioid** dependence

> EXCLUDES1 *opioid abuse (F11.1-)*
>
> *opioid use, unspecified (F11.9-)*
>
> EXCLUDES2 *opioid poisoning (T40.0-T40.2-)*

F11.20 **Opioid dependence,** uncomplicated cᶜ HCC

Opioid use disorder, moderate

Opioid use disorder, severe

F11.21 **Opioid dependence,** in remission HCC

Opioid use disorder, moderate, in early remission

Opioid use disorder, moderate, in sustained remission

Opioid use disorder, severe, in early remission

Opioid use disorder, severe, in sustained remission

6ᵗʰ F11.22 **Opioid dependence** with intoxication

> EXCLUDES1 *opioid dependence with withdrawal (F11.23)*

F11.220 **Opioid dependence with intoxication, uncomplicated** HCC

F11.221 **Opioid dependence with intoxication delirium** cᶜ HCC cc/mcc Exc

F11.222 **Opioid dependence with intoxication with perceptual disturbance** cᶜ HCC

F11.229 **Opioid dependence with intoxication, unspecified** HCC

F11.23 **Opioid dependence** with withdrawal cᶜ HCC cc/mcc Exc

> EXCLUDES1 *opioid dependence with intoxication (F11.22-)*

F11.24 **Opioid dependence with opioid-induced** mood disorder HCC

Opioid use disorder, moderate, with opioid induced depressive disorder

6ᵗʰ F11.25 **Opioid dependence with opioid-induced** psychotic disorder

F11.250 **Opioid dependence with opioid-induced psychotic disorder with delusions** cᶜ HCC cc/mcc Exc

F11.251 **Opioid dependence with opioid-induced psychotic disorder with hallucinations** cᶜ HCC cc/mcc Exc

F11.259 **Opioid dependence with opioid-induced psychotic disorder, unspecified** cᶜ HCC

ᴾᴰˣ Unacceptable principal diagnosis symbol per Medicare code edits   ᴾᴼᴬ Code exempt from diagnosis present on admission requirement
❓ Questionable admission   cᶜ Complication or comorbidity   cc/mcc Exc CC/MCC exclusion   mcᶜ Major complication or comorbidity
ᴾᴰˣ Principal diagnosis as its own CC   ᴾᴰˣ Principal diagnosis as its own MCC   HCC HCC diagnosis code   RxHCC RxHCC diagnosis code
MACRA code   Z1 Z code as first-listed diagnosis

546   When symbols appear on a code that requires a 7th character extension, refer to Appendix B to identify applicable 7th character codes.   **2018 ICD-10-CM**

[6th] **F11.28 Opioid dependence with** other opioid-induced disorder
- **F11.281 Opioid dependence with opioid-induced** sexual dysfunction CC [HCC]
- **F11.282 Opioid dependence with opioid-induced** sleep disorder CC [HCC]
- **F11.288 Opioid dependence with other opioid-induced disorder** CC [HCC]

F11.29 Opioid dependence with unspecified opioid-induced disorder [HCC]

[5th] **F11.9 Opioid** use, **unspecified**

[EXCLUDES1] *opioid abuse (F11.1-)*
opioid dependence (F11.2-)

F11.90 Opioid use, unspecified, uncomplicated

[6th] **F11.92 Opioid use, unspecified** with intoxication

[EXCLUDES1] *opioid use, unspecified with withdrawal (F11.93)*

- **F11.920 Opioid use, unspecified with intoxication,** uncomplicated [HCC]
- **F11.921 Opioid use, unspecified with intoxication** delirium CC [HCC] CC/MCC Exc
  Opioid-induced delirium
- **F11.922 Opioid use, unspecified with intoxication with** perceptual disturbance [HCC]
- **F11.929 Opioid use, unspecified with intoxication, unspecified** [HCC]

F11.93 Opioid use, unspecified with withdrawal CC [HCC] CC/MCC Exc

[EXCLUDES1] *opioid use, unspecified with intoxication (F11.92-)*

F11.94 Opioid use, unspecified with opioid-induced mood disorder [HCC]
Opioid induced depressive disorder, without use disorder

[6th] **F11.95 Opioid use, unspecified with opioid-induced** psychotic disorder
- **F11.950 Opioid use, unspecified with opioid-induced psychotic disorder with** delusions CC [HCC] CC/MCC Exc
- **F11.951 Opioid use, unspecified with opioid-induced psychotic disorder with** hallucinations CC [HCC] CC/MCC Exc
- **F11.959 Opioid use, unspecified with opioid-induced psychotic disorder, unspecified** [HCC]

[6th] **F11.98 Opioid use, unspecified with** other specified opioid-induced disorder
- **F11.981 Opioid use, unspecified with opioid-induced** sexual dysfunction [HCC]
  Opioid induced sexual dysfunction, without use disorder
- **F11.982 Opioid use, unspecified with opioid-induced** sleep disorder [HCC]
  Opioid induced sleep disorder, without use disorder
- **F11.988 Opioid use, unspecified with other opioid-induced disorder** [HCC]
  Opioid induced anxiety disorder, without use disorder

F11.99 Opioid use, unspecified with unspecified opioid-induced disorder [HCC]

[4th] **F12** Cannabis **related disorders**

[INCLUDES] *marijuana*

[5th] **F12.1 Cannabis** abuse

[EXCLUDES1] *cannabis dependence (F12.2-)*
cannabis use, unspecified (F12.9-)

F12.10 Cannabis abuse, uncomplicated
Cannabis use disorder, mild

● **F12.11 Cannabis** abuse, **in remission**
Cannabis use disorder, mild, in early remission
Cannabis use disorder, mild, in sustained remission

[6th] **F12.12 Cannabis abuse** with intoxication
- **F12.120 Cannabis abuse with intoxication,** uncomplicated [HCC]
- **F12.121 Cannabis abuse with intoxication** delirium CC [HCC] CC/MCC Exc
- **F12.122 Cannabis abuse with intoxication with** perceptual disturbance [HCC]
- **F12.129 Cannabis abuse with intoxication, unspecified** [HCC]

[6th] **F12.15 Cannabis abuse with psychotic disorder**
- **F12.150 Cannabis abuse with psychotic disorder with** delusions CC [HCC] CC/MCC Exc
- **F12.151 Cannabis abuse with psychotic disorder with** hallucinations CC [HCC] CC/MCC Exc
- **F12.159 Cannabis abuse with psychotic disorder, unspecified** [HCC]

[6th] **F12.18 Cannabis abuse with** other cannabis-induced disorder
- **F12.180 Cannabis abuse with cannabis-induced** anxiety disorder [HCC]
- **F12.188 Cannabis abuse with other cannabis-induced disorder** [HCC]
  Cannabis use disorder, mild, with cannabis-induced sleep disorder

F12.19 Cannabis abuse with unspecified cannabis-induced disorder [HCC]

[5th] **F12.2 Cannabis** dependence

[EXCLUDES1] *cannabis abuse (F12.1-)*
cannabis use, unspecified (F12.9-)

[EXCLUDES2] *cannabis poisoning (T40.7-)*

F12.20 Cannabis dependence, uncomplicated [HCC]
Cannabis use disorder, moderate
Cannabis use disorder, severe

F12.21 Cannabis dependence, in remission [HCC]
Cannabis use disorder, moderate, in early remission
Cannabis use disorder, moderate, in sustained remission
Cannabis use disorder, severe, in early remission
Cannabis use disorder, severe, in sustained remission

[6th] **F12.22 Cannabis dependence** with intoxication
- **F12.220 Cannabis dependence with intoxication,** uncomplicated [HCC]
- **F12.221 Cannabis dependence with intoxication** delirium CC [HCC] CC/MCC Exc
- **F12.222 Cannabis dependence with intoxication with** perceptual disturbance [HCC]
- **F12.229 Cannabis dependence with intoxication, unspecified** [HCC]

[6th] **F12.25 Cannabis dependence** with psychotic disorder
- **F12.250 Cannabis dependence with psychotic disorder with** delusions CC [HCC] CC/MCC Exc
- **F12.251 Cannabis dependence with psychotic disorder with** hallucinations CC [HCC] CC/MCC Exc
- **F12.259 Cannabis dependence with psychotic disorder, unspecified** [HCC]

[6th] **F12.28 Cannabis dependence with** other cannabis-induced disorder
- **F12.280 Cannabis dependence with cannabis-induced** anxiety disorder [HCC]
- **F12.288 Cannabis dependence with other cannabis-induced disorder** [HCC]
  Cannabis use disorder, moderate, with cannabis-induced sleep disorder
  Cannabis use disorder, severe, with cannabis-induced sleep disorder
  Cannabis withdrawal

F12.29 Cannabis dependence with unspecified cannabis-induced disorder [HCC]

[5th] **F12.9 Cannabis** use, **unspecified**

[EXCLUDES1] *cannabis abuse (F12.1-)*
cannabis dependence (F12.2-)

Unspecified Code | Other Specified Code | Manifestation Code | [N] Newborn | [P] Pediatric | [M] Maternity | [A] Adult | ♂ Male | ♀ Female
● New Code | ▲ Revised Code Title | ►◄ Revised Text | [NOTES] | [INCLUDES] | [EXCLUDES1] Not coded here | [EXCLUDES2] Not included here
[4th] 4th character required | [5th] 5th character required | [6th] 6th character required | [7th] 7th character required
[x7th] Extension 'X' Alert | [HAC] Hospital-acquired condition (HAC) alert | AHA AHA Coding Clinic©

F12.90 Cannabis use, unspecified, uncomplicated

🔳 F12.92 Cannabis use, unspecified with intoxication

F12.920 **Cannabis use, unspecified with intoxication,** uncomplicated `HCC`

F12.921 **Cannabis use, unspecified with intoxication** delirium `CC HCC CC/MCC Exc`

F12.922 **Cannabis use, unspecified with intoxication with** perceptual disturbance `HCC`

F12.929 **Cannabis use, unspecified with intoxication,** unspecified `HCC`

🔳 F12.95 Cannabis use, unspecified with psychotic disorder

F12.950 **Cannabis use, unspecified with psychotic disorder with** delusions `CC HCC CC/MCC Exc`

F12.951 **Cannabis use, unspecified with psychotic disorder with** hallucinations `CC HCC CC/MCC Exc`

F12.959 **Cannabis use, unspecified with psychotic disorder, unspecified** `HCC`
Cannabis induced psychotic disorder, without use disorder

🔳 F12.98 Cannabis use, unspecified with other cannabis-induced disorder

F12.980 **Cannabis use, unspecified with** anxiety disorder `HCC`
Cannabis induced anxiety disorder, without use disorder

F12.988 **Cannabis use, unspecified with other cannabis-induced disorder** `HCC`
Cannabis induced sleep disorder, without use disorder

F12.99 **Cannabis use, unspecified with unspecified cannabis-induced disorder** `HCC`

🔳 F13 Sedative, hypnotic, or anxiolytic related disorders

🔳 F13.1 Sedative, hypnotic or anxiolytic-related abuse

EXCLUDES1 sedative, hypnotic or anxiolytic-related dependence (F13.2-)

sedative, hypnotic, or anxiolytic use, unspecified (F13.9-)

F13.10 **Sedative, hypnotic or anxiolytic abuse,** uncomplicated
Sedative, hypnotic, or anxiolytic use disorder, mild

● F13.11 **Sedative, hypnotic or anxiolytic** abuse, **in remission**
Sedative, hypnotic or anxiolytic use disorder, mild, in early remission
Sedative, hypnotic or anxiolytic use disorder, mild, in sustained remission

🔳 F13.12 Sedative, hypnotic or anxiolytic abuse with intoxication

F13.120 **Sedative, hypnotic or anxiolytic abuse with intoxication,** uncomplicated `HCC`

F13.121 **Sedative, hypnotic or anxiolytic abuse with intoxication** delirium `CC HCC CC/MCC Exc`

F13.129 **Sedative, hypnotic or anxiolytic abuse with intoxication, unspecified** `HCC`

F13.14 **Sedative, hypnotic or anxiolytic abuse with sedative, hypnotic or anxiolytic-induced** mood disorder `HCC`
Sedative, hypnotic, or anxiolytic use disorder, mild, with sedative, hypnotic, or ▶anxiolytic-induced◀ bipolar or related disorder
Sedative, hypnotic, or anxiolytic use disorder, mild, with sedative, hypnotic, or ▶anxiolytic-induced◀ depressive disorder

🔳 F13.15 Sedative, hypnotic or anxiolytic abuse with sedative, hypnotic or anxiolytic-induced psychotic disorder

F13.150 **Sedative, hypnotic or anxiolytic abuse with sedative, hypnotic or anxiolytic-induced psychotic disorder with** delusions `CC HCC CC/MCC Exc`

F13.151 **Sedative, hypnotic or anxiolytic abuse with sedative, hypnotic or anxiolytic-induced psychotic disorder with** hallucinations `CC HCC CC/MCC Exc`

F13.159 **Sedative, hypnotic or anxiolytic abuse with sedative, hypnotic or anxiolytic-induced psychotic disorder, unspecified** `HCC`

🔳 F13.18 Sedative, hypnotic or anxiolytic abuse with other sedative, hypnotic or anxiolytic-induced disorders

F13.180 **Sedative, hypnotic or anxiolytic abuse with sedative, hypnotic or anxiolytic-induced** anxiety disorder `HCC`

F13.181 **Sedative, hypnotic or anxiolytic abuse with sedative, hypnotic or anxiolytic-induced** sexual dysfunction `HCC`

F13.182 **Sedative, hypnotic or anxiolytic abuse with sedative, hypnotic or anxiolytic-induced** sleep disorder `HCC`

F13.188 **Sedative, hypnotic or anxiolytic abuse with other sedative, hypnotic or anxiolytic-induced disorder** `HCC`

F13.19 **Sedative, hypnotic or anxiolytic abuse with unspecified sedative, hypnotic or anxiolytic-induced disorder** `HCC`

🔳 F13.2 Sedative, hypnotic or anxiolytic-related dependence

EXCLUDES1 sedative, hypnotic or anxiolytic-related abuse (F13.1-)

sedative, hypnotic, or anxiolytic use, unspecified (F13.9-)

EXCLUDES2 sedative, hypnotic, or anxiolytic poisoning (T42.-)

F13.20 **Sedative, hypnotic or anxiolytic dependence,** uncomplicated `CC HCC`

F13.21 **Sedative, hypnotic or anxiolytic dependence, in** remission `HCC`
Sedative, hypnotic or anxiolytic use disorder, moderate, in early remission
Sedative, hypnotic or anxiolytic use disorder, moderate, in sustained remission
Sedative, hypnotic or anxiolytic use disorder, severe, in early remission
Sedative, hypnotic or anxiolytic use disorder, severe, in sustained remission

🔳 F13.22 Sedative, hypnotic or anxiolytic dependence with intoxication

EXCLUDES1 sedative, hypnotic or anxiolytic dependence with withdrawal (F13.23-)

F13.220 **Sedative, hypnotic or anxiolytic dependence with intoxication,** uncomplicated `HCC`

F13.221 **Sedative, hypnotic or anxiolytic dependence with intoxication** delirium `CC HCC CC/MCC Exc`

F13.229 **Sedative, hypnotic or anxiolytic dependence with intoxication, unspecified** `HCC`

🔳 F13.23 Sedative, hypnotic or anxiolytic dependence with withdrawal
Sedative, hypnotic, or anxiolytic use disorder, moderate
Sedative, hypnotic, or anxiolytic use disorder, severe

EXCLUDES1 sedative, hypnotic or anxiolytic dependence with intoxication (F13.22-)

F13.230 **Sedative, hypnotic or anxiolytic dependence with withdrawal,** uncomplicated `CC HCC CC/MCC Exc`

F13.231 **Sedative, hypnotic or anxiolytic dependence with withdrawal** delirium `CC HCC CC/MCC Exc`

F13.232 **Sedative, hypnotic or anxiolytic dependence with withdrawal with** perceptual disturbance `CC HCC CC/MCC Exc`
Sedative, hypnotic, or anxiolytic withdrawal with perceptual disturbances

---

😳 Unacceptable principal diagnosis symbol per Medicare code edits   😳 Code exempt from diagnosis present on admission requirement
❓ Questionable admission   `CC` Complication or comorbidity   `CC/MCC` CC/MCC exclusion   `MCC` Major complication or comorbidity
📘 Principal diagnosis as its own CC   📘 Principal diagnosis as its own MCC   `HCC` HCC diagnosis code   `RxHCC` RxHCC diagnosis code
MACRA code   `Z` Z code as first-listed diagnosis

548   When symbols appear on a code that requires a 7th character extension, refer to Appendix B to identify applicable 7th character codes.   **2018 ICD-10-CM**

F13.239 **Sedative, hypnotic or anxiolytic dependence with withdrawal, unspecified** CC HCC CC/MCC Exc
Sedative, hypnotic, or anxiolytic withdrawal without perceptual disturbances

F13.24 **Sedative, hypnotic or anxiolytic dependence with sedative, hypnotic or anxiolytic-induced mood disorder** HCC
Sedative, hypnotic, or anxiolytic use disorder, moderate, with sedative, hypnotic, or ▶anxiolytic-induced◀ bipolar or related disorder
Sedative, hypnotic, or anxiolytic use disorder, moderate, with sedative, hypnotic, or ▶anxiolytic-induced◀ depressive disorder
Sedative, hypnotic, or anxiolytic use disorder, severe, with sedative, hypnotic, or ▶anxiolytic-induced◀ bipolar or related disorder
Sedative, hypnotic, or anxiolytic use disorder, severe, with sedative, hypnotic, or ▶anxiolytic-induced◀ depressive disorder

[6th] F13.25 **Sedative, hypnotic or anxiolytic dependence with sedative, hypnotic or anxiolytic-induced psychotic disorder**

F13.250 **Sedative, hypnotic or anxiolytic dependence with sedative, hypnotic or anxiolytic-induced psychotic disorder with delusions** CC HCC CC/MCC Exc

F13.251 **Sedative, hypnotic or anxiolytic dependence with sedative, hypnotic or anxiolytic-induced psychotic disorder with hallucinations** CC HCC CC/MCC Exc

F13.259 **Sedative, hypnotic or anxiolytic dependence with sedative, hypnotic or anxiolytic-induced psychotic disorder, unspecified** CC HCC

F13.26 **Sedative, hypnotic or anxiolytic dependence with sedative, hypnotic or anxiolytic-induced persisting amnestic disorder** CC HCC

F13.27 **Sedative, hypnotic or anxiolytic dependence with sedative, hypnotic or anxiolytic-induced persisting dementia** CC HCC CC/MCC Exc
Sedative, hypnotic, or anxiolytic use disorder, moderate, with sedative, hypnotic, or ▶anxiolytic-induced◀ major neurocognitive disorder
Sedative, hypnotic, or anxiolytic use disorder, severe, with sedative, hypnotic, or anxiolytic-induced major neurocognitive disorder

[6th] F13.28 **Sedative, hypnotic or anxiolytic dependence with other sedative, hypnotic or anxiolytic-induced disorders**

F13.280 **Sedative, hypnotic or anxiolytic dependence with sedative, hypnotic or anxiolytic-induced anxiety disorder** CC HCC

F13.281 **Sedative, hypnotic or anxiolytic dependence with sedative, hypnotic or anxiolytic-induced sexual dysfunction** CC HCC

F13.282 **Sedative, hypnotic or anxiolytic dependence with sedative, hypnotic or anxiolytic-induced sleep disorder** CC HCC

F13.288 **Sedative, hypnotic or anxiolytic dependence with other sedative, hypnotic or anxiolytic-induced disorder** CC HCC
Sedative, hypnotic, or anxiolytic use disorder, moderate, with sedative, hypnotic, or ▶anxiolytic-induced◀ mild neurocognitive disorder
Sedative, hypnotic, or anxiolytic use disorder, severe, with sedative, hypnotic, or ▶anxiolytic-induced◀ mild neurocognitive disorder

F13.29 **Sedative, hypnotic or anxiolytic dependence with unspecified sedative, hypnotic or anxiolytic-induced disorder** HCC

[5th] F13.9 **Sedative, hypnotic or anxiolytic-related use, unspecified**
[EXCLUDES1] *sedative, hypnotic or anxiolytic-related abuse (F13.1-)*
sedative, hypnotic or anxiolytic-related dependence (F13.2-)

F13.90 **Sedative, hypnotic, or anxiolytic use, unspecified, uncomplicated**

[6th] F13.92 **Sedative, hypnotic or anxiolytic use, unspecified with intoxication**
[EXCLUDES1] *sedative, hypnotic or anxiolytic use, unspecified with withdrawal (F13.93-)*

F13.920 **Sedative, hypnotic or anxiolytic use, unspecified with intoxication, uncomplicated** HCC

F13.921 **Sedative, hypnotic or anxiolytic use, unspecified with intoxication delirium** CC HCC CC/MCC Exc
Sedative, hypnotic, or anxiolytic-induced delirium

F13.929 **Sedative, hypnotic or anxiolytic use, unspecified with intoxication, unspecified** HCC

[6th] F13.93 **Sedative, hypnotic or anxiolytic use, unspecified with withdrawal**
[EXCLUDES1] *sedative, hypnotic or anxiolytic use, unspecified with intoxication (F13.92-)*

F13.930 **Sedative, hypnotic or anxiolytic use, unspecified with withdrawal, uncomplicated** CC HCC CC/MCC Exc

F13.931 **Sedative, hypnotic or anxiolytic use, unspecified with withdrawal delirium** CC HCC CC/MCC Exc

F13.932 **Sedative, hypnotic or anxiolytic use, unspecified with withdrawal with perceptual disturbances** CC HCC CC/MCC Exc

F13.939 **Sedative, hypnotic or anxiolytic use, unspecified with withdrawal, unspecified** CC HCC CC/MCC Exc

F13.94 **Sedative, hypnotic or anxiolytic use, unspecified with sedative, hypnotic or anxiolytic-induced mood disorder** HCC
Sedative, hypnotic, or anxiolytic-induced bipolar or related disorder, without use disorder
Sedative, hypnotic, or anxiolytic-induced depressive disorder, without use disorder

[6th] F13.95 **Sedative, hypnotic or anxiolytic use, unspecified with sedative, hypnotic or anxiolytic-induced psychotic disorder**

F13.950 **Sedative, hypnotic or anxiolytic use, unspecified with sedative, hypnotic or anxiolytic-induced psychotic disorder with delusions** CC HCC CC/MCC Exc

F13.951 **Sedative, hypnotic or anxiolytic use, unspecified with sedative, hypnotic or anxiolytic-induced psychotic disorder with hallucinations** CC HCC CC/MCC Exc

F13.959 **Sedative, hypnotic or anxiolytic use, unspecified with sedative, hypnotic or anxiolytic-induced psychotic disorder, unspecified** HCC
Sedative, hypnotic, or ▶anxiolytic-induced◀ psychotic disorder, without use disorder

F13.96 **Sedative, hypnotic or anxiolytic use, unspecified with sedative, hypnotic or anxiolytic-induced persisting amnestic disorder** HCC

F13.97 **Sedative, hypnotic or anxiolytic use, unspecified with sedative, hypnotic or anxiolytic-induced persisting dementia** CC HCC CC/MCC Exc
Sedative, hypnotic, or ▶anxiolytic-induced◀ major neurocognitive disorder, without use disorder

[6th] F13.98 **Sedative, hypnotic or anxiolytic use, unspecified with other sedative, hypnotic or anxiolytic-induced disorders**

F13.980 **Sedative, hypnotic or anxiolytic use, unspecified with sedative, hypnotic or anxiolytic-induced** anxiety disorder **HCC**
Sedative, hypnotic, or ▶anxiolytic-induced◀ anxiety disorder, without use disorder

F13.981 **Sedative, hypnotic or anxiolytic use, unspecified with sedative, hypnotic or anxiolytic-induced** sexual dysfunction **HCC**
Sedative, hypnotic, or ▶anxiolytic-induced◀ sexual dysfunction disorder, without use disorder

F13.982 **Sedative, hypnotic or anxiolytic use, unspecified with sedative, hypnotic or anxiolytic-induced** sleep disorder **HCC**
Sedative, hypnotic, or ▶anxiolytic-induced◀ sleep disorder, without use disorder

F13.988 **Sedative, hypnotic or anxiolytic use, unspecified with other sedative, hypnotic or anxiolytic-induced disorder** **HCC**
Sedative, hypnotic, or ▶anxiolytic-induced◀ mild neurocognitive disorder

F13.99 **Sedative, hypnotic or anxiolytic use, unspecified with unspecified sedative, hypnotic or anxiolytic-induced disorder** **HCC**

F14 Cocaine related disorders
EXCLUDES2 other stimulant-related disorders (F15.-)

F14.1 Cocaine abuse
EXCLUDES1 cocaine dependence (F14.2-)
cocaine use, unspecified (F14.9-)

F14.10 **Cocaine abuse,** uncomplicated
Cocaine use disorder, mild

● F14.11 **Cocaine** abuse, in remission
Cocaine use disorder, mild, in early remission
Cocaine use disorder, mild, in sustained remission

F14.12 **Cocaine abuse** with intoxication
F14.120 **Cocaine abuse with intoxication,** uncomplicated **HCC**
F14.121 **Cocaine abuse with intoxication with** delirium ᴄᴄ HCC ᴄᴄ/ᴍᴄᴄ ᴇ̶ˣ̶ᴄ̶
F14.122 **Cocaine abuse with intoxication with** perceptual disturbance **HCC**
F14.129 **Cocaine abuse with intoxication, unspecified** **HCC**

F14.14 **Cocaine abuse with cocaine-induced** mood disorder **HCC**
Cocaine use disorder, mild, with cocaine-induced bipolar or related disorder
Cocaine use disorder, mild, with cocaine-induced depressive disorder

F14.15 **Cocaine abuse with cocaine-induced** psychotic disorder
F14.150 **Cocaine abuse with cocaine-induced psychotic disorder with** delusions ᴄᴄ HCC ᴄᴄ/ᴍᴄᴄ ᴇ̶ˣ̶ᴄ̶
F14.151 **Cocaine abuse with cocaine-induced psychotic disorder with** hallucinations ᴄᴄ HCC ᴄᴄ/ᴍᴄᴄ ᴇ̶ˣ̶ᴄ̶
F14.159 **Cocaine abuse with cocaine-induced psychotic disorder, unspecified** **HCC**

F14.18 **Cocaine abuse with other cocaine-induced disorder**
F14.180 **Cocaine abuse with cocaine-induced** anxiety disorder **HCC**
F14.181 **Cocaine abuse with cocaine-induced** sexual dysfunction **HCC**
F14.182 **Cocaine abuse with cocaine-induced** sleep disorder **HCC**
F14.188 **Cocaine abuse with other cocaine-induced disorder** **HCC**
Cocaine use disorder, mild, with cocaine-induced obsessive compulsive or related disorder

F14.19 **Cocaine abuse with unspecified cocaine-induced disorder** **HCC**

F14.2 Cocaine dependence
EXCLUDES1 cocaine abuse (F14.1-)
cocaine use, unspecified (F14.9-)
EXCLUDES2 cocaine poisoning (T40.5-)

F14.20 **Cocaine dependence,** uncomplicated ᴄᴄ HCC
Cocaine use disorder, moderate
Cocaine use disorder, severe

F14.21 **Cocaine dependence,** in remission **HCC**
AHA: Q2 2017
Cocaine use disorder, moderate, in early remission
Cocaine use disorder, moderate, in sustained remission
Cocaine use disorder, severe, in early remission
Cocaine use disorder, severe, in sustained remission

F14.22 **Cocaine dependence with intoxication**
EXCLUDES1 cocaine dependence with withdrawal (F14.23)
F14.220 **Cocaine dependence with intoxication,** uncomplicated **HCC**
F14.221 **Cocaine dependence with intoxication** delirium ᴄᴄ HCC ᴄᴄ/ᴍᴄᴄ ᴇ̶ˣ̶ᴄ̶
F14.222 **Cocaine dependence with intoxication with** perceptual disturbance ᴄᴄ HCC
F14.229 **Cocaine dependence with intoxication, unspecified** ᴄᴄ HCC

F14.23 **Cocaine dependence** with withdrawal ᴄᴄ HCC ᴄᴄ/ᴍᴄᴄ ᴇ̶ˣ̶ᴄ̶
EXCLUDES1 cocaine dependence with intoxication (F14.22-)

F14.24 **Cocaine dependence with cocaine-induced** mood disorder **HCC**
Cocaine use disorder, moderate, with cocaine-induced bipolar or related disorder
Cocaine use disorder, moderate, with cocaine-induced depressive disorder
Cocaine use disorder, severe, with cocaine-induced bipolar or related disorder
Cocaine use disorder, severe, with cocaine-induced depressive disorder

F14.25 **Cocaine dependence with cocaine-induced** psychotic disorder
F14.250 **Cocaine dependence with cocaine-induced psychotic disorder with** delusions ᴄᴄ HCC ᴄᴄ/ᴍᴄᴄ ᴇ̶ˣ̶ᴄ̶
F14.251 **Cocaine dependence with cocaine-induced psychotic disorder with** hallucinations ᴄᴄ HCC ᴄᴄ/ᴍᴄᴄ ᴇ̶ˣ̶ᴄ̶
F14.259 **Cocaine dependence with cocaine-induced psychotic disorder, unspecified** ᴄᴄ HCC

F14.28 **Cocaine dependence with other cocaine-induced disorder**
F14.280 **Cocaine dependence with cocaine-induced** anxiety disorder ᴄᴄ HCC
F14.281 **Cocaine dependence with cocaine-induced** sexual dysfunction ᴄᴄ HCC
F14.282 **Cocaine dependence with cocaine-induced** sleep disorder ᴄᴄ HCC
F14.288 **Cocaine dependence with other cocaine-induced disorder** ᴄᴄ HCC
Cocaine use disorder, moderate, with cocaine-induced obsessive compulsive or related disorder
Cocaine use disorder, severe, with cocaine-induced obsessive compulsive or related disorder

F14.29 **Cocaine dependence with unspecified cocaine-induced disorder** **HCC**

F14.9 Cocaine use, unspecified
EXCLUDES1 cocaine abuse (F14.1-)
cocaine dependence (F14.2-)

F14.90 **Cocaine use, unspecified,** uncomplicated

F14.92 **Cocaine use, unspecified** with intoxication

ᴘᴅˣ Unacceptable principal diagnosis symbol per Medicare code edits   ᴘᴏ̸ᴀ Code exempt from diagnosis present on admission requirement
? Questionable admission   ᴄᴄ Complication or comorbidity   ᴄᴄ/ᴍᴄᴄ ᴇˣᴄ CC/MCC exclusion   ᴍᴄᴄ Major complication or comorbidity
ᴘᴅˣ Principal diagnosis as its own CC   ᴘᴅˣ Principal diagnosis as its own MCC   HCC HCC diagnosis code   ʀˣʜᴄᴄ RxHCC diagnosis code
MACRA code   Z₁ Z code as first-listed diagnosis

F14.920 Cocaine use, unspecified with intoxication, uncomplicated

F14.921 Cocaine use, unspecified with intoxication delirium cc⊘ HCC CC/MCC Exc

F14.922 Cocaine use, unspecified with intoxication with perceptual disturbance HCC

F14.929 Cocaine use, unspecified with intoxication, unspecified HCC

F14.94 Cocaine use, unspecified with cocaine-induced mood disorder HCC

Cocaine induced bipolar or related disorder, without use disorder

Cocaine induced depressive disorder, without use disorder

6ᵗʰ F14.95 Cocaine use, unspecified with cocaine-induced psychotic disorder

F14.950 Cocaine use, unspecified with cocaine-induced psychotic disorder with delusions cc⊘ HCC CC/MCC Exc

F14.951 Cocaine use, unspecified with cocaine-induced psychotic disorder with hallucinations cc⊘ HCC CC/MCC Exc

F14.959 Cocaine use, unspecified with cocaine-induced psychotic disorder, unspecified HCC

Cocaine induced psychotic disorder, without use disorder

6ᵗʰ F14.98 Cocaine use, unspecified with other specified cocaine-induced disorder

F14.980 Cocaine use, unspecified with cocaine-induced anxiety disorder HCC

Cocaine induced anxiety disorder, without use disorder

F14.981 Cocaine use, unspecified with cocaine-induced sexual dysfunction HCC

Cocaine induced sexual dysfunction, without use disorder

F14.982 Cocaine use, unspecified with cocaine-induced sleep disorder HCC

Cocaine induced sleep disorder, without use disorder

F14.988 Cocaine use, unspecified with other cocaine-induced disorder HCC

Cocaine induced obsessive compulsive or related disorder

F14.99 Cocaine use, unspecified with unspecified cocaine-induced disorder HCC

4ᵗʰ F15 Other stimulant related disorders

INCLUDES amphetamine-related disorders
caffeine

EXCLUDES2 cocaine-related disorders (F14.-)

5ᵗʰ F15.1 Other stimulant abuse

EXCLUDES1 other stimulant dependence (F15.2-)
other stimulant use, unspecified (F15.9-)

F15.10 Other stimulant abuse, uncomplicated

Amphetamine type substance use disorder, mild
Other or unspecified stimulant use disorder, mild

● F15.11 Other stimulant abuse, in remission

Amphetamine type substance use disorder, mild, in early remission

Amphetamine type substance use disorder, mild, in sustained remission

Other or unspecified stimulant use disorder, mild, in early remission

Other or unspecified stimulant use disorder, mild, in sustained remission

6ᵗʰ F15.12 Other stimulant abuse with intoxication

F15.120 Other stimulant abuse with intoxication, uncomplicated HCC

F15.121 Other stimulant abuse with intoxication delirium cc⊘ HCC CC/MCC Exc

F15.122 Other stimulant abuse with intoxication with perceptual disturbance HCC

Amphetamine or other stimulant use disorder, mild, with amphetamine or other stimulant intoxication, with perceptual disturbances

F15.129 Other stimulant abuse with intoxication, unspecified HCC

Amphetamine or other stimulant use disorder, mild, with amphetamine or other stimulant intoxication, without perceptual disturbances

F15.14 Other stimulant abuse with stimulant-induced mood disorder HCC

Amphetamine or other stimulant use disorder, mild, with amphetamine or other stimulant induced bipolar or related disorder

Amphetamine or other stimulant use disorder, mild, with amphetamine or other stimulant induced depressive disorder

6ᵗʰ F15.15 Other stimulant abuse with stimulant-induced psychotic disorder

F15.150 Other stimulant abuse with stimulant-induced psychotic disorder with delusions cc⊘ HCC CC/MCC Exc

F15.151 Other stimulant abuse with stimulant-induced psychotic disorder with hallucinations cc⊘ HCC CC/MCC Exc

F15.159 Other stimulant abuse with stimulant-induced psychotic disorder, unspecified HCC

6ᵗʰ F15.18 Other stimulant abuse with other stimulant-induced disorder

F15.180 Other stimulant abuse with stimulant-induced anxiety disorder HCC

F15.181 Other stimulant abuse with stimulant-induced sexual dysfunction HCC

F15.182 Other stimulant abuse with stimulant-induced sleep disorder HCC

F15.188 Other stimulant abuse with other stimulant-induced disorder HCC

Amphetamine or other stimulant use disorder, mild, with amphetamine or other stimulant induced obsessive-compulsive or related disorder

F15.19 Other stimulant abuse with unspecified stimulant-induced disorder HCC

5ᵗʰ F15.2 Other stimulant dependence

EXCLUDES1 other stimulant abuse (F15.1-)
other stimulant use, unspecified (F15.9-)

F15.20 Other stimulant dependence, uncomplicated cc⊘ HCC

Amphetamine type substance use disorder, moderate
Amphetamine type substance use disorder, severe
Other or unspecified stimulant use disorder, moderate
Other or unspecified stimulant use disorder, severe

F15.21 Other stimulant dependence, in remission HCC

Amphetamine type substance use disorder, moderate, in early remission

Amphetamine type substance use disorder, moderate, in sustained remission

Amphetamine type substance use disorder, severe, in early remission

Amphetamine type substance use disorder, severe, in sustained remission

Other or unspecified stimulant use disorder, moderate, in early remission

Other or unspecified stimulant use disorder, moderate, in sustained remission

Other or unspecified stimulant use disorder, severe, in early remission

Other or unspecified stimulant use disorder, severe, in sustained remission

---

Unspecified Code   Other Specified Code   Manifestation Code   N Newborn   P Pediatric   M Maternity   A Adult   ♂ Male   ♀ Female
● New Code   ▲ Revised Code Title   ►◄ Revised Text   NOTES   INCLUDES   EXCLUDES 1 Not coded here   EXCLUDES 2 Not included here
4ᵗʰ 4ᵗʰ character required   5ᵗʰ 5ᵗʰ character required   6ᵗʰ 6ᵗʰ character required   7ᵗʰ 7ᵗʰ character required
Extension 'X' Alert   HCC Hospital-acquired condition (HAC) alert   AHA AHA Coding Clinic

F15.22 Other stimulant dependence with intoxication

EXCLUDES1 other stimulant dependence with withdrawal (F15.23)

F15.220 Other stimulant dependence with intoxication, uncomplicated HCC

F15.221 Other stimulant dependence with intoxication delirium cc HCC cc/mcc Exc

F15.222 Other stimulant dependence with intoxication with perceptual disturbance cc HCC

Amphetamine or other stimulant use disorder, moderate, with amphetamine or other stimulant intoxication, with perceptual disturbances

Amphetamine or other stimulant use disorder, severe, with amphetamine or other stimulant intoxication, with perceptual disturbances

F15.229 Other stimulant dependence with intoxication, unspecified HCC

Amphetamine or other stimulant use disorder, moderate, with amphetamine or other stimulant intoxication, without perceptual disturbances

Amphetamine or other stimulant use disorder, severe, with amphetamine or other stimulant intoxication, without perceptual disturbances

F15.23 Other stimulant dependence with withdrawal cc HCC cc/mcc Exc

Amphetamine or other stimulant withdrawal

EXCLUDES1 other stimulant dependence with intoxication (F15.22-)

F15.24 Other stimulant dependence with stimulant-induced mood disorder HCC

Amphetamine or other stimulant use disorder, moderate, with amphetamine or other stimulant-induced bipolar or related disorder

Amphetamine or other stimulant use disorder, moderate, with amphetamine or other stimulant induced depressive disorder

Amphetamine or other stimulant use disorder, severe, with amphetamine or other stimulant-induced bipolar or related disorder

Amphetamine or other stimulant use disorder, severe, with amphetamine or other stimulant-induced depressive disorder

F15.25 Other stimulant dependence with stimulant-induced psychotic disorder

F15.250 Other stimulant dependence with stimulant-induced psychotic disorder with delusions cc HCC cc/mcc Exc

F15.251 Other stimulant dependence with stimulant-induced psychotic disorder with hallucinations cc HCC cc/mcc Exc

F15.259 Other stimulant dependence with stimulant-induced psychotic disorder, unspecified cc HCC

F15.28 Other stimulant dependence with other stimulant-induced disorder

F15.280 Other stimulant dependence with stimulant-induced anxiety disorder cc HCC

F15.281 Other stimulant dependence with stimulant-induced sexual dysfunction cc HCC

F15.282 Other stimulant dependence with stimulant-induced sleep disorder cc HCC

F15.288 Other stimulant dependence with other stimulant-induced disorder cc HCC

Amphetamine or other stimulant use disorder, moderate, with amphetamine or other stimulant induced obsessive ▶compulsive or◀ related disorder

Amphetamine or other stimulant use disorder, severe, with amphetamine or other stimulant induced obsessive ▶compulsive or◀ related disorder

F15.29 Other stimulant dependence with unspecified stimulant-induced disorder HCC

F15.9 Other stimulant use, unspecified

EXCLUDES1 other stimulant abuse (F15.1-)

other stimulant dependence (F15.2-)

F15.90 Other stimulant use, unspecified, uncomplicated

F15.92 Other stimulant use, unspecified with intoxication

EXCLUDES1 other stimulant use, unspecified with withdrawal (F15.93)

F15.920 Other stimulant use, unspecified with intoxication, uncomplicated HCC

F15.921 Other stimulant use, unspecified with intoxication delirium cc HCC cc/mcc Exc

Amphetamine or other stimulant-induced delirium

F15.922 Other stimulant use, unspecified with intoxication with perceptual disturbance HCC

F15.929 Other stimulant use, unspecified with intoxication, unspecified HCC

Caffeine intoxication

F15.93 Other stimulant use, unspecified with withdrawal cc HCC cc/mcc Exc

Caffeine withdrawal

EXCLUDES1 other stimulant use, unspecified with intoxication (F15.92-)

F15.94 Other stimulant use, unspecified with stimulant-induced mood disorder HCC

Amphetamine or other stimulant-induced bipolar or related disorder, without use disorder

Amphetamine or other stimulant-induced depressive disorder, without use disorder

F15.95 Other stimulant use, unspecified with stimulant-induced psychotic disorder

F15.950 Other stimulant use, unspecified with stimulant-induced psychotic disorder with delusions cc HCC cc/mcc Exc

F15.951 Other stimulant use, unspecified with stimulant-induced psychotic disorder with hallucinations cc HCC cc/mcc Exc

F15.959 Other stimulant use, unspecified with stimulant-induced psychotic disorder, unspecified HCC

Amphetamine or other ▶stimulant-induced psychotic disorder,◀ without use disorder

F15.98 Other stimulant use, unspecified with other stimulant-induced disorder

F15.980 Other stimulant use, unspecified with stimulant-induced anxiety disorder HCC

Amphetamine or other stimulant-induced anxiety disorder, without use disorder

Caffeine induced anxiety disorder, without use disorder

F15.981 Other stimulant use, unspecified with stimulant-induced sexual dysfunction HCC

Amphetamine or other stimulant-induced sexual dysfunction, without use disorder

F15.982 Other stimulant use, unspecified with stimulant-induced sleep disorder HCC

Amphetamine or other stimulant-induced sleep disorder, without use disorder

Caffeine induced sleep disorder, without use disorder

F15.988 Other stimulant use, unspecified with other stimulant-induced disorder HCC

Amphetamine or other stimulant-induced obsessive compulsive or related disorder, without use disorder

PDx Unacceptable principal diagnosis symbol per Medicare code edits POA Code exempt from diagnosis present on admission requirement

? Questionable admission cc Complication or comorbidity cc/mcc Exc CC/MCC exclusion mcc Major complication or comorbidity

Principal diagnosis as its own CC Principal diagnosis as its own MCC HCC HCC diagnosis code RxHCC RxHCC diagnosis code

MACRA code Z Z code as first-listed diagnosis

552 When symbols appear on a code that requires a 7th character extension, refer to Appendix B to identify applicable 7th character codes. 2018 ICD-10-CM

F15.99 **Other stimulant use, unspecified with unspecified stimulant-induced disorder** HCC

F16 Hallucinogen related disorders

INCLUDES ecstasy
PCP
phencyclidine

F16.1 **Hallucinogen** abuse

EXCLUDES1 *hallucinogen dependence (F16.2-)*
hallucinogen use, unspecified (F16.9-)

F16.10 **Hallucinogen abuse, uncomplicated**
Other hallucinogen use disorder, mild
Phencyclidine use disorder, mild

● F16.11 **Hallucinogen** abuse, in remission
Other hallucinogen use disorder, mild, in early remission
Other hallucinogen use disorder, mild, in sustained remission
Phencyclidine use disorder, mild, in early remission
Phencyclidine use disorder, mild, in sustained remission

F16.12 **Hallucinogen abuse** with intoxication

F16.120 **Hallucinogen abuse with intoxication, uncomplicated** HCC
F16.121 **Hallucinogen abuse with intoxication with** delirium cc⊘ HCC CC/MCC Exc
F16.122 **Hallucinogen abuse with intoxication with** perceptual disturbance HCC
F16.129 **Hallucinogen abuse with intoxication, unspecified** HCC

F16.14 **Hallucinogen abuse with hallucinogen-induced** mood disorder HCC
Other hallucinogen use disorder, mild, with other hallucinogen induced bipolar or related disorder
Other hallucinogen use disorder, mild, with other hallucinogen induced depressive disorder
Phencyclidine use disorder, mild, with phencyclidine induced bipolar or related disorder
Phencyclidine use disorder, mild, with phencyclidine induced depressive disorder

F16.15 **Hallucinogen abuse with hallucinogen-induced** psychotic disorder
F16.150 **Hallucinogen abuse with hallucinogen-induced psychotic disorder with** delusions cc⊘ HCC CC/MCC Exc
F16.151 **Hallucinogen abuse with hallucinogen-induced psychotic disorder with** hallucinations cc⊘ HCC CC/MCC Exc
F16.159 **Hallucinogen abuse with hallucinogen-induced psychotic disorder, unspecified** HCC

F16.18 **Hallucinogen abuse with** other hallucinogen-induced disorder
F16.180 **Hallucinogen abuse with hallucinogen-induced** anxiety disorder HCC
F16.183 **Hallucinogen abuse with hallucinogen persisting** perception disorder (flashbacks) HCC
F16.188 **Hallucinogen abuse with other hallucinogen-induced disorder** HCC

F16.19 **Hallucinogen abuse with unspecified hallucinogen-induced disorder** HCC

F16.2 **Hallucinogen** dependence

EXCLUDES1 *hallucinogen abuse (F16.1-)*
hallucinogen use, unspecified (F16.9-)

F16.20 **Hallucinogen dependence, uncomplicated** cc⊘ HCC
Other hallucinogen use disorder, moderate
Other hallucinogen use disorder, severe
Phencyclidine use disorder, moderate
Phencyclidine use disorder, severe

F16.21 **Hallucinogen dependence, in remission** HCC
Other hallucinogen use disorder, moderate, in early remission

Other hallucinogen use disorder, moderate, in sustained remission
Other hallucinogen use disorder, severe, in early remission
Other hallucinogen use disorder, severe, in sustained remission
Phencyclidine use disorder, moderate, in early remission
Phencyclidine use disorder, moderate, in sustained remission
Phencyclidine use disorder, severe, in early remission
Phencyclidine use disorder, severe, in sustained remission

F16.22 **Hallucinogen dependence** with intoxication
F16.220 **Hallucinogen dependence with intoxication, uncomplicated** HCC
F16.221 **Hallucinogen dependence with intoxication with** delirium cc⊘ HCC CC/MCC Exc
F16.229 **Hallucinogen dependence with intoxication, unspecified** HCC

F16.24 **Hallucinogen dependence with hallucinogen-induced** mood disorder HCC
Other hallucinogen use disorder, moderate, with other hallucinogen induced bipolar or related disorder
Other hallucinogen use disorder, moderate, with other hallucinogen induced depressive disorder
Other hallucinogen use disorder, severe, with other hallucinogen-induced bipolar or related disorder
Other hallucinogen use disorder, severe, with other hallucinogen-induced depressive disorder
Phencyclidine use disorder, moderate, with phencyclidine induced bipolar or related disorder
Phencyclidine use disorder, moderate, with phencyclidine induced depressive disorder
Phencyclidine use disorder, severe, with phencyclidine induced bipolar or related disorder
Phencyclidine use disorder, severe, with phencyclidine-induced depressive disorder

F16.25 **Hallucinogen dependence with hallucinogen-induced** psychotic disorder
F16.250 **Hallucinogen dependence with hallucinogen-induced psychotic disorder with** delusions cc⊘ HCC CC/MCC Exc
F16.251 **Hallucinogen dependence with hallucinogen-induced psychotic disorder with** hallucinations cc⊘ HCC CC/MCC Exc
F16.259 **Hallucinogen dependence with hallucinogen-induced psychotic disorder, unspecified** cc⊘ HCC

F16.28 **Hallucinogen dependence with** other hallucinogen-induced disorder
F16.280 **Hallucinogen dependence with hallucinogen-induced** anxiety disorder cc⊘ HCC
F16.283 **Hallucinogen dependence with hallucinogen persisting** perception disorder (flashbacks) cc⊘ HCC
F16.288 **Hallucinogen dependence with other hallucinogen-induced disorder** cc⊘ HCC

F16.29 **Hallucinogen dependence with unspecified hallucinogen-induced disorder** HCC

F16.9 **Hallucinogen** use, unspecified

EXCLUDES1 *hallucinogen abuse (F16.1-)*
hallucinogen dependence (F16.2-)

F16.90 **Hallucinogen use, unspecified, uncomplicated**
F16.92 **Hallucinogen use, unspecified** with intoxication
F16.920 **Hallucinogen use, unspecified with intoxication, uncomplicated** HCC
F16.921 **Hallucinogen use, unspecified with intoxication with** delirium cc⊘ HCC CC/MCC Exc
Other hallucinogen intoxication delirium

Unspecified Code   Other Specified Code   Manifestation Code   N Newborn   P Pediatric   M Maternity   A Adult   ♂ Male   ♀ Female
● New Code   ▲ Revised Code Title   ▶◀ Revised Text   NOTES   INCLUDES   EXCLUDES 1 Not coded here   EXCLUDES 2 Not included here
4th character required   5th character required   6th character required   7th character required
Extension 'X' Alert   HAC Hospital-acquired condition (HAC) alert   AHA AHA Coding Clinic©

F16.929 **Hallucinogen use, unspecified with intoxication, unspecified** HCC

F16.94 **Hallucinogen use, unspecified with hallucinogen-induced** mood disorder HCC

Other hallucinogen induced bipolar or related disorder, without use disorder

Other hallucinogen induced depressive disorder, without use disorder

Phencyclidine induced bipolar or related disorder, without use disorder

Phencyclidine induced depressive disorder, without use disorder

F16.95 **Hallucinogen use, unspecified with hallucinogen-induced** psychotic disorder

F16.950 **Hallucinogen use, unspecified with hallucinogen-induced psychotic disorder with** delusions CC HCC CC/MCC Exc

F16.951 **Hallucinogen use, unspecified with hallucinogen-induced psychotic disorder with** hallucinations CC HCC CC/MCC Exc

F16.959 **Hallucinogen use, unspecified with hallucinogen-induced psychotic disorder, unspecified** HCC

Other hallucinogen induced psychotic disorder, without use disorder

Phencyclidine induced psychotic disorder, without use disorder

F16.98 **Hallucinogen use, unspecified with** other specified hallucinogen-induced disorder

F16.980 **Hallucinogen use, unspecified with hallucinogen-induced** anxiety disorder HCC

Other hallucinogen-induced anxiety disorder, without use disorder

Phencyclidine induced anxiety disorder, without use disorder

F16.983 **Hallucinogen use, unspecified with hallucinogen persisting** perception disorder **(flashbacks)** HCC

F16.988 **Hallucinogen use, unspecified with other hallucinogen-induced disorder** HCC

F16.99 **Hallucinogen use, unspecified with unspecified hallucinogen-induced disorder** HCC

F17 **Nicotine dependence**

EXCLUDES1 history of tobacco dependence (Z87.891)

tobacco use NOS (Z72.0)

EXCLUDES2 tobacco use (smoking) during pregnancy, childbirth and the puerperium (O99.33-)

toxic effect of nicotine (T65.2-)

F17.2 **Nicotine** dependence

F17.20 **Nicotine dependence, unspecified**

F17.200 **Nicotine dependence, unspecified,** uncomplicated PDxIn

AHA: Q1 2016, Q4 2013

Tobacco use disorder, mild

Tobacco use disorder, moderate

Tobacco use disorder, severe

F17.201 **Nicotine dependence, unspecified, in** remission PDxIn

Tobacco use disorder, mild, in early remission

Tobacco use disorder, mild, in sustained remission

Tobacco use disorder, moderate, in early remission

Tobacco use disorder, moderate, in sustained remission

Tobacco use disorder, severe, in early remission

Tobacco use disorder, severe, in sustained remission

F17.203 **Nicotine dependence unspecified, with** withdrawal CC CC/MCC Exc

Tobacco withdrawal

F17.208 **Nicotine dependence, unspecified, with** other **nicotine-induced disorders**

F17.209 **Nicotine dependence, unspecified, with unspecified nicotine-induced disorders**

F17.21 **Nicotine dependence,** cigarettes

F17.210 **Nicotine dependence, cigarettes,** uncomplicated PDxIn

AHA: Q2 2017, Q4 2013

F17.211 **Nicotine dependence, cigarettes, in** remission PDxIn

Tobacco use disorder, cigarettes, mild, in early remission

Tobacco use disorder, cigarettes, mild, in sustained remission

Tobacco use disorder, cigarettes, moderate, in early remission

Tobacco use disorder, cigarettes, moderate, in sustained remission

Tobacco use disorder, cigarettes, severe, in early remission

Tobacco use disorder, cigarettes, severe, in sustained remission

F17.213 **Nicotine dependence, cigarettes, with** withdrawal CC CC/MCC Exc

F17.218 **Nicotine dependence, cigarettes, with other nicotine-induced disorders**

AHA: Q4 2013

F17.219 **Nicotine dependence, cigarettes, with unspecified nicotine-induced disorders**

F17.22 **Nicotine dependence,** chewing tobacco

F17.220 **Nicotine dependence, chewing tobacco,** uncomplicated PDxIn

F17.221 **Nicotine dependence, chewing tobacco, in** remission PDxIn

Tobacco use disorder, chewing tobacco, mild, in early remission

Tobacco use disorder, chewing tobacco, mild, in sustained remission

Tobacco use disorder, chewing tobacco, moderate, in early remission

Tobacco use disorder, chewing tobacco, moderate, in sustained remission

Tobacco use disorder, chewing tobacco, severe, in early remission

Tobacco use disorder, chewing tobacco, severe, in sustained remission

F17.223 **Nicotine dependence, chewing tobacco, with withdrawal** CC CC/MCC Exc

F17.228 **Nicotine dependence, chewing tobacco, with other nicotine-induced disorders**

F17.229 **Nicotine dependence, chewing tobacco, with unspecified nicotine-induced disorders**

F17.29 **Nicotine dependence,** other tobacco product

F17.290 **Nicotine dependence, other tobacco product,** uncomplicated PDxIn

AHA: Q2 2017

F17.291 **Nicotine dependence, other tobacco product, in** remission PDxIn

Tobacco use disorder, other tobacco product, mild, in early remission

Tobacco use disorder, other tobacco product, mild, in sustained remission

Tobacco use disorder, other tobacco product, moderate, in early remission

Tobacco use disorder, other tobacco product, moderate, in sustained remission

Tobacco use disorder, other tobacco product, severe, in early remission

Tobacco use disorder, other tobacco product, severe, in sustained remission

PDxIn Unacceptable principal diagnosis symbol per Medicare code edits   POA Code exempt from diagnosis present on admission requirement

❓ Questionable admission   CC Complication or comorbidity   CC/MCC Exc CC/MCC exclusion   MCC Major complication or comorbidity

PDx CC Principal diagnosis as its own CC   PDx MCC Principal diagnosis as its own MCC   HCC HCC diagnosis code   RxHCC RxHCC diagnosis code

MACRA code   Z1 Z code as first-listed diagnosis

554

When symbols appear on a code that requires a 7th character extension, refer to Appendix B to identify applicable 7th character codes.

2018 ICD-10-CM

F17.293 **Nicotine dependence, other tobacco product, with withdrawal** CC CC/MCC Exc

F17.298 **Nicotine dependence, other tobacco product, with other nicotine-induced disorders**

F17.299 **Nicotine dependence, other tobacco product, with unspecified nicotine-induced disorders**

[4th] **F18 Inhalant related disorders**

INCLUDES *volatile solvents*

[5th] **F18.1 Inhalant abuse**

EXCLUDES1 *inhalant dependence (F18.2-)*
inhalant use, unspecified (F18.9-)

F18.10 **Inhalant abuse, uncomplicated**
Inhalant use disorder, mild

● F18.11 **Inhalant abuse, in remission**
Inhalant use disorder, mild, in early remission
Inhalant use disorder, mild, in sustained remission

[6th] F18.12 **Inhalant abuse with intoxication**

F18.120 **Inhalant abuse with intoxication, uncomplicated** HCC

F18.121 **Inhalant abuse with intoxication delirium** CC HCC CC/MCC Exc

F18.129 **Inhalant abuse with intoxication, unspecified** HCC

F18.14 **Inhalant abuse with inhalant-induced mood disorder** HCC
Inhalant use disorder, mild, with inhalant induced depressive disorder

[6th] F18.15 **Inhalant abuse with inhalant-induced psychotic disorder**

F18.150 **Inhalant abuse with inhalant-induced psychotic disorder with delusions** CC HCC CC/MCC Exc

F18.151 **Inhalant abuse with inhalant-induced psychotic disorder with hallucinations** CC HCC CC/MCC Exc

F18.159 **Inhalant abuse with inhalant-induced psychotic disorder, unspecified** HCC

F18.17 **Inhalant abuse with inhalant-induced dementia** CC HCC CC/MCC Exc
Inhalant use disorder, mild, with inhalant induced major neurocognitive disorder

[6th] F18.18 **Inhalant abuse with other inhalant-induced disorders**

F18.180 **Inhalant abuse with inhalant-induced anxiety disorder** HCC

F18.188 **Inhalant abuse with other inhalant-induced disorder** HCC
Inhalant use disorder, mild, with inhalant induced mild neurocognitive disorder

F18.19 **Inhalant abuse with unspecified inhalant-induced disorder** HCC

[5th] **F18.2 Inhalant dependence**

EXCLUDES1 *inhalant abuse (F18.1-)*
inhalant use, unspecified (F18.9-)

F18.20 **Inhalant dependence, uncomplicated** CC HCC
Inhalant use disorder, moderate
Inhalant use disorder, severe

F18.21 **Inhalant dependence, in remission** HCC
Inhalant use disorder, moderate, in early remission
Inhalant use disorder, moderate, in sustained remission
Inhalant use disorder, severe, in early remission
Inhalant use disorder, severe, in sustained remission

[6th] F18.22 **Inhalant dependence with intoxication**

F18.220 **Inhalant dependence with intoxication, uncomplicated** HCC

F18.221 **Inhalant dependence with intoxication delirium** CC HCC CC/MCC Exc

F18.229 **Inhalant dependence with intoxication, unspecified** HCC

F18.24 **Inhalant dependence with inhalant-induced mood disorder** HCC
Inhalant use disorder, moderate, with inhalant induced depressive disorder
Inhalant use disorder, severe, with inhalant induced depressive disorder

[6th] F18.25 **Inhalant dependence with inhalant-induced psychotic disorder**

F18.250 **Inhalant dependence with inhalant-induced psychotic disorder with delusions** CC HCC CC/MCC Exc

F18.251 **Inhalant dependence with inhalant-induced psychotic disorder with hallucinations** CC HCC CC/MCC Exc

F18.259 **Inhalant dependence with inhalant-induced psychotic disorder, unspecified** CC HCC

F18.27 **Inhalant dependence with inhalant-induced dementia** CC HCC CC/MCC Exc
Inhalant use disorder, moderate, with inhalant induced major neurocognitive disorder
Inhalant use disorder, severe, with inhalant induced major neurocognitive disorder

[6th] F18.28 **Inhalant dependence with other inhalant-induced disorders**

F18.280 **Inhalant dependence with inhalant-induced anxiety disorder** CC HCC

F18.288 **Inhalant dependence with other inhalant-induced disorder** CC HCC
Inhalant use disorder, moderate, with inhalant-induced mild neurocognitive disorder
Inhalant use disorder, severe, with inhalant-induced mild neurocognitive disorder

F18.29 **Inhalant dependence with unspecified inhalant-induced disorder** HCC

[5th] **F18.9 Inhalant use, unspecified**

EXCLUDES1 *inhalant abuse (F18.1-)*
inhalant dependence (F18.2-)

F18.90 **Inhalant use, unspecified, uncomplicated**

[6th] F18.92 **Inhalant use, unspecified with intoxication**

F18.920 **Inhalant use, unspecified with intoxication, uncomplicated** HCC

F18.921 **Inhalant use, unspecified with intoxication with delirium** CC HCC CC/MCC Exc

F18.929 **Inhalant use, unspecified with intoxication, unspecified** HCC

F18.94 **Inhalant use, unspecified with inhalant-induced mood disorder** HCC
Inhalant induced depressive disorder

[6th] F18.95 **Inhalant use, unspecified with inhalant-induced psychotic disorder**

F18.950 **Inhalant use, unspecified with inhalant-induced psychotic disorder with delusions** CC HCC CC/MCC Exc

F18.951 **Inhalant use, unspecified with inhalant-induced psychotic disorder with hallucinations** CC HCC CC/MCC Exc

F18.959 **Inhalant use, unspecified with inhalant-induced psychotic disorder, unspecified** HCC

F18.97 **Inhalant use, unspecified with inhalant-induced persisting dementia** CC HCC CC/MCC Exc
Inhalant-induced major neurocognitive disorder

[6th] F18.98 **Inhalant use, unspecified with other inhalant-induced disorders**

F18.980 **Inhalant use, unspecified with inhalant-induced anxiety disorder** HCC

F18.988 **Inhalant use, unspecified with other inhalant-induced disorder** HCC
Inhalant-induced mild neurocognitive disorder

F18.99   **Inhalant use, unspecified with unspecified inhalant-induced disorder** HCC

⁴ᵗʰ F19   Other psychoactive substance related disorders

INCLUDES   polysubstance drug use (indiscriminate drug use)

⁵ᵗʰ F19.1   Other psychoactive substance abuse

EXCLUDES1   other psychoactive substance dependence (F19.2-)

other psychoactive substance use, unspecified (F19.9-)

F19.10   **Other psychoactive substance abuse, uncomplicated**

Other (or unknown) substance use disorder, mild

● F19.11   **Other psychoactive substance abuse, in remission**

Other (or unknown) substance use disorder, mild, in early remission

Other (or unknown) substance use disorder, mild, in sustained remission

⁶ᵗʰ F19.12   **Other psychoactive substance abuse with intoxication**

F19.120   **Other psychoactive substance abuse with intoxication, uncomplicated**

F19.121   **Other psychoactive substance abuse with intoxication delirium** cᶜ HCC CC/MCC Exc

F19.122   **Other psychoactive substance abuse with intoxication with perceptual disturbances** HCC

F19.129   **Other psychoactive substance abuse with intoxication, unspecified** HCC

F19.14   **Other psychoactive substance abuse with psychoactive substance-induced mood disorder** HCC

Other (or unknown) substance use disorder, mild, with other (or unknown) substance-induced bipolar or related disorder

Other (or unknown) substance use disorder, mild, with other (or unknown) substance-induced depressive disorder

⁶ᵗʰ F19.15   **Other psychoactive substance abuse with psychoactive substance-induced psychotic disorder**

F19.150   **Other psychoactive substance abuse with psychoactive substance-induced psychotic disorder with delusions** cᶜ HCC CC/MCC Exc

F19.151   **Other psychoactive substance abuse with psychoactive substance-induced psychotic disorder with hallucinations** cᶜ HCC CC/MCC Exc

F19.159   **Other psychoactive substance abuse with psychoactive substance-induced psychotic disorder, unspecified** HCC

F19.16   **Other psychoactive substance abuse with psychoactive substance-induced persisting amnestic disorder** HCC

F19.17   **Other psychoactive substance abuse with psychoactive substance-induced persisting dementia** cᶜ HCC CC/MCC Exc

Other (or unknown) substance use disorder, mild, with other (or unknown) substance-induced major neurocognitive disorder

⁶ᵗʰ F19.18   **Other psychoactive substance abuse with other psychoactive substance-induced disorders**

F19.180   **Other psychoactive substance abuse with psychoactive substance-induced anxiety disorder** HCC

F19.181   **Other psychoactive substance abuse with psychoactive substance-induced sexual dysfunction** HCC

F19.182   **Other psychoactive substance abuse with psychoactive substance-induced sleep disorder** HCC

F19.188   **Other psychoactive substance abuse with other psychoactive substance-induced disorder** HCC

Other (or unknown) substance use disorder, mild, with other (or unknown) substance induced mild neurocognitive disorder

Other (or unknown) substance use disorder, mild, with other (or unknown) substance induced obsessive-compulsive or related disorder

F19.19   **Other psychoactive substance abuse with unspecified psychoactive substance-induced disorder** HCC

⁵ᵗʰ F19.2   Other psychoactive substance dependence

EXCLUDES1   other psychoactive substance abuse (F19.1-)

other psychoactive substance use, unspecified (F19.9-)

F19.20   **Other psychoactive substance dependence, uncomplicated** cᶜ HCC

Other (or unknown) substance use disorder, moderate

Other (or unknown) substance use disorder, severe

F19.21   **Other psychoactive substance dependence, in remission** HCC

Other (or unknown) substance use disorder, moderate, in early remission

Other (or unknown) substance use disorder, moderate, in sustained remission

Other (or unknown) substance use disorder, severe, in early remission

Other (or unknown) substance use, severe, in sustained remission

⁶ᵗʰ F19.22   **Other psychoactive substance dependence with intoxication**

EXCLUDES1   other psychoactive substance dependence with withdrawal (F19.23-)

F19.220   **Other psychoactive substance dependence with intoxication, uncomplicated** HCC

F19.221   **Other psychoactive substance dependence with intoxication delirium** cᶜ HCC CC/MCC Exc

F19.222   **Other psychoactive substance dependence with intoxication with perceptual disturbance** cᶜ HCC

F19.229   **Other psychoactive substance dependence with intoxication, unspecified** HCC

⁶ᵗʰ F19.23   **Other psychoactive substance dependence with withdrawal**

EXCLUDES1   other psychoactive substance dependence with intoxication (F19.22-)

F19.230   **Other psychoactive substance dependence with withdrawal, uncomplicated** cᶜ HCC CC/MCC Exc

F19.231   **Other psychoactive substance dependence with withdrawal delirium** cᶜ HCC CC/MCC Exc

F19.232   **Other psychoactive substance dependence with withdrawal with perceptual disturbance** cᶜ HCC CC/MCC Exc

F19.239   **Other psychoactive substance dependence with withdrawal, unspecified** cᶜ HCC CC/MCC Exc

F19.24   **Other psychoactive substance dependence with psychoactive substance-induced mood disorder** HCC

Other (or unknown) substance use disorder, moderate, with other (or unknown) substance induced bipolar or related disorder

Other (or unknown) substance use disorder, moderate, with other (or unknown) substance induced depressive disorder

Other (or unknown) substance use disorder, severe, with other (or unknown) substance induced bipolar or related disorder

Other (or unknown) substance use disorder, severe, with other (or unknown) substance induced depressive disorder

---

PDxᴹ Unacceptable principal diagnosis symbol per Medicare code edits   ₌ₐ Code exempt from diagnosis present on admission requirement
🅀 Questionable admission   cᶜ Complication or comorbidity   CC/MCC Exc CC/MCC exclusion   MCC Major complication or comorbidity
🄿🄲🄲 Principal diagnosis as its own CC   🄿🄼🄲 Principal diagnosis as its own MCC   HCC HCC diagnosis code   RxHCC RxHCC diagnosis code
MACRA code   🅉🄰 Z code as first-listed diagnosis

6ᵗʰ F19.25 Other psychoactive substance dependence with psychoactive substance-induced psychotic disorder

    F19.250 Other psychoactive substance dependence with psychoactive substance-induced psychotic disorder with delusions cc HCC CC/MCC Exc

    F19.251 Other psychoactive substance dependence with psychoactive substance-induced psychotic disorder with hallucinations cc HCC CC/MCC Exc

    F19.259 Other psychoactive substance dependence with psychoactive substance-induced psychotic disorder, unspecified cc HCC

F19.26 Other psychoactive substance dependence with psychoactive substance-induced persisting amnestic disorder cc HCC

F19.27 Other psychoactive substance dependence with psychoactive substance-induced persisting dementia cc HCC CC/MCC

Other (or unknown) substance use disorder, moderate, with other (or unknown) substance induced major neurocognitive disorder

Other (or unknown) substance use disorder, severe, with other (or unknown) substance induced major neurocognitive disorder

6ᵗʰ F19.28 Other psychoactive substance dependence with other psychoactive substance-induced disorders

    F19.280 Other psychoactive substance dependence with psychoactive substance-induced anxiety disorder cc HCC

    F19.281 Other psychoactive substance dependence with psychoactive substance-induced sexual dysfunction cc HCC

    F19.282 Other psychoactive substance dependence with psychoactive substance-induced sleep disorder cc HCC

    F19.288 Other psychoactive substance dependence with other psychoactive substance-induced disorder cc HCC

Other (or unknown) substance use disorder, moderate, with other (or unknown) substance induced mild neurocognitive disorder

Other (or unknown) substance use disorder, severe, with other (or unknown) substance induced mild neurocognitive disorder

Other (or unknown) substance use disorder, moderate, with other (or unknown) substance induced obsessive compulsive or related disorder

Other (or unknown) substance use disorder, severe, with other (or unknown) substance induced obsessive-compulsive or related disorder

F19.29 Other psychoactive substance dependence with unspecified psychoactive substance-induced disorder HCC

5ᵗʰ F19.9 Other psychoactive substance use, unspecified

    EXCLUDES1 other psychoactive substance abuse (F19.1-)

               other psychoactive substance dependence (F19.2-)

    F19.90 Other psychoactive substance use, unspecified, uncomplicated

    6ᵗʰ F19.92 Other psychoactive substance use, unspecified with intoxication

        EXCLUDES1 other psychoactive substance use, unspecified with withdrawal (F19.93)

        F19.920 Other psychoactive substance use, unspecified with intoxication, uncomplicated HCC

        F19.921 Other psychoactive substance use, unspecified with intoxication with delirium cc HCC CC/MCC Exc

        Other (or unknown) substance-induced delirium

        F19.922 Other psychoactive substance use, unspecified with intoxication with perceptual disturbance HCC

        F19.929 Other psychoactive substance use, unspecified with intoxication, unspecified HCC

6ᵗʰ F19.93 Other psychoactive substance use, unspecified with withdrawal

    EXCLUDES1 other psychoactive substance use, unspecified with intoxication (F19.92-)

    F19.930 Other psychoactive substance use, unspecified with withdrawal, uncomplicated cc HCC CC/MCC Exc

    F19.931 Other psychoactive substance use, unspecified with withdrawal delirium cc HCC CC/MCC Exc

    F19.932 Other psychoactive substance use, unspecified with withdrawal with perceptual disturbance cc HCC CC/MCC Exc

    F19.939 Other psychoactive substance use, unspecified with withdrawal, unspecified cc HCC CC/MCC Exc

F19.94 Other psychoactive substance use, unspecified with psychoactive substance-induced mood disorder HCC

Other (or unknown) substance-induced bipolar or related disorder, without use disorder

Other (or unknown) substance-induced depressive disorder, without use disorder

6ᵗʰ F19.95 Other psychoactive substance use, unspecified with psychoactive substance-induced psychotic disorder

    F19.950 Other psychoactive substance use, unspecified with psychoactive substance-induced psychotic disorder with delusions cc HCC CC/MCC Exc

    F19.951 Other psychoactive substance use, unspecified with psychoactive substance-induced psychotic disorder with hallucinations cc HCC CC/MCC Exc

    F19.959 Other psychoactive substance use, unspecified with psychoactive substance-induced psychotic disorder, unspecified HCC

    Other or unknown substance-induced psychotic disorder, without use disorder

F19.96 Other psychoactive substance use, unspecified with psychoactive substance-induced persisting amnestic disorder HCC

F19.97 Other psychoactive substance use, unspecified with psychoactive substance-induced persisting dementia cc HCC CC/MCC Exc

Other (or unknown) substance-induced major neurocognitive disorder, without use disorder

6ᵗʰ F19.98 Other psychoactive substance use, unspecified with other psychoactive substance-induced disorders

    F19.980 Other psychoactive substance use, unspecified with psychoactive substance-induced anxiety disorder HCC

    Other (or unknown) substance-induced anxiety disorder, without use disorder

    F19.981 Other psychoactive substance use, unspecified with psychoactive substance-induced sexual dysfunction HCC

    Other (or unknown) substance-induced sexual dysfunction, without use disorder

---

Unspecified Code   Other Specified Code   Manifestation Code   N Newborn   P Pediatric   M Maternity   A Adult   ♂ Male   ♀ Female
● New Code   ▲ Revised Code Title   ►◄ Revised Text   **NOTES**   *INCLUDES*   *EXCLUDES 1* Not coded here   *EXCLUDES 2* Not included here
4ᵗʰ character required   5ᵗʰ character required   6ᵗʰ character required   7ᵗʰ character required
Extension 'X' Alert   HAC Hospital-acquired condition (HAC) alert   **AHA** AHA Coding Clinic©

NOTES

Chapter 6: Diseases of the Nervous System (G00-G99)
Anatomy of the Nervous System

The nervous system constitutes the body's control center and the communication network and directs the functions of multiple body organs and systems. It helps the individual to interpret external environmental events and respond to various environmental stimuli. The nervous system includes the following types and components:

1. The Central Nervous System (CNS)

The central nervous system is regarded as the control center of the entire nervous system. It is composed of the brain and the spinal cord. The CNS receives the body's sensations and information about the external environmental changes via receptors and sense organs, and directs the body to act accordingly in response to these external environmental stimuli.

Human Nervous System

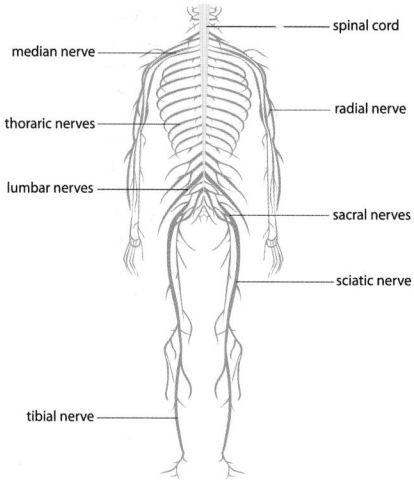

2. The Peripheral Nervous System (PNS)

The peripheral nervous system is composed of the nerves that connect the brain and spinal cord with the glands, muscles and sensory receptors. The PNS can be further divided into the following subcategories:

a) The Afferent Peripheral System

The afferent peripheral system is composed of sensory (or afferent) neurons that transfer information to the brain and spinal cord via peripheral receptors.

b) The Efferent Peripheral System

The efferent peripheral system consists of the motor (or efferent) neurons that form a communication channel (for information transfer) between the brain, spinal cord, muscles and glands. This system of neurons is further divided into the following subcategories:

i) Somatic Nervous System

The somatic nervous system helps the individual to respond to the changes in the external environment by conducting the impulses from the brain and spinal cord to the skeletal muscle.

ii) Autonomic Nervous System

The autonomic nervous system (ANS) is an involuntary system of nerves that conduct impulses from the brain and spinal cord to the smooth muscles of the intestine, the cardiac muscles of the heart, and the endocrine glands. The organs of this particular system receive nerve fibers from the following divisions of the ANS:

(a) Sympathetic Division

The sympathetic division acts to mobilize the body's resources and induce the fight-or-flight response. This system uses norepinephrine as a neurotransmitter to speed up its activity through energy expenditure.

(b) Parasympathetic Division

The parasympathetic division facilitates the vegetative activities of human body (like digestion, urination and defecation).

3. The Spinal Cord (or Medulla Spinalis)

The spinal cord initiates as a continuation of the medulla oblongata of the brainstem. Its length varies between 16 to 18 inches and is made up of a series of 31 segments, each of which gives rise to a pair of spinal nerves. The human spinal cord is further protected by a series of connective tissue membranes that are known as the spinal meninges.

4. The Brain or Encephalon

The brain is regarded as one of the largest organs of the body and weighs about 3 pounds in an average adult. The major parts of the human brain are described as follows:

a) The Brainstem

The brainstem is regarded as the posterior portion of the brain, which is structurally continuous with the spinal cord. It is composed of the medulla oblongata, the pons Varolii, and the midbrain.

b) The Diencephalon

The diencephalon is located between the two cerebral hemispheres, and superiorly to the midbrain. It surrounds the third ventricle of the brain and consists of the thalamus and hypothalamus regions.

c) The Cerebrum (or Telencephalon)

The cerebrum constitutes the bulk of the brain and is composed of the gray matter (or cerebral cortex), longitudinal fissure, and the right and left cerebral hemispheres. It is further subdivided into the frontal, parietal, occipital and temporal lobes.

d) The Cerebellum

The cerebellum is regarded as the second largest portion of the brain. It is located under the occipital lobes of the cerebrum, and behind the pons and medulla oblongata of brainstem. The two partially separated hemispheres of the cerebellum are connected together by a centrally constricted structure, which is known as the vermis. The cerebellum is constituted primarily by the white matter and a thin layer of gray matter on its surface, which is known as the cerebellar cortex. The cerebrospinal fluid (CSF) is a colorless fluid that fills up the subarachnoid space (or interval between the arachnoid membrane and pia mater) and the ventricular system inside and around the spinal cord and brain.

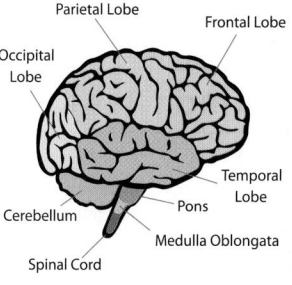

5. The Cranial Nerves

The cranial nerves are based on 12 pairs that remain attached to the brain and leave the skull through various foramina in the cranial base. The names of the various cranial nerves are listed below:

a) Olfactory (1st cranial nerve)

b) Optic (2nd cranial nerve)

c) Oculomotor (3rd cranial nerve)

d) Trochlear (4th cranial nerve)

e) Trigeminal (5th cranial nerve)

f) Abducens (6th cranial nerve)

g) The Facial (7th cranial nerve)

h) Acoustic (8th cranial nerve)

i) Glossopharyngeal (9th cranial nerve)

j) Vagus/Pneumogastric (10th cranial nerve)

k) Accessory (11th cranial nerve)

l) Hypoglossal (12th cranial nerve)

The Cranial Nerves

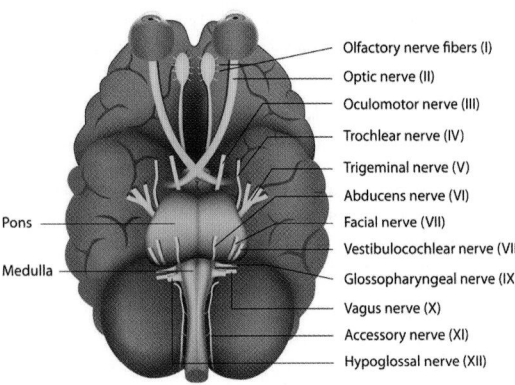

- Olfactory nerve fibers (I)
- Optic nerve (II)
- Oculomotor nerve (III)
- Trochlear nerve (IV)
- Trigeminal nerve (V)
- Abducens nerve (VI)
- Facial nerve (VII)
- Vestibulocochlear nerve (VIII)
- Glossopharyngeal nerve (IX)
- Vagus nerve (X)
- Accessory nerve (XI)
- Hypoglossal nerve (XII)

Pons

Medulla

6. **The Spinal Nerves**

The 31 pairs of spinal nerves originate from the integration of the dorsal and ventral roots of the spinal nerves. These nerves carry the motor, sensory and the autonomic signals between the spinal cord and the body. They are also called mixed nerves as they consist of both motor and sensory fibers. The spinal nerves exit the vertebral column between the adjacent vertebrae. The naming convention of the spinal nerves is based on the region and level of the spinal cord from which these nerves arise. The division of the spinal nerves is documented below:

a) 8 pairs of cervical nerves (C1-C8)

b) 12 pairs of thoracic nerves (T1-T12)

c) 5 pairs of lumbar nerves (L1-L5)

d) 5 pairs of sacral nerves (S1-S5)

e) 1 pair of coccygeal nerves (Cx)

7. **The Sympathetic Nerves**

The sympathetic nerves are a part of the sympathetic nervous system, which innervates the striated muscles of the heart, the smooth muscles, and multiple glands of the body. The sympathetic nervous system is that division of the autonomic nervous system which prepares the body for stressful conditions requiring energy expenditure. The nerve fibers of this system originate from the thoracic and lumbar regions of the spinal cord. The axons of these nerves leave the spinal cord via the anterior root. They further pass near the spinal ganglion and integrate with the anterior rami of the spinal nerves.

Common Pathologies

Muscular dystrophy (MD)

This is characterized by progressive muscle weakness, abnormal muscle protein, and death of muscle tissues and cells.

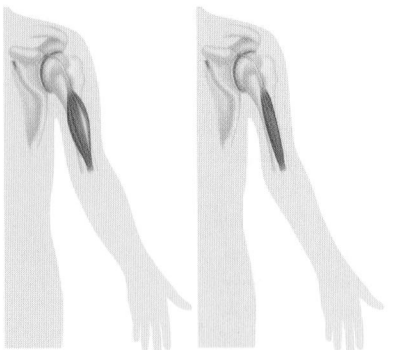

Normal biceps   Muscular dystrophy

Spina Bifida

This is a type of birth defect of the brain, spine, or spinal cord, also known as the neural tube defect. It happens if the spinal column of the fetus doesn't close completely during the first month of pregnancy.

Parkinson's Disease (PD)

This is a progressive disorder of the nervous system that affects the movement and is known as a movement disorder.

Alzheimer's Disease (AD)

This is a brain disorder that seriously affects a person's ability to carry out daily activities. Alzheimer's disease is the most common form of dementia.

Strokes

This is a condition in which, due to lack of oxygen, the sudden death of brain cells occurs and can be caused by an obstruction in the blood flow to the brain. The more common kind, called ischemic stroke, is caused by a blood clot that blocks or plugs a blood vessel in the brain. The other kind, called hemorrhagic stroke, is caused by a blood vessel that breaks and bleeds into the brain. "Mini-strokes" or transient ischemic attacks (TIAs), occur when the blood supply to the brain is briefly interrupted.

Hemorrhagic Stroke

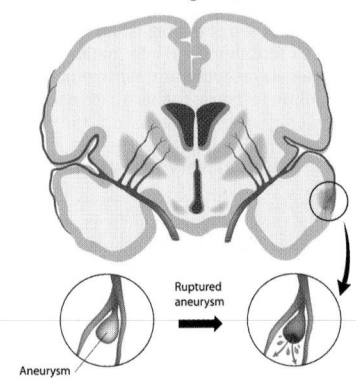

Ruptured aneurysm

Aneurysm

Malignant Brain Tumor

Cancer of the brain is usually called a malignant brain tumor.

Meningitis

The inflammation of the thin tissue that surrounds the brain and spinal cord, called the meninges, is known as Meningitis.

Epilepsy

This is a neurological condition that affects the nervous system. Epilepsy is also known as a seizure disorder that causes people to have recurring seizures.

Bell's Palsy

This condition occurs due to compression of a facial nerve.

Diseases of the nervous system (G00-G99)

EXCLUDES2 *certain conditions originating in the perinatal period (P04-P96)*

certain infectious and parasitic diseases (A00-B99)

complications of pregnancy, childbirth and the puerperium (O00-O9A)

congenital malformations, deformations, and chromosomal abnormalities (Q00-Q99)

endocrine, nutritional and metabolic diseases (E00-E88)

injury, poisoning and certain other consequences of external causes (S00-T88)

neoplasms (C00-D49)

symptoms, signs and abnormal clinical and laboratory findings, not elsewhere classified (R00-R94)

This chapter contains the following blocks:

G00-G09 Inflammatory diseases of the central nervous system

G10-G14 Systemic atrophies primarily affecting the central nervous system

G20-G26 Extrapyramidal and movement disorders

G30-G32 Other degenerative diseases of the nervous system

G35-G37 Demyelinating diseases of the central nervous system

G40-G47 Episodic and paroxysmal disorders

G50-G59 Nerve, nerve root and plexus disorders

G60-G65 Polyneuropathies and other disorders of the peripheral nervous system

G70-G73 Diseases of myoneural junction and muscle

G80-G83 Cerebral palsy and other paralytic syndromes

G89-G99 Other disorders of the nervous system

Inflammatory diseases of the central nervous system (G00-G09)

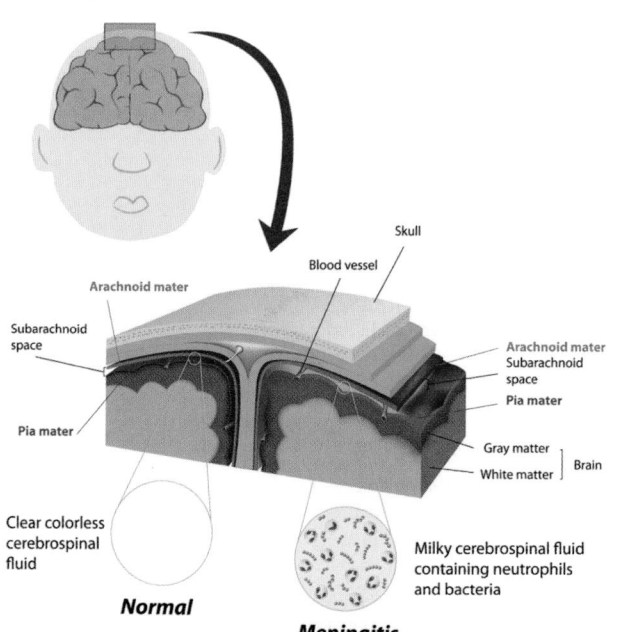

Skull
Blood vessel
Arachnoid mater
Subarachnoid space
Arachnoid mater
Subarachnoid space
Pia mater
Pia mater
Gray matter
White matter
Brain
Clear colorless cerebrospinal fluid
Milky cerebrospinal fluid containing neutrophils and bacteria
Normal
Meningitis

Figure 6.1 Meningitis

4ᵗʰ **G00 Bacterial meningitis, not elsewhere classified**

INCLUDES *bacterial arachnoiditis*

bacterial leptomeningitis

bacterial meningitis

bacterial pachymeningitis

EXCLUDES1 ▶*bacterial meningoencephalitis (G04.2)*◀

▶*bacterial meningomyelitis (G04.2)*◀

G00.0 Hemophilus meningitis MCC CC/MCC Exc
Meningitis due to Hemophilus influenzae

G00.1 Pneumococcal meningitis MCC CC/MCC Exc
Meningtitis due to Streptococcal pneumoniae

G00.2 Streptococcal meningitis MCC CC/MCC Exc
Use additional code to further identify organism (B95.0-B95.5)

G00.3 Staphylococcal meningitis MCC CC/MCC Exc
Use additional code to further identify organism (B95.61-B95.8)

G00.8 Other bacterial meningitis MCC CC/MCC Exc
Meningitis due to Escherichia coli
Meningitis due to Friedländer's bacillus
Meningitis due to Klebsiella
Use additional code to further identify organism (B96.-)

G00.9 Bacterial meningitis, unspecified MCC CC/MCC Exc
Meningitis due to gram-negative bacteria, unspecified
Purulent meningitis NOS
Pyogenic meningitis NOS
Suppurative meningitis NOS

G01 Meningitis in bacterial diseases classified elsewhere MCC CC/MCC Exc
Code first underlying disease

EXCLUDES1 *meningitis (in):*

gonococcal (A54.81)

leptospirosis (A27.81)

listeriosis (A32.11)

Lyme disease (A69.21)

meningococcal (A39.0)

neurosyphilis (A52.13)

tuberculosis (A17.0)

meningoencephalitis and meningomyelitis in bacterial diseases classified elsewhere (G05)

G02 Meningitis in other infectious and parasitic diseases classified elsewhere MCC CC/MCC Exc
Code first underlying disease, such as:
African trypanosomiasis (B56.-)
poliovirus infection (A80.-)

EXCLUDES1 *candidal meningitis (B37.5)*

coccidioidomycosis meningitis (B38.4)

cryptococcal meningitis (B45.1)

herpesviral [herpes simplex] meningitis (B00.3)

infectious mononucleosis complicated by meningitis (B27.- with fourth character 2)

measles complicated by meningitis (B05.1)

meningoencephalitis and meningomyelitis in other infectious and parasitic diseases classified elsewhere (G05)

mumps meningitis (B26.1)

rubella meningitis (B06.02)

varicella [chickenpox] meningitis (B01.0)

zoster meningitis (B02.1)

4ᵗʰ **G03 Meningitis due to other and unspecified causes**

INCLUDES *arachnoiditis NOS*

leptomeningitis NOS

meningitis NOS

pachymeningitis NOS

EXCLUDES1 *meningoencephalitis (G04.-)*

meningomyelitis (G04.-)

G03.0 Nonpyogenic meningitis MCC CC/MCC Exc
Aseptic meningitis
Nonbacterial meningitis

G03.1 Chronic meningitis CC CC/MCC Exc

G03.2 Benign recurrent meningitis [Mollaret] CC CC/MCC Exc

G03.8 Meningitis due to other specified causes MCC CC/MCC Exc

G03.9 Meningitis, unspecified MCC CC/MCC Exc
Arachnoiditis (spinal) NOS

Unspecified Code   Other Specified Code   Manifestation Code   Ⓝ Newborn   Ⓟ Pediatric   Ⓜ Maternity   Ⓐ Adult   ♂ Male   ♀ Female
● New Code   ▲ Revised Code Title   ▶◀ Revised Text   **NOTES** INCLUDES EXCLUDES 1 Not coded here EXCLUDES 2 Not included here
④ᵗʰ 4ᵗʰ character required   ⑤ᵗʰ 5ᵗʰ character required   ⑥ᵗʰ 6ᵗʰ character required   ⑦ᵗʰ 7ᵗʰ character required
⑦ Extension 'X' Alert   HAC Hospital-acquired condition (HAC) alert   **AHA** AHA Coding Clinic©

🔵 **G04 Encephalitis, myelitis and encephalomyelitis**

    INCLUDES   acute ascending myelitis

              meningoencephalitis

              meningomyelitis

    EXCLUDES1 encephalopathy NOS (G93.40)

    EXCLUDES2 acute transverse myelitis (G37.3-)

              alcoholic encephalopathy (G31.2)

              benign myalgic encephalomyelitis (G93.3)

              multiple sclerosis (G35)

              subacute necrotizing myelitis (G37.4)

              toxic encephalitis (G92)

              toxic encephalopathy (G92)

  🔵 **G04.0 Acute disseminated encephalitis and encephalomyelitis (ADEM)**

      EXCLUDES1 acute necrotizing hemorrhagic encephalopathy (G04.3-)

              other noninfectious acute disseminated encephalomyelitis (noninfectious ADEM) (G04.81)

      G04.00 Acute disseminated encephalitis and encephalomyelitis, unspecified MCC CC/MCC Exc

      G04.01 Postinfectious acute disseminated encephalitis and encephalomyelitis (postinfectious ADEM) MCC CC/MCC Exc

        EXCLUDES1 post chickenpox encephalitis (B01.1)

                post measles encephalitis (B05.0)

                post measles myelitis (B05.1)

      G04.02 Postimmunization acute disseminated encephalitis, myelitis and encephalomyelitis MCC

        Encephalitis, post immunization

        Encephalomyelitis, post immunization

        Use additional code to identify the vaccine (T50.A-, T50.B-, T50.Z-)

  G04.1 Tropical spastic paraplegia CC HCC RxHCC CC/MCC Exc

  G04.2 Bacterial meningoencephalitis and meningomyelitis, not elsewhere classified MCC CC/MCC Exc

  🔵 **G04.3 Acute necrotizing hemorrhagic encephalopathy**

      EXCLUDES1 acute disseminated encephalitis and encephalomyelitis (G04.0-)

      G04.30 Acute necrotizing hemorrhagic encephalopathy, unspecified MCC

      G04.31 Postinfectious acute necrotizing hemorrhagic encephalopathy MCC CC/MCC Exc

      G04.32 Postimmunization acute necrotizing hemorrhagic encephalopathy MCC

        Use additional code to identify the vaccine (T50.A-, T50.B-, T50.Z-)

      G04.39 Other acute necrotizing hemorrhagic encephalopathy MCC

        Code also underlying etiology, if applicable

  🔵 **G04.8 Other encephalitis, myelitis and encephalomyelitis**

      Code also any associated seizure (G40.-, R56.9)

      G04.81 Other encephalitis and encephalomyelitis MCC CC/MCC Exc

        Noninfectious acute disseminated encephalomyelitis (noninfectious ADEM)

      G04.89 Other myelitis HCC MCC RxHCC CC/MCC Exc

  🔵 **G04.9 Encephalitis, myelitis and encephalomyelitis, unspecified**

      G04.90 Encephalitis and encephalomyelitis, unspecified MCC CC/MCC Exc

        Ventriculitis (cerebral) NOS

      G04.91 Myelitis, unspecified HCC MCC RxHCC CC/MCC Exc

🔵 **G05 Encephalitis, myelitis and encephalomyelitis in diseases classified elsewhere**

    Code first underlying disease, such as:

    human immunodeficiency virus [HIV] disease (B20)

    poliovirus (A80.-)

    suppurative otitis media (H66.01-H66.4)

    trichinellosis (B75)

    EXCLUDES1 adenoviral encephalitis, myelitis and encephalomyelitis (A85.1)

              congenital toxoplasmosis encephalitis, myelitis and encephalomyelitis (P37.1)

              cytomegaloviral encephalitis, myelitis and encephalomyelitis (B25.8)

              encephalitis, myelitis and encephalomyelitis (in) measles (B05.0)

              encephalitis, myelitis and encephalomyelitis (in) systemic lupus erythematosus (M32.19)

              enteroviral encephalitis, myelitis and encephalomyelitis (A85.0)

              eosinophilic meningoencephalitis (B83.2)

              herpesviral [herpes simplex] encephalitis, myelitis and encephalomyelitis (B00.4)

              listerial encephalitis, myelitis and encephalomyelitis (A32.12)

              meningococcal encephalitis, myelitis and encephalomyelitis (A39.81)

              mumps encephalitis, myelitis and encephalomyelitis (B26.2)

              postchickenpox encephalitis, myelitis and encephalomyelitis (B01.1-)

              rubella encephalitis, myelitis and encephalomyelitis (B06.01)

              toxoplasmosis encephalitis, myelitis and encephalomyelitis (B58.2)

              zoster encephalitis, myelitis and encephalomyelitis (B02.0)

  G05.3 Encephalitis and encephalomyelitis in diseases classified elsewhere MCC CC/MCC Exc

    Meningoencephalitis in diseases classified elsewhere

  G05.4 Myelitis in diseases classified elsewhere HCC MCC RxHCC CC/MCC Exc

    Meningomyelitis in diseases classified elsewhere

🔵 **G06 Intracranial and intraspinal abscess and granuloma**

    Use additional code (B95-B97) to identify infectious agent.

  G06.0 Intracranial abscess and granuloma MCC CC/MCC Exc

    Brain [any part] abscess (embolic)

    Cerebellar abscess (embolic)

    Cerebral abscess (embolic)

    Intracranial epidural abscess or granuloma

    Intracranial extradural abscess or granuloma

    Intracranial subdural abscess or granuloma

    Otogenic abscess (embolic)

    EXCLUDES1 tuberculous intracranial abscess and granuloma (A17.81)

  G06.1 Intraspinal abscess and granuloma MCC CC/MCC Exc

    Abscess (embolic) of spinal cord [any part]

    Intraspinal epidural abscess or granuloma

    Intraspinal extradural abscess or granuloma

    Intraspinal subdural abscess or granuloma

    EXCLUDES1 tuberculous intraspinal abscess and granuloma (A17.81)

  G06.2 Extradural and subdural abscess, unspecified MCC CC/MCC Exc

G07 Intracranial and intraspinal abscess and granuloma in diseases classified elsewhere MCC CC/MCC Exc

    Code first underlying disease, such as:

    schistosomiasis granuloma of brain (B65.-)

    EXCLUDES1 abscess of brain:

              amebic (A06.6)

              chromomycotic (B43.1)

              gonococcal (A54.82)

              tuberculous (A17.81)

              tuberculoma of meninges (A17.1)

G08 Intracranial and intraspinal phlebitis and thrombophlebitis MCC CC/MCC Exc

    Septic embolism of intracranial or intraspinal venous sinuses and veins

    Septic endophlebitis of intracranial or intraspinal venous sinuses and veins

    Septic phlebitis of intracranial or intraspinal venous sinuses and veins

    Septic thrombophlebitis of intracranial or intraspinal venous sinuses and veins

    Septic thrombosis of intracranial or intraspinal venous sinuses and veins

    EXCLUDES1 intracranial phlebitis and thrombophlebitis complicating:

PDx Unacceptable principal diagnosis symbol per Medicare code edits   POA Code exempt from diagnosis present on admission requirement

? Questionable admission   CC Complication or comorbidity   CC/MCC Exc CC/MCC exclusion   MCC Major complication or comorbidity

CC Principal diagnosis as its own CC   MCC Principal diagnosis as its own MCC   HCC HCC diagnosis code   RxHCC RxHCC diagnosis code

MACRA code   Z1 Z code as first-listed diagnosis

572   When symbols appear on a code that requires a 7th character extension, refer to Appendix B to identify applicable 7th character codes.   **2018 ICD-10-CM**

abortion, ectopic or molar pregnancy (O00-O07, O08.7)
pregnancy, childbirth and the puerperium (O22.5, O87.3)
nonpyogenic intracranial phlebitis and thrombophlebitis (I67.6)

EXCLUDES2 *intracranial phlebitis and thrombophlebitis complicating nonpyogenic intraspinal phlebitis and thrombophlebitis (G95.1)*

G09 Sequelae of inflammatory diseases of central nervous system
NOTES Category G09 is to be used to indicate conditions whose primary classification is to G00-G08 as the cause of sequelae, themselves classifiable elsewhere. The 'sequelae' include conditions specified as residuals.
Code first condition resulting from (sequela) of inflammatory diseases of central nervous system

Systemic atrophies primarily affecting the central nervous system (G10-G14)

G10 Huntington's disease   cc⊘ HCC RxHCC CC/MCC Exc
Huntington's chorea
Huntington's dementia
Code also dementia in other diseases classified elsewhere without behavioral disturbance (F02.80)

4th **G11 Hereditary ataxia**
EXCLUDES2 *cerebral palsy (G80.-)*
hereditary and idiopathic neuropathy (G60.-)
metabolic disorders (E70-E88)

G11.0 Congenital nonprogressive ataxia   cc⊘ HCC CC/MCC Exc
G11.1 Early-onset cerebellar ataxia   cc⊘ HCC CC/MCC Exc
Early-onset cerebellar ataxia with essential tremor
Early-onset cerebellar ataxia with myoclonus [Hunt's ataxia]
Early-onset cerebellar ataxia with retained tendon reflexes
Friedreich's ataxia (autosomal recessive)
X-linked recessive spinocerebellar ataxia
G11.2 Late-onset cerebellar ataxia   A cc⊘ HCC CC/MCC Exc
G11.3 Cerebellar ataxia with defective DNA repair   cc⊘ HCC CC/MCC Exc
Ataxia telangiectasia [Louis-Bar]
EXCLUDES2 *Cockayne's syndrome (Q87.1)*
other disorders of purine and pyrimidine metabolism (E79.-)
xeroderma pigmentosum (Q82.1)
G11.4 Hereditary spastic paraplegia   cc⊘ HCC CC/MCC Exc
G11.8 Other hereditary ataxias   cc⊘ HCC CC/MCC Exc
G11.9 Hereditary ataxia, unspecified   cc⊘ HCC CC/MCC Exc
Hereditary cerebellar ataxia NOS
Hereditary cerebellar degeneration
Hereditary cerebellar disease
Hereditary cerebellar syndrome

4th **G12 Spinal muscular atrophy and related syndromes**
G12.0 Infantile spinal muscular atrophy, type I [Werdnig-Hoffman]   cc⊘ HCC RxHCC CC/MCC Exc
G12.1 Other inherited spinal muscular atrophy   cc⊘ HCC RxHCC CC/MCC Exc
Adult form spinal muscular atrophy
Childhood form, type II spinal muscular atrophy
Distal spinal muscular atrophy
Juvenile form, type III spinal muscular atrophy [Kugelberg-Welander]
Progressive bulbar palsy of childhood [Fazio-Londe]
Scapuloperoneal form spinal muscular atrophy
5th **G12.2 Motor neuron disease**
G12.20 Motor neuron disease, unspecified   cc⊘ HCC RxHCC CC/MCC Exc
G12.21 Amyotrophic lateral sclerosis   A cc⊘ HCC RxHCC CC/MCC Exc
G12.22 Progressive bulbar palsy   cc⊘ HCC CC/MCC Exc
● **G12.23 Primary lateral sclerosis**   cc⊘ CC/MCC Exc
● **G12.24 Familial motor neuron disease**   cc⊘ CC/MCC Exc
● **G12.25 Progressive spinal muscle atrophy**   cc⊘ CC/MCC Exc
G12.29 Other motor neuron disease   cc⊘ HCC RxHCC CC/MCC Exc
G12.8 Other spinal muscular atrophies and related syndromes   cc⊘ HCC CC/MCC Exc
G12.9 Spinal muscular atrophy, unspecified   cc⊘ HCC RxHCC CC/MCC Exc

4th **G13 Systemic atrophies primarily affecting central nervous system in diseases classified elsewhere**
G13.0 Paraneoplastic neuromyopathy and neuropathy   HCC RxHCC
Carcinomatous neuromyopathy
Sensorial paraneoplastic neuropathy [Denny Brown]
Code first underlying neoplasm (C00-D49)
G13.1 Other systemic atrophy primarily affecting central nervous system in neoplastic disease   HCC RxHCC
Paraneoplastic limbic encephalopathy
Code first underlying neoplasm (C00-D49)
G13.2 Systemic atrophy primarily affecting the central nervous system in myxedema   RxHCC
Code first underlying disease, such as:
hypothyroidism (E03.-)
myxedematous congenital iodine deficiency (E00.1)
G13.8 Systemic atrophy primarily affecting central nervous system in other diseases classified elsewhere   RxHCC
Code first underlying disease

G14 Postpolio syndrome
INCLUDES *postpolio myelitic syndrome*
EXCLUDES1 *sequelae of poliomyelitis (B91)*

Extrapyramidal and movement disorders (G20-G26)

G20 Parkinson's disease   HCC RxHCC
AHA: Q2 2017, Q2 2016
Hemiparkinsonism
Idiopathic Parkinsonism or Parkinson's disease
Paralysis agitans
Parkinsonism or Parkinson's disease NOS
Primary Parkinsonism or Parkinson's disease
EXCLUDES1 *dementia with Parkinsonism (G31.83)*
4th **G21 Secondary parkinsonism**
EXCLUDES1 *dementia with Parkinsonism (G31.83)*
Huntington's disease (G10)
Shy-Drager syndrome (G90.3)
syphilitic Parkinsonism (A52.19)
G21.0 Malignant neuroleptic syndrome   MCC⊘ CC/MCC Exc
Use additional code for adverse effect, if applicable, to identify drug (T43.3X5, T43.4X5, T43.505, T43.595)
EXCLUDES1 *neuroleptic induced parkinsonism (G21.11)*
5th **G21.1 Other drug-induced secondary parkinsonism**
G21.11 Neuroleptic induced parkinsonism   cc⊘ HCC RxHCC CC/MCC Exc
Use additional code for adverse effect, if applicable, to identify drug (T43.3X5, T43.4X5, T43.505, T43.595)
EXCLUDES1 *malignant neuroleptic syndrome (G21.0)*
G21.19 Other drug induced secondary parkinsonism   cc⊘ HCC RxHCC CC/MCC Exc
Other medication-induced parkinsonism
Use additional code for adverse effect, if applicable, to identify drug (T36-T50 with fifth or sixth character 5)
G21.2 Secondary parkinsonism due to other external agents   cc⊘ HCC RxHCC CC/MCC Exc
Code first (T51-T65) to identify external agent
G21.3 Postencephalitic parkinsonism   cc⊘ HCC RxHCC CC/MCC Exc
G21.4 Vascular parkinsonism   HCC RxHCC
G21.8 Other secondary parkinsonism   cc⊘ HCC RxHCC CC/MCC Exc
G21.9 Secondary parkinsonism, unspecified   cc⊘ HCC RxHCC CC/MCC Exc
4th **G23 Other degenerative diseases of basal ganglia**
EXCLUDES2 *multi-system degeneration of the autonomic nervous system (G90.3)*
G23.0 Hallervorden-Spatz disease   cc⊘ HCC CC/MCC Exc
Pigmentary pallidal degeneration
G23.1 Progressive supranuclear ophthalmoplegia [Steele-Richardson-Olszewski]   cc⊘ HCC CC/MCC Exc
Progressive supranuclear palsy
G23.2 Striatonigral degeneration   cc⊘ HCC CC/MCC Exc

Unspecified Code   Other Specified Code   Manifestation Code   N Newborn   P Pediatric   M Maternity   A Adult   ♂ Male   ♀ Female
● New Code   ▲ Revised Code Title   ►◄ Revised Text   NOTES   INCLUDES   EXCLUDES 1 Not coded here   EXCLUDES 2 Not included here
4th 4th character required   5th 5th character required   6th 6th character required   7th 7th character required
7th Extension 'X' Alert   HAC Hospital-acquired condition (HAC) alert   AHA AHA Coding Clinic©

G23.8 Other specified degenerative diseases of basal ganglia ⚄ HCC CC/MCC Exc
Calcification of basal ganglia

G23.9 Degenerative disease of basal ganglia, unspecified ⚄ HCC CC/MCC Exc

G24 Dystonia

INCLUDES dyskinesia

EXCLUDES2 athetoid cerebral palsy (G80.3)

G24.0 Drug induced dystonia
Use additional code for adverse effect, if applicable, to identify drug (T36-T50 with fifth or sixth character 5)

G24.01 Drug induced subacute dyskinesia
Drug induced blepharospasm
Drug induced orofacial dyskinesia
Neuroleptic induced tardive dyskinesia
Tardive dyskinesia

G24.02 Drug induced acute dystonia ⚄ CC/MCC Exc
Acute dystonic reaction to drugs
Neuroleptic induced acute dystonia

G24.09 Other drug induced dystonia ⚄ CC/MCC Exc

G24.1 Genetic torsion dystonia
Dystonia deformans progressiva
Dystonia musculorum deformans
Familial torsion dystonia
Idiopathic familial dystonia
Idiopathic (torsion) dystonia NOS
(Schwalbe-) Ziehen-Oppenheim disease

G24.2 Idiopathic nonfamilial dystonia ⚄ CC/MCC Exc

G24.3 Spasmodic torticollis

EXCLUDES1 congenital torticollis (Q68.0)
hysterical torticollis (F44.4)
ocular torticollis (R29.891)
psychogenic torticollis (F45.8)
torticollis NOS (M43.6)
traumatic recurrent torticollis (S13.4)

G24.4 Idiopathic orofacial dystonia
Orofacial dyskinesia

EXCLUDES1 drug induced orofacial dyskinesia (G24.01)

G24.5 Blepharospasm

EXCLUDES1 drug induced blepharospasm (G24.01)

G24.8 Other dystonia ⚄ CC/MCC Exc
Acquired torsion dystonia NOS

G24.9 Dystonia, unspecified
Dyskinesia NOS

G25 Other extrapyramidal and movement disorders

EXCLUDES2 sleep related movement disorders (G47.6-)

G25.0 Essential tremor
Familial tremor

EXCLUDES1 tremor NOS (R25.1)

G25.1 Drug-induced tremor
Use additional code for adverse effect, if applicable, to identify drug (T36-T50 with fifth or sixth character 5)

G25.2 Other specified forms of tremor
Intention tremor

G25.3 Myoclonus
Drug-induced myoclonus
Palatal myoclonus
Use additional code for adverse effect, if applicable, to identify drug (T36-T50 with fifth or sixth character 5)

EXCLUDES1 facial myokymia (G51.4)
myoclonic epilepsy (G40.-)

G25.4 Drug-induced chorea
Use additional code for adverse effect, if applicable, to identify drug (T36-T50 with fifth or sixth character 5)

G25.5 Other chorea
Chorea NOS

EXCLUDES1 chorea NOS with heart involvement (I02.0)
Huntington's chorea (G10)
rheumatic chorea (I02.-)
Sydenham's chorea (I02.-)

G25.6 Drug induced tics and other tics of organic origin

G25.61 Drug induced tics
Use additional code for adverse effect, if applicable, to identify drug (T36-T50 with fifth or sixth character 5)

G25.69 Other tics of organic origin

EXCLUDES1 habit spasm (F95.9)
tic NOS (F95.9)
Tourette's syndrome (F95.2)

G25.7 Other and unspecified drug induced movement disorders
Use additional code for adverse effect, if applicable, to identify drug (T36-T50 with fifth or sixth character 5)

G25.70 Drug induced movement disorder, unspecified

G25.71 Drug induced akathisia
Drug induced acathisia
Neuroleptic induced acute akathisia
Tardive akathisia

G25.79 Other drug induced movement disorders

G25.8 Other specified extrapyramidal and movement disorders

G25.81 Restless legs syndrome

G25.82 Stiff-man syndrome ⚄ CC/MCC Exc

G25.83 Benign shuddering attacks

G25.89 Other specified extrapyramidal and movement disorders

G25.9 Extrapyramidal and movement disorder, unspecified ⚄ CC/MCC Exc

G26 Extrapyramidal and movement disorders in diseases classified elsewhere
Code first underlying disease

Other degenerative diseases of the nervous system (G30-G32)

G30 Alzheimer's disease

INCLUDES Alzheimer's dementia senile and presenile forms

Use additional code to identify:
delirium, if applicable (F05)
dementia with behavioral disturbance (F02.81)
dementia without behavioral disturbance (F02.80)

EXCLUDES1 senile degeneration of brain NEC (G31.1)
senile dementia NOS (F03)
senility NOS (R41.81)

G30.0 Alzheimer's disease with early onset RxHCC

G30.1 Alzheimer's disease with late onset A RxHCC

G30.8 Other Alzheimer's disease RxHCC

G30.9 Alzheimer's disease, unspecified RxHCC
AHA: Q1 2017, Q2 2016, Q4 2012

G31 Other degenerative diseases of nervous system, not elsewhere classified
Use additional code to identify:
dementia with behavioral disturbance (F02.81)
dementia without behavioral disturbance (F02.80)

EXCLUDES2 Reye's syndrome (G93.7)

G31.0 Frontotemporal dementia

G31.01 Pick's disease RxHCC
Primary progressive aphasia
Progressive isolated aphasia

G31.09 Other frontotemporal dementia RxHCC
Frontal dementia

G31.1 Senile degeneration of brain, not elsewhere classified RxHCC

EXCLUDES1 Alzheimer's disease (G30.-)
senility NOS (R41.81)

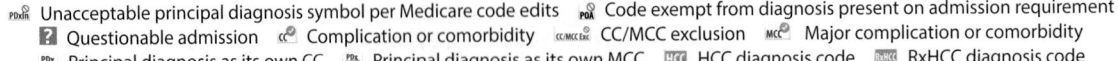

PDIn Unacceptable principal diagnosis symbol per Medicare code edits POA Code exempt from diagnosis present on admission requirement
❓ Questionable admission ⚄ Complication or comorbidity CC/MCC Exc CC/MCC exclusion MCC Major complication or comorbidity
Principal diagnosis as its own CC Principal diagnosis as its own MCC HCC HCC diagnosis code RxHCC RxHCC diagnosis code
MACRA code Z1 Z code as first-listed diagnosis

G31.2 **Degeneration of nervous system due to alcohol** RxHCC
  Alcoholic cerebellar ataxia
  Alcoholic cerebellar degeneration
  Alcoholic cerebral degeneration
  Alcoholic encephalopathy
  Dysfunction of the autonomic nervous system due to alcohol
  Code also associated alcoholism (F10.-)

5ᵗʰ G31.8 **Other specified degenerative diseases of nervous system**

  G31.81 **Alpers disease** ccᴼ RxHCC CC/MCC Exc
    AHA: Q2 2017
    Grey-matter degeneration
  G31.82 **Leigh's disease** ccᴼ RxHCC CC/MCC Exc
    Subacute necrotizing encephalopathy
  G31.83 **Dementia with Lewy bodies** RxHCC
    AHA: Q2 2017, Q4 2016
    Dementia with Parkinsonism
    Lewy body dementia
    Lewy body disease
  G31.84 **Mild cognitive impairment, so stated**
    Mild neurocognitive disorder
    EXCLUDES1 age related cognitive decline (R41.81)
      altered mental status (R41.82)
      cerebral degeneration (G31.9)
      change in mental status (R41.82)
      cognitive deficits following (sequelae of) cerebral hemorrhage or infarction (I69.01-, I69.11-, I69.21-, I69.31-, I69.81-, I69.91-)
      cognitive impairment due to intracranial or head injury (S06.-)
      dementia (F01.-, F02.-, F03)
      mild memory disturbance (F06.8)
      neurologic neglect syndrome (R41.4)
      personality change, nonpsychotic (F68.8)
  G31.85 **Corticobasal degeneration** RxHCC
  G31.89 **Other specified degenerative diseases of nervous system** RxHCC
  G31.9 **Degenerative disease of nervous system, unspecified** RxHCC

4ᵗʰ G32 **Other degenerative disorders of nervous system in diseases classified elsewhere**

  G32.0 **Subacute combined degeneration of spinal cord in diseases classified elsewhere** ccᴼ HCC RxHCC CC/MCC Exc
    Dana-Putnam syndrome
    Sclerosis of spinal cord (combined) (dorsolateral) (posterolateral)
    Code first underlying disease, such as:
    anemia (D51.9)
    dietary (D51.3)
    pernicious (D51.0)
    vitamin B12 deficiency (E53.8)
    EXCLUDES1 syphilitic combined degeneration of spinal cord (A52.11)

  5ᵗʰ G32.8 **Other specified degenerative disorders of nervous system in diseases classified elsewhere**
    Code first underlying disease, such as:
    amyloidosis cerebral degeneration (E85.-)
    cerebral degeneration (due to) hypothyroidism (E00.0-E03.9)
    cerebral degeneration (due to) neoplasm (C00-D49)
    cerebral degeneration (due to) vitamin B deficiency, except thiamine (E52-E53.-)
    EXCLUDES1 superior hemorrhagic polioencephalitis [Wernicke's encephalopathy] (E51.2)

  G32.81 **Cerebellar ataxia in diseases classified elsewhere** ccᴼ HCC CC/MCC Exc
    Code first underlying disease, such as:
    celiac disease (with gluten ataxia) (K90.0)
    cerebellar ataxia (in) neoplastic disease (paraneoplastic cerebellar degeneration) (C00-D49)
    non-celiac gluten ataxia (M35.9)

EXCLUDES1 systemic atrophy primarily affecting the central nervous system in alcoholic cerebellar ataxia (G31.2)
  systemic atrophy primarily affecting the central nervous system in myxedema (G13.2)

  G32.89 **Other specified degenerative disorders of nervous system in diseases classified elsewhere**
    Degenerative encephalopathy in diseases classified elsewhere

Demyelinating diseases of the central nervous system (G35-G37)

  G35 **Multiple sclerosis** HCC RxHCC
    Disseminated multiple sclerosis
    Generalized multiple sclerosis
    Multiple sclerosis NOS
    Multiple sclerosis of brain stem
    Multiple sclerosis of cord

4ᵗʰ G36 **Other acute disseminated demyelination**
    EXCLUDES1 postinfectious encephalitis and encephalomyelitis NOS (G04.01)

  G36.0 **Neuromyelitis optica [Devic]** ccᴼ HCC RxHCC CC/MCC Exc
    Demyelination in optic neuritis
    EXCLUDES1 optic neuritis NOS (H46)
  G36.1 **Acute and subacute hemorrhagic leukoencephalitis [Hurst]** ccᴼ HCC CC/MCC Exc
  G36.8 **Other specified acute disseminated demyelination** ccᴼ HCC CC/MCC Exc
  G36.9 **Acute disseminated demyelination, unspecified** ccᴼ HCC CC/MCC Exc

4ᵗʰ G37 **Other demyelinating diseases of central nervous system**
  G37.0 **Diffuse sclerosis of central nervous system** ccᴼ HCC RxHCC CC/MCC Exc
    Periaxial encephalitis
    Schilder's disease
    EXCLUDES1 X linked adrenoleukodystrophy (E71.52-)
  G37.1 **Central demyelination of corpus callosum** ccᴼ HCC CC/MCC Exc
  G37.2 **Central pontine myelinolysis** ccᴼ HCC CC/MCC Exc
  G37.3 **Acute transverse myelitis in demyelinating disease of central nervous system** ccᴼ HCC RxHCC CC/MCC Exc
    Acute transverse myelitis NOS
    Acute transverse myelopathy
    EXCLUDES1 multiple sclerosis (G35)
      neuromyelitis optica [Devic] (G36.0)
  G37.4 **Subacute necrotizing myelitis of central nervous system** HCC MCCᴼ RxHCC CC/MCC Exc
  G37.5 **Concentric sclerosis [Balo] of central nervous system** ccᴼ HCC RxHCC CC/MCC Exc
  G37.8 **Other specified demyelinating diseases of central nervous system** ccᴼ HCC CC/MCC Exc
  G37.9 **Demyelinating disease of central nervous system, unspecified** ccᴼ HCC CC/MCC Exc

Episodic and paroxysmal disorders (G40-G47)

4ᵗʰ G40 **Epilepsy and recurrent seizures**
    NOTES the following terms are to be considered equivalent to intractable: pharmacoresistant (pharmacologically resistant), treatment resistant, refractory (medically) and poorly controlled
    EXCLUDES1 conversion disorder with seizures (F44.5)
      convulsions NOS (R56.9)
      post traumatic seizures (R56.1)
      seizure (convulsive) NOS (R56.9)
      seizure of newborn (P90)
    EXCLUDES2 hippocampal sclerosis (G93.81)
      mesial temporal sclerosis (G93.81)
      temporal sclerosis (G93.81)
      Todd's paralysis (G83.84)

Unspecified Code   Other Specified Code   Manifestation Code   N Newborn   P Pediatric   M Maternity   A Adult   ♂ Male   ♀ Female
● New Code   ▲ Revised Code Title   ►◄ Revised Text   **NOTES**   INCLUDES   EXCLUDES 1 Not coded here   EXCLUDES 2 Not included here
4ᵗʰ 4ᵗʰ character required   5ᵗʰ 5ᵗʰ character required   6ᵗʰ 6ᵗʰ character required   7ᵗʰ 7ᵗʰ character required
7ᵗʰ Extension 'X' Alert   HAC Hospital-acquired condition (HAC) alert   **AHA** AHA Coding Clinic©

5ᵗʰ G40.0 Localization-related (focal) (partial) idiopathic epilepsy and epileptic syndromes with seizures of localized onset

Benign childhood epilepsy with centrotemporal EEG spikes

Childhood epilepsy with occipital EEG paroxysms

EXCLUDES1 *adult onset localization-related epilepsy (G40.1-, G40.2-)*

6ᵗʰ G40.00 Localization-related (focal) (partial) idiopathic epilepsy and epileptic syndromes with seizures of localized onset, not intractable

Localization-related (focal) (partial) idiopathic epilepsy and epileptic syndromes with seizures of localized onset without intractability

G40.001 Localization-related (focal) (partial) idiopathic epilepsy and epileptic syndromes with seizures of localized onset, not intractable, with status epilepticus c♥ HCC RxHCC CC/MCC Exc

G40.009 Localization-related (focal) (partial) idiopathic epilepsy and epileptic syndromes with seizures of localized onset, not intractable, without status epilepticus c♥ HCC RxHCC CC/MCC Exc

Localization-related (focal) (partial) idiopathic epilepsy and epileptic syndromes with seizures of localized onset NOS

6ᵗʰ G40.01 Localization-related (focal) (partial) idiopathic epilepsy and epileptic syndromes with seizures of localized onset, intractable

G40.011 Localization-related (focal) (partial) idiopathic epilepsy and epileptic syndromes with seizures of localized onset, intractable, with status epilepticus c♥ HCC RxHCC CC/MCC Exc

G40.019 Localization-related (focal) (partial) idiopathic epilepsy and epileptic syndromes with seizures of localized onset, intractable, without status epilepticus c♥ HCC RxHCC CC/MCC Exc

5ᵗʰ G40.1 Localization-related (focal) (partial) symptomatic epilepsy and epileptic syndromes with simple partial seizures

Attacks without alteration of consciousness

Epilepsia partialis continua [Kozhevnikof]

Simple partial seizures developing into secondarily generalized seizures

6ᵗʰ G40.10 Localization-related (focal) (partial) symptomatic epilepsy and epileptic syndromes with simple partial seizures, not intractable

Localization-related (focal) (partial) symptomatic epilepsy and epileptic syndromes with simple partial seizures without intractability

G40.101 Localization-related (focal) (partial) symptomatic epilepsy and epileptic syndromes with simple partial seizures, not intractable, with status epilepticus c♥ HCC RxHCC CC/MCC Exc

G40.109 Localization-related (focal) (partial) symptomatic epilepsy and epileptic syndromes with simple partial seizures, not intractable, without status epilepticus c♥ HCC RxHCC CC/MCC Exc

Localization-related (focal) (partial) symptomatic epilepsy and epileptic syndromes with simple partial seizures NOS

6ᵗʰ G40.11 Localization-related (focal) (partial) symptomatic epilepsy and epileptic syndromes with simple partial seizures, intractable

G40.111 Localization-related (focal) (partial) symptomatic epilepsy and epileptic syndromes with simple partial seizures, intractable, with status epilepticus c♥ HCC RxHCC CC/MCC Exc

G40.119 Localization-related (focal) (partial) symptomatic epilepsy and epileptic syndromes with simple partial seizures, intractable, without status epilepticus c♥ HCC RxHCC CC/MCC Exc

5ᵗʰ G40.2 Localization-related (focal) (partial) symptomatic epilepsy and epileptic syndromes with complex partial seizures

Attacks with alteration of consciousness, often with automatisms

Complex partial seizures developing into secondarily generalized seizures

6ᵗʰ G40.20 Localization-related (focal) (partial) symptomatic epilepsy and epileptic syndromes with complex partial seizures, not intractable

Localization-related (focal) (partial) symptomatic epilepsy and epileptic syndromes with complex partial seizures without intractability

G40.201 Localization-related (focal) (partial) symptomatic epilepsy and epileptic syndromes with complex partial seizures, not intractable, with status epilepticus c♥ HCC RxHCC CC/MCC Exc

G40.209 Localization-related (focal) (partial) symptomatic epilepsy and epileptic syndromes with complex partial seizures, not intractable, without status epilepticus c♥ HCC RxHCC CC/MCC Exc

Localization-related (focal) (partial) symptomatic epilepsy and epileptic syndromes with complex partial seizures NOS

6ᵗʰ G40.21 Localization-related (focal) (partial) symptomatic epilepsy and epileptic syndromes with complex partial seizures, intractable

G40.211 Localization-related (focal) (partial) symptomatic epilepsy and epileptic syndromes with complex partial seizures, intractable, with status epilepticus c♥ HCC RxHCC CC/MCC Exc

G40.219 Localization-related (focal) (partial) symptomatic epilepsy and epileptic syndromes with complex partial seizures, intractable, without status epilepticus c♥ HCC RxHCC CC/MCC Exc

5ᵗʰ G40.3 Generalized idiopathic epilepsy and epileptic syndromes

Code also MERRF syndrome, if applicable (E88.42)

6ᵗʰ G40.30 Generalized idiopathic epilepsy and epileptic syndromes, not intractable

Generalized idiopathic epilepsy and epileptic syndromes without intractability

G40.301 Generalized idiopathic epilepsy and epileptic syndromes, not intractable, with status epilepticus HCC MCC RxHCC CC/MCC Exc

G40.309 Generalized idiopathic epilepsy and epileptic syndromes, not intractable, without status epilepticus HCC RxHCC

Generalized idiopathic epilepsy and epileptic syndromes NOS

6ᵗʰ G40.31 Generalized idiopathic epilepsy and epileptic syndromes, intractable

G40.311 Generalized idiopathic epilepsy and epileptic syndromes, intractable, with status epilepticus HCC MCC RxHCC CC/MCC Exc

G40.319 Generalized idiopathic epilepsy and epileptic syndromes, intractable, without status epilepticus HCC MCC RxHCC CC/MCC Exc

5ᵗʰ G40.A Absence epileptic syndrome

Childhood absence epilepsy [pyknolepsy]

Juvenile absence epilepsy

Absence epileptic syndrome, NOS

6ᵗʰ G40.A0 Absence epileptic syndrome, not intractable

G40.A01 Absence epileptic syndrome, not intractable, with status epilepticus HCC RxHCC

PDx Unacceptable principal diagnosis symbol per Medicare code edits   POA Code exempt from diagnosis present on admission requirement

❓ Questionable admission   c♥ Complication or comorbidity   CC/MCC Exc CC/MCC exclusion   MCC Major complication or comorbidity

Principal diagnosis as its own CC   Principal diagnosis as its own MCC   HCC HCC diagnosis code   RxHCC RxHCC diagnosis code

MACRA code   Z1 Z code as first-listed diagnosis

576   When symbols appear on a code that requires a 7th character extension, refer to Appendix B to identify applicable 7th character codes.   2018 ICD-10-CM

G40.A09 **Absence epileptic syndrome, not intractable, without status epilepticus** [HCC] [RxHCC]

[6th] G40.A1 **Absence epileptic syndrome, intractable**

G40.A11 **Absence epileptic syndrome, intractable, with status epilepticus** [CC] [HCC] [RxHCC] [CC/MCC Exc]

G40.A19 **Absence epileptic syndrome, intractable, without status epilepticus** [CC] [HCC] [RxHCC] [CC/MCC Exc]

[5th] G40.B **Juvenile myoclonic epilepsy [impulsive petit mal]**

[6th] G40.B0 **Juvenile myoclonic epilepsy, not intractable**

G40.B01 **Juvenile myoclonic epilepsy, not intractable, with status epilepticus** [CC] [HCC] [RxHCC] [CC/MCC Exc]

G40.B09 **Juvenile myoclonic epilepsy, not intractable, without status epilepticus** [CC] [HCC] [RxHCC] [CC/MCC Exc]

[6th] G40.B1 **Juvenile myoclonic epilepsy, intractable**

G40.B11 **Juvenile myoclonic epilepsy, intractable, with status epilepticus** [CC] [HCC] [RxHCC] [CC/MCC Exc]

G40.B19 **Juvenile myoclonic epilepsy, intractable, without status epilepticus** [CC] [HCC] [RxHCC] [CC/MCC Exc]

[5th] G40.4 **Other generalized epilepsy and epileptic syndromes**

Epilepsy with grand mal seizures on awakening
Epilepsy with myoclonic absences
Epilepsy with myoclonic-astatic seizures
Grand mal seizure NOS
Nonspecific atonic epileptic seizures
Nonspecific clonic epileptic seizures
Nonspecific myoclonic epileptic seizures
Nonspecific tonic epileptic seizures
Nonspecific tonic-clonic epileptic seizures
Symptomatic early myoclonic encephalopathy

[6th] G40.40 **Other generalized epilepsy and epileptic syndromes, not intractable**

Other generalized epilepsy and epileptic syndromes without intractability
Other generalized epilepsy and epileptic syndromes NOS

G40.401 **Other generalized epilepsy and epileptic syndromes, not intractable, with status epilepticus** [HCC] [RxHCC]

G40.409 **Other generalized epilepsy and epileptic syndromes, not intractable, without status epilepticus** [HCC] [RxHCC]

[6th] G40.41 **Other generalized epilepsy and epileptic syndromes, intractable**

G40.411 **Other generalized epilepsy and epileptic syndromes, intractable, with status epilepticus** [CC] [HCC] [RxHCC] [CC/MCC Exc]

G40.419 **Other generalized epilepsy and epileptic syndromes, intractable, without status epilepticus** [CC] [HCC] [RxHCC] [CC/MCC Exc]

[5th] G40.5 **Epileptic seizures related to external causes**

Epileptic seizures related to alcohol
Epileptic seizures related to drugs
Epileptic seizures related to hormonal changes
Epileptic seizures related to sleep deprivation
Epileptic seizures related to stress

Code also, if applicable, associated epilepsy and recurrent seizures (G40.-)

Use additional code for adverse effect, if applicable, to identify drug (T36-T50 with fifth or sixth character 5)

[6th] G40.50 **Epileptic seizures related to external causes, not intractable**

G40.501 **Epileptic seizures related to external causes, not intractable, with status epilepticus** [CC] [HCC] [RxHCC] [CC/MCC Exc]

G40.509 **Epileptic seizures related to external causes, not intractable, without status epilepticus** [CC] [HCC] [RxHCC] [CC/MCC Exc]

Epileptic seizures related to external causes, NOS

[5th] G40.8 **Other epilepsy and recurrent seizures**

Epilepsies and epileptic syndromes undetermined as to whether they are focal or generalized
Landau-Kleffner syndrome

[6th] G40.80 **Other epilepsy**

G40.801 **Other epilepsy, not intractable, with status epilepticus** [CC] [HCC] [RxHCC] [CC/MCC Exc]

Other epilepsy without intractability with status epilepticus

G40.802 **Other epilepsy, not intractable, without status epilepticus** [CC] [HCC] [RxHCC] [CC/MCC Exc]

Other epilepsy NOS
Other epilepsy without intractability without status epilepticus

G40.803 **Other epilepsy, intractable, with status epilepticus** [CC] [HCC] [RxHCC] [CC/MCC Exc]

G40.804 **Other epilepsy, intractable, without status epilepticus** [CC] [HCC] [RxHCC] [CC/MCC Exc]

[6th] G40.81 **Lennox-Gastaut syndrome**

G40.811 **Lennox-Gastaut syndrome, not intractable, with status epilepticus** [CC] [HCC] [RxHCC] [CC/MCC Exc]

G40.812 **Lennox-Gastaut syndrome, not intractable, without status epilepticus** [CC] [HCC] [RxHCC] [CC/MCC Exc]

G40.813 **Lennox-Gastaut syndrome, intractable, with status epilepticus** [CC] [HCC] [RxHCC] [CC/MCC Exc]

G40.814 **Lennox-Gastaut syndrome, intractable, without status epilepticus** [CC] [HCC] [RxHCC] [CC/MCC Exc]

[6th] G40.82 **Epileptic spasms**

Infantile spasms
Salaam attacks
West's syndrome

G40.821 **Epileptic spasms, not intractable, with status epilepticus** [CC] [HCC] [RxHCC] [CC/MCC Exc]

G40.822 **Epileptic spasms, not intractable, without status epilepticus** [CC] [HCC] [RxHCC] [CC/MCC Exc]

G40.823 **Epileptic spasms, intractable, with status epilepticus** [CC] [HCC] [RxHCC] [CC/MCC Exc]

G40.824 **Epileptic spasms, intractable, without status epilepticus** [CC] [HCC] [RxHCC] [CC/MCC Exc]

G40.89 **Other seizures** [CC] [HCC] [RxHCC] [CC/MCC Exc]

[EXCLUDES1] *post traumatic seizures (R56.1)*
recurrent seizures NOS (G40.909)
seizure NOS (R56.9)

[5th] G40.9 **Epilepsy, unspecified**

[6th] G40.90 **Epilepsy, unspecified, not intractable**

Epilepsy, unspecified, without intractability

G40.901 **Epilepsy, unspecified, not intractable, with status epilepticus** [HCC] [RxHCC]

G40.909 **Epilepsy, unspecified, not intractable, without status epilepticus** [HCC] [RxHCC]

Epilepsy NOS
Epileptic convulsions NOS
Epileptic fits NOS
Epileptic seizures NOS
Recurrent seizures NOS
Seizure disorder NOS

[6th] G40.91 **Epilepsy, unspecified, intractable**

Intractable seizure disorder NOS

G40.911 **Epilepsy, unspecified, intractable, with status epilepticus** [CC] [HCC] [RxHCC] [CC/MCC Exc]

G40.919 **Epilepsy, unspecified, intractable, without status epilepticus** [CC] [HCC] [RxHCC] [CC/MCC Exc]

[4th] G43 **Migraine**

[NOTES] the following terms are to be considered equivalent to intractable: pharmacoresistant (pharmacologically resistant), treatment resistant, refractory (medically) and poorly controlled

Use additional code for adverse effect, if applicable, to identify drug (T36-T50 with fifth or sixth character 5)

EXCLUDES1 headache NOS (R51)
    lower half migraine (G44.00)

EXCLUDES2 headache syndromes (G44.-)

5th **G43.0** **Migraine** without aura
Common migraine
EXCLUDES1 chronic migraine without aura (G43.7-)

6th **G43.00** **Migraine without aura,** not intractable
Migraine without aura without mention of refractory migraine

    G43.001 **Migraine without aura, not intractable, with status migrainosus** RxHCC

    G43.009 **Migraine without aura, not intractable, without status migrainosus** RxHCC
    Migraine without aura NOS

6th **G43.01** **Migraine without aura,** intractable
Migraine without aura with refractory migraine

    G43.011 **Migraine without aura, intractable, with status migrainosus** RxHCC

    G43.019 **Migraine without aura, intractable, without status migrainosus** RxHCC

5th **G43.1** **Migraine** with aura
Basilar migraine
Classical migraine
Migraine equivalents
Migraine preceded or accompanied by transient focal neurological phenomena
Migraine triggered seizures
Migraine with acute-onset aura
Migraine with aura without headache (migraine equivalents)
Migraine with prolonged aura
Migraine with typical aura
Retinal migraine
Code also any associated seizure (G40.-, R56.9)
EXCLUDES1 persistent migraine aura (G43.5-, G43.6-)

6th **G43.10** **Migraine with aura,** not intractable
Migraine with aura without mention of refractory migraine

    G43.101 **Migraine with aura, not intractable, with status migrainosus** RxHCC

    G43.109 **Migraine with aura, not intractable, without status migrainosus** RxHCC
    Migraine with aura NOS

6th **G43.11** **Migraine with aura,** intractable
Migraine with aura with refractory migraine

    G43.111 **Migraine with aura, intractable, with status migrainosus** RxHCC

    G43.119 **Migraine with aura, intractable, without status migrainosus** RxHCC

5th **G43.4** Hemiplegic **migraine**
Familial migraine
Sporadic migraine

6th **G43.40** **Hemiplegic migraine,** not intractable
Hemiplegic migraine without refractory migraine

    G43.401 **Hemiplegic migraine, not intractable, with status migrainosus** RxHCC

    G43.409 **Hemiplegic migraine, not intractable, without status migrainosus** RxHCC
    Hemiplegic migraine NOS

6th **G43.41** **Hemiplegic migraine,** intractable
Hemiplegic migraine with refractory migraine

    G43.411 **Hemiplegic migraine, intractable, with status migrainosus** RxHCC

    G43.419 **Hemiplegic migraine, intractable, without status migrainosus** RxHCC

5th **G43.5** Persistent **migraine aura** without cerebral infarction

6th **G43.50** **Persistent migraine aura without cerebral infarction,** not intractable
Persistent migraine aura without cerebral infarction, without refractory migraine

    G43.501 **Persistent migraine aura without cerebral infarction, not intractable,** with status migrainosus RxHCC

    G43.509 **Persistent migraine aura without cerebral infarction, not intractable,** without status migrainosus RxHCC
    Persistent migraine aura NOS

6th **G43.51** **Persistent migraine aura without cerebral infarction,** intractable
Persistent migraine aura without cerebral infarction, with refractory migraine

    G43.511 **Persistent migraine aura without cerebral infarction, intractable,** with status migrainosus RxHCC

    G43.519 **Persistent migraine aura without cerebral infarction, intractable,** without status migrainosus RxHCC

5th **G43.6** **Persistent migraine aura** with cerebral infarction
Code also the type of cerebral infarction (I63.-)

6th **G43.60** **Persistent migraine aura with cerebral infarction,** not intractable
Persistent migraine aura with cerebral infarction, without refractory migraine

    G43.601 **Persistent migraine aura with cerebral infarction, not intractable,** with status migrainosus CC RxHCC CC/MCC Exc

    G43.609 **Persistent migraine aura with cerebral infarction, not intractable,** without status migrainosus CC RxHCC CC/MCC Exc

6th **G43.61** **Persistent migraine aura with cerebral infarction,** intractable
Persistent migraine aura with cerebral infarction, with refractory migraine

    G43.611 **Persistent migraine aura with cerebral infarction, intractable,** with status migrainosus CC RxHCC CC/MCC Exc

    G43.619 **Persistent migraine aura with cerebral infarction, intractable,** without status migrainosus CC RxHCC CC/MCC Exc

5th **G43.7** Chronic **migraine** without aura
Transformed migraine
EXCLUDES1 migraine without aura (G43.0-)

6th **G43.70** **Chronic migraine without aura,** not intractable
Chronic migraine without aura, without refractory migraine

    G43.701 **Chronic migraine without aura, not intractable,** with status migrainosus RxHCC

    G43.709 **Chronic migraine without aura, not intractable,** without status migrainosus RxHCC
    Chronic migraine without aura NOS

6th **G43.71** **Chronic migraine without aura,** intractable
Chronic migraine without aura, with refractory migraine

    G43.711 **Chronic migraine without aura, intractable,** with status migrainosus RxHCC

    G43.719 **Chronic migraine without aura, intractable,** without status migrainosus RxHCC

5th **G43.A** Cyclical vomiting

    G43.A0 **Cyclical vomiting,** not intractable RxHCC
    Cyclical vomiting, without refractory migraine

    G43.A1 **Cyclical vomiting,** intractable RxHCC
    Cyclical vomiting, with refractory migraine

5th **G43.B** Ophthalmoplegic **migraine**

    G43.B0 **Ophthalmoplegic migraine,** not intractable RxHCC
    Ophthalmoplegic migraine, without refractory migraine

    G43.B1 **Ophthalmoplegic migraine,** intractable RxHCC
    Ophthalmoplegic migraine, with refractory migraine

5th **G43.C** Periodic **headache syndromes in** child or adult

    G43.C0 **Periodic headache syndromes in child or adult,** not intractable RxHCC
    Periodic headache syndromes in child or adult, without refractory migraine

---

PDx Unacceptable principal diagnosis symbol per Medicare code edits   POA Code exempt from diagnosis present on admission requirement
? Questionable admission   CC Complication or comorbidity   CC/MCC Exc CC/MCC exclusion   MCC Major complication or comorbidity
PDx Principal diagnosis as its own CC   Principal diagnosis as its own MCC   HCC HCC diagnosis code   RxHCC RxHCC diagnosis code
MACRA code   Z Z code as first-listed diagnosis

G43.C1 **Periodic headache syndromes in child or adult,** intractable `RxHCC`
Periodic headache syndromes in child or adult, with refractory migraine

5ᵗʰ G43.D Abdominal **migraine**

G43.D0 **Abdominal migraine,** not intractable `RxHCC`
Abdominal migraine, without refractory migraine

G43.D1 **Abdominal migraine,** intractable `RxHCC`
Abdominal migraine, with refractory migraine

5ᵗʰ G43.8 Other **migraine**

6ᵗʰ G43.80 **Other migraine,** not intractable
Other migraine, without refractory migraine

G43.801 **Other migraine, not intractable, with** status migrainosus `RxHCC`

G43.809 **Other migraine, not intractable, without** status migrainosus `RxHCC`

6ᵗʰ G43.81 **Other migraine,** intractable
Other migraine, with refractory migraine

G43.811 **Other migraine, intractable, with status** migrainosus `RxHCC`

G43.819 **Other migraine, intractable, without** status migrainosus `RxHCC`

6ᵗʰ G43.82 **Menstrual migraine,** not intractable
Menstrual headache, not intractable
Menstrual migraine, without refractory migraine
Menstrually related migraine, not intractable
Pre-menstrual headache, not intractable
Pre-menstrual migraine, not intractable
Pure menstrual migraine, not intractable
Code also associated premenstrual tension syndrome (N94.3)

G43.821 **Menstrual migraine, not intractable, with** status migrainosus `RxHCC` ♀

G43.829 **Menstrual migraine, not intractable,** without status migrainosus `RxHCC` ♀
Menstrual migraine NOS

6ᵗʰ G43.83 **Menstrual migraine,** intractable
Menstrual headache, intractable
Menstrual migraine, with refractory migraine
Menstrually related migraine, intractable
Pre-menstrual headache, intractable
Pre-menstrual migraine, intractable
Pure menstrual migraine, intractable
Code also associated premenstrual tension syndrome (N94.3)

G43.831 **Menstrual migraine, intractable, with** status migrainosus `RxHCC` ♀

G43.839 **Menstrual migraine, intractable, without** status migrainosus `RxHCC` ♀

5ᵗʰ G43.9 Migraine, unspecified

6ᵗʰ G43.90 **Migraine, unspecified,** not intractable
Migraine, unspecified, without refractory migraine

G43.901 **Migraine, unspecified, not intractable, with status migrainosus** `RxHCC`
Status migrainosus NOS

G43.909 **Migraine, unspecified, not intractable, without status migrainosus** `RxHCC`
Migraine NOS

6ᵗʰ G43.91 **Migraine, unspecified,** intractable
Migraine, unspecified, with refractory migraine

G43.911 **Migraine, unspecified, intractable, with** status migrainosus `RxHCC`

G43.919 **Migraine, unspecified, intractable, without** status migrainosus `RxHCC`

4ᵗʰ G44 Other **headache syndromes**

EXCLUDES1 headache NOS (R51)

EXCLUDES2 atypical facial pain (G50.1)
headache due to lumbar puncture (G97.1)
migraines (G43.-)
trigeminal neuralgia (G50.0)

5ᵗʰ G44.0 **Cluster headaches and other trigeminal autonomic cephalgias (TAC)**

6ᵗʰ G44.00 **Cluster headache syndrome,** unspecified
Ciliary neuralgia
Cluster headache NOS
Histamine cephalgia
Lower half migraine
Migrainous neuralgia

G44.001 **Cluster headache syndrome, unspecified, intractable**

G44.009 **Cluster headache syndrome, unspecified, not intractable**
Cluster headache syndrome NOS

6ᵗʰ G44.01 Episodic **cluster headache**

G44.011 **Episodic cluster headache,** intractable

G44.019 **Episodic cluster headache,** not intractable
Episodic cluster headache NOS

6ᵗʰ G44.02 Chronic **cluster headache**

G44.021 **Chronic cluster headache,** intractable

G44.029 **Chronic cluster headache,** not intractable
Chronic cluster headache NOS

6ᵗʰ G44.03 Episodic **paroxysmal hemicrania**
Paroxysmal hemicrania NOS

G44.031 **Episodic paroxysmal hemicrania, intractable**

G44.039 **Episodic paroxysmal hemicrania,** not intractable
Episodic paroxysmal hemicrania NOS

6ᵗʰ G44.04 Chronic **paroxysmal hemicrania**

G44.041 **Chronic paroxysmal hemicrania, intractable**

G44.049 **Chronic paroxysmal hemicrania,** not intractable
Chronic paroxysmal hemicrania NOS

6ᵗʰ G44.05 Short lasting unilateral neuralgiform headache with conjunctival injection and tearing (SUNCT)

G44.051 **Short lasting unilateral neuralgiform headache with conjunctival injection and tearing (SUNCT),** intractable

G44.059 **Short lasting unilateral neuralgiform headache with conjunctival injection and tearing (SUNCT),** not intractable
Short lasting unilateral neuralgiform headache with conjunctival injection and tearing (SUNCT) NOS

6ᵗʰ G44.09 Other **trigeminal autonomic cephalgias (TAC)**

G44.091 **Other trigeminal autonomic cephalgias (TAC),** intractable

G44.099 **Other trigeminal autonomic cephalgias (TAC),** not intractable

G44.1 Vascular **headache, not elsewhere classified**

EXCLUDES2 cluster headache (G44.0)
complicated headache syndromes (G44.5-)
drug-induced headache (G44.4-)
migraine (G43.-)
other specified headache syndromes (G44.8-)
post-traumatic headache (G44.3-)
tension-type headache (G44.2-)

5ᵗʰ G44.2 Tension-type **headache**

6ᵗʰ G44.20 **Tension-type headache,** unspecified

G44.201 **Tension-type headache, unspecified, intractable**

G44.209 **Tension-type headache, unspecified, not intractable**
Tension headache NOS

6ᵗʰ G44.21 Episodic **tension-type headache**

G44.211 **Episodic tension-type headache, intractable**

G44.219 **Episodic tension-type headache,** not intractable
Episodic tension-type headache NOS

6ᵗʰ G44.22 Chronic tension-type **headache**

Unspecified Code   Other Specified Code   Manifestation Code   Ⓝ Newborn   Ⓟ Pediatric   Ⓜ Maternity   Ⓐ Adult   ♂ Male   ♀ Female
● New Code   ▲ Revised Code Title   ▶◀ Revised Text   NOTES   INCLUDES   EXCLUDES 1 Not coded here   EXCLUDES 2 Not included here
4ᵗʰ 4ᵗʰ character required   5ᵗʰ 5ᵗʰ character required   6ᵗʰ 6ᵗʰ character required   7ᵗʰ 7ᵗʰ character required
Ⓧ Extension 'X' Alert   HAC Hospital-acquired condition (HAC) alert   AHA AHA Coding Clinic©

G44.221 **Chronic tension-type headache, intractable**

G44.229 **Chronic tension-type headache,** not intractable

Chronic tension-type headache NOS

5ᵗʰ G44.3 Post-traumatic **headache**

6ᵗʰ G44.30 **Post-traumatic headache,** unspecified

G44.301 **Post-traumatic headache, unspecified, intractable**

G44.309 **Post-traumatic headache, unspecified, not intractable**

Post-traumatic headache NOS

6ᵗʰ G44.31 Acute post-traumatic **headache**

G44.311 **Acute post-traumatic headache, intractable**

G44.319 **Acute post-traumatic headache,** not intractable

Acute post-traumatic headache NOS

6ᵗʰ G44.32 Chronic post-traumatic **headache**

G44.321 **Chronic post-traumatic headache, intractable**

G44.329 **Chronic post-traumatic headache, not intractable**

Chronic post-traumatic headache NOS

5ᵗʰ G44.4 Drug-induced **headache,** not elsewhere classified

Medication overuse headache

Use additional code for adverse effect, if applicable, to identify drug (T36-T50 with fifth or sixth character 5)

G44.40 **Drug-induced headache, not elsewhere classified, not intractable**

G44.41 **Drug-induced headache, not elsewhere classified, intractable**

5ᵗʰ G44.5 Complicated **headache syndromes**

G44.51 **Hemicrania continua**

G44.52 **New daily persistent headache (NDPH)**

G44.53 **Primary thunderclap headache**

G44.59 **Other complicated headache syndrome**

5ᵗʰ G44.8 Other specified **headache syndromes**

G44.81 **Hypnic headache**

G44.82 **Headache associated** with sexual activity

Orgasmic headache
Preorgasmic headache

G44.83 **Primary cough headache**

G44.84 **Primary exertional headache**

G44.85 **Primary stabbing headache**

G44.89 **Other headache syndrome**

4ᵗʰ G45 Transient cerebral ischemic attacks and related syndromes

EXCLUDES1 neonatal cerebral ischemia (P91.0)

transient retinal artery occlusion (H34.0-)

G45.0 Vertebro-basilar artery **syndrome**   CC   RxHCC   CC/MCC Exc

G45.1 Carotid artery **syndrome (hemispheric)**   CC   RxHCC   CC/MCC Exc

G45.2 Multiple and bilateral precerebral artery **syndromes**   CC   RxHCC   CC/MCC Exc

G45.3 **Amaurosis fugax**   CC   CC/MCC Exc

G45.4 Transient global amnesia

EXCLUDES1 amnesia NOS (R41.3)

G45.8 **Other transient cerebral ischemic attacks and related syndromes**   CC   RxHCC   CC/MCC Exc

G45.9 **Transient cerebral ischemic attack, unspecified**   CC   RxHCC   CC/MCC Exc

Spasm of cerebral artery
TIA
Transient cerebral ischemia NOS

4ᵗʰ G46 Vascular syndromes of brain in cerebrovascular diseases

Code first underlying cerebrovascular disease (I60-I69)

G46.0 Middle **cerebral artery syndrome**   CC   RxHCC   CC/MCC Exc

G46.1 Anterior **cerebral artery syndrome**   CC   RxHCC   CC/MCC Exc

G46.2 Posterior **cerebral artery syndrome**   CC   RxHCC   CC/MCC Exc

G46.3 Brain stem stroke **syndrome**   RxHCC

Benedikt syndrome
Claude syndrome
Foville syndrome

Millard-Gubler syndrome
Wallenberg syndrome
Weber syndrome

G46.4 Cerebellar stroke **syndrome**   RxHCC

G46.5 Pure motor lacunar **syndrome**   RxHCC

G46.6 Pure sensory lacunar **syndrome**   RxHCC

G46.7 Other lacunar **syndromes**   RxHCC

G46.8 Other vascular syndromes of brain in cerebrovascular diseases   RxHCC

4ᵗʰ G47 Sleep disorders

EXCLUDES2 nightmares (F51.5)

nonorganic sleep disorders (F51.-)

sleep terrors (F51.4)

sleepwalking (F51.3)

5ᵗʰ G47.0 Insomnia

EXCLUDES2 alcohol related insomnia (F10.182, F10.282, F10.982)

drug-related insomnia (F11.182, F11.282, F11.982, F13.182, F13.282, F13.982, F14.182, F14.282, F14.982, F15.182, F15.282, F15.982, F19.182, F19.282, F19.982)

idiopathic insomnia (F51.01)

insomnia due to a mental disorder (F51.05)

insomnia not due to a substance or known physiological condition (F51.0-)

nonorganic insomnia (F51.0-)

primary insomnia (F51.01)

sleep apnea (G47.3-)

G47.00 **Insomnia, unspecified**

Insomnia NOS

G47.01 **Insomnia due to medical condition**

Code also associated medical condition

G47.09 **Other insomnia**

5ᵗʰ G47.1 Hypersomnia

EXCLUDES2 alcohol-related hypersomnia (F10.182, F10.282, F10.982)

drug-related hypersomnia (F11.182, F11.282, F11.982, F13.182, F13.282, F13.982, F14.182, F14.282, F14.982, F15.182, F15.282, F15.982, F19.182, F19.282, F19.982)

hypersomnia due to a mental disorder (F51.13)

hypersomnia not due to a substance or known physiological condition (F51.1-)

primary hypersomnia (F51.11)

sleep apnea (G47.3-)

G47.10 **Hypersomnia, unspecified**

Hypersomnia NOS

G47.11 **Idiopathic hypersomnia** with long sleep time

Idiopathic hypersomnia NOS

G47.12 **Idiopathic hypersomnia** without long sleep time

G47.13 **Recurrent hypersomnia**

Kleine-Levin syndrome
Menstrual related hypersomnia

G47.14 **Hypersomnia** due to medical condition

Code also associated medical condition

G47.19 **Other hypersomnia**

5ᵗʰ G47.2 Circadian rhythm sleep disorders

Disorders of the sleep wake schedule
Inversion of nyctohemeral rhythm
Inversion of sleep rhythm

G47.20 **Circadian rhythm sleep disorder, unspecified type**

Sleep wake schedule disorder NOS

G47.21 **Circadian rhythm sleep disorder,** delayed sleep phase type

Delayed sleep phase syndrome

G47.22 **Circadian rhythm sleep disorder,** advanced sleep phase type

G47.23 **Circadian rhythm sleep disorder,** irregular sleep wake type

Irregular sleep-wake pattern

PDx Unacceptable principal diagnosis symbol per Medicare code edits   POA Code exempt from diagnosis present on admission requirement

❓ Questionable admission   CC Complication or comorbidity   CC/MCC Exc CC/MCC exclusion   MCC Major complication or comorbidity

CC Principal diagnosis as its own CC   MCC Principal diagnosis as its own MCC   HCC HCC diagnosis code   RxHCC RxHCC diagnosis code

MACRA code   Z Z code as first-listed diagnosis

580   When symbols appear on a code that requires a 7th character extension, refer to Appendix B to identify applicable 7th character codes.   **2018 ICD-10-CM**

G47.24 **Circadian rhythm sleep disorder,** free running type
Circadian rhythm sleep disorder, non-24-hour sleep-wake type

G47.25 **Circadian rhythm sleep disorder,** jet lag type

G47.26 **Circadian rhythm sleep disorder,** shift work type

G47.27 **Circadian rhythm sleep disorder in conditions classified elsewhere**
Code first underlying condition

G47.29 **Other** circadian rhythm sleep disorder

⑤ G47.3 **Sleep apnea**
Code also any associated underlying condition

EXCLUDES1 apnea NOS (R06.81)

Cheyne-Stokes breathing (R06.3)

pickwickian syndrome (E66.2)

sleep apnea of newborn (P28.3)

G47.30 **Sleep apnea, unspecified**
Sleep apnea NOS

G47.31 **Primary central sleep apnea**
Idiopathic central sleep apnea

G47.32 **High altitude periodic breathing**

G47.33 **Obstructive sleep apnea (adult) (pediatric)**
Obstructive sleep apnea hypopnea

EXCLUDES1 obstructive sleep apnea of newborn (P28.3)

G47.34 **Idiopathic sleep related nonobstructive alveolar hypoventilation**
Sleep related hypoxia

G47.35 **Congenital central alveolar hypoventilation syndrome**

G47.36 **Sleep related hypoventilation in conditions classified elsewhere**
Sleep related hypoxemia in conditions classified elsewhere
Code first underlying condition

G47.37 **Central sleep apnea in conditions classified elsewhere**
Code first underlying condition

G47.39 **Other sleep apnea**

⑤ G47.4 **Narcolepsy and cataplexy**

⑥ G47.41 **Narcolepsy**

G47.411 **Narcolepsy with cataplexy** RxHCC

G47.419 **Narcolepsy without cataplexy** RxHCC
Narcolepsy NOS

⑥ G47.42 **Narcolepsy in conditions classified elsewhere**
Code first underlying condition

G47.421 **Narcolepsy in conditions classified elsewhere with cataplexy** RxHCC

G47.429 **Narcolepsy in conditions classified elsewhere without cataplexy** RxHCC

⑤ G47.5 **Parasomnia**

EXCLUDES1 alcohol induced parasomnia (F10.182, F10.282, F10.982)

drug induced parasomnia (F11.182, F11.282, F11.982, F13.182, F13.282, F13.982, F14.182, F14.282, F14.982, F15.182, F15.282, F15.982, F19.182, F19.282, F19.982)

parasomnia not due to a substance or known physiological condition (F51.8)

G47.50 **Parasomnia, unspecified**
Parasomnia NOS

G47.51 **Confusional arousals**

G47.52 **REM sleep behavior disorder**

G47.53 **Recurrent isolated sleep paralysis**

G47.54 **Parasomnia in conditions classified elsewhere**
Code first underlying condition

G47.59 **Other parasomnia**

⑤ G47.6 **Sleep related movement disorders**

EXCLUDES2 restless legs syndrome (G25.81)

G47.61 **Periodic limb movement disorder**

G47.62 **Sleep related** leg cramps

G47.63 **Sleep related** bruxism
AHA: Q4 2016

EXCLUDES1 psychogenic bruxism (F45.8)

G47.69 **Other** sleep related movement disorders

G47.8 **Other** sleep disorders
Other specified sleep-wake disorder

G47.9 **Sleep disorder, unspecified**
Sleep disorder NOS
Unspecified sleep-wake disorder

Nerve, nerve root and plexus disorders (G50-G59)

EXCLUDES1 current traumatic nerve, nerve root and plexus disorders - see Injury, nerve by body region

neuralgia NOS (M79.2)

neuritis NOS (M79.2)

peripheral neuritis in pregnancy (O26.82-)

radiculitis NOS (M54.1-)

④ G50 **Disorders of** trigeminal nerve

INCLUDES disorders of 5th cranial nerve

G50.0 **Trigeminal** neuralgia RxHCC
Syndrome of paroxysmal facial pain
Tic douloureux

G50.1 **Atypical facial pain** RxHCC

G50.8 **Other disorders** of trigeminal nerve RxHCC

G50.9 **Disorder of trigeminal nerve, unspecified** RxHCC

④ G51 **Facial nerve** disorders

INCLUDES disorders of 7th cranial nerve

G51.0 **Bell's palsy**
Facial palsy

G51.1 **Geniculate ganglionitis**

EXCLUDES1 postherpetic geniculate ganglionitis (B02.21)

G51.2 **Melkersson's syndrome**
Melkersson-Rosenthal syndrome

G51.3 **Clonic hemifacial spasm**

G51.4 **Facial myokymia**

G51.8 **Other disorders of facial nerve**

G51.9 **Disorder of facial nerve, unspecified**

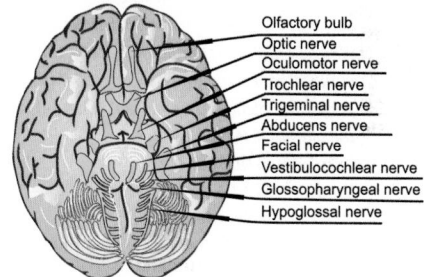

Olfactory bulb
Optic nerve
Oculomotor nerve
Trochlear nerve
Trigeminal nerve
Abducens nerve
Facial nerve
Vestibulocochlear nerve
Glossopharyngeal nerve
Hypoglossal nerve

Figure 6.2 The Cranial nerves

④ G52 **Disorders of** other cranial nerves

EXCLUDES2 disorders of acoustic [8th] nerve (H93.3)

disorders of optic [2nd] nerve (H46, H47.0)

paralytic strabismus due to nerve palsy (H49.0-H49.2)

G52.0 **Disorders of** olfactory **nerve**
Disorders of 1st cranial nerve

G52.1 **Disorders of** glossopharyngeal **nerve**
Disorder of 9th cranial nerve
Glossopharyngeal neuralgia

G52.2 **Disorders of** vagus **nerve**
Disorders of pneumogastric [10th] nerve

G52.3 **Disorders of** hypoglossal **nerve**
Disorders of 12th cranial nerve

G52.7 **Disorders of** multiple cranial **nerves**
Polyneuritis cranialis

G52.8 **Disorders of** other specified cranial nerves

G52.9 **Cranial nerve disorder, unspecified**

Unspecified Code   Other Specified Code   Manifestation Code   Ⓝ Newborn   Ⓟ Pediatric   Ⓜ Maternity   Ⓐ Adult   ♂ Male   ♀ Female
● New Code   ▲ Revised Code Title   ▶◀ Revised Text   **NOTES**   INCLUDES   EXCLUDES 1   Not coded here   EXCLUDES 2   Not included here
④ 4th character required   ⑤ 5th character required   ⑥ 6th character required   ⑦ 7th character required
⑦ Extension 'X' Alert   HAC Hospital-acquired condition (HAC) alert   **AHA** AHA Coding Clinic©

G53 **Cranial nerve disorders in diseases classified elsewhere**
 Code first underlying disease, such as:
 neoplasm (C00-D49)
 EXCLUDES1 *multiple cranial nerve palsy in sarcoidosis (D86.82)*
  multiple cranial nerve palsy in syphilis (A52.15)
  postherpetic geniculate ganglionitis (B02.21)
  postherpetic trigeminal neuralgia (B02.22)

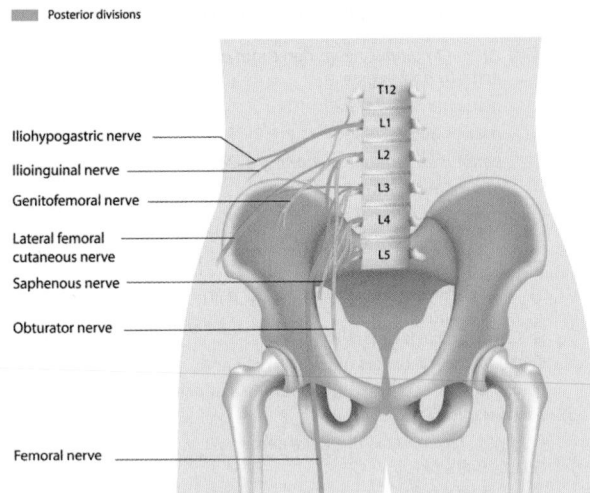

Anterior divisions
Posterior divisions

Iliohypogastric nerve
Ilioinguinal nerve
Genitofemoral nerve
Lateral femoral cutaneous nerve
Saphenous nerve
Obturator nerve
Femoral nerve

T12
L1
L2
L3
L4
L5

Figure 6.3 The Lumbar plexus

G54 **Nerve root and plexus disorders**
 EXCLUDES1 *current traumatic nerve root and plexus disorders - see nerve injury by body region*
  intervertebral disc disorders (M50-M51)
  neuralgia or neuritis NOS (M79.2)
  neuritis or radiculitis brachial NOS (M54.13)
  neuritis or radiculitis lumbar NOS (M54.16)
  neuritis or radiculitis lumbosacral NOS (M54.17)
  neuritis or radiculitis thoracic NOS (M54.14)
  radiculitis NOS (M54.10)
  radiculopathy NOS (M54.10)
  spondylosis (M47.-)
 G54.0 **Brachial plexus disorders**
  Thoracic outlet syndrome
 G54.1 **Lumbosacral plexus disorders**
 G54.2 **Cervical root disorders, not elsewhere classified**
 G54.3 **Thoracic root disorders, not elsewhere classified**   PDxIn
 G54.4 **Lumbosacral root disorders, not elsewhere classified**
 G54.5 **Neuralgic amyotrophy**
  Parsonage-Aldren-Turner syndrome
  Shoulder-girdle neuritis
  EXCLUDES1 *neuralgic amyotrophy in diabetes mellitus (E08-E13 with .44)*
 G54.6 **Phantom limb syndrome with pain**   HCC
 G54.7 **Phantom limb syndrome without pain**   HCC
  Phantom limb syndrome NOS
 G54.8 **Other nerve root and plexus disorders**
 G54.9 **Nerve root and plexus disorder, unspecified**
G55 **Nerve root and plexus compressions in diseases classified elsewhere**
 Code first underlying disease, such as:
 neoplasm (C00-D49)

 EXCLUDES1 *nerve root compression (due to) (in) ankylosing spondylitis (M45.-)*
  nerve root compression (due to) (in) dorsopathies (M53.-, M54.-)
  nerve root compression (due to) (in) intervertebral disc disorders (M50.1.-, M51.1.-)
  nerve root compression (due to) (in) spondylopathies (M46.-, M48.-)
  nerve root compression (due to) (in) spondylosis (M47.0-M47.2.-)
G56 **Mononeuropathies of upper limb**
 EXCLUDES1 *current traumatic nerve disorder - see nerve injury by body region*
 G56.0 **Carpal tunnel syndrome**
  G56.00 **Carpal tunnel syndrome, unspecified upper limb**
  G56.01 **Carpal tunnel syndrome, right upper limb**
  G56.02 **Carpal tunnel syndrome, left upper limb**
  G56.03 **Carpal tunnel syndrome, bilateral upper limbs**
   AHA: Q4 2016
 G56.1 **Other lesions of median nerve**
  G56.10 **Other lesions of median nerve, unspecified upper limb**
  G56.11 **Other lesions of median nerve, right upper limb**
  G56.12 **Other lesions of median nerve, left upper limb**
  G56.13 **Other lesions of median nerve, bilateral upper limbs**
   AHA: Q4 2016
 G56.2 **Lesion of ulnar nerve**
  Tardy ulnar nerve palsy
  G56.20 **Lesion of ulnar nerve, unspecified upper limb**
  G56.21 **Lesion of ulnar nerve, right upper limb**
  G56.22 **Lesion of ulnar nerve, left upper limb**
  G56.23 **Lesion of ulnar nerve, bilateral upper limbs**
   AHA: Q4 2016
 G56.3 **Lesion of radial nerve**
  G56.30 **Lesion of radial nerve, unspecified upper limb**
  G56.31 **Lesion of radial nerve, right upper limb**
  G56.32 **Lesion of radial nerve, left upper limb**
  G56.33 **Lesion of radial nerve, bilateral upper limbs**
   AHA: Q4 2016
 G56.4 **Causalgia of upper limb**
  Complex regional pain syndrome II of upper limb
  EXCLUDES1 *complex regional pain syndrome I of lower limb (G90.52-)*
   complex regional pain syndrome I of upper limb (G90.51-)
   complex regional pain syndrome II of lower limb (G57.7-)
   reflex sympathetic dystrophy of lower limb (G90.52-)
   reflex sympathetic dystrophy of upper limb (G90.51-)
  G56.40 **Causalgia of unspecified upper limb**
  G56.41 **Causalgia of right upper limb**
  G56.42 **Causalgia of left upper limb**
  G56.43 **Causalgia of bilateral upper limbs**
   AHA: Q4 2016
 G56.8 **Other specified mononeuropathies of upper limb**
  Interdigital neuroma of upper limb
  G56.80 **Other specified mononeuropathies of unspecified upper limb**
  G56.81 **Other specified mononeuropathies of right upper limb**
  G56.82 **Other specified mononeuropathies of left upper limb**
  G56.83 **Other specified mononeuropathies of bilateral upper limbs**
   AHA: Q4 2016
 G56.9 **Unspecified mononeuropathy of upper limb**
  G56.90 **Unspecified mononeuropathy of unspecified upper limb**
  G56.91 **Unspecified mononeuropathy of right upper limb**
  G56.92 **Unspecified mononeuropathy of left upper limb**

 PDxIn Unacceptable principal diagnosis symbol per Medicare code edits   PoA Code exempt from diagnosis present on admission requirement
 ❓ Questionable admission   cc Complication or comorbidity   cc/MCC Exc CC/MCC exclusion   MCC Major complication or comorbidity
 PDxCC Principal diagnosis as its own CC   PDxMCC Principal diagnosis as its own MCC   HCC HCC diagnosis code   RxHCC RxHCC diagnosis code
 MACRA code   Z1 Z code as first-listed diagnosis

G56.93 Unspecified mononeuropathy of bilateral upper limbs

AHA: Q4 2016

🔵 G57 Mononeuropathies of lower limb

EXCLUDES1 current traumatic nerve disorder - see nerve injury by body region

🔵 G57.0 Lesion of sciatic nerve

EXCLUDES1 sciatica NOS (M54.3-)

EXCLUDES2 sciatica attributed to intervertebral disc disorder (M51.1.-)

G57.00 Lesion of sciatic nerve, unspecified lower limb

G57.01 Lesion of sciatic nerve, right lower limb

G57.02 Lesion of sciatic nerve, left lower limb

G57.03 Lesion of sciatic nerve, bilateral lower limbs

AHA: Q4 2016

🔵 G57.1 Meralgia paresthetica

Lateral cutaneous nerve of thigh syndrome

G57.10 Meralgia paresthetica, unspecified lower limb

G57.11 Meralgia paresthetica, right lower limb

G57.12 Meralgia paresthetica, left lower limb

G57.13 Meralgia paresthetica, bilateral lower limbs

AHA: Q4 2016

🔵 G57.2 Lesion of femoral nerve

G57.20 Lesion of femoral nerve, unspecified lower limb

G57.21 Lesion of femoral nerve, right lower limb

G57.22 Lesion of femoral nerve, left lower limb

G57.23 Lesion of femoral nerve, bilateral lower limbs

AHA: Q4 2016

🔵 G57.3 Lesion of lateral popliteal nerve

Peroneal nerve palsy

G57.30 Lesion of lateral popliteal nerve, unspecified lower limb

G57.31 Lesion of lateral popliteal nerve, right lower limb

G57.32 Lesion of lateral popliteal nerve, left lower limb

G57.33 Lesion of lateral popliteal nerve, bilateral lower limbs

AHA: Q4 2016

🔵 G57.4 Lesion of medial popliteal nerve

G57.40 Lesion of medial popliteal nerve, unspecified lower limb

G57.41 Lesion of medial popliteal nerve, right lower limb

G57.42 Lesion of medial popliteal nerve, left lower limb

G57.43 Lesion of medial popliteal nerve, bilateral lower limbs

AHA: Q4 2016

🔵 G57.5 Tarsal tunnel syndrome

G57.50 Tarsal tunnel syndrome, unspecified lower limb

G57.51 Tarsal tunnel syndrome, right lower limb

G57.52 Tarsal tunnel syndrome, left lower limb

G57.53 Tarsal tunnel syndrome, bilateral lower limbs

AHA: Q4 2016

🔵 G57.6 Lesion of plantar nerve

Morton's metatarsalgia

G57.60 Lesion of plantar nerve, unspecified lower limb

G57.61 Lesion of plantar nerve, right lower limb

G57.62 Lesion of plantar nerve, left lower limb

G57.63 Lesion of plantar nerve, bilateral lower limbs

AHA: Q4 2016

🔵 G57.7 Causalgia of lower limb

Complex regional pain syndrome II of lower limb

EXCLUDES1 complex regional pain syndrome I of lower limb (G90.52-)

complex regional pain syndrome I of upper limb (G90.51-)

complex regional pain syndrome II of upper limb (G56.4-)

reflex sympathetic dystrophy of lower limb (G90.52-)

reflex sympathetic dystrophy of upper limb (G90.51-)

G57.70 Causalgia of unspecified lower limb

G57.71 Causalgia of right lower limb

G57.72 Causalgia of left lower limb

G57.73 Causalgia of bilateral lower limbs

AHA: Q4 2016

🔵 G57.8 Other specified mononeuropathies of lower limb

Interdigital neuroma of lower limb

G57.80 Other specified mononeuropathies of unspecified lower limb

G57.81 Other specified mononeuropathies of right lower limb

G57.82 Other specified mononeuropathies of left lower limb

G57.83 Other specified mononeuropathies of bilateral lower limbs

AHA: Q4 2016

🔵 G57.9 Unspecified mononeuropathy of lower limb

G57.90 Unspecified mononeuropathy of unspecified lower limb

G57.91 Unspecified mononeuropathy of right lower limb

G57.92 Unspecified mononeuropathy of left lower limb

G57.93 Unspecified mononeuropathy of bilateral lower limbs

AHA: Q4 2016

🔵 G58 Other mononeuropathies

G58.0 Intercostal neuropathy

G58.7 Mononeuritis multiplex

G58.8 Other specified mononeuropathies

G58.9 Mononeuropathy, unspecified

G59 Mononeuropathy in diseases classified elsewhere

Code first underlying disease

EXCLUDES1 diabetic mononeuropathy (E08-E13 with .41)

syphilitic nerve paralysis (A52.19)

syphilitic neuritis (A52.15)

tuberculous mononeuropathy (A17.83)

Polyneuropathies and other disorders of the peripheral nervous system (G60-G65)

EXCLUDES1 neuralgia NOS (M79.2)

neuritis NOS (M79.2)

peripheral neuritis in pregnancy (O26.82-)

radiculitis NOS (M54.10)

🔵 G60 Hereditary and idiopathic neuropathy

G60.0 Hereditary motor and sensory neuropathy

Charcot-Marie-Tooth disease

Déjérine-Sottas disease

Hereditary motor and sensory neuropathy, types I-IV

Hypertrophic neuropathy of infancy

Peroneal muscular atrophy (axonal type) (hypertrophic type)

Roussy-Levy syndrome

G60.1 Refsum's disease ♂ CC/MCC Exc

Infantile Refsum disease

G60.2 Neuropathy in association with hereditary ataxia

G60.3 Idiopathic progressive neuropathy

G60.8 Other hereditary and idiopathic neuropathies

Dominantly inherited sensory neuropathy

Morvan's disease

Nelaton's syndrome

Recessively inherited sensory neuropathy

G60.9 Hereditary and idiopathic neuropathy, unspecified

🔵 G61 Inflammatory polyneuropathy

G61.0 Guillain-Barre syndrome ♂ HCC RxHCC CC/MCC Exc

Acute (post-)infective polyneuritis

Miller Fisher Syndrome

G61.1 Serum neuropathy HCC RxHCC

Use additional code for adverse effect, if applicable, to identify serum (T50.-)

🔵 G61.8 Other inflammatory polyneuropathies

G61.81 Chronic inflammatory demyelinating polyneuritis ♂ HCC RxHCC CC/MCC Exc

---

Unspecified Code	Other Specified Code	Manifestation Code ℕ Newborn ℙ Pediatric ℳ Maternity 🅰 Adult ♂ Male ♀ Female

● New Code ▲ Revised Code Title ▶◀ Revised Text **NOTES** *INCLUDES* *EXCLUDES 1* Not coded here *EXCLUDES 2* Not included here

🔵 4th character required 🔵 5th character required 🔵 6th character required 🔵 7th character required

🔵 Extension 'X' Alert HAC Hospital-acquired condition (HAC) alert **AHA** AHA Coding Clinic©

G61.82 Multifocal motor neuropathy `HCC` `RxHCC`
AHA: Q4 2016
MMN
G61.89 Other **inflammatory polyneuropathies** `HCC` `RxHCC`
G61.9 **Inflammatory polyneuropathy, unspecified** `HCC` `RxHCC`
G62 Other and unspecified **polyneuropathies**
G62.0 Drug-induced **polyneuropathy** `HCC` `RxHCC`
Use additional code for adverse effect, if applicable, to identify drug (T36-T50 with fifth or sixth character 5)
G62.1 Alcoholic **polyneuropathy** `HCC` `RxHCC`
G62.2 Polyneuropathy due to other toxic agents `HCC` `RxHCC`
Code first (T51-T65) to identify toxic agent
G62.8 Other specified **polyneuropathies**
G62.81 Critical illness **polyneuropathy** `CC` `HCC` `RxHCC` `CC/MCC Exc`
Acute motor neuropathy
G62.82 Radiation-induced **polyneuropathy** `HCC` `RxHCC`
Use additional external cause code (W88-W90, X39.0-) to identify cause
G62.89 Other specified **polyneuropathies**
AHA: Q2 2016
G62.9 **Polyneuropathy, unspecified**
Neuropathy NOS
G63 **Polyneuropathy in diseases classified elsewhere** `HCC` `RxHCC`
AHA: Q4 2012
Code first underlying disease, such as:
amyloidosis (E85.-)
endocrine disease, except diabetes (E00-E07, E15-E16, E20-E34)
metabolic diseases (E70-E88)
neoplasm (C00-D49)
nutritional deficiency (E40-E64)
EXCLUDES1 polyneuropathy (in):
diabetes mellitus (E08-E13 with .42)
diphtheria (A36.83)
infectious mononucleosis (B27.0-B27.9 with 1)
Lyme disease (A69.22)
mumps (B26.84)
postherpetic (B02.23)
rheumatoid arthritis (M05.33)
scleroderma (M34.83)
systemic lupus erythematosus (M32.19)
G64 **Other disorders of peripheral nervous system**
Disorder of peripheral nervous system NOS
G65 **Sequelae of inflammatory and toxic polyneuropathies**
Code first condition resulting from (sequela) of inflammatory and toxic polyneuropathies
G65.0 Sequelae of Guillain-Barré syndrome `HCC` `RxHCC`
G65.1 Sequelae of other inflammatory **polyneuropathy** `HCC` `RxHCC`
G65.2 Sequelae of toxic **polyneuropathy** `HCC` `RxHCC`

Diseases of myoneural junction and muscle (G70-G73)

G70 **Myasthenia gravis and other myoneural disorders**
EXCLUDES1 botulism (A05.1, A48.51-A48.52)
transient neonatal myasthenia gravis (P94.0)
G70.0 **Myasthenia gravis**
G70.00 **Myasthenia gravis** without (acute) exacerbation `HCC` `RxHCC`
Myasthenia gravis NOS
G70.01 **Myasthenia gravis** with (acute) exacerbation `HCC` `MCC` `RxHCC` `CC/MCC Exc`
Myasthenia gravis in crisis
G70.1 **Toxic myoneural disorders** `HCC` `RxHCC`
Code first (T51-T65) to identify toxic agent
G70.2 **Congenital and developmental myasthenia** `HCC` `RxHCC`
G70.8 Other specified **myoneural disorders**
G70.80 **Lambert-Eaton syndrome, unspecified** `CC` `HCC` `RxHCC` `CC/MCC Exc`
Lambert-Eaton syndrome NOS

G70.81 **Lambert-Eaton syndrome in disease classified elsewhere** `CC` `HCC` `RxHCC` `CC/MCC Exc`
Code first underlying disease
EXCLUDES1 Lambert-Eaton syndrome in neoplastic disease (G73.1)
G70.89 Other specified **myoneural disorders** `HCC` `RxHCC`
G70.9 **Myoneural disorder, unspecified** `HCC` `RxHCC`
G71 **Primary disorders of muscles**
EXCLUDES2 arthrogryposis multiplex congenita (Q74.3)
metabolic disorders (E70-E88)
myositis (M60.-)
G71.0 **Muscular dystrophy** `CC` `HCC` `CC/MCC Exc`
Autosomal recessive, childhood type, muscular dystrophy resembling Duchenne or Becker muscular dystrophy
Benign [Becker] muscular dystrophy
Benign scapuloperoneal muscular dystrophy with early contractures [Emery-Dreifuss]
Congenital muscular dystrophy NOS
Congenital muscular dystrophy with specific morphological abnormalities of the muscle fiber
Distal muscular dystrophy
Facioscapulohumeral muscular dystrophy
Limb-girdle muscular dystrophy
Ocular muscular dystrophy
Oculopharyngeal muscular dystrophy
Scapuloperoneal muscular dystrophy
Severe [Duchenne] muscular dystrophy
G71.1 **Myotonic disorders**
G71.11 **Myotonic muscular dystrophy** `HCC`
Dystrophia myotonica [Steinert]
Myotonia atrophica
Myotonic dystrophy
Proximal myotonic myopathy (PROMM)
Steinert disease
G71.12 **Myotonia** congenita
Acetazolamide responsive myotonia congenita
Dominant myotonia congenita [Thomsen disease]
Myotonia levior
Recessive myotonia congenita [Becker disease]
G71.13 **Myotonic** chondrodystrophy
Chondrodystrophic myotonia
Congenital myotonic chondrodystrophy
Schwartz-Jampel disease
G71.14 Drug induced **myotonia**
Use additional code for adverse effect, if applicable, to identify drug (T36-T50 with fifth or sixth character 5)
G71.19 Other specified **myotonic disorders**
Myotonia fluctuans
Myotonia permanens
Neuromyotonia [Isaacs]
Paramyotonia congenita (of von Eulenburg)
Pseudomyotonia
Symptomatic myotonia
G71.2 Congenital myopathies `CC` `HCC` `CC/MCC Exc`
Central core disease
Fiber-type disproportion
Minicore disease
Multicore disease
Myotubular (centronuclear) myopathy
Nemaline myopathy
EXCLUDES1 arthrogryposis multiplex congenita (Q74.3)
G71.3 Mitochondrial **myopathy, not elsewhere classified**
EXCLUDES1 Kearns-Sayre syndrome (H49.81)
Leber's disease (H47.21)
Leigh's encephalopathy (G31.82)
mitochondrial metabolism disorders (E88.4.-)
Reye's syndrome (G93.7)
G71.8 Other primary **disorders of muscles**
G71.9 **Primary disorder of muscle, unspecified**
Hereditary myopathy NOS

`PDx` Unacceptable principal diagnosis symbol per Medicare code edits   `PDx` Code exempt from diagnosis present on admission requirement
`?` Questionable admission   `CC` Complication or comorbidity   `CC/MCC Exc` CC/MCC exclusion   `MCC` Major complication or comorbidity
`CC` Principal diagnosis as its own CC   `MCC` Principal diagnosis as its own MCC   `HCC` HCC diagnosis code   `RxHCC` RxHCC diagnosis code
MACRA code   `Z1` Z code as first-listed diagnosis

When symbols appear on a code that requires a 7th character extension, refer to Appendix B to identify applicable 7th character codes.
2018 ICD-10-CM

G72 Other and unspecified **myopathies**

EXCLUDES1 arthrogryposis multiplex congenita (Q74.3)

dermatopolymyositis (M33.-)

ischemic infarction of muscle (M62.2-)

myositis (M60.-)

polymyositis (M33.2.-)

G72.0 Drug-induced **myopathy**

Use additional code for adverse effect, if applicable, to identify drug (T36-T50 with fifth or sixth character 5)

G72.1 Alcoholic **myopathy**

Use additional code to identify alcoholism (F10.-)

G72.2 Myopathy due to other toxic agents

Code first (T51-T65) to identify toxic agent

G72.3 Periodic paralysis

Familial periodic paralysis

Hyperkalemic periodic paralysis (familial)

Hypokalemic periodic paralysis (familial)

Myotonic periodic paralysis (familial)

Normokalemic paralysis (familial)

Potassium sensitive periodic paralysis

EXCLUDES1 paramyotonia congenita (of von Eulenburg) (G71.19)

G72.4 Inflammatory and immune **myopathies, not elsewhere classified**

G72.41 Inclusion body myositis [IBM]

G72.49 Other **inflammatory and immune myopathies, not elsewhere classified**

Inflammatory myopathy NOS

G72.8 Other specified **myopathies**

G72.81 Critical illness **myopathy**

Acute necrotizing myopathy

Acute quadriplegic myopathy

Intensive care (ICU) myopathy

Myopathy of critical illness

G72.89 Other specified myopathies

G72.9 Myopathy, unspecified

G73 Disorders of myoneural junction and muscle in diseases classified elsewhere

G73.1 Lambert-Eaton syndrome in neoplastic disease

Code first underlying neoplasm (C00-D49)

EXCLUDES1 Lambert-Eaton syndrome not associated with neoplasm (G70.80-G70.81)

G73.3 Myasthenic syndromes in other diseases classified elsewhere

Code first underlying disease, such as:

neoplasm (C00-D49)

thyrotoxicosis (E05.-)

G73.7 Myopathy in diseases classified elsewhere

Code first underlying disease, such as:

hyperparathyroidism (E21.0, E21.3)

hypoparathyroidism (E20.-)

glycogen storage disease (E74.0)

lipid storage disorders (E75.-)

EXCLUDES1 myopathy in:

rheumatoid arthritis (M05.32)

sarcoidosis (D86.87)

scleroderma (M34.82)

sicca syndrome [Sjögren] (M35.03)

systemic lupus erythematosus (M32.19)

Cerebral palsy and other paralytic syndromes (G80-G83)

G80 Cerebral palsy

EXCLUDES1 hereditary spastic paraplegia (G11.4)

G80.0 Spastic quadriplegic **cerebral palsy**

Congenital spastic paralysis (cerebral)

G80.1 Spastic diplegic **cerebral palsy**

Spastic cerebral palsy NOS

G80.2 Spastic hemiplegic **cerebral palsy**

G80.3 Athetoid **cerebral palsy**

Double athetosis (syndrome)

Dyskinetic cerebral palsy

Dystonic cerebral palsy

Vogt disease

G80.4 Ataxic **cerebral palsy**

G80.8 Other **cerebral palsy**

Mixed cerebral palsy syndromes

G80.9 Cerebral palsy, unspecified

Cerebral palsy NOS

G81 Hemiplegia and hemiparesis

NOTES This category is to be used only when hemiplegia (complete)(incomplete) is reported without further specification, or is stated to be old or longstanding but of unspecified cause. The category is also for use in multiple coding to identify these types of hemiplegia resulting from any cause.

EXCLUDES1 congenital cerebral palsy (G80.-)

hemiplegia and hemiparesis due to sequela of cerebrovascular disease (I69.05-, I69.15-, I69.25-, I69.35-, I69.85-, I69.95-)

G81.0 Flaccid hemiplegia

G81.00 Flaccid hemiplegia affecting unspecified side

G81.01 Flaccid hemiplegia affecting right **dominant side**

G81.02 Flaccid hemiplegia affecting left **dominant side**

G81.03 Flaccid hemiplegia affecting right **nondominant side**

G81.04 Flaccid hemiplegia affecting left **nondominant side**

G81.1 Spastic hemiplegia

G81.10 Spastic hemiplegia affecting unspecified side

G81.11 Spastic hemiplegia affecting right **dominant side**

G81.12 Spastic hemiplegia affecting left **dominant side**

G81.13 Spastic hemiplegia affecting right **nondominant side**

G81.14 Spastic hemiplegia affecting left **nondominant side**

G81.9 Hemiplegia, unspecified

G81.90 Hemiplegia, unspecified affecting unspecified side

G81.91 Hemiplegia, unspecified affecting right **dominant side**

G81.92 Hemiplegia, unspecified affecting left **dominant side**

G81.93 Hemiplegia, unspecified affecting right **nondominant side**

G81.94 Hemiplegia, unspecified affecting left **nondominant side**

AHA: Q1 2015

G82 Paraplegia (paraparesis) and quadriplegia (quadriparesis)

NOTES This category is to be used only when the listed conditions are reported without further specification, or are stated to be old or longstanding but of unspecified cause. The category is also for use in multiple coding to identify these conditions resulting from any cause

EXCLUDES1 congenital cerebral palsy (G80.-)

functional quadriplegia (R53.2)

hysterical paralysis (F44.4)

G82.2 Paraplegia

Paralysis of both lower limbs NOS

Paraparesis (lower) NOS

Paraplegia (lower) NOS

G82.20 Paraplegia, unspecified

G82.21 Paraplegia, complete

G82.22 Paraplegia, incomplete

Unspecified Code   Other Specified Code   Manifestation Code   N Newborn   P Pediatric   M Maternity   A Adult   ♂ Male   ♀ Female

● New Code   ▲ Revised Code Title   ►◄ Revised Text   **NOTES** *INCLUDES* *EXCLUDES 1* Not coded here   *EXCLUDES 2* Not included here

4th character required   5th character required   6th character required   7th character required

Extension 'X' Alert   **HAC** Hospital-acquired condition (HAC) alert   **AHA** AHA Coding Clinic©

G82.5 - G89.3

CHAPTER 6: DISEASES OF THE NERVOUS SYSTEM (G00-G99)

G82.5 Quadriplegia
- **G82.50** Quadriplegia, unspecified ⬛HCC MCC CC/MCC Exc
- **G82.51** Quadriplegia, C1-C4 complete ⬛HCC MCC CC/MCC Exc
- **G82.52** Quadriplegia, C1-C4 incomplete ⬛HCC MCC CC/MCC Exc
- **G82.53** Quadriplegia, C5-C7 complete ⬛HCC MCC CC/MCC Exc
- **G82.54** Quadriplegia, C5-C7 incomplete ⬛HCC MCC CC/MCC Exc

G83 Other **paralytic syndromes**

NOTES This category is to be used only when the listed conditions are reported without further specification, or are stated to be old or longstanding but of unspecified cause. The category is also for use in multiple coding to identify these conditions resulting from any cause.

INCLUDES paralysis (complete) (incomplete), except as in G80-G82

G83.0 Diplegia **of upper limbs** CC HCC CC/MCC Exc
Diplegia (upper)
Paralysis of both upper limbs

G83.1 Monoplegia **of lower limb**
Paralysis of lower limb
EXCLUDES1 monoplegia of lower limbs due to sequela of cerebrovascular disease (I69.04-, I69.14-, I69.24-, I69.34-, I69.84-, I69.94-)
- **G83.10** Monoplegia of lower limb affecting unspecified side HCC
- **G83.11** Monoplegia of lower limb affecting right dominant side HCC
- **G83.12** Monoplegia of lower limb affecting left dominant side HCC
- **G83.13** Monoplegia of lower limb affecting right nondominant side HCC
- **G83.14** Monoplegia of lower limb affecting left nondominant side HCC

G83.2 Monoplegia **of upper limb**
Paralysis of upper limb
EXCLUDES1 monoplegia of upper limbs due to sequela of cerebrovascular disease (I69.03-, I69.13-, I69.23-, I69.33-, I69.83-, I69.93-)
- **G83.20** Monoplegia of upper limb affecting unspecified side HCC
- **G83.21** Monoplegia of upper limb affecting right dominant side HCC
- **G83.22** Monoplegia of upper limb affecting left dominant side HCC
- **G83.23** Monoplegia of upper limb affecting right nondominant side HCC
- **G83.24** Monoplegia of upper limb affecting left nondominant side HCC

G83.3 Monoplegia, unspecified
- **G83.30** Monoplegia, unspecified affecting unspecified side HCC
- **G83.31** Monoplegia, unspecified affecting right dominant side HCC
- **G83.32** Monoplegia, unspecified affecting left dominant side HCC
- **G83.33** Monoplegia, unspecified affecting right nondominant side HCC
- **G83.34** Monoplegia, unspecified affecting left nondominant side HCC

G83.4 Cauda equina **syndrome** CC HCC RxHCC CC/MCC Exc
Neurogenic bladder due to cauda equina syndrome
EXCLUDES1 cord bladder NOS (G95.89)
neurogenic bladder NOS (N31.9)

G83.5 Locked-in state HCC MCC CC/MCC Exc

G83.8 Other specified **paralytic syndromes**
EXCLUDES1 paralytic syndromes due to current spinal cord injury- code to spinal cord injury (S14, S24, S34)
- **G83.81** Brown-Séquard syndrome HCC
- **G83.82** Anterior cord syndrome HCC
- **G83.83** Posterior cord syndrome HCC
- **G83.84** Todd's paralysis (postepileptic) HCC
- **G83.89** Other specified paralytic syndromes HCC

G83.9 Paralytic syndrome, unspecified HCC

Other disorders of the nervous system (G89-G99)

G89 Pain, not elsewhere classified
Code also related psychological factors associated with pain (F45.42)
EXCLUDES1 generalized pain NOS (R52)
pain disorders exclusively related to psychological factors (F45.41)
pain NOS (R52)
EXCLUDES2 atypical face pain (G50.1)
headache syndromes (G44.-)
localized pain, unspecified type - code to pain by site, such as:
abdomen pain (R10.-)
back pain (M54.9)
breast pain (N64.4)
chest pain (R07.1-R07.9)
ear pain (H92.0-)
eye pain (H57.1)
headache (R51)
joint pain (M25.5-)
limb pain (M79.6-)
lumbar region pain (M54.5)
painful urination (R30.9)
pelvic and perineal pain (R10.2)
shoulder pain (M25.51-)
spine pain (M54.-)
throat pain (R07.0)
tongue pain (K14.6)
tooth pain (K08.8)
renal colic (N23)
migraines (G43.-)
myalgia (M79.1)
pain from prosthetic devices, implants, and grafts (T82.84, T83.84, T84.84, T85.84-)
phantom limb syndrome with pain (G54.6)
vulvar vestibulitis (N94.810)
vulvodynia (N94.81-)

G89.0 Central pain **syndrome**
Déjérine-Roussy syndrome
Myelopathic pain syndrome
Thalamic pain syndrome (hyperesthetic)

G89.1 Acute pain, **not elsewhere classified**
- **G89.11** Acute pain due to trauma
- **G89.12** Acute post-thoracotomy pain
Post-thoracotomy pain NOS
- **G89.18** Other acute postprocedural pain
Postoperative pain NOS
Postprocedural pain NOS

G89.2 Chronic pain, **not elsewhere classified**
EXCLUDES1 causalgia, lower limb (G57.7-)
causalgia, upper limb (G56.4-)
central pain syndrome (G89.0)
chronic pain syndrome (G89.4)
complex regional pain syndrome II, lower limb (G57.7-)
complex regional pain syndrome II, upper limb (G56.4-)
neoplasm related chronic pain (G89.3)
reflex sympathetic dystrophy (G90.5-)
- **G89.21** Chronic pain due to trauma
- **G89.22** Chronic post-thoracotomy pain
- **G89.28** Other chronic postprocedural pain
Other chronic postoperative pain
- **G89.29** Other chronic pain

G89.3 Neoplasm related **pain (acute) (chronic)**
Cancer associated pain
Pain due to malignancy (primary) (secondary)
Tumor associated pain

PDx Unacceptable principal diagnosis symbol per Medicare code edits   POA Code exempt from diagnosis present on admission requirement
❓ Questionable admission   CC Complication or comorbidity   CC/MCC Exc CC/MCC exclusion   MCC Major complication or comorbidity
Principal diagnosis as its own CC   Principal diagnosis as its own MCC   HCC HCC diagnosis code   RxHCC RxHCC diagnosis code
MACRA code   Z1 Z code as first-listed diagnosis

G89.4 Chronic **pain syndrome**

Chronic pain associated with significant psychosocial dysfunction

G90 Disorders of autonomic **nervous system**

EXCLUDES1 *dysfunction of the autonomic nervous system due to alcohol (G31.2)*

G90.0 **Idiopathic** peripheral **autonomic neuropathy**

G90.01 Carotid sinus syncope

Carotid sinus syndrome

G90.09 Other idiopathic **peripheral autonomic neuropathy**

Idiopathic peripheral autonomic neuropathy NOS

G90.1 Familial dysautonomia **[Riley-Day]**   HCC RxHCC

G90.2 Horner's **syndrome**

Bernard(-Horner) syndrome

Cervical sympathetic dystrophy or paralysis

G90.3 Multi-system degeneration **of the autonomic nervous system**   CC HCC CC/MCC Exc

Neurogenic orthostatic hypotension [Shy-Drager]

EXCLUDES1 *orthostatic hypotension NOS (I95.1)*

G90.4 **Autonomic** dysreflexia

Use additional code to identify the cause, such as:

fecal impaction (K56.41)

pressure ulcer (pressure area) (L89.-)

urinary tract infection (N39.0)

G90.5 Complex regional **pain syndrome I (CRPS I)**

Reflex sympathetic dystrophy

EXCLUDES1 *causalgia of lower limb (G57.7-)*

causalgia of upper limb (G56.4-)

complex regional pain syndrome II of lower limb (G57.7-)

complex regional pain syndrome II of upper limb (G56.4-)

G90.50 **Complex regional pain syndrome I, unspecified**   CC CC/MCC Exc

G90.51 Complex regional pain syndrome I of upper limb

G90.511 **Complex regional pain syndrome I of** right **upper limb**   CC CC/MCC Exc

G90.512 **Complex regional pain syndrome I of** left **upper limb**   CC CC/MCC Exc

G90.513 **Complex regional pain syndrome I of upper limb,** bilateral   CC CC/MCC Exc

G90.519 **Complex regional pain syndrome I of unspecified upper limb**   CC CC/MCC Exc

G90.52 Complex regional pain syndrome I of lower limb

G90.521 **Complex regional pain syndrome I of** right **lower limb**   CC CC/MCC Exc

G90.522 **Complex regional pain syndrome I of** left **lower limb**   CC CC/MCC Exc

G90.523 **Complex regional pain syndrome I of lower limb,** bilateral   CC CC/MCC Exc

G90.529 **Complex regional pain syndrome I of unspecified lower limb**   CC CC/MCC Exc

G90.59 Complex regional pain syndrome I of other specified site   CC CC/MCC Exc

G90.8 Other disorders of autonomic nervous system

G90.9 **Disorder of the autonomic nervous system, unspecified**

G91 **Hydrocephalus**

INCLUDES *acquired hydrocephalus*

EXCLUDES1 *Arnold-Chiari syndrome with hydrocephalus (Q07.-)*

congenital hydrocephalus (Q03.-)

spina bifida with hydrocephalus (Q05.-)

G91.0 Communicating **hydrocephalus**   CC CC/MCC Exc

Secondary normal pressure hydrocephalus

G91.1 Obstructive **hydrocephalus**   CC CC/MCC Exc

G91.2 (Idiopathic) normal pressure **hydrocephalus**   CC CC/MCC Exc

Normal pressure hydrocephalus NOS

G91.3 Post-traumatic **hydrocephalus, unspecified**   CC CC/MCC Exc

G91.4 **Hydrocephalus in diseases classified elsewhere**

Code first underlying condition, such as:

congenital syphilis (A50.4-)

neoplasm (C00-D49)

EXCLUDES1 *hydrocephalus due to congenital toxoplasmosis (P37.1)*

G91.8 Other **hydrocephalus**   CC CC/MCC Exc

G91.9 Hydrocephalus, unspecified   CC CC/MCC Exc

G92 Toxic **encephalopathy**   MCC CC/MCC Exc

AHA: Q1 2017

Toxic encephalitis

Toxic metabolic encephalopathy

Code first, if applicable, drug induced (T36-T50) (T51-T65) to identify toxic agent

G93 **Other** disorders of brain

G93.0 Cerebral cysts

Arachnoid cyst

Porencephalic cyst, acquired

EXCLUDES1 *acquired periventricular cysts of newborn (P91.1)*

congenital cerebral cysts (Q04.6)

G93.1 Anoxic brain damage, **not elsewhere classified**   CC HCC CC/MCC Exc

EXCLUDES1 *cerebral anoxia due to anesthesia during labor and delivery (O74.3)*

cerebral anoxia due to anesthesia during the puerperium (O89.2)

neonatal anoxia (P84)

G93.2 Benign intracranial hypertension

EXCLUDES1 *hypertensive encephalopathy (I67.4)*

G93.3 Postviral fatigue **syndrome**

Benign myalgic encephalomyelitis

EXCLUDES1 *chronic fatigue syndrome NOS (R53.82)*

G93.4 **Other and unspecified** encephalopathy

EXCLUDES1 *alcoholic encephalopathy (G31.2)*

encephalopathy in diseases classified elsewhere (G94)

hypertensive encephalopathy (I67.4)

toxic (metabolic) encephalopathy (G92)

G93.40 **Encephalopathy, unspecified**   MCC CC/MCC Exc

AHA: Q2 2017

G93.41 Metabolic **encephalopathy**   MCC CC/MCC Exc

AHA: Q2 2017, Q3 2016, Q3 2015

Septic encephalopathy

G93.49 Other **encephalopathy**   MCC CC/MCC Exc

AHA: Q2 2017

Encephalopathy NEC

G93.5 Compression of brain   HCC MCC CC/MCC Exc

Arnold-Chiari type 1 compression of brain

Compression of brain (stem)

Herniation of brain (stem)

EXCLUDES1 *diffuse traumatic compression of brain (S06.2-)*

focal traumatic compression of brain (S06.3-)

G93.6 Cerebral edema   HCC MCC CC/MCC Exc

EXCLUDES1 *cerebral edema due to birth injury (P11.0)*

traumatic cerebral edema (S06.1-)

G93.7 Reye's syndrome   P MCC RxHCC CC/MCC Exc

Code first poisoning due to salicylates, if applicable (T39.0-, with sixth character 1-4)

Use additional code for adverse effect due to salicylates, if applicable (T39.0-, with sixth character 5)

G93.8 Other specified **disorders of brain**

G93.81 **Temporal sclerosis**

Hippocampal sclerosis

Mesial temporal sclerosis

G93.82 Brain death   MCC CC/MCC Exc

G93.89 Other specified disorders of brain

AHA: Q4 2016

Postradiation encephalopathy

G93.9 **Disorder of brain, unspecified**

G94 Other disorders of brain in diseases classified elsewhere

AHA: Q2 2017

Code first underlying disease

Unspecified Code   Other Specified Code   Manifestation Code   N Newborn   P Pediatric   M Maternity   A Adult   ♂ Male   ♀ Female

● New Code   ▲ Revised Code Title   ►◄ Revised Text   **NOTES**   *INCLUDES*   *EXCLUDES 1* Not coded here   *EXCLUDES 2* Not included here

4th character required   5th character required   6th character required   7th character required

Extension 'X' Alert   HAC Hospital-acquired condition (HAC) alert   **AHA** AHA Coding Clinic©

Common Pathologies

Cataract

Cataracts are an eye disorder in which clouding of the lens occurs, which leads to blurry vision. It is an aging disorder. This disorder leads to dimness in eye vision, and if not treated can lead to blindness.

Cataract Surgery

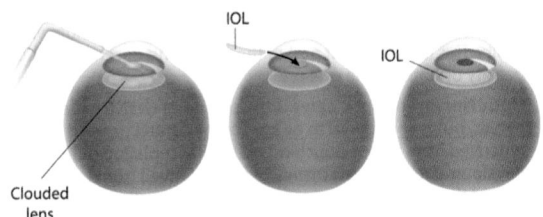

Clouded lens

Clouded lens removed

Intraocular lens (IOL) implanted in place

Glaucoma

In this disease, damage occurs to optic nerves due to increased intraocular pressure and leads to blindness.

Development of Glaucoma

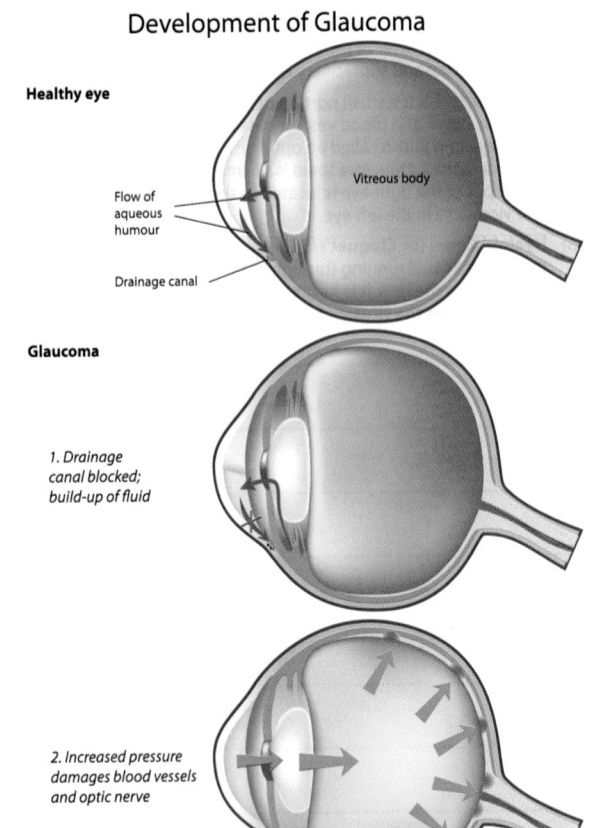

Healthy eye

Flow of aqueous humour

Vitreous body

Drainage canal

Glaucoma

1. Drainage canal blocked; build-up of fluid

2. Increased pressure damages blood vessels and optic nerve

Strabismus

A condition of eye in which there is nonalignment between both eyes. This condition is commonly called squint.

Strabismus

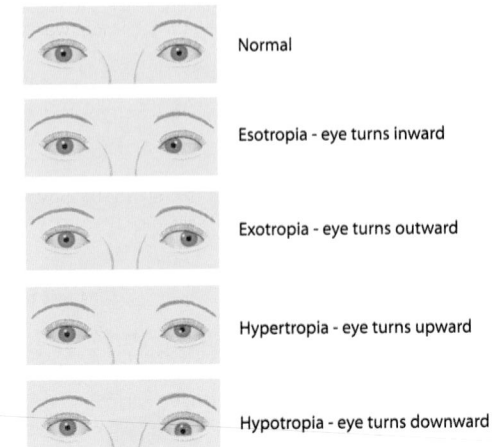

Normal

Esotropia - eye turns inward

Exotropia - eye turns outward

Hypertropia - eye turns upward

Hypotropia - eye turns downward

Macular Degeneration

This condition occurs because of degeneration in the macula of the eye due to aging and leads to blurry vision. It is a disease that destroys sharp, central vision. Central vision is required to see objects clearly and to do tasks such as reading and driving.

Conjunctivitis

An infection in the eye. The conjunctiva in the eye gets exposed to bacteria and other allergic irritants, which can lead to inflammation and infection. It is also known as pinkeye.

Optic Neuritis

This disorder occurs due to inflammation of the optic nerve. Pain and temporary vision loss are common.

Diseases of the eye and adnexa (H00-H59)

NOTES Use an external cause code following the code for the eye condition, if applicable, to identify the cause of the eye condition

EXCLUDES2 certain conditions originating in the perinatal period (P04-P96)

certain infectious and parasitic diseases (A00-B99)

complications of pregnancy, childbirth and the puerperium (O00-O9A)

congenital malformations, deformations, and chromosomal abnormalities (Q00-Q99)

diabetes mellitus related eye conditions (E09.3-, E10.3-, E11.3-, E13.3-)

endocrine, nutritional and metabolic diseases (E00-E88)

injury (trauma) of eye and orbit (S05.-)

injury, poisoning and certain other consequences of external causes (S00-T88)

neoplasms (C00-D49)

symptoms, signs and abnormal clinical and laboratory findings, not elsewhere classified (R00-R94)

syphilis related eye disorders (A50.01, A50.3-, A51.43, A52.71)

This chapter contains the following blocks:

H00-H05	Disorders of eyelid, lacrimal system and orbit
H10-H11	Disorders of conjunctiva
H15-H22	Disorders of sclera, cornea, iris and ciliary body
H25-H28	Disorders of lens
H30-H36	Disorders of choroid and retina
H40-H42	Glaucoma
H43-H44	Disorders of vitreous body and globe
H46-H47	Disorders of optic nerve and visual pathways
H49-H52	Disorders of ocular muscles, binocular movement, accommodation and refraction
H53-H54	Visual disturbances and blindness
H55-H57	Other disorders of eye and adnexa
H59	Intraoperative and postprocedural complications and disorders of eye and adnexa, not elsewhere classified

Disorders of eyelid, lacrimal system and orbit (H00-H05)

EXCLUDES2 open wound of eyelid (S01.1-)

superficial injury of eyelid (S00.1-, S00.2-)

🔟 **H00** Hordeolum and chalazion

  5️⃣ **H00.0** Hordeolum (externum) (internum) of eyelid

    6️⃣ **H00.01** Hordeolum externum

      Hordeolum NOS
      Stye

      H00.011 Hordeolum externum right upper eyelid
      H00.012 Hordeolum externum right lower eyelid
      H00.013 Hordeolum externum right eye, unspecified eyelid
      H00.014 Hordeolum externum left upper eyelid
      H00.015 Hordeolum externum left lower eyelid
      H00.016 Hordeolum externum left eye, unspecified eyelid
      H00.019 Hordeolum externum unspecified eye, unspecified eyelid

    6️⃣ **H00.02** Hordeolum internum

      Infection of meibomian gland

      H00.021 Hordeolum internum right upper eyelid
      H00.022 Hordeolum internum right lower eyelid
      H00.023 Hordeolum internum right eye, unspecified eyelid
      H00.024 Hordeolum internum left upper eyelid
      H00.025 Hordeolum internum left lower eyelid
      H00.026 Hordeolum internum left eye, unspecified eyelid
      H00.029 Hordeolum internum unspecified eye, unspecified eyelid

    6️⃣ **H00.03** Abscess of eyelid

      Furuncle of eyelid

      H00.031 Abscess of right upper eyelid

H00.032 Abscess of right lower eyelid
H00.033 Abscess of eyelid right eye, unspecified eyelid
H00.034 Abscess of left upper eyelid
H00.035 Abscess of left lower eyelid
H00.036 Abscess of eyelid left eye, unspecified eyelid
H00.039 Abscess of eyelid unspecified eye, unspecified eyelid

  5️⃣ **H00.1** Chalazion

    Meibomian (gland) cyst

    EXCLUDES2 infected meibomian gland (H00.02-)

    H00.11 Chalazion right upper eyelid
    H00.12 Chalazion right lower eyelid
    H00.13 Chalazion right eye, unspecified eyelid
    H00.14 Chalazion left upper eyelid
    H00.15 Chalazion left lower eyelid
    H00.16 Chalazion left eye, unspecified eyelid
    H00.19 Chalazion unspecified eye, unspecified eyelid

🔟 **H01** Other inflammation of eyelid

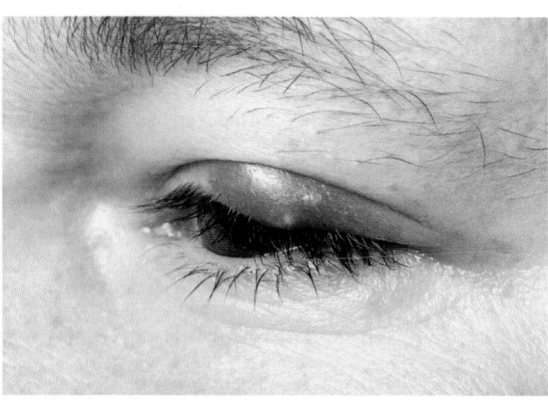

Figure 7.1 Blepharitis

  5️⃣ **H01.0** Blepharitis

    EXCLUDES1 blepharoconjunctivitis (H10.5-)

    6️⃣ **H01.00** Unspecified blepharitis

      H01.001 Unspecified blepharitis right upper eyelid
      H01.002 Unspecified blepharitis right lower eyelid
      H01.003 Unspecified blepharitis right eye, unspecified eyelid
      H01.004 Unspecified blepharitis left upper eyelid
      H01.005 Unspecified blepharitis left lower eyelid
      H01.006 Unspecified blepharitis left eye, unspecified eyelid
      H01.009 Unspecified blepharitis unspecified eye, unspecified eyelid

    6️⃣ **H01.01** Ulcerative blepharitis

      H01.011 Ulcerative blepharitis right upper eyelid
      H01.012 Ulcerative blepharitis right lower eyelid
      H01.013 Ulcerative blepharitis right eye, unspecified eyelid
      H01.014 Ulcerative blepharitis left upper eyelid
      H01.015 Ulcerative blepharitis left lower eyelid
      H01.016 Ulcerative blepharitis left eye, unspecified eyelid
      H01.019 Ulcerative blepharitis unspecified eye, unspecified eyelid

    6️⃣ **H01.02** Squamous blepharitis

      H01.021 Squamous blepharitis right upper eyelid
      H01.022 Squamous blepharitis right lower eyelid
      H01.023 Squamous blepharitis right eye, unspecified eyelid
      H01.024 Squamous blepharitis left upper eyelid
      H01.025 Squamous blepharitis left lower eyelid
      H01.026 Squamous blepharitis left eye, unspecified eyelid

---

Unspecified Code Other Specified Code Manifestation Code Ⓝ Newborn Ⓟ Pediatric Ⓜ Maternity Ⓐ Adult ♂ Male ♀ Female
  ● New Code ▲ Revised Code Title ►◄ Revised Text **NOTES** *INCLUDES* *EXCLUDES 1* Not coded here *EXCLUDES 2* Not included here
  4️⃣ 4th character required 5️⃣ 5th character required 6️⃣ 6th character required 7️⃣ 7th character required
  7️⃣ₓ Extension 'X' Alert **HAC** Hospital-acquired condition (HAC) alert **AHA** AHA Coding Clinic©

H01.029 Squamous blepharitis unspecified eye, unspecified eyelid

H01.1 Noninfectious dermatoses of eyelid

H01.11 Allergic dermatitis of eyelid
Contact dermatitis of eyelid

H01.111 Allergic dermatitis of right upper eyelid

H01.112 Allergic dermatitis of right lower eyelid

H01.113 Allergic dermatitis of right eye, unspecified eyelid

H01.114 Allergic dermatitis of left upper eyelid

H01.115 Allergic dermatitis of left lower eyelid

H01.116 Allergic dermatitis of left eye, unspecified eyelid

H01.119 Allergic dermatitis of unspecified eye, unspecified eyelid

H01.12 Discoid lupus erythematosus of eyelid

H01.121 Discoid lupus erythematosus of right upper eyelid

H01.122 Discoid lupus erythematosus of right lower eyelid

H01.123 Discoid lupus erythematosus of right eye, unspecified eyelid

H01.124 Discoid lupus erythematosus of left upper eyelid

H01.125 Discoid lupus erythematosus of left lower eyelid

H01.126 Discoid lupus erythematosus of left eye, unspecified eyelid

H01.129 Discoid lupus erythematosus of unspecified eye, unspecified eyelid

H01.13 Eczematous dermatitis of eyelid

H01.131 Eczematous dermatitis of right upper eyelid

H01.132 Eczematous dermatitis of right lower eyelid

H01.133 Eczematous dermatitis of right eye, unspecified eyelid

H01.134 Eczematous dermatitis of left upper eyelid

H01.135 Eczematous dermatitis of left lower eyelid

H01.136 Eczematous dermatitis of left eye, unspecified eyelid

H01.139 Eczematous dermatitis of unspecified eye, unspecified eyelid

H01.14 Xeroderma of eyelid

H01.141 Xeroderma of right upper eyelid

H01.142 Xeroderma of right lower eyelid

H01.143 Xeroderma of right eye, unspecified eyelid

H01.144 Xeroderma of left upper eyelid

H01.145 Xeroderma of left lower eyelid

H01.146 Xeroderma of left eye, unspecified eyelid

H01.149 Xeroderma of unspecified eye, unspecified eyelid

H01.8 Other specified inflammations of eyelid

H01.9 Unspecified inflammation of eyelid
Inflammation of eyelid NOS

H02 Other disorders of eyelid

EXCLUDES1 congenital malformations of eyelid (Q10.0-Q10.3)

H02.0 Entropion and trichiasis of eyelid

H02.00 Unspecified entropion of eyelid

H02.001 Unspecified entropion of right upper eyelid

H02.002 Unspecified entropion of right lower eyelid

H02.003 Unspecified entropion of right eye, unspecified eyelid

H02.004 Unspecified entropion of left upper eyelid

H02.005 Unspecified entropion of left lower eyelid

H02.006 Unspecified entropion of left eye, unspecified eyelid

H02.009 Unspecified entropion of unspecified eye, unspecified eyelid

H02.01 Cicatricial entropion of eyelid

H02.011 Cicatricial entropion of right upper eyelid

H02.012 Cicatricial entropion of right lower eyelid

H02.013 Cicatricial entropion of right eye, unspecified eyelid

H02.014 Cicatricial entropion of left upper eyelid

H02.015 Cicatricial entropion of left lower eyelid

H02.016 Cicatricial entropion of left eye, unspecified eyelid

H02.019 Cicatricial entropion of unspecified eye, unspecified eyelid

H02.02 Mechanical entropion of eyelid

H02.021 Mechanical entropion of right upper eyelid

H02.022 Mechanical entropion of right lower eyelid

H02.023 Mechanical entropion of right eye, unspecified eyelid

H02.024 Mechanical entropion of left upper eyelid

H02.025 Mechanical entropion of left lower eyelid

H02.026 Mechanical entropion of left eye, unspecified eyelid

H02.029 Mechanical entropion of unspecified eye, unspecified eyelid

H02.03 Senile entropion of eyelid

H02.031 Senile entropion of right upper eyelid A

H02.032 Senile entropion of right lower eyelid A

H02.033 Senile entropion of right eye, unspecified eyelid A

H02.034 Senile entropion of left upper eyelid A

H02.035 Senile entropion of left lower eyelid A

H02.036 Senile entropion of left eye, unspecified eyelid A

H02.039 Senile entropion of unspecified eye, unspecified eyelid A

H02.04 Spastic entropion of eyelid

H02.041 Spastic entropion of right upper eyelid

H02.042 Spastic entropion of right lower eyelid

H02.043 Spastic entropion of right eye, unspecified eyelid

H02.044 Spastic entropion of left upper eyelid

H02.045 Spastic entropion of left lower eyelid

H02.046 Spastic entropion of left eye, unspecified eyelid

H02.049 Spastic entropion of unspecified eye, unspecified eyelid

▲ H02.05 Trichiasis without ▶entropion◀

▲ H02.051 Trichiasis without ▶entropion◀ right upper eyelid

▲ H02.052 Trichiasis without ▶entropion◀ right lower eyelid

▲ H02.053 Trichiasis without ▶entropion◀ right eye, unspecified eyelid

▲ H02.054 Trichiasis without ▶entropion◀ left upper eyelid

▲ H02.055 Trichiasis without ▶entropion◀ left lower eyelid

▲ H02.056 Trichiasis without ▶entropion◀ left eye, unspecified eyelid

▲ H02.059 Trichiasis without ▶entropion◀ unspecified eye, unspecified eyelid

H02.1 Ectropion of eyelid

H02.10 Unspecified ectropion of eyelid

H02.101 Unspecified ectropion of right upper eyelid

H02.102 Unspecified ectropion of right lower eyelid

H02.103 Unspecified ectropion of right eye, unspecified eyelid

H02.104 Unspecified ectropion of left upper eyelid

H02.105 Unspecified ectropion of left lower eyelid

PDxⁿ Unacceptable principal diagnosis symbol per Medicare code edits   POA Code exempt from diagnosis present on admission requirement
❓ Questionable admission   CC Complication or comorbidity   CC/MCC Exd CC/MCC exclusion   MCC Major complication or comorbidity
CC Principal diagnosis as its own CC   MCC Principal diagnosis as its own MCC   HCC HCC diagnosis code   RxHCC RxHCC diagnosis code
MACRA code   Z1 Z code as first-listed diagnosis

H02.106 Unspecified ectropion of left eye, unspecified eyelid
H02.109 Unspecified ectropion of unspecified eye, unspecified eyelid

[6th] H02.11 Cicatricial ectropion of eyelid
H02.111 Cicatricial ectropion of right upper eyelid
H02.112 Cicatricial ectropion of right lower eyelid
H02.113 Cicatricial ectropion of right eye, unspecified eyelid
H02.114 Cicatricial ectropion of left upper eyelid
H02.115 Cicatricial ectropion of left lower eyelid
H02.116 Cicatricial ectropion of left eye, unspecified eyelid
H02.119 Cicatricial ectropion of unspecified eye, unspecified eyelid

[6th] H02.12 Mechanical ectropion of eyelid
H02.121 Mechanical ectropion of right upper eyelid
H02.122 Mechanical ectropion of right lower eyelid
H02.123 Mechanical ectropion of right eye, unspecified eyelid
H02.124 Mechanical ectropion of left upper eyelid
H02.125 Mechanical ectropion of left lower eyelid
H02.126 Mechanical ectropion of left eye, unspecified eyelid
H02.129 Mechanical ectropion of unspecified eye, unspecified eyelid

[6th] H02.13 Senile ectropion of eyelid
H02.131 Senile ectropion of right upper eyelid [A]
H02.132 Senile ectropion of right lower eyelid [A]
H02.133 Senile ectropion of right eye, unspecified eyelid [A]
H02.134 Senile ectropion of left upper eyelid [A]
H02.135 Senile ectropion of left lower eyelid [A]
H02.136 Senile ectropion of left eye, unspecified eyelid [A]
H02.139 Senile ectropion of unspecified eye, unspecified eyelid [A]

[6th] H02.14 Spastic ectropion of eyelid
H02.141 Spastic ectropion of right upper eyelid
H02.142 Spastic ectropion of right lower eyelid
H02.143 Spastic ectropion of right eye, unspecified eyelid
H02.144 Spastic ectropion of left upper eyelid
H02.145 Spastic ectropion of left lower eyelid
H02.146 Spastic ectropion of left eye, unspecified eyelid
H02.149 Spastic ectropion of unspecified eye, unspecified eyelid

[5th] H02.2 Lagophthalmos

[6th] H02.20 Unspecified lagophthalmos
H02.201 Unspecified lagophthalmos right upper eyelid
H02.202 Unspecified lagophthalmos right lower eyelid
H02.203 Unspecified lagophthalmos right eye, unspecified eyelid
H02.204 Unspecified lagophthalmos left upper eyelid
H02.205 Unspecified lagophthalmos left lower eyelid
H02.206 Unspecified lagophthalmos left eye, unspecified eyelid
H02.209 Unspecified lagophthalmos unspecified eye, unspecified eyelid

[6th] H02.21 Cicatricial lagophthalmos
H02.211 Cicatricial lagophthalmos right upper eyelid
H02.212 Cicatricial lagophthalmos right lower eyelid
H02.213 Cicatricial lagophthalmos right eye, unspecified eyelid
H02.214 Cicatricial lagophthalmos left upper eyelid
H02.215 Cicatricial lagophthalmos left lower eyelid
H02.216 Cicatricial lagophthalmos left eye, unspecified eyelid
H02.219 Cicatricial lagophthalmos unspecified eye, unspecified eyelid

[6th] H02.22 Mechanical lagophthalmos
H02.221 Mechanical lagophthalmos right upper eyelid
H02.222 Mechanical lagophthalmos right lower eyelid
H02.223 Mechanical lagophthalmos right eye, unspecified eyelid
H02.224 Mechanical lagophthalmos left upper eyelid
H02.225 Mechanical lagophthalmos left lower eyelid
H02.226 Mechanical lagophthalmos left eye, unspecified eyelid
H02.229 Mechanical lagophthalmos unspecified eye, unspecified eyelid

[6th] H02.23 Paralytic lagophthalmos
H02.231 Paralytic lagophthalmos right upper eyelid
H02.232 Paralytic lagophthalmos right lower eyelid
H02.233 Paralytic lagophthalmos right eye, unspecified eyelid
H02.234 Paralytic lagophthalmos left upper eyelid
H02.235 Paralytic lagophthalmos left lower eyelid
H02.236 Paralytic lagophthalmos left eye, unspecified eyelid
H02.239 Paralytic lagophthalmos unspecified eye, unspecified eyelid

[5th] H02.3 Blepharochalasis
Pseudoptosis
H02.30 Blepharochalasis unspecified eye, unspecified eyelid
H02.31 Blepharochalasis right upper eyelid
H02.32 Blepharochalasis right lower eyelid
H02.33 Blepharochalasis right eye, unspecified eyelid
H02.34 Blepharochalasis left upper eyelid
H02.35 Blepharochalasis left lower eyelid
H02.36 Blepharochalasis left eye, unspecified eyelid

[5th] H02.4 Ptosis of eyelid

[6th] H02.40 Unspecified ptosis of eyelid
H02.401 Unspecified ptosis of right eyelid
H02.402 Unspecified ptosis of left eyelid
H02.403 Unspecified ptosis of bilateral eyelids
H02.409 Unspecified ptosis of unspecified eyelid

[6th] H02.41 Mechanical ptosis of eyelid
H02.411 Mechanical ptosis of right eyelid
H02.412 Mechanical ptosis of left eyelid
H02.413 Mechanical ptosis of bilateral eyelids
H02.419 Mechanical ptosis of unspecified eyelid

[6th] H02.42 Myogenic ptosis of eyelid
H02.421 Myogenic ptosis of right eyelid
H02.422 Myogenic ptosis of left eyelid
H02.423 Myogenic ptosis of bilateral eyelids
H02.429 Myogenic ptosis of unspecified eyelid

[6th] H02.43 Paralytic ptosis of eyelid
Neurogenic ptosis of eyelid
H02.431 Paralytic ptosis of right eyelid
H02.432 Paralytic ptosis of left eyelid
H02.433 Paralytic ptosis of bilateral eyelids
H02.439 Paralytic ptosis unspecified eyelid

[5th] H02.5 Other disorders affecting eyelid function
[EXCLUDES2] *blepharospasm (G24.5)*
organic tic (G25.69)
psychogenic tic (F95.-)

Unspecified Code Other Specified Code Manifestation Code [N] Newborn [P] Pediatric [M] Maternity [A] Adult ♂ Male ♀ Female
● New Code ▲ Revised Code Title ►◄ Revised Text [NOTES] [INCLUDES] [EXCLUDES1] Not coded here [EXCLUDES2] Not included here
[4th] 4th character required [5th] 5th character required [6th] 6th character required [7th] 7th character required
[7th] Extension 'X' Alert [HAC] Hospital-acquired condition (HAC) alert AHA AHA Coding Clinic©

When symbols appear on a code that requires a 7th character extension, refer to Appendix B to identify applicable 7th character codes.

H02.51 Abnormal innervation syndrome
    H02.511 Abnormal innervation syndrome right upper eyelid
    H02.512 Abnormal innervation syndrome right lower eyelid
    H02.513 Abnormal innervation syndrome right eye, unspecified eyelid
    H02.514 Abnormal innervation syndrome left upper eyelid
    H02.515 Abnormal innervation syndrome left lower eyelid
    H02.516 Abnormal innervation syndrome left eye, unspecified eyelid
    H02.519 Abnormal innervation syndrome unspecified eye, unspecified eyelid

H02.52 Blepharophimosis
Ankyloblepharon
    H02.521 Blepharophimosis right upper eyelid
    H02.522 Blepharophimosis right lower eyelid
    H02.523 Blepharophimosis right eye, unspecified eyelid
    H02.524 Blepharophimosis left upper eyelid
    H02.525 Blepharophimosis left lower eyelid
    H02.526 Blepharophimosis left eye, unspecified eyelid
    H02.529 Blepharophimosis unspecified eye, unspecified lid

H02.53 Eyelid retraction
Eyelid lag
    H02.531 Eyelid retraction right upper eyelid
    H02.532 Eyelid retraction right lower eyelid
    H02.533 Eyelid retraction right eye, unspecified eyelid
    H02.534 Eyelid retraction left upper eyelid
    H02.535 Eyelid retraction left lower eyelid
    H02.536 Eyelid retraction left eye, unspecified eyelid
    H02.539 Eyelid retraction unspecified eye, unspecified lid

H02.59 Other disorders affecting eyelid function
Deficient blink reflex
Sensory disorders

H02.6 Xanthelasma of eyelid
    H02.60 Xanthelasma of unspecified eye, unspecified eyelid
    H02.61 Xanthelasma of right upper eyelid
    H02.62 Xanthelasma of right lower eyelid
    H02.63 Xanthelasma of right eye, unspecified eyelid
    H02.64 Xanthelasma of left upper eyelid
    H02.65 Xanthelasma of left lower eyelid
    H02.66 Xanthelasma of left eye, unspecified eyelid

H02.7 Other and unspecified degenerative disorders of eyelid and periocular area
    H02.70 Unspecified degenerative disorders of eyelid and periocular area

H02.71 Chloasma of eyelid and periocular area
Dyspigmentation of eyelid
Hyperpigmentation of eyelid
    H02.711 Chloasma of right upper eyelid and periocular area
    H02.712 Chloasma of right lower eyelid and periocular area
    H02.713 Chloasma of right eye, unspecified eyelid and periocular area
    H02.714 Chloasma of left upper eyelid and periocular area
    H02.715 Chloasma of left lower eyelid and periocular area
    H02.716 Chloasma of left eye, unspecified eyelid and periocular area
    H02.719 Chloasma of unspecified eye, unspecified eyelid and periocular area

H02.72 Madarosis of eyelid and periocular area
Hypotrichosis of eyelid
    H02.721 Madarosis of right upper eyelid and periocular area
    H02.722 Madarosis of right lower eyelid and periocular area
    H02.723 Madarosis of right eye, unspecified eyelid and periocular area
    H02.724 Madarosis of left upper eyelid and periocular area
    H02.725 Madarosis of left lower eyelid and periocular area
    H02.726 Madarosis of left eye, unspecified eyelid and periocular area
    H02.729 Madarosis of unspecified eye, unspecified eyelid and periocular area

H02.73 Vitiligo of eyelid and periocular area
Hypopigmentation of eyelid
    H02.731 Vitiligo of right upper eyelid and periocular area
    H02.732 Vitiligo of right lower eyelid and periocular area
    H02.733 Vitiligo of right eye, unspecified eyelid and periocular area
    H02.734 Vitiligo of left upper eyelid and periocular area
    H02.735 Vitiligo of left lower eyelid and periocular area
    H02.736 Vitiligo of left eye, unspecified eyelid and periocular area
    H02.739 Vitiligo of unspecified eye, unspecified eyelid and periocular area

H02.79 Other degenerative disorders of eyelid and periocular area

H02.8 Other specified disorders of eyelid

H02.81 Retained foreign body in eyelid
Use additional code to identify the type of retained foreign body (Z18.-)
    EXCLUDES1 laceration of eyelid with foreign body (S01.12-)
            retained intraocular foreign body (H44.6-, H44.7-)
            superficial foreign body of eyelid and periocular area (S00.25-)
    H02.811 Retained foreign body in right upper eyelid
    H02.812 Retained foreign body in right lower eyelid
    H02.813 Retained foreign body in right eye, unspecified eyelid
    H02.814 Retained foreign body in left upper eyelid
    H02.815 Retained foreign body in left lower eyelid
    H02.816 Retained foreign body in left eye, unspecified eyelid
    H02.819 Retained foreign body in unspecified eye, unspecified eyelid

H02.82 Cysts of eyelid
Sebaceous cyst of eyelid
    H02.821 Cysts of right upper eyelid
    H02.822 Cysts of right lower eyelid
    H02.823 Cysts of right eye, unspecified eyelid
    H02.824 Cysts of left upper eyelid
    H02.825 Cysts of left lower eyelid
    H02.826 Cysts of left eye, unspecified eyelid
    H02.829 Cysts of unspecified eye, unspecified eyelid

H02.83 Dermatochalasis of eyelid
    H02.831 Dermatochalasis of right upper eyelid
    H02.832 Dermatochalasis of right lower eyelid
    H02.833 Dermatochalasis of right eye, unspecified eyelid
    H02.834 Dermatochalasis of left upper eyelid

PDAB Unacceptable principal diagnosis symbol per Medicare code edits   POA Code exempt from diagnosis present on admission requirement
? Questionable admission   CC Complication or comorbidity   CC/MCC excl CC/MCC exclusion   MCC Major complication or comorbidity
CC Principal diagnosis as its own CC   MCC Principal diagnosis as its own MCC   HCC HCC diagnosis code   RxHCC RxHCC diagnosis code
MACRA code   Z1 Z code as first-listed diagnosis

596   When symbols appear on a code that requires a 7th character extension, refer to Appendix B to identify applicable 7th character codes.   2018 ICD-10-CM

H02.835 Dermatochalasis of left lower eyelid
H02.836 Dermatochalasis of left eye, unspecified eyelid
H02.839 Dermatochalasis of unspecified eye, unspecified eyelid
H02.84 Edema of eyelid
Hyperemia of eyelid
H02.841 Edema of right upper eyelid
H02.842 Edema of right lower eyelid
H02.843 Edema of right eye, unspecified eyelid
H02.844 Edema of left upper eyelid
H02.845 Edema of left lower eyelid
H02.846 Edema of left eye, unspecified eyelid
H02.849 Edema of unspecified eye, unspecified eyelid
H02.85 Elephantiasis of eyelid
H02.851 Elephantiasis of right upper eyelid
H02.852 Elephantiasis of right lower eyelid
H02.853 Elephantiasis of right eye, unspecified eyelid
H02.854 Elephantiasis of left upper eyelid
H02.855 Elephantiasis of left lower eyelid
H02.856 Elephantiasis of left eye, unspecified eyelid
H02.859 Elephantiasis of unspecified eye, unspecified eyelid
H02.86 Hypertrichosis of eyelid
H02.861 Hypertrichosis of right upper eyelid
H02.862 Hypertrichosis of right lower eyelid
H02.863 Hypertrichosis of right eye, unspecified eyelid
H02.864 Hypertrichosis of left upper eyelid
H02.865 Hypertrichosis of left lower eyelid
H02.866 Hypertrichosis of left eye, unspecified eyelid
H02.869 Hypertrichosis of unspecified eye, unspecified eyelid
H02.87 Vascular anomalies of eyelid
H02.871 Vascular anomalies of right upper eyelid
H02.872 Vascular anomalies of right lower eyelid
H02.873 Vascular anomalies of right eye, unspecified eyelid
H02.874 Vascular anomalies of left upper eyelid
H02.875 Vascular anomalies of left lower eyelid
H02.876 Vascular anomalies of left eye, unspecified eyelid
H02.879 Vascular anomalies of unspecified eye, unspecified eyelid
H02.89 Other specified disorders of eyelid
Hemorrhage of eyelid
H02.9 Unspecified disorder of eyelid
Disorder of eyelid NOS

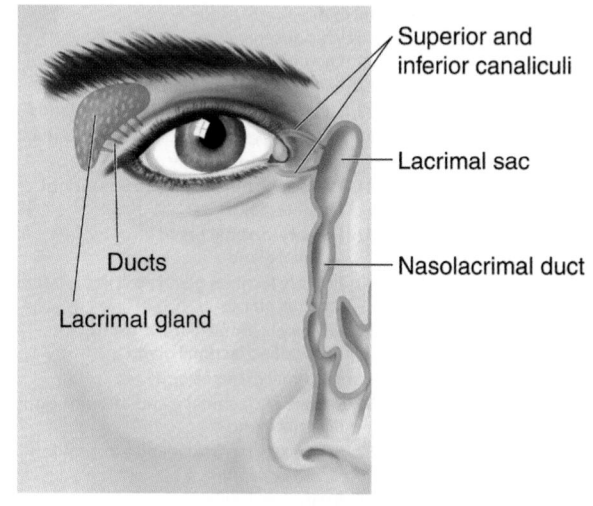

Figure 7.2 Lacrimal system

H04 Disorders of lacrimal system
EXCLUDES1 congenital malformations of lacrimal system (Q10.4-Q10.6)
H04.0 Dacryoadenitis
H04.00 Unspecified dacryoadenitis
H04.001 Unspecified dacryoadenitis, right lacrimal gland
H04.002 Unspecified dacryoadenitis, left lacrimal gland
H04.003 Unspecified dacryoadenitis, bilateral lacrimal glands
H04.009 Unspecified dacryoadenitis, unspecified lacrimal gland
H04.01 Acute dacryoadenitis
H04.011 Acute dacryoadenitis, right lacrimal gland
H04.012 Acute dacryoadenitis, left lacrimal gland
H04.013 Acute dacryoadenitis, bilateral lacrimal glands
H04.019 Acute dacryoadenitis, unspecified lacrimal gland
H04.02 Chronic dacryoadenitis
H04.021 Chronic dacryoadenitis, right lacrimal gland
H04.022 Chronic dacryoadenitis, left lacrimal gland
H04.023 Chronic dacryoadenitis, bilateral lacrimal gland
H04.029 Chronic dacryoadenitis, unspecified lacrimal gland
H04.03 Chronic enlargement of lacrimal gland
H04.031 Chronic enlargement of right lacrimal gland
H04.032 Chronic enlargement of left lacrimal gland
H04.033 Chronic enlargement of bilateral lacrimal glands
H04.039 Chronic enlargement of unspecified lacrimal gland
H04.1 Other disorders of lacrimal gland
H04.11 Dacryops
H04.111 Dacryops of right lacrimal gland
H04.112 Dacryops of left lacrimal gland
H04.113 Dacryops of bilateral lacrimal glands
H04.119 Dacryops of unspecified lacrimal gland
H04.12 Dry eye syndrome
Tear film insufficiency, NOS
H04.121 Dry eye syndrome of right lacrimal gland
H04.122 Dry eye syndrome of left lacrimal gland
H04.123 Dry eye syndrome of bilateral lacrimal glands
H04.129 Dry eye syndrome of unspecified lacrimal gland

Unspecified Code   Other Specified Code   Manifestation Code   Ⓝ Newborn   Ⓟ Pediatric   Ⓜ Maternity   Ⓐ Adult   ♂ Male   ♀ Female
● New Code   ▲ Revised Code Title   ►◄ Revised Text   NOTES   INCLUDES   EXCLUDES 1 Not coded here   EXCLUDES 2 Not included here
4th character required   5th character required   6th character required   7th character required
Extension 'X' Alert   HAC Hospital-acquired condition (HAC) alert   AHA AHA Coding Clinic©

H04.13 Lacrimal cyst
      Lacrimal cystic degeneration
      H04.131 Lacrimal cyst, right lacrimal gland
      H04.132 Lacrimal cyst, left lacrimal gland
      H04.133 Lacrimal cyst, bilateral lacrimal glands
      H04.139 Lacrimal cyst, unspecified lacrimal gland

H04.14 Primary lacrimal gland atrophy
      H04.141 Primary lacrimal gland atrophy, right lacrimal gland
      H04.142 Primary lacrimal gland atrophy, left lacrimal gland
      H04.143 Primary lacrimal gland atrophy, bilateral lacrimal glands
      H04.149 Primary lacrimal gland atrophy, unspecified lacrimal gland

H04.15 Secondary lacrimal gland atrophy
      H04.151 Secondary lacrimal gland atrophy, right lacrimal gland
      H04.152 Secondary lacrimal gland atrophy, left lacrimal gland
      H04.153 Secondary lacrimal gland atrophy, bilateral lacrimal glands
      H04.159 Secondary lacrimal gland atrophy, unspecified lacrimal gland

H04.16 Lacrimal gland dislocation
      H04.161 Lacrimal gland dislocation, right lacrimal gland
      H04.162 Lacrimal gland dislocation, left lacrimal gland
      H04.163 Lacrimal gland dislocation, bilateral lacrimal glands
      H04.169 Lacrimal gland dislocation, unspecified lacrimal gland

H04.19 Other specified disorders of lacrimal gland

H04.2 Epiphora
  H04.20 Unspecified epiphora
      H04.201 Unspecified epiphora, right lacrimal gland
      H04.202 Unspecified epiphora, left lacrimal gland
      H04.203 Unspecified epiphora, bilateral lacrimal glands
      H04.209 Unspecified epiphora, unspecified lacrimal gland
  H04.21 Epiphora due to excess lacrimation
      H04.211 Epiphora due to excess lacrimation, right lacrimal gland
      H04.212 Epiphora due to excess lacrimation, left lacrimal gland
      H04.213 Epiphora due to excess lacrimation, bilateral lacrimal glands
      H04.219 Epiphora due to excess lacrimation, unspecified lacrimal gland
  H04.22 Epiphora due to insufficient drainage
      H04.221 Epiphora due to insufficient drainage, right lacrimal gland
      H04.222 Epiphora due to insufficient drainage, left lacrimal gland
      H04.223 Epiphora due to insufficient drainage, bilateral lacrimal glands
      H04.229 Epiphora due to insufficient drainage, unspecified lacrimal gland

H04.3 Acute and unspecified inflammation of lacrimal passages
  EXCLUDES1 neonatal dacryocystitis (P39.1)
  H04.30 Unspecified dacryocystitis
      H04.301 Unspecified dacryocystitis of right lacrimal passage
      H04.302 Unspecified dacryocystitis of left lacrimal passage
      H04.303 Unspecified dacryocystitis of bilateral lacrimal passages
      H04.309 Unspecified dacryocystitis of unspecified lacrimal passage

H04.31 Phlegmonous dacryocystitis
      H04.311 Phlegmonous dacryocystitis of right lacrimal passage
      H04.312 Phlegmonous dacryocystitis of left lacrimal passage
      H04.313 Phlegmonous dacryocystitis of bilateral lacrimal passages
      H04.319 Phlegmonous dacryocystitis of unspecified lacrimal passage

H04.32 Acute dacryocystitis
      Acute dacryopericystitis
      H04.321 Acute dacryocystitis of right lacrimal passage
      H04.322 Acute dacryocystitis of left lacrimal passage
      H04.323 Acute dacryocystitis of bilateral lacrimal passages
      H04.329 Acute dacryocystitis of unspecified lacrimal passage

H04.33 Acute lacrimal canaliculitis
      H04.331 Acute lacrimal canaliculitis of right lacrimal passage
      H04.332 Acute lacrimal canaliculitis of left lacrimal passage
      H04.333 Acute lacrimal canaliculitis of bilateral lacrimal passages
      H04.339 Acute lacrimal canaliculitis of unspecified lacrimal passage

H04.4 Chronic inflammation of lacrimal passages
  H04.41 Chronic dacryocystitis
      H04.411 Chronic dacryocystitis of right lacrimal passage
      H04.412 Chronic dacryocystitis of left lacrimal passage
      H04.413 Chronic dacryocystitis of bilateral lacrimal passages
      H04.419 Chronic dacryocystitis of unspecified lacrimal passage
  H04.42 Chronic lacrimal canaliculitis
      H04.421 Chronic lacrimal canaliculitis of right lacrimal passage
      H04.422 Chronic lacrimal canaliculitis of left lacrimal passage
      H04.423 Chronic lacrimal canaliculitis of bilateral lacrimal passages
      H04.429 Chronic lacrimal canaliculitis of unspecified lacrimal passage
  H04.43 Chronic lacrimal mucocele
      H04.431 Chronic lacrimal mucocele of right lacrimal passage
      H04.432 Chronic lacrimal mucocele of left lacrimal passage
      H04.433 Chronic lacrimal mucocele of bilateral lacrimal passages
      H04.439 Chronic lacrimal mucocele of unspecified lacrimal passage

H04.5 Stenosis and insufficiency of lacrimal passages
  H04.51 Dacryolith
      H04.511 Dacryolith of right lacrimal passage
      H04.512 Dacryolith of left lacrimal passage
      H04.513 Dacryolith of bilateral lacrimal passages
      H04.519 Dacryolith of unspecified lacrimal passage
  H04.52 Eversion of lacrimal punctum
      H04.521 Eversion of right lacrimal punctum
      H04.522 Eversion of left lacrimal punctum
      H04.523 Eversion of bilateral lacrimal punctum
      H04.529 Eversion of unspecified lacrimal punctum
  H04.53 Neonatal obstruction of nasolacrimal duct
      EXCLUDES1 congenital stenosis and stricture of lacrimal duct (Q10.5)

PDx Unacceptable principal diagnosis symbol per Medicare code edits   PoA Code exempt from diagnosis present on admission requirement
? Questionable admission   CC Complication or comorbidity   CC/MCC CC/MCC exclusion   MCC Major complication or comorbidity
CC Principal diagnosis as its own CC   MCC Principal diagnosis as its own MCC   HCC HCC diagnosis code   RxHCC RxHCC diagnosis code
MACRA code   Z1 Z code as first-listed diagnosis

When symbols appear on a code that requires a 7th character extension, refer to Appendix B to identify applicable 7th character codes.
2018 ICD-10-CM

H04.531 Neonatal obstruction of right nasolacrimal duct N

H04.532 Neonatal obstruction of left nasolacrimal duct N

H04.533 Neonatal obstruction of bilateral nasolacrimal duct N

H04.539 Neonatal obstruction of unspecified nasolacrimal duct N

Ⓡ H04.54 Stenosis of lacrimal canaliculi

H04.541 Stenosis of right lacrimal canaliculi

H04.542 Stenosis of left lacrimal canaliculi

H04.543 Stenosis of bilateral lacrimal canaliculi

H04.549 Stenosis of unspecified lacrimal canaliculi

Ⓡ H04.55 Acquired stenosis of nasolacrimal duct

H04.551 Acquired stenosis of right nasolacrimal duct

H04.552 Acquired stenosis of left nasolacrimal duct

H04.553 Acquired stenosis of bilateral nasolacrimal duct

H04.559 Acquired stenosis of unspecified nasolacrimal duct

Ⓡ H04.56 Stenosis of lacrimal punctum

H04.561 Stenosis of right lacrimal punctum

H04.562 Stenosis of left lacrimal punctum

H04.563 Stenosis of bilateral lacrimal punctum

H04.569 Stenosis of unspecified lacrimal punctum

Ⓡ H04.57 Stenosis of lacrimal sac

H04.571 Stenosis of right lacrimal sac

H04.572 Stenosis of left lacrimal sac

H04.573 Stenosis of bilateral lacrimal sac

H04.579 Stenosis of unspecified lacrimal sac

Ⓟ H04.6 Other changes of lacrimal passages

Ⓡ H04.61 Lacrimal fistula

H04.611 Lacrimal fistula right lacrimal passage

H04.612 Lacrimal fistula left lacrimal passage

H04.613 Lacrimal fistula bilateral lacrimal passages

H04.619 Lacrimal fistula unspecified lacrimal passage

H04.69 Other changes of lacrimal passages

Ⓟ H04.8 Other disorders of lacrimal system

Ⓡ H04.81 Granuloma of lacrimal passages

H04.811 Granuloma of right lacrimal passage

H04.812 Granuloma of left lacrimal passage

H04.813 Granuloma of bilateral lacrimal passages

H04.819 Granuloma of unspecified lacrimal passage

H04.89 Other disorders of lacrimal system

H04.9 Disorder of lacrimal system, unspecified

Ⓝ H05 Disorders of orbit

EXCLUDES1 congenital malformation of orbit (Q10.7)

Ⓟ H05.0 Acute inflammation of orbit

H05.00 Unspecified acute inflammation of orbit

Ⓡ H05.01 Cellulitis of orbit

Abscess of orbit

H05.011 Cellulitis of right orbit CⓇ CC/MCC ExcⓇ

H05.012 Cellulitis of left orbit CⓇ CC/MCC ExcⓇ

H05.013 Cellulitis of bilateral orbits CⓇ CC/MCC ExcⓇ

H05.019 Cellulitis of unspecified orbit CⓇ CC/MCC ExcⓇ

Ⓡ H05.02 Osteomyelitis of orbit

H05.021 Osteomyelitis of right orbit CⓇ CC/MCC ExcⓇ

H05.022 Osteomyelitis of left orbit CⓇ CC/MCC ExcⓇ

H05.023 Osteomyelitis of bilateral orbits CⓇ CC/MCC ExcⓇ

H05.029 Osteomyelitis of unspecified orbit CⓇ CC/MCC ExcⓇ

Ⓡ H05.03 Periostitis of orbit

H05.031 Periostitis of right orbit CⓇ CC/MCC ExcⓇ

H05.032 Periostitis of left orbit CⓇ CC/MCC ExcⓇ

H05.033 Periostitis of bilateral orbits CⓇ CC/MCC ExcⓇ

H05.039 Periostitis of unspecified orbit CⓇ CC/MCC ExcⓇ

Ⓡ H05.04 Tenonitis of orbit

H05.041 Tenonitis of right orbit

H05.042 Tenonitis of left orbit

H05.043 Tenonitis of bilateral orbits

H05.049 Tenonitis of unspecified orbit

Ⓟ H05.1 Chronic inflammatory disorders of orbit

H05.10 Unspecified chronic inflammatory disorders of orbit

Ⓡ H05.11 Granuloma of orbit

Pseudotumor (inflammatory) of orbit

H05.111 Granuloma of right orbit

H05.112 Granuloma of left orbit

H05.113 Granuloma of bilateral orbits

H05.119 Granuloma of unspecified orbit

Ⓡ H05.12 Orbital myositis

H05.121 Orbital myositis, right orbit

H05.122 Orbital myositis, left orbit

H05.123 Orbital myositis, bilateral

H05.129 Orbital myositis, unspecified orbit

Ⓟ H05.2 Exophthalmic conditions

H05.20 Unspecified exophthalmos

Ⓡ H05.21 Displacement (lateral) of globe

H05.211 Displacement (lateral) of globe, right eye

H05.212 Displacement (lateral) of globe, left eye

H05.213 Displacement (lateral) of globe, bilateral

H05.219 Displacement (lateral) of globe, unspecified eye

Ⓡ H05.22 Edema of orbit

Orbital congestion

H05.221 Edema of right orbit

H05.222 Edema of left orbit

H05.223 Edema of bilateral orbit

H05.229 Edema of unspecified orbit

Ⓡ H05.23 Hemorrhage of orbit

H05.231 Hemorrhage of right orbit

H05.232 Hemorrhage of left orbit

H05.233 Hemorrhage of bilateral orbit

H05.239 Hemorrhage of unspecified orbit

Ⓡ H05.24 Constant exophthalmos

H05.241 Constant exophthalmos, right eye

H05.242 Constant exophthalmos, left eye

H05.243 Constant exophthalmos, bilateral

H05.249 Constant exophthalmos, unspecified eye

Ⓡ H05.25 Intermittent exophthalmos

H05.251 Intermittent exophthalmos, right eye

H05.252 Intermittent exophthalmos, left eye

H05.253 Intermittent exophthalmos, bilateral

H05.259 Intermittent exophthalmos, unspecified eye

Ⓡ H05.26 Pulsating exophthalmos

H05.261 Pulsating exophthalmos, right eye

H05.262 Pulsating exophthalmos, left eye

H05.263 Pulsating exophthalmos, bilateral

H05.269 Pulsating exophthalmos, unspecified eye

Ⓟ H05.3 Deformity of orbit

EXCLUDES1 congenital deformity of orbit (Q10.7)

hypertelorism (Q75.2)

H05.30 Unspecified deformity of orbit

Ⓡ H05.31 Atrophy of orbit

H05.311 Atrophy of right orbit

H05.312 Atrophy of left orbit

H05.313 Atrophy of bilateral orbit

H05.319 Atrophy of unspecified orbit

Ⓡ H05.32 Deformity of orbit due to bone disease

Code also associated bone disease

H05.321 Deformity of right orbit due to bone disease

H05.322 Deformity of left orbit due to bone disease

H05.323 Deformity of bilateral orbits due to bone disease

Unspecified Code   Other Specified Code   Manifestation Code   N Newborn   P Pediatric   M Maternity   A Adult   ♂ Male   ♀ Female
● New Code   ▲ Revised Code Title   ►◄ Revised Text   NOTES   INCLUDES   EXCLUDES 1   Not coded here   EXCLUDES 2   Not included here
Ⓝ 4th character required   Ⓟ 5th character required   Ⓡ 6th character required   Ⓣ 7th character required
Ⓣ Extension 'X' Alert   HAC Hospital-acquired condition (HAC) alert   AHA AHA Coding Clinic©

2018 ICD-10-CM   When symbols appear on a code that requires a 7th character extension, refer to Appendix B to identify applicable 7th character codes.   599

H05.329 Deformity of unspecified orbit due to bone disease
[6th] H05.33 Deformity of orbit due to trauma or surgery
H05.331 Deformity of right orbit due to trauma or surgery
H05.332 Deformity of left orbit due to trauma or surgery
H05.333 Deformity of bilateral orbits due to trauma or surgery
H05.339 Deformity of unspecified orbit due to trauma or surgery
[6th] H05.34 Enlargement of orbit
H05.341 Enlargement of right orbit
H05.342 Enlargement of left orbit
H05.343 Enlargement of bilateral orbits
H05.349 Enlargement of unspecified orbit
[6th] H05.35 Exostosis of orbit
H05.351 Exostosis of right orbit
H05.352 Exostosis of left orbit
H05.353 Exostosis of bilateral orbits
H05.359 Exostosis of unspecified orbit
[5th] H05.4 Enophthalmos
[6th] H05.40 Unspecified enophthalmos
H05.401 Unspecified enophthalmos, right eye
H05.402 Unspecified enophthalmos, left eye
H05.403 Unspecified enophthalmos, bilateral
H05.409 Unspecified enophthalmos, unspecified eye
[6th] H05.41 Enophthalmos due to atrophy of orbital tissue
H05.411 Enophthalmos due to atrophy of orbital tissue, right eye
H05.412 Enophthalmos due to atrophy of orbital tissue, left eye
H05.413 Enophthalmos due to atrophy of orbital tissue, bilateral
H05.419 Enophthalmos due to atrophy of orbital tissue, unspecified eye
[6th] H05.42 Enophthalmos due to trauma or surgery
H05.421 Enophthalmos due to trauma or surgery, right eye
H05.422 Enophthalmos due to trauma or surgery, left eye
H05.423 Enophthalmos due to trauma or surgery, bilateral
H05.429 Enophthalmos due to trauma or surgery, unspecified eye
[5th] H05.5 Retained (old) foreign body following penetrating wound of orbit
Retrobulbar foreign body
Use additional code to identify the type of retained foreign body (Z18.-)
[EXCLUDES1] *current penetrating wound of orbit (S05.4-)*
[EXCLUDES2] *retained foreign body of eyelid (H02.81-)*
retained intraocular foreign body (H44.6-, H44.7-)
H05.50 Retained (old) foreign body following penetrating wound of unspecified orbit
H05.51 Retained (old) foreign body following penetrating wound of right orbit
H05.52 Retained (old) foreign body following penetrating wound of left orbit
H05.53 Retained (old) foreign body following penetrating wound of bilateral orbits
[5th] H05.8 Other disorders of orbit
[6th] H05.81 Cyst of orbit
Encephalocele of orbit
H05.811 Cyst of right orbit
H05.812 Cyst of left orbit
H05.813 Cyst of bilateral orbits
H05.819 Cyst of unspecified orbit
[6th] H05.82 Myopathy of extraocular muscles
H05.821 Myopathy of extraocular muscles, right orbit
H05.822 Myopathy of extraocular muscles, left orbit
H05.823 Myopathy of extraocular muscles, bilateral
H05.829 Myopathy of extraocular muscles, unspecified orbit
H05.89 Other disorders of orbit
H05.9 Unspecified disorder of orbit

Disorders of conjunctiva (H10-H11)

[4th] H10 Conjunctivitis
[EXCLUDES1] *keratoconjunctivitis (H16.2-)*
[5th] H10.0 Mucopurulent conjunctivitis
[6th] H10.01 Acute follicular conjunctivitis
H10.011 Acute follicular conjunctivitis, right eye
H10.012 Acute follicular conjunctivitis, left eye
H10.013 Acute follicular conjunctivitis, bilateral
H10.019 Acute follicular conjunctivitis, unspecified eye
[6th] H10.02 Other mucopurulent conjunctivitis
H10.021 Other mucopurulent conjunctivitis, right eye
H10.022 Other mucopurulent conjunctivitis, left eye
H10.023 Other mucopurulent conjunctivitis, bilateral
H10.029 Other mucopurulent conjunctivitis, unspecified eye
[5th] H10.1 Acute atopic conjunctivitis
Acute papillary conjunctivitis
H10.10 Acute atopic conjunctivitis, unspecified eye
H10.11 Acute atopic conjunctivitis, right eye
H10.12 Acute atopic conjunctivitis, left eye
H10.13 Acute atopic conjunctivitis, bilateral
[5th] H10.2 Other acute conjunctivitis
[6th] H10.21 Acute toxic conjunctivitis
Acute chemical conjunctivitis
Code first (T51-T65) to identify chemical and intent
[EXCLUDES1] *burn and corrosion of eye and adnexa (T26.-)*
H10.211 Acute toxic conjunctivitis, right eye
H10.212 Acute toxic conjunctivitis, left eye
H10.213 Acute toxic conjunctivitis, bilateral
H10.219 Acute toxic conjunctivitis, unspecified eye
[6th] H10.22 Pseudomembranous conjunctivitis
H10.221 Pseudomembranous conjunctivitis, right eye
H10.222 Pseudomembranous conjunctivitis, left eye
H10.223 Pseudomembranous conjunctivitis, bilateral
H10.229 Pseudomembranous conjunctivitis, unspecified eye
[6th] H10.23 Serous conjunctivitis, except viral
[EXCLUDES1] *viral conjunctivitis (B30.-)*
H10.231 Serous conjunctivitis, except viral, right eye
H10.232 Serous conjunctivitis, except viral, left eye
H10.233 Serous conjunctivitis, except viral, bilateral
H10.239 Serous conjunctivitis, except viral, unspecified eye
[5th] H10.3 Unspecified acute conjunctivitis
[EXCLUDES1] *ophthalmia neonatorum NOS (P39.1)*
H10.30 Unspecified acute conjunctivitis, unspecified eye
H10.31 Unspecified acute conjunctivitis, right eye
H10.32 Unspecified acute conjunctivitis, left eye
H10.33 Unspecified acute conjunctivitis, bilateral
[5th] H10.4 Chronic conjunctivitis

[PDx] Unacceptable principal diagnosis symbol per Medicare code edits [POA] Code exempt from diagnosis present on admission requirement
[Q] Questionable admission [CC] Complication or comorbidity [CC/MCC Exc] CC/MCC exclusion [MCC] Major complication or comorbidity
[PDx CC] Principal diagnosis as its own CC [PDx MCC] Principal diagnosis as its own MCC [HCC] HCC diagnosis code [RxHCC] RxHCC diagnosis code
MACRA code [Z1] Z code as first-listed diagnosis

⑤ᵗʰ H10.40　Unspecified chronic conjunctivitis
　　　　H10.401　Unspecified chronic conjunctivitis, right eye
　　　　H10.402　Unspecified chronic conjunctivitis, left eye
　　　　H10.403　Unspecified chronic conjunctivitis, bilateral
　　　　H10.409　Unspecified chronic conjunctivitis, unspecified eye
⑥ᵗʰ H10.41　Chronic giant papillary conjunctivitis
　　　　H10.411　Chronic giant papillary conjunctivitis, right eye
　　　　H10.412　Chronic giant papillary conjunctivitis, left eye
　　　　H10.413　Chronic giant papillary conjunctivitis, bilateral
　　　　H10.419　Chronic giant papillary conjunctivitis, unspecified eye
⑥ᵗʰ H10.42　Simple chronic conjunctivitis
　　　　H10.421　Simple chronic conjunctivitis, right eye
　　　　H10.422　Simple chronic conjunctivitis, left eye
　　　　H10.423　Simple chronic conjunctivitis, bilateral
　　　　H10.429　Simple chronic conjunctivitis, unspecified eye
⑥ᵗʰ H10.43　Chronic follicular conjunctivitis
　　　　H10.431　Chronic follicular conjunctivitis, right eye
　　　　H10.432　Chronic follicular conjunctivitis, left eye
　　　　H10.433　Chronic follicular conjunctivitis, bilateral
　　　　H10.439　Chronic follicular conjunctivitis, unspecified eye
　　H10.44　Vernal conjunctivitis
　　　　EXCLUDES1　vernal keratoconjunctivitis with limbar and corneal involvement (H16.26-)
　　H10.45　Other chronic allergic conjunctivitis
⑤ᵗʰ H10.5　Blepharoconjunctivitis
　⑥ᵗʰ H10.50　Unspecified blepharoconjunctivitis
　　　　H10.501　Unspecified blepharoconjunctivitis, right eye
　　　　H10.502　Unspecified blepharoconjunctivitis, left eye
　　　　H10.503　Unspecified blepharoconjunctivitis, bilateral
　　　　H10.509　Unspecified blepharoconjunctivitis, unspecified eye
　⑥ᵗʰ H10.51　Ligneous conjunctivitis
　　　　H10.511　Ligneous conjunctivitis, right eye
　　　　H10.512　Ligneous conjunctivitis, left eye
　　　　H10.513　Ligneous conjunctivitis, bilateral
　　　　H10.519　Ligneous conjunctivitis, unspecified eye
　⑥ᵗʰ H10.52　Angular blepharoconjunctivitis
　　　　H10.521　Angular blepharoconjunctivitis, right eye
　　　　H10.522　Angular blepharoconjunctivitis, left eye
　　　　H10.523　Angular blepharoconjunctivitis, bilateral
　　　　H10.529　Angular blepharoconjunctivitis, unspecified eye
　⑥ᵗʰ H10.53　Contact blepharoconjunctivitis
　　　　H10.531　Contact blepharoconjunctivitis, right eye
　　　　H10.532　Contact blepharoconjunctivitis, left eye
　　　　H10.533　Contact blepharoconjunctivitis, bilateral
　　　　H10.539　Contact blepharoconjunctivitis, unspecified eye
⑤ᵗʰ H10.8　Other conjunctivitis
　⑥ᵗʰ H10.81　Pingueculitis
　　　　EXCLUDES1　pinguecula (H11.15-)
　　　　H10.811　Pingueculitis, right eye
　　　　H10.812　Pingueculitis, left eye
　　　　H10.813　Pingueculitis, bilateral
　　　　H10.819　Pingueculitis, unspecified eye
　　H10.89　Other conjunctivitis
　H10.9　Unspecified conjunctivitis
④ᵗʰ H11　Other disorders of conjunctiva

EXCLUDES1　keratoconjunctivitis (H16.2-)

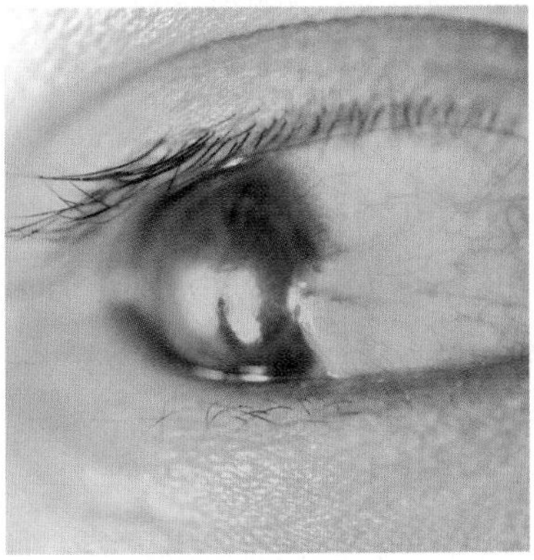

Figure 7.3　Pterygium

⑤ᵗʰ H11.0　Pterygium of eye
　　　　EXCLUDES1　pseudopterygium (H11.81-)
　⑥ᵗʰ H11.00　Unspecified pterygium of eye
　　　　H11.001　Unspecified pterygium of right eye
　　　　H11.002　Unspecified pterygium of left eye
　　　　H11.003　Unspecified pterygium of eye, bilateral
　　　　H11.009　Unspecified pterygium of unspecified eye
　⑥ᵗʰ H11.01　Amyloid pterygium
　　　　H11.011　Amyloid pterygium of right eye
　　　　H11.012　Amyloid pterygium of left eye
　　　　H11.013　Amyloid pterygium of eye, bilateral
　　　　H11.019　Amyloid pterygium of unspecified eye
　⑥ᵗʰ H11.02　Central pterygium of eye
　　　　H11.021　Central pterygium of right eye
　　　　H11.022　Central pterygium of left eye
　　　　H11.023　Central pterygium of eye, bilateral
　　　　H11.029　Central pterygium of unspecified eye
　⑥ᵗʰ H11.03　Double pterygium of eye
　　　　H11.031　Double pterygium of right eye
　　　　H11.032　Double pterygium of left eye
　　　　H11.033　Double pterygium of eye, bilateral
　　　　H11.039　Double pterygium of unspecified eye
　⑥ᵗʰ H11.04　Peripheral pterygium of eye, stationary
　　　　H11.041　Peripheral pterygium, stationary, right eye
　　　　H11.042　Peripheral pterygium, stationary, left eye
　　　　H11.043　Peripheral pterygium, stationary, bilateral
　　　　H11.049　Peripheral pterygium, stationary, unspecified eye
　⑥ᵗʰ H11.05　Peripheral pterygium of eye, progressive
　　　　H11.051　Peripheral pterygium, progressive, right eye
　　　　H11.052　Peripheral pterygium, progressive, left eye
　　　　H11.053　Peripheral pterygium, progressive, bilateral
　　　　H11.059　Peripheral pterygium, progressive, unspecified eye
　⑥ᵗʰ H11.06　Recurrent pterygium of eye
　　　　H11.061　Recurrent pterygium of right eye
　　　　H11.062　Recurrent pterygium of left eye
　　　　H11.063　Recurrent pterygium of eye, bilateral
　　　　H11.069　Recurrent pterygium of unspecified eye
⑤ᵗʰ H11.1　Conjunctival degenerations and deposits
　　　　EXCLUDES2　pseudopterygium (H11.81)
　　H11.10　Unspecified conjunctival degenerations
　⑥ᵗʰ H11.11　Conjunctival deposits
　　　　H11.111　Conjunctival deposits, right eye
　　　　H11.112　Conjunctival deposits, left eye
　　　　H11.113　Conjunctival deposits, bilateral
　　　　H11.119　Conjunctival deposits, unspecified eye
　⑥ᵗʰ H11.12　Conjunctival concretions

Unspecified Code　　Other Specified Code　　Manifestation Code　　Ⓝ Newborn　Ⓟ Pediatric　Ⓜ Maternity　Ⓐ Adult　♂ Male　♀ Female
● New Code　▲ Revised Code Title　▶◀ Revised Text　NOTES　INCLUDES　EXCLUDES 1 Not coded here　EXCLUDES 2 Not included here
④ᵗʰ 4ᵗʰ character required　⑤ᵗʰ 5ᵗʰ character required　⑥ᵗʰ 6ᵗʰ character required　⑦ᵗʰ 7ᵗʰ character required
⑦ Extension 'X' Alert　HAC Hospital-acquired condition (HAC) alert　AHA AHA Coding Clinic©

H11.121 Conjunctival concretions, right eye
H11.122 Conjunctival concretions, left eye
H11.123 Conjunctival concretions, bilateral
H11.129 Conjunctival concretions, unspecified eye
6️⃣ H11.13 Conjunctival pigmentations
Conjunctival argyrosis [argyria]
H11.131 Conjunctival pigmentations, right eye
H11.132 Conjunctival pigmentations, left eye
H11.133 Conjunctival pigmentations, bilateral
H11.139 Conjunctival pigmentations, unspecified eye
6️⃣ H11.14 Conjunctival xerosis, unspecified
EXCLUDES1 xerosis of conjunctiva due to vitamin A deficiency (E50.0, E50.1)
H11.141 Conjunctival xerosis, unspecified, right eye
H11.142 Conjunctival xerosis, unspecified, left eye
H11.143 Conjunctival xerosis, unspecified, bilateral
H11.149 Conjunctival xerosis, unspecified, unspecified eye
6️⃣ H11.15 Pinguecula
EXCLUDES1 pingueculitis (H10.81-)
H11.151 Pinguecula, right eye
H11.152 Pinguecula, left eye
H11.153 Pinguecula, bilateral
H11.159 Pinguecula, unspecified eye
5️⃣ H11.2 Conjunctival scars
6️⃣ H11.21 Conjunctival adhesions and strands (localized)
H11.211 Conjunctival adhesions and strands (localized), right eye
H11.212 Conjunctival adhesions and strands (localized), left eye
H11.213 Conjunctival adhesions and strands (localized), bilateral
H11.219 Conjunctival adhesions and strands (localized), unspecified eye
6️⃣ H11.22 Conjunctival granuloma
H11.221 Conjunctival granuloma, right eye
H11.222 Conjunctival granuloma, left eye
H11.223 Conjunctival granuloma, bilateral
H11.229 Conjunctival granuloma, unspecified
6️⃣ H11.23 Symblepharon
H11.231 Symblepharon, right eye
H11.232 Symblepharon, left eye
H11.233 Symblepharon, bilateral
H11.239 Symblepharon, unspecified eye
6️⃣ H11.24 Scarring of conjunctiva
H11.241 Scarring of conjunctiva, right eye
H11.242 Scarring of conjunctiva, left eye
H11.243 Scarring of conjunctiva, bilateral
H11.249 Scarring of conjunctiva, unspecified eye
5️⃣ H11.3 Conjunctival hemorrhage
Subconjunctival hemorrhage
H11.30 Conjunctival hemorrhage, unspecified eye
H11.31 Conjunctival hemorrhage, right eye
H11.32 Conjunctival hemorrhage, left eye
H11.33 Conjunctival hemorrhage, bilateral
5️⃣ H11.4 Other conjunctival vascular disorders and cysts
6️⃣ H11.41 Vascular abnormalities of conjunctiva
Conjunctival aneurysm
H11.411 Vascular abnormalities of conjunctiva, right eye
H11.412 Vascular abnormalities of conjunctiva, left eye
H11.413 Vascular abnormalities of conjunctiva, bilateral
H11.419 Vascular abnormalities of conjunctiva, unspecified eye
6️⃣ H11.42 Conjunctival edema
H11.421 Conjunctival edema, right eye

H11.422 Conjunctival edema, left eye
H11.423 Conjunctival edema, bilateral
H11.429 Conjunctival edema, unspecified eye
6️⃣ H11.43 Conjunctival hyperemia
H11.431 Conjunctival hyperemia, right eye
H11.432 Conjunctival hyperemia, left eye
H11.433 Conjunctival hyperemia, bilateral
H11.439 Conjunctival hyperemia, unspecified eye
6️⃣ H11.44 Conjunctival cysts
H11.441 Conjunctival cysts, right eye
H11.442 Conjunctival cysts, left eye
H11.443 Conjunctival cysts, bilateral
H11.449 Conjunctival cysts, unspecified eye
5️⃣ H11.8 Other specified disorders of conjunctiva
6️⃣ H11.81 Pseudopterygium of conjunctiva
H11.811 Pseudopterygium of conjunctiva, right eye
H11.812 Pseudopterygium of conjunctiva, left eye
H11.813 Pseudopterygium of conjunctiva, bilateral
H11.819 Pseudopterygium of conjunctiva, unspecified eye
6️⃣ H11.82 Conjunctivochalasis
H11.821 Conjunctivochalasis, right eye
H11.822 Conjunctivochalasis, left eye
H11.823 Conjunctivochalasis, bilateral
H11.829 Conjunctivochalasis, unspecified eye
H11.89 Other specified disorders of conjunctiva
H11.9 Unspecified disorder of conjunctiva

Disorders of sclera, cornea, iris and ciliary body (H15-H22)

4️⃣ H15 Disorders of sclera
5️⃣ H15.0 Scleritis
6️⃣ H15.00 Unspecified scleritis
H15.001 Unspecified scleritis, right eye
H15.002 Unspecified scleritis, left eye
H15.003 Unspecified scleritis, bilateral
H15.009 Unspecified scleritis, unspecified eye
6️⃣ H15.01 Anterior scleritis
H15.011 Anterior scleritis, right eye
H15.012 Anterior scleritis, left eye
H15.013 Anterior scleritis, bilateral
H15.019 Anterior scleritis, unspecified eye
6️⃣ H15.02 Brawny scleritis
H15.021 Brawny scleritis, right eye
H15.022 Brawny scleritis, left eye
H15.023 Brawny scleritis, bilateral
H15.029 Brawny scleritis, unspecified eye
6️⃣ H15.03 Posterior scleritis
Sclerotenonitis
H15.031 Posterior scleritis, right eye
H15.032 Posterior scleritis, left eye
H15.033 Posterior scleritis, bilateral
H15.039 Posterior scleritis, unspecified eye
6️⃣ H15.04 Scleritis with corneal involvement
H15.041 Scleritis with corneal involvement, right eye
H15.042 Scleritis with corneal involvement, left eye
H15.043 Scleritis with corneal involvement, bilateral
H15.049 Scleritis with corneal involvement, unspecified eye
6️⃣ H15.05 Scleromalacia perforans
H15.051 Scleromalacia perforans, right eye
H15.052 Scleromalacia perforans, left eye
H15.053 Scleromalacia perforans, bilateral
H15.059 Scleromalacia perforans, unspecified eye
6️⃣ H15.09 Other scleritis
Scleral abscess

PDxⁿ Unacceptable principal diagnosis symbol per Medicare code edits   PDx Code exempt from diagnosis present on admission requirement
❓ Questionable admission   cc Complication or comorbidity   cc/Mcc Exc CC/MCC exclusion   Mcc Major complication or comorbidity
Principal diagnosis as its own CC   Principal diagnosis as its own MCC   HCC HCC diagnosis code   RxHCC RxHCC diagnosis code
MACRA code   Z code as first-listed diagnosis

H15.091 Other scleritis, right eye
H15.092 Other scleritis, left eye
H15.093 Other scleritis, bilateral
H15.099 Other scleritis, unspecified eye

[5th] H15.1 Episcleritis
[6th] H15.10 Unspecified episcleritis
H15.101 Unspecified episcleritis, right eye
H15.102 Unspecified episcleritis, left eye
H15.103 Unspecified episcleritis, bilateral
H15.109 Unspecified episcleritis, unspecified eye
[6th] H15.11 Episcleritis periodica fugax
H15.111 Episcleritis periodica fugax, right eye
H15.112 Episcleritis periodica fugax, left eye
H15.113 Episcleritis periodica fugax, bilateral
H15.119 Episcleritis periodica fugax, unspecified eye
[6th] H15.12 Nodular episcleritis
H15.121 Nodular episcleritis, right eye
H15.122 Nodular episcleritis, left eye
H15.123 Nodular episcleritis, bilateral
H15.129 Nodular episcleritis, unspecified eye

[5th] H15.8 Other disorders of sclera
[EXCLUDES2] *blue sclera (Q13.5)*
degenerative myopia (H44.2-)
[6th] H15.81 Equatorial staphyloma
H15.811 Equatorial staphyloma, right eye
H15.812 Equatorial staphyloma, left eye
H15.813 Equatorial staphyloma, bilateral
H15.819 Equatorial staphyloma, unspecified eye
[6th] H15.82 Localized anterior staphyloma
H15.821 Localized anterior staphyloma, right eye
H15.822 Localized anterior staphyloma, left eye
H15.823 Localized anterior staphyloma, bilateral
H15.829 Localized anterior staphyloma, unspecified eye
[6th] H15.83 Staphyloma posticum
H15.831 Staphyloma posticum, right eye
H15.832 Staphyloma posticum, left eye
H15.833 Staphyloma posticum, bilateral
H15.839 Staphyloma posticum, unspecified eye
[6th] H15.84 Scleral ectasia
H15.841 Scleral ectasia, right eye
H15.842 Scleral ectasia, left eye
H15.843 Scleral ectasia, bilateral
H15.849 Scleral ectasia, unspecified eye
[6th] H15.85 Ring staphyloma
H15.851 Ring staphyloma, right eye
H15.852 Ring staphyloma, left eye
H15.853 Ring staphyloma, bilateral
H15.859 Ring staphyloma, unspecified eye
H15.89 Other disorders of sclera
H15.9 Unspecified disorder of sclera

[4th] H16 Keratitis
[5th] H16.0 Corneal ulcer
[6th] H16.00 Unspecified corneal ulcer
H16.001 Unspecified corneal ulcer, right eye
H16.002 Unspecified corneal ulcer, left eye
H16.003 Unspecified corneal ulcer, bilateral
H16.009 Unspecified corneal ulcer, unspecified eye
[6th] H16.01 Central corneal ulcer
H16.011 Central corneal ulcer, right eye
H16.012 Central corneal ulcer, left eye
H16.013 Central corneal ulcer, bilateral
H16.019 Central corneal ulcer, unspecified eye
[6th] H16.02 Ring corneal ulcer
H16.021 Ring corneal ulcer, right eye
H16.022 Ring corneal ulcer, left eye
H16.023 Ring corneal ulcer, bilateral
H16.029 Ring corneal ulcer, unspecified eye
[6th] H16.03 Corneal ulcer with hypopyon
H16.031 Corneal ulcer with hypopyon, right eye
H16.032 Corneal ulcer with hypopyon, left eye
H16.033 Corneal ulcer with hypopyon, bilateral
H16.039 Corneal ulcer with hypopyon, unspecified eye
[6th] H16.04 Marginal corneal ulcer
H16.041 Marginal corneal ulcer, right eye
H16.042 Marginal corneal ulcer, left eye
H16.043 Marginal corneal ulcer, bilateral
H16.049 Marginal corneal ulcer, unspecified eye
[6th] H16.05 Mooren's corneal ulcer
H16.051 Mooren's corneal ulcer, right eye
H16.052 Mooren's corneal ulcer, left eye
H16.053 Mooren's corneal ulcer, bilateral
H16.059 Mooren's corneal ulcer, unspecified eye
[6th] H16.06 Mycotic corneal ulcer
H16.061 Mycotic corneal ulcer, right eye
H16.062 Mycotic corneal ulcer, left eye
H16.063 Mycotic corneal ulcer, bilateral
H16.069 Mycotic corneal ulcer, unspecified eye
[6th] H16.07 Perforated corneal ulcer
H16.071 Perforated corneal ulcer, right eye
H16.072 Perforated corneal ulcer, left eye
H16.073 Perforated corneal ulcer, bilateral
H16.079 Perforated corneal ulcer, unspecified eye

[5th] H16.1 Other and unspecified superficial keratitis without conjunctivitis
[6th] H16.10 Unspecified superficial keratitis
H16.101 Unspecified superficial keratitis, right eye
H16.102 Unspecified superficial keratitis, left eye
H16.103 Unspecified superficial keratitis, bilateral
H16.109 Unspecified superficial keratitis, unspecified eye
[6th] H16.11 Macular keratitis
Areolar keratitis
Nummular keratitis
Stellate keratitis
Striate keratitis
H16.111 Macular keratitis, right eye
H16.112 Macular keratitis, left eye
H16.113 Macular keratitis, bilateral
H16.119 Macular keratitis, unspecified eye
[6th] H16.12 Filamentary keratitis
H16.121 Filamentary keratitis, right eye
H16.122 Filamentary keratitis, left eye
H16.123 Filamentary keratitis, bilateral
H16.129 Filamentary keratitis, unspecified eye
[6th] H16.13 Photokeratitis
Snow blindness
Welders keratitis
H16.131 Photokeratitis, right eye
H16.132 Photokeratitis, left eye
H16.133 Photokeratitis, bilateral
H16.139 Photokeratitis, unspecified eye
[6th] H16.14 Punctate keratitis
H16.141 Punctate keratitis, right eye
H16.142 Punctate keratitis, left eye
H16.143 Punctate keratitis, bilateral
H16.149 Punctate keratitis, unspecified eye

[5th] H16.2 Keratoconjunctivitis
[6th] H16.20 Unspecified keratoconjunctivitis
Superficial keratitis with conjunctivitis NOS
H16.201 Unspecified keratoconjunctivitis, right eye
H16.202 Unspecified keratoconjunctivitis, left eye
H16.203 Unspecified keratoconjunctivitis, bilateral
H16.209 Unspecified keratoconjunctivitis, unspecified eye

⑥ **H16.21** Exposure keratoconjunctivitis
- H16.211 Exposure keratoconjunctivitis, right eye
- H16.212 Exposure keratoconjunctivitis, left eye
- H16.213 Exposure keratoconjunctivitis, bilateral
- H16.219 Exposure keratoconjunctivitis, unspecified eye

⑥ **H16.22** Keratoconjunctivitis sicca, not specified as Sjögren's
> EXCLUDES1 *Sjögren's syndrome (M35.01)*
- H16.221 Keratoconjunctivitis sicca, not specified as Sjögren's, right eye
- H16.222 Keratoconjunctivitis sicca, not specified as Sjögren's, left eye
- H16.223 Keratoconjunctivitis sicca, not specified as Sjögren's, bilateral
- H16.229 Keratoconjunctivitis sicca, not specified as Sjögren's, unspecified eye

⑥ **H16.23** Neurotrophic keratoconjunctivitis
- H16.231 Neurotrophic keratoconjunctivitis, right eye
- H16.232 Neurotrophic keratoconjunctivitis, left eye
- H16.233 Neurotrophic keratoconjunctivitis, bilateral
- H16.239 Neurotrophic keratoconjunctivitis, unspecified eye

⑥ **H16.24** Ophthalmia nodosa
- H16.241 Ophthalmia nodosa, right eye
- H16.242 Ophthalmia nodosa, left eye
- H16.243 Ophthalmia nodosa, bilateral
- H16.249 Ophthalmia nodosa, unspecified eye

⑥ **H16.25** Phlyctenular keratoconjunctivitis
- H16.251 Phlyctenular keratoconjunctivitis, right eye
- H16.252 Phlyctenular keratoconjunctivitis, left eye
- H16.253 Phlyctenular keratoconjunctivitis, bilateral
- H16.259 Phlyctenular keratoconjunctivitis, unspecified eye

⑥ **H16.26** Vernal keratoconjunctivitis, with limbar and corneal involvement
> EXCLUDES1 *vernal conjunctivitis without limbar and corneal involvement (H10.44)*
- H16.261 Vernal keratoconjunctivitis, with limbar and corneal involvement, right eye
- H16.262 Vernal keratoconjunctivitis, with limbar and corneal involvement, left eye
- H16.263 Vernal keratoconjunctivitis, with limbar and corneal involvement, bilateral
- H16.269 Vernal keratoconjunctivitis, with limbar and corneal involvement, unspecified eye

⑥ **H16.29** Other keratoconjunctivitis
- H16.291 Other keratoconjunctivitis, right eye
- H16.292 Other keratoconjunctivitis, left eye
- H16.293 Other keratoconjunctivitis, bilateral
- H16.299 Other keratoconjunctivitis, unspecified eye

⑤ **H16.3** Interstitial and deep keratitis
⑥ **H16.30** Unspecified interstitial keratitis
- H16.301 Unspecified interstitial keratitis, right eye
- H16.302 Unspecified interstitial keratitis, left eye
- H16.303 Unspecified interstitial keratitis, bilateral
- H16.309 Unspecified interstitial keratitis, unspecified eye

⑥ **H16.31** Corneal abscess
- H16.311 Corneal abscess, right eye
- H16.312 Corneal abscess, left eye
- H16.313 Corneal abscess, bilateral
- H16.319 Corneal abscess, unspecified eye

⑥ **H16.32** Diffuse interstitial keratitis
Cogan's syndrome
- H16.321 Diffuse interstitial keratitis, right eye
- H16.322 Diffuse interstitial keratitis, left eye
- H16.323 Diffuse interstitial keratitis, bilateral
- H16.329 Diffuse interstitial keratitis, unspecified eye

⑥ **H16.33** Sclerosing keratitis
- H16.331 Sclerosing keratitis, right eye
- H16.332 Sclerosing keratitis, left eye
- H16.333 Sclerosing keratitis, bilateral
- H16.339 Sclerosing keratitis, unspecified eye

⑥ **H16.39** Other interstitial and deep keratitis
- H16.391 Other interstitial and deep keratitis, right eye
- H16.392 Other interstitial and deep keratitis, left eye
- H16.393 Other interstitial and deep keratitis, bilateral
- H16.399 Other interstitial and deep keratitis, unspecified eye

⑤ **H16.4** Corneal neovascularization
⑥ **H16.40** Unspecified corneal neovascularization
- H16.401 Unspecified corneal neovascularization, right eye
- H16.402 Unspecified corneal neovascularization, left eye
- H16.403 Unspecified corneal neovascularization, bilateral
- H16.409 Unspecified corneal neovascularization, unspecified eye

⑥ **H16.41** Ghost vessels (corneal)
- H16.411 Ghost vessels (corneal), right eye
- H16.412 Ghost vessels (corneal), left eye
- H16.413 Ghost vessels (corneal), bilateral
- H16.419 Ghost vessels (corneal), unspecified eye

⑥ **H16.42** Pannus (corneal)
- H16.421 Pannus (corneal), right eye
- H16.422 Pannus (corneal), left eye
- H16.423 Pannus (corneal), bilateral
- H16.429 Pannus (corneal), unspecified eye

⑤ **H16.43** Localized vascularization of cornea
- H16.431 Localized vascularization of cornea, right eye
- H16.432 Localized vascularization of cornea, left eye
- H16.433 Localized vascularization of cornea, bilateral
- H16.439 Localized vascularization of cornea, unspecified eye

⑥ **H16.44** Deep vascularization of cornea
- H16.441 Deep vascularization of cornea, right eye
- H16.442 Deep vascularization of cornea, left eye
- H16.443 Deep vascularization of cornea, bilateral
- H16.449 Deep vascularization of cornea, unspecified eye

H16.8 Other keratitis   PDxⁿ̲ᵣ

H16.9 Unspecified keratitis

④ **H17** Corneal scars and opacities
⑤ **H17.0** Adherent leukoma
- H17.00 Adherent leukoma, unspecified eye
- H17.01 Adherent leukoma, right eye
- H17.02 Adherent leukoma, left eye
- H17.03 Adherent leukoma, bilateral

⑤ **H17.1** Central corneal opacity
- H17.10 Central corneal opacity, unspecified eye
- H17.11 Central corneal opacity, right eye
- H17.12 Central corneal opacity, left eye
- H17.13 Central corneal opacity, bilateral

⑤ **H17.8** Other corneal scars and opacities
⑥ **H17.81** Minor opacity of cornea
Corneal nebula
- H17.811 Minor opacity of cornea, right eye
- H17.812 Minor opacity of cornea, left eye

PDxⁿ̲ᵣ Unacceptable principal diagnosis symbol per Medicare code edits POA Code exempt from diagnosis present on admission requirement
❓ Questionable admission ℅ᴸ Complication or comorbidity CC/MCC Excl CC/MCC exclusion MCC℗ Major complication or comorbidity
℅ᵇ Principal diagnosis as its own CC ᴹᶜᶜᵇ Principal diagnosis as its own MCC HCC HCC diagnosis code RxHCC RxHCC diagnosis code
MACRA code ☑ Z code as first-listed diagnosis

When symbols appear on a code that requires a 7th character extension, refer to Appendix B to identify applicable 7th character codes.

H17.813 Minor opacity of cornea, bilateral
H17.819 Minor opacity of cornea, unspecified eye
[6th] H17.82 Peripheral opacity of cornea
H17.821 Peripheral opacity of cornea, right eye
H17.822 Peripheral opacity of cornea, left eye
H17.823 Peripheral opacity of cornea, bilateral
H17.829 Peripheral opacity of cornea, unspecified eye
H17.89 Other corneal scars and opacities
H17.9 Unspecified corneal scar and opacity
[4th] H18 Other disorders of cornea
[5th] H18.0 Corneal pigmentations and deposits
[6th] H18.00 Unspecified corneal deposit
H18.001 Unspecified corneal deposit, right eye
H18.002 Unspecified corneal deposit, left eye
H18.003 Unspecified corneal deposit, bilateral
H18.009 Unspecified corneal deposit, unspecified eye
[6th] H18.01 Anterior corneal pigmentations
Staehli's line
H18.011 Anterior corneal pigmentations, right eye
H18.012 Anterior corneal pigmentations, left eye
H18.013 Anterior corneal pigmentations, bilateral
H18.019 Anterior corneal pigmentations, unspecified eye
[6th] H18.02 Argentous corneal deposits
H18.021 Argentous corneal deposits, right eye
H18.022 Argentous corneal deposits, left eye
H18.023 Argentous corneal deposits, bilateral
H18.029 Argentous corneal deposits, unspecified eye
[6th] H18.03 Corneal deposits in metabolic disorders
Code also associated metabolic disorder
H18.031 Corneal deposits in metabolic disorders, right eye
H18.032 Corneal deposits in metabolic disorders, left eye
H18.033 Corneal deposits in metabolic disorders, bilateral
H18.039 Corneal deposits in metabolic disorders, unspecified eye
[6th] H18.04 Kayser-Fleischer ring
Code also associated Wilson's disease (E83.01)
H18.041 Kayser-Fleischer ring, right eye
H18.042 Kayser-Fleischer ring, left eye
H18.043 Kayser-Fleischer ring, bilateral
H18.049 Kayser-Fleischer ring, unspecified eye
[6th] H18.05 Posterior corneal pigmentations
Krukenberg's spindle
H18.051 Posterior corneal pigmentations, right eye
H18.052 Posterior corneal pigmentations, left eye
H18.053 Posterior corneal pigmentations, bilateral
H18.059 Posterior corneal pigmentations, unspecified eye
[6th] H18.06 Stromal corneal pigmentations
Hematocornea
H18.061 Stromal corneal pigmentations, right eye
H18.062 Stromal corneal pigmentations, left eye
H18.063 Stromal corneal pigmentations, bilateral
H18.069 Stromal corneal pigmentations, unspecified eye
[5th] H18.1 Bullous keratopathy
H18.10 Bullous keratopathy, unspecified eye
H18.11 Bullous keratopathy, right eye
H18.12 Bullous keratopathy, left eye
H18.13 Bullous keratopathy, bilateral
[5th] H18.2 Other and unspecified corneal edema
H18.20 Unspecified corneal edema
[6th] H18.21 Corneal edema secondary to contact lens
[EXCLUDES2] *other corneal disorders due to contact lens (H18.82-)*
H18.211 Corneal edema secondary to contact lens, right eye
H18.212 Corneal edema secondary to contact lens, left eye
H18.213 Corneal edema secondary to contact lens, bilateral
H18.219 Corneal edema secondary to contact lens, unspecified eye
[6th] H18.22 Idiopathic corneal edema
H18.221 Idiopathic corneal edema, right eye
H18.222 Idiopathic corneal edema, left eye
H18.223 Idiopathic corneal edema, bilateral
H18.229 Idiopathic corneal edema, unspecified eye
[6th] H18.23 Secondary corneal edema
H18.231 Secondary corneal edema, right eye
H18.232 Secondary corneal edema, left eye
H18.233 Secondary corneal edema, bilateral
H18.239 Secondary corneal edema, unspecified eye
[5th] H18.3 Changes of corneal membranes
H18.30 Unspecified corneal membrane change
[6th] H18.31 Folds and rupture in Bowman's membrane
H18.311 Folds and rupture in Bowman's membrane, right eye
H18.312 Folds and rupture in Bowman's membrane, left eye
H18.313 Folds and rupture in Bowman's membrane, bilateral
H18.319 Folds and rupture in Bowman's membrane, unspecified eye
[6th] H18.32 Folds in Descemet's membrane
H18.321 Folds in Descemet's membrane, right eye
H18.322 Folds in Descemet's membrane, left eye
H18.323 Folds in Descemet's membrane, bilateral
H18.329 Folds in Descemet's membrane, unspecified eye
[6th] H18.33 Rupture in Descemet's membrane
H18.331 Rupture in Descemet's membrane, right eye
H18.332 Rupture in Descemet's membrane, left eye
H18.333 Rupture in Descemet's membrane, bilateral
H18.339 Rupture in Descemet's membrane, unspecified eye
[5th] H18.4 Corneal degeneration
[EXCLUDES1] *Mooren's ulcer (H16.0-)*
recurrent erosion of cornea (H18.83-)
H18.40 Unspecified corneal degeneration
[6th] H18.41 Arcus senilis
Senile corneal changes
H18.411 Arcus senilis, right eye
H18.412 Arcus senilis, left eye
H18.413 Arcus senilis, bilateral
H18.419 Arcus senilis, unspecified eye
[6th] H18.42 Band keratopathy
H18.421 Band keratopathy, right eye
H18.422 Band keratopathy, left eye
H18.423 Band keratopathy, bilateral
H18.429 Band keratopathy, unspecified eye
H18.43 Other calcerous corneal degeneration
[6th] H18.44 Keratomalacia
[EXCLUDES1] *keratomalacia due to vitamin A deficiency (E50.4)*
H18.441 Keratomalacia, right eye
H18.442 Keratomalacia, left eye
H18.443 Keratomalacia, bilateral
H18.449 Keratomalacia, unspecified eye
[6th] H18.45 Nodular corneal degeneration

H18.451 Nodular corneal degeneration, right eye
H18.452 Nodular corneal degeneration, left eye
H18.453 Nodular corneal degeneration, bilateral
H18.459 Nodular corneal degeneration, unspecified eye
[6th] H18.46 Peripheral corneal degeneration
H18.461 Peripheral corneal degeneration, right eye
H18.462 Peripheral corneal degeneration, left eye
H18.463 Peripheral corneal degeneration, bilateral
H18.469 Peripheral corneal degeneration, unspecified eye
H18.49 Other corneal degeneration
[5th] H18.5 Hereditary corneal dystrophies
H18.50 Unspecified hereditary corneal dystrophies
H18.51 Endothelial corneal dystrophy
Fuchs' dystrophy
H18.52 Epithelial (juvenile) corneal dystrophy
H18.53 Granular corneal dystrophy
H18.54 Lattice corneal dystrophy
H18.55 Macular corneal dystrophy
H18.59 Other hereditary corneal dystrophies
[5th] H18.6 Keratoconus
[6th] H18.60 Keratoconus, unspecified
H18.601 Keratoconus, unspecified, right eye
H18.602 Keratoconus, unspecified, left eye
H18.603 Keratoconus, unspecified, bilateral
H18.609 Keratoconus, unspecified, unspecified eye
[6th] H18.61 Keratoconus, stable
H18.611 Keratoconus, stable, right eye
H18.612 Keratoconus, stable, left eye
H18.613 Keratoconus, stable, bilateral
H18.619 Keratoconus, stable, unspecified eye
[6th] H18.62 Keratoconus, unstable
Acute hydrops
H18.621 Keratoconus, unstable, right eye
H18.622 Keratoconus, unstable, left eye
H18.623 Keratoconus, unstable, bilateral
H18.629 Keratoconus, unstable, unspecified eye
[5th] H18.7 Other and unspecified corneal deformities
[EXCLUDES1] *congenital malformations of cornea (Q13.3-Q13.4)*
H18.70 Unspecified corneal deformity
[6th] H18.71 Corneal ectasia
H18.711 Corneal ectasia, right eye
H18.712 Corneal ectasia, left eye
H18.713 Corneal ectasia, bilateral
H18.719 Corneal ectasia, unspecified eye
[6th] H18.72 Corneal staphyloma
H18.721 Corneal staphyloma, right eye
H18.722 Corneal staphyloma, left eye
H18.723 Corneal staphyloma, bilateral
H18.729 Corneal staphyloma, unspecified eye
[6th] H18.73 Descemetocele
H18.731 Descemetocele, right eye
H18.732 Descemetocele, left eye
H18.733 Descemetocele, bilateral
H18.739 Descemetocele, unspecified eye
[6th] H18.79 Other corneal deformities
H18.791 Other corneal deformities, right eye
H18.792 Other corneal deformities, left eye
H18.793 Other corneal deformities, bilateral
H18.799 Other corneal deformities, unspecified eye
[5th] H18.8 Other specified disorders of cornea
[6th] H18.81 Anesthesia and hypoesthesia of cornea
H18.811 Anesthesia and hypoesthesia of cornea, right eye
H18.812 Anesthesia and hypoesthesia of cornea, left eye
H18.813 Anesthesia and hypoesthesia of cornea, bilateral
H18.819 Anesthesia and hypoesthesia of cornea, unspecified eye
[6th] H18.82 Corneal disorder due to contact lens
[EXCLUDES2] *corneal edema due to contact lens (H18.21-)*
H18.821 Corneal disorder due to contact lens, right eye
H18.822 Corneal disorder due to contact lens, left eye
H18.823 Corneal disorder due to contact lens, bilateral
H18.829 Corneal disorder due to contact lens, unspecified eye
[6th] H18.83 Recurrent erosion of cornea
H18.831 Recurrent erosion of cornea, right eye
H18.832 Recurrent erosion of cornea, left eye
H18.833 Recurrent erosion of cornea, bilateral
H18.839 Recurrent erosion of cornea, unspecified eye
[6th] H18.89 Other specified disorders of cornea
H18.891 Other specified disorders of cornea, right eye
H18.892 Other specified disorders of cornea, left eye
H18.893 Other specified disorders of cornea, bilateral
H18.899 Other specified disorders of cornea, unspecified eye
H18.9 Unspecified disorder of cornea
[4th] H20 Iridocyclitis
[5th] H20.0 Acute and subacute iridocyclitis
Acute anterior uveitis
Acute cyclitis
Acute iritis
Subacute anterior uveitis
Subacute cyclitis
Subacute iritis
[EXCLUDES1] *iridocyclitis, iritis, uveitis (due to) (in) diabetes mellitus (E08-E13 with .39)*
iridocyclitis, iritis, uveitis (due to) (in) diphtheria (A36.89)
iridocyclitis, iritis, uveitis (due to) (in) gonococcal (A54.32)
iridocyclitis, iritis, uveitis (due to) (in) herpes (simplex) (B00.51)
iridocyclitis, iritis, uveitis (due to) (in) herpes zoster (B02.32)
iridocyclitis, iritis, uveitis (due to) (in) late congenital syphilis (A50.39)
iridocyclitis, iritis, uveitis (due to) (in) late syphilis (A52.71)
iridocyclitis, iritis, uveitis (due to) (in) sarcoidosis (D86.83)
iridocyclitis, iritis, uveitis (due to) (in) syphilis (A51.43)
iridocyclitis, iritis, uveitis (due to) (in) toxoplasmosis (B58.09)
iridocyclitis, iritis, uveitis (due to) (in) tuberculosis (A18.54)
H20.00 Unspecified acute and subacute iridocyclitis [CC] [CC/MCC Exc]
[6th] H20.01 Primary iridocyclitis
H20.011 Primary iridocyclitis, right eye [CC] [CC/MCC Exc]
H20.012 Primary iridocyclitis, left eye [CC] [CC/MCC Exc]
H20.013 Primary iridocyclitis, bilateral [CC] [CC/MCC Exc]
H20.019 Primary iridocyclitis, unspecified eye [CC] [CC/MCC Exc]
[6th] H20.02 Recurrent acute iridocyclitis
H20.021 Recurrent acute iridocyclitis, right eye [CC] [CC/MCC Exc]
H20.022 Recurrent acute iridocyclitis, left eye [CC] [CC/MCC Exc]
H20.023 Recurrent acute iridocyclitis, bilateral [CC] [CC/MCC Exc]

[PDx] Unacceptable principal diagnosis symbol per Medicare code edits [POA] Code exempt from diagnosis present on admission requirement
[?] Questionable admission [CC] Complication or comorbidity [CC/MCC Exc] CC/MCC exclusion [MCC] Major complication or comorbidity
[PDx CC] Principal diagnosis as its own CC [PDx MCC] Principal diagnosis as its own MCC [HCC] HCC diagnosis code [RxHCC] RxHCC diagnosis code
MACRA code [Z1] Z code as first-listed diagnosis

H20.029 Recurrent acute iridocyclitis, unspecified eye [CC] [CC/MCC Exc]

[6th] H20.03 Secondary infectious iridocyclitis
- H20.031 Secondary infectious iridocyclitis, right eye [CC] [CC/MCC Exc]
- H20.032 Secondary infectious iridocyclitis, left eye [CC] [CC/MCC Exc]
- H20.033 Secondary infectious iridocyclitis, bilateral [CC] [CC/MCC Exc]
- H20.039 Secondary infectious iridocyclitis, unspecified eye [CC] [CC/MCC Exc]

[6th] H20.04 Secondary noninfectious iridocyclitis
- H20.041 Secondary noninfectious iridocyclitis, right eye
- H20.042 Secondary noninfectious iridocyclitis, left eye
- H20.043 Secondary noninfectious iridocyclitis, bilateral
- H20.049 Secondary noninfectious iridocyclitis, unspecified eye

[6th] H20.05 Hypopyon
- H20.051 Hypopyon, right eye
- H20.052 Hypopyon, left eye
- H20.053 Hypopyon, bilateral
- H20.059 Hypopyon, unspecified eye

[5th] H20.1 Chronic iridocyclitis

Use additional code for any associated cataract (H26.21-)

[EXCLUDES2] *posterior cyclitis (H30.2-)*
- H20.10 Chronic iridocyclitis, unspecified eye
- H20.11 Chronic iridocyclitis, right eye
- H20.12 Chronic iridocyclitis, left eye
- H20.13 Chronic iridocyclitis, bilateral

[5th] H20.2 Lens-induced iridocyclitis
- H20.20 Lens-induced iridocyclitis, unspecified eye
- H20.21 Lens-induced iridocyclitis, right eye
- H20.22 Lens-induced iridocyclitis, left eye
- H20.23 Lens-induced iridocyclitis, bilateral

[5th] H20.8 Other iridocyclitis

[EXCLUDES2] *glaucomatocyclitis crises (H40.4-)*
posterior cyclitis (H30.2-)
sympathetic uveitis (H44.13-)

[6th] H20.81 Fuchs' heterochromic cyclitis
- H20.811 Fuchs' heterochromic cyclitis, right eye
- H20.812 Fuchs' heterochromic cyclitis, left eye
- H20.813 Fuchs' heterochromic cyclitis, bilateral
- H20.819 Fuchs' heterochromic cyclitis, unspecified eye

[6th] H20.82 Vogt-Koyanagi syndrome
- H20.821 Vogt-Koyanagi syndrome, right eye
- H20.822 Vogt-Koyanagi syndrome, left eye
- H20.823 Vogt-Koyanagi syndrome, bilateral
- H20.829 Vogt-Koyanagi syndrome, unspecified eye

H20.9 Unspecified iridocyclitis [CC] [CC/MCC Exc]

Uveitis NOS

[4th] H21 Other disorders of iris and ciliary body

[EXCLUDES2] *sympathetic uveitis (H44.1-)*

[5th] H21.0 Hyphema

[EXCLUDES1] *traumatic hyphema (S05.1-)*
- H21.00 Hyphema, unspecified eye
- H21.01 Hyphema, right eye
- H21.02 Hyphema, left eye
- H21.03 Hyphema, bilateral

[5th] H21.1 Other vascular disorders of iris and ciliary body

Neovascularization of iris or ciliary body
Rubeosis iridis
Rubeosis of iris

[6th] H21.1X Other vascular disorders of iris and ciliary body
- H21.1X1 Other vascular disorders of iris and ciliary body, right eye
- H21.1X2 Other vascular disorders of iris and ciliary body, left eye
- H21.1X3 Other vascular disorders of iris and ciliary body, bilateral
- H21.1X9 Other vascular disorders of iris and ciliary body, unspecified eye

[5th] H21.2 Degeneration of iris and ciliary body

[6th] H21.21 Degeneration of chamber angle
- H21.211 Degeneration of chamber angle, right eye
- H21.212 Degeneration of chamber angle, left eye
- H21.213 Degeneration of chamber angle, bilateral
- H21.219 Degeneration of chamber angle, unspecified eye

[6th] H21.22 Degeneration of ciliary body
- H21.221 Degeneration of ciliary body, right eye
- H21.222 Degeneration of ciliary body, left eye
- H21.223 Degeneration of ciliary body, bilateral
- H21.229 Degeneration of ciliary body, unspecified eye

[6th] H21.23 Degeneration of iris (pigmentary)

Translucency of iris
- H21.231 Degeneration of iris (pigmentary), right eye
- H21.232 Degeneration of iris (pigmentary), left eye
- H21.233 Degeneration of iris (pigmentary), bilateral
- H21.239 Degeneration of iris (pigmentary), unspecified eye

[6th] H21.24 Degeneration of pupillary margin
- H21.241 Degeneration of pupillary margin, right eye
- H21.242 Degeneration of pupillary margin, left eye
- H21.243 Degeneration of pupillary margin, bilateral
- H21.249 Degeneration of pupillary margin, unspecified eye

[6th] H21.25 Iridoschisis
- H21.251 Iridoschisis, right eye
- H21.252 Iridoschisis, left eye
- H21.253 Iridoschisis, bilateral
- H21.259 Iridoschisis, unspecified eye

[6th] H21.26 Iris atrophy (essential) (progressive)
- H21.261 Iris atrophy (essential) (progressive), right eye
- H21.262 Iris atrophy (essential) (progressive), left eye
- H21.263 Iris atrophy (essential) (progressive), bilateral
- H21.269 Iris atrophy (essential) (progressive), unspecified eye

[6th] H21.27 Miotic pupillary cyst
- H21.271 Miotic pupillary cyst, right eye
- H21.272 Miotic pupillary cyst, left eye
- H21.273 Miotic pupillary cyst, bilateral
- H21.279 Miotic pupillary cyst, unspecified eye

H21.29 Other iris atrophy

[5th] H21.3 Cyst of iris, ciliary body and anterior chamber

[EXCLUDES2] *miotic pupillary cyst (H21.27-)*

[6th] H21.30 Idiopathic cysts of iris, ciliary body or anterior chamber

Cyst of iris, ciliary body or anterior chamber NOS
- H21.301 Idiopathic cysts of iris, ciliary body or anterior chamber, right eye
- H21.302 Idiopathic cysts of iris, ciliary body or anterior chamber, left eye
- H21.303 Idiopathic cysts of iris, ciliary body or anterior chamber, bilateral
- H21.309 Idiopathic cysts of iris, ciliary body or anterior chamber, unspecified eye

[6th] H21.31 Exudative cysts of iris or anterior chamber

H21.311 Exudative cysts of iris or anterior chamber, right eye

H21.312 Exudative cysts of iris or anterior chamber, left eye

H21.313 Exudative cysts of iris or anterior chamber, bilateral

H21.319 Exudative cysts of iris or anterior chamber, unspecified eye

5ᵗʰ H21.32 Implantation cysts of iris, ciliary body or anterior chamber

H21.321 Implantation cysts of iris, ciliary body or anterior chamber, right eye

H21.322 Implantation cysts of iris, ciliary body or anterior chamber, left eye

H21.323 Implantation cysts of iris, ciliary body or anterior chamber, bilateral

H21.329 Implantation cysts of iris, ciliary body or anterior chamber, unspecified eye

5ᵗʰ H21.33 Parasitic cyst of iris, ciliary body or anterior chamber

H21.331 Parasitic cyst of iris, ciliary body or anterior chamber, right eye   cc CC/MCC Exc

H21.332 Parasitic cyst of iris, ciliary body or anterior chamber, left eye   cc CC/MCC Exc

H21.333 Parasitic cyst of iris, ciliary body or anterior chamber, bilateral   cc CC/MCC Exc

H21.339 Parasitic cyst of iris, ciliary body or anterior chamber, unspecified eye   cc CC/MCC Exc

5ᵗʰ H21.34 Primary cyst of pars plana

H21.341 Primary cyst of pars plana, right eye

H21.342 Primary cyst of pars plana, left eye

H21.343 Primary cyst of pars plana, bilateral

H21.349 Primary cyst of pars plana, unspecified eye

5ᵗʰ H21.35 Exudative cyst of pars plana

H21.351 Exudative cyst of pars plana, right eye

H21.352 Exudative cyst of pars plana, left eye

H21.353 Exudative cyst of pars plana, bilateral

H21.359 Exudative cyst of pars plana, unspecified eye

5ᵗʰ H21.4 Pupillary membranes

Iris bombé
Pupillary occlusion
Pupillary seclusion
EXCLUDES1 congenital pupillary membranes (Q13.8)

H21.40 Pupillary membranes, unspecified eye

H21.41 Pupillary membranes, right eye

H21.42 Pupillary membranes, left eye

H21.43 Pupillary membranes, bilateral

5ᵗʰ H21.5 Other and unspecified adhesions and disruptions of iris and ciliary body

EXCLUDES1 corectopia (Q13.2)

5ᵗʰ H21.50 Unspecified adhesions of iris

Synechia (iris) NOS

H21.501 Unspecified adhesions of iris, right eye

H21.502 Unspecified adhesions of iris, left eye

H21.503 Unspecified adhesions of iris, bilateral

H21.509 Unspecified adhesions of iris and ciliary body, unspecified eye

5ᵗʰ H21.51 Anterior synechiae (iris)

H21.511 Anterior synechiae (iris), right eye

H21.512 Anterior synechiae (iris), left eye

H21.513 Anterior synechiae (iris), bilateral

H21.519 Anterior synechiae (iris), unspecified eye

5ᵗʰ H21.52 Goniosynechiae

H21.521 Goniosynechiae, right eye

H21.522 Goniosynechiae, left eye

H21.523 Goniosynechiae, bilateral

H21.529 Goniosynechiae, unspecified eye

5ᵗʰ H21.53 Iridodialysis

H21.531 Iridodialysis, right eye

H21.532 Iridodialysis, left eye

H21.533 Iridodialysis, bilateral

H21.539 Iridodialysis, unspecified eye

6ᵗʰ H21.54 Posterior synechiae (iris)

H21.541 Posterior synechiae (iris), right eye

H21.542 Posterior synechiae (iris), left eye

H21.543 Posterior synechiae (iris), bilateral

H21.549 Posterior synechiae (iris), unspecified eye

6ᵗʰ H21.55 Recession of chamber angle

H21.551 Recession of chamber angle, right eye

H21.552 Recession of chamber angle, left eye

H21.553 Recession of chamber angle, bilateral

H21.559 Recession of chamber angle, unspecified eye

6ᵗʰ H21.56 Pupillary abnormalities

Deformed pupil
Ectopic pupil
Rupture of sphincter, pupil
EXCLUDES1 congenital deformity of pupil (Q13.2-)

H21.561 Pupillary abnormality, right eye

H21.562 Pupillary abnormality, left eye

H21.563 Pupillary abnormality, bilateral

H21.569 Pupillary abnormality, unspecified eye

5ᵗʰ H21.8 Other specified disorders of iris and ciliary body

H21.81 Floppy iris syndrome

Intraoperative floppy iris syndrome (IFIS)
Use additional code for adverse effect, if applicable, to identify drug (T36-T50 with fifth or sixth character 5)

H21.82 Plateau iris syndrome (post-iridectomy) (postprocedural)

H21.89 Other specified disorders of iris and ciliary body

H21.9 Unspecified disorder of iris and ciliary body

H22 Disorders of iris and ciliary body in diseases classified elsewhere

Code first underlying disease, such as:
gout (M1A.-, M10.-)
leprosy (A30.-)
parasitic disease (B89)

Disorders of lens (H25-H28)

4ᵗʰ H25 Age-related cataract

Senile cataract
EXCLUDES2 capsular glaucoma with pseudoexfoliation of lens (H40.1-)

5ᵗʰ H25.0 Age-related incipient cataract

6ᵗʰ H25.01 Cortical age-related cataract

H25.011 Cortical age-related cataract, right eye   A

H25.012 Cortical age-related cataract, left eye   A

H25.013 Cortical age-related cataract, bilateral   A

H25.019 Cortical age-related cataract, unspecified eye   A

6ᵗʰ H25.03 Anterior subcapsular polar age-related cataract

H25.031 Anterior subcapsular polar age-related cataract, right eye   A

H25.032 Anterior subcapsular polar age-related cataract, left eye   A

H25.033 Anterior subcapsular polar age-related cataract, bilateral   A

H25.039 Anterior subcapsular polar age-related cataract, unspecified eye   A

6ᵗʰ H25.04 Posterior subcapsular polar age-related cataract

H25.041 Posterior subcapsular polar age-related cataract, right eye   A

H25.042 Posterior subcapsular polar age-related cataract, left eye   A

H25.043 Posterior subcapsular polar age-related cataract, bilateral   A

H25.049 Posterior subcapsular polar age-related cataract, unspecified eye   A

PDₓ Unacceptable principal diagnosis symbol per Medicare code edits   Code exempt from diagnosis present on admission requirement
? Questionable admission   cc Complication or comorbidity   CC/MCC Exc CC/MCC exclusion   MCC Major complication or comorbidity
Principal diagnosis as its own CC   Principal diagnosis as its own MCC   HCC HCC diagnosis code   RxHCC RxHCC diagnosis code
MACRA code   Z1 Z code as first-listed diagnosis

[6th] H25.09 Other age-related incipient cataract
Coronary age-related cataract
Punctate age-related cataract
Water clefts
H25.091 Other age-related incipient cataract, right eye [A]
H25.092 Other age-related incipient cataract, left eye [A]
H25.093 Other age-related incipient cataract, bilateral [A]
H25.099 Other age-related incipient cataract, unspecified eye [A]

[5th] H25.1 Age-related nuclear cataract
Cataracta brunescens
Nuclear sclerosis cataract
H25.10 Age-related nuclear cataract, unspecified eye [A]
H25.11 Age-related nuclear cataract, right eye [A]
H25.12 Age-related nuclear cataract, left eye [A]
AHA: Q1 2016
H25.13 Age-related nuclear cataract, bilateral [A]
AHA: Q1 2016

[5th] H25.2 Age-related cataract, morgagnian type
Age-related hypermature cataract
H25.20 Age-related cataract, morgagnian type, unspecified eye [A]
H25.21 Age-related cataract, morgagnian type, right eye [A]
H25.22 Age-related cataract, morgagnian type, left eye [A]
H25.23 Age-related cataract, morgagnian type, bilateral [A]

[5th] H25.8 Other age-related cataract
[6th] H25.81 Combined forms of age-related cataract
H25.811 Combined forms of age-related cataract, right eye [A]
H25.812 Combined forms of age-related cataract, left eye [A]
H25.813 Combined forms of age-related cataract, bilateral [A]
H25.819 Combined forms of age-related cataract, unspecified eye [A]
H25.89 Other age-related cataract [A]
H25.9 Unspecified age-related cataract [A]

[4th] H26 Other cataract
EXCLUDES1 *congenital cataract (Q12.0)*

[5th] H26.0 Infantile and juvenile cataract
[6th] H26.00 Unspecified infantile and juvenile cataract
H26.001 Unspecified infantile and juvenile cataract, right eye [P]
H26.002 Unspecified infantile and juvenile cataract, left eye [P]
H26.003 Unspecified infantile and juvenile cataract, bilateral [P]
H26.009 Unspecified infantile and juvenile cataract, unspecified eye [P]
[6th] H26.01 Infantile and juvenile cortical, lamellar, or zonular cataract
H26.011 Infantile and juvenile cortical, lamellar, or zonular cataract, right eye [P]
H26.012 Infantile and juvenile cortical, lamellar, or zonular cataract, left eye [P]
H26.013 Infantile and juvenile cortical, lamellar, or zonular cataract, bilateral [P]
H26.019 Infantile and juvenile cortical, lamellar, or zonular cataract, unspecified eye [P]
[6th] H26.03 Infantile and juvenile nuclear cataract
H26.031 Infantile and juvenile nuclear cataract, right eye [P]
H26.032 Infantile and juvenile nuclear cataract, left eye [P]
H26.033 Infantile and juvenile nuclear cataract, bilateral [P]
H26.039 Infantile and juvenile nuclear cataract, unspecified eye [P]
[6th] H26.04 Anterior subcapsular polar infantile and juvenile cataract
H26.041 Anterior subcapsular polar infantile and juvenile cataract, right eye [P]
H26.042 Anterior subcapsular polar infantile and juvenile cataract, left eye [P]
H26.043 Anterior subcapsular polar infantile and juvenile cataract, bilateral [P]
H26.049 Anterior subcapsular polar infantile and juvenile cataract, unspecified eye [P]
[6th] H26.05 Posterior subcapsular polar infantile and juvenile cataract
H26.051 Posterior subcapsular polar infantile and juvenile cataract, right eye [P]
H26.052 Posterior subcapsular polar infantile and juvenile cataract, left eye [P]
H26.053 Posterior subcapsular polar infantile and juvenile cataract, bilateral [P]
H26.059 Posterior subcapsular polar infantile and juvenile cataract, unspecified eye [P]
[6th] H26.06 Combined forms of infantile and juvenile cataract
H26.061 Combined forms of infantile and juvenile cataract, right eye [P]
H26.062 Combined forms of infantile and juvenile cataract, left eye [P]
H26.063 Combined forms of infantile and juvenile cataract, bilateral [P]
H26.069 Combined forms of infantile and juvenile cataract, unspecified eye [P]
H26.09 Other infantile and juvenile cataract [P]

[5th] H26.1 Traumatic cataract
Use additional code (Chapter 20) to identify external cause
[6th] H26.10 Unspecified traumatic cataract
H26.101 Unspecified traumatic cataract, right eye
H26.102 Unspecified traumatic cataract, left eye
H26.103 Unspecified traumatic cataract, bilateral
H26.109 Unspecified traumatic cataract, unspecified eye
[6th] H26.11 Localized traumatic opacities
H26.111 Localized traumatic opacities, right eye
H26.112 Localized traumatic opacities, left eye
H26.113 Localized traumatic opacities, bilateral
H26.119 Localized traumatic opacities, unspecified eye
[6th] H26.12 Partially resolved traumatic cataract
H26.121 Partially resolved traumatic cataract, right eye
H26.122 Partially resolved traumatic cataract, left eye
H26.123 Partially resolved traumatic cataract, bilateral
H26.129 Partially resolved traumatic cataract, unspecified eye
[6th] H26.13 Total traumatic cataract
H26.131 Total traumatic cataract, right eye
H26.132 Total traumatic cataract, left eye
H26.133 Total traumatic cataract, bilateral
H26.139 Total traumatic cataract, unspecified eye

[5th] H26.2 Complicated cataract
H26.20 Unspecified complicated cataract
Cataracta complicata NOS
[6th] H26.21 Cataract with neovascularization
Code also associated condition, such as:
chronic iridocyclitis (H20.1-)
H26.211 Cataract with neovascularization, right eye
H26.212 Cataract with neovascularization, left eye
H26.213 Cataract with neovascularization, bilateral
H26.219 Cataract with neovascularization, unspecified eye

Unspecified Code | Other Specified Code | Manifestation Code | [N] Newborn | [P] Pediatric | [M] Maternity | [A] Adult | ♂ Male | ♀ Female
● New Code ▲ Revised Code Title ►◄ Revised Text NOTES INCLUDES EXCLUDES1 Not coded here EXCLUDES2 Not included here
[4th] 4th character required [5th] 5th character required [6th] 6th character required [7th] 7th character required
[x] Extension 'X' Alert [HAC] Hospital-acquired condition (HAC) alert AHA AHA Coding Clinic©

When symbols appear on a code that requires a 7th character extension, refer to Appendix B to identify applicable 7th character codes.

H35.439 Paving stone degeneration of retina, unspecified eye

🔵 H35.44 Age-related reticular degeneration of retina

H35.441 Age-related reticular degeneration of retina, right eye Ⓐ

H35.442 Age-related reticular degeneration of retina, left eye Ⓐ

H35.443 Age-related reticular degeneration of retina, bilateral Ⓐ

H35.449 Age-related reticular degeneration of retina, unspecified eye Ⓐ

🔵 H35.45 Secondary pigmentary degeneration

H35.451 Secondary pigmentary degeneration, right eye

H35.452 Secondary pigmentary degeneration, left eye

H35.453 Secondary pigmentary degeneration, bilateral

H35.459 Secondary pigmentary degeneration, unspecified eye

🔵 H35.46 Secondary vitreoretinal degeneration

H35.461 Secondary vitreoretinal degeneration, right eye

H35.462 Secondary vitreoretinal degeneration, left eye

H35.463 Secondary vitreoretinal degeneration, bilateral

H35.469 Secondary vitreoretinal degeneration, unspecified eye

🔵 H35.5 Hereditary retinal dystrophy

EXCLUDES1 dystrophies primarily involving Bruch's membrane (H31.1-)

H35.50 Unspecified hereditary retinal dystrophy

H35.51 Vitreoretinal dystrophy

H35.52 Pigmentary retinal dystrophy

Albipunctate retinal dystrophy
Retinitis pigmentosa
Tapetoretinal dystrophy

H35.53 Other dystrophies primarily involving the sensory retina

Stargardt's disease

H35.54 Dystrophies primarily involving the retinal pigment epithelium

Vitelliform retinal dystrophy

🔵 H35.6 Retinal hemorrhage

H35.60 Retinal hemorrhage, unspecified eye

H35.61 Retinal hemorrhage, right eye

H35.62 Retinal hemorrhage, left eye

H35.63 Retinal hemorrhage, bilateral

🔵 H35.7 Separation of retinal layers

EXCLUDES1 retinal detachment (serous) (H33.2-)

rhegmatogenous retinal detachment (H33.0-)

H35.70 Unspecified separation of retinal layers CC CC/MCC Exc

🔵 H35.71 Central serous chorioretinopathy

H35.711 Central serous chorioretinopathy, right eye

H35.712 Central serous chorioretinopathy, left eye

H35.713 Central serous chorioretinopathy, bilateral

H35.719 Central serous chorioretinopathy, unspecified eye

🔵 H35.72 Serous detachment of retinal pigment epithelium

H35.721 Serous detachment of retinal pigment epithelium, right eye CC CC/MCC Exc

H35.722 Serous detachment of retinal pigment epithelium, left eye CC CC/MCC Exc

H35.723 Serous detachment of retinal pigment epithelium, bilateral CC CC/MCC Exc

H35.729 Serous detachment of retinal pigment epithelium, unspecified eye CC CC/MCC Exc

🔵 H35.73 Hemorrhagic detachment of retinal pigment epithelium

H35.731 Hemorrhagic detachment of retinal pigment epithelium, right eye CC CC/MCC Exc

H35.732 Hemorrhagic detachment of retinal pigment epithelium, left eye CC CC/MCC Exc

H35.733 Hemorrhagic detachment of retinal pigment epithelium, bilateral CC CC/MCC Exc

H35.739 Hemorrhagic detachment of retinal pigment epithelium, unspecified eye CC CC/MCC Exc

🔵 H35.8 Other specified retinal disorders

EXCLUDES2 retinal hemorrhage (H35.6-)

H35.81 Retinal edema

Retinal cotton wool spots

H35.82 Retinal ischemia CC CC/MCC Exc

H35.89 Other specified retinal disorders

H35.9 Unspecified retinal disorder

H36 Retinal disorders in diseases classified elsewhere

Code first underlying disease, such as:
lipid storage disorders (E75.-)
sickle-cell disorders (D57.-)

EXCLUDES1 arteriosclerotic retinopathy (H35.0-)

diabetic retinopathy (E08.3-, E09.3-, E10.3-, E11.3-, E13.3-)

Glaucoma (H40-H42)

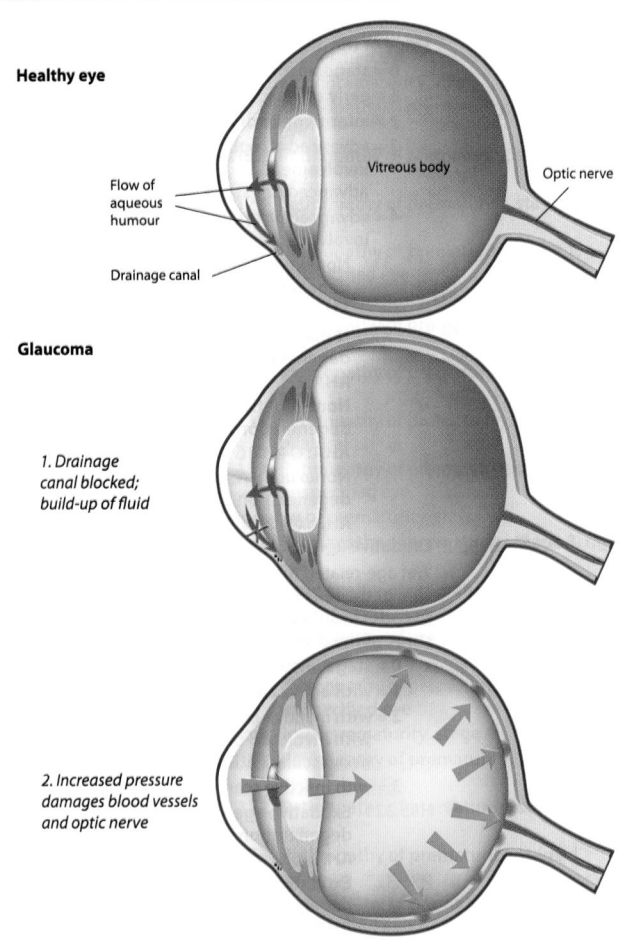

Healthy eye

Flow of aqueous humour

Drainage canal

Vitreous body

Optic nerve

Glaucoma

1. Drainage canal blocked; build-up of fluid

2. Increased pressure damages blood vessels and optic nerve

Figure 7.4 Development of glaucoma

🔵 H40 Glaucoma

EXCLUDES1 absolute glaucoma (H44.51-)

congenital glaucoma (Q15.0)

traumatic glaucoma due to birth injury (P15.3)

PDxₐ Unacceptable principal diagnosis symbol per Medicare code edits   POA Code exempt from diagnosis present on admission requirement
❓ Questionable admission   CC Complication or comorbidity   CC/MCC Exc CC/MCC exclusion   MCC Major complication or comorbidity
CC Principal diagnosis as its own CC   MCC Principal diagnosis as its own MCC   HCC HCC diagnosis code   RxHCC RxHCC diagnosis code
MACRA code   Z1 Z code as first-listed diagnosis

When symbols appear on a code that requires a 7th character extension, refer to Appendix B to identify applicable 7th character codes.

[5th] H40.0 Glaucoma suspect
- [6th] H40.00 Preglaucoma, unspecified
  - H40.001 Preglaucoma, unspecified, right eye
  - H40.002 Preglaucoma, unspecified, left eye
  - H40.003 Preglaucoma, unspecified, bilateral
  - H40.009 Preglaucoma, unspecified, unspecified eye
- [6th] H40.01 Open angle with borderline findings, low risk
  Open angle, low risk
  - H40.011 Open angle with borderline findings, low risk, right eye
  - H40.012 Open angle with borderline findings, low risk, left eye
  - H40.013 Open angle with borderline findings, low risk, bilateral
  - H40.019 Open angle with borderline findings, low risk, unspecified eye
- [6th] H40.02 Open angle with borderline findings, high risk
  Open angle, high risk
  - H40.021 Open angle with borderline findings, high risk, right eye
  - H40.022 Open angle with borderline findings, high risk, left eye
  - H40.023 Open angle with borderline findings, high risk, bilateral
  - H40.029 Open angle with borderline findings, high risk, unspecified eye
- [6th] H40.03 Anatomical narrow angle
  Primary angle closure suspect
  - H40.031 Anatomical narrow angle, right eye
  - H40.032 Anatomical narrow angle, left eye
  - H40.033 Anatomical narrow angle, bilateral
  - H40.039 Anatomical narrow angle, unspecified eye
- [6th] H40.04 Steroid responder
  - H40.041 Steroid responder, right eye
  - H40.042 Steroid responder, left eye
  - H40.043 Steroid responder, bilateral
  - H40.049 Steroid responder, unspecified eye
- [6th] H40.05 Ocular hypertension
  - H40.051 Ocular hypertension, right eye
  - H40.052 Ocular hypertension, left eye
  - H40.053 Ocular hypertension, bilateral
  - H40.059 Ocular hypertension, unspecified eye
- [6th] H40.06 Primary angle closure without glaucoma damage
  - H40.061 Primary angle closure without glaucoma damage, right eye
  - H40.062 Primary angle closure without glaucoma damage, left eye
  - H40.063 Primary angle closure without glaucoma damage, bilateral
  - H40.069 Primary angle closure without glaucoma damage, unspecified eye

[5th] H40.1 Open-angle glaucoma
- [7th] H40.10 Unspecified open-angle glaucoma [RxHCC]
  One of the following 7th characters is to be assigned to code H40.10 to designate the stage of glaucoma
  - 0 = stage unspecified
  - 1 = mild stage
  - 2 = moderate stage
  - 3 = severe stage
  - 4 = indeterminate stage
- [6th] H40.11 Primary open-angle glaucoma [RxHCC]
  Chronic simple glaucoma
  One of the following 7th characters is to be assigned to each code in subcategory H40.11 to designate the stage of glaucoma
  - 0 = stage unspecified
  - 1 = mild stage
  - 2 = moderate stage
  - 3 = severe stage
  - 4 = indeterminate stage
  - [7th] H40.111 Primary open-angle glaucoma, right eye [RxHCC]
    AHA: Q4 2016
  - [7th] H40.112 Primary open-angle glaucoma, left eye [RxHCC]
    AHA: Q4 2016
  - [7th] H40.113 Primary open-angle glaucoma, bilateral [RxHCC]
    AHA: Q4 2016
  - [7th] H40.119 Primary open-angle glaucoma, unspecified eye [RxHCC]
    AHA: Q4 2016
- [6th] H40.12 Low-tension glaucoma
  One of the following 7th characters is to be assigned to each code in subcategory H40.12 to designate the stage of glaucoma
  - 0 = stage unspecified
  - 1 = mild stage
  - 2 = moderate stage
  - 3 = severe stage
  - 4 = indeterminate stage
  - [7th] H40.121 Low-tension glaucoma, right eye [RxHCC] [PDx]
  - [7th] H40.122 Low-tension glaucoma, left eye [RxHCC] [PDx]
  - [7th] H40.123 Low-tension glaucoma, bilateral [RxHCC] [PDx]
  - [7th] H40.129 Low-tension glaucoma, unspecified eye [RxHCC] [PDx]
- [6th] H40.13 Pigmentary glaucoma
  One of the following 7th characters is to be assigned to each code in subcategory H40.13 to designate the stage of glaucoma
  - 0 = stage unspecified
  - 1 = mild stage
  - 2 = moderate stage
  - 3 = severe stage
  - 4 = indeterminate stage
  - [7th] H40.131 Pigmentary glaucoma, right eye [RxHCC] [PDx]
  - [7th] H40.132 Pigmentary glaucoma, left eye [RxHCC] [PDx]
  - [7th] H40.133 Pigmentary glaucoma, bilateral [RxHCC] [PDx]
  - [7th] H40.139 Pigmentary glaucoma, unspecified eye [RxHCC] [PDx]
- [6th] H40.14 Capsular glaucoma with pseudoexfoliation of lens
  One of the following 7th characters is to be assigned to each code in subcategory H40.14 to designate the stage of glaucoma
  - 0 = stage unspecified
  - 1 = mild stage
  - 2 = moderate stage
  - 3 = severe stage
  - 4 = indeterminate stage
  - [7th] H40.141 Capsular glaucoma with pseudoexfoliation of lens, right eye
  - [7th] H40.142 Capsular glaucoma with pseudoexfoliation of lens, left eye
  - [7th] H40.143 Capsular glaucoma with pseudoexfoliation of lens, bilateral
  - [7th] H40.149 Capsular glaucoma with pseudoexfoliation of lens, unspecified eye
- [6th] H40.15 Residual stage of open-angle glaucoma
  - H40.151 Residual stage of open-angle glaucoma, right eye [RxHCC] [PDx]
  - H40.152 Residual stage of open-angle glaucoma, left eye [RxHCC] [PDx]
  - H40.153 Residual stage of open-angle glaucoma, bilateral [RxHCC] [PDx]
  - H40.159 Residual stage of open-angle glaucoma, unspecified eye [RxHCC] [PDx]

[5th] H40.2 Primary angle-closure glaucoma

[EXCLUDES1] *aqueous misdirection (H40.83-)*
malignant glaucoma (H40.83-)

Unspecified Code | Other Specified Code | Manifestation Code | [N] Newborn | [P] Pediatric | [M] Maternity | [A] Adult | ♂ Male | ♀ Female
● New Code | ▲ Revised Code Title | ►◄ Revised Text | [NOTES] | [INCLUDES] | [EXCLUDES1] Not coded here | [EXCLUDES2] Not included here
[4th] 4th character required | [5th] 5th character required | [6th] 6th character required | [7th] 7th character required
[x7th] Extension 'X' Alert | [HAC] Hospital-acquired condition (HAC) alert | AHA AHA Coding Clinic©

7ᵗʰ **H40.20 Unspecified primary angle-closure glaucoma**
    One of the following 7th characters is to be assigned to code H40.20 to designate the stage of glaucoma
        0 = stage unspecified
        1 = mild stage
        2 = moderate stage
        3 = severe stage
        4 = indeterminate stage

6ᵗʰ **H40.21** Acute angle-closure glaucoma
    Acute angle-closure glaucoma attack
    Acute angle-closure glaucoma crisis
    H40.211 Acute angle-closure glaucoma, right eye   CC CC/MCC Exc
    H40.212 Acute angle-closure glaucoma, left eye   CC CC/MCC Exc
    H40.213 Acute angle-closure glaucoma, bilateral   CC CC/MCC Exc
    H40.219 Acute angle-closure glaucoma, unspecified eye   CC CC/MCC Exc

6ᵗʰ **H40.22** Chronic angle-closure glaucoma
    Chronic primary angle closure glaucoma
    One of the following 7th characters is to be assigned to each code in subcategory H40.22 to designate the stage of glaucoma
        0 = stage unspecified
        1 = mild stage
        2 = moderate stage
        3 = severe stage
        4 = indeterminate stage
  7ᵗʰ H40.221 Chronic angle-closure glaucoma, right eye
  7ᵗʰ H40.222 Chronic angle-closure glaucoma, left eye
  7ᵗʰ H40.223 Chronic angle-closure glaucoma, bilateral
  7ᵗʰ H40.229 Chronic angle-closure glaucoma, unspecified eye

6ᵗʰ **H40.23** Intermittent angle-closure glaucoma
    H40.231 Intermittent angle-closure glaucoma, right eye
    H40.232 Intermittent angle-closure glaucoma, left eye
    H40.233 Intermittent angle-closure glaucoma, bilateral
    H40.239 Intermittent angle-closure glaucoma, unspecified eye

6ᵗʰ **H40.24** Residual stage of angle-closure glaucoma
    H40.241 Residual stage of angle-closure glaucoma, right eye
    H40.242 Residual stage of angle-closure glaucoma, left eye
    H40.243 Residual stage of angle-closure glaucoma, bilateral
    H40.249 Residual stage of angle-closure glaucoma, unspecified eye

5ᵗʰ **H40.3** Glaucoma secondary to eye trauma
    Code also underlying condition
    One of the following 7th characters is to be assigned to each code in subcategory H40.3 to designate the stage of glaucoma
        0 = stage unspecified
        1 = mild stage
        2 = moderate stage
        3 = severe stage
        4 = indeterminate stage
  7ᵗʰ H40.30 Glaucoma secondary to eye trauma, unspecified eye
  7ᵗʰ H40.31 Glaucoma secondary to eye trauma, right eye
  7ᵗʰ H40.32 Glaucoma secondary to eye trauma, left eye
  7ᵗʰ H40.33 Glaucoma secondary to eye trauma, bilateral

5ᵗʰ **H40.4** Glaucoma secondary to eye inflammation
    Code also underlying condition
    One of the following 7th characters is to be assigned to each code in subcategory H40.4 to designate the stage of glaucoma

        0 = stage unspecified
        1 = mild stage
        2 = moderate stage
        3 = severe stage
        4 = indeterminate stage
  7ᵗʰ **H40.40 Glaucoma secondary to eye inflammation, unspecified eye**
  7ᵗʰ H40.41 Glaucoma secondary to eye inflammation, right eye
  7ᵗʰ H40.42 Glaucoma secondary to eye inflammation, left eye
  7ᵗʰ H40.43 Glaucoma secondary to eye inflammation, bilateral

5ᵗʰ **H40.5** Glaucoma secondary to other eye disorders
    Code also underlying eye disorder
    One of the following 7th characters is to be assigned to each code in subcategory H40.5 to designate the stage of glaucoma
        0 = stage unspecified
        1 = mild stage
        2 = moderate stage
        3 = severe stage
        4 = indeterminate stage
  7ᵗʰ **H40.50 Glaucoma secondary to other eye disorders, unspecified eye**
  7ᵗʰ H40.51 Glaucoma secondary to other eye disorders, right eye
  7ᵗʰ H40.52 Glaucoma secondary to other eye disorders, left eye
  7ᵗʰ H40.53 Glaucoma secondary to other eye disorders, bilateral

5ᵗʰ **H40.6** Glaucoma secondary to drugs
    Use additional code for adverse effect, if applicable, to identify drug (T36-T50 with fifth or sixth character 5)
    One of the following 7th characters is to be assigned to each code in subcategory H40.6 to designate the stage of glaucoma
        0 = stage unspecified
        1 = mild stage
        2 = moderate stage
        3 = severe stage
        4 = indeterminate stage
  7ᵗʰ **H40.60 Glaucoma secondary to drugs, unspecified eye**
  7ᵗʰ H40.61 Glaucoma secondary to drugs, right eye
  7ᵗʰ H40.62 Glaucoma secondary to drugs, left eye
  7ᵗʰ H40.63 Glaucoma secondary to drugs, bilateral

5ᵗʰ **H40.8** Other glaucoma
  6ᵗʰ **H40.81** Glaucoma with increased episcleral venous pressure
    H40.811 Glaucoma with increased episcleral venous pressure, right eye
    H40.812 Glaucoma with increased episcleral venous pressure, left eye
    H40.813 Glaucoma with increased episcleral venous pressure, bilateral
    H40.819 Glaucoma with increased episcleral venous pressure, unspecified eye
  6ᵗʰ **H40.82** Hypersecretion glaucoma
    H40.821 Hypersecretion glaucoma, right eye
    H40.822 Hypersecretion glaucoma, left eye
    H40.823 Hypersecretion glaucoma, bilateral
    H40.829 **Hypersecretion glaucoma, unspecified eye**
  6ᵗʰ **H40.83** Aqueous misdirection
    Malignant glaucoma
    H40.831 Aqueous misdirection, right eye
    H40.832 Aqueous misdirection, left eye
    H40.833 Aqueous misdirection, bilateral
    H40.839 **Aqueous misdirection, unspecified eye**
  H40.89 **Other specified glaucoma**

H40.9 **Unspecified glaucoma**

H42 Glaucoma in diseases classified elsewhere
  Code first underlying condition, such as:
  amyloidosis (E85.-)
  aniridia (Q13.1)
  glaucoma (in) diabetes mellitus (E08.39, E09.39, E10.39, E11.39, E13.39)

PDx Unacceptable principal diagnosis symbol per Medicare code edits   POA Code exempt from diagnosis present on admission requirement
❓ Questionable admission   CC Complication or comorbidity   CC/MCC Exc CC/MCC exclusion   MCC Major complication or comorbidity
PDx CC Principal diagnosis as its own CC   PDx MCC Principal diagnosis as its own MCC   HCC HCC diagnosis code   RxHCC RxHCC diagnosis code
MACRA code   Z1 Z code as first-listed diagnosis

Lowe's syndrome (E72.03)

Reiger's anomaly (Q13.81)

specified metabolic disorder (E70-E88)

    EXCLUDES1 *glaucoma (in) onchocerciasis (B73.02)*

        glaucoma (in) syphilis (A52.71)

        glaucoma (in) tuberculous (A18.59)

Disorders of vitreous body and globe (H43-H44)

H43 Disorders of vitreous body

  H43.0 Vitreous prolapse

    EXCLUDES1 *vitreous syndrome following cataract surgery (H59.0-)*

        traumatic vitreous prolapse (S05.2-)

    H43.00 **Vitreous prolapse, unspecified eye**

    H43.01 **Vitreous prolapse, right** eye

    H43.02 **Vitreous prolapse, left** eye

    H43.03 **Vitreous prolapse, bilateral**

  H43.1 Vitreous hemorrhage

    H43.10 **Vitreous hemorrhage, unspecified eye**   HCC

    H43.11 **Vitreous hemorrhage, right** eye   HCC

    H43.12 **Vitreous hemorrhage, left** eye   HCC

    H43.13 **Vitreous hemorrhage, bilateral**   HCC

  H43.2 Crystalline deposits in vitreous body

    H43.20 **Crystalline deposits in vitreous body, unspecified eye**

    H43.21 **Crystalline deposits in vitreous body, right** eye

    H43.22 **Crystalline deposits in vitreous body, left** eye

    H43.23 **Crystalline deposits in vitreous body, bilateral**

  H43.3 Other vitreous opacities

    H43.31 Vitreous membranes and strands

      H43.311 **Vitreous membranes and strands, right** eye

      H43.312 **Vitreous membranes and strands, left** eye

      H43.313 **Vitreous membranes and strands, bilateral**

      H43.319 **Vitreous membranes and strands, unspecified eye**

    H43.39 Other vitreous opacities

      Vitreous floaters

      H43.391 **Other vitreous opacities, right** eye

      H43.392 **Other vitreous opacities, left** eye

      H43.393 **Other vitreous opacities, bilateral**

      H43.399 **Other vitreous opacities, unspecified eye**

  H43.8 Other disorders of vitreous body

    EXCLUDES1 *proliferative vitreo-retinopathy with retinal detachment (H33.4-)*

    EXCLUDES2 *vitreous abscess (H44.02-)*

    H43.81 Vitreous degeneration

      Vitreous detachment

      H43.811 **Vitreous degeneration, right** eye

      H43.812 **Vitreous degeneration, left** eye

      H43.813 **Vitreous degeneration, bilateral**

      H43.819 **Vitreous degeneration, unspecified eye**

    H43.82 Vitreomacular adhesion

      Vitreomacular traction

      H43.821 **Vitreomacular adhesion, right** eye   A

      H43.822 **Vitreomacular adhesion, left** eye   A

      H43.823 **Vitreomacular adhesion, bilateral**   A

      H43.829 **Vitreomacular adhesion, unspecified eye**   A

    H43.89 **Other disorders of vitreous body**

  H43.9 **Unspecified disorder of vitreous body**

H44 Disorders of globe

  INCLUDES *disorders affecting multiple structures of eye*

  H44.0 Purulent endophthalmitis

    Use additional code to identify organism

    EXCLUDES1 *bleb associated endophthalmitis (H59.4-)*

    H44.00 Unspecified purulent endophthalmitis

      H44.001 **Unspecified purulent endophthalmitis, right eye**   CC CC/MCC Exc

      H44.002 **Unspecified purulent endophthalmitis, left eye**   CC CC/MCC Exc

      H44.003 **Unspecified purulent endophthalmitis, bilateral**   CC CC/MCC Exc

      H44.009 **Unspecified purulent endophthalmitis, unspecified eye**   CC CC/MCC Exc

    H44.01 Panophthalmitis (acute)

      H44.011 **Panophthalmitis (acute), right** eye   CC CC/MCC Exc

      H44.012 **Panophthalmitis (acute), left** eye   CC CC/MCC Exc

      H44.013 **Panophthalmitis (acute), bilateral**   CC CC/MCC Exc

      H44.019 **Panophthalmitis (acute), unspecified eye**   CC CC/MCC Exc

    H44.02 Vitreous abscess (chronic)

      H44.021 **Vitreous abscess (chronic), right** eye   CC CC/MCC Exc

      H44.022 **Vitreous abscess (chronic), left** eye   CC CC/MCC Exc

      H44.023 **Vitreous abscess (chronic), bilateral**   CC CC/MCC Exc

      H44.029 **Vitreous abscess (chronic), unspecified eye**   CC CC/MCC Exc

  H44.1 Other endophthalmitis

    EXCLUDES1 *bleb associated endophthalmitis (H59.4-)*

    EXCLUDES2 *ophthalmia nodosa (H16.2-)*

    H44.11 Panuveitis

      H44.111 **Panuveitis, right** eye   CC CC/MCC Exc

      H44.112 **Panuveitis, left** eye   CC CC/MCC Exc

      H44.113 **Panuveitis, bilateral**   CC CC/MCC Exc

      H44.119 **Panuveitis, unspecified eye**   CC CC/MCC Exc

    H44.12 Parasitic endophthalmitis, unspecified

      H44.121 **Parasitic endophthalmitis, unspecified, right eye**   CC CC/MCC Exc

      H44.122 **Parasitic endophthalmitis, unspecified, left eye**   CC CC/MCC Exc

      H44.123 **Parasitic endophthalmitis, unspecified, bilateral**   CC CC/MCC Exc

      H44.129 **Parasitic endophthalmitis, unspecified, unspecified eye**   CC CC/MCC Exc

    H44.13 Sympathetic uveitis

      H44.131 **Sympathetic uveitis, right** eye   CC CC/MCC Exc

      H44.132 **Sympathetic uveitis, left** eye   CC CC/MCC Exc

      H44.133 **Sympathetic uveitis, bilateral**   CC CC/MCC Exc

      H44.139 **Sympathetic uveitis, unspecified eye**   CC CC/MCC Exc

    H44.19 **Other endophthalmitis**

  H44.2 Degenerative myopia

    Malignant myopia

    H44.20 **Degenerative myopia, unspecified eye**

    H44.21 **Degenerative myopia, right** eye

    H44.22 **Degenerative myopia, left** eye

    H44.23 **Degenerative myopia, bilateral**

    ● **H44.2A** Degenerative myopia with choroidal neovascularization

      Use additional code for any associated choroid disorders (H31.-)

      ● H44.2A1 **Degenerative myopia with choroidal neovascularization, right** eye

      ● H44.2A2 **Degenerative myopia with choroidal neovascularization, left** eye

      ● H44.2A3 **Degenerative myopia with choroidal neovascularization, bilateral** eye

      ● H44.2A9 **Degenerative myopia with choroidal neovascularization, unspecified eye**

    ● **H44.2B** Degenerative myopia with macular hole

      ● H44.2B1 **Degenerative myopia with macular hole, right** eye

      ● H44.2B2 **Degenerative myopia with macular hole, left** eye

      ● H44.2B3 **Degenerative myopia with macular hole, bilateral** eye

---

Unspecified Code   Other Specified Code   Manifestation Code   N Newborn   P Pediatric   M Maternity   A Adult   ♂ Male   ♀ Female

● New Code   ▲ Revised Code Title   ▶◀ Revised Text   **NOTES**   *INCLUDES*   *EXCLUDES 1* Not coded here   *EXCLUDES 2* Not included here

4th character required   5th character required   6th character required   7th character required

Extension 'X' Alert   HAC Hospital-acquired condition (HAC) alert   **AHA** AHA Coding Clinic©

- H44.2B9 **Degenerative myopia with macular hole, unspecified eye**
- 6ᵗʰ H44.2C Degenerative myopia with retinal detachment
  Use additional code to identify the retinal detachment (H33.-)
  - H44.2C1 Degenerative myopia with retinal detachment, right eye
  - H44.2C2 Degenerative myopia with retinal detachment, left eye
  - H44.2C3 Degenerative myopia with retinal detachment, bilateral eye
  - H44.2C9 **Degenerative myopia with retinal detachment, unspecified eye**
- 6ᵗʰ H44.2D Degenerative myopia with foveoschisis
  - H44.2D1 Degenerative myopia with foveoschisis, right eye
  - H44.2D2 Degenerative myopia with foveoschisis, left eye
  - H44.2D3 Degenerative myopia with foveoschisis, bilateral eye
  - H44.2D9 **Degenerative myopia with foveoschisis, unspecified eye**
- 6ᵗʰ H44.2E Degenerative myopia with other maculopathy
  - H44.2E1 Degenerative myopia with other maculopathy, right eye
  - H44.2E2 Degenerative myopia with other maculopathy, left eye
  - H44.2E3 Degenerative myopia with other maculopathy, bilateral eye
  - H44.2E9 **Degenerative myopia with other maculopathy, unspecified eye**

5ᵗʰ H44.3 Other and unspecified degenerative disorders of globe

H44.30 **Unspecified degenerative disorder of globe**

6ᵗʰ H44.31 Chalcosis

H44.311 Chalcosis, right eye

H44.312 Chalcosis, left eye

H44.313 Chalcosis, bilateral

H44.319 **Chalcosis, unspecified eye**

6ᵗʰ H44.32 Siderosis of eye

H44.321 Siderosis of eye, right eye

H44.322 Siderosis of eye, left eye

H44.323 Siderosis of eye, bilateral

H44.329 **Siderosis of eye, unspecified eye**

6ᵗʰ H44.39 Other degenerative disorders of globe

H44.391 Other degenerative disorders of globe, right eye

H44.392 Other degenerative disorders of globe, left eye

H44.393 Other degenerative disorders of globe, bilateral

H44.399 **Other degenerative disorders of globe, unspecified eye**

5ᵗʰ H44.4 Hypotony of eye

H44.40 **Unspecified hypotony of eye**

6ᵗʰ H44.41 Flat anterior chamber hypotony of eye

H44.411 Flat anterior chamber hypotony of right eye

H44.412 Flat anterior chamber hypotony of left eye

H44.413 Flat anterior chamber hypotony of eye, bilateral

H44.419 **Flat anterior chamber hypotony of unspecified eye**

6ᵗʰ H44.42 Hypotony of eye due to ocular fistula

H44.421 Hypotony of right eye due to ocular fistula

H44.422 Hypotony of left eye due to ocular fistula

H44.423 Hypotony of eye due to ocular fistula, bilateral

H44.429 **Hypotony of unspecified eye due to ocular fistula**

6ᵗʰ H44.43 Hypotony of eye due to other ocular disorders

H44.431 Hypotony of eye due to other ocular disorders, right eye

H44.432 Hypotony of eye due to other ocular disorders, left eye

H44.433 Hypotony of eye due to other ocular disorders, bilateral

H44.439 **Hypotony of eye due to other ocular disorders, unspecified eye**

6ᵗʰ H44.44 Primary hypotony of eye

H44.441 Primary hypotony of right eye

H44.442 Primary hypotony of left eye

H44.443 Primary hypotony of eye, bilateral

H44.449 **Primary hypotony of unspecified eye**

5ᵗʰ H44.5 Degenerated conditions of globe

H44.50 **Unspecified degenerated conditions of globe**

6ᵗʰ H44.51 Absolute glaucoma

H44.511 Absolute glaucoma, right eye

H44.512 Absolute glaucoma, left eye

H44.513 Absolute glaucoma, bilateral

H44.519 **Absolute glaucoma, unspecified eye**

6ᵗʰ H44.52 Atrophy of globe
Phthisis bulbi

H44.521 Atrophy of globe, right eye

H44.522 Atrophy of globe, left eye

H44.523 Atrophy of globe, bilateral

H44.529 **Atrophy of globe, unspecified eye**

6ᵗʰ H44.53 Leucocoria

H44.531 Leucocoria, right eye

H44.532 Leucocoria, left eye

H44.533 Leucocoria, bilateral

H44.539 **Leucocoria, unspecified eye**

5ᵗʰ H44.6 Retained (old) intraocular foreign body, magnetic
Use additional code to identify magnetic foreign body (Z18.11)

EXCLUDES1 current intraocular foreign body (S05.-)

EXCLUDES2 retained foreign body in eyelid (H02.81-)

retained (old) foreign body following penetrating wound of orbit (H05.5-)

retained (old) intraocular foreign body, nonmagnetic (H44.7-)

6ᵗʰ H44.60 Unspecified retained (old) intraocular foreign body, magnetic

H44.601 **Unspecified retained (old) intraocular foreign body, magnetic, right eye**

H44.602 **Unspecified retained (old) intraocular foreign body, magnetic, left eye**

H44.603 **Unspecified retained (old) intraocular foreign body, magnetic, bilateral**

H44.609 **Unspecified retained (old) intraocular foreign body, magnetic, unspecified eye**

6ᵗʰ H44.61 Retained (old) magnetic foreign body in anterior chamber

H44.611 Retained (old) magnetic foreign body in anterior chamber, right eye

H44.612 Retained (old) magnetic foreign body in anterior chamber, left eye

H44.613 Retained (old) magnetic foreign body in anterior chamber, bilateral

H44.619 **Retained (old) magnetic foreign body in anterior chamber, unspecified eye**

6ᵗʰ H44.62 Retained (old) magnetic foreign body in iris or ciliary body

H44.621 Retained (old) magnetic foreign body in iris or ciliary body, right eye

H44.622 Retained (old) magnetic foreign body in iris or ciliary body, left eye

H44.623 Retained (old) magnetic foreign body in iris or ciliary body, bilateral

H44.629 **Retained (old) magnetic foreign body in iris or ciliary body, unspecified eye**

Unacceptable principal diagnosis symbol per Medicare code edits   Code exempt from diagnosis present on admission requirement
? Questionable admission   Complication or comorbidity   CC/MCC exclusion   Major complication or comorbidity
Principal diagnosis as its own CC   Principal diagnosis as its own MCC   HCC diagnosis code   RxHCC diagnosis code
MACRA code   Z code as first-listed diagnosis

6ᵗʰ H44.63 Retained (old) magnetic foreign body in lens

H44.631 Retained (old) magnetic foreign body in lens, right eye

H44.632 Retained (old) magnetic foreign body in lens, left eye

H44.633 Retained (old) magnetic foreign body in lens, bilateral

H44.639 Retained (old) magnetic foreign body in lens, unspecified eye

6ᵗʰ H44.64 Retained (old) magnetic foreign body in posterior wall of globe

H44.641 Retained (old) magnetic foreign body in posterior wall of globe, right eye

H44.642 Retained (old) magnetic foreign body in posterior wall of globe, left eye

H44.643 Retained (old) magnetic foreign body in posterior wall of globe, bilateral

H44.649 Retained (old) magnetic foreign body in posterior wall of globe, unspecified eye

6ᵗʰ H44.65 Retained (old) magnetic foreign body in vitreous body

H44.651 Retained (old) magnetic foreign body in vitreous body, right eye

H44.652 Retained (old) magnetic foreign body in vitreous body, left eye

H44.653 Retained (old) magnetic foreign body in vitreous body, bilateral

H44.659 Retained (old) magnetic foreign body in vitreous body, unspecified eye

6ᵗʰ H44.69 Retained (old) intraocular foreign body, magnetic, in other or multiple sites

H44.691 Retained (old) intraocular foreign body, magnetic, in other or multiple sites, right eye

H44.692 Retained (old) intraocular foreign body, magnetic, in other or multiple sites, left eye

H44.693 Retained (old) intraocular foreign body, magnetic, in other or multiple sites, bilateral

H44.699 Retained (old) intraocular foreign body, magnetic, in other or multiple sites, unspecified eye

5ᵗʰ H44.7 Retained (old) intraocular foreign body, nonmagnetic

Use additional code to identify nonmagnetic foreign body (Z18.01-Z18.10, Z18.12, Z18.2-Z18.9)

EXCLUDES1 current intraocular foreign body (S05.-)

EXCLUDES2 retained foreign body in eyelid (H02.81-)

retained (old) foreign body following penetrating wound of orbit (H05.5-)

retained (old) intraocular foreign body, magnetic (H44.6-)

6ᵗʰ H44.70 Unspecified retained (old) intraocular foreign body, nonmagnetic

H44.701 Unspecified retained (old) intraocular foreign body, nonmagnetic, right eye

H44.702 Unspecified retained (old) intraocular foreign body, nonmagnetic, left eye

H44.703 Unspecified retained (old) intraocular foreign body, nonmagnetic, bilateral

H44.709 Unspecified retained (old) intraocular foreign body, nonmagnetic, unspecified eye

Retained (old) intraocular foreign body NOS

5ᵗʰ H44.71 Retained (nonmagnetic) (old) foreign body in anterior chamber

H44.711 Retained (nonmagnetic) (old) foreign body in anterior chamber, right eye

H44.712 Retained (nonmagnetic) (old) foreign body in anterior chamber, left eye

H44.713 Retained (nonmagnetic) (old) foreign body in anterior chamber, bilateral

H44.719 Retained (nonmagnetic) (old) foreign body in anterior chamber, unspecified eye

6ᵗʰ H44.72 Retained (nonmagnetic) (old) foreign body in iris or ciliary body

H44.721 Retained (nonmagnetic) (old) foreign body in iris or ciliary body, right eye

H44.722 Retained (nonmagnetic) (old) foreign body in iris or ciliary body, left eye

H44.723 Retained (nonmagnetic) (old) foreign body in iris or ciliary body, bilateral

H44.729 Retained (nonmagnetic) (old) foreign body in iris or ciliary body, unspecified eye

6ᵗʰ H44.73 Retained (nonmagnetic) (old) foreign body in lens

H44.731 Retained (nonmagnetic) (old) foreign body in lens, right eye

H44.732 Retained (nonmagnetic) (old) foreign body in lens, left eye

H44.733 Retained (nonmagnetic) (old) foreign body in lens, bilateral

H44.739 Retained (nonmagnetic) (old) foreign body in lens, unspecified eye

6ᵗʰ H44.74 Retained (nonmagnetic) (old) foreign body in posterior wall of globe

H44.741 Retained (nonmagnetic) (old) foreign body in posterior wall of globe, right eye

H44.742 Retained (nonmagnetic) (old) foreign body in posterior wall of globe, left eye

H44.743 Retained (nonmagnetic) (old) foreign body in posterior wall of globe, bilateral

H44.749 Retained (nonmagnetic) (old) foreign body in posterior wall of globe, unspecified eye

6ᵗʰ H44.75 Retained (nonmagnetic) (old) foreign body in vitreous body

H44.751 Retained (nonmagnetic) (old) foreign body in vitreous body, right eye

H44.752 Retained (nonmagnetic) (old) foreign body in vitreous body, left eye

H44.753 Retained (nonmagnetic) (old) foreign body in vitreous body, bilateral

H44.759 Retained (nonmagnetic) (old) foreign body in vitreous body, unspecified eye

6ᵗʰ H44.79 Retained (old) intraocular foreign body, nonmagnetic, in other or multiple sites

H44.791 Retained (old) intraocular foreign body, nonmagnetic, in other or multiple sites, right eye

H44.792 Retained (old) intraocular foreign body, nonmagnetic, in other or multiple sites, left eye

H44.793 Retained (old) intraocular foreign body, nonmagnetic, in other or multiple sites, bilateral

H44.799 Retained (old) intraocular foreign body, nonmagnetic, in other or multiple sites, unspecified eye

5ᵗʰ H44.8 Other disorders of globe

6ᵗʰ H44.81 Hemophthalmos

H44.811 Hemophthalmos, right eye

H44.812 Hemophthalmos, left eye

H44.813 Hemophthalmos, bilateral

H44.819 Hemophthalmos, unspecified eye

6ᵗʰ H44.82 Luxation of globe

H44.821 Luxation of globe, right eye

H44.822 Luxation of globe, left eye

H44.823 Luxation of globe, bilateral

H44.829 Luxation of globe, unspecified eye

H44.89 Other disorders of globe

H44.9 Unspecified disorder of globe

Unspecified Code   Other Specified Code   Manifestation Code   N Newborn   P Pediatric   M Maternity   A Adult   ♂ Male   ♀ Female

● New Code   ▲ Revised Code Title   ►◄ Revised Text   NOTES   INCLUDES   EXCLUDES 1 Not coded here   EXCLUDES 2 Not included here

4ᵗʰ character required   5ᵗʰ character required   6ᵗʰ character required   7ᵗʰ character required

7ᵗʰ Extension 'X' Alert   HAC Hospital-acquired condition (HAC) alert   AHA AHA Coding Clinic©

Disorders of optic nerve and visual pathways (H46-H47)

[4th] **H46 Optic neuritis**
EXCLUDES2 ischemic optic neuropathy (H47.01-)
neuromyelitis optica [Devic] (G36.0)

[5th] **H46.0 Optic papillitis**
- H46.00 Optic papillitis, unspecified eye CC CC/MCC Exc
- H46.01 Optic papillitis, right eye CC CC/MCC Exc
- H46.02 Optic papillitis, left eye CC CC/MCC Exc
- H46.03 Optic papillitis, bilateral CC CC/MCC Exc

[5th] **H46.1 Retrobulbar neuritis**
Retrobulbar neuritis NOS
EXCLUDES1 syphilitic retrobulbar neuritis (A52.15)
- H46.10 Retrobulbar neuritis, unspecified eye CC CC/MCC Exc
- H46.11 Retrobulbar neuritis, right eye CC CC/MCC Exc
- H46.12 Retrobulbar neuritis, left eye CC CC/MCC Exc
- H46.13 Retrobulbar neuritis, bilateral CC CC/MCC Exc

H46.2 Nutritional optic neuropathy

H46.3 Toxic optic neuropathy
Code first (T51-T65) to identify cause

H46.8 Other optic neuritis CC CC/MCC Exc

H46.9 Unspecified optic neuritis CC CC/MCC Exc

[4th] **H47 Other disorders of optic [2nd] nerve and visual pathways**

[5th] **H47.0 Disorders of optic nerve, not elsewhere classified**

[6th] **H47.01 Ischemic optic neuropathy**
- H47.011 Ischemic optic neuropathy, right eye
- H47.012 Ischemic optic neuropathy, left eye
- H47.013 Ischemic optic neuropathy, bilateral
- H47.019 Ischemic optic neuropathy, unspecified eye

[6th] **H47.02 Hemorrhage in optic nerve sheath**
- H47.021 Hemorrhage in optic nerve sheath, right eye
- H47.022 Hemorrhage in optic nerve sheath, left eye
- H47.023 Hemorrhage in optic nerve sheath, bilateral
- H47.029 Hemorrhage in optic nerve sheath, unspecified eye

[6th] **H47.03 Optic nerve hypoplasia**
- H47.031 Optic nerve hypoplasia, right eye
- H47.032 Optic nerve hypoplasia, left eye
- H47.033 Optic nerve hypoplasia, bilateral
- H47.039 Optic nerve hypoplasia, unspecified eye

[6th] **H47.09 Other disorders of optic nerve, not elsewhere classified**
Compression of optic nerve
- H47.091 Other disorders of optic nerve, not elsewhere classified, right eye
- H47.092 Other disorders of optic nerve, not elsewhere classified, left eye
- H47.093 Other disorders of optic nerve, not elsewhere classified, bilateral
- H47.099 Other disorders of optic nerve, not elsewhere classified, unspecified eye

[5th] **H47.1 Papilledema**
- H47.10 Unspecified papilledema CC CC/MCC Exc
- H47.11 Papilledema associated with increased intracranial pressure CC CC/MCC Exc
- H47.12 Papilledema associated with decreased ocular pressure
- H47.13 Papilledema associated with retinal disorder

[6th] **H47.14 Foster-Kennedy syndrome**
- H47.141 Foster-Kennedy syndrome, right eye
- H47.142 Foster-Kennedy syndrome, left eye
- H47.143 Foster-Kennedy syndrome, bilateral
- H47.149 Foster-Kennedy syndrome, unspecified eye

[5th] **H47.2 Optic atrophy**
- H47.20 Unspecified optic atrophy

[6th] **H47.21 Primary optic atrophy**
- H47.211 Primary optic atrophy, right eye
- H47.212 Primary optic atrophy, left eye
- H47.213 Primary optic atrophy, bilateral
- H47.219 Primary optic atrophy, unspecified eye

H47.22 Hereditary optic atrophy
Leber's optic atrophy

[6th] **H47.23 Glaucomatous optic atrophy**
- H47.231 Glaucomatous optic atrophy, right eye
- H47.232 Glaucomatous optic atrophy, left eye
- H47.233 Glaucomatous optic atrophy, bilateral
- H47.239 Glaucomatous optic atrophy, unspecified eye

[6th] **H47.29 Other optic atrophy**
Temporal pallor of optic disc
- H47.291 Other optic atrophy, right eye
- H47.292 Other optic atrophy, left eye
- H47.293 Other optic atrophy, bilateral
- H47.299 Other optic atrophy, unspecified eye

[5th] **H47.3 Other disorders of optic disc**

[6th] **H47.31 Coloboma of optic disc**
- H47.311 Coloboma of optic disc, right eye
- H47.312 Coloboma of optic disc, left eye
- H47.313 Coloboma of optic disc, bilateral
- H47.319 Coloboma of optic disc, unspecified eye

[6th] **H47.32 Drusen of optic disc**
- H47.321 Drusen of optic disc, right eye
- H47.322 Drusen of optic disc, left eye
- H47.323 Drusen of optic disc, bilateral
- H47.329 Drusen of optic disc, unspecified eye

[6th] **H47.33 Pseudopapilledema of optic disc**
- H47.331 Pseudopapilledema of optic disc, right eye
- H47.332 Pseudopapilledema of optic disc, left eye
- H47.333 Pseudopapilledema of optic disc, bilateral
- H47.339 Pseudopapilledema of optic disc, unspecified eye

[6th] **H47.39 Other disorders of optic disc**
- H47.391 Other disorders of optic disc, right eye
- H47.392 Other disorders of optic disc, left eye
- H47.393 Other disorders of optic disc, bilateral
- H47.399 Other disorders of optic disc, unspecified eye

[5th] **H47.4 Disorders of optic chiasm**
Code also underlying condition
- H47.41 Disorders of optic chiasm in (due to) inflammatory disorders CC CC/MCC Exc
- H47.42 Disorders of optic chiasm in (due to) neoplasm CC CC/MCC Exc
- H47.43 Disorders of optic chiasm in (due to) vascular disorders CC CC/MCC Exc
- H47.49 Disorders of optic chiasm in (due to) other disorders CC CC/MCC Exc

[5th] **H47.5 Disorders of other visual pathways**
Disorders of optic tracts, geniculate nuclei and optic radiations
Code also underlying condition

[6th] **H47.51 Disorders of visual pathways in (due to) inflammatory disorders**
- H47.511 Disorders of visual pathways in (due to) inflammatory disorders, right side CC CC/MCC Exc
- H47.512 Disorders of visual pathways in (due to) inflammatory disorders, left side CC CC/MCC Exc
- H47.519 Disorders of visual pathways in (due to) inflammatory disorders, unspecified side CC CC/MCC Exc

[6th] **H47.52 Disorders of visual pathways in (due to) neoplasm**
- H47.521 Disorders of visual pathways in (due to) neoplasm, right side CC CC/MCC Exc
- H47.522 Disorders of visual pathways in (due to) neoplasm, left side CC CC/MCC Exc

Unacceptable principal diagnosis symbol per Medicare code edits · Code exempt from diagnosis present on admission requirement · Questionable admission · Complication or comorbidity · CC/MCC exclusion · Major complication or comorbidity · Principal diagnosis as its own CC · Principal diagnosis as its own MCC · HCC diagnosis code · RxHCC diagnosis code · MACRA code · Z code as first-listed diagnosis

H47.529 Disorders of visual pathways in (due to) neoplasm, unspecified side

🔵 H47.53 Disorders of visual pathways in (due to) vascular disorders

    H47.531 Disorders of visual pathways in (due to) vascular disorders, right side CC CC/MCC Exc

    H47.532 Disorders of visual pathways in (due to) vascular disorders, left side CC CC/MCC Exc

    H47.539 Disorders of visual pathways in (due to) vascular disorders, unspecified side CC CC/MCC Exc

🔵 H47.6 Disorders of visual cortex

    Code also underlying condition

    EXCLUDES1 injury to visual cortex S04.04

🔵 H47.61 Cortical blindness

    H47.611 Cortical blindness, right side of brain

    H47.612 Cortical blindness, left side of brain

    H47.619 Cortical blindness, unspecified side of brain

🔵 H47.62 Disorders of visual cortex in (due to) inflammatory disorders

    H47.621 Disorders of visual cortex in (due to) inflammatory disorders, right side of brain CC CC/MCC Exc

    H47.622 Disorders of visual cortex in (due to) inflammatory disorders, left side of brain CC CC/MCC Exc

    H47.629 Disorders of visual cortex in (due to) inflammatory disorders, unspecified side of brain CC CC/MCC Exc

🔵 H47.63 Disorders of visual cortex in (due to) neoplasm

    H47.631 Disorders of visual cortex in (due to) neoplasm, right side of brain CC CC/MCC Exc

    H47.632 Disorders of visual cortex in (due to) neoplasm, left side of brain CC CC/MCC Exc

    H47.639 Disorders of visual cortex in (due to) neoplasm, unspecified side of brain CC CC/MCC Exc

🔵 H47.64 Disorders of visual cortex in (due to) vascular disorders

    H47.641 Disorders of visual cortex in (due to) vascular disorders, right side of brain CC CC/MCC Exc

    H47.642 Disorders of visual cortex in (due to) vascular disorders, left side of brain CC CC/MCC Exc

    H47.649 Disorders of visual cortex in (due to) vascular disorders, unspecified side of brain CC CC/MCC Exc

H47.9 Unspecified disorder of visual pathways

Disorders of ocular muscles, binocular movement, accommodation and refraction (H49-H52)

    EXCLUDES2 nystagmus and other irregular eye movements (H55)

🔵 H49 Paralytic strabismus

    EXCLUDES2 internal ophthalmoplegia (H52.51-)

             internuclear ophthalmoplegia (H51.2-)

             progressive supranuclear ophthalmoplegia (G23.1)

🔵 H49.0 Third [oculomotor] nerve palsy

    H49.00 Third [oculomotor] nerve palsy, unspecified eye

    H49.01 Third [oculomotor] nerve palsy, right eye

    H49.02 Third [oculomotor] nerve palsy, left eye

    H49.03 Third [oculomotor] nerve palsy, bilateral

🔵 H49.1 Fourth [trochlear] nerve palsy

    H49.10 Fourth [trochlear] nerve palsy, unspecified eye

    H49.11 Fourth [trochlear] nerve palsy, right eye

    H49.12 Fourth [trochlear] nerve palsy, left eye

    H49.13 Fourth [trochlear] nerve palsy, bilateral

🔵 H49.2 Sixth [abducent] nerve palsy

    H49.20 Sixth [abducent] nerve palsy, unspecified eye

    H49.21 Sixth [abducent] nerve palsy, right eye

    H49.22 Sixth [abducent] nerve palsy, left eye

    H49.23 Sixth [abducent] nerve palsy, bilateral

🔵 H49.3 Total (external) ophthalmoplegia

    H49.30 Total (external) ophthalmoplegia, unspecified eye

    H49.31 Total (external) ophthalmoplegia, right eye

    H49.32 Total (external) ophthalmoplegia, left eye

    H49.33 Total (external) ophthalmoplegia, bilateral

🔵 H49.4 Progressive external ophthalmoplegia

    EXCLUDES1 Kearns-Sayre syndrome (H49.81-)

    H49.40 Progressive external ophthalmoplegia, unspecified eye

    H49.41 Progressive external ophthalmoplegia, right eye

    H49.42 Progressive external ophthalmoplegia, left eye

    H49.43 Progressive external ophthalmoplegia, bilateral

🔵 H49.8 Other paralytic strabismus

🔵 H49.81 Kearns-Sayre syndrome

    Progressive external ophthalmoplegia with pigmentary retinopathy

    Use additional code for other manifestation, such as:

    heart block (I45.9)

    H49.811 Kearns-Sayre syndrome, right eye CC HCC RxHCC CC/MCC Exc

    H49.812 Kearns-Sayre syndrome, left eye CC HCC RxHCC CC/MCC Exc

    H49.813 Kearns-Sayre syndrome, bilateral CC HCC RxHCC CC/MCC Exc

    H49.819 Kearns-Sayre syndrome, unspecified eye CC HCC RxHCC CC/MCC Exc

🔵 H49.88 Other paralytic strabismus

    External ophthalmoplegia NOS

    H49.881 Other paralytic strabismus, right eye

    H49.882 Other paralytic strabismus, left eye

    H49.883 Other paralytic strabismus, bilateral

    H49.889 Other paralytic strabismus, unspecified eye

H49.9 Unspecified paralytic strabismus

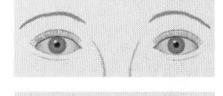 Normal

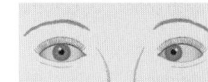 Esotropia - eye turns inward

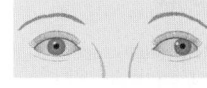 Exotropia - eye turns outward

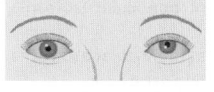 Hypertropia - eye turns upward

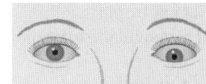 Hypotropia - eye turns downward

Figure 7.5 Types of Strabismus

🔵 H50 Other strabismus

🔵 H50.0 Esotropia

    Convergent concomitant strabismus

    EXCLUDES1 intermittent esotropia (H50.31-, H50.32)

    H50.00 Unspecified esotropia

🔵 H50.01 Monocular esotropia

    H50.011 Monocular esotropia, right eye

    H50.012 Monocular esotropia, left eye

Unspecified Code Other Specified Code Manifestation Code N Newborn P Pediatric M Maternity A Adult ♂ Male ♀ Female
● New Code ▲ Revised Code Title ►◄ Revised Text NOTES INCLUDES EXCLUDES 1 Not coded here EXCLUDES 2 Not included here
4th character required 5th character required 6th character required 7th character required
Extension 'X' Alert HAC Hospital-acquired condition (HAC) alert AHA AHA Coding Clinic©

H50.02 Monocular esotropia with A pattern
    H50.021 Monocular esotropia with A pattern, right eye
    H50.022 Monocular esotropia with A pattern, left eye
H50.03 Monocular esotropia with V pattern
    H50.031 Monocular esotropia with V pattern, right eye
    H50.032 Monocular esotropia with V pattern, left eye
H50.04 Monocular esotropia with other noncomitancies
    H50.041 Monocular esotropia with other noncomitancies, right eye
    H50.042 Monocular esotropia with other noncomitancies, left eye
H50.05 Alternating esotropia
H50.06 Alternating esotropia with A pattern
H50.07 Alternating esotropia with V pattern
H50.08 Alternating esotropia with other noncomitancies

H50.1 Exotropia
Divergent concomitant strabismus
EXCLUDES1 intermittent exotropia (H50.33-, H50.34)
H50.10 Unspecified exotropia
H50.11 Monocular exotropia
    H50.111 Monocular exotropia, right eye
    H50.112 Monocular exotropia, left eye
H50.12 Monocular exotropia with A pattern
    H50.121 Monocular exotropia with A pattern, right eye
    H50.122 Monocular exotropia with A pattern, left eye
H50.13 Monocular exotropia with V pattern
    H50.131 Monocular exotropia with V pattern, right eye
    H50.132 Monocular exotropia with V pattern, left eye
H50.14 Monocular exotropia with other noncomitancies
    H50.141 Monocular exotropia with other noncomitancies, right eye
    H50.142 Monocular exotropia with other noncomitancies, left eye
H50.15 Alternating exotropia
H50.16 Alternating exotropia with A pattern
H50.17 Alternating exotropia with V pattern
H50.18 Alternating exotropia with other noncomitancies

H50.2 Vertical strabismus
Hypertropia
H50.21 Vertical strabismus, right eye
H50.22 Vertical strabismus, left eye

H50.3 Intermittent heterotropia
H50.30 Unspecified intermittent heterotropia
H50.31 Intermittent monocular esotropia
    H50.311 Intermittent monocular esotropia, right eye
    H50.312 Intermittent monocular esotropia, left eye
H50.32 Intermittent alternating esotropia
H50.33 Intermittent monocular exotropia
    H50.331 Intermittent monocular exotropia, right eye
    H50.332 Intermittent monocular exotropia, left eye
H50.34 Intermittent alternating exotropia

H50.4 Other and unspecified heterotropia
H50.40 Unspecified heterotropia
H50.41 Cyclotropia
    H50.411 Cyclotropia, right eye
    H50.412 Cyclotropia, left eye
H50.42 Monofixation syndrome
H50.43 Accommodative component in esotropia

H50.5 Heterophoria
H50.50 Unspecified heterophoria
H50.51 Esophoria
H50.52 Exophoria
H50.53 Vertical heterophoria
H50.54 Cyclophoria
H50.55 Alternating heterophoria

H50.6 Mechanical strabismus
H50.60 Mechanical strabismus, unspecified
H50.61 Brown's sheath syndrome
    H50.611 Brown's sheath syndrome, right eye
    H50.612 Brown's sheath syndrome, left eye
H50.69 Other mechanical strabismus
Strabismus due to adhesions
Traumatic limitation of duction of eye muscle

H50.8 Other specified strabismus
H50.81 Duane's syndrome
    H50.811 Duane's syndrome, right eye
    H50.812 Duane's syndrome, left eye
H50.89 Other specified strabismus

H50.9 Unspecified strabismus

H51 Other disorders of binocular movement
H51.0 Palsy (spasm) of conjugate gaze
H51.1 Convergence insufficiency and excess
H51.11 Convergence insufficiency
H51.12 Convergence excess
H51.2 Internuclear ophthalmoplegia
H51.20 Internuclear ophthalmoplegia, unspecified eye
H51.21 Internuclear ophthalmoplegia, right eye
H51.22 Internuclear ophthalmoplegia, left eye
H51.23 Internuclear ophthalmoplegia, bilateral
H51.8 Other specified disorders of binocular movement
H51.9 Unspecified disorder of binocular movement

H52 Disorders of refraction and accommodation
H52.0 Hypermetropia
H52.00 Hypermetropia, unspecified eye
H52.01 Hypermetropia, right eye
H52.02 Hypermetropia, left eye
H52.03 Hypermetropia, bilateral
H52.1 Myopia
EXCLUDES1 degenerative myopia (H44.2-)
H52.10 Myopia, unspecified eye
H52.11 Myopia, right eye
H52.12 Myopia, left eye
H52.13 Myopia, bilateral
H52.2 Astigmatism
H52.20 Unspecified astigmatism
    H52.201 Unspecified astigmatism, right eye
    H52.202 Unspecified astigmatism, left eye
    H52.203 Unspecified astigmatism, bilateral
    H52.209 Unspecified astigmatism, unspecified eye
H52.21 Irregular astigmatism
    H52.211 Irregular astigmatism, right eye
    H52.212 Irregular astigmatism, left eye
    H52.213 Irregular astigmatism, bilateral
    H52.219 Irregular astigmatism, unspecified eye
H52.22 Regular astigmatism
    H52.221 Regular astigmatism, right eye
    H52.222 Regular astigmatism, left eye
    H52.223 Regular astigmatism, bilateral
    H52.229 Regular astigmatism, unspecified eye
H52.3 Anisometropia and aniseikonia
H52.31 Anisometropia
H52.32 Aniseikonia
H52.4 Presbyopia
H52.5 Disorders of accommodation
H52.51 Internal ophthalmoplegia (complete) (total)
    H52.511 Internal ophthalmoplegia (complete) (total), right eye
    H52.512 Internal ophthalmoplegia (complete) (total), left eye

---

PDxIN Unacceptable principal diagnosis symbol per Medicare code edits   POA Code exempt from diagnosis present on admission requirement
? Questionable admission   CC Complication or comorbidity   CC-MCC Exc CC/MCC exclusion   MCC Major complication or comorbidity
PCC Principal diagnosis as its own CC   PMCC Principal diagnosis as its own MCC   HCC HCC diagnosis code   RxHCC RxHCC diagnosis code
MACRA code   Z1 Z code as first-listed diagnosis

H52.513 **Internal ophthalmoplegia (complete) (total), bilateral**

H52.519 **Internal ophthalmoplegia (complete) (total), unspecified eye**

6th H52.52 Paresis of accommodation

H52.521 Paresis of accommodation, right eye

H52.522 Paresis of accommodation, left eye

H52.523 Paresis of accommodation, bilateral

H52.529 **Paresis of accommodation, unspecified eye**

6th H52.53 Spasm of accommodation

H52.531 Spasm of accommodation, right eye

H52.532 Spasm of accommodation, left eye

H52.533 Spasm of accommodation, bilateral

H52.539 **Spasm of accommodation, unspecified eye**

H52.6 Other disorders of refraction

H52.7 **Unspecified disorder of refraction**

Visual disturbances and blindness (H53-H54)

4th H53 Visual disturbances

5th H53.0 Amblyopia ex anopsia

EXCLUDES1 *amblyopia due to vitamin A deficiency (E50.5)*

6th H53.00 Unspecified amblyopia

H53.001 Unspecified amblyopia, right eye

H53.002 Unspecified amblyopia, left eye

H53.003 Unspecified amblyopia, bilateral

H53.009 **Unspecified amblyopia, unspecified eye**

6th H53.01 Deprivation amblyopia

H53.011 Deprivation amblyopia, right eye

H53.012 Deprivation amblyopia, left eye

H53.013 Deprivation amblyopia, bilateral

H53.019 **Deprivation amblyopia, unspecified eye**

6th H53.02 Refractive amblyopia

H53.021 Refractive amblyopia, right eye

H53.022 Refractive amblyopia, left eye

H53.023 Refractive amblyopia, bilateral

H53.029 **Refractive amblyopia, unspecified eye**

6th H53.03 Strabismic amblyopia

EXCLUDES1 *strabismus (H50.-)*

H53.031 Strabismic amblyopia, right eye

H53.032 Strabismic amblyopia, left eye

H53.033 Strabismic amblyopia, bilateral

H53.039 **Strabismic amblyopia, unspecified eye**

6th H53.04 Amblyopia suspect

H53.041 Amblyopia suspect, right eye
AHA: Q4 2016

H53.042 Amblyopia suspect, left eye
AHA: Q4 2016

H53.043 Amblyopia suspect, bilateral
AHA: Q4 2016

H53.049 **Amblyopia suspect, unspecified eye**
AHA: Q4 2016

5th H53.1 Subjective visual disturbances

EXCLUDES1 *subjective visual disturbances due to vitamin A deficiency (E50.5)*

visual hallucinations (R44.1)

H53.10 **Unspecified subjective visual disturbances**

H53.11 Day blindness
Hemeralopia

6th H53.12 Transient visual loss
Scintillating scotoma

EXCLUDES1 *amaurosis fugax (G45.3-)*

transient retinal artery occlusion (H34.0-)

H53.121 Transient visual loss, right eye cc cc/MCC Exc

H53.122 Transient visual loss, left eye cc cc/MCC Exc

H53.123 Transient visual loss, bilateral cc cc/MCC Exc

H53.129 **Transient visual loss, unspecified eye** cc cc/MCC Exc

6th H53.13 Sudden visual loss

H53.131 Sudden visual loss, right eye cc cc/MCC Exc

H53.132 Sudden visual loss, left eye cc cc/MCC Exc

H53.133 Sudden visual loss, bilateral cc cc/MCC Exc

H53.139 **Sudden visual loss, unspecified eye** cc cc/MCC Exc

6th H53.14 Visual discomfort
Asthenopia
Photophobia

H53.141 Visual discomfort, right eye

H53.142 Visual discomfort, left eye

H53.143 Visual discomfort, bilateral

H53.149 **Visual discomfort, unspecified**

H53.15 Visual distortions of shape and size
Metamorphopsia

H53.16 Psychophysical visual disturbances

H53.19 Other subjective visual disturbances
Visual halos

H53.2 Diplopia
Double vision

5th H53.3 Other and unspecified disorders of binocular vision

H53.30 **Unspecified disorder of binocular vision**

H53.31 Abnormal retinal correspondence

H53.32 Fusion with defective stereopsis

H53.33 Simultaneous visual perception without fusion

H53.34 Suppression of binocular vision

5th H53.4 Visual field defects

H53.40 **Unspecified visual field defects**

6th H53.41 Scotoma involving central area
Central scotoma

H53.411 Scotoma involving central area, right eye

H53.412 Scotoma involving central area, left eye

H53.413 Scotoma involving central area, bilateral

H53.419 **Scotoma involving central area, unspecified eye**

6th H53.42 Scotoma of blind spot area
Enlarged blind spot

H53.421 Scotoma of blind spot area, right eye

H53.422 Scotoma of blind spot area, left eye

H53.423 Scotoma of blind spot area, bilateral

H53.429 **Scotoma of blind spot area, unspecified eye**

6th H53.43 Sector or arcuate defects
Arcuate scotoma
Bjerrum scotoma

H53.431 Sector or arcuate defects, right eye

H53.432 Sector or arcuate defects, left eye

H53.433 Sector or arcuate defects, bilateral

H53.439 **Sector or arcuate defects, unspecified eye**

6th H53.45 Other localized visual field defect
Peripheral visual field defect
Ring scotoma NOS
Scotoma NOS

H53.451 Other localized visual field defect, right eye

H53.452 Other localized visual field defect, left eye

H53.453 Other localized visual field defect, bilateral

H53.459 **Other localized visual field defect, unspecified eye**

6th H53.46 Homonymous bilateral field defects
Homonymous hemianopia
Homonymous hemianopsia
Quadrant anopia
Quadrant anopsia

H53.461 Homonymous bilateral field defects, right side

H53.462 Homonymous bilateral field defects, left side

Unspecified Code   Other Specified Code   Manifestation Code   N Newborn   P Pediatric   M Maternity   A Adult   ♂ Male   ♀ Female
● New Code   ▲ Revised Code Title   ►◄ Revised Text   NOTES   INCLUDES   EXCLUDES 1   Not coded here   EXCLUDES 2   Not included here
4th 4th character required   5th 5th character required   6th 6th character required   7th 7th character required
Extension 'X' Alert   HAC Hospital-acquired condition (HAC) alert   AHA AHA Coding Clinic©

H53.469 **Homonymous bilateral field defects, unspecified side**
Homonymous bilateral field defects NOS

H53.47 Heteronymous **bilateral field defects**
Heteronymous hemianop(s)ia

6ᵗʰ H53.48 Generalized contraction of visual field

H53.481 **Generalized contraction of visual field,** right **eye**

H53.482 **Generalized contraction of visual field,** left **eye**

H53.483 **Generalized contraction of visual field, bilateral**

H53.489 **Generalized contraction of visual field, unspecified eye**

5ᵗʰ H53.5 Color vision deficiencies
Color blindness
EXCLUDES2 *day blindness (H53.11)*

H53.50 **Unspecified color vision deficiencies**
Color blindness NOS

H53.51 **Achromatopsia**

H53.52 **Acquired color vision deficiency**

H53.53 **Deuteranomaly**
Deuteranopia

H53.54 **Protanomaly**
Protanopia

H53.55 **Tritanomaly**
Tritanopia

H53.59 **Other color vision deficiencies**

5ᵗʰ H53.6 Night blindness
EXCLUDES1 *night blindness due to vitamin A deficiency (E50.5)*

H53.60 **Unspecified night blindness**

H53.61 Abnormal dark adaptation curve

H53.62 Acquired **night blindness**

H53.63 Congenital **night blindness**

H53.69 Other **night blindness**

5ᵗʰ H53.7 Vision sensitivity deficiencies

H53.71 Glare **sensitivity**

H53.72 Impaired contrast **sensitivity**

H53.8 **Other visual disturbances**

H53.9 **Unspecified visual disturbance**

4ᵗʰ H54 Blindness and low vision
NOTES For definition of visual impairment categories see table below
Code first any associated underlying cause of the blindness
EXCLUDES1 *amaurosis fugax (G45.3)*

5ᵗʰ H54.0 **Blindness,** both eyes
Visual impairment categories 3, 4, 5 in both eyes.

● 6ᵗʰ H54.0X **Blindness,** both eyes, different category levels

● 7ᵗʰ H54.0X3 **Blindness** right **eye, category 3**

● 7ᵗʰ H54.0X4 **Blindness** right **eye, category 4**

● 7ᵗʰ H54.0X5 **Blindness** right **eye, category 5**

5ᵗʰ H54.1 **Blindness,** one eye, low vision other eye
Visual impairment categories 3, 4, 5 in one eye, with categories 1 or 2 in the other eye.

H54.10 **Blindness, one eye, low vision other eye, unspecified eyes**

6ᵗʰ H54.11 **Blindness,** right **eye, low vision** left **eye**

● 7ᵗʰ H54.113 **Blindness** right **eye category 3, low vision** left **eye**

● 7ᵗʰ H54.114 **Blindness** right **eye category 4, low vision** left **eye**

● 7ᵗʰ H54.115 **Blindness** right **eye category 5, low vision** left **eye**

6ᵗʰ H54.12 **Blindness,** left **eye, low vision** right **eye**

● 7ᵗʰ H54.121 **Low vision** right **eye category 1, blindness** left **eye**

● 7ᵗʰ H54.122 **Low vision** right **eye category 2, blindness** left **eye**

5ᵗʰ H54.2 **Low vision,** both eyes
Visual impairment categories 1 or 2 in both eyes.

● 6ᵗʰ H54.2X **Low vision,** both eyes, different category levels

● 7ᵗʰ H54.2X1 **Low vision,** right **eye, category 1**

● 7ᵗʰ H54.2X2 **Low vision,** right **eye, category 2**

H54.3 Unqualified **visual loss, both eyes**
Visual impairment category 9 in both eyes.

5ᵗʰ H54.4 Blindness, **one eye**
Visual impairment categories 3, 4, 5 in one eye [normal vision in other eye]

H54.40 **Blindness, one eye, unspecified eye**

6ᵗʰ H54.41 **Blindness,** right **eye, normal vision** left **eye**

● 7ᵗʰ H54.413 **Blindness,** right **eye, category 3**

● 7ᵗʰ H54.414 **Blindness,** right **eye, category 4**

● 7ᵗʰ H54.415 **Blindness,** right **eye, category 5**

6ᵗʰ H54.42 **Blindness,** left **eye, normal vision** right **eye**

● 7ᵗʰ H54.42A **Blindness,** left **eye, category 3-5**

5ᵗʰ H54.5 **Low vision,** one eye
Visual impairment categories 1 or 2 in one eye [normal vision in other eye].

H54.50 **Low vision, one eye, unspecified eye**

6ᵗʰ H54.51 **Low vision,** right **eye, normal vision** left **eye**

● 7ᵗʰ H54.511 **Low vision,** right **eye, category 1-2**

6ᵗʰ H54.52 **Low vision,** left **eye, normal vision** right **eye**

● 7ᵗʰ H54.52A **Low vision,** left **eye, category 1-2**

5ᵗʰ H54.6 Unqualified **visual loss,** one eye
Visual impairment category 9 in one eye [normal vision in other eye].

H54.60 **Unqualified visual loss, one eye, unspecified**

H54.61 **Unqualified visual loss,** right **eye, normal vision** left **eye**

H54.62 **Unqualified visual loss,** left **eye, normal vision** right **eye**

H54.7 Unspecified visual loss   PDxₐ

Visual impairment category 9 NOS

H54.8 Legal blindness, **as defined in USA**
Blindness NOS according to USA definition
EXCLUDES1 *legal blindness with specification of impairment level (H54.0-H54.7)*

NOTES   The table below gives a classification of severity of visual impairment recommended by a WHO Study Group on the Prevention of Blindness, Geneva, 6-10 November 1972.
The term 'low vision' in category H54 comprises categories 1 and 2 of the table, the term 'blindness' categories 3, 4 and 5, and the term 'unqualified visual loss' category 9.
If the extent of the visual field is taken into account, patients with a field no greater than 10 but greater than 5 around central fixation should be placed in category 3 and patients with a field no greater than 5 around central fixation should be placed in category 4, even if the central acuity is not impaired.

Category of visual impairment	Visual acuity with best possible correction	
	Maximum less than:	Minimum equal to or better than:
	6/18	6/60
3/10(0.3)	1/10(0.1)	-
20/70	20/200	-
	6/60	3/60
1/10(0.1)	1/20(0.05)	-
20/200	20/400	-
	3/60	1/60 (finger counting at one meter)
1/20(0.05)	1/50(0.02)	-
20/400	5/300(20/1200)	-
	1/60 (finger counting at one meter)	Light perception
1/50(0.02)		-
5/300		-
	No light perception	-
	Undetermined or unspecified	-

PDxₐ Unacceptable principal diagnosis symbol per Medicare code edits   PDxₐ Code exempt from diagnosis present on admission requirement
❓ Questionable admission   ℅ Complication or comorbidity   ℅/MCC Exc CC/MCC exclusion   MCC℗ Major complication or comorbidity
℗ℂℂ Principal diagnosis as its own CC   ℗ℳℂℂ Principal diagnosis as its own MCC   HCC HCC diagnosis code   RxHCC RxHCC diagnosis code
MACRA code   Ⓩ Z code as first-listed diagnosis

Other disorders of eye and adnexa (H55-H57)

- H55 **Nystagmus and other** irregular eye movements
  - H55.0 **Nystagmus**
    - H55.00 **Unspecified nystagmus**
    - H55.01 Congenital **nystagmus**
    - H55.02 Latent **nystagmus**
    - H55.03 Visual deprivation **nystagmus**
    - H55.04 Dissociated **nystagmus**
    - H55.09 Other forms of nystagmus
  - H55.8 Other irregular eye movements
    - H55.81 Saccadic **eye movements**
    - H55.89 Other irregular eye movements
- H57 Other disorders **of eye and adnexa**
  - H57.0 **Anomalies of pupillary function**
    - H57.00 **Unspecified anomaly of pupillary function**
    - H57.01 Argyll Robertson pupil, atypical
      - EXCLUDES1 *syphilitic Argyll Robertson pupil (A52.19)*
    - H57.02 **Anisocoria**
    - H57.03 **Miosis**
    - H57.04 **Mydriasis**
    - H57.05 **Tonic pupil**
      - H57.051 **Tonic pupil,** right **eye**
      - H57.052 **Tonic pupil,** left **eye**
      - H57.053 **Tonic pupil,** bilateral
      - H57.059 Tonic pupil, unspecified eye
    - H57.09 **Other anomalies of pupillary function**
  - H57.1 **Ocular pain**
    - H57.10 **Ocular pain, unspecified eye**
    - H57.11 **Ocular pain,** right **eye**
    - H57.12 **Ocular pain,** left **eye**
    - H57.13 **Ocular pain,** bilateral
  - H57.8 Other specified disorders of eye and adnexa
  - H57.9 **Unspecified disorder of eye and adnexa** PDxIn

Intraoperative and postprocedural complications and disorders of eye and adnexa, not elsewhere classified (H59)

- H59 **Intraoperative and postprocedural complications and disorders of eye and adnexa, not elsewhere classified**
  - EXCLUDES1 *mechanical complication of intraocular lens (T85.2)*
    - *mechanical complication of other ocular prosthetic devices, implants and grafts (T85.3)*
    - *pseudophakia (Z96.1)*
    - *secondary cataracts (H26.4-)*
  - H59.0 **Disorders of the eye** following cataract surgery
    - H59.01 Keratopathy (bullous aphakic) following cataract surgery
      - Vitreal corneal syndrome
      - Vitreous (touch) syndrome
      - H59.011 **Keratopathy (bullous aphakic) following cataract surgery,** right **eye** CC CC/MCC Exc
      - H59.012 **Keratopathy (bullous aphakic) following cataract surgery,** left **eye** CC CC/MCC Exc
      - H59.013 **Keratopathy (bullous aphakic) following cataract surgery,** bilateral CC CC/MCC Exc
      - H59.019 Keratopathy (bullous aphakic) following cataract surgery, unspecified eye CC CC/MCC Exc
    - H59.02 Cataract (lens) fragments in eye following cataract surgery
      - H59.021 Cataract (lens) fragments in eye following cataract surgery, right eye
      - H59.022 Cataract (lens) fragments in eye following cataract surgery, left eye
      - H59.023 Cataract (lens) fragments in eye following cataract surgery, bilateral
      - H59.029 Cataract (lens) fragments in eye following cataract surgery, unspecified eye
    - H59.03 Cystoid macular edema following cataract surgery
      - H59.031 Cystoid macular edema following cataract surgery, right eye CC CC/MCC Exc
      - H59.032 Cystoid macular edema following cataract surgery, left eye CC CC/MCC Exc
      - H59.033 Cystoid macular edema following cataract surgery, bilateral CC CC/MCC Exc
      - H59.039 Cystoid macular edema following cataract surgery, unspecified eye CC CC/MCC Exc
    - H59.09 Other disorders of the eye following cataract surgery
      - H59.091 Other disorders of the right eye following cataract surgery CC CC/MCC Exc
      - H59.092 Other disorders of the left eye following cataract surgery CC CC/MCC Exc
      - H59.093 Other disorders of the eye following cataract surgery, bilateral CC CC/MCC Exc
      - H59.099 Other disorders of unspecified eye following cataract surgery CC CC/MCC Exc
  - H59.1 Intraoperative hemorrhage and hematoma of eye and adnexa complicating a procedure
    - EXCLUDES1 *intraoperative hemorrhage and hematoma of eye and adnexa due to accidental puncture or laceration during a procedure (H59.2-)*
    - H59.11 Intraoperative hemorrhage and hematoma of eye and adnexa complicating an ophthalmic procedure
      - H59.111 Intraoperative hemorrhage and hematoma of right eye and adnexa complicating an ophthalmic procedure CC CC/MCC Exc
      - H59.112 Intraoperative hemorrhage and hematoma of left eye and adnexa complicating an ophthalmic procedure CC CC/MCC Exc
      - H59.113 Intraoperative hemorrhage and hematoma of eye and adnexa complicating an ophthalmic procedure, bilateral CC CC/MCC Exc
      - H59.119 Intraoperative hemorrhage and hematoma of unspecified eye and adnexa complicating an ophthalmic procedure CC CC/MCC Exc
    - H59.12 Intraoperative hemorrhage and hematoma of eye and adnexa complicating other procedure
      - H59.121 Intraoperative hemorrhage and hematoma of right eye and adnexa complicating other procedure CC CC/MCC Exc
      - H59.122 Intraoperative hemorrhage and hematoma of left eye and adnexa complicating other procedure CC CC/MCC Exc
      - H59.123 Intraoperative hemorrhage and hematoma of eye and adnexa complicating other procedure, bilateral CC CC/MCC Exc
      - H59.129 Intraoperative hemorrhage and hematoma of unspecified eye and adnexa complicating other procedure CC CC/MCC Exc
  - H59.2 Accidental puncture and laceration of eye and adnexa during a procedure
    - H59.21 Accidental puncture and laceration of eye and adnexa during an ophthalmic procedure
      - H59.211 Accidental puncture and laceration of right eye and adnexa during an ophthalmic procedure CC CC/MCC Exc
      - H59.212 Accidental puncture and laceration of left eye and adnexa during an ophthalmic procedure CC CC/MCC Exc
      - H59.213 Accidental puncture and laceration of eye and adnexa during an ophthalmic procedure, bilateral CC CC/MCC Exc
      - H59.219 Accidental puncture and laceration of unspecified eye and adnexa during an ophthalmic procedure CC CC/MCC Exc

| Unspecified Code | Other Specified Code | Manifestation Code | N Newborn | P Pediatric | M Maternity | A Adult | ♂ Male | ♀ Female |

● New Code   ▲ Revised Code Title   ►◄ Revised Text   NOTES   *INCLUDES*   EXCLUDES 1 Not coded here   EXCLUDES 2 Not included here
4th character required   5th character required   6th character required   7th character required
7th Extension 'X' Alert   HAC Hospital-acquired condition (HAC) alert   AHA AHA Coding Clinic©

2018 ICD-10-CM   When symbols appear on a code that requires a 7th character extension, refer to Appendix B to identify applicable 7th character codes.   **627**

6ᵗʰ H59.22 Accidental puncture and laceration of eye and adnexa during other procedure

H59.221 Accidental puncture and laceration of right eye and adnexa during other procedure　CC CC/MCC Exc

H59.222 Accidental puncture and laceration of left eye and adnexa during other procedure　CC CC/MCC Exc

H59.223 Accidental puncture and laceration of eye and adnexa during other procedure, bilateral　CC CC/MCC Exc

H59.229 Accidental puncture and laceration of unspecified eye and adnexa during other procedure　CC CC/MCC Exc

5ᵗʰ H59.3 Postprocedural hemorrhage, hematoma, and seroma of eye and adnexa following a procedure

6ᵗʰ H59.31 Postprocedural hemorrhage of eye and adnexa following an ophthalmic procedure

H59.311 Postprocedural hemorrhage of right eye and adnexa following an ophthalmic procedure　CC CC/MCC Exc

H59.312 Postprocedural hemorrhage of left eye and adnexa following an ophthalmic procedure　CC CC/MCC Exc

H59.313 Postprocedural hemorrhage of eye and adnexa following an ophthalmic procedure, bilateral　CC CC/MCC Exc

H59.319 Postprocedural hemorrhage of unspecified eye and adnexa following an ophthalmic procedure　CC CC/MCC Exc

6ᵗʰ H59.32 Postprocedural hemorrhage of eye and adnexa following other procedure

H59.321 Postprocedural hemorrhage of right eye and adnexa following other procedure　CC CC/MCC Exc

H59.322 Postprocedural hemorrhage of left eye and adnexa following other procedure　CC CC/MCC Exc

H59.323 Postprocedural hemorrhage of eye and adnexa following other procedure, bilateral　CC CC/MCC Exc

H59.329 Postprocedural hemorrhage of unspecified eye and adnexa following other procedure　CC CC/MCC Exc

6ᵗʰ H59.33 Postprocedural hematoma of eye and adnexa following an ophthalmic procedure

H59.331 Postprocedural hematoma of right eye and adnexa following an ophthalmic procedure　CC CC/MCC Exc

H59.332 Postprocedural hematoma of left eye and adnexa following an ophthalmic procedure　CC CC/MCC Exc

H59.333 Postprocedural hematoma of eye and adnexa following an ophthalmic procedure, bilateral　CC CC/MCC Exc

H59.339 Postprocedural hematoma of unspecified eye and adnexa following an ophthalmic procedure　CC CC/MCC Exc

6ᵗʰ H59.34 Postprocedural hematoma of eye and adnexa following other procedure

H59.341 Postprocedural hematoma of right eye and adnexa following other procedure　CC CC/MCC Exc

H59.342 Postprocedural hematoma of left eye and adnexa following other procedure　CC CC/MCC Exc

H59.343 Postprocedural hematoma of eye and adnexa following other procedure, bilateral　CC CC/MCC Exc

H59.349 Postprocedural hematoma of unspecified eye and adnexa following other procedure　CC CC/MCC Exc

6ᵗʰ H59.35 Postprocedural seroma of eye and adnexa following an ophthalmic procedure

H59.351 Postprocedural seroma of right eye and adnexa following an ophthalmic procedure　CC CC/MCC Exc

H59.352 Postprocedural seroma of left eye and adnexa following an ophthalmic procedure　CC CC/MCC Exc

H59.353 Postprocedural seroma of eye and adnexa following an ophthalmic procedure, bilateral　CC CC/MCC Exc

H59.359 Postprocedural seroma of unspecified eye and adnexa following an ophthalmic procedure　CC CC/MCC Exc

6ᵗʰ H59.36 Postprocedural seroma of eye and adnexa following other procedure

H59.361 Postprocedural seroma of right eye and adnexa following other procedure　CC CC/MCC Exc

H59.362 Postprocedural seroma of left eye and adnexa following other procedure　CC CC/MCC Exc

H59.363 Postprocedural seroma of eye and adnexa following other procedure, bilateral　CC CC/MCC Exc

H59.369 Postprocedural seroma of unspecified eye and adnexa following other procedure　CC CC/MCC Exc

5ᵗʰ H59.4 Inflammation (infection) of postprocedural bleb

Postprocedural blebitis

EXCLUDES1 filtering (vitreous) bleb after glaucoma surgery status (Z98.83)

H59.40 Inflammation (infection) of postprocedural bleb, unspecified

H59.41 Inflammation (infection) of postprocedural bleb, stage 1

H59.42 Inflammation (infection) of postprocedural bleb, stage 2

H59.43 Inflammation (infection) of postprocedural bleb, stage 3

Bleb endophthalmitis

5ᵗʰ H59.8 Other intraoperative and postprocedural complications and disorders of eye and adnexa, not elsewhere classified

6ᵗʰ H59.81 Chorioretinal scars after surgery for detachment

H59.811 Chorioretinal scars after surgery for detachment, right eye　CC CC/MCC Exc

H59.812 Chorioretinal scars after surgery for detachment, left eye　CC CC/MCC Exc

H59.813 Chorioretinal scars after surgery for detachment, bilateral　CC CC/MCC Exc

H59.819 Chorioretinal scars after surgery for detachment, unspecified eye　CC CC/MCC Exc

H59.88 Other intraoperative complications of eye and adnexa, not elsewhere classified　CC CC/MCC Exc

H59.89 Other postprocedural complications and disorders of eye and adnexa, not elsewhere classified　CC CC/MCC Exc

---

PDxⁿ Unacceptable principal diagnosis symbol per Medicare code edits　PDx Code exempt from diagnosis present on admission requirement

❓ Questionable admission　CC Complication or comorbidity　CC/MCC Exc CC/MCC exclusion　MCC Major complication or comorbidity

CC Principal diagnosis as its own CC　MCC Principal diagnosis as its own MCC　HCC HCC diagnosis code　RxHCC RxHCC diagnosis code

MACRA code　Z1 Z code as first-listed diagnosis

When symbols appear on a code that requires a 7th character extension, refer to Appendix B to identify applicable 7th character codes.

2018 ICD-10-CM

NOTES

NOTES

Chapter 8: Diseases of the Ear and Mastoid Process (H60-H95)
Anatomy of the Ear

The Organ of Hearing

The external, inner and middle ear contain the organs of hearing and balance. The external ear extends from outside of the head to the eardrum. The middle ear is the air-filled chamber and located medially to the eardrum. It contains the auditory ossicles (the malleus, incus, and stapes). The external and middle ears are primarily involved in the process of hearing. The inner ear comprises of fluid-filled chambers, which serve to maintain balance (or equilibrium) and hearing. The various organs of a typical human ear are listed below:

1. **The External Ear**
   a) Auricle (or Pinna)
   b) External Auditory (or Auricular) Canal (or Ear Canal/External Auditory Meatus/External Acoustic Meatus)
   c) Surface of Eardrum

2. **The Middle Ear**
   a) Malleus
   b) Incus
   c) Stapes
   d) Tympanic Membrane (or Eardrum)
   e) Auditory/Eustachian Tube (or Pharyngotympanic Tube)

3. **The Inner Ear**
   a) Cochlea
   b) Vestibule
   c) Semicircular Canals

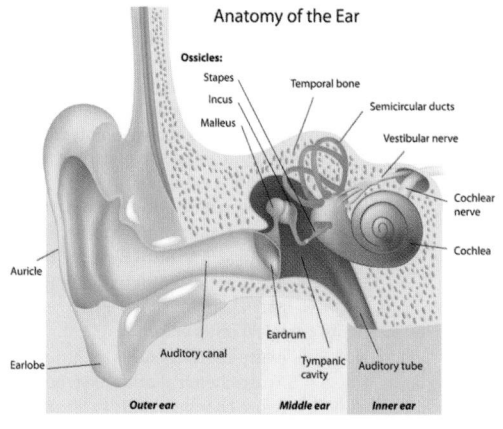
Anatomy of the Ear

Common Pathologies

Swimmer's ear
Swimmer's ear is an inflammation, irritation, or infection of the outer ear and ear canal. The medical term for swimmer's ear is otitis externa. Acute external otitis is commonly a bacterial infection caused by streptococcus, staphylococcus, or pseudomonas types of bacteria.

Otitis media
Otitis media is the medical term for middle ear infection. One symptom of acute otitis media is ear pain; other possible symptoms include fever and irritability (in infants) often with drainage of purulent material. After an acute infection, fluid (an effusion) may remain behind the ear drum (tympanic membrane) leading to otitis media with effusion chronic suppurative otitis media.

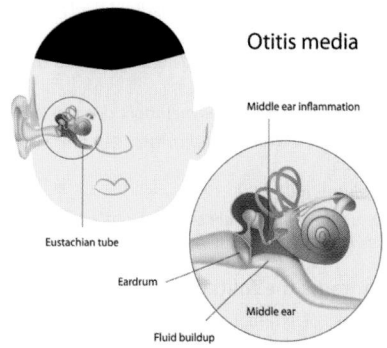
Otitis media

Ménière's disease
Ménière's disease is a disorder of the inner ear that can affect hearing. It causes severe dizziness and a feeling of ear pressure or pain. It is characterized by episodes of vertigo, low-pitched tinnitus, and hearing loss. It usually affects just one ear. It may occur when the pressure of the fluid in part of the inner ear gets too high. The inner ear contains fluid-filled tubes called semicircular canals. These canals help to maintain position and balance.

Vestibular neuritis
Vestibular neuritis is a disorder resulting from an acute infection of the nerves in the inner ear. This disrupts transmission of sensory information. Its main symptom is vertigo, which appears suddenly, often with nausea and vomiting. This can be made worse by head movement. Vertigo usually lasts for several days or weeks. In rare cases it can take months to go away entirely. Vestibular neuritis does not lead to loss of hearing.

Cholesteatoma
Cholesteatoma can be congenital, but it more commonly occurs as a complication of chronic ear infection. An abnormal skin growth in the middle ear behind the eardrum is called cholesteatoma. Poor function in the eustachian tube leads to negative pressure in the middle ear. Over time, the cholesteatoma can increase in size and destroy the surrounding delicate bones of the middle ear leading to hearing loss.

Otosclerosis
Otosclerosis is an abnormal bone growth in the middle ear that causes hearing loss. This bone prevents structures within the ear from working properly and causes hearing loss. It is a condition that mainly affects the stapes, one of the tiny bony ossicles in the middle ear. It significantly involves the bone that surrounds the inner ear, called the otic capsule, and a sensory-type hearing loss occurs.

Acoustic Neuroma
An acoustic neuroma is a benign tumor of the nerve that connects the ear to the brain. This nerve is called the vestibular cochlear nerve. It is also called vestibular schwannoma. The cause is generally unknown. If an acoustic tumor becomes large it will push on the surface of the brainstem but not really grow into brain tissue. Symptoms of acoustic neuroma are loss of hearing on one side, ringing in ears, dizziness and balance problems.

Acoustic Neuroma

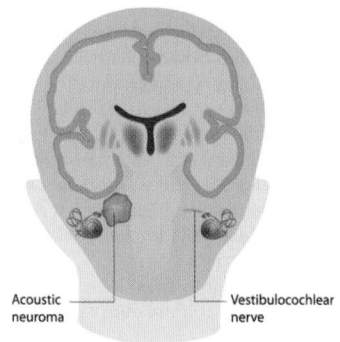

Diseases of the ear and mastoid process (H60-H95)

NOTES Use an external cause code following the code for the ear condition, if applicable, to identify the cause of the ear condition

EXCLUDES2 certain conditions originating in the perinatal period (P04-P96)

certain infectious and parasitic diseases (A00-B99)

complications of pregnancy, childbirth and the puerperium (O00-O9A)

congenital malformations, deformations and chromosomal abnormalities (Q00-Q99)

endocrine, nutritional and metabolic diseases (E00-E88)

injury, poisoning and certain other consequences of external causes (S00-T88)

neoplasms (C00-D49)

symptoms, signs and abnormal clinical and laboratory findings, not elsewhere classified (R00-R94)

This chapter contains the following blocks:

H60-H62 Diseases of external ear

H65-H75 Diseases of middle ear and mastoid

H80-H83 Diseases of inner ear

H90-H94 Other disorders of ear

H95 Intraoperative and postprocedural complications and disorders of ear and mastoid process, not elsewhere classified

Diseases of external ear (H60-H62)

Anatomy of the Ear

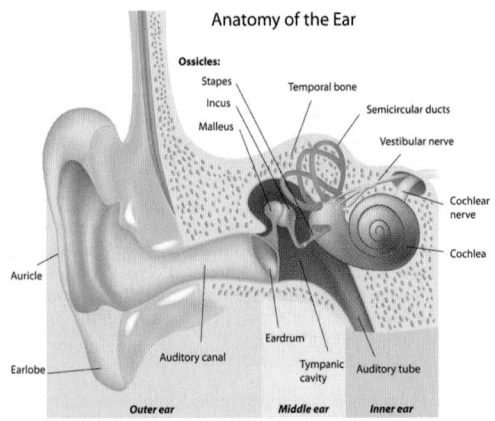

Figure 8.1 Anatomy of the ear

🔵 **H60** Otitis externa

  🔵 **H60.0** Abscess of external ear

    Boil of external ear

    Carbuncle of auricle or external auditory canal

    Furuncle of external ear

    H60.00 Abscess of external ear, unspecified ear

    H60.01 Abscess of right external ear

    H60.02 Abscess of left external ear

    H60.03 Abscess of external ear, bilateral

  🔵 **H60.1** Cellulitis of external ear

    Cellulitis of auricle

    Cellulitis of external auditory canal

    H60.10 Cellulitis of external ear, unspecified ear

    H60.11 Cellulitis of right external ear

    H60.12 Cellulitis of left external ear

    H60.13 Cellulitis of external ear, bilateral

  🔵 **H60.2** Malignant otitis externa

    H60.20 Malignant otitis externa, unspecified ear CC CC/MCC Exc

    H60.21 Malignant otitis externa, right ear CC CC/MCC Exc

    H60.22 Malignant otitis externa, left ear CC CC/MCC Exc

    H60.23 Malignant otitis externa, bilateral CC CC/MCC Exc

  🔵 **H60.3** Other infective otitis externa

    🔵 **H60.31** Diffuse otitis externa

      H60.311 Diffuse otitis externa, right ear

      H60.312 Diffuse otitis externa, left ear

      H60.313 Diffuse otitis externa, bilateral

      H60.319 Diffuse otitis externa, unspecified ear

    🔵 **H60.32** Hemorrhagic otitis externa

      H60.321 Hemorrhagic otitis externa, right ear

      H60.322 Hemorrhagic otitis externa, left ear

      H60.323 Hemorrhagic otitis externa, bilateral

      H60.329 Hemorrhagic otitis externa, unspecified ear

    🔵 **H60.33** Swimmer's ear

      H60.331 Swimmer's ear, right ear

      H60.332 Swimmer's ear, left ear

      H60.333 Swimmer's ear, bilateral

      H60.339 Swimmer's ear, unspecified ear

    🔵 **H60.39** Other infective otitis externa

      H60.391 Other infective otitis externa, right ear

      H60.392 Other infective otitis externa, left ear

      H60.393 Other infective otitis externa, bilateral

      H60.399 Other infective otitis externa, unspecified ear

  🔵 **H60.4** Cholesteatoma of external ear

    Keratosis obturans of external ear (canal)

    EXCLUDES2 cholesteatoma of middle ear (H71.-)

      recurrent cholesteatoma of postmastoidectomy cavity (H95.0-)

    H60.40 Cholesteatoma of external ear, unspecified ear

    H60.41 Cholesteatoma of right external ear

    H60.42 Cholesteatoma of left external ear

    H60.43 Cholesteatoma of external ear, bilateral

  🔵 **H60.5** Acute noninfective otitis externa

    🔵 **H60.50** Unspecified acute noninfective otitis externa

      Acute otitis externa NOS

      H60.501 Unspecified acute noninfective otitis externa, right ear

      H60.502 Unspecified acute noninfective otitis externa, left ear

      H60.503 Unspecified acute noninfective otitis externa, bilateral

      H60.509 Unspecified acute noninfective otitis externa, unspecified ear

    🔵 **H60.51** Acute actinic otitis externa

      H60.511 Acute actinic otitis externa, right ear

      H60.512 Acute actinic otitis externa, left ear

      H60.513 Acute actinic otitis externa, bilateral

      H60.519 Acute actinic otitis externa, unspecified ear

    🔵 **H60.52** Acute chemical otitis externa

      H60.521 Acute chemical otitis externa, right ear

      H60.522 Acute chemical otitis externa, left ear

      H60.523 Acute chemical otitis externa, bilateral

      H60.529 Acute chemical otitis externa, unspecified ear

    🔵 **H60.53** Acute contact otitis externa

      H60.531 Acute contact otitis externa, right ear

      H60.532 Acute contact otitis externa, left ear

      H60.533 Acute contact otitis externa, bilateral

      H60.539 Acute contact otitis externa, unspecified ear

    🔵 **H60.54** Acute eczematoid otitis externa

      H60.541 Acute eczematoid otitis externa, right ear

      H60.542 Acute eczematoid otitis externa, left ear

      H60.543 Acute eczematoid otitis externa, bilateral

      H60.549 Acute eczematoid otitis externa, unspecified ear

    🔵 **H60.55** Acute reactive otitis externa

      H60.551 Acute reactive otitis externa, right ear

      H60.552 Acute reactive otitis externa, left ear

      H60.553 Acute reactive otitis externa, bilateral

PDxₐ Unacceptable principal diagnosis symbol per Medicare code edits POA Code exempt from diagnosis present on admission requirement

❓ Questionable admission CC Complication or comorbidity CC/MCC Exc CC/MCC exclusion MCC Major complication or comorbidity

CC Principal diagnosis as its own CC MCC Principal diagnosis as its own MCC HCC HCC diagnosis code RxHCC RxHCC diagnosis code

MACRA code Z1 Z code as first-listed diagnosis

When symbols appear on a code that requires a 7th character extension, refer to Appendix B to identify applicable 7th character codes.

2018 ICD-10-CM

H60.559   Acute reactive otitis externa, unspecified ear
5ᵗʰ H60.59 Other noninfective acute otitis externa
H60.591   Other noninfective acute otitis externa, right ear
H60.592   Other noninfective acute otitis externa, left ear
H60.593   Other noninfective acute otitis externa, bilateral
H60.599   Other noninfective acute otitis externa, unspecified ear
5ᵗʰ H60.6 Unspecified chronic otitis externa
H60.60   Unspecified chronic otitis externa, unspecified ear
H60.61   Unspecified chronic otitis externa, right ear
H60.62   Unspecified chronic otitis externa, left ear
H60.63   Unspecified chronic otitis externa, bilateral
5ᵗʰ H60.8 Other otitis externa
6ᵗʰ H60.8X   Other otitis externa
H60.8X1   Other otitis externa, right ear
H60.8X2   Other otitis externa, left ear
H60.8X3   Other otitis externa, bilateral
H60.8X9   Other otitis externa, unspecified ear
5ᵗʰ H60.9 Unspecified otitis externa
H60.90   Unspecified otitis externa, unspecified ear
H60.91   Unspecified otitis externa, right ear
H60.92   Unspecified otitis externa, left ear
H60.93   Unspecified otitis externa, bilateral
4ᵗʰ H61 Other disorders of external ear
5ᵗʰ H61.0 Chondritis and perichondritis of external ear
Chondrodermatitis nodularis chronica helicis
Perichondritis of auricle
Perichondritis of pinna
6ᵗʰ H61.00   Unspecified perichondritis of external ear
H61.001   Unspecified perichondritis of right external ear
H61.002   Unspecified perichondritis of left external ear
H61.003   Unspecified perichondritis of external ear, bilateral
H61.009   Unspecified perichondritis of external ear, unspecified ear
6ᵗʰ H61.01   Acute perichondritis of external ear
H61.011   Acute perichondritis of right external ear
H61.012   Acute perichondritis of left external ear
H61.013   Acute perichondritis of external ear, bilateral
H61.019   Acute perichondritis of external ear, unspecified ear
6ᵗʰ H61.02   Chronic perichondritis of external ear
H61.021   Chronic perichondritis of right external ear
H61.022   Chronic perichondritis of left external ear
H61.023   Chronic perichondritis of external ear, bilateral
H61.029   Chronic perichondritis of external ear, unspecified ear
6ᵗʰ H61.03   Chondritis of external ear
Chondritis of auricle
Chondritis of pinna
H61.031   Chondritis of right external ear
H61.032   Chondritis of left external ear
AHA: Q1 2015
H61.033   Chondritis of external ear, bilateral
H61.039   Chondritis of external ear, unspecified ear
5ᵗʰ H61.1 Noninfective disorders of pinna
EXCLUDES2 cauliflower ear (M95.1-)
gouty tophi of ear (M1A.-)
6ᵗʰ H61.10   Unspecified noninfective disorders of pinna
Disorder of pinna NOS

H61.101   Unspecified noninfective disorders of pinna, right ear
H61.102   Unspecified noninfective disorders of pinna, left ear
H61.103   Unspecified noninfective disorders of pinna, bilateral
H61.109   Unspecified noninfective disorders of pinna, unspecified ear
6ᵗʰ H61.11   Acquired deformity of pinna
Acquired deformity of auricle
EXCLUDES2 cauliflower ear (M95.1-)
H61.111   Acquired deformity of pinna, right ear
H61.112   Acquired deformity of pinna, left ear
H61.113   Acquired deformity of pinna, bilateral
H61.119   Acquired deformity of pinna, unspecified ear
6ᵗʰ H61.12   Hematoma of pinna
Hematoma of auricle
H61.121   Hematoma of pinna, right ear
H61.122   Hematoma of pinna, left ear
H61.123   Hematoma of pinna, bilateral
H61.129   Hematoma of pinna, unspecified ear
6ᵗʰ H61.19   Other noninfective disorders of pinna
H61.191   Noninfective disorders of pinna, right ear
H61.192   Noninfective disorders of pinna, left ear
H61.193   Noninfective disorders of pinna, bilateral
H61.199   Noninfective disorders of pinna, unspecified ear
5ᵗʰ H61.2 Impacted cerumen
Wax in ear
H61.20   Impacted cerumen, unspecified ear   ❓
H61.21   Impacted cerumen, right ear   ❓
H61.22   Impacted cerumen, left ear   ❓
H61.23   Impacted cerumen, bilateral   ❓
5ᵗʰ H61.3 Acquired stenosis of external ear canal
Collapse of external ear canal
EXCLUDES1 postprocedural stenosis of external ear canal (H95.81-)
6ᵗʰ H61.30   Acquired stenosis of external ear canal, unspecified
H61.301   Acquired stenosis of right external ear canal, unspecified
H61.302   Acquired stenosis of left external ear canal, unspecified
H61.303   Acquired stenosis of external ear canal, unspecified, bilateral
H61.309   Acquired stenosis of external ear canal, unspecified, unspecified ear
6ᵗʰ H61.31   Acquired stenosis of external ear canal secondary to trauma
H61.311   Acquired stenosis of right external ear canal secondary to trauma
H61.312   Acquired stenosis of left external ear canal secondary to trauma
H61.313   Acquired stenosis of external ear canal secondary to trauma, bilateral
H61.319   Acquired stenosis of external ear canal secondary to trauma, unspecified ear
6ᵗʰ H61.32   Acquired stenosis of external ear canal secondary to inflammation and infection
H61.321   Acquired stenosis of right external ear canal secondary to inflammation and infection
H61.322   Acquired stenosis of left external ear canal secondary to inflammation and infection
H61.323   Acquired stenosis of external ear canal secondary to inflammation and infection, bilateral
H61.329   Acquired stenosis of external ear canal secondary to inflammation and infection, unspecified ear
6ᵗʰ H61.39   Other acquired stenosis of external ear canal

Unspecified Code   Other Specified Code   Manifestation Code   N Newborn   P Pediatric   M Maternity   A Adult   ♂ Male   ♀ Female
● New Code   ▲ Revised Code Title   ▶◀ Revised Text   NOTES   INCLUDES   EXCLUDES1 Not coded here   EXCLUDES2 Not included here
4ᵗʰ character required   5ᵗʰ character required   6ᵗʰ character required   7ᵗʰ character required
7ᵗʰ Extension 'X' Alert   HAC Hospital-acquired condition (HAC) alert   AHA AHA Coding Clinic©

2018 ICD-10-CM   When symbols appear on a code that requires a 7th character extension, refer to Appendix B to identify applicable 7th character codes.   633

H61.391 Other acquired stenosis of right external ear canal

H61.392 Other acquired stenosis of left external ear canal

H61.393 Other acquired stenosis of external ear canal, bilateral

H61.399 Other acquired stenosis of external ear canal, unspecified ear

� H61.8 Other specified disorders of external ear

🔟 H61.81 Exostosis of external canal

H61.811 Exostosis of right external canal

H61.812 Exostosis of left external canal

H61.813 Exostosis of external canal, bilateral

H61.819 Exostosis of external canal, unspecified ear

🔟 H61.89 Other specified disorders of external ear

H61.891 Other specified disorders of right external ear

H61.892 Other specified disorders of left external ear

H61.893 Other specified disorders of external ear, bilateral

H61.899 Other specified disorders of external ear, unspecified ear

� H61.9 Disorder of external ear, unspecified

H61.90 Disorder of external ear, unspecified, unspecified ear

H61.91 Disorder of right external ear, unspecified

H61.92 Disorder of left external ear, unspecified

H61.93 Disorder of external ear, unspecified, bilateral

🔴 H62 Disorders of external ear in diseases classified elsewhere

🔟 H62.4 Otitis externa in other diseases classified elsewhere

Code first underlying disease, such as:

erysipelas (A46)

impetigo (L01.0)

EXCLUDES1 otitis externa (in):

candidiasis (B37.84)

herpes viral [herpes simplex] (B00.1)

herpes zoster (B02.8)

H62.40 Otitis externa in other diseases classified elsewhere, unspecified ear

H62.41 Otitis externa in other diseases classified elsewhere, right ear

H62.42 Otitis externa in other diseases classified elsewhere, left ear

H62.43 Otitis externa in other diseases classified elsewhere, bilateral

🔟 H62.8 Other disorders of external ear in diseases classified elsewhere

Code first underlying disease, such as:

gout (M1A.-, M10.-)

🔟 H62.8X Other disorders of external ear in diseases classified elsewhere

H62.8X1 Other disorders of right external ear in diseases classified elsewhere

H62.8X2 Other disorders of left external ear in diseases classified elsewhere

H62.8X3 Other disorders of external ear in diseases classified elsewhere, bilateral

H62.8X9 Other disorders of external ear in diseases classified elsewhere, unspecified ear

Diseases of middle ear and mastoid (H65-H75)

🔴 H65 Nonsuppurative otitis media

INCLUDES nonsuppurative otitis media with myringitis

Use additional code for any associated perforated tympanic membrane (H72.-)

Use additional code to identify:

exposure to environmental tobacco smoke (Z77.22)

exposure to tobacco smoke in the perinatal period (P96.81)

history of tobacco dependence (Z87.891)

occupational exposure to environmental tobacco smoke (Z57.31)

tobacco dependence (F17.-)

tobacco use (Z72.0)

🔟 H65.0 Acute serous otitis media

Acute and subacute secretory otitis

H65.00 Acute serous otitis media, unspecified ear

H65.01 Acute serous otitis media, right ear

H65.02 Acute serous otitis media, left ear

H65.03 Acute serous otitis media, bilateral

H65.04 Acute serous otitis media, recurrent, right ear

H65.05 Acute serous otitis media, recurrent, left ear

H65.06 Acute serous otitis media, recurrent, bilateral

H65.07 Acute serous otitis media, recurrent, unspecified ear

🔟 H65.1 Other acute nonsuppurative otitis media

EXCLUDES1 otitic barotrauma (T70.0)

otitis media (acute) NOS (H66.9)

🔟 H65.11 Acute and subacute allergic otitis media (mucoid) (sanguinous) (serous)

H65.111 Acute and subacute allergic otitis media (mucoid) (sanguinous) (serous), right ear

H65.112 Acute and subacute allergic otitis media (mucoid) (sanguinous) (serous), left ear

H65.113 Acute and subacute allergic otitis media (mucoid) (sanguinous) (serous), bilateral

H65.114 Acute and subacute allergic otitis media (mucoid) (sanguinous) (serous), recurrent, right ear

H65.115 Acute and subacute allergic otitis media (mucoid) (sanguinous) (serous), recurrent, left ear

H65.116 Acute and subacute allergic otitis media (mucoid) (sanguinous) (serous), recurrent, bilateral

H65.117 Acute and subacute allergic otitis media (mucoid) (sanguinous) (serous), recurrent, unspecified ear

H65.119 Acute and subacute allergic otitis media (mucoid) (sanguinous) (serous), unspecified ear

🔟 H65.19 Other acute nonsuppurative otitis media

Acute and subacute mucoid otitis media

Acute and subacute nonsuppurative otitis media NOS

Acute and subacute sanguinous otitis media

Acute and subacute seromucinous otitis media

H65.191 Other acute nonsuppurative otitis media, right ear

H65.192 Other acute nonsuppurative otitis media, left ear

H65.193 Other acute nonsuppurative otitis media, bilateral

H65.194 Other acute nonsuppurative otitis media, recurrent, right ear

H65.195 Other acute nonsuppurative otitis media, recurrent, left ear

H65.196 Other acute nonsuppurative otitis media, recurrent, bilateral

H65.197 Other acute nonsuppurative otitis media recurrent, unspecified ear

H65.199 Other acute nonsuppurative otitis media, unspecified ear

🔟 H65.2 Chronic serous otitis media

Chronic tubotympanal catarrh

H65.20 Chronic serous otitis media, unspecified ear

H65.21 Chronic serous otitis media, right ear

H65.22 Chronic serous otitis media, left ear

H65.23 Chronic serous otitis media, bilateral

🔟 H65.3 Chronic mucoid otitis media

Chronic mucinous otitis media

Chronic secretory otitis media

PDx Unacceptable principal diagnosis symbol per Medicare code edits   PDx Code exempt from diagnosis present on admission requirement

❓ Questionable admission   ↩ Complication or comorbidity   CC/MCC Excl. CC/MCC exclusion   MCC Major complication or comorbidity

Principal diagnosis as its own CC   Principal diagnosis as its own MCC   HCC HCC diagnosis code   RxHCC RxHCC diagnosis code

MACRA code   Z Z code as first-listed diagnosis

When symbols appear on a code that requires a 7th character extension, refer to Appendix B to identify applicable 7th character codes.

2018 ICD-10-CM

Chronic transudative otitis media
Glue ear
EXCLUDES1 adhesive middle ear disease (H74.1)

H65.30 **Chronic mucoid otitis media, unspecified ear**

H65.31 **Chronic mucoid otitis media, right ear**

H65.32 **Chronic mucoid otitis media, left ear**

H65.33 **Chronic mucoid otitis media, bilateral**

5ᵗʰ H65.4 **Other chronic nonsuppurative otitis media**

  6ᵗʰ H65.41 **Chronic allergic otitis media**

    H65.411 **Chronic allergic otitis media, right ear**

    H65.412 **Chronic allergic otitis media, left ear**

    H65.413 **Chronic allergic otitis media, bilateral**

    H65.419 **Chronic allergic otitis media, unspecified ear**

  6ᵗʰ H65.49 **Other chronic nonsuppurative otitis media**

    Chronic exudative otitis media
    Chronic nonsuppurative otitis media NOS
    Chronic otitis media with effusion (nonpurulent)
    Chronic seromucinous otitis media

    H65.491 **Other chronic nonsuppurative otitis media, right ear**

    H65.492 **Other chronic nonsuppurative otitis media, left ear**

    H65.493 **Other chronic nonsuppurative otitis media, bilateral**

    H65.499 **Other chronic nonsuppurative otitis media, unspecified ear**

5ᵗʰ H65.9 **Unspecified nonsuppurative otitis media**

  Allergic otitis media NOS
  Catarrhal otitis media NOS
  Exudative otitis media NOS
  Mucoid otitis media NOS
  Otitis media with effusion (nonpurulent) NOS
  Secretory otitis media NOS
  Seromucinous otitis media NOS
  Serous otitis media NOS
  Transudative otitis media NOS

  H65.90 **Unspecified nonsuppurative otitis media, unspecified ear**

  H65.91 **Unspecified nonsuppurative otitis media, right ear**

  H65.92 **Unspecified nonsuppurative otitis media, left ear**

  H65.93 **Unspecified nonsuppurative otitis media, bilateral**

4ᵗʰ **H66 Suppurative and unspecified otitis media**

INCLUDES suppurative and unspecified otitis media with myringitis

Use additional code to identify:
exposure to environmental tobacco smoke (Z77.22)
exposure to tobacco smoke in the perinatal period (P96.81)
history of tobacco dependence (Z87.891)
occupational exposure to environmental tobacco smoke (Z57.31)
tobacco dependence (F17.-)
tobacco use (Z72.0)

5ᵗʰ H66.0 **Acute suppurative otitis media**

  6ᵗʰ H66.00 **Acute suppurative otitis media without spontaneous rupture of ear drum**

    H66.001 **Acute suppurative otitis media without spontaneous rupture of ear drum, right ear**
      AHA: Q1 2016

    H66.002 **Acute suppurative otitis media without spontaneous rupture of ear drum, left ear**

    H66.003 **Acute suppurative otitis media without spontaneous rupture of ear drum, bilateral**

    H66.004 **Acute suppurative otitis media without spontaneous rupture of ear drum, recurrent, right ear**

    H66.005 **Acute suppurative otitis media without spontaneous rupture of ear drum, recurrent, left ear**

    H66.006 **Acute suppurative otitis media without spontaneous rupture of ear drum, recurrent, bilateral**

    H66.007 **Acute suppurative otitis media without spontaneous rupture of ear drum, recurrent, unspecified ear**

    H66.009 **Acute suppurative otitis media without spontaneous rupture of ear drum, unspecified ear**

  6ᵗʰ H66.01 **Acute suppurative otitis media with spontaneous rupture of ear drum**

    H66.011 **Acute suppurative otitis media with spontaneous rupture of ear drum, right ear**

    H66.012 **Acute suppurative otitis media with spontaneous rupture of ear drum, left ear**

    H66.013 **Acute suppurative otitis media with spontaneous rupture of ear drum, bilateral**

    H66.014 **Acute suppurative otitis media with spontaneous rupture of ear drum, recurrent, right ear**

    H66.015 **Acute suppurative otitis media with spontaneous rupture of ear drum, recurrent, left ear**

    H66.016 **Acute suppurative otitis media with spontaneous rupture of ear drum, recurrent, bilateral**

    H66.017 **Acute suppurative otitis media with spontaneous rupture of ear drum, recurrent, unspecified ear**

    H66.019 **Acute suppurative otitis media with spontaneous rupture of ear drum, unspecified ear**

5ᵗʰ H66.1 **Chronic tubotympanic suppurative otitis media**

  Benign chronic suppurative otitis media
  Chronic tubotympanic disease
  Use additional code for any associated perforated tympanic membrane (H72.-)

  H66.10 **Chronic tubotympanic suppurative otitis media, unspecified**

  H66.11 **Chronic tubotympanic suppurative otitis media, right ear**

  H66.12 **Chronic tubotympanic suppurative otitis media, left ear**

  H66.13 **Chronic tubotympanic suppurative otitis media, bilateral**

5ᵗʰ H66.2 **Chronic atticoantral suppurative otitis media**

  Chronic atticoantral disease
  Use additional code for any associated perforated tympanic membrane (H72.-)

  H66.20 **Chronic atticoantral suppurative otitis media, unspecified ear**

  H66.21 **Chronic atticoantral suppurative otitis media, right ear**

  H66.22 **Chronic atticoantral suppurative otitis media, left ear**

  H66.23 **Chronic atticoantral suppurative otitis media, bilateral**

5ᵗʰ H66.3 **Other chronic suppurative otitis media**

  Chronic suppurative otitis media NOS
  Use additional code for any associated perforated tympanic membrane (H72.-)
  EXCLUDES1 tuberculous otitis media (A18.6)

  6ᵗʰ H66.3X **Other chronic suppurative otitis media**

    H66.3X1 **Other chronic suppurative otitis media, right ear**

    H66.3X2 **Other chronic suppurative otitis media, left ear**

    H66.3X3 **Other chronic suppurative otitis media, bilateral**

    H66.3X9 **Other chronic suppurative otitis media, unspecified ear**

Unspecified Code Other Specified Code Manifestation Code N Newborn P Pediatric M Maternity A Adult ♂ Male ♀ Female
● New Code ▲ Revised Code Title ►◄ Revised Text NOTES INCLUDES EXCLUDES 1 Not coded here EXCLUDES 2 Not included here
4ᵗʰ 4ᵗʰ character required 5ᵗʰ 5ᵗʰ character required 6ᵗʰ 6ᵗʰ character required 7ᵗʰ 7ᵗʰ character required
7ᵗʰ Extension 'X' Alert HAC Hospital-acquired condition (HAC) alert AHA AHA Coding Clinic©

H66.4 Suppurative otitis media, unspecified
Purulent otitis media NOS
Use additional code for any associated perforated tympanic membrane (H72.-)

H66.40 Suppurative otitis media, unspecified, unspecified ear

H66.41 Suppurative otitis media, unspecified, right ear

H66.42 Suppurative otitis media, unspecified, left ear

H66.43 Suppurative otitis media, unspecified, bilateral

H66.9 Otitis media, unspecified
Otitis media NOS
Acute otitis media NOS
Chronic otitis media NOS
Use additional code for any associated perforated tympanic membrane (H72.-)

H66.90 Otitis media, unspecified, unspecified ear

H66.91 Otitis media, unspecified, right ear

H66.92 Otitis media, unspecified, left ear

H66.93 Otitis media, unspecified, bilateral

H67 Otitis media in diseases classified elsewhere
Code first underlying disease, such as:
viral disease NEC (B00-B34)
Use additional code for any associated perforated tympanic membrane (H72.-)

EXCLUDES1 otitis media in:
influenza (J09.X9, J10.83, J11.83)
measles (B05.3)
scarlet fever (A38.0)
tuberculosis (A18.6)

H67.1 Otitis media in diseases classified elsewhere, right ear

H67.2 Otitis media in diseases classified elsewhere, left ear

H67.3 Otitis media in diseases classified elsewhere, bilateral

H67.9 Otitis media in diseases classified elsewhere, unspecified ear

H68 Eustachian salpingitis and obstruction

H68.0 Eustachian salpingitis

H68.00 Unspecified Eustachian salpingitis

H68.001 Unspecified Eustachian salpingitis, right ear

H68.002 Unspecified Eustachian salpingitis, left ear

H68.003 Unspecified Eustachian salpingitis, bilateral

H68.009 Unspecified Eustachian salpingitis, unspecified ear

H68.01 Acute Eustachian salpingitis

H68.011 Acute Eustachian salpingitis, right ear

H68.012 Acute Eustachian salpingitis, left ear

H68.013 Acute Eustachian salpingitis, bilateral

H68.019 Acute Eustachian salpingitis, unspecified ear

H68.02 Chronic Eustachian salpingitis

H68.021 Chronic Eustachian salpingitis, right ear

H68.022 Chronic Eustachian salpingitis, left ear

H68.023 Chronic Eustachian salpingitis, bilateral

H68.029 Chronic Eustachian salpingitis, unspecified ear

H68.1 Obstruction of Eustachian tube
Stenosis of Eustachian tube
Stricture of Eustachian tube

H68.10 Unspecified obstruction of Eustachian tube

H68.101 Unspecified obstruction of Eustachian tube, right ear

H68.102 Unspecified obstruction of Eustachian tube, left ear

H68.103 Unspecified obstruction of Eustachian tube, bilateral

H68.109 Unspecified obstruction of Eustachian tube, unspecified ear

H68.11 Osseous obstruction of Eustachian tube

H68.111 Osseous obstruction of Eustachian tube, right ear

H68.112 Osseous obstruction of Eustachian tube, left ear

H68.113 Osseous obstruction of Eustachian tube, bilateral

H68.119 Osseous obstruction of Eustachian tube, unspecified ear

H68.12 Intrinsic cartilagenous obstruction of Eustachian tube

H68.121 Intrinsic cartilagenous obstruction of Eustachian tube, right ear

H68.122 Intrinsic cartilagenous obstruction of Eustachian tube, left ear

H68.123 Intrinsic cartilagenous obstruction of Eustachian tube, bilateral

H68.129 Intrinsic cartilagenous obstruction of Eustachian tube, unspecified ear

H68.13 Extrinsic cartilagenous obstruction of Eustachian tube
Compression of Eustachian tube

H68.131 Extrinsic cartilagenous obstruction of Eustachian tube, right ear

H68.132 Extrinsic cartilagenous obstruction of Eustachian tube, left ear

H68.133 Extrinsic cartilagenous obstruction of Eustachian tube, bilateral

H68.139 Extrinsic cartilagenous obstruction of Eustachian tube, unspecified ear

H69 Other and unspecified disorders of Eustachian tube

H69.0 Patulous Eustachian tube

H69.00 Patulous Eustachian tube, unspecified ear

H69.01 Patulous Eustachian tube, right ear

H69.02 Patulous Eustachian tube, left ear

H69.03 Patulous Eustachian tube, bilateral

H69.8 Other specified disorders of Eustachian tube

H69.80 Other specified disorders of Eustachian tube, unspecified ear

H69.81 Other specified disorders of Eustachian tube, right ear

H69.82 Other specified disorders of Eustachian tube, left ear

H69.83 Other specified disorders of Eustachian tube, bilateral

H69.9 Unspecified Eustachian tube disorder

H69.90 Unspecified Eustachian tube disorder, unspecified ear

H69.91 Unspecified Eustachian tube disorder, right ear

H69.92 Unspecified Eustachian tube disorder, left ear

H69.93 Unspecified Eustachian tube disorder, bilateral

H70 Mastoiditis and related conditions

H70.0 Acute mastoiditis
Abscess of mastoid
Empyema of mastoid

H70.00 Acute mastoiditis without complications

H70.001 Acute mastoiditis without complications, right ear

H70.002 Acute mastoiditis without complications, left ear

H70.003 Acute mastoiditis without complications, bilateral

H70.009 Acute mastoiditis without complications, unspecified ear

H70.01 Subperiosteal abscess of mastoid

H70.011 Subperiosteal abscess of mastoid, right ear

H70.012 Subperiosteal abscess of mastoid, left ear

H70.013 Subperiosteal abscess of mastoid, bilateral

H70.019 Subperiosteal abscess of mastoid, unspecified ear

H70.09 Acute mastoiditis with other complications

Unacceptable principal diagnosis symbol per Medicare code edits Code exempt from diagnosis present on admission requirement
Questionable admission Complication or comorbidity CC/MCC exclusion Major complication or comorbidity
Principal diagnosis as its own CC Principal diagnosis as its own MCC HCC diagnosis code RxHCC diagnosis code
MACRA code Z code as first-listed diagnosis

636 When symbols appear on a code that requires a 7th character extension, refer to Appendix B to identify applicable 7th character codes. 2018 ICD-10-CM

H70.091 Acute mastoiditis with other complications, right ear CC☑ CC/MCC Exc

H70.092 Acute mastoiditis with other complications, left ear CC☑ CC/MCC Exc

H70.093 Acute mastoiditis with other complications, bilateral CC☑ CC/MCC Exc

H70.099 Acute mastoiditis with other complications, unspecified ear CC☑ CC/MCC Exc

5ᵗʰ H70.1 Chronic mastoiditis

Caries of mastoid

Fistula of mastoid

EXCLUDES1 tuberculous mastoiditis (A18.03)

H70.10 Chronic mastoiditis, unspecified ear

H70.11 Chronic mastoiditis, right ear

H70.12 Chronic mastoiditis, left ear

H70.13 Chronic mastoiditis, bilateral

5ᵗʰ H70.2 Petrositis

Inflammation of petrous bone

6ᵗʰ H70.20 Unspecified petrositis

H70.201 Unspecified petrositis, right ear

H70.202 Unspecified petrositis, left ear

H70.203 Unspecified petrositis, bilateral

H70.209 Unspecified petrositis, unspecified ear

6ᵗʰ H70.21 Acute petrositis

H70.211 Acute petrositis, right ear

H70.212 Acute petrositis, left ear

H70.213 Acute petrositis, bilateral

H70.219 Acute petrositis, unspecified ear

6ᵗʰ H70.22 Chronic petrositis

H70.221 Chronic petrositis, right ear

H70.222 Chronic petrositis, left ear

H70.223 Chronic petrositis, bilateral

H70.229 Chronic petrositis, unspecified ear

5ᵗʰ H70.8 Other mastoiditis and related conditions

EXCLUDES1 preauricular sinus and cyst (Q18.1)

sinus, fistula, and cyst of branchial cleft (Q18.0)

6ᵗʰ H70.81 Postauricular fistula

H70.811 Postauricular fistula, right ear

H70.812 Postauricular fistula, left ear

H70.813 Postauricular fistula, bilateral

H70.819 Postauricular fistula, unspecified ear

6ᵗʰ H70.89 Other mastoiditis and related conditions

H70.891 Other mastoiditis and related conditions, right ear

H70.892 Other mastoiditis and related conditions, left ear

H70.893 Other mastoiditis and related conditions, bilateral

H70.899 Other mastoiditis and related conditions, unspecified ear

5ᵗʰ H70.9 Unspecified mastoiditis

H70.90 Unspecified mastoiditis, unspecified ear

H70.91 Unspecified mastoiditis, right ear

H70.92 Unspecified mastoiditis, left ear

H70.93 Unspecified mastoiditis, bilateral

4ᵗʰ H71 Cholesteatoma of middle ear

EXCLUDES2 cholesteatoma of external ear (H60.4-)

recurrent cholesteatoma of postmastoidectomy cavity (H95.0-)

5ᵗʰ H71.0 Cholesteatoma of attic

H71.00 Cholesteatoma of attic, unspecified ear

H71.01 Cholesteatoma of attic, right ear

H71.02 Cholesteatoma of attic, left ear

H71.03 Cholesteatoma of attic, bilateral

5ᵗʰ H71.1 Cholesteatoma of tympanum

H71.10 Cholesteatoma of tympanum, unspecified ear

H71.11 Cholesteatoma of tympanum, right ear

H71.12 Cholesteatoma of tympanum, left ear

H71.13 Cholesteatoma of tympanum, bilateral

5ᵗʰ H71.2 Cholesteatoma of mastoid

H71.20 Cholesteatoma of mastoid, unspecified ear

H71.21 Cholesteatoma of mastoid, right ear

H71.22 Cholesteatoma of mastoid, left ear

H71.23 Cholesteatoma of mastoid, bilateral

5ᵗʰ H71.3 Diffuse cholesteatosis

H71.30 Diffuse cholesteatosis, unspecified ear

H71.31 Diffuse cholesteatosis, right ear

H71.32 Diffuse cholesteatosis, left ear

H71.33 Diffuse cholesteatosis, bilateral

5ᵗʰ H71.9 Unspecified cholesteatoma

H71.90 Unspecified cholesteatoma, unspecified ear

H71.91 Unspecified cholesteatoma, right ear

H71.92 Unspecified cholesteatoma, left ear

H71.93 Unspecified cholesteatoma, bilateral

4ᵗʰ H72 Perforation of tympanic membrane

INCLUDES persistent post-traumatic perforation of ear drum

postinflammatory perforation of ear drum

Code first any associated otitis media (H65.-, H66.1-, H66.2-, H66.3-, H66.4-, H66.9-, H67.-)

EXCLUDES1 acute suppurative otitis media with rupture of the tympanic membrane (H66.01-)

traumatic rupture of ear drum (S09.2-)

5ᵗʰ H72.0 Central perforation of tympanic membrane

H72.00 Central perforation of tympanic membrane, unspecified ear

H72.01 Central perforation of tympanic membrane, right ear

H72.02 Central perforation of tympanic membrane, left ear

H72.03 Central perforation of tympanic membrane, bilateral

5ᵗʰ H72.1 Attic perforation of tympanic membrane

Perforation of pars flaccida

H72.10 Attic perforation of tympanic membrane, unspecified ear

H72.11 Attic perforation of tympanic membrane, right ear

H72.12 Attic perforation of tympanic membrane, left ear

H72.13 Attic perforation of tympanic membrane, bilateral

5ᵗʰ H72.2 Other marginal perforations of tympanic membrane

6ᵗʰ H72.2X Other marginal perforations of tympanic membrane

H72.2X1 Other marginal perforations of tympanic membrane, right ear

H72.2X2 Other marginal perforations of tympanic membrane, left ear

H72.2X3 Other marginal perforations of tympanic membrane, bilateral

H72.2X9 Other marginal perforations of tympanic membrane, unspecified ear

5ᵗʰ H72.8 Other perforations of tympanic membrane

6ᵗʰ H72.81 Multiple perforations of tympanic membrane

H72.811 Multiple perforations of tympanic membrane, right ear

H72.812 Multiple perforations of tympanic membrane, left ear

H72.813 Multiple perforations of tympanic membrane, bilateral

H72.819 Multiple perforations of tympanic membrane, unspecified ear

6ᵗʰ H72.82 Total perforations of tympanic membrane

H72.821 Total perforations of tympanic membrane, right ear

H72.822 Total perforations of tympanic membrane, left ear

H72.823 Total perforations of tympanic membrane, bilateral

H72.829 Total perforations of tympanic membrane, unspecified ear

5ᵗʰ H72.9 Unspecified perforation of tympanic membrane

H72.90 Unspecified perforation of tympanic membrane, unspecified ear

Unspecified Code   Other Specified Code   Manifestation Code   N Newborn   P Pediatric   M Maternity   A Adult   ♂ Male   ♀ Female
● New Code   ▲ Revised Code Title   ▶◀ Revised Text   NOTES   INCLUDES   EXCLUDES 1 Not coded here   EXCLUDES 2 Not included here
4ᵗʰ 4ᵗʰ character required   5ᵗʰ 5ᵗʰ character required   6ᵗʰ 6ᵗʰ character required   7ᵗʰ 7ᵗʰ character required
7ᵗʰ Extension 'X' Alert   HAC Hospital-acquired condition (HAC) alert   AHA AHA Coding Clinic©

H72.91 Unspecified perforation of tympanic membrane, right ear
H72.92 Unspecified perforation of tympanic membrane, left ear
H72.93 Unspecified perforation of tympanic membrane, bilateral

[4th] H73 Other disorders of tympanic membrane

[5th] H73.0 Acute myringitis

[EXCLUDES1] *acute myringitis with otitis media (H65, H66)*

[6th] H73.00 Unspecified acute myringitis
Acute tympanitis NOS
H73.001 Acute myringitis, right ear
H73.002 Acute myringitis, left ear
H73.003 Acute myringitis, bilateral
H73.009 Acute myringitis, unspecified ear

[6th] H73.01 Bullous myringitis
H73.011 Bullous myringitis, right ear
H73.012 Bullous myringitis, left ear
H73.013 Bullous myringitis, bilateral
H73.019 Bullous myringitis, unspecified ear

[6th] H73.09 Other acute myringitis
H73.091 Other acute myringitis, right ear
H73.092 Other acute myringitis, left ear
H73.093 Other acute myringitis, bilateral
H73.099 Other acute myringitis, unspecified ear

[5th] H73.1 Chronic myringitis
Chronic tympanitis

[EXCLUDES1] *chronic myringitis with otitis media (H65, H66)*

H73.10 Chronic myringitis, unspecified ear
H73.11 Chronic myringitis, right ear
H73.12 Chronic myringitis, left ear
H73.13 Chronic myringitis, bilateral

[5th] H73.2 Unspecified myringitis
H73.20 Unspecified myringitis, unspecified ear
H73.21 Unspecified myringitis, right ear
H73.22 Unspecified myringitis, left ear
H73.23 Unspecified myringitis, bilateral

[5th] H73.8 Other specified disorders of tympanic membrane

[6th] H73.81 Atrophic flaccid tympanic membrane
H73.811 Atrophic flaccid tympanic membrane, right ear
H73.812 Atrophic flaccid tympanic membrane, left ear
H73.813 Atrophic flaccid tympanic membrane, bilateral
H73.819 Atrophic flaccid tympanic membrane, unspecified ear

[6th] H73.82 Atrophic nonflaccid tympanic membrane
H73.821 Atrophic nonflaccid tympanic membrane, right ear
H73.822 Atrophic nonflaccid tympanic membrane, left ear
H73.823 Atrophic nonflaccid tympanic membrane, bilateral
H73.829 Atrophic nonflaccid tympanic membrane, unspecified ear

[6th] H73.89 Other specified disorders of tympanic membrane
H73.891 Other specified disorders of tympanic membrane, right ear
H73.892 Other specified disorders of tympanic membrane, left ear
H73.893 Other specified disorders of tympanic membrane, bilateral
H73.899 Other specified disorders of tympanic membrane, unspecified ear

[5th] H73.9 Unspecified disorder of tympanic membrane
H73.90 Unspecified disorder of tympanic membrane, unspecified ear
H73.91 Unspecified disorder of tympanic membrane, right ear
H73.92 Unspecified disorder of tympanic membrane, left ear
H73.93 Unspecified disorder of tympanic membrane, bilateral

[4th] H74 Other disorders of middle ear mastoid

[EXCLUDES2] *mastoiditis (H70.-)*

[5th] H74.0 Tympanosclerosis
H74.01 Tympanosclerosis, right ear
H74.02 Tympanosclerosis, left ear
H74.03 Tympanosclerosis, bilateral
H74.09 Tympanosclerosis, unspecified ear

[5th] H74.1 Adhesive middle ear disease
Adhesive otitis

[EXCLUDES1] *glue ear (H65.3-)*

H74.11 Adhesive right middle ear disease
H74.12 Adhesive left middle ear disease
H74.13 Adhesive middle ear disease, bilateral
H74.19 Adhesive middle ear disease, unspecified ear

[5th] H74.2 Discontinuity and dislocation of ear ossicles
H74.20 Discontinuity and dislocation of ear ossicles, unspecified ear
H74.21 Discontinuity and dislocation of right ear ossicles
H74.22 Discontinuity and dislocation of left ear ossicles
H74.23 Discontinuity and dislocation of ear ossicles, bilateral

[5th] H74.3 Other acquired abnormalities of ear ossicles

[6th] H74.31 Ankylosis of ear ossicles
H74.311 Ankylosis of ear ossicles, right ear
H74.312 Ankylosis of ear ossicles, left ear
H74.313 Ankylosis of ear ossicles, bilateral
H74.319 Ankylosis of ear ossicles, unspecified ear

[6th] H74.32 Partial loss of ear ossicles
H74.321 Partial loss of ear ossicles, right ear
H74.322 Partial loss of ear ossicles, left ear
H74.323 Partial loss of ear ossicles, bilateral
H74.329 Partial loss of ear ossicles, unspecified ear

[6th] H74.39 Other acquired abnormalities of ear ossicles
H74.391 Other acquired abnormalities of right ear ossicles
H74.392 Other acquired abnormalities of left ear ossicles
H74.393 Other acquired abnormalities of ear ossicles, bilateral
H74.399 Other acquired abnormalities of ear ossicles, unspecified ear

[5th] H74.4 Polyp of middle ear
H74.40 Polyp of middle ear, unspecified ear
H74.41 Polyp of right middle ear
H74.42 Polyp of left middle ear
H74.43 Polyp of middle ear, bilateral

[5th] H74.8 Other specified disorders of middle ear and mastoid

[6th] H74.8X Other specified disorders of middle ear and mastoid
H74.8X1 Other specified disorders of right middle ear and mastoid
H74.8X2 Other specified disorders of left middle ear and mastoid
H74.8X3 Other specified disorders of middle ear and mastoid, bilateral
H74.8X9 Other specified disorders of middle ear and mastoid, unspecified ear

[5th] H74.9 Unspecified disorder of middle ear and mastoid
H74.90 Unspecified disorder of middle ear and mastoid, unspecified ear
H74.91 Unspecified disorder of right middle ear and mastoid
H74.92 Unspecified disorder of left middle ear and mastoid
H74.93 Unspecified disorder of middle ear and mastoid, bilateral

[PDx] Unacceptable principal diagnosis symbol per Medicare code edits [POA] Code exempt from diagnosis present on admission requirement
[?] Questionable admission [CC] Complication or comorbidity [CC/MCC Exc] CC/MCC exclusion [MCC] Major complication or comorbidity
[PDx CC] Principal diagnosis as its own CC [PDx MCC] Principal diagnosis as its own MCC [HCC] HCC diagnosis code [RxHCC] RxHCC diagnosis code
MACRA code [Z1] Z code as first-listed diagnosis

🔵⁴ᵗʰ **H75** Other disorders of middle ear and mastoid in diseases classified elsewhere
Code first underlying disease
🔵⁵ᵗʰ **H75.0** Mastoiditis in infectious and parasitic diseases classified elsewhere
EXCLUDES1 mastoiditis (in):
syphilis (A52.77)
tuberculosis (A18.03)
H75.00 Mastoiditis in infectious and parasitic diseases classified elsewhere, unspecified ear
H75.01 Mastoiditis in infectious and parasitic diseases classified elsewhere, right ear
H75.02 Mastoiditis in infectious and parasitic diseases classified elsewhere, left ear
H75.03 Mastoiditis in infectious and parasitic diseases classified elsewhere, bilateral
🔵⁵ᵗʰ **H75.8** Other specified disorders of middle ear and mastoid in diseases classified elsewhere
H75.80 Other specified disorders of middle ear and mastoid in diseases classified elsewhere, unspecified ear
H75.81 Other specified disorders of right middle ear and mastoid in diseases classified elsewhere
H75.82 Other specified disorders of left middle ear and mastoid in diseases classified elsewhere
H75.83 Other specified disorders of middle ear and mastoid in diseases classified elsewhere, bilateral

Diseases of inner ear (H80-H83)

🔵⁴ᵗʰ **H80** Otosclerosis
INCLUDES Otospongiosis
🔵⁵ᵗʰ **H80.0** Otosclerosis involving oval window, nonobliterative
H80.00 Otosclerosis involving oval window, nonobliterative, unspecified ear
H80.01 Otosclerosis involving oval window, nonobliterative, right ear
H80.02 Otosclerosis involving oval window, nonobliterative, left ear
H80.03 Otosclerosis involving oval window, nonobliterative, bilateral
🔵⁵ᵗʰ **H80.1** Otosclerosis involving oval window, obliterative
H80.10 Otosclerosis involving oval window, obliterative, unspecified ear
H80.11 Otosclerosis involving oval window, obliterative, right ear
H80.12 Otosclerosis involving oval window, obliterative, left ear
H80.13 Otosclerosis involving oval window, obliterative, bilateral
🔵⁵ᵗʰ **H80.2** Cochlear otosclerosis
Otosclerosis involving otic capsule
Otosclerosis involving round window
H80.20 Cochlear otosclerosis, unspecified ear
H80.21 Cochlear otosclerosis, right ear
H80.22 Cochlear otosclerosis, left ear
H80.23 Cochlear otosclerosis, bilateral
🔵⁵ᵗʰ **H80.8** Other otosclerosis
H80.80 Other otosclerosis, unspecified ear
H80.81 Other otosclerosis, right ear
H80.82 Other otosclerosis, left ear
H80.83 Other otosclerosis, bilateral
🔵⁵ᵗʰ **H80.9** Unspecified otosclerosis
H80.90 Unspecified otosclerosis, unspecified ear
H80.91 Unspecified otosclerosis, right ear
H80.92 Unspecified otosclerosis, left ear
H80.93 Unspecified otosclerosis, bilateral
🔵⁴ᵗʰ **H81** Disorders of vestibular function
EXCLUDES1 epidemic vertigo (A88.1)
vertigo NOS (R42)

🔵⁵ᵗʰ **H81.0** Ménière's disease
Labyrinthine hydrops
Ménière's syndrome or vertigo
H81.01 Ménière's disease, right ear
H81.02 Ménière's disease, left ear
H81.03 Ménière's disease, bilateral
H81.09 Ménière's disease, unspecified ear
🔵⁵ᵗʰ **H81.1** Benign paroxysmal vertigo
H81.10 Benign paroxysmal vertigo, unspecified ear
H81.11 Benign paroxysmal vertigo, right ear
H81.12 Benign paroxysmal vertigo, left ear
H81.13 Benign paroxysmal vertigo, bilateral
🔵⁵ᵗʰ **H81.2** Vestibular neuronitis
H81.20 Vestibular neuronitis, unspecified ear
H81.21 Vestibular neuronitis, right ear
H81.22 Vestibular neuronitis, left ear
H81.23 Vestibular neuronitis, bilateral
🔵⁵ᵗʰ **H81.3** Other peripheral vertigo
🔵⁶ᵗʰ **H81.31** Aural vertigo
H81.311 Aural vertigo, right ear
H81.312 Aural vertigo, left ear
H81.313 Aural vertigo, bilateral
H81.319 Aural vertigo, unspecified ear
🔵⁶ᵗʰ **H81.39** Other peripheral vertigo
Lermoyez' syndrome
Otogenic vertigo
Peripheral vertigo NOS
H81.391 Other peripheral vertigo, right ear
H81.392 Other peripheral vertigo, left ear
H81.393 Other peripheral vertigo, bilateral
H81.399 Other peripheral vertigo, unspecified ear
🔵⁵ᵗʰ **H81.4** Vertigo of central origin
Central positional nystagmus
H81.41 Vertigo of central origin, right ear
H81.42 Vertigo of central origin, left ear
H81.43 Vertigo of central origin, bilateral
H81.49 Vertigo of central origin, unspecified ear
🔵⁵ᵗʰ **H81.8** Other disorders of vestibular function
🔵⁶ᵗʰ **H81.8X** Other disorders of vestibular function
H81.8X1 Other disorders of vestibular function, right ear
H81.8X2 Other disorders of vestibular function, left ear
H81.8X3 Other disorders of vestibular function, bilateral
H81.8X9 Other disorders of vestibular function, unspecified ear
🔵⁵ᵗʰ **H81.9** Unspecified disorder of vestibular function
Vertiginous syndrome NOS
H81.90 Unspecified disorder of vestibular function, unspecified ear
H81.91 Unspecified disorder of vestibular function, right ear
H81.92 Unspecified disorder of vestibular function, left ear
H81.93 Unspecified disorder of vestibular function, bilateral
🔵⁴ᵗʰ **H82** Vertiginous syndromes in diseases classified elsewhere
Code first underlying disease
EXCLUDES1 epidemic vertigo (A88.1)
H82.1 Vertiginous syndromes in diseases classified elsewhere, right ear
H82.2 Vertiginous syndromes in diseases classified elsewhere, left ear
H82.3 Vertiginous syndromes in diseases classified elsewhere, bilateral
H82.9 Vertiginous syndromes in diseases classified elsewhere, unspecified ear
🔵⁴ᵗʰ **H83** Other diseases of inner ear
🔵⁵ᵗʰ **H83.0** Labyrinthitis
H83.01 Labyrinthitis, right ear
H83.02 Labyrinthitis, left ear

Unspecified Code   Other Specified Code   Manifestation Code   🅽 Newborn   🅿 Pediatric   🅼 Maternity   🄰 Adult   ♂ Male   ♀ Female
● New Code   ▲ Revised Code Title   ►◄ Revised Text   **NOTES**   *INCLUDES*   *EXCLUDES 1* Not coded here   *EXCLUDES 2* Not included here
4ᵗʰ character required   5ᵗʰ character required   6ᵗʰ character required   7ᵗʰ character required
7ᵗʰ Extension 'X' Alert   HAC Hospital-acquired condition (HAC) alert   **AHA** AHA Coding Clinic©

H83.03 Labyrinthitis, bilateral
H83.09 Labyrinthitis, unspecified ear
5ᵗʰ H83.1 Labyrinthine fistula
H83.11 Labyrinthine fistula, right ear
H83.12 Labyrinthine fistula, left ear
H83.13 Labyrinthine fistula, bilateral
H83.19 Labyrinthine fistula, unspecified ear
5ᵗʰ H83.2 Labyrinthine dysfunction
Labyrinthine hypersensitivity
Labyrinthine hypofunction
Labyrinthine loss of function
6ᵗʰ H83.2X Labyrinthine dysfunction
H83.2X1 Labyrinthine dysfunction, right ear
H83.2X2 Labyrinthine dysfunction, left ear
H83.2X3 Labyrinthine dysfunction, bilateral
H83.2X9 Labyrinthine dysfunction, unspecified ear
5ᵗʰ H83.3 Noise effects on inner ear
Acoustic trauma of inner ear
Noise-induced hearing loss of inner ear
6ᵗʰ H83.3X Noise effects on inner ear
H83.3X1 Noise effects on right inner ear
H83.3X2 Noise effects on left inner ear
H83.3X3 Noise effects on inner ear, bilateral
H83.3X9 Noise effects on inner ear, unspecified ear
5ᵗʰ H83.8 Other specified diseases of inner ear
6ᵗʰ H83.8X Other specified diseases of inner ear
H83.8X1 Other specified diseases of right inner ear
H83.8X2 Other specified diseases of left inner ear
H83.8X3 Other specified diseases of inner ear, bilateral
H83.8X9 Other specified diseases of inner ear, unspecified ear
5ᵗʰ H83.9 Unspecified disease of inner ear
H83.90 Unspecified disease of inner ear, unspecified ear
H83.91 Unspecified disease of right inner ear
H83.92 Unspecified disease of left inner ear
H83.93 Unspecified disease of inner ear, bilateral

Other disorders of ear (H90-H94)

4ᵗʰ H90 Conductive and sensorineural hearing loss
EXCLUDES1 deaf nonspeaking NEC (H91.3)
deafness NOS (H91.9-)
hearing loss NOS (H91.9-)
noise-induced hearing loss (H83.3-)
ototoxic hearing loss (H91.0-)
sudden (idiopathic) hearing loss (H91.2-)
H90.0 Conductive hearing loss, bilateral
5ᵗʰ H90.1 Conductive hearing loss, unilateral with unrestricted hearing on the contralateral side
H90.11 Conductive hearing loss, unilateral, right ear, with unrestricted hearing on the contralateral side
H90.12 Conductive hearing loss, unilateral, left ear, with unrestricted hearing on the contralateral side
H90.2 Conductive hearing loss, unspecified
Conductive deafness NOS
H90.3 Sensorineural hearing loss, bilateral
5ᵗʰ H90.4 Sensorineural hearing loss, unilateral with unrestricted hearing on the contralateral side
H90.41 Sensorineural hearing loss, unilateral, right ear, with unrestricted hearing on the contralateral side
H90.42 Sensorineural hearing loss, unilateral, left ear, with unrestricted hearing on the contralateral side
H90.5 Unspecified sensorineural hearing loss
Central hearing loss NOS
Congenital deafness NOS
Neural hearing loss NOS
Perceptive hearing loss NOS
Sensorineural deafness NOS
Sensory hearing loss NOS

EXCLUDES1 abnormal auditory perception (H93.2-)
psychogenic deafness (F44.6)
H90.6 Mixed conductive and sensorineural hearing loss, bilateral
5ᵗʰ H90.7 Mixed conductive and sensorineural hearing loss, unilateral with unrestricted hearing on the contralateral side
H90.71 Mixed conductive and sensorineural hearing loss, unilateral, right ear, with unrestricted hearing on the contralateral side
H90.72 Mixed conductive and sensorineural hearing loss, unilateral, left ear, with unrestricted hearing on the contralateral side
H90.8 Mixed conductive and sensorineural hearing loss, unspecified
5ᵗʰ H90.A Conductive and sensorineural hearing loss with restricted hearing on the contralateral side
6ᵗʰ H90.A1 Conductive hearing loss, unilateral, with restricted hearing on the contralateral side
H90.A11 Conductive hearing loss, unilateral, right ear with restricted hearing on the contralateral side
AHA: Q4 2016
H90.A12 Conductive hearing loss, unilateral, left ear with restricted hearing on the contralateral side
AHA: Q4 2016
6ᵗʰ H90.A2 Sensorineural hearing loss, unilateral, with restricted hearing on the contralateral side
H90.A21 Sensorineural hearing loss, unilateral, right ear, with restricted hearing on the contralateral side
AHA: Q4 2016
H90.A22 Sensorineural hearing loss, unilateral, left ear, with restricted hearing on the contralateral side
AHA: Q4 2016
6ᵗʰ H90.A3 Mixed conductive and sensorineural hearing loss, unilateral with restricted hearing on the contralateral side
H90.A31 Mixed conductive and sensorineural hearing loss, unilateral, right ear with restricted hearing on the contralateral side
AHA: Q4 2016
H90.A32 Mixed conductive and sensorineural hearing loss, unilateral, left ear with restricted hearing on the contralateral side
AHA: Q4 2016
4ᵗʰ H91 Other and unspecified hearing loss
EXCLUDES1 abnormal auditory perception (H93.2-)
hearing loss as classified in H90.-
impacted cerumen (H61.2-)
noise-induced hearing loss (H83.3-)
psychogenic deafness (F44.6)
transient ischemic deafness (H93.01-)
5ᵗʰ H91.0 Ototoxic hearing loss
Code first poisoning due to drug or toxin, if applicable (T36-T65 with fifth or sixth character 1-4 or 6)
Use additional code for adverse effect, if applicable, to identify drug (T36-T50 with fifth or sixth character 5)
H91.01 Ototoxic hearing loss, right ear
H91.02 Ototoxic hearing loss, left ear
H91.03 Ototoxic hearing loss, bilateral
H91.09 Ototoxic hearing loss, unspecified ear
5ᵗʰ H91.1 Presbycusis
Presbyacusia
H91.10 Presbycusis, unspecified ear
H91.11 Presbycusis, right ear
H91.12 Presbycusis, left ear
H91.13 Presbycusis, bilateral

ᴾᴰˣ Unacceptable principal diagnosis symbol per Medicare code edits ᴾᴼᴬ Code exempt from diagnosis present on admission requirement
❓ Questionable admission 🄲 Complication or comorbidity 🄲🄲/🄼🄲🄲🄴ˣ CC/MCC exclusion ᴹᶜᶜ Major complication or comorbidity
🄿🄲 Principal diagnosis as its own CC 🄿🄼🄲 Principal diagnosis as its own MCC 🄷🄲🄲 HCC diagnosis code 🅁🄷🄲🄲 RxHCC diagnosis code
MACRA code 🅉¹ Z code as first-listed diagnosis

[5th] H91.2 Sudden idiopathic hearing loss
Sudden hearing loss NOS
H91.20 Sudden idiopathic hearing loss, unspecified ear
H91.21 Sudden idiopathic hearing loss, right ear
H91.22 Sudden idiopathic hearing loss, left ear
H91.23 Sudden idiopathic hearing loss, bilateral
H91.3 Deaf nonspeaking, not elsewhere classified
[5th] H91.8 Other specified hearing loss
[6th] H91.8X Other specified hearing loss
H91.8X1 Other specified hearing loss, right ear
H91.8X2 Other specified hearing loss, left ear
H91.8X3 Other specified hearing loss, bilateral
H91.8X9 Other specified hearing loss, unspecified ear
[5th] H91.9 Unspecified hearing loss
Deafness NOS
High frequency deafness
Low frequency deafness
H91.90 Unspecified hearing loss, unspecified ear
H91.91 Unspecified hearing loss, right ear
H91.92 Unspecified hearing loss, left ear
H91.93 Unspecified hearing loss, bilateral
[4th] H92 Otalgia and effusion of ear
[5th] H92.0 Otalgia
H92.01 Otalgia, right ear
H92.02 Otalgia, left ear
H92.03 Otalgia, bilateral
H92.09 Otalgia, unspecified ear
[5th] H92.1 Otorrhea
[EXCLUDES1] *leakage of cerebrospinal fluid through ear (G96.0)*
H92.10 Otorrhea, unspecified ear
H92.11 Otorrhea, right ear
H92.12 Otorrhea, left ear
H92.13 Otorrhea, bilateral
[5th] H92.2 Otorrhagia
[EXCLUDES1] *traumatic otorrhagia - code to injury*
H92.20 Otorrhagia, unspecified ear
H92.21 Otorrhagia, right ear
H92.22 Otorrhagia, left ear
H92.23 Otorrhagia, bilateral
[4th] H93 Other disorders of ear, not elsewhere classified
[5th] H93.0 Degenerative and vascular disorders of ear
[EXCLUDES1] *presbycusis (H91.1)*
[6th] H93.01 Transient ischemic deafness
H93.011 Transient ischemic deafness, right ear
H93.012 Transient ischemic deafness, left ear
H93.013 Transient ischemic deafness, bilateral
H93.019 Transient ischemic deafness, unspecified ear
[6th] H93.09 Unspecified degenerative and vascular disorders of ear
H93.091 Unspecified degenerative and vascular disorders of right ear
H93.092 Unspecified degenerative and vascular disorders of left ear
H93.093 Unspecified degenerative and vascular disorders of ear, bilateral
H93.099 Unspecified degenerative and vascular disorders of unspecified ear
[5th] H93.1 Tinnitus
H93.11 Tinnitus, right ear
H93.12 Tinnitus, left ear
H93.13 Tinnitus, bilateral
H93.19 Tinnitus, unspecified ear
[5th] H93.A Pulsatile tinnitus
H93.A1 Pulsatile tinnitus, right ear
AHA: Q4 2016
H93.A2 Pulsatile tinnitus, left ear
AHA: Q4 2016
H93.A3 Pulsatile tinnitus, bilateral
AHA: Q4 2016
H93.A9 Pulsatile tinnitus, unspecified ear
AHA: Q4 2016
[5th] H93.2 Other abnormal auditory perceptions
[EXCLUDES2] *auditory hallucinations (R44.0)*
[6th] H93.21 Auditory recruitment
H93.211 Auditory recruitment, right ear
H93.212 Auditory recruitment, left ear
H93.213 Auditory recruitment, bilateral
H93.219 Auditory recruitment, unspecified ear
[6th] H93.22 Diplacusis
H93.221 Diplacusis, right ear
H93.222 Diplacusis, left ear
H93.223 Diplacusis, bilateral
H93.229 Diplacusis, unspecified ear
[6th] H93.23 Hyperacusis
H93.231 Hyperacusis, right ear
H93.232 Hyperacusis, left ear
H93.233 Hyperacusis, bilateral
H93.239 Hyperacusis, unspecified ear
[6th] H93.24 Temporary auditory threshold shift
H93.241 Temporary auditory threshold shift, right ear
H93.242 Temporary auditory threshold shift, left ear
H93.243 Temporary auditory threshold shift, bilateral
H93.249 Temporary auditory threshold shift, unspecified ear
H93.25 Central auditory processing disorder
Congenital auditory imperception
Word deafness
[EXCLUDES1] *mixed receptive-expressive language disorder (F80.2)*
[6th] H93.29 Other abnormal auditory perceptions
H93.291 Other abnormal auditory perceptions, right ear
H93.292 Other abnormal auditory perceptions, left ear
H93.293 Other abnormal auditory perceptions, bilateral
H93.299 Other abnormal auditory perceptions, unspecified ear
[5th] H93.3 Disorders of acoustic nerve
Disorder of 8th cranial nerve
[EXCLUDES1] *acoustic neuroma (D33.3)*
syphilitic acoustic neuritis (A52.15)
[6th] H93.3X Disorders of acoustic nerve
H93.3X1 Disorders of right acoustic nerve
H93.3X2 Disorders of left acoustic nerve
H93.3X3 Disorders of bilateral acoustic nerves
H93.3X9 Disorders of unspecified acoustic nerve
[5th] H93.8 Other specified disorders of ear
[6th] H93.8X Other specified disorders of ear
H93.8X1 Other specified disorders of right ear
H93.8X2 Other specified disorders of left ear
H93.8X3 Other specified disorders of ear, bilateral
H93.8X9 Other specified disorders of ear, unspecified ear
[5th] H93.9 Unspecified disorder of ear
H93.90 Unspecified disorder of ear, unspecified ear [PDx]
H93.91 Unspecified disorder of right ear [PDx]
H93.92 Unspecified disorder of left ear [PDx]
H93.93 Unspecified disorder of ear, bilateral [PDx]
[4th] H94 Other disorders of ear in diseases classified elsewhere
[5th] H94.0 Acoustic neuritis in infectious and parasitic diseases classified elsewhere
Code first underlying disease, such as:
parasitic disease (B65-B89)

Unspecified Code | Other Specified Code | Manifestation Code | [N] Newborn | [P] Pediatric | [M] Maternity | [A] Adult | ♂ Male | ♀ Female
● New Code | ▲ Revised Code Title | ►◄ Revised Text | [NOTES] | [INCLUDES] | [EXCLUDES1] Not coded here | [EXCLUDES2] Not included here
[4th] 4th character required | [5th] 5th character required | [6th] 6th character required | [7th] 7th character required
[X] Extension 'X' Alert | [HAC] Hospital-acquired condition (HAC) alert | AHA AHA Coding Clinic©

When symbols appear on a code that requires a 7th character extension, refer to Appendix B to identify applicable 7th character codes.

H94.00 - H95.89

> EXCLUDES1 acoustic neuritis (in):
> herpes zoster (B02.29)
> syphilis (A52.15)

H94.00 **Acoustic neuritis in infectious and parasitic diseases classified elsewhere, unspecified ear**

H94.01 **Acoustic neuritis in infectious and parasitic diseases classified elsewhere, right ear**

H94.02 **Acoustic neuritis in infectious and parasitic diseases classified elsewhere, left ear**

H94.03 **Acoustic neuritis in infectious and parasitic diseases classified elsewhere, bilateral**

H94.8 **Other specified disorders of ear in diseases classified elsewhere**

Code first underlying disease, such as:
congenital syphilis (A50.0)

> EXCLUDES1 aural myiasis (B87.4)
> syphilitic labyrinthitis (A52.79)

H94.80 **Other specified disorders of ear in diseases classified elsewhere, unspecified ear**

H94.81 **Other specified disorders of right ear in diseases classified elsewhere**

H94.82 **Other specified disorders of left ear in diseases classified elsewhere**

H94.83 **Other specified disorders of ear in diseases classified elsewhere, bilateral**

Intraoperative and postprocedural complications and disorders of ear and mastoid process, not elsewhere classified (H95)

H95 Intraoperative and postprocedural complications and disorders of ear and mastoid process, not elsewhere classified

H95.0 Recurrent cholesteatoma of postmastoidectomy cavity

H95.00 **Recurrent cholesteatoma of postmastoidectomy cavity, unspecified ear**

H95.01 Recurrent cholesteatoma of postmastoidectomy cavity, right ear

H95.02 Recurrent cholesteatoma of postmastoidectomy cavity, left ear

H95.03 Recurrent cholesteatoma of postmastoidectomy cavity, bilateral ears

H95.1 Other disorders of ear and mastoid process following mastoidectomy

H95.11 Chronic inflammation of postmastoidectomy cavity

H95.111 Chronic inflammation of postmastoidectomy cavity, right ear

H95.112 Chronic inflammation of postmastoidectomy cavity, left ear

H95.113 Chronic inflammation of postmastoidectomy cavity, bilateral ears

H95.119 **Chronic inflammation of postmastoidectomy cavity, unspecified ear**

H95.12 Granulation of postmastoidectomy cavity

H95.121 Granulation of postmastoidectomy cavity, right ear

H95.122 Granulation of postmastoidectomy cavity, left ear

H95.123 Granulation of postmastoidectomy cavity, bilateral ears

H95.129 **Granulation of postmastoidectomy cavity, unspecified ear**

H95.13 Mucosal cyst of postmastoidectomy cavity

H95.131 Mucosal cyst of postmastoidectomy cavity, right ear

H95.132 Mucosal cyst of postmastoidectomy cavity, left ear

H95.133 Mucosal cyst of postmastoidectomy cavity, bilateral ears

H95.139 **Mucosal cyst of postmastoidectomy cavity, unspecified ear**

H95.19 Other disorders following mastoidectomy

H95.191 Other disorders following mastoidectomy, right ear

H95.192 Other disorders following mastoidectomy, left ear

H95.193 Other disorders following mastoidectomy, bilateral ears

H95.199 **Other disorders following mastoidectomy, unspecified ear**

H95.2 Intraoperative hemorrhage and hematoma of ear and mastoid process complicating a procedure

> EXCLUDES1 intraoperative hemorrhage and hematoma of ear and mastoid process due to accidental puncture or laceration during a procedure (H95.3-)

H95.21 Intraoperative hemorrhage and hematoma of ear and mastoid process complicating a procedure on the ear and mastoid process CC CC/MCC Exc

H95.22 Intraoperative hemorrhage and hematoma of ear and mastoid process complicating other procedure CC CC/MCC Exc

H95.3 Accidental puncture and laceration of ear and mastoid process during a procedure

H95.31 Accidental puncture and laceration of the ear and mastoid process during a procedure on the ear and mastoid process CC CC/MCC Exc

H95.32 Accidental puncture and laceration of the ear and mastoid process during other procedure CC CC/MCC Exc

H95.4 Postprocedural hemorrhage of ear and mastoid process following a procedure

H95.41 Postprocedural hemorrhage of ear and mastoid process following a procedure on the ear and mastoid process CC CC/MCC Exc

H95.42 Postprocedural hemorrhage of ear and mastoid process following other procedure CC CC/MCC Exc

H95.5 Postprocedural hematoma and seroma of ear and mastoid process following a procedure

H95.51 Postprocedural hematoma of ear and mastoid process following a procedure on the ear and mastoid process CC CC/MCC Exc

H95.52 Postprocedural hematoma of ear and mastoid process following other procedure CC CC/MCC Exc

H95.53 Postprocedural seroma of ear and mastoid process following a procedure on the ear and mastoid process CC CC/MCC Exc

H95.54 Postprocedural seroma of ear and mastoid process following other procedure CC CC/MCC Exc

H95.8 Other intraoperative and postprocedural complications and disorders of the ear and mastoid process, not elsewhere classified

> EXCLUDES2 postprocedural complications and disorders following mastoidectomy (H95.0-, H95.1-)

H95.81 Postprocedural stenosis of external ear canal

H95.811 Postprocedural stenosis of right external ear canal CC CC/MCC Exc

H95.812 Postprocedural stenosis of left external ear canal CC CC/MCC Exc

H95.813 Postprocedural stenosis of external ear canal, bilateral CC CC/MCC Exc

H95.819 **Postprocedural stenosis of unspecified external ear canal** CC CC/MCC Exc

H95.88 Other intraoperative complications and disorders of the ear and mastoid process, not elsewhere classified CC CC/MCC Exc

Use additional code, if applicable, to further specify disorder

H95.89 Other postprocedural complications and disorders of the ear and mastoid process, not elsewhere classified CC CC/MCC Exc

Use additional code, if applicable, to further specify disorder

---

PDxR Unacceptable principal diagnosis symbol per Medicare code edits   PDxA Code exempt from diagnosis present on admission requirement
❓ Questionable admission   CC Complication or comorbidity   CC/MCC Exc CC/MCC exclusion   MCC Major complication or comorbidity
🅒 Principal diagnosis as its own CC   🅜 Principal diagnosis as its own MCC   HCC HCC diagnosis code   RxHCC RxHCC diagnosis code
MACRA code   Z1 Z code as first-listed diagnosis

642   When symbols appear on a code that requires a 7th character extension, refer to Appendix B to identify applicable 7th character codes.   **2018 ICD-10-CM**

NOTES

NOTES

Chapter 9: Diseases of the Circulatory System (I00-I99)

Anatomy of the Cardiovascular System

Introduction

The human vascular system comprises a series of tubes (which are known as vessels) that travel in almost all parts of the human body. It is categorized into the following two classes:

1. **Blood Vascular System**
   The blood vascular system includes the heart and blood vessels required to facilitate the circulation of the colored fluid (blood) inside the body.

   a) The Structure of Arteries

   The arteries possess stronger and thicker walls than the corresponding veins and are based on the following components:

   i) Tunica Intima

   ii) Tunica Media

   iii) Tunica Externa

   b. The Structure of Veins

   The veins have a similar structure as that of the arteries. The components of a typical vein are described below:

   i) Tunica Intima

   ii) Tunica Media

   iii) Tunica Externa

   c. The Blood

   The blood is considered a uniquely specialized connective tissue that is composed of the formed elements (or the blood cells) and the fluid portion (or plasma). The formed elements of blood are based on the red blood cells (RBCs or erythrocytes), the white blood cells (WBCs or leukocytes) and the platelets (or thrombocytes). The blood contributes to about 8% of total body weight. The quantity of blood in an average human varies between 5 to 6 liters. The elements of blood are categorized below:

   d. Erythrocytes or Red Blood Cells: The red blood cells are the most common type of blood cells that contribute to about 95% of the blood cell volume.

   e. Leukocytes or White Blood Cells: The white blood cells can be divided into the following subcategories:

   f. Granular Leukocytes: The granular leukocytes contain granules in their cytoplasm and can be further classified into the following three types:

   i) neutrophils constitute about 60% to 70% of the white blood cells.

   ii) eosinophils constitute about 2% to 4% of the white blood cells.

   iii) basophils constitute about 0.5% to 1% of the white blood cells.

   g. Agranular Leukocytes: The agranular leukocytes do not contain granules in their cytoplasm and can be further classified into the following two types:

   i) monocytes constitute about 3% to 8% of the white blood cells.

   ii) lymphocytes constitute about 20% to 25% of the white blood cells.

   h. Thrombocytes or Platelets: The platelets are small cell fragments that do not contain nucleus in their cytoplasm.

   i. Blood Plasma

   The plasma is the fluid component of blood in which the blood cells usually remain suspended. The blood plasma is composed of 91% water, 7% proteins, and 2% solutes.

2. **Lymph Vascular System**
   The lymph vascular system includes the lymph glands and lymphatic vessels for circulating the colorless fluid (lymph) throughout the human body. Both of the blood vascular and the lymph vascular systems work in close association with each other for sustaining the human life cycle.

3. **The Thoracic Cavity**
   The thoracic cavity is enclosed by the thoracic wall and primarily contains the structures of the cardiovascular and respiratory systems.

   a) The Pericardium

   The heart and the roots of the great vessels are contained within the conical and fibro-serous sac, which is known as the pericardium. It is composed of two closely connected sacs, which are known as the fibrous pericardium (or the outer sac) and the serous pericardium (the inner sac).

b) The Heart

The heart is a hollow muscular organ that remains enclosed in the fibro-serous sac (or the pericardium) and is regarded as the central organ of the cardiovascular system. It lies between the lungs in the middle mediastinum and receives blood from the veins.

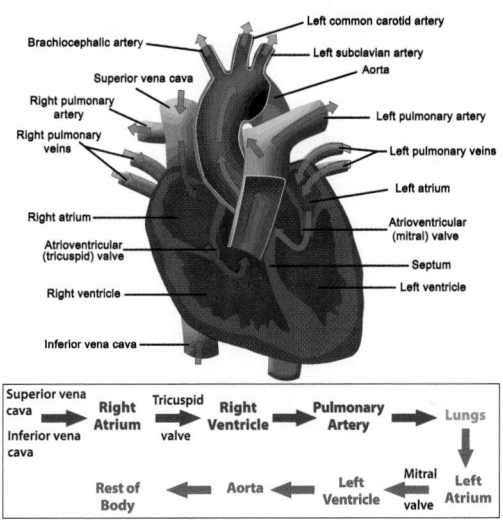

CIRCULATION OF BLOOD THROUGH THE HEART

4. **The Chambers of the Heart**
   The human heart is based on the following four chambers:

   a) The Right Atrium: The right border of the human heart is formed by the right atrium. The superior vena cava, inferior vena cava and coronary sinus provide venous blood supply to the right atrium of the heart.

   The right atrium contains the following elements inside it:

   i) Sinus Venarum

   ii) Pectinate Muscles

   iii) Opening of Superior Vena Cava

   iv) Opening of Inferior Vena Cava

   v) Opening of Coronary Sinus

   vi) The Right Atrioventricular Orifice

   vii) Interatrial Septum

   b) The Right Ventricle: The inferior border of the human heart is constituted by the right ventricle.

   c) The Left Atrium: The left atrium chiefly constitutes the base of the heart and utilizes the mitral valve to pump the oxygenated blood received from the pulmonary veins into the left ventricle of the heart. The interior of the left atrium is based on the following components:

   i) Two superior and two inferior pulmonary veins that enter the posterior wall of the left atrium.

   ii) A posteriorly directed interatrial septum that separates the right atrium from the left atrium of the heart.

   iii) A smooth walled portion and a muscular auricle containing pectinate muscles.

   iv) A comparatively thicker wall than the corresponding right atrium.

   v) A left atrioventricular orifice that facilitates the discharge of oxygenated blood into the left ventricle.

   d) The Left Ventricle: The left ventricle pumps the oxygenated blood (through the aortic valve) to the whole body through the aorta. The interior of the left ventricle is based on the following elements:

   i) a double-leaflet/dual-flap mitral (bicuspid or left atrioventricular) valve, which is located between the left atrium and ventricle for guarding the left atrioventricular orifice.

   ii) walls of the left ventricle, which are comparatively thicker than the corresponding right ventricle.

iii) conical cavity of the left ventricle that is comparatively longer than the corresponding right ventricle.

iv) anterior and posterior left ventricular papillary muscles that get attached to the cusps of the mitral valve through the tendinous cords (or the chordae tendineae).

v) aortic vestibule, which is a smooth-walled, nonmuscular, superoanterior outflow portion of the left ventricle that lies inferior to the aortic orifice and possesses fibrous walls.

vi) aortic orifice (or opening) is an opening of the left ventricle into the aorta. This valve is usually tricuspid (with three leaflets) and located posterior to the left side of the sternum at the level of the third intercostal space.

vii) inner surface of the left ventricle gives rise to the irregular, rounded and thick muscular ridges that are termed as the trabeculae carneae.

5. **The Cardiac Cycle:**
The cardiac cycle is based on the synchronous pumping of the right and left chambers of the heart.

a) The Arterial Supply of the Heart

The heart is supplied by the following arteries:

i) right coronary artery (RCA)

ii) sino-atrial nodal artery

iii) right marginal artery

iv) posterior interventricular artery

v) atrio-ventricular nodal artery

vi) left coronary artery

vii) anterior interventricular artery (or Left Anterior Descending Artery)

viii) circumflex artery

ix) left marginal artery

x) posterior interventricular artery

b) The Arteries

The major types of arteries are described below:

i) pulmonary arteries- pulmonary arteries carry the oxygen deficient blood from the heart to the lungs for attaining oxygen.

ii) systemic arteries- systemic arteries transport the oxygenated blood to the rest of the body.

c) The Aorta

The aorta is divided into the following components:

i) ascending aorta

ii) arch of aorta

iii) descending aorta

d) Thoracic Aorta

i) aortic intercostal arteries (nine pairs)

ii) left bronchial arteries (two in number)

iii) posterior mediastinal arteries

iv) pericardial arteries

v) superior phrenic arteries

e) The Abdominal Aorta

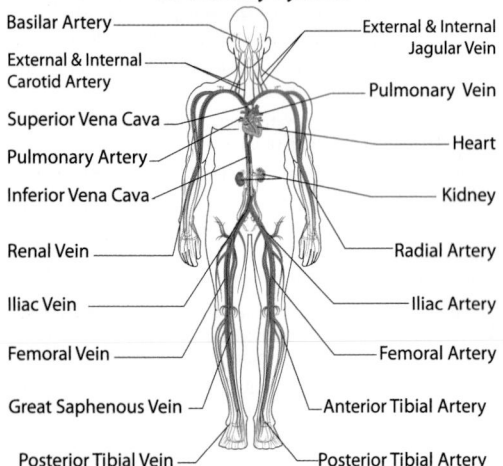

Circulatory System

Basilar Artery

External & Internal Carotid Artery

Superior Vena Cava

Pulmonary Artery

Inferior Vena Cava

Renal Vein

Iliac Vein

Femoral Vein

Great Saphenous Vein

Posterior Tibial Vein

External & Internal Jagular Vein

Pulmonary Vein

Heart

Kidney

Radial Artery

Iliac Artery

Femoral Artery

Anterior Tibial Artery

Posterior Tibial Artery

6. **The Arteries of the Head and Neck**
The major arteries that supply blood to the head and neck regions are the two common carotid arteries. These arteries travel through the neck and each one of them gets divided into the following branches:

a) External Carotid Arteries

b) Ascending Pharyngeal Artery

c) Occipital Artery

i) muscular branches

ii) sternocleidomastoid branch/sternocleidomastoid artery

iii) auricular branch

iv) meningeal or dural branch

v) descending branch

d) Posterior Auricular Artery

i) stylomastoid branch/stylomastoid artery

ii) auricular branch

iii) occipital branch

e) Superior Thyroid Artery

i) hyoid branch

ii) sternocleidomastoid branch/sternocleidomastoid artery

iii) superior laryngeal branch/superior laryngeal artery

iv) cricothyroid branch

f) Lingual Artery

i) hyoid branch

ii) dorsal lingual branches

iii) sublingual branch/sublingual artery

iv) deep lingual branch/deep lingual artery

g) Facial (or External Maxillary) Artery

Cervical Branches		Facial Branches	
i)	ascending palatine artery	i)	inferior labial artery
ii)	tonsillar branch	ii)	superior labial artery
iii)	glandular branches	iii)	lateral nasal branch
iv)	submental artery	iv)	angular artery
v)	muscular branches	v)	muscular branches

7. **The Internal Carotid Arteries:** The internal carotid arteries are the direct continuation of the common carotid arteries. However, the other portions of these arteries extend into the following arterial branches:

a) The petrous portion of the internal carotid arteries gives rise to the following branches:

i) caroticotympanic artery

ii) artery of the pterygoid canal (or vidian artery)

b) The cavernous portion of the internal carotid arteries gives rise to the following branches:

i) cavernous artery

ii) hypophyseal artery

iii) semilunar arterial branches

iv) anterior meningeal artery

v) ophthalmic artery

c) Anterior Cerebral Artery

i) anteromedial ganglionic branches

ii) inferior branches

iii) anterior branches

iv) middle branches

v) posterior branches

d) The Middle Cerebral Artery

i) anterolateral ganglionic branches

ii) inferior lateral frontal branch

iii) ascending frontal branch

iv) ascending parietal branch

v) parietotemporal branch

vi) temporal branches

e) Posterior Communicating Artery

f) Anterior Choroidal Artery (or Choroid Artery)

8. **The Arteries of the Upper Extremity:** The Subclavian Artery divides into the following branches:

   a) Vertebral Artery: The vertebral artery is divided into the following branches:

Cervical Branches		Cranial Branches
i) spinal branches	i)	posterior meningeal branch
ii) muscular branches	ii)	posterior/dorsal spinal artery
	iii)	anterior/ventral spinal artery
	iv)	posterior inferior cerebellar artery
	v)	medullary arteries

   b) Internal Thoracic (or Internal Mammary) Artery
      i) pericardiacophrenic artery
      ii) anterior mediastinal arteries
      iii) pericardial branches
      iv) sternal branches
      v) anterior intercostal arteries
      vi) perforating branches
      vii) musculophrenic artery
      viii) superior epigastric artery

   c) Thyrocervical trunk (or Thyroid axis)
      i) inferior thyroid artery
      ii) inferior laryngeal artery
      iii) esophageal branches
      iv) tracheal artery
      v) ascending cervical artery
      vi) muscular branches

   d) Suprascapular (or Transverse Scapular) Artery
      i) suprasternal branch
      ii) acromial branch

   e) Transverse Cervical Artery (or Transverse Artery of Neck)
      i) ascending branch
      ii) descending branch

   f) The costocervical trunk is the highest intercostal artery (superior intercostal), and it includes:
      i) first posterior intercostal artery
      ii) second posterior intercostal artery
      iii) deep cervical artery
      iv) third arterial part

   g) Axillary Artery
      i) first part
      ii) second part
      iii) third part

   h) Brachial Artery
      i) muscular branches
      ii) human nutrient artery
      iii) profunda brachii artery (deep artery of the arm/superior profunda artery)
      iv) superior ulnar collateral artery (or inferior profunda artery)
      v) inferior ulnar collateral artery (or anastomotica magna artery)

   i) Radial Artery

Branches of the Radial Artery in Forearm	Branches of the Radial Artery in Wrist	Branches of the Radial Artery in Hand
The Radial Recurrent Artery	The Posterior Radial Carpal Artery (The Dorsal Carpal Branch)	The Princeps Pollicis Artery
The Muscular (Arterial) Branches	The First Dorsal Metacarpal Artery	The Radialis Indicis Artery

Branches of the Radial Artery in Forearm	Branches of the Radial Artery in Wrist	Branches of the Radial Artery in Hand
The Anterior Radial Carpal Artery (The Volar Carpal Branch)		The Deep Palmar/ Volar Arch
The Superficial Volar Artery (The Superficial Palmar Branch of Radial Artery)		The Palmar Interosseous (or Volar Metacarpal) Arteries
		The Perforating (Arterial) Branches
		The Recurrent (Arterial) Branches

   j) Ulnar Artery- The ulnar artery originates from the brachial artery and runs along the medial aspect (or ulnar side) of the forearm. A tabular representation of the arterial branches of ulnar artery is provided below:

Branches of the Ulnar Artery in Forearm	Branches of the Ulnar Artery in Wrist	Branches of the Ulnar Artery in Hand
The Anterior Ulnar Recurrent Artery	The Volar Carpal Branch (or Anterior Ulnar Carpal Artery)	The Deep Volar Branch (or Profunda Branch)
The Posterior Ulnar Recurrent Artery	The Dorsal Carpal Branch (or Posterior Ulnar Carpal Artery)	The Superficial Volar Arch (or Superficial Palmar Arch)
The Common Interosseous Artery (divides into the following two branches) ➲ The Volar Interosseous Artery (or Anterior Interosseous Artery) ➲ The Dorsal Interosseous Artery (or Posterior Interosseous Artery)		
The Muscular (Arterial) Branches		

9. **Arteries of the Trunk**
   Arteries of the trunk are based on the following arteries:

   a) The Descending Aorta
      i) thoracic aorta
      ii) abdominal aorta

   b) The Common Iliac Arteries

   c) Internal Iliac (or Hypogastric) Artery

The Anterior Trunk	The Posterior Trunk
The Superior Vesical Artery	The Iliolumbar Artery-with the following branches:
The Middle Vesical Artery	
The Inferior Vesical Artery	- The Lumbar (Arterial) Branch - The Iliac (Arterial) Branch
The Middle Hemorrhoidal Artery	The Superior and Inferior Lateral Sacral Arteries
The Uterine Artery (In Female)	
The Vaginal Artery (In Female)	The Superior Gluteal Artery (or Gluteal Artery)-with the following branches:
The Obturator Artery	- The Superficial (Arterial) Branch - The Deep (Arterial) Branch

The Anterior Trunk	The Posterior Trunk
The Internal Pudendal Artery (Internal Pubic Artery)-with the following branches:	
The Muscular (Arterial) Branches	
The Inferior Hemorrhoidal Artery	
The Perineal (or Superficial Perineal) Artery	
The Artery of the Urethral Bulb	
The Urethral Artery	
The Deep Artery of the Penis (or Artery to the Corpus Cavernosum)	
The Dorsal Artery of the Penis	
The Inferior Gluteal Artery (Sciatic Artery)-with the following branches:	
The Muscular (Arterial) Branches	
The Coccygeal (Arterial) Branches	
The Arteria Comitans Nervi Ischiadici	
The Anastomotic (Arterial) Branch	
The Articular (Arterial) Branch	
The Cutaneous (Arterial) Branches	

d) The External Iliac Artery divides into the inferior epigastric artery, which includes:

   i)   muscular branches
   ii) cutaneous branches
   iii) external spermatic branch (in males) and artery of round ligament of uterus (in females)
   iv) pubic branch

e) Deep Iliac Circumflex Artery

   i)   muscular branch
   ii) cutaneous branch

10. The Arteries of the Lower Extremity

   a) Femoral Artery- The branches of the femoral artery are presented below in a tabular format:

The Branches of the Femoral Artery		
The Superficial Epigastric Artery		
The Superficial Iliac Circumflex Artery		
The Superficial External Pudendal Artery (or Superficial External Pubic Artery)		
The Deep External Pudendal Artery (or Deep External Pubic Artery)		
The Muscular (Arterial) Branches		
The Profunda Femoris Artery (or Deep Femoral Artery)		
Branches and Subordinate Branches of the Profunda Femoris Artery	The Lateral Femoral Circumflex Artery	
	Sub-Branches	The Ascending (Arterial) Branch
		The Descending (Arterial) Branch
		The Transverse (Arterial) Branch
	The Medial Femoral Circumflex Artery (or Internal Circumflex Artery)	
	Sub-Branches	The Superficial (Arterial) Branch
		The Deep (Arterial) Branch
		The Acetabular (Arterial) Branch
	The Perforating Arteries	
	Sub-Branches	The First Perforating Artery
		The Second Perforating Artery
		The Third Perforating Artery
	The Muscular (Arterial) Branches	
The Highest Genicular Artery (or Anastomotica Magna Artery)		

The Branches of the Femoral Artery	
Branches of the Highest Genicular Artery	The Saphenous (Arterial) Branch
	The Musculoarticular (Arterial) Branch

b) Popliteal Artery- A tabular presentation of the branches of the popliteal artery is given below:

Branches of the Popliteal Artery	
The Superior Muscular Branches	
The Sural Arteries (or Inferior Muscular Arteries)	
The Cutaneous Branches	
The Superior Genicular Arteries (or Superior Articular Arteries)	
Branches of the Superior Genicular Arteries	The Medial Superior Genicular Artery
	The Lateral Superior Genicular Artery
The Middle Genicular Artery (or Azygos Articular Artery)	
The Inferior Genicular Arteries (or Inferior Articular Arteries)	
Branches of the Inferior Genicular Arteries	The Medial Inferior Genicular Artery
	The Lateral Inferior Genicular Artery

c) Anterior Tibial Artery

   i)   Posterior Tibial Recurrent Artery
   ii)   Fibular Artery
   iii) Anterior Tibial Recurrent Artery
   iv)   Muscular (Arterial) Branches
   v)   Anterior Medial Malleolar Artery (or Internal Malleolar Artery)
   vi)   Anterior Lateral Malleolar Artery (or External Malleolar Artery)

d) Dorsalis Pedis Artery (or Dorsal Artery of Foot)- A tabular presentation of the branches of the dorsalis pedis artery is given below:

Branches of the Dorsalis Pedis Artery	
The lateral Tarsal Artery (or Tarsal Artery)	
The Medial Tarsal Arteries	
The Arcuate Artery (or Metatarsal Artery)	
Branches of Arcuate Artery	The Second Dorsal Metatarsal Artery
	The Third Dorsal Metatarsal Artery
	The Fourth Dorsal Metatarsal Artery
The First Dorsal Metatarsal Artery	
The Deep Plantar Artery (or Communicating Artery)	

e) Posterior Tibial Artery- The branching tree of the posterior tibial artery is presented below:

Branches of the Posterior Tibial Artery	
The Peroneal Artery	
Branches of Peroneal Artery	The Muscular (Arterial) Branches
	The Nutrient Artery of Fibula
	The Perforating Branch (or Anterior Peroneal Artery)
	The Communicating Branch of Peroneal Artery
	The Lateral Calcaneal Arteries (or External Calcaneal Arteries)
The Nutrient Artery of Tibia	
The Muscular Branches of the Posterior Tibial Artery	
The Posterior Medial Malleolar Artery (or Internal Malleolar Artery)	
The Communicating Branch of Posterior Tibial Artery	
The Medial Calcaneal Arteries (or Internal Calcaneal Arteries)	
The Medial Plantar Artery (or Internal Plantar Artery)	
The Lateral Plantar Artery (or External Plantar Artery)	

11. The Veins

The veins are the blood vessels that carry deoxygenated blood from the body tissues towards the heart via capillaries. The veins can be categorized into the following classes:

a) Pulmonary Veins: The pulmonary veins carry oxygenated blood from the lungs to the left atrium of the heart. The pulmonary veins are of the following types:

   i) right inferior pulmonary vein
   ii) right superior pulmonary vein
   iii) left inferior pulmonary vein
   iv) left superior pulmonary vein

b) Systemic Veins: The systemic veins deliver deoxygenated blood from the body tissues to the right atrium of the human heart.

c) Superficial (or Cutaneous) Veins: The superficial veins are found immediately beneath the skin between the layers of the superficial fascia.

d) Deep Veins: The deep veins are located under the deep fascia with their corresponding arteries.

e) Systemic Veins

   The systemic veins are divided into the following groups:

   i) veins of the heart
   ii) veins of the head and neck
   iii) veins of the upper extremity and thorax
   iv) veins of the lower extremity, abdomen, and pelvis

f) Veins of the Heart

   i) great cardiac vein
   ii) small cardiac vein
   iii) middle cardiac vein
   iv) posterior vein of the left ventricle
   v) oblique vein of the left atrium

g) Veins of the Head and Neck

   i) frontal vein (or supratrochlear vein)
   ii) supraorbital vein
   iii) angular vein
   iv) anterior facial vein (or facial vein)
   v) superficial temporal vein
   vi) parotid veins
   vii) articular veins (from temporomandibular joint)
   viii) anterior auricular veins
   ix) transverse facial veins
   x) internal maxillary vein
   xi) posterior facial vein (or temporomaxillary vein)
   xii) posterior auricular vein
   xiii) occipital vein

h) Veins of the Neck

   i) external jugular vein
   ii) posterior external jugular vein
   iii) anterior jugular vein
   iv) internal jugular vein
   v) vertebral vein
   vi) diploic veins
      (a) frontal diploic vein
      (b) anterior temporal diploic vein
      (c) posterior temporal diploic vein
      (d) occipital diploic vein

12. Veins of the Brain

a) External Cerebral Veins
   i) superior cerebral veins
   ii) middle cerebral vein (or superficial sylvian vein)
   iii) inferior cerebral veins
b) Internal Cerebral Veins (or deep cerebral veins)
c) Terminal Vein
d) Great Cerebral Veins (or Great Vein of Galen)

e) Cerebellar Veins
   i) superior cerebellar veins
   ii) inferior cerebellar veins

f) Ophthalmic and Emissary Veins
   i) Ophthalmic veins are the veins that serve to perform the venous drainage of the orbit and pass through the superior orbital fissure to enter into the cavernous sinus.
   ii) superior ophthalmic veins
   iii) inferior ophthalmic veins
   iv) Emissary veins are those valveless veins that connect the dural venous sinuses with veins outside the cranium.

g) Sinuses of the Dura Mater
   i) posterosuperior sinuses
   ii) superior sagittal sinus (or superior longitudinal sinus)
   iii) inferior sagittal sinus (or inferior sagittal sinus)
   iv) straight sinus (or tentorial sinus)
   v) transverse sinuses (or lateral sinuses)

h) Occipital Sinuses
   i) anteroinferior sinuses
   ii) cavernous sinuses
   iii) intercavernous sinuses
   iv) superior petrosal sinuses
   v) inferior petrosal sinuses
   vi) basilar plexus (or transverse/basilar sinus)

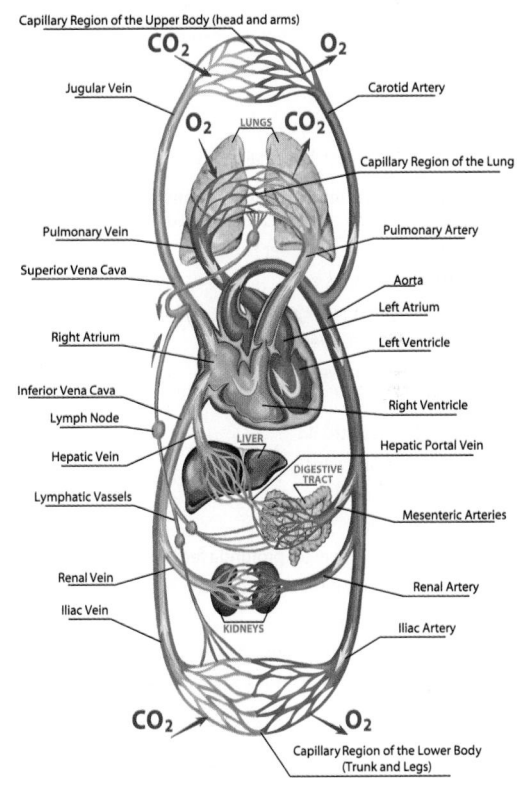

Capillary Region of the Upper Body (head and arms)
CO_2 O_2
Jugular Vein — Carotid Artery
O_2 LUNGS CO_2
Capillary Region of the Lung
Pulmonary Vein — Pulmonary Artery
Superior Vena Cava — Aorta
Left Atrium
Right Atrium — Left Ventricle
Inferior Vena Cava — Right Ventricle
Lymph Node
LIVER
Hepatic Vein — Hepatic Portal Vein
DIGESTIVE TRACT
Lymphatic Vessels — Mesenteric Arteries
Renal Vein — Renal Artery
Iliac Vein — Iliac Artery
KIDNEYS
CO_2 O_2
Capillary Region of the Lower Body (Trunk and Legs)

13. Veins of the Upper Extremity, Thorax and Vertebral Column

The veins of the upper extremity are divided into the following two major groups:

a) Superficial Veins of the Upper Extremity
   i) cephalic vein (or antecubital vein)
   ii) accessory cephalic vein
   iii) median cubital vein (or median basilic vein/antecubital vein)
   iv) basilic vein
   v) median antebrachial vein
   vi) dorsal venous network of the hand
   vii) intercapitular veins

viii) dorsal metacarpal veins

ix) dorsal digital veins

b) Deep Veins of the Upper Extremity

   i) radial veins

   ii) ulnar veins

   iii) brachial veins

   iv) axillary veins

   v) subclavian veins

   vi) deep palmar venous arch

c) Veins of the thorax

   i) innominate veins (or brachiocephalic veins)

   ii) internal mammary veins (or internal thoracic veins)

   iii) inferior thyroid veins

   iv) highest intercostal vein (or superior intercostal vein)

   v) right superior intercostal vein

   vi) left superior intercostal vein

   vii) superior vena cava

   viii) azygos vein

   ix) hemiazygos vein

   x) accessory hemiazygos vein (or vena azygos minor superior)

   xi) bronchial veins

d) Veins of the vertebral column

   i) external vertebral venous plexuses (or extraspinal veins)

   ii) anterior external vertebral plexuses

   iii) posterior external vertebral plexuses

   iv) internal vertebral venous plexus (or intraspinal veins)

   v) basivertebral veins

   vi) intervertebral veins

   vii) veins of the medulla spinalis (or veins of spinal cord)

14. Veins of the Lower Extremity, Abdomen, and Pelvis

The veins of the lower extremity are arranged into the following groups:

a. Superficial Veins of the Lower Extremity

   i) great saphenous vein

   ii) small saphenous vein (or lesser saphenous vein)

b. Deep Veins of the Lower Extremity

   i) posterior tibial veins

   ii) peroneal veins

   iii) tibioperoneal trunk

   iv) anterior tibial veins

   v) popliteal vein

   vi) femoral vein

   vii) deep femoral vein (or profunda femoris vein)

   viii) common femoral vein

   ix) external iliac vein

b) Major Veins of Abdomen and Pelvis

   i) ascending lumbar vein

   ii) left gastric vein

   iii) right gastric vein

   iv) left gastro-omental vein

   v) right gastro-omental vein

   vi) left hepatic vein

   vii) middle hepatic vein

   viii) right hepatic vein

   ix) superior mesenteric vein

   x) inferior phrenic veins

   xi) inferior vena cava

   xii) left renal vein

   xiii) right renal vein

xiv) splenic vein

xv) suprarenal veins

xvi) deep dorsal vein of clitoris

xvii) deep dorsal vein of penis

xviii) external pudendal veins

xix) internal pudendal vein

xx) ovarian vein

xxi) pampiniform venous plexus

xxii) prostatic venous plexus

xxiii) rectal venous plexus

xxiv) uterine venous plexus

xxv) vaginal venous plexus

xxvi) common iliac veins

xxvii) middle sacral veins

xxviii) vesical venous plexus

15. The Portal System of Veins

The hepatic portal system of the veins is responsible for the portal circulation, which denotes the passage of blood from the gastrointestinal tract and spleen through the portal vein to the liver.

The tributaries and sub-tributaries of the portal vein are presented below:

The Tributaries and Subtributaries of the Portal Vein		
The Lienal Vein		
The Tributaries of Lienal Vein	The Short Gastric Veins	
	The Left Gastroepiploic Vein	
	The Pancreatic Veins	
	The Inferior Mesenteric Vein	
	The Tributaries of Inferior Mesenteric Vein	The Sigmoid Veins
		The Left Colic Vein
The Superior Mesenteric Vein		
The Tributaries of Superior Mesenteric Vein	The Right Gastroepiploic Vein	
	The Pancreaticoduodenal Veins	
The Coronary Vein		
The Pyloric Vein		
The Cystic Vein		
The Paraumbilical Veins		

Common Pathologies

Angina pectoris
Commonly known as angina, angina pectoris chest pain is due to ischemia of the heart muscle, generally due to obstruction or spasm of the coronary arteries. The main cause of angina pectoris is coronary artery disease, due to atherosclerosis of the arteries feeding the heart.

Cardiomyopathy
Cardiomyopathy is a chronic disease of the heart muscle, in which the muscle is abnormally enlarged, thickened, and/or stiffened. The weakened heart muscle loses the ability to pump blood effectively, resulting in irregular heartbeats (arrhythmias) and possibly even heart failure.

Rheumatic Heart Disease
Rheumatic heart disease is a condition in which permanent damage to heart valves is caused by rheumatic fever. The heart valve is damaged by a disease process that generally begins with a strep throat caused by bacteria called Streptococcus, and may eventually cause rheumatic fever.

Arrhythmia
An arrhythmia is an abnormal rate or rhythm of the heart beat. It can beat too fast, too slow, or with an irregular rhythm. If the heart beat is fast it is called tachycardia and if is too slow, it is referred to as bradycardia.

Congenital Heart Defects
Congenital heart defects are abnormalities in the morphological or physiological functioning of the heart that are present at the time of birth. The primary cause is the incomplete or abnormal development of the fetal heart during the early weeks of pregnancy.

Hypertension
Hypertension, also referred to as high blood pressure, is a condition in which the arteries have persistently elevated blood pressure. Every time the human heart beats, it pumps blood to the whole body through the arteries. The pumping through the narrowed vessel consistently increases the systolic and diastolic pressure above normal reference range.

Main complications of hypertension

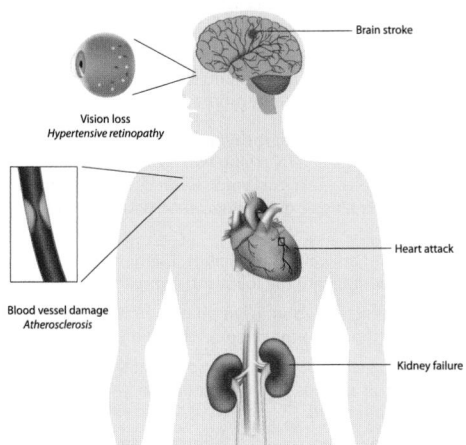

Aortic Aneurysm
An aneurysm is an abnormal bulging or swelling of a portion of a blood vessel. The aorta, which can develop these abnormal bulges, is the large blood vessel that carries oxygen-rich blood away from the heart to the rest of the body.

Atherosclerosis
Atherosclerosis is a disease of the arterial blood vessels (arteries), in which the walls of the blood vessels become thickened and hardened by "plaques." The plaques are composed of cholesterol and other lipids, inflammatory cells, and calcium deposits.

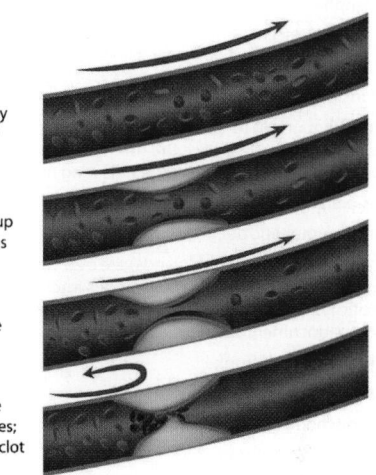

STAGES OF ATHEROSCLEROSIS

Deep Vein Thrombosis
Deep vein thrombosis (DVT) is a blood clot in a major vein that usually develops in the legs and/or pelvis.

Coronary Artery Disease
Coronary artery disease (CAD) is one of the common vascular diseases marked by accumulation of atherosclerotic plaque in the coronary blood vessels. As the plaque thickens, secondary changes may take place like enlargement of size and calcification that may lead to complete occlusion of the lumen of the coronary artery, resulting in inadequate supply of oxygen to the heart muscle.

Peripheral Vascular Disease
Peripheral vascular disease is a narrowing of blood vessels that restricts blood flow. It mostly occurs in the legs, but is sometimes seen in the arms.

Hypercholesterolemia
Hypercholesterolemia is the presence of high levels of cholesterol in the blood. It is a form of "hyperlipidemia" (elevated levels of lipids in the blood) and "hyperlipoproteinemia" (elevated levels of lipoproteins in the blood).

Lymphedema
A condition in which excess fluid collects in tissue and causes swelling. Lymphedema may occur in the arm or leg after lymph vessels or lymph nodes in the underarm or groin are removed.

Hodgkin's Lymphoma
This is a type of cancer of the lymphatic system. It can start almost anywhere in the body. It's believed to be caused by HIV, Epstein-Barr Syndrome, age, and family history.

Non-Hodgkin's Lymphoma
Non-Hodgkin's lymphoma is a cancer of the lymphoid system. It is divided into three types: high-grade, intermediate-grade and low-grade.

Lymphangitis
Lymphangitis is an inflammation of the lymphatics (lymph channels) due to an infection by a microbe or some chemical irritant. It occurs when an infection or inflammation occurs somewhere else and the microbe or the irritant is transported along with lymph fluid through the lymphatics.

Splenomegaly
Splenomegaly is a condition in which the spleen becomes enlarged, tender and painful. It can occur due to a number of reasons, ranging from certain infections to cancers.

1. **Introduction**
   The human lymphatic system is closely linked with the blood and the vascular system. Both of these systems work in an intimate association with each other and transport vital fluids throughout the body via a system of vessels. The lymph capillaries and lymphatics are the special vessels that serve to transport a fluid (called lymph). The human lymphatic system consists of the below mentioned components:

   a) The Lymph
   b) The Lymph Vessels
   c) The Lymph Nodes
   d) The Tonsils, Spleen, Thymus Gland and Peyer's Patches

   The most important function of the lymphatic system is to drain the protein containing fluid from the tissue spaces. The entire lymphatics of the body converge into one of the following major channels:

   i) thoracic duct (or the main collecting channel)
   ii) right lymphatic duct

   e) The lymph nodes (or lymph glands) are oval structures that are found along the length of lymphatics at various intervals. The lymph trunk is a specific lymph vessel containing lymph. The various types of lymph trunks are documented below:

   i) jugular lymph trunk
   ii) subclavian lymph trunk
   iii) bronchomediastinal lymph trunk
   iv) lumbar lymph trunk
   v) intestinal lymph trunk

The Lymphatic System

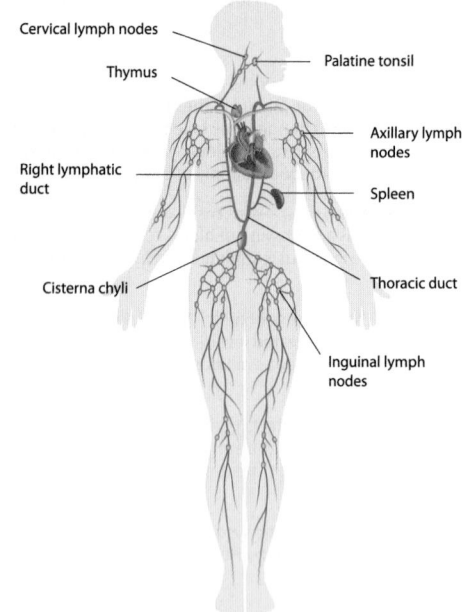

Cervical lymph nodes

Thymus

Palatine tonsil

Axillary lymph nodes

Right lymphatic duct

Spleen

Cisterna chyli

Thoracic duct

Inguinal lymph nodes

2. **Thoracic Duct**
   The thoracic duct is the largest lymphatic vessel in the body and constitutes an essential part of the lymphatic system. It is also called the alimentary duct, chyliferous duct, left lymphatic duct or Van Hoorne's canal.

3. **Lymphatics of the Head, Face and Neck**
   The entire lymph glands of the head are mostly extra-cranial, and arranged in the following groups:

   a) Occipital Lymph Glands: The occipital lymph glands are two or three in number and located on the back of the head.
   b) Posterior Auricular Lymph Glands (or Mastoid Glands): The posterior auricular lymph glands are two in number and exist on the upper part of the sternomastoid muscle and mastoid portion of the temporal bone.

   c) Anterior Auricular Lymph Glands (or Superficial Parotid/Preauricular Glands): The superficial parotid glands are present on the lateral surface of the parotid gland.
   d) Parotid Lymph Glands (or Deep Parotid Glands): The parotid lymph glands remain embedded in the deeper portions of the parotid gland.
   e) Superficial Facial Lymph Glands: The superficial facial lymph glands are based on several lymph glands in the region of face. However, the major ones are described below:

   i) Infraorbital Lymph Glands (or Maxillary Glands): The infraorbital lymph glands remain scattered along the angle between the nose and cheek, and below the margin of the orbit.
   ii) Buccinator Lymph Glands: The buccinator lymph glands are found on the superficial surface of the anterior part of buccinator muscle, opposite to the angle of the mouth.
   iii) Supramandibular Lymph Glands: The supramandibular lymph glands lie on the outer surface of the mandible at the anterior border of the masseter muscle, between the external maxillary artery and the anterior facial vein.

   f) The Deep Facial Lymph Glands (or Internal Maxillary Glands): The deep facial lymph glands are found in association with the internal maxillary artery, on the outer surface of the external pterygoid muscle.
   g) The Lingual Lymph Glands: The lingual lymph glands are based on two or three small nodules that exist on the lateral surfaces of the hypoglossal and genioglossus muscles.
   h) The Retropharyngeal Glands: The retropharyngeal glands are located in the buccopharyngeal fascia behind the upper part of the pharynx.

4. **The Lymph Glands of the Neck:** The lymph glands of the neck are divided into the following major groups:
   a) The Submaxillary Glands: The submaxillary glands are a pair of salivary glands located on each side under the body of the mandible.
   b) The Submental (or Suprahyoid Glands): The submental glands are located beneath the chin, and between the anterior bellies of the two digastric muscles.
   c) The Superficial Cervical Glands: The superficial cervical glands remain embedded in the deep fascia along the course of the external jugular vein, and superficial to the sternomastoid muscle.

5. **The Anterior Cervical Glands:** The lymph glands of the anterior neck region are divisible into the following two groups:
   a) Superficial Anterior Cervical Lymph Glands- The superficial anterior cervical lymph glands exist in association with the anterior jugular veins.
   b) Deep Anterior Cervical Lymph Glands: The deep anterior cervical lymph glands are divisible into the following groups/types:

   i) infrahyoid glands obtain lymph fluid from the region of epiglottis and transport it to the deep cervical glands.
   ii) prelaryngeal gland obtains lymph from the anterior portion of the larynx, the isthmus, and the portions of the right and left lobes of the thyroid gland.
   iii) pretracheal lymph glands are the numerous small nodules that follow the course of the inferior thyroid veins.
   iv) paratracheal lymph glands lie in association with the branches of the superior and inferior thyroid arteries and the recurrent nerves.

   c) Deep Cervical Glands: The deep cervical glands are the intercommunicating lymph vessels that remain positioned in the anterior and posterior triangles of the neck, and under the cover of the sternomastoid muscle. These glands are divisible into the following groups:

   i) superior deep cervical glands are located under the cover of the sternomastoid muscle, and lie in close association with the accessory nerve and internal jugular vein.
   ii) inferior deep cervical glands are located below the level of the omohyoid muscle.

   d) Lymphatic vessels of the scalp are distributed in the soft tissue envelope of the frontal, temporoparietal and the occipital regions of the cranium.
   e) Lymphatic Vessels of the Ear divide into upper and lateral portions of the auricle and terminate into the anterior auricular glands.

f) Lymphatic vessels of the face are more widely distributed than the scalp vessels, and can be divided into the following groups:

6. **Lymphatic Vessels of the Eyelids and Conjunctiva:** The lymphatic vessels of the eyelids and conjunctiva form the following two groups:
   a) Medial Lymph Vessels: The medial lymph vessels travel from the medial portions of the superior and inferior eyelids, and terminate to the submaxillary lymph glands.
   b) Lateral Lymph Vessels: The lateral lymph vessels arise from the lateral parts of the eyelids, and terminate into the anterior auricular and the parotid lymph glands.
   c) Lymphatic Vessels of the Cheeks: The superficial and deep lymphatic vessels of the cheeks usually communicate with the submaxillary glands.
   d) Lymphatic Vessels of the Lips: The lymphatic vessels of the lips drain lymph fluid to the submental and submaxillary glands.
   e) Lymphatic Vessels of the Nose: The lymphatic vessels from the external part of the nose drain lymph fluid to the anterior auricular and submaxillary glands.
   f) Lymphatic Vessels of the Nasal Cavities: The lymphatic vessels from the anterior and posterior portions of the nasal cavities drain lymph fluid to the submaxillary, the retropharyngeal, and the superior deep cervical glands.
   g) Lymphatic Vessels of the Mouth: The lymphatic vessels of the mouth can be divided into the following groups:
   h) Lymphatic Vessels of the Palatine Tonsil: The lymphatic vessels of the palatine tonsil arise from the buccopharyngeal fascia and constrictor pharyngis superior and meet with the superior deep cervical glands.
   i) Lymphatic Vessels of the Tongue: The lymphatic vessels of the tongue are divided into the following three groups:
      i) anterior lymph vessels of the tongue drain lymph fluid from the tip and lower surface of the tongue to the submental glands.
      ii) middle lymph vessels of the tongue drain lymph fluid from the anterior two third portion of the tongue to the submaxillary and medial superior deep cervical glands.
      iii) posterior lymph vessels of the tongue drain lymph fluid from the portion of the tongue, which lies in the anterior wall of pharynx.
   j) Lymphatic Vessels of the Gums: The lymph vessels of the anterior portion of mandibular gum drain lymph fluid to the submandibular gland. The lymph vessels from the inner portion of the mandibular gum also drain lymph fluid to the submaxillary glands.
   k) Lymphatic Vessels of the Teeth: The lymph vessels of the teeth and mandible transport lymph fluid to the sub maxillary or the superior deep cervical glands.

7. **The Lymphatics of the Upper Extremity:** The lymph glands of the upper extremity are divisible into the following two groups:
   a) The Superficial Lymph Glands- The superficial lymph glands of the upper extremity are of the following types:
      i) supratrochlear lymph glands are situated above the medial epicondyle of humerus, and drain lymph fluid from the middle, ring and little fingers, and the portions of the hand and forearm.
      ii) deltoideopectoral lymph glands are located in the groove between the pectoralis major and deltoid muscles.
   b) The Deep Lymph Glands: The deep lymph glands are chiefly found in the axillary region, where they constitute several constant as well as variable groups.
      i) lateral group of axillary lymph glands lies along the line of the great axillary vessels. These glands drain lymph fluid from the greater part of the upper extremity to the central and inferior deep cervical glands.
      ii) anterior group of axillary lymph glands travels from third to sixth intercostal space, along the line of the lateral thoracic artery.
      iii) posterior group of axillary lymph glands lies along the posterior wall of axilla, and follow the course of the subscapular vessels.
      iv) central group of axillary lymph glands are located in the central part of the axilla, and along the line of the intercosto-brachial nerve.
      v) infra-clavicular group of axillary lymph glands is found between the upper border of the pectoralis minor muscle and the clavicle, along the medial side of the axillary artery.
   c) The Lymphatic Vessels of the Upper Extremity: The lymphatic vessels of the upper extremity are divisible into the following two groups:

   i) superficial lymph vessels of the upper extremity are located in the skin and subcutaneous tissues, and commence in the cutaneous plexuses on the volar aspects of the fingers and hand.
   ii) deep lymph vessels of the upper extremity follow the course of the deeper blood vessels in the regions of the forearm and hand.

8. **Lymphatics of the Lower Extremity:** The lymph glands of the lower extremity are divisible into the following groups:
   a) The Superficial Lymph Glands- superficial lymph glands are found in the superficial fascia in subinguinal and inguinal regions. These glands are separable into the following groups:
      i) inguinal lymph glands are located above the level of the inguinal ligament.
      ii) superficial sublingual lymph glands are divisible into the proximal and distal groups.
   b) Deep Lymph Glands: The deep lymph glands of the inferior extremity are divided into the following two groups:
      i) popliteal lymph glands are located in the popliteal fossa.
      ii) deep sublingual lymph glands are located in the femoral trigone.
   c) Lymphatic Vessels of the Lower Extremity: The lymphatic vessels of the lower extremity are based on the following two groups:
      i) superficial lymphatic vessels are located in the superficial fascia and divided into vessels of the medial group arises on the tibial side and dorsum of the foot, and terminates in the distal group of superficial subinguinal glands and vessels of the lateral group commences from the fibular side of the foot.
      ii) deep lymphatic vessels of the lower extremity follow the course of the deep blood vessels, and terminate into the deep subinguinal and hypogastric glands.

9. **The Lymphatics of the Abdomen and Pelvis:** The lymph glands of the abdomen and pelvis are divisible into parietal lymph glands and visceral lymph glands.
   a) External Iliac Glands: The external iliac group of glands pertains to the pelvic region, located along the course of the external iliac vessels, and constitutes the lateral, intermediate and medial chains.
   b) Common Iliac Glands: The common iliac glands of the pelvis are located on the sides of the common iliac artery and below the bifurcation of aorta.
   c) Epigastric Glands: The epigastric glands of the anterior abdominal wall are divisible into the following types:
      i) superior epigastric gland is located in the superficial fascia of the median part of the epigastric region.
      ii) inferior epigastric glands are located along the course of the inferior epigastric artery.
   d) Circumflex Iliac Glands: The circumflex iliac glands of the anterior abdominal wall follow the course of the deep circumflex iliac artery in the lateral aspect of groin.
   e) Hypogastric Glands: The hypogastric glands of the pelvis are located along the course of the hypogastric vessels.
      i) gluteal lymph glands
      ii) pubo-gluteal lymph glands
      iii) middle hemorrhoidal gland
      iv) inter-iliac glands
      v) obturator gland
   f) Sacral Glands: The sacral lymph glands of the pelvis are located along the anterior aspect of sacrum, between the anterior sacral foramina.
   g) Lumbar Glands: The lumbar lymph glands are located behind the peritoneum of the posterior wall of the abdomen. The lumbar lymph glands are further separable into the following groups:
      i) right lateral aortic glands
      ii) left lateral aortic glands
      iii) preaortic glands
      iv) retroaortic glands
   h) Superior Gastric Glands: The superior gastric glands exist in association with the left gastric artery and constitute the following subdivisions:
      i) anterior left gastric glands (or lower coronary glands)
      ii) right paracardial glands
      iii) left paracardial glands
      iv) posterior paracardial glands

v)　posterior left gastric glands (or upper coronary glands)

vi)　right gastric gland (or pyloric gland)

vii)　left suprapancreatic glands

viii)　right suprapancreatic glands

ix)　subpyloric glands

x)　biliary lymph glands

i)　Inferior Gastric Glands (or Right Gastroepiploic Glands): The inferior gastric glands are associated with the greater curvature of the stomach and follow the course of the right gastroepiploic artery.

j)　Hepatic Glands: The hepatic lymph glands exist in the region of porta hepatis (or transverse fissure of the liver), between the layers of the lesser omentum.

k)　Pancreaticolienal Glands (or Splenic Glands): The pancreaticolienal glands are positioned in relation to the posterior surface and upper border of pancreas, and follow the course of the lienal (or splenic) artery.

l)　Mesenteric Glands: The mesenteric lymph glands are located between the layers of the mesentery.

m)　Ileocolic glands: The ileocolic glands are located around the ileocolic artery and form the following major groups:

i)　ileal glands

ii)　anterior ileocolic glands

iii)　posterior ileocolic glands

iv)　right colic glands

n)　Mesocolic Glands: The mesocolic glands exist in close association with the transverse colon.

o)　Inferior Mesenteric Glands- The inferior mesenteric glands are located on the branches of the left colic and sigmoid arteries, the superior hemorrhoidal artery, and the muscular coat of the rectum.

10. **The Lymphatic Vessels of the Abdominal Viscera and the Superior and Posterior Walls of the Abdomen**

a)　Lymphatic Vessels of the Abdominal Part of the Alimentary Canal

b)　Lymphatic Vessels of the Stomach

c)　Lymphatic Vessels of the Duodenum

d)　Lymphatic Vessels of the Jejunum and Ileum (or the Lacteals)

e)　Lymphatic Vessels of the Cecum, Vermiform Process, and the Ascending Colon

f)　Lymphatic Vessels of the Right Colic Flexure and the Transverse Colon

g)　Lymphatic Vessels of the Left Colic Flexure, Descending Colon, Iliac Colon, and Pelvic Colon

h)　Lymphatic Vessels of the Liver

i)　Lymphatic Vessels of the Gall Bladder

j)　Lymphatic Vessels of the Pancreas

k)　Lymphatic Vessels of the Spleen

l)　Lymphatic Vessels of the Kidneys

m)　Lymphatic Vessels of the Ureters

n)　Lymphatic Vessels of the Suprarenal Glands

o)　Lymphatic Vessels of the Diaphragm

11. **The Lymphatic Vessels of the Pelvic Viscera**

a)　lymphatic Vessels of the Male Urethra

b)　Lymphatic Vessels of the Prostate

c)　Lymphatic Vessels of the Female Urethra

d)　Lymphatic Vessels of the Seminal Vesicle

e)　Lymphatic Vessels of the Ductus Deferens

f)　Lymphatic Vessels of the Urinary Bladder

g)　Lymphatic Vessels of the Ureter

h)　Lymphatic Vessels of the Vagina

i)　Lymphatic Vessels of the Uterus

j)　Lymphatic Vessels of the Uterine Tube

k)　Lymphatic Vessels of the Ovaries

l)　Lymphatic Vessels of the Testis and Epididymis

m)　Lymphatic Vessels of the Anus, Anal Canal and Rectum

12. **The Lymphatics of the Thorax**

The Lymph Glands of the thorax are separable into the following groups:

a)　Sternal Lymph Glands- The sternal lymph glands are located at the margins of the sternum along the side of the internal mammary artery.

b)　Intercostal Lymph Glands- The intercostal lymph glands are situated in the posterior portions of the intercostal spaces (in relation to the intercostal vessels), and in front of the heads of the ribs.

c)　Anterior Mediastinal Lymph Glands- The anterior mediastinal lymph glands are located in the lower portion of the anterior mediastinum, and the anterior part of the superior mediastinal cavity.

d)　Posterior Mediastinal Lymph Glands- The posterior mediastinal lymph glands exist along the thoracic part of the esophagus and the descending thoracic aorta.

e)　Bronchial Lymph Glands- The bronchial lymph glands lie along the walls of the intrathoracic of the trachea, the bronchi and their intrapulmonary branches. These glands are further categorized into the following groups:

i)　tracheobronchial lymph glands

ii)　lymph glands of the bifurcation (or intertracheobronchial lymph glands)

iii)　bronchopulmonary lymph glands

iv)　pulmonary lymph glands

13. **The Lymphatic Vessels of the Thorax**

These vessels are divisible into the following groups:

a)　Intercostal Lymph Vessels

b)　Lymph Vessels of the Diaphragm

c)　Lymphatic Vessels of the Contents of the Thorax: The lymphatic vessels of the contents of the thorax are divisible into the following groups:

i)　lymph vessels of the heart

ii)　lymph vessels of the pericardium

iii)　lymph vessels of the thymus

iv)　lymph vessels of the thoracic part of esophagus

v)　lymph vessels of the pleura

vi)　lymph vessels of the lungs

Diseases of the circulatory system (I00-I99)

EXCLUDES2 certain conditions originating in the perinatal period (P04-P96)

certain infectious and parasitic diseases (A00-B99)

complications of pregnancy, childbirth and the puerperium (O00-O9A)

congenital malformations, deformations, and chromosomal abnormalities (Q00-Q99)

endocrine, nutritional and metabolic diseases (E00-E88)

injury, poisoning and certain other consequences of external causes (S00-T88)

neoplasms (C00-D49)

symptoms, signs and abnormal clinical and laboratory findings, not elsewhere classified (R00-R94)

systemic connective tissue disorders (M30-M36)

transient cerebral ischemic attacks and related syndromes (G45.-)

This chapter contains the following blocks:

I00-I02	Acute rheumatic fever
I05-I09	Chronic rheumatic heart diseases
I10-I16	Hypertensive diseases
I20-I25	Ischemic heart diseases
I26-I28	Pulmonary heart disease and diseases of pulmonary circulation
I30-I52	Other forms of heart disease
I60-I69	Cerebrovascular diseases
I70-I79	Diseases of arteries, arterioles and capillaries
I80-I89	Diseases of veins, lymphatic vessels and lymph nodes, not elsewhere classified
I95-I99	Other and unspecified disorders of the circulatory system

Acute rheumatic fever (I00-I02)

I00   Rheumatic fever without heart involvement

AHA: Q4 2016

INCLUDES   arthritis, rheumatic, acute or subacute

EXCLUDES1 rheumatic fever with heart involvement (I01.0 -I01.9)

I01   Rheumatic fever with heart involvement

EXCLUDES1 chronic diseases of rheumatic origin (I05-I09) unless rheumatic fever is also present or there is evidence of reactivation or activity of the rheumatic process.

I01.0   Acute rheumatic pericarditis   cc CC/MCC Exc

Any condition in I00 with pericarditis

Rheumatic pericarditis (acute)

EXCLUDES1 acute pericarditis not specified as rheumatic (I30.-)

I01.1   Acute rheumatic endocarditis   cc CC/MCC Exc

Any condition in I00 with endocarditis or valvulitis

Acute rheumatic valvulitis

I01.2   Acute rheumatic myocarditis   cc CC/MCC Exc

Any condition in I00 with myocarditis

I01.8   Other acute rheumatic heart disease   cc CC/MCC Exc

Any condition in I00 with other or multiple types of heart involvement

Acute rheumatic pancarditis

I01.9   Acute rheumatic heart disease, unspecified   cc CC/MCC Exc

Any condition in I00 with unspecified type of heart involvement

Rheumatic carditis, acute

Rheumatic heart disease, active or acute

I02   Rheumatic chorea

INCLUDES   Sydenham's chorea

EXCLUDES1 chorea NOS (G25.5)

Huntington's chorea (G10)

I02.0   Rheumatic chorea with heart involvement   cc CC/MCC Exc

Chorea NOS with heart involvement

Rheumatic chorea with heart involvement of any type classifiable under I01.-

I02.9   Rheumatic chorea without heart involvement   cc CC/MCC Exc

Rheumatic chorea NOS

Chronic rheumatic heart diseases (I05-I09)

I05   Rheumatic mitral valve **diseases**

INCLUDES   conditions classifiable to both I05.0 and I05.2-I05.9, whether specified as rheumatic or not

EXCLUDES1 mitral valve disease specified as nonrheumatic (I34.-)

mitral valve disease with aortic and/or tricuspid valve involvement (I08.-)

I05.0   Rheumatic mitral stenosis

Mitral (valve) obstruction (rheumatic)

I05.1   Rheumatic mitral insufficiency

Rheumatic mitral incompetence

Rheumatic mitral regurgitation

EXCLUDES1 mitral insufficiency not specified as rheumatic (I34.0)

I05.2   Rheumatic mitral stenosis with insufficiency

Rheumatic mitral stenosis with incompetence or regurgitation

I05.8   Other rheumatic mitral valve diseases

Rheumatic mitral (valve) failure

I05.9   Rheumatic mitral valve disease, unspecified

Rheumatic mitral (valve) disorder (chronic) NOS

I06   Rheumatic aortic valve **diseases**

EXCLUDES1 aortic valve disease not specified as rheumatic (I35.-)

aortic valve disease with mitral and/or tricuspid valve involvement (I08.-)

I06.0   Rheumatic aortic stenosis

Rheumatic aortic (valve) obstruction

I06.1   Rheumatic aortic insufficiency

Rheumatic aortic incompetence

Rheumatic aortic regurgitation

I06.2   Rheumatic aortic stenosis with insufficiency

Rheumatic aortic stenosis with incompetence or regurgitation

I06.8   Other rheumatic aortic valve diseases

I06.9   Rheumatic aortic valve disease, unspecified

Rheumatic aortic (valve) disease NOS

I07   Rheumatic tricuspid valve **diseases**

INCLUDES   rheumatic tricuspid valve diseases specified as rheumatic or unspecified

EXCLUDES1 tricuspid valve disease specified as nonrheumatic (I36.-)

tricuspid valve disease with aortic and/or mitral valve involvement (I08.-)

I07.0   Rheumatic tricuspid stenosis

Tricuspid (valve) stenosis (rheumatic)

I07.1   Rheumatic tricuspid insufficiency

Tricuspid (valve) insufficiency (rheumatic)

I07.2   Rheumatic tricuspid stenosis and insufficiency

I07.8   Other rheumatic tricuspid valve diseases

I07.9   Rheumatic tricuspid valve disease, unspecified

Rheumatic tricuspid valve disorder NOS

I08   Multiple valve diseases

INCLUDES   multiple valve diseases specified as rheumatic or unspecified

EXCLUDES1 endocarditis, valve unspecified (I38)

multiple valve disease specified a nonrheumatic (I34.-, I35.-, I36.-, I37.-, I38.-, Q22.-, Q23.-, Q24.8-)

rheumatic valve disease NOS (I09.1)

I08.0   Rheumatic disorders of both mitral **and** aortic **valves**

Involvement of both mitral and aortic valves specified as rheumatic or unspecified

I08.1   Rheumatic disorders of both mitral **and** tricuspid **valves**

I08.2   Rheumatic disorders of both aortic **and** tricuspid **valves**

I08.3   Combined rheumatic disorders of mitral, aortic **and** tricuspid **valves**

I08.8   Other rheumatic multiple valve diseases

I08.9   Rheumatic multiple valve disease, unspecified

I09   Other rheumatic heart diseases

I09.0   Rheumatic myocarditis   cc CC/MCC Exc

EXCLUDES1 myocarditis not specified as rheumatic (I51.4)

I09.1   Rheumatic diseases of endocardium, valve unspecified

Rheumatic endocarditis (chronic)

Rheumatic valvulitis (chronic)

EXCLUDES1 endocarditis, valve unspecified (I38)

Unspecified Code   Other Specified Code   Manifestation Code   N Newborn   P Pediatric   M Maternity   A Adult   ♂ Male   ♀ Female

● New Code   ▲ Revised Code Title   ►◄ Revised Text   *NOTES*   *INCLUDES*   *EXCLUDES 1*   Not coded here   *EXCLUDES 2*   Not included here

4th character required   5th character required   6th character required   7th character required

Extension 'X' Alert   *HAC* Hospital-acquired condition (HAC) alert   **AHA** AHA Coding Clinic©

I09.2 Chronic **rheumatic** pericarditis [CC] [CC/MCC Exc]
Adherent pericardium, rheumatic
Chronic rheumatic mediastinopericarditis
Chronic rheumatic myopericarditis
[EXCLUDES1] *chronic pericarditis not specified as rheumatic (I31.-)*

[5th] **I09.8 Other specified rheumatic heart diseases**
I09.81 Rheumatic heart failure [CC] [HCC] [RxHCC] [CC/MCC Exc]
Use additional code to identify type of heart failure (I50.-)

I09.89 Other specified rheumatic heart diseases
Rheumatic disease of pulmonary valve

I09.9 Rheumatic heart disease, unspecified
Rheumatic carditis
[EXCLUDES1] *rheumatoid carditis (M05.31)*

Hypertensive diseases (I10-I16)

Use additional code to identify:
exposure to environmental tobacco smoke (Z77.22)
history of tobacco dependence (Z87.891)
occupational exposure to environmental tobacco smoke (Z57.31)
tobacco dependence (F17.-)
tobacco use (Z72.0)
[EXCLUDES1] *neonatal hypertension (P29.2)*
primary pulmonary hypertension (I27.0)
[EXCLUDES2] *hypertensive disease complicating pregnancy, childbirth and the puerperium (O10-O11, O13-O16)*

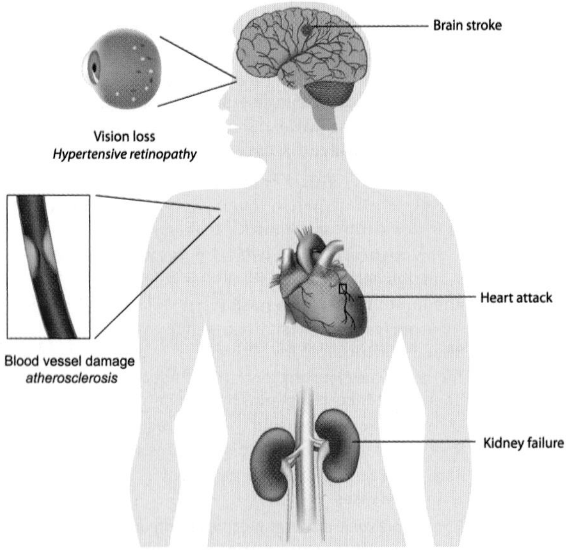

Figure 9.1 Main complications of hypertension

I10 Essential **(primary) hypertension** [?] [RxHCC]
AHA: Q4 2016, Q4 2013
[INCLUDES] *high blood pressure*
hypertension (arterial) (benign) (essential) (malignant) (primary) (systemic)
[EXCLUDES1] *hypertensive disease complicating pregnancy, childbirth and the puerperium (O10-O11, O13-O16)*
[EXCLUDES2] *essential (primary) hypertension involving vessels of brain (I60-I69)*
essential (primary) hypertension involving vessels of eye (H35.0-)

[4th] **I11 Hypertensive** heart **disease**
[INCLUDES] *any condition in ►I50.-, I51.4-I51.9◄ due to hypertension*

I11.0 Hypertensive heart disease with heart failure [HCC] [RxHCC]
AHA: Q1 2017
Hypertensive heart failure
Use additional code to identify type of heart failure (I50.-)

I11.9 Hypertensive heart disease without heart failure [RxHCC]
Hypertensive heart disease NOS

[4th] **I12 Hypertensive** chronic kidney **disease**
[INCLUDES] *any condition in N18 and N26 - due to hypertension*
arteriosclerosis of kidney
arteriosclerotic nephritis (chronic) (interstitial)
hypertensive nephropathy
nephrosclerosis
[EXCLUDES1] *hypertension due to kidney disease (I15.0, I15.1)*
renovascular hypertension (I15.0)
secondary hypertension (I15.-)
[EXCLUDES2] *acute kidney failure (N17.-)*

I12.0 Hypertensive chronic kidney disease with stage 5 **chronic kidney disease or** end stage renal disease [CC] [HCC] [RxHCC] [CC/MCC Exc]
AHA: Q3 2016
Use additional code to identify the stage of chronic kidney disease (N18.5, N18.6)

I12.9 Hypertensive chronic kidney disease with stage 1 through stage 4 **chronic kidney disease, or unspecified chronic kidney disease** [RxHCC]
Hypertensive chronic kidney disease NOS
Hypertensive renal disease NOS
Use additional code to identify the stage of chronic kidney disease (N18.1-N18.4, N18.9)

[4th] **I13 Hypertensive** heart **and** chronic kidney **disease**
[INCLUDES] *any condition in I11.- with any condition in I12.-*
cardiorenal disease
cardiovascular renal disease

I13.0 Hypertensive heart and chronic kidney disease with heart failure and stage 1 through stage 4 **chronic kidney disease, or unspecified chronic kidney disease** [CC] [HCC] [RxHCC] [CC/MCC Exc]
Use additional code to identify type of heart failure (I50.-)
Use additional code to identify stage of chronic kidney disease (N18.1-N18.4, N18.9)

[5th] **I13.1 Hypertensive** heart **and** chronic kidney **disease** without heart **failure**

I13.10 Hypertensive heart and chronic kidney disease without heart failure, with stage 1 through stage 4 **chronic kidney disease, or unspecified chronic kidney disease** [RxHCC]
Hypertensive heart disease and hypertensive chronic kidney disease NOS
Use additional code to identify the stage of chronic kidney disease (N18.1-N18.4, N18.9)

I13.11 Hypertensive heart and chronic kidney disease without heart failure, with stage 5 **chronic kidney disease, or** end stage renal disease [CC] [HCC] [RxHCC] [CC/MCC Exc]
Use additional code to identify the stage of chronic kidney disease (N18.5, N18.6)

I13.2 Hypertensive heart and chronic kidney disease with heart failure **and with** stage 5 **chronic kidney disease, or** end stage renal disease [CC] [HCC] [RxHCC] [CC/MCC Exc]
Use additional code to identify type of heart failure (I50.-)
Use additional code to identify the stage of chronic kidney disease (N18.5, N18.6)

[4th] **I15** Secondary **hypertension**
Code also underlying condition
[EXCLUDES1] *postprocedural hypertension (I97.3)*
[EXCLUDES2] *secondary hypertension involving vessels of brain (I60-I69)*
secondary hypertension involving vessels of eye (H35.0-)

I15.0 Renovascular **hypertension** [RxHCC]
I15.1 Hypertension secondary to other renal disorders [RxHCC]
AHA: Q3 2016
I15.2 Hypertension secondary to endocrine disorders [RxHCC]
I15.8 Other **secondary hypertension** [RxHCC]
I15.9 Secondary hypertension, unspecified [RxHCC]

[4th] **I16 Hypertensive** crisis
Code also any identified hypertensive disease (I10-I15)

[PDx] Unacceptable principal diagnosis symbol per Medicare code edits [POA] Code exempt from diagnosis present on admission requirement
[?] Questionable admission [CC] Complication or comorbidity [CC/MCC Exc] CC/MCC exclusion [MCC] Major complication or comorbidity
[PDx CC] Principal diagnosis as its own CC [PDx MCC] Principal diagnosis as its own MCC [HCC] HCC diagnosis code [RxHCC] RxHCC diagnosis code
MACRA code [Z1] Z code as first-listed diagnosis

I16.0 **Hypertensive** urgency [RxHCC]
AHA: Q4 2016
I16.1 **Hypertensive** emergency [RxHCC]
AHA: Q4 2016
I16.9 **Hypertensive crisis,** unspecified [RxHCC]
AHA: Q4 2016

Ischemic heart diseases (I20-I25)

Use additional code to identify presence of hypertension (I10-I16)

[4th] I20 **Angina pectoris**
Use additional code to identify:
exposure to environmental tobacco smoke (Z77.22)
history of tobacco dependence (Z87.891)
occupational exposure to environmental tobacco smoke (Z57.31)
tobacco dependence (F17.-)
tobacco use (Z72.0)
[EXCLUDES1] *angina pectoris with atherosclerotic heart disease of native coronary arteries (I25.1-)*
atherosclerosis of coronary artery bypass graft(s) and coronary artery of transplanted heart with angina pectoris (I25.7-)
postinfarction angina (I23.7)

I20.0 Unstable **angina** [CC] [HCC] [RxHCC] [CC/MCC Exc]
Accelerated angina
Crescendo angina
De novo effort angina
Intermediate coronary syndrome
Preinfarction syndrome
Worsening effort angina

I20.1 **Angina pectoris** with documented spasm [CC] [HCC] [RxHCC] [CC/MCC Exc]
Angiospastic angina
Prinzmetal angina
Spasm-induced angina
Variant angina

I20.8 **Other forms of angina pectoris** [HCC] [RxHCC]
Angina equivalent
Angina of effort
Coronary slow flow syndrome
Stenocardia
Stable angina
Use additional code(s) for symptoms associated with angina equivalent

I20.9 **Angina pectoris, unspecified** [HCC] [RxHCC]
Angina NOS
Anginal syndrome
Cardiac angina
Ischemic chest pain

▲ [4th] I21 **►Acute◄ myocardial infarction**
[INCLUDES] *cardiac infarction*
coronary (artery) embolism
coronary (artery) occlusion
coronary (artery) rupture
coronary (artery) thrombosis
infarction of heart, myocardium, or ventricle
myocardial infarction specified as acute or with a stated duration of 4 weeks (28 days) or less from onset
Use additional code, if applicable, to identify:
exposure to environmental tobacco smoke (Z77.22)
history of tobacco dependence (Z87.891)
occupational exposure to environmental tobacco smoke (Z57.31)
status post administration of tPA (rtPA) in a different facility within the last 24 hours prior to admission to current facility (Z92.82)
tobacco dependence (F17.-)
tobacco use (Z72.0)
[EXCLUDES2] *old myocardial infarction (I25.2)*
postmyocardial infarction syndrome (I24.1)
subsequent type 1 myocardial infarction (I22.-)

[5th] I21.0 ST elevation **(STEMI) myocardial infarction of** anterior wall
Type 1 ST elevation myocardial infarction of anterior wall

I21.01 **ST elevation (STEMI) myocardial infarction involving** left main coronary artery [HCC] [MCC] [RxHCC] [CC/MCC Exc]

I21.02 **ST elevation (STEMI) myocardial infarction involving** left anterior descending coronary artery [HCC] [MCC] [RxHCC] [CC/MCC Exc]
AHA: Q1 2013
ST elevation (STEMI) myocardial infarction involving diagonal coronary artery

I21.09 **ST elevation (STEMI) myocardial infarction involving** other coronary artery **of anterior wall** [HCC] [MCC] [RxHCC] [CC/MCC Exc]
AHA: Q4 2012
Acute transmural myocardial infarction of anterior wall
Anteroapical transmural (Q wave) infarction (acute)
Anterolateral transmural (Q wave) infarction (acute)
Anteroseptal transmural (Q wave) infarction (acute)
Transmural (Q wave) infarction (acute) (of) anterior (wall) NOS

[5th] I21.1 ST elevation **(STEMI) myocardial infarction of** inferior wall
Type 1 ST elevation myocardial infarction of inferior wall

I21.11 **ST elevation (STEMI) myocardial infarction involving** right coronary artery [HCC] [MCC] [RxHCC] [CC/MCC Exc]
Inferoposterior transmural (Q wave) infarction (acute)

I21.19 **ST elevation (STEMI) myocardial infarction involving** other coronary artery **of inferior wall** [HCC] [MCC] [RxHCC] [CC/MCC Exc]
AHA: Q4 2012
Acute transmural myocardial infarction of inferior wall
Inferolateral transmural (Q wave) infarction (acute)
Transmural (Q wave) infarction (acute) (of) diaphragmatic wall
Transmural (Q wave) infarction (acute) (of) inferior (wall) NOS
[EXCLUDES2] *ST elevation (STEMI) myocardial infarction involving left circumflex coronary artery (I21.21)*

[5th] I21.2 ST elevation **(STEMI) myocardial infarction of** other sites
Type 1 ST elevation myocardial infarction of other sites

I21.21 **ST elevation (STEMI) myocardial infarction involving** left circumflex coronary artery [HCC] [MCC] [RxHCC] [CC/MCC Exc]
ST elevation (STEMI) myocardial infarction involving oblique marginal coronary artery

I21.29 **ST elevation (STEMI) myocardial infarction involving** other sites [HCC] [MCC] [RxHCC] [CC/MCC Exc]
Acute transmural myocardial infarction of other sites
Apical-lateral transmural (Q wave) infarction (acute)
Basal-lateral transmural (Q wave) infarction (acute)
High lateral transmural (Q wave) infarction (acute)
Lateral (wall) NOS transmural (Q wave) infarction (acute)
Posterior (true) transmural (Q wave) infarction (acute)
Posterobasal transmural (Q wave) infarction (acute)
Posterolateral transmural (Q wave) infarction (acute)
Posteroseptal transmural (Q wave) infarction (acute)
Septal transmural (Q wave) infarction (acute) NOS

I21.3 ST elevation **(STEMI) myocardial infarction of** unspecified site [HCC] [MCC] [RxHCC] [CC/MCC Exc]
AHA: Q1 2013
Acute transmural myocardial infarction of unspecified site
Transmural (Q wave) myocardial infarction NOS
Type 1 ST elevation myocardial infarction of unspecified site

I21.4 Non-ST elevation **(NSTEMI) myocardial infarction** [HCC] [MCC] [RxHCC] [CC/MCC Exc]
AHA: Q1 2017
Acute subendocardial myocardial infarction
Non-Q wave myocardial infarction NOS
Nontransmural myocardial infarction NOS
Type 1 non-ST elevation myocardial infarction

● I21.9 Acute **myocardial infarction,** unspecified
Myocardial infarction (acute) NOS

● [5th] I21.A Other **type of myocardial infarction**

● I21.A1 **Myocardial infarction** type 2
Myocardial infarction due to demand ischemia
Myocardial infarction secondary to ischemic imbalance

Unspecified Code Other Specified Code Manifestation Code [N] Newborn [P] Pediatric [M] Maternity [A] Adult ♂ Male ♀ Female
● New Code ▲ Revised Code Title ►◄ Revised Text [NOTES] [INCLUDES] [EXCLUDES1] Not coded here [EXCLUDES2] Not included here
[4th] 4th character required [5th] 5th character required [6th] 6th character required [7th] 7th character required
[x] Extension 'X' Alert [HAC] Hospital-acquired condition (HAC) alert AHA AHA Coding Clinic©

polymyositis (M33.2-)
portal hypertension (K76.6)
rheumatoid arthritis (M05.-)
schistosomiasis (B65.-)
Sjögren syndrome (M35.0-)
systemic sclerosis (M34.-)

● I27.22 **Pulmonary hypertension due to left heart disease**
Group 2 pulmonary hypertension
Code also associated left heart disease, if known, such as:
multiple valve disease (I08.-)
rheumatic mitral valve diseases (I05.-)
rheumatic aortic valve diseases (I06.-)

● I27.23 **Pulmonary hypertension due to lung diseases and hypoxia**
Group 3 pulmonary hypertension
Code also associated lung disease, if known, such as:
bronchiectasis (J47.-)
cystic fibrosis with pulmonary manifestations (E84.0)
interstitial lung disease (J84.-)
pleural effusion (J90)
sleep apnea (G47.3-)

● I27.24 **Chronic thromboembolic pulmonary hypertension**
Group 4 pulmonary hypertension
Code also associated pulmonary embolism, if applicable (I26.-, I27.82)

● I27.29 **Other secondary pulmonary hypertension**
Group 5 pulmonary hypertension
Pulmonary hypertension with unclear multifactorial mechanisms
Pulmonary hypertension due to hematologic disorders
Pulmonary hypertension due to metabolic disorders
Pulmonary hypertension due to other systemic disorders
Code also other associated disorders, if known, such as:
chronic myeloid leukemia (C92.10- C92.22)
essential thrombocythemia (D47.3)
Gaucher disease (E75.22)
hypertensive chronic kidney disease with end stage renal disease (I12.0, I12.11, I13.2)
hyperthyroidism (E05.-)
hypothyroidism (E00-E03)
polycythemia vera (D45)
sarcoidosis (D86.-)

I27.8 **Other specified pulmonary heart diseases**

I27.81 **Cor pulmonale (chronic)**   HCC RxHCC
Cor pulmonale NOS
EXCLUDES1 acute cor pulmonale (I26.0-)

I27.82 **Chronic pulmonary embolism**   HCC RxHCC CC/MCC Exc
Use additional code, if applicable, for associated long-term (current) use of anticoagulants (Z79.01)
EXCLUDES1 personal history of pulmonary embolism (Z86.711)

● I27.83 **Eisenmenger's syndrome**
Eisenmenger's complex
(Irreversible) Eisenmenger's disease
Pulmonary hypertension with right to left shunt related to congenital heart disease
Code also underlying heart defect, if known, such as:
atrial septal defect (Q21.1)
Eisenmenger's defect (Q21.8)
patent ductus arteriosus (Q25.0)
ventricular septal defect (Q21.0)

I27.89 **Other specified pulmonary heart diseases**   HCC RxHCC

I27.9 **Pulmonary heart disease, unspecified**   HCC RxHCC
Chronic cardiopulmonary disease

I28 **Other diseases of pulmonary vessels**

I28.0 **Arteriovenous fistula of pulmonary vessels**   HCC RxHCC CC/MCC Exc
EXCLUDES1 congenital arteriovenous fistula (Q25.72)

I28.1 **Aneurysm of pulmonary artery**   HCC RxHCC CC/MCC Exc
EXCLUDES1 congenital aneurysm (Q25.79)
congenital arteriovenous aneurysm (Q25.72)

I28.8 **Other diseases of pulmonary vessels**   HCC RxHCC
Pulmonary arteritis
Pulmonary endarteritis
Rupture of pulmonary vessels
Stenosis of pulmonary vessels
Stricture of pulmonary vessels

I28.9 **Disease of pulmonary vessels, unspecified**   HCC RxHCC

Other forms of heart disease (I30-I52)

I30 **Acute pericarditis**
INCLUDES acute mediastinopericarditis
acute myopericarditis
acute pericardial effusion
acute pleuropericarditis
acute pneumopericarditis
EXCLUDES1 Dressler's syndrome (I24.1)
rheumatic pericarditis (acute) (I01.0)
viral pericarditis due to Coxsakie virus (B33.23)

I30.0 **Acute nonspecific idiopathic pericarditis**   CC/MCC Exc

I30.1 **Infective pericarditis**   CC/MCC Exc
Pneumococcal pericarditis
Pneumopyopericardium
Purulent pericarditis
Pyopericarditis
Pyopericardium
Pyopneumopericardium
Staphylococcal pericarditis
Streptococcal pericarditis
Suppurative pericarditis
Viral pericarditis
Use additional code (B95-B97) to identify infectious agent

I30.8 **Other forms of acute pericarditis**   CC/MCC Exc

I30.9 **Acute pericarditis, unspecified**   CC/MCC Exc

I31 **Other diseases of pericardium**
EXCLUDES1 diseases of pericardium specified as rheumatic (I09.2)
postcardiotomy syndrome (I97.0)
traumatic injury to pericardium (S26.-)

I31.0 **Chronic adhesive pericarditis**   CC/MCC Exc
Accretio cordis
Adherent pericardium
Adhesive mediastinopericarditis

I31.1 **Chronic constrictive pericarditis**   CC/MCC Exc
Concretio cordis
Pericardial calcification

I31.2 **Hemopericardium, not elsewhere classified**   CC/MCC Exc
EXCLUDES1 hemopericardium as current complication following acute myocardial infarction (I23.0)

I31.3 **Pericardial effusion (noninflammatory)**   CC/MCC Exc
Chylopericardium
EXCLUDES1 acute pericardial effusion (I30.9)

I31.4 **Cardiac tamponade**   PDxIn CC/MCC Exc
Code first underlying cause

I31.8 **Other specified diseases of pericardium**   CC/MCC Exc
Epicardial plaques
Focal pericardial adhesions

I31.9 **Disease of pericardium, unspecified**   CC/MCC Exc
Pericarditis (chronic) NOS

I32 **Pericarditis in diseases classified elsewhere**   CC/MCC Exc
Code first underlying disease
EXCLUDES1 pericarditis (in):
coxsackie (virus) (B33.23)
gonococcal (A54.83)
meningococcal (A39.53)
rheumatoid (arthritis) (M05.31)
syphilitic (A52.06)
systemic lupus erythematosus (M32.12)
tuberculosis (A18.84)

PDxIn Unacceptable principal diagnosis symbol per Medicare code edits   POA Code exempt from diagnosis present on admission requirement
❓ Questionable admission   Complication or comorbidity   CC/MCC Exc CC/MCC exclusion   MCC Major complication or comorbidity
Principal diagnosis as its own CC   Principal diagnosis as its own MCC   HCC HCC diagnosis code   RxHCC RxHCC diagnosis code
MACRA code   Z1 Z code as first-listed diagnosis

[4th] **I33 Acute and subacute endocarditis**

[EXCLUDES1] *acute rheumatic endocarditis (I01.1)*
endocarditis NOS (I38)

I33.0 Acute and subacute infective endocarditis MCC CC/MCC Exc
Bacterial endocarditis (acute) (subacute)
Infective endocarditis (acute) (subacute) NOS
Endocarditis lenta (acute) (subacute)
Malignant endocarditis (acute) (subacute)
Purulent endocarditis (acute) (subacute)
Septic endocarditis (acute) (subacute)
Ulcerative endocarditis (acute) (subacute)
Vegetative endocarditis (acute) (subacute)
Use additional code (B95-B97) to identify infectious agent

I33.9 Acute and subacute endocarditis, unspecified MCC CC/MCC Exc
Acute endocarditis NOS
Acute myoendocarditis NOS
Acute periendocarditis NOS
Subacute endocarditis NOS
Subacute myoendocarditis NOS
Subacute periendocarditis NOS

[4th] **I34 Nonrheumatic mitral valve disorders**

[EXCLUDES1] *mitral valve disease (I05.9)*
mitral valve failure (I05.8)
mitral valve stenosis (I05.0)
mitral valve disorder of unspecified cause with diseases of aortic and/or tricuspid valve(s) (I08.-)
mitral valve disorder of unspecified cause with mitral stenosis or obstruction (I05.0)
mitral valve disorder specified as congenital ►(Q23.2, Q23.9)◄
mitral valve disorder specified as rheumatic (I05.-)

I34.0 Nonrheumatic mitral (valve) insufficiency
Nonrheumatic mitral (valve) incompetence NOS
Nonrheumatic mitral (valve) regurgitation NOS

I34.1 Nonrheumatic mitral (valve) prolapse
Floppy nonrheumatic mitral valve syndrome
[EXCLUDES1] *Marfan's syndrome (Q87.4-)*

I34.2 Nonrheumatic mitral (valve) stenosis

I34.8 Other nonrheumatic mitral valve disorders

I34.9 Nonrheumatic mitral valve disorder, unspecified

[4th] **I35 Nonrheumatic aortic valve disorders**

[EXCLUDES1] *aortic valve disorder of unspecified cause but with diseases of mitral and/or tricuspid valve(s) (I08.-)*
aortic valve disorder specified as congenital (Q23.0, Q23.1)
aortic valve disorder specified as rheumatic (I06.-)
hypertrophic subaortic stenosis (I42.1)

I35.0 Nonrheumatic aortic (valve) stenosis

I35.1 Nonrheumatic aortic (valve) insufficiency
Nonrheumatic aortic (valve) incompetence NOS
Nonrheumatic aortic (valve) regurgitation NOS

I35.2 Nonrheumatic aortic (valve) stenosis with insufficiency

I35.8 Other nonrheumatic aortic valve disorders

I35.9 Nonrheumatic aortic valve disorder, unspecified

[4th] **I36 Nonrheumatic tricuspid valve disorders**

[EXCLUDES1] *tricuspid valve disorders of unspecified cause (I07.-)*
tricuspid valve disorders specified as congenital (Q22.4, Q22.8, Q22.9)
tricuspid valve disorders specified as rheumatic (I07.-)
tricuspid valve disorders with aortic and/or mitral valve involvement (I08.-)

I36.0 Nonrheumatic tricuspid (valve) stenosis

I36.1 Nonrheumatic tricuspid (valve) insufficiency
Nonrheumatic tricuspid (valve) incompetence
Nonrheumatic tricuspid (valve) regurgitation

I36.2 Nonrheumatic tricuspid (valve) stenosis with insufficiency

I36.8 Other nonrheumatic tricuspid valve disorders

I36.9 Nonrheumatic tricuspid valve disorder, unspecified

[4th] **I37 Nonrheumatic pulmonary valve disorders**

[EXCLUDES1] *pulmonary valve disorder specified as congenital (Q22.1, Q22.2, Q22.3)*
pulmonary valve disorder specified as rheumatic (I09.89)

I37.0 Nonrheumatic pulmonary valve stenosis

I37.1 Nonrheumatic pulmonary valve insufficiency
Nonrheumatic pulmonary valve incompetence
Nonrheumatic pulmonary valve regurgitation

I37.2 Nonrheumatic pulmonary valve stenosis with insufficiency

I37.8 Other nonrheumatic pulmonary valve disorders

I37.9 Nonrheumatic pulmonary valve disorder, unspecified

I38 Endocarditis, valve unspecified CC CC/MCC Exc

[INCLUDES] *endocarditis (chronic) NOS*
valvular incompetence NOS
valvular insufficiency NOS
valvular regurgitation NOS
valvular stenosis NOS
valvulitis (chronic) NOS

[EXCLUDES1] *congenital insufficiency of cardiac valve NOS (Q24.8)*
congenital stenosis of cardiac valve NOS (Q24.8)
endocardial fibroelastosis (I42.4)
endocarditis specified as rheumatic (I09.1)

I39 Endocarditis and heart valve disorders in diseases classified elsewhere CC CC/MCC Exc

Code first underlying disease, such as:
Q fever (A78)

[EXCLUDES1] *endocardial involvement in:*
candidiasis (B37.6)
gonococcal infection (A54.83)
Libman-Sacks disease (M32.11)
listerosis (A32.82)
meningococcal infection (A39.51)
rheumatoid arthritis (M05.31)
syphilis (A52.03)
tuberculosis (A18.84)
typhoid fever (A01.02)

[4th] **I40 Acute myocarditis**

[INCLUDES] *subacute myocarditis*

[EXCLUDES1] *acute rheumatic myocarditis (I01.2)*

I40.0 Infective myocarditis MCC CC/MCC Exc
Septic myocarditis
Use additional code (B95-B97) to identify infectious agent

I40.1 Isolated myocarditis MCC CC/MCC Exc
Fiedler's myocarditis
Giant cell myocarditis
Idiopathic myocarditis

I40.8 Other acute myocarditis MCC CC/MCC Exc

I40.9 Acute myocarditis, unspecified MCC CC/MCC Exc

I41 Myocarditis in diseases classified elsewhere MCC CC/MCC Exc

Code first underlying disease, such as:
typhus (A75.0-A75.9)

[EXCLUDES1] *myocarditis (in):*
Chagas' disease (chronic) (B57.2)
acute (B57.0)
coxsackie (virus) infection (B33.22)
diphtheritic (A36.81)
gonococcal (A54.83)
influenzal (J09.X9, J10.82, J11.82)
meningococcal (A39.52)
mumps (B26.82)
rheumatoid arthritis (M05.31)
sarcoid (D86.85)
syphilis (A52.06)
toxoplasmosis (B58.81)
tuberculous (A18.84)

Unspecified Code | Other Specified Code | Manifestation Code | [N] Newborn | [P] Pediatric | [M] Maternity | [A] Adult | ♂ Male | ♀ Female
● New Code | ▲ Revised Code Title | ►◄ Revised Text | [NOTES] | [INCLUDES] | [EXCLUDES1] Not coded here | [EXCLUDES2] Not included here
[4th] 4th character required | [5th] 5th character required | [6th] 6th character required | [7th] 7th character required
[7x] Extension 'X' Alert | [HAC] Hospital-acquired condition (HAC) alert | AHA AHA Coding Clinic©

When symbols appear on a code that requires a 7th character extension, refer to Appendix B to identify applicable 7th character codes.

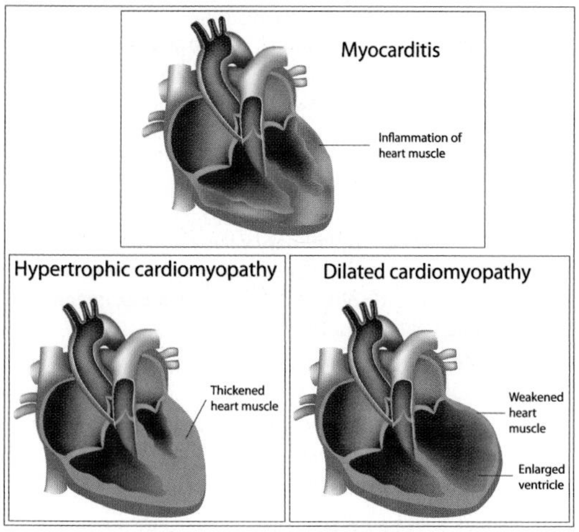

Figure 9.2 Heart muscle disease

[4th] **I42 Cardiomyopathy**
[INCLUDES] *myocardiopathy*
Code first pre-existing cardiomyopathy complicating pregnancy and puerperium (O99.4)
[EXCLUDES2] *ischemic cardiomyopathy (I25.5)*
peripartum cardiomyopathy (O90.3)
ventricular hypertrophy (I51.7)

I42.0 Dilated **cardiomyopathy** [CC] [HCC] [RxHCC] [CC/MCC Exc]
Congestive cardiomyopathy

I42.1 Obstructive hypertrophic **cardiomyopathy** [CC] [HCC] [RxHCC] [CC/MCC Exc]
Hypertrophic subaortic stenosis (idiopathic)

I42.2 Other hypertrophic **cardiomyopathy** [CC] [HCC] [RxHCC] [CC/MCC Exc]
Nonobstructive hypertrophic cardiomyopathy

I42.3 Endomyocardial (eosinophilic) disease [CC] [HCC] [RxHCC] [CC/MCC Exc]
Endomyocardial (tropical) fibrosis
Löffler's endocarditis

I42.4 Endocardial fibroelastosis [CC] [HCC] [RxHCC] [CC/MCC Exc]
Congenital cardiomyopathy
Elastomyofibrosis

I42.5 Other restrictive **cardiomyopathy** [CC] [HCC] [RxHCC] [CC/MCC Exc]
Constrictive cardiomyopathy NOS

I42.6 Alcoholic **cardiomyopathy** [CC] [HCC] [RxHCC] [CC/MCC Exc]
Code also presence of alcoholism (F10.-)

I42.7 **Cardiomyopathy** due to drug and external agent [CC] [HCC] [RxHCC] [CC/MCC Exc]
Code first poisoning due to drug or toxin, if applicable (T36-T65 with fifth or sixth character 1-4 or 6)
Use additional code for adverse effect, if applicable, to identify drug (T36-T50 with fifth or sixth character 5)

I42.8 **Other cardiomyopathies** [CC] [HCC] [RxHCC] [CC/MCC Exc]

I42.9 **Cardiomyopathy, unspecified** [CC] [HCC] [RxHCC] [CC/MCC Exc]
Cardiomyopathy (primary) (secondary) NOS

I43 **Cardiomyopathy in diseases classified elsewhere** [CC] [HCC] [RxHCC] [CC/MCC Exc]
Code first underlying disease, such as:
amyloidosis (E85.-)
glycogen storage disease (E74.0)
gout (M10.0-)
thyrotoxicosis (E05.0-E05.9-)
[EXCLUDES1] *cardiomyopathy (in):*
coxsackie (virus) (B33.24)
diphtheria (A36.81)
sarcoidosis (D86.85)
tuberculosis (A18.84)

[4th] **I44** Atrioventricular **and left bundle-branch block**

I44.0 **Atrioventricular block,** first degree

I44.1 **Atrioventricular block,** second degree
Atrioventricular block, type I and II
Möbitz block block, type I and II
Second degree block, type I and II
Wenckebach's block

I44.2 **Atrioventricular block,** complete [CC] [HCC] [CC/MCC Exc]
Complete heart block NOS
Third degree block

[5th] **I44.3** Other and unspecified **atrioventricular block**
Atrioventricular block NOS

I44.30 **Unspecified atrioventricular block**

I44.39 **Other atrioventricular block**

I44.4 Left anterior **fascicular block** [?]

I44.5 Left posterior **fascicular block** [?]

[5th] **I44.6** Other and unspecified **fascicular block**

I44.60 **Unspecified fascicular block** [?]
Left bundle-branch hemiblock NOS

I44.69 **Other fascicular block** [?]

I44.7 **Left bundle-branch block, unspecified** [?]

[4th] **I45** **Other conduction disorders**

I45.0 Right **fascicular block** [?]

[5th] **I45.1** **Other and unspecified** right bundle-branch block

I45.10 **Unspecified right bundle-branch block** [?]
Right bundle-branch block NOS

I45.19 **Other right bundle-branch block** [?]

I45.2 Bifascicular **block** [CC] [CC/MCC Exc]

I45.3 Trifascicular **block** [CC] [CC/MCC Exc]

I45.4 Nonspecific intraventricular **block**
Bundle-branch block NOS

I45.5 **Other specified heart block**
Sinoatrial block
Sinoauricular block
[EXCLUDES1] *heart block NOS (I45.9)*

I45.6 **Pre-excitation syndrome**
Accelerated atrioventricular conduction
Accessory atrioventricular conduction
Anomalous atrioventricular excitation
Lown-Ganong-Levine syndrome
Pre-excitation atrioventricular conduction
Wolff-Parkinson-White syndrome

[5th] **I45.8** **Other specified conduction disorders**

I45.81 **Long QT syndrome**

I45.89 **Other specified conduction disorders** [CC] [CC/MCC Exc]
Atrioventricular [AV] dissociation
Interference dissociation
Isorhythmic dissociation
Nonparoxysmal AV nodal tachycardia

I45.9 **Conduction disorder, unspecified**
Heart block NOS
Stokes-Adams syndrome

[4th] **I46** **Cardiac arrest**
[EXCLUDES1] *cardiogenic shock (R57.0)*

I46.2 **Cardiac arrest due to underlying cardiac condition** [HCC] [MCC] [CC/MCC Exc]
Code first underlying cardiac condition

I46.8 **Cardiac arrest due to other underlying condition** [HCC] [MCC] [CC/MCC Exc]
Code first underlying condition

I46.9 **Cardiac arrest, cause unspecified** [HCC] [MCC] [CC/MCC Exc]

[4th] **I47** **Paroxysmal** tachycardia
Code first tachycardia complicating:
abortion or ectopic or molar pregnancy (O00-O07, O08.8)
obstetric surgery and procedures (O75.4)
[EXCLUDES1] *tachycardia NOS (R00.0)*
sinoauricular tachycardia NOS (R00.0)
sinus [sinusal] tachycardia NOS (R00.0)

I47.0 **Re-entry ventricular arrhythmia** [CC] [HCC] [CC/MCC Exc]

I47.1 Supraventricular **tachycardia** [CC] [HCC] [RxHCC] [CC/MCC Exc]
Atrial (paroxysmal) tachycardia
Atrioventricular [AV] (paroxysmal) tachycardia
Atrioventricular re-entrant (nodal) tachycardia [AVNRT] [AVRT]
Junctional (paroxysmal) tachycardia
Nodal (paroxysmal) tachycardia

I47.2 Ventricular **tachycardia** [CC] [HCC] [CC/MCC Exc]
AHA: Q3 2013

I47.9 **Paroxysmal tachycardia, unspecified** [HCC] [RxHCC]
Bouveret (-Hoffman) syndrome

[PDx] Unacceptable principal diagnosis symbol per Medicare code edits [POA] Code exempt from diagnosis present on admission requirement
[?] Questionable admission [CC] Complication or comorbidity [CC/MCC Exc] CC/MCC exclusion [MCC] Major complication or comorbidity
[PDx CC] Principal diagnosis as its own CC [PDx MCC] Principal diagnosis as its own MCC [HCC] HCC diagnosis code [RxHCC] RxHCC diagnosis code
MACRA code [Z] Z code as first-listed diagnosis

[4th] **I48 Atrial fibrillation and flutter**

I48.0 **Paroxysmal atrial fibrillation** [HCC] [RxHCC]

I48.1 **Persistent atrial fibrillation** [CC] [HCC] [RxHCC] [CC/MCC Exc]

I48.2 **Chronic atrial fibrillation** [HCC] [RxHCC]
AHA: Q4 2013
Permanent atrial fibrillation

I48.3 **Typical atrial flutter** [CC] [HCC] [RxHCC] [CC/MCC Exc]
Type I atrial flutter

I48.4 **Atypical atrial flutter** [CC] [HCC] [RxHCC] [CC/MCC Exc]
Type II atrial flutter

[5th] **I48.9 Unspecified atrial fibrillation and atrial flutter**

I48.91 **Unspecified atrial fibrillation** [HCC] [RxHCC]

I48.92 **Unspecified atrial flutter** [CC] [HCC] [RxHCC] [CC/MCC Exc]

[4th] **I49 Other cardiac arrhythmias**
Code first cardiac arrhythmia complicating:
abortion or ectopic or molar pregnancy (O00-O07, O08.8)
obstetric surgery and procedures (O75.4)

[EXCLUDES1] *neonatal dysrhythmia (P29.1-)*
sinoatrial bradycardia (R00.1)
sinus bradycardia (R00.1)
vagal bradycardia (R00.1)

[EXCLUDES2] *bradycardia NOS (R00.1)*

[5th] **I49.0 Ventricular fibrillation and flutter**

I49.01 **Ventricular fibrillation** [HCC] [MCC] [CC/MCC Exc]

I49.02 **Ventricular flutter** [HCC] [MCC] [CC/MCC Exc]

I49.1 **Atrial premature depolarization**
Atrial premature beats

I49.2 **Junctional premature depolarization** [CC] [HCC] [RxHCC] [CC/MCC Exc]

I49.3 **Ventricular premature depolarization**

[5th] **I49.4 Other and unspecified premature depolarization**

I49.40 **Unspecified premature depolarization**
Premature beats NOS

I49.49 **Other premature depolarization**
Ectopic beats
Extrasystoles
Extrasystolic arrhythmias
Premature contractions

I49.5 **Sick sinus syndrome** [HCC]
Tachycardia-bradycardia syndrome

I49.8 **Other specified cardiac arrhythmias**
Brugada syndrome
Coronary sinus rhythm disorder
Ectopic rhythm disorder
Nodal rhythm disorder

I49.9 **Cardiac arrhythmia, unspecified**
Arrhythmia (cardiac) NOS

[4th] **I50 Heart failure**
Code first heart failure complicating abortion or ectopic or molar pregnancy (O00-O07, O08.8)
heart failure due to hypertension (I11.0)
heart failure due to hypertension with chronic kidney disease (I13.-)
heart failure following surgery (I97.13-)
obstetric surgery and procedures (O75.4)
rheumatic heart failure (I09.81)

[EXCLUDES1] *neonatal cardiac failure (P29.0)*

[EXCLUDES2] *cardiac arrest (I46.-)*

▲ I50.1 **Left ventricular failure, ▶unspecified◀** [CC] [HCC] [RxHCC] [CC/MCC Exc]
Cardiac asthma
Edema of lung with heart disease NOS
Edema of lung with heart failure
Left heart failure
Pulmonary edema with heart disease NOS
Pulmonary edema with heart failure

[EXCLUDES1] *edema of lung without heart disease or heart failure (J81.-)*
pulmonary edema without heart disease or failure (J81.-)

[5th] **I50.2 Systolic (congestive) heart failure**
Heart failure with reduced ejection fraction [HFrEF]
Systolic left ventricular heart failure
Code also end stage heart failure, if applicable (I50.84)

[EXCLUDES1] *combined systolic (congestive) and diastolic (congestive) heart failure (I50.4-)*

I50.20 **Unspecified systolic (congestive) heart failure** [CC] [HCC] [RxHCC] [CC/MCC Exc]

I50.21 **Acute systolic (congestive) heart failure** [HCC] [MCC] [RxHCC] [CC/MCC Exc]

I50.22 **Chronic systolic (congestive) heart failure** [CC] [HCC] [RxHCC] [CC/MCC Exc]

I50.23 **Acute on chronic systolic (congestive) heart failure** [HCC] [MCC] [RxHCC] [CC/MCC Exc]

[5th] **I50.3 Diastolic (congestive) heart failure**
Diastolic left ventricular heart failure
Heart failure with normal ejection fraction
Heart failure with preserved ejection fraction [HFpEF]
Code also end stage heart failure, if applicable (I50.84)

[EXCLUDES1] *combined systolic (congestive) and diastolic (congestive) heart failure (I50.4-)*

I50.30 **Unspecified diastolic (congestive) heart failure** [CC] [HCC] [RxHCC] [CC/MCC Exc]

I50.31 **Acute diastolic (congestive) heart failure** [HCC] [MCC] [RxHCC] [CC/MCC Exc]
AHA: Q1 2017

I50.32 **Chronic diastolic (congestive) heart failure** [CC] [HCC] [RxHCC] [CC/MCC Exc]

I50.33 **Acute on chronic diastolic (congestive) heart failure** [HCC] [MCC] [RxHCC] [CC/MCC Exc]

[5th] **I50.4 Combined systolic (congestive) and diastolic (congestive) heart failure**
Combined systolic and diastolic left ventricular heart failure
Heart failure with reduced ejection fraction and diastolic dysfunction
Code also end stage heart failure, if applicable (I50.84)

I50.40 **Unspecified combined systolic (congestive) and diastolic (congestive) heart failure** [CC] [HCC] [RxHCC] [CC/MCC Exc]

I50.41 **Acute combined systolic (congestive) and diastolic (congestive) heart failure** [HCC] [MCC] [RxHCC] [CC/MCC Exc]

I50.42 **Chronic combined systolic (congestive) and diastolic (congestive) heart failure** [CC] [HCC] [RxHCC] [CC/MCC Exc]

I50.43 **Acute on chronic combined systolic (congestive) and diastolic (congestive) heart failure** [HCC] [MCC] [RxHCC] [CC/MCC Exc]

● [5th] **I50.8 Other heart failure**

● [6th] **I50.81 Right heart failure**
Right ventricular failure

● I50.810 **Right heart failure, unspecified**
Right heart failure without mention of left heart failure
Right ventricular failure NOS

● I50.811 **Acute right heart failure**
Acute isolated right heart failure
Acute (isolated) right ventricular failure

● I50.812 **Chronic right heart failure**
Chronic isolated right heart failure
Chronic (isolated) right ventricular failure

● I50.813 **Acute on chronic right heart failure**
Acute on chronic isolated right heart failure
Acute on chronic (isolated) right ventricular failure
Acute decompensation of chronic (isolated) right ventricular failure
Acute exacerbation of chronic (isolated) right ventricular failure

● I50.814 **Right heart failure due to left heart failure**
Right ventricular failure secondary to left ventricular failure
Code also the type of left ventricular failure, if known (I50.2-I50.43)

[EXCLUDES1] *Right heart failure with but not due to left heart failure (I50.82)*

● I50.82 **Biventricular heart failure**
Code also the type of left ventricular failure as systolic, diastolic, or combined, if known (I50.2-I50.43)

Unspecified Code | Other Specified Code | Manifestation Code | [N] Newborn | [P] Pediatric | [M] Maternity | [A] Adult | ♂ Male | ♀ Female
● New Code | ▲ Revised Code Title | ▶◀ Revised Text | [NOTES] | [INCLUDES] | [EXCLUDES1] Not coded here | [EXCLUDES2] Not included here
[4th] 4th character required | [5th] 5th character required | [6th] 6th character required | [7th] 7th character required
[x] Extension 'X' Alert | [HAC] Hospital-acquired condition (HAC) alert | AHA AHA Coding Clinic©

When symbols appear on a code that requires a 7th character extension, refer to Appendix B to identify applicable 7th character codes.

- **I50.83** High **output heart failure**
- **I50.84** End stage **heart failure**
  Stage D heart failure
  Code also the type of heart failure as systolic, diastolic, or combined, if known (I50.2-I50.43)
- **I50.89** Other **heart failure**

I50.9 **Heart failure, unspecified** 〔HCC〕〔RxHCC〕
  AHA: Q1 2017
  Cardiac, heart or myocardial failure NOS
  Congestive heart disease
  Congestive heart failure NOS
  EXCLUDES2 fluid overload (E87.70)

I51 **Complications and ill-defined descriptions of heart disease**
  EXCLUDES1 any condition in I51.4-I51.9 due to hypertension (I11.-)
    any condition in I51.4-I51.9 due to hypertension and chronic kidney disease (I13.-)
    heart disease specified as rheumatic (I00-I09)

I51.0 **Cardiac septal defect, acquired** 〔A〕〔CC〕〔CC/MCC Exc〕
  Acquired septal atrial defect (old)
  Acquired septal auricular defect (old)
  Acquired septal ventricular defect (old)
  EXCLUDES1 cardiac septal defect as current complication following acute myocardial infarction (I23.1, I23.2)

I51.1 **Rupture of chordae tendineae, not elsewhere classified** 〔HCC〕〔MCC〕〔RxHCC〕〔CC/MCC Exc〕
  EXCLUDES1 rupture of chordae tendineae as current complication following acute myocardial infarction (I23.4)

I51.2 **Rupture of papillary muscle, not elsewhere classified** 〔HCC〕〔MCC〕〔RxHCC〕〔CC/MCC Exc〕
  EXCLUDES1 rupture of papillary muscle as current complication following acute myocardial infarction (I23.5)

I51.3 **Intracardiac thrombosis, not elsewhere classified**
  AHA: Q1 2013
  Apical thrombosis (old)
  Atrial thrombosis (old)
  Auricular thrombosis (old)
  Mural thrombosis (old)
  Ventricular thrombosis (old)
  EXCLUDES1 intracardiac thrombosis as current complication following acute myocardial infarction (I23.6)

I51.4 **Myocarditis, unspecified** 〔HCC〕〔RxHCC〕
  AHA: Q4 2016
  Chronic (interstitial) myocarditis
  Myocardial fibrosis
  Myocarditis NOS
  EXCLUDES1 acute or subacute myocarditis (I40.-)

I51.5 **Myocardial degeneration** 〔HCC〕〔RxHCC〕
  AHA: Q4 2016
  Fatty degeneration of heart or myocardium
  Myocardial disease
  Senile degeneration of heart or myocardium

I51.7 **Cardiomegaly**
  AHA: Q4 2016
  Cardiac dilatation
  Cardiac hypertrophy
  Ventricular dilatation

I51.8 **Other ill-defined heart diseases**
  I51.81 **Takotsubo syndrome** 〔CC〕〔CC/MCC Exc〕
    AHA: Q4 2016
    Reversible left ventricular dysfunction following sudden emotional stress
    Stress induced cardiomyopathy
    Takotsubo cardiomyopathy
    Transient left ventricular apical ballooning syndrome
  I51.89 **Other ill-defined heart diseases**
    AHA: Q4 2016
    Carditis (acute)(chronic)
    Pancarditis (acute)(chronic)

I51.9 **Heart disease, unspecified**
  AHA: Q4 2016

I52 **Other heart disorders in diseases classified elsewhere**
  Code first underlying disease, such as:

congenital syphilis (A50.5)
mucopolysaccharidosis (E76.3)
schistosomiasis (B65.0-B65.9)
EXCLUDES1 heart disease (in):
  gonococcal infection (A54.83)
  meningococcal infection (A39.50)
  rheumatoid arthritis (M05.31)
  syphilis (A52.06)

Cerebrovascular diseases (I60-I69)

Use additional code to identify presence of:
alcohol abuse and dependence (F10.-)
exposure to environmental tobacco smoke (Z77.22)
history of tobacco dependence (Z87.891)
hypertension (I10-I15)
occupational exposure to environmental tobacco smoke (Z57.31)
tobacco dependence (F17.-)
tobacco use (Z72.0)
EXCLUDES1 traumatic intracranial hemorrhage (S06.-)

I60 **Nontraumatic** subarachnoid **hemorrhage**
  EXCLUDES1 syphilitic ruptured cerebral aneurysm (A52.05)
  EXCLUDES2 sequelae of subarachnoid hemorrhage (I69.0-)

I60.0 **Nontraumatic subarachnoid hemorrhage from** carotid siphon and bifurcation
  I60.00 **Nontraumatic subarachnoid hemorrhage from** unspecified **carotid siphon and bifurcation** 〔HCC〕〔MCC〕〔CC/MCC Exc〕
  I60.01 **Nontraumatic subarachnoid hemorrhage from** right **carotid siphon and bifurcation** 〔HCC〕〔MCC〕〔CC/MCC Exc〕
  I60.02 **Nontraumatic subarachnoid hemorrhage from** left **carotid siphon and bifurcation** 〔HCC〕〔MCC〕〔CC/MCC Exc〕

I60.1 **Nontraumatic subarachnoid hemorrhage from** middle cerebral artery
  I60.10 **Nontraumatic subarachnoid hemorrhage from** unspecified **middle cerebral artery** 〔HCC〕〔MCC〕〔CC/MCC Exc〕
  I60.11 **Nontraumatic subarachnoid hemorrhage from** right **middle cerebral artery** 〔HCC〕〔MCC〕〔CC/MCC Exc〕
  I60.12 **Nontraumatic subarachnoid hemorrhage from** left **middle cerebral artery** 〔HCC〕〔MCC〕〔CC/MCC Exc〕

I60.2 **Nontraumatic subarachnoid hemorrhage** from anterior communicating artery

I60.3 **Nontraumatic subarachnoid hemorrhage from** posterior communicating artery
  I60.30 **Nontraumatic subarachnoid hemorrhage from** unspecified **posterior communicating artery** 〔HCC〕〔MCC〕〔CC/MCC Exc〕
  I60.31 **Nontraumatic subarachnoid hemorrhage from** right **posterior communicating artery** 〔HCC〕〔MCC〕〔CC/MCC Exc〕
  I60.32 **Nontraumatic subarachnoid hemorrhage from** left **posterior communicating artery** 〔HCC〕〔MCC〕〔CC/MCC Exc〕

I60.4 **Nontraumatic subarachnoid hemorrhage from basilar artery** 〔HCC〕〔MCC〕〔CC/MCC Exc〕

I60.5 **Nontraumatic subarachnoid hemorrhage from** vertebral artery
  I60.50 **Nontraumatic subarachnoid hemorrhage from** unspecified **vertebral artery** 〔HCC〕〔MCC〕〔CC/MCC Exc〕
  I60.51 **Nontraumatic subarachnoid hemorrhage from** right **vertebral artery** 〔HCC〕〔MCC〕〔CC/MCC Exc〕
  I60.52 **Nontraumatic subarachnoid hemorrhage from** left **vertebral artery** 〔HCC〕〔MCC〕〔CC/MCC Exc〕

I60.6 **Nontraumatic subarachnoid hemorrhage from** other intracranial arteries 〔HCC〕〔MCC〕〔CC/MCC Exc〕

I60.7 **Nontraumatic subarachnoid hemorrhage from** unspecified intracranial artery 〔HCC〕〔MCC〕〔CC/MCC Exc〕
  Ruptured (congenital) berry aneurysm
  Ruptured (congenital) cerebral aneurysm
  Subarachnoid hemorrhage (nontraumatic) from cerebral artery NOS
  Subarachnoid hemorrhage (nontraumatic) from communicating artery NOS
  EXCLUDES1 berry aneurysm, nonruptured (I67.1)

〔PDx〕 Unacceptable principal diagnosis symbol per Medicare code edits 〔 〕 Code exempt from diagnosis present on admission requirement
〔?〕 Questionable admission 〔CC〕 Complication or comorbidity 〔CC/MCC Exc〕 CC/MCC exclusion 〔MCC〕 Major complication or comorbidity
〔 〕 Principal diagnosis as its own CC 〔 〕 Principal diagnosis as its own MCC 〔HCC〕 HCC diagnosis code 〔RxHCC〕 RxHCC diagnosis code
MACRA code 〔Z1〕 Z code as first-listed diagnosis

666

When symbols appear on a code that requires a 7th character extension, refer to Appendix B to identify applicable 7th character codes.

2018 ICD-10-CM

I60.8 Other nontraumatic subarachnoid hemorrhage `HCC` `MCC` `CC/MCC Exc`
Meningeal hemorrhage
Rupture of cerebral arteriovenous malformation

I60.9 **Nontraumatic subarachnoid hemorrhage, unspecified** `HCC` `MCC` `CC/MCC Exc`

4ᵗʰ **I61** Nontraumatic intracerebral hemorrhage
EXCLUDES2 sequelae of intracerebral hemorrhage (I69.1-)

I61.0 **Nontraumatic intracerebral hemorrhage** in hemisphere, subcortical `HCC` `MCC` `CC/MCC Exc`
AHA: Q4 2016
Deep intracerebral hemorrhage (nontraumatic)

I61.1 **Nontraumatic intracerebral hemorrhage** in hemisphere, cortical `HCC` `MCC` `CC/MCC Exc`
Cerebral lobe hemorrhage (nontraumatic)
Superficial intracerebral hemorrhage (nontraumatic)

I61.2 **Nontraumatic intracerebral hemorrhage** in hemisphere, unspecified `HCC` `MCC` `CC/MCC Exc`

I61.3 **Nontraumatic intracerebral hemorrhage** in brain stem `HCC` `MCC` `CC/MCC Exc`

I61.4 **Nontraumatic intracerebral hemorrhage** in cerebellum `HCC` `MCC` `CC/MCC Exc`

I61.5 **Nontraumatic intracerebral hemorrhage, intraventricular** `HCC` `MCC` `CC/MCC Exc`

I61.6 **Nontraumatic intracerebral hemorrhage, multiple localized** `HCC` `MCC` `CC/MCC Exc`

I61.8 Other nontraumatic intracerebral hemorrhage `HCC` `MCC` `CC/MCC Exc`

I61.9 **Nontraumatic intracerebral hemorrhage, unspecified** `HCC` `MCC` `CC/MCC Exc`

4ᵗʰ **I62** Other and unspecified nontraumatic intracranial hemorrhage
EXCLUDES2 sequelae of intracranial hemorrhage (I69.2)

5ᵗʰ I62.0 Nontraumatic subdural hemorrhage

I62.00 **Nontraumatic subdural hemorrhage, unspecified** `HCC` `MCC` `CC/MCC Exc`

I62.01 **Nontraumatic acute subdural hemorrhage** `HCC` `MCC` `CC/MCC Exc`

I62.02 **Nontraumatic subacute subdural hemorrhage** `HCC` `MCC` `CC/MCC Exc`

I62.03 **Nontraumatic chronic subdural hemorrhage** `HCC` `MCC` `CC/MCC Exc`

I62.1 **Nontraumatic extradural hemorrhage** `HCC` `MCC` `CC/MCC Exc`
Nontraumatic epidural hemorrhage

I62.9 **Nontraumatic intracranial hemorrhage, unspecified** `CC` `HCC` `CC/MCC Exc`

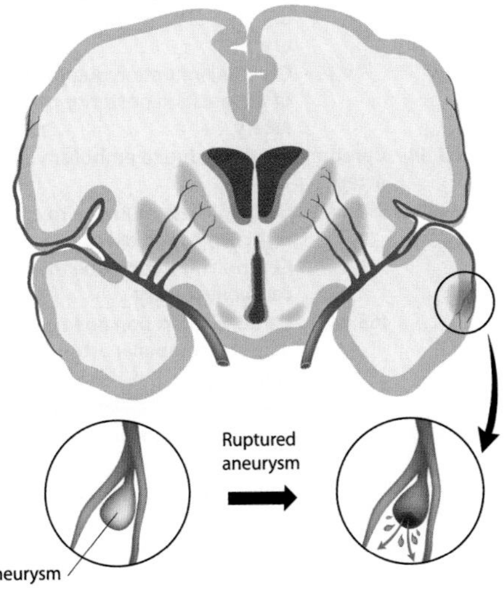

Figure 9.3 Hemorrhagic stroke

4ᵗʰ **I63** Cerebral infarction
INCLUDES occlusion and stenosis of cerebral and precerebral arteries, resulting in cerebral infarction

Use additional code, if applicable, to identify status post administration of tPA (rtPA) in a different facility within the last 24 hours prior to admission to current facility (Z92.82)
Use additional code, if known, to indicate National Institutes of Health Stroke Scale (NIHSS) score (R29.7-)
EXCLUDES2 sequelae of cerebral infarction (I69.3-)

5ᵗʰ I63.0 Cerebral infarction due to thrombosis of precerebral arteries

I63.00 **Cerebral infarction due to thrombosis of unspecified precerebral artery** `HCC` `MCC` `RxHCC` `CC/MCC Exc`

6ᵗʰ I63.01 Cerebral infarction due to thrombosis of vertebral artery

I63.011 Cerebral infarction due to thrombosis of right vertebral artery `HCC` `MCC` `RxHCC` `CC/MCC Exc`

I63.012 Cerebral infarction due to thrombosis of left vertebral artery `HCC` `MCC` `RxHCC` `CC/MCC Exc`

I63.013 Cerebral infarction due to thrombosis of bilateral vertebral arteries `HCC` `MCC` `RxHCC` `CC/MCC Exc`

I63.019 **Cerebral infarction due to thrombosis of unspecified vertebral artery** `HCC` `MCC` `RxHCC` `CC/MCC Exc`

I63.02 Cerebral infarction due to thrombosis of basilar artery `HCC` `MCC` `RxHCC` `CC/MCC Exc`

6ᵗʰ I63.03 Cerebral infarction due to thrombosis of carotid artery

I63.031 Cerebral infarction due to thrombosis of right carotid artery

I63.032 Cerebral infarction due to thrombosis of left carotid artery

I63.033 Cerebral infarction due to thrombosis of bilateral carotid arteries

I63.039 **Cerebral infarction due to thrombosis of unspecified carotid artery** `HCC` `MCC` `RxHCC` `CC/MCC Exc`

I63.09 Cerebral infarction due to thrombosis of other precerebral artery `HCC` `MCC` `RxHCC` `CC/MCC Exc`

5ᵗʰ I63.1 Cerebral infarction due to embolism of precerebral arteries

I63.10 **Cerebral infarction due to embolism of unspecified precerebral artery** `HCC` `MCC` `RxHCC` `CC/MCC Exc`

6ᵗʰ I63.11 Cerebral infarction due to embolism of vertebral artery

I63.111 Cerebral infarction due to embolism of right vertebral artery `HCC` `MCC` `RxHCC` `CC/MCC Exc`

I63.112 Cerebral infarction due to embolism of left vertebral artery `HCC` `MCC` `RxHCC` `CC/MCC Exc`

I63.113 Cerebral infarction due to embolism of bilateral vertebral arteries `HCC` `MCC` `RxHCC` `CC/MCC Exc`

I63.119 **Cerebral infarction due to embolism of unspecified vertebral artery** `HCC` `MCC` `RxHCC` `CC/MCC Exc`

I63.12 Cerebral infarction due to embolism of basilar artery `HCC` `MCC` `RxHCC` `CC/MCC Exc`

6ᵗʰ I63.13 Cerebral infarction due to embolism of carotid artery

I63.131 Cerebral infarction due to embolism of right carotid artery `HCC` `MCC` `RxHCC` `CC/MCC Exc`

I63.132 Cerebral infarction due to embolism of left carotid artery `HCC` `MCC` `RxHCC` `CC/MCC Exc`

I63.133 Cerebral infarction due to embolism of bilateral carotid arteries `HCC` `MCC` `RxHCC` `CC/MCC Exc`

I63.139 **Cerebral infarction due to embolism of unspecified carotid artery** `HCC` `MCC` `RxHCC` `CC/MCC Exc`

I63.19 Cerebral infarction due to embolism of other precerebral artery `HCC` `MCC` `RxHCC` `CC/MCC Exc`

5ᵗʰ I63.2 Cerebral infarction due to unspecified occlusion or stenosis of precerebral arteries

I63.20 **Cerebral infarction due to unspecified occlusion or stenosis of unspecified precerebral arteries** `HCC` `MCC` `RxHCC` `CC/MCC Exc`

6ᵗʰ I63.21 Cerebral infarction due to unspecified occlusion or stenosis of vertebral arteries

▲ I63.211 **Cerebral infarction due to unspecified occlusion or stenosis of right vertebral ►artery◄** `HCC` `MCC` `RxHCC` `CC/MCC Exc`

| Unspecified Code | Other Specified Code | Manifestation Code | Ⓝ Newborn | Ⓟ Pediatric | Ⓜ Maternity | Ⓐ Adult | ♂ Male | ♀ Female |

● New Code ▲ Revised Code Title ►◄ Revised Text **NOTES** INCLUDES EXCLUDES1 Not coded here EXCLUDES2 Not included here
4ᵗʰ 4ᵗʰ character required 5ᵗʰ 5ᵗʰ character required 6ᵗʰ 6ᵗʰ character required 7ᵗʰ 7ᵗʰ character required
7ᵗʰ Extension 'X' Alert `HAC` Hospital-acquired condition (HAC) alert **AHA** AHA Coding Clinic©

▲   I63.212   Cerebral infarction due to unspecified occlusion or stenosis of left vertebral ►artery◄   HCC MCC RxHCC CC/MCC Exc

I63.213   Cerebral infarctiondue to unspecified occlusion or stenosis of bilateral vertebral arteries   HCC MCC RxHCC CC/MCC Exc

I63.219   Cerebral infarction due to unspecified occlusion or stenosis of unspecified vertebral arteries   HCC MCC RxHCC CC/MCC Exc

▲   I63.22   Cerebral infarction due to unspecified occlusion or stenosis of basilar ►artery◄   HCC MCC RxHCC CC/MCC Exc

6ᵗʰ   I63.23   Cerebral infarction due to unspecified occlusion or stenosis of carotid arteries

I63.231   Cerebral infarction due to unspecified occlusion or stenosis of right carotid arteries   HCC MCC RxHCC CC/MCC Exc

I63.232   Cerebral infarction due to unspecified occlusion or stenosis of left carotid arteries   HCC MCC RxHCC CC/MCC Exc

I63.233   Cerebral infarction due to unspecified occlusion or stenosis of bilateral carotid arteries   HCC MCC RxHCC CC/MCC Exc

I63.239   Cerebral infarction due to unspecified occlusion or stenosis of unspecified carotid arteries   HCC MCC RxHCC CC/MCC Exc

I63.29   Cerebral infarction due to unspecified occlusion or stenosis of other precerebral arteries   HCC MCC RxHCC CC/MCC Exc

5ᵗʰ   I63.3   Cerebral infarction due to thrombosis of cerebral arteries

I63.30   Cerebral infarction due to thrombosis of unspecified cerebral artery   HCC MCC RxHCC CC/MCC Exc

6ᵗʰ   I63.31   Cerebral infarction due to thrombosis of middle cerebral artery

I63.311   Cerebral infarction due to thrombosis of right middle cerebral artery   HCC MCC RxHCC CC/MCC Exc

I63.312   Cerebral infarction due to thrombosis of left middle cerebral artery   HCC MCC RxHCC CC/MCC Exc

I63.313   Cerebral infarction due to thrombosis of bilateral middle cerebral arteries   HCC MCC RxHCC CC/MCC Exc

I63.319   Cerebral infarction due to thrombosis of unspecified middle cerebral artery   HCC MCC RxHCC CC/MCC Exc

6ᵗʰ   I63.32   Cerebral infarction due to thrombosis of anterior cerebral artery

I63.321   Cerebral infarction due to thrombosis of right anterior cerebral artery   HCC MCC RxHCC CC/MCC Exc

I63.322   Cerebral infarction due to thrombosis of left anterior cerebral artery   HCC MCC RxHCC CC/MCC Exc

▲   I63.323   Cerebral infarction due to thrombosis of bilateral anterior ►cerebral◄ arteries   HCC MCC RxHCC CC/MCC Exc

I63.329   Cerebral infarction due to thrombosis of unspecified anterior cerebral artery   HCC MCC RxHCC CC/MCC Exc

6ᵗʰ   I63.33   Cerebral infarction due to thrombosis of posterior cerebral artery

I63.331   Cerebral infarction due to thrombosis of right posterior cerebral artery   HCC MCC RxHCC CC/MCC Exc

I63.332   Cerebral infarction due to thrombosis of left posterior cerebral artery   HCC MCC RxHCC CC/MCC Exc

▲   I63.333   Cerebral infarction to thrombosis of bilateral posterior ►cerebral◄ arteries   HCC MCC RxHCC CC/MCC Exc

I63.339   Cerebral infarction due to thrombosis of unspecified posterior cerebral artery   HCC MCC RxHCC CC/MCC Exc

6ᵗʰ   I63.34   Cerebral infarction due to thrombosis of cerebellar artery

I63.341   Cerebral infarction due to thrombosis of right cerebellar artery   HCC MCC RxHCC CC/MCC Exc

I63.342   Cerebral infarction due to thrombosis of left cerebellar artery   HCC MCC RxHCC CC/MCC Exc

I63.343   Cerebral infarction to thrombosis of bilateral cerebellar arteries   HCC MCC RxHCC CC/MCC Exc

I63.349   Cerebral infarction due to thrombosis of unspecified cerebellar artery   HCC MCC RxHCC CC/MCC Exc

I63.39   Cerebral infarction due to thrombosis of other cerebral artery

5ᵗʰ   I63.4   Cerebral infarction due to embolism of cerebral arteries

I63.40   Cerebral infarction due to embolism of unspecified cerebral artery   HCC MCC RxHCC CC/MCC Exc

6ᵗʰ   I63.41   Cerebral infarction due to embolism of middle cerebral artery

I63.411   Cerebral infarction due to embolism of right middle cerebral artery   HCC MCC RxHCC CC/MCC Exc

I63.412   Cerebral infarction due to embolism of left middle cerebral artery   HCC MCC RxHCC CC/MCC Exc

I63.413   Cerebral infarction due to embolism of bilateral middle cerebral arteries   HCC MCC RxHCC CC/MCC Exc

I63.419   Cerebral infarction due to embolism of unspecified middle cerebral artery   HCC MCC RxHCC CC/MCC Exc

6ᵗʰ   I63.42   Cerebral infarction due to embolism of anterior cerebral artery

I63.421   Cerebral infarction due to embolism of right anterior cerebral artery   HCC MCC RxHCC CC/MCC Exc

I63.422   Cerebral infarction due to embolism of left anterior cerebral artery   HCC MCC RxHCC CC/MCC Exc

I63.423   Cerebral infarction due to embolism of bilateral anterior cerebral arteries   HCC MCC RxHCC CC/MCC Exc

I63.429   Cerebral infarction due to embolism of unspecified anterior cerebral artery   HCC MCC RxHCC CC/MCC Exc

6ᵗʰ   I63.43   Cerebral infarction due to embolism of posterior cerebral artery

I63.431   Cerebral infarction due to embolism of right posterior cerebral artery   HCC MCC RxHCC CC/MCC Exc

I63.432   Cerebral infarction due to embolism of left posterior cerebral artery   HCC MCC RxHCC CC/MCC Exc

I63.433   Cerebral infarction due to embolism of bilateral posterior cerebral arteries   HCC MCC RxHCC CC/MCC Exc

I63.439   Cerebral infarction due to embolism of unspecified posterior cerebral artery   HCC MCC RxHCC CC/MCC Exc

6ᵗʰ   I63.44   Cerebral infarction due to embolism of cerebellar artery

I63.441   Cerebral infarction due to embolism of right cerebellar artery   HCC MCC RxHCC CC/MCC Exc

I63.442   Cerebral infarction due to embolism of left cerebellar artery   HCC MCC RxHCC CC/MCC Exc

I63.443   Cerebral infarction due to embolism of bilateral cerebellar arteries   HCC MCC RxHCC CC/MCC Exc

I63.449   Cerebral infarction due to embolism of unspecified cerebellar artery   HCC MCC RxHCC CC/MCC Exc

I63.49   Cerebral infarction due to embolism of other cerebral artery   HCC MCC RxHCC CC/MCC Exc

5ᵗʰ   I63.5   Cerebral infarction due to unspecified occlusion or stenosis of cerebral arteries

I63.50   Cerebral infarction due to unspecified occlusion or stenosis of unspecified cerebral artery   HCC MCC RxHCC CC/MCC Exc

6ᵗʰ   I63.51   Cerebral infarction due to unspecified occlusion or stenosis of middle cerebral artery

I63.511   Cerebral infarction due to unspecified occlusion or stenosis of right middle cerebral artery   HCC MCC RxHCC CC/MCC Exc

---

PDᴅx Unacceptable principal diagnosis symbol per Medicare code edits   POA Code exempt from diagnosis present on admission requirement   ❓ Questionable admission   ᶜ Complication or comorbidity   CC/MCC Exc CC/MCC exclusion   MCC Major complication or comorbidity   ᴄᴄ Principal diagnosis as its own CC   ᴍᴄᴄ Principal diagnosis as its own MCC   HCC HCC diagnosis code   RxHCC RxHCC diagnosis code   MACRA code   Z1 Z code as first-listed diagnosis

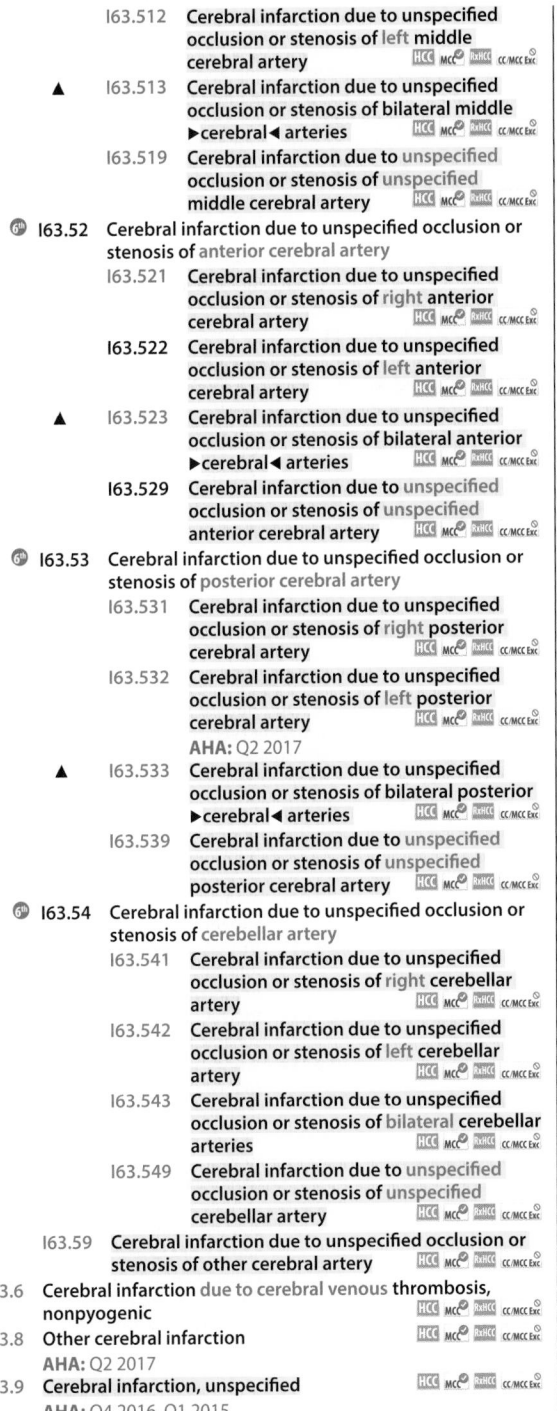

I63.512 **Cerebral infarction due to unspecified occlusion or stenosis of left middle cerebral artery** HCC MCC° RxHCC CC/MCC Exc°

▲ I63.513 **Cerebral infarction due to unspecified occlusion or stenosis of bilateral middle ►cerebral◄ arteries** HCC MCC° RxHCC CC/MCC Exc°

I63.519 **Cerebral infarction due to unspecified occlusion or stenosis of unspecified middle cerebral artery** HCC MCC° RxHCC CC/MCC Exc°

6ᵗʰ I63.52 Cerebral infarction due to unspecified occlusion or stenosis of anterior cerebral artery

I63.521 **Cerebral infarction due to unspecified occlusion or stenosis of right anterior cerebral artery** HCC MCC° RxHCC CC/MCC Exc°

I63.522 **Cerebral infarction due to unspecified occlusion or stenosis of left anterior cerebral artery** HCC MCC° RxHCC CC/MCC Exc°

▲ I63.523 **Cerebral infarction due to unspecified occlusion or stenosis of bilateral anterior ►cerebral◄ arteries** HCC MCC° RxHCC CC/MCC Exc°

I63.529 **Cerebral infarction due to unspecified occlusion or stenosis of unspecified anterior cerebral artery** HCC MCC° RxHCC CC/MCC Exc°

6ᵗʰ I63.53 Cerebral infarction due to unspecified occlusion or stenosis of posterior cerebral artery

I63.531 **Cerebral infarction due to unspecified occlusion or stenosis of right posterior cerebral artery** HCC MCC° RxHCC CC/MCC Exc°

I63.532 **Cerebral infarction due to unspecified occlusion or stenosis of left posterior cerebral artery** HCC MCC° RxHCC CC/MCC Exc°
AHA: Q2 2017

▲ I63.533 **Cerebral infarction due to unspecified occlusion or stenosis of bilateral posterior ►cerebral◄ arteries** HCC MCC° RxHCC CC/MCC Exc°

I63.539 **Cerebral infarction due to unspecified occlusion or stenosis of unspecified posterior cerebral artery** HCC MCC° RxHCC CC/MCC Exc°

6ᵗʰ I63.54 Cerebral infarction due to unspecified occlusion or stenosis of cerebellar artery

I63.541 **Cerebral infarction due to unspecified occlusion or stenosis of right cerebellar artery** HCC MCC° RxHCC CC/MCC Exc°

I63.542 **Cerebral infarction due to unspecified occlusion or stenosis of left cerebellar artery** HCC MCC° RxHCC CC/MCC Exc°

I63.543 **Cerebral infarction due to unspecified occlusion or stenosis of bilateral cerebellar arteries** HCC MCC° RxHCC CC/MCC Exc°

I63.549 **Cerebral infarction due to unspecified occlusion or stenosis of unspecified cerebellar artery** HCC MCC° RxHCC CC/MCC Exc°

I63.59 **Cerebral infarction due to unspecified occlusion or stenosis of other cerebral artery** HCC MCC° RxHCC CC/MCC Exc°

I63.6 **Cerebral infarction due to cerebral venous thrombosis, nonpyogenic** HCC MCC° RxHCC CC/MCC Exc°

I63.8 **Other cerebral infarction** HCC MCC° RxHCC CC/MCC Exc°
AHA: Q2 2017

I63.9 **Cerebral infarction, unspecified** HCC MCC° RxHCC CC/MCC Exc°
AHA: Q4 2016, Q1 2015
Stroke NOS
EXCLUDES2 *transient cerebral ischemic attacks and related syndromes (G45.-)*

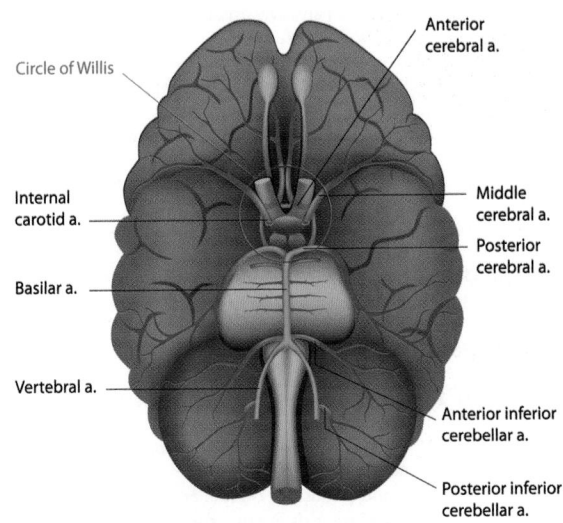

Figure 9.4 Blood supply of the brain

4ᵗʰ **I65 Occlusion and stenosis of precerebral arteries, not resulting in cerebral infarction**
INCLUDES embolism of precerebral artery
narrowing of precerebral artery
obstruction (complete) (partial) of precerebral artery
thrombosis of precerebral artery
EXCLUDES1 insufficiency, NOS, of precerebral artery (G45.-)
insufficiency of precerebral arteries causing cerebral infarction (I63.0-I63.2)

5ᵗʰ **I65.0 Occlusion and stenosis of vertebral artery**
I65.01 **Occlusion and stenosis of right vertebral artery** RxHCC
I65.02 **Occlusion and stenosis of left vertebral artery** RxHCC
I65.03 **Occlusion and stenosis of bilateral vertebral arteries** RxHCC
I65.09 **Occlusion and stenosis of unspecified vertebral artery** RxHCC

I65.1 **Occlusion and stenosis of basilar artery** RxHCC

5ᵗʰ **I65.2 Occlusion and stenosis of carotid artery**
I65.21 **Occlusion and stenosis of right carotid artery** RxHCC
I65.22 **Occlusion and stenosis of left carotid artery** RxHCC
I65.23 **Occlusion and stenosis of bilateral carotid arteries** RxHCC
I65.29 **Occlusion and stenosis of unspecified carotid artery** RxHCC

I65.8 **Occlusion and stenosis of other precerebral arteries** RxHCC
I65.9 **Occlusion and stenosis of unspecified precerebral artery** RxHCC
Occlusion and stenosis of precerebral artery NOS

4ᵗʰ **I66 Occlusion and stenosis of cerebral arteries, not resulting in cerebral infarction**
INCLUDES embolism of cerebral artery
narrowing of cerebral artery
obstruction (complete) (partial) of cerebral artery
thrombosis of cerebral artery
EXCLUDES1 Occlusion and stenosis of cerebral artery causing cerebral infarction (I63.3-I63.5)

5ᵗʰ **I66.0 Occlusion and stenosis of middle cerebral artery**
I66.01 **Occlusion and stenosis of right middle cerebral artery** RxHCC
I66.02 **Occlusion and stenosis of left middle cerebral artery** RxHCC
I66.03 **Occlusion and stenosis of bilateral middle cerebral arteries** RxHCC

Unspecified Code   Other Specified Code   Manifestation Code   Ⓝ Newborn   Ⓟ Pediatric   Ⓜ Maternity   Ⓐ Adult   ♂ Male   ♀ Female
● New Code   ▲ Revised Code Title   ►◄ Revised Text   **NOTES**   *INCLUDES*   *EXCLUDES 1* Not coded here   *EXCLUDES 2* Not included here
4ᵗʰ character required   5ᵗʰ character required   6ᵗʰ character required   7ᵗʰ character required
7ᵗʰ Extension 'X' Alert   HAC Hospital-acquired condition (HAC) alert   **AHA** AHA Coding Clinic©

I66.09   **Occlusion and stenosis of unspecified middle cerebral artery**   RxHCC

5ᵗʰ I66.1   Occlusion and stenosis of anterior cerebral artery

    I66.11   **Occlusion and stenosis of right anterior cerebral artery**   RxHCC

    I66.12   **Occlusion and stenosis of left anterior cerebral artery**   RxHCC

    I66.13   **Occlusion and stenosis of bilateral anterior cerebral arteries**   RxHCC

    I66.19   **Occlusion and stenosis of unspecified anterior cerebral artery**   RxHCC

5ᵗʰ I66.2   Occlusion and stenosis of posterior cerebral artery

    I66.21   **Occlusion and stenosis of right posterior cerebral artery**   RxHCC

    I66.22   **Occlusion and stenosis of left posterior cerebral artery**   RxHCC

    I66.23   **Occlusion and stenosis of bilateral posterior cerebral arteries**   RxHCC

    I66.29   **Occlusion and stenosis of unspecified posterior cerebral artery**   RxHCC

   I66.3   **Occlusion and stenosis of cerebellar arteries**   RxHCC

   I66.8   **Occlusion and stenosis of other cerebral arteries**   RxHCC
     Occlusion and stenosis of perforating arteries

   I66.9   **Occlusion and stenosis of unspecified cerebral artery**   RxHCC

4ᵗʰ I67   **Other cerebrovascular diseases**
    EXCLUDES2 sequelae of the listed conditions (I69.8)

   I67.0   **Dissection of cerebral arteries, nonruptured**   HCC MCC🅐 CC/MCC Exc
     EXCLUDES1 ruptured cerebral arteries (I60.7)

   I67.1   **Cerebral aneurysm, nonruptured**
     Cerebral aneurysm NOS
     Cerebral arteriovenous fistula, acquired
     Internal carotid artery aneurysm, intracranial portion
     Internal carotid artery aneurysm, NOS
     EXCLUDES1 congenital cerebral aneurysm, nonruptured (Q28.-)
        ruptured cerebral aneurysm (I60.7)

   I67.2   **Cerebral atherosclerosis**   A RxHCC
     Atheroma of cerebral and precerebral arteries

   I67.3   **Progressive vascular leukoencephalopathy**   CC🅐 RxHCC CC/MCC Exc
     Binswanger's disease

   I67.4   **Hypertensive encephalopathy**   CC🅐 RxHCC CC/MCC Exc
     EXCLUDES2 insufficiency, NOS, of precerebral arteries (G45.2)

   I67.5   **Moyamoya disease**

   I67.6   **Nonpyogenic thrombosis of intracranial venous system**   CC🅐 RxHCC CC/MCC Exc
     Nonpyogenic thrombosis of cerebral vein
     Nonpyogenic thrombosis of intracranial venous sinus
     EXCLUDES1 nonpyogenic thrombosis of intracranial venous system causing infarction (I63.6)

   I67.7   **Cerebral arteritis, not elsewhere classified**   CC🅐 RxHCC CC/MCC Exc
     Granulomatous angiitis of the nervous system
     EXCLUDES1 allergic granulomatous angiitis (M30.1)

5ᵗʰ I67.8   **Other specified cerebrovascular diseases**

    I67.81   **Acute cerebrovascular insufficiency**   CC🅐 RxHCC CC/MCC Exc
      Acute cerebrovascular insufficiency unspecified as to location or reversibility

    I67.82   **Cerebral ischemia**   CC🅐 RxHCC CC/MCC Exc
      Chronic cerebral ischemia

    I67.83   **Posterior reversible encephalopathy syndrome**   MCC🅐 CC/MCC Exc
      PRES

    6ᵗʰ I67.84   **Cerebral vasospasm and vasoconstriction**

      I67.841   **Reversible cerebrovascular vasoconstriction syndrome**   CC🅐 RxHCC CC/MCC Exc
        Call-Fleming syndrome
        Code first underlying condition, if applicable, such as eclampsia (O15.00-O15.9)

      I67.848   **Other cerebrovascular vasospasm and vasoconstriction**   CC🅐 RxHCC CC/MCC Exc

    I67.89   **Other cerebrovascular disease**   CC🅐 RxHCC CC/MCC Exc

   I67.9   **Cerebrovascular disease, unspecified**   RxHCC

4ᵗʰ I68   Cerebrovascular disorders in diseases classified elsewhere

   I68.0   **Cerebral amyloid angiopathy**   RxHCC
     Code first underlying amyloidosis (E85.-)

   I68.2   **Cerebral arteritis in other diseases classified elsewhere**   CC🅐 RxHCC CC/MCC Exc
     Code first underlying disease
     EXCLUDES1 cerebral arteritis (in):
        listerosis (A32.89)
        systemic lupus erythematosus (M32.19)
        syphilis (A52.04)
        tuberculosis (A18.89)

   I68.8   **Other cerebrovascular disorders in diseases classified elsewhere**   RxHCC
     Code first underlying disease
     EXCLUDES1 syphilitic cerebral aneurysm (A52.05)

4ᵗʰ I69   **Sequelae of cerebrovascular disease**
    NOTES   Category I69 is to be used to indicate conditions in I60-I67 as the cause of sequelae. The 'sequelae' include conditions specified as such or as residuals which may occur at any time after the onset of the causal condition
    EXCLUDES1 personal history of cerebral infarction without residual deficit (Z86.73)
       personal history of prolonged reversible ischemic neurologic deficit (PRIND) (Z86.73)
       personal history of reversible ischemic neurologcial deficit (RIND) (Z86.73)
       sequelae of traumatic intracranial injury (S06.-)

5ᵗʰ I69.0   **Sequelae of nontraumatic subarachnoid hemorrhage**

    I69.00   **Unspecified sequelae of nontraumatic subarachnoid hemorrhage**   POA

    6ᵗʰ I69.01   Cognitive deficits following nontraumatic subarachnoid hemorrhage

      I69.010   Attention and concentration deficit following nontraumatic subarachnoid hemorrhage   POA

      I69.011   Memory deficit following nontraumatic subarachnoid hemorrhage   POA

      I69.012   Visuospatial deficit and spatial neglect following nontraumatic subarachnoid hemorrhage   POA

      I69.013   Psychomotor deficit following nontraumatic subarachnoid hemorrhage   POA

      I69.014   Frontal lobe and executive function deficit following nontraumatic subarachnoid hemorrhage   POA

      I69.015   Cognitive social or emotional deficit following nontraumatic subarachnoid hemorrhage   POA

      I69.018   Other symptoms and signs involving cognitive functions following nontraumatic subarachnoid hemorrhage   POA

      I69.019   Unspecified symptoms and signs involving cognitive functions following nontraumatic subarachnoid hemorrhage   POA

    6ᵗʰ I69.02   Speech and language deficits following nontraumatic subarachnoid hemorrhage

      I69.020   Aphasia following nontraumatic subarachnoid hemorrhage   POA

      I69.021   Dysphasia following nontraumatic subarachnoid hemorrhage   POA

      I69.022   Dysarthria following nontraumatic subarachnoid hemorrhage   POA

      I69.023   Fluency disorder following nontraumatic subarachnoid hemorrhage   POA
        Stuttering following nontraumatic subarachnoid hemorrhage

      I69.028   Other speech and language deficits following nontraumatic subarachnoid hemorrhage   POA

    6ᵗʰ I69.03   Monoplegia of upper limb following nontraumatic subarachnoid hemorrhage

---

POA Unacceptable principal diagnosis symbol per Medicare code edits   POA Code exempt from diagnosis present on admission requirement
  ❓ Questionable admission   CC🅐 Complication or comorbidity   CC/MCC Exc CC/MCC exclusion   MCC🅐 Major complication or comorbidity
  🅒 Principal diagnosis as its own CC   🅜 Principal diagnosis as its own MCC   HCC HCC diagnosis code   RxHCC RxHCC diagnosis code
         MACRA code   Z1 Z code as first-listed diagnosis

When symbols appear on a code that requires a 7th character extension, refer to Appendix B to identify applicable 7th character codes.

I69.031 Monoplegia of upper limb following nontraumatic subarachnoid hemorrhage affecting right dominant side POA HCC

I69.032 Monoplegia of upper limb following nontraumatic subarachnoid hemorrhage affecting left dominant side POA HCC

I69.033 Monoplegia of upper limb following nontraumatic subarachnoid hemorrhage affecting right non-dominant side POA HCC

I69.034 Monoplegia of upper limb following nontraumatic subarachnoid hemorrhage affecting left non-dominant side POA HCC

I69.039 Monoplegia of upper limb following nontraumatic subarachnoid hemorrhage affecting unspecified side POA HCC

6ᵗʰ I69.04 Monoplegia of lower limb following nontraumatic subarachnoid hemorrhage

I69.041 Monoplegia of lower limb following nontraumatic subarachnoid hemorrhage affecting right dominant side POA HCC

I69.042 Monoplegia of lower limb following nontraumatic subarachnoid hemorrhage affecting left dominant side POA HCC

I69.043 Monoplegia of lower limb following nontraumatic subarachnoid hemorrhage affecting right non-dominant side POA HCC

I69.044 Monoplegia of lower limb following nontraumatic subarachnoid hemorrhage affecting left non-dominant side POA HCC

I69.049 Monoplegia of lower limb following nontraumatic subarachnoid hemorrhage affecting unspecified side POA HCC

6ᵗʰ I69.05 Hemiplegia and hemiparesis following nontraumatic subarachnoid hemorrhage

I69.051 Hemiplegia and hemiparesis following nontraumatic subarachnoid hemorrhage affecting right dominant side CC POA HCC CC/MCC Exc

I69.052 Hemiplegia and hemiparesis following nontraumatic subarachnoid hemorrhage affecting left dominant side CC POA HCC CC/MCC Exc

I69.053 Hemiplegia and hemiparesis following nontraumatic subarachnoid hemorrhage affecting right non-dominant side CC POA HCC CC/MCC Exc

I69.054 Hemiplegia and hemiparesis following nontraumatic subarachnoid hemorrhage affecting left non-dominant side CC POA HCC CC/MCC Exc

I69.059 Hemiplegia and hemiparesis following nontraumatic subarachnoid hemorrhage affecting unspecified side CC POA HCC CC/MCC Exc

6ᵗʰ I69.06 Other paralytic syndrome following nontraumatic subarachnoid hemorrhage

Use additional code to identify type of paralytic syndrome, such as:
locked-in state (G83.5)
quadriplegia (G82.5-)

EXCLUDES1 hemiplegia/hemiparesis following nontraumatic subarachnoid hemorrhage (I69.05-)

monoplegia of lower limb following nontraumatic subarachnoid hemorrhage (I69.04-)

monoplegia of upper limb following nontraumatic subarachnoid hemorrhage (I69.03-)

I69.061 Other paralytic syndrome following nontraumatic subarachnoid hemorrhage affecting right dominant side POA HCC

I69.062 Other paralytic syndrome following nontraumatic subarachnoid hemorrhage affecting left dominant side POA HCC

I69.063 Other paralytic syndrome following nontraumatic subarachnoid hemorrhage affecting right non-dominant side POA HCC

I69.064 Other paralytic syndrome following nontraumatic subarachnoid hemorrhage affecting left non-dominant side POA HCC

I69.065 Other paralytic syndrome following nontraumatic subarachnoid hemorrhage, bilateral POA HCC

I69.069 Other paralytic syndrome following nontraumatic subarachnoid hemorrhage affecting unspecified side POA HCC

6ᵗʰ I69.09 Other sequelae of nontraumatic subarachnoid hemorrhage

I69.090 Apraxia following nontraumatic subarachnoid hemorrhage POA

I69.091 Dysphagia following nontraumatic subarachnoid hemorrhage POA
Use additional code to identify the type of dysphagia, if known (R13.1-)

I69.092 Facial weakness following nontraumatic subarachnoid hemorrhage POA
Facial droop following nontraumatic subarachnoid hemorrhage

I69.093 Ataxia following nontraumatic subarachnoid hemorrhage POA

I69.098 Other sequelae following nontraumatic subarachnoid hemorrhage POA
Alterations of sensation following nontraumatic subarachnoid hemorrhage
Disturbance of vision following nontraumatic subarachnoid hemorrhage
Use additional code to identify the sequelae

5ᵗʰ I69.1 Sequelae of nontraumatic intracerebral hemorrhage

I69.10 Unspecified sequelae of nontraumatic intracerebral hemorrhage POA

6ᵗʰ I69.11 Cognitive deficits following nontraumatic intracerebral hemorrhage

I69.110 Attention and concentration deficit following nontraumatic intracerebral hemorrhage POA

I69.111 Memory deficit following nontraumatic intracerebral hemorrhage POA

I69.112 Visuospatial deficit and spatial neglect following nontraumatic intracerebral hemorrhage POA

I69.113 Psychomotor deficit following nontraumatic intracerebral hemorrhage POA

I69.114 Frontal lobe and executive function deficit following nontraumatic intracerebral hemorrhage POA

I69.115 Cognitive social or emotional deficit following nontraumatic intracerebral hemorrhage POA

I69.118 Other symptoms and signs involving cognitive functions following nontraumatic intracerebral hemorrhage POA

I69.119 Unspecified symptoms and signs involving cognitive functions following nontraumatic intracerebral hemorrhage POA

6ᵗʰ I69.12 Speech and language deficits following nontraumatic intracerebral hemorrhage

I69.120 Aphasia following nontraumatic intracerebral hemorrhage POA

I69.121 Dysphasia following nontraumatic intracerebral hemorrhage POA

I69.122 Dysarthria following nontraumatic intracerebral hemorrhage POA

I69.123 Fluency disorder following nontraumatic intracerebral hemorrhage POA
Stuttering following nontraumatic intracerebral hemorrhage

Unspecified Code   Other Specified Code   Manifestation Code   Ⓝ Newborn   Ⓟ Pediatric   Ⓜ Maternity   Ⓐ Adult   ♂ Male   ♀ Female
● New Code   ▲ Revised Code Title   ▶◀ Revised Text   NOTES   INCLUDES   EXCLUDES 1 Not coded here   EXCLUDES 2 Not included here
4ᵗʰ 4th character required   5ᵗʰ 5th character required   6ᵗʰ 6th character required   7ᵗʰ 7th character required
7ˣ Extension 'X' Alert   HAC Hospital-acquired condition (HAC) alert   AHA AHA Coding Clinic©

I69.128 Other speech and language deficits following nontraumatic intracerebral hemorrhage ᴘᴏᴀ

🄶 **I69.13** Monoplegia of upper limb following nontraumatic intracerebral hemorrhage

I69.131 Monoplegia of upper limb following nontraumatic intracerebral hemorrhage affecting right dominant side ᴘᴏᴀ HCC

I69.132 Monoplegia of upper limb following nontraumatic intracerebral hemorrhage affecting left dominant side ᴘᴏᴀ HCC

I69.133 Monoplegia of upper limb following nontraumatic intracerebral hemorrhage affecting right non-dominant side ᴘᴏᴀ HCC

I69.134 Monoplegia of upper limb following nontraumatic intracerebral hemorrhage affecting left non-dominant side ᴘᴏᴀ HCC

I69.139 Monoplegia of upper limb following nontraumatic intracerebral hemorrhage affecting unspecified side ᴘᴏᴀ HCC

🄶 **I69.14** Monoplegia of lower limb following nontraumatic intracerebral hemorrhage

I69.141 Monoplegia of lower limb following nontraumatic intracerebral hemorrhage affecting right dominant side ᴘᴏᴀ HCC

I69.142 Monoplegia of lower limb following nontraumatic intracerebral hemorrhage affecting left dominant side ᴘᴏᴀ HCC

I69.143 Monoplegia of lower limb following nontraumatic intracerebral hemorrhage affecting right non-dominant side ᴘᴏᴀ HCC

I69.144 Monoplegia of lower limb following nontraumatic intracerebral hemorrhage affecting left non-dominant side ᴘᴏᴀ HCC

I69.149 Monoplegia of lower limb following nontraumatic intracerebral hemorrhage affecting unspecified side ᴘᴏᴀ HCC

🄶 **I69.15** Hemiplegia and hemiparesis following nontraumatic intracerebral hemorrhage

I69.151 Hemiplegia and hemiparesis following nontraumatic intracerebral hemorrhage affecting right dominant side cc ᴘᴏᴀ HCC cc/mcc Exc

I69.152 Hemiplegia and hemiparesis following nontraumatic intracerebral hemorrhage affecting left dominant side cc ᴘᴏᴀ HCC cc/mcc Exc

I69.153 Hemiplegia and hemiparesis following nontraumatic intracerebral hemorrhage affecting right non-dominant side cc ᴘᴏᴀ HCC cc/mcc Exc

I69.154 Hemiplegia and hemiparesis following nontraumatic intracerebral hemorrhage affecting left non-dominant side cc ᴘᴏᴀ HCC cc/mcc Exc

I69.159 Hemiplegia and hemiparesis following nontraumatic intracerebral hemorrhage affecting unspecified side cc ᴘᴏᴀ HCC cc/mcc Exc

🄶 **I69.16** Other paralytic syndrome following nontraumatic intracerebral hemorrhage

Use additional code to identify type of paralytic syndrome, such as:

locked-in state (G83.5)

quadriplegia (G82.5-)

EXCLUDES1 *hemiplegia/hemiparesis following nontraumatic intracerebral hemorrhage (I69.15-)*

monoplegia of lower limb following nontraumatic intracerebral hemorrhage (I69.14-)

monoplegia of upper limb following nontraumatic intracerebral hemorrhage (I69.13-)

I69.161 Other paralytic syndrome following nontraumatic intracerebral hemorrhage affecting right dominant side ᴘᴏᴀ HCC

I69.162 Other paralytic syndrome following nontraumatic intracerebral hemorrhage affecting left dominant side ᴘᴏᴀ HCC

I69.163 Other paralytic syndrome following nontraumatic intracerebral hemorrhage affecting right non-dominant side ᴘᴏᴀ HCC

I69.164 Other paralytic syndrome following nontraumatic intracerebral hemorrhage affecting left non-dominant side ᴘᴏᴀ HCC

I69.165 Other paralytic syndrome following nontraumatic intracerebral hemorrhage, bilateral ᴘᴏᴀ HCC

I69.169 Other paralytic syndrome following nontraumatic intracerebral hemorrhage affecting unspecified side ᴘᴏᴀ HCC

🄶 **I69.19** Other sequelae of nontraumatic intracerebral hemorrhage

I69.190 Apraxia following nontraumatic intracerebral hemorrhage ᴘᴏᴀ

I69.191 Dysphagia following nontraumatic intracerebral hemorrhage ᴘᴏᴀ

Use additional code to identify the type of dysphagia, if known (R13.1-)

I69.192 Facial weakness following nontraumatic intracerebral hemorrhage ᴘᴏᴀ

Facial droop following nontraumatic intracerebral hemorrhage

I69.193 Ataxia following nontraumatic intracerebral hemorrhage ᴘᴏᴀ

I69.198 Other sequelae of nontraumatic intracerebral hemorrhage ᴘᴏᴀ

Alteration of sensations following nontraumatic intracerebral hemorrhage

Disturbance of vision following nontraumatic intracerebral hemorrhage

Use additional code to identify the sequelae

🄢 **I69.2** Sequelae of other nontraumatic intracranial hemorrhage

I69.20 Unspecified sequelae of other nontraumatic intracranial hemorrhage ᴘᴏᴀ

🄶 **I69.21** Cognitive deficits following other nontraumatic intracranial hemorrhage

I69.210 Attention and concentration deficit following other nontraumatic intracranial hemorrhage ᴘᴏᴀ

I69.211 Memory deficit following other nontraumatic intracranial hemorrhage ᴘᴏᴀ

I69.212 Visuospatial deficit and spatial neglect following other nontraumatic intracranial hemorrhage ᴘᴏᴀ

I69.213 Psychomotor deficit following other nontraumatic intracranial hemorrhage ᴘᴏᴀ

I69.214 Frontal lobe and executive function deficit following other nontraumatic intracranial hemorrhage ᴘᴏᴀ

I69.215 Cognitive social or emotional deficit following other nontraumatic intracranial hemorrhage ᴘᴏᴀ

I69.218 Other symptoms and signs involving cognitive functions following other nontraumatic intracranial hemorrhage ᴘᴏᴀ

I69.219 Unspecified symptoms and signs involving cognitive functions following other nontraumatic intracranial hemorrhage ᴘᴏᴀ

🄶 **I69.22** Speech and language deficits following other nontraumatic intracranial hemorrhage

I69.220 Aphasia following other nontraumatic intracranial hemorrhage ᴘᴏᴀ

ᴘᴏᴀ Unacceptable principal diagnosis symbol per Medicare code edits   ᴘᴏᴀ Code exempt from diagnosis present on admission requirement
🄿 Questionable admission   cc Complication or comorbidity   cc/mcc Exc CC/MCC exclusion   mcc Major complication or comorbidity
🄿🄲 Principal diagnosis as its own CC   🄿🄼 Principal diagnosis as its own MCC   HCC HCC diagnosis code   RxHCC RxHCC diagnosis code
MACRA code   🄩🄵 Z code as first-listed diagnosis

I69.221 **Dysphasia** following other nontraumatic intracranial hemorrhage POA

I69.222 **Dysarthria** following other nontraumatic intracranial hemorrhage POA

I69.223 **Fluency disorder** following other nontraumatic intracranial hemorrhage POA

Stuttering following other nontraumatic intracranial hemorrhage

I69.228 **Other speech and language deficits** following other nontraumatic intracranial hemorrhage POA

5ᵗʰ I69.23 Monoplegia of upper limb following other nontraumatic intracranial hemorrhage

I69.231 Monoplegia of upper limb following other nontraumatic intracranial hemorrhage affecting right dominant side POA HCC

I69.232 Monoplegia of upper limb following other nontraumatic intracranial hemorrhage affecting left dominant side POA HCC

I69.233 Monoplegia of upper limb following other nontraumatic intracranial hemorrhage affecting right non-dominant side POA HCC

I69.234 Monoplegia of upper limb following other nontraumatic intracranial hemorrhage affecting left non-dominant side POA HCC

I69.239 **Monoplegia of upper limb following other nontraumatic intracranial hemorrhage affecting unspecified side** POA HCC

5ᵗʰ I69.24 Monoplegia of lower limb following other nontraumatic intracranial hemorrhage

I69.241 Monoplegia of lower limb following other nontraumatic intracranial hemorrhage affecting right dominant side POA HCC

I69.242 Monoplegia of lower limb following other nontraumatic intracranial hemorrhage affecting left dominant side POA HCC

I69.243 Monoplegia of lower limb following other nontraumatic intracranial hemorrhage affecting right non-dominant side POA HCC

I69.244 Monoplegia of lower limb following other nontraumatic intracranial hemorrhage affecting left non-dominant side POA HCC

I69.249 **Monoplegia of lower limb following other nontraumatic intracranial hemorrhage affecting unspecified side** POA HCC

5ᵗʰ I69.25 Hemiplegia and hemiparesis following other nontraumatic intracranial hemorrhage

I69.251 Hemiplegia and hemiparesis following other nontraumatic intracranial hemorrhage affecting right dominant side CC POA HCC CC.MCC Exc

I69.252 Hemiplegia and hemiparesis following other nontraumatic intracranial hemorrhage affecting left dominant side CC POA HCC CC.MCC Exc

I69.253 Hemiplegia and hemiparesis following other nontraumatic intracranial hemorrhage affecting right non-dominant side CC POA HCC CC.MCC Exc

I69.254 Hemiplegia and hemiparesis following other nontraumatic intracranial hemorrhage affecting left non-dominant side CC POA HCC CC.MCC Exc

I69.259 **Hemiplegia and hemiparesis following other nontraumatic intracranial hemorrhage affecting unspecified side** CC POA HCC CC.MCC Exc

6ᵗʰ I69.26 Other paralytic syndrome following other nontraumatic intracranial hemorrhage

Use additional code to identify type of paralytic syndrome, such as:
locked-in state (G83.5)
quadriplegia (G82.5-)

EXCLUDES1 hemiplegia/hemiparesis following other nontraumatic intracranial hemorrhage (I69.25-)

monoplegia of lower limb following other nontraumatic intracranial hemorrhage (I69.24-)

monoplegia of upper limb following other nontraumatic intracranial hemorrhage (I69.23-)

I69.261 **Other paralytic syndrome following other nontraumatic intracranial hemorrhage affecting right dominant side** POA HCC

I69.262 **Other paralytic syndrome following other nontraumatic intracranial hemorrhage affecting left dominant side** POA HCC

I69.263 **Other paralytic syndrome following other nontraumatic intracranial hemorrhage affecting right non-dominant side** POA HCC

I69.264 **Other paralytic syndrome following other nontraumatic intracranial hemorrhage affecting left non-dominant side** POA HCC

I69.265 **Other paralytic syndrome following other nontraumatic intracranial hemorrhage, bilateral** POA HCC

I69.269 **Other paralytic syndrome following other nontraumatic intracranial hemorrhage affecting unspecified side** POA HCC

6ᵗʰ I69.29 Other sequelae of other nontraumatic intracranial hemorrhage

I69.290 **Apraxia** following other nontraumatic intracranial hemorrhage POA

I69.291 **Dysphagia** following other nontraumatic intracranial hemorrhage POA

Use additional code to identify the type of dysphagia, if known (R13.1-)

I69.292 **Facial weakness** following other nontraumatic intracranial hemorrhage POA

Facial droop following other nontraumatic intracranial hemorrhage

I69.293 **Ataxia** following other nontraumatic intracranial hemorrhage POA

I69.298 **Other sequelae** of other nontraumatic intracranial hemorrhage POA

Alteration of sensation following other nontraumatic intracranial hemorrhage
Disturbance of vision following other nontraumatic intracranial hemorrhage
Use additional code to identify the sequelae

5ᵗʰ I69.3 Sequelae of cerebral infarction

Sequelae of stroke NOS

I69.30 **Unspecified sequelae of cerebral infarction** POA

6ᵗʰ I69.31 Cognitive deficits following cerebral infarction

I69.310 **Attention and concentration deficit** following cerebral infarction POA

I69.311 **Memory deficit** following cerebral infarction POA

I69.312 **Visuospatial deficit and spatial neglect** following cerebral infarction POA

I69.313 **Psychomotor deficit** following cerebral infarction POA

I69.314 **Frontal lobe and executive function deficit** following cerebral infarction POA

I69.315 **Cognitive social or emotional deficit** following cerebral infarction POA

I69.318 **Other symptoms and signs** involving cognitive functions following cerebral infarction POA

I69.319 **Unspecified symptoms and signs involving cognitive functions following cerebral infarction** POA

6ᵗʰ I69.32 Speech and language deficits following cerebral infarction

---

Unspecified Code   Other Specified Code   Manifestation Code   Ⓝ Newborn   Ⓟ Pediatric   Ⓜ Maternity   Ⓐ Adult   ♂ Male   ♀ Female
● New Code   ▲ Revised Code Title   ▶◀ Revised Text   **NOTES**   *INCLUDES*   *EXCLUDES 1* Not coded here   *EXCLUDES 2* Not included here
4ᵗʰ character required   5ᵗʰ character required   6ᵗʰ character required   7ᵗʰ character required
Extension 'X' Alert   HAC Hospital-acquired condition (HAC) alert   **AHA** AHA Coding Clinic©

I69.320 Aphasia **following cerebral infarction** POA
AHA: Q4 2013

I69.321 Dysphasia **following cerebral infarction** POA

I69.322 Dysarthria **following cerebral infarction** POA
EXCLUDES2 *transient ischemic attack (TIA) (G45.9)*

I69.323 Fluency disorder **following cerebral infarction** POA
Stuttering following cerebral infarction

I69.328 Other speech and language deficits **following cerebral infarction** POA

6ᵗʰ I69.33 Monoplegia of upper limb **following cerebral infarction**

I69.331 **Monoplegia of upper limb following cerebral infarction affecting** right **dominant side** POA HCC

I69.332 **Monoplegia of upper limb following cerebral infarction affecting** left dominant **side** POA HCC

I69.333 **Monoplegia of upper limb following cerebral infarction affecting** right non-**dominant side** POA HCC

I69.334 **Monoplegia of upper limb following cerebral infarction affecting** left non-**dominant side** POA HCC

I69.339 **Monoplegia of upper limb following cerebral infarction affecting** unspecified **side** POA HCC

6ᵗʰ I69.34 Monoplegia of lower limb **following cerebral infarction**

I69.341 **Monoplegia of lower limb following cerebral infarction affecting** right **dominant side** POA HCC

I69.342 **Monoplegia of lower limb following cerebral infarction affecting** left dominant **side** POA HCC

I69.343 **Monoplegia of lower limb following cerebral infarction affecting** right non-**dominant side** POA HCC

I69.344 **Monoplegia of lower limb following cerebral infarction affecting** left non-**dominant side** POA HCC

I69.349 **Monoplegia of lower limb following cerebral infarction affecting** unspecified **side** POA HCC

6ᵗʰ I69.35 Hemiplegia and hemiparesis **following cerebral infarction**

I69.351 **Hemiplegia and hemiparesis following cerebral infarction affecting** right **dominant side** CC POA HCC CC/MCC Exc
AHA: Q1 2015, Q4 2013
EXCLUDES2 *transient ischemic attack (TIA) (G45.9)*

I69.352 **Hemiplegia and hemiparesis following cerebral infarction affecting** left dominant **side** CC POA HCC CC/MCC Exc

I69.353 **Hemiplegia and hemiparesis following cerebral infarction affecting** right non-**dominant side** CC POA HCC CC/MCC Exc

I69.354 **Hemiplegia and hemiparesis following cerebral infarction affecting** left non-**dominant side** CC POA HCC CC/MCC Exc

I69.359 **Hemiplegia and hemiparesis following cerebral infarction affecting** unspecified **side** CC POA HCC CC/MCC Exc

6ᵗʰ I69.36 Other paralytic syndrome **following cerebral infarction**
Use additional code to identify type of paralytic syndrome, such as:
locked-in state (G83.5)
quadriplegia (G82.5-)

EXCLUDES1 *hemiplegia/hemiparesis following cerebral infarction (I69.35-)*
monoplegia of lower limb following cerebral infarction (I69.34-)
monoplegia of upper limb following cerebral infarction (I69.33-)

I69.361 **Other paralytic syndrome following cerebral infarction affecting** right **dominant side** POA HCC

I69.362 **Other paralytic syndrome following cerebral infarction affecting** left dominant **side** POA HCC

I69.363 **Other paralytic syndrome following cerebral infarction affecting** right non-**dominant side** POA HCC

I69.364 **Other paralytic syndrome following cerebral infarction affecting** left non-**dominant side** POA HCC

I69.365 **Other paralytic syndrome following cerebral infarction,** bilateral POA HCC

I69.369 **Other paralytic syndrome following cerebral infarction affecting** unspecified **side** POA HCC

6ᵗʰ I69.39 Other sequelae **of cerebral infarction**

I69.390 Apraxia **following cerebral infarction** POA

I69.391 Dysphagia **following cerebral infarction** POA
Use additional code to identify the type of dysphagia, if known (R13.1-)

I69.392 Facial weakness **following cerebral infarction** POA
Facial droop following cerebral infarction

I69.393 Ataxia **following cerebral infarction** POA

I69.398 **Other sequelae of cerebral infarction** POA
Alteration of sensation following cerebral infarction
Disturbance of vision following cerebral infarction
Use additional code to identify the sequelae

5ᵗʰ I69.8 Sequelae of **other cerebrovascular diseases**
EXCLUDES1 *sequelae of traumatic intracranial injury (S06.-)*

I69.80 **Unspecified sequelae of other cerebrovascular disease** POA

6ᵗʰ I69.81 Cognitive deficits following other cerebrovascular disease

I69.810 Attention and concentration **deficit following other cerebrovascular disease** POA

I69.811 Memory deficit **following other cerebrovascular disease** POA

I69.812 Visuospatial deficit and spatial neglect **following other cerebrovascular disease** POA

I69.813 Psychomotor deficit **following other cerebrovascular disease** POA

I69.814 Frontal lobe and executive function deficit **following other cerebrovascular disease** POA

I69.815 Cognitive social or emotional **deficit following other cerebrovascular disease** POA

I69.818 Other symptoms and signs **involving cognitive functions following other cerebrovascular disease** POA

I69.819 Unspecified symptoms and signs **involving cognitive functions following other cerebrovascular disease** POA

6ᵗʰ I69.82 Speech and language deficits **following other cerebrovascular disease**

I69.820 Aphasia **following other cerebrovascular disease** POA

I69.821 Dysphasia **following other cerebrovascular disease** POA

I69.822 Dysarthria **following other cerebrovascular disease** POA

POA Unacceptable principal diagnosis Symbol per Medicare code edits   POA Code exempt from diagnosis present on admission requirement
❓ Questionable admission   CC Complication or comorbidity   CC/MCC Exc CC/MCC exclusion   MCC Major complication or comorbidity
Principal diagnosis as its own CC   Principal diagnosis as its own MCC   HCC HCC diagnosis code   RxHCC RxHCC diagnosis code
MACRA code   Z1 Z code as first-listed diagnosis

I69.823   Fluency disorder **following other cerebrovascular disease** POA

    Stuttering following other cerebrovascular disease

I69.828   **Other speech and language deficits following other cerebrovascular disease** POA

6ᵀᴴ   I69.83   Monoplegia of upper limb **following other cerebrovascular disease**

I69.831   **Monoplegia of upper limb following other cerebrovascular disease affecting** right **dominant side** POA HCC

I69.832   **Monoplegia of upper limb following other cerebrovascular disease affecting** left **dominant side** POA HCC

I69.833   **Monoplegia of upper limb following other cerebrovascular disease affecting** right **non-dominant side** POA HCC

I69.834   **Monoplegia of upper limb following other cerebrovascular disease affecting** left **non-dominant side** POA HCC

I69.839   **Monoplegia of upper limb following other cerebrovascular disease affecting unspecified side** POA HCC

6ᵀᴴ   I69.84   Monoplegia of lower limb **following other cerebrovascular disease**

I69.841   **Monoplegia of lower limb following other cerebrovascular disease affecting** right **dominant side** POA HCC

I69.842   **Monoplegia of lower limb following other cerebrovascular disease affecting** left **dominant side** POA HCC

I69.843   **Monoplegia of lower limb following other cerebrovascular disease affecting** right **non-dominant side** POA HCC

I69.844   **Monoplegia of lower limb following other cerebrovascular disease affecting** left **non-dominant side** POA HCC

I69.849   **Monoplegia of lower limb following other cerebrovascular disease affecting unspecified side** POA HCC

6ᵀᴴ   I69.85   Hemiplegia and hemiparesis **following other cerebrovascular disease**

I69.851   **Hemiplegia and hemiparesis following other cerebrovascular disease affecting** right dominant side   CC POA HCC CC/MCC Exc

I69.852   **Hemiplegia and hemiparesis following other cerebrovascular disease affecting** left dominant side   CC POA HCC CC/MCC Exc

I69.853   **Hemiplegia and hemiparesis following other cerebrovascular disease affecting** right non-dominant side   CC POA HCC CC/MCC Exc

I69.854   **Hemiplegia and hemiparesis following other cerebrovascular disease affecting** left non-dominant side   CC POA HCC CC/MCC Exc

I69.859   **Hemiplegia and hemiparesis following other cerebrovascular disease affecting unspecified side**   CC POA HCC CC/MCC Exc

6ᵀᴴ   I69.86   Other paralytic syndrome **following other cerebrovascular disease**

    Use additional code to identify type of paralytic syndrome, such as:

    locked-in state (G83.5)

    quadriplegia (G82.5-)

    EXCLUDES1   hemiplegia/hemiparesis following other cerebrovascular disease (I69.85-)

      monoplegia of lower limb following other cerebrovascular disease (I69.84-)

      monoplegia of upper limb following other cerebrovascular disease (I69.83-)

I69.861   **Other paralytic syndrome following other cerebrovascular disease affecting** right **dominant side** POA HCC

I69.862   **Other paralytic syndrome following other cerebrovascular disease affecting** left **dominant side** POA HCC

I69.863   **Other paralytic syndrome following other cerebrovascular disease affecting** right **non-dominant side** POA HCC

I69.864   **Other paralytic syndrome following other cerebrovascular disease affecting** left **non-dominant side** POA HCC

I69.865   **Other paralytic syndrome following other cerebrovascular disease,** bilateral POA HCC

I69.869   **Other paralytic syndrome following other cerebrovascular disease affecting unspecified side** POA HCC

6ᵀᴴ   I69.89   Other sequelae **of other cerebrovascular disease**

I69.890   **Apraxia following other cerebrovascular disease** POA

I69.891   **Dysphagia following other cerebrovascular disease** POA

    Use additional code to identify the type of dysphagia, if known (R13.1-)

I69.892   **Facial weakness following other cerebrovascular disease** POA

    Facial droop following other cerebrovascular disease

I69.893   **Ataxia following other cerebrovascular disease** POA

I69.898   **Other sequelae of other cerebrovascular disease** POA

    Alteration of sensation following other cerebrovascular disease

    Disturbance of vision following other cerebrovascular disease

    Use additional code to identify the sequelae

5ᵀᴴ   I69.9   Sequelae of **unspecified cerebrovascular diseases**

    EXCLUDES1   sequelae of stroke (I69.3)

      sequelae of traumatic intracranial injury (S06.-)

I69.90   **Unspecified sequelae of unspecified cerebrovascular disease** POA

6ᵀᴴ   I69.91   Cognitive deficits **following unspecified cerebrovascular disease**

I69.910   Attention and concentration **deficit following unspecified cerebrovascular disease**

I69.911   Memory deficit **following unspecified cerebrovascular disease**

I69.912   Visuospatial deficit and spatial neglect **following unspecified cerebrovascular disease**

I69.913   Psychomotor deficit **following unspecified cerebrovascular disease**

I69.914   Frontal lobe and executive function **deficit following unspecified cerebrovascular disease**

I69.915   Cognitive social or emotional **deficit following unspecified cerebrovascular disease**

I69.918   Other symptoms and signs **involving cognitive functions following unspecified cerebrovascular disease**

I69.919   Unspecified symptoms and signs **involving cognitive functions following unspecified cerebrovascular disease**

6ᵀᴴ   I69.92   Speech and language deficits **following unspecified cerebrovascular disease**

I69.920   Aphasia **following unspecified cerebrovascular disease** POA

I69.921   Dysphasia **following unspecified cerebrovascular disease** POA

I69.922   Dysarthria **following unspecified cerebrovascular disease** POA

Unspecified Code   Other Specified Code   Manifestation Code   N Newborn   P Pediatric   M Maternity   A Adult   ♂ Male   ♀ Female
   ● New Code   ▲ Revised Code Title   ▶◀ Revised Text   **NOTES**   *INCLUDES*   *EXCLUDES 1*   Not coded here   *EXCLUDES 2*   Not included here
     4ᵀᴴ 4ᵗʰ character required   5ᵀᴴ 5ᵗʰ character required   6ᵀᴴ 6ᵗʰ character required   7ᵀᴴ 7ᵗʰ character required
      7ᵀᴴ Extension 'X' Alert   HAC Hospital-acquired condition (HAC) alert   **AHA** AHA Coding Clinic©

I69.923 **Fluency disorder** following unspecified cerebrovascular disease POA

Stuttering following unspecified cerebrovascular disease

I69.928 **Other speech and language deficits following unspecified cerebrovascular disease** POA

6⁷ I69.93 Monoplegia of upper limb following unspecified cerebrovascular disease

I69.931 **Monoplegia of upper limb following unspecified cerebrovascular disease affecting** right dominant side POA HCC

I69.932 **Monoplegia of upper limb following unspecified cerebrovascular disease affecting** left dominant side POA HCC

I69.933 **Monoplegia of upper limb following unspecified cerebrovascular disease affecting** right non-dominant side POA HCC

I69.934 **Monoplegia of upper limb following unspecified cerebrovascular disease affecting** left non-dominant side POA HCC

I69.939 **Monoplegia of upper limb following unspecified cerebrovascular disease affecting** unspecified side POA HCC

6⁷ I69.94 Monoplegia of lower limb following unspecified cerebrovascular disease

I69.941 **Monoplegia of lower limb following unspecified cerebrovascular disease affecting** right dominant side POA HCC

I69.942 **Monoplegia of lower limb following unspecified cerebrovascular disease affecting** left dominant side POA HCC

I69.943 **Monoplegia of lower limb following unspecified cerebrovascular disease affecting** right non-dominant side POA HCC

I69.944 **Monoplegia of lower limb following unspecified cerebrovascular disease affecting** left non-dominant side POA HCC

I69.949 **Monoplegia of lower limb following unspecified cerebrovascular disease affecting** unspecified side POA HCC

6⁷ I69.95 Hemiplegia and hemiparesis following unspecified cerebrovascular disease

I69.951 **Hemiplegia and hemiparesis following unspecified cerebrovascular disease affecting** right dominant side CC POA HCC CC/MCC Exc

I69.952 **Hemiplegia and hemiparesis following unspecified cerebrovascular disease affecting** left dominant side CC POA HCC CC/MCC Exc

I69.953 **Hemiplegia and hemiparesis following unspecified cerebrovascular disease affecting** right non-dominant side CC POA HCC CC/MCC Exc

I69.954 **Hemiplegia and hemiparesis following unspecified cerebrovascular disease affecting** left non-dominant side CC POA HCC CC/MCC Exc

I69.959 **Hemiplegia and hemiparesis following unspecified cerebrovascular disease affecting** unspecified side CC POA HCC CC/MCC Exc

6⁷ I69.96 Other paralytic syndrome following unspecified cerebrovascular disease

Use additional code to identify type of paralytic syndrome, such as:

locked-in state (G83.5)

quadriplegia (G82.5-)

EXCLUDES1 hemiplegia/hemiparesis following unspecified cerebrovascular disease (I69.95-)

monoplegia of lower limb following unspecified cerebrovascular disease (I69.94-)

monoplegia of upper limb following unspecified cerebrovascular disease (I69.93-)

I69.961 **Other paralytic syndrome following unspecified cerebrovascular disease affecting** right dominant side POA HCC

I69.962 **Other paralytic syndrome following unspecified cerebrovascular disease affecting** left dominant side POA HCC

I69.963 **Other paralytic syndrome following unspecified cerebrovascular disease affecting** right non-dominant side POA HCC

I69.964 **Other paralytic syndrome following unspecified cerebrovascular disease affecting** left non-dominant side POA HCC

I69.965 **Other paralytic syndrome following unspecified cerebrovascular disease, bilateral** POA HCC

I69.969 **Other paralytic syndrome following unspecified cerebrovascular disease affecting** unspecified side POA HCC

5⁷ I69.99 Other sequelae of unspecified cerebrovascular disease

I69.990 **Apraxia following unspecified cerebrovascular disease** POA

I69.991 **Dysphagia following unspecified cerebrovascular disease** POA

Use additional code to identify the type of dysphagia, if known (R13.1-)

I69.992 **Facial weakness following unspecified cerebrovascular disease** POA

Facial droop following unspecified cerebrovascular disease

I69.993 **Ataxia following unspecified cerebrovascular disease** POA

I69.998 **Other sequelae following unspecified cerebrovascular disease** POA

Alteration in sensation following unspecified cerebrovascular disease

Disturbance of vision following unspecified cerebrovascular disease

Use additional code to identify the sequelae

Diseases of arteries, arterioles and capillaries (I70-I79)

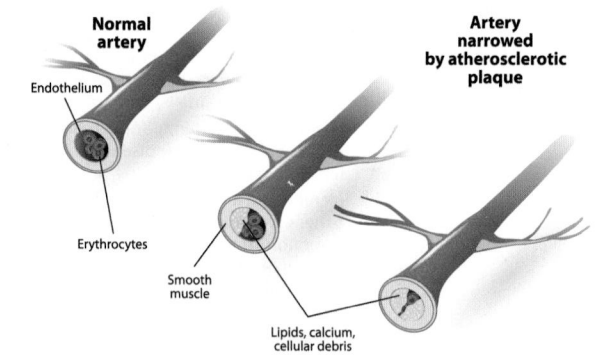

Figure 9.5 Atherosclerosis

4⁷ I70 **Atherosclerosis**

INCLUDES arteriolosclerosis

arterial degeneration

arteriosclerosis

arteriosclerotic vascular disease

arteriovascular degeneration

atheroma

endarteritis deformans or obliterans

senile arteritis

senile endarteritis

vascular degeneration

POA Unacceptable principal diagnosis symbol per Medicare code edits   POA Code exempt from diagnosis present on admission requirement
? Questionable admission   CC Complication or comorbidity   CC/MCC Exc CC/MCC exclusion   MCC Major complication or comorbidity
Principal diagnosis as its own CC   Principal diagnosis as its own MCC   HCC HCC diagnosis code   RxHCC RxHCC diagnosis code
MACRA code   Z1 Z code as first-listed diagnosis

676   When symbols appear on a code that requires a 7th character extension, refer to Appendix B to identify applicable 7th character codes.   **2018 ICD-10-CM**

Use additional code to identify:
exposure to environmental tobacco smoke (Z77.22)
history of tobacco dependence (Z87.891)
occupational exposure to environmental tobacco smoke (Z57.31)
tobacco dependence (F17.-)
tobacco use (Z72.0)
EXCLUDES2 *arteriosclerotic cardiovascular disease (I25.1-)*
     arteriosclerotic heart disease (I25.1-)
     atheroembolism (I75.-)
     cerebral atherosclerosis (I67.2)
     coronary atherosclerosis (I25.1-)
     mesenteric atherosclerosis (K55.1)
     precerebral atherosclerosis (I67.2)
     primary pulmonary atherosclerosis (I27.0)

I70.0 **Atherosclerosis of** aorta   A HCC RxHCC

I70.1 **Atherosclerosis of** renal artery   A HCC RxHCC
Goldblatt's kidney
EXCLUDES2 *atherosclerosis of renal arterioles (I12.-)*

5ᵗʰ **I70.2** **Atherosclerosis of** native arteries of the extremities
Mönckeberg's (medial) sclerosis
Use additional code, if applicable, to identify chronic total occlusion of artery of extremity (I70.92)
EXCLUDES2 *atherosclerosis of bypass graft of extremities (I70.30-I70.79)*

6ᵗʰ **I70.20** Unspecified atherosclerosis of native arteries of extremities

    I70.201 Unspecified atherosclerosis of native arteries of extremities, right leg   A HCC RxHCC

    I70.202 Unspecified atherosclerosis of native arteries of extremities, left leg   A HCC RxHCC

    I70.203 Unspecified atherosclerosis of native arteries of extremities, bilateral legs   A HCC RxHCC

    I70.208 Unspecified atherosclerosis of native arteries of extremities, other extremity   A HCC RxHCC

    I70.209 Unspecified atherosclerosis of native arteries of extremities, unspecified extremity   A HCC RxHCC

6ᵗʰ **I70.21** Atherosclerosis of native arteries of extremities with intermittent claudication

    I70.211 Atherosclerosis of native arteries of extremities with intermittent claudication, right leg   A HCC RxHCC

    I70.212 Atherosclerosis of native arteries of extremities with intermittent claudication, left leg   A HCC RxHCC

    I70.213 Atherosclerosis of native arteries of extremities with intermittent claudication, bilateral legs   A HCC RxHCC

    I70.218 Atherosclerosis of native arteries of extremities with intermittent claudication, other extremity   A HCC RxHCC

    I70.219 Atherosclerosis of native arteries of extremities with intermittent claudication, unspecified extremity   A HCC RxHCC

6ᵗʰ **I70.22** Atherosclerosis of native arteries of extremities with rest pain
INCLUDES *any condition classifiable to I70.21-*

    I70.221 Atherosclerosis of native arteries of extremities with rest pain, right leg A HCC RxHCC

    I70.222 Atherosclerosis of native arteries of extremities with rest pain, left leg A HCC RxHCC

    I70.223 Atherosclerosis of native arteries of extremities with rest pain, bilateral legs   A HCC RxHCC

    I70.228 Atherosclerosis of native arteries of extremities with rest pain, other extremity   A HCC RxHCC

    I70.229 Atherosclerosis of native arteries of extremities with rest pain, unspecified extremity   A HCC RxHCC

6ᵗʰ **I70.23** **Atherosclerosis of** native arteries of right leg with ulceration
INCLUDES *any condition classifiable to I70.211 and I70.221*
Use additional code to identify severity of ulcer (L97.-)

    I70.231 Atherosclerosis of native arteries of right leg with ulceration of thigh   A HCC RxHCC

    I70.232 Atherosclerosis of native arteries of right leg with ulceration of calf   A HCC RxHCC

    I70.233 Atherosclerosis of native arteries of right leg with ulceration of ankle   A HCC RxHCC

    I70.234 Atherosclerosis of native arteries of right leg with ulceration of heel and midfoot   A HCC RxHCC
Atherosclerosis of native arteries of right leg with ulceration of plantar surface of midfoot

    I70.235 Atherosclerosis of native arteries of right leg with ulceration of other part of foot   A HCC RxHCC
Atherosclerosis of native arteries of right leg extremities with ulceration of toe

    I70.238 Atherosclerosis of native arteries of right leg with ulceration of other part of lower right leg   A HCC RxHCC

    I70.239 Atherosclerosis of native arteries of right leg with ulceration of unspecified site   A HCC RxHCC

6ᵗʰ **I70.24** **Atherosclerosis of** native arteries of left leg with ulceration
INCLUDES *any condition classifiable to I70.212 and I70.222*
Use additional code to identify severity of ulcer (L97.-)

    I70.241 Atherosclerosis of native arteries of left leg with ulceration of thigh   A HCC RxHCC

    I70.242 Atherosclerosis of native arteries of left leg with ulceration of calf   A HCC RxHCC

    I70.243 Atherosclerosis of native arteries of left leg with ulceration of ankle   A HCC RxHCC

    I70.244 Atherosclerosis of native arteries of left leg with ulceration of heel and midfoot   A HCC RxHCC
Atherosclerosis of native arteries of left leg with ulceration of plantar surface of midfoot

    I70.245 Atherosclerosis of native arteries of left leg with ulceration of other part of foot   A HCC RxHCC
Atherosclerosis of native arteries of left leg extremities with ulceration of toe

    I70.248 Atherosclerosis of native arteries of left leg with ulceration of other part of lower left leg   A HCC RxHCC

    I70.249 Atherosclerosis of native arteries of left leg with ulceration of unspecified site   A HCC RxHCC

I70.25 **Atherosclerosis of** native arteries of other extremities with ulceration   A HCC RxHCC
INCLUDES *any condition classifiable to I70.218 and I70.228*
Use additional code to identify the severity of the ulcer (L98.49-)

6ᵗʰ **I70.26** **Atherosclerosis of** native arteries of extremities with gangrene
INCLUDES *any condition classifiable to I70.21-, I70.22-, I70.23-, I70.24-, and I70.25-*
Use additional code to identify the severity of any ulcer (L97.-, L98.49-), if applicable

    I70.261 Atherosclerosis of native arteries of extremities with gangrene, right leg   A cc HCC CC/MCC Exc

---

Unspecified Code   Other Specified Code   Manifestation Code   N Newborn P Pediatric M Maternity A Adult ♂ Male ♀ Female
● New Code   ▲ Revised Code Title   ▶◀ Revised Text **NOTES** *INCLUDES* *EXCLUDES 1* Not coded here *EXCLUDES 2* Not included here
4ᵗʰ 4ᵗʰ character required 5ᵗʰ 5ᵗʰ character required 6ᵗʰ 6ᵗʰ character required 7ᵗʰ 7ᵗʰ character required
7ˣ Extension 'X' Alert HAC Hospital-acquired condition (HAC) alert **AHA** AHA Coding Clinic©

I70.262   Atherosclerosis of native arteries of extremities with gangrene, left leg   A c⊘ HCC CC/MCC Exc

I70.263   Atherosclerosis of native arteries of extremities with gangrene, bilateral legs   A c⊘ HCC CC/MCC Exc

I70.268   Atherosclerosis of native arteries of extremities with gangrene, other extremity   A c⊘ HCC CC/MCC Exc

I70.269   Atherosclerosis of native arteries of extremities with gangrene, unspecified extremity   A c⊘ HCC CC/MCC Exc

6ᵗʰ   I70.29   Other atherosclerosis of native arteries of extremities

   I70.291   Other atherosclerosis of native arteries of extremities, right leg   A HCC RxHCC

   I70.292   Other atherosclerosis of native arteries of extremities, left leg   A HCC RxHCC

   I70.293   Other atherosclerosis of native arteries of extremities, bilateral legs   A HCC RxHCC

   I70.298   Other atherosclerosis of native arteries of extremities, other extremity   A HCC RxHCC

   I70.299   Other atherosclerosis of native arteries of extremities, unspecified extremity   A HCC RxHCC

5ᵗʰ   I70.3   Atherosclerosis of unspecified type of bypass graft(s) of the extremities

Use additional code, if applicable, to identify chronic total occlusion of artery of extremity (I70.92)

EXCLUDES1   embolism or thrombus of bypass graft(s) of extremities (T82.8-)

6ᵗʰ   I70.30   Unspecified atherosclerosis of unspecified type of bypass graft(s) of the extremities

   I70.301   Unspecified atherosclerosis of unspecified type of bypass graft(s) of the extremities, right leg   A HCC RxHCC

   I70.302   Unspecified atherosclerosis of unspecified type of bypass graft(s) of the extremities, left leg   A HCC RxHCC

   I70.303   Unspecified atherosclerosis of unspecified type of bypass graft(s) of the extremities, bilateral legs   A HCC RxHCC

   I70.308   Unspecified atherosclerosis of unspecified type of bypass graft(s) of the extremities, other extremity   A HCC RxHCC

   I70.309   Unspecified atherosclerosis of unspecified type of bypass graft(s) of the extremities, unspecified extremity   A HCC RxHCC

6ᵗʰ   I70.31   Atherosclerosis of unspecified type of bypass graft(s) of the extremities with intermittent claudication

   I70.311   Atherosclerosis of unspecified type of bypass graft(s) of the extremities with intermittent claudication, right leg   A HCC RxHCC

   I70.312   Atherosclerosis of unspecified type of bypass graft(s) of the extremities with intermittent claudication, left leg   A HCC RxHCC

   I70.313   Atherosclerosis of unspecified type of bypass graft(s) of the extremities with intermittent claudication, bilateral legs   A HCC RxHCC

   I70.318   Atherosclerosis of unspecified type of bypass graft(s) of the extremities with intermittent claudication, other extremity   A HCC RxHCC

   I70.319   Atherosclerosis of unspecified type of bypass graft(s) of the extremities with intermittent claudication, unspecified extremity   A HCC RxHCC

6ᵗʰ   I70.32   Atherosclerosis of unspecified type of bypass graft(s) of the extremities with rest pain

INCLUDES   any condition classifiable to I70.31-

I70.321   Atherosclerosis of unspecified type of bypass graft(s) of the extremities with rest pain, right leg   A HCC RxHCC

I70.322   Atherosclerosis of unspecified type of bypass graft(s) of the extremities with rest pain, left leg   A HCC RxHCC

I70.323   Atherosclerosis of unspecified type of bypass graft(s) of the extremities with rest pain, bilateral legs   A HCC RxHCC

I70.328   Atherosclerosis of unspecified type of bypass graft(s) of the extremities with rest pain, other extremity   A HCC RxHCC

I70.329   Atherosclerosis of unspecified type of bypass graft(s) of the extremities with rest pain, unspecified extremity   A HCC RxHCC

5ᵗʰ   I70.33   Atherosclerosis of unspecified type of bypass graft(s) of the right leg with ulceration

INCLUDES   any condition classifiable to I70.311 and I70.321

Use additional code to identify severity of ulcer (L97.-)

I70.331   Atherosclerosis of unspecified type of bypass graft(s) of the right leg with ulceration of thigh   A c⊘ HCC PDx RxHCC CC/MCC Exc

I70.332   Atherosclerosis of unspecified type of bypass graft(s) of the right leg with ulceration of calf   A c⊘ HCC PDx RxHCC CC/MCC Exc

I70.333   Atherosclerosis of unspecified type of bypass graft(s) of the right leg with ulceration of ankle   A c⊘ HCC PDx RxHCC CC/MCC Exc

I70.334   Atherosclerosis of unspecified type of bypass graft(s) of the right leg with ulceration of heel and midfoot   A c⊘ HCC PDx RxHCC CC/MCC Exc

Atherosclerosis of unspecified type of bypass graft(s) of right leg with ulceration of plantar surface of midfoot

I70.335   Atherosclerosis of unspecified type of bypass graft(s) of the right leg with ulceration of other part of foot   A HCC RxHCC

Atherosclerosis of unspecified type of bypass graft(s) of the right leg with ulceration of toe

I70.338   Atherosclerosis of unspecified type of bypass graft(s) of the right leg with ulceration of other part of lower leg   A c⊘ HCC PDx RxHCC CC/MCC Exc

I70.339   Atherosclerosis of unspecified type of bypass graft(s) of the right leg with ulceration of unspecified site   A c⊘ HCC PDx RxHCC CC/MCC Exc

5ᵗʰ   I70.34   Atherosclerosis of unspecified type of bypass graft(s) of the left leg with ulceration

INCLUDES   any condition classifiable to I70.312 and I70.322

Use additional code to identify severity of ulcer (L97.-)

I70.341   Atherosclerosis of unspecified type of bypass graft(s) of the left leg with ulceration of thigh   A c⊘ HCC PDx RxHCC CC/MCC Exc

I70.342   Atherosclerosis of unspecified type of bypass graft(s) of the left leg with ulceration of calf   A c⊘ HCC PDx RxHCC CC/MCC Exc

I70.343   Atherosclerosis of unspecified type of bypass graft(s) of the left leg with ulceration of ankle   A c⊘ HCC PDx RxHCC CC/MCC Exc

I70.344   Atherosclerosis of unspecified type of bypass graft(s) of the left leg with ulceration of heel and midfoot   A c⊘ HCC PDx RxHCC CC/MCC Exc

Atherosclerosis of unspecified type of bypass graft(s) of left leg with ulceration of plantar surface of midfoot

---

PDx Unacceptable principal diagnosis symbol per Medicare code edits   POA Code exempt from diagnosis present on admission requirement
❓ Questionable admission   c⊘ Complication or comorbidity   CC/MCC Exc CC/MCC exclusion   MCC Major complication or comorbidity
PDx CC Principal diagnosis as its own CC   PDx MCC Principal diagnosis as its own MCC   HCC HCC diagnosis code   RxHCC RxHCC diagnosis code
MACRA code   Z1 Z code as first-listed diagnosis

When symbols appear on a code that requires a 7th character extension, refer to Appendix B to identify applicable 7th character codes.   2018 ICD-10-CM

I70.345 Atherosclerosis of unspecified type of bypass graft(s) of the left leg with ulceration of other part of foot   A HCC RxHCC

Atherosclerosis of unspecified type of bypass graft(s) of the left leg with ulceration of toe

I70.348 Atherosclerosis of unspecified type of bypass graft(s) of the left leg with ulceration of other part of lower leg   A CC HCC PD₂ RxHCC CC/MCC Exc

I70.349 Atherosclerosis of unspecified type of bypass graft(s) of the left leg with ulceration of unspecified site   A CC HCC PD₂ RxHCC CC/MCC Exc

I70.35 Atherosclerosis of unspecified type of bypass graft(s) of other extremity with ulceration   A HCC RxHCC

INCLUDES   any condition classifiable to I70.318 and I70.328

Use additional code to identify severity of ulcer (L98.49-)

6ᵗʰ **I70.36** Atherosclerosis of unspecified type of bypass graft(s) of the extremities with gangrene

INCLUDES   any condition classifiable to I70.31-, I70.32-, I70.33-, I70.34-, I70.35

Use additional code to identify the severity of any ulcer (L97.-, L98.49-), if applicable

I70.361 Atherosclerosis of unspecified type of bypass graft(s) of the extremities with gangrene, right leg   A CC HCC PD₂ CC/MCC Exc

I70.362 Atherosclerosis of unspecified type of bypass graft(s) of the extremities with gangrene, left leg   A CC HCC PD₂ CC/MCC Exc

I70.363 Atherosclerosis of unspecified type of bypass graft(s) of the extremities with gangrene, bilateral legs   A CC HCC PD₂ CC/MCC Exc

I70.368 Atherosclerosis of unspecified type of bypass graft(s) of the extremities with gangrene, other extremity   A CC HCC PD₂ CC/MCC Exc

I70.369 Atherosclerosis of unspecified type of bypass graft(s) of the extremities with gangrene, unspecified extremity   A CC HCC PD₂ CC/MCC Exc

6ᵗʰ **I70.39** Other atherosclerosis of unspecified type of bypass graft(s) of the extremities

I70.391 Other atherosclerosis of unspecified type of bypass graft(s) of the extremities, right leg   A HCC RxHCC

I70.392 Other atherosclerosis of unspecified type of bypass graft(s) of the extremities, left leg   A HCC RxHCC

I70.393 Other atherosclerosis of unspecified type of bypass graft(s) of the extremities, bilateral legs   A HCC RxHCC

I70.398 Other atherosclerosis of unspecified type of bypass graft(s) of the extremities, other extremity   A HCC RxHCC

I70.399 Other atherosclerosis of unspecified type of bypass graft(s) of the extremities, unspecified extremity   A HCC RxHCC

5ᵗʰ **I70.4** Atherosclerosis of autologous vein bypass graft(s) of the extremities

Use additional code, if applicable, to identify chronic total occlusion of artery of extremity (I70.92)

6ᵗʰ **I70.40** Unspecified atherosclerosis of autologous vein bypass graft(s) of the extremities

I70.401 Unspecified atherosclerosis of autologous vein bypass graft(s) of the extremities, right leg   A HCC RxHCC

I70.402 Unspecified atherosclerosis of autologous vein bypass graft(s) of the extremities, left leg   A HCC RxHCC

I70.403 Unspecified atherosclerosis of autologous vein bypass graft(s) of the extremities, bilateral legs   A HCC RxHCC

I70.408 Unspecified atherosclerosis of autologous vein bypass graft(s) of the extremities, other extremity   A HCC RxHCC

I70.409 Unspecified atherosclerosis of autologous vein bypass graft(s) of the extremities, unspecified extremity   A HCC RxHCC

6ᵗʰ **I70.41** Atherosclerosis of autologous vein bypass graft(s) of the extremities with intermittent claudication

I70.411 Atherosclerosis of autologous vein bypass graft(s) of the extremities with intermittent claudication, right leg   A HCC RxHCC

I70.412 Atherosclerosis of autologous vein bypass graft(s) of the extremities with intermittent claudication, left leg   A HCC RxHCC

I70.413 Atherosclerosis of autologous vein bypass graft(s) of the extremities with intermittent claudication, bilateral legs   A HCC RxHCC

I70.418 Atherosclerosis of autologous vein bypass graft(s) of the extremities with intermittent claudication, other extremity   A HCC RxHCC

I70.419 Atherosclerosis of autologous vein bypass graft(s) of the extremities with intermittent claudication, unspecified extremity   A HCC RxHCC

6ᵗʰ **I70.42** Atherosclerosis of autologous vein bypass graft(s) of the extremities with rest pain

INCLUDES   any condition classifiable to I70.41-

I70.421 Atherosclerosis of autologous vein bypass graft(s) of the extremities with rest pain, right leg   A HCC RxHCC

I70.422 Atherosclerosis of autologous vein bypass graft(s) of the extremities with rest pain, left leg   A HCC RxHCC

I70.423 Atherosclerosis of autologous vein bypass graft(s) of the extremities with rest pain, bilateral legs   A HCC RxHCC

I70.428 Atherosclerosis of autologous vein bypass graft(s) of the extremities with rest pain, other extremity   A HCC RxHCC

I70.429 Atherosclerosis of autologous vein bypass graft(s) of the extremities with rest pain, unspecified extremity   A HCC RxHCC

6ᵗʰ **I70.43** Atherosclerosis of autologous vein bypass graft(s) of the right leg with ulceration

INCLUDES   any condition classifiable to I70.411 and I70.421

Use additional code to identify severity of ulcer (L97.-)

I70.431 Atherosclerosis of autologous vein bypass graft(s) of the right leg with ulceration of thigh   A CC HCC PD₂ RxHCC CC/MCC Exc

I70.432 Atherosclerosis of autologous vein bypass graft(s) of the right leg with ulceration of calf   A CC HCC PD₂ RxHCC CC/MCC Exc

I70.433 Atherosclerosis of autologous vein bypass graft(s) of the right leg with ulceration of ankle   A CC HCC PD₂ RxHCC CC/MCC Exc

I70.434 Atherosclerosis of autologous vein bypass graft(s) of the right leg with ulceration of heel and midfoot   A CC HCC PD₂ RxHCC CC/MCC Exc

Atherosclerosis of autologous vein bypass graft(s) of right leg with ulceration of plantar surface of midfoot

I70.435 Atherosclerosis of autologous vein bypass graft(s) of the right leg with ulceration of other part of foot   A HCC RxHCC

Atherosclerosis of autologous vein bypass graft(s) of right leg with ulceration of toe

---

Unspecified Code   Other Specified Code   Manifestation Code   N Newborn   P Pediatric   M Maternity   A Adult   ♂ Male   ♀ Female
● New Code   ▲ Revised Code Title   ▶◀ Revised Text   NOTES   INCLUDES   EXCLUDES 1   Not coded here   EXCLUDES 2   Not included here
4ᵗʰ 4ᵗʰ character required   5ᵗʰ 5ᵗʰ character required   6ᵗʰ 6ᵗʰ character required   7ᵗʰ 7ᵗʰ character required
X Extension 'X' Alert   HAC Hospital-acquired condition (HAC) alert   AHA AHA Coding Clinic©

I70.438   Atherosclerosis of autologous vein bypass graft(s) of the right leg with ulceration of other part of lower leg [A] [C] [HCC] [RxHCC] [CC/MCC Exc]

I70.439   **Atherosclerosis of autologous vein bypass graft(s) of the left leg with ulceration of unspecified site** [A] [C] [HCC] [RxHCC] [CC/MCC Exc]

🔵 I70.44   Atherosclerosis of autologous vein bypass graft(s) of the left leg with ulceration

     INCLUDES   *any condition classifiable to I70.412 and I70.422*

     Use additional code to identify severity of ulcer (L97.-)

I70.441   Atherosclerosis of autologous vein bypass graft(s) of the left leg with ulceration of thigh [A] [C] [HCC] [RxHCC] [CC/MCC Exc]

I70.442   Atherosclerosis of autologous vein bypass graft(s) of the left leg with ulceration of calf [A] [C] [HCC] [RxHCC] [CC/MCC Exc]

I70.443   Atherosclerosis of autologous vein bypass graft(s) of the left leg with ulceration of ankle [A] [C] [HCC] [RxHCC] [CC/MCC Exc]

I70.444   Atherosclerosis of autologous vein bypass graft(s) of the left leg with ulceration of heel and midfoot [A] [C] [HCC] [RxHCC] [CC/MCC Exc]

     Atherosclerosis of autologous vein bypass graft(s) of left leg with ulceration of plantar surface of midfoot

I70.445   Atherosclerosis of autologous vein bypass graft(s) of the left leg with ulceration of other part of foot [A] [HCC] [RxHCC]

     Atherosclerosis of autologous vein bypass graft(s) of left leg with ulceration of toe

I70.448   Atherosclerosis of autologous vein bypass graft(s) of the left leg with ulceration of other part of lower leg [A] [C] [HCC] [RxHCC] [CC/MCC Exc]

I70.449   **Atherosclerosis of autologous vein bypass graft(s) of the left leg with ulceration of unspecified site** [A] [C] [HCC] [RxHCC] [CC/MCC Exc]

I70.45   Atherosclerosis of autologous vein bypass graft(s) of other extremity with ulceration [A] [HCC] [RxHCC]

     INCLUDES   *any condition classifiable to I70.418, I70.428, and I70.438*

     Use additional code to identify severity of ulcer (L98.49)

🔵 I70.46   Atherosclerosis of autologous vein bypass graft(s) of the extremities with gangrene

     INCLUDES   *any condition classifiable to I70.41-, I70.42-, and I70.43-, I70.44-, I70.45*

     Use additional code to identify the severity of any ulcer (L97.-, L98.49-), if applicable

I70.461   Atherosclerosis of autologous vein bypass graft(s) of the extremities with gangrene, right leg [A] [C] [HCC] [RxHCC] [CC/MCC Exc]

I70.462   Atherosclerosis of autologous vein bypass graft(s) of the extremities with gangrene, left leg [A] [C] [HCC] [RxHCC] [CC/MCC Exc]

I70.463   Atherosclerosis of autologous vein bypass graft(s) of the extremities with gangrene, bilateral legs [A] [C] [HCC] [RxHCC] [CC/MCC Exc]

I70.468   Atherosclerosis of autologous vein bypass graft(s) of the extremities with gangrene, other extremity [A] [C] [HCC] [RxHCC] [CC/MCC Exc]

I70.469   **Atherosclerosis of autologous vein bypass graft(s) of the extremities with gangrene, unspecified extremity** [A] [C] [HCC] [RxHCC] [CC/MCC Exc]

🔵 I70.49   Other atherosclerosis of autologous vein bypass graft(s) of the extremities

I70.491   Other atherosclerosis of autologous vein bypass graft(s) of the extremities, right leg [A] [HCC] [RxHCC]

I70.492   Other atherosclerosis of autologous vein bypass graft(s) of the extremities, left leg [A] [HCC] [RxHCC]

I70.493   Other atherosclerosis of autologous vein bypass graft(s) of the extremities, bilateral legs [A] [HCC] [RxHCC]

I70.498   Other atherosclerosis of autologous vein bypass graft(s) of the extremities, other extremity [A] [HCC] [RxHCC]

I70.499   **Other atherosclerosis of autologous vein bypass graft(s) of the extremities, unspecified extremity** [A] [HCC] [RxHCC]

🔵 I70.5   Atherosclerosis of nonautologous biological bypass graft(s) of the extremities

     Use additional code, if applicable, to identify chronic total occlusion of artery of extremity (I70.92)

🔵 I70.50   Unspecified atherosclerosis of nonautologous biological bypass graft(s) of the extremities

I70.501   **Unspecified atherosclerosis of nonautologous biological bypass graft(s) of the extremities, right leg** [A] [HCC] [RxHCC]

I70.502   **Unspecified atherosclerosis of nonautologous biological bypass graft(s) of the extremities, left leg** [A] [HCC] [RxHCC]

I70.503   **Unspecified atherosclerosis of nonautologous biological bypass graft(s) of the extremities, bilateral legs** [A] [HCC] [RxHCC]

I70.508   **Unspecified atherosclerosis of nonautologous biological bypass graft(s) of the extremities, other extremity** [A] [HCC] [RxHCC]

I70.509   **Unspecified atherosclerosis of nonautologous biological bypass graft(s) of the extremities, unspecified extremity** [A] [HCC] [RxHCC]

🔵 I70.51   Atherosclerosis of nonautologous biological bypass graft(s) of the extremities intermittent claudication

I70.511   Atherosclerosis of nonautologous biological bypass graft(s) of the extremities with intermittent claudication, right leg [A] [HCC] [RxHCC]

I70.512   Atherosclerosis of nonautologous biological bypass graft(s) of the extremities with intermittent claudication, left leg [A] [HCC] [RxHCC]

I70.513   Atherosclerosis of nonautologous biological bypass graft(s) of the extremities with intermittent claudication, bilateral legs [A] [HCC] [RxHCC]

I70.518   Atherosclerosis of nonautologous biological bypass graft(s) of the extremities with intermittent claudication, other extremity [A] [HCC] [RxHCC]

I70.519   **Atherosclerosis of nonautologous biological bypass graft(s) of the extremities with intermittent claudication, unspecified extremity** [A] [HCC] [RxHCC]

🔵 I70.52   Atherosclerosis of nonautologous biological bypass graft(s) of the extremities with rest pain

     INCLUDES   *any condition classifiable to I70.51-*

I70.521   Atherosclerosis of nonautologous biological bypass graft(s) of the extremities with rest pain, right leg [A] [HCC] [RxHCC]

I70.522   Atherosclerosis of nonautologous biological bypass graft(s) of the extremities with rest pain, left leg [A] [HCC] [RxHCC]

I70.523   Atherosclerosis of nonautologous biological bypass graft(s) of the extremities with rest pain, bilateral legs [A] [HCC] [RxHCC]

I70.528   Atherosclerosis of nonautologous biological bypass graft(s) of the extremities with rest pain, other extremity [A] [HCC] [RxHCC]

I70.529   **Atherosclerosis of nonautologous biological bypass graft(s) of the extremities with rest pain, unspecified extremity** [A] [HCC] [RxHCC]

Unacceptable principal diagnosis symbol per Medicare code edits   Code exempt from diagnosis present on admission requirement

? Questionable admission   Complication or comorbidity   CC/MCC exclusion   Major complication or comorbidity

Principal diagnosis as its own CC   Principal diagnosis as its own MCC   HCC HCC diagnosis code   RxHCC RxHCC diagnosis code

MACRA code   Z code as first-listed diagnosis

When symbols appear on a code that requires a 7th character extension, refer to Appendix B to identify applicable 7th character codes.

2018 ICD-10-CM

6ᵗʰ I70.53 Atherosclerosis of nonautologous biological bypass graft(s) of the right leg with ulceration

> INCLUDES   any condition classifiable to I70.511 and I70.521

Use additional code to identify severity of ulcer (L97.-)

I70.531 Atherosclerosis of nonautologous biological bypass graft(s) of the right leg with ulceration of thigh 🅰 ℅ HCC PDₓ RxHCC CC/MCC Exc

I70.532 Atherosclerosis of nonautologous biological bypass graft(s) of the right leg with ulceration of calf 🅰 ℅ HCC PDₓ RxHCC CC/MCC Exc

I70.533 Atherosclerosis of nonautologous biological bypass graft(s) of the right leg with ulceration of ankle 🅰 ℅ HCC PDₓ RxHCC CC/MCC Exc

I70.534 Atherosclerosis of nonautologous biological bypass graft(s) of the right leg with ulceration of heel and midfoot 🅰 ℅ HCC PDₓ RxHCC CC/MCC Exc

Atherosclerosis of nonautologous biological bypass graft(s) of right leg with ulceration of plantar surface of midfoot

I70.535 Atherosclerosis of nonautologous biological bypass graft(s) of the right leg with ulceration of other part of foot 🅰 HCC RxHCC

Atherosclerosis of nonautologous biological bypass graft(s) of the right leg with ulceration of toe

I70.538 Atherosclerosis of nonautologous biological bypass graft(s) of the right leg with ulceration of other part of lower leg 🅰 ℅ HCC PDₓ RxHCC CC/MCC Exc

I70.539 Atherosclerosis of nonautologous biological bypass graft(s) of the right leg with ulceration of unspecified site 🅰 ℅ HCC PDₓ RxHCC CC/MCC Exc

6ᵗʰ I70.54 Atherosclerosis of nonautologous biological bypass graft(s) of the left leg with ulceration

> INCLUDES   any condition classifiable to I70.512 and I70.522

Use additional code to identify severity of ulcer (L97.-)

I70.541 Atherosclerosis of nonautologous biological bypass graft(s) of the left leg with ulceration of thigh 🅰 ℅ HCC PDₓ RxHCC CC/MCC Exc

I70.542 Atherosclerosis of nonautologous biological bypass graft(s) of the left leg with ulceration of calf 🅰 ℅ HCC PDₓ RxHCC CC/MCC Exc

I70.543 Atherosclerosis of nonautologous biological bypass graft(s) of the left leg with ulceration of ankle 🅰 ℅ HCC PDₓ RxHCC CC/MCC Exc

I70.544 Atherosclerosis of nonautologous biological bypass graft(s) of the left leg with ulceration of heel and midfoot 🅰 ℅ HCC PDₓ RxHCC CC/MCC Exc

Atherosclerosis of nonautologous biological bypass graft(s) of left leg with ulceration of plantar surface of midfoot

I70.545 Atherosclerosis of nonautologous biological bypass graft(s) of the left leg with ulceration of other part of foot 🅰 HCC RxHCC

Atherosclerosis of nonautologous biological bypass graft(s) of the left leg with ulceration of toe

I70.548 Atherosclerosis of nonautologous biological bypass graft(s) of the left leg with ulceration of other part of lower leg 🅰 ℅ HCC PDₓ RxHCC CC/MCC Exc

I70.549 Atherosclerosis of nonautologous biological bypass graft(s) of the left leg with ulceration of unspecified site 🅰 ℅ HCC PDₓ RxHCC CC/MCC Exc

I70.55 Atherosclerosis of nonautologous biological bypass graft(s) of other extremity with ulceration 🅰 HCC RxHCC

> INCLUDES   any condition classifiable to I70.518, I70.528, and I70.538

Use additional code to identify severity of ulcer (L98.49)

6ᵗʰ I70.56 Atherosclerosis of nonautologous biological bypass graft(s) of the extremities with gangrene

> INCLUDES   any condition classifiable to I70.51-, I70.52-, and I70.53-, I70.54-, I70.55

Use additional code to identify the severity of any ulcer (L97.-, L98.49-), if applicable

I70.561 Atherosclerosis of nonautologous biological bypass graft(s) of the extremities with gangrene, right leg 🅰 ℅ HCC PDₓ CC/MCC Exc

I70.562 Atherosclerosis of nonautologous biological bypass graft(s) of the extremities with gangrene, left leg 🅰 ℅ HCC PDₓ CC/MCC Exc

I70.563 Atherosclerosis of nonautologous biological bypass graft(s) of the extremities with gangrene, bilateral legs 🅰 ℅ HCC PDₓ CC/MCC Exc

I70.568 Atherosclerosis of nonautologous biological bypass graft(s) of the extremities with gangrene, other extremity 🅰 ℅ HCC PDₓ CC/MCC Exc

I70.569 Atherosclerosis of nonautologous biological bypass graft(s) of the extremities with gangrene, unspecified extremity 🅰 ℅ HCC PDₓ CC/MCC Exc

6ᵗʰ I70.59 Other atherosclerosis of nonautologous biological bypass graft(s) of the extremities

I70.591 Other atherosclerosis of nonautologous biological bypass graft(s) of the extremities, right leg 🅰 HCC RxHCC

I70.592 Other atherosclerosis of nonautologous biological bypass graft(s) of the extremities, left leg 🅰 HCC RxHCC

I70.593 Other atherosclerosis of nonautologous biological bypass graft(s) of the extremities, bilateral legs 🅰 HCC RxHCC

I70.598 Other atherosclerosis of nonautologous biological bypass graft(s) of the extremities, other extremity 🅰 HCC RxHCC

I70.599 Other atherosclerosis of nonautologous biological bypass graft(s) of the extremities, unspecified extremity 🅰 HCC RxHCC

5ᵗʰ I70.6 Atherosclerosis of nonbiological bypass graft(s) of the extremities

Use additional code, if applicable, to identify chronic total occlusion of artery of extremity (I70.92)

6ᵗʰ I70.60 Unspecified atherosclerosis of nonbiological bypass graft(s) of the extremities

I70.601 Unspecified atherosclerosis of nonbiological bypass graft(s) of the extremities, right leg 🅰 HCC RxHCC

I70.602 Unspecified atherosclerosis of nonbiological bypass graft(s) of the extremities, left leg 🅰 HCC RxHCC

I70.603 Unspecified atherosclerosis of nonbiological bypass graft(s) of the extremities, bilateral legs 🅰 HCC RxHCC

I70.608 Unspecified atherosclerosis of nonbiological bypass graft(s) of the extremities, other extremity 🅰 HCC RxHCC

Unspecified Code   Other Specified Code   Manifestation Code   Ⓝ Newborn   Ⓟ Pediatric   Ⓜ Maternity   🅰 Adult   ♂ Male   ♀ Female
   ● New Code   ▲ Revised Code Title   ▶◀ Revised Text   **NOTES**   *INCLUDES*   *EXCLUDES 1* Not coded here   *EXCLUDES 2* Not included here
      4ᵗʰ 4ᵗʰ character required   5ᵗʰ 5ᵗʰ character required   6ᵗʰ 6ᵗʰ character required   7ᵗʰ 7ᵗʰ character required
         Extension 'X' Alert   HAC Hospital-acquired condition (HAC) alert   **AHA** AHA Coding Clinic©

I82.493 **Acute embolism and thrombosis of other specified deep vein of lower extremity, bilateral** [CC] [HAC] [HCC] [RxHCC] [CC/MCC Exc]

I82.499 **Acute embolism and thrombosis of other specified deep vein of unspecified lower extremity** [CC] [HAC] [HCC] [RxHCC] [CC/MCC Exc]

[6th] I82.4Y **Acute embolism and thrombosis of unspecified deep veins of proximal lower extremity**

Acute embolism and thrombosis of deep vein of thigh NOS

Acute embolism and thrombosis of deep vein of upper leg NOS

I82.4Y1 **Acute embolism and thrombosis of unspecified deep veins of right proximal lower extremity** [CC] [HAC] [HCC] [RxHCC] [CC/MCC Exc]

I82.4Y2 **Acute embolism and thrombosis of unspecified deep veins of left proximal lower extremity** [CC] [HAC] [HCC] [RxHCC] [CC/MCC Exc]

I82.4Y3 **Acute embolism and thrombosis of unspecified deep veins of proximal lower extremity, bilateral** [CC] [HAC] [HCC] [RxHCC] [CC/MCC Exc]

I82.4Y9 **Acute embolism and thrombosis of unspecified deep veins of unspecified proximal lower extremity** [CC] [HAC] [HCC] [RxHCC] [CC/MCC Exc]

[6th] I82.4Z **Acute embolism and thrombosis of unspecified deep veins of distal lower extremity**

Acute embolism and thrombosis of deep vein of calf NOS

Acute embolism and thrombosis of deep vein of lower leg NOS

I82.4Z1 **Acute embolism and thrombosis of unspecified deep veins of right distal lower extremity** [CC] [HAC] [HCC] [RxHCC] [CC/MCC Exc]

I82.4Z2 **Acute embolism and thrombosis of unspecified deep veins of left distal lower extremity** [CC] [HAC] [HCC] [RxHCC] [CC/MCC Exc]

I82.4Z3 **Acute embolism and thrombosis of unspecified deep veins of distal lower extremity, bilateral** [CC] [HAC] [HCC] [RxHCC] [CC/MCC Exc]

I82.4Z9 **Acute embolism and thrombosis of unspecified deep veins of unspecified distal lower extremity** [CC] [HAC] [HCC] [RxHCC] [CC/MCC Exc]

[5th] I82.5 **Chronic embolism and thrombosis of deep veins of lower extremity**

Use additional code, if applicable, for associated long-term (current) use of anticoagulants (Z79.01)

[EXCLUDES1] *personal history of venous embolism and thrombosis (Z86.718)*

[6th] I82.50 **Chronic embolism and thrombosis of unspecified deep veins of lower extremity**

[EXCLUDES1] *chronic embolism and thrombosis of unspecified deep veins of distal lower extremity (I82.5Z-)*

chronic embolism and thrombosis of unspecified deep veins of proximal lower extremity (I82.5Y-)

I82.501 **Chronic embolism and thrombosis of unspecified deep veins of right lower extremity** [CC] [HCC] [RxHCC] [CC/MCC Exc]

I82.502 **Chronic embolism and thrombosis of unspecified deep veins of left lower extremity** [CC] [HCC] [RxHCC] [CC/MCC Exc]

I82.503 **Chronic embolism and thrombosis of unspecified deep veins of lower extremity, bilateral** [CC] [HCC] [RxHCC] [CC/MCC Exc]

I82.509 **Chronic embolism and thrombosis of unspecified deep veins of unspecified lower extremity** [CC] [HCC] [RxHCC] [CC/MCC Exc]

[6th] I82.51 **Chronic embolism and thrombosis of femoral vein**

I82.511 **Chronic embolism and thrombosis of right femoral vein** [CC] [HCC] [RxHCC] [CC/MCC Exc]

I82.512 **Chronic embolism and thrombosis of left femoral vein** [CC] [HCC] [RxHCC] [CC/MCC Exc]

I82.513 **Chronic embolism and thrombosis of femoral vein, bilateral** [CC] [HCC] [RxHCC] [CC/MCC Exc]

I82.519 **Chronic embolism and thrombosis of unspecified femoral vein** [CC] [HCC] [RxHCC] [CC/MCC Exc]

[6th] I82.52 **Chronic embolism and thrombosis of iliac vein**

I82.521 **Chronic embolism and thrombosis of right iliac vein** [CC] [HCC] [RxHCC] [CC/MCC Exc]

I82.522 **Chronic embolism and thrombosis of left iliac vein** [CC] [HCC] [RxHCC] [CC/MCC Exc]

I82.523 **Chronic embolism and thrombosis of iliac vein, bilateral** [CC] [HCC] [RxHCC] [CC/MCC Exc]

I82.529 **Chronic embolism and thrombosis of unspecified iliac vein** [CC] [HCC] [RxHCC] [CC/MCC Exc]

[6th] I82.53 **Chronic embolism and thrombosis of popliteal vein**

I82.531 **Chronic embolism and thrombosis of right popliteal vein** [CC] [HCC] [RxHCC] [CC/MCC Exc]

I82.532 **Chronic embolism and thrombosis of left popliteal vein** [CC] [HCC] [RxHCC] [CC/MCC Exc]

I82.533 **Chronic embolism and thrombosis of popliteal vein, bilateral** [CC] [HCC] [RxHCC] [CC/MCC Exc]

I82.539 **Chronic embolism and thrombosis of unspecified popliteal vein** [CC] [HCC] [RxHCC] [CC/MCC Exc]

[6th] I82.54 **Chronic embolism and thrombosis of tibial vein**

I82.541 **Chronic embolism and thrombosis of right tibial vein** [CC] [HCC] [RxHCC] [CC/MCC Exc]

I82.542 **Chronic embolism and thrombosis of left tibial vein** [CC] [HCC] [RxHCC] [CC/MCC Exc]

I82.543 **Chronic embolism and thrombosis of tibial vein, bilateral** [CC] [HCC] [RxHCC] [CC/MCC Exc]

I82.549 **Chronic embolism and thrombosis of unspecified tibial vein** [CC] [HCC] [RxHCC] [CC/MCC Exc]

[6th] I82.59 **Chronic embolism and thrombosis of other specified deep vein of lower extremity**

I82.591 **Chronic embolism and thrombosis of other specified deep vein of right lower extremity** [CC] [HCC] [RxHCC] [CC/MCC Exc]

I82.592 **Chronic embolism and thrombosis of other specified deep vein of left lower extremity** [CC] [HCC] [RxHCC] [CC/MCC Exc]

I82.593 **Chronic embolism and thrombosis of other specified deep vein of lower extremity, bilateral** [CC] [HCC] [RxHCC] [CC/MCC Exc]

I82.599 **Chronic embolism and thrombosis of other specified deep vein of unspecified lower extremity** [CC] [HCC] [RxHCC] [CC/MCC Exc]

[6th] I82.5Y **Chronic embolism and thrombosis of unspecified deep veins of proximal lower extremity**

Chronic embolism and thrombosis of deep veins of thigh NOS

Chronic embolism and thrombosis of deep veins of upper leg NOS

I82.5Y1 **Chronic embolism and thrombosis of unspecified deep veins of right proximal lower extremity** [CC] [HCC] [RxHCC] [CC/MCC Exc]

I82.5Y2 **Chronic embolism and thrombosis of unspecified deep veins of left proximal lower extremity** [CC] [HCC] [RxHCC] [CC/MCC Exc]

I82.5Y3 **Chronic embolism and thrombosis of unspecified deep veins of proximal lower extremity, bilateral** [CC] [HCC] [RxHCC] [CC/MCC Exc]

I82.5Y9 **Chronic embolism and thrombosis of unspecified deep veins of unspecified proximal lower extremity** [CC] [HCC] [RxHCC] [CC/MCC Exc]

[6th] I82.5Z **Chronic embolism and thrombosis of unspecified deep veins of distal lower extremity**

Chronic embolism and thrombosis of deep veins of calf NOS

Chronic embolism and thrombosis of deep veins of lower leg NOS

I82.5Z1 **Chronic embolism and thrombosis of unspecified deep veins of right distal lower extremity** [CC] [HCC] [RxHCC] [CC/MCC Exc]

[PDx] Unacceptable principal diagnosis symbol per Medicare code edits [POA] Code exempt from diagnosis present on admission requirement
[?] Questionable admission [CC] Complication or comorbidity [CC/MCC Exc] CC/MCC exclusion [MCC] Major complication or comorbidity
[PDx CC] Principal diagnosis as its own CC [PDx MCC] Principal diagnosis as its own MCC [HCC] HCC diagnosis code [RxHCC] RxHCC diagnosis code
MACRA code [Z1] Z code as first-listed diagnosis

 When symbols appear on a code that requires a 7th character extension, refer to Appendix B to identify applicable 7th character codes.

I82.5Z2 **Chronic embolism and thrombosis of unspecified deep veins of** left **distal lower extremity** cc HCC RxHCC CC/MCC Exc

I82.5Z3 **Chronic embolism and thrombosis of unspecified deep veins of distal lower extremity,** bilateral cc HCC RxHCC CC/MCC Exc

I82.5Z9 **Chronic embolism and thrombosis of unspecified deep veins of unspecified distal lower extremity** HCC RxHCC CC/MCC Exc

🄳 I82.6 **Acute** embolism and thrombosis of veins of upper extremity

🄴 I82.60 **Acute embolism and thrombosis of** unspecified **veins of upper extremity**

I82.601 **Acute embolism and thrombosis of unspecified veins of** right **upper extremity** cc CC/MCC Exc

I82.602 **Acute embolism and thrombosis of unspecified veins of** left **upper extremity** cc CC/MCC Exc

I82.603 **Acute embolism and thrombosis of unspecified veins of upper extremity,** bilateral cc CC/MCC Exc

I82.609 **Acute embolism and thrombosis of unspecified veins of unspecified upper extremity** cc CC/MCC Exc

🄴 I82.61 **Acute embolism and thrombosis of** superficial **veins of upper extremity**

Acute embolism and thrombosis of antecubital vein
Acute embolism and thrombosis of basilic vein
Acute embolism and thrombosis of cephalic vein

I82.611 **Acute embolism and thrombosis of superficial veins of** right **upper extremity** cc CC/MCC Exc

I82.612 **Acute embolism and thrombosis of superficial veins of** left **upper extremity** cc CC/MCC Exc

I82.613 **Acute embolism and thrombosis of superficial veins of upper extremity,** bilateral cc CC/MCC Exc

I82.619 **Acute embolism and thrombosis of superficial veins of unspecified upper extremity** cc CC/MCC Exc

🄴 I82.62 **Acute embolism and thrombosis of** deep **veins of upper extremity**

Acute embolism and thrombosis of brachial vein
Acute embolism and thrombosis of radial vein
Acute embolism and thrombosis of ulnar vein

I82.621 **Acute embolism and thrombosis of deep veins of** right **upper extremity** cc HCC RxHCC CC/MCC Exc

I82.622 **Acute embolism and thrombosis of deep veins of** left **upper extremity** cc HCC RxHCC CC/MCC Exc

I82.623 **Acute embolism and thrombosis of deep veins of upper extremity,** bilateral cc HCC RxHCC CC/MCC Exc

I82.629 **Acute embolism and thrombosis of deep veins of unspecified upper extremity** cc HCC RxHCC CC/MCC Exc

🄳 I82.7 **Chronic** embolism and thrombosis of veins of upper extremity

Use additional code, if applicable, for associated long-term (current) use of anticoagulants (Z79.01)

EXCLUDES1 *personal history of venous embolism and thrombosis (Z86.718)*

🄴 I82.70 **Chronic embolism and thrombosis of** unspecified **veins of upper extremity**

I82.701 **Chronic embolism and thrombosis of unspecified veins of** right **upper extremity** cc CC/MCC Exc

I82.702 **Chronic embolism and thrombosis of unspecified veins of** left **upper extremity** cc CC/MCC Exc

I82.703 **Chronic embolism and thrombosis of unspecified veins of upper extremity,** bilateral cc CC/MCC Exc

I82.709 **Chronic embolism and thrombosis of unspecified veins of unspecified upper extremity** cc CC/MCC Exc

🄴 I82.71 **Chronic embolism and thrombosis of** superficial **veins of upper extremity**

Chronic embolism and thrombosis of antecubital vein
Chronic embolism and thrombosis of basilic vein
Chronic embolism and thrombosis of cephalic vein

I82.711 **Chronic embolism and thrombosis of superficial veins of** right **upper extremity** cc CC/MCC Exc

I82.712 **Chronic embolism and thrombosis of superficial veins of** left **upper extremity** cc CC/MCC Exc

I82.713 **Chronic embolism and thrombosis of superficial veins of upper extremity,** bilateral cc CC/MCC Exc

I82.719 **Chronic embolism and thrombosis of superficial veins of unspecified upper extremity** cc CC/MCC Exc

🄴 I82.72 **Chronic embolism and thrombosis of** deep **veins of upper extremity**

Chronic embolism and thrombosis of brachial vein
Chronic embolism and thrombosis of radial vein
Chronic embolism and thrombosis of ulnar vein

I82.721 **Chronic embolism and thrombosis of deep veins of** right **upper extremity** cc HCC RxHCC CC/MCC Exc

I82.722 **Chronic embolism and thrombosis of deep veins of** left **upper extremity** cc HCC RxHCC CC/MCC Exc

I82.723 **Chronic embolism and thrombosis of deep veins of upper extremity,** bilateral cc HCC RxHCC CC/MCC Exc

I82.729 **Chronic embolism and thrombosis of deep veins of unspecified upper extremity** cc HCC RxHCC CC/MCC Exc

🄳 I82.A **Embolism and thrombosis of** axillary vein

🄴 I82.A1 **Acute** embolism and thrombosis of axillary vein

I82.A11 **Acute embolism and thrombosis of** right **axillary vein** cc HCC RxHCC CC/MCC Exc

I82.A12 **Acute embolism and thrombosis of** left **axillary vein** cc HCC RxHCC CC/MCC Exc

I82.A13 **Acute embolism and thrombosis of axillary vein,** bilateral cc HCC RxHCC CC/MCC Exc

I82.A19 **Acute embolism and thrombosis of unspecified axillary vein** cc HCC RxHCC CC/MCC Exc

🄴 I82.A2 **Chronic** embolism and thrombosis of axillary vein

I82.A21 **Chronic embolism and thrombosis of** right **axillary vein** cc HCC RxHCC CC/MCC Exc

I82.A22 **Chronic embolism and thrombosis of** left **axillary vein** cc HCC RxHCC CC/MCC Exc

I82.A23 **Chronic embolism and thrombosis of axillary vein,** bilateral cc HCC RxHCC CC/MCC Exc

I82.A29 **Chronic embolism and thrombosis of unspecified axillary vein** cc HCC RxHCC CC/MCC Exc

🄳 I82.B **Embolism and thrombosis of** subclavian vein

🄴 I82.B1 **Acute** embolism and thrombosis of subclavian vein

I82.B11 **Acute embolism and thrombosis of** right **subclavian vein** cc HCC RxHCC CC/MCC Exc

I82.B12 **Acute embolism and thrombosis of** left **subclavian vein** cc HCC RxHCC CC/MCC Exc

I82.B13 **Acute embolism and thrombosis of subclavian vein,** bilateral cc HCC RxHCC CC/MCC Exc

I82.B19 **Acute embolism and thrombosis of unspecified subclavian vein** cc HCC RxHCC CC/MCC Exc

🄴 I82.B2 **Chronic** embolism and thrombosis of subclavian vein

I82.B21 **Chronic embolism and thrombosis of** right **subclavian vein** cc HCC RxHCC CC/MCC Exc

---

| Unspecified Code | Other Specified Code | Manifestation Code | N Newborn | P Pediatric | M Maternity | A Adult | ♂ Male | ♀ Female |

● New Code ▲ Revised Code Title ►◄ Revised Text **NOTES** *INCLUDES* *EXCLUDES 1* Not coded here *EXCLUDES 2* Not included here

🄴 4th character required 🄳 5th character required 🄵 6th character required 🄶 7th character required

🄾 Extension 'X' Alert **HAC** Hospital-acquired condition (HAC) alert **AHA** AHA Coding Clinic©

NOTES

Chapter 10: Diseases of the Respiratory System (J00-J99)
Anatomy of the Respiratory System

1. **An Outline of the Respiratory System**
   a) The human respiratory system is based on the following organs:
      i) nose
      ii) pharynx
      iii) larynx
      iv) trachea
      v) bronchi
      vi) lungs
   b) The process of respiration involves the exchange of oxygen and carbon dioxide between the atmosphere, blood and cells.

The Respiratory System

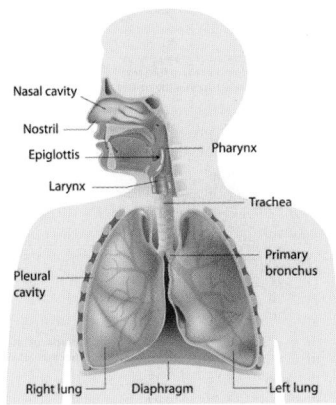

2. **The Anatomy of the Nose**
   a) The nostrils or external nares are openings into the external nose.
   b) The internal nares serve to connect the internal nose with the throat or pharynx.
   c) The nasal septum divides the nose into the right and left nasal cavities.
   d) The internal nose contains three turbinate bones (superior, middle and inferior meatus).
   e) The olfactory receptors are located in the superior meatus.

3. **The Anatomy of the Pharynx**
   a) The pharynx is a resonating chamber for speech sounds and also provides a passage to both air and food.
   b) The nasopharynx, oropharynx and laryngopharynx are the parts of the pharynx.
   c) The nasopharynx surrounds the pharyngeal tonsils. It contains two internal nares and the openings of the eustachian tubes.
   d) The oropharynx surrounds the palatine and lingual tonsils and its opening (or fauces) provides connection to the mouth.
   e) The laryngopharynx gets connected with the larynx on anterior aspect and the esophagus posteriorly.

4. **The Anatomy of the Larynx**
   a) The larynx is also known as the voice box.
   b) The skeleton of the larynx is made up of nine cartilages. Three of them are single (thyroid, cricoid, and epiglottis) and the remaining three (arytenoid, corniculate, and cuneiform) are paired cartilages.
   c) The thyroid cartilage is also known as the Adam's apple. It is the largest single cartilage of the laryngeal skeleton.
   d) The cricoid cartilage connects with the first tracheal ring and is made up of a single ring of cartilage.
   e) The epiglottis is a large and single leaf-shaped flap of elastic cartilage. It is lined with the mucous membrane and remains attached to the entrance of larynx. It pulls down over the glottis during the process of swallowing to obstruct the entrance of the fluids and food in the trachea.
   f) The arytenoid cartilages are formed by a pair of three ladle-shaped pyramids that remain attached to the laryngeal muscles and the vocal cords.

   g) The corniculate cartilages are based on two cone-shaped nodules of yellow elastic cartilage.
   h) The cuneiform cartilages are also known as the cartilages of Wrisberg. They are based on two rod-shaped pieces of yellow elastic cartilage.
   i) The mucous membrane of the larynx is divided into two pairs of folds. The vestibular folds (or false vocal cords) constitute the upper pair, while the vocal folds (or true vocal cords) form the lower pair of fold.
   j) The opening over the true vocal cords is known as the glottis.

5. **The Anatomy of the Trachea**
   a) The trachea is also known as the windpipe and located anteriorly to the esophagus.
   b) It begins at the larynx and gets divided into primary bronchi at the level of T4/T5 vertebrae.
   c) The trachea is lined by the respiratory epithelium and consists of a series of incomplete C-shaped cartilaginous rings.

6. **The Anatomy of the Bronchial Tree**
   a) The bronchial tree is based on right and left primary bronchi, secondary and tertiary bronchi, and the bronchioles.
   b) The right and left primary bronchi emanate from the trachea and merge with the right and left lungs.
   c) The primary bronchi further get branched into the secondary (or lobar) bronchi that penetrate into the lobes of the lungs.
   d) The secondary bronchi further get divided into the tertiary or segmental bronchi that penetrate into the segments of the lobes of the lungs.
   e) The bronchioles are the branches that emanate from the tertiary bronchi.

7. **The Anatomy of the Lungs**
   a) The lungs are the human organs of respiration.
   b) The right and left lungs are based on multiple lobes. The right lung contains three lobes, while the left lung is based on two lobes.
   c) The lungs are protected by the pleural membrane. The pleural membrane is further made up of two layers of serous membranes. The outer layer is known as the parietal pleura, while the inner layer is termed as the visceral pleura.
   d) The bronchopulmonary segment is a segment of lung tissue that is supplied by each of the tertiary bronchi. It is divided into multiple lobules that remain covered with the elastic connective tissue.
   e) A terminal bronchiole exists at the end of the conducting zone of the respiratory system.
   f) The microscopic respiratory bronchioles are the subdivisions of the terminal bronchioles. The atria or the alveolar ducts emanate from these respiratory bronchioles.
   g) The alveoli and alveolar sacs lie around the circumference of the alveolar ducts.
   h) The alveolar sac is made up of two or more alveoli with a common opening.
   i) The respiratory (or the alveolar capillary) membrane is a membrane that provides a medium for the movement of respiratory gases.

8. **The Process of Respiration**
   a) The respiration in humans is based on the following stages:
      i) Ventilation is also known as the breathing, which involves the movement of the ambient air into the alveoli of the lungs.
      ii) The process of pulmonary gas exchange is based on the exchange of respiratory gases between the alveoli and the pulmonary capillaries.
      iii) The gas process involves the transport of respiratory gases from the pulmonary capillaries to the peripheral capillaries in the organs via circulation.
      iv) Peripheral gas exchange is the process of exchange of respiratory gases between the tissue capillaries and the cells and mitochondria.
   b) Nasal breathing is the process of respiration that involves the inhalation and exhalation of the respiratory gases through the nose.

Common Pathologies

Sinusitis
Inflammation of mucous membrane lining that lines the paranasal sinuses. This inflammation dries out the sinuses and can also cause dizziness and difficulty breathing. Using a humidifier can alleviate symptoms

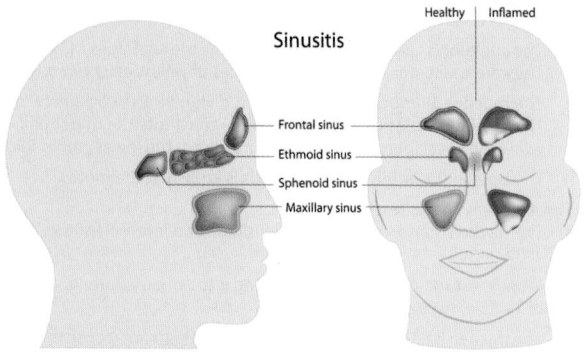

Epiglottitis
Inflammation of the epiglottis caused by H. Influenzae type B; characterized by fever and a severe sore throat and difficulty in swallowing.

Laryngitis
Inflammation of the larynx and vocal cords resulting in hoarseness of the voice (Dysphonia), and difficulty in swallowing (Dysphagia).

Pharyngitis
Inflammation of the pharynx, usually causing a sore throat. Acute Pharyngitis is a sudden, severe inflammation of the pharynx. Chronic Pharyngitis is a persistent throat inflammation that may be associated with the lymphoid granules in the pharyngeal mucosa.

Acute Bronchitis
Inflammation of the mucous membrane lining the bronchus, involves the trachea resulting in tracheobronchitis, chest tightness, fever, and a cough that progresses from nonproductive to productive.

Chronic Bronchitis
Inflammation of the bronchial mucous membrane characterized by cough, hyper-secretion of mucus, and expectoration of sputum over a long period of time and associated with increased vulnerability to bronchial infection.

Influenza
Influenza is a highly infectious respiratory disease. The disease is caused by certain strains of the influenza virus.

Pneumonia
Pneumonia is an infection of the lung that can be caused by nearly any class of organism known to cause human infections. These include bacteria, amoebae, viruses, fungi, and parasites.

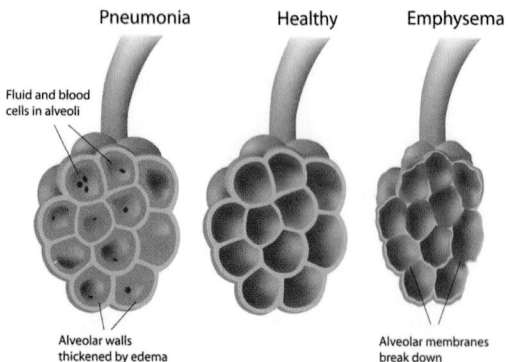

Pulmonary Abscess
Lung abscess that is a collection of infectious material contained within a capsule in the lung, which results in coughing of bloody or foul-smelling sputum (breath foul-smelling). The most important preventative measure to avoid pulmonary abscess is to prevent aspiration.

Pulmonary TB
Pulmonary tuberculosis is an infection (inflammation) caused by mycobacterium tuberculosis.Pathologic changes depend on the type of infection or "exposure" given below:Primary pulmonary TB (Primary Exposure), Secondary pulmonary TB(Reactivation) and Progressive pulmonary TB.

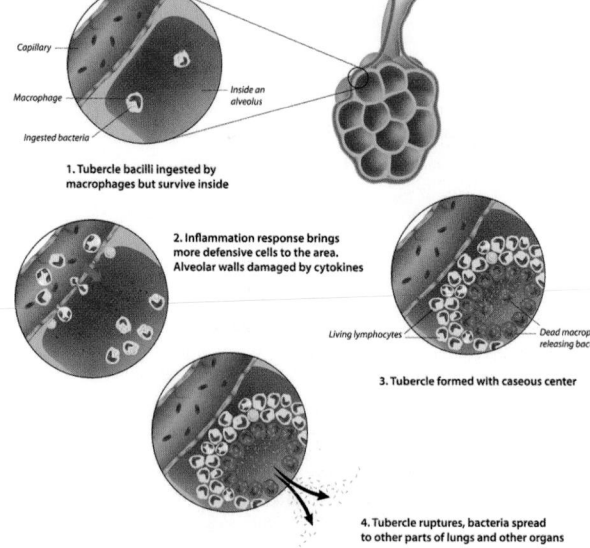

Asthma
Asthma is a common chronic inflammatory disease of the airways characterized by variable and recurring symptoms, reversible airflow obstruction, and bronchospasm. Common symptoms include wheezing, coughing, chest tightness, and shortness of breath.

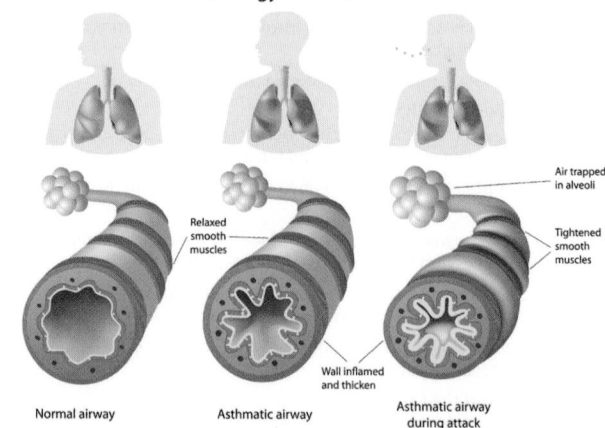

Cystic Fibrosis
Cystic Fibrosis is an autosomal recessive genetic disorder that affects most critically the lungs, and also the pancreas, liver, and intestine. It is characterized by abnormal transport of chloride and sodium across an epithelium, leading to thick, viscous secretions.

CHAPTER 10: DISEASES OF THE RESPIRATORY SYSTEM (J00-J99)

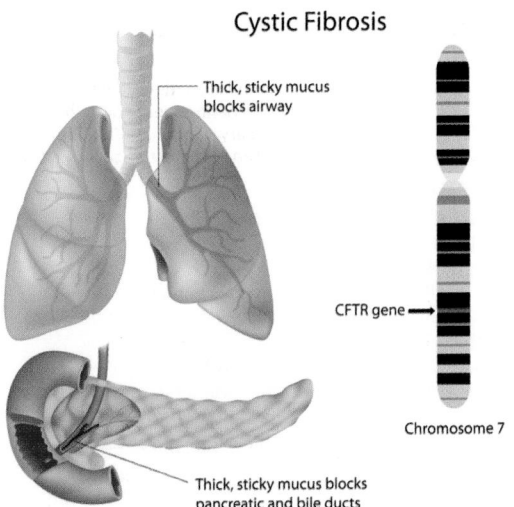

Cystic Fibrosis

Thick, sticky mucus blocks airway

CFTR gene →

Chromosome 7

Thick, sticky mucus blocks pancreatic and bile ducts

Chronic Obstructive Pulmonary Disease (COPD)
Chronic obstructive pulmonary disease (COPD) is a lung disease characterized by chronic obstruction of lung airflow that interferes with normal breathing and is not fully reversible. The more familiar terms 'chronic bronchitis' and 'emphysema' are no longer used, but are now included within the COPD diagnosis.

Emphysema
Emphysema is a chronic lung disease caused by damage to the alveoli, the tiny air sacs in the lung where exchange of oxygen and carbon dioxide takes place. With emphysema, damage to the alveoli results in air becoming trapped, causing them to expand and rupture.

Bronchiectasis
Bronchiectasis is a disease state defined by localized, irreversible dilation of part of the bronchial tree caused by destruction of the muscle and elastic tissue. It is classified as an obstructive lung disease, along with emphysema, bronchitis, asthma, and cystic fibrosis.

Diseases of the respiratory system (J00-J99)

[NOTES] When a respiratory condition is described as occurring in more than one site and is not specifically indexed, it should be classified to the lower anatomic site (e.g. tracheobronchitis to bronchitis in J40).

Use additional code, where applicable, to identify:
exposure to environmental tobacco smoke (Z77.22)
exposure to tobacco smoke in the perinatal period (P96.81)
history of tobacco dependence (Z87.891)
occupational exposure to environmental tobacco smoke (Z57.31)
tobacco dependence (F17.-)
tobacco use (Z72.0)

[EXCLUDES2] *certain conditions originating in the perinatal period (P04-P96)*
certain infectious and parasitic diseases (A00-B99)
complications of pregnancy, childbirth and the puerperium (O00-O9A)
congenital malformations, deformations and chromosomal abnormalities (Q00-Q99)
endocrine, nutritional and metabolic diseases (E00-E88)
injury, poisoning and certain other consequences of external causes (S00-T88)
neoplasms (C00-D49)
smoke inhalation (T59.81-)
symptoms, signs and abnormal clinical and laboratory findings, not elsewhere classified (R00-R94)

This chapter contains the following blocks:

J00-J06	Acute upper respiratory infections
J09-J18	Influenza and pneumonia
J20-J22	Other acute lower respiratory infections
J30-J39	Other diseases of upper respiratory tract
J40-J47	Chronic lower respiratory diseases
J60-J70	Lung diseases due to external agents
J80-J84	Other respiratory diseases principally affecting the interstitium
J85-J86	Suppurative and necrotic conditions of the lower respiratory tract
J90-J94	Other diseases of the pleura
J95	Intraoperative and postprocedural complications and disorders of respiratory system, not elsewhere classified
J96-J99	Other diseases of the respiratory system

Acute upper respiratory infections (J00-J06)

[EXCLUDES1] *chronic obstructive pulmonary disease with acute lower respiratory infection (J44.0)*
influenza virus with other respiratory manifestations (J09.X2, J10.1, J11.1)

J00 Acute nasopharyngitis [common cold]
Acute rhinitis
Coryza (acute)
Infective nasopharyngitis NOS
Infective rhinitis
Nasal catarrh, acute
Nasopharyngitis NOS
[EXCLUDES1] *acute pharyngitis (J02.-)*
acute sore throat NOS (J02.9)
pharyngitis NOS (J02.9)
rhinitis NOS (J31.0)
sore throat NOS (J02.9)
[EXCLUDES2] *allergic rhinitis (J30.1-J30.9)*
chronic pharyngitis (J31.2)
chronic rhinitis (J31.0)
chronic sore throat (J31.2)
nasopharyngitis, chronic (J31.1)
vasomotor rhinitis (J30.0)

[4th] **J01 Acute sinusitis**
[INCLUDES] *acute abscess of sinus*
acute empyema of sinus
acute infection of sinus
acute inflammation of sinus
acute suppuration of sinus
Use additional code (B95-B97) to identify infectious agent.
[EXCLUDES1] *sinusitis NOS (J32.9)*
[EXCLUDES2] *chronic sinusitis (J32.0-J32.8)*

[5th] **J01.0 Acute maxillary sinusitis**
Acute antritis
J01.00 Acute maxillary sinusitis, unspecified
J01.01 Acute recurrent maxillary sinusitis

[5th] **J01.1 Acute frontal sinusitis**
J01.10 Acute frontal sinusitis, unspecified
J01.11 Acute recurrent frontal sinusitis

[5th] **J01.2 Acute ethmoidal sinusitis**
J01.20 Acute ethmoidal sinusitis, unspecified
J01.21 Acute recurrent ethmoidal sinusitis

[5th] **J01.3 Acute sphenoidal sinusitis**
J01.30 Acute sphenoidal sinusitis, unspecified
J01.31 Acute recurrent sphenoidal sinusitis

[5th] **J01.4 Acute pansinusitis**
J01.40 Acute pansinusitis, unspecified
J01.41 Acute recurrent pansinusitis

[5th] **J01.8 Other acute sinusitis**
J01.80 Other acute sinusitis
Acute sinusitis involving more than one sinus but not pansinusitis
J01.81 Other acute recurrent sinusitis
Acute recurrent sinusitis involving more than one sinus but not pansinusitis

[5th] **J01.9 Acute sinusitis, unspecified**
J01.90 Acute sinusitis, unspecified
J01.91 Acute recurrent sinusitis, unspecified

[4th] **J02 Acute pharyngitis**
[INCLUDES] *acute sore throat*
[EXCLUDES1] *acute laryngopharyngitis (J06.0)*
peritonsillar abscess (J36)
pharyngeal abscess (J39.1)
retropharyngeal abscess (J39.0)
[EXCLUDES2] *chronic pharyngitis (J31.2)*

J02.0 Streptococcal pharyngitis
Septic pharyngitis
Streptococcal sore throat
[EXCLUDES2] *scarlet fever (A38.-)*

J02.8 Acute pharyngitis due to other specified organisms
Use additional code (B95-B97) to identify infectious agent
[EXCLUDES1] *acute pharyngitis due to coxsackie virus (B08.5)*
acute pharyngitis due to gonococcus (A54.5)
acute pharyngitis due to herpes [simplex] virus (B00.2)
acute pharyngitis due to infectious mononucleosis (B27.-)
enteroviral vesicular pharyngitis (B08.5)

J02.9 Acute pharyngitis, unspecified
Gangrenous pharyngitis (acute)
Infective pharyngitis (acute) NOS
Pharyngitis (acute) NOS
Sore throat (acute) NOS
Suppurative pharyngitis (acute)
Ulcerative pharyngitis (acute)

[4th] **J03 Acute tonsillitis**
[EXCLUDES1] *acute sore throat (J02.-)*
hypertrophy of tonsils (J35.1)
peritonsillar abscess (J36)
sore throat NOS (J02.9)
streptococcal sore throat (J02.0)
[EXCLUDES2] *chronic tonsillitis (J35.0)*

[PDx] Unacceptable principal diagnosis symbol per Medicare code edits [POA] Code exempt from diagnosis present on admission requirement
[?] Questionable admission [CC] Complication or comorbidity [CC/MCC Exc] CC/MCC exclusion [MCC] Major complication or comorbidity
[PDx CC] Principal diagnosis as its own CC [PDx MCC] Principal diagnosis as its own MCC [HCC] HCC diagnosis code [RxHCC] RxHCC diagnosis code
MACRA code [Z-1] Z code as first-listed diagnosis

J03.0 Streptococcal tonsillitis

J03.00 Acute streptococcal tonsillitis, unspecified

J03.01 Acute recurrent streptococcal tonsillitis

J03.8 Acute tonsillitis due to other specified organisms

Use additional code (B95-B97) to identify infectious agent.

EXCLUDES1 diphtheritic tonsillitis (A36.0)

herpesviral pharyngotonsillitis (B00.2)

streptococcal tonsillitis (J03.0)

tuberculous tonsillitis (A15.8)

Vincent's tonsillitis (A69.1)

J03.80 Acute tonsillitis due to other specified organisms

J03.81 Acute recurrent tonsillitis due to other specified organisms

J03.9 Acute tonsillitis, unspecified

Follicular tonsillitis (acute)

Gangrenous tonsillitis (acute)

Infective tonsillitis (acute)

Tonsillitis (acute) NOS

Ulcerative tonsillitis (acute)

J03.90 Acute tonsillitis, unspecified

J03.91 Acute recurrent tonsillitis, unspecified

J04 Acute laryngitis and tracheitis

Use additional code (B95-B97) to identify infectious agent.

EXCLUDES1 acute obstructive laryngitis [croup] and epiglottitis (J05.-)

EXCLUDES2 laryngismus (stridulus) (J38.5)

J04.0 Acute laryngitis

Edematous laryngitis (acute)

Laryngitis (acute) NOS

Subglottic laryngitis (acute)

Suppurative laryngitis (acute)

Ulcerative laryngitis (acute)

EXCLUDES1 acute obstructive laryngitis (J05.0)

EXCLUDES2 chronic laryngitis (J37.0)

J04.1 Acute tracheitis

Acute viral tracheitis

Catarrhal tracheitis (acute)

Tracheitis (acute) NOS

EXCLUDES2 chronic tracheitis (J42)

J04.10 Acute tracheitis without obstruction

J04.11 Acute tracheitis with obstruction MCC© CC/MCC Exc

J04.2 Acute laryngotracheitis

Laryngotracheitis NOS

Tracheitis (acute) with laryngitis (acute)

EXCLUDES1 acute obstructive laryngotracheitis (J05.0)

EXCLUDES2 chronic laryngotracheitis (J37.1)

J04.3 Supraglottis, unspecified

J04.30 Supraglottitis, unspecified, without obstruction

J04.31 Supraglottitis, unspecified, with obstruction MCC© CC/MCC Exc

J05 Acute obstructive laryngitis [croup] and epiglottitis

Use additional code (B95-B97) to identify infectious agent.

J05.0 Acute obstructive laryngitis [croup]

Obstructive laryngitis (acute) NOS

Obstructive laryngotracheitis NOS

J05.1 Acute epiglottitis

EXCLUDES2 epiglottitis, chronic (J37.0)

J05.10 Acute epiglottitis without obstruction

Epiglottitis NOS

J05.11 Acute epiglottitis with obstruction MCC© CC/MCC Exc

J06 Acute upper respiratory infections of multiple and unspecified sites

EXCLUDES1 acute respiratory infection NOS (J22)

streptococcal pharyngitis (J02.0)

J06.0 Acute laryngopharyngitis

J06.9 Acute upper respiratory infection, unspecified

Upper respiratory disease, acute

Upper respiratory infection NOS

Influenza and pneumonia (J09-J18)

EXCLUDES2 allergic or eosinophilic pneumonia (J82)

aspiration pneumonia NOS (J69.0)

meconium pneumonia (P24.01)

neonatal aspiration pneumonia (P24.-)

pneumonia due to solids and liquids (J69.-)

congenital pneumonia (P23.9)

lipid pneumonia (J69.1)

rheumatic pneumonia (I00)

ventilator associated pneumonia (J95.851)

J09 Influenza due to certain identified influenza viruses

EXCLUDES1 influenza A/H1N1 (J10.-)

influenza due to other identified influenza virus (J10.-)

influenza due to unidentified influenza virus (J11.-)

seasonal influenza due to other identified influenza virus (J10.-)

seasonal influenza due to unidentified influenza virus (J11.-)

J09.X Influenza due to identified novel influenza A virus

Avian influenza

Bird influenza

Influenza A/H5N1

Influenza of other animal origin, not bird or swine

Swine influenza virus (viruses that normally cause infections in pigs)

J09.X1 Influenza due to identified novel influenza A virus with pneumonia MCC© CC/MCC Exc

Code also, if applicable, associated:

lung abscess (J85.1)

other specified type of pneumonia

J09.X2 Influenza due to identified novel influenza A virus with other respiratory manifestations

Influenza due to identified novel influenza A virus NOS

Influenza due to identified novel influenza A virus with laryngitis

Influenza due to identified novel influenza A virus with pharyngitis

Influenza due to identified novel influenza A virus with upper respiratory symptoms

Use additional code, if applicable, for associated:

pleural effusion (J91.8)

sinusitis (J01.-)

J09.X3 Influenza due to identified novel influenza A virus with gastrointestinal manifestations

Influenza due to identified novel influenza A virus gastroenteritis

EXCLUDES1 'intestinal flu' [viral gastroenteritis] (A08.-)

J09.X9 Influenza due to identified novel influenza A virus with other manifestations

Influenza due to identified novel influenza A virus with encephalopathy

Influenza due to identified novel influenza A virus with myocarditis

Influenza due to identified novel influenza A virus with otitis media

Use additional code to identify manifestation

J10 Influenza due to other identified influenza virus

EXCLUDES1 influenza due to avian influenza virus (J09.X-)

influenza due to swine flu (J09.X-)

influenza due to unidentifed influenza virus (J11.-)

J10.0 Influenza due to other identified influenza virus with pneumonia

Code also associated lung abscess, if applicable (J85.1)

J10.00 Influenza due to other identified influenza virus with unspecified type of pneumonia MCC© CC/MCC Exc

J10.01 Influenza due to other identified influenza virus with the same other identified influenza virus pneumonia MCC© CC/MCC Exc

---

Unspecified Code   Other Specified Code   Manifestation Code   N Newborn   P Pediatric   M Maternity   A Adult   ♂ Male   ♀ Female

● New Code   ▲ Revised Code Title   ►◄ Revised Text   **NOTES**   *INCLUDES*   *EXCLUDES 1* Not coded here   *EXCLUDES 2* Not included here

4ᵗʰ 4th character required   5ᵗʰ 5th character required   6ᵗʰ 6th character required   7ᵗʰ 7th character required

7ᵗʰ Extension 'X' Alert   HAC Hospital-acquired condition (HAC) alert   AHA AHA Coding Clinic©

J10.08 Influenza due to other identified influenza virus with other specified pneumonia MCC CC/MCC Exc
   Code also other specified type of pneumonia

J10.1 Influenza due to other identified influenza virus with other respiratory manifestations
   AHA: Q3 2016
   Influenza due to other identified influenza virus NOS
   Influenza due to other identified influenza virus with laryngitis
   Influenza due to other identified influenza virus with pharyngitis
   Influenza due to other identified influenza virus with upper respiratory symptoms
   Use additional code for associated pleural effusion, if applicable (J91.8)
   Use additional code for associated sinusitis, if applicable (J01.-)

J10.2 Influenza due to other identified influenza virus with gastrointestinal manifestations
   Influenza due to other identified influenza virus gastroenteritis
   EXCLUDES1 'intestinal flu' [viral gastroenteritis] (A08.-)

5ᵗʰ **J10.8** Influenza due to other identified influenza virus with other manifestations

   J10.81 Influenza due to other identified influenza virus with encephalopathy

   J10.82 Influenza due to other identified influenza virus with myocarditis

   J10.83 Influenza due to other identified influenza virus with otitis media
      Use additional code for any associated perforated tympanic membrane (H72.-)

   J10.89 Influenza due to other identified influenza virus with other manifestations
      Use additional codes to identify the manifestations

4ᵗʰ **J11** Influenza due to unidentified influenza virus

5ᵗʰ **J11.0** Influenza due to unidentified influenza virus with pneumonia
   Code also associated lung abscess, if applicable (J85.1)

   J11.00 Influenza due to unidentified influenza virus with unspecified type of pneumonia MCC CC/MCC Exc
      AHA: Q3 2016
      Influenza with pneumonia NOS

   J11.08 Influenza due to unidentified influenza virus with specified pneumonia MCC CC/MCC Exc
      Code also other specified type of pneumonia

J11.1 Influenza due to unidentified influenza virus with other respiratory manifestations
   Influenza NOS
   Influenzal laryngitis NOS
   Influenzal pharyngitis NOS
   Influenza with upper respiratory symptoms NOS
   Use additional code for associated pleural effusion, if applicable (J91.8)
   Use additional code for associated sinusitis, if applicable (J01.-)

J11.2 Influenza due to unidentified influenza virus with gastrointestinal manifestations
   Influenza gastroenteritis NOS
   EXCLUDES1 'intestinal flu' [viral gastroenteritis] (A08.-)

5ᵗʰ **J11.8** Influenza due to unidentified influenza virus with other manifestations

   J11.81 Influenza due to unidentified influenza virus with encephalopathy
      Influenzal encephalopathy NOS

   J11.82 Influenza due to unidentified influenza virus with myocarditis
      Influenzal myocarditis NOS

   J11.83 Influenza due to unidentified influenza virus with otitis media
      Influenzal otitis media NOS
      Use additional code for any associated perforated tympanic membrane (H72.-)

J11.89 Influenza due to unidentified influenza virus with other manifestations
   Use additional codes to identify the manifestations

4ᵗʰ **J12** Viral pneumonia, **not elsewhere classified**
   INCLUDES bronchopneumonia due to viruses other than influenza viruses
   Code first associated influenza, if applicable (J09.X1, J10.0-, J11.0-)
   Code also associated abscess, if applicable (J85.1)
   EXCLUDES1 aspiration pneumonia due to anesthesia during labor and delivery (O74.0)
      aspiration pneumonia due to anesthesia during pregnancy (O29)
      aspiration pneumonia due to anesthesia during puerperium (O89.0)
      aspiration pneumonia due to solids and liquids (J69.-)
      aspiration pneumonia NOS (J69.0)
      congenital pneumonia (P23.0)
      congenital rubella pneumonitis (P35.0)
      interstitial pneumonia NOS (J84.9)
      lipid pneumonia (J69.1)
      neonatal aspiration pneumonia (P24.-)

J12.0 Adenoviral **pneumonia** MCC CC/MCC Exc

J12.1 Respiratory syncytial virus **pneumonia** MCC CC/MCC Exc

J12.2 Parainfluenza virus **pneumonia** MCC CC/MCC Exc

J12.3 Human metapneumovirus **pneumonia** MCC CC/MCC Exc

5ᵗʰ **J12.8** Other **viral pneumonia**

   J12.81 **Pneumonia** due to SARS-associated coronavirus MCC CC/MCC Exc
      Severe acute respiratory syndrome NOS

   J12.89 Other **viral pneumonia** MCC CC/MCC Exc

J12.9 **Viral pneumonia, unspecified** MCC CC/MCC Exc

J13 **Pneumonia due to** Streptococcus pneumoniae HCC MCC CC/MCC Exc
   Bronchopneumonia due to S. pneumoniae
   Code first associated influenza, if applicable (J09.X1, J10.0-, J11.0-)
   Code also associated abscess, if applicable (J85.1)
   EXCLUDES1 congenital pneumonia due to S. pneumoniae (P23.6)
      lobar pneumonia, unspecified organism (J18.1)
      pneumonia due to other streptococci (J15.3-J15.4)

J14 **Pneumonia due to** Hemophilus influenzae HCC MCC CC/MCC Exc
   Bronchopneumonia due to H. influenzae
   Code first associated influenza, if applicable (J09.X1, J10.0-, J11.0-)
   Code also associated abscess, if applicable (J85.1)
   EXCLUDES1 congenital pneumonia due to H. influenzae (P23.6)

4ᵗʰ **J15** Bacterial **pneumonia, not elsewhere classified**
   INCLUDES bronchopneumonia due to bacteria other than S. pneumoniae and H. influenzae
   Code first associated influenza, if applicable (J09.X1, J10.0-, J11.0-)
   Code also associated abscess, if applicable (J85.1)
   EXCLUDES1 chlamydial pneumonia (J16.0)
      congenital pneumonia (P23.-)
      Legionnaires' disease (A48.1)
      spirochetal pneumonia (A69.8)

J15.0 **Pneumonia due to** Klebsiella pneumoniae HCC MCC CC/MCC Exc

J15.1 **Pneumonia due to** Pseudomonas HCC MCC CC/MCC Exc

5ᵗʰ **J15.2** **Pneumonia due to** staphylococcus

   J15.20 **Pneumonia due to staphylococcus, unspecified** HCC MCC CC/MCC Exc

6ᵗʰ **J15.21** **Pneumonia due to** staphylococcus aureus

      J15.211 **Pneumonia due to** Methicillin susceptible Staphylococcus aureus HCC MCC CC/MCC Exc
         MSSA pneumonia
         Pneumonia due to Staphylococcus aureus NOS

      J15.212 **Pneumonia due to** Methicillin resistant Staphylococcus aureus HCC MCC CC/MCC Exc

   J15.29 **Pneumonia due to** other staphylococcus HCC MCC CC/MCC Exc

J15.3 **Pneumonia due to** streptococcus, group B HCC MCC CC/MCC Exc

---

PDx Unacceptable principal diagnosis symbol per Medicare code edits   POA Code exempt from diagnosis present on admission requirement
? Questionable admission   Complication or comorbidity   CC/MCC Exc CC/MCC exclusion   MCC Major complication or comorbidity
Principal diagnosis as its own CC   Principal diagnosis as its own MCC   HCC HCC diagnosis code   RxHCC RxHCC diagnosis code
MACRA code   Z1 Z code as first-listed diagnosis

J15.4 Pneumonia due to other streptococci [HCC] [MCC] [CC/MCC Exc]
[EXCLUDES1] *pneumonia due to streptococcus, group B (J15.3)*
pneumonia due to Streptococcus pneumoniae (J13)

J15.5 Pneumonia due to Escherichia coli [HCC] [MCC] [CC/MCC Exc]

▲ J15.6 Pneumonia due to other Gram-negative bacteria [HCC] [MCC] [CC/MCC Exc]
Pneumonia due to other aerobic Gram-negative bacteria
Pneumonia due to Serratia marcescens

J15.7 Pneumonia due to Mycoplasma pneumoniae [MCC] [CC/MCC Exc]

J15.8 Pneumonia due to other specified bacteria [HCC] [MCC] [CC/MCC Exc]

J15.9 Unspecified bacterial pneumonia [MCC] [CC/MCC Exc]
Pneumonia due to gram-positive bacteria

[4th] **J16 Pneumonia due to other infectious organisms, not elsewhere classified**
Code first associated influenza, if applicable (J09.X1, J10.0-, J11.0-)
Code also associated abscess, if applicable (J85.1)
[EXCLUDES1] *congenital pneumonia (P23.-)*
ornithosis (A70)
pneumocystosis (B59)
pneumonia NOS (J18.9)

J16.0 Chlamydial pneumonia [MCC] [CC/MCC Exc]

J16.8 Pneumonia due to other specified infectious organisms [MCC] [CC/MCC Exc]

J17 Pneumonia in diseases classified elsewhere [MCC] [CC/MCC Exc]
Code first underlying disease, such as:
Q fever (A78)
rheumatic fever (I00)
schistosomiasis (B65.0-B65.9)
[EXCLUDES1] *candidial pneumonia (B37.1)*
chlamydial pneumonia (J16.0)
gonorrheal pneumonia (A54.84)
histoplasmosis pneumonia (B39.0-B39.2)
measles pneumonia (B05.2)
nocardiosis pneumonia (A43.0)
pneumocystosis (B59)
pneumonia due to Pneumocystis carinii (B59)
pneumonia due to Pneumocystis jiroveci (B59)
pneumonia in actinomycosis (A42.0)
pneumonia in anthrax (A22.1)
pneumonia in ascariasis (B77.81)
pneumonia in aspergillosis (B44.0-B44.1)
pneumonia in coccidioidomycosis (B38.0-B38.2)
pneumonia in cytomegalovirus disease (B25.0)
pneumonia in toxoplasmosis (B58.3)
rubella pneumonia (B06.81)
salmonella pneumonia (A02.22)
spirochetal infection NEC with pneumonia (A69.8)
tularemia pneumonia (A21.2)
typhoid fever with pneumonia (A01.03)
varicella pneumonia (B01.2)
whooping cough with pneumonia (A37 with fifth-character 1)

[4th] **J18 Pneumonia, unspecified organism**
Code first associated influenza, if applicable (J09.X1, J10.0-, J11.0-)
[EXCLUDES1] *abscess of lung with pneumonia (J85.1)*
aspiration pneumonia due to anesthesia during labor and delivery (O74.0)
aspiration pneumonia due to anesthesia during pregnancy (O29)
aspiration pneumonia due to anesthesia during puerperium (O89.0)
aspiration pneumonia due to solids and liquids (J69.-)
aspiration pneumonia NOS (J69.0)
congenital pneumonia (P23.0)
drug-induced interstitial lung disorder (J70.2-J70.4)
interstitial pneumonia NOS (J84.9)
lipid pneumonia (J69.1)
neonatal aspiration pneumonia (P24.-)
pneumonitis due to external agents (J67-J70)
pneumonitis due to fumes and vapors (J68.0)
usual interstitial pneumonia (J84.17)

J18.0 Bronchopneumonia, unspecified organism [MCC] [CC/MCC Exc]
[EXCLUDES1] *hypostatic bronchopneumonia (J18.2)*
lipid pneumonia (J69.1)
[EXCLUDES2] *acute bronchiolitis (J21.-)*
chronic bronchiolitis (J44.9)

J18.1 Lobar pneumonia, unspecified organism [HCC] [MCC] [CC/MCC Exc]
AHA: Q3 2016

J18.2 Hypostatic pneumonia, unspecified organism [CC] [CC/MCC Exc]
Hypostatic bronchopneumonia
Passive pneumonia

J18.8 Other pneumonia, unspecified organism [MCC] [CC/MCC Exc]

J18.9 Pneumonia, unspecified organism [MCC] [CC/MCC Exc]
AHA: Q3 2016, Q4 2013

Other acute lower respiratory infections (J20-J22)

[EXCLUDES2] *chronic obstructive pulmonary disease with acute lower respiratory infection (J44.0)*

[4th] **J20 Acute bronchitis**
[INCLUDES] *acute and subacute bronchitis (with) bronchospasm*
acute and subacute bronchitis (with) tracheitis
acute and subacute bronchitis (with) tracheobronchitis, acute
acute and subacute fibrinous bronchitis
acute and subacute membranous bronchitis
acute and subacute purulent bronchitis
acute and subacute septic bronchitis
[EXCLUDES1] *bronchitis NOS (J40)*
tracheobronchitis NOS (J40)
[EXCLUDES2] *acute bronchitis with bronchiectasis (J47.0)*
acute bronchitis with chronic obstructive asthma (J44.0)
acute bronchitis with chronic obstructive pulmonary disease (J44.0)
allergic bronchitis NOS (J45.909-)
bronchitis due to chemicals, fumes and vapors (J68.0)
chronic bronchitis NOS (J42)
chronic mucopurulent bronchitis (J41.1)
chronic obstructive bronchitis (J44.-)
chronic obstructive tracheobronchitis (J44.-)
chronic simple bronchitis (J41.0)
chronic tracheobronchitis (J42)

J20.0 Acute bronchitis due to Mycoplasma pneumoniae

J20.1 Acute bronchitis due to Hemophilus influenzae

J20.2 Acute bronchitis due to streptococcus

J20.3 Acute bronchitis due to coxsackievirus

J20.4 Acute bronchitis due to parainfluenza virus

J20.5 Acute bronchitis due to respiratory syncytial virus

J20.6 Acute bronchitis due to rhinovirus
AHA: Q3 2016

J20.7 Acute bronchitis due to echovirus

J20.8 Acute bronchitis due to other specified organisms
AHA: Q3 2016

J20.9 Acute bronchitis, unspecified
AHA: Q3 2016

[4th] **J21 Acute bronchiolitis**
[INCLUDES] *acute bronchiolitis with bronchospasm*
[EXCLUDES2] *respiratory bronchiolitis interstitial lung disease (J84.115)*

J21.0 Acute bronchiolitis due to respiratory syncytial virus [CC] [CC/MCC Exc]

J21.1 Acute bronchiolitis due to human metapneumovirus [CC] [CC/MCC Exc]

J21.8 Acute bronchiolitis due to other specified organisms [CC] [CC/MCC Exc]

J21.9 **Acute bronchiolitis, unspecified**
Bronchiolitis (acute)
EXCLUDES1 *chronic bronchiolitis (J44.-)*

J22 **Unspecified acute lower respiratory infection**
Acute (lower) respiratory (tract) infection NOS
EXCLUDES1 *upper respiratory infection (acute) (J06.9)*

Other diseases of upper respiratory tract (J30-J39)

J30 **Vasomotor and allergic rhinitis**
INCLUDES spasmodic rhinorrhea
EXCLUDES1 *allergic rhinitis with asthma (bronchial) (J45.909)*
rhinitis NOS (J31.0)

J30.0 **Vasomotor rhinitis**

J30.1 **Allergic rhinitis due to pollen**
Allergy NOS due to pollen
Hay fever
Pollinosis

J30.2 **Other seasonal allergic rhinitis**

J30.5 **Allergic rhinitis due to food**

J30.8 **Other allergic rhinitis**

J30.81 **Allergic rhinitis due to animal (cat) (dog) hair and dander**

J30.89 **Other allergic rhinitis**
Perennial allergic rhinitis

J30.9 **Allergic rhinitis, unspecified**

J31 **Chronic rhinitis, nasopharyngitis and pharyngitis**
Use additional code to identify:
exposure to environmental tobacco smoke (Z77.22)
exposure to tobacco smoke in the perinatal period (P96.81)
history of tobacco dependence (Z87.891)
occupational exposure to environmental tobacco smoke (Z57.31)
tobacco dependence (F17.-)
tobacco use (Z72.0)

J31.0 **Chronic rhinitis**
Atrophic rhinitis (chronic)
Granulomatous rhinitis (chronic)
Hypertrophic rhinitis (chronic)
Obstructive rhinitis (chronic)
Ozena
Purulent rhinitis (chronic)
Rhinitis (chronic) NOS
Ulcerative rhinitis (chronic)
EXCLUDES1 *allergic rhinitis (J30.1-J30.9)*
vasomotor rhinitis (J30.0)

J31.1 **Chronic nasopharyngitis**
EXCLUDES2 *acute nasopharyngitis (J00)*

J31.2 **Chronic pharyngitis**
Chronic sore throat
Atrophic pharyngitis (chronic)
Granular pharyngitis (chronic)
Hypertrophic pharyngitis (chronic)
EXCLUDES2 *acute pharyngitis (J02.9)*

J32 **Chronic sinusitis**
INCLUDES sinus abscess
sinus empyema
sinus infection
sinus suppuration
Use additional code to identify:
exposure to environmental tobacco smoke (Z77.22)
exposure to tobacco smoke in the perinatal period (P96.81)
history of tobacco dependence (Z87.891)
infectious agent (B95-B97)
occupational exposure to environmental tobacco smoke (Z57.31)
tobacco dependence (F17.-)
tobacco use (Z72.0)
EXCLUDES2 *acute sinusitis (J01.-)*

J32.0 **Chronic maxillary sinusitis**
Antritis (chronic)
Maxillary sinusitis NOS

J32.1 **Chronic frontal sinusitis**
Frontal sinusitis NOS

J32.2 **Chronic ethmoidal sinusitis**
Ethmoidal sinusitis NOS
EXCLUDES1 *Woakes' ethmoiditis (J33.1)*

J32.3 **Chronic sphenoidal sinusitis**
Sphenoidal sinusitis NOS

J32.4 **Chronic pansinusitis**
Pansinusitis NOS

J32.8 **Other chronic sinusitis**
Sinusitis (chronic) involving more than one sinus but not pansinusitis

J32.9 **Chronic sinusitis, unspecified**
Sinusitis (chronic) NOS

J33 **Nasal polyp**
Use additional code to identify:
exposure to environmental tobacco smoke (Z77.22)
exposure to tobacco smoke in the perinatal period (P96.81)
history of tobacco dependence (Z87.891)
occupational exposure to environmental tobacco smoke (Z57.31)
tobacco dependence (F17.-)
tobacco use (Z72.0)
EXCLUDES1 *adenomatous polyps (D14.0)*

J33.0 **Polyp of nasal cavity**
Choanal polyp
Nasopharyngeal polyp

J33.1 **Polypoid sinus degeneration**
Woakes' syndrome or ethmoiditis

J33.8 **Other polyp of sinus**
Accessory polyp of sinus
Ethmoidal polyp of sinus
Maxillary polyp of sinus
Sphenoidal polyp of sinus

J33.9 **Nasal polyp, unspecified**

J34 **Other and unspecified disorders of nose and nasal sinuses**
EXCLUDES2 *varicose ulcer of nasal septum (I86.8)*

J34.0 **Abscess, furuncle and carbuncle of nose**
Cellulitis of nose
Necrosis of nose
Ulceration of nose

J34.1 **Cyst and mucocele of nose and nasal sinus**

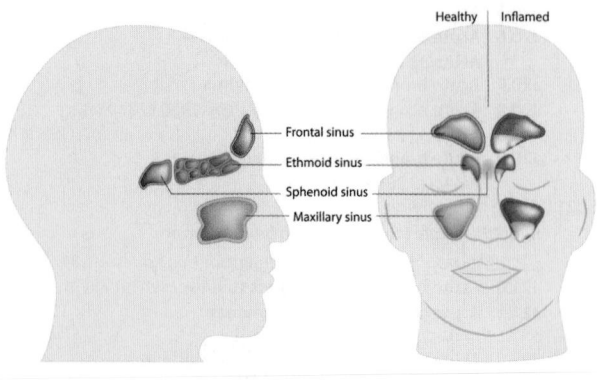

Healthy | Inflamed

Frontal sinus
Ethmoid sinus
Sphenoid sinus
Maxillary sinus

Figure 10.1 Sinusitis

POA Unacceptable principal diagnosis symbol per Medicare code edits   POA Code exempt from diagnosis present on admission requirement
? Questionable admission   CC Complication or comorbidity   CC/MCC CC/MCC exclusion   MCC Major complication or comorbidity
Principal diagnosis as its own CC   Principal diagnosis as its own MCC   HCC HCC diagnosis code   RxHCC RxHCC diagnosis code
MACRA code   Z1 Z code as first-listed diagnosis

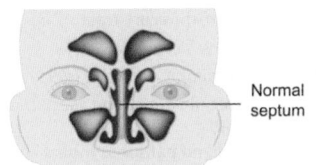

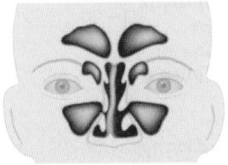

Figure 10.2 Deviated nasal septum

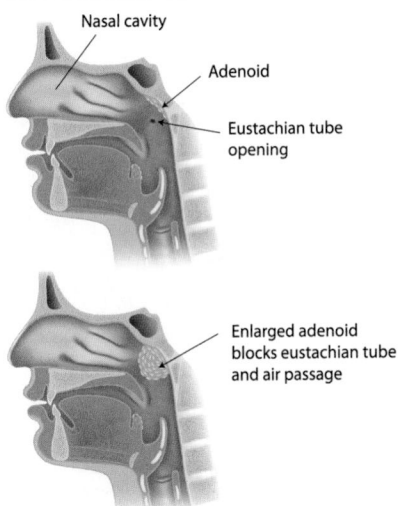

Figure 10.3 Adenoid hypertrophy

J34.2 **Deviated nasal septum**
Deflection or deviation of septum (nasal) (acquired)
EXCLUDES1 *congenital deviated nasal septum (Q67.4)*

J34.3 **Hypertrophy of nasal turbinates**

🔟 J34.8 **Other specified disorders of nose and nasal sinuses**

J34.81 **Nasal mucositis (ulcerative)**
Code also type of associated therapy, such as:
antineoplastic and immunosuppressive drugs
(T45.1X-)
radiological procedure and radiotherapy (Y84.2)
EXCLUDES2 *gastrointestinal mucositis (ulcerative)*
(K92.81)
mucositis (ulcerative) of vagina and vulva
(N76.81)
oral mucositis (ulcerative) (K12.3-)

J34.89 **Other specified disorders of nose and nasal sinuses**
Perforation of nasal septum NOS
Rhinolith

J34.9 **Unspecified disorder of nose and nasal sinuses**

🔟 J35 **Chronic diseases of tonsils and adenoids**
Use additional code to identify:
exposure to environmental tobacco smoke (Z77.22)
exposure to tobacco smoke in the perinatal period (P96.81)
history of tobacco dependence (Z87.891)
occupational exposure to environmental tobacco smoke (Z57.31)
tobacco dependence (F17.-)
tobacco use (Z72.0)

🔟 J35.0 **Chronic tonsillitis and adenoiditis**
EXCLUDES2 *acute tonsillitis (J03.-)*

J35.01 **Chronic tonsillitis**

J35.02 **Chronic adenoiditis**

J35.03 **Chronic tonsillitis and adenoiditis**

J35.1 **Hypertrophy of tonsils**
Enlargement of tonsils
EXCLUDES1 *hypertrophy of tonsils with tonsillitis (J35.0-)*

J35.2 **Hypertrophy of adenoids**
Enlargement of adenoids
EXCLUDES1 *hypertrophy of adenoids with adenoiditis (J35.0-)*

J35.3 **Hypertrophy of tonsils with hypertrophy of adenoids**
EXCLUDES1 *hypertrophy of tonsils and adenoids with tonsillitis and*
adenoiditis (J35.03)

J35.8 **Other chronic diseases of tonsils and adenoids**
Adenoid vegetations
Amygdalolith
Calculus, tonsil
Cicatrix of tonsil (and adenoid)
Tonsillar tag
Ulcer of tonsil

J35.9 **Chronic disease of tonsils and adenoids, unspecified**
Disease (chronic) of tonsils and adenoids NOS

J36 **Peritonsillar abscess** cc CC/MCC Exc
INCLUDES *abscess of tonsil*
peritonsillar cellulitis
quinsy
Use additional code (B95-B97) to identify infectious agent.
EXCLUDES1 *acute tonsillitis (J03.-)*
chronic tonsillitis (J35.0)
retropharyngeal abscess (J39.0)
tonsillitis NOS (J03.9-)

🔟 J37 **Chronic laryngitis and laryngotracheitis**
Use additional code to identify:
exposure to environmental tobacco smoke (Z77.22)
exposure to tobacco smoke in the perinatal period (P96.81)
history of tobacco dependence (Z87.891)
infectious agent (B95-B97)
occupational exposure to environmental tobacco smoke (Z57.31)
tobacco dependence (F17.-)
tobacco use (Z72.0)

J37.0 **Chronic laryngitis**
Catarrhal laryngitis
Hypertrophic laryngitis
Sicca laryngitis
EXCLUDES2 *acute laryngitis (J04.0)*
obstructive (acute) laryngitis (J05.0)

J37.1 **Chronic laryngotracheitis**
Laryngitis, chronic, with tracheitis (chronic)
Tracheitis, chronic, with laryngitis
EXCLUDES1 *chronic tracheitis (J42)*
EXCLUDES2 *acute laryngotracheitis (J04.2)*
acute tracheitis (J04.1)

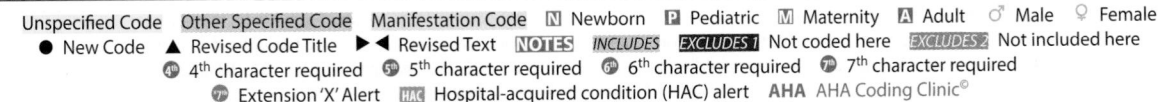

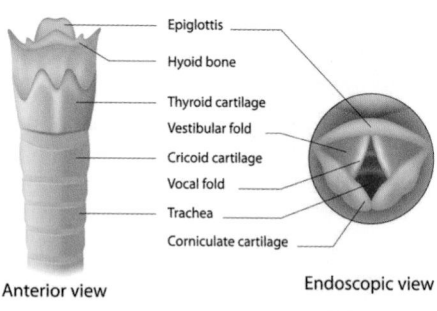

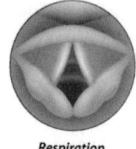

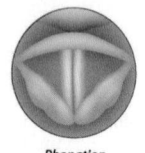

Figure 10.4 Larynx

🌐 **J38 Diseases of vocal cords and larynx, not elsewhere classified**
Use additional code to identify:
exposure to environmental tobacco smoke (Z77.22)
exposure to tobacco smoke in the perinatal period (P96.81)
history of tobacco dependence (Z87.891)
occupational exposure to environmental tobacco smoke (Z57.31)
tobacco dependence (F17.-)
tobacco use (Z72.0)
EXCLUDES1 congenital laryngeal stridor (P28.89)
obstructive laryngitis (acute) (J05.0)
postprocedural subglottic stenosis (J95.5)
stridor (R06.1)
ulcerative laryngitis (J04.0)

🔵 **J38.0 Paralysis of vocal cords and larynx**
Laryngoplegia
Paralysis of glottis
J38.00 Paralysis of vocal cords and larynx, unspecified
J38.01 Paralysis of vocal cords and larynx, unilateral
J38.02 Paralysis of vocal cords and larynx, bilateral

J38.1 Polyp of vocal cord and larynx
EXCLUDES1 adenomatous polyps (D14.1)

J38.2 Nodules of vocal cords
Chorditis (fibrinous)(nodosa)(tuberosa)
Singer's nodes
Teacher's nodes

J38.3 Other diseases of vocal cords
Abscess of vocal cords
Cellulitis of vocal cords
Granuloma of vocal cords
Leukokeratosis of vocal cords
Leukoplakia of vocal cords

J38.4 Edema of larynx
Edema (of) glottis
Subglottic edema
Supraglottic edema
EXCLUDES1 acute obstructive laryngitis [croup] (J05.0)
edematous laryngitis (J04.0)

J38.5 Laryngeal spasm
Laryngismus (stridulus)

J38.6 Stenosis of larynx

J38.7 Other diseases of larynx
Abscess of larynx
Cellulitis of larynx
Disease of larynx NOS
Necrosis of larynx
Pachyderma of larynx
Perichondritis of larynx
Ulcer of larynx

🌐 **J39 Other diseases of upper respiratory tract**
EXCLUDES1 acute respiratory infection NOS (J22)
acute upper respiratory infection (J06.9)
upper respiratory inflammation due to chemicals, gases, fumes or vapors (J68.2)

J39.0 Retropharyngeal and parapharyngeal abscess cc⊘ CC/MCC Exc
Peripharyngeal abscess
EXCLUDES1 peritonsillar abscess (J36)

J39.1 Other abscess of pharynx cc⊘ CC/MCC Exc
Cellulitis of pharynx
Nasopharyngeal abscess

J39.2 Other diseases of pharynx
Cyst of pharynx
Edema of pharynx
EXCLUDES2 chronic pharyngitis (J31.2)
ulcerative pharyngitis (J02.9)

J39.3 Upper respiratory tract hypersensitivity reaction, site unspecified
EXCLUDES1 hypersensitivity reaction of upper respiratory tract, such as:
extrinsic allergic alveolitis (J67.9)
pneumoconiosis (J60-J67.9)

J39.8 Other specified diseases of upper respiratory tract

J39.9 Disease of upper respiratory tract, unspecified

Chronic lower respiratory diseases (J40-J47)

EXCLUDES1 bronchitis due to chemicals, gases, fumes and vapors (J68.0)
EXCLUDES2 cystic fibrosis (E84.-)

J40 Bronchitis, not specified as acute or chronic
Bronchitis NOS
Bronchitis with tracheitis NOS
Catarrhal bronchitis
Tracheobronchitis NOS
Use additional code to identify:
exposure to environmental tobacco smoke (Z77.22)
exposure to tobacco smoke in the perinatal period (P96.81)
history of tobacco dependence (Z87.891)
occupational exposure to environmental tobacco smoke (Z57.31)
tobacco dependence (F17.-)
tobacco use (Z72.0)
EXCLUDES1 acute bronchitis (J20.-)
allergic bronchitis NOS (J45.909-)
asthmatic bronchitis NOS (J45.9-)
bronchitis due to chemicals, gases, fumes and vapors (J68.0)

🌐 **J41 Simple and mucopurulent chronic bronchitis**
Use additional code to identify:
exposure to environmental tobacco smoke (Z77.22)
exposure to tobacco smoke in the perinatal period (P96.81)
history of tobacco dependence (Z87.891)
occupational exposure to environmental tobacco smoke (Z57.31)
tobacco dependence (F17.-)
tobacco use (Z72.0)
EXCLUDES1 chronic bronchitis NOS (J42)
chronic obstructive bronchitis (J44.-)

J41.0 Simple chronic bronchitis HCC RxHCC
J41.1 Mucopurulent chronic bronchitis HCC RxHCC
J41.8 Mixed simple and mucopurulent chronic bronchitis HCC RxHCC

J42 Unspecified chronic bronchitis HCC RxHCC
Chronic bronchitis NOS
Chronic tracheitis
Chronic tracheobronchitis
Use additional code to identify:
exposure to environmental tobacco smoke (Z77.22)
exposure to tobacco smoke in the perinatal period (P96.81)
history of tobacco dependence (Z87.891)
occupational exposure to environmental tobacco smoke (Z57.31)
tobacco dependence (F17.-)
tobacco use (Z72.0)

PDiR Unacceptable principal diagnosis symbol per Medicare code edits   POA Code exempt from diagnosis present on admission requirement
❓ Questionable admission   cc⊘ Complication or comorbidity   cc/mcc Exc CC/MCC exclusion   mcc⊘ Major complication or comorbidity
🅰 Principal diagnosis as its own CC   🅱 Principal diagnosis as its own MCC   HCC HCC diagnosis code   RxHCC RxHCC diagnosis code
MACRA code   🆉 Z code as first-listed diagnosis

EXCLUDES1 *chronic asthmatic bronchitis (J44.-)*

chronic bronchitis with airways obstruction (J44.-)

chronic emphysematous bronchitis (J44.-)

chronic obstructive pulmonary disease NOS (J44.9)

simple and mucopurulent chronic bronchitis (J41.-)

J43 Emphysema

Use additional code to identify:

exposure to environmental tobacco smoke (Z77.22)

history of tobacco dependence (Z87.891)

occupational exposure to environmental tobacco smoke (Z57.31)

tobacco dependence (F17.-)

tobacco use (Z72.0)

EXCLUDES1 *compensatory emphysema (J98.3)*

emphysema due to inhalation of chemicals, gases, fumes or vapors (J68.4)

emphysema with chronic (obstructive) bronchitis (J44.-)

emphysematous (obstructive) bronchitis (J44.-)

interstitial emphysema (J98.2)

mediastinal emphysema (J98.2)

neonatal interstitial emphysema (P25.0)

surgical (subcutaneous) emphysema (T81.82)

traumatic subcutaneous emphysema (T79.7)

J43.0 Unilateral pulmonary **emphysema** [MacLeod's syndrome] `HCC` `RxHCC`

Swyer-James syndrome

Unilateral emphysema

Unilateral hyperlucent lung

Unilateral pulmonary artery functional hypoplasia

Unilateral transparency of lung

J43.1 Panlobular **emphysema** `HCC` `RxHCC`

Panacinar emphysema

J43.2 Centrilobular **emphysema** `HCC` `RxHCC`

J43.8 Other **emphysema** `HCC` `RxHCC`

J43.9 **Emphysema, unspecified** `HCC` `RxHCC`

Bullous emphysema (lung)(pulmonary)

Emphysema (lung)(pulmonary) NOS

Emphysematous bleb

Vesicular emphysema (lung)(pulmonary)

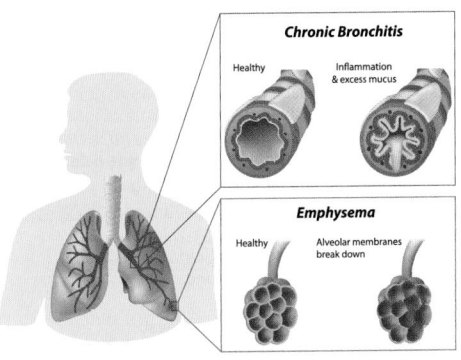

Figure 10.5 Chronic obstructive pulmonary disease (COPD): chronic bronchitis and emphysema

J44 Other **chronic obstructive pulmonary disease**

INCLUDES *asthma with chronic obstructive pulmonary disease*

chronic asthmatic (obstructive) bronchitis

chronic bronchitis with airways obstruction

chronic bronchitis with emphysema

chronic emphysematous bronchitis

chronic obstructive asthma

chronic obstructive bronchitis

chronic obstructive tracheobronchitis

Code also type of asthma, if applicable (J45.-)

Use additional code to identify:

exposure to environmental tobacco smoke (Z77.22)

history of tobacco dependence (Z87.891)

occupational exposure to environmental tobacco smoke (Z57.31)

tobacco dependence (F17.-)

tobacco use (Z72.0)

EXCLUDES1 *bronchiectasis (J47.-)*

chronic bronchitis NOS (J42)

chronic simple and mucopurulent bronchitis (J41.-)

chronic tracheitis (J42)

chronic tracheobronchitis (J42)

emphysema without chronic bronchitis (J43.-)

J44.0 **Chronic obstructive pulmonary disease** with acute lower respiratory infection `CC` `HCC` `RxHCC` `CC/MCC Exc`

AHA: Q1 2017, Q2 2017, Q3 2016

Code also to identify the infection

J44.1 **Chronic obstructive pulmonary disease** with (acute) exacerbation `CC` `HCC` `RxHCC` `CC/MCC Exc`

AHA: Q1 2017, Q3 2016

Decompensated COPD

Decompensated COPD with (acute) exacerbation

EXCLUDES2 *chronic obstructive pulmonary disease [COPD] with acute bronchitis (J44.0)*

lung diseases due to external agents (J60-J70)

J44.9 **Chronic obstructive pulmonary disease, unspecified** `HCC` `RxHCC`

AHA: Q1 2017, Q1 2016, Q4 2013

Chronic obstructive airway disease NOS

Chronic obstructive lung disease NOS

EXCLUDES2 *lung diseases due to external agents (J60-J70)*

J45 Asthma

INCLUDES *allergic (predominantly) asthma*

allergic bronchitis NOS

allergic rhinitis with asthma

atopic asthma

extrinsic allergic asthma

hay fever with asthma

idiosyncratic asthma

intrinsic nonallergic asthma

nonallergic asthma

Use additional code to identify:

exposure to environmental tobacco smoke (Z77.22)

exposure to tobacco smoke in the perinatal period (P96.81)

history of tobacco dependence (Z87.891)

occupational exposure to environmental tobacco smoke (Z57.31)

tobacco dependence (F17.-)

tobacco use (Z72.0)

EXCLUDES1 *detergent asthma (J69.8)*

eosinophilic asthma (J82)

miner's asthma (J60)

wheezing NOS (R06.2)

wood asthma (J67.8)

EXCLUDES2 *asthma with chronic obstructive pulmonary disease (J44.9)*

chronic asthmatic (obstructive) bronchitis (J44.9)

chronic obstructive asthma (J44.9)

J45.2 Mild intermittent **asthma**

J45.20 **Mild intermittent asthma,** uncomplicated `RxHCC`

Mild intermittent asthma NOS

J45.21 **Mild intermittent asthma** with (acute) exacerbation `CC` `RxHCC` `CC/MCC Exc`

J45.22 **Mild intermittent asthma** with status asthmaticus `CC` `RxHCC` `CC/MCC Exc`

J45.3 Mild persistent **asthma**

J45.30 **Mild persistent asthma,** uncomplicated `RxHCC`

Mild persistent asthma NOS

J45.31 **Mild persistent asthma** with (acute) exacerbation `CC` `RxHCC` `CC/MCC Exc`

J45.32 **Mild persistent asthma** with status asthmaticus `CC` `RxHCC` `CC/MCC Exc`

Unspecified Code   Other Specified Code   Manifestation Code   Ⓝ Newborn   Ⓟ Pediatric   Ⓜ Maternity   Ⓐ Adult   ♂ Male   ♀ Female

● New Code   ▲ Revised Code Title   ►◄ Revised Text   **NOTES**   *INCLUDES*   *EXCLUDES 1* Not coded here   *EXCLUDES 2* Not included here

④ 4th character required   ⑤ 5th character required   ⑥ 6th character required   ⑦ 7th character required

Ⓧ Extension 'X' Alert   **HAC** Hospital-acquired condition (HAC) alert   **AHA** AHA Coding Clinic©

EXCLUDES1 *aspiration pneumonitis due to anesthesia complicating labor and delivery (O74.0)*

aspiration pneumonitis due to anesthesia complicating pregnancy (O29)

aspiration pneumonitis due to anesthesia complicating the puerperium (O89.01)

J95.5 Postprocedural subglottic stenosis   cc⊘ cc/mcc Exc

J95.6 Intraoperative hemorrhage and hematoma of a respiratory system organ or structure complicating a procedure

EXCLUDES1 *intraoperative hemorrhage and hematoma of a respiratory system organ or structure due to accidental puncture and laceration during procedure (J95.7-)*

J95.61 Intraoperative hemorrhage and hematoma of a respiratory system organ or structure complicating a respiratory system procedure   cc⊘ cc/mcc Exc

J95.62 Intraoperative hemorrhage and hematoma of a respiratory system organ or structure complicating other procedure   cc⊘ cc/mcc Exc

J95.7 Accidental puncture and laceration of a respiratory system organ or structure during a procedure

EXCLUDES2 *postprocedural pneumothorax (J95.811)*

J95.71 Accidental puncture and laceration of a respiratory system organ or structure during a respiratory system procedure   cc⊘ cc/mcc Exc

J95.72 Accidental puncture and laceration of a respiratory system organ or structure during other procedure   cc⊘ cc/mcc Exc

J95.8 Other intraoperative and postprocedural complications and disorders of respiratory system, not elsewhere classified

J95.81 Postprocedural pneumothorax and air leak

J95.811 Postprocedural pneumothorax   cc⊘ HAC cc/mcc Exc

J95.812 Postprocedural air leak   cc⊘ cc/mcc Exc

J95.82 Postprocedural respiratory failure

EXCLUDES1 *Respiratory failure in other conditions (J96.-)*

J95.821 Acute postprocedural respiratory failure   HCC mcc⊘ cc/mcc Exc

Postprocedural respiratory failure NOS

J95.822 Acute and chronic postprocedural respiratory failure   HCC mcc⊘ cc/mcc Exc

J95.83 Postprocedural hemorrhage of a respiratory system organ or structure following a procedure

J95.830 Postprocedural hemorrhage of a respiratory system organ or structure following a respiratory system procedure   cc⊘ cc/mcc Exc

J95.831 Postprocedural hemorrhage of a respiratory system organ or structure following other procedure   cc⊘ cc/mcc Exc

J95.84 Transfusion-related acute lung injury (TRALI)   cc⊘ cc/mcc Exc

J95.85 Complication of respirator [ventilator]

J95.850 Mechanical complication of respirator   cc⊘ HCC cc/mcc Exc

EXCLUDES1 *encounter for respirator [ventilator] dependence during power failure (Z99.12)*

J95.851 Ventilator associated pneumonia   cc⊘ HCC cc/mcc Exc

AHA: Q1 2017

Ventilator associated pneumonitis

Use additional code to identify the organism, if known (B95.-, B96.-, B97.-)

EXCLUDES1 *ventilator lung in newborn (P27.8)*

J95.859 Other complication of respirator [ventilator]   cc⊘ HCC cc/mcc Exc

J95.86 Postprocedural hematoma and seroma of a respiratory system organ or structure following a procedure

J95.860 Postprocedural hematoma of a respiratory system organ or structure following a respiratory system procedure   cc⊘ cc/mcc Exc

J95.861 Postprocedural hematoma of a respiratory system organ or structure following other procedure   cc⊘ cc/mcc Exc

J95.862 Postprocedural seroma of a respiratory system organ or structure following a respiratory system procedure   cc⊘ cc/mcc Exc

J95.863 Postprocedural seroma of a respiratory system organ or structure following other procedure   cc⊘ cc/mcc Exc

J95.88 Other intraoperative complications of respiratory system, not elsewhere classified   cc⊘ cc/mcc Exc

J95.89 Other postprocedural complications and disorders of respiratory system, not elsewhere classified   cc⊘ cc/mcc Exc

Use additional code to identify disorder, such as:

aspiration pneumonia (J69.-)

bacterial or viral pneumonia (J12-J18)

EXCLUDES2 *acute pulmonary insufficiency following thoracic surgery (J95.1)*

postprocedural subglottic stenosis (J95.5)

Other diseases of the respiratory system (J96-J99)

J96 Respiratory failure, not elsewhere classified

EXCLUDES1 *acute respiratory distress syndrome (J80)*

cardiorespiratory failure (R09.2)

newborn respiratory distress syndrome (P22.0)

postprocedural respiratory failure (J95.82-)

respiratory arrest (R09.2)

respiratory arrest of newborn (P28.81)

respiratory failure of newborn (P28.5)

J96.0 Acute respiratory failure

J96.00 Acute respiratory failure, unspecified whether with hypoxia or hypercapnia   HCC mcc⊘ cc/mcc Exc

AHA: Q3 2016, Q4 2013

J96.01 Acute respiratory failure with hypoxia   HCC mcc⊘ cc/mcc Exc

J96.02 Acute respiratory failure with hypercapnia   HCC mcc⊘ cc/mcc Exc

J96.1 Chronic respiratory failure

J96.10 Chronic respiratory failure, unspecified whether with hypoxia or hypercapnia   cc⊘ HCC cc/mcc Exc

AHA: Q1 2016, Q1 2015

J96.11 Chronic respiratory failure with hypoxia   cc⊘ HCC cc/mcc Exc

AHA: Q4 2013

J96.12 Chronic respiratory failure with hypercapnia   cc⊘ HCC cc/mcc Exc

J96.2 Acute and chronic respiratory failure

Acute on chronic respiratory failure

J96.20 Acute and chronic respiratory failure, unspecified whether with hypoxia or hypercapnia   HCC mcc⊘ cc/mcc Exc

J96.21 Acute and chronic respiratory failure with hypoxia   HCC mcc⊘ cc/mcc Exc

J96.22 Acute and chronic respiratory failure with hypercapnia   HCC mcc⊘ cc/mcc Exc

J96.9 Respiratory failure, unspecified

J96.90 Respiratory failure, unspecified, unspecified whether with hypoxia or hypercapnia   HCC mcc⊘ cc/mcc Exc

J96.91 Respiratory failure, unspecified with hypoxia   HCC mcc⊘ cc/mcc Exc

J96.92 Respiratory failure, unspecified with hypercapnia   HCC mcc⊘ cc/mcc Exc

J98 Other respiratory disorders

Use additional code to identify:

exposure to environmental tobacco smoke (Z77.22)

exposure to tobacco smoke in the perinatal period (P96.81)

history of tobacco dependence (Z87.891)

occupational exposure to environmental tobacco smoke (Z57.31)

tobacco dependence (F17.-)

tobacco use (Z72.0)

PDx⊘ Unacceptable principal diagnosis symbol per Medicare code edits   Code exempt from diagnosis present on admission requirement

❓ Questionable admission   cc⊘ Complication or comorbidity   cc/mcc Exc CC/MCC exclusion   mcc⊘ Major complication or comorbidity

Principal diagnosis as its own CC   Principal diagnosis as its own MCC   HCC HCC diagnosis code   RxHCC RxHCC diagnosis code

MACRA code   Z Z code as first-listed diagnosis

When symbols appear on a code that requires a 7th character extension, refer to Appendix B to identify applicable 7th character codes.

2018 ICD-10-CM

EXCLUDES1 *newborn apnea (P28.4)*
      newborn sleep apnea (P28.3)
EXCLUDES2 *apnea NOS (R06.81)*
      sleep apnea (G47.3-)

5ᵗʰ **J98.0** **Diseases of bronchus, not elsewhere classified**

    J98.01 Acute **bronchospasm**

        EXCLUDES1 *acute bronchiolitis with bronchospasm (J21.-)*
           acute bronchitis with bronchospasm (J20.-)
           asthma (J45.-)
           exercise induced bronchospasm (J45.990)

    J98.09 **Other diseases of bronchus, not elsewhere classified**
        Broncholithiasis
        Calcification of bronchus
        Stenosis of bronchus
        Tracheobronchial collapse
        Tracheobronchial dyskinesia
        Ulcer of bronchus

5ᵗʰ **J98.1** **Pulmonary** collapse

    EXCLUDES1 *therapeutic collapse of lung status (Z98.3)*

    J98.11 Atelectasis   CC CC/MCC Exc

        EXCLUDES1 *newborn atelectasis*
           tuberculous atelectasis (current disease) (A15)

    J98.19 Other pulmonary **collapse**   CC CC/MCC Exc

J98.2 Interstitial **emphysema**   HCC RxHCC
    Mediastinal emphysema
    EXCLUDES1 *emphysema NOS (J43.9)*
        emphysema in newborn (P25.0)
        surgical emphysema (subcutaneous) (T81.82)
        traumatic subcutaneous emphysema (T79.7)

J98.3 Compensatory **emphysema**   HCC RxHCC

J98.4 Other **disorders of lung**
    Calcification of lung
    Cystic lung disease (acquired)
    Lung disease NOS
    Pulmolithiasis
    EXCLUDES1 *acute interstitial pneumonitis (J84.114)*
        pulmonary insufficiency following surgery (J95.1-J95.2)

5ᵗʰ **J98.5** **Diseases of** mediastinum, **not elsewhere classified**

    EXCLUDES2 *abscess of mediastinum (J85.3)*

    J98.51 Mediastinitis   MCC CC/MCC Exc
        AHA: Q4 2016
        Code first underlying condition, if applicable, such
        as postoperative mediastinitis (T81.-)

    J98.59 Other **diseases of mediastinum, not elsewhere**
        classified   MCC CC/MCC Exc
        AHA: Q4 2016
        Fibrosis of mediastinum
        Hernia of mediastinum
        Retraction of mediastinum

J98.6 **Disorders of diaphragm**
    Diaphragmatitis
    Paralysis of diaphragm
    Relaxation of diaphragm
    EXCLUDES1 *congenital malformation of diaphragm NEC (Q79.1)*
        congenital diaphragmatic hernia (Q79.0)
    EXCLUDES2 *diaphragmatic hernia (K44.-)*

J98.8 **Other specified respiratory disorders**

J98.9 **Respiratory disorder, unspecified**
    Respiratory disease (chronic) NOS

J99 **Respiratory disorders in diseases classified elsewhere**   HCC RxHCC
    Code first underlying disease, such as:
    amyloidosis (E85.-)
    ankylosing spondylitis (M45)
    congenital syphilis (A50.5)
    cryoglobulinemia (D89.1)
    early congenital syphilis (A50.0)
    schistosomiasis (B65.0-B65.9)
    EXCLUDES1 *respiratory disorders in:*
        amebiasis (A06.5)
        blastomycosis (B40.0-B40.2)
        candidiasis (B37.1)
        coccidioidomycosis (B38.0-B38.2)
        cystic fibrosis with pulmonary manifestations (E84.0)
        dermatomyositis (M33.01, M33.11)
        histoplasmosis (B39.0-B39.2)
        late syphilis (A52.72, A52.73)
        polymyositis (M33.21)
        sicca syndrome (M35.02)
        systemic lupus erythematosus (M32.13)
        systemic sclerosis (M34.81)
        Wegener's granulomatosis (M31.30-M31.31)

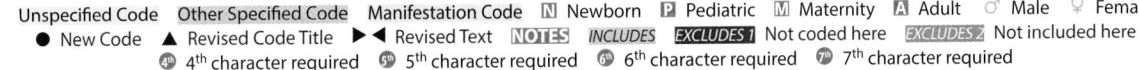

Unspecified Code   Other Specified Code   Manifestation Code   N Newborn   P Pediatric   M Maternity   A Adult   ♂ Male   ♀ Female
● New Code   ▲ Revised Code Title   ►◄ Revised Text   NOTES   *INCLUDES*   EXCLUDES 1 Not coded here   EXCLUDES 2 Not included here
4ᵗʰ character required   5ᵗʰ character required   6ᵗʰ character required   7ᵗʰ character required
Ⓧ Extension 'X' Alert   HAC Hospital-acquired condition (HAC) alert   **AHA** AHA Coding Clinic©

d) The Kupffer cells (or stellate macrophages) of the liver perform phagocytosis of the bacteria and the worn out blood cells.

e) The liver stores various elements like copper, iron, and vitamins A, D, E, and K. It also helps to detoxify the poisonous substances in the human body, and produces bile salts for the emulsification (or break down) of the body fats.

f) The liver lobules facilitate the production of bile, which is then stored and concentrated in gall bladder.

g) The common bile duct carries the bile from the liver and gallbladder to the duodenum. It is formed by the union of the cystic and hepatic ducts.

h) The porta hepatis is a transverse fissure in the middle visceral surface of the liver that gives passage to the hepatic portal vein, hepatic artery, hepatic nerve plexus, hepatic ducts, and the lymphatic vessels.

Liver Anatomy

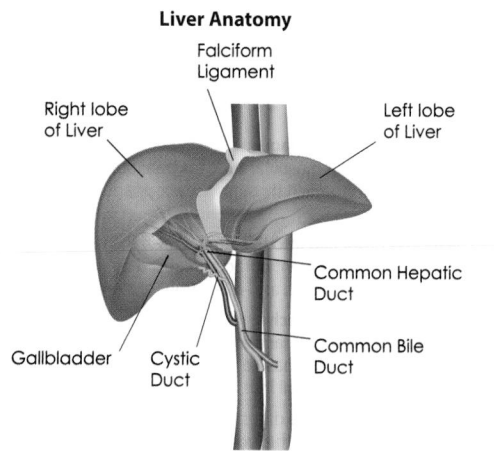

8. **The Anatomy of the Small Intestine**
   a) The small intestine extends from the pylorus of the stomach to the ileocecal junction. It is divided into the duodenum, jejunum and ileum.
   b) The ileocecal valve serves to connect the small intestine with the large intestine.
   c) The small intestine is involved in the completion of absorption of the digested food through the intestinal digestive enzymes, which are secreted by the intestinal glands (or the crypts of Lieberkuhn).
   d) The Brunner's glands (or pancreal glands/duodenal glands) are the compound tubular submucosal glands of the duodenum that secrete alkaline mucus.

9. **The Anatomy of the Large Intestine**
   a) The large intestine performs the following functions:
      i) reabsorption of water.
      ii) absorption and manufacture of vitamins.
      iii) formation and expulsion of feces.
   b) The large intestine is based on cecum, colon, rectum, and anus.
   c) The colon is divided into the following parts:
      i) ascending colon
      ii) right colic (or hepatic) flexure
      iii) transverse colon
      iv) left colic (or splenic) flexure
      v) descending colon
      vi) sigmoid colon
   d) The rectum terminates at the anus. The dilated portion of the rectum where feces are stored (before their elimination through the anal canal) is termed as the rectal ampulla.

Common Pathologies

Appendicitis
Inflammation of the appendix, which is usually acute and caused by the blocking of the appendix.

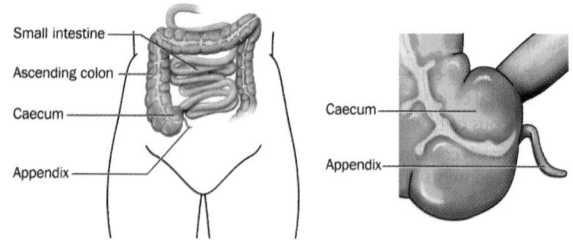

Ascites
Condition of abnormal accumulation of serous fluid in the peritoneal cavity.

Cirrhosis of Liver
This is a chronic liver disease, which is characterized by destruction of liver cells that ultimately leads to ineffective liver function and jaundice.

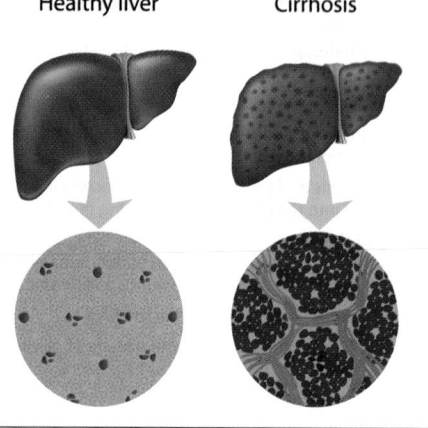

Diverticular Disease
This is a condition in which bulging pouches (known as diverticula) in the gastrointestinal (GI) tract push the mucosal lining through the surrounding muscle.

Dysentery
This is a condition that leads to inflammation of the intestine, especially of the colon, which may be caused by chemical irritants, bacteria, protozoa, or parasites.

Fistula
This is a condition in which there is an abnormal passage from one organ to another, or from a hollow organ to the surface.

Gastroesophageal Reflux Disease (GERD)
This is a condition that causes backflow (reflux) of gastric contents into the esophagus due to malfunction of the lower esophageal sphincter (LES).

Hematochezia
This is a condition marked by the passage of stools containing bright red blood.

Hemorrhoid
This is a condition that causes a mass of enlarged, twisted varicose veins in the mucous membrane inside (internal) or just outside (external) the rectum; also known as piles.

Hemorrhoid

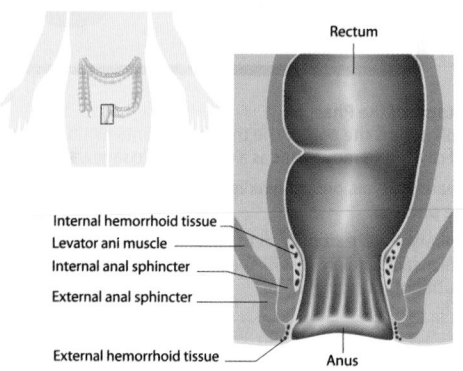

Hernia
This is a condition caused by the protrusion or projection of an organ or a part of an organ through the wall of the cavity that normally contains it.

Hiatus Hernia

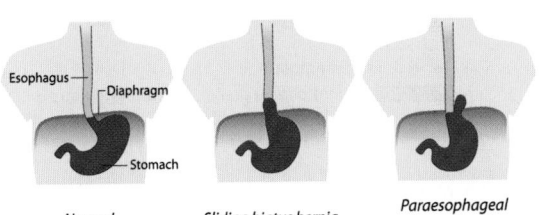

| Normal | Sliding hiatus hernia | Paraesophageal hiatus hernia |

Inflammatory Bowel Disease (IBD)
This is a condition in which ulceration of the colon mucosa occurs.Ulcerative colitis and Crohn's disease are forms of IBD.

Crohn's Disease
This is the condition of chronic IBD that usually affects the ileum but may affect any portion of the intestinal tract.

Inflammatory Bowel Disease

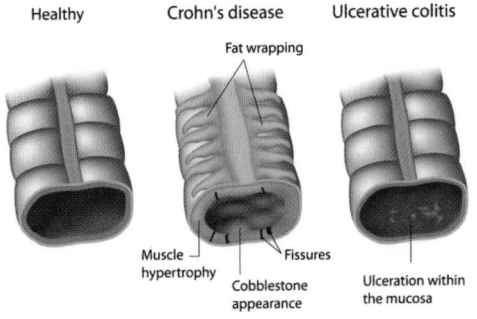

Ulcerative Colitis
This is the condition of chronic IBD of the colon characterized by episodes of diarrhea, rectal bleeding, and pain.

Irritable Bowel Syndrome (IBS)
This is the condition characterized by gastrointestinal signs and symptoms, including constipation, diarrhea, gas, and bloating, all in the absence of organic pathology; also called spastic colon.

Jaundice
This is the condition in which yellow discoloration of the skin, mucous membranes, and sclerae of the eyes is caused by excessive levels of bilirubin in the blood (hyperbilirubinemia).

Obesity
This is the condition in which a person accumulates an amount of fat that exceeds the body's skeletal and physical standards, usually an increase of 20 percent or more above ideal body weight.

Morbid Obesity
Condition of more severe obesity in which a person has a body mass index (BMI) of 40 or greater, which is generally 100 or more pounds over ideal body weight.

Polyp
A polyp is a small tumorlike, benign growth that projects from a mucous membrane surface.

Polyposis
This is a condition in which polyps develop in the intestinal tract.

Peptic Ulcer
This condition is also known as peptic ulcer disease; these are the painful ulcers that usually arise in duodenum.

Peptic Ulcer

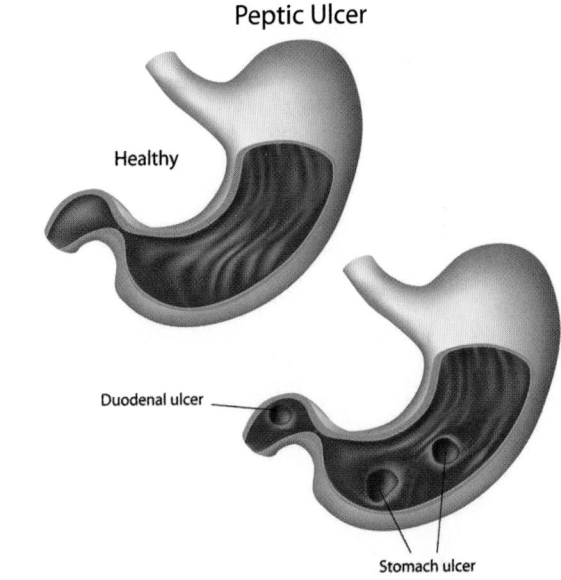

Volvulus
This is a condition in which the bowel twists on itself, causing obstruction.

Diseases of the digestive system (K00-K95)

EXCLUDES2 *certain conditions originating in the perinatal period (P04-P96)*

certain infectious and parasitic diseases (A00-B99)

complications of pregnancy, childbirth and the puerperium (O00-O9A)

congenital malformations, deformations and chromosomal abnormalities (Q00-Q99)

endocrine, nutritional and metabolic diseases (E00-E88)

injury, poisoning and certain other consequences of external causes (S00-T88)

neoplasms (C00-D49)

symptoms, signs and abnormal clinical and laboratory findings, not elsewhere classified (R00-R94)

This chapter contains the following blocks:

K00-K14	Diseases of oral cavity and salivary glands
K20-K31	Diseases of esophagus, stomach and duodenum
K35-K38	Diseases of appendix
K40-K46	Hernia
K50-K52	Noninfective enteritis and colitis
K55-K64	Other diseases of intestines
K65-K68	Diseases of peritoneum and retroperitoneum
K70-K77	Diseases of liver
K80-K87	Disorders of gallbladder, biliary tract and pancreas
K90-K95	Other diseases of the digestive system

Diseases of oral cavity and salivary glands (K00-K14)

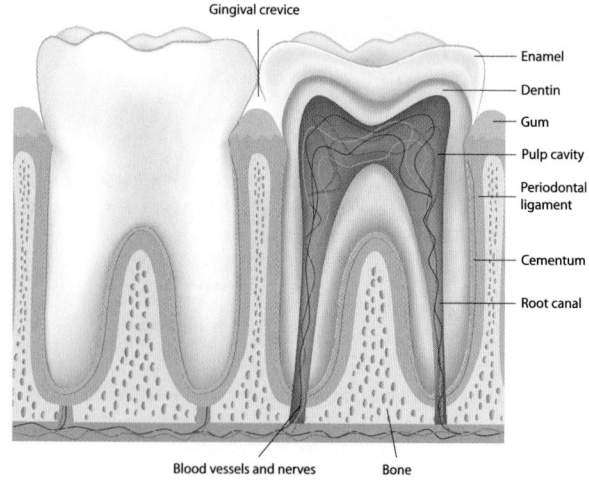

Gingival crevice

Enamel

Dentin

Gum

Pulp cavity

Periodontal ligament

Cementum

Root canal

Blood vessels and nerves   Bone

Figure 11.1 Tooth anatomy

K00 **Disorders of tooth development and eruption**

EXCLUDES2 *embedded and impacted teeth (K01.-)*

K00.0 **Anodontia**
Hypodontia
Oligodontia
EXCLUDES1 *acquired absence of teeth (K08.1-)*

K00.1 **Supernumerary teeth**
Distomolar
Fourth molar
Mesiodens
Paramolar
Supplementary teeth
EXCLUDES2 *supernumerary roots (K00.2)*

K00.2 **Abnormalities of size and form of teeth**
Concrescence of teeth
Fusion of teeth
Gemination of teeth
Dens evaginatus

Dens in dente
Dens invaginatus
Enamel pearls
Macrodontia
Microdontia
Peg-shaped [conical] teeth
Supernumerary roots
Taurodontism
Tuberculum paramolare
EXCLUDES1 *abnormalities of teeth due to congenital syphilis (A50.5)*

tuberculum Carabelli, which is regarded as a normal variation and should not be coded

K00.3 **Mottled teeth**
Dental fluorosis
Mottling of enamel
Nonfluoride enamel opacities
EXCLUDES2 *deposits [accretions] on teeth (K03.6)*

K00.4 **Disturbances in tooth formation**
Aplasia and hypoplasia of cementum
Dilaceration of tooth
Enamel hypoplasia (neonatal) (postnatal) (prenatal)
Regional odontodysplasia
Turner's tooth
EXCLUDES1 *Hutchinson's teeth and mulberry molars in congenital syphilis (A50.5)*
EXCLUDES2 *mottled teeth (K00.3)*

K00.5 **Hereditary disturbances in tooth structure, not elsewhere classified**
Amelogenesis imperfecta
Dentinogenesis imperfecta
Odontogenesis imperfecta
Dentinal dysplasia
Shell teeth

K00.6 **Disturbances in tooth eruption**
Dentia praecox
Natal tooth
Neonatal tooth
Premature eruption of tooth
Premature shedding of primary [deciduous] tooth
Prenatal teeth
Retained [persistent] primary tooth
EXCLUDES2 *embedded and impacted teeth (K01.-)*

K00.7 **Teething syndrome**

K00.8 **Other disorders of tooth development**
Color changes during tooth formation
Intrinsic staining of teeth NOS
EXCLUDES2 *posteruptive color changes (K03.7)*

K00.9 **Disorder of tooth development, unspecified**
Disorder of odontogenesis NOS

K01 **Embedded and impacted teeth**
EXCLUDES1 *abnormal position of fully erupted teeth (M26.3-)*

K01.0 **Embedded teeth**

K01.1 **Impacted teeth**

K02 **Dental caries**

INCLUDES *caries of dentine*

dental cavities

early childhood caries

pre-eruptive caries

recurrent caries (dentino enamel junction) (enamel) (to the pulp)

tooth decay

K02.3 Arrested **dental caries**
Arrested coronal and root caries

K02.5 **Dental caries on** pit and fissure surface
Dental caries on chewing surface of tooth

K02.51 **Dental caries on pit and fissure surface** limited to enamel
White spot lesions [initial caries] on pit and fissure surface of tooth

PDₓ Unacceptable principal diagnosis symbol per Medicare code edits   POA Code exempt from diagnosis present on admission requirement

？ Questionable admission   CC Complication or comorbidity   CC/MCC Exc CC/MCC exclusion   MCC Major complication or comorbidity

Principal diagnosis as its own CC   Principal diagnosis as its own MCC   HCC HCC diagnosis code   RxHCC RxHCC diagnosis code

MACRA code   Z1 Z code as first-listed diagnosis

K02.52 **Dental caries on pit and fissure surface** penetrating into dentin
Primary dental caries, cervical origin

K02.53 **Dental caries on pit and fissure surface** penetrating into pulp

🔟 K02.6 **Dental caries on** smooth surface

K02.61 **Dental caries on smooth surface** limited to enamel
White spot lesions [initial caries] on smooth surface of tooth

K02.62 **Dental caries on smooth surface** penetrating into dentin

K02.63 **Dental caries on smooth surface** penetrating into pulp

K02.7 **Dental** root **caries**

K02.9 **Dental caries, unspecified**

🔟 K03 **Other diseases of hard tissues of teeth**

EXCLUDES2 bruxism (F45.8)

dental caries (K02.-)

teeth-grinding NOS (F45.8)

K03.0 **Excessive attrition of teeth**
Approximal wear of teeth
Occlusal wear of teeth

K03.1 **Abrasion of teeth**
Dentifrice abrasion of teeth
Habitual abrasion of teeth
Occupational abrasion of teeth
Ritual abrasion of teeth
Traditional abrasion of teeth
Wedge defect NOS

K03.2 **Erosion of teeth**
Erosion of teeth due to diet
Erosion of teeth due to drugs and medicaments
Erosion of teeth due to persistent vomiting
Erosion of teeth NOS
Idiopathic erosion of teeth
Occupational erosion of teeth

K03.3 **Pathological resorption of teeth**
Internal granuloma of pulp
Resorption of teeth (external)

K03.4 **Hypercementosis**
Cementation hyperplasia

K03.5 **Ankylosis of teeth**

K03.6 **Deposits [accretions] on teeth**
Betel deposits [accretions] on teeth
Black deposits [accretions] on teeth
Extrinsic staining of teeth NOS
Green deposits [accretions] on teeth
Materia alba deposits [accretions] on teeth
Orange deposits [accretions] on teeth
Staining of teeth NOS
Subgingival dental calculus
Supragingival dental calculus
Tobacco deposits [accretions] on teeth

K03.7 **Posteruptive color changes of dental hard tissues**
EXCLUDES2 deposits [accretions] on teeth (K03.6)

🔟 K03.8 **Other specified diseases of hard tissues of teeth**

K03.81 **Cracked tooth**
EXCLUDES1 asymptomatic craze lines in enamel - omit code
broken or fractured tooth due to trauma (S02.5)

K03.89 **Other specified diseases of hard tissues of teeth**

K03.9 **Disease of hard tissues of teeth, unspecified**

🔟 K04 **Diseases of pulp and periapical tissues**

🔟 K04.0 **Pulpitis**
Acute pulpitis
Chronic (hyperplastic) (ulcerative) pulpitis

K04.01 **Reversible pulpitis** CC CC/MCC Exc

K04.02 **Irreversible pulpitis** CC CC/MCC Exc

K04.1 **Necrosis of pulp**
Pulpal gangrene

K04.2 **Pulp degeneration**
Denticles
Pulpal calcifications
Pulpal stones

K04.3 **Abnormal hard tissue formation in pulp**
Secondary or irregular dentine

K04.4 **Acute apical periodontitis of pulpal origin** CC CC/MCC Exc
Acute apical periodontitis NOS
EXCLUDES1 acute periodontitis (K05.2-)

K04.5 **Chronic apical periodontitis**
Apical or periapical granuloma
Apical periodontitis NOS
EXCLUDES1 chronic periodontitis (K05.3-)

K04.6 **Periapical abscess with sinus**
Dental abscess with sinus
Dentoalveolar abscess with sinus

K04.7 **Periapical abscess without sinus**
Dental abscess without sinus
Dentoalveolar abscess without sinus

K04.8 **Radicular cyst**
Apical (periodontal) cyst
Periapical cyst
Residual radicular cyst
EXCLUDES2 lateral periodontal cyst (K09.0)

🔟 K04.9 **Other and unspecified diseases of pulp and periapical tissues**

K04.90 **Unspecified diseases of pulp and periapical tissues**

K04.99 **Other diseases of pulp and periapical tissues**

🔟 K05 **Gingivitis and periodontal diseases**
Use additional code to identify:
alcohol abuse and dependence (F10.-)
exposure to environmental tobacco smoke (Z77.22)
exposure to tobacco smoke in the perinatal period (P96.81)
history of tobacco dependence (Z87.891)
occupational exposure to environmental tobacco smoke (Z57.31)
tobacco dependence (F17.-)
tobacco use (Z72.0)

🔟 K05.0 **Acute gingivitis**
EXCLUDES1 acute necrotizing ulcerative gingivitis (A69.1)
herpesviral [herpes simplex] gingivostomatitis (B00.2)

K05.00 **Acute gingivitis,** plaque induced
Acute gingivitis NOS
Plaque induced gingival disease

K05.01 **Acute gingivitis,** non-plaque induced

🔟 K05.1 **Chronic gingivitis**
Desquamative gingivitis (chronic)
Gingivitis (chronic) NOS
Hyperplastic gingivitis (chronic)
Pregnancy associated gingivitis
Simple marginal gingivitis (chronic)
Ulcerative gingivitis (chronic)
Code first, if applicable, diseases of the digestive system complicating pregnancy (O99.61-)

K05.10 **Chronic gingivitis,** plaque induced
Chronic gingivitis NOS
Gingivitis NOS

K05.11 **Chronic gingivitis,** non-plaque induced

🔟 K05.2 **Aggressive periodontitis**
Acute pericoronitis
EXCLUDES1 acute apical periodontitis (K04.4)
periapical abscess (K04.7)
periapical abscess with sinus (K04.6)

K05.20 **Aggressive periodontitis, unspecified**

6️⃣ K05.21 **Aggressive periodontitis,** localized
Periodontal abscess

K05.211 **Aggressive periodontitis, localized,** slight

K05.212 **Aggressive periodontitis, localized,** moderate

K05.213 **Aggressive periodontitis, localized,** severe

Unspecified Code   Other Specified Code   Manifestation Code   Ⓝ Newborn   Ⓟ Pediatric   Ⓜ Maternity   Ⓐ Adult   ♂ Male   ♀ Female
● New Code   ▲ Revised Code Title   ►◄ Revised Text   **NOTES**   *INCLUDES*   *EXCLUDES 1* Not coded here   *EXCLUDES 2* Not included here
4️⃣ 4ᵗʰ character required   5️⃣ 5ᵗʰ character required   6️⃣ 6ᵗʰ character required   7️⃣ 7ᵗʰ character required
7️⃣ Extension 'X' Alert   **HAC** Hospital-acquired condition (HAC) alert   **AHA** AHA Coding Clinic©

K05.219 **Aggressive periodontitis, localized,** unspecified severity

K05.22 Aggressive periodontitis, generalized

    K05.221 **Aggressive periodontitis, generalized,** slight

    K05.222 **Aggressive periodontitis, generalized,** moderate

    K05.223 **Aggressive periodontitis, generalized,** severe

    K05.229 **Aggressive periodontitis, generalized,** unspecified severity

K05.3 Chronic periodontitis
  Chronic pericoronitis
  Complex periodontitis
  Periodontitis NOS
  Simplex periodontitis
  EXCLUDES1 chronic apical periodontitis (K04.5)

  K05.30 **Chronic periodontitis, unspecified**

  K05.31 Chronic periodontitis, localized

    K05.311 **Chronic periodontitis, localized,** slight

    K05.312 **Chronic periodontitis, localized,** moderate

    K05.313 **Chronic periodontitis, localized,** severe

    K05.319 **Chronic periodontitis, localized,** unspecified severity

  K05.32 Chronic periodontitis, generalized

    K05.321 **Chronic periodontitis, generalized,** slight

    K05.322 **Chronic periodontitis, generalized,** moderate

    K05.323 **Chronic periodontitis, generalized,** severe

    K05.329 **Chronic periodontitis, generalized,** unspecified severity

K05.4 **Periodontosis**
  Juvenile periodontosis

K05.5 **Other periodontal diseases**
  Combined periodontic-endodontic lesion
  Narrow gingival width (of periodontal soft tissue)
  EXCLUDES2 leukoplakia of gingiva (K13.21)

K05.6 **Periodontal disease, unspecified**

K06 Other disorders of gingiva and edentulous alveolar ridge
  EXCLUDES2 acute gingivitis (K05.0)
    atrophy of edentulous alveolar ridge (K08.2)
    chronic gingivitis (K05.1)
    gingivitis NOS (K05.1)

K06.0 Gingival recession
  Gingival recession (postinfective) (postprocedural)

  K06.01 Gingival recession, localized

    ● K06.010 **Localized gingival recession,** unspecified
      Localized gingival recession, NOS

    ● K06.011 **Localized gingival recession,** minimal

    ● K06.012 **Localized gingival recession,** moderate

    ● K06.013 **Localized gingival recession,** severe

  ● K06.02 Gingival recession, generalized

    ● K06.020 **Generalized gingival recession,** unspecified
      Generalized gingival recession, NOS

    ● K06.021 **Generalized gingival recession,** minimal

    ● K06.022 **Generalized gingival recession,** moderate

    ● K06.023 **Generalized gingival recession,** severe

K06.1 Gingival enlargement
  Gingival fibromatosis

K06.2 Gingival and edentulous alveolar ridge lesions associated with trauma
  Irritative hyperplasia of edentulous ridge [denture hyperplasia]
  Use additional code (Chapter 20) to identify external cause or denture status (Z97.2)

K06.3 **Horizontal alveolar bone loss**

K06.8 **Other specified disorders of gingiva and edentulous alveolar ridge**
  Fibrous epulis
  Flabby alveolar ridge

  Giant cell epulis
  Peripheral giant cell granuloma of gingiva
  Pyogenic granuloma of gingiva
  Vertical ridge deficiency
  EXCLUDES2 gingival cyst (K09.0)

K06.9 **Disorder of gingiva and edentulous alveolar ridge, unspecified**

K08 Other disorders of teeth and supporting structures
  EXCLUDES2 dentofacial anomalies [including malocclusion] (M26.-)
    disorders of jaw (M27.-)

K08.0 Exfoliation of teeth due to systemic causes
  Code also underlying systemic condition

K08.1 Complete loss of teeth
  Acquired loss of teeth, complete
  EXCLUDES1 congenital absence of teeth (K00.0)
    exfoliation of teeth due to systemic causes (K08.0)
    partial loss of teeth (K08.4-)

  K08.10 Complete loss of teeth, unspecified cause

    K08.101 **Complete loss of teeth, unspecified cause,** class I

    K08.102 **Complete loss of teeth, unspecified cause,** class II

    K08.103 **Complete loss of teeth, unspecified cause,** class III

    K08.104 **Complete loss of teeth, unspecified cause,** class IV

    K08.109 **Complete loss of teeth, unspecified cause, unspecified class**
      Edentulism NOS

  K08.11 Complete loss of teeth due to trauma

    K08.111 **Complete loss of teeth due to trauma,** class I

    K08.112 **Complete loss of teeth due to trauma,** class II

    K08.113 **Complete loss of teeth due to trauma,** class III

    K08.114 **Complete loss of teeth due to trauma,** class IV

    K08.119 **Complete loss of teeth due to trauma, unspecified class**

  K08.12 Complete loss of teeth due to periodontal diseases

    K08.121 **Complete loss of teeth due to periodontal diseases,** class I

    K08.122 **Complete loss of teeth due to periodontal diseases,** class II

    K08.123 **Complete loss of teeth due to periodontal diseases,** class III

    K08.124 **Complete loss of teeth due to periodontal diseases,** class IV

    K08.129 **Complete loss of teeth due to periodontal diseases, unspecified class**

  K08.13 Complete loss of teeth due to caries

    K08.131 **Complete loss of teeth due to caries, class I**

    K08.132 **Complete loss of teeth due to caries, class II**

    K08.133 **Complete loss of teeth due to caries,** class III

    K08.134 **Complete loss of teeth due to caries,** class IV

    K08.139 **Complete loss of teeth due to caries, unspecified class**

  K08.19 Complete loss of teeth due to other specified cause

    K08.191 **Complete loss of teeth due to other specified cause, class I**

    K08.192 **Complete loss of teeth due to other specified cause, class II**

    K08.193 **Complete loss of teeth due to other specified cause, class III**

    K08.194 **Complete loss of teeth due to other specified cause, class IV**

    K08.199 **Complete loss of teeth due to other specified cause, unspecified class**

ᴾᴰˣ Unacceptable principal diagnosis symbol per Medicare code edits   ᴾᴼᴬ Code exempt from diagnosis present on admission requirement
❓ Questionable admission ᶜᶜ Complication or comorbidity ᶜᶜ⁻ᴹᶜᶜ ᴱˣᶜ CC/MCC exclusion ᴹᶜᶜ Major complication or comorbidity
ᴾᶜᶜ Principal diagnosis as its own CC ᴾᴹᶜᶜ Principal diagnosis as its own MCC ᴴᶜᶜ HCC diagnosis code ᴿˣᴴᶜᶜ RxHCC diagnosis code
MACRA code Z1 Z code as first-listed diagnosis

720   When symbols appear on a code that requires a 7th character extension, refer to Appendix B to identify applicable 7th character codes.   **2018 ICD-10-CM**

5ᵗʰ K08.2 **Atrophy of edentulous alveolar ridge**
    K08.20 **Unspecified atrophy of edentulous alveolar ridge**
        Atrophy of the mandible NOS
        Atrophy of the maxilla NOS
    K08.21 Minimal **atrophy of the** mandible
        Minimal atrophy of the edentulous mandible
    K08.22 Moderate **atrophy of the** mandible
        Moderate atrophy of the edentulous mandible
    K08.23 Severe **atrophy of the** mandible
        Severe atrophy of the edentulous mandible
    K08.24 Minimal **atrophy of** maxilla
        Minimal atrophy of the edentulous maxilla
    K08.25 Moderate **atrophy of the** maxilla
        Moderate atrophy of the edentulous maxilla
    K08.26 Severe **atrophy of the** maxilla
        Severe atrophy of the edentulous maxilla

K08.3 **Retained dental root**

5ᵗʰ K08.4 **Partial loss of teeth**
    Acquired loss of teeth, partial
    EXCLUDES1 complete loss of teeth (K08.1-)
        congenital absence of teeth (K00.0)
    EXCLUDES2 exfoliation of teeth due to systemic causes (K08.0)
   6ᵗʰ K08.40 **Partial loss of teeth,** unspecified cause
      K08.401 **Partial loss of teeth, unspecified cause, class I**
      K08.402 **Partial loss of teeth, unspecified cause, class II**
      K08.403 **Partial loss of teeth, unspecified cause, class III**
      K08.404 **Partial loss of teeth, unspecified cause, class IV**
      K08.409 **Partial loss of teeth, unspecified cause, unspecified class**
        Tooth extraction status NOS
   6ᵗʰ K08.41 **Partial loss of teeth due to** trauma
      K08.411 **Partial loss of teeth due to trauma,** class I
      K08.412 **Partial loss of teeth due to trauma,** class II
      K08.413 **Partial loss of teeth due to trauma,** class III
      K08.414 **Partial loss of teeth due to trauma,** class IV
      K08.419 **Partial loss of teeth due to trauma, unspecified class**
   6ᵗʰ K08.42 **Partial loss of teeth due to** periodontal diseases
      K08.421 **Partial loss of teeth due to periodontal diseases,** class I
      K08.422 **Partial loss of teeth due to periodontal diseases,** class II
      K08.423 **Partial loss of teeth due to periodontal diseases,** class III
      K08.424 **Partial loss of teeth due to periodontal diseases,** class IV
      K08.429 **Partial loss of teeth due to periodontal diseases, unspecified class**
   6ᵗʰ K08.43 **Partial loss of teeth due to** caries
      K08.431 **Partial loss of teeth due to caries,** class I
      K08.432 **Partial loss of teeth due to caries,** class II
      K08.433 **Partial loss of teeth due to caries,** class III
      K08.434 **Partial loss of teeth due to caries,** class IV
      K08.439 **Partial loss of teeth due to caries, unspecified class**
   6ᵗʰ K08.49 **Partial loss of teeth due to** other specified cause
      K08.491 **Partial loss of teeth due to other specified cause, class I**
      K08.492 **Partial loss of teeth due to other specified cause, class II**
      K08.493 **Partial loss of teeth due to other specified cause, class III**
      K08.494 **Partial loss of teeth due to other specified cause, class IV**
      K08.499 **Partial loss of teeth due to other specified cause, unspecified class**

5ᵗʰ K08.5 **Unsatisfactory restoration of tooth**
    Defective bridge, crown, filling
    Defective dental restoration
    EXCLUDES1 dental restoration status (Z98.811)
    EXCLUDES2 endosseous dental implant failure (M27.6-)
        unsatisfactory endodontic treatment (M27.5-)
    K08.50 **Unsatisfactory restoration of tooth, unspecified**
        Defective dental restoration NOS
    K08.51 Open **restoration margins of tooth**
        Dental restoration failure of marginal integrity
        Open margin on tooth restoration
        Poor gingival margin to tooth restoration
    K08.52 **Unrepairable overhanging of dental restorative materials**
        Overhanging of tooth restoration
   6ᵗʰ K08.53 **Fractured dental restorative material**
      EXCLUDES1 cracked tooth (K03.81)
        traumatic fracture of tooth (S02.5)
      K08.530 **Fractured dental restorative material** without loss of material
      K08.531 **Fractured dental restorative material** with loss of material
      K08.539 **Fractured dental restorative material, unspecified**
    K08.54 **Contour of existing restoration of tooth biologically incompatible with oral health**
        Dental restoration failure of periodontal anatomical integrity
        Unacceptable contours of existing restoration of tooth
        Unacceptable morphology of existing restoration of tooth
    K08.55 **Allergy to existing dental restorative material**
        Use additional code to identify the specific type of allergy
    K08.56 **Poor aesthetic of existing restoration of tooth**
        Dental restoration aesthetically inadequate or displeasing
    K08.59 **Other unsatisfactory restoration of tooth**
        Other defective dental restoration

5ᵗʰ K08.8 **Other specified disorders of teeth and supporting structures**
    K08.81 Primary occlusal trauma
    K08.82 Secondary occlusal trauma
    K08.89 **Other specified disorders of teeth and supporting structures**
        Enlargement of alveolar ridge NOS
        Insufficient anatomic crown height
        Insufficient clinical crown length
        Irregular alveolar process
        Toothache NOS

K08.9 **Disorder of teeth and supporting structures, unspecified**

4ᵗʰ K09 **Cysts of oral region, not elsewhere classified**
    INCLUDES lesions showing histological features both of aneurysmal cyst and of another fibro-osseous lesion
    EXCLUDES2 cysts of jaw (M27.0-, M27.4-)
        radicular cyst (K04.8)
    K09.0 Developmental odontogenic **cysts**
        Dentigerous cyst
        Eruption cyst
        Follicular cyst
        Gingival cyst
        Lateral periodontal cyst
        Primordial cyst
      EXCLUDES2 keratocysts (D16.4, D16.5)
        odontogenic keratocystic tumors (D16.4, D16.5)
    K09.1 Developmental (nonodontogenic) **cysts of oral region**
        Cyst (of) incisive canal
        Cyst (of) palatine of papilla
        Globulomaxillary cyst
        Median palatal cyst
        Nasoalveolar cyst
        Nasolabial cyst
        Nasopalatine duct cyst

● Unspecified Code   Other Specified Code   Manifestation Code   Ⓝ Newborn   Ⓟ Pediatric   Ⓜ Maternity   Ⓐ Adult   ♂ Male   ♀ Female
● New Code   ▲ Revised Code Title   ▶◀ Revised Text   **NOTES**   *INCLUDES*   *EXCLUDES 1* Not coded here   *EXCLUDES 2* Not included here
4ᵗʰ character required   5ᵗʰ character required   6ᵗʰ character required   7ᵗʰ character required
7ᵗʰ Extension 'X' Alert   HAC Hospital-acquired condition (HAC) alert   **AHA** AHA Coding Clinic©

K09.8 Other cysts of oral region, not elsewhere classified
Dermoid cyst
Epidermoid cyst
Lymphoepithelial cyst
Epstein's pearl

K09.9 Cyst of oral region, unspecified

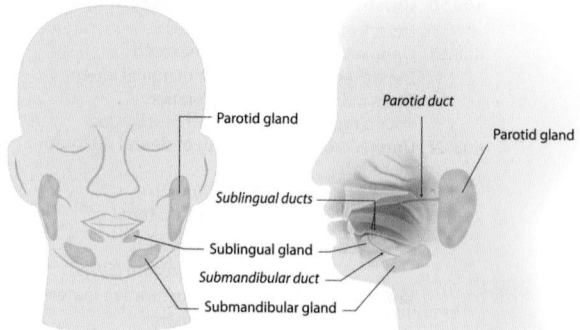

Figure 11.2 Salivary glands

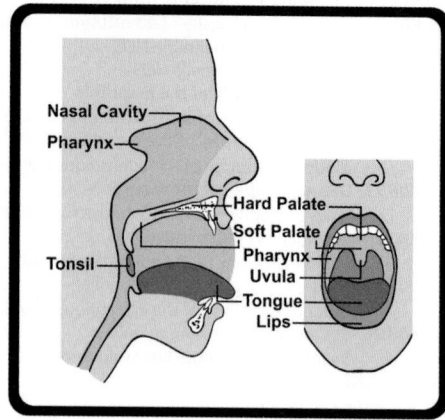

Figure 11.3 Mouth

K11 Diseases of salivary glands
Use additional code to identify:
alcohol abuse and dependence (F10.-)
exposure to environmental tobacco smoke (Z77.22)
exposure to tobacco smoke in the perinatal period (P96.81)
history of tobacco dependence (Z87.891)
occupational exposure to environmental tobacco smoke (Z57.31)
tobacco dependence (F17.-)
tobacco use (Z72.0)

K11.0 Atrophy of salivary gland

K11.1 Hypertrophy of salivary gland

K11.2 Sialoadenitis
Parotitis
EXCLUDES1 epidemic parotitis (B26.-)
mumps (B26.-)
uveoparotid fever [Heerfordt] (D86.89)

K11.20 Sialoadenitis, unspecified

K11.21 Acute sialoadenitis
EXCLUDES1 acute recurrent sialoadenitis (K11.22)

K11.22 Acute recurrent sialoadenitis

K11.23 Chronic sialoadenitis

K11.3 Abscess of salivary gland   cc CC/MCC Exc

K11.4 Fistula of salivary gland   cc CC/MCC Exc
EXCLUDES1 congenital fistula of salivary gland (Q38.4)

K11.5 Sialolithiasis
Calculus of salivary gland or duct
Stone of salivary gland or duct

K11.6 Mucocele of salivary gland
Mucous extravasation cyst of salivary gland
Mucous retention cyst of salivary gland
Ranula

K11.7 Disturbances of salivary secretion
Hypoptyalism
Ptyalism
Xerostomia
EXCLUDES2 dry mouth NOS (R68.2)

K11.8 Other diseases of salivary glands
Benign lymphoepithelial lesion of salivary gland
Mikulicz' disease
Necrotizing sialometaplasia
Sialectasia
Stenosis of salivary duct
Stricture of salivary duct
EXCLUDES1 sicca syndrome [Sjögren] (M35.0-)

K11.9 Disease of salivary gland, unspecified
Sialoadenopathy NOS

K12 Stomatitis and related lesions
Use additional code to identify:
alcohol abuse and dependence (F10.-)
exposure to environmental tobacco smoke (Z77.22)
exposure to tobacco smoke in the perinatal period (P96.81)
history of tobacco dependence (Z87.891)
occupational exposure to environmental tobacco smoke (Z57.31)
tobacco dependence (F17.-)
tobacco use (Z72.0)
EXCLUDES1 cancrum oris (A69.0)
cheilitis (K13.0)
gangrenous stomatitis (A69.0)
herpesviral [herpes simplex] gingivostomatitis (B00.2)
noma (A69.0)

K12.0 Recurrent oral aphthae
Aphthous stomatitis (major) (minor)
Bednar's aphthae
Periadenitis mucosa necrotica recurrens
Recurrent aphthous ulcer
Stomatitis herpetiformis

K12.1 Other forms of stomatitis
Stomatitis NOS
Denture stomatitis
Ulcerative stomatitis
Vesicular stomatitis
EXCLUDES1 acute necrotizing ulcerative stomatitis (A69.1)
Vincent's stomatitis (A69.1)

K12.2 Cellulitis and abscess of mouth   cc CC/MCC Exc
Cellulitis of mouth (floor)
Submandibular abscess
EXCLUDES2 abscess of salivary gland (K11.3)
abscess of tongue (K14.0)
periapical abscess (K04.6-K04.7)
periodontal abscess (K05.21)
peritonsillar abscess (J36)

K12.3 Oral mucositis (ulcerative)
Mucositis (oral) (oropharyneal)
EXCLUDES2 gastrointestinal mucositis (ulcerative) (K92.81)
mucositis (ulcerative) of vagina and vulva (N76.81)
nasal mucositis (ulcerative) (J34.81)

K12.30 Oral mucositis (ulcerative), unspecified

K12.31 Oral mucositis (ulcerative) due to antineoplastic therapy
Use additional code for adverse effect, if applicable, to identify antineoplastic and immunosuppressive drugs (T45.1X5)
Use additional code for other antineoplastic therapy, such as:
radiological procedure and radiotherapy (Y84.2)

PDxM Unacceptable principal diagnosis symbol per Medicare code edits   POA Code exempt from diagnosis present on admission requirement
❓ Questionable admission   cc Complication or comorbidity   cc/mcc Exc CC/MCC exclusion   mcc Major complication or comorbidity
Principal diagnosis as its own CC   Principal diagnosis as its own MCC   HCC HCC diagnosis code   RxHCC RxHCC diagnosis code
MACRA code   Z Z code as first-listed diagnosis

722
When symbols appear on a code that requires a 7th character extension, refer to Appendix B to identify applicable 7th character codes.
2018 ICD-10-CM

K12.32 **Oral mucositis (ulcerative) due to** other drugs
Use additional code for adverse effect, if applicable, to identify drug (T36-T50 with fifth or sixth character 5)

K12.33 **Oral mucositis (ulcerative) due to** radiation
Use additional external cause code (W88-W90, X39.0-) to identify cause

K12.39 **Other oral mucositis (ulcerative)**
Viral oral mucositis (ulcerative)

K13 **Other diseases of lip and oral mucosa**
INCLUDES epithelial disturbances of tongue
Use additional code to identify:
alcohol abuse and dependence (F10.-)
exposure to environmental tobacco smoke (Z77.22)
exposure to tobacco smoke in the perinatal period (P96.81)
history of tobacco dependence (Z87.891)
occupational exposure to environmental tobacco smoke (Z57.31)
tobacco dependence (F17.-)
tobacco use (Z72.0)
EXCLUDES2 certain disorders of gingiva and edentulous alveolar ridge (K05-K06)
cysts of oral region (K09.-)
diseases of tongue (K14.-)
stomatitis and related lesions (K12.-)

K13.0 **Diseases of lips**
Abscess of lips
Angular cheilitis
Cellulitis of lips
Cheilitis NOS
Cheilodynia
Cheilosis
Exfoliative cheilitis
Fistula of lips
Glandular cheilitis
Hypertrophy of lips
Perlèche NEC
EXCLUDES1 ariboflavinosis (E53.0)
cheilitis due to radiation-related disorders (L55-L59)
congenital fistula of lips (Q38.0)
congenital hypertrophy of lips (Q18.6)
Perlèche due to candidiasis (B37.83)
Perlèche due to riboflavin deficiency (E53.0)

K13.1 **Cheek and lip biting**

K13.2 **Leukoplakia and other disturbances of oral epithelium, including tongue**
EXCLUDES1 carcinoma in situ of oral epithelium (D00.0-)
hairy leukoplakia (K13.3)

K13.21 **Leukoplakia of** oral mucosa, **including tongue**
Leukokeratosis of oral mucosa
Leukoplakia of gingiva, lips, tongue
EXCLUDES1 hairy leukoplakia (K13.3)
leukokeratosis nicotina palati (K13.24)

K13.22 **Minimal keratinized residual ridge mucosa**
Minimal keratinization of alveolar ridge mucosa

K13.23 **Excessive keratinized residual ridge mucosa**
Excessive keratinization of alveolar ridge mucosa

K13.24 **Leukokeratosis nicotina palati**
Smoker's palate

K13.29 **Other disturbances of oral epithelium, including tongue**
Erythroplakia of mouth or tongue
Focal epithelial hyperplasia of mouth or tongue
Leukoedema of mouth or tongue
Other oral epithelium disturbances

K13.3 **Hairy leukoplakia**

K13.4 **Granuloma and granuloma-like lesions of oral mucosa**
Eosinophilic granuloma
Granuloma pyogenicum
Verrucous xanthoma

K13.5 **Oral submucous fibrosis**
Submucous fibrosis of tongue

K13.6 **Irritative hyperplasia of oral mucosa**
EXCLUDES2 irritative hyperplasia of edentulous ridge [denture hyperplasia] (K06.2)

K13.7 **Other and unspecified lesions of oral mucosa**

K13.70 **Unspecified lesions of oral mucosa**

K13.79 **Other lesions of oral mucosa**
Focal oral mucinosis

K14 **Diseases of tongue**
Use additional code to identify:
alcohol abuse and dependence (F10.-)
exposure to environmental tobacco smoke (Z77.22)
history of tobacco dependence (Z87.891)
occupational exposure to environmental tobacco smoke (Z57.31)
tobacco dependence (F17.-)
tobacco use (Z72.0)
EXCLUDES2 erythroplakia (K13.29)
focal epithelial hyperplasia (K13.29)
leukedema of tongue (K13.29)
leukoplakia of tongue (K13.21)
hairy leukoplakia (K13.3)
macroglossia (congenital) (Q38.2)
submucous fibrosis of tongue (K13.5)

K14.0 **Glossitis**
Abscess of tongue
Ulceration (traumatic) of tongue
EXCLUDES1 atrophic glossitis (K14.4)

K14.1 **Geographic tongue**
Benign migratory glossitis
Glossitis areata exfoliativa

K14.2 **Median rhomboid glossitis**

K14.3 **Hypertrophy of tongue papillae**
Black hairy tongue
Coated tongue
Hypertrophy of foliate papillae
Lingua villosa nigra

K14.4 **Atrophy of tongue papillae**
Atrophic glossitis

K14.5 **Plicated tongue**
Fissured tongue
Furrowed tongue
Scrotal tongue
EXCLUDES1 fissured tongue, congenital (Q38.3)

K14.6 **Glossodynia**
Glossopyrosis
Painful tongue

K14.8 **Other diseases of tongue**
Atrophy of tongue
Crenated tongue
Enlargement of tongue
Glossocele
Glossoptosis
Hypertrophy of tongue

K14.9 **Disease of tongue, unspecified**
Glossopathy NOS

Diseases of esophagus, stomach and duodenum (K20-K31)

EXCLUDES2 hiatus hernia (K44.-)

K20 **Esophagitis**
Use additional code to identify:
alcohol abuse and dependence (F10.-)
EXCLUDES1 erosion of esophagus (K22.1-)
esophagitis with gastro-esophageal reflux disease (K21.0)
reflux esophagitis (K21.0)
ulcerative esophagitis (K22.1-)
EXCLUDES2 eosinophilic gastritis or gastroenteritis (K52.81)

| Unspecified Code | Other Specified Code | Manifestation Code | N Newborn | P Pediatric | M Maternity | A Adult | ♂ Male | ♀ Female |

● New Code ▲ Revised Code Title ▶◀ Revised Text NOTES INCLUDES EXCLUDES 1 Not coded here EXCLUDES 2 Not included here
4th character required 5th character required 6th character required 7th character required
Extension 'X' Alert HAC Hospital-acquired condition (HAC) alert AHA AHA Coding Clinic©

K20.0 Eosinophilic esophagitis `RxHCC`

K20.8 Other esophagitis `RxHCC`

Abscess of esophagus

K20.9 Esophagitis, unspecified `RxHCC`

Esophagitis NOS

4ᵗʰ **K21 Gastro-esophageal reflux disease**

EXCLUDES1 *newborn esophageal reflux (P78.83)*

K21.0 Gastro-esophageal reflux disease with esophagitis `RxHCC`

Reflux esophagitis

K21.9 Gastro-esophageal reflux disease without esophagitis `RxHCC`

AHA: Q1 2016

Esophageal reflux NOS

4ᵗʰ **K22 Other diseases of esophagus**

EXCLUDES2 *esophageal varices (I85.-)*

K22.0 Achalasia of cardia `RxHCC`

Achalasia NOS

Cardiospasm

EXCLUDES1 *congenital cardiospasm (Q39.5)*

5ᵗʰ **K22.1 Ulcer of esophagus**

Barrett's ulcer

Erosion of esophagus

Fungal ulcer of esophagus

Peptic ulcer of esophagus

Ulcer of esophagus due to ingestion of chemicals

Ulcer of esophagus due to ingestion of drugs and medicaments

Ulcerative esophagitis

Code first poisoning due to drug or toxin, if applicable (T36-T65 with fifth or sixth character 1-4 or 6)

Use additional code for adverse effect, if applicable, to identify drug (T36-T50 with fifth or sixth character 5)

EXCLUDES1 *Barrett's esophagus (K22.7-)*

K22.10 Ulcer of esophagus without bleeding `CC` `CC/MCC Exc`

Ulcer of esophagus NOS

K22.11 Ulcer of esophagus with bleeding `MCC` `CC/MCC Exc`

EXCLUDES2 *bleeding esophageal varices (I85.01, I85.11)*

K22.2 Esophageal obstruction `RxHCC`

Compression of esophagus

Constriction of esophagus

Stenosis of esophagus

Stricture of esophagus

EXCLUDES1 *congenital stenosis or stricture of esophagus (Q39.3)*

K22.3 Perforation of esophagus `MCC` `RxHCC` `CC/MCC Exc`

Rupture of esophagus

EXCLUDES1 *traumatic perforation of (thoracic) esophagus (S27.8-)*

K22.4 Dyskinesia of esophagus `RxHCC`

Corkscrew esophagus

Diffuse esophageal spasm

Spasm of esophagus

EXCLUDES1 *cardiospasm (K22.0)*

K22.5 Diverticulum of esophagus, acquired `RxHCC`

Esophageal pouch, acquired

EXCLUDES1 *diverticulum of esophagus (congenital) (Q39.6)*

K22.6 Gastro-esophageal laceration-hemorrhage syndrome `MCC` `CC/MCC Exc`

Mallory-Weiss syndrome

5ᵗʰ **K22.7 Barrett's esophagus**

Barrett's disease

Barrett's syndrome

EXCLUDES1 *Barrett's ulcer (K22.1)*

malignant neoplasm of esophagus (C15.-)

K22.70 Barrett's esophagus without dysplasia `RxHCC`

Barrett's esophagus NOS

6ᵗʰ **K22.71 Barrett's esophagus** with dysplasia

K22.710 Barrett's esophagus with low grade **dysplasia** `RxHCC`

K22.711 Barrett's esophagus with high grade **dysplasia** `RxHCC`

K22.719 Barrett's esophagus with dysplasia, unspecified `RxHCC`

K22.8 Other specified diseases of esophagus `RxHCC`

Hemorrhage of esophagus NOS

EXCLUDES2 *esophageal varices (I85.-)*

Paterson-Kelly syndrome (D50.1)

K22.9 Disease of esophagus, unspecified `RxHCC`

K23 Disorders of esophagus in diseases classified elsewhere `RxHCC`

Code first underlying disease, such as:

congenital syphilis (A50.5)

EXCLUDES1 *late syphilis (A52.79)*

megaesophagus due to Chagas' disease (B57.31)

tuberculosis (A18.83)

4ᵗʰ **K25 Gastric ulcer**

INCLUDES erosion (acute) of stomach

pylorus ulcer (peptic)

stomach ulcer (peptic)

Use additional code to identify:

alcohol abuse and dependence (F10.-)

EXCLUDES1 *acute gastritis (K29.0-)*

peptic ulcer NOS (K27.-)

K25.0 Acute gastric ulcer with hemorrhage `MCC` `CC/MCC Exc`

K25.1 Acute gastric ulcer with perforation `HCC` `MCC` `CC/MCC Exc`

K25.2 Acute gastric ulcer with both hemorrhage and perforation `HCC` `MCC` `CC/MCC Exc`

K25.3 Acute gastric ulcer without hemorrhage or perforation `CC` `CC/MCC Exc`

K25.4 Chronic or unspecified gastric ulcer with hemorrhage `MCC` `CC/MCC Exc`

K25.5 Chronic or unspecified gastric ulcer with perforation `HCC` `MCC` `CC/MCC Exc`

K25.6 Chronic or unspecified gastric ulcer with both hemorrhage and perforation `HCC` `MCC` `CC/MCC Exc`

K25.7 Chronic gastric ulcer without hemorrhage or perforation

K25.9 Gastric ulcer, unspecified as acute or chronic, without hemorrhage or perforation

4ᵗʰ **K26 Duodenal ulcer**

INCLUDES erosion (acute) of duodenum

duodenum ulcer (peptic)

postpyloric ulcer (peptic)

Use additional code to identify:

alcohol abuse and dependence (F10.-)

EXCLUDES1 *peptic ulcer NOS (K27.-)*

K26.0 Acute duodenal ulcer with hemorrhage `MCC` `CC/MCC Exc`

K26.1 Acute duodenal ulcer with perforation `HCC` `MCC` `CC/MCC Exc`

K26.2 Acute duodenal ulcer with both hemorrhage and perforation `HCC` `MCC` `CC/MCC Exc`

K26.3 Acute duodenal ulcer without hemorrhage or perforation `CC` `CC/MCC Exc`

K26.4 Chronic or unspecified duodenal ulcer with hemorrhage `MCC` `CC/MCC Exc`

AHA: Q1 2016

K26.5 Chronic or unspecified duodenal ulcer with perforation `HCC` `MCC` `CC/MCC Exc`

K26.6 Chronic or unspecified duodenal ulcer with both hemorrhage and perforation `HCC` `MCC` `CC/MCC Exc`

K26.7 Chronic duodenal ulcer without hemorrhage or perforation

K26.9 Duodenal ulcer, unspecified as acute or chronic, without hemorrhage or perforation

4ᵗʰ **K27 Peptic ulcer, site unspecified**

INCLUDES gastroduodenal ulcer NOS

peptic ulcer NOS

Use additional code to identify:

alcohol abuse and dependence (F10.-)

EXCLUDES1 *peptic ulcer of newborn (P78.82)*

K27.0 Acute peptic ulcer, site unspecified, with hemorrhage `MCC` `CC/MCC Exc`

K27.1 Acute peptic ulcer, site unspecified, with perforation `HCC` `MCC` `CC/MCC Exc`

PDx Unacceptable principal diagnosis symbol per Medicare code edits   POA Code exempt from diagnosis present on admission requirement

? Questionable admission   `CC` Complication or comorbidity   `CC/MCC Exc` CC/MCC exclusion   `MCC` Major complication or comorbidity

Principal diagnosis as its own CC   Principal diagnosis as its own MCC   `HCC` HCC diagnosis code   `RxHCC` RxHCC diagnosis code

MACRA code   Z Z code as first-listed diagnosis

K27.2 **Acute peptic ulcer, site unspecified,** with both hemorrhage and perforation `HCC` `MCC` `CC/MCC Exc`

K27.3 **Acute peptic ulcer, site unspecified,** without hemorrhage or perforation `CC` `CC/MCC Exc`

K27.4 **Chronic or unspecified peptic ulcer, site unspecified,** with hemorrhage `MCC` `CC/MCC Exc`

K27.5 **Chronic or unspecified peptic ulcer, site unspecified,** with perforation `HCC` `MCC` `CC/MCC Exc`

K27.6 **Chronic or unspecified peptic ulcer, site unspecified,** with both hemorrhage and perforation `HCC` `MCC` `CC/MCC Exc`

K27.7 **Chronic peptic ulcer, site unspecified,** without hemorrhage or perforation

K27.9 **Peptic ulcer, site unspecified, unspecified as acute or chronic, without hemorrhage or perforation**

K28 **Gastrojejunal ulcer**

INCLUDES anastomotic ulcer (peptic) or erosion
gastrocolic ulcer (peptic) or erosion
gastrointestinal ulcer (peptic) or erosion
gastrojejunal ulcer (peptic) or erosion
jejunal ulcer (peptic) or erosion
marginal ulcer (peptic) or erosion
stomal ulcer (peptic) or erosion

Use additional code to identify:
alcohol abuse and dependence (F10.-)

EXCLUDES1 primary ulcer of small intestine (K63.3)

K28.0 **Acute gastrojejunal ulcer** with hemorrhage `MCC` `CC/MCC Exc`

K28.1 **Acute gastrojejunal ulcer** with perforation `HCC` `MCC` `CC/MCC Exc`

K28.2 **Acute gastrojejunal ulcer** with both hemorrhage and perforation `HCC` `MCC` `CC/MCC Exc`

K28.3 **Acute gastrojejunal ulcer** without hemorrhage or perforation `CC` `CC/MCC Exc`

K28.4 **Chronic or unspecified gastrojejunal ulcer** with hemorrhage `MCC` `CC/MCC Exc`

K28.5 **Chronic or unspecified gastrojejunal ulcer** with perforation `HCC` `MCC` `CC/MCC Exc`

K28.6 **Chronic or unspecified gastrojejunal ulcer** with both hemorrhage and perforation `HCC` `MCC` `CC/MCC Exc`

K28.7 **Chronic gastrojejunal ulcer** without hemorrhage or perforation

K28.9 **Gastrojejunal ulcer, unspecified as acute or chronic, without hemorrhage or perforation**

K29 **Gastritis and duodenitis**

EXCLUDES1 eosinophilic gastritis or gastroenteritis (K52.81)
Zollinger-Ellison syndrome (E16.4)

K29.0 **Acute gastritis**
Use additional code to identify:
alcohol abuse and dependence (F10.-)
EXCLUDES1 erosion (acute) of stomach (K25.-)
K29.00 **Acute gastritis** without bleeding
K29.01 **Acute gastritis** with bleeding `MCC` `CC/MCC Exc`

K29.2 **Alcoholic gastritis**
Use additional code to identify:
alcohol abuse and dependence (F10.-)
K29.20 **Alcoholic gastritis** without bleeding
K29.21 **Alcoholic gastritis** with bleeding `MCC` `CC/MCC Exc`

K29.3 **Chronic superficial gastritis**
K29.30 **Chronic superficial gastritis** without bleeding
K29.31 **Chronic superficial gastritis** with bleeding `MCC` `CC/MCC Exc`

K29.4 **Chronic atrophic gastritis**
Gastric atrophy
K29.40 **Chronic atrophic gastritis** without bleeding
K29.41 **Chronic atrophic gastritis** with bleeding `MCC` `CC/MCC Exc`

K29.5 **Unspecified chronic gastritis**
Chronic antral gastritis
Chronic fundal gastritis
K29.50 **Unspecified chronic gastritis** without bleeding
K29.51 **Unspecified chronic gastritis** with bleeding `MCC` `CC/MCC Exc`

K29.6 **Other gastritis**
Giant hypertrophic gastritis
Granulomatous gastritis
Ménétrier's disease
K29.60 **Other gastritis** without bleeding
K29.61 **Other gastritis** with bleeding `MCC` `CC/MCC Exc`

K29.7 **Gastritis, unspecified**
K29.70 **Gastritis, unspecified,** without bleeding
K29.71 **Gastritis, unspecified,** with bleeding `MCC` `CC/MCC Exc`

K29.8 **Duodenitis**
K29.80 **Duodenitis** without bleeding
K29.81 **Duodenitis** with bleeding `MCC` `CC/MCC Exc`

K29.9 **Gastroduodenitis, unspecified**
K29.90 **Gastroduodenitis, unspecified,** without bleeding
K29.91 **Gastroduodenitis, unspecified, with bleeding** `MCC` `CC/MCC Exc`

K30 **Functional dyspepsia**
Indigestion
EXCLUDES1 dyspepsia NOS (R10.13)
heartburn (R12)
nervous dyspepsia (F45.8)
neurotic dyspepsia (F45.8)
psychogenic dyspepsia (F45.8)

K31 **Other diseases of stomach and duodenum**
INCLUDES functional disorders of stomach
EXCLUDES2 diabetic gastroparesis (E08.43, E09.43, E10.43, E11.43, E13.43)
diverticulum of duodenum (K57.00-K57.13)

K31.0 **Acute dilatation of stomach** `CC` `CC/MCC Exc`
Acute distention of stomach

K31.1 **Adult hypertrophic pyloric stenosis** `A` `CC` `CC/MCC Exc`
Pyloric stenosis NOS
EXCLUDES1 congenital or infantile pyloric stenosis (Q40.0)

K31.2 **Hourglass stricture and stenosis of stomach**
EXCLUDES1 congenital hourglass stomach (Q40.2)
hourglass contraction of stomach (K31.89)

K31.3 **Pylorospasm, not elsewhere classified**
EXCLUDES1 congenital or infantile pylorospasm (Q40.0)
neurotic pylorospasm (F45.8)
psychogenic pylorospasm (F45.8)

K31.4 **Gastric diverticulum**
EXCLUDES1 congenital diverticulum of stomach (Q40.2)

K31.5 **Obstruction of duodenum** `CC` `CC/MCC Exc`
Constriction of duodenum
Duodenal ileus (chronic)
Stenosis of duodenum
Stricture of duodenum
Volvulus of duodenum
EXCLUDES1 congenital stenosis of duodenum (Q41.0)

K31.6 **Fistula of stomach and duodenum** `CC` `CC/MCC Exc`
Gastrocolic fistula
Gastrojejunocolic fistula

K31.7 **Polyp of stomach and duodenum**
EXCLUDES1 adenomatous polyp of stomach (D13.1)

K31.8 **Other specified diseases of stomach and duodenum**
K31.81 **Angiodysplasia of stomach and duodenum**
K31.811 **Angiodysplasia of stomach and duodenum with bleeding** `MCC` `CC/MCC Exc`
K31.819 **Angiodysplasia of stomach and duodenum without bleeding**
Angiodysplasia of stomach and duodenum NOS

K31.82 **Dieulafoy lesion (hemorrhagic) of stomach and duodenum** `MCC` `CC/MCC Exc`
EXCLUDES2 Dieulafoy lesion of intestine (K63.81)

K31.83 **Achlorhydria**

K31.84 **Gastroparesis**
AHA: Q4 2013
Gastroparalysis

Unspecified Code   Other Specified Code   Manifestation Code   `N` Newborn   `P` Pediatric   `M` Maternity   `A` Adult   `♂` Male   `♀` Female
● New Code   ▲ Revised Code Title   ►◄ Revised Text   NOTES   INCLUDES   EXCLUDES 1 Not coded here   EXCLUDES 2 Not included here
`4ᵗʰ` 4th character required   `5ᵗʰ` 5th character required   `6ᵗʰ` 6th character required   `7ᵗʰ` 7th character required
`X` Extension 'X' Alert   `HAC` Hospital-acquired condition (HAC) alert   AHA AHA Coding Clinic©

Code first underlying disease, if known, such as:
anorexia nervosa (F50.0-)
diabetes mellitus (E08.43, E09.43, E10.43, E11.43, E13.43)
scleroderma (M34.-)

K31.89 Other diseases of stomach and duodenum
AHA: Q1 2017

K31.9 Disease of stomach and duodenum, unspecified

Diseases of appendix (K35-K38)

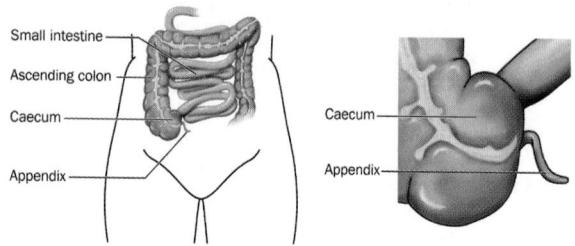

Figure 11.4 Vermiform appendix

4ᵗʰ **K35 Acute appendicitis**

K35.2 Acute appendicitis with generalized peritonitis   MCC✓ CC/MCC Exc⊘
Appendicitis (acute) with generalized (diffuse) peritonitis following rupture or perforation of appendix
Perforated appendix NOS
Ruptured appendix NOS

K35.3 Acute appendicitis with localized peritonitis   MCC✓ CC/MCC Exc⊘
Acute appendicitis with or without perforation or rupture with peritonitis NOS
Acute appendicitis with or without perforation or rupture with localized peritonitis
Acute appendicitis with peritoneal abscess

5ᵗʰ **K35.8 Other and unspecified acute appendicitis**

K35.80 Unspecified acute appendicitis   CC✓ CC/MCC Exc⊘
Acute appendicitis NOS
Acute appendicitis without (localized) (generalized) peritonitis

K35.89 Other acute appendicitis   CC✓ CC/MCC Exc⊘

K36 Other appendicitis
Chronic appendicitis
Recurrent appendicitis

K37 Unspecified appendicitis
EXCLUDES1 *unspecified appendicitis with peritonitis (K35.2-K35.3)*

4ᵗʰ **K38 Other diseases of appendix**

K38.0 Hyperplasia of appendix

K38.1 Appendicular concretions
Fecalith of appendix
Stercolith of appendix

K38.2 Diverticulum of appendix

K38.3 Fistula of appendix

K38.8 Other specified diseases of appendix
Intussusception of appendix

K38.9 Disease of appendix, unspecified

Hernia (K40-K46)

NOTES   Hernia with both gangrene and obstruction is classified to hernia with gangrene.
INCLUDES *acquired hernia*
congenital [except diaphragmatic or hiatus] hernia
recurrent hernia

4ᵗʰ **K40 Inguinal hernia**
INCLUDES *bubonocele*
direct inguinal hernia
double inguinal hernia
indirect inguinal hernia
inguinal hernia NOS
oblique inguinal hernia
scrotal hernia

5ᵗʰ **K40.0 Bilateral inguinal hernia, with obstruction, without gangrene**
Inguinal hernia (bilateral) causing obstruction without gangrene
Incarcerated inguinal hernia (bilateral) without gangrene
Irreducible inguinal hernia (bilateral) without gangrene
Strangulated inguinal hernia (bilateral) without gangrene

K40.00 Bilateral inguinal hernia, with obstruction, without gangrene, not specified as recurrent   CC✓ CC/MCC Exc⊘
Bilateral inguinal hernia, with obstruction, without gangrene NOS

K40.01 Bilateral inguinal hernia, with obstruction, without gangrene, recurrent   CC✓ CC/MCC Exc⊘

5ᵗʰ **K40.1 Bilateral inguinal hernia, with gangrene**

K40.10 Bilateral inguinal hernia, with gangrene, not specified as recurrent   MCC✓ CC/MCC Exc⊘
Bilateral inguinal hernia, with gangrene NOS

K40.11 Bilateral inguinal hernia, with gangrene, recurrent   MCC✓ CC/MCC Exc⊘

5ᵗʰ **K40.2 Bilateral inguinal hernia, without obstruction or gangrene**

K40.20 Bilateral inguinal hernia, without obstruction or gangrene, not specified as recurrent
Bilateral inguinal hernia NOS

K40.21 Bilateral inguinal hernia, without obstruction or gangrene, recurrent

5ᵗʰ **K40.3 Unilateral inguinal hernia, with obstruction, without gangrene**
Inguinal hernia (unilateral) causing obstruction without gangrene
Incarcerated inguinal hernia (unilateral) without gangrene
Irreducible inguinal hernia (unilateral) without gangrene
Strangulated inguinal hernia (unilateral) without gangrene

K40.30 Unilateral inguinal hernia, with obstruction, without gangrene, not specified as recurrent   CC✓ CC/MCC Exc⊘
Inguinal hernia, with obstruction NOS
Unilateral inguinal hernia, with obstruction, without gangrene NOS

K40.31 Unilateral inguinal hernia, with obstruction, without gangrene, recurrent   CC✓ CC/MCC Exc⊘

5ᵗʰ **K40.4 Unilateral inguinal hernia, with gangrene**

K40.40 Unilateral inguinal hernia, with gangrene, not specified as recurrent   MCC✓ CC/MCC Exc⊘
Inguinal hernia with gangrene NOS
Unilateral inguinal hernia with gangrene NOS

K40.41 Unilateral inguinal hernia, with gangrene, recurrent   MCC✓ CC/MCC Exc⊘

5ᵗʰ **K40.9 Unilateral inguinal hernia, without obstruction or gangrene**

K40.90 Unilateral inguinal hernia, without obstruction or gangrene, not specified as recurrent
Inguinal hernia NOS
Unilateral inguinal hernia NOS

K40.91 Unilateral inguinal hernia, without obstruction or gangrene, recurrent

4ᵗʰ **K41 Femoral hernia**

5ᵗʰ **K41.0 Bilateral femoral hernia, with obstruction, without gangrene**
Femoral hernia (bilateral) causing obstruction, without gangrene
Incarcerated femoral hernia (bilateral), without gangrene
Irreducible femoral hernia (bilateral), without gangrene
Strangulated femoral hernia (bilateral), without gangrene

K41.00 Bilateral femoral hernia, with obstruction, without gangrene, not specified as recurrent   CC✓ CC/MCC Exc⊘
Bilateral femoral hernia, with obstruction, without gangrene NOS

K41.01 Bilateral femoral hernia, with obstruction, without gangrene, recurrent   CC✓ CC/MCC Exc⊘

5ᵗʰ **K41.1 Bilateral femoral hernia, with gangrene**

K41.10 Bilateral femoral hernia, with gangrene, not specified as recurrent   MCC✓ CC/MCC Exc⊘
Bilateral femoral hernia, with gangrene NOS

ᴘᴅx Unacceptable principal diagnosis symbol per Medicare code edits   ᴘᴏᴀ Code exempt from diagnosis present on admission requirement
❓ Questionable admission   ᴄᵉ Complication or comorbidity   ᴄᴄ/ᴍᴄᴄ Exᶜ CC/MCC exclusion   ᴍᴄᶜ Major complication or comorbidity
ᴄᴄ Principal diagnosis as its own CC   ᴍᴄᴄ Principal diagnosis as its own MCC   ʜᴄᴄ HCC diagnosis code   ʀʜᴄᴄ RxHCC diagnosis code
MACRA code   Zᴬ¹ Z code as first-listed diagnosis

When symbols appear on a code that requires a 7th character extension, refer to Appendix B to identify applicable 7th character codes.

2018 ICD-10-CM

K41.11   **Bilateral femoral hernia, with gangrene, recurrent**   MCC CC/MCC Exc

5ᵗʰ K41.2   Bilateral **femoral hernia,** without obstruction or gangrene

    K41.20   **Bilateral femoral hernia, without obstruction or gangrene,** not specified as recurrent
      Bilateral femoral hernia NOS
    K41.21   **Bilateral femoral hernia, without obstruction or gangrene,** recurrent

5ᵗʰ K41.3   Unilateral **femoral hernia, with obstruction, without gangrene**
      Femoral hernia (unilateral) causing obstruction, without gangrene
      Incarcerated femoral hernia (unilateral), without gangrene
      Irreducible femoral hernia (unilateral), without gangrene
      Strangulated femoral hernia (unilateral), without gangrene
    K41.30   **Unilateral femoral hernia, with obstruction, without gangrene,** not specified as recurrent   CC CC/MCC Exc
      Femoral hernia, with obstruction NOS
      Unilateral femoral hernia, with obstruction NOS
    K41.31   **Unilateral femoral hernia, with obstruction, without gangrene,** recurrent   CC CC/MCC Exc

5ᵗʰ K41.4   Unilateral **femoral hernia, with gangrene**
    K41.40   **Unilateral femoral hernia, with gangrene,** not specified as recurrent   MCC CC/MCC Exc
      Femoral hernia, with gangrene NOS
      Unilateral femoral hernia, with gangrene NOS
    K41.41   **Unilateral femoral hernia, with gangrene,** recurrent   MCC CC/MCC Exc

5ᵗʰ K41.9   Unilateral **femoral hernia,** without obstruction or gangrene
    K41.90   **Unilateral femoral hernia, without obstruction or gangrene,** not specified as recurrent
      Femoral hernia NOS
      Unilateral femoral hernia NOS
    K41.91   **Unilateral femoral hernia, without obstruction or gangrene,** recurrent

4ᵗʰ K42   Umbilical **hernia**

    INCLUDES   paraumbilical hernia
    EXCLUDES1   omphalocele (Q79.2)

    K42.0   **Umbilical hernia** with obstruction, without gangrene   CC CC/MCC Exc
      Umbilical hernia causing obstruction, without gangrene
      Incarcerated umbilical hernia, without gangrene
      Irreducible umbilical hernia, without gangrene
      Strangulated umbilical hernia, without gangrene
    K42.1   **Umbilical hernia** with gangrene   MCC CC/MCC Exc
      Gangrenous umbilical hernia
    K42.9   **Umbilical hernia** without obstruction or gangrene
      Umbilical hernia NOS

4ᵗʰ K43   Ventral **hernia**

    K43.0   Incisional **hernia** with obstruction, without gangrene   CC CC/MCC Exc
      Incisional hernia causing obstruction, without gangrene
      Incarcerated incisional hernia, without gangrene
      Irreducible incisional hernia, without gangrene
      Strangulated incisional hernia, without gangrene
    K43.1   Incisional **hernia** with gangrene   MCC CC/MCC Exc
      Gangrenous incisional hernia
    K43.2   Incisional **hernia** without obstruction or gangrene
      Incisional hernia NOS
    K43.3   Parastomal **hernia** with obstruction, without gangrene   CC CC/MCC Exc
      Incarcerated parastomal hernia, without gangrene
      Irreducible parastomal hernia, without gangrene
      Parastomal hernia causing obstruction, without gangrene
      Strangulated parastomal hernia, without gangrene
    K43.4   Parastomal **hernia** with gangrene   MCC CC/MCC Exc
      Gangrenous parastomal hernia
    K43.5   Parastomal **hernia** without obstruction or gangrene
      Parastomal hernia NOS
    K43.6   Other and unspecified ventral hernia with obstruction, without gangrene   CC CC/MCC Exc
      Epigastric hernia causing obstruction, without gangrene
      Hypogastric hernia causing obstruction, without gangrene

      Incarcerated epigastric hernia without gangrene
      Incarcerated hypogastric hernia without gangrene
      Incarcerated midline hernia without gangrene
      Incarcerated spigelian hernia without gangrene
      Incarcerated subxiphoid hernia without gangrene
      Irreducible epigastric hernia without gangrene
      Irreducible hypogastric hernia without gangrene
      Irreducible midline hernia without gangrene
      Irreducible spigelian hernia without gangrene
      Irreducible subxiphoid hernia without gangrene
      Midline hernia causing obstruction, without gangrene
      Spigelian hernia causing obstruction, without gangrene
      Strangulated epigastric hernia without gangrene
      Strangulated hypogastric hernia without gangrene
      Strangulated midline hernia without gangrene
      Strangulated spigelian hernia without gangrene
      Strangulated subxiphoid hernia without gangrene
      Subxiphoid hernia causing obstruction, without gangrene
    K43.7   **Other and unspecified ventral hernia** with gangrene   MCC CC/MCC Exc
      Any condition listed under K43.6 specified as gangrenous
    K43.9   **Ventral hernia** without obstruction or gangrene
      Epigastric hernia
      Ventral hernia NOS

4ᵗʰ K44   Diaphragmatic **hernia**

    INCLUDES   hiatus hernia (esophageal) (sliding)
          paraesophageal hernia

    EXCLUDES1   congenital diaphragmatic hernia (Q79.0)
          congenital hiatus hernia (Q40.1)

    K44.0   **Diaphragmatic hernia** with obstruction, without gangrene   CC CC/MCC Exc
      Diaphragmatic hernia causing obstruction
      Incarcerated diaphragmatic hernia
      Irreducible diaphragmatic hernia
      Strangulated diaphragmatic hernia
    K44.1   **Diaphragmatic hernia** with gangrene   MCC CC/MCC Exc
      Gangrenous diaphragmatic hernia
    K44.9   **Diaphragmatic hernia** without obstruction or gangrene
      Diaphragmatic hernia NOS

4ᵗʰ K45   Other abdominal **hernia**

    INCLUDES   abdominal hernia, specified site NEC
          lumbar hernia
          obturator hernia
          pudendal hernia
          retroperitoneal hernia
          sciatic hernia

    K45.0   Other specified abdominal hernia with obstruction, without gangrene   CC CC/MCC Exc
      Other specified abdominal hernia causing obstruction
      Other specified incarcerated abdominal hernia
      Other specified irreducible abdominal hernia
      Other specified strangulated abdominal hernia
    K45.1   Other specified abdominal hernia with gangrene   MCC CC/MCC Exc
      Any condition listed under K45 specified as gangrenous
    K45.8   Other specified abdominal hernia without obstruction or gangrene

4ᵗʰ K46   Unspecified abdominal **hernia**

    INCLUDES   enterocele
          epiplocele
          hernia NOS
          interstitial hernia
          intestinal hernia
          intra-abdominal hernia

    EXCLUDES1   vaginal enterocele (N81.5)

    K46.0   **Unspecified abdominal hernia with obstruction, without gangrene**   CC CC/MCC Exc
      Unspecified abdominal hernia causing obstruction
      Unspecified incarcerated abdominal hernia
      Unspecified irreducible abdominal hernia
      Unspecified strangulated abdominal hernia
    K46.1   **Unspecified abdominal hernia with gangrene**   MCC CC/MCC Exc
      Any condition listed under K46 specified as gangrenous

Unspecified Code   Other Specified Code   Manifestation Code   N Newborn   P Pediatric   M Maternity   A Adult   ♂ Male   ♀ Female
● New Code   ▲ Revised Code Title   ▶◀ Revised Text   **NOTES**   *INCLUDES*   *EXCLUDES 1* Not coded here   *EXCLUDES 2* Not included here
4ᵗʰ 4ᵗʰ character required   5ᵗʰ 5ᵗʰ character required   6ᵗʰ 6ᵗʰ character required   7ᵗʰ 7ᵗʰ character required
7ᵗʰ Extension 'X' Alert   **HAC** Hospital-acquired condition (HAC) alert   **AHA** AHA Coding Clinic©

K46.9 **Unspecified abdominal hernia without obstruction or gangrene**
Abdominal hernia NOS

Noninfective enteritis and colitis (K50-K52)

INCLUDES   noninfective inflammatory bowel disease
EXCLUDES1 irritable bowel syndrome (K58.-)
megacolon (K59.3-)

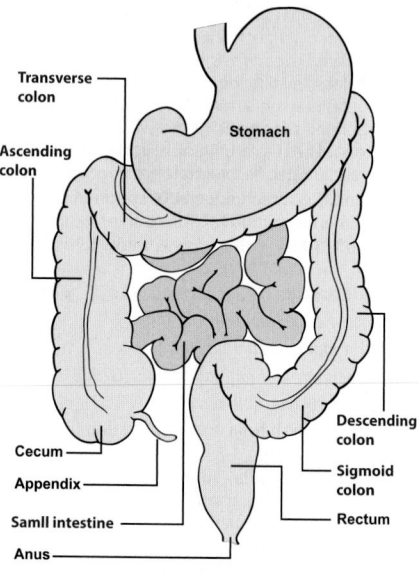

Figure 11.5 Large and small intestine

4ᵗʰ K50   **Crohn's disease [regional enteritis]**
INCLUDES   granulomatous enteritis
Use additional code to identify manifestations, such as:
pyoderma gangrenosum (L88)
EXCLUDES1 ulcerative colitis (K51.-)

5ᵗʰ K50.0   **Crohn's disease of** small intestine
Crohn's disease [regional enteritis] of duodenum
Crohn's disease [regional enteritis] of ileum
Crohn's disease [regional enteritis] of jejunum
Regional ileitis
Terminal ileitis
EXCLUDES1 Crohn's disease of both small and large intestine (K50.8-)
K50.00   **Crohn's disease of small intestine** without complications   CC HCC RxHCC CC/MCC Exc

6ᵗʰ K50.01   **Crohn's disease of small intestine** with complications
K50.011   **Crohn's disease of small intestine with** rectal bleeding   CC HCC RxHCC CC/MCC Exc
K50.012   **Crohn's disease of small intestine with** intestinal obstruction   CC HCC PDx RxHCC CC/MCC Exc
K50.013   **Crohn's disease of small intestine with** fistula   CC HCC PDx RxHCC CC/MCC Exc
K50.014   **Crohn's disease of small intestine with** abscess   CC HCC PDx RxHCC CC/MCC Exc
AHA: Q4 2012
K50.018   **Crohn's disease of small intestine with** other complication   CC HCC RxHCC CC/MCC Exc
K50.019   **Crohn's disease of small intestine with** unspecified complications   CC HCC RxHCC CC/MCC Exc

5ᵗʰ K50.1   **Crohn's disease of** large intestine
Crohn's disease [regional enteritis] of colon
Crohn's disease [regional enteritis] of large bowel
Crohn's disease [regional enteritis] of rectum
Granulomatous colitis
Regional colitis

EXCLUDES1 Crohn's disease of both small and large intestine (K50.8)
K50.10   **Crohn's disease of large intestine** without complications   CC HCC RxHCC CC/MCC Exc
6ᵗʰ K50.11   **Crohn's disease of large intestine** with complications
K50.111   **Crohn's disease of large intestine with** rectal bleeding   CC HCC RxHCC CC/MCC Exc
K50.112   **Crohn's disease of large intestine with** intestinal obstruction   CC HCC PDx RxHCC CC/MCC Exc
K50.113   **Crohn's disease of large intestine with** fistula   CC HCC PDx RxHCC CC/MCC Exc
K50.114   **Crohn's disease of large intestine with** abscess   CC HCC PDx RxHCC CC/MCC Exc
AHA: Q4 2012
K50.118   **Crohn's disease of large intestine with** other complication   CC HCC RxHCC CC/MCC Exc
K50.119   **Crohn's disease of large intestine with** unspecified complications   CC HCC RxHCC CC/MCC Exc

5ᵗʰ K50.8   **Crohn's disease of** both small and large intestine
K50.80   **Crohn's disease of both small and large intestine** without complications   CC HCC RxHCC CC/MCC Exc
6ᵗʰ K50.81   **Crohn's disease of both small and large intestine** with complications
K50.811   **Crohn's disease of both small and large intestine with** rectal bleeding   CC HCC RxHCC CC/MCC Exc
K50.812   **Crohn's disease of both small and large intestine with** intestinal obstruction   CC HCC PDx RxHCC CC/MCC Exc
K50.813   **Crohn's disease of both small and large intestine with** fistula   CC HCC PDx RxHCC CC/MCC Exc
K50.814   **Crohn's disease of both small and large intestine with** abscess   CC HCC PDx RxHCC CC/MCC Exc
AHA: Q4 2012
K50.818   **Crohn's disease of both small and large intestine with** other complication   CC HCC RxHCC CC/MCC Exc
K50.819   **Crohn's disease of both small and large intestine with** unspecified complications   CC HCC RxHCC CC/MCC Exc

5ᵗʰ K50.9   **Crohn's disease, unspecified**
K50.90   **Crohn's disease, unspecified,** without complications   CC HCC RxHCC CC/MCC Exc
Crohn's disease NOS
Regional enteritis NOS
6ᵗʰ K50.91   **Crohn's disease, unspecified, with complications**
K50.911   **Crohn's disease, unspecified, with rectal** bleeding   CC HCC RxHCC CC/MCC Exc
K50.912   **Crohn's disease, unspecified, with** intestinal obstruction   CC HCC PDx RxHCC CC/MCC Exc
K50.913   **Crohn's disease, unspecified, with fistula**   CC HCC PDx RxHCC CC/MCC Exc
K50.914   **Crohn's disease, unspecified, with abscess**   CC HCC PDx RxHCC CC/MCC Exc
AHA: Q4 2012
K50.918   **Crohn's disease, unspecified, with other complication**   CC HCC RxHCC CC/MCC Exc
K50.919   **Crohn's disease, unspecified, with unspecified complications**   CC HCC RxHCC CC/MCC Exc

4ᵗʰ K51   **Ulcerative colitis**
Use additional code to identify manifestations, such as:
pyoderma gangrenosum (L88)
EXCLUDES1 Crohn's disease [regional enteritis] (K50.-)
5ᵗʰ K51.0   **Ulcerative (chronic)** pancolitis
Backwash ileitis
K51.00   **Ulcerative (chronic) pancolitis without** complications   CC HCC RxHCC CC/MCC Exc
Ulcerative (chronic) pancolitis NOS
6ᵗʰ K51.01   **Ulcerative (chronic) pancolitis** with complications
K51.011   **Ulcerative (chronic) pancolitis with** rectal bleeding   CC HCC RxHCC CC/MCC Exc
K51.012   **Ulcerative (chronic) pancolitis with** intestinal obstruction   CC HCC PDx RxHCC CC/MCC Exc

---

PDx   Unacceptable principal diagnosis symbol per Medicare code edits   Code exempt from diagnosis present on admission requirement
?   Questionable admission   CC   Complication or comorbidity   CC/MCC Exc   CC/MCC exclusion   MCC   Major complication or comorbidity
PDx   Principal diagnosis as its own CC   PMCC   Principal diagnosis as its own MCC   HCC   HCC diagnosis code   RxHCC   RxHCC diagnosis code
MACRA code   Z1   Z code as first-listed diagnosis

K51.013   Ulcerative (chronic) pancolitis with fistula   ♂ HCC ℞ ℞HCC CC/MCC Exc

K51.014   Ulcerative (chronic) pancolitis with abscess   ♂ HCC ℞ ℞HCC CC/MCC Exc

K51.018   Ulcerative (chronic) pancolitis with other complication   ♂ HCC ℞HCC CC/MCC Exc

K51.019   Ulcerative (chronic) pancolitis with unspecified complications   ♂ HCC ℞HCC CC/MCC Exc

5ᵗʰ K51.2   Ulcerative (chronic) proctitis

    K51.20   Ulcerative (chronic) proctitis without complications   ♂ HCC ℞HCC CC/MCC Exc

      Ulcerative (chronic) proctitis NOS

   6ᵗʰ K51.21   Ulcerative (chronic) proctitis with complications

      K51.211   Ulcerative (chronic) proctitis with rectal bleeding   ♂ HCC ℞HCC CC/MCC Exc

      K51.212   Ulcerative (chronic) proctitis with intestinal obstruction   ♂ HCC ℞ ℞HCC CC/MCC Exc

      K51.213   Ulcerative (chronic) proctitis with fistula   ♂ HCC ℞ ℞HCC CC/MCC Exc

      K51.214   Ulcerative (chronic) proctitis with abscess   ♂ HCC ℞ ℞HCC CC/MCC Exc

      K51.218   Ulcerative (chronic) proctitis with other complication   ♂ HCC ℞HCC CC/MCC Exc

      K51.219   Ulcerative (chronic) proctitis with unspecified complications   ♂ HCC ℞HCC CC/MCC Exc

5ᵗʰ K51.3   Ulcerative (chronic) rectosigmoiditis

    K51.30   Ulcerative (chronic) rectosigmoiditis without complications   ♂ HCC ℞HCC CC/MCC Exc

      Ulcerative (chronic) rectosigmoiditis NOS

   6ᵗʰ K51.31   Ulcerative (chronic) rectosigmoiditis with complications

      K51.311   Ulcerative (chronic) rectosigmoiditis with rectal bleeding   ♂ HCC ℞HCC CC/MCC Exc

      K51.312   Ulcerative (chronic) rectosigmoiditis with intestinal obstruction   ♂ HCC ℞ ℞HCC CC/MCC Exc

      K51.313   Ulcerative (chronic) rectosigmoiditis with fistula   ♂ HCC ℞ ℞HCC CC/MCC Exc

      K51.314   Ulcerative (chronic) rectosigmoiditis with abscess   ♂ HCC ℞ ℞HCC CC/MCC Exc

      K51.318   Ulcerative (chronic) rectosigmoiditis with other complication   ♂ HCC ℞HCC CC/MCC Exc

      K51.319   Ulcerative (chronic) rectosigmoiditis with unspecified complications   ♂ HCC ℞HCC CC/MCC Exc

5ᵗʰ K51.4   Inflammatory polyps of colon

    EXCLUDES1   adenomatous polyp of colon (D12.6)
             polyposis of colon (D12.6)
             polyps of colon NOS (K63.5)

    K51.40   Inflammatory polyps of colon without complications   ♂ HCC ℞HCC CC/MCC Exc

      Inflammatory polyps of colon NOS

   6ᵗʰ K51.41   Inflammatory polyps of colon with complications

      K51.411   Inflammatory polyps of colon with rectal bleeding   ♂ HCC ℞HCC CC/MCC Exc

      K51.412   Inflammatory polyps of colon with intestinal obstruction   ♂ HCC ℞ ℞HCC CC/MCC Exc

      K51.413   Inflammatory polyps of colon with fistula   ♂ HCC ℞ ℞HCC CC/MCC Exc

      K51.414   Inflammatory polyps of colon with abscess   ♂ HCC ℞ ℞HCC CC/MCC Exc

      K51.418   Inflammatory polyps of colon with other complication   ♂ HCC ℞HCC CC/MCC Exc

      K51.419   Inflammatory polyps of colon with unspecified complications   ♂ HCC ℞HCC CC/MCC Exc

5ᵗʰ K51.5   Left sided colitis

    Left hemicolitis

    K51.50   Left sided colitis without complications   ♂ HCC ℞HCC CC/MCC Exc

      Left sided colitis NOS

   6ᵗʰ K51.51   Left sided colitis with complications

      K51.511   Left sided colitis with rectal bleeding   ♂ HCC ℞HCC CC/MCC Exc

      K51.512   Left sided colitis with intestinal obstruction   ♂ HCC ℞ ℞HCC CC/MCC Exc

      K51.513   Left sided colitis with fistula   ♂ HCC ℞ ℞HCC CC/MCC Exc

      K51.514   Left sided colitis with abscess   ♂ HCC ℞ ℞HCC CC/MCC Exc

      K51.518   Left sided colitis with other complication   ♂ HCC ℞HCC CC/MCC Exc

      K51.519   Left sided colitis with unspecified complications   ♂ HCC ℞HCC CC/MCC Exc

5ᵗʰ K51.8   Other ulcerative colitis

    K51.80   Other ulcerative colitis without complications   ♂ HCC ℞HCC CC/MCC Exc

   6ᵗʰ K51.81   Other ulcerative colitis with complications

      K51.811   Other ulcerative colitis with rectal bleeding   ♂ HCC ℞HCC CC/MCC Exc

      K51.812   Other ulcerative colitis with intestinal obstruction   ♂ HCC ℞ ℞HCC CC/MCC Exc

      K51.813   Other ulcerative colitis with fistula   ♂ HCC ℞ ℞HCC CC/MCC Exc

      K51.814   Other ulcerative colitis with abscess   ♂ HCC ℞ ℞HCC CC/MCC Exc

      K51.818   Other ulcerative colitis with other complication   ♂ HCC ℞HCC CC/MCC Exc

      K51.819   Other ulcerative colitis with unspecified complications   ♂ HCC ℞HCC CC/MCC Exc

5ᵗʰ K51.9   Ulcerative colitis, unspecified

    K51.90   Ulcerative colitis, unspecified, without complications   ♂ HCC ℞HCC CC/MCC Exc

   6ᵗʰ K51.91   Ulcerative colitis, unspecified, with complications

      K51.911   Ulcerative colitis, unspecified with rectal bleeding   ♂ HCC ℞HCC CC/MCC Exc

      K51.912   Ulcerative colitis, unspecified with intestinal obstruction   ♂ HCC ℞ ℞HCC CC/MCC Exc

      K51.913   Ulcerative colitis, unspecified with fistula   ♂ HCC ℞ ℞HCC CC/MCC Exc

      K51.914   Ulcerative colitis, unspecified with abscess   ♂ HCC ℞ ℞HCC CC/MCC Exc

      K51.918   Ulcerative colitis, unspecified with other complication   ♂ HCC ℞HCC CC/MCC Exc

      K51.919   Ulcerative colitis, unspecified with unspecified complications   ♂ HCC ℞HCC CC/MCC Exc

4ᵗʰ K52   Other and unspecified noninfective gastroenteritis and colitis

    K52.0   Gastroenteritis and colitis due to radiation   ♂ CC/MCC Exc

    K52.1   Toxic gastroenteritis and colitis   ♂ CC/MCC Exc

      Drug-induced gastroenteritis and colitis

      Code first (T51-T65) to identify toxic agent

      Use additional code for adverse effect, if applicable, to identify drug (T36-T50 with fifth or sixth character 5)

   5ᵗʰ K52.2   Allergic and dietetic gastroenteritis and colitis

      Food hypersensitivity gastroenteritis or colitis

      Use additional code to identify type of food allergy (Z91.01-, Z91.02-)

      EXCLUDES2   allergic eosinophilic colitis (K52.82)
               allergic eosinophilic esophagitis (K20.0)
               allergic eosinophilic gastritis (K52.81)
               allergic eosinophilic gastroenteritis (K52.81)
               food protein-induced proctocolitis (K52.82)

      K52.21   Food protein-induced enterocolitis syndrome
        AHA: Q4 2016
        Use additional code for hypovolemic shock, if present (R57.1)

      K52.22   Food protein-induced enteropathy
        AHA: Q4 2016

      K52.29   Other allergic and dietetic gastroenteritis and colitis
        AHA: Q4 2016
        Food hypersensitivity gastroenteritis or colitis
        Immediate gastrointestinal hypersensitivity

Unspecified Code   Other Specified Code   Manifestation Code   Ⓝ Newborn   Ⓟ Pediatric   Ⓜ Maternity   Ⓐ Adult   ♂ Male   ♀ Female
   ● New Code   ▲ Revised Code Title   ▶◀ Revised Text   NOTES   INCLUDES   EXCLUDES 1 Not coded here   EXCLUDES 2 Not included here
   4ᵗʰ character required   5ᵗʰ character required   6ᵗʰ character required   7ᵗʰ character required
   7ᵗʰ Extension 'X' Alert   HAC Hospital-acquired condition (HAC) alert   AHA AHA Coding Clinic©

K52.3 Indeterminate **colitis**
AHA: Q4 2016
Colonic inflammatory bowel disease unclassified (IBDU)
EXCLUDES1 unspecified colitis (K52.9)

K52.8 Other specified noninfective gastroenteritis and colitis
  K52.81 Eosinophilic gastritis or gastroenteritis
    Eosinophilic enteritis
    EXCLUDES2 eosinophilic esophagitis (K20.0)
  K52.82 Eosinophilic colitis
    Allergic proctocolitis
    Food-induced eosinophilic proctocolitis
    Food protein-induced proctocolitis
    Milk protein-induced proctocolitis
  K52.83 Microscopic **colitis**
    K52.831 Collagenous **colitis**
      AHA: Q4 2016
    K52.832 Lymphocytic **colitis**
      AHA: Q4 2016
    K52.838 Other **microscopic colitis**
      AHA: Q4 2016
    K52.839 Microscopic colitis, unspecified
      AHA: Q4 2016
  K52.89 Other specified noninfective gastroenteritis and colitis

K52.9 Noninfective gastroenteritis and colitis, unspecified
  Colitis NOS
  Enteritis NOS
  Gastroenteritis NOS
  Ileitis NOS
  Jejunitis NOS
  Sigmoiditis NOS
  EXCLUDES1 diarrhea NOS (R19.7)
    functional diarrhea (K59.1)
    infectious gastroenteritis and colitis NOS (A09)
    neonatal diarrhea (noninfective) (P78.3)
    psychogenic diarrhea (F45.8)

Other diseases of intestines (K55-K64)

K55 Vascular disorders of intestine   HCC
  EXCLUDES1 necrotizing enterocolitis of newborn (P77.-)

K55.0 Acute **vascular disorders of intestine**
  Infarction of appendices epiploicae
  Mesenteric (artery) (vein) embolism
  Mesenteric (artery) (vein) infarction
  Mesenteric (artery) (vein) thrombosis
  K55.01 Acute (reversible) ischemia of small **intestine**
    K55.011 Focal (segmental) acute (reversible) ischemia of small intestine HCC MCC CC/MCC Exc
    K55.012 Diffuse acute (reversible) ischemia of small intestine HCC MCC CC/MCC Exc
    K55.019 Acute (reversible) ischemia of small intestine, extent unspecified HCC MCC CC/MCC Exc
  K55.02 Acute infarction of small **intestine**
    Gangrene of small intestine
    Necrosis of small intestine
    K55.021 Focal (segmental) acute infarction of small intestine HCC MCC CC/MCC Exc
    K55.022 Diffuse acute infarction of small intestine HCC MCC CC/MCC Exc
    K55.029 Acute infarction of small intestine, extent unspecified HCC MCC CC/MCC Exc
  K55.03 Acute (reversible) ischemia of large **intestine**
    Acute fulminant ischemic colitis
    Subacute ischemic colitis
    K55.031 Focal (segmental) acute (reversible) ischemia of large intestine HCC MCC CC/MCC Exc
    K55.032 Diffuse acute (reversible) ischemia of large intestine HCC MCC CC/MCC Exc
    K55.039 Acute (reversible) ischemia of large intestine, extent unspecified HCC MCC CC/MCC Exc

K55.04 Acute infarction of large **intestine**
  Gangrene of large intestine
  Necrosis of large intestine
  K55.041 Focal (segmental) acute infarction of large intestine HCC MCC CC/MCC Exc
  K55.042 Diffuse acute infarction of large intestine HCC MCC CC/MCC Exc
  K55.049 Acute infarction of large intestine, extent unspecified HCC MCC CC/MCC Exc

K55.05 Acute (reversible) ischemia **of intestine, part unspecified**
  K55.051 Focal (segmental) acute (reversible) ischemia of intestine, part unspecified HCC MCC CC/MCC Exc
  K55.052 Diffuse acute (reversible) ischemia of intestine, part unspecified HCC MCC CC/MCC Exc
  K55.059 Acute (reversible) ischemia of intestine, part and extent unspecified HCC MCC CC/MCC Exc

K55.06 Acute infarction **of intestine, part unspecified**
  Acute intestinal infarction
  Gangrene of intestine
  Necrosis of intestine
  K55.061 Focal (segmental) acute infarction of intestine, part unspecified HCC MCC CC/MCC Exc
  K55.062 Diffuse acute infarction of intestine, part unspecified HCC MCC CC/MCC Exc
  K55.069 Acute infarction of intestine, part and extent unspecified HCC MCC CC/MCC Exc

K55.1 Chronic **vascular disorders of intestine** CC HCC CC/MCC Exc
  Chronic ischemic colitis
  Chronic ischemic enteritis
  Chronic ischemic enterocolitis
  Ischemic stricture of intestine
  Mesenteric atherosclerosis
  Mesenteric vascular insufficiency

K55.2 Angiodysplasia **of colon**
  K55.20 Angiodysplasia of colon without hemorrhage
  K55.21 Angiodysplasia of colon with hemorrhage MCC CC/MCC Exc

K55.3 Necrotizing enterocolitis
  EXCLUDES1 necrotizing enterocolitis of newborn (P77.-)
  EXCLUDES2 necrotizing enterocolitis due to Clostridium difficile ▶(A04.7-)◀
  K55.30 Necrotizing enterocolitis, unspecified HCC MCC CC/MCC Exc
    AHA: Q4 2016
    Necrotizing enterocolitis, NOS
  K55.31 Stage 1 **necrotizing enterocolitis** HCC MCC CC/MCC Exc
    AHA: Q4 2016
    Necrotizing enterocolitis without pneumatosis, without perforation
  K55.32 Stage 2 **necrotizing enterocolitis** HCC MCC CC/MCC Exc
    AHA: Q4 2016
    Necrotizing enterocolitis with pneumatosis, without perforation
  K55.33 Stage 3 **necrotizing enterocolitis** HCC MCC CC/MCC Exc
    AHA: Q4 2016
    Necrotizing enterocolitis with perforation
    Necrotizing enterocolitis with pneumatosis and perforation

K55.8 Other vascular disorders of intestine CC HCC CC/MCC Exc

K55.9 Vascular disorder of intestine, unspecified CC HCC CC/MCC Exc
  Ischemic colitis
  Ischemic enteritis
  Ischemic enterocolitis

K56 Paralytic ileus and intestinal obstruction without hernia
  EXCLUDES1 congenital stricture or stenosis of intestine (Q41-Q42)
    cystic fibrosis with meconium ileus (E84.11)
    ischemic stricture of intestine (K55.1)
    meconium ileus NOS (P76.0)
    neonatal intestinal obstructions classifiable to P76.-
    obstruction of duodenum (K31.5)
    postprocedural intestinal obstruction ▶(K91.3-)◀
    stenosis of anus or rectum (K62.4)

PDxⁿ Unacceptable principal diagnosis symbol per Medicare code edits   POA Code exempt from diagnosis present on admission requirement
? Questionable admission   CC Complication or comorbidity   CC/MCC Exc CC/MCC exclusion   MCC Major complication or comorbidity
CC Principal diagnosis as its own CC   MCC Principal diagnosis as its own MCC   HCC HCC diagnosis code   RxHCC RxHCC diagnosis code
MACRA code   Z1 Z code as first-listed diagnosis

730   When symbols appear on a code that requires a 7th character extension, refer to Appendix B to identify applicable 7th character codes.   **2018 ICD-10-CM**

K56.0 Paralytic ileus [CC] [HCC] [CC/MCC Exc]
Paralysis of bowel
Paralysis of colon
Paralysis of intestine
[EXCLUDES1] *gallstone ileus (K56.3)*
ileus NOS (K56.7)
obstructive ileus NOS ►(K56.69-)◄

K56.1 Intussusception [CC] [HCC] [CC/MCC Exc]
Intussusception or invagination of bowel
Intussusception or invagination of colon
Intussusception or invagination of intestine
Intussusception or invagination of rectum
[EXCLUDES2] *intussusception of appendix (K38.8)*

K56.2 Volvulus [HCC] [MCC] [CC/MCC Exc]
Strangulation of colon or intestine
Torsion of colon or intestine
Twist of colon or intestine
[EXCLUDES2] *volvulus of duodenum (K31.5)*

K56.3 Gallstone ileus [CC] [HCC] [CC/MCC Exc]
Obstruction of intestine by gallstone

[5th] **K56.4 Other impaction of intestine**

K56.41 Fecal impaction [HCC]
[EXCLUDES1] *constipation (K59.0-)*
incomplete defecation (R15.0)

K56.49 Other impaction of intestine [CC] [HCC] [CC/MCC Exc]

▲ [5th] **K56.5 Intestinal adhesions [bands] with obstruction (postinfection)** [HCC]
Abdominal hernia due to adhesions with obstruction
Peritoneal adhesions [bands] with intestinal obstruction (postinfection)

● **K56.50 Intestinal adhesions [bands], unspecified as to partial versus complete obstruction** [CC] [CC/MCC Exc]
Intestinal adhesions with obstruction NOS

● **K56.51 Intestinal adhesions [bands], with partial obstruction** [CC] [CC/MCC Exc]
Intestinal adhesions with incomplete obstruction

● **K56.52 Intestinal adhesions [bands] with complete obstruction** [CC] [CC/MCC Exc]

[5th] **K56.6 Other and unspecified intestinal obstruction**

[6th] **K56.60 Unspecified intestinal obstruction** [HCC]
[EXCLUDES1] *intestinal obstruction due to specified condition-code to condition*

● **K56.600 Partial intestinal obstruction, unspecified as to cause** [CC] [CC/MCC Exc]
Incomplete intestinal obstruction, NOS

● **K56.601 Complete intestinal obstruction, unspecified as to cause** [CC] [CC/MCC Exc]

● **K56.609 Unspecified intestinal obstruction, unspecified as to partial versus complete obstruction** [CC] [CC/MCC Exc]
Intestinal obstruction NOS

[6th] **K56.69 Other intestinal obstruction** [HCC]
Enterostenosis NOS
Obstructive ileus NOS
Occlusion of colon or intestine NOS
Stenosis of colon or intestine NOS
Stricture of colon or intestine NOS
[EXCLUDES1] *intestinal obstruction due to specified condition-code to condition*

● **K56.690 Other partial intestinal obstruction** [CC] [CC/MCC Exc]
Other incomplete intestinal obstruction

● **K56.691 Other complete intestinal obstruction** [CC] [CC/MCC Exc]

● **K56.699 Other intestinal obstruction unspecified as to partial versus complete obstruction** [CC] [CC/MCC Exc]
Other intestinal obstruction, NEC

K56.7 Ileus, unspecified [CC] [HCC] [CC/MCC Exc]
AHA: Q1 2017
[EXCLUDES1] *obstructive ileus ►(K56.69-)◄*
[EXCLUDES2] *intestinal obstruction with hernia (K40-K46)*

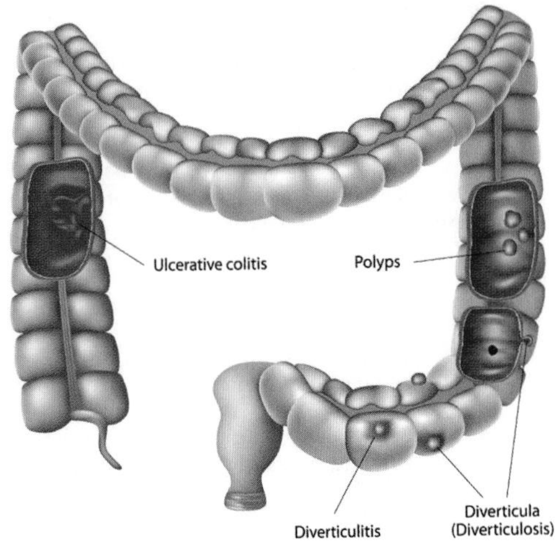

Figure 11.6 Noncancerous colon disorders

[4th] **K57 Diverticular disease of intestine**
[EXCLUDES1] *congenital diverticulum of intestine (Q43.8)*
Meckel's diverticulum (Q43.0)
[EXCLUDES2] *diverticulum of appendix (K38.2)*

[5th] **K57.0 Diverticulitis of small intestine with perforation and abscess**
Diverticulitis of small intestine with peritonitis
[EXCLUDES1] *diverticulitis of both small and large intestine with perforation and abscess (K57.4-)*

K57.00 Diverticulitis of small intestine with perforation and abscess without bleeding [CC] [PDx] [CC/MCC Exc]

K57.01 Diverticulitis of small intestine with perforation and abscess with bleeding [MCC] [PDx] [CC/MCC Exc]

[5th] **K57.1 Diverticular disease of small intestine without perforation or abscess**
[EXCLUDES1] *diverticular disease of both small and large intestine without perforation or abscess (K57.5-)*

K57.10 Diverticulosis of small intestine without perforation or abscess without bleeding
Diverticular disease of small intestine NOS

K57.11 Diverticulosis of small intestine without perforation or abscess with bleeding [MCC] [CC/MCC Exc]

K57.12 Diverticulitis of small intestine without perforation or abscess without bleeding [CC] [CC/MCC Exc]

K57.13 Diverticulitis of small intestine without perforation or abscess with bleeding [MCC] [CC/MCC Exc]

[5th] **K57.2 Diverticulitis of large intestine with perforation and abscess**
Diverticulitis of colon with peritonitis
[EXCLUDES1] *diverticulitis of both small and large intestine with perforation and abscess (K57.4-)*

K57.20 Diverticulitis of large intestine with perforation and abscess without bleeding [CC] [PDx] [CC/MCC Exc]

K57.21 Diverticulitis of large intestine with perforation and abscess with bleeding [MCC] [PDx] [CC/MCC Exc]

[5th] **K57.3 Diverticular disease of large intestine without perforation or abscess**
[EXCLUDES1] *diverticular disease of both small and large intestine without perforation or abscess (K57.5-)*

K57.30 Diverticulosis of large intestine without perforation or abscess without bleeding
Diverticular disease of colon NOS

K57.31 Diverticulosis of large intestine without perforation or abscess with bleeding [MCC] [CC/MCC Exc]

Unspecified Code Other Specified Code Manifestation Code [N] Newborn [P] Pediatric [M] Maternity [A] Adult ♂ Male ♀ Female
● New Code ▲ Revised Code Title ►◄ Revised Text [NOTES] [INCLUDES] [EXCLUDES1] Not coded here [EXCLUDES2] Not included here
[4th] 4th character required [5th] 5th character required [6th] 6th character required [7th] 7th character required
[7th] Extension 'X' Alert [HAC] Hospital-acquired condition (HAC) alert **AHA** AHA Coding Clinic©

When symbols appear on a code that requires a 7th character extension, refer to Appendix B to identify applicable 7th character codes.

K57.32 Diverticulitis of large intestine without perforation or abscess without bleeding CC CC/MCC Exc

K57.33 Diverticulitis of large intestine without perforation or abscess with bleeding MCC CC/MCC Exc

K57.4 Diverticulitis of both small and large intestine with perforation and abscess
Diverticulitis of both small and large intestine with peritonitis

K57.40 Diverticulitis of both small and large intestine with perforation and abscess without bleeding CC PDx CC/MCC Exc

K57.41 Diverticulitis of both small and large intestine with perforation and abscess with bleeding MCC PDx CC/MCC Exc

K57.5 Diverticular disease of both small and large intestine without perforation or abscess

K57.50 Diverticulosis of both small and large intestine without perforation or abscess without bleeding
Diverticular disease of both small and large intestine NOS

K57.51 Diverticulosis of both small and large intestine without perforation or abscess with bleeding MCC CC/MCC Exc

K57.52 Diverticulitis of both small and large intestine without perforation or abscess without bleeding CC PDx CC/MCC Exc

K57.53 Diverticulitis of both small and large intestine without perforation or abscess with bleeding MCC CC/MCC Exc

K57.8 Diverticulitis of intestine, part unspecified, with perforation and abscess
Diverticulitis of intestine NOS with peritonitis

K57.80 Diverticulitis of intestine, part unspecified, with perforation and abscess without bleeding CC PDx CC/MCC Exc

K57.81 Diverticulitis of intestine, part unspecified, with perforation and abscess with bleeding MCC PDx CC/MCC Exc

K57.9 Diverticular disease of intestine, part unspecified, without perforation or abscess

K57.90 Diverticulosis of intestine, part unspecified, without perforation or abscess without bleeding
Diverticular disease of intestine NOS

K57.91 Diverticulosis of intestine, part unspecified, without perforation or abscess with bleeding MCC CC/MCC Exc

K57.92 Diverticulitis of intestine, part unspecified, without perforation or abscess without bleeding CC CC/MCC Exc

K57.93 Diverticulitis of intestine, part unspecified, without perforation or abscess with bleeding MCC CC/MCC Exc

K58 Irritable bowel syndrome
INCLUDES   irritable colon
spastic colon

K58.0 Irritable bowel syndrome with diarrhea

K58.1 Irritable bowel syndrome with constipation
AHA: Q4 2016

K58.2 Mixed irritable bowel syndrome
AHA: Q4 2016

K58.8 Other irritable bowel syndrome
AHA: Q4 2016

K58.9 Irritable bowel syndrome without diarrhea
Irritable bowel syndrome NOS

K59 Other functional intestinal disorders
EXCLUDES1 change in bowel habit NOS (R19.4)
intestinal malabsorption (K90.-)
psychogenic intestinal disorders (F45.8)
EXCLUDES2 functional disorders of stomach (K31.-)

K59.0 Constipation
Use additional code for adverse effect, if applicable, to identify drug (T36-T50 with fifth or sixth character 5)
EXCLUDES1 fecal impaction (K56.41)
incomplete defecation (R15.0)

K59.00 Constipation, unspecified

K59.01 Slow transit constipation

K59.02 Outlet dysfunction constipation

K59.03 Drug induced constipation
AHA: Q4 2016
Use additional code for adverse effect, if applicable, to identify drug (T36-T50 with fifth or sixth character 5

K59.04 Chronic idiopathic constipation
AHA: Q4 2016
Functional constipation

K59.09 Other constipation
Chronic constipation

K59.1 Functional diarrhea
EXCLUDES1 diarrhea NOS (R19.7)
irritable bowel syndrome with diarrhea (K58.0)

K59.2 Neurogenic bowel, not elsewhere classified CC CC/MCC Exc

K59.3 Megacolon, not elsewhere classified
Dilatation of colon
Code first, if applicable (T51-T65) to identify toxic agent
EXCLUDES1 congenital megacolon (aganglionic) (Q43.1)
megacolon (due to) (in) Chagas' disease (B57.32)
megacolon (due to) (in) Clostridium difficile ▶(A04.7-)◀
megacolon (due to) (in) Hirschsprung's disease (Q43.1)

K59.31 Toxic megacolon CC HCC CC/MCC Exc
AHA: Q4 2016

K59.39 Other megacolon CC CC/MCC Exc
AHA: Q4 2016
Megacolon NOS

K59.4 Anal spasm
Proctalgia fugax

K59.8 Other specified functional intestinal disorders
Atony of colon
Pseudo-obstruction (acute) (chronic) of intestine

K59.9 Functional intestinal disorder, unspecified

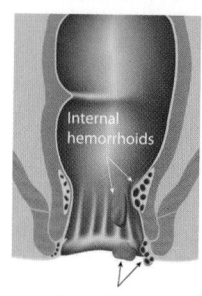
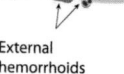
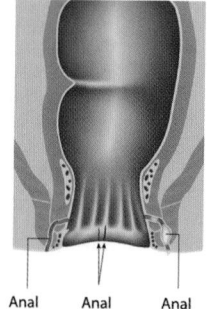

Internal hemorrhoids

External hemorrhoids

Anal fistula   Anal fissures   Anal abscess

Figure 11.7 Anal disorders

K60 Fissure and fistula of anal and rectal regions
EXCLUDES1 fissure and fistula of anal and rectal regions with abscess or cellulitis (K61.-)
EXCLUDES2 anal sphincter tear (healed) (nontraumatic) (old) (K62.81)

K60.0 Acute anal fissure

K60.1 Chronic anal fissure

K60.2 Anal fissure, unspecified

K60.3 Anal fistula

K60.4 Rectal fistula
Fistula of rectum to skin
EXCLUDES1 rectovaginal fistula (N82.3)
vesicorectal fistual (N32.1)

K60.5 Anorectal fistula

K61 Abscess of anal and rectal regions
INCLUDES   abscess of anal and rectal regions
cellulitis of anal and rectal regions

K61.0 Anal abscess CC CC/MCC Exc
Perianal abscess
EXCLUDES1 intrasphincteric abscess (K61.4)

PDx Unacceptable principal diagnosis symbol per Medicare code edits   POA Code exempt from diagnosis present on admission requirement
? Questionable admission   CC Complication or comorbidity   CC/MCC Exc CC/MCC exclusion   MCC Major complication or comorbidity
PDx Principal diagnosis as its own CC   MDx Principal diagnosis as its own MCC   HCC HCC diagnosis code   RxHCC RxHCC diagnosis code
MACRA code   Z Z code as first-listed diagnosis

K61.1 Rectal **abscess**   CC CC/MCC Exc
   AHA: Q4 2012
   Perirectal abscess
   EXCLUDES1 ischiorectal abscess (K61.3)
K61.2 Anorectal **abscess**   CC CC/MCC Exc
K61.3 Ischiorectal **abscess**   CC
   Abscess of ischiorectal fossa
K61.4 Intrasphincteric **abscess**   CC CC/MCC Exc
K62 Other diseases of anus and rectum
   INCLUDES   anal canal
   EXCLUDES2 colostomy and enterostomy malfunction (K94.0-, K94.1-)
           fecal incontinence (R15.-)
           hemorrhoids (K64.-)
K62.0 Anal polyp
K62.1 Rectal polyp
   EXCLUDES1 adenomatous polyp (D12.8)
K62.2 Anal prolapse
   Prolapse of anal canal
K62.3 Rectal prolapse
   Prolapse of rectal mucosa
K62.4 Stenosis of anus and rectum
   Stricture of anus (sphincter)
K62.5 Hemorrhage of anus and rectum   CC CC/MCC Exc
   EXCLUDES1 gastrointestinal bleeding NOS (K92.2)
           melena (K92.1)
           neonatal rectal hemorrhage (P54.2)
K62.6 Ulcer of anus and rectum   CC CC/MCC Exc
   Solitary ulcer of anus and rectum
   Stercoral ulcer of anus and rectum
   EXCLUDES1 fissure and fistula of anus and rectum (K60.-)
           ulcerative colitis (K51.-)
K62.7 Radiation proctitis
   Use additional code to identify the type of radiation (W90.-)
K62.8 Other specified diseases of anus and rectum
   EXCLUDES2 ulcerative proctitis (K51.2)
   K62.81 **Anal sphincter tear (healed) (nontraumatic) (old)**
           Tear of anus, nontraumatic
           Use additional code for any associated fecal
           incontinence (R15.-)
           EXCLUDES2 anal fissure (K60.-)
                   anal sphincter tear (healed) (old)
                   complicating delivery (O34.7-)
                   traumatic tear of anal sphincter (S31.831)
   K62.82 **Dysplasia of anus**
           Anal intraepithelial neoplasia I and II (AIN I and II)
             (histologically confirmed)
           Dysplasia of anus NOS
           Mild and moderate dysplasia of anus (histologically
             confirmed)
           EXCLUDES1 abnormal results from anal cytologic
                   examination without histologic confirmation
                   (R85.61-)
                   anal intraepithelial neoplasia III (D01.3)
                   carcinoma in situ of anus (D01.3)
                   HGSIL of anus (R85.613)
                   severe dysplasia of anus (D01.3)
   K62.89 Other specified diseases of anus and rectum
           Proctitis NOS
           Use additional code for any associated fecal
           incontinence (R15.-)
K62.9 Disease of anus and rectum, unspecified
K63 Other diseases of intestine
K63.0 Abscess of intestine   CC CC/MCC Exc
   EXCLUDES1 abscess of intestine with Crohn's disease (K50.014,
           K50.114, K50.814, K50.914,)
           abscess of intestine with diverticular disease (K57.0,
           K57.2, K57.4, K57.8)

abscess of intestine with ulcerative colitis (K51.014,
K51.214, K51.314, K51.414, K51.514, K51.814, K51.914)
   EXCLUDES2 abscess of anal and rectal regions (K61.-)
           abscess of appendix (K35.3)
K63.1 Perforation of intestine (nontraumatic)   HCC MCC CC/MCC Exc
   Perforation (nontraumatic) of rectum
   EXCLUDES1 perforation (nontraumatic) of duodenum (K26.-)
           perforation (nontraumatic) of intestine with
           diverticular disease (K57.0, K57.2, K57.4, K57.8)
   EXCLUDES2 perforation (nontraumatic) of appendix (K35.2, K35.3)
K63.2 Fistula of intestine   CC CC/MCC Exc
   EXCLUDES1 fistula of duodenum (K31.6)
           fistula of intestine with Crohn's disease (K50.013,
           K50.113, K50.813, K50.913,)
           fistula of intestine with ulcerative colitis (K51.013,
           K51.213, K51.313, K51.413, K51.513, K51.813, K51.913)
   EXCLUDES2 fistula of anal and rectal regions (K60.-)
           fistula of appendix (K38.3)
           intestinal-genital fistula, female (N82.2-N82.4)
           vesicointestinal fistula (N32.1)
K63.3 Ulcer of intestine   CC CC/MCC Exc
   Primary ulcer of small intestine
   EXCLUDES1 duodenal ulcer (K26.-)
           gastrointestinal ulcer (K28.-)
           gastrojejunal ulcer (K28.-)
           jejunal ulcer (K28.-)
           peptic ulcer, site unspecified (K27.-)
           ulcer of intestine with perforation (K63.1)
           ulcer of anus or rectum (K62.6)
           ulcerative colitis (K51.-)
K63.4 Enteroptosis
K63.5 Polyp of colon
   AHA: Q1 2017
   EXCLUDES1 adenomatous polyp of colon (D12.6)
           inflammatory polyp of colon (K51.4-)
           polyposis of colon (D12.6)
K63.8 Other specified diseases of intestine
   K63.81 Dieulafoy lesion of intestine   MCC CC/MCC Exc
           EXCLUDES2 Dieulafoy lesion of stomach and duodenum
                   (K31.82)
   K63.89 Other specified diseases of intestine
K63.9 Disease of intestine, unspecified
K64 Hemorrhoids and perianal venous thrombosis
   INCLUDES   piles
   EXCLUDES1 hemorrhoids complicating childbirth and the puerperium
           (O87.2)
           hemorrhoids complicating pregnancy (O22.4)
K64.0 First degree hemorrhoids
   Grade/stage I hemorrhoids
   Hemorrhoids (bleeding) without prolapse outside of anal canal
K64.1 Second degree hemorrhoids
   Grade/stage II hemorrhoids
   Hemorrhoids (bleeding) that prolapse with straining, but
     retract spontaneously
K64.2 Third degree hemorrhoids
   Grade/stage III hemorrhoids
   Hemorrhoids (bleeding) that prolapse with straining and
     require manual replacement back inside anal canal
K64.3 Fourth degree hemorrhoids
   Grade/stage IV hemorrhoids
   Hemorrhoids (bleeding) with prolapsed tissue that cannot be
     manually replaced
K64.4 Residual hemorrhoidal skin tags
   External hemorrhoids, NOS
   Skin tags of anus

Unspecified Code   Other Specified Code   Manifestation Code   N Newborn   P Pediatric   M Maternity   A Adult   ♂ Male   ♀ Female
● New Code   ▲ Revised Code Title   ►◄ Revised Text   NOTES   *INCLUDES*   *EXCLUDES 1* Not coded here   *EXCLUDES2* Not included here
4ᵗʰ character required   5ᵗʰ character required   6ᵗʰ character required   7ᵗʰ character required
7ᵗʰ Extension 'X' Alert   HAC Hospital-acquired condition (HAC) alert   AHA AHA Coding Clinic©

K64.5 Perianal venous thrombosis
External hemorrhoids with thrombosis
Perianal hematoma
Thrombosed hemorrhoids NOS

K64.8 Other hemorrhoids
Internal hemorrhoids, without mention of degree
Prolapsed hemorrhoids, degree not specified

K64.9 Unspecified hemorrhoids
Hemorrhoids (bleeding) NOS
Hemorrhoids (bleeding) without mention of degree

Diseases of peritoneum and retroperitoneum (K65-K68)

K65 Peritonitis
Use additional code (B95-B97), to identify infectious agent
EXCLUDES1 *acute appendicitis with generalized peritonitis (K35.2)*
aseptic peritonitis (T81.6)
benign paroxysmal peritonitis (E85.0)
chemical peritonitis (T81.6)
diverticulitis of both small and large intestine with peritonitis (K57.4-)
diverticulitis of colon with peritonitis (K57.2-)
diverticulitis of intestine, NOS, with peritonitis (K57.8-)
diverticulitis of small intestine with peritonitis (K57.0-)
gonococcal peritonitis (A54.85)
neonatal peritonitis (P78.0-P78.1)
pelvic peritonitis, female (N73.3-N73.5)
periodic familial peritonitis (E85.0)
peritonitis due to talc or other foreign substance (T81.6)
peritonitis in chlamydia (A74.81)
peritonitis in diphtheria (A36.89)
peritonitis in syphilis (late) (A52.74)
peritonitis in tuberculosis (A18.31)
peritonitis with or following abortion or ectopic or molar pregnancy (O00-O07, O08.0)
peritonitis with or following appendicitis (K35.-)
peritonitis with or following diverticular disease of intestine (K57.-)
puerperal peritonitis (O85)
retroperitoneal infections (K68.-)

K65.0 Generalized (acute) peritonitis — HCC MCC CC/MCC Exc
Pelvic peritonitis (acute), male
Subphrenic peritonitis (acute)
Suppurative peritonitis (acute)

K65.1 Peritoneal abscess — HCC MCC CC/MCC Exc
Abdominopelvic abscess
Abscess (of) omentum
Abscess (of) peritoneum
Mesenteric abscess
Retrocecal abscess
Subdiaphragmatic abscess
Subhepatic abscess
Subphrenic abscess

K65.2 Spontaneous bacterial peritonitis — HCC MCC CC/MCC Exc
EXCLUDES1 *bacterial peritonitis NOS (K65.9)*

K65.3 Choleperitonitis — HCC MCC CC/MCC Exc
Peritonitis due to bile

K65.4 Sclerosing mesenteritis — CC HCC CC/MCC Exc
Fat necrosis of peritoneum
(Idiopathic) sclerosing mesenteric fibrosis
Mesenteric lipodystrophy
Mesenteric panniculitis
Retractile mesenteritis

K65.8 Other peritonitis — HCC MCC CC/MCC Exc
Chronic proliferative peritonitis
Peritonitis due to urine

K65.9 Peritonitis, unspecified — HCC MCC CC/MCC Exc
Bacterial peritonitis NOS

K66 Other disorders of peritoneum
EXCLUDES2 *ascites (R18.-)*
peritoneal effusion (chronic) (R18.8)

K66.0 Peritoneal adhesions (postprocedural) (postinfection)
Adhesions (of) abdominal (wall)
Adhesions (of) diaphragm
Adhesions (of) intestine
Adhesions (of) male pelvis
Adhesions (of) omentum
Adhesions (of) stomach
Adhesive bands
Mesenteric adhesions
EXCLUDES1 *female pelvic adhesions [bands] (N73.6)*
peritoneal adhesions with intestinal obstruction ►*(K56.5-)*◄

K66.1 Hemoperitoneum — MCC CC/MCC Exc
EXCLUDES1 *traumatic hemoperitoneum (S36.8-)*

K66.8 Other specified disorders of peritoneum

K66.9 Disorder of peritoneum, unspecified

K67 Disorders of peritoneum in infectious diseases classified elsewhere — HCC MCC CC/MCC Exc
Code first underlying disease, such as :
congenital syphilis (A50.0)
helminthiasis (B65.0 -B83.9)
EXCLUDES1 *peritonitis in chlamydia (A74.81)*
peritonitis in diphtheria (A36.89)
peritonitis in gonococcal (A54.85)
peritonitis in syphilis (late) (A52.74)
peritonitis in tuberculosis (A18.31)

K68 Disorders of retroperitoneum

K68.1 Retroperitoneal abscess
K68.11 Postprocedural retroperitoneal abscess — CC HAC CC/MCC Exc
K68.12 Psoas muscle abscess — HCC MCC CC/MCC Exc
K68.19 Other retroperitoneal abscess — HCC MCC CC/MCC Exc

K68.9 Other disorders of retroperitoneum — MCC CC/MCC Exc

Diseases of liver (K70-K77)

EXCLUDES1 *jaundice NOS (R17)*
EXCLUDES2 *hemochromatosis (E83.11-)*
Reye's syndrome (G93.7)
viral hepatitis (B15-B19)
Wilson's disease (E83.0)

K70 Alcoholic liver disease
Use additional code to identify:
alcohol abuse and dependence (F10.-)

K70.0 Alcoholic fatty liver — A

K70.1 Alcoholic hepatitis — A
K70.10 Alcoholic hepatitis without ascites — A
K70.11 Alcoholic hepatitis with ascites — A

K70.2 Alcoholic fibrosis and sclerosis of liver — A

K70.3 Alcoholic cirrhosis of liver
Alcoholic cirrhosis NOS
K70.30 Alcoholic cirrhosis of liver without ascites — A HCC
K70.31 Alcoholic cirrhosis of liver with ascites — A HCC

K70.4 Alcoholic hepatic failure
Acute alcoholic hepatic failure
Alcoholic hepatic failure NOS
Chronic alcoholic hepatic failure
Subacute alcoholic hepatic failure
K70.40 Alcoholic hepatic failure without coma — A HCC
K70.41 Alcoholic hepatic failure with coma — A HCC MCC PDx MCC CC/MCC Exc

K70.9 Alcoholic liver disease, unspecified — A HCC

K71 Toxic liver disease
INCLUDES *drug-induced idiosyncratic (unpredictable) liver disease*
drug-induced toxic (predictable) liver disease
Code first poisoning due to drug or toxin, if applicable (T36-T65 with fifth or sixth character 1-4 or 6)

PDx Unacceptable principal diagnosis symbol per Medicare code edits   POA Code exempt from diagnosis present on admission requirement
? Questionable admission   CC Complication or comorbidity   CC/MCC CC/MCC exclusion   MCC Major complication or comorbidity
PDx CC Principal diagnosis as its own CC   PDx MCC Principal diagnosis as its own MCC   HCC HCC diagnosis code   RxHCC RxHCC diagnosis code
MACRA code   Z1 Z code as first-listed diagnosis

734

When symbols appear on a code that requires a 7th character extension, refer to Appendix B to identify applicable 7th character codes.

2018 ICD-10-CM

Use additional code for adverse effect, if applicable, to identify drug (T36-T50 with fifth or sixth character 5)

EXCLUDES2 *alcoholic liver disease (K70.-)*

Budd-Chiari syndrome (I82.0)

K71.0 Toxic liver disease with cholestasis

Cholestasis with hepatocyte injury

'Pure' cholestasis

🄢 **K71.1 Toxic liver disease with** hepatic necrosis

Hepatic failure (acute) (chronic) due to drugs

K71.10 Toxic liver disease with hepatic necrosis, without coma

K71.11 Toxic liver disease with hepatic necrosis, with coma HCC MCC PDx CC/MCC Exc

K71.2 Toxic liver disease with acute hepatitis

K71.3 Toxic liver disease with chronic persistent hepatitis

K71.4 Toxic liver disease with chronic lobular hepatitis

🄢 **K71.5 Toxic liver disease with** chronic active hepatitis

Toxic liver disease with lupoid hepatitis

K71.50 Toxic liver disease with chronic active hepatitis without ascites

K71.51 Toxic liver disease with chronic active hepatitis with ascites

K71.6 Toxic liver disease with hepatitis, not elsewhere classified

K71.7 Toxic liver disease with fibrosis and cirrhosis **of liver**

K71.8 Toxic liver disease with other disorders of liver

Toxic liver disease with focal nodular hyperplasia

Toxic liver disease with hepatic granulomas

Toxic liver disease with peliosis hepatis

Toxic liver disease with veno-occlusive disease of liver

K71.9 Toxic liver disease, unspecified

🄠 **K72 Hepatic failure, not elsewhere classified**

INCLUDES fulminant hepatitis NEC, with hepatic failure

hepatic encephalopathy NOS

liver (cell) necrosis with hepatic failure

malignant hepatitis NEC, with hepatic failure

yellow liver atrophy or dystrophy

EXCLUDES1 *alcoholic hepatic failure (K70.4)*

hepatic failure with toxic liver disease (K71.1-)

icterus of newborn (P55-P59)

postprocedural hepatic failure (K91.82)

EXCLUDES2 *hepatic failure complicating abortion or ectopic or molar pregnancy (O00-O07, O08.8)*

hepatic failure complicating pregnancy, childbirth and the puerperium (O26.6-)

viral hepatitis with hepatic coma (B15-B19)

🄢 **K72.0 Acute and subacute** hepatic failure

Acute non-viral hepatitis NOS

K72.00 Acute and subacute hepatic failure without coma MCC CC/MCC Exc

K72.01 Acute and subacute hepatic failure with coma HCC MCC PDx CC/MCC Exc

🄢 **K72.1 Chronic** hepatic failure

K72.10 Chronic hepatic failure without coma HCC

AHA: Q1 2017

K72.11 Chronic hepatic failure with coma HCC MCC PDx CC/MCC Exc

🄢 **K72.9 Hepatic failure, unspecified**

K72.90 Hepatic failure, unspecified without coma HCC

AHA: Q2 2016

K72.91 Hepatic failure, unspecified with coma HCC MCC CC/MCC Exc

Hepatic coma NOS

🄠 **K73 Chronic hepatitis, not elsewhere classified**

EXCLUDES1 *alcoholic hepatitis (chronic) (K70.1-)*

drug-induced hepatitis (chronic) (K71.-)

granulomatous hepatitis (chronic) NEC (K75.3)

reactive, nonspecific hepatitis (chronic) (K75.2)

viral hepatitis (chronic) (B15-B19)

K73.0 Chronic persistent **hepatitis, not elsewhere classified** HCC

K73.1 Chronic lobular **hepatitis, not elsewhere classified** HCC

K73.2 Chronic active **hepatitis, not elsewhere classified** HCC

K73.8 Other chronic hepatitis, not elsewhere classified HCC

K73.9 Chronic hepatitis, unspecified HCC

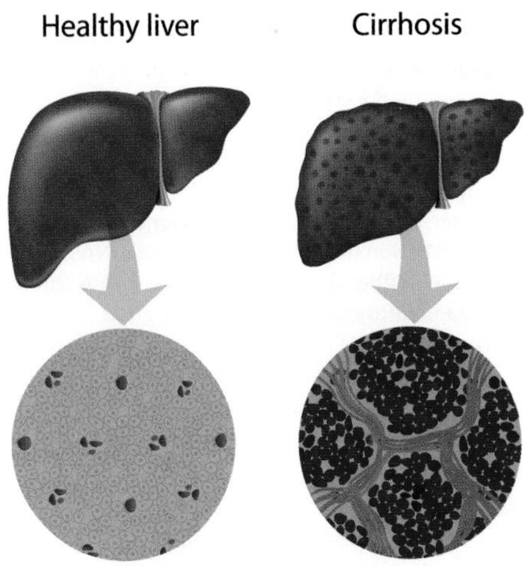

Healthy liver   Cirrhosis

Figure 11.8 Cirrhosis of the liver

🄠 **K74 Fibrosis and cirrhosis of liver**

Code also, if applicable, viral hepatitis (acute) (chronic) (B15-B19)

EXCLUDES1 *alcoholic cirrhosis (of liver) (K70.3)*

alcoholic fibrosis of liver (K70.2)

cardiac sclerosis of liver (K76.1)

cirrhosis (of liver) with toxic liver disease (K71.7)

congenital cirrhosis (of liver) (P78.81)

pigmentary cirrhosis (of liver) (E83.110)

K74.0 Hepatic fibrosis

K74.1 Hepatic sclerosis

K74.2 Hepatic fibrosis with hepatic sclerosis

K74.3 Primary biliary cirrhosis HCC

Chronic nonsuppurative destructive cholangitis

K74.4 Secondary biliary cirrhosis HCC

K74.5 Biliary cirrhosis, unspecified HCC

🄢 **K74.6 Other and unspecified cirrhosis of liver**

K74.60 Unspecified cirrhosis of liver HCC

Cirrhosis (of liver) NOS

K74.69 Other cirrhosis of liver HCC

Cryptogenic cirrhosis (of liver)

Macronodular cirrhosis (of liver)

Micronodular cirrhosis (of liver)

Mixed type cirrhosis (of liver)

Portal cirrhosis (of liver)

Postnecrotic cirrhosis (of liver)

🄠 **K75 Other inflammatory liver diseases**

EXCLUDES2 *toxic liver disease (K71.-)*

K75.0 Abscess of liver MCC CC/MCC Exc

Cholangitic hepatic abscess

Hematogenic hepatic abscess

Hepatic abscess NOS

Lymphogenic hepatic abscess

Pylephlebitic hepatic abscess

EXCLUDES1 *amebic liver abscess (A06.4)*

cholangitis without liver abscess (K83.0)

pylephlebitis without liver abscess (K75.1)

EXCLUDES2 *acute or subacute hepatitis NOS (B17.9)*

acute or subacute non-viral hepatitis (K72.0)

chronic hepatitis NEC (K73.8)

K75.1 Phlebitis of portal vein MCC CC/MCC Exc

Pylephlebitis

EXCLUDES1 *pylephlebitic liver abscess (K75.0)*

Unspecified Code   Other Specified Code   Manifestation Code   Ⓝ Newborn   Ⓟ Pediatric   Ⓜ Maternity   Ⓐ Adult   ♂ Male   ♀ Female
● New Code   ▲ Revised Code Title   ▶◀ Revised Text   **NOTES** *INCLUDES* *EXCLUDES 1* Not coded here   *EXCLUDES 2* Not included here
🄠 4th character required   🄢 5th character required   🄤 6th character required   🄥 7th character required
🄦 Extension 'X' Alert   HAC Hospital-acquired condition (HAC) alert   **AHA** AHA Coding Clinic©

K75.2 **Nonspecific reactive hepatitis**
  EXCLUDES1 *acute or subacute hepatitis (K72.0-)*
      chronic hepatitis NEC (K73.-)
      viral hepatitis (B15-B19)
K75.3 **Granulomatous hepatitis, not elsewhere classified**
  EXCLUDES1 *acute or subacute hepatitis (K72.0-)*
      chronic hepatitis NEC (K73.-)
      viral hepatitis (B15-B19)
K75.4 **Autoimmune hepatitis** ⬛HCC
  Lupoid hepatitis NEC
5ᵗʰ K75.8 **Other specified inflammatory liver diseases**
  K75.81 **Nonalcoholic steatohepatitis (NASH)**
  K75.89 Other specified inflammatory liver diseases
K75.9 **Inflammatory liver disease, unspecified**
  Hepatitis NOS
  EXCLUDES1 *acute or subacute hepatitis (K72.0-)*
      chronic hepatitis NEC (K73.-)
      viral hepatitis (B15-B19)
4ᵗʰ K76 **Other diseases of liver**
  EXCLUDES2 *alcoholic liver disease (K70.-)*
      amyloid degeneration of liver (E85.-)
      cystic disease of liver (congenital) (Q44.6)
      hepatic vein thrombosis (I82.0)
      hepatomegaly NOS (R16.0)
      pigmentary cirrhosis (of liver) (E83.110)
      portal vein thrombosis (I81)
      toxic liver disease (K71.-)
  K76.0 **Fatty (change of) liver, not elsewhere classified**
    Nonalcoholic fatty liver disease (NAFLD)
    EXCLUDES1 *nonalcoholic steatohepatitis (NASH) (K75.81)*
  K76.1 **Chronic passive congestion of liver**
    Cardiac cirrhosis
    Cardiac sclerosis
  K76.2 **Central hemorrhagic necrosis of liver** MCC CC/MCC Exc.
    EXCLUDES1 *liver necrosis with hepatic failure (K72.-)*
  K76.3 **Infarction of liver** MCC CC/MCC Exc.
  K76.4 **Peliosis hepatis**
    Hepatic angiomatosis
  K76.5 **Hepatic veno-occlusive disease**
    EXCLUDES1 *Budd-Chiari syndrome (I82.0)*
  K76.6 **Portal hypertension** CC HCC CC/MCC Exc.
    Use additional code for any associated complications, such as:
    portal hypertensive gastropathy (K31.89)
  K76.7 **Hepatorenal syndrome** HCC MCC CC/MCC Exc.
    EXCLUDES1 *hepatorenal syndrome following labor and delivery (O90.4)*
      postprocedural hepatorenal syndrome (K91.83)
5ᵗʰ K76.8 **Other specified diseases of liver**
  K76.81 **Hepatopulmonary syndrome** HCC PDxIn
    Code first underlying liver disease, such as:
    alcoholic cirrhosis of liver (K70.3-)
    cirrhosis of liver without mention of alcohol (K74.6-)
  K76.89 Other specified diseases of liver
    Cyst (simple) of liver
    Focal nodular hyperplasia of liver
    Hepatoptosis
  K76.9 **Liver disease, unspecified**
K77 **Liver disorders in diseases classified elsewhere** CC CC/MCC Exc.
  Code first underlying disease, such as:
  amyloidosis (E85.-)
  congenital syphilis (A50.0, A50.5)
  congenital toxoplasmosis (P37.1)
  schistosomiasis (B65.0-B65.9)
  EXCLUDES1 *alcoholic hepatitis (K70.1-)*
      alcoholic liver disease (K70.-)
      cytomegaloviral hepatitis (B25.1)

herpesviral [herpes simplex] hepatitis (B00.81)
infectious mononucleosis with liver disease (B27.0-B27.9 with .9)
mumps hepatitis (B26.81)
sarcoidosis with liver disease (D86.89)
secondary syphilis with liver disease (A51.45)
syphilis (late) with liver disease (A52.74)
toxoplasmosis (acquired) hepatitis (B58.1)
tuberculosis with liver disease (A18.83)

Disorders of gallbladder, biliary tract and pancreas (K80-K87)

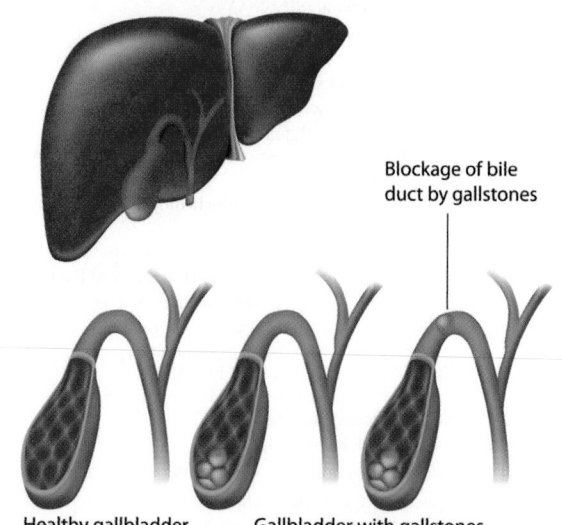

Blockage of bile duct by gallstones

Healthy gallbladder   Gallbladder with gallstones

Figure 11.9 Illustration showing normal and obstructed gallbladder

4ᵗʰ K80 **Cholelithiasis**
  EXCLUDES1 *retained cholelithiasis following cholecystectomy (K91.86)*
5ᵗʰ K80.0 **Calculus of** gallbladder with acute cholecystitis
    Any condition listed in K80.2 with acute cholecystitis
    K80.00 **Calculus of gallbladder with acute cholecystitis without obstruction** CC CC/MCC Exc.
    K80.01 **Calculus of gallbladder with acute cholecystitis** with **obstruction** CC CC/MCC Exc.
5ᵗʰ K80.1 **Calculus of** gallbladder with other cholecystitis
    K80.10 **Calculus of gallbladder with** chronic **cholecystitis without obstruction** CC CC/MCC Exc.
      Cholelithiasis with cholecystitis NOS
    K80.11 **Calculus of gallbladder with** chronic **cholecystitis with obstruction** CC CC/MCC Exc.
    K80.12 **Calculus of gallbladder with** acute and chronic **cholecystitis** without obstruction CC CC/MCC Exc.
    K80.13 **Calculus of gallbladder with** acute and chronic **cholecystitis** with obstruction CC CC/MCC Exc.
    K80.18 **Calculus of gallbladder with other cholecystitis without obstruction** CC CC/MCC Exc.
    K80.19 **Calculus of gallbladder with other cholecystitis** with **obstruction** CC CC/MCC Exc.
5ᵗʰ K80.2 **Calculus of** gallbladder without cholecystitis
    Cholecystolithiasis without cholecystitis
    Cholelithiasis (without cholecystitis)
    Colic (recurrent) of gallbladder (without cholecystitis)
    Gallstone (impacted) of cystic duct (without cholecystitis)
    Gallstone (impacted) of gallbladder (without cholecystitis)
    K80.20 **Calculus of gallbladder without cholecystitis without obstruction**
    K80.21 **Calculus of gallbladder without cholecystitis with obstruction** CC CC/MCC Exc.
5ᵗʰ K80.3 **Calculus of** bile duct with cholangitis
    Any condition listed in K80.5 with cholangitis

PDxIn Unacceptable principal diagnosis symbol per Medicare code edits   POA Code exempt from diagnosis present on admission requirement
❓ Questionable admission   CC Complication or comorbidity   CC/MCC Exc. CC/MCC exclusion   MCC Major complication or comorbidity
PDxCC Principal diagnosis as its own CC   PDxMCC Principal diagnosis as its own MCC   HCC HCC diagnosis code   RHCC RxHCC diagnosis code
MACRA code   Z1 Z code as first-listed diagnosis

K80.30 **Calculus of bile duct with cholangitis, unspecified, without obstruction** [CC] [PDx] [CC/MCC Exc]

K80.31 **Calculus of bile duct with cholangitis, unspecified, with obstruction** [CC] [PDx] [CC/MCC Exc]

K80.32 **Calculus of bile duct with acute cholangitis without obstruction** [CC] [PDx] [CC/MCC Exc]

K80.33 **Calculus of bile duct with acute cholangitis with obstruction** [CC] [PDx] [CC/MCC Exc]

K80.34 **Calculus of bile duct with chronic cholangitis without obstruction** [CC] [PDx] [CC/MCC Exc]

K80.35 **Calculus of bile duct with chronic cholangitis with obstruction** [CC] [PDx] [CC/MCC Exc]

K80.36 **Calculus of bile duct with acute and chronic cholangitis without obstruction** [CC] [PDx] [CC/MCC Exc]

K80.37 **Calculus of bile duct with acute and chronic cholangitis with obstruction** [CC] [PDx] [CC/MCC Exc]

[5th] K80.4 **Calculus of bile duct with cholecystitis**

Any condition listed in K80.5 with cholecystitis (with cholangitis)

K80.40 **Calculus of bile duct with cholecystitis, unspecified, without obstruction** [CC] [CC/MCC Exc]

K80.41 **Calculus of bile duct with cholecystitis, unspecified, with obstruction** [CC] [CC/MCC Exc]

K80.42 **Calculus of bile duct with acute cholecystitis without obstruction** [CC] [CC/MCC Exc]

K80.43 **Calculus of bile duct with acute cholecystitis with obstruction** [CC] [CC/MCC Exc]

K80.44 **Calculus of bile duct with chronic cholecystitis without obstruction** [CC] [CC/MCC Exc]

K80.45 **Calculus of bile duct with chronic cholecystitis with obstruction** [CC] [CC/MCC Exc]

K80.46 **Calculus of bile duct with acute and chronic cholecystitis without obstruction** [CC] [CC/MCC Exc]

K80.47 **Calculus of bile duct with acute and chronic cholecystitis with obstruction** [CC] [CC/MCC Exc]

[5th] K80.5 **Calculus of bile duct without cholangitis or cholecystitis**

Choledocholithiasis (without cholangitis or cholecystitis)
Gallstone (impacted) of bile duct NOS (without cholangitis or cholecystitis)
Gallstone (impacted) of common duct (without cholangitis or cholecystitis)
Gallstone (impacted) of hepatic duct (without cholangitis or cholecystitis)
Hepatic cholelithiasis (without cholangitis or cholecystitis)
Hepatic colic (recurrent) (without cholangitis or cholecystitis)

K80.50 **Calculus of bile duct without cholangitis or cholecystitis without obstruction**

K80.51 **Calculus of bile duct without cholangitis or cholecystitis with obstruction** [CC] [CC/MCC Exc]

[5th] K80.6 **Calculus of gallbladder and bile duct with cholecystitis**

K80.60 **Calculus of gallbladder and bile duct with cholecystitis, unspecified, without obstruction** [CC] [CC/MCC Exc]

K80.61 **Calculus of gallbladder and bile duct with cholecystitis, unspecified, with obstruction** [CC] [CC/MCC Exc]

K80.62 **Calculus of gallbladder and bile duct with acute cholecystitis without obstruction** [CC] [CC/MCC Exc]

K80.63 **Calculus of gallbladder and bile duct with acute cholecystitis with obstruction** [CC] [CC/MCC Exc]

K80.64 **Calculus of gallbladder and bile duct with chronic cholecystitis without obstruction** [CC] [CC/MCC Exc]

K80.65 **Calculus of gallbladder and bile duct with chronic cholecystitis with obstruction** [CC] [CC/MCC Exc]

K80.66 **Calculus of gallbladder and bile duct with acute and chronic cholecystitis without obstruction** [CC] [CC/MCC Exc]

K80.67 **Calculus of gallbladder and bile duct with acute and chronic cholecystitis with obstruction** [MCC] [CC/MCC Exc]

[5th] K80.7 **Calculus of gallbladder and bile duct without cholecystitis**

K80.70 **Calculus of gallbladder and bile duct without cholecystitis without obstruction**

K80.71 **Calculus of gallbladder and bile duct without cholecystitis with obstruction** [CC] [CC/MCC Exc]

[5th] K80.8 **Other cholelithiasis**

K80.80 **Other cholelithiasis without obstruction**

K80.81 **Other cholelithiasis with obstruction** [CC] [CC/MCC Exc]

[4th] K81 **Cholecystitis**

[EXCLUDES1] *cholecystitis with cholelithiasis (K80.-)*

K81.0 **Acute cholecystitis** [CC] [CC/MCC Exc]

Abscess of gallbladder
Angiocholecystitis
Emphysematous (acute) cholecystitis
Empyema of gallbladder
Gangrene of gallbladder
Gangrenous cholecystitis
Suppurative cholecystitis

K81.1 **Chronic cholecystitis**

K81.2 **Acute cholecystitis with chronic cholecystitis** [CC] [CC/MCC Exc]

K81.9 **Cholecystitis, unspecified**

[4th] K82 **Other diseases of gallbladder**

[EXCLUDES1] *nonvisualization of gallbladder (R93.2)*
postcholecystectomy syndrome (K91.5)

K82.0 **Obstruction of gallbladder** [CC] [CC/MCC Exc]

Occlusion of cystic duct or gallbladder without cholelithiasis
Stenosis of cystic duct or gallbladder without cholelithiasis
Stricture of cystic duct or gallbladder without cholelithiasis

[EXCLUDES1] *obstruction of gallbladder with cholelithiasis (K80.-)*

K82.1 **Hydrops of gallbladder** [CC] [CC/MCC Exc]

Mucocele of gallbladder

K82.2 **Perforation of gallbladder** [MCC] [CC/MCC Exc]

Rupture of cystic duct or gallbladder

K82.3 **Fistula of gallbladder** [CC] [CC/MCC Exc]

Cholecystocolic fistula
Cholecystoduodenal fistula

K82.4 **Cholesterolosis of gallbladder**

Strawberry gallbladder

[EXCLUDES1] *cholesterolosis of gallbladder with cholecystitis (K81.-)*
cholesterolosis of gallbladder with cholelithiasis (K80.-)

K82.8 **Other specified diseases of gallbladder**

Adhesions of cystic duct or gallbladder
Atrophy of cystic duct or gallbladder
Cyst of cystic duct or gallbladder
Dyskinesia of cystic duct or gallbladder
Hypertrophy of cystic duct or gallbladder
Nonfunctioning of cystic duct or gallbladder
Ulcer of cystic duct or gallbladder

K82.9 **Disease of gallbladder, unspecified**

[4th] K83 **Other diseases of biliary tract**

[EXCLUDES1] *postcholecystectomy syndrome (K91.5)*

[EXCLUDES2] *conditions involving the gallbladder (K81-K82)*
conditions involving the cystic duct (K81-K82)

K83.0 **Cholangitis** [CC] [CC/MCC Exc]

Ascending cholangitis
Cholangitis NOS
Primary cholangitis
Recurrent cholangitis
Sclerosing cholangitis
Secondary cholangitis
Stenosing cholangitis
Suppurative cholangitis

[EXCLUDES1] *cholangitic liver abscess (K75.0)*
cholangitis with choledocholithiasis (K80.3-, K80.4-)
chronic nonsuppurative destructive cholangitis (K74.3)

K83.1 **Obstruction of bile duct** [MCC] [CC/MCC Exc]

AHA: Q1 2016

Occlusion of bile duct without cholelithiasis
Stenosis of bile duct without cholelithiasis
Stricture of bile duct without cholelithiasis

[EXCLUDES1] *congenital obstruction of bile duct (Q44.3)*
obstruction of bile duct with cholelithiasis (K80.-)

K83.2 **Perforation of bile duct** [MCC] [CC/MCC Exc]

Rupture of bile duct

Unspecified Code | Other Specified Code | Manifestation Code | [N] Newborn | [P] Pediatric | [M] Maternity | [A] Adult | ♂ Male | ♀ Female
● New Code | ▲ Revised Code Title | ►◄ Revised Text | [NOTES] | [INCLUDES] | [EXCLUDES1] Not coded here | [EXCLUDES2] Not included here
[4th] 4th character required | [5th] 5th character required | [6th] 6th character required | [7th] 7th character required
[x7] Extension 'X' Alert | [HAC] Hospital-acquired condition (HAC) alert | AHA AHA Coding Clinic©

When symbols appear on a code that requires a 7th character extension, refer to Appendix B to identify applicable 7th character codes.

Psoriasis

Psoriasis is a chronic skin problem that causes skin cells to grow too quickly, resulting in thick, white, silvery patches of skin. This occurs when the immune system mistakenly attacks and destroys healthy body tissue. Bacteria or viral infections, stress, dry air, injury to the skin and some medicines may trigger the condition. It is a noncontagious skin condition that produces red papules that merge together into plaques of thickened scaling skin. Psoriasis commonly affects the skin of the elbows, knees, and scalp. Psoriasis symptoms improve or can go into remission.

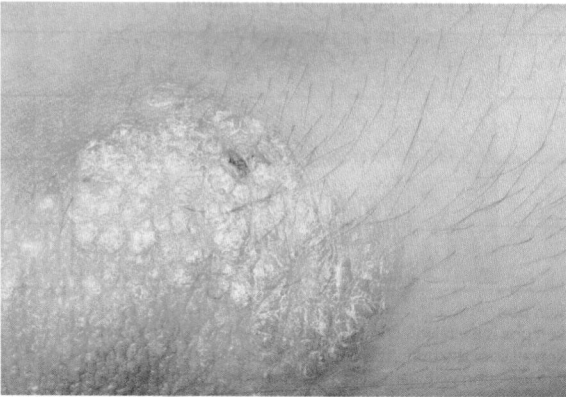

Ringworm

Ringworm is a type of fungal skin infection which is caused by fungi called tinea. It is a common highly contagious skin infection that causes a ring-like red rash on the skin. The rash can appear almost anywhere on the body, with the scalp, feet and groin being most common sites.

Diseases of the skin and subcutaneous tissue (L00-L99)

EXCLUDES2 *certain conditions originating in the perinatal period (P04-P96)*

certain infectious and parasitic diseases (A00-B99)

complications of pregnancy, childbirth and the puerperium (O00-O9A)

congenital malformations, deformations, and chromosomal abnormalities (Q00-Q99)

endocrine, nutritional and metabolic diseases (E00-E88)

lipomelanotic reticulosis (I89.8)

neoplasms (C00-D49)

symptoms, signs and abnormal clinical and laboratory findings, not elsewhere classified (R00-R94)

systemic connective tissue disorders (M30-M36)

viral warts (B07.-)

This chapter contains the following blocks:

L00-L08	Infections of the skin and subcutaneous tissue
L10-L14	Bullous disorders
L20-L30	Dermatitis and eczema
L40-L45	Papulosquamous disorders
L49-L54	Urticaria and erythema
L55-L59	Radiation-related disorders of the skin and subcutaneous tissue
L60-L75	Disorders of skin appendages
L76	Intraoperative and postprocedural complications of skin and subcutaneous tissue
L80-L99	Other disorders of the skin and subcutaneous tissue

Infections of the skin and subcutaneous tissue (L00-L08)

Use additional code (B95-B97) to identify infectious agent.

EXCLUDES2 *hordeolum (H00.0)*

infective dermatitis (L30.3)

local infections of skin classified in Chapter 1

lupus panniculitis (L93.2)

panniculitis NOS (M79.3)

panniculitis of neck and back (M54.0-)

Perlèche NOS (K13.0)

Perlèche due to candidiasis (B37.0)

Perlèche due to riboflavin deficiency (E53.0)

pyogenic granuloma (L98.0)

relapsing panniculitis [Weber-Christian] (M35.6)

viral warts (B07.-)

zoster (B02.-)

L00 **Staphylococcal scalded skin syndrome**
AHA: Q4 2016
Ritter's disease
Use additional code to identify percentage of skin exfoliation (L49.-)
EXCLUDES1 *bullous impetigo (L01.03)*
pemphigus neonatorum (L01.03)
toxic epidermal necrolysis [Lyell] (L51.2)

4️⃣ L01 **Impetigo**
EXCLUDES1 *impetigo herpetiformis (L40.1)*
5️⃣ L01.0 **Impetigo**
Impetigo contagiosa
Impetigo vulgaris
L01.00 **Impetigo, unspecified**
Impetigo NOS
L01.01 **Non-bullous impetigo**
L01.02 **Bockhart's impetigo**
Impetigo follicularis
Perifolliculitis NOS
Superficial pustular perifolliculitis
L01.03 **Bullous impetigo**
Impetigo neonatorum
Pemphigus neonatorum
L01.09 **Other impetigo**
Ulcerative impetigo

L01.1 **Impetiginization of other dermatoses**
4️⃣ L02 **Cutaneous abscess, furuncle and carbuncle**
Use additional code to identify organism (B95-B96)
EXCLUDES2 *abscess of anus and rectal regions (K61.-)*
abscess of female genital organs (external) (N76.4)
abscess of male genital organs (external) (N48.2, N49.-)
5️⃣ L02.0 **Cutaneous abscess, furuncle and carbuncle of** face
EXCLUDES2 *abscess of ear, external (H60.0)*
abscess of eyelid (H00.0)
abscess of head [any part, except face] (L02.8)
abscess of lacrimal gland (H04.0)
abscess of lacrimal passages (H04.3)
abscess of mouth (K12.2)
abscess of nose (J34.0)
abscess of orbit (H05.0)
submandibular abscess (K12.2)
L02.01 **Cutaneous abscess of** face   CC CC/MCC Exc
L02.02 **Furuncle of** face
Boil of face
Folliculitis of face
L02.03 **Carbuncle of** face
5️⃣ L02.1 **Cutaneous abscess, furuncle and carbuncle of** neck
L02.11 **Cutaneous abscess of** neck   CC CC/MCC Exc
L02.12 **Furuncle of** neck
Boil of neck
Folliculitis of neck
L02.13 **Carbuncle of** neck
5️⃣ L02.2 **Cutaneous abscess, furuncle and carbuncle of** trunk
EXCLUDES1 *non-newborn omphalitis (L08.82)*
omphalitis of newborn (P38.-)
EXCLUDES2 *abscess of breast (N61.1)*
abscess of buttocks (L02.3)
abscess of female external genital organs (N76.4)
abscess of male external genital organs (N48.2, N49.-)
abscess of hip (L02.4)
6️⃣ L02.21 **Cutaneous abscess of** trunk
L02.211 **Cutaneous abscess of** abdominal wall CC CC/MCC Exc
L02.212 **Cutaneous abscess of** back [any part, except buttock] CC CC/MCC Exc
L02.213 **Cutaneous abscess of** chest wall CC CC/MCC Exc
L02.214 **Cutaneous abscess of** groin CC CC/MCC Exc
L02.215 **Cutaneous abscess of** perineum CC CC/MCC Exc
L02.216 **Cutaneous abscess of** umbilicus CC CC/MCC Exc
L02.219 **Cutaneous abscess of trunk, unspecified** CC CC/MCC Exc
6️⃣ L02.22 **Furuncle of** trunk
Boil of trunk
Folliculitis of trunk
L02.221 **Furuncle of** abdominal wall
L02.222 **Furuncle of** back [any part, except buttock]
L02.223 **Furuncle of** chest wall
L02.224 **Furuncle of** groin
L02.225 **Furuncle of** perineum
L02.226 **Furuncle of** umbilicus
L02.229 **Furuncle of trunk, unspecified**
6️⃣ L02.23 **Carbuncle of** trunk
L02.231 **Carbuncle of** abdominal wall
L02.232 **Carbuncle of** back [any part, except buttock]
L02.233 **Carbuncle of** chest wall
L02.234 **Carbuncle of** groin
L02.235 **Carbuncle of** perineum
L02.236 **Carbuncle of** umbilicus
L02.239 **Carbuncle of trunk, unspecified**

Unspecified Code	Other Specified Code	Manifestation Code	Ⓝ Newborn	Ⓟ Pediatric	Ⓜ Maternity	Ⓐ Adult	♂ Male	♀ Female

● New Code   ▲ Revised Code Title   ►◄ Revised Text   **NOTES**   *INCLUDES*   *EXCLUDES 1* Not coded here   *EXCLUDES 2* Not included here

4️⃣ 4th character required   5️⃣ 5th character required   6️⃣ 6th character required   7️⃣ 7th character required

7️⃣ Extension 'X' Alert   HAC Hospital-acquired condition (HAC) alert   **AHA** AHA Coding Clinic©

L29.2 Pruritus vulvae ♀
L29.3 Anogenital pruritus, unspecified
L29.8 Other pruritus
L29.9 Pruritus, unspecified
Itch NOS

[4th] L30 Other and unspecified dermatitis
[EXCLUDES2] *contact dermatitis (L23-L25)*
dry skin dermatitis (L85.3)
small plaque parapsoriasis (L41.3)
stasis dermatitis (I87.2)
L30.0 Nummular dermatitis
L30.1 Dyshidrosis [pompholyx]
L30.2 Cutaneous autosensitization
Candidid [levurid]
Dermatophytid
Eczematid
L30.3 Infective dermatitis
Infectious eczematoid dermatitis
L30.4 Erythema intertrigo
L30.5 Pityriasis alba
L30.8 Other specified dermatitis
L30.9 Dermatitis, unspecified
Eczema NOS

Papulosquamous disorders (L40-L45)

[4th] L40 Psoriasis
L40.0 Psoriasis vulgaris [RxHCC]
Nummular psoriasis
Plaque psoriasis
L40.1 Generalized pustular psoriasis [RxHCC]
Impetigo herpetiformis
Von Zumbusch's disease
L40.2 Acrodermatitis continua [RxHCC]
L40.3 Pustulosis palmaris et plantaris [RxHCC]
L40.4 Guttate psoriasis [RxHCC]
[5th] L40.5 Arthropathic psoriasis
L40.50 Arthropathic psoriasis, unspecified [HCC] [RxHCC]
L40.51 Distal interphalangeal psoriatic arthropathy [HCC] [RxHCC]
L40.52 Psoriatic arthritis mutilans [HCC] [RxHCC]
L40.53 Psoriatic spondylitis [HCC] [RxHCC]
L40.54 Psoriatic juvenile arthropathy [HCC] [RxHCC]
L40.59 Other psoriatic arthropathy [HCC] [RxHCC]
L40.8 Other psoriasis [RxHCC]
Flexural psoriasis
L40.9 Psoriasis, unspecified [RxHCC]

[4th] L41 Parapsoriasis
[EXCLUDES1] *poikiloderma vasculare atrophicans (L94.5)*
L41.0 Pityriasis lichenoides et varioliformis acuta [RxHCC]
Mucha-Habermann disease
L41.1 Pityriasis lichenoides chronica [RxHCC]
L41.3 Small plaque parapsoriasis [RxHCC]
L41.4 Large plaque parapsoriasis [RxHCC]
L41.5 Retiform parapsoriasis [RxHCC]
L41.8 Other parapsoriasis [RxHCC]
L41.9 Parapsoriasis, unspecified [RxHCC]

L42 Pityriasis rosea

[4th] L43 Lichen planus
[EXCLUDES1] *lichen planopilaris (L66.1)*
L43.0 Hypertrophic lichen planus
L43.1 Bullous lichen planus
L43.2 Lichenoid drug reaction
Use additional code for adverse effect, if applicable, to identify drug (T36-T50 with fifth or sixth character 5)
L43.3 Subacute (active) lichen planus
Lichen planus tropicus
L43.8 Other lichen planus
L43.9 Lichen planus, unspecified

[4th] L44 Other papulosquamous disorders
L44.0 Pityriasis rubra pilaris
L44.1 Lichen nitidus
L44.2 Lichen striatus
L44.3 Lichen ruber moniliformis
L44.4 Infantile papular acrodermatitis [Gianotti-Crosti] [P]
L44.8 Other specified papulosquamous disorders
L44.9 Papulosquamous disorder, unspecified

L45 Papulosquamous disorders in diseases classified elsewhere
Code first underlying disease.

Urticaria and erythema (L49-L54)

[EXCLUDES1] *Lyme disease (A69.2-)*
rosacea (L71.-)

[4th] L49 Exfoliation due to erythematous conditions according to extent of body surface involved
Code first erythematous condition causing exfoliation, such as:
Ritter's disease (L00)
(Staphylococcal) scalded skin syndrom (L00)
Stevens-Johnson syndrome (L51.1)
Stevens-Johnson syndrome-toxic epidermal necrolysis overlap syndrome (L51.3)
Toxic epidermal necrolysis (L51.2)
L49.0 Exfoliation due to erythematous condition involving less than 10 percent of body surface [PDxIn]
Exfoliation due to erythematous condition NOS
L49.1 Exfoliation due to erythematous condition involving 10-19 percent of body surface [PDxIn]
L49.2 Exfoliation due to erythematous condition involving 20-29 percent of body surface [PDxIn]
L49.3 Exfoliation due to erythematous condition involving 30-39 percent of body surface [CC] [PDxIn] [CC/MCC Exc]
L49.4 Exfoliation due to erythematous condition involving 40-49 percent of body surface [CC] [PDxIn] [CC/MCC Exc]
L49.5 Exfoliation due to erythematous condition involving 50-59 percent of body surface [CC] [PDxIn] [CC/MCC Exc]
L49.6 Exfoliation due to erythematous condition involving 60-69 percent of body surface [CC] [PDxIn] [CC/MCC Exc]
L49.7 Exfoliation due to erythematous condition involving 70-79 percent of body surface [CC] [PDxIn] [CC/MCC Exc]
L49.8 Exfoliation due to erythematous condition involving 80-89 percent of body surface [CC] [PDxIn] [CC/MCC Exc]
L49.9 Exfoliation due to erythematous condition involving 90 or more percent of body surface [CC] [PDxIn] [CC/MCC Exc]

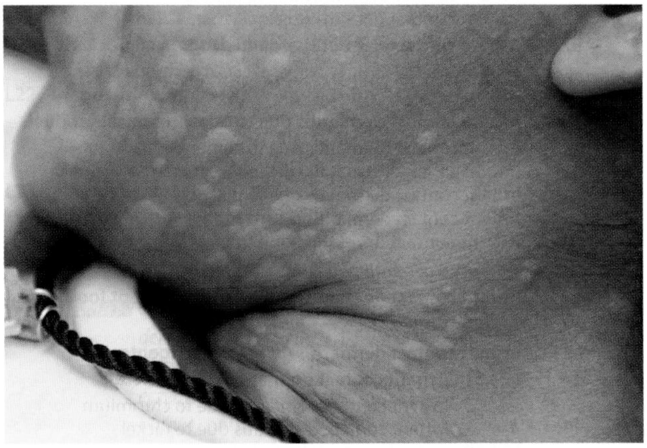

Figure 12.1 Urticaria

[4th] L50 Urticaria
[EXCLUDES1] *allergic contact dermatitis (L23.-)*
angioneurotic edema (T78.3)
giant urticaria (T78.3)
hereditary angio-edema (D84.1)

[PDxIn] Unacceptable principal diagnosis symbol per Medicare code edits [POA] Code exempt from diagnosis present on admission requirement
[?] Questionable admission [CC] Complication or comorbidity [CC/MCC Exc] CC/MCC exclusion [MCC] Major complication or comorbidity
[PDx CC] Principal diagnosis as its own CC [PDx MCC] Principal diagnosis as its own MCC [HCC] HCC diagnosis code [RxHCC] RxHCC diagnosis code
MACRA code [Z1] Z code as first-listed diagnosis

Quincke's edema (T78.3)

serum urticaria (T80.6-)

solar urticaria (L56.3)

urticaria neonatorum (P83.8)

urticaria papulosa (L28.2)

urticaria pigmentosa (Q82.2)

L50.0   Allergic **urticaria**

L50.1   Idiopathic **urticaria**

L50.2   **Urticaria** due to cold and heat

     EXCLUDES2 *familial cold urticaria (M04.2)*

L50.3   Dermatographic **urticaria**

L50.4   Vibratory **urticaria**

L50.5   Cholinergic **urticaria**

L50.6   Contact **urticaria**

L50.8   **Other urticaria**

     Chronic urticaria

     Recurrent periodic urticaria

L50.9   **Urticaria, unspecified**

🔵 **L51**   **Erythema multiforme**

Use additional code for adverse effect, if applicable, to identify drug (T36-T50 with fifth or sixth character 5)

Use additional code to identify associated manifestations, such as: arthropathy associated with dermatological disorders (M14.8-)

conjunctival edema (H11.42)

conjunctivitis (H10.22-)

corneal scars and opacities (H17.-)

corneal ulcer (H16.0-)

edema of eyelid (H02.84)

inflammation of eyelid (H01.8)

keratoconjunctivitis sicca (H16.22-)

mechanical lagophthalmos (H02.22-)

stomatitis (K12.-)

symblepharon (H11.23-)

Use additional code to identify percentage of skin exfoliation (L49.-)

     EXCLUDES1 *staphylococcal scalded skin syndrome (L00)*

       Ritter's disease (L00)

L51.0   **Nonbullous erythema multiforme**

L51.1   **Stevens-Johnson syndrome**   CC HCC CC/MCC Exc

L51.2   **Toxic epidermal necrolysis [Lyell]**   CC HCC CC/MCC Exc

L51.3   **Stevens-Johnson syndrome-toxic epidermal necrolysis overlap syndrome**   CC HCC CC/MCC Exc

     SJS-TEN overlap syndrome

L51.8   **Other erythema multiforme**

L51.9   **Erythema multiforme, unspecified**

     Erythema iris

     Erythema multiforme major NOS

     Erythema multiforme minor NOS

     Herpes iris

L52   **Erythema nodosum**

     EXCLUDES1 *tuberculous erythema nodosum (A18.4)*

🔵 **L53**   Other erythematous **conditions**

     EXCLUDES1 *erythema ab igne (L59.0)*

       erythema due to external agents in contact with skin (L23-L25)

       erythema intertrigo (L30.4)

L53.0   Toxic **erythema**   CC CC/MCC Exc

     Code first poisoning due to drug or toxin, if applicable (T36-T65 with fifth or sixth character 1-4 or 6)

     Use additional code for adverse effect, if applicable, to identify drug (T36-T50 with fifth or sixth character 5)

     EXCLUDES1 *neonatal erythema toxicum (P83.1)*

L53.1   **Erythema** annulare centrifugum   CC CC/MCC Exc

L53.2   **Erythema** marginatum   CC CC/MCC Exc

L53.3   **Other chronic figurate erythema**   CC CC/MCC Exc

L53.8   Other specified erythematous conditions

L53.9   **Erythematous condition, unspecified**

     Erythema NOS

     Erythroderma NOS

L54   **Erythema in diseases classified elsewhere**

     Code first underlying disease.

Radiation-related disorders of the skin and subcutaneous tissue (L55-L59)

🔵 **L55**   **Sunburn**

L55.0   **Sunburn of** first **degree**

L55.1   **Sunburn of** second **degree**

L55.2   **Sunburn of** third **degree**

L55.9   **Sunburn, unspecified**

🔵 **L56**   **Other acute skin changes due to ultraviolet radiation**

Use additional code to identify the source of the ultraviolet radiation (W89, X32)

L56.0   **Drug phototoxic response**

     Use additional code for adverse effect, if applicable, to identify drug (T36-T50 with fifth or sixth character 5)

L56.1   **Drug photoallergic response**

     Use additional code for adverse effect, if applicable, to identify drug (T36-T50 with fifth or sixth character 5)

L56.2   **Photocontact dermatitis [berloque dermatitis]**

L56.3   **Solar urticaria**

L56.4   **Polymorphous light eruption**

L56.5   **Disseminated superficial actinic porokeratosis (DSAP)**

L56.8   Other specified acute skin changes due to ultraviolet radiation

L56.9   **Acute skin change due to ultraviolet radiation, unspecified**

🔵 **L57**   **Skin changes due to chronic exposure to nonionizing radiation**

Use additional code to identify the source of the ultraviolet radiation (W89)

L57.0   **Actinic keratosis**

     Keratosis NOS

     Senile keratosis

     Solar keratosis

L57.1   **Actinic reticuloid**

L57.2   **Cutis rhomboidalis nuchae**

L57.3   **Poikiloderma of Civatte**

L57.4   **Cutis laxa senilis**

     Elastosis senilis

L57.5   **Actinic granuloma**

L57.8   **Other skin changes due to chronic exposure to nonionizing radiation**

     Farmer's skin

     Sailor's skin

     Solar dermatitis

L57.9   Skin changes due to chronic exposure to nonionizing radiation, unspecified

🔵 **L58**   **Radiodermatitis**

Use additional code to identify the source of the radiation (W88, W90)

L58.0   Acute **radiodermatitis**

L58.1   Chronic **radiodermatitis**

L58.9   **Radiodermatitis, unspecified**

🔵 **L59**   **Other disorders of skin and subcutaneous tissue related to radiation**

L59.0   **Erythema ab igne [dermatitis ab igne]**

L59.8   Other specified disorders of the skin and subcutaneous tissue related to radiation

     AHA: Q1 2017

L59.9   **Disorder of the skin and subcutaneous tissue related to radiation, unspecified**

Disorders of skin appendages (L60-L75)

     EXCLUDES1 *congenital malformations of integument (Q84.-)*

🔵 **L60**   **Nail disorders**

     EXCLUDES2 *clubbing of nails (R68.3)*

       onychia and paronychia (L03.0-)

L60.0   **Ingrowing nail**

L60.1   **Onycholysis**

L60.2   **Onychogryphosis**

L60.3   **Nail dystrophy**

L60.4   **Beau's lines**

L60.5   **Yellow nail syndrome**

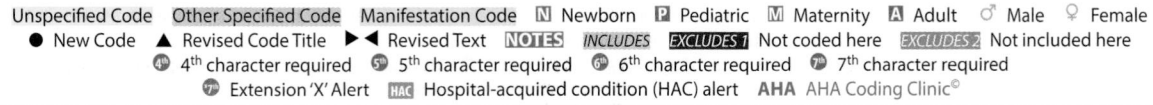

Unspecified Code   Other Specified Code   Manifestation Code   Ⓝ Newborn   Ⓟ Pediatric   Ⓜ Maternity   Ⓐ Adult   ♂ Male   ♀ Female

● New Code   ▲ Revised Code Title   ►◄ Revised Text   **NOTES**   *INCLUDES*   **EXCLUDES 1** Not coded here   **EXCLUDES 2** Not included here

🔵 4th character required   🔵 5th character required   🔵 6th character required   🔵 7th character required

🔵 Extension 'X' Alert   **HAC** Hospital-acquired condition (HAC) alert   **AHA** AHA Coding Clinic©

L60.8 Other nail disorders
L60.9 Nail disorder, unspecified

L62 Nail disorders in diseases classified elsewhere
Code first underlying disease, such as:
pachydermoperiostosis (M89.4-)

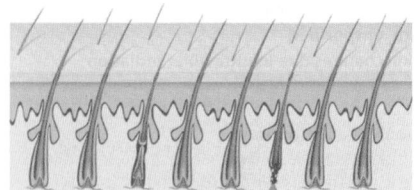

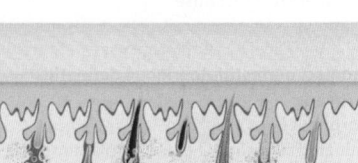

Healthy

Unhealthy hair
roots and follicles

Figure 12.2 Alopecia areata

L63 Alopecia areata
L63.0 Alopecia (capitis) totalis
L63.1 Alopecia universalis
L63.2 Ophiasis
L63.8 Other alopecia areata
L63.9 Alopecia areata, unspecified

L64 Androgenic alopecia
INCLUDES male-pattern baldness
L64.0 Drug-induced androgenic alopecia
Use additional code for adverse effect, if applicable, to
identify drug (T36-T50 with fifth or sixth character 5)
L64.8 Other androgenic alopecia
L64.9 Androgenic alopecia, unspecified

L65 Other nonscarring hair loss
Use additional code for adverse effect, if applicable, to identify drug
(T36-T50 with fifth or sixth character 5)
EXCLUDES1 trichotillomania (F63.3)
L65.0 Telogen effluvium
L65.1 Anagen effluvium
L65.2 Alopecia mucinosa
L65.8 Other specified nonscarring hair loss
L65.9 Nonscarring hair loss, unspecified
Alopecia NOS

L66 Cicatricial alopecia [scarring hair loss]
L66.0 Pseudopelade
L66.1 Lichen planopilaris
Follicular lichen planus
L66.2 Folliculitis decalvans
L66.3 Perifolliculitis capitis abscedens
L66.4 Folliculitis ulerythematosa reticulata
L66.8 Other cicatricial alopecia
AHA: Q1 2015
L66.9 Cicatricial alopecia, unspecified

L67 Hair color and hair shaft abnormalities
EXCLUDES1 monilethrix (Q84.1)
pili annulati (Q84.1)
telogen effluvium (L65.0)
L67.0 Trichorrhexis nodosa
L67.1 Variations in hair color
Canities
Greyness, hair (premature)
Heterochromia of hair
Poliosis circumscripta, acquired
Poliosis NOS
L67.8 Other hair color and hair shaft abnormalities
Fragilitas crinium

L67.9 Hair color and hair shaft abnormality, unspecified

L68 Hypertrichosis
INCLUDES excess hair
EXCLUDES1 congenital hypertrichosis (Q84.2)
persistent lanugo (Q84.2)
L68.0 Hirsutism
L68.1 Acquired hypertrichosis lanuginosa
L68.2 Localized hypertrichosis
L68.3 Polytrichia
L68.8 Other hypertrichosis
L68.9 Hypertrichosis, unspecified

L70 Acne
EXCLUDES2 acne keloid (L73.0)
L70.0 Acne vulgaris
L70.1 Acne conglobata
L70.2 Acne varioliformis
Acne necrotica miliaris
L70.3 Acne tropica
L70.4 Infantile acne ℗
L70.5 Acné excoriée
Acné excoriée des jeunes filles
Picker's acne
L70.8 Other acne
L70.9 Acne, unspecified

L71 Rosacea
Use additional code for adverse effect, if applicable, to identify drug
(T36-T50 with fifth or sixth character 5)
L71.0 Perioral dermatitis
L71.1 Rhinophyma
L71.8 Other rosacea
L71.9 Rosacea, unspecified

L72 Follicular cysts of skin and subcutaneous tissue
L72.0 Epidermal cyst
L72.1 Pilar and trichodermal cyst
L72.11 Pilar cyst
L72.12 Trichodermal cyst
Trichilemmal (proliferating) cyst
L72.2 Steatocystoma multiplex
L72.3 Sebaceous cyst
EXCLUDES2 pilar cyst (L72.11)
trichilemmal (proliferating) cyst (L72.12)
L72.8 Other follicular cysts of the skin and subcutaneous tissue
L72.9 Follicular cyst of the skin and subcutaneous tissue,
unspecified

L73 Other follicular disorders
L73.0 Acne keloid
L73.1 Pseudofolliculitis barbae
L73.2 Hidradenitis suppurativa
L73.8 Other specified follicular disorders
Sycosis barbae
L73.9 Follicular disorder, unspecified

L74 Eccrine sweat disorders
EXCLUDES2 generalized hyperhidrosis (R61)
L74.0 Miliaria rubra
L74.1 Miliaria crystallina
L74.2 Miliaria profunda
Miliaria tropicalis
L74.3 Miliaria, unspecified
L74.4 Anhidrosis
Hypohidrosis
L74.5 Focal hyperhidrosis
L74.51 Primary focal hyperhidrosis
L74.510 Primary focal hyperhidrosis, axilla
L74.511 Primary focal hyperhidrosis, face
L74.512 Primary focal hyperhidrosis, palms
L74.513 Primary focal hyperhidrosis, soles
L74.519 Primary focal hyperhidrosis, unspecified
L74.52 Secondary focal hyperhidrosis
Frey's syndrome

Unacceptable principal diagnosis symbol per Medicare code edits   Code exempt from diagnosis present on admission requirement
Questionable admission   Complication or comorbidity   CC/MCC exclusion   Major complication or comorbidity
Principal diagnosis as its own CC   Principal diagnosis as its own MCC   HCC diagnosis code   RxHCC diagnosis code
MACRA code   Z code as first-listed diagnosis

L74.8 Other eccrine sweat disorders

L74.9 Eccrine sweat disorder, unspecified
Sweat gland disorder NOS

⁴ᵗʰ L75 Apocrine sweat disorders

EXCLUDES1 dyshidrosis (L30.1)

hidradenitis suppurativa (L73.2)

L75.0 Bromhidrosis

L75.1 Chromhidrosis

L75.2 Apocrine miliaria
Fox-Fordyce disease

L75.8 Other apocrine sweat disorders

L75.9 Apocrine sweat disorder, unspecified

Intraoperative and postprocedural complications of skin and subcutaneous tissue (L76)

⁴ᵗʰ L76 Intraoperative and postprocedural complications of skin and subcutaneous tissue

⁵ᵗʰ L76.0 Intraoperative hemorrhage and hematoma of skin and subcutaneous tissue complicating a procedure

EXCLUDES1 intraoperative hemorrhage and hematoma of skin and subcutaneous tissue due to accidental puncture and laceration during a procedure (L76.1-)

L76.01 Intraoperative hemorrhage and hematoma of skin and subcutaneous tissue complicating a dermatologic procedure   CC² CC/MCC Exc○

L76.02 Intraoperative hemorrhage and hematoma of skin and subcutaneous tissue complicating other procedure   CC² CC/MCC Exc○

⁵ᵗʰ L76.1 Accidental puncture and laceration of skin and subcutaneous tissue during a procedure

L76.11 Accidental puncture and laceration of skin and subcutaneous tissue during a dermatologic procedure   CC² CC/MCC Exc○

L76.12 Accidental puncture and laceration of skin and subcutaneous tissue during other procedure   CC² CC/MCC Exc○

⁵ᵗʰ L76.2 Postprocedural hemorrhage of skin and subcutaneous tissue following a procedure

L76.21 Postprocedural hemorrhage of skin and subcutaneous tissue following a dermatologic procedure   CC² CC/MCC Exc○

L76.22 Postprocedural hemorrhage of skin and subcutaneous tissue following other procedure   CC² CC/MCC Exc○

⁵ᵗʰ L76.3 Postprocedural hematoma and seroma of skin and subcutaneous tissue following a procedure

L76.31 Postprocedural hematoma of skin and subcutaneous tissue following a dermatologic procedure   CC² CC/MCC Exc○

L76.32 Postprocedural hematoma of skin and subcutaneous tissue following other procedure   CC² CC/MCC Exc○

L76.33 Postprocedural seroma of skin and subcutaneous tissue following a dermatologic procedure   CC² CC/MCC Exc○

L76.34 Postprocedural seroma of skin and subcutaneous tissue following other procedure   CC² CC/MCC Exc○

⁵ᵗʰ L76.8 Other intraoperative and postprocedural complications of skin and subcutaneous tissue
Use additional code, if applicable, to further specify disorder

L76.81 Other intraoperative complications of skin and subcutaneous tissue

L76.82 Other postprocedural complications of skin and subcutaneous tissue

Other disorders of the skin and subcutaneous tissue (L80-L99)

L80 Vitiligo

EXCLUDES2 vitiligo of eyelids (H02.73-)

vitiligo of vulva (N90.89)

⁴ᵗʰ L81 Other disorders of pigmentation

EXCLUDES1 birthmark NOS (Q82.5)

Peutz-Jeghers syndrome (Q85.8)

EXCLUDES2 nevus - see Alphabetical Index

L81.0 Postinflammatory hyperpigmentation

L81.1 Chloasma

L81.2 Freckles

L81.3 Café au lait spots

L81.4 Other melanin hyperpigmentation
Lentigo

L81.5 Leukoderma, not elsewhere classified

L81.6 Other disorders of diminished melanin formation

L81.7 Pigmented purpuric dermatosis
Angioma serpiginosum

L81.8 Other specified disorders of pigmentation
Iron pigmentation
Tattoo pigmentation

L81.9 Disorder of pigmentation, unspecified

⁴ᵗʰ L82 Seborrheic keratosis

INCLUDES basal cell papilloma

dermatosis papulosa nigra

Leser-Trélat disease

EXCLUDES2 seborrheic dermatitis (L21.-)

L82.0 Inflamed seborrheic keratosis

L82.1 Other seborrheic keratosis
Seborrheic keratosis NOS

L83 Acanthosis nigricans
Confluent and reticulated papillomatosis

L84 Corns and callosities
Callus
Clavus

⁴ᵗʰ L85 Other epidermal thickening

EXCLUDES2 hypertrophic disorders of the skin (L91.-)

L85.0 Acquired ichthyosis

EXCLUDES1 congenital ichthyosis (Q80.-)

L85.1 Acquired keratosis [keratoderma] palmaris et plantaris

EXCLUDES1 inherited keratosis palmaris et plantaris (Q82.8)

L85.2 Keratosis punctata (palmaris et plantaris)

L85.3 Xerosis cutis
Dry skin dermatitis

L85.8 Other specified epidermal thickening
Cutaneous horn

L85.9 Epidermal thickening, unspecified

L86 Keratoderma in diseases classified elsewhere
Code first underlying disease, such as:
Reiter's disease (M02.3-)

EXCLUDES1 gonococcal keratoderma (A54.89)

gonococcal keratosis (A54.89)

keratoderma due to vitamin A deficiency (E50.8)

keratosis due to vitamin A deficiency (E50.8)

xeroderma due to vitamin A deficiency (E50.8)

⁴ᵗʰ L87 Transepidermal elimination disorders

EXCLUDES1 granuloma annulare (perforating) (L92.0)

L87.0 Keratosis follicularis et parafollicularis in cutem penetrans
Kyrle disease
Hyperkeratosis follicularis penetrans

L87.1 Reactive perforating collagenosis

L87.2 Elastosis perforans serpiginosa

L87.8 Other transepidermal elimination disorders

L87.9 Transepidermal elimination disorder, unspecified

L88 Pyoderma gangrenosum   CC² CC/MCC Exc○
Phagedenic pyoderma

EXCLUDES1 dermatitis gangrenosa (L08.0)

⁴ᵗʰ L89 Pressure ulcer

INCLUDES bed sore

decubitus ulcer

plaster ulcer

Unspecified Code   Other Specified Code   Manifestation Code   Ⓝ Newborn   Ⓟ Pediatric   Ⓜ Maternity   Ⓐ Adult   ♂ Male   ♀ Female
● New Code   ▲ Revised Code Title   ►◄ Revised Text   **NOTES**   *INCLUDES*   *EXCLUDES1* Not coded here   *EXCLUDES2* Not included here
⁴ᵗʰ 4ᵗʰ character required   ⁵ᵗʰ 5ᵗʰ character required   ⁶ᵗʰ 6ᵗʰ character required   ⁷ᵗʰ 7ᵗʰ character required
⁷ˣ Extension 'X' Alert   **HAC** Hospital-acquired condition (HAC) alert   **AHA** AHA Coding Clinic©

Pressure ulcer with abrasion, blister, partial thickness skin loss involving epidermis and/or dermis, sacral region

L89.153 **Pressure ulcer of sacral region, stage 3** HAC HCC MCC PDx CC/MCC Exc

Healing pressure ulcer of sacral region, stage 3

Pressure ulcer with full thickness skin loss involving damage or necrosis of subcutaneous tissue, sacral region

L89.154 **Pressure ulcer of sacral region, stage 4** HAC HCC MCC PDx CC/MCC Exc

Healing pressure ulcer of sacral region, stage 4

Pressure ulcer with necrosis of soft tissues through to underlying muscle, tendon, or bone, sacral region

L89.159 **Pressure ulcer of sacral region, unspecified stage**

Healing pressure ulcer of sacral region NOS

Healing pressure ulcer of sacral region, unspecified stage

5th **L89.2 Pressure ulcer of hip**

6th **L89.20 Pressure ulcer of unspecified hip**

L89.200 **Pressure ulcer of unspecified hip, unstageable** HCC

L89.201 **Pressure ulcer of unspecified hip, stage 1**

Healing pressure ulcer of unspecified hip back, stage 1

Pressure pre-ulcer skin changes limited to persistent focal edema, unspecified hip

L89.202 **Pressure ulcer of unspecified hip, stage 2**

Healing pressure ulcer of unspecified hip, stage 2

Pressure ulcer with abrasion, blister, partial thickness skin loss involving epidermis and/or dermis, unspecified hip

L89.203 **Pressure ulcer of unspecified hip, stage 3** HAC HCC MCC PDx CC/MCC Exc

Healing pressure ulcer of unspecified hip, stage 3

Pressure ulcer with full thickness skin loss involving damage or necrosis of subcutaneous tissue, unspecified hip

L89.204 **Pressure ulcer of unspecified hip, stage 4** HAC HCC MCC PDx CC/MCC Exc

Healing pressure ulcer of unspecified hip, stage 4

Pressure ulcer with necrosis of soft tissues through to underlying muscle, tendon, or bone, unspecified hip

L89.209 **Pressure ulcer of unspecified hip, unspecified stage**

Healing pressure ulcer of unspecified hip NOS

Healing pressure ulcer of unspecified hip, unspecified stage

6th **L89.21 Pressure ulcer of right hip**

L89.210 **Pressure ulcer of right hip, unstageable** HCC

L89.211 **Pressure ulcer of right hip, stage 1**

Healing pressure ulcer of right hip back, stage 1

Pressure pre-ulcer skin changes limited to persistent focal edema, right hip

L89.212 **Pressure ulcer of right hip, stage 2**

Healing pressure ulcer of right hip, stage 2

Pressure ulcer with abrasion, blister, partial thickness skin loss involving epidermis and/or dermis, right hip

L89.213 **Pressure ulcer of right hip, stage 3** HAC HCC MCC PDx CC/MCC Exc

Healing pressure ulcer of right hip, stage 3

Pressure ulcer with full thickness skin loss involving damage or necrosis of subcutaneous tissue, right hip

L89.214 **Pressure ulcer of right hip, stage 4** HAC HCC MCC PDx CC/MCC Exc

Healing pressure ulcer of right hip, stage 4

Pressure ulcer with necrosis of soft tissues through to underlying muscle, tendon, or bone, right hip

L89.219 **Pressure ulcer of right hip, unspecified stage**

Healing pressure ulcer of right hip NOS

Healing pressure ulcer of right hip, unspecified stage

6th **L89.22 Pressure ulcer of left hip**

L89.220 **Pressure ulcer of left hip, unstageable** HCC

L89.221 **Pressure ulcer of left hip, stage 1**

Healing pressure ulcer of left hip back, stage 1

Pressure pre-ulcer skin changes limited to persistent focal edema, left hip

L89.222 **Pressure ulcer of left hip, stage 2**

Healing pressure ulcer of left hip, stage 2

Pressure ulcer with abrasion, blister, partial thickness skin loss involving epidermis and/or dermis, left hip

L89.223 **Pressure ulcer of left hip, stage 3** HAC HCC MCC PDx CC/MCC Exc

Healing pressure ulcer of left hip, stage 3

Pressure ulcer with full thickness skin loss involving damage or necrosis of subcutaneous tissue, left hip

L89.224 **Pressure ulcer of left hip, stage 4** HAC HCC MCC PDx CC/MCC Exc

Healing pressure ulcer of left hip, stage 4

Pressure ulcer with necrosis of soft tissues through to underlying muscle, tendon, or bone, left hip

L89.229 **Pressure ulcer of left hip, unspecified stage**

Healing pressure ulcer of left hip NOS

Healing pressure ulcer of left hip, unspecified stage

5th **L89.3 Pressure ulcer of buttock**

6th **L89.30 Pressure ulcer of unspecified buttock**

L89.300 **Pressure ulcer of unspecified buttock, unstageable** HCC

L89.301 **Pressure ulcer of unspecified buttock, stage 1**

Healing pressure ulcer of unspecified buttock, stage 1

Pressure pre-ulcer skin changes limited to persistent focal edema, unspecified buttock

L89.302 **Pressure ulcer of unspecified buttock, stage 2**

Healing pressure ulcer of unspecified buttock, stage 2

Pressure ulcer with abrasion, blister, partial thickness skin loss involving epidermis and/or dermis, unspecified buttock

L89.303 **Pressure ulcer of unspecified buttock, stage 3** HAC HCC MCC PDx CC/MCC Exc

Healing pressure ulcer of unspecified buttock, stage 3

Pressure ulcer with full thickness skin loss involving damage or necrosis of subcutaneous tissue, unspecified buttock

L89.304 **Pressure ulcer of unspecified buttock, stage 4** HAC HCC MCC PDx CC/MCC Exc

Healing pressure ulcer of unspecified buttock, stage 4

Pressure ulcer with necrosis of soft tissues through to underlying muscle, tendon, or bone, unspecified buttock

---

PDx Unacceptable principal diagnosis symbol per Medicare code edits   POA Code exempt from diagnosis present on admission requirement
? Questionable admission   CC Complication or comorbidity   CC/MCC Exc CC/MCC exclusion   MCC Major complication or comorbidity
PDx Principal diagnosis as its own CC   MCC Principal diagnosis as its own MCC   HCC HCC diagnosis code   RxHCC RxHCC diagnosis code
MACRA code   Z1 Z code as first-listed diagnosis

L89.309 Pressure ulcer of unspecified buttock, unspecified stage
Healing pressure ulcer of unspecified buttock NOS
Healing pressure ulcer of unspecified buttock, unspecified stage

L89.31 **Pressure ulcer of right buttock**

L89.310 Pressure ulcer of right buttock, unstageable `HCC`

L89.311 Pressure ulcer of right buttock, stage 1
Healing pressure ulcer of right buttock, stage 1
Pressure pre-ulcer skin changes limited to persistent focal edema, right buttock

L89.312 Pressure ulcer of right buttock, stage 2
Healing pressure ulcer of right buttock, stage 2
Pressure ulcer with abrasion, blister, partial thickness skin loss involving epidermis and/or dermis, right buttock

L89.313 Pressure ulcer of right buttock, stage 3 `HAC` `HCC` `MCC` `PDx MCCb` `CC/MCC Exc`
Healing pressure ulcer of right buttock, stage 3
Pressure ulcer with full thickness skin loss involving damage or necrosis of subcutaneous tissue, right buttock

L89.314 Pressure ulcer of right buttock, stage 4 `HAC` `HCC` `MCC` `PDx MCCb` `CC/MCC Exc`
Healing pressure ulcer of right buttock, stage 4
Pressure ulcer with necrosis of soft tissues through to underlying muscle, tendon, or bone, right buttock

L89.319 Pressure ulcer of right buttock, unspecified stage
Healing pressure ulcer of right buttock NOS
Healing pressure ulcer of right buttock, unspecified stage

L89.32 **Pressure ulcer of left buttock**

L89.320 Pressure ulcer of left buttock, unstageable `HCC`

L89.321 Pressure ulcer of left buttock, stage 1
Healing pressure ulcer of left buttock, stage 1
Pressure pre-ulcer skin changes limited to persistent focal edema, left buttock

L89.322 Pressure ulcer of left buttock, stage 2
Healing pressure ulcer of left buttock, stage 2
Pressure ulcer with abrasion, blister, partial thickness skin loss involving epidermis and/or dermis, left buttock

L89.323 Pressure ulcer of left buttock, stage 3 `HAC` `HCC` `MCC` `PDx MCCb` `CC/MCC Exc`
Healing pressure ulcer of left buttock, stage 3
Pressure ulcer with full thickness skin loss involving damage or necrosis of subcutaneous tissue, left buttock

L89.324 Pressure ulcer of left buttock, stage 4 `HAC` `HCC` `MCC` `PDx MCCb` `CC/MCC Exc`
Healing pressure ulcer of left buttock, stage 4
Pressure ulcer with necrosis of soft tissues through to underlying muscle, tendon, or bone, left buttock

L89.329 Pressure ulcer of left buttock, unspecified stage
Healing pressure ulcer of left buttock NOS
Healing pressure ulcer of left buttock, unspecified stage

L89.4 **Pressure ulcer of contiguous site of back, buttock and hip**

L89.40 Pressure ulcer of contiguous site of back, buttock and hip, unspecified stage
Healing pressure ulcer of contiguous site of back, buttock and hip NOS
Healing pressure ulcer of contiguous site of back, buttock and hip, unspecified stage

L89.41 Pressure ulcer of contiguous site of back, buttock and hip, stage 1
Healing pressure ulcer of contiguous site of back, buttock and hip, stage 1
Pressure pre-ulcer skin changes limited to persistent focal edema, contiguous site of back, buttock and hip

L89.42 Pressure ulcer of contiguous site of back, buttock and hip, stage 2
Healing pressure ulcer of contiguous site of back, buttock and hip, stage 2
Pressure ulcer with abrasion, blister, partial thickness skin loss involving epidermis and/or dermis, contiguous site of back, buttock and hip

L89.43 Pressure ulcer of contiguous site of back, buttock and hip, stage 3 `HAC` `HCC` `MCC` `PDx MCCb` `CC/MCC Exc`
Healing pressure ulcer of contiguous site of back, buttock and hip, stage 3
Pressure ulcer with full thickness skin loss involving damage or necrosis of subcutaneous tissue, contiguous site of back, buttock and hip

L89.44 Pressure ulcer of contiguous site of back, buttock and hip, stage 4 `HAC` `HCC` `MCC` `PDx MCCb` `CC/MCC Exc`
Healing pressure ulcer of contiguous site of back, buttock and hip, stage 4
Pressure ulcer with necrosis of soft tissues through to underlying muscle, tendon, or bone, contiguous site of back, buttock and hip

L89.45 Pressure ulcer of contiguous site of back, buttock and hip, unstageable `HCC`

L89.5 **Pressure ulcer of ankle**

L89.50 **Pressure ulcer of unspecified ankle**

L89.500 Pressure ulcer of unspecified ankle, unstageable `HCC`

L89.501 Pressure ulcer of unspecified ankle, stage 1
Healing pressure ulcer of unspecified ankle, stage 1
Pressure pre-ulcer skin changes limited to persistent focal edema, unspecified ankle

L89.502 Pressure ulcer of unspecified ankle, stage 2
Healing pressure ulcer of unspecified ankle, stage 2
Pressure ulcer with abrasion, blister, partial thickness skin loss involving epidermis and/or dermis, unspecified ankle

L89.503 Pressure ulcer of unspecified ankle, stage 3 `HAC` `HCC` `MCC` `PDx MCCb` `CC/MCC Exc`
Healing pressure ulcer of unspecified ankle, stage 3
Pressure ulcer with full thickness skin loss involving damage or necrosis of subcutaneous tissue, unspecified ankle

L89.504 Pressure ulcer of unspecified ankle, stage 4 `HAC` `HCC` `MCC` `PDx MCCb` `CC/MCC Exc`
Healing pressure ulcer of unspecified ankle, stage 4
Pressure ulcer with necrosis of soft tissues through to underlying muscle, tendon, or bone, unspecified ankle

L89.509 Pressure ulcer of unspecified ankle, unspecified stage
Healing pressure ulcer of unspecified ankle NOS
Healing pressure ulcer of unspecified ankle, unspecified stage

L89.51 **Pressure ulcer of right ankle**

L89.510 Pressure ulcer of right ankle, unstageable `HCC`

L89.511 Pressure ulcer of right ankle, stage 1
Healing pressure ulcer of right ankle, stage 1
Pressure pre-ulcer skin changes limited to persistent focal edema, right ankle

---

Unspecified Code   Other Specified Code   Manifestation Code   Ⓝ Newborn   Ⓟ Pediatric   Ⓜ Maternity   Ⓐ Adult   ♂ Male   ♀ Female
● New Code   ▲ Revised Code Title   ▶◀ Revised Text   **NOTES**   *INCLUDES*   *EXCLUDES 1* Not coded here   *EXCLUDES 2* Not included here
4th character required   5th character required   6th character required   7th character required
7th Extension 'X' Alert   `HAC` Hospital-acquired condition (HAC) alert   **AHA** AHA Coding Clinic©

L89.512 Pressure ulcer of right ankle, stage 2
Healing pressure ulcer of right ankle, stage 2
Pressure ulcer with abrasion, blister, partial thickness skin loss involving epidermis and/or dermis, right ankle

L89.513 Pressure ulcer of right ankle, stage 3 [HAC] [HCC] [MCC] [PDx MCC] [CC/MCC Exc]
Healing pressure ulcer of right ankle, stage 3
Pressure ulcer with full thickness skin loss involving damage or necrosis of subcutaneous tissue, right ankle

L89.514 Pressure ulcer of right ankle, stage 4 [HAC] [HCC] [MCC] [PDx MCC] [CC/MCC Exc]
Healing pressure ulcer of right ankle, stage 4
Pressure ulcer with necrosis of soft tissues through to underlying muscle, tendon, or bone, right ankle

L89.519 Pressure ulcer of right ankle, unspecified stage
Healing pressure ulcer of right ankle NOS
Healing pressure ulcer of right ankle, unspecified stage

[6th] **L89.52 Pressure ulcer of left ankle**

L89.520 Pressure ulcer of left ankle, unstageable [HCC]

L89.521 Pressure ulcer of left ankle, stage 1
Healing pressure ulcer of left ankle, stage 1
Pressure pre-ulcer skin changes limited to persistent focal edema, left ankle

L89.522 Pressure ulcer of left ankle, stage 2
Healing pressure ulcer of left ankle, stage 2
Pressure ulcer with abrasion, blister, partial thickness skin loss involving epidermis and/or dermis, left ankle

L89.523 Pressure ulcer of left ankle, stage 3 [HAC] [HCC] [MCC] [PDx MCC] [CC/MCC Exc]
Healing pressure ulcer of left ankle, stage 3
Pressure ulcer with full thickness skin loss involving damage or necrosis of subcutaneous tissue, left ankle

L89.524 Pressure ulcer of left ankle, stage 4 [HAC] [HCC] [MCC] [PDx MCC] [CC/MCC Exc]
Healing pressure ulcer of left ankle, stage 4
Pressure ulcer with necrosis of soft tissues through to underlying muscle, tendon, or bone, left ankle

L89.529 Pressure ulcer of left ankle, unspecified stage
Healing pressure ulcer of left ankle NOS
Healing pressure ulcer of left ankle, unspecified stage

[5th] **L89.6 Pressure ulcer of heel**

[6th] **L89.60 Pressure ulcer of unspecified heel**

L89.600 Pressure ulcer of unspecified heel, unstageable [HCC]

L89.601 Pressure ulcer of unspecified heel, stage 1
Healing pressure ulcer of unspecified heel, stage 1
Pressure pre-ulcer skin changes limited to persistent focal edema, unspecified heel

L89.602 Pressure ulcer of unspecified heel, stage 2
Healing pressure ulcer of unspecified heel, stage 2
Pressure ulcer with abrasion, blister, partial thickness skin loss involving epidermis and/or dermis, unspecified heel

L89.603 Pressure ulcer of unspecified heel, stage 3 [HAC] [HCC] [MCC] [PDx MCC] [CC/MCC Exc]
Healing pressure ulcer of unspecified heel, stage 3
Pressure ulcer with full thickness skin loss involving damage or necrosis of subcutaneous tissue, unspecified heel

L89.604 Pressure ulcer of unspecified heel, stage 4 [HAC] [HCC] [MCC] [PDx MCC] [CC/MCC Exc]
Healing pressure ulcer of unspecified heel, stage 4
Pressure ulcer with necrosis of soft tissues through to underlying muscle, tendon, or bone, unspecified heel

L89.609 Pressure ulcer of unspecified heel, unspecified stage
Healing pressure ulcer of unspecified heel NOS
Healing pressure ulcer of unspecified heel, unspecified stage

[6th] **L89.61 Pressure ulcer of right heel**

L89.610 Pressure ulcer of right heel, unstageable [HCC]

L89.611 Pressure ulcer of right heel, stage 1
Healing pressure ulcer of right heel, stage 1
Pressure pre-ulcer skin changes limited to persistent focal edema, right heel

L89.612 Pressure ulcer of right heel, stage 2
Healing pressure ulcer of right heel, stage 2
Pressure ulcer with abrasion, blister, partial thickness skin loss involving epidermis and/or dermis, right heel

L89.613 Pressure ulcer of right heel, stage 3 [HAC] [HCC] [MCC] [PDx MCC] [CC/MCC Exc]
Healing pressure ulcer of right heel, stage 3
Pressure ulcer with full thickness skin loss involving damage or necrosis of subcutaneous tissue, right heel

L89.614 Pressure ulcer of right heel, stage 4 [HAC] [HCC] [MCC] [PDx MCC] [CC/MCC Exc]
Healing pressure ulcer of right heel, stage 4
Pressure ulcer with necrosis of soft tissues through to underlying muscle, tendon, or bone, right heel

L89.619 Pressure ulcer of right heel, unspecified stage
Healing pressure ulcer of right heel NOS
Healing pressure ulcer of ►right heel◄, unspecified stage

[6th] **L89.62 Pressure ulcer of left heel**

L89.620 Pressure ulcer of left heel, unstageable [HCC]

L89.621 Pressure ulcer of left heel, stage 1
Healing pressure ulcer of left heel, stage 1
Pressure pre-ulcer skin changes limited to persistent focal edema, left heel

L89.622 Pressure ulcer of left heel, stage 2
AHA: Q4 2016
Healing pressure ulcer of left heel, stage 2
Pressure ulcer with abrasion, blister, partial thickness skin loss involving epidermis and/or dermis, left heel

L89.623 Pressure ulcer of left heel, stage 3 [HAC] [HCC] [MCC] [PDx MCC] [CC/MCC Exc]
AHA: Q4 2016
Healing pressure ulcer of left heel, stage 3
Pressure ulcer with full thickness skin loss involving damage or necrosis of subcutaneous tissue, left heel

L89.624 Pressure ulcer of left heel, stage 4 [HAC] [HCC] [MCC] [PDx MCC] [CC/MCC Exc]
Healing pressure ulcer of left heel, stage 4
Pressure ulcer with necrosis of soft tissues through to underlying muscle, tendon, or bone, left heel

L89.629 Pressure ulcer of left heel, unspecified stage
Healing pressure ulcer of left heel NOS
Healing pressure ulcer of left heel, unspecified stage

[PDx] Unacceptable principal diagnosis symbol per Medicare code edits [POA] Code exempt from diagnosis present on admission requirement
[?] Questionable admission [CC] Complication or comorbidity [CC/MCC Exc] CC/MCC exclusion [MCC] Major complication or comorbidity
[PDx CC] Principal diagnosis as its own CC [PDx MCC] Principal diagnosis as its own MCC [HCC] HCC diagnosis code [RxHCC] RxHCC diagnosis code
MACRA code [Z1] Z code as first-listed diagnosis

5ᵗʰ L89.8 **Pressure ulcer of** other site

  6ᵗʰ L89.81 **Pressure ulcer of** head

    Pressure ulcer of face

    L89.810 **Pressure ulcer of head,** unstageable HCC

    L89.811 **Pressure ulcer of head,** stage 1

      Healing pressure ulcer of head, stage 1

      Pressure pre-ulcer skin changes limited to persistent focal edema, head

    L89.812 **Pressure ulcer of head,** stage 2

      Healing pressure ulcer of head, stage 2

      Pressure ulcer with abrasion, blister, partial thickness skin loss involving epidermis and/or dermis, head

    L89.813 **Pressure ulcer of head, stage 3** HAC HCC MCC⁰ PDx MCC⁰ CC/MCC Exc

      Healing pressure ulcer of head, stage 3

      Pressure ulcer with full thickness skin loss involving damage or necrosis of subcutaneous tissue, head

    L89.814 **Pressure ulcer of head, stage 4** HAC HCC MCC⁰ PDx MCC⁰ CC/MCC Exc

      Healing pressure ulcer of head, stage 4

      Pressure ulcer with necrosis of soft tissues through to underlying muscle, tendon, or bone, head

    L89.819 **Pressure ulcer of head, unspecified stage**

      Healing pressure ulcer of head NOS

      Healing pressure ulcer of head, unspecified stage

  6ᵗʰ L89.89 **Pressure ulcer of** other site

    L89.890 **Pressure ulcer of other site,** unstageable HCC

    L89.891 **Pressure ulcer of other site,** stage 1

      Healing pressure ulcer of other site, stage 1

      Pressure pre-ulcer skin changes limited to persistent focal edema, other site

    L89.892 **Pressure ulcer of other site,** stage 2

      Healing pressure ulcer of other site, stage 2

      Pressure ulcer with abrasion, blister, partial thickness skin loss involving epidermis and/or dermis, other site

    L89.893 **Pressure ulcer of other site, stage 3** HAC HCC MCC⁰ PDx MCC⁰ CC/MCC Exc

      Healing pressure ulcer of other site, stage 3

      Pressure ulcer with full thickness skin loss involving damage or necrosis of subcutaneous tissue, other site

    L89.894 **Pressure ulcer of other site, stage 4** HAC HCC MCC⁰ PDx MCC⁰ CC/MCC Exc

      Healing pressure ulcer of other site, stage 4

      Pressure ulcer with necrosis of soft tissues through to underlying muscle, tendon, or bone, other site

    L89.899 **Pressure ulcer of other site, unspecified stage**

      Healing pressure ulcer of other site NOS

      Healing pressure ulcer of other site, unspecified stage

5ᵗʰ L89.9 **Pressure ulcer of** unspecified site

  L89.90 **Pressure ulcer of unspecified site,** unspecified stage

    Healing pressure ulcer of unspecified site NOS

    Healing pressure ulcer of unspecified site, unspecified stage

  L89.91 **Pressure ulcer of unspecified site,** stage 1

    Healing pressure ulcer of unspecified site, stage 1

    Pressure pre-ulcer skin changes limited to persistent focal edema, unspecified site

  L89.92 **Pressure ulcer of unspecified site,** stage 2

    Healing pressure ulcer of unspecified site, stage 2

    Pressure ulcer with abrasion, blister, partial thickness skin loss involving epidermis and/or dermis, unspecified site

  L89.93 **Pressure ulcer of unspecified site, stage 3** HAC HCC MCC⁰ PDx MCC⁰ CC/MCC Exc

    Healing pressure ulcer of unspecified site, stage 3

    Pressure ulcer with full thickness skin loss involving damage or necrosis of subcutaneous tissue, unspecified site

  L89.94 **Pressure ulcer of unspecified site, stage 4** HAC HCC MCC⁰ PDx MCC⁰ CC/MCC Exc

    Healing pressure ulcer of unspecified site, stage 4

    Pressure ulcer with necrosis of soft tissues through to underlying muscle, tendon, or bone, unspecified site

  L89.95 **Pressure ulcer of unspecified site, unstageable** HCC

4ᵗʰ L90 **Atrophic disorders of skin**

  L90.0 **Lichen sclerosus et atrophicus**

    EXCLUDES2 *lichen sclerosus of external female genital organs (N90.4)*

      lichen sclerosus of external male genital organs (N48.0)

  L90.1 **Anetoderma of Schweninger-Buzzi**

  L90.2 **Anetoderma of Jadassohn-Pellizzari**

  L90.3 **Atrophoderma of Pasini and Pierini**

  L90.4 **Acrodermatitis chronica atrophicans**

  L90.5 **Scar conditions and fibrosis of skin**

    AHA: Q2 2016, Q1 2015

    Adherent scar (skin)

    Cicatrix

    Disfigurement of skin due to scar

    Fibrosis of skin NOS

    Scar NOS

    EXCLUDES2 *hypertrophic scar (L91.0)*

      keloid scar (L91.0)

  L90.6 **Striae atrophicae**

  L90.8 **Other atrophic disorders of skin**

  L90.9 **Atrophic disorder of skin, unspecified**

4ᵗʰ L91 **Hypertrophic disorders of skin**

  L91.0 **Hypertrophic scar**

    Keloid

    Keloid scar

    EXCLUDES2 *acne keloid (L73.0)*

      scar NOS (L90.5)

  L91.8 **Other hypertrophic disorders of the skin**

  L91.9 **Hypertrophic disorder of the skin, unspecified**

4ᵗʰ L92 **Granulomatous disorders of skin and subcutaneous tissue**

  EXCLUDES2 *actinic granuloma (L57.5)*

  L92.0 **Granuloma annulare**

    Perforating granuloma annulare

  L92.1 **Necrobiosis lipoidica, not elsewhere classified**

    EXCLUDES1 *necrobiosis lipoidica associated with diabetes mellitus (E08-E13 with .620)*

  L92.2 **Granuloma faciale [eosinophilic granuloma of skin]**

  L92.3 **Foreign body granuloma of the skin and subcutaneous tissue**

    Use additional code to identify the type of retained foreign body (Z18.-)

  L92.8 **Other granulomatous disorders of the skin and subcutaneous tissue**

  L92.9 **Granulomatous disorder of the skin and subcutaneous tissue, unspecified**

    EXCLUDES2 *umbilical granuloma (P83.81)*

4ᵗʰ L93 **Lupus erythematosus**

  Use additional code for adverse effect, if applicable, to identify drug (T36-T50 with fifth or sixth character 5)

  EXCLUDES1 *lupus exedens (A18.4)*

    lupus vulgaris (A18.4)

    scleroderma (M34.-)

    systemic lupus erythematosus (M32.-)

  L93.0 **Discoid lupus erythematosus**

    Lupus erythematosus NOS

  L93.1 **Subacute cutaneous lupus erythematosus**

  L93.2 **Other local lupus erythematosus**

    Lupus erythematosus profundus

    Lupus panniculitis

Unspecified Code   Other Specified Code   Manifestation Code   Ⓝ Newborn   Ⓟ Pediatric   Ⓜ Maternity   Ⓐ Adult   ♂ Male   ♀ Female

● New Code   ▲ Revised Code Title   ▶◀ Revised Text   NOTES   INCLUDES   EXCLUDES 1 Not coded here   EXCLUDES 2 Not included here

4ᵗʰ 4ᵗʰ character required   **5ᵗʰ** 5ᵗʰ character required   **6ᵗʰ** 6ᵗʰ character required   **7ᵗʰ** 7ᵗʰ character required

7ᵗʰ Extension 'X' Alert   HAC Hospital-acquired condition (HAC) alert   **AHA** AHA Coding Clinic©

L94 - L97.209

CHAPTER 12: DISEASES OF THE SKIN AND SUBCUTANEOUS TISSUE (L00-L99)

L94 Other localized connective tissue disorders

EXCLUDES1 systemic connective tissue disorders (M30-M36)

L94.0 Localized scleroderma [morphea]

Circumscribed scleroderma

L94.1 Linear scleroderma

En coup de sabre lesion

L94.2 Calcinosis cutis

L94.3 Sclerodactyly

L94.4 Gottron's papules

L94.5 Poikiloderma vasculare atrophicans   RxHCC

L94.6 Ainhum

L94.8 Other specified localized connective tissue disorders

L94.9 Localized connective tissue disorder, unspecified

L95 Vasculitis limited to skin, not elsewhere classified

EXCLUDES1 angioma serpiginosum (L81.7)

Henoch(-Schönlein) purpura (D69.0)

hypersensitivity angiitis (M31.0)

lupus panniculitis (L93.2)

panniculitis NOS (M79.3)

panniculitis of neck and back (M54.0-)

polyarteritis nodosa (M30.0)

relapsing panniculitis (M35.6)

rheumatoid vasculitis (M05.2)

serum sickness (T80.6-)

urticaria (L50.-)

Wegener's granulomatosis (M31.3-)

L95.0 Livedoid vasculitis

Atrophie blanche (en plaque)

L95.1 Erythema elevatum diutinum

L95.8 Other vasculitis limited to the skin

L95.9 Vasculitis limited to the skin, unspecified

L97 Non-pressure chronic ulcer of lower limb, not elsewhere classified

INCLUDES chronic ulcer of skin of lower limb NOS

non-healing ulcer of skin

non-infected sinus of skin

trophic ulcer NOS

tropical ulcer NOS

ulcer of skin of lower limb NOS

Code first any associated underlying condition, such as:
any associated gangrene (I96)
atherosclerosis of the lower extremities (I70.23-, I70.24-, I70.33-, I70.34-, I70.43-, I70.44-, I70.53-, I70.54-, I70.63-, I70.64-, I70.73-, I70.74-)
chronic venous hypertension (I87.31-, I87.33-)
diabetic ulcers (E08.621, E08.622, E09.621, E09.622, E10.621, E10.622, E11.621, E11.622, E13.621, E13.622)
postphlebitic syndrome (I87.01-, I87.03-)
postthrombotic syndrome (I87.01-, I87.03-)
varicose ulcer (I83.0-, I83.2-)

EXCLUDES2 pressure ulcer (pressure area) (L89.-)

skin infections (L00-L08)

specific infections classified to A00-B99

L97.1 Non-pressure chronic ulcer of thigh

L97.10 Non-pressure chronic ulcer of unspecified thigh

L97.101 Non-pressure chronic ulcer of unspecified thigh limited to breakdown of skin   HCC RxHCC CC/MCC Exc

L97.102 Non-pressure chronic ulcer of unspecified thigh with fat layer exposed   HCC RxHCC CC/MCC Exc

L97.103 Non-pressure chronic ulcer of unspecified thigh with necrosis of muscle   HCC RxHCC CC/MCC Exc

L97.104 Non-pressure chronic ulcer of unspecified thigh with necrosis of bone   HCC RxHCC CC/MCC Exc

● **L97.105** Non-pressure chronic ulcer of unspecified thigh with muscle involvement without evidence of necrosis   CC/MCC Exc

● **L97.106** Non-pressure chronic ulcer of unspecified thigh with bone involvement without evidence of necrosis   CC/MCC Exc

● **L97.108** Non-pressure chronic ulcer of unspecified thigh with other specified severity   CC/MCC Exc

L97.109 Non-pressure chronic ulcer of unspecified thigh with unspecified severity   HCC RxHCC CC/MCC Exc

L97.11 Non-pressure chronic ulcer of right thigh

L97.111 Non-pressure chronic ulcer of right thigh limited to breakdown of skin   HCC RxHCC CC/MCC Exc

L97.112 Non-pressure chronic ulcer of right thigh with fat layer exposed   HCC RxHCC CC/MCC Exc

L97.113 Non-pressure chronic ulcer of right thigh with necrosis of muscle   HCC RxHCC CC/MCC Exc

L97.114 Non-pressure chronic ulcer of right thigh with necrosis of bone   HCC RxHCC CC/MCC Exc

● **L97.115** Non-pressure chronic ulcer of right thigh with muscle involvement without evidence of necrosis   CC/MCC Exc

● **L97.116** Non-pressure chronic ulcer of right thigh with bone involvement without evidence of necrosis   CC/MCC Exc

● **L97.118** Non-pressure chronic ulcer of right thigh with other specified severity   CC/MCC Exc

L97.119 Non-pressure chronic ulcer of right thigh with unspecified severity   HCC RxHCC CC/MCC Exc

L97.12 Non-pressure chronic ulcer of left thigh

L97.121 Non-pressure chronic ulcer of left thigh limited to breakdown of skin   HCC RxHCC CC/MCC Exc

L97.122 Non-pressure chronic ulcer of left thigh with fat layer exposed   HCC RxHCC CC/MCC Exc

L97.123 Non-pressure chronic ulcer of left thigh with necrosis of muscle   HCC RxHCC CC/MCC Exc

L97.124 Non-pressure chronic ulcer of left thigh with necrosis of bone   HCC RxHCC CC/MCC Exc

● **L97.125** Non-pressure chronic ulcer of left thigh with muscle involvement without evidence of necrosis   CC/MCC Exc

● **L97.126** Non-pressure chronic ulcer of left thigh with bone involvement without evidence of necrosis   CC/MCC Exc

● **L97.128** Non-pressure chronic ulcer of left thigh with other specified severity   CC/MCC Exc

L97.129 Non-pressure chronic ulcer of left thigh with unspecified severity   HCC RxHCC CC/MCC Exc

L97.2 Non-pressure chronic ulcer of calf

L97.20 Non-pressure chronic ulcer of unspecified calf

L97.201 Non-pressure chronic ulcer of unspecified calf limited to breakdown of skin   HCC RxHCC CC/MCC Exc

L97.202 Non-pressure chronic ulcer of unspecified calf with fat layer exposed   HCC RxHCC CC/MCC Exc

L97.203 Non-pressure chronic ulcer of unspecified calf with necrosis of muscle   HCC RxHCC CC/MCC Exc

L97.204 Non-pressure chronic ulcer of unspecified calf with necrosis of bone   HCC RxHCC CC/MCC Exc

● **L97.205** Non-pressure chronic ulcer of unspecified calf with muscle involvement without evidence of necrosis   CC/MCC Exc

● **L97.206** Non-pressure chronic ulcer of unspecified calf with bone involvement without evidence of necrosis   CC/MCC Exc

● **L97.208** Non-pressure chronic ulcer of unspecified calf with other specified severity   CC/MCC Exc

L97.209 Non-pressure chronic ulcer of unspecified calf with unspecified severity   HCC RxHCC CC/MCC Exc

---

PDx Unacceptable principal diagnosis symbol per Medicare code edits   POA Code exempt from diagnosis present on admission requirement   ? Questionable admission   CC Complication or comorbidity   CC/MCC Exc CC/MCC exclusion   MCC Major complication or comorbidity   PCC Principal diagnosis as its own CC   PMCC Principal diagnosis as its own MCC   HCC HCC diagnosis code   RxHCC RxHCC diagnosis code   MACRA code   Z1 Z code as first-listed diagnosis

L97.21 Non-pressure chronic ulcer of right calf

L97.211 Non-pressure chronic ulcer of right calf limited to breakdown of skin `CC` `HCC` `RxHCC` `CC/MCC Exc`

L97.212 Non-pressure chronic ulcer of right calf with fat layer exposed `CC` `HCC` `RxHCC` `CC/MCC Exc`

L97.213 Non-pressure chronic ulcer of right calf with necrosis of muscle `CC` `HCC` `RxHCC` `CC/MCC Exc`

L97.214 Non-pressure chronic ulcer of right calf with necrosis of bone `CC` `HCC` `RxHCC` `CC/MCC Exc`

● **L97.215** Non-pressure chronic ulcer of right calf with muscle involvement without evidence of necrosis `CC` `CC/MCC Exc`

● **L97.216** Non-pressure chronic ulcer of right calf with bone involvement without evidence of necrosis `CC` `CC/MCC Exc`

● **L97.218** Non-pressure chronic ulcer of right calf with other specified severity `CC` `CC/MCC Exc`

L97.219 Non-pressure chronic ulcer of right calf with unspecified severity `CC` `HCC` `RxHCC` `CC/MCC Exc`

L97.22 Non-pressure chronic ulcer of left calf

L97.221 Non-pressure chronic ulcer of left calf limited to breakdown of skin `CC` `HCC` `RxHCC` `CC/MCC Exc`

L97.222 Non-pressure chronic ulcer of left calf with fat layer exposed `CC` `HCC` `RxHCC` `CC/MCC Exc`

L97.223 Non-pressure chronic ulcer of left calf with necrosis of muscle `CC` `HCC` `RxHCC` `CC/MCC Exc`

L97.224 Non-pressure chronic ulcer of left calf with necrosis of bone `CC` `HCC` `RxHCC` `CC/MCC Exc`

● **L97.225** Non-pressure chronic ulcer of left calf with muscle involvement without evidence of necrosis `CC` `CC/MCC Exc`

● **L97.226** Non-pressure chronic ulcer of left calf with bone involvement without evidence of necrosis `CC` `CC/MCC Exc`

● **L97.228** Non-pressure chronic ulcer of left calf with other specified severity `CC` `CC/MCC Exc`

L97.229 Non-pressure chronic ulcer of left calf with unspecified severity `CC` `HCC` `RxHCC` `CC/MCC Exc`

L97.3 Non-pressure chronic ulcer of ankle

L97.30 Non-pressure chronic ulcer of unspecified ankle

L97.301 Non-pressure chronic ulcer of unspecified ankle limited to breakdown of skin `CC` `HCC` `RxHCC` `CC/MCC Exc`

L97.302 Non-pressure chronic ulcer of unspecified ankle with fat layer exposed `CC` `HCC` `RxHCC` `CC/MCC Exc`

L97.303 Non-pressure chronic ulcer of unspecified ankle with necrosis of muscle `CC` `HCC` `RxHCC` `CC/MCC Exc`

L97.304 Non-pressure chronic ulcer of unspecified ankle with necrosis of bone `CC` `HCC` `RxHCC` `CC/MCC Exc`

● **L97.305** Non-pressure chronic ulcer of unspecified ankle with muscle involvement without evidence of necrosis `CC` `CC/MCC Exc`

● **L97.306** Non-pressure chronic ulcer of unspecified ankle with bone involvement without evidence of necrosis `CC` `CC/MCC Exc`

● **L97.308** Non-pressure chronic ulcer of unspecified ankle with other specified severity `CC` `CC/MCC Exc`

L97.309 Non-pressure chronic ulcer of unspecified ankle with unspecified severity `CC` `HCC` `RxHCC` `CC/MCC Exc`

L97.31 Non-pressure chronic ulcer of right ankle

L97.311 Non-pressure chronic ulcer of right ankle limited to breakdown of skin `CC` `HCC` `RxHCC` `CC/MCC Exc`

L97.312 Non-pressure chronic ulcer of right ankle with fat layer exposed `CC` `HCC` `RxHCC` `CC/MCC Exc`

L97.313 Non-pressure chronic ulcer of right ankle with necrosis of muscle `CC` `HCC` `RxHCC` `CC/MCC Exc`

L97.314 Non-pressure chronic ulcer of right ankle with necrosis of bone `CC` `HCC` `RxHCC` `CC/MCC Exc`

● **L97.315** Non-pressure chronic ulcer of right ankle with muscle involvement without evidence of necrosis `CC` `CC/MCC Exc`

● **L97.316** Non-pressure chronic ulcer of right ankle with bone involvement without evidence of necrosis `CC` `CC/MCC Exc`

● **L97.318** Non-pressure chronic ulcer of right ankle with other specified severity `CC` `CC/MCC Exc`

L97.319 Non-pressure chronic ulcer of right ankle with unspecified severity `CC` `HCC` `RxHCC` `CC/MCC Exc`

L97.32 Non-pressure chronic ulcer of left ankle

L97.321 Non-pressure chronic ulcer of left ankle limited to breakdown of skin `CC` `HCC` `RxHCC` `CC/MCC Exc`

L97.322 Non-pressure chronic ulcer of left ankle with fat layer exposed `CC` `HCC` `RxHCC` `CC/MCC Exc`

L97.323 Non-pressure chronic ulcer of left ankle with necrosis of muscle `CC` `HCC` `RxHCC` `CC/MCC Exc`

L97.324 Non-pressure chronic ulcer of left ankle with necrosis of bone `CC` `HCC` `RxHCC` `CC/MCC Exc`

● **L97.325** Non-pressure chronic ulcer of left ankle with muscle involvement without evidence of necrosis `CC` `CC/MCC Exc`

● **L97.326** Non-pressure chronic ulcer of left ankle with bone involvement without evidence of necrosis `CC` `CC/MCC Exc`

● **L97.328** Non-pressure chronic ulcer of left ankle with other specified severity `CC` `CC/MCC Exc`

L97.329 Non-pressure chronic ulcer of left ankle with unspecified severity `CC` `HCC` `RxHCC` `CC/MCC Exc`

L97.4 Non-pressure chronic ulcer of heel and midfoot
Non-pressure chronic ulcer of plantar surface of midfoot

L97.40 Non-pressure chronic ulcer of unspecified heel and midfoot

L97.401 Non-pressure chronic ulcer of unspecified heel and midfoot limited to breakdown of skin `CC` `HCC` `RxHCC` `CC/MCC Exc`

L97.402 Non-pressure chronic ulcer of unspecified heel and midfoot with fat layer exposed `CC` `HCC` `RxHCC` `CC/MCC Exc`

L97.403 Non-pressure chronic ulcer of unspecified heel and midfoot with necrosis of muscle `CC` `HCC` `RxHCC` `CC/MCC Exc`

L97.404 Non-pressure chronic ulcer of unspecified heel and midfoot with necrosis of bone `CC` `HCC` `RxHCC` `CC/MCC Exc`

● **L97.405** Non-pressure chronic ulcer of unspecified heel and midfoot with muscle involvement without evidence of necrosis `CC` `CC/MCC Exc`

● **L97.406** Non-pressure chronic ulcer of unspecified heel and midfoot with bone involvement without evidence of necrosis `CC` `CC/MCC Exc`

● **L97.408** Non-pressure chronic ulcer of unspecified heel and midfoot with other specified severity `CC` `CC/MCC Exc`

L97.409 Non-pressure chronic ulcer of unspecified heel and midfoot with unspecified severity `CC` `HCC` `RxHCC` `CC/MCC Exc`

L97.41 Non-pressure chronic ulcer of right heel and midfoot

L97.411 Non-pressure chronic ulcer of right heel and midfoot limited to breakdown of skin `CC` `HCC` `RxHCC` `CC/MCC Exc`

L97.412 Non-pressure chronic ulcer of right heel and midfoot with fat layer exposed `CC` `HCC` `RxHCC` `CC/MCC Exc`

L97.413 Non-pressure chronic ulcer of right heel and midfoot with necrosis of muscle `CC` `HCC` `RxHCC` `CC/MCC Exc`

Unspecified Code   Other Specified Code   Manifestation Code   N Newborn   P Pediatric   M Maternity   A Adult   ♂ Male   ♀ Female
● New Code   ▲ Revised Code Title   ▶◀ Revised Text   NOTES   INCLUDES   EXCLUDES 1 Not coded here   EXCLUDES 2 Not included here
④ 4th character required   ⑤ 5th character required   ⑥ 6th character required   ⑦ 7th character required
Ⓧ Extension 'X' Alert   HAC Hospital-acquired condition (HAC) alert   AHA AHA Coding Clinic©

L97.414 Non-pressure chronic ulcer of right heel and midfoot with necrosis of bone HCC RxHCC

● L97.415 Non-pressure chronic ulcer of right heel and midfoot with muscle involvement without evidence of necrosis CC CC/MCC Exc

● L97.416 Non-pressure chronic ulcer of right heel and midfoot with bone involvement without evidence of necrosis CC CC/MCC Exc

● L97.418 Non-pressure chronic ulcer of right heel and midfoot with other specified severity CC CC/MCC Exc

L97.419 Non-pressure chronic ulcer of right heel and midfoot with unspecified severity CC HCC RxHCC CC/MCC Exc

6th L97.42 Non-pressure chronic ulcer of left heel and midfoot

L97.421 Non-pressure chronic ulcer of left heel and midfoot limited to breakdown of skin CC HCC RxHCC CC/MCC Exc
AHA: Q1 2016

L97.422 Non-pressure chronic ulcer of left heel and midfoot with fat layer exposed CC HCC RxHCC CC/MCC Exc

L97.423 Non-pressure chronic ulcer of left heel and midfoot with necrosis of muscle CC HCC RxHCC CC/MCC Exc

L97.424 Non-pressure chronic ulcer of left heel and midfoot with necrosis of bone CC HCC RxHCC CC/MCC Exc

● L97.425 Non-pressure chronic ulcer of left heel and midfoot with muscle involvement without evidence of necrosis CC CC/MCC Exc

● L97.426 Non-pressure chronic ulcer of left heel and midfoot with bone involvement without evidence of necrosis CC CC/MCC Exc

● L97.428 Non-pressure chronic ulcer of left heel and midfoot with other specified severity CC CC/MCC Exc

L97.429 Non-pressure chronic ulcer of left heel and midfoot with unspecified severity CC HCC RxHCC CC/MCC Exc

5th L97.5 Non-pressure chronic ulcer of other part of foot
Non-pressure chronic ulcer of toe

6th L97.50 Non-pressure chronic ulcer of other part of unspecified foot

L97.501 Non-pressure chronic ulcer of other part of unspecified foot limited to breakdown of skin HCC RxHCC

L97.502 Non-pressure chronic ulcer of other part of unspecified foot with fat layer exposed HCC RxHCC

L97.503 Non-pressure chronic ulcer of other part of unspecified foot with necrosis of muscle HCC RxHCC

L97.504 Non-pressure chronic ulcer of other part of unspecified foot with necrosis of bone HCC RxHCC

● L97.505 Non-pressure chronic ulcer of other part of unspecified foot with muscle involvement without evidence of necrosis CC CC/MCC Exc

● L97.506 Non-pressure chronic ulcer of other part of unspecified foot with bone involvement without evidence of necrosis CC CC/MCC Exc

● L97.508 Non-pressure chronic ulcer of other part of unspecified foot with other specified severity CC CC/MCC Exc

L97.509 Non-pressure chronic ulcer of other part of unspecified foot with unspecified severity HCC RxHCC

6th L97.51 Non-pressure chronic ulcer of other part of right foot

L97.511 Non-pressure chronic ulcer of other part of right foot limited to breakdown of skin HCC RxHCC

L97.512 Non-pressure chronic ulcer of other part of right foot with fat layer exposed HCC RxHCC

L97.513 Non-pressure chronic ulcer of other part of right foot with necrosis of muscle HCC RxHCC

L97.514 Non-pressure chronic ulcer of other part of right foot with necrosis of bone HCC RxHCC

● L97.515 Non-pressure chronic ulcer of other part of right foot with muscle involvement without evidence of necrosis CC CC/MCC Exc

● L97.516 Non-pressure chronic ulcer of other part of right foot with bone involvement without evidence of necrosis CC CC/MCC Exc

● L97.518 Non-pressure chronic ulcer of other part of right foot with other specified severity CC CC/MCC Exc

L97.519 Non-pressure chronic ulcer of other part of right foot with unspecified severity HCC RxHCC

6th L97.52 Non-pressure chronic ulcer of other part of left foot

L97.521 Non-pressure chronic ulcer of other part of left foot limited to breakdown of skin HCC RxHCC

L97.522 Non-pressure chronic ulcer of other part of left foot with fat layer exposed HCC RxHCC

L97.523 Non-pressure chronic ulcer of other part of left foot with necrosis of muscle HCC RxHCC

L97.524 Non-pressure chronic ulcer of other part of left foot with necrosis of bone HCC RxHCC

● L97.525 Non-pressure chronic ulcer of other part of left foot with muscle involvement without evidence of necrosis CC CC/MCC Exc

● L97.526 Non-pressure chronic ulcer of other part of left foot with bone involvement without evidence of necrosis CC CC/MCC Exc

● L97.528 Non-pressure chronic ulcer of other part of left foot with other specified severity CC CC/MCC Exc

L97.529 Non-pressure chronic ulcer of other part of left foot with unspecified severity HCC RxHCC

5th L97.8 Non-pressure chronic ulcer of other part of lower leg

6th L97.80 Non-pressure chronic ulcer of other part of unspecified lower leg

L97.801 Non-pressure chronic ulcer of other part of unspecified lower leg limited to breakdown of skin CC HCC RxHCC CC/MCC Exc

L97.802 Non-pressure chronic ulcer of other part of unspecified lower leg with fat layer exposed CC HCC RxHCC CC/MCC Exc

L97.803 Non-pressure chronic ulcer of other part of unspecified lower leg with necrosis of muscle CC HCC RxHCC CC/MCC Exc

L97.804 Non-pressure chronic ulcer of other part of unspecified lower leg with necrosis of bone CC HCC RxHCC CC/MCC Exc

● L97.805 Non-pressure chronic ulcer of other part of unspecified lower leg with muscle involvement without evidence of necrosis CC CC/MCC Exc

● L97.806 Non-pressure chronic ulcer of other part of unspecified lower leg with bone involvement without evidence of necrosis CC CC/MCC Exc

● L97.808 Non-pressure chronic ulcer of other part of unspecified lower leg with other specified severity CC CC/MCC Exc

L97.809 Non-pressure chronic ulcer of other part of unspecified lower leg with unspecified severity CC HCC RxHCC CC/MCC Exc

6th L97.81 Non-pressure chronic ulcer of other part of right lower leg

L97.811 Non-pressure chronic ulcer of other part of right lower leg limited to breakdown of skin CC HCC RxHCC CC/MCC Exc

---

PDxIn Unacceptable principal diagnosis symbol per Medicare code edits   PDx Code exempt from diagnosis present on admission requirement
? Questionable admission   CC Complication or comorbidity   CC/MCC Exc CC/MCC exclusion   MCC Major complication or comorbidity
PDx CC Principal diagnosis as its own CC   PDx MCC Principal diagnosis as its own MCC   HCC HCC diagnosis code   RxHCC RxHCC diagnosis code
MACRA code   Z1 Z code as first-listed diagnosis

762

When symbols appear on a code that requires a 7th character extension, refer to Appendix B to identify applicable 7th character codes.

2018 ICD-10-CM

L97.812 Non-pressure chronic ulcer of other part of right lower leg with fat layer exposed [CC] [HCC] [RxHCC] [CC/MCC Exc]

L97.813 Non-pressure chronic ulcer of other part of right lower leg with necrosis of muscle [CC] [HCC] [RxHCC] [CC/MCC Exc]

L97.814 Non-pressure chronic ulcer of other part of right lower leg with necrosis of bone [CC] [HCC] [RxHCC] [CC/MCC Exc]

● L97.815 Non-pressure chronic ulcer of other part of right lower leg with muscle involvement without evidence of necrosis [CC] [CC/MCC Exc]

● L97.816 Non-pressure chronic ulcer of other part of right lower leg with bone involvement without evidence of necrosis [CC] [CC/MCC Exc]

● L97.818 Non-pressure chronic ulcer of other part of right lower leg with other specified severity [CC] [CC/MCC Exc]

L97.819 Non-pressure chronic ulcer of other part of right lower leg with unspecified severity [CC] [HCC] [RxHCC] [CC/MCC Exc]

[6th] L97.82 Non-pressure chronic ulcer of other part of left lower leg

L97.821 Non-pressure chronic ulcer of other part of left lower leg limited to breakdown of skin [CC] [HCC] [RxHCC] [CC/MCC Exc]

L97.822 Non-pressure chronic ulcer of other part of left lower leg with fat layer exposed [CC] [HCC] [RxHCC] [CC/MCC Exc]

L97.823 Non-pressure chronic ulcer of other part of left lower leg with necrosis of muscle [CC] [HCC] [RxHCC] [CC/MCC Exc]

L97.824 Non-pressure chronic ulcer of other part of left lower leg with necrosis of bone [CC] [HCC] [RxHCC] [CC/MCC Exc]

● L97.825 Non-pressure chronic ulcer of other part of left lower leg with muscle involvement without evidence of necrosis [CC] [CC/MCC Exc]

● L97.826 Non-pressure chronic ulcer of other part of left lower leg with bone involvement without evidence of necrosis [CC] [CC/MCC Exc]

● L97.828 Non-pressure chronic ulcer of other part of left lower leg with other specified severity [CC] [CC/MCC Exc]

L97.829 Non-pressure chronic ulcer of other part of left lower leg with unspecified severity [CC] [HCC] [RxHCC] [CC/MCC Exc]

[5th] L97.9 Non-pressure chronic ulcer of unspecified part of lower leg

[6th] L97.90 Non-pressure chronic ulcer of unspecified part of unspecified lower leg

L97.901 Non-pressure chronic ulcer of unspecified part of unspecified lower leg limited to breakdown of skin [CC] [HCC] [RxHCC] [CC/MCC Exc]

L97.902 Non-pressure chronic ulcer of unspecified part of unspecified lower leg with fat layer exposed [CC] [HCC] [RxHCC] [CC/MCC Exc]

L97.903 Non-pressure chronic ulcer of unspecified part of unspecified lower leg with necrosis of muscle [CC] [HCC] [RxHCC] [CC/MCC Exc]

L97.904 Non-pressure chronic ulcer of unspecified part of unspecified lower leg with necrosis of bone [CC] [HCC] [RxHCC] [CC/MCC Exc]

● L97.905 Non-pressure chronic ulcer of unspecified part of unspecified lower leg with muscle involvement without evidence of necrosis [CC] [CC/MCC Exc]

● L97.906 Non-pressure chronic ulcer of unspecified part of unspecified lower leg with bone involvement without evidence of necrosis [CC] [CC/MCC Exc]

● L97.908 Non-pressure chronic ulcer of unspecified part of unspecified lower leg with other specified severity [CC] [CC/MCC Exc]

L97.909 Non-pressure chronic ulcer of unspecified part of unspecified lower leg with unspecified severity [CC] [HCC] [RxHCC] [CC/MCC Exc]

[6th] L97.91 Non-pressure chronic ulcer of unspecified part of right lower leg

L97.911 Non-pressure chronic ulcer of unspecified part of right lower leg limited to breakdown of skin [CC] [HCC] [RxHCC] [CC/MCC Exc]

L97.912 Non-pressure chronic ulcer of unspecified part of right lower leg with fat layer exposed [CC] [HCC] [RxHCC] [CC/MCC Exc]

L97.913 Non-pressure chronic ulcer of unspecified part of right lower leg with necrosis of muscle [CC] [HCC] [RxHCC] [CC/MCC Exc]

L97.914 Non-pressure chronic ulcer of unspecified part of right lower leg with necrosis of bone [CC] [HCC] [RxHCC] [CC/MCC Exc]

● L97.915 Non-pressure chronic ulcer of unspecified part of right lower leg with muscle involvement without evidence of necrosis [CC] [CC/MCC Exc]

● L97.916 Non-pressure chronic ulcer of unspecified part of right lower leg with bone involvement without evidence of necrosis [CC] [CC/MCC Exc]

● L97.918 Non-pressure chronic ulcer of unspecified part of right lower leg with other specified severity [CC] [CC/MCC Exc]

L97.919 Non-pressure chronic ulcer of unspecified part of right lower leg with unspecified severity [CC] [HCC] [RxHCC] [CC/MCC Exc]

[6th] L97.92 Non-pressure chronic ulcer of unspecified part of left lower leg

L97.921 Non-pressure chronic ulcer of unspecified part of left lower leg limited to breakdown of skin [CC] [HCC] [RxHCC] [CC/MCC Exc]

L97.922 Non-pressure chronic ulcer of unspecified part of left lower leg with fat layer exposed [CC] [HCC] [RxHCC] [CC/MCC Exc]

L97.923 Non-pressure chronic ulcer of unspecified part of left lower leg with necrosis of muscle [CC] [HCC] [RxHCC] [CC/MCC Exc]

L97.924 Non-pressure chronic ulcer of unspecified part of left lower leg with necrosis of bone [CC] [HCC] [RxHCC] [CC/MCC Exc]

● L97.925 Non-pressure chronic ulcer of unspecified part of left lower leg with muscle involvement without evidence of necrosis [CC] [CC/MCC Exc]

● L97.926 Non-pressure chronic ulcer of unspecified part of left lower leg with bone involvement without evidence of necrosis [CC] [CC/MCC Exc]

● L97.928 Non-pressure chronic ulcer of unspecified part of left lower leg with other specified severity [CC] [CC/MCC Exc]

L97.929 Non-pressure chronic ulcer of unspecified part of left lower leg with unspecified severity [CC] [HCC] [RxHCC] [CC/MCC Exc]

[4th] **L98 Other disorders of skin and subcutaneous tissue, not elsewhere classified**

L98.0 Pyogenic granuloma

[EXCLUDES2] *pyogenic granuloma of gingiva (K06.8)*
pyogenic granuloma of maxillary alveolar ridge (K04.5)
pyogenic granuloma of oral mucosa (K13.4)

L98.1 Factitial dermatitis

AHA: Q4 2016

Neurotic excoriation

[EXCLUDES1] *Excoriation (skin-picking) disorder (F42.4)*

L98.2 Febrile neutrophilic dermatosis [Sweet]

L98.3 Eosinophilic cellulitis [Wells] [CC] [CC/MCC Exc]

[5th] L98.4 Non-pressure chronic ulcer of skin, not elsewhere classified

Chronic ulcer of skin NOS

Tropical ulcer NOS

Ulcer of skin NOS

EXCLUDES2 pressure ulcer (pressure area) (L89.-)

　　gangrene (I96)

　　skin infections (L00-L08)

　　specific infections classified to A00-B99

　　ulcer of lower limb NEC (L97.-)

　　varicose ulcer (I83.0-I82.2)

⑥ **L98.41 Non-pressure chronic ulcer of** buttock

　　L98.411 **Non-pressure chronic ulcer of buttock limited** to breakdown of skin HCC RxHCC

　　L98.412 **Non-pressure chronic ulcer of buttock with fat layer exposed** HCC RxHCC

　　L98.413 **Non-pressure chronic ulcer of buttock with necrosis of muscle** HCC RxHCC

　　L98.414 **Non-pressure chronic ulcer of buttock with necrosis of bone** HCC RxHCC

● 　L98.415 **Non-pressure chronic ulcer of buttock with muscle involvement** without evidence of necrosis CC CC/MCC Exc

● 　L98.416 **Non-pressure chronic ulcer of buttock with bone involvement** without evidence of necrosis CC CC/MCC Exc

● 　L98.418 **Non-pressure chronic ulcer of buttock with other specified severity** CC CC/MCC Exc

　　L98.419 **Non-pressure chronic ulcer of buttock with unspecified severity** HCC RxHCC

⑥ **L98.42 Non-pressure chronic ulcer of** back

　　L98.421 **Non-pressure chronic ulcer of back limited** to breakdown of skin HCC RxHCC

　　L98.422 **Non-pressure chronic ulcer of back with** fat layer exposed HCC RxHCC

　　L98.423 **Non-pressure chronic ulcer of back with** necrosis of muscle HCC RxHCC

　　L98.424 **Non-pressure chronic ulcer of back with** necrosis of bone HCC RxHCC

● 　L98.425 **Non-pressure chronic ulcer of back with muscle involvement** without evidence of necrosis CC CC/MCC Exc

● 　L98.426 **Non-pressure chronic ulcer of back with bone involvement** without evidence of necrosis CC CC/MCC Exc

● 　L98.428 **Non-pressure chronic ulcer of back with other specified severity** CC CC/MCC Exc

　　L98.429 **Non-pressure chronic ulcer of back with unspecified severity** HCC RxHCC

⑥ **L98.49 Non-pressure chronic ulcer of skin of other sites**

　　Non-pressure chronic ulcer of skin NOS

　　L98.491 **Non-pressure chronic ulcer of skin of other sites limited** to breakdown of skin HCC RxHCC

　　L98.492 **Non-pressure chronic ulcer of skin of other sites with fat layer exposed** HCC RxHCC

　　L98.493 **Non-pressure chronic ulcer of skin of other sites** with necrosis of muscle HCC RxHCC

　　L98.494 **Non-pressure chronic ulcer of skin of other sites** with necrosis of bone HCC RxHCC

● 　L98.495 **Non-pressure chronic ulcer of other sites with muscle involvement** without evidence of necrosis CC CC/MCC Exc

● 　L98.496 **Non-pressure chronic ulcer of other sites with bone involvement** without evidence of necrosis CC CC/MCC Exc

● 　L98.498 **Non-pressure chronic ulcer of other sites with other specified severity** CC CC/MCC Exc

　　L98.499 **Non-pressure chronic ulcer of skin of other sites** with unspecified severity HCC RxHCC

L98.5 Mucinosis of the skin

Focal mucinosis

Lichen myxedematosus

Reticular erythematous mucinosis

EXCLUDES1 focal oral mucinosis (K13.79)

　　myxedema (E03.9)

L98.6 Other infiltrative disorders of the skin and subcutaneous tissue

EXCLUDES1 hyalinosis cutis et mucosae (E78.89)

L98.7 Excessive and redundant skin and subcutaneous tissue

AHA: Q4 2016

Loose or sagging skin following bariatric surgery weight loss

Loose or sagging skin following dietary weight loss

Loose or sagging skin, NOS

EXCLUDES2 acquired excess or redundant skin of eyelid (H02.3-)

　　congenital excess or redundant skin of eyelid (Q10.3)

　　skin changes due to chronic exposure to nonionizing radiation (L57.-)

L98.8 Other specified disorders of the skin and subcutaneous tissue

L98.9 Disorder of the skin and subcutaneous tissue, unspecified

L99 Other disorders of skin and subcutaneous tissue in diseases classified elsewhere

AHA: Q4 2016

Code first underlying disease, such as:

amyloidosis (E85.-)

EXCLUDES1 skin disorders in diabetes (E08-E13 with .62)

　　skin disorders in gonorrhea (A54.89)

　　skin disorders in syphilis (A51.31, A52.79)

PDxG Unacceptable principal diagnosis symbol per Medicare code edits 　PDxG Code exempt from diagnosis present on admission requirement

❓ Questionable admission 　CC Complication or comorbidity 　CC/MCC Exc CC/MCC exclusion 　MCC Major complication or comorbidity

PDxCC Principal diagnosis as its own CC 　PDxMCC Principal diagnosis as its own MCC 　HCC HCC diagnosis code 　RxHCC RxHCC diagnosis code

MACRA code 　Z1 Z code as first-listed diagnosis

When symbols appear on a code that requires a 7th character extension, refer to Appendix B to identify applicable 7th character codes. 　**2018 ICD-10-CM**

NOTES

NOTES

Anatomy of the Musculoskeletal System

Introduction

Osteology (Osteo: bone; logy: study) is the branch of anatomy that deals with the detailed analysis of structure, function and diseases of the skeletal elements. It constitutes the bony framework of the body. The human bony skeleton is composed of the below mentioned components (and is derived from the mesoderm, which is the primary germ cell layer).

Skeletal Region	Body Structure	Quantity of bones
Axial Skeleton (the trunk)	Skull	22
	Hyoid Bone	1
	Ribs & Sternum	25
	Vertebral Column	26
Appendicular Skeleton (the limbs)	Upper Extremities	64
	Lower Extremities	62
Auditory Ossicles		6

1. **Structure of a Normal Human Bone:** Bone is comprised of a rigid structure, which is based on dense connective tissue. A normal human bone is made up of the following essential macro and micro elements:
    a) Periosteum
    b) Medullary Membrane
    c) Marrow
    d) Blood Vessels and Nerves of Bone
    e) Haversian Canals (Canals of Havers)
    f) Lamellae
    g) Lacunae
    h) Canaliculi
    i) Perichondrium
    j) Osteoblasts
    k) Osteoclasts
    l) Medullary spaces
    m) Epiphysis
    n) Diaphysis
    o) Metaphysis

2. **The Vertebral Column**
    a) Anatomical Detail: The vertebral column is composed of a continuous series of compact bones that articulate with each other via intervertebral discs, and are called vertebrae. The structure forms the dorsal aspect of the trunk. The vertebral column is also called spine. The spinal cord traverses through the spinal canal of the vertebral column. The individual vertebrae remain connected together by intervertebral discs. The cervical, thoracic, and lumbar vertebrae are termed true vertebrae. However, sacral and coccygeal ones are false vertebrae. The concept behind considering them as true or false is based on mobility of the individual vertebrae through intervertebral discs. Cervical, thoracic and lumbar vertebrae are moveable to some extent and therefore termed as true vertebral bodies. In contrast, the sacral-coccygeal section is rather fixed and thus not categorized as true vertebrae. Each vertebral segment is associated with a portion of spinal cord, which travels the entire vertebral column, and each spinal cord segment has specific physiology and functions. The vertebral bodies communicate with each other through the pads of elastic fibro-cartilage. These flexible pads constitute the intervertebral discs, which help in the movement of vertebral bodies and provide protection from trauma or shocks. However, the length of the adult vertebral column ranges from 60-70 cm. The entire vertebral column is based on a total of 33 vertebrae that are categorized (below) in accordance with the occupied region.
        i) neck or the cervical region is composed of seven cervical vertebrae.
        ii) back or thorax region contains 12 thoracic vertebrae.
        iii) loin or lumbar region is based on five lumbar vertebrae.
        iv) sacrum forms five (fused) sacral vertebrae.
        v) coccyx (tail) has usually four (fused) coccygeal vertebrae.
    b) Cervical Vertebrae

        These are small and delicate bones, which are marked by the existence of a foramen in every transverse process. The cervical region is based on the seven cervical bones (C1-C7). However, the first cervical vertebra is known as Atlas and the second one is Axis.
    c) Thoracic Vertebrae

        Thoracic vertebrae are 12 in quantity (T1–T12), and communicate with the head (tubercles) of ribs in the thoracic region through articular facets of the transverse processes. Their body structure is similar to the shape of the heart, with nearly circular vertebral foramina.
    d) Lumbar Vertebrae

        These are five vertebrae (L1-L5), with kidney shaped bodies. Lumbar vertebrae are in fact the most toughest and robust in configuration. These are enlarged in size and marked by the absence of a transverse process foramen and vertebral facets. They are true vertebrae, thereby allowing flexion and extension movements via flexible intervertebral discs. Their broad lamellae, large bodies, long transverse processes, and strong pedicles make them suitable to support additional body weight as compared to other similar vertebrae.
    e) Sacral Vertebrae

        These are five vertebral bodies (S1-S5), which constitute a portion of the pelvic cavity. Sacral vertebral bodies consist of five separate segments that get fused together at maturity. As a matter of fact, these vertebrae lack intervertebral discs, which restrict their mobility and put them into the category of false vertebrae.
    f) Coccygeal Vertebrae

        The four coccygeal vertebrae constitute the human vestigial tail bone, in which vertebral bodies are fused together without the existence of any intervertebral disc. Movement of the individual vertebral bodies is restricted due to their interfusion. Hence, these are considered as false vertebrae. The number of bones in the coccygeal region may rarely vary between three to five vertebrae, in few individuals.

3. **Thorax; Anatomical Detail**
    The part of the trunk situated between the neck and abdomen constitutes the thorax. The thoracic cavity is bounded by ribs, sternum, costal cartilages, and the thoracic vertebrae. The thorax is also known as the chest region. The osseocartilaginous cage of the thorax covers and protects the prime organs of circulation and respiration. Furthermore, this osseocartilaginous cage is composed mainly of the ribcage, shoulder girdle, and spine.

    The 12 thoracic vertebrae and certain component of the ribs constitute the posterior (back) wall of the thoracic cavity. However, the anterior (front) region is composed of sternum and the costal cartilages. The entire human chest (thorax) region contains multiple organs, muscles, bones, vasculature, internal and external structures. These contents include heart, lungs, thymus, pectoral muscles, scapula, sternum, ribs, aorta, trachea, diaphragm, and mammary glands etc.

4. **Sternum (Chest or Breast Bone)**
    a) Sternum: It is a flat and long bone situated in the center of the thorax and forms the midline of the anterior thoracic cage. It articulates with both clavicles (collar bones) through its upper ends. It is composed of the following three (interfused) components:
        i)   manubrium
        ii) body (gladiolus/corpus sterni)
        iii) xiphoid process (processus xiphoideus/ensiform or xiphoid appendix) ribs.
    b) Ribs are the elongated, flattened, lightweight, resilient, and twisted bones that are the essential constituent of the thoracic skeleton. The total number of ribs in the human body is 24 (12 on each side). The ribs can be classified as follows:
        i)   True Ribs-These are also called vertebrosternal ribs. True ribs comprise the first seven ribs that communicate (to the dorsum) with the vertebral column as well as sternum (in front) via costal cartilages.

ii) False Ribs-These are also called vertebrochondral ribs. False ribs comprise the eighth, ninth, and tenth ribs that are indirectly attached to the sternum through costal cartilages. The individual cartilages of each of these ribs are connected to the cartilage of the rib lying just above them.

iii) Floating Ribs-These are also termed vertebral ribs. These ribs include the 11th and 12th ribs that are free at their anterior extremities (without any attachment with the sternum) and are connected to the vertebral bodies on their dorsal ends.

5. **The Skull**
The human skull is based on the skeleton of the head. Several bones of the skull integrate together to form the cranium (or the skull). The skull can be categorized as follows:

a) The Brain Box or Brain Case (The Calvaria). It constitutes the upper cranium and contains the brain.

b) The Facial Skeleton comprises the portion of skull (other than the brain box) and includes the mandible bone of the face.

The Composition of Human Skull

The Calvaria			
Paired Bones		Unpaired Bones	
i)	Parietal	i)	Frontal
ii)	Temporal	ii)	Occipital
		iii)	Sphenoid
		iv)	Ethmoid
The Facial Skeleton			
Paired Bones		Unpaired Bones	
iii)	Maxilla	v)	Mandible
iv)	Zygomatic	vi)	Vomer
v)	Nasal		
vi)	Lacrimal		
vii)	Palatine		
viii)	Inferior Nasal Concha		

c. The Facial Bones- The facial skeleton comprises the lower and anterior portion of the human skull and includes the following bones:

i) nasal bones

ii) maxillae (upper jaw)

iii) lacrimal bone

iv) zygomatic bone

v) palatine bone

vi) inferior nasal concha

vii) vomer

viii) mandible (lower jaw)

ix) hyoid bone

6. **The Bones of the Upper Extremity**
a. Clavicle

The clavicle is also called the collar bone that forms the anterior portion of the shoulder girdle. The clavicles are two in number and called the right and left clavicles.

b. Scapula

The scapula is also called the shoulder blade and constitutes the back portion of the shoulder girdle. It is a flat bone that articulates with the clavicle and humerus. It also contains a triangular process that projects laterally and is called the acromion. Additionally, the upper part of the neck of the scapula contains a curved process, which is known as the coracoid process. The scapulae are two in number (right and left scapula).

c. Humerus

The humerus is the long bone of the arm that begins from the shoulder and ends up at the elbow. It is the largest bone of the upper extremity and consists of the following major components:

i) greater tubercle (greater tuberosity)

ii) lesser tubercle (lesser tuberosity)

iii) body or shaft (corpus humeri)

iv) anterior, lateral, and medial borders

v) medial and lateral epicondyles

vi) radial sulcus (musculospiral groove)

vii) lateral and medial supracondylar ridges

viii) deltoid tuberosity.

d. Ulna

The ulna is one of the two long and prismatic bones of the forearm that extends parallel with the radius. The ulna possesses a body and two extremities. The proximal or upper extremity contains olecranon and coronoid processes, and the semilunar and radial notches respectively. The body or shaft of the ulna is also known as the corpus ulnae. The lower or distal extremity is comprised of an articular eminence (the head of the ulna) and a nonarticular eminence (the styloid process).

e. Radius

The radius is one of the two long bones of the forearm that extends laterally with the ulna. Its lower end participates in the formation of the wrist joint and upper end helps to create the elbow joint. The upper or proximal extremity consists of a head, neck, and tuberosity. The body or shaft is also known as the corpus radii. The lateral surface of the lower extremity contains a conical projection, which is known as the styloid process.

f. Carpus

The carpus region of the hand contains the carpal bones, which consist of a total of eight bones positioned in proximal and distal rows to facilitate uninterrupted movement of the wrist joint. The carpal bones of the proximal row are: navicular, lunate, triangular, and pisiform. The bones of the distal row are: greater multangular, lesser multangular, capitate, and hamate.

g. Metacarpus

The metacarpus region of hand is based on cylindrical (metacarpal) bones that are five in number and constitute the intermediary portion of the bony skeleton of hand. The first through fifth metacarpal bones belong to the thumb, index, middle, ring and little fingers respectively.

h. Phalanges of the Hand

The phalanges (finger bones) of the hand constitute the fingers. These are 14 in number. Each finger consists of three phalanges. However, the thumb consists of only two phalanges. A single finger bone has a body, with two extremities. The finger bones serve to facilitate the basic functions of the hand, like-effective grasping of objects and writing, etc.

7. **The Bones of the Lower Extremity**
a. Hip Bone

The hip bone is also known as the coxal bone. It's based on three components: ilium, ischium, and pubis. The ilium holds the flank. It is the broad portion situated on top of the large cup-shaped articular cavity, the acetabulum. The ischium forms the lower back part of the hip bone that facilitates sitting. It's located downward from the acetabulum and is the strongest component of the hip bone, containing an enlarged opening, the obturator foramen. The pubis is the lower frontal portion of the hip bone, which is located medially below the acetabulum. It supports the internal organs of reproduction. The angle across the pubic symphysis is known as the pubic arch.

b. Pelvis

The pelvis consists of a bony ring that provides a connecting medium between the vertebral column and femurs. It is based on the following 4 bones:

i) The hip bones are two in number.

ii) The sacrum-The fused vertebrae that are five in number and connected to the hip bones.

iii) The coccyx-The fused vertebrae that are four in number and constitute the tailbone.

The space surrounded by the pelvic girdle is known as the pelvic cavity. The pelvic girdle bears the entire weight of the trunk and upper body while sitting and transfers this weight to the lower limbs during standing, walking, or running.

c. Femur

The femur is one of the two largest, longest, and strongest bones in the human skeleton that bears the load of the upper body via the pelvis in standing, walking, or running. It also participates in the formation of the hip and knee joints. The components of a normal femur bone are as follows:

The Upper (Proximal) Extremity consists of the following elements:

i) Head

ii) Neck

iii) Greater Trochanter

iv) Lesser Trochanter

The Body or Shaft-The body is cylindrical in shape, lies between the upper and lower extremities and is also known as corpus femoris.

The Lower (Distal) Extremity -The distal extremity is based on two projections (the lateral and medial condyles). These projections (condyles) are separated in front by an articular depression, known as the patellar surface. The same condyles are further interrupted from behind by a deep pit, which is termed as the intercondyloid fossa.

d. Patella

The knee cap (patella) is a flat, thick, circular-triangular, and dense cancellous articular bone that is situated on the frontal portion of the knee joint. The superior border is thick and forms the base of patella. The patella is further marked by medial and lateral borders. The apex of patella is a pointed region that provides attachment to the patellar ligament. The patella articulates with the femur through the patellofemoral joint.

e. Tibia

The tibia (shin bone) is located medially in the lower leg and is regarded as the largest and strongest bone of the skeleton after the femur. It also participates in the formation of the knee and ankle joints. The tibia is composed of the following elements:

i) upper (proximal) end – The proximal extremity is composed of the projections, which are known as the medial and lateral condyles. The condylar surfaces further merge to form an eminence on the frontal side, which is known as the tibial tuberosity.

ii) body or shaft of tibia – The shaft of the tibia is also known as corpus tibiae and contains the anterior crest (or border), the medial border, and the interosseous crest (or lateral border).

iii) lower (distal) end – The distal extremity contains the inferior articular surface, the anterior surface, the posterior surface, the lateral surface, and the medial surface. However, the medial surface extends medially to form a pyramidal process, which is termed as the medial malleolus.

f. Fibula

The fibula (calf bone) is located laterally in the lower leg and runs laterally with the adjacent shin bone (tibia). It's a thin and slender bone which is composed of a body with upper and lower extremities. The lower or distal extremity constitutes the lateral malleolus, which is also known as the external malleolus or malleolus lateralis.

g. Tarsus

The tarsus region of foot is based on the following seven tarsal bones:

i) calcaneus

ii) talus

iii) cuboid

iv) navicular

v) three cuneiforms

h. Phalanges of the Foot

The phalanges of the foot constitute the region of forefoot. These are also known as the toe bones. The great toe (hallux) contains two phalanges (proximal and distal). The proximal and distal phalangeal bones of the great toe articulate with each other to form the first interphalangeal joint. The proximal phalanges of the other toes articulate with their respective metatarsal heads to form the metatarsophalangeal joints.

8. **Syndesmology (The Articulations or Joints)**
Syndesmology is defined as the branch of anatomy that deals with the joints and their components (including ligaments). The junctions of bones, where multiple parts of the individual bones connect together, are called articulations or joints. These articulations are further supported by sheets of tough fibrous tissue that connect the joint bones together and are termed ligaments. Various components of the joints are listed below:

a) Bones

b) Cartilages

The cartilages are flexible nonvascular structures composed of connective tissue and found mainly in joints. A cartilage can be categorized into the following elements:

c) Hyaline cartilage

d) White fibrocartilage

The white fibrocartilage can further be categorized into four subcategories:

i) interarticular fibrocartilage

ii) connecting fibrocartilage

iii) circumferential fibrocartilage

iv) stratiform fibrocartilage

e) Yellow or elastic fibrocartilage

f) Articular Capsule

The articular capsule is also known as the joint capsule that completely covers and protects the freely movable (synovial) joints.

g) Mucous Sheaths

The mucous sheaths cover a part of the fibroosseous canals and surface of the tendons that glide upon these canals to facilitate the movement of these tendons on their respective canals.

9. **Classification of Joints**
The joints can be classified into the following three classes:

a) Synarthroses (Immovable Joints)

b) Amphiarthroses (Slightly Movable Joints)

c) Diarthroses (Freely Movable Joints)

10. **Joints of the Trunk**

a) Joints between Vertebral Bodies

The articulations between the individual vertebral bodies are based on the amphiarthrodial (slightly movable) intervertebral joints that possess only a very slight degree of mobility.

b) Joints between Vertebral Arches

The articulations between the individual vertebral arches are carried out through the two pairs of articular processes. The articular processes of a typical vertebral arch connect together with the articular processes of the adjacent vertebral arch to form true diarthrosis of arthrodial variety.

c) Joints of the Atlas with the Axis

The atlas forms three diarthroses with the axis. Moreover, the articulations of the axis with the atlas are known as the Atlantoaxial articulations.

d) Joints of the Vertebral Column with the Cranium

The atlas forms two articulations (known as diarthrosis) with the occipital bone. The occipital condyles interact with the articular surfaces of the atlas to constitute diarthroses. The synovial stratum covers the articular capsules around the condyles of the occipital bone.

e) Joints of the Mandible

The temporomandibular articulation forms an arthrodial diarthrosis. The temporal mandibular fossa and mandibular condyle interact together to constitute the temporomandibular articulation.

f) Joints of the Ribs with the Vertebrae

The head and tubercle of a typical rib articulates with the vertebral column to form a costovertebral articulation.

g) Joints of the Vertebral Column with the Pelvis

The fifth lumbar vertebra connects with the sacrum to form the lumbosacral articulation. The inner lip of the iliac crest connects with the transverse processes of the fifth lumbar vertebra through iliolumbar ligament.

h) Joints of the Pelvis

The articulations of the pelvis are mainly based on the following types of joints:

i) symphysis pubis

The two pubic bones articulate with each other to constitute a joint, which is known as the symphysis pubis.

ii) sacroiliac articulation

The auricular surfaces of sacrum and ilium connect with each other to form an amphiarthrodial joint, which is termed as the sacroiliac articulation.

iii) sacrococcygeal symphysis

The apex of the sacrum and base of the coccyx articulate with each other to form an amphiarthrodial joint, which is known as the sacrococcygeal symphysis.

11. Joints of Upper Extremity

a) The Acromioclavicular Joint

The medial aspect of the acromion (of the scapula) connects with the acromial end of the clavicle to constitute the acromioclavicular articulation. However, this type of joint is categorized as an arthrodial diarthrosis.

b) The Shoulder Joint

The humeral articulation constitutes the shoulder joint, which is an enarthrodial (ball and socket) joint and considered as the largest joint of the upper limb. The shoulder joint offers an extended range of movement and is composed of the articular head of humerus and the shallow glenoid cavity of the scapula. The ligaments of the shoulder joint include the articular capsule (capsular ligament), glenoid labrum (glenoid ligament) as well as the glenohumeral, coracohumeral, and transverse humeral ligaments.

c) The Elbow Joint

The elbow articulation falls under the category of hinge joint (ginglymus diarthrosis). The elbow joint performs the flexion and extension movements around a transversely placed single axis. The elbow joint consists of the humerus, ulna, and radius bones. An elbow joint is formed when the trochlea of humerus connects with the semilunar notch of ulna and the capitulum of humerus interacts with the cup (shallow-depression or fovea) on the proximal aspect of the head of the radius. The articular surfaces of the elbow joint are enclosed by and interact with each other through a well defined articular capsule.

d) The Radioulnar Joint

The radioulnar joint is based on two articulations positioned at the proximal and distal ends of the radius and ulna. These articulations facilitate the rotational movements of the radius around its longitudinal axis to constitute a uniaxial diarthrosis, which is known as lateral ginglymus.

e) The Radiocarpal Joint

The radiocarpal articulation is also known as the wrist joint, which is a type of condyloid articulation. The distal (lower) end of radius, discus articularis (the articular disc), and the proximal articular surfaces of navicular, lunate and triquetral bones (including their interosseous ligaments) together constitute the wrist articulation. Moreover, the wrist joint is completely encapsulated by the articular capsule.

f) The Intercarpal Joint

The carpal joints are based on the articulations between the carpal bones with limited range of movement. These joints consist of the arthrodial diarthroses and are therefore known as the gliding joints. The carpal bone articulations are characterized as follows:

i) Proximal Row (Carpal) Joint

ii) Distal Row (Carpal) Joint

iii) Transverse (Carpal) Joint

g) The Carpometacarpal joint

The Carpometacarpal (CMC) joints are based on the interaction between the carpal and metacarpal bones. However, the carpometacarpal articulation of the thumb region differs from the articulations of the other four metacarpal bones with the carpus. Therefore, the carpometacarpal articulations can be categorized as follows:

h) The Joints of the other Four Metacarpal Bones with the Carpus

These types of carpometacarpal articulations are formed by the connections between the bases of the second, third, fourth, and fifth medial metacarpal bones and the four bones of the distal carpal row.

i) The Intermetacarpal Joints

The four medial metacarpal bones articulate with each other to form the arthrodial diarthroses, which are known as the intermetacarpal joints.

j) The Metacarpophalangeal Joints

With the exception of the thumb, the spherical head of each metacarpal bone articulates with the shallow oval cavity on the base of the first phalanx to constitute the metacarpophalangeal joints. The metacarpophalangeal articulations facilitate flexion, extension, adduction, abduction, and circumduction type of joint movements.

k) The Joints of the Digits

The interphalangeal joints are categorized as hinge joints that are two in number for each finger and only one for the thumb. The interphalangeal joints can perform movements like flexion and extension.

12. Joints of the Lower Extremity

a) The Hip Joint

The coxal articulation constitutes the hip joint, which is a type of enarthrodial diarthrosis (ball and socket joint). The articular surfaces of the hip joint consist of the head of the femur and a cup shaped cavity (acetabulum) that connect together to constitute the coxal articulation. The hip joint can perform multi-axial movements like rotation, flexion, extension, abduction, and adduction. The hip joint cavity is completely encapsulated by an articular capsule or the capsular ligament. Other ligaments of the hip joint are described below:

i) iliofemoral ligament (ligamentum iliofemorale/Y-ligament/ligament of Bigelow)

ii) pubocapsular ligament (ligamentum pubocapsulare/pubofemoral ligament)

iii) ischiocapsular ligament (ligamentum ischiocapsulare/ischiocapsular band/ligament of Bertin)

iv) ligamentum teres femoris

v) glenoidal labrum (labrum glenoidale/cotyloid ligament)

vi) transverse acetabular ligament (ligamentum transversum acetabuli/transverse ligament)

b) The Knee Joint

The knee articulation/joint is considered as the largest articulation in the human body and related to the ginglymus (hinge) variety of diarthroses. However, its structure is more elaborate and complicated. The articular surfaces of the knee joint pertain to specific portions of the femur, tibia and patella bones. The ligaments associated with the knee joint are as follows:

i) articular capsule (capsula articularis/capsular ligament)

ii) ligamentum patellae (anterior ligament)

iii) oblique popliteal ligament (ligamentum popliteum obliquum/posterior ligament)

iv) tibial collateral ligament (ligamentum collaterale tibiale/internal lateral ligament)

v) fibular collateral ligament (ligamentum collaterale fibulare/external lateral or long external lateral ligament)

vi) anterior cruciate ligament (ligamentum cruciatum anterius/external crucial ligament)

vii) posterior cruciate ligament (ligamentum cruciatum posterius/internal crucial ligament)

viii) medial meniscus (meniscus medialis/internal semilunar fibrocartilage)

ix) lateral meniscus (meniscus lateralis/external semilunar fibrocartilage)

x) transverse ligament (ligamentum transversum genu)

xi) coronary ligaments

xii) synovial membrane encapsulates the upper border of the patella and the lower portion of the front of the femur. The movements associated with the knee joint are flexion, extension, internal, and external rotation.

c) The Joints between Tibia and Fibula

The articulations between the tibia and fibula constitute the tibiofibular joints. The fibula articulates with the tibia through its proximal and distal ends. The proximal tibiofibular joint is an arthrodial articulation between head of the fibula and lateral condyle of the tibia. The interosseous membrane acts as an accessory ligament to bind the shafts of tibia and fibula together. However, the tibiofibular syndesmosis constitutes the distal tibiofibular joint, which presents a series of ligaments that are accessory to the ankle joint.

d) The Talocrural Joint

The talocrural articulation constitutes the ankle joint, which is a ginglymus variety of diarthrosis. In other words, the ankle joint is a type of hinge joint. The ankle joint facilitates the movements like dorsiflexion and extension.

e) The Intertarsal Joints

The intertarsal articulations (joints) are diarthroses that facilitate the gliding movements of the foot. These joints can be categorized in the following manner:

i) talocalcaneal joint

ii) talocalcaneonavicular joint

iii) calcaneocuboid joint

　　iv)　cuneonavicular joint

　　v)　cuboideonavicular joint

　　vi)　intercuneiform and cuneocuboid joint

f)　The Tarsometatarsal Joint

The tarsometatarsal joints include the articular surfaces of the cuneiform, the cuboid, and the metatarsal bones. The articular facets of the three cuneiform and cuboid bones connect with the bases of the five metatarsal bones to constitute the tarsometatarsal articulations.

g)　The Intermetatarsal Joint

The articular facets on the bases of the four metatarsal bones connect with each other via dorsal, plantar, and interosseous ligaments to form the intermetatarsal joints. However, no ligament acts to connect the first metatarsal base with the second one.

h)　The Metatarsophalangeal Joint

The metatarsophalangeal joints are types of modified ball and socket articulations, wherein globular heads of metatarsal bones articulate with the shallow cups upon the bases of the first phalanges via plantar and collateral ligaments. These joints are encapsulated by an articular capsule.

i)　The Joints of the Digits

The articulations between the digits constitute the interphalangeal joints. The phalanges of the toes connect with each other to form the interphalangeal articulations. The great toe possesses only one interphalangeal joint. However, every other toe (except great toe) comprises of two interphalangeal joints.

13. The Muscular System

Introduction

The muscle cells of the human body facilitate the movements of various body parts through their special function of contraction in response to a requisite external or internal stimulus. These muscle cells can be characterized under the below mentioned three different classes:

a)　Striated Muscle Cells

The striated muscle cells are those voluntary muscle cells that constitute the skeletal muscular system.

b)　Non Striated Muscle Cells

The nonstriated muscle cells are those involuntary muscle cells that occur in the vessel walls and hollow viscera.

c)　Cardiac Muscle Cells

The cardiac muscle cells consist of those striated cells that constitute the substance of the heart. However, these muscle cells are involuntary in nature.

14. The Muscles of the Trunk

The muscles of the back are based on the following group of muscles:

a)　Splenius

The splenius muscles constitute the superficial layer of the intrinsic back muscles that occupy the back of neck and upper portion of the thoracic region. The splenius muscles overlap the vertical muscles like a bandage and have the following two types:

　　i)　splenius capitis

　　ii)　splenius cervicis

b)　Sacrospinalis (Erector Spinae)

The erector spinae muscles are positioned in a groove between the angle of the ribs and spinal processes on each side of the vertebral column. The erector spinae is divided into the following three muscle columns:

c)　Iliocostalis

The lateral column is further divided into the following muscle components:

　　i)　iliocostalis lumborum (iliocostalis/sacrolumbalis muscle)

　　ii)　iliocostalis dorsi (musculus accessorius)

　　iii)　iliocostalis cervicis (cervicalis ascendens)

d)　Longissimus

　　i)　longissimus dorsi

　　ii)　longissimus cervicis (transversalis cervicis)

　　iii)　longissimus capitis (trachelomastoid muscle)

e)　Spinalis

　　i)　spinalis dorsi

　　ii)　spinalis cervicis (spinalis coli)

　　iii)　spinalis capitis (biventer cervicis)

f)　Semispinalis

The semispinalis constitute the deeper layer of intrinsic back muscles. These muscles originate from half of the vertebral column and are categorized into three distinct parts:

　　i)　semispinalis dorsi

　　ii)　semispinalis cervicis (semispinalis colli)

　　iii)　semispinalis capitis (complexus)

g)　Multifidus (Multifidus Spinae)

The multifidus consists of short triangular muscular bundles that remain apparent from sacrum to the axis.

h)　Rotatores (Rotatores Spinae)

It remains confined in the thoracic region.

　　i)　Interspinales and Intertransversarii (Intertransversales) are best developed and most distinct in the cervical region and considered as the smallest of the deep back muscles.

15. The Muscles of the Pelvis

The muscles of the pelvis include the following:

a)　Obturator Internus

b)　Piriformis

c)　Levator Ani (Pubococcygeus and Iliococcygeus)

d)　Coccygeus (Ischiococcygeus)

16. The Muscles of the Upper Extremity

a)　The muscles that connect the upper extremity to the vertebral column are defined below:

　　i)　trapezius

　　ii)　rhomboideus major

　　iii)　latissimus dorsi

　　iv)　rhomboideus minor

　　v)　levator scapulae

b)　The Muscles Connecting the Upper Extremity to the Anterior and Lateral Thoracic Walls

　　i)　pectoralis major

　　ii)　subclavius

　　iii)　pectoralis minor

　　iv)　serratus anterior

c)　The Muscles of the Shoulder

　　i)　Deltoid muscle originates from the lateral third portion of clavicle, the acromion, and the spine of scapula. However, it gets inserted into the deltoid tuberosity of humerus. This muscle facilitates the abduction and medial and lateral rotation of the arm.

　　ii)　Subscapularis muscle originates from the subscapular fossa that forms the ventral surface of scapula. However, it gets inserted into the lesser tubercle of humerus. The subscapularis helps to medially rotate and adduct the arm and fixes the humeral head in the glenoid cavity (of the scapula).

　　iii)　Supraspinatus muscle originates from the supraspinatous fossa of scapula and gets inserted into the superior facet of greater tubercle of humerus. This muscle assists the deltoid in the abduction of the arm.

　　iv)　Infraspinatus muscle arises from the infraspinatous fossa of scapula and gets inserted into the middle facet of the greater tubercle of humerus. This muscle helps in the lateral rotation of the arm and fixes the head of humerus into the glenoid cavity of scapula.

　　v)　Teres Minor muscle originates from the middle portion of lateral border of scapula and gets inserted into the inferior facet of greater tubercle of humerus. Like infraspinatus, teres minor muscle also helps in the lateral rotation of the arm and fixes the head of humerus into the glenoid cavity of scapula.

　　vi)　Teres Major muscle arises from the posterior surface of the inferior angle of scapula and gets inserted into the medial lip of the intertubercular groove of humerus. This muscle facilitates the adduction and medial rotation of the arm.

d)　The Muscles of the Arm

　　i)　coracobrachialis

　　ii)　biceps brachii

　　iii)　brachialis

　　iv)　triceps brachii

Diseases of the musculoskeletal system and connective tissue (M00-M99)

NOTES Use an external cause code following the code for the musculoskeletal condition, if applicable, to identify the cause of the musculoskeletal condition

EXCLUDES2 arthropathic psoriasis (L40.5-)

certain conditions originating in the perinatal period (P04-P96)

certain infectious and parasitic diseases (A00-B99)

compartment syndrome (traumatic) (T79.A-)

complications of pregnancy, childbirth and the puerperium (O00-O9A)

congenital malformations, deformations, and chromosomal abnormalities (Q00-Q99)

endocrine, nutritional and metabolic diseases (E00-E88)

injury, poisoning and certain other consequences of external causes (S00-T88)

neoplasms (C00-D49)

symptoms, signs and abnormal clinical and laboratory findings, not elsewhere classified (R00-R94)

This chapter contains the following blocks:

M00-M02	Infectious arthropathies
M04	Autoinflammatory syndromes
	Editor's Note: At press time, CMS deleted this block for 2018 even though there are valid codes within the block. The block has been left here because it includes valid codes. Check www.cms.gov for further updates.
M05-M14	Inflammatory polyarthropathies
M15-M19	Osteoarthritis
M20-M25	Other joint disorders
M26-M27	Dentofacial anomalies [including malocclusion] and other disorders of jaw
M30-M36	Systemic connective tissue disorders
M40-M43	Deforming dorsopathies
M45-M49	Spondylopathies
M50-M54	Other dorsopathies
M60-M63	Disorders of muscles
M65-M67	Disorders of synovium and tendon
M70-M79	Other soft tissue disorders
M80-M85	Disorders of bone density and structure
M86-M90	Other osteopathies
M91-M94	Chondropathies
M95	Other disorders of the musculoskeletal system and connective tissue
M96	Intraoperative and postprocedural complications and disorders of musculoskeletal system, not elsewhere classified
M97	Periprosthetic fracture around internal prosthetic joint
	Editor's Note: At press time, CMS deleted this block for 2018 even though there are valid codes within the block. The block has been left here because it includes valid codes. Check www.cms.gov for further updates.
M99	Biomechanical lesions, not elsewhere classified

Arthropathies (M00-M25)

INCLUDES *Disorders affecting predominantly peripheral (limb) joints*

Infectious arthropathies (M00-M02)

NOTES This block comprises arthropathies due to microbiological agents. Distinction is made between the following types of etiological relationship:
a) direct infection of joint, where organisms invade synovial tissue and microbial antigen is present in the joint;
b) indirect infection, which may be of two types: a reactive arthropathy, where microbial infection of the body is established but neither organisms nor antigens can be identified in the joint, and a postinfective arthropathy, where microbial antigen is present but recovery of an organism is inconstant and evidence of local multiplication is lacking.

M00 Pyogenic arthritis

M00.0 Staphylococcal **arthritis and polyarthritis**

Use additional code (B95.61-B95.8) to identify bacterial agent

EXCLUDES2 *infection and inflammatory reaction due to internal joint prosthesis (T84.5-)*

M00.00 **Staphylococcal arthritis, unspecified joint**

M00.01 Staphylococcal arthritis, shoulder

    M00.011 Staphylococcal arthritis, right shoulder

    M00.012 Staphylococcal arthritis, left shoulder

    M00.019 **Staphylococcal arthritis, unspecified shoulder**

M00.02 Staphylococcal arthritis, elbow

    M00.021 Staphylococcal arthritis, right elbow

    M00.022 Staphylococcal arthritis, left elbow

    M00.029 **Staphylococcal arthritis, unspecified elbow**

M00.03 Staphylococcal arthritis, wrist

    Staphylococcal arthritis of carpal bones

    M00.031 Staphylococcal arthritis, right wrist

    M00.032 Staphylococcal arthritis, left wrist

    M00.039 **Staphylococcal arthritis, unspecified wrist**

M00.04 Staphylococcal arthritis, hand

    Staphylococcal arthritis of metacarpus and phalanges

    M00.041 Staphylococcal arthritis, right hand

    M00.042 Staphylococcal arthritis, left hand

    M00.049 **Staphylococcal arthritis, unspecified hand**

M00.05 Staphylococcal arthritis, hip

    M00.051 Staphylococcal arthritis, right hip

    M00.052 Staphylococcal arthritis, left hip

    M00.059 **Staphylococcal arthritis, unspecified hip**

M00.06 Staphylococcal arthritis, knee

    M00.061 Staphylococcal arthritis, right knee

    M00.062 Staphylococcal arthritis, left knee

    M00.069 **Staphylococcal arthritis, unspecified knee**

M00.07 Staphylococcal arthritis, ankle and foot

    Staphylococcal arthritis, tarsus, metatarsus and phalanges

    M00.071 Staphylococcal arthritis, right ankle and foot

    M00.072 Staphylococcal arthritis, left ankle and foot

    M00.079 **Staphylococcal arthritis, unspecified ankle and foot**

M00.08 Staphylococcal arthritis, vertebrae

M00.09 Staphylococcal polyarthritis

M00.1 Pneumococcal arthritis and polyarthritis

    M00.10 **Pneumococcal arthritis, unspecified joint**

M00.11 Pneumococcal arthritis, shoulder

    M00.111 Pneumococcal arthritis, right shoulder

    M00.112 Pneumococcal arthritis, left shoulder

    M00.119 **Pneumococcal arthritis, unspecified shoulder**

M00.12 Pneumococcal arthritis, elbow

    M00.121 Pneumococcal arthritis, right elbow

PDₓ Unacceptable principal diagnosis symbol per Medicare code edits   **PDₓ** Code exempt from diagnosis present on admission requirement   **?** Questionable admission   **cc** Complication or comorbidity   **CC/MCC Exc** CC/MCC exclusion   **mcc** Major complication or comorbidity   **PDₓ** Principal diagnosis as its own CC   **PDₓ** Principal diagnosis as its own MCC   **HCC** HCC diagnosis code   **RxHCC** RxHCC diagnosis code   MACRA code   **Z** Z code as first-listed diagnosis

M00.122 Pneumococcal arthritis,
         left elbow   cc HCC CC/MCC Exc

M00.129 Pneumococcal arthritis, unspecified
         elbow   cc HCC CC/MCC Exc

6ᵗʰ M00.13 Pneumococcal arthritis, wrist
         Pneumococcal arthritis of carpal bones

M00.131 Pneumococcal arthritis,
         right wrist   cc HCC CC/MCC Exc

M00.132 Pneumococcal arthritis,
         left wrist   cc HCC CC/MCC Exc

M00.139 Pneumococcal arthritis, unspecified
         wrist   cc HCC CC/MCC Exc

6ᵗʰ M00.14 Pneumococcal arthritis, hand
         Pneumococcal arthritis of metacarpus and phalanges

M00.141 Pneumococcal arthritis,
         right hand   cc HCC CC/MCC Exc

M00.142 Pneumococcal arthritis,
         left hand   cc HCC CC/MCC Exc

M00.149 Pneumococcal arthritis, unspecified
         hand   cc HCC CC/MCC Exc

6ᵗʰ M00.15 Pneumococcal arthritis, hip

M00.151 Pneumococcal arthritis,
         right hip   cc HCC CC/MCC Exc

M00.152 Pneumococcal arthritis, left hip   cc HCC CC/MCC Exc

M00.159 Pneumococcal arthritis, unspecified
         hip   cc HCC CC/MCC Exc

6ᵗʰ M00.16 Pneumococcal arthritis, knee

M00.161 Pneumococcal arthritis,
         right knee   cc HCC CC/MCC Exc

M00.162 Pneumococcal arthritis,
         left knee   cc HCC CC/MCC Exc

M00.169 Pneumococcal arthritis, unspecified
         knee   cc HCC CC/MCC Exc

6ᵗʰ M00.17 Pneumococcal arthritis, ankle and foot
         Pneumococcal arthritis, tarsus, metatarsus and
         phalanges

M00.171 Pneumococcal arthritis, right ankle and
         foot   cc HCC CC/MCC Exc

M00.172 Pneumococcal arthritis, left
         ankle and foot   cc HCC CC/MCC Exc

M00.179 Pneumococcal arthritis, unspecified ankle
         and foot   cc HCC CC/MCC Exc

M00.18   Pneumococcal arthritis, vertebrae   cc HCC CC/MCC Exc

M00.19   Pneumococcal polyarthritis   cc HCC CC/MCC Exc

5ᵗʰ M00.2 Other streptococcal arthritis and polyarthritis
         Use additional code (B95.0-B95.2, B95.4-B95.5) to identify
         bacterial agent

M00.20   Other streptococcal arthritis,
         unspecified joint   cc HCC CC/MCC Exc

6ᵗʰ M00.21 Other streptococcal arthritis, shoulder

M00.211 Other streptococcal arthritis, right
         shoulder   cc HCC CC/MCC Exc

M00.212 Other streptococcal arthritis,
         left shoulder   cc HCC CC/MCC Exc

M00.219 Other streptococcal arthritis, unspecified
         shoulder   cc HCC CC/MCC Exc

6ᵗʰ M00.22 Other streptococcal arthritis, elbow

M00.221 Other streptococcal arthritis,
         right elbow   cc HCC CC/MCC Exc

M00.222 Other streptococcal arthritis,
         left elbow   cc HCC CC/MCC Exc

M00.229 Other streptococcal arthritis, unspecified
         elbow   cc HCC CC/MCC Exc

6ᵗʰ M00.23 Other streptococcal arthritis, wrist
         Other streptococcal arthritis of carpal bones

M00.231 Other streptococcal arthritis,
         right wrist   cc HCC CC/MCC Exc

M00.232 Other streptococcal arthritis,
         left wrist   cc HCC CC/MCC Exc

M00.239 Other streptococcal arthritis, unspecified
         wrist   cc HCC CC/MCC Exc

6ᵗʰ M00.24 Other streptococcal arthritis, hand
         Other streptococcal arthritis metacarpus and
         phalanges

M00.241 Other streptococcal arthritis,
         right hand   cc HCC CC/MCC Exc

M00.242 Other streptococcal arthritis,
         left hand   cc HCC CC/MCC Exc

M00.249 Other streptococcal arthritis, unspecified
         hand   cc HCC CC/MCC Exc

6ᵗʰ M00.25 Other streptococcal arthritis, hip

M00.251 Other streptococcal arthritis,
         right hip   cc HCC CC/MCC Exc

M00.252 Other streptococcal arthritis,
         left hip   cc HCC CC/MCC Exc

M00.259 Other streptococcal arthritis, unspecified
         hip   cc HCC CC/MCC Exc

6ᵗʰ M00.26 Other streptococcal arthritis, knee

M00.261 Other streptococcal arthritis,
         right knee   cc HCC CC/MCC Exc

M00.262 Other streptococcal arthritis,
         left knee   cc HCC CC/MCC Exc

M00.269 Other streptococcal arthritis, unspecified
         knee   cc HCC CC/MCC Exc

6ᵗʰ M00.27 Other streptococcal arthritis,
         ankle and foot
         Other streptococcal arthritis, tarsus, metatarsus and
         phalanges

M00.271 Other streptococcal arthritis, right ankle
         and foot   cc HCC CC/MCC Exc

M00.272 Other streptococcal arthritis, left ankle
         and foot   cc HCC CC/MCC Exc

M00.279 Other streptococcal arthritis, unspecified
         ankle and foot   cc HCC CC/MCC Exc

M00.28   Other streptococcal arthritis, vertebrae   cc HCC CC/MCC Exc

M00.29   Other streptococcal polyarthritis   cc HCC CC/MCC Exc

5ᵗʰ M00.8 Arthritis and polyarthritis due to other bacteria
         Use additional code (B96) to identify bacteria

M00.80   Arthritis due to other bacteria,
         unspecified joint   cc HCC CC/MCC Exc

6ᵗʰ M00.81 Arthritis due to other bacteria, shoulder

M00.811 Arthritis due to other bacteria, right
         shoulder   cc HCC CC/MCC Exc

M00.812 Arthritis due to other bacteria, left
         shoulder   cc HCC CC/MCC Exc

M00.819 Arthritis due to other bacteria, unspecified
         shoulder   cc HCC CC/MCC Exc

6ᵗʰ M00.82 Arthritis due to other bacteria, elbow

M00.821 Arthritis due to other bacteria,
         right elbow   cc HCC CC/MCC Exc

M00.822 Arthritis due to other bacteria,
         left elbow   cc HCC CC/MCC Exc

M00.829 Arthritis due to other bacteria, unspecified
         elbow   cc HCC CC/MCC Exc

6ᵗʰ M00.83 Arthritis due to other bacteria, wrist
         Arthritis due to other bacteria, carpal bones

M00.831 Arthritis due to other bacteria,
         right wrist   cc HCC CC/MCC Exc

M00.832 Arthritis due to other bacteria, left
         wrist   cc HCC CC/MCC Exc

M00.839 Arthritis due to other bacteria, unspecified
         wrist   cc HCC CC/MCC Exc

6ᵗʰ M00.84 Arthritis due to other bacteria, hand
         Arthritis due to other bacteria, metacarpus and
         phalanges

M00.841 Arthritis due to other bacteria,
         right hand   cc HCC CC/MCC Exc

M00.842 Arthritis due to other bacteria,
         left hand   cc HCC CC/MCC Exc

M00.849 Arthritis due to other bacteria, unspecified
         hand   cc HCC CC/MCC Exc

6ᵗʰ M00.85 Arthritis due to other bacteria, hip

Unspecified Code   Other Specified Code   Manifestation Code   Ⓝ Newborn   Ⓟ Pediatric   Ⓜ Maternity   Ⓐ Adult   ♂ Male   ♀ Female
● New Code   ▲ Revised Code Title   ►◄ Revised Text   NOTES   INCLUDES   EXCLUDES 1   Not coded here   EXCLUDES 2   Not included here
4ᵗʰ character required   5ᵗʰ character required   6ᵗʰ character required   7ᵗʰ character required
Extension 'X' Alert   HAC Hospital-acquired condition (HAC) alert   AHA AHA Coding Clinic©

M00.851 **Arthritis due to other bacteria, right hip** [CC] [HCC] [CC/MCC Exc]

M00.852 **Arthritis due to other bacteria, left hip** [CC] [HCC] [CC/MCC Exc]

M00.859 **Arthritis due to other bacteria, unspecified hip** [CC] [HCC] [CC/MCC Exc]

[6th] M00.86 **Arthritis due to other bacteria, knee**

M00.861 **Arthritis due to other bacteria, right knee** [CC] [HCC] [CC/MCC Exc]

M00.862 **Arthritis due to other bacteria, left knee** [CC] [HCC] [CC/MCC Exc]

M00.869 **Arthritis due to other bacteria, unspecified knee** [CC] [HCC] [CC/MCC Exc]

[6th] M00.87 **Arthritis due to other bacteria, ankle and foot**

Arthritis due to other bacteria, tarsus, metatarsus, and phalanges

M00.871 **Arthritis due to other bacteria, right ankle and foot** [CC] [HCC] [CC/MCC Exc]

M00.872 **Arthritis due to other bacteria, left ankle and foot** [CC] [HCC] [CC/MCC Exc]

M00.879 **Arthritis due to other bacteria, unspecified ankle and foot** [CC] [HCC] [CC/MCC Exc]

M00.88 **Arthritis due to other bacteria, vertebrae** [CC] [HCC] [CC/MCC Exc]

M00.89 **Polyarthritis due to other bacteria** [CC] [HCC] [CC/MCC Exc]

M00.9 **Pyogenic arthritis, unspecified** [CC] [HCC] [CC/MCC Exc]

Infective arthritis NOS

[4th] M01 **Direct infections of joint in infectious and parasitic diseases classified elsewhere**

Code first underlying disease, such as:
leprosy [Hansen's disease] (A30.-)
mycoses (B35-B49)
O'nyong-nyong fever (A92.1)
paratyphoid fever (A01.1-A01.4)

[EXCLUDES1] *arthropathy in Lyme disease (A69.23)*
gonococcal arthritis (A54.42)
meningococcal arthritis (A39.83)
mumps arthritis (B26.85)
postinfective arthropathy (M02.-)
postmeningococcal arthritis (A39.84)
reactive arthritis (M02.3)
rubella arthritis (B06.82)
sarcoidosis arthritis (D86.86)
typhoid fever arthritis (A01.04)
tuberculosis arthritis (A18.01-A18.02)

[5th] M01.X **Direct infection of joint in infectious and parasitic diseases classified elsewhere**

M01.X0 **Direct infection of unspecified joint in infectious and parasitic diseases classified elsewhere** [CC] [HCC] [CC/MCC Exc]

[6th] M01.X1 **Direct infection of shoulder joint in infectious and parasitic diseases classified elsewhere**

M01.X11 **Direct infection of right shoulder in infectious and parasitic diseases classified elsewhere** [CC] [HCC] [CC/MCC Exc]

M01.X12 **Direct infection of left shoulder in infectious and parasitic diseases classified elsewhere** [CC] [HCC] [CC/MCC Exc]

M01.X19 **Direct infection of unspecified shoulder in infectious and parasitic diseases classified elsewhere** [CC] [HCC] [CC/MCC Exc]

[6th] M01.X2 **Direct infection of elbow in infectious and parasitic diseases classified elsewhere**

M01.X21 **Direct infection of right elbow in infectious and parasitic diseases classified elsewhere** [CC] [HCC] [CC/MCC Exc]

M01.X22 **Direct infection of left elbow in infectious and parasitic diseases classified elsewhere** [CC] [HCC] [CC/MCC Exc]

M01.X29 **Direct infection of unspecified elbow in infectious and parasitic diseases classified elsewhere** [CC] [HCC] [CC/MCC Exc]

[6th] M01.X3 **Direct infection of wrist in infectious and parasitic diseases classified elsewhere**

Direct infection of carpal bones in infectious and parasitic diseases classified elsewhere

M01.X31 **Direct infection of right wrist in infectious and parasitic diseases classified elsewhere** [CC] [HCC] [CC/MCC Exc]

M01.X32 **Direct infection of left wrist in infectious and parasitic diseases classified elsewhere** [CC] [HCC] [CC/MCC Exc]

M01.X39 **Direct infection of unspecified wrist in infectious and parasitic diseases classified elsewhere** [CC] [HCC] [CC/MCC Exc]

[6th] M01.X4 **Direct infection of hand in infectious and parasitic diseases classified elsewhere**

Direct infection of metacarpus and phalanges in infectious and parasitic diseases classified elsewhere

M01.X41 **Direct infection of right hand in infectious and parasitic diseases classified elsewhere** [CC] [HCC] [CC/MCC Exc]

M01.X42 **Direct infection of left hand in infectious and parasitic diseases classified elsewhere** [CC] [HCC] [CC/MCC Exc]

M01.X49 **Direct infection of unspecified hand in infectious and parasitic diseases classified elsewhere** [CC] [HCC] [CC/MCC Exc]

[6th] M01.X5 **Direct infection of hip in infectious and parasitic diseases classified elsewhere**

M01.X51 **Direct infection of right hip in infectious and parasitic diseases classified elsewhere** [CC] [HCC] [CC/MCC Exc]

M01.X52 **Direct infection of left hip in infectious and parasitic diseases classified elsewhere** [CC] [HCC] [CC/MCC Exc]

M01.X59 **Direct infection of unspecified hip in infectious and parasitic diseases classified elsewhere** [CC] [HCC] [CC/MCC Exc]

[6th] M01.X6 **Direct infection of knee in infectious and parasitic diseases classified elsewhere**

M01.X61 **Direct infection of right knee in infectious and parasitic diseases classified elsewhere** [CC] [HCC] [CC/MCC Exc]

M01.X62 **Direct infection of left knee in infectious and parasitic diseases classified elsewhere** [CC] [HCC] [CC/MCC Exc]

M01.X69 **Direct infection of unspecified knee in infectious and parasitic diseases classified elsewhere** [CC] [HCC] [CC/MCC Exc]

[6th] M01.X7 **Direct infection of ankle and foot in infectious and parasitic diseases classified elsewhere**

Direct infection of tarsus, metatarsus and phalanges in infectious and parasitic diseases classified elsewhere

M01.X71 **Direct infection of right ankle and foot in infectious and parasitic diseases classified elsewhere** [CC] [HCC] [CC/MCC Exc]

M01.X72 **Direct infection of left ankle and foot in infectious and parasitic diseases classified elsewhere** [CC] [HCC] [CC/MCC Exc]

M01.X79 **Direct infection of unspecified ankle and foot in infectious and parasitic diseases classified elsewhere** [CC] [HCC] [CC/MCC Exc]

M01.X8 **Direct infection of vertebrae in infectious and parasitic diseases classified elsewhere** [CC] [HCC] [CC/MCC Exc]

M01.X9 **Direct infection of multiple joints in infectious and parasitic diseases classified elsewhere** [CC] [HCC] [CC/MCC Exc]

[4th] M02 **Postinfective and reactive arthropathies**

Code first underlying disease, such as:
congenital syphilis [Clutton's joints] (A50.5)
enteritis due to Yersinia enterocolitica (A04.6)
infective endocarditis (I33.0)
viral hepatitis (B15-B19)

[EXCLUDES1] *Behçet's disease (M35.2)*

[PDx] Unacceptable principal diagnosis symbol per Medicare code edits; [POA] Code exempt from diagnosis present on admission requirement; [?] Questionable admission; [CC] Complication or comorbidity; [CC/MCC Exc] CC/MCC exclusion; [MCC] Major complication or comorbidity; [PDx CC] Principal diagnosis as its own CC; [PDx MCC] Principal diagnosis as its own MCC; [HCC] HCC diagnosis code; [RxHCC] RxHCC diagnosis code; MACRA code; [Z-1] Z code as first-listed diagnosis

direct infections of joint in infectious and parasitic diseases classified elsewhere (M01.-)

postmeningococcal arthritis (A39.84)

mumps arthritis (B26.85)

rubella arthritis (B06.82)

syphilis arthritis (late) (A52.77)

rheumatic fever (I00)

tabetic arthropathy [Charcôt's] (A52.16)

M02.0 Arthropathy following intestinal bypass

    M02.00 Arthropathy following intestinal bypass, unspecified site

    M02.01 Arthropathy following intestinal bypass, shoulder

        M02.011 Arthropathy following intestinal bypass, right shoulder

        M02.012 Arthropathy following intestinal bypass, left shoulder

        M02.019 Arthropathy following intestinal bypass, unspecified shoulder

    M02.02 Arthropathy following intestinal bypass, elbow

        M02.021 Arthropathy following intestinal bypass, right elbow

        M02.022 Arthropathy following intestinal bypass, left elbow

        M02.029 Arthropathy following intestinal bypass, unspecified elbow

    M02.03 Arthropathy following intestinal bypass, wrist

        Arthropathy following intestinal bypass, carpal bones

        M02.031 Arthropathy following intestinal bypass, right wrist

        M02.032 Arthropathy following intestinal bypass, left wrist

        M02.039 Arthropathy following intestinal bypass, unspecified wrist

    M02.04 Arthropathy following intestinal bypass, hand

        Arthropathy following intestinal bypass, metacarpals and phalanges

        M02.041 Arthropathy following intestinal bypass, right hand

        M02.042 Arthropathy following intestinal bypass, left hand

        M02.049 Arthropathy following intestinal bypass, unspecified hand

    M02.05 Arthropathy following intestinal bypass, hip

        M02.051 Arthropathy following intestinal bypass, right hip

        M02.052 Arthropathy following intestinal bypass, left hip

        M02.059 Arthropathy following intestinal bypass, unspecified hip

    M02.06 Arthropathy following intestinal bypass, knee

        M02.061 Arthropathy following intestinal bypass, right knee

        M02.062 Arthropathy following intestinal bypass, left knee

        M02.069 Arthropathy following intestinal bypass, unspecified knee

    M02.07 Arthropathy following intestinal bypass, ankle and foot

        Arthropathy following intestinal bypass, tarsus, metatarsus and phalanges

        M02.071 Arthropathy following intestinal bypass, right ankle and foot

        M02.072 Arthropathy following intestinal bypass, left ankle and foot

        M02.079 Arthropathy following intestinal bypass, unspecified ankle and foot

    M02.08 Arthropathy following intestinal bypass, vertebrae

    M02.09 Arthropathy following intestinal bypass, multiple sites

M02.1 Postdysenteric arthropathy

M02.10 Postdysenteric arthropathy, unspecified site

M02.11 Postdysenteric arthropathy, shoulder

    M02.111 Postdysenteric arthropathy, right shoulder

    M02.112 Postdysenteric arthropathy, left shoulder

    M02.119 Postdysenteric arthropathy, unspecified shoulder

M02.12 Postdysenteric arthropathy, elbow

    M02.121 Postdysenteric arthropathy, right elbow

    M02.122 Postdysenteric arthropathy, left elbow

    M02.129 Postdysenteric arthropathy, unspecified elbow

M02.13 Postdysenteric arthropathy, wrist

    Postdysenteric arthropathy, carpal bones

    M02.131 Postdysenteric arthropathy, right wrist

    M02.132 Postdysenteric arthropathy, left wrist

    M02.139 Postdysenteric arthropathy, unspecified wrist

M02.14 Postdysenteric arthropathy, hand

    Postdysenteric arthropathy, metacarpus and phalanges

    M02.141 Postdysenteric arthropathy, right hand

    M02.142 Postdysenteric arthropathy, left hand

    M02.149 Postdysenteric arthropathy, unspecified hand

M02.15 Postdysenteric arthropathy, hip

    M02.151 Postdysenteric arthropathy, right hip

    M02.152 Postdysenteric arthropathy, left hip

    M02.159 Postdysenteric arthropathy, unspecified hip

M02.16 Postdysenteric arthropathy, knee

    M02.161 Postdysenteric arthropathy, right knee

    M02.162 Postdysenteric arthropathy, left knee

    M02.169 Postdysenteric arthropathy, unspecified knee

M02.17 Postdysenteric arthropathy, ankle and foot

    Postdysenteric arthropathy, tarsus, metatarsus and phalanges

    M02.171 Postdysenteric arthropathy, right ankle and foot

    M02.172 Postdysenteric arthropathy, left ankle and foot

    M02.179 Postdysenteric arthropathy, unspecified ankle and foot

M02.18 Postdysenteric arthropathy, vertebrae

M02.19 Postdysenteric arthropathy, multiple sites

M02.2 Postimmunization arthropathy

    M02.20 Postimmunization arthropathy, unspecified site

M02.21 Postimmunization arthropathy, shoulder

    M02.211 Postimmunization arthropathy, right shoulder

    M02.212 Postimmunization arthropathy, left shoulder

    M02.219 Postimmunization arthropathy, unspecified shoulder

M02.22 Postimmunization arthropathy, elbow

    M02.221 Postimmunization arthropathy, right elbow

    M02.222 Postimmunization arthropathy, left elbow

    M02.229 Postimmunization arthropathy, unspecified elbow

Unspecified Code Other Specified Code Manifestation Code N Newborn P Pediatric M Maternity A Adult ♂ Male ♀ Female
● New Code ▲ Revised Code Title ►◄ Revised Text NOTES *INCLUDES* *EXCLUDES 1* Not coded here *EXCLUDES 2* Not included here
4th character required 5th character required 6th character required 7th character required
Extension 'X' Alert HAC Hospital-acquired condition (HAC) alert **AHA** AHA Coding Clinic©

M02.23 **Postimmunization arthropathy,** wrist
Postimmunization arthropathy, carpal bones
M02.231 **Postimmunization arthropathy,** right **wrist**
M02.232 **Postimmunization arthropathy,** left **wrist**
M02.239 **Postimmunization arthropathy, unspecified wrist**

M02.24 **Postimmunization arthropathy,** hand
Postimmunization arthropathy, metacarpus and phalanges
M02.241 **Postimmunization arthropathy,** right **hand**
M02.242 **Postimmunization arthropathy,** left **hand**
M02.249 **Postimmunization arthropathy, unspecified hand**

M02.25 **Postimmunization arthropathy,** hip
M02.251 **Postimmunization arthropathy,** right **hip**
M02.252 **Postimmunization arthropathy,** left **hip**
M02.259 **Postimmunization arthropathy, unspecified hip**

M02.26 **Postimmunization arthropathy,** knee
M02.261 **Postimmunization arthropathy,** right **knee**
M02.262 **Postimmunization arthropathy,** left **knee**
M02.269 **Postimmunization arthropathy, unspecified knee**

M02.27 **Postimmunization arthropathy,** ankle and foot
Postimmunization arthropathy, tarsus, metatarsus and phalanges
M02.271 **Postimmunization arthropathy,** right **ankle and foot**
M02.272 **Postimmunization arthropathy,** left **ankle and foot**
M02.279 **Postimmunization arthropathy, unspecified ankle and foot**

M02.28 **Postimmunization arthropathy,** vertebrae
M02.29 **Postimmunization arthropathy,** multiple sites

M02.3 **Reiter's disease**
Reactive arthritis
M02.30 **Reiter's disease, unspecified site** HCC CC/MCC Exc
M02.31 **Reiter's disease,** shoulder
M02.311 **Reiter's disease,** right **shoulder** HCC CC/MCC Exc
M02.312 **Reiter's disease,** left **shoulder** HCC CC/MCC Exc
M02.319 **Reiter's disease, unspecified shoulder** HCC CC/MCC Exc

M02.32 **Reiter's disease,** elbow
M02.321 **Reiter's disease,** right **elbow** HCC CC/MCC Exc
M02.322 **Reiter's disease,** left **elbow** HCC CC/MCC Exc
M02.329 **Reiter's disease, unspecified elbow** HCC CC/MCC Exc

M02.33 **Reiter's disease,** wrist
Reiter's disease, carpal bones
M02.331 **Reiter's disease,** right **wrist** HCC CC/MCC Exc
M02.332 **Reiter's disease,** left **wrist** HCC CC/MCC Exc
M02.339 **Reiter's disease, unspecified wrist** HCC CC/MCC Exc

M02.34 **Reiter's disease,** hand
Reiter's disease, metacarpus and phalanges
M02.341 **Reiter's disease,** right **hand** HCC CC/MCC Exc
M02.342 **Reiter's disease,** left **hand** HCC CC/MCC Exc
M02.349 **Reiter's disease, unspecified hand** HCC CC/MCC Exc

M02.35 **Reiter's disease,** hip
M02.351 **Reiter's disease,** right **hip** HCC CC/MCC Exc
M02.352 **Reiter's disease,** left **hip** HCC CC/MCC Exc
M02.359 **Reiter's disease, unspecified hip** HCC CC/MCC Exc

M02.36 **Reiter's disease,** knee
M02.361 **Reiter's disease,** right **knee** HCC CC/MCC Exc
M02.362 **Reiter's disease,** left **knee** HCC CC/MCC Exc
M02.369 **Reiter's disease, unspecified knee** HCC CC/MCC Exc

M02.37 **Reiter's disease,** ankle and foot
Reiter's disease, tarsus, metatarsus and phalanges
M02.371 **Reiter's disease,** right **ankle and foot** HCC CC/MCC Exc
M02.372 **Reiter's disease,** left **ankle and foot** HCC CC/MCC Exc
M02.379 **Reiter's disease, unspecified ankle and foot** HCC CC/MCC Exc

M02.38 **Reiter's disease,** vertebrae HCC CC/MCC Exc
M02.39 **Reiter's disease,** multiple sites HCC CC/MCC Exc

M02.8 Other reactive arthropathies
M02.80 **Other reactive arthropathies, unspecified site** HCC CC/MCC Exc
M02.81 **Other reactive arthropathies,** shoulder
M02.811 **Other reactive arthropathies, right shoulder** HCC CC/MCC Exc
M02.812 **Other reactive arthropathies, left shoulder** HCC CC/MCC Exc
M02.819 **Other reactive arthropathies, unspecified shoulder** HCC CC/MCC Exc

M02.82 **Other reactive arthropathies,** elbow
M02.821 **Other reactive arthropathies, right elbow** HCC CC/MCC Exc
M02.822 **Other reactive arthropathies, left elbow** HCC CC/MCC Exc
M02.829 **Other reactive arthropathies, unspecified elbow** HCC CC/MCC Exc

M02.83 **Other reactive arthropathies,** wrist
Other reactive arthropathies, carpal bones
M02.831 **Other reactive arthropathies, right wrist** HCC CC/MCC Exc
M02.832 **Other reactive arthropathies, left wrist** HCC CC/MCC Exc
M02.839 **Other reactive arthropathies, unspecified wrist** HCC CC/MCC Exc

M02.84 **Other reactive arthropathies,** hand
Other reactive arthropathies, metacarpus and phalanges
M02.841 **Other reactive arthropathies, right hand** HCC CC/MCC Exc
M02.842 **Other reactive arthropathies, left hand** HCC CC/MCC Exc
M02.849 **Other reactive arthropathies, unspecified hand** HCC CC/MCC Exc

M02.85 **Other reactive arthropathies,** hip
M02.851 **Other reactive arthropathies, right hip** HCC CC/MCC Exc
M02.852 **Other reactive arthropathies, left hip** HCC CC/MCC Exc
M02.859 **Other reactive arthropathies, unspecified hip** HCC CC/MCC Exc

M02.86 **Other reactive arthropathies,** knee
M02.861 **Other reactive arthropathies, right knee** HCC CC/MCC Exc
M02.862 **Other reactive arthropathies, left knee** HCC CC/MCC Exc
M02.869 **Other reactive arthropathies, unspecified knee** HCC CC/MCC Exc

M02.87 **Other reactive arthropathies,** ankle and foot
Other reactive arthropathies, tarsus, metatarsus and phalanges
M02.871 **Other reactive arthropathies, right ankle and foot** HCC CC/MCC Exc
M02.872 **Other reactive arthropathies, left ankle and foot** HCC CC/MCC Exc

PDx Unacceptable principal diagnosis symbol per Medicare code edits   POA Code exempt from diagnosis present on admission requirement
Questionable admission   Complication or comorbidity   CC/MCC Exc CC/MCC exclusion   MCC Major complication or comorbidity
PDx Principal diagnosis as its own CC   Principal diagnosis as its own MCC   HCC HCC diagnosis code   RxHCC RxHCC diagnosis code
MACRA code   Z1 Z code as first-listed diagnosis

778

When symbols appear on a code that requires a 7th character extension, refer to Appendix B to identify applicable 7th character codes.

2018 ICD-10-CM

M02.879 Other reactive arthropathies, unspecified ankle and foot [CC] [HCC] [CC/MCC Exc]
M02.88 Other reactive arthropathies, vertebrae [CC] [HCC] [CC/MCC Exc]
M02.89 Other reactive arthropathies, multiple sites [CC] [HCC] [CC/MCC Exc]
M02.9 Reactive arthropathy, unspecified [HCC]

Autoinflammatory syndromes (M04)

[4th] M04 Autoinflammatory syndromes
[EXCLUDES2] *Crohn's disease (K50.-)*
M04.1 Periodic fever syndromes [HCC] [RxHCC]
AHA: Q4 2016
Familial Mediterranean fever
Hyperimmunoglobin D syndrome
Mevalonate kinase deficiency
Tumor necrosis factor receptor associated periodic syndrome [TRAPS]
M04.2 Cryopyrin-associated periodic syndromes [HCC] [RxHCC]
AHA: Q4 2016
Chronic infantile neurological, cutaneous and articular syndrome [CINCA]
Familial cold autoinflammatory syndrome
Familial cold urticaria
Muckle-Wells syndrome
Neonatal onset multisystemic inflammatory disorder [NOMID]
M04.8 Other autoinflammatory syndromes [HCC] [RxHCC]
AHA: Q4 2016
Blau syndrome
Deficiency of interleukin 1 receptor antagonist [DIRA]
Majeed syndrome
Periodic fever, aphthous stomatitis, pharyngitis, and adenopathy syndrome [PFAPA]
Pyogenic arthritis, pyoderma gangrenosum, and acne syndrome [PAPA]
M04.9 Autoinflammatory syndrome, unspecified [HCC] [RxHCC]
AHA: Q4 2016

Inflammatory polyarthropathies (M05-M14)

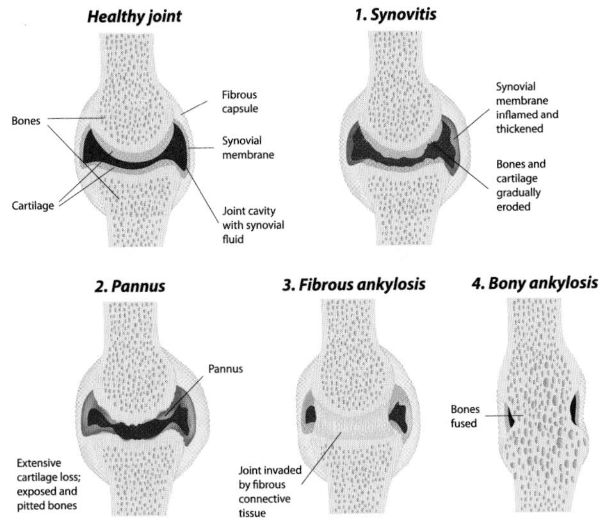
Healthy joint
1. Synovitis
Bones
Fibrous capsule
Synovial membrane
Cartilage
Joint cavity with synovial fluid
Synovial membrane inflamed and thickened
Bones and cartilage gradually eroded
2. Pannus
3. Fibrous ankylosis
4. Bony ankylosis
Pannus
Extensive cartilage loss; exposed and pitted bones
Joint invaded by fibrous connective tissue
Bones fused

Figure 13.1 Stages of rheumatoid arthritis

[4th] M05 Rheumatoid arthritis with rheumatoid factor
[EXCLUDES1] *rheumatic fever (I00)*
juvenile rheumatoid arthritis (M08.-)
rheumatoid arthritis of spine (M45.-)
[5th] M05.0 Felty's syndrome
Rheumatoid arthritis with splenoadenomegaly and leukopenia
M05.00 Felty's syndrome, unspecified site [HCC] [RxHCC]
[6th] M05.01 Felty's syndrome, shoulder
M05.011 Felty's syndrome, right shoulder [HCC] [RxHCC]
M05.012 Felty's syndrome, left shoulder [HCC] [RxHCC]
M05.019 Felty's syndrome, unspecified shoulder [HCC] [RxHCC]
[6th] M05.02 Felty's syndrome, elbow
M05.021 Felty's syndrome, right elbow [HCC] [RxHCC]
M05.022 Felty's syndrome, left elbow [HCC] [RxHCC]
M05.029 Felty's syndrome, unspecified elbow [HCC] [RxHCC]
[6th] M05.03 Felty's syndrome, wrist
Felty's syndrome, carpal bones
M05.031 Felty's syndrome, right wrist [HCC] [RxHCC]
M05.032 Felty's syndrome, left wrist [HCC] [RxHCC]
M05.039 Felty's syndrome, unspecified wrist [HCC] [RxHCC]
[6th] M05.04 Felty's syndrome, hand
Felty's syndrome, metacarpus and phalanges
M05.041 Felty's syndrome, right hand [HCC] [RxHCC]
M05.042 Felty's syndrome, left hand [HCC] [RxHCC]
M05.049 Felty's syndrome, unspecified hand [HCC] [RxHCC]
[6th] M05.05 Felty's syndrome, hip
M05.051 Felty's syndrome, right hip [HCC] [RxHCC]
M05.052 Felty's syndrome, left hip [HCC] [RxHCC]
M05.059 Felty's syndrome, unspecified hip [HCC] [RxHCC]
[6th] M05.06 Felty's syndrome, knee
M05.061 Felty's syndrome, right knee [HCC] [RxHCC]
M05.062 Felty's syndrome, left knee [HCC] [RxHCC]
M05.069 Felty's syndrome, unspecified knee [HCC] [RxHCC]
[6th] M05.07 Felty's syndrome, ankle and foot
Felty's syndrome, tarsus, metatarsus and phalanges
M05.071 Felty's syndrome, right ankle and foot [HCC] [RxHCC]
M05.072 Felty's syndrome, left ankle and foot [HCC] [RxHCC]
M05.079 Felty's syndrome, unspecified ankle and foot [HCC] [RxHCC]
M05.09 Felty's syndrome, multiple sites [HCC] [RxHCC]
[5th] M05.1 Rheumatoid lung disease with rheumatoid arthritis
M05.10 Rheumatoid lung disease with rheumatoid arthritis of unspecified site [HCC] [RxHCC]
[6th] M05.11 Rheumatoid lung disease with rheumatoid arthritis of shoulder
M05.111 Rheumatoid lung disease with rheumatoid arthritis of right shoulder [HCC] [RxHCC]
M05.112 Rheumatoid lung disease with rheumatoid arthritis of left shoulder [HCC] [RxHCC]
M05.119 Rheumatoid lung disease with rheumatoid arthritis of unspecified shoulder [HCC] [RxHCC]
[6th] M05.12 Rheumatoid lung disease with rheumatoid arthritis of elbow
M05.121 Rheumatoid lung disease with rheumatoid arthritis of right elbow [HCC] [RxHCC]
M05.122 Rheumatoid lung disease with rheumatoid arthritis of left elbow [HCC] [RxHCC]
M05.129 Rheumatoid lung disease with rheumatoid arthritis of unspecified elbow [HCC] [RxHCC]
[6th] M05.13 Rheumatoid lung disease with rheumatoid arthritis of wrist
Rheumatoid lung disease with rheumatoid arthritis, carpal bones
M05.131 Rheumatoid lung disease with rheumatoid arthritis of right wrist [HCC] [RxHCC]
M05.132 Rheumatoid lung disease with rheumatoid arthritis of left wrist [HCC] [RxHCC]
M05.139 Rheumatoid lung disease with rheumatoid arthritis of unspecified wrist [HCC] [RxHCC]
[6th] M05.14 Rheumatoid lung disease with rheumatoid arthritis of hand
Rheumatoid lung disease with rheumatoid arthritis, metacarpus and phalanges
M05.141 Rheumatoid lung disease with rheumatoid arthritis of right hand [HCC] [RxHCC]

M05.142 Rheumatoid lung disease with rheumatoid arthritis of left hand HCC RxHCC

M05.149 Rheumatoid lung disease with rheumatoid arthritis of unspecified hand HCC RxHCC

M05.15 Rheumatoid lung disease with rheumatoid arthritis of hip

M05.151 Rheumatoid lung disease with rheumatoid arthritis of right hip HCC RxHCC

M05.152 Rheumatoid lung disease with rheumatoid arthritis of left hip HCC RxHCC

M05.159 Rheumatoid lung disease with rheumatoid arthritis of unspecified hip HCC RxHCC

M05.16 Rheumatoid lung disease with rheumatoid arthritis of knee

M05.161 Rheumatoid lung disease with rheumatoid arthritis of right knee HCC RxHCC

M05.162 Rheumatoid lung disease with rheumatoid arthritis of left knee HCC RxHCC

M05.169 Rheumatoid lung disease with rheumatoid arthritis of unspecified knee HCC RxHCC

M05.17 Rheumatoid lung disease with rheumatoid arthritis of ankle and foot
Rheumatoid lung disease with rheumatoid arthritis, tarsus, metatarsus and phalanges

M05.171 Rheumatoid lung disease with rheumatoid arthritis of right ankle and foot HCC RxHCC

M05.172 Rheumatoid lung disease with rheumatoid arthritis of left ankle and foot HCC RxHCC

M05.179 Rheumatoid lung disease with rheumatoid arthritis of unspecified ankle and foot HCC RxHCC

M05.19 Rheumatoid lung disease with rheumatoid arthritis of multiple sites HCC RxHCC

M05.2 Rheumatoid vasculitis with rheumatoid arthritis

M05.20 Rheumatoid vasculitis with rheumatoid arthritis of unspecified site HCC RxHCC

M05.21 Rheumatoid vasculitis with rheumatoid arthritis of shoulder

M05.211 Rheumatoid vasculitis with rheumatoid arthritis of right shoulder HCC RxHCC

M05.212 Rheumatoid vasculitis with rheumatoid arthritis of left shoulder HCC RxHCC

M05.219 Rheumatoid vasculitis with rheumatoid arthritis of unspecified shoulder HCC RxHCC

M05.22 Rheumatoid vasculitis with rheumatoid arthritis of elbow

M05.221 Rheumatoid vasculitis with rheumatoid arthritis of right elbow HCC RxHCC

M05.222 Rheumatoid vasculitis with rheumatoid arthritis of left elbow HCC RxHCC

M05.229 Rheumatoid vasculitis with rheumatoid arthritis of unspecified elbow HCC RxHCC

M05.23 Rheumatoid vasculitis with rheumatoid arthritis of wrist
Rheumatoid vasculitis with rheumatoid arthritis, carpal bones

M05.231 Rheumatoid vasculitis with rheumatoid arthritis of right wrist HCC RxHCC

M05.232 Rheumatoid vasculitis with rheumatoid arthritis of left wrist HCC RxHCC

M05.239 Rheumatoid vasculitis with rheumatoid arthritis of unspecified wrist HCC RxHCC

M05.24 Rheumatoid vasculitis with rheumatoid arthritis of hand
Rheumatoid vasculitis with rheumatoid arthritis, metacarpus and phalanges

M05.241 Rheumatoid vasculitis with rheumatoid arthritis of right hand HCC RxHCC

M05.242 Rheumatoid vasculitis with rheumatoid arthritis of left hand HCC RxHCC

M05.249 Rheumatoid vasculitis with rheumatoid arthritis of unspecified hand HCC RxHCC

M05.25 Rheumatoid vasculitis with rheumatoid arthritis of hip

M05.251 Rheumatoid vasculitis with rheumatoid arthritis of right hip HCC RxHCC

M05.252 Rheumatoid vasculitis with rheumatoid arthritis of left hip HCC RxHCC

M05.259 Rheumatoid vasculitis with rheumatoid arthritis of unspecified hip HCC RxHCC

M05.26 Rheumatoid vasculitis with rheumatoid arthritis of knee

M05.261 Rheumatoid vasculitis with rheumatoid arthritis of right knee HCC RxHCC

M05.262 Rheumatoid vasculitis with rheumatoid arthritis of left knee HCC RxHCC

M05.269 Rheumatoid vasculitis with rheumatoid arthritis of unspecified knee HCC RxHCC

M05.27 Rheumatoid vasculitis with rheumatoid arthritis of ankle and foot
Rheumatoid vasculitis with rheumatoid arthritis, tarsus, metatarsus and phalanges

M05.271 Rheumatoid vasculitis with rheumatoid arthritis of right ankle and foot HCC RxHCC

M05.272 Rheumatoid vasculitis with rheumatoid arthritis of left ankle and foot HCC RxHCC

M05.279 Rheumatoid vasculitis with rheumatoid arthritis of unspecified ankle and foot HCC RxHCC

M05.29 Rheumatoid vasculitis with rheumatoid arthritis of multiple sites HCC RxHCC

M05.3 Rheumatoid heart disease with rheumatoid arthritis
Rheumatoid carditis
Rheumatoid endocarditis
Rheumatoid myocarditis
Rheumatoid pericarditis

M05.30 Rheumatoid heart disease with rheumatoid arthritis of unspecified site HCC RxHCC

M05.31 Rheumatoid heart disease with rheumatoid arthritis of shoulder

M05.311 Rheumatoid heart disease with rheumatoid arthritis of right shoulder HCC RxHCC

M05.312 Rheumatoid heart disease with rheumatoid arthritis of left shoulder HCC RxHCC

M05.319 Rheumatoid heart disease with rheumatoid arthritis of unspecified shoulder HCC RxHCC

M05.32 Rheumatoid heart disease with rheumatoid arthritis of elbow

M05.321 Rheumatoid heart disease with rheumatoid arthritis of right elbow HCC RxHCC

M05.322 Rheumatoid heart disease with rheumatoid arthritis of left elbow HCC RxHCC

M05.329 Rheumatoid heart disease with rheumatoid arthritis of unspecified elbow HCC RxHCC

M05.33 Rheumatoid heart disease with rheumatoid arthritis of wrist
Rheumatoid heart disease with rheumatoid arthritis, carpal bones

M05.331 Rheumatoid heart disease with rheumatoid arthritis of right wrist HCC RxHCC

M05.332 Rheumatoid heart disease with rheumatoid arthritis of left wrist HCC RxHCC

M05.339 Rheumatoid heart disease with rheumatoid arthritis of unspecified wrist HCC RxHCC

M05.34 Rheumatoid heart disease with rheumatoid arthritis of hand
Rheumatoid heart disease with rheumatoid arthritis, metacarpus and phalanges

M05.341 Rheumatoid heart disease with rheumatoid arthritis of right hand HCC RxHCC

M05.342 Rheumatoid heart disease with rheumatoid arthritis of left hand HCC RxHCC

PDx Unacceptable principal diagnosis symbol per Medicare code edits   Code exempt from diagnosis present on admission requirement
Questionable admission   CC Complication or comorbidity   CC/MCC CC/MCC exclusion   MCC Major complication or comorbidity
Principal diagnosis as its own CC   Principal diagnosis as its own MCC   HCC HCC diagnosis code   RxHCC RxHCC diagnosis code
MACRA code   Z1 Z code as first-listed diagnosis

780   When symbols appear on a code that requires a 7th character extension, refer to Appendix B to identify applicable 7th character codes.   2018 ICD-10-CM

M05.349 Rheumatoid heart disease with rheumatoid arthritis of unspecified hand `HCC` `RxHCC`

6️⃣ M05.35 Rheumatoid heart disease with rheumatoid arthritis of hip

M05.351 Rheumatoid heart disease with rheumatoid arthritis of right hip `HCC` `RxHCC`

M05.352 Rheumatoid heart disease with rheumatoid arthritis of left hip `HCC` `RxHCC`

M05.359 Rheumatoid heart disease with rheumatoid arthritis of unspecified hip `HCC` `RxHCC`

6️⃣ M05.36 Rheumatoid heart disease with rheumatoid arthritis of knee

M05.361 Rheumatoid heart disease with rheumatoid arthritis of right knee `HCC` `RxHCC`

M05.362 Rheumatoid heart disease with rheumatoid arthritis of left knee `HCC` `RxHCC`

M05.369 Rheumatoid heart disease with rheumatoid arthritis of unspecified knee `HCC` `RxHCC`

6️⃣ M05.37 Rheumatoid heart disease with rheumatoid arthritis of ankle and foot

Rheumatoid heart disease with rheumatoid arthritis, tarsus, metatarsus and phalanges

M05.371 Rheumatoid heart disease with rheumatoid arthritis of right ankle and foot `HCC` `RxHCC`

M05.372 Rheumatoid heart disease with rheumatoid arthritis of left ankle and foot `HCC` `RxHCC`

M05.379 Rheumatoid heart disease with rheumatoid arthritis of unspecified ankle and foot `HCC` `RxHCC`

M05.39 Rheumatoid heart disease with rheumatoid arthritis of multiple sites `HCC` `RxHCC`

5️⃣ M05.4 Rheumatoid myopathy with rheumatoid arthritis

M05.40 Rheumatoid myopathy with rheumatoid arthritis of unspecified site `♂️` `HCC` `♀️` `RxHCC` `CC/MCC Exc`

6️⃣ M05.41 Rheumatoid myopathy with rheumatoid arthritis of shoulder

M05.411 Rheumatoid myopathy with rheumatoid arthritis of right shoulder `♂️` `HCC` `♀️` `RxHCC` `CC/MCC Exc`

M05.412 Rheumatoid myopathy with rheumatoid arthritis of left shoulder `♂️` `HCC` `♀️` `RxHCC` `CC/MCC Exc`

M05.419 Rheumatoid myopathy with rheumatoid arthritis of unspecified shoulder `♂️` `HCC` `♀️` `RxHCC` `CC/MCC Exc`

6️⃣ M05.42 Rheumatoid myopathy with rheumatoid arthritis of elbow

M05.421 Rheumatoid myopathy with rheumatoid arthritis of right elbow `♂️` `HCC` `♀️` `RxHCC` `CC/MCC Exc`

M05.422 Rheumatoid myopathy with rheumatoid arthritis of left elbow `♂️` `HCC` `♀️` `RxHCC` `CC/MCC Exc`

M05.429 Rheumatoid myopathy with rheumatoid arthritis of unspecified elbow `♂️` `HCC` `♀️` `RxHCC` `CC/MCC Exc`

6️⃣ M05.43 Rheumatoid myopathy with rheumatoid arthritis of wrist

Rheumatoid myopathy with rheumatoid arthritis, carpal bones

M05.431 Rheumatoid myopathy with rheumatoid arthritis of right wrist `♂️` `HCC` `♀️` `RxHCC` `CC/MCC Exc`

M05.432 Rheumatoid myopathy with rheumatoid arthritis of left wrist `♂️` `HCC` `♀️` `RxHCC` `CC/MCC Exc`

M05.439 Rheumatoid myopathy with rheumatoid arthritis of unspecified wrist `♂️` `HCC` `♀️` `RxHCC` `CC/MCC Exc`

6️⃣ M05.44 Rheumatoid myopathy with rheumatoid arthritis of hand

Rheumatoid myopathy with rheumatoid arthritis, metacarpus and phalanges

M05.441 Rheumatoid myopathy with rheumatoid arthritis of right hand `♂️` `HCC` `♀️` `RxHCC` `CC/MCC Exc`

M05.442 Rheumatoid myopathy with rheumatoid arthritis of left hand `♂️` `HCC` `♀️` `RxHCC` `CC/MCC Exc`

M05.449 Rheumatoid myopathy with rheumatoid arthritis of unspecified hand `♂️` `HCC` `♀️` `RxHCC` `CC/MCC Exc`

6️⃣ M05.45 Rheumatoid myopathy with rheumatoid arthritis of hip

M05.451 Rheumatoid myopathy with rheumatoid arthritis of right hip `♂️` `HCC` `♀️` `RxHCC` `CC/MCC Exc`

M05.452 Rheumatoid myopathy with rheumatoid arthritis of left hip `♂️` `HCC` `♀️` `RxHCC` `CC/MCC Exc`

M05.459 Rheumatoid myopathy with rheumatoid arthritis of unspecified hip `♂️` `HCC` `♀️` `RxHCC` `CC/MCC Exc`

6️⃣ M05.46 Rheumatoid myopathy with rheumatoid arthritis of knee

M05.461 Rheumatoid myopathy with rheumatoid arthritis of right knee `♂️` `HCC` `♀️` `RxHCC` `CC/MCC Exc`

M05.462 Rheumatoid myopathy with rheumatoid arthritis of left knee `♂️` `HCC` `♀️` `RxHCC` `CC/MCC Exc`

M05.469 Rheumatoid myopathy with rheumatoid arthritis of unspecified knee `♂️` `HCC` `♀️` `RxHCC` `CC/MCC Exc`

6️⃣ M05.47 Rheumatoid myopathy with rheumatoid arthritis of ankle and foot

Rheumatoid myopathy with rheumatoid arthritis, tarsus, metatarsus and phalanges

M05.471 Rheumatoid myopathy with rheumatoid arthritis of right ankle and foot `♂️` `HCC` `♀️` `RxHCC` `CC/MCC Exc`

M05.472 Rheumatoid myopathy with rheumatoid arthritis of left ankle and foot `♂️` `HCC` `♀️` `RxHCC` `CC/MCC Exc`

M05.479 Rheumatoid myopathy with rheumatoid arthritis of unspecified ankle and foot `♂️` `HCC` `♀️` `RxHCC` `CC/MCC Exc`

M05.49 Rheumatoid myopathy with rheumatoid arthritis of multiple sites `♂️` `HCC` `♀️` `RxHCC` `CC/MCC Exc`

5️⃣ M05.5 Rheumatoid polyneuropathy with rheumatoid arthritis

M05.50 Rheumatoid polyneuropathy with rheumatoid arthritis of unspecified site `HCC` `RxHCC`

6️⃣ M05.51 Rheumatoid polyneuropathy with rheumatoid arthritis of shoulder

M05.511 Rheumatoid polyneuropathy with rheumatoid arthritis of right shoulder `HCC` `RxHCC`

M05.512 Rheumatoid polyneuropathy with rheumatoid arthritis of left shoulder `HCC` `RxHCC`

M05.519 Rheumatoid polyneuropathy with rheumatoid arthritis of unspecified shoulder `HCC` `RxHCC`

6️⃣ M05.52 Rheumatoid polyneuropathy with rheumatoid arthritis of elbow

M05.521 Rheumatoid polyneuropathy with rheumatoid arthritis of right elbow `HCC` `RxHCC`

M05.522 Rheumatoid polyneuropathy with rheumatoid arthritis of left elbow `HCC` `RxHCC`

M05.529 Rheumatoid polyneuropathy with rheumatoid arthritis of unspecified elbow `HCC` `RxHCC`

6️⃣ M05.53 Rheumatoid polyneuropathy with rheumatoid arthritis of wrist

Rheumatoid polyneuropathy with rheumatoid arthritis, carpal bones

M05.531 Rheumatoid polyneuropathy with rheumatoid arthritis of right wrist `HCC` `RxHCC`

M05.532 Rheumatoid polyneuropathy with rheumatoid arthritis of left wrist `HCC` `RxHCC`

M05.539 Rheumatoid polyneuropathy with rheumatoid arthritis of unspecified wrist `HCC` `RxHCC`

Unspecified Code   Other Specified Code   Manifestation Code   Ⓝ Newborn   Ⓟ Pediatric   Ⓜ Maternity   Ⓐ Adult   ♂ Male   ♀ Female
● New Code   ▲ Revised Code Title   ►◄ Revised Text   **NOTES**   *INCLUDES*   *EXCLUDES 1* Not coded here   *EXCLUDES 2* Not included here
4th character required   5th character required   6th character required   7th character required
Extension 'X' Alert   **HAC** Hospital-acquired condition (HAC) alert   **AHA** AHA Coding Clinic©

M10.142 Lead-induced gout, left hand

M10.149 Lead-induced gout, unspecified hand

6️⃣ M10.15 Lead-induced gout, hip

    M10.151 Lead-induced gout, right hip

    M10.152 Lead-induced gout, left hip

    M10.159 Lead-induced gout, unspecified hip

6️⃣ M10.16 Lead-induced gout, knee

    M10.161 Lead-induced gout, right knee

    M10.162 Lead-induced gout, left knee

    M10.169 Lead-induced gout, unspecified knee

6️⃣ M10.17 Lead-induced gout, ankle and foot

    M10.171 Lead-induced gout, right ankle and foot

    M10.172 Lead-induced gout, left ankle and foot

    M10.179 Lead-induced gout, unspecified ankle and foot

M10.18 Lead-induced gout, vertebrae

M10.19 Lead-induced gout, multiple sites

5️⃣ M10.2 Drug-induced gout

Use additional code for adverse effect, if applicable, to identify drug (T36-T50 with fifth or sixth character 5)

M10.20 Drug-induced gout, unspecified site

6️⃣ M10.21 Drug-induced gout, shoulder

    M10.211 Drug-induced gout, right shoulder

    M10.212 Drug-induced gout, left shoulder

    M10.219 Drug-induced gout, unspecified shoulder

6️⃣ M10.22 Drug-induced gout, elbow

    M10.221 Drug-induced gout, right elbow

    M10.222 Drug-induced gout, left elbow

    M10.229 Drug-induced gout, unspecified elbow

6️⃣ M10.23 Drug-induced gout, wrist

    M10.231 Drug-induced gout, right wrist

    M10.232 Drug-induced gout, left wrist

    M10.239 Drug-induced gout, unspecified wrist

6️⃣ M10.24 Drug-induced gout, hand

    M10.241 Drug-induced gout, right hand

    M10.242 Drug-induced gout, left hand

    M10.249 Drug-induced gout, unspecified hand

6️⃣ M10.25 Drug-induced gout, hip

    M10.251 Drug-induced gout, right hip

    M10.252 Drug-induced gout, left hip

    M10.259 Drug-induced gout, unspecified hip

6️⃣ M10.26 Drug-induced gout, knee

    M10.261 Drug-induced gout, right knee

    M10.262 Drug-induced gout, left knee

    M10.269 Drug-induced gout, unspecified knee

6️⃣ M10.27 Drug-induced gout, ankle and foot

    M10.271 Drug-induced gout, right ankle and foot

    M10.272 Drug-induced gout, left ankle and foot

    M10.279 Drug-induced gout, unspecified ankle and foot

M10.28 Drug-induced gout, vertebrae

M10.29 Drug-induced gout, multiple sites

5️⃣ M10.3 Gout due to renal impairment

Code first associated renal disease

M10.30 Gout due to renal impairment, unspecified site

6️⃣ M10.31 Gout due to renal impairment, shoulder

    M10.311 Gout due to renal impairment, right shoulder

    M10.312 Gout due to renal impairment, left shoulder

    M10.319 Gout due to renal impairment, unspecified shoulder

6️⃣ M10.32 Gout due to renal impairment, elbow

    M10.321 Gout due to renal impairment, right elbow

    M10.322 Gout due to renal impairment, left elbow

    M10.329 Gout due to renal impairment, unspecified elbow

6️⃣ M10.33 Gout due to renal impairment, wrist

    M10.331 Gout due to renal impairment, right wrist

M10.332 Gout due to renal impairment, left wrist

M10.339 Gout due to renal impairment, unspecified wrist

6️⃣ M10.34 Gout due to renal impairment, hand

    M10.341 Gout due to renal impairment, right hand

    M10.342 Gout due to renal impairment, left hand

    M10.349 Gout due to renal impairment, unspecified hand

6️⃣ M10.35 Gout due to renal impairment, hip

    M10.351 Gout due to renal impairment, right hip

    M10.352 Gout due to renal impairment, left hip

    M10.359 Gout due to renal impairment, unspecified hip

6️⃣ M10.36 Gout due to renal impairment, knee

    M10.361 Gout due to renal impairment, right knee

    M10.362 Gout due to renal impairment, left knee

    M10.369 Gout due to renal impairment, unspecified knee

6️⃣ M10.37 Gout due to renal impairment, ankle and foot

    M10.371 Gout due to renal impairment, right ankle and foot

    M10.372 Gout due to renal impairment, left ankle and foot

    M10.379 Gout due to renal impairment, unspecified ankle and foot

M10.38 Gout due to renal impairment, vertebrae

M10.39 Gout due to renal impairment, multiple sites

5️⃣ M10.4 Other secondary gout

Code first associated condition

M10.40 Other secondary gout, unspecified site

6️⃣ M10.41 Other secondary gout, shoulder

    M10.411 Other secondary gout, right shoulder

    M10.412 Other secondary gout, left shoulder

    M10.419 Other secondary gout, unspecified shoulder

6️⃣ M10.42 Other secondary gout, elbow

    M10.421 Other secondary gout, right elbow

    M10.422 Other secondary gout, left elbow

    M10.429 Other secondary gout, unspecified elbow

6️⃣ M10.43 Other secondary gout, wrist

    M10.431 Other secondary gout, right wrist

    M10.432 Other secondary gout, left wrist

    M10.439 Other secondary gout, unspecified wrist

6️⃣ M10.44 Other secondary gout, hand

    M10.441 Other secondary gout, right hand

    M10.442 Other secondary gout, left hand

    M10.449 Other secondary gout, unspecified hand

6️⃣ M10.45 Other secondary gout, hip

    M10.451 Other secondary gout, right hip

    M10.452 Other secondary gout, left hip

    M10.459 Other secondary gout, unspecified hip

6️⃣ M10.46 Other secondary gout, knee

    M10.461 Other secondary gout, right knee

    M10.462 Other secondary gout, left knee

    M10.469 Other secondary gout, unspecified knee

6️⃣ M10.47 Other secondary gout, ankle and foot

    M10.471 Other secondary gout, right ankle and foot

    M10.472 Other secondary gout, left ankle and foot

    M10.479 Other secondary gout, unspecified ankle and foot

M10.48 Other secondary gout, vertebrae

M10.49 Other secondary gout, multiple sites

M10.9 Gout, unspecified

Gout NOS

4️⃣ M11 Other crystal arthropathies

5️⃣ M11.0 Hydroxyapatite deposition disease

M11.00 Hydroxyapatite deposition disease, unspecified site

6️⃣ M11.01 Hydroxyapatite deposition disease, shoulder

PDxⁿ Unacceptable principal diagnosis symbol per Medicare code edits   PDx Code exempt from diagnosis present on admission requirement

❓ Questionable admission   CC Complication or comorbidity   CC/MCC CC/MCC exclusion   MCC Major complication or comorbidity

CC Principal diagnosis as its own CC   MCC Principal diagnosis as its own MCC   HCC HCC diagnosis code   RxHCC RxHCC diagnosis code

MACRA code   Z Z code as first-listed diagnosis

790   When symbols appear on a code that requires a 7th character extension, refer to Appendix B to identify applicable 7th character codes.   **2018 ICD-10-CM**

M11.011 Hydroxyapatite deposition disease, right shoulder
M11.012 Hydroxyapatite deposition disease, left shoulder
M11.019 Hydroxyapatite deposition disease, unspecified shoulder
6️⃣ M11.02 Hydroxyapatite deposition disease, elbow
M11.021 Hydroxyapatite deposition disease, right elbow
M11.022 Hydroxyapatite deposition disease, left elbow
M11.029 Hydroxyapatite deposition disease, unspecified elbow
6️⃣ M11.03 Hydroxyapatite deposition disease, wrist
M11.031 Hydroxyapatite deposition disease, right wrist
M11.032 Hydroxyapatite deposition disease, left wrist
M11.039 Hydroxyapatite deposition disease, unspecified wrist
6️⃣ M11.04 Hydroxyapatite deposition disease, hand
M11.041 Hydroxyapatite deposition disease, right hand
M11.042 Hydroxyapatite deposition disease, left hand
M11.049 Hydroxyapatite deposition disease, unspecified hand
6️⃣ M11.05 Hydroxyapatite deposition disease, hip
M11.051 Hydroxyapatite deposition disease, right hip
M11.052 Hydroxyapatite deposition disease, left hip
M11.059 Hydroxyapatite deposition disease, unspecified hip
6️⃣ M11.06 Hydroxyapatite deposition disease, knee
M11.061 Hydroxyapatite deposition disease, right knee
M11.062 Hydroxyapatite deposition disease, left knee
M11.069 Hydroxyapatite deposition disease, unspecified knee
6️⃣ M11.07 Hydroxyapatite deposition disease, ankle and foot
M11.071 Hydroxyapatite deposition disease, right ankle and foot
M11.072 Hydroxyapatite deposition disease, left ankle and foot
M11.079 Hydroxyapatite deposition disease, unspecified ankle and foot
M11.08 Hydroxyapatite deposition disease, vertebrae
M11.09 Hydroxyapatite deposition disease, multiple sites
5️⃣ M11.1 Familial chondrocalcinosis
M11.10 Familial chondrocalcinosis, unspecified site
6️⃣ M11.11 Familial chondrocalcinosis, shoulder
M11.111 Familial chondrocalcinosis, right shoulder
M11.112 Familial chondrocalcinosis, left shoulder
M11.119 Familial chondrocalcinosis, unspecified shoulder
6️⃣ M11.12 Familial chondrocalcinosis, elbow
M11.121 Familial chondrocalcinosis, right elbow
M11.122 Familial chondrocalcinosis, left elbow
M11.129 Familial chondrocalcinosis, unspecified elbow
6️⃣ M11.13 Familial chondrocalcinosis, wrist
M11.131 Familial chondrocalcinosis, right wrist
M11.132 Familial chondrocalcinosis, left wrist
M11.139 Familial chondrocalcinosis, unspecified wrist
6️⃣ M11.14 Familial chondrocalcinosis, hand
M11.141 Familial chondrocalcinosis, right hand
M11.142 Familial chondrocalcinosis, left hand

M11.149 Familial chondrocalcinosis, unspecified hand
6️⃣ M11.15 Familial chondrocalcinosis, hip
M11.151 Familial chondrocalcinosis, right hip
M11.152 Familial chondrocalcinosis, left hip
M11.159 Familial chondrocalcinosis, unspecified hip
6️⃣ M11.16 Familial chondrocalcinosis, knee
M11.161 Familial chondrocalcinosis, right knee
M11.162 Familial chondrocalcinosis, left knee
M11.169 Familial chondrocalcinosis, unspecified knee
6️⃣ M11.17 Familial chondrocalcinosis, ankle and foot
M11.171 Familial chondrocalcinosis, right ankle and foot
M11.172 Familial chondrocalcinosis, left ankle and foot
M11.179 Familial chondrocalcinosis, unspecified ankle and foot
M11.18 Familial chondrocalcinosis, vertebrae
M11.19 Familial chondrocalcinosis, multiple sites
5️⃣ M11.2 Other chondrocalcinosis
Chondrocalcinosis NOS
M11.20 Other chondrocalcinosis, unspecified site
6️⃣ M11.21 Other chondrocalcinosis, shoulder
M11.211 Other chondrocalcinosis, right shoulder
M11.212 Other chondrocalcinosis, left shoulder
M11.219 Other chondrocalcinosis, unspecified shoulder
6️⃣ M11.22 Other chondrocalcinosis, elbow
M11.221 Other chondrocalcinosis, right elbow
M11.222 Other chondrocalcinosis, left elbow
M11.229 Other chondrocalcinosis, unspecified elbow
6️⃣ M11.23 Other chondrocalcinosis, wrist
M11.231 Other chondrocalcinosis, right wrist
M11.232 Other chondrocalcinosis, left wrist
M11.239 Other chondrocalcinosis, unspecified wrist
6️⃣ M11.24 Other chondrocalcinosis, hand
M11.241 Other chondrocalcinosis, right hand
M11.242 Other chondrocalcinosis, left hand
M11.249 Other chondrocalcinosis, unspecified hand
6️⃣ M11.25 Other chondrocalcinosis, hip
M11.251 Other chondrocalcinosis, right hip
M11.252 Other chondrocalcinosis, left hip
M11.259 Other chondrocalcinosis, unspecified hip
6️⃣ M11.26 Other chondrocalcinosis, knee
M11.261 Other chondrocalcinosis, right knee
M11.262 Other chondrocalcinosis, left knee
M11.269 Other chondrocalcinosis, unspecified knee
6️⃣ M11.27 Other chondrocalcinosis, ankle and foot
M11.271 Other chondrocalcinosis, right ankle and foot
M11.272 Other chondrocalcinosis, left ankle and foot
M11.279 Other chondrocalcinosis, unspecified ankle and foot
M11.28 Other chondrocalcinosis, vertebrae
M11.29 Other chondrocalcinosis, multiple sites
5️⃣ M11.8 Other specified crystal arthropathies
M11.80 Other specified crystal arthropathies, unspecified site
6️⃣ M11.81 Other specified crystal arthropathies, shoulder
M11.811 Other specified crystal arthropathies, right shoulder
M11.812 Other specified crystal arthropathies, left shoulder
M11.819 Other specified crystal arthropathies, unspecified shoulder

---

Unspecified Code   Other Specified Code   Manifestation Code   N Newborn   P Pediatric   M Maternity   A Adult   ♂ Male   ♀ Female
● New Code   ▲ Revised Code Title   ▶◀ Revised Text   NOTES   *INCLUDES*   *EXCLUDES 1* Not coded here   *EXCLUDES 2* Not included here
4️⃣ 4th character required   5️⃣ 5th character required   6️⃣ 6th character required   7️⃣ 7th character required
7️⃣ Extension 'X' Alert   HAC Hospital-acquired condition (HAC) alert   AHA AHA Coding Clinic©

6ᵗʰ M11.82 Other specified crystal arthropathies, elbow
  M11.821 Other specified crystal arthropathies, right elbow
  M11.822 Other specified crystal arthropathies, left elbow
  M11.829 Other specified crystal arthropathies, unspecified elbow

6ᵗʰ M11.83 Other specified crystal arthropathies, wrist
  M11.831 Other specified crystal arthropathies, right wrist
  M11.832 Other specified crystal arthropathies, left wrist
  M11.839 Other specified crystal arthropathies, unspecified wrist

6ᵗʰ M11.84 Other specified crystal arthropathies, hand
  M11.841 Other specified crystal arthropathies, right hand
  M11.842 Other specified crystal arthropathies, left hand
  M11.849 Other specified crystal arthropathies, unspecified hand

6ᵗʰ M11.85 Other specified crystal arthropathies, hip
  M11.851 Other specified crystal arthropathies, right hip
  M11.852 Other specified crystal arthropathies, left hip
  M11.859 Other specified crystal arthropathies, unspecified hip

6ᵗʰ M11.86 Other specified crystal arthropathies, knee
  M11.861 Other specified crystal arthropathies, right knee
  M11.862 Other specified crystal arthropathies, left knee
  M11.869 Other specified crystal arthropathies, unspecified knee

6ᵗʰ M11.87 Other specified crystal arthropathies, ankle and foot
  M11.871 Other specified crystal arthropathies, right ankle and foot
  M11.872 Other specified crystal arthropathies, left ankle and foot
  M11.879 Other specified crystal arthropathies, unspecified ankle and foot

M11.88 Other specified crystal arthropathies, vertebrae
M11.89 Other specified crystal arthropathies, multiple sites
M11.9 Crystal arthropathy, unspecified

4ᵗʰ M12 Other and unspecified arthropathy
EXCLUDES1 arthrosis (M15-M19)
    cricoarytenoid arthropathy (J38.7)

5ᵗʰ M12.0 Chronic postrheumatic arthropathy [Jaccoud]
  M12.00 Chronic postrheumatic arthropathy [Jaccoud], unspecified site   HCC RxHCC

  6ᵗʰ M12.01 Chronic postrheumatic arthropathy [Jaccoud], shoulder
    M12.011 Chronic postrheumatic arthropathy [Jaccoud], right shoulder   HCC RxHCC
    M12.012 Chronic postrheumatic arthropathy [Jaccoud], left shoulder   HCC RxHCC
    M12.019 Chronic postrheumatic arthropathy [Jaccoud], unspecified shoulder   HCC RxHCC

  6ᵗʰ M12.02 Chronic postrheumatic arthropathy [Jaccoud], elbow
    M12.021 Chronic postrheumatic arthropathy [Jaccoud], right elbow   HCC RxHCC
    M12.022 Chronic postrheumatic arthropathy [Jaccoud], left elbow   HCC RxHCC
    M12.029 Chronic postrheumatic arthropathy [Jaccoud], unspecified elbow   HCC RxHCC

  6ᵗʰ M12.03 Chronic postrheumatic arthropathy [Jaccoud], wrist
    M12.031 Chronic postrheumatic arthropathy [Jaccoud], right wrist   HCC RxHCC

  M12.032 Chronic postrheumatic arthropathy [Jaccoud], left wrist   HCC RxHCC
  M12.039 Chronic postrheumatic arthropathy [Jaccoud], unspecified wrist   HCC RxHCC

6ᵗʰ M12.04 Chronic postrheumatic arthropathy [Jaccoud], hand
  M12.041 Chronic postrheumatic arthropathy [Jaccoud], right hand   HCC RxHCC
  M12.042 Chronic postrheumatic arthropathy [Jaccoud], left hand   HCC RxHCC
  M12.049 Chronic postrheumatic arthropathy [Jaccoud], unspecified hand   HCC RxHCC

6ᵗʰ M12.05 Chronic postrheumatic arthropathy [Jaccoud], hip
  M12.051 Chronic postrheumatic arthropathy [Jaccoud], right hip   HCC RxHCC
  M12.052 Chronic postrheumatic arthropathy [Jaccoud], left hip   HCC RxHCC
  M12.059 Chronic postrheumatic arthropathy [Jaccoud], unspecified hip   HCC RxHCC

6ᵗʰ M12.06 Chronic postrheumatic arthropathy [Jaccoud], knee
  M12.061 Chronic postrheumatic arthropathy [Jaccoud], right knee   HCC RxHCC
  M12.062 Chronic postrheumatic arthropathy [Jaccoud], left knee   HCC RxHCC
  M12.069 Chronic postrheumatic arthropathy [Jaccoud], unspecified knee   HCC RxHCC

6ᵗʰ M12.07 Chronic postrheumatic arthropathy [Jaccoud], ankle and foot
  M12.071 Chronic postrheumatic arthropathy [Jaccoud], right ankle and foot   HCC RxHCC
  M12.072 Chronic postrheumatic arthropathy [Jaccoud], left ankle and foot   HCC RxHCC
  M12.079 Chronic postrheumatic arthropathy [Jaccoud], unspecified ankle and foot   HCC RxHCC

M12.08 Chronic postrheumatic arthropathy [Jaccoud], other specified site   HCC RxHCC
  Chronic postrheumatic arthropathy [Jaccoud], vertebrae

M12.09 Chronic postrheumatic arthropathy [Jaccoud], multiple sites   HCC RxHCC

5ᵗʰ M12.1 Kaschin-Beck disease
  Osteochondroarthrosis deformans endemica
  M12.10 Kaschin-Beck disease, unspecified site

6ᵗʰ M12.11 Kaschin-Beck disease, shoulder
  M12.111 Kaschin-Beck disease, right shoulder
  M12.112 Kaschin-Beck disease, left shoulder
  M12.119 Kaschin-Beck disease, unspecified shoulder

6ᵗʰ M12.12 Kaschin-Beck disease, elbow
  M12.121 Kaschin-Beck disease, right elbow
  M12.122 Kaschin-Beck disease, left elbow
  M12.129 Kaschin-Beck disease, unspecified elbow

6ᵗʰ M12.13 Kaschin-Beck disease, wrist
  M12.131 Kaschin-Beck disease, right wrist
  M12.132 Kaschin-Beck disease, left wrist
  M12.139 Kaschin-Beck disease, unspecified wrist

6ᵗʰ M12.14 Kaschin-Beck disease, hand
  M12.141 Kaschin-Beck disease, right hand
  M12.142 Kaschin-Beck disease, left hand
  M12.149 Kaschin-Beck disease, unspecified hand

6ᵗʰ M12.15 Kaschin-Beck disease, hip
  M12.151 Kaschin-Beck disease, right hip
  M12.152 Kaschin-Beck disease, left hip
  M12.159 Kaschin-Beck disease, unspecified hip

6ᵗʰ M12.16 Kaschin-Beck disease, knee
  M12.161 Kaschin-Beck disease, right knee
  M12.162 Kaschin-Beck disease, left knee
  M12.169 Kaschin-Beck disease, unspecified knee

6ᵗʰ M12.17 Kaschin-Beck disease, ankle and foot
  M12.171 Kaschin-Beck disease, right ankle and foot
  M12.172 Kaschin-Beck disease, left ankle and foot

PDxR Unacceptable principal diagnosis symbol per Medicare code edits   PO̷A Code exempt from diagnosis present on admission requirement
❓ Questionable admission   cc Complication or comorbidity   CC/MCC Exc. CC/MCC exclusion   MCC Major complication or comorbidity
PDx Principal diagnosis as its own CC   PDx Principal diagnosis as its own MCC   HCC HCC diagnosis code   RxHCC RxHCC diagnosis code
MACRA code   Z1 Z code as first-listed diagnosis

792

When symbols appear on a code that requires a 7th character extension, refer to Appendix B to identify applicable 7th character codes.

2018 ICD-10-CM

M12.179 Kaschin-Beck disease, unspecified ankle and foot
M12.18 Kaschin-Beck disease, vertebrae
M12.19 Kaschin-Beck disease, multiple sites
5ᵗʰ M12.2 Villonodular synovitis (pigmented)
M12.20 Villonodular synovitis (pigmented), unspecified site
6ᵗʰ M12.21 Villonodular synovitis (pigmented), shoulder
M12.211 Villonodular synovitis (pigmented), right shoulder
M12.212 Villonodular synovitis (pigmented), left shoulder
M12.219 Villonodular synovitis (pigmented), unspecified shoulder
6ᵗʰ M12.22 Villonodular synovitis (pigmented), elbow
M12.221 Villonodular synovitis (pigmented), right elbow
M12.222 Villonodular synovitis (pigmented), left elbow
M12.229 Villonodular synovitis (pigmented), unspecified elbow
6ᵗʰ M12.23 Villonodular synovitis (pigmented), wrist
M12.231 Villonodular synovitis (pigmented), right wrist
M12.232 Villonodular synovitis (pigmented), left wrist
M12.239 Villonodular synovitis (pigmented), unspecified wrist
6ᵗʰ M12.24 Villonodular synovitis (pigmented), hand
M12.241 Villonodular synovitis (pigmented), right hand
M12.242 Villonodular synovitis (pigmented), left hand
M12.249 Villonodular synovitis (pigmented), unspecified hand
6ᵗʰ M12.25 Villonodular synovitis (pigmented), hip
M12.251 Villonodular synovitis (pigmented), right hip
M12.252 Villonodular synovitis (pigmented), left hip
M12.259 Villonodular synovitis (pigmented), unspecified hip
6ᵗʰ M12.26 Villonodular synovitis (pigmented), knee
M12.261 Villonodular synovitis (pigmented), right knee
M12.262 Villonodular synovitis (pigmented), left knee
M12.269 Villonodular synovitis (pigmented), unspecified knee
6ᵗʰ M12.27 Villonodular synovitis (pigmented), ankle and foot
M12.271 Villonodular synovitis (pigmented), right ankle and foot
M12.272 Villonodular synovitis (pigmented), left ankle and foot
M12.279 Villonodular synovitis (pigmented), unspecified ankle and foot
M12.28 Villonodular synovitis (pigmented), other specified site
Villonodular synovitis (pigmented), vertebrae
M12.29 Villonodular synovitis (pigmented), multiple sites
5ᵗʰ M12.3 Palindromic rheumatism
M12.30 Palindromic rheumatism, unspecified site
6ᵗʰ M12.31 Palindromic rheumatism, shoulder
M12.311 Palindromic rheumatism, right shoulder
M12.312 Palindromic rheumatism, left shoulder
M12.319 Palindromic rheumatism, unspecified shoulder
6ᵗʰ M12.32 Palindromic rheumatism, elbow
M12.321 Palindromic rheumatism, right elbow
M12.322 Palindromic rheumatism, left elbow
M12.329 Palindromic rheumatism, unspecified elbow

6ᵗʰ M12.33 Palindromic rheumatism, wrist
M12.331 Palindromic rheumatism, right wrist
M12.332 Palindromic rheumatism, left wrist
M12.339 Palindromic rheumatism, unspecified wrist
6ᵗʰ M12.34 Palindromic rheumatism, hand
M12.341 Palindromic rheumatism, right hand
M12.342 Palindromic rheumatism, left hand
M12.349 Palindromic rheumatism, unspecified hand
6ᵗʰ M12.35 Palindromic rheumatism, hip
M12.351 Palindromic rheumatism, right hip
M12.352 Palindromic rheumatism, left hip
M12.359 Palindromic rheumatism, unspecified hip
6ᵗʰ M12.36 Palindromic rheumatism, knee
M12.361 Palindromic rheumatism, right knee
M12.362 Palindromic rheumatism, left knee
M12.369 Palindromic rheumatism, unspecified knee
6ᵗʰ M12.37 Palindromic rheumatism, ankle and foot
M12.371 Palindromic rheumatism, right ankle and foot
M12.372 Palindromic rheumatism, left ankle and foot
M12.379 Palindromic rheumatism, unspecified ankle and foot
M12.38 Palindromic rheumatism, other specified site
Palindromic rheumatism, vertebrae
M12.39 Palindromic rheumatism, multiple sites
5ᵗʰ M12.4 Intermittent hydrarthrosis
M12.40 Intermittent hydrarthrosis, unspecified site
6ᵗʰ M12.41 Intermittent hydrarthrosis, shoulder
M12.411 Intermittent hydrarthrosis, right shoulder
M12.412 Intermittent hydrarthrosis, left shoulder
M12.419 Intermittent hydrarthrosis, unspecified shoulder
6ᵗʰ M12.42 Intermittent hydrarthrosis, elbow
M12.421 Intermittent hydrarthrosis, right elbow
M12.422 Intermittent hydrarthrosis, left elbow
M12.429 Intermittent hydrarthrosis, unspecified elbow
6ᵗʰ M12.43 Intermittent hydrarthrosis, wrist
M12.431 Intermittent hydrarthrosis, right wrist
M12.432 Intermittent hydrarthrosis, left wrist
M12.439 Intermittent hydrarthrosis, unspecified wrist
6ᵗʰ M12.44 Intermittent hydrarthrosis, hand
M12.441 Intermittent hydrarthrosis, right hand
M12.442 Intermittent hydrarthrosis, left hand
M12.449 Intermittent hydrarthrosis, unspecified hand
6ᵗʰ M12.45 Intermittent hydrarthrosis, hip
M12.451 Intermittent hydrarthrosis, right hip
M12.452 Intermittent hydrarthrosis, left hip
M12.459 Intermittent hydrarthrosis, unspecified hip
6ᵗʰ M12.46 Intermittent hydrarthrosis, knee
M12.461 Intermittent hydrarthrosis, right knee
M12.462 Intermittent hydrarthrosis, left knee
M12.469 Intermittent hydrarthrosis, unspecified knee
6ᵗʰ M12.47 Intermittent hydrarthrosis, ankle and foot
M12.471 Intermittent hydrarthrosis, right ankle and foot
M12.472 Intermittent hydrarthrosis, left ankle and foot
M12.479 Intermittent hydrarthrosis, unspecified ankle and foot
M12.48 Intermittent hydrarthrosis, other site
M12.49 Intermittent hydrarthrosis, multiple sites

Unspecified Code	Other Specified Code	Manifestation Code	N Newborn	P Pediatric	M Maternity	A Adult	♂ Male	♀ Female

● New Code ▲ Revised Code Title ▶◀ Revised Text **NOTES** *INCLUDES* *EXCLUDES 1* Not coded here *EXCLUDES 2* Not included here
4ᵗʰ 4ᵗʰ character required 5ᵗʰ 5ᵗʰ character required 6ᵗʰ 6ᵗʰ character required 7ᵗʰ 7ᵗʰ character required
7ᵗʰ Extension 'X' Alert **HAC** Hospital-acquired condition (HAC) alert **AHA** AHA Coding Clinic©

5ᵗʰ **M12.5** Traumatic arthropathy

EXCLUDES1 current injury-see Alphabetic Index

post-traumatic osteoarthritis of first carpometacarpal joint (M18.2-M18.3)

post-traumatic osteoarthritis of hip (M16.4-M16.5)

post-traumatic osteoarthritis of knee (M17.2-M17.3)

post-traumatic osteoarthritis NOS (M19.1-)

post-traumatic osteoarthritis of other single joints (M19.1-)

    M12.50 Traumatic arthropathy, unspecified site

6ᵗʰ **M12.51** Traumatic arthropathy, shoulder

    M12.511 Traumatic arthropathy, right shoulder

    M12.512 Traumatic arthropathy, left shoulder

    M12.519 Traumatic arthropathy, unspecified shoulder

6ᵗʰ **M12.52** Traumatic arthropathy, elbow

    M12.521 Traumatic arthropathy, right elbow

    M12.522 Traumatic arthropathy, left elbow

    M12.529 Traumatic arthropathy, unspecified elbow

6ᵗʰ **M12.53** Traumatic arthropathy, wrist

    M12.531 Traumatic arthropathy, right wrist

    M12.532 Traumatic arthropathy, left wrist

    M12.539 Traumatic arthropathy, unspecified wrist

6ᵗʰ **M12.54** Traumatic arthropathy, hand

    M12.541 Traumatic arthropathy, right hand

    M12.542 Traumatic arthropathy, left hand

    M12.549 Traumatic arthropathy, unspecified hand

6ᵗʰ **M12.55** Traumatic arthropathy, hip

    M12.551 Traumatic arthropathy, right hip

    M12.552 Traumatic arthropathy, left hip

      AHA: Q1 2015

    M12.559 Traumatic arthropathy, unspecified hip

6ᵗʰ **M12.56** Traumatic arthropathy, knee

    M12.561 Traumatic arthropathy, right knee

    M12.562 Traumatic arthropathy, left knee

    M12.569 Traumatic arthropathy, unspecified knee

6ᵗʰ **M12.57** Traumatic arthropathy, ankle and foot

    M12.571 Traumatic arthropathy, right ankle and foot

    M12.572 Traumatic arthropathy, left ankle and foot

    M12.579 Traumatic arthropathy, unspecified ankle and foot

    M12.58 Traumatic arthropathy, other specified site

Traumatic arthropathy, vertebrae

    M12.59 Traumatic arthropathy, multiple sites

5ᵗʰ **M12.8** Other specific arthropathies, not elsewhere classified

Transient arthropathy

    M12.80 Other specific arthropathies, not elsewhere classified, unspecified site

6ᵗʰ **M12.81** Other specific arthropathies, not elsewhere classified, shoulder

    M12.811 Other specific arthropathies, not elsewhere classified, right shoulder

    M12.812 Other specific arthropathies, not elsewhere classified, left shoulder

    M12.819 Other specific arthropathies, not elsewhere classified, unspecified shoulder

6ᵗʰ **M12.82** Other specific arthropathies, not elsewhere classified, elbow

    M12.821 Other specific arthropathies, not elsewhere classified, right elbow

    M12.822 Other specific arthropathies, not elsewhere classified, left elbow

    M12.829 Other specific arthropathies, not elsewhere classified, unspecified elbow

6ᵗʰ **M12.83** Other specific arthropathies, not elsewhere classified, wrist

    M12.831 Other specific arthropathies, not elsewhere classified, right wrist

    M12.832 Other specific arthropathies, not elsewhere classified, left wrist

    M12.839 Other specific arthropathies, not elsewhere classified, unspecified wrist

6ᵗʰ **M12.84** Other specific arthropathies, not elsewhere classified, hand

    M12.841 Other specific arthropathies, not elsewhere classified, right hand

    M12.842 Other specific arthropathies, not elsewhere classified, left hand

    M12.849 Other specific arthropathies, not elsewhere classified, unspecified hand

6ᵗʰ **M12.85** Other specific arthropathies, not elsewhere classified, hip

    M12.851 Other specific arthropathies, not elsewhere classified, right hip

    M12.852 Other specific arthropathies, not elsewhere classified, left hip

    M12.859 Other specific arthropathies, not elsewhere classified, unspecified hip

6ᵗʰ **M12.86** Other specific arthropathies, not elsewhere classified, knee

    M12.861 Other specific arthropathies, not elsewhere classified, right knee

    M12.862 Other specific arthropathies, not elsewhere classified, left knee

    M12.869 Other specific arthropathies, not elsewhere classified, unspecified knee

6ᵗʰ **M12.87** Other specific arthropathies, not elsewhere classified, ankle and foot

    M12.871 Other specific arthropathies, not elsewhere classified, right ankle and foot

    M12.872 Other specific arthropathies, not elsewhere classified, left ankle and foot

    M12.879 Other specific arthropathies, not elsewhere classified, unspecified ankle and foot

    M12.88 Other specific arthropathies, not elsewhere classified, other specified site

Other specific arthropathies, not elsewhere classified, vertebrae

    M12.89 Other specific arthropathies, not elsewhere classified, multiple sites

    M12.9 Arthropathy, unspecified

4ᵗʰ **M13** Other arthritis

EXCLUDES1 arthrosis (M15-M19)

osteoarthritis (M15-M19)

    M13.0 Polyarthritis, unspecified

5ᵗʰ **M13.1** Monoarthritis, not elsewhere classified

    M13.10 Monoarthritis, not elsewhere classified, unspecified site

6ᵗʰ **M13.11** Monoarthritis, not elsewhere classified, shoulder

    M13.111 Monoarthritis, not elsewhere classified, right shoulder

    M13.112 Monoarthritis, not elsewhere classified, left shoulder

    M13.119 Monoarthritis, not elsewhere classified, unspecified shoulder

6ᵗʰ **M13.12** Monoarthritis, not elsewhere classified, elbow

    M13.121 Monoarthritis, not elsewhere classified, right elbow

    M13.122 Monoarthritis, not elsewhere classified, left elbow

    M13.129 Monoarthritis, not elsewhere classified, unspecified elbow

6ᵗʰ **M13.13** Monoarthritis, not elsewhere classified, wrist

    M13.131 Monoarthritis, not elsewhere classified, right wrist

    M13.132 Monoarthritis, not elsewhere classified, left wrist

---

PDx Unacceptable principal diagnosis symbol per Medicare code edits   Code exempt from diagnosis present on admission requirement   ? Questionable admission   CC Complication or comorbidity   CC/MCC CC/MCC exclusion   MCC Major complication or comorbidity   Principal diagnosis as its own CC   Principal diagnosis as its own MCC   HCC HCC diagnosis code   RxHCC RxHCC diagnosis code   MACRA code   Z1 Z code as first-listed diagnosis

794

When symbols appear on a code that requires a 7th character extension, refer to Appendix B to identify applicable 7th character codes.

2018 ICD-10-CM

M13.139 Monoarthritis, not elsewhere classified, unspecified wrist

6th M13.14 Monoarthritis, not elsewhere classified, hand
   M13.141 Monoarthritis, not elsewhere classified, right hand
   M13.142 Monoarthritis, not elsewhere classified, left hand
   M13.149 Monoarthritis, not elsewhere classified, unspecified hand

6th M13.15 Monoarthritis, not elsewhere classified, hip
   M13.151 Monoarthritis, not elsewhere classified, right hip
   M13.152 Monoarthritis, not elsewhere classified, left hip
   M13.159 Monoarthritis, not elsewhere classified, unspecified hip

6th M13.16 Monoarthritis, not elsewhere classified, knee
   M13.161 Monoarthritis, not elsewhere classified, right knee
   M13.162 Monoarthritis, not elsewhere classified, left knee
   M13.169 Monoarthritis, not elsewhere classified, unspecified knee

6th M13.17 Monoarthritis, not elsewhere classified, ankle and foot
   M13.171 Monoarthritis, not elsewhere classified, right ankle and foot
   M13.172 Monoarthritis, not elsewhere classified, left ankle and foot
   M13.179 Monoarthritis, not elsewhere classified, unspecified ankle and foot

5th M13.8 Other specified arthritis
   Allergic arthritis
   EXCLUDES1 osteoarthritis (M15-M19)
   M13.80 Other specified arthritis, unspecified site

6th M13.81 Other specified arthritis, shoulder
   M13.811 Other specified arthritis, right shoulder
   M13.812 Other specified arthritis, left shoulder
   M13.819 Other specified arthritis, unspecified shoulder

6th M13.82 Other specified arthritis, elbow
   M13.821 Other specified arthritis, right elbow
   M13.822 Other specified arthritis, left elbow
   M13.829 Other specified arthritis, unspecified elbow

6th M13.83 Other specified arthritis, wrist
   M13.831 Other specified arthritis, right wrist
   M13.832 Other specified arthritis, left wrist
   M13.839 Other specified arthritis, unspecified wrist

6th M13.84 Other specified arthritis, hand
   M13.841 Other specified arthritis, right hand
   M13.842 Other specified arthritis, left hand
   M13.849 Other specified arthritis, unspecified hand

6th M13.85 Other specified arthritis, hip
   M13.851 Other specified arthritis, right hip
   M13.852 Other specified arthritis, left hip
   M13.859 Other specified arthritis, unspecified hip

6th M13.86 Other specified arthritis, knee
   M13.861 Other specified arthritis, right knee
   M13.862 Other specified arthritis, left knee
   M13.869 Other specified arthritis, unspecified knee

6th M13.87 Other specified arthritis, ankle and foot
   M13.871 Other specified arthritis, right ankle and foot
   M13.872 Other specified arthritis, left ankle and foot
   M13.879 Other specified arthritis, unspecified ankle and foot

   M13.88 Other specified arthritis, other site
   M13.89 Other specified arthritis, multiple sites

4th M14 Arthropathies in other diseases classified elsewhere
   EXCLUDES1 arthropathy in:
      diabetes mellitus (E08-E13 with .61-)
      hematological disorders (M36.2-M36.3)
      hypersensitivity reactions (M36.4)
      neoplastic disease (M36.1)
      neurosyphillis (A52.16)
      sarcoidosis (D86.86)
      enteropathic arthropathies (M07.-)
      juvenile psoriatic arthropathy (L40.54)
      lipoid dermatoarthritis (E78.81)

5th M14.6 Charcôt's joint
   Neuropathic arthropathy
   EXCLUDES1 Charcôt's joint in diabetes mellitus (E08-E13 with .610)
      Charcôt's joint in tabes dorsalis (A52.16)
   M14.60 Charcôt's joint, unspecified site

6th M14.61 Charcôt's joint, shoulder
   M14.611 Charcôt's joint, right shoulder
   M14.612 Charcôt's joint, left shoulder
   M14.619 Charcôt's joint, unspecified shoulder

6th M14.62 Charcôt's joint, elbow
   M14.621 Charcôt's joint, right elbow
   M14.622 Charcôt's joint, left elbow
   M14.629 Charcôt's joint, unspecified elbow

6th M14.63 Charcôt's joint, wrist
   M14.631 Charcôt's joint, right wrist
   M14.632 Charcôt's joint, left wrist
   M14.639 Charcôt's joint, unspecified wrist

6th M14.64 Charcôt's joint, hand
   M14.641 Charcôt's joint, right hand
   M14.642 Charcôt's joint, left hand
   M14.649 Charcôt's joint, unspecified hand

6th M14.65 Charcôt's joint, hip
   M14.651 Charcôt's joint, right hip
   M14.652 Charcôt's joint, left hip
   M14.659 Charcôt's joint, unspecified hip

6th M14.66 Charcôt's joint, knee
   M14.661 Charcôt's joint, right knee
   M14.662 Charcôt's joint, left knee
   M14.669 Charcôt's joint, unspecified knee

6th M14.67 Charcôt's joint, ankle and foot
   M14.671 Charcôt's joint, right ankle and foot
   M14.672 Charcôt's joint, left ankle and foot
   M14.679 Charcôt's joint, unspecified ankle and foot

   M14.68 Charcôt's joint, vertebrae
   M14.69 Charcôt's joint, multiple sites

5th M14.8 Arthropathies in other specified diseases classified elsewhere
   Code first underlying disease, such as:
   amyloidosis (E85.-)
   erythema multiforme (L51.-)
   erythema nodosum (L52)
   hemochromatosis (E83.11-)
   hyperparathyroidism (E21.-)
   hypothyroidism (E00-E03)
   sickle-cell disorders (D57.-)
   thyrotoxicosis [hyperthyroidism] (E05.-)
   Whipple's disease (K90.81)
   M14.80 Arthropathies in other specified diseases classified elsewhere, unspecified site

6th M14.81 Arthropathies in other specified diseases classified elsewhere, shoulder
   M14.811 Arthropathies in other specified diseases classified elsewhere, right shoulder
   M14.812 Arthropathies in other specified diseases classified elsewhere, left shoulder
   M14.819 Arthropathies in other specified diseases classified elsewhere, unspecified shoulder

Unspecified Code Other Specified Code Manifestation Code N Newborn P Pediatric M Maternity A Adult ♂ Male ♀ Female
● New Code ▲ Revised Code Title ►◄ Revised Text NOTES INCLUDES EXCLUDES 1 Not coded here EXCLUDES 2 Not included here
4th character required 5th character required 6th character required 7th character required
Extension 'X' Alert HAC Hospital-acquired condition (HAC) alert AHA AHA Coding Clinic©

M14.82 Arthropathies in other specified diseases classified elsewhere, elbow
- M14.821 Arthropathies in other specified diseases classified elsewhere, right elbow
- M14.822 Arthropathies in other specified diseases classified elsewhere, left elbow
- M14.829 Arthropathies in other specified diseases classified elsewhere, unspecified elbow

M14.83 Arthropathies in other specified diseases classified elsewhere, wrist
- M14.831 Arthropathies in other specified diseases classified elsewhere, right wrist
- M14.832 Arthropathies in other specified diseases classified elsewhere, left wrist
- M14.839 Arthropathies in other specified diseases classified elsewhere, unspecified wrist

M14.84 Arthropathies in other specified diseases classified elsewhere, hand
- M14.841 Arthropathies in other specified diseases classified elsewhere, right hand
- M14.842 Arthropathies in other specified diseases classified elsewhere, left hand
- M14.849 Arthropathies in other specified diseases classified elsewhere, unspecified hand

M14.85 Arthropathies in other specified diseases classified elsewhere, hip
- M14.851 Arthropathies in other specified diseases classified elsewhere, right hip
- M14.852 Arthropathies in other specified diseases classified elsewhere, left hip
- M14.859 Arthropathies in other specified diseases classified elsewhere, unspecified hip

M14.86 Arthropathies in other specified diseases classified elsewhere, knee
- M14.861 Arthropathies in other specified diseases classified elsewhere, right knee
- M14.862 Arthropathies in other specified diseases classified elsewhere, left knee
- M14.869 Arthropathies in other specified diseases classified elsewhere, unspecified knee

M14.87 Arthropathies in other specified diseases classified elsewhere, ankle and foot
- M14.871 Arthropathies in other specified diseases classified elsewhere, right ankle and foot
- M14.872 Arthropathies in other specified diseases classified elsewhere, left ankle and foot
- M14.879 Arthropathies in other specified diseases classified elsewhere, unspecified ankle and foot

M14.88 Arthropathies in other specified diseases classified elsewhere, vertebrae

M14.89 Arthropathies in other specified diseases classified elsewhere, multiple sites

Osteoarthritis (M15-M19)

EXCLUDES2 osteoarthritis of spine (M47.-)

M15 Polyosteoarthritis

INCLUDES arthritis of multiple sites

EXCLUDES1 bilateral involvement of single joint (M16-M19)

- M15.0 Primary generalized (osteo)arthritis
- M15.1 Heberden's nodes (with arthropathy)
  Interphalangeal distal osteoarthritis
- M15.2 Bouchard's nodes (with arthropathy)
  Juxtaphalangeal distal osteoarthritis
- M15.3 Secondary multiple arthritis
  Post-traumatic polyosteoarthritis
- M15.4 Erosive (osteo)arthritis
- M15.8 Other polyosteoarthritis
- M15.9 Polyosteoarthritis, unspecified
  Generalized osteoarthritis NOS

M16 Osteoarthritis of hip
- M16.0 Bilateral primary osteoarthritis of hip
  AHA: Q4 2016
- M16.1 Unilateral primary osteoarthritis of hip
  Primary osteoarthritis of hip NOS
  - M16.10 Unilateral primary osteoarthritis, unspecified hip
  - M16.11 Unilateral primary osteoarthritis, right hip
  - M16.12 Unilateral primary osteoarthritis, left hip
- M16.2 Bilateral osteoarthritis resulting from hip dysplasia
- M16.3 Unilateral osteoarthritis resulting from hip dysplasia
  Dysplastic osteoarthritis of hip NOS
  - M16.30 Unilateral osteoarthritis resulting from hip dysplasia, unspecified hip
  - M16.31 Unilateral osteoarthritis resulting from hip dysplasia, right hip
  - M16.32 Unilateral osteoarthritis resulting from hip dysplasia, left hip
- M16.4 Bilateral post-traumatic osteoarthritis of hip
- M16.5 Unilateral post-traumatic osteoarthritis of hip
  Post-traumatic osteoarthritis of hip NOS
  - M16.50 Unilateral post-traumatic osteoarthritis, unspecified hip
  - M16.51 Unilateral post-traumatic osteoarthritis, right hip
  - M16.52 Unilateral post-traumatic osteoarthritis, left hip
- M16.6 Other bilateral secondary osteoarthritis of hip
- M16.7 Other unilateral secondary osteoarthritis of hip
  Secondary osteoarthritis of hip NOS
- M16.9 Osteoarthritis of hip, unspecified

M17 Osteoarthritis of knee
- M17.0 Bilateral primary osteoarthritis of knee
- M17.1 Unilateral primary osteoarthritis of knee
  Primary osteoarthritis of knee NOS
  - M17.10 Unilateral primary osteoarthritis, unspecified knee
    AHA: Q4 2016
  - M17.11 Unilateral primary osteoarthritis, right knee
  - M17.12 Unilateral primary osteoarthritis, left knee
    AHA: Q4 2016
- M17.2 Bilateral post-traumatic osteoarthritis of knee
- M17.3 Unilateral post-traumatic osteoarthritis of knee
  Post-traumatic osteoarthritis of knee NOS
  - M17.30 Unilateral post-traumatic osteoarthritis, unspecified knee
  - M17.31 Unilateral post-traumatic osteoarthritis, right knee
  - M17.32 Unilateral post-traumatic osteoarthritis, left knee
- M17.4 Other bilateral secondary osteoarthritis of knee
- M17.5 Other unilateral secondary osteoarthritis of knee
  Secondary osteoarthritis of knee NOS
- M17.9 Osteoarthritis of knee, unspecified
  AHA: Q4 2016

M18 Osteoarthritis of first carpometacarpal joint
- M18.0 Bilateral primary osteoarthritis of first carpometacarpal joints
- M18.1 Unilateral primary osteoarthritis of first carpometacarpal joint
  Primary osteoarthritis of first carpometacarpal joint NOS
  - M18.10 Unilateral primary osteoarthritis of first carpometacarpal joint, unspecified hand
  - M18.11 Unilateral primary osteoarthritis of first carpometacarpal joint, right hand
  - M18.12 Unilateral primary osteoarthritis of first carpometacarpal joint, left hand
- M18.2 Bilateral post-traumatic osteoarthritis of first carpometacarpal joints
- M18.3 Unilateral post-traumatic osteoarthritis of first carpometacarpal joint
  Post-traumatic osteoarthritis of first carpometacarpal joint NOS
  - M18.30 Unilateral post-traumatic osteoarthritis of first carpometacarpal joint, unspecified hand
  - M18.31 Unilateral post-traumatic osteoarthritis of first carpometacarpal joint, right hand

---

PDxR Unacceptable principal diagnosis symbol per Medicare code edits   PoA Code exempt from diagnosis present on admission requirement
❓ Questionable admission   cc Complication or comorbidity   CC/MCC Exc CC/MCC exclusion   MCC Major complication or comorbidity
Principal diagnosis as its own CC   Principal diagnosis as its own MCC   HCC HCC diagnosis code   RxHCC RxHCC diagnosis code
MACRA code   Z1 Z code as first-listed diagnosis

M18.32 Unilateral post-traumatic osteoarthritis of first carpometacarpal joint, left hand

M18.4 Other bilateral secondary osteoarthritis of first carpometacarpal joints

5️⃣ M18.5 Other unilateral secondary osteoarthritis of first carpometacarpal joint

Secondary osteoarthritis of first carpometacarpal joint NOS

M18.50 Other unilateral secondary osteoarthritis of first carpometacarpal joint, unspecified hand

M18.51 Other unilateral secondary osteoarthritis of first carpometacarpal joint, right hand

M18.52 Other unilateral secondary osteoarthritis of first carpometacarpal joint, left hand

M18.9 Osteoarthritis of first carpometacarpal joint, unspecified

4️⃣ M19 Other and unspecified osteoarthritis

EXCLUDES1 polyarthritis (M15.-)

EXCLUDES2 arthrosis of spine (M47.-)

hallux rigidus (M20.2)

osteoarthritis of spine (M47.-)

5️⃣ M19.0 Primary osteoarthritis of other joints

6️⃣ M19.01 Primary osteoarthritis, shoulder

M19.011 Primary osteoarthritis, right shoulder

AHA: Q4 2016

M19.012 Primary osteoarthritis, left shoulder

M19.019 Primary osteoarthritis, unspecified shoulder

6️⃣ M19.02 Primary osteoarthritis, elbow

M19.021 Primary osteoarthritis, right elbow

M19.022 Primary osteoarthritis, left elbow

M19.029 Primary osteoarthritis, unspecified elbow

6️⃣ M19.03 Primary osteoarthritis, wrist

M19.031 Primary osteoarthritis, right wrist

M19.032 Primary osteoarthritis, left wrist

M19.039 Primary osteoarthritis, unspecified wrist

6️⃣ M19.04 Primary osteoarthritis, hand

EXCLUDES2 primary osteoarthritis of first carpometacarpal joint (M18.0-, M18.1-)

M19.041 Primary osteoarthritis, right hand

M19.042 Primary osteoarthritis, left hand

M19.049 Primary osteoarthritis, unspecified hand

6️⃣ M19.07 Primary osteoarthritis ankle and foot

M19.071 Primary osteoarthritis, right ankle and foot

M19.072 Primary osteoarthritis, left ankle and foot

M19.079 Primary osteoarthritis, unspecified ankle and foot

5️⃣ M19.1 Post-traumatic osteoarthritis of other joints

6️⃣ M19.11 Post-traumatic osteoarthritis, shoulder

M19.111 Post-traumatic osteoarthritis, right shoulder

M19.112 Post-traumatic osteoarthritis, left shoulder

M19.119 Post-traumatic osteoarthritis, unspecified shoulder

6️⃣ M19.12 Post-traumatic osteoarthritis, elbow

M19.121 Post-traumatic osteoarthritis, right elbow

M19.122 Post-traumatic osteoarthritis, left elbow

M19.129 Post-traumatic osteoarthritis, unspecified elbow

6️⃣ M19.13 Post-traumatic osteoarthritis, wrist

M19.131 Post-traumatic osteoarthritis, right wrist

M19.132 Post-traumatic osteoarthritis, left wrist

M19.139 Post-traumatic osteoarthritis, unspecified wrist

6️⃣ M19.14 Post-traumatic osteoarthritis, hand

EXCLUDES2 post-traumatic osteoarthritis of first carpometacarpal joint (M18.2-, M18.3-)

M19.141 Post-traumatic osteoarthritis, right hand

M19.142 Post-traumatic osteoarthritis, left hand

M19.149 Post-traumatic osteoarthritis, unspecified hand

6️⃣ M19.17 Post-traumatic osteoarthritis, ankle and foot

M19.171 Post-traumatic osteoarthritis, right ankle and foot

M19.172 Post-traumatic osteoarthritis, left ankle and foot

M19.179 Post-traumatic osteoarthritis, unspecified ankle and foot

5️⃣ M19.2 Secondary osteoarthritis of other joints

6️⃣ M19.21 Secondary osteoarthritis, shoulder

M19.211 Secondary osteoarthritis, right shoulder

M19.212 Secondary osteoarthritis, left shoulder

M19.219 Secondary osteoarthritis, unspecified shoulder

6️⃣ M19.22 Secondary osteoarthritis, elbow

M19.221 Secondary osteoarthritis, right elbow

M19.222 Secondary osteoarthritis, left elbow

M19.229 Secondary osteoarthritis, unspecified elbow

6️⃣ M19.23 Secondary osteoarthritis, wrist

M19.231 Secondary osteoarthritis, right wrist

M19.232 Secondary osteoarthritis, left wrist

M19.239 Secondary osteoarthritis, unspecified wrist

6️⃣ M19.24 Secondary osteoarthritis, hand

M19.241 Secondary osteoarthritis, right hand

M19.242 Secondary osteoarthritis, left hand

M19.249 Secondary osteoarthritis, unspecified hand

6️⃣ M19.27 Secondary osteoarthritis, ankle and foot

M19.271 Secondary osteoarthritis, right ankle and foot

M19.272 Secondary osteoarthritis, left ankle and foot

M19.279 Secondary osteoarthritis, unspecified ankle and foot

5️⃣ M19.9 Osteoarthritis, unspecified site

M19.90 Unspecified osteoarthritis, unspecified site

AHA: Q4 2016

Arthrosis NOS

Arthritis NOS

Osteoarthritis NOS

M19.91 Primary osteoarthritis, unspecified site

Primary osteoarthritis NOS

M19.92 Post-traumatic osteoarthritis, unspecified site

Post-traumatic osteoarthritis NOS

M19.93 Secondary osteoarthritis, unspecified site

Secondary osteoarthritis NOS

Other joint disorders (M20-M25)

EXCLUDES2 joints of the spine (M40-M54)

4️⃣ M20 Acquired deformities of fingers and toes

EXCLUDES1 acquired absence of fingers and toes (Z89.-)

congenital absence of fingers and toes (Q71.3-, Q72.3-)

congenital deformities and malformations of fingers and toes (Q66.-, Q68-Q70, Q74.-)

5️⃣ M20.0 Deformity of finger(s)

EXCLUDES1 clubbing of fingers (R68.3)

palmar fascial fibromatosis [Dupuytren] (M72.0)

trigger finger (M65.3)

6️⃣ M20.00 Unspecified deformity of finger(s)

M20.001 Unspecified deformity of right finger(s)

M20.002 Unspecified deformity of left finger(s)

M20.009 Unspecified deformity of unspecified finger(s)

6️⃣ M20.01 Mallet finger

M20.011 Mallet finger of right finger(s)

M20.012 Mallet finger of left finger(s)

Unspecified Code   Other Specified Code   Manifestation Code   Ⓝ Newborn   Ⓟ Pediatric   Ⓜ Maternity   Ⓐ Adult   ♂ Male   ♀ Female
● New Code   ▲ Revised Code Title   ►◄ Revised Text   NOTES   INCLUDES   EXCLUDES 1 Not coded here   EXCLUDES 2 Not included here
4️⃣ 4th character required   5️⃣ 5th character required   6️⃣ 6th character required   7️⃣ 7th character required
7️⃣ Extension 'X' Alert   HAC Hospital-acquired condition (HAC) alert   AHA AHA Coding Clinic©

M20.019 Mallet finger of unspecified finger(s)
6ᵗʰ M20.02 Boutonnière deformity
    M20.021 Boutonnière deformity of right finger(s)
    M20.022 Boutonnière deformity of left finger(s)
    M20.029 Boutonnière deformity of unspecified finger(s)
6ᵗʰ M20.03 Swan-neck deformity
    M20.031 Swan-neck deformity of right finger(s)
    M20.032 Swan-neck deformity of left finger(s)
    M20.039 Swan-neck deformity of unspecified finger(s)
6ᵗʰ M20.09 Other deformity of finger(s)
    M20.091 Other deformity of right finger(s)
    M20.092 Other deformity of left finger(s)
    M20.099 Other deformity of finger(s), unspecified finger(s)

Normal   Bunion

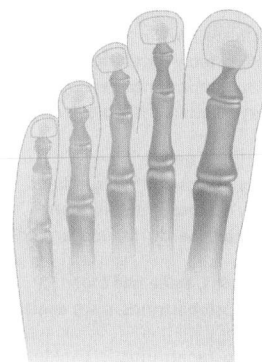 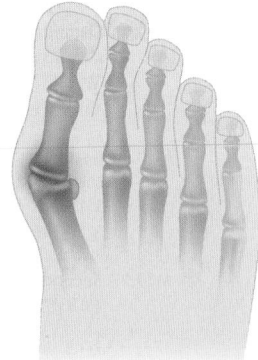

Figure 13.2 Bunion

5ᵗʰ M20.1 Hallux valgus (acquired)
    EXCLUDES2 bunion (M21.6-)
    M20.10 Hallux valgus (acquired), unspecified foot
    M20.11 Hallux valgus (acquired), right foot
    M20.12 Hallux valgus (acquired), left foot
5ᵗʰ M20.2 Hallux rigidus
    M20.20 Hallux rigidus, unspecified foot
    M20.21 Hallux rigidus, right foot
    M20.22 Hallux rigidus, left foot
5ᵗʰ M20.3 Hallux varus (acquired)
    M20.30 Hallux varus (acquired), unspecified foot
    M20.31 Hallux varus (acquired), right foot
    M20.32 Hallux varus (acquired), left foot
5ᵗʰ M20.4 Other hammer toe(s) (acquired)
    M20.40 Other hammer toe(s) (acquired), unspecified foot
    M20.41 Other hammer toe(s) (acquired), right foot
    M20.42 Other hammer toe(s) (acquired), left foot
5ᵗʰ M20.5 Other deformities of toe(s) (acquired)
  6ᵗʰ M20.5X Other deformities of toe(s) (acquired)
    M20.5X1 Other deformities of toe(s) (acquired), right foot
    M20.5X2 Other deformities of toe(s) (acquired), left foot
    M20.5X9 Other deformities of toe(s) (acquired), unspecified foot
5ᵗʰ M20.6 Acquired deformities of toe(s), unspecified
    M20.60 Acquired deformities of toe(s), unspecified, unspecified foot
    M20.61 Acquired deformities of toe(s), unspecified, right foot
    M20.62 Acquired deformities of toe(s), unspecified, left foot
4ᵗʰ M21 Other acquired deformities of limbs
    EXCLUDES1 acquired absence of limb (Z89.-)
      congenital absence of limbs (Q71-Q73)

congenital deformities and malformations of limbs (Q65-Q66, Q68-Q74)
    EXCLUDES2 acquired deformities of fingers or toes (M20.-)
      coxa plana (M91.2)
5ᵗʰ M21.0 Valgus deformity, not elsewhere classified
    EXCLUDES1 metatarsus valgus (Q66.6)
      talipes calcaneovalgus (Q66.4)
    M21.00 Valgus deformity, not elsewhere classified, unspecified site
  6ᵗʰ M21.02 Valgus deformity, not elsewhere classified, elbow
    Cubitus valgus
    M21.021 Valgus deformity, not elsewhere classified, right elbow
    M21.022 Valgus deformity, not elsewhere classified, left elbow
    M21.029 Valgus deformity, not elsewhere classified, unspecified elbow
  6ᵗʰ M21.05 Valgus deformity, not elsewhere classified, hip
    M21.051 Valgus deformity, not elsewhere classified, right hip
    M21.052 Valgus deformity, not elsewhere classified, left hip
    M21.059 Valgus deformity, not elsewhere classified, unspecified hip
  6ᵗʰ M21.06 Valgus deformity, not elsewhere classified, knee
    Genu valgum
    Knock knee
    M21.061 Valgus deformity, not elsewhere classified, right knee
    M21.062 Valgus deformity, not elsewhere classified, left knee
    M21.069 Valgus deformity, not elsewhere classified, unspecified knee
  6ᵗʰ M21.07 Valgus deformity, not elsewhere classified, ankle
    M21.071 Valgus deformity, not elsewhere classified, right ankle
    M21.072 Valgus deformity, not elsewhere classified, left ankle
    M21.079 Valgus deformity, not elsewhere classified, unspecified ankle
5ᵗʰ M21.1 Varus deformity, not elsewhere classified
    EXCLUDES1 metatarsus varus (Q66.22)
      tibia vara (M92.5)
    M21.10 Varus deformity, not elsewhere classified, unspecified site
  6ᵗʰ M21.12 Varus deformity, not elsewhere classified, elbow
    Cubitus varus, elbow
    M21.121 Varus deformity, not elsewhere classified, right elbow
    M21.122 Varus deformity, not elsewhere classified, left elbow
    M21.129 Varus deformity, not elsewhere classified, unspecified elbow
  6ᵗʰ M21.15 Varus deformity, not elsewhere classified, hip
    M21.151 Varus deformity, not elsewhere classified, right hip
    M21.152 Varus deformity, not elsewhere classified, left hip
    M21.159 Varus deformity, not elsewhere classified, unspecified
  6ᵗʰ M21.16 Varus deformity, not elsewhere classified, knee
    Bow leg
    Genu varum
    M21.161 Varus deformity, not elsewhere classified, right knee
    M21.162 Varus deformity, not elsewhere classified, left knee
    M21.169 Varus deformity, not elsewhere classified, unspecified knee
  6ᵗʰ M21.17 Varus deformity, not elsewhere classified, ankle
    M21.171 Varus deformity, not elsewhere classified, right ankle

ᴾᴰˣ Unacceptable principal diagnosis symbol per Medicare code edits   ᴾᴼᴬ Code exempt from diagnosis present on admission requirement
❓ Questionable admission   ᶜᶜ Complication or comorbidity   ᶜᶜ/ᴹᶜᶜ ᴱˣ CC/MCC exclusion   ᴹᶜᶜ Major complication or comorbidity
ᴾᴰˣ Principal diagnosis as its own CC   ᴾᴰˣ Principal diagnosis as its own MCC   ᴴᶜᶜ HCC diagnosis code   ᴿˣ RxHCC diagnosis code
MACRA code   Z₁ Z code as first-listed diagnosis

When symbols appear on a code that requires a 7th character extension, refer to Appendix B to identify applicable 7th character codes.

M21.172 Varus deformity, not elsewhere classified, left **ankle**

M21.179 **Varus deformity, not elsewhere classified, unspecified ankle**

⑤ M21.2 Flexion deformity

M21.20 **Flexion deformity, unspecified site**

⑥ M21.21 Flexion deformity, shoulder

M21.211 Flexion deformity, right **shoulder**

M21.212 Flexion deformity, left **shoulder**

M21.219 **Flexion deformity, unspecified shoulder**

⑥ M21.22 Flexion deformity, elbow

M21.221 Flexion deformity, right **elbow**

M21.222 Flexion deformity, left **elbow**

M21.229 **Flexion deformity, unspecified elbow**

⑥ M21.23 Flexion deformity, wrist

M21.231 Flexion deformity, right **wrist**

M21.232 Flexion deformity, left **wrist**

M21.239 **Flexion deformity, unspecified wrist**

⑥ M21.24 Flexion deformity, finger joints

M21.241 Flexion deformity, right **finger joints**

M21.242 Flexion deformity, left **finger joints**

M21.249 **Flexion deformity, unspecified finger joints**

⑥ M21.25 Flexion deformity, hip

M21.251 Flexion deformity, right **hip**

M21.252 Flexion deformity, left **hip**

M21.259 **Flexion deformity, unspecified hip**

⑥ M21.26 Flexion deformity, knee

M21.261 Flexion deformity, right **knee**

M21.262 Flexion deformity, left **knee**

M21.269 **Flexion deformity, unspecified knee**

⑥ M21.27 Flexion deformity, ankle and toes

M21.271 Flexion deformity, right **ankle and toes**

M21.272 Flexion deformity, left **ankle and toes**

M21.279 **Flexion deformity, unspecified ankle and toes**

⑤ M21.3 Wrist or foot drop (acquired)

⑥ M21.33 Wrist drop (acquired)

M21.331 Wrist drop, right **wrist**

M21.332 Wrist drop, left **wrist**

M21.339 **Wrist drop, unspecified wrist**

⑥ M21.37 Foot drop (acquired)

M21.371 Foot drop, right **foot**

M21.372 Foot drop, left **foot**

M21.379 **Foot drop, unspecified foot**

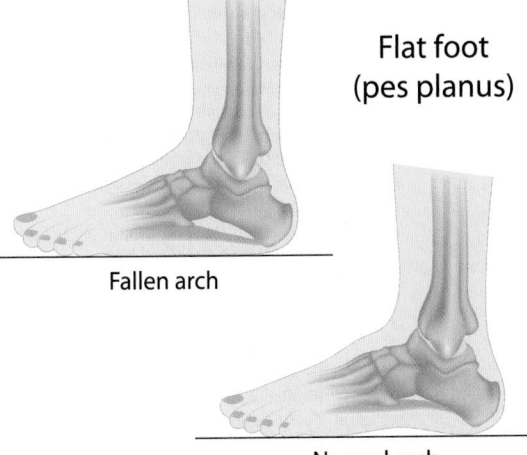

Flat foot
(pes planus)

Fallen arch

Normal arch

Figure 13.3 Illustration showing normal and flat foot

⑤ M21.4 Flat foot [pes planus] (acquired)

EXCLUDES1 congenital pes planus (Q66.5-)

M21.40 **Flat foot [pes planus] (acquired), unspecified foot**

M21.41 Flat foot [pes planus] (acquired), right **foot**

M21.42 Flat foot [pes planus] (acquired), left **foot**

⑤ M21.5 Acquired clawhand, clubhand, clawfoot and clubfoot

EXCLUDES1 clubfoot, not specified as acquired (Q66.89)

⑥ M21.51 Acquired clawhand

M21.511 Acquired clawhand, right **hand**

M21.512 Acquired clawhand, left **hand**

M21.519 **Acquired clawhand, unspecified hand**

⑥ M21.52 Acquired clubhand

M21.521 Acquired clubhand, right **hand**

M21.522 Acquired clubhand, left **hand**

M21.529 **Acquired clubhand, unspecified hand**

⑥ M21.53 Acquired clawfoot

M21.531 Acquired clawfoot, right **foot**

M21.532 Acquired clawfoot, left **foot**

M21.539 **Acquired clawfoot, unspecified foot**

⑥ M21.54 Acquired clubfoot

M21.541 Acquired clubfoot, right **foot**

M21.542 Acquired clubfoot, left **foot**

M21.549 **Acquired clubfoot, unspecified foot**

⑤ M21.6 Other acquired deformities of foot

EXCLUDES2 deformities of toe (acquired) (M20.1-M20.6-)

⑥ M21.61 Bunion

M21.611 Bunion of right **foot**

AHA: Q4 2016

M21.612 Bunion of left **foot**

AHA: Q4 2016

M21.619 Bunion of unspecified **foot**

AHA: Q4 2016

⑥ M21.62 Bunionette

M21.621 Bunionette of right **foot**

AHA: Q4 2016

M21.622 Bunionette of left **foot**

AHA: Q4 2016

M21.629 Bunionette of unspecified **foot**

AHA: Q4 2016

⑥ M21.6X Other acquired deformities of foot

M21.6X1 Other acquired deformities of right **foot**

M21.6X2 Other acquired deformities of left **foot**

M21.6X9 **Other acquired deformities of unspecified foot**

⑤ M21.7 Unequal limb length (acquired)

NOTES The site used should correspond to the shorter limb

M21.70 **Unequal limb length (acquired), unspecified site**

⑥ M21.72 Unequal limb length (acquired), humerus

M21.721 Unequal limb length (acquired), right **humerus**

M21.722 Unequal limb length (acquired), left **humerus**

M21.729 **Unequal limb length (acquired), unspecified humerus**

⑥ M21.73 Unequal limb length (acquired), ulna and radius

M21.731 Unequal limb length (acquired), right **ulna**

M21.732 Unequal limb length (acquired), left **ulna**

M21.733 Unequal limb length (acquired), right **radius**

M21.734 Unequal limb length (acquired), left **radius**

M21.739 **Unequal limb length (acquired), unspecified ulna and radius**

⑥ M21.75 Unequal limb length (acquired), femur

M21.751 Unequal limb length (acquired), right **femur**

M21.752 Unequal limb length (acquired), left **femur**

M21.759 **Unequal limb length (acquired), unspecified femur**

⑥ M21.76 Unequal limb length (acquired), tibia and fibula

● Unspecified Code	Other Specified Code	Manifestation Code	Ⓝ Newborn	Ⓟ Pediatric	Ⓜ Maternity	Ⓐ Adult	♂ Male	♀ Female

● New Code ▲ Revised Code Title ►◄ Revised Text **NOTES** *INCLUDES* *EXCLUDES 1* Not coded here *EXCLUDES 2* Not included here

④ 4th character required ⑤ 5th character required ⑥ 6th character required ⑦ 7th character required

⑦ Extension 'X' Alert **HAC** Hospital-acquired condition (HAC) alert **AHA** AHA Coding Clinic©

M21.761 Unequal limb length (acquired), right tibia
M21.762 Unequal limb length (acquired), left tibia
M21.763 Unequal limb length (acquired), right fibula
M21.764 Unequal limb length (acquired), left fibula
M21.769 Unequal limb length (acquired), unspecified tibia and fibula

[5th] M21.8 Other specified acquired deformities of limbs
[EXCLUDES2] *coxa plana (M91.2)*
M21.80 Other specified acquired deformities of unspecified limb
[6th] M21.82 Other specified acquired deformities of upper arm
M21.821 Other specified acquired deformities of right upper arm
M21.822 Other specified acquired deformities of left upper arm
M21.829 Other specified acquired deformities of unspecified upper arm
[6th] M21.83 Other specified acquired deformities of forearm
M21.831 Other specified acquired deformities of right forearm
M21.832 Other specified acquired deformities of left forearm
M21.839 Other specified acquired deformities of unspecified forearm
[6th] M21.85 Other specified acquired deformities of thigh
M21.851 Other specified acquired deformities of right thigh
M21.852 Other specified acquired deformities of left thigh
M21.859 Other specified acquired deformities of unspecified thigh
[6th] M21.86 Other specified acquired deformities of lower leg
M21.861 Other specified acquired deformities of right lower leg
M21.862 Other specified acquired deformities of left lower leg
M21.869 Other specified acquired deformities of unspecified lower leg

[5th] M21.9 Unspecified acquired deformity of limb and hand
M21.90 Unspecified acquired deformity of unspecified limb
[6th] M21.92 Unspecified acquired deformity of upper arm
M21.921 Unspecified acquired deformity of right upper arm
M21.922 Unspecified acquired deformity of left upper arm
M21.929 Unspecified acquired deformity of unspecified upper arm
[6th] M21.93 Unspecified acquired deformity of forearm
M21.931 Unspecified acquired deformity of right forearm
M21.932 Unspecified acquired deformity of left forearm
M21.939 Unspecified acquired deformity of unspecified forearm
[6th] M21.94 Unspecified acquired deformity of hand
M21.941 Unspecified acquired deformity of hand, right hand
M21.942 Unspecified acquired deformity of hand, left hand
M21.949 Unspecified acquired deformity of hand, unspecified hand
[6th] M21.95 Unspecified acquired deformity of thigh
M21.951 Unspecified acquired deformity of right thigh
M21.952 Unspecified acquired deformity of left thigh
M21.959 Unspecified acquired deformity of unspecified thigh
[6th] M21.96 Unspecified acquired deformity of lower leg
M21.961 Unspecified acquired deformity of right lower leg
M21.962 Unspecified acquired deformity of left lower leg
M21.969 Unspecified acquired deformity of unspecified lower leg

[4th] M22 Disorder of patella
[EXCLUDES1] *traumatic dislocation of patella (S83.0-)*

[5th] M22.0 Recurrent dislocation of patella
M22.00 Recurrent dislocation of patella, unspecified knee
M22.01 Recurrent dislocation of patella, right knee
M22.02 Recurrent dislocation of patella, left knee

[5th] M22.1 Recurrent subluxation of patella
Incomplete dislocation of patella
M22.10 Recurrent subluxation of patella, unspecified knee
M22.11 Recurrent subluxation of patella, right knee
M22.12 Recurrent subluxation of patella, left knee

[5th] M22.2 Patellofemoral disorders
[6th] M22.2X Patellofemoral disorders
M22.2X1 Patellofemoral disorders, right knee
M22.2X2 Patellofemoral disorders, left knee
M22.2X9 Patellofemoral disorders, unspecified knee

[5th] M22.3 Other derangements of patella
[6th] M22.3X Other derangements of patella
M22.3X1 Other derangements of patella, right knee
M22.3X2 Other derangements of patella, left knee
M22.3X9 Other derangements of patella, unspecified knee

[5th] M22.4 Chondromalacia patellae
M22.40 Chondromalacia patellae, unspecified knee
M22.41 Chondromalacia patellae, right knee
M22.42 Chondromalacia patellae, left knee

[5th] M22.8 Other disorders of patella
[6th] M22.8X Other disorders of patella
M22.8X1 Other disorders of patella, right knee
M22.8X2 Other disorders of patella, left knee
M22.8X9 Other disorders of patella, unspecified knee

[5th] M22.9 Unspecified disorder of patella
M22.90 Unspecified disorder of patella, unspecified knee
M22.91 Unspecified disorder of patella, right knee
M22.92 Unspecified disorder of patella, left knee

[4th] M23 Internal derangement of knee
[EXCLUDES1] *ankylosis (M24.66)*
current injury - see injury of knee and lower leg (S80-S89)
deformity of knee (M21.-)
osteochondritis dissecans (M93.2)
recurrent dislocation or subluxation of joints (M24.4)
recurrent dislocation or subluxation of patella (M22.0-M22.1)

[5th] M23.0 Cystic meniscus
[6th] M23.00 Cystic meniscus, unspecified meniscus
Cystic meniscus, unspecified lateral meniscus
Cystic meniscus, unspecified medial meniscus
M23.000 Cystic meniscus, unspecified lateral meniscus, right knee
M23.001 Cystic meniscus, unspecified lateral meniscus, left knee
M23.002 Cystic meniscus, unspecified lateral meniscus, unspecified knee
M23.003 Cystic meniscus, unspecified medial meniscus, right knee
M23.004 Cystic meniscus, unspecified medial meniscus, left knee
M23.005 Cystic meniscus, unspecified medial meniscus, unspecified knee
M23.006 Cystic meniscus, unspecified meniscus, right knee
M23.007 Cystic meniscus, unspecified meniscus, left knee
M23.009 Cystic meniscus, unspecified meniscus, unspecified knee

Unacceptable principal diagnosis symbol per Medicare code edits — Code exempt from diagnosis present on admission requirement
Questionable admission — Complication or comorbidity — CC/MCC exclusion — Major complication or comorbidity
Principal diagnosis as its own CC — Principal diagnosis as its own MCC — [HCC] HCC diagnosis code — [RxHCC] RxHCC diagnosis code
MACRA code — [Z1] Z code as first-listed diagnosis

When symbols appear on a code that requires a 7th character extension, refer to Appendix B to identify applicable 7th character codes.

6️⃣ M23.01 Cystic meniscus, anterior horn of medial meniscus
- M23.011 Cystic meniscus, anterior horn of medial meniscus, right knee
- M23.012 Cystic meniscus, anterior horn of medial meniscus, left knee
- M23.019 Cystic meniscus, anterior horn of medial meniscus, unspecified knee

6️⃣ M23.02 Cystic meniscus, posterior horn of medial meniscus
- M23.021 Cystic meniscus, posterior horn of medial meniscus, right knee
- M23.022 Cystic meniscus, posterior horn of medial meniscus, left knee
- M23.029 Cystic meniscus, posterior horn of medial meniscus, unspecified knee

6️⃣ M23.03 Cystic meniscus, other medial meniscus
- M23.031 Cystic meniscus, other medial meniscus, right knee
- M23.032 Cystic meniscus, other medial meniscus, left knee
- M23.039 Cystic meniscus, other medial meniscus, unspecified knee

6️⃣ M23.04 Cystic meniscus, anterior horn of lateral meniscus
- M23.041 Cystic meniscus, anterior horn of lateral meniscus, right knee
- M23.042 Cystic meniscus, anterior horn of lateral meniscus, left knee
- M23.049 Cystic meniscus, anterior horn of lateral meniscus, unspecified knee

6️⃣ M23.05 Cystic meniscus, posterior horn of lateral meniscus
- M23.051 Cystic meniscus, posterior horn of lateral meniscus, right knee
- M23.052 Cystic meniscus, posterior horn of lateral meniscus, left knee
- M23.059 Cystic meniscus, posterior horn of lateral meniscus, unspecified knee

6️⃣ M23.06 Cystic meniscus, other lateral meniscus
- M23.061 Cystic meniscus, other lateral meniscus, right knee
- M23.062 Cystic meniscus, other lateral meniscus, left knee
- M23.069 Cystic meniscus, other lateral meniscus, unspecified knee

5️⃣ M23.2 Derangement of meniscus due to old tear or injury
Old bucket-handle tear

6️⃣ M23.20 Derangement of unspecified meniscus due to old tear or injury
Derangement of unspecified lateral meniscus due to old tear or injury
Derangement of unspecified medial meniscus due to old tear or injury
- M23.200 Derangement of unspecified lateral meniscus due to old tear or injury, right knee
- M23.201 Derangement of unspecified lateral meniscus due to old tear or injury, left knee
- M23.202 Derangement of unspecified lateral meniscus due to old tear or injury, unspecified knee
- M23.203 Derangement of unspecified medial meniscus due to old tear or injury, right knee
- M23.204 Derangement of unspecified medial meniscus due to old tear or injury, left knee
- M23.205 Derangement of unspecified medial meniscus due to old tear or injury, unspecified knee
- M23.206 Derangement of unspecified meniscus due to old tear or injury, right knee
- M23.207 Derangement of unspecified meniscus due to old tear or injury, left knee
- M23.209 Derangement of unspecified meniscus due to old tear or injury, unspecified knee

6️⃣ M23.21 Derangement of anterior horn of medial meniscus due to old tear or injury
- M23.211 Derangement of anterior horn of medial meniscus due to old tear or injury, right knee
- M23.212 Derangement of anterior horn of medial meniscus due to old tear or injury, left knee
- M23.219 Derangement of anterior horn of medial meniscus due to old tear or injury, unspecified knee

6️⃣ M23.22 Derangement of posterior horn of medial meniscus due to old tear or injury
- M23.221 Derangement of posterior horn of medial meniscus due to old tear or injury, right knee
- M23.222 Derangement of posterior horn of medial meniscus due to old tear or injury, left knee
- M23.229 Derangement of posterior horn of medial meniscus due to old tear or injury, unspecified knee

6️⃣ M23.23 Derangement of other medial meniscus due to old tear or injury
- M23.231 Derangement of other medial meniscus due to old tear or injury, right knee
- M23.232 Derangement of other medial meniscus due to old tear or injury, left knee
- M23.239 Derangement of other medial meniscus due to old tear or injury, unspecified knee

6️⃣ M23.24 Derangement of anterior horn of lateral meniscus due to old tear or injury
- M23.241 Derangement of anterior horn of lateral meniscus due to old tear or injury, right knee
- M23.242 Derangement of anterior horn of lateral meniscus due to old tear or injury, left knee
- M23.249 Derangement of anterior horn of lateral meniscus due to old tear or injury, unspecified knee

6️⃣ M23.25 Derangement of posterior horn of lateral meniscus due to old tear or injury
- M23.251 Derangement of posterior horn of lateral meniscus due to old tear or injury, right knee
- M23.252 Derangement of posterior horn of lateral meniscus due to old tear or injury, left knee
- M23.259 Derangement of posterior horn of lateral meniscus due to old tear or injury, unspecified knee

6️⃣ M23.26 Derangement of other lateral meniscus due to old tear or injury
- M23.261 Derangement of other lateral meniscus due to old tear or injury, right knee
- M23.262 Derangement of other lateral meniscus due to old tear or injury, left knee
- M23.269 Derangement of other lateral meniscus due to old tear or injury, unspecified knee

5️⃣ M23.3 Other meniscus derangements
Degenerate meniscus
Detached meniscus
Retained meniscus

6️⃣ M23.30 Other meniscus derangements, unspecified meniscus
Other meniscus derangements, unspecified lateral meniscus
Other meniscus derangements, unspecified medial meniscus

Unspecified Code   Other Specified Code   Manifestation Code   N Newborn   P Pediatric   M Maternity   A Adult   ♂ Male   ♀ Female
● New Code   ▲ Revised Code Title   ▶◀ Revised Text   **NOTES**   *INCLUDES*   *EXCLUDES 1* Not coded here   *EXCLUDES 2* Not included here
4️⃣ 4th character required   5️⃣ 5th character required   6️⃣ 6th character required   7️⃣ 7th character required
7️⃣ Extension 'X' Alert   **HAC** Hospital-acquired condition (HAC) alert   **AHA** AHA Coding Clinic©

M23.300 Other meniscus derangements, unspecified lateral meniscus, right knee
M23.301 Other meniscus derangements, unspecified lateral meniscus, left knee
M23.302 Other meniscus derangements, unspecified lateral meniscus, unspecified knee
M23.303 Other meniscus derangements, unspecified medial meniscus, right knee
M23.304 Other meniscus derangements, unspecified medial meniscus, left knee
M23.305 Other meniscus derangements, unspecified medial meniscus, unspecified knee
M23.306 Other meniscus derangements, unspecified meniscus, right knee
M23.307 Other meniscus derangements, unspecified meniscus, left knee
M23.309 Other meniscus derangements, unspecified meniscus, unspecified knee

[6th] M23.31 Other meniscus derangements, anterior horn of medial meniscus
M23.311 Other meniscus derangements, anterior horn of medial meniscus, right knee
M23.312 Other meniscus derangements, anterior horn of medial meniscus, left knee
M23.319 Other meniscus derangements, anterior horn of medial meniscus, unspecified knee

[6th] M23.32 Other meniscus derangements, posterior horn of medial meniscus
M23.321 Other meniscus derangements, posterior horn of medial meniscus, right knee
M23.322 Other meniscus derangements, posterior horn of medial meniscus, left knee
M23.329 Other meniscus derangements, posterior horn of medial meniscus, unspecified knee

[6th] M23.33 Other meniscus derangements, other medial meniscus
M23.331 Other meniscus derangements, other medial meniscus, right knee
M23.332 Other meniscus derangements, other medial meniscus, left knee
M23.339 Other meniscus derangements, other medial meniscus, unspecified knee

[6th] M23.34 Other meniscus derangements, anterior horn of lateral meniscus
M23.341 Other meniscus derangements, anterior horn of lateral meniscus, right knee
M23.342 Other meniscus derangements, anterior horn of lateral meniscus, left knee
M23.349 Other meniscus derangements, anterior horn of lateral meniscus, unspecified knee

[6th] M23.35 Other meniscus derangements, posterior horn of lateral meniscus
M23.351 Other meniscus derangements, posterior horn of lateral meniscus, right knee
M23.352 Other meniscus derangements, posterior horn of lateral meniscus, left knee
M23.359 Other meniscus derangements, posterior horn of lateral meniscus, unspecified knee

[6th] M23.36 Other meniscus derangements, other lateral meniscus
M23.361 Other meniscus derangements, other lateral meniscus, right knee
M23.362 Other meniscus derangements, other lateral meniscus, left knee
M23.369 Other meniscus derangements, other lateral meniscus, unspecified knee

[5th] M23.4 Loose body in knee
M23.40 Loose body in knee, unspecified knee
M23.41 Loose body in knee, right knee
M23.42 Loose body in knee, left knee

[5th] M23.5 Chronic instability of knee
M23.50 Chronic instability of knee, unspecified knee
M23.51 Chronic instability of knee, right knee
M23.52 Chronic instability of knee, left knee

[5th] M23.6 Other spontaneous disruption of ligament(s) of knee

[6th] M23.60 Other spontaneous disruption of unspecified ligament of knee
M23.601 Other spontaneous disruption of unspecified ligament of right knee
M23.602 Other spontaneous disruption of unspecified ligament of left knee
M23.609 Other spontaneous disruption of unspecified ligament of unspecified knee

[6th] M23.61 Other spontaneous disruption of anterior cruciate ligament of knee
M23.611 Other spontaneous disruption of anterior cruciate ligament of right knee
M23.612 Other spontaneous disruption of anterior cruciate ligament of left knee
M23.619 Other spontaneous disruption of anterior cruciate ligament of unspecified knee

[6th] M23.62 Other spontaneous disruption of posterior cruciate ligament of knee
M23.621 Other spontaneous disruption of posterior cruciate ligament of right knee
M23.622 Other spontaneous disruption of posterior cruciate ligament of left knee
M23.629 Other spontaneous disruption of posterior cruciate ligament of unspecified knee

[6th] M23.63 Other spontaneous disruption of medial collateral ligament of knee
M23.631 Other spontaneous disruption of medial collateral ligament of right knee
M23.632 Other spontaneous disruption of medial collateral ligament of left knee
M23.639 Other spontaneous disruption of medial collateral ligament of unspecified knee

[6th] M23.64 Other spontaneous disruption of lateral collateral ligament of knee
M23.641 Other spontaneous disruption of lateral collateral ligament of right knee
M23.642 Other spontaneous disruption of lateral collateral ligament of left knee
M23.649 Other spontaneous disruption of lateral collateral ligament of unspecified knee

[6th] M23.67 Other spontaneous disruption of capsular ligament of knee
M23.671 Other spontaneous disruption of capsular ligament of right knee
M23.672 Other spontaneous disruption of capsular ligament of left knee
M23.679 Other spontaneous disruption of capsular ligament of unspecified knee

[5th] M23.8 Other internal derangements of knee
Laxity of ligament of knee
Snapping knee

[6th] M23.8X Other internal derangements of knee
M23.8X1 Other internal derangements of right knee
M23.8X2 Other internal derangements of left knee
M23.8X9 Other internal derangements of unspecified knee

[5th] M23.9 Unspecified internal derangement of knee
M23.90 Unspecified internal derangement of unspecified knee
M23.91 Unspecified internal derangement of right knee
M23.92 Unspecified internal derangement of left knee

[4th] M24 Other specific joint derangements
[EXCLUDES1] *current injury - see injury of joint by body region*
[EXCLUDES2] *ganglion (M67.4)*
snapping knee (M23.8-)
temporomandibular joint disorders (M26.6-)

Unacceptable principal diagnosis symbol per Medicare code edits · Code exempt from diagnosis present on admission requirement · Questionable admission · Complication or comorbidity · CC/MCC exclusion · Major complication or comorbidity · Principal diagnosis as its own CC · Principal diagnosis as its own MCC · HCC diagnosis code · RxHCC diagnosis code · MACRA code · Z code as first-listed diagnosis

M24.0 Loose body in joint
EXCLUDES2 *loose body in knee (M23.4)*
    M24.00 Loose body in unspecified joint
M24.01 Loose body in shoulder
    M24.011 Loose body in right shoulder
    M24.012 Loose body in left shoulder
    M24.019 Loose body in unspecified shoulder
M24.02 Loose body in elbow
    M24.021 Loose body in right elbow
    M24.022 Loose body in left elbow
    M24.029 Loose body in unspecified elbow
M24.03 Loose body in wrist
    M24.031 Loose body in right wrist
    M24.032 Loose body in left wrist
    M24.039 Loose body in unspecified wrist
M24.04 Loose body in finger joints
    M24.041 Loose body in right finger joint(s)
    M24.042 Loose body in left finger joint(s)
    M24.049 Loose body in unspecified finger joint(s)
M24.05 Loose body in hip
    M24.051 Loose body in right hip
    M24.052 Loose body in left hip
    M24.059 Loose body in unspecified hip
M24.07 Loose body in ankle and toe joints
    M24.071 Loose body in right ankle
    M24.072 Loose body in left ankle
    M24.073 Loose body in unspecified ankle
    M24.074 Loose body in right toe joint(s)
    M24.075 Loose body in left toe joint(s)
    M24.076 Loose body in unspecified toe joints
    M24.08 Loose body, other site
M24.1 Other articular cartilage disorders
EXCLUDES2 *chondrocalcinosis (M11.1, M11.2-)*
    internal derangement of knee (M23.-)
    metastatic calcification (E83.5)
    ochronosis (E70.2)
    M24.10 Other articular cartilage disorders, unspecified site
M24.11 Other articular cartilage disorders, shoulder
    M24.111 Other articular cartilage disorders, right shoulder
    M24.112 Other articular cartilage disorders, left shoulder
    M24.119 Other articular cartilage disorders, unspecified shoulder
M24.12 Other articular cartilage disorders, elbow
    M24.121 Other articular cartilage disorders, right elbow
    M24.122 Other articular cartilage disorders, left elbow
    M24.129 Other articular cartilage disorders, unspecified elbow
M24.13 Other articular cartilage disorders, wrist
    M24.131 Other articular cartilage disorders, right wrist
    M24.132 Other articular cartilage disorders, left wrist
    M24.139 Other articular cartilage disorders, unspecified wrist
M24.14 Other articular cartilage disorders, hand
    M24.141 Other articular cartilage disorders, right hand
    M24.142 Other articular cartilage disorders, left hand
    M24.149 Other articular cartilage disorders, unspecified hand
M24.15 Other articular cartilage disorders, hip
    M24.151 Other articular cartilage disorders, right hip
    M24.152 Other articular cartilage disorders, left hip

    M24.159 Other articular cartilage disorders, unspecified hip
M24.17 Other articular cartilage disorders, ankle and foot
    M24.171 Other articular cartilage disorders, right ankle
    M24.172 Other articular cartilage disorders, left ankle
    M24.173 Other articular cartilage disorders, unspecified ankle
    M24.174 Other articular cartilage disorders, right foot
    M24.175 Other articular cartilage disorders, left foot
    M24.176 Other articular cartilage disorders, unspecified foot
M24.2 Disorder of ligament
Instability secondary to old ligament injury
Ligamentous laxity NOS
EXCLUDES1 *familial ligamentous laxity (M35.7)*
EXCLUDES2 *internal derangement of knee (M23.5-M23.89)*
    M24.20 Disorder of ligament, unspecified site
M24.21 Disorder of ligament, shoulder
    M24.211 Disorder of ligament, right shoulder
    M24.212 Disorder of ligament, left shoulder
    M24.219 Disorder of ligament, unspecified shoulder
M24.22 Disorder of ligament, elbow
    M24.221 Disorder of ligament, right elbow
    M24.222 Disorder of ligament, left elbow
    M24.229 Disorder of ligament, unspecified elbow
M24.23 Disorder of ligament, wrist
    M24.231 Disorder of ligament, right wrist
    M24.232 Disorder of ligament, left wrist
    M24.239 Disorder of ligament, unspecified wrist
M24.24 Disorder of ligament, hand
    M24.241 Disorder of ligament, right hand
    M24.242 Disorder of ligament, left hand
    M24.249 Disorder of ligament, unspecified hand
M24.25 Disorder of ligament, hip
    M24.251 Disorder of ligament, right hip
    M24.252 Disorder of ligament, left hip
    M24.259 Disorder of ligament, unspecified hip
M24.27 Disorder of ligament, ankle and foot
    M24.271 Disorder of ligament, right ankle
    M24.272 Disorder of ligament, left ankle
    M24.273 Disorder of ligament, unspecified ankle
    M24.274 Disorder of ligament, right foot
    M24.275 Disorder of ligament, left foot
    M24.276 Disorder of ligament, unspecified foot
    M24.28 Disorder of ligament, vertebrae
M24.3 Pathological dislocation of joint, not elsewhere classified
EXCLUDES1 *congenital dislocation or displacement of joint- see congenital malformations and deformations of the musculoskeletal system (Q65-Q79)*
    current injury - see injury of joints and ligaments by body region
    recurrent dislocation of joint (M24.4-)
    M24.30 Pathological dislocation of unspecified joint, not elsewhere classified
M24.31 Pathological dislocation of shoulder, not elsewhere classified
    M24.311 Pathological dislocation of right shoulder, not elsewhere classified
    M24.312 Pathological dislocation of left shoulder, not elsewhere classified
    M24.319 Pathological dislocation of unspecified shoulder, not elsewhere classified
M24.32 Pathological dislocation of elbow, not elsewhere classified

---

Unspecified Code   Other Specified Code   Manifestation Code   N Newborn   P Pediatric   M Maternity   A Adult   ♂ Male   ♀ Female
● New Code   ▲ Revised Code Title   ▶◀ Revised Text   **NOTES**   *INCLUDES*   *EXCLUDES 1* Not coded here   *EXCLUDES 2* Not included here
4th character required   5th character required   6th character required   7th character required
Extension 'X' Alert   HAC Hospital-acquired condition (HAC) alert   **AHA** AHA Coding Clinic©

M24.321 Pathological dislocation of right elbow, not elsewhere classified
M24.322 Pathological dislocation of left elbow, not elsewhere classified
M24.329 Pathological dislocation of unspecified elbow, not elsewhere classified

[6th] M24.33 Pathological dislocation of wrist, not elsewhere classified
M24.331 Pathological dislocation of right wrist, not elsewhere classified
M24.332 Pathological dislocation of left wrist, not elsewhere classified
M24.339 Pathological dislocation of unspecified wrist, not elsewhere classified

[6th] M24.34 Pathological dislocation of hand, not elsewhere classified
M24.341 Pathological dislocation of right hand, not elsewhere classified
M24.342 Pathological dislocation of left hand, not elsewhere classified
M24.349 Pathological dislocation of unspecified hand, not elsewhere classified

[6th] M24.35 Pathological dislocation of hip, not elsewhere classified
M24.351 Pathological dislocation of right hip, not elsewhere classified
M24.352 Pathological dislocation of left hip, not elsewhere classified
M24.359 Pathological dislocation of unspecified hip, not elsewhere classified

[6th] M24.36 Pathological dislocation of knee, not elsewhere classified
M24.361 Pathological dislocation of right knee, not elsewhere classified
M24.362 Pathological dislocation of left knee, not elsewhere classified
M24.369 Pathological dislocation of unspecified knee, not elsewhere classified

[6th] M24.37 Pathological dislocation of ankle and foot, not elsewhere classified
M24.371 Pathological dislocation of right ankle, not elsewhere classified
M24.372 Pathological dislocation of left ankle, not elsewhere classified
M24.373 Pathological dislocation of unspecified ankle, not elsewhere classified
M24.374 Pathological dislocation of right foot, not elsewhere classified
M24.375 Pathological dislocation of left foot, not elsewhere classified
M24.376 Pathological dislocation of unspecified foot, not elsewhere classified

[5th] M24.4 Recurrent dislocation of joint
Recurrent subluxation of joint
[EXCLUDES2] *recurrent dislocation of patella (M22.0-M22.1)*
recurrent vertebral dislocation (M43.3-, M43.4, M43.5-)
M24.40 Recurrent dislocation, unspecified joint

[6th] M24.41 Recurrent dislocation, shoulder
M24.411 Recurrent dislocation, right shoulder
M24.412 Recurrent dislocation, left shoulder
M24.419 Recurrent dislocation, unspecified shoulder

[6th] M24.42 Recurrent dislocation, elbow
M24.421 Recurrent dislocation, right elbow
M24.422 Recurrent dislocation, left elbow
M24.429 Recurrent dislocation, unspecified elbow

[6th] M24.43 Recurrent dislocation, wrist
M24.431 Recurrent dislocation, right wrist
M24.432 Recurrent dislocation, left wrist
M24.439 Recurrent dislocation, unspecified wrist

[6th] M24.44 Recurrent dislocation, hand and finger(s)
M24.441 Recurrent dislocation, right hand
M24.442 Recurrent dislocation, left hand
M24.443 Recurrent dislocation, unspecified hand
M24.444 Recurrent dislocation, right finger
M24.445 Recurrent dislocation, left finger
M24.446 Recurrent dislocation, unspecified finger

[6th] M24.45 Recurrent dislocation, hip
M24.451 Recurrent dislocation, right hip
M24.452 Recurrent dislocation, left hip
M24.459 Recurrent dislocation, unspecified hip

[6th] M24.46 Recurrent dislocation, knee
M24.461 Recurrent dislocation, right knee
M24.462 Recurrent dislocation, left knee
M24.469 Recurrent dislocation, unspecified knee

[6th] M24.47 Recurrent dislocation, ankle, foot and toes
M24.471 Recurrent dislocation, right ankle
M24.472 Recurrent dislocation, left ankle
M24.473 Recurrent dislocation, unspecified ankle
M24.474 Recurrent dislocation, right foot
M24.475 Recurrent dislocation, left foot
M24.476 Recurrent dislocation, unspecified foot
M24.477 Recurrent dislocation, right toe(s)
M24.478 Recurrent dislocation, left toe(s)
M24.479 Recurrent dislocation, unspecified toe(s)

[5th] M24.5 Contracture of joint
[EXCLUDES1] *contracture of muscle without contracture of joint (M62.4-)*
contracture of tendon (sheath) without contracture of joint (M62.4-)
Dupuytren's contracture (M72.0)
[EXCLUDES2] *acquired deformities of limbs (M20-M21)*
M24.50 Contracture, unspecified joint

[6th] M24.51 Contracture, shoulder
M24.511 Contracture, right shoulder
M24.512 Contracture, left shoulder
M24.519 Contracture, unspecified shoulder

[6th] M24.52 Contracture, elbow
M24.521 Contracture, right elbow
M24.522 Contracture, left elbow
M24.529 Contracture, unspecified elbow

[6th] M24.53 Contracture, wrist
M24.531 Contracture, right wrist
M24.532 Contracture, left wrist
M24.539 Contracture, unspecified wrist

[6th] M24.54 Contracture, hand
M24.541 Contracture, right hand
M24.542 Contracture, left hand
M24.549 Contracture, unspecified hand

[6th] M24.55 Contracture, hip
M24.551 Contracture, right hip
AHA: Q2 2016
M24.552 Contracture, left hip
AHA: Q2 2016
M24.559 Contracture, unspecified hip

[6th] M24.56 Contracture, knee
M24.561 Contracture, right knee
AHA: Q2 2016
M24.562 Contracture, left knee
AHA: Q2 2016
M24.569 Contracture, unspecified knee

[6th] M24.57 Contracture, ankle and foot
M24.571 Contracture, right ankle
M24.572 Contracture, left ankle
M24.573 Contracture, unspecified ankle
M24.574 Contracture, right foot
M24.575 Contracture, left foot
M24.576 Contracture, unspecified foot

[PDx] Unacceptable principal diagnosis symbol per Medicare code edits [POA] Code exempt from diagnosis present on admission requirement
[Q] Questionable admission [CC] Complication or comorbidity [CC/MCC Exc] CC/MCC exclusion [MCC] Major complication or comorbidity
[PDx CC] Principal diagnosis as its own CC [PDx MCC] Principal diagnosis as its own MCC [HCC] HCC diagnosis code [RxHCC] RxHCC diagnosis code
MACRA code [Z-1] Z code as first-listed diagnosis

When symbols appear on a code that requires a 7th character extension, refer to Appendix B to identify applicable 7th character codes.

5ᵗʰ **M24.6 Ankylosis** of joint
   EXCLUDES1 *stiffness of joint without ankylosis (M25.6-)*
   EXCLUDES2 *spine (M43.2-)*
   M24.60 Ankylosis, unspecified joint
6ᵗʰ **M24.61 Ankylosis,** shoulder
   M24.611 Ankylosis, right **shoulder**
   M24.612 Ankylosis, left **shoulder**
   M24.619 Ankylosis, unspecified shoulder
6ᵗʰ **M24.62 Ankylosis,** elbow
   M24.621 Ankylosis, right **elbow**
   M24.622 Ankylosis, left **elbow**
   M24.629 Ankylosis, unspecified elbow
6ᵗʰ **M24.63 Ankylosis,** wrist
   M24.631 Ankylosis, right **wrist**
   M24.632 Ankylosis, left **wrist**
   M24.639 Ankylosis, unspecified wrist
6ᵗʰ **M24.64 Ankylosis,** hand
   M24.641 Ankylosis, right **hand**
   M24.642 Ankylosis, left **hand**
   M24.649 Ankylosis, unspecified hand
6ᵗʰ **M24.65 Ankylosis,** hip
   M24.651 Ankylosis, right **hip**
   M24.652 Ankylosis, left **hip**
   M24.659 Ankylosis, unspecified hip
6ᵗʰ **M24.66 Ankylosis,** knee
   M24.661 Ankylosis, right **knee**
   M24.662 Ankylosis, left **knee**
   M24.669 Ankylosis, unspecified knee
6ᵗʰ **M24.67 Ankylosis,** ankle and foot
   M24.671 Ankylosis, right **ankle**
   M24.672 Ankylosis, left **ankle**
   M24.673 Ankylosis, unspecified ankle
   M24.674 Ankylosis, right **foot**
   M24.675 Ankylosis, left **foot**
   M24.676 Ankylosis, unspecified foot
M24.7 Protrusio acetabuli
5ᵗʰ **M24.8 Other specific joint derangements, not elsewhere classified**
   EXCLUDES2 *iliotibial band syndrome (M76.3)*
   M24.80 Other specific joint derangements of unspecified joint, not elsewhere classified
6ᵗʰ **M24.81 Other specific joint derangements of** shoulder, **not elsewhere classified**
   M24.811 Other specific joint derangements of right **shoulder, not elsewhere classified**
   M24.812 Other specific joint derangements of left **shoulder, not elsewhere classified**
   M24.819 Other specific joint derangements of unspecified shoulder, not elsewhere classified
6ᵗʰ **M24.82 Other specific joint derangements of** elbow, **not elsewhere classified**
   M24.821 Other specific joint derangements of right **elbow, not elsewhere classified**
   M24.822 Other specific joint derangements of left **elbow, not elsewhere classified**
   M24.829 Other specific joint derangements of unspecified elbow, not elsewhere classified
6ᵗʰ **M24.83 Other specific joint derangements of** wrist, **not elsewhere classified**
   M24.831 Other specific joint derangements of right **wrist, not elsewhere classified**
   M24.832 Other specific joint derangements of left **wrist, not elsewhere classified**
   M24.839 Other specific joint derangements of unspecified wrist, not elsewhere classified
6ᵗʰ **M24.84 Other specific joint derangements of** hand, **not elsewhere classified**
   M24.841 Other specific joint derangements of right **hand, not elsewhere classified**

   M24.842 Other specific joint derangements of left **hand, not elsewhere classified**
   M24.849 Other specific joint derangements of unspecified hand, not elsewhere classified
6ᵗʰ **M24.85 Other specific joint derangements of** hip, **not elsewhere classified**
   Irritable hip
   M24.851 Other specific joint derangements of right **hip, not elsewhere classified**
   M24.852 Other specific joint derangements of left **hip, not elsewhere classified**
   M24.859 Other specific joint derangements of unspecified hip, not elsewhere classified
6ᵗʰ **M24.87 Other specific joint derangements of** ankle and foot, **not elsewhere classified**
   M24.871 Other specific joint derangements of right **ankle, not elsewhere classified**
   M24.872 Other specific joint derangements of left **ankle, not elsewhere classified**
   M24.873 Other specific joint derangements of unspecified ankle, not elsewhere classified
   M24.874 Other specific joint derangements of right **foot, not elsewhere classified**
   M24.875 Other specific joint derangements left **foot, not elsewhere classified**
   M24.876 Other specific joint derangements of unspecified foot, not elsewhere classified
M24.9 Joint derangement, unspecified
4ᵗʰ **M25 Other joint disorder, not elsewhere classified**
   EXCLUDES2 *abnormality of gait and mobility (R26.-)*
      acquired deformities of limb (M20-M21)
      calcification of bursa (M71.4-)
      calcification of shoulder (joint) (M75.3)
      calcification of tendon (M65.2-)
      difficulty in walking (R26.2)
      temporomandibular joint disorder (M26.6-)
5ᵗʰ **M25.0 Hemarthrosis**
   EXCLUDES1 *current injury - see injury of joint by body region*
      hemophilic arthropathy (M36.2)
   M25.00 Hemarthrosis, unspecified joint CC/MCC Exc
6ᵗʰ **M25.01 Hemarthrosis,** shoulder
   M25.011 Hemarthrosis, right **shoulder** CC/MCC Exc
   M25.012 Hemarthrosis, left **shoulder** CC/MCC Exc
   M25.019 Hemarthrosis, unspecified shoulder CC/MCC Exc
6ᵗʰ **M25.02 Hemarthrosis,** elbow
   M25.021 Hemarthrosis, right **elbow** CC/MCC Exc
   M25.022 Hemarthrosis, left **elbow** CC/MCC Exc
   M25.029 Hemarthrosis, unspecified elbow CC/MCC Exc
6ᵗʰ **M25.03 Hemarthrosis,** wrist
   M25.031 Hemarthrosis, right **wrist** CC/MCC Exc
   M25.032 Hemarthrosis, left **wrist** CC/MCC Exc
   M25.039 Hemarthrosis, unspecified wrist CC/MCC Exc
6ᵗʰ **M25.04 Hemarthrosis,** hand
   M25.041 Hemarthrosis, right **hand** CC/MCC Exc
   M25.042 Hemarthrosis, left **hand** CC/MCC Exc
   M25.049 Hemarthrosis, unspecified hand CC/MCC Exc
6ᵗʰ **M25.05 Hemarthrosis,** hip
   M25.051 Hemarthrosis, right **hip** CC/MCC Exc
   M25.052 Hemarthrosis, left **hip** CC/MCC Exc
   M25.059 Hemarthrosis, unspecified hip CC/MCC Exc
6ᵗʰ **M25.06 Hemarthrosis,** knee
   M25.061 Hemarthrosis, right **knee** CC/MCC Exc
   M25.062 Hemarthrosis, left **knee** CC/MCC Exc
   M25.069 Hemarthrosis, unspecified knee CC/MCC Exc
6ᵗʰ **M25.07 Hemarthrosis,** ankle and foot
   M25.071 Hemarthrosis, right **ankle** CC/MCC Exc
   M25.072 Hemarthrosis, left **ankle** CC/MCC Exc
   M25.073 Hemarthrosis, unspecified ankle CC/MCC Exc

Unspecified Code Other Specified Code Manifestation Code N Newborn P Pediatric M Maternity A Adult ♂ Male ♀ Female
● New Code ▲ Revised Code Title ►◄ Revised Text **NOTES** *INCLUDES* EXCLUDES 1 Not coded here EXCLUDES 2 Not included here
4ᵗʰ character required 5ᵗʰ character required 6ᵗʰ character required 7ᵗʰ character required
7ᵗʰ Extension 'X' Alert HAC Hospital-acquired condition (HAC) alert **AHA** AHA Coding Clinic©

M25.074 Hemarthrosis, right foot [CC] [CC/MCC Exc]
M25.075 Hemarthrosis, left foot [CC] [CC/MCC Exc]
M25.076 Hemarthrosis, unspecified foot [CC] [CC/MCC Exc]
M25.08 Hemarthrosis, other specified site [CC] [CC/MCC Exc]
Hemarthrosis, vertebrae

[5th] M25.1 Fistula of joint
M25.10 Fistula, unspecified joint
[6th] M25.11 Fistula, shoulder
M25.111 Fistula, right shoulder
M25.112 Fistula, left shoulder
M25.119 Fistula, unspecified shoulder
[6th] M25.12 Fistula, elbow
M25.121 Fistula, right elbow
M25.122 Fistula, left elbow
M25.129 Fistula, unspecified elbow
[6th] M25.13 Fistula, wrist
M25.131 Fistula, right wrist
M25.132 Fistula, left wrist
M25.139 Fistula, unspecified wrist
[6th] M25.14 Fistula, hand
M25.141 Fistula, right hand
M25.142 Fistula, left hand
M25.149 Fistula, unspecified hand
[6th] M25.15 Fistula, hip
M25.151 Fistula, right hip
M25.152 Fistula, left hip
M25.159 Fistula, unspecified hip
[6th] M25.16 Fistula, knee
M25.161 Fistula, right knee
M25.162 Fistula, left knee
M25.169 Fistula, unspecified knee
[6th] M25.17 Fistula, ankle and foot
M25.171 Fistula, right ankle
M25.172 Fistula, left ankle
M25.173 Fistula, unspecified ankle
M25.174 Fistula, right foot
M25.175 Fistula, left foot
M25.176 Fistula, unspecified foot
M25.18 Fistula, other specified site
Fistula, vertebrae

[5th] M25.2 Flail joint
M25.20 Flail joint, unspecified joint
[6th] M25.21 Flail joint, shoulder
M25.211 Flail joint, right shoulder
M25.212 Flail joint, left shoulder
M25.219 Flail joint, unspecified shoulder
[6th] M25.22 Flail joint, elbow
M25.221 Flail joint, right elbow
M25.222 Flail joint, left elbow
M25.229 Flail joint, unspecified elbow
[6th] M25.23 Flail joint, wrist
M25.231 Flail joint, right wrist
M25.232 Flail joint, left wrist
M25.239 Flail joint, unspecified wrist
[6th] M25.24 Flail joint, hand
M25.241 Flail joint, right hand
M25.242 Flail joint, left hand
M25.249 Flail joint, unspecified hand
[6th] M25.25 Flail joint, hip
M25.251 Flail joint, right hip
M25.252 Flail joint, left hip
M25.259 Flail joint, unspecified hip
[6th] M25.26 Flail joint, knee
M25.261 Flail joint, right knee
M25.262 Flail joint, left knee
M25.269 Flail joint, unspecified knee
[6th] M25.27 Flail joint, ankle and foot
M25.271 Flail joint, right ankle and foot
M25.272 Flail joint, left ankle and foot
M25.279 Flail joint, unspecified ankle and foot
M25.28 Flail joint, other site

[5th] M25.3 Other instability of joint
[EXCLUDES1] *instability of joint secondary to old ligament injury (M24.2-)*
instability of joint secondary to removal of joint prosthesis (M96.8-)
[EXCLUDES2] *spinal instabilities (M53.2-)*
M25.30 Other instability, unspecified joint
[6th] M25.31 Other instability, shoulder
M25.311 Other instability, right shoulder
M25.312 Other instability, left shoulder
M25.319 Other instability, unspecified shoulder
[6th] M25.32 Other instability, elbow
M25.321 Other instability, right elbow
M25.322 Other instability, left elbow
M25.329 Other instability, unspecified elbow
[6th] M25.33 Other instability, wrist
M25.331 Other instability, right wrist
M25.332 Other instability, left wrist
M25.339 Other instability, unspecified wrist
[6th] M25.34 Other instability, hand
M25.341 Other instability, right hand
M25.342 Other instability, left hand
M25.349 Other instability, unspecified hand
[6th] M25.35 Other instability, hip
M25.351 Other instability, right hip
M25.352 Other instability, left hip
M25.359 Other instability, unspecified hip
[6th] M25.36 Other instability, knee
M25.361 Other instability, right knee
M25.362 Other instability, left knee
M25.369 Other instability, unspecified knee
[6th] M25.37 Other instability, ankle and foot
M25.371 Other instability, right ankle
M25.372 Other instability, left ankle
M25.373 Other instability, unspecified ankle
M25.374 Other instability, right foot
M25.375 Other instability, left foot
M25.376 Other instability, unspecified foot

[5th] M25.4 Effusion of joint
[EXCLUDES1] *hydrarthrosis in yaws (A66.6)*
intermittent hydrarthrosis (M12.4-)
other infective (teno)synovitis (M65.1-)
M25.40 Effusion, unspecified joint
[6th] M25.41 Effusion, shoulder
M25.411 Effusion, right shoulder
M25.412 Effusion, left shoulder
M25.419 Effusion, unspecified shoulder
[6th] M25.42 Effusion, elbow
M25.421 Effusion, right elbow
M25.422 Effusion, left elbow
M25.429 Effusion, unspecified elbow
[6th] M25.43 Effusion, wrist
M25.431 Effusion, right wrist
M25.432 Effusion, left wrist
M25.439 Effusion, unspecified wrist
[6th] M25.44 Effusion, hand
M25.441 Effusion, right hand
M25.442 Effusion, left hand
M25.449 Effusion, unspecified hand
[6th] M25.45 Effusion, hip
M25.451 Effusion, right hip
M25.452 Effusion, left hip
M25.459 Effusion, unspecified hip
[6th] M25.46 Effusion, knee
M25.461 Effusion, right knee

[PDx] Unacceptable principal diagnosis symbol per Medicare code edits [POA] Code exempt from diagnosis present on admission requirement
[?] Questionable admission [CC] Complication or comorbidity [CC/MCC Exc] CC/MCC exclusion [MCC] Major complication or comorbidity
[PDx CC] Principal diagnosis as its own CC [PDx MCC] Principal diagnosis as its own MCC [HCC] HCC diagnosis code [RxHCC] RxHCC diagnosis code
MACRA code [Z-1] Z code as first-listed diagnosis

When symbols appear on a code that requires a 7th character extension, refer to Appendix B to identify applicable 7th character codes.

M25.462 Effusion, left knee
M25.469 Effusion, unspecified knee
6ᵗʰ M25.47 Effusion, ankle and foot
M25.471 Effusion, right ankle
M25.472 Effusion, left ankle
M25.473 Effusion, unspecified ankle
M25.474 Effusion, right foot
M25.475 Effusion, left foot
M25.476 Effusion, unspecified foot
M25.48 Effusion, other site
5ᵗʰ M25.5 Pain in joint
EXCLUDES2 pain in hand (M79.64-)
pain in fingers (M79.64-)
pain in foot (M79.67-)
pain in limb (M79.6-)
pain in toes (M79.67-)
M25.50 Pain in unspecified joint
6ᵗʰ M25.51 Pain in shoulder
M25.511 Pain in right shoulder
M25.512 Pain in left shoulder
M25.519 Pain in unspecified shoulder
6ᵗʰ M25.52 Pain in elbow
M25.521 Pain in right elbow
M25.522 Pain in left elbow
M25.529 Pain in unspecified elbow
5ᵗʰ M25.53 Pain in wrist
M25.531 Pain in right wrist
M25.532 Pain in left wrist
M25.539 Pain in unspecified wrist
6ᵗʰ M25.54 Pain in joints of hand
M25.541 Pain in joints of right hand
AHA: Q4 2016
M25.542 Pain in joints of left hand
AHA: Q4 2016
M25.549 Pain in joints of unspecified hand
AHA: Q4 2016
Pain in joints of hand NOS
6ᵗʰ M25.55 Pain in hip
M25.551 Pain in right hip
M25.552 Pain in left hip
M25.559 Pain in unspecified hip
6ᵗʰ M25.56 Pain in knee
M25.561 Pain in right knee
M25.562 Pain in left knee
M25.569 Pain in unspecified knee
6ᵗʰ M25.57 Pain in ankle and joints of foot
M25.571 Pain in right ankle and joints of right foot
M25.572 Pain in left ankle and joints of left foot
M25.579 Pain in unspecified ankle and joints of unspecified foot
5ᵗʰ M25.6 Stiffness of joint, not elsewhere classified
EXCLUDES1 ankylosis of joint (M24.6-)
contracture of joint (M24.5-)
M25.60 Stiffness of unspecified joint, not elsewhere classified
6ᵗʰ M25.61 Stiffness of shoulder, not elsewhere classified
M25.611 Stiffness of right shoulder, not elsewhere classified
M25.612 Stiffness of left shoulder, not elsewhere classified
M25.619 Stiffness of unspecified shoulder, not elsewhere classified
6ᵗʰ M25.62 Stiffness of elbow, not elsewhere classified
M25.621 Stiffness of right elbow, not elsewhere classified
M25.622 Stiffness of left elbow, not elsewhere classified
M25.629 Stiffness of unspecified elbow, not elsewhere classified

6ᵗʰ M25.63 Stiffness of wrist, not elsewhere classified
M25.631 Stiffness of right wrist, not elsewhere classified
M25.632 Stiffness of left wrist, not elsewhere classified
M25.639 Stiffness of unspecified wrist, not elsewhere classified
6ᵗʰ M25.64 Stiffness of hand, not elsewhere classified
M25.641 Stiffness of right hand, not elsewhere classified
M25.642 Stiffness of left hand, not elsewhere classified
M25.649 Stiffness of unspecified hand, not elsewhere classified
6ᵗʰ M25.65 Stiffness of hip, not elsewhere classified
M25.651 Stiffness of right hip, not elsewhere classified
M25.652 Stiffness of left hip, not elsewhere classified
M25.659 Stiffness of unspecified hip, not elsewhere classified
6ᵗʰ M25.66 Stiffness of knee, not elsewhere classified
M25.661 Stiffness of right knee, not elsewhere classified
M25.662 Stiffness of left knee, not elsewhere classified
M25.669 Stiffness of unspecified knee, not elsewhere classified
6ᵗʰ M25.67 Stiffness of ankle and foot, not elsewhere classified
M25.671 Stiffness of right ankle, not elsewhere classified
M25.672 Stiffness of left ankle, not elsewhere classified
M25.673 Stiffness of unspecified ankle, not elsewhere classified
M25.674 Stiffness of right foot, not elsewhere classified
M25.675 Stiffness of left foot, not elsewhere classified
M25.676 Stiffness of unspecified foot, not elsewhere classified
5ᵗʰ M25.7 Osteophyte
M25.70 Osteophyte, unspecified joint
6ᵗʰ M25.71 Osteophyte, shoulder
M25.711 Osteophyte, right shoulder
M25.712 Osteophyte, left shoulder
M25.719 Osteophyte, unspecified shoulder
6ᵗʰ M25.72 Osteophyte, elbow
M25.721 Osteophyte, right elbow
M25.722 Osteophyte, left elbow
M25.729 Osteophyte, unspecified elbow
6ᵗʰ M25.73 Osteophyte, wrist
M25.731 Osteophyte, right wrist
M25.732 Osteophyte, left wrist
M25.739 Osteophyte, unspecified wrist
6ᵗʰ M25.74 Osteophyte, hand
M25.741 Osteophyte, right hand
M25.742 Osteophyte, left hand
M25.749 Osteophyte, unspecified hand
6ᵗʰ M25.75 Osteophyte, hip
M25.751 Osteophyte, right hip
M25.752 Osteophyte, left hip
M25.759 Osteophyte, unspecified hip
6ᵗʰ M25.76 Osteophyte, knee
M25.761 Osteophyte, right knee
M25.762 Osteophyte, left knee
M25.769 Osteophyte, unspecified knee
6ᵗʰ M25.77 Osteophyte, ankle and foot
M25.771 Osteophyte, right ankle
M25.772 Osteophyte, left ankle

Unspecified Code   Other Specified Code   Manifestation Code   Ⓝ Newborn   Ⓟ Pediatric   Ⓜ Maternity   Ⓐ Adult   ♂ Male   ♀ Female
● New Code   ▲ Revised Code Title   ▶◀ Revised Text   NOTES   INCLUDES   EXCLUDES 1   Not coded here   EXCLUDES 2   Not included here
4ᵗʰ character required   5ᵗʰ character required   6ᵗʰ character required   7ᵗʰ character required
7ᵗʰ Extension 'X' Alert   HAC Hospital-acquired condition (HAC) alert   AHA AHA Coding Clinic©

M25.773 Osteophyte, unspecified ankle
M25.774 Osteophyte, right foot
M25.775 Osteophyte, left foot
M25.776 Osteophyte, unspecified foot
M25.78 Osteophyte, vertebrae
M25.8 Other specified joint disorders
M25.80 Other specified joint disorders, unspecified joint
M25.81 Other specified joint disorders, shoulder
M25.811 Other specified joint disorders, right shoulder
M25.812 Other specified joint disorders, left shoulder
M25.819 Other specified joint disorders, unspecified shoulder
M25.82 Other specified joint disorders, elbow
M25.821 Other specified joint disorders, right elbow
M25.822 Other specified joint disorders, left elbow
M25.829 Other specified joint disorders, unspecified elbow
M25.83 Other specified joint disorders, wrist
M25.831 Other specified joint disorders, right wrist
M25.832 Other specified joint disorders, left wrist
M25.839 Other specified joint disorders, unspecified wrist
M25.84 Other specified joint disorders, hand
M25.841 Other specified joint disorders, right hand
M25.842 Other specified joint disorders, left hand
M25.849 Other specified joint disorders, unspecified hand
M25.85 Other specified joint disorders, hip
M25.851 Other specified joint disorders, right hip
M25.852 Other specified joint disorders, left hip
M25.859 Other specified joint disorders, unspecified hip
M25.86 Other specified joint disorders, knee
M25.861 Other specified joint disorders, right knee
M25.862 Other specified joint disorders, left knee
M25.869 Other specified joint disorders, unspecified knee
M25.87 Other specified joint disorders, ankle and foot
M25.871 Other specified joint disorders, right ankle and foot
M25.872 Other specified joint disorders, left ankle and foot
M25.879 Other specified joint disorders, unspecified ankle and foot
M25.9 Joint disorder, unspecified

Dentofacial anomalies [including malocclusion] and other disorders of jaw (M26-M27)

EXCLUDES1 hemifacial atrophy or hypertrophy (Q67.4)
unilateral condylar hyperplasia or hypoplasia (M27.8)
M26 Dentofacial anomalies [including malocclusion]
M26.0 Major anomalies of jaw size
EXCLUDES1 acromegaly (E22.0)
Robin's syndrome (Q87.0)
M26.00 Unspecified anomaly of jaw size
M26.01 Maxillary hyperplasia
M26.02 Maxillary hypoplasia
M26.03 Mandibular hyperplasia
M26.04 Mandibular hypoplasia
M26.05 Macrogenia
M26.06 Microgenia
M26.07 Excessive tuberosity of jaw
Entire maxillary tuberosity
M26.09 Other specified anomalies of jaw size
M26.1 Anomalies of jaw-cranial base relationship

M26.10 Unspecified anomaly of jaw-cranial base relationship
M26.11 Maxillary asymmetry
M26.12 Other jaw asymmetry
M26.19 Other specified anomalies of jaw-cranial base relationship
M26.2 Anomalies of dental arch relationship
M26.20 Unspecified anomaly of dental arch relationship
M26.21 Malocclusion, Angle's class
M26.211 Malocclusion, Angle's class I
Neutro-occlusion
M26.212 Malocclusion, Angle's class II
Disto-occlusion Division I
Disto-occlusion Division II
M26.213 Malocclusion, Angle's class III
Mesio-occlusion
M26.219 Malocclusion, Angle's class, unspecified
M26.22 Open occlusal relationship
M26.220 Open anterior occlusal relationship
Anterior openbite
M26.221 Open posterior occlusal relationship
Posterior openbite
M26.23 Excessive horizontal overlap
Excessive horizontal overjet
M26.24 Reverse articulation
Crossbite (anterior) (posterior)
M26.25 Anomalies of interarch distance
M26.29 Other anomalies of dental arch relationship
Midline deviation of dental arch
Overbite (excessive) deep
Overbite (excessive) horizontal
Overbite (excessive) vertical
Posterior lingual occlusion of mandibular teeth
M26.3 Anomalies of tooth position of fully erupted tooth or teeth
EXCLUDES2 embedded and impacted teeth (K01.-)
M26.30 Unspecified anomaly of tooth position of fully erupted tooth or teeth
Abnormal spacing of fully erupted tooth or teeth NOS
Displacement of fully erupted tooth or teeth NOS
Transposition of fully erupted tooth or teeth NOS
M26.31 Crowding of fully erupted teeth
M26.32 Excessive spacing of fully erupted teeth
Diastema of fully erupted tooth or teeth NOS
M26.33 Horizontal displacement of fully erupted tooth or teeth
Tipped tooth or teeth
Tipping of fully erupted tooth
M26.34 Vertical displacement of fully erupted tooth or teeth
Extruded tooth
Infraeruption of tooth or teeth
Supraeruption of tooth or teeth
M26.35 Rotation of fully erupted tooth or teeth
M26.36 Insufficient interocclusal distance of fully erupted teeth (ridge)
Lack of adequate intermaxillary vertical dimension of fully erupted teeth
M26.37 Excessive interocclusal distance of fully erupted teeth
Excessive intermaxillary vertical dimension of fully erupted teeth
Loss of occlusal vertical dimension of fully erupted teeth
M26.39 Other anomalies of tooth position of fully erupted tooth or teeth
M26.4 Malocclusion, unspecified
M26.5 Dentofacial functional abnormalities
EXCLUDES1 bruxism (F45.8)
teeth-grinding NOS (F45.8)
M26.50 Dentofacial functional abnormalities, unspecified
M26.51 Abnormal jaw closure
M26.52 Limited mandibular range of motion
M26.53 Deviation in opening and closing of the mandible

PDx Unacceptable principal diagnosis symbol per Medicare code edits   POA Code exempt from diagnosis present on admission requirement
? Questionable admission   cc Complication or comorbidity   cc/mcc exc CC/MCC exclusion   mcc Major complication or comorbidity
Principal diagnosis as its own CC   Principal diagnosis as its own MCC   HCC HCC diagnosis code   RxHCC RxHCC diagnosis code
MACRA code   Z1 Z code as first-listed diagnosis

When symbols appear on a code that requires a 7th character extension, refer to Appendix B to identify applicable 7th character codes.

2018 ICD-10-CM

M26.54 **Insufficient anterior guidance**
Insufficient anterior occlusal guidance
M26.55 **Centric occlusion maximum intercuspation discrepancy**
EXCLUDES1 *centric occlusion NOS (M26.59)*
M26.56 **Non-working side interference**
Balancing side interference
M26.57 **Lack of posterior occlusal support**
M26.59 **Other dentofacial functional abnormalities**
Centric occlusion (of teeth) NOS
Malocclusion due to abnormal swallowing
Malocclusion due to mouth breathing
Malocclusion due to tongue, lip or finger habits

🇸 M26.6 **Temporomandibular joint disorders**
EXCLUDES2 *current temporomandibular joint dislocation (S03.0)*
current temporomandibular joint sprain (S03.4)
🇶 M26.60 **Temporomandibular joint disorder,** unspecified
M26.601 Right **temporomandibular joint disorder, unspecified**
M26.602 Left **temporomandibular joint disorder, unspecified**
M26.603 Bilateral **temporomandibular joint disorder, unspecified**
M26.609 **Unspecified temporomandibular joint disorder,** unspecified side
Temporomandibular joint disorder NOS
🇶 M26.61 Adhesions and ankylosis of **temporomandibular joint**
M26.611 **Adhesions and ankylosis of** right **temporomandibular joint**
M26.612 **Adhesions and ankylosis of** left **temporomandibular joint**
M26.613 **Adhesions and ankylosis of** bilateral **temporomandibular joint**
M26.619 **Adhesions and ankylosis of temporomandibular joint,** unspecified side
🇶 M26.62 Arthralgia of temporomandibular joint
M26.621 **Arthralgia of** right **temporomandibular joint**
M26.622 **Arthralgia of** left **temporomandibular joint**
M26.623 **Arthralgia of** bilateral **temporomandibular joint**
M26.629 **Arthralgia of temporomandibular joint,** unspecified side
🇶 M26.63 Articular disc disorder **of temporomandibular joint**
M26.631 **Articular disc disorder of** right **temporomandibular joint**
M26.632 **Articular disc disorder of** left **temporomandibular joint**
M26.633 **Articular disc disorder of** bilateral **temporomandibular joint**
M26.639 **Articular disc disorder of temporomandibular joint,** unspecified side
M26.69 **Other specified disorders of temporomandibular joint**
🇸 M26.7 **Dental alveolar anomalies**
M26.70 **Unspecified alveolar anomaly**
M26.71 **Alveolar** maxillary hyperplasia
M26.72 **Alveolar** mandibular hyperplasia
M26.73 **Alveolar** maxillary hypoplasia
M26.74 **Alveolar** mandibular hypoplasia
M26.79 **Other specified alveolar anomalies**
🇸 M26.8 **Other dentofacial anomalies**
M26.81 Anterior **soft tissue impingement**
Anterior soft tissue impingement on teeth
M26.82 Posterior **soft tissue impingement**
Posterior soft tissue impingement on teeth
M26.89 **Other dentofacial anomalies**
M26.9 **Dentofacial anomaly, unspecified**

🇶 M27 **Other diseases of jaws**
M27.0 **Developmental disorders of jaws**
Latent bone cyst of jaw
Stafne's cyst
Torus mandibularis
Torus palatinus
M27.1 **Giant cell granuloma, central**
Giant cell granuloma NOS
EXCLUDES1 *peripheral giant cell granuloma (K06.8)*
M27.2 **Inflammatory conditions of jaws**
Osteitis of jaw(s)
Osteomyelitis (neonatal) jaw(s)
Osteoradionecrosis jaw(s)
Periostitis jaw(s)
Sequestrum of jaw bone
Use additional code (W88-W90, X39.0) to identify radiation, if radiation-induced
EXCLUDES2 *osteonecrosis of jaw due to drug (M87.180)*
M27.3 **Alveolitis of jaws**
Alveolar osteitis
Dry socket
🇸 M27.4 **Other and unspecified cysts of jaw**
EXCLUDES1 *cysts of oral region (K09.-)*
latent bone cyst of jaw (M27.0)
Stafne's cyst (M27.0)
M27.40 **Unspecified cyst of jaw**
Cyst of jaw NOS
M27.49 **Other cysts of jaw**
Aneurysmal cyst of jaw
Hemorrhagic cyst of jaw
Traumatic cyst of jaw
🇸 M27.5 **Periradicular pathology associated with previous endodontic treatment**
M27.51 **Perforation of root canal space due to endodontic treatment**
M27.52 **Endodontic overfill**
M27.53 **Endodontic underfill**
M27.59 **Other periradicular pathology associated with previous endodontic treatment**
🇸 M27.6 **Endosseous dental implant failure**
M27.61 **Osseointegration failure of dental implant**
Hemorrhagic complications of dental implant placement
Iatrogenic osseointegration failure of dental implant
Osseointegration failure of dental implant due to complications of systemic disease
Osseointegration failure of dental implant due to poor bone quality
Pre-integration failure of dental implant NOS
Pre-osseointegration failure of dental implant
M27.62 **Post-osseointegration biological failure of dental implant**
Failure of dental implant due to lack of attached gingiva
Failure of dental implant due to occlusal trauma (caused by poor prosthetic design)
Failure of dental implant due to parafunctional habits
Failure of dental implant due to periodontal infection (peri-implantitis)
Failure of dental implant due to poor oral hygiene
Iatrogenic post-osseointegration failure of dental implant
Post-osseointegration failure of dental implant due to complications of systemic disease
M27.63 **Post-osseointegration mechanical failure of dental implant**
Failure of dental prosthesis causing loss of dental implant
Fracture of dental implant
EXCLUDES2 *cracked tooth (K03.81)*
fractured dental restorative material with loss of material (K08.531)

Unspecified Code   Other Specified Code   Manifestation Code   Ⓝ Newborn   Ⓟ Pediatric   Ⓜ Maternity   Ⓐ Adult   ♂ Male   ♀ Female
● New Code   ▲ Revised Code Title   ▶◀ Revised Text   **NOTES**   *INCLUDES*   *EXCLUDES 1* Not coded here   *EXCLUDES 2* Not included here
🇶 4th character required   🇸 5th character required   🇶 6th character required   🇶 7th character required
🇶 Extension 'X' Alert   **HAC** Hospital-acquired condition (HAC) alert   **AHA** AHA Coding Clinic©

2018 | **2018 ICD-10-CM**   When symbols appear on a code that requires a 7th character extension, refer to Appendix B to identify applicable 7th character codes.   **809**

M62.10 **Other rupture of muscle (nontraumatic), unspecified site**

⑥ M62.11 Other rupture of muscle (nontraumatic), shoulder

M62.111 Other rupture of muscle (nontraumatic), right shoulder

M62.112 Other rupture of muscle (nontraumatic), left shoulder

M62.119 **Other rupture of muscle (nontraumatic), unspecified shoulder**

⑥ M62.12 Other rupture of muscle (nontraumatic), upper arm

M62.121 Other rupture of muscle (nontraumatic), right upper arm

M62.122 Other rupture of muscle (nontraumatic), left upper arm

M62.129 **Other rupture of muscle (nontraumatic), unspecified upper arm**

⑥ M62.13 Other rupture of muscle (nontraumatic), forearm

M62.131 Other rupture of muscle (nontraumatic), right forearm

M62.132 Other rupture of muscle (nontraumatic), left forearm

M62.139 **Other rupture of muscle (nontraumatic), unspecified forearm**

⑥ M62.14 Other rupture of muscle (nontraumatic), hand

M62.141 Other rupture of muscle (nontraumatic), right hand

M62.142 Other rupture of muscle (nontraumatic), left hand

M62.149 **Other rupture of muscle (nontraumatic), unspecified hand**

⑥ M62.15 Other rupture of muscle (nontraumatic), thigh

M62.151 Other rupture of muscle (nontraumatic), right thigh

M62.152 Other rupture of muscle (nontraumatic), left thigh

M62.159 **Other rupture of muscle (nontraumatic), unspecified thigh**

⑥ M62.16 Other rupture of muscle (nontraumatic), lower leg

M62.161 Other rupture of muscle (nontraumatic), right lower leg

M62.162 Other rupture of muscle (nontraumatic), left lower leg

M62.169 **Other rupture of muscle (nontraumatic), unspecified lower leg**

⑥ M62.17 Other rupture of muscle (nontraumatic), ankle and foot

M62.171 Other rupture of muscle (nontraumatic), right ankle and foot

M62.172 Other rupture of muscle (nontraumatic), left ankle and foot

M62.179 **Other rupture of muscle (nontraumatic), unspecified ankle and foot**

M62.18 Other rupture of muscle (nontraumatic), other site

⑤ M62.2 Nontraumatic ischemic infarction of muscle

EXCLUDES1 compartment syndrome (traumatic) (T79.A-)

nontraumatic compartment syndrome (M79.A-)

traumatic ischemia of muscle (T79.6)

rhabdomyolysis (M62.82)

Volkmann's ischemic contracture (T79.6)

M62.20 **Nontraumatic ischemic infarction of muscle, unspecified site**

⑥ M62.21 Nontraumatic ischemic infarction of muscle, shoulder

M62.211 Nontraumatic ischemic infarction of muscle, right shoulder

M62.212 Nontraumatic ischemic infarction of muscle, left shoulder

M62.219 **Nontraumatic ischemic infarction of muscle, unspecified shoulder**

⑥ M62.22 Nontraumatic ischemic infarction of muscle, upper arm

M62.221 Nontraumatic ischemic infarction of muscle, right upper arm

M62.222 Nontraumatic ischemic infarction of muscle, left upper arm

M62.229 **Nontraumatic ischemic infarction of muscle, unspecified upper arm**

⑥ M62.23 Nontraumatic ischemic infarction of muscle, forearm

M62.231 Nontraumatic ischemic infarction of muscle, right forearm

M62.232 Nontraumatic ischemic infarction of muscle, left forearm

M62.239 **Nontraumatic ischemic infarction of muscle, unspecified forearm**

⑥ M62.24 Nontraumatic ischemic infarction of muscle, hand

M62.241 Nontraumatic ischemic infarction of muscle, right hand

M62.242 Nontraumatic ischemic infarction of muscle, left hand

M62.249 **Nontraumatic ischemic infarction of muscle, unspecified hand**

⑥ M62.25 Nontraumatic ischemic infarction of muscle, thigh

M62.251 Nontraumatic ischemic infarction of muscle, right thigh

M62.252 Nontraumatic ischemic infarction of muscle, left thigh

M62.259 **Nontraumatic ischemic infarction of muscle, unspecified thigh**

⑥ M62.26 Nontraumatic ischemic infarction of muscle, lower leg

M62.261 Nontraumatic ischemic infarction of muscle, right lower leg

M62.262 Nontraumatic ischemic infarction of muscle, left lower leg

M62.269 **Nontraumatic ischemic infarction of muscle, unspecified lower leg**

⑥ M62.27 Nontraumatic ischemic infarction of muscle, ankle and foot

M62.271 Nontraumatic ischemic infarction of muscle, right ankle and foot

M62.272 Nontraumatic ischemic infarction of muscle, left ankle and foot

M62.279 **Nontraumatic ischemic infarction of muscle, unspecified ankle and foot**

M62.28 Nontraumatic ischemic infarction of muscle, other site

M62.3 Immobility syndrome (paraplegic)

⑤ M62.4 Contracture of muscle

Contracture of tendon (sheath)

EXCLUDES1 contracture of joint (M24.5-)

M62.40 **Contracture of muscle, unspecified site**

⑥ M62.41 Contracture of muscle, shoulder

M62.411 Contracture of muscle, right shoulder

M62.412 Contracture of muscle, left shoulder

M62.419 **Contracture of muscle, unspecified shoulder**

⑥ M62.42 Contracture of muscle, upper arm

M62.421 Contracture of muscle, right upper arm

M62.422 Contracture of muscle, left upper arm

M62.429 **Contracture of muscle, unspecified upper arm**

⑥ M62.43 Contracture of muscle, forearm

M62.431 Contracture of muscle, right forearm

M62.432 Contracture of muscle, left forearm

M62.439 **Contracture of muscle, unspecified forearm**

⑥ M62.44 Contracture of muscle, hand

M62.441 Contracture of muscle, right hand

M62.442 Contracture of muscle, left hand

M62.449 **Contracture of muscle, unspecified hand**

🄿🄳🅇 Unacceptable principal diagnosis symbol per Medicare code edits   🄿🅇 Code exempt from diagnosis present on admission requirement

❓ Questionable admission   ᶜᶜ Complication or comorbidity   ᶜᶜ/ᴹᶜᶜ ᴱˣᶜ CC/MCC exclusion   ᴹᶜᶜ Major complication or comorbidity

🄿ᶜ Principal diagnosis as its own CC   🄿ᴹ Principal diagnosis as its own MCC   ᴴᶜᶜ HCC diagnosis code   ᴿˣᴴᶜᶜ RxHCC diagnosis code

ᴹᴬᶜᴿᴬ MACRA code   🅉 Z code as first-listed diagnosis

When symbols appear on a code that requires a 7th character extension, refer to Appendix B to identify applicable 7th character codes.

2018 ICD-10-C

[6th] M62.45 Contracture of muscle, thigh
M62.451 Contracture of muscle, right thigh
M62.452 Contracture of muscle, left thigh
M62.459 Contracture of muscle, unspecified thigh
[6th] M62.46 Contracture of muscle, lower leg
M62.461 Contracture of muscle, right lower leg
M62.462 Contracture of muscle, left lower leg
M62.469 Contracture of muscle, unspecified lower leg
[6th] M62.47 Contracture of muscle, ankle and foot
M62.471 Contracture of muscle, right ankle and foot
M62.472 Contracture of muscle, left ankle and foot
M62.479 Contracture of muscle, unspecified ankle and foot
M62.48 Contracture of muscle, other site
M62.49 Contracture of muscle, multiple sites
[5th] M62.5 Muscle wasting and atrophy, not elsewhere classified
Disuse atrophy NEC
[EXCLUDES1] *neuralgic amyotrophy (G54.5)*
progressive muscular atrophy ▶(G12.21)◀
sarcopenia (M62.84)
[EXCLUDES2] *pelvic muscle wasting (N81.84)*
M62.50 Muscle wasting and atrophy, not elsewhere classified, unspecified site
[6th] M62.51 Muscle wasting and atrophy, not elsewhere classified, shoulder
M62.511 Muscle wasting and atrophy, not elsewhere classified, right shoulder
M62.512 Muscle wasting and atrophy, not elsewhere classified, left shoulder
M62.519 Muscle wasting and atrophy, not elsewhere classified, unspecified shoulder
[6th] M62.52 Muscle wasting and atrophy, not elsewhere classified, upper arm
M62.521 Muscle wasting and atrophy, not elsewhere classified, right upper arm
M62.522 Muscle wasting and atrophy, not elsewhere classified, left upper arm
M62.529 Muscle wasting and atrophy, not elsewhere classified, unspecified upper arm
[6th] M62.53 Muscle wasting and atrophy, not elsewhere classified, forearm
M62.531 Muscle wasting and atrophy, not elsewhere classified, right forearm
M62.532 Muscle wasting and atrophy, not elsewhere classified, left forearm
M62.539 Muscle wasting and atrophy, not elsewhere classified, unspecified forearm
[6th] M62.54 Muscle wasting and atrophy, not elsewhere classified, hand
M62.541 Muscle wasting and atrophy, not elsewhere classified, right hand
M62.542 Muscle wasting and atrophy, not elsewhere classified, left hand
M62.549 Muscle wasting and atrophy, not elsewhere classified, unspecified hand
[6th] M62.55 Muscle wasting and atrophy, not elsewhere classified, thigh
M62.551 Muscle wasting and atrophy, not elsewhere classified, right thigh
M62.552 Muscle wasting and atrophy, not elsewhere classified, left thigh
M62.559 Muscle wasting and atrophy, not elsewhere classified, unspecified thigh
[6th] M62.56 Muscle wasting and atrophy, not elsewhere classified, lower leg
M62.561 Muscle wasting and atrophy, not elsewhere classified, right lower leg
M62.562 Muscle wasting and atrophy, not elsewhere classified, left lower leg
M62.569 Muscle wasting and atrophy, not elsewhere classified, unspecified lower leg
[6th] M62.57 Muscle wasting and atrophy, not elsewhere classified, ankle and foot
M62.571 Muscle wasting and atrophy, not elsewhere classified, right ankle and foot
M62.572 Muscle wasting and atrophy, not elsewhere classified, left ankle and foot
M62.579 Muscle wasting and atrophy, not elsewhere classified, unspecified ankle and foot
M62.58 Muscle wasting and atrophy, not elsewhere classified, other site
M62.59 Muscle wasting and atrophy, not elsewhere classified, multiple sites
[5th] M62.8 Other specified disorders of muscle
[EXCLUDES2] *nontraumatic hematoma of muscle (M79.81)*
M62.81 Muscle weakness (generalized)
[EXCLUDES1] *muscle weakness in sarcopenia (M62.84)*
M62.82 Rhabdomyolysis CC CC/MCC Exc
[EXCLUDES1] *traumatic rhabdomyolysis (T79.6)*
[6th] M62.83 Muscle spasm
M62.830 Muscle spasm of back
M62.831 Muscle spasm of calf
Charley-horse
M62.838 Other muscle spasm
M62.84 Sarcopenia
Age-related sarcopenia
Code first underlying disease, if applicable, such as:
disorders of myoneural junction and muscle disease in diseases classified elsewhere (G73.-)
other and unspecified myopathies (G72.-)
primary disorders of muscles (G71.-)
M62.89 Other specified disorders of muscle
Muscle (sheath) hernia
M62.9 Disorder of muscle, unspecified
[4th] M63 Disorders of muscle in diseases classified elsewhere
Code first underlying disease, such as:
leprosy (A30.-)
neoplasm (C49.-, C79.89, D21.-, D48.1)
schistosomiasis (B65.-)
trichinellosis (B75)
[EXCLUDES1] *myopathy in cysticercosis (B69.81)*
myopathy in endocrine diseases (G73.7)
myopathy in metabolic diseases (G73.7)
myopathy in sarcoidosis (D86.87)
myopathy in secondary syphilis (A51.49)
myopathy in syphilis (late) (A52.78)
myopathy in toxoplasmosis (B58.82)
myopathy in tuberculosis (A18.09)
[5th] M63.8 Disorders of muscle in diseases classified elsewhere
M63.80 Disorders of muscle in diseases classified elsewhere, unspecified site
[6th] M63.81 Disorders of muscle in diseases classified elsewhere, shoulder
M63.811 Disorders of muscle in diseases classified elsewhere, right shoulder
M63.812 Disorders of muscle in diseases classified elsewhere, left shoulder
M63.819 Disorders of muscle in diseases classified elsewhere, unspecified shoulder
[6th] M63.82 Disorders of muscle in diseases classified elsewhere, upper arm
M63.821 Disorders of muscle in diseases classified elsewhere, right upper arm
M63.822 Disorders of muscle in diseases classified elsewhere, left upper arm

M63.829 Disorders of muscle in diseases classified elsewhere, unspecified upper arm
6️⃣ M63.83 Disorders of muscle in diseases classified elsewhere, forearm
   M63.831 Disorders of muscle in diseases classified elsewhere, right forearm
   M63.832 Disorders of muscle in diseases classified elsewhere, left forearm
   M63.839 Disorders of muscle in diseases classified elsewhere, unspecified forearm
6️⃣ M63.84 Disorders of muscle in diseases classified elsewhere, hand
   M63.841 Disorders of muscle in diseases classified elsewhere, right hand
   M63.842 Disorders of muscle in diseases classified elsewhere, left hand
   M63.849 Disorders of muscle in diseases classified elsewhere, unspecified hand
6️⃣ M63.85 Disorders of muscle in diseases classified elsewhere, thigh
   M63.851 Disorders of muscle in diseases classified elsewhere, right thigh
   M63.852 Disorders of muscle in diseases classified elsewhere, left thigh
   M63.859 Disorders of muscle in diseases classified elsewhere, unspecified thigh
6️⃣ M63.86 Disorders of muscle in diseases classified elsewhere, lower leg
   M63.861 Disorders of muscle in diseases classified elsewhere, right lower leg
   M63.862 Disorders of muscle in diseases classified elsewhere, left lower leg
   M63.869 Disorders of muscle in diseases classified elsewhere, unspecified lower leg
6️⃣ M63.87 Disorders of muscle in diseases classified elsewhere, ankle and foot
   M63.871 Disorders of muscle in diseases classified elsewhere, right ankle and foot
   M63.872 Disorders of muscle in diseases classified elsewhere, left ankle and foot
   M63.879 Disorders of muscle in diseases classified elsewhere, unspecified ankle and foot
M63.88 Disorders of muscle in diseases classified elsewhere, other site
M63.89 Disorders of muscle in diseases classified elsewhere, multiple sites

Disorders of synovium and tendon (M65-M67)

4️⃣ M65 Synovitis and tenosynovitis
   EXCLUDES1 chronic crepitant synovitis of hand and wrist (M70.0-)
      current injury - see injury of ligament or tendon by body region
      soft tissue disorders related to use, overuse and pressure (M70.-)
  5️⃣ M65.0 Abscess of tendon sheath
    Use additional code (B95-B96) to identify bacterial agent.
    M65.00 Abscess of tendon sheath, unspecified site
  6️⃣ M65.01 Abscess of tendon sheath, shoulder
    M65.011 Abscess of tendon sheath, right shoulder
    M65.012 Abscess of tendon sheath, left shoulder
    M65.019 Abscess of tendon sheath, unspecified shoulder
  6️⃣ M65.02 Abscess of tendon sheath, upper arm
    M65.021 Abscess of tendon sheath, right upper arm
    M65.022 Abscess of tendon sheath, left upper arm
    M65.029 Abscess of tendon sheath, unspecified upper arm
  6️⃣ M65.03 Abscess of tendon sheath, forearm
    M65.031 Abscess of tendon sheath, right forearm
    M65.032 Abscess of tendon sheath, left forearm
    M65.039 Abscess of tendon sheath, unspecified forearm

6️⃣ M65.04 Abscess of tendon sheath, hand
   M65.041 Abscess of tendon sheath, right hand
   M65.042 Abscess of tendon sheath, left hand
   M65.049 Abscess of tendon sheath, unspecified hand
6️⃣ M65.05 Abscess of tendon sheath, thigh
   M65.051 Abscess of tendon sheath, right thigh
   M65.052 Abscess of tendon sheath, left thigh
   M65.059 Abscess of tendon sheath, unspecified thigh
6️⃣ M65.06 Abscess of tendon sheath, lower leg
   M65.061 Abscess of tendon sheath, right lower leg
   M65.062 Abscess of tendon sheath, left lower leg
   M65.069 Abscess of tendon sheath, unspecified lower leg
6️⃣ M65.07 Abscess of tendon sheath, ankle and foot
   M65.071 Abscess of tendon sheath, right ankle and foot
   M65.072 Abscess of tendon sheath, left ankle and foot
   M65.079 Abscess of tendon sheath, unspecified ankle and foot
M65.08 Abscess of tendon sheath, other site
5️⃣ M65.1 Other infective (teno)synovitis
  M65.10 Other infective (teno)synovitis, unspecified site
6️⃣ M65.11 Other infective (teno)synovitis, shoulder
   M65.111 Other infective (teno)synovitis, right shoulder
   M65.112 Other infective (teno)synovitis, left shoulder
   M65.119 Other infective (teno)synovitis, unspecified shoulder
6️⃣ M65.12 Other infective (teno)synovitis, elbow
   M65.121 Other infective (teno)synovitis, right elbow
   M65.122 Other infective (teno)synovitis, left elbow
   M65.129 Other infective (teno)synovitis, unspecified elbow
6️⃣ M65.13 Other infective (teno)synovitis, wrist
   M65.131 Other infective (teno)synovitis, right wrist
   M65.132 Other infective (teno)synovitis, left wrist
   M65.139 Other infective (teno)synovitis, unspecified wrist
6️⃣ M65.14 Other infective (teno)synovitis, hand
   M65.141 Other infective (teno)synovitis, right hand
   M65.142 Other infective (teno)synovitis, left hand
   M65.149 Other infective (teno)synovitis, unspecified hand
6️⃣ M65.15 Other infective (teno)synovitis, hip
   M65.151 Other infective (teno)synovitis, right hip
   M65.152 Other infective (teno)synovitis, left hip
   M65.159 Other infective (teno)synovitis, unspecified hip
6️⃣ M65.16 Other infective (teno)synovitis, knee
   M65.161 Other infective (teno)synovitis, right knee
   M65.162 Other infective (teno)synovitis, left knee
   M65.169 Other infective (teno)synovitis, unspecified knee
6️⃣ M65.17 Other infective (teno)synovitis, ankle and foot
   M65.171 Other infective (teno)synovitis, right ankle and foot
   M65.172 Other infective (teno)synovitis, left ankle and foot
   M65.179 Other infective (teno)synovitis, unspecified ankle and foot
M65.18 Other infective (teno)synovitis, other site
M65.19 Other infective (teno)synovitis, multiple sites
5️⃣ M65.2 Calcific tendinitis
  EXCLUDES1 tendinitis as classified in M75-M77
    calcified tendinitis of shoulder (M75.3)
M65.20 Calcific tendinitis, unspecified site

📛 Unacceptable principal diagnosis symbol per Medicare code edits   📛 Code exempt from diagnosis present on admission requirement
❓ Questionable admission   🔵 Complication or comorbidity   CC/MCC exclusion   🔵 Major complication or comorbidity
🔵 Principal diagnosis as its own CC   🔵 Principal diagnosis as its own MCC   HCC HCC diagnosis code   RxHCC RxHCC diagnosis code
MACRA code   Z Z code as first-listed diagnosis

⑥ M65.22 Calcific tendinitis, upper arm
    M65.221 Calcific tendinitis, right upper arm
    M65.222 Calcific tendinitis, left upper arm
    M65.229 Calcific tendinitis, unspecified upper arm
⑥ M65.23 Calcific tendinitis, forearm
    M65.231 Calcific tendinitis, right forearm
    M65.232 Calcific tendinitis, left forearm
    M65.239 Calcific tendinitis, unspecified forearm
⑥ M65.24 Calcific tendinitis, hand
    M65.241 Calcific tendinitis, right hand
    M65.242 Calcific tendinitis, left hand
    M65.249 Calcific tendinitis, unspecified hand
⑥ M65.25 Calcific tendinitis, thigh
    M65.251 Calcific tendinitis, right thigh
    M65.252 Calcific tendinitis, left thigh
    M65.259 Calcific tendinitis, unspecified thigh
⑥ M65.26 Calcific tendinitis, lower leg
    M65.261 Calcific tendinitis, right lower leg
    M65.262 Calcific tendinitis, left lower leg
    M65.269 Calcific tendinitis, unspecified lower leg
⑥ M65.27 Calcific tendinitis, ankle and foot
    M65.271 Calcific tendinitis, right ankle and foot
    M65.272 Calcific tendinitis, left ankle and foot
    M65.279 Calcific tendinitis, unspecified ankle and foot
    M65.28 Calcific tendinitis, other site
    M65.29 Calcific tendinitis, multiple sites
⑤ M65.3 Trigger finger
    Nodular tendinous disease
    M65.30 Trigger finger, unspecified finger
⑥ M65.31 Trigger thumb
    M65.311 Trigger thumb, right thumb
    M65.312 Trigger thumb, left thumb
    M65.319 Trigger thumb, unspecified thumb
⑥ M65.32 Trigger finger, index finger
    M65.321 Trigger finger, right index finger
    M65.322 Trigger finger, left index finger
    M65.329 Trigger finger, unspecified index finger
⑥ M65.33 Trigger finger, middle finger
    M65.331 Trigger finger, right middle finger
    M65.332 Trigger finger, left middle finger
    M65.339 Trigger finger, unspecified middle finger
⑥ M65.34 Trigger finger, ring finger
    M65.341 Trigger finger, right ring finger
    M65.342 Trigger finger, left ring finger
    M65.349 Trigger finger, unspecified ring finger
⑥ M65.35 Trigger finger, little finger
    M65.351 Trigger finger, right little finger
    M65.352 Trigger finger, left little finger
    M65.359 Trigger finger, unspecified little finger
    M65.4 Radial styloid tenosynovitis [de Quervain]
⑤ M65.8 Other synovitis and tenosynovitis
    M65.80 Other synovitis and tenosynovitis, unspecified site
⑥ M65.81 Other synovitis and tenosynovitis, shoulder
    M65.811 Other synovitis and tenosynovitis, right shoulder
    M65.812 Other synovitis and tenosynovitis, left shoulder
    M65.819 Other synovitis and tenosynovitis, unspecified shoulder
⑥ M65.82 Other synovitis and tenosynovitis, upper arm
    M65.821 Other synovitis and tenosynovitis, right upper arm
    M65.822 Other synovitis and tenosynovitis, left upper arm
    M65.829 Other synovitis and tenosynovitis, unspecified upper arm
⑥ M65.83 Other synovitis and tenosynovitis, forearm

    M65.831 Other synovitis and tenosynovitis, right forearm
    M65.832 Other synovitis and tenosynovitis, left forearm
    M65.839 Other synovitis and tenosynovitis, unspecified forearm
⑥ M65.84 Other synovitis and tenosynovitis, hand
    M65.841 Other synovitis and tenosynovitis, right hand
    M65.842 Other synovitis and tenosynovitis, left hand
    M65.849 Other synovitis and tenosynovitis, unspecified hand
⑥ M65.85 Other synovitis and tenosynovitis, thigh
    M65.851 Other synovitis and tenosynovitis, right thigh
    M65.852 Other synovitis and tenosynovitis, left thigh
    M65.859 Other synovitis and tenosynovitis, unspecified thigh
⑥ M65.86 Other synovitis and tenosynovitis, lower leg
    M65.861 Other synovitis and tenosynovitis, right lower leg
    M65.862 Other synovitis and tenosynovitis, left lower leg
    M65.869 Other synovitis and tenosynovitis, unspecified lower leg
⑥ M65.87 Other synovitis and tenosynovitis, ankle and foot
    M65.871 Other synovitis and tenosynovitis, right ankle and foot
    M65.872 Other synovitis and tenosynovitis, left ankle and foot
    M65.879 Other synovitis and tenosynovitis, unspecified ankle and foot
    M65.88 Other synovitis and tenosynovitis, other site
    M65.89 Other synovitis and tenosynovitis, multiple sites
    M65.9 Synovitis and tenosynovitis, unspecified
④ M66 Spontaneous rupture of synovium and tendon

    INCLUDES   *rupture that occurs when a normal force is applied to tissues that are inferred to have less than normal strength*

    EXCLUDES2 *rotator cuff syndrome (M75.1-)*

        rupture where an abnormal force is applied to normal tissue - see injury of tendon by body region

    M66.0 Rupture of popliteal cyst
⑤ M66.1 Rupture of synovium
    Rupture of synovial cyst
    EXCLUDES2 *rupture of popliteal cyst (M66.0)*
    M66.10 Rupture of synovium, unspecified joint
⑥ M66.11 Rupture of synovium, shoulder
    M66.111 Rupture of synovium, right shoulder
    M66.112 Rupture of synovium, left shoulder
    M66.119 Rupture of synovium, unspecified shoulder
⑥ M66.12 Rupture of synovium, elbow
    M66.121 Rupture of synovium, right elbow
    M66.122 Rupture of synovium, left elbow
    M66.129 Rupture of synovium, unspecified elbow
⑥ M66.13 Rupture of synovium, wrist
    M66.131 Rupture of synovium, right wrist
    M66.132 Rupture of synovium, left wrist
    M66.139 Rupture of synovium, unspecified wrist
⑥ M66.14 Rupture of synovium, hand and fingers
    M66.141 Rupture of synovium, right hand
    M66.142 Rupture of synovium, left hand
    M66.143 Rupture of synovium, unspecified hand
    M66.144 Rupture of synovium, right finger(s)
    M66.145 Rupture of synovium, left finger(s)
    M66.146 Rupture of synovium, unspecified finger(s)
⑥ M66.15 Rupture of synovium, hip
    M66.151 Rupture of synovium, right hip

Unspecified Code   Other Specified Code   Manifestation Code   ℕ Newborn   ℙ Pediatric   𝕄 Maternity   𝔸 Adult   ♂ Male   ♀ Female
● New Code   ▲ Revised Code Title   ►◄ Revised Text   **NOTES**   *INCLUDES*   *EXCLUDES 1* Not coded here   *EXCLUDES 2* Not included here
④ 4th character required   ⑤ 5th character required   ⑥ 6th character required   ⑦ 7th character required
⑦ Extension 'X' Alert   **HAC** Hospital-acquired condition (HAC) alert   **AHA** AHA Coding Clinic©

M66.152 Rupture of synovium, left hip
M66.159 Rupture of synovium, unspecified hip
M66.17 Rupture of synovium, ankle, foot and toes
M66.171 Rupture of synovium, right ankle
M66.172 Rupture of synovium, left ankle
M66.173 Rupture of synovium, unspecified ankle
M66.174 Rupture of synovium, right foot
M66.175 Rupture of synovium, left foot
M66.176 Rupture of synovium, unspecified foot
M66.177 Rupture of synovium, right toe(s)
M66.178 Rupture of synovium, left toe(s)
M66.179 Rupture of synovium, unspecified toe(s)
M66.18 Rupture of synovium, other site
M66.2 Spontaneous rupture of extensor tendons
M66.20 Spontaneous rupture of extensor tendons, unspecified site
M66.21 Spontaneous rupture of extensor tendons, shoulder
M66.211 Spontaneous rupture of extensor tendons, right shoulder
M66.212 Spontaneous rupture of extensor tendons, left shoulder
M66.219 Spontaneous rupture of extensor tendons, unspecified shoulder
M66.22 Spontaneous rupture of extensor tendons, upper arm
M66.221 Spontaneous rupture of extensor tendons, right upper arm
M66.222 Spontaneous rupture of extensor tendons, left upper arm
M66.229 Spontaneous rupture of extensor tendons, unspecified upper arm
M66.23 Spontaneous rupture of extensor tendons, forearm
M66.231 Spontaneous rupture of extensor tendons, right forearm
M66.232 Spontaneous rupture of extensor tendons, left forearm
M66.239 Spontaneous rupture of extensor tendons, unspecified forearm
M66.24 Spontaneous rupture of extensor tendons, hand
M66.241 Spontaneous rupture of extensor tendons, right hand
M66.242 Spontaneous rupture of extensor tendons, left hand
M66.249 Spontaneous rupture of extensor tendons, unspecified hand
M66.25 Spontaneous rupture of extensor tendons, thigh
M66.251 Spontaneous rupture of extensor tendons, right thigh
M66.252 Spontaneous rupture of extensor tendons, left thigh
M66.259 Spontaneous rupture of extensor tendons, unspecified thigh
M66.26 Spontaneous rupture of extensor tendons, lower leg
M66.261 Spontaneous rupture of extensor tendons, right lower leg
M66.262 Spontaneous rupture of extensor tendons, left lower leg
M66.269 Spontaneous rupture of extensor tendons, unspecified lower leg
M66.27 Spontaneous rupture of extensor tendons, ankle and foot
M66.271 Spontaneous rupture of extensor tendons, right ankle and foot
M66.272 Spontaneous rupture of extensor tendons, left ankle and foot
M66.279 Spontaneous rupture of extensor tendons, unspecified ankle and foot
M66.28 Spontaneous rupture of extensor tendons, other site
M66.29 Spontaneous rupture of extensor tendons, multiple sites

M66.3 Spontaneous rupture of flexor tendons
M66.30 Spontaneous rupture of flexor tendons, unspecified site
M66.31 Spontaneous rupture of flexor tendons, shoulder
M66.311 Spontaneous rupture of flexor tendons, right shoulder
M66.312 Spontaneous rupture of flexor tendons, left shoulder
M66.319 Spontaneous rupture of flexor tendons, unspecified shoulder
M66.32 Spontaneous rupture of flexor tendons, upper arm
M66.321 Spontaneous rupture of flexor tendons, right upper arm
M66.322 Spontaneous rupture of flexor tendons, left upper arm
M66.329 Spontaneous rupture of flexor tendons, unspecified upper arm
M66.33 Spontaneous rupture of flexor tendons, forearm
M66.331 Spontaneous rupture of flexor tendons, right forearm
M66.332 Spontaneous rupture of flexor tendons, left forearm
M66.339 Spontaneous rupture of flexor tendons, unspecified forearm
M66.34 Spontaneous rupture of flexor tendons, hand
M66.341 Spontaneous rupture of flexor tendons, right hand
M66.342 Spontaneous rupture of flexor tendons, left hand
M66.349 Spontaneous rupture of flexor tendons, unspecified hand
M66.35 Spontaneous rupture of flexor tendons, thigh
M66.351 Spontaneous rupture of flexor tendons, right thigh
M66.352 Spontaneous rupture of flexor tendons, left thigh
M66.359 Spontaneous rupture of flexor tendons, unspecified thigh
M66.36 Spontaneous rupture of flexor tendons, lower leg
M66.361 Spontaneous rupture of flexor tendons, right lower leg
M66.362 Spontaneous rupture of flexor tendons, left lower leg
M66.369 Spontaneous rupture of flexor tendons, unspecified lower leg
M66.37 Spontaneous rupture of flexor tendons, ankle and foot
M66.371 Spontaneous rupture of flexor tendons, right ankle and foot
M66.372 Spontaneous rupture of flexor tendons, left ankle and foot
M66.379 Spontaneous rupture of flexor tendons, unspecified ankle and foot
M66.38 Spontaneous rupture of flexor tendons, other site
M66.39 Spontaneous rupture of flexor tendons, multiple sites
M66.8 Spontaneous rupture of other tendons
M66.80 Spontaneous rupture of other tendons, unspecified site
M66.81 Spontaneous rupture of other tendons, shoulder
M66.811 Spontaneous rupture of other tendons, right shoulder
M66.812 Spontaneous rupture of other tendons, left shoulder
M66.819 Spontaneous rupture of other tendons, unspecified shoulder
M66.82 Spontaneous rupture of other tendons, upper arm
M66.821 Spontaneous rupture of other tendons, right upper arm
M66.822 Spontaneous rupture of other tendons, left upper arm

PDxᴹ Unacceptable principal diagnosis symbol per Medicare code edits   PᴏA Code exempt from diagnosis present on admission requirement
? Questionable admission   Complication or comorbidity   CC/MCC Excl. CC/MCC exclusion   MCC Major complication or comorbidity
Principal diagnosis as its own CC   Principal diagnosis as its own MCC   HCC HCC diagnosis code   RxHCC RxHCC diagnosis code
MACRA code   Z1 Z code as first-listed diagnosis

When symbols appear on a code that requires a 7th character extension, refer to Appendix B to identify applicable 7th character codes.
2018 ICD-10-CM

M66.829 Spontaneous rupture of other tendons, unspecified upper arm

[6th] M66.83 Spontaneous rupture of other tendons, forearm
M66.831 Spontaneous rupture of other tendons, right forearm
M66.832 Spontaneous rupture of other tendons, left forearm
M66.839 Spontaneous rupture of other tendons, unspecified forearm

[6th] M66.84 Spontaneous rupture of other tendons, hand
M66.841 Spontaneous rupture of other tendons, right hand
M66.842 Spontaneous rupture of other tendons, left hand
M66.849 Spontaneous rupture of other tendons, unspecified hand

[6th] M66.85 Spontaneous rupture of other tendons, thigh
M66.851 Spontaneous rupture of other tendons, right thigh
M66.852 Spontaneous rupture of other tendons, left thigh
M66.859 Spontaneous rupture of other tendons, unspecified thigh

[6th] M66.86 Spontaneous rupture of other tendons, lower leg
M66.861 Spontaneous rupture of other tendons, right lower leg
M66.862 Spontaneous rupture of other tendons, left lower leg
M66.869 Spontaneous rupture of other tendons, unspecified lower leg

[6th] M66.87 Spontaneous rupture of other tendons, ankle and foot
M66.871 Spontaneous rupture of other tendons, right ankle and foot
M66.872 Spontaneous rupture of other tendons, left ankle and foot
M66.879 Spontaneous rupture of other tendons, unspecified ankle and foot

M66.88 Spontaneous rupture of other tendons, other
M66.89 Spontaneous rupture of other tendons, multiple sites

M66.9 Spontaneous rupture of unspecified tendon
Rupture at musculotendinous junction, nontraumatic

[4th] **M67 Other disorders of synovium and tendon**
[EXCLUDES1] *palmar fascial fibromatosis [Dupuytren] (M72.0)*
tendinitis NOS (M77.9-)
xanthomatosis localized to tendons (E78.2)

[5th] M67.0 Short Achilles tendon (acquired)
M67.00 Short Achilles tendon (acquired), unspecified ankle
M67.01 Short Achilles tendon (acquired), right ankle
M67.02 Short Achilles tendon (acquired), left ankle

[5th] M67.2 Synovial hypertrophy, not elsewhere classified
[EXCLUDES1] *villonodular synovitis (pigmented) (M12.2-)*
M67.20 Synovial hypertrophy, not elsewhere classified, unspecified site

[6th] M67.21 Synovial hypertrophy, not elsewhere classified, shoulder
M67.211 Synovial hypertrophy, not elsewhere classified, right shoulder
M67.212 Synovial hypertrophy, not elsewhere classified, left shoulder
M67.219 Synovial hypertrophy, not elsewhere classified, unspecified shoulder

[6th] M67.22 Synovial hypertrophy, not elsewhere classified, upper arm
M67.221 Synovial hypertrophy, not elsewhere classified, right upper arm
M67.222 Synovial hypertrophy, not elsewhere classified, left upper arm
M67.229 Synovial hypertrophy, not elsewhere classified, unspecified upper arm

[6th] M67.23 Synovial hypertrophy, not elsewhere classified, forearm
M67.231 Synovial hypertrophy, not elsewhere classified, right forearm
M67.232 Synovial hypertrophy, not elsewhere classified, left forearm
M67.239 Synovial hypertrophy, not elsewhere classified, unspecified forearm

[6th] M67.24 Synovial hypertrophy, not elsewhere classified, hand
M67.241 Synovial hypertrophy, not elsewhere classified, right hand
M67.242 Synovial hypertrophy, not elsewhere classified, left hand
M67.249 Synovial hypertrophy, not elsewhere classified, unspecified hand

[6th] M67.25 Synovial hypertrophy, not elsewhere classified, thigh
M67.251 Synovial hypertrophy, not elsewhere classified, right thigh
M67.252 Synovial hypertrophy, not elsewhere classified, left thigh
M67.259 Synovial hypertrophy, not elsewhere classified, unspecified thigh

[6th] M67.26 Synovial hypertrophy, not elsewhere classified, lower leg
M67.261 Synovial hypertrophy, not elsewhere classified, right lower leg
M67.262 Synovial hypertrophy, not elsewhere classified, left lower leg
M67.269 Synovial hypertrophy, not elsewhere classified, unspecified lower leg

[6th] M67.27 Synovial hypertrophy, not elsewhere classified, ankle and foot
M67.271 Synovial hypertrophy, not elsewhere classified, right ankle and foot
M67.272 Synovial hypertrophy, not elsewhere classified, left ankle and foot
M67.279 Synovial hypertrophy, not elsewhere classified, unspecified ankle and foot

M67.28 Synovial hypertrophy, not elsewhere classified, other site
M67.29 Synovial hypertrophy, not elsewhere classified, multiple sites

[5th] M67.3 Transient synovitis
Toxic synovitis
[EXCLUDES1] *palindromic rheumatism (M12.3-)*
M67.30 Transient synovitis, unspecified site

[6th] M67.31 Transient synovitis, shoulder
M67.311 Transient synovitis, right shoulder
M67.312 Transient synovitis, left shoulder
M67.319 Transient synovitis, unspecified shoulder

[6th] M67.32 Transient synovitis, elbow
M67.321 Transient synovitis, right elbow
M67.322 Transient synovitis, left elbow
M67.329 Transient synovitis, unspecified elbow

[6th] M67.33 Transient synovitis, wrist
M67.331 Transient synovitis, right wrist
M67.332 Transient synovitis, left wrist
M67.339 Transient synovitis, unspecified wrist

[6th] M67.34 Transient synovitis, hand
M67.341 Transient synovitis, right hand
M67.342 Transient synovitis, left hand
M67.349 Transient synovitis, unspecified hand

[6th] M67.35 Transient synovitis, hip
M67.351 Transient synovitis, right hip
M67.352 Transient synovitis, left hip
M67.359 Transient synovitis, unspecified hip

[6th] M67.36 Transient synovitis, knee
M67.361 Transient synovitis, right knee

Unspecified Code Other Specified Code Manifestation Code [N] Newborn [P] Pediatric [M] Maternity [A] Adult ♂ Male ♀ Female
● New Code ▲ Revised Code Title ►◄ Revised Text [NOTES] [INCLUDES] [EXCLUDES1] Not coded here [EXCLUDES2] Not included here
[4th] 4th character required [5th] 5th character required [6th] 6th character required [7th] 7th character required
[x7th] Extension 'X' Alert [HAC] Hospital-acquired condition (HAC) alert AHA AHA Coding Clinic©

M67.362 Transient synovitis, left knee
M67.369 Transient synovitis, unspecified knee
[6th] M67.37 Transient synovitis, ankle and foot
M67.371 Transient synovitis, right ankle and foot
M67.372 Transient synovitis, left ankle and foot
M67.379 Transient synovitis, unspecified ankle and foot
M67.38 Transient synovitis, other site
M67.39 Transient synovitis, multiple sites
[5th] M67.4 Ganglion
Ganglion of joint or tendon (sheath)
EXCLUDES1 *ganglion in yaws (A66.6)*
EXCLUDES2 *cyst of bursa (M71.2-M71.3)*
cyst of synovium (M71.2-M71.3)
M67.40 Ganglion, unspecified site
[6th] M67.41 Ganglion, shoulder
M67.411 Ganglion, right shoulder
M67.412 Ganglion, left shoulder
M67.419 Ganglion, unspecified shoulder
[6th] M67.42 Ganglion, elbow
M67.421 Ganglion, right elbow
M67.422 Ganglion, left elbow
M67.429 Ganglion, unspecified elbow
[6th] M67.43 Ganglion, wrist
M67.431 Ganglion, right wrist
M67.432 Ganglion, left wrist
M67.439 Ganglion, unspecified wrist
[6th] M67.44 Ganglion, hand
M67.441 Ganglion, right hand
M67.442 Ganglion, left hand
M67.449 Ganglion, unspecified hand
[6th] M67.45 Ganglion, hip
M67.451 Ganglion, right hip
M67.452 Ganglion, left hip
M67.459 Ganglion, unspecified hip
[6th] M67.46 Ganglion, knee
M67.461 Ganglion, right knee
M67.462 Ganglion, left knee
M67.469 Ganglion, unspecified knee
[6th] M67.47 Ganglion, ankle and foot
M67.471 Ganglion, right ankle and foot
M67.472 Ganglion, left ankle and foot
M67.479 Ganglion, unspecified ankle and foot
M67.48 Ganglion, other site
M67.49 Ganglion, multiple sites
[5th] M67.5 Plica syndrome
Plica knee
M67.50 Plica syndrome, unspecified knee
M67.51 Plica syndrome, right knee
M67.52 Plica syndrome, left knee
[5th] M67.8 Other specified disorders of synovium and tendon
M67.80 Other specified disorders of synovium and tendon, unspecified site
[6th] M67.81 Other specified disorders of synovium and tendon, shoulder
M67.811 Other specified disorders of synovium, right shoulder
M67.812 Other specified disorders of synovium, left shoulder
M67.813 Other specified disorders of tendon, right shoulder
M67.814 Other specified disorders of tendon, left shoulder
M67.819 Other specified disorders of synovium and tendon, unspecified shoulder
[6th] M67.82 Other specified disorders of synovium and tendon, elbow
M67.821 Other specified disorders of synovium, right elbow
M67.822 Other specified disorders of synovium, left elbow
M67.823 Other specified disorders of tendon, right elbow
M67.824 Other specified disorders of tendon, left elbow
M67.829 Other specified disorders of synovium and tendon, unspecified elbow
[6th] M67.83 Other specified disorders of synovium and tendon, wrist
M67.831 Other specified disorders of synovium, right wrist
M67.832 Other specified disorders of synovium, left wrist
M67.833 Other specified disorders of tendon, right wrist
M67.834 Other specified disorders of tendon, left wrist
M67.839 Other specified disorders of synovium and tendon, unspecified forearm
[6th] M67.84 Other specified disorders of synovium and tendon, hand
M67.841 Other specified disorders of synovium, right hand
M67.842 Other specified disorders of synovium, left hand
M67.843 Other specified disorders of tendon, right hand
M67.844 Other specified disorders of tendon, left hand
M67.849 Other specified disorders of synovium and tendon, unspecified hand
[6th] M67.85 Other specified disorders of synovium and tendon, hip
M67.851 Other specified disorders of synovium, right hip
M67.852 Other specified disorders of synovium, left hip
M67.853 Other specified disorders of tendon, right hip
M67.854 Other specified disorders of tendon, left hip
M67.859 Other specified disorders of synovium and tendon, unspecified hip
[6th] M67.86 Other specified disorders of synovium and tendon, knee
M67.861 Other specified disorders of synovium, right knee
M67.862 Other specified disorders of synovium, left knee
M67.863 Other specified disorders of tendon, right knee
M67.864 Other specified disorders of tendon, left knee
M67.869 Other specified disorders of synovium and tendon, unspecified knee
[6th] M67.87 Other specified disorders of synovium and tendon, ankle and foot
M67.871 Other specified disorders of synovium, right ankle and foot
M67.872 Other specified disorders of synovium, left ankle and foot
M67.873 Other specified disorders of tendon, right ankle and foot
M67.874 Other specified disorders of tendon, left ankle and foot
M67.879 Other specified disorders of synovium and tendon, unspecified ankle and foot
M67.88 Other specified disorders of synovium and tendon, other site
M67.89 Other specified disorders of synovium and tendon, multiple sites

[PDx] Unacceptable principal diagnosis symbol per Medicare code edits [POA] Code exempt from diagnosis present on admission requirement
[?] Questionable admission [CC] Complication or comorbidity [CC/MCC Exc] CC/MCC exclusion [MCC] Major complication or comorbidity
[PDx CC] Principal diagnosis as its own CC [PDx MCC] Principal diagnosis as its own MCC [HCC] HCC diagnosis code [RxHCC] RxHCC diagnosis code
MACRA code [Z1] Z code as first-listed diagnosis

M67.9 Unspecified disorder of synovium and tendon
  M67.90 Unspecified disorder of synovium and tendon, unspecified site
  M67.91 Unspecified disorder of synovium and tendon, shoulder
    M67.911 Unspecified disorder of synovium and tendon, right shoulder
    M67.912 Unspecified disorder of synovium and tendon, left shoulder
    M67.919 Unspecified disorder of synovium and tendon, unspecified shoulder
  M67.92 Unspecified disorder of synovium and tendon, upper arm
    M67.921 Unspecified disorder of synovium and tendon, right upper arm
    M67.922 Unspecified disorder of synovium and tendon, left upper arm
    M67.929 Unspecified disorder of synovium and tendon, unspecified upper arm
  M67.93 Unspecified disorder of synovium and tendon, forearm
    M67.931 Unspecified disorder of synovium and tendon, right forearm
    M67.932 Unspecified disorder of synovium and tendon, left forearm
    M67.939 Unspecified disorder of synovium and tendon, unspecified forearm
  M67.94 Unspecified disorder of synovium and tendon, hand
    M67.941 Unspecified disorder of synovium and tendon, right hand
    M67.942 Unspecified disorder of synovium and tendon, left hand
    M67.949 Unspecified disorder of synovium and tendon, unspecified hand
  M67.95 Unspecified disorder of synovium and tendon, thigh
    M67.951 Unspecified disorder of synovium and tendon, right thigh
    M67.952 Unspecified disorder of synovium and tendon, left thigh
    M67.959 Unspecified disorder of synovium and tendon, unspecified thigh
  M67.96 Unspecified disorder of synovium and tendon, lower leg
    M67.961 Unspecified disorder of synovium and tendon, right lower leg
    M67.962 Unspecified disorder of synovium and tendon, left lower leg
    M67.969 Unspecified disorder of synovium and tendon, unspecified lower leg
  M67.97 Unspecified disorder of synovium and tendon, ankle and foot
    M67.971 Unspecified disorder of synovium and tendon, right ankle and foot
    M67.972 Unspecified disorder of synovium and tendon, left ankle and foot
    M67.979 Unspecified disorder of synovium and tendon, unspecified ankle and foot
  M67.98 Unspecified disorder of synovium and tendon, other site
  M67.99 Unspecified disorder of synovium and tendon, multiple sites

Other soft tissue disorders (M70-M79)

M70 Soft tissue disorders related to use, overuse and pressure
  INCLUDES soft tissue disorders of occupational origin
  Use additional external cause code to identify activity causing disorder (Y93.-)
  EXCLUDES1 bursitis NOS (M71.9-)
  EXCLUDES2 bursitis of shoulder (M75.5)
    enthesopathies (M76-M77)

pressure ulcer (pressure area) (L89.-)
M70.0 Crepitant synovitis (acute) (chronic) of hand and wrist
  M70.03 Crepitant synovitis (acute) (chronic), wrist
    M70.031 Crepitant synovitis (acute) (chronic), right wrist
    M70.032 Crepitant synovitis (acute) (chronic), left wrist
    M70.039 Crepitant synovitis (acute) (chronic), unspecified wrist
  M70.04 Crepitant synovitis (acute) (chronic), hand
    M70.041 Crepitant synovitis (acute) (chronic), right hand
    M70.042 Crepitant synovitis (acute) (chronic), left hand
    M70.049 Crepitant synovitis (acute) (chronic), unspecified hand
M70.1 Bursitis of hand
  M70.10 Bursitis, unspecified hand
  M70.11 Bursitis, right hand
  M70.12 Bursitis, left hand
M70.2 Olecranon bursitis
  M70.20 Olecranon bursitis, unspecified elbow
  M70.21 Olecranon bursitis, right elbow
  M70.22 Olecranon bursitis, left elbow
M70.3 Other bursitis of elbow
  M70.30 Other bursitis of elbow, unspecified elbow
  M70.31 Other bursitis of elbow, right elbow
  M70.32 Other bursitis of elbow, left elbow
M70.4 Prepatellar bursitis
  M70.40 Prepatellar bursitis, unspecified knee
  M70.41 Prepatellar bursitis, right knee
  M70.42 Prepatellar bursitis, left knee
M70.5 Other bursitis of knee
  M70.50 Other bursitis of knee, unspecified knee
  M70.51 Other bursitis of knee, right knee
  M70.52 Other bursitis of knee, left knee
M70.6 Trochanteric bursitis
  Trochanteric tendinitis
  M70.60 Trochanteric bursitis, unspecified hip
  M70.61 Trochanteric bursitis, right hip
  M70.62 Trochanteric bursitis, left hip
M70.7 Other bursitis of hip
  Ischial bursitis
  M70.70 Other bursitis of hip, unspecified hip
  M70.71 Other bursitis of hip, right hip
  M70.72 Other bursitis of hip, left hip
M70.8 Other soft tissue disorders related to use, overuse and pressure
  M70.80 Other soft tissue disorders related to use, overuse and pressure of unspecified site
  M70.81 Other soft tissue disorders related to use, overuse and pressure of shoulder
    M70.811 Other soft tissue disorders related to use, overuse and pressure, right shoulder
    M70.812 Other soft tissue disorders related to use, overuse and pressure, left shoulder
    M70.819 Other soft tissue disorders related to use, overuse and pressure, unspecified shoulder
  M70.82 Other soft tissue disorders related to use, overuse and pressure of upper arm
    M70.821 Other soft tissue disorders related to use, overuse and pressure, right upper arm
    M70.822 Other soft tissue disorders related to use, overuse and pressure, left upper arm
    M70.829 Other soft tissue disorders related to use, overuse and pressure, unspecified upper arms
  M70.83 Other soft tissue disorders related to use, overuse and pressure of forearm

Unspecified Code   Other Specified Code   Manifestation Code   N Newborn   P Pediatric   M Maternity   A Adult   ♂ Male   ♀ Female
● New Code   ▲ Revised Code Title   ►◄ Revised Text   NOTES   INCLUDES   EXCLUDES 1   Not coded here   EXCLUDES 2   Not included here
4th character required   5th character required   6th character required   7th character required
Extension 'X' Alert   HAC Hospital-acquired condition (HAC) alert   AHA AHA Coding Clinic©

M70.831 Other soft tissue disorders related to use, overuse and pressure, right forearm

M70.832 Other soft tissue disorders related to use, overuse and pressure, left forearm

M70.839 Other soft tissue disorders related to use, overuse and pressure, unspecified forearm

M70.84 Other soft tissue disorders related to use, overuse and pressure of hand

M70.841 Other soft tissue disorders related to use, overuse and pressure, right hand

M70.842 Other soft tissue disorders related to use, overuse and pressure, left hand

M70.849 Other soft tissue disorders related to use, overuse and pressure, unspecified hand

M70.85 Other soft tissue disorders related to use, overuse and pressure of thigh

M70.851 Other soft tissue disorders related to use, overuse and pressure, right thigh

M70.852 Other soft tissue disorders related to use, overuse and pressure, left thigh

M70.859 Other soft tissue disorders related to use, overuse and pressure, unspecified thigh

M70.86 Other soft tissue disorders related to use, overuse and pressure lower leg

M70.861 Other soft tissue disorders related to use, overuse and pressure, right lower leg

M70.862 Other soft tissue disorders related to use, overuse and pressure, left lower leg

M70.869 Other soft tissue disorders related to use, overuse and pressure, unspecified leg

M70.87 Other soft tissue disorders related to use, overuse and pressure of ankle and foot

M70.871 Other soft tissue disorders related to use, overuse and pressure, right ankle and foot

M70.872 Other soft tissue disorders related to use, overuse and pressure, left ankle and foot

M70.879 Other soft tissue disorders related to use, overuse and pressure, unspecified ankle and foot

M70.88 Other soft tissue disorders related to use, overuse and pressure other site

M70.89 Other soft tissue disorders related to use, overuse and pressure multiple sites

M70.9 Unspecified soft tissue disorder related to use, overuse and pressure

M70.90 Unspecified soft tissue disorder related to use, overuse and pressure of unspecified site

M70.91 Unspecified soft tissue disorder related to use, overuse and pressure of shoulder

M70.911 Unspecified soft tissue disorder related to use, overuse and pressure, right shoulder

M70.912 Unspecified soft tissue disorder related to use, overuse and pressure, left shoulder

M70.919 Unspecified soft tissue disorder related to use, overuse and pressure, unspecified shoulder

M70.92 Unspecified soft tissue disorder related to use, overuse and pressure of upper arm

M70.921 Unspecified soft tissue disorder related to use, overuse and pressure, right upper arm

M70.922 Unspecified soft tissue disorder related to use, overuse and pressure, left upper arm

M70.929 Unspecified soft tissue disorder related to use, overuse and pressure, unspecified upper arm

M70.93 Unspecified soft tissue disorder related to use, overuse and pressure of forearm

M70.931 Unspecified soft tissue disorder related to use, overuse and pressure, right forearm

M70.932 Unspecified soft tissue disorder related to use, overuse and pressure, left forearm

M70.939 Unspecified soft tissue disorder related to use, overuse and pressure, unspecified forearm

M70.94 Unspecified soft tissue disorder related to use, overuse and pressure of hand

M70.941 Unspecified soft tissue disorder related to use, overuse and pressure, right hand

M70.942 Unspecified soft tissue disorder related to use, overuse and pressure, left hand

M70.949 Unspecified soft tissue disorder related to use, overuse and pressure, unspecified hand

M70.95 Unspecified soft tissue disorder related to use, overuse and pressure of thigh

M70.951 Unspecified soft tissue disorder related to use, overuse and pressure, right thigh

M70.952 Unspecified soft tissue disorder related to use, overuse and pressure, left thigh

M70.959 Unspecified soft tissue disorder related to use, overuse and pressure, unspecified thigh

M70.96 Unspecified soft tissue disorder related to use, overuse and pressure lower leg

M70.961 Unspecified soft tissue disorder related to use, overuse and pressure, right lower leg

M70.962 Unspecified soft tissue disorder related to use, overuse and pressure, left lower leg

M70.969 Unspecified soft tissue disorder related to use, overuse and pressure, unspecified lower leg

M70.97 Unspecified soft tissue disorder related to use, overuse and pressure of ankle and foot

M70.971 Unspecified soft tissue disorder related to use, overuse and pressure, right ankle and foot

M70.972 Unspecified soft tissue disorder related to use, overuse and pressure, left ankle and foot

M70.979 Unspecified soft tissue disorder related to use, overuse and pressure, unspecified ankle and foot

M70.98 Unspecified soft tissue disorder related to use, overuse and pressure other

M70.99 Unspecified soft tissue disorder related to use, overuse and pressure multiple sites

M71 Other bursopathies

EXCLUDES1 bunion (M20.1)

bursitis related to use, overuse or pressure (M70.-)

enthesopathies (M76-M77)

M71.0 Abscess of bursa

Use additional code (B95.-, B96.-) to identify causative organism

M71.00 Abscess of bursa, unspecified site

M71.01 Abscess of bursa, shoulder

M71.011 Abscess of bursa, right shoulder

M71.012 Abscess of bursa, left shoulder

M71.019 Abscess of bursa, unspecified shoulder

M71.02 Abscess of bursa, elbow

M71.021 Abscess of bursa, right elbow

M71.022 Abscess of bursa, left elbow

M71.029 Abscess of bursa, unspecified elbow

M71.03 Abscess of bursa, wrist

M71.031 Abscess of bursa, right wrist

M71.032 Abscess of bursa, left wrist

M71.039 Abscess of bursa, unspecified wrist

M71.04 Abscess of bursa, hand

M71.041 Abscess of bursa, right hand

M71.042 Abscess of bursa, left hand

M71.049 Abscess of bursa, unspecified hand

M71.05 Abscess of bursa, hip

M71.051 Abscess of bursa, right hip

Unacceptable principal diagnosis symbol per Medicare code edits   Code exempt from diagnosis present on admission requirement
Questionable admission   Complication or comorbidity   CC/MCC exclusion   Major complication or comorbidity
Principal diagnosis as its own CC   Principal diagnosis as its own MCC   HCC HCC diagnosis code   RxHCC diagnosis code
MACRA code   Z code as first-listed diagnosis

832   When symbols appear on a code that requires a 7th character extension, refer to Appendix B to identify applicable 7th character codes.   **2018 ICD-10-CM**

M71.052 Abscess of bursa, left hip
M71.059 Abscess of bursa, unspecified hip
M71.06 Abscess of bursa, knee
    M71.061 Abscess of bursa, right knee
    M71.062 Abscess of bursa, left knee
    M71.069 Abscess of bursa, unspecified knee
M71.07 Abscess of bursa, ankle and foot
    M71.071 Abscess of bursa, right ankle and foot
    M71.072 Abscess of bursa, left ankle and foot
    M71.079 Abscess of bursa, unspecified ankle and foot
M71.08 Abscess of bursa, other site
M71.09 Abscess of bursa, multiple sites
M71.1 Other infective bursitis
    Use additional code (B95.-, B96.-) to identify causative organism
M71.10 Other infective bursitis, unspecified site
M71.11 Other infective bursitis, shoulder
    M71.111 Other infective bursitis, right shoulder
    M71.112 Other infective bursitis, left shoulder
    M71.119 Other infective bursitis, unspecified shoulder
M71.12 Other infective bursitis, elbow
    M71.121 Other infective bursitis, right elbow
    M71.122 Other infective bursitis, left elbow
    M71.129 Other infective bursitis, unspecified elbow
M71.13 Other infective bursitis, wrist
    M71.131 Other infective bursitis, right wrist
    M71.132 Other infective bursitis, left wrist
    M71.139 Other infective bursitis, unspecified wrist
M71.14 Other infective bursitis, hand
    M71.141 Other infective bursitis, right hand
    M71.142 Other infective bursitis, left hand
    M71.149 Other infective bursitis, unspecified hand
M71.15 Other infective bursitis, hip
    M71.151 Other infective bursitis, right hip
    M71.152 Other infective bursitis, left hip
    M71.159 Other infective bursitis, unspecified hip
M71.16 Other infective bursitis, knee
    M71.161 Other infective bursitis, right knee
    M71.162 Other infective bursitis, left knee
    M71.169 Other infective bursitis, unspecified knee
M71.17 Other infective bursitis, ankle and foot
    M71.171 Other infective bursitis, right ankle and foot
    M71.172 Other infective bursitis, left ankle and foot
    M71.179 Other infective bursitis, unspecified ankle and foot
M71.18 Other infective bursitis, other site
M71.19 Other infective bursitis, multiple sites
M71.2 Synovial cyst of popliteal space [Baker]
    EXCLUDES1 synovial cyst of popliteal space with rupture (M66.0)
M71.20 Synovial cyst of popliteal space [Baker], unspecified knee
M71.21 Synovial cyst of popliteal space [Baker], right knee
M71.22 Synovial cyst of popliteal space [Baker], left knee
M71.3 Other bursal cyst
    Synovial cyst NOS
    EXCLUDES1 synovial cyst with rupture (M66.1-)
M71.30 Other bursal cyst, unspecified site
M71.31 Other bursal cyst, shoulder
    M71.311 Other bursal cyst, right shoulder
    M71.312 Other bursal cyst, left shoulder
    M71.319 Other bursal cyst, unspecified shoulder
M71.32 Other bursal cyst, elbow
    M71.321 Other bursal cyst, right elbow
    M71.322 Other bursal cyst, left elbow
    M71.329 Other bursal cyst, unspecified elbow
M71.33 Other bursal cyst, wrist

M71.331 Other bursal cyst, right wrist
M71.332 Other bursal cyst, left wrist
M71.339 Other bursal cyst, unspecified wrist
M71.34 Other bursal cyst, hand
    M71.341 Other bursal cyst, right hand
    M71.342 Other bursal cyst, left hand
    M71.349 Other bursal cyst, unspecified hand
M71.35 Other bursal cyst, hip
    M71.351 Other bursal cyst, right hip
    M71.352 Other bursal cyst, left hip
    M71.359 Other bursal cyst, unspecified hip
M71.37 Other bursal cyst, ankle and foot
    M71.371 Other bursal cyst, right ankle and foot
    M71.372 Other bursal cyst, left ankle and foot
    M71.379 Other bursal cyst, unspecified ankle and foot
M71.38 Other bursal cyst, other site
M71.39 Other bursal cyst, multiple sites
M71.4 Calcium deposit in bursa
    EXCLUDES2 calcium deposit in bursa of shoulder (M75.3)
M71.40 Calcium deposit in bursa, unspecified site
M71.42 Calcium deposit in bursa, elbow
    M71.421 Calcium deposit in bursa, right elbow
    M71.422 Calcium deposit in bursa, left elbow
    M71.429 Calcium deposit in bursa, unspecified elbow
M71.43 Calcium deposit in bursa, wrist
    M71.431 Calcium deposit in bursa, right wrist
    M71.432 Calcium deposit in bursa, left wrist
    M71.439 Calcium deposit in bursa, unspecified wrist
M71.44 Calcium deposit in bursa, hand
    M71.441 Calcium deposit in bursa, right hand
    M71.442 Calcium deposit in bursa, left hand
    M71.449 Calcium deposit in bursa, unspecified hand
M71.45 Calcium deposit in bursa, hip
    M71.451 Calcium deposit in bursa, right hip
    M71.452 Calcium deposit in bursa, left hip
    M71.459 Calcium deposit in bursa, unspecified hip
M71.46 Calcium deposit in bursa, knee
    M71.461 Calcium deposit in bursa, right knee
    M71.462 Calcium deposit in bursa, left knee
    M71.469 Calcium deposit in bursa, unspecified knee
M71.47 Calcium deposit in bursa, ankle and foot
    M71.471 Calcium deposit in bursa, right ankle and foot
    M71.472 Calcium deposit in bursa, left ankle and foot
    M71.479 Calcium deposit in bursa, unspecified ankle and foot
M71.48 Calcium deposit in bursa, other site
M71.49 Calcium deposit in bursa, multiple sites
M71.5 Other bursitis, not elsewhere classified
    EXCLUDES1 bursitis NOS (M71.9-)
    EXCLUDES2 bursitis of shoulder (M75.5)
    bursitis of tibial collateral [Pellegrini-Stieda] (M76.4-)
M71.50 Other bursitis, not elsewhere classified, unspecified site
M71.52 Other bursitis, not elsewhere classified, elbow
    M71.521 Other bursitis, not elsewhere classified, right elbow
    M71.522 Other bursitis, not elsewhere classified, left elbow
    M71.529 Other bursitis, not elsewhere classified, unspecified elbow
M71.53 Other bursitis, not elsewhere classified, wrist

Unspecified Code Other Specified Code Manifestation Code N Newborn P Pediatric M Maternity A Adult ♂ Male ♀ Female
● New Code ▲ Revised Code Title ►◄ Revised Text NOTES INCLUDES EXCLUDES 1 Not coded here EXCLUDES 2 Not included here
4th character required 5th character required 6th character required 7th character required
Extension 'X' Alert HAC Hospital-acquired condition (HAC) alert AHA AHA Coding Clinic©

2018 ICD-10-CM   When symbols appear on a code that requires a 7th character extension, refer to Appendix B to identify applicable 7th character codes.   833

M84.46 Pathological fracture, tibia and fibula
- M84.461 Pathological fracture, right tibia
- M84.462 Pathological fracture, left tibia
- M84.463 Pathological fracture, right fibula
- M84.464 Pathological fracture, left fibula
- M84.469 Pathological fracture, unspecified tibia and fibula

M84.47 Pathological fracture, ankle, foot and toes
- M84.471 Pathological fracture, right ankle
- M84.472 Pathological fracture, left ankle
- M84.473 Pathological fracture, unspecified ankle
- M84.474 Pathological fracture, right foot
- M84.475 Pathological fracture, left foot
- M84.476 Pathological fracture, unspecified foot
- M84.477 Pathological fracture, right toe(s)
- M84.478 Pathological fracture, left toe(s)
- M84.479 Pathological fracture, unspecified toe(s)

M84.48 Pathological fracture, other site

M84.5 Pathological fracture in neoplastic disease
Code also underlying neoplasm

The appropriate 7th character is to be added to each code from subcategory M84.5:
- A = initial encounter for fracture
- D = subsequent encounter for fracture with routine healing
- G = subsequent encounter for fracture with delayed healing
- K = subsequent encounter for fracture with nonunion
- P = subsequent encounter for fracture with malunion
- S = sequela

M84.50 Pathological fracture in neoplastic disease, unspecified site

M84.51 Pathological fracture in neoplastic disease, shoulder
- M84.511 Pathological fracture in neoplastic disease, right shoulder
- M84.512 Pathological fracture in neoplastic disease, left shoulder
- M84.519 Pathological fracture in neoplastic disease, unspecified shoulder

M84.52 Pathological fracture in neoplastic disease, humerus
- M84.521 Pathological fracture in neoplastic disease, right humerus
- M84.522 Pathological fracture in neoplastic disease, left humerus
- M84.529 Pathological fracture in neoplastic disease, unspecified humerus

M84.53 Pathological fracture in neoplastic disease, ulna and radius
- M84.531 Pathological fracture in neoplastic disease, right ulna
- M84.532 Pathological fracture in neoplastic disease, left ulna
- M84.533 Pathological fracture in neoplastic disease, right radius
- M84.534 Pathological fracture in neoplastic disease, left radius
- M84.539 Pathological fracture in neoplastic disease, unspecified ulna and radius

M84.54 Pathological fracture in neoplastic disease, hand

M84.541 Pathological fracture in neoplastic disease, right hand
M84.542 Pathological fracture in neoplastic disease, left hand
M84.549 Pathological fracture in neoplastic disease, unspecified hand

M84.55 Pathological fracture in neoplastic disease, pelvis and femur
- M84.550 Pathological fracture in neoplastic disease, pelvis
- M84.551 Pathological fracture in neoplastic disease, right femur
- M84.552 Pathological fracture in neoplastic disease, left femur
- M84.553 Pathological fracture in neoplastic disease, unspecified femur
- M84.559 Pathological fracture in neoplastic disease, hip, unspecified

M84.56 Pathological fracture in neoplastic disease, tibia and fibula
- M84.561 Pathological fracture in neoplastic disease, right tibia
- M84.562 Pathological fracture in neoplastic disease, left tibia
- M84.563 Pathological fracture in neoplastic disease, right fibula
- M84.564 Pathological fracture in neoplastic disease, left fibula
- M84.569 Pathological fracture in neoplastic disease, unspecified tibia and fibula

M84.57 Pathological fracture in neoplastic disease, ankle and foot
- M84.571 Pathological fracture in neoplastic disease, right ankle
- M84.572 Pathological fracture in neoplastic disease, left ankle
- M84.573 Pathological fracture in neoplastic disease, unspecified ankle
- M84.574 Pathological fracture in neoplastic disease, right foot
- M84.575 Pathological fracture in neoplastic disease, left foot
- M84.576 Pathological fracture in neoplastic disease, unspecified foot

M84.58 Pathological fracture in neoplastic disease, other specified site
Pathological fracture in neoplastic disease, vertebrae

M84.6 Pathological fracture in other disease
Code also underlying condition
EXCLUDES1 pathological fracture in osteoporosis (M80.-)
The appropriate 7th character is to be added to each code from subcategory M84.6:
- A = initial encounter for fracture
- D = subsequent encounter for fracture with routine healing
- G = subsequent encounter for fracture with delayed healing
- K = subsequent encounter for fracture with nonunion
- P = subsequent encounter for fracture with malunion
- S = sequela

M84.60 Pathological fracture in other disease, unspecified site

M84.61 Pathological fracture in other disease, shoulder
- M84.611 Pathological fracture in other disease, right shoulder
- M84.612 Pathological fracture in other disease, left shoulder
- M84.619 Pathological fracture in other disease, unspecified shoulder

M84.62 Pathological fracture in other disease, humerus

PDx Unacceptable principal diagnosis symbol per Medicare code edits   POA Code exempt from diagnosis present on admission requirement
❓ Questionable admission   cc Complication or comorbidity   CC/MCC Exc CC/MCC exclusion   MCC Major complication or comorbidity
Principal diagnosis as its own CC   Principal diagnosis as its own MCC   HCC HCC diagnosis code   RxHCC RxHCC diagnosis code
MACRA code   Z1 Z code as first-listed diagnosis

840   When symbols appear on a code that requires a 7th character extension, refer to Appendix B to identify applicable 7th character codes.   2018 ICD-10-CM

M84.621 Pathological fracture in other disease, right humerus

M84.622 Pathological fracture in other disease, left humerus

M84.629 Pathological fracture in other disease, unspecified humerus

M84.63 Pathological fracture in other disease, ulna and radius

    M84.631 Pathological fracture in other disease, right ulna

    M84.632 Pathological fracture in other disease, left ulna

    M84.633 Pathological fracture in other disease, right radius

    M84.634 Pathological fracture in other disease, left radius

    M84.639 Pathological fracture in other disease, unspecified ulna and radius

M84.64 Pathological fracture in other disease, hand

    M84.641 Pathological fracture in other disease, right hand

    M84.642 Pathological fracture in other disease, left hand

    M84.649 Pathological fracture in other disease, unspecified hand

M84.65 Pathological fracture in other disease, pelvis and femur

    M84.650 Pathological fracture in other disease, pelvis

    M84.651 Pathological fracture in other disease, right femur

    M84.652 Pathological fracture in other disease, left femur

    M84.653 Pathological fracture in other disease, unspecified femur

    M84.659 Pathological fracture in other disease, hip, unspecified

M84.66 Pathological fracture in other disease, tibia and fibula

    M84.661 Pathological fracture in other disease, right tibia

    M84.662 Pathological fracture in other disease, left tibia

    M84.663 Pathological fracture in other disease, right fibula

    M84.664 Pathological fracture in other disease, left fibula

    M84.669 Pathological fracture in other disease, unspecified tibia and fibula

M84.67 Pathological fracture in other disease, ankle and foot

    M84.671 Pathological fracture in other disease, right ankle

    M84.672 Pathological fracture in other disease, left ankle

    M84.673 Pathological fracture in other disease, unspecified ankle

    M84.674 Pathological fracture in other disease, right foot

    M84.675 Pathological fracture in other disease, left foot

    M84.676 Pathological fracture in other disease, unspecified foot

M84.68 Pathological fracture in other disease, other site

M84.7 Nontraumatic fracture, not elsewhere classified

M84.75 Atypical femoral fracture

The appropriate 7th character is to be added to each code from M84.75:

A = initial encounter for fracture
D = subsequent encounter for fracture with routine healing
G = subsequent encounter for fracture with delayed healing
K = subsequent encounter for fracture with nonunion
P = subsequent encounter for fracture with malunion
S = sequela

M84.750 Atypical femoral fracture, unspecified

M84.751 Incomplete atypical femoral fracture, right leg

M84.752 Incomplete atypical femoral fracture, left leg

M84.753 Incomplete atypical femoral fracture, unspecified leg

M84.754 Complete transverse atypical femoral fracture, right leg

M84.755 Complete transverse atypical femoral fracture, left leg

M84.756 Complete transverse atypical femoral fracture, unspecified leg

M84.757 Complete oblique atypical femoral fracture, right leg

M84.758 Complete oblique atypical femoral fracture, left leg

M84.759 Complete oblique atypical femoral fracture, unspecified leg

M84.8 Other disorders of continuity of bone

M84.80 Other disorders of continuity of bone, unspecified site

M84.81 Other disorders of continuity of bone, shoulder

    M84.811 Other disorders of continuity of bone, right shoulder

    M84.812 Other disorders of continuity of bone, left shoulder

    M84.819 Other disorders of continuity of bone, unspecified shoulder

M84.82 Other disorders of continuity of bone, humerus

    M84.821 Other disorders of continuity of bone, right humerus

    M84.822 Other disorders of continuity of bone, left humerus

    M84.829 Other disorders of continuity of bone, unspecified humerus

M84.83 Other disorders of continuity of bone, ulna and radius

    M84.831 Other disorders of continuity of bone, right ulna

    M84.832 Other disorders of continuity of bone, left ulna

    M84.833 Other disorders of continuity of bone, right radius

    M84.834 Other disorders of continuity of bone, left radius

    M84.839 Other disorders of continuity of bone, unspecified ulna and radius

M84.84 Other disorders of continuity of bone, hand

    M84.841 Other disorders of continuity of bone, right hand

    M84.842 Other disorders of continuity of bone, left hand

    M84.849 Other disorders of continuity of bone, unspecified hand

M84.85 Other disorders of continuity of bone, pelvic region and thigh

    M84.851 Other disorders of continuity of bone, right pelvic region and thigh

    M84.852 Other disorders of continuity of bone, left pelvic region and thigh

    M84.859 Other disorders of continuity of bone, unspecified pelvic region and thigh

Anatomy of the Urinary System

1. An Outline of the Urinary System
a) Two Kidneys

b) Two Ureters

c) The Urinary Bladder

d) The Urethra

e) The urinary system maintains the state of homeostasis by regulating water and solutes in the human body.

f) Kidneys produce the urine and function as the major filtering organs of the urinary system.

g) Urine is composed of components like urea, water, ions, and toxic wastes that need to be regulated in the human body by the entire urinary system.

2. The Functions of Kidneys
a) Excretion

b) Maintenance of blood volume and concentration

c) pH regulation

d) Maintenance of blood pressure

e) Maintenance of erythrocyte concentration

f) The conversion of vitamin D to its active form (or calciferol).

3. The Anatomy of Kidneys
a) Kidneys are situated between the parietal peritoneum and posterior wall of abdomen.

b) There is a notch (known as hilum) located in the concave center of each kidney. The ureter exits the kidney, and blood vessels, lymph vessels and nerves enter and leave the kidney through the hilum.

c) The kidney is surrounded by the following three layers:

   i) The innermost layer of the kidney is known as the renal capsule. It acts as a barrier against trauma and infection.

   ii) Adipose capsule is the middle layer of the kidney. It is made up of fatty tissue and protects the kidney from blows.

   iii) The renal fascia is the outermost layer of the kidney. It serves to attach the kidney to the abdominal wall.

d) Cortex is the outer region of the kidney.

e) Medulla is the inner area of the kidney.

f) Renal pyramids are striated triangular structures that are found within the medulla. The bases of these pyramids face toward the cortex. However, their tips point to the center of the kidney and are known as the renal papillae.

g) The renal columns constitute the cortical material that extends between the pyramids.

h) The parenchyma of the kidney is formed by the cortex and renal pyramids.

i) The parenchyma is further composed of the microscopic units or nephrons, which are the structural and functional units of the kidneys.

j) The minor calyx is a funnel-shaped structure that surrounds the tip of each renal pyramid. The function of this minor calyx is to collect the urine from the ducts of the renal pyramids. The minor calyces integrate to constitute the major calyces.

k) The renal pelvis is the large collecting funnel that is formed by a bunch of major calyces. The renal pelvis is further narrowed and extended to constitute the ureter.

4. The Ureter
a) It is the extension of the renal pelvis of the kidney and communicates with the urinary bladder.

b) They are two in number and carry urine from the renal pelvis to the urinary bladder.

c) Urine is expelled from the bladder by the act of micturition.

5. The Urethra
a) It is a thin walled tube that connects the floor of the urinary bladder to the genitals for the expulsion of fluids (urine, semen, etc.) out of the body.

b) It is located in the wall of the vagina and above the vaginal opening in females. The female urethral orifice is the opening of the urethra and situated between the vaginal opening and clitoris.

c) It lies below the bladder in males and travels through the prostate gland and penis.

d) The opening at the tip of the male penis is known as the male urethral orifice.

e) The external urethral sphincter is a striated muscle and provides voluntary control of urination.

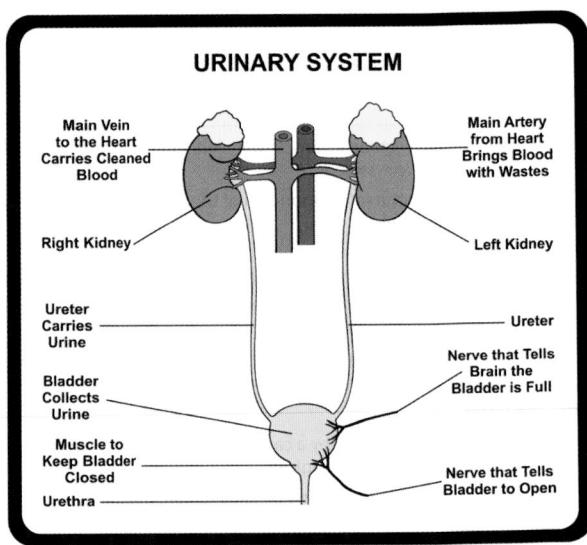

URINARY SYSTEM

Common Pathologies

Glomerulonephritis
Glomerulonephritis, also known as nephritic syndrome, is a disease of the kidney, characterized by inflammation of the glomeruli, small structures through which the kidney filters urine. Inflammation of the glomeruli prevents the kidneys from being able to filter the urine. Fluid and toxins then build up in the body and can lead to chronic renal failure, also known as chronic kidney failure (CKD).

Acute Renal Failure
Acute renal failure refers to the inability of the kidneys to filter waste products, resulting in the buildup of toxic substances in the blood.

Chronic Kidney Disease
Chronic kidney disease, or CKD, is a condition of gradual loss of kidney function, described in five stages, with stage 1 being the least severe and stage 5 being end stage renal disease, requiring dialysis or kidney transplant for treatment.

Bladder Cancer
Bladder cancer is an abnormal growth of cells in the bladder, typically beginning in the lining of the bladder and then spreading throughout the bladder and to adjacent organs.

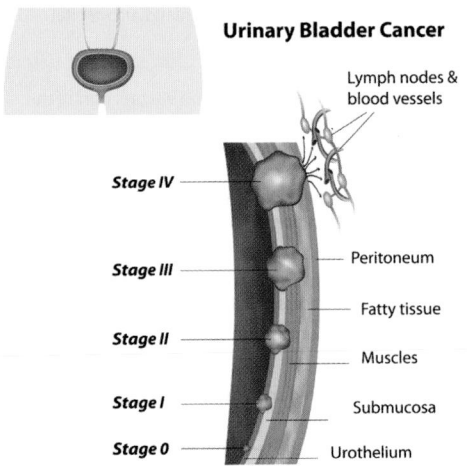

Urinary Bladder Cancer

Interstitial Cystitis
Interstitial cystitis is an inflammatory condition of the bladder that results in ongoing pain and feeling the need to urinate urgently and frequently.

Cystocele
Cystocele is a condition that occurs when the tough fibrous wall between a woman's bladder and her vagina weakens, allowing the bladder to droop into the vagina.

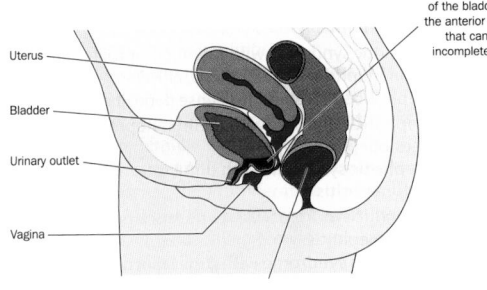

A cystocele is a bulging of the bladder through the anterior vaginal wall that can lead to incomplete emptying

Uterus

Bladder

Urinary outlet

Vagina

UTI
A urinary tract infection, or UTI, is a bacterial infection of one or more structures in the urinary tract, typically involving the bladder or urethra.

Kidney Stones
A kidney stone, also known as a calculus, results from a buildup of mineral salts or other such material in the kidney. Kidney stones vary in size. Larger stones can block the flow of urine, resulting in severe pain and blood in the urine.

N34.1 Nonspecific urethritis
Nongonococcal urethritis
Nonvenereal urethritis

N34.2 Other urethritis
Meatitis, urethral
Postmenopausal urethritis
Ulcer of urethra (meatus)
Urethritis NOS

N34.3 Urethral syndrome, unspecified

N35 **Urethral stricture**
EXCLUDES1 *congenital urethral stricture (Q64.3-)*
postprocedural urethral stricture (N99.1-)

N35.0 **Post-traumatic urethral stricture**
Urethral stricture due to injury
EXCLUDES1 *postprocedural urethral stricture (N99.1-)*

N35.01 **Post-traumatic urethral stricture, male**
N35.010 **Post-traumatic urethral stricture, male, meatal** ♂
N35.011 **Post-traumatic bulbous urethral stricture**
N35.012 **Post-traumatic membranous urethral stricture**
N35.013 **Post-traumatic anterior urethral stricture**
N35.014 **Post-traumatic urethral stricture, male, unspecified** ♂

N35.02 **Post-traumatic urethral stricture, female**
N35.021 **Urethral stricture due to childbirth** ♀
N35.028 **Other post-traumatic urethral stricture, female** ♀

N35.1 **Postinfective urethral stricture, not elsewhere classified**
EXCLUDES1 *urethral stricture associated with schistosomiasis (B65.-, N29)*
gonococcal urethral stricture (A54.01)
syphilitic urethral stricture (A52.76)

N35.11 **Postinfective urethral stricture, not elsewhere classified, male**
N35.111 **Postinfective urethral stricture, not elsewhere classified, male, meatal** ♂
▲ N35.112 **Postinfective bulbous urethral stricture, not elsewhere ►classified, male◄**
▲ N35.113 **Postinfective membranous urethral stricture, not elsewhere ►classified, male◄**
▲ N35.114 **Postinfective anterior urethral stricture, not elsewhere ►classified, male◄**
N35.119 **Postinfective urethral stricture, not elsewhere classified, male, unspecified** ♂

N35.12 **Postinfective urethral stricture, not elsewhere classified, female** ♀

N35.8 Other urethral stricture
EXCLUDES1 *postprocedural urethral stricture (N99.1-)*

N35.9 Urethral stricture, unspecified

N36 **Other disorders of urethra**

N36.0 **Urethral fistula** CC CC/MCC Exc
Urethroperineal fistula
Urethrorectal fistula
Urinary fistula NOS
EXCLUDES1 *urethroscrotal fistula (N50.89)*
urethrovaginal fistula (N82.1)
urethrovesicovaginal fistula (N82.1)

N36.1 Urethral diverticulum

N36.2 Urethral caruncle

N36.4 **Urethral functional and muscular disorders**
Use additional code to identify associated urinary stress incontinence (N39.3)
N36.41 **Hypermobility of urethra**
N36.42 **Intrinsic sphincter deficiency (ISD)**
N36.43 **Combined hypermobility of urethra and intrinsic sphincter deficiency**
N36.44 **Muscular disorders of urethra**
Bladder sphincter dyssynergy

N36.5 Urethral false passage

N36.8 **Other specified disorders of urethra**
EXCLUDES1 *congenital urethrocele (Q64.7)*
female urethrocele (N81.0)

N36.9 Urethral disorder, unspecified

N37 **Urethral disorders in diseases classified elsewhere**
Code first underlying disease
EXCLUDES1 *urethritis (in):*
candidal infection (B37.41)
chlamydial (A56.01)
gonorrhea (A54.01)
syphilis (A52.76)
trichomonal infection (A59.03)
tuberculosis (A18.13)

N39 **Other disorders of urinary system**
EXCLUDES2 *hematuria NOS (R31.-)*
recurrent or persistent hematuria (N02.-)
recurrent or persistent hematuria with specified morphological lesion (N02.-)
proteinuria NOS (R80.-)

N39.0 **Urinary tract infection, site not specified** CC HAC CC/MCC Exc
Use additional code (B95-B97), to identify infectious agent.
EXCLUDES1 *candidiasis of urinary tract (B37.4-)*
neonatal urinary tract infection (P39.3)
urinary tract infection of specified site, such as:
cystitis (N30.-)
urethritis (N34.-)

N39.3 **Stress incontinence (female) (male)**
Code also any associated overactive bladder (N32.81)
EXCLUDES1 *mixed incontinence (N39.46)*

N39.4 **Other specified urinary incontinence**
Code also any associated overactive bladder (N32.81)
EXCLUDES1 *enuresis NOS (R32)*
functional urinary incontinence (R39.81)
urinary incontinence associated with cognitive impairment (R39.81)
urinary incontinence NOS (R32)
urinary incontinence of nonorganic origin (F98.0)

N39.41 **Urge incontinence**
EXCLUDES1 *mixed incontinence (N39.46)*
N39.42 **Incontinence without sensory awareness**
AHA: Q4 2016
Insensible (urinary) incontinence
N39.43 **Post-void dribbling**
N39.44 **Nocturnal enuresis**
N39.45 **Continuous leakage**
N39.46 **Mixed incontinence**
Urge and stress incontinence

N39.49 **Other specified urinary incontinence**
N39.490 **Overflow incontinence**
N39.491 **Coital incontinence**
AHA: Q4 2016
N39.492 **Postural (urinary) incontinence**
AHA: Q4 2016
N39.498 **Other specified urinary incontinence**
Reflex incontinence
Total incontinence

N39.8 **Other specified disorders of urinary system**

N39.9 **Disorder of urinary system, unspecified**

PDMR Unacceptable principal diagnosis symbol per Medicare code edits   POA Code exempt from diagnosis present on admission requirement
? Questionable admission   CC Complication or comorbidity   CC/MCC Exc CC/MCC exclusion   MCC Major complication or comorbidity
PDx Principal diagnosis as its own CC   PDx Principal diagnosis as its own MCC   HCC HCC diagnosis code   RxHCC RxHCC diagnosis code
MACRA code   Z1 Z code as first-listed diagnosis

872

When symbols appear on a code that requires a 7th character extension, refer to Appendix B to identify applicable 7th character codes.

2018 ICD-10-CM

Diseases of male genital organs (N40-N53)

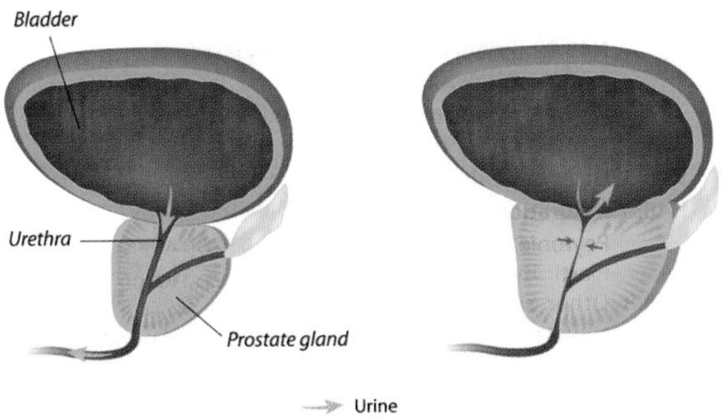
Normal
Enlarged prostate gland
Bladder
Urethra
Prostate gland
Urine

Figure 14.2 Benign prostatic hyperplasia

[4th] **N40** Benign prostatic hyperplasia
INCLUDES *adenofibromatous hypertrophy of prostate*
benign hypertrophy of the prostate
benign prostatic hypertrophy
BPH
enlarged prostate
nodular prostate
polyp of prostate
EXCLUDES1 *benign neoplasms of prostate (adenoma, benign) (fibroadenoma) (fibroma) (myoma) (D29.1)*
EXCLUDES2 *malignant neoplasm of prostate (C61)*
N40.0 **Benign prostatic hyperplasia** without lower urinary tract symptoms [A] ♂
Enlarged prostate without LUTS
Enlarged prostate NOS
N40.1 **Benign prostatic hyperplasia** with lower urinary tract symptoms [A] ♂
Enlarged prostate with LUTS
Use additional code for associated symptoms, when specified:
incomplete bladder emptying (R39.14)
nocturia (R35.1)
straining on urination (R39.16)
urinary frequency (R35.0)
urinary hesitancy (R39.11)
urinary incontinence (N39.4-)
urinary obstruction (N13.8)
urinary retention (R33.8)
urinary urgency (R39.15)
weak urinary stream (R39.12)
N40.2 Nodular **prostate** without lower urinary tract symptoms [A] ♂
Nodular prostate without LUTS
N40.3 Nodular **prostate** with lower urinary tract symptoms [A] ♂
Use additional code for associated symptoms, when specified:
incomplete bladder emptying (R39.14)
nocturia (R35.1)
straining on urination (R39.16)
urinary frequency (R35.0)
urinary hesitancy (R39.11)
urinary incontinence (N39.4-)
urinary obstruction (N13.8)
urinary retention (R33.8)
urinary urgency (R39.15)
weak urinary stream (R39.12)

[4th] **N41** Inflammatory diseases of prostate
Use additional code (B95-B97), to identify infectious agent.
N41.0 Acute prostatitis [A] [CC] ♂ [CC/MCC Exc]
N41.1 Chronic prostatitis [A] ♂
N41.2 Abscess of prostate [A] [CC] ♂ [CC/MCC Exc]
N41.3 Prostatocystitis [A] ♂
N41.4 Granulomatous prostatitis [A] ♂
N41.8 Other inflammatory diseases of prostate [A] ♂
N41.9 Inflammatory disease of prostate, unspecified [A] ♂
Prostatitis NOS

[4th] **N42** Other and unspecified disorders of prostate
N42.0 Calculus of prostate [A] ♂
Prostatic stone
N42.1 Congestion and hemorrhage of prostate [A] ♂
EXCLUDES1 *enlarged prostate (N40.-)*
hematuria (R31.-)
hyperplasia of prostate (N40.-)
inflammatory diseases of prostate (N41.-)
[5th] **N42.3** Dysplasia **of prostate**
N42.30 Unspecified dysplasia of prostate ♂
AHA: Q4 2016
N42.31 Prostatic intraepithelial neoplasia ♂
AHA: Q4 2016
PIN
Prostatic intraepithelial neoplasia I (PIN I)
Prostatic intraepithelial neoplasia II (PIN II)
EXCLUDES1 *prostatic intraepithelial neoplasia III (PIN III) (D07.5)*
N42.32 Atypical small acinar proliferation **of prostate** ♂
AHA: Q4 2016
N42.39 Other **dysplasia of prostate** ♂
AHA: Q4 2016
[5th] **N42.8** Other specified disorders of prostate
N42.81 Prostatodynia syndrome [A] ♂
Painful prostate syndrome
N42.82 Prostatosis syndrome [A] ♂
N42.83 Cyst of prostate [A] ♂
N42.89 Other specified disorders of prostate [A] ♂
N42.9 Disorder of prostate, unspecified [A] ♂

[4th] **N43** Hydrocele **and** spermatocele
INCLUDES *hydrocele of spermatic cord, testis or tunica vaginalis*
EXCLUDES1 *congenital hydrocele (P83.5)*
N43.0 Encysted **hydrocele** ♂
N43.1 Infected **hydrocele** [CC] ♂ [CC/MCC Exc]
Use additional code (B95-B97), to identify infectious agent
N43.2 Other hydrocele ♂
N43.3 Hydrocele, unspecified ♂
[5th] **N43.4** Spermatocele of epididymis
Spermatic cyst
N43.40 Spermatocele of epididymis, unspecified ♂
N43.41 Spermatocele of epididymis, single ♂
N43.42 Spermatocele of epididymis, multiple ♂

[4th] **N44** Noninflammatory disorders of testis
[5th] **N44.0** Torsion **of testis**
N44.00 Torsion of testis, unspecified [CC] ♂ [CC/MCC Exc]
N44.01 Extravaginal **torsion of spermatic cord** [CC] ♂ [CC/MCC Exc]
N44.02 Intravaginal **torsion of spermatic cord** [CC] ♂ [CC/MCC Exc]
Torsion of spermatic cord NOS
N44.03 Torsion of appendix testis [CC] ♂ [CC/MCC Exc]
N44.04 Torsion of appendix epididymis [CC] ♂ [CC/MCC Exc]
N44.1 Cyst of tunica albuginea **testis** ♂
N44.2 Benign cyst **of testis** ♂
N44.8 Other noninflammatory disorders of the testis ♂

[4th] **N45** Orchitis and epididymitis
Use additional code (B95-B97), to identify infectious agent.
N45.1 Epididymitis ♂
N45.2 Orchitis ♂
N45.3 Epididymo-orchitis ♂
N45.4 Abscess of epididymis or testis [CC] ♂ [CC/MCC Exc]

Unspecified Code | Other Specified Code | Manifestation Code | [N] Newborn | [P] Pediatric | [M] Maternity | [A] Adult | ♂ Male | ♀ Female
● New Code | ▲ Revised Code Title | ►◄ Revised Text | NOTES | INCLUDES | EXCLUDES1 Not coded here | EXCLUDES2 Not included here
[4th] 4th character required | [5th] 5th character required | [6th] 6th character required | [7th] 7th character required
[X] Extension 'X' Alert | [HAC] Hospital-acquired condition (HAC) alert | AHA AHA Coding Clinic©

N90.89 Other specified noninflammatory disorders of vulva and perineum ♀
  Adhesions of vulva
  Hypertrophy of clitoris
N90.9 Noninflammatory disorder of vulva and perineum, unspecified ♀
🔵 **N91** Absent, scanty and rare menstruation
  EXCLUDES1 ovarian dysfunction (E28.-)
N91.0 Primary amenorrhea ♀
N91.1 Secondary amenorrhea ♀
N91.2 Amenorrhea, unspecified ♀
N91.3 Primary oligomenorrhea ♀
N91.4 Secondary oligomenorrhea ♀
N91.5 Oligomenorrhea, unspecified ♀
  Hypomenorrhea NOS
🔵 **N92** Excessive, frequent and irregular menstruation
  EXCLUDES1 postmenopausal bleeding (N95.0)
    precocious puberty (menstruation) (E30.1)
N92.0 Excessive and frequent menstruation with regular cycle ♀
  Heavy periods NOS
  Menorrhagia NOS
  Polymenorrhea
N92.1 Excessive and frequent menstruation with irregular cycle ♀
  Irregular intermenstrual bleeding
  Irregular, shortened intervals between menstrual bleeding
  Menometrorrhagia
  Metrorrhagia
N92.2 Excessive menstruation at puberty 🅿 ♀
  Excessive bleeding associated with onset of menstrual periods
  Pubertal menorrhagia
  Puberty bleeding
N92.3 Ovulation bleeding ♀
  Regular intermenstrual bleeding
N92.4 Excessive bleeding in the premenopausal period ♀
  Climacteric menorrhagia or metrorrhagia
  Menopausal menorrhagia or metrorrhagia
  Preclimacteric menorrhagia or metrorrhagia
  Premenopausal menorrhagia or metrorrhagia
N92.5 Other specified irregular menstruation ♀
N92.6 Irregular menstruation, unspecified ♀
  Irregular bleeding NOS
  Irregular periods NOS
  EXCLUDES1 irregular menstruation with:
    lengthened intervals or scanty bleeding (N91.3-N91.5)
    shortened intervals or excessive bleeding (N92.1)
🔵 **N93** Other abnormal uterine and vaginal bleeding
  EXCLUDES1 neonatal vaginal hemorrhage (P54.6)
    precocious puberty (menstruation) (E30.1)
    pseudomenses (P54.6)
N93.0 Postcoital and contact bleeding ♀
N93.1 Pre-pubertal vaginal bleeding ♀
  AHA: Q4 2016
N93.8 Other specified abnormal uterine and vaginal bleeding ♀
  Dysfunctional or functional uterine or vaginal bleeding NOS
N93.9 Abnormal uterine and vaginal bleeding, unspecified ♀
🔵 **N94** Pain and other conditions associated with female genital organs and menstrual cycle
N94.0 Mittelschmerz ♀
🔵 **N94.1** Dyspareunia
  EXCLUDES1 psychogenic dyspareunia (F52.6)
  N94.10 Unspecified dyspareunia ♀
    AHA: Q4 2016
  N94.11 Superficial (introital) dyspareunia ♀
    AHA: Q4 2016
  N94.12 Deep dyspareunia ♀
    AHA: Q4 2016
  N94.19 Other specified dyspareunia ♀
    AHA: Q4 2016
N94.2 Vaginismus ♀
  EXCLUDES1 psychogenic vaginismus (F52.5)

N94.3 Premenstrual tension syndrome ♀
  AHA: Q4 2016
  Code also associated menstrual migraine (G43.82-, G43.83-)
  EXCLUDES1 Premenstrual dysphoric disorder (F32.81)
N94.4 Primary dysmenorrhea ♀
N94.5 Secondary dysmenorrhea ♀
N94.6 Dysmenorrhea, unspecified ♀
  EXCLUDES1 psychogenic dysmenorrhea (F45.8)
🔵 **N94.8** Other specified conditions associated with female genital organs and menstrual cycle
  🔵 **N94.81** Vulvodynia
    N94.810 Vulvar vestibulitis ♀
    N94.818 Other vulvodynia ♀
    N94.819 Vulvodynia, unspecified ♀
      Vulvodynia NOS
  N94.89 Other specified conditions associated with female genital organs and menstrual cycle ♀
N94.9 Unspecified condition associated with female genital organs and menstrual cycle ♀
🔵 **N95** Menopausal and other perimenopausal disorders
  Menopausal and other perimenopausal disorders due to naturally occurring (age-related) menopause and perimenopause
  EXCLUDES1 excessive bleeding in the premenopausal period (N92.4)
    menopausal and perimenopausal disorders due to artificial or premature menopause (E89.4-, E28.31-)
    premature menopause (E28.31-)
  EXCLUDES2 postmenopausal osteoporosis (M81.0-)
    postmenopausal osteoporosis with current pathological fracture (M80.0-)
    postmenopausal urethritis (N34.2)
N95.0 Postmenopausal bleeding ♀
N95.1 Menopausal and female climacteric states ♀
  Symptoms such as flushing, sleeplessness, headache, lack of concentration, associated with natural (age-related) menopause
  Use additional code for associated symptoms
  EXCLUDES1 asymptomatic menopausal state (Z78.0)
    symptoms associated with artificial menopause (E89.41)
    symptoms associated with premature menopause (E28.310)
N95.2 Postmenopausal atrophic vaginitis ♀
  Senile (atrophic) vaginitis
N95.8 Other specified menopausal and perimenopausal disorders ♀
N95.9 Unspecified menopausal and perimenopausal disorder ♀
N96 Recurrent pregnancy loss ♀
  Investigation or care in a nonpregnant woman with history of recurrent pregnancy loss
  EXCLUDES1 recurrent pregancy loss with current pregnancy (O26.2-)
🔵 **N97** Female infertility
  INCLUDES inability to achieve a pregnancy
    sterility, female NOS
  EXCLUDES1 female infertility associated with:
    hypopituitarism (E23.0)
    Stein-Leventhal syndrome (E28.2)
  EXCLUDES2 incompetence of cervix uteri (N88.3)
N97.0 Female infertility associated with anovulation ♀
N97.1 Female infertility of tubal origin ♀
  Female infertility associated with congenital anomaly of tube
  Female infertility due to tubal block
  Female infertility due to tubal occlusion
  Female infertility due to tubal stenosis
N97.2 Female infertility of uterine origin ♀
  Female infertility associated with congenital anomaly of uterus
  Female infertility due to nonimplantation of ovum
N97.8 Female infertility of other origin ♀
N97.9 Female infertility, unspecified ♀
🔵 **N98** Complications associated with artificial fertilization
  N98.0 Infection associated with artificial insemination ©© ♀ ©©/MCC Exc

---

| ₚₒₓₙ | Unacceptable principal diagnosis symbol per Medicare code edits | ₚₒₐ | Code exempt from diagnosis present on admission requirement |

🅠 Questionable admission   ©© Complication or comorbidity   ©©/MCC Exc CC/MCC exclusion   ᴹᶜᶜ Major complication or comorbidity
🅟 Principal diagnosis as its own CC   🅜 Principal diagnosis as its own MCC   ᴴᶜᶜ HCC diagnosis code   ᴿˣᴴᶜᶜ RxHCC diagnosis code
MACRA code   ☑ Z code as first-listed diagnosis

N98.1 **Hyperstimulation** of ovaries ♀ CC/MCC Exc
Hyperstimulation of ovaries NOS
Hyperstimulation of ovaries associated with induced ovulation

N98.2 **Complications of attempted** introduction of fertilized ovum **following** in vitro fertilization ♀ CC/MCC Exc

N98.3 **Complications of attempted** introduction of embryo in embryo **transfer** ♀ CC/MCC Exc

N98.8 **Other complications associated with artificial fertilization** ♀ CC/MCC Exc

N98.9 **Complication associated with artificial fertilization, unspecified** ♀ CC/MCC Exc

Intraoperative and postprocedural complications and disorders of genitourinary system, not elsewhere classified (N99)

N99 **Intraoperative and postprocedural complications and disorders of genitourinary system, not elsewhere classified**
EXCLUDES2 irradiation cystitis (N30.4-)
postoophorectomy osteoporosis with current pathological fracture (M80.8-)
postoophorectomy osteoporosis without current pathological fracture (M81.8)

N99.0 **Postprocedural (acute) (chronic)** kidney failure
Use additional code to type of kidney disease

N99.1 **Postprocedural** urethral stricture
Postcatheterization urethral stricture

N99.11 **Postprocedural urethral stricture,** male
N99.110 **Postprocedural urethral stricture, male, meatal** ♂
▲ N99.111 **Postprocedural bulbous urethral ▶stricture, male◀** ♂
▲ N99.112 **Postprocedural membranous urethral ▶stricture, male◀** ♂
▲ N99.113 **Postprocedural anterior bulbous urethral ▶stricture, male◀** ♂
AHA: Q4 2016
N99.114 **Postprocedural urethral stricture, male, unspecified** ♂
N99.115 **Postprocedural** fossa navicularis **urethral stricture**
AHA: Q4 2016

N99.12 **Postprocedural urethral stricture,** female ♀

N99.2 **Postprocedural** adhesions of vagina ♀

N99.3 **Prolapse of vaginal vault after hysterectomy** ♀

N99.4 **Postprocedural** pelvic peritoneal adhesions
EXCLUDES2 pelvic peritoneal adhesions NOS (N73.6)
postinfective pelvic peritoneal adhesions (N73.6)

N99.5 **Complications of stoma of urinary tract**
EXCLUDES2 mechanical complication of urinary catheter (T83.0-)

N99.51 **Complication of** cystostomy
N99.510 **Cystostomy** hemorrhage HCC CC/MCC Exc
N99.511 **Cystostomy** infection HCC CC/MCC Exc
N99.512 **Cystostomy** malfunction HCC CC/MCC Exc
N99.518 **Other cystostomy complication** HCC CC/MCC Exc

N99.52 **Complication of incontinent external stoma of urinary tract**
N99.520 **Hemorrhage** of incontinent external stoma of urinary tract HCC
N99.521 **Infection** of incontinent external stoma of urinary tract HCC
AHA: Q4 2016
N99.522 **Malfunction** of incontinent external stoma of urinary tract HCC
N99.523 **Herniation** of incontinent stoma of urinary tract HCC
AHA: Q4 2016
N99.524 **Stenosis** of incontinent stoma of urinary tract HCC
AHA: Q4 2016
N99.528 **Other complication** of incontinent external stoma of urinary tract HCC

N99.53 **Complication of continent stoma of urinary tract**
N99.530 **Hemorrhage** of continent stoma of urinary tract HCC
N99.531 **Infection** of continent stoma of urinary tract HCC
N99.532 **Malfunction** of continent stoma of urinary tract HCC
N99.533 **Herniation** of continent stoma of urinary tract HCC
AHA: Q4 2016
N99.534 **Stenosis** of continent stoma of urinary tract HCC
AHA: Q4 2016
N99.538 **Other complication** of continent stoma of urinary tract HCC

N99.6 **Intraoperative hemorrhage and hematoma** of a **genitourinary system organ or structure complicating a procedure**
EXCLUDES1 intraoperative hemorrhage and hematoma of a genitourinary system organ or structure due to accidental puncture or laceration during a procedure (N99.7-)
N99.61 **Intraoperative hemorrhage and hematoma of a genitourinary system organ or structure complicating a** genitourinary system procedure CC/MCC Exc
N99.62 **Intraoperative hemorrhage and hematoma of a genitourinary system organ or structure complicating** other procedure CC/MCC Exc

N99.7 **Accidental puncture and laceration** of a genitourinary system organ or structure during a procedure
N99.71 **Accidental puncture and laceration of a genitourinary system organ or structure during a** genitourinary system procedure CC/MCC Exc
N99.72 **Accidental puncture and laceration of a genitourinary system organ or structure during** other procedure CC/MCC Exc

N99.8 **Other** intraoperative and postprocedural complications and **disorders of genitourinary system**
N99.81 **Other** intraoperative complications of **genitourinary system**
N99.82 **Postprocedural** hemorrhage of a genitourinary **system organ or structure following a procedure**
N99.820 **Postprocedural hemorrhage of a genitourinary system organ or structure following a** genitourinary system procedure CC/MCC Exc
N99.821 **Postprocedural hemorrhage of a genitourinary system organ or structure following other procedure** CC/MCC Exc
N99.83 **Residual ovary syndrome** ♀
N99.84 **Postprocedural** hematoma and seroma of a **genitourinary system organ or structure following a procedure**
N99.840 **Postprocedural** hematoma of a genitourinary **system organ or structure following a** genitourinary system procedure CC/MCC Exc
N99.841 **Postprocedural** hematoma of a genitourinary system organ or structure following other procedure CC/MCC Exc
N99.842 **Postprocedural** seroma of a genitourinary system organ or structure following a genitourinary system procedure CC/MCC Exc
N99.843 **Postprocedural** seroma of a genitourinary system organ or structure following other procedure CC/MCC Exc
N99.89 **Other postprocedural complications and disorders of genitourinary system**

Unspecified Code   Other Specified Code   Manifestation Code   N Newborn   P Pediatric   M Maternity   A Adult   ♂ Male   ♀ Female
● New Code   ▲ Revised Code Title   ▶◀ Revised Text   NOTES   INCLUDES   EXCLUDES 1 Not coded here   EXCLUDES 2 Not included here
4th character required   5th character required   6th character required   7th character required
Extension 'X' Alert   HAC Hospital-acquired condition (HAC) alert   AHA AHA Coding Clinic©

[5th] **O02.8 Other specified abnormal products of conception**

[EXCLUDES1] *abnormal products of conception with blighted ovum (O02.0)*

abnormal products of conception with hydatidiform mole (O01.-)

abnormal products of conception with nonhydatidiform mole (O02.0)

O02.81 Inappropriate change in quantitative human chorionic gonadotropin (hCG) in early pregnancy [M] ♀

Biochemical pregnancy
Chemical pregnancy
Inappropriate level of quantitative human chorionic gonadotropin (hCG) for gestational age in early pregnancy

O02.89 Other abnormal products of conception [M] ♀

O02.9 Abnormal product of conception, unspecified [M] ♀

[4th] **O03 Spontaneous abortion**

[NOTES] Incomplete abortion includes retained products of conception following spontaneous abortion

INCLUDES *miscarriage*

O03.0 Genital tract and pelvic infection following incomplete spontaneous abortion [M] CC ♀ CC/MCC Exc

Endometritis following incomplete spontaneous abortion
Oophoritis following incomplete spontaneous abortion
Parametritis following incomplete spontaneous abortion
Pelvic peritonitis following incomplete spontaneous abortion
Salpingitis following incomplete spontaneous abortion
Salpingo-oophoritis following incomplete spontaneous abortion

[EXCLUDES1] *sepsis following incomplete spontaneous abortion (O03.37)*

urinary tract infection following incomplete spontaneous abortion (O03.38)

O03.1 Delayed or excessive hemorrhage following incomplete spontaneous abortion [M] ♀

Afibrinogenemia following incomplete spontaneous abortion
Defibrination syndrome following incomplete spontaneous abortion
Hemolysis following incomplete spontaneous abortion
Intravascular coagulation following incomplete spontaneous abortion

O03.2 Embolism following incomplete spontaneous abortion [M] MCC ♀ CC/MCC Exc

Air embolism following incomplete spontaneous abortion
Amniotic fluid embolism following incomplete spontaneous abortion
Blood-clot embolism following incomplete spontaneous abortion
Embolism NOS following incomplete spontaneous abortion
Fat embolism following incomplete spontaneous abortion
Pulmonary embolism following incomplete spontaneous abortion
Pyemic embolism following incomplete spontaneous abortion
Septic or septicopyemic embolism following incomplete spontaneous abortion
Soap embolism following incomplete spontaneous abortion

[5th] **O03.3 Other and unspecified complications following incomplete spontaneous abortion**

O03.30 Unspecified complication following incomplete spontaneous abortion [M] CC ♀ CC/MCC Exc

O03.31 Shock following incomplete spontaneous abortion [M] MCC ♀ CC/MCC Exc

Circulatory collapse following incomplete spontaneous abortion
Shock (postprocedural) following incomplete spontaneous abortion

[EXCLUDES1] *shock due to infection following incomplete spontaneous abortion (O03.37)*

O03.32 Renal failure following incomplete spontaneous abortion [M] MCC ♀ CC/MCC Exc

Kidney failure (acute) following incomplete spontaneous abortion
Oliguria following incomplete spontaneous abortion
Renal shutdown following incomplete spontaneous abortion
Renal tubular necrosis following incomplete spontaneous abortion
Uremia following incomplete spontaneous abortion

O03.33 Metabolic disorder following incomplete spontaneous abortion [M] CC ♀ CC/MCC Exc

O03.34 Damage to pelvic organs following incomplete spontaneous abortion [M] CC ♀ CC/MCC Exc

Laceration, perforation, tear or chemical damage of bladder following incomplete spontaneous abortion
Laceration, perforation, tear or chemical damage of bowel following incomplete spontaneous abortion
Laceration, perforation, tear or chemical damage of broad ligament following incomplete spontaneous abortion
Laceration, perforation, tear or chemical damage of cervix following incomplete spontaneous abortion
Laceration, perforation, tear or chemical damage of periurethral tissue following incomplete spontaneous abortion
Laceration, perforation, tear or chemical damage of uterus following incomplete spontaneous abortion
Laceration, perforation, tear or chemical damage of vagina following incomplete spontaneous abortion

O03.35 Other venous complications following incomplete spontaneous abortion [M] CC ♀ CC/MCC Exc

O03.36 Cardiac arrest following incomplete spontaneous abortion [M] CC ♀ CC/MCC Exc

O03.37 Sepsis following incomplete spontaneous abortion [M] CC ♀ CC/MCC Exc

Use additional code to identify infectious agent (B95-B97)

Use additional code to identify severe sepsis, if applicable (R65.2-)

[EXCLUDES1] *septic or septicopyemic embolism following incomplete spontaneous abortion (O03.2)*

O03.38 Urinary tract infection following incomplete spontaneous abortion [M] CC ♀ CC/MCC Exc

Cystitis following incomplete spontaneous abortion

O03.39 Incomplete spontaneous abortion with other complications [M] CC ♀ CC/MCC Exc

O03.4 Incomplete spontaneous abortion without complication [M] ♀

O03.5 Genital tract and pelvic infection following complete or unspecified spontaneous abortion [M] CC ♀ CC/MCC Exc

Endometritis following complete or unspecified spontaneous abortion
Oophoritis following complete or unspecified spontaneous abortion
Parametritis following complete or unspecified spontaneous abortion
Pelvic peritonitis following complete or unspecified spontaneous abortion
Salpingitis following complete or unspecified spontaneous abortion
Salpingo-oophoritis following complete or unspecified spontaneous abortion

[EXCLUDES1] *sepsis following complete or unspecified spontaneous abortion (O03.87)*

urinary tract infection following complete or unspecified spontaneous abortion (O03.88)

O03.6 Delayed or excessive hemorrhage following complete or unspecified spontaneous abortion [M] ♀

Afibrinogenemia following complete or unspecified spontaneous abortion
Defibrination syndrome following complete or unspecified spontaneous abortion
Hemolysis following complete or unspecified spontaneous abortion
Intravascular coagulation following complete or unspecified spontaneous abortion

O03.7 **Embolism following complete or unspecified spontaneous abortion** Ⓜ ♂ ♀ cc/mcc Exc

Air embolism following complete or unspecified spontaneous abortion

Amniotic fluid embolism following complete or unspecified spontaneous abortion

Blood-clot embolism following complete or unspecified spontaneous abortion

Embolism NOS following complete or unspecified spontaneous abortion

Fat embolism following complete or unspecified spontaneous abortion

Pulmonary embolism following complete or unspecified spontaneous abortion

Pyemic embolism following complete or unspecified spontaneous abortion

Septic or septicopyemic embolism following complete or unspecified spontaneous abortion

Soap embolism following complete or unspecified spontaneous abortion

🄥 O03.8 Other and unspecified complications **following** complete or unspecified **spontaneous abortion**

O03.80 **Unspecified complication following complete or unspecified spontaneous abortion** Ⓜ ♂ ♀ cc/mcc Exc

O03.81 **Shock following complete or unspecified spontaneous abortion** Ⓜ mcc ♀ cc/mcc Exc

Circulatory collapse following complete or unspecified spontaneous abortion

Shock (postprocedural) following complete or unspecified spontaneous abortion

EXCLUDES1 *shock due to infection following complete or unspecified spontaneous abortion (O03.87)*

O03.82 **Renal failure following complete or unspecified spontaneous abortion** Ⓜ mcc ♀ cc/mcc Exc

Kidney failure (acute) following complete or unspecified spontaneous abortion

Oliguria following complete or unspecified spontaneous abortion

Renal shutdown following complete or unspecified spontaneous abortion

Renal tubular necrosis following complete or unspecified spontaneous abortion

Uremia following complete or unspecified spontaneous abortion

O03.83 **Metabolic disorder following complete or unspecified spontaneous abortion** Ⓜ ♂ ♀ cc/mcc Exc

O03.84 **Damage to pelvic organs following complete or unspecified spontaneous abortion** Ⓜ ♂ ♀ cc/mcc Exc

Laceration, perforation, tear or chemical damage of bladder following complete or unspecified spontaneous abortion

Laceration, perforation, tear or chemical damage of bowel following complete or unspecified spontaneous abortion

Laceration, perforation, tear or chemical damage of broad ligament following complete or unspecified spontaneous abortion

Laceration, perforation, tear or chemical damage of cervix following complete or unspecified spontaneous abortion

Laceration, perforation, tear or chemical damage of periurethral tissue following complete or unspecified spontaneous abortion

Laceration, perforation, tear or chemical damage of uterus following complete or unspecified spontaneous abortion

Laceration, perforation, tear or chemical damage of vagina following complete or unspecified spontaneous abortion

O03.85 **Other venous complications following complete or unspecified spontaneous abortion** Ⓜ ♂ ♀ cc/mcc Exc

O03.86 **Cardiac arrest following complete or unspecified spontaneous abortion** Ⓜ ♂ ♀ cc/mcc Exc

O03.87 **Sepsis following complete or unspecified spontaneous abortion** Ⓜ ♂ ♀ cc/mcc Exc

Use additional code to identify infectious agent (B95-B97)

Use additional code to identify severe sepsis, if applicable (R65.2-)

EXCLUDES1 *septic or septicopyemic embolism following complete or unspecified spontaneous abortion (O03.7)*

O03.88 **Urinary tract infection following complete or unspecified spontaneous abortion** Ⓜ ♂ ♀ cc/mcc Exc

Cystitis following complete or unspecified spontaneous abortion

O03.89 **Complete or unspecified spontaneous abortion with other complications** Ⓜ ♂ ♀ cc/mcc Exc

O03.9 **Complete or unspecified spontaneous abortion** without **complication** Ⓜ ♀

Miscarriage NOS

Spontaneous abortion NOS

🄠 O04 Complications **following (induced) termination of pregnancy**

INCLUDES *complications following (induced) termination of pregnancy*

EXCLUDES1 *encounter for elective termination of pregnancy, uncomplicated (Z33.2)*

failed attempted termination of pregnancy (O07.-)

O04.5 Genital tract and pelvic infection **following (induced) termination of pregnancy** Ⓜ ♂ ♀ cc/mcc Exc

Endometritis following (induced) termination of pregnancy

Oophoritis following (induced) termination of pregnancy

Parametritis following (induced) termination of pregnancy

Pelvic peritonitis following (induced) termination of pregnancy

Salpingitis following (induced) termination of pregnancy

Salpingo-oophoritis following (induced) termination of pregnancy

EXCLUDES1 *sepsis following (induced) termination of pregnancy (O04.87)*

urinary tract infection following (induced) termination of pregnancy (O04.88)

O04.6 Delayed or excessive hemorrhage **following (induced) termination of pregnancy** Ⓜ ♀

Afibrinogenemia following (induced) termination of pregnancy

Defibrination syndrome following (induced) termination of pregnancy

Hemolysis following (induced) termination of pregnancy

Intravascular coagulation following (induced) termination of pregnancy

O04.7 Embolism **following (induced) termination of pregnancy** Ⓜ mcc ♀ cc/mcc Exc

Air embolism following (induced) termination of pregnancy

Amniotic fluid embolism following (induced) termination of pregnancy

Blood-clot embolism following (induced) termination of pregnancy

Embolism NOS following (induced) termination of pregnancy

Fat embolism following (induced) termination of pregnancy

Pulmonary embolism following (induced) termination of pregnancy

Pyemic embolism following (induced) termination of pregnancy

Septic or septicopyemic embolism following (induced) termination of pregnancy

Soap embolism following (induced) termination of pregnancy

🄥 O04.8 **(Induced) termination of pregnancy with** other and unspecified **complications**

O04.80 **(Induced) termination of pregnancy with unspecified complications** Ⓜ ♂ ♀ cc/mcc Exc

O04.81 Shock **following (induced) termination of pregnancy** Ⓜ mcc ♀ cc/mcc Exc

Circulatory collapse following (induced) termination of pregnancy

Shock (postprocedural) following (induced) termination of pregnancy

EXCLUDES1 *shock due to infection following (induced) termination of pregnancy (O04.87)*

Unspecified Code   Other Specified Code   Manifestation Code   Ⓝ Newborn   Ⓟ Pediatric   Ⓜ Maternity   Ⓐ Adult   ♂ Male   ♀ Female
● New Code   ▲ Revised Code Title   ▶◀ Revised Text   NOTES   INCLUDES   EXCLUDES 1   Not coded here   EXCLUDES 2   Not included here
🄠 4ᵗʰ character required   🄥 5ᵗʰ character required   🄖 6ᵗʰ character required   🄦 7ᵗʰ character required
🄫 Extension 'X' Alert   HAC Hospital-acquired condition (HAC) alert   AHA AHA Coding Clinic©

O04.82 Renal failure **following (induced) termination of pregnancy** M MCC ♀ CC/MCC Exc
Kidney failure (acute) following (induced) termination of pregnancy
Oliguria following (induced) termination of pregnancy
Renal shutdown following (induced) termination of pregnancy
Renal tubular necrosis following (induced) termination of pregnancy
Uremia following (induced) termination of pregnancy

O04.83 Metabolic disorder **following (induced) termination of pregnancy** M CC ♀ CC/MCC Exc

O04.84 Damage to pelvic organs **following (induced) termination of pregnancy** M CC ♀ CC/MCC Exc
Laceration, perforation, tear or chemical damage of bladder following (induced) termination of pregnancy
Laceration, perforation, tear or chemical damage of bowel following (induced) termination of pregnancy
Laceration, perforation, tear or chemical damage of broad ligament following (induced) termination of pregnancy
Laceration, perforation, tear or chemical damage of cervix following (induced) termination of pregnancy
Laceration, perforation, tear or chemical damage of periurethral tissue following (induced) termination of pregnancy
Laceration, perforation, tear or chemical damage of uterus following (induced) termination of pregnancy
Laceration, perforation, tear or chemical damage of vagina following (induced) termination of pregnancy

O04.85 Other venous **complications following (induced) termination of pregnancy** M CC ♀ CC/MCC Exc

O04.86 Cardiac arrest **following (induced) termination of pregnancy** M MCC ♀ CC/MCC Exc

O04.87 Sepsis **following (induced) termination of pregnancy** M CC ♀ CC/MCC Exc
Use additional code to identify infectious agent (B95-B97)
Use additional code to identify severe sepsis, if applicable (R65.2-)
EXCLUDES1 *septic or septicopyemic embolism following (induced) termination of pregnancy (O04.7)*

O04.88 Urinary tract infection **following (induced) termination of pregnancy** M CC ♀ CC/MCC Exc
Cystitis following (induced) termination of pregnancy

O04.89 (Induced) termination of pregnancy with other **complications** M CC ♀ CC/MCC Exc

O07 Failed attempted termination **of pregnancy**
INCLUDES *failure of attempted induction of termination of pregnancy*
incomplete elective abortion
EXCLUDES1 *incomplete spontaneous abortion (O03.0-)*

O07.0 Genital tract and pelvic infection **following failed attempted termination of pregnancy** M CC ♀ CC/MCC Exc
Endometritis following failed attempted termination of pregnancy
Oophoritis following failed attempted termination of pregnancy
Parametritis following failed attempted termination of pregnancy
Pelvic peritonitis following failed attempted termination of pregnancy
Salpingitis following failed attempted termination of pregnancy
Salpingo-oophoritis following failed attempted termination of pregnancy
EXCLUDES1 *sepsis following failed attempted termination of pregnancy (O07.37)*
urinary tract infection following failed attempted termination of pregnancy (O07.38)

O07.1 Delayed or excessive hemorrhage **following failed attempted termination of pregnancy** M CC ♀ CC/MCC Exc
Afibrinogenemia following failed attempted termination of pregnancy
Defibrination syndrome following failed attempted termination of pregnancy
Hemolysis following failed attempted termination of pregnancy
Intravascular coagulation following failed attempted termination of pregnancy

O07.2 Embolism **following failed attempted termination of pregnancy** M MCC ♀ CC/MCC Exc
Air embolism following failed attempted termination of pregnancy
Amniotic fluid embolism following failed attempted termination of pregnancy
Blood-clot embolism following failed attempted termination of pregnancy
Embolism NOS following failed attempted termination of pregnancy
Fat embolism following failed attempted termination of pregnancy
Pulmonary embolism following failed attempted termination of pregnancy
Pyemic embolism following failed attempted termination of pregnancy
Septic or septicopyemic embolism following failed attempted termination of pregnancy
Soap embolism following failed attempted termination of pregnancy

O07.3 Failed attempted termination of pregnancy with other and unspecified **complications**

O07.30 Failed attempted termination of pregnancy with unspecified complications M CC ♀ CC/MCC Exc

O07.31 Shock **following failed attempted termination of pregnancy** M MCC ♀ CC/MCC Exc
Circulatory collapse following failed termination of pregnancy
Shock (postprocedural) following failed attempted termination of pregnancy
EXCLUDES1 *shock due to infection following failed attempted termination of pregnancy (O07.37)*

O07.32 Renal failure **following failed attempted termination of pregnancy** M MCC ♀ CC/MCC Exc
Kidney failure (acute) following failed attempted termination of pregnancy
Oliguria following failed attempted termination of pregnancy
Renal shutdown following failed attempted termination of pregnancy
Renal tubular necrosis following failed attempted termination of pregnancy
Uremia following failed attempted termination of pregnancy

O07.33 Metabolic disorder **following failed attempted termination of pregnancy** M CC ♀ CC/MCC Exc

O07.34 Damage to pelvic organs **following failed attempted termination of pregnancy** M CC ♀ CC/MCC Exc
Laceration, perforation, tear or chemical damage of bladder following failed attempted termination of pregnancy
Laceration, perforation, tear or chemical damage of bowel following failed attempted termination of pregnancy
Laceration, perforation, tear or chemical damage of broad ligament following failed attempted termination of pregnancy
Laceration, perforation, tear or chemical damage of cervix following failed attempted termination of pregnancy
Laceration, perforation, tear or chemical damage of periurethral tissue following failed attempted termination of pregnancy

1st 1st trimester   2nd 2nd trimester   3rd 3rd trimester   PDx Unacceptable principal diagnosis symbol per Medicare code edits
POA Code exempt from diagnosis present on admission requirement   ? Questionable admission   CC Complication or comorbidity
CC/MCC Exc CC/MCC exclusion   MCC Major complication or comorbidity   Principal diagnosis as its own CC   Principal diagnosis as its own MCC
HCC HCC diagnosis code   RHCC RxHCC diagnosis code   MACRA code   Z Z code as first-listed diagnosis

888   When symbols appear on a code that requires a 7th character extension, refer to Appendix B to identify applicable 7th character codes.   **2018 ICD-10-CM**

Laceration, perforation, tear or chemical damage of uterus following failed attempted termination of pregnancy
Laceration, perforation, tear or chemical damage of vagina following failed attempted termination of pregnancy

O07.35 Other venous complications following failed attempted termination of pregnancy [M] CC ♀ CC/MCC Exc

O07.36 Cardiac arrest following failed attempted termination of pregnancy [M] CC ♀ CC/MCC Exc

O07.37 Sepsis following failed attempted termination of pregnancy [M] CC ♀ CC/MCC Exc
Use additional code (B95-B97), to identify infectious agent
Use additional code (R65.2-) to identify severe sepsis, if applicable
[EXCLUDES1] *septic or septicopyemic embolism following failed attempted termination of pregnancy (O07.2)*

O07.38 Urinary tract infection following failed attempted termination of pregnancy [M] CC ♀ CC/MCC Exc
Cystitis following failed attempted termination of pregnancy

O07.39 Failed attempted termination of pregnancy with other complications [M] CC ♀ CC/MCC Exc

O07.4 Failed attempted termination of pregnancy without complication [M] ♀

[4th] **O08 Complications following ectopic and molar pregnancy**
This category is for use with categories O00-O02 to identify any associated complications

O08.0 Genital tract and pelvic infection following ectopic and molar pregnancy [M] CC ♀ CC/MCC Exc
Endometritis following ectopic and molar pregnancy
Oophoritis following ectopic and molar pregnancy
Parametritis following ectopic and molar pregnancy
Pelvic peritonitis following ectopic and molar pregnancy
Salpingitis following ectopic and molar pregnancy
Salpingo-oophoritis following ectopic and molar pregnancy
[EXCLUDES1] *sepsis following ectopic and molar pregnancy (O08.82)*
urinary tract infection (O08.83)

O08.1 Delayed or excessive hemorrhage following ectopic and molar pregnancy [M] CC ♀ CC/MCC Exc
Afibrinogenemia following ectopic and molar pregnancy
Defibrination syndrome following ectopic and molar pregnancy
Hemolysis following ectopic and molar pregnancy
Intravascular coagulation following ectopic and molar pregnancy
[EXCLUDES1] *delayed or excessive hemorrhage due to incomplete abortion (O03.1)*

O08.2 Embolism following ectopic and molar pregnancy [M] MCC ♀ CC/MCC Exc
Air embolism following ectopic and molar pregnancy
Amniotic fluid embolism following ectopic and molar pregnancy
Blood-clot embolism following ectopic and molar pregnancy
Embolism NOS following ectopic and molar pregnancy
Fat embolism following ectopic and molar pregnancy
Pulmonary embolism following ectopic and molar pregnancy
Pyemic embolism following ectopic and molar pregnancy
Septic or septicopyemic embolism following ectopic and molar pregnancy
Soap embolism following ectopic and molar pregnancy

O08.3 Shock following ectopic and molar pregnancy [M] MCC ♀ CC/MCC Exc
Circulatory collapse following ectopic and molar pregnancy
Shock (postprocedural) following ectopic and molar pregnancy
[EXCLUDES1] *shock due to infection following ectopic and molar pregnancy (O08.82)*

O08.4 Renal failure following ectopic and molar pregnancy [M] MCC ♀ CC/MCC Exc
Kidney failure (acute) following ectopic and molar pregnancy
Oliguria following ectopic and molar pregnancy
Renal shutdown following ectopic and molar pregnancy
Renal tubular necrosis following ectopic and molar pregnancy
Uremia following ectopic and molar pregnancy

O08.5 Metabolic disorders following an ectopic and molar pregnancy [M] CC ♀ CC/MCC Exc

O08.6 Damage to pelvic organs and tissues following an ectopic and molar pregnancy [M] CC ♀ CC/MCC Exc
Laceration, perforation, tear or chemical damage of bladder following an ectopic and molar pregnancy
Laceration, perforation, tear or chemical damage of bowel following an ectopic and molar pregnancy
Laceration, perforation, tear or chemical damage of broad ligament following an ectopic and molar pregnancy
Laceration, perforation, tear or chemical damage of cervix following an ectopic and molar pregnancy
Laceration, perforation, tear or chemical damage of periurethral tissue following an ectopic and molar pregnancy
Laceration, perforation, tear or chemical damage of uterus following an ectopic and molar pregnancy
Laceration, perforation, tear or chemical damage of vagina following an ectopic and molar pregnancy

O08.7 Other venous complications following an ectopic and molar pregnancy [M] CC ♀ CC/MCC Exc

[5th] **O08.8 Other complications following an ectopic and molar pregnancy**

O08.81 Cardiac arrest following an ectopic and molar pregnancy [M] CC ♀ CC/MCC Exc

O08.82 Sepsis following ectopic and molar pregnancy [M] CC ♀ CC/MCC Exc
Use additional code (B95-B97), to identify infectious agent
Use additional code (R65.2-) to identify severe sepsis, if applicable
[EXCLUDES1] *septic or septicopyemic embolism following ectopic and molar pregnancy (O08.2)*

O08.83 Urinary tract infection following an ectopic and molar pregnancy [M] CC ♀ CC/MCC Exc
Cystitis following an ectopic and molar pregnancy

O08.89 Other complications following an ectopic and molar pregnancy [M] CC ♀ CC/MCC Exc

O08.9 Unspecified complication following an ectopic and molar pregnancy [M] CC ♀ CC/MCC Exc

Supervision of high risk pregnancy (O09)

[4th] **O09 Supervision of high risk pregnancy**

[5th] **O09.0 Supervision of pregnancy with history of infertility**

O09.00 Supervision of pregnancy with history of infertility, unspecified trimester [M] POA ♀ POA Exc

O09.01 Supervision of pregnancy with history of infertility, first trimester [1st] [M] POA ♀ POA Exc

O09.02 Supervision of pregnancy with history of infertility, second trimester [2nd] [M] POA ♀ POA Exc

O09.03 Supervision of pregnancy with history of infertility, third trimester [3rd] [M] POA ♀ POA Exc

[5th] **O09.1 Supervision of pregnancy with history of ectopic pregnancy**

O09.10 Supervision of pregnancy with history of ectopic pregnancy, unspecified trimester [M] POA ♀ POA Exc
AHA: Q4 2016

O09.11 Supervision of pregnancy with history of ectopic pregnancy, first trimester [1st] [M] POA ♀ POA Exc
AHA: Q4 2016

O09.12 Supervision of pregnancy with history of ectopic pregnancy, second trimester [2nd] [M] POA ♀ POA Exc
AHA: Q4 2016

O09.13 Supervision of pregnancy with history of ectopic pregnancy, third trimester [3rd] [M] POA ♀ POA Exc
AHA: Q4 2016

[5th] **O09.A Supervision of pregnancy with history of molar pregnancy**

O09.A0 Supervision of pregnancy with history of molar pregnancy, unspecified trimester [M] ♀ POA Exc
AHA: Q4 2016

Unspecified Code | Other Specified Code | Manifestation Code | [N] Newborn | [P] Pediatric | [M] Maternity | [A] Adult | ♂ Male | ♀ Female
● New Code | ▲ Revised Code Title | ►◄ Revised Text | [NOTES] | [INCLUDES] | [EXCLUDES1] Not coded here | [EXCLUDES2] Not included here
[4th] 4th character required | [5th] 5th character required | [6th] 6th character required | [7th] 7th character required
[X] Extension 'X' Alert | [HAC] Hospital-acquired condition (HAC) alert | **AHA** AHA Coding Clinic©

O09.A1 Supervision of pregnancy with history of molar pregnancy, first trimester [1st] [M] ♀ [PDx]
AHA: Q4 2016
O09.A2 Supervision of pregnancy with history of molar pregnancy, second trimester [2nd] [M] ♀ [PDx]
AHA: Q4 2016
O09.A3 Supervision of pregnancy with history of molar pregnancy, third trimester [3rd] [M] ♀ [PDx]
AHA: Q4 2016

[5th] O09.2 Supervision of pregnancy with other poor reproductive or obstetric history
[EXCLUDES2] *pregnancy care for patient with history of recurrent pregnancy loss (O26.2-)*

[6th] O09.21 Supervision of pregnancy with history of pre-term labor
O09.211 Supervision of pregnancy with history of pre-term labor, first trimester [1st] [M] [POA] ♀ [PDx]
O09.212 Supervision of pregnancy with history of pre-term labor, second trimester [2nd] [M] [POA] ♀ [PDx]
O09.213 Supervision of pregnancy with history of pre-term labor, third trimester [3rd] [M] [POA] ♀ [PDx]
O09.219 Supervision of pregnancy with history of pre-term labor, unspecified trimester [M] [POA] ♀ [PDx]

[6th] O09.29 Supervision of pregnancy with other poor reproductive or obstetric history
Supervision of pregnancy with history of neonatal death
Supervision of pregnancy with history of stillbirth
O09.291 Supervision of pregnancy with other poor reproductive or obstetric history, first trimester [1st] [M] [POA] ♀ [PDx]
O09.292 Supervision of pregnancy with other poor reproductive or obstetric history, second trimester [2nd] [M] [POA] ♀ [PDx]
O09.293 Supervision of pregnancy with other poor reproductive or obstetric history, third trimester [3rd] [M] [POA] ♀ [PDx]
O09.299 Supervision of pregnancy with other poor reproductive or obstetric history, unspecified trimester [M] [POA] ♀ [PDx]

[5th] O09.3 Supervision of pregnancy with insufficient antenatal care
Supervision of concealed pregnancy
Supervision of hidden pregnancy
O09.30 Supervision of pregnancy with insufficient antenatal care, unspecified trimester [M] [POA] ♀ [PDx]
O09.31 Supervision of pregnancy with insufficient antenatal care, first trimester [1st] [M] [POA] ♀ [PDx]
O09.32 Supervision of pregnancy with insufficient antenatal care, second trimester [2nd] [M] [POA] ♀ [PDx]
O09.33 Supervision of pregnancy with insufficient antenatal care, third trimester [3rd] [M] [POA] ♀ [PDx]

[5th] O09.4 Supervision of pregnancy with grand multiparity
O09.40 Supervision of pregnancy with grand multiparity, unspecified trimester [M] [POA] ♀ [PDx]
O09.41 Supervision of pregnancy with grand multiparity, first trimester [1st] [M] [POA] ♀ [PDx]
O09.42 Supervision of pregnancy with grand multiparity, second trimester [2nd] [M] [POA] ♀ [PDx]
O09.43 Supervision of pregnancy with grand multiparity, third trimester [3rd] [M] [POA] ♀ [PDx]

[5th] O09.5 Supervision of elderly primigravida and multigravida
Pregnancy for a female 35 years and older at expected date of delivery

[6th] O09.51 Supervision of elderly primigravida
O09.511 Supervision of elderly primigravida, first trimester [1st] [M] [POA] ♀ [PDx]
O09.512 Supervision of elderly primigravida, second trimester [2nd] [M] [POA] ♀ [PDx]
O09.513 Supervision of elderly primigravida, third trimester [3rd] [M] [POA] ♀ [PDx]
O09.519 Supervision of elderly primigravida, unspecified trimester [M] [POA] ♀ [PDx]

[6th] O09.52 Supervision of elderly multigravida
O09.521 Supervision of elderly multigravida, first trimester [1st] [M] [POA] ♀ [PDx]
O09.522 Supervision of elderly multigravida, second trimester [2nd] [M] [POA] ♀ [PDx]
O09.523 Supervision of elderly multigravida, third trimester [3rd] [M] [POA] ♀ [PDx]
AHA: Q4 2016
O09.529 Supervision of elderly multigravida, unspecified trimester [M] [POA] ♀ [PDx]

[5th] O09.6 Supervision of young primigravida and multigravida
Supervision of pregnancy for a female less than 16 years old at expected date of delivery

[6th] O09.61 Supervision of young primigravida
O09.611 Supervision of young primigravida, first trimester [1st] [M] [POA] ♀ [PDx]
O09.612 Supervision of young primigravida, second trimester [2nd] [M] [POA] ♀ [PDx]
O09.613 Supervision of young primigravida, third trimester [3rd] [M] [POA] ♀ [PDx]
O09.619 Supervision of young primigravida, unspecified trimester [M] [POA] ♀ [PDx]

[6th] O09.62 Supervision of young multigravida
O09.621 Supervision of young multigravida, first trimester [1st] [M] [POA] ♀ [PDx]
O09.622 Supervision of young multigravida, second trimester [2nd] [M] [POA] ♀ [PDx]
O09.623 Supervision of young multigravida, third trimester [3rd] [M] [POA] ♀ [PDx]
O09.629 Supervision of young multigravida, unspecified trimester [M] [POA] ♀ [PDx]

[5th] O09.7 Supervision of high risk pregnancy due to social problems
O09.70 Supervision of high risk pregnancy due to social problems, unspecified trimester [M] [POA] ♀ [PDx]
O09.71 Supervision of high risk pregnancy due to social problems, first trimester [1st] [M] [POA] ♀ [PDx]
O09.72 Supervision of high risk pregnancy due to social problems, second trimester [2nd] [M] [POA] ♀ [PDx]
O09.73 Supervision of high risk pregnancy due to social problems, third trimester [3rd] [M] [POA] ♀ [PDx]

[5th] O09.8 Supervision of other high risk pregnancies

[6th] O09.81 Supervision of pregnancy resulting from assisted reproductive technology
Supervision of pregnancy resulting from in-vitro fertilization
[EXCLUDES2] *gestational carrier status (Z33.3)*
O09.811 Supervision of pregnancy resulting from assisted reproductive technology, first trimester [1st] [M] [POA] ♀ [PDx]
O09.812 Supervision of pregnancy resulting from assisted reproductive technology, second trimester [2nd] [M] [POA] ♀ [PDx]
O09.813 Supervision of pregnancy resulting from assisted reproductive technology, third trimester [3rd] [M] [POA] ♀ [PDx]
O09.819 Supervision of pregnancy resulting from assisted reproductive technology, unspecified trimester [M] [POA] ♀ [PDx]

[6th] O09.82 Supervision of pregnancy with history of in utero procedure during previous pregnancy
O09.821 Supervision of pregnancy with history of in utero procedure during previous pregnancy, first trimester [1st] [M] [POA] ♀ [PDx]
O09.822 Supervision of pregnancy with history of in utero procedure during previous pregnancy, second trimester [2nd] [M] [POA] ♀ [PDx]
O09.823 Supervision of pregnancy with history of in utero procedure during previous pregnancy, third trimester [3rd] [M] [POA] ♀ [PDx]

[1st] 1st trimester [2nd] 2nd trimester [3rd] 3rd trimester [PDx] Unacceptable principal diagnosis symbol per Medicare code edits
[POA] Code exempt from diagnosis present on admission requirement [?] Questionable admission [CC] Complication or comorbidity
[CC/MCC Exc] CC/MCC exclusion [MCC] Major complication or comorbidity [PDx CC] Principal diagnosis as its own CC [PDx MCC] Principal diagnosis as its own MCC
[HCC] HCC diagnosis code [RxHCC] RxHCC diagnosis code MACRA code [Z-1] Z code as first-listed diagnosis

O09.829 **Supervision of pregnancy with history of in utero procedure during previous pregnancy, unspecified trimester** M PoA ♀ PDxIn

EXCLUDES1 *supervision of pregnancy affected by in utero procedure during current pregnancy (O35.7)*

6th O09.89 **Supervision of other high risk pregnancies**

O09.891 **Supervision of other high risk pregnancies, first trimester** 1st M PoA ♀ PDxIn

O09.892 **Supervision of other high risk pregnancies, second trimester** 2nd M PoA ♀ PDxIn

O09.893 **Supervision of other high risk pregnancies, third trimester** 3rd M PoA ♀ PDxIn

O09.899 **Supervision of other high risk pregnancies, unspecified trimester** M PoA ♀ PDxIn

5th O09.9 **Supervision of high risk pregnancy, unspecified**

O09.90 **Supervision of high risk pregnancy, unspecified, unspecified trimester** M PoA ♀ PDxIn

O09.91 **Supervision of high risk pregnancy, unspecified, first trimester** 1st M PoA ♀ PDxIn

O09.92 **Supervision of high risk pregnancy, unspecified, second trimester** 2nd M PoA ♀ PDxIn

O09.93 **Supervision of high risk pregnancy, unspecified, third trimester** 3rd M PoA ♀ PDxIn

Edema, proteinuria and hypertensive disorders in pregnancy, childbirth and the puerperium (O10-O16)

4th O10 **Pre-existing hypertension complicating pregnancy, childbirth and the puerperium**

INCLUDES *pre-existing hypertension with pre-existing proteinuria complicating pregnancy, childbirth and the puerperium*

EXCLUDES2 *pre-existing hypertension with superimposed pre-eclampsia complicating pregnancy, childbirth and the puerperium (O11.-)*

5th O10.0 **Pre-existing essential hypertension complicating pregnancy, childbirth and the puerperium**

Any condition in I10 specified as a reason for obstetric care during pregnancy, childbirth or the puerperium

6th O10.01 **Pre-existing essential hypertension complicating pregnancy**

O10.011 **Pre-existing essential hypertension complicating pregnancy, first trimester** 1st M CC ♀ CC/MCC Exc

O10.012 **Pre-existing essential hypertension complicating pregnancy, second trimester** 2nd M CC ♀ CC/MCC Exc

O10.013 **Pre-existing essential hypertension complicating pregnancy, third trimester** 3rd M CC ♀ CC/MCC Exc

O10.019 **Pre-existing essential hypertension complicating pregnancy, unspecified trimester** M ♀

O10.02 **Pre-existing essential hypertension complicating childbirth** M CC ♀ CC/MCC Exc

O10.03 **Pre-existing essential hypertension complicating the puerperium** M ♀

5th O10.1 **Pre-existing hypertensive heart disease complicating pregnancy, childbirth and the puerperium**

Any condition in I11 specified as a reason for obstetric care during pregnancy, childbirth or the puerperium

Use additional code from I11 to identify the type of hypertensive heart disease

6th O10.11 **Pre-existing hypertensive heart disease complicating pregnancy**

O10.111 **Pre-existing hypertensive heart disease complicating pregnancy, first trimester** 1st M ♀

O10.112 **Pre-existing hypertensive heart disease complicating pregnancy, second trimester** 2nd M ♀

O10.113 **Pre-existing hypertensive heart disease complicating pregnancy, third trimester** 3rd M ♀

O10.119 **Pre-existing hypertensive heart disease complicating pregnancy, unspecified trimester** M ♀

O10.12 **Pre-existing hypertensive heart disease complicating childbirth** M ♀

O10.13 **Pre-existing hypertensive heart disease complicating the puerperium** M ♀

5th O10.2 **Pre-existing hypertensive chronic kidney disease complicating pregnancy, childbirth and the puerperium**

Any condition in I12 specified as a reason for obstetric care during pregnancy, childbirth or the puerperium

Use additional code from I12 to identify the type of hypertensive chronic kidney disease

6th O10.21 **Pre-existing hypertensive chronic kidney disease complicating pregnancy**

O10.211 **Pre-existing hypertensive chronic kidney disease complicating pregnancy, first trimester** 1st M ♀

O10.212 **Pre-existing hypertensive chronic kidney disease complicating pregnancy, second trimester** 2nd M ♀

O10.213 **Pre-existing hypertensive chronic kidney disease complicating pregnancy, third trimester** 3rd M ♀

O10.219 **Pre-existing hypertensive chronic kidney disease complicating pregnancy, unspecified trimester** M ♀

O10.22 **Pre-existing hypertensive chronic kidney disease complicating childbirth** M ♀

O10.23 **Pre-existing hypertensive chronic kidney disease complicating the puerperium** M ♀

5th O10.3 **Pre-existing hypertensive heart and chronic kidney disease complicating pregnancy, childbirth and the puerperium**

Any condition in I13 specified as a reason for obstetric care during pregnancy, childbirth or the puerperium

Use additional code from I13 to identify the type of hypertensive heart and chronic kidney disease

6th O10.31 **Pre-existing hypertensive heart and chronic kidney disease complicating pregnancy**

O10.311 **Pre-existing hypertensive heart and chronic kidney disease complicating pregnancy, first trimester** 1st M

O10.312 **Pre-existing hypertensive heart and chronic kidney disease complicating pregnancy, second trimester** 2nd M

O10.313 **Pre-existing hypertensive heart and chronic kidney disease complicating pregnancy, third trimester** 3rd M

O10.319 **Pre-existing hypertensive heart and chronic kidney disease complicating pregnancy, unspecified trimester** M

O10.32 **Pre-existing hypertensive heart and chronic kidney disease complicating childbirth** M

O10.33 **Pre-existing hypertensive heart and chronic kidney disease complicating the puerperium** M

5th O10.4 **Pre-existing secondary hypertension complicating pregnancy, childbirth and the puerperium**

Any condition in I15 specified as a reason for obstetric care during pregnancy, childbirth or the puerperium

Use additional code from I15 to identify the type of secondary hypertension

6th O10.41 **Pre-existing secondary hypertension complicating pregnancy**

O10.411 **Pre-existing secondary hypertension complicating pregnancy, first trimester** 1st M CC ♀ CC/MCC Exc

O10.412 **Pre-existing secondary hypertension complicating pregnancy, second trimester** 2nd M CC ♀ CC/MCC Exc

---

Unspecified Code   Other Specified Code   Manifestation Code   N Newborn   P Pediatric   M Maternity   A Adult   ♂ Male   ♀ Female
● New Code   ▲ Revised Code Title   ▶◀ Revised Text   NOTES   INCLUDES   EXCLUDES 1 Not coded here   EXCLUDES 2 Not included here
4th 4th character required   5th 5th character required   6th 6th character required   7th 7th character required
7th Extension 'X' Alert   HAC Hospital-acquired condition (HAC) alert   AHA AHA Coding Clinic©

O10.413 Pre-existing secondary hypertension complicating pregnancy, third trimester `3rd` M cc♀ CC/MCC Exc

O10.419 Pre-existing secondary hypertension complicating pregnancy, unspecified trimester M ♀

O10.42 Pre-existing secondary hypertension complicating childbirth M MCC ♀ CC/MCC Exc

O10.43 Pre-existing secondary hypertension complicating the puerperium M cc♀ CC/MCC Exc

O10.9 Unspecified pre-existing hypertension complicating pregnancy, childbirth and the puerperium

O10.91 Unspecified pre-existing hypertension complicating pregnancy

O10.911 Unspecified pre-existing hypertension complicating pregnancy, first trimester `1st` M cc♀ CC/MCC Exc

O10.912 Unspecified pre-existing hypertension complicating pregnancy, second trimester `2nd` M cc♀ CC/MCC Exc

O10.913 Unspecified pre-existing hypertension complicating pregnancy, third trimester `3rd` M cc♀ CC/MCC Exc

O10.919 Unspecified pre-existing hypertension complicating pregnancy, unspecified trimester M ♀

O10.92 Unspecified pre-existing hypertension complicating childbirth M cc♀ CC/MCC Exc

O10.93 Unspecified pre-existing hypertension complicating the puerperium M ♀

O11 Pre-existing hypertension with pre-eclampsia

INCLUDES conditions in O10 complicated by pre-eclampsia

pre-eclampsia superimposed pre-existing hypertension

Use additional code from O10 to identify the type of hypertension

O11.1 Pre-existing hypertension with pre-eclampsia, first trimester `1st` M cc♀ CC/MCC Exc

O11.2 Pre-existing hypertension with pre-eclampsia, second trimester `2nd` M cc♀ CC/MCC Exc

O11.3 Pre-existing hypertension with pre-eclampsia, third trimester `3rd` M MCC ♀ CC/MCC Exc

O11.4 Pre-existing hypertension with pre-eclampsia, complicating childbirth M ♀

O11.5 Pre-existing hypertension with pre-eclampsia, complicating the puerperium M ♀

O11.9 Pre-existing hypertension with pre-eclampsia, unspecified trimester M ♀

O12 Gestational [pregnancy-induced] edema and proteinuria without hypertension

O12.0 Gestational edema

O12.00 Gestational edema, unspecified trimester M ♀

O12.01 Gestational edema, first trimester `1st` M ♀

O12.02 Gestational edema, second trimester `2nd` M ♀

O12.03 Gestational edema, third trimester `3rd` M ♀

O12.04 Gestational edema, complicating childbirth M ♀

O12.05 Gestational edema, complicating the puerperium M ♀

O12.1 Gestational proteinuria

O12.10 Gestational proteinuria, unspecified trimester M ♀

O12.11 Gestational proteinuria, first trimester `1st` M cc♀ CC/MCC Exc

O12.12 Gestational proteinuria, second trimester `2nd` M cc♀ CC/MCC Exc

O12.13 Gestational proteinuria, third trimester `3rd` M cc♀ CC/MCC Exc

O12.14 Gestational proteinuria, complicating childbirth M ♀

O12.15 Gestational proteinuria, complicating the puerperium M ♀

O12.2 Gestational edema with proteinuria

O12.20 Gestational edema with proteinuria, unspecified trimester M ♀

O12.21 Gestational edema with proteinuria, first trimester `1st` M cc♀ CC/MCC Exc

O12.22 Gestational edema with proteinuria, second trimester `2nd` M cc♀ CC/MCC Exc

O12.23 Gestational edema with proteinuria, third trimester `3rd` M cc♀ CC/MCC Exc

O12.24 Gestational edema with proteinuria, complicating childbirth M ♀

O12.25 Gestational edema with proteinuria, complicating the puerperium M ♀

O13 Gestational [pregnancy-induced] hypertension without significant proteinuria

INCLUDES gestational hypertension NOS

transient hypertension of pregnancy

O13.1 Gestational [pregnancy-induced] hypertension without significant proteinuria, first trimester `1st` M ♀

O13.2 Gestational [pregnancy-induced] hypertension without significant proteinuria, second trimester `2nd` M ♀

O13.3 Gestational [pregnancy-induced] hypertension without significant proteinuria, third trimester `3rd` M ♀

O13.4 Gestational [pregnancy-induced] hypertension without significant proteinuria, complicating childbirth M ♀

O13.5 Gestational [pregnancy-induced] hypertension without significant proteinuria, complicating the puerperium M ♀

O13.9 Gestational [pregnancy-induced] hypertension without significant proteinuria, unspecified trimester M ♀

O14 Pre-eclampsia

EXCLUDES1 pre-existing hypertension with pre-eclampsia (O11)

O14.0 Mild to moderate pre-eclampsia

O14.00 Mild to moderate pre-eclampsia, unspecified trimester M ♀

O14.02 Mild to moderate pre-eclampsia, second trimester `2nd` M cc♀ CC/MCC Exc

O14.03 Mild to moderate pre-eclampsia, third trimester `3rd` M cc♀ CC/MCC Exc

O14.04 Mild to moderate pre-eclampsia, complicating childbirth M ♀

O14.05 Mild to moderate pre-eclampsia, complicating the puerperium M ♀

O14.1 Severe pre-eclampsia

EXCLUDES1 HELLP syndrome (O14.2-)

O14.10 Severe pre-eclampsia, unspecified trimester M ♀

O14.12 Severe pre-eclampsia, second trimester `2nd` M MCC ♀ CC/MCC Exc

O14.13 Severe pre-eclampsia, third trimester `3rd` M MCC ♀ CC/MCC Exc

O14.14 Severe pre-eclampsia complicating childbirth M ♀

O14.15 Severe pre-eclampsia, complicating the puerperium M ♀

O14.2 HELLP syndrome

Severe pre-eclampsia with hemolysis, elevated liver enzymes and low platelet count (HELLP)

O14.20 HELLP syndrome (HELLP), unspecified trimester M ♀

O14.22 HELLP syndrome (HELLP), second trimester `2nd` M MCC ♀ CC/MCC Exc

O14.23 HELLP syndrome (HELLP), third trimester `3rd` M MCC ♀ CC/MCC Exc

O14.24 HELLP syndrome, complicating childbirth M ♀

O14.25 HELLP syndrome, complicating the puerperium M ♀

O14.9 Unspecified pre-eclampsia

O14.90 Unspecified pre-eclampsia, unspecified trimester M ♀

O14.92 Unspecified pre-eclampsia, second trimester `2nd` M cc♀ CC/MCC Exc

O14.93 Unspecified pre-eclampsia, third trimester `3rd` M cc♀ CC/MCC Exc

O14.94 Unspecified pre-eclampsia, complicating childbirth M ♀

O14.95 Unspecified pre-eclampsia, complicating the puerperium M ♀

`1st` 1st trimester　`2nd` 2nd trimester　`3rd` 3rd trimester　PDx Unacceptable principal diagnosis symbol per Medicare code edits　POA Code exempt from diagnosis present on admission requirement　? Questionable admission　cc Complication or comorbidity　CC/MCC Exc CC/MCC exclusion　MCC Major complication or comorbidity　Principal diagnosis as its own CC　Principal diagnosis as its own MCC　HCC HCC diagnosis code　RxHCC RxHCC diagnosis code　MACRA code　Z code as first-listed diagnosis

When symbols appear on a code that requires a 7th character extension, refer to Appendix B to identify applicable 7th character codes.

2018 ICD-10-CM

O15 Eclampsia

INCLUDES convulsions following conditions in O10-O14 and O16

O15.0 Eclampsia complicating pregnancy

O15.00 Eclampsia complicating pregnancy, unspecified trimester Ⓜ ♀

O15.02 Eclampsia complicating pregnancy, second trimester 2nd Ⓜ MCC ♀ CC/MCC Exc

O15.03 Eclampsia complicating pregnancy, third trimester 3rd Ⓜ MCC ♀ CC/MCC Exc

O15.1 Eclampsia complicating labor Ⓜ MCC ♀ CC/MCC Exc

O15.2 Eclampsia complicating the puerperium Ⓜ MCC ♀ CC/MCC Exc

O15.9 Eclampsia, unspecified as to time period Ⓜ ♀
Eclampsia NOS

O16 Unspecified maternal hypertension

O16.1 Unspecified maternal hypertension, first trimester 1st Ⓜ cc♀ ♀ CC/MCC Exc

O16.2 Unspecified maternal hypertension, second trimester 2nd Ⓜ cc♀ ♀ CC/MCC Exc

O16.3 Unspecified maternal hypertension, third trimester 3rd Ⓜ cc♀ ♀ CC/MCC Exc

O16.4 Unspecified maternal hypertension, complicating childbirth Ⓜ ♀

O16.5 Unspecified maternal hypertension, complicating the puerperium Ⓜ ♀

O16.9 Unspecified maternal hypertension, unspecified trimester Ⓜ ♀

Other maternal disorders predominantly related to pregnancy (O20-O29)

EXCLUDES2 maternal care related to the fetus and amniotic cavity and possible delivery problems (O30-O48)

maternal diseases classifiable elsewhere but complicating pregnancy, labor and delivery, and the puerperium (O98-O99)

O20 Hemorrhage in early pregnancy

INCLUDES hemorrhage before completion of 20 weeks gestation

EXCLUDES1 pregnancy with abortive outcome (O00-O08)

O20.0 Threatened abortion Ⓜ cc♀ ♀ CC/MCC Exc
Hemorrhage specified as due to threatened abortion

O20.8 Other hemorrhage in early pregnancy Ⓜ ♀

O20.9 Hemorrhage in early pregnancy, unspecified Ⓜ cc♀ ♀ CC/MCC Exc

O21 Excessive vomiting in pregnancy

O21.0 Mild hyperemesis gravidarum Ⓜ ♀
Hyperemesis gravidarum, mild or unspecified, starting before the end of the 20th week of gestation

O21.1 Hyperemesis gravidarum with metabolic disturbance Ⓜ ♀
Hyperemesis gravidarum, starting before the end of the 20th week of gestation, with metabolic disturbance such as carbohydrate depletion
Hyperemesis gravidarum, starting before the end of the 20th week of gestation, with metabolic disturbance such as dehydration
Hyperemesis gravidarum, starting before the end of the 20th week of gestation, with metabolic disturbance such as electrolyte imbalance

O21.2 Late vomiting of pregnancy Ⓜ ♀
Excessive vomiting starting after 20 completed weeks of gestation

O21.8 Other vomiting complicating pregnancy Ⓜ ♀
Vomiting due to diseases classified elsewhere, complicating pregnancy
Use additional code, to identify cause.

O21.9 Vomiting of pregnancy, unspecified Ⓜ ♀

O22 Venous complications and hemorrhoids in pregnancy

EXCLUDES1 venous complications of:
abortion NOS (O03.9)
ectopic or molar pregnancy (O08.7)
failed attempted abortion (O07.35)
induced abortion (O04.85)
spontaneous abortion (O03.89)

EXCLUDES2 obstetric pulmonary embolism (O88.-)
venous complications and hemorrhoids of childbirth and the puerperium (O87.-)

O22.0 Varicose veins of lower extremity in pregnancy
Varicose veins NOS in pregnancy

O22.00 Varicose veins of lower extremity in pregnancy, unspecified trimester Ⓜ ♀

O22.01 Varicose veins of lower extremity in pregnancy, first trimester 1st Ⓜ ♀

O22.02 Varicose veins of lower extremity in pregnancy, second trimester 2nd Ⓜ ♀

O22.03 Varicose veins of lower extremity in pregnancy, third trimester 3rd Ⓜ ♀

O22.1 Genital varices in pregnancy
Perineal varices in pregnancy
Vaginal varices in pregnancy
Vulval varices in pregnancy

O22.10 Genital varices in pregnancy, unspecified trimester Ⓜ ♀

O22.11 Genital varices in pregnancy, first trimester 1st Ⓜ ♀

O22.12 Genital varices in pregnancy, second trimester 2nd Ⓜ ♀

O22.13 Genital varices in pregnancy, third trimester 3rd Ⓜ ♀

O22.2 Superficial thrombophlebitis in pregnancy
Phlebitis in pregnancy NOS
Thrombophlebitis of legs in pregnancy
Thrombosis in pregnancy NOS
Use additional code to identify the superficial thrombophlebitis (I80.0-)

O22.20 Superficial thrombophlebitis in pregnancy, unspecified trimester Ⓜ cc♀ ♀ CC/MCC Exc

O22.21 Superficial thrombophlebitis in pregnancy, first trimester 1st Ⓜ cc♀ ♀ CC/MCC Exc

O22.22 Superficial thrombophlebitis in pregnancy, second trimester 2nd Ⓜ cc♀ ♀ CC/MCC Exc

O22.23 Superficial thrombophlebitis in pregnancy, third trimester 3rd Ⓜ cc♀ ♀ CC/MCC Exc

O22.3 Deep phlebothrombosis in pregnancy
Deep vein thrombosis, antepartum
Use additional code to identify the deep vein thrombosis (I82.4-, I82.5-, I82.62-. I82.72-)
Use additional code, if applicable, for associated long-term (current) use of anticoagulants (Z79.01)

O22.30 Deep phlebothrombosis in pregnancy, unspecified trimester Ⓜ cc♀ ♀ CC/MCC Exc

O22.31 Deep phlebothrombosis in pregnancy, first trimester 1st Ⓜ MCC ♀ CC/MCC Exc

O22.32 Deep phlebothrombosis in pregnancy, second trimester 2nd Ⓜ MCC ♀ CC/MCC Exc

O22.33 Deep phlebothrombosis in pregnancy, third trimester 3rd Ⓜ MCC ♀ CC/MCC Exc

O22.4 Hemorrhoids in pregnancy

O22.40 Hemorrhoids in pregnancy, unspecified trimester Ⓜ cc♀ ♀ CC/MCC Exc

O22.41 Hemorrhoids in pregnancy, first trimester 1st Ⓜ cc♀ ♀ CC/MCC Exc

O22.42 Hemorrhoids in pregnancy, second trimester 2nd Ⓜ cc♀ ♀ CC/MCC Exc

O22.43 Hemorrhoids in pregnancy, third trimester 3rd Ⓜ cc♀ ♀ CC/MCC Exc

O22.5 Cerebral venous thrombosis in pregnancy
Cerebrovenous sinus thrombosis in pregnancy

O22.50 Cerebral venous thrombosis in pregnancy, unspecified trimester Ⓜ cc♀ ♀ CC/MCC Exc

O22.51 Cerebral venous thrombosis in pregnancy, first trimester 1st Ⓜ cc♀ ♀ CC/MCC Exc

O22.52 Cerebral venous thrombosis in pregnancy, second trimester 2nd Ⓜ cc♀ ♀ CC/MCC Exc

O22.53 Cerebral venous thrombosis in pregnancy, third trimester 3rd Ⓜ cc♀ ♀ CC/MCC Exc

O22.8 Other venous complications in pregnancy

O22.8X Other venous complications in pregnancy

Unspecified Code   Other Specified Code   Manifestation Code   Ⓝ Newborn   Ⓟ Pediatric   Ⓜ Maternity   Ⓐ Adult   ♂ Male   ♀ Female
● New Code   ▲ Revised Code Title   ▶◀ Revised Text   NOTES   INCLUDES   EXCLUDES 1 Not coded here   EXCLUDES 2 Not included here
4th character required   5th character required   6th character required   7th character required
Extension 'X' Alert   HAC Hospital-acquired condition (HAC) alert   AHA AHA Coding Clinic©

O22.8X1 **Other venous complications in pregnancy, first trimester** 1st M cc ♀ CC/MCC Exc

O22.8X2 **Other venous complications in pregnancy, second trimester** 2nd M cc ♀ CC/MCC Exc

O22.8X3 **Other venous complications in pregnancy, third trimester** 3rd M cc ♀ CC/MCC Exc

O22.8X9 **Other venous complications in pregnancy, unspecified trimester** M cc ♀ CC/MCC Exc

5ᵗʰ O22.9 Venous complication in pregnancy, unspecified
Gestational phlebitis NOS
Gestational phlebopathy NOS
Gestational thrombosis NOS

O22.90 **Venous complication in pregnancy, unspecified, unspecified trimester** M cc ♀ CC/MCC Exc

O22.91 **Venous complication in pregnancy, unspecified, first trimester** 1st M ♀

O22.92 **Venous complication in pregnancy, unspecified, second trimester** 2nd M ♀

O22.93 **Venous complication in pregnancy, unspecified, third trimester** 3rd M ♀

4ᵗʰ O23 Infections of genitourinary tract in pregnancy
Use additional code to identify organism (B95.-, B96.-)

EXCLUDES2 gonococcal infections complicating pregnancy, childbirth and the puerperium (O98.2)

infections with a predominantly sexual mode of transmission NOS complicating pregnancy, childbirth and the puerperium (O98.3)

syphilis complicating pregnancy, childbirth and the puerperium (O98.1)

tuberculosis of genitourinary system complicating pregnancy, childbirth and the puerperium (O98.0)

venereal disease NOS complicating pregnancy, childbirth and the puerperium (O98.3)

5ᵗʰ O23.0 Infections of kidney in pregnancy
Pyelonephritis in pregnancy

O23.00 **Infections of kidney in pregnancy, unspecified trimester** M ♀

O23.01 **Infections of kidney in pregnancy, first trimester** 1st M cc ♀ CC/MCC Exc

O23.02 **Infections of kidney in pregnancy, second trimester** 2nd M cc ♀ CC/MCC Exc

O23.03 **Infections of kidney in pregnancy, third trimester** 3rd M cc ♀ CC/MCC Exc

5ᵗʰ O23.1 Infections of bladder in pregnancy

O23.10 **Infections of bladder in pregnancy, unspecified trimester** M ♀

O23.11 **Infections of bladder in pregnancy, first trimester** 1st M cc ♀ CC/MCC Exc

O23.12 **Infections of bladder in pregnancy, second trimester** 2nd M cc ♀ CC/MCC Exc

O23.13 **Infections of bladder in pregnancy, third trimester** 3rd M cc ♀ CC/MCC Exc

5ᵗʰ O23.2 Infections of urethra in pregnancy

O23.20 **Infections of urethra in pregnancy, unspecified trimester** M ♀

O23.21 **Infections of urethra in pregnancy, first trimester** 1st M cc ♀ CC/MCC Exc

O23.22 **Infections of urethra in pregnancy, second trimester** 2nd M cc ♀ CC/MCC Exc

O23.23 **Infections of urethra in pregnancy, third trimester** 3rd M cc ♀ CC/MCC Exc

5ᵗʰ O23.3 Infections of other parts of urinary tract in pregnancy

O23.30 **Infections of other parts of urinary tract in pregnancy, unspecified trimester** M ♀

O23.31 **Infections of other parts of urinary tract in pregnancy, first trimester** 1st M cc ♀ CC/MCC Exc

O23.32 **Infections of other parts of urinary tract in pregnancy, second trimester** 2nd M cc ♀ CC/MCC Exc

O23.33 **Infections of other parts of urinary tract in pregnancy, third trimester** 3rd M cc ♀ CC/MCC Exc

5ᵗʰ O23.4 Unspecified infection of urinary tract in pregnancy

O23.40 **Unspecified infection of urinary tract in pregnancy, unspecified trimester** M ♀

O23.41 **Unspecified infection of urinary tract in pregnancy, first trimester** 1st M cc ♀ CC/MCC Exc

O23.42 **Unspecified infection of urinary tract in pregnancy, second trimester** 2nd M cc ♀ CC/MCC Exc

O23.43 **Unspecified infection of urinary tract in pregnancy, third trimester** 3rd M cc ♀ CC/MCC Exc

5ᵗʰ O23.5 Infections of the genital tract in pregnancy

6ᵗʰ O23.51 Infection of cervix in pregnancy

O23.511 **Infections of cervix in pregnancy, first trimester** 1st M cc ♀ CC/MCC Exc

O23.512 **Infections of cervix in pregnancy, second trimester** 2nd M cc ♀ CC/MCC Exc

O23.513 **Infections of cervix in pregnancy, third trimester** 3rd M cc ♀ CC/MCC Exc

O23.519 **Infections of cervix in pregnancy, unspecified trimester** M ♀

6ᵗʰ O23.52 Salpingo-oophoritis in pregnancy
Oophoritis in pregnancy
Salpingitis in pregnancy

O23.521 **Salpingo-oophoritis in pregnancy, first trimester** 1st M cc ♀ CC/MCC Exc

O23.522 **Salpingo-oophoritis in pregnancy, second trimester** 2nd M cc ♀ CC/MCC Exc

O23.523 **Salpingo-oophoritis in pregnancy, third trimester** 3rd M cc ♀ CC/MCC Exc

O23.529 **Salpingo-oophoritis in pregnancy, unspecified trimester** M ♀

6ᵗʰ O23.59 Infection of other part of genital tract in pregnancy

O23.591 **Infection of other part of genital tract in pregnancy, first trimester** 1st M cc ♀ CC/MCC Exc

O23.592 **Infection of other part of genital tract in pregnancy, second trimester** 2nd M cc ♀ CC/MCC Exc

O23.593 **Infection of other part of genital tract in pregnancy, third trimester** 3rd M cc ♀ CC/MCC Exc

O23.599 **Infection of other part of genital tract in pregnancy, unspecified trimester** M ♀

5ᵗʰ O23.9 Unspecified genitourinary tract infection in pregnancy
Genitourinary tract infection in pregnancy NOS

O23.90 **Unspecified genitourinary tract infection in pregnancy, unspecified trimester** M ♀

O23.91 **Unspecified genitourinary tract infection in pregnancy, first trimester** 1st M cc ♀ CC/MCC Exc

O23.92 **Unspecified genitourinary tract infection in pregnancy, second trimester** 2nd M cc ♀ CC/MCC Exc

O23.93 **Unspecified genitourinary tract infection in pregnancy, third trimester** 3rd M cc ♀ CC/MCC Exc

4ᵗʰ O24 Diabetes mellitus in pregnancy, childbirth, and the puerperium

5ᵗʰ O24.0 Pre-existing type 1 diabetes mellitus, in pregnancy, childbirth and the puerperium
Juvenile onset diabetes mellitus, in pregnancy, childbirth and the puerperium
Ketosis-prone diabetes mellitus in pregnancy, childbirth and the puerperium
Use additional code from category E10 to further identify any manifestations

6ᵗʰ O24.01 Pre-existing type 1 diabetes mellitus, in pregnancy

O24.011 **Pre-existing type 1 diabetes mellitus, in pregnancy, first trimester** 1st M cc ♀ CC/MCC Exc

O24.012 **Pre-existing type 1 diabetes mellitus, in pregnancy, second trimester** 2nd M cc ♀ CC/MCC Exc

O24.013 **Pre-existing type 1 diabetes mellitus, in pregnancy, third trimester** 3rd M cc ♀ CC/MCC Exc

O24.019 **Pre-existing type 1 diabetes mellitus, in pregnancy, unspecified trimester** M cc ♀ CC/MCC Exc

O24.02 **Pre-existing type 1 diabetes mellitus, in childbirth** M MCC ♀ CC/MCC Exc

---

1st 1st trimester 2nd 2nd trimester 3rd 3rd trimester PDx Unacceptable principal diagnosis symbol per Medicare code edits PoA Code exempt from diagnosis present on admission requirement ❓ Questionable admission cc Complication or comorbidity CC/MCC CC/MCC exclusion MCC Major complication or comorbidity Px Principal diagnosis as its own CC Mx Principal diagnosis as its own MCC HCC HCC diagnosis code RxHCC RxHCC diagnosis code MACRA code Z1 Z code as first-listed diagnosis

O24.03 Pre-existing type 1 diabetes mellitus, in the puerperium Ⓜ CC/MCC Exc

Ⓢ O24.1 Pre-existing type 2 diabetes mellitus, in pregnancy, childbirth and the puerperium
Insulin-resistant diabetes mellitus in pregnancy, childbirth and the puerperium
Use additional code (for):
from category E11 to further identify any manifestations
long-term (current) use of insulin (Z79.4)

Ⓖ O24.11 Pre-existing type 2 diabetes mellitus, in pregnancy
O24.111 Pre-existing type 2 diabetes mellitus, in pregnancy, first trimester 1st Ⓜ CC ♀ CC/MCC Exc
O24.112 Pre-existing type 2 diabetes mellitus, in pregnancy, second trimester 2nd Ⓜ CC ♀ CC/MCC Exc
O24.113 Pre-existing type 2 diabetes mellitus, in pregnancy, third trimester 3rd Ⓜ CC ♀ CC/MCC Exc
O24.119 Pre-existing type 2 diabetes mellitus, in pregnancy, unspecified trimester Ⓜ CC ♀ CC/MCC Exc
O24.12 Pre-existing type 2 diabetes mellitus, in childbirth Ⓜ MCC ♀ CC/MCC Exc
O24.13 Pre-existing type 2 diabetes mellitus, in the puerperium Ⓜ CC ♀ CC/MCC Exc

Ⓢ O24.3 Unspecified pre-existing diabetes mellitus in pregnancy, childbirth and the puerperium
Use additional code (for):
from category E11 to further identify any manifestation
long-term (current) use of insulin (Z79.4)

Ⓖ O24.31 Unspecified pre-existing diabetes mellitus in pregnancy
O24.311 Unspecified pre-existing diabetes mellitus in pregnancy, first trimester 1st Ⓜ CC ♀ CC/MCC Exc
O24.312 Unspecified pre-existing diabetes mellitus in pregnancy, second trimester 2nd Ⓜ CC ♀ CC/MCC Exc
O24.313 Unspecified pre-existing diabetes mellitus in pregnancy, third trimester 3rd Ⓜ CC ♀ CC/MCC Exc
O24.319 Unspecified pre-existing diabetes mellitus in pregnancy, unspecified trimester Ⓜ CC ♀ CC/MCC Exc
O24.32 Unspecified pre-existing diabetes mellitus in childbirth Ⓜ MCC ♀ CC/MCC Exc
O24.33 Unspecified pre-existing diabetes mellitus in the puerperium Ⓜ CC ♀ CC/MCC Exc

Ⓢ O24.4 Gestational diabetes mellitus
Diabetes mellitus arising in pregnancy
Gestational diabetes mellitus NOS

Ⓖ O24.41 Gestational diabetes mellitus in pregnancy
O24.410 Gestational diabetes mellitus in pregnancy, diet controlled Ⓜ ♀
O24.414 Gestational diabetes mellitus in pregnancy, insulin controlled Ⓜ ♀
O24.415 Gestational diabetes mellitus in pregnancy, controlled by oral hypoglycemic drugs *No Z-code* Ⓜ ♀
AHA: Q4 2016
Gestational diabetes mellitus in pregnancy, controlled by oral antidiabetic drugs
O24.419 Gestational diabetes mellitus in pregnancy, unspecified control Ⓜ ♀
AHA: Q4 2015

Ⓖ O24.42 Gestational diabetes mellitus in childbirth
O24.420 Gestational diabetes mellitus in childbirth, diet controlled Ⓜ ♀
O24.424 Gestational diabetes mellitus in childbirth, insulin controlled Ⓜ ♀

O24.425 Gestational diabetes mellitus in childbirth, controlled by oral hypoglycemic drugs Ⓜ ♀
AHA: Q4 2016
Gestational diabetes mellitus in childbirth, controlled by oral antidiabetic drugs
O24.429 Gestational diabetes mellitus in childbirth, unspecified control Ⓜ ♀

Ⓖ O24.43 Gestational diabetes mellitus in the puerperium
O24.430 Gestational diabetes mellitus in the puerperium, diet controlled Ⓜ ♀
O24.434 Gestational diabetes mellitus in the puerperium, insulin controlled Ⓜ ♀
O24.435 Gestational diabetes mellitus in puerperium, controlled by oral hypoglycemic drugs Ⓜ ♀
AHA: Q4 2016
Gestational diabetes mellitus in puerperium, controlled by oral antidiabetic drugs
O24.439 Gestational diabetes mellitus in the puerperium, unspecified control Ⓜ ♀

Ⓢ O24.8 Other pre-existing diabetes mellitus in pregnancy, childbirth, and the puerperium
Use additional code (for):
from categories E08, E09 and E13 to further identify any manifestation
long-term (current) use of insulin (Z79.4)

Ⓖ O24.81 Other pre-existing diabetes mellitus in pregnancy
O24.811 Other pre-existing diabetes mellitus in pregnancy, first trimester 1st Ⓜ CC ♀ CC/MCC Exc
O24.812 Other pre-existing diabetes mellitus in pregnancy, second trimester 2nd Ⓜ CC ♀ CC/MCC Exc
O24.813 Other pre-existing diabetes mellitus in pregnancy, third trimester 3rd Ⓜ CC ♀ CC/MCC Exc
O24.819 Other pre-existing diabetes mellitus in pregnancy, unspecified trimester Ⓜ CC ♀ CC/MCC Exc
O24.82 Other pre-existing diabetes mellitus in childbirth Ⓜ MCC ♀ CC/MCC Exc
O24.83 Other pre-existing diabetes mellitus in the puerperium Ⓜ CC ♀ CC/MCC Exc

Ⓢ O24.9 Unspecified diabetes mellitus in pregnancy, childbirth and the puerperium
Use additional code for long-term (current) use of insulin (Z79.4)

Ⓖ O24.91 Unspecified diabetes mellitus in pregnancy
O24.911 Unspecified diabetes mellitus in pregnancy, first trimester 1st Ⓜ CC ♀ CC/MCC Exc
O24.912 Unspecified diabetes mellitus in pregnancy, second trimester 2nd Ⓜ CC ♀ CC/MCC Exc
O24.913 Unspecified diabetes mellitus in pregnancy, third trimester 3rd Ⓜ CC ♀ CC/MCC Exc
O24.919 Unspecified diabetes mellitus in pregnancy, unspecified trimester Ⓜ CC ♀ CC/MCC Exc
O24.92 Unspecified diabetes mellitus in childbirth Ⓜ ♀
O24.93 Unspecified diabetes mellitus in the puerperium Ⓜ CC ♀ CC/MCC Exc

Ⓠ O25 Malnutrition in pregnancy, childbirth and the puerperium
Ⓢ O25.1 Malnutrition in pregnancy
O25.10 Malnutrition in pregnancy, unspecified trimester Ⓜ ♀
O25.11 Malnutrition in pregnancy, first trimester 1st Ⓜ ♀
O25.12 Malnutrition in pregnancy, second trimester 2nd Ⓜ ♀
O25.13 Malnutrition in pregnancy, third trimester 3rd Ⓜ ♀

Unspecified Code ▐ Other Specified Code ▐ Manifestation Code Ⓝ Newborn Ⓟ Pediatric Ⓜ Maternity Ⓐ Adult ♂ Male ♀ Female
● New Code ▲ Revised Code Title ►◄ Revised Text **NOTES** *INCLUDES* *EXCLUDES1* Not coded here *EXCLUDES2* Not included here
Ⓠ 4th character required Ⓢ 5th character required Ⓖ 6th character required Ⓞ 7th character required
Ⓞ Extension 'X' Alert **HAC** Hospital-acquired condition (HAC) alert **AHA** AHA Coding Clinic©

O25.2 **Malnutrition in** childbirth M ♀

O25.3 **Malnutrition in the** puerperium M ♀

O26 Maternal care for other conditions predominantly related to pregnancy

  O26.0 Excessive weight gain in pregnancy

    EXCLUDES2 gestational edema (O12.0, O12.2)

    O26.00 **Excessive weight gain in pregnancy, unspecified trimester** M ♀

    O26.01 **Excessive weight gain in pregnancy,** first trimester 1st M ♀

    O26.02 **Excessive weight gain in pregnancy,** second trimester 2nd M ♀

    O26.03 **Excessive weight gain in pregnancy,** third trimester 3rd M ♀

  O26.1 Low weight gain in pregnancy

    O26.10 **Low weight gain in pregnancy, unspecified trimester** M ♀

    O26.11 Low weight gain in pregnancy, first trimester 1st M ♀

    O26.12 Low weight gain in pregnancy, second trimester 2nd M ♀

    O26.13 Low weight gain in pregnancy, third trimester 3rd M ♀

  O26.2 Pregnancy care for patient with recurrent pregnancy loss

    O26.20 **Pregnancy care for patient with recurrent pregnancy loss, unspecified trimester** M ♀

    O26.21 **Pregnancy care for patient with recurrent pregnancy loss,** first trimester 1st M ♀

    O26.22 **Pregnancy care for patient with recurrent pregnancy loss,** second trimester 2nd M ♀

    O26.23 **Pregnancy care for patient with recurrent pregnancy loss,** third trimester 3rd M ♀

  O26.3 Retained intrauterine contraceptive device in pregnancy

    O26.30 **Retained intrauterine contraceptive device in pregnancy, unspecified trimester** M ♀

    O26.31 **Retained intrauterine contraceptive device in pregnancy,** first trimester 1st M ♀

    O26.32 **Retained intrauterine contraceptive device in pregnancy,** second trimester 2nd M ♀

    O26.33 **Retained intrauterine contraceptive device in pregnancy,** third trimester 3rd M ♀

  O26.4 Herpes gestationis

    O26.40 **Herpes gestationis, unspecified trimester** M ♀

    O26.41 **Herpes gestationis,** first trimester 1st M ♀

    O26.42 **Herpes gestationis,** second trimester 2nd M ♀

    O26.43 **Herpes gestationis,** third trimester 3rd M ♀

  O26.5 Maternal hypotension syndrome

    Supine hypotensive syndrome

    O26.50 **Maternal hypotension syndrome, unspecified trimester** M ♀

    O26.51 **Maternal hypotension syndrome,** first trimester 1st M ♀

    O26.52 **Maternal hypotension syndrome,** second trimester 2nd M ♀

    O26.53 **Maternal hypotension syndrome,** third trimester 3rd M ♀

  O26.6 Liver and biliary tract disorders in pregnancy, childbirth and the puerperium

    Use additional code to identify the specific disorder

    EXCLUDES2 hepatorenal syndrome following labor and delivery (O90.4)

    O26.61 Liver and biliary tract disorders in pregnancy

      O26.611 **Liver and biliary tract disorders in pregnancy,** first trimester 1st M cc ♀ CC/MCC Exc

      O26.612 **Liver and biliary tract disorders in pregnancy,** second trimester 2nd M cc ♀ CC/MCC Exc

      O26.613 **Liver and biliary tract disorders in pregnancy,** third trimester 3rd M cc ♀ CC/MCC Exc

      O26.619 **Liver and biliary tract disorders in pregnancy, unspecified trimester** M ♀

O26.62 Liver and biliary tract disorders in childbirth M cc ♀ CC/MCC Exc

O26.63 Liver and biliary tract disorders in the puerperium M ♀

  O26.7 Subluxation of symphysis (pubis) in pregnancy, childbirth and the puerperium

    EXCLUDES1 traumatic separation of symphysis (pubis) during childbirth (O71.6)

    O26.71 Subluxation of symphysis (pubis) in pregnancy

      O26.711 **Subluxation of symphysis (pubis) in pregnancy,** first trimester 1st M ♀

      O26.712 **Subluxation of symphysis (pubis) in pregnancy,** second trimester 2nd M ♀

      O26.713 **Subluxation of symphysis (pubis) in pregnancy,** third trimester 3rd M ♀

      O26.719 **Subluxation of symphysis (pubis) in pregnancy, unspecified trimester** M ♀

    O26.72 Subluxation of symphysis (pubis) in childbirth M ♀

    O26.73 Subluxation of symphysis (pubis) in the puerperium M ♀

  O26.8 Other specified pregnancy related conditions

    O26.81 Pregnancy related exhaustion and fatigue

      O26.811 **Pregnancy related exhaustion and fatigue,** first trimester 1st M ♀

      O26.812 **Pregnancy related exhaustion and fatigue,** second trimester 2nd M ♀

      O26.813 **Pregnancy related exhaustion and fatigue,** third trimester 3rd M ♀

      O26.819 **Pregnancy related exhaustion and fatigue, unspecified trimester** M ♀

    O26.82 Pregnancy related peripheral neuritis

      O26.821 **Pregnancy related peripheral neuritis,** first trimester 1st M ♀

      O26.822 **Pregnancy related peripheral neuritis,** second trimester 2nd M ♀

      O26.823 **Pregnancy related peripheral neuritis,** third trimester 3rd M ♀

      O26.829 **Pregnancy related peripheral neuritis, unspecified trimester** M ♀

    O26.83 Pregnancy related renal disease

    Use additional code to identify the specific disorder

      O26.831 **Pregnancy related renal disease,** first trimester 1st M cc ♀ CC/MCC Exc

      O26.832 **Pregnancy related renal disease,** second trimester 2nd M cc ♀ CC/MCC Exc

      O26.833 **Pregnancy related renal disease,** third trimester 3rd M cc ♀ CC/MCC Exc

      O26.839 **Pregnancy related renal disease, unspecified trimester** M ♀

    O26.84 Uterine size-date discrepancy complicating pregnancy

    EXCLUDES1 encounter for suspected problem with fetal growth ruled out (Z03.74)

      O26.841 **Uterine size-date discrepancy,** first trimester 1st M ♀

      O26.842 **Uterine size-date discrepancy,** second trimester 2nd M ♀

      O26.843 **Uterine size-date discrepancy,** third trimester 3rd M ♀

      O26.849 **Uterine size-date discrepancy, unspecified trimester** M ♀

    O26.85 Spotting complicating pregnancy

      O26.851 **Spotting complicating pregnancy,** first trimester 1st M ♀

      O26.852 **Spotting complicating pregnancy,** second trimester 2nd M ♀

      O26.853 **Spotting complicating pregnancy,** third trimester 3rd M ♀

      O26.859 **Spotting complicating pregnancy, unspecified trimester** M ♀

1st 1st trimester 2nd 2nd trimester 3rd 3rd trimester Unacceptable principal diagnosis symbol per Medicare code edits Code exempt from diagnosis present on admission requirement ❓ Questionable admission cc Complication or comorbidity CC/MCC CC/MCC exclusion MCC Major complication or comorbidity Principal diagnosis as its own CC Principal diagnosis as its own MCC HCC HCC diagnosis code RxHCC RxHCC diagnosis code MACRA code Z Z code as first-listed diagnosis

When symbols appear on a code that requires a 7th character extension, refer to Appendix B to identify applicable 7th character codes. **2018 ICD-10-CM**

O26.86 **Pruritic urticarial papules and plaques of pregnancy (PUPPP)** Ⓜ ♀
Polymorphic eruption of pregnancy

6ᵗʰ O26.87 **Cervical shortening**
EXCLUDES1 encounter for suspected cervical shortening ruled out (Z03.75)

O26.872 **Cervical shortening,** second trimester 2nd Ⓜ cc ♀ CC/MCC Excl

O26.873 **Cervical shortening,** third trimester 3rd Ⓜ cc ♀ CC/MCC Excl

O26.879 **Cervical shortening, unspecified trimester** Ⓜ cc ♀ CC/MCC Excl

6ᵗʰ O26.89 Other specified **pregnancy related conditions**

O26.891 **Other specified pregnancy related conditions,** first trimester 1st Ⓜ ♀

O26.892 **Other specified pregnancy related conditions,** second trimester 2nd Ⓜ ♀

O26.893 **Other specified pregnancy related conditions,** third trimester 3rd Ⓜ ♀
AHA: Q3 2015

O26.899 **Other specified pregnancy related conditions, unspecified trimester** Ⓜ ♀

5ᵗʰ O26.9 **Pregnancy related conditions, unspecified**

O26.90 **Pregnancy related conditions, unspecified, unspecified trimester** Ⓜ ♀

O26.91 **Pregnancy related conditions, unspecified,** first trimester 1st Ⓜ ♀

O26.92 **Pregnancy related conditions, unspecified,** second trimester 2nd Ⓜ ♀

O26.93 **Pregnancy related conditions, unspecified,** third trimester 3rd Ⓜ ♀

4ᵗʰ O28 **Abnormal findings on antenatal screening of mother**
EXCLUDES1 diagnostic findings classified elsewhere -see Alphabetical Index

O28.0 **Abnormal** hematological **finding on antenatal screening of mother** Ⓜ ♀

O28.1 **Abnormal** biochemical **finding on antenatal screening of mother** Ⓜ ♀

O28.2 **Abnormal** cytological **finding on antenatal screening of mother** Ⓜ ♀

O28.3 **Abnormal** ultrasonic **finding on antenatal screening of mother** Ⓜ ♀
AHA: Q4 2016

O28.4 **Abnormal** radiological **finding on antenatal screening of mother** Ⓜ ♀

O28.5 **Abnormal** chromosomal and genetic **finding on antenatal screening of mother** Ⓜ ♀

O28.8 **Other abnormal findings on antenatal screening of mother** Ⓜ ♀

O28.9 **Unspecified abnormal findings on antenatal screening of mother** Ⓜ ♀

4ᵗʰ O29 **Complications of anesthesia during pregnancy**
INCLUDES maternal complications arising from the administration of a general, regional or local anesthetic, analgesic or other sedation during pregnancy
Use additional code, if necessary, to identify the complication
EXCLUDES2 complications of anesthesia during labor and delivery (O74.-)
complications of anesthesia during the puerperium (O89.-)

5ᵗʰ O29.0 Pulmonary **complications of anesthesia during pregnancy**

6ᵗʰ O29.01 Aspiration pneumonitis **due to anesthesia during pregnancy**
Inhalation of stomach contents or secretions NOS due to anesthesia during pregnancy
Mendelson's syndrome due to anesthesia during pregnancy

O29.011 **Aspiration pneumonitis due to anesthesia during pregnancy,** first trimester 1st Ⓜ ♀

O29.012 **Aspiration pneumonitis due to anesthesia during pregnancy,** second trimester 2nd Ⓜ ♀

O29.013 **Aspiration pneumonitis due to anesthesia during pregnancy,** third trimester 3rd Ⓜ ♀

O29.019 **Aspiration pneumonitis due to anesthesia during pregnancy, unspecified trimester** Ⓜ ♀

6ᵗʰ O29.02 Pressure collapse of lung **due to anesthesia during pregnancy**

O29.021 **Pressure collapse of lung due to anesthesia during pregnancy,** first trimester 1st Ⓜ ♀

O29.022 **Pressure collapse of lung due to anesthesia during pregnancy,** second trimester 2nd Ⓜ ♀

O29.023 **Pressure collapse of lung due to anesthesia during pregnancy,** third trimester 3rd Ⓜ ♀

O29.029 **Pressure collapse of lung due to anesthesia during pregnancy, unspecified trimester** Ⓜ ♀

6ᵗʰ O29.09 Other pulmonary complications of anesthesia during pregnancy

O29.091 **Other pulmonary complications of anesthesia during pregnancy,** first trimester 1st Ⓜ ♀

O29.092 **Other pulmonary complications of anesthesia during pregnancy,** second trimester 2nd Ⓜ ♀

O29.093 **Other pulmonary complications of anesthesia during pregnancy,** third trimester 3rd Ⓜ ♀

O29.099 **Other pulmonary complications of anesthesia during pregnancy, unspecified trimester** Ⓜ ♀

5ᵗʰ O29.1 Cardiac **complications of anesthesia during pregnancy**

6ᵗʰ O29.11 Cardiac arrest **due to anesthesia during** pregnancy

O29.111 **Cardiac arrest due to anesthesia during pregnancy,** first trimester 1st Ⓜ ♀

O29.112 **Cardiac arrest due to anesthesia during pregnancy,** second trimester 2nd Ⓜ ♀

O29.113 **Cardiac arrest due to anesthesia during pregnancy,** third trimester 3rd Ⓜ ♀

O29.119 **Cardiac arrest due to anesthesia during pregnancy, unspecified trimester** Ⓜ ♀

6ᵗʰ O29.12 Cardiac failure **due to anesthesia during** pregnancy

O29.121 **Cardiac failure due to anesthesia during pregnancy,** first trimester 1st Ⓜ ♀

O29.122 **Cardiac failure due to anesthesia during pregnancy,** second trimester 2nd Ⓜ ♀

O29.123 **Cardiac failure due to anesthesia during pregnancy,** third trimester 3rd Ⓜ ♀

O29.129 **Cardiac failure due to anesthesia during pregnancy, unspecified trimester** Ⓜ ♀

6ᵗʰ O29.19 Other cardiac complications of anesthesia during pregnancy

O29.191 **Other cardiac complications of anesthesia during pregnancy,** first trimester 1st Ⓜ ♀

O29.192 **Other cardiac complications of anesthesia during pregnancy,** second trimester 2nd Ⓜ ♀

O29.193 **Other cardiac complications of anesthesia during pregnancy,** third trimester 3rd Ⓜ ♀

O29.199 **Other cardiac complications of anesthesia during pregnancy, unspecified trimester** Ⓜ ♀

5ᵗʰ O29.2 Central nervous system **complications of anesthesia during pregnancy**

6ᵗʰ O29.21 Cerebral anoxia **due to anesthesia during** pregnancy

O29.211 **Cerebral anoxia due to anesthesia during pregnancy,** first trimester 1st Ⓜ ♀

O29.212 **Cerebral anoxia due to anesthesia during pregnancy,** second trimester 2nd Ⓜ ♀

Unspecified Code   Other Specified Code   Manifestation Code   Ⓝ Newborn   Ⓟ Pediatric   Ⓜ Maternity   Ⓐ Adult   ♂ Male   ♀ Female
● New Code   ▲ Revised Code Title   ▶◀ Revised Text   **NOTES** *INCLUDES* *EXCLUDES 1* Not coded here   *EXCLUDES 2* Not included here
4ᵗʰ 4ᵗʰ character required   5ᵗʰ 5ᵗʰ character required   6ᵗʰ 6ᵗʰ character required   7ᵗʰ 7ᵗʰ character required
7ᵗʰ Extension 'X' Alert   HAC Hospital-acquired condition (HAC) alert   **AHA** AHA Coding Clinic©

O30.8 Other specified multiple gestation
Multiple gestation pregnancy greater then quadruplets

O30.80 Other specified multiple gestation, unspecified number of placenta and unspecified number of amniotic sacs

O30.801 Other specified multiple gestation, unspecified number of placenta and unspecified number of amniotic sacs, first trimester 1st M ♀ CC/MCC Exc

O30.802 Other specified multiple gestation, unspecified number of placenta and unspecified number of amniotic sacs, second trimester 2nd M ♀ CC/MCC Exc

O30.803 Other specified multiple gestation, unspecified number of placenta and unspecified number of amniotic sacs, third trimester 3rd M ♀ CC/MCC Exc

O30.809 Other specified multiple gestation, unspecified number of placenta and unspecified number of amniotic sacs, unspecified trimester M ♀

O30.81 Other specified multiple gestation with two or more monochorionic fetuses

O30.811 Other specified multiple gestation with two or more monochorionic fetuses, first trimester 1st M ♀ CC/MCC Exc

O30.812 Other specified multiple gestation with two or more monochorionic fetuses, second trimester 2nd M ♀ CC/MCC Exc

O30.813 Other specified multiple gestation with two or more monochorionic fetuses, third trimester 3rd M ♀ CC/MCC Exc

O30.819 Other specified multiple gestation with two or more monochorionic fetuses, unspecified trimester M ♀

O30.82 Other specified multiple gestation with two or more monoamniotic fetuses

O30.821 Other specified multiple gestation with two or more monoamniotic fetuses, first trimester 1st M ♀ CC/MCC Exc

O30.822 Other specified multiple gestation with two or more monoamniotic fetuses, second trimester 2nd M ♀ CC/MCC Exc

O30.823 Other specified multiple gestation with two or more monoamniotic fetuses, third trimester 3rd M ♀ CC/MCC Exc

O30.829 Other specified multiple gestation with two or more monoamniotic fetuses, unspecified trimester M ♀

O30.89 Other specified multiple gestation, unable to determine number of placenta and number of amniotic sacs

O30.891 Other specified multiple gestation, unable to determine number of placenta and number of amniotic sacs, first trimester 1st M ♀ CC/MCC Exc

O30.892 Other specified multiple gestation, unable to determine number of placenta and number of amniotic sacs, second trimester 2nd M ♀ CC/MCC Exc

O30.893 Other specified multiple gestation, unable to determine number of placenta and number of amniotic sacs, third trimester 3rd M ♀ CC/MCC Exc

O30.899 Other specified multiple gestation, unable to determine number of placenta and number of amniotic sacs, unspecified trimester M ♀

O30.9 Multiple gestation, unspecified
Multiple pregnancy NOS

O30.90 Multiple gestation, unspecified, unspecified trimester M ♀

O30.91 Multiple gestation, unspecified, first trimester 1st M ♀

O30.92 Multiple gestation, unspecified, second trimester 2nd M ♀

O30.93 Multiple gestation, unspecified, third trimester 3rd M ♀

O31 Complications specific to multiple gestation
EXCLUDES2 delayed delivery of second twin, triplet, etc. (O63.2)
malpresentation of one fetus or more (O32.9)
placental transfusion syndromes (O43.0-)

One of the following 7th characters is to be assigned to each code under category O31. 7th character 0 is for single gestations and multiple gestations where the fetus is unspecified. 7th characters 1 through 9 are for cases of multiple gestations to identify the fetus for which the code applies. The appropriate code from category O30, Multiple gestation, must also be assigned when assigning a code from category O31 that has a 7th character of 1 through 9.

0 = not applicable or unspecified *which fetus is causing complication*
1 = fetus 1
2 = fetus 2
3 = fetus 3
4 = fetus 4
5 = fetus 5
9 = other fetus

O31.0 Papyraceous fetus
Fetus compressus

O31.00 Papyraceous fetus, unspecified trimester M ♀

O31.01 Papyraceous fetus, first trimester 1st M ♀

O31.02 Papyraceous fetus, second trimester 2nd M ♀

O31.03 Papyraceous fetus, third trimester 3rd M ♀

O31.1 Continuing pregnancy after spontaneous abortion of one fetus or more

O31.10 Continuing pregnancy after spontaneous abortion of one fetus or more, unspecified trimester M ♀

O31.11 Continuing pregnancy after spontaneous abortion of one fetus or more, first trimester 1st M ♀

O31.12 Continuing pregnancy after spontaneous abortion of one fetus or more, second trimester 2nd M ♀

O31.13 Continuing pregnancy after spontaneous abortion of one fetus or more, third trimester 3rd M ♀

O31.2 Continuing pregnancy after intrauterine death of one fetus or more

O31.20 Continuing pregnancy after intrauterine death of one fetus or more, unspecified trimester M ♀

O31.21 Continuing pregnancy after intrauterine death of one fetus or more, first trimester 1st M ♀

O31.22 Continuing pregnancy after intrauterine death of one fetus or more, second trimester 2nd M ♀

O31.23 Continuing pregnancy after intrauterine death of one fetus or more, third trimester 3rd M ♀

O31.3 Continuing pregnancy after elective fetal reduction of one fetus or more
Continuing pregnancy after selective termination of one fetus or more

O31.30 Continuing pregnancy after elective fetal reduction of one fetus or more, unspecified trimester M ♀

O31.31 Continuing pregnancy after elective fetal reduction of one fetus or more, first trimester 1st M ♀

O31.32 Continuing pregnancy after elective fetal reduction of one fetus or more, second trimester 2nd M ♀

O31.33 Continuing pregnancy after elective fetal reduction of one fetus or more, third trimester 3rd M ♀

O31.8 Other complications specific to multiple gestation

O31.8X Other complications specific to multiple gestation

O31.8X1 Other complications specific to multiple gestation, first trimester 1st M ♀ CC/MCC Exc

O31.8X2 Other complications specific to multiple gestation, second trimester 2nd M ♀ CC/MCC Exc

O31.8X3 Other complications specific to multiple gestation, third trimester 3rd M ♀ CC/MCC Exc

---

1st 1st trimester 2nd 2nd trimester 3rd 3rd trimester PDx Unacceptable principal diagnosis symbol per Medicare code edits
PDx Code exempt from diagnosis present on admission requirement ❓ Questionable admission CC Complication or comorbidity
CC/MCC Exc CC/MCC exclusion MCC Major complication or comorbidity Principal diagnosis as its own CC Principal diagnosis as its own MCC
HCC HCC diagnosis code RxHCC RxHCC diagnosis code MACRA code Z1 Z code as first-listed diagnosis

When symbols appear on a code that requires a 7th character extension, refer to Appendix B to identify applicable 7th character codes.
2018 ICD-10-CM

[7th] O31.8X9 Other complications specific to multiple gestation, unspecified trimester [M] ♀

[4th] **O32 Maternal care for malpresentation of fetus**

INCLUDES *the listed conditions as a reason for observation, hospitalization or other obstetric care of the mother, or for cesarean delivery before onset of labor*

EXCLUDES1 *malpresentation of fetus with obstructed labor (O64.-)*

One of the following 7th characters is to be assigned to each code under category O32. 7th character 0 is for single gestations and multiple gestations where the fetus is unspecified. 7th characters 1 through 9 are for cases of multiple gestations to identify the fetus for which the code applies. The appropriate code from category O30, Multiple gestation, must also be assigned when assigning a code from category O32 that has a 7th character of 1 through 9.

0 = not applicable or unspecified
1 = fetus 1
2 = fetus 2
3 = fetus 3
4 = fetus 4
5 = fetus 5
9 = other fetus

[7th] O32.0 Maternal care for unstable lie [M] ♀

[7th] O32.1 Maternal care for breech presentation [M] ♀
Maternal care for buttocks presentation
Maternal care for complete breech
Maternal care for frank breech
EXCLUDES1 *footling presentation (O32.8)*
incomplete breech (O32.8)

[7th] O32.2 Maternal care for transverse and oblique lie [M] ♀
Maternal care for oblique presentation
Maternal care for transverse presentation

[7th] O32.3 Maternal care for face, brow and chin presentation [M] ♀

[7th] O32.4 Maternal care for high head at term [M] ♀
Maternal care for failure of head to enter pelvic brim

[7th] O32.6 Maternal care for compound presentation [M] ♀

[7th] O32.8 Maternal care for other malpresentation of fetus [M] ♀
Maternal care for footling presentation
Maternal care for incomplete breech

[7th] O32.9 Maternal care for malpresentation of fetus, unspecified [M] ♀

[4th] **O33 Maternal care for disproportion**

INCLUDES *the listed conditions as a reason for observation, hospitalization or other obstetric care of the mother, or for cesarean delivery before onset of labor*

EXCLUDES1 *disproportion with obstructed labor (O65-O66)*

O33.0 Maternal care for disproportion due to deformity of maternal pelvic bones [M] CC ♀ CC/MCC Exc
Maternal care for disproportion due to pelvic deformity causing disproportion NOS

O33.1 Maternal care for disproportion due to generally contracted pelvis [M] ♀
Maternal care for disproportion due to contracted pelvis NOS causing disproportion

O33.2 Maternal care for disproportion due to inlet contraction of pelvis [M] ♀
Maternal care for disproportion due to inlet contraction (pelvis) causing disproportion

[7th] O33.3 Maternal care for disproportion due to outlet contraction of pelvis [M] ♀
Maternal care for disproportion due to mid-cavity contraction (pelvis)
Maternal care for disproportion due to outlet contraction (pelvis)

One of the following 7th characters is to be assigned to code O33.3. 7th character 0 is for single gestations and multiple gestations where the fetus is unspecified. 7th characters 1 through 9 are for cases of multiple gestations to identify the fetus for which the code applies. The appropriate code from category O30, Multiple gestation, must also be assigned when assigning code O33.3 with a 7th character of 1 through 9.

0 = not applicable or unspecified
1 = fetus 1
2 = fetus 2
3 = fetus 3
4 = fetus 4
5 = fetus 5
9 = other fetus

[7th] O33.4 Maternal care for disproportion of mixed maternal and fetal origin [M] ♀

One of the following 7th characters is to be assigned to code O33.4. 7th character 0 is for single gestations and multiple gestations where the fetus is unspecified. 7th characters 1 through 9 are for cases of multiple gestations to identify the fetus for which the code applies. The appropriate code from category O30, Multiple gestation, must also be assigned when assigning code O33.4 with a 7th character of 1 through 9.

0 = not applicable or unspecified
1 = fetus 1
2 = fetus 2
3 = fetus 3
4 = fetus 4
5 = fetus 5
9 = other fetus

[7th] O33.5 Maternal care for disproportion due to unusually large fetus [M] ♀
Maternal care for disproportion due to disproportion of fetal origin with normally formed fetus
Maternal care for disproportion due to fetal disproportion NOS

One of the following 7th characters is to be assigned to code O33.5. 7th character 0 is for single gestations and multiple gestations where the fetus is unspecified. 7th characters 1 through 9 are for cases of multiple gestations to identify the fetus for which the code applies. The appropriate code from category O30, Multiple gestation, must also be assigned when assigning code O33.5 with a 7th character of 1 through 9.

0 = not applicable or unspecified
1 = fetus 1
2 = fetus 2
3 = fetus 3
4 = fetus 4
5 = fetus 5
9 = other fetus

[7th] O33.6 Maternal care for disproportion due to hydrocephalic fetus [M] ♀

One of the following 7th characters is to be assigned to code O33.6. 7th character 0 is for single gestations and multiple gestations where the fetus is unspecified. 7th characters 1 through 9 are for cases of multiple gestations to identify the fetus for which the code applies. The appropriate code from category O30, Multiple gestation, must also be assigned when assigning code O33.6 with a 7th character of 1 through 9.

0 = not applicable or unspecified
1 = fetus 1
2 = fetus 2
3 = fetus 3
4 = fetus 4
5 = fetus 5
9 = other fetus

[7th] O33.7 Maternal care for disproportion due to other fetal deformities [M] ♀
AHA: Q4 2016
Maternal care for disproportion due to fetal ascites
Maternal care for disproportion due to fetal hydrops
Maternal care for disproportion due to fetal meningomyelocele
Maternal care for disproportion due to fetal sacral teratoma
Maternal care for disproportion due to fetal tumor

One of the following 7th characters is to be assigned to code O33.7. 7th character 0 is for single gestations and multiple gestations where the fetus is unspecified. 7th characters 1 through 9 are for cases of multiple gestations to identify

the fetus for which the code applies. The appropriate code from category O30, Multiple gestation, must also be assigned when assigning code O33.7 with a 7th character of 1 through 9.

0 = not applicable or unspecified
1 = fetus 1
2 = fetus 2
3 = fetus 3
4 = fetus 4
5 = fetus 5
9 = other fetus

[EXCLUDES1] *obstructed labor due to other fetal deformities (O66.3)*

O33.8 **Maternal care for disproportion of other origin** [M] ♀

O33.9 **Maternal care for disproportion, unspecified** [M] ♀
Maternal care for disproportion due to cephalopelvic disproportion NOS
Maternal care for disproportion due to fetopelvic disproportion NOS

[4th] O34 **Maternal care for abnormality of pelvic organs**
[INCLUDES] *the listed conditions as a reason for hospitalization or other obstetric care of the mother, or for cesarean delivery before onset of labor*
Code first any associated obstructed labor (O65.5)
Use additional code for specific condition

[5th] O34.0 **Maternal care for congenital malformation of uterus**
Maternal care for double uterus
Maternal care for uterus bicornis

O34.00 **Maternal care for unspecified congenital malformation of uterus, unspecified trimester** [M] ♀
O34.01 **Maternal care for unspecified congenital malformation of uterus, first trimester** [1st] [M] ♀
O34.02 **Maternal care for unspecified congenital malformation of uterus, second trimester** [2nd] [M] ♀
O34.03 **Maternal care for unspecified congenital malformation of uterus, third trimester** [3rd] [M] ♀

[5th] O34.1 **Maternal care for benign tumor of corpus uteri**
[EXCLUDES2] *maternal care for benign tumor of cervix (O34.4-)*
maternal care for malignant neoplasm of uterus (O9A.1-)

O34.10 **Maternal care for benign tumor of corpus uteri, unspecified trimester** [M] ♀
O34.11 **Maternal care for benign tumor of corpus uteri, first trimester** [1st] [M] ♀
O34.12 **Maternal care for benign tumor of corpus uteri, second trimester** [2nd] [M] ♀
O34.13 **Maternal care for benign tumor of corpus uteri, third trimester** [3rd] [M] ♀

[5th] O34.2 **Maternal care due to uterine scar from previous surgery**

[6th] O34.21 **Maternal care for scar from previous cesarean delivery**

O34.211 **Maternal care for low transverse scar from previous cesarean delivery** [M] ♀
AHA: Q4 2016

O34.212 **Maternal care for vertical scar from previous cesarean delivery** [M] ♀
AHA: Q4 2016
Maternal care for classical scar from previous cesarean delivery

O34.219 **Maternal care for unspecified type scar from previous cesarean delivery** [M] ♀
AHA: Q4 2016

O34.29 **Maternal care due to uterine scar from other previous surgery** [M] ♀
AHA: Q4 2016
Maternal care due to uterine scar from other transmural uterine incision

[5th] O34.3 **Maternal care for cervical incompetence**
Maternal care for cerclage with or without cervical incompetence
Maternal care for Shirodkar suture with or without cervical incompetence

O34.30 **Maternal care for cervical incompetence, unspecified trimester** [M] ♀
O34.31 **Maternal care for cervical incompetence, first trimester** [1st] [M] [MCC] ♀ [CC/MCC Exc]
O34.32 **Maternal care for cervical incompetence, second trimester** [2nd] [M] [MCC] ♀ [CC/MCC Exc]
O34.33 **Maternal care for cervical incompetence, third trimester** [3rd] [M] [MCC] ♀ [CC/MCC Exc]

[5th] O34.4 **Maternal care for other abnormalities of cervix**

O34.40 **Maternal care for other abnormalities of cervix, unspecified trimester** [M] ♀
O34.41 **Maternal care for other abnormalities of cervix, first trimester** [1st] [M] ♀
O34.42 **Maternal care for other abnormalities of cervix, second trimester** [2nd] [M] ♀
O34.43 **Maternal care for other abnormalities of cervix, third trimester** [3rd] [M] ♀

[5th] O34.5 **Maternal care for other abnormalities of gravid uterus**

[6th] O34.51 **Maternal care for incarceration of gravid uterus**

O34.511 **Maternal care for incarceration of gravid uterus, first trimester** [1st] [M] ♀
O34.512 **Maternal care for incarceration of gravid uterus, second trimester** [2nd] [M] ♀
O34.513 **Maternal care for incarceration of gravid uterus, third trimester** [3rd] [M] ♀
O34.519 **Maternal care for incarceration of gravid uterus, unspecified trimester** [M] ♀

[6th] O34.52 **Maternal care for prolapse of gravid uterus**

O34.521 **Maternal care for prolapse of gravid uterus, first trimester** [1st] [M] ♀
O34.522 **Maternal care for prolapse of gravid uterus, second trimester** [2nd] [M] ♀
O34.523 **Maternal care for prolapse of gravid uterus, third trimester** [3rd] [M] ♀
O34.529 **Maternal care for prolapse of gravid uterus, unspecified trimester** [M] ♀

[6th] O34.53 **Maternal care for retroversion of gravid uterus**

O34.531 **Maternal care for retroversion of gravid uterus, first trimester** [1st] [M] ♀
O34.532 **Maternal care for retroversion of gravid uterus, second trimester** [2nd] [M] ♀
O34.533 **Maternal care for retroversion of gravid uterus, third trimester** [3rd] [M] ♀
O34.539 **Maternal care for retroversion of gravid uterus, unspecified trimester** [M] ♀

[6th] O34.59 **Maternal care for other abnormalities of gravid uterus**

O34.591 **Maternal care for other abnormalities of gravid uterus, first trimester** [1st] [M] ♀
O34.592 **Maternal care for other abnormalities of gravid uterus, second trimester** [2nd] [M] ♀
O34.593 **Maternal care for other abnormalities of gravid uterus, third trimester** [3rd] [M] ♀
O34.599 **Maternal care for other abnormalities of gravid uterus, unspecified trimester** [M] ♀

[5th] O34.6 **Maternal care for abnormality of vagina**
[EXCLUDES2] *maternal care for vaginal varices in pregnancy (O22.1-)*

O34.60 **Maternal care for abnormality of vagina, unspecified trimester** [M] ♀
O34.61 **Maternal care for abnormality of vagina, first trimester** [1st] [M] ♀
O34.62 **Maternal care for abnormality of vagina, second trimester** [2nd] [M] ♀
O34.63 **Maternal care for abnormality of vagina, third trimester** [3rd] [M] ♀

[5th] O34.7 **Maternal care for abnormality of vulva and perineum**
[EXCLUDES2] *maternal care for perineal and vulval varices in pregnancy (O22.1-)*

O34.70 **Maternal care for abnormality of vulva and perineum, unspecified trimester** [M] ♀

[1st] 1st trimester [2nd] 2nd trimester [3rd] 3rd trimester [PDx] Unacceptable principal diagnosis symbol per Medicare code edits
[POA] Code exempt from diagnosis present on admission requirement [?] Questionable admission [CC] Complication or comorbidity
[CC/MCC Exc] CC/MCC exclusion [MCC] Major complication or comorbidity [PDx CC] Principal diagnosis as its own CC [PDx MCC] Principal diagnosis as its own MCC
[HCC] HCC diagnosis code [RxHCC] RxHCC diagnosis code MACRA code [Z-1] Z code as first-listed diagnosis

 When symbols appear on a code that requires a 7th character extension, refer to Appendix B to identify applicable 7th character codes.

O34.71 Maternal care for abnormality of vulva and perineum, first trimester [1st] M ♀

O34.72 Maternal care for abnormality of vulva and perineum, second trimester [2nd] M ♀

O34.73 Maternal care for abnormality of vulva and perineum, third trimester [3rd] M ♀

O34.8 Maternal care for other abnormalities of pelvic organs

O34.80 Maternal care for other abnormalities of pelvic organs, unspecified trimester M ♀

O34.81 Maternal care for other abnormalities of pelvic organs, first trimester [1st] M ♀

O34.82 Maternal care for other abnormalities of pelvic organs, second trimester [2nd] ♀

O34.83 Maternal care for other abnormalities of pelvic organs, third trimester [3rd] M ♀

O34.9 Maternal care for abnormality of pelvic organ, unspecified

O34.90 Maternal care for abnormality of pelvic organ, unspecified, unspecified trimester M ♀

O34.91 Maternal care for abnormality of pelvic organ, unspecified, first trimester [1st] M ♀

O34.92 Maternal care for abnormality of pelvic organ, unspecified, second trimester [2nd] M ♀

O34.93 Maternal care for abnormality of pelvic organ, unspecified, third trimester [3rd] M ♀

O35 Maternal care for known or suspected fetal abnormality and damage

INCLUDES   the listed conditions in the fetus as a reason for hospitalization or other obstetric care to the mother, or for termination of pregnancy

Code also any associated maternal condition

EXCLUDES1 encounter for suspected maternal and fetal conditions ruled out (Z03.7-)

One of the following 7th characters is to be assigned to each code under category O35. 7th character 0 is for single gestations and multiple gestations where the fetus is unspecified. 7th characters 1 through 9 are for cases of multiple gestations to identify the fetus for which the code applies. The appropriate code from category O30, Multiple gestation, must also be assigned when assigning a code from category O35 that has a 7th character of 1 through 9.

0 = not applicable or unspecified
1 = fetus 1
2 = fetus 2
3 = fetus 3
4 = fetus 4
5 = fetus 5
9 = other fetus

O35.0 Maternal care for (suspected) central nervous system malformation in fetus M ♀
Maternal care for fetal anencephaly
Maternal care for fetal hydrocephalus
Maternal care for fetal spina bifida
EXCLUDES2 chromosomal abnormality in fetus (O35.1)

O35.1 Maternal care for (suspected) chromosomal abnormality in fetus M ♀

O35.2 Maternal care for (suspected) hereditary disease in fetus M ♀
EXCLUDES2 chromosomal abnormality in fetus (O35.1)

O35.3 Maternal care for (suspected) damage to fetus from viral disease in mother M ♀
Maternal care for damage to fetus from maternal cytomegalovirus infection
Maternal care for damage to fetus from maternal rubella

O35.4 Maternal care for (suspected) damage to fetus from alcohol M ♀

O35.5 Maternal care for (suspected) damage to fetus by drugs M ♀
Maternal care for damage to fetus from drug addiction

O35.6 Maternal care for (suspected) damage to fetus by radiation M ♀

O35.7 Maternal care for (suspected) damage to fetus by other medical procedures M ♀
Maternal care for damage to fetus by amniocentesis
Maternal care for damage to fetus by biopsy procedures
Maternal care for damage to fetus by hematological investigation
Maternal care for damage to fetus by intrauterine contraceptive device
Maternal care for damage to fetus by intrauterine surgery

O35.8 Maternal care for other (suspected) fetal abnormality and damage M ♀
Maternal care for damage to fetus from maternal listeriosis
Maternal care for damage to fetus from maternal toxoplasmosis

O35.9 Maternal care for (suspected) fetal abnormality and damage, unspecified M ♀

O36 Maternal care for other fetal problems

INCLUDES   the listed conditions in the fetus as a reason for hospitalization or other obstetric care of the mother, or for termination of pregnancy

EXCLUDES1 encounter for suspected maternal and fetal conditions ruled out (Z03.7-)
placental transfusion syndromes (O43.0-)

EXCLUDES2 labor and delivery complicated by fetal stress (O77.-)

One of the following 7th characters is to be assigned to each code under category O36. 7th character 0 is for single gestations and multiple gestations where the fetus is unspecified. 7th characters 1 through 9 are for cases of multiple gestations to identify the fetus for which the code applies. The appropriate code from category O30, Multiple gestation, must also be assigned when assigning a code from category O36 that has a 7th character of 1 through 9.

0 = not applicable or unspecified
1 = fetus 1
2 = fetus 2
3 = fetus 3
4 = fetus 4
5 = fetus 5
9 = other fetus

O36.0 Maternal care for rhesus isoimmunization
Maternal care for Rh incompatibility (with hydrops fetalis)

O36.01 Maternal care for anti-D [Rh] antibodies

O36.011 Maternal care for anti-D [Rh] antibodies, first trimester [1st] M ♀ CC/MCC Exc.

O36.012 Maternal care for anti-D [Rh] antibodies, second trimester [2nd] M ♀ CC/MCC Exc.

O36.013 Maternal care for anti-D [Rh] antibodies, third trimester [3rd] M ♀ CC/MCC Exc.

O36.019 Maternal care for anti-D [Rh] antibodies, unspecified trimester M ♀

O36.09 Maternal care for other rhesus isoimmunization

O36.091 Maternal care for other rhesus isoimmunization, first trimester [1st] M ♀ CC/MCC Exc.

O36.092 Maternal care for other rhesus isoimmunization, second trimester [2nd] M ♀ CC/MCC Exc.

O36.093 Maternal care for other rhesus isoimmunization, third trimester [3rd] M ♀ CC/MCC Exc.

O36.099 Maternal care for other rhesus isoimmunization, unspecified trimester M ♀

O36.1 Maternal care for other isoimmunization
Maternal care for ABO isoimmunization

O36.11 Maternal care for Anti-A sensitization
Maternal care for isoimmunization NOS (with hydrops fetalis)

O36.111 Maternal care for Anti-A sensitization, first trimester [1st] M ♀

O36.112 Maternal care for Anti-A sensitization, second trimester [2nd] M ♀

O36.113 Maternal care for Anti-A sensitization, third trimester [3rd] M ♀

O36.119 Maternal care for Anti-A sensitization, unspecified trimester M ♀

Unspecified Code   Other Specified Code   Manifestation Code   N Newborn   P Pediatric   M Maternity   A Adult   ♂ Male   ♀ Female
● New Code   ▲ Revised Code Title   ▶◀ Revised Text   NOTES   INCLUDES   EXCLUDES 1 Not coded here   EXCLUDES 2 Not included here
4th character required   5th character required   6th character required   7th character required
Extension 'X' Alert   HAC Hospital-acquired condition (HAC) alert   AHA AHA Coding Clinic©

⑥ᵗʰ O36.19 **Maternal care for** other isoimmunization
Maternal care for Anti-B sensitization
- ⑦ᵗʰ O36.191 **Maternal care for other isoimmunization,** first trimester 1st M ♀
- ⑦ᵗʰ O36.192 **Maternal care for other isoimmunization,** second trimester 2nd M ♀
- ⑦ᵗʰ O36.193 **Maternal care for other isoimmunization,** third trimester 3rd M ♀
- ⑦ᵗʰ O36.199 **Maternal care for other isoimmunization, unspecified trimester** M ♀

⑤ᵗʰ O36.2 **Maternal care for** hydrops fetalis
Maternal care for hydrops fetalis NOS
Maternal care for hydrops fetalis not associated with isoimmunization
EXCLUDES1 hydrops fetalis associated with ABO isoimmunization (O36.1-)
hydrops fetalis associated with rhesus isoimmunization (O36.0-)
- ⑦ᵗʰ O36.20 **Maternal care for hydrops fetalis, unspecified trimester** M ♀
- ⑦ᵗʰ O36.21 **Maternal care for hydrops fetalis,** first trimester 1st M ♀
- ⑦ᵗʰ O36.22 **Maternal care for hydrops fetalis,** second trimester 2nd M ♀
- ⑦ᵗʰ O36.23 **Maternal care for hydrops fetalis,** third trimester 3rd M ♀

⑦ᵗʰ O36.4 **Maternal care for** intrauterine death M cc ♀ CC/MCC Exc
Maternal care for intrauterine fetal death NOS
Maternal care for intrauterine fetal death after completion of 20 weeks of gestation
Maternal care for late fetal death
Maternal care for missed delivery
EXCLUDES1 missed abortion (O02.1) ⟨20 weeks
stillbirth (P95)

⑤ᵗʰ O36.5 **Maternal care for** known or suspected poor fetal growth
⑥ᵗʰ O36.51 **Maternal care for known or suspected** placental insufficiency
- ⑦ᵗʰ O36.511 **Maternal care for known or suspected placental insufficiency,** first trimester 1st M ♀
- ⑦ᵗʰ O36.512 **Maternal care for known or suspected placental insufficiency,** second trimester 2nd M ♀
- ⑦ᵗʰ O36.513 **Maternal care for known or suspected placental insufficiency,** third trimester 3rd M ♀
- ⑦ᵗʰ O36.519 **Maternal care for known or suspected placental insufficiency,** unspecified trimester M ♀
⑥ᵗʰ O36.59 **Maternal care for** other known or suspected poor fetal growth
Maternal care for known or suspected light-for-dates NOS
Maternal care for known or suspected small-for-dates NOS
- ⑦ᵗʰ O36.591 **Maternal care for other known or suspected poor fetal growth,** first trimester 1st M ♀
- ⑦ᵗʰ O36.592 **Maternal care for other known or suspected poor fetal growth,** second trimester 2nd M ♀
- ⑦ᵗʰ O36.593 **Maternal care for other known or suspected poor fetal growth,** third trimester 3rd M ♀
- ⑦ᵗʰ O36.599 **Maternal care for other known or suspected poor fetal growth, unspecified trimester** M ♀

⑤ᵗʰ O36.6 **Maternal care for** excessive fetal growth
Maternal care for known or suspected large-for-dates
- ⑦ᵗʰ O36.60 **Maternal care for excessive fetal growth, unspecified trimester** M ♀

⑦ᵗʰ O36.61 **Maternal care for excessive fetal growth,** first trimester 1st M ♀
⑦ᵗʰ O36.62 **Maternal care for excessive fetal growth,** second trimester 2nd M ♀
⑦ᵗʰ O36.63 **Maternal care for excessive fetal growth,** third trimester 3rd M ♀

⑤ᵗʰ O36.7 **Maternal care for** viable fetus in abdominal pregnancy
- ⑦ᵗʰ O36.70 **Maternal care for viable fetus in abdominal pregnancy, unspecified trimester** M ♀
- ⑦ᵗʰ O36.71 **Maternal care for viable fetus in abdominal pregnancy,** first trimester 1st M ♀
- ⑦ᵗʰ O36.72 **Maternal care for viable fetus in abdominal pregnancy,** second trimester 2nd M ♀
- ⑦ᵗʰ O36.73 **Maternal care for viable fetus in abdominal pregnancy,** third trimester 3rd M ♀

⑤ᵗʰ O36.8 **Maternal care for** other specified fetal problems
- ⑦ᵗʰ O36.80 **Pregnancy with inconclusive fetal viability** M ♀ PDxIn
Encounter to determine fetal viability of pregnancy
⑥ᵗʰ O36.81 **Decreased fetal movements**
- ⑦ᵗʰ O36.812 **Decreased fetal movements,** second trimester 2nd M ♀
- ⑦ᵗʰ O36.813 **Decreased fetal movements,** third trimester 3rd M ♀
- ⑦ᵗʰ O36.819 **Decreased fetal movements, unspecified trimester** M ♀
⑥ᵗʰ O36.82 **Fetal anemia and thrombocytopenia**
- ⑦ᵗʰ O36.821 **Fetal anemia and thrombocytopenia,** first trimester 1st M ♀
- ⑦ᵗʰ O36.822 **Fetal anemia and thrombocytopenia,** second trimester 2nd M ♀
- ⑦ᵗʰ O36.823 **Fetal anemia and thrombocytopenia,** third trimester 3rd M ♀
- ⑦ᵗʰ O36.829 **Fetal anemia and thrombocytopenia, unspecified trimester** M ♀
● ⑥ᵗʰ O36.83 **Maternal care for abnormalities of the fetal heart rate or rhythm**
- ● ⑦ᵗʰ O36.831 **Maternal care for abnormalities of the fetal heart rate or rhythm,** first trimester 1st M ♀
- ● ⑦ᵗʰ O36.832 **Maternal care for abnormalities of the fetal heart rate or rhythm,** second trimester 2nd M ♀
- ● ⑦ᵗʰ O36.833 **Maternal care for abnormalities of the fetal heart rate or rhythm,** third trimester 3rd M ♀
- ● ⑦ᵗʰ O36.839 **Maternal care for abnormalities of the fetal heart rate or rhythm, unspecified trimester** M ♀
⑥ᵗʰ O36.89 **Maternal care for other specified fetal problems**
- ⑦ᵗʰ O36.891 **Maternal care for other specified fetal problems,** first trimester 1st M ♀
- ⑦ᵗʰ O36.892 **Maternal care for other specified fetal problems,** second trimester 2nd M ♀
- ⑦ᵗʰ O36.893 **Maternal care for other specified fetal problems,** third trimester 3rd M ♀
- ⑦ᵗʰ O36.899 **Maternal care for other specified fetal problems, unspecified trimester** M ♀

⑤ᵗʰ O36.9 **Maternal care for** fetal problem, unspecified
- ⑦ᵗʰ O36.90 **Maternal care for fetal problem, unspecified, unspecified trimester** M ♀
- ⑦ᵗʰ O36.91 **Maternal care for fetal problem, unspecified,** first trimester 1st M ♀
- ⑦ᵗʰ O36.92 **Maternal care for fetal problem, unspecified,** second trimester 2nd M ♀
- ⑦ᵗʰ O36.93 **Maternal care for fetal problem, unspecified,** third trimester 3rd M ♀

④ᵗʰ O40 **Polyhydramnios**
INCLUDES hydramnios
EXCLUDES1 encounter for suspected maternal and fetal conditions ruled out (Z03.7-)

1st 1st trimester 2nd 2nd trimester 3rd 3rd trimester PDx Unacceptable principal diagnosis symbol per Medicare code edits
POA Code exempt from diagnosis present on admission requirement ? Questionable admission cc Complication or comorbidity
CC/MCC Exc CC/MCC exclusion MCC Major complication or comorbidity Principal diagnosis as its own CC Principal diagnosis as its own MCC
HCC HCC diagnosis code RxHCC RxHCC diagnosis code MACRA code Z1 Z code as first-listed diagnosis

When symbols appear on a code that requires a 7th character extension, refer to Appendix B to identify applicable 7th character codes.
2018 ICD-10-CM

One of the following 7th characters is to be assigned to each code under category O40. 7th character 0 is for single gestations and multiple gestations where the fetus is unspecified. 7th characters 1 through 9 are for cases of multiple gestations to identify the fetus for which the code applies. The appropriate code from category O30, Multiple gestation, must also be assigned when assigning a code from category O40 that has a 7th character of 1 through 9.

0 = not applicable or unspecified
1 = fetus 1
2 = fetus 2
3 = fetus 3
4 = fetus 4
5 = fetus 5
9 = other fetus

7️⃣ O40.1 Polyhydramnios, first trimester   1st M ♀
7️⃣ O40.2 Polyhydramnios, second trimester   2nd M ♀
7️⃣ O40.3 Polyhydramnios, third trimester   3rd M ♀
7️⃣ O40.9 Polyhydramnios, unspecified trimester   M ♀

4️⃣ O41 Other disorders of amniotic fluid and membranes

EXCLUDES1 *encounter for suspected maternal and fetal conditions ruled out (Z03.7-)*

One of the following 7th characters is to be assigned to each code under category O41. 7th character 0 is for single gestations and multiple gestations where the fetus is unspecified. 7th characters 1 through 9 are for cases of multiple gestations to identify the fetus for which the code applies. The appropriate code from category O30, Multiple gestation, must also be assigned when assigning a code from category O41 that has a 7th character of 1 through 9.

0 = not applicable or unspecified
1 = fetus 1
2 = fetus 2
3 = fetus 3
4 = fetus 4
5 = fetus 5
9 = other fetus

5️⃣ O41.0 Oligohydramnios

Oligohydramnios without rupture of membranes

7️⃣ O41.00 Oligohydramnios, unspecified trimester   M ♀
7️⃣ O41.01 Oligohydramnios, first trimester   1st M ♀ CC/MCC Exc
7️⃣ O41.02 Oligohydramnios, second trimester   2nd M ♀ CC/MCC Exc
7️⃣ O41.03 Oligohydramnios, third trimester   3rd M ♀ CC/MCC Exc

5️⃣ O41.1 Infection of amniotic sac and membranes

6️⃣ O41.10 Infection of amniotic sac and membranes, unspecified

7️⃣ O41.101 Infection of amniotic sac and membranes, unspecified, first trimester   1st M MCC ♀ CC/MCC Exc
7️⃣ O41.102 Infection of amniotic sac and membranes, unspecified, second trimester   2nd M MCC ♀ CC/MCC Exc
7️⃣ O41.103 Infection of amniotic sac and membranes, unspecified, third trimester   3rd M MCC ♀ CC/MCC Exc
7️⃣ O41.109 Infection of amniotic sac and membranes, unspecified trimester   M ♀

6️⃣ O41.12 Chorioamnionitis

7️⃣ O41.121 Chorioamnionitis, first trimester   1st M MCC ♀ CC/MCC Exc
7️⃣ O41.122 Chorioamnionitis, second trimester   2nd M MCC ♀ CC/MCC Exc
7️⃣ O41.123 Chorioamnionitis, third trimester   3rd M MCC ♀ CC/MCC Exc
7️⃣ O41.129 Chorioamnionitis, unspecified trimester   M ♀

6️⃣ O41.14 Placentitis

7️⃣ O41.141 Placentitis, first trimester   1st M MCC ♀ CC/MCC Exc
7️⃣ O41.142 Placentitis, second trimester   2nd M MCC ♀ CC/MCC Exc
7️⃣ O41.143 Placentitis, third trimester   3rd M MCC ♀ CC/MCC Exc
7️⃣ O41.149 Placentitis, unspecified trimester   M ♀

5️⃣ O41.8 Other specified disorders of amniotic fluid and membranes

6️⃣ O41.8X Other specified disorders of amniotic fluid and membranes

7️⃣ O41.8X1 Other specified disorders of amniotic fluid and membranes, first trimester   1st M ♀
7️⃣ O41.8X2 Other specified disorders of amniotic fluid and membranes, second trimester   2nd M ♀
7️⃣ O41.8X3 Other specified disorders of amniotic fluid and membranes, third trimester   3rd M ♀
7️⃣ O41.8X9 Other specified disorders of amniotic fluid and membranes, unspecified trimester   M ♀

5️⃣ O41.9 Disorder of amniotic fluid and membranes, unspecified

7️⃣ O41.90 Disorder of amniotic fluid and membranes, unspecified, unspecified trimester   M ♀
7️⃣ O41.91 Disorder of amniotic fluid and membranes, unspecified, first trimester   1st M ♀
7️⃣ O41.92 Disorder of amniotic fluid and membranes, unspecified, second trimester   2nd M ♀
7️⃣ O41.93 Disorder of amniotic fluid and membranes, unspecified, third trimester   3rd M ♀

4️⃣ O42 Premature rupture of membranes

5️⃣ O42.0 Premature rupture of membranes, onset of labor within 24 hours of rupture

O42.00 Premature rupture of membranes, onset of labor within 24 hours of rupture, unspecified weeks of gestation   M ♀

6️⃣ O42.01 Preterm premature rupture of membranes, onset of labor within 24 hours of rupture

Premature rupture of membranes before 37 completed weeks of gestation

O42.011 Preterm premature rupture of membranes, onset of labor within 24 hours of rupture, first trimester   1st M ♀
O42.012 Preterm premature rupture of membranes, onset of labor within 24 hours of rupture, second trimester   2nd M ♀
O42.013 Preterm premature rupture of membranes, onset of labor within 24 hours of rupture, third trimester   3rd M ♀
O42.019 Preterm premature rupture of membranes, onset of labor within 24 hours of rupture, unspecified trimester   M ♀

O42.02 Full-term premature rupture of membranes, onset of labor within 24 hours of rupture   M ♀

Premature rupture of membranes at or after 37 completed weeks of gestation, onset of labor within 24 hours of rupture

5️⃣ O42.1 Premature rupture of membranes, onset of labor more than 24 hours following rupture

O42.10 Premature rupture of membranes, onset of labor more than 24 hours following rupture, unspecified weeks of gestation   M ♀

6️⃣ O42.11 Preterm premature rupture of membranes, onset of labor more than 24 hours following rupture

Premature rupture of membranes before 37 completed weeks of gestation

O42.111 Preterm premature rupture of membranes, onset of labor more than 24 hours following rupture, first trimester   1st M ♀
O42.112 Preterm premature rupture of membranes, onset of labor more than 24 hours following rupture, second trimester   2nd M ♀
O42.113 Preterm premature rupture of membranes, onset of labor more than 24 hours following rupture, third trimester   3rd M ♀
O42.119 Preterm premature rupture of membranes, onset of labor more than 24 hours following rupture, unspecified trimester   M ♀

Unspecified Code   Other Specified Code   Manifestation Code   N Newborn   P Pediatric   M Maternity   A Adult   ♂ Male   ♀ Female
● New Code   ▲ Revised Code Title   ►◄ Revised Text   NOTES   *INCLUDES*   EXCLUDES 1 Not coded here   EXCLUDES 2 Not included here
4️⃣ 4th character required   5️⃣ 5th character required   6️⃣ 6th character required   7️⃣ 7th character required
❎ Extension 'X' Alert   HAC Hospital-acquired condition (HAC) alert   **AHA** AHA Coding Clinic©

O75.3 Other infection during labor [M] MCC ♀ CC/MCC Exc
Sepsis during labor
Use additional code (B95-B97), to identify infectious agent

O75.4 Other complications of obstetric surgery and procedures [M] ♀
Cardiac arrest following obstetric surgery or procedures
Cardiac failure following obstetric surgery or procedures
Cerebral anoxia following obstetric surgery or procedures
Pulmonary edema following obstetric surgery or procedures
Use additional code to identify specific complication

[EXCLUDES2] *complications of anesthesia during labor and delivery (O74.-)*
disruption of obstetrical (surgical) wound (O90.0-O90.1)
hematoma of obstetrical (surgical) wound (O90.2)
infection of obstetrical (surgical) wound (O86.0)

O75.5 Delayed delivery after artificial rupture of membranes [M] ♀

[5th] **O75.8 Other specified complications of labor and delivery**

O75.81 Maternal exhaustion complicating labor and delivery [M] ♀

O75.82 Onset (spontaneous) of labor after 37 completed weeks of gestation but before 39 completed weeks gestation, with delivery by (planned) cesarean section [3rd] [M] ♀
Delivery by (planned) cesarean section occurring after 37 completed weeks of gestation but before 39 completed weeks gestation due to (spontaneous) onset of labor
Code first to specify reason for planned cesarean section such as:
cephalopelvic disproportion (normally formed fetus) (O33.9)
previous cesarean delivery (O34.21)

O75.89 Other specified complications of labor and delivery [M] ♀

O75.9 Complication of labor and delivery, unspecified [M] ♀

O76 Abnormality in fetal heart rate and rhythm complicating labor and delivery [M] ♀
AHA: Q4 2013
Depressed fetal heart rate tones complicating labor and delivery
Fetal bradycardia complicating labor and delivery
Fetal heart rate decelerations complicating labor and delivery
Fetal heart rate irregularity complicating labor and delivery
Fetal heart rate abnormal variability complicating labor and delivery
Fetal tachycardia complicating labor and delivery
Non-reassuring fetal heart rate or rhythm complicating labor and delivery

[EXCLUDES1] *fetal stress NOS (O77.9)*
labor and delivery complicated by electrocardiographic evidence of fetal stress (O77.8)
labor and delivery complicated by ultrasonic evidence of fetal stress (O77.8)

[EXCLUDES2] *fetal metabolic acidemia (O68)*
other fetal stress (O77.0-O77.1)

[4th] **O77 Other fetal stress complicating labor and delivery**

O77.0 Labor and delivery complicated by meconium in amniotic fluid [M] ♀
AHA: Q4 2013

O77.1 Fetal stress in labor or delivery due to drug administration [M] ♀

O77.8 Labor and delivery complicated by other evidence of fetal stress [M] ♀
Labor and delivery complicated by electrocardiographic evidence of fetal stress
Labor and delivery complicated by ultrasonic evidence of fetal stress

[EXCLUDES1] *abnormality of fetal acid-base balance (O68)*
abnormality in fetal heart rate or rhythm (O76)
fetal metabolic acidemia (O68)

O77.9 Labor and delivery complicated by fetal stress, unspecified [M] ♀

[EXCLUDES1] *abnormality of fetal acid-base balance (O68)*
abnormality in fetal heart rate or rhythm (O76)
fetal metabolic acidemia (O68)

Encounter for delivery (O80-O82)

O80 Encounter for full-term uncomplicated delivery [M] POA ♀
AHA: Q4 2016
Delivery requiring minimal or no assistance, with or without episiotomy, without fetal manipulation [e.g., rotation version] or instrumentation [forceps] of a spontaneous, cephalic, vaginal, full-term, single, live-born infant. This code is for use as a single diagnosis code and is not to be used with any other code from chapter 15.
Use additional code to indicate outcome of delivery (Z37.0)

O82 Encounter for cesarean delivery without indication [M] ♀
Use additional code to indicate outcome of delivery (Z37.0)
schedule c-section

Complications predominantly related to the puerperium (O85-O92)

[EXCLUDES2] *mental and behavioral disorders associated with the puerperium (F53)*
obstetrical tetanus (A34)
puerperal osteomalacia (M83.0)

O85 Puerperal sepsis [M] MCC ♀ CC/MCC Exc
Postpartum sepsis
Puerperal peritonitis
Puerperal pyemia
Use additional code (B95-B97), to identify infectious agent
Use additional code (R65.2-) to identify severe sepsis, if applicable

[EXCLUDES1] *fever of unknown origin following delivery (O86.4)*
genital tract infection following delivery (O86.1-)
obstetric pyemic and septic embolism (O88.3-)
puerperal septic thrombophlebitis (O86.81)
urinary tract infection following delivery (O86.2-)

[EXCLUDES2] *sepsis during labor (O75.3)*

[4th] **O86 Other puerperal infections**
Use additional code (B95-B97), to identify infectious agent

[EXCLUDES2] *infection during labor (O75.3)*
obstetrical tetanus (A34)

O86.0 Infection of obstetric surgical wound [M] ♀
Infected cesarean delivery wound following delivery
Infected perineal repair following delivery

[5th] **O86.1 Other infection of genital tract following delivery**

O86.11 Cervicitis following delivery [M] CC ♀ CC/MCC Exc
O86.12 Endometritis following delivery [M] CC ♀ CC/MCC Exc
O86.13 Vaginitis following delivery [M] CC ♀ CC/MCC Exc
O86.19 Other infection of genital tract following delivery [M] CC ♀ CC/MCC Exc

[5th] **O86.2 Urinary tract infection following delivery**

O86.20 Urinary tract infection following delivery, unspecified [M] CC ♀ CC/MCC Exc
Puerperal urinary tract infection NOS
O86.21 Infection of kidney following delivery [M] CC ♀ CC/MCC Exc
O86.22 Infection of bladder following delivery [M] CC ♀ CC/MCC Exc
Infection of urethra following delivery
O86.29 Other urinary tract infection following delivery [M] CC ♀ CC/MCC Exc

O86.4 Pyrexia of unknown origin following delivery [M] CC ♀ CC/MCC Exc
Puerperal infection NOS following delivery
Puerperal pyrexia NOS following delivery

[EXCLUDES2] *pyrexia during labor (O75.2)*

[5th] **O86.8 Other specified puerperal infections**

O86.81 Puerperal septic thrombophlebitis [M] MCC ♀ CC/MCC Exc
O86.89 Other specified puerperal infections [M] MCC ♀ CC/MCC Exc

[4th] **O87 Venous complications and hemorrhoids in the puerperium**

[INCLUDES] *venous complications in labor, delivery and the puerperium*

[EXCLUDES2] *obstetric embolism (O88.-)*
puerperal septic thrombophlebitis (O86.81)
venous complications in pregnancy (O22.-)

[1st] 1st trimester [2nd] 2nd trimester [3rd] 3rd trimester PDx Unacceptable principal diagnosis symbol per Medicare code edits
POA Code exempt from diagnosis present on admission requirement [?] Questionable admission CC Complication or comorbidity
CC/MCC Exc CC/MCC exclusion MCC Major complication or comorbidity PDx CC Principal diagnosis as its own CC PDx MCC Principal diagnosis as its own MCC
[HCC] HCC diagnosis code [RxHCC] RxHCC diagnosis code MACRA code [Z1] Z code as first-listed diagnosis

 When symbols appear on a code that requires a 7th character extension, refer to Appendix B to identify applicable 7th character codes.

O87.0 Superficial thrombophlebitis in the puerperium [M] CC ♀ CC/MCC Exc
Puerperal phlebitis NOS
Puerperal thrombosis NOS

O87.1 Deep phlebothrombosis in the puerperium [M] MCC ♀ CC/MCC Exc
Deep vein thrombosis, postpartum
Pelvic thrombophlebitis, postpartum
Use additional code to identify the deep vein thrombosis (I82.4-, I82.5-, I82.62-. I82.72-)
Use additional code, if applicable, for associated long-term (current) use of anticoagulants (Z79.01)

O87.2 Hemorrhoids in the puerperium [M] CC ♀ CC/MCC Exc

O87.3 Cerebral venous thrombosis in the puerperium [M] CC ♀ CC/MCC Exc
Cerebrovenous sinus thrombosis in the puerperium

O87.4 Varicose veins of lower extremity in the puerperium [M] ♀

O87.8 Other venous complications in the puerperium [M] CC ♀ CC/MCC Exc
Genital varices in the puerperium

O87.9 Venous complication in the puerperium, unspecified [M] ♀
Puerperal phlebopathy NOS

[4th] O88 Obstetric embolism

[EXCLUDES1] *embolism complicating abortion NOS (O03.2)*
embolism complicating ectopic or molar pregnancy (O08.2)
embolism complicating failed attempted abortion (O07.2)
embolism complicating induced abortion (O04.7)
embolism complicating spontaneous abortion (O03.2, O03.7)

[5th] O88.0 Obstetric air embolism

[6th] O88.01 Obstetric air embolism in pregnancy
O88.011 Air embolism in pregnancy, first trimester [1st] [M] MCC ♀ CC/MCC Exc
O88.012 Air embolism in pregnancy, second trimester [2nd] [M] MCC ♀ CC/MCC Exc
O88.013 Air embolism in pregnancy, third trimester [3rd] [M] MCC ♀ CC/MCC Exc
O88.019 Air embolism in pregnancy, unspecified trimester [M] ♀

O88.02 Air embolism in childbirth [M] MCC ♀ CC/MCC Exc
O88.03 Air embolism in the puerperium [M] MCC ♀ CC/MCC Exc

[5th] O88.1 Amniotic fluid embolism
Anaphylactoid syndrome in pregnancy

[6th] O88.11 Amniotic fluid embolism in pregnancy
O88.111 Amniotic fluid embolism in pregnancy, first trimester [1st] [M] MCC ♀ CC/MCC Exc
O88.112 Amniotic fluid embolism in pregnancy, second trimester [2nd] [M] MCC ♀ CC/MCC Exc
O88.113 Amniotic fluid embolism in pregnancy, third trimester [3rd] [M] MCC ♀ CC/MCC Exc
O88.119 Amniotic fluid embolism in pregnancy, unspecified trimester [M] ♀

O88.12 Amniotic fluid embolism in childbirth [M] MCC ♀ CC/MCC Exc
O88.13 Amniotic fluid embolism in the puerperium [M] MCC ♀ CC/MCC Exc

[5th] O88.2 Obstetric thromboembolism

[6th] O88.21 Thromboembolism in pregnancy
Obstetric (pulmonary) embolism NOS
O88.211 Thromboembolism in pregnancy, first trimester [1st] [M] MCC ♀ CC/MCC Exc
O88.212 Thromboembolism in pregnancy, second trimester [2nd] [M] MCC ♀ CC/MCC Exc
O88.213 Thromboembolism in pregnancy, third trimester [3rd] [M] MCC ♀ CC/MCC Exc
O88.219 Thromboembolism in pregnancy, unspecified trimester [M] ♀

O88.22 Thromboembolism in childbirth [M] MCC ♀ CC/MCC Exc
O88.23 Thromboembolism in the puerperium [M] MCC ♀ CC/MCC Exc
Puerperal (pulmonary) embolism NOS

[5th] O88.3 Obstetric pyemic and septic embolism

[6th] O88.31 Pyemic and septic embolism in pregnancy
O88.311 Pyemic and septic embolism in pregnancy, first trimester [1st] [M] MCC ♀ CC/MCC Exc
O88.312 Pyemic and septic embolism in pregnancy, second trimester [2nd] [M] MCC ♀ CC/MCC Exc
O88.313 Pyemic and septic embolism in pregnancy, third trimester [3rd] [M] MCC ♀ CC/MCC Exc
O88.319 Pyemic and septic embolism in pregnancy, unspecified trimester [M] CC ♀ CC/MCC Exc

O88.32 Pyemic and septic embolism in childbirth [M] MCC ♀ CC/MCC Exc
O88.33 Pyemic and septic embolism in the puerperium [M] MCC ♀ CC/MCC Exc

[5th] O88.8 Other obstetric embolism
Obstetric fat embolism

[6th] O88.81 Other embolism in pregnancy
O88.811 Other embolism in pregnancy, first trimester [1st] [M] MCC ♀ CC/MCC Exc
O88.812 Other embolism in pregnancy, second trimester [2nd] [M] MCC ♀ CC/MCC Exc
O88.813 Other embolism in pregnancy, third trimester [3rd] [M] MCC ♀ CC/MCC Exc
O88.819 Other embolism in pregnancy, unspecified trimester [M] ♀

O88.82 Other embolism in childbirth [M] MCC ♀ CC/MCC Exc
O88.83 Other embolism in the puerperium [M] MCC ♀ CC/MCC Exc

[4th] O89 Complications of anesthesia during the puerperium

[INCLUDES] *maternal complications arising from the administration of a general, regional or local anesthetic, analgesic or other sedation during the puerperium*

Use additional code, if applicable, to identify specific complication

[5th] O89.0 Pulmonary complications of anesthesia during the puerperium

O89.01 Aspiration pneumonitis due to anesthesia during the puerperium [M] ♀
Inhalation of stomach contents or secretions NOS due to anesthesia during the puerperium
Mendelson's syndrome due to anesthesia during the puerperium

O89.09 Other pulmonary complications of anesthesia during the puerperium [M] ♀

O89.1 Cardiac complications of anesthesia during the puerperium [M] ♀

O89.2 Central nervous system complications of anesthesia during the puerperium [M] ♀

O89.3 Toxic reaction to local anesthesia during the puerperium [M] ♀

O89.4 Spinal and epidural anesthesia-induced headache during the puerperium [M] ♀

O89.5 Other complications of spinal and epidural anesthesia during the puerperium [M] ♀

O89.6 Failed or difficult intubation for anesthesia during the puerperium [M] ♀

O89.8 Other complications of anesthesia during the puerperium [M] ♀

O89.9 Complication of anesthesia during the puerperium, unspecified [M] ♀

[4th] O90 Complications of the puerperium, not elsewhere classified

O90.0 Disruption of cesarean delivery wound [M] ♀
Dehiscence of cesarean delivery wound
[EXCLUDES1] *rupture of uterus (spontaneous) before onset of labor (O71.0-)*
rupture of uterus during labor (O71.1)

O90.1 Disruption of perineal obstetric wound [M] ♀
Disruption of wound of episiotomy
Disruption of wound of perineal laceration
Secondary perineal tear

O90.2 Hematoma of obstetric wound [M] ♀

O90.3 Peripartum cardiomyopathy [M] MCC ♀ CC/MCC Exc
Conditions in I42.- arising during pregnancy and the puerperium
[EXCLUDES1] *pre-existing heart disease complicating pregnancy and the puerperium (O99.4-)*

O90.4 Postpartum acute kidney failure [M] MCC ♀ CC/MCC Exc
Hepatorenal syndrome following labor and delivery

O90.5 Postpartum thyroiditis [M] ♀

P56.9 Hydrops fetalis due to other and unspecified hemolytic disease

P56.90 Hydrops fetalis due to unspecified hemolytic disease `MCC` `CC/MCC Exc`

P56.99 Hydrops fetalis due to other hemolytic disease `MCC` `CC/MCC Exc`

P57 Kernicterus

P57.0 Kernicterus due to isoimmunization `MCC` `CC/MCC Exc`

P57.8 Other specified kernicterus `MCC` `CC/MCC Exc`

EXCLUDES1 *Crigler-Najjar syndrome (E80.5)*

P57.9 Kernicterus, unspecified `MCC` `CC/MCC Exc`

P58 Neonatal jaundice due to other excessive hemolysis

EXCLUDES1 *jaundice due to isoimmunization (P55-P57)*

P58.0 Neonatal jaundice due to bruising

P58.1 Neonatal jaundice due to bleeding

P58.2 Neonatal jaundice due to infection

P58.3 Neonatal jaundice due to polycythemia

P58.4 Neonatal jaundice due to drugs or toxins transmitted from mother or given to newborn

Code first poisoning due to drug or toxin, if applicable (T36-T65 with fifth or sixth character 1-4 or 6)

Use additional code for adverse effect, if applicable, to identify drug (T36-T50 with fifth or sixth character 5)

P58.41 Neonatal jaundice due to drugs or toxins transmitted from mother

P58.42 Neonatal jaundice due to drugs or toxins given to newborn

P58.5 Neonatal jaundice due to swallowed maternal blood

P58.8 Neonatal jaundice due to other specified excessive hemolysis

P58.9 Neonatal jaundice due to excessive hemolysis, unspecified

P59 Neonatal jaundice from other and unspecified causes

EXCLUDES1 *jaundice due to inborn errors of metabolism (E70-E88)*

kernicterus (P57.-)

P59.0 Neonatal jaundice associated with preterm delivery

Hyperbilirubinemia of prematurity

Jaundice due to delayed conjugation associated with preterm delivery

P59.1 Inspissated bile syndrome `MCC` `CC/MCC Exc`

P59.2 Neonatal jaundice from other and unspecified hepatocellular damage

EXCLUDES1 *congenital viral hepatitis (P35.3)*

P59.20 Neonatal jaundice from unspecified hepatocellular damage `MCC` `CC/MCC Exc`

P59.29 Neonatal jaundice from other hepatocellular damage

Neonatal giant cell hepatitis

Neonatal (idiopathic) hepatitis

P59.3 Neonatal jaundice from breast milk inhibitor

P59.8 Neonatal jaundice from other specified causes

P59.9 Neonatal jaundice, unspecified

AHA: Q3 2015

Neonatal physiological jaundice (intense)(prolonged) NOS

P60 Disseminated intravascular coagulation of newborn `MCC` `CC/MCC Exc`

Defibrination syndrome of newborn

P61 Other perinatal hematological disorders

EXCLUDES1 *transient hypogammaglobulinemia of infancy (D80.7)*

P61.0 Transient neonatal thrombocytopenia `MCC` `CC/MCC Exc`

Neonatal thrombocytopenia due to exchange transfusion

Neonatal thrombocytopenia due to idiopathic maternal thrombocytopenia

Neonatal thrombocytopenia due to isoimmunization

P61.1 Polycythemia neonatorum

P61.2 Anemia of prematurity `CC` `CC/MCC Exc`

P61.3 Congenital anemia from fetal blood loss `CC` `CC/MCC Exc`

P61.4 Other congenital anemias, not elsewhere classified `CC` `CC/MCC Exc`

Congenital anemia NOS

P61.5 Transient neonatal neutropenia `MCC` `CC/MCC Exc`

EXCLUDES1 *congenital neutropenia (nontransient) (D70.0)*

P61.6 Other transient neonatal disorders of coagulation `CC` `CC/MCC Exc`

P61.8 Other specified perinatal hematological disorders

P61.9 Perinatal hematological disorder, unspecified

Transitory endocrine and metabolic disorders specific to newborn (P70-P74)

INCLUDES *transitory endocrine and metabolic disturbances caused by the infant's response to maternal endocrine and metabolic factors, or its adjustment to extrauterine environment*

P70 Transitory disorders of carbohydrate metabolism specific to newborn

P70.0 Syndrome of infant of mother with gestational diabetes

Newborn (with hypoglycemia) affected by maternal gestational diabetes

EXCLUDES1 *newborn (with hypoglycemia) affected by maternal (pre-existing) diabetes mellitus (P70.1)*

syndrome of infant of a diabetic mother (P70.1)

P70.1 Syndrome of infant of a diabetic mother

Newborn (with hypoglycemia) affected by maternal (pre-existing) diabetes mellitus

EXCLUDES1 *newborn (with hypoglycemia) affected by maternal gestational diabetes (P70.0)*

syndrome of infant of mother with gestational diabetes (P70.0)

P70.2 Neonatal diabetes mellitus `CC` `CC/MCC Exc`

P70.3 Iatrogenic neonatal hypoglycemia

P70.4 Other neonatal hypoglycemia

Transitory neonatal hypoglycemia

P70.8 Other transitory disorders of carbohydrate metabolism of newborn `CC` `CC/MCC Exc`

P70.9 Transitory disorder of carbohydrate metabolism of newborn, unspecified

P71 Transitory neonatal disorders of calcium and magnesium metabolism

P71.0 Cow's milk hypocalcemia in newborn `CC` `CC/MCC Exc`

P71.1 Other neonatal hypocalcemia `CC` `CC/MCC Exc`

EXCLUDES1 *neonatal hypoparathyroidism (P71.4)*

P71.2 Neonatal hypomagnesemia `CC` `CC/MCC Exc`

P71.3 Neonatal tetany without calcium or magnesium deficiency `CC` `CC/MCC Exc`

Neonatal tetany NOS

P71.4 Transitory neonatal hypoparathyroidism `CC` `CC/MCC Exc`

P71.8 Other transitory neonatal disorders of calcium and magnesium metabolism `CC` `CC/MCC Exc`

AHA: Q4 2016

P71.9 Transitory neonatal disorder of calcium and magnesium metabolism, unspecified `CC` `CC/MCC Exc`

P72 Other transitory neonatal endocrine disorders

EXCLUDES1 *congenital hypothyroidism with or without goiter (E03.0-E03.1)*

dyshormogenetic goiter (E07.1)

Pendred's syndrome (E07.1)

P72.0 Neonatal goiter, not elsewhere classified `CC` `CC/MCC Exc`

Transitory congenital goiter with normal functioning

P72.1 Transitory neonatal hyperthyroidism `CC` `CC/MCC Exc`

Neonatal thyrotoxicosis

P72.2 Other transitory neonatal disorders of thyroid function, not elsewhere classified `CC` `CC/MCC Exc`

Transitory neonatal hypothyroidism

P72.8 Other specified transitory neonatal endocrine disorders `CC` `CC/MCC Exc`

P72.9 Transitory neonatal endocrine disorder, unspecified

P74 Other transitory neonatal electrolyte and metabolic disturbances

P74.0 Late metabolic acidosis of newborn `MCC` `CC/MCC Exc`

EXCLUDES1 *(fetal) metabolic acidosis of newborn (P19)*

P74.1 Dehydration of newborn

P74.2 Disturbances of sodium balance of newborn

P74.3 Disturbances of potassium balance of newborn

P74.4 Other transitory electrolyte disturbances of newborn

P74.5 Transitory tyrosinemia of newborn `CC` `CC/MCC Exc`

P74.6 Transitory hyperammonemia of newborn `CC` `CC/MCC Exc`

`PDx` Unacceptable principal diagnosis symbol per Medicare code edits   `POA` Code exempt from diagnosis present on admission requirement
`?` Questionable admission   `CC` Complication or comorbidity   `CC/MCC Exc` CC/MCC exclusion   `MCC` Major complication or comorbidity
`PDx CC` Principal diagnosis as its own CC   `PDx MCC` Principal diagnosis as its own MCC   `HCC` HCC diagnosis code   `RxHCC` RxHCC diagnosis code
MACRA code   `Z` Z code as first-listed diagnosis

P74.8 Other transitory metabolic disturbances of newborn CC CC/MCC Exc
Amino-acid metabolic disorders described as transitory

P74.9 **Transitory metabolic disturbance of newborn, unspecified**

Digestive system disorders of newborn (P76-P78)

P76 Other intestinal obstruction of newborn

P76.0 **Meconium plug syndrome**
Meconium ileus NOS
EXCLUDES1 *meconium ileus in cystic fibrosis (E84.11)*

P76.1 **Transitory ileus of newborn** CC CC/MCC Exc
EXCLUDES1 *Hirschsprung's disease (Q43.1)*

P76.2 **Intestinal obstruction due to inspissated milk**

P76.8 Other specified intestinal obstruction of newborn
EXCLUDES1 *intestinal obstruction classifiable to K56.-*

P76.9 **Intestinal obstruction of newborn, unspecified**

P77 Necrotizing enterocolitis of newborn

P77.1 Stage 1 necrotizing enterocolitis in newborn MCC CC/MCC Exc
Necrotizing enterocolitis without pneumatosis, without perforation

P77.2 Stage 2 necrotizing enterocolitis in newborn MCC CC/MCC Exc
Necrotizing enterocolitis with pneumatosis, without perforation

P77.3 Stage 3 necrotizing enterocolitis in newborn MCC CC/MCC Exc
Necrotizing enterocolitis with perforation
Necrotizing enterocolitis with pneumatosis and perforation

P77.9 **Necrotizing enterocolitis in newborn, unspecified** MCC CC/MCC Exc
Necrotizing enterocolitis in newborn, NOS

P78 Other perinatal digestive system disorders
EXCLUDES1 *cystic fibrosis (E84.0-E84.9)*
neonatal gastrointestinal hemorrhages (P54.0-P54.3)

P78.0 **Perinatal intestinal perforation** MCC CC/MCC Exc
Meconium peritonitis

P78.1 **Other neonatal peritonitis**
Neonatal peritonitis NOS

P78.2 **Neonatal hematemesis and melena due to swallowed maternal blood**

P78.3 **Noninfective neonatal diarrhea**
Neonatal diarrhea NOS

P78.8 Other specified perinatal digestive system disorders

P78.81 **Congenital cirrhosis (of liver)**

P78.82 **Peptic ulcer of newborn**

P78.83 **Newborn esophageal reflux**
Neonatal esophageal reflux

● P78.84 **Gestational alloimmune liver disease**
GALD
Neonatal hemochromatosis
EXCLUDES 1 *hemochromatosis (E83.11-)*

P78.89 Other specified perinatal digestive system disorders

P78.9 **Perinatal digestive system disorder, unspecified**

Conditions involving the integument and temperature regulation of newborn (P80-P83)

P80 Hypothermia of newborn

P80.0 **Cold injury syndrome**
Severe and usually chronic hypothermia associated with a pink flushed appearance, edema and neurological and biochemical abnormalities.
EXCLUDES1 *mild hypothermia of newborn (P80.8)*

P80.8 **Other hypothermia of newborn**
Mild hypothermia of newborn

P80.9 **Hypothermia of newborn, unspecified**

P81 Other disturbances of temperature regulation of newborn

P81.0 **Environmental hyperthermia of newborn**

P81.8 Other specified disturbances of temperature regulation of newborn

P81.9 **Disturbance of temperature regulation of newborn, unspecified**
Fever of newborn NOS

P83 Other conditions of integument specific to newborn
EXCLUDES1 *congenital malformations of skin and integument (Q80-Q84)*
hydrops fetalis due to hemolytic disease (P56.-)
neonatal skin infection (P39.4)
staphylococcal scalded skin syndrome (L00)
EXCLUDES2 *cradle cap (L21.0)*
diaper [napkin] dermatitis (L22)

P83.0 **Sclerema neonatorum** CC CC/MCC Exc

P83.1 **Neonatal erythema toxicum**

P83.2 **Hydrops fetalis not due to hemolytic disease** MCC CC/MCC Exc
Hydrops fetalis NOS

P83.3 Other and unspecified edema specific to newborn CC CC/MCC Exc

P83.30 **Unspecified edema specific to newborn** CC CC/MCC Exc

P83.39 **Other edema specific to newborn** CC CC/MCC Exc

P83.4 **Breast engorgement of newborn**
Noninfective mastitis of newborn

P83.5 **Congenital hydrocele** ♂

P83.6 **Umbilical polyp of newborn**

P83.8 Other specified conditions of integument specific to newborn

● P83.81 Umbilical granuloma N
EXCLUDES2 *:Granulomatous disorder of the skin and subcutaneous tissue, unspecified (L92.9)*

● P83.88 Other specified conditions of integument specific to newborn N
Bronze baby syndrome
Neonatal scleroderma
Urticaria neonatorum

P83.9 **Condition of the integument specific to newborn, unspecified**

Other problems with newborn (P84)

P84 **Other problems with newborn**
Acidemia of newborn
Acidosis of newborn
Anoxia of newborn NOS
Asphyxia of newborn NOS
Hypercapnia of newborn
Hypoxemia of newborn
Hypoxia of newborn NOS
Mixed metabolic and respiratory acidosis of newborn
EXCLUDES1 *intracranial hemorrhage due to anoxia or hypoxia (P52.-)*
hypoxic ischemic encephalopathy [HIE] (P91.6-)
late metabolic acidosis of newborn (P74.0)

Other disorders originating in the perinatal period (P90-P96)

P90 **Convulsions of newborn** MCC CC/MCC Exc
EXCLUDES1 *benign myoclonic epilepsy in infancy (G40.3-)*
benign neonatal convulsions (familial) (G40.3-)

P91 Other disturbances of cerebral status of newborn

P91.0 **Neonatal cerebral ischemia** MCC CC/MCC Exc

P91.1 **Acquired periventricular cysts of newborn** MCC CC/MCC Exc

P91.2 **Neonatal cerebral leukomalacia** MCC CC/MCC Exc
Periventricular leukomalacia

P91.3 **Neonatal cerebral irritability** MCC CC/MCC Exc

P91.4 **Neonatal cerebral depression** MCC CC/MCC Exc

P91.5 **Neonatal coma** MCC CC/MCC Exc

P91.6 Hypoxic ischemic encephalopathy [HIE]
EXCLUDES1 *Neonatal cerebral depression (P91.4)*
Neonatal cerebral irritability (P91.3)
Neonatal coma (P91.5)

P91.60 **Hypoxic ischemic encephalopathy [HIE], unspecified** CC CC/MCC Exc

P91.61 Mild **hypoxic ischemic encephalopathy [HIE]** CC CC/MCC Exc

P91.62 Moderate **hypoxic ischemic encephalopathy [HIE]** CC CC/MCC Exc

---

Unspecified Code	Other Specified Code	Manifestation Code	N Newborn	P Pediatric	M Maternity	A Adult	♂ Male	♀ Female

● New Code ▲ Revised Code Title ►◄ Revised Text **NOTES** *INCLUDES* EXCLUDES 1 Not coded here EXCLUDES 2 Not included here

4th character required 5th character required 6th character required 7th character required

Extension 'X' Alert HAC Hospital-acquired condition (HAC) alert **AHA** AHA Coding Clinic©

Q05.7 Lumbar **spina bifida** without hydrocephalus POA HCC RxHCC
Lumbosacral spina bifida NOS

Q05.8 Sacral **spina bifida** without hydrocephalus POA HCC RxHCC

Q05.9 **Spina bifida, unspecified** POA HCC RxHCC

Q06 Other **congenital malformations of** spinal cord

Q06.0 **Amyelia** POA HCC RxHCC

Q06.1 **Hypoplasia and dysplasia of spinal cord** POA HCC RxHCC
Atelomyelia
Myelatelia
Myelodysplasia of spinal cord

Q06.2 **Diastematomyelia** POA HCC RxHCC

Q06.3 **Other congenital cauda equina malformations** POA HCC RxHCC

Q06.4 **Hydromyelia** POA HCC RxHCC
Hydrorachis

Q06.8 **Other specified congenital malformations of spinal cord** POA HCC RxHCC

Q06.9 **Congenital malformation of spinal cord, unspecified** POA HCC RxHCC
Congenital anomaly NOS of spinal cord
Congenital deformity NOS of spinal cord
Congenital disease or lesion NOS of spinal cord

Q07 Other **congenital malformations of** nervous system

EXCLUDES2 *congenital central alveolar hypoventilation syndrome (G47.35)*
familial dysautonomia [Riley-Day] (G90.1)
neurofibromatosis (nonmalignant) (Q85.0-)

Q07.0 **Arnold-Chiari syndrome**
Arnold-Chiari syndrome, type II
EXCLUDES1 *Arnold-Chiari syndrome, type III (Q01.-)*
Arnold-Chiari syndrome, type IV (Q04.8)

Q07.00 **Arnold-Chiari syndrome** without spina bifida or hydrocephalus POA HCC RxHCC

Q07.01 **Arnold-Chiari syndrome** with spina bifida POA HCC RxHCC

Q07.02 **Arnold-Chiari syndrome** with hydrocephalus CC POA HCC RxHCC CC/MCC Exc

Q07.03 **Arnold-Chiari syndrome** with spina bifida and hydrocephalus CC POA HCC RxHCC CC/MCC Exc

Q07.8 **Other specified congenital malformations of nervous system** POA HCC RxHCC
Agenesis of nerve
Displacement of brachial plexus
Jaw-winking syndrome
Marcus Gunn's syndrome

Q07.9 **Congenital malformation of nervous system, unspecified** POA HCC RxHCC
Congenital anomaly NOS of nervous system
Congenital deformity NOS of nervous system
Congenital disease or lesion NOS of nervous system

Congenital malformations of eye, ear, face and neck (Q10-Q18)

EXCLUDES2 *cleft lip and cleft palate (Q35-Q37)*
congenital malformation of cervical spine (Q05.0, Q05.5, Q67.5, Q76.0-Q76.4)
congenital malformation of larynx (Q31.-)
congenital malformation of lip NEC (Q38.0)
congenital malformation of nose (Q30.-)
congenital malformation of parathyroid gland (Q89.2)
congenital malformation of thyroid gland (Q89.2)

Q10 **Congenital malformations of** eyelid, lacrimal apparatus and orbit
EXCLUDES1 *cryptophthalmos NOS (Q11.2)*
cryptophthalmos syndrome (Q87.0)

Q10.0 **Congenital** ptosis POA

Q10.1 **Congenital** ectropion POA

Q10.2 **Congenital** entropion POA

Q10.3 Other **congenital malformations of eyelid** POA
Ablepharon
Blepharophimosis, congenital
Coloboma of eyelid

Congenital absence or agenesis of cilia
Congenital absence or agenesis of eyelid
Congenital accessory eyelid
Congenital accessory eye muscle
Congenital malformation of eyelid NOS

Q10.4 **Absence and agenesis of lacrimal apparatus** POA
Congenital absence of punctum lacrimale

Q10.5 **Congenital** stenosis and stricture of lacrimal duct POA

Q10.6 Other **congenital malformations of lacrimal apparatus** POA
Congenital malformation of lacrimal apparatus NOS

Q10.7 **Congenital malformation of** orbit POA

Q11 **Anophthalmos, microphthalmos and macrophthalmos**

Q11.0 **Cystic eyeball** POA

Q11.1 **Other anophthalmos** POA
Anophthalmos NOS
Agenesis of eye
Aplasia of eye

Q11.2 **Microphthalmos** POA
AHA: Q4 2004
Cryptophthalmos NOS
Dysplasia of eye
Hypoplasia of eye
Rudimentary eye
EXCLUDES1 *cryptophthalmos syndrome (Q87.0)*

Q11.3 **Macrophthalmos** POA
EXCLUDES1 *macrophthalmos in congenital glaucoma (Q15.0)*

Q12 **Congenital** lens malformations

Q12.0 **Congenital** cataract POA

Q12.1 **Congenital** displaced lens POA

Q12.2 Coloboma of lens POA

Q12.3 **Congenital** aphakia POA

Q12.4 Spherophakia POA

Q12.8 Other **congenital lens malformations** POA
Microphakia

Q12.9 **Congenital lens malformation, unspecified** POA

Q13 **Congenital malformations of** anterior segment of eye

Q13.0 Coloboma of iris POA
Coloboma NOS

Q13.1 Absence of iris POA
Aniridia
Use additional code for associated glaucoma (H42)

Q13.2 Other **congenital malformations of iris** POA
Anisocoria, congenital
Atresia of pupil
Congenital malformation of iris NOS
Corectopia

Q13.3 **Congenital** corneal opacity POA

Q13.4 **Other congenital corneal malformations** POA
Congenital malformation of cornea NOS
Microcornea
Peter's anomaly

Q13.5 **Blue sclera** POA

Q13.8 Other **congenital malformations of anterior segment of eye**

Q13.81 **Rieger's anomaly** POA
Use additional code for associated glaucoma (H42)

Q13.89 **Other congenital malformations of anterior segment of eye** POA

Q13.9 **Congenital malformation of anterior segment of eye, unspecified** POA

Q14 **Congenital malformations of** posterior segment of eye
EXCLUDES2 *optic nerve hypoplasia (H47.03-)*

Q14.0 **Congenital malformation of** vitreous humor POA
Congenital vitreous opacity

Q14.1 **Congenital malformation of** retina POA
Congenital retinal aneurysm

Q14.2 **Congenital malformation of** optic disc POA
Coloboma of optic disc

Q14.3 **Congenital malformation of** choroid POA

Q14.8 Other **congenital malformations of posterior segment of eye** POA
Coloboma of the fundus

POADx Unacceptable principal diagnosis symbol per Medicare code edits   POA Code exempt from diagnosis present on admission requirement
❓ Questionable admission   CC Complication or comorbidity   CC/MCC Exc CC/MCC exclusion   MCC Major complication or comorbidity
PCC Principal diagnosis as its own CC   PMCC Principal diagnosis as its own MCC   HCC HCC diagnosis code   RxHCC RxHCC diagnosis code
MACRA code   Z Z code as first-listed diagnosis

Q14.9 **Congenital malformation of posterior segment of eye, unspecified** POA

4ᵗʰ **Q15** Other **congenital malformations of** eye

EXCLUDES1 *congenital nystagmus (H55.01)*

ocular albinism (E70.31-)

optic nerve hypoplasia (H47.03-)

retinitis pigmentosa (H35.52)

Q15.0 **Congenital** glaucoma POA

Axenfeld's anomaly

Buphthalmos

Glaucoma of childhood

Glaucoma of newborn

Hydrophthalmos

Keratoglobus, congenital, with glaucoma

Macrocornea with glaucoma

Macrophthalmos in congenital glaucoma

Megalocornea with glaucoma

Q15.8 Other specified congenital malformations of eye POA

Q15.9 **Congenital malformation of eye, unspecified** POA

Congenital anomaly of eye

Congenital deformity of eye

4ᵗʰ **Q16** Congenital malformations of ear causing impairment of hearing

EXCLUDES1 *congenital deafness (H90.-)*

Q16.0 **Congenital** absence of (ear) auricle POA

Q16.1 **Congenital** absence, atresia and stricture of auditory canal (external) (openly) POA

Congenital atresia or stricture of osseous meatus

Q16.2 Absence of eustachian tube POA

Q16.3 **Congenital malformation of** ear ossicles POA

Congenital fusion of ear ossicles

Q16.4 **Other congenital malformations of middle ear** POA

Congenital malformation of middle ear NOS

Q16.5 **Congenital malformation of** inner ear POA

Congenital anomaly of membranous labyrinth

Congenital anomaly of organ of Corti

Q16.9 Congenital malformation of ear causing impairment of hearing, unspecified POA

Congenital absence of ear NOS

4ᵗʰ **Q17** Other congenital malformations of ear

EXCLUDES1 *congenital malformations of ear with impairment of hearing (Q16.0-Q16.9)*

preauricular sinus (Q18.1)

Q17.0 **Accessory auricle** POA

Accessory tragus

Polyotia

Preauricular appendage or tag

Supernumerary ear

Supernumerary lobule

Q17.1 **Macrotia** POA

Q17.2 **Microtia** POA

Q17.3 **Other misshapen ear**

Pointed ear

Q17.4 **Misplaced ear** POA

Low-set ears

EXCLUDES1 *cervical auricle (Q18.2)*

Q17.5 **Prominent ear** POA

Bat ear

Q17.8 Other specified congenital malformations of ear POA

Congenital absence of lobe of ear

Q17.9 Congenital malformation of ear, unspecified POA

Congenital anomaly of ear NOS

4ᵗʰ **Q18** Other **congenital malformations of** face and neck

EXCLUDES1 *cleft lip and cleft palate (Q35-Q37)*

conditions classified to Q67.0-Q67.4

congenital malformations of skull and face bones (Q75.-)

cyclopia (Q87.0)

dentofacial anomalies [including malocclusion] (M26.-)

malformation syndromes affecting facial appearance (Q87.0)

persistent thyroglossal duct (Q89.2)

Q18.0 **Sinus, fistula and cyst of branchial** cleft POA

Branchial vestige

Q18.1 **Preauricular sinus and cyst** POA

Fistula of auricle, congenital

Cervicoaural fistula

Q18.2 **Other branchial** cleft **malformations** POA

Branchial cleft malformation NOS

Cervical auricle

Otocephaly

Q18.3 **Webbing of neck** POA

Pterygium colli

Q18.4 **Macrostomia** POA

Q18.5 **Microstomia** POA

Q18.6 **Macrocheilia** POA

Hypertrophy of lip, congenital

Q18.7 **Microcheilia** POA

Q18.8 Other specified congenital malformations of face and neck POA

Medial cyst of face and neck

Medial fistula of face and neck

Medial sinus of face and neck

Q18.9 Congenital malformation of face and neck, unspecified POA

Congenital anomaly NOS of face and neck

Congenital malformations of the circulatory system (Q20-Q28)

4ᵗʰ **Q20** Congenital malformations of cardiac chambers and connections

EXCLUDES1 *dextrocardia with situs inversus (Q89.3)*

mirror-image atrial arrangement with situs inversus (Q89.3)

Q20.0 **Common arterial trunk** POA MCC CC/MCC Exc

Persistent truncus arteriosus

EXCLUDES1 *aortic septal defect (Q21.4)*

Q20.1 **Double** outlet right **ventricle** POA MCC CC/MCC Exc

Taussig-Bing syndrome

Q20.2 **Double** outlet left **ventricle** POA MCC CC/MCC Exc

Q20.3 **Discordant ventriculoarterial connection** POA MCC CC/MCC Exc

Dextrotransposition of aorta

Transposition of great vessels (complete)

Q20.4 **Double** inlet **ventricle** POA MCC CC/MCC Exc

Common ventricle

Cor triloculare biatriatum

Single ventricle

Q20.5 **Discordant** atrioventricular **connection** CC POA CC/MCC Exc

Corrected transposition

Levotransposition

Ventricular inversion

Q20.6 **Isomerism of atrial appendages** POA

Isomerism of atrial appendages with asplenia or polysplenia

Q20.8 **Other congenital malformations of cardiac chambers and connections** POA

Cor binoculare

Q20.9 Congenital malformation of cardiac chambers and connections, unspecified POA

4ᵗʰ **Q21** Congenital malformations of cardiac septa

EXCLUDES1 *acquired cardiac septal defect (I51.0)*

Q21.0 Ventricular **septal defect** CC POA CC/MCC Exc

Roger's disease

Q21.1 Atrial **septal defect** CC POA CC/MCC Exc

Coronary sinus defect

Patent or persistent foramen ovale

Patent or persistent ostium secundum defect (type II)

Patent or persistent sinus venosus defect

Q21.2 Atrioventricular **septal defect** CC POA CC/MCC Exc

Common atrioventricular canal

Endocardial cushion defect

Ostium primum atrial septal defect (type I)

Q21.3 **Tetralogy of Fallot** POA MCC CC/MCC Exc

Ventricular septal defect with pulmonary stenosis or atresia, dextroposition of aorta and hypertrophy of right ventricle.

Unspecified Code   Other Specified Code   Manifestation Code   Ⓝ Newborn   Ⓟ Pediatric   Ⓜ Maternity   Ⓐ Adult   ♂ Male   ♀ Female

● New Code   ▲ Revised Code Title   ▶◀ Revised Text   NOTES   INCLUDES   EXCLUDES 1 Not coded here   EXCLUDES 2 Not included here

4ᵗʰ 4ᵗʰ character required   5ᵗʰ 5ᵗʰ character required   6ᵗʰ 6ᵗʰ character required   7ᵗʰ 7ᵗʰ character required

7ˣ Extension 'X' Alert   HAC Hospital-acquired condition (HAC) alert   AHA AHA Coding Clinic©

Q21.4 **Aortopulmonary** septal defect POA
Aortic septal defect
Aortopulmonary window

Q21.8 **Other congenital malformations of cardiac septa** POA
Eisenmenger's defect
Pentalogy of Fallot
Code also if applicable:
Eisenmenger's complex (I27.83)
Eisenmenger's syndrome (I27.83)

Q21.9 **Congenital malformation of cardiac septum, unspecified** POA
Septal (heart) defect NOS

Q22 **Congenital malformations of** pulmonary and tricuspid valves
Q22.0 **Pulmonary** valve atresia POA MCC CC/MCC Exc
Q22.1 **Congenital pulmonary valve** stenosis CC POA CC/MCC Exc
Q22.2 **Congenital pulmonary valve** insufficiency CC POA CC/MCC Exc
Congenital pulmonary valve regurgitation
Q22.3 **Other congenital malformations of pulmonary valve** CC POA CC/MCC Exc
Congenital malformation of pulmonary valve NOS
Supernumerary cusps of pulmonary valve
Q22.4 **Congenital** tricuspid stenosis POA MCC CC/MCC Exc
Congenital tricuspid atresia
Q22.5 **Ebstein's anomaly** POA MCC CC/MCC Exc
Q22.6 **Hypoplastic** right heart syndrome POA MCC CC/MCC Exc
Q22.8 **Other congenital malformations of tricuspid valve** POA MCC CC/MCC Exc
Q22.9 **Congenital malformation of tricuspid valve, unspecified** POA MCC CC/MCC Exc

Q23 **Congenital malformations of** aortic and mitral valves
Q23.0 **Congenital** stenosis of aortic valve CC POA CC/MCC Exc
Congenital aortic atresia
Congenital aortic stenosis NOS
EXCLUDES1 congenital stenosis of aortic valve in hypoplastic left heart syndrome (Q23.4)
congenital subaortic stenosis (Q24.4)
supravalvular aortic stenosis (congenital) (Q25.3)
Q23.1 **Congenital** insufficiency of aortic valve CC POA CC/MCC Exc
Bicuspid aortic valve
Congenital aortic insufficiency
Q23.2 **Congenital** mitral stenosis CC POA CC/MCC Exc
Congenital mitral atresia
Q23.3 **Congenital** mitral insufficiency CC POA CC/MCC Exc
Q23.4 **Hypoplastic** left heart syndrome POA MCC CC/MCC Exc
Q23.8 **Other congenital malformations of aortic and mitral valves** POA
Q23.9 **Congenital malformation of aortic and mitral valves, unspecified** POA

Q24 **Other** congenital malformations of heart
EXCLUDES1 endocardial fibroelastosis (I42.4)
Q24.0 **Dextrocardia** CC POA CC/MCC Exc
EXCLUDES1 dextrocardia with situs inversus (Q89.3)
isomerism of atrial appendages (with asplenia or polysplenia) (Q20.6)
mirror-image atrial arrangement with situs inversus (Q89.3)
Q24.1 **Levocardia** CC POA CC/MCC Exc
Q24.2 **Cor triatriatum** POA MCC CC/MCC Exc
Q24.3 **Pulmonary infundibular** stenosis CC POA CC/MCC Exc
Subvalvular pulmonic stenosis
Q24.4 **Congenital subaortic** stenosis POA MCC CC/MCC Exc
Q24.5 **Malformation of coronary vessels** CC POA RxHCC CC/MCC Exc
Congenital coronary (artery) aneurysm
Q24.6 **Congenital heart block** POA MCC CC/MCC Exc
Q24.8 **Other specified congenital malformations of heart** POA
Congenital diverticulum of left ventricle
Congenital malformation of myocardium
Congenital malformation of pericardium
Malposition of heart
Uhl's disease

Q24.9 **Congenital malformation of heart, unspecified** POA
Congenital anomaly of heart
Congenital disease of heart

Q25 **Congenital malformations of** great arteries
Q25.0 **Patent ductus** arteriosus CC POA CC/MCC Exc
Patent ductus Botallo
Persistent ductus arteriosus
Q25.1 **Coarctation** of aorta CC POA CC/MCC Exc
AHA: Q4 2016
Coarctation of aorta (preductal) (postductal)
Stenosis of aorta
Q25.2 **Atresia** of aorta
Q25.21 **Interruption of aortic** arch CC POA CC/MCC Exc
AHA: Q4 2016
Atresia of aortic arch
Q25.29 **Other** atresia of aorta CC POA CC/MCC Exc
AHA: Q4 2016
Atresia of aorta
Q25.3 **Supravalvular** aortic stenosis CC POA CC/MCC Exc
EXCLUDES1 congenital aortic stenosis NOS (Q23.0)
congenital stenosis of aortic valve (Q23.0)
Q25.4 **Other congenital malformations of aorta**
EXCLUDES1 hypoplasia of aorta in hypoplastic left heart syndrome (Q23.4)
Q25.40 **Congenital malformation of aorta unspecified** CC POA CC/MCC Exc
AHA: Q4 2016
Q25.41 **Absence and aplasia** of aorta CC POA CC/MCC Exc
AHA: Q4 2016
Q25.42 **Hypoplasia** of aorta CC POA CC/MCC Exc
AHA: Q4 2016
Q25.43 **Congenital aneurysm** of aorta CC POA CC/MCC Exc
AHA: Q4 2016
Congenital aneurysm of aortic root
Congenital aneurysm of aortic sinus
Q25.44 **Congenital dilation** of aorta CC POA CC/MCC Exc
AHA: Q4 2016
Q25.45 **Double aortic arch** CC POA CC/MCC Exc
AHA: Q4 2016
Vascular ring of aorta
Q25.46 **Tortuous** aortic arch CC POA CC/MCC Exc
AHA: Q4 2016
Persistent convolutions of aortic arch
Q25.47 **Right** aortic arch CC POA CC/MCC Exc
AHA: Q4 2016
Persistent right aortic arch
Q25.48 **Anomalous origin of subclavian artery** CC POA CC/MCC Exc
AHA: Q4 2016
Q25.49 **Other** congenital malformations of aorta CC POA CC/MCC Exc
AHA: Q4 2016
Aortic arch
Bovine arch
Q25.5 **Atresia** of pulmonary artery POA MCC CC/MCC Exc
Q25.6 **Stenosis** of pulmonary artery POA MCC CC/MCC Exc
Supravalvular pulmonary stenosis
Q25.7 **Other congenital malformations of** pulmonary artery
Q25.71 **Coarctation** of pulmonary artery POA MCC CC/MCC Exc
Q25.72 **Congenital pulmonary** arteriovenous malformation POA MCC CC/MCC Exc
Congenital pulmonary arteriovenous aneurysm
Q25.79 **Other congenital malformations of pulmonary artery** POA MCC CC/MCC Exc
Aberrant pulmonary artery
Agenesis of pulmonary artery
Congenital aneurysm of pulmonary artery
Congenital anomaly of pulmonary artery
Hypoplasia of pulmonary artery
Q25.8 **Other congenital malformations of other great arteries** CC POA CC/MCC Exc
Q25.9 **Congenital malformation of great arteries, unspecified** CC POA CC/MCC Exc

---

POA Unacceptable principal diagnosis symbol per Medicare code edits   POA Code exempt from diagnosis present on admission requirement
? Questionable admission   CC Complication or comorbidity   CC/MCC Exc CC/MCC exclusion   MCC Major complication or comorbidity
Principal diagnosis as its own CC   Principal diagnosis as its own MCC   HCC HCC diagnosis code   RxHCC RxHCC diagnosis code
MACRA code   Z code as first-listed diagnosis

Q26 Congenital malformations of great veins

Q26.0 **Congenital stenosis of vena cava** CC POA CC/MCC Exc
Congenital stenosis of vena cava (inferior)(superior)

Q26.1 Persistent left **superior vena cava** CC POA CC/MCC Exc

Q26.2 Total anomalous **pulmonary venous connection** CC POA CC/MCC Exc
Total anomalous pulmonary venous return [TAPVR], subdiaphragmatic
Total anomalous pulmonary venous return [TAPVR], supradiaphragmatic

Q26.3 Partial anomalous **pulmonary venous connection** CC POA CC/MCC Exc
Partial anomalous pulmonary venous return

Q26.4 **Anomalous pulmonary venous connection, unspecified** CC POA CC/MCC Exc

Q26.5 Anomalous **portal venous connection** POA

Q26.6 Portal vein-hepatic artery fistula POA

Q26.8 **Other congenital malformations of great veins** CC POA CC/MCC Exc
Absence of vena cava (inferior) (superior)
Azygos continuation of inferior vena cava
Persistent left posterior cardinal vein
Scimitar syndrome

Q26.9 **Congenital malformation of great vein, unspecified** CC POA CC/MCC Exc
Congenital anomaly of vena cava (inferior) (superior) NOS

Q27 Other congenital malformations of peripheral vascular system

EXCLUDES2 *anomalies of cerebral and precerebral vessels (Q28.0-Q28.3)*
anomalies of coronary vessels (Q24.5)
anomalies of pulmonary artery (Q25.5-Q25.7)
congenital retinal aneurysm (Q14.1)
hemangioma and lymphangioma (D18.-)

Q27.0 **Congenital absence and hypoplasia of umbilical artery** POA
Single umbilical artery

Q27.1 **Congenital renal artery stenosis** POA

Q27.2 **Other congenital malformations of renal artery** POA
Congenital malformation of renal artery NOS
Multiple renal arteries

Q27.3 **Arteriovenous malformation (peripheral)**
Arteriovenous aneurysm
EXCLUDES1 *acquired arteriovenous aneurysm (I77.0)*
EXCLUDES2 *arteriovenous malformation of cerebral vessels (Q28.2)*
arteriovenous malformation of precerebral vessels (Q28.0)

Q27.30 **Arteriovenous malformation, site unspecified** CC POA CC/MCC Exc

Q27.31 **Arteriovenous malformation of vessel of upper limb** POA

Q27.32 **Arteriovenous malformation of vessel of lower limb** POA

Q27.33 **Arteriovenous malformation of digestive system vessel** POA

Q27.34 **Arteriovenous malformation of renal vessel** POA

Q27.39 **Arteriovenous malformation, other site** POA

Q27.4 **Congenital phlebectasia** CC POA CC/MCC Exc

Q27.8 Other specified congenital malformations of peripheral vascular system POA
Absence of peripheral vascular system
Atresia of peripheral vascular system
Congenital aneurysm (peripheral)
Congenital stricture, artery
Congenital varix
EXCLUDES1 *arteriovenous malformation (Q27.3-)*

Q27.9 **Congenital malformation of peripheral vascular system, unspecified** POA
Anomaly of artery or vein NOS

Q28 Other congenital malformations of circulatory system

EXCLUDES1 *congenital aneurysm NOS (Q27.8)*
congenital coronary aneurysm (Q24.5)
ruptured cerebral arteriovenous malformation (I60.8)
ruptured malformation of precerebral vessels (I72.0)

EXCLUDES2 *congenital peripheral aneurysm (Q27.8)*
congenital pulmonary aneurysm (Q25.79)
congenital retinal aneurysm (Q14.1)

Q28.0 **Arteriovenous malformation of precerebral vessels** CC POA CC/MCC Exc
Congenital arteriovenous precerebral aneurysm (nonruptured)

Q28.1 **Other malformations of precerebral vessels** CC POA CC/MCC Exc
Congenital malformation of precerebral vessels NOS
Congenital precerebral aneurysm (nonruptured)

Q28.2 **Arteriovenous malformation of cerebral vessels** POA MCC CC/MCC Exc
Arteriovenous malformation of brain NOS
Congenital arteriovenous cerebral aneurysm (nonruptured)

Q28.3 Other **malformations of cerebral vessels** POA MCC CC/MCC Exc
Congenital cerebral aneurysm (nonruptured)
Congenital malformation of cerebral vessels NOS
Developmental venous anomaly

Q28.8 Other specified congenital malformations of circulatory system CC POA CC/MCC Exc
Congenital aneurysm, specified site NEC
Spinal vessel anomaly

Q28.9 **Congenital malformation of circulatory system, unspecified** CC POA CC/MCC Exc

Congenital malformations of the respiratory system (Q30-Q34)

Q30 Congenital malformations of nose

EXCLUDES1 *congenital deviation of nasal septum (Q67.4)*

Q30.0 Choanal atresia POA
Atresia of nares (anterior) (posterior)
Congenital stenosis of nares (anterior) (posterior)

Q30.1 Agenesis and underdevelopment **of nose** POA
Congenital absent of nose

Q30.2 Fissured, notched and cleft **nose** POA

Q30.3 Congenital perforated **nasal septum** POA

Q30.8 **Other congenital malformations of nose**
Accessory nose
Congenital anomaly of nasal sinus wall

Q30.9 **Congenital malformation of nose, unspecified** POA

Q31 Congenital malformations of larynx

EXCLUDES1 *congenital laryngeal stridor NOS (P28.89)*

Q31.0 Web **of larynx** POA
Glottic web of larynx
Subglottic web of larynx
Web of larynx NOS

Q31.1 Congenital subglottic stenosis CC POA CC/MCC Exc

Q31.2 Laryngeal hypoplasia CC POA CC/MCC Exc

Q31.3 Laryngocele CC POA CC/MCC Exc

Q31.5 Congenital laryngomalacia CC POA CC/MCC Exc

Q31.8 **Other congenital malformations of larynx** CC POA CC/MCC Exc
Absence of larynx
Agenesis of larynx
Atresia of larynx
Congenital cleft thyroid cartilage
Congenital fissure of epiglottis
Congenital stenosis of larynx NEC
Posterior cleft of cricoid cartilage

Q31.9 **Congenital malformation of larynx, unspecified** CC POA CC/MCC Exc

Q32 Congenital malformations of trachea and bronchus

EXCLUDES1 *congenital bronchiectasis (Q33.4)*

Q32.0 **Congenital tracheomalacia** CC POA CC/MCC Exc

Q32.1 **Other congenital malformations of trachea** CC POA CC/MCC Exc
Atresia of trachea
Congenital anomaly of tracheal cartilage
Congenital dilatation of trachea
Congenital malformation of trachea
Congenital stenosis of trachea
Congenital tracheocele

Q32.2 **Congenital bronchomalacia** CC POA CC/MCC Exc

Q32.3 **Congenital stenosis of bronchus** CC POA CC/MCC Exc

Q32.4 **Other congenital malformations of bronchus** CC POA CC/MCC Exc

---

Unspecified Code   Other Specified Code   Manifestation Code   N Newborn   P Pediatric   M Maternity   A Adult   ♂ Male   ♀ Female
● New Code   ▲ Revised Code Title   ▶◀ Revised Text   NOTES   INCLUDES   EXCLUDES 1 Not coded here   EXCLUDES 2 Not included here
4th character required   5th character required   6th character required   7th character required
Extension 'X' Alert   HAC Hospital-acquired condition (HAC) alert   AHA AHA Coding Clinic©

EXCLUDES1 *congenital diabetes mellitus (E10.-)*

cystic fibrosis (E84.0-E84.9)

fibrocystic disease of pancreas (E84.-)

neonatal diabetes mellitus (P70.2)

Q45.8 **Other specified congenital malformations of digestive system**

Absence (complete) (partial) of alimentary tract NOS

Duplication of digestive system

Malposition, congenital of digestive system

Q45.9 **Congenital malformation of digestive system, unspecified**

Congenital anomaly of digestive system

Congenital deformity of digestive system

Congenital malformations of genital organs (Q50-Q56)

EXCLUDES1 *androgen insensitivity syndrome (E34.5-)*

syndromes associated with anomalies in the number and form of chromosomes (Q90-Q99)

Q50 **Congenital malformations of** ovaries, fallopian tubes and broad ligaments

Q50.0 **Congenital absence of** ovary

EXCLUDES1 *Turner's syndrome (Q96.-)*

Q50.01 **Congenital absence of ovary,** unilateral

Q50.02 **Congenital absence of ovary,** bilateral

Q50.1 **Developmental ovarian** cyst

Q50.2 **Congenital** torsion **of ovary**

Q50.3 **Other** congenital malformations of ovary

Q50.31 **Accessory** ovary

Q50.32 **Ovarian** streak

46, XX with streak gonads

Q50.39 **Other congenital malformation of ovary**

Congenital malformation of ovary NOS

Q50.4 **Embryonic cyst of** fallopian tube

Fimbrial cyst

Q50.5 **Embryonic cyst of** broad ligament

Epoophoron cyst

Parovarian cyst

Q50.6 **Other congenital malformations of fallopian tube and broad ligament**

Absence of fallopian tube and broad ligament

Accessory fallopian tube and broad ligament

Atresia of fallopian tube and broad ligament

Congenital malformation of fallopian tube or broad ligament NOS

Q51 **Congenital malformations of** uterus and cervix

Q51.0 Agenesis and aplasia **of** uterus

Congenital absence of uterus

Q51.1 Doubling **of uterus** with doubling of cervix and vagina

Q51.10 **Doubling of uterus with doubling of cervix and vagina** without obstruction

Doubling of uterus with doubling of cervix and vagina NOS

Q51.11 **Doubling of uterus with doubling of cervix and vagina** with obstruction

Q51.2 Other doubling **of uterus**

Doubling of uterus NOS

Septate uterus, complete or partial

Q51.3 Bicornate **uterus**

Bicornate uterus, complete or partial

Q51.4 Unicornate **uterus**

Unicornate uterus with or without a separate uterine horn

Uterus with only one functioning horn

Q51.5 Agenesis and aplasia **of cervix**

Congenital absence of cervix

Q51.6 Embryonic cyst **of cervix**

Q51.7 **Congenital** fistulae **between** uterus and digestive and urinary tracts

Q51.8 Other **congenital malformations of uterus and cervix**

Q51.81 **Other congenital malformations of uterus**

Q51.810 **Arcuate uterus**

Arcuatus uterus

Q51.811 **Hypoplasia** of uterus

Q51.818 **Other congenital malformations of uterus**

Müllerian anomaly of uterus NEC

Q51.82 **Other congenital malformations of** cervix

Q51.820 **Cervical** duplication

Q51.821 **Hypoplasia** of cervix

Q51.828 **Other congenital malformations of cervix**

Q51.9 **Congenital malformation of uterus and cervix, unspecified**

Q52 Other congenital malformations of female genitalia

Q52.0 **Congenital** absence of vagina

Vaginal agenesis, total or partial

Q52.1 Doubling of vagina

EXCLUDES1 *doubling of vagina with doubling of uterus and cervix (Q51.1-)*

Q52.10 **Doubling of vagina, unspecified**

Septate vagina NOS

Q52.11 **Transverse** vaginal septum

Q52.12 Longitudinal vaginal septum

Q52.120 **Longitudinal vaginal septum, nonobstructing**

AHA: Q4 2016

Q52.121 **Longitudinal vaginal septum,** obstructing, right side

AHA: Q4 2016

Q52.122 **Longitudinal vaginal septum,** obstructing, left side

AHA: Q4 2016

Q52.123 **Longitudinal vaginal septum, microperforate, right side**

AHA: Q4 2016

Q52.124 **Longitudinal vaginal septum, microperforate, left side**

AHA: Q4 2016

Q52.129 Other and unspecified longitudinal **vaginal septum**

AHA: Q4 2016

Q52.2 **Congenital** rectovaginal fistula

EXCLUDES1 *cloaca (Q43.7)*

Q52.3 Imperforate hymen

Q52.4 **Other congenital malformations of vagina**

Canal of Nuck cyst, congenital

Congenital malformation of vagina NOS

Embryonic vaginal cyst

Gartner's duct cyst

Q52.5 **Fusion of labia**

Q52.6 **Congenital malformation of** clitoris

Q52.7 Other and unspecified congenital malformations of vulva

Q52.70 **Unspecified congenital malformations of vulva**

Congenital malformation of vulva NOS

Q52.71 **Congenital** absence **of vulva**

Q52.79 **Other congenital malformations of vulva**

Congenital cyst of vulva

Q52.8 **Other specified congenital malformations of female genitalia**

Q52.9 **Congenital malformation of female genitalia, unspecified**

Q53 Undescended and ectopic testicle

Q53.0 Ectopic testis

Q53.00 **Ectopic testis, unspecified**

Q53.01 **Ectopic testis,** unilateral

Q53.02 **Ectopic testes,** bilateral

Q53.1 Undescended testicle, unilateral

Q53.10 **Unspecified undescended testicle, unilateral**

PDx Unacceptable principal diagnosis symbol per Medicare code edits | POA Code exempt from diagnosis present on admission requirement

❓ Questionable admission | ☞ Complication or comorbidity | CC-MCC Exc CC/MCC exclusion | MCC Major complication or comorbidity

PDx CC Principal diagnosis as its own CC | PDx MCC Principal diagnosis as its own MCC | HCC HCC diagnosis code | RxHCC RxHCC diagnosis code

MACRA code | Z1 Z code as first-listed diagnosis

[6th] Q53.11 Abdominal testis, unilateral
- ● Q53.111 Unilateral intraabdominal testis ♂
- ● Q53.112 Unilateral inguinal testis ♂

Q53.12 Ectopic perineal testis, unilateral POA ♂

● Q53.13 Unilateral high scrotal testis ♂

[5th] Q53.2 Undescended testicle, bilateral

Q53.20 Undescended testicle, unspecified, bilateral POA ♂

[6th] Q53.21 Abdominal testis, bilateral
- ● Q53.211 Bilateral intraabdominal testes ♂
- ● Q53.212 Bilateral inguinal testes ♂

Q53.22 Ectopic perineal testis, bilateral POA ♂

● Q53.23 Bilateral high scrotal testes ♂

Q53.9 Undescended testicle, unspecified POA ♂
Cryptorchism NOS

[4th] **Q54 Hypospadias**
[EXCLUDES1] *epispadias (Q64.0)*

Q54.0 Hypospadias, balanic POA ♂
Hypospadias, coronal
Hypospadias, glandular

Q54.1 Hypospadias, penile POA ♂

Q54.2 Hypospadias, penoscrotal POA ♂

Q54.3 Hypospadias, perineal POA ♂

Q54.4 Congenital chordee POA ♂
Chordee without hypospadias

Q54.8 Other hypospadias POA ♂
Hypospadias with intersex state

Q54.9 Hypospadias, unspecified POA ♂

[4th] **Q55 Other congenital malformations of male genital organs**
[EXCLUDES1] *congenital hydrocele (P83.5)*
hypospadias (Q54.-)

Q55.0 Absence and aplasia of testis POA ♂
Monorchism

Q55.1 Hypoplasia of testis and scrotum POA ♂
Fusion of testes

[5th] Q55.2 Other and unspecified congenital malformations of testis and scrotum

Q55.20 Unspecified congenital malformations of testis and scrotum POA ♂
Congenital malformation of testis or scrotum NOS

Q55.21 Polyorchism POA ♂

Q55.22 Retractile testis POA ♂

Q55.23 Scrotal transposition POA ♂

Q55.29 Other congenital malformations of testis and scrotum POA ♂

Q55.3 Atresia of vas deferens POA ♂
Code first any associated cystic fibrosis (E84.-)

Q55.4 Other congenital malformations of vas deferens, epididymis, seminal vesicles and prostate POA ♂
Absence or aplasia of prostate
Absence or aplasia of spermatic cord
Congenital malformation of vas deferens, epididymis, seminal vesicles or prostate NOS

Q55.5 Congenital absence and aplasia of penis POA ♂

[5th] Q55.6 Other congenital malformations of penis

Q55.61 Curvature of penis (lateral) POA ♂

Q55.62 Hypoplasia of penis POA ♂
Micropenis

Q55.63 Congenital torsion of penis POA ♂
[EXCLUDES1] *acquired torsion of penis (N48.82)*

Q55.64 Hidden penis POA ♂
Buried penis
Concealed penis
[EXCLUDES1] *acquired buried penis (N48.83)*

Q55.69 Other congenital malformation of penis POA ♂
Congenital malformation of penis NOS

Q55.7 Congenital vasocutaneous fistula POA ♂

Q55.8 Other specified congenital malformations of male genital organs POA ♂

Q55.9 Congenital malformation of male genital organ, unspecified POA ♂
Congenital anomaly of male genital organ
Congenital deformity of male genital organ

[4th] **Q56 Indeterminate sex and pseudohermaphroditism**
[EXCLUDES1] *46,XX true hermaphrodite (Q99.1)*
androgen insensitivity syndrome (E34.5-)
chimera 46,XX/46,XY true hermaphrodite (Q99.0)
female pseudohermaphroditism with adrenocortical disorder (E25.-)
pseudohermaphroditism with specified chromosomal anomaly (Q96-Q99)
pure gonadal dysgenesis (Q99.1)

Q56.0 Hermaphroditism, not elsewhere classified POA
Ovotestis

Q56.1 Male pseudohermaphroditism, not elsewhere classified POA ♂
46, XY with streak gonads
Male pseudohermaphroditism NOS

Q56.2 Female pseudohermaphroditism, not elsewhere classified POA ♀
Female pseudohermaphroditism NOS

Q56.3 Pseudohermaphroditism, unspecified POA

Q56.4 Indeterminate sex, unspecified POA
Ambiguous genitalia

Congenital malformations of the urinary system (Q60-Q64)

[4th] **Q60 Renal agenesis and other reduction defects of kidney**
[INCLUDES] *congenital absence of kidney*
congenital atrophy of kidney
infantile atrophy of kidney

Q60.0 Renal agenesis, unilateral CC POA CC/MCC Exc

Q60.1 Renal agenesis, bilateral CC POA CC/MCC Exc

Q60.2 Renal agenesis, unspecified CC POA CC/MCC Exc

Q60.3 Renal hypoplasia, unilateral CC POA CC/MCC Exc

Q60.4 Renal hypoplasia, bilateral CC POA CC/MCC Exc

Q60.5 Renal hypoplasia, unspecified CC POA CC/MCC Exc

Q60.6 Potter's syndrome CC POA CC/MCC Exc

[4th] **Q61 Cystic kidney disease**
[EXCLUDES1] *acquired cyst of kidney (N28.1)*
Potter's syndrome (Q60.6)

[5th] Q61.0 Congenital renal cyst

Q61.00 Congenital renal cyst, unspecified CC POA CC/MCC Exc
Cyst of kidney NOS (congenital)

Q61.01 Congenital single renal cyst CC POA CC/MCC Exc

Q61.02 Congenital multiple renal cysts CC POA CC/MCC Exc

[5th] Q61.1 Polycystic kidney, infantile type
Polycystic kidney, autosomal recessive

Q61.11 Cystic dilatation of collecting ducts CC POA CC/MCC Exc

Q61.19 Other polycystic kidney, infantile type CC POA CC/MCC Exc

Q61.2 Polycystic kidney, adult type CC POA CC/MCC Exc
Polycystic kidney, autosomal dominant

Q61.3 Polycystic kidney, unspecified CC POA CC/MCC Exc
AHA: Q3 2016

Q61.4 Renal dysplasia CC POA CC/MCC Exc
Multicystic dysplastic kidney
Multicystic kidney (development)
Multicystic kidney disease
Multicystic renal dysplasia
[EXCLUDES1] *polycystic kidney disease (Q61.11-Q61.3)*

Q61.5 Medullary cystic kidney CC POA CC/MCC Exc
Nephronopthisis
Sponge kidney NOS

Q61.8 Other cystic kidney diseases CC POA CC/MCC Exc
Fibrocystic kidney
Fibrocystic renal degeneration or disease

Q61.9 Cystic kidney disease, unspecified CC POA CC/MCC Exc
Meckel-Gruber syndrome

[4th] **Q62 Congenital obstructive defects of renal pelvis and congenital malformations of ureter**

Q62.0 Congenital hydronephrosis · CC · POA · CC/MCC Exc

5ᵗʰ Q62.1 Congenital occlusion of ureter
Atresia and stenosis of ureter

    Q62.10 Congenital occlusion of ureter, unspecified · CC · POA · CC/MCC Exc

    Q62.11 Congenital occlusion of ureteropelvic junction · CC · POA · CC/MCC Exc

    Q62.12 Congenital occlusion of ureterovesical orifice · CC · POA · CC/MCC Exc

Q62.2 Congenital megaureter · CC · POA · CC/MCC Exc
Congenital dilatation of ureter

5ᵗʰ Q62.3 Other obstructive defects of renal pelvis and ureter

    Q62.31 Congenital ureterocele, orthotopic · CC · POA · CC/MCC Exc

    Q62.32 Cecoureterocele · CC · POA · CC/MCC Exc
Ectopic ureterocele

    Q62.39 Other obstructive defects of renal pelvis and ureter · CC · POA · CC/MCC Exc
Ureteropelvic junction obstruction NOS

Q62.4 Agenesis of ureter · POA
Congenital absence ureter

Q62.5 Duplication of ureter · POA
Accessory ureter
Double ureter

5ᵗʰ Q62.6 Malposition of ureter

    Q62.60 Malposition of ureter, unspecified · POA

    Q62.61 Deviation of ureter · POA

    Q62.62 Displacement of ureter · POA

    Q62.63 Anomalous implantation of ureter · POA
Ectopia of ureter
Ectopic ureter

    Q62.69 Other malposition of ureter · POA

Q62.7 Congenital vesico-uretero-renal reflux · POA

Q62.8 Other congenital malformations of ureter · POA
Anomaly of ureter NOS

4ᵗʰ Q63 Other congenital malformations of kidney
EXCLUDES1 congenital nephrotic syndrome (N04.-)

Q63.0 Accessory kidney · POA

Q63.1 Lobulated, fused and horseshoe kidney · POA

Q63.2 Ectopic kidney · POA
Congenital displaced kidney
Malrotation of kidney

Q63.3 Hyperplastic and giant kidney · POA
Compensatory hypertrophy of kidney

Q63.8 Other specified congenital malformations of kidney · POA
Congenital renal calculi

Q63.9 Congenital malformation of kidney, unspecified · POA

4ᵗʰ Q64 Other congenital malformations of urinary system

Q64.0 Epispadias · POA · ♂
EXCLUDES1 hypospadias (Q54.-)

5ᵗʰ Q64.1 Exstrophy of urinary bladder

    Q64.10 Exstrophy of urinary bladder, unspecified · CC · POA · CC/MCC Exc
Ectopia vesicae

    Q64.11 Supravesical fissure of urinary bladder · CC · POA · CC/MCC Exc

▲ Q64.12 Cloacal ►exstrophy◄ of urinary bladder · CC · POA · CC/MCC Exc

    Q64.19 Other exstrophy of urinary bladder · CC · POA · CC/MCC Exc
Extroversion of bladder

Q64.2 Congenital posterior urethral valves · CC · POA · CC/MCC Exc

5ᵗʰ Q64.3 Other atresia and stenosis of urethra and bladder neck

    Q64.31 Congenital bladder neck obstruction · CC · POA · CC/MCC Exc
Congenital obstruction of vesicourethral orifice

    Q64.32 Congenital stricture of urethra · CC · POA · CC/MCC Exc

    Q64.33 Congenital stricture of urinary meatus · CC · POA · CC/MCC Exc

    Q64.39 Other atresia and stenosis of urethra and bladder neck · CC · POA · CC/MCC Exc
Atresia and stenosis of urethra and bladder neck NOS

Q64.4 Malformation of urachus · POA
Cyst of urachus
Patent urachus
Prolapse of urachus

Q64.5 Congenital absence of bladder and urethra · POA

Q64.6 Congenital diverticulum of bladder · POA

5ᵗʰ Q64.7 Other and unspecified congenital malformations of bladder and urethra

    EXCLUDES1 congenital prolapse of bladder (mucosa) (Q79.4)

    Q64.70 Unspecified congenital malformation of bladder and urethra · POA
Malformation of bladder or urethra NOS

    Q64.71 Congenital prolapse of urethra · POA

    Q64.72 Congenital prolapse of urinary meatus · POA

    Q64.73 Congenital urethrorectal fistula · POA

    Q64.74 Double urethra · POA

    Q64.75 Double urinary meatus · POA

    Q64.79 Other congenital malformations of bladder and urethra · POA

Q64.8 Other specified congenital malformations of urinary system · POA

Q64.9 Congenital malformation of urinary system, unspecified · POA
Congenital anomaly NOS of urinary system
Congenital deformity NOS of urinary system

Congenital malformations and deformations of the musculoskeletal system (Q65-Q79)

4ᵗʰ Q65 Congenital deformities of hip
EXCLUDES1 clicking hip (R29.4)

5ᵗʰ Q65.0 Congenital dislocation of hip, unilateral

    Q65.00 Congenital dislocation of unspecified hip, unilateral · POA

    Q65.01 Congenital dislocation of right hip, unilateral · POA

    Q65.02 Congenital dislocation of left hip, unilateral · POA

Q65.1 Congenital dislocation of hip, bilateral · POA

Q65.2 Congenital dislocation of hip, unspecified · POA

5ᵗʰ Q65.3 Congenital partial dislocation of hip, unilateral

    Q65.30 Congenital partial dislocation of unspecified hip, unilateral · POA

    Q65.31 Congenital partial dislocation of right hip, unilateral · POA

    Q65.32 Congenital partial dislocation of left hip, unilateral · POA

Q65.4 Congenital partial dislocation of hip, bilateral · POA

Q65.5 Congenital partial dislocation of hip, unspecified · POA

Q65.6 Congenital unstable hip · POA
Congenital dislocatable hip

5ᵗʰ Q65.8 Other congenital deformities of hip

    Q65.81 Congenital coxa valga · POA

    Q65.82 Congenital coxa vara · POA

    Q65.89 Other specified congenital deformities of hip · POA
Anteversion of femoral neck
Congenital acetabular dysplasia

Q65.9 Congenital deformity of hip, unspecified · POA

4ᵗʰ Q66 Congenital deformities of feet
EXCLUDES1 reduction defects of feet (Q72.-)
valgus deformities (acquired) (M21.0-)
varus deformities (acquired) (M21.1-)

Q66.0 Congenital talipes equinovarus · POA

Q66.1 Congenital talipes calcaneovarus · POA

5ᵗʰ Q66.2 Congenital metatarsus (primus) varus

    Q66.21 Congenital metatarsus primus varus · POA
AHA: Q4 2016

    Q66.22 Congenital metatarsus adductus · POA
AHA: Q4 2016
Congenital metatarsus varus

Q66.3 Other congenital varus deformities of feet · POA
Hallux varus, congenital

Q66.4 Congenital talipes calcaneovalgus · POA

5ᵗʰ Q66.5 Congenital pes planus
Congenital flat foot
Congenital rigid flat foot
Congenital spastic (everted) flat foot
EXCLUDES1 pes planus, acquired (M21.4)

    Q66.50 Congenital pes planus, unspecified foot · POA

POA Unacceptable principal diagnosis symbol per Medicare code edits   POA Code exempt from diagnosis present on admission requirement
? Questionable admission   CC Complication or comorbidity   CC/MCC Exc CC/MCC exclusion   MCC Major complication or comorbidity
Principal diagnosis as its own CC   Principal diagnosis as its own MCC   HCC HCC diagnosis code   RxHCC RxHCC diagnosis code
MACRA code   Z Z code as first-listed diagnosis

Q66.51 Congenital pes planus, right foot · POA
Q66.52 Congenital pes planus, left foot · POA
Q66.6 Other congenital valgus deformities of feet · POA
Congenital metatarsus valgus
Q66.7 Congenital pes cavus · POA
Q66.8 Other congenital deformities of feet
Q66.80 Congenital vertical talus deformity, unspecified foot · POA
Q66.81 Congenital vertical talus deformity, right foot · POA
Q66.82 Congenital vertical talus deformity, left foot · POA
Q66.89 Other specified congenital deformities of feet · POA
Congenital asymmetric talipes
Congenital clubfoot NOS
Congenital talipes NOS
Congenital tarsal coalition
Hammer toe, congenital
Q66.9 Congenital deformity of feet, unspecified · POA

Q67 Congenital musculoskeletal deformities of head, face, spine and chest
EXCLUDES1 congenital malformation syndromes classified to Q87.-
Potter's syndrome (Q60.6)
Q67.0 Congenital facial asymmetry · POA
Q67.1 Congenital compression facies · POA
Q67.2 Dolichocephaly · POA
Q67.3 Plagiocephaly · POA
Q67.4 Other congenital deformities of skull, face and jaw · POA
Congenital depressions in skull
Congenital hemifacial atrophy or hypertrophy
Deviation of nasal septum, congenital
Squashed or bent nose, congenital
EXCLUDES1 dentofacial anomalies [including malocclusion] (M26.-)
syphilitic saddle nose (A50.5)
Q67.5 Congenital deformity of spine · CC POA CC/MCC Exc
Congenital postural scoliosis
Congenital scoliosis NOS
EXCLUDES1 infantile idiopathic scoliosis (M41.0)
scoliosis due to congenital bony malformation (Q76.3)
Q67.6 Pectus excavatum · POA
Congenital funnel chest
Q67.7 Pectus carinatum · POA
Congenital pigeon chest
Q67.8 Other congenital deformities of chest · CC POA CC/MCC Exc
Congenital deformity of chest wall NOS

Q68 Other congenital musculoskeletal deformities
EXCLUDES1 reduction defects of limb(s) (Q71-Q73)
EXCLUDES2 congenital myotonic chondrodystrophy (G71.13)
Q68.0 Congenital deformity of sternocleidomastoid muscle · POA
Congenital contracture of sternocleidomastoid (muscle)
Congenital (sternomastoid) torticollis
Sternomastoid tumor (congenital)
Q68.1 Congenital deformity of finger(s) and hand · CC POA CC/MCC Exc
Congenital clubfinger
Spade-like hand (congenital)
Q68.2 Congenital deformity of knee · POA
Congenital dislocation of knee
Congenital genu recurvatum
Q68.3 Congenital bowing of femur · POA
EXCLUDES1 anteversion of femur (neck) (Q65.89)
Q68.4 Congenital bowing of tibia and fibula · POA
Q68.5 Congenital bowing of long bones of leg, unspecified · POA
Q68.6 Discoid meniscus · POA
Q68.8 Other specified congenital musculoskeletal deformities · POA
Congenital deformity of clavicle
Congenital deformity of elbow
Congenital deformity of forearm
Congenital deformity of scapula
Congenital deformity of wrist
Congenital dislocation of elbow
Congenital dislocation of shoulder
Congenital dislocation of wrist

Q69 Polydactyly
Q69.0 Accessory finger(s) · POA
Q69.1 Accessory thumb(s) · POA
Q69.2 Accessory toe(s) · POA
Accessory hallux
Q69.9 Polydactyly, unspecified · POA
Supernumerary digit(s) NOS

Q70 Syndactyly
Q70.0 Fused fingers
Complex syndactyly of fingers with synostosis
Q70.00 Fused fingers, unspecified hand · POA
Q70.01 Fused fingers, right hand · POA
Q70.02 Fused fingers, left hand · POA
Q70.03 Fused fingers, bilateral · POA
Q70.1 Webbed fingers
Simple syndactyly of fingers without synostosis
Q70.10 Webbed fingers, unspecified hand · POA
Q70.11 Webbed fingers, right hand · POA
Q70.12 Webbed fingers, left hand · POA
Q70.13 Webbed fingers, bilateral · POA
Q70.2 Fused toes
Complex syndactyly of toes with synostosis
Q70.20 Fused toes, unspecified foot · POA
Q70.21 Fused toes, right foot · POA
Q70.22 Fused toes, left foot · POA
Q70.23 Fused toes, bilateral · POA
Q70.3 Webbed toes
Simple syndactyly of toes without synostosis
Q70.30 Webbed toes, unspecified foot · POA
Q70.31 Webbed toes, right foot · POA
Q70.32 Webbed toes, left foot · POA
Q70.33 Webbed toes, bilateral · POA
Q70.4 Polysyndactyly, unspecified · POA
EXCLUDES1 specified syndactyly of hand and feet - code to specified conditions (Q70.0- -Q70.3-)
Q70.9 Syndactyly, unspecified · POA
Symphalangy NOS

Q71 Reduction defects of upper limb
Q71.0 Congenital complete absence of upper limb
Q71.00 Congenital complete absence of unspecified upper limb · POA
Q71.01 Congenital complete absence of right upper limb · POA
Q71.02 Congenital complete absence of left upper limb · POA
Q71.03 Congenital complete absence of upper limb, bilateral · POA
Q71.1 Congenital absence of upper arm and forearm with hand present
Q71.10 Congenital absence of unspecified upper arm and forearm with hand present · POA
Q71.11 Congenital absence of right upper arm and forearm with hand present · POA
Q71.12 Congenital absence of left upper arm and forearm with hand present · POA
Q71.13 Congenital absence of upper arm and forearm with hand present, bilateral · POA
Q71.2 Congenital absence of both forearm and hand
Q71.20 Congenital absence of both forearm and hand, unspecified upper limb · POA
Q71.21 Congenital absence of both forearm and hand, right upper limb · POA
Q71.22 Congenital absence of both forearm and hand, left upper limb · POA
Q71.23 Congenital absence of both forearm and hand, bilateral · POA
Q71.3 Congenital absence of hand and finger
Q71.30 Congenital absence of unspecified hand and finger · POA
Q71.31 Congenital absence of right hand and finger · POA
Q71.32 Congenital absence of left hand and finger · POA
Q71.33 Congenital absence of hand and finger, bilateral · POA

Unspecified Code   Other Specified Code   Manifestation Code   N Newborn   P Pediatric   M Maternity   A Adult   ♂ Male   ♀ Female
● New Code   ▲ Revised Code Title   ▶◀ Revised Text   NOTES   INCLUDES   EXCLUDES1 Not coded here   EXCLUDES2 Not included here
4ᵗʰ 4th character required   5ᵗʰ 5th character required   6ᵗʰ 6th character required   7ᵗʰ 7th character required
Extension 'X' Alert   HAC Hospital-acquired condition (HAC) alert   AHA AHA Coding Clinic©

⑤ **Q71.4** Longitudinal reduction defect of radius
Clubhand (congenital)
Radial clubhand

Q71.40 **Longitudinal reduction defect of unspecified radius** ᴘᴏᴬ

Q71.41 Longitudinal reduction defect of right radius ᴘᴏᴬ

Q71.42 Longitudinal reduction defect of left radius ᴘᴏᴬ

Q71.43 Longitudinal reduction defect of radius, bilateral ᴘᴏᴬ

⑤ **Q71.5** Longitudinal reduction defect of ulna

Q71.50 **Longitudinal reduction defect of unspecified ulna** ᴘᴏᴬ

Q71.51 Longitudinal reduction defect of right ulna ᴘᴏᴬ

Q71.52 Longitudinal reduction defect of left ulna ᴘᴏᴬ

Q71.53 Longitudinal reduction defect of ulna, bilateral ᴘᴏᴬ

⑤ **Q71.6** Lobster-claw hand

Q71.60 **Lobster-claw hand, unspecified hand** ᴘᴏᴬ

Q71.61 Lobster-claw right hand ᴘᴏᴬ

Q71.62 Lobster-claw left hand ᴘᴏᴬ

Q71.63 Lobster-claw hand, bilateral ᴘᴏᴬ

⑤ **Q71.8** Other reduction defects of upper limb

⑥ **Q71.81** Congenital shortening of upper limb

Q71.811 Congenital shortening of right upper limb ᴘᴏᴬ

Q71.812 Congenital shortening of left upper limb ᴘᴏᴬ

Q71.813 Congenital shortening of upper limb, bilateral ᴘᴏᴬ

Q71.819 **Congenital shortening of unspecified upper limb** ᴘᴏᴬ

⑥ **Q71.89** Other reduction defects of upper limb

Q71.891 Other reduction defects of right upper limb ᴘᴏᴬ

Q71.892 Other reduction defects of left upper limb ᴘᴏᴬ

Q71.893 Other reduction defects of upper limb, bilateral ᴘᴏᴬ

Q71.899 **Other reduction defects of unspecified upper limb** ᴘᴏᴬ

⑤ **Q71.9** Unspecified reduction defect of upper limb

Q71.90 Unspecified reduction defect of unspecified upper limb ᴘᴏᴬ

Q71.91 Unspecified reduction defect of right upper limb ᴘᴏᴬ

Q71.92 Unspecified reduction defect of left upper limb ᴘᴏᴬ

Q71.93 Unspecified reduction defect of upper limb, bilateral ᴘᴏᴬ

④ **Q72** Reduction defects of lower limb

⑤ **Q72.0** Congenital complete absence of lower limb

Q72.00 **Congenital complete absence of unspecified lower limb** ᴘᴏᴬ

Q72.01 Congenital complete absence of right lower limb ᴘᴏᴬ

Q72.02 Congenital complete absence of left lower limb ᴘᴏᴬ

Q72.03 Congenital complete absence of lower limb, bilateral ᴘᴏᴬ

⑤ **Q72.1** Congenital absence of thigh and lower leg with foot present

Q72.10 **Congenital absence of unspecified thigh and lower leg with foot present** ᴘᴏᴬ

Q72.11 Congenital absence of right thigh and lower leg with foot present ᴘᴏᴬ

Q72.12 Congenital absence of left thigh and lower leg with foot present ᴘᴏᴬ

Q72.13 Congenital absence of thigh and lower leg with foot present, bilateral ᴘᴏᴬ

⑤ **Q72.2** Congenital absence of both lower leg and foot

Q72.20 **Congenital absence of both lower leg and foot, unspecified lower limb** ᴘᴏᴬ

Q72.21 Congenital absence of both lower leg and foot, right lower limb ᴘᴏᴬ

Q72.22 Congenital absence of both lower leg and foot, left lower limb ᴘᴏᴬ

Q72.23 Congenital absence of both lower leg and foot, bilateral ᴘᴏᴬ

⑤ **Q72.3** Congenital absence of foot and toe(s)

Q72.30 **Congenital absence of unspecified foot and toe(s)** ᴘᴏᴬ

Q72.31 Congenital absence of right foot and toe(s) ᴘᴏᴬ

Q72.32 Congenital absence of left foot and toe(s) ᴘᴏᴬ

Q72.33 Congenital absence of foot and toe(s), bilateral ᴘᴏᴬ

⑤ **Q72.4** Longitudinal reduction defect of femur
Proximal femoral focal deficiency

Q72.40 **Longitudinal reduction defect of unspecified femur** ᴘᴏᴬ

Q72.41 Longitudinal reduction defect of right femur ᴘᴏᴬ

Q72.42 Longitudinal reduction defect of left femur ᴘᴏᴬ

Q72.43 Longitudinal reduction defect of femur, bilateral ᴘᴏᴬ

⑤ **Q72.5** Longitudinal reduction defect of tibia

Q72.50 **Longitudinal reduction defect of unspecified tibia** ᴘᴏᴬ

Q72.51 Longitudinal reduction defect of right tibia ᴘᴏᴬ

Q72.52 Longitudinal reduction defect of left tibia ᴘᴏᴬ

Q72.53 Longitudinal reduction defect of tibia, bilateral ᴘᴏᴬ

⑤ **Q72.6** Longitudinal reduction defect of fibula

Q72.60 **Longitudinal reduction defect of unspecified fibula** ᴘᴏᴬ

Q72.61 Longitudinal reduction defect of right fibula ᴘᴏᴬ

Q72.62 Longitudinal reduction defect of left fibula ᴘᴏᴬ

Q72.63 Longitudinal reduction defect of fibula, bilateral ᴘᴏᴬ

⑤ **Q72.7** Split foot

Q72.70 Split foot, unspecified lower limb ᴘᴏᴬ

Q72.71 Split foot, right lower limb ᴘᴏᴬ

Q72.72 Split foot, left lower limb ᴘᴏᴬ

Q72.73 Split foot, bilateral ᴘᴏᴬ

⑤ **Q72.8** Other reduction defects of lower limb

⑥ **Q72.81** Congenital shortening of lower limb

Q72.811 Congenital shortening of right lower limb ᴘᴏᴬ

Q72.812 Congenital shortening of left lower limb ᴘᴏᴬ

Q72.813 Congenital shortening of lower limb, bilateral ᴘᴏᴬ

Q72.819 **Congenital shortening of unspecified lower limb** ᴘᴏᴬ

⑥ **Q72.89** Other reduction defects of lower limb

Q72.891 Other reduction defects of right lower limb ᴘᴏᴬ

Q72.892 Other reduction defects of left lower limb ᴘᴏᴬ

Q72.893 Other reduction defects of lower limb, bilateral ᴘᴏᴬ

Q72.899 **Other reduction defects of unspecified lower limb** ᴘᴏᴬ

⑤ **Q72.9** Unspecified reduction defect of lower limb

Q72.90 **Unspecified reduction defect of unspecified lower limb** ᴘᴏᴬ

Q72.91 Unspecified reduction defect of right lower limb ᴘᴏᴬ

Q72.92 Unspecified reduction defect of left lower limb ᴘᴏᴬ

Q72.93 Unspecified reduction defect of lower limb, bilateral ᴘᴏᴬ

④ **Q73** Reduction defects of unspecified limb

Q73.0 **Congenital absence of unspecified limb(s)** ᴘᴏᴬ
Amelia NOS

Q73.1 **Phocomelia, unspecified limb(s)** ᴘᴏᴬ
Phocomelia NOS

Q73.8 Other reduction defects of unspecified limb(s) ᴘᴏᴬ
Longitudinal reduction deformity of unspecified limb(s)
Ectromelia of limb NOS
Hemimelia of limb NOS
Reduction defect of limb NOS

④ **Q74** Other congenital malformations of limb(s)

EXCLUDES1 polydactyly (Q69.-)

reduction defect of limb (Q71-Q73)

syndactyly (Q70.-)

Q74.0 Other congenital malformations of upper limb(s), including shoulder girdle ᴘᴏᴬ

ᴘᴏᴬ Unacceptable principal diagnosis symbol per Medicare code edits   ᴘᴏᴬ Code exempt from diagnosis present on admission requirement   ❓ Questionable admission   ᶜᶜ Complication or comorbidity   ᶜᶜ⁄ᴹᶜᶜ Eₓ CC/MCC exclusion   ᴹᶜᶜ Major complication or comorbidity   ᴾ𝒸ᶜ Principal diagnosis as its own CC   ᴾᴹᶜᶜ Principal diagnosis as its own MCC   ʜᴄᴄ HCC diagnosis code   ᴿˣʜᴄᴄ RxHCC diagnosis code   MACRA code   Zₗ Z code as first-listed diagnosis

When symbols appear on a code that requires a 7th character extension, refer to Appendix B to identify applicable 7th character codes.

2018 ICD-10-CM

Accessory carpal bones
Cleidocranial dysostosis
Congenital pseudarthrosis of clavicle
Macrodactylia (fingers)
Madelung's deformity
Radioulnar synostosis
Sprengel's deformity
Triphalangeal thumb

Q74.1 Congenital malformation of knee   POA
Congenital absence of patella
Congenital dislocation of patella
Congenital genu valgum
Congenital genu varum
Rudimentary patella
EXCLUDES1 congenital dislocation of knee (Q68.2)
congenital genu recurvatum (Q68.2)
nail patella syndrome (Q87.2)

Q74.2 Other congenital malformations of lower limb(s), including pelvic girdle   POA
Congenital fusion of sacroiliac joint
Congenital malformation of ankle joint
Congenital malformation of sacroiliac joint
EXCLUDES1 anteversion of femur (neck) (Q65.89)

Q74.3 Arthrogryposis multiplex congenita   CC POA CC/MCC Exc

Q74.8 Other specified congenital malformations of limb(s)   POA

Q74.9 Unspecified congenital malformation of limb(s)   POA
Congenital anomaly of limb(s) NOS

4ᵗʰ **Q75 Other congenital malformations of** skull and face bones
EXCLUDES1 congenital malformation of face NOS (Q18.-)
congenital malformation syndromes classified to Q87.-
dentofacial anomalies [including malocclusion] (M26.-)
musculoskeletal deformities of head and face (Q67.0-Q67.4)
skull defects associated with congenital anomalies of brain such as:
anencephaly (Q00.0)
encephalocele (Q01.-)
hydrocephalus (Q03.-)
microcephaly (Q02)

Q75.0 Craniosynostosis   POA
Acrocephaly
Imperfect fusion of skull
Oxycephaly
Trigonocephaly

Q75.1 Craniofacial dysostosis   POA
Crouzon's disease

Q75.2 Hypertelorism   POA

Q75.3 Macrocephaly   POA

Q75.4 Mandibulofacial dysostosis   POA
Franceschetti syndrome
Treacher Collins syndrome

Q75.5 Oculomandibular dysostosis   POA

Q75.8 Other specified congenital malformations of skull and face bones
Absence of skull bone, congenital
Congenital deformity of forehead
Platybasia

Q75.9 Congenital malformation of skull and face bones, unspecified   POA
Congenital anomaly of face bones NOS
Congenital anomaly of skull NOS

4ᵗʰ **Q76 Congenital malformations of** spine and bony thorax
EXCLUDES1 congenital musculoskeletal deformities of spine and chest (Q67.5-Q67.8)

Q76.0 Spina bifida occulta   POA
EXCLUDES1 meningocele (spinal) (Q05.-)
spina bifida (aperta) (cystica) (Q05.-)

Q76.1 Klippel-Feil syndrome   POA
Cervical fusion syndrome

Q76.2 Congenital spondylolisthesis   POA
Congenital spondylolysis

EXCLUDES1 spondylolisthesis (acquired) (M43.1-)
spondylolysis (acquired) (M43.0-)

Q76.3 Congenital scoliosis due to congenital bony malformation   CC POA CC/MCC Exc
Hemivertebra fusion or failure of segmentation with scoliosis

5ᵗʰ **Q76.4 Other congenital malformations of** spine, not associated with scoliosis

6ᵗʰ **Q76.41 Congenital** kyphosis
Q76.411 Congenital kyphosis, occipito-atlanto-axial region   POA
Q76.412 Congenital kyphosis, cervical region   POA
Q76.413 Congenital kyphosis, cervicothoracic region   POA
Q76.414 Congenital kyphosis, thoracic region   POA
Q76.415 Congenital kyphosis, thoracolumbar region   POA
Q76.419 Congenital kyphosis, unspecified region   POA

6ᵗʰ **Q76.42 Congenital** lordosis
Q76.425 Congenital lordosis, thoracolumbar region   CC POA CC/MCC Exc
Q76.426 Congenital lordosis, lumbar region   CC POA CC/MCC Exc
Q76.427 Congenital lordosis, lumbosacral region   CC POA CC/MCC Exc
Q76.428 Congenital lordosis, sacral and sacrococcygeal region   CC POA CC/MCC Exc
Q76.429 Congenital lordosis, unspecified region   CC POA CC/MCC Exc

Q76.49 Other congenital malformations of spine, not associated with scoliosis   POA
Congenital absence of vertebra NOS
Congenital fusion of spine NOS
Congenital malformation of lumbosacral (joint) (region) NOS
Congenital malformation of spine NOS
Hemivertebra NOS
Malformation of spine NOS
Platyspondylisis NOS
Supernumerary vertebra NOS

Q76.5 Cervical rib   POA
Supernumerary rib in cervical region

Q76.6 Other congenital malformations of ribs   CC POA CC/MCC Exc
Accessory rib
Congenital absence of rib
Congenital fusion of ribs
Congenital malformation of ribs NOS
EXCLUDES1 short rib syndrome (Q77.2)

Q76.7 Congenital malformation of sternum   CC POA CC/MCC Exc
Congenital absence of sternum
Sternum bifidum

Q76.8 Other congenital malformations of bony thorax   CC POA CC/MCC Exc

Q76.9 Congenital malformation of bony thorax, unspecified   CC POA CC/MCC Exc

4ᵗʰ **Q77 Osteochondrodysplasia with defects of growth of tubular bones and spine**
EXCLUDES1 mucopolysaccharidosis (E76.0-E76.3)
EXCLUDES2 congenital myotonic chondrodystrophy (G71.13)

Q77.0 Achondrogenesis   POA
Hypochondrogenesis

Q77.1 Thanatophoric short stature   POA

Q77.2 Short rib syndrome   CC POA CC/MCC Exc
Asphyxiating thoracic dysplasia [Jeune]

Q77.3 Chondrodysplasia punctata   POA
EXCLUDES1 Rhizomelic chondrodysplasia punctata (E71.43)

Q77.4 Achondroplasia   POA
Hypochondroplasia
Osteosclerosis congenita

Q77.5 Diastrophic dysplasia   POA

Q77.6 Chondroectodermal dysplasia   POA
Ellis-van Creveld syndrome

Q77.7 Spondyloepiphyseal dysplasia   POA

Unspecified Code   Other Specified Code   Manifestation Code   Ⓝ Newborn   Ⓟ Pediatric   Ⓜ Maternity   Ⓐ Adult   ♂ Male   ♀ Female
● New Code   ▲ Revised Code Title   ►◄ Revised Text   NOTES   *INCLUDES*   *EXCLUDES 1* Not coded here   *EXCLUDES 2* Not included here
4ᵗʰ 4ᵗʰ character required   5ᵗʰ 5ᵗʰ character required   6ᵗʰ 6ᵗʰ character required   7ᵗʰ 7ᵗʰ character required
Extension 'X' Alert   HAC Hospital-acquired condition (HAC) alert   **AHA** AHA Coding Clinic©

Q77.8 **Other osteochondrodysplasia with defects of growth of tubular bones and spine**

Q77.9 Osteochondrodysplasia with defects of growth of tubular bones and spine, unspecified

Q78 Other osteochondrodysplasias

EXCLUDES2 *congenital myotonic chondrodystrophy (G71.13)*

Q78.0 **Osteogenesis imperfecta**
Fragilitas ossium
Osteopsathyrosis

Q78.1 **Polyostotic fibrous dysplasia**
Albright(-McCune)(-Sternberg) syndrome

Q78.2 **Osteopetrosis**
Albers-Schönberg syndrome
Osteosclerosis NOS

Q78.3 **Progressive diaphyseal dysplasia**
Camurati-Engelmann syndrome

Q78.4 **Enchondromatosis**
Maffucci's syndrome
Ollier's disease

Q78.5 **Metaphyseal dysplasia**
Pyle's syndrome

Q78.6 **Multiple congenital exostoses**
Diaphyseal aclasis

Q78.8 Other specified osteochondrodysplasias
Osteopoikilosis

Q78.9 **Osteochondrodysplasia, unspecified**
Chondrodystrophy NOS
Osteodystrophy NOS

Q79 **Congenital malformations of musculoskeletal system, not elsewhere classified**

EXCLUDES2 *congenital (sternomastoid) torticollis (Q68.0)*

Q79.0 **Congenital diaphragmatic hernia**

EXCLUDES1 *congenital hiatus hernia (Q40.1)*

Q79.1 **Other congenital malformations of diaphragm**
Absence of diaphragm
Congenital malformation of diaphragm NOS
Eventration of diaphragm

Q79.2 **Exomphalos**
Omphalocele

EXCLUDES1 *umbilical hernia (K42.-)*

Q79.3 **Gastroschisis**

Q79.4 **Prune belly syndrome**
Congenital prolapse of bladder mucosa
Eagle-Barrett syndrome

Q79.5 Other **congenital malformations of** abdominal wall

EXCLUDES1 *umbilical hernia (K42.-)*

Q79.51 **Congenital hernia of bladder**

Q79.59 **Other congenital malformations of abdominal wall**

Q79.6 **Ehlers-Danlos syndrome**

Q79.8 **Other congenital malformations of musculoskeletal system**
Absence of muscle
Absence of tendon
Accessory muscle
Amyotrophia congenita
Congenital constricting bands
Congenital shortening of tendon
Poland syndrome

Q79.9 Congenital malformation of musculoskeletal system, unspecified
Congenital anomaly of musculoskeletal system NOS
Congenital deformity of musculoskeletal system NOS

Other congenital malformations (Q80-Q89)

Q80 **Congenital ichthyosis**

EXCLUDES1 *Refsum's disease (G60.1)*

Q80.0 **Ichthyosis** vulgaris

Q80.1 X-linked **ichthyosis**

Q80.2 Lamellar **ichthyosis**
Collodion baby

Q80.3 Congenital bullous **ichthyosiform erythroderma**

Q80.4 Harlequin fetus

Q80.8 **Other congenital ichthyosis**

Q80.9 **Congenital ichthyosis, unspecified**

Q81 Epidermolysis bullosa

Q81.0 **Epidermolysis bullosa** simplex

EXCLUDES1 *Cockayne's syndrome (Q87.1)*

Q81.1 **Epidermolysis bullosa** letalis
Herlitz' syndrome

Q81.2 **Epidermolysis bullosa** dystrophica

Q81.8 **Other epidermolysis bullosa**

Q81.9 **Epidermolysis bullosa, unspecified**

Q82 Other congenital malformations of skin

EXCLUDES1 *acrodermatitis enteropathica (E83.2)*
congenital erythropoietic porphyria (E80.0)
pilonidal cyst or sinus (L05.-)
Sturge-Weber (-Dimitri) syndrome (Q85.8)

Q82.0 **Hereditary lymphedema**

Q82.1 **Xeroderma pigmentosum**

▲ Q82.2 ▶Congenital cutaneous◀ **mastocytosis**
Congenital diffuse cutaneous mastocytosis
Congenital maculopapular cutaneous mastocytosis
Congenital urticaria pigmentosa

EXCLUDES1 *cutaneous mastocytosis NOS (D47.01)*
diffuse cutaneous mastocytosis (with onset after newborn period) (D47.01)
malignant mastocytosis (C96.2-)
systemic mastocytosis (D47.02)
urticaria pigmentosa (non-congenital) (with onset after newborn period) (D47.01)

Q82.3 **Incontinentia pigmenti**

Q82.4 **Ectodermal dysplasia (anhidrotic)**

EXCLUDES1 *Ellis-van Creveld syndrome (Q77.6)*

Q82.5 **Congenital non-neoplastic nevus**
Birthmark NOS
Flammeus Nevus
Portwine Nevus
Sanguineous Nevus
Strawberry Nevus
Vascular Nevus NOS
Verrucous Nevus

EXCLUDES2 *Café au lait spots (L81.3)*
lentigo (L81.4)
nevus NOS (D22.-)
araneus nevus (I78.1)
melanocytic nevus (D22.-)
pigmented nevus (D22.-)
spider nevus (I78.1)
stellar nevus (I78.1)

Q82.6 **Congenital** sacral dimple
AHA: Q4 2016
Parasacral dimple

EXCLUDES2 *pilonidal cyst with abscess (L05.01)*
pilonidal cyst without abscess (L05.91)

Q82.8 Other specified congenital malformations of skin
AHA: Q1 2016
Abnormal palmar creases
Accessory skin tags
Benign familial pemphigus [Hailey-Hailey]
Congenital poikiloderma
Cutis laxa (hyperelastica)
Dermatoglyphic anomalies
Inherited keratosis palmaris et plantaris
Keratosis follicularis [Darier-White]

EXCLUDES1 *Ehlers-Danlos syndrome (Q79.6)*

Q82.9 **Congenital malformation of skin, unspecified**

PDX Unacceptable principal diagnosis symbol per Medicare code edits   POA Code exempt from diagnosis present on admission requirement
❓ Questionable admission   CC Complication or comorbidity   CC-MCC Exc CC/MCC exclusion   MCC Major complication or comorbidity
Principal diagnosis as its own CC   Principal diagnosis as its own MCC   HCC HCC diagnosis code   RxHCC RxHCC diagnosis code
MACRA code   Z1 Z code as first-listed diagnosis

When symbols appear on a code that requires a 7th character extension, refer to Appendix B to identify applicable 7th character codes.

Q83 Congenital malformations of breast

EXCLUDES2 absence of pectoral muscle (Q79.8)

hypoplasia of breast (N64.82)

micromastia (N64.82)

Q83.0 Congenital absence of breast with absent nipple POA

Q83.1 Accessory breast
Supernumerary breast

Q83.2 Absent nipple POA

Q83.3 Accessory nipple POA
Supernumerary nipple

Q83.8 Other congenital malformations of breast POA

Q83.9 Congenital malformation of breast, unspecified POA

Q84 Other congenital malformations of integument

Q84.0 Congenital alopecia POA
Congenital atrichosis

Q84.1 Congenital morphological disturbances of hair, not elsewhere classified POA
Beaded hair
Monilethrix
Pili annulati
EXCLUDES1 Menkes' kinky hair syndrome (E83.0)

Q84.2 Other congenital malformations of hair POA
Congenital hypertrichosis
Congenital malformation of hair NOS
Persistent lanugo

Q84.3 Anonychia POA
EXCLUDES1 nail patella syndrome (Q87.2)

Q84.4 Congenital leukonychia POA

Q84.5 Enlarged and hypertrophic nails POA
Congenital onychauxis
Pachyonychia

Q84.6 Other congenital malformations of nails POA
Congenital clubnail
Congenital koilonychia
Congenital malformation of nail NOS

Q84.8 Other specified congenital malformations of integument POA
Aplasia cutis congenita

Q84.9 Congenital malformation of integument, unspecified POA
Congenital anomaly of integument NOS
Congenital deformity of integument NOS

Q85 Phakomatoses, not elsewhere classified

EXCLUDES1 ataxia telangiectasia [Louis-Bar] (G11.3)

familial dysautonomia [Riley-Day] (G90.1)

Q85.0 Neurofibromatosis (nonmalignant)

Q85.00 Neurofibromatosis, unspecified POA HCC

Q85.01 Neurofibromatosis, type 1 POA HCC
Von Recklinghausen disease

Q85.02 Neurofibromatosis, type 2 POA HCC
Acoustic neurofibromatosis

Q85.03 Schwannomatosis POA HCC

Q85.09 Other neurofibromatosis POA HCC

Q85.1 Tuberous sclerosis CC POA HCC RxHCC CC/MCC Exc
Bourneville's disease
Epiloia

Q85.8 Other phakomatoses, not elsewhere classified CC POA HCC RxHCC CC/MCC Exc
Peutz-Jeghers Syndrome
Sturge-Weber(-Dimitri) syndrome
von Hippel-Lindau syndrome
EXCLUDES1 Meckel-Gruber syndrome (Q61.9)

Q85.9 Phakomatosis, unspecified CC POA HCC RxHCC CC/MCC Exc
Hamartosis NOS

Q86 Congenital malformation syndromes due to known exogenous causes, not elsewhere classified

EXCLUDES2 iodine-deficiency-related hypothyroidism (E00-E02)

nonteratogenic effects of substances transmitted via placenta or breast milk (P04.-)

Q86.0 Fetal alcohol syndrome (dysmorphic) POA

Q86.1 Fetal hydantoin syndrome POA
Meadow's syndrome

Q86.2 Dysmorphism due to warfarin POA

Q86.8 Other congenital malformation syndromes due to known exogenous causes POA

Q87 Other specified congenital malformation syndromes affecting multiple systems
Use additional code(s) to identify all associated manifestations

Q87.0 Congenital malformation syndromes predominantly affecting facial appearance POA
Acrocephalopolysyndactyly
Acrocephalosyndactyly [Apert]
Cryptophthalmos syndrome
Cyclopia
Goldenhar syndrome
Moebius syndrome
Oro-facial-digital syndrome
Robin syndrome
Whistling face

Q87.1 Congenital malformation syndromes predominantly associated with short stature CC POA CC/MCC Exc
Aarskog syndrome
Cockayne syndrome
De Lange syndrome
Dubowitz syndrome
Noonan syndrome
Prader-Willi syndrome
Robinow-Silverman-Smith syndrome
Russell-Silver syndrome
Seckel syndrome
EXCLUDES1 Ellis-van Creveld syndrome (Q77.6)

Smith-Lemli-Opitz syndrome (E78.72)

Q87.2 Congenital malformation syndromes predominantly involving limbs CC POA CC/MCC Exc
Holt-Oram syndrome
Klippel-Trenaunay-Weber syndrome
Nail patella syndrome
Rubinstein-Taybi syndrome
Sirenomelia syndrome
Thrombocytopenia with absent radius [TAR] syndrome
VATER syndrome

Q87.3 Congenital malformation syndromes involving early overgrowth CC POA CC/MCC Exc
Beckwith-Wiedemann syndrome
Sotos syndrome
Weaver syndrome

Q87.4 Marfan's syndrome

Q87.40 Marfan's syndrome, unspecified CC POA RxHCC CC/MCC Exc

Q87.41 Marfan's syndrome with cardiovascular manifestations

Q87.410 Marfan's syndrome with aortic dilation CC POA RxHCC CC/MCC Exc

Q87.418 Marfan's syndrome with other cardiovascular manifestations CC POA RxHCC CC/MCC Exc

Q87.42 Marfan's syndrome with ocular manifestations CC POA RxHCC CC/MCC Exc

Q87.43 Marfan's syndrome with skeletal manifestation CC POA RxHCC CC/MCC Exc

Q87.5 Other congenital malformation syndromes with other skeletal changes

Q87.8 Other specified congenital malformation syndromes, not elsewhere classified

EXCLUDES1 Zellweger syndrome (E71.510)

Q87.81 Alport syndrome CC POA CC/MCC Exc
Use additional code to identify stage of chronic kidney disease (N18.1-N18.6)

Q87.82 Arterial tortuosity syndrome CC POA RxHCC CC/MCC Exc
AHA: Q4 2016

Q87.89 Other specified congenital malformation syndromes, not elsewhere classified CC POA CC/MCC Exc
Laurence-Moon (-Bardet)-Biedl syndrome

Unspecified Code Other Specified Code Manifestation Code N Newborn P Pediatric M Maternity A Adult ♂ Male ♀ Female
● New Code ▲ Revised Code Title ▶◀ Revised Text NOTES INCLUDES EXCLUDES 1 Not coded here EXCLUDES 2 Not included here
④ 4th character required ⑤ 5th character required ⑥ 6th character required ⑦ 7th character required
⑦ Extension 'X' Alert HAC Hospital-acquired condition (HAC) alert AHA AHA Coding Clinic©

Q89 Other congenital malformations, not elsewhere classified

Q89.0 Congenital absence and malformations of spleen

EXCLUDES1 isomerism of atrial appendages (with asplenia or polysplenia) (Q20.6)

Q89.01 Asplenia (congenital) CC POA CC/MCC Exc

Q89.09 Congenital malformations of spleen CC POA CC/MCC Exc
Congenital splenomegaly

Q89.1 Congenital malformations of adrenal gland POA

EXCLUDES1 adrenogenital disorders (E25.-)
congenital adrenal hyperplasia (E25.0)

Q89.2 Congenital malformations of other endocrine glands POA
Congenital malformation of parathyroid or thyroid gland
Persistent thyroglossal duct
Thyroglossal cyst

EXCLUDES1 congenital goiter (E03.0)
congenital hypothyroidism (E03.1)

Q89.3 Situs inversus CC POA CC/MCC Exc
Dextrocardia with situs inversus
Mirror-image atrial arrangement with situs inversus
Situs inversus or transversus abdominalis
Situs inversus or transversus thoracis
Transposition of abdominal viscera
Transposition of thoracic viscera

EXCLUDES1 dextrocardia NOS (Q24.0)

Q89.4 Conjoined twins POA MCC CC/MCC Exc
Craniopagus
Dicephaly
Pygopagus
Thoracopagus

Q89.7 Multiple congenital malformations, not elsewhere classified CC POA CC/MCC Exc
Multiple congenital anomalies NOS
Multiple congenital deformities NOS

EXCLUDES1 congenital malformation syndromes affecting multiple systems (Q87.-)

Q89.8 Other specified congenital malformations CC POA CC/MCC Exc
Use additional code(s) to identify all associated manifestations

Q89.9 Congenital malformation, unspecified POA
Congenital anomaly NOS
Congenital deformity NOS

Chromosomal abnormalities, not elsewhere classified (Q90-Q99)

EXCLUDES2 mitochondrial metabolic disorders (E88.4-)

Q90 Down syndrome
Use additional code(s) to identify any associated physical conditions and degree of intellectual disabilities (F70-F79)

Q90.0 Trisomy 21, nonmosaicism (meiotic nondisjunction) POA

Q90.1 Trisomy 21, mosaicism (mitotic nondisjunction) POA

Q90.2 Trisomy 21, translocation POA

Q90.9 Down syndrome, unspecified POA
Trisomy 21 NOS

Q91 Trisomy 18 and Trisomy 13

Q91.0 Trisomy 18, nonmosaicism (meiotic nondisjunction) CC POA RxHCC CC/MCC Exc

Q91.1 Trisomy 18, mosaicism (mitotic nondisjunction) CC POA RxHCC CC/MCC Exc

Q91.2 Trisomy 18, translocation CC POA RxHCC CC/MCC Exc

Q91.3 Trisomy 18, unspecified CC POA RxHCC CC/MCC Exc

Q91.4 Trisomy 13, nonmosaicism (meiotic nondisjunction) CC POA RxHCC CC/MCC Exc

Q91.5 Trisomy 13, mosaicism (mitotic nondisjunction) CC POA RxHCC CC/MCC Exc

Q91.6 Trisomy 13, translocation CC POA RxHCC CC/MCC Exc

Q91.7 Trisomy 13, unspecified CC POA RxHCC CC/MCC Exc

Q92 Other trisomies and partial trisomies of the autosomes, not elsewhere classified

INCLUDES unbalanced translocations and insertions

EXCLUDES1 trisomies of chromosomes 13, 18, 21 (Q90-Q91)

Q92.0 Whole chromosome trisomy, nonmosaicism (meiotic nondisjunction) POA RxHCC

Q92.1 Whole chromosome trisomy, mosaicism (mitotic nondisjunction) POA RxHCC

Q92.2 Partial trisomy POA RxHCC
Less than whole arm duplicated
Whole arm or more duplicated

EXCLUDES1 partial trisomy due to unbalanced translocation (Q92.5)

Q92.5 Duplications with other complex rearrangements POA RxHCC
Partial trisomy due to unbalanced translocations
Code also any associated deletions due to unbalanced translocations, inversions and insertions (Q93.7)

Q92.6 Marker chromosomes
Trisomies due to dicentrics
Trisomies due to extra rings
Trisomies due to isochromosomes
Individual with marker heterochromatin

Q92.61 Marker chromosomes in normal individual POA RxHCC

Q92.62 Marker chromosomes in abnormal individual POA RxHCC

Q92.7 Triploidy and polyploidy POA RxHCC

Q92.8 Other specified trisomies and partial trisomies of autosomes POA RxHCC
Duplications identified by fluorescence in situ hybridization (FISH)
Duplications identified by in situ hybridization (ISH)
Duplications seen only at prometaphase

Q92.9 Trisomy and partial trisomy of autosomes, unspecified POA RxHCC

Q93 Monosomies and deletions from the autosomes, not elsewhere classified

Q93.0 Whole chromosome monosomy, nonmosaicism (meiotic nondisjunction) POA RxHCC

Q93.1 Whole chromosome monosomy, mosaicism (mitotic nondisjunction) POA RxHCC

Q93.2 Chromosome replaced with ring, dicentric or isochromosome POA RxHCC

Q93.3 Deletion of short arm of chromosome 4 CC POA RxHCC CC/MCC Exc
Wolff-Hirschorn syndrome

Q93.4 Deletion of short arm of chromosome 5 CC POA RxHCC CC/MCC Exc
Cri-du-chat syndrome

Q93.5 Other deletions of part of a chromosome CC POA RxHCC CC/MCC Exc
Angelman syndrome

Q93.7 Deletions with other complex rearrangements CC POA RxHCC CC/MCC Exc
Deletions due to unbalanced translocations, inversions and insertions
Code also any associated duplications due to unbalanced translocations, inversions and insertions (Q92.5)

Q93.8 Other deletions from the autosomes

Q93.81 Velo-cardio-facial syndrome POA MCC RxHCC CC/MCC Exc
Deletion 22q11.2

Q93.88 Other microdeletions CC POA RxHCC CC/MCC Exc
Miller-Dieker syndrome
Smith-Magenis syndrome

Q93.89 Other deletions from the autosomes CC POA RxHCC CC/MCC Exc
Deletions identified by fluorescence in situ hybridization (FISH)
Deletions identified by in situ hybridization (ISH)
Deletions seen only at prometaphase

Q93.9 Deletion from autosomes, unspecified CC POA RxHCC CC/MCC Exc

Q95 Balanced rearrangements and structural markers, not elsewhere classified

INCLUDES Robertsonian and balanced reciprocal translocations and insertions

Q95.0 Balanced translocation and insertion in normal individual POA

Q95.1 Chromosome inversion in normal individual POA

Q95.2 Balanced autosomal rearrangement in abnormal individual POA RxHCC

Q95.3 Balanced sex/autosomal rearrangement in abnormal individual POA RxHCC

Q95.5 Individual with autosomal fragile site POA

PDia Unacceptable principal diagnosis symbol per Medicare code edits POA Code exempt from diagnosis present on admission requirement ? Questionable admission CC Complication or comorbidity CC/MCC Exc CC/MCC exclusion MCC Major complication or comorbidity Principal diagnosis as its own CC Principal diagnosis as its own MCC HCC HCC diagnosis code RxHCC RxHCC diagnosis code MACRA code Z Z code as first-listed diagnosis

948

When symbols appear on a code that requires a 7th character extension, refer to Appendix B to identify applicable 7th character codes.

2018 ICD-10-CM

Q95.8 Other balanced rearrangements and structural markers POA

Q95.9 **Balanced rearrangement and structural marker, unspecified** POA

4th Q96 Turner's syndrome

EXCLUDES1 *Noonan syndrome (Q87.1)*

Q96.0 **Karyotype** 45, X POA ♀

Q96.1 **Karyotype** 46, X iso (Xq) POA ♀

Karyotype 46, isochromosome Xq

Q96.2 **Karyotype** 46, X with abnormal sex chromosome, except iso (Xq) POA ♀

Karyotype 46, X with abnormal sex chromosome, except isochromosome Xq

Q96.3 **Mosaicism,** 45, X/46, XX or XY POA ♀

Q96.4 **Mosaicism,** 45, X/other cell line(s) with abnormal sex chromosome POA ♀

Q96.8 Other variants of Turner's syndrome POA ♀

Q96.9 Turner's syndrome, unspecified POA ♀

4th Q97 Other sex chromosome abnormalities, female phenotype, **not elsewhere classified**

EXCLUDES1 *Turner's syndrome (Q96.-)*

Q97.0 **Karyotype** 47, XXX POA ♀

Q97.1 Female with more than three X chromosomes POA ♀

Q97.2 Mosaicism, lines with various numbers of X chromosomes POA ♀

Q97.3 Female with 46, XY karyotype POA ♀

Q97.8 **Other specified sex chromosome abnormalities, female phenotype** POA ♀

Q97.9 **Sex chromosome abnormality, female phenotype, unspecified** POA ♀

4th Q98 Other sex chromosome abnormalities, male phenotype, **not elsewhere classified**

Q98.0 Klinefelter syndrome karyotype 47, XXY POA ♂

Q98.1 Klinefelter syndrome, male with more than two X chromosomes POA ♂

Q98.3 Other male with 46, XX karyotype POA ♂

Q98.4 **Klinefelter syndrome, unspecified** POA ♂

Q98.5 **Karyotype** 47, XYY POA

Q98.6 Male with structurally abnormal sex chromosome POA ♂

Q98.7 Male with sex chromosome mosaicism POA ♂

Q98.8 **Other specified sex chromosome abnormalities, male phenotype** POA ♂

Q98.9 **Sex chromosome abnormality, male phenotype, unspecified** POA ♂

4th Q99 Other chromosome abnormalities, **not elsewhere classified**

Q99.0 **Chimera** 46, XX/46, XY POA

Chimera 46, XX/46, XY true hermaphrodite

Q99.1 **46, XX true hermaphrodite** POA

46, XX with streak gonads

46, XY with streak gonads

Pure gonadal dysgenesis

Q99.2 **Fragile X chromosome** POA RxHCC

Fragile X syndrome

Q99.8 **Other specified chromosome abnormalities** POA

Q99.9 **Chromosomal abnormality, unspecified** POA

Unspecified Code   Other Specified Code   Manifestation Code   N Newborn   P Pediatric   M Maternity   A Adult   ♂ Male   ♀ Female
● New Code   ▲ Revised Code Title   ►◄ Revised Text   NOTES   INCLUDES   EXCLUDES1 Not coded here   EXCLUDES2 Not included here
4th 4th character required   5th 5th character required   6th 6th character required   7th 7th character required
Extension 'X' Alert   HAC Hospital-acquired condition (HAC) alert   AHA AHA Coding Clinic©

NOTES

Chapter 18: Symptoms, Signs, and Abnormal Clinical and Laboratory Findings, Not Elsewhere Classified (R00-R99)

DO NOT INCLUDE IF IN DIAGNOSIS

Symptoms, signs and abnormal clinical and laboratory findings, not elsewhere classified (R00-R99)

[NOTES] This chapter includes symptoms, signs, abnormal results of clinical or other investigative procedures, and ill-defined conditions regarding which no diagnosis classifiable elsewhere is recorded.

Signs and symptoms that point rather definitely to a given diagnosis have been assigned to a category in other chapters of the classification. In general, categories in this chapter include the less well-defined conditions and symptoms that, without the necessary study of the case to establish a final diagnosis, point perhaps equally to two or more diseases or to two or more systems of the body. Practically all categories in the chapter could be designated 'not otherwise specified', 'unknown etiology' or 'transient'. The Alphabetical Index should be consulted to determine which symptoms and signs are to be allocated here and which to other chapters. The residual subcategories, numbered .8, are generally provided for other relevant symptoms that cannot be allocated elsewhere in the classification.

The conditions and signs or symptoms included in categories R00-R94 consist of:

(a) cases for which no more specific diagnosis can be made even after all the facts bearing on the case have been investigated;

(b) signs or symptoms existing at the time of initial encounter that proved to be transient and whose causes could not be determined;

(c) provisional diagnosis in a patient who failed to return for further investigation or care;

(d) cases referred elsewhere for investigation or treatment before the diagnosis was made;

(e) cases in which a more precise diagnosis was not available for any other reason;

(f) certain symptoms, for which supplementary information is provided, that represent important problems in medical care in their own right.

[EXCLUDES2] *abnormal findings on antenatal screening of mother (O28.-)*
certain conditions originating in the perinatal period (P04-P96)
signs and symptoms classified in the body system chapters
signs and symptoms of breast (N63, N64.5)

This chapter contains the following blocks:

R00-R09	Symptoms and signs involving the circulatory and respiratory systems
R10-R19	Symptoms and signs involving the digestive system and abdomen
R20-R23	Symptoms and signs involving the skin and subcutaneous tissue
R25-R29	Symptoms and signs involving the nervous and musculoskeletal systems
R30-R39	Symptoms and signs involving the genitourinary system
R40-R46	Symptoms and signs involving cognition, perception, emotional state and behavior
R47-R49	Symptoms and signs involving speech and voice
R50-R69	General symptoms and signs
R70-R79	Abnormal findings on examination of blood, without diagnosis
R80-R82	Abnormal findings on examination of urine, without diagnosis
R83-R89	Abnormal findings on examination of other body fluids, substances and tissues, without diagnosis
R90-R94	Abnormal findings on diagnostic imaging and in function studies, without diagnosis
R97	Abnormal tumor markers
R99	Ill-defined and unknown cause of mortality

Symptoms and signs involving the circulatory and respiratory systems (R00-R09)

[4th] **R00 Abnormalities of heart beat**
[EXCLUDES1] *abnormalities originating in the perinatal period (P29.1-)*
[EXCLUDES2] *specified arrhythmias (I47-I49)*

R00.0 Tachycardia, unspecified
Rapid heart beat
Sinoauricular tachycardia NOS
Sinus [sinusal] tachycardia NOS
[EXCLUDES1] *neonatal tachycardia (P29.11)*
paroxysmal tachycardia (I47.-)

R00.1 Bradycardia, unspecified
Sinoatrial bradycardia
Sinus bradycardia
Slow heart beat
Vagal bradycardia
Use additional code for adverse effect, if applicable, to identify drug (T36-T50 with fifth or sixth character 5)
[EXCLUDES1] *neonatal bradycardia (P29.12)*

R00.2 Palpitations
Awareness of heart beat

R00.8 Other abnormalities of heart beat

R00.9 Unspecified abnormalities of heart beat

[4th] **R01 Cardiac murmurs and other cardiac sounds**
[EXCLUDES1] *cardiac murmurs and sounds originating in the perinatal period (P29.8)*

R01.0 Benign and innocent cardiac murmurs
Functional cardiac murmur

R01.1 Cardiac murmur, unspecified
Cardiac bruit NOS
Heart murmur NOS
Systolic murmur NOS

R01.2 Other cardiac sounds
Cardiac dullness, increased or decreased
Precordial friction

[4th] **R03 Abnormal blood-pressure reading, without diagnosis**

R03.0 Elevated blood-pressure reading, without diagnosis of hypertension [?]
[NOTES] This category is to be used to record an episode of elevated blood pressure in a patient in whom no formal diagnosis of hypertension has been made, or as an isolated incidental finding.

R03.1 Nonspecific low blood-pressure reading
[EXCLUDES1] *hypotension (I95.-)*
maternal hypotension syndrome (O26.5-)
neurogenic orthostatic hypotension (G90.3)

[4th] **R04 Hemorrhage from respiratory passages**

R04.0 Epistaxis
Hemorrhage from nose
Nosebleed

R04.1 Hemorrhage from throat
[EXCLUDES2] *hemoptysis (R04.2)*

R04.2 Hemoptysis CC CC/MCC Exc
AHA: Q4 2013
Blood-stained sputum
Cough with hemorrhage

[5th] **R04.8 Hemorrhage from other sites in respiratory passages**

R04.81 Acute idiopathic pulmonary hemorrhage in infants [P] CC CC/MCC Exc
AIPHI
Acute idiopathic hemorrhage in infants over 28 days old
[EXCLUDES1] *perinatal pulmonary hemorrhage (P26.-)*
von Willebrand's disease (D68.0)

Unspecified Code | Other Specified Code | Manifestation Code | [N] Newborn | [P] Pediatric | [M] Maternity | [A] Adult | ♂ Male | ♀ Female
● New Code | ▲ Revised Code Title | ►◄ Revised Text | [NOTES] | [INCLUDES] | [EXCLUDES1] Not coded here | [EXCLUDES2] Not included here
[4th] 4th character required | [5th] 5th character required | [6th] 6th character required | [7th] 7th character required
[7th] Extension 'X' Alert | [HAC] Hospital-acquired condition (HAC) alert | AHA AHA Coding Clinic©

When symbols appear on a code that requires a 7th character extension, refer to Appendix B to identify applicable 7th character codes.

CHAPTER 18: SYMPTOMS, SIGNS, AND ABNORMAL CLINICAL AND LABORATORY FINDINGS, NOT ELSEWHERE CLASSIFIED (R00-R99) R04.89 – R09.89

R04.89 **Hemorrhage from other sites in respiratory passages**
Pulmonary hemorrhage NOS

R04.9 **Hemorrhage from respiratory passages, unspecified**

R05 **Cough**
AHA: Q2 2016
EXCLUDES1 cough with hemorrhage (R04.2)
smoker's cough (J41.0)

R06 **Abnormalities of breathing**
EXCLUDES1 acute respiratory distress syndrome (J80)
respiratory arrest (R09.2)
respiratory arrest of newborn (P28.81)
respiratory distress syndrome of newborn (P22.-)
respiratory failure (J96.-)
respiratory failure of newborn (P28.5)

R06.0 **Dyspnea**
EXCLUDES1 tachypnea NOS (R06.82)
transient tachypnea of newborn (P22.1)

R06.00 **Dyspnea, unspecified**
AHA: Q1 2017

R06.01 **Orthopnea**

R06.02 **Shortness of breath**

● R06.03 **Acute respiratory distress**

R06.09 **Other forms of dyspnea**

R06.1 **Stridor**
EXCLUDES1 congenital laryngeal stridor (P28.89)
laryngismus (stridulus) (J38.5)

R06.2 **Wheezing**
AHA: Q2 2016
EXCLUDES1 Asthma (J45.-)

R06.3 **Periodic breathing**
Cheyne-Stokes breathing

R06.4 **Hyperventilation**
EXCLUDES1 psychogenic hyperventilation (F45.8)

R06.5 **Mouth breathing**
EXCLUDES2 dry mouth NOS (R68.2)

R06.6 **Hiccough**
EXCLUDES1 psychogenic hiccough (F45.8)

R06.7 **Sneezing**

R06.8 **Other abnormalities of breathing**

R06.81 **Apnea, not elsewhere classified**
Apnea NOS
EXCLUDES1 apnea (of) newborn (P28.4)
sleep apnea (G47.3-)
sleep apnea of newborn (primary) (P28.3)

R06.82 **Tachypnea, not elsewhere classified**
Tachypnea NOS
EXCLUDES1 transitory tachypnea of newborn (P22.1)

R06.83 **Snoring**

R06.89 **Other abnormalities of breathing**
Breath-holding (spells)
Sighing

R06.9 **Unspecified abnormalities of breathing**

R07 **Pain in throat and chest**
EXCLUDES1 epidemic myalgia (B33.0)
EXCLUDES2 jaw pain R68.84
pain in breast (N64.4)

R07.0 **Pain in throat**
EXCLUDES1 chronic sore throat (J31.2)
sore throat (acute) NOS (J02.9)
EXCLUDES2 dysphagia (R13.1-)
pain in neck (M54.2)

R07.1 **Chest pain on breathing**
Painful respiration

R07.2 **Precordial pain**

R07.8 **Other chest pain**

R07.81 **Pleurodynia**
Pleurodynia NOS

EXCLUDES1 epidemic pleurodynia (B33.0)

R07.82 **Intercostal pain**

R07.89 **Other chest pain**
Anterior chest-wall pain NOS

R07.9 **Chest pain, unspecified**

R09 **Other symptoms and signs involving the circulatory and respiratory system**
EXCLUDES1 acute respiratory distress syndrome (J80)
respiratory arrest of newborn (P28.81)
respiratory distress syndrome of newborn (P22.0)
respiratory failure (J96.-)
respiratory failure of newborn (P28.5)

R09.0 **Asphyxia and hypoxemia**
EXCLUDES1 asphyxia due to carbon monoxide (T58.-)
asphyxia due to foreign body in respiratory tract (T17.-)
birth (intrauterine) asphyxia (P84)
hyperventilation (R06.4)
traumatic asphyxia (T71.-)
EXCLUDES2 hypercapnia (R06.89)

R09.01 **Asphyxia**

R09.02 **Hypoxemia**

R09.1 **Pleurisy**
EXCLUDES1 pleurisy with effusion (J90)

R09.2 **Respiratory arrest**
Cardiorespiratory failure
EXCLUDES1 cardiac arrest (I46.-)
respiratory arrest of newborn (P28.81)
respiratory distress of newborn (P22.0)
respiratory failure (J96.-)
respiratory failure of newborn (P28.5)
respiratory insufficiency (R06.89)
respiratory insufficiency of newborn (P28.5)

R09.3 **Abnormal sputum**
Abnormal amount of sputum
Abnormal color of sputum
Abnormal odor of sputum
Excessive sputum
EXCLUDES1 blood-stained sputum (R04.2)

R09.8 **Other specified symptoms and signs involving the circulatory and respiratory systems**

R09.81 **Nasal congestion**

R09.82 **Postnasal drip**

R09.89 **Other specified symptoms and signs involving the circulatory and respiratory systems**
Bruit (arterial)
Abnormal chest percussion
Feeling of foreign body in throat
Friction sounds in chest
Chest tympany
Choking sensation
Rales
Weak pulse
EXCLUDES2 foreign body in throat (T17.2-)
wheezing (R06.2)

Symptoms and signs involving the digestive system and abdomen (R10-R19)

EXCLUDES2 congenital or infantile pylorospasm (Q40.0)
gastrointestinal hemorrhage (K92.0-K92.2)
intestinal obstruction (K56.-)
newborn gastrointestinal hemorrhage (P54.0-P54.3)
newborn intestinal obstruction (P76.-)
pylorospasm (K31.3)
signs and symptoms involving the urinary system (R30-R39)
symptoms referable to female genital organs (N94.-)
symptoms referable to male genital organs (N48-N50)

Unacceptable principal diagnosis symbol per Medicare code edits   Code exempt from diagnosis present on admission requirement
Questionable admission   Complication or comorbidity   CC/MCC exclusion   Major complication or comorbidity
Principal diagnosis as its own CC   Principal diagnosis as its own MCC   HCC HCC diagnosis code   RxHCC RxHCC diagnosis code
MACRA code   Z code as first-listed diagnosis

952   When symbols appear on a code that requires a 7th character extension, refer to Appendix B to identify applicable 7th character codes.   2018 ICD-10-CM

🔟 R10 **Abdominal and pelvic pain**
  EXCLUDES1 *renal colic (N23)*
  EXCLUDES2 *dorsalgia (M54.-)*
    flatulence and related conditions (R14.-)
  R10.0 **Acute** abdomen
    Severe abdominal pain (generalized) (with abdominal rigidity)
    EXCLUDES1 *abdominal rigidity NOS (R19.3)*
      generalized abdominal pain NOS (R10.84)
      localized abdominal pain (R10.1-R10.3-)
  🔟 R10.1 **Pain** localized to upper abdomen
    R10.10 **Upper abdominal pain, unspecified**
    R10.11 **Right** upper quadrant pain
    R10.12 **Left** upper quadrant pain
    R10.13 **Epigastric** pain
      Dyspepsia
      EXCLUDES1 *functional dyspepsia (K30)*
  R10.2 **Pelvic** and perineal pain
    EXCLUDES1 *vulvodynia (N94.81)*
  🔟 R10.3 **Pain** localized to other parts of lower abdomen
    R10.30 **Lower abdominal pain, unspecified**
    R10.31 **Right** lower quadrant pain
    R10.32 **Left** lower quadrant pain
    R10.33 **Periumbilical** pain
  🔟 R10.8 **Other** abdominal pain
    🔟 R10.81 **Abdominal** tenderness
      Abdominal tenderness NOS
      R10.811 **Right upper** quadrant abdominal tenderness
      R10.812 **Left upper** quadrant abdominal tenderness
      R10.813 **Right lower** quadrant abdominal tenderness
      R10.814 **Left lower** quadrant abdominal tenderness
      R10.815 **Periumbilic** abdominal tenderness
      R10.816 **Epigastric** abdominal tenderness
      R10.817 **Generalized** abdominal tenderness
      R10.819 **Abdominal tenderness, unspecified site**
    🔟 R10.82 **Rebound** abdominal tenderness
      R10.821 **Right upper** quadrant rebound abdominal tenderness
      R10.822 **Left upper** quadrant rebound abdominal tenderness
      R10.823 **Right lower** quadrant rebound abdominal tenderness
      R10.824 **Left lower** quadrant rebound abdominal tenderness
      R10.825 **Periumbilic** rebound abdominal tenderness
      R10.826 **Epigastric** rebound abdominal tenderness
      R10.827 **Generalized** rebound abdominal tenderness
      R10.829 **Rebound abdominal tenderness, unspecified site**
    R10.83 **Colic**   P
      Colic NOS
      Infantile colic
      EXCLUDES1 *colic in adult and child over 12 months old (R10.84)*
    R10.84 **Generalized** abdominal pain
      EXCLUDES1 *generalized abdominal pain associated with acute abdomen (R10.0)*
  R10.9 **Unspecified abdominal pain**
🔟 R11 **Nausea and vomiting**
  EXCLUDES1 *cyclical vomiting associated with migraine (G43.A-)*
    excessive vomiting in pregnancy (O21.-)
    hematemesis (K92.0)
    neonatal hematemesis (P54.0)
    newborn vomiting (P92.0-)
    psychogenic vomiting (F50.89)
    vomiting associated with bulimia nervosa (F50.2)
    vomiting following gastrointestinal surgery (K91.0)

  R11.0 **Nausea**
    Nausea NOS
    Nausea without vomiting
  🔟 R11.1 **Vomiting**
    R11.10 **Vomiting, unspecified**
      Vomiting NOS
    R11.11 **Vomiting** without nausea
    R11.12 **Projectile vomiting**
    R11.13 **Vomiting of** fecal matter
    R11.14 **Bilious** vomiting
      Bilious emesis
    R11.2 **Nausea with vomiting, unspecified**
      Persistent nausea with vomiting NOS
R12 **Heartburn**
  EXCLUDES1 *dyspepsia NOS (R10.13)*
    functional dyspepsia (K30)
🔟 R13 **Aphagia and dysphagia**
  R13.0 **Aphagia**
    Inability to swallow
    EXCLUDES1 *psychogenic aphagia (F50.9)*
  🔟 R13.1 **Dysphagia**
    Code first, if applicable, dysphagia following cerebrovascular disease (I69. with final characters -91)
    EXCLUDES1 *psychogenic dysphagia (F45.8)*
    R13.10 **Dysphagia, unspecified**
      Difficulty in swallowing NOS
    R13.11 **Dysphagia, oral** phase
    R13.12 **Dysphagia, oropharyngeal** phase
    R13.13 **Dysphagia, pharyngeal** phase
    R13.14 **Dysphagia, pharyngoesophageal** phase
    R13.19 **Other dysphagia**
      Cervical dysphagia
      Neurogenic dysphagia
🔟 R14 **Flatulence and related conditions**
  EXCLUDES1 *psychogenic aerophagy (F45.8)*
  R14.0 **Abdominal distension (gaseous)**
    Bloating
    Tympanites (abdominal) (intestinal)
  R14.1 **Gas pain**
  R14.2 **Eructation**
  R14.3 **Flatulence**
🔟 R15 **Fecal incontinence**
  INCLUDES encopresis NOS
  EXCLUDES1 *fecal incontinence of nonorganic origin (F98.1)*
  R15.0 **Incomplete defecation**
    EXCLUDES1 *constipation (K59.0-)*
      fecal impaction (K56.41)
  R15.1 **Fecal smearing**
    Fecal soiling
  R15.2 **Fecal urgency**
  R15.9 **Full incontinence of feces**
    Fecal incontinence NOS
🔟 R16 **Hepatomegaly and splenomegaly, not elsewhere classified**
  R16.0 **Hepatomegaly, not elsewhere classified**
    Hepatomegaly NOS
  R16.1 **Splenomegaly, not elsewhere classified**
    Splenomegaly NOS
  R16.2 **Hepatomegaly with splenomegaly, not elsewhere classified**
    Hepatosplenomegaly NOS
R17 **Unspecified jaundice**   CC CC/MCC Exc
  EXCLUDES1 *neonatal jaundice (P55, P57-P59)*
🔟 R18 **Ascites**
  INCLUDES fluid in peritoneal cavity
  EXCLUDES1 *ascites in alcoholic cirrhosis (K70.31)*
    ascites in alcoholic hepatitis (K70.11)
    ascites in toxic liver disease with chronic active hepatitis (K71.51)

Unspecified Code   Other Specified Code   Manifestation Code   Ⓝ Newborn   Ⓟ Pediatric   Ⓜ Maternity   Ⓐ Adult   ♂ Male   ♀ Female
● New Code   ▲ Revised Code Title   ►◄ Revised Text   NOTES   INCLUDES   EXCLUDES1 Not coded here   EXCLUDES2 Not included here
🔟 4th character required   🔟 5th character required   🔟 6th character required   🔟 7th character required
Ⓧ Extension 'X' Alert   HAC Hospital-acquired condition (HAC) alert   AHA AHA Coding Clinic©

R18.0 **Malignant** ascites   CC PDxIn CC/MCC Exc
Code first malignancy, such as:
malignant neoplasm of ovary (C56.-)
secondary malignant neoplasm of retroperitoneum and peritoneum (C78.6)

R18.8 **Other ascites**   CC CC/MCC Exc
Ascites NOS
Peritoneal effusion (chronic)

R19 Other symptoms and signs involving the digestive system and abdomen
EXCLUDES1 acute abdomen (R10.0)

R19.0 **Intra-abdominal and pelvic swelling, mass and lump**
EXCLUDES1 abdominal distension (gaseous) (R14.-)
ascites (R18.-)

R19.00 **Intra-abdominal and pelvic swelling, mass and lump, unspecified site**

R19.01 **Right upper quadrant** abdominal swelling, mass and lump

R19.02 **Left upper quadrant** abdominal swelling, mass and lump

R19.03 **Right lower quadrant** abdominal swelling, mass and lump

R19.04 **Left lower quadrant** abdominal swelling, mass and lump

R19.05 **Periumbilic** swelling, mass or lump
Diffuse or generalized umbilical swelling or mass

R19.06 **Epigastric** swelling, mass or lump

R19.07 **Generalized intra-abdominal and pelvic swelling, mass and lump**
Diffuse or generalized intra-abdominal swelling or mass NOS
Diffuse or generalized pelvic swelling or mass NOS

R19.09 **Other intra-abdominal and pelvic swelling, mass and lump**

R19.1 **Abnormal bowel sounds**

R19.11 **Absent** bowel sounds

R19.12 **Hyperactive** bowel sounds

R19.15 **Other abnormal bowel sounds**
Abnormal bowel sounds NOS

R19.2 **Visible peristalsis**
Hyperperistalsis

R19.3 **Abdominal rigidity**
EXCLUDES1 abdominal rigidity with severe abdominal pain (R10.0)

R19.30 **Abdominal rigidity, unspecified site**

R19.31 **Right upper quadrant** abdominal rigidity

R19.32 **Left upper quadrant** abdominal rigidity

R19.33 **Right lower quadrant** abdominal rigidity

R19.34 **Left lower quadrant** abdominal rigidity

R19.35 **Periumbilic** abdominal rigidity

R19.36 **Epigastric** abdominal rigidity

R19.37 **Generalized** abdominal rigidity

R19.4 **Change in bowel habit**
EXCLUDES1 constipation (K59.0-)
functional diarrhea (K59.1)

R19.5 **Other fecal abnormalities**
Abnormal stool color
Bulky stools
Mucus in stools
Occult blood in feces
Occult blood in stools
EXCLUDES1 melena (K92.1)
neonatal melena (P54.1)

R19.6 **Halitosis**

R19.7 **Diarrhea, unspecified**
Diarrhea NOS
EXCLUDES1 functional diarrhea (K59.1)
neonatal diarrhea (P78.3)
psychogenic diarrhea (F45.8)

R19.8 **Other specified symptoms and signs involving the digestive system and abdomen**

Symptoms and signs involving the skin and subcutaneous tissue (R20-R23)

EXCLUDES2 symptoms relating to breast (N64.4-N64.5)

R20 **Disturbances of skin sensation**
EXCLUDES1 dissociative anesthesia and sensory loss (F44.6)
psychogenic disturbances (F45.8)

R20.0 **Anesthesia** of skin

R20.1 **Hypoesthesia** of skin

R20.2 **Paresthesia** of skin
Formication
Pins and needles
Tingling skin
EXCLUDES1 acroparesthesia (I73.8)

R20.3 **Hyperesthesia**

R20.8 **Other disturbances of skin sensation**

R20.9 **Unspecified disturbances of skin sensation**

R21 **Rash and other nonspecific skin eruption**
INCLUDES rash NOS
EXCLUDES1 specified type of rash- code to condition
vesicular eruption (R23.8)

R22 **Localized swelling, mass and lump of skin and subcutaneous tissue**
INCLUDES subcutaneous nodules (localized)(superficial)
EXCLUDES1 abnormal findings on diagnostic imaging (R90-R93)
edema (R60.-)
enlarged lymph nodes (R59.-)
localized adiposity (E65)
swelling of joint (M25.4-)

R22.0 **Localized swelling, mass and lump, head**

R22.1 **Localized swelling, mass and lump, neck**

R22.2 **Localized swelling, mass and lump, trunk**
EXCLUDES1 intra-abdominal or pelvic mass and lump (R19.0-)
intra-abdominal or pelvic swelling (R19.0-)
EXCLUDES2 breast mass and lump (N63)

R22.3 **Localized swelling, mass and lump, upper limb**

R22.30 **Localized swelling, mass and lump, unspecified upper limb**

R22.31 **Localized swelling, mass and lump, right upper limb**

R22.32 **Localized swelling, mass and lump, left upper limb**

R22.33 **Localized swelling, mass and lump, upper limb, bilateral**

R22.4 **Localized swelling, mass and lump, lower limb**

R22.40 **Localized swelling, mass and lump, unspecified lower limb**

R22.41 **Localized swelling, mass and lump, right lower limb**

R22.42 **Localized swelling, mass and lump, left lower limb**

R22.43 **Localized swelling, mass and lump, lower limb, bilateral**

R22.9 **Localized swelling, mass and lump, unspecified**

R23 **Other skin changes**

R23.0 **Cyanosis**
EXCLUDES1 acrocyanosis (I73.8)
cyanotic attacks of newborn (P28.2)

R23.1 **Pallor**
Clammy skin

R23.2 **Flushing**
Excessive blushing
Code first, if applicable, menopausal and female climacteric states (N95.1)

R23.3 **Spontaneous ecchymoses**
Petechiae
EXCLUDES1 ecchymoses of newborn (P54.5)
purpura (D69.-)

PDxIn Unacceptable principal diagnosis symbol per Medicare code edits   POA Code exempt from diagnosis present on admission requirement
? Questionable admission   CC Complication or comorbidity   CC/MCC Exc CC/MCC exclusion   MCC Major complication or comorbidity
Principal diagnosis as its own CC   Principal diagnosis as its own MCC   HCC HCC diagnosis code   RxHCC RxHCC diagnosis code
MACRA code   Z Z code as first-listed diagnosis

When symbols appear on a code that requires a 7th character extension, refer to Appendix B to identify applicable 7th character codes.

2018 ICD-10-CM

R23.4 **Changes in skin texture**
Desquamation of skin
Induration of skin
Scaling of skin
EXCLUDES1 *epidermal thickening NOS (L85.9)*

R23.8 **Other skin changes**

R23.9 **Unspecified skin changes**

Symptoms and signs involving the nervous and musculoskeletal systems (R25-R29)

R25 **Abnormal involuntary movements**
EXCLUDES1 *specific movement disorders (G20-G26)*
stereotyped movement disorders (F98.4)
tic disorders (F95.-)

R25.0 **Abnormal head movements**

R25.1 **Tremor, unspecified**
EXCLUDES1 *chorea NOS (G25.5)*
essential tremor (G25.0)
hysterical tremor (F44.4)
intention tremor (G25.2)

R25.2 **Cramp and spasm**
EXCLUDES2 *carpopedal spasm (R29.0)*
charley-horse (M62.831)
infantile spasms (G40.4-)
muscle spasm of back (M62.830)
muscle spasm of calf (M62.831)

R25.3 **Fasciculation**
Twitching NOS

R25.8 **Other abnormal involuntary movements**

R25.9 **Unspecified abnormal involuntary movements**

R26 **Abnormalities of gait and mobility**
EXCLUDES1 *ataxia NOS (R27.0)*
hereditary ataxia (G11.-)
locomotor (syphilitic) ataxia (A52.11)
immobility syndrome (paraplegic) (M62.3)

R26.0 **Ataxic gait**
Staggering gait

R26.1 **Paralytic gait**
Spastic gait

R26.2 **Difficulty in walking, not elsewhere classified**
AHA: Q2 2016
EXCLUDES1 *falling (R29.6)*
unsteadiness on feet (R26.81)

R26.8 **Other abnormalities of gait and mobility**
R26.81 **Unsteadiness on feet**
R26.89 **Other abnormalities of gait and mobility**

R26.9 **Unspecified abnormalities of gait and mobility**

R27 **Other lack of coordination**
EXCLUDES1 *ataxic gait (R26.0)*
hereditary ataxia (G11.-)
vertigo NOS (R42)

R27.0 **Ataxia, unspecified**
EXCLUDES1 *ataxia following cerebrovascular disease (I69. with final characters -93)*

R27.8 **Other lack of coordination**

R27.9 **Unspecified lack of coordination**

R29 **Other symptoms and signs involving the nervous and musculoskeletal systems**
R29.0 **Tetany** CC CC/MCC Exc
Carpopedal spasm
EXCLUDES1 *hysterical tetany (F44.5)*
neonatal tetany (P71.3)
parathyroid tetany (E20.9)
post-thyroidectomy tetany (E89.2)

R29.1 **Meningismus** CC CC/MCC Exc

R29.2 **Abnormal reflex**
EXCLUDES2 *abnormal pupillary reflex (H57.0)*
hyperactive gag reflex (J39.2)
vasovagal reaction or syncope (R55)

R29.3 **Abnormal posture**

R29.4 **Clicking hip**
EXCLUDES1 *congenital deformities of hip (Q65.-)*

R29.5 **Transient paralysis** CC CC/MCC Exc
Code first any associated spinal cord injury (S14.0, S14.1-, S24.0, S24.1-, S34.0-, S34.1-)
EXCLUDES1 *transient ischemic attack (G45.9)*

R29.6 **Repeated falls**
AHA: Q2 2016
Falling
Tendency to fall
EXCLUDES2 *at risk for falling (Z91.81)*
history of falling (Z91.81)

R29.7 National Institutes of Health Stroke Scale (NIHSS) score
Code first the type of cerebral infarction (I63-) *[handwritten: Not Primary Code]*

R29.70 **NIHSS score** 0-9
R29.700 **NIHSS score 0** PDx in
R29.701 **NIHSS score 1** PDx in
R29.702 **NIHSS score 2** PDx in
R29.703 **NIHSS score 3** PDx in
R29.704 **NIHSS score 4** PDx in
R29.705 **NIHSS score 5** PDx in
R29.706 **NIHSS score 6** PDx in
R29.707 **NIHSS score 7** PDx in
R29.708 **NIHSS score 8** PDx in
R29.709 **NIHSS score 9** PDx in

R29.71 **NIHSS score** 10-19
R29.710 **NIHSS score 10** PDx in
R29.711 **NIHSS score 11** PDx in
R29.712 **NIHSS score 12** PDx in
R29.713 **NIHSS score 13** PDx in
R29.714 **NIHSS score 14** PDx in
R29.715 **NIHSS score 15** PDx in
R29.716 **NIHSS score 16** PDx in
R29.717 **NIHSS score 17** PDx in
R29.718 **NIHSS score 18** PDx in
R29.719 **NIHSS score 19** PDx in

R29.72 **NIHSS score** 20-29
R29.720 **NIHSS score 20** PDx in
R29.721 **NIHSS score 21** PDx in
R29.722 **NIHSS score 22** PDx in
R29.723 **NIHSS score 23** PDx in
R29.724 **NIHSS score 24** PDx in
R29.725 **NIHSS score 25** PDx in
R29.726 **NIHSS score 26** PDx in
R29.727 **NIHSS score 27** PDx in
R29.728 **NIHSS score 28** PDx in
R29.729 **NIHSS score 29** PDx in

R29.73 **NIHSS score** 30-39
R29.730 **NIHSS score 30** PDx in
AHA: Q4 2016
R29.731 **NIHSS score 31** PDx in
R29.732 **NIHSS score 32** PDx in
R29.733 **NIHSS score 33** PDx in
R29.734 **NIHSS score 34** PDx in
R29.735 **NIHSS score 35** PDx in
R29.736 **NIHSS score 36** PDx in
R29.737 **NIHSS score 37** PDx in
R29.738 **NIHSS score 38** PDx in
R29.739 **NIHSS score 39** PDx in

R29.74 **NIHSS score** 40-42
R29.740 **NIHSS score 40** PDx in
R29.741 **NIHSS score 41** PDx in

Unspecified Code   Other Specified Code   Manifestation Code   N Newborn   P Pediatric   M Maternity   A Adult   ♂ Male   ♀ Female
● New Code   ▲ Revised Code Title   ►◄ Revised Text   NOTES   INCLUDES   EXCLUDES 1 Not coded here   EXCLUDES 2 Not included here
4th character required   5th character required   6th character required   7th character required
Extension 'X' Alert   HAC Hospital-acquired condition (HAC) alert   AHA AHA Coding Clinic©

R29.742 NIHSS score 42   PDxⓧ

- R29.8 Other **symptoms and signs involving the nervous and musculoskeletal systems**
  - R29.81 **Other symptoms and signs involving the** nervous system
    - R29.810 **Facial weakness**
      Facial droop
      EXCLUDES1 Bell's palsy (G51.0)
          facial weakness following cerebrovascular disease (I69. with final characters -92)
    - R29.818 **Other symptoms and signs involving the nervous system**
  - R29.89 **Other symptoms and signs involving the** musculoskeletal system
    - *EXCLUDES2* pain in limb (M79.6-)
    - R29.890 **Loss of height**
      EXCLUDES1 osteoporosis (M80-M81)
    - R29.891 **Ocular torticollis**
      EXCLUDES1 congenital (sternomastoid) torticollis Q68.0
          psychogenic torticollis (F45.8)
          spasmodic torticollis (G24.3)
          torticollis due to birth injury (P15.8)
          torticollis NOS M43.6
    - R29.898 **Other symptoms and signs involving the musculoskeletal system**
- R29.9 **Unspecified symptoms and signs involving the nervous and musculoskeletal systems**
  - R29.90 **Unspecified symptoms and signs involving the nervous system**
  - R29.91 **Unspecified symptoms and signs involving the musculoskeletal system**

Symptoms and signs involving the genitourinary system (R30-R39)

- R30 **Pain associated with micturition**
  EXCLUDES1 psychogenic pain associated with micturition (F45.8)
  - R30.0 **Dysuria**
    Strangury
  - R30.1 **Vesical tenesmus**
  - R30.9 **Painful micturition, unspecified**
    Painful urination NOS
- R31 **Hematuria**
  EXCLUDES1 hematuria included with underlying conditions, such as:
      acute cystitis with hematuria (N30.01)
      recurrent and persistent hematuria in glomerular diseases (N02.-)
  - R31.0 Gross **hematuria**
    AHA: Q1 2017
  - R31.1 Benign **essential microscopic hematuria**
  - R31.2 **Other microscopic hematuria**
    - R31.21 Asymptomatic **microscopic hematuria**
      AHA: Q4 2016
      AMH
    - R31.29 **Other microscopic hematuria**
      AHA: Q4 2016
  - R31.9 **Hematuria, unspecified**
- R32 **Unspecified urinary incontinence**
  Enuresis NOS
  EXCLUDES1 functional urinary incontinence (R39.81)
      nonorganic enuresis (F98.0)
      stress incontinence and other specified urinary incontinence (N39.3-N39.4-)
      urinary incontinence associated with cognitive impairment (R39.81)
- R33 **Retention of urine**
  EXCLUDES1 psychogenic retention of urine (F45.8)

- R33.0 Drug induced **retention of urine**
  Use additional code for adverse effect, if applicable, to identify drug (T36-T50 with fifth or sixth character 5)
- R33.8 **Other retention of urine**
  Code first, if applicable, any causal condition, such as:
  enlarged prostate (N40.1)
- R33.9 **Retention of urine, unspecified**
- R34 **Anuria and oliguria**
  EXCLUDES1 anuria and oliguria complicating abortion or ectopic or molar pregnancy (O00-O07, O08.4)
      anuria and oliguria complicating pregnancy (O26.83-)
      anuria and oliguria complicating the puerperium (O90.4)
- R35 **Polyuria**
  Code first, if applicable, any causal condition, such as:
  enlarged prostate (N40.1)
  EXCLUDES1 psychogenic polyuria (F45.8)
  - R35.0 **Frequency of micturition**
  - R35.1 **Nocturia**
  - R35.8 **Other polyuria**
    Polyuria NOS
- R36 **Urethral discharge**
  - R36.0 **Urethral discharge without blood**
  - R36.1 **Hematospermia** ♂
  - R36.9 **Urethral discharge, unspecified**
    Penile discharge NOS
    Urethrorrhea
- R37 **Sexual dysfunction, unspecified**
- R39 **Other and unspecified symptoms and signs involving the genitourinary system**
  - R39.0 **Extravasation of urine**   CC CC/MCC Exc
  - R39.1 **Other difficulties with micturition**
    Code first, if applicable, any causal condition, such as: enlarged prostate (N40.1)
    - R39.11 **Hesitancy of micturition**
    - R39.12 **Poor urinary stream**
      Weak urinary steam
    - R39.13 **Splitting of urinary stream**
    - R39.14 **Feeling of incomplete bladder emptying**
    - R39.15 **Urgency of urination**
      EXCLUDES1 urge incontinence (N39.41, N39.46)
    - R39.16 **Straining to void**
    - R39.19 **Other difficulties with micturition**
      - R39.191 Need to immediately re-void
        AHA: Q4 2016
      - R39.192 Position dependent **micturition**
        AHA: Q4 2016
      - R39.198 **Other difficulties with micturition**
        AHA: Q4 2016
  - R39.2 **Extrarenal uremia**
    Prerenal uremia
    EXCLUDES1 uremia NOS (N19)
  - R39.8 **Other symptoms and signs involving the genitourinary system**
    - R39.81 **Functional urinary incontinence**
      Urinary incontinence due to cognitive impairment, or severe physical disability or immobility
      EXCLUDES1 stress incontinence and other specified urinary incontinence (N39.3-N39.4-)
          urinary incontinence NOS (R32)
    - R39.82 **Chronic bladder pain**
      AHA: Q4 2016
    - R39.83 Unilateral **non-palpable testicle** ♂
    - R39.84 Bilateral **non-palpable testicles** ♂
    - R39.89 **Other symptoms and signs involving the genitourinary system**
      AHA: Q4 2016
  - R39.9 **Unspecified symptoms and signs involving the genitourinary system**

PDxⓧ Unacceptable principal diagnosis symbol per Medicare code edits   Code exempt from diagnosis present on admission requirement
❓ Questionable admission   CC Complication or comorbidity   CC/MCC Exc CC/MCC exclusion   MCC Major complication or comorbidity
Principal diagnosis as its own CC   Principal diagnosis as its own MCC   HCC HCC diagnosis code   RxHCC RxHCC diagnosis code
MACRA code   Z code as first-listed diagnosis

Symptoms and signs involving cognition, perception, emotional state and behavior (R40-R46)

EXCLUDES2 *symptoms and signs constituting part of a pattern of mental disorder (F01-F99)*

R40 Somnolence, stupor and coma
EXCLUDES1 *neonatal coma (P91.5)*
somnolence, stupor and coma in diabetes (E08-E13)
somnolence, stupor and coma in hepatic failure (K72.-)
somnolence, stupor and coma in hypoglycemia (nondiabetic) (E15)

R40.0 Somnolence
Drowsiness
EXCLUDES1 *coma (R40.2-)*

R40.1 Stupor
Catatonic stupor
Semicoma
EXCLUDES1 *catatonic schizophrenia (F20.2)*
coma (R40.2-)
depressive stupor (F31-F33)
dissociative stupor (F44.2)
manic stupor (F30.2)

R40.2 Coma   *Never primary code*
Code first any associated:
fracture of skull (S02.-)
intracranial injury (S06.-)
NOTES One code from each subcategory, R40.21-R40.23, is required to complete the coma scale

R40.20 Unspecified coma HCC MCC PDxIn CC/MCC Exc
Coma NOS
Unconsciousness NOS

R40.21 Coma scale, eyes open
The following appropriate 7th character is to be added to subcategory R40.21-:
0 = unspecified time
1 = in the field [EMT or ambulance]
2 = at arrival to emergency department
3 = at hospital admission
4 = 24 hours or more after hospital admission

R40.211 Coma scale, eyes open, never HCC MCC PDxIn CC/MCC Exc

R40.212 Coma scale, eyes open, to pain HCC MCC PDxIn CC/MCC Exc

R40.213 Coma scale, eyes open, to sound PDxIn

R40.214 Coma scale, eyes open, spontaneous PDxIn

R40.22 Coma scale, best verbal response
The following appropriate 7th character is to be added to subcategory R40.22-:
0 = unspecified time
1 = in the field [EMT or ambulance]
2 = at arrival to emergency department
3 = at hospital admission
4 = 24 hours or more after hospital admission

R40.221 Coma scale, best verbal response, none HCC MCC PDxIn CC/MCC Exc

R40.222 Coma scale, best verbal response, incomprehensible words HCC MCC PDxIn CC/MCC Exc
Incomprehensible sounds (2-5 years of age)
Moans/grunts to pain; restless (<2 years old)

R40.223 Coma scale, best verbal response, inappropriate words PDxIn
Inappropriate crying or screaming (< 2 years of age)
Screaming (2-5 years of age)

R40.224 Coma scale, best verbal response, confused conversation PDxIn
Inappropriate words (2-5 years of age)
Irritable cries (< 2 years of age)

R40.225 Coma scale, best verbal response, oriented PDxIn
Cooing or babbling or crying appropriately (< 2 years of age)
Uses appropriate words (2- 5 years of age)

R40.23 Coma scale, best motor response
The following appropriate 7th character is to be added to subcategory R40.23-:
0 = unspecified time
1 = in the field [EMT or ambulance]
2 = at arrival to emergency department
3 = at hospital admission
4 = 24 hours or more after hospital admission

R40.231 Coma scale, best motor response, none HCC MCC PDxIn CC/MCC Exc

R40.232 Coma scale, best motor response, extension HCC MCC PDxIn CC/MCC Exc
Abnormal extensor posturing to pain or noxious stimuli (< 2 years of age)
Extensor posturing to pain or noxious stimuli (2-5 years of age)

R40.233 Coma scale, best motor response, abnormal PDxIn
Abnormal flexure posturing to pain or noxious stimuli (0-5 years of age)
Flexion/decorticate posturing (< 2 years of age)

R40.234 Coma scale, best motor response, flexion withdrawal HCC MCC PDxIn CC/MCC Exc
Withdraws from pain or noxious stimuli (0-5 years of age)

R40.235 Coma scale, best motor response, localizes pain PDxIn
Localizes pain (2-5 years of age)
Withdraws to touch (< 2 years of age)

R40.236 Coma scale, best motor response, obeys commands PDxIn
Normal or spontaneous movement (< 2 years of age)
Obeys commands (2-5 years of age)

R40.24 Glasgow coma scale, total score
NOTES Assign a code from subcategory R40.24, when only the total coma score is documented
The following appropriate 7th character is to be added to subcategory R40.24-:
0 = unspecified time
1 = in the field [EMT or ambulance]
2 = at arrival to emergency department
3 = at hospital admission
4 = 24 hours or more after hospital admission

R40.241 Glasgow coma scale score 13-15 PDxIn

R40.242 Glasgow coma scale score 9-12 PDxIn

R40.243 Glasgow coma scale score 3-8 HCC PDxIn

R40.244 Other coma, without documented Glasgow coma scale score, or with partial score reported HCC CC/MCC Exc

R40.3 Persistent vegetative state CC HCC CC/MCC Exc

R40.4 Transient alteration of awareness

R41 Other symptoms and signs involving cognitive functions and awareness
EXCLUDES1 *dissociative [conversion] disorders (F44.-)*
mild cognitive impairment, so stated (G31.84)

R41.0 Disorientation, unspecified
AHA: Q4 2016
Confusion NOS
Delirium NOS

R41.1 Anterograde amnesia

R41.2 Retrograde amnesia

R41.3 Other amnesia
Amnesia NOS
Memory loss NOS

Unspecified Code Other Specified Code Manifestation Code N Newborn P Pediatric M Maternity A Adult ♂ Male ♀ Female
● New Code ▲ Revised Code Title ▶◀ Revised Text NOTES INCLUDES EXCLUDES 1 Not coded here EXCLUDES 2 Not included here
4th character required 5th character required 6th character required 7th character required
Extension 'X' Alert HAC Hospital-acquired condition (HAC) alert AHA AHA Coding Clinic©

2018 ICD-10-CM When symbols appear on a code that requires a 7th character extension, refer to Appendix B to identify applicable 7th character codes. **957**

EXCLUDES1 *amnestic disorder due to known physiologic condition (F04)*

amnestic syndrome due to psychoactive substance use (F10-F19 with 5th character .6)

mild memory disturbance due to known physiological condition (F06.8)

transient global amnesia (G45.4)

R41.4 Neurologic neglect syndrome CC CC/MCC Exc
Asomatognosia
Hemi-akinesia
Hemi-inattention
Hemispatial neglect
Left-sided neglect
Sensory neglect
Visuospatial neglect
EXCLUDES1 *visuospatial deficit (R41.842)*

R41.8 Other symptoms and signs involving cognitive functions and awareness

R41.81 Age-related **cognitive decline** A
Senility NOS

R41.82 Altered mental status, unspecified
Change in mental status NOS
EXCLUDES1 *altered level of consciousness (R40.-)*

altered mental status due to known condition - code to condition

delirium NOS (R41.0)

R41.83 Borderline intellectual **functioning** PDxIn
IQ level 71 to 84
EXCLUDES1 *intellectual disabilities (F70-F79)*

R41.84 Other **specified** cognitive deficit
EXCLUDES1 *cognitive deficits as sequelae of cerebrovascular disease (I69.01-, I69.11-, I69.21-, I69.31-, I69.81-, I69.91-)*

R41.840 Attention and concentration **deficit**
EXCLUDES1 *attention-deficit hyperactivity disorders (F90.-)*

R41.841 Cognitive communication **deficit**

R41.842 Visuospatial **deficit**

R41.843 Psychomotor **deficit**

R41.844 Frontal lobe and executive function **deficit**

R41.89 Other symptoms and signs involving cognitive functions and awareness
Anosognosia

R41.9 Unspecified symptoms and signs involving cognitive functions and awareness
Unspecified neurocognitive disorder

R42 Dizziness and giddiness
AHA: Q4 2015
Light-headedness
Vertigo NOS
EXCLUDES1 *vertiginous syndromes (H81.-)*

vertigo from infrasound (T75.23)

R43 Disturbances of smell and taste
R43.0 Anosmia
R43.1 Parosmia
R43.2 Parageusia
R43.8 Other disturbances of smell and taste
Mixed disturbance of smell and taste
R43.9 Unspecified disturbances of smell and taste

R44 Other symptoms and signs involving general sensations and perceptions
EXCLUDES1 *alcoholic hallucinations (F1.5)*

hallucinations in drug psychosis (F11-F19 with .5)

hallucinations in mood disorders with psychotic symptoms (F30.2, F31.5, F32.3, F33.3)

hallucinations in schizophrenia, schizotypal and delusional disorders (F20-F29)

EXCLUDES2 *disturbances of skin sensation (R20.-)*

R44.0 Auditory **hallucinations** CC CC/MCC Exc

R44.1 Visual **hallucinations**

R44.2 Other hallucinations CC CC/MCC Exc
R44.3 Hallucinations, unspecified CC CC/MCC Exc
R44.8 Other symptoms and signs involving general sensations and perceptions
R44.9 Unspecified symptoms and signs involving general sensations and perceptions

R45 Symptoms and signs involving emotional state
R45.0 Nervousness
Nervous tension
R45.1 Restlessness and agitation
R45.2 Unhappiness
R45.3 Demoralization and apathy
EXCLUDES1 *anhedonia (R45.84)*

R45.4 Irritability and anger
R45.5 Hostility
R45.6 Violent behavior
R45.7 State of emotional shock and stress, unspecified
R45.8 Other symptoms and signs involving emotional state
R45.81 Low self-esteem
R45.82 Worries
R45.83 Excessive crying of child, adolescent or adult
EXCLUDES1 *excessive crying of infant (baby) R68.11*

R45.84 Anhedonia
R45.85 Homicidal and suicidal ideations
EXCLUDES1 *suicide attempt (T14.91)*

R45.850 Homicidal **ideations** PDxIn
R45.851 Suicidal **ideations** CC CC/MCC Exc

R45.86 Emotional lability
R45.87 Impulsiveness
R45.89 Other symptoms and signs involving emotional state

R46 Symptoms and signs involving appearance and behavior
EXCLUDES1 *appearance and behavior in schizophrenia, schizotypal and delusional disorders (F20-F29)*

mental and behavioral disorders (F01-F99)

R46.0 Very low level of personal hygiene
R46.1 Bizarre personal appearance
R46.2 Strange and inexplicable behavior
R46.3 Overactivity
R46.4 Slowness and poor responsiveness
EXCLUDES1 *stupor (R40.1)*

R46.5 Suspiciousness and marked evasiveness
R46.6 Undue concern and preoccupation with stressful events
R46.7 Verbosity and circumstantial detail obscuring reason for contact
R46.8 Other symptoms and signs involving appearance and behavior
R46.81 Obsessive-compulsive behavior PDxIn
EXCLUDES1 *obsessive-compulsive disorder (F42-)*

R46.89 Other symptoms and signs involving appearance and behavior PDxIn

Symptoms and signs involving speech and voice (R47-R49)

R47 Speech disturbances, not elsewhere classified
EXCLUDES1 *autism (F84.0)*

cluttering (F80.81)

specific developmental disorders of speech and language (F80.-)

stuttering (F80.81)

R47.0 Dysphasia and aphasia
R47.01 Aphasia CC CC/MCC Exc
EXCLUDES1 *aphasia following cerebrovascular disease (I69. with final characters -20)*

progressive isolated aphasia (G31.01)

R47.02 Dysphasia
EXCLUDES1 *dysphasia following cerebrovascular disease (I69. with final characters -21)*

PDxIn Unacceptable principal diagnosis symbol per Medicare code edits | PoA Code exempt from diagnosis present on admission requirement
? Questionable admission | CC Complication or comorbidity | CC/MCC Exc CC/MCC exclusion | MCC Major complication or comorbidity
Principal diagnosis as its own CC | Principal diagnosis as its own MCC | HCC HCC diagnosis code | RxHCC RxHCC diagnosis code
MACRA code | Z code as first-listed diagnosis

R47.1 **Dysarthria and anarthria**
  EXCLUDES1 *dysarthria following cerebrovascular disease (I69. with final characters -22)*

5ᵗʰ R47.8 **Other speech disturbances**
  EXCLUDES1 *dysarthria following cerebrovascular disease (I69. with final characters -28)*

  R47.81 **Slurred speech**
  R47.82 **Fluency disorder in conditions classified elsewhere**
    Stuttering in conditions classified elsewhere
    Code first underlying disease or condition, such as:
    Parkinson's disease (G20)
    EXCLUDES1 *adult onset fluency disorder (F98.5)*
      childhood onset fluency disorder (F80.81)
      fluency disorder (stuttering) following cerebrovascular disease (I69. with final characters -23)
  R47.89 **Other speech disturbances**
  R47.9 **Unspecified speech disturbances**

4ᵗʰ R48 **Dyslexia and other symbolic dysfunctions, not elsewhere classified**
  EXCLUDES1 *specific developmental disorders of scholastic skills (F81.-)*

  R48.0 **Dyslexia and alexia**
  R48.1 **Agnosia**
    Astereognosia (astereognosis)
    Autotopagnosia
    EXCLUDES1 *visual object agnosia (R48.3)*
  R48.2 **Apraxia**
    EXCLUDES1 *apraxia following cerebrovascular disease (I69. with final characters -90)*
  R48.3 **Visual agnosia**
    Prosopagnosia
    Simultanagnosia (asimultagnosia)
  R48.8 **Other symbolic dysfunctions**
    AHA: Q1 2017
    Acalculia
    Agraphia
  R48.9 **Unspecified symbolic dysfunctions**

4ᵗʰ R49 **Voice and resonance disorders**
  EXCLUDES1 *psychogenic voice and resonance disorders (F44.4)*

  R49.0 **Dysphonia**
    Hoarseness
  R49.1 **Aphonia**
    Loss of voice
  5ᵗʰ R49.2 **Hypernasality and hyponasality**
    R49.21 **Hypernasality**
    R49.22 **Hyponasality**
  R49.8 **Other voice and resonance disorders**
  R49.9 **Unspecified voice and resonance disorder**
    Change in voice NOS
    Resonance disorder NOS

General symptoms and signs (R50-R69)

4ᵗʰ R50 **Fever of other and unknown origin**
  EXCLUDES1 *chills without fever (R68.83)*
    febrile convulsions (R56.0-)
    fever of unknown origin during labor (O75.2)
    fever of unknown origin in newborn (P81.9)
    hypothermia due to illness (R68.0)
    malignant hyperthermia due to anesthesia (T88.3)
    puerperal pyrexia NOS (O86.4)
  R50.2 **Drug induced fever**
    Use additional code for adverse effect, if applicable, to identify drug (T36-T50 with fifth or sixth character 5)
    EXCLUDES1 *postvaccination (postimmunization) fever (R50.83)*
  5ᵗʰ R50.8 **Other specified fever**
    R50.81 **Fever presenting with conditions classified elsewhere**
      Code first underlying condition when associated fever is present, such as with:

      leukemia (C91-C95)
      neutropenia (D70.-)
      sickle-cell disease (D57.-)
    R50.82 **Postprocedural fever**
      EXCLUDES1 *postprocedural infection (T81.4-)*
        posttransfusion fever (R50.84)
        postvaccination (postimmunization) fever (R50.83)
    R50.83 **Postvaccination fever**
      Postimmunization fever
    R50.84 **Febrile nonhemolytic transfusion reaction**
      FNHTR
      Posttransfusion fever
  R50.9 **Fever, unspecified**
    Fever NOS
    Fever of unknown origin [FUO]
    Fever with chills
    Fever with rigors
    Hyperpyrexia NOS
    Persistent fever
    Pyrexia NOS

R51 **Headache**
  Facial pain NOS
  EXCLUDES1 *atypical face pain (G50.1)*
    migraine and other headache syndromes (G43-G44)
    trigeminal neuralgia (G50.0)

R52 **Pain, unspecified**
  Acute pain NOS
  Generalized pain NOS
  Pain NOS
  EXCLUDES1 *acute and chronic pain, not elsewhere classified (G89.-)*
    localized pain, unspecified type - code to pain by site, such as:
    abdomen pain (R10.-)
    back pain (M54.9)
    breast pain (N64.4)
    chest pain (R07.1-R07.9)
    ear pain (H92.0-)
    eye pain (H57.1)
    headache (R51)
    joint pain (M25.5-)
    limb pain (M79.6-)
    lumbar region pain (M54.5)
    pelvic and perineal pain (R10.2)
    shoulder pain (M25.51-)
    spine pain (M54.-)
    throat pain (R07.0)
    tongue pain (K14.6)
    tooth pain (K08.8)
    renal colic (N23)
    pain disorders exclusively related to psychological factors (F45.41)

4ᵗʰ R53 **Malaise and fatigue**
  R53.0 **Neoplastic (malignant) related fatigue**
    Code first associated neoplasm
  R53.1 **Weakness**
    Asthenia NOS
    EXCLUDES1 *age-related weakness (R54)*
      muscle weakness (M62.8-)
      sarcopenia (M62.84)
      senile asthenia (R54)
  R53.2 **Functional quadriplegia**   HCC MCC✓ CC/MCC Exc ©
    AHA: Q2 2016
    Complete immobility due to severe physical disability or frailty
    EXCLUDES1 *frailty NOS (R54)*
      hysterical paralysis (F44.4)
      immobility syndrome (M62.3)
      neurologic quadriplegia (G82.5-)
      quadriplegia (G82.50)

Unspecified Code Other Specified Code Manifestation Code Ⓝ Newborn Ⓟ Pediatric Ⓜ Maternity Ⓐ Adult ♂ Male ♀ Female
● New Code ▲ Revised Code Title ►◄ Revised Text NOTES *INCLUDES* EXCLUDES1 Not coded here EXCLUDES2 Not included here
4ᵗʰ 4ᵗʰ character required 5ᵗʰ 5ᵗʰ character required 6ᵗʰ 6ᵗʰ character required 7ᵗʰ 7ᵗʰ character required
7ₓ Extension 'X' Alert HAC Hospital-acquired condition (HAC) alert AHA AHA Coding Clinic©

[5th] **R53.8 Other malaise and fatigue**

[EXCLUDES1] *combat exhaustion and fatigue (F43.0)*
congenital debility (P96.9)
exhaustion and fatigue due to excessive exertion (T73.3)
exhaustion and fatigue due to exposure (T73.2)
exhaustion and fatigue due to heat (T67.-)
exhaustion and fatigue due to pregnancy (O26.8-)
exhaustion and fatigue due to recurrent depressive episode (F33)
exhaustion and fatigue due to senile debility (R54)

R53.81 Other malaise
Chronic debility
Debility NOS
General physical deterioration
Malaise NOS
Nervous debility
[EXCLUDES1] *age-related physical debility (R54)*

R53.82 Chronic fatigue, unspecified
Chronic fatigue syndrome NOS
[EXCLUDES1] *postviral fatigue syndrome (G93.3)*

R53.83 Other fatigue
Fatigue NOS
Lack of energy
Lethargy
Tiredness
[EXCLUDES2] *exhaustion and fatigue due to depressive episode (F32.-)*

R54 Age-related physical debility [A]
Frailty
Old age
Senescence
Senile asthenia
Senile debility
[EXCLUDES1] *age-related cognitive decline (R41.81)*
sarcopenia (M62.84)
senile psychosis (F03)
senility NOS (R41.81)

R55 Syncope and collapse
Blackout
Fainting
Vasovagal attack
[EXCLUDES1] *cardiogenic shock (R57.0)*
carotid sinus syncope (G90.01)
heat syncope (T67.1)
neurocirculatory asthenia (F45.8)
neurogenic orthostatic hypotension (G90.3)
orthostatic hypotension (I95.1)
postprocedural shock (T81.1-)
psychogenic syncope (F48.8)
shock NOS (R57.9)
shock complicating or following abortion or ectopic or molar pregnancy (O00-O07, O08.3)
shock complicating or following labor and delivery (O75.1)
Stokes-Adams attack (I45.9)
unconsciousness NOS (R40.2-)

[4th] **R56 Convulsions, not elsewhere classified**
[EXCLUDES1] *dissociative convulsions and seizures (F44.5)*
epileptic convulsions and seizures (G40.-)
newborn convulsions and seizures (P90)

[5th] **R56.0 Febrile convulsions**

R56.00 Simple febrile convulsions [CC] [HCC] [RxHCC] [CC/MCC Exc]
Febrile convulsion NOS
Febrile seizure NOS

R56.01 Complex febrile convulsions [CC] [HCC] [RxHCC] [CC/MCC Exc]
Atypical febrile seizure
Complex febrile seizure
Complicated febrile seizure
[EXCLUDES1] *status epilepticus (G40.901)*

R56.1 Post traumatic seizures [CC] [HCC] [RxHCC] [CC/MCC Exc]
[EXCLUDES1] *post traumatic epilepsy (G40.-)*

R56.9 Unspecified convulsions [HCC] [RxHCC]
Convulsion disorder
Fit NOS
Recurrent convulsions
Seizure(s) (convulsive) NOS

[4th] **R57 Shock, not elsewhere classified**
[EXCLUDES1] *anaphylactic shock NOS (T78.2)*
anaphylactic reaction or shock due to adverse food reaction (T78.0-)
anaphylactic shock due to adverse effect of correct drug or medicament properly administered (T88.6)
anaphylactic shock due to serum (T80.5-)
anesthetic shock (T88.3)
electric shock (T75.4)
obstetric shock (O75.1)
postprocedural shock (T81.1-)
psychic shock (F43.0)
shock complicating or following ectopic or molar pregnancy (O00-O07, O08.3)
shock due to lightning (T75.01)
traumatic shock (T79.4)
toxic shock syndrome (A48.3)

R57.0 Cardiogenic shock [HCC] [MCC] [CC/MCC Exc]
[EXCLUDES2] *septic shock (R65.21)*

R57.1 Hypovolemic shock [HCC] [MCC] [CC/MCC Exc]

R57.8 Other shock [HCC] [MCC] [CC/MCC Exc]

R57.9 Shock, unspecified [CC] [HCC] [CC/MCC Exc]
Failure of peripheral circulation NOS

R58 Hemorrhage, not elsewhere classified
Hemorrhage NOS
[EXCLUDES1] *hemorrhage included with underlying conditions, such as:*
acute duodenal ulcer with hemorrhage (K26.0)
acute gastritis with bleeding (K29.01)
ulcerative enterocolitis with rectal bleeding (K51.01)

[4th] **R59 Enlarged lymph nodes**
[INCLUDES] *swollen glands*
[EXCLUDES1] *lymphadenitis NOS (I88.9)*
acute lymphadenitis (L04.-)
chronic lymphadenitis (I88.1)
mesenteric (acute) (chronic) lymphadenitis (I88.0)

R59.0 Localized enlarged lymph nodes

R59.1 Generalized enlarged lymph nodes
Lymphadenopathy NOS

R59.9 Enlarged lymph nodes, unspecified

[4th] **R60 Edema, not elsewhere classified**
[EXCLUDES1] *angioneurotic edema (T78.3)*
ascites (R18.-)
cerebral edema (G93.6)
cerebral edema due to birth injury (P11.0)
edema of larynx (J38.4)
edema of nasopharynx (J39.2)
edema of pharynx (J39.2)
gestational edema (O12.0-)
hereditary edema (Q82.0)
hydrops fetalis NOS (P83.2)
hydrothorax (J94.8)
hydrops fetalis NOS (P83.2)
newborn edema (P83.3)
pulmonary edema (J81.-)

R60.0 Localized edema

R60.1 Generalized edema
[EXCLUDES2] *nutritional edema (E40-E46)*

[PDx] Unacceptable principal diagnosis symbol per Medicare code edits [POA] Code exempt from diagnosis present on admission requirement
[?] Questionable admission [CC] Complication or comorbidity [CC/MCC Exc] CC/MCC exclusion [MCC] Major complication or comorbidity
[PDx CC] Principal diagnosis as its own CC [PDx MCC] Principal diagnosis as its own MCC [HCC] HCC diagnosis code [RxHCC] RxHCC diagnosis code
MACRA code [Z1] Z code as first-listed diagnosis

R60.9 **Edema, unspecified**
Fluid retention NOS

R61 **Generalized hyperhidrosis**
Excessive sweating
Night sweats
Secondary hyperhidrosis
Code first, if applicable, menopausal and female climacteric states
(N95.1)

EXCLUDES1 *focal (primary) (secondary) hyperhidrosis (L74.5-)*
Frey's syndrome (L74.52)
localized (primary) (secondary) hyperhidrosis (L74.5-)

R62 **Lack of expected normal physiological development in childhood and adults**

EXCLUDES1 *delayed puberty (E30.0)*
gonadal dysgenesis (Q99.1)
hypopituitarism (E23.0)

R62.0 **Delayed milestone in childhood**   P
Delayed attainment of expected physiological developmental
stage
Late talker
Late walker

R62.5 **Other and unspecified lack of expected normal physiological
development in childhood**

EXCLUDES1 *HIV disease resulting in failure to thrive (B20)*
physical retardation due to malnutrition (E45)

R62.50 **Unspecified lack of expected normal physiological
development in childhood**
Infantilism NOS

R62.51 **Failure to thrive (child)**   P
Failure to gain weight

EXCLUDES1 *failure to thrive in child under 28 days old (P92.6)*

R62.52 **Short stature (child)**
Lack of growth
Physical retardation
Short stature NOS

EXCLUDES1 *short stature due to endocrine disorder (E34.3)*

R62.59 **Other lack of expected normal physiological
development in childhood**

R62.7 **Adult failure to thrive**   A

R63 **Symptoms and signs concerning food and fluid intake**

EXCLUDES1 *bulimia NOS (F50.2)*
eating disorders of nonorganic origin (F50.-)
malnutrition (E40-E46)

R63.0 **Anorexia**
Loss of appetite

EXCLUDES1 *anorexia nervosa (F50.0-)*
loss of appetite of nonorganic origin (F50.89)

R63.1 **Polydipsia**
Excessive thirst

R63.2 **Polyphagia**
Excessive eating
Hyperalimentation NOS

R63.3 **Feeding difficulties**
AHA: Q1 2017, Q3 2016
Feeding problem (elderly) (infant) NOS
Picky eater

EXCLUDES1 *eating disorders (F50.-)*
feeding problems of newborn (P92.-)
infant feeding disorder of nonorganic origin (F98.2-)

R63.4 **Abnormal weight loss**

R63.5 **Abnormal weight gain**

EXCLUDES1 *excessive weight gain in pregnancy (O26.0-)*
obesity (E66.-)

R63.6 **Underweight**
Use additional code to identify body mass index (BMI), if
known (Z68.-)

EXCLUDES1 *abnormal weight loss (R63.4)*
anorexia nervosa (F50.0-)
malnutrition (E40-E46)

R63.8 **Other symptoms and signs concerning food and fluid intake**

R64 **Cachexia**   CC HCC CC/MCC Exc
Wasting syndrome
Code first underlying condition, if known

EXCLUDES1 *abnormal weight loss (R63.4)*
nutritional marasmus (E41)

R65 **Symptoms and signs specifically associated with systemic
inflammation and infection**

R65.1 **Systemic inflammatory response syndrome (SIRS) of** non-
infectious origin
Code first underlying condition, such as:
heatstroke (T67.0)
injury and trauma (S00-T88)

EXCLUDES1 *sepsis- code to infection*
severe sepsis (R65.2)

R65.10 **Systemic inflammatory response syndrome (SIRS)
of non-infectious origin** without acute organ
dysfunction   CC HCC CC/MCC Exc
Systemic inflammatory response syndrome (SIRS) NOS

R65.11 **Systemic inflammatory response syndrome (SIRS)
of non-infectious origin with acute organ
dysfunction**   HCC MCC CC/MCC Exc
Use additional code to identify specific acute organ
dysfunction, such as:
acute kidney failure (N17.-)
acute respiratory failure (J96.0-)
critical illness myopathy (G72.81)
critical illness polyneuropathy (G62.81)
disseminated intravascular coagulopathy [DIC] (D65)
encephalopathy (metabolic) (septic) (G93.41)
hepatic failure (K72.0-)

R65.2 **Severe sepsis**
Infection with associated acute organ dysfunction
Sepsis with acute organ dysfunction
Sepsis with multiple organ dysfunction
Systemic inflammatory response syndrome due to infectious
process with acute organ dysfunction
Code first underlying infection, such as:
infection following a procedure (T81.4-)
infections following infusion, transfusion and therapeutic
injection (T80.2-)
puerperal sepsis (O85)
sepsis following complete or unspecified spontaneous
abortion (O03.87)
sepsis following ectopic and molar pregnancy (O08.82)
sepsis following incomplete spontaneous abortion (O03.37)
sepsis following (induced) termination of pregnancy (O04.87)
sepsis NOS (A41.9)
Use additional code to identify specific acute organ
dysfunction, such as:
acute kidney failure (N17.-)
acute respiratory failure (J96.0-)
critical illness myopathy (G72.81)
critical illness polyneuropathy (G62.81)
disseminated intravascular coagulopathy [DIC] (D65)
encephalopathy (metabolic) (septic) (G93.41)
hepatic failure (K72.0-)

R65.20 **Severe sepsis** without septic shock   HCC MCC CC/MCC Exc
AHA: Q3 2016, Q4 2013
Severe sepsis NOS

R65.21 **Severe sepsis** with septic shock   HCC MCC PDx CC/MCC Exc

R68 **Other general symptoms and signs**

R68.0 **Hypothermia, not associated with low environmental
temperature**

EXCLUDES1 *hypothermia NOS (accidental) (T68)*
hypothermia due to anesthesia (T88.51)
hypothermia due to low environmental temperature (T68)
newborn hypothermia (P80.-)

Unspecified Code   Other Specified Code   Manifestation Code   N Newborn   P Pediatric   M Maternity   A Adult   ♂ Male   ♀ Female
● New Code   ▲ Revised Code Title   ►◄ Revised Text   NOTES   *INCLUDES*   EXCLUDES 1 Not coded here   EXCLUDES 2 Not included here
4ᵗʰ 4th character required   5ᵗʰ 5th character required   6ᵗʰ 6th character required   7ᵗʰ 7th character required
7ᵗʰ Extension 'X' Alert   HAC Hospital-acquired condition (HAC) alert   AHA AHA Coding Clinic©

R68.1 **Nonspecific symptoms peculiar to infancy**
　　EXCLUDES1 colic, infantile (R10.83)
　　　　neonatal cerebral irritability (P91.3)
　　　　teething syndrome (K00.7)

　R68.11 **Excessive crying of infant (baby)** P
　　EXCLUDES1 excessive crying of child, adolescent, or adult (R45.83)

　R68.12 **Fussy infant (baby)** P
　　Irritable infant

　R68.13 **Apparent life threatening event in infant (ALTE)** P
　　Apparent life threatening event in newborn
　　Brief resolved unexplained event (BRUE)
　　Code first confirmed diagnosis, if known
　　Use additional code(s) for associated signs and symptoms if no confirmed diagnosis established, or if signs and symptoms are not associated routinely with confirmed diagnosis, or provide additional information for cause of ALTE

　R68.19 **Other nonspecific symptoms peculiar to infancy** P

R68.2 **Dry mouth, unspecified**
　　EXCLUDES1 dry mouth due to dehydration (E86.0)
　　　　dry mouth due to sicca syndrome [Sjögren] (M35.0-)
　　　　salivary gland hyposecretion (K11.7)

R68.3 **Clubbing of fingers**
　　Clubbing of nails
　　EXCLUDES1 congenital clubfinger (Q68.1)

R68.8 **Other general symptoms and signs**
　R68.81 **Early satiety**
　R68.82 **Decreased libido** A
　　Decreased sexual desire
　R68.83 **Chills (without fever)**
　　Chills NOS
　　EXCLUDES1 chills with fever (R50.9)
　R68.84 **Jaw pain**
　　Mandibular pain
　　Maxilla pain
　　EXCLUDES1 temporomandibular joint arthralgia (M26.62-)
　R68.89 **Other general symptoms and signs**

R69 **Illness, unspecified**
　　Unknown and unspecified cases of morbidity

Abnormal findings on examination of blood, without diagnosis (R70-R79)

EXCLUDES2 abnormal findings on antenatal screening of mother (O28.-)
　　abnormalities of lipids (E78.-)
　　abnormalities of platelets and thrombocytes (D69.-)
　　abnormalities of white blood cells classified elsewhere (D70-D72)
　　coagulation hemorrhagic disorders (D65-D68)
　　diagnostic abnormal findings classified elsewhere - see Alphabetical Index
　　hemorrhagic and hematological disorders of newborn (P50-P61)

R70 **Elevated erythrocyte sedimentation rate and abnormality of plasma viscosity**
　R70.0 **Elevated erythrocyte sedimentation rate**
　R70.1 **Abnormal plasma viscosity**

R71 **Abnormality of red blood cells**
　　EXCLUDES1 anemias (D50-D64)
　　　　anemia of premature infant (P61.2)
　　　　benign (familial) polycythemia (D75.0)
　　　　congenital anemias (P61.2-P61.4)
　　　　newborn anemia due to isoimmunization (P55.-)
　　　　polycythemia neonatorum (P61.1)
　　　　polycythemia NOS (D75.1)
　　　　polycythemia vera (D45)
　　　　secondary polycythemia (D75.1)

R71.0 **Precipitous drop in hematocrit** CC CC/MCC Exc
　　Drop (precipitous) in hemoglobin
　　Drop in hematocrit

R71.8 **Other abnormality of red blood cells**
　　Abnormal red-cell morphology NOS
　　Abnormal red-cell volume NOS
　　Anisocytosis
　　Poikilocytosis

R73 **Elevated blood glucose level**
　　EXCLUDES1 diabetes mellitus (E08-E13)
　　　　diabetes mellitus in pregnancy, childbirth and the puerperium (O24.-)
　　　　neonatal disorders (P70.0-P70.2)
　　　　postsurgical hypoinsulinemia (E89.1)

R73.0 **Abnormal glucose**
　　EXCLUDES1 abnormal glucose in pregnancy (O99.81-)
　　　　diabetes mellitus (E08-E13)
　　　　dysmetabolic syndrome X (E88.81)
　　　　gestational diabetes (O24.4-)
　　　　glycosuria (R81)
　　　　hypoglycemia (E16.2)

　R73.01 **Impaired fasting glucose**
　　Elevated fasting glucose

　R73.02 **Impaired glucose tolerance (oral)**
　　Elevated glucose tolerance

　R73.03 **Prediabetes**
　　AHA: Q4 2016
　　Latent diabetes

　R73.09 **Other abnormal glucose**
　　AHA: Q4 2016
　　Abnormal glucose NOS
　　Abnormal non-fasting glucose tolerance

R73.9 **Hyperglycemia, unspecified**

R74 **Abnormal serum enzyme levels**
　R74.0 **Nonspecific elevation of levels of transaminase and lactic acid dehydrogenase [LDH]**
　R74.8 **Abnormal levels of other serum enzymes**
　　Abnormal level of acid phosphatase
　　Abnormal level of alkaline phosphatase
　　Abnormal level of amylase
　　Abnormal level of lipase [triacylglycerol lipase]
　R74.9 **Abnormal serum enzyme level, unspecified**

R75 **Inconclusive laboratory evidence of human immunodeficiency virus [HIV]**
　　Nonconclusive HIV-test finding in infants
　　EXCLUDES1 asymptomatic human immunodeficiency virus [HIV] infection status (Z21)
　　　　human immunodeficiency virus [HIV] disease (B20)

R76 **Other abnormal immunological findings in serum**
　R76.0 **Raised antibody titer**
　　EXCLUDES1 isoimmunization in pregnancy (O36.0-O36.1)
　　　　isoimmunization affecting newborn (P55.-)

　R76.1 **Nonspecific reaction to test for tuberculosis**
　　R76.11 **Nonspecific reaction to tuberculin skin test without active tuberculosis**
　　　Abnormal result of Mantoux test
　　　PPD positive
　　　Tuberculin (skin test) positive
　　　Tuberculin (skin test) reactor
　　　EXCLUDES1 nonspecific reaction to cell mediated immunity measurement of gamma interferon antigen response without active tuberculosis (R76.12)

　　R76.12 **Nonspecific reaction to cell mediated immunity measurement of gamma interferon antigen response without active tuberculosis**
　　　Nonspecific reaction to QuantiFERON-TB test (QFT) without active tuberculosis
　　　EXCLUDES1 nonspecific reaction to tuberculin skin test without active tuberculosis (R76.11)
　　　　positive tuberculin skin test (R76.11)

PDx Unacceptable principal diagnosis symbol per Medicare code edits　　POA Code exempt from diagnosis present on admission requirement
❓ Questionable admission　　CC Complication or comorbidity　　CC/MCC Exc CC/MCC exclusion　　MCC Major complication or comorbidity
Principal diagnosis as its own CC　　Principal diagnosis as its own MCC　　HCC HCC diagnosis code　　RxHCC RxHCC diagnosis code
MACRA code　　Z Z code as first-listed diagnosis

962　　When symbols appear on a code that requires a 7th character extension, refer to Appendix B to identify applicable 7th character codes.　　**2018 ICD-10-CM**

R76.8 Other specified abnormal immunological findings in serum
Raised level of immunoglobulins NOS
R76.9 Abnormal immunological finding in serum, unspecified

[4th] **R77 Other abnormalities of plasma proteins**
[EXCLUDES1] *disorders of plasma-protein metabolism (E88.0)*
R77.0 Abnormality of albumin
R77.1 Abnormality of globulin
Hyperglobulinemia NOS
R77.2 Abnormality of alphafetoprotein
R77.8 Other specified abnormalities of plasma proteins
R77.9 Abnormality of plasma protein, unspecified

[4th] **R78 Findings of drugs and other substances, not normally found in blood**
Use additional code to identify the any retained foreign body, if applicable (Z18.-)
[EXCLUDES1] *mental or behavioral disorders due to psychoactive substance use (F10-F19)*
R78.0 Finding of alcohol in blood
Use additional external cause code (Y90.-), for detail regarding alcohol level.
R78.1 Finding of opiate drug in blood
R78.2 Finding of cocaine in blood
R78.3 Finding of hallucinogen in blood
R78.4 Finding of other drugs of addictive potential in blood
R78.5 Finding of other psychotropic drug in blood
R78.6 Finding of steroid agent in blood
[5th] R78.7 Finding of abnormal level of heavy metals in blood
R78.71 Abnormal lead level in blood
[EXCLUDES1] *lead poisoning (T56.0-)*
R78.79 Finding of abnormal level of heavy metals in blood
[5th] R78.8 Finding of other specified substances, not normally found in blood
R78.81 Bacteremia [CC] [CC/MCC Exc]
[EXCLUDES1] *sepsis-code to specified infection*
R78.89 Finding of other specified substances, not normally found in blood
Finding of abnormal level of lithium in blood
R78.9 Finding of unspecified substance, not normally found in blood

[4th] **R79 Other abnormal findings of blood chemistry**
Use additional code to identify any retained foreign body, if applicable (Z18.-)
[EXCLUDES1] *asymptomatic hyperuricemia (E79.0)*
hyperglycemia NOS (R73.9)
hypoglycemia NOS (E16.2)
neonatal hypoglycemia (P70.3-P70.4)
specific findings indicating disorder of amino-acid metabolism (E70-E72)
specific findings indicating disorder of carbohydrate metabolism (E73-E74)
specific findings indicating disorder of lipid metabolism (E75.-)
R79.0 Abnormal level of blood mineral
Abnormal blood level of cobalt
Abnormal blood level of copper
Abnormal blood level of iron
Abnormal blood level of magnesium
Abnormal blood level of mineral NEC
Abnormal blood level of zinc
[EXCLUDES1] *abnormal level of lithium (R78.89)*
disorders of mineral metabolism (E83.-)
neonatal hypomagnesemia (P71.2)
nutritional mineral deficiency (E58-E61)
R79.1 Abnormal coagulation profile
Abnormal or prolonged bleeding time
Abnormal or prolonged coagulation time
Abnormal or prolonged partial thromboplastin time [PTT]
Abnormal or prolonged prothrombin time [PT]
[EXCLUDES1] *coagulation defects (D68.-)*
[EXCLUDES2] *abnormality of fluid, electrolyte or acid-base balance (E86-E87)*
[5th] R79.8 Other specified abnormal findings of blood chemistry
R79.81 Abnormal blood-gas level
R79.82 Elevated C-reactive protein (CRP)
R79.89 Other specified abnormal findings of blood chemistry
R79.9 Abnormal finding of blood chemistry, unspecified

Abnormal findings on examination of urine, without diagnosis (R80-R82)

[EXCLUDES1] *abnormal findings on antenatal screening of mother (O28.-)*
diagnostic abnormal findings classified elsewhere - see Alphabetical Index
specific findings indicating disorder of amino-acid metabolism (E70-E72)
specific findings indicating disorder of carbohydrate metabolism (E73-E74)

[4th] **R80 Proteinuria**
[EXCLUDES1] *gestational proteinuria (O12.1-)*
R80.0 Isolated proteinuria
Idiopathic proteinuria
[EXCLUDES1] *isolated proteinuria with specific morphological lesion (N06.-)*
R80.1 Persistent proteinuria, unspecified
R80.2 Orthostatic proteinuria, unspecified
Postural proteinuria
R80.3 Bence Jones proteinuria
R80.8 Other proteinuria
R80.9 Proteinuria, unspecified
Albuminuria NOS

R81 Glycosuria
[EXCLUDES1] *renal glycosuria (E74.8)*

[4th] **R82 Other and unspecified abnormal findings in urine**
[INCLUDES] *chromoabnormalities in urine*
Use additional code to identify any retained foreign body, if applicable (Z18.-)
[EXCLUDES2] *hematuria (R31.-)*
R82.0 Chyluria [CC] [CC/MCC Exc]
[EXCLUDES1] *filarial chyluria (B74.-)*
R82.1 Myoglobinuria [CC] [CC/MCC Exc]
R82.2 Biliuria
R82.3 Hemoglobinuria
[EXCLUDES1] *hemoglobinuria due to hemolysis from external causes NEC (D59.6)*
hemoglobinuria due to paroxysmal nocturnal [Marchiafava-Micheli] (D59.5)
R82.4 Acetonuria
Ketonuria
R82.5 Elevated urine levels of drugs, medicaments and biological substances
Elevated urine levels of catecholamines
Elevated urine levels of indoleacetic acid
Elevated urine levels of 17-ketosteroids
Elevated urine levels of steroids
R82.6 Abnormal urine levels of substances chiefly nonmedicinal as to source
Abnormal urine level of heavy metals
[5th] R82.7 Abnormal findings on microbiological examination of urine
[EXCLUDES1] *colonization status (Z22.-)*
R82.71 Bacteriuria
AHA: Q4 2016
R82.79 Other abnormal findings on microbiological examination of urine
AHA: Q4 2016
Positive culture findings of urine
R82.8 Abnormal findings on cytological and histological examination of urine

R82.9 **Other and unspecified abnormal findings in urine**

R82.90 **Unspecified abnormal findings in urine**

R82.91 **Other chromoabnormalities of urine**
Chromoconversion (dipstick)
Idiopathic dipstick converts positive for blood with no cellular forms in sediment
EXCLUDES1 *hemoglobinuria (R82.3)*
myoglobinuria (R82.1)

R82.99 **Other abnormal findings in urine**
Cells and casts in urine
Crystalluria
Melanuria

Abnormal findings on examination of other body fluids, substances and tissues, without diagnosis (R83-R89)

EXCLUDES1 *abnormal findings on antenatal screening of mother (O28.-)*
diagnostic abnormal findings classified elsewhere - see Alphabetical Index

EXCLUDES2 *abnormal findings on examination of blood, without diagnosis (R70-R79)*
abnormal findings on examination of urine, without diagnosis (R80-R82)
abnormal tumor markers (R97.-)

R83 **Abnormal findings in** cerebrospinal fluid

R83.0 **Abnormal level of** enzymes **in cerebrospinal fluid**

R83.1 **Abnormal level of** hormones **in cerebrospinal fluid**

R83.2 **Abnormal level of other drugs, medicaments and biological substances in cerebrospinal fluid**

R83.3 **Abnormal level of** substances chiefly nonmedicinal **as to source in cerebrospinal fluid**

R83.4 **Abnormal** immunological **findings in cerebrospinal fluid**

R83.5 **Abnormal** microbiological **findings in cerebrospinal fluid**
Positive culture findings in cerebrospinal fluid
EXCLUDES1 *colonization status (Z22.-)*

R83.6 **Abnormal** cytological **findings in cerebrospinal fluid**

R83.8 **Other abnormal findings in cerebrospinal fluid**
Abnormal chromosomal findings in cerebrospinal fluid

R83.9 **Unspecified abnormal finding in cerebrospinal fluid**

R84 **Abnormal findings in specimens from** respiratory organs and thorax

INCLUDES *abnormal findings in bronchial washings*
abnormal findings in nasal secretions
abnormal findings in pleural fluid
abnormal findings in sputum
abnormal findings in throat scrapings

EXCLUDES1 *blood-stained sputum (R04.2)*

R84.0 **Abnormal level of** enzymes **in specimens from respiratory organs and thorax**

R84.1 **Abnormal level of** hormones **in specimens from respiratory organs and thorax**

R84.2 **Abnormal level of other** drugs, medicaments and biological **substances in specimens from respiratory organs and thorax**

R84.3 **Abnormal level of** substances chiefly nonmedicinal **as to source in specimens from respiratory organs and thorax**

R84.4 **Abnormal** immunological **findings in specimens from respiratory organs and thorax**

R84.5 **Abnormal** microbiological **findings in specimens from respiratory organs and thorax**
Positive culture findings in specimens from respiratory organs and thorax
EXCLUDES1 *colonization status (Z22.-)*

R84.6 **Abnormal** cytological **findings in specimens from respiratory organs and thorax**

R84.7 **Abnormal** histological **findings in specimens from respiratory organs and thorax**

R84.8 **Other abnormal findings in specimens from respiratory organs and thorax**
Abnormal chromosomal findings in specimens from respiratory organs and thorax

R84.9 **Unspecified abnormal finding in specimens from respiratory organs and thorax**

R85 **Abnormal findings in** specimens **from** digestive organs and abdominal cavity

INCLUDES *abnormal findings in peritoneal fluid*
abnormal findings in saliva

EXCLUDES1 *cloudy peritoneal dialysis effluent (R88.0)*
fecal abnormalities (R19.5)

R85.0 **Abnormal level of** enzymes **in specimens from digestive organs and abdominal cavity**

R85.1 **Abnormal level of** hormones **in specimens from digestive organs and abdominal cavity**

R85.2 **Abnormal level of other drugs, medicaments and biological substances in specimens from digestive organs and abdominal cavity**

R85.3 **Abnormal level of** substances chiefly nonmedicinal **as to source in specimens from digestive organs and abdominal cavity**

R85.4 **Abnormal** immunological **findings in specimens from digestive organs and abdominal cavity**

R85.5 **Abnormal** microbiological **findings in specimens from digestive organs and abdominal cavity**
Positive culture findings in specimens from digestive organs and abdominal cavity
EXCLUDES1 *colonization status (Z22.-)*

R85.6 **Abnormal** cytological **findings in specimens from digestive organs and abdominal cavity**

R85.61 **Abnormal cytologic smear of** anus
EXCLUDES1 *abnormal cytological findings in specimens from other digestive organs and abdominal cavity (R85.69)*
carcinoma in situ of anus (histologically confirmed) (D01.3)
anal intraepithelial neoplasia I [AIN I] (K62.82)
anal intraepithelial neoplasia II [AIN II] (K62.82)
anal intraepithelial neoplasia III [AIN III] (D01.3)
dysplasia (mild) (moderate) of anus (histologically confirmed) (K62.82)
severe dysplasia of anus (histologically confirmed) (D01.3)
EXCLUDES2 *anal high risk human papillomavirus (HPV) DNA test positive (R85.81)*
anal low risk human papillomavirus (HPV) DNA test positive (R85.82)

R85.610 **Atypical squamous cells of undetermined significance on cytologic smear of anus** (ASC-US)

R85.611 **Atypical squamous cells cannot exclude high grade squamous intraepithelial lesion on cytologic smear of anus** (ASC-H)

R85.612 **Low grade squamous intraepithelial lesion on cytologic smear of anus** (LGSIL)

R85.613 **High grade squamous intraepithelial lesion on cytologic smear of anus** (HGSIL)

R85.614 **Cytologic evidence of** malignancy on **smear of anus**

R85.615 Unsatisfactory **cytologic smear of anus**
Inadequate sample of cytologic smear of anus

R85.616 Satisfactory **anal smear but** lacking transformation zone

R85.618 **Other abnormal cytological findings on specimens from anus**

R85.619 **Unspecified abnormal cytological findings in specimens from anus**
Abnormal anal cytology NOS
Atypical glandular cells of anus NOS

R85.69 **Abnormal cytological findings in specimens from other digestive organs and abdominal cavity**

PDxₐ Unacceptable principal diagnosis symbol per Medicare code edits   PDxₐ Code exempt from diagnosis present on admission requirement
❓ Questionable admission   cc Complication or comorbidity   cc-mcc Exc CC/MCC exclusion   mcc Major complication or comorbidity
Principal diagnosis as its own CC   Principal diagnosis as its own MCC   HCC HCC diagnosis code   RxHCC RxHCC diagnosis code
MACRA code   Z1 Z code as first-listed diagnosis

964   When symbols appear on a code that requires a 7th character extension, refer to Appendix B to identify applicable 7th character codes.   2018 ICD-10-CM

R85.7 Abnormal histological findings in specimens from digestive organs and abdominal cavity

[5th] **R85.8 Other abnormal findings in specimens from digestive organs and abdominal cavity**

R85.81 Anal high risk human papillomavirus (HPV) DNA test positive

[EXCLUDES1] *anogenital warts due to human papillomavirus (HPV) (A63.0)*

condyloma acuminatum (A63.0)

R85.82 Anal low risk human papillomavirus (HPV) DNA test positive

Use additional code for associated human papillomavirus (B97.7)

R85.89 Other abnormal findings in specimens from digestive organs and abdominal cavity

Abnormal chromosomal findings in specimens from digestive organs and abdominal cavity

R85.9 Unspecified abnormal finding in specimens from digestive organs and abdominal cavity

[4th] **R86 Abnormal findings in specimens from male genital organs**

[INCLUDES] *abnormal findings in prostatic secretions*

abnormal findings in semen, seminal fluid

abnormal spermatozoa

[EXCLUDES1] *azoospermia (N46.0-)*

oligospermia (N46.1-)

R86.0 Abnormal level of enzymes in specimens from male genital organs ♂

R86.1 Abnormal level of hormones in specimens from male genital organs ♂

R86.2 Abnormal level of other drugs, medicaments and biological substances in specimens from male genital organs ♂

R86.3 Abnormal level of substances chiefly nonmedicinal as to source in specimens from male genital organs ♂

R86.4 Abnormal immunological findings in specimens from male genital organs ♂

R86.5 Abnormal microbiological findings in specimens from male genital organs ♂

Positive culture findings in specimens from male genital organs

[EXCLUDES1] *colonization status (Z22.-)*

R86.6 Abnormal cytological findings in specimens from male genital organs ♂

R86.7 Abnormal histological findings in specimens from male genital organs ♂

R86.8 Other abnormal findings in specimens from male genital organs ♂

Abnormal chromosomal findings in specimens from male genital organs

R86.9 Unspecified abnormal finding in specimens from male genital organs ♂

[4th] **R87 Abnormal findings in specimens from female genital organs**

[INCLUDES] *abnormal findings in secretion and smears from cervix uteri*

abnormal findings in secretion and smears from vagina

abnormal findings in secretion and smears from vulva

R87.0 Abnormal level of enzymes in specimens from female genital organs ♀

R87.1 Abnormal level of hormones in specimens from female genital organs ♀

R87.2 Abnormal level of other drugs, medicaments and biological substances in specimens from female genital organs ♀

R87.3 Abnormal level of substances chiefly nonmedicinal as to source in specimens from female genital organs ♀

R87.4 Abnormal immunological findings in specimens from female genital organs ♀

R87.5 Abnormal microbiological findings in specimens from female genital organs ♀

Positive culture findings in specimens from female genital organs

[EXCLUDES1] *colonization status (Z22.-)*

[5th] **R87.6 Abnormal cytological findings in specimens from female genital organs**

[6th] **R87.61 Abnormal cytological findings in specimens from cervix uteri**

[EXCLUDES1] *abnormal cytological findings in specimens from other female genital organs (R87.69)*

abnormal cytological findings in specimens from vagina (R87.62-)

carcinoma in situ of cervix uteri (histologically confirmed) (D06.-)

cervical intraepithelial neoplasia I [CIN I] (N87.0)

cervical intraepithelial neoplasia II [CIN II] (N87.1)

cervical intraepithelial neoplasia III [CIN III] (D06.-)

dysplasia (mild) (moderate) of cervix uteri (histologically confirmed) (N87.-)

severe dysplasia of cervix uteri (histologically confirmed) (D06.-)

[EXCLUDES2] *cervical high risk human papillomavirus (HPV) DNA test positive (R87.810)*

cervical low risk human papillomavirus (HPV) DNA test positive (R87.820)

R87.610 Atypical squamous cells of undetermined significance on cytologic smear of cervix (ASC-US) ♀

R87.611 Atypical squamous cells cannot exclude high grade squamous intraepithelial lesion on cytologic smear of cervix (ASC-H) ♀

R87.612 Low grade squamous intraepithelial lesion on cytologic smear of cervix (LGSIL) ♀

R87.613 High grade squamous intraepithelial lesion on cytologic smear of cervix (HGSIL) ♀

R87.614 Cytologic evidence of malignancy on smear of cervix ♀

R87.615 Unsatisfactory cytologic smear of cervix ♀

Inadequate sample of cytologic smear of cervix

R87.616 Satisfactory cervical smear but lacking transformation zone ♀

R87.618 Other abnormal cytological findings on specimens from cervix uteri ♀

R87.619 Unspecified abnormal cytological findings in specimens from cervix uteri ♀

Abnormal cervical cytology NOS

Abnormal Papanicolaou smear of cervix NOS

Abnormal thin preparation smear of cervix NOS

Atypical endocervical cells of cervix NOS

Atypical endometrial cells of cervix NOS

Atypical glandular cells of cervix NOS

[6th] **R87.62 Abnormal cytological findings in specimens from vagina**

Use additional code to identify acquired absence of uterus and cervix, if applicable (Z90.71-)

[EXCLUDES1] *abnormal cytological findings in specimens from cervix uteri (R87.61-)*

abnormal cytological findings in specimens from other female genital organs (R87.69)

carcinoma in situ of vagina (histologically confirmed) (D07.2)

vaginal intraepithelial neoplasia I [VAIN I] (N89.0)

vaginal intraepithelial neoplasia II [VAIN II] (N89.1)

vaginal intraepithelial neoplasia III [VAIN III] (D07.2)

Unspecified Code | Other Specified Code | Manifestation Code | [N] Newborn | [P] Pediatric | [M] Maternity | [A] Adult | ♂ Male | ♀ Female
● New Code | ▲ Revised Code Title | ►◄ Revised Text | [NOTES] | [INCLUDES] | [EXCLUDES1] Not coded here | [EXCLUDES2] Not included here
[4th] 4th character required | [5th] 5th character required | [6th] 6th character required | [7th] 7th character required
[x] Extension 'X' Alert | [HAC] Hospital-acquired condition (HAC) alert | AHA AHA Coding Clinic©

When symbols appear on a code that requires a 7th character extension, refer to Appendix B to identify applicable 7th character codes.

dysplasia (mild) (moderate) of vagina (histologically confirmed) (N89.-)

severe dysplasia of vagina (histologically confirmed) (D07.2)

EXCLUDES2 vaginal high risk human papillomavirus (HPV) DNA test positive (R87.811)

vaginal low risk human papillomavirus (HPV) DNA test positive (R87.821)

R87.620 Atypical squamous cells of undetermined significance on cytologic smear of vagina (ASC-US) ♀

R87.621 Atypical squamous cells cannot exclude high grade squamous intraepithelial lesion on cytologic smear of vagina (ASC-H) ♀

R87.622 Low grade squamous intraepithelial lesion on cytologic smear of vagina (LGSIL) ♀

R87.623 High grade squamous intraepithelial lesion on cytologic smear of vagina (HGSIL) ♀

R87.624 Cytologic evidence of malignancy on smear of vagina ♀

R87.625 Unsatisfactory cytologic smear of vagina ♀

Inadequate sample of cytologic smear of vagina

R87.628 Other abnormal cytological findings on specimens from vagina ♀

R87.629 Unspecified abnormal cytological findings in specimens from vagina ♀

Abnormal Papanicolaou smear of vagina NOS

Abnormal thin preparation smear of vagina NOS

Abnormal vaginal cytology NOS

Atypical endocervical cells of vagina NOS

Atypical endometrial cells of vagina NOS

Atypical glandular cells of vagina NOS

R87.69 Abnormal cytological findings in specimens from other female genital organs ♀

Abnormal cytological findings in specimens from female genital organs NOS

EXCLUDES1 dysplasia of vulva (histologically confirmed) (N90.0-N90.3)

R87.7 Abnormal histological findings in specimens from female genital organs ♀

EXCLUDES1 carcinoma in situ (histologically confirmed) of female genital organs (D06-D07.3)

cervical intraepithelial neoplasia I [CIN I] (N87.0)

cervical intraepithelial neoplasia II [CIN II] (N87.1)

cervical intraepithelial neoplasia III [CIN III] (D06.-)

dysplasia (mild) (moderate) of cervix uteri (histologically confirmed) (N87.-)

dysplasia (mild) (moderate) of vagina (histologically confirmed) (N89.-)

vaginal intraepithelial neoplasia I [VAIN I] (N89.0)

vaginal intraepithelial neoplasia II [VAIN II] (N89.1)

vaginal intraepithelial neoplasia III [VAIN III] (D07.2)

severe dysplasia of cervix uteri (histologically confirmed) (D06.-)

severe dysplasia of vagina (histologically confirmed) (D07.2)

5ᵗʰ R87.8 Other abnormal findings in specimens from female genital organs

6ᵗʰ R87.81 High risk human papillomavirus (HPV) DNA test positive from female genital organs

EXCLUDES1 anogenital warts due to human papillomavirus (HPV) (A63.0)

condyloma acuminatum (A63.0)

R87.810 Cervical high risk human papillomavirus (HPV) DNA test positive ♀

R87.811 Vaginal high risk human papillomavirus (HPV) DNA test positive ♀

6ᵗʰ R87.82 Low risk human papillomavirus (HPV) DNA test positive from female genital organs

Use additional code for associated human papillomavirus (B97.7)

R87.820 Cervical low risk human papillomavirus (HPV) DNA test positive ♀

R87.821 Vaginal low risk human papillomavirus (HPV) DNA test positive ♀

R87.89 Other abnormal findings in specimens from female genital organs ♀

Abnormal chromosomal findings in specimens from female genital organs

R87.9 Unspecified abnormal finding in specimens from female genital organs ♀

4ᵗʰ R88 Abnormal findings in other body fluids and substances

R88.0 Cloudy (hemodialysis) (peritoneal) dialysis effluent

R88.8 Abnormal findings in other body fluids and substances

4ᵗʰ R89 Abnormal findings in specimens from other organs, systems and tissues

INCLUDES abnormal findings in nipple discharge

abnormal findings in synovial fluid

abnormal findings in wound secretions

R89.0 Abnormal level of enzymes in specimens from other organs, systems and tissues

R89.1 Abnormal level of hormones in specimens from other organs, systems and tissues

R89.2 Abnormal level of other drugs, medicaments and biological substances in specimens from other organs, systems and tissues

R89.3 Abnormal level of substances chiefly nonmedicinal as to source in specimens from other organs, systems and tissues

R89.4 Abnormal immunological findings in specimens from other organs, systems and tissues

R89.5 Abnormal microbiological findings in specimens from other organs, systems and tissues

Positive culture findings in specimens from other organs, systems and tissues

EXCLUDES1 colonization status (Z22.-)

R89.6 Abnormal cytological findings in specimens from other organs, systems and tissues

R89.7 Abnormal histological findings in specimens from other organs, systems and tissues

R89.8 Other abnormal findings in specimens from other organs, systems and tissues

Abnormal chromosomal findings in specimens from other organs, systems and tissues

R89.9 Unspecified abnormal finding in specimens from other organs, systems and tissues

Abnormal findings on diagnostic imaging and in function studies, without diagnosis (R90-R94)

INCLUDES nonspecific abnormal findings on diagnostic imaging by computerized axial tomography [CAT scan]

nonspecific abnormal findings on diagnostic imaging by magnetic resonance imaging [MRI][NMR]

nonspecific abnormal findings on diagnostic imaging by positron emission tomography [PET scan]

nonspecific abnormal findings on diagnostic imaging by thermography

nonspecific abnormal findings on diagnostic imaging by ultrasound [echogram]

nonspecific abnormal findings on diagnostic imaging by X-ray examination

EXCLUDES1 abnormal findings on antenatal screening of mother (O28.-)

diagnostic abnormal findings classified elsewhere - see Alphabetical Index

PDₓ Unacceptable principal diagnosis symbol per Medicare code edits   Code exempt from diagnosis present on admission requirement

? Questionable admission   Complication or comorbidity   CC/MCC EXC CC/MCC exclusion   MCC Major complication or comorbidity

Principal diagnosis as its own CC   Principal diagnosis as its own MCC   HCC HCC diagnosis code   RxHCC RxHCC diagnosis code

MACRA code   Z Z code as first-listed diagnosis

When symbols appear on a code that requires a 7th character extension, refer to Appendix B to identify applicable 7th character codes.

2018 ICD-10-CM

R90 **Abnormal findings on** diagnostic imaging of central nervous system

  R90.0 **Intracranial** space-occupying lesion found on diagnostic imaging of central nervous system

  R90.8 **Other abnormal findings on diagnostic imaging of** central nervous system

    R90.81 **Abnormal echoencephalogram**

    R90.82 **White matter disease, unspecified**

    R90.89 **Other abnormal findings on diagnostic imaging of central nervous system**

      Other cerebrovascular abnormality found on diagnostic imaging of central nervous system

R91 **Abnormal findings on diagnostic imaging of** lung

  R91.1 **Solitary pulmonary nodule**

    Coin lesion lung

    Solitary pulmonary nodule, subsegmental branch of the bronchial tree

  R91.8 **Other nonspecific abnormal finding of lung field**

    Lung mass NOS found on diagnostic imaging of lung

    Pulmonary infiltrate NOS

    Shadow, lung

R92 **Abnormal and inconclusive findings on diagnostic imaging of** breast

  R92.0 **Mammographic** microcalcification **found on diagnostic imaging of breast**

    EXCLUDES2 mammographic calcification (calculus) found on diagnostic imaging of breast (R92.1)

  R92.1 **Mammographic** calcification **found on diagnostic imaging of breast**

    Mammographic calculus found on diagnostic imaging of breast

  R92.2 Inconclusive **mammogram**

    AHA: Q1 2015

    Dense breasts NOS

    Inconclusive mammogram NEC

    Inconclusive mammography due to dense breasts

    Inconclusive mammography NEC

  R92.8 **Other abnormal and inconclusive findings on diagnostic imaging of breast**

R93 **Abnormal findings on diagnostic imaging of** other body structures

  R93.0 **Abnormal findings on diagnostic imaging of** skull and head, **not elsewhere classified**

    EXCLUDES1 intracranial space-occupying lesion found on diagnostic imaging (R90.0)

  R93.1 **Abnormal findings on diagnostic imaging of** heart and coronary **circulation**

    Abnormal echocardiogram NOS

    Abnormal heart shadow

  R93.2 **Abnormal findings on diagnostic imaging of** liver and biliary tract

    Nonvisualization of gallbladder

  R93.3 **Abnormal findings on diagnostic imaging of** other parts of digestive tract

  R93.4 **Abnormal findings on diagnostic imaging of** urinary organs

    EXCLUDES2 hypertrophy of kidney (N28.81)

    R93.41 **Abnormal radiologic findings on diagnostic imaging of** renal pelvis, ureter, or bladder

      AHA: Q4 2016

      Filling defect of bladder found on diagnostic imaging

      Filling defect of renal pelvis found on diagnostic imaging

      Filling defect of ureter found on diagnostic imaging

    R93.42 **Abnormal radiologic findings on diagnostic imaging of kidney**

      R93.421 **Abnormal radiologic findings on diagnostic imaging of** right **kidney**

        AHA: Q4 2016

      R93.422 **Abnormal radiologic findings on diagnostic imaging of** left **kidney**

        AHA: Q4 2016

      R93.429 **Abnormal radiologic findings on diagnostic imaging of** unspecified **kidney**

        AHA: Q4 2016

    R93.49 **Abnormal radiologic findings on diagnostic imaging of** other urinary organs

      AHA: Q4 2016

  R93.5 **Abnormal findings on diagnostic imaging of** other abdominal regions, including retroperitoneum

  R93.6 **Abnormal findings on diagnostic imaging of** limbs

    EXCLUDES2 abnormal finding in skin and subcutaneous tissue (R93.8)

  R93.7 **Abnormal findings on diagnostic imaging of** other parts of musculoskeletal system

    EXCLUDES2 abnormal findings on diagnostic imaging of skull (R93.0)

  R93.8 **Abnormal findings on diagnostic imaging of other specified body structures**

    Abnormal finding by radioisotope localization of placenta

    Abnormal radiological finding in skin and subcutaneous tissue

    Mediastinal shift

  R93.9 **Diagnostic imaging inconclusive due to** excess body fat of patient

R94 **Abnormal results of function studies**

  INCLUDES abnormal results of radionuclide [radioisotope] uptake studies

    abnormal results of scintigraphy

  R94.0 **Abnormal results of function studies of** central nervous system

    R94.01 **Abnormal** electroencephalogram [EEG]

    R94.02 **Abnormal** brain scan

    R94.09 **Abnormal results of other function studies of central nervous system**

  R94.1 **Abnormal results of function studies of** peripheral nervous system and special senses

    R94.11 **Abnormal results of function studies of** eye

      R94.110 **Abnormal** electro-oculogram [EOG]

      R94.111 **Abnormal** electroretinogram [ERG]

        Abnormal retinal function study

      R94.112 **Abnormal** visually evoked potential [VEP]

      R94.113 **Abnormal** oculomotor **study**

      R94.118 **Abnormal results of other function studies of eye**

    R94.12 **Abnormal results of function studies of** ear and other special senses

      R94.120 **Abnormal** auditory **function study**

        AHA: Q3 2016

      R94.121 **Abnormal** vestibular **function study**

      R94.128 **Abnormal results of other function studies of ear and other special senses**

    R94.13 **Abnormal results of function studies of** peripheral nervous system

      R94.130 **Abnormal response to nerve stimulation, unspecified**

      R94.131 **Abnormal** electromyogram [EMG]

        EXCLUDES1 electromyogram of eye (R94.113)

      R94.138 **Abnormal results of other function studies of peripheral nervous system**

  R94.2 **Abnormal results of** pulmonary function **studies**

    Reduced ventilatory capacity

    Reduced vital capacity

  R94.3 **Abnormal results of** cardiovascular function **studies**

    R94.30 **Abnormal result of cardiovascular function study, unspecified**

    R94.31 **Abnormal** electrocardiogram [ECG] [EKG]

      EXCLUDES1 long QT syndrome (I45.81)

    R94.39 **Abnormal result of other cardiovascular function study**

      Abnormal electrophysiological intracardiac studies

      Abnormal phonocardiogram

      Abnormal vectorcardiogram

  R94.4 **Abnormal results of** kidney function **studies**

    Abnormal renal function test

  R94.5 **Abnormal results of** liver function **studies**

  R94.6 **Abnormal results of** thyroid function **studies**

Unspecified Code   Other Specified Code   Manifestation Code   N Newborn   P Pediatric   M Maternity   A Adult   ♂ Male   ♀ Female

● New Code   ▲ Revised Code Title   ►◄ Revised Text   **NOTES**   *INCLUDES*   *EXCLUDES 1*   Not coded here   *EXCLUDES 2*   Not included here

4th character required   5th character required   6th character required   7th character required

Extension 'X' Alert   **HAC** Hospital-acquired condition (HAC) alert   **AHA** AHA Coding Clinic©

R94.7   **Abnormal results of** other endocrine function **studies**
        EXCLUDES2 *abnormal glucose (R73.0-)*
R94.8   **Abnormal results of function studies of** other organs and systems
        Abnormal basal metabolic rate [BMR]
        Abnormal bladder function test
        Abnormal splenic function test

Abnormal tumor markers (R97)

R97   **Abnormal tumor markers**
      Elevated tumor associated antigens [TAA]
      Elevated tumor specific antigens [TSA]
      R97.0   **Elevated carcinoembryonic antigen [CEA]**
      R97.1   **Elevated cancer antigen 125 [CA 125]**   ♀
      R97.2   **Elevated prostate specific antigen [PSA]**
              R97.20   **Elevated prostate specific antigen [PSA]**   🅰 ❓ ♂
                       AHA: Q4 2016
              R97.21   **Rising PSA** following treatment for malignant
                       neoplasm of prostate   🅰 ❓ ♂
                       AHA: Q4 2016
      R97.8   **Other abnormal tumor markers**

Ill-defined and unknown cause of mortality (R99)

R99   **Ill-defined and unknown cause of mortality**
      AHA: Q4 2016
      Death (unexplained) NOS
      Unspecified cause of mortality

Unacceptable principal diagnosis symbol per Medicare code edits   Code exempt from diagnosis present on admission requirement
❓ Questionable admission   Complication or comorbidity   CC/MCC exclusion   Major complication or comorbidity
Principal diagnosis as its own CC   Principal diagnosis as its own MCC   HCC HCC diagnosis code   RxHCC RxHCC diagnosis code
MACRA code   Z code as first-listed diagnosis

968   When symbols appear on a code that requires a 7th character extension, refer to Appendix B to identify applicable 7th character codes.   **2018 ICD-10-CM**

NOTES

NOTES

Active treatment - first time seen for treatment

after care Z codes should NOT be used for aftercare for conditions such as injuries or person

Chapter 19: Injury, Poisoning, and Certain Other Consequences of External Causes (S00-T88)

Injury, poisoning and certain other consequences of external causes (S00-T88)

NOTES Use secondary code(s) from Chapter 20, External causes of morbidity, to indicate cause of injury. Codes within the T section that include the external cause do not require an additional external cause code

Use additional code to identify any retained foreign body, if applicable (Z18.-)

EXCLUDES1 birth trauma (P10-P15)

obstetric trauma (O70-O71)

This chapter contains the following blocks:

S00-S09	Injuries to the head
S10-S19	Injuries to the neck
S20-S29	Injuries to the thorax
S30-S39	Injuries to the abdomen, lower back, lumbar spine, pelvis and external genitals
S40-S49	Injuries to the shoulder and upper arm
S50-S59	Injuries to the elbow and forearm
S60-S69	Injuries to the wrist, hand and fingers
S70-S79	Injuries to the hip and thigh
S80-S89	Injuries to the knee and lower leg
S90-S99	Injuries to the ankle and foot
T07	Injuries involving multiple body regions
T14	Injury of unspecified body region
T15-T19	Effects of foreign body entering through natural orifice
T20-T32	Burns and corrosions

Editor's Note: At press time, CMS deleted this block for 2018 even though there are valid codes within the block. The block has been left here because it includes valid codes. Check www.cms.gov for further updates.

T20-T25	Burns and corrosions of external body surface, specified by site
T26-T28	Burns and corrosions confined to eye and internal organs
T30-T32	Burns and corrosions of multiple and unspecified body regions
T33-T34	Frostbite
T36-T50	Poisoning by, adverse effect of and underdosing of drugs, medicaments and biological substances
T51-T65	Toxic effects of substances chiefly nonmedicinal as to source
T66-T78	Other and unspecified effects of external causes
T79	Certain early complications of trauma
T80-T88	Complications of surgical and medical care, not elsewhere classified

NOTES The chapter uses the S-section for coding different types of injuries related to single body regions and the T-section to cover injuries to unspecified body regions as well as poisoning and certain other consequences of external causes.

Injuries to the head (S00-S09)

INCLUDES injuries of ear

injuries of eye

injuries of face [any part]

injuries of gum

injuries of jaw

injuries of oral cavity

injuries of palate

injuries of periocular area

injuries of scalp

injuries of temporomandibular joint area

injuries of tongue

injuries of tooth

Code also for any associated infection

EXCLUDES2 burns and corrosions (T20-T32)

effects of foreign body in ear (T16)

effects of foreign body in larynx (T17.3)

effects of foreign body in mouth NOS (T18.0)

effects of foreign body in nose (T17.0-T17.1)

effects of foreign body in pharynx (T17.2)

effects of foreign body on external eye (T15.-)

frostbite (T33-T34)

insect bite or sting, venomous (T63.4)

S00 Superficial injury of head

EXCLUDES1 diffuse cerebral contusion (S06.2-)

focal cerebral contusion (S06.3-)

injury of eye and orbit (S05.-)

open wound of head (S01.-)

The appropriate 7th character is to be added to each code from category S00

A = initial encounter

D = subsequent encounter

S = sequela

S00.0 Superficial injury of scalp

S00.00 Unspecified superficial injury of scalp

S00.01 Abrasion of scalp

S00.02 Blister (nonthermal) of scalp

S00.03 Contusion of scalp

Bruise of scalp

Hematoma of scalp

S00.04 External constriction of part of scalp

S00.05 Superficial foreign body of scalp

Splinter in the scalp

S00.06 Insect bite (nonvenomous) of scalp

S00.07 Other superficial bite of scalp

EXCLUDES1 open bite of scalp (S01.05)

S00.1 Contusion of eyelid and periocular area

Black eye

EXCLUDES2 contusion of eyeball and orbital tissues (S05.1)

S00.10 Contusion of unspecified eyelid and periocular area

S00.11 Contusion of right eyelid and periocular area

S00.12 Contusion of left eyelid and periocular area

S00.2 Other and unspecified superficial injuries of eyelid and periocular area

EXCLUDES2 superficial injury of conjunctiva and cornea (S05.0-)

S00.20 Unspecified superficial injury of eyelid and periocular area

S00.201 Unspecified superficial injury of right eyelid and periocular area

S00.202 Unspecified superficial injury of left eyelid and periocular area

S00.209 Unspecified superficial injury of unspecified eyelid and periocular area

S00.21 Abrasion of eyelid and periocular area

S00.211 Abrasion of right eyelid and periocular area

S00.212 Abrasion of left eyelid and periocular area

S00.219 Abrasion of unspecified eyelid and periocular area

S00.22 Blister (nonthermal) of eyelid and periocular area

S00.221 Blister (nonthermal) of right eyelid and periocular area

S00.222 Blister (nonthermal) of left eyelid and periocular area

S00.229 Blister (nonthermal) of unspecified eyelid and periocular area

S00.24 External constriction of eyelid and periocular area

S00.241 External constriction of right eyelid and periocular area

---

Unspecified Code	Other Specified Code Manifestation Code N Newborn P Pediatric M Maternity A Adult ♂ Male ♀ Female

● New Code   ▲ Revised Code Title   ►◄ Revised Text   **NOTES**   *INCLUDES*   **EXCLUDES 1** Not coded here   **EXCLUDES 2** Not included here

④ᵗʰ 4th character required   ⑤ᵗʰ 5th character required   ⑥ᵗʰ 6th character required   ⑦ᵗʰ 7th character required

⑦ˣ Extension 'X' Alert   **HAC** Hospital-acquired condition (HAC) alert   **AHA** AHA Coding Clinic©

7ᵗʰ **S00.242** External constriction of left eyelid and periocular area POA

7ᵗʰ **S00.249** External constriction of unspecified eyelid and periocular area POA

6ᵗʰ **S00.25** Superficial foreign body of eyelid and periocular area

Splinter of eyelid and periocular area

EXCLUDES2 retained foreign body in eyelid (H02.81-)

7ᵗʰ **S00.251** Superficial foreign body of right eyelid and periocular area

7ᵗʰ **S00.252** Superficial foreign body of left eyelid and periocular area POA

7ᵗʰ **S00.259** Superficial foreign body of unspecified eyelid and periocular area POA

6ᵗʰ **S00.26** Insect bite (nonvenomous) of eyelid and periocular area

7ᵗʰ **S00.261** Insect bite (nonvenomous) of right eyelid and periocular area

7ᵗʰ **S00.262** Insect bite (nonvenomous) of left eyelid and periocular area POA

7ᵗʰ **S00.269** Insect bite (nonvenomous) of unspecified eyelid and periocular area POA

6ᵗʰ **S00.27** Other superficial bite of eyelid and periocular area

EXCLUDES1 open bite of eyelid and periocular area (S01.15)

7ᵗʰ **S00.271** Other superficial bite of right eyelid and periocular area POA

7ᵗʰ **S00.272** Other superficial bite of left eyelid and periocular area POA

7ᵗʰ **S00.279** Other superficial bite of unspecified eyelid and periocular area POA

5ᵗʰ **S00.3** Superficial injury of nose

7ᵗʰ **S00.30** Unspecified superficial injury of nose POA

7ᵗʰ **S00.31** Abrasion of nose POA

7ᵗʰ **S00.32** Blister (nonthermal) of nose POA

7ᵗʰ **S00.33** Contusion of nose POA

Bruise of nose
Hematoma of nose

7ᵗʰ **S00.34** External constriction of nose POA

7ᵗʰ **S00.35** Superficial foreign body of nose POA

Splinter in the nose

7ᵗʰ **S00.36** Insect bite (nonvenomous) of nose POA

7ᵗʰ **S00.37** Other superficial bite of nose POA

EXCLUDES1 open bite of nose (S01.25)

5ᵗʰ **S00.4** Superficial injury of ear

6ᵗʰ **S00.40** Unspecified superficial injury of ear

7ᵗʰ **S00.401** Unspecified superficial injury of right ear POA

7ᵗʰ **S00.402** Unspecified superficial injury of left ear POA

7ᵗʰ **S00.409** Unspecified superficial injury of unspecified ear POA

6ᵗʰ **S00.41** Abrasion of ear

7ᵗʰ **S00.411** Abrasion of right ear POA

7ᵗʰ **S00.412** Abrasion of left ear POA

7ᵗʰ **S00.419** Abrasion of unspecified ear POA

6ᵗʰ **S00.42** Blister (nonthermal) of ear

7ᵗʰ **S00.421** Blister (nonthermal) of right ear POA

7ᵗʰ **S00.422** Blister (nonthermal) of left ear POA

7ᵗʰ **S00.429** Blister (nonthermal) of unspecified ear POA

6ᵗʰ **S00.43** Contusion of ear

Bruise of ear
Hematoma of ear

7ᵗʰ **S00.431** Contusion of right ear POA

7ᵗʰ **S00.432** Contusion of left ear POA

7ᵗʰ **S00.439** Contusion of unspecified ear POA

6ᵗʰ **S00.44** External constriction of ear

7ᵗʰ **S00.441** External constriction of right ear POA

7ᵗʰ **S00.442** External constriction of left ear POA

7ᵗʰ **S00.449** External constriction of unspecified ear POA

6ᵗʰ **S00.45** Superficial foreign body of ear

Splinter in the ear

7ᵗʰ **S00.451** Superficial foreign body of right ear POA

7ᵗʰ **S00.452** Superficial foreign body of left ear POA

7ᵗʰ **S00.459** Superficial foreign body of unspecified ear POA

6ᵗʰ **S00.46** Insect bite (nonvenomous) of ear

7ᵗʰ **S00.461** Insect bite (nonvenomous) of right ear POA

7ᵗʰ **S00.462** Insect bite (nonvenomous) of left ear POA

7ᵗʰ **S00.469** Insect bite (nonvenomous) of unspecified ear POA

6ᵗʰ **S00.47** Other superficial bite of ear

EXCLUDES1 open bite of ear (S01.35)

7ᵗʰ **S00.471** Other superficial bite of right ear POA

7ᵗʰ **S00.472** Other superficial bite of left ear POA

7ᵗʰ **S00.479** Other superficial bite of unspecified ear POA

5ᵗʰ **S00.5** Superficial injury of lip and oral cavity

6ᵗʰ **S00.50** Unspecified superficial injury of lip and oral cavity

7ᵗʰ **S00.501** Unspecified superficial injury of lip POA

7ᵗʰ **S00.502** Unspecified superficial injury of oral cavity POA

6ᵗʰ **S00.51** Abrasion of lip and oral cavity

7ᵗʰ **S00.511** Abrasion of lip POA

7ᵗʰ **S00.512** Abrasion of oral cavity POA

6ᵗʰ **S00.52** Blister (nonthermal) of lip and oral cavity

7ᵗʰ **S00.521** Blister (nonthermal) of lip POA

7ᵗʰ **S00.522** Blister (nonthermal) of oral cavity POA

6ᵗʰ **S00.53** Contusion of lip and oral cavity

7ᵗʰ **S00.531** Contusion of lip POA

Bruise of lip
Hematoma of ▶lip◀

7ᵗʰ **S00.532** Contusion of oral cavity POA

Bruise of oral cavity
Hematoma of ▶oral cavity◀

6ᵗʰ **S00.54** External constriction of lip and oral cavity

7ᵗʰ **S00.541** External constriction of lip POA

7ᵗʰ **S00.542** External constriction of oral cavity POA

6ᵗʰ **S00.55** Superficial foreign body of lip and oral cavity

7ᵗʰ **S00.551** Superficial foreign body of lip POA

Splinter of lip and oral cavity

7ᵗʰ **S00.552** Superficial foreign body of oral cavity POA

Splinter of lip and oral cavity

6ᵗʰ **S00.56** Insect bite (nonvenomous) of lip and oral cavity

7ᵗʰ **S00.561** Insect bite (nonvenomous) of lip POA

7ᵗʰ **S00.562** Insect bite (nonvenomous) of oral cavity POA

6ᵗʰ **S00.57** Other superficial bite of lip and oral cavity

7ᵗʰ **S00.571** Other superficial bite of lip POA

EXCLUDES1 open bite of lip (S01.551)

7ᵗʰ **S00.572** Other superficial bite of oral cavity POA

EXCLUDES1 open bite of oral cavity (S01.552)

5ᵗʰ **S00.8** Superficial injury of other parts of head

Superficial injuries of face [any part]

7ᵗʰ **S00.80** Unspecified superficial injury of other part of head POA

7ᵗʰ **S00.81** Abrasion of other part of head POA

7ᵗʰ **S00.82** Blister (nonthermal) of other part of head POA

7ᵗʰ **S00.83** Contusion of other part of head POA

Bruise of other part of head
Hematoma of other part of head

7ᵗʰ **S00.84** External constriction of other part of head POA

7ᵗʰ **S00.85** Superficial foreign body of other part of head POA

Splinter in other part of head

7ᵗʰ **S00.86** Insect bite (nonvenomous) of other part of head POA

7ᵗʰ **S00.87** Other superficial bite of other part of head POA

EXCLUDES1 open bite of other part of head (S01.85)

5ᵗʰ **S00.9** Superficial injury of unspecified part of head

7ᵗʰ **S00.90** Unspecified superficial injury of unspecified part of head POA

7ᵗʰ **S00.91** Abrasion of unspecified part of head POA

POA Unacceptable principal diagnosis symbol per Medicare code edits   Code exempt from diagnosis present on admission requirement

❓ Questionable admission   cc Complication or comorbidity   cc/mcc Excl. CC/MCC exclusion   mcc Major complication or comorbidity

Principal diagnosis as its own CC   Principal diagnosis as its own MCC   HCC HCC diagnosis code   RxHCC RxHCC diagnosis code

MACRA code   Z code as first-listed diagnosis

S00.92 Blister (nonthermal) of unspecified part of head
S00.93 Contusion of unspecified part of head
Bruise of head
Hematoma of head
S00.94 External constriction of unspecified part of head
S00.95 Superficial foreign body of unspecified part of head
Splinter of head
S00.96 Insect bite (nonvenomous) of unspecified part of head
S00.97 Other superficial bite of unspecified part of head
EXCLUDES1 open bite of head (S01.95)

S01 Open wound of head
Code also any associated:
injury of cranial nerve (S04.-)
injury of muscle and tendon of head (S09.1-)
intracranial injury (S06.-)
wound infection
EXCLUDES1 open skull fracture (S02.- with 7th character B)
EXCLUDES2 injury of eye and orbit (S05.-)
traumatic amputation of part of head (S08.-)
The appropriate 7th character is to be added to each code from category S01
A = initial encounter
D = subsequent encounter
S = sequela

S01.0 Open wound of scalp
EXCLUDES1 avulsion of scalp (S08.0)
S01.00 Unspecified open wound of scalp
S01.01 Laceration without foreign body of scalp
S01.02 Laceration with foreign body of scalp
S01.03 Puncture wound without foreign body of scalp
S01.04 Puncture wound with foreign body of scalp
S01.05 Open bite of scalp
Bite of scalp NOS
EXCLUDES1 superficial bite of scalp (S00.06, S00.07-)

S01.1 Open wound of eyelid and periocular area
Open wound of eyelid and periocular area with or without involvement of lacrimal passages
S01.10 Unspecified open wound of eyelid and periocular area
S01.101 Unspecified open wound of right eyelid and periocular area
S01.102 Unspecified open wound of left eyelid and periocular area
S01.109 Unspecified open wound of unspecified eyelid and periocular area
S01.11 Laceration without foreign body of eyelid and periocular area
S01.111 Laceration without foreign body of right eyelid and periocular area
S01.112 Laceration without foreign body of left eyelid and periocular area
S01.119 Laceration without foreign body of unspecified eyelid and periocular area
S01.12 Laceration with foreign body of eyelid and periocular area
S01.121 Laceration with foreign body of right eyelid and periocular area
S01.122 Laceration with foreign body of left eyelid and periocular area
S01.129 Laceration with foreign body of unspecified eyelid and periocular area
S01.13 Puncture wound without foreign body of eyelid and periocular area
S01.131 Puncture wound without foreign body of right eyelid and periocular area
S01.132 Puncture wound without foreign body of left eyelid and periocular area

S01.139 Puncture wound without foreign body of unspecified eyelid and periocular area
S01.14 Puncture wound with foreign body of eyelid and periocular area
S01.141 Puncture wound with foreign body of right eyelid and periocular area
S01.142 Puncture wound with foreign body of left eyelid and periocular area
S01.149 Puncture wound with foreign body of unspecified eyelid and periocular area
S01.15 Open bite of eyelid and periocular area
Bite of eyelid and periocular area NOS
EXCLUDES1 superficial bite of eyelid and periocular area (S00.26, S00.27)
S01.151 Open bite of right eyelid and periocular area
S01.152 Open bite of left eyelid and periocular area
S01.159 Open bite of unspecified eyelid and periocular area

S01.2 Open wound of nose
S01.20 Unspecified open wound of nose
S01.21 Laceration without foreign body of nose
S01.22 Laceration with foreign body of nose
S01.23 Puncture wound without foreign body of nose
S01.24 Puncture wound with foreign body of nose
S01.25 Open bite of nose
Bite of nose NOS
EXCLUDES1 superficial bite of nose (S00.36, S00.37)

S01.3 Open wound of ear
S01.30 Unspecified open wound of ear
S01.301 Unspecified open wound of right ear
S01.302 Unspecified open wound of left ear
S01.309 Unspecified open wound of unspecified ear
S01.31 Laceration without foreign body of ear
S01.311 Laceration without foreign body of right ear
S01.312 Laceration without foreign body of left ear
S01.319 Laceration without foreign body of unspecified ear
S01.32 Laceration with foreign body of ear
S01.321 Laceration with foreign body of right ear
S01.322 Laceration with foreign body of left ear
S01.329 Laceration with foreign body of unspecified ear
S01.33 Puncture wound without foreign body of ear
S01.331 Puncture wound without foreign body of right ear
S01.332 Puncture wound without foreign body of left ear
S01.339 Puncture wound without foreign body of unspecified ear
S01.34 Puncture wound with foreign body of ear
S01.341 Puncture wound with foreign body of right ear
S01.342 Puncture wound with foreign body of left ear
S01.349 Puncture wound with foreign body of unspecified ear
S01.35 Open bite of ear
Bite of ear NOS
EXCLUDES1 superficial bite of ear (S00.46, S00.47)
S01.351 Open bite of right ear
S01.352 Open bite of left ear
S01.359 Open bite of unspecified ear
S01.4 Open wound of cheek and temporomandibular area
S01.40 Unspecified open wound of cheek and temporomandibular area

Unspecified Code   Other Specified Code   Manifestation Code   N Newborn   P Pediatric   M Maternity   A Adult   ♂ Male   ♀ Female
● New Code   ▲ Revised Code Title   ►◄ Revised Text   NOTES   INCLUDES   EXCLUDES 1 Not coded here   EXCLUDES 2 Not included here
4th character required   5th character required   6th character required   7th character required
Extension 'X' Alert   HAC Hospital-acquired condition (HAC) alert   AHA AHA Coding Clinic©

[7th] S01.401 Unspecified open wound of right cheek and temporomandibular area [POA]

[7th] S01.402 Unspecified open wound of left cheek and temporomandibular area [POA]

[7th] S01.409 Unspecified open wound of unspecified cheek and temporomandibular area [POA]

[6th] S01.41 Laceration without foreign body of cheek and temporomandibular area

[7th] S01.411 Laceration without foreign body of right cheek and temporomandibular area [POA]

[7th] S01.412 Laceration without foreign body of left cheek and temporomandibular area [POA]

[7th] S01.419 Laceration without foreign body of unspecified cheek and temporomandibular area [POA]

[6th] S01.42 Laceration with foreign body of cheek and temporomandibular area

[7th] S01.421 Laceration with foreign body of right cheek and temporomandibular area [POA]

[7th] S01.422 Laceration with foreign body of left cheek and temporomandibular area [POA]

[7th] S01.429 Laceration with foreign body of unspecified cheek and temporomandibular area [POA]

[6th] S01.43 Puncture wound without foreign body of cheek and temporomandibular area

[7th] S01.431 Puncture wound without foreign body of right cheek and temporomandibular area [POA]

[7th] S01.432 Puncture wound without foreign body of left cheek and temporomandibular area [POA]

[7th] S01.439 Puncture wound without foreign body of unspecified cheek and temporomandibular area [POA]

[6th] S01.44 Puncture wound with foreign body of cheek and temporomandibular area

[7th] S01.441 Puncture wound with foreign body of right cheek and temporomandibular area [POA]

[7th] S01.442 Puncture wound with foreign body of left cheek and temporomandibular area [POA]

[7th] S01.449 Puncture wound with foreign body of unspecified cheek and temporomandibular area [POA]

[6th] S01.45 Open bite of cheek and temporomandibular area

Bite of cheek and temporomandibular area NOS

[EXCLUDES2] *superficial bite of cheek and temporomandibular area (S00.86, S00.87)*

[7th] S01.451 Open bite of right cheek and temporomandibular area [POA]

[7th] S01.452 Open bite of left cheek and temporomandibular area [POA]

[7th] S01.459 Open bite of unspecified cheek and temporomandibular area [POA]

[5th] S01.5 Open wound of lip and oral cavity

[EXCLUDES2] *tooth dislocation (S03.2)*
tooth fracture (S02.5)

[6th] S01.50 Unspecified open wound of lip and oral cavity

[7th] S01.501 Unspecified open wound of lip [POA]

[7th] S01.502 Unspecified open wound of oral cavity [POA]

[6th] S01.51 Laceration of lip and oral cavity without foreign body

[7th] S01.511 Laceration without foreign body of lip [POA]

[7th] S01.512 Laceration without foreign body of oral cavity [POA]

[6th] S01.52 Laceration of lip and oral cavity with foreign body

[7th] S01.521 Laceration with foreign body of lip [POA]

[7th] S01.522 Laceration with foreign body of oral cavity [POA]

[6th] S01.53 Puncture wound of lip and oral cavity without foreign body

[7th] S01.531 Puncture wound without foreign body of lip [POA]

[7th] S01.532 Puncture wound without foreign body of oral cavity [POA]

[6th] S01.54 Puncture wound of lip and oral cavity with foreign body

[7th] S01.541 Puncture wound with foreign body of lip [POA]

[7th] S01.542 Puncture wound with foreign body of oral cavity [POA]

[6th] S01.55 Open bite of lip and oral cavity

[7th] S01.551 Open bite of lip [POA]

Bite of lip NOS

[EXCLUDES1] *superficial bite of lip (S00.571)*

[7th] S01.552 Open bite of oral cavity [POA]

Bite of oral cavity NOS

[EXCLUDES1] *superficial bite of oral cavity (S00.572)*

[5th] S01.8 Open wound of other parts of head

[7th] S01.80 Unspecified open wound of other part of head [POA]

[7th] S01.81 Laceration without foreign body of other part of head [POA]

[7th] S01.82 Laceration with foreign body of other part of head [POA]

[7th] S01.83 Puncture wound without foreign body of other part of head [POA]

[7th] S01.84 Puncture wound with foreign body of other part of head [POA]

[7th] S01.85 Open bite of other part of head [POA]

Bite of other part of head NOS

[EXCLUDES1] *superficial bite of other part of head ►(S00.87)◄*

[5th] S01.9 Open wound of unspecified part of head

[7th] S01.90 Unspecified open wound of unspecified part of head [POA]

[7th] S01.91 Laceration without foreign body of unspecified part of head [POA]

[7th] S01.92 Laceration with foreign body of unspecified part of head [POA]

[7th] S01.93 Puncture wound without foreign body of unspecified part of head [POA]

[7th] S01.94 Puncture wound with foreign body of unspecified part of head [POA]

[7th] S01.95 Open bite of unspecified part of head [POA]

Bite of head NOS

[EXCLUDES1] *superficial bite of head NOS (S00.97)*

[4th] S02 Fracture of skull and facial bones

[NOTES] A fracture not indicated as open or closed should be coded to closed

Code also any associated intracranial injury (S06.-)

The appropriate 7th character is to be added to each code from category S02

- A = initial encounter for closed fracture
- B = initial encounter for open fracture
- D = subsequent encounter for fracture with routine healing
- G = subsequent encounter for fracture with delayed healing
- K = subsequent encounter for fracture with nonunion
- S = sequela

[7th] S02.0 Fracture of vault of skull [CC] [POA] [HAC] [HCC] [MCC] [CC/MCC Exc]

Fracture of frontal bone
Fracture of parietal bone

[5th] S02.1 Fracture of base of skull

[EXCLUDES1] *orbit NOS (S02.8)*

[EXCLUDES2] *orbital floor (S02.3-)*

[6th] S02.10 Unspecified fracture of base of skull [HCC]

[7th] S02.101 Fracture of base of skull, right side [CC] [POA] [HCC] [MCC] [CC/MCC Exc]

[7th] S02.102 Fracture of base of skull, left side [CC] [POA] [HCC] [MCC] [CC/MCC Exc]

[7th] S02.109 Fracture of base of skull, unspecified side [CC] [POA] [HCC] [MCC] [CC/MCC Exc]

[PDx] Unacceptable principal diagnosis symbol per Medicare code edits [POA] Code exempt from diagnosis present on admission requirement
[?] Questionable admission [CC] Complication or comorbidity [CC/MCC Exc] CC/MCC exclusion [MCC] Major complication or comorbidity
[PDx CC] Principal diagnosis as its own CC [PDx MCC] Principal diagnosis as its own MCC [HCC] HCC diagnosis code [RxHCC] RxHCC diagnosis code
MACRA code [Z-1] Z code as first-listed diagnosis

[6th] **S02.11 Fracture of occiput**
- [7th] S02.110 Type I occipital condyle fracture, unspecified side [CC] [POA] [HAC] [HCC] [MCC] [CC/MCC Exc]
- [7th] S02.111 Type II occipital condyle fracture, unspecified side [CC] [POA] [HAC] [HCC] [MCC] [CC/MCC Exc]
- [7th] S02.112 Type III occipital condyle fracture, unspecified side [CC] [POA] [HAC] [HCC] [MCC] [CC/MCC Exc]
- [7th] S02.113 Unspecified occipital condyle fracture [CC] [POA] [HAC] [HCC] [MCC] [CC/MCC Exc]
- [7th] S02.118 Other fracture of occiput, unspecified side [CC] [POA] [HAC] [HCC] [MCC] [CC/MCC Exc]
- [7th] S02.119 Unspecified fracture of occiput [CC] [POA] [HAC] [HCC] [MCC] [CC/MCC Exc]
- [7th] S02.11A Type I occipital condyle fracture, right side [CC] [POA] [HCC] [MCC] [CC/MCC Exc]
- [7th] S02.11B Type I occipital condyle fracture, left side [CC] [POA] [HCC] [MCC] [CC/MCC Exc]
- [7th] S02.11C Type II occipital condyle fracture, right side [CC] [POA] [HCC] [MCC] [CC/MCC Exc]
- [7th] S02.11D Type II occipital condyle fracture, left side [CC] [POA] [HCC] [MCC] [CC/MCC Exc]
- [7th] S02.11E Type III occipital condyle fracture, right side [CC] [POA] [HCC] [MCC] [CC/MCC Exc]
- [7th] S02.11F Type III occipital condyle fracture, left side [CC] [POA] [HCC] [MCC] [CC/MCC Exc]
- [7th] S02.11G Other fracture of occiput, right side [CC] [POA] [HCC] [MCC] [CC/MCC Exc]
- [7th] S02.11H Other fracture of occiput, left side [CC] [POA] [HCC] [MCC] [CC/MCC Exc]

[7th] **S02.19 Other fracture of base of skull** [CC] [POA] [HAC] [HCC] [MCC] [CC/MCC Exc]
Fracture of anterior fossa of base of skull
Fracture of ethmoid sinus
Fracture of frontal sinus
Fracture of middle fossa of base of skull
Fracture of orbital roof
Fracture of posterior fossa of base of skull
Fracture of sphenoid
Fracture of temporal bone

[7th] **S02.2 Fracture of nasal bones** [CC] [POA] [HAC] [CC/MCC Exc]

[5th] **S02.3 Fracture of orbital floor** [HCC]
[EXCLUDES1] *orbit NOS (S02.8)*
[EXCLUDES2] *orbital roof (S02.1-)*
- [7th] S02.30 Fracture of orbital floor, unspecified side [CC] [POA] [HCC] [CC/MCC Exc]
- [7th] S02.31 Fracture of orbital floor, right side [CC] [POA] [HCC] [CC/MCC Exc]
- [7th] S02.32 Fracture of orbital floor, left side [CC] [POA] [HCC] [CC/MCC Exc]

[5th] **S02.4 Fracture of malar, maxillary and zygoma bones**
Fracture of superior maxilla
Fracture of upper jaw (bone)
Fracture of zygomatic process of temporal bone

[6th] **S02.40 Fracture of malar, maxillary and zygoma bones, unspecified**
- [7th] S02.400 Malar fracture, unspecified side [CC] [POA] [HAC] [HCC] [CC/MCC Exc]
- [7th] S02.401 Maxillary fracture, unspecified side [CC] [POA] [HAC] [HCC] [CC/MCC Exc]
- [7th] S02.402 Zygomatic fracture, unspecified side [CC] [POA] [HAC] [HCC] [CC/MCC Exc]
- [7th] S02.40A Malar fracture, right side [CC] [POA] [HCC] [CC/MCC Exc]
- [7th] S02.40B Malar fracture, left side [CC] [POA] [HCC] [CC/MCC Exc]
- [7th] S02.40C Maxillary fracture, right side [CC] [POA] [HCC] [CC/MCC Exc]
- [7th] S02.40D Maxillary fracture, left side [CC] [POA] [HCC] [CC/MCC Exc]
- [7th] S02.40E Zygomatic fracture, right side [CC] [POA] [HCC] [CC/MCC Exc]
- [7th] S02.40F Zygomatic fracture, left side [CC] [POA] [HCC] [CC/MCC Exc]

[6th] **S02.41 LeFort fracture**
- [7th] S02.411 LeFort I fracture [CC] [POA] [HAC] [HCC] [CC/MCC Exc]
- [7th] S02.412 LeFort II fracture [CC] [POA] [HAC] [HCC] [CC/MCC Exc]
- [7th] S02.413 LeFort III fracture [CC] [POA] [HAC] [HCC] [CC/MCC Exc]

[7th] **S02.42 Fracture of alveolus of maxilla** [CC] [POA] [HAC] [HCC] [CC/MCC Exc]

[7th] **S02.5 Fracture of tooth (traumatic)** [CC] [POA] [CC/MCC Exc]
Broken tooth
[EXCLUDES1] *cracked tooth (nontraumatic) (K03.81)*

[5th] **S02.6 Fracture of mandible**
Fracture of lower jaw (bone)

[6th] **S02.60 Fracture of mandible, unspecified**
- [7th] S02.600 Fracture of unspecified part of body of mandible, unspecified side [CC] [POA] [HAC] [HCC] [CC/MCC Exc]
- [7th] S02.601 Fracture of unspecified part of body of right mandible [CC] [POA] [HCC] [CC/MCC Exc]
- [7th] S02.602 Fracture of unspecified part of body of left mandible [CC] [POA] [HCC] [CC/MCC Exc]
- [7th] S02.609 Fracture of mandible, unspecified [CC] [POA] [HAC] [HCC] [CC/MCC Exc]

[6th] **S02.61 Fracture of condylar process of mandible** [HCC]
- [7th] S02.610 Fracture of condylar process of mandible, unspecified side [CC] [POA] [HCC] [CC/MCC Exc]
- [7th] S02.611 Fracture of condylar process of right mandible [CC] [POA] [HCC] [CC/MCC Exc]
- [7th] S02.612 Fracture of condylar process of left mandible [CC] [POA] [HCC] [CC/MCC Exc]

[6th] **S02.62 Fracture of subcondylar process of mandible** [HCC]
- [7th] S02.620 Fracture of subcondylar process of mandible, unspecified side [CC] [POA] [HCC] [CC/MCC Exc]
- [7th] S02.621 Fracture of subcondylar process of right mandible [CC] [POA] [HCC] [CC/MCC Exc]
- [7th] S02.622 Fracture of subcondylar process of left mandible [CC] [POA] [HCC] [CC/MCC Exc]

[6th] **S02.63 Fracture of coronoid process of mandible** [HCC]
- [7th] S02.630 Fracture of coronoid process of mandible, unspecified side [CC] [POA] [HCC] [CC/MCC Exc]
- [7th] S02.631 Fracture of coronoid process of right mandible [CC] [POA] [HCC] [CC/MCC Exc]
- [7th] S02.632 Fracture of coronoid process of left mandible [CC] [POA] [HCC] [CC/MCC Exc]

[6th] **S02.64 Fracture of ramus of mandible** [HCC]
- [7th] S02.640 Fracture of ramus of mandible, unspecified side [CC] [POA] [HCC] [CC/MCC Exc]
- [7th] S02.641 Fracture of ramus of right mandible [CC] [POA] [HCC] [CC/MCC Exc]
- [7th] S02.642 Fracture of ramus of left mandible [CC] [POA] [HCC] [CC/MCC Exc]

[6th] **S02.65 Fracture of angle of mandible** [HCC]
- [7th] S02.650 Fracture of angle of mandible, unspecified side [CC] [POA] [HCC] [CC/MCC Exc]
- [7th] S02.651 Fracture of angle of right mandible [CC] [POA] [HCC] [CC/MCC Exc]
- [7th] S02.652 Fracture of angle of left mandible [CC] [POA] [HCC] [CC/MCC Exc]

[7th] **S02.66 Fracture of symphysis of mandible** [CC] [POA] [HAC] [HCC] [CC/MCC Exc]

[6th] **S02.67 Fracture of alveolus of mandible** [HCC]
- [7th] S02.670 Fracture of alveolus of mandible, unspecified side [CC] [POA] [HCC] [CC/MCC Exc]
- [7th] S02.671 Fracture of alveolus of right mandible [CC] [POA] [HCC] [CC/MCC Exc]
- [7th] S02.672 Fracture of alveolus of left mandible [CC] [POA] [HCC] [CC/MCC Exc]

[7th] **S02.69 Fracture of mandible of other specified site** [CC] [POA] [HAC] [HCC] [CC/MCC Exc]

[5th] **S02.8 Fractures of other specified skull and facial bones** [HCC]
Fracture of orbit NOS
Fracture of palate
[EXCLUDES1] *fracture of orbital floor (S02.3-)*
fracture of orbital roof (S02.1-)
- [7th] S02.80 Fracture of other specified skull and facial bones, unspecified side [CC] [POA] [HCC] [CC/MCC Exc]
- [7th] S02.81 Fracture of other specified skull and facial bones, right side [CC] [POA] [HCC] [CC/MCC Exc]
- [7th] S02.82 Fracture of other specified skull and facial bones, left side [CC] [POA] [HCC] [CC/MCC Exc]

Unspecified Code | Other Specified Code | Manifestation Code | [N] Newborn | [P] Pediatric | [M] Maternity | [A] Adult | ♂ Male | ♀ Female
● New Code | ▲ Revised Code Title | ►◄ Revised Text | [NOTES] | [INCLUDES] | [EXCLUDES1] Not coded here | [EXCLUDES2] Not included here
[4th] 4th character required | [5th] 5th character required | [6th] 6th character required | [7th] 7th character required
[7th] Extension 'X' Alert | [HAC] Hospital-acquired condition (HAC) alert | AHA AHA Coding Clinic©

S02.9 Fracture of unspecified skull and facial bones
- **S02.91** Unspecified fracture of skull `cc` `POA` `HAC` `HCC` `MCC` `CC/MCC Exc`
- **S02.92** Unspecified fracture of facial bones `cc` `POA` `HAC` `HCC` `CC/MCC Exc`

S03 Dislocation and sprain of joints and ligaments of head
INCLUDES avulsion of joint (capsule) or ligament of head
laceration of cartilage, joint (capsule) or ligament of head
sprain of cartilage, joint (capsule) or ligament of head
traumatic hemarthrosis of joint or ligament of head
traumatic rupture of joint or ligament of head
traumatic subluxation of joint or ligament of head
traumatic tear of joint or ligament of head

Code also any associated open wound
EXCLUDES2 Strain of muscle or tendon of head (S09.1)

The appropriate 7th character is to be added to each code from category S03
A = initial encounter
D = subsequent encounter
S = sequela

S03.0 Dislocation of jaw
Dislocation of jaw (cartilage) (meniscus)
Dislocation of mandible
Dislocation of temporomandibular (joint)
- **S03.00** Dislocation of jaw, unspecified side `POA`
- **S03.01** Dislocation of jaw, right side `POA`
- **S03.02** Dislocation of jaw, left side `POA`
- **S03.03** Dislocation of jaw, bilateral `POA`
S03.1 Dislocation of septal cartilage of nose `POA`
S03.2 Dislocation of tooth `POA`
S03.4 Sprain of jaw
Sprain of temporomandibular (joint) (ligament)
- **S03.40** Sprain of jaw, unspecified side `POA`
- **S03.41** Sprain of jaw, right side `POA`
- **S03.42** Sprain of jaw, left side `POA`
- **S03.43** Sprain of jaw, bilateral `POA`
S03.8 Sprain of joints and ligaments of other parts of head `POA`
S03.9 Sprain of joints and ligaments of unspecified parts of head `POA`

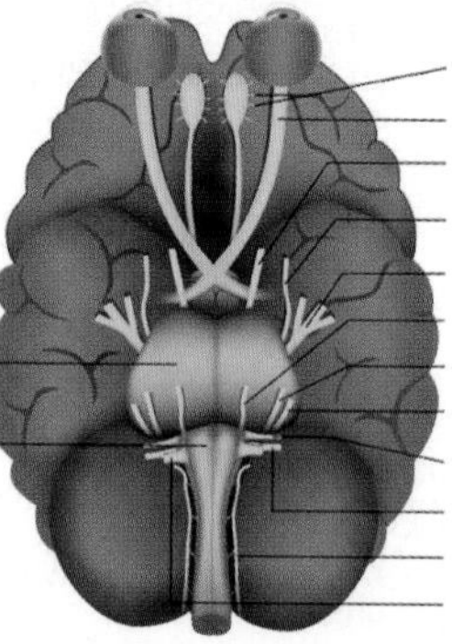

Figure 19.1 Cranial nerves

Olfactory nerve fibers (I)
Optic nerve (II)
Oculomotor nerve (III)
Trochlear nerve (IV)
Trigeminal nerve (V)
Abducens nerve (VI)
Facial nerve (VII)
Vestibulocochlear nerve (VIII)
Glossopharyngeal nerve (IX)
Vagus nerve (X)
Accessory nerve (XI)
Hypoglossal nerve (XII)
Pons
Medulla

S04 Injury of cranial nerve
The selection of side should be based on the side of the body being affected
Code first any associated intracranial injury (S06.-)
Code also any associated:
open wound of head (S01.-)
skull fracture (S02.-)

The appropriate 7th character is to be added to each code from category S04
A = initial encounter
D = subsequent encounter
S = sequela

S04.0 Injury of optic nerve and pathways
Use additional code to identify any visual field defect or blindness ▶(H53.4-, H54.-)◀

S04.01 Injury of optic nerve
Injury of 2nd cranial nerve
- **S04.011** Injury of optic nerve, right eye `cc` `POA` `CC/MCC Exc`
- **S04.012** Injury of optic nerve, left eye `cc` `POA` `CC/MCC Exc`
- **S04.019** Injury of optic nerve, unspecified eye `cc` `POA` `CC/MCC Exc`
Injury of optic nerve NOS
S04.02 Injury of optic chiasm `cc` `POA` `CC/MCC Exc`
S04.03 Injury of optic tract and pathways
Injury of optic radiation
- ▲ **S04.031** Injury of optic tract and pathways, right ▶side◀ `cc` `POA` `CC/MCC Exc`
- ▲ **S04.032** Injury of optic tract and pathways, left ▶side◀ `cc` `POA` `CC/MCC Exc`
- ▲ **S04.039** Injury of optic tract and pathways, unspecified ▶side◀ `cc` `POA` `CC/MCC Exc`
Injury of optic tract and pathways NOS
S04.04 Injury of visual cortex
- ▲ **S04.041** Injury of visual cortex, right ▶side◀ `cc` `POA` `CC/MCC Exc`
- ▲ **S04.042** Injury of visual cortex, left ▶side◀ `cc` `POA` `CC/MCC Exc`
- ▲ **S04.049** Injury of visual cortex, unspecified ▶side◀ `cc` `POA` `CC/MCC Exc`
Injury of visual cortex NOS

S04.1 Injury of oculomotor nerve
Injury of 3rd cranial nerve
- **S04.10** Injury of oculomotor nerve, unspecified side `cc` `POA` `CC/MCC Exc`
- **S04.11** Injury of oculomotor nerve, right side `cc` `POA` `CC/MCC Exc`
- **S04.12** Injury of oculomotor nerve, left side `cc` `POA` `CC/MCC Exc`
S04.2 Injury of trochlear nerve
Injury of 4th cranial nerve
- **S04.20** Injury of trochlear nerve, unspecified side `cc` `POA` `CC/MCC Exc`
- **S04.21** Injury of trochlear nerve, right side `cc` `POA` `CC/MCC Exc`
- **S04.22** Injury of trochlear nerve, left side `cc` `POA` `CC/MCC Exc`
S04.3 Injury of trigeminal nerve
Injury of 5th cranial nerve
- **S04.30** Injury of trigeminal nerve, unspecified side `cc` `POA` `CC/MCC Exc`
- **S04.31** Injury of trigeminal nerve, right side `cc` `POA` `CC/MCC Exc`
- **S04.32** Injury of trigeminal nerve, left side `cc` `POA` `CC/MCC Exc`
S04.4 Injury of abducent nerve
Injury of 6th cranial nerve
- **S04.40** Injury of abducent nerve, unspecified side `cc` `POA` `CC/MCC Exc`
- **S04.41** Injury of abducent nerve, right side `cc` `POA` `CC/MCC Exc`
- **S04.42** Injury of abducent nerve, left side `cc` `POA` `CC/MCC Exc`
S04.5 Injury of facial nerve
Injury of 7th cranial nerve
- **S04.50** Injury of facial nerve, unspecified side `cc` `POA` `CC/MCC Exc`
- **S04.51** Injury of facial nerve, right side `cc` `POA` `CC/MCC Exc`
- **S04.52** Injury of facial nerve, left side `cc` `POA` `CC/MCC Exc`
S04.6 Injury of acoustic nerve
Injury of auditory nerve
Injury of 8th cranial nerve
- **S04.60** Injury of acoustic nerve, unspecified side `cc` `POA` `CC/MCC Exc`
- **S04.61** Injury of acoustic nerve, right side `cc` `POA` `CC/MCC Exc`
- **S04.62** Injury of acoustic nerve, left side `cc` `POA` `CC/MCC Exc`
S04.7 Injury of accessory nerve
Injury of 11th cranial nerve
- **S04.70** Injury of accessory nerve, unspecified side `cc` `POA` `CC/MCC Exc`
- **S04.71** Injury of accessory nerve, right side `cc` `POA` `CC/MCC Exc`
- **S04.72** Injury of accessory nerve, left side `cc` `POA` `CC/MCC Exc`
S04.8 Injury of other cranial nerves
S04.81 Injury of olfactory [1st] nerve
- **S04.811** Injury of olfactory [1st] nerve, right side `cc` `POA` `CC/MCC Exc`
- **S04.812** Injury of olfactory [1st] nerve, left side `cc` `POA` `CC/MCC Exc`

`POA≡` Unacceptable principal diagnosis symbol per Medicare code edits   `POA` Code exempt from diagnosis present on admission requirement   `?` Questionable admission   `cc` Complication or comorbidity   `CC/MCC Exc` CC/MCC exclusion   `MCC` Major complication or comorbidity   `≡CC` Principal diagnosis as its own CC   `≡MCC` Principal diagnosis as its own MCC   `HCC` HCC diagnosis code   `RxHCC` RxHCC diagnosis code   MACRA code   `Z1` Z code as first-listed diagnosis

S04.819   **Injury of olfactory [1st] nerve, unspecified side**   CC POA CC/MCC Exc

S04.89   **Injury of other cranial nerves**
Injury of vagus [10th] nerve

S04.891   **Injury of other cranial nerves, right side**   CC POA CC/MCC Exc

S04.892   **Injury of other cranial nerves, left side**   CC POA CC/MCC Exc

S04.899   **Injury of other cranial nerves, unspecified side**   CC POA CC/MCC Exc

S04.9   **Injury of unspecified cranial nerve**   CC POA CC/MCC Exc

S05   **Injury of eye and orbit**

INCLUDES   *open wound of eye and orbit*

EXCLUDES2   *2nd cranial [optic] nerve injury (S04.0-)*

3rd cranial [oculomotor] nerve injury (S04.1-)

open wound of eyelid and periocular area (S01.1-)

orbital bone fracture (S02.1-, S02.3-, S02.8-)

superficial injury of eyelid (S00.1-S00.2)

The appropriate 7th character is to be added to each code from category S05

A = initial encounter

D = subsequent encounter

S = sequela

S05.0   **Injury of conjunctiva and corneal abrasion without foreign body**

EXCLUDES1   *foreign body in conjunctival sac (T15.1)*

foreign body in cornea (T15.0)

S05.00   **Injury of conjunctiva and corneal abrasion without foreign body, unspecified eye**   POA

S05.01   **Injury of conjunctiva and corneal abrasion without foreign body, right eye**   POA

S05.02   **Injury of conjunctiva and corneal abrasion without foreign body, left eye**   POA

S05.1   **Contusion of eyeball and orbital tissues**
Traumatic hyphema

EXCLUDES2   *black eye NOS (S00.1)*

contusion of eyelid and periocular area (S00.1)

S05.10   **Contusion of eyeball and orbital tissues, unspecified eye**   POA

S05.11   **Contusion of eyeball and orbital tissues, right eye**   POA

S05.12   **Contusion of eyeball and orbital tissues, left eye**   POA

S05.2   **Ocular laceration and rupture with prolapse or loss of intraocular tissue**

S05.20   **Ocular laceration and rupture with prolapse or loss of intraocular tissue, unspecified eye**   CC POA CC/MCC Exc

S05.21   **Ocular laceration and rupture with prolapse or loss of intraocular tissue, right eye**   CC POA CC/MCC Exc

S05.22   **Ocular laceration and rupture with prolapse or loss of intraocular tissue, left eye**   CC POA CC/MCC Exc

S05.3   **Ocular laceration without prolapse or loss of intraocular tissue**
Laceration of eye NOS

S05.30   **Ocular laceration without prolapse or loss of intraocular tissue, unspecified eye**   CC POA CC/MCC Exc

S05.31   **Ocular laceration without prolapse or loss of intraocular tissue, right eye**   CC POA CC/MCC Exc

S05.32   **Ocular laceration without prolapse or loss of intraocular tissue, left eye**   CC POA CC/MCC Exc

S05.4   **Penetrating wound of orbit with or without foreign body**

EXCLUDES2   *retained (old) foreign body following penetrating wound in orbit (H05.5-)*

S05.40   **Penetrating wound of orbit with or without foreign body, unspecified eye**   CC POA CC/MCC Exc

S05.41   **Penetrating wound of orbit with or without foreign body, right eye**   CC POA CC/MCC Exc

S05.42   **Penetrating wound of orbit with or without foreign body, left eye**   CC POA CC/MCC Exc

S05.5   **Penetrating wound with foreign body of eyeball**

EXCLUDES2   *retained (old) intraocular foreign body (H44.6-, H44.7)*

S05.50   **Penetrating wound with foreign body of unspecified eyeball**   CC POA CC/MCC Exc

S05.51   **Penetrating wound with foreign body of right eyeball**   CC POA CC/MCC Exc

S05.52   **Penetrating wound with foreign body of left eyeball**   CC POA CC/MCC Exc

S05.6   **Penetrating wound without foreign body of eyeball**
Ocular penetration NOS

S05.60   **Penetrating wound without foreign body of unspecified eyeball**   POA

S05.61   **Penetrating wound without foreign body of right eyeball**   POA

S05.62   **Penetrating wound without foreign body of left eyeball**   POA

S05.7   **Avulsion of eye**
Traumatic enucleation

S05.70   **Avulsion of unspecified eye**   CC POA CC/MCC Exc

S05.71   **Avulsion of right eye**   CC POA CC/MCC Exc

S05.72   **Avulsion of left eye**   CC POA CC/MCC Exc

S05.8   **Other injuries of eye and orbit**
Lacrimal duct injury

S05.8X   **Other injuries of eye and orbit**

S05.8X1   **Other injuries of right eye and orbit**   CC POA CC/MCC Exc

S05.8X2   **Other injuries of left eye and orbit**   CC POA CC/MCC Exc

S05.8X9   **Other injuries of unspecified eye and orbit**   CC POA CC/MCC Exc

S05.9   **Unspecified injury of eye and orbit**
Injury of eye NOS

S05.90   **Unspecified injury of unspecified eye and orbit**   POA

S05.91   **Unspecified injury of right eye and orbit**   CC POA CC/MCC Exc

S05.92   **Unspecified injury of left eye and orbit**   CC POA CC/MCC Exc

S06   **Intracranial injury**

INCLUDES   *traumatic brain injury*

Code also any associated:

open wound of head (S01.-)

skull fracture (S02.-)

EXCLUDES1   *head injury NOS (S09.90)*

The appropriate 7th character is to be added to each code from category S06

A = initial encounter

D = subsequent encounter

S = sequela

NOTES   7th characters D and S do not apply to codes in category S06 with 6th character 7 - death due to brain injury prior to regaining consciousness, or 8 - death due to other cause prior to regaining consciousness.

S06.0   **Concussion**
Commotio cerebri

EXCLUDES1   *concussion with other intracranial injuries classified in subcategories S06.1- to S06.6-, S06.81- and S06.82- code to specified intracranial injury*

S06.0X   **Concussion**

S06.0X0   **Concussion without loss of consciousness**   POA HCC

S06.0X1   **Concussion with loss of consciousness of 30 minutes or less**   CC POA HAC HCC CC/MCC Exc

S06.0X9   **Concussion with loss of consciousness of unspecified duration**   CC POA HAC HCC CC/MCC Exc
AHA: Q4 2016
Concussion NOS

S06.1   **Traumatic cerebral edema**
Diffuse traumatic cerebral edema
Focal traumatic cerebral edema

S06.1X   **Traumatic cerebral edema**

S06.1X0   **Traumatic cerebral edema without loss of consciousness**   POA HCC MCC CC/MCC Exc

S06.1X1   **Traumatic cerebral edema with loss of consciousness of 30 minutes or less**   POA HAC HCC MCC CC/MCC Exc

---

Unspecified Code   Other Specified Code   Manifestation Code   N Newborn   P Pediatric   M Maternity   A Adult   ♂ Male   ♀ Female
● New Code   ▲ Revised Code Title   ►◄ Revised Text   NOTES   INCLUDES   EXCLUDES 1 Not coded here   EXCLUDES 2 Not included here
4th character required   5th character required   6th character required   7th character required
Extension 'X' Alert   HAC Hospital-acquired condition (HAC) alert   AHA AHA Coding Clinic©

7️⃣ **S06.355** **Traumatic hemorrhage of left cerebrum with loss of consciousness** greater than 24 hours with return to pre-existing conscious level ⓟⓞⓐ HAC HCC MCC CC/MCC Exc

7️⃣ **S06.356** **Traumatic hemorrhage of left cerebrum with loss of consciousness greater than 24 hours** without **return to pre-existing conscious level with patient surviving** ⓟⓞⓐ HAC HCC MCC CC/MCC Exc

7️⃣ **S06.357** **Traumatic hemorrhage of left cerebrum with loss of consciousness of** any duration with death due to brain injury prior to regaining consciousness ⓟⓞⓐ HAC MCC CC/MCC Exc

7️⃣ **S06.358** **Traumatic hemorrhage of left cerebrum with loss of consciousness of any duration with death due to** other **cause prior to regaining consciousness** ⓟⓞⓐ HAC MCC CC/MCC Exc

7️⃣ S06.359 Traumatic hemorrhage of left cerebrum with loss of consciousness of unspecified duration ⓟⓞⓐ HAC HCC MCC CC/MCC Exc

Traumatic hemorrhage of left cerebrum NOS

6️⃣ **S06.36** **Traumatic hemorrhage of cerebrum, unspecified**

Traumatic intracerebral hemorrhage and hematoma, unspecified

7️⃣ S06.360 **Traumatic hemorrhage of cerebrum, unspecified, without loss of consciousness** ⓟⓞⓐ HAC HCC MCC CC/MCC Exc

7️⃣ S06.361 **Traumatic hemorrhage of cerebrum, unspecified,** with loss of consciousness of 30 minutes or less ⓟⓞⓐ HAC HCC MCC CC/MCC Exc

7️⃣ S06.362 **Traumatic hemorrhage of cerebrum, unspecified, with loss of consciousness of** 31 minutes to 59 minutes ⓟⓞⓐ HAC HCC MCC CC/MCC Exc

7️⃣ S06.363 **Traumatic hemorrhage of cerebrum, unspecified, with loss of consciousness of** 1 hours to 5 hours 59 minutes ⓟⓞⓐ HAC HCC MCC CC/MCC Exc

7️⃣ S06.364 **Traumatic hemorrhage of cerebrum, unspecified, with loss of consciousness of** 6 hours to 24 hours ⓟⓞⓐ HAC HCC MCC CC/MCC Exc

7️⃣ S06.365 **Traumatic hemorrhage of cerebrum, unspecified, with loss of consciousness** greater than 24 hours with return to pre-existing conscious level HAC HCC MCC CC/MCC Exc

7️⃣ S06.366 **Traumatic hemorrhage of cerebrum, unspecified, with loss of consciousness greater than 24 hours** without **return to pre-existing conscious level with patient surviving** ⓟⓞⓐ HAC HCC MCC CC/MCC Exc

7️⃣ S06.367 **Traumatic hemorrhage of cerebrum, unspecified, with loss of consciousness of any duration with death due to brain injury prior to regaining consciousness** ⓟⓞⓐ HAC MCC CC/MCC Exc

7️⃣ S06.368 **Traumatic hemorrhage of cerebrum, unspecified, with loss of consciousness of any duration with death due to** other **cause prior to regaining consciousness** ⓟⓞⓐ HAC MCC CC/MCC Exc

7️⃣ S06.369 **Traumatic hemorrhage of cerebrum, unspecified, with loss of consciousness of unspecified duration** ⓟⓞⓐ HAC HCC MCC CC/MCC Exc

Traumatic hemorrhage of cerebrum NOS

6️⃣ **S06.37** **Contusion, laceration, and hemorrhage of cerebellum**

7️⃣ S06.370 **Contusion, laceration, and hemorrhage of cerebellum without loss of consciousness** ⓟⓞⓐ HAC HCC MCC CC/MCC Exc

7️⃣ S06.371 **Contusion, laceration, and hemorrhage of cerebellum** with loss of consciousness of 30 minutes or less ⓒⓒ ⓟⓞⓐ HAC HCC CC/MCC Exc

7️⃣ S06.372 Contusion, laceration, and hemorrhage of cerebellum with loss of consciousness of 31 minutes to 59 minutes ⓒⓒ ⓟⓞⓐ HAC HCC CC/MCC Exc

7️⃣ S06.373 Contusion, laceration, and hemorrhage of cerebellum with loss of consciousness of 1 hour to 5 hours 59 minutes ⓒⓒ ⓟⓞⓐ HAC HCC CC/MCC Exc

7️⃣ S06.374 Contusion, laceration, and hemorrhage of cerebellum with loss of consciousness of 6 hours to 24 hours ⓒⓒ ⓟⓞⓐ HAC HCC CC/MCC Exc

7️⃣ S06.375 Contusion, laceration, and hemorrhage of cerebellum with loss of consciousness greater than 24 hours with return to pre-existing conscious level ⓒⓒ ⓟⓞⓐ HAC HCC CC/MCC Exc

7️⃣ S06.376 Contusion, laceration, and hemorrhage of cerebellum with loss of consciousness greater than 24 hours without **return to pre-existing conscious level** with patient surviving ⓟⓞⓐ HAC HCC MCC CC/MCC Exc

7️⃣ S06.377 Contusion, laceration, and hemorrhage of cerebellum with loss of consciousness of any duration with death due to brain injury prior to regaining consciousness ⓟⓞⓐ HAC MCC CC/MCC Exc

7️⃣ S06.378 Contusion, laceration, and hemorrhage of cerebellum with loss of consciousness of any duration with death due to other cause prior to regaining consciousness ⓟⓞⓐ HAC MCC CC/MCC Exc

7️⃣ S06.379 Contusion, laceration, and hemorrhage of cerebellum with loss of consciousness of unspecified duration ⓒⓒ ⓟⓞⓐ HAC HCC CC/MCC Exc

Contusion, laceration, and hemorrhage of cerebellum NOS

6️⃣ **S06.38** **Contusion, laceration, and hemorrhage of brainstem**

7️⃣ S06.380 Contusion, laceration, and hemorrhage of brainstem without loss of consciousness ⓟⓞⓐ HAC HCC MCC CC/MCC Exc

7️⃣ S06.381 Contusion, laceration, and hemorrhage of brainstem with loss of consciousness of 30 minutes or less ⓒⓒ ⓟⓞⓐ HAC HCC CC/MCC Exc

7️⃣ S06.382 Contusion, laceration, and hemorrhage of brainstem with loss of consciousness of 31 minutes to 59 minutes ⓒⓒ ⓟⓞⓐ HAC HCC CC/MCC Exc

7️⃣ S06.383 Contusion, laceration, and hemorrhage of brainstem with loss of consciousness of 1 hour to 5 hours 59 minutes ⓒⓒ ⓟⓞⓐ HAC HCC CC/MCC Exc

7️⃣ S06.384 Contusion, laceration, and hemorrhage of brainstem with loss of consciousness of 6 hours to 24 hours ⓒⓒ ⓟⓞⓐ HAC HCC CC/MCC Exc

7️⃣ S06.385 Contusion, laceration, and hemorrhage of brainstem with loss of consciousness greater than 24 hours with return to pre-existing conscious level ⓒⓒ ⓟⓞⓐ HAC HCC CC/MCC Exc

7️⃣ S06.386 Contusion, laceration, and hemorrhage of brainstem with loss of consciousness greater than 24 hours without **return to pre-existing conscious level** with patient surviving ⓟⓞⓐ HAC HCC MCC CC/MCC Exc

7️⃣ S06.387 Contusion, laceration, and hemorrhage of brainstem with loss of consciousness of any duration with death due to brain injury prior to regaining consciousness ⓟⓞⓐ HAC MCC CC/MCC Exc

7️⃣ S06.388 Contusion, laceration, and hemorrhage of brainstem with loss of consciousness of any duration with death due to other cause prior to regaining consciousness ⓟⓞⓐ HAC MCC CC/MCC Exc

---

ⓟⓞⓐ Unacceptable principal diagnosis symbol per Medicare code edits   ⓟⓞⓐ Code exempt from diagnosis present on admission requirement
❓ Questionable admission   ⓒⓒ Complication or comorbidity   CC/MCC Exc CC/MCC exclusion   MCC Major complication or comorbidity
Principal diagnosis as its own CC   Principal diagnosis as its own MCC   HCC HCC diagnosis code   RxHCC RxHCC diagnosis code
MACRA code   Z1 Z code as first-listed diagnosis

[7th] S06.389 **Contusion, laceration, and hemorrhage of brainstem with loss of consciousness of unspecified duration** CC POA HAC HCC CC/MCC Exc
Contusion, laceration, and hemorrhage of brainstem NOS

[5th] **S06.4 Epidural hemorrhage**
Extradural hemorrhage NOS
Extradural hemorrhage (traumatic)

[6th] **S06.4X Epidural hemorrhage**

[7th] S06.4X0 **Epidural hemorrhage without loss of consciousness** POA HAC HCC MCC CC/MCC Exc

[7th] S06.4X1 **Epidural hemorrhage with loss of consciousness of 30 minutes or less** POA HAC HCC MCC CC/MCC Exc

[7th] S06.4X2 **Epidural hemorrhage with loss of consciousness of 31 minutes to 59 minutes** POA HAC HCC MCC CC/MCC Exc

[7th] S06.4X3 **Epidural hemorrhage with loss of consciousness of 1 hour to 5 hours 59 minutes** POA HAC HCC CC/MCC Exc

[7th] S06.4X4 **Epidural hemorrhage with loss of consciousness of 6 hours to 24 hours** POA HAC HCC MCC CC/MCC Exc

[7th] S06.4X5 **Epidural hemorrhage with loss of consciousness greater than 24 hours with return to pre-existing conscious level** POA HAC HCC MCC CC/MCC Exc

[7th] S06.4X6 **Epidural hemorrhage with loss of consciousness greater than 24 hours without return to pre-existing conscious level with patient surviving** POA HAC HCC MCC CC/MCC Exc

[7th] S06.4X7 **Epidural hemorrhage with loss of consciousness of any duration with death due to brain injury prior to regaining consciousness** POA HAC MCC CC/MCC Exc

[7th] S06.4X8 **Epidural hemorrhage with loss of consciousness of any duration with death due to other causes prior to regaining consciousness** POA HAC MCC CC/MCC Exc

[7th] S06.4X9 **Epidural hemorrhage with loss of consciousness of unspecified duration** POA HAC HCC MCC CC/MCC Exc
Epidural hemorrhage NOS

[5th] **S06.5 Traumatic subdural hemorrhage**

[6th] **S06.5X Traumatic subdural hemorrhage**

[7th] S06.5X0 **Traumatic subdural hemorrhage without loss of consciousness** POA HAC HCC MCC CC/MCC Exc

[7th] S06.5X1 **Traumatic subdural hemorrhage with loss of consciousness of 30 minutes or less** POA HAC HCC MCC CC/MCC Exc

[7th] S06.5X2 **Traumatic subdural hemorrhage with loss of consciousness of 31 minutes to 59 minutes** POA HAC HCC MCC CC/MCC Exc

[7th] S06.5X3 **Traumatic subdural hemorrhage with loss of consciousness of 1 hour to 5 hours 59 minutes** POA HAC HCC MCC CC/MCC Exc

[7th] S06.5X4 **Traumatic subdural hemorrhage with loss of consciousness of 6 hours to 24 hours** POA HAC HCC MCC CC/MCC Exc

[7th] S06.5X5 **Traumatic subdural hemorrhage with loss of consciousness greater than 24 hours with return to pre-existing conscious level** POA HAC HCC MCC CC/MCC Exc

[7th] S06.5X6 **Traumatic subdural hemorrhage with loss of consciousness greater than 24 hours without return to pre-existing conscious level with patient surviving** POA HAC HCC MCC CC/MCC Exc

[7th] S06.5X7 **Traumatic subdural hemorrhage with loss of consciousness of any duration with death due to brain injury before regaining consciousness** POA HAC MCC CC/MCC Exc

[7th] S06.5X8 **Traumatic subdural hemorrhage with loss of consciousness of any duration with death due to other cause before regaining consciousness** POA HAC MCC CC/MCC Exc

[7th] S06.5X9 **Traumatic subdural hemorrhage with loss of consciousness of unspecified duration** POA HAC HCC MCC CC/MCC Exc
Traumatic subdural hemorrhage NOS

[5th] **S06.6 Traumatic subarachnoid hemorrhage**

[6th] **S06.6X Traumatic subarachnoid hemorrhage**

[7th] S06.6X0 **Traumatic subarachnoid hemorrhage without loss of consciousness** POA HAC HCC MCC CC/MCC Exc

[7th] S06.6X1 **Traumatic subarachnoid hemorrhage with loss of consciousness of 30 minutes or less** POA HAC HCC MCC CC/MCC Exc

[7th] S06.6X2 **Traumatic subarachnoid hemorrhage with loss of consciousness of 31 minutes to 59 minutes** POA HAC HCC MCC CC/MCC Exc

[7th] S06.6X3 **Traumatic subarachnoid hemorrhage with loss of consciousness of 1 hour to 5 hours 59 minutes** POA HAC HCC MCC CC/MCC Exc

[7th] S06.6X4 **Traumatic subarachnoid hemorrhage with loss of consciousness of 6 hours to 24 hours** POA HAC HCC MCC CC/MCC Exc

[7th] S06.6X5 **Traumatic subarachnoid hemorrhage with loss of consciousness greater than 24 hours with return to pre-existing conscious level** POA HAC HCC MCC CC/MCC Exc

[7th] S06.6X6 **Traumatic subarachnoid hemorrhage with loss of consciousness greater than 24 hours without return to pre-existing conscious level with patient surviving** POA HAC HCC MCC CC/MCC Exc

[7th] S06.6X7 **Traumatic subarachnoid hemorrhage with loss of consciousness of any duration with death due to brain injury prior to regaining consciousness** POA HAC MCC CC/MCC Exc

[7th] S06.6X8 **Traumatic subarachnoid hemorrhage with loss of consciousness of any duration with death due to other cause prior to regaining consciousness** POA HAC MCC CC/MCC Exc

[7th] S06.6X9 **Traumatic subarachnoid hemorrhage with loss of consciousness of unspecified duration** POA HAC HCC MCC CC/MCC Exc
Traumatic subarachnoid hemorrhage NOS

[5th] **S06.8 Other specified intracranial injuries**

[6th] **S06.81 Injury of right internal carotid artery, intracranial portion, not elsewhere classified**

[7th] S06.810 **Injury of right internal carotid artery, intracranial portion, not elsewhere classified without loss of consciousness** POA HCC

[7th] S06.811 **Injury of right internal carotid artery, intracranial portion, not elsewhere classified with loss of consciousness of 30 minutes or less** CC POA HAC HCC CC/MCC Exc

[7th] S06.812 **Injury of right internal carotid artery, intracranial portion, not elsewhere classified with loss of consciousness of 31 minutes to 59 minutes** CC POA HAC HCC CC/MCC Exc

[7th] S06.813 **Injury of right internal carotid artery, intracranial portion, not elsewhere classified with loss of consciousness of 1 hour to 5 hours 59 minutes** CC POA HAC HCC CC/MCC Exc

[7th] S06.814 **Injury of right internal carotid artery, intracranial portion, not elsewhere classified with loss of consciousness of 6 hours to 24 hours** CC POA HAC HCC CC/MCC Exc

7th **S06.815** Injury of right internal carotid artery, intracranial portion, not elsewhere classified with loss of consciousness greater than 24 hours with return to pre-existing conscious level POA HAC HCC CC/MCC Exc

7th **S06.816** Injury of right internal carotid artery, intracranial portion, not elsewhere classified with loss of consciousness greater than 24 hours without return to pre-existing conscious level with patient surviving POA HAC MCC CC/MCC Exc

7th **S06.817** Injury of right internal carotid artery, intracranial portion, not elsewhere classified with loss of consciousness of any duration with death due to brain injury prior to regaining consciousness POA HAC MCC CC/MCC Exc

7th **S06.818** Injury of right internal carotid artery, intracranial portion, not elsewhere classified with loss of consciousness of any duration with death due to other cause prior to regaining consciousness POA HAC MCC CC/MCC Exc

7th **S06.819** Injury of right internal carotid artery, intracranial portion, not elsewhere classified with loss of consciousness of unspecified duration CC POA HAC HCC CC/MCC Exc

Injury of right internal carotid artery, intracranial portion, not elsewhere classified NOS

6th **S06.82** Injury of left internal carotid artery, intracranial portion, not elsewhere classified

7th **S06.820** Injury of left internal carotid artery, intracranial portion, not elsewhere classified without loss of consciousness POA HCC

7th **S06.821** Injury of left internal carotid artery, intracranial portion, not elsewhere classified with loss of consciousness of 30 minutes or less CC POA HAC HCC CC/MCC Exc

7th **S06.822** Injury of left internal carotid artery, intracranial portion, not elsewhere classified with loss of consciousness of 31 minutes to 59 minutes CC POA HAC HCC CC/MCC Exc

7th **S06.823** Injury of left internal carotid artery, intracranial portion, not elsewhere classified with loss of consciousness of 1 hour to 5 hours 59 minutes CC POA HAC HCC CC/MCC Exc

7th **S06.824** Injury of left internal carotid artery, intracranial portion, not elsewhere classified with loss of consciousness of 6 hours to 24 hours CC POA HAC HCC CC/MCC Exc

7th **S06.825** Injury of left internal carotid artery, intracranial portion, not elsewhere classified with loss of consciousness greater than 24 hours with return to pre-existing conscious level CC POA HAC HCC CC/MCC Exc

7th **S06.826** Injury of left internal carotid artery, intracranial portion, not elsewhere classified with loss of consciousness greater than 24 hours without return to pre-existing conscious level with patient surviving POA HAC HCC MCC CC/MCC Exc

7th **S06.827** Injury of left internal carotid artery, intracranial portion, not elsewhere classified with loss of consciousness of any duration with death due to brain injury prior to regaining consciousness POA HAC MCC CC/MCC Exc

7th **S06.828** Injury of left internal carotid artery, intracranial portion, not elsewhere classified with loss of consciousness of any duration with death due to other cause prior to regaining consciousness POA HAC MCC CC/MCC Exc

7th **S06.829** Injury of left internal carotid artery, intracranial portion, not elsewhere classified with loss of consciousness of unspecified duration CC POA HAC HCC CC/MCC Exc

Injury of left internal carotid artery, intracranial portion, not elsewhere classified NOS

6th **S06.89** Other specified intracranial injury

EXCLUDES1 concussion (S06.0X-)

7th **S06.890** Other specified intracranial injury without loss of consciousness POA HCC

7th **S06.891** Other specified intracranial injury with loss of consciousness of 30 minutes or less CC POA HAC HCC CC/MCC Exc

7th **S06.892** Other specified intracranial injury with loss of consciousness of 31 minutes to 59 minutes CC POA HAC HCC CC/MCC Exc

7th **S06.893** Other specified intracranial injury with loss of consciousness of 1 hour to 5 hours 59 minutes CC POA HAC HCC CC/MCC Exc

7th **S06.894** Other specified intracranial injury with loss of consciousness of 6 hours to 24 hours CC POA HAC HCC CC/MCC Exc

7th **S06.895** Other specified intracranial injury with loss of consciousness greater than 24 hours with return to pre-existing conscious level CC POA HAC HCC CC/MCC Exc

7th **S06.896** Other specified intracranial injury with loss of consciousness greater than 24 hours without return to pre-existing conscious level with patient surviving POA HAC HCC MCC CC/MCC Exc

7th **S06.897** Other specified intracranial injury with loss of consciousness of any duration with death due to brain injury prior to regaining consciousness POA HAC MCC CC/MCC Exc

7th **S06.898** Other specified intracranial injury with loss of consciousness of any duration with death due to other cause prior to regaining consciousness POA HAC MCC CC/MCC Exc

7th **S06.899** Other specified intracranial injury with loss of consciousness of unspecified duration CC POA HAC HCC CC/MCC Exc

5th **S06.9** Unspecified intracranial injury

Brain injury NOS

Head injury NOS with loss of consciousness

Traumatic brain injury NOS

EXCLUDES1 conditions classifiable to S06.0- to S06.8-code to specified intracranial injury

head injury NOS (S09.90)

6th **S06.9X** Unspecified intracranial injury

7th **S06.9X0** Unspecified intracranial injury without loss of consciousness POA HCC

7th **S06.9X1** Unspecified intracranial injury with loss of consciousness of 30 minutes or less CC POA HAC HCC CC/MCC Exc

7th **S06.9X2** Unspecified intracranial injury with loss of consciousness of 31 minutes to 59 minutes CC POA HAC HCC CC/MCC Exc

7th **S06.9X3** Unspecified intracranial injury with loss of consciousness of 1 hour to 5 hours 59 minutes CC POA HAC HCC CC/MCC Exc

7th **S06.9X4** Unspecified intracranial injury with loss of consciousness of 6 hours to 24 hours CC POA HAC HCC CC/MCC Exc

7th **S06.9X5** Unspecified intracranial injury with loss of consciousness greater than 24 hours with return to pre-existing conscious level CC POA HAC HCC CC/MCC Exc

PDx Unacceptable principal diagnosis symbol per Medicare code edits   Code exempt from diagnosis present on admission requirement

? Questionable admission   CC Complication or comorbidity   CC/MCC Exc CC/MCC exclusion   MCC Major complication or comorbidity

Principal diagnosis as its own CC   Principal diagnosis as its own MCC   HCC HCC diagnosis code   RxHCC RxHCC diagnosis code

MACRA code   Z Z code as first-listed diagnosis

982

When symbols appear on a code that requires a 7th character extension, refer to Appendix B to identify applicable 7th character codes.

2018 ICD-10-CM

[7th] **S06.9X6 Unspecified intracranial injury with loss of consciousness greater than 24 hours without return to pre-existing conscious level with patient surviving** POA HAC HCC MCC CC/MCC Exc

[7th] **S06.9X7 Unspecified intracranial injury with loss of consciousness of any duration with death due to brain injury prior to regaining consciousness** POA HAC MCC CC/MCC Exc

[7th] **S06.9X8 Unspecified intracranial injury with loss of consciousness of any duration with death due to other cause prior to regaining consciousness** POA HAC MCC CC/MCC Exc

[7th] **S06.9X9 Unspecified intracranial injury with loss of consciousness of unspecified duration** CC POA HAC HCC CC/MCC Exc

[4th] **S07 Crushing injury of head**
Use additional code for all associated injuries, such as:
intracranial injuries (S06.-)
skull fractures (S02.-)
The appropriate 7th character is to be added to each code from category S07
A = initial encounter
D = subsequent encounter
S = sequela

[7th] **S07.0 Crushing injury of face** CC POA HAC CC/MCC Exc
[7th] **S07.1 Crushing injury of skull** CC POA HAC CC/MCC Exc
[7th] **S07.8 Crushing injury of other parts of head** CC POA HAC CC/MCC Exc
[7th] **S07.9 Crushing injury of head, part unspecified** CC POA HAC CC/MCC Exc

[4th] **S08 Avulsion and traumatic amputation of part of head**
An amputation not identified as partial or complete should be coded to complete
The appropriate 7th character is to be added to each code from category S08
A = initial encounter
D = subsequent encounter
S = sequela

[7th] **S08.0 Avulsion of scalp** POA
[5th] **S08.1 Traumatic amputation of ear**
[6th] **S08.11 Complete traumatic amputation of ear**
[7th] **S08.111 Complete traumatic amputation of right ear** POA
[7th] **S08.112 Complete traumatic amputation of left ear** POA
[7th] **S08.119 Complete traumatic amputation of unspecified ear** POA
[6th] **S08.12 Partial traumatic amputation of ear**
[7th] **S08.121 Partial traumatic amputation of right ear** POA
[7th] **S08.122 Partial traumatic amputation of left ear** POA
[7th] **S08.129 Partial traumatic amputation of unspecified ear** POA
[5th] **S08.8 Traumatic amputation of other parts of head**
[6th] **S08.81 Traumatic amputation of nose**
[7th] **S08.811 Complete traumatic amputation of nose** POA
[7th] **S08.812 Partial traumatic amputation of nose** POA
[7th] **S08.89 Traumatic amputation of other parts of head** POA

[4th] **S09 Other and unspecified injuries of head**
The appropriate 7th character is to be added to each code from category S09
A = initial encounter
D = subsequent encounter
S = sequela

[7th] **S09.0 Injury of blood vessels of head, not elsewhere classified** CC POA CC/MCC Exc
[EXCLUDES1] *injury of cerebral blood vessels (S06.-)*
injury of precerebral blood vessels (S15.-)

[5th] **S09.1 Injury of muscle and tendon of head**
Code also any associated open wound (S01.-)
[EXCLUDES2] *sprain to joints and ligament of head (S03.9)*

[7th] **S09.10 Unspecified injury of muscle and tendon of head** POA
Injury of muscle and tendon of head NOS
[7th] **S09.11 Strain of muscle and tendon of head** POA
[7th] **S09.12 Laceration of muscle and tendon of head** POA
[7th] **S09.19 Other specified injury of muscle and tendon of head** POA

[5th] **S09.2 Traumatic rupture of ear drum**
[EXCLUDES1] *traumatic rupture of ear drum due to blast injury (S09.31-)*
[7th] **S09.20 Traumatic rupture of unspecified ear drum** CC POA CC/MCC Exc
[7th] **S09.21 Traumatic rupture of right ear drum** CC POA CC/MCC Exc
[7th] **S09.22 Traumatic rupture of left ear drum** CC POA CC/MCC Exc

[5th] **S09.3 Other specified and unspecified injury of middle and inner ear**
[EXCLUDES1] *injury to ear NOS (S09.91-)*
[EXCLUDES2] *injury to external ear (S00.4-, S01.3-, S08.1-)*
[6th] **S09.30 Unspecified injury of middle and inner ear**
[7th] **S09.301 Unspecified injury of right middle and inner ear** CC POA CC/MCC Exc
[7th] **S09.302 Unspecified injury of left middle and inner ear** CC POA CC/MCC Exc
[7th] **S09.309 Unspecified injury of unspecified middle and inner ear** CC POA CC/MCC Exc
[6th] **S09.31 Primary blast injury of ear**
Blast injury of ear NOS
[7th] **S09.311 Primary blast injury of right ear** CC POA CC/MCC Exc
[7th] **S09.312 Primary blast injury of left ear** CC POA CC/MCC Exc
[7th] **S09.313 Primary blast injury of ear, bilateral** CC POA CC/MCC Exc
[7th] **S09.319 Primary blast injury of unspecified ear** CC POA CC/MCC Exc
[6th] **S09.39 Other specified injury of middle and inner ear**
Secondary blast injury to ear
[7th] **S09.391 Other specified injury of right middle and inner ear** CC POA CC/MCC Exc
[7th] **S09.392 Other specified injury of left middle and inner ear** CC POA CC/MCC Exc
[7th] **S09.399 Other specified injury of unspecified middle and inner ear** CC POA CC/MCC Exc

[7th] **S09.8 Other specified injuries of head** POA
[5th] **S09.9 Unspecified injury of face and head**
[7th] **S09.90 Unspecified injury of head** POA
Head injury NOS
[EXCLUDES1] *brain injury NOS (S06.9-)*
head injury NOS with loss of consciousness (S06.9-)
intracranial injury NOS (S06.9-)
[7th] **S09.91 Unspecified injury of ear** POA
Injury of ear NOS
[7th] **S09.92 Unspecified injury of nose** POA
Injury of nose NOS
[7th] **S09.93 Unspecified injury of face** POA
Injury of face NOS

Injuries to the neck (S10-S19)

[INCLUDES] *injuries of nape*
injuries of supraclavicular region
injuries of throat
[EXCLUDES2] *burns and corrosions (T20-T32)*
effects of foreign body in esophagus (T18.1)
effects of foreign body in larynx (T17.3)
effects of foreign body in pharynx (T17.2)
effects of foreign body in trachea (T17.4)
frostbite (T33-T34)
insect bite or sting, venomous (T63.4)

Unspecified Code | Other Specified Code | Manifestation Code | [N] Newborn | [P] Pediatric | [M] Maternity | [A] Adult | ♂ Male | ♀ Female
● New Code | ▲ Revised Code Title | ►◄ Revised Text | [NOTES] | [INCLUDES] | [EXCLUDES1] Not coded here | [EXCLUDES2] Not included here
[4th] 4th character required | [5th] 5th character required | [6th] 6th character required | [7th] 7th character required
[7th] Extension 'X' Alert | [HAC] Hospital-acquired condition (HAC) alert | AHA AHA Coding Clinic©

[4th] **S10 Superficial injury of neck**
The appropriate 7th character is to be added to each code from category S10
A = initial encounter
D = subsequent encounter
S = sequela

[7th] S10.0 **Contusion of throat** [POA]
Contusion of cervical esophagus
Contusion of larynx
Contusion of pharynx
Contusion of trachea

[5th] S10.1 **Other and unspecified superficial injuries of throat**
[7th] S10.10 **Unspecified superficial injuries of throat** [POA]
[7th] S10.11 **Abrasion of throat** [POA]
[7th] S10.12 **Blister (nonthermal) of throat** [POA]
[7th] S10.14 **External constriction of part of throat** [POA]
[7th] S10.15 **Superficial foreign body of throat** [POA]
Splinter in the throat
[7th] S10.16 **Insect bite (nonvenomous) of throat** [POA]
[7th] S10.17 **Other superficial bite of throat** [POA]
[EXCLUDES1] *open bite of throat (S11.85)*

[5th] S10.8 **Superficial injury of other specified parts of neck**
[7th] S10.80 **Unspecified superficial injury of other specified part of neck** [POA]
[7th] S10.81 **Abrasion of other specified part of neck** [POA]
[7th] S10.82 **Blister (nonthermal) of other specified part of neck** [POA]
[7th] S10.83 **Contusion of other specified part of neck** [POA]
[7th] S10.84 **External constriction of other specified part of neck** [POA]
[7th] S10.85 **Superficial foreign body of other specified part of neck** [POA]
Splinter in other specified part of neck
[7th] S10.86 **Insect bite of other specified part of neck** [POA]
[7th] S10.87 **Other superficial bite of other specified part of neck** [POA]
[EXCLUDES1] *open bite of other specified parts of neck (S11.85)*

[5th] S10.9 **Superficial injury of unspecified part of neck**
[7th] S10.90 **Unspecified superficial injury of unspecified part of neck** [POA]
[7th] S10.91 **Abrasion of unspecified part of neck** [POA]
[7th] S10.92 **Blister (nonthermal) of unspecified part of neck** [POA]
[7th] S10.93 **Contusion of unspecified part of neck** [POA]
[7th] S10.94 **External constriction of unspecified part of neck** [POA]
[7th] S10.95 **Superficial foreign body of unspecified part of neck** [POA]
[7th] S10.96 **Insect bite of unspecified part of neck** [POA]
[7th] S10.97 **Other superficial bite of unspecified part of neck** [POA]

[4th] **S11 Open wound of neck**
Code also any associated:
spinal cord injury (S14.0, S14.1-)
wound infection
[EXCLUDES2] *open fracture of vertebra (S12.- with 7th character B)*
The appropriate 7th character is to be added to each code from category S11
A = initial encounter
D = subsequent encounter
S = sequela

[5th] S11.0 **Open wound of larynx and trachea**
[6th] S11.01 **Open wound of larynx**
[EXCLUDES2] *open wound of vocal cord (S11.03)*
[7th] S11.011 **Laceration without foreign body of larynx** [POA] [MCC] [CC/MCC Exc]
[7th] S11.012 **Laceration with foreign body of larynx** [POA] [MCC] [CC/MCC Exc]
[7th] S11.013 **Puncture wound without foreign body of larynx** [POA] [MCC] [CC/MCC Exc]
[7th] S11.014 **Puncture wound with foreign body of larynx** [POA] [MCC] [CC/MCC Exc]
[7th] S11.015 **Open bite of larynx** [POA] [MCC] [CC/MCC Exc]
Bite of larynx NOS
[7th] S11.019 **Unspecified open wound of larynx** [POA] [MCC] [CC/MCC Exc]
[6th] S11.02 **Open wound of trachea**
Open wound of cervical trachea
Open wound of trachea NOS
[EXCLUDES2] *open wound of thoracic trachea (S27.5-)*
[7th] S11.021 **Laceration without foreign body of trachea** [POA] [MCC] [CC/MCC Exc]
[7th] S11.022 **Laceration with foreign body of trachea** [POA] [MCC] [CC/MCC Exc]
[7th] S11.023 **Puncture wound without foreign body of trachea** [POA] [MCC] [CC/MCC Exc]
[7th] S11.024 **Puncture wound with foreign body of trachea** [POA] [MCC] [CC/MCC Exc]
[7th] S11.025 **Open bite of trachea** [POA] [MCC] [CC/MCC Exc]
Bite of trachea NOS
[7th] S11.029 **Unspecified open wound of trachea** [POA] [MCC] [CC/MCC Exc]
[6th] S11.03 **Open wound of vocal cord**
[7th] S11.031 **Laceration without foreign body of vocal cord** [POA] [MCC] [CC/MCC Exc]
[7th] S11.032 **Laceration with foreign body of vocal cord** [POA] [MCC] [CC/MCC Exc]
[7th] S11.033 **Puncture wound without foreign body of vocal cord** [POA] [MCC] [CC/MCC Exc]
[7th] S11.034 **Puncture wound with foreign body of vocal cord** [POA] [MCC] [CC/MCC Exc]
[7th] S11.035 **Open bite of vocal cord** [POA] [MCC] [CC/MCC Exc]
Bite of vocal cord NOS
[7th] S11.039 **Unspecified open wound of vocal cord** [POA] [MCC] [CC/MCC Exc]

[5th] S11.1 **Open wound of thyroid gland**
[7th] S11.10 **Unspecified open wound of thyroid gland** [CC] [POA] [CC/MCC Exc]
[7th] S11.11 **Laceration without foreign body of thyroid gland** [CC] [POA] [CC/MCC Exc]
[7th] S11.12 **Laceration with foreign body of thyroid gland** [CC] [POA] [CC/MCC Exc]
[7th] S11.13 **Puncture wound without foreign body of thyroid gland** [CC] [POA] [CC/MCC Exc]
[7th] S11.14 **Puncture wound with foreign body of thyroid gland** [CC] [POA] [CC/MCC Exc]
[7th] S11.15 **Open bite of thyroid gland** [CC] [POA] [CC/MCC Exc]
Bite of thyroid gland NOS

[5th] S11.2 **Open wound of pharynx and cervical esophagus**
[EXCLUDES1] *open wound of esophagus NOS (S27.8-)*
[7th] S11.20 **Unspecified open wound of pharynx and cervical esophagus** [CC] [POA] [CC/MCC Exc]
[7th] S11.21 **Laceration without foreign body of pharynx and cervical esophagus** [CC] [POA] [CC/MCC Exc]
[7th] S11.22 **Laceration with foreign body of pharynx and cervical esophagus** [CC] [POA] [CC/MCC Exc]
[7th] S11.23 **Puncture wound without foreign body of pharynx and cervical esophagus** [CC] [POA] [CC/MCC Exc]
[7th] S11.24 **Puncture wound with foreign body of pharynx and cervical esophagus** [CC] [POA] [CC/MCC Exc]
[7th] S11.25 **Open bite of pharynx and cervical esophagus** [CC] [POA] [CC/MCC Exc]
Bite of pharynx and cervical esophagus NOS

[5th] S11.8 **Open wound of other specified parts of neck**
[7th] S11.80 **Unspecified open wound of other specified part of neck** [POA]
[7th] S11.81 **Laceration without foreign body of other specified part of neck** [POA]
[7th] S11.82 **Laceration with foreign body of other specified part of neck** [POA]
[7th] S11.83 **Puncture wound without foreign body of other specified part of neck** [POA]
[7th] S11.84 **Puncture wound with foreign body of other specified part of neck** [POA]

[PDx] Unacceptable principal diagnosis symbol per Medicare code edits [POA] Code exempt from diagnosis present on admission requirement
[?] Questionable admission [CC] Complication or comorbidity [CC/MCC Exc] CC/MCC exclusion [MCC] Major complication or comorbidity
[PDx CC] Principal diagnosis as its own CC [PDx MCC] Principal diagnosis as its own MCC [HCC] HCC diagnosis code [RxHCC] RxHCC diagnosis code
MACRA code [Z-1] Z code as first-listed diagnosis

When symbols appear on a code that requires a 7th character extension, refer to Appendix B to identify applicable 7th character codes.

[7th] S11.85 Open bite of other specified part of neck POA
Bite of other specified part of neck NOS
[EXCLUDES1] *superficial bite of other specified part of neck (S10.87)*

[7th] S11.89 Other open wound of other specified part of neck POA

[5th] S11.9 Open wound of unspecified part of neck

[7th] S11.90 Unspecified open wound of unspecified part of neck POA

[7th] S11.91 Laceration without foreign body of unspecified part of neck POA

[7th] S11.92 Laceration with foreign body of unspecified part of neck POA

[7th] S11.93 Puncture wound without foreign body of unspecified part of neck POA

[7th] S11.94 Puncture wound with foreign body of unspecified part of neck POA

[7th] S11.95 Open bite of unspecified part of neck POA
Bite of neck NOS
[EXCLUDES1] *superficial bite of neck (S10.97)*

[4th] S12 Fracture of cervical vertebra and other parts of neck

[NOTES] A fracture not indicated as displaced or nondisplaced should be coded to displaced
A fracture not indicated as open or closed should be coded to closed

INCLUDES *fracture of cervical neural arch*
fracture of cervical spine
fracture of cervical spinous process
fracture of cervical transverse process
fracture of cervical vertebral arch
fracture of neck

Code first any associated cervical spinal cord injury (S14.0, S14.1-)

The appropriate 7th character is to be added to all codes from subcategories S12.0-S12.6
- A = initial encounter for closed fracture
- B = initial encounter for open fracture
- D = subsequent encounter for fracture with routine healing
- G = subsequent encounter for fracture with delayed healing
- K = subsequent encounter for fracture with nonunion
- S = sequela

[5th] S12.0 Fracture of first cervical vertebra
Atlas

[6th] S12.00 Unspecified fracture of first cervical vertebra

[7th] S12.000 Unspecified displaced fracture of first cervical vertebra CC POA HAC HCC MCC CC/MCC Exc

[7th] S12.001 Unspecified nondisplaced fracture of first cervical vertebra CC POA HAC HCC MCC CC/MCC Exc

[7th] S12.01 Stable burst fracture of first cervical vertebra CC POA HAC HCC MCC CC/MCC Exc

[7th] S12.02 Unstable burst fracture of first cervical vertebra CC POA HAC HCC MCC CC/MCC Exc

[6th] S12.03 Posterior arch fracture of first cervical vertebra

[7th] S12.030 Displaced posterior arch fracture of first cervical vertebra CC POA HAC HCC MCC CC/MCC Exc

[7th] S12.031 Nondisplaced posterior arch fracture of first cervical vertebra CC POA HAC HCC MCC CC/MCC Exc

[6th] S12.04 Lateral mass fracture of first cervical vertebra

[7th] S12.040 Displaced lateral mass fracture of first cervical vertebra CC POA HAC HCC MCC CC/MCC Exc

[7th] S12.041 Nondisplaced lateral mass fracture of first cervical vertebra CC POA HAC HCC MCC CC/MCC Exc

[6th] S12.09 Other fracture of first cervical vertebra

[7th] S12.090 Other displaced fracture of first cervical vertebra CC POA HAC HCC MCC CC/MCC Exc

[7th] S12.091 Other nondisplaced fracture of first cervical vertebra CC POA HAC HCC MCC CC/MCC Exc

[5th] S12.1 Fracture of second cervical vertebra
Axis

[6th] S12.10 Unspecified fracture of second cervical vertebra

[7th] S12.100 Unspecified displaced fracture of second cervical vertebra CC POA HAC HCC MCC CC/MCC Exc

[7th] S12.101 Unspecified nondisplaced fracture of second cervical vertebra CC POA HAC HCC MCC CC/MCC Exc

[6th] S12.11 Type II dens fracture

[7th] S12.110 Anterior displaced Type II dens fracture CC POA HAC HCC MCC CC/MCC Exc

[7th] S12.111 Posterior displaced Type II dens fracture CC POA HAC HCC MCC CC/MCC Exc

[7th] S12.112 Nondisplaced Type II dens fracture CC POA HAC HCC MCC CC/MCC Exc

[6th] S12.12 Other dens fracture

[7th] S12.120 Other displaced dens fracture CC POA HAC HCC MCC CC/MCC Exc

[7th] S12.121 Other nondisplaced dens fracture CC POA HAC HCC MCC CC/MCC Exc

[6th] S12.13 Unspecified traumatic spondylolisthesis of second cervical vertebra

[7th] S12.130 Unspecified traumatic displaced spondylolisthesis of second cervical vertebra CC POA HAC HCC MCC CC/MCC Exc

[7th] S12.131 Unspecified traumatic nondisplaced spondylolisthesis of second cervical vertebra CC POA HAC HCC MCC CC/MCC Exc

[7th] S12.14 Type III traumatic spondylolisthesis of second cervical vertebra CC POA HAC HCC MCC CC/MCC Exc

[6th] S12.15 Other traumatic spondylolisthesis of second cervical vertebra

[7th] S12.150 Other traumatic displaced spondylolisthesis of second cervical vertebra CC POA HAC HCC MCC CC/MCC Exc

[7th] S12.151 Other traumatic nondisplaced spondylolisthesis of second cervical vertebra CC POA HAC HCC MCC CC/MCC Exc

[6th] S12.19 Other fracture of second cervical vertebra

[7th] S12.190 Other displaced fracture of second cervical vertebra CC POA HAC HCC MCC CC/MCC Exc

[7th] S12.191 Other nondisplaced fracture of second cervical vertebra CC POA HAC HCC MCC CC/MCC Exc

[5th] S12.2 Fracture of third cervical vertebra

[6th] S12.20 Unspecified fracture of third cervical vertebra

[7th] S12.200 Unspecified displaced fracture of third cervical vertebra CC POA HAC HCC MCC CC/MCC Exc

[7th] S12.201 Unspecified nondisplaced fracture of third cervical vertebra CC POA HAC HCC MCC CC/MCC Exc

[6th] S12.23 Unspecified traumatic spondylolisthesis of third cervical vertebra

[7th] S12.230 Unspecified traumatic displaced spondylolisthesis of third cervical vertebra CC POA HAC HCC MCC CC/MCC Exc

[7th] S12.231 Unspecified traumatic nondisplaced spondylolisthesis of third cervical vertebra CC POA HAC HCC MCC CC/MCC Exc

[7th] S12.24 Type III traumatic spondylolisthesis of third cervical vertebra CC POA HAC HCC MCC CC/MCC Exc

[6th] S12.25 Other traumatic spondylolisthesis of third cervical vertebra

[7th] S12.250 Other traumatic displaced spondylolisthesis of third cervical vertebra CC POA HAC HCC MCC CC/MCC Exc

[7th] S12.251 Other traumatic nondisplaced spondylolisthesis of third cervical vertebra CC POA HAC HCC MCC CC/MCC Exc

[6th] S12.29 Other fracture of third cervical vertebra

[7th] S12.290 Other displaced fracture of third cervical vertebra CC POA HAC HCC MCC CC/MCC Exc

[7th] S12.291 Other nondisplaced fracture of third cervical vertebra CC POA HAC HCC MCC CC/MCC Exc

[5th] S12.3 Fracture of fourth cervical vertebra

[6th] S12.30 Unspecified fracture of fourth cervical vertebra

[7th] S12.300 Unspecified displaced fracture of fourth cervical vertebra CC POA HAC HCC MCC CC/MCC Exc

S12.301 Unspecified nondisplaced fracture of fourth cervical vertebra CC POA HAC HCC MCC CC/MCC Exc

S12.33 Unspecified traumatic spondylolisthesis of fourth cervical vertebra

  S12.330 Unspecified traumatic displaced spondylolisthesis of fourth cervical vertebra CC POA HAC HCC MCC CC/MCC Exc

  S12.331 Unspecified traumatic nondisplaced spondylolisthesis of fourth cervical vertebra CC POA HAC HCC MCC CC/MCC Exc

S12.34 Type III traumatic spondylolisthesis of fourth cervical vertebra CC POA HAC HCC MCC CC/MCC Exc

S12.35 Other traumatic spondylolisthesis of fourth cervical vertebra

  S12.350 Other traumatic displaced spondylolisthesis of fourth cervical vertebra CC POA HAC HCC MCC CC/MCC Exc

  S12.351 Other traumatic nondisplaced spondylolisthesis of fourth cervical vertebra CC POA HAC HCC MCC CC/MCC Exc

S12.39 Other fracture of fourth cervical vertebra

  S12.390 Other displaced fracture of fourth cervical vertebra CC POA HAC HCC MCC CC/MCC Exc

  S12.391 Other nondisplaced fracture of fourth cervical vertebra CC POA HAC HCC MCC CC/MCC Exc

S12.4 Fracture of fifth cervical vertebra

  S12.40 Unspecified fracture of fifth cervical vertebra

    S12.400 Unspecified displaced fracture of fifth cervical vertebra CC POA HAC HCC MCC CC/MCC Exc

    S12.401 Unspecified nondisplaced fracture of fifth cervical vertebra CC POA HAC HCC MCC CC/MCC Exc

  S12.43 Unspecified traumatic spondylolisthesis of fifth cervical vertebra

    S12.430 Unspecified traumatic displaced spondylolisthesis of fifth cervical vertebra CC POA HAC HCC MCC CC/MCC Exc

    S12.431 Unspecified traumatic nondisplaced spondylolisthesis of fifth cervical vertebra CC POA HAC HCC MCC CC/MCC Exc

  S12.44 Type III traumatic spondylolisthesis of fifth cervical vertebra CC POA HAC HCC MCC CC/MCC Exc

  S12.45 Other traumatic spondylolisthesis of fifth cervical vertebra

    S12.450 Other traumatic displaced spondylolisthesis of fifth cervical vertebra CC POA HAC HCC MCC CC/MCC Exc

    S12.451 Other traumatic nondisplaced spondylolisthesis of fifth cervical vertebra CC POA HAC HCC MCC CC/MCC Exc

  S12.49 Other fracture of fifth cervical vertebra

    S12.490 Other displaced fracture of fifth cervical vertebra CC POA HAC HCC MCC CC/MCC Exc

    S12.491 Other nondisplaced fracture of fifth cervical vertebra CC POA HAC HCC MCC CC/MCC Exc

S12.5 Fracture of sixth cervical vertebra

  S12.50 Unspecified fracture of sixth cervical vertebra

    S12.500 Unspecified displaced fracture of sixth cervical vertebra CC POA HAC HCC CC/MCC Exc

    S12.501 Unspecified nondisplaced fracture of sixth cervical vertebra CC POA HAC HCC CC/MCC Exc

  S12.53 Unspecified traumatic spondylolisthesis of sixth cervical vertebra

    S12.530 Unspecified traumatic displaced spondylolisthesis of sixth cervical vertebra CC POA HAC HCC MCC CC/MCC Exc

    S12.531 Unspecified traumatic nondisplaced spondylolisthesis of sixth cervical vertebra CC POA HAC HCC MCC CC/MCC Exc

  S12.54 Type III traumatic spondylolisthesis of sixth cervical vertebra CC POA HAC HCC MCC CC/MCC Exc

S12.55 Other traumatic spondylolisthesis of sixth cervical vertebra

  S12.550 Other traumatic displaced spondylolisthesis of sixth cervical vertebra CC POA HAC HCC MCC CC/MCC Exc

  S12.551 Other traumatic nondisplaced spondylolisthesis of sixth cervical vertebra CC POA HAC HCC MCC CC/MCC Exc

S12.59 Other fracture of sixth cervical vertebra

  S12.590 Other displaced fracture of sixth cervical vertebra CC POA HAC HCC MCC CC/MCC Exc

  S12.591 Other nondisplaced fracture of sixth cervical vertebra CC POA HAC HCC MCC CC/MCC Exc

S12.6 Fracture of seventh cervical vertebra

  S12.60 Unspecified fracture of seventh cervical vertebra

    S12.600 Unspecified displaced fracture of seventh cervical vertebra CC POA HAC HCC MCC CC/MCC Exc

    S12.601 Unspecified nondisplaced fracture of seventh cervical vertebra CC POA HAC HCC MCC CC/MCC Exc

  S12.63 Unspecified traumatic spondylolisthesis of seventh cervical vertebra

    S12.630 Unspecified traumatic displaced spondylolisthesis of seventh cervical vertebra CC POA HAC HCC MCC CC/MCC Exc

    S12.631 Unspecified traumatic nondisplaced spondylolisthesis of seventh cervical vertebra CC POA HAC HCC MCC CC/MCC Exc

  S12.64 Type III traumatic spondylolisthesis of seventh cervical vertebra CC POA HAC HCC MCC CC/MCC Exc

  S12.65 Other traumatic spondylolisthesis of seventh cervical vertebra

    S12.650 Other traumatic displaced spondylolisthesis of seventh cervical vertebra CC POA HAC HCC MCC CC/MCC Exc

    S12.651 Other traumatic nondisplaced spondylolisthesis of seventh cervical vertebra CC POA HAC HCC MCC CC/MCC Exc

  S12.69 Other fracture of seventh cervical vertebra

    S12.690 Other displaced fracture of seventh cervical vertebra CC POA HAC HCC MCC CC/MCC Exc

    S12.691 Other nondisplaced fracture of seventh cervical vertebra CC POA HAC HCC MCC CC/MCC Exc

S12.8 Fracture of other parts of neck POA HAC HCC MCC CC/MCC Exc
Hyoid bone
Larynx
Thyroid cartilage
Trachea
The appropriate 7th character is to be added to code S12.8
  A = initial encounter
  D = subsequent encounter
  S = sequela

S12.9 Fracture of neck, unspecified CC POA HAC HCC CC/MCC Exc
Fracture of neck NOS
Fracture of cervical spine NOS
Fracture of cervical vertebra NOS
The appropriate 7th character is to be added to code S12.9
  A = initial encounter
  D = subsequent encounter
  S = sequela

S13 Dislocation and sprain of joints and ligaments at neck level
  INCLUDES avulsion of joint or ligament at neck level
    laceration of cartilage, joint or ligament at neck level
    sprain of cartilage, joint or ligament at neck level
    traumatic hemarthrosis of joint or ligament at neck level
    traumatic rupture of joint or ligament at neck level
    traumatic subluxation of joint or ligament at neck level
    traumatic tear of joint or ligament at neck level
  Code also any associated open wound

POA Unacceptable principal diagnosis symbol per Medicare code edits POA Code exempt from diagnosis present on admission requirement
? Questionable admission CC Complication or comorbidity CC/MCC Exc CC/MCC exclusion MCC Major complication or comorbidity
CC Principal diagnosis as its own CC MCC Principal diagnosis as its own MCC HCC HCC diagnosis code RxHCC RxHCC diagnosis code
MACRA code Z1 Z code as first-listed diagnosis

When symbols appear on a code that requires a 7th character extension, refer to Appendix B to identify applicable 7th character codes.

2018 ICD-10-CM

EXCLUDES2 *strain of muscle or tendon at neck level (S16.1)*

The appropriate 7th character is to be added to each code from category S13

> **A = initial encounter**
> **D = subsequent encounter**
> **S = sequela**

S13.0 Traumatic rupture of cervical intervertebral disc cc POA HAC CC/MCC Exc

> EXCLUDES1 *rupture or displacement (nontraumatic) of cervical intervertebral disc NOS (M50.-)*

S13.1 Subluxation and dislocation of cervical vertebrae

> Code also any associated:
>> open wound of neck (S11.-)
>> spinal cord injury (S14.1-)

> EXCLUDES2 *fracture of cervical vertebrae (S12.0-S12.3-)*

S13.10 Subluxation and dislocation of unspecified **cervical vertebrae**

> **S13.100** Subluxation **of unspecified cervical vertebrae** cc POA HAC CC/MCC Exc

> **S13.101** Dislocation **of unspecified cervical vertebrae** cc POA HAC CC/MCC Exc

S13.11 Subluxation and dislocation of C0/C1 **cervical vertebrae**

> Subluxation and dislocation of atlantooccipital joint
> Subluxation and dislocation of atloidooccipital joint
> Subluxation and dislocation of occipitoatloid joint

> **S13.110** Subluxation **of C0/C1 cervical vertebrae** cc POA HAC CC/MCC Exc

> **S13.111** Dislocation **of C0/C1 cervical vertebrae** cc POA HAC CC/MCC Exc

S13.12 Subluxation and dislocation of C1/C2 **cervical vertebrae**

> Subluxation and dislocation of atlantoaxial joint

> **S13.120** Subluxation **of C1/C2 cervical vertebrae** cc POA HAC CC/MCC Exc

> **S13.121** Dislocation **of C1/C2 cervical vertebrae** cc POA HAC CC/MCC Exc

S13.13 Subluxation and dislocation of C2/C3 **cervical vertebrae**

> **S13.130** Subluxation **of C2/C3 cervical vertebrae** cc POA HAC CC/MCC Exc

> **S13.131** Dislocation **of C2/C3 cervical vertebrae** cc POA HAC CC/MCC Exc

S13.14 Subluxation and dislocation of C3/C4 **cervical vertebrae**

> **S13.140** Subluxation **of C3/C4 cervical vertebrae** cc POA HAC CC/MCC Exc

> **S13.141** Dislocation **of C3/C4 cervical vertebrae** cc POA HAC CC/MCC Exc

S13.15 Subluxation and dislocation of C4/C5 **cervical vertebrae**

> **S13.150** Subluxation **of C4/C5 cervical vertebrae** cc POA HAC CC/MCC Exc

> **S13.151** Dislocation **of C4/C5 cervical vertebrae** cc POA HAC CC/MCC Exc

S13.16 Subluxation and dislocation of C5/C6 **cervical vertebrae**

> **S13.160** Subluxation **of C5/C6 cervical vertebrae** cc POA HAC CC/MCC Exc

> **S13.161** Dislocation **of C5/C6 cervical vertebrae** cc POA HAC CC/MCC Exc

S13.17 Subluxation and dislocation of C6/C7 **cervical vertebrae**

> **S13.170** Subluxation **of C6/C7 cervical vertebrae** cc POA HAC CC/MCC Exc

> **S13.171** Dislocation **of C6/C7 cervical vertebrae** cc POA HAC CC/MCC Exc

S13.18 Subluxation and dislocation of C7/T1 **cervical vertebrae**

> **S13.180** Subluxation **of C7/T1 cervical vertebrae** cc POA HAC CC/MCC Exc

> **S13.181** Dislocation **of C7/T1 cervical vertebrae** cc POA HAC CC/MCC Exc

S13.2 Dislocation of other and unspecified parts of neck

> **S13.20 Dislocation of unspecified parts of neck** cc POA HAC CC/MCC Exc

> **S13.29 Dislocation of other parts of neck** cc POA HAC CC/MCC Exc

S13.4 Sprain of ligaments of cervical spine POA

> Sprain of anterior longitudinal (ligament), cervical
> Sprain of atlanto-axial (joints)
> Sprain of atlanto-occipital (joints)
> Whiplash injury of cervical spine

S13.5 Sprain of thyroid region POA

> Sprain of cricoarytenoid (joint) (ligament)
> Sprain of cricothyroid (joint) (ligament)
> Sprain of thyroid cartilage

S13.8 Sprain of joints and ligaments of other parts of neck POA

S13.9 Sprain of joints and ligaments of unspecified parts of neck POA

S14 Injury of nerves and spinal cord at neck level

> NOTES Code to highest level of cervical cord injury
> Code also any associated:
>> fracture of cervical vertebra (S12.0--S12.6.-)
>> open wound of neck (S11.-)
>> transient paralysis (R29.5)

The appropriate 7th character is to be added to each code from category S14

> **A = initial encounter**
> **D = subsequent encounter**
> **S = sequela**

S14.0 Concussion and edema of cervical spinal cord POA HCC MCC CC/MCC Exc

S14.1 Other and unspecified injuries of cervical spinal cord

> **S14.10** Unspecified injury **of cervical spinal cord**

>> **S14.101 Unspecified injury at** C1 level **of cervical spinal cord** POA HAC HCC CC/MCC Exc

>> **S14.102 Unspecified injury at** C2 level **of cervical spinal cord** POA HAC HCC CC/MCC Exc

>> **S14.103 Unspecified injury at** C3 level **of cervical spinal cord** POA HAC HCC CC/MCC Exc

>> **S14.104 Unspecified injury at** C4 level **of cervical spinal cord** POA HAC HCC CC/MCC Exc

>> **S14.105 Unspecified injury at** C5 level **of cervical spinal cord** POA HAC HCC MCC CC/MCC Exc

>> **S14.106 Unspecified injury at** C6 level **of cervical spinal cord** POA HAC HCC MCC CC/MCC Exc

>> **S14.107 Unspecified injury at** C7 level **of cervical spinal cord** POA HAC HCC MCC CC/MCC Exc

>> **S14.108 Unspecified injury at** C8 level **of cervical spinal cord** POA HCC MCC CC/MCC Exc

>> **S14.109 Unspecified injury at** unspecified **level of cervical spinal cord** POA HAC HCC

>>> Injury of cervical spinal cord NOS

> **S14.11** Complete lesion **of cervical spinal cord**

>> **S14.111 Complete lesion at** C1 level **of cervical spinal cord** POA HAC HCC MCC CC/MCC Exc

>> **S14.112 Complete lesion at** C2 level **of cervical spinal cord** POA HAC HCC MCC CC/MCC Exc

>> **S14.113 Complete lesion at** C3 level **of cervical spinal cord** POA HAC HCC MCC CC/MCC Exc

>> **S14.114 Complete lesion at** C4 level **of cervical spinal cord** POA HAC HCC MCC CC/MCC Exc

>> **S14.115 Complete lesion at** C5 level **of cervical spinal cord** POA HAC HCC MCC CC/MCC Exc

>> **S14.116 Complete lesion at** C6 level **of cervical spinal cord** POA HAC HCC MCC CC/MCC Exc

>> **S14.117 Complete lesion at** C7 level **of cervical spinal cord** POA HAC HCC MCC CC/MCC Exc

>> **S14.118 Complete lesion at** C8 level **of cervical spinal cord** POA HCC MCC CC/MCC Exc

>> **S14.119 Complete lesion at unspecified level of cervical spinal cord** POA HCC

> **S14.12** Central cord syndrome **of cervical spinal cord**

Unspecified Code	Other Specified Code	Manifestation Code	N Newborn	P Pediatric	M Maternity	A Adult	♂ Male	♀ Female

● New Code ▲ Revised Code Title ▶◀ Revised Text NOTES *INCLUDES* EXCLUDES 1 Not coded here EXCLUDES 2 Not included here

4th character required 5th character required 6th character required 7th character required

Extension 'X' Alert HAC Hospital-acquired condition (HAC) alert AHA AHA Coding Clinic©

S14.121 Central cord syndrome at C1 level of cervical spinal cord POA HAC HCC MCC CC/MCC Exc

S14.122 Central cord syndrome at C2 level of cervical spinal cord POA HAC HCC MCC CC/MCC Exc

S14.123 Central cord syndrome at C3 level of cervical spinal cord POA HAC HCC MCC CC/MCC Exc

S14.124 Central cord syndrome at C4 level of cervical spinal cord POA HAC HCC MCC CC/MCC Exc

S14.125 Central cord syndrome at C5 level of cervical spinal cord POA HAC HCC MCC CC/MCC Exc

S14.126 Central cord syndrome at C6 level of cervical spinal cord POA HAC HCC MCC CC/MCC Exc

S14.127 Central cord syndrome at C7 level of cervical spinal cord POA HAC HCC MCC CC/MCC Exc

S14.128 Central cord syndrome at C8 level of cervical spinal cord POA HCC MCC CC/MCC Exc

S14.129 Central cord syndrome at unspecified level of cervical spinal cord POA HCC

S14.13 Anterior cord syndrome of cervical spinal cord

S14.131 Anterior cord syndrome at C1 level of cervical spinal cord POA HAC HCC MCC CC/MCC Exc

S14.132 Anterior cord syndrome at C2 level of cervical spinal cord POA HAC HCC MCC CC/MCC Exc

S14.133 Anterior cord syndrome at C3 level of cervical spinal cord POA HAC HCC MCC CC/MCC Exc

S14.134 Anterior cord syndrome at C4 level of cervical spinal cord POA HAC HCC MCC CC/MCC Exc

S14.135 Anterior cord syndrome at C5 level of cervical spinal cord POA HAC HCC MCC CC/MCC Exc

S14.136 Anterior cord syndrome at C6 level of cervical spinal cord POA HAC HCC MCC CC/MCC Exc

S14.137 Anterior cord syndrome at C7 level of cervical spinal cord POA HAC HCC MCC CC/MCC Exc

S14.138 Anterior cord syndrome at C8 level of cervical spinal cord POA HCC MCC CC/MCC Exc

S14.139 Anterior cord syndrome at unspecified level of cervical spinal cord POA HCC

S14.14 Brown-Séquard syndrome of cervical spinal cord

S14.141 Brown-Séquard syndrome at C1 level of cervical spinal cord POA HCC MCC CC/MCC Exc

S14.142 Brown-Séquard syndrome at C2 level of cervical spinal cord POA HCC MCC CC/MCC Exc

S14.143 Brown-Séquard syndrome at C3 level of cervical spinal cord POA HCC MCC CC/MCC Exc

S14.144 Brown-Séquard syndrome at C4 level of cervical spinal cord POA HCC MCC CC/MCC Exc

S14.145 Brown-Séquard syndrome at C5 level of cervical spinal cord POA HCC MCC CC/MCC Exc

S14.146 Brown-Séquard syndrome at C6 level of cervical spinal cord POA HCC MCC CC/MCC Exc

S14.147 Brown-Séquard syndrome at C7 level of cervical spinal cord POA HCC MCC CC/MCC Exc

S14.148 Brown-Séquard syndrome at C8 level of cervical spinal cord POA HCC MCC CC/MCC Exc

S14.149 Brown-Séquard syndrome at unspecified level of cervical spinal cord POA HCC

S14.15 Other incomplete lesions of cervical spinal cord

Incomplete lesion of cervical spinal cord NOS
Posterior cord syndrome of cervical spinal cord

S14.151 Other incomplete lesion at C1 level of cervical spinal cord POA HAC HCC MCC CC/MCC Exc

S14.152 Other incomplete lesion at C2 level of cervical spinal cord POA HAC HCC MCC CC/MCC Exc

S14.153 Other incomplete lesion at C3 level of cervical spinal cord POA HAC HCC MCC CC/MCC Exc

S14.154 Other incomplete lesion at C4 level of cervical spinal cord POA HAC HCC MCC CC/MCC Exc

S14.155 Other incomplete lesion at C5 level of cervical spinal cord POA HAC HCC MCC CC/MCC Exc

S14.156 Other incomplete lesion at C6 level of cervical spinal cord POA HAC HCC MCC CC/MCC Exc

S14.157 Other incomplete lesion at C7 level of cervical spinal cord POA HAC HCC MCC CC/MCC Exc

S14.158 Other incomplete lesion at C8 level of cervical spinal cord POA HCC MCC CC/MCC Exc

S14.159 Other incomplete lesion at unspecified level of cervical spinal cord POA HCC

S14.2 Injury of nerve root of cervical spine POA

S14.3 Injury of brachial plexus POA

S14.4 Injury of peripheral nerves of neck POA

S14.5 Injury of cervical sympathetic nerves POA

S14.8 Injury of other specified nerves of neck POA

S14.9 Injury of unspecified nerves of neck POA

S15 Injury of blood vessels at neck level

Code also any associated open wound (S11.-)

The appropriate 7th character is to be added to each code from category S15

A = initial encounter
D = subsequent encounter
S = sequela

S15.0 Injury of carotid artery of neck

Injury of carotid artery (common) (external) (internal, extracranial portion)
Injury of carotid artery NOS

EXCLUDES1 injury of internal carotid artery, intracranial portion (S06.8)

S15.00 Unspecified injury of carotid artery

S15.001 Unspecified injury of right carotid artery CC POA CC/MCC Exc

S15.002 Unspecified injury of left carotid artery CC POA CC/MCC Exc

S15.009 Unspecified injury of unspecified carotid artery CC POA CC/MCC Exc

S15.01 Minor laceration of carotid artery

Incomplete transection of carotid artery
Laceration of carotid artery NOS
Superficial laceration of carotid artery

S15.011 Minor laceration of right carotid artery CC POA CC/MCC Exc

S15.012 Minor laceration of left carotid artery CC POA CC/MCC Exc

S15.019 Minor laceration of unspecified carotid artery CC POA CC/MCC Exc

S15.02 Major laceration of carotid artery

Complete transection of carotid artery
Traumatic rupture of carotid artery

S15.021 Major laceration of right carotid artery CC POA CC/MCC Exc

S15.022 Major laceration of left carotid artery CC POA CC/MCC Exc

S15.029 Major laceration of unspecified carotid artery CC POA CC/MCC Exc

S15.09 Other specified injury of carotid artery

S15.091 Other specified injury of right carotid artery CC POA CC/MCC Exc

S15.092 Other specified injury of left carotid artery CC POA CC/MCC Exc

S15.099 Other specified injury of unspecified carotid artery CC POA CC/MCC Exc

S15.1 Injury of vertebral artery

S15.10 Unspecified injury of vertebral artery

S15.101 Unspecified injury of right vertebral artery CC POA CC/MCC Exc

S15.102 Unspecified injury of left vertebral artery CC POA CC/MCC Exc

S15.109 Unspecified injury of unspecified vertebral artery CC POA CC/MCC Exc

S15.11 Minor laceration of vertebral artery

Incomplete transection of vertebral artery
Laceration of vertebral artery NOS
Superficial laceration of vertebral artery

PDxExc: Unacceptable principal diagnosis symbol per Medicare code edits   POA Code exempt from diagnosis present on admission requirement
? Questionable admission   CC Complication or comorbidity   CC/MCC Exc CC/MCC exclusion   MCC Major complication or comorbidity
PDxCC Principal diagnosis as its own CC   PDxMCC Principal diagnosis as its own MCC   HCC HCC diagnosis code   RxHCC RxHCC diagnosis code
MACRA code   Z1 Z code as first-listed diagnosis

988

When symbols appear on a code that requires a 7th character extension, refer to Appendix B to identify applicable 7th character codes.

2018 ICD-10-CM

⑦ S15.111 Minor laceration of right vertebral artery CC POA CC/MCC Exc

⑦ S15.112 Minor laceration of left vertebral artery CC POA CC/MCC Exc

⑦ S15.119 Minor laceration of unspecified vertebral artery CC POA CC/MCC Exc

⑥ S15.12 Major laceration of vertebral artery
Complete transection of vertebral artery
Traumatic rupture of vertebral artery

⑦ S15.121 Major laceration of right vertebral artery CC POA CC/MCC Exc

⑦ S15.122 Major laceration of left vertebral artery CC POA CC/MCC Exc

⑦ S15.129 Major laceration of unspecified vertebral artery CC POA CC/MCC Exc

⑥ S15.19 Other specified injury of vertebral artery

⑦ S15.191 Other specified injury of right vertebral artery CC POA CC/MCC Exc

⑦ S15.192 Other specified injury of left vertebral artery CC POA CC/MCC Exc

⑦ S15.199 Other specified injury of unspecified vertebral artery CC POA CC/MCC Exc

⑤ S15.2 Injury of external jugular vein

⑥ S15.20 Unspecified injury of external jugular vein

⑦ S15.201 Unspecified injury of right external jugular vein CC POA CC/MCC Exc

⑦ S15.202 Unspecified injury of left external jugular vein CC POA CC/MCC Exc

⑦ S15.209 Unspecified injury of unspecified external jugular vein CC POA CC/MCC Exc

⑥ S15.21 Minor laceration of external jugular vein
Incomplete transection of external jugular vein
Laceration of external jugular vein NOS
Superficial laceration of external jugular vein

⑦ S15.211 Minor laceration of right external jugular vein CC POA CC/MCC Exc

⑦ S15.212 Minor laceration of left external jugular vein CC POA CC/MCC Exc

⑦ S15.219 Minor laceration of unspecified external jugular vein CC POA CC/MCC Exc

⑥ S15.22 Major laceration of external jugular vein
Complete transection of external jugular vein
Traumatic rupture of external jugular vein

⑦ S15.221 Major laceration of right external jugular vein CC POA CC/MCC Exc

⑦ S15.222 Major laceration of left external jugular vein CC POA CC/MCC Exc

⑦ S15.229 Major laceration of unspecified external jugular vein CC POA CC/MCC Exc

⑥ S15.29 Other specified injury of external jugular vein

⑦ S15.291 Other specified injury of right external jugular vein CC POA CC/MCC Exc

⑦ S15.292 Other specified injury of left external jugular vein CC POA CC/MCC Exc

⑦ S15.299 Other specified injury of unspecified external jugular vein CC POA CC/MCC Exc

⑤ S15.3 Injury of internal jugular vein

⑥ S15.30 Unspecified injury of internal jugular vein

⑦ S15.301 Unspecified injury of right internal jugular vein CC POA CC/MCC Exc

⑦ S15.302 Unspecified injury of left internal jugular vein CC POA CC/MCC Exc

⑦ S15.309 Unspecified injury of unspecified internal jugular vein CC POA CC/MCC Exc

⑥ S15.31 Minor laceration of internal jugular vein
Incomplete transection of internal jugular vein
Laceration of internal jugular vein NOS
Superficial laceration of internal jugular vein

⑦ S15.311 Minor laceration of right internal jugular vein CC POA CC/MCC Exc

⑦ S15.312 Minor laceration of left internal jugular vein CC POA CC/MCC Exc

⑦ S15.319 Minor laceration of unspecified internal jugular vein CC POA CC/MCC Exc

⑥ S15.32 Major laceration of internal jugular vein
Complete transection of internal jugular vein
Traumatic rupture of internal jugular vein

⑦ S15.321 Major laceration of right internal jugular vein CC POA CC/MCC Exc

⑦ S15.322 Major laceration of left internal jugular vein CC POA CC/MCC Exc

⑦ S15.329 Major laceration of unspecified internal jugular vein CC POA CC/MCC Exc

⑥ S15.39 Other specified injury of internal jugular vein

⑦ S15.391 Other specified injury of right internal jugular vein CC POA CC/MCC Exc

⑦ S15.392 Other specified injury of left internal jugular vein CC POA CC/MCC Exc

⑦ S15.399 Other specified injury of unspecified internal jugular vein CC POA CC/MCC Exc

⑦ S15.8 Injury of other specified blood vessels at neck level CC POA CC/MCC Exc

⑦ S15.9 Injury of unspecified blood vessel at neck level CC POA CC/MCC Exc

④ S16 Injury of muscle, fascia and tendon at neck level
Code also any associated open wound (S11.-)
EXCLUDES2 sprain of joint or ligament at neck level (S13.9)
The appropriate 7th character is to be added to each code from category S16
   A = initial encounter
   D = subsequent encounter
   S = sequela

⑦ S16.1 Strain of muscle, fascia and tendon at neck level POA

⑦ S16.2 Laceration of muscle, fascia and tendon at neck level POA

⑦ S16.8 Other specified injury of muscle, fascia and tendon at neck level POA

⑦ S16.9 Unspecified injury of muscle, fascia and tendon at neck level POA

④ S17 Crushing injury of neck
Use additional code for all associated injuries, such as:
injury of blood vessels (S15.-)
open wound of neck (S11.-)
spinal cord injury (S14.0, S14.1-)
vertebral fracture (S12.0--S12.3-)
The appropriate 7th character is to be added to each code from category S17
   A = initial encounter
   D = subsequent encounter
   S = sequela

⑦ S17.0 Crushing injury of larynx and trachea CC POA HAC CC/MCC Exc

⑦ S17.8 Crushing injury of other specified parts of neck CC POA HAC CC/MCC Exc

⑦ S17.9 Crushing injury of neck, part unspecified CC POA HAC CC/MCC Exc

④ S19 Other specified and unspecified injuries of neck
The appropriate 7th character is to be added to each code from category S19
   A = initial encounter
   D = subsequent encounter
   S = sequela

⑤ S19.8 Other specified injuries of neck

⑦ S19.80 Other specified injuries of unspecified part of neck POA

⑦ S19.81 Other specified injuries of larynx POA

⑦ S19.82 Other specified injuries of cervical trachea POA
EXCLUDES2 other specified injury of thoracic trachea (S27.5-)

⑦ S19.83 Other specified injuries of vocal cord POA

⑦ S19.84 Other specified injuries of thyroid gland POA

⑦ S19.85 Other specified injuries of pharynx and cervical esophagus POA

⑦ S19.89 Other specified injuries of other specified part of neck POA

⑦ S19.9 Unspecified injury of neck POA

| Unspecified Code | Other Specified Code | Manifestation Code | N Newborn | P Pediatric | M Maternity | A Adult | ♂ Male | ♀ Female |

● New Code ▲ Revised Code Title ▶◀ Revised Text NOTES INCLUDES EXCLUDES 1 Not coded here EXCLUDES 2 Not included here
④ 4th character required ⑤ 5th character required ⑥ 6th character required ⑦ 7th character required
⑦ Extension 'X' Alert HAC Hospital-acquired condition (HAC) alert AHA AHA Coding Clinic©

Injuries to the thorax (S20-S29)

INCLUDES
- injuries of breast
- injuries of chest (wall)
- injuries of interscapular area

EXCLUDES2
- burns and corrosions (T20-T32)
- effects of foreign body in bronchus (T17.5)
- effects of foreign body in esophagus (T18.1)
- effects of foreign body in lung (T17.8)
- effects of foreign body in trachea (T17.4)
- frostbite (T33-T34)
- injuries of axilla
- injuries of clavicle
- injuries of scapular region
- injuries of shoulder
- insect bite or sting, venomous (T63.4)

S20 **Superficial injury of thorax**

The appropriate 7th character is to be added to each code from category S20
- A = initial encounter
- D = subsequent encounter
- S = sequela

S20.0 **Contusion of breast**
- S20.00 **Contusion of breast, unspecified breast**
- S20.01 **Contusion of right breast**
- S20.02 **Contusion of left breast**

S20.1 **Other and unspecified superficial injuries of breast**
- S20.10 Unspecified superficial injuries of breast
  - S20.101 **Unspecified superficial injuries of breast, right breast**
  - S20.102 **Unspecified superficial injuries of breast, left breast**
  - S20.109 **Unspecified superficial injuries of breast, unspecified breast**
- S20.11 Abrasion of breast
  - S20.111 **Abrasion of breast, right breast**
  - S20.112 **Abrasion of breast, left breast**
  - S20.119 **Abrasion of breast, unspecified breast**
- S20.12 Blister (nonthermal) of breast
  - S20.121 **Blister (nonthermal) of breast, right breast**
  - S20.122 **Blister (nonthermal) of breast, left breast**
  - S20.129 **Blister (nonthermal) of breast, unspecified breast**
- S20.14 External constriction of part of breast
  - S20.141 **External constriction of part of breast, right breast**
  - S20.142 **External constriction of part of breast, left breast**
  - S20.149 **External constriction of part of breast, unspecified breast**
- S20.15 Superficial foreign body of breast
  Splinter in the breast
  - S20.151 **Superficial foreign body of breast, right breast**
  - S20.152 **Superficial foreign body of breast, left breast**
  - S20.159 **Superficial foreign body of breast, unspecified breast**
- S20.16 Insect bite (nonvenomous) of breast
  - S20.161 **Insect bite (nonvenomous) of breast, right breast**
  - S20.162 **Insect bite (nonvenomous) of breast, left breast**
  - S20.169 **Insect bite (nonvenomous) of breast, unspecified breast**
- S20.17 Other superficial bite of breast
  EXCLUDES1 open bite of breast (S21.05-)
  - S20.171 **Other superficial bite of breast, right breast**
  - S20.172 **Other superficial bite of breast, left breast**
  - S20.179 **Other superficial bite of breast, unspecified breast**

S20.2 **Contusion of thorax**
- S20.20 **Contusion of thorax, unspecified**
- S20.21 Contusion of front wall of thorax
  - S20.211 **Contusion of right front wall of thorax**
  - S20.212 **Contusion of left front wall of thorax**
  - S20.219 **Contusion of unspecified front wall of thorax**
- S20.22 Contusion of back wall of thorax
  - S20.221 **Contusion of right back wall of thorax**
  - S20.222 **Contusion of left back wall of thorax**
  - S20.229 **Contusion of unspecified back wall of thorax**

S20.3 **Other and unspecified superficial injuries of front wall of thorax**
- S20.30 Unspecified superficial injuries of front wall of thorax
  - S20.301 **Unspecified superficial injuries of right front wall of thorax**
  - S20.302 **Unspecified superficial injuries of left front wall of thorax**
  - S20.309 **Unspecified superficial injuries of unspecified front wall of thorax**
- S20.31 Abrasion of front wall of thorax
  - S20.311 **Abrasion of right front wall of thorax**
  - S20.312 **Abrasion of left front wall of thorax**
  - S20.319 **Abrasion of unspecified front wall of thorax**
- S20.32 Blister (nonthermal) of front wall of thorax
  - S20.321 **Blister (nonthermal) of right front wall of thorax**
  - S20.322 **Blister (nonthermal) of left front wall of thorax**
  - S20.329 **Blister (nonthermal) of unspecified front wall of thorax**
- S20.34 External constriction of front wall of thorax
  - S20.341 **External constriction of right front wall of thorax**
  - S20.342 **External constriction of left front wall of thorax**
  - S20.349 **External constriction of unspecified front wall of thorax**
- S20.35 Superficial foreign body of front wall of thorax
  Splinter in front wall of thorax
  - S20.351 **Superficial foreign body of right front wall of thorax**
  - S20.352 **Superficial foreign body of left front wall of thorax**
  - S20.359 **Superficial foreign body of unspecified front wall of thorax**
- S20.36 Insect bite (nonvenomous) of front wall of thorax
  - S20.361 **Insect bite (nonvenomous) of right front wall of thorax**
  - S20.362 **Insect bite (nonvenomous) of left front wall of thorax**
  - S20.369 **Insect bite (nonvenomous) of unspecified front wall of thorax**
- S20.37 Other superficial bite of front wall of thorax
  EXCLUDES1 open bite of front wall of thorax (S21.14)
  - S20.371 **Other superficial bite of right front wall of thorax**
  - S20.372 **Other superficial bite of left front wall of thorax**
  - S20.379 **Other superficial bite of unspecified front wall of thorax**

POADit Unacceptable principal diagnosis symbol per Medicare code edits   Code exempt from diagnosis present on admission requirement
? Questionable admission   CC Complication or comorbidity   CC/MCC CC/MCC exclusion   MCC Major complication or comorbidity
PDCC Principal diagnosis as its own CC   PDMCC Principal diagnosis as its own MCC   HCC HCC diagnosis code   RxHCC RxHCC diagnosis code
MACRA code   Z Z code as first-listed diagnosis

5ᵗʰ **S20.4** Other and unspecified superficial injuries of back wall of thorax

   6ᵗʰ **S20.40** Unspecified superficial injuries of back wall of thorax

      7ᵗʰ **S20.401** Unspecified superficial injuries of right back wall of thorax POA

      7ᵗʰ **S20.402** Unspecified superficial injuries of left back wall of thorax POA

      7ᵗʰ **S20.409** Unspecified superficial injuries of unspecified back wall of thorax POA

   6ᵗʰ **S20.41** Abrasion of back wall of thorax

      7ᵗʰ **S20.411** Abrasion of right back wall of thorax POA

      7ᵗʰ **S20.412** Abrasion of left back wall of thorax POA

      7ᵗʰ **S20.419** Abrasion of unspecified back wall of thorax POA

   6ᵗʰ **S20.42** Blister (nonthermal) of back wall of thorax

      7ᵗʰ **S20.421** Blister (nonthermal) of right back wall of thorax POA

      7ᵗʰ **S20.422** Blister (nonthermal) of left back wall of thorax POA

      7ᵗʰ **S20.429** Blister (nonthermal) of unspecified back wall of thorax POA

   6ᵗʰ **S20.44** External constriction of back wall of thorax

      7ᵗʰ **S20.441** External constriction of right back wall of thorax POA

      7ᵗʰ **S20.442** External constriction of left back wall of thorax POA

      7ᵗʰ **S20.449** External constriction of unspecified back wall of thorax POA

   6ᵗʰ **S20.45** Superficial foreign body of back wall of thorax
      Splinter of back wall of thorax

      7ᵗʰ **S20.451** Superficial foreign body of right back wall of thorax POA

      7ᵗʰ **S20.452** Superficial foreign body of left back wall of thorax POA

      7ᵗʰ **S20.459** Superficial foreign body of unspecified back wall of thorax POA

   6ᵗʰ **S20.46** Insect bite (nonvenomous) of back wall of thorax

      7ᵗʰ **S20.461** Insect bite (nonvenomous) of right back wall of thorax POA

      7ᵗʰ **S20.462** Insect bite (nonvenomous) of left back wall of thorax POA

      7ᵗʰ **S20.469** Insect bite (nonvenomous) of unspecified back wall of thorax POA

   6ᵗʰ **S20.47** Other superficial bite of back wall of thorax
      EXCLUDES1 open bite of back wall of thorax (S21.24)

      7ᵗʰ **S20.471** Other superficial bite of right back wall of thorax POA

      7ᵗʰ **S20.472** Other superficial bite of left back wall of thorax POA

      7ᵗʰ **S20.479** Other superficial bite of unspecified back wall of thorax POA

5ᵗʰ **S20.9** Superficial injury of unspecified parts of thorax
   EXCLUDES1 contusion of thorax NOS (S20.20)

   7ᵗʰ **S20.90** Unspecified superficial injury of unspecified parts of thorax POA
      Superficial injury of thoracic wall NOS

   7ᵗʰ **S20.91** Abrasion of unspecified parts of thorax POA

   7ᵗʰ **S20.92** Blister (nonthermal) of unspecified parts of thorax POA

   7ᵗʰ **S20.94** External constriction of unspecified parts of thorax POA

   7ᵗʰ **S20.95** Superficial foreign body of unspecified parts of thorax POA
      Splinter in thorax NOS

   7ᵗʰ **S20.96** Insect bite (nonvenomous) of unspecified parts of thorax POA

   7ᵗʰ **S20.97** Other superficial bite of unspecified parts of thorax POA
      EXCLUDES1 open bite of thorax NOS (S21.95)

4ᵗʰ **S21** Open wound of thorax
   Code also any associated injury, such as:
      injury of heart (S26.-)
      injury of intrathoracic organs (S27.-)
      rib fracture (S22.3-, S22.4-)
      spinal cord injury (S24.0-, S24.1-)
      traumatic hemopneumothorax (S27.3)
      traumatic hemothorax (S27.1)
      traumatic pneumothorax (S27.0)
      wound infection
   EXCLUDES1 traumatic amputation (partial) of thorax (S28.1)
   The appropriate 7th character is to be added to each code from category S21
      A = initial encounter
      D = subsequent encounter
      S = sequela

5ᵗʰ **S21.0** Open wound of breast

   6ᵗʰ **S21.00** Unspecified open wound of breast

      7ᵗʰ **S21.001** Unspecified open wound of right breast POA

      7ᵗʰ **S21.002** Unspecified open wound of left breast POA

      7ᵗʰ **S21.009** Unspecified open wound of unspecified breast POA

   6ᵗʰ **S21.01** Laceration without foreign body of breast

      7ᵗʰ **S21.011** Laceration without foreign body of right breast POA

      7ᵗʰ **S21.012** Laceration without foreign body of left breast POA

      7ᵗʰ **S21.019** Laceration without foreign body of unspecified breast POA

   6ᵗʰ **S21.02** Laceration with foreign body of breast

      7ᵗʰ **S21.021** Laceration with foreign body of right breast POA

      7ᵗʰ **S21.022** Laceration with foreign body of left breast POA

      7ᵗʰ **S21.029** Laceration with foreign body of unspecified breast POA

   6ᵗʰ **S21.03** Puncture wound without foreign body of breast

      7ᵗʰ **S21.031** Puncture wound without foreign body of right breast POA

      7ᵗʰ **S21.032** Puncture wound without foreign body of left breast POA

      7ᵗʰ **S21.039** Puncture wound without foreign body of unspecified breast POA

   6ᵗʰ **S21.04** Puncture wound with foreign body of breast

      7ᵗʰ **S21.041** Puncture wound with foreign body of right breast POA

      7ᵗʰ **S21.042** Puncture wound with foreign body of left breast POA

      7ᵗʰ **S21.049** Puncture wound with foreign body of unspecified breast POA

   6ᵗʰ **S21.05** Open bite of breast
      Bite of breast NOS
      EXCLUDES1 superficial bite of breast (S20.17)

      7ᵗʰ **S21.051** Open bite of right breast POA

      7ᵗʰ **S21.052** Open bite of left breast POA

      7ᵗʰ **S21.059** Open bite of unspecified breast POA

5ᵗʰ **S21.1** Open wound of front wall of thorax without penetration into thoracic cavity
   Open wound of chest without penetration into thoracic cavity

   6ᵗʰ **S21.10** Unspecified open wound of front wall of thorax without penetration into thoracic cavity

      7ᵗʰ **S21.101** Unspecified open wound of right front wall of thorax without penetration into thoracic cavity CC POA CC/MCC Exc

      7ᵗʰ **S21.102** Unspecified open wound of left front wall of thorax without penetration into thoracic cavity CC POA CC/MCC Exc

      7ᵗʰ **S21.109** Unspecified open wound of unspecified front wall of thorax without penetration into thoracic cavity CC POA CC/MCC Exc

---

Unspecified Code	Other Specified Code	Manifestation Code	N Newborn	P Pediatric	M Maternity	A Adult	♂ Male	♀ Female

● New Code   ▲ Revised Code Title   ▶◀ Revised Text   **NOTES**   *INCLUDES*   *EXCLUDES 1* Not coded here   *EXCLUDES 2* Not included here
4ᵗʰ 4ᵗʰ character required   5ᵗʰ 5ᵗʰ character required   6ᵗʰ 6ᵗʰ character required   7ᵗʰ 7ᵗʰ character required
7ᵗʰ Extension 'X' Alert   HAC Hospital-acquired condition (HAC) alert   **AHA** AHA Coding Clinic©

S21.11 Laceration without foreign body of front wall of thorax without penetration into thoracic cavity

    S21.111 Laceration without foreign body of right front wall of thorax without penetration into thoracic cavity ⒸⒸ POA CC/MCC Exc

    S21.112 Laceration without foreign body of left front wall of thorax without penetration into thoracic cavity ⒸⒸ POA CC/MCC Exc

    S21.119 Laceration without foreign body of unspecified front wall of thorax without penetration into thoracic cavity ⒸⒸ POA CC/MCC Exc

S21.12 Laceration with foreign body of front wall of thorax without penetration into thoracic cavity

    S21.121 Laceration with foreign body of right front wall of thorax without penetration into thoracic cavity ⒸⒸ POA CC/MCC Exc

    S21.122 Laceration with foreign body of left front wall of thorax without penetration into thoracic cavity ⒸⒸ POA CC/MCC Exc

    S21.129 Laceration with foreign body of unspecified front wall of thorax without penetration into thoracic cavity ⒸⒸ POA CC/MCC Exc

S21.13 Puncture wound without foreign body of front wall of thorax without penetration into thoracic cavity

    S21.131 Puncture wound without foreign body of right front wall of thorax without penetration into thoracic cavity ⒸⒸ POA CC/MCC Exc

    S21.132 Puncture wound without foreign body of left front wall of thorax without penetration into thoracic cavity ⒸⒸ POA CC/MCC Exc

    S21.139 Puncture wound without foreign body of unspecified front wall of thorax without penetration into thoracic cavity ⒸⒸ POA CC/MCC Exc

S21.14 Puncture wound with foreign body of front wall of thorax without penetration into thoracic cavity

    S21.141 Puncture wound with foreign body of right front wall of thorax without penetration into thoracic cavity ⒸⒸ POA CC/MCC Exc

    S21.142 Puncture wound with foreign body of left front wall of thorax without penetration into thoracic cavity ⒸⒸ POA CC/MCC Exc

    S21.149 Puncture wound with foreign body of unspecified front wall of thorax without penetration into thoracic cavity ⒸⒸ POA CC/MCC Exc

S21.15 Open bite of front wall of thorax without penetration into thoracic cavity

    Bite of front wall of thorax NOS

    EXCLUDES1 *superficial bite of front wall of thorax (S20.37)*

    S21.151 Open bite of right front wall of thorax without penetration into thoracic cavity ⒸⒸ POA CC/MCC Exc

    S21.152 Open bite of left front wall of thorax without penetration into thoracic cavity ⒸⒸ POA CC/MCC Exc

    S21.159 Open bite of unspecified front wall of thorax without penetration into thoracic cavity ⒸⒸ POA CC/MCC Exc

S21.2 Open wound of back wall of thorax without penetration into thoracic cavity

  S21.20 Unspecified open wound of back wall of thorax without penetration into thoracic cavity

    S21.201 Unspecified open wound of right back wall of thorax without penetration into thoracic cavity POA

    S21.202 Unspecified open wound of left back wall of thorax without penetration into thoracic cavity POA

    S21.209 Unspecified open wound of unspecified back wall of thorax without penetration into thoracic cavity POA

  S21.21 Laceration without foreign body of back wall of thorax without penetration into thoracic cavity

    S21.211 Laceration without foreign body of right back wall of thorax without penetration into thoracic cavity POA

    S21.212 Laceration without foreign body of left back wall of thorax without penetration into thoracic cavity POA

    S21.219 Laceration without foreign body of unspecified back wall of thorax without penetration into thoracic cavity POA

  S21.22 Laceration with foreign body of back wall of thorax without penetration into thoracic cavity

    S21.221 Laceration with foreign body of right back wall of thorax without penetration into thoracic cavity POA

    S21.222 Laceration with foreign body of left back wall of thorax without penetration into thoracic cavity POA

    S21.229 Laceration with foreign body of unspecified back wall of thorax without penetration into thoracic cavity POA

  S21.23 Puncture wound without foreign body of back wall of thorax without penetration into thoracic cavity

    S21.231 Puncture wound without foreign body of right back wall of thorax without penetration into thoracic cavity POA

    S21.232 Puncture wound without foreign body of left back wall of thorax without penetration into thoracic cavity POA

    S21.239 Puncture wound without foreign body of unspecified back wall of thorax without penetration into thoracic cavity POA

  S21.24 Puncture wound with foreign body of back wall of thorax without penetration into thoracic cavity

    S21.241 Puncture wound with foreign body of right back wall of thorax without penetration into thoracic cavity POA

    S21.242 Puncture wound with foreign body of left back wall of thorax without penetration into thoracic cavity POA

    S21.249 Puncture wound with foreign body of unspecified back wall of thorax without penetration into thoracic cavity POA

  S21.25 Open bite of back wall of thorax without penetration into thoracic cavity

    Bite of back wall of thorax NOS

    EXCLUDES1 *superficial bite of back wall of thorax (S20.47)*

    S21.251 Open bite of right back wall of thorax without penetration into thoracic cavity POA

    S21.252 Open bite of left back wall of thorax without penetration into thoracic cavity POA

    S21.259 Open bite of unspecified back wall of thorax without penetration into thoracic cavity POA

S21.3 Open wound of front wall of thorax with penetration into thoracic cavity

  Open wound of chest with penetration into thoracic cavity

  S21.30 Unspecified open wound of front wall of thorax with penetration into thoracic cavity

    S21.301 Unspecified open wound of right front wall of thorax with penetration into thoracic cavity POA MCC CC/MCC Exc

    S21.302 Unspecified open wound of left front wall of thorax with penetration into thoracic cavity POA MCC CC/MCC Exc

    S21.309 Unspecified open wound of unspecified front wall of thorax with penetration into thoracic cavity POA MCC CC/MCC Exc

  S21.31 Laceration without foreign body of front wall of thorax with penetration into thoracic cavity

    S21.311 Laceration without foreign body of right front wall of thorax with penetration into thoracic cavity POA MCC CC/MCC Exc

POA Unacceptable principal diagnosis symbol per Medicare code edits   POA Code exempt from diagnosis present on admission requirement   ❓ Questionable admission   ⒸⒸ Complication or comorbidity   CC/MCC Exc CC/MCC exclusion   MCC Major complication or comorbidity   Principal diagnosis as its own CC   Principal diagnosis as its own MCC   HCC HCC diagnosis code   RxHCC RxHCC diagnosis code   MACRA code   Z Z code as first-listed diagnosis

When symbols appear on a code that requires a 7th character extension, refer to Appendix B to identify applicable 7th character codes.   **2018 ICD-10-CM**

S21.312 Laceration without foreign body of left front wall of thorax with penetration into thoracic cavity POA MCC CC/MCC Exc

S21.319 Laceration without foreign body of unspecified front wall of thorax with penetration into thoracic cavity POA MCC CC/MCC Exc

S21.32 Laceration with foreign body of front wall of thorax with penetration into thoracic cavity

S21.321 Laceration with foreign body of right front wall of thorax with penetration into thoracic cavity POA MCC CC/MCC Exc

S21.322 Laceration with foreign body of left front wall of thorax with penetration into thoracic cavity POA MCC CC/MCC Exc

S21.329 Laceration with foreign body of unspecified front wall of thorax with penetration into thoracic cavity POA MCC CC/MCC Exc

S21.33 Puncture wound without foreign body of front wall of thorax with penetration into thoracic cavity

S21.331 Puncture wound without foreign body of right front wall of thorax with penetration into thoracic cavity POA MCC CC/MCC Exc

S21.332 Puncture wound without foreign body of left front wall of thorax with penetration into thoracic cavity POA MCC CC/MCC Exc

S21.339 Puncture wound without foreign body of unspecified front wall of thorax with penetration into thoracic cavity POA MCC CC/MCC Exc

S21.34 Puncture wound with foreign body of front wall of thorax with penetration into thoracic cavity

S21.341 Puncture wound with foreign body of right front wall of thorax with penetration into thoracic cavity POA MCC CC/MCC Exc

S21.342 Puncture wound with foreign body of left front wall of thorax with penetration into thoracic cavity POA MCC CC/MCC Exc

S21.349 Puncture wound with foreign body of unspecified front wall of thorax with penetration into thoracic cavity POA MCC CC/MCC Exc

S21.35 Open bite of front wall of thorax with penetration into thoracic cavity
EXCLUDES1 superficial bite of front wall of thorax (S20.37)

S21.351 Open bite of right front wall of thorax with penetration into thoracic cavity POA MCC CC/MCC Exc

S21.352 Open bite of left front wall of thorax with penetration into thoracic cavity POA MCC CC/MCC Exc

S21.359 Open bite of unspecified front wall of thorax with penetration into thoracic cavity POA MCC CC/MCC Exc

S21.4 Open wound of back wall of thorax with penetration into thoracic cavity

S21.40 Unspecified open wound of back wall of thorax with penetration into thoracic cavity

S21.401 Unspecified open wound of right back wall of thorax with penetration into thoracic cavity POA MCC CC/MCC Exc

S21.402 Unspecified open wound of left back wall of thorax with penetration into thoracic cavity POA MCC CC/MCC Exc

S21.409 Unspecified open wound of unspecified back wall of thorax with penetration into thoracic cavity POA MCC CC/MCC Exc

S21.41 Laceration without foreign body of back wall of thorax with penetration into thoracic cavity

S21.411 Laceration without foreign body of right back wall of thorax with penetration into thoracic cavity POA MCC CC/MCC Exc

S21.412 Laceration without foreign body of left back wall of thorax with penetration into thoracic cavity POA MCC CC/MCC Exc

S21.419 Laceration without foreign body of unspecified back wall of thorax with penetration into thoracic cavity POA MCC CC/MCC Exc

S21.42 Laceration with foreign body of back wall of thorax with penetration into thoracic cavity

S21.421 Laceration with foreign body of right back wall of thorax with penetration into thoracic cavity POA MCC CC/MCC Exc

S21.422 Laceration with foreign body of left back wall of thorax with penetration into thoracic cavity POA MCC CC/MCC Exc

S21.429 Laceration with foreign body of unspecified back wall of thorax with penetration into thoracic cavity POA MCC CC/MCC Exc

S21.43 Puncture wound without foreign body of back wall of thorax with penetration into thoracic cavity

S21.431 Puncture wound without foreign body of right back wall of thorax with penetration into thoracic cavity POA MCC CC/MCC Exc

S21.432 Puncture wound without foreign body of left back wall of thorax with penetration into thoracic cavity POA MCC CC/MCC Exc

S21.439 Puncture wound without foreign body of unspecified back wall of thorax with penetration into thoracic cavity POA MCC CC/MCC Exc

S21.44 Puncture wound with foreign body of back wall of thorax with penetration into thoracic cavity

S21.441 Puncture wound with foreign body of right back wall of thorax with penetration into thoracic cavity POA MCC CC/MCC Exc

S21.442 Puncture wound with foreign body of left back wall of thorax with penetration into thoracic cavity POA MCC CC/MCC Exc

S21.449 Puncture wound with foreign body of unspecified back wall of thorax with penetration into thoracic cavity POA MCC CC/MCC Exc

S21.45 Open bite of back wall of thorax with penetration into thoracic cavity
Bite of back wall of thorax NOS
EXCLUDES1 superficial bite of back wall of thorax (S20.47)

S21.451 Open bite of right back wall of thorax with penetration into thoracic cavity POA MCC CC/MCC Exc

S21.452 Open bite of left back wall of thorax with penetration into thoracic cavity POA MCC CC/MCC Exc

S21.459 Open bite of unspecified back wall of thorax with penetration into thoracic cavity POA MCC CC/MCC Exc

S21.9 Open wound of unspecified part of thorax
Open wound of thoracic wall NOS

S21.90 Unspecified open wound of unspecified part of thorax CC POA CC/MCC Exc

S21.91 Laceration without foreign body of unspecified part of thorax CC POA CC/MCC Exc

S21.92 Laceration with foreign body of unspecified part of thorax CC POA CC/MCC Exc

S21.93 Puncture wound without foreign body of unspecified part of thorax CC POA CC/MCC Exc

S21.94 Puncture wound with foreign body of unspecified part of thorax CC POA CC/MCC Exc

S21.95 Open bite of unspecified part of thorax CC POA CC/MCC Exc
EXCLUDES1 superficial bite of thorax (S20.97)

Unspecified Code   Other Specified Code   Manifestation Code   N Newborn   P Pediatric   M Maternity   A Adult   ♂ Male   ♀ Female
● New Code   ▲ Revised Code Title   ►◄ Revised Text   NOTES   INCLUDES   EXCLUDES 1 Not coded here   EXCLUDES 2 Not included here
4th character required   5th character required   6th character required   7th character required
Extension 'X' Alert   HAC Hospital-acquired condition (HAC) alert   AHA AHA Coding Clinic©

S22 **Fracture of rib(s), sternum and thoracic spine**

NOTES A fracture not indicated as displaced or nondisplaced should be coded to displaced

A fracture not indicated as open or closed should be coded to closed

INCLUDES *fracture of thoracic neural arch*

fracture of thoracic spinous process

fracture of thoracic transverse process

fracture of thoracic vertebra

fracture of thoracic vertebral arch

Code first any associated:

injury of intrathoracic organ (S27.-)

spinal cord injury (S24.0-, S24.1-)

EXCLUDES1 *transection of thorax (S28.1)*

EXCLUDES2 *fracture of clavicle (S42.0-)*

fracture of scapula (S42.1-)

The appropriate 7th character is to be added to each code from category S22

A = initial encounter for closed fracture

B = initial encounter for open fracture

D = subsequent encounter for fracture with routine healing

G = subsequent encounter for fracture with delayed healing

K = subsequent encounter for fracture with nonunion

S = sequela

S22.0 **Fracture of thoracic vertebra**

  S22.00 **Fracture of unspecified thoracic vertebra**

    S22.000 Wedge compression **fracture of unspecified thoracic vertebra** CC POA HAC HCC MCC CC/MCC Exc

    S22.001 Stable burst **fracture of unspecified thoracic vertebra** CC POA HAC HCC MCC CC/MCC Exc

    S22.002 Unstable burst **fracture of unspecified thoracic vertebra** CC POA HAC HCC MCC CC/MCC Exc

    S22.008 Other **fracture of unspecified thoracic vertebra** CC POA HAC HCC MCC CC/MCC Exc

    S22.009 Unspecified **fracture of unspecified thoracic vertebra** CC POA HAC HCC MCC CC/MCC Exc

  S22.01 **Fracture of first thoracic vertebra**

    S22.010 Wedge compression **fracture of first thoracic vertebra** CC POA HAC HCC MCC CC/MCC Exc

    S22.011 Stable **burst fracture of first thoracic vertebra** CC POA HAC HCC MCC CC/MCC Exc

    S22.012 Unstable **burst fracture of first thoracic vertebra** CC POA HAC HCC MCC CC/MCC Exc

    S22.018 Other **fracture of first thoracic vertebra** CC POA HAC HCC MCC CC/MCC Exc

    S22.019 Unspecified **fracture of first thoracic vertebra** CC POA HAC HCC MCC CC/MCC Exc

  S22.02 **Fracture of second thoracic vertebra**

    S22.020 Wedge compression **fracture of second thoracic vertebra** CC POA HAC HCC MCC CC/MCC Exc

    S22.021 Stable **burst fracture of second thoracic vertebra** CC POA HAC HCC MCC CC/MCC Exc

    S22.022 Unstable **burst fracture of second thoracic vertebra** CC POA HAC HCC MCC CC/MCC Exc

    S22.028 Other **fracture of second thoracic vertebra** CC POA HAC HCC MCC CC/MCC Exc

    S22.029 Unspecified **fracture of second thoracic vertebra** CC POA HAC HCC MCC CC/MCC Exc

  S22.03 **Fracture of third thoracic vertebra**

    S22.030 Wedge compression **fracture of third thoracic vertebra** CC POA HAC HCC MCC CC/MCC Exc

    S22.031 Stable **burst fracture of third thoracic vertebra** CC POA HAC HCC MCC CC/MCC Exc

    S22.032 Unstable **burst fracture of third thoracic vertebra** CC POA HAC HCC MCC CC/MCC Exc

    S22.038 Other **fracture of third thoracic vertebra** CC POA HAC HCC MCC CC/MCC Exc

    S22.039 Unspecified **fracture of third thoracic vertebra** CC POA HAC HCC MCC CC/MCC Exc

S22.04 **Fracture of fourth thoracic vertebra**

    S22.040 Wedge compression **fracture of fourth thoracic vertebra** CC POA HAC HCC MCC CC/MCC Exc

    S22.041 Stable **burst fracture of fourth thoracic vertebra** CC POA HAC HCC MCC CC/MCC Exc

    S22.042 Unstable **burst fracture of fourth thoracic vertebra** CC POA HAC HCC MCC CC/MCC Exc

    S22.048 Other **fracture of fourth thoracic vertebra** CC POA HAC HCC MCC CC/MCC Exc

    S22.049 Unspecified **fracture of fourth thoracic vertebra** CC POA HAC HCC MCC CC/MCC Exc

S22.05 **Fracture of T5-T6 vertebra**

    S22.050 Wedge compression **fracture of T5-T6 vertebra** CC POA HAC HCC MCC CC/MCC Exc

    S22.051 Stable **burst fracture of T5-T6 vertebra** CC POA HAC HCC MCC CC/MCC Exc

    S22.052 Unstable **burst fracture of T5-T6 vertebra** CC POA HAC HCC MCC CC/MCC Exc

    S22.058 Other **fracture of T5-T6 vertebra** CC POA HAC HCC MCC CC/MCC Exc

    S22.059 Unspecified **fracture of T5-T6 vertebra** CC POA HAC HCC MCC CC/MCC Exc

S22.06 **Fracture of T7-T8 vertebra**

    S22.060 Wedge compression **fracture of T7-T8 vertebra** CC POA HAC HCC MCC CC/MCC Exc

    S22.061 Stable **burst fracture of T7-T8 vertebra** CC POA HAC HCC MCC CC/MCC Exc

    S22.062 Unstable **burst fracture of T7-T8 vertebra** CC POA HAC HCC MCC CC/MCC Exc

    S22.068 Other **fracture of T7-T8 thoracic vertebra** CC POA HAC HCC MCC CC/MCC Exc

    S22.069 Unspecified **fracture of T7-T8 vertebra** CC POA HAC HCC MCC CC/MCC Exc

S22.07 **Fracture of T9-T10 vertebra**

    S22.070 Wedge compression **fracture of T9-T10 vertebra** CC POA HAC HCC MCC CC/MCC Exc

    S22.071 Stable **burst fracture of T9-T10 vertebra** CC POA HAC HCC MCC CC/MCC Exc

    S22.072 Unstable **burst fracture of T9-T10 vertebra** CC POA HAC HCC MCC CC/MCC Exc

    S22.078 Other **fracture of T9-T10 vertebra** CC POA HAC HCC MCC CC/MCC Exc

    S22.079 Unspecified **fracture of T9-T10 vertebra** CC POA HAC HCC MCC CC/MCC Exc

S22.08 **Fracture of T11-T12 vertebra**

    S22.080 Wedge compression **fracture of T11-T12 vertebra** CC POA HAC HCC MCC CC/MCC Exc

    S22.081 Stable **burst fracture of T11-T12 vertebra** CC POA HAC HCC MCC CC/MCC Exc

    S22.082 Unstable **burst fracture of T11-T12 vertebra** CC POA HAC HCC MCC CC/MCC Exc

    S22.088 Other **fracture of T11-T12 vertebra** CC POA HAC HCC MCC CC/MCC Exc

    S22.089 Unspecified **fracture of T11-T12 vertebra** CC POA HAC HCC MCC CC/MCC Exc

S22.2 **Fracture of sternum**

    S22.20 Unspecified **fracture of sternum** CC POA HAC MCC CC/MCC Exc

    S22.21 **Fracture of** manubrium CC POA HAC MCC CC/MCC Exc

    S22.22 **Fracture of body of** sternum CC POA HAC MCC CC/MCC Exc

    S22.23 **Sternal** manubrial dissociation CC POA HAC MCC CC/MCC Exc

    S22.24 **Fracture of** xiphoid process CC POA HAC MCC CC/MCC Exc

S22.3 **Fracture of one rib**

    S22.31 **Fracture of one rib,** right side CC POA HAC MCC CC/MCC Exc

    S22.32 **Fracture of one rib,** left side CC POA HAC MCC CC/MCC Exc

    S22.39 **Fracture of one rib, unspecified side** CC POA HAC MCC CC/MCC Exc

S22.4 **Multiple fractures of ribs**

Fractures of two or more ribs

EXCLUDES1 *flail chest (S22.5-)*

    S22.41 **Multiple fractures of ribs,** right side CC POA HAC MCC CC/MCC Exc

---

POA Unacceptable principal diagnosis symbol per Medicare code edits   POA Code exempt from diagnosis present on admission requirement
? Questionable admission   CC Complication or comorbidity   CC/MCC Exc CC/MCC exclusion   MCC Major complication or comorbidity
PDx CC Principal diagnosis as its own CC   PDx MCC Principal diagnosis as its own MCC   HCC HCC diagnosis code   RxHCC RxHCC diagnosis code
MACRA code   Z1 Z code as first-listed diagnosis

[7th] **S22.42 Multiple fractures of ribs, left side** [CC] [POA] [HAC] [MCC] [CC/MCC Excl]
[7th] **S22.43 Multiple fractures of ribs, bilateral** [CC] [POA] [HAC] [MCC] [CC/MCC Excl]
[7th] **S22.49 Multiple fractures of ribs, unspecified side** [CC] [POA] [HAC] [MCC] [CC/MCC Excl]
[7th] **S22.5 Flail chest** [CC] [POA] [HAC] [MCC] [CC/MCC Excl]
[7th] **S22.9 Fracture of bony thorax, part unspecified** [CC] [POA] [HAC] [MCC] [CC/MCC Excl]

[4th] **S23 Dislocation and sprain of joints and ligaments of thorax**

[INCLUDES] *avulsion of joint or ligament of thorax*
laceration of cartilage, joint or ligament of thorax
sprain of cartilage, joint or ligament of thorax
traumatic hemarthrosis of joint or ligament of thorax
traumatic rupture of joint or ligament of thorax
traumatic subluxation of joint or ligament of thorax
traumatic tear of joint or ligament of thorax

Code also any associated open wound

[EXCLUDES2] *dislocation, sprain of sternoclavicular joint (S43.2, S43.6)*
strain of muscle or tendon of thorax (S29.01-)

The appropriate 7th character is to be added to each code from category S23
A = initial encounter
D = subsequent encounter
S = sequela

[7th] **S23.0 Traumatic rupture of thoracic intervertebral disc** [POA]
[EXCLUDES1] *rupture or displacement (nontraumatic) of thoracic intervertebral disc NOS (M51.- with fifth character 4)*

[5th] **S23.1 Subluxation and dislocation of thoracic vertebra**
Code also any associated
open wound of thorax (S21.-)
spinal cord injury (S24.0-, S24.1-)
[EXCLUDES2] *fracture of thoracic vertebrae (S22.0-)*

[6th] **S23.10 Subluxation and dislocation of unspecified thoracic vertebra**
[7th] **S23.100 Subluxation of unspecified thoracic vertebra** [POA]
[7th] **S23.101 Dislocation of unspecified thoracic vertebra** [POA]

[6th] **S23.11 Subluxation and dislocation of T1/T2 thoracic vertebra**
[7th] **S23.110 Subluxation of T1/T2 thoracic vertebra** [POA]
[7th] **S23.111 Dislocation of T1/T2 thoracic vertebra** [POA]

[6th] **S23.12 Subluxation and dislocation of T2/T3-T3/T4 thoracic vertebra**
[7th] **S23.120 Subluxation of T2/T3 thoracic vertebra** [POA]
[7th] **S23.121 Dislocation of T2/T3 thoracic vertebra** [POA]
[7th] **S23.122 Subluxation of T3/T4 thoracic vertebra** [POA]
[7th] **S23.123 Dislocation of T3/T4 thoracic vertebra** [POA]

[6th] **S23.13 Subluxation and dislocation of T4/T5-T5/T6 thoracic vertebra**
[7th] **S23.130 Subluxation of T4/T5 thoracic vertebra** [POA]
[7th] **S23.131 Dislocation of T4/T5 thoracic vertebra** [POA]
[7th] **S23.132 Subluxation of T5/T6 thoracic vertebra** [POA]
[7th] **S23.133 Dislocation of T5/T6 thoracic vertebra** [POA]

[6th] **S23.14 Subluxation and dislocation of T6/T7-T7/T8 thoracic vertebra**
[7th] **S23.140 Subluxation of T6/T7 thoracic vertebra** [POA]
[7th] **S23.141 Dislocation of T6/T7 thoracic vertebra** [POA]
[7th] **S23.142 Subluxation of T7/T8 thoracic vertebra** [POA]
[7th] **S23.143 Dislocation of T7/T8 thoracic vertebra** [POA]

[6th] **S23.15 Subluxation and dislocation of T8/T9-T9/T10 thoracic vertebra**
[7th] **S23.150 Subluxation of T8/T9 thoracic vertebra** [POA]
[7th] **S23.151 Dislocation of T8/T9 thoracic vertebra** [POA]
[7th] **S23.152 Subluxation of T9/T10 thoracic vertebra** [POA]
[7th] **S23.153 Dislocation of T9/T10 thoracic vertebra** [POA]

[6th] **S23.16 Subluxation and dislocation of T10/T11-T11/T12 thoracic vertebra**
[7th] **S23.160 Subluxation of T10/T11 thoracic vertebra** [POA]
[7th] **S23.161 Dislocation of T10/T11 thoracic vertebra** [POA]
[7th] **S23.162 Subluxation of T11/T12 thoracic vertebra** [POA]
[7th] **S23.163 Dislocation of T11/T12 thoracic vertebra** [POA]

[6th] **S23.17 Subluxation and dislocation of T12/L1 thoracic vertebra**
[7th] **S23.170 Subluxation of T12/L1 thoracic vertebra** [POA]
[7th] **S23.171 Dislocation of T12/L1 thoracic vertebra** [POA]

[5th] **S23.2 Dislocation of other and unspecified parts of thorax**
[7th] **S23.20 Dislocation of unspecified part of thorax** [POA]
[7th] **S23.29 Dislocation of other parts of thorax** [POA]

[7th] **S23.3 Sprain of ligaments of thoracic spine** [POA]

[5th] **S23.4 Sprain of ribs and sternum**
[7th] **S23.41 Sprain of ribs** [POA]
[6th] **S23.42 Sprain of sternum**
[7th] **S23.420 Sprain of sternoclavicular (joint) (ligament)** [POA]
[7th] **S23.421 Sprain of chondrosternal joint** [POA]
[7th] **S23.428 Other sprain of sternum** [POA]
[7th] **S23.429 Unspecified sprain of sternum** [POA]

[7th] **S23.8 Sprain of other specified parts of thorax** [POA]
[7th] **S23.9 Sprain of unspecified parts of thorax** [POA]

[4th] **S24 Injury of nerves and spinal cord at thorax level**

[NOTES] Code to highest level of thoracic spinal cord injury
Injuries to the spinal cord (S24.0 and S24.1) refer to the cord level and not bone level injury, and can affect nerve roots at and below the level given.

Code also any associated:
fracture of thoracic vertebra (S22.0-)
open wound of thorax (S21.-)
transient paralysis (R29.5)

[EXCLUDES2] *injury of brachial plexus (S14.3)*

The appropriate 7th character is to be added to each code from category S24
A = initial encounter
D = subsequent encounter
S = sequela

[7th] **S24.0 Concussion and edema of thoracic spinal cord** [POA] [HCC] [MCC] [CC/MCC Excl]

[5th] **S24.1 Other and unspecified injuries of thoracic spinal cord**

[6th] **S24.10 Unspecified injury of thoracic spinal cord**
[7th] **S24.101 Unspecified injury at T1 level of thoracic spinal cord** [POA] [HAC] [HCC] [MCC] [CC/MCC Excl]
[7th] **S24.102 Unspecified injury at T2-T6 level of thoracic spinal cord** [POA] [HAC] [HCC] [MCC] [CC/MCC Excl]
[7th] **S24.103 Unspecified injury at T7-T10 level of thoracic spinal cord** [POA] [HAC] [HCC] [MCC] [CC/MCC Excl]
[7th] **S24.104 Unspecified injury at T11-T12 level of thoracic spinal cord** [POA] [HAC] [HCC] [MCC] [CC/MCC Excl]
[7th] **S24.109 Unspecified injury at unspecified level of thoracic spinal cord** [POA] [HAC] [HCC]
Injury of thoracic spinal cord NOS

[6th] **S24.11 Complete lesion of thoracic spinal cord**
[7th] **S24.111 Complete lesion at T1 level of thoracic spinal cord** [POA] [HAC] [HCC] [MCC] [CC/MCC Excl]
[7th] **S24.112 Complete lesion at T2-T6 level of thoracic spinal cord** [POA] [HAC] [HCC] [MCC] [CC/MCC Excl]
[7th] **S24.113 Complete lesion at T7-T10 level of thoracic spinal cord** [POA] [HAC] [HCC] [MCC] [CC/MCC Excl]
[7th] **S24.114 Complete lesion at T11-T12 level of thoracic spinal cord** [POA] [HAC] [HCC] [MCC] [CC/MCC Excl]
[7th] **S24.119 Complete lesion at unspecified level of thoracic spinal cord** [POA] [HCC]

[6th] **S24.13 Anterior cord syndrome of thoracic spinal cord**
[7th] **S24.131 Anterior cord syndrome at T1 level of thoracic spinal cord** [POA] [HAC] [HCC] [MCC] [CC/MCC Excl]
[7th] **S24.132 Anterior cord syndrome at T2-T6 level of thoracic spinal cord** [POA] [HAC] [HCC] [MCC] [CC/MCC Excl]
[7th] **S24.133 Anterior cord syndrome at T7-T10 level of thoracic spinal cord** [POA] [HAC] [HCC] [MCC] [CC/MCC Excl]
[7th] **S24.134 Anterior cord syndrome at T11-T12 level of thoracic spinal cord** [POA] [HAC] [HCC] [MCC] [CC/MCC Excl]

Unspecified Code Other Specified Code Manifestation Code [N] Newborn [P] Pediatric [M] Maternity [A] Adult ♂ Male ♀ Female
● New Code ▲ Revised Code Title ►◄ Revised Text [NOTES] [INCLUDES] [EXCLUDES1] Not coded here [EXCLUDES2] Not included here
[4th] 4th character required [5th] 5th character required [6th] 6th character required [7th] 7th character required
[X] Extension 'X' Alert [HAC] Hospital-acquired condition (HAC) alert AHA AHA Coding Clinic©

When symbols appear on a code that requires a 7th character extension, refer to Appendix B to identify applicable 7th character codes.

S24.139 Anterior cord syndrome at unspecified level of thoracic spinal cord `POA` `HCC`

S24.14 Brown-Séquard syndrome of thoracic spinal cord
  S24.141 Brown-Séquard syndrome at T1 level of thoracic spinal cord `POA` `HCC` `MCC` `CC/MCC Exc`
  S24.142 Brown-Séquard syndrome at T2-T6 level of thoracic spinal cord `POA` `HCC` `MCC` `CC/MCC Exc`
  S24.143 Brown-Séquard syndrome at T7-T10 level of thoracic spinal cord `POA` `HCC` `MCC` `CC/MCC Exc`
  S24.144 Brown-Séquard syndrome at T11-T12 level of thoracic spinal cord `POA` `HCC` `MCC` `CC/MCC Exc`
  S24.149 Brown-Séquard syndrome at unspecified level of thoracic spinal cord `POA` `HCC`

S24.15 Other incomplete lesions of thoracic spinal cord
  Incomplete lesion of thoracic spinal cord NOS
  Posterior cord syndrome of thoracic spinal cord
  S24.151 Other incomplete lesion at T1 level of thoracic spinal cord `POA` `HAC` `HCC` `MCC` `CC/MCC Exc`
  S24.152 Other incomplete lesion at T2-T6 level of thoracic spinal cord `POA` `HAC` `HCC` `MCC` `CC/MCC Exc`
  S24.153 Other incomplete lesion at T7-T10 level of thoracic spinal cord `POA` `HAC` `HCC` `MCC` `CC/MCC Exc`
  S24.154 Other incomplete lesion at T11-T12 level of thoracic spinal cord `POA` `HAC` `HCC` `MCC` `CC/MCC Exc`
  S24.159 Other incomplete lesion at unspecified level of thoracic spinal cord `POA` `HCC`

S24.2 Injury of nerve root of thoracic spine `POA`
S24.3 Injury of peripheral nerves of thorax `POA`
S24.4 Injury of thoracic sympathetic nervous system `POA`
  Injury of cardiac plexus
  Injury of esophageal plexus
  Injury of pulmonary plexus
  Injury of stellate ganglion
  Injury of thoracic sympathetic ganglion
S24.8 Injury of other specified nerves of thorax `POA`
S24.9 Injury of unspecified nerve of thorax `POA`

S25 Injury of blood vessels of thorax
  Code also any associated open wound (S21.-)

  The appropriate 7th character is to be added to each code from category S25.
  A = initial encounter
  D = subsequent encounter
  S = sequela

S25.0 Injury of thoracic aorta
  Injury of aorta NOS
  S25.00 Unspecified injury of thoracic aorta `POA` `MCC` `CC/MCC Exc`
  S25.01 Minor laceration of thoracic aorta `POA` `MCC` `CC/MCC Exc`
    Incomplete transection of thoracic aorta
    Laceration of thoracic aorta NOS
    Superficial laceration of thoracic aorta
  S25.02 Major laceration of thoracic aorta `POA` `MCC` `CC/MCC Exc`
    Complete transection of thoracic aorta
    Traumatic rupture of thoracic aorta
  S25.09 Other specified injury of thoracic aorta `POA` `MCC` `CC/MCC Exc`

S25.1 Injury of innominate or subclavian artery
  S25.10 Unspecified injury of innominate or subclavian artery
    S25.101 Unspecified injury of right innominate or subclavian artery `POA` `MCC` `CC/MCC Exc`
    S25.102 Unspecified injury of left innominate or subclavian artery `POA` `MCC` `CC/MCC Exc`
    S25.109 Unspecified injury of unspecified innominate or subclavian artery `POA` `MCC` `CC/MCC Exc`
  S25.11 Minor laceration of innominate or subclavian artery
    Incomplete transection of innominate or subclavian artery
    Laceration of innominate or subclavian artery NOS
    Superficial laceration of innominate or subclavian artery
    S25.111 Minor laceration of right innominate or subclavian artery `POA` `MCC` `CC/MCC Exc`
    S25.112 Minor laceration of left innominate or subclavian artery `POA` `MCC` `CC/MCC Exc`
    S25.119 Minor laceration of unspecified innominate or subclavian artery `POA` `MCC` `CC/MCC Exc`
  S25.12 Major laceration of innominate or subclavian artery
    Complete transection of innominate or subclavian artery
    Traumatic rupture of innominate or subclavian artery
    S25.121 Major laceration of right innominate or subclavian artery `POA` `MCC` `CC/MCC Exc`
    S25.122 Major laceration of left innominate or subclavian artery `POA` `MCC` `CC/MCC Exc`
    S25.129 Major laceration of unspecified innominate or subclavian artery `POA` `MCC` `CC/MCC Exc`
  S25.19 Other specified injury of innominate or subclavian artery
    S25.191 Other specified injury of right innominate or subclavian artery `POA` `MCC` `CC/MCC Exc`
    S25.192 Other specified injury of left innominate or subclavian artery `POA` `MCC` `CC/MCC Exc`
    S25.199 Other specified injury of unspecified innominate or subclavian artery `POA` `MCC` `CC/MCC Exc`

S25.2 Injury of superior vena cava
  Injury of vena cava NOS
  S25.20 Unspecified injury of superior vena cava `POA` `MCC` `CC/MCC Exc`
  S25.21 Minor laceration of superior vena cava `POA` `MCC` `CC/MCC Exc`
    Incomplete transection of superior vena cava
    Laceration of superior vena cava NOS
    Superficial laceration of superior vena cava
  S25.22 Major laceration of superior vena cava `POA` `MCC` `CC/MCC Exc`
    Complete transection of superior vena cava
    Traumatic rupture of superior vena cava
  S25.29 Other specified injury of superior vena cava `POA` `MCC` `CC/MCC Exc`

S25.3 Injury of innominate or subclavian vein
  S25.30 Unspecified injury of innominate or subclavian vein
    S25.301 Unspecified injury of right innominate or subclavian vein `POA` `MCC` `CC/MCC Exc`
    S25.302 Unspecified injury of left innominate or subclavian vein `POA` `MCC` `CC/MCC Exc`
    S25.309 Unspecified injury of unspecified innominate or subclavian vein `POA` `MCC` `CC/MCC Exc`
  S25.31 Minor laceration of innominate or subclavian vein
    Incomplete transection of innominate or subclavian vein
    Laceration of innominate or subclavian vein NOS
    Superficial laceration of innominate or subclavian vein
    S25.311 Minor laceration of right innominate or subclavian vein `POA` `MCC` `CC/MCC Exc`
    S25.312 Minor laceration of left innominate or subclavian vein `POA` `MCC` `CC/MCC Exc`
    S25.319 Minor laceration of unspecified innominate or subclavian vein `POA` `MCC` `CC/MCC Exc`
  S25.32 Major laceration of innominate or subclavian vein
    Complete transection of innominate or subclavian vein
    Traumatic rupture of innominate or subclavian vein
    S25.321 Major laceration of right innominate or subclavian vein `POA` `MCC` `CC/MCC Exc`
    S25.322 Major laceration of left innominate or subclavian vein `POA` `MCC` `CC/MCC Exc`
    S25.329 Major laceration of unspecified innominate or subclavian vein `POA` `MCC` `CC/MCC Exc`
  S25.39 Other specified injury of innominate or subclavian vein
    S25.391 Other specified injury of right innominate or subclavian vein `POA` `MCC` `CC/MCC Exc`
    S25.392 Other specified injury of left innominate or subclavian vein `POA` `MCC` `CC/MCC Exc`

Unacceptable principal diagnosis symbol per Medicare code edits   Code exempt from diagnosis present on admission requirement
❓ Questionable admission   Complication or comorbidity   CC/MCC CC/MCC exclusion   MCC Major complication or comorbidity
Principal diagnosis as its own CC   Principal diagnosis as its own MCC   HCC HCC diagnosis code   RxHCC RxHCC diagnosis code
MACRA code   Z Z code as first-listed diagnosis

S25.399 **Other specified injury of unspecified innominate or subclavian vein** POA MCC CC/MCC Exc

5ᵗʰ **S25.4 Injury of pulmonary blood vessels**

6ᵗʰ S25.40 **Unspecified injury of** pulmonary **blood vessels**

7ᵗʰ S25.401 **Unspecified injury of** right **pulmonary blood vessels** POA MCC CC/MCC Exc

7ᵗʰ S25.402 **Unspecified injury of** left **pulmonary blood vessels** POA MCC CC/MCC Exc

7ᵗʰ S25.409 **Unspecified injury of unspecified pulmonary blood vessels** POA MCC CC/MCC Exc

6ᵗʰ S25.41 **Minor laceration of pulmonary blood vessels**
Incomplete transection of pulmonary blood vessels
Laceration of pulmonary blood vessels NOS
Superficial laceration of pulmonary blood vessels

7ᵗʰ S25.411 **Minor laceration of** right **pulmonary blood vessels** POA MCC CC/MCC Exc

7ᵗʰ S25.412 **Minor laceration of** left **pulmonary blood vessels** POA MCC CC/MCC Exc

7ᵗʰ S25.419 **Minor laceration of unspecified pulmonary blood vessels** POA MCC CC/MCC Exc

6ᵗʰ S25.42 **Major laceration of pulmonary blood vessels**
Complete transection of pulmonary blood vessels
Traumatic rupture of pulmonary blood vessels

7ᵗʰ S25.421 **Major laceration of** right **pulmonary blood vessels** POA MCC CC/MCC Exc

7ᵗʰ S25.422 **Major laceration of** left **pulmonary blood vessels** POA MCC CC/MCC Exc

7ᵗʰ S25.429 **Major laceration of unspecified pulmonary blood vessels** POA MCC CC/MCC Exc

6ᵗʰ S25.49 **Other specified injury of pulmonary blood vessels**

7ᵗʰ S25.491 **Other specified injury of** right **pulmonary blood vessels** POA MCC CC/MCC Exc

7ᵗʰ S25.492 **Other specified injury of** left **pulmonary blood vessels** POA MCC CC/MCC Exc

7ᵗʰ S25.499 **Other specified injury of unspecified pulmonary blood vessels** POA MCC CC/MCC Exc

5ᵗʰ **S25.5 Injury of intercostal blood vessels**

6ᵗʰ S25.50 **Unspecified injury of intercostal blood vessels**

7ᵗʰ S25.501 **Unspecified injury of intercostal blood vessels,** right **side** CC POA CC/MCC Exc

7ᵗʰ S25.502 **Unspecified injury of intercostal blood vessels,** left **side** CC POA CC/MCC Exc

7ᵗʰ S25.509 **Unspecified injury of intercostal blood vessels, unspecified side** CC POA CC/MCC Exc

6ᵗʰ S25.51 **Laceration of intercostal blood vessels**

7ᵗʰ S25.511 **Laceration of intercostal blood vessels,** right **side** CC POA CC/MCC Exc

7ᵗʰ S25.512 **Laceration of intercostal blood vessels,** left **side** CC POA CC/MCC Exc

7ᵗʰ S25.519 **Laceration of intercostal blood vessels, unspecified side** CC POA CC/MCC Exc

6ᵗʰ S25.59 **Other specified injury of intercostal blood vessels**

7ᵗʰ S25.591 **Other specified injury of intercostal blood vessels,** right **side** CC POA CC/MCC Exc

7ᵗʰ S25.592 **Other specified injury of intercostal blood vessels,** left **side** CC POA CC/MCC Exc

7ᵗʰ S25.599 **Other specified injury of intercostal blood vessels, unspecified side** CC POA CC/MCC Exc

5ᵗʰ **S25.8 Injury of other blood vessels of thorax**
Injury of azygos vein
Injury of mammary artery or vein

6ᵗʰ S25.80 **Unspecified injury of other blood vessels of thorax**

7ᵗʰ S25.801 **Unspecified injury of other blood vessels of thorax,** right **side** CC POA CC/MCC Exc

7ᵗʰ S25.802 **Unspecified injury of other blood vessels of thorax,** left **side** CC POA CC/MCC Exc

7ᵗʰ S25.809 **Unspecified injury of other blood vessels of thorax, unspecified side** CC POA CC/MCC Exc

6ᵗʰ S25.81 **Laceration of other blood vessels of thorax**

7ᵗʰ S25.811 **Laceration of other blood vessels of thorax,** right **side** CC POA CC/MCC Exc

7ᵗʰ S25.812 **Laceration of other blood vessels of thorax,** left **side** CC POA CC/MCC Exc

7ᵗʰ S25.819 **Laceration of other blood vessels of thorax, unspecified side** CC POA CC/MCC Exc

6ᵗʰ S25.89 **Other specified injury of other blood vessels of thorax**

7ᵗʰ S25.891 **Other specified injury of other blood vessels of thorax,** right **side** CC POA CC/MCC Exc

7ᵗʰ S25.892 **Other specified injury of other blood vessels of thorax,** left **side** CC POA CC/MCC Exc

7ᵗʰ S25.899 **Other specified injury of other blood vessels of thorax, unspecified side** CC POA CC/MCC Exc

5ᵗʰ **S25.9 Injury of unspecified blood vessel of thorax**

7ᵗʰ S25.90 **Unspecified injury of unspecified blood vessel of thorax** CC POA CC/MCC Exc

7ᵗʰ S25.91 **Laceration of unspecified blood vessel of thorax** CC POA CC/MCC Exc

7ᵗʰ S25.99 **Other specified injury of unspecified blood vessel of thorax** CC POA CC/MCC Exc

4ᵗʰ **S26 Injury of heart**
Code also any associated:
open wound of thorax (S21.-)
traumatic hemopneumothorax (S27.2)
traumatic hemothorax (S27.1)
traumatic pneumothorax (S27.0)

The appropriate 7th character is to be added to each code from category S26
A = initial encounter
D = subsequent encounter
S = sequela

5ᵗʰ **S26.0 Injury of heart with hemopericardium**

7ᵗʰ S26.00 **Unspecified injury of heart with hemopericardium** CC POA CC/MCC Exc

7ᵗʰ S26.01 **Contusion of heart with hemopericardium** CC POA CC/MCC Exc

6ᵗʰ S26.02 **Laceration of heart with hemopericardium**

7ᵗʰ S26.020 **Mild laceration of heart with hemopericardium** POA MCC CC/MCC Exc
Laceration of heart without penetration of heart chamber

7ᵗʰ S26.021 **Moderate laceration of heart with hemopericardium** POA MCC CC/MCC Exc
Laceration of heart with penetration of heart chamber

7ᵗʰ S26.022 **Major laceration of heart with hemopericardium** POA MCC CC/MCC Exc
Laceration of heart with penetration of multiple heart chambers

7ᵗʰ S26.09 **Other injury of heart with hemopericardium** CC POA CC/MCC Exc

5ᵗʰ **S26.1 Injury of heart without hemopericardium**

7ᵗʰ S26.10 **Unspecified injury of heart without hemopericardium** CC POA CC/MCC Exc

7ᵗʰ S26.11 **Contusion of heart without hemopericardium** CC POA CC/MCC Exc

7ᵗʰ S26.12 **Laceration of heart without hemopericardium** POA MCC CC/MCC Exc

7ᵗʰ S26.19 **Other injury of heart without hemopericardium** CC POA CC/MCC Exc

5ᵗʰ **S26.9 Injury of heart, unspecified with or without hemopericardium**

7ᵗʰ S26.90 **Unspecified injury of heart, unspecified with or without hemopericardium** CC POA CC/MCC Exc

7ᵗʰ S26.91 **Contusion of heart, unspecified with or without hemopericardium** CC POA CC/MCC Exc

7ᵗʰ S26.92 **Laceration of heart, unspecified with or without hemopericardium** POA MCC CC/MCC Exc
Laceration of heart NOS

7ᵗʰ S26.99 **Other injury of heart, unspecified with or without hemopericardium** CC POA CC/MCC Exc

---

| Unspecified Code | Other Specified Code | Manifestation Code | N Newborn | P Pediatric | M Maternity | A Adult | ♂ Male | ♀ Female |

● New Code ▲ Revised Code Title ▶◀ Revised Text **NOTES** *INCLUDES* EXCLUDES1 Not coded here EXCLUDES2 Not included here

4ᵗʰ 4ᵗʰ character required 5ᵗʰ 5ᵗʰ character required 6ᵗʰ 6ᵗʰ character required 7ᵗʰ 7ᵗʰ character required

Extension 'X' Alert HAC Hospital-acquired condition (HAC) alert **AHA** AHA Coding Clinic©

S27 **Injury of other and unspecified intrathoracic organs**
Code also any associated open wound of thorax (S21.-)
EXCLUDES2 injury of cervical esophagus (S10-S19)
injury of trachea (cervical) (S10-S19)
The appropriate 7th character is to be added to each code from category S27
A = initial encounter
D = subsequent encounter
S = sequela

S27.0 **Traumatic** pneumothorax
EXCLUDES1 spontaneous pneumothorax (J93.-)

S27.1 **Traumatic** hemothorax

S27.2 **Traumatic** hemopneumothorax

S27.3 **Other and unspecified injuries of lung**
- S27.30 Unspecified injury of lung
  - S27.301 **Unspecified injury of lung,** unilateral
  - S27.302 **Unspecified injury of lung,** bilateral
  - S27.309 **Unspecified injury of lung,** unspecified
- S27.31 Primary **blast injury of lung**
  Blast injury of lung NOS
  - S27.311 **Primary blast injury of lung,** unilateral
  - S27.312 **Primary blast injury of lung,** bilateral
  - S27.319 **Primary blast injury of lung,** unspecified
- S27.32 Contusion **of lung**
  - S27.321 **Contusion of lung,** unilateral
  - S27.322 **Contusion of lung,** bilateral
  - S27.329 **Contusion of lung,** unspecified
- S27.33 Laceration **of lung**
  - S27.331 **Laceration of lung,** unilateral
  - S27.332 **Laceration of lung,** bilateral
  - S27.339 **Laceration of lung,** unspecified
- S27.39 Other injuries of lung
  Secondary blast injury of lung
  - S27.391 **Other injuries of lung,** unilateral
  - S27.392 **Other injuries of lung,** bilateral
  - S27.399 **Other injuries of lung,** unspecified

S27.4 **Injury of bronchus**
- S27.40 Unspecified injury of bronchus
  - S27.401 **Unspecified injury of bronchus,** unilateral
  - S27.402 **Unspecified injury of bronchus,** bilateral
  - S27.409 **Unspecified injury of bronchus,** unspecified
- S27.41 Primary blast injury of bronchus
  Blast injury of bronchus NOS
  - S27.411 **Primary blast injury of bronchus,** unilateral
  - S27.412 **Primary blast injury of bronchus,** bilateral
  - S27.419 **Primary blast injury of bronchus,** unspecified
- S27.42 Contusion of bronchus
  - S27.421 **Contusion of bronchus,** unilateral
  - S27.422 **Contusion of bronchus,** bilateral
  - S27.429 **Contusion of bronchus,** unspecified
- S27.43 Laceration of bronchus
  - S27.431 **Laceration of bronchus,** unilateral
  - S27.432 **Laceration of bronchus,** bilateral
  - S27.439 **Laceration of bronchus,** unspecified
- S27.49 Other injury of bronchus
  Secondary blast injury of bronchus
  - S27.491 **Other injury of bronchus,** unilateral
  - S27.492 **Other injury of bronchus,** bilateral
  - S27.499 **Other injury of bronchus,** unspecified

S27.5 **Injury of thoracic trachea**
- S27.50 **Unspecified injury of thoracic trachea**
- S27.51 **Primary blast injury of thoracic trachea**
  Blast injury of thoracic trachea NOS
- S27.52 **Contusion of thoracic trachea**
- S27.53 **Laceration of thoracic trachea**
- S27.59 **Other injury of thoracic trachea**
  Secondary blast injury of thoracic trachea

S27.6 **Injury of pleura**
- S27.60 **Unspecified injury of pleura**
- S27.63 **Laceration of pleura**
- S27.69 **Other injury of pleura**

S27.8 **Injury of other specified intrathoracic organs**
- S27.80 Injury of diaphragm
  - S27.802 **Contusion of diaphragm**
  - S27.803 **Laceration of diaphragm**
  - S27.808 **Other injury of diaphragm**
  - S27.809 **Unspecified injury of diaphragm**
- S27.81 Injury of esophagus (thoracic part)
  - S27.812 **Contusion of esophagus (thoracic part)**
  - S27.813 **Laceration of esophagus (thoracic part)**
  - S27.818 **Other injury of esophagus (thoracic part)**
  - S27.819 **Unspecified injury of esophagus (thoracic part)**
- S27.89 Injury of other specified intrathoracic organs
  Injury of lymphatic thoracic duct
  Injury of thymus gland
  - S27.892 **Contusion of other specified intrathoracic organs**
  - S27.893 **Laceration of other specified intrathoracic organs**
  - S27.898 **Other injury of other specified intrathoracic organs**
  - S27.899 **Unspecified injury of other specified intrathoracic organs**

S27.9 **Injury of unspecified intrathoracic organ**

S28 **Crushing injury of thorax, and traumatic amputation of part of thorax**
The appropriate 7th character is to be added to each code from category S28
A = initial encounter
D = subsequent encounter
S = sequela

S28.0 **Crushed chest**
Use additional code for all associated injuries
EXCLUDES1 flail chest (S22.5)

S28.1 **Traumatic amputation (partial) of part of thorax,** except breast

S28.2 **Traumatic amputation of breast**
- S28.21 Complete traumatic amputation of breast
  Traumatic amputation of breast NOS
  - S28.211 **Complete traumatic amputation of right breast**

PDx̄ Unacceptable principal diagnosis symbol per Medicare code edits   Code exempt from diagnosis present on admission requirement
? Questionable admission   CC Complication or comorbidity   CC/MCC Exc CC/MCC exclusion   MCC Major complication or comorbidity
PDx Principal diagnosis as its own CC   Principal diagnosis as its own MCC   HCC HCC diagnosis code   RxHCC RxHCC diagnosis code
MACRA code   Z1 Z code as first-listed diagnosis

When symbols appear on a code that requires a 7th character extension, refer to Appendix B to identify applicable 7th character codes.

2018 ICD-10-CM

    7ᵗʰ **S28.212** Complete traumatic amputation of left breast   POA

    7ᵗʰ **S28.219** Complete traumatic amputation of unspecified breast   POA

   6ᵗʰ **S28.22** Partial traumatic amputation of breast

    7ᵗʰ **S28.221** Partial traumatic amputation of right breast   POA

    7ᵗʰ **S28.222** Partial traumatic amputation of left breast   POA

    7ᵗʰ **S28.229** Partial traumatic amputation of unspecified breast   POA

4ᵗʰ **S29** Other and unspecified injuries of thorax

   Code also any associated open wound (S21.-)

   The appropriate 7th character is to be added to each code from category S29

    A = initial encounter
    D = subsequent encounter
    S = sequela

  5ᵗʰ **S29.0** Injury of muscle and tendon at thorax level

   6ᵗʰ **S29.00** Unspecified injury of muscle and tendon of thorax

    7ᵗʰ **S29.001** Unspecified injury of muscle and tendon of front wall of thorax   POA

    7ᵗʰ **S29.002** Unspecified injury of muscle and tendon of back wall of thorax   POA

    7ᵗʰ **S29.009** Unspecified injury of muscle and tendon of unspecified wall of thorax   POA

   6ᵗʰ **S29.01** Strain of muscle and tendon of thorax

    7ᵗʰ **S29.011** Strain of muscle and tendon of front wall of thorax   POA

    7ᵗʰ **S29.012** Strain of muscle and tendon of back wall of thorax   POA

    7ᵗʰ **S29.019** Strain of muscle and tendon of unspecified wall of thorax   POA

   6ᵗʰ **S29.02** Laceration of muscle and tendon of thorax

    7ᵗʰ **S29.021** Laceration of muscle and tendon of front wall of thorax   CC POA CC/MCC Exc

    7ᵗʰ **S29.022** Laceration of muscle and tendon of back wall of thorax   POA

    7ᵗʰ **S29.029** Laceration of muscle and tendon of unspecified wall of thorax   CC POA CC/MCC Exc

   6ᵗʰ **S29.09** Other injury of muscle and tendon of thorax

    7ᵗʰ **S29.091** Other injury of muscle and tendon of front wall of thorax   POA

    7ᵗʰ **S29.092** Other injury of muscle and tendon of back wall of thorax   POA

    7ᵗʰ **S29.099** Other injury of muscle and tendon of unspecified wall of thorax   POA

  7ᵗʰ **S29.8** Other specified injuries of thorax   POA

  7ᵗʰ **S29.9** Unspecified injury of thorax   POA

Injuries to the abdomen, lower back, lumbar spine, pelvis and external genitals (S30-S39)

INCLUDES   injuries to the abdominal wall

     injuries to the anus

     injuries to the buttock

     injuries to the external genitalia

     injuries to the flank

     injuries to the groin

EXCLUDES2   burns and corrosions (T20-T32)

     effects of foreign body in anus and rectum (T18.5)

     effects of foreign body in genitourinary tract (T19.-)

     effects of foreign body in stomach, small intestine and colon (T18.2-T18.4)

     frostbite (T33-T34)

     insect bite or sting, venomous (T63.4)

4ᵗʰ **S30** Superficial injury of abdomen, lower back, pelvis and external genitals

   EXCLUDES2 superficial injury of hip (S70.-)

   The appropriate 7th character is to be added to each code from category S30

    A = initial encounter
    D = subsequent encounter
    S = sequela

  7ᵗʰ **S30.0** Contusion of lower back and pelvis   POA

   Contusion of buttock

  7ᵗʰ **S30.1** Contusion of abdominal wall   POA

   Contusion of flank

   Contusion of groin

  5ᵗʰ **S30.2** Contusion of external genital organs

   6ᵗʰ **S30.20** Contusion of unspecified external genital organ

    7ᵗʰ **S30.201** Contusion of unspecified external genital organ, male   POA ♂

    7ᵗʰ **S30.202** Contusion of unspecified external genital organ, female   POA ♀

   7ᵗʰ **S30.21** Contusion of penis   POA ♂

   7ᵗʰ **S30.22** Contusion of scrotum and testes   POA ♂

   7ᵗʰ **S30.23** Contusion of vagina and vulva   POA ♀

  7ᵗʰ **S30.3** Contusion of anus   POA

  5ᵗʰ **S30.8** Other superficial injuries of abdomen, lower back, pelvis and external genitals

   6ᵗʰ **S30.81** Abrasion of abdomen, lower back, pelvis and external genitals

    7ᵗʰ **S30.810** Abrasion of lower back and pelvis   POA

    7ᵗʰ **S30.811** Abrasion of abdominal wall   POA

    7ᵗʰ **S30.812** Abrasion of penis   POA ♂

    7ᵗʰ **S30.813** Abrasion of scrotum and testes   POA ♂

    7ᵗʰ **S30.814** Abrasion of vagina and vulva   POA ♀

    7ᵗʰ **S30.815** Abrasion of unspecified external genital organs, male   POA ♂

    7ᵗʰ **S30.816** Abrasion of unspecified external genital organs, female   POA ♀

    7ᵗʰ **S30.817** Abrasion of anus   POA

   6ᵗʰ **S30.82** Blister (nonthermal) of abdomen, lower back, pelvis and external genitals

    7ᵗʰ **S30.820** Blister (nonthermal) of lower back and pelvis   POA

    7ᵗʰ **S30.821** Blister (nonthermal) of abdominal wall   POA

    7ᵗʰ **S30.822** Blister (nonthermal) of penis   POA ♂

    7ᵗʰ **S30.823** Blister (nonthermal) of scrotum and testes   POA ♂

    7ᵗʰ **S30.824** Blister (nonthermal) of vagina and vulva   POA ♀

    7ᵗʰ **S30.825** Blister (nonthermal) of unspecified external genital organs, male   POA ♂

    7ᵗʰ **S30.826** Blister (nonthermal) of unspecified external genital organs, female   POA ♀

    7ᵗʰ **S30.827** Blister (nonthermal) of anus   POA

   6ᵗʰ **S30.84** External constriction of abdomen, lower back, pelvis and external genitals

    7ᵗʰ **S30.840** External constriction of lower back and pelvis   POA

    7ᵗʰ **S30.841** External constriction of abdominal wall   POA

    7ᵗʰ **S30.842** External constriction of penis   POA ♂

     Hair tourniquet syndrome of penis

     Use additional cause code to identify the constricting item (W49.0-)

    7ᵗʰ **S30.843** External constriction of scrotum and testes   POA ♂

    7ᵗʰ **S30.844** External constriction of vagina and vulva   POA ♀

    7ᵗʰ **S30.845** External constriction of unspecified external genital organs, male   POA ♂

    7ᵗʰ **S30.846** External constriction of unspecified external genital organs, female   POA ♀

Unspecified Code   Other Specified Code   Manifestation Code   Ⓝ Newborn   Ⓟ Pediatric   Ⓜ Maternity   Ⓐ Adult   ♂ Male   ♀ Female
   ● New Code   ▲ Revised Code Title   ▶◀ Revised Text   **NOTES**   *INCLUDES*   *EXCLUDES 1* Not coded here   *EXCLUDES 2* Not included here
   4ᵗʰ character required   5ᵗʰ character required   6ᵗʰ character required   7ᵗʰ character required
   Extension 'X' Alert   **HAC** Hospital-acquired condition (HAC) alert   **AHA** AHA Coding Clinic©

S30.85 **Superficial** foreign body **of abdomen, lower back, pelvis and external genitals**
  Splinter in the abdomen, lower back, pelvis and external genitals

  S30.850 **Superficial foreign body of** lower back and pelvis POA

  S30.851 **Superficial foreign body of** abdominal wall POA

  S30.852 **Superficial foreign body of** penis POA ♂

  S30.853 **Superficial foreign body of** scrotum and testes POA ♂

  S30.854 **Superficial foreign body of** vagina and vulva POA ♀

  S30.855 **Superficial foreign body of unspecified external genital organs, male** POA ♂

  S30.856 **Superficial foreign body of unspecified external genital organs, female** POA ♀

  S30.857 **Superficial foreign body of anus** POA

S30.86 Insect bite **(nonvenomous) of** abdomen, lower back, pelvis and external genitals

  S30.860 **Insect bite (nonvenomous) of** lower back and pelvis POA

  S30.861 **Insect bite (nonvenomous) of** abdominal wall POA

  S30.862 **Insect bite (nonvenomous) of** penis POA ♂

  S30.863 **Insect bite (nonvenomous) of** scrotum and testes POA ♂

  S30.864 **Insect bite (nonvenomous) of** vagina and vulva POA ♀

  S30.865 **Insect bite (nonvenomous) of unspecified external genital organs, male** POA ♂

  S30.866 **Insect bite (nonvenomous) of unspecified external genital organs, female** POA ♀

  S30.867 **Insect bite (nonvenomous) of anus** POA

S30.87 Other superficial bite **of abdomen, lower back, pelvis and external genitals**

  EXCLUDES1 open bite of abdomen, lower back, pelvis and external genitals (S31.05, S31.15, S31.25, S31.35, S31.45, S31.55)

  S30.870 **Other superficial bite of** lower back and pelvis POA

  S30.871 **Other superficial bite of** abdominal wall POA

  S30.872 **Other superficial bite of** penis POA ♂

  S30.873 **Other superficial bite of** scrotum and testes POA ♂

  S30.874 **Other superficial bite of vagina and vulva** POA ♀

  S30.875 **Other superficial bite of unspecified external genital organs, male** POA ♂

  S30.876 **Other superficial bite of unspecified external genital organs, female** POA ♀

  S30.877 **Other superficial bite of anus** POA

S30.9 Unspecified superficial injury of abdomen, lower back, pelvis and external genitals

  S30.91 **Unspecified superficial injury of** lower back and pelvis POA

  S30.92 **Unspecified superficial injury of** abdominal wall POA

  S30.93 **Unspecified superficial injury of** penis POA ♂

  S30.94 **Unspecified superficial injury of** scrotum and testes POA ♂

  S30.95 **Unspecified superficial injury of** vagina and vulva POA ♀

  S30.96 **Unspecified superficial injury of unspecified** external genital organs, male POA ♂

  S30.97 **Unspecified superficial injury of unspecified** external genital organs, female POA ♀

  S30.98 **Unspecified superficial injury of** anus POA

S31 **Open wound of** abdomen, lower back, pelvis and external genitals
  Code also any associated:
    spinal cord injury (S24.0, S24.1-, S34.0-, S34.1-)
    wound infection
  EXCLUDES1 traumatic amputation of part of abdomen, lower back and pelvis (S38.2-, S38.3)
  EXCLUDES2 open wound of hip (S71.00-S71.02)
    open fracture of pelvis (S32.1--S32.9 with 7th character B)
  The appropriate 7th character is to be added to each code from category S31
    A = initial encounter
    D = subsequent encounter
    S = sequela

S31.0 **Open wound of** lower back and pelvis

  S31.00 **Unspecified open wound of lower back and pelvis**

    S31.000 **Unspecified open wound of lower back and pelvis** without penetration into retroperitoneum POA
      Unspecified open wound of lower back and pelvis NOS

    S31.001 **Unspecified open wound of lower back and pelvis** with penetration into retroperitoneum POA MCC CC/MCC Exc

  S31.01 Laceration without foreign body **of lower back and pelvis**

    S31.010 **Laceration without foreign body of lower back and pelvis** without penetration into retroperitoneum POA
      Laceration without foreign body of lower back and pelvis NOS

    S31.011 **Laceration without foreign body of lower back and pelvis with penetration into retroperitoneum** POA MCC CC/MCC Exc

  S31.02 Laceration with foreign body **of lower back and pelvis**

    S31.020 **Laceration with foreign body of lower back and pelvis** without penetration into retroperitoneum POA
      Laceration with foreign body of lower back and pelvis NOS

    S31.021 **Laceration with foreign body of lower back and pelvis** with penetration into retroperitoneum POA MCC CC/MCC Exc

  S31.03 Puncture wound without foreign body **of lower back and pelvis**

    S31.030 **Puncture wound without foreign body of lower back and pelvis** without penetration into retroperitoneum POA
      Puncture wound without foreign body of lower back and pelvis NOS

    S31.031 **Puncture wound without foreign body of lower back and pelvis** with penetration into retroperitoneum POA MCC CC/MCC Exc

  S31.04 Puncture wound with foreign body **of lower back and pelvis**

    S31.040 **Puncture wound with foreign body of lower back and pelvis** without penetration into retroperitoneum POA
      Puncture wound with foreign body of lower back and pelvis NOS

    S31.041 **Puncture wound with foreign body of lower back and pelvis** with penetration into retroperitoneum POA MCC CC/MCC Exc

  S31.05 Open bite **of lower back and pelvis**
    Bite of lower back and pelvis NOS
    EXCLUDES1 superficial bite of lower back and pelvis (S30.860, S30.870)

PDx Unacceptable principal diagnosis symbol per Medicare code edits   POA Code exempt from diagnosis present on admission requirement
? Questionable admission   CC Complication or comorbidity   CC/MCC Exc CC/MCC exclusion   MCC Major complication or comorbidity
CC Principal diagnosis as its own CC   MCC Principal diagnosis as its own MCC   HCC HCC diagnosis code   RxHCC RxHCC diagnosis code
MACRA code   Z1 Z code as first-listed diagnosis

7ᵗʰ S31.050 **Open bite of lower back and pelvis** without penetration into retroperitoneum
Open bite of lower back and pelvis NOS POA

7ᵗʰ S31.051 **Open bite of lower back and pelvis** with penetration into retroperitoneum POA MCC CC-MCC Exc

5ᵗʰ S31.1 **Open wound of abdominal wall without penetration into peritoneal cavity**
Open wound of abdominal wall NOS
EXCLUDES2 open wound of abdominal wall with penetration into peritoneal cavity (S31.6-)

6ᵗʰ S31.10 **Unspecified open wound of abdominal wall without penetration into peritoneal cavity**

7ᵗʰ S31.100 **Unspecified open wound of abdominal wall, right upper quadrant without penetration into peritoneal cavity** POA

7ᵗʰ S31.101 **Unspecified open wound of abdominal wall, left upper quadrant without penetration into peritoneal cavity** POA

7ᵗʰ S31.102 **Unspecified open wound of abdominal wall, epigastric region without penetration into peritoneal cavity** POA

7ᵗʰ S31.103 **Unspecified open wound of abdominal wall, right lower quadrant without penetration into peritoneal cavity** POA

7ᵗʰ S31.104 **Unspecified open wound of abdominal wall, left lower quadrant without penetration into peritoneal cavity** POA

7ᵗʰ S31.105 **Unspecified open wound of abdominal wall, periumbilic region without penetration into peritoneal cavity** POA

7ᵗʰ S31.109 **Unspecified open wound of abdominal wall, unspecified quadrant without penetration into peritoneal cavity**
Unspecified open wound of abdominal wall NOS POA

6ᵗʰ S31.11 **Laceration without foreign body of abdominal wall without penetration into peritoneal cavity**

7ᵗʰ S31.110 **Laceration without foreign body of abdominal wall, right upper quadrant without penetration into peritoneal cavity** POA

7ᵗʰ S31.111 **Laceration without foreign body of abdominal wall, left upper quadrant without penetration into peritoneal cavity** POA

7ᵗʰ S31.112 **Laceration without foreign body of abdominal wall, epigastric region without penetration into peritoneal cavity** POA

7ᵗʰ S31.113 **Laceration without foreign body of abdominal wall, right lower quadrant without penetration into peritoneal cavity** POA

7ᵗʰ S31.114 **Laceration without foreign body of abdominal wall, left lower quadrant without penetration into peritoneal cavity** POA

7ᵗʰ S31.115 **Laceration without foreign body of abdominal wall, periumbilic region without penetration into peritoneal cavity** POA

7ᵗʰ S31.119 **Laceration without foreign body of abdominal wall, unspecified quadrant without penetration into peritoneal cavity** POA

6ᵗʰ S31.12 **Laceration with foreign body of abdominal wall without penetration into peritoneal cavity**

7ᵗʰ S31.120 **Laceration of abdominal wall with foreign body, right upper quadrant without penetration into peritoneal cavity** POA

7ᵗʰ S31.121 **Laceration of abdominal wall with foreign body, left upper quadrant without penetration into peritoneal cavity** POA

7ᵗʰ S31.122 **Laceration of abdominal wall with foreign body, epigastric region without penetration into peritoneal cavity** POA

7ᵗʰ S31.123 **Laceration of abdominal wall with foreign body, right lower quadrant without penetration into peritoneal cavity** POA

7ᵗʰ S31.124 **Laceration of abdominal wall with foreign body, left lower quadrant without penetration into peritoneal cavity** POA

7ᵗʰ S31.125 **Laceration of abdominal wall with foreign body, periumbilic region without penetration into peritoneal cavity** POA

7ᵗʰ S31.129 **Laceration of abdominal wall with foreign body, unspecified quadrant without penetration into peritoneal cavity** POA

5ᵗʰ S31.13 **Puncture wound of abdominal wall without foreign body without penetration into peritoneal cavity**

7ᵗʰ S31.130 **Puncture wound of abdominal wall without foreign body, right upper quadrant without penetration into peritoneal cavity** POA

7ᵗʰ S31.131 **Puncture wound of abdominal wall without foreign body, left upper quadrant without penetration into peritoneal cavity** POA

7ᵗʰ S31.132 **Puncture wound of abdominal wall without foreign body, epigastric region without penetration into peritoneal cavity** POA

7ᵗʰ S31.133 **Puncture wound of abdominal wall without foreign body, right lower quadrant without penetration into peritoneal cavity** POA

7ᵗʰ S31.134 **Puncture wound of abdominal wall without foreign body, left lower quadrant without penetration into peritoneal cavity** POA

7ᵗʰ S31.135 **Puncture wound of abdominal wall without foreign body, periumbilic region without penetration into peritoneal cavity** POA

7ᵗʰ S31.139 **Puncture wound of abdominal wall without foreign body, unspecified quadrant without penetration into peritoneal cavity** POA

5ᵗʰ S31.14 **Puncture wound of abdominal wall with foreign body without penetration into peritoneal cavity**

7ᵗʰ S31.140 **Puncture wound of abdominal wall with foreign body, right upper quadrant without penetration into peritoneal cavity** POA

7ᵗʰ S31.141 **Puncture wound of abdominal wall with foreign body, left upper quadrant without penetration into peritoneal cavity** POA

7ᵗʰ S31.142 **Puncture wound of abdominal wall with foreign body, epigastric region without penetration into peritoneal cavity** POA

7ᵗʰ S31.143 **Puncture wound of abdominal wall with foreign body, right lower quadrant without penetration into peritoneal cavity** POA

7ᵗʰ S31.144 **Puncture wound of abdominal wall with foreign body, left lower quadrant without penetration into peritoneal cavity** POA

7ᵗʰ S31.145 **Puncture wound of abdominal wall with foreign body, periumbilic region without penetration into peritoneal cavity** POA

7ᵗʰ S31.149 **Puncture wound of abdominal wall with foreign body, unspecified quadrant without penetration into peritoneal cavity** POA

Unspecified Code   Other Specified Code   Manifestation Code   Ⓝ Newborn   Ⓟ Pediatric   Ⓜ Maternity   Ⓐ Adult   ♂ Male   ♀ Female
● New Code   ▲ Revised Code Title   ▶◀ Revised Text   NOTES   INCLUDES   EXCLUDES 1 Not coded here   EXCLUDES 2 Not included here
4ᵗʰ 4ᵗʰ character required   5ᵗʰ 5ᵗʰ character required   6ᵗʰ 6ᵗʰ character required   7ᵗʰ 7ᵗʰ character required
Ⓧ Extension 'X' Alert   HAC Hospital-acquired condition (HAC) alert   **AHA** AHA Coding Clinic©

S31.15 **Open bite of abdominal wall without penetration into peritoneal cavity**
Bite of abdominal wall NOS
EXCLUDES1 superficial bite of abdominal wall (S30.871)

S31.150 Open bite of abdominal wall, right upper quadrant without penetration into peritoneal cavity

S31.151 Open bite of abdominal wall, left upper quadrant without penetration into peritoneal cavity

S31.152 Open bite of abdominal wall, epigastric region without penetration into peritoneal cavity

S31.153 Open bite of abdominal wall, right lower quadrant without penetration into peritoneal cavity

S31.154 Open bite of abdominal wall, left lower quadrant without penetration into peritoneal cavity

S31.155 Open bite of abdominal wall, periumbilic region without penetration into peritoneal cavity

S31.159 **Open bite of abdominal wall, unspecified quadrant without penetration into peritoneal cavity**

S31.2 Open wound of penis

S31.20 **Unspecified open wound of penis**

S31.21 Laceration without foreign body of penis

S31.22 Laceration with foreign body of penis

S31.23 Puncture wound without foreign body of penis

S31.24 Puncture wound with foreign body of penis

S31.25 Open bite of penis
Bite of penis NOS
EXCLUDES1 superficial bite of penis (S30.862, S30.872)

S31.3 Open wound of scrotum and testes

S31.30 **Unspecified open wound of scrotum and testes**

S31.31 Laceration without foreign body of scrotum and testes

S31.32 Laceration with foreign body of scrotum and testes

S31.33 Puncture wound without foreign body of scrotum and testes

S31.34 Puncture wound with foreign body of scrotum and testes

S31.35 Open bite of scrotum and testes
Bite of scrotum and testes NOS
EXCLUDES1 superficial bite of scrotum and testes (S30.863, S30.873)

S31.4 Open wound of vagina and vulva
EXCLUDES1 injury to vagina and vulva during delivery (O70.-, O71.4)

S31.40 **Unspecified open wound of vagina and vulva**

S31.41 Laceration without foreign body of vagina and vulva

S31.42 Laceration with foreign body of vagina and vulva

S31.43 Puncture wound without foreign body of vagina and vulva

S31.44 Puncture wound with foreign body of vagina and vulva

S31.45 Open bite of vagina and vulva
Bite of vagina and vulva NOS
EXCLUDES1 superficial bite of vagina and vulva (S30.864, S30.874)

S31.5 Open wound of unspecified external genital organs
EXCLUDES1 traumatic amputation of external genital organs (S38.21, S38.22)

S31.50 Unspecified open wound of unspecified external genital organs

S31.501 **Unspecified open wound of unspecified external genital organs, male**

S31.502 **Unspecified open wound of unspecified external genital organs, female**

S31.51 Laceration without foreign body of unspecified external genital organs

S31.511 **Laceration without foreign body of unspecified external genital organs, male**

S31.512 **Laceration without foreign body of unspecified external genital organs, female**

S31.52 Laceration with foreign body of unspecified external genital organs

S31.521 **Laceration with foreign body of unspecified external genital organs, male**

S31.522 **Laceration with foreign body of unspecified external genital organs, female**

S31.53 Puncture wound without foreign body of unspecified external genital organs

S31.531 **Puncture wound without foreign body of unspecified external genital organs, male**

S31.532 **Puncture wound without foreign body of unspecified external genital organs, female**

S31.54 Puncture wound with foreign body of unspecified external genital organs

S31.541 **Puncture wound with foreign body of unspecified external genital organs, male**

S31.542 **Puncture wound with foreign body of unspecified external genital organs, female**

S31.55 Open bite of unspecified external genital organs
Bite of unspecified external genital organs NOS
EXCLUDES1 superficial bite of unspecified external genital organs (S30.865, S30.866, S30.875, S30.876)

S31.551 **Open bite of unspecified external genital organs, male**

S31.552 **Open bite of unspecified external genital organs, female**

S31.6 Open wound of abdominal wall with penetration into peritoneal cavity

S31.60 Unspecified open wound of abdominal wall with penetration into peritoneal cavity

S31.600 **Unspecified open wound of abdominal wall, right upper quadrant with penetration into peritoneal cavity**

S31.601 Unspecified open wound of abdominal wall, left upper quadrant with penetration into peritoneal cavity

S31.602 Unspecified open wound of abdominal wall, epigastric region with penetration into peritoneal cavity

S31.603 Unspecified open wound of abdominal wall, right lower quadrant with penetration into peritoneal cavity

S31.604 Unspecified open wound of abdominal wall, left lower quadrant with penetration into peritoneal cavity

S31.605 Unspecified open wound of abdominal wall, periumbilic region with penetration into peritoneal cavity

S31.609 Unspecified open wound of abdominal wall, unspecified quadrant with penetration into peritoneal cavity

S31.61 Laceration without foreign body of abdominal wall with penetration into peritoneal cavity

Unacceptable principal diagnosis symbol per Medicare code edits   Code exempt from diagnosis present on admission requirement
❓ Questionable admission   ᶜᶜ Complication or comorbidity   CC/MCC Exc CC/MCC exclusion   MCC Major complication or comorbidity
Principal diagnosis as its own CC   Principal diagnosis as its own MCC   HCC HCC diagnosis code   RxHCC RxHCC diagnosis code
MACRA code   Z Z code as first-listed diagnosis

1002   When symbols appear on a code that requires a 7th character extension, refer to Appendix B to identify applicable 7th character codes.   **2018 ICD-10-CM**

S31.610 Laceration without foreign body of abdominal wall, right upper quadrant with penetration into peritoneal cavity POA MCC CC/MCC Exc

S31.611 Laceration without foreign body of abdominal wall, left upper quadrant with penetration into peritoneal cavity POA MCC CC/MCC Exc

S31.612 Laceration without foreign body of abdominal wall, epigastric region with penetration into peritoneal cavity POA MCC CC/MCC Exc

S31.613 Laceration without foreign body of abdominal wall, right lower quadrant with penetration into peritoneal cavity POA MCC CC/MCC Exc

S31.614 Laceration without foreign body of abdominal wall, left lower quadrant with penetration into peritoneal cavity POA MCC CC/MCC Exc

S31.615 Laceration without foreign body of abdominal wall, periumbilic region with penetration into peritoneal cavity POA MCC CC/MCC Exc

S31.619 Laceration without foreign body of abdominal wall, unspecified quadrant with penetration into peritoneal cavity POA MCC CC/MCC Exc

S31.62 Laceration with foreign body of abdominal wall with penetration into peritoneal cavity

S31.620 Laceration with foreign body of abdominal wall, right upper quadrant with penetration into peritoneal cavity POA MCC CC/MCC Exc

S31.621 Laceration with foreign body of abdominal wall, left upper quadrant with penetration into peritoneal cavity POA MCC CC/MCC Exc

S31.622 Laceration with foreign body of abdominal wall, epigastric region with penetration into peritoneal cavity POA MCC CC/MCC Exc

S31.623 Laceration with foreign body of abdominal wall, right lower quadrant with penetration into peritoneal cavity POA MCC CC/MCC Exc

S31.624 Laceration with foreign body of abdominal wall, left lower quadrant with penetration into peritoneal cavity POA MCC CC/MCC Exc

S31.625 Laceration with foreign body of abdominal wall, periumbilic region with penetration into peritoneal cavity POA MCC CC/MCC Exc

S31.629 Laceration with foreign body of abdominal wall, unspecified quadrant with penetration into peritoneal cavity POA MCC CC/MCC Exc

S31.63 Puncture wound without foreign body of abdominal wall with penetration into peritoneal cavity

S31.630 Puncture wound without foreign body of abdominal wall, right upper quadrant with penetration into peritoneal cavity POA MCC CC/MCC Exc

S31.631 Puncture wound without foreign body of abdominal wall, left upper quadrant with penetration into peritoneal cavity POA MCC CC/MCC Exc

S31.632 Puncture wound without foreign body of abdominal wall, epigastric region with penetration into peritoneal cavity POA MCC CC/MCC Exc

S31.633 Puncture wound without foreign body of abdominal wall, right lower quadrant with penetration into peritoneal cavity POA MCC CC/MCC Exc

S31.634 Puncture wound without foreign body of abdominal wall, left lower quadrant with penetration into peritoneal cavity POA MCC CC/MCC Exc

S31.635 Puncture wound without foreign body of abdominal wall, periumbilic region with penetration into peritoneal cavity POA MCC CC/MCC Exc

S31.639 Puncture wound without foreign body of abdominal wall, unspecified quadrant with penetration into peritoneal cavity POA MCC CC/MCC Exc

S31.64 Puncture wound with foreign body of abdominal wall with penetration into peritoneal cavity

S31.640 Puncture wound with foreign body of abdominal wall, right upper quadrant with penetration into peritoneal cavity POA MCC CC/MCC Exc

S31.641 Puncture wound with foreign body of abdominal wall, left upper quadrant with penetration into peritoneal cavity POA MCC CC/MCC Exc

S31.642 Puncture wound with foreign body of abdominal wall, epigastric region with penetration into peritoneal cavity POA MCC CC/MCC Exc

S31.643 Puncture wound with foreign body of abdominal wall, right lower quadrant with penetration into peritoneal cavity POA MCC CC/MCC Exc

S31.644 Puncture wound with foreign body of abdominal wall, left lower quadrant with penetration into peritoneal cavity POA MCC CC/MCC Exc

S31.645 Puncture wound with foreign body of abdominal wall, periumbilic region with penetration into peritoneal cavity POA MCC CC/MCC Exc

S31.649 Puncture wound with foreign body of abdominal wall, unspecified quadrant with penetration into peritoneal cavity POA MCC CC/MCC Exc

S31.65 Open bite of abdominal wall with penetration into peritoneal cavity

EXCLUDES1 superficial bite of abdominal wall (S30.861, S30.871)

S31.650 Open bite of abdominal wall, right upper quadrant with penetration into peritoneal cavity POA MCC CC/MCC Exc

S31.651 Open bite of abdominal wall, left upper quadrant with penetration into peritoneal cavity POA MCC CC/MCC Exc

S31.652 Open bite of abdominal wall, epigastric region with penetration into peritoneal cavity POA MCC CC/MCC Exc

S31.653 Open bite of abdominal wall, right lower quadrant with penetration into peritoneal cavity POA MCC CC/MCC Exc

S31.654 Open bite of abdominal wall, left lower quadrant with penetration into peritoneal cavity POA MCC CC/MCC Exc

S31.655 Open bite of abdominal wall, periumbilic region with penetration into peritoneal cavity POA MCC CC/MCC Exc

S31.659 Open bite of abdominal wall, unspecified quadrant with penetration into peritoneal cavity POA MCC CC/MCC Exc

---

Unspecified Code   Other Specified Code   Manifestation Code   N Newborn   P Pediatric   M Maternity   A Adult   ♂ Male   ♀ Female
● New Code   ▲ Revised Code Title   ►◄ Revised Text   NOTES   INCLUDES   EXCLUDES 1   Not coded here   EXCLUDES 2   Not included here
4th character required   5th character required   6th character required   7th character required
Extension 'X' Alert   HAC Hospital-acquired condition (HAC) alert   AHA AHA Coding Clinic©

6️⃣ **S32.44** Fracture of posterior column [ilioischial] of acetabulum

7️⃣ S32.441 Displaced fracture of posterior column [ilioischial] of right acetabulum `cc̄ POA HAC HCC McC CC/MCC Exc`

7️⃣ S32.442 Displaced fracture of posterior column [ilioischial] of left acetabulum `cc̄ POA HAC HCC McC CC/MCC Exc`

7️⃣ S32.443 Displaced fracture of posterior column [ilioischial] of unspecified acetabulum `cc̄ POA HAC HCC McC CC/MCC Exc`

7️⃣ S32.444 Nondisplaced fracture of posterior column [ilioischial] of right acetabulum `cc̄ POA HAC HCC McC CC/MCC Exc`

7️⃣ S32.445 Nondisplaced fracture of posterior column [ilioischial] of left acetabulum `cc̄ POA HAC HCC McC CC/MCC Exc`

7️⃣ S32.446 Nondisplaced fracture of posterior column [ilioischial] of unspecified acetabulum `cc̄ POA HAC HCC McC CC/MCC Exc`

6️⃣ **S32.45** Transverse fracture of acetabulum

7️⃣ S32.451 Displaced transverse fracture of right acetabulum `cc̄ POA HAC HCC McC CC/MCC Exc`

7️⃣ S32.452 Displaced transverse fracture of left acetabulum `cc̄ POA HAC HCC McC CC/MCC Exc`

7️⃣ S32.453 Displaced transverse fracture of unspecified acetabulum `cc̄ POA HAC HCC McC CC/MCC Exc`

7️⃣ S32.454 Nondisplaced transverse fracture of right acetabulum `cc̄ POA HAC HCC McC CC/MCC Exc`

7️⃣ S32.455 Nondisplaced transverse fracture of left acetabulum `cc̄ POA HAC HCC McC CC/MCC Exc`

7️⃣ S32.456 Nondisplaced transverse fracture of unspecified acetabulum `cc̄ POA HAC HCC McC CC/MCC Exc`

6️⃣ **S32.46** Associated transverse-posterior fracture of acetabulum

7️⃣ S32.461 Displaced associated transverse-posterior fracture of right acetabulum `cc̄ POA HAC HCC McC CC/MCC Exc`

7️⃣ S32.462 Displaced associated transverse-posterior fracture of left acetabulum `cc̄ POA HAC HCC McC CC/MCC Exc`

7️⃣ S32.463 Displaced associated transverse-posterior fracture of unspecified acetabulum `cc̄ POA HAC HCC McC CC/MCC Exc`

7️⃣ S32.464 Nondisplaced associated transverse-posterior fracture of right acetabulum `cc̄ POA HAC HCC McC CC/MCC Exc`

7️⃣ S32.465 Nondisplaced associated transverse-posterior fracture of left acetabulum `cc̄ POA HAC HCC McC CC/MCC Exc`

7️⃣ S32.466 Nondisplaced associated transverse-posterior fracture of unspecified acetabulum `cc̄ POA HAC HCC McC CC/MCC Exc`

6️⃣ **S32.47** Fracture of medial wall of acetabulum

7️⃣ S32.471 Displaced fracture of medial wall of right acetabulum `cc̄ POA HAC HCC McC CC/MCC Exc`

7️⃣ S32.472 Displaced fracture of medial wall of left acetabulum `cc̄ POA HAC HCC McC CC/MCC Exc`

7️⃣ S32.473 Displaced fracture of medial wall of unspecified acetabulum `cc̄ POA HAC HCC McC CC/MCC Exc`

7️⃣ S32.474 Nondisplaced fracture of medial wall of right acetabulum `cc̄ POA HAC HCC McC CC/MCC Exc`

7️⃣ S32.475 Nondisplaced fracture of medial wall of left acetabulum `cc̄ POA HAC HCC McC CC/MCC Exc`

7️⃣ S32.476 Nondisplaced fracture of medial wall of unspecified acetabulum `cc̄ POA HAC HCC McC CC/MCC Exc`

6️⃣ **S32.48** Dome fracture of acetabulum

7️⃣ S32.481 Displaced dome fracture of right acetabulum `cc̄ POA HAC HCC McC CC/MCC Exc`

7️⃣ S32.482 Displaced dome fracture of left acetabulum `cc̄ POA HAC HCC McC CC/MCC Exc`

7️⃣ S32.483 Displaced dome fracture of unspecified acetabulum `cc̄ POA HAC HCC McC CC/MCC Exc`

7️⃣ S32.484 Nondisplaced dome fracture of right acetabulum `cc̄ POA HAC HCC McC CC/MCC Exc`

7️⃣ S32.485 Nondisplaced dome fracture of left acetabulum `cc̄ POA HAC HCC McC CC/MCC Exc`

7️⃣ S32.486 Nondisplaced dome fracture of unspecified acetabulum `cc̄ POA HAC HCC McC CC/MCC Exc`

6️⃣ **S32.49** Other specified fracture of acetabulum

7️⃣ S32.491 Other specified fracture of right acetabulum `cc̄ POA HAC HCC McC CC/MCC Exc`

7️⃣ S32.492 Other specified fracture of left acetabulum `cc̄ POA HAC HCC McC CC/MCC Exc`

7️⃣ S32.499 Other specified fracture of unspecified acetabulum `cc̄ POA HAC HCC McC CC/MCC Exc`

5️⃣ **S32.5** Fracture of pubis

EXCLUDES1 fracture of pubis with associated disruption of pelvic ring (S32.8-)

6️⃣ **S32.50** Unspecified fracture of pubis

7️⃣ S32.501 Unspecified fracture of right pubis `cc̄ POA HAC HCC McC CC/MCC Exc`

7️⃣ S32.502 Unspecified fracture of left pubis `cc̄ POA HAC HCC McC CC/MCC Exc`

7️⃣ S32.509 Unspecified fracture of unspecified pubis `cc̄ POA HAC HCC McC CC/MCC Exc`

6️⃣ **S32.51** Fracture of superior rim of pubis

7️⃣ S32.511 Fracture of superior rim of right pubis `cc̄ POA HAC HCC McC CC/MCC Exc`

7️⃣ S32.512 Fracture of superior rim of left pubis `cc̄ POA HAC HCC McC CC/MCC Exc`

7️⃣ S32.519 Fracture of superior rim of unspecified pubis `cc̄ POA HAC HCC McC CC/MCC Exc`

6️⃣ **S32.59** Other specified fracture of pubis

7️⃣ S32.591 Other specified fracture of right pubis `cc̄ POA HAC HCC McC CC/MCC Exc`

7️⃣ S32.592 Other specified fracture of left pubis `cc̄ POA HAC HCC McC CC/MCC Exc`

7️⃣ S32.599 Other specified fracture of unspecified pubis `cc̄ POA HAC HCC McC CC/MCC Exc`

5️⃣ **S32.6** Fracture of ischium

EXCLUDES1 fracture of ischium with associated disruption of pelvic ring (S32.8-)

6️⃣ **S32.60** Unspecified fracture of ischium

7️⃣ S32.601 Unspecified fracture of right ischium `cc̄ POA HAC HCC McC CC/MCC Exc`

7️⃣ S32.602 Unspecified fracture of left ischium `cc̄ POA HAC HCC McC CC/MCC Exc`

7️⃣ S32.609 Unspecified fracture of unspecified ischium `cc̄ POA HAC HCC McC CC/MCC Exc`

6️⃣ **S32.61** Avulsion fracture of ischium

7️⃣ S32.611 Displaced avulsion fracture of right ischium `cc̄ POA HAC HCC McC CC/MCC Exc`

7️⃣ S32.612 Displaced avulsion fracture of left ischium `cc̄ POA HAC HCC McC CC/MCC Exc`

7️⃣ S32.613 Displaced avulsion fracture of unspecified ischium `cc̄ POA HAC HCC McC CC/MCC Exc`

7️⃣ S32.614 Nondisplaced avulsion fracture of right ischium `cc̄ POA HAC HCC McC CC/MCC Exc`

7️⃣ S32.615 Nondisplaced avulsion fracture of left ischium `cc̄ POA HAC HCC McC CC/MCC Exc`

7️⃣ S32.616 Nondisplaced avulsion fracture of unspecified ischium `cc̄ POA HAC HCC McC CC/MCC Exc`

6️⃣ **S32.69** Other specified fracture of ischium

7️⃣ S32.691 Other specified fracture of right ischium `cc̄ POA HAC HCC McC CC/MCC Exc`

7️⃣ S32.692 Other specified fracture of left ischium `cc̄ POA HAC HCC McC CC/MCC Exc`

POxÃ Unacceptable principal diagnosis symbol per Medicare code edits   POA Code exempt from diagnosis present on admission requirement

❓ Questionable admission   cc̄ Complication or comorbidity   CC/MCC Exc CC/MCC exclusion   McC Major complication or comorbidity

Principal diagnosis as its own CC   Principal diagnosis as its own MCC   HCC HCC diagnosis code   RxHCC RxHCC diagnosis code

MACRA code   Z1 Z code as first-listed diagnosis

S32.699 Other specified fracture of unspecified ischium cc⊘ POA HAC HCC MCC⊘ CC/MCC Exc

S32.8 Fracture of other parts of pelvis
Code also any associated:
fracture of acetabulum (S32.4-)
sacral fracture (S32.1-)

S32.81 Multiple fractures of pelvis with disruption of pelvic ring
Multiple pelvic fractures with disruption of pelvic circle

S32.810 Multiple fractures of pelvis with stable disruption of pelvic ring cc⊘ POA HAC HCC MCC⊘ CC/MCC Exc

S32.811 Multiple fractures of pelvis with unstable disruption of pelvic ring cc⊘ POA HAC HCC MCC⊘ CC/MCC Exc

S32.82 Multiple fractures of pelvis without disruption of pelvic ring cc⊘ POA HAC HCC MCC⊘ CC/MCC Exc
Multiple pelvic fractures without disruption of pelvic circle

S32.89 Fracture of other parts of pelvis cc⊘ POA HAC HCC MCC⊘ CC/MCC Exc

S32.9 Fracture of unspecified parts of lumbosacral spine and pelvis cc⊘ POA HAC HCC MCC⊘ CC/MCC Exc
Fracture of lumbosacral spine NOS
Fracture of pelvis NOS

S33 Dislocation and sprain of joints and ligaments of lumbar spine and pelvis

INCLUDES avulsion of joint or ligament of lumbar spine and pelvis
laceration of cartilage, joint or ligament of lumbar spine and pelvis
sprain of cartilage, joint or ligament of lumbar spine and pelvis
traumatic hemarthrosis of joint or ligament of lumbar spine and pelvis
traumatic rupture of joint or ligament of lumbar spine and pelvis
traumatic subluxation of joint or ligament of lumbar spine and pelvis
traumatic tear of joint or ligament of lumbar spine and pelvis

Code also any associated open wound

EXCLUDES1 nontraumatic rupture or displacement of lumbar intervertebral disc NOS (M51.-)
obstetric damage to pelvic joints and ligaments (O71.6)

EXCLUDES2 dislocation and sprain of joints and ligaments of hip (S73.-)
strain of muscle of lower back and pelvis (S39.01-)

The appropriate 7th character is to be added to each code from category S33
A = initial encounter
D = subsequent encounter
S = sequela

S33.0 Traumatic rupture of lumbar intervertebral disc POA
EXCLUDES1 rupture or displacement (nontraumatic) of lumbar intervertebral disc NOS (M51.- with fifth character 6)

S33.1 Subluxation and dislocation of lumbar vertebra
Code also any associated:
open wound of abdomen, lower back and pelvis (S31)
spinal cord injury (S24.0, S24.1-, S34.0-, S34.1-)
EXCLUDES2 fracture of lumbar vertebrae (S32.0-)

S33.10 Subluxation and dislocation of unspecified lumbar vertebra

S33.100 Subluxation of unspecified lumbar vertebra POA

S33.101 Dislocation of unspecified lumbar vertebra POA

S33.11 Subluxation and dislocation of L1/L2 lumbar vertebra

S33.110 Subluxation of L1/L2 lumbar vertebra POA

S33.111 Dislocation of L1/L2 lumbar vertebra POA

S33.12 Subluxation and dislocation of L2/L3 lumbar vertebra

S33.120 Subluxation of L2/L3 lumbar vertebra POA

S33.121 Dislocation of L2/L3 lumbar vertebra POA

S33.13 Subluxation and dislocation of L3/L4 lumbar vertebra

S33.130 Subluxation of L3/L4 lumbar vertebra POA

S33.131 Dislocation of L3/L4 lumbar vertebra POA

S33.14 Subluxation and dislocation of L4/L5 lumbar vertebra

S33.140 Subluxation of L4/L5 lumbar vertebra POA

S33.141 Dislocation of L4/L5 lumbar vertebra POA

S33.2 Dislocation of sacroiliac and sacrococcygeal joint POA

S33.3 Dislocation of other and unspecified parts of lumbar spine and pelvis

S33.30 Dislocation of unspecified parts of lumbar spine and pelvis POA

S33.39 Dislocation of other parts of lumbar spine and pelvis POA

S33.4 Traumatic rupture of symphysis pubis POA

S33.5 Sprain of ligaments of lumbar spine POA

S33.6 Sprain of sacroiliac joint POA

S33.8 Sprain of other parts of lumbar spine and pelvis POA

S33.9 Sprain of unspecified parts of lumbar spine and pelvis POA

S34 Injury of lumbar and sacral spinal cord and nerves at abdomen, lower back and pelvis level
NOTES Code to highest level of lumbar cord injury
Injuries to the spinal cord (S34.0 and S34.1) refer to the cord level and not bone level injury, and can affect nerve roots at and below the level given.
Code also any associated:
fracture of vertebra (S22.0-, S32.0-)
open wound of abdomen, lower back and pelvis (S31.-)
transient paralysis (R29.5)

The appropriate 7th character is to be added to each code from category S34
A = initial encounter
D = subsequent encounter
S = sequela

S34.0 Concussion and edema of lumbar and sacral spinal cord

S34.01 Concussion and edema of lumbar spinal cord POA HCC MCC⊘ CC/MCC Exc

S34.02 Concussion and edema of sacral spinal cord POA HCC MCC⊘ CC/MCC Exc
Concussion and edema of conus medullaris

S34.1 Other and unspecified injury of lumbar and sacral spinal cord

S34.10 Unspecified injury to lumbar spinal cord

S34.101 Unspecified injury to L1 level of lumbar spinal cord POA HAC HCC MCC⊘ CC/MCC Exc
Unspecified injury to lumbar spinal cord level 1

S34.102 Unspecified injury to L2 level of lumbar spinal cord POA HAC HCC MCC⊘ CC/MCC Exc
Unspecified injury to lumbar spinal cord level 2

S34.103 Unspecified injury to L3 level of lumbar spinal cord POA HAC HCC MCC⊘ CC/MCC Exc
Unspecified injury to lumbar spinal cord level 3

S34.104 Unspecified injury to L4 level of lumbar spinal cord POA HAC HCC MCC⊘ CC/MCC Exc
Unspecified injury to lumbar spinal cord level 4

S34.105 Unspecified injury to L5 level of lumbar spinal cord POA HAC HCC MCC⊘ CC/MCC Exc
Unspecified injury to lumbar spinal cord level 5

S34.109 Unspecified injury to unspecified level of lumbar spinal cord POA HAC HCC MCC⊘ CC/MCC Exc

S34.11 Complete lesion of lumbar spinal cord

Unspecified Code   Other Specified Code   Manifestation Code   N Newborn   P Pediatric   M Maternity   A Adult   ♂ Male   ♀ Female
● New Code   ▲ Revised Code Title   ►◄ Revised Text   NOTES   INCLUDES   EXCLUDES 1 Not coded here   EXCLUDES 2 Not included here
4ᵗʰ 4th character required   5ᵗʰ 5th character required   6ᵗʰ 6th character required   7ᵗʰ 7th character required
Extension 'X' Alert   HAC Hospital-acquired condition (HAC) alert   AHA AHA Coding Clinic©

2018 ICD-10-CM   When symbols appear on a code that requires a 7th character extension, refer to Appendix B to identify applicable 7th character codes.   1007

7ᵗʰ **S34.111** **Complete lesion of** L1 level **of lumbar spinal cord** POA HAC HCC MCC CC/MCC Exc
　　Complete lesion of lumbar spinal cord level 1

7ᵗʰ **S34.112** **Complete lesion of** L2 level **of lumbar spinal cord** POA HAC HCC MCC CC/MCC Exc
　　Complete lesion of lumbar spinal cord level 2

7ᵗʰ **S34.113** **Complete lesion of** L3 level **of lumbar spinal cord** POA HAC HCC MCC CC/MCC Exc
　　Complete lesion of lumbar spinal cord level 3

7ᵗʰ **S34.114** **Complete lesion of** L4 level **of lumbar spinal cord** POA HAC HCC MCC CC/MCC Exc
　　Complete lesion of lumbar spinal cord level 4

7ᵗʰ **S34.115** **Complete lesion of** L5 level **of lumbar spinal cord** POA HAC HCC MCC CC/MCC Exc
　　Complete lesion of lumbar spinal cord level 5

7ᵗʰ **S34.119** **Complete lesion of unspecified level of lumbar spinal cord** POA HAC HCC MCC CC/MCC Exc

6ᵗʰ **S34.12** Incomplete lesion **of lumbar spinal cord**

7ᵗʰ **S34.121** **Incomplete lesion of** L1 level **of lumbar spinal cord** POA HAC HCC MCC CC/MCC Exc
　　Incomplete lesion of lumbar spinal cord level 1

7ᵗʰ **S34.122** **Incomplete lesion of** L2 level **of lumbar spinal cord** POA HAC HCC MCC CC/MCC Exc
　　Incomplete lesion of lumbar spinal cord level 2

7ᵗʰ **S34.123** **Incomplete lesion of** L3 level **of lumbar spinal cord** POA HAC HCC MCC CC/MCC Exc
　　Incomplete lesion of lumbar spinal cord level 3

7ᵗʰ **S34.124** **Incomplete lesion of** L4 level **of lumbar spinal cord** POA HAC HCC MCC CC/MCC Exc
　　Incomplete lesion of lumbar spinal cord level 4

7ᵗʰ **S34.125** **Incomplete lesion of** L5 level **of lumbar spinal cord** POA HAC HCC MCC CC/MCC Exc
　　Incomplete lesion of lumbar spinal cord level 5

7ᵗʰ **S34.129** **Incomplete lesion of unspecified level of lumbar spinal cord** POA HAC HCC MCC CC/MCC Exc

6ᵗʰ **S34.13** **Other and unspecified injury to sacral spinal cord**
　　Other injury to conus medullaris

7ᵗʰ **S34.131** Complete **lesion of sacral spinal cord** POA HAC HCC MCC CC/MCC Exc
　　Complete lesion of conus medullaris

7ᵗʰ **S34.132** Incomplete **lesion of sacral spinal cord** POA HAC HCC MCC CC/MCC Exc
　　Incomplete lesion of conus medullaris

7ᵗʰ **S34.139** **Unspecified injury to sacral spinal cord** POA HAC HCC MCC CC/MCC Exc
　　Unspecified injury of conus medullaris

5ᵗʰ **S34.2** **Injury of nerve root of lumbar and** sacral spine

7ᵗʰ **S34.21** **Injury of nerve root of** lumbar spine POA

7ᵗʰ **S34.22** **Injury of nerve root of** sacral spine POA

7ᵗʰ **S34.3** **Injury of cauda equina** POA HAC HCC MCC CC/MCC Exc

7ᵗʰ **S34.4** **Injury of lumbosacral plexus** POA

7ᵗʰ **S34.5** **Injury of lumbar, sacral and pelvic sympathetic nerves** POA
　　Injury of celiac ganglion or plexus
　　Injury of hypogastric plexus
　　Injury of mesenteric plexus (inferior) (superior)
　　Injury of splanchnic nerve

7ᵗʰ **S34.6** **Injury of peripheral nerve(s) at abdomen, lower back and pelvis level** POA

7ᵗʰ **S34.8** **Injury of other nerves at abdomen, lower back and pelvis level** POA

7ᵗʰ **S34.9** **Injury of unspecified nerves at abdomen, lower back and pelvis level** POA

4ᵗʰ **S35** **Injury of blood vessels at abdomen, lower back and pelvis level**
　Code also any associated open wound (S31.-)
　The appropriate 7th character is to be added to each code from category S35
　　A = initial encounter
　　D = subsequent encounter
　　S = sequela

5ᵗʰ **S35.0** **Injury of** abdominal aorta
　　EXCLUDES1 injury of aorta NOS (S25.0)

7ᵗʰ **S35.00** **Unspecified injury of abdominal aorta** POA MCC CC/MCC Exc

7ᵗʰ **S35.01** Minor laceration **of abdominal aorta** POA MCC CC/MCC Exc
　　Incomplete transection of abdominal aorta
　　Laceration of abdominal aorta NOS
　　Superficial laceration of abdominal aorta

7ᵗʰ **S35.02** Major laceration **of abdominal aorta** POA MCC CC/MCC Exc
　　Complete transection of abdominal aorta
　　Traumatic rupture of abdominal aorta

7ᵗʰ **S35.09** **Other injury of abdominal aorta** POA MCC CC/MCC Exc

5ᵗʰ **S35.1** **Injury of inferior vena cava**
　　Injury of hepatic vein
　　EXCLUDES1 injury of vena cava NOS (S25.2)

7ᵗʰ **S35.10** **Unspecified injury of inferior vena cava** POA MCC CC/MCC Exc

7ᵗʰ **S35.11** Minor laceration **of inferior vena cava** POA MCC CC/MCC Exc
　　Incomplete transection of inferior vena cava
　　Laceration of inferior vena cava NOS
　　Superficial laceration of inferior vena cava

7ᵗʰ **S35.12** Major laceration **of inferior vena cava** POA MCC CC/MCC Exc
　　Complete transection of inferior vena cava
　　Traumatic rupture of inferior vena cava

7ᵗʰ **S35.19** **Other injury of inferior vena cava** POA MCC CC/MCC Exc

5ᵗʰ **S35.2** **Injury of** celiac or mesenteric artery **and branches**

6ᵗʰ **S35.21** **Injury of celiac artery**

7ᵗʰ **S35.211** Minor laceration **of celiac artery** POA MCC CC/MCC Exc
　　Incomplete transection of celiac artery
　　Laceration of celiac artery NOS
　　Superficial laceration of celiac artery

7ᵗʰ **S35.212** Major laceration **of celiac artery** POA MCC CC/MCC Exc
　　Complete transection of celiac artery
　　Traumatic rupture of celiac artery

7ᵗʰ **S35.218** **Other injury of celiac artery** POA MCC CC/MCC Exc

7ᵗʰ **S35.219** **Unspecified injury of celiac artery** POA MCC CC/MCC Exc

6ᵗʰ **S35.22** **Injury of** superior mesenteric artery

7ᵗʰ **S35.221** Minor laceration **of superior mesenteric artery** POA MCC CC/MCC Exc
　　Incomplete transection of superior mesenteric artery
　　Laceration of superior mesenteric artery NOS
　　Superficial laceration of superior mesenteric artery

7ᵗʰ **S35.222** Major laceration **of superior mesenteric artery** POA MCC CC/MCC Exc
　　Complete transection of superior mesenteric artery
　　Traumatic rupture of superior mesenteric artery

7ᵗʰ **S35.228** **Other injury of superior mesenteric artery** POA MCC CC/MCC Exc

7ᵗʰ **S35.229** **Unspecified injury of superior mesenteric artery** POA MCC CC/MCC Exc

6ᵗʰ **S35.23** **Injury of** inferior mesenteric artery

7ᵗʰ **S35.231** Minor laceration **of inferior mesenteric artery** POA MCC CC/MCC Exc
　　Incomplete transection of inferior mesenteric artery
　　Laceration of inferior mesenteric artery NOS
　　Superficial laceration of inferior mesenteric artery

POA⃠ Unacceptable principal diagnosis symbol per Medicare code edits　POA Code exempt from diagnosis present on admission requirement
❓ Questionable admission　cc Complication or comorbidity　cc/mcc Exc CC/MCC exclusion　MCC Major complication or comorbidity
Principal diagnosis as its own CC　Principal diagnosis as its own MCC　HCC HCC diagnosis code　RxHCC RxHCC diagnosis code
MACRA code　Z1 Z code as first-listed diagnosis

[7th] S35.232 Major laceration of inferior mesenteric artery POA MCC CC/MCC Exc
Complete transection of inferior mesenteric artery
Traumatic rupture of inferior mesenteric artery

[7th] S35.238 Other injury of inferior mesenteric artery POA MCC CC/MCC Exc

[7th] S35.239 Unspecified injury of inferior mesenteric artery POA MCC CC/MCC Exc

[6th] S35.29 Injury of branches of celiac and mesenteric artery
Injury of gastric artery
Injury of gastroduodenal artery
Injury of hepatic artery
Injury of splenic artery

[7th] S35.291 Minor laceration of branches of celiac and mesenteric artery POA MCC CC/MCC Exc
Incomplete transection of branches of celiac and mesenteric artery
Laceration of branches of celiac and mesenteric artery NOS
Superficial laceration of branches of celiac and mesenteric artery

[7th] S35.292 Major laceration of branches of celiac and mesenteric artery POA MCC CC/MCC Exc
Complete transection of branches of celiac and mesenteric artery
Traumatic rupture of branches of celiac and mesenteric artery

[7th] S35.298 Other injury of branches of celiac and mesenteric artery POA MCC CC/MCC Exc

[7th] S35.299 Unspecified injury of branches of celiac and mesenteric artery POA MCC CC/MCC Exc

[5th] S35.3 Injury of portal or splenic vein and branches

[6th] S35.31 Injury of portal vein

[7th] S35.311 Laceration of portal vein POA MCC CC/MCC Exc

[7th] S35.318 Other specified injury of portal vein POA MCC CC/MCC Exc

[7th] S35.319 Unspecified injury of portal vein POA MCC CC/MCC Exc

[6th] S35.32 Injury of splenic vein

[7th] S35.321 Laceration of splenic vein POA MCC CC/MCC Exc

[7th] S35.328 Other specified injury of splenic vein POA MCC CC/MCC Exc

[7th] S35.329 Unspecified injury of splenic vein POA MCC CC/MCC Exc

[6th] S35.33 Injury of superior mesenteric vein

[7th] S35.331 Laceration of superior mesenteric vein POA MCC CC/MCC Exc

[7th] S35.338 Other specified injury of superior mesenteric vein POA MCC CC/MCC Exc

[7th] S35.339 Unspecified injury of superior mesenteric vein POA MCC CC/MCC Exc

[6th] S35.34 Injury of inferior mesenteric vein

[7th] S35.341 Laceration of inferior mesenteric vein POA MCC CC/MCC Exc

[7th] S35.348 Other specified injury of inferior mesenteric vein POA MCC CC/MCC Exc

[7th] S35.349 Unspecified injury of inferior mesenteric vein POA MCC CC/MCC Exc

[5th] S35.4 Injury of renal blood vessels

[6th] S35.40 Unspecified injury of renal blood vessel

[7th] S35.401 Unspecified injury of right renal artery POA MCC CC/MCC Exc

[7th] S35.402 Unspecified injury of left renal artery POA MCC CC/MCC Exc

[7th] S35.403 Unspecified injury of unspecified renal artery POA MCC CC/MCC Exc

[7th] S35.404 Unspecified injury of right renal vein POA MCC CC/MCC Exc

[7th] S35.405 Unspecified injury of left renal vein POA MCC CC/MCC Exc

[7th] S35.406 Unspecified injury of unspecified renal vein POA MCC CC/MCC Exc

[6th] S35.41 Laceration of renal blood vessel

[7th] S35.411 Laceration of right renal artery POA MCC CC/MCC Exc

[7th] S35.412 Laceration of left renal artery POA MCC CC/MCC Exc

[7th] S35.413 Laceration of unspecified renal artery POA MCC CC/MCC Exc

[7th] S35.414 Laceration of right renal vein POA MCC CC/MCC Exc

[7th] S35.415 Laceration of left renal vein POA MCC CC/MCC Exc

[7th] S35.416 Laceration of unspecified renal vein POA MCC CC/MCC Exc

[6th] S35.49 Other specified injury of renal blood vessel

[7th] S35.491 Other specified injury of right renal artery POA MCC CC/MCC Exc

[7th] S35.492 Other specified injury of left renal artery POA MCC CC/MCC Exc

[7th] S35.493 Other specified injury of unspecified renal artery POA MCC CC/MCC Exc

[7th] S35.494 Other specified injury of right renal vein POA MCC CC/MCC Exc

[7th] S35.495 Other specified injury of left renal vein POA MCC CC/MCC Exc

[7th] S35.496 Other specified injury of unspecified renal vein POA MCC CC/MCC Exc

[5th] S35.5 Injury of iliac blood vessels

[7th] S35.50 Injury of unspecified iliac blood vessel(s) POA MCC CC/MCC Exc

[6th] S35.51 Injury of iliac artery or vein
Injury of hypogastric artery or vein

[7th] S35.511 Injury of right iliac artery POA MCC CC/MCC Exc

[7th] S35.512 Injury of left iliac artery POA MCC CC/MCC Exc

[7th] S35.513 Injury of unspecified iliac artery POA MCC CC/MCC Exc

[7th] S35.514 Injury of right iliac vein POA MCC CC/MCC Exc

[7th] S35.515 Injury of left iliac vein POA MCC CC/MCC Exc

[7th] S35.516 Injury of unspecified iliac vein POA MCC CC/MCC Exc

[6th] S35.53 Injury of uterine artery or vein

[7th] S35.531 Injury of right uterine artery CC POA ♀ CC/MCC Exc

[7th] S35.532 Injury of left uterine artery CC POA ♀ CC/MCC Exc

[7th] S35.533 Injury of unspecified uterine artery CC POA ♀ CC/MCC Exc

[7th] S35.534 Injury of right uterine vein CC POA ♀ CC/MCC Exc

[7th] S35.535 Injury of left uterine vein CC POA ♀ CC/MCC Exc

[7th] S35.536 Injury of unspecified uterine vein CC POA ♀ CC/MCC Exc

[7th] S35.59 Injury of other iliac blood vessels POA MCC CC/MCC Exc

[5th] S35.8 Injury of other blood vessels at abdomen, lower back and pelvis level
Injury of ovarian artery or vein

[6th] S35.8X Injury of other blood vessels at abdomen, lower back and pelvis level

[7th] S35.8X1 Laceration of other blood vessels at abdomen, lower back and pelvis level CC POA CC/MCC Exc

[7th] S35.8X8 Other specified injury of other blood vessels at abdomen, lower back and pelvis level CC POA CC/MCC Exc

[7th] S35.8X9 Unspecified injury of other blood vessels at abdomen, lower back and pelvis level CC POA CC/MCC Exc

[5th] S35.9 Injury of unspecified blood vessel at abdomen, lower back and pelvis level

[7th] S35.90 Unspecified injury of unspecified blood vessel at abdomen, lower back and pelvis level CC POA CC/MCC Exc

[7th] S35.91 Laceration of unspecified blood vessel at abdomen, lower back and pelvis level CC POA CC/MCC Exc

[7th] S35.99 Other specified injury of unspecified blood vessel at abdomen, lower back and pelvis level CC POA CC/MCC Exc

Unspecified Code Other Specified Code Manifestation Code [N] Newborn [P] Pediatric [M] Maternity [A] Adult ♂ Male ♀ Female
● New Code ▲ Revised Code Title ►◄ Revised Text [NOTES] [INCLUDES] [EXCLUDES 1] Not coded here [EXCLUDES 2] Not included here
[4th] 4th character required [5th] 5th character required [6th] 6th character required [7th] 7th character required
[7th] Extension 'X' Alert [HAC] Hospital-acquired condition (HAC) alert AHA AHA Coding Clinic©

When symbols appear on a code that requires a 7th character extension, refer to Appendix B to identify applicable 7th character codes.

S36 Injury of intra-abdominal organs
Code also any associated open wound (S31.-)
The appropriate 7th character is to be added to each code from category S36
A = initial encounter
D = subsequent encounter
S = sequela

S36.0 Injury of spleen
- S36.00 Unspecified injury of spleen
- S36.02 Contusion of spleen
  - S36.020 Minor contusion of spleen
    Contusion of spleen less than 2 cm
  - S36.021 Major contusion of spleen
    Contusion of spleen greater than 2 cm
  - S36.029 Unspecified contusion of spleen
- S36.03 Laceration of spleen
  - S36.030 Superficial (capsular) laceration of spleen
    Laceration of spleen less than 1 cm
    Minor laceration of spleen
  - S36.031 Moderate laceration of spleen
    Laceration of spleen 1 to 3 cm
  - S36.032 Major laceration of spleen
    Avulsion of spleen
    Laceration of spleen greater than 3 cm
    Massive laceration of spleen
    Multiple moderate lacerations of spleen
    Stellate laceration of spleen
  - S36.039 Unspecified laceration of spleen
- S36.09 Other injury of spleen

S36.1 Injury of liver and gallbladder and bile duct
- S36.11 Injury of liver
  - S36.112 Contusion of liver
  - S36.113 Laceration of liver, unspecified degree
  - S36.114 Minor laceration of liver
    Laceration involving capsule only, or, without significant involvement of hepatic parenchyma [i.e., less than 1 cm deep]
  - S36.115 Moderate laceration of liver
    Laceration involving parenchyma but without major disruption of parenchyma [i.e., less than 10 cm long and less than 3 cm deep]
  - S36.116 Major laceration of liver
    Laceration with significant disruption of hepatic parenchyma [i.e., greater than 10 cm long and 3 cm deep]
    Multiple moderate lacerations, with or without hematoma
    Stellate laceration of liver
  - S36.118 Other injury of liver
  - S36.119 Unspecified injury of liver
- S36.12 Injury of gallbladder
  - S36.122 Contusion of gallbladder
  - S36.123 Laceration of gallbladder
  - S36.128 Other injury of gallbladder
  - S36.129 Unspecified injury of gallbladder
- S36.13 Injury of bile duct

S36.2 Injury of pancreas
- S36.20 Unspecified injury of pancreas
  - S36.200 Unspecified injury of head of pancreas
  - S36.201 Unspecified injury of body of pancreas
  - S36.202 Unspecified injury of tail of pancreas
  - S36.209 Unspecified injury of unspecified part of pancreas

S36.22 Contusion of pancreas
- S36.220 Contusion of head of pancreas
- S36.221 Contusion of body of pancreas
- S36.222 Contusion of tail of pancreas
- S36.229 Contusion of unspecified part of pancreas

S36.23 Laceration of pancreas, unspecified degree
- S36.230 Laceration of head of pancreas, unspecified degree
- S36.231 Laceration of body of pancreas, unspecified degree
- S36.232 Laceration of tail of pancreas, unspecified degree
- S36.239 Laceration of unspecified part of pancreas, unspecified degree

S36.24 Minor laceration of pancreas
- S36.240 Minor laceration of head of pancreas
- S36.241 Minor laceration of body of pancreas
- S36.242 Minor laceration of tail of pancreas
- S36.249 Minor laceration of unspecified part of pancreas

S36.25 Moderate laceration of pancreas
- S36.250 Moderate laceration of head of pancreas
- S36.251 Moderate laceration of body of pancreas
- S36.252 Moderate laceration of tail of pancreas
- S36.259 Moderate laceration of unspecified part of pancreas

S36.26 Major laceration of pancreas
- S36.260 Major laceration of head of pancreas
- S36.261 Major laceration of body of pancreas
- S36.262 Major laceration of tail of pancreas
- S36.269 Major laceration of unspecified part of pancreas

S36.29 Other injury of pancreas
- S36.290 Other injury of head of pancreas
- S36.291 Other injury of body of pancreas
- S36.292 Other injury of tail of pancreas
- S36.299 Other injury of unspecified part of pancreas

S36.3 Injury of stomach
- S36.30 Unspecified injury of stomach
- S36.32 Contusion of stomach
- S36.33 Laceration of stomach
- S36.39 Other injury of stomach

S36.4 Injury of small intestine
- S36.40 Unspecified injury of small intestine
  - S36.400 Unspecified injury of duodenum
  - S36.408 Unspecified injury of other part of small intestine
  - S36.409 Unspecified injury of unspecified part of small intestine
- S36.41 Primary blast injury of small intestine
  Blast injury of small intestine NOS
  - S36.410 Primary blast injury of duodenum
  - S36.418 Primary blast injury of other part of small intestine
  - S36.419 Primary blast injury of unspecified part of small intestine

PDₓ Unacceptable principal diagnosis symbol per Medicare code edits   POA Code exempt from diagnosis present on admission requirement
? Questionable admission   CC Complication or comorbidity   CC/MCC Exc CC/MCC exclusion   MCC Major complication or comorbidity
Principal diagnosis as its own CC   Principal diagnosis as its own MCC   HCC HCC diagnosis code   RxHCC RxHCC diagnosis code
MACRA code   Z1 Z code as first-listed diagnosis

1010   When symbols appear on a code that requires a 7th character extension, refer to Appendix B to identify applicable 7th character codes.   2018 ICD-10-CM

⑥ **S36.42** Contusion of small intestine
- ⑦ **S36.420** Contusion of duodenum · CC POA CC/MCC Exc
- ⑦ **S36.428** Contusion of other part of small intestine · CC POA CC/MCC Exc
- ⑦ **S36.429** Contusion of unspecified part of small intestine · CC POA CC/MCC Exc

⑥ **S36.43** Laceration of small intestine
- ⑦ **S36.430** Laceration of duodenum · CC POA CC/MCC Exc
- ⑦ **S36.438** Laceration of other part of small intestine · CC POA CC/MCC Exc
- ⑦ **S36.439** Laceration of unspecified part of small intestine · CC POA CC/MCC Exc

⑥ **S36.49** Other injury of small intestine
- ⑦ **S36.490** Other injury of duodenum · CC POA CC/MCC Exc
- ⑦ **S36.498** Other injury of other part of small intestine · CC POA CC/MCC Exc
- ⑦ **S36.499** Other injury of unspecified part of small intestine · CC POA CC/MCC Exc

⑤ **S36.5** Injury of colon
  EXCLUDES2 injury of rectum (S36.6-)
- ⑥ **S36.50** Unspecified injury of colon
  - ⑦ **S36.500** Unspecified injury of ascending [right] colon · CC POA CC/MCC Exc
  - ⑦ **S36.501** Unspecified injury of transverse colon · CC POA CC/MCC Exc
  - ⑦ **S36.502** Unspecified injury of descending [left] colon · CC POA CC/MCC Exc
  - ⑦ **S36.503** Unspecified injury of sigmoid colon · CC POA CC/MCC Exc
  - ⑦ **S36.508** Unspecified injury of other part of colon · CC POA CC/MCC Exc
  - ⑦ **S36.509** Unspecified injury of unspecified part of colon · CC POA CC/MCC Exc
- ⑥ **S36.51** Primary blast injury of colon
  Blast injury of colon NOS
  - ⑦ **S36.510** Primary blast injury of ascending [right] colon · CC POA CC/MCC Exc
  - ⑦ **S36.511** Primary blast injury of transverse colon · CC POA CC/MCC Exc
  - ⑦ **S36.512** Primary blast injury of descending [left] colon · CC POA CC/MCC Exc
  - ⑦ **S36.513** Primary blast injury of sigmoid colon · CC POA CC/MCC Exc
  - ⑦ **S36.518** Primary blast injury of other part of colon · CC POA CC/MCC Exc
  - ⑦ **S36.519** Primary blast injury of unspecified part of colon · CC POA CC/MCC Exc
- ⑥ **S36.52** Contusion of colon
  - ⑦ **S36.520** Contusion of ascending [right] colon · CC POA CC/MCC Exc
  - ⑦ **S36.521** Contusion of transverse colon · CC POA CC/MCC Exc
  - ⑦ **S36.522** Contusion of descending [left] colon · CC POA CC/MCC Exc
  - ⑦ **S36.523** Contusion of sigmoid colon · CC POA CC/MCC Exc
  - ⑦ **S36.528** Contusion of other part of colon · CC POA CC/MCC Exc
  - ⑦ **S36.529** Contusion of unspecified part of colon · CC POA CC/MCC Exc
- ⑥ **S36.53** Laceration of colon
  - ⑦ **S36.530** Laceration of ascending [right] colon · CC POA CC/MCC Exc
  - ⑦ **S36.531** Laceration of transverse colon · CC POA CC/MCC Exc
  - ⑦ **S36.532** Laceration of descending [left] colon · CC POA CC/MCC Exc
  - ⑦ **S36.533** Laceration of sigmoid colon · CC POA CC/MCC Exc
  - ⑦ **S36.538** Laceration of other part of colon · CC POA CC/MCC Exc
  - ⑦ **S36.539** Laceration of unspecified part of colon · CC POA CC/MCC Exc
- ⑥ **S36.59** Other injury of colon
  Secondary blast injury of colon

- ⑦ **S36.590** Other injury of ascending [right] colon · CC POA CC/MCC Exc
- ⑦ **S36.591** Other injury of transverse colon · CC POA CC/MCC Exc
- ⑦ **S36.592** Other injury of descending [left] colon · CC POA CC/MCC Exc
- ⑦ **S36.593** Other injury of sigmoid colon · CC POA CC/MCC Exc
- ⑦ **S36.598** Other injury of other part of colon · CC POA CC/MCC Exc
- ⑦ **S36.599** Other injury of unspecified part of colon · CC POA CC/MCC Exc

⑤ **S36.6** Injury of rectum
- ⑦ **S36.60** Unspecified injury of rectum · CC POA CC/MCC Exc
- ⑦ **S36.61** Primary blast injury of rectum · CC POA CC/MCC Exc
  Blast injury of rectum NOS
- ⑦ **S36.62** Contusion of rectum · CC POA CC/MCC Exc
- ⑦ **S36.63** Laceration of rectum · CC POA CC/MCC Exc
- ⑦ **S36.69** Other injury of rectum · CC POA CC/MCC Exc
  Secondary blast injury of rectum

⑤ **S36.8** Injury of other intra-abdominal organs
- ⑦ **S36.81** Injury of peritoneum · CC POA CC/MCC Exc
- ⑥ **S36.89** Injury of other intra-abdominal organs
  Injury of retroperitoneum
  - ⑦ **S36.892** Contusion of other intra-abdominal organs · CC POA CC/MCC Exc
  - ⑦ **S36.893** Laceration of other intra-abdominal organs · CC POA CC/MCC Exc
  - ⑦ **S36.898** Other injury of other intra-abdominal organs · CC POA CC/MCC Exc
  - ⑦ **S36.899** Unspecified injury of other intra-abdominal organs · CC POA CC/MCC Exc

⑤ **S36.9** Injury of unspecified intra-abdominal organ
- ⑦ **S36.90** Unspecified injury of unspecified intra-abdominal organ · CC POA CC/MCC Exc
- ⑦ **S36.92** Contusion of unspecified intra-abdominal organ · CC POA CC/MCC Exc
- ⑦ **S36.93** Laceration of unspecified intra-abdominal organ · CC POA CC/MCC Exc
- ⑦ **S36.99** Other injury of unspecified intra-abdominal organ · CC POA CC/MCC Exc

④ **S37** Injury of urinary and pelvic organs
  Code also any associated open wound (S31.-)
  EXCLUDES1 obstetric trauma to pelvic organs (O71.-)
  EXCLUDES2 injury of peritoneum (S36.81)
    injury of retroperitoneum (S36.89-)
  The appropriate 7th character is to be added to each code from category S37
  A = initial encounter
  D = subsequent encounter
  S = sequela

⑤ **S37.0** Injury of kidney
  EXCLUDES2 acute kidney injury (nontraumatic) (N17.9)
- ⑥ **S37.00** Unspecified injury of kidney
  - ⑦ **S37.001** Unspecified injury of right kidney · CC POA CC/MCC Exc
  - ⑦ **S37.002** Unspecified injury of left kidney · CC POA CC/MCC Exc
  - ⑦ **S37.009** Unspecified injury of unspecified kidney · CC POA CC/MCC Exc
- ⑥ **S37.01** Minor contusion of kidney
  Contusion of kidney less than 2 cm
  Contusion of kidney NOS
  - ⑦ **S37.011** Minor contusion of right kidney · CC POA CC/MCC Exc
  - ⑦ **S37.012** Minor contusion of left kidney · CC POA CC/MCC Exc
  - ⑦ **S37.019** Minor contusion of unspecified kidney · CC POA CC/MCC Exc
- ⑥ **S37.02** Major contusion of kidney
  Contusion of kidney greater than 2 cm
  - ⑦ **S37.021** Major contusion of right kidney · CC POA CC/MCC Exc
  - ⑦ **S37.022** Major contusion of left kidney · CC POA CC/MCC Exc
  - ⑦ **S37.029** Major contusion of unspecified kidney · CC POA CC/MCC Exc

---

Unspecified Code · Other Specified Code · Manifestation Code · N Newborn · P Pediatric · M Maternity · A Adult · ♂ Male · ♀ Female
● New Code · ▲ Revised Code Title · ▶◀ Revised Text · NOTES · INCLUDES · EXCLUDES 1 Not coded here · EXCLUDES 2 Not included here
④ 4th character required · ⑤ 5th character required · ⑥ 6th character required · ⑦ 7th character required
⑦ Extension 'X' Alert · HAC Hospital-acquired condition (HAC) alert · AHA AHA Coding Clinic©

- [7th] **S40.219 Abrasion of unspecified shoulder** [POA]
- [6th] **S40.22** Blister **(nonthermal) of shoulder**
  - [7th] **S40.221 Blister (nonthermal) of** right **shoulder** [POA]
  - [7th] **S40.222 Blister (nonthermal) of** left **shoulder** [POA]
  - [7th] **S40.229 Blister (nonthermal) of unspecified shoulder** [POA]
- [6th] **S40.24** External constriction **of shoulder**
  - [7th] **S40.241 External constriction of** right **shoulder** [POA]
  - [7th] **S40.242 External constriction of** left **shoulder** [POA]
  - [7th] **S40.249 External constriction of unspecified shoulder** [POA]
- [6th] **S40.25** Superficial foreign body **of shoulder**
  - Splinter in the shoulder
  - [7th] **S40.251 Superficial foreign body of** right **shoulder** [POA]
  - [7th] **S40.252 Superficial foreign body of** left **shoulder** [POA]
  - [7th] **S40.259 Superficial foreign body of unspecified shoulder** [POA]
- [6th] **S40.26** Insect bite **(nonvenomous) of shoulder**
  - [7th] **S40.261 Insect bite (nonvenomous) of** right **shoulder** [POA]
  - [7th] **S40.262 Insect bite (nonvenomous) of** left **shoulder** [POA]
  - [7th] **S40.269 Insect bite (nonvenomous) of unspecified shoulder** [POA]
- [6th] **S40.27 Other superficial bite of shoulder**
  - [EXCLUDES1] *open bite of shoulder (S41.05)*
  - [7th] **S40.271 Other superficial bite of** right **shoulder** [POA]
  - [7th] **S40.272 Other superficial bite of** left **shoulder** [POA]
  - [7th] **S40.279 Other superficial bite of unspecified shoulder** [POA]

[5th] **S40.8 Other superficial injuries of upper arm**
- [6th] **S40.81** Abrasion **of upper arm**
  - [7th] **S40.811 Abrasion of** right **upper arm** [POA]
  - [7th] **S40.812 Abrasion of** left **upper arm** [POA]
  - [7th] **S40.819 Abrasion of unspecified upper arm** [POA]
- [6th] **S40.82** Blister **(nonthermal) of upper arm**
  - [7th] **S40.821 Blister (nonthermal) of** right **upper arm** [POA]
  - [7th] **S40.822 Blister (nonthermal) of** left **upper arm** [POA]
  - [7th] **S40.829 Blister (nonthermal) of unspecified upper arm** [POA]
- [6th] **S40.84** External constriction **of upper arm**
  - [7th] **S40.841 External constriction of** right **upper arm** [POA]
  - [7th] **S40.842 External constriction of** left **upper arm** [POA]
  - [7th] **S40.849 External constriction of unspecified upper arm** [POA]
- [6th] **S40.85** Superficial foreign body **of upper arm**
  - Splinter in the upper arm
  - [7th] **S40.851 Superficial foreign body of** right **upper arm** [POA]
  - [7th] **S40.852 Superficial foreign body of** left **upper arm** [POA]
  - [7th] **S40.859 Superficial foreign body of unspecified upper arm** [POA]
- [6th] **S40.86** Insect bite **(nonvenomous) of upper arm**
  - [7th] **S40.861 Insect bite (nonvenomous) of** right **upper arm** [POA]
  - [7th] **S40.862 Insect bite (nonvenomous) of** left **upper arm** [POA]
  - [7th] **S40.869 Insect bite (nonvenomous) of unspecified upper arm** [POA]
- [6th] **S40.87** Other **superficial bite of upper arm**
  - [EXCLUDES1] *open bite of upper arm (S41.14)*
  - [EXCLUDES2] *other superficial bite of shoulder (S40.27-)*
  - [7th] **S40.871 Other superficial bite of** right **upper arm** [POA]
  - [7th] **S40.872 Other superficial bite of** left **upper arm** [POA]
  - [7th] **S40.879 Other superficial bite of unspecified upper arm** [POA]

[5th] **S40.9 Unspecified superficial injury of shoulder and upper arm**
- [6th] **S40.91** Unspecified **superficial injury of shoulder**
  - [7th] **S40.911 Unspecified superficial injury of** right **shoulder** [POA]
  - [7th] **S40.912 Unspecified superficial injury of** left **shoulder** [POA]
  - [7th] **S40.919 Unspecified superficial injury of unspecified shoulder** [POA]
- [6th] **S40.92 Unspecified superficial injury of upper arm**
  - [7th] **S40.921 Unspecified superficial injury of** right **upper arm** [POA]
  - [7th] **S40.922 Unspecified superficial injury of** left **upper arm** [POA]
  - [7th] **S40.929 Unspecified superficial injury of unspecified upper arm** [POA]

[4th] **S41 Open wound of shoulder and upper arm**

Code also any associated wound infection

[EXCLUDES1] *traumatic amputation of shoulder and upper arm (S48.-)*

[EXCLUDES2] *open fracture of shoulder and upper arm (S42.- with 7th character B or C)*

The appropriate 7th character is to be added to each code from category S41
- **A = initial encounter**
- **D = subsequent encounter**
- **S = sequela**

[5th] **S41.0 Open wound of** shoulder
- [6th] **S41.00** Unspecified **open wound of shoulder**
  - [7th] **S41.001 Unspecified open wound of** right **shoulder** [POA]
  - [7th] **S41.002 Unspecified open wound of** left **shoulder** [POA]
  - [7th] **S41.009 Unspecified open wound of unspecified shoulder** [POA]
- [6th] **S41.01** Laceration without foreign body **of shoulder**
  - [7th] **S41.011 Laceration without foreign body of** right **shoulder** [POA]
  - [7th] **S41.012 Laceration without foreign body of** left **shoulder** [POA]
  - [7th] **S41.019 Laceration without foreign body of unspecified shoulder** [POA]
- [6th] **S41.02** Laceration with foreign body **of shoulder**
  - [7th] **S41.021 Laceration with foreign body of** right **shoulder** [POA]
  - [7th] **S41.022 Laceration with foreign body of** left **shoulder** [POA]
  - [7th] **S41.029 Laceration with foreign body of unspecified shoulder** [POA]
- [6th] **S41.03** Puncture wound without foreign body **of shoulder**
  - [7th] **S41.031 Puncture wound without foreign body of** right **shoulder** [POA]
  - [7th] **S41.032 Puncture wound without foreign body of** left **shoulder** [POA]
  - [7th] **S41.039 Puncture wound without foreign body of unspecified shoulder** [POA]
- [6th] **S41.04** Puncture wound with foreign body **of shoulder**
  - [7th] **S41.041 Puncture wound with foreign body of** right **shoulder** [POA]
  - [7th] **S41.042 Puncture wound with foreign body of** left **shoulder** [POA]
  - [7th] **S41.049 Puncture wound with foreign body of unspecified shoulder** [POA]
- [6th] **S41.05** Open bite **of shoulder**
  - Bite of shoulder NOS
  - [EXCLUDES1] *superficial bite of shoulder (S40.27)*
  - [7th] **S41.051 Open bite of** right **shoulder** [POA]
  - [7th] **S41.052 Open bite of** left **shoulder** [POA]
  - [7th] **S41.059 Open bite of unspecified shoulder** [POA]

[5th] **S41.1 Open wound of** upper arm
- [6th] **S41.10** Unspecified **open wound of upper arm**
  - [7th] **S41.101 Unspecified open wound of** right **upper arm** [POA]
  - [7th] **S41.102 Unspecified open wound of** left **upper arm** [POA]

[PDx] Unacceptable principal diagnosis symbol per Medicare code edits [POA] Code exempt from diagnosis present on admission requirement [?] Questionable admission [CC] Complication or comorbidity [CC/MCC Exc] CC/MCC exclusion [MCC] Major complication or comorbidity [PDx CC] Principal diagnosis as its own CC [PDx MCC] Principal diagnosis as its own MCC [HCC] HCC diagnosis code [RxHCC] RxHCC diagnosis code MACRA code [Z] Z code as first-listed diagnosis

When symbols appear on a code that requires a 7th character extension, refer to Appendix B to identify applicable 7th character codes.

[7th] S41.109 Unspecified open wound of unspecified upper arm [POA]

[6th] S41.11 Laceration without foreign body of upper arm
- [7th] S41.111 Laceration without foreign body of right upper arm [POA]
- [7th] S41.112 Laceration without foreign body of left upper arm [POA]
- [7th] S41.119 Laceration without foreign body of unspecified upper arm [POA]

[6th] S41.12 Laceration with foreign body of upper arm
- [7th] S41.121 Laceration with foreign body of right upper arm [POA]
- [7th] S41.122 Laceration with foreign body of left upper arm [POA]
- [7th] S41.129 Laceration with foreign body of unspecified upper arm [POA]

[6th] S41.13 Puncture wound without foreign body of upper arm
- [7th] S41.131 Puncture wound without foreign body of right upper arm [POA]
- [7th] S41.132 Puncture wound without foreign body of left upper arm [POA]
- [7th] S41.139 Puncture wound without foreign body of unspecified upper arm [POA]

[6th] S41.14 Puncture wound with foreign body of upper arm
- [7th] S41.141 Puncture wound with foreign body of right upper arm [POA]
- [7th] S41.142 Puncture wound with foreign body of left upper arm [POA]
- [7th] S41.149 Puncture wound with foreign body of unspecified upper arm [POA]

[6th] S41.15 Open bite of upper arm

Bite of upper arm NOS

[EXCLUDES1] *superficial bite of upper arm (S40.87)*

- [7th] S41.151 Open bite of right upper arm [POA]
- [7th] S41.152 Open bite of left upper arm [POA]
- [7th] S41.159 Open bite of unspecified upper arm [POA]

[4th] **S42 Fracture of shoulder and upper arm**

[NOTES] A fracture not indicated as displaced or nondisplaced should be coded to displaced

A fracture not indicated as open or closed should be coded to closed

[EXCLUDES1] *traumatic amputation of shoulder and upper arm (S48.-)*

The appropriate 7th character is to be added to all codes from category S42

- A = initial encounter for closed fracture
- B = initial encounter for open fracture
- D = subsequent encounter for fracture with routine healing
- G = subsequent encounter for fracture with delayed healing
- K = subsequent encounter for fracture with nonunion
- P = subsequent encounter for fracture with malunion
- S = sequela

[5th] S42.0 Fracture of clavicle

[6th] S42.00 Fracture of unspecified part of clavicle
- [7th] S42.001 Fracture of unspecified part of right clavicle [CC] [POA] [HAC] [CC/MCC Exc]
- [7th] S42.002 Fracture of unspecified part of left clavicle [CC] [POA] [HAC] [CC/MCC Exc]
- [7th] S42.009 Fracture of unspecified part of unspecified clavicle [CC] [POA] [HAC] [CC/MCC Exc]

[6th] S42.01 Fracture of sternal end of clavicle
- [7th] S42.011 Anterior displaced fracture of sternal end of right clavicle [CC] [POA] [HAC] [CC/MCC Exc]
- [7th] S42.012 Anterior displaced fracture of sternal end of left clavicle [CC] [POA] [HAC] [CC/MCC Exc]
- [7th] S42.013 Anterior displaced fracture of sternal end of unspecified clavicle [CC] [POA] [HAC] [CC/MCC Exc]
  Displaced fracture of sternal end of clavicle NOS
- [7th] S42.014 Posterior displaced fracture of sternal end of right clavicle [CC] [POA] [HAC] [CC/MCC Exc]
- [7th] S42.015 Posterior displaced fracture of sternal end of left clavicle [CC] [POA] [HAC] [CC/MCC Exc]
- [7th] S42.016 Posterior displaced fracture of sternal end of unspecified clavicle [CC] [POA] [HAC] [CC/MCC Exc]
- [7th] S42.017 Nondisplaced fracture of sternal end of right clavicle [CC] [POA] [HAC] [CC/MCC Exc]
- [7th] S42.018 Nondisplaced fracture of sternal end of left clavicle [CC] [POA] [HAC] [CC/MCC Exc]
- [7th] S42.019 Nondisplaced fracture of sternal end of unspecified clavicle [CC] [POA] [HAC] [CC/MCC Exc]

[6th] S42.02 Fracture of shaft of clavicle
- [7th] S42.021 Displaced fracture of shaft of right clavicle [CC] [POA] [HAC] [CC/MCC Exc]
- [7th] S42.022 Displaced fracture of shaft of left clavicle [CC] [POA] [HAC] [CC/MCC Exc]
- [7th] S42.023 Displaced fracture of shaft of unspecified clavicle [CC] [POA] [HAC] [CC/MCC Exc]
- [7th] S42.024 Nondisplaced fracture of shaft of right clavicle [CC] [POA] [HAC] [CC/MCC Exc]
- [7th] S42.025 Nondisplaced fracture of shaft of left clavicle [CC] [POA] [HAC] [CC/MCC Exc]
- [7th] S42.026 Nondisplaced fracture of shaft of unspecified clavicle [CC] [POA] [HAC] [CC/MCC Exc]

[6th] S42.03 Fracture of lateral end of clavicle

Fracture of acromial end of clavicle
- [7th] S42.031 Displaced fracture of lateral end of right clavicle [CC] [POA] [HAC] [CC/MCC Exc]
- [7th] S42.032 Displaced fracture of lateral end of left clavicle [CC] [POA] [HAC] [CC/MCC Exc]
- [7th] S42.033 Displaced fracture of lateral end of unspecified clavicle [CC] [POA] [HAC] [CC/MCC Exc]
- [7th] S42.034 Nondisplaced fracture of lateral end of right clavicle [CC] [POA] [HAC] [CC/MCC Exc]
- [7th] S42.035 Nondisplaced fracture of lateral end of left clavicle [CC] [POA] [HAC] [CC/MCC Exc]
- [7th] S42.036 Nondisplaced fracture of lateral end of unspecified clavicle [CC] [POA] [HAC] [CC/MCC Exc]

[5th] S42.1 Fracture of scapula

[6th] S42.10 Fracture of unspecified part of scapula
- [7th] S42.101 Fracture of unspecified part of scapula, right shoulder [CC] [POA] [HAC] [CC/MCC Exc]
- [7th] S42.102 Fracture of unspecified part of scapula, left shoulder [CC] [POA] [HAC] [CC/MCC Exc]
- [7th] S42.109 Fracture of unspecified part of scapula, unspecified shoulder [CC] [POA] [HAC] [CC/MCC Exc]

[6th] S42.11 Fracture of body of scapula
- [7th] S42.111 Displaced fracture of body of scapula, right shoulder [CC] [POA] [HAC] [CC/MCC Exc]
- [7th] S42.112 Displaced fracture of body of scapula, left shoulder [CC] [POA] [HAC] [CC/MCC Exc]
- [7th] S42.113 Displaced fracture of body of scapula, unspecified shoulder [CC] [POA] [HAC] [CC/MCC Exc]
- [7th] S42.114 Nondisplaced fracture of body of scapula, right shoulder [CC] [POA] [HAC] [CC/MCC Exc]
- [7th] S42.115 Nondisplaced fracture of body of scapula, left shoulder [CC] [POA] [HAC] [CC/MCC Exc]
- [7th] S42.116 Nondisplaced fracture of body of scapula, unspecified shoulder [CC] [POA] [HAC] [CC/MCC Exc]

[6th] S42.12 Fracture of acromial process
- [7th] S42.121 Displaced fracture of acromial process, right shoulder [CC] [POA] [HAC] [CC/MCC Exc]
- [7th] S42.122 Displaced fracture of acromial process, left shoulder [CC] [POA] [HAC] [CC/MCC Exc]
- [7th] S42.123 Displaced fracture of acromial process, unspecified shoulder [CC] [POA] [HAC] [CC/MCC Exc]
- [7th] S42.124 Nondisplaced fracture of acromial process, right shoulder [CC] [POA] [HAC] [CC/MCC Exc]
- [7th] S42.125 Nondisplaced fracture of acromial process, left shoulder [CC] [POA] [HAC] [CC/MCC Exc]
- [7th] S42.126 Nondisplaced fracture of acromial process, unspecified shoulder [CC] [POA] [HAC] [CC/MCC Exc]

[6th] S42.13 Fracture of coracoid process

- 7ᵗʰ **S42.131** Displaced fracture of coracoid process, right shoulder `CC` `POA` `HAC` `CC/MCC Exc`
- 7ᵗʰ **S42.132** Displaced fracture of coracoid process, left shoulder `CC` `POA` `HAC` `CC/MCC Exc`
- 7ᵗʰ **S42.133** Displaced fracture of coracoid process, unspecified shoulder `CC` `POA` `HAC` `CC/MCC Exc`
- 7ᵗʰ **S42.134** Nondisplaced fracture of coracoid process, right shoulder `CC` `POA` `HAC` `CC/MCC Exc`
- 7ᵗʰ **S42.135** Nondisplaced fracture of coracoid process, left shoulder `CC` `POA` `HAC` `CC/MCC Exc`
- 7ᵗʰ **S42.136** Nondisplaced fracture of coracoid process, unspecified shoulder `CC` `POA` `HAC` `CC/MCC Exc`

6ᵗʰ **S42.14** Fracture of glenoid cavity of scapula
- 7ᵗʰ **S42.141** Displaced fracture of glenoid cavity of scapula, right shoulder `CC` `POA` `HAC` `CC/MCC Exc`
- 7ᵗʰ **S42.142** Displaced fracture of glenoid cavity of scapula, left shoulder `CC` `POA` `HAC` `CC/MCC Exc`
- 7ᵗʰ **S42.143** Displaced fracture of glenoid cavity of scapula, unspecified shoulder `CC` `POA` `HAC` `CC/MCC Exc`
- 7ᵗʰ **S42.144** Nondisplaced fracture of glenoid cavity of scapula, right shoulder `CC` `POA` `HAC` `CC/MCC Exc`
- 7ᵗʰ **S42.145** Nondisplaced fracture of glenoid cavity of scapula, left shoulder `CC` `POA` `HAC` `CC/MCC Exc`
- 7ᵗʰ **S42.146** Nondisplaced fracture of glenoid cavity of scapula, unspecified shoulder `CC` `POA` `HAC` `CC/MCC Exc`

6ᵗʰ **S42.15** Fracture of neck of scapula
- 7ᵗʰ **S42.151** Displaced fracture of neck of scapula, right shoulder `CC` `POA` `HAC` `CC/MCC Exc`
- 7ᵗʰ **S42.152** Displaced fracture of neck of scapula, left shoulder `CC` `POA` `HAC` `CC/MCC Exc`
- 7ᵗʰ **S42.153** Displaced fracture of neck of scapula, unspecified shoulder `CC` `POA` `HAC` `CC/MCC Exc`
- 7ᵗʰ **S42.154** Nondisplaced fracture of neck of scapula, right shoulder `CC` `POA` `HAC` `CC/MCC Exc`
- 7ᵗʰ **S42.155** Nondisplaced fracture of neck of scapula, left shoulder `CC` `POA` `HAC` `CC/MCC Exc`
- 7ᵗʰ **S42.156** Nondisplaced fracture of neck of scapula, unspecified shoulder `CC` `POA` `HAC` `CC/MCC Exc`

6ᵗʰ **S42.19** Fracture of other part of scapula
- 7ᵗʰ **S42.191** Fracture of other part of scapula, right shoulder `CC` `POA` `HAC` `CC/MCC Exc`
- 7ᵗʰ **S42.192** Fracture of other part of scapula, left shoulder `CC` `POA` `HAC` `CC/MCC Exc`
- 7ᵗʰ **S42.199** Fracture of other part of scapula, unspecified shoulder `CC` `POA` `HAC` `CC/MCC Exc`

5ᵗʰ **S42.2** Fracture of upper end of humerus
Fracture of proximal end of humerus
EXCLUDES2 fracture of shaft of humerus (S42.3-)
physeal fracture of upper end of humerus (S49.0-)

6ᵗʰ **S42.20** Unspecified fracture of upper end of humerus
- 7ᵗʰ **S42.201** Unspecified fracture of upper end of right humerus `CC` `POA` `HAC` `MCC` `CC/MCC Exc`
- 7ᵗʰ **S42.202** Unspecified fracture of upper end of left humerus `CC` `POA` `HAC` `MCC` `CC/MCC Exc`
- 7ᵗʰ **S42.209** Unspecified fracture of upper end of unspecified humerus `CC` `POA` `HAC` `MCC` `CC/MCC Exc`

6ᵗʰ **S42.21** Unspecified fracture of surgical neck of humerus
Fracture of neck of humerus NOS
- 7ᵗʰ **S42.211** Unspecified displaced fracture of surgical neck of right humerus `CC` `POA` `HAC` `MCC` `CC/MCC Exc`
- 7ᵗʰ **S42.212** Unspecified displaced fracture of surgical neck of left humerus `CC` `POA` `HAC` `MCC` `CC/MCC Exc`
- 7ᵗʰ **S42.213** Unspecified displaced fracture of surgical neck of unspecified humerus `CC` `POA` `HAC` `MCC` `CC/MCC Exc`
- 7ᵗʰ **S42.214** Unspecified nondisplaced fracture of surgical neck of right humerus `CC` `POA` `HAC` `MCC` `CC/MCC Exc`
- 7ᵗʰ **S42.215** Unspecified nondisplaced fracture of surgical neck of left humerus `CC` `POA` `HAC` `MCC` `CC/MCC Exc`
- 7ᵗʰ **S42.216** Unspecified nondisplaced fracture of surgical neck of unspecified humerus `CC` `POA` `HAC` `MCC` `CC/MCC Exc`

6ᵗʰ **S42.22** 2-part fracture of surgical neck of humerus
- 7ᵗʰ **S42.221** 2-part displaced fracture of surgical neck of right humerus `CC` `POA` `HAC` `MCC` `CC/MCC Exc`
- 7ᵗʰ **S42.222** 2-part displaced fracture of surgical neck of left humerus `CC` `POA` `HAC` `MCC` `CC/MCC Exc`
- 7ᵗʰ **S42.223** 2-part displaced fracture of surgical neck of unspecified humerus `CC` `POA` `HAC` `MCC` `CC/MCC Exc`
- 7ᵗʰ **S42.224** 2-part nondisplaced fracture of surgical neck of right humerus `CC` `POA` `HAC` `MCC` `CC/MCC Exc`
- 7ᵗʰ **S42.225** 2-part nondisplaced fracture of surgical neck of left humerus `CC` `POA` `HAC` `MCC` `CC/MCC Exc`
- 7ᵗʰ **S42.226** 2-part nondisplaced fracture of surgical neck of unspecified humerus `CC` `POA` `HAC` `MCC` `CC/MCC Exc`

6ᵗʰ **S42.23** 3-part fracture of surgical neck of humerus
- 7ᵗʰ **S42.231** 3-part fracture of surgical neck of right humerus `CC` `POA` `HAC` `MCC` `CC/MCC Exc`
- 7ᵗʰ **S42.232** 3-part fracture of surgical neck of left humerus `CC` `POA` `HAC` `MCC` `CC/MCC Exc`
- 7ᵗʰ **S42.239** 3-part fracture of surgical neck of unspecified humerus `CC` `POA` `HAC` `MCC` `CC/MCC Exc`

6ᵗʰ **S42.24** 4-part fracture of surgical neck of humerus
- 7ᵗʰ **S42.241** 4-part fracture of surgical neck of right humerus `CC` `POA` `HAC` `MCC` `CC/MCC Exc`
- 7ᵗʰ **S42.242** 4-part fracture of surgical neck of left humerus `CC` `POA` `HAC` `MCC` `CC/MCC Exc`
- 7ᵗʰ **S42.249** 4-part fracture of surgical neck of unspecified humerus `CC` `POA` `HAC` `MCC` `CC/MCC Exc`

6ᵗʰ **S42.25** Fracture of greater tuberosity of humerus
- 7ᵗʰ **S42.251** Displaced fracture of greater tuberosity of right humerus `CC` `POA` `HAC` `MCC` `CC/MCC Exc`
- 7ᵗʰ **S42.252** Displaced fracture of greater tuberosity of left humerus `CC` `POA` `HAC` `MCC` `CC/MCC Exc`
- 7ᵗʰ **S42.253** Displaced fracture of greater tuberosity of unspecified humerus `CC` `POA` `HAC` `MCC` `CC/MCC Exc`
- 7ᵗʰ **S42.254** Nondisplaced fracture of greater tuberosity of right humerus `CC` `POA` `HAC` `MCC` `CC/MCC Exc`
- 7ᵗʰ **S42.255** Nondisplaced fracture of greater tuberosity of left humerus `CC` `POA` `HAC` `MCC` `CC/MCC Exc`
- 7ᵗʰ **S42.256** Nondisplaced fracture of greater tuberosity of unspecified humerus `CC` `POA` `HAC` `MCC` `CC/MCC Exc`

6ᵗʰ **S42.26** Fracture of lesser tuberosity of humerus
- 7ᵗʰ **S42.261** Displaced fracture of lesser tuberosity of right humerus `CC` `POA` `HAC` `MCC` `CC/MCC Exc`
- 7ᵗʰ **S42.262** Displaced fracture of lesser tuberosity of left humerus `CC` `POA` `HAC` `MCC` `CC/MCC Exc`
- 7ᵗʰ **S42.263** Displaced fracture of lesser tuberosity of unspecified humerus `CC` `POA` `HAC` `MCC` `CC/MCC Exc`
- 7ᵗʰ **S42.264** Nondisplaced fracture of lesser tuberosity of right humerus `CC` `POA` `HAC` `MCC` `CC/MCC Exc`
- 7ᵗʰ **S42.265** Nondisplaced fracture of lesser tuberosity of left humerus `CC` `POA` `HAC` `MCC` `CC/MCC Exc`
- 7ᵗʰ **S42.266** Nondisplaced fracture of lesser tuberosity of unspecified humerus `CC` `POA` `HAC` `MCC` `CC/MCC Exc`

6ᵗʰ **S42.27** Torus fracture of upper end of humerus
The appropriate 7th character is to be added to all codes in subcategory S42.27
  A = initial encounter for closed fracture
  D = subsequent encounter for fracture with routine healing
  G = subsequent encounter for fracture with delayed healing

`POA⌐` Unacceptable principal diagnosis symbol per Medicare code edits `POA` Code exempt from diagnosis present on admission requirement `?` Questionable admission `CC` Complication or comorbidity `CC/MCC Exc` CC/MCC exclusion `MCC` Major complication or comorbidity `PDx CC` Principal diagnosis as its own CC `PDx MCC` Principal diagnosis as its own MCC `HCC` HCC diagnosis code `RxHCC` RxHCC diagnosis code `MACRA` MACRA code `Z1` Z code as first-listed diagnosis

1016 When symbols appear on a code that requires a 7th character extension, refer to Appendix B to identify applicable 7th character codes. **2018 ICD-10-CM**

K = subsequent encounter for fracture with nonunion

P = subsequent encounter for fracture with malunion

S = sequela

⑦ S42.271 Torus fracture of upper end of right humerus ✓⁷ POA HAC CC/MCC Exc

⑦ S42.272 Torus fracture of upper end of left humerus ✓⁷ POA HAC CC/MCC Exc

⑦ S42.279 Torus fracture of upper end of unspecified humerus ✓⁷ POA HAC CC/MCC Exc

⑥ S42.29 Other fracture of upper end of humerus
Fracture of anatomical neck of humerus
Fracture of articular head of humerus

⑦ S42.291 Other displaced fracture of upper end of right humerus CC POA HAC MCC CC/MCC Exc

⑦ S42.292 Other displaced fracture of upper end of left humerus CC POA HAC MCC CC/MCC Exc

⑦ S42.293 Other displaced fracture of upper end of unspecified humerus CC POA HAC MCC CC/MCC Exc

⑦ S42.294 Other nondisplaced fracture of upper end of right humerus CC POA HAC MCC CC/MCC Exc

⑦ S42.295 Other nondisplaced fracture of upper end of left humerus CC POA HAC MCC CC/MCC Exc

⑦ S42.296 Other nondisplaced fracture of upper end of unspecified humerus CC POA HAC MCC CC/MCC Exc

⑤ S42.3 Fracture of shaft of humerus
Fracture of humerus NOS
Fracture of upper arm NOS
EXCLUDES2 physeal fractures of upper end of humerus (S49.0-)
physeal fractures of lower end of humerus (S49.1-)

⑥ S42.30 Unspecified fracture of shaft of humerus

⑦ S42.301 Unspecified fracture of shaft of humerus, right arm CC POA HAC MCC CC/MCC Exc

⑦ S42.302 Unspecified fracture of shaft of humerus, left arm CC POA HAC MCC CC/MCC Exc

⑦ S42.309 Unspecified fracture of shaft of humerus, unspecified arm CC POA HAC MCC CC/MCC Exc

⑥ S42.31 Greenstick fracture of shaft of humerus
The appropriate 7th character is to be added to all codes in subcategory S42.31

A = initial encounter for closed fracture

D = subsequent encounter for fracture with routine healing

G = subsequent encounter for fracture with delayed healing

K = subsequent encounter for fracture with nonunion

P = subsequent encounter for fracture with malunion

S = sequela

⑦ S42.311 Greenstick fracture of shaft of humerus, right arm CC POA HAC CC/MCC Exc

⑦ S42.312 Greenstick fracture of shaft of humerus, left arm CC POA HAC CC/MCC Exc

⑦ S42.319 Greenstick fracture of shaft of humerus, unspecified arm CC POA HAC CC/MCC Exc

⑥ S42.32 Transverse fracture of shaft of humerus

⑦ S42.321 Displaced transverse fracture of shaft of humerus, right arm CC POA HAC MCC CC/MCC Exc

⑦ S42.322 Displaced transverse fracture of shaft of humerus, left arm CC POA HAC MCC CC/MCC Exc

⑦ S42.323 Displaced transverse fracture of shaft of humerus, unspecified arm CC POA HAC MCC CC/MCC Exc

⑦ S42.324 Nondisplaced transverse fracture of shaft of humerus, right arm CC POA HAC MCC CC/MCC Exc

⑦ S42.325 Nondisplaced transverse fracture of shaft of humerus, left arm CC POA HAC MCC CC/MCC Exc

⑦ S42.326 Nondisplaced transverse fracture of shaft of humerus, unspecified arm CC POA HAC MCC CC/MCC Exc

⑥ S42.33 Oblique fracture of shaft of humerus

⑦ S42.331 Displaced oblique fracture of shaft of humerus, right arm CC POA HAC MCC CC/MCC Exc

⑦ S42.332 Displaced oblique fracture of shaft of humerus, left arm CC POA HAC MCC CC/MCC Exc

⑦ S42.333 Displaced oblique fracture of shaft of humerus, unspecified arm CC POA HAC MCC CC/MCC Exc

⑦ S42.334 Nondisplaced oblique fracture of shaft of humerus, right arm CC POA HAC MCC CC/MCC Exc

⑦ S42.335 Nondisplaced oblique fracture of shaft of humerus, left arm CC POA HAC MCC CC/MCC Exc

⑦ S42.336 Nondisplaced oblique fracture of shaft of humerus, unspecified arm CC POA HAC MCC CC/MCC Exc

⑥ S42.34 Spiral fracture of shaft of humerus

⑦ S42.341 Displaced spiral fracture of shaft of humerus, right arm CC POA HAC MCC CC/MCC Exc

⑦ S42.342 Displaced spiral fracture of shaft of humerus, left arm CC POA HAC MCC CC/MCC Exc

⑦ S42.343 Displaced spiral fracture of shaft of humerus, unspecified arm CC POA HAC MCC CC/MCC Exc

⑦ S42.344 Nondisplaced spiral fracture of shaft of humerus, right arm CC POA HAC MCC CC/MCC Exc

⑦ S42.345 Nondisplaced spiral fracture of shaft of humerus, left arm CC POA HAC MCC CC/MCC Exc

⑦ S42.346 Nondisplaced spiral fracture of shaft of humerus, unspecified arm CC POA HAC MCC CC/MCC Exc

⑥ S42.35 Comminuted fracture of shaft of humerus

⑦ S42.351 Displaced comminuted fracture of shaft of humerus, right arm CC POA HAC MCC CC/MCC Exc

⑦ S42.352 Displaced comminuted fracture of shaft of humerus, left arm CC POA HAC MCC CC/MCC Exc

⑦ S42.353 Displaced comminuted fracture of shaft of humerus, unspecified arm CC POA HAC MCC CC/MCC Exc

⑦ S42.354 Nondisplaced comminuted fracture of shaft of humerus, right arm CC POA HAC MCC CC/MCC Exc

⑦ S42.355 Nondisplaced comminuted fracture of shaft of humerus, left arm CC POA HAC MCC CC/MCC Exc

⑦ S42.356 Nondisplaced comminuted fracture of shaft of humerus, unspecified arm CC POA HAC MCC CC/MCC Exc

⑥ S42.36 Segmental fracture of shaft of humerus

⑦ S42.361 Displaced segmental fracture of shaft of humerus, right arm CC POA HAC MCC CC/MCC Exc

⑦ S42.362 Displaced segmental fracture of shaft of humerus, left arm CC POA HAC MCC CC/MCC Exc

⑦ S42.363 Displaced segmental fracture of shaft of humerus, unspecified arm CC POA HAC MCC CC/MCC Exc

⑦ S42.364 Nondisplaced segmental fracture of shaft of humerus, right arm CC POA HAC MCC CC/MCC Exc

⑦ S42.365 Nondisplaced segmental fracture of shaft of humerus, left arm CC POA HAC MCC CC/MCC Exc

⑦ S42.366 Nondisplaced segmental fracture of shaft of humerus, unspecified arm CC POA HAC MCC CC/MCC Exc

⑥ S42.39 Other fracture of shaft of humerus

⑦ S42.391 Other fracture of shaft of right humerus CC POA HAC MCC CC/MCC Exc

⑦ S42.392 Other fracture of shaft of left humerus CC POA HAC MCC CC/MCC Exc

⑦ S42.399 Other fracture of shaft of unspecified humerus CC POA HAC MCC CC/MCC Exc

Unspecified Code	Other Specified Code	Manifestation Code	N Newborn	P Pediatric	M Maternity	A Adult	♂ Male	♀ Female

● New Code ▲ Revised Code Title ▶◀ Revised Text **NOTES** *INCLUDES* *EXCLUDES 1* Not coded here *EXCLUDES 2* Not included here

④ 4th character required ⑤ 5th character required ⑥ 6th character required ⑦ 7th character required

⑦ Extension 'X' Alert HAC Hospital-acquired condition (HAC) alert **AHA** AHA Coding Clinic©

S42.4 Fracture of lower end of humerus
Fracture of distal end of humerus
EXCLUDES2 fracture of shaft of humerus (S42.3-)
physeal fracture of lower end of humerus (S49.1-)

S42.40 Unspecified fracture of lower end of humerus
Fracture of elbow NOS

S42.401 Unspecified fracture of lower end of right humerus cc̊ pöa̋ HAC mcc̊ cc/mcc Exc

S42.402 Unspecified fracture of lower end of left humerus cc̊ pöa̋ HAC mcc̊ cc/mcc Exc

S42.409 Unspecified fracture of lower end of unspecified humerus cc̊ pöa̋ HAC mcc̊ cc/mcc Exc

S42.41 Simple supracondylar fracture without intercondylar fracture of humerus

S42.411 Displaced simple supracondylar fracture without intercondylar fracture of right humerus cc̊ pöa̋ HAC mcc̊ cc/mcc Exc

S42.412 Displaced simple supracondylar fracture without intercondylar fracture of left humerus cc̊ pöa̋ HAC mcc̊ cc/mcc Exc

S42.413 Displaced simple supracondylar fracture without intercondylar fracture of unspecified humerus cc̊ pöa̋ HAC mcc̊ cc/mcc Exc

S42.414 Nondisplaced simple supracondylar fracture without intercondylar fracture of right humerus cc̊ pöa̋ HAC mcc̊ cc/mcc Exc

S42.415 Nondisplaced simple supracondylar fracture without intercondylar fracture of left humerus cc̊ pöa̋ HAC mcc̊ cc/mcc Exc

S42.416 Nondisplaced simple supracondylar fracture without intercondylar fracture of unspecified humerus cc̊ pöa̋ HAC mcc̊ cc/mcc Exc

S42.42 Comminuted supracondylar fracture without intercondylar fracture of humerus

S42.421 Displaced comminuted supracondylar fracture without intercondylar fracture of right humerus cc̊ pöa̋ HAC mcc̊ cc/mcc Exc

S42.422 Displaced comminuted supracondylar fracture without intercondylar fracture of left humerus cc̊ pöa̋ HAC mcc̊ cc/mcc Exc

S42.423 Displaced comminuted supracondylar fracture without intercondylar fracture of unspecified humerus cc̊ pöa̋ HAC mcc̊ cc/mcc Exc

S42.424 Nondisplaced comminuted supracondylar fracture without intercondylar fracture of right humerus cc̊ pöa̋ HAC mcc̊ cc/mcc Exc

S42.425 Nondisplaced comminuted supracondylar fracture without intercondylar fracture of left humerus cc̊ pöa̋ HAC mcc̊ cc/mcc Exc

S42.426 Nondisplaced comminuted supracondylar fracture without intercondylar fracture of unspecified humerus cc̊ pöa̋ HAC mcc̊ cc/mcc Exc

S42.43 Fracture (avulsion) of lateral epicondyle of humerus

S42.431 Displaced fracture (avulsion) of lateral epicondyle of right humerus cc̊ pöa̋ HAC mcc̊ cc/mcc Exc

S42.432 Displaced fracture (avulsion) of lateral epicondyle of left humerus cc̊ pöa̋ HAC mcc̊ cc/mcc Exc

S42.433 Displaced fracture (avulsion) of lateral epicondyle of unspecified humerus cc̊ pöa̋ HAC mcc̊ cc/mcc Exc

S42.434 Nondisplaced fracture (avulsion) of lateral epicondyle of right humerus cc̊ pöa̋ HAC mcc̊ cc/mcc Exc

S42.435 Nondisplaced fracture (avulsion) of lateral epicondyle of left humerus cc̊ pöa̋ HAC mcc̊ cc/mcc Exc

S42.436 Nondisplaced fracture (avulsion) of lateral epicondyle of unspecified humerus cc̊ pöa̋ HAC mcc̊ cc/mcc Exc

S42.44 Fracture (avulsion) of medial epicondyle of humerus

S42.441 Displaced fracture (avulsion) of medial epicondyle of right humerus cc̊ pöa̋ HAC mcc̊ cc/mcc Exc

S42.442 Displaced fracture (avulsion) of medial epicondyle of left humerus cc̊ pöa̋ HAC mcc̊ cc/mcc Exc

S42.443 Displaced fracture (avulsion) of medial epicondyle of unspecified humerus cc̊ pöa̋ HAC mcc̊ cc/mcc Exc

S42.444 Nondisplaced fracture (avulsion) of medial epicondyle of right humerus cc̊ pöa̋ HAC mcc̊ cc/mcc Exc

S42.445 Nondisplaced fracture (avulsion) of medial epicondyle of left humerus cc̊ pöa̋ HAC mcc̊ cc/mcc Exc

S42.446 Nondisplaced fracture (avulsion) of medial epicondyle of unspecified humerus cc̊ pöa̋ HAC mcc̊ cc/mcc Exc

S42.447 Incarcerated fracture (avulsion) of medial epicondyle of right humerus cc̊ pöa̋ HAC mcc̊ cc/mcc Exc

S42.448 Incarcerated fracture (avulsion) of medial epicondyle of left humerus cc̊ pöa̋ HAC mcc̊ cc/mcc Exc

S42.449 Incarcerated fracture (avulsion) of medial epicondyle of unspecified humerus cc̊ pöa̋ HAC mcc̊ cc/mcc Exc

S42.45 Fracture of lateral condyle of humerus
Fracture of capitellum of humerus

S42.451 Displaced fracture of lateral condyle of right humerus cc̊ pöa̋ HAC mcc̊ cc/mcc Exc

S42.452 Displaced fracture of lateral condyle of left humerus cc̊ pöa̋ HAC mcc̊ cc/mcc Exc

S42.453 Displaced fracture of lateral condyle of unspecified humerus cc̊ pöa̋ HAC mcc̊ cc/mcc Exc

S42.454 Nondisplaced fracture of lateral condyle of right humerus cc̊ pöa̋ HAC mcc̊ cc/mcc Exc

S42.455 Nondisplaced fracture of lateral condyle of left humerus cc̊ pöa̋ HAC mcc̊ cc/mcc Exc

S42.456 Nondisplaced fracture of lateral condyle of unspecified humerus cc̊ pöa̋ HAC mcc̊ cc/mcc Exc

S42.46 Fracture of medial condyle of humerus
Trochlea fracture of humerus

S42.461 Displaced fracture of medial condyle of right humerus cc̊ pöa̋ HAC mcc̊ cc/mcc Exc

S42.462 Displaced fracture of medial condyle of left humerus cc̊ pöa̋ HAC mcc̊ cc/mcc Exc

S42.463 Displaced fracture of medial condyle of unspecified humerus cc̊ pöa̋ HAC mcc̊ cc/mcc Exc

S42.464 Nondisplaced fracture of medial condyle of right humerus cc̊ pöa̋ HAC mcc̊ cc/mcc Exc

S42.465 Nondisplaced fracture of medial condyle of left humerus cc̊ pöa̋ HAC mcc̊ cc/mcc Exc

S42.466 Nondisplaced fracture of medial condyle of unspecified humerus cc̊ pöa̋ HAC mcc̊ cc/mcc Exc

S42.47 Transcondylar fracture of humerus

S42.471 Displaced transcondylar fracture of right humerus cc̊ pöa̋ HAC mcc̊ cc/mcc Exc

S42.472 Displaced transcondylar fracture of left humerus cc̊ pöa̋ HAC mcc̊ cc/mcc Exc

S42.473 Displaced transcondylar fracture of unspecified humerus cc̊ pöa̋ HAC mcc̊ cc/mcc Exc

S42.474 Nondisplaced transcondylar fracture of right humerus cc̊ pöa̋ HAC mcc̊ cc/mcc Exc

S42.475 Nondisplaced transcondylar fracture of left humerus cc̊ pöa̋ HAC mcc̊ cc/mcc Exc

S42.476 Nondisplaced transcondylar fracture of unspecified humerus cc̊ pöa̋ HAC mcc̊ cc/mcc Exc

---

pöa̋ Unacceptable principal diagnosis symbol per Medicare code edits   pöa Code exempt from diagnosis present on admission requirement
? Questionable admission   cc̊ Complication or comorbidity   cc/mcc Exc CC/MCC exclusion   mcc̊ Major complication or comorbidity
Principal diagnosis as its own CC   Principal diagnosis as its own MCC   HCC HCC diagnosis code   RxHCC RxHCC diagnosis code
MACRA code   Z1 Z code as first-listed diagnosis

6ᵗʰ S42.48 Torus fracture of lower end of humerus

The appropriate 7th character is to be added to all codes in subcategory S42.48

A = initial encounter for closed fracture

D = subsequent encounter for fracture with routine healing

G = subsequent encounter for fracture with delayed healing

K = subsequent encounter for fracture with nonunion

P = subsequent encounter for fracture with malunion

S = sequela

7ᵗʰ S42.481 Torus fracture of lower end of right humerus cᶜ POA HAC CC/MCC Exc

7ᵗʰ S42.482 Torus fracture of lower end of left humerus cᶜ POA HAC CC/MCC Exc

7ᵗʰ S42.489 Torus fracture of lower end of unspecified humerus cᶜ POA HAC CC/MCC Exc

6ᵗʰ S42.49 Other fracture of lower end of humerus

7ᵗʰ S42.491 Other displaced fracture of lower end of right humerus cᶜ POA HAC MCC CC/MCC Exc

7ᵗʰ S42.492 Other displaced fracture of lower end of left humerus cᶜ POA HAC MCC CC/MCC Exc

7ᵗʰ S42.493 Other displaced fracture of lower end of unspecified humerus cᶜ POA HAC MCC CC/MCC Exc

7ᵗʰ S42.494 Other nondisplaced fracture of lower end of right humerus cᶜ POA HAC MCC CC/MCC Exc

7ᵗʰ S42.495 Other nondisplaced fracture of lower end of left humerus cᶜ POA HAC MCC CC/MCC Exc

7ᵗʰ S42.496 Other nondisplaced fracture of lower end of unspecified humerus cᶜ POA HAC MCC CC/MCC Exc

5ᵗʰ S42.9 Fracture of shoulder girdle, part unspecified

Fracture of shoulder NOS

6ᵗʰ S42.90 Fracture of unspecified shoulder girdle, part unspecified cᶜ POA HAC MCC CC/MCC Exc

6ᵗʰ S42.91 Fracture of right shoulder girdle, part unspecified cᶜ POA HAC MCC CC/MCC Exc

6ᵗʰ S42.92 Fracture of left shoulder girdle, part unspecified cᶜ POA HAC MCC CC/MCC Exc

4ᵗʰ S43 Dislocation and sprain of joints and ligaments of shoulder girdle

INCLUDES   avulsion of joint or ligament of shoulder girdle

laceration of cartilage, joint or ligament of shoulder girdle

sprain of cartilage, joint or ligament of shoulder girdle

traumatic hemarthrosis of joint or ligament of shoulder girdle

traumatic rupture of joint or ligament of shoulder girdle

traumatic subluxation of joint or ligament of shoulder girdle

traumatic tear of joint or ligament of shoulder girdle

Code also any associated open wound

EXCLUDES2 strain of muscle, fascia and tendon of shoulder and upper arm (S46.-)

The appropriate 7th character is to be added to each code from category S43

A = initial encounter

D = subsequent encounter

S = sequela

5ᵗʰ S43.0 Subluxation and dislocation of shoulder joint

Dislocation of glenohumeral joint

Subluxation of glenohumeral joint

6ᵗʰ S43.00 Unspecified subluxation and dislocation of shoulder joint

Dislocation of humerus NOS

Subluxation of humerus NOS

7ᵗʰ S43.001 Unspecified subluxation of right shoulder joint POA

7ᵗʰ S43.002 Unspecified subluxation of left shoulder joint POA

7ᵗʰ S43.003 Unspecified subluxation of unspecified shoulder joint POA

7ᵗʰ S43.004 Unspecified dislocation of right shoulder joint POA

7ᵗʰ S43.005 Unspecified dislocation of left shoulder joint POA

7ᵗʰ S43.006 Unspecified dislocation of unspecified shoulder joint POA

6ᵗʰ S43.01 Anterior subluxation and dislocation of humerus

7ᵗʰ S43.011 Anterior subluxation of right humerus POA

7ᵗʰ S43.012 Anterior subluxation of left humerus POA

7ᵗʰ S43.013 Anterior subluxation of unspecified humerus POA

7ᵗʰ S43.014 Anterior dislocation of right humerus POA

7ᵗʰ S43.015 Anterior dislocation of left humerus POA

7ᵗʰ S43.016 Anterior dislocation of unspecified humerus POA

6ᵗʰ S43.02 Posterior subluxation and dislocation of humerus

7ᵗʰ S43.021 Posterior subluxation of right humerus POA

7ᵗʰ S43.022 Posterior subluxation of left humerus POA

7ᵗʰ S43.023 Posterior subluxation of unspecified humerus POA

7ᵗʰ S43.024 Posterior dislocation of right humerus POA

7ᵗʰ S43.025 Posterior dislocation of left humerus POA

7ᵗʰ S43.026 Posterior dislocation of unspecified humerus POA

6ᵗʰ S43.03 Inferior subluxation and dislocation of humerus

7ᵗʰ S43.031 Inferior subluxation of right humerus POA

7ᵗʰ S43.032 Inferior subluxation of left humerus POA

7ᵗʰ S43.033 Inferior subluxation of unspecified humerus POA

7ᵗʰ S43.034 Inferior dislocation of right humerus POA

7ᵗʰ S43.035 Inferior dislocation of left humerus POA

7ᵗʰ S43.036 Inferior dislocation of unspecified humerus POA

6ᵗʰ S43.08 Other subluxation and dislocation of shoulder joint

7ᵗʰ S43.081 Other subluxation of right shoulder joint POA

7ᵗʰ S43.082 Other subluxation of left shoulder joint POA

7ᵗʰ S43.083 Other subluxation of unspecified shoulder joint POA

7ᵗʰ S43.084 Other dislocation of right shoulder joint POA

7ᵗʰ S43.085 Other dislocation of left shoulder joint POA

7ᵗʰ S43.086 Other dislocation of unspecified shoulder joint POA

5ᵗʰ S43.1 Subluxation and dislocation of acromioclavicular joint

6ᵗʰ S43.10 Unspecified dislocation of acromioclavicular joint

7ᵗʰ S43.101 Unspecified dislocation of right acromioclavicular joint POA

7ᵗʰ S43.102 Unspecified dislocation of left acromioclavicular joint POA

7ᵗʰ S43.109 Unspecified dislocation of unspecified acromioclavicular joint POA

6ᵗʰ S43.11 Subluxation of acromioclavicular joint

7ᵗʰ S43.111 Subluxation of right acromioclavicular joint POA

7ᵗʰ S43.112 Subluxation of left acromioclavicular joint POA

7ᵗʰ S43.119 Subluxation of unspecified acromioclavicular joint POA

6ᵗʰ S43.12 Dislocation of acromioclavicular joint, 100%-200% displacement

7ᵗʰ S43.121 Dislocation of right acromioclavicular joint, 100%-200% displacement POA

7ᵗʰ S43.122 Dislocation of left acromioclavicular joint, 100%-200% displacement POA

7ᵗʰ S43.129 Dislocation of unspecified acromioclavicular joint, 100%-200% displacement POA

6ᵗʰ S43.13 Dislocation of acromioclavicular joint, greater than 200% displacement

7ᵗʰ S43.131 Dislocation of right acromioclavicular joint, greater than 200% displacement POA

Unspecified Code   Other Specified Code   Manifestation Code   Ⓝ Newborn   Ⓟ Pediatric   Ⓜ Maternity   Ⓐ Adult   ♂ Male   ♀ Female
● New Code   ▲ Revised Code Title   ►◄ Revised Text   NOTES   INCLUDES   EXCLUDES 1 Not coded here   EXCLUDES 2 Not included here
4ᵗʰ character required   5ᵗʰ character required   6ᵗʰ character required   7ᵗʰ character required
Extension 'X' Alert   HAC Hospital-acquired condition (HAC) alert   AHA AHA Coding Clinic©

S43.132 - S43.6

CHAPTER 19: INJURY, POISONING, AND CERTAIN OTHER CONSEQUENCES OF EXTERNAL CAUSES (S00-T88)

S43.132 Dislocation of left acromioclavicular joint, greater than 200% displacement

S43.139 Dislocation of unspecified acromioclavicular joint, greater than 200% displacement

S43.14 Inferior dislocation of acromioclavicular joint
- S43.141 Inferior dislocation of right acromioclavicular joint
- S43.142 Inferior dislocation of left acromioclavicular joint
- S43.149 Inferior dislocation of unspecified acromioclavicular joint

S43.15 Posterior dislocation of acromioclavicular joint
- S43.151 Posterior dislocation of right acromioclavicular joint
- S43.152 Posterior dislocation of left acromioclavicular joint
- S43.159 Posterior dislocation of unspecified acromioclavicular joint

S43.2 Subluxation and dislocation of sternoclavicular joint

S43.20 Unspecified subluxation and dislocation of sternoclavicular joint
- S43.201 Unspecified subluxation of right sternoclavicular joint
- S43.202 Unspecified subluxation of left sternoclavicular joint
- S43.203 Unspecified subluxation of unspecified sternoclavicular joint
- S43.204 Unspecified dislocation of right sternoclavicular joint
- S43.205 Unspecified dislocation of left sternoclavicular joint
- S43.206 Unspecified dislocation of unspecified sternoclavicular joint

S43.21 Anterior subluxation and dislocation of sternoclavicular joint
- S43.211 Anterior subluxation of right sternoclavicular joint
- S43.212 Anterior subluxation of left sternoclavicular joint
- S43.213 Anterior subluxation of unspecified sternoclavicular joint
- S43.214 Anterior dislocation of right sternoclavicular joint
- S43.215 Anterior dislocation of left sternoclavicular joint
- S43.216 Anterior dislocation of unspecified sternoclavicular joint

S43.22 Posterior subluxation and dislocation of sternoclavicular joint
- S43.221 Posterior subluxation of right sternoclavicular joint
- S43.222 Posterior subluxation of left sternoclavicular joint
- S43.223 Posterior subluxation of unspecified sternoclavicular joint
- S43.224 Posterior dislocation of right sternoclavicular joint
- S43.225 Posterior dislocation of left sternoclavicular joint
- S43.226 Posterior dislocation of unspecified sternoclavicular joint

S43.3 Subluxation and dislocation of other and unspecified parts of shoulder girdle

S43.30 Subluxation and dislocation of unspecified parts of shoulder girdle
  Dislocation of shoulder girdle NOS
  Subluxation of shoulder girdle NOS
- S43.301 Subluxation of unspecified parts of right shoulder girdle
- S43.302 Subluxation of unspecified parts of left shoulder girdle

S43.303 Subluxation of unspecified parts of unspecified shoulder girdle

S43.304 Dislocation of unspecified parts of right shoulder girdle

S43.305 Dislocation of unspecified parts of left shoulder girdle

S43.306 Dislocation of unspecified parts of unspecified shoulder girdle

S43.31 Subluxation and dislocation of scapula
- S43.311 Subluxation of right scapula
- S43.312 Subluxation of left scapula
- S43.313 Subluxation of unspecified scapula
- S43.314 Dislocation of right scapula
- S43.315 Dislocation of left scapula
- S43.316 Dislocation of unspecified scapula

S43.39 Subluxation and dislocation of other parts of shoulder girdle
- S43.391 Subluxation of other parts of right shoulder girdle
- S43.392 Subluxation of other parts of left shoulder girdle
- S43.393 Subluxation of other parts of unspecified shoulder girdle
- S43.394 Dislocation of other parts of right shoulder girdle
- S43.395 Dislocation of other parts of left shoulder girdle
- S43.396 Dislocation of other parts of unspecified shoulder girdle

S43.4 Sprain of shoulder joint

S43.40 Unspecified sprain of shoulder joint
- S43.401 Unspecified sprain of right shoulder joint
- S43.402 Unspecified sprain of left shoulder joint
- S43.409 Unspecified sprain of unspecified shoulder joint

S43.41 Sprain of coracohumeral (ligament)
- S43.411 Sprain of right coracohumeral (ligament)
- S43.412 Sprain of left coracohumeral (ligament)
- S43.419 Sprain of unspecified coracohumeral (ligament)

S43.42 Sprain of rotator cuff capsule
  EXCLUDES1 rotator cuff syndrome (complete) (incomplete), not specified as traumatic (M75.1-)
  EXCLUDES2 injury of tendon of rotator cuff (S46.0-)
- S43.421 Sprain of right rotator cuff capsule
- S43.422 Sprain of left rotator cuff capsule
- S43.429 Sprain of unspecified rotator cuff capsule

S43.43 Superior glenoid labrum lesion
  SLAP lesion
- S43.431 Superior glenoid labrum lesion of right shoulder
- S43.432 Superior glenoid labrum lesion of left shoulder
- S43.439 Superior glenoid labrum lesion of unspecified shoulder

S43.49 Other sprain of shoulder joint
- S43.491 Other sprain of right shoulder joint
- S43.492 Other sprain of left shoulder joint
- S43.499 Other sprain of unspecified shoulder joint

S43.5 Sprain of acromioclavicular joint
  Sprain of acromioclavicular ligament
- S43.50 Sprain of unspecified acromioclavicular joint
- S43.51 Sprain of right acromioclavicular joint
- S43.52 Sprain of left acromioclavicular joint

S43.6 Sprain of sternoclavicular joint

POA Unacceptable principal diagnosis symbol per Medicare code edits   Code exempt from diagnosis present on admission requirement
?? Questionable admission   Complication or comorbidity   CC/MCC exclusion   Major complication or comorbidity
Principal diagnosis as its own CC   Principal diagnosis as its own MCC   HCC diagnosis code   RxHCC diagnosis code
MACRA code   Z code as first-listed diagnosis

When symbols appear on a code that requires a 7th character extension, refer to Appendix B to identify applicable 7th character codes.

5ᵗʰ S43.60 Sprain of unspecified sternoclavicular joint `POA`

7ᵗʰ S43.61 Sprain of right sternoclavicular joint `POA`

7ᵗʰ S43.62 Sprain of left sternoclavicular joint `POA`

5ᵗʰ S43.8 Sprain of other specified parts of shoulder girdle

7ᵗʰ S43.80 Sprain of other specified parts of unspecified shoulder girdle `POA`

7ᵗʰ S43.81 Sprain of other specified parts of right shoulder girdle `POA`

7ᵗʰ S43.82 Sprain of other specified parts of left shoulder girdle `POA`

5ᵗʰ S43.9 Sprain of unspecified parts of shoulder girdle

7ᵗʰ S43.90 Sprain of unspecified parts of unspecified shoulder girdle `POA`

Sprain of shoulder girdle NOS

7ᵗʰ S43.91 Sprain of unspecified parts of right shoulder girdle `POA`

7ᵗʰ S43.92 Sprain of unspecified parts of left shoulder girdle `POA`

4ᵗʰ S44 Injury of nerves at shoulder and upper arm level

Code also any associated open wound (S41.-)

EXCLUDES2 injury of brachial plexus (S14.3-)

The appropriate 7th character is to be added to each code from category S44

A = initial encounter

D = subsequent encounter

S = sequela

5ᵗʰ S44.0 Injury of ulnar nerve at upper arm level

EXCLUDES1 ulnar nerve NOS (S54.0)

7ᵗʰ S44.00 Injury of ulnar nerve at upper arm level, unspecified arm `POA`

7ᵗʰ S44.01 Injury of ulnar nerve at upper arm level, right arm `POA`

7ᵗʰ S44.02 Injury of ulnar nerve at upper arm level, left arm `POA`

5ᵗʰ S44.1 Injury of median nerve at upper arm level

EXCLUDES1 median nerve NOS (S54.1)

7ᵗʰ S44.10 Injury of median nerve at upper arm level, unspecified arm `POA`

7ᵗʰ S44.11 Injury of median nerve at upper arm level, right arm `POA`

7ᵗʰ S44.12 Injury of median nerve at upper arm level, left arm `POA`

5ᵗʰ S44.2 Injury of radial nerve at upper arm level

EXCLUDES1 radial nerve NOS (S54.2)

7ᵗʰ S44.20 Injury of radial nerve at upper arm level, unspecified arm `POA`

7ᵗʰ S44.21 Injury of radial nerve at upper arm level, right arm `POA`

7ᵗʰ S44.22 Injury of radial nerve at upper arm level, left arm `POA`

5ᵗʰ S44.3 Injury of axillary nerve

7ᵗʰ S44.30 Injury of axillary nerve, unspecified arm `POA`

7ᵗʰ S44.31 Injury of axillary nerve, right arm `POA`

7ᵗʰ S44.32 Injury of axillary nerve, left arm `POA`

5ᵗʰ S44.4 Injury of musculocutaneous nerve

7ᵗʰ S44.40 Injury of musculocutaneous nerve, unspecified arm `POA`

7ᵗʰ S44.41 Injury of musculocutaneous nerve, right arm `POA`

7ᵗʰ S44.42 Injury of musculocutaneous nerve, left arm `POA`

5ᵗʰ S44.5 Injury of cutaneous sensory nerve at shoulder and upper arm level

7ᵗʰ S44.50 Injury of cutaneous sensory nerve at shoulder and upper arm level, unspecified arm `POA`

7ᵗʰ S44.51 Injury of cutaneous sensory nerve at shoulder and upper arm level, right arm `POA`

7ᵗʰ S44.52 Injury of cutaneous sensory nerve at shoulder and upper arm level, left arm `POA`

5ᵗʰ S44.8 Injury of other nerves at shoulder and upper arm level

S44.8X Injury of other nerves at shoulder and upper arm level

7ᵗʰ S44.8X1 Injury of other nerves at shoulder and upper arm level, right arm `POA`

7ᵗʰ S44.8X2 Injury of other nerves at shoulder and upper arm level, left arm `POA`

7ᵗʰ S44.8X9 Injury of other nerves at shoulder and upper arm level, unspecified arm `POA`

5ᵗʰ S44.9 Injury of unspecified nerve at shoulder and upper arm level

7ᵗʰ S44.90 Injury of unspecified nerve at shoulder and upper arm level, unspecified arm `POA`

7ᵗʰ S44.91 Injury of unspecified nerve at shoulder and upper arm level, right arm `POA`

7ᵗʰ S44.92 Injury of unspecified nerve at shoulder and upper arm level, left arm `POA`

4ᵗʰ S45 Injury of blood vessels at shoulder and upper arm level

Code also any associated open wound (S41.-)

EXCLUDES2 injury of subclavian artery (S25.1)

injury of subclavian vein (S25.3)

The appropriate 7th character is to be added to each code from category S45

A = initial encounter

D = subsequent encounter

S = sequela

5ᵗʰ S45.0 Injury of axillary artery

6ᵗʰ S45.00 Unspecified injury of axillary artery

7ᵗʰ S45.001 Unspecified injury of axillary artery, right side `POA` `MCC` `CC/MCC Exc`

7ᵗʰ S45.002 Unspecified injury of axillary artery, left side `POA` `MCC` `CC/MCC Exc`

7ᵗʰ S45.009 Unspecified injury of axillary artery, unspecified side `POA` `MCC` `CC/MCC Exc`

6ᵗʰ S45.01 Laceration of axillary artery

7ᵗʰ S45.011 Laceration of axillary artery, right side `POA` `MCC` `CC/MCC Exc`

7ᵗʰ S45.012 Laceration of axillary artery, left side `POA` `MCC` `CC/MCC Exc`

7ᵗʰ S45.019 Laceration of axillary artery, unspecified side `POA` `MCC` `CC/MCC Exc`

6ᵗʰ S45.09 Other specified injury of axillary artery

7ᵗʰ S45.091 Other specified injury of axillary artery, right side `POA` `MCC` `CC/MCC Exc`

7ᵗʰ S45.092 Other specified injury of axillary artery, left side `POA` `MCC` `CC/MCC Exc`

7ᵗʰ S45.099 Other specified injury of axillary artery, unspecified side `POA` `MCC` `CC/MCC Exc`

5ᵗʰ S45.1 Injury of brachial artery

6ᵗʰ S45.10 Unspecified injury of brachial artery

7ᵗʰ S45.101 Unspecified injury of brachial artery, right side `CC` `POA` `CC/MCC Exc`

7ᵗʰ S45.102 Unspecified injury of brachial artery, left side `CC` `POA` `CC/MCC Exc`

7ᵗʰ S45.109 Unspecified injury of brachial artery, unspecified side `CC` `POA` `CC/MCC Exc`

6ᵗʰ S45.11 Laceration of brachial artery

7ᵗʰ S45.111 Laceration of brachial artery, right side `CC` `POA` `CC/MCC Exc`

7ᵗʰ S45.112 Laceration of brachial artery, left side `CC` `POA` `CC/MCC Exc`

7ᵗʰ S45.119 Laceration of brachial artery, unspecified side `CC` `POA` `CC/MCC Exc`

6ᵗʰ S45.19 Other specified injury of brachial artery

7ᵗʰ S45.191 Other specified injury of brachial artery, right side `CC` `POA` `CC/MCC Exc`

7ᵗʰ S45.192 Other specified injury of brachial artery, left side `CC` `POA` `CC/MCC Exc`

7ᵗʰ S45.199 Other specified injury of brachial artery, unspecified side `CC` `POA` `CC/MCC Exc`

5ᵗʰ S45.2 Injury of axillary or brachial vein

6ᵗʰ S45.20 Unspecified injury of axillary or brachial vein

7ᵗʰ S45.201 Unspecified injury of axillary or brachial vein, right side `CC` `POA` `CC/MCC Exc`

7ᵗʰ S45.202 Unspecified injury of axillary or brachial vein, left side `CC` `POA` `CC/MCC Exc`

7ᵗʰ S45.209 Unspecified injury of axillary or brachial vein, unspecified side `CC` `POA` `CC/MCC Exc`

Unspecified Code	Other Specified Code	Manifestation Code	Ⓝ Newborn	Ⓟ Pediatric	Ⓜ Maternity	Ⓐ Adult	♂ Male	♀ Female

● New Code   ▲ Revised Code Title   ▶◀ Revised Text   *NOTES*   *INCLUDES*   *EXCLUDES 1* Not coded here   *EXCLUDES 2* Not included here

4ᵗʰ character required   5ᵗʰ character required   6ᵗʰ character required   7ᵗʰ character required

Extension 'X' Alert   *HAC* Hospital-acquired condition (HAC) alert   **AHA** AHA Coding Clinic©

S46.819 Strain of other muscles, fascia and tendons at shoulder and upper arm level, unspecified arm POA

S46.82 Laceration of other muscles, fascia and tendons at shoulder and upper arm level

S46.821 Laceration of other muscles, fascia and tendons at shoulder and upper arm level, right arm CC/MCC Exc POA

S46.822 Laceration of other muscles, fascia and tendons at shoulder and upper arm level, left arm CC/MCC Exc POA

S46.829 Laceration of other muscles, fascia and tendons at shoulder and upper arm level, unspecified arm POA CC/MCC Exc

S46.89 Other injury of other muscles, fascia and tendons at shoulder and upper arm level

S46.891 Other injury of other muscles, fascia and tendons at shoulder and upper arm level, right arm POA

S46.892 Other injury of other muscles, fascia and tendons at shoulder and upper arm level, left arm POA

S46.899 Other injury of other muscles, fascia and tendons at shoulder and upper arm level, unspecified arm POA

S46.9 Injury of unspecified muscle, fascia and tendon at shoulder and upper arm level

S46.90 Unspecified injury of unspecified muscle, fascia and tendon at shoulder and upper arm level

S46.901 Unspecified injury of unspecified muscle, fascia and tendon at shoulder and upper arm level, right arm POA

S46.902 Unspecified injury of unspecified muscle, fascia and tendon at shoulder and upper arm level, left arm POA

S46.909 Unspecified injury of unspecified muscle, fascia and tendon at shoulder and upper arm level, unspecified arm POA

S46.91 Strain of unspecified muscle, fascia and tendon at shoulder and upper arm level

S46.911 Strain of unspecified muscle, fascia and tendon at shoulder and upper arm level, right arm POA

S46.912 Strain of unspecified muscle, fascia and tendon at shoulder and upper arm level, left arm POA

S46.919 Strain of unspecified muscle, fascia and tendon at shoulder and upper arm level, unspecified arm POA

S46.92 Laceration of unspecified muscle, fascia and tendon at shoulder and upper arm level

S46.921 Laceration of unspecified muscle, fascia and tendon at shoulder and upper arm level, right arm CC/MCC Exc POA

S46.922 Laceration of unspecified muscle, fascia and tendon at shoulder and upper arm level, left arm CC/MCC Exc POA

S46.929 Laceration of unspecified muscle, fascia and tendon at shoulder and upper arm level, unspecified arm CC/MCC Exc POA

S46.99 Other injury of unspecified muscle, fascia and tendon at shoulder and upper arm level

S46.991 Other injury of unspecified muscle, fascia and tendon at shoulder and upper arm level, right arm POA

S46.992 Other injury of unspecified muscle, fascia and tendon at shoulder and upper arm level, left arm POA

S46.999 Other injury of unspecified muscle, fascia and tendon at shoulder and upper arm level, unspecified arm POA

S47 Crushing injury of shoulder and upper arm

Use additional code for all associated injuries

EXCLUDES2 crushing injury of elbow (S57.0-)

The appropriate 7th character is to be added to each code from category S47

A = initial encounter

D = subsequent encounter

S = sequela

S47.1 Crushing injury of right shoulder and upper arm POA

S47.2 Crushing injury of left shoulder and upper arm POA

S47.9 Crushing injury of shoulder and upper arm, unspecified arm POA

S48 Traumatic amputation of shoulder and upper arm

An amputation not identified as partial or complete should be coded to complete

EXCLUDES1 traumatic amputation at elbow level (S58.0)

The appropriate 7th character is to be added to each code from category S48

A = initial encounter

D = subsequent encounter

S = sequela

S48.0 Traumatic amputation at shoulder joint

S48.01 Complete traumatic amputation at shoulder joint

S48.011 Complete traumatic amputation at right shoulder joint POA HCC CC/MCC Exc

S48.012 Complete traumatic amputation at left shoulder joint POA HCC CC/MCC Exc

S48.019 Complete traumatic amputation at unspecified shoulder joint POA HCC CC/MCC Exc

S48.02 Partial traumatic amputation at shoulder joint

S48.021 Partial traumatic amputation at right shoulder joint POA HCC CC/MCC Exc

S48.022 Partial traumatic amputation at left shoulder joint POA HCC CC/MCC Exc

S48.029 Partial traumatic amputation at unspecified shoulder joint POA HCC CC/MCC Exc

S48.1 Traumatic amputation at level between shoulder and elbow

S48.11 Complete traumatic amputation at level between shoulder and elbow

S48.111 Complete traumatic amputation at level between right shoulder and elbow POA HCC CC/MCC Exc

S48.112 Complete traumatic amputation at level between left shoulder and elbow POA HCC CC/MCC Exc

S48.119 Complete traumatic amputation at level between unspecified shoulder and elbow POA HCC CC/MCC Exc

S48.12 Partial traumatic amputation at level between shoulder and elbow

S48.121 Partial traumatic amputation at level between right shoulder and elbow POA HCC CC/MCC Exc

S48.122 Partial traumatic amputation at level between left shoulder and elbow POA HCC CC/MCC Exc

S48.129 Partial traumatic amputation at level between unspecified shoulder and elbow POA HCC CC/MCC Exc

S48.9 Traumatic amputation of shoulder and upper arm, level unspecified

S48.91 Complete traumatic amputation of shoulder and upper arm, level unspecified

S48.911 Complete traumatic amputation of right shoulder and upper arm, level unspecified POA HCC CC/MCC Exc

S48.912 Complete traumatic amputation of left shoulder and upper arm, level unspecified POA HCC CC/MCC Exc

---

PDx Unacceptable principal diagnosis symbol per Medicare code edits   POA Code exempt from diagnosis present on admission requirement
? Questionable admission   CC Complication or comorbidity   CC/MCC Exc CC/MCC exclusion   MCC Major complication or comorbidity
CC Principal diagnosis as its own CC   MCC Principal diagnosis as its own MCC   HCC HCC diagnosis code   RxHCC RxHCC diagnosis code
MACRA code   Z1 Z code as first-listed diagnosis

S48.919 Complete traumatic amputation of unspecified shoulder and upper arm, level unspecified `CC POA HCC CC/MCC Exc`

6ᵗʰ S48.92 Partial traumatic amputation of shoulder and upper arm, level unspecified

S48.921 Partial traumatic amputation of right shoulder and upper arm, level unspecified `CC POA HCC CC/MCC Exc`

S48.922 Partial traumatic amputation of left shoulder and upper arm, level unspecified `CC POA HCC CC/MCC Exc`

S48.929 Partial traumatic amputation of unspecified shoulder and upper arm, level unspecified `CC POA HCC CC/MCC Exc`

4ᵗʰ S49 Other and unspecified injuries of shoulder and upper arm

The appropriate 7th character is to be added to each code from subcategories S49.0 and S49.1

A = initial encounter for closed fracture
D = subsequent encounter for fracture with routine healing
G = subsequent encounter for fracture with delayed healing
K = subsequent encounter for fracture with nonunion
P = subsequent encounter for fracture with malunion
S = sequela

5ᵗʰ S49.0 Physeal fracture of upper end of humerus

6ᵗʰ S49.00 Unspecified physeal fracture of upper end of humerus

S49.001 Unspecified physeal fracture of upper end of humerus, right arm `CC POA HAC CC/MCC Exc`

S49.002 Unspecified physeal fracture of upper end of humerus, left arm `CC POA HAC CC/MCC Exc`

S49.009 Unspecified physeal fracture of upper end of humerus, unspecified arm `CC POA HAC CC/MCC Exc`

6ᵗʰ S49.01 Salter-Harris Type I physeal fracture of upper end of humerus

S49.011 Salter-Harris Type I physeal fracture of upper end of humerus, right arm `CC POA HAC CC/MCC Exc`

S49.012 Salter-Harris Type I physeal fracture of upper end of humerus, left arm `CC POA HAC CC/MCC Exc`

S49.019 Salter-Harris Type I physeal fracture of upper end of humerus, unspecified arm `CC POA HAC CC/MCC Exc`

6ᵗʰ S49.02 Salter-Harris Type II physeal fracture of upper end of humerus

S49.021 Salter-Harris Type II physeal fracture of upper end of humerus, right arm `CC POA HAC CC/MCC Exc`

S49.022 Salter-Harris Type II physeal fracture of upper end of humerus, left arm `CC POA HAC CC/MCC Exc`

S49.029 Salter-Harris Type II physeal fracture of upper end of humerus, unspecified arm `CC POA HAC CC/MCC Exc`

6ᵗʰ S49.03 Salter-Harris Type III physeal fracture of upper end of humerus

S49.031 Salter-Harris Type III physeal fracture of upper end of humerus, right arm `CC POA HAC CC/MCC Exc`

S49.032 Salter-Harris Type III physeal fracture of upper end of humerus, left arm `CC POA HAC CC/MCC Exc`

S49.039 Salter-Harris Type III physeal fracture of upper end of humerus, unspecified arm `CC POA HAC CC/MCC Exc`

6ᵗʰ S49.04 Salter-Harris Type IV physeal fracture of upper end of humerus

S49.041 Salter-Harris Type IV physeal fracture of upper end of humerus, right arm `CC POA HAC CC/MCC Exc`

S49.042 Salter-Harris Type IV physeal fracture of upper end of humerus, left arm `CC POA HAC CC/MCC Exc`

S49.049 Salter-Harris Type IV physeal fracture of upper end of humerus, unspecified arm `CC POA HAC CC/MCC Exc`

6ᵗʰ S49.09 Other physeal fracture of upper end of humerus

S49.091 Other physeal fracture of upper end of humerus, right arm `CC POA HAC CC/MCC Exc`

S49.092 Other physeal fracture of upper end of humerus, left arm `CC POA HAC CC/MCC Exc`

S49.099 Other physeal fracture of upper end of humerus, unspecified arm `CC POA HAC CC/MCC Exc`

5ᵗʰ S49.1 Physeal fracture of lower end of humerus

6ᵗʰ S49.10 Unspecified physeal fracture of lower end of humerus

S49.101 Unspecified physeal fracture of lower end of humerus, right arm `CC POA HAC CC/MCC Exc`

S49.102 Unspecified physeal fracture of lower end of humerus, left arm `CC POA HAC CC/MCC Exc`

S49.109 Unspecified physeal fracture of lower end of humerus, unspecified arm `CC POA HAC CC/MCC Exc`

6ᵗʰ S49.11 Salter-Harris Type I physeal fracture of lower end of humerus

S49.111 Salter-Harris Type I physeal fracture of lower end of humerus, right arm `CC POA HAC CC/MCC Exc`

S49.112 Salter-Harris Type I physeal fracture of lower end of humerus, left arm `CC POA HAC CC/MCC Exc`

S49.119 Salter-Harris Type I physeal fracture of lower end of humerus, unspecified arm `CC POA HAC CC/MCC Exc`

6ᵗʰ S49.12 Salter-Harris Type II physeal fracture of lower end of humerus

S49.121 Salter-Harris Type II physeal fracture of lower end of humerus, right arm `CC POA HAC CC/MCC Exc`

S49.122 Salter-Harris Type II physeal fracture of lower end of humerus, left arm `CC POA HAC CC/MCC Exc`

S49.129 Salter-Harris Type II physeal fracture of lower end of humerus, unspecified arm `CC POA HAC CC/MCC Exc`

6ᵗʰ S49.13 Salter-Harris Type III physeal fracture of lower end of humerus

S49.131 Salter-Harris Type III physeal fracture of lower end of humerus, right arm `CC POA HAC CC/MCC Exc`

S49.132 Salter-Harris Type III physeal fracture of lower end of humerus, left arm `CC POA HAC CC/MCC Exc`

S49.139 Salter-Harris Type III physeal fracture of lower end of humerus, unspecified arm `CC POA HAC CC/MCC Exc`

6ᵗʰ S49.14 Salter-Harris Type IV physeal fracture of lower end of humerus

S49.141 Salter-Harris Type IV physeal fracture of lower end of humerus, right arm `CC POA HAC CC/MCC Exc`

S49.142 Salter-Harris Type IV physeal fracture of lower end of humerus, left arm `CC POA HAC CC/MCC Exc`

S49.149 Salter-Harris Type IV physeal fracture of lower end of humerus, unspecified arm `CC POA HAC CC/MCC Exc`

6ᵗʰ S49.19 Other physeal fracture of lower end of humerus

S49.191 Other physeal fracture of lower end of humerus, right arm `CC POA HAC CC/MCC Exc`

S49.192 Other physeal fracture of lower end of humerus, left arm `CC POA HAC CC/MCC Exc`

Unspecified Code   Other Specified Code   Manifestation Code   Ⓝ Newborn   Ⓟ Pediatric   Ⓜ Maternity   Ⓐ Adult   ♂ Male   ♀ Female
● New Code   ▲ Revised Code Title   ►◄ Revised Text   **NOTES**   *INCLUDES*   *EXCLUDES 1* Not coded here   *EXCLUDES 2* Not included here
4ᵗʰ character required   5ᵗʰ character required   6ᵗʰ character required   7ᵗʰ character required
Extension 'X' Alert   **HAC** Hospital-acquired condition (HAC) alert   **AHA** AHA Coding Clinic©

S52.01 Torus fracture of upper end of ulna

The appropriate 7th character is to be added to all codes in subcategory S52.01

- A = initial encounter for closed fracture
- D = subsequent encounter for fracture with routine healing
- G = subsequent encounter for fracture with delayed healing
- K = subsequent encounter for fracture with nonunion
- P = subsequent encounter for fracture with malunion
- S = sequela

S52.011 Torus fracture of upper end of right ulna

S52.012 Torus fracture of upper end of left ulna

S52.019 Torus fracture of upper end of unspecified ulna

S52.02 Fracture of olecranon process without intraarticular extension of ulna

S52.021 Displaced fracture of olecranon process without intraarticular extension of right ulna

S52.022 Displaced fracture of olecranon process without intraarticular extension of left ulna

S52.023 Displaced fracture of olecranon process without intraarticular extension of unspecified ulna

S52.024 Nondisplaced fracture of olecranon process without intraarticular extension of right ulna

S52.025 Nondisplaced fracture of olecranon process without intraarticular extension of left ulna

S52.026 Nondisplaced fracture of olecranon process without intraarticular extension of unspecified ulna

S52.03 Fracture of olecranon process with intraarticular extension of ulna

S52.031 Displaced fracture of olecranon process with intraarticular extension of right ulna

S52.032 Displaced fracture of olecranon process with intraarticular extension of left ulna

S52.033 Displaced fracture of olecranon process with intraarticular extension of unspecified ulna

S52.034 Nondisplaced fracture of olecranon process with intraarticular extension of right ulna

S52.035 Nondisplaced fracture of olecranon process with intraarticular extension of left ulna

S52.036 Nondisplaced fracture of olecranon process with intraarticular extension of unspecified ulna

S52.04 Fracture of coronoid process of ulna

S52.041 Displaced fracture of coronoid process of right ulna

S52.042 Displaced fracture of coronoid process of left ulna

S52.043 Displaced fracture of coronoid process of unspecified ulna

S52.044 Nondisplaced fracture of coronoid process of right ulna

S52.045 Nondisplaced fracture of coronoid process of left ulna

S52.046 Nondisplaced fracture of coronoid process of unspecified ulna

S52.09 Other fracture of upper end of ulna

S52.091 Other fracture of upper end of right ulna

S52.092 Other fracture of upper end of left ulna

S52.099 Other fracture of upper end of unspecified ulna

S52.1 Fracture of upper end of radius

Fracture of proximal end of radius

EXCLUDES2 physeal fractures of upper end of radius (S59.2-)

fracture of shaft of radius (S52.3-)

S52.10 Unspecified fracture of upper end of radius

S52.101 Unspecified fracture of upper end of right radius

S52.102 Unspecified fracture of upper end of left radius

S52.109 Unspecified fracture of upper end of unspecified radius

S52.11 Torus fracture of upper end of radius

The appropriate 7th character is to be added to all codes in subcategory S52.11

- A = initial encounter for closed fracture
- D = subsequent encounter for fracture with routine healing
- G = subsequent encounter for fracture with delayed healing
- K = subsequent encounter for fracture with nonunion
- P = subsequent encounter for fracture with malunion
- S = sequela

S52.111 Torus fracture of upper end of right radius

S52.112 Torus fracture of upper end of left radius

S52.119 Torus fracture of upper end of unspecified radius

S52.12 Fracture of head of radius

S52.121 Displaced fracture of head of right radius

S52.122 Displaced fracture of head of left radius

S52.123 Displaced fracture of head of unspecified radius

S52.124 Nondisplaced fracture of head of right radius

S52.125 Nondisplaced fracture of head of left radius

S52.126 Nondisplaced fracture of head of unspecified radius

S52.13 Fracture of neck of radius

S52.131 Displaced fracture of neck of right radius

S52.132 Displaced fracture of neck of left radius

S52.133 Displaced fracture of neck of unspecified radius

S52.134 Nondisplaced fracture of neck of right radius

S52.135 Nondisplaced fracture of neck of left radius

S52.136 Nondisplaced fracture of neck of unspecified radius

S52.18 Other fracture of upper end of radius

S52.181 Other fracture of upper end of right radius

S52.182 Other fracture of upper end of left radius

S52.189 Other fracture of upper end of unspecified radius

S52.2 Fracture of shaft of ulna

PDXLN Unacceptable principal diagnosis symbol per Medicare code edits   POA Code exempt from diagnosis present on admission requirement
❓ Questionable admission   CC Complication or comorbidity   CC/MCC Exc CC/MCC exclusion   MCC Major complication or comorbidity
CC Principal diagnosis as its own CC   MCC Principal diagnosis as its own MCC   HCC HCC diagnosis code   RxHCC RxHCC diagnosis code
MACRA code   Z Z code as first-listed diagnosis

6ᵗʰ S52.20 Unspecified fracture of shaft of ulna
Fracture of ulna NOS

7ᵗʰ S52.201 Unspecified fracture of shaft of right ulna cc POA HAC MCC CC/MCC Exc

7ᵗʰ S52.202 Unspecified fracture of shaft of left ulna cc POA HAC MCC CC/MCC Exc

7ᵗʰ S52.209 Unspecified fracture of shaft of unspecified ulna cc POA HAC MCC CC/MCC Exc

6ᵗʰ S52.21 Greenstick fracture of shaft of ulna
The appropriate 7th character is to be added to all codes in subcategory S52.21
A = initial encounter for closed fracture
D = subsequent encounter for fracture with routine healing
G = subsequent encounter for fracture with delayed healing
K = subsequent encounter for fracture with nonunion
P = subsequent encounter for fracture with malunion
S = sequela

7ᵗʰ S52.211 Greenstick fracture of shaft of right ulna cc POA HAC CC/MCC Exc

7ᵗʰ S52.212 Greenstick fracture of shaft of left ulna cc POA HAC CC/MCC Exc

7ᵗʰ S52.219 Greenstick fracture of shaft of unspecified ulna cc POA HAC CC/MCC Exc

6ᵗʰ S52.22 Transverse fracture of shaft of ulna

7ᵗʰ S52.221 Displaced transverse fracture of shaft of right ulna cc POA HAC MCC CC/MCC Exc

7ᵗʰ S52.222 Displaced transverse fracture of shaft of left ulna cc POA HAC MCC CC/MCC Exc

7ᵗʰ S52.223 Displaced transverse fracture of shaft of unspecified ulna cc POA HAC MCC CC/MCC Exc

7ᵗʰ S52.224 Nondisplaced transverse fracture of shaft of right ulna cc POA HAC MCC CC/MCC Exc

7ᵗʰ S52.225 Nondisplaced transverse fracture of shaft of left ulna cc POA HAC MCC CC/MCC Exc

7ᵗʰ S52.226 Nondisplaced transverse fracture of shaft of unspecified ulna cc POA HAC MCC CC/MCC Exc

6ᵗʰ S52.23 Oblique fracture of shaft of ulna

7ᵗʰ S52.231 Displaced oblique fracture of shaft of right ulna cc POA HAC MCC CC/MCC Exc

7ᵗʰ S52.232 Displaced oblique fracture of shaft of left ulna cc POA HAC MCC CC/MCC Exc

7ᵗʰ S52.233 Displaced oblique fracture of shaft of unspecified ulna cc POA HAC MCC CC/MCC Exc

7ᵗʰ S52.234 Nondisplaced oblique fracture of shaft of right ulna cc POA HAC MCC CC/MCC Exc

7ᵗʰ S52.235 Nondisplaced oblique fracture of shaft of left ulna cc POA HAC MCC CC/MCC Exc

7ᵗʰ S52.236 Nondisplaced oblique fracture of shaft of unspecified ulna cc POA HAC MCC CC/MCC Exc

6ᵗʰ S52.24 Spiral fracture of shaft of ulna

7ᵗʰ S52.241 Displaced spiral fracture of shaft of ulna, right arm cc POA HAC MCC CC/MCC Exc

7ᵗʰ S52.242 Displaced spiral fracture of shaft of ulna, left arm cc POA HAC MCC CC/MCC Exc

7ᵗʰ S52.243 Displaced spiral fracture of shaft of ulna, unspecified arm cc POA HAC MCC CC/MCC Exc

7ᵗʰ S52.244 Nondisplaced spiral fracture of shaft of ulna, right arm cc POA HAC MCC CC/MCC Exc

7ᵗʰ S52.245 Nondisplaced spiral fracture of shaft of ulna, left arm cc POA HAC MCC CC/MCC Exc

7ᵗʰ S52.246 Nondisplaced spiral fracture of shaft of ulna, unspecified arm cc POA HAC MCC CC/MCC Exc

6ᵗʰ S52.25 Comminuted fracture of shaft of ulna

7ᵗʰ S52.251 Displaced comminuted fracture of shaft of ulna, right arm cc POA HAC MCC CC/MCC Exc

7ᵗʰ S52.252 Displaced comminuted fracture of shaft of ulna, left arm cc POA HAC MCC CC/MCC Exc

7ᵗʰ S52.253 Displaced comminuted fracture of shaft of ulna, unspecified arm cc POA HAC MCC CC/MCC Exc

7ᵗʰ S52.254 Nondisplaced comminuted fracture of shaft of ulna, right arm cc POA HAC MCC CC/MCC Exc

7ᵗʰ S52.255 Nondisplaced comminuted fracture of shaft of ulna, left arm cc POA HAC MCC CC/MCC Exc

7ᵗʰ S52.256 Nondisplaced comminuted fracture of shaft of ulna, unspecified arm cc POA HAC MCC CC/MCC Exc

6ᵗʰ S52.26 Segmental fracture of shaft of ulna

7ᵗʰ S52.261 Displaced segmental fracture of shaft of ulna, right arm cc POA HAC MCC CC/MCC Exc

7ᵗʰ S52.262 Displaced segmental fracture of shaft of ulna, left arm cc POA HAC MCC CC/MCC Exc

7ᵗʰ S52.263 Displaced segmental fracture of shaft of ulna, unspecified arm cc POA HAC MCC CC/MCC Exc

7ᵗʰ S52.264 Nondisplaced segmental fracture of shaft of ulna, right arm cc POA HAC MCC CC/MCC Exc

7ᵗʰ S52.265 Nondisplaced segmental fracture of shaft of ulna, left arm cc POA HAC MCC CC/MCC Exc

7ᵗʰ S52.266 Nondisplaced segmental fracture of shaft of ulna, unspecified arm cc POA HAC MCC CC/MCC Exc

6ᵗʰ S52.27 Monteggia's fracture of ulna
Fracture of upper shaft of ulna with dislocation of radial head

7ᵗʰ S52.271 Monteggia's fracture of right ulna cc POA HAC MCC CC/MCC Exc

7ᵗʰ S52.272 Monteggia's fracture of left ulna cc POA HAC MCC CC/MCC Exc

7ᵗʰ S52.279 Monteggia's fracture of unspecified ulna cc POA HAC MCC CC/MCC Exc

6ᵗʰ S52.28 Bent bone of ulna

7ᵗʰ S52.281 Bent bone of right ulna cc POA HAC MCC CC/MCC Exc

7ᵗʰ S52.282 Bent bone of left ulna cc POA HAC MCC CC/MCC Exc

7ᵗʰ S52.283 Bent bone of unspecified ulna cc POA HAC MCC CC/MCC Exc

6ᵗʰ S52.29 Other fracture of shaft of ulna

7ᵗʰ S52.291 Other fracture of shaft of right ulna cc POA HAC MCC CC/MCC Exc

7ᵗʰ S52.292 Other fracture of shaft of left ulna cc POA HAC MCC CC/MCC Exc

7ᵗʰ S52.299 Other fracture of shaft of unspecified ulna cc POA HAC MCC CC/MCC Exc

5ᵗʰ S52.3 Fracture of shaft of radius

6ᵗʰ S52.30 Unspecified fracture of shaft of radius

7ᵗʰ S52.301 Unspecified fracture of shaft of right radius cc POA HAC MCC CC/MCC Exc

7ᵗʰ S52.302 Unspecified fracture of shaft of left radius cc POA HAC MCC CC/MCC Exc

7ᵗʰ S52.309 Unspecified fracture of shaft of unspecified radius cc POA HAC MCC CC/MCC Exc

6ᵗʰ S52.31 Greenstick fracture of shaft of radius
The appropriate 7th character is to be added to all codes in subcategory S52.31
A = initial encounter for closed fracture
D = subsequent encounter for fracture with routine healing
G = subsequent encounter for fracture with delayed healing
K = subsequent encounter for fracture with nonunion
P = subsequent encounter for fracture with malunion
S = sequela

7ᵗʰ S52.311 Greenstick fracture of shaft of radius, right arm cc POA HAC CC/MCC Exc

7ᵗʰ S52.312 Greenstick fracture of shaft of radius, left arm cc POA HAC CC/MCC Exc

7ᵗʰ S52.319 Greenstick fracture of shaft of radius, unspecified arm cc POA HAC CC/MCC Exc

6ᵗʰ S52.32 Transverse fracture of shaft of radius

Unspecified Code   Other Specified Code   Manifestation Code   N Newborn   P Pediatric   M Maternity   A Adult   ♂ Male   ♀ Female
● New Code   ▲ Revised Code Title   ►◄ Revised Text   NOTES   INCLUDES   EXCLUDES 1 Not coded here   EXCLUDES 2 Not included here
4ᵗʰ 4th character required   5ᵗʰ 5th character required   6ᵗʰ 6th character required   7ᵗʰ 7th character required
7ᵉˣ Extension 'X' Alert   HAC Hospital-acquired condition (HAC) alert   AHA AHA Coding Clinic©

7ᵗʰ S52.321 Displaced transverse fracture of shaft of right radius CC POA HAC MCC CC/MCC Exc

7ᵗʰ S52.322 Displaced transverse fracture of shaft of left radius CC POA HAC MCC CC/MCC Exc

7ᵗʰ S52.323 Displaced transverse fracture of shaft of unspecified radius CC POA HAC MCC CC/MCC Exc

7ᵗʰ S52.324 Nondisplaced transverse fracture of shaft of right radius CC POA HAC MCC CC/MCC Exc

7ᵗʰ S52.325 Nondisplaced transverse fracture of shaft of left radius CC POA HAC MCC CC/MCC Exc

7ᵗʰ S52.326 Nondisplaced transverse fracture of shaft of unspecified radius CC POA HAC MCC CC/MCC Exc

6ᵗʰ S52.33 Oblique fracture of shaft of radius

7ᵗʰ S52.331 Displaced oblique fracture of shaft of right radius CC POA HAC MCC CC/MCC Exc

7ᵗʰ S52.332 Displaced oblique fracture of shaft of left radius CC POA HAC MCC CC/MCC Exc

7ᵗʰ S52.333 Displaced oblique fracture of shaft of unspecified radius CC POA HAC MCC CC/MCC Exc

7ᵗʰ S52.334 Nondisplaced oblique fracture of shaft of right radius CC POA HAC MCC CC/MCC Exc

7ᵗʰ S52.335 Nondisplaced oblique fracture of shaft of left radius CC POA HAC MCC CC/MCC Exc

7ᵗʰ S52.336 Nondisplaced oblique fracture of shaft of unspecified radius CC POA HAC MCC CC/MCC Exc

6ᵗʰ S52.34 Spiral fracture of shaft of radius

7ᵗʰ S52.341 Displaced spiral fracture of shaft of radius, right arm CC POA HAC MCC CC/MCC Exc

7ᵗʰ S52.342 Displaced spiral fracture of shaft of radius, left arm CC POA HAC MCC CC/MCC Exc

7ᵗʰ S52.343 Displaced spiral fracture of shaft of radius, unspecified arm CC POA HAC MCC CC/MCC Exc

7ᵗʰ S52.344 Nondisplaced spiral fracture of shaft of radius, right arm CC POA HAC MCC CC/MCC Exc

7ᵗʰ S52.345 Nondisplaced spiral fracture of shaft of radius, left arm CC POA HAC MCC CC/MCC Exc

7ᵗʰ S52.346 Nondisplaced spiral fracture of shaft of radius, unspecified arm CC POA HAC MCC CC/MCC Exc

6ᵗʰ S52.35 Comminuted fracture of shaft of radius

7ᵗʰ S52.351 Displaced comminuted fracture of shaft of radius, right arm CC POA HAC MCC CC/MCC Exc

7ᵗʰ S52.352 Displaced comminuted fracture of shaft of radius, left arm CC POA HAC MCC CC/MCC Exc

7ᵗʰ S52.353 Displaced comminuted fracture of shaft of radius, unspecified arm CC POA HAC MCC CC/MCC Exc

7ᵗʰ S52.354 Nondisplaced comminuted fracture of shaft of radius, right arm CC POA HAC MCC CC/MCC Exc

7ᵗʰ S52.355 Nondisplaced comminuted fracture of shaft of radius, left arm CC POA HAC MCC CC/MCC Exc

7ᵗʰ S52.356 Nondisplaced comminuted fracture of shaft of radius, unspecified arm CC POA HAC MCC CC/MCC Exc

6ᵗʰ S52.36 Segmental fracture of shaft of radius

7ᵗʰ S52.361 Displaced segmental fracture of shaft of radius, right arm CC POA HAC MCC CC/MCC Exc

7ᵗʰ S52.362 Displaced segmental fracture of shaft of radius, left arm CC POA HAC MCC CC/MCC Exc

7ᵗʰ S52.363 Displaced segmental fracture of shaft of radius, unspecified arm CC POA HAC MCC CC/MCC Exc

7ᵗʰ S52.364 Nondisplaced segmental fracture of radius, right arm CC POA HAC MCC CC/MCC Exc

7ᵗʰ S52.365 Nondisplaced segmental fracture of shaft of radius, left arm CC POA HAC MCC CC/MCC Exc

7ᵗʰ S52.366 Nondisplaced segmental fracture of shaft of radius, unspecified arm CC POA HAC MCC CC/MCC Exc

6ᵗʰ S52.37 Galeazzi's fracture

Fracture of lower shaft of radius with radioulnar joint dislocation

7ᵗʰ S52.371 Galeazzi's fracture of right radius CC POA HAC MCC CC/MCC Exc

7ᵗʰ S52.372 Galeazzi's fracture of left radius CC POA HAC MCC CC/MCC Exc

7ᵗʰ S52.379 Galeazzi's fracture of unspecified radius CC POA HAC MCC CC/MCC Exc

6ᵗʰ S52.38 Bent bone of radius

7ᵗʰ S52.381 Bent bone of right radius CC POA HAC MCC CC/MCC Exc

7ᵗʰ S52.382 Bent bone of left radius CC POA HAC MCC CC/MCC Exc

7ᵗʰ S52.389 Bent bone of unspecified radius CC POA HAC MCC CC/MCC Exc

6ᵗʰ S52.39 Other fracture of shaft of radius

7ᵗʰ S52.391 Other fracture of shaft of radius, right arm CC POA HAC MCC CC/MCC Exc

7ᵗʰ S52.392 Other fracture of shaft of radius, left arm CC POA HAC MCC CC/MCC Exc

7ᵗʰ S52.399 Other fracture of shaft of radius, unspecified arm CC POA HAC MCC CC/MCC Exc

5ᵗʰ S52.5 Fracture of lower end of radius

Fracture of distal end of radius

EXCLUDES2 physeal fractures of lower end of radius (S59.2-)

6ᵗʰ S52.50 Unspecified fracture of the lower end of radius

7ᵗʰ S52.501 Unspecified fracture of the lower end of right radius CC POA HAC MCC CC/MCC Exc

7ᵗʰ S52.502 Unspecified fracture of the lower end of left radius CC POA HAC MCC CC/MCC Exc

7ᵗʰ S52.509 Unspecified fracture of the lower end of unspecified radius CC POA HAC MCC CC/MCC Exc

6ᵗʰ S52.51 Fracture of radial styloid process

7ᵗʰ S52.511 Displaced fracture of right radial styloid process CC POA HAC MCC CC/MCC Exc

7ᵗʰ S52.512 Displaced fracture of left radial styloid process CC POA HAC MCC CC/MCC Exc

7ᵗʰ S52.513 Displaced fracture of unspecified radial styloid process CC POA HAC MCC CC/MCC Exc

7ᵗʰ S52.514 Nondisplaced fracture of right radial styloid process CC POA HAC MCC CC/MCC Exc

7ᵗʰ S52.515 Nondisplaced fracture of left radial styloid process CC POA HAC MCC CC/MCC Exc

7ᵗʰ S52.516 Nondisplaced fracture of unspecified radial styloid process CC POA HAC MCC CC/MCC Exc

6ᵗʰ S52.52 Torus fracture of lower end of radius

The appropriate 7th character is to be added to all codes in subcategory S52.52

A = initial encounter for closed fracture

D = subsequent encounter for fracture with routine healing

G = subsequent encounter for fracture with delayed healing

K = subsequent encounter for fracture with nonunion

P = subsequent encounter for fracture with malunion

S = sequela

7ᵗʰ S52.521 Torus fracture of lower end of right radius CC POA HAC CC/MCC Exc

7ᵗʰ S52.522 Torus fracture of lower end of left radius CC POA HAC CC/MCC Exc

7ᵗʰ S52.529 Torus fracture of lower end of unspecified radius CC POA HAC CC/MCC Exc

5ᵗʰ S52.53 Colles' fracture

7ᵗʰ S52.531 Colles' fracture of right radius CC POA HAC MCC CC/MCC Exc

7ᵗʰ S52.532 Colles' fracture of left radius CC POA HAC MCC CC/MCC Exc

7ᵗʰ S52.539 Colles' fracture of unspecified radius CC POA HAC MCC CC/MCC Exc

---

PDxᵣ Unacceptable principal diagnosis symbol per Medicare code edits   POA Code exempt from diagnosis present on admission requirement

❓ Questionable admission   CC Complication or comorbidity   CC/MCC Exc CC/MCC exclusion   MCC Major complication or comorbidity

CC Principal diagnosis as its own CC   MCC Principal diagnosis as its own MCC   HCC HCC diagnosis code   RxHCC RxHCC diagnosis code

MACRA code   Z1 Z code as first-listed diagnosis

[6th] S52.54 Smith's fracture
- [7th] S52.541 Smith's fracture of right radius [CC] [POA] [HAC] [MCC] [CC/MCC Exc]
- [7th] S52.542 Smith's fracture of left radius [CC] [POA] [HAC] [MCC] [CC/MCC Exc]
- [7th] S52.549 Smith's fracture of unspecified radius [CC] [POA] [HAC] [MCC] [CC/MCC Exc]

[6th] S52.55 Other extraarticular fracture of lower end of radius
- [7th] S52.551 Other extraarticular fracture of lower end of right radius [CC] [POA] [HAC] [MCC] [CC/MCC Exc]
- [7th] S52.552 Other extraarticular fracture of lower end of left radius [CC] [POA] [HAC] [MCC] [CC/MCC Exc]
- [7th] S52.559 Other extraarticular fracture of lower end of unspecified radius [CC] [POA] [HAC] [MCC] [CC/MCC Exc]

[6th] S52.56 Barton's fracture
- [7th] S52.561 Barton's fracture of right radius [CC] [POA] [HAC] [MCC] [CC/MCC Exc]
- [7th] S52.562 Barton's fracture of left radius [CC] [POA] [HAC] [MCC] [CC/MCC Exc]
- [7th] S52.569 Barton's fracture of unspecified radius [CC] [POA] [HAC] [MCC] [CC/MCC Exc]

[6th] S52.57 Other intraarticular fracture of lower end of radius
- [7th] S52.571 Other intraarticular fracture of lower end of right radius [CC] [POA] [HAC] [MCC] [CC/MCC Exc]
- [7th] S52.572 Other intraarticular fracture of lower end of left radius [CC] [POA] [HAC] [MCC] [CC/MCC Exc]
- [7th] S52.579 Other intraarticular fracture of lower end of unspecified radius [CC] [POA] [HAC] [MCC] [CC/MCC Exc]

[6th] S52.59 Other fractures of lower end of radius
- [7th] S52.591 Other fractures of lower end of right radius [CC] [POA] [HAC] [MCC] [CC/MCC Exc]
- [7th] S52.592 Other fractures of lower end of left radius [CC] [POA] [HAC] [MCC] [CC/MCC Exc]
- [7th] S52.599 Other fractures of lower end of unspecified radius [CC] [POA] [HAC] [MCC] [CC/MCC Exc]

[5th] S52.6 Fracture of lower end of ulna

[6th] S52.60 Unspecified fracture of lower end of ulna
- [7th] S52.601 Unspecified fracture of lower end of right ulna [CC] [POA] [HAC] [MCC] [CC/MCC Exc]
- [7th] S52.602 Unspecified fracture of lower end of left ulna [CC] [POA] [HAC] [MCC] [CC/MCC Exc]
- [7th] S52.609 Unspecified fracture of lower end of unspecified ulna [CC] [POA] [HAC] [MCC] [CC/MCC Exc]

[6th] S52.61 Fracture of ulna styloid process
- [7th] S52.611 Displaced fracture of right ulna styloid process [CC] [POA] [HAC] [MCC] [CC/MCC Exc]
- [7th] S52.612 Displaced fracture of left ulna styloid process [CC] [POA] [HAC] [MCC] [CC/MCC Exc]
- [7th] S52.613 Displaced fracture of unspecified ulna styloid process [CC] [POA] [HAC] [MCC] [CC/MCC Exc]
- [7th] S52.614 Nondisplaced fracture of right ulna styloid process [CC] [POA] [HAC] [MCC] [CC/MCC Exc]
- [7th] S52.615 Nondisplaced fracture of left ulna styloid process [CC] [POA] [HAC] [MCC] [CC/MCC Exc]
- [7th] S52.616 Nondisplaced fracture of unspecified ulna styloid process [CC] [POA] [HAC] [MCC] [CC/MCC Exc]

[6th] S52.62 Torus fracture of lower end of ulna

The appropriate 7th character is to be added to all codes in subcategory S52.62
- A = initial encounter for closed fracture
- D = subsequent encounter for fracture with routine healing
- G = subsequent encounter for fracture with delayed healing
- K = subsequent encounter for fracture with nonunion
- P = subsequent encounter for fracture with malunion
- S = sequela

- [7th] S52.621 Torus fracture of lower end of right ulna [CC] [POA] [HAC] [CC/MCC Exc]
- [7th] S52.622 Torus fracture of lower end of left ulna [CC] [POA] [HAC] [CC/MCC Exc]
- [7th] S52.629 Torus fracture of lower end of unspecified ulna [CC] [POA] [HAC] [CC/MCC Exc]

[6th] S52.69 Other fracture of lower end of ulna
- [7th] S52.691 Other fracture of lower end of right ulna [CC] [POA] [HAC] [MCC] [CC/MCC Exc]
- [7th] S52.692 Other fracture of lower end of left ulna [CC] [POA] [HAC] [MCC] [CC/MCC Exc]
- [7th] S52.699 Other fracture of lower end of unspecified ulna [CC] [POA] [HAC] [MCC] [CC/MCC Exc]

[5th] S52.9 Unspecified fracture of forearm
- [7th X] S52.90 Unspecified fracture of unspecified forearm [CC] [POA] [HAC] [MCC] [CC/MCC Exc]
- [7th X] S52.91 Unspecified fracture of right forearm [CC] [POA] [HAC] [MCC] [CC/MCC Exc]
- [7th X] S52.92 Unspecified fracture of left forearm [CC] [POA] [HAC] [MCC] [CC/MCC Exc]

[4th] S53 Dislocation and sprain of joints and ligaments of elbow

[INCLUDES] *avulsion of joint or ligament of elbow*
laceration of cartilage, joint or ligament of elbow
sprain of cartilage, joint or ligament of elbow
traumatic hemarthrosis of joint or ligament of elbow
traumatic rupture of joint or ligament of elbow
traumatic subluxation of joint or ligament of elbow
traumatic tear of joint or ligament of elbow

Code also any associated open wound

[EXCLUDES2] *strain of muscle, fascia and tendon at forearm level (S56.-)*

The appropriate 7th character is to be added to each code from category S53
- A = initial encounter
- D = subsequent encounter
- S = sequela

[5th] S53.0 Subluxation and dislocation of radial head

Dislocation of radiohumeral joint
Subluxation of radiohumeral joint

[EXCLUDES1] *Monteggia's fracture-dislocation (S52.27-)*

[6th] S53.00 Unspecified subluxation and dislocation of radial head
- [7th] S53.001 Unspecified subluxation of right radial head [POA]
- [7th] S53.002 Unspecified subluxation of left radial head [POA]
- [7th] S53.003 Unspecified subluxation of unspecified radial head [POA]
- [7th] S53.004 Unspecified dislocation of right radial head [POA]
- [7th] S53.005 Unspecified dislocation of left radial head [POA]
- [7th] S53.006 Unspecified dislocation of unspecified radial head [POA]

[6th] S53.01 Anterior subluxation and dislocation of radial head

Anteriomedial subluxation and dislocation of radial head
- [7th] S53.011 Anterior subluxation of right radial head [POA]
- [7th] S53.012 Anterior subluxation of left radial head [POA]
- [7th] S53.013 Anterior subluxation of unspecified radial head [POA]
- [7th] S53.014 Anterior dislocation of right radial head [POA]
- [7th] S53.015 Anterior dislocation of left radial head [POA]
- [7th] S53.016 Anterior dislocation of unspecified radial head [POA]

[6th] S53.02 Posterior subluxation and dislocation of radial head

Posteriolateral subluxation and dislocation of radial head

S53.021 Posterior subluxation of right radial head

S53.022 Posterior subluxation of left radial head

S53.023 Posterior subluxation of unspecified radial head

S53.024 Posterior dislocation of right radial head

S53.025 Posterior dislocation of left radial head

S53.026 Posterior dislocation of unspecified radial head

S53.03 Nursemaid's elbow

S53.031 Nursemaid's elbow, right elbow

S53.032 Nursemaid's elbow, left elbow

S53.033 Nursemaid's elbow, unspecified elbow

S53.09 Other subluxation and dislocation of radial head

S53.091 Other subluxation of right radial head

S53.092 Other subluxation of left radial head

S53.093 Other subluxation of unspecified radial head

S53.094 Other dislocation of right radial head

S53.095 Other dislocation of left radial head

S53.096 Other dislocation of unspecified radial head

S53.1 Subluxation and dislocation of ulnohumeral joint

Subluxation and dislocation of elbow NOS

EXCLUDES1 dislocation of radial head alone (S53.0-)

S53.10 Unspecified subluxation and dislocation of ulnohumeral joint

S53.101 Unspecified subluxation of right ulnohumeral joint

S53.102 Unspecified subluxation of left ulnohumeral joint

S53.103 Unspecified subluxation of unspecified ulnohumeral joint

S53.104 Unspecified dislocation of right ulnohumeral joint

S53.105 Unspecified dislocation of left ulnohumeral joint

S53.106 Unspecified dislocation of unspecified ulnohumeral joint

S53.11 Anterior subluxation and dislocation of ulnohumeral joint

S53.111 Anterior subluxation of right ulnohumeral joint

S53.112 Anterior subluxation of left ulnohumeral joint

S53.113 Anterior subluxation of unspecified ulnohumeral joint

S53.114 Anterior dislocation of right ulnohumeral joint

S53.115 Anterior dislocation of left ulnohumeral joint

S53.116 Anterior dislocation of unspecified ulnohumeral joint

S53.12 Posterior subluxation and dislocation of ulnohumeral joint

S53.121 Posterior subluxation of right ulnohumeral joint

S53.122 Posterior subluxation of left ulnohumeral joint

S53.123 Posterior subluxation of unspecified ulnohumeral joint

S53.124 Posterior dislocation of right ulnohumeral joint

S53.125 Posterior dislocation of left ulnohumeral joint

S53.126 Posterior dislocation of unspecified ulnohumeral joint

S53.13 Medial subluxation and dislocation of ulnohumeral joint

S53.131 Medial subluxation of right ulnohumeral joint

S53.132 Medial subluxation of left ulnohumeral joint

S53.133 Medial subluxation of unspecified ulnohumeral joint

S53.134 Medial dislocation of right ulnohumeral joint

S53.135 Medial dislocation of left ulnohumeral joint

S53.136 Medial dislocation of unspecified ulnohumeral joint

S53.14 Lateral subluxation and dislocation of ulnohumeral joint

S53.141 Lateral subluxation of right ulnohumeral joint

S53.142 Lateral subluxation of left ulnohumeral joint

S53.143 Lateral subluxation of unspecified ulnohumeral joint

S53.144 Lateral dislocation of right ulnohumeral joint

S53.145 Lateral dislocation of left ulnohumeral joint

S53.146 Lateral dislocation of unspecified ulnohumeral joint

S53.19 Other subluxation and dislocation of ulnohumeral joint

S53.191 Other subluxation of right ulnohumeral joint

S53.192 Other subluxation of left ulnohumeral joint

S53.193 Other subluxation of unspecified ulnohumeral joint

S53.194 Other dislocation of right ulnohumeral joint

S53.195 Other dislocation of left ulnohumeral joint

S53.196 Other dislocation of unspecified ulnohumeral joint

S53.2 Traumatic rupture of radial collateral ligament

EXCLUDES1 sprain of radial collateral ligament NOS (S53.43-)

S53.20 Traumatic rupture of unspecified radial collateral ligament

S53.21 Traumatic rupture of right radial collateral ligament

S53.22 Traumatic rupture of left radial collateral ligament

S53.3 Traumatic rupture of ulnar collateral ligament

EXCLUDES1 sprain of ulnar collateral ligament (S53.44-)

S53.30 Traumatic rupture of unspecified ulnar collateral ligament

S53.31 Traumatic rupture of right ulnar collateral ligament

S53.32 Traumatic rupture of left ulnar collateral ligament

S53.4 Sprain of elbow

EXCLUDES2 traumatic rupture of radial collateral ligament (S53.2-)

traumatic rupture of ulnar collateral ligament (S53.3-)

S53.40 Unspecified sprain of elbow

S53.401 Unspecified sprain of right elbow

S53.402 Unspecified sprain of left elbow

S53.409 Unspecified sprain of unspecified elbow

Sprain of elbow NOS

S53.41 Radiohumeral (joint) sprain

S53.411 Radiohumeral (joint) sprain of right elbow

S53.412 Radiohumeral (joint) sprain of left elbow

S53.419 Radiohumeral (joint) sprain of unspecified elbow

POA Unacceptable principal diagnosis symbol per Medicare code edits   POA Code exempt from diagnosis present on admission requirement
? Questionable admission   CC Complication or comorbidity   CC·MCC·Exc CC/MCC exclusion   MCC Major complication or comorbidity
Principal diagnosis as its own CC   Principal diagnosis as its own MCC   HCC HCC diagnosis code   HCC RxHCC diagnosis code
MACRA code   Z Z code as first-listed diagnosis

1032   When symbols appear on a code that requires a 7th character extension, refer to Appendix B to identify applicable 7th character codes.   2018 ICD-10-CM

6ᵗʰ **S53.42** Ulnohumeral (joint) sprain
    7ᵗʰ **S53.421** Ulnohumeral (joint) sprain of right elbow POA
    7ᵗʰ **S53.422** Ulnohumeral (joint) sprain of left elbow POA
    7ᵗʰ **S53.429** Ulnohumeral (joint) sprain of unspecified elbow POA

6ᵗʰ **S53.43** Radial collateral ligament sprain
    7ᵗʰ **S53.431** Radial collateral ligament sprain of right elbow POA
    7ᵗʰ **S53.432** Radial collateral ligament sprain of left elbow POA
    7ᵗʰ **S53.439** Radial collateral ligament sprain of unspecified elbow POA

6ᵗʰ **S53.44** Ulnar collateral ligament sprain
    7ᵗʰ **S53.441** Ulnar collateral ligament sprain of right elbow POA
    7ᵗʰ **S53.442** Ulnar collateral ligament sprain of left elbow POA
    7ᵗʰ **S53.449** Ulnar collateral ligament sprain of unspecified elbow POA

6ᵗʰ **S53.49** Other sprain of elbow
    7ᵗʰ **S53.491** Other sprain of right elbow POA
    7ᵗʰ **S53.492** Other sprain of left elbow POA
    7ᵗʰ **S53.499** Other sprain of unspecified elbow POA

4ᵗʰ **S54** Injury of nerves at forearm level
Code also any associated open wound (S51.-)
EXCLUDES2 injury of nerves at wrist and hand level (S64.-)
The appropriate 7th character is to be added to each code from category S54
    A = initial encounter
    D = subsequent encounter
    S = sequela

5ᵗʰ **S54.0** Injury of ulnar nerve at forearm level
Injury of ulnar nerve NOS
    7ᵗʰ **S54.00** Injury of ulnar nerve at forearm level, unspecified arm POA
    7ᵗʰ **S54.01** Injury of ulnar nerve at forearm level, right arm POA
    7ᵗʰ **S54.02** Injury of ulnar nerve at forearm level, left arm POA

5ᵗʰ **S54.1** Injury of median nerve at forearm level
Injury of median nerve NOS
    7ᵗʰ **S54.10** Injury of median nerve at forearm level, unspecified arm POA
    7ᵗʰ **S54.11** Injury of median nerve at forearm level, right arm POA
    7ᵗʰ **S54.12** Injury of median nerve at forearm level, left arm POA

5ᵗʰ **S54.2** Injury of radial nerve at forearm level
Injury of radial nerve NOS
    7ᵗʰ **S54.20** Injury of radial nerve at forearm level, unspecified arm POA
    7ᵗʰ **S54.21** Injury of radial nerve at forearm level, right arm POA
    7ᵗʰ **S54.22** Injury of radial nerve at forearm level, left arm POA

5ᵗʰ **S54.3** Injury of cutaneous sensory nerve at forearm level
    7ᵗʰ **S54.30** Injury of cutaneous sensory nerve at forearm level, unspecified arm POA
    7ᵗʰ **S54.31** Injury of cutaneous sensory nerve at forearm level, right arm POA
    7ᵗʰ **S54.32** Injury of cutaneous sensory nerve at forearm level, left arm POA

5ᵗʰ **S54.8** Injury of other nerves at forearm level
  6ᵗʰ **S54.8X** Injury of other nerves at forearm level
    7ᵗʰ **S54.8X1** Injury of other nerves at forearm level, right arm POA
    7ᵗʰ **S54.8X2** Injury of other nerves at forearm level, left arm POA
    7ᵗʰ **S54.8X9** Injury of other nerves at forearm level, unspecified arm POA

5ᵗʰ **S54.9** Injury of unspecified nerve at forearm level
    7ᵗʰ **S54.90** Injury of unspecified nerve at forearm level, unspecified arm POA

    7ᵗʰ **S54.91** Injury of unspecified nerve at forearm level, right arm POA
    7ᵗʰ **S54.92** Injury of unspecified nerve at forearm level, left arm POA

4ᵗʰ **S55** Injury of blood vessels at forearm level
Code also any associated open wound (S51.-)
EXCLUDES2 injury of blood vessels at wrist and hand level (S65.-)
    injury of brachial vessels (S45.1-S45.2)
The appropriate 7th character is to be added to each code from category S55
    A = initial encounter
    D = subsequent encounter
    S = sequela

5ᵗʰ **S55.0** Injury of ulnar artery at forearm level
  6ᵗʰ **S55.00** Unspecified injury of ulnar artery at forearm level
    7ᵗʰ **S55.001** Unspecified injury of ulnar artery at forearm level, right arm CC POA CC/MCC Exc
    7ᵗʰ **S55.002** Unspecified injury of ulnar artery at forearm level, left arm CC POA CC/MCC Exc
    7ᵗʰ **S55.009** Unspecified injury of ulnar artery at forearm level, unspecified arm CC POA CC/MCC Exc
  6ᵗʰ **S55.01** Laceration of ulnar artery at forearm level
    7ᵗʰ **S55.011** Laceration of ulnar artery at forearm level, right arm CC POA CC/MCC Exc
    7ᵗʰ **S55.012** Laceration of ulnar artery at forearm level, left arm CC POA CC/MCC Exc
    7ᵗʰ **S55.019** Laceration of ulnar artery at forearm level, unspecified arm CC POA CC/MCC Exc
  6ᵗʰ **S55.09** Other specified injury of ulnar artery at forearm level
    7ᵗʰ **S55.091** Other specified injury of ulnar artery at forearm level, right arm CC POA CC/MCC Exc
    7ᵗʰ **S55.092** Other specified injury of ulnar artery at forearm level, left arm CC POA CC/MCC Exc
    7ᵗʰ **S55.099** Other specified injury of ulnar artery at forearm level, unspecified arm CC POA CC/MCC Exc

5ᵗʰ **S55.1** Injury of radial artery at forearm level
  6ᵗʰ **S55.10** Unspecified injury of radial artery at forearm level
    7ᵗʰ **S55.101** Unspecified injury of radial artery at forearm level, right arm CC POA CC/MCC Exc
    7ᵗʰ **S55.102** Unspecified injury of radial artery at forearm level, left arm CC POA CC/MCC Exc
    7ᵗʰ **S55.109** Unspecified injury of radial artery at forearm level, unspecified arm CC POA CC/MCC Exc
  6ᵗʰ **S55.11** Laceration of radial artery at forearm level
    7ᵗʰ **S55.111** Laceration of radial artery at forearm level, right arm CC POA CC/MCC Exc
    7ᵗʰ **S55.112** Laceration of radial artery at forearm level, left arm CC POA CC/MCC Exc
    7ᵗʰ **S55.119** Laceration of radial artery at forearm level, unspecified arm CC POA CC/MCC Exc
  6ᵗʰ **S55.19** Other specified injury of radial artery at forearm level
    7ᵗʰ **S55.191** Other specified injury of radial artery at forearm level, right arm CC POA CC/MCC Exc
    7ᵗʰ **S55.192** Other specified injury of radial artery at forearm level, left arm CC POA CC/MCC Exc
    7ᵗʰ **S55.199** Other specified injury of radial artery at forearm level, unspecified arm CC POA CC/MCC Exc

5ᵗʰ **S55.2** Injury of vein at forearm level
  6ᵗʰ **S55.20** Unspecified injury of vein at forearm level
    7ᵗʰ **S55.201** Unspecified injury of vein at forearm level, right arm CC POA CC/MCC Exc
    7ᵗʰ **S55.202** Unspecified injury of vein at forearm level, left arm CC POA CC/MCC Exc
    7ᵗʰ **S55.209** Unspecified injury of vein at forearm level, unspecified arm CC POA CC/MCC Exc

---

Unspecified Code   Other Specified Code   Manifestation Code   Ⓝ Newborn   Ⓟ Pediatric   Ⓜ Maternity   Ⓐ Adult   ♂ Male   ♀ Female
  ● New Code   ▲ Revised Code Title   ▶◀ Revised Text   **NOTES**   *INCLUDES*   *EXCLUDES 1* Not coded here   *EXCLUDES 2* Not included here
    4ᵗʰ character required   5ᵗʰ character required   6ᵗʰ character required   7ᵗʰ character required
    7ᵗʰ Extension 'X' Alert   **HAC** Hospital-acquired condition (HAC) alert   **AHA** AHA Coding Clinic©

S55.21 Laceration of vein at forearm level
- S55.211 Laceration of vein at forearm level, right arm CC POA CC/MCC Exc
- S55.212 Laceration of vein at forearm level, left arm CC POA CC/MCC Exc
- S55.219 Laceration of vein at forearm level, unspecified arm CC POA CC/MCC Exc

S55.29 Other specified injury of vein at forearm level
- S55.291 Other specified injury of vein at forearm level, right arm CC POA CC/MCC Exc
- S55.292 Other specified injury of vein at forearm level, left arm CC POA CC/MCC Exc
- S55.299 Other specified injury of vein at forearm level, unspecified arm CC POA CC/MCC Exc

S55.8 Injury of other blood vessels at forearm level
- S55.80 Unspecified injury of other blood vessels at forearm level
  - S55.801 Unspecified injury of other blood vessels at forearm level, right arm CC POA CC/MCC Exc
  - S55.802 Unspecified injury of other blood vessels at forearm level, left arm CC POA CC/MCC Exc
  - S55.809 Unspecified injury of other blood vessels at forearm level, unspecified arm CC POA CC/MCC Exc
- S55.81 Laceration of other blood vessels at forearm level
  - S55.811 Laceration of other blood vessels at forearm level, right arm CC POA CC/MCC Exc
  - S55.812 Laceration of other blood vessels at forearm level, left arm CC POA CC/MCC Exc
  - S55.819 Laceration of other blood vessels at forearm level, unspecified arm CC POA CC/MCC Exc
- S55.89 Other specified injury of other blood vessels at forearm level
  - S55.891 Other specified injury of other blood vessels at forearm level, right arm CC POA CC/MCC Exc
  - S55.892 Other specified injury of other blood vessels at forearm level, left arm CC POA CC/MCC Exc
  - S55.899 Other specified injury of other blood vessels at forearm level, unspecified arm CC POA CC/MCC Exc

S55.9 Injury of unspecified blood vessel at forearm level
- S55.90 Unspecified injury of unspecified blood vessel at forearm level
  - S55.901 Unspecified injury of unspecified blood vessel at forearm level, right arm CC POA CC/MCC Exc
  - S55.902 Unspecified injury of unspecified blood vessel at forearm level, left arm CC POA CC/MCC Exc
  - S55.909 Unspecified injury of unspecified blood vessel at forearm level, unspecified arm CC POA CC/MCC Exc
- S55.91 Laceration of unspecified blood vessel at forearm level
  - S55.911 Laceration of unspecified blood vessel at forearm level, right arm CC POA CC/MCC Exc
  - S55.912 Laceration of unspecified blood vessel at forearm level, left arm CC POA CC/MCC Exc
  - S55.919 Laceration of unspecified blood vessel at forearm level, unspecified arm CC POA CC/MCC Exc
- S55.99 Other specified injury of unspecified blood vessel at forearm level
  - S55.991 Other specified injury of unspecified blood vessel at forearm level, right arm CC POA CC/MCC Exc
  - S55.992 Other specified injury of unspecified blood vessel at forearm level, left arm CC POA CC/MCC Exc
  - S55.999 Other specified injury of unspecified blood vessel at forearm level, unspecified arm CC POA CC/MCC Exc

S56 Injury of muscle, fascia and tendon at forearm level
Code also any associated open wound (S51.-)
EXCLUDES2 injury of muscle, fascia and tendon at or below wrist (S66.-)
sprain of joints and ligaments of elbow (S53.4-)
The appropriate 7th character is to be added to each code from category S56
A = initial encounter
D = subsequent encounter
S = sequela

S56.0 Injury of flexor muscle, fascia and tendon of thumb at forearm level
- S56.00 Unspecified injury of flexor muscle, fascia and tendon of thumb at forearm level
  - S56.001 Unspecified injury of flexor muscle, fascia and tendon of right thumb at forearm level POA
  - S56.002 Unspecified injury of flexor muscle, fascia and tendon of left thumb at forearm level POA
  - S56.009 Unspecified injury of flexor muscle, fascia and tendon of unspecified thumb at forearm level POA
- S56.01 Strain of flexor muscle, fascia and tendon of thumb at forearm level
  - S56.011 Strain of flexor muscle, fascia and tendon of right thumb at forearm level POA
  - S56.012 Strain of flexor muscle, fascia and tendon of left thumb at forearm level POA
  - S56.019 Strain of flexor muscle, fascia and tendon of unspecified thumb at forearm level POA
- S56.02 Laceration of flexor muscle, fascia and tendon of thumb at forearm level
  - S56.021 Laceration of flexor muscle, fascia and tendon of right thumb at forearm level CC POA CC/MCC Exc
  - S56.022 Laceration of flexor muscle, fascia and tendon of left thumb at forearm level CC POA CC/MCC Exc
  - S56.029 Laceration of flexor muscle, fascia and tendon of unspecified thumb at forearm level CC POA CC/MCC Exc
- S56.09 Other injury of flexor muscle, fascia and tendon of thumb at forearm level
  - S56.091 Other injury of flexor muscle, fascia and tendon of right thumb at forearm level POA
  - S56.092 Other injury of flexor muscle, fascia and tendon of left thumb at forearm level POA
  - S56.099 Other injury of flexor muscle, fascia and tendon of unspecified thumb at forearm level POA

S56.1 Injury of flexor muscle, fascia and tendon of other and unspecified finger at forearm level
- S56.10 Unspecified injury of flexor muscle, fascia and tendon of other and unspecified finger at forearm level
  - S56.101 Unspecified injury of flexor muscle, fascia and tendon of right index finger at forearm level POA
  - S56.102 Unspecified injury of flexor muscle, fascia and tendon of left index finger at forearm level POA
  - S56.103 Unspecified injury of flexor muscle, fascia and tendon of right middle finger at forearm level POA
  - S56.104 Unspecified injury of flexor muscle, fascia and tendon of left middle finger at forearm level POA
  - S56.105 Unspecified injury of flexor muscle, fascia and tendon of right ring finger at forearm level POA

POA Unacceptable principal diagnosis symbol per Medicare code edits POA Code exempt from diagnosis present on admission requirement
? Questionable admission CC Complication or comorbidity CC/MCC Exc CC/MCC exclusion MCC Major complication or comorbidity
Principal diagnosis as its own CC Principal diagnosis as its own MCC HCC HCC diagnosis code RxHCC RxHCC diagnosis code
MACRA code Z Z code as first-listed diagnosis

1034

When symbols appear on a code that requires a 7th character extension, refer to Appendix B to identify applicable 7th character codes.

2018 ICD-10-CM

S56.106 Unspecified injury of flexor muscle, fascia and tendon of left ring finger at forearm level POA

S56.107 Unspecified injury of flexor muscle, fascia and tendon of right little finger at forearm level POA

S56.108 Unspecified injury of flexor muscle, fascia and tendon of left little finger at forearm level POA

S56.109 Unspecified injury of flexor muscle, fascia and tendon of unspecified finger at forearm level POA

S56.11 Strain of flexor muscle, fascia and tendon of other and unspecified finger at forearm level

S56.111 Strain of flexor muscle, fascia and tendon of right index finger at forearm level POA

S56.112 Strain of flexor muscle, fascia and tendon of left index finger at forearm level POA

S56.113 Strain of flexor muscle, fascia and tendon of right middle finger at forearm level POA

S56.114 Strain of flexor muscle, fascia and tendon of left middle finger at forearm level POA

S56.115 Strain of flexor muscle, fascia and tendon of right ring finger at forearm level POA

S56.116 Strain of flexor muscle, fascia and tendon of left ring finger at forearm level POA

S56.117 Strain of flexor muscle, fascia and tendon of right little finger at forearm level POA

S56.118 Strain of flexor muscle, fascia and tendon of left little finger at forearm level POA

S56.119 Strain of flexor muscle, fascia and tendon of finger of unspecified finger at forearm level POA

S56.12 Laceration of flexor muscle, fascia and tendon of other and unspecified finger at forearm level

S56.121 Laceration of flexor muscle, fascia and tendon of right index finger at forearm level CC POA CC/MCC Exc

S56.122 Laceration of flexor muscle, fascia and tendon of left index finger at forearm level CC POA CC/MCC Exc

S56.123 Laceration of flexor muscle, fascia and tendon of right middle finger at forearm level CC POA CC/MCC Exc

S56.124 Laceration of flexor muscle, fascia and tendon of left middle finger at forearm level CC POA CC/MCC Exc

S56.125 Laceration of flexor muscle, fascia and tendon of right ring finger at forearm level CC POA CC/MCC Exc

S56.126 Laceration of flexor muscle, fascia and tendon of left ring finger at forearm level CC POA CC/MCC Exc

S56.127 Laceration of flexor muscle, fascia and tendon of right little finger at forearm level CC POA CC/MCC Exc

S56.128 Laceration of flexor muscle, fascia and tendon of left little finger at forearm level CC POA CC/MCC Exc

S56.129 Laceration of flexor muscle, fascia and tendon of unspecified finger at forearm level CC POA CC/MCC Exc

S56.19 Other injury of flexor muscle, fascia and tendon of other and unspecified finger at forearm level

S56.191 Other injury of flexor muscle, fascia and tendon of right index finger at forearm level POA

S56.192 Other injury of flexor muscle, fascia and tendon of left index finger at forearm level POA

S56.193 Other injury of flexor muscle, fascia and tendon of right middle finger at forearm level POA

S56.194 Other injury of flexor muscle, fascia and tendon of left middle finger at forearm level POA

S56.195 Other injury of flexor muscle, fascia and tendon of right ring finger at forearm level POA

S56.196 Other injury of flexor muscle, fascia and tendon of left ring finger at forearm level POA

S56.197 Other injury of flexor muscle, fascia and tendon of right little finger at forearm level POA

S56.198 Other injury of flexor muscle, fascia and tendon of left little finger at forearm level POA

S56.199 Other injury of flexor muscle, fascia and tendon of unspecified finger at forearm level POA

S56.2 Injury of other flexor muscle, fascia and tendon at forearm level

S56.20 Unspecified injury of other flexor muscle, fascia and tendon at forearm level

S56.201 Unspecified injury of other flexor muscle, fascia and tendon at forearm level, right arm POA

S56.202 Unspecified injury of other flexor muscle, fascia and tendon at forearm level, left arm POA

S56.209 Unspecified injury of other flexor muscle, fascia and tendon at forearm level, unspecified arm POA

S56.21 Strain of other flexor muscle, fascia and tendon at forearm level

S56.211 Strain of other flexor muscle, fascia and tendon at forearm level, right arm POA

S56.212 Strain of other flexor muscle, fascia and tendon at forearm level, left arm POA

S56.219 Strain of other flexor muscle, fascia and tendon at forearm level, unspecified arm POA

S56.22 Laceration of other flexor muscle, fascia and tendon at forearm level

S56.221 Laceration of other flexor muscle, fascia and tendon at forearm level, right arm CC POA CC/MCC Exc

S56.222 Laceration of other flexor muscle, fascia and tendon at forearm level, left arm CC POA CC/MCC Exc

S56.229 Laceration of other flexor muscle, fascia and tendon at forearm level, unspecified arm CC POA CC/MCC Exc

S56.29 Other injury of other flexor muscle, fascia and tendon at forearm level

S56.291 Other injury of other flexor muscle, fascia and tendon at forearm level, right arm POA

S56.292 Other injury of other flexor muscle, fascia and tendon at forearm level, left arm POA

S56.299 Other injury of other flexor muscle, fascia and tendon at forearm level, unspecified arm POA

S56.3 Injury of extensor or abductor muscles, fascia and tendons of thumb at forearm level

S56.30 Unspecified injury of extensor or abductor muscles, fascia and tendons of thumb at forearm level

S56.301 Unspecified injury of extensor or abductor muscles, fascia and tendons of right thumb at forearm level POA

S56.302 Unspecified injury of extensor or abductor muscles, fascia and tendons of left thumb at forearm level POA

S56.309 Unspecified injury of extensor or abductor muscles, fascia and tendons of unspecified thumb at forearm level POA

Unspecified Code   Other Specified Code   Manifestation Code   N Newborn   P Pediatric   M Maternity   A Adult   ♂ Male   ♀ Female
● New Code   ▲ Revised Code Title   ►◄ Revised Text   NOTES   INCLUDES   EXCLUDES 1 Not coded here   EXCLUDES 2 Not included here
4ᵗʰ 4th character required   5ᵗʰ 5th character required   6ᵗʰ 6th character required   7ᵗʰ 7th character required
Extension 'X' Alert   HAC Hospital-acquired condition (HAC) alert   AHA AHA Coding Clinic©

6ᵗʰ S56.31 Strain of extensor or abductor muscles, fascia and tendons of thumb at forearm level

   7ᵗʰ S56.311 Strain of extensor or abductor muscles, fascia and tendons of right thumb at forearm level ᴘᴏᴀ

   7ᵗʰ S56.312 Strain of extensor or abductor muscles, fascia and tendons of left thumb at forearm level ᴘᴏᴀ

   7ᵗʰ S56.319 Strain of extensor or abductor muscles, fascia and tendons of unspecified thumb at forearm level ᴘᴏᴀ

6ᵗʰ S56.32 Laceration of extensor or abductor muscles, fascia and tendons of thumb at forearm level

   7ᵗʰ S56.321 Laceration of extensor or abductor muscles, fascia and tendons of right thumb at forearm level ᴄᴄ ᴘᴏᴀ ᴄᴄ/ᴍᴄᴄ Exc

   7ᵗʰ S56.322 Laceration of extensor or abductor muscles, fascia and tendons of left thumb at forearm level ᴄᴄ ᴘᴏᴀ ᴄᴄ/ᴍᴄᴄ Exc

   7ᵗʰ S56.329 Laceration of extensor or abductor muscles, fascia and tendons of unspecified thumb at forearm level ᴄᴄ ᴘᴏᴀ ᴄᴄ/ᴍᴄᴄ Exc

6ᵗʰ S56.39 Other injury of extensor or abductor muscles, fascia and tendons of thumb at forearm level

   7ᵗʰ S56.391 Other injury of extensor or abductor muscles, fascia and tendons of right thumb at forearm level ᴘᴏᴀ

   7ᵗʰ S56.392 Other injury of extensor or abductor muscles, fascia and tendons of left thumb at forearm level ᴘᴏᴀ

   7ᵗʰ S56.399 Other injury of extensor or abductor muscles, fascia and tendons of unspecified thumb at forearm level ᴘᴏᴀ

5ᵗʰ S56.4 Injury of extensor muscle, fascia and tendon of other and unspecified finger at forearm level

6ᵗʰ S56.40 Unspecified injury of extensor muscle, fascia and tendon of other and unspecified finger at forearm level

   7ᵗʰ S56.401 Unspecified injury of extensor muscle, fascia and tendon of right index finger at forearm level ᴘᴏᴀ

   7ᵗʰ S56.402 Unspecified injury of extensor muscle, fascia and tendon of left index finger at forearm level ᴘᴏᴀ

   7ᵗʰ S56.403 Unspecified injury of extensor muscle, fascia and tendon of right middle finger at forearm level ᴘᴏᴀ

   7ᵗʰ S56.404 Unspecified injury of extensor muscle, fascia and tendon of left middle finger at forearm level ᴘᴏᴀ

   7ᵗʰ S56.405 Unspecified injury of extensor muscle, fascia and tendon of right ring finger at forearm level ᴘᴏᴀ

   7ᵗʰ S56.406 Unspecified injury of extensor muscle, fascia and tendon of left ring finger at forearm level ᴘᴏᴀ

   7ᵗʰ S56.407 Unspecified injury of extensor muscle, fascia and tendon of right little finger at forearm level ᴘᴏᴀ

   7ᵗʰ S56.408 Unspecified injury of extensor muscle, fascia and tendon of left little finger at forearm level ᴘᴏᴀ

   7ᵗʰ S56.409 Unspecified injury of extensor muscle, fascia and tendon of unspecified finger at forearm level ᴘᴏᴀ

6ᵗʰ S56.41 Strain of extensor muscle, fascia and tendon of other and unspecified finger at forearm level

   7ᵗʰ S56.411 Strain of extensor muscle, fascia and tendon of right index finger at forearm level ᴘᴏᴀ

   7ᵗʰ S56.412 Strain of extensor muscle, fascia and tendon of left index finger at forearm level ᴘᴏᴀ

7ᵗʰ S56.413 Strain of extensor muscle, fascia and tendon of right middle finger at forearm level ᴘᴏᴀ

7ᵗʰ S56.414 Strain of extensor muscle, fascia and tendon of left middle finger at forearm level ᴘᴏᴀ

7ᵗʰ S56.415 Strain of extensor muscle, fascia and tendon of right ring finger at forearm level ᴘᴏᴀ

7ᵗʰ S56.416 Strain of extensor muscle, fascia and tendon of left ring finger at forearm level ᴘᴏᴀ

7ᵗʰ S56.417 Strain of extensor muscle, fascia and tendon of right little finger at forearm level ᴘᴏᴀ

7ᵗʰ S56.418 Strain of extensor muscle, fascia and tendon of left little finger at forearm level ᴘᴏᴀ

7ᵗʰ S56.419 Strain of extensor muscle, fascia and tendon of finger, unspecified finger at forearm level ᴘᴏᴀ

6ᵗʰ S56.42 Laceration of extensor muscle, fascia and tendon of other and unspecified finger at forearm level

   7ᵗʰ S56.421 Laceration of extensor muscle, fascia and tendon of right index finger at forearm level ᴄᴄ ᴘᴏᴀ ᴄᴄ/ᴍᴄᴄ Exc

   7ᵗʰ S56.422 Laceration of extensor muscle, fascia and tendon of left index finger at forearm level ᴄᴄ ᴘᴏᴀ ᴄᴄ/ᴍᴄᴄ Exc

   7ᵗʰ S56.423 Laceration of extensor muscle, fascia and tendon of right middle finger at forearm level ᴄᴄ ᴘᴏᴀ ᴄᴄ/ᴍᴄᴄ Exc

   7ᵗʰ S56.424 Laceration of extensor muscle, fascia and tendon of left middle finger at forearm level ᴄᴄ ᴘᴏᴀ ᴄᴄ/ᴍᴄᴄ Exc

   7ᵗʰ S56.425 Laceration of extensor muscle, fascia and tendon of right ring finger at forearm level ᴄᴄ ᴘᴏᴀ ᴄᴄ/ᴍᴄᴄ Exc

   7ᵗʰ S56.426 Laceration of extensor muscle, fascia and tendon of left ring finger at forearm level ᴄᴄ ᴘᴏᴀ ᴄᴄ/ᴍᴄᴄ Exc

   7ᵗʰ S56.427 Laceration of extensor muscle, fascia and tendon of right little finger at forearm level ᴄᴄ ᴘᴏᴀ ᴄᴄ/ᴍᴄᴄ Exc

   7ᵗʰ S56.428 Laceration of extensor muscle, fascia and tendon of left little finger at forearm level ᴄᴄ ᴘᴏᴀ ᴄᴄ/ᴍᴄᴄ Exc

   7ᵗʰ S56.429 Laceration of extensor muscle, fascia and tendon of unspecified finger at forearm level ᴄᴄ ᴘᴏᴀ ᴄᴄ/ᴍᴄᴄ Exc

6ᵗʰ S56.49 Other injury of extensor muscle, fascia and tendon of other and unspecified finger at forearm level

   7ᵗʰ S56.491 Other injury of extensor muscle, fascia and tendon of right index finger at forearm level ᴘᴏᴀ

   7ᵗʰ S56.492 Other injury of extensor muscle, fascia and tendon of left index finger at forearm level ᴘᴏᴀ

   7ᵗʰ S56.493 Other injury of extensor muscle, fascia and tendon of right middle finger at forearm level ᴘᴏᴀ

   7ᵗʰ S56.494 Other injury of extensor muscle, fascia and tendon of left middle finger at forearm level ᴘᴏᴀ

   7ᵗʰ S56.495 Other injury of extensor muscle, fascia and tendon of right ring finger at forearm level ᴘᴏᴀ

   7ᵗʰ S56.496 Other injury of extensor muscle, fascia and tendon of left ring finger at forearm level ᴘᴏᴀ

   7ᵗʰ S56.497 Other injury of extensor muscle, fascia and tendon of right little finger at forearm level ᴘᴏᴀ

ᴘᴏᴀ Unacceptable principal diagnosis symbol per Medicare code edits   ᴘᴏᴀ Code exempt from diagnosis present on admission requirement
❓ Questionable admission   ᴄᴄ Complication or comorbidity   ᴄᴄ/ᴍᴄᴄ Exc CC/MCC exclusion   ᴍᴄᴄ Major complication or comorbidity
🅐 Principal diagnosis as its own CC   🅑 Principal diagnosis as its own MCC   ʜᴄᴄ HCC diagnosis code   ʀxʜᴄᴄ RxHCC diagnosis code
MACRA code   🆉 Z code as first-listed diagnosis

When symbols appear on a code that requires a 7th character extension, refer to Appendix B to identify applicable 7th character codes.

2018 ICD-10-CM

7ᵗʰ S56.498 Other injury of extensor muscle, fascia and tendon of left little finger at forearm level

7ᵗʰ S56.499 Other injury of extensor muscle, fascia and tendon of unspecified finger at forearm level POA

5ᵗʰ S56.5 Injury of other extensor muscle, fascia and tendon at forearm level

6ᵗʰ S56.50 Unspecified injury of other extensor muscle, fascia and tendon at forearm level

7ᵗʰ S56.501 Unspecified injury of other extensor muscle, fascia and tendon at forearm level, right arm POA

7ᵗʰ S56.502 Unspecified injury of other extensor muscle, fascia and tendon at forearm level, left arm POA

7ᵗʰ S56.509 Unspecified injury of other extensor muscle, fascia and tendon at forearm level, unspecified arm POA

6ᵗʰ S56.51 Strain of other extensor muscle, fascia and tendon at forearm level

7ᵗʰ S56.511 Strain of other extensor muscle, fascia and tendon at forearm level, right arm POA

7ᵗʰ S56.512 Strain of other extensor muscle, fascia and tendon at forearm level, left arm POA

7ᵗʰ S56.519 Strain of other extensor muscle, fascia and tendon at forearm level, unspecified arm POA

6ᵗʰ S56.52 Laceration of other extensor muscle, fascia and tendon at forearm level

7ᵗʰ S56.521 Laceration of other extensor muscle, fascia and tendon at forearm level, right arm CC POA CC/MCC Exc

7ᵗʰ S56.522 Laceration of other extensor muscle, fascia and tendon at forearm level, left arm CC POA CC/MCC Exc

7ᵗʰ S56.529 Laceration of other extensor muscle, fascia and tendon at forearm level, unspecified arm CC POA CC/MCC Exc

6ᵗʰ S56.59 Other injury of other extensor muscle, fascia and tendon at forearm level

7ᵗʰ S56.591 Other injury of other extensor muscle, fascia and tendon at forearm level, right arm POA

7ᵗʰ S56.592 Other injury of other extensor muscle, fascia and tendon at forearm level, left arm POA

7ᵗʰ S56.599 Other injury of other extensor muscle, fascia and tendon at forearm level, unspecified arm POA

5ᵗʰ S56.8 Injury of other muscles, fascia and tendons at forearm level

6ᵗʰ S56.80 Unspecified injury of other muscles, fascia and tendons at forearm level

7ᵗʰ S56.801 Unspecified injury of other muscles, fascia and tendons at forearm level, right arm POA

7ᵗʰ S56.802 Unspecified injury of other muscles, fascia and tendons at forearm level, left arm POA

7ᵗʰ S56.809 Unspecified injury of other muscles, fascia and tendons at forearm level, unspecified arm POA

6ᵗʰ S56.81 Strain of other muscles, fascia and tendons at forearm level

7ᵗʰ S56.811 Strain of other muscles, fascia and tendons at forearm level, right arm POA

7ᵗʰ S56.812 Strain of other muscles, fascia and tendons at forearm level, left arm POA

7ᵗʰ S56.819 Strain of other muscles, fascia and tendons at forearm level, unspecified arm POA

6ᵗʰ S56.82 Laceration of other muscles, fascia and tendons at forearm level

7ᵗʰ S56.821 Laceration of other muscles, fascia and tendons at forearm level, right arm CC POA CC/MCC Exc

7ᵗʰ S56.822 Laceration of other muscles, fascia and tendons at forearm level, left arm CC POA CC/MCC Exc

7ᵗʰ S56.829 Laceration of other muscles, fascia and tendons at forearm level, unspecified arm CC POA CC/MCC Exc

6ᵗʰ S56.89 Other injury of other muscles, fascia and tendons at forearm level

7ᵗʰ S56.891 Other injury of other muscles, fascia and tendons at forearm level, right arm POA

7ᵗʰ S56.892 Other injury of other muscles, fascia and tendons at forearm level, left arm POA

7ᵗʰ S56.899 Other injury of other muscles, fascia and tendons at forearm level, unspecified arm POA

5ᵗʰ S56.9 Injury of unspecified muscles, fascia and tendons at forearm level

6ᵗʰ S56.90 Unspecified injury of unspecified muscles, fascia and tendons at forearm level

7ᵗʰ S56.901 Unspecified injury of unspecified muscles, fascia and tendons at forearm level, right arm POA

7ᵗʰ S56.902 Unspecified injury of unspecified muscles, fascia and tendons at forearm level, left arm POA

7ᵗʰ S56.909 Unspecified injury of unspecified muscles, fascia and tendons at forearm level, unspecified arm POA

6ᵗʰ S56.91 Strain of unspecified muscles, fascia and tendons at forearm level

7ᵗʰ S56.911 Strain of unspecified muscles, fascia and tendons at forearm level, right arm POA

7ᵗʰ S56.912 Strain of unspecified muscles, fascia and tendons at forearm level, left arm POA

7ᵗʰ S56.919 Strain of unspecified muscles, fascia and tendons at forearm level, unspecified arm POA

6ᵗʰ S56.92 Laceration of unspecified muscles, fascia and tendons at forearm level

7ᵗʰ S56.921 Laceration of unspecified muscles, fascia and tendons at forearm level, right arm CC POA CC/MCC Exc

7ᵗʰ S56.922 Laceration of unspecified muscles, fascia and tendons at forearm level, left arm CC POA CC/MCC Exc

7ᵗʰ S56.929 Laceration of unspecified muscles, fascia and tendons at forearm level, unspecified arm CC POA CC/MCC Exc

6ᵗʰ S56.99 Other injury of unspecified muscles, fascia and tendons at forearm level

7ᵗʰ S56.991 Other injury of unspecified muscles, fascia and tendons at forearm level, right arm POA

7ᵗʰ S56.992 Other injury of unspecified muscles, fascia and tendons at forearm level, left arm POA

7ᵗʰ S56.999 Other injury of unspecified muscles, fascia and tendons at forearm level, unspecified arm POA

4ᵗʰ S57 Crushing injury of elbow and forearm
Use additional code(s) for all associated injuries
EXCLUDES2 crushing injury of wrist and hand (S67.-)
The appropriate 7th character is to be added to each code from category S57
A = initial encounter
D = subsequent encounter
S = sequela

2018 ICD-10-CM

When symbols appear on a code that requires a 7th character extension, refer to Appendix B to identify applicable 7th character codes.

1037

Unspecified Code   Other Specified Code   Manifestation Code   N Newborn   P Pediatric   M Maternity   A Adult   ♂ Male   ♀ Female
● New Code   ▲ Revised Code Title   ►◄ Revised Text   NOTES   INCLUDES   EXCLUDES 1 Not coded here   EXCLUDES 2 Not included here
4ᵗʰ 4ᵗʰ character required   5ᵗʰ 5ᵗʰ character required   6ᵗʰ 6ᵗʰ character required   7ᵗʰ 7ᵗʰ character required
7ᵗʰ Extension 'X' Alert   HAC Hospital-acquired condition (HAC) alert   AHA AHA Coding Clinic©

S57.0 Crushing injury of elbow
- **S57.00** Crushing injury of unspecified elbow POA
- **S57.01** Crushing injury of right elbow POA
- **S57.02** Crushing injury of left elbow POA

S57.8 Crushing injury of forearm
- **S57.80** Crushing injury of unspecified forearm POA
- **S57.81** Crushing injury of right forearm POA
- **S57.82** Crushing injury of left forearm POA

S58 Traumatic amputation of elbow and forearm

An amputation not identified as partial or complete should be coded to complete

EXCLUDES1 traumatic amputation of wrist and hand (S68.-)

The appropriate 7th character is to be added to each code from category S58

A = initial encounter
D = subsequent encounter
S = sequela

S58.0 Traumatic amputation at elbow level
- **S58.01** Complete traumatic amputation at elbow level
  - **S58.011** Complete traumatic amputation at elbow level, right arm CC POA HCC CC/MCC Exc
  - **S58.012** Complete traumatic amputation at elbow level, left arm CC POA HCC CC/MCC Exc
  - **S58.019** Complete traumatic amputation at elbow level, unspecified arm CC POA HCC CC/MCC Exc
- **S58.02** Partial traumatic amputation at elbow level
  - **S58.021** Partial traumatic amputation at elbow level, right arm CC POA HCC CC/MCC Exc
  - **S58.022** Partial traumatic amputation at elbow level, left arm CC POA HCC CC/MCC Exc
  - **S58.029** Partial traumatic amputation at elbow level, unspecified arm CC POA HCC CC/MCC Exc

S58.1 Traumatic amputation at level between elbow and wrist
- **S58.11** Complete traumatic amputation at level between elbow and wrist
  - **S58.111** Complete traumatic amputation at level between elbow and wrist, right arm CC POA HCC CC/MCC Exc
  - **S58.112** Complete traumatic amputation at level between elbow and wrist, left arm CC POA HCC CC/MCC Exc
  - **S58.119** Complete traumatic amputation at level between elbow and wrist, unspecified arm CC POA HCC CC/MCC Exc
- **S58.12** Partial traumatic amputation at level between elbow and wrist
  - **S58.121** Partial traumatic amputation at level between elbow and wrist, right arm CC POA HCC CC/MCC Exc
  - **S58.122** Partial traumatic amputation at level between elbow and wrist, left arm CC POA HCC CC/MCC Exc
  - **S58.129** Partial traumatic amputation at level between elbow and wrist, unspecified arm CC POA HCC CC/MCC Exc

S58.9 Traumatic amputation of forearm, level unspecified

EXCLUDES1 traumatic amputation of wrist (S68.-)

- **S58.91** Complete traumatic amputation of forearm, level unspecified
  - **S58.911** Complete traumatic amputation of right forearm, level unspecified CC POA HCC CC/MCC Exc
  - **S58.912** Complete traumatic amputation of left forearm, level unspecified CC POA HCC CC/MCC Exc
  - **S58.919** Complete traumatic amputation of unspecified forearm, level unspecified CC POA HCC CC/MCC Exc
- **S58.92** Partial traumatic amputation of forearm, level unspecified

- **S58.921** Partial traumatic amputation of right forearm, level unspecified CC POA HCC CC/MCC Exc
- **S58.922** Partial traumatic amputation of left forearm, level unspecified CC POA HCC CC/MCC Exc
- **S58.929** Partial traumatic amputation of unspecified forearm, level unspecified CC POA HCC CC/MCC Exc

S59 Other and unspecified injuries of elbow and forearm

EXCLUDES2 other and unspecified injuries of wrist and hand (S69.-)

The appropriate 7th character is to be added to each code from subcategories S59.0, S59.1, and S59.2

A = initial encounter for closed fracture
D = subsequent encounter for fracture with routine healing
G = subsequent encounter for fracture with delayed healing
K = subsequent encounter for fracture with nonunion
P = subsequent encounter for fracture with malunion
S = sequela

S59.0 Physeal fracture of lower end of ulna
- **S59.00** Unspecified physeal fracture of lower end of ulna
  - **S59.001** Unspecified physeal fracture of lower end of ulna, right arm CC POA HAC CC/MCC Exc
  - **S59.002** Unspecified physeal fracture of lower end of ulna, left arm CC POA HAC CC/MCC Exc
  - **S59.009** Unspecified physeal fracture of lower end of ulna, unspecified arm CC POA HAC CC/MCC Exc
- **S59.01** Salter-Harris Type I physeal fracture of lower end of ulna
  - **S59.011** Salter-Harris Type I physeal fracture of lower end of ulna, right arm CC POA HAC CC/MCC Exc
  - **S59.012** Salter-Harris Type I physeal fracture of lower end of ulna, left arm CC POA HAC CC/MCC Exc
  - **S59.019** Salter-Harris Type I physeal fracture of lower end of ulna, unspecified arm CC POA HAC CC/MCC Exc
- **S59.02** Salter-Harris Type II physeal fracture of lower end of ulna
  - **S59.021** Salter-Harris Type II physeal fracture of lower end of ulna, right arm CC POA HAC CC/MCC Exc
  - **S59.022** Salter-Harris Type II physeal fracture of lower end of ulna, left arm CC POA HAC CC/MCC Exc
  - **S59.029** Salter-Harris Type II physeal fracture of lower end of ulna, unspecified arm CC POA HAC CC/MCC Exc
- **S59.03** Salter-Harris Type III physeal fracture of lower end of ulna
  - **S59.031** Salter-Harris Type III physeal fracture of lower end of ulna, right arm CC POA HAC CC/MCC Exc
  - **S59.032** Salter-Harris Type III physeal fracture of lower end of ulna, left arm CC POA HAC CC/MCC Exc
  - **S59.039** Salter-Harris Type III physeal fracture of lower end of ulna, unspecified arm CC POA HAC CC/MCC Exc
- **S59.04** Salter-Harris Type IV physeal fracture of lower end of ulna
  - **S59.041** Salter-Harris Type IV physeal fracture of lower end of ulna, right arm CC POA HAC CC/MCC Exc
  - **S59.042** Salter-Harris Type IV physeal fracture of lower end of ulna, left arm CC POA HAC CC/MCC Exc
  - **S59.049** Salter-Harris Type IV physeal fracture of lower end of ulna, unspecified arm CC POA HAC CC/MCC Exc
- **S59.09** Other physeal fracture of lower end of ulna
  - **S59.091** Other physeal fracture of lower end of ulna, right arm CC POA HAC CC/MCC Exc
  - **S59.092** Other physeal fracture of lower end of ulna, left arm CC POA HAC CC/MCC Exc
  - **S59.099** Other physeal fracture of lower end of ulna, unspecified arm CC POA HAC CC/MCC Exc

---

POA⊘ Unacceptable principal diagnosis symbol per Medicare code edits   POA Code exempt from diagnosis present on admission requirement
❓ Questionable admission   CC Complication or comorbidity   CC/MCC Exc CC/MCC exclusion   MCC Major complication or comorbidity
Principal diagnosis as its own CC   Principal diagnosis as its own MCC   HCC HCC diagnosis code   RxHCC RxHCC diagnosis code
MACRA code   Z1 Z code as first-listed diagnosis

5ᵗʰ **S59.1 Physeal fracture of** upper end of radius

   6ᵗʰ **S59.10 Unspecified** physeal fracture of upper end of radius

      7ᵗʰ **S59.101 Unspecified physeal fracture of upper end of radius, right arm** cc POA CC/MCC Exc

      7ᵗʰ **S59.102 Unspecified physeal fracture of upper end of radius, left arm** cc POA CC/MCC Exc

      7ᵗʰ **S59.109 Unspecified physeal fracture of upper end of radius, unspecified arm** cc POA CC/MCC Exc

   6ᵗʰ **S59.11 Salter-Harris Type I physeal fracture of upper end of radius**

      7ᵗʰ **S59.111 Salter-Harris Type I physeal fracture of upper end of radius, right arm** cc POA CC/MCC Exc

      7ᵗʰ **S59.112 Salter-Harris Type I physeal fracture of upper end of radius, left arm** cc POA CC/MCC Exc

      7ᵗʰ **S59.119 Salter-Harris Type I physeal fracture of upper end of radius, unspecified arm** cc POA CC/MCC Exc

   6ᵗʰ **S59.12 Salter-Harris Type II physeal fracture of upper end of radius**

      7ᵗʰ **S59.121 Salter-Harris Type II physeal fracture of upper end of radius, right arm** cc POA CC/MCC Exc

      7ᵗʰ **S59.122 Salter-Harris Type II physeal fracture of upper end of radius, left arm** cc POA CC/MCC Exc

      7ᵗʰ **S59.129 Salter-Harris Type II physeal fracture of upper end of radius, unspecified arm** cc POA CC/MCC Exc

   6ᵗʰ **S59.13 Salter-Harris Type III physeal fracture of upper end of radius**

      7ᵗʰ **S59.131 Salter-Harris Type III physeal fracture of upper end of radius, right arm** cc POA CC/MCC Exc

      7ᵗʰ **S59.132 Salter-Harris Type III physeal fracture of upper end of radius, left arm** cc POA CC/MCC Exc

      7ᵗʰ **S59.139 Salter-Harris Type III physeal fracture of upper end of radius, unspecified arm** cc POA CC/MCC Exc

   6ᵗʰ **S59.14 Salter-Harris Type IV physeal fracture of upper end of radius**

      7ᵗʰ **S59.141 Salter-Harris Type IV physeal fracture of upper end of radius, right arm** cc POA CC/MCC Exc

      7ᵗʰ **S59.142 Salter-Harris Type IV physeal fracture of upper end of radius, left arm** cc POA CC/MCC Exc

      7ᵗʰ **S59.149 Salter-Harris Type IV physeal fracture of upper end of radius, unspecified arm** cc POA CC/MCC Exc

   6ᵗʰ **S59.19 Other physeal fracture of upper end of radius**

      7ᵗʰ **S59.191 Other physeal fracture of upper end of radius, right arm** cc POA CC/MCC Exc

      7ᵗʰ **S59.192 Other physeal fracture of upper end of radius, left arm** cc POA CC/MCC Exc

      7ᵗʰ **S59.199 Other physeal fracture of upper end of radius, unspecified arm** cc POA CC/MCC Exc

5ᵗʰ **S59.2 Physeal fracture of lower end of radius**

   6ᵗʰ **S59.20 Unspecified physeal fracture of lower end of radius**

      7ᵗʰ **S59.201 Unspecified physeal fracture of lower end of radius, right arm** cc POA HAC CC/MCC Exc

      7ᵗʰ **S59.202 Unspecified physeal fracture of lower end of radius, left arm** cc POA HAC CC/MCC Exc

      7ᵗʰ **S59.209 Unspecified physeal fracture of lower end of radius, unspecified arm** cc POA HAC CC/MCC Exc

   6ᵗʰ **S59.21 Salter-Harris Type I physeal fracture of lower end of radius**

      7ᵗʰ **S59.211 Salter-Harris Type I physeal fracture of lower end of radius, right arm** cc POA HAC CC/MCC Exc

      7ᵗʰ **S59.212 Salter-Harris Type I physeal fracture of lower end of radius, left arm** cc POA HAC CC/MCC Exc

      7ᵗʰ **S59.219 Salter-Harris Type I physeal fracture of lower end of radius, unspecified arm** cc POA HAC CC/MCC Exc

   6ᵗʰ **S59.22 Salter-Harris Type II physeal fracture of lower end of radius**

      7ᵗʰ **S59.221 Salter-Harris Type II physeal fracture of lower end of radius, right arm** cc POA HAC CC/MCC Exc

      7ᵗʰ **S59.222 Salter-Harris Type II physeal fracture of lower end of radius, left arm** cc POA HAC CC/MCC Exc

      7ᵗʰ **S59.229 Salter-Harris Type II physeal fracture of lower end of radius, unspecified arm** cc POA HAC CC/MCC Exc

   6ᵗʰ **S59.23 Salter-Harris Type III physeal fracture of lower end of radius**

      7ᵗʰ **S59.231 Salter-Harris Type III physeal fracture of lower end of radius, right arm** cc POA HAC CC/MCC Exc

      7ᵗʰ **S59.232 Salter-Harris Type III physeal fracture of lower end of radius, left arm** cc POA HAC CC/MCC Exc

      7ᵗʰ **S59.239 Salter-Harris Type III physeal fracture of lower end of radius, unspecified arm** cc POA HAC CC/MCC Exc

   6ᵗʰ **S59.24 Salter-Harris Type IV physeal fracture of lower end of radius**

      7ᵗʰ **S59.241 Salter-Harris Type IV physeal fracture of lower end of radius, right arm** cc POA HAC CC/MCC Exc

      7ᵗʰ **S59.242 Salter-Harris Type IV physeal fracture of lower end of radius, left arm** cc POA HAC CC/MCC Exc

      7ᵗʰ **S59.249 Salter-Harris Type IV physeal fracture of lower end of radius, unspecified arm** cc POA HAC CC/MCC Exc

   6ᵗʰ **S59.29 Other physeal fracture of lower end of radius**

      7ᵗʰ **S59.291 Other physeal fracture of lower end of radius, right arm** cc POA HAC CC/MCC Exc

      7ᵗʰ **S59.292 Other physeal fracture of lower end of radius, left arm** cc POA HAC CC/MCC Exc

      7ᵗʰ **S59.299 Other physeal fracture of lower end of radius, unspecified arm** cc POA HAC CC/MCC Exc

5ᵗʰ **S59.8 Other specified injuries of elbow and forearm**

   The appropriate 7th character is to be added to each code in subcategory S59.8

     A = initial encounter

     D = subsequent encounter

     S = sequela

   6ᵗʰ **S59.80 Other specified injuries of elbow**

      7ᵗʰ **S59.801 Other specified injuries of right elbow** POA

      7ᵗʰ **S59.802 Other specified injuries of left elbow** POA

      7ᵗʰ **S59.809 Other specified injuries of unspecified elbow** POA

   6ᵗʰ **S59.81 Other specified injuries of forearm**

      7ᵗʰ **S59.811 Other specified injuries right forearm** POA

      7ᵗʰ **S59.812 Other specified injuries left forearm** POA

      7ᵗʰ **S59.819 Other specified injuries unspecified forearm** POA

5ᵗʰ **S59.9 Unspecified injury of elbow and forearm**

   The appropriate 7th character is to be added to each code in subcategory S59.9

     A = initial encounter

     D = subsequent encounter

     S = sequela

   6ᵗʰ **S59.90 Unspecified injury of elbow**

      7ᵗʰ **S59.901 Unspecified injury of right elbow** POA

      7ᵗʰ **S59.902 Unspecified injury of left elbow** POA

      7ᵗʰ **S59.909 Unspecified injury of unspecified elbow** POA

   6ᵗʰ **S59.91 Unspecified injury of forearm**

      7ᵗʰ **S59.911 Unspecified injury of right forearm** POA

      7ᵗʰ **S59.912 Unspecified injury of left forearm** POA

      7ᵗʰ **S59.919 Unspecified injury of unspecified forearm** POA

Unspecified Code Other Specified Code Manifestation Code Ⓝ Newborn Ⓟ Pediatric Ⓜ Maternity Ⓐ Adult ♂ Male ♀ Female
● New Code ▲ Revised Code Title ▶◀ Revised Text **NOTES** *INCLUDES* *EXCLUDES 1* Not coded here *EXCLUDES 2* Not included here
4ᵗʰ character required 5ᵗʰ character required 6ᵗʰ character required 7ᵗʰ character required
Ⓧ Extension 'X' Alert **HAC** Hospital-acquired condition (HAC) alert **AHA** AHA Coding Clinic©

Injuries to the wrist, hand and fingers (S60-S69)

EXCLUDES2   burns and corrosions (T20-T32)

frostbite (T33-T34)

insect bite or sting, venomous (T63.4)

S60   **Superficial injury of wrist, hand and fingers**

The appropriate 7th character is to be added to each code from category S60

A = initial encounter

D = subsequent encounter

S = sequela

S60.0   Contusion of finger without damage to nail

EXCLUDES1   contusion involving nail (matrix) (S60.1)

S60.00   Contusion of unspecified finger without damage to nail   POA

Contusion of finger(s) NOS

S60.01   Contusion of thumb without damage to nail

S60.011   Contusion of right thumb without damage to nail   POA

S60.012   Contusion of left thumb without damage to nail   POA

S60.019   Contusion of unspecified thumb without damage to nail   POA

S60.02   Contusion of index finger without damage to nail

S60.021   Contusion of right index finger without damage to nail   POA

S60.022   Contusion of left index finger without damage to nail   POA

S60.029   Contusion of unspecified index finger without damage to nail   POA

S60.03   Contusion of middle finger without damage to nail

S60.031   Contusion of right middle finger without damage to nail   POA

S60.032   Contusion of left middle finger without damage to nail   POA

S60.039   Contusion of unspecified middle finger without damage to nail   POA

S60.04   Contusion of ring finger without damage to nail

S60.041   Contusion of right ring finger without damage to nail   POA

S60.042   Contusion of left ring finger without damage to nail   POA

S60.049   Contusion of unspecified ring finger without damage to nail   POA

S60.05   Contusion of little finger without damage to nail

S60.051   Contusion of right little finger without damage to nail   POA

S60.052   Contusion of left little finger without damage to nail   POA

S60.059   Contusion of unspecified little finger without damage to nail   POA

S60.1   Contusion of finger with damage to nail

S60.10   Contusion of unspecified finger with damage to nail   POA

S60.11   Contusion of thumb with damage to nail

S60.111   Contusion of right thumb with damage to nail   POA

S60.112   Contusion of left thumb with damage to nail   POA

S60.119   Contusion of unspecified thumb with damage to nail   POA

S60.12   Contusion of index finger with damage to nail

S60.121   Contusion of right index finger with damage to nail   POA

S60.122   Contusion of left index finger with damage to nail   POA

S60.129   Contusion of unspecified index finger with damage to nail   POA

S60.13   Contusion of middle finger with damage to nail

S60.131   Contusion of right middle finger with damage to nail   POA

S60.132   Contusion of left middle finger with damage to nail   POA

S60.139   Contusion of unspecified middle finger with damage to nail   POA

S60.14   Contusion of ring finger with damage to nail

S60.141   Contusion of right ring finger with damage to nail   POA

S60.142   Contusion of left ring finger with damage to nail   POA

S60.149   Contusion of unspecified ring finger with damage to nail   POA

S60.15   Contusion of little finger with damage to nail

S60.151   Contusion of right little finger with damage to nail   POA

S60.152   Contusion of left little finger with damage to nail   POA

S60.159   Contusion of unspecified little finger with damage to nail   POA

S60.2   Contusion of wrist and hand

EXCLUDES2   contusion of fingers (S60.0-, S60.1-)

S60.21   Contusion of wrist

S60.211   Contusion of right wrist   POA

S60.212   Contusion of left wrist   POA

S60.219   Contusion of unspecified wrist   POA

S60.22   Contusion of hand

S60.221   Contusion of right hand   POA

S60.222   Contusion of left hand   POA

S60.229   Contusion of unspecified hand   POA

S60.3   Other superficial injuries of thumb

S60.31   Abrasion of thumb

S60.311   Abrasion of right thumb   POA

S60.312   Abrasion of left thumb   POA

S60.319   Abrasion of unspecified thumb   POA

S60.32   Blister (nonthermal) of thumb

S60.321   Blister (nonthermal) of right thumb   POA

S60.322   Blister (nonthermal) of left thumb   POA

S60.329   Blister (nonthermal) of unspecified thumb   POA

S60.34   External constriction of thumb

Hair tourniquet syndrome of thumb

Use additional cause code to identify the constricting item (W49.0-)

S60.341   External constriction of right thumb   POA

S60.342   External constriction of left thumb   POA

S60.349   External constriction of unspecified thumb   POA

S60.35   Superficial foreign body of thumb

Splinter in the thumb

S60.351   Superficial foreign body of right thumb   POA

S60.352   Superficial foreign body of left thumb   POA

S60.359   Superficial foreign body of unspecified thumb   POA

S60.36   Insect bite (nonvenomous) of thumb

S60.361   Insect bite (nonvenomous) of right thumb   POA

S60.362   Insect bite (nonvenomous) of left thumb   POA

S60.369   Insect bite (nonvenomous) of unspecified thumb   POA

S60.37   Other superficial bite of thumb

EXCLUDES1   open bite of thumb (S61.05-, S61.15-)

S60.371   Other superficial bite of right thumb   POA

S60.372   Other superficial bite of left thumb   POA

S60.379   Other superficial bite of unspecified thumb   POA

S60.39   Other superficial injuries of thumb

S60.391   Other superficial injuries of right thumb   POA

S60.392   Other superficial injuries of left thumb   POA

S60.399   Other superficial injuries of unspecified thumb   POA

POA Unacceptable principal diagnosis symbol per Medicare code edits   POA Code exempt from diagnosis present on admission requirement
❓ Questionable admission   CC Complication or comorbidity   CC-MCC Exc CC/MCC exclusion   MCC Major complication or comorbidity
CC Principal diagnosis as its own CC   MCC Principal diagnosis as its own MCC   HCC HCC diagnosis code   RHCC RxHCC diagnosis code
MACRA code   Z1 Z code as first-listed diagnosis

1040   When symbols appear on a code that requires a 7th character extension, refer to Appendix B to identify applicable 7th character codes.   **2018 ICD-10-CM**

S60.4 Other superficial injuries of other fingers
- S60.41 Abrasion of fingers
  - S60.410 Abrasion of right index finger POA
  - S60.411 Abrasion of left index finger POA
  - S60.412 Abrasion of right middle finger POA
  - S60.413 Abrasion of left middle finger POA
  - S60.414 Abrasion of right ring finger POA
  - S60.415 Abrasion of left ring finger POA
  - S60.416 Abrasion of right little finger POA
  - S60.417 Abrasion of left little finger POA
  - S60.418 Abrasion of other finger POA
    Abrasion of specified finger with unspecified laterality
  - S60.419 Abrasion of unspecified finger POA
- S60.42 Blister (nonthermal) of fingers
  - S60.420 Blister (nonthermal) of right index finger POA
  - S60.421 Blister (nonthermal) of left index finger POA
  - S60.422 Blister (nonthermal) of right middle finger POA
  - S60.423 Blister (nonthermal) of left middle finger POA
  - S60.424 Blister (nonthermal) of right ring finger POA
  - S60.425 Blister (nonthermal) of left ring finger POA
  - S60.426 Blister (nonthermal) of right little finger POA
  - S60.427 Blister (nonthermal) of left little finger POA
  - S60.428 Blister (nonthermal) of other finger POA
    Blister (nonthermal) of specified finger with unspecified laterality
  - S60.429 Blister (nonthermal) of unspecified finger POA
- S60.44 External constriction of fingers
  Hair tourniquet syndrome of finger
  Use additional cause code to identify the constricting item (W49.0-)
  - S60.440 External constriction of right index finger POA
  - S60.441 External constriction of left index finger POA
  - S60.442 External constriction of right middle finger POA
  - S60.443 External constriction of left middle finger POA
  - S60.444 External constriction of right ring finger POA
  - S60.445 External constriction of left ring finger POA
  - S60.446 External constriction of right little finger POA
  - S60.447 External constriction of left little finger POA
  - S60.448 External constriction of other finger POA
    External constriction of specified finger with unspecified laterality
  - S60.449 External constriction of unspecified finger POA
- S60.45 Superficial foreign body of fingers
  Splinter in the finger(s)
  - S60.450 Superficial foreign body of right index finger POA
  - S60.451 Superficial foreign body of left index finger POA
  - S60.452 Superficial foreign body of right middle finger POA
  - S60.453 Superficial foreign body of left middle finger POA
  - S60.454 Superficial foreign body of right ring finger POA
  - S60.455 Superficial foreign body of left ring finger POA
  - S60.456 Superficial foreign body of right little finger POA
  - S60.457 Superficial foreign body of left little finger POA
  - S60.458 Superficial foreign body of other finger POA
    Superficial foreign body of specified finger with unspecified laterality
  - S60.459 Superficial foreign body of unspecified finger POA
- S60.46 Insect bite (nonvenomous) of fingers
  - S60.460 Insect bite (nonvenomous) of right index finger POA
  - S60.461 Insect bite (nonvenomous) of left index finger POA
  - S60.462 Insect bite (nonvenomous) of right middle finger POA
  - S60.463 Insect bite (nonvenomous) of left middle finger POA
  - S60.464 Insect bite (nonvenomous) of right ring finger POA
  - S60.465 Insect bite (nonvenomous) of left ring finger POA
  - S60.466 Insect bite (nonvenomous) of right little finger POA
  - S60.467 Insect bite (nonvenomous) of left little finger POA
  - S60.468 Insect bite (nonvenomous) of other finger POA
    Insect bite (nonvenomous) of specified finger with unspecified laterality
  - S60.469 Insect bite (nonvenomous) of unspecified finger POA
- S60.47 Other superficial bite of fingers
  EXCLUDES1 open bite of fingers (S61.25-, S61.35-)
  - S60.470 Other superficial bite of right index finger POA
  - S60.471 Other superficial bite of left index finger POA
  - S60.472 Other superficial bite of right middle finger POA
  - S60.473 Other superficial bite of left middle finger POA
  - S60.474 Other superficial bite of right ring finger POA
  - S60.475 Other superficial bite of left ring finger POA
  - S60.476 Other superficial bite of right little finger POA
  - S60.477 Other superficial bite of left little finger POA
  - S60.478 Other superficial bite of other finger POA
    Other superficial bite of specified finger with unspecified laterality
  - S60.479 Other superficial bite of unspecified finger POA
S60.5 Other superficial injuries of hand
  EXCLUDES2 superficial injuries of fingers (S60.3-, S60.4-)
- S60.51 Abrasion of hand
  - S60.511 Abrasion of right hand POA
  - S60.512 Abrasion of left hand POA
  - S60.519 Abrasion of unspecified hand POA
- S60.52 Blister (nonthermal) of hand
  - S60.521 Blister (nonthermal) of right hand POA
  - S60.522 Blister (nonthermal) of left hand POA
  - S60.529 Blister (nonthermal) of unspecified hand POA
- S60.54 External constriction of hand
  - S60.541 External constriction of right hand POA
  - S60.542 External constriction of left hand POA
  - S60.549 External constriction of unspecified hand POA
- S60.55 Superficial foreign body of hand
  Splinter in the hand
  - S60.551 Superficial foreign body of right hand POA
  - S60.552 Superficial foreign body of left hand POA
  - S60.559 Superficial foreign body of unspecified hand POA

Unspecified Code	Other Specified Code	Manifestation Code	N Newborn	P Pediatric	M Maternity	A Adult	♂ Male	♀ Female

● New Code   ▲ Revised Code Title   ▶◀ Revised Text   NOTES   INCLUDES   EXCLUDES 1 Not coded here   EXCLUDES 2 Not included here
4th character required   5th character required   6th character required   7th character required
Extension 'X' Alert   HAC Hospital-acquired condition (HAC) alert   AHA AHA Coding Clinic©

[6th] S60.56 Insect bite (nonvenomous) of hand
[7th] S60.561 Insect bite (nonvenomous) of right hand [POA]
[7th] S60.562 Insect bite (nonvenomous) of left hand [POA]
[7th] S60.569 Insect bite (nonvenomous) of unspecified hand [POA]

[6th] S60.57 Other superficial bite of hand
[EXCLUDES1] *open bite of hand (S61.45-)*
[7th] S60.571 Other superficial bite of hand of right hand [POA]
[7th] S60.572 Other superficial bite of hand of left hand [POA]
[7th] S60.579 Other superficial bite of hand of unspecified hand [POA]

[5th] S60.8 Other superficial injuries of wrist
[6th] S60.81 Abrasion of wrist
[7th] S60.811 Abrasion of right wrist [POA]
[7th] S60.812 Abrasion of left wrist [POA]
[7th] S60.819 Abrasion of unspecified wrist [POA]

[6th] S60.82 Blister (nonthermal) of wrist
[7th] S60.821 Blister (nonthermal) of right wrist [POA]
[7th] S60.822 Blister (nonthermal) of left wrist [POA]
[7th] S60.829 Blister (nonthermal) of unspecified wrist [POA]

[6th] S60.84 External constriction of wrist
[7th] S60.841 External constriction of right wrist [POA]
[7th] S60.842 External constriction of left wrist [POA]
[7th] S60.849 External constriction of unspecified wrist [POA]

[6th] S60.85 Superficial foreign body of wrist
Splinter in the wrist
[7th] S60.851 Superficial foreign body of right wrist [POA]
[7th] S60.852 Superficial foreign body of left wrist [POA]
[7th] S60.859 Superficial foreign body of unspecified wrist [POA]

[6th] S60.86 Insect bite (nonvenomous) of wrist
[7th] S60.861 Insect bite (nonvenomous) of right wrist [POA]
[7th] S60.862 Insect bite (nonvenomous) of left wrist [POA]
[7th] S60.869 Insect bite (nonvenomous) of unspecified wrist [POA]

[6th] S60.87 Other superficial bite of wrist
[EXCLUDES1] *open bite of wrist (S61.55)*
[7th] S60.871 Other superficial bite of right wrist [POA]
[7th] S60.872 Other superficial bite of left wrist [POA]
[7th] S60.879 Other superficial bite of unspecified wrist [POA]

[5th] S60.9 Unspecified superficial injury of wrist, hand and fingers
[6th] S60.91 Unspecified superficial injury of wrist
[7th] S60.911 Unspecified superficial injury of right wrist [POA]
[7th] S60.912 Unspecified superficial injury of left wrist [POA]
[7th] S60.919 Unspecified superficial injury of unspecified wrist [POA]

[6th] S60.92 Unspecified superficial injury of hand
[7th] S60.921 Unspecified superficial injury of right hand [POA]
[7th] S60.922 Unspecified superficial injury of left hand [POA]
[7th] S60.929 Unspecified superficial injury of unspecified hand [POA]

[6th] S60.93 Unspecified superficial injury of thumb
[7th] S60.931 Unspecified superficial injury of right thumb [POA]
[7th] S60.932 Unspecified superficial injury of left thumb [POA]
[7th] S60.939 Unspecified superficial injury of unspecified thumb [POA]

[6th] S60.94 Unspecified superficial injury of other fingers
[7th] S60.940 Unspecified superficial injury of right index finger [POA]
[7th] S60.941 Unspecified superficial injury of left index finger [POA]
[7th] S60.942 Unspecified superficial injury of right middle finger [POA]
[7th] S60.943 Unspecified superficial injury of left middle finger [POA]
[7th] S60.944 Unspecified superficial injury of right ring finger [POA]
[7th] S60.945 Unspecified superficial injury of left ring finger [POA]
[7th] S60.946 Unspecified superficial injury of right little finger [POA]
[7th] S60.947 Unspecified superficial injury of left little finger [POA]
[7th] S60.948 Unspecified superficial injury of other finger [POA]
Unspecified superficial injury of specified finger with unspecified laterality
[7th] S60.949 Unspecified superficial injury of unspecified finger [POA]

[4th] S61 Open wound of wrist, hand and fingers
Code also any associated wound infection
[EXCLUDES1] *open fracture of wrist, hand and finger (S62.- with 7th character B)*
traumatic amputation of wrist and hand (S68.-)
The appropriate 7th character is to be added to each code from category S61
A = initial encounter
D = subsequent encounter
S = sequela

[5th] S61.0 Open wound of thumb without damage to nail
[EXCLUDES1] *open wound of thumb with damage to nail (S61.1-)*
[6th] S61.00 Unspecified open wound of thumb without damage to nail
[7th] S61.001 Unspecified open wound of right thumb without damage to nail [POA]
[7th] S61.002 Unspecified open wound of left thumb without damage to nail [POA]
[7th] S61.009 Unspecified open wound of unspecified thumb without damage to nail [POA]

[6th] S61.01 Laceration without foreign body of thumb without damage to nail
[7th] S61.011 Laceration without foreign body of right thumb without damage to nail [POA]
[7th] S61.012 Laceration without foreign body of left thumb without damage to nail [POA]
[7th] S61.019 Laceration without foreign body of unspecified thumb without damage to nail [POA]

[6th] S61.02 Laceration with foreign body of thumb without damage to nail
[7th] S61.021 Laceration with foreign body of right thumb without damage to nail [POA]
[7th] S61.022 Laceration with foreign body of left thumb without damage to nail [POA]
[7th] S61.029 Laceration with foreign body of unspecified thumb without damage to nail [POA]

[6th] S61.03 Puncture wound without foreign body of thumb without damage to nail
[7th] S61.031 Puncture wound without foreign body of right thumb without damage to nail [POA]
[7th] S61.032 Puncture wound without foreign body of left thumb without damage to nail [POA]
[7th] S61.039 Puncture wound without foreign body of unspecified thumb without damage to nail [POA]

[6th] S61.04 Puncture wound with foreign body of thumb without damage to nail

[PDx] Unacceptable principal diagnosis symbol per Medicare code edits [POA] Code exempt from diagnosis present on admission requirement
[?] Questionable admission [CC] Complication or comorbidity [CC/MCC Exc] CC/MCC exclusion [MCC] Major complication or comorbidity
[PDx CC] Principal diagnosis as its own CC [PDx MCC] Principal diagnosis as its own MCC [HCC] HCC diagnosis code [RxHCC] RxHCC diagnosis code
MACRA code [Z1] Z code as first-listed diagnosis

When symbols appear on a code that requires a 7th character extension, refer to Appendix B to identify applicable 7th character codes.

7️⃣ S61.041 Puncture wound with foreign body of right thumb without damage to nail ᴾᴼᴬ

7️⃣ S61.042 Puncture wound with foreign body of left thumb without damage to nail ᴾᴼᴬ

7️⃣ S61.049 Puncture wound with foreign body of unspecified thumb without damage to nail ᴾᴼᴬ

6️⃣ S61.05 Open bite of thumb without damage to nail
Bite of thumb NOS
EXCLUDES1 superficial bite of thumb (S60.36-, S60.37-)

7️⃣ S61.051 Open bite of right thumb without damage to nail ᴾᴼᴬ

7️⃣ S61.052 Open bite of left thumb without damage to nail ᴾᴼᴬ

7️⃣ S61.059 Open bite of unspecified thumb without damage to nail ᴾᴼᴬ

5️⃣ S61.1 Open wound of thumb with damage to nail

6️⃣ S61.10 Unspecified open wound of thumb with damage to nail

7️⃣ S61.101 Unspecified open wound of right thumb with damage to nail ᴾᴼᴬ

7️⃣ S61.102 Unspecified open wound of left thumb with damage to nail ᴾᴼᴬ

7️⃣ S61.109 Unspecified open wound of unspecified thumb with damage to nail ᴾᴼᴬ

6️⃣ S61.11 Laceration without foreign body of thumb with damage to nail

7️⃣ S61.111 Laceration without foreign body of right thumb with damage to nail ᴾᴼᴬ

7️⃣ S61.112 Laceration without foreign body of left thumb with damage to nail ᴾᴼᴬ

7️⃣ S61.119 Laceration without foreign body of unspecified thumb with damage to nail ᴾᴼᴬ

6️⃣ S61.12 Laceration with foreign body of thumb with damage to nail

7️⃣ S61.121 Laceration with foreign body of right thumb with damage to nail ᴾᴼᴬ

7️⃣ S61.122 Laceration with foreign body of left thumb with damage to nail ᴾᴼᴬ

7️⃣ S61.129 Laceration with foreign body of unspecified thumb with damage to nail ᴾᴼᴬ

6️⃣ S61.13 Puncture wound without foreign body of thumb with damage to nail

7️⃣ S61.131 Puncture wound without foreign body of right thumb with damage to nail ᴾᴼᴬ

7️⃣ S61.132 Puncture wound without foreign body of left thumb with damage to nail ᴾᴼᴬ

7️⃣ S61.139 Puncture wound without foreign body of unspecified thumb with damage to nail ᴾᴼᴬ

6️⃣ S61.14 Puncture wound with foreign body of thumb with damage to nail

7️⃣ S61.141 Puncture wound with foreign body of right thumb with damage to nail ᴾᴼᴬ

7️⃣ S61.142 Puncture wound with foreign body of left thumb with damage to nail ᴾᴼᴬ

7️⃣ S61.149 Puncture wound with foreign body of unspecified thumb with damage to nail ᴾᴼᴬ

6️⃣ S61.15 Open bite of thumb with damage to nail
Bite of thumb with damage to nail NOS
EXCLUDES1 superficial bite of thumb (S60.36-, S60.37-)

7️⃣ S61.151 Open bite of right thumb with damage to nail ᴾᴼᴬ

7️⃣ S61.152 Open bite of left thumb with damage to nail ᴾᴼᴬ

7️⃣ S61.159 Open bite of unspecified thumb with damage to nail ᴾᴼᴬ

5️⃣ S61.2 Open wound of other finger without damage to nail
EXCLUDES1 open wound of finger involving nail (matrix) (S61.3-)
EXCLUDES2 open wound of thumb without damage to nail (S61.0-)

6️⃣ S61.20 Unspecified open wound of other finger without damage to nail

7️⃣ S61.200 Unspecified open wound of right index finger without damage to nail ᴾᴼᴬ

7️⃣ S61.201 Unspecified open wound of left index finger without damage to nail ᴾᴼᴬ

7️⃣ S61.202 Unspecified open wound of right middle finger without damage to nail ᴾᴼᴬ

7️⃣ S61.203 Unspecified open wound of left middle finger without damage to nail ᴾᴼᴬ

7️⃣ S61.204 Unspecified open wound of right ring finger without damage to nail ᴾᴼᴬ

7️⃣ S61.205 Unspecified open wound of left ring finger without damage to nail ᴾᴼᴬ

7️⃣ S61.206 Unspecified open wound of right little finger without damage to nail ᴾᴼᴬ

7️⃣ S61.207 Unspecified open wound of left little finger without damage to nail ᴾᴼᴬ

7️⃣ S61.208 Unspecified open wound of other finger without damage to nail ᴾᴼᴬ
Unspecified open wound of specified finger with unspecified laterality without damage to nail

7️⃣ S61.209 Unspecified open wound of unspecified finger without damage to nail ᴾᴼᴬ

6️⃣ S61.21 Laceration without foreign body of finger without damage to nail

7️⃣ S61.210 Laceration without foreign body of right index finger without damage to nail ᴾᴼᴬ

7️⃣ S61.211 Laceration without foreign body of left index finger without damage to nail ᴾᴼᴬ

7️⃣ S61.212 Laceration without foreign body of right middle finger without damage to nail ᴾᴼᴬ

7️⃣ S61.213 Laceration without foreign body of left middle finger without damage to nail ᴾᴼᴬ

7️⃣ S61.214 Laceration without foreign body of right ring finger without damage to nail ᴾᴼᴬ

7️⃣ S61.215 Laceration without foreign body of left ring finger without damage to nail ᴾᴼᴬ

7️⃣ S61.216 Laceration without foreign body of right little finger without damage to nail ᴾᴼᴬ

7️⃣ S61.217 Laceration without foreign body of left little finger without damage to nail ᴾᴼᴬ

7️⃣ S61.218 Laceration without foreign body of other finger without damage to nail ᴾᴼᴬ
Laceration without foreign body of specified finger with unspecified laterality without damage to nail

7️⃣ S61.219 Laceration without foreign body of unspecified finger without damage to nail ᴾᴼᴬ

6️⃣ S61.22 Laceration with foreign body of finger without damage to nail

7️⃣ S61.220 Laceration with foreign body of right index finger without damage to nail ᴾᴼᴬ

7️⃣ S61.221 Laceration with foreign body of left index finger without damage to nail ᴾᴼᴬ

7️⃣ S61.222 Laceration with foreign body of right middle finger without damage to nail ᴾᴼᴬ

7️⃣ S61.223 Laceration with foreign body of left middle finger without damage to nail ᴾᴼᴬ

7️⃣ S61.224 Laceration with foreign body of right ring finger without damage to nail ᴾᴼᴬ

7️⃣ S61.225 Laceration with foreign body of left ring finger without damage to nail ᴾᴼᴬ

7️⃣ S61.226 Laceration with foreign body of right little finger without damage to nail ᴾᴼᴬ

7️⃣ S61.227 Laceration with foreign body of left little finger without damage to nail ᴾᴼᴬ

7️⃣ S61.228 Laceration with foreign body of other finger without damage to nail ᴾᴼᴬ
Laceration with foreign body of specified finger with unspecified laterality without damage to nail

---

Unspecified Code   Other Specified Code   Manifestation Code   N Newborn   P Pediatric   M Maternity   A Adult   ♂ Male   ♀ Female
● New Code   ▲ Revised Code Title   ▶◀ Revised Text   NOTES   INCLUDES   EXCLUDES 1 Not coded here   EXCLUDES 2 Not included here
4️⃣ 4th character required   5️⃣ 5th character required   6️⃣ 6th character required   7️⃣ 7th character required
Ⓧ Extension 'X' Alert   HAC Hospital-acquired condition (HAC) alert   AHA AHA Coding Clinic©

S61.229 Laceration with foreign body of unspecified finger without damage to nail

6ᵗʰ S61.23 Puncture wound without foreign body of finger without damage to nail

S61.230 Puncture wound without foreign body of right index finger without damage to nail

S61.231 Puncture wound without foreign body of left index finger without damage to nail

S61.232 Puncture wound without foreign body of right middle finger without damage to nail

S61.233 Puncture wound without foreign body of left middle finger without damage to nail

S61.234 Puncture wound without foreign body of right ring finger without damage to nail

S61.235 Puncture wound without foreign body of left ring finger without damage to nail

S61.236 Puncture wound without foreign body of right little finger without damage to nail

S61.237 Puncture wound without foreign body of left little finger without damage to nail

S61.238 Puncture wound without foreign body of other finger without damage to nail

Puncture wound without foreign body of specified finger with unspecified laterality without damage to nail

S61.239 Puncture wound without foreign body of unspecified finger without damage to nail

6ᵗʰ S61.24 Puncture wound with foreign body of finger without damage to nail

S61.240 Puncture wound with foreign body of right index finger without damage to nail

S61.241 Puncture wound with foreign body of left index finger without damage to nail

S61.242 Puncture wound with foreign body of right middle finger without damage to nail

S61.243 Puncture wound with foreign body of left middle finger without damage to nail

S61.244 Puncture wound with foreign body of right ring finger without damage to nail

S61.245 Puncture wound with foreign body of left ring finger without damage to nail

S61.246 Puncture wound with foreign body of right little finger without damage to nail

S61.247 Puncture wound with foreign body of left little finger without damage to nail

S61.248 Puncture wound with foreign body of other finger without damage to nail

Puncture wound with foreign body of specified finger with unspecified laterality without damage to nail

S61.249 Puncture wound with foreign body of unspecified finger without damage to nail

5ᵗʰ S61.25 Open bite of finger without damage to nail

Bite of finger without damage to nail NOS

EXCLUDES1 superficial bite of finger (S60.46-, S60.47-)

S61.250 Open bite of right index finger without damage to nail

S61.251 Open bite of left index finger without damage to nail

S61.252 Open bite of right middle finger without damage to nail

S61.253 Open bite of left middle finger without damage to nail

S61.254 Open bite of right ring finger without damage to nail

S61.255 Open bite of left ring finger without damage to nail

S61.256 Open bite of right little finger without damage to nail

S61.257 Open bite of left little finger without damage to nail

S61.258 Open bite of other finger without damage to nail

Open bite of specified finger with unspecified laterality without damage to nail

S61.259 Open bite of unspecified finger without damage to nail

5ᵗʰ S61.3 Open wound of other finger with damage to nail

6ᵗʰ S61.30 Unspecified open wound of finger with damage to nail

S61.300 Unspecified open wound of right index finger with damage to nail

S61.301 Unspecified open wound of left index finger with damage to nail

S61.302 Unspecified open wound of right middle finger with damage to nail

S61.303 Unspecified open wound of left middle finger with damage to nail

S61.304 Unspecified open wound of right ring finger with damage to nail

S61.305 Unspecified open wound of left ring finger with damage to nail

S61.306 Unspecified open wound of right little finger with damage to nail

S61.307 Unspecified open wound of left little finger with damage to nail

S61.308 Unspecified open wound of other finger with damage to nail

Unspecified open wound of specified finger with unspecified laterality with damage to nail

S61.309 Unspecified open wound of unspecified finger with damage to nail

6ᵗʰ S61.31 Laceration without foreign body of finger with damage to nail

S61.310 Laceration without foreign body of right index finger with damage to nail

S61.311 Laceration without foreign body of left index finger with damage to nail

S61.312 Laceration without foreign body of right middle finger with damage to nail

S61.313 Laceration without foreign body of left middle finger with damage to nail

S61.314 Laceration without foreign body of right ring finger with damage to nail

S61.315 Laceration without foreign body of left ring finger with damage to nail

S61.316 Laceration without foreign body of right little finger with damage to nail

S61.317 Laceration without foreign body of left little finger with damage to nail

S61.318 Laceration without foreign body of other finger with damage to nail

Laceration without foreign body of specified finger with unspecified laterality with damage to nail

S61.319 Laceration without foreign body of unspecified finger with damage to nail

6ᵗʰ S61.32 Laceration with foreign body of finger with damage to nail

S61.320 Laceration with foreign body of right index finger with damage to nail

S61.321 Laceration with foreign body of left index finger with damage to nail

S61.322 Laceration with foreign body of right middle finger with damage to nail

---

PDⁿ Unacceptable principal diagnosis symbol per Medicare code edits   Code exempt from diagnosis present on admission requirement
? Questionable admission   CC Complication or comorbidity   CC/MCC CC/MCC exclusion   MCC Major complication or comorbidity
Principal diagnosis as its own CC   Principal diagnosis as its own MCC   HCC HCC diagnosis code   RxHCC RxHCC diagnosis code
MACRA code   Z Z code as first-listed diagnosis

1044   When symbols appear on a code that requires a 7th character extension, refer to Appendix B to identify applicable 7th character codes.   **2018 ICD-10-CM**

S61.323 Laceration with foreign body of left middle finger with damage to nail

S61.324 Laceration with foreign body of right ring finger with damage to nail

S61.325 Laceration with foreign body of left ring finger with damage to nail

S61.326 Laceration with foreign body of right little finger with damage to nail

S61.327 Laceration with foreign body of left little finger with damage to nail

S61.328 Laceration with foreign body of other finger with damage to nail
Laceration with foreign body of specified finger with unspecified laterality with damage to nail

S61.329 **Laceration with foreign body of unspecified finger with damage to nail**

S61.33 Puncture wound without foreign body of finger with damage to nail

S61.330 Puncture wound without foreign body of right index finger with damage to nail

S61.331 Puncture wound without foreign body of left index finger with damage to nail

S61.332 Puncture wound without foreign body of right middle finger with damage to nail

S61.333 Puncture wound without foreign body of left middle finger with damage to nail

S61.334 Puncture wound without foreign body of right ring finger with damage to nail

S61.335 Puncture wound without foreign body of left ring finger with damage to nail

S61.336 Puncture wound without foreign body of right little finger with damage to nail

S61.337 Puncture wound without foreign body of left little finger with damage to nail

S61.338 Puncture wound without foreign body of other finger with damage to nail
Puncture wound without foreign body of specified finger with unspecified laterality with damage to nail

S61.339 **Puncture wound without foreign body of unspecified finger with damage to nail**

S61.34 Puncture wound with foreign body of finger with damage to nail

S61.340 Puncture wound with foreign body of right index finger with damage to nail

S61.341 Puncture wound with foreign body of left index finger with damage to nail

S61.342 Puncture wound with foreign body of right middle finger with damage to nail

S61.343 Puncture wound with foreign body of left middle finger with damage to nail

S61.344 Puncture wound with foreign body of right ring finger with damage to nail

S61.345 Puncture wound with foreign body of left ring finger with damage to nail

S61.346 Puncture wound with foreign body of right little finger with damage to nail

S61.347 Puncture wound with foreign body of left little finger with damage to nail

S61.348 Puncture wound with foreign body of other finger with damage to nail
Puncture wound with foreign body of specified finger with unspecified laterality with damage to nail

S61.349 **Puncture wound with foreign body of unspecified finger with damage to nail**

S61.35 Open bite of finger with damage to nail
Bite of finger with damage to nail NOS
EXCLUDES1 superficial bite of finger (S60.46-, S60.47-)

S61.350 Open bite of right index finger with damage to nail

S61.351 Open bite of left index finger with damage to nail

S61.352 Open bite of right middle finger with damage to nail

S61.353 Open bite of left middle finger with damage to nail

S61.354 Open bite of right ring finger with damage to nail

S61.355 Open bite of left ring finger with damage to nail

S61.356 Open bite of right little finger with damage to nail

S61.357 Open bite of left little finger with damage to nail

S61.358 Open bite of other finger with damage to nail
Open bite of specified finger with unspecified laterality with damage to nail

S61.359 **Open bite of unspecified finger with damage to nail**

S61.4 Open wound of hand

S61.40 Unspecified open wound of hand

S61.401 Unspecified open wound of right hand

S61.402 Unspecified open wound of left hand

S61.409 Unspecified open wound of unspecified hand

S61.41 Laceration without foreign body of hand

S61.411 Laceration without foreign body of right hand

S61.412 Laceration without foreign body of left hand

S61.419 **Laceration without foreign body of unspecified hand**

S61.42 Laceration with foreign body of hand

S61.421 Laceration with foreign body of right hand

S61.422 Laceration with foreign body of left hand

S61.429 **Laceration with foreign body of unspecified hand**

S61.43 Puncture wound without foreign body of hand

S61.431 Puncture wound without foreign body of right hand

S61.432 Puncture wound without foreign body of left hand

S61.439 **Puncture wound without foreign body of unspecified hand**

S61.44 Puncture wound with foreign body of hand

S61.441 Puncture wound with foreign body of right hand

S61.442 Puncture wound with foreign body of left hand

S61.449 **Puncture wound with foreign body of unspecified hand**

S61.45 Open bite of hand
Bite of hand NOS
EXCLUDES1 superficial bite of hand (S60.56-, S60.57-)

S61.451 Open bite of right hand

S61.452 Open bite of left hand

S61.459 **Open bite of unspecified hand**

S61.5 Open wound of wrist

S61.50 Unspecified open wound of wrist

S61.501 Unspecified open wound of right wrist

S61.502 Unspecified open wound of left wrist

S61.509 **Unspecified open wound of unspecified wrist**

S61.51 Laceration without foreign body of wrist

S61.511 Laceration without foreign body of right wrist

S61.512 Laceration without foreign body of left wrist

Unspecified Code   Other Specified Code   Manifestation Code   N Newborn   P Pediatric   M Maternity   A Adult   ♂ Male   ♀ Female
● New Code   ▲ Revised Code Title   ►◄ Revised Text   **NOTES**   *INCLUDES*   *EXCLUDES1* Not coded here   *EXCLUDES2* Not included here
4th character required   5th character required   6th character required   7th character required
Extension 'X' Alert   HAC Hospital-acquired condition (HAC) alert   **AHA** AHA Coding Clinic©

S61.519 Laceration without foreign body of unspecified wrist

S61.52 Laceration with foreign body of wrist

S61.521 Laceration with foreign body of right wrist

S61.522 Laceration with foreign body of left wrist

S61.529 Laceration with foreign body of unspecified wrist

S61.53 Puncture wound without foreign body of wrist

S61.531 Puncture wound without foreign body of right wrist

S61.532 Puncture wound without foreign body of left wrist

S61.539 Puncture wound without foreign body of unspecified wrist

S61.54 Puncture wound with foreign body of wrist

S61.541 Puncture wound with foreign body of right wrist

S61.542 Puncture wound with foreign body of left wrist

S61.549 Puncture wound with foreign body of unspecified wrist

S61.55 Open bite of wrist
Bite of wrist NOS
EXCLUDES1 superficial bite of wrist (S60.86-, S60.87-)

S61.551 Open bite of right wrist

S61.552 Open bite of left wrist

S61.559 Open bite of unspecified wrist

S62 Fracture at wrist and hand level
NOTES A fracture not indicated as displaced or nondisplaced should be coded to displaced
A fracture not indicated as open or closed should be coded to closed
EXCLUDES1 traumatic amputation of wrist and hand (S68.-)
EXCLUDES2 fracture of distal parts of ulna and radius (S52.-)

The appropriate 7th character is to be added to each code from category S62
A = initial encounter for closed fracture
B = initial encounter for open fracture
D = subsequent encounter for fracture with routine healing
G = subsequent encounter for fracture with delayed healing
K = subsequent encounter for fracture with nonunion
P = subsequent encounter for fracture with malunion
S = sequela

S62.0 Fracture of navicular [scaphoid] bone of wrist

S62.00 Unspecified fracture of navicular [scaphoid] bone of wrist

S62.001 Unspecified fracture of navicular [scaphoid] bone of right wrist

S62.002 Unspecified fracture of navicular [scaphoid] bone of left wrist

S62.009 Unspecified fracture of navicular [scaphoid] bone of unspecified wrist

S62.01 Fracture of distal pole of navicular [scaphoid] bone of wrist
Fracture of volar tuberosity of navicular [scaphoid] bone of wrist

S62.011 Displaced fracture of distal pole of navicular [scaphoid] bone of right wrist

S62.012 Displaced fracture of distal pole of navicular [scaphoid] bone of left wrist

S62.013 Displaced fracture of distal pole of navicular [scaphoid] bone of unspecified wrist

S62.014 Nondisplaced fracture of distal pole of navicular [scaphoid] bone of right wrist

S62.015 Nondisplaced fracture of distal pole of navicular [scaphoid] bone of left wrist

S62.016 Nondisplaced fracture of distal pole of navicular [scaphoid] bone of unspecified wrist

S62.02 Fracture of middle third of navicular [scaphoid] bone of wrist

S62.021 Displaced fracture of middle third of navicular [scaphoid] bone of right wrist

S62.022 Displaced fracture of middle third of navicular [scaphoid] bone of left wrist

S62.023 Displaced fracture of middle third of navicular [scaphoid] bone of unspecified wrist

S62.024 Nondisplaced fracture of middle third of navicular [scaphoid] bone of right wrist

S62.025 Nondisplaced fracture of middle third of navicular [scaphoid] bone of left wrist

S62.026 Nondisplaced fracture of middle third of navicular [scaphoid] bone of unspecified wrist

S62.03 Fracture of proximal third of navicular [scaphoid] bone of wrist

S62.031 Displaced fracture of proximal third of navicular [scaphoid] bone of right wrist

S62.032 Displaced fracture of proximal third of navicular [scaphoid] bone of left wrist

S62.033 Displaced fracture of proximal third of navicular [scaphoid] bone of unspecified wrist

S62.034 Nondisplaced fracture of proximal third of navicular [scaphoid] bone of right wrist

S62.035 Nondisplaced fracture of proximal third of navicular [scaphoid] bone of left wrist

S62.036 Nondisplaced fracture of proximal third of navicular [scaphoid] bone of unspecified wrist

S62.1 Fracture of other and unspecified carpal bone(s)
EXCLUDES2 fracture of scaphoid of wrist (S62.0-)

S62.10 Fracture of unspecified carpal bone
Fracture of wrist NOS

S62.101 Fracture of unspecified carpal bone, right wrist

S62.102 Fracture of unspecified carpal bone, left wrist

S62.109 Fracture of unspecified carpal bone, unspecified wrist

S62.11 Fracture of triquetrum [cuneiform] bone of wrist

S62.111 Displaced fracture of triquetrum [cuneiform] bone, right wrist

S62.112 Displaced fracture of triquetrum [cuneiform] bone, left wrist

S62.113 Displaced fracture of triquetrum [cuneiform] bone, unspecified wrist

S62.114 Nondisplaced fracture of triquetrum [cuneiform] bone, right wrist

S62.115 Nondisplaced fracture of triquetrum [cuneiform] bone, left wrist

---

PDx Unacceptable principal diagnosis symbol per Medicare code edits   Code exempt from diagnosis present on admission requirement
? Questionable admission   Complication or comorbidity   CC/MCC exclusion   MCC Major complication or comorbidity
Principal diagnosis as its own CC   Principal diagnosis as its own MCC   HCC HCC diagnosis code   RxHCC RxHCC diagnosis code
MACRA code   Z1 Z code as first-listed diagnosis

[7th] S62.116 Nondisplaced fracture of triquetrum [cuneiform] bone, unspecified wrist [CC] [POA] [HAC] [CC/MCC Exc]

[6th] S62.12 Fracture of lunate [semilunar]
- [7th] S62.121 Displaced fracture of lunate [semilunar], right wrist [CC] [POA] [HAC] [CC/MCC Exc]
- [7th] S62.122 Displaced fracture of lunate [semilunar], left wrist [CC] [POA] [HAC] [CC/MCC Exc]
- [7th] S62.123 Displaced fracture of lunate [semilunar], unspecified wrist [CC] [POA] [HAC] [CC/MCC Exc]
- [7th] S62.124 Nondisplaced fracture of lunate [semilunar], right wrist [CC] [POA] [HAC] [CC/MCC Exc]
- [7th] S62.125 Nondisplaced fracture of lunate [semilunar], left wrist [CC] [POA] [HAC] [CC/MCC Exc]
- [7th] S62.126 Nondisplaced fracture of lunate [semilunar], unspecified wrist [CC] [POA] [HAC] [CC/MCC Exc]

[6th] S62.13 Fracture of capitate [os magnum] bone
- [7th] S62.131 Displaced fracture of capitate [os magnum] bone, right wrist [CC] [POA] [HAC] [CC/MCC Exc]
- [7th] S62.132 Displaced fracture of capitate [os magnum] bone, left wrist [CC] [POA] [HAC] [CC/MCC Exc]
- [7th] S62.133 Displaced fracture of capitate [os magnum] bone, unspecified wrist [CC] [POA] [HAC] [CC/MCC Exc]
- [7th] S62.134 Nondisplaced fracture of capitate [os magnum] bone, right wrist [CC] [POA] [HAC] [CC/MCC Exc]
- [7th] S62.135 Nondisplaced fracture of capitate [os magnum] bone, left wrist [CC] [POA] [HAC] [CC/MCC Exc]
- [7th] S62.136 Nondisplaced fracture of capitate [os magnum] bone, unspecified wrist [CC] [POA] [HAC] [CC/MCC Exc]

[6th] S62.14 Fracture of body of hamate [unciform] bone
Fracture of hamate [unciform] bone NOS
- [7th] S62.141 Displaced fracture of body of hamate [unciform] bone, right wrist [CC] [POA] [HAC] [CC/MCC Exc]
- [7th] S62.142 Displaced fracture of body of hamate [unciform] bone, left wrist [CC] [POA] [HAC] [CC/MCC Exc]
- [7th] S62.143 Displaced fracture of body of hamate [unciform] bone, unspecified wrist [CC] [POA] [HAC] [CC/MCC Exc]
- [7th] S62.144 Nondisplaced fracture of body of hamate [unciform] bone, right wrist [CC] [POA] [HAC] [CC/MCC Exc]
- [7th] S62.145 Nondisplaced fracture of body of hamate [unciform] bone, left wrist [CC] [POA] [HAC] [CC/MCC Exc]
- [7th] S62.146 Nondisplaced fracture of body of hamate [unciform] bone, unspecified wrist [CC] [POA] [HAC] [CC/MCC Exc]

[6th] S62.15 Fracture of hook process of hamate [unciform] bone
Fracture of unciform process of hamate [unciform] bone
- [7th] S62.151 Displaced fracture of hook process of hamate [unciform] bone, right wrist [CC] [POA] [HAC] [CC/MCC Exc]
- [7th] S62.152 Displaced fracture of hook process of hamate [unciform] bone, left wrist [CC] [POA] [HAC] [CC/MCC Exc]
- [7th] S62.153 Displaced fracture of hook process of hamate [unciform] bone, unspecified wrist [CC] [POA] [HAC] [CC/MCC Exc]
- [7th] S62.154 Nondisplaced fracture of hook process of hamate [unciform] bone, right wrist [CC] [POA] [HAC] [CC/MCC Exc]
- [7th] S62.155 Nondisplaced fracture of hook process of hamate [unciform] bone, left wrist [CC] [POA] [HAC] [CC/MCC Exc]
- [7th] S62.156 Nondisplaced fracture of hook process of hamate [unciform] bone, unspecified wrist [CC] [POA] [HAC] [CC/MCC Exc]

[6th] S62.16 Fracture of pisiform
- [7th] S62.161 Displaced fracture of pisiform, right wrist [CC] [POA] [HAC] [CC/MCC Exc]
- [7th] S62.162 Displaced fracture of pisiform, left wrist [CC] [POA] [HAC] [CC/MCC Exc]
- [7th] S62.163 Displaced fracture of pisiform, unspecified wrist [CC] [POA] [HAC] [CC/MCC Exc]
- [7th] S62.164 Nondisplaced fracture of pisiform, right wrist [CC] [POA] [HAC] [CC/MCC Exc]
- [7th] S62.165 Nondisplaced fracture of pisiform, left wrist [CC] [POA] [HAC] [CC/MCC Exc]
- [7th] S62.166 Nondisplaced fracture of pisiform, unspecified wrist [CC] [POA] [HAC] [CC/MCC Exc]

[6th] S62.17 Fracture of trapezium [larger multangular]
- [7th] S62.171 Displaced fracture of trapezium [larger multangular], right wrist [CC] [POA] [HAC] [CC/MCC Exc]
- [7th] S62.172 Displaced fracture of trapezium [larger multangular], left wrist [CC] [POA] [HAC] [CC/MCC Exc]
- [7th] S62.173 Displaced fracture of trapezium [larger multangular], unspecified wrist [CC] [POA] [HAC] [CC/MCC Exc]
- [7th] S62.174 Nondisplaced fracture of trapezium [larger multangular], right wrist [CC] [POA] [HAC] [CC/MCC Exc]
- [7th] S62.175 Nondisplaced fracture of trapezium [larger multangular], left wrist [CC] [POA] [HAC] [CC/MCC Exc]
- [7th] S62.176 Nondisplaced fracture of trapezium [larger multangular], unspecified wrist [CC] [POA] [HAC] [CC/MCC Exc]

[6th] S62.18 Fracture of trapezoid [smaller multangular]
- [7th] S62.181 Displaced fracture of trapezoid [smaller multangular], right wrist [CC] [POA] [HAC] [CC/MCC Exc]
- [7th] S62.182 Displaced fracture of trapezoid [smaller multangular], left wrist [CC] [POA] [HAC] [CC/MCC Exc]
- [7th] S62.183 Displaced fracture of trapezoid [smaller multangular], unspecified wrist [CC] [POA] [HAC] [CC/MCC Exc]
- [7th] S62.184 Nondisplaced fracture of trapezoid [smaller multangular], right wrist [CC] [POA] [HAC] [CC/MCC Exc]
- [7th] S62.185 Nondisplaced fracture of trapezoid [smaller multangular], left wrist [CC] [POA] [HAC] [CC/MCC Exc]
- [7th] S62.186 Nondisplaced fracture of trapezoid [smaller multangular], unspecified wrist [CC] [POA] [HAC] [CC/MCC Exc]

[5th] S62.2 Fracture of first metacarpal bone

[6th] S62.20 Unspecified fracture of first metacarpal bone
- [7th] S62.201 Unspecified fracture of first metacarpal bone, right hand [CC] [POA] [HAC] [CC/MCC Exc]
- [7th] S62.202 Unspecified fracture of first metacarpal bone, left hand [CC] [POA] [HAC] [CC/MCC Exc]
- [7th] S62.209 Unspecified fracture of first metacarpal bone, unspecified hand [CC] [POA] [HAC] [CC/MCC Exc]

[6th] S62.21 Bennett's fracture
- [7th] S62.211 Bennett's fracture, right hand [CC] [POA] [HAC] [CC/MCC Exc]
- [7th] S62.212 Bennett's fracture, left hand [CC] [POA] [HAC] [CC/MCC Exc]
- [7th] S62.213 Bennett's fracture, unspecified hand [CC] [POA] [HAC] [CC/MCC Exc]

[6th] S62.22 Rolando's fracture
- [7th] S62.221 Displaced Rolando's fracture, right hand [CC] [POA] [HAC] [CC/MCC Exc]
- [7th] S62.222 Displaced Rolando's fracture, left hand [CC] [POA] [HAC] [CC/MCC Exc]
- [7th] S62.223 Displaced Rolando's fracture, unspecified hand [CC] [POA] [HAC] [CC/MCC Exc]
- [7th] S62.224 Nondisplaced Rolando's fracture, right hand [CC] [POA] [HAC] [CC/MCC Exc]
- [7th] S62.225 Nondisplaced Rolando's fracture, left hand [CC] [POA] [HAC] [CC/MCC Exc]
- [7th] S62.226 Nondisplaced Rolando's fracture, unspecified hand [CC] [POA] [HAC] [CC/MCC Exc]

[6th] S62.23 Other fracture of base of first metacarpal bone

7ᵗʰ **S62.231** Other displaced fracture of base of first metacarpal bone, right hand cc POA HAC CC/MCC Exc

7ᵗʰ **S62.232** Other displaced fracture of base of first metacarpal bone, left hand cc POA HAC CC/MCC Exc

7ᵗʰ **S62.233** Other displaced fracture of base of first metacarpal bone, unspecified hand cc POA HAC CC/MCC Exc

7ᵗʰ **S62.234** Other nondisplaced fracture of base of first metacarpal bone, right hand cc POA HAC CC/MCC Exc

7ᵗʰ **S62.235** Other nondisplaced fracture of base of first metacarpal bone, left hand cc POA HAC CC/MCC Exc

7ᵗʰ **S62.236** Other nondisplaced fracture of base of first metacarpal bone, unspecified hand cc POA HAC CC/MCC Exc

6ᵗʰ **S62.24** Fracture of shaft of first metacarpal bone

7ᵗʰ **S62.241** Displaced fracture of shaft of first metacarpal bone, right hand cc POA HAC CC/MCC Exc

7ᵗʰ **S62.242** Displaced fracture of shaft of first metacarpal bone, left hand cc POA HAC CC/MCC Exc

7ᵗʰ **S62.243** Displaced fracture of shaft of first metacarpal bone, unspecified hand cc POA HAC CC/MCC Exc

7ᵗʰ **S62.244** Nondisplaced fracture of shaft of first metacarpal bone, right hand cc POA HAC CC/MCC Exc

7ᵗʰ **S62.245** Nondisplaced fracture of shaft of first metacarpal bone, left hand cc POA HAC CC/MCC Exc

7ᵗʰ **S62.246** Nondisplaced fracture of shaft of first metacarpal bone, unspecified hand cc POA HAC CC/MCC Exc

6ᵗʰ **S62.25** Fracture of neck of first metacarpal bone

7ᵗʰ **S62.251** Displaced fracture of neck of first metacarpal bone, right hand cc POA HAC CC/MCC Exc

7ᵗʰ **S62.252** Displaced fracture of neck of first metacarpal bone, left hand cc POA HAC CC/MCC Exc

7ᵗʰ **S62.253** Displaced fracture of neck of first metacarpal bone, unspecified hand cc POA HAC CC/MCC Exc

7ᵗʰ **S62.254** Nondisplaced fracture of neck of first metacarpal bone, right hand cc POA HAC CC/MCC Exc

7ᵗʰ **S62.255** Nondisplaced fracture of neck of first metacarpal bone, left hand cc POA HAC CC/MCC Exc

7ᵗʰ **S62.256** Nondisplaced fracture of neck of first metacarpal bone, unspecified hand cc POA HAC CC/MCC Exc

6ᵗʰ **S62.29** Other fracture of first metacarpal bone

7ᵗʰ **S62.291** Other fracture of first metacarpal bone, right hand cc POA HAC CC/MCC Exc

7ᵗʰ **S62.292** Other fracture of first metacarpal bone, left hand cc POA HAC CC/MCC Exc

7ᵗʰ **S62.299** Other fracture of first metacarpal bone, unspecified hand cc POA HAC CC/MCC Exc

5ᵗʰ **S62.3** Fracture of other and unspecified metacarpal bone

EXCLUDES2 fracture of first metacarpal bone (S62.2-)

6ᵗʰ **S62.30** Unspecified fracture of other metacarpal bone

7ᵗʰ **S62.300** Unspecified fracture of second metacarpal bone, right hand cc POA HAC CC/MCC Exc

7ᵗʰ **S62.301** Unspecified fracture of second metacarpal bone, left hand cc POA HAC CC/MCC Exc

7ᵗʰ **S62.302** Unspecified fracture of third metacarpal bone, right hand cc POA HAC CC/MCC Exc

7ᵗʰ **S62.303** Unspecified fracture of third metacarpal bone, left hand cc POA HAC CC/MCC Exc

7ᵗʰ **S62.304** Unspecified fracture of fourth metacarpal bone, right hand cc POA HAC CC/MCC Exc

7ᵗʰ **S62.305** Unspecified fracture of fourth metacarpal bone, left hand cc POA HAC CC/MCC Exc

7ᵗʰ **S62.306** Unspecified fracture of fifth metacarpal bone, right hand cc POA HAC CC/MCC Exc

7ᵗʰ **S62.307** Unspecified fracture of fifth metacarpal bone, left hand cc POA HAC CC/MCC Exc

7ᵗʰ **S62.308** Unspecified fracture of other metacarpal bone cc POA HAC CC/MCC Exc

Unspecified fracture of specified metacarpal bone with unspecified laterality

7ᵗʰ **S62.309** Unspecified fracture of unspecified metacarpal bone cc POA HAC CC/MCC Exc

6ᵗʰ **S62.31** Displaced fracture of base of other metacarpal bone

7ᵗʰ **S62.310** Displaced fracture of base of second metacarpal bone, right hand cc POA HAC CC/MCC Exc

▲ 7ᵗʰ **S62.311** Displaced fracture of base of second metacarpal ▶bone,◀ left hand cc POA HAC CC/MCC Exc

7ᵗʰ **S62.312** Displaced fracture of base of third metacarpal bone, right hand cc POA HAC CC/MCC Exc

7ᵗʰ **S62.313** Displaced fracture of base of third metacarpal bone, left hand cc POA HAC CC/MCC Exc

7ᵗʰ **S62.314** Displaced fracture of base of fourth metacarpal bone, right hand cc POA HAC CC/MCC Exc

7ᵗʰ **S62.315** Displaced fracture of base of fourth metacarpal bone, left hand cc POA HAC CC/MCC Exc

7ᵗʰ **S62.316** Displaced fracture of base of fifth metacarpal bone, right hand cc POA HAC CC/MCC Exc

▲ 7ᵗʰ **S62.317** Displaced fracture of base of fifth metacarpal ▶bone,◀ left hand cc POA HAC CC/MCC Exc

7ᵗʰ **S62.318** Displaced fracture of base of other metacarpal bone cc POA HAC CC/MCC Exc

Displaced fracture of base of specified metacarpal bone with unspecified laterality

7ᵗʰ **S62.319** Displaced fracture of base of unspecified metacarpal bone cc POA HAC CC/MCC Exc

6ᵗʰ **S62.32** Displaced fracture of shaft of other metacarpal bone

7ᵗʰ **S62.320** Displaced fracture of shaft of second metacarpal bone, right hand cc POA HAC CC/MCC Exc

7ᵗʰ **S62.321** Displaced fracture of shaft of second metacarpal bone, left hand cc POA HAC CC/MCC Exc

7ᵗʰ **S62.322** Displaced fracture of shaft of third metacarpal bone, right hand cc POA HAC CC/MCC Exc

7ᵗʰ **S62.323** Displaced fracture of shaft of third metacarpal bone, left hand cc POA HAC CC/MCC Exc

7ᵗʰ **S62.324** Displaced fracture of shaft of fourth metacarpal bone, right hand cc POA HAC CC/MCC Exc

7ᵗʰ **S62.325** Displaced fracture of shaft of fourth metacarpal bone, left hand cc POA HAC CC/MCC Exc

7ᵗʰ **S62.326** Displaced fracture of shaft of fifth metacarpal bone, right hand cc POA HAC CC/MCC Exc

7ᵗʰ **S62.327** Displaced fracture of shaft of fifth metacarpal bone, left hand cc POA HAC CC/MCC Exc

7ᵗʰ **S62.328** Displaced fracture of shaft of other metacarpal bone cc POA HAC CC/MCC Exc

Displaced fracture of shaft of specified metacarpal bone with unspecified laterality

7ᵗʰ **S62.329** Displaced fracture of shaft of unspecified metacarpal bone cc POA HAC CC/MCC Exc

6ᵗʰ **S62.33** Displaced fracture of neck of other metacarpal bone

PDx Unacceptable principal diagnosis symbol per Medicare code edits   POA Code exempt from diagnosis present on admission requirement

❓ Questionable admission   cc Complication or comorbidity   CC/MCC Exc CC/MCC exclusion   MCC Major complication or comorbidity

Principal diagnosis as its own CC   Principal diagnosis as its own MCC   HCC HCC diagnosis code   RxHCC RxHCC diagnosis code

MACRA code   Z1 Z code as first-listed diagnosis

1048   When symbols appear on a code that requires a 7th character extension, refer to Appendix B to identify applicable 7th character codes.   **2018 ICD-10-CM**

S62.330 Displaced fracture of neck of second metacarpal bone, right hand

S62.331 Displaced fracture of neck of second metacarpal bone, left hand

S62.332 Displaced fracture of neck of third metacarpal bone, right hand

S62.333 Displaced fracture of neck of third metacarpal bone, left hand

S62.334 Displaced fracture of neck of fourth metacarpal bone, right hand

S62.335 Displaced fracture of neck of fourth metacarpal bone, left hand

S62.336 Displaced fracture of neck of fifth metacarpal bone, right hand

S62.337 Displaced fracture of neck of fifth metacarpal bone, left hand

S62.338 Displaced fracture of neck of other metacarpal bone
   Displaced fracture of neck of specified metacarpal bone with unspecified laterality

S62.339 Displaced fracture of neck of unspecified metacarpal bone

S62.34 Nondisplaced fracture of base of other metacarpal bone

S62.340 Nondisplaced fracture of base of second metacarpal bone, right hand

▲ S62.341 Nondisplaced fracture of base of second metacarpal ▶bone,◀ left hand

S62.342 Nondisplaced fracture of base of third metacarpal bone, right hand

S62.343 Nondisplaced fracture of base of third metacarpal bone, left hand

S62.344 Nondisplaced fracture of base of fourth metacarpal bone, right hand

S62.345 Nondisplaced fracture of base of fourth metacarpal bone, left hand

S62.346 Nondisplaced fracture of base of fifth metacarpal bone, right hand

▲ S62.347 Nondisplaced fracture of base of fifth metacarpal ▶bone,◀ left hand

S62.348 Nondisplaced fracture of base of other metacarpal bone
   Nondisplaced fracture of base of specified metacarpal bone with unspecified laterality

S62.349 Nondisplaced fracture of base of unspecified metacarpal bone

S62.35 Nondisplaced fracture of shaft of other metacarpal bone

S62.350 Nondisplaced fracture of shaft of second metacarpal bone, right hand

S62.351 Nondisplaced fracture of shaft of second metacarpal bone, left hand

S62.352 Nondisplaced fracture of shaft of third metacarpal bone, right hand

S62.353 Nondisplaced fracture of shaft of third metacarpal bone, left hand

S62.354 Nondisplaced fracture of shaft of fourth metacarpal bone, right hand

S62.355 Nondisplaced fracture of shaft of fourth metacarpal bone, left hand

S62.356 Nondisplaced fracture of shaft of fifth metacarpal bone, right hand

S62.357 Nondisplaced fracture of shaft of fifth metacarpal bone, left hand

S62.358 Nondisplaced fracture of shaft of other metacarpal bone
   Nondisplaced fracture of shaft of specified metacarpal bone with unspecified laterality

S62.359 Nondisplaced fracture of shaft of unspecified metacarpal bone

S62.36 Nondisplaced fracture of neck of other metacarpal bone

S62.360 Nondisplaced fracture of neck of second metacarpal bone, right hand

S62.361 Nondisplaced fracture of neck of second metacarpal bone, left hand

S62.362 Nondisplaced fracture of neck of third metacarpal bone, right hand

S62.363 Nondisplaced fracture of neck of third metacarpal bone, left hand

S62.364 Nondisplaced fracture of neck of fourth metacarpal bone, right hand

S62.365 Nondisplaced fracture of neck of fourth metacarpal bone, left hand

S62.366 Nondisplaced fracture of neck of fifth metacarpal bone, right hand

S62.367 Nondisplaced fracture of neck of fifth metacarpal bone, left hand

S62.368 Nondisplaced fracture of neck of other metacarpal bone
   Nondisplaced fracture of neck of specified metacarpal bone with unspecified laterality

S62.369 Nondisplaced fracture of neck of unspecified metacarpal bone

S62.39 Other fracture of other metacarpal bone

S62.390 Other fracture of second metacarpal bone, right hand

S62.391 Other fracture of second metacarpal bone, left hand

S62.392 Other fracture of third metacarpal bone, right hand

S62.393 Other fracture of third metacarpal bone, left hand

S62.394 Other fracture of fourth metacarpal bone, right hand

S62.395 Other fracture of fourth metacarpal bone, left hand

S62.396 Other fracture of fifth metacarpal bone, right hand

S62.397 Other fracture of fifth metacarpal bone, left hand

S62.398 Other fracture of other metacarpal bone
   Other fracture of specified metacarpal bone with unspecified laterality

S62.399 Other fracture of unspecified metacarpal bone

S62.5 Fracture of thumb

| Unspecified Code | Other Specified Code | Manifestation Code | N Newborn | P Pediatric | M Maternity | A Adult | ♂ Male | ♀ Female |

● New Code   ▲ Revised Code Title   ▶◀ Revised Text   **NOTES**   *INCLUDES*   *EXCLUDES 1* Not coded here   *EXCLUDES 2* Not included here

4th character required   5th character required   6th character required   7th character required

Ⓧ Extension 'X' Alert   **HAC** Hospital-acquired condition (HAC) alert   **AHA** AHA Coding Clinic©

6ᵗʰ **S62.50** Fracture of unspecified phalanx of thumb
- 7ᵗʰ **S62.501** Fracture of unspecified phalanx of right thumb CC POA HAC CC/MCC Exc
- 7ᵗʰ **S62.502** Fracture of unspecified phalanx of left thumb CC POA HAC CC/MCC Exc
- 7ᵗʰ **S62.509** Fracture of unspecified phalanx of unspecified thumb CC POA HAC CC/MCC Exc

6ᵗʰ **S62.51** Fracture of proximal phalanx of thumb
- 7ᵗʰ **S62.511** Displaced fracture of proximal phalanx of right thumb CC POA HAC CC/MCC Exc
- 7ᵗʰ **S62.512** Displaced fracture of proximal phalanx of left thumb CC POA HAC CC/MCC Exc
- 7ᵗʰ **S62.513** Displaced fracture of proximal phalanx of unspecified thumb CC POA HAC CC/MCC Exc
- 7ᵗʰ **S62.514** Nondisplaced fracture of proximal phalanx of right thumb CC POA HAC CC/MCC Exc
- 7ᵗʰ **S62.515** Nondisplaced fracture of proximal phalanx of left thumb CC POA HAC CC/MCC Exc
- 7ᵗʰ **S62.516** Nondisplaced fracture of proximal phalanx of unspecified thumb CC POA HAC CC/MCC Exc

6ᵗʰ **S62.52** Fracture of distal phalanx of thumb
- 7ᵗʰ **S62.521** Displaced fracture of distal phalanx of right thumb CC POA HAC CC/MCC Exc
- 7ᵗʰ **S62.522** Displaced fracture of distal phalanx of left thumb CC POA HAC CC/MCC Exc
- 7ᵗʰ **S62.523** Displaced fracture of distal phalanx of unspecified thumb CC POA HAC CC/MCC Exc
- 7ᵗʰ **S62.524** Nondisplaced fracture of distal phalanx of right thumb CC POA HAC CC/MCC Exc
- 7ᵗʰ **S62.525** Nondisplaced fracture of distal phalanx of left thumb CC POA HAC CC/MCC Exc
- 7ᵗʰ **S62.526** Nondisplaced fracture of distal phalanx of unspecified thumb CC POA HAC CC/MCC Exc

5ᵗʰ **S62.6** Fracture of other and unspecified finger(s)
> EXCLUDES2 fracture of thumb (S62.5-)

6ᵗʰ **S62.60** Fracture of unspecified phalanx of finger
- 7ᵗʰ **S62.600** Fracture of unspecified phalanx of right index finger CC POA HAC CC/MCC Exc
- 7ᵗʰ **S62.601** Fracture of unspecified phalanx of left index finger CC POA HAC CC/MCC Exc
- 7ᵗʰ **S62.602** Fracture of unspecified phalanx of right middle finger CC POA HAC CC/MCC Exc
- 7ᵗʰ **S62.603** Fracture of unspecified phalanx of left middle finger CC POA HAC CC/MCC Exc
- 7ᵗʰ **S62.604** Fracture of unspecified phalanx of right ring finger CC POA HAC CC/MCC Exc
- 7ᵗʰ **S62.605** Fracture of unspecified phalanx of left ring finger CC POA HAC CC/MCC Exc
- 7ᵗʰ **S62.606** Fracture of unspecified phalanx of right little finger CC POA HAC CC/MCC Exc
- 7ᵗʰ **S62.607** Fracture of unspecified phalanx of left little finger CC POA HAC CC/MCC Exc
- 7ᵗʰ **S62.608** Fracture of unspecified phalanx of other finger CC POA HAC CC/MCC Exc
  Fracture of unspecified phalanx of specified finger with unspecified laterality
- 7ᵗʰ **S62.609** Fracture of unspecified phalanx of unspecified finger CC POA HAC CC/MCC Exc

6ᵗʰ **S62.61** Displaced fracture of proximal phalanx of finger
- 7ᵗʰ **S62.610** Displaced fracture of proximal phalanx of right index finger CC POA HAC CC/MCC Exc
- 7ᵗʰ **S62.611** Displaced fracture of proximal phalanx of left index finger CC POA HAC CC/MCC Exc
- 7ᵗʰ **S62.612** Displaced fracture of proximal phalanx of right middle finger CC POA HAC CC/MCC Exc
- 7ᵗʰ **S62.613** Displaced fracture of proximal phalanx of left middle finger CC POA HAC CC/MCC Exc
- 7ᵗʰ **S62.614** Displaced fracture of proximal phalanx of right ring finger CC POA HAC CC/MCC Exc
- 7ᵗʰ **S62.615** Displaced fracture of proximal phalanx of left ring finger CC POA HAC CC/MCC Exc

- 7ᵗʰ **S62.616** Displaced fracture of proximal phalanx of right little finger CC POA HAC CC/MCC Exc
- 7ᵗʰ **S62.617** Displaced fracture of proximal phalanx of left little finger CC POA HAC CC/MCC Exc
- 7ᵗʰ **S62.618** Displaced fracture of proximal phalanx of other finger CC POA HAC CC/MCC Exc
  Displaced fracture of proximal phalanx of specified finger with unspecified laterality
- 7ᵗʰ **S62.619** Displaced fracture of proximal phalanx of unspecified finger CC POA HAC CC/MCC Exc

▲ 6ᵗʰ **S62.62** Displaced fracture of ▶middle◀ phalanx of finger
- ▲ 7ᵗʰ **S62.620** Displaced fracture of ▶middle◀ phalanx of right index finger CC POA HAC CC/MCC Exc
- ▲ 7ᵗʰ **S62.621** Displaced fracture of ▶middle◀ phalanx of left index finger CC POA HAC CC/MCC Exc
- ▲ 7ᵗʰ **S62.622** Displaced fracture of ▶middle◀ phalanx of right middle finger CC POA HAC CC/MCC Exc
- ▲ 7ᵗʰ **S62.623** Displaced fracture of ▶middle◀ phalanx of left middle finger CC POA HAC CC/MCC Exc
- ▲ 7ᵗʰ **S62.624** Displaced fracture of ▶middle◀ phalanx of right ring finger CC POA HAC CC/MCC Exc
- ▲ 7ᵗʰ **S62.625** Displaced fracture of ▶middle◀ phalanx of left ring finger CC POA HAC CC/MCC Exc
- 7ᵗʰ **S62.626** Displaced fracture of medial phalanx of right little finger CC POA HAC CC/MCC Exc
- 7ᵗʰ **S62.627** Displaced fracture of medial phalanx of left little finger CC POA HAC CC/MCC Exc
- 7ᵗʰ **S62.628** Displaced fracture of medial phalanx of other finger CC POA HAC CC/MCC Exc
  Displaced fracture of medial phalanx of specified finger with unspecified laterality
- 7ᵗʰ **S62.629** Displaced fracture of medial phalanx of unspecified finger CC POA HAC CC/MCC Exc

6ᵗʰ **S62.63** Displaced fracture of distal phalanx of finger
- 7ᵗʰ **S62.630** Displaced fracture of distal phalanx of right index finger CC POA HAC CC/MCC Exc
- 7ᵗʰ **S62.631** Displaced fracture of distal phalanx of left index finger CC POA HAC CC/MCC Exc
- 7ᵗʰ **S62.632** Displaced fracture of distal phalanx of right middle finger CC POA HAC CC/MCC Exc
- 7ᵗʰ **S62.633** Displaced fracture of distal phalanx of left middle finger CC POA HAC CC/MCC Exc
- 7ᵗʰ **S62.634** Displaced fracture of distal phalanx of right ring finger CC POA HAC CC/MCC Exc
- 7ᵗʰ **S62.635** Displaced fracture of distal phalanx of left ring finger CC POA HAC CC/MCC Exc
- 7ᵗʰ **S62.636** Displaced fracture of distal phalanx of right little finger CC POA HAC CC/MCC Exc
- 7ᵗʰ **S62.637** Displaced fracture of distal phalanx of left little finger CC POA HAC CC/MCC Exc
- 7ᵗʰ **S62.638** Displaced fracture of distal phalanx of other finger CC POA HAC CC/MCC Exc
  Displaced fracture of distal phalanx of specified finger with unspecified laterality
- 7ᵗʰ **S62.639** Displaced fracture of distal phalanx of unspecified finger CC POA HAC CC/MCC Exc

6ᵗʰ **S62.64** Nondisplaced fracture of proximal phalanx of finger
- 7ᵗʰ **S62.640** Nondisplaced fracture of proximal phalanx of right index finger CC POA HAC CC/MCC Exc
- 7ᵗʰ **S62.641** Nondisplaced fracture of proximal phalanx of left index finger CC POA HAC CC/MCC Exc
- 7ᵗʰ **S62.642** Nondisplaced fracture of proximal phalanx of right middle finger CC POA HAC CC/MCC Exc
- 7ᵗʰ **S62.643** Nondisplaced fracture of proximal phalanx of left middle finger CC POA HAC CC/MCC Exc
- 7ᵗʰ **S62.644** Nondisplaced fracture of proximal phalanx of right ring finger CC POA HAC CC/MCC Exc
- 7ᵗʰ **S62.645** Nondisplaced fracture of proximal phalanx of left ring finger CC POA HAC CC/MCC Exc

---

POA⊘ Unacceptable principal diagnosis symbol per Medicare code edits   POA Code exempt from diagnosis present on admission requirement
❓ Questionable admission   CC Complication or comorbidity   CC/MCC Exc CC/MCC exclusion   MCC Major complication or comorbidity
CC Principal diagnosis as its own CC   MCC Principal diagnosis as its own MCC   HCC HCC diagnosis code   RxHCC RxHCC diagnosis code
MACRA code   Z1 Z code as first-listed diagnosis

7ᵀ S62.646 Nondisplaced fracture of proximal phalanx of right little finger cc꜀ POA HAC CC/MCC Exc

7ᵀ S62.647 Nondisplaced fracture of proximal phalanx of left little finger cc꜀ POA HAC CC/MCC Exc

7ᵀ S62.648 Nondisplaced fracture of proximal phalanx of other finger cc꜀ POA HAC CC/MCC Exc
Nondisplaced fracture of proximal phalanx of specified finger with unspecified laterality

7ᵀ S62.649 Nondisplaced fracture of proximal phalanx of unspecified finger cc꜀ POA HAC CC/MCC Exc

▲ 6ᵀ S62.65 Nondisplaced fracture of ▶middle◀ phalanx of finger

▲ 7ᵀ S62.650 Nondisplaced fracture of ▶middle◀ phalanx of right index finger cc꜀ POA HAC CC/MCC Exc

▲ 7ᵀ S62.651 Nondisplaced fracture of ▶middle◀ phalanx of left index finger cc꜀ POA HAC CC/MCC Exc

▲ 7ᵀ S62.652 Nondisplaced fracture of ▶middle◀ phalanx of right middle finger cc꜀ POA HAC CC/MCC Exc

▲ 7ᵀ S62.653 Nondisplaced fracture of ▶middle◀ phalanx of left middle finger cc꜀ POA HAC CC/MCC Exc

7ᵀ S62.654 Nondisplaced fracture of medial phalanx of right ring finger cc꜀ POA HAC CC/MCC Exc

7ᵀ S62.655 Nondisplaced fracture of medial phalanx of left ring finger cc꜀ POA HAC CC/MCC Exc

7ᵀ S62.656 Nondisplaced fracture of medial phalanx of right little finger cc꜀ POA HAC CC/MCC Exc

7ᵀ S62.657 Nondisplaced fracture of medial phalanx of left little finger cc꜀ POA HAC CC/MCC Exc

7ᵀ S62.658 Nondisplaced fracture of medial phalanx of other finger cc꜀ POA HAC CC/MCC Exc
Nondisplaced fracture of medial phalanx of specified finger with unspecified laterality

7ᵀ S62.659 Nondisplaced fracture of medial phalanx of unspecified finger cc꜀ POA HAC CC/MCC Exc

6ᵀ S62.66 Nondisplaced fracture of distal phalanx of finger

7ᵀ S62.660 Nondisplaced fracture of distal phalanx of right index finger cc꜀ POA HAC CC/MCC Exc

7ᵀ S62.661 Nondisplaced fracture of distal phalanx of left index finger cc꜀ POA HAC CC/MCC Exc

7ᵀ S62.662 Nondisplaced fracture of distal phalanx of right middle finger cc꜀ POA HAC CC/MCC Exc

7ᵀ S62.663 Nondisplaced fracture of distal phalanx of left middle finger cc꜀ POA HAC CC/MCC Exc

7ᵀ S62.664 Nondisplaced fracture of distal phalanx of right ring finger cc꜀ POA HAC CC/MCC Exc

7ᵀ S62.665 Nondisplaced fracture of distal phalanx of left ring finger cc꜀ POA HAC CC/MCC Exc

7ᵀ S62.666 Nondisplaced fracture of distal phalanx of right little finger cc꜀ POA HAC CC/MCC Exc

7ᵀ S62.667 Nondisplaced fracture of distal phalanx of left little finger cc꜀ POA HAC CC/MCC Exc

7ᵀ S62.668 Nondisplaced fracture of distal phalanx of other finger cc꜀ POA HAC CC/MCC Exc
Nondisplaced fracture of distal phalanx of specified finger with unspecified laterality

7ᵀ S62.669 Nondisplaced fracture of distal phalanx of unspecified finger cc꜀ POA HAC CC/MCC Exc

5ᵀ S62.9 Unspecified fracture of wrist and hand

7ᵀ S62.90 Unspecified fracture of unspecified wrist and hand cc꜀ POA HAC CC/MCC Exc

7ᵀ S62.91 Unspecified fracture of right wrist and hand cc꜀ POA HAC CC/MCC Exc

7ᵀ S62.92 Unspecified fracture of left wrist and hand cc꜀ POA HAC CC/MCC Exc

4ᵀ S63 Dislocation and sprain of joints and ligaments at wrist and hand level

INCLUDES avulsion of joint or ligament at wrist and hand level

laceration of cartilage, joint or ligament at wrist and hand level

sprain of cartilage, joint or ligament at wrist and hand level

traumatic hemarthrosis of joint or ligament at wrist and hand level

traumatic rupture of joint or ligament at wrist and hand level

traumatic subluxation of joint or ligament at wrist and hand level

traumatic tear of joint or ligament at wrist and hand level

Code also any associated open wound

EXCLUDES2 strain of muscle, fascia and tendon of wrist and hand (S66.-)

The appropriate 7th character is to be added to each code from category S63

A = initial encounter
D = subsequent encounter
S = sequela

5ᵀ S63.0 Subluxation and dislocation of wrist and hand joints

6ᵀ S63.00 Unspecified subluxation and dislocation of wrist and hand
Dislocation of carpal bone NOS
Dislocation of distal end of radius NOS
Subluxation of carpal bone NOS
Subluxation of distal end of radius NOS

7ᵀ S63.001 Unspecified subluxation of right wrist and hand POA

7ᵀ S63.002 Unspecified subluxation of left wrist and hand POA

7ᵀ S63.003 Unspecified subluxation of unspecified wrist and hand POA

7ᵀ S63.004 Unspecified dislocation of right wrist and hand POA

7ᵀ S63.005 Unspecified dislocation of left wrist and hand POA

7ᵀ S63.006 Unspecified dislocation of unspecified wrist and hand POA

6ᵀ S63.01 Subluxation and dislocation of distal radioulnar joint

7ᵀ S63.011 Subluxation of distal radioulnar joint of right wrist POA

7ᵀ S63.012 Subluxation of distal radioulnar joint of left wrist POA

7ᵀ S63.013 Subluxation of distal radioulnar joint of unspecified wrist POA

7ᵀ S63.014 Dislocation of distal radioulnar joint of right wrist POA

7ᵀ S63.015 Dislocation of distal radioulnar joint of left wrist POA

7ᵀ S63.016 Dislocation of distal radioulnar joint of unspecified wrist POA

6ᵀ S63.02 Subluxation and dislocation of radiocarpal joint

7ᵀ S63.021 Subluxation of radiocarpal joint of right wrist POA

7ᵀ S63.022 Subluxation of radiocarpal joint of left wrist POA

7ᵀ S63.023 Subluxation of radiocarpal joint of unspecified wrist POA

7ᵀ S63.024 Dislocation of radiocarpal joint of right wrist POA

7ᵀ S63.025 Dislocation of radiocarpal joint of left wrist POA

7ᵀ S63.026 Dislocation of radiocarpal joint of unspecified wrist POA

6ᵀ S63.03 Subluxation and dislocation of midcarpal joint

7ᵀ S63.031 Subluxation of midcarpal joint of right wrist POA

7ᵀ S63.032 Subluxation of midcarpal joint of left wrist POA

7ᵀ S63.033 Subluxation of midcarpal joint of unspecified wrist POA

7ᵀ S63.034 Dislocation of midcarpal joint of right wrist POA

Unspecified Code   Other Specified Code   Manifestation Code   Ⓝ Newborn   Ⓟ Pediatric   Ⓜ Maternity   Ⓐ Adult   ♂ Male   ♀ Female
● New Code   ▲ Revised Code Title   ▶◀ Revised Text   **NOTES**   *INCLUDES*   *EXCLUDES 1* Not coded here   *EXCLUDES 2* Not included here
4ᵀ 4th character required   5ᵀ 5th character required   6ᵀ 6th character required   7ᵀ 7th character required
7ᵀ Extension 'X' Alert   HAC Hospital-acquired condition (HAC) alert   AHA AHA Coding Clinic©

7ᵗʰ **S63.035** Dislocation of midcarpal joint of left wrist POA

7ᵗʰ **S63.036** Dislocation of midcarpal joint of unspecified wrist POA

6ᵗʰ **S63.04** Subluxation and dislocation of carpometacarpal joint of thumb

EXCLUDES2 interphalangeal subluxation and dislocation of thumb (S63.1-)

7ᵗʰ **S63.041** Subluxation of carpometacarpal joint of right thumb POA

7ᵗʰ **S63.042** Subluxation of carpometacarpal joint of left thumb POA

7ᵗʰ **S63.043** Subluxation of carpometacarpal joint of unspecified thumb POA

7ᵗʰ **S63.044** Dislocation of carpometacarpal joint of right thumb POA

7ᵗʰ **S63.045** Dislocation of carpometacarpal joint of left thumb POA

7ᵗʰ **S63.046** Dislocation of carpometacarpal joint of unspecified thumb POA

6ᵗʰ **S63.05** Subluxation and dislocation of other carpometacarpal joint

EXCLUDES2 subluxation and dislocation of carpometacarpal joint of thumb (S63.04-)

7ᵗʰ **S63.051** Subluxation of other carpometacarpal joint of right hand POA

7ᵗʰ **S63.052** Subluxation of other carpometacarpal joint of left hand POA

7ᵗʰ **S63.053** Subluxation of other carpometacarpal joint of unspecified hand POA

7ᵗʰ **S63.054** Dislocation of other carpometacarpal joint of right hand POA

7ᵗʰ **S63.055** Dislocation of other carpometacarpal joint of left hand POA

7ᵗʰ **S63.056** Dislocation of other carpometacarpal joint of unspecified hand POA

6ᵗʰ **S63.06** Subluxation and dislocation of metacarpal (bone), proximal end

7ᵗʰ **S63.061** Subluxation of metacarpal (bone), proximal end of right hand POA

7ᵗʰ **S63.062** Subluxation of metacarpal (bone), proximal end of left hand POA

7ᵗʰ **S63.063** Subluxation of metacarpal (bone), proximal end of unspecified hand POA

7ᵗʰ **S63.064** Dislocation of metacarpal (bone), proximal end of right hand POA

7ᵗʰ **S63.065** Dislocation of metacarpal (bone), proximal end of left hand POA

7ᵗʰ **S63.066** Dislocation of metacarpal (bone), proximal end of unspecified hand POA

6ᵗʰ **S63.07** Subluxation and dislocation of distal end of ulna

7ᵗʰ **S63.071** Subluxation of distal end of right ulna POA

7ᵗʰ **S63.072** Subluxation of distal end of left ulna POA

7ᵗʰ **S63.073** Subluxation of distal end of unspecified ulna POA

7ᵗʰ **S63.074** Dislocation of distal end of right ulna POA

7ᵗʰ **S63.075** Dislocation of distal end of left ulna POA

7ᵗʰ **S63.076** Dislocation of distal end of unspecified ulna POA

6ᵗʰ **S63.09** Other subluxation and dislocation of wrist and hand

7ᵗʰ **S63.091** Other subluxation of right wrist and hand POA

7ᵗʰ **S63.092** Other subluxation of left wrist and hand POA

7ᵗʰ **S63.093** Other subluxation of unspecified wrist and hand POA

7ᵗʰ **S63.094** Other dislocation of right wrist and hand POA

7ᵗʰ **S63.095** Other dislocation of left wrist and hand POA

7ᵗʰ **S63.096** Other dislocation of unspecified wrist and hand POA

5ᵗʰ **S63.1** Subluxation and dislocation of thumb

6ᵗʰ **S63.10** Unspecified subluxation and dislocation of thumb

7ᵗʰ **S63.101** Unspecified subluxation of right thumb POA

7ᵗʰ **S63.102** Unspecified subluxation of left thumb POA

7ᵗʰ **S63.103** Unspecified subluxation of unspecified thumb POA

7ᵗʰ **S63.104** Unspecified dislocation of right thumb POA

7ᵗʰ **S63.105** Unspecified dislocation of left thumb POA

7ᵗʰ **S63.106** Unspecified dislocation of unspecified thumb POA

6ᵗʰ **S63.11** Subluxation and dislocation of metacarpophalangeal joint of thumb

7ᵗʰ **S63.111** Subluxation of metacarpophalangeal joint of right thumb POA

7ᵗʰ **S63.112** Subluxation of metacarpophalangeal joint of left thumb POA

7ᵗʰ **S63.113** Subluxation of metacarpophalangeal joint of unspecified thumb POA

7ᵗʰ **S63.114** Dislocation of metacarpophalangeal joint of right thumb POA

7ᵗʰ **S63.115** Dislocation of metacarpophalangeal joint of left thumb POA

7ᵗʰ **S63.116** Dislocation of metacarpophalangeal joint of unspecified thumb POA

▲ 6ᵗʰ **S63.12** Subluxation and dislocation of interphalangeal joint of thumb

▲ 7ᵗʰ **S63.121** Subluxation of interphalangeal joint of right thumb POA

▲ 7ᵗʰ **S63.122** Subluxation of interphalangeal joint of left thumb POA

▲ 7ᵗʰ **S63.123** Subluxation of interphalangeal joint of unspecified thumb POA

▲ 7ᵗʰ **S63.124** Dislocation of interphalangeal joint of right thumb POA

▲ 7ᵗʰ **S63.125** Dislocation of interphalangeal joint of left thumb POA

▲ 7ᵗʰ **S63.126** Dislocation of interphalangeal joint of unspecified thumb POA

5ᵗʰ **S63.2** Subluxation and dislocation of other finger(s)

EXCLUDES2 subluxation and dislocation of thumb (S63.1-)

6ᵗʰ **S63.20** Unspecified subluxation of other finger

7ᵗʰ **S63.200** Unspecified subluxation of right index finger POA

7ᵗʰ **S63.201** Unspecified subluxation of left index finger POA

7ᵗʰ **S63.202** Unspecified subluxation of right middle finger POA

7ᵗʰ **S63.203** Unspecified subluxation of left middle finger POA

7ᵗʰ **S63.204** Unspecified subluxation of right ring finger POA

7ᵗʰ **S63.205** Unspecified subluxation of left ring finger POA

7ᵗʰ **S63.206** Unspecified subluxation of right little finger POA

7ᵗʰ **S63.207** Unspecified subluxation of left little finger POA

7ᵗʰ **S63.208** Unspecified subluxation of other finger POA
  Unspecified subluxation of specified finger with unspecified laterality

7ᵗʰ **S63.209** Unspecified subluxation of unspecified finger POA

6ᵗʰ **S63.21** Subluxation of metacarpophalangeal joint of finger

7ᵗʰ **S63.210** Subluxation of metacarpophalangeal joint of right index finger POA

7ᵗʰ **S63.211** Subluxation of metacarpophalangeal joint of left index finger POA

7ᵗʰ **S63.212** Subluxation of metacarpophalangeal joint of right middle finger POA

7ᵗʰ **S63.213** Subluxation of metacarpophalangeal joint of left middle finger POA

PDxⁿ Unacceptable principal diagnosis symbol per Medicare code edits POA Code exempt from diagnosis present on admission requirement
❓ Questionable admission ᶜᶜ Complication or comorbidity CC/MCC Excl CC/MCC exclusion MCC Major complication or comorbidity
CC Principal diagnosis as its own CC MCC Principal diagnosis as its own MCC HCC HCC diagnosis code RxHCC RxHCC diagnosis code
MACRA code Z1 Z code as first-listed diagnosis

When symbols appear on a code that requires a 7th character extension, refer to Appendix B to identify applicable 7th character codes.

2018 ICD-10-CM

7️⃣ S63.214 Subluxation of metacarpophalangeal joint of right ring finger ᴾᴼᴬ

7️⃣ S63.215 Subluxation of metacarpophalangeal joint of left ring finger ᴾᴼᴬ

7️⃣ S63.216 Subluxation of metacarpophalangeal joint of right little finger ᴾᴼᴬ

7️⃣ S63.217 Subluxation of metacarpophalangeal joint of left little finger ᴾᴼᴬ

7️⃣ S63.218 Subluxation of metacarpophalangeal joint of other finger ᴾᴼᴬ
　　　Subluxation of metacarpophalangeal joint of specified finger with unspecified laterality

7️⃣ S63.219 Subluxation of metacarpophalangeal joint of unspecified finger ᴾᴼᴬ

6️⃣ S63.22 Subluxation of unspecified interphalangeal joint of finger

　7️⃣ S63.220 Subluxation of unspecified interphalangeal joint of right index finger ᴾᴼᴬ

　7️⃣ S63.221 Subluxation of unspecified interphalangeal joint of left index finger ᴾᴼᴬ

　7️⃣ S63.222 Subluxation of unspecified interphalangeal joint of right middle finger ᴾᴼᴬ

　7️⃣ S63.223 Subluxation of unspecified interphalangeal joint of left middle finger ᴾᴼᴬ

　7️⃣ S63.224 Subluxation of unspecified interphalangeal joint of right ring finger ᴾᴼᴬ

　7️⃣ S63.225 Subluxation of unspecified interphalangeal joint of left ring finger ᴾᴼᴬ

　7️⃣ S63.226 Subluxation of unspecified interphalangeal joint of right little finger ᴾᴼᴬ

　7️⃣ S63.227 Subluxation of unspecified interphalangeal joint of left little finger ᴾᴼᴬ

　7️⃣ S63.228 Subluxation of unspecified interphalangeal joint of other finger ᴾᴼᴬ
　　　　Subluxation of unspecified interphalangeal joint of specified finger with unspecified laterality

　7️⃣ S63.229 Subluxation of unspecified interphalangeal joint of unspecified finger ᴾᴼᴬ

6️⃣ S63.23 Subluxation of proximal interphalangeal joint of finger

　7️⃣ S63.230 Subluxation of proximal interphalangeal joint of right index finger ᴾᴼᴬ

　7️⃣ S63.231 Subluxation of proximal interphalangeal joint of left index finger ᴾᴼᴬ

　7️⃣ S63.232 Subluxation of proximal interphalangeal joint of right middle finger ᴾᴼᴬ

　7️⃣ S63.233 Subluxation of proximal interphalangeal joint of left middle finger ᴾᴼᴬ

　7️⃣ S63.234 Subluxation of proximal interphalangeal joint of right ring finger ᴾᴼᴬ

　7️⃣ S63.235 Subluxation of proximal interphalangeal joint of left ring finger ᴾᴼᴬ

　7️⃣ S63.236 Subluxation of proximal interphalangeal joint of right little finger ᴾᴼᴬ

　7️⃣ S63.237 Subluxation of proximal interphalangeal joint of left little finger ᴾᴼᴬ

　7️⃣ S63.238 Subluxation of proximal interphalangeal joint of other finger ᴾᴼᴬ
　　　　Subluxation of proximal interphalangeal joint of specified finger with unspecified laterality

　7️⃣ S63.239 Subluxation of proximal interphalangeal joint of unspecified finger ᴾᴼᴬ

6️⃣ S63.24 Subluxation of distal interphalangeal joint of finger

　7️⃣ S63.240 Subluxation of distal interphalangeal joint of right index finger

7️⃣ S63.241 Subluxation of distal interphalangeal joint of left index finger ᴾᴼᴬ

7️⃣ S63.242 Subluxation of distal interphalangeal joint of right middle finger ᴾᴼᴬ

7️⃣ S63.243 Subluxation of distal interphalangeal joint of left middle finger ᴾᴼᴬ

7️⃣ S63.244 Subluxation of distal interphalangeal joint of right ring finger ᴾᴼᴬ

7️⃣ S63.245 Subluxation of distal interphalangeal joint of left ring finger ᴾᴼᴬ

7️⃣ S63.246 Subluxation of distal interphalangeal joint of right little finger ᴾᴼᴬ

7️⃣ S63.247 Subluxation of distal interphalangeal joint of left little finger ᴾᴼᴬ

7️⃣ S63.248 Subluxation of distal interphalangeal joint of other finger ᴾᴼᴬ
　　　Subluxation of distal interphalangeal joint of specified finger with unspecified laterality

7️⃣ S63.249 Subluxation of distal interphalangeal joint of unspecified finger ᴾᴼᴬ

6️⃣ S63.25 Unspecified dislocation of other finger

　7️⃣ S63.250 Unspecified dislocation of right index finger ᴾᴼᴬ

　7️⃣ S63.251 Unspecified dislocation of left index finger ᴾᴼᴬ

　7️⃣ S63.252 Unspecified dislocation of right middle finger ᴾᴼᴬ

　7️⃣ S63.253 Unspecified dislocation of left middle finger ᴾᴼᴬ

　7️⃣ S63.254 Unspecified dislocation of right ring finger ᴾᴼᴬ

　7️⃣ S63.255 Unspecified dislocation of left ring finger ᴾᴼᴬ

　7️⃣ S63.256 Unspecified dislocation of right little finger ᴾᴼᴬ

　7️⃣ S63.257 Unspecified dislocation of left little finger ᴾᴼᴬ

　7️⃣ S63.258 Unspecified dislocation of other finger ᴾᴼᴬ
　　　　Unspecified dislocation of specified finger with unspecified laterality

　7️⃣ S63.259 Unspecified dislocation of unspecified finger ᴾᴼᴬ
　　　　Unspecified dislocation of ▶unspecified◀ finger with unspecified laterality

6️⃣ S63.26 Dislocation of metacarpophalangeal joint of finger

　7️⃣ S63.260 Dislocation of metacarpophalangeal joint of right index finger ᴾᴼᴬ

　7️⃣ S63.261 Dislocation of metacarpophalangeal joint of left index finger ᴾᴼᴬ

　7️⃣ S63.262 Dislocation of metacarpophalangeal joint of right middle finger ᴾᴼᴬ

　7️⃣ S63.263 Dislocation of metacarpophalangeal joint of left middle finger ᴾᴼᴬ

　7️⃣ S63.264 Dislocation of metacarpophalangeal joint of right ring finger ᴾᴼᴬ

　7️⃣ S63.265 Dislocation of metacarpophalangeal joint of left ring finger ᴾᴼᴬ

　7️⃣ S63.266 Dislocation of metacarpophalangeal joint of right little finger ᴾᴼᴬ

　7️⃣ S63.267 Dislocation of metacarpophalangeal joint of left little finger ᴾᴼᴬ

　7️⃣ S63.268 Dislocation of metacarpophalangeal joint of other finger ᴾᴼᴬ
　　　　Dislocation of metacarpophalangeal joint of specified finger with unspecified laterality

　7️⃣ S63.269 Dislocation of metacarpophalangeal joint of unspecified finger ᴾᴼᴬ

6️⃣ S63.27 Dislocation of unspecified interphalangeal joint of finger

　7️⃣ S63.270 Dislocation of unspecified interphalangeal joint of right index finger ᴾᴼᴬ

Unspecified Code　Other Specified Code　Manifestation Code　🅽 Newborn　🅿 Pediatric　🅼 Maternity　🅰 Adult　♂ Male　♀ Female
● New Code　▲ Revised Code Title　▶◀ Revised Text　**NOTES**　*INCLUDES*　*EXCLUDES 1* Not coded here　*EXCLUDES 2* Not included here
4️⃣ 4ᵗʰ character required　5️⃣ 5ᵗʰ character required　6️⃣ 6ᵗʰ character required　7️⃣ 7ᵗʰ character required
7️⃣ Extension 'X' Alert　🅷🅰🅲 Hospital-acquired condition (HAC) alert　**AHA** AHA Coding Clinic©

(7ᵗʰ) **S63.271 Dislocation of unspecified interphalangeal joint of left index finger** POA

(7ᵗʰ) **S63.272 Dislocation of unspecified interphalangeal joint of right middle finger** POA

(7ᵗʰ) **S63.273 Dislocation of unspecified interphalangeal joint of left middle finger** POA

(7ᵗʰ) **S63.274 Dislocation of unspecified interphalangeal joint of right ring finger** POA

(7ᵗʰ) **S63.275 Dislocation of unspecified interphalangeal joint of left ring finger** POA

(7ᵗʰ) **S63.276 Dislocation of unspecified interphalangeal joint of right little finger** POA

(7ᵗʰ) **S63.277 Dislocation of unspecified interphalangeal joint of left little finger** POA

(7ᵗʰ) **S63.278 Dislocation of unspecified interphalangeal joint of other finger** POA

Dislocation of unspecified interphalangeal joint of specified finger with unspecified laterality

(7ᵗʰ) **S63.279 Dislocation of unspecified interphalangeal joint of unspecified finger** POA

Dislocation of unspecified interphalangeal joint of ▶unspecified◀ finger without specified laterality

(6ᵗʰ) **S63.28 Dislocation of proximal interphalangeal joint of finger**

(7ᵗʰ) **S63.280 Dislocation of proximal interphalangeal joint of right index finger** POA

(7ᵗʰ) **S63.281 Dislocation of proximal interphalangeal joint of left index finger** POA

(7ᵗʰ) **S63.282 Dislocation of proximal interphalangeal joint of right middle finger** POA

(7ᵗʰ) **S63.283 Dislocation of proximal interphalangeal joint of left middle finger** POA

(7ᵗʰ) **S63.284 Dislocation of proximal interphalangeal joint of right ring finger** POA

(7ᵗʰ) **S63.285 Dislocation of proximal interphalangeal joint of left ring finger** POA

(7ᵗʰ) **S63.286 Dislocation of proximal interphalangeal joint of right little finger** POA

(7ᵗʰ) **S63.287 Dislocation of proximal interphalangeal joint of left little finger** POA

(7ᵗʰ) **S63.288 Dislocation of proximal interphalangeal joint of other finger** POA

Dislocation of proximal interphalangeal joint of specified finger with unspecified laterality

(7ᵗʰ) **S63.289 Dislocation of proximal interphalangeal joint of unspecified finger** POA

(6ᵗʰ) **S63.29 Dislocation of distal interphalangeal joint of finger**

(7ᵗʰ) **S63.290 Dislocation of distal interphalangeal joint of right index finger** POA

(7ᵗʰ) **S63.291 Dislocation of distal interphalangeal joint of left index finger** POA

(7ᵗʰ) **S63.292 Dislocation of distal interphalangeal joint of right middle finger** POA

(7ᵗʰ) **S63.293 Dislocation of distal interphalangeal joint of left middle finger** POA

(7ᵗʰ) **S63.294 Dislocation of distal interphalangeal joint of right ring finger** POA

(7ᵗʰ) **S63.295 Dislocation of distal interphalangeal joint of left ring finger** POA

(7ᵗʰ) **S63.296 Dislocation of distal interphalangeal joint of right little finger** POA

(7ᵗʰ) **S63.297 Dislocation of distal interphalangeal joint of left little finger** POA

(7ᵗʰ) **S63.298 Dislocation of distal interphalangeal joint of other finger** POA

Dislocation of distal interphalangeal joint of specified finger with unspecified laterality

(7ᵗʰ) **S63.299 Dislocation of distal interphalangeal joint of unspecified finger** POA

(5ᵗʰ) **S63.3 Traumatic rupture of ligament of wrist**

(6ᵗʰ) **S63.30 Traumatic rupture of unspecified ligament of wrist**

(7ᵗʰ) **S63.301 Traumatic rupture of unspecified ligament of right wrist** POA

(7ᵗʰ) **S63.302 Traumatic rupture of unspecified ligament of left wrist** POA

(7ᵗʰ) **S63.309 Traumatic rupture of unspecified ligament of unspecified wrist** POA

(6ᵗʰ) **S63.31 Traumatic rupture of collateral ligament of wrist**

(7ᵗʰ) **S63.311 Traumatic rupture of collateral ligament of right wrist** POA

(7ᵗʰ) **S63.312 Traumatic rupture of collateral ligament of left wrist** POA

(7ᵗʰ) **S63.319 Traumatic rupture of collateral ligament of unspecified wrist** POA

(5ᵗʰ) **S63.32 Traumatic rupture of radiocarpal ligament**

(7ᵗʰ) **S63.321 Traumatic rupture of right radiocarpal ligament** POA

(7ᵗʰ) **S63.322 Traumatic rupture of left radiocarpal ligament** POA

(7ᵗʰ) **S63.329 Traumatic rupture of unspecified radiocarpal ligament** POA

(6ᵗʰ) **S63.33 Traumatic rupture of ulnocarpal (palmar) ligament**

(7ᵗʰ) **S63.331 Traumatic rupture of right ulnocarpal (palmar) ligament** POA

(7ᵗʰ) **S63.332 Traumatic rupture of left ulnocarpal (palmar) ligament** POA

(7ᵗʰ) **S63.339 Traumatic rupture of unspecified ulnocarpal (palmar) ligament** POA

(6ᵗʰ) **S63.39 Traumatic rupture of other ligament of wrist**

(7ᵗʰ) **S63.391 Traumatic rupture of other ligament of right wrist** POA

(7ᵗʰ) **S63.392 Traumatic rupture of other ligament of left wrist** POA

(7ᵗʰ) **S63.399 Traumatic rupture of other ligament of unspecified wrist** POA

(5ᵗʰ) **S63.4 Traumatic rupture of ligament of finger at metacarpophalangeal and interphalangeal joint(s)**

(6ᵗʰ) **S63.40 Traumatic rupture of unspecified ligament of finger at metacarpophalangeal and interphalangeal joint**

(7ᵗʰ) **S63.400 Traumatic rupture of unspecified ligament of right index finger at metacarpophalangeal and interphalangeal joint** POA

(7ᵗʰ) **S63.401 Traumatic rupture of unspecified ligament of left index finger at metacarpophalangeal and interphalangeal joint** POA

(7ᵗʰ) **S63.402 Traumatic rupture of unspecified ligament of right middle finger at metacarpophalangeal and interphalangeal joint** POA

(7ᵗʰ) **S63.403 Traumatic rupture of unspecified ligament of left middle finger at metacarpophalangeal and interphalangeal joint** POA

(7ᵗʰ) **S63.404 Traumatic rupture of unspecified ligament of right ring finger at metacarpophalangeal and interphalangeal joint** POA

(7ᵗʰ) **S63.405 Traumatic rupture of unspecified ligament of left ring finger at metacarpophalangeal and interphalangeal joint** POA

(7ᵗʰ) **S63.406 Traumatic rupture of unspecified ligament of right little finger at metacarpophalangeal and interphalangeal joint** POA

(7ᵗʰ) **S63.407 Traumatic rupture of unspecified ligament of left little finger at metacarpophalangeal and interphalangeal joint** POA

(7ᵗʰ) **S63.408 Traumatic rupture of unspecified ligament of other finger at metacarpophalangeal and interphalangeal joint** POA

PDxⁿ Unacceptable principal diagnosis symbol per Medicare code edits   POA Code exempt from diagnosis present on admission requirement
❓ Questionable admission   cc Complication or comorbidity   CC-MCC Excl CC/MCC exclusion   MCC Major complication or comorbidity
PDx CC Principal diagnosis as its own CC   PDx MCC Principal diagnosis as its own MCC   HCC HCC diagnosis code   RxHCC RxHCC diagnosis code
MACRA code   Z1 Z code as first-listed diagnosis

1054

When symbols appear on a code that requires a 7th character extension, refer to Appendix B to identify applicable 7th character codes.

2018 ICD-10-CM

Traumatic rupture of unspecified ligament of specified finger with unspecified laterality at metacarpophalangeal and interphalangeal joint

7ᵀ **S63.409** **Traumatic rupture of unspecified ligament of unspecified finger at metacarpophalangeal and interphalangeal joint** POA

6ᵀ S63.41 Traumatic rupture of collateral ligament of finger at metacarpophalangeal and interphalangeal joint

7ᵀ **S63.410** Traumatic rupture of collateral ligament of right index finger at metacarpophalangeal and interphalangeal joint POA

7ᵀ **S63.411** Traumatic rupture of collateral ligament of left index finger at metacarpophalangeal and interphalangeal joint POA

7ᵀ **S63.412** Traumatic rupture of collateral ligament of right middle finger at metacarpophalangeal and interphalangeal joint POA

7ᵀ **S63.413** Traumatic rupture of collateral ligament of left middle finger at metacarpophalangeal and interphalangeal joint POA

7ᵀ **S63.414** Traumatic rupture of collateral ligament of right ring finger at metacarpophalangeal and interphalangeal joint POA

7ᵀ **S63.415** Traumatic rupture of collateral ligament of left ring finger at metacarpophalangeal and interphalangeal joint POA

7ᵀ **S63.416** Traumatic rupture of collateral ligament of right little finger at metacarpophalangeal and interphalangeal joint POA

7ᵀ **S63.417** Traumatic rupture of collateral ligament of left little finger at metacarpophalangeal and interphalangeal joint POA

7ᵀ **S63.418** Traumatic rupture of collateral ligament of other finger at metacarpophalangeal and interphalangeal joint POA

Traumatic rupture of collateral ligament of specified finger with unspecified laterality at metacarpophalangeal and interphalangeal joint

7ᵀ **S63.419** **Traumatic rupture of collateral ligament of unspecified finger at metacarpophalangeal and interphalangeal joint** POA

6ᵀ S63.42 Traumatic rupture of palmar ligament of finger at metacarpophalangeal and interphalangeal joint

7ᵀ **S63.420** Traumatic rupture of palmar ligament of right index finger at metacarpophalangeal and interphalangeal joint POA

7ᵀ **S63.421** Traumatic rupture of palmar ligament of left index finger at metacarpophalangeal and interphalangeal joint POA

7ᵀ **S63.422** Traumatic rupture of palmar ligament of right middle finger at metacarpophalangeal and interphalangeal joint POA

7ᵀ **S63.423** Traumatic rupture of palmar ligament of left middle finger at metacarpophalangeal and interphalangeal joint POA

7ᵀ **S63.424** Traumatic rupture of palmar ligament of right ring finger at metacarpophalangeal and interphalangeal joint POA

7ᵀ **S63.425** Traumatic rupture of palmar ligament of left ring finger at metacarpophalangeal and interphalangeal joint POA

7ᵀ **S63.426** Traumatic rupture of palmar ligament of right little finger at metacarpophalangeal and interphalangeal joint POA

7ᵀ **S63.427** Traumatic rupture of palmar ligament of left little finger at metacarpophalangeal and interphalangeal joint POA

7ᵀ **S63.428** Traumatic rupture of palmar ligament of other finger at metacarpophalangeal and interphalangeal joint POA

Traumatic rupture of palmar ligament of specified finger with unspecified laterality at metacarpophalangeal and interphalangeal joint

7ᵀ **S63.429** **Traumatic rupture of palmar ligament of unspecified finger at metacarpophalangeal and interphalangeal joint** POA

6ᵀ S63.43 Traumatic rupture of volar plate of finger at metacarpophalangeal and interphalangeal joint

7ᵀ **S63.430** Traumatic rupture of volar plate of right index finger at metacarpophalangeal and interphalangeal joint POA

7ᵀ **S63.431** Traumatic rupture of volar plate of left index finger at metacarpophalangeal and interphalangeal joint POA

7ᵀ **S63.432** Traumatic rupture of volar plate of right middle finger at metacarpophalangeal and interphalangeal joint POA

7ᵀ **S63.433** Traumatic rupture of volar plate of left middle finger at metacarpophalangeal and interphalangeal joint POA

7ᵀ **S63.434** Traumatic rupture of volar plate of right ring finger at metacarpophalangeal and interphalangeal joint POA

7ᵀ **S63.435** Traumatic rupture of volar plate of left ring finger at metacarpophalangeal and interphalangeal joint POA

7ᵀ **S63.436** Traumatic rupture of volar plate of right little finger at metacarpophalangeal and interphalangeal joint POA

7ᵀ **S63.437** Traumatic rupture of volar plate of left little finger at metacarpophalangeal and interphalangeal joint POA

7ᵀ **S63.438** Traumatic rupture of volar plate of other finger at metacarpophalangeal and interphalangeal joint POA

Traumatic rupture of volar plate of specified finger with unspecified laterality at metacarpophalangeal and interphalangeal joint

7ᵀ **S63.439** **Traumatic rupture of volar plate of unspecified finger at metacarpophalangeal and interphalangeal joint** POA

6ᵀ S63.49 Traumatic rupture of other ligament of finger at metacarpophalangeal and interphalangeal joint

7ᵀ **S63.490** Traumatic rupture of other ligament of right index finger at metacarpophalangeal and interphalangeal joint POA

7ᵀ **S63.491** Traumatic rupture of other ligament of left index finger at metacarpophalangeal and interphalangeal joint POA

7ᵀ **S63.492** Traumatic rupture of other ligament of right middle finger at metacarpophalangeal and interphalangeal joint POA

7ᵀ **S63.493** Traumatic rupture of other ligament of left middle finger at metacarpophalangeal and interphalangeal joint POA

7ᵀ **S63.494** Traumatic rupture of other ligament of right ring finger at metacarpophalangeal and interphalangeal joint POA

7ᵀ **S63.495** Traumatic rupture of other ligament of left ring finger at metacarpophalangeal and interphalangeal joint POA

7ᵀ **S63.496** Traumatic rupture of other ligament of right little finger at metacarpophalangeal and interphalangeal joint POA

Unspecified Code	Other Specified Code	Manifestation Code
N Newborn	P Pediatric	M Maternity	A Adult	♂ Male	♀ Female

● New Code ▲ Revised Code Title ▶◀ Revised Text **NOTES** *INCLUDES* **EXCLUDES 1** Not coded here *EXCLUDES 2* Not included here

4ᵗʰ 4th character required 5ᵗʰ 5th character required 6ᵗʰ 6th character required 7ᵗʰ 7th character required

7ˣ Extension 'X' Alert HAC Hospital-acquired condition (HAC) alert **AHA** AHA Coding Clinic©

S63.497 Traumatic rupture of other ligament of left little finger at metacarpophalangeal and interphalangeal joint POA

S63.498 Traumatic rupture of other ligament of other finger at metacarpophalangeal and interphalangeal joint POA

Traumatic rupture of ligament of specified finger with unspecified laterality at metacarpophalangeal and interphalangeal joint

S63.499 Traumatic rupture of other ligament of unspecified finger at metacarpophalangeal and interphalangeal joint POA

S63.5 Other and unspecified sprain of wrist

S63.50 Unspecified sprain of wrist

S63.501 Unspecified sprain of right wrist POA

S63.502 Unspecified sprain of left wrist POA

S63.509 Unspecified sprain of unspecified wrist POA

S63.51 Sprain of carpal (joint)

S63.511 Sprain of carpal joint of right wrist POA

S63.512 Sprain of carpal joint of left wrist POA

S63.519 Sprain of carpal joint of unspecified wrist POA

S63.52 Sprain of radiocarpal joint

EXCLUDES1 traumatic rupture of radiocarpal ligament (S63.32-)

S63.521 Sprain of radiocarpal joint of right wrist POA

S63.522 Sprain of radiocarpal joint of left wrist POA

S63.529 Sprain of radiocarpal joint of unspecified wrist POA

S63.59 Other specified sprain of wrist

S63.591 Other specified sprain of right wrist POA

S63.592 Other specified sprain of left wrist POA

S63.599 Other specified sprain of unspecified wrist POA

S63.6 Other and unspecified sprain of finger(s)

EXCLUDES1 traumatic rupture of ligament of finger at metacarpophalangeal and interphalangeal joint(s) (S63.4-)

S63.60 Unspecified sprain of thumb

S63.601 Unspecified sprain of right thumb POA

S63.602 Unspecified sprain of left thumb POA

S63.609 Unspecified sprain of unspecified thumb POA

S63.61 Unspecified sprain of other and unspecified finger(s)

S63.610 Unspecified sprain of right index finger POA

S63.611 Unspecified sprain of left index finger POA

S63.612 Unspecified sprain of right middle finger POA

S63.613 Unspecified sprain of left middle finger POA

S63.614 Unspecified sprain of right ring finger POA

S63.615 Unspecified sprain of left ring finger POA

S63.616 Unspecified sprain of right little finger POA

S63.617 Unspecified sprain of left little finger POA

S63.618 Unspecified sprain of other finger

Unspecified sprain of specified finger with unspecified laterality

S63.619 Unspecified sprain of unspecified finger POA

S63.62 Sprain of interphalangeal joint of thumb

S63.621 Sprain of interphalangeal joint of right thumb POA

S63.622 Sprain of interphalangeal joint of left thumb POA

S63.629 Sprain of interphalangeal joint of unspecified thumb POA

S63.63 Sprain of interphalangeal joint of other and unspecified finger(s)

S63.630 Sprain of interphalangeal joint of right index finger POA

S63.631 Sprain of interphalangeal joint of left index finger POA

S63.632 Sprain of interphalangeal joint of right middle finger POA

S63.633 Sprain of interphalangeal joint of left middle finger POA

S63.634 Sprain of interphalangeal joint of right ring finger POA

S63.635 Sprain of interphalangeal joint of left ring finger POA

S63.636 Sprain of interphalangeal joint of right little finger POA

S63.637 Sprain of interphalangeal joint of left little finger POA

S63.638 Sprain of interphalangeal joint of other finger POA

S63.639 Sprain of interphalangeal joint of unspecified finger POA

S63.64 Sprain of metacarpophalangeal joint of thumb

S63.641 Sprain of metacarpophalangeal joint of right thumb POA

S63.642 Sprain of metacarpophalangeal joint of left thumb POA

S63.649 Sprain of metacarpophalangeal joint of unspecified thumb POA

S63.65 Sprain of metacarpophalangeal joint of other and unspecified finger(s)

S63.650 Sprain of metacarpophalangeal joint of right index finger POA

S63.651 Sprain of metacarpophalangeal joint of left index finger POA

S63.652 Sprain of metacarpophalangeal joint of right middle finger POA

S63.653 Sprain of metacarpophalangeal joint of left middle finger POA

S63.654 Sprain of metacarpophalangeal joint of right ring finger POA

S63.655 Sprain of metacarpophalangeal joint of left ring finger POA

S63.656 Sprain of metacarpophalangeal joint of right little finger POA

S63.657 Sprain of metacarpophalangeal joint of left little finger POA

S63.658 Sprain of metacarpophalangeal joint of other finger POA

Sprain of metacarpophalangeal joint of specified finger with unspecified laterality

S63.659 Sprain of metacarpophalangeal joint of unspecified finger POA

S63.68 Other sprain of thumb

S63.681 Other sprain of right thumb POA

S63.682 Other sprain of left thumb POA

S63.689 Other sprain of unspecified thumb POA

S63.69 Other sprain of other and unspecified finger(s)

S63.690 Other sprain of right index finger POA

S63.691 Other sprain of left index finger POA

S63.692 Other sprain of right middle finger POA

S63.693 Other sprain of left middle finger POA

S63.694 Other sprain of right ring finger POA

S63.695 Other sprain of left ring finger POA

S63.696 Other sprain of right little finger POA

S63.697 Other sprain of left little finger POA

S63.698 Other sprain of other finger POA

Other sprain of specified finger with unspecified laterality

S63.699 Other sprain of unspecified finger POA

S63.8 Sprain of other part of wrist and hand

S63.8X Sprain of other part of wrist and hand

S63.8X1 Sprain of other part of right wrist and hand POA

S63.8X2 Sprain of other part of left wrist and hand POA

PDXᴺᴸ Unacceptable principal diagnosis symbol per Medicare code edits   Code exempt from diagnosis present on admission requirement
❓ Questionable admission   ᶜᶜ Complication or comorbidity   ᶜᶜ·ᴹᶜᶜ ᴱˣᶜ CC/MCC exclusion   ᴹᶜᶜ Major complication or comorbidity
Principal diagnosis as its own CC   Principal diagnosis as its own MCC   HCC HCC diagnosis code   RxHCC RxHCC diagnosis code
MACRA code   Z Z code as first-listed diagnosis

7ᵗʰ **S63.8X9** Sprain of other part of unspecified wrist and hand ᴾᴼᴬ

5ᵗʰ **S63.9** Sprain of unspecified part of wrist and hand

7ᵗʰ **S63.90** Sprain of unspecified part of unspecified wrist and hand ᴾᴼᴬ

7ᵗʰ **S63.91** Sprain of unspecified part of right wrist and hand ᴾᴼᴬ

7ᵗʰ **S63.92** Sprain of unspecified part of left wrist and hand ᴾᴼᴬ

4ᵗʰ **S64** Injury of nerves at wrist and hand level

Code also any associated open wound (S61.-)

The appropriate 7th character is to be added to each code from category S64

A = initial encounter
D = subsequent encounter
S = sequela

5ᵗʰ **S64.0** Injury of ulnar nerve at wrist and hand level

7ᵗʰ **S64.00** Injury of ulnar nerve at wrist and hand level of unspecified arm ᴾᴼᴬ

7ᵗʰ **S64.01** Injury of ulnar nerve at wrist and hand level of right arm ᴾᴼᴬ

7ᵗʰ **S64.02** Injury of ulnar nerve at wrist and hand level of left arm ᴾᴼᴬ

5ᵗʰ **S64.1** Injury of median nerve at wrist and hand level

7ᵗʰ **S64.10** Injury of median nerve at wrist and hand level of unspecified arm ᴾᴼᴬ

7ᵗʰ **S64.11** Injury of median nerve at wrist and hand level of right arm ᴾᴼᴬ

7ᵗʰ **S64.12** Injury of median nerve at wrist and hand level of left arm ᴾᴼᴬ

5ᵗʰ **S64.2** Injury of radial nerve at wrist and hand level

7ᵗʰ **S64.20** Injury of radial nerve at wrist and hand level of unspecified arm ᴾᴼᴬ

7ᵗʰ **S64.21** Injury of radial nerve at wrist and hand level of right arm ᴾᴼᴬ

7ᵗʰ **S64.22** Injury of radial nerve at wrist and hand level of left arm ᴾᴼᴬ

5ᵗʰ **S64.3** Injury of digital nerve of thumb

7ᵗʰ **S64.30** Injury of digital nerve of unspecified thumb ᴾᴼᴬ

7ᵗʰ **S64.31** Injury of digital nerve of right thumb ᴾᴼᴬ

7ᵗʰ **S64.32** Injury of digital nerve of left thumb ᴾᴼᴬ

5ᵗʰ **S64.4** Injury of digital nerve of other and unspecified finger

7ᵗʰ **S64.40** Injury of digital nerve of unspecified finger ᴾᴼᴬ

6ᵗʰ **S64.49** Injury of digital nerve of other finger

7ᵗʰ **S64.490** Injury of digital nerve of right index finger ᴾᴼᴬ

7ᵗʰ **S64.491** Injury of digital nerve of left index finger ᴾᴼᴬ

7ᵗʰ **S64.492** Injury of digital nerve of right middle finger ᴾᴼᴬ

7ᵗʰ **S64.493** Injury of digital nerve of left middle finger ᴾᴼᴬ

7ᵗʰ **S64.494** Injury of digital nerve of right ring finger ᴾᴼᴬ

7ᵗʰ **S64.495** Injury of digital nerve of left ring finger ᴾᴼᴬ

7ᵗʰ **S64.496** Injury of digital nerve of right little finger ᴾᴼᴬ

7ᵗʰ **S64.497** Injury of digital nerve of left little finger ᴾᴼᴬ

7ᵗʰ **S64.498** Injury of digital nerve of other finger

Injury of digital nerve of specified finger with unspecified laterality

5ᵗʰ **S64.8** Injury of other nerves at wrist and hand level

6ᵗʰ **S64.8X** Injury of other nerves at wrist and hand level

7ᵗʰ **S64.8X1** Injury of other nerves at wrist and hand level of right arm ᴾᴼᴬ

7ᵗʰ **S64.8X2** Injury of other nerves at wrist and hand level of left arm ᴾᴼᴬ

7ᵗʰ **S64.8X9** Injury of other nerves at wrist and hand level of unspecified arm ᴾᴼᴬ

5ᵗʰ **S64.9** Injury of unspecified nerve at wrist and hand level

7ᵗʰ **S64.90** Injury of unspecified nerve at wrist and hand level of unspecified arm ᴾᴼᴬ

7ᵗʰ **S64.91** Injury of unspecified nerve at wrist and hand level of right arm ᴾᴼᴬ

7ᵗʰ **S64.92** Injury of unspecified nerve at wrist and hand level of left arm ᴾᴼᴬ

4ᵗʰ **S65** Injury of blood vessels at wrist and hand level

Code also any associated open wound (S61.-)

The appropriate 7th character is to be added to each code from category S65

A = initial encounter
D = subsequent encounter
S = sequela

5ᵗʰ **S65.0** Injury of ulnar artery at wrist and hand level

6ᵗʰ **S65.00** Unspecified injury of ulnar artery at wrist and hand level

7ᵗʰ **S65.001** Unspecified injury of ulnar artery at wrist and hand level of right arm CC ᴾᴼᴬ CC/MCC Exc

7ᵗʰ **S65.002** Unspecified injury of ulnar artery at wrist and hand level of left arm CC ᴾᴼᴬ CC/MCC Exc

7ᵗʰ **S65.009** Unspecified injury of ulnar artery at wrist and hand level of unspecified arm CC ᴾᴼᴬ CC/MCC Exc

6ᵗʰ **S65.01** Laceration of ulnar artery at wrist and hand level

7ᵗʰ **S65.011** Laceration of ulnar artery at wrist and hand level of right arm CC ᴾᴼᴬ CC/MCC Exc

7ᵗʰ **S65.012** Laceration of ulnar artery at wrist and hand level of left arm CC ᴾᴼᴬ CC/MCC Exc

7ᵗʰ **S65.019** Laceration of ulnar artery at wrist and hand level of unspecified arm CC ᴾᴼᴬ CC/MCC Exc

6ᵗʰ **S65.09** Other specified injury of ulnar artery at wrist and hand level

7ᵗʰ **S65.091** Other specified injury of ulnar artery at wrist and hand level of right arm CC ᴾᴼᴬ CC/MCC Exc

7ᵗʰ **S65.092** Other specified injury of ulnar artery at wrist and hand level of left arm CC ᴾᴼᴬ CC/MCC Exc

7ᵗʰ **S65.099** Other specified injury of ulnar artery at wrist and hand level of unspecified arm CC ᴾᴼᴬ CC/MCC Exc

5ᵗʰ **S65.1** Injury of radial artery at wrist and hand level

6ᵗʰ **S65.10** Unspecified injury of radial artery at wrist and hand level

7ᵗʰ **S65.101** Unspecified injury of radial artery at wrist and hand level of right arm CC ᴾᴼᴬ CC/MCC Exc

7ᵗʰ **S65.102** Unspecified injury of radial artery at wrist and hand level of left arm CC ᴾᴼᴬ CC/MCC Exc

7ᵗʰ **S65.109** Unspecified injury of radial artery at wrist and hand level of unspecified arm CC ᴾᴼᴬ CC/MCC Exc

6ᵗʰ **S65.11** Laceration of radial artery at wrist and hand level

7ᵗʰ **S65.111** Laceration of radial artery at wrist and hand level of right arm CC ᴾᴼᴬ CC/MCC Exc

7ᵗʰ **S65.112** Laceration of radial artery at wrist and hand level of left arm CC ᴾᴼᴬ CC/MCC Exc

7ᵗʰ **S65.119** Laceration of radial artery at wrist and hand level of unspecified arm CC ᴾᴼᴬ CC/MCC Exc

6ᵗʰ **S65.19** Other specified injury of radial artery at wrist and hand level

7ᵗʰ **S65.191** Other specified injury of radial artery at wrist and hand level of right arm CC ᴾᴼᴬ CC/MCC Exc

7ᵗʰ **S65.192** Other specified injury of radial artery at wrist and hand level of left arm CC ᴾᴼᴬ CC/MCC Exc

7ᵗʰ **S65.199** Other specified injury of radial artery at wrist and hand level of unspecified arm CC ᴾᴼᴬ CC/MCC Exc

5ᵗʰ **S65.2** Injury of superficial palmar arch

6ᵗʰ **S65.20** Unspecified injury of superficial palmar arch

7ᵗʰ **S65.201** Unspecified injury of superficial palmar arch of right hand CC ᴾᴼᴬ CC/MCC Exc

7ᵗʰ **S65.202** Unspecified injury of superficial palmar arch of left hand CC ᴾᴼᴬ CC/MCC Exc

---

Unspecified Code   Other Specified Code   Manifestation Code   Ⓝ Newborn   Ⓟ Pediatric   Ⓜ Maternity   Ⓐ Adult   ♂ Male   ♀ Female

● New Code   ▲ Revised Code Title   ►◄ Revised Text   **NOTES**   *INCLUDES*   *EXCLUDES 1* Not coded here   *EXCLUDES 2* Not included here

4ᵗʰ 4th character required   5ᵗʰ 5th character required   6ᵗʰ 6th character required   7ᵗʰ 7th character required

7ᵗʰ Extension 'X' Alert   **HAC** Hospital-acquired condition (HAC) alert   **AHA** AHA Coding Clinic©

7ᵗʰ S65.209 Unspecified injury of superficial palmar arch of unspecified hand ⁍ ᴘᴏᴀ ᴄᴄ/ᴍᴄᴄ ᴇxᴄ

6ᵗʰ S65.21 Laceration of superficial palmar arch
  7ᵗʰ S65.211 Laceration of superficial palmar arch of right hand ⁍ ᴘᴏᴀ ᴄᴄ/ᴍᴄᴄ ᴇxᴄ
  7ᵗʰ S65.212 Laceration of superficial palmar arch of left hand ⁍ ᴘᴏᴀ ᴄᴄ/ᴍᴄᴄ ᴇxᴄ
  7ᵗʰ S65.219 Laceration of superficial palmar arch of unspecified hand ⁍ ᴘᴏᴀ ᴄᴄ/ᴍᴄᴄ ᴇxᴄ

6ᵗʰ S65.29 Other specified injury of superficial palmar arch
  7ᵗʰ S65.291 Other specified injury of superficial palmar arch of right hand ⁍ ᴘᴏᴀ ᴄᴄ/ᴍᴄᴄ ᴇxᴄ
  7ᵗʰ S65.292 Other specified injury of superficial palmar arch of left hand ⁍ ᴘᴏᴀ ᴄᴄ/ᴍᴄᴄ ᴇxᴄ
  7ᵗʰ S65.299 Other specified injury of superficial palmar arch of unspecified hand ⁍ ᴘᴏᴀ ᴄᴄ/ᴍᴄᴄ ᴇxᴄ

5ᵗʰ S65.3 Injury of deep palmar arch
  6ᵗʰ S65.30 Unspecified injury of deep palmar arch
    7ᵗʰ S65.301 Unspecified injury of deep palmar arch of right hand ⁍ ᴘᴏᴀ ᴄᴄ/ᴍᴄᴄ ᴇxᴄ
    7ᵗʰ S65.302 Unspecified injury of deep palmar arch of left hand ⁍ ᴘᴏᴀ ᴄᴄ/ᴍᴄᴄ ᴇxᴄ
    7ᵗʰ S65.309 Unspecified injury of deep palmar arch of unspecified hand ⁍ ᴘᴏᴀ ᴄᴄ/ᴍᴄᴄ ᴇxᴄ

  6ᵗʰ S65.31 Laceration of deep palmar arch
    7ᵗʰ S65.311 Laceration of deep palmar arch of right hand ⁍ ᴘᴏᴀ ᴄᴄ/ᴍᴄᴄ ᴇxᴄ
    7ᵗʰ S65.312 Laceration of deep palmar arch of left hand ⁍ ᴘᴏᴀ ᴄᴄ/ᴍᴄᴄ ᴇxᴄ
    7ᵗʰ S65.319 Laceration of deep palmar arch of unspecified hand ⁍ ᴘᴏᴀ ᴄᴄ/ᴍᴄᴄ ᴇxᴄ

  6ᵗʰ S65.39 Other specified injury of deep palmar arch
    7ᵗʰ S65.391 Other specified injury of deep palmar arch of right hand ⁍ ᴘᴏᴀ ᴄᴄ/ᴍᴄᴄ ᴇxᴄ
    7ᵗʰ S65.392 Other specified injury of deep palmar arch of left hand ⁍ ᴘᴏᴀ ᴄᴄ/ᴍᴄᴄ ᴇxᴄ
    7ᵗʰ S65.399 Other specified injury of deep palmar arch of unspecified hand ⁍ ᴘᴏᴀ ᴄᴄ/ᴍᴄᴄ ᴇxᴄ

5ᵗʰ S65.4 Injury of blood vessel of thumb
  6ᵗʰ S65.40 Unspecified injury of blood vessel of thumb
    7ᵗʰ S65.401 Unspecified injury of blood vessel of right thumb ⁍ ᴘᴏᴀ ᴄᴄ/ᴍᴄᴄ ᴇxᴄ
    7ᵗʰ S65.402 Unspecified injury of blood vessel of left thumb ⁍ ᴘᴏᴀ ᴄᴄ/ᴍᴄᴄ ᴇxᴄ
    7ᵗʰ S65.409 Unspecified injury of blood vessel of unspecified thumb ⁍ ᴘᴏᴀ ᴄᴄ/ᴍᴄᴄ ᴇxᴄ

  6ᵗʰ S65.41 Laceration of blood vessel of thumb
    7ᵗʰ S65.411 Laceration of blood vessel of right thumb ⁍ ᴘᴏᴀ ᴄᴄ/ᴍᴄᴄ ᴇxᴄ
    7ᵗʰ S65.412 Laceration of blood vessel of left thumb ⁍ ᴘᴏᴀ ᴄᴄ/ᴍᴄᴄ ᴇxᴄ
    7ᵗʰ S65.419 Laceration of blood vessel of unspecified thumb ⁍ ᴘᴏᴀ ᴄᴄ/ᴍᴄᴄ ᴇxᴄ

  6ᵗʰ S65.49 Other specified injury of blood vessel of thumb
    7ᵗʰ S65.491 Other specified injury of blood vessel of right thumb ⁍ ᴘᴏᴀ ᴄᴄ/ᴍᴄᴄ ᴇxᴄ
    7ᵗʰ S65.492 Other specified injury of blood vessel of left thumb ⁍ ᴘᴏᴀ ᴄᴄ/ᴍᴄᴄ ᴇxᴄ
    7ᵗʰ S65.499 Other specified injury of blood vessel of unspecified thumb ⁍ ᴘᴏᴀ ᴄᴄ/ᴍᴄᴄ ᴇxᴄ

5ᵗʰ S65.5 Injury of blood vessel of other and unspecified finger
  6ᵗʰ S65.50 Unspecified injury of blood vessel of other and unspecified finger
    7ᵗʰ S65.500 Unspecified injury of blood vessel of right index finger ⁍ ᴘᴏᴀ ᴄᴄ/ᴍᴄᴄ ᴇxᴄ
    7ᵗʰ S65.501 Unspecified injury of blood vessel of left index finger ⁍ ᴘᴏᴀ ᴄᴄ/ᴍᴄᴄ ᴇxᴄ
    7ᵗʰ S65.502 Unspecified injury of blood vessel of right middle finger ⁍ ᴘᴏᴀ ᴄᴄ/ᴍᴄᴄ ᴇxᴄ

7ᵗʰ S65.503 Unspecified injury of blood vessel of left middle finger ⁍ ᴘᴏᴀ ᴄᴄ/ᴍᴄᴄ ᴇxᴄ
7ᵗʰ S65.504 Unspecified injury of blood vessel of right ring finger ⁍ ᴘᴏᴀ ᴄᴄ/ᴍᴄᴄ ᴇxᴄ
7ᵗʰ S65.505 Unspecified injury of blood vessel of left ring finger ⁍ ᴘᴏᴀ ᴄᴄ/ᴍᴄᴄ ᴇxᴄ
7ᵗʰ S65.506 Unspecified injury of blood vessel of right little finger ⁍ ᴘᴏᴀ ᴄᴄ/ᴍᴄᴄ ᴇxᴄ
7ᵗʰ S65.507 Unspecified injury of blood vessel of left little finger ⁍ ᴘᴏᴀ ᴄᴄ/ᴍᴄᴄ ᴇxᴄ
7ᵗʰ S65.508 Unspecified injury of blood vessel of other finger ⁍ ᴘᴏᴀ ᴄᴄ/ᴍᴄᴄ ᴇxᴄ

Unspecified injury of blood vessel of specified finger with unspecified laterality
7ᵗʰ S65.509 Unspecified injury of blood vessel of unspecified finger ⁍ ᴘᴏᴀ ᴄᴄ/ᴍᴄᴄ ᴇxᴄ

6ᵗʰ S65.51 Laceration of blood vessel of other and unspecified finger
  7ᵗʰ S65.510 Laceration of blood vessel of right index finger ⁍ ᴘᴏᴀ ᴄᴄ/ᴍᴄᴄ ᴇxᴄ
  7ᵗʰ S65.511 Laceration of blood vessel of left index finger ⁍ ᴘᴏᴀ ᴄᴄ/ᴍᴄᴄ ᴇxᴄ
  7ᵗʰ S65.512 Laceration of blood vessel of right middle finger ⁍ ᴘᴏᴀ ᴄᴄ/ᴍᴄᴄ ᴇxᴄ
  7ᵗʰ S65.513 Laceration of blood vessel of left middle finger ⁍ ᴘᴏᴀ ᴄᴄ/ᴍᴄᴄ ᴇxᴄ
  7ᵗʰ S65.514 Laceration of blood vessel of right ring finger ⁍ ᴘᴏᴀ ᴄᴄ/ᴍᴄᴄ ᴇxᴄ
  7ᵗʰ S65.515 Laceration of blood vessel of left ring finger ⁍ ᴘᴏᴀ ᴄᴄ/ᴍᴄᴄ ᴇxᴄ
  7ᵗʰ S65.516 Laceration of blood vessel of right little finger ⁍ ᴘᴏᴀ ᴄᴄ/ᴍᴄᴄ ᴇxᴄ
  7ᵗʰ S65.517 Laceration of blood vessel of left little finger ⁍ ᴘᴏᴀ ᴄᴄ/ᴍᴄᴄ ᴇxᴄ
  7ᵗʰ S65.518 Laceration of blood vessel of other finger ⁍ ᴘᴏᴀ ᴄᴄ/ᴍᴄᴄ ᴇxᴄ

  Laceration of blood vessel of specified finger with unspecified laterality
  7ᵗʰ S65.519 Laceration of blood vessel of unspecified finger ⁍ ᴘᴏᴀ ᴄᴄ/ᴍᴄᴄ ᴇxᴄ

6ᵗʰ S65.59 Other specified injury of blood vessel of other and unspecified finger
  7ᵗʰ S65.590 Other specified injury of blood vessel of right index finger ⁍ ᴘᴏᴀ ᴄᴄ/ᴍᴄᴄ ᴇxᴄ
  7ᵗʰ S65.591 Other specified injury of blood vessel of left index finger ⁍ ᴘᴏᴀ ᴄᴄ/ᴍᴄᴄ ᴇxᴄ
  7ᵗʰ S65.592 Other specified injury of blood vessel of right middle finger ⁍ ᴘᴏᴀ ᴄᴄ/ᴍᴄᴄ ᴇxᴄ
  7ᵗʰ S65.593 Other specified injury of blood vessel of left middle finger ⁍ ᴘᴏᴀ ᴄᴄ/ᴍᴄᴄ ᴇxᴄ
  7ᵗʰ S65.594 Other specified injury of blood vessel of right ring finger ⁍ ᴘᴏᴀ ᴄᴄ/ᴍᴄᴄ ᴇxᴄ
  7ᵗʰ S65.595 Other specified injury of blood vessel of left ring finger ⁍ ᴘᴏᴀ ᴄᴄ/ᴍᴄᴄ ᴇxᴄ
  7ᵗʰ S65.596 Other specified injury of blood vessel of right little finger ⁍ ᴘᴏᴀ ᴄᴄ/ᴍᴄᴄ ᴇxᴄ
  7ᵗʰ S65.597 Other specified injury of blood vessel of left little finger ⁍ ᴘᴏᴀ ᴄᴄ/ᴍᴄᴄ ᴇxᴄ
  7ᵗʰ S65.598 Other specified injury of blood vessel of other finger ⁍ ᴘᴏᴀ ᴄᴄ/ᴍᴄᴄ ᴇxᴄ

  Other specified injury of blood vessel of specified finger with unspecified laterality
  7ᵗʰ S65.599 Other specified injury of blood vessel of unspecified finger ⁍ ᴘᴏᴀ ᴄᴄ/ᴍᴄᴄ ᴇxᴄ

5ᵗʰ S65.8 Injury of other blood vessels at wrist and hand level
  6ᵗʰ S65.80 Unspecified injury of other blood vessels at wrist and hand level
    7ᵗʰ S65.801 Unspecified injury of other blood vessels at wrist and hand level of right arm ⁍ ᴘᴏᴀ ᴄᴄ/ᴍᴄᴄ ᴇxᴄ

ᴘᴅx Unacceptable principal diagnosis symbol per Medicare code edits ᴘᴏᴀ Code exempt from diagnosis present on admission requirement
? Questionable admission ⁍ Complication or comorbidity ᴄᴄ/ᴍᴄᴄ ᴇxᴄ CC/MCC exclusion ᴍᴄᴄ Major complication or comorbidity
Principal diagnosis as its own CC Principal diagnosis as its own MCC ʜᴄᴄ HCC diagnosis code ʀxʜᴄᴄ RxHCC diagnosis code
MACRA code Z1 Z code as first-listed diagnosis

7ᵗʰ **S65.802** Unspecified injury of other blood vessels at wrist and hand level of left arm CC POA CC/MCC Exc

7ᵗʰ **S65.809** Unspecified injury of other blood vessels at wrist and hand level of unspecified arm CC POA CC/MCC Exc

6ᵗʰ **S65.81** Laceration of other blood vessels at wrist and hand level

7ᵗʰ **S65.811** Laceration of other blood vessels at wrist and hand level of right arm CC POA CC/MCC Exc

7ᵗʰ **S65.812** Laceration of other blood vessels at wrist and hand level of left arm CC POA CC/MCC Exc

7ᵗʰ **S65.819** Laceration of other blood vessels at wrist and hand level of unspecified arm CC POA CC/MCC Exc

6ᵗʰ **S65.89** Other specified injury of other blood vessels at wrist and hand level

7ᵗʰ **S65.891** Other specified injury of other blood vessels at wrist and hand level of right arm CC POA CC/MCC Exc

7ᵗʰ **S65.892** Other specified injury of other blood vessels at wrist and hand level of left arm CC POA CC/MCC Exc

7ᵗʰ **S65.899** Other specified injury of other blood vessels at wrist and hand level of unspecified arm CC POA CC/MCC Exc

5ᵗʰ **S65.9** Injury of unspecified blood vessel at wrist and hand level

6ᵗʰ **S65.90** Unspecified injury of unspecified blood vessel at wrist and hand level

7ᵗʰ **S65.901** Unspecified injury of unspecified blood vessel at wrist and hand level of right arm CC POA CC/MCC Exc

7ᵗʰ **S65.902** Unspecified injury of unspecified blood vessel at wrist and hand level of left arm CC POA CC/MCC Exc

7ᵗʰ **S65.909** Unspecified injury of unspecified blood vessel at wrist and hand level of unspecified arm CC POA CC/MCC Exc

6ᵗʰ **S65.91** Laceration of unspecified blood vessel at wrist and hand level

7ᵗʰ **S65.911** Laceration of unspecified blood vessel at wrist and hand level of right arm CC POA CC/MCC Exc

7ᵗʰ **S65.912** Laceration of unspecified blood vessel at wrist and hand level of left arm CC POA CC/MCC Exc

7ᵗʰ **S65.919** Laceration of unspecified blood vessel at wrist and hand level of unspecified arm CC POA CC/MCC Exc

6ᵗʰ **S65.99** Other specified injury of unspecified blood vessel at wrist and hand level

7ᵗʰ **S65.991** Other specified injury of unspecified blood vessel at wrist and hand of right arm CC POA CC/MCC Exc

7ᵗʰ **S65.992** Other specified injury of unspecified blood vessel at wrist and hand of left arm CC POA CC/MCC Exc

7ᵗʰ **S65.999** Other specified injury of unspecified blood vessel at wrist and hand of unspecified arm CC POA CC/MCC Exc

4ᵗʰ **S66** Injury of muscle, fascia and tendon at wrist and hand level

Code also any associated open wound (S61.-)

EXCLUDES2 sprain of joints and ligaments of wrist and hand (S63.-)

The appropriate 7th character is to be added to each code from category S66

A = initial encounter
D = subsequent encounter
S = sequela

5ᵗʰ **S66.0** Injury of long flexor muscle, fascia and tendon of thumb at wrist and hand level

6ᵗʰ **S66.00** Unspecified injury of long flexor muscle, fascia and tendon of thumb at wrist and hand level

7ᵗʰ **S66.001** Unspecified injury of long flexor muscle, fascia and tendon of right thumb at wrist and hand level POA

7ᵗʰ **S66.002** Unspecified injury of long flexor muscle, fascia and tendon of left thumb at wrist and hand level POA

7ᵗʰ **S66.009** Unspecified injury of long flexor muscle, fascia and tendon of unspecified thumb at wrist and hand level POA

6ᵗʰ **S66.01** Strain of long flexor muscle, fascia and tendon of thumb at wrist and hand level

7ᵗʰ **S66.011** Strain of long flexor muscle, fascia and tendon of right thumb at wrist and hand level POA

7ᵗʰ **S66.012** Strain of long flexor muscle, fascia and tendon of left thumb at wrist and hand level POA

7ᵗʰ **S66.019** Strain of long flexor muscle, fascia and tendon of unspecified thumb at wrist and hand level POA

6ᵗʰ **S66.02** Laceration of long flexor muscle, fascia and tendon of thumb at wrist and hand level

7ᵗʰ **S66.021** Laceration of long flexor muscle, fascia and tendon of right thumb at wrist and hand level CC POA CC/MCC Exc

7ᵗʰ **S66.022** Laceration of long flexor muscle, fascia and tendon of left thumb at wrist and hand level CC POA CC/MCC Exc

7ᵗʰ **S66.029** Laceration of long flexor muscle, fascia and tendon of unspecified thumb at wrist and hand level CC POA CC/MCC Exc

6ᵗʰ **S66.09** Other specified injury of long flexor muscle, fascia and tendon of thumb at wrist and hand level

7ᵗʰ **S66.091** Other specified injury of long flexor muscle, fascia and tendon of right thumb at wrist and hand level POA

7ᵗʰ **S66.092** Other specified injury of long flexor muscle, fascia and tendon of left thumb at wrist and hand level POA

7ᵗʰ **S66.099** Other specified injury of long flexor muscle, fascia and tendon of unspecified thumb at wrist and hand level POA

5ᵗʰ **S66.1** Injury of flexor muscle, fascia and tendon of other and unspecified finger at wrist and hand level

EXCLUDES2 Injury of long flexor muscle, fascia and tendon of thumb at wrist and hand level (S66.0-)

6ᵗʰ **S66.10** Unspecified injury of flexor muscle, fascia and tendon of other and unspecified finger at wrist and hand level

7ᵗʰ **S66.100** Unspecified injury of flexor muscle, fascia and tendon of right index finger at wrist and hand level POA

7ᵗʰ **S66.101** Unspecified injury of flexor muscle, fascia and tendon of left index finger at wrist and hand level POA

7ᵗʰ **S66.102** Unspecified injury of flexor muscle, fascia and tendon of right middle finger at wrist and hand level POA

7ᵗʰ **S66.103** Unspecified injury of flexor muscle, fascia and tendon of left middle finger at wrist and hand level POA

7ᵗʰ **S66.104** Unspecified injury of flexor muscle, fascia and tendon of right ring finger at wrist and hand level POA

7ᵗʰ **S66.105** Unspecified injury of flexor muscle, fascia and tendon of left ring finger at wrist and hand level POA

7ᵗʰ **S66.106** Unspecified injury of flexor muscle, fascia and tendon of right little finger at wrist and hand level POA

7ᵗʰ **S66.107** Unspecified injury of flexor muscle, fascia and tendon of left little finger at wrist and hand level POA

Unspecified Code   Other Specified Code   Manifestation Code   N Newborn   P Pediatric   M Maternity   A Adult   ♂ Male   ♀ Female
● New Code   ▲ Revised Code Title   ▶◀ Revised Text   NOTES   INCLUDES   EXCLUDES 1   Not coded here   EXCLUDES 2   Not included here
4ᵗʰ 4th character required   5ᵗʰ 5th character required   6ᵗʰ 6th character required   7ᵗʰ 7th character required
7ˣ Extension 'X' Alert   HAC Hospital-acquired condition (HAC) alert   AHA AHA Coding Clinic©

7ᵗʰ **S66.108 Unspecified injury of flexor muscle, fascia and tendon of other finger at wrist and hand level** POA

Unspecified injury of flexor muscle, fascia and tendon of specified finger with unspecified laterality at wrist and hand level

7ᵗʰ **S66.109 Unspecified injury of flexor muscle, fascia and tendon of unspecified finger at wrist and hand level** POA

6ᵗʰ S66.11 Strain of flexor muscle, fascia and tendon of other and unspecified finger at wrist and hand level

7ᵗʰ S66.110 Strain of flexor muscle, fascia and tendon of right index finger at wrist and hand level POA

7ᵗʰ S66.111 Strain of flexor muscle, fascia and tendon of left index finger at wrist and hand level POA

7ᵗʰ S66.112 Strain of flexor muscle, fascia and tendon of right middle finger at wrist and hand level POA

7ᵗʰ S66.113 Strain of flexor muscle, fascia and tendon of left middle finger at wrist and hand level POA

7ᵗʰ S66.114 Strain of flexor muscle, fascia and tendon of right ring finger at wrist and hand level POA

7ᵗʰ S66.115 Strain of flexor muscle, fascia and tendon of left ring finger at wrist and hand level POA

7ᵗʰ S66.116 Strain of flexor muscle, fascia and tendon of right little finger at wrist and hand level POA

7ᵗʰ S66.117 Strain of flexor muscle, fascia and tendon of left little finger at wrist and hand level POA

7ᵗʰ S66.118 Strain of flexor muscle, fascia and tendon of other finger at wrist and hand level POA

Strain of flexor muscle, fascia and tendon of specified finger with unspecified laterality at wrist and hand level

7ᵗʰ **S66.119 Strain of flexor muscle, fascia and tendon of unspecified finger at wrist and hand level** POA

6ᵗʰ S66.12 Laceration of flexor muscle, fascia and tendon of other and unspecified finger at wrist and hand level

7ᵗʰ S66.120 Laceration of flexor muscle, fascia and tendon of right index finger at wrist and hand level CC POA CC/MCC Exc

7ᵗʰ S66.121 Laceration of flexor muscle, fascia and tendon of left index finger at wrist and hand level CC POA CC/MCC Exc

7ᵗʰ S66.122 Laceration of flexor muscle, fascia and tendon of right middle finger at wrist and hand level CC POA CC/MCC Exc

7ᵗʰ S66.123 Laceration of flexor muscle, fascia and tendon of left middle finger at wrist and hand level CC POA CC/MCC Exc

7ᵗʰ S66.124 Laceration of flexor muscle, fascia and tendon of right ring finger at wrist and hand level CC POA CC/MCC Exc

7ᵗʰ S66.125 Laceration of flexor muscle, fascia and tendon of left ring finger at wrist and hand level CC POA CC/MCC Exc

7ᵗʰ S66.126 Laceration of flexor muscle, fascia and tendon of right little finger at wrist and hand level CC POA CC/MCC Exc

7ᵗʰ S66.127 Laceration of flexor muscle, fascia and tendon of left little finger at wrist and hand level CC POA CC/MCC Exc

7ᵗʰ S66.128 Laceration of flexor muscle, fascia and tendon of other finger at wrist and hand level CC POA CC/MCC Exc

Laceration of flexor muscle, fascia and tendon of specified finger with unspecified laterality at wrist and hand level

7ᵗʰ S66.129 Laceration of flexor muscle, fascia and tendon of unspecified finger at wrist and hand level CC POA CC/MCC Exc

6ᵗʰ S66.19 Other injury of flexor muscle, fascia and tendon of other and unspecified finger at wrist and hand level

7ᵗʰ S66.190 Other injury of flexor muscle, fascia and tendon of right index finger at wrist and hand level POA

7ᵗʰ S66.191 Other injury of flexor muscle, fascia and tendon of left index finger at wrist and hand level POA

7ᵗʰ S66.192 Other injury of flexor muscle, fascia and tendon of right middle finger at wrist and hand level POA

7ᵗʰ S66.193 Other injury of flexor muscle, fascia and tendon of left middle finger at wrist and hand level POA

7ᵗʰ S66.194 Other injury of flexor muscle, fascia and tendon of right ring finger at wrist and hand level POA

7ᵗʰ S66.195 Other injury of flexor muscle, fascia and tendon of left ring finger at wrist and hand level POA

7ᵗʰ S66.196 Other injury of flexor muscle, fascia and tendon of right little finger at wrist and hand level POA

7ᵗʰ S66.197 Other injury of flexor muscle, fascia and tendon of left little finger at wrist and hand level POA

7ᵗʰ S66.198 Other injury of flexor muscle, fascia and tendon of other finger at wrist and hand level POA

Other injury of flexor muscle, fascia and tendon of specified finger with unspecified laterality at wrist and hand level

7ᵗʰ **S66.199 Other injury of flexor muscle, fascia and tendon of unspecified finger at wrist and hand level** POA

5ᵗʰ S66.2 Injury of extensor muscle, fascia and tendon of thumb at wrist and hand level

6ᵗʰ S66.20 Unspecified injury of extensor muscle, fascia and tendon of thumb at wrist and hand level

7ᵗʰ **S66.201 Unspecified injury of extensor muscle, fascia and tendon of right thumb at wrist and hand level** POA

7ᵗʰ **S66.202 Unspecified injury of extensor muscle, fascia and tendon of left thumb at wrist and hand level** POA

7ᵗʰ **S66.209 Unspecified injury of extensor muscle, fascia and tendon of unspecified thumb at wrist and hand level** POA

6ᵗʰ S66.21 Strain of extensor muscle, fascia and tendon of thumb at wrist and hand level

7ᵗʰ S66.211 Strain of extensor muscle, fascia and tendon of right thumb at wrist and hand level POA

7ᵗʰ S66.212 Strain of extensor muscle, fascia and tendon of left thumb at wrist and hand level POA

7ᵗʰ **S66.219 Strain of extensor muscle, fascia and tendon of unspecified thumb at wrist and hand level** POA

6ᵗʰ S66.22 Laceration of extensor muscle, fascia and tendon of thumb at wrist and hand level

7ᵗʰ S66.221 Laceration of extensor muscle, fascia and tendon of right thumb at wrist and hand level CC POA CC/MCC Exc

---

PDx Unacceptable principal diagnosis symbol per Medicare code edits   Code exempt from diagnosis present on admission requirement
? Questionable admission   CC Complication or comorbidity   CC/MCC Exc CC/MCC exclusion   MCC Major complication or comorbidity
Principal diagnosis as its own CC   Principal diagnosis as its own MCC   HCC HCC diagnosis code   RxHCC RxHCC diagnosis code
MACRA code   Z1 Z code as first-listed diagnosis

[7th] S66.222 Laceration of extensor muscle, fascia and tendon of left thumb at wrist and hand level CC POA CC/MCC Exc

[7th] S66.229 Laceration of extensor muscle, fascia and tendon of unspecified thumb at wrist and hand level CC POA CC/MCC Exc

[6th] S66.29 Other specified injury of extensor muscle, fascia and tendon of thumb at wrist and hand level

[7th] S66.291 Other specified injury of extensor muscle, fascia and tendon of right thumb at wrist and hand level POA

[7th] S66.292 Other specified injury of extensor muscle, fascia and tendon of left thumb at wrist and hand level POA

[7th] S66.299 Other specified injury of extensor muscle, fascia and tendon of unspecified thumb at wrist and hand level POA

[5th] S66.3 Injury of extensor muscle, fascia and tendon of other and unspecified finger at wrist and hand level

[EXCLUDES2] *Injury of extensor muscle, fascia and tendon of thumb at wrist and hand level (S66.2-)*

[6th] S66.30 Unspecified injury of extensor muscle, fascia and tendon of other and unspecified finger at wrist and hand level

[7th] S66.300 Unspecified injury of extensor muscle, fascia and tendon of right index finger at wrist and hand level POA

[7th] S66.301 Unspecified injury of extensor muscle, fascia and tendon of left index finger at wrist and hand level POA

[7th] S66.302 Unspecified injury of extensor muscle, fascia and tendon of right middle finger at wrist and hand level POA

[7th] S66.303 Unspecified injury of extensor muscle, fascia and tendon of left middle finger at wrist and hand level POA

[7th] S66.304 Unspecified injury of extensor muscle, fascia and tendon of right ring finger at wrist and hand level POA

[7th] S66.305 Unspecified injury of extensor muscle, fascia and tendon of left ring finger at wrist and hand level POA

[7th] S66.306 Unspecified injury of extensor muscle, fascia and tendon of right little finger at wrist and hand level POA

[7th] S66.307 Unspecified injury of extensor muscle, fascia and tendon of left little finger at wrist and hand level POA

[7th] S66.308 Unspecified injury of extensor muscle, fascia and tendon of other finger at wrist and hand level POA

Unspecified injury of extensor muscle, fascia and tendon of specified finger with unspecified laterality at wrist and hand level

[7th] S66.309 Unspecified injury of extensor muscle, fascia and tendon of unspecified finger at wrist and hand level POA

[6th] S66.31 Strain of extensor muscle, fascia and tendon of other and unspecified finger at wrist and hand level

[7th] S66.310 Strain of extensor muscle, fascia and tendon of right index finger at wrist and hand level POA

[7th] S66.311 Strain of extensor muscle, fascia and tendon of left index finger at wrist and hand level POA

[7th] S66.312 Strain of extensor muscle, fascia and tendon of right middle finger at wrist and hand level POA

[7th] S66.313 Strain of extensor muscle, fascia and tendon of left middle finger at wrist and hand level POA

[7th] S66.314 Strain of extensor muscle, fascia and tendon of right ring finger at wrist and hand level POA

[7th] S66.315 Strain of extensor muscle, fascia and tendon of left ring finger at wrist and hand level POA

[7th] S66.316 Strain of extensor muscle, fascia and tendon of right little finger at wrist and hand level POA

[7th] S66.317 Strain of extensor muscle, fascia and tendon of left little finger at wrist and hand level POA

[7th] S66.318 Strain of extensor muscle, fascia and tendon of other finger at wrist and hand level POA

Strain of extensor muscle, fascia and tendon of specified finger with unspecified laterality at wrist and hand level

[7th] S66.319 Strain of extensor muscle, fascia and tendon of unspecified finger at wrist and hand level POA

[6th] S66.32 Laceration of extensor muscle, fascia and tendon of other and unspecified finger at wrist and hand level

[7th] S66.320 Laceration of extensor muscle, fascia and tendon of right index finger at wrist and hand level CC POA CC/MCC Exc

[7th] S66.321 Laceration of extensor muscle, fascia and tendon of left index finger at wrist and hand level CC POA CC/MCC Exc

[7th] S66.322 Laceration of extensor muscle, fascia and tendon of right middle finger at wrist and hand level CC POA CC/MCC Exc

[7th] S66.323 Laceration of extensor muscle, fascia and tendon of left middle finger at wrist and hand level CC POA CC/MCC Exc

[7th] S66.324 Laceration of extensor muscle, fascia and tendon of right ring finger at wrist and hand level CC POA CC/MCC Exc

[7th] S66.325 Laceration of extensor muscle, fascia and tendon of left ring finger at wrist and hand level CC POA CC/MCC Exc

[7th] S66.326 Laceration of extensor muscle, fascia and tendon of right little finger at wrist and hand level CC POA CC/MCC Exc

[7th] S66.327 Laceration of extensor muscle, fascia and tendon of left little finger at wrist and hand level CC POA CC/MCC Exc

[7th] S66.328 Laceration of extensor muscle, fascia and tendon of other finger at wrist and hand level CC POA CC/MCC Exc

Laceration of extensor muscle, fascia and tendon of specified finger with unspecified laterality at wrist and hand level

[7th] S66.329 Laceration of extensor muscle, fascia and tendon of unspecified finger at wrist and hand level CC POA CC/MCC Exc

[6th] S66.39 Other injury of extensor muscle, fascia and tendon of other and unspecified finger at wrist and hand level

[7th] S66.390 Other injury of extensor muscle, fascia and tendon of right index finger at wrist and hand level POA

[7th] S66.391 Other injury of extensor muscle, fascia and tendon of left index finger at wrist and hand level POA

[7th] S66.392 Other injury of extensor muscle, fascia and tendon of right middle finger at wrist and hand level POA

[7th] S66.393 Other injury of extensor muscle, fascia and tendon of left middle finger at wrist and hand level POA

Unspecified Code | Other Specified Code | Manifestation Code | [N] Newborn | [P] Pediatric | [M] Maternity | [A] Adult | ♂ Male | ♀ Female
● New Code | ▲ Revised Code Title | ►◄ Revised Text | [NOTES] | [INCLUDES] | [EXCLUDES1] Not coded here | [EXCLUDES2] Not included here
[4th] 4th character required | [5th] 5th character required | [6th] 6th character required | [7th] 7th character required
[x7th] Extension 'X' Alert | [HAC] Hospital-acquired condition (HAC) alert | AHA AHA Coding Clinic©

- 7th **S72.031** Displaced midcervical fracture of right femur
- 7th **S72.032** Displaced midcervical fracture of left femur
- 7th **S72.033** Displaced midcervical fracture of unspecified femur
- 7th **S72.034** Nondisplaced midcervical fracture of right femur
- 7th **S72.035** Nondisplaced midcervical fracture of left femur
- 7th **S72.036** Nondisplaced midcervical fracture of unspecified femur
- 6th **S72.04** Fracture of base of neck of femur
  Cervicotrochanteric fracture of femur
  - 7th **S72.041** Displaced fracture of base of neck of right femur
  - 7th **S72.042** Displaced fracture of base of neck of left femur
  - 7th **S72.043** Displaced fracture of base of neck of unspecified femur
  - 7th **S72.044** Nondisplaced fracture of base of neck of right femur
  - 7th **S72.045** Nondisplaced fracture of base of neck of left femur
  - 7th **S72.046** Nondisplaced fracture of base of neck of unspecified femur
- 6th **S72.05** Unspecified fracture of head of femur
  Fracture of head of femur NOS
  - 7th **S72.051** Unspecified fracture of head of right femur
  - 7th **S72.052** Unspecified fracture of head of left femur
  - 7th **S72.059** Unspecified fracture of head of unspecified femur
- 6th **S72.06** Articular fracture of head of femur
  - 7th **S72.061** Displaced articular fracture of head of right femur
  - 7th **S72.062** Displaced articular fracture of head of left femur
  - 7th **S72.063** Displaced articular fracture of head of unspecified femur
  - 7th **S72.064** Nondisplaced articular fracture of head of right femur
  - 7th **S72.065** Nondisplaced articular fracture of head of left femur
  - 7th **S72.066** Nondisplaced articular fracture of head of unspecified femur
- 6th **S72.09** Other fracture of head and neck of femur
  - 7th **S72.091** Other fracture of head and neck of right femur
  - 7th **S72.092** Other fracture of head and neck of left femur
  - 7th **S72.099** Other fracture of head and neck of unspecified femur
- 5th **S72.1** Pertrochanteric fracture
  - 6th **S72.10** Unspecified trochanteric fracture of femur
    Fracture of trochanter NOS
    - 7th **S72.101** Unspecified trochanteric fracture of right femur
    - 7th **S72.102** Unspecified trochanteric fracture of left femur
    - 7th **S72.109** Unspecified trochanteric fracture of unspecified femur
  - 6th **S72.11** Fracture of greater trochanter of femur
    - 7th **S72.111** Displaced fracture of greater trochanter of right femur
    - 7th **S72.112** Displaced fracture of greater trochanter of left femur
    - 7th **S72.113** Displaced fracture of greater trochanter of unspecified femur
    - 7th **S72.114** Nondisplaced fracture of greater trochanter of right femur
    - 7th **S72.115** Nondisplaced fracture of greater trochanter of left femur
    - 7th **S72.116** Nondisplaced fracture of greater trochanter of unspecified femur
  - 6th **S72.12** Fracture of lesser trochanter of femur
    - 7th **S72.121** Displaced fracture of lesser trochanter of right femur
    - 7th **S72.122** Displaced fracture of lesser trochanter of left femur
    - 7th **S72.123** Displaced fracture of lesser trochanter of unspecified femur
    - 7th **S72.124** Nondisplaced fracture of lesser trochanter of right femur
    - 7th **S72.125** Nondisplaced fracture of lesser trochanter of left femur
    - 7th **S72.126** Nondisplaced fracture of lesser trochanter of unspecified femur
  - 5th **S72.13** Apophyseal fracture of femur
    EXCLUDES1 chronic (nontraumatic) slipped upper femoral epiphysis (M93.0-)
    - 7th **S72.131** Displaced apophyseal fracture of right femur
    - 7th **S72.132** Displaced apophyseal fracture of left femur
    - 7th **S72.133** Displaced apophyseal fracture of unspecified femur
    - 7th **S72.134** Nondisplaced apophyseal fracture of right femur
    - 7th **S72.135** Nondisplaced apophyseal fracture of left femur
    - 7th **S72.136** Nondisplaced apophyseal fracture of unspecified femur
  - 6th **S72.14** Intertrochanteric fracture of femur
    - 7th **S72.141** Displaced intertrochanteric fracture of right femur
    - 7th **S72.142** Displaced intertrochanteric fracture of left femur
    - 7th **S72.143** Displaced intertrochanteric fracture of unspecified femur
    - 7th **S72.144** Nondisplaced intertrochanteric fracture of right femur
    - 7th **S72.145** Nondisplaced intertrochanteric fracture of left femur
    - 7th **S72.146** Nondisplaced intertrochanteric fracture of unspecified femur
- 5th **S72.2** Subtrochanteric fracture of femur
  - 7th **S72.21** Displaced subtrochanteric fracture of right femur
  - 7th **S72.22** Displaced subtrochanteric fracture of left femur
  - 7th **S72.23** Displaced subtrochanteric fracture of unspecified femur
  - 7th **S72.24** Nondisplaced subtrochanteric fracture of right femur
  - 7th **S72.25** Nondisplaced subtrochanteric fracture of left femur
  - 7th **S72.26** Nondisplaced subtrochanteric fracture of unspecified femur
- 5th **S72.3** Fracture of shaft of femur
  - 6th **S72.30** Unspecified fracture of shaft of femur
    - 7th **S72.301** Unspecified fracture of shaft of right femur
    - 7th **S72.302** Unspecified fracture of shaft of left femur
    - 7th **S72.309** Unspecified fracture of shaft of unspecified femur
  - 6th **S72.32** Transverse fracture of shaft of femur

PDxⁿ Unacceptable principal diagnosis symbol per Medicare code edits   POA Code exempt from diagnosis present on admission requirement
🄰 Questionable admission   CC Complication or comorbidity   CC/MCC Exc CC/MCC exclusion   MCC Major complication or comorbidity
PDx/CC Principal diagnosis as its own CC   PDx/MCC Principal diagnosis as its own MCC   HCC HCC diagnosis code   RxHCC RxHCC diagnosis code
MACRA code   Z1 Z code as first-listed diagnosis

S72.321 Displaced transverse fracture of shaft of right femur
S72.322 Displaced transverse fracture of shaft of left femur
S72.323 Displaced transverse fracture of shaft of unspecified femur
S72.324 Nondisplaced transverse fracture of shaft of right femur
S72.325 Nondisplaced transverse fracture of shaft of left femur
S72.326 Nondisplaced transverse fracture of shaft of unspecified femur

S72.33 Oblique fracture of shaft of femur
S72.331 Displaced oblique fracture of shaft of right femur
S72.332 Displaced oblique fracture of shaft of left femur
S72.333 Displaced oblique fracture of shaft of unspecified femur
S72.334 Nondisplaced oblique fracture of shaft of right femur
S72.335 Nondisplaced oblique fracture of shaft of left femur
S72.336 Nondisplaced oblique fracture of shaft of unspecified femur

S72.34 Spiral fracture of shaft of femur
S72.341 Displaced spiral fracture of shaft of right femur
S72.342 Displaced spiral fracture of shaft of left femur
S72.343 Displaced spiral fracture of shaft of unspecified femur
S72.344 Nondisplaced spiral fracture of shaft of right femur
S72.345 Nondisplaced spiral fracture of shaft of left femur
S72.346 Nondisplaced spiral fracture of shaft of unspecified femur

S72.35 Comminuted fracture of shaft of femur
S72.351 Displaced comminuted fracture of shaft of right femur
S72.352 Displaced comminuted fracture of shaft of left femur
S72.353 Displaced comminuted fracture of shaft of unspecified femur
S72.354 Nondisplaced comminuted fracture of shaft of right femur
S72.355 Nondisplaced comminuted fracture of shaft of left femur
S72.356 Nondisplaced comminuted fracture of shaft of unspecified femur

S72.36 Segmental fracture of shaft of femur
S72.361 Displaced segmental fracture of shaft of right femur
S72.362 Displaced segmental fracture of shaft of left femur
S72.363 Displaced segmental fracture of shaft of unspecified femur
S72.364 Nondisplaced segmental fracture of shaft of right femur
S72.365 Nondisplaced segmental fracture of shaft of left femur
S72.366 Nondisplaced segmental fracture of shaft of unspecified femur

S72.39 Other fracture of shaft of femur
S72.391 Other fracture of shaft of right femur
S72.392 Other fracture of shaft of left femur
S72.399 Other fracture of shaft of unspecified femur

S72.4 Fracture of lower end of femur
Fracture of distal end of femur
EXCLUDES2 fracture of shaft of femur (S72.3-)
physeal fracture of lower end of femur (S79.1-)

S72.40 Unspecified fracture of lower end of femur
S72.401 Unspecified fracture of lower end of right femur
S72.402 Unspecified fracture of lower end of left femur
S72.409 Unspecified fracture of lower end of unspecified femur

S72.41 Unspecified condyle fracture of lower end of femur
Condyle fracture of femur NOS
S72.411 Displaced unspecified condyle fracture of lower end of right femur
S72.412 Displaced unspecified condyle fracture of lower end of left femur
S72.413 Displaced unspecified condyle fracture of lower end of unspecified femur
S72.414 Nondisplaced unspecified condyle fracture of lower end of right femur
S72.415 Nondisplaced unspecified condyle fracture of lower end of left femur
S72.416 Nondisplaced unspecified condyle fracture of lower end of unspecified femur

S72.42 Fracture of lateral condyle of femur
S72.421 Displaced fracture of lateral condyle of right femur
S72.422 Displaced fracture of lateral condyle of left femur
S72.423 Displaced fracture of lateral condyle of unspecified femur
S72.424 Nondisplaced fracture of lateral condyle of right femur
S72.425 Nondisplaced fracture of lateral condyle of left femur
S72.426 Nondisplaced fracture of lateral condyle of unspecified femur

S72.43 Fracture of medial condyle of femur
S72.431 Displaced fracture of medial condyle of right femur
S72.432 Displaced fracture of medial condyle of left femur
S72.433 Displaced fracture of medial condyle of unspecified femur
S72.434 Nondisplaced fracture of medial condyle of right femur
S72.435 Nondisplaced fracture of medial condyle of left femur
S72.436 Nondisplaced fracture of medial condyle of unspecified femur

S72.44 Fracture of lower epiphysis (separation) of femur
EXCLUDES1 Salter-Harris Type I physeal fracture of lower end of femur (S79.11-)
S72.441 Displaced fracture of lower epiphysis (separation) of right femur
S72.442 Displaced fracture of lower epiphysis (separation) of left femur
S72.443 Displaced fracture of lower epiphysis (separation) of unspecified femur
S72.444 Nondisplaced fracture of lower epiphysis (separation) of right femur

---

Unspecified Code Other Specified Code Manifestation Code N Newborn P Pediatric M Maternity A Adult ♂ Male ♀ Female
● New Code ▲ Revised Code Title ▶◀ Revised Text NOTES INCLUDES EXCLUDES 1 Not coded here EXCLUDES 2 Not included here
4th character required 5th character required 6th character required 7th character required
Extension 'X' Alert HAC Hospital-acquired condition (HAC) alert AHA AHA Coding Clinic©

S72.445 **Nondisplaced** fracture of lower epiphysis (separation) of left femur CC POA HAC HCC MCC CC/MCC Exc

S72.446 **Nondisplaced** fracture of lower epiphysis (separation) of unspecified femur CC POA HAC HCC MCC CC/MCC Exc

S72.45 Supracondylar **fracture** without intracondylar **extension** of lower end of femur
Supracondylar fracture of lower end of femur NOS
EXCLUDES1 supracondylar fracture with intracondylar extension of lower end of femur (S72.46-)

S72.451 **Displaced** supracondylar fracture without intracondylar extension of lower end of right femur CC POA HAC HCC MCC CC/MCC Exc

S72.452 **Displaced** supracondylar fracture without intracondylar extension of lower end of left femur CC POA HAC HCC MCC CC/MCC Exc

S72.453 **Displaced** supracondylar fracture without intracondylar extension of lower end of unspecified femur CC POA HAC HCC MCC CC/MCC Exc

S72.454 **Nondisplaced** supracondylar fracture without intracondylar extension of lower end of right femur CC POA HAC HCC MCC CC/MCC Exc

S72.455 **Nondisplaced** supracondylar fracture without intracondylar extension of lower end of left femur CC POA HAC HCC MCC CC/MCC Exc

S72.456 **Nondisplaced** supracondylar fracture without intracondylar extension of lower end of unspecified femur CC POA HAC HCC MCC CC/MCC Exc

S72.46 Supracondylar **fracture** with intracondylar extension of lower end of femur
EXCLUDES1 supracondylar fracture without intracondylar extension of lower end of femur (S72.45-)

S72.461 **Displaced** supracondylar fracture with intracondylar extension of lower end of right femur CC POA HAC HCC MCC CC/MCC Exc

S72.462 **Displaced** supracondylar fracture with intracondylar extension of lower end of left femur CC POA HAC HCC MCC CC/MCC Exc

S72.463 **Displaced** supracondylar fracture with intracondylar extension of lower end of unspecified femur CC POA HAC HCC MCC CC/MCC Exc

S72.464 **Nondisplaced** supracondylar fracture with intracondylar extension of lower end of right femur CC POA HAC HCC MCC CC/MCC Exc

S72.465 **Nondisplaced** supracondylar fracture with intracondylar extension of lower end of left femur CC POA HAC HCC MCC CC/MCC Exc

S72.466 **Nondisplaced** supracondylar fracture with intracondylar extension of lower end of unspecified femur CC POA HAC HCC MCC CC/MCC Exc

S72.47 Torus **fracture** of lower end of femur
The appropriate 7th character is to be added to all codes in subcategory S72.47
A = initial encounter for closed fracture
D = subsequent encounter for fracture with routine healing
G = subsequent encounter for fracture with delayed healing
K = subsequent encounter for fracture with nonunion
P = subsequent encounter for fracture with malunion
S = sequela

S72.471 **Torus** fracture of lower end of right femur CC POA HAC HCC CC/MCC Exc

S72.472 **Torus** fracture of lower end of left femur CC POA HAC HCC CC/MCC Exc

S72.479 **Torus** fracture of lower end of unspecified femur CC POA HAC HCC CC/MCC Exc

S72.49 Other **fracture** of lower end of femur

S72.491 **Other** fracture of lower end of right femur CC POA HAC HCC MCC CC/MCC Exc

S72.492 **Other** fracture of lower end of left femur CC POA HAC HCC MCC CC/MCC Exc

S72.499 **Other** fracture of lower end of unspecified femur CC POA HAC HCC MCC CC/MCC Exc

S72.8 Other fracture of femur

S72.8X Other fracture of femur

S72.8X1 Other fracture of right femur CC POA HAC HCC MCC CC/MCC Exc

S72.8X2 Other fracture of left femur CC POA HAC HCC MCC CC/MCC Exc

S72.8X9 **Other fracture** of unspecified femur CC POA HAC HCC MCC CC/MCC Exc

S72.9 Unspecified fracture of femur
Fracture of thigh NOS
Fracture of upper leg NOS
EXCLUDES1 fracture of hip NOS (S72.00-, S72.01-)

S72.90 **Unspecified** fracture of unspecified femur CC POA HAC HCC MCC CC/MCC Exc

S72.91 **Unspecified** fracture of right femur CC POA HAC HCC MCC CC/MCC Exc

S72.92 **Unspecified** fracture of left femur CC POA HAC HCC MCC CC/MCC Exc

S73 Dislocation and sprain of joint and ligaments of hip

INCLUDES avulsion of joint or ligament of hip
laceration of cartilage, joint or ligament of hip
sprain of cartilage, joint or ligament of hip
traumatic hemarthrosis of joint or ligament of hip
traumatic rupture of joint or ligament of hip
traumatic subluxation of joint or ligament of hip
traumatic tear of joint or ligament of hip

Code also any associated open wound
EXCLUDES2 strain of muscle, fascia and tendon of hip and thigh (S76.-)

The appropriate 7th character is to be added to each code from category S73
A = initial encounter
D = subsequent encounter
S = sequela

S73.0 Subluxation and dislocation of hip
EXCLUDES2 dislocation and subluxation of hip prosthesis (T84.020, T84.021)

S73.00 **Unspecified** subluxation and dislocation of hip
Dislocation of hip NOS
Subluxation of hip NOS

S73.001 **Unspecified** subluxation of right hip CC POA HAC HCC CC/MCC Exc

S73.002 **Unspecified** subluxation of left hip CC POA HAC HCC CC/MCC Exc

S73.003 **Unspecified** subluxation of unspecified hip CC POA HAC HCC CC/MCC Exc

S73.004 **Unspecified** dislocation of right hip CC POA HAC HCC CC/MCC Exc

S73.005 **Unspecified** dislocation of left hip CC POA HAC HCC CC/MCC Exc

S73.006 **Unspecified** dislocation of unspecified hip CC POA HAC HCC CC/MCC Exc

S73.01 **Posterior** subluxation and dislocation of hip

S73.011 **Posterior** subluxation of right hip CC POA HAC HCC CC/MCC Exc

S73.012 **Posterior** subluxation of left hip CC POA HAC HCC CC/MCC Exc

S73.013 **Posterior** subluxation of unspecified hip CC POA HAC HCC CC/MCC Exc

S73.014 **Posterior** dislocation of right hip CC POA HAC HCC CC/MCC Exc

S73.015 **Posterior** dislocation of left hip CC POA HAC HCC CC/MCC Exc

S73.016 **Posterior** dislocation of unspecified hip CC POA HAC HCC CC/MCC Exc

---

POA Unacceptable principal diagnosis symbol per Medicare code edits   POA Code exempt from diagnosis present on admission requirement
? Questionable admission   CC Complication or comorbidity   CC/MCC Exc CC/MCC exclusion   MCC Major complication or comorbidity
CC Principal diagnosis as its own CC   MCC Principal diagnosis as its own MCC   HCC HCC diagnosis code   RxHCC RxHCC diagnosis code
MACRA code   Z1 Z code as first-listed diagnosis

S73.02 Obturator subluxation and dislocation of hip

S73.021 Obturator subluxation of right hip ◌⁷ POA HAC HCC CC/MCC Exc

S73.022 Obturator subluxation of left hip CC POA HAC HCC CC/MCC Exc

S73.023 Obturator subluxation of unspecified hip CC POA HAC HCC CC/MCC Exc

S73.024 Obturator dislocation of right hip ◌⁷ POA HAC HCC CC/MCC Exc

S73.025 Obturator dislocation of left hip CC POA HAC HCC CC/MCC Exc

S73.026 Obturator dislocation of unspecified hip CC POA HAC HCC CC/MCC Exc

▲ S73.03 Other anterior ▶subluxation and◀ dislocation of hip

S73.031 Other anterior subluxation of right hip CC POA HAC HCC CC/MCC Exc

S73.032 Other anterior subluxation of left hip CC POA HAC HCC CC/MCC Exc

S73.033 Other anterior subluxation of unspecified hip CC POA HAC HCC CC/MCC Exc

S73.034 Other anterior dislocation of right hip CC POA HAC HCC CC/MCC Exc

S73.035 Other anterior dislocation of left hip CC POA HAC HCC CC/MCC Exc

S73.036 Other anterior dislocation of unspecified hip CC POA HAC HCC CC/MCC Exc

▲ S73.04 Central ▶subluxation and◀ dislocation of hip

S73.041 Central subluxation of right hip CC POA HAC HCC CC/MCC Exc

S73.042 Central subluxation of left hip CC POA HAC HCC CC/MCC Exc

S73.043 Central subluxation of unspecified hip CC POA HAC HCC CC/MCC Exc

S73.044 Central dislocation of right hip CC POA HAC HCC CC/MCC Exc

S73.045 Central dislocation of left hip CC POA HAC HCC CC/MCC Exc

S73.046 Central dislocation of unspecified hip CC POA HAC HCC CC/MCC Exc

S73.1 Sprain of hip

S73.10 Unspecified sprain of hip

S73.101 Unspecified sprain of right hip POA

S73.102 Unspecified sprain of left hip POA

S73.109 Unspecified sprain of unspecified hip POA

S73.11 Iliofemoral ligament sprain of hip

S73.111 Iliofemoral ligament sprain of right hip POA

S73.112 Iliofemoral ligament sprain of left hip POA

S73.119 Iliofemoral ligament sprain of unspecified hip POA

S73.12 Ischiocapsular (ligament) sprain of hip

S73.121 Ischiocapsular ligament sprain of right hip POA

S73.122 Ischiocapsular ligament sprain of left hip POA

S73.129 Ischiocapsular ligament sprain of unspecified hip POA

S73.19 Other sprain of hip

S73.191 Other sprain of right hip POA

S73.192 Other sprain of left hip POA

S73.199 Other sprain of unspecified hip POA

S74 Injury of nerves at hip and thigh level

Code also any associated open wound (S71.-)

EXCLUDES2 injury of nerves at ankle and foot level (S94.-)

injury of nerves at lower leg level (S84.-)

The appropriate 7th character is to be added to each code from category S74

A = initial encounter

D = subsequent encounter

S = sequela

S74.0 Injury of sciatic nerve at hip and thigh level

S74.00 Injury of sciatic nerve at hip and thigh level, unspecified leg POA

S74.01 Injury of sciatic nerve at hip and thigh level, right leg POA

S74.02 Injury of sciatic nerve at hip and thigh level, left leg POA

S74.1 Injury of femoral nerve at hip and thigh level

S74.10 Injury of femoral nerve at hip and thigh level, unspecified leg POA

S74.11 Injury of femoral nerve at hip and thigh level, right leg POA

S74.12 Injury of femoral nerve at hip and thigh level, left leg POA

S74.2 Injury of cutaneous sensory nerve at hip and thigh level

S74.20 Injury of cutaneous sensory nerve at hip and thigh level, unspecified leg POA

S74.21 Injury of cutaneous sensory nerve at hip and high level, right leg POA

S74.22 Injury of cutaneous sensory nerve at hip and thigh level, left leg POA

S74.8 Injury of other nerves at hip and thigh level

S74.8X Injury of other nerves at hip and thigh level

S74.8X1 Injury of other nerves at hip and thigh level, right leg POA

S74.8X2 Injury of other nerves at hip and thigh level, left leg POA

S74.8X9 Injury of other nerves at hip and thigh level, unspecified leg POA

S74.9 Injury of unspecified nerve at hip and thigh level

S74.90 Injury of unspecified nerve at hip and thigh level, unspecified leg POA

S74.91 Injury of unspecified nerve at hip and thigh level, right leg POA

S74.92 Injury of unspecified nerve at hip and thigh level, left leg POA

S75 Injury of blood vessels at hip and thigh level

Code also any associated open wound (S71.-)

EXCLUDES2 injury of blood vessels at lower leg level (S85.-)

injury of popliteal artery (S85.0)

The appropriate 7th character is to be added to each code from category S75

A = initial encounter

D = subsequent encounter

S = sequela

S75.0 Injury of femoral artery

S75.00 Unspecified injury of femoral artery

S75.001 Unspecified injury of femoral artery, right leg POA MCC CC/MCC Exc

S75.002 Unspecified injury of femoral artery, left leg POA MCC CC/MCC Exc

S75.009 Unspecified injury of femoral artery, unspecified leg POA MCC CC/MCC Exc

S75.01 Minor laceration of femoral artery

Incomplete transection of femoral artery

Laceration of femoral artery NOS

Superficial laceration of femoral artery

S75.011 Minor laceration of femoral artery, right leg POA MCC CC/MCC Exc

S75.012 Minor laceration of femoral artery, left leg POA MCC CC/MCC Exc

S75.019 Minor laceration of femoral artery, unspecified leg POA MCC CC/MCC Exc

S75.02 Major laceration of femoral artery

Complete transection of femoral artery

Traumatic rupture of femoral artery

S75.021 Major laceration of femoral artery, right leg POA MCC CC/MCC Exc

S75.022 Major laceration of femoral artery, left leg POA MCC CC/MCC Exc

S75.029 Major laceration of femoral artery, unspecified leg POA MCC CC/MCC Exc

---

Unspecified Code Other Specified Code Manifestation Code Ⓝ Newborn Ⓟ Pediatric Ⓜ Maternity Ⓐ Adult ♂ Male ♀ Female
● New Code ▲ Revised Code Title ▶◀ Revised Text NOTES INCLUDES EXCLUDES 1 Not coded here EXCLUDES 2 Not included here
4th character required 5th character required 6th character required 7th character required
Extension 'X' Alert HAC Hospital-acquired condition (HAC) alert AHA AHA Coding Clinic©

7ᵗʰ S82.002 **Unspecified** fracture of left patella ⌐ᵖᴼᴬ HAC CC/MCC Exc

7ᵗʰ S82.009 **Unspecified** fracture of unspecified patella ⌐ᵖᴼᴬ HAC CC/MCC Exc

6ᵗʰ S82.01 **Osteochondral** fracture of patella

7ᵗʰ S82.011 **Displaced** osteochondral fracture of right patella ⌐ᵖᴼᴬ HAC CC/MCC Exc

7ᵗʰ S82.012 **Displaced** osteochondral fracture of left patella ⌐ᵖᴼᴬ HAC CC/MCC Exc

7ᵗʰ S82.013 **Displaced** osteochondral fracture of unspecified patella ⌐ᵖᴼᴬ HAC CC/MCC Exc

7ᵗʰ S82.014 **Nondisplaced** osteochondral fracture of right patella ⌐ᵖᴼᴬ HAC CC/MCC Exc

7ᵗʰ S82.015 **Nondisplaced** osteochondral fracture of left patella ⌐ᵖᴼᴬ HAC CC/MCC Exc

7ᵗʰ S82.016 **Nondisplaced** osteochondral fracture of unspecified patella ⌐ᵖᴼᴬ HAC CC/MCC Exc

6ᵗʰ S82.02 **Longitudinal** fracture of patella

7ᵗʰ S82.021 **Displaced** longitudinal fracture of right patella ⌐ᵖᴼᴬ HAC CC/MCC Exc

7ᵗʰ S82.022 **Displaced** longitudinal fracture of left patella ⌐ᵖᴼᴬ HAC CC/MCC Exc

7ᵗʰ S82.023 **Displaced** longitudinal fracture of unspecified patella ⌐ᵖᴼᴬ HAC CC/MCC Exc

7ᵗʰ S82.024 **Nondisplaced** longitudinal fracture of right patella ⌐ᵖᴼᴬ HAC CC/MCC Exc

7ᵗʰ S82.025 **Nondisplaced** longitudinal fracture of left patella ⌐ᵖᴼᴬ HAC CC/MCC Exc

7ᵗʰ S82.026 **Nondisplaced** longitudinal fracture of unspecified patella ⌐ᵖᴼᴬ HAC CC/MCC Exc

6ᵗʰ S82.03 **Transverse** fracture of patella

7ᵗʰ S82.031 **Displaced** transverse fracture of right patella ⌐ᵖᴼᴬ HAC CC/MCC Exc

7ᵗʰ S82.032 **Displaced** transverse fracture of left patella ⌐ᵖᴼᴬ HAC CC/MCC Exc

7ᵗʰ S82.033 **Displaced** transverse fracture of unspecified patella ⌐ᵖᴼᴬ HAC CC/MCC Exc

7ᵗʰ S82.034 **Nondisplaced** transverse fracture of right patella ⌐ᵖᴼᴬ HAC CC/MCC Exc

7ᵗʰ S82.035 **Nondisplaced** transverse fracture of left patella ⌐ᵖᴼᴬ HAC CC/MCC Exc

7ᵗʰ S82.036 **Nondisplaced** transverse fracture of unspecified patella ⌐ᵖᴼᴬ HAC CC/MCC Exc

6ᵗʰ S82.04 **Comminuted** fracture of patella

7ᵗʰ S82.041 **Displaced** comminuted fracture of right patella ⌐ᵖᴼᴬ HAC CC/MCC Exc

7ᵗʰ S82.042 **Displaced** comminuted fracture of left patella ⌐ᵖᴼᴬ HAC CC/MCC Exc

7ᵗʰ S82.043 **Displaced** comminuted fracture of unspecified patella ⌐ᵖᴼᴬ HAC CC/MCC Exc

7ᵗʰ S82.044 **Nondisplaced** comminuted fracture of right patella ⌐ᵖᴼᴬ HAC CC/MCC Exc

7ᵗʰ S82.045 **Nondisplaced** comminuted fracture of left patella ⌐ᵖᴼᴬ HAC CC/MCC Exc

7ᵗʰ S82.046 **Nondisplaced** comminuted fracture of unspecified patella ⌐ᵖᴼᴬ HAC CC/MCC Exc

6ᵗʰ S82.09 **Other** fracture of patella

7ᵗʰ S82.091 **Other** fracture of right patella ⌐ᵖᴼᴬ HAC CC/MCC Exc

7ᵗʰ S82.092 **Other** fracture of left patella ⌐ᵖᴼᴬ HAC CC/MCC Exc

7ᵗʰ S82.099 **Other** fracture of unspecified patella ⌐ᵖᴼᴬ HAC CC/MCC Exc

5ᵗʰ S82.1 **Fracture of** upper end of tibia

Fracture of proximal end of tibia

EXCLUDES2 fracture of shaft of tibia (S82.2-)

physeal fracture of upper end of tibia (S89.0-)

5ᵗʰ S82.10 **Unspecified** fracture of upper end of tibia

7ᵗʰ S82.101 **Unspecified** fracture of upper end of right tibia ⌐ᵖᴼᴬ HAC MCC CC/MCC Exc

7ᵗʰ S82.102 **Unspecified** fracture of upper end of left tibia ⌐ᵖᴼᴬ HAC MCC CC/MCC Exc

7ᵗʰ S82.109 **Unspecified** fracture of upper end of unspecified tibia ⌐ᵖᴼᴬ HAC MCC CC/MCC Exc

6ᵗʰ S82.11 **Fracture of** tibial spine

7ᵗʰ S82.111 **Displaced** fracture of right tibial spine ⌐ᵖᴼᴬ HAC CC/MCC Exc

7ᵗʰ S82.112 **Displaced** fracture of left tibial spine ⌐ᵖᴼᴬ HAC CC/MCC Exc

7ᵗʰ S82.113 **Displaced** fracture of unspecified tibial spine ⌐ᵖᴼᴬ HAC CC/MCC Exc

7ᵗʰ S82.114 **Nondisplaced** fracture of right tibial spine ⌐ᵖᴼᴬ HAC MCC CC/MCC Exc

7ᵗʰ S82.115 **Nondisplaced** fracture of left tibial spine ⌐ᵖᴼᴬ HAC CC/MCC Exc

7ᵗʰ S82.116 **Nondisplaced** fracture of unspecified tibial spine ⌐ᵖᴼᴬ HAC CC/MCC Exc

6ᵗʰ S82.12 **Fracture of** lateral condyle of tibia

7ᵗʰ S82.121 **Displaced** fracture of lateral condyle of right tibia ⌐ᵖᴼᴬ HAC CC/MCC Exc

7ᵗʰ S82.122 **Displaced** fracture of lateral condyle of left tibia ⌐ᵖᴼᴬ HAC MCC CC/MCC Exc

7ᵗʰ S82.123 **Displaced** fracture of lateral condyle of unspecified tibia ⌐ᵖᴼᴬ HAC CC/MCC Exc

7ᵗʰ S82.124 **Nondisplaced** fracture of lateral condyle of right tibia ⌐ᵖᴼᴬ HAC CC/MCC Exc

7ᵗʰ S82.125 **Nondisplaced** fracture of lateral condyle of left tibia ⌐ᵖᴼᴬ HAC MCC CC/MCC Exc

7ᵗʰ S82.126 **Nondisplaced** fracture of lateral condyle of unspecified tibia ⌐ᵖᴼᴬ HAC MCC CC/MCC Exc

6ᵗʰ S82.13 **Fracture of** medial condyle of tibia

7ᵗʰ S82.131 **Displaced** fracture of medial condyle of right tibia ⌐ᵖᴼᴬ HAC CC/MCC Exc

7ᵗʰ S82.132 **Displaced** fracture of medial condyle of left tibia ⌐ᵖᴼᴬ HAC MCC CC/MCC Exc

7ᵗʰ S82.133 **Displaced** fracture of medial condyle of unspecified tibia ⌐ᵖᴼᴬ HAC MCC CC/MCC Exc

7ᵗʰ S82.134 **Nondisplaced** fracture of medial condyle of right tibia ⌐ᵖᴼᴬ HAC CC/MCC Exc

7ᵗʰ S82.135 **Nondisplaced** fracture of medial condyle of left tibia ⌐ᵖᴼᴬ HAC CC/MCC Exc

7ᵗʰ S82.136 **Nondisplaced** fracture of medial condyle of unspecified tibia ⌐ᵖᴼᴬ HAC MCC CC/MCC Exc

6ᵗʰ S82.14 **Bicondylar** fracture of tibia

Fracture of tibial plateau NOS

7ᵗʰ S82.141 **Displaced** bicondylar fracture of right tibia ⌐ᵖᴼᴬ HAC MCC CC/MCC Exc

7ᵗʰ S82.142 **Displaced** bicondylar fracture of left tibia ⌐ᵖᴼᴬ HAC MCC CC/MCC Exc

7ᵗʰ S82.143 **Displaced** bicondylar fracture of unspecified tibia ⌐ᵖᴼᴬ HAC MCC CC/MCC Exc

7ᵗʰ S82.144 **Nondisplaced** bicondylar fracture of right tibia ⌐ᵖᴼᴬ HAC MCC CC/MCC Exc

7ᵗʰ S82.145 **Nondisplaced** bicondylar fracture of left tibia ⌐ᵖᴼᴬ HAC MCC CC/MCC Exc

7ᵗʰ S82.146 **Nondisplaced** bicondylar fracture of unspecified tibia ⌐ᵖᴼᴬ HAC MCC CC/MCC Exc

6ᵗʰ S82.15 **Fracture of** tibial tuberosity

7ᵗʰ S82.151 **Displaced** fracture of right tibial tuberosity ⌐ᵖᴼᴬ HAC MCC CC/MCC Exc

7ᵗʰ S82.152 **Displaced** fracture of left tibial tuberosity ⌐ᵖᴼᴬ HAC MCC CC/MCC Exc

7ᵗʰ S82.153 **Displaced** fracture of unspecified tibial tuberosity ⌐ᵖᴼᴬ HAC MCC CC/MCC Exc

7ᵗʰ S82.154 **Nondisplaced** fracture of right tibial tuberosity ⌐ᵖᴼᴬ HAC MCC CC/MCC Exc

7ᵗʰ S82.155 **Nondisplaced** fracture of left tibial tuberosity ⌐ᵖᴼᴬ HAC MCC CC/MCC Exc

7ᵗʰ S82.156 **Nondisplaced** fracture of unspecified tibial tuberosity ⌐ᵖᴼᴬ HAC MCC CC/MCC Exc

6ᵗʰ S82.16 **Torus** fracture of upper end of tibia

The appropriate 7th character is to be added to all codes in subcategory S82.16

A = initial encounter for closed fracture

ᵖᴼᴬ Unacceptable principal diagnosis symbol per Medicare code edits   Code exempt from diagnosis present on admission requirement

❓ Questionable admission   ⌐ Complication or comorbidity   CC/MCC Exc CC/MCC exclusion   MCC Major complication or comorbidity

Principal diagnosis as its own CC   Principal diagnosis as its own MCC   HCC HCC diagnosis code   RxHCC RxHCC diagnosis code

MACRA code   Z1 Z code as first-listed diagnosis

1078   When symbols appear on a code that requires a 7th character extension, refer to Appendix B to identify applicable 7th character codes.   **2018 ICD-10-CM**

D = subsequent encounter for fracture with routine healing
G = subsequent encounter for fracture with delayed healing
K = subsequent encounter for fracture with nonunion
P = subsequent encounter for fracture with malunion
S = sequela

[7th] S82.161 Torus fracture of upper end of right tibia [CC] [POA] [HAC] [CC/MCC Exc]
[7th] S82.162 Torus fracture of upper end of left tibia [CC] [POA] [HAC] [CC/MCC Exc]
[7th] S82.169 Torus fracture of upper end of unspecified tibia [CC] [POA] [HAC] [CC/MCC Exc]

[6th] S82.19 Other fracture of upper end of tibia
[7th] S82.191 Other fracture of upper end of right tibia [CC] [POA] [HAC] [MCC] [CC/MCC Exc]
[7th] S82.192 Other fracture of upper end of left tibia [CC] [POA] [HAC] [MCC] [CC/MCC Exc]
[7th] S82.199 Other fracture of upper end of unspecified tibia [CC] [POA] [HAC] [MCC] [CC/MCC Exc]

[5th] S82.2 Fracture of shaft of tibia

[6th] S82.20 Unspecified fracture of shaft of tibia
Fracture of tibia NOS
[7th] S82.201 Unspecified fracture of shaft of right tibia [CC] [POA] [HAC] [MCC] [CC/MCC Exc]
[7th] S82.202 Unspecified fracture of shaft of left tibia [CC] [POA] [HAC] [MCC] [CC/MCC Exc]
[7th] S82.209 Unspecified fracture of shaft of unspecified tibia [CC] [POA] [HAC] [MCC] [CC/MCC Exc]

[6th] S82.22 Transverse fracture of shaft of tibia
[7th] S82.221 Displaced transverse fracture of shaft of right tibia [CC] [POA] [HAC] [MCC] [CC/MCC Exc]
[7th] S82.222 Displaced transverse fracture of shaft of left tibia [CC] [POA] [HAC] [MCC] [CC/MCC Exc]
[7th] S82.223 Displaced transverse fracture of shaft of unspecified tibia [CC] [POA] [HAC] [MCC] [CC/MCC Exc]
[7th] S82.224 Nondisplaced transverse fracture of shaft of right tibia [CC] [POA] [HAC] [MCC] [CC/MCC Exc]
[7th] S82.225 Nondisplaced transverse fracture of shaft of left tibia [CC] [POA] [HAC] [MCC] [CC/MCC Exc]
[7th] S82.226 Nondisplaced transverse fracture of shaft of unspecified tibia [CC] [POA] [HAC] [MCC] [CC/MCC Exc]

[6th] S82.23 Oblique fracture of shaft of tibia
[7th] S82.231 Displaced oblique fracture of shaft of right tibia [CC] [POA] [HAC] [MCC] [CC/MCC Exc]
[7th] S82.232 Displaced oblique fracture of shaft of left tibia [CC] [POA] [HAC] [MCC] [CC/MCC Exc]
[7th] S82.233 Displaced oblique fracture of shaft of unspecified tibia [CC] [POA] [HAC] [MCC] [CC/MCC Exc]
[7th] S82.234 Nondisplaced oblique fracture of shaft of right tibia [CC] [POA] [HAC] [MCC] [CC/MCC Exc]
[7th] S82.235 Nondisplaced oblique fracture of shaft of left tibia [CC] [POA] [HAC] [MCC] [CC/MCC Exc]
[7th] S82.236 Nondisplaced oblique fracture of shaft of unspecified tibia [CC] [POA] [HAC] [MCC] [CC/MCC Exc]

[6th] S82.24 Spiral fracture of shaft of tibia
Toddler fracture
[7th] S82.241 Displaced spiral fracture of shaft of right tibia [CC] [POA] [HAC] [MCC] [CC/MCC Exc]
[7th] S82.242 Displaced spiral fracture of shaft of left tibia [CC] [POA] [HAC] [MCC] [CC/MCC Exc]
[7th] S82.243 Displaced spiral fracture of shaft of unspecified tibia [CC] [POA] [HAC] [MCC] [CC/MCC Exc]
[7th] S82.244 Nondisplaced spiral fracture of shaft of right tibia [CC] [POA] [HAC] [MCC] [CC/MCC Exc]
[7th] S82.245 Nondisplaced spiral fracture of shaft of left tibia [CC] [POA] [HAC] [MCC] [CC/MCC Exc]
[7th] S82.246 Nondisplaced spiral fracture of shaft of unspecified tibia [CC] [POA] [HAC] [MCC] [CC/MCC Exc]

[6th] S82.25 Comminuted fracture of shaft of tibia
[7th] S82.251 Displaced comminuted fracture of shaft of right tibia [CC] [POA] [HAC] [MCC] [CC/MCC Exc]
[7th] S82.252 Displaced comminuted fracture of shaft of left tibia [CC] [POA] [HAC] [MCC] [CC/MCC Exc]
[7th] S82.253 Displaced comminuted fracture of shaft of unspecified tibia [CC] [POA] [HAC] [MCC] [CC/MCC Exc]
[7th] S82.254 Nondisplaced comminuted fracture of shaft of right tibia [CC] [POA] [HAC] [MCC] [CC/MCC Exc]
[7th] S82.255 Nondisplaced comminuted fracture of shaft of left tibia [CC] [POA] [HAC] [MCC] [CC/MCC Exc]
[7th] S82.256 Nondisplaced comminuted fracture of shaft of unspecified tibia [CC] [POA] [HAC] [MCC] [CC/MCC Exc]

[6th] S82.26 Segmental fracture of shaft of tibia
[7th] S82.261 Displaced segmental fracture of shaft of right tibia [CC] [POA] [HAC] [MCC] [CC/MCC Exc]
[7th] S82.262 Displaced segmental fracture of shaft of left tibia [CC] [POA] [HAC] [MCC] [CC/MCC Exc]
[7th] S82.263 Displaced segmental fracture of shaft of unspecified tibia [CC] [POA] [HAC] [MCC] [CC/MCC Exc]
[7th] S82.264 Nondisplaced segmental fracture of shaft of right tibia [CC] [POA] [HAC] [MCC] [CC/MCC Exc]
[7th] S82.265 Nondisplaced segmental fracture of shaft of left tibia [CC] [POA] [HAC] [MCC] [CC/MCC Exc]
[7th] S82.266 Nondisplaced segmental fracture of shaft of unspecified tibia [CC] [POA] [HAC] [MCC] [CC/MCC Exc]

[6th] S82.29 Other fracture of shaft of tibia
[7th] S82.291 Other fracture of shaft of right tibia [CC] [POA] [HAC] [MCC] [CC/MCC Exc]
[7th] S82.292 Other fracture of shaft of left tibia [CC] [POA] [HAC] [MCC] [CC/MCC Exc]
[7th] S82.299 Other fracture of shaft of unspecified tibia [CC] [POA] [HAC] [MCC] [CC/MCC Exc]

[5th] S82.3 Fracture of lower end of tibia
[EXCLUDES1] *bimalleolar fracture of lower leg (S82.84-)*
fracture of medial malleolus alone (S82.5-)
Maisonneuve's fracture (S82.86-)
pilon fracture of distal tibia (S82.87-)
trimalleolar fractures of lower leg (S82.85-)

[6th] S82.30 Unspecified fracture of lower end of tibia
[7th] S82.301 Unspecified fracture of lower end of right tibia [CC] [POA] [HAC] [CC/MCC Exc]
[7th] S82.302 Unspecified fracture of lower end of left tibia [CC] [POA] [HAC] [CC/MCC Exc]
[7th] S82.309 Unspecified fracture of lower end of unspecified tibia [CC] [POA] [HAC] [CC/MCC Exc]

[6th] S82.31 Torus fracture of lower end of tibia
The appropriate 7th character is to be added to all codes in subcategory S82.31
A = initial encounter for closed fracture
D = subsequent encounter for fracture with routine healing
G = subsequent encounter for fracture with delayed healing
K = subsequent encounter for fracture with nonunion
P = subsequent encounter for fracture with malunion
S = sequela
[7th] S82.311 Torus fracture of lower end of right tibia [CC] [POA] [HAC] [CC/MCC Exc]
[7th] S82.312 Torus fracture of lower end of left tibia [CC] [POA] [HAC] [CC/MCC Exc]
[7th] S82.319 Torus fracture of lower end of unspecified tibia [CC] [POA] [HAC] [CC/MCC Exc]

[6th] S82.39 Other fracture of lower end of tibia
[7th] S82.391 Other fracture of lower end of right tibia [CC] [POA] [HAC] [CC/MCC Exc]
[7th] S82.392 Other fracture of lower end of left tibia [CC] [POA] [HAC] [CC/MCC Exc]
[7th] S82.399 Other fracture of lower end of unspecified tibia [CC] [POA] [HAC] [CC/MCC Exc]

[5th] S82.4 Fracture of shaft of fibula
EXCLUDES2 *fracture of lateral malleolus alone (S82.6-)*

[6th] S82.40 Unspecified fracture of shaft of fibula
[7th] S82.401 Unspecified fracture of shaft of right fibula [CC] [POA] [HAC] [MCC] [CC/MCC Exc]
[7th] S82.402 Unspecified fracture of shaft of left fibula [CC] [POA] [HAC] [MCC] [CC/MCC Exc]
[7th] S82.409 Unspecified fracture of shaft of unspecified fibula [CC] [POA] [HAC] [MCC] [CC/MCC Exc]

[6th] S82.42 Transverse fracture of shaft of fibula
[7th] S82.421 Displaced transverse fracture of shaft of right fibula [CC] [POA] [HAC] [MCC] [CC/MCC Exc]
[7th] S82.422 Displaced transverse fracture of shaft of left fibula [CC] [POA] [HAC] [MCC] [CC/MCC Exc]
[7th] S82.423 Displaced transverse fracture of shaft of unspecified fibula [CC] [POA] [HAC] [MCC] [CC/MCC Exc]
[7th] S82.424 Nondisplaced transverse fracture of shaft of right fibula [CC] [POA] [HAC] [MCC] [CC/MCC Exc]
[7th] S82.425 Nondisplaced transverse fracture of shaft of left fibula [CC] [POA] [HAC] [MCC] [CC/MCC Exc]
[7th] S82.426 Nondisplaced transverse fracture of shaft of unspecified fibula [CC] [POA] [HAC] [MCC] [CC/MCC Exc]

[6th] S82.43 Oblique fracture of shaft of fibula
[7th] S82.431 Displaced oblique fracture of shaft of right fibula [CC] [POA] [HAC] [MCC] [CC/MCC Exc]
[7th] S82.432 Displaced oblique fracture of shaft of left fibula [CC] [POA] [HAC] [MCC] [CC/MCC Exc]
[7th] S82.433 Displaced oblique fracture of shaft of unspecified fibula [CC] [POA] [HAC] [MCC] [CC/MCC Exc]
[7th] S82.434 Nondisplaced oblique fracture of shaft of right fibula [CC] [POA] [HAC] [MCC] [CC/MCC Exc]
[7th] S82.435 Nondisplaced oblique fracture of shaft of left fibula [CC] [POA] [HAC] [MCC] [CC/MCC Exc]
[7th] S82.436 Nondisplaced oblique fracture of shaft of unspecified fibula [CC] [POA] [HAC] [MCC] [CC/MCC Exc]

[6th] S82.44 Spiral fracture of shaft of fibula
[7th] S82.441 Displaced spiral fracture of shaft of right fibula [CC] [POA] [HAC] [MCC] [CC/MCC Exc]
[7th] S82.442 Displaced spiral fracture of shaft of left fibula [CC] [POA] [HAC] [MCC] [CC/MCC Exc]
[7th] S82.443 Displaced spiral fracture of shaft of unspecified fibula [CC] [POA] [HAC] [MCC] [CC/MCC Exc]
[7th] S82.444 Nondisplaced spiral fracture of shaft of right fibula [CC] [POA] [HAC] [MCC] [CC/MCC Exc]
[7th] S82.445 Nondisplaced spiral fracture of shaft of left fibula [CC] [POA] [HAC] [MCC] [CC/MCC Exc]
[7th] S82.446 Nondisplaced spiral fracture of shaft of unspecified fibula [CC] [POA] [HAC] [MCC] [CC/MCC Exc]

[6th] S82.45 Comminuted fracture of shaft of fibula
[7th] S82.451 Displaced comminuted fracture of shaft of right fibula [CC] [POA] [HAC] [MCC] [CC/MCC Exc]
[7th] S82.452 Displaced comminuted fracture of shaft of left fibula [CC] [POA] [HAC] [MCC] [CC/MCC Exc]
[7th] S82.453 Displaced comminuted fracture of shaft of unspecified fibula [CC] [POA] [HAC] [MCC] [CC/MCC Exc]
[7th] S82.454 Nondisplaced comminuted fracture of shaft of right fibula [CC] [POA] [HAC] [MCC] [CC/MCC Exc]
[7th] S82.455 Nondisplaced comminuted fracture of shaft of left fibula [CC] [POA] [HAC] [MCC] [CC/MCC Exc]
[7th] S82.456 Nondisplaced comminuted fracture of shaft of unspecified fibula [CC] [POA] [HAC] [MCC] [CC/MCC Exc]

[6th] S82.46 Segmental fracture of shaft of fibula
[7th] S82.461 Displaced segmental fracture of shaft of right fibula [CC] [POA] [HAC] [MCC] [CC/MCC Exc]
[7th] S82.462 Displaced segmental fracture of shaft of left fibula [CC] [POA] [HAC] [MCC] [CC/MCC Exc]
[7th] S82.463 Displaced segmental fracture of shaft of unspecified fibula [CC] [POA] [HAC] [MCC] [CC/MCC Exc]
[7th] S82.464 Nondisplaced segmental fracture of shaft of right fibula [CC] [POA] [HAC] [MCC] [CC/MCC Exc]
[7th] S82.465 Nondisplaced segmental fracture of shaft of left fibula [CC] [POA] [HAC] [MCC] [CC/MCC Exc]
[7th] S82.466 Nondisplaced segmental fracture of shaft of unspecified fibula [CC] [POA] [HAC] [MCC] [CC/MCC Exc]

[6th] S82.49 Other fracture of shaft of fibula
[7th] S82.491 Other fracture of shaft of right fibula [CC] [POA] [HAC] [MCC] [CC/MCC Exc]
[7th] S82.492 Other fracture of shaft of left fibula [CC] [POA] [HAC] [MCC] [CC/MCC Exc]
[7th] S82.499 Other fracture of shaft of unspecified fibula [CC] [POA] [HAC] [MCC] [CC/MCC Exc]

[5th] S82.5 Fracture of medial malleolus
EXCLUDES1 *pilon fracture of distal tibia (S82.87-)*
Salter-Harris type III of lower end of tibia (S89.13-)
Salter-Harris type IV of lower end of tibia (S89.14-)

[7th] S82.51 Displaced fracture of medial malleolus of right tibia [CC] [POA] [HAC] [CC/MCC Exc]
[7th] S82.52 Displaced fracture of medial malleolus of left tibia [CC] [POA] [HAC] [CC/MCC Exc]
[7th] S82.53 Displaced fracture of medial malleolus of unspecified tibia [CC] [POA] [HAC] [CC/MCC Exc]
[7th] S82.54 Nondisplaced fracture of medial malleolus of right tibia [CC] [POA] [HAC] [CC/MCC Exc]
[7th] S82.55 Nondisplaced fracture of medial malleolus of left tibia [CC] [POA] [HAC] [CC/MCC Exc]
[7th] S82.56 Nondisplaced fracture of medial malleolus of unspecified tibia [CC] [POA] [HAC] [CC/MCC Exc]

[5th] S82.6 Fracture of lateral malleolus
EXCLUDES1 *pilon fracture of distal tibia (S82.87-)*

[7th] S82.61 Displaced fracture of lateral malleolus of right fibula [CC] [POA] [HAC] [CC/MCC Exc]
[7th] S82.62 Displaced fracture of lateral malleolus of left fibula [CC] [POA] [HAC] [CC/MCC Exc]
[7th] S82.63 Displaced fracture of lateral malleolus of unspecified fibula [CC] [POA] [HAC] [CC/MCC Exc]
[7th] S82.64 Nondisplaced fracture of lateral malleolus of right fibula [CC] [POA] [HAC] [CC/MCC Exc]
[7th] S82.65 Nondisplaced fracture of lateral malleolus of left fibula [CC] [POA] [HAC] [CC/MCC Exc]
[7th] S82.66 Nondisplaced fracture of lateral malleolus of unspecified fibula [CC] [POA] [HAC] [CC/MCC Exc]

[5th] S82.8 Other fractures of lower leg

[6th] S82.81 Torus fracture of upper end of fibula
The appropriate 7th character is to be added to all codes in subcategory S82.81
A = initial encounter for closed fracture
D = subsequent encounter for fracture with routine healing
G = subsequent encounter for fracture with delayed healing
K = subsequent encounter for fracture with nonunion
P = subsequent encounter for fracture with malunion
S = sequela

[7th] S82.811 Torus fracture of upper end of right fibula [CC] [POA] [CC/MCC Exc]
[7th] S82.812 Torus fracture of upper end of left fibula [CC] [POA] [CC/MCC Exc]
[7th] S82.819 Torus fracture of upper end of unspecified fibula [CC] [POA] [CC/MCC Exc]

[6th] S82.82 Torus fracture of lower end of fibula
The appropriate 7th character is to be added to all codes in subcategory S82.82
A = initial encounter for closed fracture
D = subsequent encounter for fracture with routine healing
G = subsequent encounter for fracture with delayed healing
K = subsequent encounter for fracture with nonunion

[PDx] Unacceptable principal diagnosis symbol per Medicare code edits [POA] Code exempt from diagnosis present on admission requirement
[?] Questionable admission [CC] Complication or comorbidity [CC/MCC Exc] CC/MCC exclusion [MCC] Major complication or comorbidity
[PDx CC] Principal diagnosis as its own CC [PDx MCC] Principal diagnosis as its own MCC [HCC] HCC diagnosis code [RxHCC] RxHCC diagnosis code
MACRA code [Z1] Z code as first-listed diagnosis

P = subsequent encounter for fracture with malunion

S = sequela

7ᵗʰ **S82.821** Torus fracture of lower end of right fibula CC⁰ POA CC/MCC Exc

7ᵗʰ **S82.822** Torus fracture of lower end of left fibula CC⁰ POA CC/MCC Exc

7ᵗʰ **S82.829** Torus fracture of lower end of unspecified fibula CC⁰ POA CC/MCC Exc

6ᵗʰ **S82.83** Other fracture of upper and lower end of fibula

7ᵗʰ **S82.831** Other fracture of upper and lower end of right fibula CC⁰ POA HAC MCC⁰ CC/MCC Exc

7ᵗʰ **S82.832** Other fracture of upper and lower end of left fibula CC⁰ POA HAC MCC⁰ CC/MCC Exc

7ᵗʰ **S82.839** Other fracture of upper and lower end of unspecified fibula CC⁰ POA HAC MCC⁰ CC/MCC Exc

6ᵗʰ **S82.84** Bimalleolar fracture of lower leg

7ᵗʰ **S82.841** Displaced bimalleolar fracture of right lower leg CC⁰ POA HAC CC/MCC Exc

7ᵗʰ **S82.842** Displaced bimalleolar fracture of left lower leg CC⁰ POA HAC CC/MCC Exc

7ᵗʰ **S82.843** Displaced bimalleolar fracture of unspecified lower leg CC⁰ POA HAC CC/MCC Exc

7ᵗʰ **S82.844** Nondisplaced bimalleolar fracture of right lower leg CC⁰ POA HAC CC/MCC Exc

7ᵗʰ **S82.845** Nondisplaced bimalleolar fracture of left lower leg CC⁰ POA HAC CC/MCC Exc

7ᵗʰ **S82.846** Nondisplaced bimalleolar fracture of unspecified lower leg CC⁰ POA HAC CC/MCC Exc

6ᵗʰ **S82.85** Trimalleolar fracture of lower leg

7ᵗʰ **S82.851** Displaced trimalleolar fracture of right lower leg CC⁰ POA HAC CC/MCC Exc

7ᵗʰ **S82.852** Displaced trimalleolar fracture of left lower leg CC⁰ POA HAC CC/MCC Exc

7ᵗʰ **S82.853** Displaced trimalleolar fracture of unspecified lower leg CC⁰ POA HAC CC/MCC Exc

7ᵗʰ **S82.854** Nondisplaced trimalleolar fracture of right lower leg CC⁰ POA HAC CC/MCC Exc

7ᵗʰ **S82.855** Nondisplaced trimalleolar fracture of left lower leg CC⁰ POA HAC CC/MCC Exc

7ᵗʰ **S82.856** Nondisplaced trimalleolar fracture of unspecified lower leg CC⁰ POA HAC CC/MCC Exc

6ᵗʰ **S82.86** Maisonneuve's fracture

7ᵗʰ **S82.861** Displaced Maisonneuve's fracture of right leg CC⁰ POA HAC MCC⁰ CC/MCC Exc

7ᵗʰ **S82.862** Displaced Maisonneuve's fracture of left leg CC⁰ POA HAC MCC⁰ CC/MCC Exc

7ᵗʰ **S82.863** Displaced Maisonneuve's fracture of unspecified leg CC⁰ POA HAC MCC⁰ CC/MCC Exc

7ᵗʰ **S82.864** Nondisplaced Maisonneuve's fracture of right leg CC⁰ POA HAC MCC⁰ CC/MCC Exc

7ᵗʰ **S82.865** Nondisplaced Maisonneuve's fracture of left leg CC⁰ POA HAC MCC⁰ CC/MCC Exc

7ᵗʰ **S82.866** Nondisplaced Maisonneuve's fracture of unspecified leg CC⁰ POA HAC MCC⁰ CC/MCC Exc

6ᵗʰ **S82.87** Pilon fracture of tibia

7ᵗʰ **S82.871** Displaced pilon fracture of right tibia CC⁰ POA HAC CC/MCC Exc

7ᵗʰ **S82.872** Displaced pilon fracture of left tibia CC⁰ POA HAC CC/MCC Exc

7ᵗʰ **S82.873** Displaced pilon fracture of unspecified tibia CC⁰ POA HAC CC/MCC Exc

7ᵗʰ **S82.874** Nondisplaced pilon fracture of right tibia CC⁰ POA HAC CC/MCC Exc

7ᵗʰ **S82.875** Nondisplaced pilon fracture of left tibia CC⁰ POA HAC CC/MCC Exc

7ᵗʰ **S82.876** Nondisplaced pilon fracture of unspecified tibia CC⁰ POA HAC CC/MCC Exc

6ᵗʰ **S82.89** Other fractures of lower leg

Fracture of ankle NOS

7ᵗʰ **S82.891** Other fracture of right lower leg CC⁰ POA HAC CC/MCC Exc

7ᵗʰ **S82.892** Other fracture of left lower leg CC⁰ POA HAC CC/MCC Exc

7ᵗʰ **S82.899** Other fracture of unspecified lower leg CC⁰ POA HAC CC/MCC Exc

5ᵗʰ **S82.9** Unspecified fracture of lower leg

7ᵗʰ **S82.90** Unspecified fracture of unspecified lower leg CC⁰ POA HAC CC/MCC Exc

S82.91 Unspecified fracture of right lower leg CC⁰ POA HAC CC/MCC Exc

S82.92 Unspecified fracture of left lower leg CC⁰ POA HAC CC/MCC Exc

4ᵗʰ **S83** Dislocation and sprain of joints and ligaments of knee

INCLUDES avulsion of joint or ligament of knee
laceration of cartilage, joint or ligament of knee
sprain of cartilage, joint or ligament of knee
traumatic hemarthrosis of joint or ligament of knee
traumatic rupture of joint or ligament of knee
traumatic subluxation of joint or ligament of knee
traumatic tear of joint or ligament of knee

Code also any associated open wound

EXCLUDES1 derangement of patella (M22.0-M22.3)
injury of patellar ligament (tendon) (S76.1-)
internal derangement of knee (M23.-)
old dislocation of knee (M24.36)
pathological dislocation of knee (M24.36)
recurrent dislocation of knee (M22.0)

EXCLUDES2 strain of muscle, fascia and tendon of lower leg (S86.-)

The appropriate 7th character is to be added to each code from category S83

A = initial encounter

D = subsequent encounter

S = sequela

5ᵗʰ **S83.0** Subluxation and dislocation of patella

6ᵗʰ **S83.00** Unspecified subluxation and dislocation of patella

7ᵗʰ **S83.001** Unspecified subluxation of right patella POA

7ᵗʰ **S83.002** Unspecified subluxation of left patella POA

7ᵗʰ **S83.003** Unspecified subluxation of unspecified patella POA

7ᵗʰ **S83.004** Unspecified dislocation of right patella POA

7ᵗʰ **S83.005** Unspecified dislocation of left patella POA

7ᵗʰ **S83.006** Unspecified dislocation of unspecified patella POA

6ᵗʰ **S83.01** Lateral subluxation and dislocation of patella

7ᵗʰ **S83.011** Lateral subluxation of right patella POA

7ᵗʰ **S83.012** Lateral subluxation of left patella POA

7ᵗʰ **S83.013** Lateral subluxation of unspecified patella POA

7ᵗʰ **S83.014** Lateral dislocation of right patella POA

7ᵗʰ **S83.015** Lateral dislocation of left patella POA

7ᵗʰ **S83.016** Lateral dislocation of unspecified patella POA

6ᵗʰ **S83.09** Other subluxation and dislocation of patella

7ᵗʰ **S83.091** Other subluxation of right patella POA

7ᵗʰ **S83.092** Other subluxation of left patella POA

7ᵗʰ **S83.093** Other subluxation of unspecified patella POA

7ᵗʰ **S83.094** Other dislocation of right patella POA

7ᵗʰ **S83.095** Other dislocation of left patella POA

7ᵗʰ **S83.096** Other dislocation of unspecified patella POA

5ᵗʰ **S83.1** Subluxation and dislocation of knee

EXCLUDES2 instability of knee prosthesis (T84.022, T84.023)

6ᵗʰ **S83.10** Unspecified subluxation and dislocation of knee

7ᵗʰ **S83.101** Unspecified subluxation of right knee POA

7ᵗʰ **S83.102** Unspecified subluxation of left knee POA

7ᵗʰ **S83.103** Unspecified subluxation of unspecified knee POA

7ᵗʰ **S83.104** Unspecified dislocation of right knee POA

7ᵗʰ **S83.105** Unspecified dislocation of left knee POA

7ᵗʰ **S83.106** Unspecified dislocation of unspecified knee POA

6ᵗʰ **S83.11** Anterior subluxation and dislocation of proximal end of tibia

---

Unspecified Code   Other Specified Code   Manifestation Code   Ⓝ Newborn   Ⓟ Pediatric   Ⓜ Maternity   Ⓐ Adult   ♂ Male   ♀ Female
● New Code   ▲ Revised Code Title   ▶◀ Revised Text   **NOTES**   *INCLUDES*   *EXCLUDES 1* Not coded here   *EXCLUDES 2* Not included here
4ᵗʰ 4ᵗʰ character required   5ᵗʰ 5ᵗʰ character required   6ᵗʰ 6ᵗʰ character required   7ᵗʰ 7ᵗʰ character required
7ᵗʰ Extension 'X' Alert   **HAC** Hospital-acquired condition (HAC) alert   **AHA** AHA Coding Clinic©

S85.092 Other specified injury of popliteal artery, left leg

S85.099 Other specified injury of popliteal artery, unspecified leg

S85.1 Injury of tibial artery

S85.10 Unspecified injury of unspecified tibial artery
Injury of tibial artery NOS

S85.101 Unspecified injury of unspecified tibial artery, right leg

S85.102 Unspecified injury of unspecified tibial artery, left leg

S85.109 Unspecified injury of unspecified tibial artery, unspecified leg

S85.11 Laceration of unspecified tibial artery

S85.111 Laceration of unspecified tibial artery, right leg

S85.112 Laceration of unspecified tibial artery, left leg

S85.119 Laceration of unspecified tibial artery, unspecified leg

S85.12 Other specified injury of unspecified tibial artery

S85.121 Other specified injury of unspecified tibial artery, right leg

S85.122 Other specified injury of unspecified tibial artery, left leg

S85.129 Other specified injury of unspecified tibial artery, unspecified leg

S85.13 Unspecified injury of anterior tibial artery

S85.131 Unspecified injury of anterior tibial artery, right leg

S85.132 Unspecified injury of anterior tibial artery, left leg

S85.139 Unspecified injury of anterior tibial artery, unspecified leg

S85.14 Laceration of anterior tibial artery

S85.141 Laceration of anterior tibial artery, right leg

S85.142 Laceration of anterior tibial artery, left leg

S85.149 Laceration of anterior tibial artery, unspecified leg

S85.15 Other specified injury of anterior tibial artery

S85.151 Other specified injury of anterior tibial artery, right leg

S85.152 Other specified injury of anterior tibial artery, left leg

S85.159 Other specified injury of anterior tibial artery, unspecified leg

S85.16 Unspecified injury of posterior tibial artery

S85.161 Unspecified injury of posterior tibial artery, right leg

S85.162 Unspecified injury of posterior tibial artery, left leg

S85.169 Unspecified injury of posterior tibial artery, unspecified leg

S85.17 Laceration of posterior tibial artery

S85.171 Laceration of posterior tibial artery, right leg

S85.172 Laceration of posterior tibial artery, left leg

S85.179 Laceration of posterior tibial artery, unspecified leg

S85.18 Other specified injury of posterior tibial artery

S85.181 Other specified injury of posterior tibial artery, right leg

S85.182 Other specified injury of posterior tibial artery, left leg

S85.189 Other specified injury of posterior tibial artery, unspecified leg

S85.2 Injury of peroneal artery

S85.20 Unspecified injury of peroneal artery

S85.201 Unspecified injury of peroneal artery, right leg

S85.202 Unspecified injury of peroneal artery, left leg

S85.209 Unspecified injury of peroneal artery, unspecified leg

S85.21 Laceration of peroneal artery

S85.211 Laceration of peroneal artery, right leg

S85.212 Laceration of peroneal artery, left leg

S85.219 Laceration of peroneal artery, unspecified leg

S85.29 Other specified injury of peroneal artery

S85.291 Other specified injury of peroneal artery, right leg

S85.292 Other specified injury of peroneal artery, left leg

S85.299 Other specified injury of peroneal artery, unspecified leg

S85.3 Injury of greater saphenous vein at lower leg level
Injury of greater saphenous vein NOS
Injury of saphenous vein NOS

S85.30 Unspecified injury of greater saphenous vein at lower leg level

S85.301 Unspecified injury of greater saphenous vein at lower leg level, right leg

S85.302 Unspecified injury of greater saphenous vein at lower leg level, left leg

S85.309 Unspecified injury of greater saphenous vein at lower leg level, unspecified leg

S85.31 Laceration of greater saphenous vein at lower leg level

S85.311 Laceration of greater saphenous vein at lower leg level, right leg

S85.312 Laceration of greater saphenous vein at lower leg level, left leg

S85.319 Laceration of greater saphenous vein at lower leg level, unspecified leg

S85.39 Other specified injury of greater saphenous vein at lower leg level

S85.391 Other specified injury of greater saphenous vein at lower leg level, right leg

S85.392 Other specified injury of greater saphenous vein at lower leg level, left leg

S85.399 Other specified injury of greater saphenous vein at lower leg level, unspecified leg

S85.4 Injury of lesser saphenous vein at lower leg level

S85.40 Unspecified injury of lesser saphenous vein at lower leg level

S85.401 Unspecified injury of lesser saphenous vein at lower leg level, right leg

S85.402 Unspecified injury of lesser saphenous vein at lower leg level, left leg

S85.409 Unspecified injury of lesser saphenous vein at lower leg level, unspecified leg

S85.41 Laceration of lesser saphenous vein at lower leg level

S85.411 Laceration of lesser saphenous vein at lower leg level, right leg

S85.412 Laceration of lesser saphenous vein at lower leg level, left leg

S85.419 Laceration of lesser saphenous vein at lower leg level, unspecified leg

S85.49 Other specified injury of lesser saphenous vein at lower leg level

---

Unacceptable principal diagnosis symbol per Medicare code edits   Code exempt from diagnosis present on admission requirement
Questionable admission   Complication or comorbidity   CC/MCC exclusion   Major complication or comorbidity
Principal diagnosis as its own CC   Principal diagnosis as its own MCC   HCC diagnosis code   RxHCC diagnosis code
MACRA code   Z code as first-listed diagnosis

[7th] S85.491 Other specified injury of lesser saphenous vein at lower leg level, right leg CC POA CC/MCC Exc
[7th] S85.492 Other specified injury of lesser saphenous vein at lower leg level, left leg CC POA CC/MCC Exc
[7th] S85.499 Other specified injury of lesser saphenous vein at lower leg level, unspecified leg CC POA CC/MCC Exc

[5th] S85.5 Injury of popliteal vein
[6th] S85.50 Unspecified injury of popliteal vein
[7th] S85.501 Unspecified injury of popliteal vein, right leg POA MCC CC/MCC Exc
[7th] S85.502 Unspecified injury of popliteal vein, left leg POA MCC CC/MCC Exc
[7th] S85.509 Unspecified injury of popliteal vein, unspecified leg POA MCC CC/MCC Exc
[6th] S85.51 Laceration of popliteal vein
[7th] S85.511 Laceration of popliteal vein, right leg POA MCC CC/MCC Exc
[7th] S85.512 Laceration of popliteal vein, left leg POA MCC CC/MCC Exc
[7th] S85.519 Laceration of popliteal vein, unspecified leg POA MCC CC/MCC Exc
[6th] S85.59 Other specified injury of popliteal vein
[7th] S85.591 Other specified injury of popliteal vein, right leg POA MCC CC/MCC Exc
[7th] S85.592 Other specified injury of popliteal vein, left leg POA MCC CC/MCC Exc
[7th] S85.599 Other specified injury of popliteal vein, unspecified leg POA MCC CC/MCC Exc

[5th] S85.8 Injury of other blood vessels at lower leg level
[6th] S85.80 Unspecified injury of other blood vessels at lower leg level
[7th] S85.801 Unspecified injury of other blood vessels at lower leg level, right leg CC POA CC/MCC Exc
[7th] S85.802 Unspecified injury of other blood vessels at lower leg level, left leg CC POA CC/MCC Exc
[7th] S85.809 Unspecified injury of other blood vessels at lower leg level, unspecified leg CC POA CC/MCC Exc
[6th] S85.81 Laceration of other blood vessels at lower leg level
[7th] S85.811 Laceration of other blood vessels at lower leg level, right leg CC POA CC/MCC Exc
[7th] S85.812 Laceration of other blood vessels at lower leg level, left leg CC POA CC/MCC Exc
[7th] S85.819 Laceration of other blood vessels at lower leg level, unspecified leg CC POA CC/MCC Exc
[6th] S85.89 Other specified injury of other blood vessels at lower leg level
[7th] S85.891 Other specified injury of other blood vessels at lower leg level, right leg CC POA CC/MCC Exc
[7th] S85.892 Other specified injury of other blood vessels at lower leg level, left leg CC POA CC/MCC Exc
[7th] S85.899 Other specified injury of other blood vessels at lower leg level, unspecified leg CC POA CC/MCC Exc

[5th] S85.9 Injury of unspecified blood vessel at lower leg level
[6th] S85.90 Unspecified injury of unspecified blood vessel at lower leg level
[7th] S85.901 Unspecified injury of unspecified blood vessel at lower leg level, right leg CC POA CC/MCC Exc
[7th] S85.902 Unspecified injury of unspecified blood vessel at lower leg level, left leg CC POA CC/MCC Exc
[7th] S85.909 Unspecified injury of unspecified blood vessel at lower leg level, unspecified leg CC POA CC/MCC Exc
[6th] S85.91 Laceration of unspecified blood vessel at lower leg level
[7th] S85.911 Laceration of unspecified blood vessel at lower leg level, right leg CC POA CC/MCC Exc
[7th] S85.912 Laceration of unspecified blood vessel at lower leg level, left leg CC POA CC/MCC Exc
[7th] S85.919 Laceration of unspecified blood vessel at lower leg level, unspecified leg CC POA CC/MCC Exc
[6th] S85.99 Other specified injury of unspecified blood vessel at lower leg level
[7th] S85.991 Other specified injury of unspecified blood vessel at lower leg level, right leg CC POA CC/MCC Exc
[7th] S85.992 Other specified injury of unspecified blood vessel at lower leg level, left leg CC POA CC/MCC Exc
[7th] S85.999 Other specified injury of unspecified blood vessel at lower leg level, unspecified leg CC POA CC/MCC Exc

[4th] S86 Injury of muscle, fascia and tendon at lower leg level

Code also any associated open wound (S81.-)

EXCLUDES2 *injury of muscle, fascia and tendon at ankle (S96.-)*
injury of patellar ligament (tendon) (S76.1-)
sprain of joints and ligaments of knee (S83.-)

The appropriate 7th character is to be added to each code from category S86

A = initial encounter
D = subsequent encounter
S = sequela

[5th] S86.0 Injury of Achilles tendon
[6th] S86.00 Unspecified injury of Achilles tendon
[7th] S86.001 Unspecified injury of right Achilles tendon POA
[7th] S86.002 Unspecified injury of left Achilles tendon POA
[7th] S86.009 Unspecified injury of unspecified Achilles tendon POA
[6th] S86.01 Strain of Achilles tendon
[7th] S86.011 Strain of right Achilles tendon POA
[7th] S86.012 Strain of left Achilles tendon POA
[7th] S86.019 Strain of unspecified Achilles tendon POA
[6th] S86.02 Laceration of Achilles tendon
[7th] S86.021 Laceration of right Achilles tendon CC POA CC/MCC Exc
[7th] S86.022 Laceration of left Achilles tendon CC POA CC/MCC Exc
[7th] S86.029 Laceration of unspecified Achilles tendon CC POA CC/MCC Exc
[6th] S86.09 Other specified injury of Achilles tendon
[7th] S86.091 Other specified injury of right Achilles tendon POA
[7th] S86.092 Other specified injury of left Achilles tendon POA
[7th] S86.099 Other specified injury of unspecified Achilles tendon POA

[5th] S86.1 Injury of other muscle(s) and tendon(s) of posterior muscle group at lower leg level
[6th] S86.10 Unspecified injury of other muscle(s) and tendon(s) of posterior muscle group at lower leg level
[7th] S86.101 Unspecified injury of other muscle(s) and tendon(s) of posterior muscle group at lower leg level, right leg POA
[7th] S86.102 Unspecified injury of other muscle(s) and tendon(s) of posterior muscle group at lower leg level, left leg POA
[7th] S86.109 Unspecified injury of other muscle(s) and tendon(s) of posterior muscle group at lower leg level, unspecified leg POA
[6th] S86.11 Strain of other muscle(s) and tendon(s) of posterior muscle group at lower leg level
[7th] S86.111 Strain of other muscle(s) and tendon(s) of posterior muscle group at lower leg level, right leg POA

S86.112 Strain of other muscle(s) and tendon(s) of posterior muscle group at lower leg level, left leg

S86.119 Strain of other muscle(s) and tendon(s) of posterior muscle group at lower leg level, unspecified leg

S86.12 Laceration of other muscle(s) and tendon(s) of posterior muscle group at lower leg level

　S86.121 Laceration of other muscle(s) and tendon(s) of posterior muscle group at lower leg level, right leg

　S86.122 Laceration of other muscle(s) and tendon(s) of posterior muscle group at lower leg level, left leg

　S86.129 Laceration of other muscle(s) and tendon(s) of posterior muscle group at lower leg level, unspecified leg

S86.19 Other injury of other muscle(s) and tendon(s) of posterior muscle group at lower leg level

　S86.191 Other injury of other muscle(s) and tendon(s) of posterior muscle group at lower leg level, right leg

　S86.192 Other injury of other muscle(s) and tendon(s) of posterior muscle group at lower leg level, left leg

　S86.199 Other injury of other muscle(s) and tendon(s) of posterior muscle group at lower leg level, unspecified leg

S86.2 Injury of muscle(s) and tendon(s) of anterior muscle group at lower leg level

　S86.20 Unspecified injury of muscle(s) and tendon(s) of anterior muscle group at lower leg level

　　S86.201 Unspecified injury of muscle(s) and tendon(s) of anterior muscle group at lower leg level, right leg

　　S86.202 Unspecified injury of muscle(s) and tendon(s) of anterior muscle group at lower leg level, left leg

　　S86.209 Unspecified injury of muscle(s) and tendon(s) of anterior muscle group at lower leg level, unspecified leg

　S86.21 Strain of muscle(s) and tendon(s) of anterior muscle group at lower leg level

　　S86.211 Strain of muscle(s) and tendon(s) of anterior muscle group at lower leg level, right leg

　　S86.212 Strain of muscle(s) and tendon(s) of anterior muscle group at lower leg level, left leg

　　S86.219 Strain of muscle(s) and tendon(s) of anterior muscle group at lower leg level, unspecified leg

　S86.22 Laceration of muscle(s) and tendon(s) of anterior muscle group at lower leg level

　　S86.221 Laceration of muscle(s) and tendon(s) of anterior muscle group at lower leg level, right leg

　　S86.222 Laceration of muscle(s) and tendon(s) of anterior muscle group at lower leg level, left leg

　　S86.229 Laceration of muscle(s) and tendon(s) of anterior muscle group at lower leg level, unspecified leg

　S86.29 Other injury of muscle(s) and tendon(s) of anterior muscle group at lower leg level

　　S86.291 Other injury of muscle(s) and tendon(s) of anterior muscle group at lower leg level, right leg

　　S86.292 Other injury of muscle(s) and tendon(s) of anterior muscle group at lower leg level, left leg

S86.299 Other injury of muscle(s) and tendon(s) of anterior muscle group at lower leg level, unspecified leg

S86.3 Injury of muscle(s) and tendon(s) of peroneal muscle group at lower leg level

　S86.30 Unspecified injury of muscle(s) and tendon(s) of peroneal muscle group at lower leg level

　　S86.301 Unspecified injury of muscle(s) and tendon(s) of peroneal muscle group at lower leg level, right leg

　　S86.302 Unspecified injury of muscle(s) and tendon(s) of peroneal muscle group at lower leg level, left leg

　　S86.309 Unspecified injury of muscle(s) and tendon(s) of peroneal muscle group at lower leg level, unspecified leg

　S86.31 Strain of muscle(s) and tendon(s) of peroneal muscle group at lower leg level

　　S86.311 Strain of muscle(s) and tendon(s) of peroneal muscle group at lower leg level, right leg

　　S86.312 Strain of muscle(s) and tendon(s) of peroneal muscle group at lower leg level, left leg

　　S86.319 Strain of muscle(s) and tendon(s) of peroneal muscle group at lower leg level, unspecified leg

　S86.32 Laceration of muscle(s) and tendon(s) of peroneal muscle group at lower leg level

　　S86.321 Laceration of muscle(s) and tendon(s) of peroneal muscle group at lower leg level, right leg

　　S86.322 Laceration of muscle(s) and tendon(s) of peroneal muscle group at lower leg level, left leg

　　S86.329 Laceration of muscle(s) and tendon(s) of peroneal muscle group at lower leg level, unspecified leg

　S86.39 Other injury of muscle(s) and tendon(s) of peroneal muscle group at lower leg level

　　S86.391 Other injury of muscle(s) and tendon(s) of peroneal muscle group at lower leg level, right leg

　　S86.392 Other injury of muscle(s) and tendon(s) of peroneal muscle group at lower leg level, left leg

　　S86.399 Other injury of muscle(s) and tendon(s) of peroneal muscle group at lower leg level, unspecified leg

S86.8 Injury of other muscles and tendons at lower leg level

　S86.80 Unspecified injury of other muscles and tendons at lower leg level

　　S86.801 Unspecified injury of other muscle(s) and tendon(s) at lower leg level, right leg

　　S86.802 Unspecified injury of other muscle(s) and tendon(s) at lower leg level, left leg

　　S86.809 Unspecified injury of other muscle(s) and tendon(s) at lower leg level, unspecified leg

　S86.81 Strain of other muscles and tendons at lower leg level

　　S86.811 Strain of other muscle(s) and tendon(s) at lower leg level, right leg

　　S86.812 Strain of other muscle(s) and tendon(s) at lower leg level, left leg

　　S86.819 Strain of other muscle(s) and tendon(s) at lower leg level, unspecified leg

　S86.82 Laceration of other muscles and tendons at lower leg level

　　S86.821 Laceration of other muscle(s) and tendon(s) at lower leg level, right leg

---

PDᵃⁿ Unacceptable principal diagnosis symbol per Medicare code edits　　POA Code exempt from diagnosis present on admission requirement
❓ Questionable admission　　cc Complication or comorbidity　　cc/mcc Exc. CC/MCC exclusion　　mcc Major complication or comorbidity
Principal diagnosis as its own CC　　Principal diagnosis as its own MCC　　HCC HCC diagnosis code　　RxHCC RxHCC diagnosis code
MACRA code　　Z Z code as first-listed diagnosis

[7th] S86.822 Laceration of other muscle(s) and tendon(s) at lower leg level, left leg [CC] [POA] [CC/MCC Exc]

[7th] S86.829 Laceration of other muscle(s) and tendon(s) at lower leg level, unspecified leg [CC] [POA] [CC/MCC Exc]

[6th] S86.89 Other injury of other muscles and tendons at lower leg level

[7th] S86.891 Other injury of other muscle(s) and tendon(s) at lower leg level, right leg [POA]

[7th] S86.892 Other injury of other muscle(s) and tendon(s) at lower leg level, left leg [POA]

[7th] S86.899 Other injury of other muscle(s) and tendon(s) at lower leg level, unspecified leg [POA]

[5th] S86.9 Injury of unspecified muscle and tendon at lower leg level

[6th] S86.90 Unspecified injury of unspecified muscle and tendon at lower leg level

[7th] S86.901 Unspecified injury of unspecified muscle(s) and tendon(s) at lower leg level, right leg [POA]

[7th] S86.902 Unspecified injury of unspecified muscle(s) and tendon(s) at lower leg level, left leg [POA]

[7th] S86.909 Unspecified injury of unspecified muscle(s) and tendon(s) at lower leg level, unspecified leg [POA]

[6th] S86.91 Strain of unspecified muscle and tendon at lower leg level

[7th] S86.911 Strain of unspecified muscle(s) and tendon(s) at lower leg level, right leg [POA]

[7th] S86.912 Strain of unspecified muscle(s) and tendon(s) at lower leg level, left leg [POA]

[7th] S86.919 Strain of unspecified muscle(s) and tendon(s) at lower leg level, unspecified leg [POA]

[6th] S86.92 Laceration of unspecified muscle and tendon at lower leg level

[7th] S86.921 Laceration of unspecified muscle(s) and tendon(s) at lower leg level, right leg [CC] [POA] [CC/MCC Exc]

[7th] S86.922 Laceration of unspecified muscle(s) and tendon(s) at lower leg level, left leg [CC] [POA] [CC/MCC Exc]

[7th] S86.929 Laceration of unspecified muscle(s) and tendon(s) at lower leg level, unspecified leg [CC] [POA] [CC/MCC Exc]

[6th] S86.99 Other injury of unspecified muscle and tendon at lower leg level

[7th] S86.991 Other injury of unspecified muscle(s) and tendon(s) at lower leg level, right leg [POA]

[7th] S86.992 Other injury of unspecified muscle(s) and tendon(s) at lower leg level, left leg [POA]

[7th] S86.999 Other injury of unspecified muscle(s) and tendon(s) at lower leg level, unspecified leg [POA]

[4th] S87 Crushing injury of lower leg

Use additional code(s) for all associated injuries

[EXCLUDES2] *crushing injury of ankle and foot (S97.-)*

The appropriate 7th character is to be added to each code from category S87

A = initial encounter
D = subsequent encounter
S = sequela

[5th] S87.0 Crushing injury of knee

[7th] S87.00 Crushing injury of unspecified knee [POA]

[7th] S87.01 Crushing injury of right knee [POA]

[7th] S87.02 Crushing injury of left knee [POA]

[5th] S87.8 Crushing injury of lower leg

[7th] S87.80 Crushing injury of unspecified lower leg [POA]

[7th] S87.81 Crushing injury of right lower leg [POA]

[7th] S87.82 Crushing injury of left lower leg [POA]

[4th] S88 Traumatic amputation of lower leg

An amputation not identified as partial or complete should be coded to complete

[EXCLUDES1] *traumatic amputation of ankle and foot (S98.-)*

The appropriate 7th character is to be added to each code from category S88

A = initial encounter
D = subsequent encounter
S = sequela

[5th] S88.0 Traumatic amputation at knee level

[6th] S88.01 Complete traumatic amputation at knee level

[7th] S88.011 Complete traumatic amputation at knee level, right lower leg [CC] [POA] [HCC] [CC/MCC Exc]

[7th] S88.012 Complete traumatic amputation at knee level, left lower leg [CC] [POA] [HCC] [CC/MCC Exc]

[7th] S88.019 Complete traumatic amputation at knee level, unspecified lower leg [CC] [POA] [HCC] [CC/MCC Exc]

[6th] S88.02 Partial traumatic amputation at knee level

[7th] S88.021 Partial traumatic amputation at knee level, right lower leg [CC] [POA] [HCC] [CC/MCC Exc]

[7th] S88.022 Partial traumatic amputation at knee level, left lower leg [CC] [POA] [HCC] [CC/MCC Exc]

[7th] S88.029 Partial traumatic amputation at knee level, unspecified lower leg [CC] [POA] [HCC] [CC/MCC Exc]

[5th] S88.1 Traumatic amputation at level between knee and ankle

[6th] S88.11 Complete traumatic amputation at level between knee and ankle

[7th] S88.111 Complete traumatic amputation at level between knee and ankle, right lower leg [CC] [POA] [HCC] [CC/MCC Exc]

[7th] S88.112 Complete traumatic amputation at level between knee and ankle, left lower leg [CC] [POA] [HCC] [CC/MCC Exc]

[7th] S88.119 Complete traumatic amputation at level between knee and ankle, unspecified lower leg [CC] [POA] [HCC] [CC/MCC Exc]

[6th] S88.12 Partial traumatic amputation at level between knee and ankle

[7th] S88.121 Partial traumatic amputation at level between knee and ankle, right lower leg [CC] [POA] [HCC] [CC/MCC Exc]

[7th] S88.122 Partial traumatic amputation at level between knee and ankle, left lower leg [CC] [POA] [HCC] [CC/MCC Exc]

[7th] S88.129 Partial traumatic amputation at level between knee and ankle, unspecified lower leg [CC] [POA] [HCC] [CC/MCC Exc]

[5th] S88.9 Traumatic amputation of lower leg, level unspecified

[6th] S88.91 Complete traumatic amputation of lower leg, level unspecified

[7th] S88.911 Complete traumatic amputation of right lower leg, level unspecified [CC] [POA] [HCC] [CC/MCC Exc]

[7th] S88.912 Complete traumatic amputation of left lower leg, level unspecified [CC] [POA] [HCC] [CC/MCC Exc]

[7th] S88.919 Complete traumatic amputation of unspecified lower leg, level unspecified [CC] [POA] [HCC] [CC/MCC Exc]

[6th] S88.92 Partial traumatic amputation of lower leg, level unspecified

[7th] S88.921 Partial traumatic amputation of right lower leg, level unspecified [CC] [POA] [HCC] [CC/MCC Exc]

[7th] S88.922 Partial traumatic amputation of left lower leg, level unspecified [CC] [POA] [HCC] [CC/MCC Exc]

[7th] S88.929 Partial traumatic amputation of unspecified lower leg, level unspecified [CC] [POA] [HCC] [CC/MCC Exc]

[4th] S89 Other and unspecified injuries of lower leg

[NOTES] A fracture not indicated as open or closed should be coded to closed

[EXCLUDES2] *other and unspecified injuries of ankle and foot (S99.-)*

The appropriate 7th character is to be added to each code from subcategories S89.0, S89.1, S89.2, and S89.3

Unspecified Code | Other Specified Code | Manifestation Code | [N] Newborn | [P] Pediatric | [M] Maternity | [A] Adult | ♂ Male | ♀ Female
● New Code | ▲ Revised Code Title | ►◄ Revised Text | [NOTES] | [INCLUDES] | [EXCLUDES1] Not coded here | [EXCLUDES2] Not included here
[4th] 4th character required | [5th] 5th character required | [6th] 6th character required | [7th] 7th character required
[X] Extension 'X' Alert | [HAC] Hospital-acquired condition (HAC) alert | AHA AHA Coding Clinic©

A = initial encounter for closed fracture
D = subsequent encounter for fracture with routine healing
G = subsequent encounter for fracture with delayed healing
K = subsequent encounter for fracture with nonunion
P = subsequent encounter for fracture with malunion
S = sequela

[5th] **S89.0** Physeal fracture of upper end of tibia

[6th] **S89.00** Unspecified physeal fracture of upper end of tibia
- [7th] S89.001 Unspecified physeal fracture of upper end of right tibia [CC] [POA] [HAC] [CC/MCC Exc]
- [7th] S89.002 Unspecified physeal fracture of upper end of left tibia [CC] [POA] [HAC] [CC/MCC Exc]
- [7th] S89.009 Unspecified physeal fracture of upper end of unspecified tibia [CC] [POA] [HAC] [CC/MCC Exc]

[6th] **S89.01** Salter-Harris Type I physeal fracture of upper end of tibia
- [7th] S89.011 Salter-Harris Type I physeal fracture of upper end of right tibia [CC] [POA] [HAC] [CC/MCC Exc]
- [7th] S89.012 Salter-Harris Type I physeal fracture of upper end of left tibia [CC] [POA] [HAC] [CC/MCC Exc]
- [7th] S89.019 Salter-Harris Type I physeal fracture of upper end of unspecified tibia [CC] [POA] [HAC] [CC/MCC Exc]

[6th] **S89.02** Salter-Harris Type II physeal fracture of upper end of tibia
- [7th] S89.021 Salter-Harris Type II physeal fracture of upper end of right tibia [CC] [POA] [HAC] [CC/MCC Exc]
- [7th] S89.022 Salter-Harris Type II physeal fracture of upper end of left tibia [CC] [POA] [HAC] [CC/MCC Exc]
- [7th] S89.029 Salter-Harris Type II physeal fracture of upper end of unspecified tibia [CC] [POA] [HAC] [CC/MCC Exc]

[6th] **S89.03** Salter-Harris Type III physeal fracture of upper end of tibia
- [7th] S89.031 Salter-Harris Type III physeal fracture of upper end of right tibia [CC] [POA] [HAC] [CC/MCC Exc]
- [7th] S89.032 Salter-Harris Type III physeal fracture of upper end of left tibia [CC] [POA] [HAC] [CC/MCC Exc]
- [7th] S89.039 Salter-Harris Type III physeal fracture of upper end of unspecified tibia [CC] [POA] [HAC] [CC/MCC Exc]

[6th] **S89.04** Salter-Harris Type IV physeal fracture of upper end of tibia
- [7th] S89.041 Salter-Harris Type IV physeal fracture of upper end of right tibia [CC] [POA] [HAC] [CC/MCC Exc]
- [7th] S89.042 Salter-Harris Type IV physeal fracture of upper end of left tibia [CC] [POA] [HAC] [CC/MCC Exc]
- [7th] S89.049 Salter-Harris Type IV physeal fracture of upper end of unspecified tibia [CC] [POA] [HAC] [CC/MCC Exc]

[6th] **S89.09** Other physeal fracture of upper end of tibia
- [7th] S89.091 Other physeal fracture of upper end of right tibia [CC] [POA] [HAC] [CC/MCC Exc]
- [7th] S89.092 Other physeal fracture of upper end of left tibia [CC] [POA] [HAC] [CC/MCC Exc]
- [7th] S89.099 Other physeal fracture of upper end of unspecified tibia [CC] [POA] [HAC] [CC/MCC Exc]

[5th] **S89.1** Physeal fracture of lower end of tibia

[6th] **S89.10** Unspecified physeal fracture of lower end of tibia
- [7th] S89.101 Unspecified physeal fracture of lower end of right tibia [CC] [POA] [CC/MCC Exc]
- [7th] S89.102 Unspecified physeal fracture of lower end of left tibia [CC] [POA] [CC/MCC Exc]
- [7th] S89.109 Unspecified physeal fracture of lower end of unspecified tibia [CC] [POA] [CC/MCC Exc]

[6th] **S89.11** Salter-Harris Type I physeal fracture of lower end of tibia
- [7th] S89.111 Salter-Harris Type I physeal fracture of lower end of right tibia [CC] [POA] [CC/MCC Exc]
- [7th] S89.112 Salter-Harris Type I physeal fracture of lower end of left tibia [CC] [POA] [CC/MCC Exc]
- [7th] S89.119 Salter-Harris Type I physeal fracture of lower end of unspecified tibia [CC] [POA] [CC/MCC Exc]

[6th] **S89.12** Salter-Harris Type II physeal fracture of lower end of tibia
- [7th] S89.121 Salter-Harris Type II physeal fracture of lower end of right tibia [CC] [POA] [CC/MCC Exc]
- [7th] S89.122 Salter-Harris Type II physeal fracture of lower end of left tibia [CC] [POA] [CC/MCC Exc]
- [7th] S89.129 Salter-Harris Type II physeal fracture of lower end of unspecified tibia [CC] [POA] [CC/MCC Exc]

[6th] **S89.13** Salter-Harris Type III physeal fracture of lower end of tibia

[EXCLUDES1] *fracture of medial malleolus (adult) (S82.5-)*
- [7th] S89.131 Salter-Harris Type III physeal fracture of lower end of right tibia [CC] [POA] [CC/MCC Exc]
- [7th] S89.132 Salter-Harris Type III physeal fracture of lower end of left tibia [CC] [POA] [CC/MCC Exc]
- [7th] S89.139 Salter-Harris Type III physeal fracture of lower end of unspecified tibia [CC] [POA] [CC/MCC Exc]

[6th] **S89.14** Salter-Harris Type IV physeal fracture of lower end of tibia

[EXCLUDES1] *fracture of medial malleolus (adult) (S82.5-)*
- [7th] S89.141 Salter-Harris Type IV physeal fracture of lower end of right tibia [CC] [POA] [CC/MCC Exc]
- [7th] S89.142 Salter-Harris Type IV physeal fracture of lower end of left tibia [CC] [POA] [CC/MCC Exc]
- [7th] S89.149 Salter-Harris Type IV physeal fracture of lower end of unspecified tibia [CC] [POA] [CC/MCC Exc]

[6th] **S89.19** Other physeal fracture of lower end of tibia
- [7th] S89.191 Other physeal fracture of lower end of right tibia [CC] [POA] [CC/MCC Exc]
- [7th] S89.192 Other physeal fracture of lower end of left tibia [CC] [POA] [CC/MCC Exc]
- [7th] S89.199 Other physeal fracture of lower end of unspecified tibia [CC] [POA] [CC/MCC Exc]

[5th] **S89.2** Physeal fracture of upper end of fibula

[6th] **S89.20** Unspecified physeal fracture of upper end of fibula
- [7th] S89.201 Unspecified physeal fracture of upper end of right fibula [CC] [POA] [CC/MCC Exc]
- [7th] S89.202 Unspecified physeal fracture of upper end of left fibula [CC] [POA] [CC/MCC Exc]
- [7th] S89.209 Unspecified physeal fracture of upper end of unspecified fibula [CC] [POA] [CC/MCC Exc]

[6th] **S89.21** Salter-Harris Type I physeal fracture of upper end of fibula
- [7th] S89.211 Salter-Harris Type I physeal fracture of upper end of right fibula [CC] [POA] [CC/MCC Exc]
- [7th] S89.212 Salter-Harris Type I physeal fracture of upper end of left fibula [CC] [POA] [CC/MCC Exc]
- [7th] S89.219 Salter-Harris Type I physeal fracture of upper end of unspecified fibula [CC] [POA] [CC/MCC Exc]

[6th] **S89.22** Salter-Harris Type II physeal fracture of upper end of fibula
- [7th] S89.221 Salter-Harris Type II physeal fracture of upper end of right fibula [CC] [POA] [CC/MCC Exc]
- [7th] S89.222 Salter-Harris Type II physeal fracture of upper end of left fibula [CC] [POA] [CC/MCC Exc]
- [7th] S89.229 Salter-Harris Type II physeal fracture of upper end of unspecified fibula [CC] [POA] [CC/MCC Exc]

[6th] **S89.29** Other physeal fracture of upper end of fibula
- [7th] S89.291 Other physeal fracture of upper end of right fibula [CC] [POA] [CC/MCC Exc]
- [7th] S89.292 Other physeal fracture of upper end of left fibula [CC] [POA] [CC/MCC Exc]
- [7th] S89.299 Other physeal fracture of upper end of unspecified fibula [CC] [POA] [CC/MCC Exc]

[5th] **S89.3** Physeal fracture of lower end of fibula

[6th] **S89.30** Unspecified physeal fracture of lower end of fibula
- [7th] S89.301 Unspecified physeal fracture of lower end of right fibula [CC] [POA] [CC/MCC Exc]

[PDx] Unacceptable principal diagnosis symbol per Medicare code edits [POA] Code exempt from diagnosis present on admission requirement
[?] Questionable admission [CC] Complication or comorbidity [CC/MCC Exc] CC/MCC exclusion [MCC] Major complication or comorbidity
[PDx CC] Principal diagnosis as its own CC [PDx MCC] Principal diagnosis as its own MCC [HCC] HCC diagnosis code [RxHCC] RxHCC diagnosis code
MACRA code [Z1] Z code as first-listed diagnosis

[7th] S89.302 Unspecified physeal fracture of lower end of left fibula [CC] [POA] [CC/MCC Exc]
[7th] S89.309 Unspecified physeal fracture of lower end of unspecified fibula [CC] [POA] [CC/MCC Exc]
[6th] S89.31 Salter-Harris Type I physeal fracture of lower end of fibula
[7th] S89.311 Salter-Harris Type I physeal fracture of lower end of right fibula [CC] [POA] [CC/MCC Exc]
[7th] S89.312 Salter-Harris Type I physeal fracture of lower end of left fibula [CC] [POA] [CC/MCC Exc]
[7th] S89.319 Salter-Harris Type I physeal fracture of lower end of unspecified fibula [CC] [POA] [CC/MCC Exc]
[6th] S89.32 Salter-Harris Type II physeal fracture of lower end of fibula
[7th] S89.321 Salter-Harris Type II physeal fracture of lower end of right fibula [CC] [POA] [CC/MCC Exc]
[7th] S89.322 Salter-Harris Type II physeal fracture of lower end of left fibula [CC] [POA] [CC/MCC Exc]
[7th] S89.329 Salter-Harris Type II physeal fracture of lower end of unspecified fibula [CC] [POA] [CC/MCC Exc]
[6th] S89.39 Other physeal fracture of lower end of fibula
[7th] S89.391 Other physeal fracture of lower end of right fibula [CC] [POA] [CC/MCC Exc]
[7th] S89.392 Other physeal fracture of lower end of left fibula [CC] [POA] [CC/MCC Exc]
[7th] S89.399 Other physeal fracture of lower end of unspecified fibula [CC] [POA] [CC/MCC Exc]
[5th] S89.8 Other specified injuries of lower leg
The appropriate 7th character is to be added to each code in subcategory S89.8
A = initial encounter
D = subsequent encounter
S = sequela
[7th] S89.80 Other specified injuries of unspecified lower leg [POA]
[7th] S89.81 Other specified injuries of right lower leg [POA]
[7th] S89.82 Other specified injuries of left lower leg [POA]
[5th] S89.9 Unspecified injury of lower leg
The appropriate 7th character is to be added to each code in subcategory S89.9
A = initial encounter
D = subsequent encounter
S = sequela
[7th] S89.90 Unspecified injury of unspecified lower leg [POA]
[7th] S89.91 Unspecified injury of right lower leg [POA]
[7th] S89.92 Unspecified injury of left lower leg [POA]

Injuries to the ankle and foot (S90-S99)

[EXCLUDES2] *burns and corrosions (T20-T32)*
fracture of ankle and malleolus (S82.-)
frostbite (T33-T34)
insect bite or sting, venomous (T63.4)

[4th] S90 Superficial injury of ankle, foot and toes
The appropriate 7th character is to be added to each code from category S90
A = initial encounter
D = subsequent encounter
S = sequela
[5th] S90.0 Contusion of ankle
[7th] S90.00 Contusion of unspecified ankle [POA]
[7th] S90.01 Contusion of right ankle [POA]
[7th] S90.02 Contusion of left ankle [POA]
[5th] S90.1 Contusion of toe without damage to nail
[6th] S90.11 Contusion of great toe without damage to nail
[7th] S90.111 Contusion of right great toe without damage to nail [POA]
[7th] S90.112 Contusion of left great toe without damage to nail [POA]
[7th] S90.119 Contusion of unspecified great toe without damage to nail [POA]
[6th] S90.12 Contusion of lesser toe without damage to nail
[7th] S90.121 Contusion of right lesser toe(s) without damage to nail [POA]
[7th] S90.122 Contusion of left lesser toe(s) without damage to nail [POA]
[7th] S90.129 Contusion of unspecified lesser toe(s) without damage to nail [POA]
Contusion of toe NOS
[5th] S90.2 Contusion of toe with damage to nail
[6th] S90.21 Contusion of great toe with damage to nail
[7th] S90.211 Contusion of right great toe with damage to nail [POA]
[7th] S90.212 Contusion of left great toe with damage to nail [POA]
[7th] S90.219 Contusion of unspecified great toe with damage to nail [POA]
[6th] S90.22 Contusion of lesser toe with damage to nail
[7th] S90.221 Contusion of right lesser toe(s) with damage to nail [POA]
[7th] S90.222 Contusion of left lesser toe(s) with damage to nail [POA]
[7th] S90.229 Contusion of unspecified lesser toe(s) with damage to nail [POA]
[5th] S90.3 Contusion of foot
[EXCLUDES2] *contusion of toes (S90.1-, S90.2-)*
[7th] S90.30 Contusion of unspecified foot [POA]
Contusion of foot NOS
[7th] S90.31 Contusion of right foot [POA]
[7th] S90.32 Contusion of left foot [POA]
[5th] S90.4 Other superficial injuries of toe
[6th] S90.41 Abrasion of toe
[7th] S90.411 Abrasion, right great toe [POA]
[7th] S90.412 Abrasion, left great toe [POA]
[7th] S90.413 Abrasion, unspecified great toe [POA]
[7th] S90.414 Abrasion, right lesser toe(s) [POA]
[7th] S90.415 Abrasion, left lesser toe(s) [POA]
[7th] S90.416 Abrasion, unspecified lesser toe(s) [POA]
[6th] S90.42 Blister (nonthermal) of toe
[7th] S90.421 Blister (nonthermal), right great toe [POA]
[7th] S90.422 Blister (nonthermal), left great toe [POA]
[7th] S90.423 Blister (nonthermal), unspecified great toe [POA]
[7th] S90.424 Blister (nonthermal), right lesser toe(s) [POA]
[7th] S90.425 Blister (nonthermal), left lesser toe(s) [POA]
[7th] S90.426 Blister (nonthermal), unspecified lesser toe(s) [POA]
[6th] S90.44 External constriction of toe
Hair tourniquet syndrome of toe
[7th] S90.441 External constriction, right great toe [POA]
[7th] S90.442 External constriction, left great toe [POA]
[7th] S90.443 External constriction, unspecified great toe [POA]
[7th] S90.444 External constriction, right lesser toe(s) [POA]
[7th] S90.445 External constriction, left lesser toe(s) [POA]
[7th] S90.446 External constriction, unspecified lesser toe(s) [POA]
[6th] S90.45 Superficial foreign body of toe
Splinter in the toe
[7th] S90.451 Superficial foreign body, right great toe [POA]
[7th] S90.452 Superficial foreign body, left great toe [POA]
[7th] S90.453 Superficial foreign body, unspecified great toe [POA]
[7th] S90.454 Superficial foreign body, right lesser toe(s) [POA]
[7th] S90.455 Superficial foreign body, left lesser toe(s) [POA]
[7th] S90.456 Superficial foreign body, unspecified lesser toe(s) [POA]
[6th] S90.46 Insect bite (nonvenomous) of toe

Unspecified Code | Other Specified Code | Manifestation Code | [N] Newborn | [P] Pediatric | [M] Maternity | [A] Adult | ♂ Male | ♀ Female
● New Code | ▲ Revised Code Title | ►◄ Revised Text | [NOTES] | [INCLUDES] | [EXCLUDES1] Not coded here | [EXCLUDES2] Not included here
[4th] 4th character required | [5th] 5th character required | [6th] 6th character required | [7th] 7th character required
[X] Extension 'X' Alert | [HAC] Hospital-acquired condition (HAC) alert | AHA AHA Coding Clinic©

When symbols appear on a code that requires a 7th character extension, refer to Appendix B to identify applicable 7th character codes.

- S90.461 Insect bite (nonvenomous), right great toe
- S90.462 Insect bite (nonvenomous), left great toe
- S90.463 Insect bite (nonvenomous), unspecified great toe
- S90.464 Insect bite (nonvenomous), right lesser toe(s)
- S90.465 Insect bite (nonvenomous), left lesser toe(s)
- S90.466 Insect bite (nonvenomous), unspecified lesser toe(s)
- S90.47 Other superficial bite of toe
  - EXCLUDES1 open bite of toe (S91.15-, S91.25-)
  - S90.471 Other superficial bite of right great toe
  - S90.472 Other superficial bite of left great toe
  - S90.473 Other superficial bite of unspecified great toe
  - S90.474 Other superficial bite of right lesser toe(s)
  - S90.475 Other superficial bite of left lesser toe(s)
  - S90.476 Other superficial bite of unspecified lesser toe(s)
- S90.5 Other superficial injuries of ankle
  - S90.51 Abrasion of ankle
    - S90.511 Abrasion, right ankle
    - S90.512 Abrasion, left ankle
    - S90.519 Abrasion, unspecified ankle
  - S90.52 Blister (nonthermal) of ankle
    - S90.521 Blister (nonthermal), right ankle
    - S90.522 Blister (nonthermal), left ankle
    - S90.529 Blister (nonthermal), unspecified ankle
  - S90.54 External constriction of ankle
    - S90.541 External constriction, right ankle
    - S90.542 External constriction, left ankle
    - S90.549 External constriction, unspecified ankle
  - S90.55 Superficial foreign body of ankle
    - Splinter in the ankle
    - S90.551 Superficial foreign body, right ankle
    - S90.552 Superficial foreign body, left ankle
    - S90.559 Superficial foreign body, unspecified ankle
  - S90.56 Insect bite (nonvenomous) of ankle
    - S90.561 Insect bite (nonvenomous), right ankle
    - S90.562 Insect bite (nonvenomous), left ankle
    - S90.569 Insect bite (nonvenomous), unspecified ankle
  - S90.57 Other superficial bite of ankle
    - EXCLUDES1 open bite of ankle (S91.05-)
    - S90.571 Other superficial bite of ankle, right ankle
    - S90.572 Other superficial bite of ankle, left ankle
    - S90.579 Other superficial bite of ankle, unspecified ankle
- S90.8 Other superficial injuries of foot
  - S90.81 Abrasion of foot
    - S90.811 Abrasion, right foot
    - S90.812 Abrasion, left foot
    - S90.819 Abrasion, unspecified foot
  - S90.82 Blister (nonthermal) of foot
    - S90.821 Blister (nonthermal), right foot
    - S90.822 Blister (nonthermal), left foot
    - S90.829 Blister (nonthermal), unspecified foot
  - S90.84 External constriction of foot
    - S90.841 External constriction, right foot
    - S90.842 External constriction, left foot
    - S90.849 External constriction, unspecified foot
  - S90.85 Superficial foreign body of foot
    - Splinter in the foot
    - S90.851 Superficial foreign body, right foot
    - S90.852 Superficial foreign body, left foot
    - S90.859 Superficial foreign body, unspecified foot
  - S90.86 Insect bite (nonvenomous) of foot
    - S90.861 Insect bite (nonvenomous), right foot
    - S90.862 Insect bite (nonvenomous), left foot
    - S90.869 Insect bite (nonvenomous), unspecified foot
  - S90.87 Other superficial bite of foot
    - EXCLUDES1 open bite of foot (S91.35-)
    - S90.871 Other superficial bite of right foot
    - S90.872 Other superficial bite of left foot
    - S90.879 Other superficial bite of unspecified foot
- S90.9 Unspecified superficial injury of ankle, foot and toe
  - S90.91 Unspecified superficial injury of ankle
    - S90.911 Unspecified superficial injury of right ankle
    - S90.912 Unspecified superficial injury of left ankle
    - S90.919 Unspecified superficial injury of unspecified ankle
  - S90.92 Unspecified superficial injury of foot
    - S90.921 Unspecified superficial injury of right foot
    - S90.922 Unspecified superficial injury of left foot
    - S90.929 Unspecified superficial injury of unspecified foot
  - S90.93 Unspecified superficial injury of toes
    - S90.931 Unspecified superficial injury of right great toe
    - S90.932 Unspecified superficial injury of left great toe
    - S90.933 Unspecified superficial injury of unspecified great toe
    - S90.934 Unspecified superficial injury of right lesser toe(s)
    - S90.935 Unspecified superficial injury of left lesser toe(s)
    - S90.936 Unspecified superficial injury of unspecified lesser toe(s)
- S91 Open wound of ankle, foot and toes
  - Code also any associated wound infection
  - EXCLUDES1 open fracture of ankle, foot and toes (S92.-with 7th character B)
  - traumatic amputation of ankle and foot (S98.-)
  - The appropriate 7th character is to be added to each code from category S91
    - A = initial encounter
    - D = subsequent encounter
    - S = sequela
  - S91.0 Open wound of ankle
    - S91.00 Unspecified open wound of ankle
      - S91.001 Unspecified open wound, right ankle
      - S91.002 Unspecified open wound, left ankle
      - S91.009 Unspecified open wound, unspecified ankle
    - S91.01 Laceration without foreign body of ankle
      - S91.011 Laceration without foreign body, right ankle
      - S91.012 Laceration without foreign body, left ankle
      - S91.019 Laceration without foreign body, unspecified ankle
    - S91.02 Laceration with foreign body of ankle
      - S91.021 Laceration with foreign body, right ankle
      - S91.022 Laceration with foreign body, left ankle
      - S91.029 Laceration with foreign body, unspecified ankle

PDDx Unacceptable principal diagnosis symbol per Medicare code edits   POA Code exempt from diagnosis present on admission requirement
❓ Questionable admission   cc Complication or comorbidity   cc/mcc exc CC/MCC exclusion   mcc Major complication or comorbidity
Principal diagnosis as its own CC   Principal diagnosis as its own MCC   HCC HCC diagnosis code   RxHCC RxHCC diagnosis code
MACRA code   Z1 Z code as first-listed diagnosis

1090   When symbols appear on a code that requires a 7th character extension, refer to Appendix B to identify applicable 7th character codes.   2018 ICD-10-CM

6ᵗʰ S91.03 Puncture wound without foreign body of ankle
  7ᵗʰ S91.031 Puncture wound without foreign body, right ankle POA
  7ᵗʰ S91.032 Puncture wound without foreign body, left ankle POA
  7ᵗʰ S91.039 Puncture wound without foreign body, unspecified ankle POA

6ᵗʰ S91.04 Puncture wound with foreign body of ankle
  7ᵗʰ S91.041 Puncture wound with foreign body, right ankle POA
  7ᵗʰ S91.042 Puncture wound with foreign body, left ankle POA
  7ᵗʰ S91.049 Puncture wound with foreign body, unspecified ankle POA

6ᵗʰ S91.05 Open bite of ankle
    EXCLUDES1 superficial bite of ankle (S90.56-, S90.57-)
  7ᵗʰ S91.051 Open bite, right ankle POA
  7ᵗʰ S91.052 Open bite, left ankle POA
  7ᵗʰ S91.059 Open bite, unspecified ankle POA

5ᵗʰ S91.1 Open wound of toe without damage to nail
  6ᵗʰ S91.10 Unspecified open wound of toe without damage to nail
    7ᵗʰ S91.101 Unspecified open wound of right great toe without damage to nail POA
    7ᵗʰ S91.102 Unspecified open wound of left great toe without damage to nail POA
    7ᵗʰ S91.103 Unspecified open wound of unspecified great toe without damage to nail POA
    7ᵗʰ S91.104 Unspecified open wound of right lesser toe(s) without damage to nail POA
    7ᵗʰ S91.105 Unspecified open wound of left lesser toe(s) without damage to nail POA
    7ᵗʰ S91.106 Unspecified open wound of unspecified lesser toe(s) without damage to nail POA
    7ᵗʰ S91.109 Unspecified open wound of unspecified toe(s) without damage to nail POA

  6ᵗʰ S91.11 Laceration without foreign body of toe without damage to nail
    7ᵗʰ S91.111 Laceration without foreign body of right great toe without damage to nail POA
    7ᵗʰ S91.112 Laceration without foreign body of left great toe without damage to nail POA
    7ᵗʰ S91.113 Laceration without foreign body of unspecified great toe without damage to nail POA
    7ᵗʰ S91.114 Laceration without foreign body of right lesser toe(s) without damage to nail POA
    7ᵗʰ S91.115 Laceration without foreign body of left lesser toe(s) without damage to nail POA
    7ᵗʰ S91.116 Laceration without foreign body of unspecified lesser toe(s) without damage to nail POA
    7ᵗʰ S91.119 Laceration without foreign body of unspecified toe without damage to nail POA

  6ᵗʰ S91.12 Laceration with foreign body of toe without damage to nail
    7ᵗʰ S91.121 Laceration with foreign body of right great toe without damage to nail POA
    7ᵗʰ S91.122 Laceration with foreign body of left great toe without damage to nail POA
    7ᵗʰ S91.123 Laceration with foreign body of unspecified great toe without damage to nail POA
    7ᵗʰ S91.124 Laceration with foreign body of right lesser toe(s) without damage to nail POA
    7ᵗʰ S91.125 Laceration with foreign body of left lesser toe(s) without damage to nail POA
    7ᵗʰ S91.126 Laceration with foreign body of unspecified lesser toe(s) without damage to nail POA

    7ᵗʰ S91.129 Laceration with foreign body of unspecified toe(s) without damage to nail POA

6ᵗʰ S91.13 Puncture wound without foreign body of toe without damage to nail
  7ᵗʰ S91.131 Puncture wound without foreign body of right great toe without damage to nail POA
  7ᵗʰ S91.132 Puncture wound without foreign body of left great toe without damage to nail POA
  7ᵗʰ S91.133 Puncture wound without foreign body of unspecified great toe without damage to nail POA
  7ᵗʰ S91.134 Puncture wound without foreign body of right lesser toe(s) without damage to nail POA
  7ᵗʰ S91.135 Puncture wound without foreign body of left lesser toe(s) without damage to nail POA
  7ᵗʰ S91.136 Puncture wound without foreign body of unspecified lesser toe(s) without damage to nail POA
  7ᵗʰ S91.139 Puncture wound without foreign body of unspecified toe(s) without damage to nail POA

6ᵗʰ S91.14 Puncture wound with foreign body of toe without damage to nail
  7ᵗʰ S91.141 Puncture wound with foreign body of right great toe without damage to nail POA
  7ᵗʰ S91.142 Puncture wound with foreign body of left great toe without damage to nail POA
  7ᵗʰ S91.143 Puncture wound with foreign body of unspecified great toe without damage to nail POA
  7ᵗʰ S91.144 Puncture wound with foreign body of right lesser toe(s) without damage to nail POA
  7ᵗʰ S91.145 Puncture wound with foreign body of left lesser toe(s) without damage to nail POA
  7ᵗʰ S91.146 Puncture wound with foreign body of unspecified lesser toe(s) without damage to nail POA
  7ᵗʰ S91.149 Puncture wound with foreign body of unspecified toe(s) without damage to nail POA

6ᵗʰ S91.15 Open bite of toe without damage to nail
    Bite of toe NOS
    EXCLUDES1 superficial bite of toe (S90.46-, S90.47-)
  7ᵗʰ S91.151 Open bite of right great toe without damage to nail POA
  7ᵗʰ S91.152 Open bite of left great toe without damage to nail POA
  7ᵗʰ S91.153 Open bite of unspecified great toe without damage to nail POA
  7ᵗʰ S91.154 Open bite of right lesser toe(s) without damage to nail POA
  7ᵗʰ S91.155 Open bite of left lesser toe(s) without damage to nail POA
  7ᵗʰ S91.156 Open bite of unspecified lesser toe(s) without damage to nail POA
  7ᵗʰ S91.159 Open bite of unspecified toe(s) without damage to nail POA

5ᵗʰ S91.2 Open wound of toe with damage to nail
  6ᵗʰ S91.20 Unspecified open wound of toe with damage to nail
    7ᵗʰ S91.201 Unspecified open wound of right great toe with damage to nail POA
    7ᵗʰ S91.202 Unspecified open wound of left great toe with damage to nail POA
    7ᵗʰ S91.203 Unspecified open wound of unspecified great toe with damage to nail POA
    7ᵗʰ S91.204 Unspecified open wound of right lesser toe(s) with damage to nail POA
    7ᵗʰ S91.205 Unspecified open wound of left lesser toe(s) with damage to nail POA

Unspecified Code   Other Specified Code   Manifestation Code   Ⓝ Newborn   Ⓟ Pediatric   Ⓜ Maternity   Ⓐ Adult   ♂ Male   ♀ Female
● New Code   ▲ Revised Code Title   ▶◀ Revised Text   NOTES   INCLUDES   EXCLUDES 1 Not coded here   EXCLUDES 2 Not included here
4ᵗʰ 4ᵗʰ character required   5ᵗʰ 5ᵗʰ character required   6ᵗʰ 6ᵗʰ character required   7ᵗʰ 7ᵗʰ character required
Ⓧ Extension 'X' Alert   HAC Hospital-acquired condition (HAC) alert   AHA AHA Coding Clinic©

S91.206 Unspecified open wound of unspecified lesser toe(s) with damage to nail POA

S91.209 Unspecified open wound of unspecified toe(s) with damage to nail POA

S91.21 Laceration without foreign body of toe with damage to nail

　S91.211 Laceration without foreign body of right great toe with damage to nail POA

　S91.212 Laceration without foreign body of left great toe with damage to nail POA

　S91.213 Laceration without foreign body of unspecified great toe with damage to nail POA

　S91.214 Laceration without foreign body of right lesser toe(s) with damage to nail POA

　S91.215 Laceration without foreign body of left lesser toe(s) with damage to nail POA

　S91.216 Laceration without foreign body of unspecified lesser toe(s) with damage to nail POA

　S91.219 Laceration without foreign body of unspecified toe(s) with damage to nail POA

S91.22 Laceration with foreign body of toe with damage to nail

　S91.221 Laceration with foreign body of right great toe with damage to nail POA

　S91.222 Laceration with foreign body of left great toe with damage to nail POA

　S91.223 Laceration with foreign body of unspecified great toe with damage to nail POA

　S91.224 Laceration with foreign body of right lesser toe(s) with damage to nail POA

　S91.225 Laceration with foreign body of left lesser toe(s) with damage to nail POA

　S91.226 Laceration with foreign body of unspecified lesser toe(s) with damage to nail POA

　S91.229 Laceration with foreign body of unspecified toe(s) with damage to nail POA

S91.23 Puncture wound without foreign body of toe with damage to nail

　S91.231 Puncture wound without foreign body of right great toe with damage to nail POA

　S91.232 Puncture wound without foreign body of left great toe with damage to nail POA

　S91.233 Puncture wound without foreign body of unspecified great toe with damage to nail POA

　S91.234 Puncture wound without foreign body of right lesser toe(s) with damage to nail POA

　S91.235 Puncture wound without foreign body of left lesser toe(s) with damage to nail POA

　S91.236 Puncture wound without foreign body of unspecified lesser toe(s) with damage to nail POA

　S91.239 Puncture wound without foreign body of unspecified toe(s) with damage to nail POA

S91.24 Puncture wound with foreign body of toe with damage to nail

　S91.241 Puncture wound with foreign body of right great toe with damage to nail POA

　S91.242 Puncture wound with foreign body of left great toe with damage to nail POA

　S91.243 Puncture wound with foreign body of unspecified great toe with damage to nail POA

　S91.244 Puncture wound with foreign body of right lesser toe(s) with damage to nail POA

　S91.245 Puncture wound with foreign body of left lesser toe(s) with damage to nail POA

S91.246 Puncture wound with foreign body of unspecified lesser toe(s) with damage to nail POA

S91.249 Puncture wound with foreign body of unspecified toe(s) with damage to nail POA

S91.25 Open bite of toe with damage to nail
Bite of toe with damage to nail NOS
EXCLUDES1 superficial bite of toe (S90.46-, S90.47-)

　S91.251 Open bite of right great toe with damage to nail POA

　S91.252 Open bite of left great toe with damage to nail POA

　S91.253 Open bite of unspecified great toe with damage to nail POA

　S91.254 Open bite of right lesser toe(s) with damage to nail POA

　S91.255 Open bite of left lesser toe(s) with damage to nail POA

　S91.256 Open bite of unspecified lesser toe(s) with damage to nail POA

　S91.259 Open bite of unspecified toe(s) with damage to nail POA

S91.3 Open wound of foot

S91.30 Unspecified open wound of foot

　S91.301 Unspecified open wound, right foot POA

　S91.302 Unspecified open wound, left foot POA

　S91.309 Unspecified open wound, unspecified foot

S91.31 Laceration without foreign body of foot

　S91.311 Laceration without foreign body, right foot POA

　S91.312 Laceration without foreign body, left foot POA

　S91.319 Laceration without foreign body, unspecified foot POA

S91.32 Laceration with foreign body of foot

　S91.321 Laceration with foreign body, right foot POA

　S91.322 Laceration with foreign body, left foot POA

　S91.329 Laceration with foreign body, unspecified foot POA

S91.33 Puncture wound without foreign body of foot

　S91.331 Puncture wound without foreign body, right foot POA

　S91.332 Puncture wound without foreign body, left foot POA

　S91.339 Puncture wound without foreign body, unspecified foot POA

S91.34 Puncture wound with foreign body of foot

　S91.341 Puncture wound with foreign body, right foot POA

　S91.342 Puncture wound with foreign body, left foot POA

　S91.349 Puncture wound with foreign body, unspecified foot POA

S91.35 Open bite of foot
EXCLUDES1 superficial bite of foot (S90.86-, S90.87-)

　S91.351 Open bite, right foot POA

　S91.352 Open bite, left foot POA

　S91.359 Open bite, unspecified foot POA

S92 Fracture of foot and toe, except ankle

NOTES A fracture not indicated as displaced or nondisplaced should be coded to displaced
A fracture not indicated as open or closed should be coded to closed

EXCLUDES1 traumatic amputation of ankle and foot (S98.-)

EXCLUDES2 fracture of ankle (S82.-)
fracture of malleolus (S82.-)

The appropriate 7th character is to be added to each code from category S92

A = initial encounter for closed fracture

POA Unacceptable principal diagnosis symbol per Medicare code edits　　Code exempt from diagnosis present on admission requirement
❓ Questionable admission　　cc Complication or comorbidity　　cc-mcc exc CC/MCC exclusion　　mcc Major complication or comorbidity
PDx Principal diagnosis as its own CC　　PDx Principal diagnosis as its own MCC　　HCC HCC diagnosis code　　RxHCC RxHCC diagnosis code
MACRA code　　🅩 Z code as first-listed diagnosis

B = initial encounter for open fracture
D = subsequent encounter for fracture with routine healing
G = subsequent encounter for fracture with delayed healing
K = subsequent encounter for fracture with nonunion
P = subsequent encounter for fracture with malunion
S = sequela

- 5ᵗʰ **S92.0** **Fracture of** calcaneus
  Heel bone
  Os calcis
  EXCLUDES2 Physeal fracture of calcaneus (S99.0-)
  - 6ᵗʰ **S92.00** Unspecified **fracture of calcaneus**
    - 7ᵗʰ **S92.001** **Unspecified fracture of** right **calcaneus** CC POA HAC CC/MCC Exc
    - 7ᵗʰ **S92.002** **Unspecified fracture of** left **calcaneus** CC POA HAC CC/MCC Exc
    - 7ᵗʰ **S92.009** **Unspecified fracture of unspecified calcaneus** CC POA HAC CC/MCC Exc
  - 6ᵗʰ **S92.01** **Fracture of** body of calcaneus
    - 7ᵗʰ **S92.011** Displaced **fracture of body of** right **calcaneus** CC POA HAC CC/MCC Exc
    - 7ᵗʰ **S92.012** Displaced **fracture of body of** left **calcaneus** CC POA HAC CC/MCC Exc
    - 7ᵗʰ **S92.013** Displaced **fracture of body of unspecified calcaneus** CC POA HAC CC/MCC Exc
    - 7ᵗʰ **S92.014** Nondisplaced **fracture of body of** right **calcaneus** CC POA HAC CC/MCC Exc
    - 7ᵗʰ **S92.015** Nondisplaced **fracture of body of** left **calcaneus** CC POA HAC CC/MCC Exc
    - 7ᵗʰ **S92.016** Nondisplaced **fracture of body of unspecified calcaneus** CC POA HAC CC/MCC Exc
  - 6ᵗʰ **S92.02** **Fracture of** anterior process of calcaneus
    - 7ᵗʰ **S92.021** Displaced **fracture of anterior process of** right **calcaneus** CC POA HAC CC/MCC Exc
    - 7ᵗʰ **S92.022** Displaced **fracture of anterior process of** left **calcaneus** CC POA HAC CC/MCC Exc
    - 7ᵗʰ **S92.023** Displaced **fracture of anterior process of unspecified calcaneus** CC POA HAC CC/MCC Exc
    - 7ᵗʰ **S92.024** Nondisplaced **fracture of anterior process of** right **calcaneus** CC POA HAC CC/MCC Exc
    - 7ᵗʰ **S92.025** Nondisplaced **fracture of anterior process of** left **calcaneus** CC POA HAC CC/MCC Exc
    - 7ᵗʰ **S92.026** Nondisplaced **fracture of anterior process of unspecified calcaneus** CC POA HAC CC/MCC Exc
  - 6ᵗʰ **S92.03** Avulsion **fracture of** tuberosity **of calcaneus**
    - 7ᵗʰ **S92.031** Displaced **avulsion fracture of tuberosity of** right **calcaneus** CC POA HAC CC/MCC Exc
    - 7ᵗʰ **S92.032** Displaced **avulsion fracture of tuberosity of** left **calcaneus** CC POA HAC CC/MCC Exc
    - 7ᵗʰ **S92.033** Displaced **avulsion fracture of tuberosity of unspecified calcaneus** CC POA HAC CC/MCC Exc
    - 7ᵗʰ **S92.034** Nondisplaced **avulsion fracture of tuberosity of** right **calcaneus** CC POA HAC CC/MCC Exc
    - 7ᵗʰ **S92.035** Nondisplaced **avulsion fracture of tuberosity of** left **calcaneus** CC POA HAC CC/MCC Exc
    - 7ᵗʰ **S92.036** Nondisplaced **avulsion fracture of tuberosity of unspecified calcaneus** CC POA HAC CC/MCC Exc
  - 6ᵗʰ **S92.04** Other **fracture of** tuberosity **of calcaneus**
    - 7ᵗʰ **S92.041** Displaced **other fracture of tuberosity of** right **calcaneus** CC POA HAC CC/MCC Exc
    - 7ᵗʰ **S92.042** Displaced **other fracture of tuberosity of** left **calcaneus** CC POA HAC CC/MCC Exc
    - 7ᵗʰ **S92.043** Displaced **other fracture of tuberosity of unspecified calcaneus** CC POA HAC CC/MCC Exc
    - 7ᵗʰ **S92.044** Nondisplaced **other fracture of tuberosity of** right **calcaneus** CC POA HAC CC/MCC Exc
    - 7ᵗʰ **S92.045** Nondisplaced **other fracture of tuberosity of** left **calcaneus** CC POA HAC CC/MCC Exc
    - 7ᵗʰ **S92.046** Nondisplaced **other fracture of tuberosity of unspecified calcaneus** CC POA HAC CC/MCC Exc

- 6ᵗʰ **S92.05** Other extraarticular **fracture of calcaneus**
  - 7ᵗʰ **S92.051** Displaced **other extraarticular fracture of** right **calcaneus** CC POA HAC CC/MCC Exc
  - 7ᵗʰ **S92.052** Displaced **other extraarticular fracture of** left **calcaneus** CC POA HAC CC/MCC Exc
  - 7ᵗʰ **S92.053** Displaced **other extraarticular fracture of unspecified calcaneus** CC POA HAC CC/MCC Exc
  - 7ᵗʰ **S92.054** Nondisplaced **other extraarticular fracture of** right **calcaneus** CC POA HAC CC/MCC Exc
  - 7ᵗʰ **S92.055** Nondisplaced **other extraarticular fracture of** left **calcaneus** CC POA HAC CC/MCC Exc
  - 7ᵗʰ **S92.056** Nondisplaced **other extraarticular fracture of unspecified calcaneus** CC POA HAC CC/MCC Exc
- 6ᵗʰ **S92.06** Intraarticular **fracture of calcaneus**
  - 7ᵗʰ **S92.061** Displaced **intraarticular fracture of** right **calcaneus** CC POA HAC CC/MCC Exc
  - 7ᵗʰ **S92.062** Displaced **intraarticular fracture of** left **calcaneus** CC POA HAC CC/MCC Exc
  - 7ᵗʰ **S92.063** Displaced **intraarticular fracture of unspecified calcaneus** CC POA HAC CC/MCC Exc
  - 7ᵗʰ **S92.064** Nondisplaced **intraarticular fracture of** right **calcaneus** CC POA HAC CC/MCC Exc
  - 7ᵗʰ **S92.065** Nondisplaced **intraarticular fracture of** left **calcaneus** CC POA HAC CC/MCC Exc
  - 7ᵗʰ **S92.066** Nondisplaced **intraarticular fracture of unspecified calcaneus** CC POA HAC CC/MCC Exc

- 5ᵗʰ **S92.1** **Fracture of** talus
  Astragalus
  - 6ᵗʰ **S92.10** Unspecified **fracture of talus**
    - 7ᵗʰ **S92.101** **Unspecified fracture of** right **talus** CC POA HAC CC/MCC Exc
    - 7ᵗʰ **S92.102** **Unspecified fracture of** left **talus** CC POA HAC CC/MCC Exc
    - 7ᵗʰ **S92.109** **Unspecified fracture of unspecified talus** CC POA HAC CC/MCC Exc
  - 6ᵗʰ **S92.11** **Fracture of** neck of talus
    - 7ᵗʰ **S92.111** Displaced **fracture of neck of** right **talus** CC POA HAC CC/MCC Exc
    - 7ᵗʰ **S92.112** Displaced **fracture of neck of** left **talus** CC POA HAC CC/MCC Exc
    - 7ᵗʰ **S92.113** Displaced **fracture of neck of unspecified talus** CC POA HAC CC/MCC Exc
    - 7ᵗʰ **S92.114** Nondisplaced **fracture of neck of** right **talus** CC POA HAC CC/MCC Exc
    - 7ᵗʰ **S92.115** Nondisplaced **fracture of neck of** left **talus** CC POA HAC CC/MCC Exc
    - 7ᵗʰ **S92.116** Nondisplaced **fracture of neck of unspecified talus** CC POA HAC CC/MCC Exc
  - 6ᵗʰ **S92.12** **Fracture of** body of talus
    - 7ᵗʰ **S92.121** Displaced **fracture of body of** right **talus** CC POA HAC CC/MCC Exc
    - 7ᵗʰ **S92.122** Displaced **fracture of body of** left **talus** CC POA HAC CC/MCC Exc
    - 7ᵗʰ **S92.123** Displaced **fracture of body of unspecified talus** CC POA HAC CC/MCC Exc
    - 7ᵗʰ **S92.124** Nondisplaced **fracture of body of** right **talus** CC POA HAC CC/MCC Exc
    - 7ᵗʰ **S92.125** Nondisplaced **fracture of body of** left **talus** CC POA HAC CC/MCC Exc
    - 7ᵗʰ **S92.126** Nondisplaced **fracture of body of unspecified talus** CC POA HAC CC/MCC Exc
  - 6ᵗʰ **S92.13** **Fracture of** posterior process of talus
    - 7ᵗʰ **S92.131** Displaced **fracture of posterior process of** right **talus** CC POA HAC CC/MCC Exc
    - 7ᵗʰ **S92.132** Displaced **fracture of posterior process of** left **talus** CC POA HAC CC/MCC Exc
    - 7ᵗʰ **S92.133** Displaced **fracture of posterior process of unspecified talus** CC POA HAC CC/MCC Exc
    - 7ᵗʰ **S92.134** Nondisplaced **fracture of posterior process of** right **talus** CC POA HAC CC/MCC Exc
    - 7ᵗʰ **S92.135** Nondisplaced **fracture of posterior process of** left **talus** CC POA HAC CC/MCC Exc

---

Unspecified Code   Other Specified Code   Manifestation Code   N Newborn   P Pediatric   M Maternity   A Adult   ♂ Male   ♀ Female
● New Code   ▲ Revised Code Title   ►◄ Revised Text   NOTES   *INCLUDES*   *EXCLUDES 1*   Not coded here   *EXCLUDES 2*   Not included here
4ᵗʰ 4ᵗʰ character required   5ᵗʰ 5ᵗʰ character required   6ᵗʰ 6ᵗʰ character required   7ᵗʰ 7ᵗʰ character required
Extension 'X' Alert   HAC Hospital-acquired condition (HAC) alert   AHA AHA Coding Clinic©

7️⃣ S92.136 Nondisplaced **fracture of posterior process of unspecified talus** ⓒ ᴘᴏᴀ HAC CC/MCC Exc

6️⃣ S92.14 Dome **fracture of talus**

EXCLUDES1 *osteochondritis dissecans (M93.2)*

7️⃣ S92.141 Displaced **dome fracture of right talus** ⓒ ᴘᴏᴀ HAC CC/MCC Exc

7️⃣ S92.142 Displaced **dome fracture of left talus** ⓒ ᴘᴏᴀ HAC CC/MCC Exc

7️⃣ S92.143 Displaced **dome fracture of unspecified talus** ⓒ ᴘᴏᴀ HAC CC/MCC Exc

7️⃣ S92.144 Nondisplaced **dome fracture of right talus** ⓒ ᴘᴏᴀ HAC CC/MCC Exc

7️⃣ S92.145 Nondisplaced **dome fracture of left talus** ⓒ ᴘᴏᴀ HAC CC/MCC Exc

7️⃣ S92.146 Nondisplaced **dome fracture of unspecified talus** ⓒ ᴘᴏᴀ HAC CC/MCC Exc

6️⃣ S92.15 Avulsion fracture (chip fracture) of talus

7️⃣ S92.151 Displaced **avulsion fracture (chip fracture) of right talus** ⓒ ᴘᴏᴀ HAC CC/MCC Exc

7️⃣ S92.152 Displaced **avulsion fracture (chip fracture) of left talus** ⓒ ᴘᴏᴀ HAC CC/MCC Exc

7️⃣ S92.153 Displaced **avulsion fracture (chip fracture) of unspecified talus** ⓒ ᴘᴏᴀ HAC CC/MCC Exc

7️⃣ S92.154 Nondisplaced **avulsion fracture (chip fracture) of right talus** ⓒ ᴘᴏᴀ HAC CC/MCC Exc

7️⃣ S92.155 Nondisplaced **avulsion fracture (chip fracture) of left talus** ⓒ ᴘᴏᴀ HAC CC/MCC Exc

7️⃣ S92.156 Nondisplaced **avulsion fracture (chip fracture) of unspecified talus** ⓒ ᴘᴏᴀ HAC CC/MCC Exc

6️⃣ S92.19 Other fracture of talus

7️⃣ S92.191 Other **fracture of right talus** ⓒ ᴘᴏᴀ HAC CC/MCC Exc

7️⃣ S92.192 Other **fracture of left talus** ⓒ ᴘᴏᴀ HAC CC/MCC Exc

7️⃣ S92.199 Other **fracture of unspecified talus** ⓒ ᴘᴏᴀ HAC CC/MCC Exc

5️⃣ S92.2 Fracture of other and unspecified tarsal bone(s)

6️⃣ S92.20 Fracture of unspecified tarsal bone(s)

7️⃣ S92.201 **Fracture of unspecified tarsal bone(s) of right foot** ⓒ ᴘᴏᴀ HAC CC/MCC Exc

7️⃣ S92.202 **Fracture of unspecified tarsal bone(s) of left foot** ⓒ ᴘᴏᴀ HAC CC/MCC Exc

7️⃣ S92.209 **Fracture of unspecified tarsal bone(s) of unspecified foot** ⓒ ᴘᴏᴀ HAC CC/MCC Exc

6️⃣ S92.21 Fracture of cuboid bone

7️⃣ S92.211 Displaced **fracture of cuboid bone of right foot** ⓒ ᴘᴏᴀ HAC CC/MCC Exc

7️⃣ S92.212 Displaced **fracture of cuboid bone of left foot** ⓒ ᴘᴏᴀ HAC CC/MCC Exc

7️⃣ S92.213 Displaced **fracture of cuboid bone of unspecified foot** ⓒ ᴘᴏᴀ HAC CC/MCC Exc

7️⃣ S92.214 Nondisplaced **fracture of cuboid bone of right foot** ⓒ ᴘᴏᴀ HAC CC/MCC Exc

7️⃣ S92.215 Nondisplaced **fracture of cuboid bone of left foot** ⓒ ᴘᴏᴀ HAC CC/MCC Exc

7️⃣ S92.216 Nondisplaced **fracture of cuboid bone of unspecified foot** ⓒ ᴘᴏᴀ HAC CC/MCC Exc

6️⃣ S92.22 Fracture of lateral cuneiform

7️⃣ S92.221 Displaced **fracture of lateral cuneiform of right foot** ⓒ ᴘᴏᴀ HAC CC/MCC Exc

7️⃣ S92.222 Displaced **fracture of lateral cuneiform of left foot** ⓒ ᴘᴏᴀ HAC CC/MCC Exc

7️⃣ S92.223 Displaced **fracture of lateral cuneiform of unspecified foot** ⓒ ᴘᴏᴀ HAC CC/MCC Exc

7️⃣ S92.224 Nondisplaced **fracture of lateral cuneiform of right foot** ⓒ ᴘᴏᴀ HAC CC/MCC Exc

7️⃣ S92.225 Nondisplaced **fracture of lateral cuneiform of left foot** ⓒ ᴘᴏᴀ HAC CC/MCC Exc

7️⃣ S92.226 Nondisplaced **fracture of lateral cuneiform of unspecified foot** ⓒ ᴘᴏᴀ HAC CC/MCC Exc

6️⃣ S92.23 Fracture of intermediate cuneiform

7️⃣ S92.231 Displaced **fracture of intermediate cuneiform of right foot** ⓒ ᴘᴏᴀ HAC CC/MCC Exc

7️⃣ S92.232 Displaced **fracture of intermediate cuneiform of left foot** ⓒ ᴘᴏᴀ HAC CC/MCC Exc

7️⃣ S92.233 Displaced **fracture of intermediate cuneiform of unspecified foot** ⓒ ᴘᴏᴀ HAC CC/MCC Exc

7️⃣ S92.234 Nondisplaced **fracture of intermediate cuneiform of right foot** ⓒ ᴘᴏᴀ HAC CC/MCC Exc

7️⃣ S92.235 Nondisplaced **fracture of intermediate cuneiform of left foot** ⓒ ᴘᴏᴀ HAC CC/MCC Exc

7️⃣ S92.236 Nondisplaced **fracture of intermediate cuneiform of unspecified foot** ⓒ ᴘᴏᴀ HAC CC/MCC Exc

6️⃣ S92.24 Fracture of medial cuneiform

7️⃣ S92.241 Displaced **fracture of medial cuneiform of right foot** ⓒ ᴘᴏᴀ HAC CC/MCC Exc

7️⃣ S92.242 Displaced **fracture of medial cuneiform of left foot** ⓒ ᴘᴏᴀ HAC CC/MCC Exc

7️⃣ S92.243 Displaced **fracture of medial cuneiform of unspecified foot** ⓒ ᴘᴏᴀ HAC CC/MCC Exc

7️⃣ S92.244 Nondisplaced **fracture of medial cuneiform of right foot** ⓒ ᴘᴏᴀ HAC CC/MCC Exc

7️⃣ S92.245 Nondisplaced **fracture of medial cuneiform of left foot** ⓒ ᴘᴏᴀ HAC CC/MCC Exc

7️⃣ S92.246 Nondisplaced **fracture of medial cuneiform of unspecified foot** ⓒ ᴘᴏᴀ HAC CC/MCC Exc

6️⃣ S92.25 Fracture of navicular [scaphoid] of foot

7️⃣ S92.251 Displaced **fracture of navicular [scaphoid] of right foot** ⓒ ᴘᴏᴀ HAC CC/MCC Exc

7️⃣ S92.252 Displaced **fracture of navicular [scaphoid] of left foot** ⓒ ᴘᴏᴀ HAC CC/MCC Exc

7️⃣ S92.253 Displaced **fracture of navicular [scaphoid] of unspecified foot** ⓒ ᴘᴏᴀ HAC CC/MCC Exc

7️⃣ S92.254 Nondisplaced **fracture of navicular [scaphoid] of right foot** ⓒ ᴘᴏᴀ HAC CC/MCC Exc

7️⃣ S92.255 Nondisplaced **fracture of navicular [scaphoid] of left foot** ⓒ ᴘᴏᴀ HAC CC/MCC Exc

7️⃣ S92.256 Nondisplaced **fracture of navicular [scaphoid] of unspecified foot** ⓒ ᴘᴏᴀ HAC CC/MCC Exc

5️⃣ S92.3 Fracture of metatarsal bone(s)

EXCLUDES2 *Physeal fracture of metatarsal (S99.1-)*

6️⃣ S92.30 Fracture of unspecified metatarsal bone(s)

7️⃣ S92.301 **Fracture of unspecified metatarsal bone(s), right foot** ⓒ ᴘᴏᴀ HAC CC/MCC Exc

7️⃣ S92.302 **Fracture of unspecified metatarsal bone(s), left foot** ⓒ ᴘᴏᴀ HAC CC/MCC Exc

7️⃣ S92.309 **Fracture of unspecified metatarsal bone(s), unspecified foot** ⓒ ᴘᴏᴀ HAC CC/MCC Exc

6️⃣ S92.31 Fracture of first metatarsal bone

7️⃣ S92.311 Displaced **fracture of first metatarsal bone, right foot** ⓒ ᴘᴏᴀ HAC CC/MCC Exc

7️⃣ S92.312 Displaced **fracture of first metatarsal bone, left foot** ⓒ ᴘᴏᴀ HAC CC/MCC Exc

7️⃣ S92.313 Displaced **fracture of first metatarsal bone, unspecified foot** ⓒ ᴘᴏᴀ HAC CC/MCC Exc

7️⃣ S92.314 Nondisplaced **fracture of first metatarsal bone, right foot** ⓒ ᴘᴏᴀ HAC CC/MCC Exc

7️⃣ S92.315 Nondisplaced **fracture of first metatarsal bone, left foot** ⓒ ᴘᴏᴀ HAC CC/MCC Exc

7️⃣ S92.316 Nondisplaced **fracture of first metatarsal bone, unspecified foot** ⓒ ᴘᴏᴀ HAC CC/MCC Exc

6️⃣ S92.32 Fracture of second metatarsal bone

7️⃣ S92.321 Displaced **fracture of second metatarsal bone, right foot** ⓒ ᴘᴏᴀ HAC CC/MCC Exc

7️⃣ S92.322 Displaced **fracture of second metatarsal bone, left foot** ⓒ ᴘᴏᴀ HAC CC/MCC Exc

7️⃣ S92.323 Displaced **fracture of second metatarsal bone, unspecified foot** ⓒ ᴘᴏᴀ HAC CC/MCC Exc

---

ᴘᴏᴀ Unacceptable principal diagnosis symbol per Medicare code edits   ᴘᴏᴀ Code exempt from diagnosis present on admission requirement
❓ Questionable admission   ⓒ Complication or comorbidity   CC/MCC Exc CC/MCC exclusion   MCC Major complication or comorbidity
PDx Principal diagnosis as its own CC   PDx Principal diagnosis as its own MCC   HCC HCC diagnosis code   RxHCC RxHCC diagnosis code
MACRA code   Z1 Z code as first-listed diagnosis

[7th] S92.324 Nondisplaced fracture of second metatarsal bone, right foot [CC] [POA] [HAC] [CC/MCC Exc]
[7th] S92.325 Nondisplaced fracture of second metatarsal bone, left foot [CC] [POA] [HAC] [CC/MCC Exc]
[7th] S92.326 Nondisplaced fracture of second metatarsal bone, unspecified foot [CC] [POA] [HAC] [CC/MCC Exc]

[6th] S92.33 Fracture of third metatarsal bone
[7th] S92.331 Displaced fracture of third metatarsal bone, right foot [CC] [POA] [HAC] [CC/MCC Exc]
[7th] S92.332 Displaced fracture of third metatarsal bone, left foot [CC] [POA] [HAC] [CC/MCC Exc]
[7th] S92.333 Displaced fracture of third metatarsal bone, unspecified foot [CC] [POA] [HAC] [CC/MCC Exc]
[7th] S92.334 Nondisplaced fracture of third metatarsal bone, right foot [CC] [POA] [HAC] [CC/MCC Exc]
[7th] S92.335 Nondisplaced fracture of third metatarsal bone, left foot [CC] [POA] [HAC] [CC/MCC Exc]
[7th] S92.336 Nondisplaced fracture of third metatarsal bone, unspecified foot [CC] [POA] [HAC] [CC/MCC Exc]

[6th] S92.34 Fracture of fourth metatarsal bone
[7th] S92.341 Displaced fracture of fourth metatarsal bone, right foot [CC] [POA] [HAC] [CC/MCC Exc]
[7th] S92.342 Displaced fracture of fourth metatarsal bone, left foot [CC] [POA] [HAC] [CC/MCC Exc]
[7th] S92.343 Displaced fracture of fourth metatarsal bone, unspecified foot [CC] [POA] [HAC] [CC/MCC Exc]
[7th] S92.344 Nondisplaced fracture of fourth metatarsal bone, right foot [CC] [POA] [HAC] [CC/MCC Exc]
[7th] S92.345 Nondisplaced fracture of fourth metatarsal bone, left foot [CC] [POA] [HAC] [CC/MCC Exc]
[7th] S92.346 Nondisplaced fracture of fourth metatarsal bone, unspecified foot [CC] [POA] [HAC] [CC/MCC Exc]

[6th] S92.35 Fracture of fifth metatarsal bone
[7th] S92.351 Displaced fracture of fifth metatarsal bone, right foot [CC] [POA] [HAC] [CC/MCC Exc]
[7th] S92.352 Displaced fracture of fifth metatarsal bone, left foot [CC] [POA] [HAC] [CC/MCC Exc]
[7th] S92.353 Displaced fracture of fifth metatarsal bone, unspecified foot [CC] [POA] [HAC] [CC/MCC Exc]
[7th] S92.354 Nondisplaced fracture of fifth metatarsal bone, right foot [CC] [POA] [HAC] [CC/MCC Exc]
[7th] S92.355 Nondisplaced fracture of fifth metatarsal bone, left foot [CC] [POA] [HAC] [CC/MCC Exc]
[7th] S92.356 Nondisplaced fracture of fifth metatarsal bone, unspecified foot [CC] [POA] [HAC] [CC/MCC Exc]

[5th] S92.4 Fracture of great toe
[EXCLUDES2] *Physeal fracture of phalanx of toe (S99.2-)*

[6th] S92.40 Unspecified fracture of great toe
[7th] S92.401 Displaced unspecified fracture of right great toe [CC] [POA] [CC/MCC Exc]
[7th] S92.402 Displaced unspecified fracture of left great toe [CC] [POA] [CC/MCC Exc]
[7th] S92.403 Displaced unspecified fracture of unspecified great toe [CC] [POA] [CC/MCC Exc]
[7th] S92.404 Nondisplaced unspecified fracture of right great toe [CC] [POA] [CC/MCC Exc]
[7th] S92.405 Nondisplaced unspecified fracture of left great toe [CC] [POA] [CC/MCC Exc]
[7th] S92.406 Nondisplaced unspecified fracture of unspecified great toe [CC] [POA] [CC/MCC Exc]

[6th] S92.41 Fracture of proximal phalanx of great toe
[7th] S92.411 Displaced fracture of proximal phalanx of right great toe [CC] [POA] [CC/MCC Exc]
[7th] S92.412 Displaced fracture of proximal phalanx of left great toe [CC] [POA] [CC/MCC Exc]
[7th] S92.413 Displaced fracture of proximal phalanx of unspecified great toe [CC] [POA] [CC/MCC Exc]
[7th] S92.414 Nondisplaced fracture of proximal phalanx of right great toe [CC] [POA] [CC/MCC Exc]
[7th] S92.415 Nondisplaced fracture of proximal phalanx of left great toe [CC] [POA] [CC/MCC Exc]
[7th] S92.416 Nondisplaced fracture of proximal phalanx of unspecified great toe [CC] [POA] [CC/MCC Exc]

[6th] S92.42 Fracture of distal phalanx of great toe
[7th] S92.421 Displaced fracture of distal phalanx of right great toe [CC] [POA] [CC/MCC Exc]
[7th] S92.422 Displaced fracture of distal phalanx of left great toe [CC] [POA] [CC/MCC Exc]
[7th] S92.423 Displaced fracture of distal phalanx of unspecified great toe [CC] [POA] [CC/MCC Exc]
[7th] S92.424 Nondisplaced fracture of distal phalanx of right great toe [CC] [POA] [CC/MCC Exc]
[7th] S92.425 Nondisplaced fracture of distal phalanx of left great toe [CC] [POA] [CC/MCC Exc]
[7th] S92.426 Nondisplaced fracture of distal phalanx of unspecified great toe [CC] [POA] [CC/MCC Exc]

[6th] S92.49 Other fracture of great toe
[7th] S92.491 Other fracture of right great toe [CC] [POA] [CC/MCC Exc]
[7th] S92.492 Other fracture of left great toe [CC] [POA] [CC/MCC Exc]
[7th] S92.499 Other fracture of unspecified great toe [CC] [POA] [CC/MCC Exc]

[5th] S92.5 Fracture of lesser toe(s)
[EXCLUDES2] *Physeal fracture of phalanx of toe (S99.2-)*

[6th] S92.50 Unspecified fracture of lesser toe(s)
[7th] S92.501 Displaced unspecified fracture of right lesser toe(s) [CC] [POA] [CC/MCC Exc]
[7th] S92.502 Displaced unspecified fracture of left lesser toe(s) [CC] [POA] [CC/MCC Exc]
[7th] S92.503 Displaced unspecified fracture of unspecified lesser toe(s) [CC] [POA] [CC/MCC Exc]
[7th] S92.504 Nondisplaced unspecified fracture of right lesser toe(s) [CC] [POA] [CC/MCC Exc]
[7th] S92.505 Nondisplaced unspecified fracture of left lesser toe(s) [CC] [POA] [CC/MCC Exc]
[7th] S92.506 Nondisplaced unspecified fracture of unspecified lesser toe(s) [CC] [POA] [CC/MCC Exc]

[6th] S92.51 Fracture of proximal phalanx of lesser toe(s)
[7th] S92.511 Displaced fracture of proximal phalanx of right lesser toe(s) [CC] [POA] [CC/MCC Exc]
[7th] S92.512 Displaced fracture of proximal phalanx of left lesser toe(s) [CC] [POA] [CC/MCC Exc]
[7th] S92.513 Displaced fracture of proximal phalanx of unspecified lesser toe(s) [CC] [POA] [CC/MCC Exc]
[7th] S92.514 Nondisplaced fracture of proximal phalanx of right lesser toe(s) [CC] [POA] [CC/MCC Exc]
[7th] S92.515 Nondisplaced fracture of proximal phalanx of left lesser toe(s) [CC] [POA] [CC/MCC Exc]
[7th] S92.516 Nondisplaced fracture of proximal phalanx of unspecified lesser toe(s) [CC] [POA] [CC/MCC Exc]

▲ [6th] S92.52 Fracture of ▶middle◀ phalanx of lesser toe(s)
▲ [7th] S92.521 Displaced fracture of ▶middle◀ phalanx of right lesser toe(s) [CC] [POA] [CC/MCC Exc]
▲ [7th] S92.522 Displaced fracture of ▶middle◀ phalanx of left lesser toe(s) [CC] [POA] [CC/MCC Exc]
▲ [7th] S92.523 Displaced fracture of ▶middle◀ phalanx of unspecified lesser toe(s) [CC] [POA] [CC/MCC Exc]
▲ [7th] S92.524 Nondisplaced fracture of ▶middle◀ phalanx of right lesser toe(s) [CC] [POA] [CC/MCC Exc]
▲ [7th] S92.525 Nondisplaced fracture of ▶middle◀ phalanx of left lesser toe(s) [CC] [POA] [CC/MCC Exc]
▲ [7th] S92.526 Nondisplaced fracture of ▶middle◀ phalanx of unspecified lesser toe(s) [CC] [POA] [CC/MCC Exc]

[6th] S92.53 Fracture of distal phalanx of lesser toe(s)
[7th] S92.531 Displaced fracture of distal phalanx of right lesser toe(s) [CC] [POA] [CC/MCC Exc]
[7th] S92.532 Displaced fracture of distal phalanx of left lesser toe(s) [CC] [POA] [CC/MCC Exc]

[7th] S92.533 Displaced fracture of distal phalanx of unspecified lesser toe(s) [CC] [POA] [CC/MCC Exc]
[7th] S92.534 Nondisplaced fracture of distal phalanx of right lesser toe(s) [CC] [POA] [CC/MCC Exc]
[7th] S92.535 Nondisplaced fracture of distal phalanx of left lesser toe(s) [CC] [POA] [CC/MCC Exc]
[7th] S92.536 Nondisplaced fracture of distal phalanx of unspecified lesser toe(s) [CC] [POA] [CC/MCC Exc]
[6th] S92.59 Other fracture of lesser toe(s)
[7th] S92.591 Other fracture of right lesser toe(s) [CC] [POA] [CC/MCC Exc]
[7th] S92.592 Other fracture of left lesser toe(s) [CC] [POA] [CC/MCC Exc]
[7th] S92.599 Other fracture of unspecified lesser toe(s) [CC] [POA] [CC/MCC Exc]
[5th] S92.8 Other fracture of foot, except ankle
[6th] S92.81 Other fracture of foot
Sesamoid fracture of foot
[7th] S92.811 Other fracture of right foot [CC] [POA] [CC/MCC Exc]
[7th] S92.812 Other fracture of left foot [CC] [POA] [CC/MCC Exc]
[7th] S92.819 Other fracture of unspecified foot [CC] [POA] [CC/MCC Exc]
[5th] S92.9 Unspecified fracture of foot and toe
[6th] S92.90 Unspecified fracture of foot
[7th] S92.901 Unspecified fracture of right foot [CC] [POA] [HAC] [CC/MCC Exc]
[7th] S92.902 Unspecified fracture of left foot [CC] [POA] [HAC] [CC/MCC Exc]
[7th] S92.909 Unspecified fracture of unspecified foot [CC] [POA] [HAC] [CC/MCC Exc]
[6th] S92.91 Unspecified fracture of toe
[7th] S92.911 Unspecified fracture of right toe(s) [CC] [POA] [CC/MCC Exc]
[7th] S92.912 Unspecified fracture of left toe(s) [CC] [POA] [CC/MCC Exc]
[7th] S92.919 Unspecified fracture of unspecified toe(s) [CC] [POA] [CC/MCC Exc]

[4th] S93 Dislocation and sprain of joints and ligaments at ankle, foot and toe level

[INCLUDES] *avulsion of joint or ligament of ankle, foot and toe*
laceration of cartilage, joint or ligament of ankle, foot and toe
sprain of cartilage, joint or ligament of ankle, foot and toe
traumatic hemarthrosis of joint or ligament of ankle, foot and toe
traumatic rupture of joint or ligament of ankle, foot and toe
traumatic subluxation of joint or ligament of ankle, foot and toe
traumatic tear of joint or ligament of ankle, foot and toe

Code also any associated open wound

[EXCLUDES2] *strain of muscle and tendon of ankle and foot (S96.-)*

The appropriate 7th character is to be added to each code from category S93
A = initial encounter
D = subsequent encounter
S = sequela

[5th] S93.0 Subluxation and dislocation of ankle joint
Subluxation and dislocation of astragalus
Subluxation and dislocation of fibula, lower end
Subluxation and dislocation of talus
Subluxation and dislocation of tibia, lower end
[7th] S93.01 Subluxation of right ankle joint [POA]
[7th] S93.02 Subluxation of left ankle joint [POA]
[7th] S93.03 Subluxation of unspecified ankle joint [POA]
[7th] S93.04 Dislocation of right ankle joint [POA]
[7th] S93.05 Dislocation of left ankle joint [POA]
[7th] S93.06 Dislocation of unspecified ankle joint [POA]
[5th] S93.1 Subluxation and dislocation of toe
[6th] S93.10 Unspecified subluxation and dislocation of toe
Dislocation of toe NOS
Subluxation of toe NOS
[7th] S93.101 Unspecified subluxation of right toe(s) [POA]
[7th] S93.102 Unspecified subluxation of left toe(s) [POA]
[7th] S93.103 Unspecified subluxation of unspecified toe(s) [POA]
[7th] S93.104 Unspecified dislocation of right toe(s) [POA]
[7th] S93.105 Unspecified dislocation of left toe(s) [POA]
[7th] S93.106 Unspecified dislocation of unspecified toe(s) [POA]
[6th] S93.11 Dislocation of interphalangeal joint
[7th] S93.111 Dislocation of interphalangeal joint of right great toe [POA]
[7th] S93.112 Dislocation of interphalangeal joint of left great toe [POA]
[7th] S93.113 Dislocation of interphalangeal joint of unspecified great toe [POA]
[7th] S93.114 Dislocation of interphalangeal joint of right lesser toe(s) [POA]
[7th] S93.115 Dislocation of interphalangeal joint of left lesser toe(s) [POA]
[7th] S93.116 Dislocation of interphalangeal joint of unspecified lesser toe(s) [POA]
[7th] S93.119 Dislocation of interphalangeal joint of unspecified toe(s) [POA]
[6th] S93.12 Dislocation of metatarsophalangeal joint
[7th] S93.121 Dislocation of metatarsophalangeal joint of right great toe [POA]
[7th] S93.122 Dislocation of metatarsophalangeal joint of left great toe [POA]
[7th] S93.123 Dislocation of metatarsophalangeal joint of unspecified great toe [POA]
[7th] S93.124 Dislocation of metatarsophalangeal joint of right lesser toe(s) [POA]
[7th] S93.125 Dislocation of metatarsophalangeal joint of left lesser toe(s) [POA]
[7th] S93.126 Dislocation of metatarsophalangeal joint of unspecified lesser toe(s) [POA]
[7th] S93.129 Dislocation of metatarsophalangeal joint of unspecified toe(s) [POA]
[6th] S93.13 Subluxation of interphalangeal joint
[7th] S93.131 Subluxation of interphalangeal joint of right great toe [POA]
[7th] S93.132 Subluxation of interphalangeal joint of left great toe [POA]
[7th] S93.133 Subluxation of interphalangeal joint of unspecified great toe [POA]
[7th] S93.134 Subluxation of interphalangeal joint of right lesser toe(s) [POA]
[7th] S93.135 Subluxation of interphalangeal joint of left lesser toe(s) [POA]
[7th] S93.136 Subluxation of interphalangeal joint of unspecified lesser toe(s) [POA]
[7th] S93.139 Subluxation of interphalangeal joint of unspecified toe(s) [POA]
[6th] S93.14 Subluxation of metatarsophalangeal joint
[7th] S93.141 Subluxation of metatarsophalangeal joint of right great toe [POA]
[7th] S93.142 Subluxation of metatarsophalangeal joint of left great toe [POA]
[7th] S93.143 Subluxation of metatarsophalangeal joint of unspecified great toe [POA]
[7th] S93.144 Subluxation of metatarsophalangeal joint of right lesser toe(s) [POA]
[7th] S93.145 Subluxation of metatarsophalangeal joint of left lesser toe(s) [POA]
[7th] S93.146 Subluxation of metatarsophalangeal joint of unspecified lesser toe(s) [POA]
[7th] S93.149 Subluxation of metatarsophalangeal joint of unspecified toe(s) [POA]
[5th] S93.3 Subluxation and dislocation of foot
[EXCLUDES2] *dislocation of toe (S93.1-)*
[6th] S93.30 Unspecified subluxation and dislocation of foot

[PDx] Unacceptable principal diagnosis symbol per Medicare code edits [POA] Code exempt from diagnosis present on admission requirement
[?] Questionable admission [CC] Complication or comorbidity [CC/MCC Exc] CC/MCC exclusion [MCC] Major complication or comorbidity
[PDx CC] Principal diagnosis as its own CC [PDx MCC] Principal diagnosis as its own MCC [HCC] HCC diagnosis code [RxHCC] RxHCC diagnosis code
MACRA code [Z1] Z code as first-listed diagnosis

Dislocation of foot NOS
Subluxation of foot NOS

- ⑦ **S93.301** Unspecified subluxation of right foot POA
- ⑦ **S93.302** Unspecified subluxation of left foot POA
- ⑦ **S93.303** Unspecified subluxation of unspecified foot POA
- ⑦ **S93.304** Unspecified dislocation of right foot POA
- ⑦ **S93.305** Unspecified dislocation of left foot POA
- ⑦ **S93.306** Unspecified dislocation of unspecified foot POA
- ⑥ **S93.31** Subluxation and dislocation of tarsal joint
  - ⑦ **S93.311** Subluxation of tarsal joint of right foot POA
  - ⑦ **S93.312** Subluxation of tarsal joint of left foot POA
  - ⑦ **S93.313** Subluxation of tarsal joint of unspecified foot POA
  - ⑦ **S93.314** Dislocation of tarsal joint of right foot POA
  - ⑦ **S93.315** Dislocation of tarsal joint of left foot POA
  - ⑦ **S93.316** Dislocation of tarsal joint of unspecified foot POA
- ⑥ **S93.32** Subluxation and dislocation of tarsometatarsal joint
  - ⑦ **S93.321** Subluxation of tarsometatarsal joint of right foot POA
  - ⑦ **S93.322** Subluxation of tarsometatarsal joint of left foot POA
  - ⑦ **S93.323** Subluxation of tarsometatarsal joint of unspecified foot POA
  - ⑦ **S93.324** Dislocation of tarsometatarsal joint of right foot POA
  - ⑦ **S93.325** Dislocation of tarsometatarsal joint of left foot POA
  - ⑦ **S93.326** Dislocation of tarsometatarsal joint of unspecified foot POA
- ⑥ **S93.33** Other subluxation and dislocation of foot
  - ⑦ **S93.331** Other subluxation of right foot POA
  - ⑦ **S93.332** Other subluxation of left foot POA
  - ⑦ **S93.333** Other subluxation of unspecified foot POA
  - ⑦ **S93.334** Other dislocation of right foot POA
  - ⑦ **S93.335** Other dislocation of left foot POA
  - ⑦ **S93.336** Other dislocation of unspecified foot POA
- ⑤ **S93.4** Sprain of ankle
  - *EXCLUDES2* injury of Achilles tendon (S86.0-)
  - ⑥ **S93.40** Sprain of unspecified ligament of ankle
    Sprain of ankle NOS
    Sprained ankle NOS
    - ⑦ **S93.401** Sprain of unspecified ligament of right ankle POA
    - ⑦ **S93.402** Sprain of unspecified ligament of left ankle POA
    - ⑦ **S93.409** Sprain of unspecified ligament of unspecified ankle POA
  - ⑥ **S93.41** Sprain of calcaneofibular ligament
    - ⑦ **S93.411** Sprain of calcaneofibular ligament of right ankle POA
    - ⑦ **S93.412** Sprain of calcaneofibular ligament of left ankle POA
    - ⑦ **S93.419** Sprain of calcaneofibular ligament of unspecified ankle POA
  - ⑥ **S93.42** Sprain of deltoid ligament
    - ⑦ **S93.421** Sprain of deltoid ligament of right ankle POA
    - ⑦ **S93.422** Sprain of deltoid ligament of left ankle POA
    - ⑦ **S93.429** Sprain of deltoid ligament of unspecified ankle POA
  - ⑥ **S93.43** Sprain of tibiofibular ligament
    - ⑦ **S93.431** Sprain of tibiofibular ligament of right ankle POA
    - ⑦ **S93.432** Sprain of tibiofibular ligament of left ankle POA
    - ⑦ **S93.439** Sprain of tibiofibular ligament of unspecified ankle POA
  - ⑥ **S93.49** Sprain of other ligament of ankle
    Sprain of internal collateral ligament

Sprain of talofibular ligament
- ⑦ **S93.491** Sprain of other ligament of right ankle POA
- ⑦ **S93.492** Sprain of other ligament of left ankle POA
- ⑦ **S93.499** Sprain of other ligament of unspecified ankle POA
- ⑤ **S93.5** Sprain of toe
  - ⑥ **S93.50** Unspecified sprain of toe
    - ⑦ **S93.501** Unspecified sprain of right great toe POA
    - ⑦ **S93.502** Unspecified sprain of left great toe POA
    - ⑦ **S93.503** Unspecified sprain of unspecified great toe POA
    - ⑦ **S93.504** Unspecified sprain of right lesser toe(s) POA
    - ⑦ **S93.505** Unspecified sprain of left lesser toe(s) POA
    - ⑦ **S93.506** Unspecified sprain of unspecified lesser toe(s) POA
    - ⑦ **S93.509** Unspecified sprain of unspecified toe(s) POA
  - ⑥ **S93.51** Sprain of interphalangeal joint of toe
    - ⑦ **S93.511** Sprain of interphalangeal joint of right great toe POA
    - ⑦ **S93.512** Sprain of interphalangeal joint of left great toe POA
    - ⑦ **S93.513** Sprain of interphalangeal joint of unspecified great toe POA
    - ⑦ **S93.514** Sprain of interphalangeal joint of right lesser toe(s) POA
    - ⑦ **S93.515** Sprain of interphalangeal joint of left lesser toe(s) POA
    - ⑦ **S93.516** Sprain of interphalangeal joint of unspecified lesser toe(s) POA
    - ⑦ **S93.519** Sprain of interphalangeal joint of unspecified toe(s) POA
  - ⑥ **S93.52** Sprain of metatarsophalangeal joint of toe
    - ⑦ **S93.521** Sprain of metatarsophalangeal joint of right great toe POA
    - ⑦ **S93.522** Sprain of metatarsophalangeal joint of left great toe POA
    - ⑦ **S93.523** Sprain of metatarsophalangeal joint of unspecified great toe POA
    - ⑦ **S93.524** Sprain of metatarsophalangeal joint of right lesser toe(s) POA
    - ⑦ **S93.525** Sprain of metatarsophalangeal joint of left lesser toe(s) POA
    - ⑦ **S93.526** Sprain of metatarsophalangeal joint of unspecified lesser toe(s) POA
    - ⑦ **S93.529** Sprain of metatarsophalangeal joint of unspecified toe(s) POA
- ⑤ **S93.6** Sprain of foot
  - *EXCLUDES2* sprain of metatarsophalangeal joint of toe (S93.52-)
    sprain of toe (S93.5-)
  - ⑥ **S93.60** Unspecified sprain of foot
    - ⑦ **S93.601** Unspecified sprain of right foot POA
    - ⑦ **S93.602** Unspecified sprain of left foot POA
    - ⑦ **S93.609** Unspecified sprain of unspecified foot POA
  - ⑥ **S93.61** Sprain of tarsal ligament of foot
    - ⑦ **S93.611** Sprain of tarsal ligament of right foot POA
    - ⑦ **S93.612** Sprain of tarsal ligament of left foot POA
    - ⑦ **S93.619** Sprain of tarsal ligament of unspecified foot POA
  - ⑥ **S93.62** Sprain of tarsometatarsal ligament of foot
    - ⑦ **S93.621** Sprain of tarsometatarsal ligament of right foot POA
    - ⑦ **S93.622** Sprain of tarsometatarsal ligament of left foot POA
    - ⑦ **S93.629** Sprain of tarsometatarsal ligament of unspecified foot POA
  - ⑥ **S93.69** Other sprain of foot
    - ⑦ **S93.691** Other sprain of right foot POA
    - ⑦ **S93.692** Other sprain of left foot POA
    - ⑦ **S93.699** Other sprain of unspecified foot POA

Unspecified Code   Other Specified Code   Manifestation Code   Ⓝ Newborn   Ⓟ Pediatric   Ⓜ Maternity   Ⓐ Adult   ♂ Male   ♀ Female
● New Code   ▲ Revised Code Title   ►◄ Revised Text   **NOTES**   *INCLUDES*   *EXCLUDES1* Not coded here   *EXCLUDES2* Not included here
④ 4th character required   ⑤ 5th character required   ⑥ 6th character required   ⑦ 7th character required
Ⓧ Extension 'X' Alert   HAC Hospital-acquired condition (HAC) alert   **AHA** AHA Coding Clinic©

S94 **Injury of nerves at ankle and foot level**
Code also any associated open wound (S91.-)
The appropriate 7th character is to be added to each code from category S94
A = initial encounter
D = subsequent encounter
S = sequela

S94.0 **Injury of lateral plantar nerve**
- S94.00 Injury of lateral plantar nerve, unspecified leg
- S94.01 Injury of lateral plantar nerve, right leg
- S94.02 Injury of lateral plantar nerve, left leg

S94.1 **Injury of medial plantar nerve**
- S94.10 Injury of medial plantar nerve, unspecified leg
- S94.11 Injury of medial plantar nerve, right leg
- S94.12 Injury of medial plantar nerve, left leg

S94.2 **Injury of deep peroneal nerve at ankle and foot level**
Injury of terminal, lateral branch of deep peroneal nerve
- S94.20 Injury of deep peroneal nerve at ankle and foot level, unspecified leg
- S94.21 Injury of deep peroneal nerve at ankle and foot level, right leg
- S94.22 Injury of deep peroneal nerve at ankle and foot level, left leg

S94.3 **Injury of cutaneous sensory nerve at ankle and foot level**
- S94.30 Injury of cutaneous sensory nerve at ankle and foot level, unspecified leg
- S94.31 Injury of cutaneous sensory nerve at ankle and foot level, right leg
- S94.32 Injury of cutaneous sensory nerve at ankle and foot level, left leg

S94.8 **Injury of other nerves at ankle and foot level**
- S94.8X Injury of other nerves at ankle and foot level
  - S94.8X1 Injury of other nerves at ankle and foot level, right leg
  - S94.8X2 Injury of other nerves at ankle and foot level, left leg
  - S94.8X9 Injury of other nerves at ankle and foot level, unspecified leg

S94.9 **Injury of unspecified nerve at ankle and foot level**
- S94.90 Injury of unspecified nerve at ankle and foot level, unspecified leg
- S94.91 Injury of unspecified nerve at ankle and foot level, right leg
- S94.92 Injury of unspecified nerve at ankle and foot level, left leg

S95 **Injury of blood vessels at ankle and foot level**
Code also any associated open wound (S91.-)
EXCLUDES2 injury of posterior tibial artery and vein (S85.1-, S85.8-)
The appropriate 7th character is to be added to each code from category S95
A = initial encounter
D = subsequent encounter
S = sequela

S95.0 **Injury of dorsal artery of foot**
- S95.00 Unspecified injury of dorsal artery of foot
  - S95.001 Unspecified injury of dorsal artery of right foot
  - S95.002 Unspecified injury of dorsal artery of left foot
  - S95.009 Unspecified injury of dorsal artery of unspecified foot
- S95.01 Laceration of dorsal artery of foot
  - S95.011 Laceration of dorsal artery of right foot
  - S95.012 Laceration of dorsal artery of left foot
  - S95.019 Laceration of dorsal artery of unspecified foot
- S95.09 Other specified injury of dorsal artery of foot
  - S95.091 Other specified injury of dorsal artery of right foot
  - S95.092 Other specified injury of dorsal artery of left foot
  - S95.099 Other specified injury of dorsal artery of unspecified foot

S95.1 **Injury of plantar artery of foot**
- S95.10 Unspecified injury of plantar artery of foot
  - S95.101 Unspecified injury of plantar artery of right foot
  - S95.102 Unspecified injury of plantar artery of left foot
  - S95.109 Unspecified injury of plantar artery of unspecified foot
- S95.11 Laceration of plantar artery of foot
  - S95.111 Laceration of plantar artery of right foot
  - S95.112 Laceration of plantar artery of left foot
  - S95.119 Laceration of plantar artery of unspecified foot
- S95.19 Other specified injury of plantar artery of foot
  - S95.191 Other specified injury of plantar artery of right foot
  - S95.192 Other specified injury of plantar artery of left foot
  - S95.199 Other specified injury of plantar artery of unspecified foot

S95.2 **Injury of dorsal vein of foot**
- S95.20 Unspecified injury of dorsal vein of foot
  - S95.201 Unspecified injury of dorsal vein of right foot
  - S95.202 Unspecified injury of dorsal vein of left foot
  - S95.209 Unspecified injury of dorsal vein of unspecified foot
- S95.21 Laceration of dorsal vein of foot
  - S95.211 Laceration of dorsal vein of right foot
  - S95.212 Laceration of dorsal vein of left foot
  - S95.219 Laceration of dorsal vein of unspecified foot
- S95.29 Other specified injury of dorsal vein of foot
  - S95.291 Other specified injury of dorsal vein of right foot
  - S95.292 Other specified injury of dorsal vein of left foot
  - S95.299 Other specified injury of dorsal vein of unspecified foot

S95.8 **Injury of other blood vessels at ankle and foot level**
- S95.80 Unspecified injury of other blood vessels at ankle and foot level
  - S95.801 Unspecified injury of other blood vessels at ankle and foot level, right leg
  - S95.802 Unspecified injury of other blood vessels at ankle and foot level, left leg
  - S95.809 Unspecified injury of other blood vessels at ankle and foot level, unspecified leg
- S95.81 Laceration of other blood vessels at ankle and foot level
  - S95.811 Laceration of other blood vessels at ankle and foot level, right leg
  - S95.812 Laceration of other blood vessels at ankle and foot level, left leg
  - S95.819 Laceration of other blood vessels at ankle and foot level, unspecified leg
- S95.89 Other specified injury of other blood vessels at ankle and foot level
  - S95.891 Other specified injury of other blood vessels at ankle and foot level, right leg

---

PDxⁿ Unacceptable principal diagnosis symbol per Medicare code edits   POA Code exempt from diagnosis present on admission requirement
❓ Questionable admission   CC Complication or comorbidity   CC/MCC Exc CC/MCC exclusion   MCC Major complication or comorbidity
Principal diagnosis as its own CC   Principal diagnosis as its own MCC   HCC HCC diagnosis code   RxHCC RxHCC diagnosis code
MACRA code   Z Z code as first-listed diagnosis

[7th] S95.892 Other specified injury of other blood vessels at ankle and foot level, left leg CC POA CC/MCC Exc

[7th] S95.899 Other specified injury of other blood vessels at ankle and foot level, unspecified leg CC POA CC/MCC Exc

[5th] S95.9 Injury of unspecified blood vessel at ankle and foot level

[6th] S95.90 Unspecified injury of unspecified blood vessel at ankle and foot level

[7th] S95.901 Unspecified injury of unspecified blood vessel at ankle and foot level, right leg CC POA CC/MCC Exc

[7th] S95.902 Unspecified injury of unspecified blood vessel at ankle and foot level, left leg CC POA CC/MCC Exc

[7th] S95.909 Unspecified injury of unspecified blood vessel at ankle and foot level, unspecified leg CC POA CC/MCC Exc

[6th] S95.91 Laceration of unspecified blood vessel at ankle and foot level

[7th] S95.911 Laceration of unspecified blood vessel at ankle and foot level, right leg CC POA CC/MCC Exc

[7th] S95.912 Laceration of unspecified blood vessel at ankle and foot level, left leg CC POA CC/MCC Exc

[7th] S95.919 Laceration of unspecified blood vessel at ankle and foot level, unspecified leg CC POA CC/MCC Exc

[6th] S95.99 Other specified injury of unspecified blood vessel at ankle and foot level

[7th] S95.991 Other specified injury of unspecified blood vessel at ankle and foot level, right leg CC POA CC/MCC Exc

[7th] S95.992 Other specified injury of unspecified blood vessel at ankle and foot level, left leg CC POA CC/MCC Exc

[7th] S95.999 Other specified injury of unspecified blood vessel at ankle and foot level, unspecified leg CC POA CC/MCC Exc

[4th] S96 Injury of muscle and tendon at ankle and foot level

Code also any associated open wound (S91.-)

EXCLUDES2 *injury of Achilles tendon (S86.0-)*

sprain of joints and ligaments of ankle and foot (S93.-)

The appropriate 7th character is to be added to each code from category S96

A = initial encounter

D = subsequent encounter

S = sequela

[5th] S96.0 Injury of muscle and tendon of long flexor muscle of toe at ankle and foot level

[6th] S96.00 Unspecified injury of muscle and tendon of long flexor muscle of toe at ankle and foot level

[7th] S96.001 Unspecified injury of muscle and tendon of long flexor muscle of toe at ankle and foot level, right foot POA

[7th] S96.002 Unspecified injury of muscle and tendon of long flexor muscle of toe at ankle and foot level, left foot POA

[7th] S96.009 Unspecified injury of muscle and tendon of long flexor muscle of toe at ankle and foot level, unspecified foot POA

[6th] S96.01 Strain of muscle and tendon of long flexor muscle of toe at ankle and foot level

[7th] S96.011 Strain of muscle and tendon of long flexor muscle of toe at ankle and foot level, right foot POA

[7th] S96.012 Strain of muscle and tendon of long flexor muscle of toe at ankle and foot level, left foot POA

[7th] S96.019 Strain of muscle and tendon of long flexor muscle of toe at ankle and foot level, unspecified foot POA

[6th] S96.02 Laceration of muscle and tendon of long flexor muscle of toe at ankle and foot level

[7th] S96.021 Laceration of muscle and tendon of long flexor muscle of toe at ankle and foot level, right foot CC POA CC/MCC Exc

[7th] S96.022 Laceration of muscle and tendon of long flexor muscle of toe at ankle and foot level, left foot CC POA CC/MCC Exc

[7th] S96.029 Laceration of muscle and tendon of long flexor muscle of toe at ankle and foot level, unspecified foot CC POA CC/MCC Exc

[6th] S96.09 Other injury of muscle and tendon of long flexor muscle of toe at ankle and foot level

[7th] S96.091 Other injury of muscle and tendon of long flexor muscle of toe at ankle and foot level, right foot POA

[7th] S96.092 Other injury of muscle and tendon of long flexor muscle of toe at ankle and foot level, left foot POA

[7th] S96.099 Other injury of muscle and tendon of long flexor muscle of toe at ankle and foot level, unspecified foot POA

[5th] S96.1 Injury of muscle and tendon of long extensor muscle of toe at ankle and foot level

[6th] S96.10 Unspecified injury of muscle and tendon of long extensor muscle of toe at ankle and foot level

[7th] S96.101 Unspecified injury of muscle and tendon of long extensor muscle of toe at ankle and foot level, right foot POA

[7th] S96.102 Unspecified injury of muscle and tendon of long extensor muscle of toe at ankle and foot level, left foot POA

[7th] S96.109 Unspecified injury of muscle and tendon of long extensor muscle of toe at ankle and foot level, unspecified foot POA

[6th] S96.11 Strain of muscle and tendon of long extensor muscle of toe at ankle and foot level

[7th] S96.111 Strain of muscle and tendon of long extensor muscle of toe at ankle and foot level, right foot POA

[7th] S96.112 Strain of muscle and tendon of long extensor muscle of toe at ankle and foot level, left foot POA

[7th] S96.119 Strain of muscle and tendon of long extensor muscle of toe at ankle and foot level, unspecified foot POA

[6th] S96.12 Laceration of muscle and tendon of long extensor muscle of toe at ankle and foot level

[7th] S96.121 Laceration of muscle and tendon of long extensor muscle of toe at ankle and foot level, right foot CC POA CC/MCC Exc

[7th] S96.122 Laceration of muscle and tendon of long extensor muscle of toe at ankle and foot level, left foot CC POA CC/MCC Exc

[7th] S96.129 Laceration of muscle and tendon of long extensor muscle of toe at ankle and foot level, unspecified foot CC POA CC/MCC Exc

[6th] S96.19 Other specified injury of muscle and tendon of long extensor muscle of toe at ankle and foot level

[7th] S96.191 Other specified injury of muscle and tendon of long extensor muscle of toe at ankle and foot level, right foot POA

[7th] S96.192 Other specified injury of muscle and tendon of long extensor muscle of toe at ankle and foot level, left foot POA

[7th] S96.199 Other specified injury of muscle and tendon of long extensor muscle of toe at ankle and foot level, unspecified foot POA

[5th] S96.2 Injury of intrinsic muscle and tendon at ankle and foot level

[6th] S96.20 Unspecified injury of intrinsic muscle and tendon at ankle and foot level

[7th] S96.201 Unspecified injury of intrinsic muscle and tendon at ankle and foot level, right foot POA

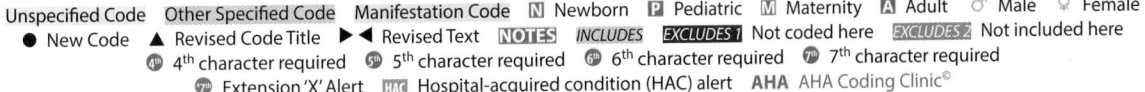

S96.202 Unspecified injury of intrinsic muscle and tendon at ankle and foot level, left foot

S96.209 Unspecified injury of intrinsic muscle and tendon at ankle and foot level, unspecified foot

S96.21 Strain of intrinsic muscle and tendon at ankle and foot level

S96.211 Strain of intrinsic muscle and tendon at ankle and foot level, right foot

S96.212 Strain of intrinsic muscle and tendon at ankle and foot level, left foot

S96.219 Strain of intrinsic muscle and tendon at ankle and foot level, unspecified foot

S96.22 Laceration of intrinsic muscle and tendon at ankle and foot level

S96.221 Laceration of intrinsic muscle and tendon at ankle and foot level, right foot

S96.222 Laceration of intrinsic muscle and tendon at ankle and foot level, left foot

S96.229 Laceration of intrinsic muscle and tendon at ankle and foot level, unspecified foot

S96.29 Other specified injury of intrinsic muscle and tendon at ankle and foot level

S96.291 Other specified injury of intrinsic muscle and tendon at ankle and foot level, right foot

S96.292 Other specified injury of intrinsic muscle and tendon at ankle and foot level, left foot

S96.299 Other specified injury of intrinsic muscle and tendon at ankle and foot level, unspecified foot

S96.8 Injury of other specified muscles and tendons at ankle and foot level

S96.80 Unspecified injury of other specified muscles and tendons at ankle and foot level

S96.801 Unspecified injury of other specified muscles and tendons at ankle and foot level, right foot

S96.802 Unspecified injury of other specified muscles and tendons at ankle and foot level, left foot

S96.809 Unspecified injury of other specified muscles and tendons at ankle and foot level, unspecified foot

S96.81 Strain of other specified muscles and tendons at ankle and foot level

S96.811 Strain of other specified muscles and tendons at ankle and foot level, right foot

S96.812 Strain of other specified muscles and tendons at ankle and foot level, left foot

S96.819 Strain of other specified muscles and tendons at ankle and foot level, unspecified foot

S96.82 Laceration of other specified muscles and tendons at ankle and foot level

S96.821 Laceration of other specified muscles and tendons at ankle and foot level, right foot

S96.822 Laceration of other specified muscles and tendons at ankle and foot level, left foot

S96.829 Laceration of other specified muscles and tendons at ankle and foot level, unspecified foot

S96.89 Other specified injury of other specified muscles and tendons at ankle and foot level

S96.891 Other specified injury of other specified muscles and tendons at ankle and foot level, right foot

S96.892 Other specified injury of other specified muscles and tendons at ankle and foot level, left foot

S96.899 Other specified injury of other specified muscles and tendons at ankle and foot level, unspecified foot

S96.9 Injury of unspecified muscle and tendon at ankle and foot level

S96.90 Unspecified injury of unspecified muscle and tendon at ankle and foot level

S96.901 Unspecified injury of unspecified muscle and tendon at ankle and foot level, right foot

S96.902 Unspecified injury of unspecified muscle and tendon at ankle and foot level, left foot

S96.909 Unspecified injury of unspecified muscle and tendon at ankle and foot level, unspecified foot

S96.91 Strain of unspecified muscle and tendon at ankle and foot level

S96.911 Strain of unspecified muscle and tendon at ankle and foot level, right foot

S96.912 Strain of unspecified muscle and tendon at ankle and foot level, left foot

S96.919 Strain of unspecified muscle and tendon at ankle and foot level, unspecified foot

S96.92 Laceration of unspecified muscle and tendon at ankle and foot level

S96.921 Laceration of unspecified muscle and tendon at ankle and foot level, right foot

S96.922 Laceration of unspecified muscle and tendon at ankle and foot level, left foot

S96.929 Laceration of unspecified muscle and tendon at ankle and foot level, unspecified foot

S96.99 Other specified injury of unspecified muscle and tendon at ankle and foot level

S96.991 Other specified injury of unspecified muscle and tendon at ankle and foot level, right foot

S96.992 Other specified injury of unspecified muscle and tendon at ankle and foot level, left foot

S96.999 Other specified injury of unspecified muscle and tendon at ankle and foot level, unspecified foot

S97 Crushing injury of ankle and foot

Use additional code(s) for all associated injuries

The appropriate 7th character is to be added to each code from category S97

A = initial encounter

D = subsequent encounter

S = sequela

S97.0 Crushing injury of ankle

S97.00 Crushing injury of unspecified ankle

S97.01 Crushing injury of right ankle

S97.02 Crushing injury of left ankle

S97.1 Crushing injury of toe

S97.10 Crushing injury of unspecified toe(s)

S97.101 Crushing injury of unspecified right toe(s)

S97.102 Crushing injury of unspecified left toe(s)

S97.109 Crushing injury of unspecified toe(s)

Crushing injury of toe NOS

S97.11 Crushing injury of great toe

S97.111 Crushing injury of right great toe

POA Unacceptable principal diagnosis symbol per Medicare code edits   POA Code exempt from diagnosis present on admission requirement
? Questionable admission   CC Complication or comorbidity   CC/MCC Exc CC/MCC exclusion   MCC Major complication or comorbidity
Principal diagnosis as its own CC   Principal diagnosis as its own MCC   HCC HCC diagnosis code   RxHCC RxHCC diagnosis code
MACRA code   Z code as first-listed diagnosis

When symbols appear on a code that requires a 7th character extension, refer to Appendix B to identify applicable 7th character codes.
2018 ICD-10-CM

7️⃣ S97.112 Crushing injury of left great toe POA
7️⃣ S97.119 Crushing injury of unspecified great toe POA
6️⃣ S97.12 Crushing injury of lesser toe(s)
7️⃣ S97.121 Crushing injury of right lesser toe(s) POA
7️⃣ S97.122 Crushing injury of left lesser toe(s) POA
7️⃣ S97.129 Crushing injury of unspecified lesser toe(s) POA
5️⃣ S97.8 Crushing injury of foot
7️⃣ S97.80 Crushing injury of unspecified foot POA
Crushing injury of foot NOS
7️⃣ S97.81 Crushing injury of right foot POA
7️⃣ S97.82 Crushing injury of left foot POA
4️⃣ S98 Traumatic amputation of ankle and foot
An amputation not identified as partial or complete should be coded to complete
The appropriate 7th character is to be added to each code from category S98
A = initial encounter
D = subsequent encounter
S = sequela
5️⃣ S98.0 Traumatic amputation of foot at ankle level
6️⃣ S98.01 Complete traumatic amputation of foot at ankle level
7️⃣ S98.011 Complete traumatic amputation of right foot at ankle level CC POA HCC CC/MCC Exc
7️⃣ S98.012 Complete traumatic amputation of left foot at ankle level CC POA HCC CC/MCC Exc
7️⃣ S98.019 Complete traumatic amputation of unspecified foot at ankle level CC POA HCC CC/MCC Exc
6️⃣ S98.02 Partial traumatic amputation of foot at ankle level
7️⃣ S98.021 Partial traumatic amputation of right foot at ankle level CC POA HCC CC/MCC Exc
7️⃣ S98.022 Partial traumatic amputation of left foot at ankle level CC POA HCC CC/MCC Exc
7️⃣ S98.029 Partial traumatic amputation of unspecified foot at ankle level CC POA HCC CC/MCC Exc
5️⃣ S98.1 Traumatic amputation of one toe
6️⃣ S98.11 Complete traumatic amputation of great toe
7️⃣ S98.111 Complete traumatic amputation of right great toe POA HCC
7️⃣ S98.112 Complete traumatic amputation of left great toe POA HCC
7️⃣ S98.119 Complete traumatic amputation of unspecified great toe POA HCC
6️⃣ S98.12 Partial traumatic amputation of great toe
7️⃣ S98.121 Partial traumatic amputation of right great toe POA HCC
7️⃣ S98.122 Partial traumatic amputation of left great toe POA HCC
7️⃣ S98.129 Partial traumatic amputation of unspecified great toe POA HCC
6️⃣ S98.13 Complete traumatic amputation of one lesser toe
Traumatic amputation of toe NOS
S98.131 Complete traumatic amputation of one right lesser toe POA HCC
7️⃣ S98.132 Complete traumatic amputation of one left lesser toe POA HCC
7️⃣ S98.139 Complete traumatic amputation of one unspecified lesser toe POA HCC
6️⃣ S98.14 Partial traumatic amputation of one lesser toe
7️⃣ S98.141 Partial traumatic amputation of one right lesser toe POA HCC
7️⃣ S98.142 Partial traumatic amputation of one left lesser toe POA HCC
7️⃣ S98.149 Partial traumatic amputation of one unspecified lesser toe POA HCC
5️⃣ S98.2 Traumatic amputation of two or more lesser toes
6️⃣ S98.21 Complete traumatic amputation of two or more lesser toes

7️⃣ S98.211 Complete traumatic amputation of two or more right lesser toes POA HCC
7️⃣ S98.212 Complete traumatic amputation of two or more left lesser toes POA HCC
7️⃣ S98.219 Complete traumatic amputation of two or more unspecified lesser toes POA HCC
6️⃣ S98.22 Partial traumatic amputation of two or more lesser toes
7️⃣ S98.221 Partial traumatic amputation of two or more right lesser toes POA HCC
7️⃣ S98.222 Partial traumatic amputation of two or more left lesser toes POA HCC
7️⃣ S98.229 Partial traumatic amputation of two or more unspecified lesser toes POA HCC
5️⃣ S98.3 Traumatic amputation of midfoot
6️⃣ S98.31 Complete traumatic amputation of midfoot
7️⃣ S98.311 Complete traumatic amputation of right midfoot CC POA HCC CC/MCC Exc
7️⃣ S98.312 Complete traumatic amputation of left midfoot CC POA HCC CC/MCC Exc
7️⃣ S98.319 Complete traumatic amputation of unspecified midfoot CC POA HCC CC/MCC Exc
6️⃣ S98.32 Partial traumatic amputation of midfoot
7️⃣ S98.321 Partial traumatic amputation of right midfoot CC POA HCC CC/MCC Exc
7️⃣ S98.322 Partial traumatic amputation of left midfoot CC POA HCC CC/MCC Exc
7️⃣ S98.329 Partial traumatic amputation of unspecified midfoot CC POA HCC CC/MCC Exc
5️⃣ S98.9 Traumatic amputation of foot, level unspecified
6️⃣ S98.91 Complete traumatic amputation of foot, level unspecified
7️⃣ S98.911 Complete traumatic amputation of right foot, level unspecified CC POA HCC CC/MCC Exc
7️⃣ S98.912 Complete traumatic amputation of left foot, level unspecified CC POA HCC CC/MCC Exc
7️⃣ S98.919 Complete traumatic amputation of unspecified foot, level unspecified CC POA HCC CC/MCC Exc
6️⃣ S98.92 Partial traumatic amputation of foot, level unspecified
7️⃣ S98.921 Partial traumatic amputation of right foot, level unspecified CC POA HCC CC/MCC Exc
7️⃣ S98.922 Partial traumatic amputation of left foot, level unspecified CC POA HCC CC/MCC Exc
7️⃣ S98.929 Partial traumatic amputation of unspecified foot, level unspecified CC POA HCC CC/MCC Exc
4️⃣ S99 Other and unspecified injuries of ankle and foot
5️⃣ S99.0 Physeal fracture of calcaneus
The appropriate 7th character is to be added to each code from subcategories S99.0
A = initial encounter for closed fracture
B = initial encounter for open fracture
D = subsequent encounter for fracture with routine healing
G = subsequent encounter for fracture with delayed healing
K = subsequent encounter for fracture with nonunion
P = subsequent encounter for fracture with malunion
S = sequela
6️⃣ S99.00 Unspecified physeal fracture of calcaneus
7️⃣ S99.001 Unspecified physeal fracture of right calcaneus POA
7️⃣ S99.002 Unspecified physeal fracture of left calcaneus POA
7️⃣ S99.009 Unspecified physeal fracture of unspecified calcaneus POA
6️⃣ S99.01 Salter-Harris Type I physeal fracture of calcaneus
7️⃣ S99.011 Salter-Harris Type I physeal fracture of right calcaneus POA

Unspecified Code Other Specified Code Manifestation Code N Newborn P Pediatric M Maternity A Adult ♂ Male ♀ Female
● New Code ▲ Revised Code Title ►◄ Revised Text NOTES INCLUDES EXCLUDES 1 Not coded here EXCLUDES 2 Not included here
4️⃣ 4th character required 5️⃣ 5th character required 6️⃣ 6th character required 7️⃣ 7th character required
7️⃣ Extension 'X' Alert HAC Hospital-acquired condition (HAC) alert AHA AHA Coding Clinic©

S99.012 - S99.299

CHAPTER 19: INJURY, POISONING, AND CERTAIN OTHER CONSEQUENCES OF EXTERNAL CAUSES (S00-T88)

7ᵗʰ S99.012 Salter-Harris Type I physeal fracture of left calcaneus

7ᵗʰ S99.019 Salter-Harris Type I physeal fracture of unspecified calcaneus

6ᵗʰ S99.02 Salter-Harris Type II physeal fracture of calcaneus

   7ᵗʰ S99.021 Salter-Harris Type II physeal fracture of right calcaneus

   7ᵗʰ S99.022 Salter-Harris Type II physeal fracture of left calcaneus

   7ᵗʰ S99.029 Salter-Harris Type II physeal fracture of unspecified calcaneus

6ᵗʰ S99.03 Salter-Harris Type III physeal fracture of calcaneus

   7ᵗʰ S99.031 Salter-Harris Type III physeal fracture of right calcaneus

   7ᵗʰ S99.032 Salter-Harris Type III physeal fracture of left calcaneus

   7ᵗʰ S99.039 Salter-Harris Type III physeal fracture of unspecified calcaneus

6ᵗʰ S99.04 Salter-Harris Type IV physeal fracture of calcaneus

   7ᵗʰ S99.041 Salter-Harris Type IV physeal fracture of right calcaneus

   7ᵗʰ S99.042 Salter-Harris Type IV physeal fracture of left calcaneus

   7ᵗʰ S99.049 Salter-Harris Type IV physeal fracture of unspecified calcaneus

6ᵗʰ S99.09 Other physeal fracture of calcaneus

   7ᵗʰ S99.091 Other physeal fracture of right calcaneus

   7ᵗʰ S99.092 Other physeal fracture of left calcaneus

   7ᵗʰ S99.099 Other physeal fracture of unspecified calcaneus

5ᵗʰ S99.1 Physeal fracture of metatarsal

The appropriate 7th character is to be added to each code from subcategories S99.1

A = initial encounter for closed fracture

B = initial encounter for open fracture

D = subsequent encounter for fracture with routine healing

G = subsequent encounter for fracture with delayed healing

K = subsequent encounter for fracture with nonunion

P = subsequent encounter for fracture with malunion

S = sequela

6ᵗʰ S99.10 Unspecified physeal fracture of metatarsal

   7ᵗʰ S99.101 Unspecified physeal fracture of right metatarsal

   7ᵗʰ S99.102 Unspecified physeal fracture of left metatarsal

   7ᵗʰ S99.109 Unspecified physeal fracture of unspecified metatarsal

6ᵗʰ S99.11 Salter-Harris Type I physeal fracture of metatarsal

   7ᵗʰ S99.111 Salter-Harris Type I physeal fracture of right metatarsal

   7ᵗʰ S99.112 Salter-Harris Type I physeal fracture of left metatarsal

   7ᵗʰ S99.119 Salter-Harris Type I physeal fracture of unspecified metatarsal

6ᵗʰ S99.12 Salter-Harris Type II physeal fracture of metatarsal

   7ᵗʰ S99.121 Salter-Harris Type II physeal fracture of right metatarsal

   7ᵗʰ S99.122 Salter-Harris Type II physeal fracture of left metatarsal

   7ᵗʰ S99.129 Salter-Harris Type II physeal fracture of unspecified metatarsal

6ᵗʰ S99.13 Salter-Harris Type III physeal fracture of metatarsal

   7ᵗʰ S99.131 Salter-Harris Type III physeal fracture of right metatarsal

   7ᵗʰ S99.132 Salter-Harris Type III physeal fracture of left metatarsal

   7ᵗʰ S99.139 Salter-Harris Type III physeal fracture of unspecified metatarsal

6ᵗʰ S99.14 Salter-Harris Type IV physeal fracture of metatarsal

   7ᵗʰ S99.141 Salter-Harris Type IV physeal fracture of right metatarsal

   7ᵗʰ S99.142 Salter-Harris Type IV physeal fracture of left metatarsal

   7ᵗʰ S99.149 Salter-Harris Type IV physeal fracture of unspecified metatarsal

6ᵗʰ S99.19 Other physeal fracture of metatarsal

   7ᵗʰ S99.191 Other physeal fracture of right metatarsal

   7ᵗʰ S99.192 Other physeal fracture of left metatarsal

   7ᵗʰ S99.199 Other physeal fracture of unspecified metatarsal

5ᵗʰ S99.2 Physeal fracture of phalanx of toe

The appropriate 7th character is to be added to each code from subcategories S99.2

A = initial encounter for closed fracture

B = initial encounter for open fracture

D = subsequent encounter for fracture with routine healing

G = subsequent encounter for fracture with delayed healing

K = subsequent encounter for fracture with nonunion

P = subsequent encounter for fracture with malunion

S = sequela

6ᵗʰ S99.20 Unspecified physeal fracture of phalanx of toe

   7ᵗʰ S99.201 Unspecified physeal fracture of phalanx of right toe

   7ᵗʰ S99.202 Unspecified physeal fracture of phalanx of left toe

   7ᵗʰ S99.209 Unspecified physeal fracture of phalanx of unspecified toe

6ᵗʰ S99.21 Salter-Harris Type I physeal fracture of phalanx of toe

   7ᵗʰ S99.211 Salter-Harris Type I physeal fracture of phalanx of right toe

   7ᵗʰ S99.212 Salter-Harris Type I physeal fracture of phalanx of left toe

   7ᵗʰ S99.219 Salter-Harris Type I physeal fracture of phalanx of unspecified toe

6ᵗʰ S99.22 Salter-Harris Type II physeal fracture of phalanx of toe

   7ᵗʰ S99.221 Salter-Harris Type II physeal fracture of phalanx of right toe

   7ᵗʰ S99.222 Salter-Harris Type II physeal fracture of phalanx of left toe

   7ᵗʰ S99.229 Salter-Harris Type II physeal fracture of phalanx of unspecified toe

6ᵗʰ S99.23 Salter-Harris Type III physeal fracture of phalanx of toe

   7ᵗʰ S99.231 Salter-Harris Type III physeal fracture of phalanx of right toe

   7ᵗʰ S99.232 Salter-Harris Type III physeal fracture of phalanx of left toe

   7ᵗʰ S99.239 Salter-Harris Type III physeal fracture of phalanx of unspecified toe

6ᵗʰ S99.24 Salter-Harris Type IV physeal fracture of phalanx of toe

   7ᵗʰ S99.241 Salter-Harris Type IV physeal fracture of phalanx of right toe

   7ᵗʰ S99.242 Salter-Harris Type IV physeal fracture of phalanx of left toe

   7ᵗʰ S99.249 Salter-Harris Type IV physeal fracture of phalanx of unspecified toe

6ᵗʰ S99.29 Other physeal fracture of phalanx of toe

   7ᵗʰ S99.291 Other physeal fracture of phalanx of right toe

   7ᵗʰ S99.292 Other physeal fracture of phalanx of left toe

   7ᵗʰ S99.299 Other physeal fracture of phalanx of unspecified toe

---

Unacceptable principal diagnosis symbol per Medicare code edits   Code exempt from diagnosis present on admission requirement

❓ Questionable admission   Complication or comorbidity   CC/MCC exclusion   Major complication or comorbidity

Principal diagnosis as its own CC   Principal diagnosis as its own MCC   HCC HCC diagnosis code   RxHCC RxHCC diagnosis code

MACRA code   Z1 Z code as first-listed diagnosis

When symbols appear on a code that requires a 7th character extension, refer to Appendix B to identify applicable 7th character codes.

2018 ICD-10-CM

5ᵗʰ **S99.8** Other specified injuries of ankle and foot
The appropriate 7th character is to be added to each code from subcategory S99.8
A = initial encounter
D = subsequent encounter
S = sequela

6ᵗʰ **S99.81** Other specified injuries of ankle
7ᵗʰ **S99.811** Other specified injuries of right ankle POA
7ᵗʰ **S99.812** Other specified injuries of left ankle POA
7ᵗʰ **S99.819** Other specified injuries of unspecified ankle POA

6ᵗʰ **S99.82** Other specified injuries of foot
7ᵗʰ **S99.821** Other specified injuries of right foot POA
7ᵗʰ **S99.822** Other specified injuries of left foot POA
7ᵗʰ **S99.829** Other specified injuries of unspecified foot POA

5ᵗʰ **S99.9** Unspecified injury of ankle and foot
The appropriate 7th character is to be added to each code from subcategory S99.9
A = initial encounter
D = subsequent encounter
S = sequela

6ᵗʰ **S99.91** Unspecified injury of ankle
7ᵗʰ **S99.911** Unspecified injury of right ankle POA
7ᵗʰ **S99.912** Unspecified injury of left ankle POA
7ᵗʰ **S99.919** Unspecified injury of unspecified ankle POA

6ᵗʰ **S99.92** Unspecified injury of foot
7ᵗʰ **S99.921** Unspecified injury of right foot POA
7ᵗʰ **S99.922** Unspecified injury of left foot POA
7ᵗʰ **S99.929** Unspecified injury of unspecified foot POA

Injury, poisoning and certain other consequences of external causes (T07-T88)

Injuries involving multiple body regions (T07)

EXCLUDES1 burns and corrosions (T20-T32)
frostbite (T33-T34)
insect bite or sting, venomous (T63.4)
sunburn (L55.-)

7ᵗʰ **T07** Unspecified multiple injuries   *DO NOT USE CODE*
The appropriate 7th character is to be added to code T07
A = initial encounter
D = subsequent encounter
S = sequela
EXCLUDES1 injury NOS ▶(T14.90)◀

Injury of unspecified body region (T14)

4ᵗʰ **T14** Injury of unspecified body region
The appropriate 7th character is to be added to each code from category T14
A = initial encounter
D = subsequent encounter
S = sequela
EXCLUDES1 multiple unspecified injuries (T07)

7ᵗʰ **T14.8** Other injury of unspecified body region
Abrasion NOS
Contusion NOS
Crush injury NOS
Fracture NOS
Skin injury NOS
Vascular injury NOS
Wound NOS

5ᵗʰ **T14.9** Unspecified injury
7ᵗʰ **T14.90** Injury, unspecified
Injury NOS
7ᵗʰ **T14.91** Suicide attempt   HCC
Attempted suicide NOS

Effects of foreign body entering through natural orifice (T15-T19)

EXCLUDES2 foreign body accidentally left in operation wound (T81.5-)
foreign body in penetrating wound - See open wound by body region
residual foreign body in soft tissue (M79.5)
splinter, without open wound - See superficial injury by body region

4ᵗʰ **T15** Foreign body on external eye
EXCLUDES2 foreign body in penetrating wound of orbit and eye ball (S05.4-, S05.5-)
open wound of eyelid and periocular area (S01.1-)
retained foreign body in eyelid (H02.8-)
retained (old) foreign body in penetrating wound of orbit and eye ball (H05.5-, H44.6-, H44.7-)
superficial foreign body of eyelid and periocular area (S00.25-)

The appropriate 7th character is to be added to each code from category T15
A = initial encounter
D = subsequent encounter
S = sequela

5ᵗʰ **T15.0** Foreign body in cornea
7ᵗʰ **T15.00** Foreign body in cornea, unspecified eye POA
7ᵗʰ **T15.01** Foreign body in cornea, right eye POA
7ᵗʰ **T15.02** Foreign body in cornea, left eye POA

5ᵗʰ **T15.1** Foreign body in conjunctival sac
7ᵗʰ **T15.10** Foreign body in conjunctival sac, unspecified eye POA
7ᵗʰ **T15.11** Foreign body in conjunctival sac, right eye POA
7ᵗʰ **T15.12** Foreign body in conjunctival sac, left eye POA

5ᵗʰ **T15.8** Foreign body in other and multiple parts of external eye
Foreign body in lacrimal punctum
7ᵗʰ **T15.80** Foreign body in other and multiple parts of external eye, unspecified eye POA
7ᵗʰ **T15.81** Foreign body in other and multiple parts of external eye, right eye POA
7ᵗʰ **T15.82** Foreign body in other and multiple parts of external eye, left eye POA

5ᵗʰ **T15.9** Foreign body on external eye, part unspecified
7ᵗʰ **T15.90** Foreign body on external eye, part unspecified, unspecified eye POA
7ᵗʰ **T15.91** Foreign body on external eye, part unspecified, right eye POA
7ᵗʰ **T15.92** Foreign body on external eye, part unspecified, left eye POA

4ᵗʰ **T16** Foreign body in ear
INCLUDES foreign body in auditory canal
The appropriate 7th character is to be added to each code from category T16
A = initial encounter
D = subsequent encounter
S = sequela
7ᵗʰ **T16.1** Foreign body in right ear POA
7ᵗʰ **T16.2** Foreign body in left ear POA
7ᵗʰ **T16.9** Foreign body in ear, unspecified ear POA

4ᵗʰ **T17** Foreign body in respiratory tract
The appropriate 7th character is to be added to each code from category T17
A = initial encounter
D = subsequent encounter
S = sequela
7ᵗʰ **T17.0** Foreign body in nasal sinus POA
7ᵗʰ **T17.1** Foreign body in nostril POA
Foreign body in nose NOS
5ᵗʰ **T17.2** Foreign body in pharynx
Foreign body in nasopharynx
Foreign body in throat NOS
6ᵗʰ **T17.20** Unspecified foreign body in pharynx
7ᵗʰ **T17.200** Unspecified foreign body in pharynx causing asphyxiation POA

Unspecified Code   Other Specified Code   Manifestation Code   N Newborn   P Pediatric   M Maternity   A Adult   ♂ Male   ♀ Female
● New Code   ▲ Revised Code Title   ▶◀ Revised Text   NOTES   INCLUDES   EXCLUDES 1 Not coded here   EXCLUDES 2 Not included here
4ᵗʰ 4th character required   5ᵗʰ 5th character required   6ᵗʰ 6th character required   7ᵗʰ 7th character required
7ᵗʰX Extension 'X' Alert   HAC Hospital-acquired condition (HAC) alert   AHA AHA Coding Clinic©

7️⃣ **T17.208 Unspecified foreign body in pharynx causing other injury** POA

6️⃣ T17.21 Gastric contents in pharynx
- Aspiration of gastric contents into pharynx
- Vomitus in pharynx
  - 7️⃣ T17.210 Gastric contents in pharynx causing asphyxiation POA
  - 7️⃣ T17.218 Gastric contents in pharynx causing other injury POA

6️⃣ T17.22 Food in pharynx
- Bones in pharynx
- Seeds in pharynx
  - 7️⃣ T17.220 Food in pharynx causing asphyxiation POA
  - 7️⃣ T17.228 Food in pharynx causing other injury POA

6️⃣ T17.29 Other foreign object in pharynx
  - 7️⃣ T17.290 Other foreign object in pharynx causing asphyxiation POA
  - 7️⃣ T17.298 Other foreign object in pharynx causing other injury POA

5️⃣ T17.3 Foreign body in larynx
- 6️⃣ T17.30 Unspecified foreign body in larynx
  - 7️⃣ **T17.300 Unspecified foreign body in larynx causing asphyxiation** POA
  - 7️⃣ **T17.308 Unspecified foreign body in larynx causing other injury** POA

6️⃣ T17.31 Gastric contents in larynx
- Aspiration of gastric contents into larynx
- Vomitus in larynx
  - 7️⃣ T17.310 Gastric contents in larynx causing asphyxiation POA
  - 7️⃣ T17.318 Gastric contents in larynx causing other injury POA

6️⃣ T17.32 Food in larynx
- Bones in larynx
- Seeds in larynx
  - 7️⃣ T17.320 Food in larynx causing asphyxiation POA
  - 7️⃣ T17.328 Food in larynx causing other injury POA

6️⃣ T17.39 Other foreign object in larynx
  - 7️⃣ T17.390 Other foreign object in larynx causing asphyxiation POA
  - 7️⃣ T17.398 Other foreign object in larynx causing other injury POA

5️⃣ T17.4 Foreign body in trachea
- 6️⃣ T17.40 Unspecified foreign body in trachea
  - 7️⃣ **T17.400 Unspecified foreign body in trachea causing asphyxiation** CC POA CC/MCC Exc
  - 7️⃣ **T17.408 Unspecified foreign body in trachea causing other injury** CC POA CC/MCC Exc

6️⃣ T17.41 Gastric contents in trachea
- Aspiration of gastric contents into trachea
- Vomitus in trachea
  - 7️⃣ T17.410 Gastric contents in trachea causing asphyxiation CC POA CC/MCC Exc
  - 7️⃣ T17.418 Gastric contents in trachea causing other injury CC POA CC/MCC Exc

6️⃣ T17.42 Food in trachea
- Bones in trachea
- Seeds in trachea
  - 7️⃣ T17.420 Food in trachea causing asphyxiation CC POA CC/MCC Exc
  - 7️⃣ T17.428 Food in trachea causing other injury CC POA CC/MCC Exc

6️⃣ T17.49 Other foreign object in trachea
  - 7️⃣ T17.490 Other foreign object in trachea causing asphyxiation CC POA CC/MCC Exc
  - 7️⃣ T17.498 Other foreign object in trachea causing other injury CC POA CC/MCC Exc

5️⃣ T17.5 Foreign body in bronchus
- 6️⃣ T17.50 Unspecified foreign body in bronchus
  - 7️⃣ **T17.500 Unspecified foreign body in bronchus causing asphyxiation** CC POA CC/MCC Exc

7️⃣ T17.508 Unspecified foreign body in bronchus causing other injury CC POA CC/MCC Exc

6️⃣ T17.51 Gastric contents in bronchus
- Aspiration of gastric contents into bronchus
- Vomitus in bronchus
  - 7️⃣ T17.510 Gastric contents in bronchus causing asphyxiation CC POA CC/MCC Exc
  - 7️⃣ T17.518 Gastric contents in bronchus causing other injury CC POA CC/MCC Exc

6️⃣ T17.52 Food in bronchus
- Bones in bronchus
- Seeds in bronchus
  - 7️⃣ T17.520 Food in bronchus causing asphyxiation CC POA CC/MCC Exc
  - 7️⃣ T17.528 Food in bronchus causing other injury CC POA CC/MCC Exc

6️⃣ T17.59 Other foreign object in bronchus
  - 7️⃣ T17.590 Other foreign object in bronchus causing asphyxiation CC POA CC/MCC Exc
  - 7️⃣ T17.598 Other foreign object in bronchus causing other injury CC POA CC/MCC Exc

5️⃣ T17.8 Foreign body in other parts of respiratory tract
- Foreign body in bronchioles
- Foreign body in lung
  - 6️⃣ T17.80 Unspecified foreign body in other parts of respiratory tract
    - 7️⃣ **T17.800 Unspecified foreign body in other parts of respiratory tract causing asphyxiation** CC POA CC/MCC Exc
    - 7️⃣ **T17.808 Unspecified foreign body in other parts of respiratory tract causing other injury** CC POA CC/MCC Exc

6️⃣ T17.81 Gastric contents in other parts of respiratory tract
- Aspiration of gastric contents into other parts of respiratory tract
- Vomitus in other parts of respiratory tract
  - 7️⃣ T17.810 Gastric contents in other parts of respiratory tract causing asphyxiation CC POA CC/MCC Exc
  - 7️⃣ T17.818 Gastric contents in other parts of respiratory tract causing other injury CC POA CC/MCC Exc

6️⃣ T17.82 Food in other parts of respiratory tract
- Bones in other parts of respiratory tract
- Seeds in other parts of respiratory tract
  - 7️⃣ T17.820 Food in other parts of respiratory tract causing asphyxiation CC POA CC/MCC Exc
  - 7️⃣ T17.828 Food in other parts of respiratory tract causing other injury CC POA CC/MCC Exc

6️⃣ T17.89 Other foreign object in other parts of respiratory tract
  - 7️⃣ T17.890 Other foreign object in other parts of respiratory tract causing asphyxiation CC POA CC/MCC Exc
  - 7️⃣ T17.898 Other foreign object in other parts of respiratory tract causing other injury CC POA CC/MCC Exc

5️⃣ T17.9 Foreign body in respiratory tract, part unspecified
- 6️⃣ T17.90 Unspecified foreign body in respiratory tract, part unspecified
  - 7️⃣ **T17.900 Unspecified foreign body in respiratory tract, part unspecified causing asphyxiation** POA
  - 7️⃣ **T17.908 Unspecified foreign body in respiratory tract, part unspecified causing other injury** POA

6️⃣ T17.91 Gastric contents in respiratory tract, part unspecified
- Aspiration of gastric contents into respiratory tract, part unspecified
- Vomitus in trachea respiratory tract, part unspecified
  - 7️⃣ T17.910 Gastric contents in respiratory tract, part unspecified causing asphyxiation POA

POA Unacceptable principal diagnosis symbol per Medicare code edits   POA Code exempt from diagnosis present on admission requirement
❓ Questionable admission   CC Complication or comorbidity   CC/MCC Exc CC/MCC exclusion   MCC Major complication or comorbidity
Principal diagnosis as its own CC   Principal diagnosis as its own MCC   HCC HCC diagnosis code   RxHCC RxHCC diagnosis code
MACRA code   Z1 Z code as first-listed diagnosis

When symbols appear on a code that requires a 7th character extension, refer to Appendix B to identify applicable 7th character codes.
2018 ICD-10-CM

[7th] T17.918 **Gastric contents in respiratory tract, part unspecified causing other injury** [POA]

[6th] T17.92 **Food in respiratory tract, part unspecified**
Bones in respiratory tract, part unspecified
Seeds in respiratory tract, part unspecified

[7th] T17.920 **Food in respiratory tract, part unspecified causing asphyxiation** [POA]

[7th] T17.928 **Food in respiratory tract, part unspecified causing other injury** [POA]

[6th] T17.99 **Other foreign object in respiratory tract, part unspecified**

[7th] T17.990 **Other foreign object in respiratory tract, part unspecified in causing asphyxiation** [POA]

[7th] T17.998 **Other foreign object in respiratory tract, part unspecified causing other injury** [POA]

[4th] T18 **Foreign body in alimentary tract**
[EXCLUDES2] *foreign body in pharynx (T17.2-)*
The appropriate 7th character is to be added to each code from category T18
A = initial encounter
D = subsequent encounter
S = sequela

[7th] T18.0 **Foreign body in mouth** [POA]

[5th] T18.1 **Foreign body in esophagus**
[EXCLUDES2] *foreign body in respiratory tract (T17.-)*

[6th] T18.10 **Unspecified foreign body in esophagus**

[7th] T18.100 **Unspecified foreign body in esophagus causing compression of trachea** [POA]
Unspecified foreign body in esophagus causing obstruction of respiration

[7th] T18.108 **Unspecified foreign body in esophagus causing other injury** [POA]

[6th] T18.11 **Gastric contents in esophagus**
Vomitus in esophagus

[7th] T18.110 **Gastric contents in esophagus causing compression of trachea** [POA]
Gastric contents in esophagus causing obstruction of respiration

[7th] T18.118 **Gastric contents in esophagus causing other injury** [POA]

[6th] T18.12 **Food in esophagus**
Bones in esophagus
Seeds in esophagus

[7th] T18.120 **Food in esophagus causing compression of trachea** [POA]
Food in esophagus causing obstruction of respiration

[7th] T18.128 **Food in esophagus causing other injury** [POA]

[6th] T18.19 **Other foreign object in esophagus**

[7th] T18.190 **Other foreign object in esophagus causing compression of trachea** [POA]
Other foreign body in esophagus causing obstruction of respiration

[7th] T18.198 **Other foreign object in esophagus causing other injury** [POA]

[7th] T18.2 **Foreign body in stomach** [POA]

[7th] T18.3 **Foreign body in small intestine** [POA]

[7th] T18.4 **Foreign body in colon** [POA]

[7th] T18.5 **Foreign body in anus and rectum** [POA]
Foreign body in rectosigmoid (junction)

[7th] T18.8 **Foreign body in other parts of alimentary tract** [POA]

[7th] T18.9 **Foreign body of alimentary tract, part unspecified** [POA]
Foreign body in digestive system NOS
Swallowed foreign body NOS

[4th] T19 **Foreign body in genitourinary tract**
[EXCLUDES2] *complications due to implanted mesh (T83.7-)*
mechanical complications of contraceptive device (intrauterine) (vaginal) (T83.3-)
presence of contraceptive device (intrauterine) (vaginal) (Z97.5)
The appropriate 7th character is to be added to each code from category T19
A = initial encounter
D = subsequent encounter
S = sequela

[7th] T19.0 **Foreign body in urethra** [POA]

[7th] T19.1 **Foreign body in bladder** [POA]

[7th] T19.2 **Foreign body in vulva and vagina** [POA] ♀

[7th] T19.3 **Foreign body in uterus** [POA] ♀

[7th] T19.4 **Foreign body in penis** [POA] ♂

[7th] T19.8 **Foreign body in other parts of genitourinary tract** [POA]

[7th] T19.9 **Foreign body in genitourinary tract, part unspecified** [POA]

Burns and corrosions (T20-T32)

[INCLUDES] *burns (thermal) from electrical heating appliances*
burns (thermal) from electricity
burns (thermal) from flame
burns (thermal) from friction
burns (thermal) from hot air and hot gases
burns (thermal) from hot objects
burns (thermal) from lightning
burns (thermal) from radiation
chemical burn [corrosion] (external) (internal)
scalds

[EXCLUDES2] *erythema [dermatitis] ab igne (L59.0)*
radiation-related disorders of the skin and subcutaneous tissue (L55-L59)
sunburn (L55.-)

Burns and corrosions of external body surface, specified by site (T20-T25)

[INCLUDES] *burns and corrosions of first degree [erythema]*
burns and corrosions of second degree [blisters][epidermal loss]
burns and corrosions of third degree [deep necrosis of underlying tissue] [full- thickness skin loss]

Use additional code from category T31 or T32 to identify extent of body surface involved

[4th] T20 **Burn and corrosion of head, face, and neck**
[EXCLUDES2] *burn and corrosion of ear drum (T28.41, T28.91)*
burn and corrosion of eye and adnexa (T26.-)
burn and corrosion of mouth and pharynx (T28.0)
The appropriate 7th character is to be added to each code from category T20
A = initial encounter
D = subsequent encounter
S = sequela

[5th] T20.0 **Burn of unspecified degree of head, face, and neck**
Use additional external cause code to identify the source, place and intent of the burn (X00-X19, X75-X77, X96-X98, Y92)

[7th] T20.00 **Burn of unspecified degree of head, face, and neck, unspecified site** [POA]

[6th] T20.01 **Burn of unspecified degree of ear [any part, except ear drum]**
[EXCLUDES2] *burn of ear drum (T28.41-)*

[7th] T20.011 **Burn of unspecified degree of right ear [any part, except ear drum]** [POA]

[7th] T20.012 **Burn of unspecified degree of left ear [any part, except ear drum]** [POA]

[7th] T20.019 **Burn of unspecified degree of unspecified ear [any part, except ear drum]** [POA]

[7th] T20.02 **Burn of unspecified degree of lip(s)** [POA]

[7th] T20.03 **Burn of unspecified degree of chin** [POA]

[7th] T20.04 **Burn of unspecified degree of nose (septum)** [POA]

Unspecified Code Other Specified Code Manifestation Code [N] Newborn [P] Pediatric [M] Maternity [A] Adult ♂ Male ♀ Female
● New Code ▲ Revised Code Title ►◄ Revised Text [NOTES] [INCLUDES] [EXCLUDES1] Not coded here [EXCLUDES2] Not included here
[4th] 4th character required [5th] 5th character required [6th] 6th character required [7th] 7th character required
[X] Extension 'X' Alert [HAC] Hospital-acquired condition (HAC) alert AHA AHA Coding Clinic©

When symbols appear on a code that requires a 7th character extension, refer to Appendix B to identify applicable 7th character codes.

CHAPTER 19: INJURY, POISONING, AND CERTAIN OTHER CONSEQUENCES OF EXTERNAL CAUSES (S00-T88)

T20.05 - T20.67

handwritten notes in left margin:
- if person has multiple burns more location, code highest degree
- a healing burn you code for

T20.05 Burn of unspecified degree of scalp [any part]

T20.06 Burn of unspecified degree of forehead and cheek

T20.07 Burn of unspecified degree of neck

T20.09 Burn of unspecified degree of multiple sites of head, face, and neck

T20.1 Burn of first degree of head, face, and neck
Use additional external cause code to identify the source, place and intent of the burn (X00-X19, X75-X77, X96-X98, Y92)

T20.10 Burn of first degree of head, face, and neck, unspecified site

T20.11 Burn of first degree of ear [any part, except ear drum]
EXCLUDES2 burn of ear drum (T28.41-)

T20.111 Burn of first degree of right ear [any part, except ear drum]

T20.112 Burn of first degree of left ear [any part, except ear drum]

T20.119 Burn of first degree of unspecified ear [any part, except ear drum]

T20.12 Burn of first degree of lip(s)

T20.13 Burn of first degree of chin

T20.14 Burn of first degree of nose (septum)

T20.15 Burn of first degree of scalp [any part]

T20.16 Burn of first degree of forehead and cheek

T20.17 Burn of first degree of neck

T20.19 Burn of first degree of multiple sites of head, face, and neck

T20.2 Burn of second degree of head, face, and neck
Use additional external cause code to identify the source, place and intent of the burn (X00-X19, X75-X77, X96-X98, Y92)

T20.20 Burn of second degree of head, face, and neck, unspecified site

T20.21 Burn of second degree of ear [any part, except ear drum]
EXCLUDES2 burn of ear drum (T28.41-)

T20.211 Burn of second degree of right ear [any part, except ear drum]

T20.212 Burn of second degree of left ear [any part, except ear drum]

T20.219 Burn of second degree of unspecified ear [any part, except ear drum]

T20.22 Burn of second degree of lip(s)

T20.23 Burn of second degree of chin

T20.24 Burn of second degree of nose (septum)

T20.25 Burn of second degree of scalp [any part]

T20.26 Burn of second degree of forehead and cheek

T20.27 Burn of second degree of neck

T20.29 Burn of second degree of multiple sites of head, face, and neck

T20.3 Burn of third degree of head, face, and neck
Use additional external cause code to identify the source, place and intent of the burn (X00-X19, X75-X77, X96-X98, Y92)

T20.30 Burn of third degree of head, face, and neck, unspecified site

T20.31 Burn of third degree of ear [any part, except ear drum]
EXCLUDES2 burn of ear drum (T28.41-)

T20.311 Burn of third degree of right ear [any part, except ear drum]

T20.312 Burn of third degree of left ear [any part, except ear drum]

T20.319 Burn of third degree of unspecified ear [any part, except ear drum]

T20.32 Burn of third degree of lip(s)

T20.33 Burn of third degree of chin

T20.34 Burn of third degree of nose (septum)

T20.35 Burn of third degree of scalp [any part]

T20.36 Burn of third degree of forehead and cheek

T20.37 Burn of third degree of neck

T20.39 Burn of third degree of multiple sites of head, face, and neck

T20.4 Corrosion of unspecified degree of head, face, and neck
Code first (T51-T65) to identify chemical and intent
Use additional external cause code to identify place (Y92)

T20.40 Corrosion of unspecified degree of head, face, and neck, unspecified site

T20.41 Corrosion of unspecified degree of ear [any part, except ear drum]
EXCLUDES2 corrosion of ear drum (T28.91-)

T20.411 Corrosion of unspecified degree of right ear [any part, except ear drum]

T20.412 Corrosion of unspecified degree of left ear [any part, except ear drum]

T20.419 Corrosion of unspecified degree of unspecified ear [any part, except ear drum]

T20.42 Corrosion of unspecified degree of lip(s)

T20.43 Corrosion of unspecified degree of chin

T20.44 Corrosion of unspecified degree of nose (septum)

T20.45 Corrosion of unspecified degree of scalp [any part]

T20.46 Corrosion of unspecified degree of forehead and cheek

T20.47 Corrosion of unspecified degree of neck

T20.49 Corrosion of unspecified degree of multiple sites of head, face, and neck

T20.5 Corrosion of first degree of head, face, and neck
Code first (T51-T65) to identify chemical and intent
Use additional external cause code to identify place (Y92)

T20.50 Corrosion of first degree of head, face, and neck, unspecified site

T20.51 Corrosion of first degree of ear [any part, except ear drum]
EXCLUDES2 corrosion of ear drum (T28.91-)

T20.511 Corrosion of first degree of right ear [any part, except ear drum]

T20.512 Corrosion of first degree of left ear [any part, except ear drum]

T20.519 Corrosion of first degree of unspecified ear [any part, except ear drum]

T20.52 Corrosion of first degree of lip(s)

T20.53 Corrosion of first degree of chin

T20.54 Corrosion of first degree of nose (septum)

T20.55 Corrosion of first degree of scalp [any part]

T20.56 Corrosion of first degree of forehead and cheek

T20.57 Corrosion of first degree of neck

T20.59 Corrosion of first degree of multiple sites of head, face, and neck

T20.6 Corrosion of second degree of head, face, and neck
Code first (T51-T65) to identify chemical and intent
Use additional external cause code to identify place (Y92)

T20.60 Corrosion of second degree of head, face, and neck, unspecified site

T20.61 Corrosion of second degree of ear [any part, except ear drum]
EXCLUDES2 corrosion of ear drum (T28.91-)

T20.611 Corrosion of second degree of right ear [any part, except ear drum]

T20.612 Corrosion of second degree of left ear [any part, except ear drum]

T20.619 Corrosion of second degree of unspecified ear [any part, except ear drum]

T20.62 Corrosion of second degree of lip(s)

T20.63 Corrosion of second degree of chin

T20.64 Corrosion of second degree of nose (septum)

T20.65 Corrosion of second degree of scalp [any part]

T20.66 Corrosion of second degree of forehead and cheek

T20.67 Corrosion of second degree of neck

POA~ Unacceptable principal diagnosis symbol per Medicare code edits   POA Code exempt from diagnosis present on admission requirement
? Questionable admission   cc Complication or comorbidity   CC/MCC Exc CC/MCC exclusion   MCC Major complication or comorbidity
Principal diagnosis as its own CC   Principal diagnosis as its own MCC   HCC HCC diagnosis code   RxHCC RxHCC diagnosis code
MACRA code   Z1 Z code as first-listed diagnosis

[7th] **T20.69** Corrosion of second degree of multiple sites of head, face, and neck POA

[5th] **T20.7** Corrosion of third degree of head, face, and neck
Code first (T51-T65) to identify chemical and intent
Use additional external cause code to identify place (Y92)

[7th] **T20.70** Corrosion of third degree of head, face, and neck, unspecified site CC POA HAC CC/MCC Exc

[6th] **T20.71** Corrosion of third degree of ear [any part, except ear drum]
EXCLUDES2 *corrosion of ear drum (T28.91-)*

[7th] **T20.711** Corrosion of third degree of right ear [any part, except ear drum] CC POA HAC CC/MCC Exc

[7th] **T20.712** Corrosion of third degree of left ear [any part, except ear drum] CC POA HAC CC/MCC Exc

[7th] **T20.719** Corrosion of third degree of unspecified ear [any part, except ear drum] CC POA HAC CC/MCC Exc

[7th] **T20.72** Corrosion of third degree of lip(s) CC POA HAC CC/MCC Exc

[7th] **T20.73** Corrosion of third degree of chin CC POA HAC CC/MCC Exc

[7th] **T20.74** Corrosion of third degree of nose (septum) CC POA HAC CC/MCC Exc

[7th] **T20.75** Corrosion of third degree of scalp [any part] CC POA HAC CC/MCC Exc

[7th] **T20.76** Corrosion of third degree of forehead and cheek CC POA HAC CC/MCC Exc

[7th] **T20.77** Corrosion of third degree of neck CC POA HAC CC/MCC Exc

[7th] **T20.79** Corrosion of third degree of multiple sites of head, face, and neck CC POA HAC CC/MCC Exc

[4th] **T21** Burn and corrosion of trunk
INCLUDES *burns and corrosion of hip region*
EXCLUDES2 *burns and corrosion of axilla (T22.- with fifth character 4)*
burns and corrosion of scapular region (T22.- with fifth character 6)
burns and corrosion of shoulder (T22.- with fifth character 5)

The appropriate 7th character is to be added to each code from category T21
A = initial encounter
D = subsequent encounter
S = sequela

[5th] **T21.0** Burn of unspecified degree of trunk
Use additional external cause code to identify the source, place and intent of the burn (X00-X19, X75-X77, X96-X98, Y92)

[7th] **T21.00** Burn of unspecified degree of trunk, unspecified site POA

[7th] **T21.01** Burn of unspecified degree of chest wall POA
Burn of of unspecified degree of breast

[7th] **T21.02** Burn of unspecified degree of abdominal wall POA
Burn of unspecified degree of flank
Burn of unspecified degree of groin

[7th] **T21.03** Burn of unspecified degree of upper back POA
Burn of unspecified degree of interscapular region

[7th] **T21.04** Burn of unspecified degree of lower back POA

[7th] **T21.05** Burn of unspecified degree of buttock POA
Burn of unspecified degree of anus

[7th] **T21.06** Burn of unspecified degree of male genital region POA ♂
Burn of unspecified degree of penis
Burn of unspecified degree of scrotum
Burn of unspecified degree of testis

[7th] **T21.07** Burn of unspecified degree of female genital region POA ♀
Burn of unspecified degree of labium (majus) (minus)
Burn of unspecified degree of perineum
Burn of unspecified degree of vulva
EXCLUDES2 *burn of vagina (T28.3)*

[7th] **T21.09** Burn of unspecified degree of other site of trunk POA

[5th] **T21.1** Burn of first degree of trunk
Use additional external cause code to identify the source, place and intent of the burn (X00-X19, X75-X77, X96-X98, Y92)

[7th] **T21.10** Burn of first degree of trunk, unspecified site POA

[7th] **T21.11** Burn of first degree of chest wall POA
Burn of first degree of breast

[7th] **T21.12** Burn of first degree of abdominal wall POA
Burn of first degree of flank
Burn of first degree of groin

[7th] **T21.13** Burn of first degree of upper back POA
Burn of first degree of interscapular region

[7th] **T21.14** Burn of first degree of lower back POA

[7th] **T21.15** Burn of first degree of buttock POA
Burn of first degree of anus

[7th] **T21.16** Burn of first degree of male genital region POA ♂
Burn of first degree of penis
Burn of first degree of scrotum
Burn of first degree of testis

[7th] **T21.17** Burn of first degree of female genital region POA ♀
Burn of first degree of labium (majus) (minus)
Burn of first degree of perineum
Burn of first degree of vulva
EXCLUDES2 *burn of vagina (T28.3)*

[7th] **T21.19** Burn of first degree of other site of trunk POA

[5th] **T21.2** Burn of second degree of trunk
Use additional external cause code to identify the source, place and intent of the burn (X00-X19, X75-X77, X96-X98, Y92)

[7th] **T21.20** Burn of second degree of trunk, unspecified site POA

[7th] **T21.21** Burn of second degree of chest wall POA
Burn of second degree of breast

[7th] **T21.22** Burn of second degree of abdominal wall POA
Burn of second degree of flank
Burn of second degree of groin

[7th] **T21.23** Burn of second degree of upper back POA
Burn of second degree of interscapular region

[7th] **T21.24** Burn of second degree of lower back POA

[7th] **T21.25** Burn of second degree of buttock POA
Burn of second degree of anus

[7th] **T21.26** Burn of second degree of male genital region POA ♂
Burn of second degree of penis
Burn of second degree of scrotum
Burn of second degree of testis

[7th] **T21.27** Burn of second degree of female genital region POA ♀
Burn of second degree of labium (majus) (minus)
Burn of second degree of perineum
Burn of second degree of vulva
EXCLUDES2 *burn of vagina (T28.3)*

[7th] **T21.29** Burn of second degree of other site of trunk POA

[5th] **T21.3** Burn of third degree of trunk
Use additional external cause code to identify the source, place and intent of the burn (X00-X19, X75-X77, X96-X98, Y92)

[7th] **T21.30** Burn of third degree of trunk, unspecified site CC POA HAC CC/MCC Exc

[7th] **T21.31** Burn of third degree of chest wall CC POA HAC CC/MCC Exc
Burn of third degree of breast

[7th] **T21.32** Burn of third degree of abdominal wall CC POA HAC CC/MCC Exc
Burn of third degree of flank
Burn of third degree of groin

[7th] **T21.33** Burn of third degree of upper back CC POA HAC CC/MCC Exc
Burn of third degree of interscapular region

[7th] **T21.34** Burn of third degree of lower back CC POA HAC CC/MCC Exc

[7th] **T21.35** Burn of third degree of buttock CC POA HAC CC/MCC Exc
Burn of third degree of anus

[7th] **T21.36** Burn of third degree of male genital region CC POA HAC ♂ CC/MCC Exc
Burn of third degree of penis
Burn of third degree of scrotum
Burn of third degree of testis

[7th] **T21.37** Burn of third degree of female genital region CC POA HAC ♀ CC/MCC Exc
Burn of third degree of labium (majus) (minus)
Burn of third degree of perineum
Burn of third degree of vulva
EXCLUDES2 *burn of vagina (T28.3)*

[7th] **T21.39** Burn of third degree of other site of trunk CC POA HAC CC/MCC Exc

Unspecified Code   Other Specified Code   Manifestation Code   [N] Newborn   [P] Pediatric   [M] Maternity   [A] Adult   ♂ Male   ♀ Female
● New Code   ▲ Revised Code Title   ►◄ Revised Text   NOTES   INCLUDES   EXCLUDES1 Not coded here   EXCLUDES2 Not included here
[4th] 4th character required   [5th] 5th character required   [6th] 6th character required   [7th] 7th character required
[7th] Extension 'X' Alert   HAC Hospital-acquired condition (HAC) alert   AHA AHA Coding Clinic©

T21.4 **Corrosion of** unspecified degree **of trunk**
　　Code first (T51-T65) to identify chemical and intent
　　Use additional external cause code to identify place (Y92)

　　T21.40 **Corrosion of unspecified degree of trunk, unspecified site** POA

　　T21.41 **Corrosion of unspecified degree of** chest wall POA
　　　　Corrosion of unspecified degree of breast

　　T21.42 **Corrosion of unspecified degree of** abdominal wall POA
　　　　Corrosion of unspecified degree of flank
　　　　Corrosion of unspecified degree of groin

　　T21.43 **Corrosion of unspecified degree of** upper back POA
　　　　Corrosion of unspecified degree of interscapular region

　　T21.44 **Corrosion of unspecified degree of** lower back POA

　　T21.45 **Corrosion of unspecified degree of** buttock POA
　　　　Corrosion of unspecified degree of anus

　　T21.46 **Corrosion of unspecified degree of** male genital region POA ♂
　　　　Corrosion of unspecified degree of penis
　　　　Corrosion of unspecified degree of scrotum
　　　　Corrosion of unspecified degree of testis

　　T21.47 **Corrosion of unspecified degree of** female genital region POA ♀
　　　　Corrosion of unspecified degree of labium (majus) (minus)
　　　　Corrosion of unspecified degree of perineum
　　　　Corrosion of unspecified degree of vulva
　　　　EXCLUDES2 corrosion of vagina (T28.8)

　　T21.49 **Corrosion of unspecified degree of other site of trunk** POA

T21.5 **Corrosion of** first degree **of trunk**
　　Code first (T51-T65) to identify chemical and intent
　　Use additional external cause code to identify place (Y92)

　　T21.50 **Corrosion of first degree of trunk, unspecified site** POA

　　T21.51 **Corrosion of first degree of** chest wall POA
　　　　Corrosion of first degree of breast

　　T21.52 **Corrosion of first degree of** abdominal wall POA
　　　　Corrosion of first degree of flank
　　　　Corrosion of first degree of groin

　　T21.53 **Corrosion of first degree of** upper back POA
　　　　Corrosion of first degree of interscapular region

　　T21.54 **Corrosion of first degree of** lower back POA

　　T21.55 **Corrosion of first degree of** buttock POA
　　　　Corrosion of first degree of anus

　　T21.56 **Corrosion of first degree of** male genital region POA ♂
　　　　Corrosion of first degree of penis
　　　　Corrosion of first degree of scrotum
　　　　Corrosion of first degree of testis

　　T21.57 **Corrosion of first degree of** female genital region POA ♀
　　　　Corrosion of first degree of labium (majus) (minus)
　　　　Corrosion of first degree of perineum
　　　　Corrosion of first degree of vulva
　　　　EXCLUDES2 corrosion of vagina (T28.8)

　　T21.59 **Corrosion of first degree of other site of trunk** POA

T21.6 **Corrosion of** second degree **of trunk**
　　Code first (T51-T65) to identify chemical and intent
　　Use additional external cause code to identify place (Y92)

　　T21.60 **Corrosion of second degree of trunk, unspecified site** POA

　　T21.61 **Corrosion of second degree of** chest wall POA
　　　　Corrosion of second degree of breast

　　T21.62 **Corrosion of second degree of** abdominal wall POA
　　　　Corrosion of second degree of flank
　　　　Corrosion of second degree of groin

　　T21.63 **Corrosion of second degree of** upper back POA
　　　　Corrosion of second degree of interscapular region

　　T21.64 **Corrosion of second degree of** lower back POA

　　T21.65 **Corrosion of second degree of** buttock POA
　　　　Corrosion of second degree of anus

　　T21.66 **Corrosion of second degree of** male genital region POA ♂
　　　　Corrosion of second degree of penis
　　　　Corrosion of second degree of scrotum
　　　　Corrosion of second degree of testis

　　T21.67 **Corrosion of second degree of female genital region** POA ♀
　　　　Corrosion of second degree of labium (majus) (minus)
　　　　Corrosion of second degree of perineum
　　　　Corrosion of second degree of vulva
　　　　EXCLUDES2 corrosion of vagina (T28.8)

　　T21.69 **Corrosion of second degree of other site of trunk** POA

T21.7 **Corrosion of** third degree **of trunk**
　　Code first (T51-T65) to identify chemical and intent
　　Use additional external cause code to identify place (Y92)

　　T21.70 **Corrosion of third degree of trunk, unspecified site** CC POA HAC CC/MCC Exc

　　T21.71 **Corrosion of third degree of** chest wall CC POA HAC CC/MCC Exc
　　　　Corrosion of third degree of breast

　　T21.72 **Corrosion of third degree of** abdominal wall CC POA HAC CC/MCC Exc
　　　　Corrosion of third degree of flank
　　　　Corrosion of third degree of groin

　　T21.73 **Corrosion of third degree of** upper back CC POA HAC CC/MCC Exc
　　　　Corrosion of third degree of interscapular region

　　T21.74 **Corrosion of third degree of** lower back CC POA HAC CC/MCC Exc

　　T21.75 **Corrosion of third degree of** buttock CC POA HAC CC/MCC Exc
　　　　Corrosion of third degree of anus

　　T21.76 **Corrosion of third degree of male genital region** CC POA HAC ♂ CC/MCC Exc
　　　　Corrosion of third degree of penis
　　　　Corrosion of third degree of scrotum
　　　　Corrosion of third degree of testis

　　T21.77 **Corrosion of third degree of female genital region** CC POA HAC ♀ CC/MCC Exc
　　　　Corrosion of third degree of labium (majus) (minus)
　　　　Corrosion of third degree of perineum
　　　　Corrosion of third degree of vulva
　　　　EXCLUDES2 corrosion of vagina (T28.8)

　　T21.79 **Corrosion of third degree of other site of trunk** CC POA HAC CC/MCC Exc

T22 **Burn and corrosion of shoulder and upper limb, except wrist and hand**
　　EXCLUDES2 burn and corrosion of interscapular region (T21.-)
　　　　　　　burn and corrosion of wrist and hand (T23.-)

　　The appropriate 7th character is to be added to each code from category T22
　　　　A = initial encounter
　　　　D = subsequent encounter
　　　　S = sequela

T22.0 **Burn of** unspecified degree **of shoulder and upper limb, except wrist and hand**
　　Use additional external cause code to identify the source, place and intent of the burn (X00-X19, X75-X77, X96-X98, Y92)

　　T22.00 **Burn of unspecified degree of shoulder and upper limb, except wrist and hand, unspecified site** POA

　　T22.01 **Burn of unspecified degree of** forearm

　　　　T22.011 **Burn of unspecified degree of** right forearm POA

　　　　T22.012 **Burn of unspecified degree of** left forearm POA

　　　　T22.019 **Burn of unspecified degree of unspecified forearm** POA

　　T22.02 **Burn of unspecified degree of** elbow

　　　　T22.021 **Burn of unspecified degree of** right elbow POA

　　　　T22.022 **Burn of unspecified degree of left elbow** POA

POA Unacceptable principal diagnosis symbol per Medicare code edits　　POA Code exempt from diagnosis present on admission requirement
? Questionable admission　　CC Complication or comorbidity　　CC/MCC Exc CC/MCC exclusion　　MCC Major complication or comorbidity
CC Principal diagnosis as its own CC　　MCC Principal diagnosis as its own MCC　　HCC HCC diagnosis code　　RxHCC RxHCC diagnosis code
MACRA code　　Z Z code as first-listed diagnosis

6ᵗ T22.029 Burn of unspecified degree of unspecified elbow POA

6ᵗ T22.03 Burn of unspecified degree of upper arm
   7ᵗ T22.031 Burn of unspecified degree of right upper arm POA
   7ᵗ T22.032 Burn of unspecified degree of left upper arm POA
   7ᵗ T22.039 Burn of unspecified degree of unspecified upper arm POA

6ᵗ T22.04 Burn of unspecified degree of axilla
   7ᵗ T22.041 Burn of unspecified degree of right axilla POA
   7ᵗ T22.042 Burn of unspecified degree of left axilla POA
   7ᵗ T22.049 Burn of unspecified degree of unspecified axilla POA

6ᵗ T22.05 Burn of unspecified degree of shoulder
   7ᵗ T22.051 Burn of unspecified degree of right shoulder POA
   7ᵗ T22.052 Burn of unspecified degree of left shoulder POA
   7ᵗ T22.059 Burn of unspecified degree of unspecified shoulder POA

6ᵗ T22.06 Burn of unspecified degree of scapular region
   7ᵗ T22.061 Burn of unspecified degree of right scapular region POA
   7ᵗ T22.062 Burn of unspecified degree of left scapular region POA
   7ᵗ T22.069 Burn of unspecified degree of unspecified scapular region POA

6ᵗ T22.09 Burn of unspecified degree of multiple sites of shoulder and upper limb, except wrist and hand
   7ᵗ T22.091 Burn of unspecified degree of multiple sites of right shoulder and upper limb, except wrist and hand POA
   7ᵗ T22.092 Burn of unspecified degree of multiple sites of left shoulder and upper limb, except wrist and hand POA
   7ᵗ T22.099 Burn of unspecified degree of multiple sites of unspecified shoulder and upper limb, except wrist and hand POA

5ᵗ T22.1 Burn of first degree of shoulder and upper limb, except wrist and hand
Use additional external cause code to identify the source, place and intent of the burn (X00-X19, X75-X77, X96-X98, Y92)
   7ᵗ T22.10 Burn of first degree of shoulder and upper limb, except wrist and hand, unspecified site POA

6ᵗ T22.11 Burn of first degree of forearm
   7ᵗ T22.111 Burn of first degree of right forearm POA
   7ᵗ T22.112 Burn of first degree of left forearm POA
   7ᵗ T22.119 Burn of first degree of unspecified forearm POA

6ᵗ T22.12 Burn of first degree of elbow
   7ᵗ T22.121 Burn of first degree of right elbow POA
   7ᵗ T22.122 Burn of first degree of left elbow POA
   7ᵗ T22.129 Burn of first degree of unspecified elbow POA

6ᵗ T22.13 Burn of first degree of upper arm
   7ᵗ T22.131 Burn of first degree of right upper arm POA
   7ᵗ T22.132 Burn of first degree of left upper arm POA
   7ᵗ T22.139 Burn of first degree of unspecified upper arm POA

6ᵗ T22.14 Burn of first degree of axilla
   7ᵗ T22.141 Burn of first degree of right axilla POA
   7ᵗ T22.142 Burn of first degree of left axilla POA
   7ᵗ T22.149 Burn of first degree of unspecified axilla POA

6ᵗ T22.15 Burn of first degree of shoulder
   7ᵗ T22.151 Burn of first degree of right shoulder POA
   7ᵗ T22.152 Burn of first degree of left shoulder POA
   7ᵗ T22.159 Burn of first degree of unspecified shoulder POA

6ᵗ T22.16 Burn of first degree of scapular region
   7ᵗ T22.161 Burn of first degree of right scapular region POA
   7ᵗ T22.162 Burn of first degree of left scapular region POA
   7ᵗ T22.169 Burn of first degree of unspecified scapular region POA

6ᵗ T22.19 Burn of first degree of multiple sites of shoulder and upper limb, except wrist and hand
   7ᵗ T22.191 Burn of first degree of multiple sites of right shoulder and upper limb, except wrist and hand POA
   7ᵗ T22.192 Burn of first degree of multiple sites of left shoulder and upper limb, except wrist and hand POA
   7ᵗ T22.199 Burn of first degree of multiple sites of unspecified shoulder and upper limb, except wrist and hand POA

5ᵗ T22.2 Burn of second degree of shoulder and upper limb, except wrist and hand
Use additional external cause code to identify the source, place and intent of the burn (X00-X19, X75-X77, X96-X98, Y92)
   7ᵗ T22.20 Burn of second degree of shoulder and upper limb, except wrist and hand, unspecified site POA

6ᵗ T22.21 Burn of second degree of forearm
   7ᵗ T22.211 Burn of second degree of right forearm POA
   7ᵗ T22.212 Burn of second degree of left forearm POA
   7ᵗ T22.219 Burn of second degree of unspecified forearm POA

6ᵗ T22.22 Burn of second degree of elbow
   7ᵗ T22.221 Burn of second degree of right elbow POA
   7ᵗ T22.222 Burn of second degree of left elbow POA
   7ᵗ T22.229 Burn of second degree of unspecified elbow POA

6ᵗ T22.23 Burn of second degree of upper arm
   7ᵗ T22.231 Burn of second degree of right upper arm POA
   7ᵗ T22.232 Burn of second degree of left upper arm POA
   7ᵗ T22.239 Burn of second degree of unspecified upper arm POA

6ᵗ T22.24 Burn of second degree of axilla
   7ᵗ T22.241 Burn of second degree of right axilla POA
   7ᵗ T22.242 Burn of second degree of left axilla POA
   7ᵗ T22.249 Burn of second degree of unspecified axilla POA

6ᵗ T22.25 Burn of second degree of shoulder
   7ᵗ T22.251 Burn of second degree of right shoulder POA
   7ᵗ T22.252 Burn of second degree of left shoulder POA
   7ᵗ T22.259 Burn of second degree of unspecified shoulder POA

6ᵗ T22.26 Burn of second degree of scapular region
   7ᵗ T22.261 Burn of second degree of right scapular region POA
   7ᵗ T22.262 Burn of second degree of left scapular region POA
   7ᵗ T22.269 Burn of second degree of unspecified scapular region POA

6ᵗ T22.29 Burn of second degree of multiple sites of shoulder and upper limb, except wrist and hand
   7ᵗ T22.291 Burn of second degree of multiple sites of right shoulder and upper limb, except wrist and hand POA
   7ᵗ T22.292 Burn of second degree of multiple sites of left shoulder and upper limb, except wrist and hand POA
   7ᵗ T22.299 Burn of second degree of multiple sites of unspecified shoulder and upper limb, except wrist and hand POA

Unspecified Code   Other Specified Code   Manifestation Code   N Newborn   P Pediatric   M Maternity   A Adult   ♂ Male   ♀ Female
● New Code   ▲ Revised Code Title   ▶◀ Revised Text   NOTES   INCLUDES   EXCLUDES 1 Not coded here   EXCLUDES 2 Not included here
4ᵗ 4th character required   5ᵗ 5th character required   6ᵗ 6th character required   7ᵗ 7th character required
7ᵗ Extension 'X' Alert   HAC Hospital-acquired condition (HAC) alert   AHA AHA Coding Clinic©

T22.3 Burn of third degree of shoulder and upper limb, except wrist and hand
Use additional external cause code to identify the source, place and intent of the burn (X00-X19, X75-X77, X96-X98, Y92)

T22.30 Burn of third degree of shoulder and upper limb, except wrist and hand, unspecified site

T22.31 Burn of third degree of forearm
T22.311 Burn of third degree of right forearm
T22.312 Burn of third degree of left forearm
T22.319 Burn of third degree of unspecified forearm

T22.32 Burn of third degree of elbow
T22.321 Burn of third degree of right elbow
T22.322 Burn of third degree of left elbow
T22.329 Burn of third degree of unspecified elbow

T22.33 Burn of third degree of upper arm
T22.331 Burn of third degree of right upper arm
T22.332 Burn of third degree of left upper arm
T22.339 Burn of third degree of unspecified upper arm

T22.34 Burn of third degree of axilla
T22.341 Burn of third degree of right axilla
T22.342 Burn of third degree of left axilla
T22.349 Burn of third degree of unspecified axilla

T22.35 Burn of third degree of shoulder
T22.351 Burn of third degree of right shoulder
T22.352 Burn of third degree of left shoulder
T22.359 Burn of third degree of unspecified shoulder

T22.36 Burn of third degree of scapular region
T22.361 Burn of third degree of right scapular region
T22.362 Burn of third degree of left scapular region
T22.369 Burn of third degree of unspecified scapular region

T22.39 Burn of third degree of multiple sites of shoulder and upper limb, except wrist and hand
T22.391 Burn of third degree of multiple sites of right shoulder and upper limb, except wrist and hand
T22.392 Burn of third degree of multiple sites of left shoulder and upper limb, except wrist and hand
T22.399 Burn of third degree of multiple sites of unspecified shoulder and upper limb, except wrist and hand

T22.4 Corrosion of unspecified degree of shoulder and upper limb, except wrist and hand
Code first (T51-T65) to identify chemical and intent
Use additional external cause code to identify place (Y92)

T22.40 Corrosion of unspecified degree of shoulder and upper limb, except wrist and hand, unspecified site

T22.41 Corrosion of unspecified degree of forearm
T22.411 Corrosion of unspecified degree of right forearm
T22.412 Corrosion of unspecified degree of left forearm

T22.419 Corrosion of unspecified degree of unspecified forearm

T22.42 Corrosion of unspecified degree of elbow
T22.421 Corrosion of unspecified degree of right elbow
T22.422 Corrosion of unspecified degree of left elbow
T22.429 Corrosion of unspecified degree of unspecified elbow

T22.43 Corrosion of unspecified degree of upper arm
T22.431 Corrosion of unspecified degree of right upper arm
T22.432 Corrosion of unspecified degree of left upper arm
T22.439 Corrosion of unspecified degree of unspecified upper arm

T22.44 Corrosion of unspecified degree of axilla
T22.441 Corrosion of unspecified degree of right axilla
T22.442 Corrosion of unspecified degree of left axilla
T22.449 Corrosion of unspecified degree of unspecified axilla

T22.45 Corrosion of unspecified degree of shoulder
T22.451 Corrosion of unspecified degree of right shoulder
T22.452 Corrosion of unspecified degree of left shoulder
T22.459 Corrosion of unspecified degree of unspecified shoulder

T22.46 Corrosion of unspecified degree of scapular region
T22.461 Corrosion of unspecified degree of right scapular region
T22.462 Corrosion of unspecified degree of left scapular region
T22.469 Corrosion of unspecified degree of unspecified scapular region

T22.49 Corrosion of unspecified degree of multiple sites of shoulder and upper limb, except wrist and hand
T22.491 Corrosion of unspecified degree of multiple sites of right shoulder and upper limb, except wrist and hand
T22.492 Corrosion of unspecified degree of multiple sites of left shoulder and upper limb, except wrist and hand
T22.499 Corrosion of unspecified degree of multiple sites of unspecified shoulder and upper limb, except wrist and hand

T22.5 Corrosion of first degree of shoulder and upper limb, except wrist and hand
Code first (T51-T65) to identify chemical and intent
Use additional external cause code to identify place (Y92)

T22.50 Corrosion of first degree of shoulder and upper limb, except wrist and hand unspecified site

T22.51 Corrosion of first degree of forearm
T22.511 Corrosion of first degree of right forearm
T22.512 Corrosion of first degree of left forearm
T22.519 Corrosion of first degree of unspecified forearm

T22.52 Corrosion of first degree of elbow
T22.521 Corrosion of first degree of right elbow
T22.522 Corrosion of first degree of left elbow
T22.529 Corrosion of first degree of unspecified elbow

T22.53 Corrosion of first degree of upper arm
T22.531 Corrosion of first degree of right upper arm
T22.532 Corrosion of first degree of left upper arm
T22.539 Corrosion of first degree of unspecified upper arm

POA̸ Unacceptable principal diagnosis symbol per Medicare code edits   POA̸ Code exempt from diagnosis present on admission requirement
❓ Questionable admission   ᴄᴄ Complication or comorbidity   ᴄᴄ/ᴍᴄᴄ ᴇˣᶜ CC/MCC exclusion   ᴍᴄᴄ Major complication or comorbidity
Principal diagnosis as its own CC   Principal diagnosis as its own MCC   ʜᴄᴄ HCC diagnosis code   ʀₓʜᴄᴄ RxHCC diagnosis code
MACRA code   Z1 Z code as first-listed diagnosis

1110   When symbols appear on a code that requires a 7th character extension, refer to Appendix B to identify applicable 7th character codes.   **2018 ICD-10-CM**

6th T22.54 Corrosion of first degree of axilla
   7th T22.541 Corrosion of first degree of right axilla POA
   7th T22.542 Corrosion of first degree of left axilla POA
   7th T22.549 **Corrosion of first degree of unspecified axilla** POA

6th T22.55 Corrosion of first degree of shoulder
   7th T22.551 Corrosion of first degree of right shoulder POA
   7th T22.552 Corrosion of first degree of left shoulder POA
   7th T22.559 **Corrosion of first degree of unspecified shoulder** POA

6th T22.56 Corrosion of first degree of scapular region
   7th T22.561 Corrosion of first degree of right scapular region POA
   7th T22.562 Corrosion of first degree of left scapular region POA
   7th T22.569 **Corrosion of first degree of unspecified scapular region** POA

6th T22.59 Corrosion of first degree of multiple sites of shoulder and upper limb, except wrist and hand
   7th T22.591 Corrosion of first degree of multiple sites of right shoulder and upper limb, except wrist and hand POA
   7th T22.592 Corrosion of first degree of multiple sites of left shoulder and upper limb, except wrist and hand POA
   7th T22.599 **Corrosion of first degree of multiple sites of unspecified shoulder and upper limb, except wrist and hand** POA

5th T22.6 Corrosion of second degree of shoulder and upper limb, except wrist and hand
   Code first (T51-T65) to identify chemical and intent
   Use additional external cause code to identify place (Y92)
  7th T22.60 **Corrosion of second degree of shoulder and upper limb, except wrist and hand, unspecified site** POA
  6th T22.61 Corrosion of second degree of forearm
   7th T22.611 Corrosion of second degree of right forearm POA
   7th T22.612 Corrosion of second degree of left forearm POA
   7th T22.619 **Corrosion of second degree of unspecified forearm** POA
  6th T22.62 Corrosion of second degree of elbow
   7th T22.621 Corrosion of second degree of right elbow POA
   7th T22.622 Corrosion of second degree of left elbow POA
   7th T22.629 **Corrosion of second degree of unspecified elbow** POA
  6th T22.63 Corrosion of second degree of upper arm
   7th T22.631 Corrosion of second degree of right upper arm POA
   7th T22.632 Corrosion of second degree of left upper arm POA
   7th T22.639 **Corrosion of second degree of unspecified upper arm** POA
  6th T22.64 Corrosion of second degree of axilla
   7th T22.641 Corrosion of second degree of right axilla POA
   7th T22.642 Corrosion of second degree of left axilla POA
   7th T22.649 **Corrosion of second degree of unspecified axilla** POA
  6th T22.65 Corrosion of second degree of shoulder
   7th T22.651 Corrosion of second degree of right shoulder POA
   7th T22.652 Corrosion of second degree of left shoulder POA
   7th T22.659 **Corrosion of second degree of unspecified shoulder** POA
  6th T22.66 Corrosion of second degree of scapular region
   7th T22.661 Corrosion of second degree of right scapular region POA

6th T22.662 Corrosion of second degree of left scapular region POA
   7th T22.669 **Corrosion of second degree of unspecified scapular region** POA

6th T22.69 Corrosion of second degree of multiple sites of shoulder and upper limb, except wrist and hand
   7th T22.691 Corrosion of second degree of multiple sites of right shoulder and upper limb, except wrist and hand POA
   7th T22.692 Corrosion of second degree of multiple sites of left shoulder and upper limb, except wrist and hand POA
   7th T22.699 **Corrosion of second degree of multiple sites of unspecified shoulder and upper limb, except wrist and hand** POA

5th T22.7 Corrosion of third degree of shoulder and upper limb, except wrist and hand
   Code first (T51-T65) to identify chemical and intent
   Use additional external cause code to identify place (Y92)
  7th T22.70 **Corrosion of third degree of shoulder and upper limb, except wrist and hand, unspecified site** CC POA HAC CC/MCC Exc
  6th T22.71 Corrosion of third degree of forearm
   7th T22.711 Corrosion of third degree of right forearm CC POA HAC CC/MCC Exc
   7th T22.712 Corrosion of third degree of left forearm CC POA HAC CC/MCC Exc
   7th T22.719 **Corrosion of third degree of unspecified forearm** CC POA HAC CC/MCC Exc
  6th T22.72 Corrosion of third degree of elbow
   7th T22.721 Corrosion of third degree of right elbow CC POA HAC CC/MCC Exc
   7th T22.722 Corrosion of third degree of left elbow CC POA HAC CC/MCC Exc
   7th T22.729 **Corrosion of third degree of unspecified elbow** CC POA HAC CC/MCC Exc
  6th T22.73 Corrosion of third degree of upper arm
   7th T22.731 Corrosion of third degree of right upper arm CC POA HAC CC/MCC Exc
   7th T22.732 Corrosion of third degree of left upper arm CC POA HAC CC/MCC Exc
   7th T22.739 **Corrosion of third degree of unspecified upper arm** CC POA HAC CC/MCC Exc
  6th T22.74 Corrosion of third degree of axilla
   7th T22.741 Corrosion of third degree of right axilla CC POA HAC CC/MCC Exc
   7th T22.742 Corrosion of third degree of left axilla CC POA HAC CC/MCC Exc
   7th T22.749 **Corrosion of third degree of unspecified axilla** CC POA HAC CC/MCC Exc
  6th T22.75 Corrosion of third degree of shoulder
   7th T22.751 Corrosion of third degree of right shoulder CC POA HAC CC/MCC Exc
   7th T22.752 Corrosion of third degree of left shoulder CC POA HAC CC/MCC Exc
   7th T22.759 **Corrosion of third degree of unspecified shoulder** CC POA HAC CC/MCC Exc
  6th T22.76 Corrosion of third degree of scapular region
   7th T22.761 Corrosion of third degree of right scapular region CC POA HAC CC/MCC Exc
   7th T22.762 Corrosion of third degree of left scapular region CC POA HAC CC/MCC Exc
   7th T22.769 **Corrosion of third degree of unspecified scapular region** CC POA HAC CC/MCC Exc
  6th T22.79 Corrosion of third degree of multiple sites of shoulder and upper limb, except wrist and hand
   7th T22.791 Corrosion of third degree of multiple sites of right shoulder and upper limb, except wrist and hand CC POA HAC CC/MCC Exc
   7th T22.792 Corrosion of third degree of multiple sites of left shoulder and upper limb, except wrist and hand CC POA HAC CC/MCC Exc

---

Unspecified Code Other Specified Code Manifestation Code N Newborn P Pediatric M Maternity A Adult ♂ Male ♀ Female
● New Code ▲ Revised Code Title ▶◀ Revised Text NOTES INCLUDES EXCLUDES 1 Not coded here EXCLUDES 2 Not included here
4th 4th character required 5th 5th character required 6th 6th character required 7th 7th character required
7th Extension 'X' Alert HAC Hospital-acquired condition (HAC) alert AHA AHA Coding Clinic©

T22.799 **Corrosion of third degree of multiple sites of unspecified shoulder and upper limb, except wrist and hand** POA HAC CC/MCC Exc

T23 **Burn and corrosion of wrist and hand**
The appropriate 7th character is to be added to each code from category T23
A = initial encounter
D = subsequent encounter
S = sequela

T23.0 **Burn of** unspecified degree **of wrist and hand**
Use additional external cause code to identify the source, place and intent of the burn (X00-X19, X75-X77, X96-X98, Y92)

T23.00 **Burn of unspecified degree of hand,** unspecified site
T23.001 **Burn of unspecified degree of** right **hand, unspecified site** POA
T23.002 **Burn of unspecified degree of** left **hand, unspecified site** POA
T23.009 **Burn of unspecified degree of unspecified hand, unspecified site** POA

T23.01 **Burn of unspecified degree of** thumb (nail)
T23.011 **Burn of unspecified degree of** right **thumb (nail)** POA
T23.012 **Burn of unspecified degree of** left **thumb (nail)** POA
T23.019 **Burn of unspecified degree of unspecified thumb (nail)** POA

T23.02 **Burn of unspecified degree of** single finger (nail) except thumb
T23.021 **Burn of unspecified degree of single** right **finger (nail) except thumb** POA
T23.022 **Burn of unspecified degree of single** left **finger (nail) except thumb** POA
T23.029 **Burn of unspecified degree of unspecified single finger (nail) except thumb** POA

T23.03 **Burn of unspecified degree of** multiple fingers (nail), not including thumb
T23.031 **Burn of unspecified degree of multiple** right **fingers (nail), not including thumb** POA
T23.032 **Burn of unspecified degree of multiple** left **fingers (nail), not including thumb** POA
T23.039 **Burn of unspecified degree of unspecified multiple fingers (nail), not including thumb** POA

T23.04 **Burn of unspecified degree of** multiple fingers (nail), including thumb
T23.041 **Burn of unspecified degree of multiple** right **fingers (nail), including thumb** POA
T23.042 **Burn of unspecified degree of multiple** left **fingers (nail), including thumb** POA
T23.049 **Burn of unspecified degree of unspecified multiple fingers (nail), including thumb** POA

T23.05 **Burn of unspecified degree of** palm
T23.051 **Burn of unspecified degree of** right **palm** POA
T23.052 **Burn of unspecified degree of** left **palm** POA
T23.059 **Burn of unspecified degree of unspecified palm** POA

T23.06 **Burn of unspecified degree of** back of hand
T23.061 **Burn of unspecified degree of back of** right **hand** POA
T23.062 **Burn of unspecified degree of back of** left **hand** POA
T23.069 **Burn of unspecified degree of back of unspecified hand** POA

T23.07 **Burn of unspecified degree of** wrist
T23.071 **Burn of unspecified degree of** right **wrist** POA
T23.072 **Burn of unspecified degree of** left **wrist** POA
T23.079 **Burn of unspecified degree of unspecified wrist** POA

T23.09 **Burn of unspecified degree of** multiple sites **of wrist and hand**

T23.091 **Burn of unspecified degree of multiple sites of** right **wrist and hand** POA
T23.092 **Burn of unspecified degree of multiple sites of** left **wrist and hand** POA
T23.099 **Burn of unspecified degree of multiple sites of unspecified wrist and hand** POA

T23.1 **Burn of** first degree **of wrist and hand**
Use additional external cause code to identify the source, place and intent of the burn (X00-X19, X75-X77, X96-X98, Y92)

T23.10 **Burn of first degree of hand,** unspecified site
T23.101 **Burn of first degree of** right **hand, unspecified site** POA
T23.102 **Burn of first degree of** left **hand, unspecified site** POA
T23.109 **Burn of first degree of unspecified hand, unspecified site** POA

T23.11 **Burn of first degree of** thumb (nail)
T23.111 **Burn of first degree of** right **thumb (nail)** POA
T23.112 **Burn of first degree of** left **thumb (nail)** POA
T23.119 **Burn of first degree of unspecified thumb (nail)** POA

T23.12 **Burn of first degree of** single finger (nail) except thumb
T23.121 **Burn of first degree of single** right **finger (nail) except thumb** POA
T23.122 **Burn of first degree of single** left **finger (nail) except thumb** POA
T23.129 **Burn of first degree of unspecified single finger (nail) except thumb** POA

T23.13 **Burn of first degree of** multiple fingers (nail), not including thumb
T23.131 **Burn of first degree of multiple** right **fingers (nail), not including thumb** POA
T23.132 **Burn of first degree of multiple** left **fingers (nail), not including thumb** POA
T23.139 **Burn of first degree of unspecified multiple fingers (nail), not including thumb** POA

T23.14 **Burn of first degree of** multiple fingers (nail), including thumb
T23.141 **Burn of first degree of multiple** right **fingers (nail), including thumb** POA
T23.142 **Burn of first degree of multiple** left **fingers (nail), including thumb** POA
T23.149 **Burn of first degree of unspecified multiple fingers (nail), including thumb** POA

T23.15 **Burn of first degree of** palm
T23.151 **Burn of first degree of** right **palm** POA
T23.152 **Burn of first degree of** left **palm** POA
T23.159 **Burn of first degree of unspecified palm** POA

T23.16 **Burn of first degree of** back of hand
T23.161 **Burn of first degree of back of** right **hand** POA
T23.162 **Burn of first degree of back of** left **hand** POA
T23.169 **Burn of first degree of back of unspecified hand** POA

T23.17 **Burn of first degree of** wrist
T23.171 **Burn of first degree of** right **wrist** POA
T23.172 **Burn of first degree of** left **wrist** POA
T23.179 **Burn of first degree of unspecified wrist** POA

T23.19 **Burn of first degree of** multiple sites of wrist and hand
T23.191 **Burn of first degree of multiple sites of** right **wrist and hand** POA
T23.192 **Burn of first degree of multiple sites of** left **wrist and hand** POA
T23.199 **Burn of first degree of multiple sites of unspecified wrist and hand** POA

T23.2 **Burn of** second degree **of wrist and hand**
Use additional external cause code to identify the source, place and intent of the burn (X00-X19, X75-X77, X96-X98, Y92)

POA Unacceptable principal diagnosis symbol per Medicare code edits   Code exempt from diagnosis present on admission requirement
❓ Questionable admission   CC Complication or comorbidity   CC/MCC Exc CC/MCC exclusion   MCC Major complication or comorbidity
Principal diagnosis as its own CC   Principal diagnosis as its own MCC   HCC HCC diagnosis code   RxHCC RxHCC diagnosis code
MACRA code   Z1 Z code as first-listed diagnosis

When symbols appear on a code that requires a 7th character extension, refer to Appendix B to identify applicable 7th character codes.
2018 ICD-10-CM

6ᵗʰ **T23.20** Burn of second degree of hand, unspecified site

7ᵗʰ **T23.201** Burn of second degree of right hand, unspecified site POA

7ᵗʰ **T23.202** Burn of second degree of left hand, unspecified site POA

7ᵗʰ **T23.209** Burn of second degree of unspecified hand, unspecified site POA

6ᵗʰ **T23.21** Burn of second degree of thumb (nail)

7ᵗʰ **T23.211** Burn of second degree of right thumb (nail) POA

7ᵗʰ **T23.212** Burn of second degree of left thumb (nail) POA

7ᵗʰ **T23.219** Burn of second degree of unspecified thumb (nail) POA

6ᵗʰ **T23.22** Burn of second degree of single finger (nail) except thumb

7ᵗʰ **T23.221** Burn of second degree of single right finger (nail) except thumb POA

7ᵗʰ **T23.222** Burn of second degree of single left finger (nail) except thumb POA

7ᵗʰ **T23.229** Burn of second degree of unspecified single finger (nail) except thumb POA

6ᵗʰ **T23.23** Burn of second degree of multiple fingers (nail), not including thumb

7ᵗʰ **T23.231** Burn of second degree of multiple right fingers (nail), not including thumb POA

7ᵗʰ **T23.232** Burn of second degree of multiple left fingers (nail), not including thumb POA

7ᵗʰ **T23.239** Burn of second degree of unspecified multiple fingers (nail), not including thumb POA

6ᵗʰ **T23.24** Burn of second degree of multiple fingers (nail), including thumb

7ᵗʰ **T23.241** Burn of second degree of multiple right fingers (nail), including thumb POA

7ᵗʰ **T23.242** Burn of second degree of multiple left fingers (nail), including thumb POA

7ᵗʰ **T23.249** Burn of second degree of unspecified multiple fingers (nail), including thumb POA

6ᵗʰ **T23.25** Burn of second degree of palm

7ᵗʰ **T23.251** Burn of second degree of right palm POA

7ᵗʰ **T23.252** Burn of second degree of left palm POA

7ᵗʰ **T23.259** Burn of second degree of unspecified palm POA

6ᵗʰ **T23.26** Burn of second degree of back of hand

7ᵗʰ **T23.261** Burn of second degree of back of right hand POA

7ᵗʰ **T23.262** Burn of second degree of back of left hand POA

7ᵗʰ **T23.269** Burn of second degree of back of unspecified hand POA

6ᵗʰ **T23.27** Burn of second degree of wrist

7ᵗʰ **T23.271** Burn of second degree of right wrist POA

7ᵗʰ **T23.272** Burn of second degree of left wrist POA

7ᵗʰ **T23.279** Burn of second degree of unspecified wrist POA

6ᵗʰ **T23.29** Burn of second degree of multiple sites of wrist and hand

7ᵗʰ **T23.291** Burn of second degree of multiple sites of right wrist and hand POA

7ᵗʰ **T23.292** Burn of second degree of multiple sites of left wrist and hand POA

7ᵗʰ **T23.299** Burn of second degree of multiple sites of unspecified wrist and hand POA

5ᵗʰ **T23.3** Burn of third degree of wrist and hand

Use additional external cause code to identify the source, place and intent of the burn (X00-X19, X75-X77, X96-X98, Y92)

6ᵗʰ **T23.30** Burn of third degree of hand, unspecified site

7ᵗʰ **T23.301** Burn of third degree of right hand, unspecified site CC POA HAC CC/MCC Exc

7ᵗʰ **T23.302** Burn of third degree of left hand, unspecified site CC POA HAC CC/MCC Exc

7ᵗʰ **T23.309** Burn of third degree of unspecified hand, unspecified site CC POA HAC CC/MCC Exc

6ᵗʰ **T23.31** Burn of third degree of thumb (nail)

7ᵗʰ **T23.311** Burn of third degree of right thumb (nail) CC POA HAC CC/MCC Exc

7ᵗʰ **T23.312** Burn of third degree of left thumb (nail) CC POA HAC CC/MCC Exc

7ᵗʰ **T23.319** Burn of third degree of unspecified thumb (nail) CC POA HAC CC/MCC Exc

6ᵗʰ **T23.32** Burn of third degree of single finger (nail) except thumb

7ᵗʰ **T23.321** Burn of third degree of single right finger (nail) except thumb CC POA HAC CC/MCC Exc

7ᵗʰ **T23.322** Burn of third degree of single left finger (nail) except thumb CC POA HAC CC/MCC Exc

7ᵗʰ **T23.329** Burn of third degree of unspecified single finger (nail) except thumb CC POA HAC CC/MCC Exc

6ᵗʰ **T23.33** Burn of third degree of multiple fingers (nail), not including thumb

7ᵗʰ **T23.331** Burn of third degree of multiple right fingers (nail), not including thumb CC POA HAC CC/MCC Exc

7ᵗʰ **T23.332** Burn of third degree of multiple left fingers (nail), not including thumb CC POA HAC CC/MCC Exc

7ᵗʰ **T23.339** Burn of third degree of unspecified multiple fingers (nail), not including thumb CC POA HAC CC/MCC Exc

6ᵗʰ **T23.34** Burn of third degree of multiple fingers (nail), including thumb

7ᵗʰ **T23.341** Burn of third degree of multiple right fingers (nail), including thumb CC POA HAC CC/MCC Exc

7ᵗʰ **T23.342** Burn of third degree of multiple left fingers (nail), including thumb CC POA HAC CC/MCC Exc

7ᵗʰ **T23.349** Burn of third degree of unspecified multiple fingers (nail), including thumb CC POA HAC CC/MCC Exc

6ᵗʰ **T23.35** Burn of third degree of palm

7ᵗʰ **T23.351** Burn of third degree of right palm CC POA HAC CC/MCC Exc

7ᵗʰ **T23.352** Burn of third degree of left palm CC POA HAC CC/MCC Exc

7ᵗʰ **T23.359** Burn of third degree of unspecified palm CC POA HAC CC/MCC Exc

6ᵗʰ **T23.36** Burn of third degree of back of hand

7ᵗʰ **T23.361** Burn of third degree of back of right hand CC POA HAC CC/MCC Exc

7ᵗʰ **T23.362** Burn of third degree of back of left hand CC POA HAC CC/MCC Exc

7ᵗʰ **T23.369** Burn of third degree of back of unspecified hand CC POA HAC CC/MCC Exc

6ᵗʰ **T23.37** Burn of third degree of wrist

7ᵗʰ **T23.371** Burn of third degree of right wrist CC POA HAC CC/MCC Exc

7ᵗʰ **T23.372** Burn of third degree of left wrist CC POA HAC CC/MCC Exc

7ᵗʰ **T23.379** Burn of third degree of unspecified wrist CC POA HAC CC/MCC Exc

6ᵗʰ **T23.39** Burn of third degree of multiple sites of wrist and hand

7ᵗʰ **T23.391** Burn of third degree of multiple sites of right wrist and hand CC POA HAC CC/MCC Exc

7ᵗʰ **T23.392** Burn of third degree of multiple sites of left wrist and hand CC POA HAC CC/MCC Exc

7ᵗʰ **T23.399** Burn of third degree of multiple sites of unspecified wrist and hand CC POA HAC CC/MCC Exc

5ᵗʰ **T23.4** Corrosion of unspecified degree of wrist and hand

Code first (T51-T65) to identify chemical and intent

Unspecified Code	Other Specified Code	Manifestation Code	N Newborn	P Pediatric	M Maternity	A Adult	♂ Male	♀ Female

● New Code   ▲ Revised Code Title   ►◄ Revised Text   NOTES   *INCLUDES*   *EXCLUDES 1* Not coded here   *EXCLUDES 2* Not included here

4ᵗʰ character required   5ᵗʰ character required   6ᵗʰ character required   7ᵗʰ character required

Extension 'X' Alert   HAC Hospital-acquired condition (HAC) alert   AHA AHA Coding Clinic©

7ᵗʰ T25.639 Corrosion of second degree of unspecified toe(s) (nail) POA

6ᵗʰ T25.69 Corrosion of second degree of multiple sites of ankle and foot

  7ᵗʰ T25.691 Corrosion of second degree of right ankle and foot POA

  7ᵗʰ T25.692 Corrosion of second degree of left ankle and foot POA

  7ᵗʰ T25.699 Corrosion of second degree of unspecified ankle and foot POA

5ᵗʰ T25.7 Corrosion of third degree of ankle and foot
Code first (T51-T65) to identify chemical and intent
Use additional external cause code to identify place (Y92)

  5ᵗʰ T25.71 Corrosion of third degree of ankle

   7ᵗʰ T25.711 Corrosion of third degree of right ankle CC POA HAC CC/MCC Exc

   7ᵗʰ T25.712 Corrosion of third degree of left ankle CC POA HAC CC/MCC Exc

   7ᵗʰ T25.719 Corrosion of third degree of unspecified ankle CC POA HAC CC/MCC Exc

  6ᵗʰ T25.72 Corrosion of third degree of foot
EXCLUDES2 corrosion of third degree of toe(s) (nail) (T25.73-)

   7ᵗʰ T25.721 Corrosion of third degree of right foot CC POA HAC CC/MCC Exc

   7ᵗʰ T25.722 Corrosion of third degree of left foot CC POA HAC CC/MCC Exc

   7ᵗʰ T25.729 Corrosion of third degree of unspecified foot CC POA HAC CC/MCC Exc

  6ᵗʰ T25.73 Corrosion of third degree of toe(s) (nail)

   7ᵗʰ T25.731 Corrosion of third degree of right toe(s) (nail) CC POA HAC CC/MCC Exc

   7ᵗʰ T25.732 Corrosion of third degree of left toe(s) (nail) CC POA HAC CC/MCC Exc

   7ᵗʰ T25.739 Corrosion of third degree of unspecified toe(s) (nail) CC POA HAC CC/MCC Exc

  6ᵗʰ T25.79 Corrosion of third degree of multiple sites of ankle and foot

   7ᵗʰ T25.791 Corrosion of third degree of multiple sites of right ankle and foot CC POA HAC CC/MCC Exc

   7ᵗʰ T25.792 Corrosion of third degree of multiple sites of left ankle and foot CC POA HAC CC/MCC Exc

   7ᵗʰ T25.799 Corrosion of third degree of multiple sites of unspecified ankle and foot CC POA HAC CC/MCC Exc

Burns and corrosions confined to eye and internal organs (T26-T28)

4ᵗʰ T26 Burn and corrosion confined to eye and adnexa
The appropriate 7th character is to be added to each code from category T26
A = initial encounter
D = subsequent encounter
S = sequela

5ᵗʰ T26.0 Burn of eyelid and periocular area
Use additional external cause code to identify the source, place and intent of the burn (X00-X19, X75-X77, X96-X98, Y92)

  7ᵗʰ T26.00 Burn of unspecified eyelid and periocular area POA

  7ᵗʰ T26.01 Burn of right eyelid and periocular area POA

  7ᵗʰ T26.02 Burn of left eyelid and periocular area POA

5ᵗʰ T26.1 Burn of cornea and conjunctival sac
Use additional external cause code to identify the source, place and intent of the burn (X00-X19, X75-X77, X96-X98, Y92)

  7ᵗʰ T26.10 Burn of cornea and conjunctival sac, unspecified eye POA

  7ᵗʰ T26.11 Burn of cornea and conjunctival sac, right eye POA

  7ᵗʰ T26.12 Burn of cornea and conjunctival sac, left eye POA

5ᵗʰ T26.2 Burn with resulting rupture and destruction of eyeball
Use additional external cause code to identify the source, place and intent of the burn (X00-X19, X75-X77, X96-X98, Y92)

  7ᵗʰ T26.20 Burn with resulting rupture and destruction of unspecified eyeball CC POA HAC CC/MCC Exc

  7ᵗʰ T26.21 Burn with resulting rupture and destruction of right eyeball CC POA HAC CC/MCC Exc

  7ᵗʰ T26.22 Burn with resulting rupture and destruction of left eyeball CC POA HAC CC/MCC Exc

5ᵗʰ T26.3 Burns of other specified parts of eye and adnexa
Use additional external cause code to identify the source, place and intent of the burn (X00-X19, X75-X77, X96-X98, Y92)

  7ᵗʰ T26.30 Burns of other specified parts of unspecified eye and adnexa POA

  7ᵗʰ T26.31 Burns of other specified parts of right eye and adnexa POA

  7ᵗʰ T26.32 Burns of other specified parts of left eye and adnexa POA

5ᵗʰ T26.4 Burn of eye and adnexa, part unspecified
Use additional external cause code to identify the source, place and intent of the burn (X00-X19, X75-X77, X96-X98, Y92)

  7ᵗʰ T26.40 Burn of unspecified eye and adnexa, part unspecified POA

  7ᵗʰ T26.41 Burn of right eye and adnexa, part unspecified POA

  7ᵗʰ T26.42 Burn of left eye and adnexa, part unspecified POA

5ᵗʰ T26.5 Corrosion of eyelid and periocular area
Code first (T51-T65) to identify chemical and intent
Use additional external cause code to identify place (Y92)

  7ᵗʰ T26.50 Corrosion of unspecified eyelid and periocular area POA

  7ᵗʰ T26.51 Corrosion of right eyelid and periocular area POA

  7ᵗʰ T26.52 Corrosion of left eyelid and periocular area POA

5ᵗʰ T26.6 Corrosion of cornea and conjunctival sac
Code first (T51-T65) to identify chemical and intent
Use additional external cause code to identify place (Y92)

  7ᵗʰ T26.60 Corrosion of cornea and conjunctival sac, unspecified eye POA

  7ᵗʰ T26.61 Corrosion of cornea and conjunctival sac, right eye POA

  7ᵗʰ T26.62 Corrosion of cornea and conjunctival sac, left eye POA

5ᵗʰ T26.7 Corrosion with resulting rupture and destruction of eyeball
Code first (T51-T65) to identify chemical and intent
Use additional external cause code to identify place (Y92)

  7ᵗʰ T26.70 Corrosion with resulting rupture and destruction of unspecified eyeball CC POA HAC CC/MCC Exc

  7ᵗʰ T26.71 Corrosion with resulting rupture and destruction of right eyeball CC POA HAC CC/MCC Exc

  7ᵗʰ T26.72 Corrosion with resulting rupture and destruction of left eyeball CC POA HAC CC/MCC Exc

5ᵗʰ T26.8 Corrosions of other specified parts of eye and adnexa
Code first (T51-T65) to identify chemical and intent
Use additional external cause code to identify place (Y92)

  7ᵗʰ T26.80 Corrosions of other specified parts of unspecified eye and adnexa POA

  7ᵗʰ T26.81 Corrosions of other specified parts of right eye and adnexa POA

  7ᵗʰ T26.82 Corrosions of other specified parts of left eye and adnexa POA

5ᵗʰ T26.9 Corrosion of eye and adnexa, part unspecified
Code first (T51-T65) to identify chemical and intent
Use additional external cause code to identify place (Y92)

  7ᵗʰ T26.90 Corrosion of unspecified eye and adnexa, part unspecified POA

  7ᵗʰ T26.91 Corrosion of right eye and adnexa, part unspecified POA

  7ᵗʰ T26.92 Corrosion of left eye and adnexa, part unspecified POA

4ᵗʰ T27 Burn and corrosion of respiratory tract
Use additional external cause code to identify the source and intent of the burn (X00-X19, X75-X77, X96-X98)
Use additional external cause code to identify place (Y92)
The appropriate 7th character is to be added to each code from category T27

POA Unacceptable principal diagnosis symbol per Medicare code edits   POA Code exempt from diagnosis present on admission requirement
? Questionable admission   CC Complication or comorbidity   CC/MCC Exc CC/MCC exclusion   MCC Major complication or comorbidity
Principal diagnosis as its own CC   Principal diagnosis as its own MCC   HCC HCC diagnosis code   RxHCC RxHCC diagnosis code
MACRA code   Z1 Z code as first-listed diagnosis

A = initial encounter
D = subsequent encounter
S = sequela

🄬 T27.0 Burn of larynx and trachea cc⊘ POA HAC CC/MCC Exc
🄬 T27.1 Burn involving larynx and trachea with lung cc⊘ POA HAC CC/MCC Exc
🄬 T27.2 Burn of other parts of respiratory tract cc⊘ POA HAC CC/MCC Exc
   Burn of thoracic cavity
🄬 T27.3 Burn of respiratory tract, part unspecified cc⊘ POA HAC CC/MCC Exc
🄬 T27.4 Corrosion of larynx and trachea cc⊘ POA HAC CC/MCC Exc
   Code first (T51-T65) to identify chemical and intent
🄬 T27.5 Corrosion involving larynx and trachea with lung cc⊘ POA HAC CC/MCC Exc
🄬 T27.6 Corrosion of other parts of respiratory tract cc⊘ POA HAC CC/MCC Exc
   Code first (T51-T65) to identify chemical and intent
🄬 T27.7 Corrosion of respiratory tract, part unspecified cc⊘ POA HAC CC/MCC Exc
   Code first (T51-T65) to identify chemical and intent

🄬 T28 Burn and corrosion of other internal organs
   Use additional external cause code to identify the source and intent of the burn (X00-X19, X75-X77, X96-X98)
   Use additional external cause code to identify place (Y92)
   The appropriate 7th character is to be added to each code from category T28
      A = initial encounter
      D = subsequent encounter
      S = sequela
🄬 T28.0 Burn of mouth and pharynx POA
🄬 T28.1 Burn of esophagus cc⊘ POA HAC CC/MCC Exc
🄬 T28.2 Burn of other parts of alimentary tract cc⊘ POA HAC CC/MCC Exc
🄬 T28.3 Burn of internal genitourinary organs POA
🄬 T28.4 Burns of other and unspecified internal organs
   Code first (T51-T65) to identify chemical and intent
   🄬 T28.40 Burn of unspecified internal organ POA
   🄬 T28.41 Burn of ear drum
      🄬 T28.411 Burn of right ear drum POA
      🄬 T28.412 Burn of left ear drum POA
      🄬 T28.419 Burn of unspecified ear drum POA
   🄬 T28.49 Burn of other internal organ POA
🄬 T28.5 Corrosion of mouth and pharynx POA
   Code first (T51-T65) to identify chemical and intent
🄬 T28.6 Corrosion of esophagus cc⊘ POA HAC CC/MCC Exc
   Code first (T51-T65) to identify chemical and intent
🄬 T28.7 Corrosion of other parts of alimentary tract cc⊘ POA HAC CC/MCC Exc
   Code first (T51-T65) to identify chemical and intent
🄬 T28.8 Corrosion of internal genitourinary organs POA
   Code first (T51-T65) to identify chemical and intent
🄬 T28.9 Corrosions of other and unspecified internal organs
   Code first (T51-T65) to identify chemical and intent
   🄬 T28.90 Corrosions of unspecified internal organs POA
   🄬 T28.91 Corrosions of ear drum
      🄬 T28.911 Corrosions of right ear drum POA
      🄬 T28.912 Corrosions of left ear drum POA
      🄬 T28.919 Corrosions of unspecified ear drum POA
   🄬 T28.99 Corrosions of other internal organs POA

Burns and corrosions of multiple and unspecified body regions (T30-T32)

🄬 T30 Burn and corrosion, body region unspecified
   T30.0 Burn of unspecified body region, unspecified degree
      This code is not for inpatient use. Code to specified site and degree of burns
      Burn NOS
      Multiple burns NOS
   T30.4 Corrosion of unspecified body region, unspecified degree
      This code is not for inpatient use. Code to specified site and degree of corrosion
      Corrosion NOS
      Multiple corrosion NOS

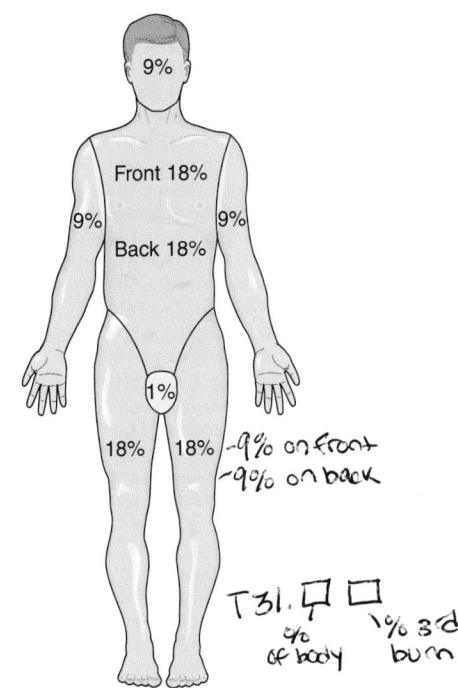

9%

Front 18%

9%   9%

Back 18%

1%

18% 18%

—9% on front
—9% on back

T31.☐☐
  %   1% 3'd
of body   burn

Figure 19.3 Rule of Nine: Percentage of burn areas

🄬 T31 Burns classified according to extent of body surface involved
   NOTES This category is to be used as the primary code only when the site of the burn is unspecified. It should be used as a supplementary code with categories T20-T25 when the site is specified.

2nd
last digit is
what % of whole
body burned

last digit
is how
much 3rd
degree burned

   T31.0 Burns involving less than 10% of body surface
   🄬 T31.1 Burns involving 10-19% of body surface
      T31.10 Burns involving 10-19% of body surface with 0% to 9% third degree burns cc⊘ HAC CC/MCC Exc
         Burns involving 10-19% of body surface NOS
      T31.11 Burns involving 10-19% of body surface with 10-19% third degree burns cc⊘ HAC HCC CC/MCC Exc
   🄬 T31.2 Burns involving 20-29% of body surface
      T31.20 Burns involving 20-29% of body surface with 0% to 9% third degree burns cc⊘ HAC CC/MCC Exc
         Burns involving 20-29% of body surface NOS
      T31.21 Burns involving 20-29% of body surface with 10-19% third degree burns HAC HCC cc⊘ CC/MCC Exc
      T31.22 Burns involving 20-29% of body surface with 20-29% third degree burns HAC HCC Mcc⊘ CC/MCC Exc
   🄬 T31.3 Burns involving 30-39% of body surface
      T31.30 Burns involving 30-39% of body surface with 0% to 9% third degree burns cc⊘ HAC CC/MCC Exc
         Burns involving 30-39% of body surface NOS
      T31.31 Burns involving 30-39% of body surface with 10-19% third degree burns HAC HCC cc⊘ CC/MCC Exc
      T31.32 Burns involving 30-39% of body surface with 20-29% third degree burns HAC HCC Mcc⊘ CC/MCC Exc
      T31.33 Burns involving 30-39% of body surface with 30-39% third degree burns HAC HCC Mcc⊘ CC/MCC Exc
   🄬 T31.4 Burns involving 40-49% of body surface
      T31.40 Burns involving 40-49% of body surface with 0% to 9% third degree burns cc⊘ HAC CC/MCC Exc
         Burns involving 40-49% of body surface NOS
      T31.41 Burns involving 40-49% of body surface with 10-19% third degree burns HAC HCC Mcc⊘ CC/MCC Exc
      T31.42 Burns involving 40-49% of body surface with 20-29% third degree burns HAC HCC Mcc⊘ CC/MCC Exc
      T31.43 Burns involving 40-49% of body surface with 30-39% third degree burns HAC HCC Mcc⊘ CC/MCC Exc

---

| Unspecified Code | Other Specified Code | Manifestation Code | N Newborn | P Pediatric | M Maternity | A Adult | ♂ Male | ♀ Female |

● New Code   ▲ Revised Code Title   ▶◀ Revised Text   **NOTES**   *INCLUDES*   *EXCLUDES 1* Not coded here   *EXCLUDES 2* Not included here
🄭 4th character required   🄮 5th character required   🄯 6th character required   🄬 7th character required
🄬 Extension 'X' Alert   HAC Hospital-acquired condition (HAC) alert   AHA AHA Coding Clinic©

T31.44 Burns involving 40-49% of body surface with 40-49% third degree burns `HAC` `HCC` `MCC` `CC/MCC Exc`

5ᵗʰ T31.5 Burns involving 50-59% of body surface

T31.50 Burns involving 50-59% of body surface with 0% to 9% third degree burns `CC` `HAC` `CC/MCC Exc`

Burns involving 50-59% of body surface NOS

T31.51 Burns involving 50-59% of body surface with 10-19% third degree burns `HAC` `HCC` `MCC` `CC/MCC Exc`

T31.52 Burns involving 50-59% of body surface with 20-29% third degree burns `HAC` `HCC` `MCC` `CC/MCC Exc`

T31.53 Burns involving 50-59% of body surface with 30-39% third degree burns `HAC` `HCC` `MCC` `CC/MCC Exc`

T31.54 Burns involving 50-59% of body surface with 40-49% third degree burns `HAC` `HCC` `MCC` `CC/MCC Exc`

T31.55 Burns involving 50-59% of body surface with 50-59% third degree burns `HAC` `HCC` `MCC` `CC/MCC Exc`

5ᵗʰ T31.6 Burns involving 60-69% of body surface

T31.60 Burns involving 60-69% of body surface with 0% to 9% third degree burns `CC` `HAC` `CC/MCC Exc`

Burns involving 60-69% of body surface NOS

T31.61 Burns involving 60-69% of body surface with 10-19% third degree burns `HAC` `HCC` `MCC` `CC/MCC Exc`

T31.62 Burns involving 60-69% of body surface with 20-29% third degree burns `HAC` `HCC` `MCC` `CC/MCC Exc`

T31.63 Burns involving 60-69% of body surface with 30-39% third degree burns `HAC` `HCC` `MCC` `CC/MCC Exc`

T31.64 Burns involving 60-69% of body surface with 40-49% third degree burns `HAC` `HCC` `MCC` `CC/MCC Exc`

T31.65 Burns involving 60-69% of body surface with 50-59% third degree burns `HAC` `HCC` `MCC` `CC/MCC Exc`

T31.66 Burns involving 60-69% of body surface with 60-69% third degree burns `HAC` `HCC` `MCC` `CC/MCC Exc`

5ᵗʰ T31.7 Burns involving 70-79% of body surface

T31.70 Burns involving 70-79% of body surface with 0% to 9% third degree burns `CC` `HAC` `CC/MCC Exc`

Burns involving 70-79% of body surface NOS

T31.71 Burns involving 70-79% of body surface with 10-19% third degree burns `HAC` `HCC` `MCC` `CC/MCC Exc`

T31.72 Burns involving 70-79% of body surface with 20-29% third degree burns `HAC` `HCC` `MCC` `CC/MCC Exc`

T31.73 Burns involving 70-79% of body surface with 30-39% third degree burns `HAC` `HCC` `MCC` `CC/MCC Exc`

T31.74 Burns involving 70-79% of body surface with 40-49% third degree burns `HAC` `HCC` `MCC` `CC/MCC Exc`

T31.75 Burns involving 70-79% of body surface with 50-59% third degree burns `HAC` `HCC` `MCC` `CC/MCC Exc`

T31.76 Burns involving 70-79% of body surface with 60-69% third degree burns `HAC` `HCC` `MCC` `CC/MCC Exc`

T31.77 Burns involving 70-79% of body surface with 70-79% third degree burns `HAC` `HCC` `MCC` `CC/MCC Exc`

5ᵗʰ T31.8 Burns involving 80-89% of body surface

T31.80 Burns involving 80-89% of body surface with 0% to 9% third degree burns `CC` `HAC` `CC/MCC Exc`

Burns involving 80-89% of body surface NOS

T31.81 Burns involving 80-89% of body surface with 10-19% third degree burns `HAC` `HCC` `MCC` `CC/MCC Exc`

T31.82 Burns involving 80-89% of body surface with 20-29% third degree burns `HAC` `HCC` `MCC` `CC/MCC Exc`

T31.83 Burns involving 80-89% of body surface with 30-39% third degree burns `HAC` `HCC` `MCC` `CC/MCC Exc`

T31.84 Burns involving 80-89% of body surface with 40-49% third degree burns `HAC` `HCC` `MCC` `CC/MCC Exc`

T31.85 Burns involving 80-89% of body surface with 50-59% third degree burns `HAC` `HCC` `MCC` `CC/MCC Exc`

T31.86 Burns involving 80-89% of body surface with 60-69% third degree burns `HAC` `HCC` `MCC` `CC/MCC Exc`

T31.87 Burns involving 80-89% of body surface with 70-79% third degree burns `HAC` `HCC` `MCC` `CC/MCC Exc`

T31.88 Burns involving 80-89% of body surface with 80-89% third degree burns `HAC` `HCC` `MCC` `CC/MCC Exc`

5ᵗʰ T31.9 Burns involving 90% or more of body surface

T31.90 Burns involving 90% or more of body surface with 0% to 9% third degree burns `CC` `HAC` `CC/MCC Exc`

Burns involving 90% or more of body surface NOS

T31.91 Burns involving 90% or more of body surface with 10-19% third degree burns `HAC` `HCC` `MCC` `CC/MCC Exc`

T31.92 Burns involving 90% or more of body surface with 20-29% third degree burns `HAC` `HCC` `MCC` `CC/MCC Exc`

T31.93 Burns involving 90% or more of body surface with 30-39% third degree burns `HAC` `HCC` `MCC` `CC/MCC Exc`

T31.94 Burns involving 90% or more of body surface with 40-49% third degree burns `HAC` `HCC` `MCC` `CC/MCC Exc`

T31.95 Burns involving 90% or more of body surface with 50-59% third degree burns `HAC` `HCC` `MCC` `CC/MCC Exc`

T31.96 Burns involving 90% or more of body surface with 60-69% third degree burns `HAC` `HCC` `MCC` `CC/MCC Exc`

T31.97 Burns involving 90% or more of body surface with 70-79% third degree burns `HAC` `HCC` `MCC` `CC/MCC Exc`

T31.98 Burns involving 90% or more of body surface with 80-89% third degree burns `HAC` `HCC` `MCC` `CC/MCC Exc`

T31.99 Burns involving 90% or more of body surface with 90% or more third degree burns `HAC` `HCC` `MCC` `CC/MCC Exc`

4ᵗʰ T32 Corrosions classified according to extent of body surface involved

`NOTES` This category is to be used as the primary code only when the site of the corrosion is unspecified. It may be used as a supplementary code with categories T20-T25 when the site is specified.

T32.0 Corrosions involving less than 10% of body surface

5ᵗʰ T32.1 Corrosions involving 10-19% of body surface

T32.10 Corrosions involving 10-19% of body surface with 0% to 9% third degree corrosion `CC` `HAC` `CC/MCC Exc`

Corrosions involving 10-19% of body surface NOS

T32.11 Corrosions involving 10-19% of body surface with 10-19% third degree corrosion `CC` `HAC` `HCC` `CC/MCC Exc`

5ᵗʰ T32.2 Corrosions involving 20-29% of body surface

T32.20 Corrosions involving 20-29% of body surface with 0% to 9% third degree corrosion `CC` `HAC` `CC/MCC Exc`

T32.21 Corrosions involving 20-29% of body surface with 10-19% third degree corrosion `HAC` `HCC` `MCC` `CC/MCC Exc`

T32.22 Corrosions involving 20-29% of body surface with 20-29% third degree corrosion `HAC` `HCC` `MCC` `CC/MCC Exc`

5ᵗʰ T32.3 Corrosions involving 30-39% of body surface

T32.30 Corrosions involving 30-39% of body surface with 0% to 9% third degree corrosion `CC` `HAC` `CC/MCC Exc`

T32.31 Corrosions involving 30-39% of body surface with 10-19% third degree corrosion `HAC` `HCC` `MCC` `CC/MCC Exc`

T32.32 Corrosions involving 30-39% of body surface with 20-29% third degree corrosion `HAC` `HCC` `MCC` `CC/MCC Exc`

T32.33 Corrosions involving 30-39% of body surface with 30-39% third degree corrosion `HAC` `HCC` `MCC` `CC/MCC Exc`

T32.4 Corrosions involving 40-49% of body surface

T32.40 Corrosions involving 40-49% of body surface with 0% to 9% third degree corrosion `CC` `HAC` `CC/MCC Exc`

T32.41 Corrosions involving 40-49% of body surface with 10-19% third degree corrosion `HAC` `HCC` `MCC` `CC/MCC Exc`

T32.42 Corrosions involving 40-49% of body surface with 20-29% third degree corrosion `HAC` `HCC` `MCC` `CC/MCC Exc`

T32.43 Corrosions involving 40-49% of body surface with 30-39% third degree corrosion `HAC` `HCC` `MCC` `CC/MCC Exc`

T32.44 Corrosions involving 40-49% of body surface with 40-49% third degree corrosion `HAC` `HCC` `MCC` `CC/MCC Exc`

5ᵗʰ T32.5 Corrosions involving 50-59% of body surface

T32.50 Corrosions involving 50-59% of body surface with 0% to 9% third degree corrosion `CC` `HAC` `CC/MCC Exc`

T32.51 Corrosions involving 50-59% of body surface with 10-19% third degree corrosion `HAC` `HCC` `MCC` `CC/MCC Exc`

T32.52 Corrosions involving 50-59% of body surface with 20-29% third degree corrosion `HAC` `HCC` `MCC` `CC/MCC Exc`

T32.53 Corrosions involving 50-59% of body surface with 30-39% third degree corrosion `HAC` `HCC` `MCC` `CC/MCC Exc`

T32.54 Corrosions involving 50-59% of body surface with 40-49% third degree corrosion `HAC` `HCC` `MCC` `CC/MCC Exc`

`PDx` Unacceptable principal diagnosis symbol per Medicare code edits   `POA` Code exempt from diagnosis present on admission requirement
`?` Questionable admission   `CC` Complication or comorbidity   `CC/MCC Exc` CC/MCC exclusion   `MCC` Major complication or comorbidity
`PCC` Principal diagnosis as its own CC   `PMCC` Principal diagnosis as its own MCC   `HCC` HCC diagnosis code   `RxHCC` RxHCC diagnosis code
MACRA code   `Z1` Z code as first-listed diagnosis

When symbols appear on a code that requires a 7th character extension, refer to Appendix B to identify applicable 7th character codes.

2018 ICD-10-CM

T32.55 Corrosions involving 50-59% of body surface with 50-59% third degree **corrosion** HAC HCC MCC⊘ CC/MCC Exc

5ᵗʰ T32.6 Corrosions involving 60-69% of body surface

T32.60 Corrosions involving 60-69% of body surface with 0% to 9% third degree **corrosion** CC⊘ HAC CC/MCC Exc

T32.61 Corrosions involving 60-69% of body surface with 10-19% third degree **corrosion** HAC HCC MCC⊘ CC/MCC Exc

T32.62 Corrosions involving 60-69% of body surface with 20-29% third degree **corrosion** HAC HCC MCC⊘ CC/MCC Exc

T32.63 Corrosions involving 60-69% of body surface with 30-39% third degree **corrosion** HAC HCC MCC⊘ CC/MCC Exc

T32.64 Corrosions involving 60-69% of body surface with 40-49% third degree **corrosion** HAC HCC MCC⊘ CC/MCC Exc

T32.65 Corrosions involving 60-69% of body surface with 50-59% third degree **corrosion** HAC HCC MCC⊘ CC/MCC Exc

T32.66 Corrosions involving 60-69% of body surface with 60-69% third degree **corrosion** HAC HCC MCC⊘ CC/MCC Exc

5ᵗʰ T32.7 Corrosions involving 70-79% of body surface

T32.70 Corrosions involving 70-79% of body surface with 0% to 9% third degree **corrosion** CC⊘ HAC CC/MCC Exc

T32.71 Corrosions involving 70-79% of body surface with 10-19% third degree **corrosion** HAC HCC MCC⊘ CC/MCC Exc

T32.72 Corrosions involving 70-79% of body surface with 20-29% third degree **corrosion** HAC HCC MCC⊘ CC/MCC Exc

T32.73 Corrosions involving 70-79% of body surface with 30-39% third degree **corrosion** HAC HCC MCC⊘ CC/MCC Exc

T32.74 Corrosions involving 70-79% of body surface with 40-49% third degree **corrosion** HAC HCC MCC⊘ CC/MCC Exc

T32.75 Corrosions involving 70-79% of body surface with 50-59% third degree **corrosion** HAC HCC MCC⊘ CC/MCC Exc

T32.76 Corrosions involving 70-79% of body surface with 60-69% third degree **corrosion** HAC HCC MCC⊘ CC/MCC Exc

T32.77 Corrosions involving 70-79% of body surface with 70-79% third degree **corrosion** HAC HCC MCC⊘ CC/MCC Exc

5ᵗʰ T32.8 Corrosions involving 80-89% of body surface

T32.80 Corrosions involving 80-89% of body surface with 0% to 9% third degree **corrosion** CC⊘ HAC CC/MCC Exc

T32.81 Corrosions involving 80-89% of body surface with 10-19% third degree **corrosion** HAC HCC MCC⊘ CC/MCC Exc

T32.82 Corrosions involving 80-89% of body surface with 20-29% third degree **corrosion** HAC HCC MCC⊘ CC/MCC Exc

T32.83 Corrosions involving 80-89% of body surface with 30-39% third degree **corrosion** HAC HCC MCC⊘ CC/MCC Exc

T32.84 Corrosions involving 80-89% of body surface with 40-49% third degree **corrosion** HAC HCC MCC⊘ CC/MCC Exc

T32.85 Corrosions involving 80-89% of body surface with 50-59% third degree **corrosion** HAC HCC MCC⊘ CC/MCC Exc

T32.86 Corrosions involving 80-89% of body surface with 60-69% third degree **corrosion** HAC HCC MCC⊘ CC/MCC Exc

T32.87 Corrosions involving 80-89% of body surface with 70-79% third degree **corrosion** HAC HCC MCC⊘ CC/MCC Exc

T32.88 Corrosions involving 80-89% of body surface with 80-89% third degree **corrosion** HAC HCC MCC⊘ CC/MCC Exc

5ᵗʰ T32.9 Corrosions involving 90% or more of body surface

T32.90 Corrosions involving 90% or more of body surface with 0% to 9% third degree **corrosion** CC⊘ HAC CC/MCC Exc

T32.91 Corrosions involving 90% or more of body surface with 10-19% third degree **corrosion** HAC HCC MCC⊘ CC/MCC Exc

T32.92 Corrosions involving 90% or more of body surface with 20-29% third degree **corrosion** HAC HCC MCC⊘ CC/MCC Exc

T32.93 Corrosions involving 90% or more of body surface with 30-39% third degree **corrosion** HAC HCC MCC⊘ CC/MCC Exc

T32.94 Corrosions involving 90% or more of body surface with 40-49% third degree **corrosion** HAC HCC MCC⊘ CC/MCC Exc

T32.95 Corrosions involving 90% or more of body surface with 50-59% third degree **corrosion** HAC HCC MCC⊘ CC/MCC Exc

T32.96 Corrosions involving 90% or more of body surface with 60-69% third degree **corrosion** HAC HCC MCC⊘ CC/MCC Exc

T32.97 Corrosions involving 90% or more of body surface with 70-79% third degree **corrosion** HAC HCC MCC⊘ CC/MCC Exc

T32.98 Corrosions involving 90% or more of body surface with 80-89% third degree **corrosion** HAC HCC MCC⊘ CC/MCC Exc

T32.99 Corrosions involving 90% or more of body surface with 90% or more third degree **corrosion** HAC HCC MCC⊘ CC/MCC Exc

Frostbite (T33-T34)

EXCLUDES2 *hypothermia and other effects of reduced temperature (T68, T69.-)*

4ᵗʰ T33 Superficial **frostbite**

INCLUDES *frostbite with partial thickness skin loss*

The appropriate 7th character is to be added to each code from category T33

A = initial encounter
D = subsequent encounter
S = sequela

5ᵗʰ T33.0 Superficial frostbite of head

6ᵗʰ T33.01 Superficial frostbite of ear

7ᵗʰ T33.011 Superficial frostbite of right ear CC⊘ POA HAC CC/MCC Exc

7ᵗʰ T33.012 Superficial frostbite of left ear CC⊘ POA HAC CC/MCC Exc

7ᵗʰ T33.019 Superficial frostbite of unspecified ear CC⊘ POA HAC CC/MCC Exc

7ᵗʰ T33.02 Superficial frostbite of nose CC⊘ POA HAC CC/MCC Exc

7ᵗʰ T33.09 Superficial frostbite of other part of head CC⊘ POA HAC CC/MCC Exc

7ᵗʰ T33.1 Superficial frostbite of neck CC⊘ POA HAC CC/MCC Exc

7ᵗʰ T33.2 Superficial frostbite of thorax CC⊘ POA HAC CC/MCC Exc

7ᵗʰ T33.3 Superficial frostbite of abdominal wall, lower back and pelvis CC⊘ POA HAC CC/MCC Exc

5ᵗʰ T33.4 Superficial frostbite of arm

EXCLUDES2 *superficial frostbite of wrist and hand (T33.5-)*

7ᵗʰ T33.40 Superficial frostbite of unspecified arm CC⊘ POA HAC CC/MCC Exc

7ᵗʰ T33.41 Superficial frostbite of right arm CC⊘ POA HAC CC/MCC Exc

7ᵗʰ T33.42 Superficial frostbite of left arm CC⊘ POA HAC CC/MCC Exc

5ᵗʰ T33.5 Superficial frostbite of wrist, hand, and fingers

6ᵗʰ T33.51 Superficial frostbite of wrist

7ᵗʰ T33.511 Superficial frostbite of right wrist CC⊘ POA HAC CC/MCC Exc

7ᵗʰ T33.512 Superficial frostbite of left wrist CC⊘ POA HAC CC/MCC Exc

7ᵗʰ T33.519 Superficial frostbite of unspecified wrist CC⊘ POA HAC CC/MCC Exc

6ᵗʰ T33.52 Superficial frostbite of hand

EXCLUDES2 *superficial frostbite of fingers (T33.53-)*

7ᵗʰ T33.521 Superficial frostbite of right hand CC⊘ POA HAC CC/MCC Exc

7ᵗʰ T33.522 Superficial frostbite of left hand CC⊘ POA HAC CC/MCC Exc

7ᵗʰ T33.529 Superficial frostbite of unspecified hand CC⊘ POA HAC CC/MCC Exc

6ᵗʰ T33.53 Superficial frostbite of finger(s)

7ᵗʰ T33.531 Superficial frostbite of right finger(s) CC⊘ POA HAC CC/MCC Exc

7ᵗʰ T33.532 Superficial frostbite of left finger(s) CC⊘ POA HAC CC/MCC Exc

7ᵗʰ T33.539 Superficial frostbite of unspecified finger(s) CC⊘ POA HAC CC/MCC Exc

5ᵗʰ T33.6 Superficial frostbite of hip and thigh

7ᵗʰ T33.60 Superficial frostbite of unspecified hip and thigh CC⊘ POA HAC CC/MCC Exc

7ᵗʰ T33.61 Superficial frostbite of right hip and thigh CC⊘ POA HAC CC/MCC Exc

7ᵗʰ T33.62 Superficial frostbite of left hip and thigh CC⊘ POA HAC CC/MCC Exc

5ᵗʰ T33.7 Superficial frostbite of knee and lower leg

EXCLUDES2 *superficial frostbite of ankle and foot (T33.8-)*

7ᵗʰ T33.70 Superficial frostbite of unspecified knee and lower leg CC⊘ POA HAC CC/MCC Exc

7ᵗʰ T33.71 Superficial frostbite of right knee and lower leg CC⊘ POA HAC CC/MCC Exc

---

Unspecified Code   Other Specified Code   Manifestation Code   N Newborn   P Pediatric   M Maternity   A Adult   ♂ Male   ♀ Female
● New Code   ▲ Revised Code Title   ▶◀ Revised Text   NOTES   INCLUDES   EXCLUDES1 Not coded here   EXCLUDES2 Not included here
4ᵗʰ 4th character required   **5ᵗʰ** 5th character required   **6ᵗʰ** 6th character required   **7ᵗʰ** 7th character required
7ᵗʰ Extension 'X' Alert   HAC Hospital-acquired condition (HAC) alert   **AHA** AHA Coding Clinic©

T33.72   Superficial frostbite of left knee and lower leg

T33.8   Superficial frostbite of ankle, foot, and toe(s)

  T33.81   Superficial frostbite of ankle

    T33.811   Superficial frostbite of right ankle   CC POA HAC CC/MCC Exc

    T33.812   Superficial frostbite of left ankle   CC POA HAC CC/MCC Exc

    T33.819   Superficial frostbite of unspecified ankle   CC POA HAC CC/MCC Exc

  T33.82   Superficial frostbite of foot

    T33.821   Superficial frostbite of right foot   CC POA HAC CC/MCC Exc

    T33.822   Superficial frostbite of left foot   CC POA HAC CC/MCC Exc

    T33.829   Superficial frostbite of unspecified foot   CC POA HAC CC/MCC Exc

  T33.83   Superficial frostbite of toe(s)

    T33.831   Superficial frostbite of right toe(s)   CC POA HAC CC/MCC Exc

    T33.832   Superficial frostbite of left toe(s)   CC POA HAC CC/MCC Exc

    T33.839   Superficial frostbite of unspecified toe(s)   CC POA HAC CC/MCC Exc

T33.9   Superficial frostbite of other and unspecified sites

  T33.90   Superficial frostbite of unspecified sites   CC POA HAC CC/MCC Exc

    Superficial frostbite NOS

  T33.99   Superficial frostbite of other sites   CC POA HAC CC/MCC Exc

    Superficial frostbite of leg NOS

    Superficial frostbite of trunk NOS

T34   Frostbite with tissue necrosis

The appropriate 7th character is to be added to each code from category T34

A = initial encounter

D = subsequent encounter

S = sequela

T34.0   Frostbite with tissue necrosis of head

  T34.01   Frostbite with tissue necrosis of ear

    T34.011   Frostbite with tissue necrosis of right ear   CC POA HAC CC/MCC Exc

    T34.012   Frostbite with tissue necrosis of left ear   CC POA HAC CC/MCC Exc

    T34.019   Frostbite with tissue necrosis of unspecified ear   CC POA HAC CC/MCC Exc

  T34.02   Frostbite with tissue necrosis of nose   CC POA HAC CC/MCC Exc

  T34.09   Frostbite with tissue necrosis of other part of head   CC POA HAC CC/MCC Exc

T34.1   Frostbite with tissue necrosis of neck   CC POA HAC CC/MCC Exc

T34.2   Frostbite with tissue necrosis of thorax   CC POA HAC CC/MCC Exc

T34.3   Frostbite with tissue necrosis of abdominal wall, lower back and pelvis   CC POA HAC CC/MCC Exc

T34.4   Frostbite with tissue necrosis of arm

  EXCLUDES2 frostbite with tissue necrosis of wrist and hand (T34.5-)

  T34.40   Frostbite with tissue necrosis of unspecified arm   CC POA HAC CC/MCC Exc

  T34.41   Frostbite with tissue necrosis of right arm   CC POA HAC CC/MCC Exc

  T34.42   Frostbite with tissue necrosis of left arm   CC POA HAC CC/MCC Exc

T34.5   Frostbite with tissue necrosis of wrist, hand, and finger(s)

  T34.51   Frostbite with tissue necrosis of wrist

    T34.511   Frostbite with tissue necrosis of right wrist   CC POA HAC CC/MCC Exc

    T34.512   Frostbite with tissue necrosis of left wrist   CC POA HAC CC/MCC Exc

    T34.519   Frostbite with tissue necrosis of unspecified wrist   CC POA HAC CC/MCC Exc

  T34.52   Frostbite with tissue necrosis of hand

    EXCLUDES2 frostbite with tissue necrosis of finger(s) (T34.53-)

    T34.521   Frostbite with tissue necrosis of right hand   CC POA HAC CC/MCC Exc

    T34.522   Frostbite with tissue necrosis of left hand   CC POA HAC CC/MCC Exc

    T34.529   Frostbite with tissue necrosis of unspecified hand   CC POA HAC CC/MCC Exc

  T34.53   Frostbite with tissue necrosis of finger(s)

    T34.531   Frostbite with tissue necrosis of right finger(s)   CC POA HAC CC/MCC Exc

    T34.532   Frostbite with tissue necrosis of left finger(s)   CC POA HAC CC/MCC Exc

    T34.539   Frostbite with tissue necrosis of unspecified finger(s)   CC POA HAC CC/MCC Exc

T34.6   Frostbite with tissue necrosis of hip and thigh

  T34.60   Frostbite with tissue necrosis of unspecified hip and thigh   CC POA HAC CC/MCC Exc

  T34.61   Frostbite with tissue necrosis of right hip and thigh   CC POA HAC CC/MCC Exc

  T34.62   Frostbite with tissue necrosis of left hip and thigh   CC POA HAC CC/MCC Exc

T34.7   Frostbite with tissue necrosis of knee and lower leg

  EXCLUDES2 frostbite with tissue necrosis of ankle and foot (T34.8-)

  T34.70   Frostbite with tissue necrosis of unspecified knee and lower leg   CC POA HAC CC/MCC Exc

  T34.71   Frostbite with tissue necrosis of right knee and lower leg   CC POA HAC CC/MCC Exc

  T34.72   Frostbite with tissue necrosis of left knee and lower leg   CC POA HAC CC/MCC Exc

T34.8   Frostbite with tissue necrosis of ankle, foot, and toe(s)

  T34.81   Frostbite with tissue necrosis of ankle

    T34.811   Frostbite with tissue necrosis of right ankle   CC POA HAC CC/MCC Exc

    T34.812   Frostbite with tissue necrosis of left ankle   CC POA HAC CC/MCC Exc

    T34.819   Frostbite with tissue necrosis of unspecified ankle   CC POA HAC CC/MCC Exc

  T34.82   Frostbite with tissue necrosis of foot

    T34.821   Frostbite with tissue necrosis of right foot   CC POA HAC CC/MCC Exc

    T34.822   Frostbite with tissue necrosis of left foot   CC POA HAC CC/MCC Exc

    T34.829   Frostbite with tissue necrosis of unspecified foot   CC POA HAC CC/MCC Exc

  T34.83   Frostbite with tissue necrosis of toe(s)

    T34.831   Frostbite with tissue necrosis of right toe(s)   CC POA HAC CC/MCC Exc

    T34.832   Frostbite with tissue necrosis of left toe(s)   CC POA HAC CC/MCC Exc

    T34.839   Frostbite with tissue necrosis of unspecified toe(s)   CC POA HAC CC/MCC Exc

T34.9   Frostbite with tissue necrosis of other and unspecified sites

  T34.90   Frostbite with tissue necrosis of unspecified sites   CC POA HAC CC/MCC Exc

    Frostbite with tissue necrosis NOS

  T34.99   Frostbite with tissue necrosis of other sites   CC POA HAC CC/MCC Exc

    Frostbite with tissue necrosis of leg NOS

    Frostbite with tissue necrosis of trunk NOS

Poisoning by, adverse effects of and underdosing of drugs, medicaments and biological substances (T36-T50)

INCLUDES   adverse effect of correct substance properly administered

    poisoning by overdose of substance

    poisoning by wrong substance given or taken in error

    underdosing by (inadvertently) (deliberately) taking less substance than prescribed or instructed

Code first, for adverse effects, the nature of the adverse effect, such as:

adverse effect NOS (T88.7)

aspirin gastritis (K29.-)

POA Unacceptable principal diagnosis symbol per Medicare code edits   POA Code exempt from diagnosis present on admission requirement

? Questionable admission   CC Complication or comorbidity   CC/MCC Exc CC/MCC exclusion   MCC Major complication or comorbidity

Principal diagnosis as its own CC   Principal diagnosis as its own MCC   HCC HCC diagnosis code   RxHCC RxHCC diagnosis code

MACRA code   Z1 Z code as first-listed diagnosis

When symbols appear on a code that requires a 7th character extension, refer to Appendix B to identify applicable 7th character codes.

blood disorders (D56-D76)

contact dermatitis (L23-L25)

dermatitis due to substances taken internally (L27.-)

nephropathy (N14.0-N14.2)

NOTES The drug giving rise to the adverse effect should be identified by use of codes from categories T36-T50 with fifth or sixth character 5.

Use additional code(s) to specify:

manifestations of poisoning

underdosing or failure in dosage during medical and surgical care (Y63.6, Y63.8-Y63.9)

underdosing of medication regimen (Z91.12-, Z91.13-)

EXCLUDES1 *toxic reaction to local anesthesia in pregnancy (O29.3-)*

EXCLUDES2 *abuse and dependence of psychoactive substances (F10-F19)*

abuse of non-dependence-producing substances (F55.-)

drug reaction and poisoning affecting newborn (P00-P96)

pathological drug intoxication (inebriation) (F10-F19)

T36 Poisoning by, adverse effect of and underdosing of systemic antibiotics

EXCLUDES1 *antineoplastic antibiotics (T45.1-)*

locally applied antibiotic NEC (T49.0)

topically used antibiotic for ear, nose and throat (T49.6)

topically used antibiotic for eye (T49.5)

The appropriate 7th character is to be added to each code from category T36

A = initial encounter

D = subsequent encounter

S = sequela

T36.0 Poisoning by, adverse effect of and underdosing of penicillins

T36.0X Poisoning by, adverse effect of and underdosing of penicillins

T36.0X1 Poisoning by penicillins, accidental (unintentional)

Poisoning by penicillins NOS

T36.0X2 Poisoning by penicillins, intentional self-harm

T36.0X3 Poisoning by penicillins, assault

T36.0X4 Poisoning by penicillins, undetermined

T36.0X5 Adverse effect of penicillins

T36.0X6 Underdosing of penicillins

T36.1 Poisoning by, adverse effect of and underdosing of cephalosporins and other beta-lactam antibiotics

T36.1X Poisoning by, adverse effect of and underdosing of cephalosporins and other beta-lactam antibiotics

T36.1X1 Poisoning by cephalosporins and other beta-lactam antibiotics, accidental (unintentional)

Poisoning by cephalosporins and other beta-lactam antibiotics NOS

T36.1X2 Poisoning by cephalosporins and other beta-lactam antibiotics, intentional self-harm

T36.1X3 Poisoning by cephalosporins and other beta-lactam antibiotics, assault

T36.1X4 Poisoning by cephalosporins and other beta-lactam antibiotics, undetermined

T36.1X5 Adverse effect of cephalosporins and other beta-lactam antibiotics

T36.1X6 Underdosing of cephalosporins and other beta-lactam antibiotics

T36.2 Poisoning by, adverse effect of and underdosing of chloramphenicol group

T36.2X Poisoning by, adverse effect of and underdosing of chloramphenicol group

T36.2X1 Poisoning by chloramphenicol group, accidental (unintentional)

Poisoning by chloramphenicol group NOS

T36.2X2 Poisoning by chloramphenicol group, intentional self-harm

T36.2X3 Poisoning by chloramphenicol group, assault

T36.2X4 Poisoning by chloramphenicol group, undetermined

T36.2X5 Adverse effect of chloramphenicol group

T36.2X6 Underdosing of chloramphenicol group

T36.3 Poisoning by, adverse effect of and underdosing of macrolides

T36.3X Poisoning by, adverse effect of and underdosing of macrolides

T36.3X1 Poisoning by macrolides, accidental (unintentional)

Poisoning by macrolides NOS

T36.3X2 Poisoning by macrolides, intentional self-harm

T36.3X3 Poisoning by macrolides, assault

T36.3X4 Poisoning by macrolides, undetermined

T36.3X5 Adverse effect of macrolides

T36.3X6 Underdosing of macrolides

T36.4 Poisoning by, adverse effect of and underdosing of tetracyclines

T36.4X Poisoning by, adverse effect of and underdosing of tetracyclines

T36.4X1 Poisoning by tetracyclines, accidental (unintentional)

Poisoning by tetracyclines NOS

T36.4X2 Poisoning by tetracyclines, intentional self-harm

T36.4X3 Poisoning by tetracyclines, assault

T36.4X4 Poisoning by tetracyclines, undetermined

T36.4X5 Adverse effect of tetracyclines

T36.4X6 Underdosing of tetracyclines

T36.5 Poisoning by, adverse effect of and underdosing of aminoglycosides

Poisoning by, adverse effect of and underdosing of streptomycin

T36.5X Poisoning by, adverse effect of and underdosing of aminoglycosides

T36.5X1 Poisoning by aminoglycosides, accidental (unintentional)

Poisoning by aminoglycosides NOS

T36.5X2 Poisoning by aminoglycosides, intentional self-harm

T36.5X3 Poisoning by aminoglycosides, assault

T36.5X4 Poisoning by aminoglycosides, undetermined

T36.5X5 Adverse effect of aminoglycosides

T36.5X6 Underdosing of aminoglycosides

T36.6 Poisoning by, adverse effect of and underdosing of rifampicins

T36.6X Poisoning by, adverse effect of and underdosing of rifampicins

T36.6X1 Poisoning by rifampicins, accidental (unintentional)

Poisoning by rifampicins NOS

T36.6X2 Poisoning by rifampicins, intentional self-harm

T36.6X3 Poisoning by rifampicins, assault

T36.6X4 Poisoning by rifampicins, undetermined

T36.6X5 Adverse effect of rifampicins

T36.6X6 Underdosing of rifampicins

T36.7 Poisoning by, adverse effect of and underdosing of antifungal antibiotics, systemically used

T36.7X Poisoning by, adverse effect of and underdosing of antifungal antibiotics, **systemically used**

T36.7X1 Poisoning by antifungal antibiotics, systemically used, accidental (unintentional)

Unspecified Code   Other Specified Code   Manifestation Code   N Newborn   P Pediatric   M Maternity   A Adult   ♂ Male   ♀ Female

● New Code   ▲ Revised Code Title   ►◄ Revised Text   **NOTES** *INCLUDES* *EXCLUDES 1* Not coded here   *EXCLUDES 2* Not included here

4th character required   5th character required   6th character required   7th character required

Extension 'X' Alert   **HAC** Hospital-acquired condition (HAC) alert   **AHA** AHA Coding Clinic©

Poisoning by antifungal antibiotics, systemically used NOS

7th T36.7X2 **Poisoning by antifungal antibiotics, systemically used,** intentional self-harm POA HCC

7th T36.7X3 **Poisoning by antifungal antibiotics, systemically used,** assault POA

7th T36.7X4 **Poisoning by antifungal antibiotics, systemically used,** undetermined POA

7th T36.7X5 Adverse effect of antifungal antibiotics, systemically used POA PDxln

7th T36.7X6 Underdosing of antifungal antibiotics, systemically used POA PDxln

5th T36.8 **Poisoning by, adverse effect of and underdosing of other systemic antibiotics**

6th T36.8X **Poisoning by, adverse effect of and underdosing of** other systemic antibiotics

7th T36.8X1 **Poisoning by other systemic antibiotics,** accidental (unintentional) POA

Poisoning by other systemic antibiotics NOS

7th T36.8X2 **Poisoning by other systemic antibiotics,** intentional self-harm POA HCC

7th T36.8X3 **Poisoning by other systemic antibiotics,** assault POA

7th T36.8X4 **Poisoning by other systemic antibiotics,** undetermined POA

7th T36.8X5 Adverse effect of other systemic antibiotics POA PDxln

7th T36.8X6 Underdosing of other systemic antibiotics POA PDxln

5th T36.9 **Poisoning by, adverse effect of and underdosing of** unspecified systemic antibiotic

7th T36.91 **Poisoning by unspecified systemic antibiotic, accidental (unintentional)** POA

Poisoning by systemic antibiotic NOS

7th T36.92 **Poisoning by unspecified systemic antibiotic,** intentional self-harm POA HCC

7th T36.93 **Poisoning by unspecified systemic antibiotic,** assault POA

7th T36.94 **Poisoning by unspecified systemic antibiotic,** undetermined POA

7th T36.95 Adverse effect of unspecified systemic antibiotic POA PDxln

7th T36.96 Underdosing of unspecified systemic antibiotic POA PDxln

4th T37 **Poisoning by, adverse effect of and underdosing of other systemic anti- infectives and antiparasitics**

EXCLUDES1 anti-infectives topically used for ear, nose and throat (T49.6-)
anti-infectives topically used for eye (T49.5-)
locally applied anti-infectives NEC (T49.0-)

The appropriate 7th character is to be added to each code from category T37

A = initial encounter
D = subsequent encounter
S = sequela

5th T37.0 **Poisoning by, adverse effect of and underdosing of sulfonamides**

6th T37.0X **Poisoning by, adverse effect of and underdosing of** sulfonamides

7th T37.0X1 **Poisoning by sulfonamides,** accidental (unintentional) POA

Poisoning by sulfonamides NOS

7th T37.0X2 **Poisoning by sulfonamides,** intentional self-harm POA HCC

7th T37.0X3 **Poisoning by sulfonamides,** assault POA

7th T37.0X4 **Poisoning by sulfonamides,** undetermined POA

7th T37.0X5 Adverse effect of sulfonamides POA PDxln

7th T37.0X6 Underdosing of sulfonamides POA PDxln

5th T37.1 **Poisoning by, adverse effect of and underdosing of antimycobacterial drugs**

EXCLUDES1 rifampicins (T36.6-)
streptomycin (T36.5-)

6th T37.1X **Poisoning by, adverse effect of and underdosing of** antimycobacterial drugs

7th T37.1X1 **Poisoning by antimycobacterial drugs, accidental (unintentional)** POA

Poisoning by antimycobacterial drugs NOS

7th T37.1X2 **Poisoning by antimycobacterial drugs, intentional self-harm** POA HCC

7th T37.1X3 **Poisoning by antimycobacterial drugs, assault** POA

7th T37.1X4 **Poisoning by antimycobacterial drugs, undetermined** POA

7th T37.1X5 Adverse effect of antimycobacterial drugs POA PDxln

7th T37.1X6 Underdosing of antimycobacterial drugs POA PDxln

5th T37.2 **Poisoning by, adverse effect of and underdosing of antimalarials and drugs acting on other blood protozoa**

EXCLUDES1 hydroxyquinoline derivatives (T37.8-)

6th T37.2X **Poisoning by, adverse effect of and underdosing of** antimalarials and drugs acting on other blood protozoa

7th T37.2X1 **Poisoning by antimalarials and drugs acting on other blood protozoa, accidental (unintentional)** POA

Poisoning by antimalarials and drugs acting on other blood protozoa NOS

7th T37.2X2 **Poisoning by antimalarials and drugs acting on other blood protozoa, intentional self-harm** POA HCC

7th T37.2X3 **Poisoning by antimalarials and drugs acting on other blood protozoa, assault** POA

7th T37.2X4 **Poisoning by antimalarials and drugs acting on other blood protozoa, undetermined** POA

7th T37.2X5 Adverse effect of antimalarials and drugs acting on other blood protozoa POA PDxln

7th T37.2X6 Underdosing of antimalarials and drugs acting on other blood protozoa POA PDxln

5th T37.3 **Poisoning by, adverse effect of and underdosing of other antiprotozoal drugs**

6th T37.3X **Poisoning by, adverse effect of and underdosing of** other antiprotozoal drugs

7th T37.3X1 **Poisoning by other antiprotozoal drugs, accidental (unintentional)** POA

Poisoning by other antiprotozoal drugs NOS

7th T37.3X2 **Poisoning by other antiprotozoal drugs, intentional self-harm** POA HCC

7th T37.3X3 **Poisoning by other antiprotozoal drugs, assault** POA

7th T37.3X4 **Poisoning by other antiprotozoal drugs, undetermined** POA

7th T37.3X5 Adverse effect of other antiprotozoal drugs POA PDxln

7th T37.3X6 Underdosing of other antiprotozoal drugs POA PDxln

5th T37.4 **Poisoning by, adverse effect of and underdosing of anthelminthics**

6th T37.4X **Poisoning by, adverse effect of and underdosing of** anthelminthics

7th T37.4X1 **Poisoning by anthelminthics, accidental (unintentional)** POA

Poisoning by anthelminthics NOS

7th T37.4X2 **Poisoning by anthelminthics, intentional self-harm** POA HCC

7th T37.4X3 **Poisoning by anthelminthics, assault** POA

7th T37.4X4 **Poisoning by anthelminthics, undetermined** POA

7th T37.4X5 Adverse effect of anthelminthics POA PDxln

7th T37.4X6 Underdosing of anthelminthics POA PDxln

PDxln Unacceptable principal diagnosis symbol per Medicare code edits   POA Code exempt from diagnosis present on admission requirement
? Questionable admission   CC Complication or comorbidity   CC/MCC excl CC/MCC exclusion   MCC Major complication or comorbidity
Principal diagnosis as its own CC   Principal diagnosis as its own MCC   HCC HCC diagnosis code   RxHCC RxHCC diagnosis code
MACRA code   Z1 Z code as first-listed diagnosis

When symbols appear on a code that requires a 7th character extension, refer to Appendix B to identify applicable 7th character codes.

5ᵈ **T37.5** Poisoning by, adverse effect of and underdosing of antiviral drugs

    EXCLUDES1 *amantadine (T42.8-)*

        cytarabine (T45.1-)

  6ᵈ **T37.5X** Poisoning by, adverse effect of and underdosing of antiviral drugs

    7ᵈ **T37.5X1** Poisoning by antiviral drugs, accidental (unintentional) POA

      Poisoning by antiviral drugs NOS

    7ᵈ **T37.5X2** Poisoning by antiviral drugs, intentional self-harm POA HCC

    7ᵈ **T37.5X3** Poisoning by antiviral drugs, assault POA

    7ᵈ **T37.5X4** Poisoning by antiviral drugs, undetermined POA

    7ᵈ **T37.5X5** Adverse effect of antiviral drugs POA PDxIn

    7ᵈ **T37.5X6** Underdosing of antiviral drugs POA PDxIn

5ᵈ **T37.8** Poisoning by, adverse effect of and underdosing of other specified systemic anti-infectives and antiparasitics

    Poisoning by, adverse effect of and underdosing of hydroxyquinoline derivatives

    EXCLUDES1 *antimalarial drugs (T37.2-)*

  6ᵈ **T37.8X** Poisoning by, adverse effect of and underdosing of other specified systemic anti-infectives and antiparasitics

    7ᵈ **T37.8X1** Poisoning by other specified systemic anti-infectives and antiparasitics, accidental (unintentional) POA

      Poisoning by other specified systemic anti-infectives and antiparasitics NOS

    7ᵈ **T37.8X2** Poisoning by other specified systemic anti-infectives and antiparasitics, intentional self-harm POA HCC

    7ᵈ **T37.8X3** Poisoning by other specified systemic anti-infectives and antiparasitics, assault POA

    7ᵈ **T37.8X4** Poisoning by other specified systemic anti-infectives and antiparasitics, undetermined POA

    7ᵈ **T37.8X5** Adverse effect of other specified systemic anti-infectives and antiparasitics POA PDxIn

    7ᵈ **T37.8X6** Underdosing of other specified systemic anti-infectives and antiparasitics POA PDxIn

5ᵈ **T37.9** Poisoning by, adverse effect of and underdosing of unspecified systemic anti-infective and antiparasitics

    7ᵈ **T37.91** Poisoning by unspecified systemic anti-infective and antiparasitics, accidental (unintentional) POA

      Poisoning by, adverse effect of and underdosing of systemic anti-infective and antiparasitics NOS

    7ᵈ **T37.92** Poisoning by unspecified systemic anti-infective and antiparasitics, intentional self-harm POA HCC

    7ᵈ **T37.93** Poisoning by unspecified systemic anti-infective and antiparasitics, assault POA

    7ᵈ **T37.94** Poisoning by unspecified systemic anti-infective and antiparasitics, undetermined POA

    7ᵈ **T37.95** Adverse effect of unspecified systemic anti-infective and antiparasitic POA PDxIn

    7ᵈ **T37.96** Underdosing of unspecified systemic anti-infectives and antiparasitics POA PDxIn

4ᵈ **T38** Poisoning by, adverse effect of and underdosing of hormones and their synthetic substitutes and antagonists, not elsewhere classified

    EXCLUDES1 *mineralocorticoids and their antagonists (T50.0-)*

        oxytocic hormones (T48.0-)

        parathyroid hormones and derivatives (T50.9-)

    The appropriate 7th character is to be added to each code from category T38

      A = initial encounter

      D = subsequent encounter

      S = sequela

  5ᵈ **T38.0** Poisoning by, adverse effect of and underdosing of glucocorticoids and synthetic analogues

    EXCLUDES1 *glucocorticoids, topically used (T49.-)*

6ᵈ **T38.0X** Poisoning by, adverse effect of and underdosing of glucocorticoids and synthetic analogues

  7ᵈ **T38.0X1** Poisoning by glucocorticoids and synthetic analogues, accidental (unintentional) POA

    Poisoning by glucocorticoids and synthetic analogues NOS

  7ᵈ **T38.0X2** Poisoning by glucocorticoids and synthetic analogues, intentional self-harm POA HCC

  7ᵈ **T38.0X3** Poisoning by glucocorticoids and synthetic analogues, assault POA

  7ᵈ **T38.0X4** Poisoning by glucocorticoids and synthetic analogues, undetermined POA

  7ᵈ **T38.0X5** Adverse effect of glucocorticoids and synthetic analogues POA PDxIn

  7ᵈ **T38.0X6** Underdosing of glucocorticoids and synthetic analogues POA PDxIn

5ᵈ **T38.1** Poisoning by, adverse effect of and underdosing of thyroid hormones and substitutes

  6ᵈ **T38.1X** Poisoning by, adverse effect of and underdosing of thyroid hormones and substitutes

    7ᵈ **T38.1X1** Poisoning by thyroid hormones and substitutes, accidental (unintentional) POA

      Poisoning by thyroid hormones and substitutes NOS

    7ᵈ **T38.1X2** Poisoning by thyroid hormones and substitutes, intentional self-harm POA HCC

    7ᵈ **T38.1X3** Poisoning by thyroid hormones and substitutes, assault POA

    7ᵈ **T38.1X4** Poisoning by thyroid hormones and substitutes, undetermined POA

    7ᵈ **T38.1X5** Adverse effect of thyroid hormones and substitutes POA PDxIn

    7ᵈ **T38.1X6** Underdosing of thyroid hormones and substitutes POA PDxIn

5ᵈ **T38.2** Poisoning by, adverse effect of and underdosing of antithyroid drugs

  6ᵈ **T38.2X** Poisoning by, adverse effect of and underdosing of antithyroid drugs

    7ᵈ **T38.2X1** Poisoning by antithyroid drugs, accidental (unintentional) POA

      Poisoning by antithyroid drugs NOS

    7ᵈ **T38.2X2** Poisoning by antithyroid drugs, intentional self-harm POA HCC

    7ᵈ **T38.2X3** Poisoning by antithyroid drugs, assault POA

    7ᵈ **T38.2X4** Poisoning by antithyroid drugs, undetermined POA

    7ᵈ **T38.2X5** Adverse effect of antithyroid drugs POA PDxIn

    7ᵈ **T38.2X6** Underdosing of antithyroid drugs POA PDxIn

5ᵈ **T38.3** Poisoning by, adverse effect of and underdosing of insulin and oral hypoglycemic [antidiabetic] drugs

  6ᵈ **T38.3X** Poisoning by, adverse effect of and underdosing of insulin and oral hypoglycemic [antidiabetic] drugs

    7ᵈ **T38.3X1** Poisoning by insulin and oral hypoglycemic [antidiabetic] drugs, accidental (unintentional) POA

      Poisoning by insulin and oral hypoglycemic [antidiabetic] drugs NOS

    7ᵈ **T38.3X2** Poisoning by insulin and oral hypoglycemic [antidiabetic] drugs, intentional self-harm POA HCC

    7ᵈ **T38.3X3** Poisoning by insulin and oral hypoglycemic [antidiabetic] drugs, assault POA

    7ᵈ **T38.3X4** Poisoning by insulin and oral hypoglycemic [antidiabetic] drugs, undetermined POA

    7ᵈ **T38.3X5** Adverse effect of insulin and oral hypoglycemic [antidiabetic] drugs POA PDxIn

    7ᵈ **T38.3X6** Underdosing of insulin and oral hypoglycemic [antidiabetic] drugs POA PDxIn

---

Unspecified Code   Other Specified Code   Manifestation Code   N Newborn   P Pediatric   M Maternity   A Adult   ♂ Male   ♀ Female

● New Code   ▲ Revised Code Title   ►◄ Revised Text   NOTES   *INCLUDES*   EXCLUDES1 Not coded here   EXCLUDES2 Not included here

4ᵈ 4th character required   5ᵈ 5th character required   6ᵈ 6th character required   7ᵈ 7th character required

Ⓧ Extension 'X' Alert   HAC Hospital-acquired condition (HAC) alert   **AHA** AHA Coding Clinic©

T38.4 **Poisoning by, adverse effect of and underdosing of oral contraceptives**

Poisoning by, adverse effect of and underdosing of multiple- and single-ingredient oral contraceptive preparations

T38.4X **Poisoning by, adverse effect of and underdosing of oral contraceptives**

T38.4X1 **Poisoning by oral contraceptives, accidental (unintentional)**

Poisoning by oral contraceptives NOS

T38.4X2 **Poisoning by oral contraceptives, intentional self-harm**

T38.4X3 **Poisoning by oral contraceptives, assault**

T38.4X4 **Poisoning by oral contraceptives, undetermined**

T38.4X5 Adverse effect of oral contraceptives

T38.4X6 Underdosing of oral contraceptives

T38.5 **Poisoning by, adverse effect of and underdosing of other estrogens and progestogens**

Poisoning by, adverse effect of and underdosing of estrogens and progestogens mixtures and substitutes

T38.5X **Poisoning by, adverse effect of and underdosing of other estrogens and progestogens**

T38.5X1 **Poisoning by other estrogens and progestogens, accidental (unintentional)**

Poisoning by other estrogens and progestogens NOS

T38.5X2 **Poisoning by other estrogens and progestogens, intentional self-harm**

T38.5X3 **Poisoning by other estrogens and progestogens, assault**

T38.5X4 **Poisoning by other estrogens and progestogens, undetermined**

T38.5X5 Adverse effect of other estrogens and progestogens

T38.5X6 Underdosing of other estrogens and progestogens

T38.6 **Poisoning by, adverse effect of and underdosing of antigonadotrophins, antiestrogens, antiandrogens, not elsewhere classified**

Poisoning by, adverse effect of and underdosing of tamoxifen

T38.6X **Poisoning by, adverse effect of and underdosing of antigonadotrophins, antiestrogens, antiandrogens, not elsewhere classified**

T38.6X1 **Poisoning by antigonadotrophins, antiestrogens, antiandrogens, not elsewhere classified, accidental (unintentional)**

Poisoning by antigonadotrophins, antiestrogens, antiandrogens, not elsewhere classified NOS

T38.6X2 **Poisoning by antigonadotrophins, antiestrogens, antiandrogens, not elsewhere classified, intentional self-harm**

T38.6X3 **Poisoning by antigonadotrophins, antiestrogens, antiandrogens, not elsewhere classified, assault**

T38.6X4 **Poisoning by antigonadotrophins, antiestrogens, antiandrogens, not elsewhere classified, undetermined**

T38.6X5 Adverse effect of antigonadotrophins, antiestrogens, antiandrogens, not elsewhere classified

T38.6X6 Underdosing of antigonadotrophins, antiestrogens, antiandrogens, not elsewhere classified

T38.7 **Poisoning by, adverse effect of and underdosing of androgens and anabolic congeners**

T38.7X **Poisoning by, adverse effect of and underdosing of androgens and anabolic congeners**

T38.7X1 **Poisoning by androgens and anabolic congeners, accidental (unintentional)**

Poisoning by androgens and anabolic congeners NOS

T38.7X2 **Poisoning by androgens and anabolic congeners, intentional self-harm**

T38.7X3 **Poisoning by androgens and anabolic congeners, assault**

T38.7X4 **Poisoning by androgens and anabolic congeners, undetermined**

T38.7X5 Adverse effect of androgens and anabolic congeners

T38.7X6 Underdosing of androgens and anabolic congeners

T38.8 **Poisoning by, adverse effect of and underdosing of other and unspecified hormones and synthetic substitutes**

T38.80 **Poisoning by, adverse effect of and underdosing of unspecified hormones and synthetic substitutes**

T38.801 **Poisoning by unspecified hormones and synthetic substitutes, accidental (unintentional)**

Poisoning by unspecified hormones and synthetic substitutes NOS

T38.802 **Poisoning by unspecified hormones and synthetic substitutes, intentional self-harm**

T38.803 **Poisoning by unspecified hormones and synthetic substitutes, assault**

T38.804 **Poisoning by unspecified hormones and synthetic substitutes, undetermined**

T38.805 Adverse effect of unspecified hormones and synthetic substitutes

T38.806 Underdosing of unspecified hormones and synthetic substitutes

T38.81 **Poisoning by, adverse effect of and underdosing of anterior pituitary [adenohypophyseal] hormones**

T38.811 **Poisoning by anterior pituitary [adenohypophyseal] hormones, accidental (unintentional)**

Poisoning by anterior pituitary [adenohypophyseal] hormones NOS

T38.812 **Poisoning by anterior pituitary [adenohypophyseal] hormones, intentional self-harm**

T38.813 **Poisoning by anterior pituitary [adenohypophyseal] hormones, assault**

T38.814 **Poisoning by anterior pituitary [adenohypophyseal] hormones, undetermined**

T38.815 Adverse effect of anterior pituitary [adenohypophyseal] hormones

T38.816 Underdosing of anterior pituitary [adenohypophyseal] hormones

T38.89 **Poisoning by, adverse effect of and underdosing of other hormones and synthetic substitutes**

T38.891 **Poisoning by other hormones and synthetic substitutes, accidental (unintentional)**

Poisoning by other hormones and synthetic substitutes NOS

T38.892 **Poisoning by other hormones and synthetic substitutes, intentional self-harm**

T38.893 **Poisoning by other hormones and synthetic substitutes, assault**

T38.894 **Poisoning by other hormones and synthetic substitutes, undetermined**

T38.895 Adverse effect of other hormones and synthetic substitutes

T38.896 Underdosing of other hormones and synthetic substitutes

T38.9 **Poisoning by, adverse effect of and underdosing of other and unspecified hormone antagonists**

Unacceptable principal diagnosis symbol per Medicare code edits   Code exempt from diagnosis present on admission requirement
? Questionable admission   Complication or comorbidity   CC/MCC exclusion   Major complication or comorbidity
Principal diagnosis as its own CC   Principal diagnosis as its own MCC   HCC HCC diagnosis code   RxHCC diagnosis code
MACRA code   Z Code as first-listed diagnosis

6️⃣ **T38.90** Poisoning by, adverse effect of and underdosing of unspecified hormone antagonists

   7️⃣ **T38.901** **Poisoning by unspecified hormone antagonists, accidental (unintentional)** POA

      Poisoning by unspecified hormone antagonists NOS

   7️⃣ **T38.902** **Poisoning by unspecified hormone antagonists, intentional self-harm** POA HCC

   7️⃣ **T38.903** **Poisoning by unspecified hormone antagonists, assault** POA

   7️⃣ **T38.904** **Poisoning by unspecified hormone antagonists, undetermined** POA

   7️⃣ **T38.905** Adverse effect of unspecified hormone antagonists POA PDxIn

   7️⃣ **T38.906** Underdosing of unspecified hormone antagonists POA PDxIn

6️⃣ **T38.99** Poisoning by, adverse effect of and underdosing of other hormone antagonists

   7️⃣ **T38.991** **Poisoning by other hormone antagonists, accidental (unintentional)** POA

      Poisoning by other hormone antagonists NOS

   7️⃣ **T38.992** **Poisoning by other hormone antagonists, intentional self-harm** POA HCC

   7️⃣ **T38.993** **Poisoning by other hormone antagonists, assault** POA

   7️⃣ **T38.994** **Poisoning by other hormone antagonists, undetermined** POA

   7️⃣ **T38.995** Adverse effect of other hormone antagonists POA PDxIn

   7️⃣ **T38.996** Underdosing of other hormone antagonists POA PDxIn

4️⃣ **T39** Poisoning by, adverse effect of and underdosing of nonopioid analgesics, antipyretics and antirheumatics

The appropriate 7th character is to be added to each code from category T39

   A = initial encounter

   D = subsequent encounter

   S = sequela

5️⃣ **T39.0** Poisoning by, adverse effect of and underdosing of salicylates

   6️⃣ **T39.01** **Poisoning by, adverse effect of and underdosing of aspirin**

      Poisoning by, adverse effect of and underdosing of acetylsalicylic acid

     7️⃣ **T39.011** **Poisoning by aspirin, accidental (unintentional)** POA

     7️⃣ **T39.012** **Poisoning by aspirin, intentional self-harm** POA HCC

     7️⃣ **T39.013** **Poisoning by aspirin, assault** POA

     7️⃣ **T39.014** **Poisoning by aspirin, undetermined** POA

     7️⃣ **T39.015** Adverse effect of aspirin POA PDxIn

     7️⃣ **T39.016** Underdosing of aspirin POA PDxIn

   6️⃣ **T39.09** **Poisoning by, adverse effect of and underdosing of other salicylates**

     7️⃣ **T39.091** **Poisoning by salicylates, accidental (unintentional)** POA

        Poisoning by salicylates NOS

     7️⃣ **T39.092** **Poisoning by salicylates, intentional self-harm** POA HCC

     7️⃣ **T39.093** **Poisoning by salicylates, assault** POA

     7️⃣ **T39.094** **Poisoning by salicylates, undetermined** POA

     7️⃣ **T39.095** Adverse effect of salicylates POA PDxIn

     7️⃣ **T39.096** Underdosing of salicylates POA PDxIn

5️⃣ **T39.1** Poisoning by, adverse effect of and underdosing of 4-Aminophenol derivatives

   6️⃣ **T39.1X** Poisoning by, adverse effect of and underdosing of 4-Aminophenol derivatives

     7️⃣ **T39.1X1** **Poisoning by 4-Aminophenol derivatives, accidental (unintentional)** POA

        Poisoning by 4-Aminophenol derivatives NOS

     7️⃣ **T39.1X2** **Poisoning by 4-Aminophenol derivatives, intentional self-harm** POA HCC

     7️⃣ **T39.1X3** **Poisoning by 4-Aminophenol derivatives, assault** POA

     7️⃣ **T39.1X4** **Poisoning by 4-Aminophenol derivatives, undetermined** POA

     7️⃣ **T39.1X5** Adverse effect of 4-Aminophenol derivatives POA PDxIn

     7️⃣ **T39.1X6** Underdosing of 4-Aminophenol derivatives POA PDxIn

5️⃣ **T39.2** Poisoning by, adverse effect of and underdosing of pyrazolone derivatives

   6️⃣ **T39.2X** Poisoning by, adverse effect of and underdosing of pyrazolone derivatives

     7️⃣ **T39.2X1** **Poisoning by pyrazolone derivatives, accidental (unintentional)** POA

        Poisoning by pyrazolone derivatives NOS

     7️⃣ **T39.2X2** **Poisoning by pyrazolone derivatives, intentional self-harm** POA HCC

     7️⃣ **T39.2X3** **Poisoning by pyrazolone derivatives, assault** POA

     7️⃣ **T39.2X4** **Poisoning by pyrazolone derivatives, undetermined** POA

     7️⃣ **T39.2X5** Adverse effect of pyrazolone derivatives POA PDxIn

     7️⃣ **T39.2X6** Underdosing of pyrazolone derivatives POA PDxIn

5️⃣ **T39.3** Poisoning by, adverse effect of and underdosing of other nonsteroidal anti-inflammatory drugs [NSAID]

   6️⃣ **T39.31** Poisoning by, adverse effect of and underdosing of propionic acid derivatives

       Poisoning by, adverse effect of and underdosing of fenoprofen

       Poisoning by, adverse effect of and underdosing of flurbiprofen

       Poisoning by, adverse effect of and underdosing of ibuprofen

       Poisoning by, adverse effect of and underdosing of ketoprofen

       Poisoning by, adverse effect of and underdosing of naproxen

       Poisoning by, adverse effect of and underdosing of oxaprozin

     7️⃣ **T39.311** **Poisoning by propionic acid derivatives, accidental (unintentional)** POA

     7️⃣ **T39.312** **Poisoning by propionic acid derivatives, intentional self-harm** POA HCC

     7️⃣ **T39.313** **Poisoning by propionic acid derivatives, assault** POA

     7️⃣ **T39.314** **Poisoning by propionic acid derivatives, undetermined** POA

     7️⃣ **T39.315** Adverse effect of propionic acid derivatives POA PDxIn

     7️⃣ **T39.316** Underdosing of propionic acid derivatives POA PDxIn

   6️⃣ **T39.39** Poisoning by, adverse effect of and underdosing of other nonsteroidal anti-inflammatory drugs [NSAID]

     7️⃣ **T39.391** **Poisoning by other nonsteroidal anti-inflammatory drugs [NSAID], accidental (unintentional)** POA

        Poisoning by other nonsteroidal anti-inflammatory drugs NOS

     7️⃣ **T39.392** **Poisoning by other nonsteroidal anti-inflammatory drugs [NSAID], intentional self-harm** POA HCC

     7️⃣ **T39.393** **Poisoning by other nonsteroidal anti-inflammatory drugs [NSAID], assault** POA

     7️⃣ **T39.394** **Poisoning by other nonsteroidal anti-inflammatory drugs [NSAID], undetermined** POA

     7️⃣ **T39.395** Adverse effect of other nonsteroidal anti-inflammatory drugs [NSAID] POA PDxIn

---

Unspecified Code   Other Specified Code   Manifestation Code   N Newborn   P Pediatric   M Maternity   A Adult   ♂ Male   ♀ Female

● New Code   ▲ Revised Code Title   ▶◀ Revised Text   **NOTES**   *INCLUDES*   *EXCLUDES 1* Not coded here   *EXCLUDES 2* Not included here

4️⃣ 4th character required   5️⃣ 5th character required   6️⃣ 6th character required   7️⃣ 7th character required

7️⃣ Extension 'X' Alert   HAC Hospital-acquired condition (HAC) alert   **AHA** AHA Coding Clinic©

T47.4X Poisoning by, adverse effect of and underdosing of other laxatives

- T47.4X1 Poisoning by other laxatives, accidental (unintentional)

  Poisoning by other laxatives NOS

- T47.4X2 Poisoning by other laxatives, intentional self-harm

- T47.4X3 Poisoning by other laxatives, assault

- T47.4X4 Poisoning by other laxatives, undetermined

- T47.4X5 Adverse effect of other laxatives

- T47.4X6 Underdosing of other laxatives

T47.5 Poisoning by, adverse effect of and underdosing of digestants

T47.5X Poisoning by, adverse effect of and underdosing of digestants

- T47.5X1 Poisoning by digestants, accidental (unintentional)

  Poisoning by digestants NOS

- T47.5X2 Poisoning by digestants, intentional self-harm

- T47.5X3 Poisoning by digestants, assault

- T47.5X4 Poisoning by digestants, undetermined

- T47.5X5 Adverse effect of digestants

- T47.5X6 Underdosing of digestants

T47.6 Poisoning by, adverse effect of and underdosing of antidiarrheal drugs

EXCLUDES2 poisoning by, adverse effect of and underdosing of systemic antibiotics and other anti-infectives (T36-T37)

T47.6X Poisoning by, adverse effect of and underdosing of antidiarrheal drugs

- T47.6X1 Poisoning by antidiarrheal drugs, accidental (unintentional)

  Poisoning by antidiarrheal drugs NOS

- T47.6X2 Poisoning by antidiarrheal drugs, intentional self-harm

- T47.6X3 Poisoning by antidiarrheal drugs, assault

- T47.6X4 Poisoning by antidiarrheal drugs, undetermined

- T47.6X5 Adverse effect of antidiarrheal drugs

- T47.6X6 Underdosing of antidiarrheal drugs

T47.7 Poisoning by, adverse effect of and underdosing of emetics

T47.7X Poisoning by, adverse effect of and underdosing of emetics

- T47.7X1 Poisoning by emetics, accidental (unintentional)

  Poisoning by emetics NOS

- T47.7X2 Poisoning by emetics, intentional self-harm

- T47.7X3 Poisoning by emetics, assault

- T47.7X4 Poisoning by emetics, undetermined

- T47.7X5 Adverse effect of emetics

- T47.7X6 Underdosing of emetics

T47.8 Poisoning by, adverse effect of and underdosing of other agents primarily affecting gastrointestinal system

T47.8X Poisoning by, adverse effect of and underdosing of other agents primarily affecting gastrointestinal system

- T47.8X1 Poisoning by other agents primarily affecting gastrointestinal system, accidental (unintentional)

  Poisoning by other agents primarily affecting gastrointestinal system NOS

- T47.8X2 Poisoning by other agents primarily affecting gastrointestinal system, intentional self-harm

- T47.8X3 Poisoning by other agents primarily affecting gastrointestinal system, assault

- T47.8X4 Poisoning by other agents primarily affecting gastrointestinal system, undetermined

- T47.8X5 Adverse effect of other agents primarily affecting gastrointestinal system

- T47.8X6 Underdosing of other agents primarily affecting gastrointestinal system

T47.9 Poisoning by, adverse effect of and underdosing of unspecified agents primarily affecting the gastrointestinal system

- T47.91 Poisoning by unspecified agents primarily affecting the gastrointestinal system, accidental (unintentional)

  Poisoning by agents primarily affecting the gastrointestinal system NOS

- T47.92 Poisoning by unspecified agents primarily affecting the gastrointestinal system, intentional self-harm

- T47.93 Poisoning by unspecified agents primarily affecting the gastrointestinal system, assault

- T47.94 Poisoning by unspecified agents primarily affecting the gastrointestinal system, undetermined

- T47.95 Adverse effect of unspecified agents primarily affecting the gastrointestinal system

- T47.96 Underdosing of unspecified agents primarily affecting the gastrointestinal system

T48 Poisoning by, adverse effect of and underdosing of agents primarily acting on smooth and skeletal muscles and the respiratory system

The appropriate 7th character is to be added to each code from category T48

A = initial encounter

D = subsequent encounter

S = sequela

T48.0 Poisoning by, adverse effect of and underdosing of oxytocic drugs

EXCLUDES1 poisoning by, adverse effect of and underdosing of estrogens, progestogens and antagonists (T38.4-T38.6)

T48.0X Poisoning by, adverse effect of and underdosing of oxytocic drugs

- T48.0X1 Poisoning by oxytocic drugs, accidental (unintentional)

  Poisoning by oxytocic drugs NOS

- T48.0X2 Poisoning by oxytocic drugs, intentional self-harm

- T48.0X3 Poisoning by oxytocic drugs, assault

- T48.0X4 Poisoning by oxytocic drugs, undetermined

- T48.0X5 Adverse effect of oxytocic drugs

- T48.0X6 Underdosing of oxytocic drugs

T48.1 Poisoning by, adverse effect of and underdosing of skeletal muscle relaxants [neuromuscular blocking agents]

T48.1X Poisoning by, adverse effect of and underdosing of skeletal muscle relaxants [neuromuscular blocking agents]

- T48.1X1 Poisoning by skeletal muscle relaxants [neuromuscular blocking agents], accidental (unintentional)

  Poisoning by skeletal muscle relaxants [neuromuscular blocking agents] NOS

- T48.1X2 Poisoning by skeletal muscle relaxants [neuromuscular blocking agents], intentional self-harm

- T48.1X3 Poisoning by skeletal muscle relaxants [neuromuscular blocking agents], assault

- T48.1X4 Poisoning by skeletal muscle relaxants [neuromuscular blocking agents], undetermined

- T48.1X5 Adverse effect of skeletal muscle relaxants [neuromuscular blocking agents]

- T48.1X6 Underdosing of skeletal muscle relaxants [neuromuscular blocking agents]

Unacceptable principal diagnosis symbol per Medicare code edits   Code exempt from diagnosis present on admission requirement   Questionable admission   Complication or comorbidity   CC/MCC exclusion   Major complication or comorbidity   Principal diagnosis as its own CC   Principal diagnosis as its own MCC   HCC diagnosis code   RxHCC diagnosis code   MACRA code   Z code as first-listed diagnosis

T48.2 Poisoning by, adverse effect of and underdosing of other and unspecified drugs acting on muscles

T48.20 Poisoning by, adverse effect of and underdosing of unspecified drugs acting on muscles

T48.201 Poisoning by unspecified drugs acting on muscles, accidental (unintentional) POA
Poisoning by unspecified drugs acting on muscles NOS

T48.202 Poisoning by unspecified drugs acting on muscles, intentional self-harm POA HCC

T48.203 Poisoning by unspecified drugs acting on muscles, assault POA

T48.204 Poisoning by unspecified drugs acting on muscles, undetermined POA

T48.205 Adverse effect of unspecified drugs acting on muscles POA PDxIn

T48.206 Underdosing of unspecified drugs acting on muscles POA PDxIn

T48.29 Poisoning by, adverse effect of and underdosing of other drugs acting on muscles

T48.291 Poisoning by other drugs acting on muscles, accidental (unintentional) POA
Poisoning by other drugs acting on muscles NOS

T48.292 Poisoning by other drugs acting on muscles, intentional self-harm POA HCC

T48.293 Poisoning by other drugs acting on muscles, assault POA

T48.294 Poisoning by other drugs acting on muscles, undetermined POA

T48.295 Adverse effect of other drugs acting on muscles POA PDxIn

T48.296 Underdosing of other drugs acting on muscles POA PDxIn

T48.3 Poisoning by, adverse effect of and underdosing of antitussives

T48.3X Poisoning by, adverse effect of and underdosing of antitussives

T48.3X1 Poisoning by antitussives, accidental (unintentional) POA
Poisoning by antitussives NOS

T48.3X2 Poisoning by antitussives, intentional self-harm POA HCC

T48.3X3 Poisoning by antitussives, assault POA

T48.3X4 Poisoning by antitussives, undetermined POA

T48.3X5 Adverse effect of antitussives POA PDxIn

T48.3X6 Underdosing of antitussives POA PDxIn

T48.4 Poisoning by, adverse effect of and underdosing of expectorants

T48.4X Poisoning by, adverse effect of and underdosing of expectorants

T48.4X1 Poisoning by expectorants, accidental (unintentional) POA
Poisoning by expectorants NOS

T48.4X2 Poisoning by expectorants, intentional self-harm POA HCC

T48.4X3 Poisoning by expectorants, assault POA

T48.4X4 Poisoning by expectorants, undetermined POA

T48.4X5 Adverse effect of expectorants POA PDxIn

T48.4X6 Underdosing of expectorants POA PDxIn

T48.5 Poisoning by, adverse effect of and underdosing of other anti-common-cold drugs
Poisoning by, adverse effect of and underdosing of decongestants

EXCLUDES2 *poisoning by, adverse effect of and underdosing of antipyretics, NEC (T39.9-)*

poisoning by, adverse effect of and underdosing of non-steroidal antiinflammatory drugs (T39.3-)

poisoning by, adverse effect of and underdosing of salicylates (T39.0-)

T48.5X Poisoning by, adverse effect of and underdosing of other anti-common-cold drugs

T48.5X1 Poisoning by other anti-common-cold drugs, accidental (unintentional) POA
Poisoning by other anti-common-cold drugs NOS

T48.5X2 Poisoning by other anti-common-cold drugs, intentional self-harm POA HCC

T48.5X3 Poisoning by other anti-common-cold drugs, assault POA

T48.5X4 Poisoning by other anti-common-cold drugs, undetermined POA

T48.5X5 Adverse effect of other anti-common-cold drugs POA

T48.5X6 Underdosing of other anti-common-cold drugs POA PDxIn

T48.6 Poisoning by, adverse effect of and underdosing of antiasthmatics, not elsewhere classified
Poisoning by, adverse effect of and underdosing of beta-adrenoreceptor agonists used in asthma therapy

EXCLUDES1 *poisoning by, adverse effect of and underdosing of beta-adrenoreceptor agonists not used in asthma therapy (T44.5)*

poisoning by, adverse effect of and underdosing of anterior pituitary [adenohypophyseal] hormones (T38.8)

T48.6X Poisoning by, adverse effect of and underdosing of antiasthmatics

T48.6X1 Poisoning by antiasthmatics, accidental (unintentional) POA
Poisoning by antiasthmatics NOS

T48.6X2 Poisoning by antiasthmatics, intentional self-harm POA HCC

T48.6X3 Poisoning by antiasthmatics, assault POA

T48.6X4 Poisoning by antiasthmatics, undetermined POA

T48.6X5 Adverse effect of antiasthmatics POA PDxIn

T48.6X6 Underdosing of antiasthmatics POA PDxIn

T48.9 Poisoning by, adverse effect of and underdosing of other and unspecified agents primarily acting on the respiratory system

T48.90 Poisoning by, adverse effect of and underdosing of unspecified agents primarily acting on the respiratory system

T48.901 Poisoning by unspecified agents primarily acting on the respiratory system, accidental (unintentional) POA

T48.902 Poisoning by unspecified agents primarily acting on the respiratory system, intentional self-harm POA HCC

T48.903 Poisoning by unspecified agents primarily acting on the respiratory system, assault POA

T48.904 Poisoning by unspecified agents primarily acting on the respiratory system, undetermined POA

T48.905 Adverse effect of unspecified agents primarily acting on the respiratory system POA PDxIn

T48.906 Underdosing of unspecified agents primarily acting on the respiratory system POA PDxIn

T48.99 Poisoning by, adverse effect of and underdosing of other agents primarily acting on the respiratory system

T48.991 Poisoning by other agents primarily acting on the respiratory system, accidental (unintentional) POA

T48.992 Poisoning by other agents primarily acting on the respiratory system, intentional self-harm POA HCC

T48.993 Poisoning by other agents primarily acting on the respiratory system, assault POA

Unspecified Code   Other Specified Code   Manifestation Code   N Newborn   P Pediatric   M Maternity   A Adult   ♂ Male   ♀ Female
● New Code   ▲ Revised Code Title   ►◄ Revised Text   NOTES   INCLUDES   EXCLUDES 1 Not coded here   EXCLUDES 2 Not included here
4th character required   5th character required   6th character required   7th character required
Extension 'X' Alert   HAC Hospital-acquired condition (HAC) alert   AHA AHA Coding Clinic©

T48.994 Poisoning by other agents primarily acting on the respiratory system, undetermined POA

T48.995 Adverse effect of other agents primarily acting on the respiratory system POA PDxIn

T48.996 Underdosing of other agents primarily acting on the respiratory system POA PDxIn

T49 Poisoning by, adverse effect of and underdosing of topical agents primarily affecting skin and mucous membrane and by ophthalmological, otorhinorlaryngological and dental drugs

INCLUDES poisoning by, adverse effect of and underdosing of glucocorticoids, topically used

The appropriate 7th character is to be added to each code from category T49

A = initial encounter
D = subsequent encounter
S = sequela

T49.0 Poisoning by, adverse effect of and underdosing of local antifungal, anti-infective and anti-inflammatory drugs

T49.0X Poisoning by, adverse effect of and underdosing of local antifungal, anti-infective and anti-inflammatory drugs

T49.0X1 Poisoning by local antifungal, anti-infective and anti-inflammatory drugs, accidental (unintentional) POA

Poisoning by local antifungal, anti-infective and anti-inflammatory drugs NOS

T49.0X2 Poisoning by local antifungal, anti-infective and anti-inflammatory drugs, intentional self-harm POA HCC

T49.0X3 Poisoning by local antifungal, anti-infective and anti-inflammatory drugs, assault POA

T49.0X4 Poisoning by local antifungal, anti-infective and anti-inflammatory drugs, undetermined POA

T49.0X5 Adverse effect of local antifungal, anti-infective and anti-inflammatory drugs POA PDxIn

T49.0X6 Underdosing of local antifungal, anti-infective and anti-inflammatory drugs POA PDxIn

T49.1 Poisoning by, adverse effect of and underdosing of antipruritics

T49.1X Poisoning by, adverse effect of and underdosing of antipruritics

T49.1X1 Poisoning by antipruritics, accidental (unintentional) POA

Poisoning by antipruritics NOS

T49.1X2 Poisoning by antipruritics, intentional self-harm POA HCC

T49.1X3 Poisoning by antipruritics, assault POA

T49.1X4 Poisoning by antipruritics, undetermined POA

T49.1X5 Adverse effect of antipruritics POA PDxIn

T49.1X6 Underdosing of antipruritics POA PDxIn

T49.2 Poisoning by, adverse effect of and underdosing of local astringents and local detergents

T49.2X Poisoning by, adverse effect of and underdosing of local astringents and local detergents

T49.2X1 Poisoning by local astringents and local detergents, accidental (unintentional) POA

Poisoning by local astringents and local detergents NOS

T49.2X2 Poisoning by local astringents and local detergents, intentional self-harm POA HCC

T49.2X3 Poisoning by local astringents and local detergents, assault POA

T49.2X4 Poisoning by local astringents and local detergents, undetermined POA

T49.2X5 Adverse effect of local astringents and local detergents POA PDxIn

T49.2X6 Underdosing of local astringents and local detergents POA PDxIn

T49.3 Poisoning by, adverse effect of and underdosing of emollients, demulcents and protectants

T49.3X Poisoning by, adverse effect of and underdosing of emollients, demulcents and protectants

T49.3X1 Poisoning by emollients, demulcents and protectants, accidental (unintentional) POA

Poisoning by emollients, demulcents and protectants NOS

T49.3X2 Poisoning by emollients, demulcents and protectants, intentional self-harm POA HCC

T49.3X3 Poisoning by emollients, demulcents and protectants, assault POA

T49.3X4 Poisoning by emollients, demulcents and protectants, undetermined POA

T49.3X5 Adverse effect of emollients, demulcents and protectants POA PDxIn

T49.3X6 Underdosing of emollients, demulcents and protectants POA PDxIn

T49.4 Poisoning by, adverse effect of and underdosing of keratolytics, keratoplastics, and other hair treatment drugs and preparations

T49.4X Poisoning by, adverse effect of and underdosing of keratolytics, keratoplastics, and other hair treatment drugs and preparations

T49.4X1 Poisoning by keratolytics, keratoplastics, and other hair treatment drugs and preparations, accidental (unintentional) POA

Poisoning by keratolytics, keratoplastics, and other hair treatment drugs and preparations NOS

T49.4X2 Poisoning by keratolytics, keratoplastics, and other hair treatment drugs and preparations, intentional self-harm POA HCC

T49.4X3 Poisoning by keratolytics, keratoplastics, and other hair treatment drugs and preparations, assault POA

T49.4X4 Poisoning by keratolytics, keratoplastics, and other hair treatment drugs and preparations, undetermined POA

T49.4X5 Adverse effect of keratolytics, keratoplastics, and other hair treatment drugs and preparations POA PDxIn

T49.4X6 Underdosing of keratolytics, keratoplastics, and other hair treatment drugs and preparations POA PDxIn

T49.5 Poisoning by, adverse effect of and underdosing of ophthalmological drugs and preparations

T49.5X Poisoning by, adverse effect of and underdosing of ophthalmological drugs and preparations

T49.5X1 Poisoning by ophthalmological drugs and preparations, accidental (unintentional) POA

Poisoning by ophthalmological drugs and preparations NOS

T49.5X2 Poisoning by ophthalmological drugs and preparations, intentional self-harm POA HCC

T49.5X3 Poisoning by ophthalmological drugs and preparations, assault POA

T49.5X4 Poisoning by ophthalmological drugs and preparations, undetermined POA

T49.5X5 Adverse effect of ophthalmological drugs and preparations POA PDxIn

T49.5X6 Underdosing of ophthalmological drugs and preparations POA PDxIn

T49.6 Poisoning by, adverse effect of and underdosing of otorhinolaryngological drugs and preparations

T49.6X Poisoning by, adverse effect of and underdosing of otorhinolaryngological drugs and preparations

T49.6X1 Poisoning by otorhinolaryngological drugs and preparations, accidental (unintentional) POA

Poisoning by otorhinolaryngological drugs and preparations NOS

PDx Unacceptable principal diagnosis symbol per Medicare code edits • POA Code exempt from diagnosis present on admission requirement • Questionable admission • CC Complication or comorbidity • CC/MCC exclusion • MCC Major complication or comorbidity • Principal diagnosis as its own CC • Principal diagnosis as its own MCC • HCC HCC diagnosis code • RxHCC RxHCC diagnosis code • MACRA code • Z1 Z code as first-listed diagnosis

T49.6X2 Poisoning by otorhinolaryngological drugs and preparations, intentional self-harm POA HCC

T49.6X3 Poisoning by otorhinolaryngological drugs and preparations, assault POA

T49.6X4 Poisoning by otorhinolaryngological drugs and preparations, undetermined POA

T49.6X5 Adverse effect of otorhinolaryngological drugs and preparations POA PDxIn

T49.6X6 Underdosing of otorhinolaryngological drugs and preparations POA PDxIn

T49.7 Poisoning by, adverse effect of and underdosing of dental drugs, topically applied

T49.7X Poisoning by, adverse effect of and underdosing of dental drugs, topically applied

T49.7X1 Poisoning by dental drugs, topically applied, accidental (unintentional) POA
Poisoning by dental drugs, topically applied NOS

T49.7X2 Poisoning by dental drugs, topically applied, intentional self-harm POA HCC

T49.7X3 Poisoning by dental drugs, topically applied, assault POA

T49.7X4 Poisoning by dental drugs, topically applied, undetermined POA

T49.7X5 Adverse effect of dental drugs, topically applied POA PDxIn

T49.7X6 Underdosing of dental drugs, topically applied POA PDxIn

T49.8 Poisoning by, adverse effect of and underdosing of other topical agents
Poisoning by, adverse effect of and underdosing of spermicides

T49.8X Poisoning by, adverse effect of and underdosing of other topical agents

T49.8X1 Poisoning by other topical agents, accidental (unintentional) POA
Poisoning by other topical agents NOS

T49.8X2 Poisoning by other topical agents, intentional self-harm POA HCC

T49.8X3 Poisoning by other topical agents, assault POA

T49.8X4 Poisoning by other topical agents, undetermined POA

T49.8X5 Adverse effect of other topical agents POA PDxIn

T49.8X6 Underdosing of other topical agents POA PDxIn

T49.9 Poisoning by, adverse effect of and underdosing of unspecified topical agent

T49.91 Poisoning by unspecified topical agent, accidental (unintentional) POA

T49.92 Poisoning by unspecified topical agent, intentional self-harm POA HCC

T49.93 Poisoning by unspecified topical agent, assault POA

T49.94 Poisoning by unspecified topical agent, undetermined POA

T49.95 Adverse effect of unspecified topical agent POA PDxIn

T49.96 Underdosing of unspecified topical agent POA PDxIn

T50 Poisoning by, adverse effect of and underdosing of diuretics and other and unspecified drugs, medicaments and biological substances
The appropriate 7th character is to be added to each code from category T50
A = initial encounter
D = subsequent encounter
S = sequela

T50.0 Poisoning by, adverse effect of and underdosing of mineralocorticoids and their antagonists

T50.0X Poisoning by, adverse effect of and underdosing of mineralocorticoids and their antagonists

T50.0X1 Poisoning by mineralocorticoids and their antagonists, accidental (unintentional) POA
Poisoning by mineralocorticoids and their antagonists NOS

T50.0X2 Poisoning by mineralocorticoids and their antagonists, intentional self-harm POA HCC

T50.0X3 Poisoning by mineralocorticoids and their antagonists, assault POA

T50.0X4 Poisoning by mineralocorticoids and their antagonists, undetermined POA

T50.0X5 Adverse effect of mineralocorticoids and their antagonists POA PDxIn

T50.0X6 Underdosing of mineralocorticoids and their antagonists POA PDxIn

T50.1 Poisoning by, adverse effect of and underdosing of loop [high-ceiling] diuretics

T50.1X Poisoning by, adverse effect of and underdosing of loop [high-ceiling] diuretics

T50.1X1 Poisoning by loop [high-ceiling] diuretics, accidental (unintentional) POA
Poisoning by loop [high-ceiling] diuretics NOS

T50.1X2 Poisoning by loop [high-ceiling] diuretics, intentional self-harm POA HCC

T50.1X3 Poisoning by loop [high-ceiling] diuretics, assault POA

T50.1X4 Poisoning by loop [high-ceiling] diuretics, undetermined POA

T50.1X5 Adverse effect of loop [high-ceiling] diuretics POA PDxIn

T50.1X6 Underdosing of loop [high-ceiling] diuretics POA PDxIn

T50.2 Poisoning by, adverse effect of and underdosing of carbonic-anhydrase inhibitors, benzothiadiazides and other diuretics
Poisoning by, adverse effect of and underdosing of acetazolamide

T50.2X Poisoning by, adverse effect of and underdosing of carbonic-anhydrase inhibitors, benzothiadiazides and other diuretics

T50.2X1 Poisoning by carbonic-anhydrase inhibitors, benzothiadiazides and other diuretics, accidental (unintentional) POA
Poisoning by carbonic-anhydrase inhibitors, benzothiadiazides and other diuretics NOS

T50.2X2 Poisoning by carbonic-anhydrase inhibitors, benzothiadiazides and other diuretics, intentional self-harm POA HCC

T50.2X3 Poisoning by carbonic-anhydrase inhibitors, benzothiadiazides and other diuretics, assault POA

T50.2X4 Poisoning by carbonic-anhydrase inhibitors, benzothiadiazides and other diuretics, undetermined POA

T50.2X5 Adverse effect of carbonic-anhydrase inhibitors, benzothiadiazides and other diuretics POA PDxIn

T50.2X6 Underdosing of carbonic-anhydrase inhibitors, benzothiadiazides and other diuretics POA PDxIn

T50.3 Poisoning by, adverse effect of and underdosing of electrolytic, caloric and water-balance agents
Poisoning by, adverse effect of and underdosing of oral rehydration salts

T50.3X Poisoning by, adverse effect of and underdosing of electrolytic, caloric and water-balance agents

T50.3X1 Poisoning by electrolytic, caloric and water-balance agents, accidental (unintentional) POA
Poisoning by electrolytic, caloric and water-balance agents NOS

Unspecified Code   Other Specified Code   Manifestation Code   N Newborn   P Pediatric   M Maternity   A Adult   ♂ Male   ♀ Female
● New Code   ▲ Revised Code Title   ►◄ Revised Text   NOTES   INCLUDES   EXCLUDES 1 Not coded here   EXCLUDES 2 Not included here
4th character required   5th character required   6th character required   7th character required
Extension 'X' Alert   HAC Hospital-acquired condition (HAC) alert   AHA AHA Coding Clinic©

- 7th T50.3X2 Poisoning by electrolytic, caloric and water-balance agents, intentional self-harm POA HCC
- 7th T50.3X3 Poisoning by electrolytic, caloric and water-balance agents, assault POA
- 7th T50.3X4 Poisoning by electrolytic, caloric and water-balance agents, undetermined POA
- 7th T50.3X5 Adverse effect of electrolytic, caloric and water-balance agents
- 7th T50.3X6 Underdosing of electrolytic, caloric and water-balance agents POA PDxIn

5th T50.4 Poisoning by, adverse effect of and underdosing of drugs affecting uric acid metabolism
- 6th T50.4X Poisoning by, adverse effect of and underdosing of drugs affecting uric acid metabolism
  - 7th T50.4X1 Poisoning by drugs affecting uric acid metabolism, accidental (unintentional) POA
    Poisoning by drugs affecting uric acid metabolism NOS
  - 7th T50.4X2 Poisoning by drugs affecting uric acid metabolism, intentional self-harm POA HCC
  - 7th T50.4X3 Poisoning by drugs affecting uric acid metabolism, assault POA
  - 7th T50.4X4 Poisoning by drugs affecting uric acid metabolism, undetermined POA
  - 7th T50.4X5 Adverse effect of drugs affecting uric acid metabolism POA PDxIn
  - 7th T50.4X6 Underdosing of drugs affecting uric acid metabolism POA PDxIn

5th T50.5 Poisoning by, adverse effect of and underdosing of appetite depressants
- 6th T50.5X Poisoning by, adverse effect of and underdosing of appetite depressants
  - 7th T50.5X1 Poisoning by appetite depressants, accidental (unintentional) POA
    Poisoning by appetite depressants NOS
  - 7th T50.5X2 Poisoning by appetite depressants, intentional self-harm POA HCC
  - 7th T50.5X3 Poisoning by appetite depressants, assault POA
  - 7th T50.5X4 Poisoning by appetite depressants, undetermined POA
  - 7th T50.5X5 Adverse effect of appetite depressants POA PDxIn
  - 7th T50.5X6 Underdosing of appetite depressants POA PDxIn

5th T50.6 Poisoning by, adverse effect of and underdosing of antidotes and chelating agents
Poisoning by, adverse effect of and underdosing of alcohol deterrents
- 6th T50.6X Poisoning by, adverse effect of and underdosing of antidotes and chelating agents
  - 7th T50.6X1 Poisoning by antidotes and chelating agents, accidental (unintentional) POA
    Poisoning by antidotes and chelating agents NOS
  - 7th T50.6X2 Poisoning by antidotes and chelating agents, intentional self-harm POA HCC
  - 7th T50.6X3 Poisoning by antidotes and chelating agents, assault POA
  - 7th T50.6X4 Poisoning by antidotes and chelating agents, undetermined POA
  - 7th T50.6X5 Adverse effect of antidotes and chelating agents POA PDxIn
  - 7th T50.6X6 Underdosing of antidotes and chelating agents POA PDxIn

5th T50.7 Poisoning by, adverse effect of and underdosing of analeptics and opioid receptor antagonists
- 6th T50.7X Poisoning by, adverse effect of and underdosing of analeptics and opioid receptor antagonists

- 7th T50.7X1 Poisoning by analeptics and opioid receptor antagonists, accidental (unintentional) POA
  Poisoning by analeptics and opioid receptor antagonists NOS
- 7th T50.7X2 Poisoning by analeptics and opioid receptor antagonists, intentional self-harm POA HCC
- 7th T50.7X3 Poisoning by analeptics and opioid receptor antagonists, assault POA
- 7th T50.7X4 Poisoning by analeptics and opioid receptor antagonists, undetermined POA
- 7th T50.7X5 Adverse effect of analeptics and opioid receptor antagonists POA PDxIn
- 7th T50.7X6 Underdosing of analeptics and opioid receptor antagonists POA PDxIn

5th T50.8 Poisoning by, adverse effect of and underdosing of diagnostic agents
- 6th T50.8X Poisoning by, adverse effect of and underdosing of diagnostic agents
  - 7th T50.8X1 Poisoning by diagnostic agents, accidental (unintentional) POA
    Poisoning by diagnostic agents NOS
  - 7th T50.8X2 Poisoning by diagnostic agents, intentional self-harm POA HCC
  - 7th T50.8X3 Poisoning by diagnostic agents, assault POA
  - 7th T50.8X4 Poisoning by diagnostic agents, undetermined POA
  - 7th T50.8X5 Adverse effect of diagnostic agents POA PDxIn
  - 7th T50.8X6 Underdosing of diagnostic agents POA PDxIn

5th T50.A Poisoning by, adverse effect of and underdosing of bacterial vaccines
- 6th T50.A1 Poisoning by, adverse effect of and underdosing of pertussis vaccine, including combinations with a pertussis component
  - 7th T50.A11 Poisoning by pertussis vaccine, including combinations with a pertussis component, accidental (unintentional) POA
  - 7th T50.A12 Poisoning by pertussis vaccine, including combinations with a pertussis component, intentional self-harm POA HCC
  - 7th T50.A13 Poisoning by pertussis vaccine, including combinations with a pertussis component, assault POA
  - 7th T50.A14 Poisoning by pertussis vaccine, including combinations with a pertussis component, undetermined POA
  - 7th T50.A15 Adverse effect of pertussis vaccine, including combinations with a pertussis component POA PDxIn
  - 7th T50.A16 Underdosing of pertussis vaccine, including combinations with a pertussis component POA PDxIn
- 6th T50.A2 Poisoning by, adverse effect of and underdosing of mixed bacterial vaccines without a pertussis component
  - 7th T50.A21 Poisoning by mixed bacterial vaccines without a pertussis component, accidental (unintentional) POA
  - 7th T50.A22 Poisoning by mixed bacterial vaccines without a pertussis component, intentional self-harm POA HCC
  - 7th T50.A23 Poisoning by mixed bacterial vaccines without a pertussis component, assault POA
  - 7th T50.A24 Poisoning by mixed bacterial vaccines without a pertussis component, undetermined POA
  - 7th T50.A25 Adverse effect of mixed bacterial vaccines without a pertussis component POA PDxIn
  - 7th T50.A26 Underdosing of mixed bacterial vaccines without a pertussis component POA PDxIn

PDxIn Unacceptable principal diagnosis symbol per Medicare code edits   POA Code exempt from diagnosis present on admission requirement
? Questionable admission   CC Complication or comorbidity   CC/MCC Excl CC/MCC exclusion   MCC Major complication or comorbidity
PDx CC Principal diagnosis as its own CC   PDx MCC Principal diagnosis as its own MCC   HCC HCC diagnosis code   RxHCC RxHCC diagnosis code
MACRA code   Z1 Z code as first-listed diagnosis

- T50.A9 Poisoning by, adverse effect of and underdosing of other bacterial vaccines
  - T50.A91 Poisoning by other bacterial vaccines, accidental (unintentional) POA
  - T50.A92 Poisoning by other bacterial vaccines, intentional self-harm POA HCC
  - T50.A93 Poisoning by other bacterial vaccines, assault POA
  - T50.A94 Poisoning by other bacterial vaccines, undetermined POA
  - T50.A95 Adverse effect of other bacterial vaccines POA PDxIn
  - T50.A96 Underdosing of other bacterial vaccines POA PDxIn
- T50.B Poisoning by, adverse effect of and underdosing of viral vaccines
  - T50.B1 Poisoning by, adverse effect of and underdosing of smallpox vaccines
    - T50.B11 Poisoning by smallpox vaccines, accidental (unintentional) POA
    - T50.B12 Poisoning by smallpox vaccines, intentional self-harm POA HCC
    - T50.B13 Poisoning by smallpox vaccines, assault POA
    - T50.B14 Poisoning by smallpox vaccines, undetermined POA
    - T50.B15 Adverse effect of smallpox vaccines POA PDxIn
    - T50.B16 Underdosing of smallpox vaccines POA PDxIn
  - T50.B9 Poisoning by, adverse effect of and underdosing of other viral vaccines
    - T50.B91 Poisoning by other viral vaccines, accidental (unintentional) POA
    - T50.B92 Poisoning by other viral vaccines, intentional self-harm POA HCC
    - T50.B93 Poisoning by other viral vaccines, assault POA
    - T50.B94 Poisoning by other viral vaccines, undetermined POA
    - T50.B95 Adverse effect of other viral vaccines POA PDxIn
    - T50.B96 Underdosing of other viral vaccines POA PDxIn
- T50.Z Poisoning by, adverse effect of and underdosing of other vaccines and biological substances
  - T50.Z1 Poisoning by, adverse effect of and underdosing of immunoglobulin
    - T50.Z11 Poisoning by immunoglobulin, accidental (unintentional) POA
    - T50.Z12 Poisoning by immunoglobulin, intentional self-harm POA HCC
    - T50.Z13 Poisoning by immunoglobulin, assault POA
    - T50.Z14 Poisoning by immunoglobulin, undetermined POA
    - T50.Z15 Adverse effect of immunoglobulin POA PDxIn
    - T50.Z16 Underdosing of immunoglobulin POA PDxIn
  - T50.Z9 Poisoning by, adverse effect of and underdosing of other vaccines and biological substances
    - T50.Z91 Poisoning by other vaccines and biological substances, accidental (unintentional) POA
    - T50.Z92 Poisoning by other vaccines and biological substances, intentional self-harm POA HCC
    - T50.Z93 Poisoning by other vaccines and biological substances, assault POA
    - T50.Z94 Poisoning by other vaccines and biological substances, undetermined POA
    - T50.Z95 Adverse effect of other vaccines and biological substances POA PDxIn
    - T50.Z96 Underdosing of other vaccines and biological substances POA PDxIn
- T50.9 Poisoning by, adverse effect of and underdosing of other and unspecified drugs, medicaments and biological substances
  - T50.90 Poisoning by, adverse effect of and underdosing of unspecified drugs, medicaments and biological substances
    - T50.901 Poisoning by unspecified drugs, medicaments and biological substances, accidental (unintentional) POA
    - T50.902 Poisoning by unspecified drugs, medicaments and biological substances, intentional self-harm POA HCC
    - T50.903 Poisoning by unspecified drugs, medicaments and biological substances, assault POA
    - T50.904 Poisoning by unspecified drugs, medicaments and biological substances, undetermined POA
    - T50.905 Adverse effect of unspecified drugs, medicaments and biological substances POA
    - T50.906 Underdosing of unspecified drugs, medicaments and biological substances POA
  - T50.99 Poisoning by, adverse effect of and underdosing of other drugs, medicaments and biological substances
    - T50.991 Poisoning by other drugs, medicaments and biological substances, accidental (unintentional) POA
    - T50.992 Poisoning by other drugs, medicaments and biological substances, intentional self-harm POA HCC
    - T50.993 Poisoning by other drugs, medicaments and biological substances, assault POA
    - T50.994 Poisoning by other drugs, medicaments and biological substances, undetermined POA
    - T50.995 Adverse effect of other drugs, medicaments and biological substances POA
    - T50.996 Underdosing of other drugs, medicaments and biological substances POA

Toxic effects of substances chiefly nonmedicinal as to source (T51-T65)

NOTES When no intent is indicated code to accidental. Undetermined intent is only for use when there is specific documentation in the record that the intent of the toxic effect cannot be determined.
Use additional code(s):
for all associated manifestations of toxic effect, such as: respiratory conditions due to external agents (J60-J70)
personal history of foreign body fully removed (Z87.821)
to identify any retained foreign body, if applicable (Z18.-)
EXCLUDES1 contact with and (suspected) exposure to toxic substances (Z77.-)

- T51 Toxic effect of alcohol
  The appropriate 7th character is to be added to each code from category T51
  A = initial encounter
  D = subsequent encounter
  S = sequela
  - T51.0 Toxic effect of ethanol
    Toxic effect of ethyl alcohol
    EXCLUDES2 acute alcohol intoxication or 'hangover' effects (F10.129, F10.229, F10.929)
    drunkenness (F10.129, F10.229, F10.929)
    pathological alcohol intoxication (F10.129, F10.229, F10.929)
    - T51.0X Toxic effect of ethanol
      - T51.0X1 Toxic effect of ethanol, accidental (unintentional) POA
        Toxic effect of ethanol NOS
      - T51.0X2 Toxic effect of ethanol, intentional self-harm POA HCC
      - T51.0X3 Toxic effect of ethanol, assault POA
      - T51.0X4 Toxic effect of ethanol, undetermined POA
  - T51.1 Toxic effect of methanol
    Toxic effect of methyl alcohol
    - T51.1X Toxic effect of methanol

Unspecified Code   Other Specified Code   Manifestation Code   N Newborn   P Pediatric   M Maternity   A Adult   ♂ Male   ♀ Female
● New Code   ▲ Revised Code Title   ▶◀ Revised Text   NOTES   INCLUDES   EXCLUDES 1 Not coded here   EXCLUDES 2 Not included here
4th character required   5th character required   6th character required   7th character required
Extension 'X' Alert   HAC Hospital-acquired condition (HAC) alert   AHA AHA Coding Clinic©

7th **T51.1X1** **Toxic effect of methanol,** accidental (unintentional) POA
Toxic effect of methanol NOS

7th **T51.1X2** **Toxic effect of methanol,** intentional self-harm POA HCC

7th **T51.1X3** **Toxic effect of methanol,** assault POA

7th **T51.1X4** **Toxic effect of methanol,** undetermined POA

5th **T51.2** **Toxic effect of 2-Propanol**
Toxic effect of isopropyl alcohol

6th **T51.2X** **Toxic effect of** 2-Propanol

7th **T51.2X1** **Toxic effect of 2-Propanol,** accidental (unintentional) POA
Toxic effect of 2-Propanol NOS

7th **T51.2X2** **Toxic effect of 2-Propanol,** intentional self-harm POA HCC

7th **T51.2X3** **Toxic effect of 2-Propanol,** assault POA

7th **T51.2X4** **Toxic effect of 2-Propanol,** undetermined POA

5th **T51.3** **Toxic effect of fusel oil**
Toxic effect of amyl alcohol
Toxic effect of butyl [1-butanol] alcohol
Toxic effect of propyl [1-propanol] alcohol

6th **T51.3X** **Toxic effect of** fusel oil

7th **T51.3X1** **Toxic effect of fusel oil,** accidental (unintentional) POA
Toxic effect of fusel oil NOS

7th **T51.3X2** **Toxic effect of fusel oil,** intentional self-harm POA HCC

7th **T51.3X3** **Toxic effect of fusel oil,** assault POA

7th **T51.3X4** **Toxic effect of fusel oil,** undetermined POA

5th **T51.8** **Toxic effect of other alcohols**

6th **T51.8X** **Toxic effect of** other alcohols

7th **T51.8X1** **Toxic effect of other alcohols,** accidental (unintentional) POA
Toxic effect of other alcohols NOS

7th **T51.8X2** **Toxic effect of other alcohols,** intentional self-harm POA HCC

7th **T51.8X3** **Toxic effect of other alcohols,** assault POA

7th **T51.8X4** **Toxic effect of other alcohols,** undetermined POA

5th **T51.9** **Toxic effect of** unspecified alcohol

7th **T51.91** **Toxic effect of unspecified alcohol,** accidental (unintentional) POA

7th **T51.92** **Toxic effect of unspecified alcohol,** intentional self-harm POA HCC

7th **T51.93** **Toxic effect of unspecified alcohol,** assault POA

7th **T51.94** **Toxic effect of unspecified alcohol,** undetermined POA

4th **T52** **Toxic effect of organic solvents**

EXCLUDES1 halogen derivatives of aliphatic and aromatic hydrocarbons (T53.-)

The appropriate 7th character is to be added to each code from category T52

A = initial encounter
D = subsequent encounter
S = sequela

5th **T52.0** **Toxic effects of petroleum products**
Toxic effects of gasoline [petrol]
Toxic effects of kerosene [paraffin oil]
Toxic effects of paraffin wax
Toxic effects of ether petroleum
Toxic effects of naphtha petroleum
Toxic effects of spirit petroleum

6th **T52.0X** **Toxic effects of** petroleum products

7th **T52.0X1** **Toxic effect of petroleum products,** accidental (unintentional) POA
Toxic effects of petroleum products NOS

7th **T52.0X2** **Toxic effect of petroleum products,** intentional self-harm POA HCC

7th **T52.0X3** **Toxic effect of petroleum products,** assault POA

7th **T52.0X4** **Toxic effect of petroleum products,** undetermined POA

5th **T52.1** **Toxic effects of benzene**

EXCLUDES1 homologues of benzene (T52.2)

nitroderivatives and aminoderivatives of benzene and its homologues (T65.3)

6th **T52.1X** **Toxic effects of** benzene

7th **T52.1X1** **Toxic effect of benzene,** accidental (unintentional) POA
Toxic effects of benzene NOS

7th **T52.1X2** **Toxic effect of benzene,** intentional self-harm POA HCC

7th **T52.1X3** **Toxic effect of benzene,** assault POA

7th **T52.1X4** **Toxic effect of benzene,** undetermined POA

5th **T52.2** **Toxic effects of homologues of benzene**
Toxic effects of toluene [methylbenzene]
Toxic effects of xylene [dimethylbenzene]

6th **T52.2X** **Toxic effects of** homologues of benzene

7th **T52.2X1** **Toxic effect of homologues of benzene, accidental (unintentional)** POA
Toxic effects of homologues of benzene NOS

7th **T52.2X2** **Toxic effect of homologues of benzene, intentional self-harm** POA HCC

7th **T52.2X3** **Toxic effect of homologues of benzene, assault** POA

7th **T52.2X4** **Toxic effect of homologues of benzene, undetermined** POA

5th **T52.3** **Toxic effects of glycols**

6th **T52.3X** **Toxic effects of** glycols

7th **T52.3X1** **Toxic effect of glycols,** accidental (unintentional) POA
Toxic effects of glycols NOS

7th **T52.3X2** **Toxic effect of glycols,** intentional self-harm POA HCC

7th **T52.3X3** **Toxic effect of glycols,** assault POA

7th **T52.3X4** **Toxic effect of glycols,** undetermined POA

5th **T52.4** **Toxic effects of ketones**

6th **T52.4X** **Toxic effects of** ketones

7th **T52.4X1** **Toxic effect of ketones,** accidental (unintentional) POA
Toxic effects of ketones NOS

7th **T52.4X2** **Toxic effect of ketones,** intentional self-harm POA HCC

7th **T52.4X3** **Toxic effect of ketones,** assault POA

7th **T52.4X4** **Toxic effect of ketones,** undetermined POA

5th **T52.8** **Toxic effects of other organic solvents**

6th **T52.8X** **Toxic effects of** other organic solvents

7th **T52.8X1** **Toxic effect of other organic solvents, accidental (unintentional)** POA
Toxic effects of other organic solvents NOS

7th **T52.8X2** **Toxic effect of other organic solvents, intentional self-harm** POA HCC

7th **T52.8X3** **Toxic effect of other organic solvents, assault** POA

7th **T52.8X4** **Toxic effect of other organic solvents, undetermined** POA

5th **T52.9** **Toxic effects of unspecified organic solvent**

7th **T52.91** **Toxic effect of unspecified organic solvent, accidental (unintentional)** POA

7th **T52.92** **Toxic effect of unspecified organic solvent, intentional self-harm** POA HCC

7th **T52.93** **Toxic effect of unspecified organic solvent,** assault POA

7th **T52.94** **Toxic effect of unspecified organic solvent, undetermined** POA

4th **T53** **Toxic effect of halogen derivatives of aliphatic and aromatic hydrocarbons**

The appropriate 7th character is to be added to each code from category T53

A = initial encounter
D = subsequent encounter
S = sequela

POA Unacceptable principal diagnosis symbol per Medicare code edits   POA Code exempt from diagnosis present on admission requirement
❓ Questionable admission   cc Complication or comorbidity   cc/mcc excl CC/MCC exclusion   mcc Major complication or comorbidity
cc Principal diagnosis as its own CC   mcc Principal diagnosis as its own MCC   HCC HCC diagnosis code   RxHCC RxHCC diagnosis code
MACRA code   Z1 Z code as first-listed diagnosis

T53.0 Toxic effects of carbon tetrachloride
Toxic effects of tetrachloromethane
  T53.0X Toxic effects of carbon tetrachloride
    T53.0X1 Toxic effect of carbon tetrachloride, accidental (unintentional) POA
      Toxic effects of carbon tetrachloride NOS
    T53.0X2 Toxic effect of carbon tetrachloride, intentional self-harm POA HCC
    T53.0X3 Toxic effect of carbon tetrachloride, assault POA
    T53.0X4 Toxic effect of carbon tetrachloride, undetermined POA

T53.1 Toxic effects of chloroform
Toxic effects of trichloromethane
  T53.1X Toxic effects of chloroform
    T53.1X1 Toxic effect of chloroform, accidental (unintentional) POA
      Toxic effects of chloroform NOS
    T53.1X2 Toxic effect of chloroform, intentional self-harm POA HCC
    T53.1X3 Toxic effect of chloroform, assault POA
    T53.1X4 Toxic effect of chloroform, undetermined POA

T53.2 Toxic effects of trichloroethylene
Toxic effects of trichloroethene
  T53.2X Toxic effects of trichloroethylene
    T53.2X1 Toxic effect of trichloroethylene, accidental (unintentional) POA
      Toxic effects of trichloroethylene NOS
    T53.2X2 Toxic effect of trichloroethylene, intentional self-harm POA HCC
    T53.2X3 Toxic effect of trichloroethylene, assault POA
    T53.2X4 Toxic effect of trichloroethylene, undetermined POA

T53.3 Toxic effects of tetrachloroethylene
Toxic effects of perchloroethylene
Toxic effect of tetrachloroethene
  T53.3X Toxic effects of tetrachloroethylene
    T53.3X1 Toxic effect of tetrachloroethylene, accidental (unintentional) POA
      Toxic effects of tetrachloroethylene NOS
    T53.3X2 Toxic effect of tetrachloroethylene, intentional self-harm POA HCC
    T53.3X3 Toxic effect of tetrachloroethylene, assault POA
    T53.3X4 Toxic effect of tetrachloroethylene, undetermined POA

T53.4 Toxic effects of dichloromethane
Toxic effects of methylene chloride
  T53.4X Toxic effects of dichloromethane
    T53.4X1 Toxic effect of dichloromethane, accidental (unintentional) POA
      Toxic effects of dichloromethane NOS
    T53.4X2 Toxic effect of dichloromethane, intentional self-harm POA HCC
    T53.4X3 Toxic effect of dichloromethane, assault POA
    T53.4X4 Toxic effect of dichloromethane, undetermined POA

T53.5 Toxic effects of chlorofluorocarbons
  T53.5X Toxic effects of chlorofluorocarbons
    T53.5X1 Toxic effect of chlorofluorocarbons, accidental (unintentional) POA
      Toxic effects of chlorofluorocarbons NOS
    T53.5X2 Toxic effect of chlorofluorocarbons, intentional self-harm POA HCC
    T53.5X3 Toxic effect of chlorofluorocarbons, assault POA
    T53.5X4 Toxic effect of chlorofluorocarbons, undetermined POA

T53.6 Toxic effects of other halogen derivatives of aliphatic hydrocarbons
  T53.6X Toxic effects of other halogen derivatives of aliphatic hydrocarbons
    T53.6X1 Toxic effect of other halogen derivatives of aliphatic hydrocarbons, accidental (unintentional) POA
      Toxic effects of other halogen derivatives of aliphatic hydrocarbons NOS
    T53.6X2 Toxic effect of other halogen derivatives of aliphatic hydrocarbons, intentional self-harm POA HCC
    T53.6X3 Toxic effect of other halogen derivatives of aliphatic hydrocarbons, assault POA
    T53.6X4 Toxic effect of other halogen derivatives of aliphatic hydrocarbons, undetermined POA

T53.7 Toxic effects of other halogen derivatives of aromatic hydrocarbons
  T53.7X Toxic effects of other halogen derivatives of aromatic hydrocarbons
    T53.7X1 Toxic effect of other halogen derivatives of aromatic hydrocarbons, accidental (unintentional) POA
      Toxic effects of other halogen derivatives of aromatic hydrocarbons NOS
    T53.7X2 Toxic effect of other halogen derivatives of aromatic hydrocarbons, intentional self-harm POA HCC
    T53.7X3 Toxic effect of other halogen derivatives of aromatic hydrocarbons, assault POA
    T53.7X4 Toxic effect of other halogen derivatives of aromatic hydrocarbons, undetermined POA

T53.9 Toxic effects of unspecified halogen derivatives of aliphatic and aromatic hydrocarbons
    T53.91 Toxic effect of unspecified halogen derivatives of aliphatic and aromatic hydrocarbons, accidental (unintentional) POA
    T53.92 Toxic effect of unspecified halogen derivatives of aliphatic and aromatic hydrocarbons, intentional self-harm POA HCC
    T53.93 Toxic effect of unspecified halogen derivatives of aliphatic and aromatic hydrocarbons, assault POA
    T53.94 Toxic effect of unspecified halogen derivatives of aliphatic and aromatic hydrocarbons, undetermined POA

T54 Toxic effect of corrosive substances
The appropriate 7th character is to be added to each code from category T54
    A = initial encounter
    D = subsequent encounter
    S = sequela

T54.0 Toxic effects of phenol and phenol homologues
  T54.0X Toxic effects of phenol and phenol homologues
    T54.0X1 Toxic effect of phenol and phenol homologues, accidental (unintentional) POA
      Toxic effects of phenol and phenol homologues NOS
    T54.0X2 Toxic effect of phenol and phenol homologues, intentional self-harm POA HCC
    T54.0X3 Toxic effect of phenol and phenol homologues, assault POA
    T54.0X4 Toxic effect of phenol and phenol homologues, undetermined POA

T54.1 Toxic effects of other corrosive organic compounds
  T54.1X Toxic effects of other corrosive organic compounds
    T54.1X1 Toxic effect of other corrosive organic compounds, accidental (unintentional) POA
      Toxic effects of other corrosive organic compounds NOS
    T54.1X2 Toxic effect of other corrosive organic compounds, intentional self-harm POA HCC

Unspecified Code Other Specified Code Manifestation Code N Newborn P Pediatric M Maternity A Adult ♂ Male ♀ Female
● New Code ▲ Revised Code Title ▶◀ Revised Text NOTES *INCLUDES* *EXCLUDES 1* Not coded here *EXCLUDES 2* Not included here
4th character required 5th character required 6th character required 7th character required
Extension 'X' Alert HAC Hospital-acquired condition (HAC) alert AHA AHA Coding Clinic©

[7th] **T54.1X3 Toxic effect of other corrosive organic compounds, assault** [POA]

[7th] **T54.1X4 Toxic effect of other corrosive organic compounds, undetermined** [POA]

[5th] **T54.2 Toxic effects of corrosive acids and acid-like substances**

Toxic effects of hydrochloric acid
Toxic effects of sulfuric acid

[6th] **T54.2X Toxic effects of corrosive acids and acid-like substances**

[7th] **T54.2X1 Toxic effect of corrosive acids and acid-like substances, accidental (unintentional)** [POA]

Toxic effects of corrosive acids and acid-like substances NOS

[7th] **T54.2X2 Toxic effect of corrosive acids and acid-like substances, intentional self-harm** [POA] [HCC]

[7th] **T54.2X3 Toxic effect of corrosive acids and acid-like substances, assault** [POA]

[7th] **T54.2X4 Toxic effect of corrosive acids and acid-like substances, undetermined** [POA]

[5th] **T54.3 Toxic effects of corrosive alkalis and alkali-like substances**

Toxic effects of potassium hydroxide
Toxic effects of sodium hydroxide

[6th] **T54.3X Toxic effects of corrosive alkalis and alkali-like substances**

[7th] **T54.3X1 Toxic effect of corrosive alkalis and alkali-like substances, accidental (unintentional)** [POA]

Toxic effects of corrosive alkalis and alkali-like substances NOS

[7th] **T54.3X2 Toxic effect of corrosive alkalis and alkali-like substances, intentional self-harm** [POA] [HCC]

[7th] **T54.3X3 Toxic effect of corrosive alkalis and alkali-like substances, assault** [POA]

[7th] **T54.3X4 Toxic effect of corrosive alkalis and alkali-like substances, undetermined** [POA]

[5th] **T54.9 Toxic effects of unspecified corrosive substance**

[7th] **T54.91 Toxic effect of unspecified corrosive substance, accidental (unintentional)** [POA]

[7th] **T54.92 Toxic effect of unspecified corrosive substance, intentional self-harm** [POA] [HCC]

[7th] **T54.93 Toxic effect of unspecified corrosive substance, assault** [POA]

[7th] **T54.94 Toxic effect of unspecified corrosive substance, undetermined** [POA]

[4th] **T55 Toxic effect of soaps and detergents**

The appropriate 7th character is to be added to each code from category T55
A = initial encounter
D = subsequent encounter
S = sequela

[5th] **T55.0 Toxic effect of soaps**

[6th] **T55.0X Toxic effect of soaps**

[7th] **T55.0X1 Toxic effect of soaps, accidental (unintentional)** [POA]

Toxic effect of soaps NOS

[7th] **T55.0X2 Toxic effect of soaps, intentional self-harm** [POA] [HCC]

[7th] **T55.0X3 Toxic effect of soaps, assault** [POA]

[7th] **T55.0X4 Toxic effect of soaps, undetermined** [POA]

[5th] **T55.1 Toxic effect of detergents**

[6th] **T55.1X Toxic effect of detergents**

[7th] **T55.1X1 Toxic effect of detergents, accidental (unintentional)** [POA]

Toxic effect of detergents NOS

[7th] **T55.1X2 Toxic effect of detergents, intentional self-harm** [POA] [HCC]

[7th] **T55.1X3 Toxic effect of detergents, assault** [POA]

[7th] **T55.1X4 Toxic effect of detergents, undetermined** [POA]

[4th] **T56 Toxic effect of metals**

[INCLUDES] *toxic effects of fumes and vapors of metals*
toxic effects of metals from all sources, except medicinal substances

Use additional code to identify any retained metal foreign body, if applicable (Z18.0-, T18.1-)

[EXCLUDES1] *arsenic and its compounds (T57.0)*
manganese and its compounds (T57.2)

The appropriate 7th character is to be added to each code from category T56
A = initial encounter
D = subsequent encounter
S = sequela

[5th] **T56.0 Toxic effects of lead and its compounds**

[6th] **T56.0X Toxic effects of lead and its compounds**

[7th] **T56.0X1 Toxic effect of lead and its compounds, accidental (unintentional)** [POA]

Toxic effects of lead and its compounds NOS

[7th] **T56.0X2 Toxic effect of lead and its compounds, intentional self-harm** [POA] [HCC]

[7th] **T56.0X3 Toxic effect of lead and its compounds, assault** [POA]

[7th] **T56.0X4 Toxic effect of lead and its compounds, undetermined** [POA]

[5th] **T56.1 Toxic effects of mercury and its compounds**

[6th] **T56.1X Toxic effects of mercury and its compounds**

[7th] **T56.1X1 Toxic effect of mercury and its compounds, accidental (unintentional)** [POA]

Toxic effects of mercury and its compounds NOS

[7th] **T56.1X2 Toxic effect of mercury and its compounds, intentional self-harm** [POA] [HCC]

[7th] **T56.1X3 Toxic effect of mercury and its compounds, assault** [POA]

[7th] **T56.1X4 Toxic effect of mercury and its compounds, undetermined** [POA]

[5th] **T56.2 Toxic effects of chromium and its compounds**

[6th] **T56.2X Toxic effects of chromium and its compounds**

[7th] **T56.2X1 Toxic effect of chromium and its compounds, accidental (unintentional)** [POA]

Toxic effects of chromium and its compounds NOS

[7th] **T56.2X2 Toxic effect of chromium and its compounds, intentional self-harm** [POA] [HCC]

[7th] **T56.2X3 Toxic effect of chromium and its compounds, assault** [POA]

[7th] **T56.2X4 Toxic effect of chromium and its compounds, undetermined** [POA]

[5th] **T56.3 Toxic effects of cadmium and its compounds**

[6th] **T56.3X Toxic effects of cadmium and its compounds**

[7th] **T56.3X1 Toxic effect of cadmium and its compounds, accidental (unintentional)** [POA]

Toxic effects of cadmium and its compounds NOS

[7th] **T56.3X2 Toxic effect of cadmium and its compounds, intentional self-harm** [POA] [HCC]

[7th] **T56.3X3 Toxic effect of cadmium and its compounds, assault** [POA]

[7th] **T56.3X4 Toxic effect of cadmium and its compounds, undetermined** [POA]

[5th] **T56.4 Toxic effects of copper and its compounds**

[6th] **T56.4X Toxic effects of copper and its compounds**

[7th] **T56.4X1 Toxic effect of copper and its compounds, accidental (unintentional)** [POA]

Toxic effects of copper and its compounds NOS

[7th] **T56.4X2 Toxic effect of copper and its compounds, intentional self-harm** [POA] [HCC]

[7th] **T56.4X3 Toxic effect of copper and its compounds, assault** [POA]

[PDx] Unacceptable principal diagnosis symbol per Medicare code edits   [POA] Code exempt from diagnosis present on admission requirement
[?] Questionable admission   [CC] Complication or comorbidity   [CC/MCC Exc] CC/MCC exclusion   [MCC] Major complication or comorbidity
[PDx CC] Principal diagnosis as its own CC   [PDx MCC] Principal diagnosis as its own MCC   [HCC] HCC diagnosis code   [RxHCC] RxHCC diagnosis code
MACRA code   [Z1] Z code as first-listed diagnosis

When symbols appear on a code that requires a 7th character extension, refer to Appendix B to identify applicable 7th character codes.

T56.4X4 Toxic effect of copper and its compounds, undetermined POA

🄢 T56.5 Toxic effects of zinc and its compounds
  🄥 T56.5X Toxic effects of zinc and its compounds
    T56.5X1 Toxic effect of zinc and its compounds, accidental (unintentional) POA
      Toxic effects of zinc and its compounds NOS
    T56.5X2 Toxic effect of zinc and its compounds, intentional self-harm POA HCC
    T56.5X3 Toxic effect of zinc and its compounds, assault POA
    T56.5X4 Toxic effect of zinc and its compounds, undetermined POA

🄢 T56.6 Toxic effects of tin and its compounds
  🄥 T56.6X Toxic effects of tin and its compounds
    T56.6X1 Toxic effect of tin and its compounds, accidental (unintentional) POA
      Toxic effects of tin and its compounds NOS
    T56.6X2 Toxic effect of tin and its compounds, intentional self-harm POA HCC
    T56.6X3 Toxic effect of tin and its compounds, assault POA
    T56.6X4 Toxic effect of tin and its compounds, undetermined POA

🄢 T56.7 Toxic effects of beryllium and its compounds
  🄥 T56.7X Toxic effects of beryllium and its compounds
    T56.7X1 Toxic effect of beryllium and its compounds, accidental (unintentional) POA
      Toxic effects of beryllium and its compounds NOS
    T56.7X2 Toxic effect of beryllium and its compounds, intentional self-harm POA HCC
    T56.7X3 Toxic effect of beryllium and its compounds, assault POA
    T56.7X4 Toxic effect of beryllium and its compounds, undetermined POA

🄢 T56.8 Toxic effects of other metals
  🄥 T56.81 Toxic effect of thallium
    T56.811 Toxic effect of thallium, accidental (unintentional) POA
      Toxic effect of thallium NOS
    T56.812 Toxic effect of thallium, intentional self-harm POA HCC
    T56.813 Toxic effect of thallium, assault POA
    T56.814 Toxic effect of thallium, undetermined POA
  🄥 T56.89 Toxic effects of other metals
    T56.891 Toxic effect of other metals, accidental (unintentional) POA
      Toxic effects of other metals NOS
    T56.892 Toxic effect of other metals, intentional self-harm POA HCC
    T56.893 Toxic effect of other metals, assault POA
    T56.894 Toxic effect of other metals, undetermined POA

🄢 T56.9 Toxic effects of unspecified metal
    T56.91 Toxic effect of unspecified metal, accidental (unintentional) POA
    T56.92 Toxic effect of unspecified metal, intentional self-harm POA HCC
    T56.93 Toxic effect of unspecified metal, assault POA
    T56.94 Toxic effect of unspecified metal, undetermined POA

🄣 T57 Toxic effect of other inorganic substances
  The appropriate 7th character is to be added to each code from category T57
    A = initial encounter
    D = subsequent encounter
    S = sequela
  🄢 T57.0 Toxic effect of arsenic and its compounds
    🄥 T57.0X Toxic effect of arsenic and its compounds

T57.0X1 Toxic effect of arsenic and its compounds, accidental (unintentional) POA
  Toxic effect of arsenic and its compounds NOS
T57.0X2 Toxic effect of arsenic and its compounds, intentional self-harm POA HCC
T57.0X3 Toxic effect of arsenic and its compounds, assault POA
T57.0X4 Toxic effect of arsenic and its compounds, undetermined POA

🄢 T57.1 Toxic effect of phosphorus and its compounds
  EXCLUDES1 organophosphate insecticides (T60.0)
  🄥 T57.1X Toxic effect of phosphorus and its compounds
    T57.1X1 Toxic effect of phosphorus and its compounds, accidental (unintentional) POA
      Toxic effect of phosphorus and its compounds NOS
    T57.1X2 Toxic effect of phosphorus and its compounds, intentional self-harm POA HCC
    T57.1X3 Toxic effect of phosphorus and its compounds, assault POA
    T57.1X4 Toxic effect of phosphorus and its compounds, undetermined POA

🄢 T57.2 Toxic effect of manganese and its compounds
  🄥 T57.2X Toxic effect of manganese and its compounds
    T57.2X1 Toxic effect of manganese and its compounds, accidental (unintentional) POA
      Toxic effect of manganese and its compounds NOS
    T57.2X2 Toxic effect of manganese and its compounds, intentional self-harm POA HCC
    T57.2X3 Toxic effect of manganese and its compounds, assault POA
    T57.2X4 Toxic effect of manganese and its compounds, undetermined POA

🄢 T57.3 Toxic effect of hydrogen cyanide
  🄥 T57.3X Toxic effect of hydrogen cyanide
    T57.3X1 Toxic effect of hydrogen cyanide, accidental (unintentional) POA
      Toxic effect of hydrogen cyanide NOS
    T57.3X2 Toxic effect of hydrogen cyanide, intentional self-harm POA HCC
    T57.3X3 Toxic effect of hydrogen cyanide, assault POA
    T57.3X4 Toxic effect of hydrogen cyanide, undetermined POA

🄢 T57.8 Toxic effect of other specified inorganic substances
  🄥 T57.8X Toxic effect of other specified inorganic substances
    T57.8X1 Toxic effect of other specified inorganic substances, accidental (unintentional) POA
      Toxic effect of other specified inorganic substances NOS
    T57.8X2 Toxic effect of other specified inorganic substances, intentional self-harm POA HCC
    T57.8X3 Toxic effect of other specified inorganic substances, assault POA
    T57.8X4 Toxic effect of other specified inorganic substances, undetermined POA

🄢 T57.9 Toxic effect of unspecified inorganic substance
    T57.91 Toxic effect of unspecified inorganic substance, accidental (unintentional) POA
    T57.92 Toxic effect of unspecified inorganic substance, intentional self-harm POA HCC
    T57.93 Toxic effect of unspecified inorganic substance, assault POA
    T57.94 Toxic effect of unspecified inorganic substance, undetermined POA

🄣 T58 Toxic effect of carbon monoxide
  INCLUDES asphyxiation from carbon monoxide
    toxic effect of carbon monoxide from all sources

Unspecified Code   Other Specified Code   Manifestation Code   Ⓝ Newborn   Ⓟ Pediatric   Ⓜ Maternity   Ⓐ Adult   ♂ Male   ♀ Female
● New Code   ▲ Revised Code Title   ▶◀ Revised Text   NOTES   INCLUDES   EXCLUDES 1   Not coded here   EXCLUDES 2   Not included here
🄣 4th character required   🄢 5th character required   🄥 6th character required   🄦 7th character required
🅧 Extension 'X' Alert   HAC Hospital-acquired condition (HAC) alert   AHA AHA Coding Clinic©

2018 ICD-10-CM   When symbols appear on a code that requires a 7th character extension, refer to Appendix B to identify applicable 7th character codes.   1151

The appropriate 7th character is to be added to each code from category T58
A = initial encounter
D = subsequent encounter
S = sequela

5ᵗʰ **T58.0 Toxic effect of carbon monoxide from motor vehicle exhaust**
Toxic effect of exhaust gas from gas engine
Toxic effect of exhaust gas from motor pump

7ᵗʰ **T58.01 Toxic effect of carbon monoxide from motor vehicle exhaust, accidental (unintentional)** POA

7ᵗʰ **T58.02 Toxic effect of carbon monoxide from motor vehicle exhaust, intentional self-harm** POA HCC

7ᵗʰ **T58.03 Toxic effect of carbon monoxide from motor vehicle exhaust, assault** POA

7ᵗʰ **T58.04 Toxic effect of carbon monoxide from motor vehicle exhaust, undetermined** POA

5ᵗʰ **T58.1 Toxic effect of carbon monoxide from utility gas**
Toxic effect of acetylene
Toxic effect of gas NOS used for lighting, heating, cooking
Toxic effect of water gas

7ᵗʰ **T58.11 Toxic effect of carbon monoxide from utility gas, accidental (unintentional)** POA

7ᵗʰ **T58.12 Toxic effect of carbon monoxide from utility gas, intentional self-harm** POA HCC

7ᵗʰ **T58.13 Toxic effect of carbon monoxide from utility gas, assault** POA

7ᵗʰ **T58.14 Toxic effect of carbon monoxide from utility gas, undetermined** POA

5ᵗʰ **T58.2 Toxic effect of carbon monoxide from incomplete combustion of other domestic fuels**
Toxic effect of carbon monoxide from incomplete combustion of coal, coke, kerosene, wood

6ᵗʰ **T58.2X Toxic effect of carbon monoxide from incomplete combustion of other domestic fuels**

7ᵗʰ **T58.2X1 Toxic effect of carbon monoxide from incomplete combustion of other domestic fuels, accidental (unintentional)** POA

7ᵗʰ **T58.2X2 Toxic effect of carbon monoxide from incomplete combustion of other domestic fuels, intentional self-harm** POA HCC

7ᵗʰ **T58.2X3 Toxic effect of carbon monoxide from incomplete combustion of other domestic fuels, assault** POA

7ᵗʰ **T58.2X4 Toxic effect of carbon monoxide from incomplete combustion of other domestic fuels, undetermined** POA

5ᵗʰ **T58.8 Toxic effect of carbon monoxide from other source**
Toxic effect of carbon monoxide from blast furnace gas
Toxic effect of carbon monoxide from fuels in industrial use
Toxic effect of carbon monoxide from kiln vapor

6ᵗʰ **T58.8X Toxic effect of carbon monoxide from other source**

7ᵗʰ **T58.8X1 Toxic effect of carbon monoxide from other source, accidental (unintentional)** POA

7ᵗʰ **T58.8X2 Toxic effect of carbon monoxide from other source, intentional self-harm** POA HCC

7ᵗʰ **T58.8X3 Toxic effect of carbon monoxide from other source, assault** POA

7ᵗʰ **T58.8X4 Toxic effect of carbon monoxide from other source, undetermined** POA

5ᵗʰ **T58.9 Toxic effect of carbon monoxide from unspecified source**

7ᵗʰ **T58.91 Toxic effect of carbon monoxide from unspecified source, accidental (unintentional)** POA

7ᵗʰ **T58.92 Toxic effect of carbon monoxide from unspecified source, intentional self-harm** POA HCC

7ᵗʰ **T58.93 Toxic effect of carbon monoxide from unspecified source, assault** POA

7ᵗʰ **T58.94 Toxic effect of carbon monoxide from unspecified source, undetermined** POA

4ᵗʰ **T59 Toxic effect of other gases, fumes and vapors**
INCLUDES aerosol propellants
EXCLUDES1 chlorofluorocarbons (T53.5)
The appropriate 7th character is to be added to each code from category T59
A = initial encounter
D = subsequent encounter
S = sequela

5ᵗʰ **T59.0 Toxic effect of nitrogen oxides**

6ᵗʰ **T59.0X Toxic effect of nitrogen oxides**

7ᵗʰ **T59.0X1 Toxic effect of nitrogen oxides, accidental (unintentional)** POA
Toxic effect of nitrogen oxides NOS

7ᵗʰ **T59.0X2 Toxic effect of nitrogen oxides, intentional self-harm** POA HCC

7ᵗʰ **T59.0X3 Toxic effect of nitrogen oxides, assault** POA

7ᵗʰ **T59.0X4 Toxic effect of nitrogen oxides, undetermined** POA

5ᵗʰ **T59.1 Toxic effect of sulfur dioxide**

6ᵗʰ **T59.1X Toxic effect of sulfur dioxide**

7ᵗʰ **T59.1X1 Toxic effect of sulfur dioxide, accidental (unintentional)** POA
Toxic effect of sulfur dioxide NOS

7ᵗʰ **T59.1X2 Toxic effect of sulfur dioxide, intentional self-harm** POA HCC

7ᵗʰ **T59.1X3 Toxic effect of sulfur dioxide, assault** POA

7ᵗʰ **T59.1X4 Toxic effect of sulfur dioxide, undetermined** POA

5ᵗʰ **T59.2 Toxic effect of formaldehyde**

6ᵗʰ **T59.2X Toxic effect of formaldehyde**

7ᵗʰ **T59.2X1 Toxic effect of formaldehyde, accidental (unintentional)** POA
Toxic effect of formaldehyde NOS

7ᵗʰ **T59.2X2 Toxic effect of formaldehyde, intentional self-harm** POA HCC

7ᵗʰ **T59.2X3 Toxic effect of formaldehyde, assault** POA

7ᵗʰ **T59.2X4 Toxic effect of formaldehyde, undetermined** POA

5ᵗʰ **T59.3 Toxic effect of lacrimogenic gas**
Toxic effect of tear gas

6ᵗʰ **T59.3X Toxic effect of lacrimogenic gas**

7ᵗʰ **T59.3X1 Toxic effect of lacrimogenic gas, accidental (unintentional)** POA
Toxic effect of lacrimogenic gas NOS

7ᵗʰ **T59.3X2 Toxic effect of lacrimogenic gas, intentional self-harm** POA HCC

7ᵗʰ **T59.3X3 Toxic effect of lacrimogenic gas, assault** POA

7ᵗʰ **T59.3X4 Toxic effect of lacrimogenic gas, undetermined** POA

5ᵗʰ **T59.4 Toxic effect of chlorine gas**

6ᵗʰ **T59.4X Toxic effect of chlorine gas**

7ᵗʰ **T59.4X1 Toxic effect of chlorine gas, accidental (unintentional)** POA
Toxic effect of chlorine gas NOS

7ᵗʰ **T59.4X2 Toxic effect of chlorine gas, intentional self-harm** POA HCC

7ᵗʰ **T59.4X3 Toxic effect of chlorine gas, assault** POA

7ᵗʰ **T59.4X4 Toxic effect of chlorine gas, undetermined** POA

5ᵗʰ **T59.5 Toxic effect of fluorine gas and hydrogen fluoride**

6ᵗʰ **T59.5X Toxic effect of fluorine gas and hydrogen fluoride**

7ᵗʰ **T59.5X1 Toxic effect of fluorine gas and hydrogen fluoride, accidental (unintentional)** POA
Toxic effect of fluorine gas and hydrogen fluoride NOS

7ᵗʰ **T59.5X2 Toxic effect of fluorine gas and hydrogen fluoride, intentional self-harm** POA HCC

7ᵗʰ **T59.5X3 Toxic effect of fluorine gas and hydrogen fluoride, assault** POA

7ᵗʰ **T59.5X4 Toxic effect of fluorine gas and hydrogen fluoride, undetermined** POA

PDX Unacceptable principal diagnosis symbol per Medicare code edits   POA Code exempt from diagnosis present on admission requirement
❓ Questionable admission   ℃ Complication or comorbidity   CC/MCC Exc. CC/MCC exclusion   MCC Major complication or comorbidity
Principal diagnosis as its own CC   Principal diagnosis as its own MCC   HCC HCC diagnosis code   RxHCC RxHCC diagnosis code
MACRA code   Z Z code as first-listed diagnosis

5ᵗʰ **T59.6 Toxic effect of hydrogen sulfide**
- 6ᵗʰ **T59.6X Toxic effect of** hydrogen sulfide
  - 7ᵗʰ **T59.6X1 Toxic effect of hydrogen sulfide, accidental (unintentional)** POA
    Toxic effect of hydrogen sulfide NOS
  - 7ᵗʰ **T59.6X2 Toxic effect of hydrogen sulfide, intentional self-harm** POA HCC
  - 7ᵗʰ **T59.6X3 Toxic effect of hydrogen sulfide, assault** POA
  - 7ᵗʰ **T59.6X4 Toxic effect of hydrogen sulfide, undetermined** POA

5ᵗʰ **T59.7 Toxic effect of carbon dioxide**
- 6ᵗʰ **T59.7X Toxic effect of** carbon dioxide
  - 7ᵗʰ **T59.7X1 Toxic effect of carbon dioxide, accidental (unintentional)** POA
    Toxic effect of carbon dioxide NOS
  - 7ᵗʰ **T59.7X2 Toxic effect of carbon dioxide, intentional self-harm** POA HCC
  - 7ᵗʰ **T59.7X3 Toxic effect of carbon dioxide, assault** POA
  - 7ᵗʰ **T59.7X4 Toxic effect of carbon dioxide, undetermined** POA

5ᵗʰ **T59.8 Toxic effect of other specified gases, fumes and vapors**
- 6ᵗʰ **T59.81 Toxic effect of** smoke
  Smoke inhalation
  EXCLUDES2 *toxic effect of cigarette (tobacco) smoke (T65.22-)*
  - 7ᵗʰ **T59.811 Toxic effect of smoke, accidental (unintentional)** POA
    Toxic effect of smoke NOS
  - 7ᵗʰ **T59.812 Toxic effect of smoke, intentional self-harm** POA HCC
  - 7ᵗʰ **T59.813 Toxic effect of smoke, assault** POA
  - 7ᵗʰ **T59.814 Toxic effect of smoke, undetermined** POA
- 6ᵗʰ **T59.89 Toxic effect of** other specified gases, fumes and vapors
  - 7ᵗʰ **T59.891 Toxic effect of other specified gases, fumes and vapors, accidental (unintentional)** POA
  - 7ᵗʰ **T59.892 Toxic effect of other specified gases, fumes and vapors, intentional self-harm** POA HCC
  - 7ᵗʰ **T59.893 Toxic effect of other specified gases, fumes and vapors, assault** POA
  - 7ᵗʰ **T59.894 Toxic effect of other specified gases, fumes and vapors, undetermined** POA

5ᵗʰ **T59.9 Toxic effect of unspecified gases, fumes and vapors**
- 7ᵗʰ **T59.91 Toxic effect of unspecified gases, fumes and vapors, accidental (unintentional)** POA
- 7ᵗʰ **T59.92 Toxic effect of unspecified gases, fumes and vapors, intentional self-harm** POA HCC
- 7ᵗʰ **T59.93 Toxic effect of unspecified gases, fumes and vapors, assault** POA
- 7ᵗʰ **T59.94 Toxic effect of unspecified gases, fumes and vapors, undetermined** POA

4ᵗʰ **T60 Toxic effect of pesticides**
  INCLUDES *toxic effect of wood preservatives*
  The appropriate 7th character is to be added to each code from category T60
  A = initial encounter
  D = subsequent encounter
  S = sequela

5ᵗʰ **T60.0 Toxic effect of organophosphate and carbamate insecticides**
- 6ᵗʰ **T60.0X Toxic effect of** organophosphate and carbamate insecticides
  - 7ᵗʰ **T60.0X1 Toxic effect of organophosphate and carbamate insecticides, accidental (unintentional)** POA
    Toxic effect of organophosphate and carbamate insecticides NOS
  - 7ᵗʰ **T60.0X2 Toxic effect of organophosphate and carbamate insecticides, intentional self-harm** POA HCC
  - 7ᵗʰ **T60.0X3 Toxic effect of organophosphate and carbamate insecticides, assault** POA

- 7ᵗʰ **T60.0X4 Toxic effect of organophosphate and carbamate insecticides, undetermined** POA

5ᵗʰ **T60.1 Toxic effect of halogenated insecticides**
  EXCLUDES1 *chlorinated hydrocarbon (T53.-)*
- 6ᵗʰ **T60.1X Toxic effect of** halogenated insecticides
  - 7ᵗʰ **T60.1X1 Toxic effect of halogenated insecticides, accidental (unintentional)** POA
    Toxic effect of halogenated insecticides NOS
  - 7ᵗʰ **T60.1X2 Toxic effect of halogenated insecticides, intentional self-harm** POA HCC
  - 7ᵗʰ **T60.1X3 Toxic effect of halogenated insecticides, assault** POA
  - 7ᵗʰ **T60.1X4 Toxic effect of halogenated insecticides, undetermined** POA

5ᵗʰ **T60.2 Toxic effect of other insecticides**
- 6ᵗʰ **T60.2X Toxic effect of** other insecticides
  - 7ᵗʰ **T60.2X1 Toxic effect of other insecticides, accidental (unintentional)** POA
    Toxic effect of other insecticides NOS
  - 7ᵗʰ **T60.2X2 Toxic effect of other insecticides, intentional self-harm** POA HCC
  - 7ᵗʰ **T60.2X3 Toxic effect of other insecticides, assault** POA
  - 7ᵗʰ **T60.2X4 Toxic effect of other insecticides, undetermined** POA

5ᵗʰ **T60.3 Toxic effect of herbicides and fungicides**
- 6ᵗʰ **T60.3X Toxic effect of** herbicides and fungicides
  - 7ᵗʰ **T60.3X1 Toxic effect of herbicides and fungicides, accidental (unintentional)** POA
    Toxic effect of herbicides and fungicides NOS
  - 7ᵗʰ **T60.3X2 Toxic effect of herbicides and fungicides, intentional self-harm** POA HCC
  - 7ᵗʰ **T60.3X3 Toxic effect of herbicides and fungicides, assault** POA
  - 7ᵗʰ **T60.3X4 Toxic effect of herbicides and fungicides, undetermined** POA

5ᵗʰ **T60.4 Toxic effect of rodenticides**
  EXCLUDES1 *strychnine and its salts (T65.1)*
          thallium (T56.81-)
- 6ᵗʰ **T60.4X Toxic effect of** rodenticides
  - 7ᵗʰ **T60.4X1 Toxic effect of rodenticides, accidental (unintentional)** POA
    Toxic effect of rodenticides NOS
  - 7ᵗʰ **T60.4X2 Toxic effect of rodenticides, intentional self-harm** POA HCC
  - 7ᵗʰ **T60.4X3 Toxic effect of rodenticides, assault** POA
  - 7ᵗʰ **T60.4X4 Toxic effect of rodenticides, undetermined** POA

5ᵗʰ **T60.8 Toxic effect of other pesticides**
- 6ᵗʰ **T60.8X Toxic effect of** other pesticides
  - 7ᵗʰ **T60.8X1 Toxic effect of other pesticides, accidental (unintentional)** POA
    Toxic effect of other pesticides NOS
  - 7ᵗʰ **T60.8X2 Toxic effect of other pesticides, intentional self-harm** POA HCC
  - 7ᵗʰ **T60.8X3 Toxic effect of other pesticides, assault** POA
  - 7ᵗʰ **T60.8X4 Toxic effect of other pesticides, undetermined** POA

5ᵗʰ **T60.9 Toxic effect of unspecified pesticide**
- 7ᵗʰ **T60.91 Toxic effect of unspecified pesticide, accidental (unintentional)** POA
- 7ᵗʰ **T60.92 Toxic effect of unspecified pesticide, intentional self-harm** POA HCC
- 7ᵗʰ **T60.93 Toxic effect of unspecified pesticide, assault** POA
- 7ᵗʰ **T60.94 Toxic effect of unspecified pesticide, undetermined** POA

4ᵗʰ **T61 Toxic effect of noxious substances eaten as seafood**
  EXCLUDES1 *allergic reaction to food, such as:*
          anaphylactic reaction or shock due to adverse food reaction (T78.0-)

| Unspecified Code | Other Specified Code | Manifestation Code | N Newborn | P Pediatric | M Maternity | A Adult | ♂ Male | ♀ Female |

● New Code   ▲ Revised Code Title   ▶◀ Revised Text   NOTES   INCLUDES   EXCLUDES 1 Not coded here   EXCLUDES 2 Not included here
4ᵗʰ 4ᵗʰ character required   5ᵗʰ 5ᵗʰ character required   6ᵗʰ 6ᵗʰ character required   7ᵗʰ 7ᵗʰ character required
7ᵖ Extension 'X' Alert   HAC Hospital-acquired condition (HAC) alert   **AHA** AHA Coding Clinic©

bacterial foodborne intoxications (A05.-)

dermatitis (L23.6, L25.4, L27.2)

food protein-induced enterocolitis syndrome (K52.21)

food protein-induced enteropathy (K52.22)

gastroenteritis (noninfective) (K52.29)

toxic effect of aflatoxin and other mycotoxins (T64)

toxic effect of cyanides (T65.0-)

toxic effect of harmful algae bloom (T65.82-)

toxic effect of hydrogen cyanide (T57.3-)

toxic effect of mercury (T56.1-)

toxic effect of red tide (T65.82-)

The appropriate 7th character is to be added to each code from category T61

A = initial encounter

D = subsequent encounter

S = sequela

- T61.0 Ciguatera fish poisoning
  - T61.01 Ciguatera fish poisoning, accidental (unintentional) POA
  - T61.02 Ciguatera fish poisoning, intentional self-harm POA HCC
  - T61.03 Ciguatera fish poisoning, assault POA
  - T61.04 Ciguatera fish poisoning, undetermined POA
- T61.1 Scombroid fish poisoning

  Histamine-like syndrome
  - T61.11 Scombroid fish poisoning, accidental (unintentional) POA
  - T61.12 Scombroid fish poisoning, intentional self-harm POA HCC
  - T61.13 Scombroid fish poisoning, assault POA
  - T61.14 Scombroid fish poisoning, undetermined POA
- T61.7 Other fish and shellfish poisoning
  - T61.77 Other fish poisoning
    - T61.771 Other fish poisoning, accidental (unintentional) POA
    - T61.772 Other fish poisoning, intentional self-harm POA HCC
    - T61.773 Other fish poisoning, assault POA
    - T61.774 Other fish poisoning, undetermined POA
  - T61.78 Other shellfish poisoning
    - T61.781 Other shellfish poisoning, accidental (unintentional) POA
    - T61.782 Other shellfish poisoning, intentional self-harm POA HCC
    - T61.783 Other shellfish poisoning, assault POA
    - T61.784 Other shellfish poisoning, undetermined POA
- T61.8 Toxic effect of other seafood
  - T61.8X Toxic effect of other seafood
    - T61.8X1 Toxic effect of other seafood, accidental (unintentional) POA
    - T61.8X2 Toxic effect of other seafood, intentional self-harm POA HCC
    - T61.8X3 Toxic effect of other seafood, assault POA
    - T61.8X4 Toxic effect of other seafood, undetermined POA
- T61.9 Toxic effect of unspecified seafood
  - T61.91 Toxic effect of unspecified seafood, accidental (unintentional) POA
  - T61.92 Toxic effect of unspecified seafood, intentional self-harm POA HCC
  - T61.93 Toxic effect of unspecified seafood, assault POA
  - T61.94 Toxic effect of unspecified seafood, undetermined POA
- T62 Toxic effect of other noxious substances eaten as food

  EXCLUDES1 allergic reaction to food, such as:

  anaphylactic shock (reaction) due to adverse food reaction (T78.0-)

  bacterial food borne intoxications (A05.-)

  dermatitis (L23.6, L25.4, L27.2)

food protein-induced enterocolitis syndrome (K52.21)

food protein-induced enteropathy (K52.22)

gastroenteritis (noninfective) (K52.29)

toxic effect of aflatoxin and other mycotoxins (T64)

toxic effect of cyanides (T65.0-)

toxic effect of hydrogen cyanide (T57.3-)

toxic effect of mercury (T56.1-)

The appropriate 7th character is to be added to each code from category T62

A = initial encounter

D = subsequent encounter

S = sequela

- T62.0 Toxic effect of ingested mushrooms
  - T62.0X Toxic effect of ingested mushrooms
    - T62.0X1 Toxic effect of ingested mushrooms, accidental (unintentional) POA

      Toxic effect of ingested mushrooms NOS
    - T62.0X2 Toxic effect of ingested mushrooms, intentional self-harm POA HCC
    - T62.0X3 Toxic effect of ingested mushrooms, assault POA
    - T62.0X4 Toxic effect of ingested mushrooms, undetermined POA
- T62.1 Toxic effect of ingested berries
  - T62.1X Toxic effect of ingested berries
    - T62.1X1 Toxic effect of ingested berries, accidental (unintentional) POA

      Toxic effect of ingested berries NOS
    - T62.1X2 Toxic effect of ingested berries, intentional self-harm POA HCC
    - T62.1X3 Toxic effect of ingested berries, assault POA
    - T62.1X4 Toxic effect of ingested berries, undetermined POA
- T62.2 Toxic effect of other ingested (parts of) plant(s)
  - T62.2X Toxic effect of other ingested (parts of) plant(s)
    - T62.2X1 Toxic effect of other ingested (parts of) plant(s), accidental (unintentional) POA

      Toxic effect of other ingested (parts of) plant(s) NOS
    - T62.2X2 Toxic effect of other ingested (parts of) plant(s), intentional self-harm POA HCC
    - T62.2X3 Toxic effect of other ingested (parts of) plant(s), assault POA
    - T62.2X4 Toxic effect of other ingested (parts of) plant(s), undetermined POA
- T62.8 Toxic effect of other specified noxious substances eaten as food
  - T62.8X Toxic effect of other specified noxious substances eaten as food
    - T62.8X1 Toxic effect of other specified noxious substances eaten as food, accidental (unintentional) POA

      Toxic effect of other specified noxious substances eaten as food NOS
    - T62.8X2 Toxic effect of other specified noxious substances eaten as food, intentional self-harm POA HCC
    - T62.8X3 Toxic effect of other specified noxious substances eaten as food, assault POA
    - T62.8X4 Toxic effect of other specified noxious substances eaten as food, undetermined POA
- T62.9 Toxic effect of unspecified noxious substance eaten as food
  - T62.91 Toxic effect of unspecified noxious substance eaten as food, accidental (unintentional) POA

    Toxic effect of unspecified noxious substance eaten as food NOS
  - T62.92 Toxic effect of unspecified noxious substance eaten as food, intentional self-harm POA HCC
  - T62.93 Toxic effect of unspecified noxious substance eaten as food, assault POA

PDxMR Unacceptable principal diagnosis symbol per Medicare code edits   POA Code exempt from diagnosis present on admission requirement

❓ Questionable admission   ᴄᴄ Complication or comorbidity   CC/MCC Excl CC/MCC exclusion   MCC Major complication or comorbidity

PDx CC Principal diagnosis as its own CC   PDx MCC Principal diagnosis as its own MCC   HCC HCC diagnosis code   RxHCC RxHCC diagnosis code

MACRA code   Z1 Z code as first-listed diagnosis

[X] T62.94 **Toxic effect of unspecified noxious substance eaten as food,** undetermined [POA]

[4th] **T63 Toxic effect of contact with venomous animals and plants**

[INCLUDES] *bite or touch of venomous animal*

pricked or stuck by thorn or leaf

[EXCLUDES2] *ingestion of toxic animal or plant (T61.-, T62.-)*

The appropriate 7th character is to be added to each code from category T63

A = initial encounter

D = subsequent encounter

S = sequela

[5th] **T63.0 Toxic effect of snake venom**

[6th] **T63.00 Toxic effect of** unspecified snake venom

[7th] T63.001 **Toxic effect of unspecified snake venom,** accidental **(unintentional)** [POA]

Toxic effect of unspecified snake venom NOS

[7th] T63.002 **Toxic effect of unspecified snake venom,** intentional self-harm [POA] [HCC]

[7th] T63.003 **Toxic effect of unspecified snake venom,** assault [POA]

[7th] T63.004 **Toxic effect of unspecified snake venom,** undetermined [POA]

[6th] **T63.01 Toxic effect of** rattlesnake venom

[7th] T63.011 **Toxic effect of rattlesnake venom,** accidental **(unintentional)** [POA]

Toxic effect of rattlesnake venom NOS

[7th] T63.012 **Toxic effect of rattlesnake venom,** intentional self-harm [POA] [HCC]

[7th] T63.013 **Toxic effect of rattlesnake venom, assault** [POA]

[7th] T63.014 **Toxic effect of rattlesnake venom,** undetermined [POA]

[6th] **T63.02 Toxic effect of** coral snake venom

[7th] T63.021 **Toxic effect of coral snake venom,** accidental **(unintentional)** [POA]

Toxic effect of coral snake venom NOS

[7th] T63.022 **Toxic effect of coral snake venom,** intentional self-harm [POA] [HCC]

[7th] T63.023 **Toxic effect of coral snake venom,** assault [POA]

[7th] T63.024 **Toxic effect of coral snake venom,** undetermined [POA]

[6th] **T63.03 Toxic effect of** taipan venom

[7th] T63.031 **Toxic effect of taipan venom,** accidental **(unintentional)** [POA]

Toxic effect of taipan venom NOS

[7th] T63.032 **Toxic effect of taipan venom,** intentional **self-harm** [POA] [HCC]

[7th] T63.033 **Toxic effect of taipan venom,** assault [POA]

[7th] T63.034 **Toxic effect of taipan venom,** undetermined [POA]

[6th] **T63.04 Toxic effect of cobra venom**

[7th] T63.041 **Toxic effect of cobra venom,** accidental **(unintentional)** [POA]

Toxic effect of cobra venom NOS

[7th] T63.042 **Toxic effect of cobra venom,** intentional **self-harm** [POA] [HCC]

[7th] T63.043 **Toxic effect of cobra venom,** assault [POA]

[7th] T63.044 **Toxic effect of cobra venom,** undetermined [POA]

[6th] **T63.06 Toxic effect of venom of other North and South** American snake

[7th] T63.061 **Toxic effect of venom of other North and South American snake,** accidental **(unintentional)** [POA]

Toxic effect of venom of other North and South American snake NOS

[7th] T63.062 **Toxic effect of venom of other North and South American snake,** intentional self-harm [POA] [HCC]

[7th] T63.063 **Toxic effect of venom of other North and South American snake,** assault [POA]

[7th] T63.064 **Toxic effect of venom of other North and South American snake,** undetermined [POA]

[6th] **T63.07 Toxic effect of venom of other** Australian snake

[7th] T63.071 **Toxic effect of venom of other Australian snake,** accidental **(unintentional)** [POA]

Toxic effect of venom of other Australian snake NOS

[7th] T63.072 **Toxic effect of venom of other Australian snake,** intentional self-harm [POA] [HCC]

[7th] T63.073 **Toxic effect of venom of other Australian snake,** assault [POA]

[7th] T63.074 **Toxic effect of venom of other Australian snake,** undetermined [POA]

[6th] **T63.08 Toxic effect of venom of** other African and Asian snake

[7th] T63.081 **Toxic effect of venom of other African and Asian snake,** accidental **(unintentional)** [POA]

Toxic effect of venom of other African and Asian snake NOS

[7th] T63.082 **Toxic effect of venom of other African and Asian snake,** intentional self-harm [POA] [HCC]

[7th] T63.083 **Toxic effect of venom of other African and Asian snake,** assault [POA]

[7th] T63.084 **Toxic effect of venom of other African and Asian snake,** undetermined [POA]

[6th] **T63.09 Toxic effect of** venom of other snake

[7th] T63.091 **Toxic effect of venom of other snake,** accidental **(unintentional)** [POA]

Toxic effect of venom of other snake NOS

[7th] T63.092 **Toxic effect of venom of other snake,** intentional self-harm [POA] [HCC]

[7th] T63.093 **Toxic effect of venom of other snake,** assault [POA]

[7th] T63.094 **Toxic effect of venom of other snake,** undetermined [POA]

[5th] **T63.1 Toxic effect of** venom of other reptiles

[6th] **T63.11 Toxic effect of** venom of gila monster

[7th] T63.111 **Toxic effect of venom of gila monster,** accidental **(unintentional)** [POA]

Toxic effect of venom of gila monster NOS

[7th] T63.112 **Toxic effect of venom of gila monster,** intentional self-harm [POA] [HCC]

[7th] T63.113 **Toxic effect of venom of gila monster,** assault [POA]

[7th] T63.114 **Toxic effect of venom of gila monster,** undetermined [POA]

[6th] **T63.12 Toxic effect of venom of** other venomous lizard

[7th] T63.121 **Toxic effect of venom of other venomous lizard,** accidental **(unintentional)** [POA]

Toxic effect of venom of other venomous lizard NOS

[7th] T63.122 **Toxic effect of venom of other venomous lizard,** intentional self-harm [POA] [HCC]

[7th] T63.123 **Toxic effect of venom of other venomous lizard,** assault [POA]

[7th] T63.124 **Toxic effect of venom of other venomous lizard,** undetermined [POA]

[6th] **T63.19 Toxic effect of** venom of other reptiles

[7th] T63.191 **Toxic effect of venom of other reptiles,** accidental **(unintentional)** [POA]

Toxic effect of venom of other reptiles NOS

[7th] T63.192 **Toxic effect of venom of other reptiles,** intentional self-harm [POA] [HCC]

[7th] T63.193 **Toxic effect of venom of other reptiles,** assault [POA]

[7th] T63.194 **Toxic effect of venom of other reptiles,** undetermined [POA]

[5th] **T63.2 Toxic effect of** venom of scorpion

[6th] **T63.2X Toxic effect of** venom of scorpion

Unspecified Code Other Specified Code Manifestation Code [N] Newborn [P] Pediatric [M] Maternity [A] Adult ♂ Male ♀ Female
● New Code ▲ Revised Code Title ▶◀ Revised Text [NOTES] [INCLUDES] [EXCLUDES1] Not coded here [EXCLUDES2] Not included here
[4th] 4th character required [5th] 5th character required [6th] 6th character required [7th] 7th character required
[X] Extension 'X' Alert [HAC] Hospital-acquired condition (HAC) alert AHA AHA Coding Clinic®

When symbols appear on a code that requires a 7th character extension, refer to Appendix B to identify applicable 7th character codes.

T63.2X1 Toxic effect of venom of scorpion, accidental (unintentional)
Toxic effect of venom of scorpion NOS

T63.2X2 Toxic effect of venom of scorpion, intentional self-harm

T63.2X3 Toxic effect of venom of scorpion, assault

T63.2X4 Toxic effect of venom of scorpion, undetermined

T63.3 Toxic effect of venom of spider

T63.30 Toxic effect of unspecified spider venom

T63.301 Toxic effect of unspecified spider venom, accidental (unintentional)

T63.302 Toxic effect of unspecified spider venom, intentional self-harm

T63.303 Toxic effect of unspecified spider venom, assault

T63.304 Toxic effect of unspecified spider venom, undetermined

T63.31 Toxic effect of venom of black widow spider

T63.311 Toxic effect of venom of black widow spider, accidental (unintentional)

T63.312 Toxic effect of venom of black widow spider, intentional self-harm

T63.313 Toxic effect of venom of black widow spider, assault

T63.314 Toxic effect of venom of black widow spider, undetermined

T63.32 Toxic effect of venom of tarantula

T63.321 Toxic effect of venom of tarantula, accidental (unintentional)

T63.322 Toxic effect of venom of tarantula, intentional self-harm

T63.323 Toxic effect of venom of tarantula, assault

T63.324 Toxic effect of venom of tarantula, undetermined

T63.33 Toxic effect of venom of brown recluse spider

T63.331 Toxic effect of venom of brown recluse spider, accidental (unintentional)

T63.332 Toxic effect of venom of brown recluse spider, intentional self-harm

T63.333 Toxic effect of venom of brown recluse spider, assault

T63.334 Toxic effect of venom of brown recluse spider, undetermined

T63.39 Toxic effect of venom of other spider

T63.391 Toxic effect of venom of other spider, accidental (unintentional)

T63.392 Toxic effect of venom of other spider, intentional self-harm

T63.393 Toxic effect of venom of other spider, assault

T63.394 Toxic effect of venom of other spider, undetermined

T63.4 Toxic effect of venom of other arthropods

T63.41 Toxic effect of venom of centipedes and venomous millipedes

T63.411 Toxic effect of venom of centipedes and venomous millipedes, accidental (unintentional)

T63.412 Toxic effect of venom of centipedes and venomous millipedes, intentional self-harm

T63.413 Toxic effect of venom of centipedes and venomous millipedes, assault

T63.414 Toxic effect of venom of centipedes and venomous millipedes, undetermined

T63.42 Toxic effect of venom of ants

T63.421 Toxic effect of venom of ants, accidental (unintentional)

T63.422 Toxic effect of venom of ants, intentional self-harm

T63.423 Toxic effect of venom of ants, assault

T63.424 Toxic effect of venom of ants, undetermined

T63.43 Toxic effect of venom of caterpillars

T63.431 Toxic effect of venom of caterpillars, accidental (unintentional)

T63.432 Toxic effect of venom of caterpillars, intentional self-harm

T63.433 Toxic effect of venom of caterpillars, assault

T63.434 Toxic effect of venom of caterpillars, undetermined

T63.44 Toxic effect of venom of bees

T63.441 Toxic effect of venom of bees, accidental (unintentional)

T63.442 Toxic effect of venom of bees, intentional self-harm

T63.443 Toxic effect of venom of bees, assault

T63.444 Toxic effect of venom of bees, undetermined

T63.45 Toxic effect of venom of hornets

T63.451 Toxic effect of venom of hornets, accidental (unintentional)

T63.452 Toxic effect of venom of hornets, intentional self-harm

T63.453 Toxic effect of venom of hornets, assault

T63.454 Toxic effect of venom of hornets, undetermined

T63.46 Toxic effect of venom of wasps
Toxic effect of yellow jacket

T63.461 Toxic effect of venom of wasps, accidental (unintentional)

T63.462 Toxic effect of venom of wasps, intentional self-harm

T63.463 Toxic effect of venom of wasps, assault

T63.464 Toxic effect of venom of wasps, undetermined

T63.48 Toxic effect of venom of other arthropod

T63.481 Toxic effect of venom of other arthropod, accidental (unintentional)

T63.482 Toxic effect of venom of other arthropod, intentional self-harm

T63.483 Toxic effect of venom of other arthropod, assault

T63.484 Toxic effect of venom of other arthropod, undetermined

T63.5 Toxic effect of contact with venomous fish
EXCLUDES2 poisoning by ingestion of fish (T61.-)

T63.51 Toxic effect of contact with stingray

T63.511 Toxic effect of contact with stingray, accidental (unintentional)

T63.512 Toxic effect of contact with stingray, intentional self-harm

T63.513 Toxic effect of contact with stingray, assault

T63.514 Toxic effect of contact with stingray, undetermined

T63.59 Toxic effect of contact with other venomous fish

T63.591 Toxic effect of contact with other venomous fish, accidental (unintentional)

T63.592 Toxic effect of contact with other venomous fish, intentional self-harm

T63.593 Toxic effect of contact with other venomous fish, assault

T63.594 Toxic effect of contact with other venomous fish, undetermined

PDx Unacceptable principal diagnosis symbol per Medicare code edits   Code exempt from diagnosis present on admission requirement
? Questionable admission   cc Complication or comorbidity   cc/mcc CC/MCC exclusion   mcc Major complication or comorbidity
Principal diagnosis as its own CC   Principal diagnosis as its own MCC   HCC HCC diagnosis code   RxHCC RxHCC diagnosis code
MACRA code   Z Z code as first-listed diagnosis

1156   When symbols appear on a code that requires a 7th character extension, refer to Appendix B to identify applicable 7th character codes.   2018 ICD-10-CM

T63.6 Toxic effect of contact with other venomous marine animals
> *EXCLUDES1* sea-snake venom (T63.09)
> *EXCLUDES2* poisoning by ingestion of shellfish (T61.78-)

 T63.61 Toxic effect of contact with Portugese Man-o-war
  Toxic effect of contact with bluebottle
  T63.611 Toxic effect of contact with Portugese Man-o-war, accidental (unintentional) POA
  T63.612 Toxic effect of contact with Portugese Man-o-war, intentional self-harm POA HCC
  T63.613 Toxic effect of contact with Portugese Man-o-war, assault POA
  T63.614 Toxic effect of contact with Portugese Man-o-war, undetermined POA

 T63.62 Toxic effect of contact with other jellyfish
  T63.621 Toxic effect of contact with other jellyfish, accidental (unintentional) POA
  T63.622 Toxic effect of contact with other jellyfish, intentional self-harm POA HCC
  T63.623 Toxic effect of contact with other jellyfish, assault POA
  T63.624 Toxic effect of contact with other jellyfish, undetermined POA

 T63.63 Toxic effect of contact with sea anemone
  T63.631 Toxic effect of contact with sea anemone, accidental (unintentional) POA
  T63.632 Toxic effect of contact with sea anemone, intentional self-harm POA HCC
  T63.633 Toxic effect of contact with sea anemone, assault POA
  T63.634 Toxic effect of contact with sea anemone, undetermined POA

 T63.69 Toxic effect of contact with other venomous marine animals
  T63.691 Toxic effect of contact with other venomous marine animals, accidental (unintentional) POA
  T63.692 Toxic effect of contact with other venomous marine animals, intentional self-harm POA HCC
  T63.693 Toxic effect of contact with other venomous marine animals, assault POA
  T63.694 Toxic effect of contact with other venomous marine animals, undetermined POA

T63.7 Toxic effect of contact with venomous plant
 T63.71 Toxic effect of contact with venomous marine plant
  T63.711 Toxic effect of contact with venomous marine plant, accidental (unintentional) POA
  T63.712 Toxic effect of contact with venomous marine plant, intentional self-harm POA HCC
  T63.713 Toxic effect of contact with venomous marine plant, assault POA
  T63.714 Toxic effect of contact with venomous marine plant, undetermined POA

 T63.79 Toxic effect of contact with other venomous plant
  T63.791 Toxic effect of contact with other venomous plant, accidental (unintentional) POA
  T63.792 Toxic effect of contact with other venomous plant, intentional self-harm POA HCC
  T63.793 Toxic effect of contact with other venomous plant, assault POA
  T63.794 Toxic effect of contact with other venomous plant, undetermined POA

T63.8 Toxic effect of contact with other venomous animals
 T63.81 Toxic effect of contact with venomous frog
  EXCLUDES1 contact with nonvenomous frog (W62.0)
  T63.811 Toxic effect of contact with venomous frog, accidental (unintentional)

  T63.812 Toxic effect of contact with venomous frog, intentional self-harm POA HCC
  T63.813 Toxic effect of contact with venomous frog, assault POA
  T63.814 Toxic effect of contact with venomous frog, undetermined POA

 T63.82 Toxic effect of contact with venomous toad
  EXCLUDES1 contact with nonvenomous toad (W62.1)
  T63.821 Toxic effect of contact with venomous toad, accidental (unintentional) POA
  T63.822 Toxic effect of contact with venomous toad, intentional self-harm POA HCC
  T63.823 Toxic effect of contact with venomous toad, assault POA
  T63.824 Toxic effect of contact with venomous toad, undetermined POA

 T63.83 Toxic effect of contact with other venomous amphibian
  EXCLUDES1 contact with nonvenomous amphibian (W62.9)
  T63.831 Toxic effect of contact with other venomous amphibian, accidental (unintentional) POA
  T63.832 Toxic effect of contact with other venomous amphibian, intentional self-harm POA HCC
  T63.833 Toxic effect of contact with other venomous amphibian, assault POA
  T63.834 Toxic effect of contact with other venomous amphibian, undetermined POA

 T63.89 Toxic effect of contact with other venomous animals
  T63.891 Toxic effect of contact with other venomous animals, accidental (unintentional) POA
  T63.892 Toxic effect of contact with other venomous animals, intentional self-harm POA HCC
  T63.893 Toxic effect of contact with other venomous animals, assault POA
  T63.894 Toxic effect of contact with other venomous animals, undetermined POA

T63.9 Toxic effect of contact with unspecified venomous animal
 T63.91 Toxic effect of contact with unspecified venomous animal, accidental (unintentional) POA
 T63.92 Toxic effect of contact with unspecified venomous animal, intentional self-harm POA HCC
 T63.93 Toxic effect of contact with unspecified venomous animal, assault POA
 T63.94 Toxic effect of contact with unspecified venomous animal, undetermined POA

T64 Toxic effect of aflatoxin and other mycotoxin food contaminants
> The appropriate 7th character is to be added to each code from category T64
> A = initial encounter
> D = subsequent encounter
> S = sequela

 T64.0 Toxic effect of aflatoxin
  T64.01 Toxic effect of aflatoxin, accidental (unintentional) POA
  T64.02 Toxic effect of aflatoxin, intentional self-harm POA HCC
  T64.03 Toxic effect of aflatoxin, assault POA
  T64.04 Toxic effect of aflatoxin, undetermined POA

 T64.8 Toxic effect of other mycotoxin food contaminants
  T64.81 Toxic effect of other mycotoxin food contaminants, accidental (unintentional) POA
  T64.82 Toxic effect of other mycotoxin food contaminants, intentional self-harm POA HCC
  T64.83 Toxic effect of other mycotoxin food contaminants, assault POA
  T64.84 Toxic effect of other mycotoxin food contaminants, undetermined POA

Unspecified Code   Other Specified Code   Manifestation Code   N Newborn   P Pediatric   M Maternity   A Adult   ♂ Male   ♀ Female
● New Code   ▲ Revised Code Title   ►◄ Revised Text   NOTES   *INCLUDES*   *EXCLUDES 1* Not coded here   *EXCLUDES 2* Not included here
4th character required   5th character required   6th character required   7th character required
Extension 'X' Alert   HAC Hospital-acquired condition (HAC) alert   AHA AHA Coding Clinic©

T65 **Toxic effect of other and unspecified substances**
The appropriate 7th character is to be added to each code from category T65
A = initial encounter
D = subsequent encounter
S = sequela

T65.0 **Toxic effect of** cyanides
EXCLUDES1 hydrogen cyanide (T57.3-)

T65.0X **Toxic effect of cyanides**
  T65.0X1 **Toxic effect of cyanides,** accidental (unintentional) POA
  Toxic effect of cyanides NOS
  T65.0X2 **Toxic effect of cyanides,** intentional self-harm POA HCC
  T65.0X3 **Toxic effect of cyanides,** assault POA
  T65.0X4 **Toxic effect of cyanides,** undetermined POA

T65.1 **Toxic effect of** strychnine and its salts
T65.1X **Toxic effect of strychnine and its salts**
  T65.1X1 **Toxic effect of strychnine and its salts,** accidental (unintentional) POA
  Toxic effect of strychnine and its salts NOS
  T65.1X2 **Toxic effect of strychnine and its salts,** intentional self-harm POA HCC
  T65.1X3 **Toxic effect of strychnine and its salts,** assault POA
  T65.1X4 **Toxic effect of strychnine and its salts,** undetermined POA

T65.2 **Toxic effect of** tobacco and nicotine
EXCLUDES2 nicotine dependence (F17.-)

T65.21 **Toxic effect of** chewing tobacco
  T65.211 **Toxic effect of chewing tobacco,** accidental (unintentional) POA
  Toxic effect of chewing tobacco NOS
  T65.212 **Toxic effect of chewing tobacco,** intentional self-harm POA HCC
  T65.213 **Toxic effect of chewing tobacco,** assault POA
  T65.214 **Toxic effect of chewing tobacco,** undetermined POA

T65.22 **Toxic effect of** tobacco cigarettes
  Toxic effect of tobacco smoke
  Use additional code for exposure to second hand tobacco smoke (Z57.31, Z77.22)
  T65.221 **Toxic effect of tobacco cigarettes,** accidental (unintentional) POA
  Toxic effect of tobacco cigarettes NOS
  T65.222 **Toxic effect of tobacco cigarettes,** intentional self-harm POA HCC
  T65.223 **Toxic effect of tobacco cigarettes,** assault POA
  T65.224 **Toxic effect of tobacco cigarettes,** undetermined POA

T65.29 **Toxic effect of** other tobacco and nicotine
  T65.291 **Toxic effect of other tobacco and nicotine,** accidental (unintentional) POA
  Toxic effect of other tobacco and nicotine NOS
  T65.292 **Toxic effect of other tobacco and nicotine,** intentional self-harm POA HCC
  T65.293 **Toxic effect of other tobacco and nicotine,** assault POA
  T65.294 **Toxic effect of other tobacco and nicotine,** undetermined POA

T65.3 **Toxic effect of** nitroderivatives and aminoderivatives of benzene and its homologues
Toxic effect of anilin [benzenamine]
Toxic effect of nitrobenzene
Toxic effect of trinitrotoluene
T65.3X **Toxic effect of nitroderivatives and aminoderivatives of benzene and its homologues**

T65.3X1 **Toxic effect of nitroderivatives and aminoderivatives of benzene and its homologues,** accidental (unintentional) POA
Toxic effect of nitroderivatives and aminoderivatives of benzene and its homologues NOS
T65.3X2 **Toxic effect of nitroderivatives and aminoderivatives of benzene and its homologues,** intentional self-harm POA HCC
T65.3X3 **Toxic effect of nitroderivatives and aminoderivatives of benzene and its homologues,** assault POA
T65.3X4 **Toxic effect of nitroderivatives and aminoderivatives of benzene and its homologues,** undetermined POA

T65.4 **Toxic effect of** carbon disulfide
T65.4X **Toxic effect of carbon disulfide**
  T65.4X1 **Toxic effect of carbon disulfide,** accidental (unintentional) POA
  Toxic effect of carbon disulfide NOS
  T65.4X2 **Toxic effect of carbon disulfide,** intentional self-harm POA HCC
  T65.4X3 **Toxic effect of carbon disulfide,** assault POA
  T65.4X4 **Toxic effect of carbon disulfide,** undetermined POA

T65.5 **Toxic effect of** nitroglycerin and other nitric acids and esters
Toxic effect of 1,2,3-Propanetriol trinitrate
T65.5X **Toxic effect of nitroglycerin and other nitric acids and esters**
  T65.5X1 **Toxic effect of nitroglycerin and other nitric acids and esters,** accidental (unintentional) POA
  Toxic effect of nitroglycerin and other nitric acids and esters NOS
  T65.5X2 **Toxic effect of nitroglycerin and other nitric acids and esters,** intentional self-harm POA HCC
  T65.5X3 **Toxic effect of nitroglycerin and other nitric acids and esters,** assault POA
  T65.5X4 **Toxic effect of nitroglycerin and other nitric acids and esters,** undetermined POA

T65.6 **Toxic effect of** paints and dyes, not elsewhere classified
T65.6X **Toxic effect of paints and dyes, not elsewhere classified**
  T65.6X1 **Toxic effect of paints and dyes, not elsewhere classified,** accidental (unintentional) POA
  Toxic effect of paints and dyes NOS
  T65.6X2 **Toxic effect of paints and dyes, not elsewhere classified,** intentional self-harm POA HCC
  T65.6X3 **Toxic effect of paints and dyes, not elsewhere classified,** assault POA
  T65.6X4 **Toxic effect of paints and dyes, not elsewhere classified,** undetermined POA

T65.8 **Toxic effect of** other specified substances
T65.81 **Toxic effect of** latex
  T65.811 **Toxic effect of latex,** accidental (unintentional) POA
  Toxic effect of latex NOS
  T65.812 **Toxic effect of latex,** intentional self-harm POA HCC
  T65.813 **Toxic effect of latex,** assault POA
  T65.814 **Toxic effect of latex,** undetermined POA

T65.82 **Toxic effect of harmful** algae **and** algae **toxins**
Toxic effect of (harmful) algae bloom NOS
Toxic effect of blue-green algae bloom
Toxic effect of brown tide
Toxic effect of cyanobacteria bloom
Toxic effect of Florida red tide
Toxic effect of pfiesteria piscicida
Toxic effect of red tide

POA Unacceptable principal diagnosis symbol per Medicare code edits   Code exempt from diagnosis present on admission requirement
❓ Questionable admission   cc Complication or comorbidity   CC/MCC CC/MCC exclusion   MCC Major complication or comorbidity
Principal diagnosis as its own CC   Principal diagnosis as its own MCC   HCC HCC diagnosis code   RxHCC RxHCC diagnosis code
MACRA code   Z1 Z code as first-listed diagnosis

[7th] **T65.821 Toxic effect of harmful algae and algae toxins, accidental (unintentional)** [POA]
Toxic effect of harmful algae and algae toxins NOS

[7th] **T65.822 Toxic effect of harmful algae and algae toxins, intentional self-harm** [POA] [HCC]

[7th] **T65.823 Toxic effect of harmful algae and algae toxins, assault** [POA]

[7th] **T65.824 Toxic effect of harmful algae and algae toxins, undetermined** [POA]

[6th] **T65.83 Toxic effect of fiberglass**

[7th] **T65.831 Toxic effect of fiberglass, accidental (unintentional)** [POA]
Toxic effect of fiberglass NOS

[7th] **T65.832 Toxic effect of fiberglass, intentional self-harm** [POA] [HCC]

[7th] **T65.833 Toxic effect of fiberglass, assault** [POA]

[7th] **T65.834 Toxic effect of fiberglass, undetermined** [POA]

[6th] **T65.89 Toxic effect of other specified substances**

[7th] **T65.891 Toxic effect of other specified substances, accidental (unintentional)** [POA]
Toxic effect of other specified substances NOS

[7th] **T65.892 Toxic effect of other specified substances, intentional self-harm** [POA] [HCC]

[7th] **T65.893 Toxic effect of other specified substances, assault** [POA]

[7th] **T65.894 Toxic effect of other specified substances, undetermined** [POA]

[5th] **T65.9 Toxic effect of unspecified substance**

[7th] **T65.91 Toxic effect of unspecified substance, accidental (unintentional)** [POA]
Poisoning NOS

[7th] **T65.92 Toxic effect of unspecified substance, intentional self-harm** [POA] [HCC]

[7th] **T65.93 Toxic effect of unspecified substance, assault** [POA]

[7th] **T65.94 Toxic effect of unspecified substance, undetermined** [POA]

Other and unspecified effects of external causes (T66-T78)

[7th] **T66 Radiation sickness, unspecified** [POA]

[EXCLUDES1] *specified adverse effects of radiation, such as:*
burns (T20-T31)
leukemia (C91-C95)
radiation gastroenteritis and colitis (K52.0)
radiation pneumonitis (J70.0)
radiation related disorders of the skin and subcutaneous tissue (L55-L59)
sunburn (L55.-)

The appropriate 7th character is to be added to code T66
A = initial encounter
D = subsequent encounter
S = sequela

[4th] **T67 Effects of heat and light**

[EXCLUDES1] *erythema [dermatitis] ab igne (L59.0)*
malignant hyperpyrexia due to anesthesia (T88.3)
radiation-related disorders of the skin and subcutaneous tissue (L55-L59)

[EXCLUDES2] *burns (T20-T31)*
sunburn (L55.-)
sweat disorder due to heat (L74-L75)

The appropriate 7th character is to be added to each code from category T67
A = initial encounter
D = subsequent encounter
S = sequela

[7th] **T67.0 Heatstroke and sunstroke** [CC] [POA] [HAC] [CC/MCC Exc]
Heat apoplexy
Heat pyrexia
Siriasis
Thermoplegia
Use additional code(s) to identify any associated complications of heatstroke, such as:
coma and stupor (R40.-)
systemic inflammatory response syndrome (R65.1-)

[7th] **T67.1 Heat syncope** [POA]
Heat collapse

[7th] **T67.2 Heat cramp** [POA]

[7th] **T67.3 Heat exhaustion, anhydrotic** [POA]
Heat prostration due to water depletion
[EXCLUDES1] *heat exhaustion due to salt depletion (T67.4)*

[7th] **T67.4 Heat exhaustion due to salt depletion** [POA]
Heat prostration due to salt (and water) depletion

[7th] **T67.5 Heat exhaustion, unspecified** [POA]
Heat prostration NOS

[7th] **T67.6 Heat fatigue, transient** [POA]

[7th] **T67.7 Heat edema** [POA]

[7th] **T67.8 Other effects of heat and light** [POA]

[7th] **T67.9 Effect of heat and light, unspecified** [POA]

[7th] **T68 Hypothermia** [POA]
Accidental hypothermia
Hypothermia NOS
Use additional code to identify source of exposure:
Exposure to excessive cold of man-made origin (W93)
Exposure to excessive cold of natural origin (X31)

[EXCLUDES1] *hypothermia following anesthesia (T88.51)*
hypothermia not associated with low environmental temperature (R68.0)
hypothermia of newborn (P80.-)

[EXCLUDES2] *frostbite (T33-T34)*

The appropriate 7th character is to be added to code T68
A = initial encounter
D = subsequent encounter
S = sequela

[4th] **T69 Other effects of reduced temperature**
Use additional code to identify source of exposure:
Exposure to excessive cold of man-made origin (W93)
Exposure to excessive cold of natural origin (X31)

[EXCLUDES2] *frostbite (T33-T34)*

The appropriate 7th character is to be added to each code from category T69
A = initial encounter
D = subsequent encounter
S = sequela

[5th] **T69.0 Immersion hand and foot**

[6th] **T69.01 Immersion hand**

[7th] **T69.011 Immersion hand, right hand** [POA]

[7th] **T69.012 Immersion hand, left hand** [POA]

[7th] **T69.019 Immersion hand, unspecified hand** [POA]

[6th] **T69.02 Immersion foot**
Trench foot

[7th] **T69.021 Immersion foot, right foot** [CC] [POA] [HAC] [CC/MCC Exc]

[7th] **T69.022 Immersion foot, left foot** [CC] [POA] [HAC] [CC/MCC Exc]

[7th] **T69.029 Immersion foot, unspecified foot** [CC] [POA] [HAC] [CC/MCC Exc]

[7th] **T69.1 Chilblains** [POA]

[7th] **T69.8 Other specified effects of reduced temperature** [POA]

[7th] **T69.9 Effect of reduced temperature, unspecified** [POA]

[4th] **T70 Effects of air pressure and water pressure**

The appropriate 7th character is to be added to each code from category T70
A = initial encounter
D = subsequent encounter
S = sequela

[7th] **T70.0 Otitic barotrauma** [POA]

Unspecified Code Other Specified Code Manifestation Code [N] Newborn [P] Pediatric [M] Maternity [A] Adult ♂ Male ♀ Female
● New Code ▲ Revised Code Title ►◄ Revised Text [NOTES] [INCLUDES] [EXCLUDES1] Not coded here [EXCLUDES2] Not included here
[4th] 4th character required [5th] 5th character required [6th] 6th character required [7th] 7th character required
[X] Extension 'X' Alert [HAC] Hospital-acquired condition (HAC) alert AHA AHA Coding Clinic©

When symbols appear on a code that requires a 7th character extension, refer to Appendix B to identify applicable 7th character codes.

Aero-otitis media
Effects of change in ambient atmospheric pressure or water pressure on ears

T70.1 Sinus barotrauma POA

Aerosinusitis
Effects of change in ambient atmospheric pressure on sinuses

T70.2 Other and unspecified effects of high altitude

EXCLUDES2 polycythemia due to high altitude (D75.1)

T70.20 Unspecified effects of high altitude POA

T70.29 Other effects of high altitude POA

Alpine sickness
Anoxia due to high altitude
Barotrauma NOS
Hypobaropathy
Mountain sickness

T70.3 Caisson disease [decompression sickness] CC POA HAC CC/MCC Exc

Compressed-air disease
Diver's palsy or paralysis

T70.4 Effects of high-pressure fluids POA

Hydraulic jet injection (industrial)
Pneumatic jet injection (industrial)
Traumatic jet injection (industrial)

T70.8 Other effects of air pressure and water pressure POA

T70.9 Effect of air pressure and water pressure, unspecified POA

T71 Asphyxiation

Mechanical suffocation
Traumatic suffocation

EXCLUDES1 acute respiratory distress (syndrome) (J80)

anoxia due to high altitude (T70.2)

asphyxia NOS (R09.01)

asphyxia from carbon monoxide (T58.-)

asphyxia from inhalation of food or foreign body (T17.-)

asphyxia from other gases, fumes and vapors (T59.-)

respiratory distress (syndrome) in newborn (P22.-)

The appropriate 7th character is to be added to each code from category T71

A = initial encounter

D = subsequent encounter

S = sequela

T71.1 Asphyxiation due to mechanical threat to breathing

Suffocation due to mechanical threat to breathing

T71.11 Asphyxiation due to smothering under pillow

T71.111 Asphyxiation due to smothering under pillow, accidental CC POA HAC CC/MCC Exc

Asphyxiation due to smothering under pillow NOS

T71.112 Asphyxiation due to smothering under pillow, intentional self-harm CC POA HAC HCC CC/MCC Exc

T71.113 Asphyxiation due to smothering under pillow, assault CC POA HAC CC/MCC Exc

T71.114 Asphyxiation due to smothering under pillow, undetermined CC POA HAC CC/MCC Exc

T71.12 Asphyxiation due to plastic bag

T71.121 Asphyxiation due to plastic bag, accidental CC POA HAC CC/MCC Exc

Asphyxiation due to plastic bag NOS

T71.122 Asphyxiation due to plastic bag, intentional self-harm CC POA HAC HCC CC/MCC Exc

T71.123 Asphyxiation due to plastic bag, assault CC POA HAC CC/MCC Exc

T71.124 Asphyxiation due to plastic bag, undetermined CC POA HAC CC/MCC Exc

T71.13 Asphyxiation due to being trapped in bed linens

T71.131 Asphyxiation due to being trapped in bed linens, accidental CC POA HAC CC/MCC Exc

Asphyxiation due to being trapped in bed linens NOS

T71.132 Asphyxiation due to being trapped in bed linens, intentional self-harm CC POA HAC HCC CC/MCC Exc

T71.133 Asphyxiation due to being trapped in bed linens, assault CC POA HAC CC/MCC Exc

T71.134 Asphyxiation due to being trapped in bed linens, undetermined CC POA HAC CC/MCC Exc

T71.14 Asphyxiation due to smothering under another person's body (in bed)

T71.141 Asphyxiation due to smothering under another person's body (in bed), accidental CC POA HAC CC/MCC Exc

Asphyxiation due to smothering under another person's body (in bed) NOS

T71.143 Asphyxiation due to smothering under another person's body (in bed), assault CC POA HAC CC/MCC Exc

T71.144 Asphyxiation due to smothering under another person's body (in bed), undetermined CC POA HAC CC/MCC Exc

T71.15 Asphyxiation due to smothering in furniture

T71.151 Asphyxiation due to smothering in furniture, accidental CC POA HAC CC/MCC Exc

Asphyxiation due to smothering in furniture NOS

T71.152 Asphyxiation due to smothering in furniture, intentional self-harm CC POA HAC HCC CC/MCC Exc

T71.153 Asphyxiation due to smothering in furniture, assault CC POA HAC CC/MCC Exc

T71.154 Asphyxiation due to smothering in furniture, undetermined CC POA HAC CC/MCC Exc

T71.16 Asphyxiation due to hanging

Hanging by window shade cord
Use additional code for any associated injuries, such as:
crushing injury of neck (S17.-)
fracture of cervical vertebrae (S12.0-S12.2-)
open wound of neck (S11.-)

T71.161 Asphyxiation due to hanging, accidental CC POA HAC CC/MCC Exc

Asphyxiation due to hanging NOS
Hanging NOS

T71.162 Asphyxiation due to hanging, intentional self-harm CC POA HAC HCC CC/MCC Exc

T71.163 Asphyxiation due to hanging, assault CC POA HAC CC/MCC Exc

T71.164 Asphyxiation due to hanging, undetermined CC POA HAC CC/MCC Exc

T71.19 Asphyxiation due to mechanical threat to breathing due to other causes

T71.191 Asphyxiation due to mechanical threat to breathing due to other causes, accidental CC POA HAC CC/MCC Exc

Asphyxiation due to other causes NOS

T71.192 Asphyxiation due to mechanical threat to breathing due to other causes, intentional self-harm CC POA HAC HCC CC/MCC Exc

T71.193 Asphyxiation due to mechanical threat to breathing due to other causes, assault CC POA HAC CC/MCC Exc

T71.194 Asphyxiation due to mechanical threat to breathing due to other causes, undetermined CC POA HAC CC/MCC Exc

T71.2 Asphyxiation due to systemic oxygen deficiency due to low oxygen content in ambient air

Suffocation due to systemic oxygen deficiency due to low oxygen content in ambient air

T71.20 Asphyxiation due to systemic oxygen deficiency due to low oxygen content in ambient air due to unspecified cause CC POA HAC CC/MCC Exc

T71.21 Asphyxiation due to cave-in or falling earth CC POA HAC CC/MCC Exc

Use additional code for any associated cataclysm (X34-X38)

T71.22 Asphyxiation due to being trapped in a car trunk

PDxIn Unacceptable principal diagnosis symbol per Medicare code edits   POA Code exempt from diagnosis present on admission requirement

? Questionable admission   CC Complication or comorbidity   CC/MCC Exc CC/MCC exclusion   MCC Major complication or comorbidity

PDx CC Principal diagnosis as its own CC   PDx MCC Principal diagnosis as its own MCC   HCC HCC diagnosis code   RxHCC RxHCC diagnosis code

MACRA code   Z Z code as first-listed diagnosis

T71.221 Asphyxiation due to being trapped in a car trunk, accidental

T71.222 Asphyxiation due to being trapped in a car trunk, intentional self-harm

T71.223 Asphyxiation due to being trapped in a car trunk, assault

T71.224 Asphyxiation due to being trapped in a car trunk, undetermined

T71.23 Asphyxiation due to being trapped in a (discarded) refrigerator

T71.231 Asphyxiation due to being trapped in a (discarded) refrigerator, accidental

T71.232 Asphyxiation due to being trapped in a (discarded) refrigerator, intentional self-harm

T71.233 Asphyxiation due to being trapped in a (discarded) refrigerator, assault

T71.234 Asphyxiation due to being trapped in a (discarded) refrigerator, undetermined

T71.29 Asphyxiation due to being trapped in other low oxygen environment

T71.9 Asphyxiation due to unspecified cause

Suffocation (by strangulation) due to unspecified cause
Suffocation NOS
Systemic oxygen deficiency due to low oxygen content in ambient air due to unspecified cause
Systemic oxygen deficiency due to mechanical threat to breathing due to unspecified cause
Traumatic asphyxia NOS

T73 Effects of other deprivation

The appropriate 7th character is to be added to each code from category T73

A = initial encounter
D = subsequent encounter
S = sequela

T73.0 Starvation

Deprivation of food

T73.1 Deprivation of water

T73.2 Exhaustion due to exposure

T73.3 Exhaustion due to excessive exertion

Exhaustion due to overexertion

T73.8 Other effects of deprivation

T73.9 Effect of deprivation, unspecified

T74 Adult and child abuse, neglect and other maltreatment, confirmed

Use additional code, if applicable, to identify any associated current injury
Use additional external cause code to identify perpetrator, if known (Y07.-)

EXCLUDES1 abuse and maltreatment in pregnancy (O9A.3-, O9A.4-, O9A.5-)
adult and child maltreatment, suspected (T76.-)

The appropriate 7th character is to be added to each code from category T74

A = initial encounter
D = subsequent encounter
S = sequela

T74.0 Neglect or abandonment, confirmed

T74.01 Adult neglect or abandonment, confirmed

T74.02 Child neglect or abandonment, confirmed

T74.1 Physical abuse, confirmed

EXCLUDES2 sexual abuse (T74.2-)

T74.11 Adult physical abuse, confirmed

T74.12 Child physical abuse, confirmed

EXCLUDES2 shaken infant syndrome (T74.4)

T74.2 Sexual abuse, confirmed

Rape, confirmed
Sexual assault, confirmed

T74.21 Adult sexual abuse, confirmed

T74.22 Child sexual abuse, confirmed

T74.3 Psychological abuse, confirmed

T74.31 Adult psychological abuse, confirmed

T74.32 Child psychological abuse, confirmed

T74.4 Shaken infant syndrome

T74.9 Unspecified maltreatment, confirmed

T74.91 Unspecified adult maltreatment, confirmed

T74.92 Unspecified child maltreatment, confirmed

T75 Other and unspecified effects of other external causes

EXCLUDES1 adverse effects NEC (T78.-)
EXCLUDES2 burns (electric) (T20-T31)

The appropriate 7th character is to be added to each code from category T75

A = initial encounter
D = subsequent encounter
S = sequela

T75.0 Effects of lightning

Struck by lightning

T75.00 Unspecified effects of lightning

Struck by lightning NOS

T75.01 Shock due to being struck by lightning

T75.09 Other effects of lightning

Use additional code for other effects of lightning

T75.1 Unspecified effects of drowning and nonfatal submersion

Immersion
EXCLUDES1 specified effects of drowning- code to effects

T75.2 Effects of vibration

T75.20 Unspecified effects of vibration

T75.21 Pneumatic hammer syndrome

T75.22 Traumatic vasospastic syndrome

T75.23 Vertigo from infrasound

EXCLUDES1 vertigo NOS (R42)

T75.29 Other effects of vibration

T75.3 Motion sickness

Airsickness
Seasickness
Travel sickness
Use additional external cause code to identify vehicle or type of motion (Y92.81-, Y93.5-)

T75.4 Electrocution

Shock from electric current
Shock from electroshock gun (taser)

T75.8 Other specified effects of external causes

T75.81 Effects of abnormal gravitation [G] forces

T75.82 Effects of weightlessness

T75.89 Other specified effects of external causes

T76 Adult and child abuse, neglect and other maltreatment, suspected

Use additional code, if applicable, to identify any associated current injury

EXCLUDES1 adult and child maltreatment, confirmed (T74.-)
suspected abuse and maltreatment in pregnancy (O9A.3-, O9A.4-, O9A.5-)
suspected adult physical abuse, ruled out (Z04.71)
suspected adult sexual abuse, ruled out (Z04.41)
suspected child physical abuse, ruled out (Z04.72)
suspected child sexual abuse, ruled out (Z04.42)

The appropriate 7th character is to be added to each code from category T76

A = initial encounter
D = subsequent encounter
S = sequela

T76.0 Neglect or abandonment, suspected

T76.01 Adult neglect or abandonment, suspected

T76.02 Child neglect or abandonment, suspected

Unspecified Code Other Specified Code Manifestation Code N Newborn P Pediatric M Maternity A Adult ♂ Male ♀ Female
● New Code ▲ Revised Code Title ►◄ Revised Text NOTES INCLUDES EXCLUDES 1 Not coded here EXCLUDES 2 Not included here
4th character required 5th character required 6th character required 7th character required
Extension 'X' Alert HAC Hospital-acquired condition (HAC) alert AHA AHA Coding Clinic©

[5th] T76.1 Physical abuse, suspected
- [7th] T76.11 Adult physical abuse, suspected [A] [CC] [POA] [CC/MCC Exc]
- [7th] T76.12 Child physical abuse, suspected [P] [CC] [POA] [CC/MCC Exc]

[5th] T76.2 Sexual abuse, suspected
Rape, suspected
[EXCLUDES1] *alleged abuse, ruled out (Z04.7)*
- [7th] T76.21 Adult sexual abuse, suspected [A] [CC] [POA] [CC/MCC Exc]
- [7th] T76.22 Child sexual abuse, suspected [P] [CC] [POA] [CC/MCC Exc]

[5th] T76.3 Psychological abuse, suspected
- [7th] T76.31 Adult psychological abuse, suspected [A] [POA]
- [7th] T76.32 Child psychological abuse, suspected [P] [CC] [POA] [CC/MCC Exc]

[5th] T76.9 Unspecified maltreatment, suspected
- [7th] T76.91 Unspecified adult maltreatment, suspected [A] [CC] [POA] [CC/MCC Exc]
- [7th] T76.92 Unspecified child maltreatment, suspected [P] [CC] [POA] [CC/MCC Exc]

[4th] T78 Adverse effects, not elsewhere classified
[EXCLUDES2] *complications of surgical and medical care NEC (T80-T88)*
The appropriate 7th character is to be added to each code from category T78
A = initial encounter
D = subsequent encounter
S = sequela

[5th] T78.0 Anaphylactic reaction due to food
Anaphylactic reaction due to adverse food reaction
Anaphylactic shock or reaction due to nonpoisonous foods
Anaphylactoid reaction due to food
- [7th] T78.00 Anaphylactic reaction due to unspecified food [CC] [POA] [CC/MCC Exc]
- [7th] T78.01 Anaphylactic reaction due to peanuts [CC] [POA] [CC/MCC Exc]
- [7th] T78.02 Anaphylactic reaction due to shellfish (crustaceans) [CC] [POA] [CC/MCC Exc]
- [7th] T78.03 Anaphylactic reaction due to other fish [CC] [POA] [CC/MCC Exc]
- [7th] T78.04 Anaphylactic reaction due to fruits and vegetables [CC] [POA] [CC/MCC Exc]
- [7th] T78.05 Anaphylactic reaction due to tree nuts and seeds [CC] [POA] [CC/MCC Exc]
  [EXCLUDES2] *anaphylactic reaction due to peanuts (T78.01)*
- [7th] T78.06 Anaphylactic reaction due to food additives [CC] [POA] [CC/MCC Exc]
- [7th] T78.07 Anaphylactic reaction due to milk and dairy products [CC] [POA] [CC/MCC Exc]
- [7th] T78.08 Anaphylactic reaction due to eggs [CC] [POA] [CC/MCC Exc]
- [7th] T78.09 Anaphylactic reaction due to other food products [CC] [POA] [CC/MCC Exc]

[7th] T78.1 Other adverse food reactions, not elsewhere classified [POA]
Use additional code to identify the type of reaction, if applicable
[EXCLUDES1] *anaphylactic reaction or shock due to adverse food reaction (T78.0-)*
anaphylactic reaction due to food (T78.0-)
bacterial food borne intoxications (A05.-)
[EXCLUDES2] *allergic and dietetic gastroenteritis and colitis (K52.29)*
allergic rhinitis due to food (J30.5)
dermatitis due to food in contact with skin (L23.6, L24.6, L25.4)
dermatitis due to ingested food (L27.2)
food protein-induced enterocolitis syndrome (K52.21)
food protein-induced enteropathy (K52.22)

[7th] T78.2 Anaphylactic shock, unspecified [CC] [POA] [CC/MCC Exc]
Allergic shock
Anaphylactic reaction
Anaphylaxis
[EXCLUDES1] *anaphylactic reaction or shock due to adverse effect of correct medicinal substance properly administered (T88.6)*
anaphylactic reaction or shock due to adverse food reaction (T78.0-)
anaphylactic reaction or shock due to serum (T80.5-)

[7th] T78.3 Angioneurotic edema [POA]
Allergic angioedema
Giant urticaria
Quincke's edema
[EXCLUDES1] *serum urticaria (T80.6-)*
urticaria (L50.-)

[5th] T78.4 Other and unspecified allergy
[EXCLUDES1] *specified types of allergic reaction such as:*
allergic diarrhea (K52.29)
allergic gastroenteritis and colitis (K52.29)
dermatitis (L23-L25, L27.-)
food protein-induced enterocolitis syndrome (K52.21)
food protein-induced enteropathy (K52.22)
hay fever (J30.1)
- [7th] T78.40 Allergy, unspecified [POA]
  Allergic reaction NOS
  Hypersensitivity NOS
- [7th] T78.41 Arthus phenomenon [POA]
  Arthus reaction
- [7th] T78.49 Other allergy [POA]

[7th] T78.8 Other adverse effects, not elsewhere classified [POA]

Certain early complications of trauma (T79)

[4th] T79 Certain early complications of trauma, not elsewhere classified
[EXCLUDES2] *acute respiratory distress syndrome (J80)*
complications occurring during or following medical procedures (T80-T88)
complications of surgical and medical care NEC (T80-T88)
newborn respiratory distress syndrome (P22.0)
The appropriate 7th character is to be added to each code from category T79
A = initial encounter
D = subsequent encounter
S = sequela

[7th] T79.0 Air embolism (traumatic) [POA] [HCC] [MCC] [CC/MCC Exc]
[EXCLUDES1] *air embolism complicating abortion or ectopic or molar pregnancy (O00-O07, O08.2)*
air embolism complicating pregnancy, childbirth and the puerperium (O88.0)
air embolism following infusion, transfusion, and therapeutic injection (T80.0)
air embolism following procedure NEC (T81.7-)

[7th] T79.1 Fat embolism (traumatic) [POA] [HCC] [MCC] [CC/MCC Exc]
[EXCLUDES1] *fat embolism complicating:*
abortion or ectopic or molar pregnancy (O00-O07, O08.2)
pregnancy, childbirth and the puerperium (O88.8)

[7th] T79.2 Traumatic secondary and recurrent hemorrhage and seroma [CC] [POA] [HCC] [CC/MCC Exc]

[7th] T79.4 Traumatic shock [POA] [HCC] [MCC] [CC/MCC Exc]
Shock (immediate) (delayed) following injury
[EXCLUDES1] *anaphylactic shock due to adverse food reaction (T78.0-)*
anaphylactic shock due to correct medicinal substance properly administered (T88.6)
anaphylactic shock due to serum (T80.5-)
anaphylactic shock NOS (T78.2)
anesthetic shock (T88.2)
electric shock (T75.4)
nontraumatic shock NEC (R57.-)
obstetric shock (O75.1)
postprocedural shock (T81.1-)
septic shock (R65.21)
shock complicating abortion or ectopic or molar pregnancy (O00-O07, O08.3)

[PDx] Unacceptable principal diagnosis symbol per Medicare code edits [POA] Code exempt from diagnosis present on admission requirement
[Q] Questionable admission [CC] Complication or comorbidity [CC/MCC Exc] CC/MCC exclusion [MCC] Major complication or comorbidity
[PDx CC] Principal diagnosis as its own CC [PDx MCC] Principal diagnosis as its own MCC [HCC] HCC diagnosis code [RxHCC] RxHCC diagnosis code
MACRA code [Z1] Z code as first-listed diagnosis

shock due to lightning (T75.01)
shock NOS (R57.9)

[7th] **T79.5 Traumatic anuria** POA HCC MCC CC/MCC Exc
Crush syndrome
Renal failure following crushing

[7th] **T79.6 Traumatic ischemia of muscle** POA HCC
Traumatic rhabdomyolysis
Volkmann's ischemic contracture
EXCLUDES2 *anterior tibial syndrome (M76.8)*
compartment syndrome (traumatic) (T79.A-)
nontraumatic ischemia of muscle (M62.2-)

[7th] **T79.7 Traumatic subcutaneous emphysema** CC POA HCC CC/MCC Exc
EXCLUDES1 *emphysema NOS (J43)*
emphysema (subcutaneous) resulting from a procedure (T81.82)

[5th] **T79.A Traumatic compartment syndrome**
EXCLUDES1 *fibromyalgia (M79.7)*
nontraumatic compartment syndrome (M79.A-)
traumatic ischemic infarction of muscle (T79.6)

[7th] **T79.A0 Compartment syndrome, unspecified** CC POA HCC CC/MCC Exc
Compartment syndrome NOS

[6th] **T79.A1 Traumatic compartment syndrome of upper extremity**
Traumatic compartment syndrome of shoulder, arm, forearm, wrist, hand, and fingers

[7th] **T79.A11 Traumatic compartment syndrome of right upper extremity** CC POA HCC CC/MCC Exc

[7th] **T79.A12 Traumatic compartment syndrome of left upper extremity** CC POA HCC CC/MCC Exc

[7th] **T79.A19 Traumatic compartment syndrome of unspecified upper extremity** CC POA HCC CC/MCC Exc

[6th] **T79.A2 Traumatic compartment syndrome of lower extremity**
Traumatic compartment syndrome of hip, buttock, thigh, leg, foot, and toes

[7th] **T79.A21 Traumatic compartment syndrome of right lower extremity** CC POA HCC CC/MCC Exc

[7th] **T79.A22 Traumatic compartment syndrome of left lower extremity** CC POA HCC CC/MCC Exc

[7th] **T79.A29 Traumatic compartment syndrome of unspecified lower extremity** CC POA HCC CC/MCC Exc

[7th] **T79.A3 Traumatic compartment syndrome of abdomen** CC POA HCC CC/MCC Exc

[7th] **T79.A9 Traumatic compartment syndrome of other sites** CC POA HCC CC/MCC Exc

[7th] **T79.8 Other early complications of trauma** POA HCC

[7th] **T79.9 Unspecified early complication of trauma** POA HCC

Complications of surgical and medical care, not elsewhere classified (T80-T88)

Use additional code for adverse effect, if applicable, to identify drug (T36-T50 with fifth or sixth character 5)
Use additional code(s) to identify the specified condition resulting from the complication
Use additional code to identify devices involved and details of circumstances (Y62-Y82)
EXCLUDES2 *any encounters with medical care for postprocedural conditions in which no complications are present, such as:*
artificial opening status (Z93.-)
closure of external stoma (Z43.-)
fitting and adjustment of external prosthetic device (Z44.-)
burns and corrosions from local applications and irradiation (T20-T32)
complications of surgical procedures during pregnancy, childbirth and the puerperium (O00-O9A)
mechanical complication of respirator [ventilator] (J95.850)
poisoning and toxic effects of drugs and chemicals (T36-T65 with fifth or sixth character 1-4 or 6)
postprocedural fever (R50.82)
specified complications classified elsewhere, such as:
cerebrospinal fluid leak from spinal puncture (G97.0)
colostomy malfunction (K94.0-)
disorders of fluid and electrolyte imbalance (E86-E87)
functional disturbances following cardiac surgery (I97.0-I97.1)
intraoperative and postprocedural complications of specified body systems (D78.-, E36.-, E89.-, G97.3-, G97.4, H59.3-, H59.-, H95.2-, H95.3, I97.4-, I97.5, J95.6-, J95.7, K91.6-, L76.-, M96.-, N99.-)
ostomy complications (J95.0-, K94.-, N99.5-)
postgastric surgery syndromes (K91.1)
postlaminectomy syndrome NEC (M96.1)
postmastectomy lymphedema syndrome (I97.2)
postsurgical blind-loop syndrome (K91.2)
ventilator associated pneumonia (J95.851)

[4th] **T80 Complications following infusion, transfusion and therapeutic injection**
INCLUDES *complications following perfusion*
EXCLUDES2 *bone marrow transplant rejection (T86.01)*
febrile nonhemolytic transfusion reaction (R50.84)
fluid overload due to transfusion (E87.71)
posttransfusion purpura (D69.51)
transfusion associated circulatory overload (TACO) (E87.71)
transfusion (red blood cell) associated hemochromatosis (E83.111)
transfusion related acute lung injury (TRALI) (J95.84)

The appropriate 7th character is to be added to each code from category T80
A = initial encounter
D = subsequent encounter
S = sequela

[7th] **T80.0 Air embolism following infusion, transfusion and therapeutic injection** POA HAC MCC CC/MCC Exc

[7th] **T80.1 Vascular complications following infusion, transfusion and therapeutic injection** CC POA CC/MCC Exc
Use additional code to identify the vascular complication
EXCLUDES2 *extravasation of vesicant agent (T80.81-)*
infiltration of vesicant agent (T80.81-)
vascular complications specified as due to prosthetic devices, implants and grafts (T82.8-, T83.8-, T84.8-, T85.8-)
postprocedural vascular complications (T81.7-)

[5th] **T80.2 Infections following infusion, transfusion and therapeutic injection**
Use additional code to identify the specific infection, such as:
sepsis (A41.9)
Use additional code (R65.2-) to identify severe sepsis, if applicable
EXCLUDES2 *infections specified as due to prosthetic devices, implants and grafts (T82.6-T82.7, T83.5-T83.6, T84.5-T84.7, T85.7)*
postprocedural infections (T81.4-)

[6th] **T80.21 Infection due to central venous catheter**
Infection due to pulmonary artery catheter (Swan-Ganz catheter)

[7th] **T80.211 Bloodstream infection due to central venous catheter** CC POA HAC CC/MCC Exc
Catheter-related bloodstream infection (CRBSI) NOS
Central line-associated bloodstream infection (CLABSI)
Bloodstream infection due to Hickman catheter
Bloodstream infection due to peripherally inserted central catheter (PICC)
Bloodstream infection due to portacath (port-a-cath)

Bloodstream infection due to pulmonary artery catheter

Bloodstream infection due to triple lumen catheter

Bloodstream infection due to umbilical venous catheter

🔢 **T80.212** Local infection **due to central venous catheter** cc 🔊 ᴘᴏᴀ HAC CC/MCC Exc

Exit or insertion site infection

Local infection due to Hickman catheter

Local infection due to peripherally inserted central catheter (PICC)

Local infection due to portacath (port-a-cath)

Local infection due to pulmonary artery catheter

Local infection due to triple lumen catheter

Local infection due to umbilical venous catheter

Port or reservoir infection

Tunnel infection

🔢 **T80.218 Other infection due to central venous catheter** cc 🔊 ᴘᴏᴀ HAC CC/MCC Exc

Other central line-associated infection

Other infection due to Hickman catheter

Other infection due to peripherally inserted central catheter (PICC)

Other infection due to portacath (port-a-cath)

Other infection due to pulmonary artery catheter

Other infection due to triple lumen catheter

Other infection due to umbilical venous catheter

🔢 **T80.219 Unspecified infection due to central venous catheter** cc 🔊 ᴘᴏᴀ HAC CC/MCC Exc

Central line-associated infection NOS

Unspecified infection due to Hickman catheter

Unspecified infection due to peripherally inserted central catheter (PICC)

Unspecified infection due to portacath (port-a-cath)

Unspecified infection due to pulmonary artery catheter

Unspecified infection due to triple lumen catheter

Unspecified infection due to umbilical venous catheter

🔢 **T80.22 Acute infection following transfusion, infusion, or injection of blood and blood products** cc 🔊 ᴘᴏᴀ CC/MCC Exc

🔢 **T80.29 Infection following other infusion, transfusion and therapeutic injection** cc 🔊 ᴘᴏᴀ CC/MCC Exc

5ᵗʰ **T80.3** ABO incompatibility **reaction due to transfusion of blood or blood products**

EXCLUDES1 *minor blood group antigens reactions (Duffy) (E) (K(ell)) (Kidd) (Lewis) (M) (N) (P) (S) (T80.A)*

🔢 **T80.30 ABO incompatibility reaction due to transfusion of blood or blood products, unspecified** cc 🔊 ᴘᴏᴀ HAC CC/MCC Exc

ABO incompatibility blood transfusion NOS

Reaction to ABO incompatibility from transfusion NOS

6ᵗʰ **T80.31 ABO incompatibility** with hemolytic transfusion reaction

🔢 **T80.310 ABO incompatibility with** acute **hemolytic transfusion reaction** cc 🔊 ᴘᴏᴀ HAC CC/MCC Exc

ABO incompatibility with hemolytic transfusion reaction less than 24 hours after transfusion

Acute hemolytic transfusion reaction (AHTR) due to ABO incompatibility

🔢 **T80.311 ABO incompatibility with** delayed **hemolytic transfusion reaction** cc 🔊 ᴘᴏᴀ HAC CC/MCC Exc

ABO incompatibility with hemolytic transfusion reaction 24 hours or more after transfusion

Delayed hemolytic transfusion reaction (DHTR) due to ABO incompatibility

🔢 **T80.319 ABO incompatibility with hemolytic transfusion reaction, unspecified** cc 🔊 ᴘᴏᴀ HAC CC/MCC Exc

ABO incompatibility with hemolytic transfusion reaction at unspecified time after transfusion

Hemolytic transfusion reaction (HTR) due to ABO incompatibility NOS

🔢 **T80.39 Other ABO incompatibility reaction due to transfusion of blood or blood products** cc 🔊 ᴘᴏᴀ HAC CC/MCC Exc

Delayed serologic transfusion reaction (DSTR) from ABO incompatibility

Other ABO incompatible blood transfusion

Other reaction to ABO incompatible blood transfusion

5ᵗʰ **T80.4** Rh incompatibility **reaction due to transfusion of blood or blood products**

Reaction due to incompatibility of Rh antigens (C) (c) (D) (E) (e)

🔢 **T80.40 Rh incompatibility reaction due to transfusion of blood or blood products, unspecified** cc 🔊 ᴘᴏᴀ CC/MCC Exc

Reaction due to Rh factor in transfusion NOS

Rh incompatible blood transfusion NOS

6ᵗʰ **T80.41 Rh incompatibility** with hemolytic transfusion reaction

🔢 **T80.410 Rh incompatibility with** acute **hemolytic transfusion reaction** cc 🔊 ᴘᴏᴀ CC/MCC Exc

Acute hemolytic transfusion reaction (AHTR) due to Rh incompatibility

Rh incompatibility with hemolytic transfusion reaction less than 24 hours after transfusion

🔢 **T80.411 Rh incompatibility with** delayed **hemolytic transfusion reaction** cc 🔊 ᴘᴏᴀ CC/MCC Exc

Delayed hemolytic transfusion reaction (DHTR) due to Rh incompatibility

Rh incompatibility with hemolytic transfusion reaction 24 hours or more after transfusion

🔢 **T80.419 Rh incompatibility with hemolytic transfusion reaction, unspecified** cc 🔊 ᴘᴏᴀ CC/MCC Exc

Rh incompatibility with hemolytic transfusion reaction at unspecified time after transfusion

Hemolytic transfusion reaction (HTR) due to Rh incompatibility NOS

🔢 **T80.49 Other Rh incompatibility reaction due to transfusion of blood or blood products** cc 🔊 ᴘᴏᴀ CC/MCC Exc

Delayed serologic transfusion reaction (DSTR) from Rh incompatibility

Other reaction to Rh incompatible blood transfusion

5ᵗʰ **T80.A** Non-ABO incompatibility **reaction due to transfusion of blood or blood products**

Reaction due to incompatibility of minor antigens (Duffy) (Kell) (Kidd) (Lewis) (M) (N) (P) (S)

🔢 **T80.A0 Non-ABO incompatibility reaction due to transfusion of blood or blood products, unspecified** cc 🔊 ᴘᴏᴀ CC/MCC Exc

Non-ABO antigen incompatibility reaction from transfusion NOS

6ᵗʰ **T80.A1 Non-ABO incompatibility** with hemolytic transfusion reaction

🔢 **T80.A10 Non-ABO incompatibility with** acute **hemolytic transfusion reaction** cc 🔊 ᴘᴏᴀ CC/MCC Exc

Acute hemolytic transfusion reaction (AHTR) due to non-ABO incompatibility

Non-ABO incompatibility with hemolytic transfusion reaction less than 24 hours after transfusion

ᴘᴏᴀ Unacceptable principal diagnosis symbol per Medicare code edits   🔊 Code exempt from diagnosis present on admission requirement

❓ Questionable admission   cc Complication or comorbidity   cc/mcc Exc CC/MCC exclusion   mcc Major complication or comorbidity

🔢 Principal diagnosis as its own CC   🔢 Principal diagnosis as its own MCC   HCC HCC diagnosis code   RxHCC RxHCC diagnosis code

MACRA code   Z1 Z code as first-listed diagnosis

1164

When symbols appear on a code that requires a 7th character extension, refer to Appendix B to identify applicable 7th character codes.

2018 ICD-10-CM

⑦ **T80.A11** **Non-ABO incompatibility with** delayed hemolytic transfusion reaction CC POA CC/MCC Exc

Delayed hemolytic transfusion reaction (DHTR) due to non-ABO incompatibility

Non-ABO incompatibility with hemolytic transfusion reaction 24 or more hours after transfusion

⑦ **T80.A19** **Non-ABO incompatibility with hemolytic transfusion reaction, unspecified** CC POA CC/MCC Exc

Hemolytic transfusion reaction (HTR) due to non-ABO incompatibility NOS

Non-ABO incompatibility with hemolytic transfusion reaction at unspecified time after transfusion

⑦ **T80.A9** **Other non-ABO incompatibility reaction due to transfusion of blood or blood products** CC POA CC/MCC Exc

Delayed serologic transfusion reaction (DSTR) from non-ABO incompatibility

Other reaction to non-ABO incompatible blood transfusion

⑤ **T80.5** **Anaphylactic reaction due to serum**

Allergic shock due to serum

Anaphylactic shock due to serum

Anaphylactoid reaction due to serum

Anaphylaxis due to serum

EXCLUDES1 *ABO incompatibility reaction due to transfusion of blood or blood products (T80.3-)*

allergic reaction or shock NOS (T78.2)

anaphylactic reaction or shock NOS (T78.2)

anaphylactic reaction or shock due to adverse effect of correct medicinal substance properly administered (T88.6)

other serum reaction (T80.6-)

⑦ **T80.51** **Anaphylactic reaction due to** administration of blood and blood products CC POA CC/MCC Exc

⑦ **T80.52** **Anaphylactic reaction due to** vaccination CC POA CC/MCC Exc

⑦ **T80.59** **Anaphylactic reaction due to other serum** CC POA CC/MCC Exc

⑤ **T80.6** **Other serum reactions**

Intoxication by serum

Protein sickness

Serum rash

Serum sickness

Serum urticaria

EXCLUDES2 *serum hepatitis (B16-B19)*

⑦ **T80.61** **Other serum reaction** due to administration of blood and blood products CC POA CC/MCC Exc

⑦ **T80.62** **Other serum reaction** due to vaccination CC POA CC/MCC Exc

⑦ **T80.69** **Other** serum **reaction due to other** serum CC POA CC/MCC Exc

Code also, if applicable, arthropathy in hypersensitivity reactions classified elsewhere (M36.4)

⑤ **T80.8** **Other complications following infusion, transfusion and therapeutic injection**

⑥ **T80.81** **Extravasation of vesicant agent**

Infiltration of vesicant agent

⑦ **T80.810** **Extravasation of vesicant antineoplastic chemotherapy** CC POA CC/MCC Exc

Infiltration of vesicant antineoplastic chemotherapy

⑦ **T80.818** **Extravasation of other vesicant agent** CC POA CC/MCC Exc

Infiltration of other vesicant agent

⑥ **T80.89** **Other complications following infusion, transfusion and therapeutic injection** POA

Delayed serologic transfusion reaction (DSTR), unspecified incompatibility

Use additional code to identify graft-versus-host reaction, if applicable, (D89.81-)

⑤ **T80.9** **Unspecified complication following infusion, transfusion and therapeutic injection**

⑦ **T80.90** **Unspecified complication** following infusion and therapeutic injection POA

⑥ **T80.91** **Hemolytic transfusion reaction, unspecified incompatibility**

EXCLUDES1 *ABO incompatibility with hemolytic transfusion reaction (T80.31-)*

Non-ABO incompatibility with hemolytic transfusion reaction (T80.A1-)

Rh incompatibility with hemolytic transfusion reaction (T80.41-)

⑦ **T80.910** **Acute** hemolytic transfusion reaction, unspecified incompatibility CC POA CC/MCC Exc

⑦ **T80.911** **Delayed** hemolytic transfusion reaction, unspecified incompatibility CC POA CC/MCC Exc

⑦ **T80.919** **Hemolytic transfusion reaction, unspecified incompatibility, unspecified as acute or delayed** CC POA CC/MCC Exc

Hemolytic transfusion reaction NOS

⑦ **T80.92** **Unspecified transfusion reaction** POA

Transfusion reaction NOS

④ **T81** **Complications of procedures, not elsewhere classified**

Use additional code for adverse effect, if applicable, to identify drug (T36-T50 with fifth or sixth character 5)

EXCLUDES2 *complications following immunization (T88.0-T88.1)*

complications following infusion, transfusion and therapeutic injection (T80.-)

complications of transplanted organs and tissue (T86.-)

specified complications classified elsewhere, such as:

complication of prosthetic devices, implants and grafts (T82-T85)

dermatitis due to drugs and medicaments (L23.3, L24.4, L25.1, L27.0-L27.1)

endosseous dental implant failure (M27.6-)

floppy iris syndrome (IFIS) (intraoperative) H21.81

intraoperative and postprocedural complications of specific body system (D78.-, E36.-, E89.-, G97.3-, G97.4, H59.3-, H59.-, H95.2-, H95.3, I97.4-, I97.5, J95, K91.-, L76.-, M96.-, N99.-)

ostomy complications (J95.0-, K94.-, N99.5-)

plateau iris syndrome (post-iridectomy) (postprocedural) H21.82

poisoning and toxic effects of drugs and chemicals (T36-T65 with fifth or sixth character 1-4 or 6)

The appropriate 7th character is to be added to each code from category T81

A = initial encounter

D = subsequent encounter

S = sequela

⑤ **T81.1** **Postprocedural shock**

Shock during or resulting from a procedure, not elsewhere classified

EXCLUDES1 *anaphylactic shock NOS (T78.2)*

anaphylactic shock due to correct substance properly administered (T88.6)

anaphylactic shock due to serum (T80.5-)

anesthetic shock (T88.2)

electric shock (T75.4)

obstetric shock (O75.1)

septic shock (R65.21)

shock following abortion or ectopic or molar pregnancy (O00-O07, O08.3)

traumatic shock (T79.4)

⑦ **T81.10** **Postprocedural shock unspecified** CC POA CC/MCC Exc

Collapse NOS during or resulting from a procedure, not elsewhere classified

Postprocedural failure of peripheral circulation

Postprocedural shock NOS

⑦ **T81.11** **Postprocedural** cardiogenic **shock** POA HCC MCC CC/MCC Exc

⑦ **T81.12** **Postprocedural** septic **shock** POA HCC MCC PDxIn CC/MCC Exc

---

Unspecified Code	Other Specified Code	Manifestation Code	Ⓝ Newborn	Ⓟ Pediatric	Ⓜ Maternity	Ⓐ Adult	♂ Male	♀ Female

● New Code ▲ Revised Code Title ►◄ Revised Text NOTES *INCLUDES* EXCLUDES1 Not coded here EXCLUDES2 Not included here

④ 4th character required ⑤ 5th character required ⑥ 6th character required ⑦ 7th character required

⑦ Extension 'X' Alert HAC Hospital-acquired condition (HAC) alert AHA AHA Coding Clinic©

Postprocedural endotoxic shock resulting from a procedure, not elsewhere classified

Postprocedural gram-negative shock resulting from a procedure, not elsewhere classified

Code first underlying infection

Use additional code, to identify any associated acute organ dysfunction, if applicable

T81.19 **Other postprocedural shock**   POA MCC CC/MCC Exc

Postprocedural hypovolemic shock

T81.3 **Disruption of wound, not elsewhere classified**

Disruption of any suture materials or other closure methods

EXCLUDES1 *breakdown (mechanical) of permanent sutures (T85.612)*

displacement of permanent sutures (T85.622)

disruption of cesarean delivery wound (O90.0)

disruption of perineal obstetric wound (O90.1)

mechanical complication of permanent sutures NEC (T85.692)

T81.30 **Disruption of wound, unspecified**   CC POA CC/MCC Exc

Disruption of wound NOS

T81.31 **Disruption of external operation (surgical) wound, not elsewhere classified**   CC POA CC/MCC Exc

Dehiscence of operation wound NOS
Disruption of operation wound NOS
Disruption or dehiscence of closure of cornea
Disruption or dehiscence of closure of mucosa
Disruption or dehiscence of closure of skin and subcutaneous tissue
Full-thickness skin disruption or dehiscence
Superficial disruption or dehiscence of operation wound

EXCLUDES1 *dehiscence of amputation stump (T87.81)*

T81.32 **Disruption of internal operation (surgical) wound, not elsewhere classified**   CC POA CC/MCC Exc

Deep disruption or dehiscence of operation wound NOS
Disruption or dehiscence of closure of internal organ or other internal tissue
Disruption or dehiscence of closure of muscle or muscle flap
Disruption or dehiscence of closure of ribs or rib cage
Disruption or dehiscence of closure of skull or craniotomy
Disruption or dehiscence of closure of sternum or sternotomy
Disruption or dehiscence of closure of tendon or ligament
Disruption or dehiscence of closure of superficial or muscular fascia

T81.33 **Disruption of traumatic injury wound repair**   CC POA CC/MCC Exc

Disruption or dehiscence of closure of traumatic laceration (external) (internal)

T81.4 **Infection following a procedure**   CC POA HAC CC/MCC Exc

Intra-abdominal abscess following a procedure
Postprocedural infection, not elsewhere classified
Sepsis following a procedure
Stitch abscess following a procedure
Subphrenic abscess following a procedure
Wound abscess following a procedure

Use additional code to identify infection

Use additional code (R65.2-) to identify severe sepsis, if applicable

EXCLUDES1 *obstetric surgical wound infection (O86.0)*

postprocedural fever NOS (R50.82)

postprocedural retroperitoneal abscess (K68.11)

EXCLUDES2 *bleb associated endophthalmitis (H59.4-)*

infection due to infusion, transfusion and therapeutic injection (T80.2-)

infection due to prosthetic devices, implants and grafts (T82.6-T82.7, T83.5-T83.6, T84.5-T84.7, T85.7)

T81.5 **Complications of** foreign body accidentally left in body following procedure

T81.50 **Unspecified complication of foreign body accidentally left in body following procedure**

T81.500 **Unspecified complication of foreign body accidentally** left in body following surgical operation   CC POA HAC CC/MCC Exc

T81.501 **Unspecified complication of foreign body accidentally** left in body following infusion or transfusion   CC POA HAC CC/MCC Exc

T81.502 **Unspecified complication of foreign body accidentally** left in body following kidney dialysis   CC POA HAC HCC RxHCC CC/MCC Exc

T81.503 **Unspecified complication of foreign body accidentally** left in body following injection or immunization   CC POA HAC CC/MCC Exc

T81.504 **Unspecified complication of foreign body accidentally** left in body following endoscopic examination   CC POA HAC CC/MCC Exc

T81.505 **Unspecified complication of foreign body accidentally** left in body following heart catheterization   CC POA HAC CC/MCC Exc

T81.506 **Unspecified complication of foreign body accidentally** left in body following aspiration, puncture or other catheterization   CC POA HAC CC/MCC Exc

T81.507 **Unspecified complication of foreign body accidentally** left in body following removal of catheter or packing   CC POA HAC CC/MCC Exc

T81.508 **Unspecified complication of foreign body accidentally** left in body following other procedure   CC POA HAC CC/MCC Exc

T81.509 **Unspecified complication of foreign body accidentally** left in body following unspecified procedure   CC POA HAC CC/MCC Exc

T81.51 **Adhesions** due to foreign body accidentally left in body following procedure

T81.510 **Adhesions due to foreign body accidentally** left in body following surgical operation   CC POA HAC CC/MCC Exc

T81.511 **Adhesions due to foreign body accidentally** left in body following infusion or transfusion   CC POA HAC CC/MCC Exc

T81.512 **Adhesions due to foreign body accidentally** left in body following kidney dialysis   CC POA HAC HCC RxHCC CC/MCC Exc

T81.513 **Adhesions due to foreign body accidentally** left in body following injection or immunization   CC POA HAC CC/MCC Exc

T81.514 **Adhesions due to foreign body accidentally** left in body following endoscopic examination   CC POA HAC CC/MCC Exc

T81.515 **Adhesions due to foreign body accidentally** left in body following heart catheterization   CC POA HAC CC/MCC Exc

T81.516 **Adhesions due to foreign body accidentally** left in body following aspiration, puncture or other catheterization   CC POA HAC CC/MCC Exc

T81.517 **Adhesions due to foreign body accidentally** left in body following removal of catheter or packing   CC POA HAC CC/MCC Exc

T81.518 **Adhesions due to foreign body accidentally** left in body following other procedure   CC POA HAC CC/MCC Exc

T81.519 **Adhesions due to foreign body accidentally** left in body following unspecified procedure   CC POA HAC CC/MCC Exc

T81.52 **Obstruction** due to foreign body accidentally left in body following procedure

T81.520 **Obstruction due to foreign body accidentally** left in body following surgical operation   CC POA HAC CC/MCC Exc

---

POA Unacceptable principal diagnosis symbol per Medicare code edits   POA Code exempt from diagnosis present on admission requirement
❓ Questionable admission   CC Complication or comorbidity   CC/MCC Exc CC/MCC exclusion   MCC Major complication or comorbidity
PDx CC Principal diagnosis as its own CC   PDx MCC Principal diagnosis as its own MCC   HCC HCC diagnosis code   RxHCC RxHCC diagnosis code
MACRA code   Z1 Z code as first-listed diagnosis

When symbols appear on a code that requires a 7th character extension, refer to Appendix B to identify applicable 7th character codes.   **2018 ICD-10-CM**

[7th] T81.521 Obstruction due to foreign body accidentally left in body following infusion or transfusion CC POA HAC CC/MCC Exc

[7th] T81.522 Obstruction due to foreign body accidentally left in body following kidney dialysis CC POA HAC HCC RxHCC CC/MCC Exc

[7th] T81.523 Obstruction due to foreign body accidentally left in body following injection or immunization CC POA HAC CC/MCC Exc

[7th] T81.524 Obstruction due to foreign body accidentally left in body following endoscopic examination CC POA HAC CC/MCC Exc

[7th] T81.525 Obstruction due to foreign body accidentally left in body following heart catheterization CC POA HAC CC/MCC Exc

[7th] T81.526 Obstruction due to foreign body accidentally left in body following aspiration, puncture or other catheterization CC POA HAC CC/MCC Exc

[7th] T81.527 Obstruction due to foreign body accidentally left in body following removal of catheter or packing CC POA HAC CC/MCC Exc

[7th] T81.528 Obstruction due to foreign body accidentally left in body following other procedure CC POA HAC CC/MCC Exc

[7th] T81.529 Obstruction due to foreign body accidentally left in body following unspecified procedure CC POA HAC CC/MCC Exc

[6th] T81.53 Perforation due to foreign body accidentally left in body following procedure

[7th] T81.530 Perforation due to foreign body accidentally left in body following surgical operation CC POA HAC CC/MCC Exc

[7th] T81.531 Perforation due to foreign body accidentally left in body following infusion or transfusion CC POA HAC CC/MCC Exc

[7th] T81.532 Perforation due to foreign body accidentally left in body following kidney dialysis CC POA HAC HCC RxHCC CC/MCC Exc

[7th] T81.533 Perforation due to foreign body accidentally left in body following injection or immunization CC POA HAC CC/MCC Exc

[7th] T81.534 Perforation due to foreign body accidentally left in body following endoscopic examination CC POA HAC CC/MCC Exc

[7th] T81.535 Perforation due to foreign body accidentally left in body following heart catheterization CC POA HAC CC/MCC Exc

[7th] T81.536 Perforation due to foreign body accidentally left in body following aspiration, puncture or other catheterization CC POA HAC CC/MCC Exc

[7th] T81.537 Perforation due to foreign body accidentally left in body following removal of catheter or packing CC POA HAC CC/MCC Exc

[7th] T81.538 Perforation due to foreign body accidentally left in body following other procedure CC POA HAC CC/MCC Exc

[7th] T81.539 Perforation due to foreign body accidentally left in body following unspecified procedure CC POA HAC CC/MCC Exc

[6th] T81.59 Other complications of foreign body accidentally left in body following procedure

EXCLUDES2 *obstruction or perforation due to prosthetic devices and implants intentionally left in body (T82.0-T82.5, T83.0-T83.4, T83.7, T84.0-T84.4, T85.0-T85.6)*

[7th] T81.590 Other complications of foreign body accidentally left in body following surgical operation CC POA HAC CC/MCC Exc

[7th] T81.591 Other complications of foreign body accidentally left in body following infusion or transfusion CC POA HAC CC/MCC Exc

[7th] T81.592 Other complications of foreign body accidentally left in body following kidney dialysis CC POA HAC HCC RxHCC CC/MCC Exc

[7th] T81.593 Other complications of foreign body accidentally left in body following injection or immunization CC POA HAC CC/MCC Exc

[7th] T81.594 Other complications of foreign body accidentally left in body following endoscopic examination CC POA HAC CC/MCC Exc

[7th] T81.595 Other complications of foreign body accidentally left in body following heart catheterization CC POA HAC CC/MCC Exc

[7th] T81.596 Other complications of foreign body accidentally left in body following aspiration, puncture or other catheterization CC POA HAC CC/MCC Exc

[7th] T81.597 Other complications of foreign body accidentally left in body following removal of catheter or packing CC POA HAC CC/MCC Exc

[7th] T81.598 Other complications of foreign body accidentally left in body following other procedure CC POA HAC CC/MCC Exc

[7th] T81.599 Other complications of foreign body accidentally left in body following unspecified procedure CC POA HAC CC/MCC Exc

[5th] T81.6 Acute reaction to foreign substance accidentally left during a procedure

EXCLUDES2 *complications of foreign body accidentally left in body cavity or operation wound following procedure (T81.5-)*

[7th] T81.60 Unspecified acute reaction to foreign substance accidentally left during a procedure CC POA HAC CC/MCC Exc

[7th] T81.61 Aseptic peritonitis due to foreign substance accidentally left during a procedure CC POA HAC CC/MCC Exc
Chemical peritonitis

[7th] T81.69 Other acute reaction to foreign substance accidentally left during a procedure CC POA HAC CC/MCC Exc

[5th] T81.7 Vascular complications following a procedure, not elsewhere classified
Air embolism following procedure NEC
Phlebitis or thrombophlebitis resulting from a procedure

EXCLUDES1 *embolism complicating abortion or ectopic or molar pregnancy (O00-O07, O08.2)*
embolism complicating pregnancy, childbirth and the puerperium (O88.-)
traumatic embolism (T79.0)

EXCLUDES2 *embolism due to prosthetic devices, implants and grafts (T82.8-, T83.81, T84.8-, T85.81-)*
embolism following infusion, transfusion and therapeutic injection (T80.0)

[6th] T81.71 Complication of artery following a procedure, not elsewhere classified

[7th] T81.710 Complication of mesenteric artery following a procedure, not elsewhere classified CC POA CC/MCC Exc

[7th] T81.711 Complication of renal artery following a procedure, not elsewhere classified CC POA CC/MCC Exc

[7th] T81.718 Complication of other artery following a procedure, not elsewhere classified CC POA CC/MCC Exc

[7th] T81.719 Complication of unspecified artery following a procedure, not elsewhere classified CC POA CC/MCC Exc

[7th] T81.72 Complication of vein following a procedure, not elsewhere classified CC POA CC/MCC Exc

[5th] T81.8 Other complications of procedures, not elsewhere classified

EXCLUDES2 *hypothermia following anesthesia (T88.51)*
malignant hyperpyrexia due to anesthesia (T88.3)

[7th] T81.81 Complication of inhalation therapy POA

[7th] T81.82 Emphysema (subcutaneous) resulting from a procedure POA

[7th] T81.83 Persistent postprocedural fistula CC POA CC/MCC Exc

T81.89 **Other complications of procedures, not elsewhere classified**

Use additional code to specify complication, such as:

postprocedural delirium (F05)

T81.9 **Unspecified complication of procedure**

T82 **Complications of cardiac and vascular prosthetic devices, implants and grafts**

EXCLUDES2 failure and rejection of transplanted organs and tissue (T86.-)

The appropriate 7th character is to be added to each code from category T82

A = initial encounter

D = subsequent encounter

S = sequela

T82.0 **Mechanical complication of heart valve prosthesis**

Mechanical complication of artificial heart valve

EXCLUDES1 mechanical complication of biological heart valve graft (T82.22-)

T82.01 **Breakdown (mechanical) of heart valve prosthesis**

T82.02 **Displacement of heart valve prosthesis**

Malposition of heart valve prosthesis

T82.03 **Leakage of heart valve prosthesis**

T82.09 **Other mechanical complication of heart valve prosthesis**

Obstruction (mechanical) of heart valve prosthesis

Perforation of heart valve prosthesis

Protrusion of heart valve prosthesis

T82.1 **Mechanical complication of cardiac electronic device**

T82.11 **Breakdown (mechanical) of cardiac electronic device**

T82.110 **Breakdown (mechanical) of cardiac electrode**

T82.111 **Breakdown (mechanical) of cardiac pulse generator (battery)**

T82.118 **Breakdown (mechanical) of other cardiac electronic device**

T82.119 **Breakdown (mechanical) of unspecified cardiac electronic device**

T82.12 **Displacement of cardiac electronic device**

Malposition of cardiac electronic device

T82.120 **Displacement of cardiac electrode**

T82.121 **Displacement of cardiac pulse generator (battery)**

T82.128 **Displacement of other cardiac electronic device**

T82.129 **Displacement of unspecified cardiac electronic device**

T82.19 **Other mechanical complication of cardiac electronic device**

Leakage of cardiac electronic device

Obstruction of cardiac electronic device

Perforation of cardiac electronic device

Protrusion of cardiac electronic device

T82.190 **Other mechanical complication of cardiac electrode**

T82.191 **Other mechanical complication of cardiac pulse generator (battery)**

T82.198 **Other mechanical complication of other cardiac electronic device**

T82.199 **Other mechanical complication of unspecified cardiac device**

T82.2 **Mechanical complication of coronary artery bypass graft and biological heart valve graft**

EXCLUDES1 mechanical complication of artificial heart valve prosthesis (T82.0-)

T82.21 **Mechanical complication of coronary artery bypass graft**

T82.211 **Breakdown (mechanical) of coronary artery bypass graft**

T82.212 **Displacement of coronary artery bypass graft**

Malposition of coronary artery bypass graft

T82.213 **Leakage of coronary artery bypass graft**

T82.218 **Other mechanical complication of coronary artery bypass graft**

Obstruction, mechanical of coronary artery bypass graft

Perforation of coronary artery bypass graft

Protrusion of coronary artery bypass graft

T82.22 **Mechanical complication of biological heart valve graft**

T82.221 **Breakdown (mechanical) of biological heart valve graft**

T82.222 **Displacement of biological heart valve graft**

Malposition of biological heart valve graft

T82.223 **Leakage of biological heart valve graft**

T82.228 **Other mechanical complication of biological heart valve graft**

Obstruction of biological heart valve graft

Perforation of biological heart valve graft

Protrusion of biological heart valve graft

T82.3 **Mechanical complication of other vascular grafts**

T82.31 **Breakdown (mechanical) of other vascular grafts**

T82.310 **Breakdown (mechanical) of aortic (bifurcation) graft (replacement)**

T82.311 **Breakdown (mechanical) of carotid arterial graft (bypass)**

T82.312 **Breakdown (mechanical) of femoral arterial graft (bypass)**

T82.318 **Breakdown (mechanical) of other vascular grafts**

T82.319 **Breakdown (mechanical) of unspecified vascular grafts**

T82.32 **Displacement of other vascular grafts**

Malposition of other vascular grafts

T82.320 **Displacement of aortic (bifurcation) graft (replacement)**

T82.321 **Displacement of carotid arterial graft (bypass)**

T82.322 **Displacement of femoral arterial graft (bypass)**

T82.328 **Displacement of other vascular grafts**

T82.329 **Displacement of unspecified vascular grafts**

T82.33 **Leakage of other vascular grafts**

T82.330 **Leakage of aortic (bifurcation) graft (replacement)**

T82.331 **Leakage of carotid arterial graft (bypass)**

T82.332 **Leakage of femoral arterial graft (bypass)**

T82.338 **Leakage of other vascular grafts**

T82.339 **Leakage of unspecified vascular graft**

T82.39 **Other mechanical complication of other vascular grafts**

Obstruction (mechanical) of other vascular grafts

Perforation of other vascular grafts

Protrusion of other vascular grafts

T82.390 **Other mechanical complication of aortic (bifurcation) graft (replacement)**

T82.391 **Other mechanical complication of carotid arterial graft (bypass)**

T82.392 **Other mechanical complication of femoral arterial graft (bypass)**

PDx Unacceptable principal diagnosis symbol per Medicare code edits POA Code exempt from diagnosis present on admission requirement
? Questionable admission CC Complication or comorbidity CC/MCC Exc CC/MCC exclusion MCC Major complication or comorbidity
PDx Principal diagnosis as its own CC PDx Principal diagnosis as its own MCC HCC HCC diagnosis code RxHCC RxHCC diagnosis code
MACRA code Z1 Z code as first-listed diagnosis

1168

When symbols appear on a code that requires a 7th character extension, refer to Appendix B to identify applicable 7th character codes.

2018 ICD-10-CM

⑦ **T82.398** Other mechanical complication of other vascular grafts CC POA HCC CC/MCC Exc

⑦ **T82.399** Other mechanical complication of unspecified vascular grafts CC POA HCC CC/MCC Exc

5ᵗʰ **T82.4** Mechanical complication of vascular dialysis catheter
Mechanical complication of hemodialysis catheter
EXCLUDES1 mechanical complication of intraperitoneal dialysis catheter (T85.62)

⑦ **T82.41** Breakdown (mechanical) of vascular dialysis catheter CC POA HCC RxHCC CC/MCC Exc

⑦ **T82.42** Displacement of vascular dialysis catheter CC POA HCC RxHCC CC/MCC Exc
Malposition of vascular dialysis catheter

⑦ **T82.43** Leakage of vascular dialysis catheter CC POA HCC RxHCC CC/MCC Exc

⑦ **T82.49** Other complication of vascular dialysis catheter CC POA HCC RxHCC CC/MCC Exc
Obstruction (mechanical) of vascular dialysis catheter
Perforation of vascular dialysis catheter
Protrusion of vascular dialysis catheter

5ᵗʰ **T82.5** Mechanical complication of other cardiac and vascular devices and implants
EXCLUDES2 mechanical complication of epidural and subdural infusion catheter (T85.61)

6ᵗʰ **T82.51** Breakdown (mechanical) of other cardiac and vascular devices and implants

⑦ **T82.510** Breakdown (mechanical) of surgically created arteriovenous fistula CC POA HCC CC/MCC Exc

⑦ **T82.511** Breakdown (mechanical) of surgically created arteriovenous shunt CC POA HCC CC/MCC Exc

⑦ **T82.512** Breakdown (mechanical) of artificial heart CC POA HCC CC/MCC Exc

⑦ **T82.513** Breakdown (mechanical) of balloon (counterpulsation) device CC POA HCC CC/MCC Exc

⑦ **T82.514** Breakdown (mechanical) of infusion catheter CC POA HCC CC/MCC Exc

⑦ **T82.515** Breakdown (mechanical) of umbrella device CC POA HCC CC/MCC Exc

⑦ **T82.518** Breakdown (mechanical) of other cardiac and vascular devices and implants CC POA HCC CC/MCC Exc

⑦ **T82.519** Breakdown (mechanical) of unspecified cardiac and vascular devices and implants CC POA CC/MCC Exc

6ᵗʰ **T82.52** Displacement of other cardiac and vascular devices and implants
Malposition of other cardiac and vascular devices and implants

⑦ **T82.520** Displacement of surgically created arteriovenous fistula CC POA HCC CC/MCC Exc

⑦ **T82.521** Displacement of surgically created arteriovenous shunt CC POA HCC CC/MCC Exc

⑦ **T82.522** Displacement of artificial heart CC POA CC/MCC Exc

⑦ **T82.523** Displacement of balloon (counterpulsation) device CC POA CC/MCC Exc

⑦ **T82.524** Displacement of infusion catheter CC POA HCC CC/MCC Exc

⑦ **T82.525** Displacement of umbrella device CC POA HCC CC/MCC Exc

⑦ **T82.528** Displacement of other cardiac and vascular devices and implants CC POA HCC CC/MCC Exc

⑦ **T82.529** Displacement of unspecified cardiac and vascular devices and implants CC POA CC/MCC Exc

6ᵗʰ **T82.53** Leakage of other cardiac and vascular devices and implants

⑦ **T82.530** Leakage of surgically created arteriovenous fistula CC POA HCC CC/MCC Exc

⑦ **T82.531** Leakage of surgically created arteriovenous shunt CC POA HCC CC/MCC Exc

⑦ **T82.532** Leakage of artificial heart CC POA CC/MCC Exc

⑦ **T82.533** Leakage of balloon (counterpulsation) device CC POA HCC CC/MCC Exc

⑦ **T82.534** Leakage of infusion catheter CC POA HCC CC/MCC Exc

⑦ **T82.535** Leakage of umbrella device CC POA HCC CC/MCC Exc

⑦ **T82.538** Leakage of other cardiac and vascular devices and implants CC POA HCC CC/MCC Exc

⑦ **T82.539** Leakage of unspecified cardiac and vascular devices and implants CC POA CC/MCC Exc

6ᵗʰ **T82.59** Other mechanical complication of other cardiac and vascular devices and implants
Obstruction (mechanical) of other cardiac and vascular devices and implants
Perforation of other cardiac and vascular devices and implants
Protrusion of other cardiac and vascular devices and implants

⑦ **T82.590** Other mechanical complication of surgically created arteriovenous fistula CC POA HCC CC/MCC Exc

⑦ **T82.591** Other mechanical complication of surgically created arteriovenous shunt CC POA HCC CC/MCC Exc

⑦ **T82.592** Other mechanical complication of artificial heart CC POA HCC CC/MCC Exc

⑦ **T82.593** Other mechanical complication of balloon (counterpulsation) device CC POA HCC CC/MCC Exc

⑦ **T82.594** Other mechanical complication of infusion catheter CC POA HCC CC/MCC Exc

⑦ **T82.595** Other mechanical complication of umbrella device CC POA HCC CC/MCC Exc

⑦ **T82.598** Other mechanical complication of other cardiac and vascular devices and implants CC POA HCC CC/MCC Exc

⑦ **T82.599** Other mechanical complication of unspecified cardiac and vascular devices and implants CC POA CC/MCC Exc

⑦ **T82.6** Infection and inflammatory reaction due to cardiac valve prosthesis CC POA HAC HCC CC/MCC Exc
Use additional code to identify infection

⑦ **T82.7** Infection and inflammatory reaction due to other cardiac and vascular devices, implants and grafts CC POA HAC HCC CC/MCC Exc
Use additional code to identify infection

5ᵗʰ **T82.8** Other specified complications of cardiac and vascular prosthetic devices, implants and grafts

6ᵗʰ **T82.81** Embolism due to cardiac and vascular prosthetic devices, implants and grafts

⑦ **T82.817** Embolism due to cardiac prosthetic devices, implants and grafts CC POA CC/MCC Exc
AHA: Q4 2016

⑦ **T82.818** Embolism due to vascular prosthetic devices, implants and grafts CC POA HCC CC/MCC Exc

6ᵗʰ **T82.82** Fibrosis due to cardiac and vascular prosthetic devices, implants and grafts

⑦ **T82.827** Fibrosis due to cardiac prosthetic devices, implants and grafts CC POA CC/MCC Exc

⑦ **T82.828** Fibrosis due to vascular prosthetic devices, implants and grafts CC POA HCC CC/MCC Exc

6ᵗʰ **T82.83** Hemorrhage due to cardiac and vascular prosthetic devices, implants and grafts

⑦ **T82.837** Hemorrhage due to cardiac prosthetic devices, implants and grafts CC POA CC/MCC Exc

⑦ **T82.838** Hemorrhage due to vascular prosthetic devices, implants and grafts CC POA HCC CC/MCC Exc

6ᵗʰ **T82.84** Pain due to cardiac and vascular prosthetic devices, implants and grafts

⑦ **T82.847** Pain due to cardiac prosthetic devices, implants and grafts CC POA CC/MCC Exc

⑦ **T82.848** Pain due to vascular prosthetic devices, implants and grafts CC POA HCC CC/MCC Exc

6ᵗʰ **T82.85** Stenosis due to cardiac and vascular prosthetic devices, implants and grafts

---

Unspecified Code Other Specified Code Manifestation Code Ⓝ Newborn Ⓟ Pediatric Ⓜ Maternity Ⓐ Adult ♂ Male ♀ Female
● New Code ▲ Revised Code Title ▶◀ Revised Text NOTES INCLUDES EXCLUDES 1 Not coded here EXCLUDES 2 Not included here
4ᵗʰ 4ᵗʰ character required 5ᵗʰ 5ᵗʰ character required 6ᵗʰ 6ᵗʰ character required 7ᵗʰ 7ᵗʰ character required
Ⓧ Extension 'X' Alert HAC Hospital-acquired condition (HAC) alert AHA AHA Coding Clinic©

[7th] **T82.855 Stenosis of coronary artery stent** [CC] [POA] [CC/MCC Exc]
AHA: Q4 2016
In-stent stenosis (restenosis) of coronary artery stent
Restenosis of coronary artery stent

[7th] **T82.856 Stenosis of peripheral vascular stent** [CC] [POA] [HCC] [CC/MCC Exc]
AHA: Q4 2016
In-stent stenosis (restenosis) of peripheral vascular stent
Restenosis of peripheral vascular stent

[7th] **T82.857 Stenosis of other cardiac prosthetic devices, implants and grafts** [CC] [POA] [CC/MCC Exc]
AHA: Q4 2016

[7th] **T82.858 Stenosis of other vascular prosthetic devices, implants and grafts** [CC] [POA] [HCC] [CC/MCC Exc]
AHA: Q4 2016

[6th] **T82.86 Thrombosis of cardiac and vascular prosthetic devices, implants and grafts**

[7th] **T82.867 Thrombosis due to cardiac prosthetic devices, implants and grafts** [CC] [POA] [CC/MCC Exc]

[7th] **T82.868 Thrombosis due to vascular prosthetic devices, implants and grafts** [CC] [POA] [HCC] [CC/MCC Exc]

[6th] **T82.89 Other specified complication of cardiac and vascular prosthetic devices, implants and grafts**

[7th] **T82.897 Other specified complication of cardiac prosthetic devices, implants and grafts** [CC] [POA] [CC/MCC Exc]

[7th] **T82.898 Other specified complication of vascular prosthetic devices, implants and grafts** [CC] [POA] [HCC] [CC/MCC Exc]

[7th] **T82.9 Unspecified complication of cardiac and vascular prosthetic device, implant and graft** [CC] [POA] [CC/MCC Exc]

[4th] **T83 Complications of genitourinary prosthetic devices, implants and grafts**
[EXCLUDES2] *failure and rejection of transplanted organs and tissue (T86.-)*
The appropriate 7th character is to be added to each code from category T83
A = initial encounter
D = subsequent encounter
S = sequela

[5th] **T83.0 Mechanical complication of urinary catheter**
[EXCLUDES2] *complications of stoma of urinary tract (N99.5-)*

[6th] **T83.01 Breakdown (mechanical) of urinary catheter**

[7th] **T83.010 Breakdown (mechanical) of cystostomy catheter** [CC] [POA] [HCC] [CC/MCC Exc]

[7th] **T83.011 Breakdown (mechanical) of indwelling urethral catheter** [POA] [HCC]

[7th] **T83.012 Breakdown (mechanical) of nephrostomy catheter** [POA] [HCC]

[7th] **T83.018 Breakdown (mechanical) of other urinary catheter** [POA] [HCC]
Breakdown (mechanical) of Hopkins catheter
Breakdown (mechanical) of ileostomy catheter
Breakdown (mechanical) urostomy catheter

[6th] **T83.02 Displacement of urinary catheter**
Malposition of urinary catheter

[7th] **T83.020 Displacement of cystostomy catheter** [CC] [POA] [HCC] [CC/MCC Exc]

[7th] **T83.021 Displacement of indwelling urethral catheter** [POA] [HCC]

[7th] **T83.022 Displacement of nephrostomy catheter** [POA] [HCC]

[7th] **T83.028 Displacement of other urinary catheter** [POA] [HCC]
Displacement of Hopkins catheter
Displacement of ileostomy catheter
Displacement of urostomy catheter

[6th] **T83.03 Leakage of urinary catheter**

[7th] **T83.030 Leakage of cystostomy catheter** [CC] [POA] [HCC] [CC/MCC Exc]

[7th] **T83.031 Leakage of indwelling urethral catheter** [POA] [HCC]

[7th] **T83.032 Leakage of nephrostomy catheter** [POA] [HCC]

[7th] **T83.038 Leakage of other urinary catheter** [POA] [HCC]
Leakage of Hopkins catheter
Leakage of ileostomy catheter
Leakage of urostomy catheter

[6th] **T83.09 Other mechanical complication of urinary catheter**
Obstruction (mechanical) of urinary catheter
Perforation of urinary catheter
Protrusion of urinary catheter

[7th] **T83.090 Other mechanical complication of cystostomy catheter** [CC] [POA] [HCC] [CC/MCC Exc]

[7th] **T83.091 Other mechanical complication of indwelling urethral catheter** [POA] [HCC]

[7th] **T83.092 Other mechanical complication of nephrostomy catheter** [POA] [HCC]

[7th] **T83.098 Other mechanical complication of other urinary catheter** [POA] [HCC]
Other mechanical complication of Hopkins catheter
Other mechanical complication of ileostomy catheter
Other mechanical complication of urostomy catheter

[5th] **T83.1 Mechanical complication of other urinary devices and implants**

[6th] **T83.11 Breakdown (mechanical) of other urinary devices and implants**

[7th] **T83.110 Breakdown (mechanical) of urinary electronic stimulator device** [CC] [POA] [HCC] [CC/MCC Exc]
[EXCLUDES2] *Breakdown (mechanical) of electrode (lead) for sacral nerve neurostimulator (T85.111)*
Breakdown (mechanical) of implanted electronic sacral neurostimulator, pulse generator or receiver (T85.113)

[7th] **T83.111 Breakdown (mechanical) of implanted urinary sphincter** [CC] [POA] [HCC] [CC/MCC Exc]

[7th] **T83.112 Breakdown (mechanical) of indwelling ureteral stent** [CC] [POA] [HCC] [CC/MCC Exc]

[7th] **T83.113 Breakdown (mechanical) of other urinary stents** [CC] [HCC] [CC/MCC Exc]
Breakdown (mechanical) of ileal conduit stent
Breakdown (mechanical) of nephroureteral stent

[7th] **T83.118 Breakdown (mechanical) of other urinary devices and implants** [CC] [POA] [HCC] [CC/MCC Exc]

[6th] **T83.12 Displacement of other urinary devices and implants**
Malposition of other urinary devices and implants

[7th] **T83.120 Displacement of urinary electronic stimulator device** [CC] [POA] [HCC] [CC/MCC Exc]
[EXCLUDES2] *Displacement of electrode (lead) for sacral nerve neurostimulator (T85.121)*
Displacement of implanted electronic sacral neurostimulator, pulse generator or receiver (T85.123)

[7th] **T83.121 Displacement of implanted urinary sphincter** [CC] [POA] [HCC] [CC/MCC Exc]

[7th] **T83.122 Displacement of indwelling ureteral stent** [CC] [POA] [HCC] [CC/MCC Exc]

[7th] **T83.123 Displacement of other urinary stents** [CC] [HCC] [CC/MCC Exc]
Displacement of ileal conduit stent
Displacement of nephroureteral stent

[7th] **T83.128 Displacement of other urinary devices and implants** [CC] [POA] [HCC] [CC/MCC Exc]

[PDx] Unacceptable principal diagnosis symbol per Medicare code edits [POA] Code exempt from diagnosis present on admission requirement
[?] Questionable admission [CC] Complication or comorbidity [CC/MCC Exc] CC/MCC exclusion [MCC] Major complication or comorbidity
[PDx CC] Principal diagnosis as its own CC [PDx MCC] Principal diagnosis as its own MCC [HCC] HCC diagnosis code [RxHCC] RxHCC diagnosis code
MACRA code [Z-1] Z code as first-listed diagnosis

⁶ᵗʰ **T83.19** Other mechanical complication of other urinary devices and implants

Leakage of other urinary devices and implants
Obstruction (mechanical) of other urinary devices and implants
Perforation of other urinary devices and implants
Protrusion of other urinary devices and implants

⁷ᵗʰ **T83.190** Other mechanical complication of urinary electronic stimulator device ㏄ ₚₒₐ HCC CC/MCC Exc

EXCLUDES2 Other mechanical complication of electrode (lead) for sacral nerve neurostimulator (T85.191)

Other mechanical complication of implanted electronic sacral neurostimulator, pulse generator or receiver (T85.193)

⁷ᵗʰ **T83.191** Other mechanical complication of implanted urinary sphincter ㏄ ₚₒₐ HCC CC/MCC Exc

⁷ᵗʰ **T83.192** Other mechanical complication of indwelling ureteral stent ㏄ ₚₒₐ HCC CC/MCC Exc

⁷ᵗʰ **T83.193** Other mechanical complication of other urinary stent ㏄ ₚₒₐ HCC CC/MCC Exc

Other mechanical complication of ileal conduit stent
Other mechanical complication of nephroureteral stent

⁷ᵗʰ **T83.198** Other mechanical complication of other urinary devices and implants ㏄ ₚₒₐ HCC CC/MCC Exc

⁵ᵗʰ **T83.2** Mechanical complication of graft of urinary organ

⁷ᵗʰ **T83.21** Breakdown (mechanical) of graft of urinary organ ㏄ ₚₒₐ HCC CC/MCC Exc

⁷ᵗʰ **T83.22** Displacement of graft of urinary organ ㏄ ₚₒₐ HCC CC/MCC Exc
Malposition of graft of urinary organ

⁷ᵗʰ **T83.23** Leakage of graft of urinary organ ㏄ ₚₒₐ HCC CC/MCC Exc

⁷ᵗʰ **T83.24** Erosion of graft of urinary organ ㏄ ₚₒₐ HCC CC/MCC Exc
AHA: Q4 2016

⁷ᵗʰ **T83.25** Exposure of graft of urinary organ ㏄ ₚₒₐ HCC CC/MCC Exc
AHA: Q4 2016

⁷ᵗʰ **T83.29** Other mechanical complication of graft of urinary organ ㏄ ₚₒₐ HCC CC/MCC Exc

Obstruction (mechanical) of graft of urinary organ
Perforation of graft of urinary organ
Protrusion of graft of urinary organ

⁵ᵗʰ **T83.3** Mechanical complication of intrauterine contraceptive device

⁷ᵗʰ **T83.31** Breakdown (mechanical) of intrauterine contraceptive device ₚₒₐ ♀

⁷ᵗʰ **T83.32** Displacement of intrauterine contraceptive device ₚₒₐ ♀

Malposition of intrauterine contraceptive device
Missing string of intrauterine contraceptive device

⁷ᵗʰ **T83.39** Other mechanical complication of intrauterine contraceptive device ₚₒₐ ♀

Leakage of intrauterine contraceptive device
Obstruction (mechanical) of intrauterine contraceptive device
Perforation of intrauterine contraceptive device
Protrusion of intrauterine contraceptive device

⁵ᵗʰ **T83.4** Mechanical complication of other prosthetic devices, implants and grafts of genital tract

⁶ᵗʰ **T83.41** Breakdown (mechanical) of other prosthetic devices, implants and grafts of genital tract

⁷ᵗʰ **T83.410** Breakdown (mechanical) of implanted penile prosthesis ㏄ ₚₒₐ HCC ♂ CC/MCC Exc

Breakdown (mechanical) of penile prosthesis cylinder
Breakdown (mechanical) of penile prosthesis pump
Breakdown (mechanical) of penile prosthesis reservoir

⁷ᵗʰ **T83.411** Breakdown (mechanical) of implanted testicular prosthesis ㏄ ₚₒₐ HCC CC/MCC Exc

⁷ᵗʰ **T83.418** Breakdown (mechanical) of other prosthetic devices, implants and grafts of genital tract ㏄ ₚₒₐ HCC CC/MCC Exc

⁶ᵗʰ **T83.42** Displacement of other prosthetic devices, implants and grafts of genital tract

Malposition of other prosthetic devices, implants and grafts of genital tract

⁷ᵗʰ **T83.420** Displacement of implanted penile prosthesis ㏄ ₚₒₐ HCC ♂ CC/MCC Exc

Displacement of penile prosthesis cylinder
Displacement of penile prosthesis pump
Displacement of penile prosthesis reservoir

⁷ᵗʰ **T83.421** Displacement of implanted testicular prosthesis ㏄ ₚₒₐ HCC CC/MCC Exc

⁷ᵗʰ **T83.428** Displacement of other prosthetic devices, implants and grafts of genital tract ㏄ ₚₒₐ HCC CC/MCC Exc

⁶ᵗʰ **T83.49** Other mechanical complication of other prosthetic devices, implants and grafts of genital tract

Leakage of other prosthetic devices, implants and grafts of genital tract
Obstruction, mechanical of other prosthetic devices, implants and grafts of genital tract
Perforation of other prosthetic devices, implants and grafts of genital tract
Protrusion of other prosthetic devices, implants and grafts of genital tract

⁷ᵗʰ **T83.490** Other mechanical complication of implanted penile prosthesis ㏄ ₚₒₐ HCC ♂ CC/MCC Exc

Other mechanical complication of penile prosthesis cylinder
Other mechanical complication of penile prosthesis pump
Other mechanical complication of penile prosthesis reservoir

⁷ᵗʰ **T83.491** Other mechanical complication of implanted testicular prosthesis ㏄ ₚₒₐ HCC CC/MCC Exc

⁷ᵗʰ **T83.498** Other mechanical complication of other prosthetic devices, implants and grafts of genital tract ㏄ ₚₒₐ HCC CC/MCC Exc

⁵ᵗʰ **T83.5** Infection and inflammatory reaction due to prosthetic device, implant and graft in urinary system

Use additional code to identify infection

⁶ᵗʰ **T83.51** Infection and inflammatory reaction due to urinary catheter HCC

EXCLUDES2 complications of stoma of urinary tract (N99.5-)

⁷ᵗʰ **T83.510** Infection and inflammatory reaction due to cystostomy catheter ㏄ ₚₒₐ HCC CC/MCC Exc

⁷ᵗʰ **T83.511** Infection and inflammatory reaction due to indwelling urethral catheter ㏄ ₚₒₐ HCC CC/MCC Exc

⁷ᵗʰ **T83.512** Infection and inflammatory reaction due to nephrostomy catheter ㏄ ₚₒₐ HCC CC/MCC Exc

⁷ᵗʰ **T83.518** Infection and inflammatory reaction due to other urinary catheter ㏄ ₚₒₐ HCC CC/MCC Exc

Infection and inflammatory reaction due to Hopkins catheter
Infection and inflammatory reaction due to ileostomy catheter
Infection and inflammatory reaction due to urostomy catheter

⁶ᵗʰ **T83.59** Infection and inflammatory reaction due to prosthetic device, implant and graft in urinary system HCC

⁷ᵗʰ **T83.590** Infection and inflammatory reaction due to implanted urinary neurostimulation device ㏄ ₚₒₐ HCC CC/MCC Exc

EXCLUDES2 Infection and inflammatory reaction due to electrode lead of sacral nerve neurostimulator (T85.732)

Unspecified Code	Other Specified Code	Manifestation Code	Ⓝ Newborn	Ⓟ Pediatric	Ⓜ Maternity	Ⓐ Adult	♂ Male	♀ Female

● New Code ▲ Revised Code Title ▶◀ Revised Text NOTES INCLUDES EXCLUDES1 Not coded here EXCLUDES2 Not included here
⁴ᵗʰ 4ᵗʰ character required ⁵ᵗʰ 5ᵗʰ character required ⁶ᵗʰ 6ᵗʰ character required ⁷ᵗʰ 7ᵗʰ character required
⁷ˣ Extension 'X' Alert HAC Hospital-acquired condition (HAC) alert AHA AHA Coding Clinic©

Infection and inflammatory reaction due to pulse generator or receiver of sacral nerve neurostimulator (T85.734)

- 7th **T83.591** Infection and inflammatory reaction due to implanted urinary sphincter ⚷ POA HCC CC/MCC Exc
- 7th **T83.592** Infection and inflammatory reaction due to indwelling ureteral stent ⚷ POA HCC CC/MCC Exc
- 7th **T83.593** Infection and inflammatory reaction due to other urinary stents ⚷ POA HCC CC/MCC Exc

  Infection and inflammatory reaction due to ileal conduit stents

  Infection and inflammatory reaction due to nephroureteral stent
- 7th **T83.598** Infection and inflammatory reaction due to other prosthetic device, implant and graft in urinary system ⚷ POA HCC CC/MCC Exc

5th **T83.6** Infection and inflammatory reaction due to prosthetic device, implant and graft in genital tract HCC

Use additional code to identify infection

- 7th **T83.61** Infection and inflammatory reaction due to implanted penile prosthesis ⚷ POA HCC CC/MCC Exc

  Infection and inflammatory reaction due to penile prosthesis cylinder

  Infection and inflammatory reaction due to penile prosthesis pump

  Infection and inflammatory reaction due to penile prosthesis reservoir
- 7th **T83.62** Infection and inflammatory reaction due to implanted testicular prosthesis ⚷ POA HCC CC/MCC Exc
- 7th **T83.69** Infection and inflammatory reaction due to other prosthetic device, implant and graft in genital tract ⚷ POA HCC CC/MCC Exc

5th **T83.7** Complications due to implanted mesh and other prosthetic materials

- 6th **T83.71** Erosion of implanted mesh and other prosthetic materials to surrounding organ or tissue
  - 7th **T83.711** Erosion of implanted vaginal mesh to surrounding organ or tissue POA HCC

    AHA: Q4 2016

    Erosion of implanted vaginal mesh into pelvic floor muscles
  - 7th **T83.712** Erosion of implanted urethral mesh to surrounding organ or tissue ⚷ POA HCC CC/MCC Exc

    Erosion of implanted female urethral sling

    Erosion of implanted male urethral sling

    Erosion of implanted urethral mesh into pelvic floor muscles
  - 7th **T83.713** Erosion of implanted urethral bulking agent to surrounding organ or tissue ⚷ POA HCC CC/MCC Exc
  - 7th **T83.714** Erosion of implanted ureteral bulking agent to surrounding organ or tissue ⚷ POA HCC CC/MCC Exc
  - 7th **T83.718** Erosion of other implanted mesh to organ or tissue ⚷ POA HCC CC/MCC Exc

    AHA: Q4 2016
  - 7th **T83.719** Erosion of other prosthetic materials to surrounding organ or tissue ⚷ POA HCC CC/MCC Exc

    AHA: Q4 2016
- 5th **T83.72** Exposure of implanted mesh and other prosthetic materials into surrounding organ or tissue

  Extrusion of implanted mesh
  - 7th **T83.721** Exposure of implanted vaginal mesh into vagina POA HCC

    Exposure of implanted vaginal mesh through vaginal wall
  - 7th **T83.722** Exposure of implanted urethral mesh into urethra ⚷ POA HCC CC/MCC Exc

    Exposure of implanted female urethral sling

    Exposure of implanted male urethral sling

    Exposure of implanted urethral mesh through urethral wall

- 7th **T83.723** Exposure of implanted urethral bulking agent into urethra ⚷ POA HCC CC/MCC Exc
- 7th **T83.724** Exposure of implanted ureteral bulking agent into ureter ⚷ POA HCC CC/MCC Exc
- 7th **T83.728** Exposure of other implanted mesh into organ or tissue ⚷ POA HCC CC/MCC Exc

  AHA: Q4 2016
- 7th **T83.729** Exposure of other prosthetic materials into organ or tissue ⚷ POA HCC CC/MCC Exc

  AHA: Q4 2016
- 7th **T83.79** Other specified complications due to other genitourinary prosthetic materials ⚷ POA HCC CC/MCC Exc

5th **T83.8** Other specified complications of genitourinary prosthetic devices, implants and grafts

- 7th **T83.81** Embolism due to genitourinary prosthetic devices, implants and grafts ⚷ POA HCC CC/MCC Exc
- 7th **T83.82** Fibrosis due to genitourinary prosthetic devices, implants and grafts ⚷ POA HCC CC/MCC Exc
- 7th **T83.83** Hemorrhage due to genitourinary prosthetic devices, implants and grafts ⚷ POA HCC CC/MCC Exc
- 7th **T83.84** Pain due to genitourinary prosthetic devices, implants and grafts ⚷ POA HCC CC/MCC Exc
- 7th **T83.85** Stenosis due to genitourinary prosthetic devices, implants and grafts ⚷ POA HCC CC/MCC Exc
- 7th **T83.86** Thrombosis due to genitourinary prosthetic devices, implants and grafts ⚷ POA HCC CC/MCC Exc
- 7th **T83.89** Other specified complication of genitourinary prosthetic devices, implants and grafts ⚷ POA HCC CC/MCC Exc

7th **T83.9** Unspecified complication of genitourinary prosthetic device, implant and graft ⚷ POA HCC CC/MCC Exc

4th **T84** Complications of internal orthopedic prosthetic devices, implants and grafts

EXCLUDES2 failure and rejection of transplanted organs and tissues (T86.-)

fracture of bone following insertion of orthopedic implant, joint prosthesis or bone plate (M96.6)

The appropriate 7th character is to be added to each code from category T84

A = initial encounter

D = subsequent encounter

S = sequela

5th **T84.0** Mechanical complication of internal joint prosthesis

- 6th **T84.01** Broken internal joint prosthesis

  Breakage (fracture) of prosthetic joint

  Broken prosthetic joint implant

  EXCLUDES1 periprosthetic joint implant fracture ▶(M97-)◀
  - 7th **T84.010** Broken internal right hip prosthesis ⚷ POA HCC CC/MCC Exc
  - 7th **T84.011** Broken internal left hip prosthesis ⚷ POA HCC CC/MCC Exc
  - 7th **T84.012** Broken internal right knee prosthesis ⚷ POA HCC CC/MCC Exc
  - 7th **T84.013** Broken internal left knee prosthesis ⚷ POA HCC CC/MCC Exc
  - 7th **T84.018** Broken internal joint prosthesis, other site ⚷ POA HCC CC/MCC Exc

    Use additional code to identify the joint (Z96.6-)
  - 7th **T84.019** Broken internal joint prosthesis, unspecified site ⚷ POA HCC CC/MCC Exc
- 6th **T84.02** Dislocation of internal joint prosthesis

  Instability of internal joint prosthesis

  Subluxation of internal joint prosthesis
  - 7th **T84.020** Dislocation of internal right hip prosthesis ⚷ POA HCC CC/MCC Exc
  - 7th **T84.021** Dislocation of internal left hip prosthesis ⚷ POA HCC CC/MCC Exc
  - 7th **T84.022** Instability of internal right knee prosthesis ⚷ POA HCC CC/MCC Exc
  - 7th **T84.023** Instability of internal left knee prosthesis ⚷ POA HCC CC/MCC Exc

---

POA^dx Unacceptable principal diagnosis symbol per Medicare code edits   POA Code exempt from diagnosis present on admission requirement
❓ Questionable admission   ⚷ Complication or comorbidity   CC/MCC Exc CC/MCC exclusion   MCC Major complication or comorbidity
Principal diagnosis as its own CC   Principal diagnosis as its own MCC   HCC HCC diagnosis code   RxHCC RxHCC diagnosis code
MACRA code   Z1 Z code as first-listed diagnosis

When symbols appear on a code that requires a 7th character extension, refer to Appendix B to identify applicable 7th character codes.

T84.028 Dislocation of other internal joint
prosthesis cc POA HCC CC/MCC Exc
Use additional code to identify the joint
(Z96.6-)

T84.029 **Dislocation of unspecified internal joint
prosthesis**

T84.03 Mechanical loosening of internal prosthetic joint
Aseptic loosening of prosthetic joint

T84.030 Mechanical loosening of internal right hip
prosthetic joint cc POA HCC CC/MCC Exc

T84.031 Mechanical loosening of internal left hip
prosthetic joint cc POA HCC CC/MCC Exc

T84.032 Mechanical loosening of internal right
knee prosthetic joint cc POA HCC CC/MCC Exc

T84.033 Mechanical loosening of internal left knee
prosthetic joint cc POA HCC CC/MCC Exc

T84.038 Mechanical loosening of other internal
prosthetic joint cc POA HCC CC/MCC Exc
Use additional code to identify the joint
(Z96.6-)

T84.039 **Mechanical loosening of unspecified
internal prosthetic joint** cc POA HCC CC/MCC Exc

T84.05 Periprosthetic osteolysis of internal prosthetic joint
Use additional code to identify major osseous
defect, if applicable (M89.7-)

T84.050 Periprosthetic osteolysis of internal
prosthetic right hip joint cc POA HCC CC/MCC Exc

T84.051 Periprosthetic osteolysis of internal
prosthetic left hip joint cc POA HCC CC/MCC Exc

T84.052 Periprosthetic osteolysis of internal
prosthetic right knee joint cc POA HCC CC/MCC Exc

T84.053 Periprosthetic osteolysis of internal
prosthetic left knee joint cc POA HCC CC/MCC Exc

T84.058 Periprosthetic osteolysis of other internal
prosthetic joint cc POA HCC CC/MCC Exc
Use additional code to identify the joint
(Z96.6-)

T84.059 **Periprosthetic osteolysis of unspecified
internal prosthetic joint** cc POA HCC CC/MCC Exc

T84.06 Wear of articular bearing surface of internal
prosthetic joint

T84.060 Wear of articular bearing surface of
internal prosthetic right hip
joint cc POA HCC CC/MCC Exc

T84.061 Wear of articular bearing surface of
internal prosthetic left hip
joint cc POA HCC CC/MCC Exc

T84.062 Wear of articular bearing surface of
internal prosthetic right knee
joint cc POA HCC CC/MCC Exc

T84.063 Wear of articular bearing surface of
internal prosthetic left knee
joint cc POA HCC CC/MCC Exc

T84.068 Wear of articular bearing surface of other
internal prosthetic joint cc POA HCC CC/MCC Exc
Use additional code to identify the joint
(Z96.6-)

T84.069 **Wear of articular bearing surface of
unspecified internal prosthetic
joint** cc POA HCC CC/MCC Exc

T84.09 Other mechanical complication of internal joint
prosthesis
Prosthetic joint implant failure NOS

T84.090 Other mechanical complication of internal
right hip prosthesis cc POA HCC CC/MCC Exc

T84.091 Other mechanical complication of internal
left hip prosthesis cc POA HCC CC/MCC Exc

T84.092 Other mechanical complication of internal
right knee prosthesis cc POA HCC CC/MCC Exc

T84.093 Other mechanical complication of internal
left knee prosthesis cc POA HCC CC/MCC Exc

T84.098 Other mechanical complication of other
internal joint prosthesis cc POA HCC CC/MCC Exc
Use additional code to identify the joint
(Z96.6-)

T84.099 **Other mechanical complication of
unspecified internal joint
prosthesis** cc POA HCC CC/MCC Exc

T84.1 Mechanical complication of internal fixation device of bones
of limb

EXCLUDES2 mechanical complication of internal fixation device of
bones of feet (T84.2-)

mechanical complication of internal fixation device of
bones of fingers (T84.2-)

mechanical complication of internal fixation device of
bones of hands (T84.2-)

mechanical complication of internal fixation device of
bones of toes (T84.2-)

T84.11 Breakdown (mechanical) of internal fixation device
of bones of limb

T84.110 Breakdown (mechanical) of internal
fixation device of right
humerus cc POA HCC CC/MCC Exc

T84.111 Breakdown (mechanical) of internal
fixation device of left
humerus cc POA HCC CC/MCC Exc

T84.112 Breakdown (mechanical) of internal
fixation device of bone of right
forearm cc POA HCC CC/MCC Exc

T84.113 Breakdown (mechanical) of internal
fixation device of bone of left
forearm cc POA HCC CC/MCC Exc

T84.114 Breakdown (mechanical) of internal
fixation device of right
femur cc POA HCC CC/MCC Exc

T84.115 Breakdown (mechanical) of internal
fixation device of left femur cc POA HCC CC/MCC Exc

T84.116 Breakdown (mechanical) of internal
fixation device of bone of
right lower leg cc POA HCC CC/MCC Exc

T84.117 Breakdown (mechanical) of internal
fixation device of bone of left
lower leg cc POA HCC CC/MCC Exc

T84.119 **Breakdown (mechanical) of internal
fixation device of unspecified
bone of limb** cc POA HCC CC/MCC Exc

T84.12 Displacement of internal fixation device of bones of
limb
Malposition of internal fixation device of bones of
limb

T84.120 Displacement of internal fixation device of
right humerus cc POA HCC CC/MCC Exc

T84.121 Displacement of internal fixation device of
left humerus cc POA HCC CC/MCC Exc

T84.122 Displacement of internal fixation device of
bone of right forearm cc POA HCC CC/MCC Exc

T84.123 Displacement of internal fixation device of
bone of left forearm cc POA HCC CC/MCC Exc

T84.124 Displacement of internal fixation device of
right femur cc POA HCC CC/MCC Exc

T84.125 Displacement of internal fixation device of
left femur cc POA HCC CC/MCC Exc

T84.126 Displacement of internal fixation device of
bone of right lower leg cc POA HCC CC/MCC Exc

T84.127 Displacement of internal fixation device of
bone of left lower leg cc POA HCC CC/MCC Exc

T84.129 **Displacement of internal fixation device of
unspecified bone of limb** cc POA HCC CC/MCC Exc

T84.19 Other mechanical complication of internal fixation
device of bones of limb
Obstruction (mechanical) of internal fixation device of
bones of limb
Perforation of internal fixation device of bones of limb

Unspecified Code Other Specified Code Manifestation Code N Newborn P Pediatric M Maternity A Adult ♂ Male ♀ Female
● New Code ▲ Revised Code Title ►◄ Revised Text NOTES *INCLUDES* *EXCLUDES 1* Not coded here *EXCLUDES 2* Not included here
4ᵗʰ character required 5ᵗʰ character required 6ᵗʰ character required 7ᵗʰ character required
Extension 'X' Alert HAC Hospital-acquired condition (HAC) alert AHA AHA Coding Clinic©

Protrusion of internal fixation device of bones of limb

7ᵈ **T84.190** Other mechanical complication of internal fixation device of right humerus

7ᵈ **T84.191** Other mechanical complication of internal fixation device of left humerus

7ᵈ **T84.192** Other mechanical complication of internal fixation device of bone of right forearm

7ᵈ **T84.193** Other mechanical complication of internal fixation device of bone of left forearm

7ᵈ **T84.194** Other mechanical complication of internal fixation device of right femur

7ᵈ **T84.195** Other mechanical complication of internal fixation device of left femur

7ᵈ **T84.196** Other mechanical complication of internal fixation device of bone of right lower leg

7ᵈ **T84.197** Other mechanical complication of internal fixation device of bone of left lower leg

7ᵈ **T84.199** Other mechanical complication of internal fixation device of unspecified bone of limb

5ᵈ **T84.2** Mechanical complication of internal fixation device of other bones

6ᵈ **T84.21** Breakdown (mechanical) of internal fixation device of other bones

7ᵈ **T84.210** Breakdown (mechanical) of internal fixation device of bones of hand and fingers

7ᵈ **T84.213** Breakdown (mechanical) of internal fixation device of bones of foot and toes

7ᵈ **T84.216** Breakdown (mechanical) of internal fixation device of vertebrae

7ᵈ **T84.218** Breakdown (mechanical) of internal fixation device of other bones

6ᵈ **T84.22** Displacement of internal fixation device of other bones

Malposition of internal fixation device of other bones

7ᵈ **T84.220** Displacement of internal fixation device of bones of hand and fingers

7ᵈ **T84.223** Displacement of internal fixation device of bones of foot and toes

7ᵈ **T84.226** Displacement of internal fixation device of vertebrae

7ᵈ **T84.228** Displacement of internal fixation device of other bones

6ᵈ **T84.29** Other mechanical complication of internal fixation device of other bones

Obstruction (mechanical) of internal fixation device of other bones

Perforation of internal fixation device of other bones

Protrusion of internal fixation device of other bones

7ᵈ **T84.290** Other mechanical complication of internal fixation device of bones of hand and fingers

7ᵈ **T84.293** Other mechanical complication of internal fixation device of bones of foot and toes

7ᵈ **T84.296** Other mechanical complication of internal fixation device of vertebrae

7ᵈ **T84.298** Other mechanical complication of internal fixation device of other bones

5ᵈ **T84.3** Mechanical complication of other bone devices, implants and grafts

EXCLUDES2 other complications of bone graft (T86.83-)

6ᵈ **T84.31** Breakdown (mechanical) of other bone devices, implants and grafts

7ᵈ **T84.310** Breakdown (mechanical) of electronic bone stimulator

7ᵈ **T84.318** Breakdown (mechanical) of other bone devices, implants and grafts

6ᵈ **T84.32** Displacement of other bone devices, implants and grafts

Malposition of other bone devices, implants and grafts

7ᵈ **T84.320** Displacement of electronic bone stimulator

7ᵈ **T84.328** Displacement of other bone devices, implants and grafts

6ᵈ **T84.39** Other mechanical complication of other bone devices, implants and grafts

Obstruction (mechanical) of other bone devices, implants and grafts

Perforation of other bone devices, implants and grafts

Protrusion of other bone devices, implants and grafts

7ᵈ **T84.390** Other mechanical complication of electronic bone stimulator

7ᵈ **T84.398** Other mechanical complication of other bone devices, implants and grafts

5ᵈ **T84.4** Mechanical complication of other internal orthopedic devices, implants and grafts

6ᵈ **T84.41** Breakdown (mechanical) of other internal orthopedic devices, implants and grafts

7ᵈ **T84.410** Breakdown (mechanical) of muscle and tendon graft

7ᵈ **T84.418** Breakdown (mechanical) of other internal orthopedic devices, implants and grafts

6ᵈ **T84.42** Displacement of other internal orthopedic devices, implants and grafts

Malposition of other internal orthopedic devices, implants and grafts

7ᵈ **T84.420** Displacement of muscle and tendon graft

7ᵈ **T84.428** Displacement of other internal orthopedic devices, implants and grafts

6ᵈ **T84.49** Other mechanical complication of other internal orthopedic devices, implants and grafts

Mechanical complication of other internal orthopedic devices, implants and grafts NOS

Obstruction (mechanical) of other internal orthopedic devices, implants and grafts

Perforation of other internal orthopedic devices, implants and grafts

Protrusion of other internal orthopedic devices, implants and grafts

7ᵈ **T84.490** Other mechanical complication of muscle and tendon graft

7ᵈ **T84.498** Other mechanical complication of other internal orthopedic devices, implants and grafts

5ᵈ **T84.5** Infection and inflammatory reaction due to internal joint prosthesis

Use additional code to identify infection

7ᵈ **T84.50** Infection and inflammatory reaction due to unspecified internal joint prosthesis

7ᵈ **T84.51** Infection and inflammatory reaction due to internal right hip prosthesis

7ᵈ **T84.52** Infection and inflammatory reaction due to internal left hip prosthesis

7ᵈ **T84.53** Infection and inflammatory reaction due to internal right knee prosthesis

7ᵈ **T84.54** Infection and inflammatory reaction due to internal left knee prosthesis

7ᵈ **T84.59** Infection and inflammatory reaction due to other internal joint prosthesis

ᴾᴰˣ Unacceptable principal diagnosis symbol per Medicare code edits — Code exempt from diagnosis present on admission requirement
? Questionable admission Complication or comorbidity CC/MCC exclusion Major complication or comorbidity
Principal diagnosis as its own CC Principal diagnosis as its own MCC HCC HCC diagnosis code RxHCC RxHCC diagnosis code
MACRA code Z code as first-listed diagnosis

1174 When symbols appear on a code that requires a 7th character extension, refer to Appendix B to identify applicable 7th character codes. **2018 ICD-10-CM**

T84.6 Infection and inflammatory reaction due to internal fixation device
Use additional code to identify infection

T84.60 Infection and inflammatory reaction due to internal fixation device of unspecified site `CC` `POA` `HAC` `HCC` CC/MCC Exc

T84.61 Infection and inflammatory reaction due to internal fixation device of arm

    T84.610 Infection and inflammatory reaction due to internal fixation device of right humerus `CC` `POA` `HAC` `HCC` CC/MCC Exc

    T84.611 Infection and inflammatory reaction due to internal fixation device of left humerus `CC` `POA` `HAC` `HCC` CC/MCC Exc

    T84.612 Infection and inflammatory reaction due to internal fixation device of right radius `CC` `POA` `HAC` `HCC` CC/MCC Exc

    T84.613 Infection and inflammatory reaction due to internal fixation device of left radius `CC` `POA` `HAC` `HCC` CC/MCC Exc

    T84.614 Infection and inflammatory reaction due to internal fixation device of right ulna `CC` `POA` `HAC` `HCC` CC/MCC Exc

    T84.615 Infection and inflammatory reaction due to internal fixation device of left ulna `CC` `POA` `HAC` `HCC` CC/MCC Exc

    T84.619 Infection and inflammatory reaction due to internal fixation device of unspecified bone of arm `CC` `POA` `HAC` `HCC` CC/MCC Exc

T84.62 Infection and inflammatory reaction due to internal fixation device of leg

    T84.620 Infection and inflammatory reaction due to internal fixation device of right femur `CC` `POA` `HCC` CC/MCC Exc

    T84.621 Infection and inflammatory reaction due to internal fixation device of left femur `CC` `POA` `HCC` CC/MCC Exc

    T84.622 Infection and inflammatory reaction due to internal fixation device of right tibia `CC` `POA` `HCC` CC/MCC Exc

    T84.623 Infection and inflammatory reaction due to internal fixation device of left tibia `CC` `POA` `HCC` CC/MCC Exc

    T84.624 Infection and inflammatory reaction due to internal fixation device of right fibula `CC` `POA` `HCC` CC/MCC Exc

    T84.625 Infection and inflammatory reaction due to internal fixation device of left fibula `CC` `POA` `HCC` CC/MCC Exc

    T84.629 Infection and inflammatory reaction due to internal fixation device of unspecified bone of leg `CC` `POA` `HCC` CC/MCC Exc

T84.63 Infection and inflammatory reaction due to internal fixation device of spine `CC` `POA` `HAC` `HCC` CC/MCC Exc

T84.69 Infection and inflammatory reaction due to internal fixation device of other site `CC` `POA` `HAC` `HCC` CC/MCC Exc

T84.7 Infection and inflammatory reaction due to other internal orthopedic prosthetic devices, implants and grafts
Use additional code to identify infection

T84.8 Other specified complications of internal orthopedic prosthetic devices, implants and grafts

T84.81 Embolism due to internal orthopedic prosthetic devices, implants and grafts `CC` `POA` CC/MCC Exc

T84.82 Fibrosis due to internal orthopedic prosthetic devices, implants and grafts `CC` `POA` `HCC` CC/MCC Exc

T84.83 Hemorrhage due to internal orthopedic prosthetic devices, implants and grafts `CC` `POA` `HCC` CC/MCC Exc

T84.84 Pain due to internal orthopedic prosthetic devices, implants and grafts `CC` `POA` `HCC` CC/MCC Exc

T84.85 Stenosis due to internal orthopedic prosthetic devices, implants and grafts `CC` `POA` `HCC` CC/MCC Exc

T84.86 Thrombosis due to internal orthopedic prosthetic devices, implants and grafts `CC` `POA` `HCC` CC/MCC Exc

T84.89 Other specified complication of internal orthopedic prosthetic devices, implants and grafts `CC` `POA` `HCC` CC/MCC Exc

T84.9 Unspecified complication of internal orthopedic prosthetic device, implant and graft `CC` `POA` `HCC` CC/MCC Exc

T85 Complications of other internal prosthetic devices, implants and grafts
EXCLUDES2 failure and rejection of transplanted organs and tissue (T86.-)
The appropriate 7th character is to be added to each code from category T85
A = initial encounter
D = subsequent encounter
S = sequela

T85.0 Mechanical complication of ventricular intracranial (communicating) shunt

T85.01 Breakdown (mechanical) of ventricular intracranial (communicating) shunt `CC` `POA` `HCC` CC/MCC Exc

T85.02 Displacement of ventricular intracranial (communicating) shunt `CC` `POA` `HCC` CC/MCC Exc
Malposition of ventricular intracranial (communicating) shunt

T85.03 Leakage of ventricular intracranial (communicating) shunt `CC` `POA` `HCC` CC/MCC Exc

T85.09 Other mechanical complication of ventricular intracranial (communicating) shunt `CC` `POA` `HCC` CC/MCC Exc
Obstruction (mechanical) of ventricular intracranial (communicating) shunt
Perforation of ventricular intracranial (communicating) shunt
Protrusion of ventricular intracranial (communicating) shunt

T85.1 Mechanical complication of implanted electronic stimulator of nervous system

T85.11 Breakdown (mechanical) of implanted electronic stimulator of nervous system

    T85.110 Breakdown (mechanical) of implanted electronic neurostimulator of brain electrode (lead) `CC` `POA` `HCC` CC/MCC Exc

    T85.111 Breakdown (mechanical) of implanted electronic neurostimulator of peripheral nerve electrode (lead) `CC` `POA` `HCC` CC/MCC Exc
Breakdown of electrode (lead) for cranial nerve neurostimulators
Breakdown of electrode (lead) for gastric neurostimulator
Breakdown of electrode (lead) for sacral nerve neurostimulator
Breakdown of electrode (lead) for vagal nerve neurostimulators

    T85.112 Breakdown (mechanical) of implanted electronic neurostimulator of spinal cord electrode (lead) `CC` `POA` `HCC` CC/MCC Exc

    T85.113 Breakdown (mechanical) of implanted electronic neurostimulator, generator `CC` `POA` `HCC` CC/MCC Exc
Breakdown (mechanical) of implanted electronic neurostimuator generator, brain, peripheral, gastric, spinal
Breakdown (mechanical) of implanted electronic sacral neurostimulator, pulse generator or receiver

    T85.118 Breakdown (mechanical) of other implanted electronic stimulator of nervous system `CC` `POA` `HCC` CC/MCC Exc

T85.12 Displacement of implanted electronic stimulator of nervous system
Malposition of implanted electronic stimulator of nervous system

    T85.120 Displacement of implanted electronic neurostimulator of brain electrode (lead) `CC` `POA` `HCC` CC/MCC Exc

---

Unspecified Code   Other Specified Code   Manifestation Code   N Newborn   P Pediatric   M Maternity   A Adult   ♂ Male   ♀ Female
● New Code   ▲ Revised Code Title   ►◄ Revised Text   NOTES   INCLUDES   EXCLUDES 1 Not coded here   EXCLUDES 2 Not included here
4th character required   5th character required   6th character required   7th character required
Extension 'X' Alert   HAC Hospital-acquired condition (HAC) alert   AHA AHA Coding Clinic©

7ᵗʰ **T85.121** **Displacement of implanted electronic neurostimulator of** peripheral nerve electrode (lead) CC POA HCC CC/MCC Exc
　Displacement of electrode (lead) for cranial nerve neurostimulators
　Displacement of electrode (lead) for gastric neurostimulator
　Displacement of electrode (lead) for sacral nerve neurostimulator
　Displacement of electrode (lead) for vagal nerve neurostimulators

7ᵗʰ **T85.122** **Displacement of implanted electronic neurostimulator of spinal cord electrode (lead)** CC POA HCC CC/MCC Exc

7ᵗʰ **T85.123** **Displacement of implanted electronic neurostimulator,** generator CC POA HCC CC/MCC Exc
　Displacement of implanted electronic neurostimulator generator, brain, peripheral, gastric, spinal
　Displacement of implanted electronic sacral neurostimulator, pulse generator or receiver

7ᵗʰ **T85.128** **Displacement of other implanted electronic stimulator of nervous system** CC POA HCC CC/MCC Exc

6ᵗʰ **T85.19** **Other** mechanical complication of implanted electronic stimulator of nervous system
　Leakage of implanted electronic stimulator of nervous system
　Obstruction (mechanical) of implanted electronic stimulator of nervous system
　Perforation of implanted electronic stimulator of nervous system
　Protrusion of implanted electronic stimulator of nervous system

7ᵗʰ **T85.190** **Other mechanical complication of implanted electronic neurostimulator of brain electrode (lead)** CC POA HCC CC/MCC Exc

7ᵗʰ **T85.191** **Other mechanical complication of implanted** electronic neurostimulator of peripheral nerve electrode (lead) CC POA HCC CC/MCC Exc
　Other mechanical complication of electrode (lead) for cranial nerve neurostimulators
　Other mechanical complication of electrode (lead) for gastric neurostimulator
　Other mechanical complication of electrode (lead) for sacral nerve neurostimulator
　Other mechanical complication of electrode (lead) for vagal nerve neurostimulators

7ᵗʰ **T85.192** **Other mechanical complication of implanted electronic neurostimulator of spinal cord electrode (lead)** CC POA HCC CC/MCC Exc

7ᵗʰ **T85.193** **Other mechanical complication of implanted electronic neurostimulator,** generator CC POA HCC CC/MCC Exc
　Other mechanical complication of implanted electronic neurostimulator generator, brain, peripheral, gastric, spinal
　Other mechanical complication of implanted electronic sacral neurostimulator, pulse generator or receiver

7ᵗʰ **T85.199** **Other mechanical complication of other implanted electronic stimulator of nervous system** CC POA HCC CC/MCC Exc

5ᵗʰ **T85.2** **Mechanical complication of** intraocular lens

7ᵗʰ **T85.21** **Breakdown** (mechanical) of intraocular lens CC POA CC/MCC Exc

7ᵗʰ **T85.22** **Displacement** of intraocular lens CC POA CC/MCC Exc
　Malposition of intraocular lens

7ᵗʰ **T85.29** **Other mechanical complication of intraocular lens** CC POA CC/MCC Exc
　Obstruction (mechanical) of intraocular lens
　Perforation of intraocular lens
　Protrusion of intraocular lens

5ᵗʰ **T85.3** **Mechanical complication of** other ocular prosthetic devices, implants and grafts
　EXCLUDES2 _other complications of corneal graft (T86.84-)_

6ᵗʰ **T85.31** **Breakdown** (mechanical) of other ocular prosthetic devices, implants and grafts

7ᵗʰ **T85.310** **Breakdown (mechanical) of prosthetic orbit of** right eye CC POA CC/MCC Exc

7ᵗʰ **T85.311** **Breakdown (mechanical) of prosthetic orbit of** left eye CC POA CC/MCC Exc

7ᵗʰ **T85.318** **Breakdown (mechanical) of other ocular prosthetic devices, implants and grafts** POA

6ᵗʰ **T85.32** **Displacement** of other ocular prosthetic devices, implants and grafts
　Malposition of other ocular prosthetic devices, implants and grafts

7ᵗʰ **T85.320** **Displacement of prosthetic orbit of** right eye CC POA CC/MCC Exc

7ᵗʰ **T85.321** **Displacement of prosthetic orbit of** left eye CC POA CC/MCC Exc

7ᵗʰ **T85.328** **Displacement of other ocular prosthetic devices, implants and grafts** POA

6ᵗʰ **T85.39** **Other** mechanical complication of other ocular prosthetic devices, implants and grafts
　Obstruction (mechanical) of other ocular prosthetic devices, implants and grafts
　Perforation of other ocular prosthetic devices, implants and grafts
　Protrusion of other ocular prosthetic devices, implants and grafts

7ᵗʰ **T85.390** **Other mechanical complication of prosthetic orbit of** right eye CC POA CC/MCC Exc

7ᵗʰ **T85.391** **Other mechanical complication of prosthetic orbit of** left eye CC POA CC/MCC Exc

7ᵗʰ **T85.398** **Other mechanical complication of other ocular prosthetic devices, implants and grafts** POA

5ᵗʰ **T85.4** **Mechanical complication of** breast prosthesis and implant

7ᵗʰ **T85.41** **Breakdown** (mechanical) of breast prosthesis and implant CC POA CC/MCC Exc

7ᵗʰ **T85.42** **Displacement** of breast prosthesis and implant CC POA CC/MCC Exc
　Malposition of breast prosthesis and implant

7ᵗʰ **T85.43** **Leakage** of breast prosthesis and implant CC POA CC/MCC Exc

7ᵗʰ **T85.44** **Capsular contracture** of breast implant CC POA CC/MCC Exc

7ᵗʰ **T85.49** **Other mechanical complication of breast prosthesis and implant** CC POA CC/MCC Exc
　Obstruction (mechanical) of breast prosthesis and implant
　Perforation of breast prosthesis and implant
　Protrusion of breast prosthesis and implant

5ᵗʰ **T85.5** **Mechanical complication of** gastrointestinal prosthetic devices, implants and grafts

6ᵗʰ **T85.51** **Breakdown** (mechanical) of gastrointestinal prosthetic devices, implants and grafts

7ᵗʰ **T85.510** **Breakdown (mechanical) of** bile duct prosthesis CC POA CC/MCC Exc

7ᵗʰ **T85.511** **Breakdown (mechanical) of** esophageal anti-reflux device CC POA CC/MCC Exc

7ᵗʰ **T85.518** **Breakdown (mechanical) of other gastrointestinal prosthetic devices, implants and grafts** CC POA CC/MCC Exc

6ᵗʰ **T85.52** **Displacement** of gastrointestinal prosthetic devices, implants and grafts
　Malposition of gastrointestinal prosthetic devices, implants and grafts

7ᵗʰ **T85.520** **Displacement of** bile duct prosthesis CC POA CC/MCC Exc

7ᵗʰ **T85.521** **Displacement of** esophageal anti-reflux device CC POA CC/MCC Exc

7ᵗʰ **T85.528** **Displacement of other gastrointestinal prosthetic devices, implants and grafts** CC POA CC/MCC Exc

---

PDxⁿ Unacceptable principal diagnosis symbol per Medicare code edits   POA Code exempt from diagnosis present on admission requirement
? Questionable admission   CC Complication or comorbidity   CC/MCC Exc CC/MCC exclusion   MCC Major complication or comorbidity
PDx Principal diagnosis as its own CC   PDx Principal diagnosis as its own MCC   HCC HCC diagnosis code   RxHCC RxHCC diagnosis code
MACRA code   Z1 Z code as first-listed diagnosis

6ᵗʰ **T85.59** Other mechanical complication of gastrointestinal prosthetic devices, implants and

Obstruction, mechanical of gastrointestinal prosthetic devices, implants and grafts

Perforation of gastrointestinal prosthetic devices, implants and grafts

Protrusion of gastrointestinal prosthetic devices, implants and grafts

7ᵗʰ **T85.590** Other mechanical complication of bile duct prosthesis   CC POA CC/MCC Exc

7ᵗʰ **T85.591** Other mechanical complication of esophageal anti-reflux device   CC POA CC/MCC Exc

7ᵗʰ **T85.598** Other mechanical complication of other gastrointestinal prosthetic devices, implants and grafts   CC POA CC/MCC Exc

5ᵗʰ **T85.6** Mechanical complication of other specified internal and external prosthetic devices, implants and grafts

6ᵗʰ **T85.61** Breakdown (mechanical) of other specified internal prosthetic devices, implants and grafts

7ᵗʰ **T85.610** Breakdown (mechanical) of cranial or spinal infusion catheter

Breakdown (mechanical) of epidural infusion catheter

Breakdown (mechanical) of intrathecal infusion catheter

Breakdown (mechanical) of subarachnoid infusion catheter

Breakdown (mechanical) of subdural infusion catheter

7ᵗʰ **T85.611** Breakdown (mechanical) of intraperitoneal dialysis catheter   CC POA HCC RxHCC CC/MCC Exc

EXCLUDES1 mechanical complication of vascular dialysis catheter (T82.4-)

7ᵗʰ **T85.612** Breakdown (mechanical) of permanent sutures   CC POA CC/MCC Exc

EXCLUDES1 mechanical complication of permanent (wire) suture used in bone repair (T84.1-T84.2)

7ᵗʰ **T85.613** Breakdown (mechanical) of artificial skin graft and decellularized allodermis   CC POA CC/MCC Exc

Failure of artificial skin graft and decellularized allodermis

Non-adherence of artificial skin graft and decellularized allodermis

Poor incorporation of artificial skin graft and decellularized allodermis

Shearing of artificial skin graft and decellularized allodermis

7ᵗʰ **T85.614** Breakdown (mechanical) of insulin pump   CC POA CC/MCC Exc

7ᵗʰ **T85.615** Breakdown (mechanical) of other nervous system device, implant or graft   CC POA HCC CC/MCC Exc

Breakdown (mechanical) of intrathecal infusion pump

7ᵗʰ **T85.618** Breakdown (mechanical) of other specified internal prosthetic devices, implants and grafts   CC POA CC/MCC Exc

6ᵗʰ **T85.62** Displacement of other specified internal prosthetic devices, implants and grafts

Malposition of other specified internal prosthetic devices, implants and grafts

7ᵗʰ **T85.620** Displacement of cranial or spinal infusion catheter   CC POA CC/MCC Exc

Displacement of epidural infusion catheter

Displacement of intrathecal infusion catheter

Displacement of subarachnoid infusion catheter

Displacement of subdural infusion catheter

7ᵗʰ **T85.621** Displacement of intraperitoneal dialysis catheter   CC POA HCC RxHCC CC/MCC Exc

EXCLUDES1 mechanical complication of vascular dialysis catheter (T82.4-)

7ᵗʰ **T85.622** Displacement of permanent sutures   CC POA CC/MCC Exc

EXCLUDES1 mechanical complication of permanent (wire) suture used in bone repair (T84.1-T84.2)

7ᵗʰ **T85.623** Displacement of artificial skin graft and decellularized allodermis   CC POA CC/MCC Exc

Dislodgement of artificial skin graft and decellularized allodermis

7ᵗʰ **T85.624** Displacement of insulin pump   CC POA CC/MCC Exc

7ᵗʰ **T85.625** Displacement of other nervous system device, implant or graft   CC POA HCC CC/MCC Exc

Displacement of intrathecal infusion pump

7ᵗʰ **T85.628** Displacement of other specified internal prosthetic devices, implants and grafts   CC POA CC/MCC Exc

6ᵗʰ **T85.63** Leakage of other specified internal prosthetic devices, implants and grafts

7ᵗʰ **T85.630** Leakage of cranial or spinal infusion catheter   CC POA CC/MCC Exc

Leakage of epidural infusion catheter

Leakage of intrathecal infusion catheter

Leakage of subdural infusion catheter

Leakage of subarachnoid infusion catheter

7ᵗʰ **T85.631** Leakage of intraperitoneal dialysis catheter   CC POA HCC RxHCC CC/MCC Exc

EXCLUDES1 mechanical complication of vascular dialysis catheter (T82.4)

7ᵗʰ **T85.633** Leakage of insulin pump   CC POA CC/MCC Exc

7ᵗʰ **T85.635** Leakage of other nervous system device, implant or graft   CC POA HCC CC/MCC Exc

Leakage of intrathecal infusion pump

7ᵗʰ **T85.638** Leakage of other specified internal prosthetic devices, implants and grafts   CC POA CC/MCC Exc

6ᵗʰ **T85.69** Other mechanical complication of other specified internal prosthetic devices, implants and grafts

Obstruction, mechanical of other specified internal prosthetic devices, implants and grafts

Perforation of other specified internal prosthetic devices, implants and grafts

Protrusion of other specified internal prosthetic devices, implants and grafts

7ᵗʰ **T85.690** Other mechanical complication of cranial or spinal infusion catheter   CC POA CC/MCC Exc

Other mechanical complication of epidural infusion catheter

Other mechanical complication of intrathecal infusion catheter

Other mechanical complication of subarachnoid infusion catheter

Other mechanical complication of subdural infusion catheter

7ᵗʰ **T85.691** Other mechanical complication of intraperitoneal dialysis catheter   CC POA HCC RxHCC CC/MCC Exc

EXCLUDES1 mechanical complication of vascular dialysis catheter (T82.4)

7ᵗʰ **T85.692** Other mechanical complication of permanent sutures   CC POA CC/MCC Exc

EXCLUDES1 mechanical complication of permanent (wire) suture used in bone repair (T84.1-T84.2)

7ᵗʰ **T85.693** Other mechanical complication of artificial skin graft and decellularized allodermis   CC POA CC/MCC Exc

7ᵗʰ **T85.694** Other mechanical complication of insulin pump   CC POA CC/MCC Exc

Unspecified Code   Other Specified Code   Manifestation Code   N Newborn   P Pediatric   M Maternity   A Adult   ♂ Male   ♀ Female
● New Code   ▲ Revised Code Title   ►◄ Revised Text   NOTES   INCLUDES   EXCLUDES 1 Not coded here   EXCLUDES 2 Not included here
4ᵗʰ character required   5ᵗʰ character required   6ᵗʰ character required   7ᵗʰ character required
7ᵗʰ Extension 'X' Alert   HAC Hospital-acquired condition (HAC) alert   AHA AHA Coding Clinic©

T85.695 Other mechanical complication of other nervous system device, implant or graft ⦿ ⚇ HCC CC/MCC Exc

Other mechanical complication of intrathecal infusion pump

T85.698 Other mechanical complication of other specified internal prosthetic devices, implants and grafts ⦿ ⚇ CC/MCC Exc

Mechanical complication of nonabsorbable surgical material NOS

T85.7 Infection and inflammatory reaction due to other internal prosthetic devices, implants and grafts

Use additional code to identify infection

T85.71 Infection and inflammatory reaction due to peritoneal dialysis catheter ⦿ ⚇ HCC RxHCC CC/MCC Exc

T85.72 Infection and inflammatory reaction due to insulin pump ⦿ ⚇ HCC CC/MCC Exc

T85.73 Infection and inflammatory reaction due to nervous system devices, implants and graft

T85.730 Infection and inflammatory reaction due to ventricular intracranial (communicating) shunt ⦿ ⚇ HCC CC/MCC Exc

T85.731 Infection and inflammatory reaction due to implanted electronic neurostimulator of brain, electrode (lead) ⦿ ⚇ HCC CC/MCC Exc

T85.732 Infection and inflammatory reaction due to implanted electronic neurostimulator of peripheral nerve, electrode (lead) ⦿ ⚇ HCC CC/MCC Exc

Infection and inflammatory reaction due to electrode (lead) for cranial nerve neurostimulators

Infection and inflammatory reaction due to electrode (lead) for gastric neurostimulator

Infection and inflammatory reaction due to electrode (lead) for sacral nerve neurostimulator

Infection and inflammatory reaction due to electrode (lead) for vagal nerve neurostimulators

T85.733 Infection and inflammatory reaction due to implanted electronic neurostimulator of spinal cord, electrode (lead) ⦿ ⚇ HCC CC/MCC Exc

T85.734 Infection and inflammatory reaction due to implanted electronic neurostimulator, generator ⦿ ⚇ CC/MCC Exc

Generator pocket infection

T85.735 Infection and inflammatory reaction due to cranial or spinal infusion catheter ⦿ ⚇ HCC CC/MCC Exc

Infection and inflammatory reaction due to epidural catheter

Infection and inflammatory reaction due to intrathecal infusion catheter

Infection and inflammatory reaction due to subarachnoid catheter

Infection and inflammatory reaction due to subdural catheter

T85.738 Infection and inflammatory reaction due to other nervous system device, implant or graft ⦿ ⚇ HCC CC/MCC Exc

Infection and inflammatory reaction due to intrathecal infusion pump

T85.79 Infection and inflammatory reaction due to other internal prosthetic devices, implants and grafts ⦿ ⚇ HCC CC/MCC Exc

AHA: Q4 2016

T85.8 Other specified complications of internal prosthetic devices, implants and grafts, not elsewhere classified

T85.81 Embolism due to internal prosthetic devices, implants and grafts, not elsewhere classified

T85.810 Embolism due to nervous system prosthetic devices, implants and grafts ⦿ ⚇ HCC CC/MCC Exc

T85.818 Embolism due to other internal prosthetic devices, implants and grafts ⚇

T85.82 Fibrosis due to internal prosthetic devices, implants and grafts, not elsewhere classified

T85.820 Fibrosis due to nervous system prosthetic devices, implants and grafts ⦿ ⚇ HCC CC/MCC Exc

T85.828 Fibrosis due to other internal prosthetic devices, implants and grafts ⚇

T85.83 Hemorrhage due to internal prosthetic devices, implants and grafts, not elsewhere classified

T85.830 Hemorrhage due to nervous system prosthetic devices, implants and grafts ⦿ ⚇ HCC CC/MCC Exc

T85.838 Hemorrhage due to other internal prosthetic devices, implants and grafts ⚇

T85.84 Pain due to internal prosthetic devices, implants and grafts, not elsewhere classified

T85.840 Pain due to nervous system prosthetic devices, implants and grafts ⦿ ⚇ HCC CC/MCC Exc

T85.848 Pain due to other internal prosthetic devices, implants and grafts ⚇

T85.85 Stenosis due to internal prosthetic devices, implants and grafts, not elsewhere classified

T85.850 Stenosis due to nervous system prosthetic devices, implants and grafts ⦿ ⚇ HCC CC/MCC Exc

T85.858 Stenosis due to other internal prosthetic devices, implants and grafts ⚇

T85.86 Thrombosis due to internal prosthetic devices, implants and grafts, not elsewhere classified

T85.860 Thrombosis due to nervous system prosthetic devices, implants and grafts ⦿ ⚇ HCC CC/MCC Exc

T85.868 Thrombosis due to other internal prosthetic devices, implants and grafts ⚇

T85.89 Other specified complication of internal prosthetic devices, implants and grafts, not elsewhere classified

Erosion or breakdown of subcutaneous device pocket

T85.890 Other specified complication of nervous system prosthetic devices, implants and grafts ⦿ ⚇ HCC CC/MCC Exc

T85.898 Other specified complication of other internal prosthetic devices, implants and grafts ⚇

T85.9 Unspecified complication of internal prosthetic device, implant and graft ⚇

Complication of internal prosthetic device, implant and graft NOS

T86 Complications of transplanted organs and tissue

Use additional code to identify other transplant complications, such as:

graft-versus-host disease (D89.81-)

malignancy associated with organ transplant (C80.2)

post-transplant lymphoproliferative disorders (PTLD) (D47.Z1)

T86.0 Complications of bone marrow transplant

T86.00 Unspecified complication of bone marrow transplant ⦿ HCC RxHCC CC/MCC Exc

T86.01 Bone marrow transplant rejection ⦿ HCC RxHCC CC/MCC Exc

T86.02 Bone marrow transplant failure ⦿ HCC RxHCC CC/MCC Exc

T86.03 Bone marrow transplant infection ⦿ HCC RxHCC CC/MCC Exc

T86.09 Other complications of bone marrow transplant ⦿ HCC RxHCC CC/MCC Exc

T86.1 Complications of kidney transplant

T86.10 Unspecified complication of kidney transplant ⦿ RxHCC CC/MCC Exc

T86.11 Kidney transplant rejection ⦿ RxHCC CC/MCC Exc

T86.12 Kidney transplant failure ⦿ RxHCC CC/MCC Exc

AHA: Q1 2013

⚇ Unacceptable principal diagnosis symbol per Medicare code edits   ⚇ Code exempt from diagnosis present on admission requirement
? Questionable admission   ⦿ Complication or comorbidity   CC/MCC CC/MCC exclusion   MCC Major complication or comorbidity
CC Principal diagnosis as its own CC   MCC Principal diagnosis as its own MCC   HCC HCC diagnosis code   RxHCC RxHCC diagnosis code
MACRA code   Z1 Z code as first-listed diagnosis

T86.13 **Kidney transplant** infection CC/MCC Exc
  Use additional code to specify infection
T86.19 **Other complication of kidney transplant** CC/MCC Exc
5th T86.2 **Complications of** heart **transplant**
  EXCLUDES1 complication of:
    artificial heart device (T82.5)
    heart-lung transplant (T86.3)
  T86.20 **Unspecified complication of heart transplant** HCC CC/MCC Exc
  T86.21 **Heart transplant** rejection HCC CC/MCC Exc
  T86.22 **Heart transplant** failure HCC CC/MCC Exc
  T86.23 **Heart transplant** infection HCC CC/MCC Exc
    Use additional code to specify infection
  6th T86.29 **Other complications of heart transplant**
    T86.290 **Cardiac allograft vasculopathy** HCC CC/MCC Exc
      EXCLUDES1 atherosclerosis of coronary arteries (I25.75-, I25.76-, I25.81-)
    T86.298 **Other complications of heart transplant** HCC CC/MCC Exc
5th T86.3 **Complications of heart-lung transplant**
  T86.30 **Unspecified complication of heart-lung transplant** HCC PDx RxHCC CC/MCC Exc
  T86.31 **Heart-lung transplant** rejection HCC PDx RxHCC CC/MCC Exc
  T86.32 **Heart-lung transplant** failure HCC PDx RxHCC CC/MCC Exc
  T86.33 **Heart-lung transplant** infection HCC PDx RxHCC CC/MCC Exc
    Use additional code to specify infection
  T86.39 **Other complications of heart-lung transplant** HCC PDx RxHCC CC/MCC Exc
5th T86.4 **Complications of** liver **transplant**
  T86.40 **Unspecified complication of liver transplant** HCC RxHCC CC/MCC Exc
  T86.41 **Liver transplant** rejection HCC RxHCC CC/MCC Exc
  T86.42 **Liver transplant** failure HCC RxHCC CC/MCC Exc
  T86.43 **Liver transplant** infection
    Use additional code to identify infection, such as:
    Cytomegalovirus (CMV) infection (B25.-)
  T86.49 **Other complications of liver transplant** HCC RxHCC CC/MCC Exc
T86.5 **Complications of** stem cell **transplant** HCC RxHCC CC/MCC Exc
  Complications from stem cells from peripheral blood
  Complications from stem cells from umbilical cord
5th T86.8 **Complications of** other **transplanted organs and tissues**
  6th T86.81 **Complications of** lung **transplant**
    EXCLUDES1 complication of heart-lung transplant (T86.3-)
    T86.810 **Lung transplant** rejection HCC RxHCC CC/MCC Exc
    T86.811 **Lung transplant** failure HCC RxHCC CC/MCC Exc
    T86.812 **Lung transplant** infection HCC RxHCC CC/MCC Exc
      Use additional code to specify infection
    T86.818 **Other complications of lung transplant** HCC RxHCC CC/MCC Exc
    T86.819 **Unspecified complication of lung transplant** HCC RxHCC CC/MCC Exc
  6th T86.82 **Complications of** skin graft (allograft) (autograft)
    EXCLUDES2 complication of artificial skin graft (T85.693)
    T86.820 **Skin graft (allograft)** rejection CC/MCC Exc
    T86.821 **Skin graft (allograft) (autograft)** failure CC/MCC Exc
    T86.822 **Skin graft (allograft) (autograft)** infection CC/MCC Exc
      Use additional code to specify infection
    T86.828 **Other complications of skin graft (allograft) (autograft)** CC/MCC Exc
    T86.829 **Unspecified complication of skin graft (allograft) (autograft)** CC/MCC Exc
  6th T86.83 **Complications of** bone graft
    EXCLUDES2 mechanical complications of bone graft (T84.3-)
    T86.830 **Bone graft** rejection CC/MCC Exc

T86.831 **Bone graft** failure CC/MCC Exc
T86.832 **Bone graft** infection CC/MCC Exc
  Use additional code to specify infection
T86.838 **Other complications of bone graft** CC/MCC Exc
T86.839 **Unspecified complication of bone graft** CC/MCC Exc
6th T86.84 **Complications of** corneal **transplant**
  EXCLUDES2 mechanical complications of corneal graft (T85.3-)
  T86.840 **Corneal transplant** rejection CC/MCC Exc
  T86.841 **Corneal transplant** failure CC/MCC Exc
  T86.842 **Corneal transplant** infection HCC CC/MCC Exc
    Use additional code to specify infection
  T86.848 **Other complications of corneal transplant** CC/MCC Exc
  T86.849 **Unspecified complication of corneal transplant** CC/MCC Exc
5th T86.85 **Complication of** intestine **transplant**
  T86.850 **Intestine transplant** rejection HCC RxHCC CC/MCC Exc
  T86.851 **Intestine transplant** failure HCC RxHCC CC/MCC Exc
  T86.852 **Intestine transplant** infection HCC RxHCC CC/MCC Exc
    Use additional code to specify infection
  T86.858 **Other complications of intestine transplant** HCC RxHCC CC/MCC Exc
  T86.859 **Unspecified complication of intestine transplant** HCC RxHCC CC/MCC Exc
6th T86.89 **Complications of** other **transplanted** tissue
  Transplant failure or rejection of pancreas
  T86.890 **Other transplanted tissue** rejection CC/MCC Exc
  T86.891 **Other transplanted tissue** failure CC/MCC Exc
  T86.892 **Other transplanted tissue** infection CC/MCC Exc
    Use additional code to specify infection
  T86.898 **Other complications of other transplanted tissue** CC/MCC Exc
  T86.899 **Unspecified complication of other transplanted tissue** CC/MCC Exc
5th T86.9 **Complication of** unspecified **transplanted** organ and tissue
  T86.90 **Unspecified complication of unspecified transplanted organ and tissue** CC/MCC Exc
  T86.91 **Unspecified transplanted organ and tissue** rejection CC/MCC Exc
  T86.92 **Unspecified transplanted organ and tissue** failure CC/MCC Exc
  T86.93 **Unspecified transplanted organ and tissue** infection CC/MCC Exc
    Use additional code to specify infection
  T86.99 **Other complications of unspecified transplanted organ and tissue** CC/MCC Exc
4th T87 **Complications peculiar to reattachment and amputation**
  5th T87.0 **Complications of reattached (part of)** upper extremity
    6th T87.0X **Complications of reattached (part of) upper extremity**
      T87.0X1 **Complications of reattached (part of)** right upper extremity HCC CC/MCC Exc
      T87.0X2 **Complications of reattached (part of)** left upper extremity HCC CC/MCC Exc
      T87.0X9 **Complications of reattached (part of) unspecified upper extremity** HCC CC/MCC Exc
  5th T87.1 **Complications of reattached (part of)** lower extremity
    6th T87.1X **Complications of reattached (part of) lower extremity**
      T87.1X1 **Complications of reattached (part of)** right lower extremity HCC CC/MCC Exc
      T87.1X2 **Complications of reattached (part of)** left lower extremity HCC CC/MCC Exc

---

Unspecified Code Other Specified Code Manifestation Code N Newborn P Pediatric M Maternity A Adult ♂ Male ♀ Female
● New Code ▲ Revised Code Title ▶◀ Revised Text NOTES INCLUDES EXCLUDES 1 Not coded here EXCLUDES 2 Not included here
4th character required 5th character required 6th character required 7th character required
7th Extension 'X' Alert HAC Hospital-acquired condition (HAC) alert AHA AHA Coding Clinic©

T87.1X9   **Complications of reattached (part of) unspecified lower extremity** HCC CC/MCC Exc

T87.2   **Complications of other reattached body part** HCC CC/MCC Exc

T87.3   Neuroma of amputation stump

    T87.30   **Neuroma of amputation stump, unspecified extremity** HCC

    T87.31   Neuroma of amputation stump, right upper extremity HCC

    T87.32   Neuroma of amputation stump, left upper extremity HCC

    T87.33   Neuroma of amputation stump, right lower extremity HCC

    T87.34   Neuroma of amputation stump, left lower extremity HCC

T87.4   Infection of amputation stump

    T87.40   **Infection of amputation stump, unspecified extremity** HCC CC/MCC Exc

    T87.41   Infection of amputation stump, right upper extremity HCC CC/MCC Exc

    T87.42   Infection of amputation stump, left upper extremity HCC CC/MCC Exc

    T87.43   Infection of amputation stump, right lower extremity HCC CC/MCC Exc

    T87.44   Infection of amputation stump, left lower extremity HCC CC/MCC Exc

T87.5   Necrosis of amputation stump

    T87.50   **Necrosis of amputation stump, unspecified extremity** HCC

    T87.51   Necrosis of amputation stump, right upper extremity HCC

    T87.52   Necrosis of amputation stump, left upper extremity HCC

    T87.53   Necrosis of amputation stump, right lower extremity HCC

    T87.54   Necrosis of amputation stump, left lower extremity HCC

T87.8   Other complications of amputation stump

    T87.81   Dehiscence of amputation stump HCC

    T87.89   Other complications of amputation stump HCC

        Amputation stump contracture
        Amputation stump contracture of next proximal joint
        Amputation stump flexion
        Amputation stump edema
        Amputation stump hematoma
        EXCLUDES2 *phantom limb syndrome (G54.6-G54.7)*

T87.9   Unspecified complications of amputation stump HCC

T88   **Other complications of surgical and medical care, not elsewhere classified**

    EXCLUDES2 *complication following infusion, transfusion and therapeutic injection (T80.-)*

        complication following procedure NEC (T81.-)

        complications of anesthesia in labor and delivery (O74.-)

        complications of anesthesia in pregnancy (O29.-)

        complications of anesthesia in puerperium (O89.-)

        complications of devices, implants and grafts (T82-T85)

        complications of obstetric surgery and procedure (O75.4)

        dermatitis due to drugs and medicaments (L23.3, L24.4, L25.1, L27.0-L27.1)

        poisoning and toxic effects of drugs and chemicals (T36-T65 with fifth or sixth character 1-4 or 6)

        specified complications classified elsewhere

    The appropriate 7th character is to be added to each code from category T88

      A = initial encounter
      D = subsequent encounter
      S = sequela

    T88.0   **Infection following immunization** CC POA CC/MCC Exc

        Sepsis following immunization

T88.1   **Other complications following immunization, not elsewhere classified** POA CC/MCC Exc

    Generalized vaccinia
    Rash following immunization
    EXCLUDES1 *vaccinia not from vaccine (B08.011)*
    EXCLUDES2 *anaphylactic shock due to serum (T80.5-)*
        other serum reactions (T80.6-)
        postimmunization arthropathy (M02.2)
        postimmunization encephalitis (G04.02)
        postimmunization fever (R50.83)

T88.2   **Shock due to anesthesia** CC POA CC/MCC Exc

    Use additional code for adverse effect, if applicable, to identify drug (T41.- with fifth or sixth character 5)
    EXCLUDES1 *complications of anesthesia (in):*
        labor and delivery (O74.-)
        pregnancy (O29.-)
        puerperium (O89.-)
        postprocedural shock NOS (T81.1-)

T88.3   **Malignant hyperthermia due to anesthesia** CC POA CC/MCC Exc

    Use additional code for adverse effect, if applicable, to identify drug (T41.- with fifth or sixth character 5)

T88.4   **Failed or difficult intubation** POA

T88.5   Other complications of anesthesia

    Use additional code for adverse effect, if applicable, to identify drug (T41.- with fifth or sixth character 5)

    T88.51   Hypothermia following anesthesia POA

    T88.52   **Failed moderate sedation during procedure** POA
        Failed conscious sedation during procedure
        EXCLUDES2 *personal history of failed moderate sedation (Z92.83)*

    T88.53   Unintended awareness under general anesthesia during procedure POA
        AHA: Q4 2016
        EXCLUDES2 *personal history of unintended awareness under general anesthesia (Z92.84)*

    T88.59   Other complications of anesthesia POA

T88.6   **Anaphylactic reaction due to adverse effect of correct drug or medicament properly administered** CC POA CC/MCC Exc

    Anaphylactic shock due to adverse effect of correct drug or medicament properly administered
    Anaphylactoid reaction NOS
    Use additional code for adverse effect, if applicable, to identify drug (T36-T50 with fifth or sixth character 5)
    EXCLUDES1 *anaphylactic reaction due to serum (T80.5-)*
        anaphylactic shock or reaction due to adverse food reaction (T78.0-)

T88.7   **Unspecified adverse effect of drug or medicament** POA

    Drug hypersensitivity NOS
    Drug reaction NOS
    Use additional code for adverse effect, if applicable, to identify drug (T36-T50 with fifth or sixth character 5)
    EXCLUDES1 *specified adverse effects of drugs and medicaments (A00-R94 and T80-T88.6, T88.8)*

T88.8   **Other specified complications of surgical and medical care, not elsewhere classified** POA

    Use additional code to identify the complication

T88.9   Complication of surgical and medical care, unspecified POA

POA Unacceptable principal diagnosis symbol per Medicare code edits   POA Code exempt from diagnosis present on admission requirement
   ? Questionable admission   CC Complication or comorbidity   CC/MCC Exc CC/MCC exclusion   MCC Major complication or comorbidity
   Principal diagnosis as its own CC   Principal diagnosis as its own MCC   HCC HCC diagnosis code   RxHCC RxHCC diagnosis code
     MACRA code   Z1 Z code as first-listed diagnosis

1180   When symbols appear on a code that requires a 7th character extension, refer to Appendix B to identify applicable 7th character codes.   **2018 ICD-10-CM**

NOTES

NOTES

External causes of morbidity (V00-Y99)

NOTES This chapter permits the classification of environmental events and circumstances as the cause of injury, and other adverse effects. Where a code from this section is applicable, it is intended that it shall be used secondary to a code from another chapter of the Classification indicating the nature of the condition. Most often, the condition will be classifiable to Chapter 19, Injury, poisoning and certain other consequences of external causes (S00-T88). Other conditions that may be stated to be due to external causes are classified in Chapters I to XVIII. For these conditions, codes from Chapter 20 should be used to provide additional information as to the cause of the condition.

This chapter contains the following blocks:

V00-X58	Accidents
V00-V99	Transport accidents
V00-V09	Pedestrian injured in transport accident
V10-V19	Pedal cycle rider injured in transport accident
V20-V29	Motorcycle rider injured in transport accident
V30-V39	Occupant of three-wheeled motor vehicle injured in transport accident
V40-V49	Car occupant injured in transport accident
V50-V59	Occupant of pick-up truck or van injured in transport accident
V60-V69	Occupant of heavy transport vehicle injured in transport accident
V70-V79	Bus occupant injured in transport accident
V80-V89	Other land transport accidents
V90-V94	Water transport accidents
V95-V97	Air and space transport accidents
V98-V99	Other and unspecified transport accidents
W00-X58	Other external causes of accidental injury
W00-W19	Slipping, tripping, stumbling and falls
W20-W49	Exposure to inanimate mechanical forces
W50-W64	Exposure to animate mechanical forces
W65-W74	Accidental non-transport drowning and submersion
W85-W99	Exposure to electric current, radiation and extreme ambient air temperature and pressure
X00-X08	Exposure to smoke, fire and flames
X10-X19	Contact with heat and hot substances
X30-X39	Exposure to forces of nature
X50	Overexertion and strenuous or repetitive movements

Editor's Note: At press time, CMS deleted this block for 2018 even though there are valid codes within the block. The block has been left here because it includes valid codes. Check www.cms.gov for further updates.

X52-X58	Accidental exposure to other specified factors
X71-X83	Intentional self-harm
X92-Y09	Assault
Y21-Y33	Event of undetermined intent
Y35-Y38	Legal intervention, operations of war, military operations, and terrorism
Y62-Y84	Complications of medical and surgical care
Y62-Y69	Misadventures to patients during surgical and medical care
Y70-Y82	Medical devices associated with adverse incidents in diagnostic and therapeutic use
Y83-Y84	Surgical and other medical procedures as the cause of abnormal reaction of the patient, or of later complication, without mention of misadventure at the time of the procedure
Y90-Y99	Supplementary factors related to causes of morbidity classified elsewhere

Accidents (V00-X58)

Transport accidents (V00-V99)

NOTES This section is structured in 12 groups. Those relating to land transport accidents (V00-V89) reflect the victim's mode of transport and are subdivided to identify the victim's 'counterpart' or the type of event. The vehicle of which the injured person is an occupant is identified in the first two characters since it is seen as the most important factor to identify for prevention purposes. A transport accident is one in which the vehicle involved must be moving or running or in use for transport purposes at the time of the accident.

Use additional code to identify:
Airbag injury (W22.1)
Type of street or road (Y92.4-)
Use of cellular telephone and other electronic equipment at the time of the transport accident (Y93.C-)

EXCLUDES1 *agricultural vehicles in stationary use or maintenance (W31.-)*
assault by crashing of motor vehicle (Y03.-)
automobile or motor cycle in stationary use or maintenance- code to type of accident
crashing of motor vehicle, undetermined intent (Y32)
intentional self-harm by crashing of motor vehicle (X82)

EXCLUDES2 *transport accidents due to cataclysm (X34-X38)*

NOTES Definitions related to transport accidents:
(a) A transport accident (V00-V99) is any accident involving a device designed primarily for, or used at the time primarily for, conveying persons or good from one place to another.
(b) A public highway [trafficway] or street is the entire width between property lines (or other boundary lines) of land open to the public as a matter of right or custom for purposes of moving persons or property from one place to another. A roadway is that part of the public highway designed, improved and customarily used for vehicular traffic.
(c) A traffic accident is any vehicle accident occurring on the public highway [i.e. originating on, terminating on, or involving a vehicle partially on the highway]. A vehicle accident is assumed to have occurred on the public highway unless another place is specified, except in the case of accidents involving only off-road motor vehicles, which are classified as nontraffic accidents unless the contrary is stated.
(d) A nontraffic accident is any vehicle accident that occurs entirely in any place other than a public highway.
(e) A pedestrian is any person involved in an accident who was not at the time of the accident riding in or on a motor vehicle, railway train, streetcar or animal-drawn or other vehicle, or on a pedal cycle or animal. This includes, a person changing a tire, working on a parked car, or a person on foot. It also includes the user of a pedestrian conveyance such as a babystroller, ice-skates, skis, sled, roller skates, a skateboard, nonmotorized or motorized wheelchair, motorized mobility scooter, or nonmotorized scooter.
(f) A driver is an occupant of a transport vehicle who is operating or intending to operate it.
(g) A passenger is any occupant of a transport vehicle other than the driver, except a person traveling on the outside of the vehicle.
(h) A person on the outside of a vehicle is any person being transported by a vehicle but not occupying the space normally reserved for the driver or passengers, or the space intended for the transport of property. This includes a person travelling on the bodywork, bumper, fender, roof, running board or step of a vehicle, as well as, hanging on the outside of the vehicle.
(i) A pedal cycle is any land transport vehicle operated solely by nonmotorized pedals including a bicycle or tricycle.
(j) A pedal cyclist is any person riding a pedal cycle or in a sidecar or trailer attached to a pedal cycle.
(k) A motorcycle is a two-wheeled motor vehicle with one or two riding saddles and sometimes with a third wheel for the support of a sidecar. The sidecar is considered part of the motorcycle. This includes a moped, motor scooter, or motorized bicycle.
(l) A motorcycle rider is any person riding a motorcycle or in a sidecar or trailer attached to the motorcycle.
(m) A three-wheeled motor vehicle is a motorized tricycle designed primarily for on-road use. This includes a motor-driven tricycle, a motorized rickshaw, or a three-wheeled motor car.

Unspecified Code	Other Specified Code	Manifestation Code	N Newborn	P Pediatric	M Maternity	A Adult	♂ Male	♀ Female

● New Code ▲ Revised Code Title ▶◀ Revised Text **NOTES** *INCLUDES* *EXCLUDES 1* Not coded here *EXCLUDES 2* Not included here
④ 4th character required ⑤ 5th character required ⑥ 6th character required ⑦ 7th character required
Ⓧ Extension 'X' Alert **HAC** Hospital-acquired condition (HAC) alert **AHA** AHA Coding Clinic©

(n) A car [automobile] is a four-wheeled motor vehicle designed primarily for carrying up to 7 persons. A trailer being towed by the car is considered part of the car. It does not include a van or minivan - see definition (o)

(o) A pick-up truck or van is a four or six-wheeled motor vehicle designed for carrying passengers as well as property or cargo weighing less than the local limit for classification as a heavy goods vehicle, and not requiring a special driver's license. This includes a minivan and a sport-utility vehicle (SUV).

(p) A heavy transport vehicle is a motor vehicle designed primarily for carrying property, meeting local criteria for classification as a heavy goods vehicle in terms of weight and requiring a special driver's license.

(q) A bus (coach) is a motor vehicle designed or adapted primarily for carrying more than 10 passengers, and requiring a special driver's license.

(r) A railway train or railway vehicle is any device, with or without freight or passenger cars couple to it, designed for traffic on a railway track. This includes subterranean (subways) or elevated trains.

(s) A streetcar, is a device designed and used primarily for transporting passengers within a municipality, running on rails, usually subject to normal traffic control signals, and operated principally on a right-of-way that forms part of the roadway. This includes a tram or trolley that runs on rails. A trailer being towed by a streetcar is considered part of the streetcar.

(t) A special vehicle mainly used on industrial premises is a motor vehicle designed primarily for use within the buildings and premises of industrial or commercial establishments. This includes battery-powered airport passenger vehicles or baggage/mail trucks, forklifts, coal-cars in a coal mine, logging cars and trucks used in mines or quarries.

(u) A special vehicle mainly used in agriculture is a motor vehicle designed specifically for use in farming and agriculture (horticulture), to work the land, tend and harvest crops and transport materials on the farm. This includes harvesters, farm machinery and tractor and trailers.

(v) A special construction vehicle is a motor vehicle designed specifically for use on construction and demolition sites. This includes bulldozers, diggers, earth levellers, dump trucks, backhoes, front-end loaders, pavers, and mechanical shovels.

(w) A special all-terrain vehicle is a motor vehicle of special design to enable it to negotiate over rough or soft terrain, snow or sand. Examples of special design are high construction, special wheels and tires, tracks, and support on a cushion of air. This includes snow mobiles, All-terrain vehicles (ATV), and dune buggies. It does not include passenger vehicle designated as Sport Utility Vehicles. (SUV)

(x) A watercraft is any device designed for transporting passengers or goods on water. This includes motor or sail boats, ships, and hovercraft.

(y) An aircraft is any device for transporting passengers or goods in the air. This includes hot-air balloons, gliders, helicopters and airplanes.

(z) A military vehicle is any motorized vehicle operating on a public roadway owned by the military and being operated by a member of the military.

Pedestrian injured in transport accident (V00-V09)

INCLUDES   person changing tire on transport vehicle
person examining engine of vehicle broken down in (on side of) road
EXCLUDES1   fall due to non-transport collision with other person (W03)
pedestrian on foot falling (slipping) on ice and snow (W00.-)
struck or bumped by another person (W51)

🌀 V00 Pedestrian conveyance accident
Use additional place of occurrence and activity external cause codes, if known (Y92.-, Y93.-)
EXCLUDES1   collision with another person without fall (W51)
fall due to person on foot colliding with another person on foot (W03)
fall from non-moving wheelchair, nonmotorized scooter and motorized mobility scooter without collision (W05.-)
pedestrian (conveyance) collision with other land transport vehicle (V01-V09)
pedestrian on foot falling (slipping) on ice and snow (W00.-)

The appropriate 7th character is to be added to each code from category V00
A = initial encounter
D = subsequent encounter
S = sequela

🌀 V00.0 Pedestrian on foot injured in collision with pedestrian conveyance
🌀 V00.01 Pedestrian on foot injured in collision with roller-skater POA
🌀 V00.02 Pedestrian on foot injured in collision with skateboarder POA
🌀 V00.09 Pedestrian on foot injured in collision with other pedestrian conveyance POA

🌀 V00.1 Rolling-type pedestrian conveyance accident
EXCLUDES1   accident with babystroller (V00.82-)
accident with wheelchair (powered) (V00.81-)
accident with motorized mobility scooter (V00.83-)
🌀 V00.11 In-line roller-skate accident
🌀 V00.111 Fall from in-line roller-skates POA
🌀 V00.112 In-line roller-skater colliding with stationary object POA
🌀 V00.118 Other in-line roller-skate accident POA
EXCLUDES1   roller-skater collision with other land transport vehicle (V01-V09 with 5th character 1)
🌀 V00.12 Non-in-line roller-skate accident
🌀 V00.121 Fall from non-in-line roller-skates POA
🌀 V00.122 Non-in-line roller-skater colliding with stationary object POA
🌀 V00.128 Other non-in-line roller-skating accident POA
EXCLUDES1   roller-skater collision with other land transport vehicle (V01-V09 with 5th character 1)
🌀 V00.13 Skateboard accident
🌀 V00.131 Fall from skateboard POA
🌀 V00.132 Skateboarder colliding with stationary object POA
🌀 V00.138 Other skateboard accident POA
EXCLUDES1   skateboarder collision with other land transport vehicle (V01-V09 with 5th character 2)
🌀 V00.14 Scooter (nonmotorized) accident
EXCLUDES1   motorscooter accident (V20-V29)
🌀 V00.141 Fall from scooter (nonmotorized) POA
🌀 V00.142 Scooter (nonmotorized) colliding with stationary object POA
🌀 V00.148 Other scooter (nonmotorized) accident POA
EXCLUDES1   scooter (nonmotorized) collision with other land transport vehicle (V01-V09 with fifth character 9)
🌀 V00.15 Heelies accident
Rolling shoe
Wheeled shoe
Wheelies accident
🌀 V00.151 Fall from heelies POA
🌀 V00.152 Heelies colliding with stationary object POA
🌀 V00.158 Other heelies accident POA
🌀 V00.18 Accident on other rolling-type pedestrian conveyance
🌀 V00.181 Fall from other rolling-type pedestrian conveyance POA
🌀 V00.182 Pedestrian on other rolling-type pedestrian conveyance colliding with stationary object POA
🌀 V00.188 Other accident on other rolling-type pedestrian conveyance POA
🌀 V00.2 Gliding-type pedestrian conveyance accident
🌀 V00.21 Ice-skates accident
🌀 V00.211 Fall from ice-skates POA

POA Unacceptable principal diagnosis symbol per Medicare code edits   Code exempt from diagnosis present on admission requirement
❓ Questionable admission   cc Complication or comorbidity   cc/mcc exc CC/MCC exclusion   mcc Major complication or comorbidity
Principal diagnosis as its own CC   Principal diagnosis as its own MCC   HCC HCC diagnosis code   RxHCC RxHCC diagnosis code
MACRA code   Z Z code as first-listed diagnosis

[7th] V00.212 Ice-skater colliding with stationary object POA

[7th] V00.218 Other ice-skates accident POA

EXCLUDES1 ice-skater collision with other land transport vehicle (V01-V09 with 5th digit 9)

[6th] V00.22 Sled accident

[7th] V00.221 Fall from sled POA

[7th] V00.222 Sledder colliding with stationary object POA

[7th] V00.228 Other sled accident POA

EXCLUDES1 sled collision with other land transport vehicle (V01-V09 with 5th digit 9)

[6th] V00.28 Other gliding-type pedestrian conveyance accident

[7th] V00.281 Fall from other gliding-type pedestrian conveyance POA

[7th] V00.282 Pedestrian on other gliding-type pedestrian conveyance colliding with stationary object POA

[7th] V00.288 Other accident on other gliding-type pedestrian conveyance POA

EXCLUDES1 gliding-type pedestrian conveyance collision with other land transport vehicle (V01-V09 with 5th digit 9)

[5th] V00.3 Flat-bottomed pedestrian conveyance accident

[6th] V00.31 Snowboard accident

[7th] V00.311 Fall from snowboard POA

[7th] V00.312 Snowboarder colliding with stationary object POA

[7th] V00.318 Other snowboard accident POA

EXCLUDES1 snowboarder collision with other land transport vehicle (V01-V09 with 5th digit 9)

[6th] V00.32 Snow-ski accident

[7th] V00.321 Fall from snow-skis POA

[7th] V00.322 Snow-skier colliding with stationary object POA

[7th] V00.328 Other snow-ski accident POA

EXCLUDES1 snow-skier collision with other land transport vehicle (V01-V09 with 5th digit 9)

[6th] V00.38 Other flat-bottomed pedestrian conveyance accident

[7th] V00.381 Fall from other flat-bottomed pedestrian conveyance POA

[7th] V00.382 Pedestrian on other flat-bottomed pedestrian conveyance colliding with stationary object POA

[7th] V00.388 Other accident on other flat-bottomed pedestrian conveyance POA

[5th] V00.8 Accident on other pedestrian conveyance

[6th] V00.81 Accident with wheelchair (powered)

[7th] V00.811 Fall from moving wheelchair (powered)

EXCLUDES1 fall from non-moving wheelchair (W05.0)

[7th] V00.812 Wheelchair (powered) colliding with stationary object

[7th] V00.818 Other accident with wheelchair (powered)

[6th] V00.82 Accident with babystroller

[7th] V00.821 Fall from babystroller POA

[7th] V00.822 Babystroller colliding with stationary object POA

[7th] V00.828 Other accident with babystroller POA

[6th] V00.83 Accident with motorized mobility scooter

[7th] V00.831 Fall from motorized mobility scooter

EXCLUDES1 fall from non-moving motorized mobility scooter (W05.2)

[7th] V00.832 Motorized mobility scooter colliding with stationary object

[7th] V00.838 Other accident with motorized mobility scooter

[6th] V00.89 Accident on other pedestrian conveyance

[7th] V00.891 Fall from other pedestrian conveyance POA

[7th] V00.892 Pedestrian on other pedestrian conveyance colliding with stationary object POA

[7th] V00.898 Other accident on other pedestrian conveyance POA

EXCLUDES1 other pedestrian (conveyance) collision with other land transport vehicle (V01-V09 with 5th digit 9)

[4th] V01 Pedestrian injured in collision with pedal cycle

The appropriate 7th character is to be added to each code from category V01

A = initial encounter

D = subsequent encounter

S = sequela

[5th] V01.0 Pedestrian injured in collision with pedal cycle in nontraffic accident

[7th] V01.00 Pedestrian on foot injured in collision with pedal cycle in nontraffic accident POA

Pedestrian NOS injured in collision with pedal cycle in nontraffic accident

[7th] V01.01 Pedestrian on roller-skates injured in collision with pedal cycle in nontraffic accident POA

[7th] V01.02 Pedestrian on skateboard injured in collision with pedal cycle in nontraffic accident POA

[7th] V01.09 Pedestrian with other conveyance injured in collision with pedal cycle in nontraffic accident POA

Pedestrian with babystroller injured in collision with pedal cycle in nontraffic accident

Pedestrian on ice-skates injured in collision with pedal cycle in nontraffic accident

Pedestrian on nonmotorized scooter injured in collision with pedal cycle in nontraffic accident

Pedestrian on sled injured in collision with pedal cycle in nontraffic accident

Pedestrian on snowboard injured in collision with pedal cycle in nontraffic accident

Pedestrian on snow-skis injured in collision with pedal cycle in nontraffic accident

Pedestrian in wheelchair (powered) injured in collision with pedal cycle in nontraffic accident

Pedestrian in motorized mobility scooter injured in collision with pedal cycle in nontraffic accident

[5th] V01.1 Pedestrian injured in collision with pedal cycle in traffic accident

[7th] V01.10 Pedestrian on foot injured in collision with pedal cycle in traffic accident POA

Pedestrian NOS injured in collision with pedal cycle in traffic accident

[7th] V01.11 Pedestrian on roller-skates injured in collision with pedal cycle in traffic accident POA

[7th] V01.12 Pedestrian on skateboard injured in collision with pedal cycle in traffic accident POA

[7th] V01.19 Pedestrian with other conveyance injured in collision with pedal cycle in traffic accident POA

Pedestrian with babystroller injured in collision with pedal cycle in traffic accident

Pedestrian on ice-skates injured in collision with pedal cycle in traffic accident

Pedestrian on nonmotorized scooter injured in collision with pedal cycle in traffic accident

Pedestrian on sled injured in collision with pedal cycle in traffic accident

Pedestrian on snowboard injured in collision with pedal cycle in traffic accident

Pedestrian on snow-skis injured in collision with pedal cycle in traffic accident

Pedestrian in wheelchair (powered) injured in collision with pedal cycle in traffic accident

Pedestrian in motorized mobility scooter injured in collision with pedal cycle in traffic accident

Unspecified Code | Other Specified Code | Manifestation Code | [N] Newborn | [P] Pediatric | [M] Maternity | [A] Adult | ♂ Male | ♀ Female
● New Code | ▲ Revised Code Title | ►◄ Revised Text | NOTES | INCLUDES | EXCLUDES1 Not coded here | EXCLUDES2 Not included here
[4th] 4th character required | [5th] 5th character required | [6th] 6th character required | [7th] 7th character required
[7th] Extension 'X' Alert | [HAC] Hospital-acquired condition (HAC) alert | AHA AHA Coding Clinic©

When symbols appear on a code that requires a 7th character extension, refer to Appendix B to identify applicable 7th character codes.

V01.9 Pedestrian injured in collision with pedal cycle, unspecified whether traffic or nontraffic accident

    V01.90 **Pedestrian on foot injured in collision with pedal cycle, unspecified whether traffic or nontraffic accident** POA

        Pedestrian NOS injured in collision with pedal cycle, unspecified whether traffic or nontraffic accident

    V01.91 **Pedestrian on roller-skates injured in collision with pedal cycle, unspecified whether traffic or nontraffic accident** POA

    V01.92 **Pedestrian on skateboard injured in collision with pedal cycle, unspecified whether traffic or nontraffic accident** POA

    V01.99 **Pedestrian with other conveyance injured in collision with pedal cycle, unspecified whether traffic or nontraffic accident** POA

        Pedestrian with babystroller injured in collision with pedal cycle, unspecified whether traffic or nontraffic accident

        Pedestrian on ice-skates injured in collision with pedal cycle unspecified, whether traffic or nontraffic accident

        Pedestrian on nonmotorized scooter injured in collision with pedal cycle, unspecified whether traffic or nontraffic accident

        Pedestrian on sled injured in collision with pedal cycle unspecified, whether traffic or nontraffic accident

        Pedestrian on snowboard injured in collision with pedal cycle, unspecified whether traffic or nontraffic accident

        Pedestrian on snow-skis injured in collision with pedal cycle, unspecified whether traffic or nontraffic accident

        Pedestrian in wheelchair (powered) injured in collision with pedal cycle, unspecified whether traffic or nontraffic accident

        Pedestrian in motorized mobility scooter injured in collision with pedal cycle, unspecified whether traffic or nontraffic accident

V02 **Pedestrian injured in collision with two- or three-wheeled motor vehicle**

    The appropriate 7th character is to be added to each code from category V02

    A = initial encounter

    D = subsequent encounter

    S = sequela

  V02.0 Pedestrian injured in collision with two- or three-wheeled motor vehicle in nontraffic accident

    V02.00 **Pedestrian on foot injured in collision with two- or three-wheeled motor vehicle in nontraffic accident** POA

        Pedestrian NOS injured in collision with two- or three-wheeled motor vehicle in nontraffic accident

    V02.01 **Pedestrian on roller-skates injured in collision with two- or three-wheeled motor vehicle in nontraffic accident** POA

    V02.02 **Pedestrian on skateboard injured in collision with two- or three-wheeled motor vehicle in nontraffic accident** POA

    V02.09 **Pedestrian with other conveyance injured in collision with two- or three-wheeled motor vehicle in nontraffic accident** POA

        Pedestrian with babystroller injured in collision with two- or three-wheeled motor vehicle in nontraffic accident

        Pedestrian on ice-skates injured in collision with two- or three-wheeled motor vehicle in nontraffic accident

        Pedestrian on nonmotorized scooter injured in collision with two- or three-wheeled motor vehicle in nontraffic accident

        Pedestrian on sled injured in collision with two- or three-wheeled motor vehicle in nontraffic accident

        Pedestrian on snowboard injured in collision with two- or three-wheeled motor vehicle in nontraffic accident

        Pedestrian on snow-skis injured in collision with two- or three-wheeled motor vehicle in nontraffic accident

        Pedestrian in wheelchair (powered) injured in collision with two- or three-wheeled motor vehicle in nontraffic accident

        Pedestrian in motorized mobility scooter injured in collision with two- or three-wheeled motor vehicle in nontraffic accident

  V02.1 Pedestrian injured in collision with two- or three-wheeled motor vehicle in traffic accident

    V02.10 **Pedestrian on foot injured in collision with two- or three-wheeled motor vehicle in traffic accident** POA

        Pedestrian NOS injured in collision with two- or three-wheeled motor vehicle in traffic accident

    V02.11 **Pedestrian on roller-skates injured in collision with two- or three-wheeled motor vehicle in traffic accident** POA

    V02.12 **Pedestrian on skateboard injured in collision with two- or three-wheeled motor vehicle in traffic accident** POA

    V02.19 **Pedestrian with other conveyance injured in collision with two- or three-wheeled motor vehicle in traffic accident** POA

        Pedestrian with babystroller injured in collision with two- or three-wheeled motor vehicle in traffic accident

        Pedestrian on ice-skates injured in collision with two- or three-wheeled motor vehicle in traffic accident

        Pedestrian on nonmotorized scooter injured in collision with two- or three-wheeled motor vehicle in traffic accident

        Pedestrian on sled injured in collision with two- or three-wheeled motor vehicle in traffic accident

        Pedestrian on snowboard injured in collision with two- or three-wheeled motor vehicle in traffic accident

        Pedestrian on snow-skis injured in collision with two- or three-wheeled motor vehicle in traffic accident

        Pedestrian in wheelchair (powered) injured in collision with two- or three-wheeled motor vehicle in traffic accident

        Pedestrian in motorized mobility scooter injured in collision with two- or three-wheeled motor vehicle in traffic accident

  V02.9 Pedestrian injured in collision with two- or three-wheeled motor vehicle, unspecified whether traffic or nontraffic accident

    V02.90 **Pedestrian on foot injured in collision with two- or three-wheeled motor vehicle, unspecified whether traffic or nontraffic accident** POA

        Pedestrian NOS injured in collision with two- or three-wheeled motor vehicle, unspecified whether traffic or nontraffic accident

    V02.91 **Pedestrian on roller-skates injured in collision with two- or three-wheeled motor vehicle, unspecified whether traffic or nontraffic accident** POA

    V02.92 **Pedestrian on skateboard injured in collision with two- or three-wheeled motor vehicle, unspecified whether traffic or nontraffic accident** POA

    V02.99 **Pedestrian with other conveyance injured in collision with two- or three-wheeled motor vehicle, unspecified whether traffic or nontraffic accident** POA

        Pedestrian with babystroller injured in collision with two- or three-wheeled motor vehicle, unspecified whether traffic or nontraffic accident

        Pedestrian on ice-skates injured in collision with two- or three-wheeled motor vehicle, unspecified whether traffic or nontraffic accident

        Pedestrian on nonmotorized scooter injured in collision with two- or three-wheeled motor vehicle, unspecified whether traffic or nontraffic accident

POAₑ Unacceptable principal diagnosis symbol per Medicare code edits   POA Code exempt from diagnosis present on admission requirement   ❓ Questionable admission   CC Complication or comorbidity   CC/MCC Exc. CC/MCC exclusion   MCC Major complication or comorbidity   Principal diagnosis as its own CC   Principal diagnosis as its own MCC   HCC HCC diagnosis code   RxHCC RxHCC diagnosis code   MACRA code   Z1 Z code as first-listed diagnosis

Pedestrian on sled injured in collision with two- or three-wheeled motor vehicle, unspecified whether traffic or nontraffic accident

Pedestrian on snowboard injured in collision with two- or three-wheeled motor vehicle, unspecified whether traffic or nontraffic accident

Pedestrian on snow-skis injured in collision with two- or three-wheeled motor vehicle, unspecified whether traffic or nontraffic accident

Pedestrian in wheelchair (powered) injured in collision with two- or three-wheeled motor vehicle, unspecified whether traffic or nontraffic accident

Pedestrian in motorized mobility scooter injured in collision with two- or three-wheeled motor vehicle, unspecified whether traffic or nontraffic accident

V03 Pedestrian injured in collision with car, pick-up truck or van

The appropriate 7th character is to be added to each code from category V03
A = initial encounter
D = subsequent encounter
S = sequela

V03.0 Pedestrian injured in collision with car, pick-up truck or van in nontraffic accident

V03.00 Pedestrian on foot **injured in collision with car, pick-up truck or van in nontraffic accident**
Pedestrian NOS injured in collision with car, pick-up truck or van in nontraffic accident

V03.01 Pedestrian on roller-skates **injured in collision with car, pick-up truck or van in nontraffic accident**

V03.02 Pedestrian on skateboard **injured in collision with car, pick-up truck or van in nontraffic accident**

V03.09 Pedestrian with other conveyance injured in collision with car, pick-up truck or van in nontraffic accident
Pedestrian with babystroller injured in collision with car, pick-up truck or van in nontraffic accident
Pedestrian on ice-skates injured in collision with car, pick-up truck or van in nontraffic accident
Pedestrian on nonmotorized scooter injured in collision with car, pick-up truck or van in nontraffic accident
Pedestrian on sled injured in collision with car, pick-up truck or van in nontraffic accident
Pedestrian on snowboard injured in collision with car, pick-up truck or van in nontraffic accident
Pedestrian on snow-skis injured in collision with car, pick-up truck or van in nontraffic accident
Pedestrian in wheelchair (powered) injured in collision with car, pick-up truck or van in nontraffic accident
Pedestrian in motorized mobility scooter injured in collision with car, pick-up truck or van in nontraffic accident

V03.1 Pedestrian injured in collision with car, pick-up truck or van in traffic accident

V03.10 Pedestrian on foot **injured in collision with car, pick-up truck or van in traffic accident**
Pedestrian NOS injured in collision with car, pick-up truck or van in traffic accident

V03.11 Pedestrian on roller-skates **injured in collision with car, pick-up truck or van in traffic accident**

V03.12 Pedestrian on skateboard **injured in collision with car, pick-up truck or van in traffic accident**

V03.19 Pedestrian with other conveyance injured in collision with car, pick-up truck or van in traffic accident
Pedestrian with babystroller injured in collision with car, pick-up truck or van in traffic accident
Pedestrian on ice-skates injured in collision with car, pick-up truck or van in traffic accident
Pedestrian on nonmotorized scooter injured in collision with car, pick-up truck or van in traffic accident
Pedestrian on sled injured in collision with car, pick-up truck or van in traffic accident

Pedestrian on snowboard injured in collision with car, pick-up truck or van in traffic accident
Pedestrian on snow-skis injured in collision with car, pick-up truck or van in traffic accident
Pedestrian in wheelchair (powered) injured in collision with car, pick-up truck or van in traffic accident
Pedestrian in motorized mobility scooter injured in collision with car, pick-up truck or van in traffic accident

V03.9 Pedestrian injured in collision with car, pick-up truck or van, unspecified whether traffic or nontraffic accident

V03.90 Pedestrian on foot injured in collision with car, pick-up truck or van, unspecified whether traffic or nontraffic accident
Pedestrian NOS injured in collision with car, pick-up truck or van, unspecified whether traffic or nontraffic accident

V03.91 Pedestrian on roller-skates injured in collision with car, pick-up truck or van, unspecified whether traffic or nontraffic accident

V03.92 Pedestrian on skateboard injured in collision with car, pick-up truck or van, unspecified whether traffic or nontraffic accident

V03.99 Pedestrian with other conveyance injured in collision with car, pick-up truck or van, unspecified whether traffic or nontraffic accident
Pedestrian with babystroller injured in collision with car, pick-up truck or van, unspecified whether traffic or nontraffic accident
Pedestrian on ice-skates injured in collision with car, pick-up truck or van, unspecified whether traffic or nontraffic accident
Pedestrian on nonmotorized scooter injured in collision with car, pick-up truck or van, unspecified whether traffic or nontraffic accident
Pedestrian on sled injured in collision with car, pick-up truck or van in nontraffic accident
Pedestrian on snowboard injured in collision with car, pick-up truck or van, unspecified whether traffic or nontraffic accident
Pedestrian on snow-skis injured in collision with car, pick-up truck or van, unspecified whether traffic or nontraffic accident
Pedestrian in wheelchair (powered) injured in collision with car, pick-up truck or van, unspecified whether traffic or nontraffic accident
Pedestrian in motorized mobility scooter injured in collision with car, pick-up truck or van, unspecified whether traffic or nontraffic accident

V04 Pedestrian injured in collision with heavy transport vehicle or bus

EXCLUDES1 pedestrian injured in collision with military vehicle (V09.01, V09.21)

The appropriate 7th character is to be added to each code from category V04
A = initial encounter
D = subsequent encounter
S = sequela

V04.0 Pedestrian injured in collision with heavy transport vehicle or bus in nontraffic accident

V04.00 Pedestrian on foot **injured in collision with heavy transport vehicle or bus in nontraffic accident**
Pedestrian NOS injured in collision with heavy transport vehicle or bus in nontraffic accident

V04.01 Pedestrian on roller-skates **injured in collision with heavy transport vehicle or bus in nontraffic accident**

V04.02 Pedestrian on skateboard **injured in collision with heavy transport vehicle or bus in nontraffic accident**

V04.09 Pedestrian with other conveyance injured in collision with heavy transport vehicle or bus in nontraffic accident
Pedestrian with babystroller injured in collision with heavy transport vehicle or bus in nontraffic accident

---

Unspecified Code   Other Specified Code   Manifestation Code   N Newborn   P Pediatric   M Maternity   A Adult   ♂ Male   ♀ Female
● New Code   ▲ Revised Code Title   ▶◀ Revised Text   *NOTES*   *INCLUDES*   *EXCLUDES 1* Not coded here   *EXCLUDES 2* Not included here
4th character required   5th character required   6th character required   7th character required
Extension 'X' Alert   HAC Hospital-acquired condition (HAC) alert   AHA AHA Coding Clinic©

Pedestrian on ice-skates injured in collision with heavy transport vehicle or bus in nontraffic accident
Pedestrian on nonmotorized scooter injured in collision with heavy transport vehicle or bus in nontraffic accident
Pedestrian on sled injured in collision with heavy transport vehicle or bus in nontraffic accident
Pedestrian on snowboard injured in collision with heavy transport vehicle or bus in nontraffic accident
Pedestrian on snow-skis injured in collision with heavy transport vehicle or bus in nontraffic accident
Pedestrian in wheelchair (powered) injured in collision with heavy transport vehicle or bus in nontraffic accident
Pedestrian in motorized mobility scooter injured in collision with heavy transport vehicle or bus in nontraffic accident

- **V04.1 Pedestrian injured in collision with heavy transport vehicle or bus** in traffic accident
  - **V04.10 Pedestrian** on foot **injured in collision with heavy transport vehicle or bus in traffic accident**
    Pedestrian NOS injured in collision with heavy transport vehicle or bus in traffic accident
  - **V04.11 Pedestrian** on roller-skates **injured in collision with heavy transport vehicle or bus in traffic accident**
  - **V04.12 Pedestrian** on skateboard **injured in collision with heavy transport vehicle or bus in traffic accident**
  - **V04.19 Pedestrian with other conveyance injured in collision with heavy transport vehicle or bus in traffic accident**
    Pedestrian with babystroller injured in collision with heavy transport vehicle or bus in traffic accident
    Pedestrian on ice-skates injured in collision with heavy transport vehicle or bus in traffic accident
    Pedestrian on nonmotorized scooter injured in collision with heavy transport vehicle or bus in traffic accident
    Pedestrian on sled injured in collision with heavy transport vehicle or bus in traffic accident
    Pedestrian on snowboard injured in collision with heavy transport vehicle or bus in traffic accident
    Pedestrian on snow-skis injured in collision with heavy transport vehicle or bus in traffic accident
    Pedestrian in wheelchair (powered) injured in collision with heavy transport vehicle or bus in traffic accident
    Pedestrian in motorized mobility scooter injured in collision with heavy transport vehicle or bus in traffic accident

- **V04.9 Pedestrian injured in collision with heavy transport vehicle or bus,** unspecified whether traffic or nontraffic accident
  - **V04.90 Pedestrian on foot injured in collision with heavy transport vehicle or bus, unspecified whether traffic or nontraffic accident**
    Pedestrian NOS injured in collision with heavy transport vehicle or bus, unspecified whether traffic or nontraffic accident
  - **V04.91 Pedestrian on roller-skates injured in collision with heavy transport vehicle or bus, unspecified whether traffic or nontraffic accident**
  - **V04.92 Pedestrian on skateboard injured in collision with heavy transport vehicle or bus, unspecified whether traffic or nontraffic accident**
  - **V04.99 Pedestrian with other conveyance injured in collision with heavy transport vehicle or bus, unspecified whether traffic or nontraffic accident**
    Pedestrian with babystroller injured in collision with heavy transport vehicle or bus, unspecified whether traffic or nontraffic accident
    Pedestrian on ice-skates injured in collision with heavy transport vehicle or bus, unspecified whether traffic or nontraffic accident
    Pedestrian on nonmotorized scooter injured in collision with heavy transport vehicle or bus, unspecified whether traffic or nontraffic accident

Pedestrian on sled injured in collision with heavy transport vehicle or bus, unspecified whether traffic or nontraffic accident
Pedestrian on snowboard injured in collision with heavy transport vehicle or bus, unspecified whether traffic or nontraffic accident
Pedestrian on snow-skis injured in collision with heavy transport vehicle or bus, unspecified whether traffic or nontraffic accident
Pedestrian in wheelchair (powered) injured in collision with heavy transport vehicle or bus, unspecified whether traffic or nontraffic accident
Pedestrian in motorized mobility scooter injured in collision with heavy transport vehicle or bus, unspecified whether traffic or nontraffic accident

- **V05 Pedestrian injured in collision** with railway train or railway vehicle
  The appropriate 7th character is to be added to each code from category V05
  - **A = initial encounter**
  - **D = subsequent encounter**
  - **S = sequela**
  - **V05.0 Pedestrian injured in collision with railway train or railway vehicle** in nontraffic accident
    - **V05.00 Pedestrian** on foot **injured in collision with railway train or railway vehicle in nontraffic accident**
      Pedestrian NOS injured in collision with railway train or railway vehicle in nontraffic accident
    - **V05.01 Pedestrian** on roller-skates **injured in collision with railway train or railway vehicle in nontraffic accident**
    - **V05.02 Pedestrian** on skateboard **injured in collision with railway train or railway vehicle in nontraffic accident**
    - **V05.09 Pedestrian with other conveyance injured in collision with railway train or railway vehicle in nontraffic accident**
      Pedestrian with babystroller injured in collision with railway train or railway vehicle in nontraffic accident
      Pedestrian on ice-skates injured in collision with railway train or railway vehicle in nontraffic accident
      Pedestrian on nonmotorized scooter injured in collision with railway train or railway vehicle in nontraffic accident
      Pedestrian on sled injured in collision with railway train or railway vehicle in nontraffic accident
      Pedestrian on snowboard injured in collision with railway train or railway vehicle in nontraffic accident
      Pedestrian on snow-skis injured in collision with railway train or railway vehicle in nontraffic accident
      Pedestrian in wheelchair (powered) injured in collision with railway train or railway vehicle in nontraffic accident
      Pedestrian in motorized mobility scooter injured in collision with railway train or railway vehicle in nontraffic accident
  - **V05.1 Pedestrian injured in collision with railway train or railway vehicle** in traffic accident
    - **V05.10 Pedestrian** on foot **injured in collision with railway train or railway vehicle in traffic accident**
      Pedestrian NOS injured in collision with railway train or railway vehicle in traffic accident
    - **V05.11 Pedestrian** on roller-skates **injured in collision with railway train or railway vehicle in traffic accident**
    - **V05.12 Pedestrian** on skateboard **injured in collision with railway train or railway vehicle in traffic accident**
    - **V05.19 Pedestrian with other conveyance injured in collision with railway train or railway vehicle in traffic accident**
      Pedestrian with babystroller injured in collision with railway train or railway vehicle in traffic accident
      Pedestrian on ice-skates injured in collision with railway train or railway vehicle in traffic accident

---

pᵒᵃ Unacceptable principal diagnosis symbol per Medicare code edits ⬚ Code exempt from diagnosis present on admission requirement
❓ Questionable admission ᶜᶜ Complication or comorbidity ᴄᴄ.ᴍᴄᴄ ᴇˣᶜ CC/MCC exclusion ᴹᶜᶜ Major complication or comorbidity
Principal diagnosis as its own CC Principal diagnosis as its own MCC HCC HCC diagnosis code RxHCC RxHCC diagnosis code
MACRA code Z1 Z code as first-listed diagnosis

1188

When symbols appear on a code that requires a 7th character extension, refer to Appendix B to identify applicable 7th character codes.

2018 ICD-10-CM

Pedestrian on nonmotorized scooter injured in collision with railway train or railway vehicle in traffic accident

Pedestrian on sled injured in collision with railway train or railway vehicle in traffic accident

Pedestrian on snowboard injured in collision with railway train or railway vehicle in traffic accident

Pedestrian on snow-skis injured in collision with railway train or railway vehicle in traffic accident

Pedestrian in wheelchair (powered) injured in collision with railway train or railway vehicle in traffic accident

Pedestrian in motorized mobility scooter injured in collision with railway train or railway vehicle in traffic accident

V05.9 **Pedestrian injured in collision with railway train or railway vehicle,** unspecified whether traffic or nontraffic accident

V05.90 **Pedestrian on foot injured in collision with railway train or railway vehicle, unspecified whether traffic or nontraffic accident** POA

Pedestrian NOS injured in collision with railway train or railway vehicle, unspecified whether traffic or nontraffic accident

V05.91 **Pedestrian on roller-skates injured in collision with railway train or railway vehicle, unspecified whether traffic or nontraffic accident** POA

V05.92 **Pedestrian on skateboard injured in collision with railway train or railway vehicle, unspecified whether traffic or nontraffic accident** POA

V05.99 **Pedestrian with other conveyance injured in collision with railway train or railway vehicle, unspecified whether traffic or nontraffic accident** POA

Pedestrian with babystroller injured in collision with railway train or railway vehicle, unspecified whether traffic or nontraffic

Pedestrian on ice-skates injured in collision with railway train or railway vehicle, unspecified whether traffic or nontraffic

Pedestrian on nonmotorized scooter injured in collision with railway train or railway vehicle, unspecified whether traffic or nontraffic

Pedestrian on sled injured in collision with railway train or railway vehicle, unspecified whether traffic or nontraffic

Pedestrian on snowboard injured in collision with railway train or railway vehicle, unspecified whether traffic or nontraffic

Pedestrian on snow-skis injured in collision with railway train or railway vehicle, unspecified whether traffic or nontraffic

Pedestrian in wheelchair (powered) injured in collision with railway train or railway vehicle, unspecified whether traffic or nontraffic

Pedestrian in motorized mobility scooter injured in collision with railway train or railway vehicle, unspecified whether traffic or nontraffic

V06 **Pedestrian injured in collision** with other nonmotor vehicle

INCLUDES collision with animal-drawn vehicle, animal being ridden, nonpowered streetcar

EXCLUDES1 pedestrian injured in collision with pedestrian conveyance (V00.0-)

The appropriate 7th character is to be added to each code from category V06

A = initial encounter

D = subsequent encounter

S = sequela

V06.0 **Pedestrian injured in collision with other nonmotor vehicle** in nontraffic accident

V06.00 **Pedestrian on foot injured in collision with other nonmotor vehicle in nontraffic accident** POA

Pedestrian NOS injured in collision with other nonmotor vehicle in nontraffic accident

V06.01 **Pedestrian on roller-skates injured in collision with other nonmotor vehicle in nontraffic accident** POA

V06.02 **Pedestrian on skateboard injured in collision with other nonmotor vehicle in nontraffic accident** POA

V06.09 **Pedestrian with other conveyance injured in collision with other nonmotor vehicle in nontraffic accident** POA

Pedestrian with babystroller injured in collision with other nonmotor vehicle in nontraffic accident

Pedestrian on ice-skates injured in collision with other nonmotor vehicle in nontraffic accident

Pedestrian on nonmotorized scooter injured in collision with other nonmotor vehicle in nontraffic accident

Pedestrian on sled injured in collision with other nonmotor vehicle in nontraffic accident

Pedestrian on snowboard injured in collision with other nonmotor vehicle in nontraffic accident

Pedestrian on snow-skis injured in collision with other nonmotor vehicle in nontraffic accident

Pedestrian in wheelchair (powered) injured in collision with other nonmotor vehicle in nontraffic accident

Pedestrian in motorized mobility scooter injured in collision with other nonmotor vehicle in nontraffic accident

V06.1 **Pedestrian injured in collision with other nonmotor vehicle** in traffic accident

V06.10 **Pedestrian on foot injured in collision with other nonmotor vehicle in traffic accident** POA

Pedestrian NOS injured in collision with other nonmotor vehicle in traffic accident

V06.11 **Pedestrian on roller-skates injured in collision with other nonmotor vehicle in traffic accident** POA

V06.12 **Pedestrian on skateboard injured in collision with other nonmotor vehicle in traffic accident** POA

V06.19 **Pedestrian with other conveyance injured in collision with other nonmotor vehicle in traffic accident** POA

Pedestrian with babystroller injured in collision with other nonmotor vehicle in nontraffic accident

Pedestrian on ice-skates injured in collision with other nonmotor vehicle in traffic accident

Pedestrian on nonmotorized scooter injured in collision with other nonmotor vehicle in traffic accident

Pedestrian on sled injured in collision with other nonmotor vehicle in traffic accident

Pedestrian on snowboard injured in collision with other nonmotor vehicle in traffic accident

Pedestrian on snow-skis injured in collision with other nonmotor vehicle in traffic accident

Pedestrian in wheelchair (powered) injured in collision with other nonmotor vehicle in traffic accident

Pedestrian in motorized mobility scooter injured in collision with other nonmotor vehicle in traffic accident

V06.9 **Pedestrian injured in collision with other nonmotor vehicle,** unspecified whether traffic or nontraffic accident

V06.90 **Pedestrian on foot injured in collision with other nonmotor vehicle, unspecified whether traffic or nontraffic accident** POA

Pedestrian NOS injured in collision with other nonmotor vehicle, unspecified whether traffic or nontraffic accident

V06.91 **Pedestrian on roller-skates injured in collision with other nonmotor vehicle, unspecified whether traffic or nontraffic accident** POA

V06.92 **Pedestrian on skateboard injured in collision with other nonmotor vehicle, unspecified whether traffic or nontraffic accident** POA

V06.99 **Pedestrian with other conveyance injured in collision with other nonmotor vehicle, unspecified whether traffic or nontraffic accident** POA

Pedestrian with babystroller injured in collision with other nonmotor vehicle, unspecified whether traffic or nontraffic accident

---

Unspecified Code   Other Specified Code   Manifestation Code   N Newborn   P Pediatric   M Maternity   A Adult   ♂ Male   ♀ Female
● New Code   ▲ Revised Code Title   ▶◀ Revised Text   NOTES   INCLUDES   EXCLUDES 1 Not coded here   EXCLUDES 2 Not included here
4th character required   5th character required   6th character required   7th character required
Extension 'X' Alert   HAC Hospital-acquired condition (HAC) alert   AHA AHA Coding Clinic©

Pedestrian on ice-skates injured in collision with other nonmotor vehicle, unspecified whether traffic or nontraffic accident

Pedestrian on nonmotorized scooter injured in collision with other nonmotor vehicle, unspecified whether traffic or nontraffic accident

Pedestrian on sled injured in collision with other nonmotor vehicle, unspecified whether traffic or nontraffic accident

Pedestrian on snowboard injured in collision with other nonmotor vehicle, unspecified whether traffic or nontraffic accident

Pedestrian on snow-skis injured in collision with other nonmotor vehicle, unspecified whether traffic or nontraffic accident

Pedestrian in wheelchair (powered) injured in collision with other nonmotor vehicle, unspecified whether traffic or nontraffic accident

Pedestrian in motorized mobility scooter injured in collision with other nonmotor vehicle, unspecified whether traffic or nontraffic accident

● V09 **Pedestrian injured in** other and unspecified transport accidents

The appropriate 7th character is to be added to each code from category V09
- A = initial encounter
- D = subsequent encounter
- S = sequela

● V09.0 **Pedestrian injured** in nontraffic accident **involving other and unspecified motor vehicles**

○ V09.00 **Pedestrian injured in nontraffic accident involving unspecified motor vehicles**

○ V09.01 **Pedestrian injured in nontraffic accident involving** military **vehicle**

○ V09.09 **Pedestrian injured in nontraffic accident involving other motor vehicles**

Pedestrian injured in nontraffic accident by special vehicle

○ V09.1 **Pedestrian injured in unspecified nontraffic accident**

● V09.2 **Pedestrian injured** in traffic accident **involving other and unspecified motor vehicles**

○ V09.20 **Pedestrian injured in traffic accident involving unspecified motor vehicles**

○ V09.21 **Pedestrian injured in traffic accident involving** military **vehicle**

○ V09.29 **Pedestrian injured in traffic accident involving other motor vehicles**

○ V09.3 **Pedestrian injured in unspecified traffic accident**

○ V09.9 **Pedestrian injured in unspecified transport accident**

Pedal cycle rider injured in transport accident (V10-V19)

INCLUDES any non-motorized vehicle, excluding an animal-drawn vehicle, or a sidecar or trailer attached to the pedal cycle

EXCLUDES2 rupture of pedal cycle tire (W37.0)

● V10 **Pedal cycle rider injured in collision with pedestrian or animal**

EXCLUDES1 pedal cycle rider collision with animal-drawn vehicle or animal being ridden (V16.-)

The appropriate 7th character is to be added to each code from category V10
- A = initial encounter
- D = subsequent encounter
- S = sequela

○ V10.0 **Pedal cycle** driver **injured in collision with pedestrian or animal** in nontraffic accident

○ V10.1 **Pedal cycle** passenger **injured in collision with pedestrian or animal** in nontraffic accident

○ V10.2 **Unspecified pedal cyclist injured in collision with pedestrian or animal in nontraffic accident**

○ V10.3 Person boarding or alighting **a pedal cycle injured in collision with pedestrian or animal**

○ V10.4 **Pedal cycle** driver **injured in collision with pedestrian or animal** in traffic accident

○ V10.5 **Pedal cycle** passenger **injured in collision with pedestrian or animal** in traffic accident

○ V10.9 **Unspecified pedal cyclist injured in collision with pedestrian or animal in traffic accident**

● V11 **Pedal cycle rider injured in** collision with other pedal cycle

The appropriate 7th character is to be added to each code from category V11
- A = initial encounter
- D = subsequent encounter
- S = sequela

○ V11.0 **Pedal cycle driver injured in collision with other pedal cycle in nontraffic accident**

○ V11.1 **Pedal cycle passenger injured in collision with other pedal cycle in nontraffic accident**

○ V11.2 **Unspecified pedal cyclist injured in collision with other pedal cycle in nontraffic accident**

○ V11.3 **Person boarding or alighting a pedal cycle injured in collision with other pedal cycle**

○ V11.4 **Pedal cycle driver injured in collision with other pedal cycle in traffic accident**

○ V11.5 **Pedal cycle passenger injured in collision with other pedal cycle in traffic accident**

○ V11.9 **Unspecified pedal cyclist injured in collision with other pedal cycle in traffic accident**

● V12 **Pedal cycle rider injured in** collision with two- or three-wheeled motor vehicle

The appropriate 7th character is to be added to each code from category V12
- A = initial encounter
- D = subsequent encounter
- S = sequela

○ V12.0 **Pedal cycle** driver **injured in collision with two- or three-wheeled motor vehicle in** nontraffic accident

○ V12.1 **Pedal cycle** passenger **injured in collision with two- or three-wheeled motor vehicle in** nontraffic accident

○ V12.2 **Unspecified pedal cyclist injured in collision with two- or three-wheeled motor vehicle in nontraffic accident**

○ V12.3 Person boarding or alighting **a pedal cycle injured in collision with two- or three-wheeled motor vehicle**

○ V12.4 **Pedal cycle** driver **injured in collision with two- or three-wheeled motor vehicle in** traffic accident

○ V12.5 **Pedal cycle** passenger **injured in collision with two- or three-wheeled motor vehicle in** traffic accident

○ V12.9 **Unspecified pedal cyclist injured in collision with two- or three-wheeled motor vehicle in traffic accident**

● V13 **Pedal cycle rider injured in** collision with car, pick-up truck or van

The appropriate 7th character is to be added to each code from category V13
- A = initial encounter
- D = subsequent encounter
- S = sequela

○ V13.0 **Pedal cycle** driver **injured in collision with car, pick-up truck or van in** nontraffic accident

○ V13.1 **Pedal cycle** passenger **injured in collision with car, pick-up truck or van in** nontraffic accident

○ V13.2 **Unspecified pedal cyclist injured in collision with car, pick-up truck or van in nontraffic accident**

○ V13.3 Person boarding or alighting **a pedal cycle injured in collision with car, pick-up truck or van**

○ V13.4 **Pedal cycle** driver **injured in collision with car, pick-up truck or van in** traffic accident

○ V13.5 **Pedal cycle** passenger **injured in collision with car, pick-up truck or van in** traffic accident

○ V13.9 **Unspecified pedal cyclist injured in collision with car, pick-up truck or van in traffic accident**

● V14 **Pedal cycle rider injured in** collision with heavy transport vehicle or bus

EXCLUDES1 pedal cycle rider injured in collision with military vehicle (V19.81)

The appropriate 7th character is to be added to each code from category V14

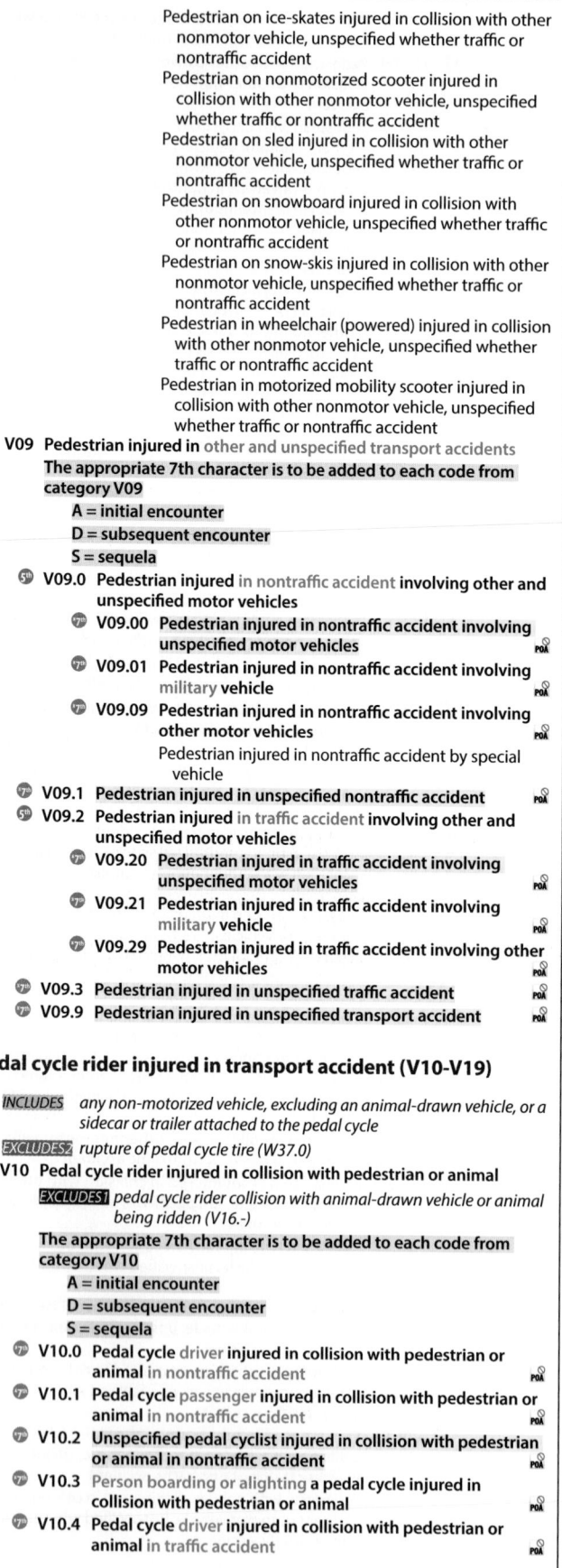

PDx Unacceptable principal diagnosis symbol per Medicare code edits   POA Code exempt from diagnosis present on admission requirement

❓ Questionable admission   CC Complication or comorbidity   CC-MCC Exc. CC/MCC exclusion   MCC Major complication or comorbidity

PDx CC Principal diagnosis as its own CC   PDx MCC Principal diagnosis as its own MCC   HCC HCC diagnosis code   RxHCC RxHCC diagnosis code

MACRA code   Z1 Z code as first-listed diagnosis

1190

When symbols appear on a code that requires a 7th character extension, refer to Appendix B to identify applicable 7th character codes.

2018 ICD-10-CM

A = initial encounter
D = subsequent encounter
S = sequela

V14.0 Pedal cycle driver injured in collision with heavy transport vehicle or bus in nontraffic accident POA

V14.1 Pedal cycle passenger injured in collision with heavy transport vehicle or bus in nontraffic accident POA

V14.2 Unspecified pedal cyclist injured in collision with heavy transport vehicle or bus in nontraffic accident POA

V14.3 Person boarding or alighting a pedal cycle injured in collision with heavy transport vehicle or bus POA

V14.4 Pedal cycle driver injured in collision with heavy transport vehicle or bus in traffic accident POA

V14.5 Pedal cycle passenger injured in collision with heavy transport vehicle or bus in traffic accident POA

V14.9 Unspecified pedal cyclist injured in collision with heavy transport vehicle or bus in traffic accident POA

V15 Pedal cycle rider injured in collision with railway train or railway vehicle

The appropriate 7th character is to be added to each code from category V15
A = initial encounter
D = subsequent encounter
S = sequela

V15.0 Pedal cycle driver injured in collision with railway train or railway vehicle in nontraffic accident POA

V15.1 Pedal cycle passenger injured in collision with railway train or railway vehicle in nontraffic accident POA

V15.2 Unspecified pedal cyclist injured in collision with railway train or railway vehicle in nontraffic accident POA

V15.3 Person boarding or alighting a pedal cycle injured in collision with railway train or railway vehicle POA

V15.4 Pedal cycle driver injured in collision with railway train or railway vehicle in traffic accident POA

V15.5 Pedal cycle passenger injured in collision with railway train or railway vehicle in traffic accident POA

V15.9 Unspecified pedal cyclist injured in collision with railway train or railway vehicle in traffic accident POA

V16 Pedal cycle rider injured in collision with other nonmotor vehicle
INCLUDES collision with animal-drawn vehicle, animal being ridden, streetcar

The appropriate 7th character is to be added to each code from category V16
A = initial encounter
D = subsequent encounter
S = sequela

V16.0 Pedal cycle driver injured in collision with other nonmotor vehicle in nontraffic accident POA

V16.1 Pedal cycle passenger injured in collision with other nonmotor vehicle in nontraffic accident POA

V16.2 Unspecified pedal cyclist injured in collision with other nonmotor vehicle in nontraffic accident POA

V16.3 Person boarding or alighting a pedal cycle injured in collision with other nonmotor vehicle in nontraffic accident POA

V16.4 Pedal cycle driver injured in collision with other nonmotor vehicle in traffic accident POA

V16.5 Pedal cycle passenger injured in collision with other nonmotor vehicle in traffic accident POA

V16.9 Unspecified pedal cyclist injured in collision with other nonmotor vehicle in traffic accident POA

V17 Pedal cycle rider injured in collision with fixed or stationary object

The appropriate 7th character is to be added to each code from category V17
A = initial encounter
D = subsequent encounter
S = sequela

V17.0 Pedal cycle driver injured in collision with fixed or stationary object in nontraffic accident POA

V17.1 Pedal cycle passenger injured in collision with fixed or stationary object in nontraffic accident

V17.2 Unspecified pedal cyclist injured in collision with fixed or stationary object in nontraffic accident POA

V17.3 Person boarding or alighting a pedal cycle injured in collision with fixed or stationary object POA

V17.4 Pedal cycle driver injured in collision with fixed or stationary object in traffic accident POA

V17.5 Pedal cycle passenger injured in collision with fixed or stationary object in traffic accident POA

V17.9 Unspecified pedal cyclist injured in collision with fixed or stationary object in traffic accident POA

V18 Pedal cycle rider injured in noncollision transport accident
INCLUDES fall or thrown from pedal cycle (without antecedent collision)
overturning pedal cycle NOS
overturning pedal cycle without collision

The appropriate 7th character is to be added to each code from category V18
A = initial encounter
D = subsequent encounter
S = sequela

V18.0 Pedal cycle driver injured in noncollision transport accident in nontraffic accident POA

V18.1 Pedal cycle passenger injured in noncollision transport accident in nontraffic accident POA

V18.2 Unspecified pedal cyclist injured in noncollision transport accident in nontraffic accident POA

V18.3 Person boarding or alighting a pedal cycle injured in noncollision transport accident POA

V18.4 Pedal cycle driver injured in noncollision transport accident in traffic accident POA

V18.5 Pedal cycle passenger injured in noncollision transport accident in traffic accident POA

V18.9 Unspecified pedal cyclist injured in noncollision transport accident in traffic accident POA

V19 Pedal cycle rider injured in other and unspecified transport accidents

The appropriate 7th character is to be added to each code from category V19
A = initial encounter
D = subsequent encounter
S = sequela

V19.0 Pedal cycle driver injured in collision with other and unspecified motor vehicles in nontraffic accident

V19.00 Pedal cycle driver injured in collision with unspecified motor vehicles in nontraffic accident POA

V19.09 Pedal cycle driver injured in collision with other motor vehicles in nontraffic accident POA

V19.1 Pedal cycle passenger injured in collision with other and unspecified motor vehicles in nontraffic accident

V19.10 Pedal cycle passenger injured in collision with unspecified motor vehicles in nontraffic accident POA

V19.19 Pedal cycle passenger injured in collision with other motor vehicles in nontraffic accident POA

V19.2 Unspecified pedal cyclist injured in collision with other and unspecified motor vehicles in nontraffic accident

V19.20 Unspecified pedal cyclist injured in collision with unspecified motor vehicles in nontraffic accident POA

Pedal cycle collision NOS, nontraffic

V19.29 Unspecified pedal cyclist injured in collision with other motor vehicles in nontraffic accident POA

V19.3 Pedal cyclist (driver) (passenger) injured in unspecified nontraffic accident POA

Pedal cycle accident NOS, nontraffic
Pedal cyclist injured in nontraffic accident NOS

V19.4 Pedal cycle driver injured in collision with other and unspecified motor vehicles in traffic accident

V19.40 Pedal cycle driver injured in collision with unspecified motor vehicles in traffic accident POA

V19.49 Pedal cycle driver injured in collision with other motor vehicles in traffic accident POA

V19.5 Pedal cycle passenger injured in collision with other and unspecified motor vehicles in traffic accident

---

Unspecified Code   Other Specified Code   Manifestation Code   N Newborn   P Pediatric   M Maternity   A Adult   ♂ Male   ♀ Female
● New Code   ▲ Revised Code Title   ▶◀ Revised Text   NOTES   INCLUDES   EXCLUDES 1 Not coded here   EXCLUDES 2 Not included here
4th character required   5th character required   6th character required   7th character required
Extension 'X' Alert   HAC Hospital-acquired condition (HAC) alert   AHA AHA Coding Clinic©

[7th] V19.50 Pedal cycle passenger injured in collision with unspecified motor vehicles in traffic accident [POA]

[7th] V19.59 Pedal cycle passenger injured in collision with other motor vehicles in traffic accident [POA]

[5th] V19.6 Unspecified pedal cyclist injured in collision with other and unspecified motor vehicles in traffic accident

[7th] V19.60 Unspecified pedal cyclist injured in collision with unspecified motor vehicles in traffic accident [POA]
Pedal cycle collision NOS (traffic)

[7th] V19.69 Unspecified pedal cyclist injured in collision with other motor vehicles in traffic accident [POA]

[5th] V19.8 Pedal cyclist (driver) (passenger) injured in other specified transport accidents

[7th] V19.81 Pedal cyclist (driver) (passenger) injured in transport accident with military vehicle [POA]

[7th] V19.88 Pedal cyclist (driver) (passenger) injured in other specified transport accidents [POA]

[7th] V19.9 Pedal cyclist (driver) (passenger) injured in unspecified traffic accident [POA]
Pedal cycle accident NOS

Motorcycle rider injured in transport accident (V20-V29)

INCLUDES *moped*
motorcycle with sidecar
motorized bicycle
motor scooter

EXCLUDES1 *three-wheeled motor vehicle (V30-V39)*

[4th] V20 Motorcycle rider injured in collision with pedestrian or animal

EXCLUDES1 *motorcycle rider collision with animal-drawn vehicle or animal being ridden (V26.-)*

The appropriate 7th character is to be added to each code from category V20
A = initial encounter
D = subsequent encounter
S = sequela

[7th] V20.0 Motorcycle driver injured in collision with pedestrian or animal in nontraffic accident [POA]

[7th] V20.1 Motorcycle passenger injured in collision with pedestrian or animal in nontraffic accident [POA]

[7th] V20.2 Unspecified motorcycle rider injured in collision with pedestrian or animal in nontraffic accident [POA]

[7th] V20.3 Person boarding or alighting a motorcycle injured in collision with pedestrian or animal [POA]

[7th] V20.4 Motorcycle driver injured in collision with pedestrian or animal in traffic accident [POA]

[7th] V20.5 Motorcycle passenger injured in collision with pedestrian or animal in traffic accident [POA]

[7th] V20.9 Unspecified motorcycle rider injured in collision with pedestrian or animal in traffic accident [POA]

[4th] V21 Motorcycle rider injured in collision with pedal cycle

The appropriate 7th character is to be added to each code from category V21
A = initial encounter
D = subsequent encounter
S = sequela

[7th] V21.0 Motorcycle driver injured in collision with pedal cycle in nontraffic accident [POA]

[7th] V21.1 Motorcycle passenger injured in collision with pedal cycle in nontraffic accident [POA]

[7th] V21.2 Unspecified motorcycle rider injured in collision with pedal cycle in nontraffic accident [POA]

[7th] V21.3 Person boarding or alighting a motorcycle injured in collision with pedal cycle [POA]

[7th] V21.4 Motorcycle driver injured in collision with pedal cycle in traffic accident [POA]

[7th] V21.5 Motorcycle passenger injured in collision with pedal cycle in traffic accident [POA]

[7th] V21.9 Unspecified motorcycle rider injured in collision with pedal cycle in traffic accident [POA]

[4th] V22 Motorcycle rider injured in collision with two- or three-wheeled motor vehicle

The appropriate 7th character is to be added to each code from category V22
A = initial encounter
D = subsequent encounter
S = sequela

[7th] V22.0 Motorcycle driver injured in collision with two- or three-wheeled motor vehicle in nontraffic accident [POA]

[7th] V22.1 Motorcycle passenger injured in collision with two- or three-wheeled motor vehicle in nontraffic accident [POA]

[7th] V22.2 Unspecified motorcycle rider injured in collision with two- or three-wheeled motor vehicle in nontraffic accident [POA]

[7th] V22.3 Person boarding or alighting a motorcycle injured in collision with two- or three-wheeled motor vehicle [POA]

[7th] V22.4 Motorcycle driver injured in collision with two- or three-wheeled motor vehicle in traffic accident [POA]

[7th] V22.5 Motorcycle passenger injured in collision with two- or three-wheeled motor vehicle in traffic accident [POA]

[7th] V22.9 Unspecified motorcycle rider injured in collision with two- or three-wheeled motor vehicle in traffic accident [POA]

[4th] V23 Motorcycle rider injured in collision with car, pick-up truck or van

The appropriate 7th character is to be added to each code from category V23
A = initial encounter
D = subsequent encounter
S = sequela

[7th] V23.0 Motorcycle driver injured in collision with car, pick-up truck or van in nontraffic accident [POA]

[7th] V23.1 Motorcycle passenger injured in collision with car, pick-up truck or van in nontraffic accident [POA]

[7th] V23.2 Unspecified motorcycle rider injured in collision with car, pick-up truck or van in nontraffic accident [POA]

[7th] V23.3 Person boarding or alighting a motorcycle injured in collision with car, pick-up truck or van [POA]

[7th] V23.4 Motorcycle driver injured in collision with car, pick-up truck or van in traffic accident [POA]

[7th] V23.5 Motorcycle passenger injured in collision with car, pick-up truck or van in traffic accident [POA]

[7th] V23.9 Unspecified motorcycle rider injured in collision with car, pick-up truck or van in traffic accident [POA]

[4th] V24 Motorcycle rider injured in collision with heavy transport vehicle or bus

EXCLUDES1 *motorcycle rider injured in collision with military vehicle (V29.81)*

The appropriate 7th character is to be added to each code from category V24
A = initial encounter
D = subsequent encounter
S = sequela

[7th] V24.0 Motorcycle driver injured in collision with heavy transport vehicle or bus in nontraffic accident [POA]

[7th] V24.1 Motorcycle passenger injured in collision with heavy transport vehicle or bus in nontraffic accident [POA]

[7th] V24.2 Unspecified motorcycle rider injured in collision with heavy transport vehicle or bus in nontraffic accident [POA]

[7th] V24.3 Person boarding or alighting a motorcycle injured in collision with heavy transport vehicle or bus [POA]

[7th] V24.4 Motorcycle driver injured in collision with heavy transport vehicle or bus in traffic accident [POA]

[7th] V24.5 Motorcycle passenger injured in collision with heavy transport vehicle or bus in traffic accident [POA]

[7th] V24.9 Unspecified motorcycle rider injured in collision with heavy transport vehicle or bus in traffic accident [POA]

[4th] V25 Motorcycle rider injured in collision with railway train or railway vehicle

The appropriate 7th character is to be added to each code from category V25
A = initial encounter
D = subsequent encounter
S = sequela

[PDx] Unacceptable principal diagnosis symbol per Medicare code edits [POA] Code exempt from diagnosis present on admission requirement
[?] Questionable admission [CC] Complication or comorbidity [CC/MCC Exc] CC/MCC exclusion [MCC] Major complication or comorbidity
[PDx] Principal diagnosis as its own CC [PDx] Principal diagnosis as its own MCC [HCC] HCC diagnosis code [RxHCC] RxHCC diagnosis code
MACRA code [Z1] Z code as first-listed diagnosis

When symbols appear on a code that requires a 7th character extension, refer to Appendix B to identify applicable 7th character codes.

- [7th] V25.0 Motorcycle driver injured in collision with railway train or railway vehicle in nontraffic accident [POA]
- [7th] V25.1 Motorcycle passenger injured in collision with railway train or railway vehicle in nontraffic accident [POA]
- [7th] V25.2 Unspecified motorcycle rider injured in collision with railway train or railway vehicle in nontraffic accident [POA]
- [7th] V25.3 Person boarding or alighting a motorcycle injured in collision with railway train or railway vehicle [POA]
- [7th] V25.4 Motorcycle driver injured in collision with railway train or railway vehicle in traffic accident [POA]
- [7th] V25.5 Motorcycle passenger injured in collision with railway train or railway vehicle in traffic accident [POA]
- [7th] V25.9 Unspecified motorcycle rider injured in collision with railway train or railway vehicle in traffic accident [POA]

[4th] V26 Motorcycle rider injured in collision with other nonmotor vehicle

INCLUDES *collision with animal-drawn vehicle, animal being ridden, streetcar*

The appropriate 7th character is to be added to each code from category V26
- A = initial encounter
- D = subsequent encounter
- S = sequela

- [7th] V26.0 Motorcycle driver injured in collision with other nonmotor vehicle in nontraffic accident [POA]
- [7th] V26.1 Motorcycle passenger injured in collision with other nonmotor vehicle in nontraffic accident [POA]
- [7th] V26.2 Unspecified motorcycle rider injured in collision with other nonmotor vehicle in nontraffic accident [POA]
- [7th] V26.3 Person boarding or alighting a motorcycle injured in collision with other nonmotor vehicle [POA]
- [7th] V26.4 Motorcycle driver injured in collision with other nonmotor vehicle in traffic accident [POA]
- [7th] V26.5 Motorcycle passenger injured in collision with other nonmotor vehicle in traffic accident [POA]
- [7th] V26.9 Unspecified motorcycle rider injured in collision with other nonmotor vehicle in traffic accident [POA]

[4th] V27 Motorcycle rider injured in collision with fixed or stationary object

The appropriate 7th character is to be added to each code from category V27
- A = initial encounter
- D = subsequent encounter
- S = sequela

- [7th] V27.0 Motorcycle driver injured in collision with fixed or stationary object in nontraffic accident [POA]
- [7th] V27.1 Motorcycle passenger injured in collision with fixed or stationary object in nontraffic accident [POA]
- [7th] V27.2 Unspecified motorcycle rider injured in collision with fixed or stationary object in nontraffic accident [POA]
- [7th] V27.3 Person boarding or alighting a motorcycle injured in collision with fixed or stationary object [POA]
- [7th] V27.4 Motorcycle driver injured in collision with fixed or stationary object in traffic accident [POA]
- [7th] V27.5 Motorcycle passenger injured in collision with fixed or stationary object in traffic accident [POA]
- [7th] V27.9 Unspecified motorcycle rider injured in collision with fixed or stationary object in traffic accident [POA]

[4th] V28 Motorcycle rider injured in noncollision transport accident

INCLUDES *fall or thrown from motorcycle (without antecedent collision)*
overturning motorcycle NOS
overturning motorcycle without collision

The appropriate 7th character is to be added to each code from category V28
- A = initial encounter
- D = subsequent encounter
- S = sequela

- [7th] V28.0 Motorcycle driver injured in noncollision transport accident in nontraffic accident [POA]
- [7th] V28.1 Motorcycle passenger injured in noncollision transport accident in nontraffic accident [POA]
- [7th] V28.2 Unspecified motorcycle rider injured in noncollision transport accident in nontraffic accident [POA]
- [7th] V28.3 Person boarding or alighting a motorcycle injured in noncollision transport accident [POA]
- [7th] V28.4 Motorcycle driver injured in noncollision transport accident in traffic accident [POA]
- [7th] V28.5 Motorcycle passenger injured in noncollision transport accident in traffic accident [POA]
- [7th] V28.9 Unspecified motorcycle rider injured in noncollision transport accident in traffic accident [POA]

[4th] V29 Motorcycle rider injured in other and unspecified transport accidents

The appropriate 7th character is to be added to each code from category V29
- A = initial encounter
- D = subsequent encounter
- S = sequela

[5th] V29.0 Motorcycle driver injured in collision with other and unspecified motor vehicles in nontraffic accident
- [7th] V29.00 Motorcycle driver injured in collision with unspecified motor vehicles in nontraffic accident [POA]
- [7th] V29.09 Motorcycle driver injured in collision with other motor vehicles in nontraffic accident [POA]

[5th] V29.1 Motorcycle passenger injured in collision with other and unspecified motor vehicles in nontraffic accident
- [7th] V29.10 Motorcycle passenger injured in collision with unspecified motor vehicles in nontraffic accident [POA]
- [7th] V29.19 Motorcycle passenger injured in collision with other motor vehicles in nontraffic accident [POA]

[5th] V29.2 Unspecified motorcycle rider injured in collision with other and unspecified motor vehicles in nontraffic accident
- [7th] V29.20 Unspecified motorcycle rider injured in collision with unspecified motor vehicles in nontraffic accident [POA]
  Motorcycle collision NOS, nontraffic
- [7th] V29.29 Unspecified motorcycle rider injured in collision with other motor vehicles in nontraffic accident [POA]

[7th] V29.3 Motorcycle rider (driver) (passenger) injured in unspecified nontraffic accident [POA]
Motorcycle accident NOS, nontraffic
Motorcycle rider injured in nontraffic accident NOS

[5th] V29.4 Motorcycle driver injured in collision with other and unspecified motor vehicles in traffic accident
- [7th] V29.40 Motorcycle driver injured in collision with unspecified motor vehicles in traffic accident [POA]
- [7th] V29.49 Motorcycle driver injured in collision with other motor vehicles in traffic accident [POA]

[5th] V29.5 Motorcycle passenger injured in collision with other and unspecified motor vehicles in traffic accident
- [7th] V29.50 Motorcycle passenger injured in collision with unspecified motor vehicles in traffic accident [POA]
- [7th] V29.59 Motorcycle passenger injured in collision with other motor vehicles in traffic accident [POA]

[5th] V29.6 Unspecified motorcycle rider injured in collision with other and unspecified motor vehicles in traffic accident
- [7th] V29.60 Unspecified motorcycle rider injured in collision with unspecified motor vehicles in traffic accident [POA]
  Motorcycle collision NOS (traffic)
- [7th] V29.69 Unspecified motorcycle rider injured in collision with other motor vehicles in traffic accident [POA]

[5th] V29.8 Motorcycle rider (driver) (passenger) injured in other specified transport accidents
- [7th] V29.81 Motorcycle rider (driver) (passenger) injured in transport accident with military vehicle [POA]
- [7th] V29.88 Motorcycle rider (driver) (passenger) injured in other specified transport accidents [POA]

[7th] V29.9 Motorcycle rider (driver) (passenger) injured in unspecified traffic accident [POA]
Motorcycle accident NOS

Unspecified Code Other Specified Code Manifestation Code [N] Newborn [P] Pediatric [M] Maternity [A] Adult ♂ Male ♀ Female
● New Code ▲ Revised Code Title ▶◀ Revised Text NOTES INCLUDES EXCLUDES1 Not coded here EXCLUDES2 Not included here
[4th] 4th character required [5th] 5th character required [6th] 6th character required [7th] 7th character required
[x7th] Extension 'X' Alert [HAC] Hospital-acquired condition (HAC) alert AHA AHA Coding Clinic©

When symbols appear on a code that requires a 7th character extension, refer to Appendix B to identify applicable 7th character codes.

Occupant of three-wheeled motor vehicle injured in transport accident (V30-V39)

INCLUDES   motorized tricycle
             motorized rickshaw
             three-wheeled motor car

EXCLUDES1   all-terrain vehicles (V86.-)
             motorcycle with sidecar (V20-V29)
             vehicle designed primarily for off-road use (V86.-)

🔵 V30 Occupant of three-wheeled motor vehicle injured in collision with pedestrian or animal

EXCLUDES1 three-wheeled motor vehicle collision with animal-drawn vehicle or animal being ridden (V36.-)

The appropriate 7th character is to be added to each code from category V30

A = initial encounter
D = subsequent encounter
S = sequela

V30.0 Driver of three-wheeled motor vehicle injured in collision with pedestrian or animal in nontraffic accident POA

V30.1 Passenger in three-wheeled motor vehicle injured in collision with pedestrian or animal in nontraffic accident POA

V30.2 Person on outside of three-wheeled motor vehicle injured in collision with pedestrian or animal in nontraffic accident POA

V30.3 Unspecified occupant of three-wheeled motor vehicle injured in collision with pedestrian or animal in nontraffic accident POA

V30.4 Person boarding or alighting a three-wheeled motor vehicle injured in collision with pedestrian or animal POA

V30.5 Driver of three-wheeled motor vehicle injured in collision with pedestrian or animal in traffic accident POA

V30.6 Passenger in three-wheeled motor vehicle injured in collision with pedestrian or animal in traffic accident POA

V30.7 Person on outside of three-wheeled motor vehicle injured in collision with pedestrian or animal in traffic accident POA

V30.9 Unspecified occupant of three-wheeled motor vehicle injured in collision with pedestrian or animal in traffic accident POA

🔵 V31 Occupant of three-wheeled motor vehicle injured in collision with pedal cycle

The appropriate 7th character is to be added to each code from category V31

A = initial encounter
D = subsequent encounter
S = sequela

V31.0 Driver of three-wheeled motor vehicle injured in collision with pedal cycle in nontraffic accident POA

V31.1 Passenger in three-wheeled motor vehicle injured in collision with pedal cycle in nontraffic accident POA

V31.2 Person on outside of three-wheeled motor vehicle injured in collision with pedal cycle in nontraffic accident POA

V31.3 Unspecified occupant of three-wheeled motor vehicle injured in collision with pedal cycle in nontraffic accident POA

V31.4 Person boarding or alighting a three-wheeled motor vehicle injured in collision with pedal cycle POA

V31.5 Driver of three-wheeled motor vehicle injured in collision with pedal cycle in traffic accident POA

V31.6 Passenger in three-wheeled motor vehicle injured in collision with pedal cycle in traffic accident POA

V31.7 Person on outside of three-wheeled motor vehicle injured in collision with pedal cycle in traffic accident POA

V31.9 Unspecified occupant of three-wheeled motor vehicle injured in collision with pedal cycle in traffic accident POA

🔵 V32 Occupant of three-wheeled motor vehicle injured in collision with two- or three-wheeled motor vehicle

The appropriate 7th character is to be added to each code from category V32

A = initial encounter
D = subsequent encounter
S = sequela

V32.0 Driver of three-wheeled motor vehicle injured in collision with two- or three-wheeled motor vehicle in nontraffic accident POA

V32.1 Passenger in three-wheeled motor vehicle injured in collision with two- or three-wheeled motor vehicle in nontraffic accident POA

V32.2 Person on outside of three-wheeled motor vehicle injured in collision with two- or three-wheeled motor vehicle in nontraffic accident POA

V32.3 Unspecified occupant of three-wheeled motor vehicle injured in collision with two- or three-wheeled motor vehicle in nontraffic accident POA

V32.4 Person boarding or alighting a three-wheeled motor vehicle injured in collision with two- or three-wheeled motor vehicle POA

V32.5 Driver of three-wheeled motor vehicle injured in collision with two- or three-wheeled motor vehicle in traffic accident POA

V32.6 Passenger in three-wheeled motor vehicle injured in collision with two- or three-wheeled motor vehicle in traffic accident POA

V32.7 Person on outside of three-wheeled motor vehicle injured in collision with two- or three-wheeled motor vehicle in traffic accident POA

V32.9 Unspecified occupant of three-wheeled motor vehicle injured in collision with two- or three-wheeled motor vehicle in traffic accident POA

🔵 V33 Occupant of three-wheeled motor vehicle injured in collision with car, pick-up truck or van

The appropriate 7th character is to be added to each code from category V33

A = initial encounter
D = subsequent encounter
S = sequela

V33.0 Driver of three-wheeled motor vehicle injured in collision with car, pick-up truck or van in nontraffic accident POA

V33.1 Passenger in three-wheeled motor vehicle injured in collision with car, pick-up truck or van in nontraffic accident POA

V33.2 Person on outside of three-wheeled motor vehicle injured in collision with car, pick-up truck or van in nontraffic accident POA

V33.3 Unspecified occupant of three-wheeled motor vehicle injured in collision with car, pick-up truck or van in nontraffic accident POA

V33.4 Person boarding or alighting a three-wheeled motor vehicle injured in collision with car, pick-up truck or van POA

V33.5 Driver of three-wheeled motor vehicle injured in collision with car, pick-up truck or van in traffic accident POA

V33.6 Passenger in three-wheeled motor vehicle injured in collision with car, pick-up truck or van in traffic accident POA

V33.7 Person on outside of three-wheeled motor vehicle injured in collision with car, pick-up truck or van in traffic accident POA

V33.9 Unspecified occupant of three-wheeled motor vehicle injured in collision with car, pick-up truck or van in traffic accident POA

🔵 V34 Occupant of three-wheeled motor vehicle injured in collision with heavy transport vehicle or bus

EXCLUDES1 occupant of three-wheeled motor vehicle injured in collision with military vehicle (V39.81)

The appropriate 7th character is to be added to each code from category V34

A = initial encounter
D = subsequent encounter
S = sequela

V34.0 Driver of three-wheeled motor vehicle injured in collision with heavy transport vehicle or bus in nontraffic accident POA

V34.1 Passenger in three-wheeled motor vehicle injured in collision with heavy transport vehicle or bus in nontraffic accident POA

POA Unacceptable principal diagnosis symbol per Medicare code edits   POA Code exempt from diagnosis present on admission requirement
❓ Questionable admission   CC Complication or comorbidity   CC-MCC Excl CC/MCC exclusion   MCC Major complication or comorbidity
PDx CC Principal diagnosis as its own CC   PDx MCC Principal diagnosis as its own MCC   HCC HCC diagnosis code   RxHCC RxHCC diagnosis code
MACRA code   Z1 Z code as first-listed diagnosis

V34.2 Person on outside of three-wheeled motor vehicle injured in collision with heavy transport vehicle or bus in nontraffic accident

V34.3 Unspecified occupant of three-wheeled motor vehicle injured in collision with heavy transport vehicle or bus in nontraffic accident

V34.4 Person boarding or alighting a three-wheeled motor vehicle injured in collision with heavy transport vehicle or bus

V34.5 Driver of three-wheeled motor vehicle injured in collision with heavy transport vehicle or bus in traffic accident

V34.6 Passenger in three-wheeled motor vehicle injured in collision with heavy transport vehicle or bus in traffic accident

V34.7 Person on outside of three-wheeled motor vehicle injured in collision with heavy transport vehicle or bus in traffic accident

V34.9 Unspecified occupant of three-wheeled motor vehicle injured in collision with heavy transport vehicle or bus in traffic accident

V35 Occupant of three-wheeled motor vehicle injured in collision with railway train or railway vehicle

The appropriate 7th character is to be added to each code from category V35
  A = initial encounter
  D = subsequent encounter
  S = sequela

V35.0 Driver of three-wheeled motor vehicle injured in collision with railway train or railway vehicle in nontraffic accident

V35.1 Passenger in three-wheeled motor vehicle injured in collision with railway train or railway vehicle in nontraffic accident

V35.2 Person on outside of three-wheeled motor vehicle injured in collision with railway train or railway vehicle in nontraffic accident

V35.3 Unspecified occupant of three-wheeled motor vehicle injured in collision with railway train or railway vehicle in nontraffic accident

V35.4 Person boarding or alighting a three-wheeled motor vehicle injured in collision with railway train or railway vehicle

V35.5 Driver of three-wheeled motor vehicle injured in collision with railway train or railway vehicle in traffic accident

V35.6 Passenger in three-wheeled motor vehicle injured in collision with railway train or railway vehicle in traffic accident

V35.7 Person on outside of three-wheeled motor vehicle injured in collision with railway train or railway vehicle in traffic accident

V35.9 Unspecified occupant of three-wheeled motor vehicle injured in collision with railway train or railway vehicle in traffic accident

V36 Occupant of three-wheeled motor vehicle injured in collision with other nonmotor vehicle

INCLUDES collision with animal-drawn vehicle, animal being ridden, streetcar

The appropriate 7th character is to be added to each code from category V36
  A = initial encounter
  D = subsequent encounter
  S = sequela

V36.0 Driver of three-wheeled motor vehicle injured in collision with other nonmotor vehicle in nontraffic accident

V36.1 Passenger in three-wheeled motor vehicle injured in collision with other nonmotor vehicle in nontraffic accident

V36.2 Person on outside of three-wheeled motor vehicle injured in collision with other nonmotor vehicle in nontraffic accident

V36.3 Unspecified occupant of three-wheeled motor vehicle injured in collision with other nonmotor vehicle in nontraffic accident

V36.4 Person boarding or alighting a three-wheeled motor vehicle injured in collision with other nonmotor vehicle

V36.5 Driver of three-wheeled motor vehicle injured in collision with other nonmotor vehicle in traffic accident

V36.6 Passenger in three-wheeled motor vehicle injured in collision with other nonmotor vehicle in traffic accident

V36.7 Person on outside of three-wheeled motor vehicle injured in collision with other nonmotor vehicle in traffic accident

V36.9 Unspecified occupant of three-wheeled motor vehicle injured in collision with other nonmotor vehicle in traffic accident

V37 Occupant of three-wheeled motor vehicle injured in collision with fixed or stationary object

The appropriate 7th character is to be added to each code from category V37
  A = initial encounter
  D = subsequent encounter
  S = sequela

V37.0 Driver of three-wheeled motor vehicle injured in collision with fixed or stationary object in nontraffic accident

V37.1 Passenger in three-wheeled motor vehicle injured in collision with fixed or stationary object in nontraffic accident

V37.2 Person on outside of three-wheeled motor vehicle injured in collision with fixed or stationary object in nontraffic accident

V37.3 Unspecified occupant of three-wheeled motor vehicle injured in collision with fixed or stationary object in nontraffic accident

V37.4 Person boarding or alighting a three-wheeled motor vehicle injured in collision with fixed or stationary object

V37.5 Driver of three-wheeled motor vehicle injured in collision with fixed or stationary object in traffic accident

V37.6 Passenger in three-wheeled motor vehicle injured in collision with fixed or stationary object in traffic accident

V37.7 Person on outside of three-wheeled motor vehicle injured in collision with fixed or stationary object in traffic accident

V37.9 Unspecified occupant of three-wheeled motor vehicle injured in collision with fixed or stationary object in traffic accident

V38 Occupant of three-wheeled motor vehicle injured in noncollision transport accident

INCLUDES fall or thrown from three-wheeled motor vehicle
  overturning of three-wheeled motor vehicle NOS
  overturning of three-wheeled motor vehicle without collision

The appropriate 7th character is to be added to each code from category V38
  A = initial encounter
  D = subsequent encounter
  S = sequela

V38.0 Driver of three-wheeled motor vehicle injured in noncollision transport accident in nontraffic accident

V38.1 Passenger in three-wheeled motor vehicle injured in noncollision transport accident in nontraffic accident

V38.2 Person on outside of three-wheeled motor vehicle injured in noncollision transport accident in nontraffic accident

V38.3 Unspecified occupant of three-wheeled motor vehicle injured in noncollision transport accident in nontraffic accident

V38.4 Person boarding or alighting a three-wheeled motor vehicle injured in noncollision transport accident

V38.5 Driver of three-wheeled motor vehicle injured in noncollision transport accident in traffic accident

V38.6 Passenger in three-wheeled motor vehicle injured in noncollision transport accident in traffic accident

V38.7 Person on outside of three-wheeled motor vehicle injured in noncollision transport accident in traffic accident

V38.9 Unspecified occupant of three-wheeled motor vehicle injured in noncollision transport accident in traffic accident

V39 Occupant of three-wheeled motor vehicle injured in other and unspecified transport accidents

Unspecified Code   Other Specified Code   Manifestation Code   N Newborn   P Pediatric   M Maternity   A Adult   ♂ Male   ♀ Female
● New Code   ▲ Revised Code Title   ►◄ Revised Text   NOTES   INCLUDES   EXCLUDES 1 Not coded here   EXCLUDES 2 Not included here
4ᵗʰ character required   5ᵗʰ character required   6ᵗʰ character required   7ᵗʰ character required
Extension 'X' Alert   HAC Hospital-acquired condition (HAC) alert   AHA AHA Coding Clinic©

2018 ICD-10-CM   When symbols appear on a code that requires a 7th character extension, refer to Appendix B to identify applicable 7th character codes.   **1195**

The appropriate 7th character is to be added to each code from category V39

A = initial encounter

D = subsequent encounter

S = sequela

5ᵗʰ **V39.0** Driver of three-wheeled motor vehicle injured in collision with other and unspecified motor vehicles in nontraffic accident

7ᵗʰ **V39.00** Driver of three-wheeled motor vehicle injured in collision with unspecified motor vehicles in nontraffic accident ᴾᴼᴬ

7ᵗʰ **V39.09** Driver of three-wheeled motor vehicle injured in collision with other motor vehicles in nontraffic accident ᴾᴼᴬ

5ᵗʰ **V39.1** Passenger in three-wheeled motor vehicle injured in collision with other and unspecified motor vehicles in nontraffic accident

7ᵗʰ **V39.10** Passenger in three-wheeled motor vehicle injured in collision with unspecified motor vehicles in nontraffic accident ᴾᴼᴬ

7ᵗʰ **V39.19** Passenger in three-wheeled motor vehicle injured in collision with other motor vehicles in nontraffic accident ᴾᴼᴬ

5ᵗʰ **V39.2** Unspecified occupant of three-wheeled motor vehicle injured in collision with other and unspecified motor vehicles in nontraffic accident

7ᵗʰ **V39.20** Unspecified occupant of three-wheeled motor vehicle injured in collision with unspecified motor vehicles in nontraffic accident ᴾᴼᴬ

Collision NOS involving three-wheeled motor vehicle, nontraffic

7ᵗʰ **V39.29** Unspecified occupant of three-wheeled motor vehicle injured in collision with other motor vehicles in nontraffic accident ᴾᴼᴬ

7ᵗʰ **V39.3** Occupant (driver) (passenger) of three-wheeled motor vehicle injured in unspecified nontraffic accident ᴾᴼᴬ

Accident NOS involving three-wheeled motor vehicle, nontraffic

Occupant of three-wheeled motor vehicle injured in nontraffic accident NOS

5ᵗʰ **V39.4** Driver of three-wheeled motor vehicle injured in collision with other and unspecified motor vehicles in traffic accident

7ᵗʰ **V39.40** Driver of three-wheeled motor vehicle injured in collision with unspecified motor vehicles in traffic accident ᴾᴼᴬ

7ᵗʰ **V39.49** Driver of three-wheeled motor vehicle injured in collision with other motor vehicles in traffic accident ᴾᴼᴬ

5ᵗʰ **V39.5** Passenger in three-wheeled motor vehicle injured in collision with other and unspecified motor vehicles in traffic accident

7ᵗʰ **V39.50** Passenger in three-wheeled motor vehicle injured in collision with unspecified motor vehicles in traffic accident ᴾᴼᴬ

7ᵗʰ **V39.59** Passenger in three-wheeled motor vehicle injured in collision with other motor vehicles in traffic accident ᴾᴼᴬ

5ᵗʰ **V39.6** Unspecified occupant of three-wheeled motor vehicle injured in collision with other and unspecified motor vehicles in traffic accident

7ᵗʰ **V39.60** Unspecified occupant of three-wheeled motor vehicle injured in collision with unspecified motor vehicles in traffic accident ᴾᴼᴬ

Collision NOS involving three-wheeled motor vehicle (traffic)

7ᵗʰ **V39.69** Unspecified occupant of three-wheeled motor vehicle injured in collision with other motor vehicles in traffic accident ᴾᴼᴬ

5ᵗʰ **V39.8** Occupant (driver) (passenger) of three-wheeled motor vehicle injured in other specified transport accidents

7ᵗʰ **V39.81** Occupant (driver) (passenger) of three-wheeled motor vehicle injured in transport accident with military vehicle ᴾᴼᴬ

7ᵗʰ **V39.89** Occupant (driver) (passenger) of three-wheeled motor vehicle injured in other specified transport accidents ᴾᴼᴬ

7ᵗʰ **V39.9** Occupant (driver) (passenger) of three-wheeled motor vehicle injured in unspecified traffic accident ᴾᴼᴬ

Accident NOS involving three-wheeled motor vehicle

Car occupant injured in transport accident (V40-V49)

INCLUDES a four-wheeled motor vehicle designed primarily for carrying passengers

automobile (pulling a trailer or camper)

EXCLUDES1 bus (V50-V59)

minibus (V50-V59)

minivan (V50-V59)

motorcoach (V70-V79)

pick-up truck (V50-V59)

sport utility vehicle (SUV) (V50-V59)

4ᵗʰ **V40** Car occupant injured in collision with pedestrian or animal

EXCLUDES1 car collision with animal-drawn vehicle or animal being ridden (V46.-)

The appropriate 7th character is to be added to each code from category V40

A = initial encounter

D = subsequent encounter

S = sequela

7ᵗʰ **V40.0** Car driver injured in collision with pedestrian or animal in nontraffic accident ᴾᴼᴬ

7ᵗʰ **V40.1** Car passenger injured in collision with pedestrian or animal in nontraffic accident ᴾᴼᴬ

7ᵗʰ **V40.2** Person on outside of car injured in collision with pedestrian or animal in nontraffic accident ᴾᴼᴬ

7ᵗʰ **V40.3** Unspecified car occupant injured in collision with pedestrian or animal in nontraffic accident ᴾᴼᴬ

7ᵗʰ **V40.4** Person boarding or alighting a car injured in collision with pedestrian or animal ᴾᴼᴬ

7ᵗʰ **V40.5** Car driver injured in collision with pedestrian or animal in traffic accident ᴾᴼᴬ

7ᵗʰ **V40.6** Car passenger injured in collision with pedestrian or animal in traffic accident ᴾᴼᴬ

7ᵗʰ **V40.7** Person on outside of car injured in collision with pedestrian or animal in traffic accident ᴾᴼᴬ

7ᵗʰ **V40.9** Unspecified car occupant injured in collision with pedestrian or animal in traffic accident ᴾᴼᴬ

4ᵗʰ **V41** Car occupant injured in collision with pedal cycle

The appropriate 7th character is to be added to each code from category V41

A = initial encounter

D = subsequent encounter

S = sequela

7ᵗʰ **V41.0** Car driver injured in collision with pedal cycle in nontraffic accident ᴾᴼᴬ

7ᵗʰ **V41.1** Car passenger injured in collision with pedal cycle in nontraffic accident ᴾᴼᴬ

7ᵗʰ **V41.2** Person on outside of car injured in collision with pedal cycle in nontraffic accident ᴾᴼᴬ

7ᵗʰ **V41.3** Unspecified car occupant injured in collision with pedal cycle in nontraffic accident ᴾᴼᴬ

7ᵗʰ **V41.4** Person boarding or alighting a car injured in collision with pedal cycle ᴾᴼᴬ

7ᵗʰ **V41.5** Car driver injured in collision with pedal cycle in traffic accident ᴾᴼᴬ

7ᵗʰ **V41.6** Car passenger injured in collision with pedal cycle in traffic accident ᴾᴼᴬ

7ᵗʰ **V41.7** Person on outside of car injured in collision with pedal cycle in traffic accident ᴾᴼᴬ

7ᵗʰ **V41.9** Unspecified car occupant injured in collision with pedal cycle in traffic accident ᴾᴼᴬ

4ᵗʰ **V42** Car occupant injured in collision with two- or three-wheeled motor vehicle

ᴾᴼᴬ Unacceptable principal diagnosis symbol per Medicare code edits ⬡ Code exempt from diagnosis present on admission requirement

❓ Questionable admission ᶜᶜ Complication or comorbidity ᶜᶜ⁻ᴹᶜᶜ CC/MCC exclusion ᴹᶜᶜ Major complication or comorbidity

Principal diagnosis as its own CC Principal diagnosis as its own MCC ᴴᶜᶜ HCC diagnosis code ᴿˣᴴᶜᶜ RxHCC diagnosis code

MACRA code Z code as first-listed diagnosis

When symbols appear on a code that requires a 7th character extension, refer to Appendix B to identify applicable 7th character codes.

2018 ICD-10-CM

The appropriate 7th character is to be added to each code from category V42

A = initial encounter
D = subsequent encounter
S = sequela

- V42.0 Car driver injured in collision with two- or three-wheeled motor vehicle in nontraffic accident POA
- V42.1 Car passenger injured in collision with two- or three-wheeled motor vehicle in nontraffic accident POA
- V42.2 Person on outside of car injured in collision with two- or three-wheeled motor vehicle in nontraffic accident POA
- V42.3 Unspecified car occupant injured in collision with two- or three-wheeled motor vehicle in nontraffic accident POA
- V42.4 Person boarding or alighting a car injured in collision with two- or three-wheeled motor vehicle POA
- V42.5 Car driver injured in collision with two- or three-wheeled motor vehicle in traffic accident POA
- V42.6 Car passenger injured in collision with two- or three-wheeled motor vehicle in traffic accident POA
- V42.7 Person on outside of car injured in collision with two- or three-wheeled motor vehicle in traffic accident POA
- V42.9 Unspecified car occupant injured in collision with two- or three-wheeled motor vehicle in traffic accident POA

- V43 Car occupant injured in collision with car, pick-up truck or van

  The appropriate 7th character is to be added to each code from category V43

  A = initial encounter
  D = subsequent encounter
  S = sequela

  - V43.0 Car driver injured in collision with car, pick-up truck or van in nontraffic accident
    - V43.01 Car driver injured in collision with sport utility vehicle in nontraffic accident POA
    - V43.02 Car driver injured in collision with other type car in nontraffic accident POA
    - V43.03 Car driver injured in collision with pick-up truck in nontraffic accident POA
    - V43.04 Car driver injured in collision with van in nontraffic accident POA
  - V43.1 Car passenger injured in collision with car, pick-up truck or van in nontraffic accident
    - V43.11 Car passenger injured in collision with sport utility vehicle in nontraffic accident POA
    - V43.12 Car passenger injured in collision with other type car in nontraffic accident POA
    - V43.13 Car passenger injured in collision with pick-up in nontraffic accident POA
    - V43.14 Car passenger injured in collision with van in nontraffic accident POA
  - V43.2 Person on outside of car injured in collision with car, pick-up truck or van in nontraffic accident
    - V43.21 Person on outside of car injured in collision with sport utility vehicle in nontraffic accident POA
    - V43.22 Person on outside of car injured in collision with other type car in nontraffic accident POA
    - V43.23 Person on outside of car injured in collision with pick-up truck in nontraffic accident POA
    - V43.24 Person on outside of car injured in collision with van in nontraffic accident POA
  - V43.3 Unspecified car occupant injured in collision with car, pick-up truck or van in nontraffic accident
    - V43.31 Unspecified car occupant injured in collision with sport utility vehicle in nontraffic accident POA
    - V43.32 Unspecified car occupant injured in collision with other type car in nontraffic accident POA
    - V43.33 Unspecified car occupant injured in collision with pick-up truck in nontraffic accident POA
    - V43.34 Unspecified car occupant injured in collision with van in nontraffic accident POA
  - V43.4 Person boarding or alighting a car injured in collision with car, pick-up truck or van
    - V43.41 Person boarding or alighting a car injured in collision with sport utility vehicle POA
    - V43.42 Person boarding or alighting a car injured in collision with other type car POA
    - V43.43 Person boarding or alighting a car injured in collision with pick-up truck POA
    - V43.44 Person boarding or alighting a car injured in collision with van POA
  - V43.5 Car driver injured in collision with car, pick-up truck or van in traffic accident
    - V43.51 Car driver injured in collision with sport utility vehicle in traffic accident POA
    - V43.52 Car driver injured in collision with other type car in traffic accident POA
    - V43.53 Car driver injured in collision with pick-up truck in traffic accident POA
    - V43.54 Car driver injured in collision with van in traffic accident POA
  - V43.6 Car passenger injured in collision with car, pick-up truck or van in traffic accident
    - V43.61 Car passenger injured in collision with sport utility vehicle in traffic accident POA
    - V43.62 Car passenger injured in collision with other type car in traffic accident POA
    - V43.63 Car passenger injured in collision with pick-up truck in traffic accident POA
    - V43.64 Car passenger injured in collision with van in traffic accident POA
  - V43.7 Person on outside of car injured in collision with car, pick-up truck or van in traffic accident
    - V43.71 Person on outside of car injured in collision with sport utility vehicle in traffic accident POA
    - V43.72 Person on outside of car injured in collision with other type car in traffic accident POA
    - V43.73 Person on outside of car injured in collision with pick-up truck in traffic accident POA
    - V43.74 Person on outside of car injured in collision with van in traffic accident POA
  - V43.9 Unspecified car occupant injured in collision with car, pick-up truck or van in traffic accident
    - V43.91 Unspecified car occupant injured in collision with sport utility vehicle in traffic accident POA
    - V43.92 Unspecified car occupant injured in collision with other type car in traffic accident POA
    - V43.93 Unspecified car occupant injured in collision with pick-up truck in traffic accident POA
    - V43.94 Unspecified car occupant injured in collision with van in traffic accident POA

- V44 Car occupant injured in collision with heavy transport vehicle or bus

  EXCLUDES1 car occupant injured in collision with military vehicle (V49.81)

  The appropriate 7th character is to be added to each code from category V44

  A = initial encounter
  D = subsequent encounter
  S = sequela

  - V44.0 Car driver injured in collision with heavy transport vehicle or bus in nontraffic accident POA
  - V44.1 Car passenger injured in collision with heavy transport vehicle or bus in nontraffic accident POA
  - V44.2 Person on outside of car injured in collision with heavy transport vehicle or bus in nontraffic accident POA
  - V44.3 Unspecified car occupant injured in collision with heavy transport vehicle or bus in nontraffic accident POA
  - V44.4 Person boarding or alighting a car injured in collision with heavy transport vehicle or bus POA
  - V44.5 Car driver injured in collision with heavy transport vehicle or bus in traffic accident POA
  - V44.6 Car passenger injured in collision with heavy transport vehicle or bus in traffic accident POA
  - V44.7 Person on outside of car injured in collision with heavy transport vehicle or bus in traffic accident POA

Unspecified Code	Other Specified Code	Manifestation Code	N Newborn	P Pediatric	M Maternity	A Adult	♂ Male	♀ Female

● New Code   ▲ Revised Code Title   ►◄ Revised Text   NOTES   *INCLUDES*   *EXCLUDES 1* Not coded here   *EXCLUDES 2* Not included here

4th character required   5th character required   6th character required   7th character required

Extension 'X' Alert   HAC Hospital-acquired condition (HAC) alert   AHA AHA Coding Clinic©

V44.9 Unspecified car occupant injured in collision with heavy transport vehicle or bus in traffic accident

V45 Car occupant injured in collision with railway train or railway vehicle

The appropriate 7th character is to be added to each code from category V45

A = initial encounter
D = subsequent encounter
S = sequela

V45.0 Car driver injured in collision with railway train or railway vehicle in nontraffic accident

V45.1 Car passenger injured in collision with railway train or railway vehicle in nontraffic accident

V45.2 Person on outside of car injured in collision with railway train or railway vehicle in nontraffic accident

V45.3 Unspecified car occupant injured in collision with railway train or railway vehicle in nontraffic accident

V45.4 Person boarding or alighting a car injured in collision with railway train or railway vehicle

V45.5 Car driver injured in collision with railway train or railway vehicle in traffic accident

V45.6 Car passenger injured in collision with railway train or railway vehicle in traffic accident

V45.7 Person on outside of car injured in collision with railway train or railway vehicle in traffic accident

V45.9 Unspecified car occupant injured in collision with railway train or railway vehicle in traffic accident

V46 Car occupant injured in collision with other nonmotor vehicle

INCLUDES collision with animal-drawn vehicle, animal being ridden, streetcar

The appropriate 7th character is to be added to each code from category V46

A = initial encounter
D = subsequent encounter
S = sequela

V46.0 Car driver injured in collision with other nonmotor vehicle in nontraffic accident

V46.1 Car passenger injured in collision with other nonmotor vehicle in nontraffic accident

V46.2 Person on outside of car injured in collision with other nonmotor vehicle in nontraffic accident

V46.3 Unspecified car occupant injured in collision with other nonmotor vehicle in nontraffic accident

V46.4 Person boarding or alighting a car injured in collision with other nonmotor vehicle

V46.5 Car driver injured in collision with other nonmotor vehicle in traffic accident

V46.6 Car passenger injured in collision with other nonmotor vehicle in traffic accident

V46.7 Person on outside of car injured in collision with other nonmotor vehicle in traffic accident

V46.9 Unspecified car occupant injured in collision with other nonmotor vehicle in traffic accident

V47 Car occupant injured in collision with fixed or stationary object

The appropriate 7th character is to be added to each code from category V47

A = initial encounter
D = subsequent encounter
S = sequela

V47.0 Car driver injured in collision with fixed or stationary object in nontraffic accident

V47.1 Car passenger injured in collision with fixed or stationary object in nontraffic accident

V47.2 Person on outside of car injured in collision with fixed or stationary object in nontraffic accident

V47.3 Unspecified car occupant injured in collision with fixed or stationary object in nontraffic accident

V47.4 Person boarding or alighting a car injured in collision with fixed or stationary object

V47.5 Car driver injured in collision with fixed or stationary object in traffic accident

V47.6 Car passenger injured in collision with fixed or stationary object in traffic accident

V47.7 Person on outside of car injured in collision with fixed or stationary object in traffic accident

V47.9 Unspecified car occupant injured in collision with fixed or stationary object in traffic accident

V48 Car occupant injured in noncollision transport accident

INCLUDES overturning car NOS
overturning car without collision

The appropriate 7th character is to be added to each code from category V48

A = initial encounter
D = subsequent encounter
S = sequela

V48.0 Car driver injured in noncollision transport accident in nontraffic accident

V48.1 Car passenger injured in noncollision transport accident in nontraffic accident

V48.2 Person on outside of car injured in noncollision transport accident in nontraffic accident

V48.3 Unspecified car occupant injured in noncollision transport accident in nontraffic accident

V48.4 Person boarding or alighting a car injured in noncollision transport accident

V48.5 Car driver injured in noncollision transport accident in traffic accident

V48.6 Car passenger injured in noncollision transport accident in traffic accident

V48.7 Person on outside of car injured in noncollision transport accident in traffic accident

V48.9 Unspecified car occupant injured in noncollision transport accident in traffic accident

V49 Car occupant injured in other and unspecified transport accidents

The appropriate 7th character is to be added to each code from category V49

A = initial encounter
D = subsequent encounter
S = sequela

V49.0 Driver injured in collision with other and unspecified motor vehicles in nontraffic accident

V49.00 Driver injured in collision with unspecified motor vehicles in nontraffic accident

V49.09 Driver injured in collision with other motor vehicles in nontraffic accident

V49.1 Passenger injured in collision with other and unspecified motor vehicles in nontraffic accident

V49.10 Passenger injured in collision with unspecified motor vehicles in nontraffic accident

V49.19 Passenger injured in collision with other motor vehicles in nontraffic accident

V49.2 Unspecified car occupant injured in collision with other and unspecified motor vehicles in nontraffic accident

V49.20 Unspecified car occupant injured in collision with unspecified motor vehicles in nontraffic accident
Car collision NOS, nontraffic

V49.29 Unspecified car occupant injured in collision with other motor vehicles in nontraffic accident

V49.3 Car occupant (driver) (passenger) injured in unspecified nontraffic accident
Car accident NOS, nontraffic
Car occupant injured in nontraffic accident NOS

V49.4 Driver injured in collision with other and unspecified motor vehicles in traffic accident

V49.40 Driver injured in collision with unspecified motor vehicles in traffic accident

V49.49 Driver injured in collision with other motor vehicles in traffic accident

V49.5 Passenger injured in collision with other and unspecified motor vehicles in traffic accident

V49.50 Passenger injured in collision with unspecified motor vehicles in traffic accident

---

Unacceptable principal diagnosis symbol per Medicare code edits Code exempt from diagnosis present on admission requirement
❓ Questionable admission ᶜᶜ Complication or comorbidity ᶜᶜ/ᴹᶜᶜ CC/MCC exclusion ᴹᶜᶜ Major complication or comorbidity
Principal diagnosis as its own CC Principal diagnosis as its own MCC ᴴᶜᶜ HCC diagnosis code ᴿˣᴴᶜᶜ RxHCC diagnosis code
MACRA code Ⓩ Z code as first-listed diagnosis

[7th] V49.59 Passenger injured in collision with other motor vehicles in traffic accident [POA]

[5th] V49.6 Unspecified car occupant injured in collision with other and unspecified motor vehicles in traffic accident

[7th] V49.60 Unspecified car occupant injured in collision with unspecified motor vehicles in traffic accident [POA]
Car collision NOS (traffic)

[7th] V49.69 Unspecified car occupant injured in collision with other motor vehicles in traffic accident [POA]

[5th] V49.8 Car occupant (driver) (passenger) injured in other specified transport accidents

[7th] V49.81 Car occupant (driver) (passenger) injured in transport accident with military vehicle [POA]

[7th] V49.88 Car occupant (driver) (passenger) injured in other specified transport accidents [POA]

[7th] V49.9 Car occupant (driver) (passenger) injured in unspecified traffic accident [POA]
Car accident NOS

Occupant of pick-up truck or van injured in transport accident (V50-V59)

[INCLUDES] *a four or six wheel motor vehicle designed primarily for carrying passengers and property but weighing less than the local limit for classification as a heavy goods vehicle*
minibus
minivan
sport utility vehicle (SUV)
truck
van

[EXCLUDES1] *heavy transport vehicle (V60-V69)*

[4th] V50 Occupant of pick-up truck or van injured in collision with pedestrian or animal
[EXCLUDES1] *pick-up truck or van collision with animal-drawn vehicle or animal being ridden (V56.-)*
The appropriate 7th character is to be added to each code from category V50
A = initial encounter
D = subsequent encounter
S = sequela

[7th] V50.0 Driver of pick-up truck or van injured in collision with pedestrian or animal in nontraffic accident [POA]

[7th] V50.1 Passenger in pick-up truck or van injured in collision with pedestrian or animal in nontraffic accident [POA]

[7th] V50.2 Person on outside of pick-up truck or van injured in collision with pedestrian or animal in nontraffic accident [POA]

[7th] V50.3 Unspecified occupant of pick-up truck or van injured in collision with pedestrian or animal in nontraffic accident [POA]

[7th] V50.4 Person boarding or alighting a pick-up truck or van injured in collision with pedestrian or animal [POA]

[7th] V50.5 Driver of pick-up truck or van injured in collision with pedestrian or animal in traffic accident [POA]

[7th] V50.6 Passenger in pick-up truck or van injured in collision with pedestrian or animal in traffic accident [POA]

[7th] V50.7 Person on outside of pick-up truck or van injured in collision with pedestrian or animal in traffic accident [POA]

[7th] V50.9 Unspecified occupant of pick-up truck or van injured in collision with pedestrian or animal in traffic accident [POA]

[4th] V51 Occupant of pick-up truck or van injured in collision with pedal cycle
The appropriate 7th character is to be added to each code from category V51
A = initial encounter
D = subsequent encounter
S = sequela

[7th] V51.0 Driver of pick-up truck or van injured in collision with pedal cycle in nontraffic accident [POA]

[7th] V51.1 Passenger in pick-up truck or van injured in collision with pedal cycle in nontraffic accident [POA]

[7th] V51.2 Person on outside of pick-up truck or van injured in collision with pedal cycle in nontraffic accident [POA]

[7th] V51.3 Unspecified occupant of pick-up truck or van injured in collision with pedal cycle in nontraffic accident [POA]

[7th] V51.4 Person boarding or alighting a pick-up truck or van injured in collision with pedal cycle [POA]

[7th] V51.5 Driver of pick-up truck or van injured in collision with pedal cycle in traffic accident [POA]

[7th] V51.6 Passenger in pick-up truck or van injured in collision with pedal cycle in traffic accident [POA]

[7th] V51.7 Person on outside of pick-up truck or van injured in collision with pedal cycle in traffic accident [POA]

[7th] V51.9 Unspecified occupant of pick-up truck or van injured in collision with pedal cycle in traffic accident [POA]

[4th] V52 Occupant of pick-up truck or van injured in collision with two- or three-wheeled motor vehicle
The appropriate 7th character is to be added to each code from category V52
A = initial encounter
D = subsequent encounter
S = sequela

[7th] V52.0 Driver of pick-up truck or van injured in collision with two- or three-wheeled motor vehicle in nontraffic accident [POA]

[7th] V52.1 Passenger in pick-up truck or van injured in collision with two- or three-wheeled motor vehicle in nontraffic accident [POA]

[7th] V52.2 Person on outside of pick-up truck or van injured in collision with two- or three-wheeled motor vehicle in nontraffic accident [POA]

[7th] V52.3 Unspecified occupant of pick-up truck or van injured in collision with two- or three-wheeled motor vehicle in nontraffic accident [POA]

[7th] V52.4 Person boarding or alighting a pick-up truck or van injured in collision with two- or three-wheeled motor vehicle [POA]

[7th] V52.5 Driver of pick-up truck or van injured in collision with two- or three-wheeled motor vehicle in traffic accident [POA]

[7th] V52.6 Passenger in pick-up truck or van injured in collision with two- or three-wheeled motor vehicle in traffic accident [POA]

[7th] V52.7 Person on outside of pick-up truck or van injured in collision with two- or three-wheeled motor vehicle in traffic accident [POA]

[7th] V52.9 Unspecified occupant of pick-up truck or van injured in collision with two- or three-wheeled motor vehicle in traffic accident [POA]

[4th] V53 Occupant of pick-up truck or van injured in collision with car, pick-up truck or van
The appropriate 7th character is to be added to each code from category V53
A = initial encounter
D = subsequent encounter
S = sequela

[7th] V53.0 Driver of pick-up truck or van injured in collision with car, pick-up truck or van in nontraffic accident [POA]

[7th] V53.1 Passenger in pick-up truck or van injured in collision with car, pick-up truck or van in nontraffic accident [POA]

[7th] V53.2 Person on outside of pick-up truck or van injured in collision with car, pick-up truck or van in nontraffic accident [POA]

[7th] V53.3 Unspecified occupant of pick-up truck or van injured in collision with car, pick-up truck or van in nontraffic accident [POA]

[7th] V53.4 Person boarding or alighting a pick-up truck or van injured in collision with car, pick-up truck or van [POA]

[7th] V53.5 Driver of pick-up truck or van injured in collision with car, pick-up truck or van in traffic accident [POA]

[7th] V53.6 Passenger in pick-up truck or van injured in collision with car, pick-up truck or van in traffic accident [POA]

[7th] V53.7 Person on outside of pick-up truck or van injured in collision with car, pick-up truck or van in traffic accident [POA]

[7th] V53.9 Unspecified occupant of pick-up truck or van injured in collision with car, pick-up truck or van in traffic accident [POA]

[4th] V54 Occupant of pick-up truck or van injured in collision with heavy transport vehicle or bus

V54.0 - V59 *(side tab)*

EXCLUDES1 *occupant of pick-up truck or van injured in collision with military vehicle (V59.81)*

The appropriate 7th character is to be added to each code from category V54

    A = initial encounter
    D = subsequent encounter
    S = sequela

V54.0 Driver of pick-up truck or van injured in collision with heavy transport vehicle or bus in nontraffic accident

V54.1 Passenger in pick-up truck or van injured in collision with heavy transport vehicle or bus in nontraffic accident

V54.2 Person on outside of pick-up truck or van injured in collision with heavy transport vehicle or bus in nontraffic accident

V54.3 Unspecified occupant of pick-up truck or van injured in collision with heavy transport vehicle or bus in nontraffic accident

V54.4 Person boarding or alighting a pick-up truck or van injured in collision with heavy transport vehicle or bus

V54.5 Driver of pick-up truck or van injured in collision with heavy transport vehicle or bus in traffic accident

V54.6 Passenger in pick-up truck or van injured in collision with heavy transport vehicle or bus in traffic accident

V54.7 Person on outside of pick-up truck or van injured in collision with heavy transport vehicle or bus in traffic accident

V54.9 Unspecified occupant of pick-up truck or van injured in collision with heavy transport vehicle or bus in traffic accident

V55 Occupant of pick-up truck or van injured in collision with railway train or railway vehicle

The appropriate 7th character is to be added to each code from category V55

    A = initial encounter
    D = subsequent encounter
    S = sequela

V55.0 Driver of pick-up truck or van injured in collision with railway train or railway vehicle in nontraffic accident

V55.1 Passenger in pick-up truck or van injured in collision with railway train or railway vehicle in nontraffic accident

V55.2 Person on outside of pick-up truck or van injured in collision with railway train or railway vehicle in nontraffic accident

V55.3 Unspecified occupant of pick-up truck or van injured in collision with railway train or railway vehicle in nontraffic accident

V55.4 Person boarding or alighting a pick-up truck or van injured in collision with railway train or railway vehicle

V55.5 Driver of pick-up truck or van injured in collision with railway train or railway vehicle in traffic accident

V55.6 Passenger in pick-up truck or van injured in collision with railway train or railway vehicle in traffic accident

V55.7 Person on outside of pick-up truck or van injured in collision with railway train or railway vehicle in traffic accident

V55.9 Unspecified occupant of pick-up truck or van injured in collision with railway train or railway vehicle in traffic accident

V56 Occupant of pick-up truck or van injured in collision with other nonmotor vehicle

INCLUDES *collision with animal-drawn vehicle, animal being ridden, streetcar*

The appropriate 7th character is to be added to each code from category V56

    A = initial encounter
    D = subsequent encounter
    S = sequela

V56.0 Driver of pick-up truck or van injured in collision with other nonmotor vehicle in nontraffic accident

V56.1 Passenger in pick-up truck or van injured in collision with other nonmotor vehicle in nontraffic accident

V56.2 Person on outside of pick-up truck or van injured in collision with other nonmotor vehicle in nontraffic accident

V56.3 Unspecified occupant of pick-up truck or van injured in collision with other nonmotor vehicle in nontraffic accident

V56.4 Person boarding or alighting a pick-up truck or van injured in collision with other nonmotor vehicle

V56.5 Driver of pick-up truck or van injured in collision with other nonmotor vehicle in traffic accident

V56.6 Passenger in pick-up truck or van injured in collision with other nonmotor vehicle in traffic accident

V56.7 Person on outside of pick-up truck or van injured in collision with other nonmotor vehicle in traffic accident

V56.9 Unspecified occupant of pick-up truck or van injured in collision with other nonmotor vehicle in traffic accident

V57 Occupant of pick-up truck or van injured in collision with fixed or stationary object

The appropriate 7th character is to be added to each code from category V57

    A = initial encounter
    D = subsequent encounter
    S = sequela

V57.0 Driver of pick-up truck or van injured in collision with fixed or stationary object in nontraffic accident

V57.1 Passenger in pick-up truck or van injured in collision with fixed or stationary object in nontraffic accident

V57.2 Person on outside of pick-up truck or van injured in collision with fixed or stationary object in nontraffic accident

V57.3 Unspecified occupant of pick-up truck or van injured in collision with fixed or stationary object in nontraffic accident

V57.4 Person boarding or alighting a pick-up truck or van injured in collision with fixed or stationary object

V57.5 Driver of pick-up truck or van injured in collision with fixed or stationary object in traffic accident

V57.6 Passenger in pick-up truck or van injured in collision with fixed or stationary object in traffic accident

V57.7 Person on outside of pick-up truck or van injured in collision with fixed or stationary object in traffic accident

V57.9 Unspecified occupant of pick-up truck or van injured in collision with fixed or stationary object in traffic accident

V58 Occupant of pick-up truck or van injured in noncollision transport accident

INCLUDES *overturning pick-up truck or van NOS*
overturning pick-up truck or van without collision

The appropriate 7th character is to be added to each code from category V58

    A = initial encounter
    D = subsequent encounter
    S = sequela

V58.0 Driver of pick-up truck or van injured in noncollision transport accident in nontraffic accident

V58.1 Passenger in pick-up truck or van injured in noncollision transport accident in nontraffic accident

V58.2 Person on outside of pick-up truck or van injured in noncollision transport accident in nontraffic accident

V58.3 Unspecified occupant of pick-up truck or van injured in noncollision transport accident in nontraffic accident

V58.4 Person boarding or alighting a pick-up truck or van injured in noncollision transport accident

V58.5 Driver of pick-up truck or van injured in noncollision transport accident in traffic accident

V58.6 Passenger in pick-up truck or van injured in noncollision transport accident in traffic accident

V58.7 Person on outside of pick-up truck or van injured in noncollision transport accident in traffic accident

V58.9 Unspecified occupant of pick-up truck or van injured in noncollision transport accident in traffic accident

V59 Occupant of pick-up truck or van injured in other and unspecified transport accidents

The appropriate 7th character is to be added to each code from category V59

    A = initial encounter
    D = subsequent encounter
    S = sequela

POA Unacceptable principal diagnosis symbol per Medicare code edits   POA Code exempt from diagnosis present on admission requirement

❓ Questionable admission cc Complication or comorbidity cc-mcc exc CC/MCC exclusion mcc Major complication or comorbidity

cc Principal diagnosis as its own CC mcc Principal diagnosis as its own MCC HCC HCC diagnosis code RxHCC RxHCC diagnosis code

MACRA code Z1 Z code as first-listed diagnosis

V59.0 Driver of pick-up truck or van injured in collision with other and unspecified motor vehicles in nontraffic accident

   V59.00 Driver of pick-up truck or van injured in collision with unspecified motor vehicles in nontraffic accident POA

   V59.09 Driver of pick-up truck or van injured in collision with other motor vehicles in nontraffic accident POA

V59.1 Passenger in pick-up truck or van injured in collision with other and unspecified motor vehicles in nontraffic accident

   V59.10 Passenger in pick-up truck or van injured in collision with unspecified motor vehicles in nontraffic accident POA

   V59.19 Passenger in pick-up truck or van injured in collision with other motor vehicles in nontraffic accident POA

V59.2 Unspecified occupant of pick-up truck or van injured in collision with other and unspecified motor vehicles in nontraffic accident

   V59.20 Unspecified occupant of pick-up truck or van injured in collision with unspecified motor vehicles in nontraffic accident POA

      Collision NOS involving pick-up truck or van, nontraffic

   V59.29 Unspecified occupant of pick-up truck or van injured in collision with other motor vehicles in nontraffic accident POA

V59.3 Occupant (driver) (passenger) of pick-up truck or van injured in unspecified nontraffic accident POA

      Accident NOS involving pick-up truck or van, nontraffic
      Occupant of pick-up truck or van injured in nontraffic accident NOS

V59.4 Driver of pick-up truck or van injured in collision with other and unspecified motor vehicles in traffic accident

   V59.40 Driver of pick-up truck or van injured in collision with unspecified motor vehicles in traffic accident POA

   V59.49 Driver of pick-up truck or van injured in collision with other motor vehicles in traffic accident POA

V59.5 Passenger in pick-up truck or van injured in collision with other and unspecified motor vehicles in traffic accident

   V59.50 Passenger in pick-up truck or van injured in collision with unspecified motor vehicles in traffic accident POA

   V59.59 Passenger in pick-up truck or van injured in collision with other motor vehicles in traffic accident POA

V59.6 Unspecified occupant of pick-up truck or van injured in collision with other and unspecified motor vehicles in traffic accident

   V59.60 Unspecified occupant of pick-up truck or van injured in collision with unspecified motor vehicles in traffic accident POA

      Collision NOS involving pick-up truck or van (traffic)

   V59.69 Unspecified occupant of pick-up truck or van injured in collision with other motor vehicles in traffic accident POA

V59.8 Occupant (driver) (passenger) of pick-up truck or van injured in other specified transport accidents

   V59.81 Occupant (driver) (passenger) of pick-up truck or van injured in transport accident with military vehicle POA

   V59.88 Occupant (driver) (passenger) of pick-up truck or van injured in other specified transport accidents POA

V59.9 Occupant (driver) (passenger) of pick-up truck or van injured in unspecified traffic accident POA

      Accident NOS involving pick-up truck or van

Occupant of heavy transport vehicle injured in transport accident (V60-V69)

INCLUDES   18 wheeler
         armored car
         panel truck

EXCLUDES1 bus
         motorcoach

V60 Occupant of heavy transport vehicle injured in collision with pedestrian or animal

   EXCLUDES1 *heavy transport vehicle collision with animal-drawn vehicle or animal being ridden (V66.-)*

   The appropriate 7th character is to be added to each code from category V60
      A = initial encounter
      D = subsequent encounter
      S = sequela

   V60.0 Driver of heavy transport vehicle injured in collision with pedestrian or animal in nontraffic accident POA

   V60.1 Passenger in heavy transport vehicle injured in collision with pedestrian or animal in nontraffic accident POA

   V60.2 Person on outside of heavy transport vehicle injured in collision with pedestrian or animal in nontraffic accident POA

   V60.3 Unspecified occupant of heavy transport vehicle injured in collision with pedestrian or animal in nontraffic accident POA

   V60.4 Person boarding or alighting a heavy transport vehicle injured in collision with pedestrian or animal POA

   V60.5 Driver of heavy transport vehicle injured in collision with pedestrian or animal in traffic accident POA

   V60.6 Passenger in heavy transport vehicle injured in collision with pedestrian or animal in traffic accident POA

   V60.7 Person on outside of heavy transport vehicle injured in collision with pedestrian or animal in traffic accident POA

   V60.9 Unspecified occupant of heavy transport vehicle injured in collision with pedestrian or animal in traffic accident POA

V61 Occupant of heavy transport vehicle injured in collision with pedal cycle

   The appropriate 7th character is to be added to each code from category V61
      A = initial encounter
      D = subsequent encounter
      S = sequela

   V61.0 Driver of heavy transport vehicle injured in collision with pedal cycle in nontraffic accident POA

   V61.1 Passenger in heavy transport vehicle injured in collision with pedal cycle in nontraffic accident POA

   V61.2 Person on outside of heavy transport vehicle injured in collision with pedal cycle in nontraffic accident POA

   V61.3 Unspecified occupant of heavy transport vehicle injured in collision with pedal cycle in nontraffic accident POA

   V61.4 Person boarding or alighting a heavy transport vehicle injured in collision with pedal cycle while boarding or alighting POA

   V61.5 Driver of heavy transport vehicle injured in collision with pedal cycle in traffic accident POA

   V61.6 Passenger in heavy transport vehicle injured in collision with pedal cycle in traffic accident POA

   V61.7 Person on outside of heavy transport vehicle injured in collision with pedal cycle in traffic accident POA

   V61.9 Unspecified occupant of heavy transport vehicle injured in collision with pedal cycle in traffic accident POA

V62 Occupant of heavy transport vehicle injured in collision with two- or three-wheeled motor vehicle

   The appropriate 7th character is to be added to each code from category V62
      A = initial encounter
      D = subsequent encounter
      S = sequela

   V62.0 Driver of heavy transport vehicle injured in collision with two- or three-wheeled motor vehicle in nontraffic accident POA

   V62.1 Passenger in heavy transport vehicle injured in collision with two- or three-wheeled motor vehicle in nontraffic accident POA

   V62.2 Person on outside of heavy transport vehicle injured in collision with two- or three-wheeled motor vehicle in nontraffic accident POA

   V62.3 Unspecified occupant of heavy transport vehicle injured in collision with two- or three-wheeled motor vehicle in nontraffic accident POA

Unspecified Code   Other Specified Code   Manifestation Code N Newborn P Pediatric M Maternity A Adult ♂ Male ♀ Female
● New Code ▲ Revised Code Title ►◄ Revised Text NOTES INCLUDES EXCLUDES1 Not coded here EXCLUDES2 Not included here
4ᵗʰ character required 5ᵗʰ character required 6ᵗʰ character required 7ᵗʰ character required
Extension 'X' Alert HAC Hospital-acquired condition (HAC) alert AHA AHA Coding Clinic©

V62.4 Person boarding or alighting a heavy transport vehicle injured in collision with two- or three-wheeled motor vehicle **POA**

V62.5 Driver of heavy transport vehicle injured in collision with two- or three-wheeled motor vehicle in traffic accident **POA**

V62.6 Passenger in heavy transport vehicle injured in collision with two- or three-wheeled motor vehicle in traffic accident **POA**

V62.7 Person on outside of heavy transport vehicle injured in collision with two- or three-wheeled motor vehicle in traffic accident **POA**

V62.9 Unspecified occupant of heavy transport vehicle injured in collision with two- or three-wheeled motor vehicle in traffic accident **POA**

V63 Occupant of heavy transport vehicle injured in collision with car, pick-up truck or van

The appropriate 7th character is to be added to each code from category V63
- A = initial encounter
- D = subsequent encounter
- S = sequela

V63.0 Driver of heavy transport vehicle injured in collision with car, pick-up truck or van in nontraffic accident **POA**

V63.1 Passenger in heavy transport vehicle injured in collision with car, pick-up truck or van in nontraffic accident **POA**

V63.2 Person on outside of heavy transport vehicle injured in collision with car, pick-up truck or van in nontraffic accident **POA**

V63.3 Unspecified occupant of heavy transport vehicle injured in collision with car, pick-up truck or van in nontraffic accident **POA**

V63.4 Person boarding or alighting a heavy transport vehicle injured in collision with car, pick-up truck or van **POA**

V63.5 Driver of heavy transport vehicle injured in collision with car, pick-up truck or van in traffic accident **POA**

V63.6 Passenger in heavy transport vehicle injured in collision with car, pick-up truck or van in traffic accident **POA**

V63.7 Person on outside of heavy transport vehicle injured in collision with car, pick-up truck or van in traffic accident **POA**

V63.9 Unspecified occupant of heavy transport vehicle injured in collision with car, pick-up truck or van in traffic accident **POA**

V64 Occupant of heavy transport vehicle injured in collision with heavy transport vehicle or bus

EXCLUDES1 occupant of heavy transport vehicle injured in collision with military vehicle (V69.81)

The appropriate 7th character is to be added to each code from category V64
- A = initial encounter
- D = subsequent encounter
- S = sequela

V64.0 Driver of heavy transport vehicle injured in collision with heavy transport vehicle or bus in nontraffic accident **POA**

V64.1 Passenger in heavy transport vehicle injured in collision with heavy transport vehicle or bus in nontraffic accident **POA**

V64.2 Person on outside of heavy transport vehicle injured in collision with heavy transport vehicle or bus in nontraffic accident **POA**

V64.3 Unspecified occupant of heavy transport vehicle injured in collision with heavy transport vehicle or bus in nontraffic accident **POA**

V64.4 Person boarding or alighting a heavy transport vehicle injured in collision with heavy transport vehicle or bus while boarding or alighting **POA**

V64.5 Driver of heavy transport vehicle injured in collision with heavy transport vehicle or bus in traffic accident **POA**

V64.6 Passenger in heavy transport vehicle injured in collision with heavy transport vehicle or bus in traffic accident **POA**

V64.7 Person on outside of heavy transport vehicle injured in collision with heavy transport vehicle or bus in traffic accident **POA**

V64.9 Unspecified occupant of heavy transport vehicle injured in collision with heavy transport vehicle or bus in traffic accident **POA**

V65 Occupant of heavy transport vehicle injured in collision with railway train or railway vehicle

The appropriate 7th character is to be added to each code from category V65
- A = initial encounter
- D = subsequent encounter
- S = sequela

V65.0 Driver of heavy transport vehicle injured in collision with railway train or railway vehicle in nontraffic accident **POA**

V65.1 Passenger in heavy transport vehicle injured in collision with railway train or railway vehicle in nontraffic accident **POA**

V65.2 Person on outside of heavy transport vehicle injured in collision with railway train or railway vehicle in nontraffic accident **POA**

V65.3 Unspecified occupant of heavy transport vehicle injured in collision with railway train or railway vehicle in nontraffic accident **POA**

V65.4 Person boarding or alighting a heavy transport vehicle injured in collision with railway train or railway vehicle **POA**

V65.5 Driver of heavy transport vehicle injured in collision with railway train or railway vehicle in traffic accident **POA**

V65.6 Passenger in heavy transport vehicle injured in collision with railway train or railway vehicle in traffic accident **POA**

V65.7 Person on outside of heavy transport vehicle injured in collision with railway train or railway vehicle in traffic accident **POA**

V65.9 Unspecified occupant of heavy transport vehicle injured in collision with railway train or railway vehicle in traffic accident **POA**

V66 Occupant of heavy transport vehicle injured in collision with other nonmotor vehicle

INCLUDES collision with animal-drawn vehicle, animal being ridden, streetcar

The appropriate 7th character is to be added to each code from category V66
- A = initial encounter
- D = subsequent encounter
- S = sequela

V66.0 Driver of heavy transport vehicle injured in collision with other nonmotor vehicle in nontraffic accident **POA**

V66.1 Passenger in heavy transport vehicle injured in collision with other nonmotor vehicle in nontraffic accident **POA**

V66.2 Person on outside of heavy transport vehicle injured in collision with other nonmotor vehicle in nontraffic accident **POA**

V66.3 Unspecified occupant of heavy transport vehicle injured in collision with other nonmotor vehicle in nontraffic accident **POA**

V66.4 Person boarding or alighting a heavy transport vehicle injured in collision with other nonmotor vehicle **POA**

V66.5 Driver of heavy transport vehicle injured in collision with other nonmotor vehicle in traffic accident **POA**

V66.6 Passenger in heavy transport vehicle injured in collision with other nonmotor vehicle in traffic accident **POA**

V66.7 Person on outside of heavy transport vehicle injured in collision with other nonmotor vehicle in traffic accident **POA**

V66.9 Unspecified occupant of heavy transport vehicle injured in collision with other nonmotor vehicle in traffic accident **POA**

V67 Occupant of heavy transport vehicle injured in collision with fixed or stationary object

The appropriate 7th character is to be added to each code from category V67
- A = initial encounter
- D = subsequent encounter
- S = sequela

V67.0 Driver of heavy transport vehicle injured in collision with fixed or stationary object in nontraffic accident **POA**

V67.1 Passenger in heavy transport vehicle injured in collision with fixed or stationary object in nontraffic accident **POA**

V67.2 Person on outside of heavy transport vehicle injured in collision with fixed or stationary object in nontraffic accident **POA**

POA Unacceptable principal diagnosis symbol per Medicare code edits   **POA** Code exempt from diagnosis present on admission requirement
? Questionable admission   **CC** Complication or comorbidity   **CC/MCC** CC/MCC exclusion   **MCC** Major complication or comorbidity
Principal diagnosis as its own CC   Principal diagnosis as its own MCC   HCC HCC diagnosis code   RxHCC RxHCC diagnosis code
MACRA code   **Z** Z code as first-listed diagnosis

[7th] V67.3 Unspecified occupant of heavy transport vehicle injured in collision with fixed or stationary object in nontraffic accident [POA]

[7th] V67.4 Person boarding or alighting a heavy transport vehicle injured in collision with fixed or stationary object [POA]

[7th] V67.5 Driver of heavy transport vehicle injured in collision with fixed or stationary object in traffic accident [POA]

[7th] V67.6 Passenger in heavy transport vehicle injured in collision with fixed or stationary object in traffic accident [POA]

[7th] V67.7 Person on outside of heavy transport vehicle injured in collision with fixed or stationary object in traffic accident [POA]

[7th] V67.9 Unspecified occupant of heavy transport vehicle injured in collision with fixed or stationary object in traffic accident [POA]

[4th] **V68 Occupant of heavy transport vehicle injured in noncollision transport accident**

INCLUDES *overturning heavy transport vehicle NOS*
overturning heavy transport vehicle without collision

The appropriate 7th character is to be added to each code from category V68
- A = initial encounter
- D = subsequent encounter
- S = sequela

[7th] V68.0 Driver of heavy transport vehicle injured in noncollision transport accident in nontraffic accident [POA]

[7th] V68.1 Passenger in heavy transport vehicle injured in noncollision transport accident in nontraffic accident [POA]

[7th] V68.2 Person on outside of heavy transport vehicle injured in noncollision transport accident in nontraffic accident [POA]

[7th] V68.3 Unspecified occupant of heavy transport vehicle injured in noncollision transport accident in nontraffic accident [POA]

[7th] V68.4 Person boarding or alighting a heavy transport vehicle injured in noncollision transport accident [POA]

[7th] V68.5 Driver of heavy transport vehicle injured in noncollision transport accident in traffic accident [POA]

[7th] V68.6 Passenger in heavy transport vehicle injured in noncollision transport accident in traffic accident [POA]

[7th] V68.7 Person on outside of heavy transport vehicle injured in noncollision transport accident in traffic accident [POA]

[7th] V68.9 Unspecified occupant of heavy transport vehicle injured in noncollision transport accident in traffic accident [POA]

[4th] **V69 Occupant of heavy transport vehicle injured in other and unspecified transport accidents**

The appropriate 7th character is to be added to each code from category V69
- A = initial encounter
- D = subsequent encounter
- S = sequela

[5th] V69.0 Driver of heavy transport vehicle injured in collision with other and unspecified motor vehicles in nontraffic accident

[7th] V69.00 Driver of heavy transport vehicle injured in collision with unspecified motor vehicles in nontraffic accident [POA]

[7th] V69.09 Driver of heavy transport vehicle injured in collision with other motor vehicles in nontraffic accident [POA]

[5th] V69.1 Passenger in heavy transport vehicle injured in collision with other and unspecified motor vehicles in nontraffic accident

[7th] V69.10 Passenger in heavy transport vehicle injured in collision with unspecified motor vehicles in nontraffic accident [POA]

[7th] V69.19 Passenger in heavy transport vehicle injured in collision with other motor vehicles in nontraffic accident [POA]

[5th] V69.2 Unspecified occupant of heavy transport vehicle injured in collision with other and unspecified motor vehicles in nontraffic accident

[7th] V69.20 Unspecified occupant of heavy transport vehicle injured in collision with unspecified motor vehicles in nontraffic accident [POA]
Collision NOS involving heavy transport vehicle, nontraffic

[7th] V69.29 Unspecified occupant of heavy transport vehicle injured in collision with other motor vehicles in nontraffic accident [POA]

[7th] V69.3 Occupant (driver) (passenger) of heavy transport vehicle injured in unspecified nontraffic accident [POA]
Accident NOS involving heavy transport vehicle, nontraffic
Occupant of heavy transport vehicle injured in nontraffic accident NOS

[5th] V69.4 Driver of heavy transport vehicle injured in collision with other and unspecified motor vehicles in traffic accident

[7th] V69.40 Driver of heavy transport vehicle injured in collision with unspecified motor vehicles in traffic accident [POA]

[7th] V69.49 Driver of heavy transport vehicle injured in collision with other motor vehicles in traffic accident [POA]

[5th] V69.5 Passenger in heavy transport vehicle injured in collision with other and unspecified motor vehicles in traffic accident

[7th] V69.50 Passenger in heavy transport vehicle injured in collision with unspecified motor vehicles in traffic accident [POA]

[7th] V69.59 Passenger in heavy transport vehicle injured in collision with other motor vehicles in traffic accident [POA]

[5th] V69.6 Unspecified occupant of heavy transport vehicle injured in collision with other and unspecified motor vehicles in traffic accident

[7th] V69.60 Unspecified occupant of heavy transport vehicle injured in collision with unspecified motor vehicles in traffic accident [POA]
Collision NOS involving heavy transport vehicle (traffic)

[7th] V69.69 Unspecified occupant of heavy transport vehicle injured in collision with other motor vehicles in traffic accident [POA]

[5th] V69.8 Occupant (driver) (passenger) of heavy transport vehicle injured in other specified transport accidents

[7th] V69.81 Occupant (driver) (passenger) of heavy transport vehicle injured in transport accidents with military vehicle [POA]

[7th] V69.88 Occupant (driver) (passenger) of heavy transport vehicle injured in other specified transport accidents [POA]

[7th] V69.9 Occupant (driver) (passenger) of heavy transport vehicle injured in unspecified traffic accident [POA]
Accident NOS involving heavy transport vehicle

Bus occupant injured in transport accident (V70-V79)

INCLUDES *motorcoach*

EXCLUDES1 *minibus (V50-V59)*

[4th] **V70 Bus occupant injured in collision with pedestrian or animal**

The appropriate 7th character is to be added to each code from category V70
- A = initial encounter
- D = subsequent encounter
- S = sequela

EXCLUDES1 *bus collision with animal-drawn vehicle or animal being ridden (V76.-)*

[7th] V70.0 Driver of bus injured in collision with pedestrian or animal in nontraffic accident [POA]

[7th] V70.1 Passenger on bus injured in collision with pedestrian or animal in nontraffic accident [POA]

[7th] V70.2 Person on outside of bus injured in collision with pedestrian or animal in nontraffic accident [POA]

[7th] V70.3 Unspecified occupant of bus injured in collision with pedestrian or animal in nontraffic accident [POA]

[7th] V70.4 Person boarding or alighting from bus injured in collision with pedestrian or animal [POA]

[7th] V70.5 Driver of bus injured in collision with pedestrian or animal in traffic accident [POA]

[7th] V70.6 Passenger on bus injured in collision with pedestrian or animal in traffic accident [POA]

V70.7 - V76.2

CHAPTER 20: EXTERNAL CAUSES OF MORBIDITY (V00-Y99)

🔟 V70.7 Person on outside of bus injured in collision with pedestrian or animal in traffic accident 🅟🅞🅐

🔟 V70.9 Unspecified occupant of bus injured in collision with pedestrian or animal in traffic accident 🅟🅞🅐

4ᵗʰ V71 Bus occupant injured in collision with pedal cycle

The appropriate 7th character is to be added to each code from category V71

   A = initial encounter
   D = subsequent encounter
   S = sequela

🔟 V71.0 Driver of bus injured in collision with pedal cycle in nontraffic accident 🅟🅞🅐

🔟 V71.1 Passenger on bus injured in collision with pedal cycle in nontraffic accident 🅟🅞🅐

🔟 V71.2 Person on outside of bus injured in collision with pedal cycle in nontraffic accident 🅟🅞🅐

🔟 V71.3 Unspecified occupant of bus injured in collision with pedal cycle in nontraffic accident 🅟🅞🅐

🔟 V71.4 Person boarding or alighting from bus injured in collision with pedal cycle 🅟🅞🅐

🔟 V71.5 Driver of bus injured in collision with pedal cycle in traffic accident 🅟🅞🅐

🔟 V71.6 Passenger on bus injured in collision with pedal cycle in traffic accident

🔟 V71.7 Person on outside of bus injured in collision with pedal cycle in traffic accident 🅟🅞🅐

🔟 V71.9 Unspecified occupant of bus injured in collision with pedal cycle in traffic accident 🅟🅞🅐

4ᵗʰ V72 Bus occupant injured in collision with two- or three-wheeled motor vehicle

The appropriate 7th character is to be added to each code from category V72

   A = initial encounter
   D = subsequent encounter
   S = sequela

🔟 V72.0 Driver of bus injured in collision with two- or three-wheeled motor vehicle in nontraffic accident 🅟🅞🅐

🔟 V72.1 Passenger on bus injured in collision with two- or three-wheeled motor vehicle in nontraffic accident 🅟🅞🅐

🔟 V72.2 Person on outside of bus injured in collision with two- or three-wheeled motor vehicle in nontraffic accident 🅟🅞🅐

🔟 V72.3 Unspecified occupant of bus injured in collision with two- or three-wheeled motor vehicle in nontraffic accident 🅟🅞🅐

🔟 V72.4 Person boarding or alighting from bus injured in collision with two- or three-wheeled motor vehicle 🅟🅞🅐

🔟 V72.5 Driver of bus injured in collision with two- or three-wheeled motor vehicle in traffic accident 🅟🅞🅐

🔟 V72.6 Passenger on bus injured in collision with two- or three-wheeled motor vehicle in traffic accident 🅟🅞🅐

🔟 V72.7 Person on outside of bus injured in collision with two- or three-wheeled motor vehicle in traffic accident 🅟🅞🅐

🔟 V72.9 Unspecified occupant of bus injured in collision with two- or three-wheeled motor vehicle in traffic accident 🅟🅞🅐

4ᵗʰ V73 Bus occupant injured in collision with car, pick-up truck or van

The appropriate 7th character is to be added to each code from category V73

   A = initial encounter
   D = subsequent encounter
   S = sequela

🔟 V73.0 Driver of bus injured in collision with car, pick-up truck or van in nontraffic accident 🅟🅞🅐

🔟 V73.1 Passenger on bus injured in collision with car, pick-up truck or van in nontraffic accident 🅟🅞🅐

🔟 V73.2 Person on outside of bus injured in collision with car, pick-up truck or van in nontraffic accident 🅟🅞🅐

🔟 V73.3 Unspecified occupant of bus injured in collision with car, pick-up truck or van in nontraffic accident 🅟🅞🅐

🔟 V73.4 Person boarding or alighting from bus injured in collision with car, pick-up truck or van 🅟🅞🅐

🔟 V73.5 Driver of bus injured in collision with car, pick-up truck or van in traffic accident 🅟🅞🅐

🔟 V73.6 Passenger on bus injured in collision with car, pick-up truck or van in traffic accident 🅟🅞🅐

🔟 V73.7 Person on outside of bus injured in collision with car, pick-up truck or van in traffic accident 🅟🅞🅐

🔟 V73.9 Unspecified occupant of bus injured in collision with car, pick-up truck or van in traffic accident 🅟🅞🅐

4ᵗʰ V74 Bus occupant injured in collision with heavy transport vehicle or bus

   EXCLUDES1 *bus occupant injured in collision with military vehicle (V79.81)*

The appropriate 7th character is to be added to each code from category V74

   A = initial encounter
   D = subsequent encounter
   S = sequela

🔟 V74.0 Driver of bus injured in collision with heavy transport vehicle or bus in nontraffic accident 🅟🅞🅐

🔟 V74.1 Passenger on bus injured in collision with heavy transport vehicle or bus in nontraffic accident 🅟🅞🅐

🔟 V74.2 Person on outside of bus injured in collision with heavy transport vehicle or bus in nontraffic accident 🅟🅞🅐

🔟 V74.3 Unspecified occupant of bus injured in collision with heavy transport vehicle or bus in nontraffic accident 🅟🅞🅐

🔟 V74.4 Person boarding or alighting from bus injured in collision with heavy transport vehicle or bus 🅟🅞🅐

🔟 V74.5 Driver of bus injured in collision with heavy transport vehicle or bus in traffic accident 🅟🅞🅐

🔟 V74.6 Passenger on bus injured in collision with heavy transport vehicle or bus in traffic accident 🅟🅞🅐

🔟 V74.7 Person on outside of bus injured in collision with heavy transport vehicle or bus in traffic accident 🅟🅞🅐

🔟 V74.9 Unspecified occupant of bus injured in collision with heavy transport vehicle or bus in traffic accident 🅟🅞🅐

4ᵗʰ V75 Bus occupant injured in collision with railway train or railway vehicle

The appropriate 7th character is to be added to each code from category V75

   A = initial encounter
   D = subsequent encounter
   S = sequela

🔟 V75.0 Driver of bus injured in collision with railway train or railway vehicle in nontraffic accident 🅟🅞🅐

🔟 V75.1 Passenger on bus injured in collision with railway train or railway vehicle in nontraffic accident 🅟🅞🅐

🔟 V75.2 Person on outside of bus injured in collision with railway train or railway vehicle in nontraffic accident 🅟🅞🅐

🔟 V75.3 Unspecified occupant of bus injured in collision with railway train or railway vehicle in nontraffic accident 🅟🅞🅐

🔟 V75.4 Person boarding or alighting from bus injured in collision with railway train or railway vehicle 🅟🅞🅐

🔟 V75.5 Driver of bus injured in collision with railway train or railway vehicle in traffic accident 🅟🅞🅐

🔟 V75.6 Passenger on bus injured in collision with railway train or railway vehicle in traffic accident 🅟🅞🅐

🔟 V75.7 Person on outside of bus injured in collision with railway train or railway vehicle in traffic accident 🅟🅞🅐

🔟 V75.9 Unspecified occupant of bus injured in collision with railway train or railway vehicle in traffic accident 🅟🅞🅐

4ᵗʰ V76 Bus occupant injured in collision with other nonmotor vehicle

   INCLUDES *collision with animal-drawn vehicle, animal being ridden, streetcar*

The appropriate 7th character is to be added to each code from category V76

   A = initial encounter
   D = subsequent encounter
   S = sequela

🔟 V76.0 Driver of bus injured in collision with other nonmotor vehicle in nontraffic accident 🅟🅞🅐

🔟 V76.1 Passenger on bus injured in collision with other nonmotor vehicle in nontraffic accident 🅟🅞🅐

🔟 V76.2 Person on outside of bus injured in collision with other nonmotor vehicle in nontraffic accident 🅟🅞🅐

🅟🅞🅐 Unacceptable principal diagnosis symbol per Medicare code edits   🅟🅞🅐 Code exempt from diagnosis present on admission requirement
❓ Questionable admission   ㏄ Complication or comorbidity   cc/mcc exc CC/MCC exclusion   mcc Major complication or comorbidity
Principal diagnosis as its own CC   Principal diagnosis as its own MCC   HCC HCC diagnosis code   RxHCC RxHCC diagnosis code
MACRA code   Ⓩ Z code as first-listed diagnosis

7️⃣ V76.3 Unspecified occupant of bus injured in collision with other nonmotor vehicle in nontraffic accident ⚕POA

7️⃣ V76.4 Person boarding or alighting from bus injured in collision with other nonmotor vehicle ⚕POA

7️⃣ V76.5 Driver of bus injured in collision with other nonmotor vehicle in traffic accident ⚕POA

7️⃣ V76.6 Passenger on bus injured in collision with other nonmotor vehicle in traffic accident ⚕POA

7️⃣ V76.7 Person on outside of bus injured in collision with other nonmotor vehicle in traffic accident ⚕POA

7️⃣ V76.9 Unspecified occupant of bus injured in collision with other nonmotor vehicle in traffic accident ⚕POA

4️⃣ V77 Bus occupant injured in collision with fixed or stationary object

The appropriate 7th character is to be added to each code from category V77

A = initial encounter
D = subsequent encounter
S = sequela

7️⃣ V77.0 Driver of bus injured in collision with fixed or stationary object in nontraffic accident ⚕POA

7️⃣ V77.1 Passenger on bus injured in collision with fixed or stationary object in nontraffic accident ⚕POA

7️⃣ V77.2 Person on outside of bus injured in collision with fixed or stationary object in nontraffic accident ⚕POA

7️⃣ V77.3 Unspecified occupant of bus injured in collision with fixed or stationary object in nontraffic accident ⚕POA

7️⃣ V77.4 Person boarding or alighting from bus injured in collision with fixed or stationary object ⚕POA

7️⃣ V77.5 Driver of bus injured in collision with fixed or stationary object in traffic accident ⚕POA

7️⃣ V77.6 Passenger on bus injured in collision with fixed or stationary object in traffic accident ⚕POA

7️⃣ V77.7 Person on outside of bus injured in collision with fixed or stationary object in traffic accident ⚕POA

7️⃣ V77.9 Unspecified occupant of bus injured in collision with fixed or stationary object in traffic accident ⚕POA

4️⃣ V78 Bus occupant injured in noncollision transport accident

INCLUDES overturning bus NOS

overturning bus without collision

The appropriate 7th character is to be added to each code from category V78

A = initial encounter
D = subsequent encounter
S = sequela

7️⃣ V78.0 Driver of bus injured in noncollision transport accident in nontraffic accident ⚕POA

7️⃣ V78.1 Passenger on bus injured in noncollision transport accident in nontraffic accident ⚕POA

7️⃣ V78.2 Person on outside of bus injured in noncollision transport accident in nontraffic accident ⚕POA

7️⃣ V78.3 Unspecified occupant of bus injured in noncollision transport accident in nontraffic accident ⚕POA

7️⃣ V78.4 Person boarding or alighting from bus injured in noncollision transport accident ⚕POA

7️⃣ V78.5 Driver of bus injured in noncollision transport accident in traffic accident ⚕POA

7️⃣ V78.6 Passenger on bus injured in noncollision transport accident in traffic accident ⚕POA

7️⃣ V78.7 Person on outside of bus injured in noncollision transport accident in traffic accident ⚕POA

7️⃣ V78.9 Unspecified occupant of bus injured in noncollision transport accident in traffic accident ⚕POA

4️⃣ V79 Bus occupant injured in other and unspecified transport accidents

The appropriate 7th character is to be added to each code from category V79

A = initial encounter
D = subsequent encounter
S = sequela

5️⃣ V79.0 Driver of bus injured in collision with other and unspecified motor vehicles in nontraffic accident

7️⃣ V79.00 Driver of bus injured in collision with unspecified motor vehicles in nontraffic accident ⚕POA

7️⃣ V79.09 Driver of bus injured in collision with other motor vehicles in nontraffic accident ⚕POA

5️⃣ V79.1 Passenger on bus injured in collision with other and unspecified motor vehicles in nontraffic accident

7️⃣ V79.10 Passenger on bus injured in collision with unspecified motor vehicles in nontraffic accident ⚕POA

7️⃣ V79.19 Passenger on bus injured in collision with other motor vehicles in nontraffic accident ⚕POA

5️⃣ V79.2 Unspecified bus occupant injured in collision with other and unspecified motor vehicles in nontraffic accident

7️⃣ V79.20 Unspecified bus occupant injured in collision with unspecified motor vehicles in nontraffic accident ⚕POA
Bus collision NOS, nontraffic

7️⃣ V79.29 Unspecified bus occupant injured in collision with other motor vehicles in nontraffic accident ⚕POA

7️⃣ V79.3 Bus occupant (driver) (passenger) injured in unspecified nontraffic accident ⚕POA
Bus accident NOS, nontraffic
Bus occupant injured in nontraffic accident NOS

5️⃣ V79.4 Driver of bus injured in collision with other and unspecified motor vehicles in traffic accident

7️⃣ V79.40 Driver of bus injured in collision with unspecified motor vehicles in traffic accident ⚕POA

7️⃣ V79.49 Driver of bus injured in collision with other motor vehicles in traffic accident ⚕POA

5️⃣ V79.5 Passenger on bus injured in collision with other and unspecified motor vehicles in traffic accident

7️⃣ V79.50 Passenger on bus injured in collision with unspecified motor vehicles in traffic accident ⚕POA

7️⃣ V79.59 Passenger on bus injured in collision with other motor vehicles in traffic accident ⚕POA

5️⃣ V79.6 Unspecified bus occupant injured in collision with other and unspecified motor vehicles in traffic accident

7️⃣ V79.60 Unspecified bus occupant injured in collision with unspecified motor vehicles in traffic accident ⚕POA
Bus collision NOS (traffic)

7️⃣ V79.69 Unspecified bus occupant injured in collision with other motor vehicles in traffic accident ⚕POA

5️⃣ V79.8 Bus occupant (driver) (passenger) injured in other specified transport accidents

7️⃣ V79.81 Bus occupant (driver) (passenger) injured in transport accidents with military vehicle ⚕POA

7️⃣ V79.88 Bus occupant (driver) (passenger) injured in other specified transport accidents ⚕POA

7️⃣ V79.9 Bus occupant (driver) (passenger) injured in unspecified traffic accident ⚕POA
Bus accident NOS

Other land transport accidents (V80-V89)

4️⃣ V80 Animal-rider or occupant of animal-drawn vehicle injured in transport accident

The appropriate 7th character is to be added to each code from category V80

A = initial encounter
D = subsequent encounter
S = sequela

5️⃣ V80.0 Animal-rider or occupant of animal drawn vehicle injured by fall from or being thrown from animal or animal-drawn vehicle in noncollision accident

6️⃣ V80.01 Animal-rider injured by fall from or being thrown from animal in noncollision accident

7️⃣ V80.010 Animal-rider injured by fall from or being thrown from horse in noncollision accident ⚕POA

7️⃣ V80.018 Animal-rider injured by fall from or being thrown from other animal in noncollision accident ⚕POA

Unspecified Code	Other Specified Code	Manifestation Code	Ⓝ Newborn	Ⓟ Pediatric	Ⓜ Maternity	Ⓐ Adult	♂ Male	♀ Female

● New Code ▲ Revised Code Title ►◄ Revised Text *NOTES* *INCLUDES* *EXCLUDES 1* Not coded here *EXCLUDES 2* Not included here

4️⃣ 4th character required 5️⃣ 5th character required 6️⃣ 6th character required 7️⃣ 7th character required

7️⃣ Extension 'X' Alert HAC Hospital-acquired condition (HAC) alert **AHA** AHA Coding Clinic©

V80.02 Occupant of animal-drawn vehicle injured by fall from or being thrown from animal-drawn vehicle in noncollision accident

Overturning animal-drawn vehicle NOS

Overturning animal-drawn vehicle without collision

V80.1 Animal-rider or occupant of animal-drawn vehicle injured in collision with pedestrian or animal

EXCLUDES1 animal-rider or animal-drawn vehicle collision with animal-drawn vehicle or animal being ridden (V80.7)

V80.11 Animal-rider injured in collision with pedestrian or animal

V80.12 Occupant of animal-drawn vehicle injured in collision with pedestrian or animal

V80.2 Animal-rider or occupant of animal-drawn vehicle injured in collision with pedal cycle

V80.21 Animal-rider injured in collision with pedal cycle

V80.22 Occupant of animal-drawn vehicle injured in collision with pedal cycle

V80.3 Animal-rider or occupant of animal-drawn vehicle injured in collision with two- or three-wheeled motor vehicle

V80.31 Animal-rider injured in collision with two- or three-wheeled motor vehicle

V80.32 Occupant of animal-drawn vehicle injured in collision with two- or three-wheeled motor vehicle

V80.4 Animal-rider or occupant of animal-drawn vehicle injured in collision with car, pick-up truck, van, heavy transport vehicle or bus

EXCLUDES1 animal-rider injured in collision with military vehicle (V80.910)

occupant of animal-drawn vehicle injured in collision with military vehicle (V80.920)

V80.41 Animal-rider injured in collision with car, pick-up truck, van, heavy transport vehicle or bus

V80.42 Occupant of animal-drawn vehicle injured in collision with car, pick-up truck, van, heavy transport vehicle or bus

V80.5 Animal-rider or occupant of animal-drawn vehicle injured in collision with other specified motor vehicle

V80.51 Animal-rider injured in collision with other specified motor vehicle

V80.52 Occupant of animal-drawn vehicle injured in collision with other specified motor vehicle

V80.6 Animal-rider or occupant of animal-drawn vehicle injured in collision with railway train or railway vehicle

V80.61 Animal-rider injured in collision with railway train or railway vehicle

V80.62 Occupant of animal-drawn vehicle injured in collision with railway train or railway vehicle

V80.7 Animal-rider or occupant of animal-drawn vehicle injured in collision with other nonmotor vehicles

V80.71 Animal-rider or occupant of animal-drawn vehicle injured in collision with animal being ridden

V80.710 Animal-rider injured in collision with other animal being ridden

V80.711 Occupant of animal-drawn vehicle injured in collision with animal being ridden

V80.72 Animal-rider or occupant of animal-drawn vehicle injured in collision with other animal-drawn vehicle

V80.720 Animal-rider injured in collision with animal-drawn vehicle

V80.721 Occupant of animal-drawn vehicle injured in collision with other animal-drawn vehicle

V80.73 Animal-rider or occupant of animal-drawn vehicle injured in collision with streetcar

V80.730 Animal-rider injured in collision with streetcar

V80.731 Occupant of animal-drawn vehicle injured in collision with streetcar

V80.79 Animal-rider or occupant of animal-drawn vehicle injured in collision with other nonmotor vehicles

V80.790 Animal-rider injured in collision with other nonmotor vehicles

V80.791 Occupant of animal-drawn vehicle injured in collision with other nonmotor vehicles

V80.8 Animal-rider or occupant of animal-drawn vehicle injured in collision with fixed or stationary object

V80.81 Animal-rider injured in collision with fixed or stationary object

V80.82 Occupant of animal-drawn vehicle injured in collision with fixed or stationary object

V80.9 Animal-rider or occupant of animal-drawn vehicle injured in other and unspecified transport accidents

V80.91 Animal-rider injured in other and unspecified transport accidents

V80.910 Animal-rider injured in transport accident with military vehicle

V80.918 Animal-rider injured in other transport accident

V80.919 Animal-rider injured in unspecified transport accident

Animal rider accident NOS

V80.92 Occupant of animal-drawn vehicle injured in other and unspecified transport accidents

V80.920 Occupant of animal-drawn vehicle injured in transport accident with military vehicle

V80.928 Occupant of animal-drawn vehicle injured in other transport accident

V80.929 Occupant of animal-drawn vehicle injured in unspecified transport accident

Animal-drawn vehicle accident NOS

V81 Occupant of railway train or railway vehicle injured in transport accident

INCLUDES derailment of railway train or railway vehicle

person on outside of train

EXCLUDES1 streetcar (V82.-)

The appropriate 7th character is to be added to each code from category V81

A = initial encounter

D = subsequent encounter

S = sequela

V81.0 Occupant of railway train or railway vehicle injured in collision with motor vehicle in nontraffic accident

EXCLUDES1 Occupant of railway train or railway vehicle injured due to collision with military vehicle (V81.83)

V81.1 Occupant of railway train or railway vehicle injured in collision with motor vehicle in traffic accident

EXCLUDES1 Occupant of railway train or railway vehicle injured due to collision with military vehicle (V81.83)

V81.2 Occupant of railway train or railway vehicle injured in collision with or hit by rolling stock

V81.3 Occupant of railway train or railway vehicle injured in collision with other object

Railway collision NOS

V81.4 Person injured while boarding or alighting from railway train or railway vehicle

V81.5 Occupant of railway train or railway vehicle injured by fall in railway train or railway vehicle

V81.6 Occupant of railway train or railway vehicle injured by fall from railway train or railway vehicle

V81.7 Occupant of railway train or railway vehicle injured in derailment without antecedent collision

V81.8 Occupant of railway train or railway vehicle injured in other specified railway accidents

V81.81 Occupant of railway train or railway vehicle injured due to explosion or fire on train

V81.82 Occupant of railway train or railway vehicle injured due to object falling onto train

Occupant of railway train or railway vehicle injured due to falling earth onto train

PDx Unacceptable principal diagnosis symbol per Medicare code edits   POA Code exempt from diagnosis present on admission requirement
? Questionable admission   CC Complication or comorbidity   CC/MCC CC/MCC exclusion   MCC Major complication or comorbidity
Principal diagnosis as its own CC   Principal diagnosis as its own MCC   HCC HCC diagnosis code   RxHCC RxHCC diagnosis code
MACRA code   Z1 Z code as first-listed diagnosis

1206   When symbols appear on a code that requires a 7th character extension, refer to Appendix B to identify applicable 7th character codes.   2018 ICD-10-CM

Occupant of railway train or railway vehicle injured
due to falling rocks onto train

Occupant of railway train or railway vehicle injured
due to falling snow onto train

Occupant of railway train or railway vehicle injured
due to falling trees onto train

⑦ V81.83 **Occupant of railway train or railway vehicle injured
due to** collision with military vehicle POA

⑦ V81.89 **Occupant of railway train or railway vehicle injured
due to other specified railway accident** POA

⑦ V81.9 **Occupant of railway train or railway vehicle injured in
unspecified railway accident** POA

Railway accident NOS

④ V82 **Occupant of powered streetcar injured in transport accident**

INCLUDES   interurban electric car

person on outside of streetcar

tram (car)

trolley (car)

EXCLUDES1   bus (V70-V79)

motorcoach (V70-V79)

nonpowered streetcar (V76.-)

train (V81.-)

The appropriate 7th character is to be added to each code from
category V82

A = initial encounter

D = subsequent encounter

S = sequela

⑦ V82.0 **Occupant of streetcar injured in collision with motor vehicle
in** nontraffic accident POA

⑦ V82.1 **Occupant of streetcar injured in collision with motor vehicle
in** traffic accident POA

⑦ V82.2 **Occupant of streetcar injured in collision with or** hit by
rolling stock POA

⑦ V82.3 **Occupant of streetcar injured in collision with other object** POA

EXCLUDES1   collision with animal-drawn vehicle or animal being
ridden (V82.8)

⑦ V82.4 **Person injured** while boarding or alighting **from streetcar** POA

⑦ V82.5 **Occupant of streetcar injured by** fall in streetcar POA

EXCLUDES1   fall in streetcar:

while boarding or alighting (V82.4)

with antecedent collision (V82.0-V82.3)

⑦ V82.6 **Occupant of streetcar injured by** fall from streetcar POA

EXCLUDES1   fall from streetcar:

while boarding or alighting (V82.4)

with antecedent collision (V82.0-V82.3)

⑦ V82.7 **Occupant of streetcar injured in** derailment without
antecedent collision POA

EXCLUDES1   occupant of streetcar injured in derailment with
antecedent collision (V82.0-V82.3)

⑦ V82.8 **Occupant of streetcar injured in other specified transport
accidents** POA

Streetcar collision with military vehicle

Streetcar collision with train or nonmotor vehicles

⑦ V82.9 **Occupant of streetcar injured in unspecified traffic
accident** POA

Streetcar accident NOS

④ V83 **Occupant of special vehicle mainly used on industrial premises
injured in transport accident**

INCLUDES   battery-powered airport passenger vehicle

battery-powered truck (baggage) (mail)

coal-car in mine

forklift (truck)

logging car

self-propelled industrial truck

station baggage truck (powered)

tram, truck, or tub (powered) in mine or quarry

EXCLUDES1   special construction vehicles (V85.-)

special industrial vehicle in stationary use or maintenance
(W31.-)

The appropriate 7th character is to be added to each code from
category V83

A = initial encounter

D = subsequent encounter

S = sequela

⑦ V83.0 **Driver** of special industrial vehicle injured in
traffic accident POA

⑦ V83.1 **Passenger** of special industrial vehicle injured in traffic
accident POA

⑦ V83.2 **Person on outside** of special industrial vehicle injured in
traffic accident POA

⑦ V83.3 **Unspecified occupant of special industrial vehicle injured in
traffic accident** POA

⑦ V83.4 **Person injured** while boarding or alighting **from special
industrial vehicle** POA

⑦ V83.5 **Driver** of special industrial vehicle injured in nontraffic
accident POA

⑦ V83.6 **Passenger** of special industrial vehicle injured in nontraffic
accident POA

⑦ V83.7 **Person on outside** of special industrial vehicle injured in
nontraffic accident POA

⑦ V83.9 **Unspecified occupant of special industrial vehicle injured in
nontraffic accident** POA

Special-industrial-vehicle accident NOS

④ V84 **Occupant of special vehicle mainly used in agriculture injured in
transport accident**

INCLUDES   self-propelled farm machinery

tractor (and trailer)

EXCLUDES1   animal-powered farm machinery accident (W30.8-)

contact with combine harvester (W30.0)

special agricultural vehicle in stationary use or maintenance
(W30.-)

The appropriate 7th character is to be added to each code from
category V84

A = initial encounter

D = subsequent encounter

S = sequela

⑦ V84.0 **Driver** of special agricultural vehicle injured in traffic
accident POA

⑦ V84.1 **Passenger** of special agricultural vehicle injured in traffic
accident POA

⑦ V84.2 **Person on outside** of special agricultural vehicle injured in
traffic accident POA

⑦ V84.3 **Unspecified occupant of special agricultural vehicle injured
in traffic accident** POA

⑦ V84.4 **Person injured** while boarding or alighting **from special
agricultural vehicle** POA

⑦ V84.5 **Driver** of special agricultural vehicle injured in nontraffic
accident POA

⑦ V84.6 **Passenger** of special agricultural vehicle injured in nontraffic
accident POA

⑦ V84.7 **Person on outside** of special agricultural vehicle injured in
nontraffic accident POA

⑦ V84.9 **Unspecified occupant of special agricultural vehicle injured
in nontraffic accident** POA

Special-agricultural vehicle accident NOS

④ V85 **Occupant of special construction vehicle injured in transport
accident**

INCLUDES   bulldozer

digger

dump truck

earth-leveller

mechanical shovel

road-roller

EXCLUDES1   special industrial vehicle (V83.-)

special construction vehicle in stationary use or maintenance
(W31.-)

Unspecified Code   Other Specified Code   Manifestation Code   N Newborn   P Pediatric   M Maternity   A Adult   ♂ Male   ♀ Female
● New Code   ▲ Revised Code Title   ►◄ Revised Text   NOTES   INCLUDES   EXCLUDES 1 Not coded here   EXCLUDES 2 Not included here
④ 4th character required   ⑤ 5th character required   ⑥ 6th character required   ⑦ 7th character required
⑦ Extension 'X' Alert   HAC Hospital-acquired condition (HAC) alert   AHA AHA Coding Clinic©

V85.0 - V86.51 *(side margin)*

The appropriate 7th character is to be added to each code from category V85
- A = initial encounter
- D = subsequent encounter
- S = sequela

V85.0 Driver of special construction vehicle injured in traffic accident

V85.1 Passenger of special construction vehicle injured in traffic accident

V85.2 Person on outside of special construction vehicle injured in traffic accident

V85.3 Unspecified occupant of special construction vehicle injured in traffic accident

V85.4 Person injured while boarding or alighting from special construction vehicle

V85.5 Driver of special construction vehicle injured in nontraffic accident

V85.6 Passenger of special construction vehicle injured in nontraffic accident

V85.7 Person on outside of special construction vehicle injured in nontraffic accident

V85.9 Unspecified occupant of special construction vehicle injured in nontraffic accident

Special-construction-vehicle accident NOS

V86 Occupant of special all-terrain or other off-road motor vehicle, injured in transport accident

EXCLUDES1 special all-terrain vehicle in stationary use or maintenance (W31.-)

sport-utility vehicle (V50-V59)

three-wheeled motor vehicle designed for on-road use (V30-V39)

The appropriate 7th character is to be added to each code from category V86
- A = initial encounter
- D = subsequent encounter
- S = sequela

V86.0 Driver of special all-terrain or other off-road motor vehicle injured in traffic accident

V86.01 Driver of ambulance or fire engine injured in traffic accident

V86.02 Driver of snowmobile injured in traffic accident

V86.03 Driver of dune buggy injured in traffic accident

V86.04 Driver of military vehicle injured in traffic accident

V86.05 Driver of 3- or 4- wheeled all-terrain vehicle (ATV) injured in traffic accident

V86.06 Driver of dirt bike or motor/cross bike injured in traffic accident

V86.09 Driver of other special all-terrain or other off-road motor vehicle injured in traffic accident

Driver of dirt bike injured in traffic accident
Driver of go cart injured in traffic accident
Driver of golf cart injured in traffic accident

V86.1 Passenger of special all-terrain or other off-road motor vehicle injured in traffic accident

V86.11 Passenger of ambulance or fire engine injured in traffic accident

V86.12 Passenger of snowmobile injured in traffic accident

V86.13 Passenger of dune buggy injured in traffic accident

V86.14 Passenger of military vehicle injured in traffic accident

V86.15 Passenger of 3- or 4- wheeled all-terrain vehicle (ATV) injured in traffic accident

V86.16 Passenger of dirt bike or motor/cross bike injured in traffic accident

V86.19 Passenger of other special all-terrain or other off-road motor vehicle injured in traffic accident

Passenger of dirt bike injured in traffic accident
Passenger of go cart injured in traffic accident
Passenger of golf cart injured in traffic accident

V86.2 Person on outside of special all-terrain or other off-road motor vehicle injured in traffic accident

V86.21 Person on outside of ambulance or fire engine injured in traffic accident

V86.22 Person on outside of snowmobile injured in traffic accident

V86.23 Person on outside of dune buggy injured in traffic accident

V86.24 Person on outside of military vehicle injured in traffic accident

V86.25 Person on outside of 3- or 4- wheeled all-terrain vehicle (ATV) injured in traffic accident

V86.26 Person on outside of dirt bike or motor/cross bike injured in traffic accident

V86.29 Person on outside of other special all-terrain or other off-road motor vehicle injured in traffic accident

Person on outside of dirt bike injured in traffic accident
Person on outside of go cart in traffic accident
Person on outside of golf cart injured in traffic accident

V86.3 Unspecified occupant of special all-terrain or other off-road motor vehicle injured in traffic accident

V86.31 Unspecified occupant of ambulance or fire engine injured in traffic accident

V86.32 Unspecified occupant of snowmobile injured in traffic accident

V86.33 Unspecified occupant of dune buggy injured in traffic accident

V86.34 Unspecified occupant of military vehicle injured in traffic accident

V86.35 Unspecified occupant of 3- or 4- wheeled all-terrain vehicle (ATV) injured in traffic accident

V86.36 Unspecified occupant of dirt bike or motor/cross bike injured in traffic accident

V86.39 Unspecified occupant of other special all-terrain or other off-road motor vehicle injured in traffic accident

Unspecified occupant of dirt bike injured in traffic accident
Unspecified occupant of go cart injured in traffic accident
Unspecified occupant of golf cart injured in traffic accident

V86.4 Person injured while boarding or alighting from special all-terrain or other off-road motor vehicle

V86.41 Person injured while boarding or alighting from ambulance or fire engine

V86.42 Person injured while boarding or alighting from snowmobile

V86.43 Person injured while boarding or alighting from dune buggy

V86.44 Person injured while boarding or alighting from military vehicle

V86.45 Person injured while boarding or alighting from a 3- or 4- wheeled all-terrain vehicle (ATV)

V86.46 Person injured while boarding or alighting from a dirt bike or motor/cross bike

V86.49 Person injured while boarding or alighting from other special all-terrain or other off-road motor vehicle

Person injured while boarding or alighting from dirt bike
Person injured while boarding or alighting from go cart
Person injured while boarding or alighting from golf cart

V86.5 Driver of special all-terrain or other off-road motor vehicle injured in nontraffic accident

V86.51 Driver of ambulance or fire engine injured in nontraffic accident

---

PDx Unacceptable principal diagnosis symbol per Medicare code edits   PDx Code exempt from diagnosis present on admission requirement
❓ Questionable admission   CC Complication or comorbidity   CC/MCC Excl. CC/MCC exclusion   MCC Major complication or comorbidity
CC Principal diagnosis as its own CC   MCC Principal diagnosis as its own MCC   HCC HCC diagnosis code   RxHCC RxHCC diagnosis code
MACRA code   Z Z code as first-listed diagnosis

7️⃣ V86.52 Driver of snowmobile injured in nontraffic accident POA

7️⃣ V86.53 Driver of dune buggy injured in nontraffic accident POA

7️⃣ V86.54 Driver of military vehicle injured in nontraffic accident POA

● 7️⃣ V86.55 Driver of 3- or 4- wheeled all-terrain vehicle (ATV) injured in nontraffic accident

● 7️⃣ V86.56 Driver of dirt bike or motor/cross bike injured in nontraffic accident

7️⃣ V86.59 Driver of other special all-terrain or other off-road motor vehicle injured in nontraffic accident POA
　　Driver of dirt bike injured in nontraffic accident
　　Driver of go cart injured in nontraffic accident
　　Driver of golf cart injured in nontraffic accident

5️⃣ V86.6 Passenger of special all-terrain or other off-road motor vehicle injured in nontraffic accident

7️⃣ V86.61 Passenger of ambulance or fire engine injured in nontraffic accident POA

7️⃣ V86.62 Passenger of snowmobile injured in nontraffic accident POA

7️⃣ V86.63 Passenger of dune buggy injured in nontraffic accident POA

7️⃣ V86.64 Passenger of military vehicle injured in nontraffic accident POA

● 7️⃣ V86.65 Passenger of 3- or 4- wheeled all-terrain vehicle (ATV) injured in nontraffic accident

● 7️⃣ V86.66 Passenger of dirt bike or motor/cross bike injured in nontraffic accident

7️⃣ V86.69 Passenger of other special all-terrain or other off-road motor vehicle injured in nontraffic accident POA
　　Passenger of dirt bike injured in nontraffic accident
　　Passenger of go cart injured in nontraffic accident
　　Passenger of golf cart injured in nontraffic accident

5️⃣ V86.7 Person on outside of special all-terrain or other off-road motor vehicle injured in nontraffic accident

7️⃣ V86.71 Person on outside of ambulance or fire engine injured in nontraffic accident POA

7️⃣ V86.72 Person on outside of snowmobile injured in nontraffic accident POA

7️⃣ V86.73 Person on outside of dune buggy injured in nontraffic accident POA

7️⃣ V86.74 Person on outside of military vehicle injured in nontraffic accident POA

● 7️⃣ V86.75 Person on outside of 3- or 4- wheeled all-terrain vehicle (ATV) injured in nontraffic accident

● 7️⃣ V86.76 Person on outside of dirt bike or motor/cross bike injured in nontraffic accident

7️⃣ V86.79 Person on outside of other special all-terrain or other off-road motor vehicles injured in nontraffic accident POA
　　Person on outside of dirt bike injured in nontraffic accident
　　Person on outside of go cart injured in nontraffic accident
　　Person on outside of golf cart injured in nontraffic accident

5️⃣ V86.9 Unspecified occupant of special all-terrain or other off-road motor vehicle injured in nontraffic accident

7️⃣ V86.91 Unspecified occupant of ambulance or fire engine injured in nontraffic accident POA

7️⃣ V86.92 Unspecified occupant of snowmobile injured in nontraffic accident POA

7️⃣ V86.93 Unspecified occupant of dune buggy injured in nontraffic accident POA

7️⃣ V86.94 Unspecified occupant of military vehicle injured in nontraffic accident POA

● 7️⃣ V86.95 Unspecified occupant of 3- or 4- wheeled all-terrain vehicle (ATV) injured in nontraffic accident

● 7️⃣ V86.96 Unspecified occupant of dirt bike or motor/cross bike injured in nontraffic accident

7️⃣ V86.99 Unspecified occupant of other special all-terrain or other off-road motor vehicle injured in nontraffic accident POA
　　Off-road motor-vehicle accident NOS
　　Other motor-vehicle accident NOS
　　Unspecified occupant of go cart injured in nontraffic accident
　　Unspecified occupant of golf cart injured in nontraffic accident

4️⃣ V87 Traffic accident of specified type but victim's mode of transport unknown
　　EXCLUDES1 collision involving:
　　　　pedal cycle (V10-V19)
　　　　pedestrian (V01-V09)

The appropriate 7th character is to be added to each code from category V87
　　A = initial encounter
　　D = subsequent encounter
　　S = sequela

7️⃣ V87.0 Person injured in collision between car and two- or three-wheeled powered vehicle (traffic) POA

7️⃣ V87.1 Person injured in collision between other motor vehicle and two- or three-wheeled motor vehicle (traffic) POA

7️⃣ V87.2 Person injured in collision between car and pick-up truck or van (traffic) POA

7️⃣ V87.3 Person injured in collision between car and bus (traffic) POA

7️⃣ V87.4 Person injured in collision between car and heavy transport vehicle (traffic) POA

7️⃣ V87.5 Person injured in collision between heavy transport vehicle and bus (traffic) POA

7️⃣ V87.6 Person injured in collision between railway train or railway vehicle and car (traffic) POA

7️⃣ V87.7 Person injured in collision between other specified motor vehicles (traffic) POA

7️⃣ V87.8 Person injured in other specified noncollision transport accidents involving motor vehicle (traffic) POA

7️⃣ V87.9 Person injured in other specified (collision)(noncollision) transport accidents involving nonmotor vehicle (traffic) POA

4️⃣ V88 Nontraffic accident of specified type but victim's mode of transport unknown
　　EXCLUDES1 collision involving:
　　　　pedal cycle (V10-V19)
　　　　pedestrian (V01-V09)

The appropriate 7th character is to be added to each code from category V88
　　A = initial encounter
　　D = subsequent encounter
　　S = sequela

7️⃣ V88.0 Person injured in collision between car and two- or three-wheeled motor vehicle, nontraffic POA

7️⃣ V88.1 Person injured in collision between other motor vehicle and two- or three-wheeled motor vehicle, nontraffic POA

7️⃣ V88.2 Person injured in collision between car and pick-up truck or van, nontraffic POA

7️⃣ V88.3 Person injured in collision between car and bus, nontraffic POA

7️⃣ V88.4 Person injured in collision between car and heavy transport vehicle, nontraffic POA

7️⃣ V88.5 Person injured in collision between heavy transport vehicle and bus, nontraffic POA

7️⃣ V88.6 Person injured in collision between railway train or railway vehicle and car, nontraffic POA

7️⃣ V88.7 Person injured in collision between other specified motor vehicle, nontraffic POA

7️⃣ V88.8 Person injured in other specified noncollision transport accidents involving motor vehicle, nontraffic POA

7️⃣ V88.9 Person injured in other specified (collision)(noncollision) transport accidents involving nonmotor vehicle, nontraffic POA

4️⃣ V89 Motor- or nonmotor-vehicle accident, type of vehicle unspecified
　　The appropriate 7th character is to be added to each code from category V89
　　A = initial encounter

Unspecified Code　Other Specified Code　Manifestation Code　Ⓝ Newborn　Ⓟ Pediatric　Ⓜ Maternity　Ⓐ Adult　♂ Male　♀ Female
● New Code　▲ Revised Code Title　▶◀ Revised Text　NOTES　INCLUDES　EXCLUDES1 Not coded here　EXCLUDES2 Not included here
4️⃣ 4th character required　5️⃣ 5th character required　6️⃣ 6th character required　7️⃣ 7th character required
7️⃣ Extension 'X' Alert　HAC Hospital-acquired condition (HAC) alert　AHA AHA Coding Clinic©

D = subsequent encounter

S = sequela

V89.0 **Person injured in unspecified motor-vehicle accident, nontraffic** POA

Motor-vehicle accident NOS, nontraffic

V89.1 **Person injured in unspecified nonmotor-vehicle accident, nontraffic** POA

Nonmotor-vehicle accident NOS (nontraffic)

V89.2 **Person injured in unspecified motor-vehicle accident, traffic** POA

Motor-vehicle accident [MVA] NOS

Road (traffic) accident [RTA] NOS

V89.3 **Person injured in unspecified nonmotor-vehicle accident, traffic** POA

Nonmotor-vehicle traffic accident NOS

V89.9 **Person injured in unspecified vehicle accident** POA

Collision NOS

Water transport accidents (V90-V94)

V90 **Drowning and submersion due to accident to watercraft**

EXCLUDES1 *civilian water transport accident involving military watercraft (V94.81-)*

fall into water not from watercraft (W16.-)

military watercraft accident in military or war operations (Y36.0-, Y37.0-)

water-transport-related drowning or submersion without accident to watercraft (V92.-)

The appropriate 7th character is to be added to each code from category V90

A = initial encounter

D = subsequent encounter

S = sequela

V90.0 **Drowning and submersion due to watercraft overturning**

V90.00 **Drowning and submersion due to merchant ship overturning** POA

V90.01 **Drowning and submersion due to passenger ship overturning** POA

Drowning and submersion due to Ferry-boat overturning

Drowning and submersion due to Liner overturning

V90.02 **Drowning and submersion due to fishing boat overturning** POA

V90.03 **Drowning and submersion due to other powered watercraft overturning** POA

Drowning and submersion due to Hovercraft (on open water) overturning

Drowning and submersion due to Jet ski overturning

V90.04 **Drowning and submersion due to sailboat overturning** POA

V90.05 **Drowning and submersion due to canoe or kayak overturning** POA

V90.06 **Drowning and submersion due to (nonpowered) inflatable craft overturning** POA

V90.08 **Drowning and submersion due to other unpowered watercraft overturning** POA

Drowning and submersion due to windsurfer overturning

V90.09 **Drowning and submersion due to unspecified watercraft overturning** POA

Drowning and submersion due to boat NOS overturning

Drowning and submersion due to ship NOS overturning

Drowning and submersion due to watercraft NOS overturning

V90.1 **Drowning and submersion due to watercraft sinking**

V90.10 **Drowning and submersion due to merchant ship sinking** POA

V90.11 **Drowning and submersion due to passenger ship sinking** POA

Drowning and submersion due to Ferry-boat sinking

Drowning and submersion due to Liner sinking

V90.12 **Drowning and submersion due to fishing boat sinking** POA

V90.13 **Drowning and submersion due to other powered watercraft sinking** POA

Drowning and submersion due to Hovercraft (on open water) sinking

Drowning and submersion due to Jet ski sinking

V90.14 **Drowning and submersion due to sailboat sinking** POA

V90.15 **Drowning and submersion due to canoe or kayak sinking** POA

V90.16 **Drowning and submersion due to (nonpowered) inflatable craft sinking** POA

V90.18 **Drowning and submersion due to other unpowered watercraft sinking** POA

V90.19 **Drowning and submersion due to unspecified watercraft sinking** POA

Drowning and submersion due to boat NOS sinking

Drowning and submersion due to ship NOS sinking

Drowning and submersion due to watercraft NOS sinking

V90.2 **Drowning and submersion due to falling or jumping from burning watercraft**

V90.20 **Drowning and submersion due to falling or jumping from burning merchant ship** POA

V90.21 **Drowning and submersion due to falling or jumping from burning passenger ship** POA

Drowning and submersion due to falling or jumping from burning Ferry-boat

Drowning and submersion due to falling or jumping from burning Liner

V90.22 **Drowning and submersion due to falling or jumping from burning fishing boat** POA

V90.23 **Drowning and submersion due to falling or jumping from other burning powered watercraft** POA

Drowning and submersion due to falling and jumping from burning Hovercraft (on open water)

Drowning and submersion due to falling and jumping from burning Jet ski

V90.24 **Drowning and submersion due to falling or jumping from burning sailboat** POA

V90.25 **Drowning and submersion due to falling or jumping from burning canoe or kayak** POA

V90.26 **Drowning and submersion due to falling or jumping from burning (nonpowered) inflatable craft** POA

V90.27 **Drowning and submersion due to falling or jumping from burning water-skis** POA

V90.28 **Drowning and submersion due to falling or jumping from other burning unpowered watercraft** POA

Drowning and submersion due to falling and jumping from burning surf-board

Drowning and submersion due to falling and jumping from burning windsurfer

V90.29 **Drowning and submersion due to falling or jumping from unspecified burning watercraft** POA

Drowning and submersion due to falling or jumping from burning boat NOS

Drowning and submersion due to falling or jumping from burning ship NOS

Drowning and submersion due to falling or jumping from burning watercraft NOS

V90.3 **Drowning and submersion due to falling or jumping from crushed watercraft**

V90.30 **Drowning and submersion due to falling or jumping from crushed merchant ship** POA

V90.31 **Drowning and submersion due to falling or jumping from crushed passenger ship** POA

Drowning and submersion due to falling and jumping from crushed Ferry boat

---

POA Unacceptable principal diagnosis symbol per Medicare code edits POA Code exempt from diagnosis present on admission requirement

? Questionable admission CC Complication or comorbidity CC/MCC CC/MCC exclusion MCC Major complication or comorbidity

PCC Principal diagnosis as its own CC PMCC Principal diagnosis as its own MCC HCC HCC diagnosis code RxHCC RxHCC diagnosis code

MACRA code Z1 Z code as first-listed diagnosis

Drowning and submersion due to falling and jumping from crushed Liner

- [7th] **V90.32 Drowning and submersion due to falling or jumping from crushed fishing boat** [POA]
- [7th] **V90.33 Drowning and submersion due to falling or jumping from other crushed powered watercraft** [POA]
  - Drowning and submersion due to falling and jumping from crushed Hovercraft
  - Drowning and submersion due to falling and jumping from crushed Jet ski
- [7th] **V90.34 Drowning and submersion due to falling or jumping from crushed sailboat** [POA]
- [7th] **V90.35 Drowning and submersion due to falling or jumping from crushed canoe or kayak** [POA]
- [7th] **V90.36 Drowning and submersion due to falling or jumping from crushed (nonpowered) inflatable craft** [POA]
- [7th] **V90.37 Drowning and submersion due to falling or jumping from crushed water-skis** [POA]
- [7th] **V90.38 Drowning and submersion due to falling or jumping from other crushed unpowered watercraft** [POA]
  - Drowning and submersion due to falling and jumping from crushed surf-board
  - Drowning and submersion due to falling and jumping from crushed windsurfer
- [7th] **V90.39 Drowning and submersion due to falling or jumping from crushed unspecified watercraft** [POA]
  - Drowning and submersion due to falling and jumping from crushed boat NOS
  - Drowning and submersion due to falling and jumping from crushed ship NOS
  - Drowning and submersion due to falling and jumping from crushed watercraft NOS

[5th] **V90.8 Drowning and submersion due to other accident to watercraft**

- [7th] **V90.80 Drowning and submersion due to other accident to merchant ship** [POA]
- [7th] **V90.81 Drowning and submersion due to other accident to passenger ship** [POA]
  - Drowning and submersion due to other accident to Ferry-boat
  - Drowning and submersion due to other accident to Liner
- [7th] **V90.82 Drowning and submersion due to other accident to fishing boat** [POA]
- [7th] **V90.83 Drowning and submersion due to other accident to other powered watercraft** [POA]
  - Drowning and submersion due to other accident to Hovercraft (on open water)
  - Drowning and submersion due to other accident to Jet ski
- [7th] **V90.84 Drowning and submersion due to other accident to sailboat** [POA]
- [7th] **V90.85 Drowning and submersion due to other accident to canoe or kayak** [POA]
- [7th] **V90.86 Drowning and submersion due to other accident to (nonpowered) inflatable craft** [POA]
- [7th] **V90.87 Drowning and submersion due to other accident to water-skis** [POA]
- [7th] **V90.88 Drowning and submersion due to other accident to other unpowered watercraft** [POA]
  - Drowning and submersion due to other accident to surf-board
  - Drowning and submersion due to other accident to windsurfer
- [7th] **V90.89 Drowning and submersion due to other accident to unspecified watercraft** [POA]
  - Drowning and submersion due to other accident to boat NOS
  - Drowning and submersion due to other accident to ship NOS
  - Drowning and submersion due to other accident to watercraft NOS

[4th] **V91 Other injury due to accident to watercraft**

[INCLUDES] *any injury except drowning and submersion as a result of an accident to watercraft*

[EXCLUDES1] *civilian water transport accident involving military watercraft (V94.81-)*
military watercraft accident in military or war operations (Y36, Y37.-)

[EXCLUDES2] *drowning and submersion due to accident to watercraft (V90.-)*

The appropriate 7th character is to be added to each code from category V91
A = initial encounter
D = subsequent encounter
S = sequela

[5th] **V91.0 Burn due to watercraft on fire**

[EXCLUDES1] *burn from localized fire or explosion on board ship without accident to watercraft (V93.-)*

- [7th] **V91.00 Burn due to merchant ship on fire** [POA]
- [7th] **V91.01 Burn due to passenger ship on fire** [POA]
  - Burn due to Ferry-boat on fire
  - Burn due to Liner on fire
- [7th] **V91.02 Burn due to fishing boat on fire** [POA]
- [7th] **V91.03 Burn due to other powered watercraft on fire** [POA]
  - Burn due to Hovercraft (on open water) on fire
  - Burn due to Jet ski on fire
- [7th] **V91.04 Burn due to sailboat on fire** [POA]
- [7th] **V91.05 Burn due to canoe or kayak on fire** [POA]
- [7th] **V91.06 Burn due to (nonpowered) inflatable craft on fire** [POA]
- [7th] **V91.07 Burn due to water-skis on fire** [POA]
- [7th] **V91.08 Burn due to other unpowered watercraft on fire** [POA]
- [7th] **V91.09 Burn due to unspecified watercraft on fire** [POA]
  - Burn due to boat NOS on fire
  - Burn due to ship NOS on fire
  - Burn due to watercraft NOS on fire

[5th] **V91.1 Crushed between watercraft and other watercraft or other object due to collision**

Crushed by lifeboat after abandoning ship in a collision

[NOTES] select the specified type of watercraft that the victim was on at the time of the collision

- [7th] **V91.10 Crushed between merchant ship and other watercraft or other object due to collision** [POA]
- [7th] **V91.11 Crushed between passenger ship and other watercraft or other object due to collision** [POA]
  - Crushed between Ferry-boat and other watercraft or other object due to collision
  - Crushed between Liner and other watercraft or other object due to collision
- [7th] **V91.12 Crushed between fishing boat and other watercraft or other object due to collision** [POA]
- [7th] **V91.13 Crushed between other powered watercraft and other watercraft or other object due to collision** [POA]
  - Crushed between Hovercraft (on open water) and other watercraft or other object due to collision
  - Crushed between Jet ski and other watercraft or other object due to collision
- [7th] **V91.14 Crushed between sailboat and other watercraft or other object due to collision** [POA]
- [7th] **V91.15 Crushed between canoe or kayak and other watercraft or other object due to collision** [POA]
- [7th] **V91.16 Crushed between (nonpowered) inflatable craft and other watercraft or other object due to collision** [POA]
- [7th] **V91.18 Crushed between other unpowered watercraft and other watercraft or other object due to collision** [POA]
  - Crushed between surfboard and other watercraft or other object due to collision
  - Crushed between windsurfer and other watercraft or other object due to collision
- [7th] **V91.19 Crushed between unspecified watercraft and other watercraft or other object due to collision** [POA]
  - Crushed between boat NOS and other watercraft or other object due to collision
  - Crushed between ship NOS and other watercraft or other object due to collision

Unspecified Code Other Specified Code Manifestation Code [N] Newborn [P] Pediatric [M] Maternity [A] Adult ♂ Male ♀ Female
● New Code ▲ Revised Code Title ►◄ Revised Text [NOTES] [INCLUDES] [EXCLUDES1] Not coded here [EXCLUDES2] Not included here
[4th] 4th character required [5th] 5th character required [6th] 6th character required [7th] 7th character required
[X] Extension 'X' Alert [HAC] Hospital-acquired condition (HAC) alert AHA AHA Coding Clinic©

Crushed between watercraft NOS and other watercraft or other object due to collision

5ᵗʰ V91.2 **Fall due to collision between watercraft and other watercraft or other object**

Fall while remaining on watercraft after collision

NOTES select the specified type of watercraft that the victim was on at the time of the collision

EXCLUDES1 crushed between watercraft and other watercraft and other object due to collision (V91.1-)

drowning and submersion due to falling from crushed watercraft (V90.3-)

7ᵗʰ V91.20 **Fall due to collision between merchant ship and other watercraft or other object** POA

7ᵗʰ V91.21 **Fall due to collision between passenger ship and other watercraft or other object** POA

Fall due to collision between Ferry-boat and other watercraft or other object

Fall due to collision between Liner and other watercraft or other object

7ᵗʰ V91.22 **Fall due to collision between fishing boat and other watercraft or other object** POA

7ᵗʰ V91.23 **Fall due to collision between other powered watercraft and other watercraft or other object** POA

Fall due to collision between Hovercraft (on open water) and other watercraft or other object

Fall due to collision between Jet ski and other watercraft or other object

7ᵗʰ V91.24 **Fall due to collision between sailboat and other watercraft or other object** POA

7ᵗʰ V91.25 **Fall due to collision between canoe or kayak and other watercraft or other object** POA

7ᵗʰ V91.26 **Fall due to collision between (nonpowered) inflatable craft and other watercraft or other object** POA

7ᵗʰ V91.29 **Fall due to collision between unspecified watercraft and other watercraft or other object** POA

Fall due to collision between boat NOS and other watercraft or other object

Fall due to collision between ship NOS and other watercraft or other object

Fall due to collision between watercraft NOS and other watercraft or other object

5ᵗʰ V91.3 **Hit or struck by falling object due to accident to watercraft**

Hit or struck by falling object (part of damaged watercraft or other object) after falling or jumping from damaged watercraft

EXCLUDES2 drowning or submersion due to fall or jumping from damaged watercraft (V90.2-, V90.3-)

7ᵗʰ V91.30 **Hit or struck by falling object due to accident to** merchant ship POA

7ᵗʰ V91.31 **Hit or struck by falling object due to accident to** passenger ship POA

Hit or struck by falling object due to accident to Ferry-boat

Hit or struck by falling object due to accident to Liner

7ᵗʰ V91.32 **Hit or struck by falling object due to accident to** fishing boat POA

7ᵗʰ V91.33 **Hit or struck by falling object due to accident to other powered watercraft** POA

Hit or struck by falling object due to accident to Hovercraft (on open water)

Hit or struck by falling object due to accident to Jet ski

7ᵗʰ V91.34 **Hit or struck by falling object due to accident to** sailboat POA

7ᵗʰ V91.35 **Hit or struck by falling object due to accident to** canoe or kayak POA

7ᵗʰ V91.36 **Hit or struck by falling object due to accident to (nonpowered)** inflatable craft POA

7ᵗʰ V91.37 **Hit or struck by falling object due to accident to** water-skis POA

Hit by water-skis after jumping off of waterskis

7ᵗʰ V91.38 **Hit or struck by falling object due to accident to other unpowered watercraft**

Hit or struck by surf-board after falling off damaged surf-board

Hit or struck by object after falling off damaged windsurfer

7ᵗʰ V91.39 **Hit or struck by falling object due to accident to unspecified watercraft** POA

Hit or struck by falling object due to accident to boat NOS

Hit or struck by falling object due to accident to ship NOS

Hit or struck by falling object due to accident to watercraft NOS

5ᵗʰ V91.8 Other **injury due to other accident to watercraft**

7ᵗʰ V91.80 **Other injury due to other accident to merchant ship** POA

7ᵗʰ V91.81 **Other injury due to other accident to passenger ship** POA

Other injury due to other accident to Ferry-boat

Other injury due to other accident to Liner

7ᵗʰ V91.82 **Other injury due to other accident to fishing boat** POA

7ᵗʰ V91.83 **Other injury due to other accident to other powered watercraft** POA

Other injury due to other accident to Hovercraft (on open water)

Other injury due to other accident to Jet ski

7ᵗʰ V91.84 **Other injury due to other accident to sailboat** POA

7ᵗʰ V91.85 **Other injury due to other accident to canoe or kayak** POA

7ᵗʰ V91.86 **Other injury due to other accident to (nonpowered) inflatable craft** POA

7ᵗʰ V91.87 **Other injury due to other accident to water-skis** POA

7ᵗʰ V91.88 **Other injury due to other accident to other unpowered watercraft** POA

Other injury due to other accident to surf-board

Other injury due to other accident to windsurfer

7ᵗʰ V91.89 **Other injury due to other accident to unspecified watercraft** POA

Other injury due to other accident to boat NOS

Other injury due to other accident to ship NOS

Other injury due to other accident to watercraft NOS

4ᵗʰ V92 **Drowning and submersion due to accident on board watercraft, without accident to watercraft**

EXCLUDES1 civilian water transport accident involving military watercraft (V94.81-)

drowning or submersion due to accident to watercraft (V90-V91)

drowning or submersion of diver who voluntarily jumps from boat not involved in an accident (W16.711, W16.721)

fall into water without watercraft (W16.-)

military watercraft accident in military or war operations (Y36, Y37)

The appropriate 7th character is to be added to each code from category V92

A = initial encounter

D = subsequent encounter

S = sequela

5ᵗʰ V92.0 **Drowning and submersion due to** fall off watercraft

Drowning and submersion due to fall from gangplank of watercraft

Drowning and submersion due to fall overboard watercraft

EXCLUDES2 hitting head on object or bottom of body of water due to fall from watercraft (V94.0-)

7ᵗʰ V92.00 **Drowning and submersion due to fall off** merchant ship POA

7ᵗʰ V92.01 **Drowning and submersion due to fall off** passenger ship POA

Drowning and submersion due to fall off Ferry-boat

Drowning and submersion due to fall off Liner

7ᵗʰ V92.02 **Drowning and submersion due to fall off** fishing boat POA

PDₓₓ Unacceptable principal diagnosis symbol per Medicare code edits   POA Code exempt from diagnosis present on admission requirement
❓ Questionable admission   ᶜᶜ Complication or comorbidity   ᶜᶜ/ᴹᶜᶜ CC/MCC exclusion   ᴹᶜᶜ Major complication or comorbidity
Principal diagnosis as its own CC   Principal diagnosis as its own MCC   HCC HCC diagnosis code   RxHCC RxHCC diagnosis code
MACRA code   Z Z code as first-listed diagnosis

CHAPTER 20: EXTERNAL CAUSES OF MORBIDITY (V00-Y99)

1212   When symbols appear on a code that requires a 7th character extension, refer to Appendix B to identify applicable 7th character codes.   **2018 ICD-10-CM**

[7th] **V92.03 Drowning and submersion due to fall off other powered watercraft** [POA]
- Drowning and submersion due to fall off Hovercraft (on open water)
- Drowning and submersion due to fall off Jet ski

[7th] **V92.04 Drowning and submersion due to fall off sailboat** [POA]

[7th] **V92.05 Drowning and submersion due to fall off canoe or kayak** [POA]

[7th] **V92.06 Drowning and submersion due to fall off (nonpowered) inflatable craft** [POA]

[7th] **V92.07 Drowning and submersion due to fall off water-skis** [POA]
- [EXCLUDES1] *drowning and submersion due to falling off burning water-skis (V90.27)*
- *drowning and submersion due to falling off crushed water-skis (V90.37)*
- *hit by boat while water-skiing NOS (V94.X)*

[7th] **V92.08 Drowning and submersion due to fall off other unpowered watercraft** [POA]
- Drowning and submersion due to fall off surf-board
- Drowning and submersion due to fall off windsurfer
- [EXCLUDES1] *drowning and submersion due to fall off burning unpowered watercraft (V90.28)*
- *drowning and submersion due to fall off crushed unpowered watercraft (V90.38)*
- *drowning and submersion due to fall off damaged unpowered watercraft (V90.88)*
- *drowning and submersion due to rider of nonpowered watercraft being hit by other watercraft (V94.-)*
- *other injury due to rider of nonpowered watercraft being hit by other watercraft (V94.-)*

[7th] **V92.09 Drowning and submersion due to fall off unspecified watercraft** [POA]
- Drowning and submersion due to fall off boat NOS
- Drowning and submersion due to fall off ship
- Drowning and submersion due to fall off watercraft NOS

[5th] **V92.1 Drowning and submersion due to being thrown overboard by motion of watercraft**
- [EXCLUDES1] *drowning and submersion due to fall off surf-board (V92.08)*
- *drowning and submersion due to fall off water-skis (V92.07)*
- *drowning and submersion due to fall off windsurfer (V92.08)*

[7th] **V92.10 Drowning and submersion due to being thrown overboard by motion of merchant ship** [POA]

[7th] **V92.11 Drowning and submersion due to being thrown overboard by motion of passenger ship** [POA]
- Drowning and submersion due to being thrown overboard by motion of Ferry-boat
- Drowning and submersion due to being thrown overboard by motion of Liner

[7th] **V92.12 Drowning and submersion due to being thrown overboard by motion of fishing boat** [POA]

[7th] **V92.13 Drowning and submersion due to being thrown overboard by motion of other powered watercraft** [POA]
- Drowning and submersion due to being thrown overboard by motion of Hovercraft

[7th] **V92.14 Drowning and submersion due to being thrown overboard by motion of sailboat** [POA]

[7th] **V92.15 Drowning and submersion due to being thrown overboard by motion of canoe or kayak** [POA]

[7th] **V92.16 Drowning and submersion due to being thrown overboard by motion of (nonpowered) inflatable craft** [POA]

[7th] **V92.19 Drowning and submersion due to being thrown overboard by motion of unspecified watercraft** [POA]
- Drowning and submersion due to being thrown overboard by motion of boat NOS
- Drowning and submersion due to being thrown overboard by motion of ship NOS
- Drowning and submersion due to being thrown overboard by motion of watercraft NOS

[5th] **V92.2 Drowning and submersion due to being washed overboard from watercraft**
- Code first any associated cataclysm (X37.0-)

[7th] **V92.20 Drowning and submersion due to being washed overboard from merchant ship** [POA]

[7th] **V92.21 Drowning and submersion due to being washed overboard from passenger ship** [POA]
- Drowning and submersion due to being washed overboard from Ferry-boat
- Drowning and submersion due to being washed overboard from Liner

[7th] **V92.22 Drowning and submersion due to being washed overboard from fishing boat** [POA]

[7th] **V92.23 Drowning and submersion due to being washed overboard from other powered watercraft** [POA]
- Drowning and submersion due to being washed overboard from Hovercraft (on open water)
- Drowning and submersion due to being washed overboard from Jet ski

[7th] **V92.24 Drowning and submersion due to being washed overboard from sailboat** [POA]

[7th] **V92.25 Drowning and submersion due to being washed overboard from canoe or kayak** [POA]

[7th] **V92.26 Drowning and submersion due to being washed overboard from (nonpowered) inflatable craft** [POA]

[7th] **V92.27 Drowning and submersion due to being washed overboard from water-skis** [POA]
- [EXCLUDES1] *drowning and submersion due to fall off water-skis (V92.07)*

[7th] **V92.28 Drowning and submersion due to being washed overboard from other unpowered watercraft** [POA]
- Drowning and submersion due to being washed overboard from surf-board
- Drowning and submersion due to being washed overboard from windsurfer

[7th] **V92.29 Drowning and submersion due to being washed overboard from unspecified watercraft** [POA]
- Drowning and submersion due to being washed overboard from boat NOS
- Drowning and submersion due to being washed overboard from ship NOS
- Drowning and submersion due to being washed overboard from watercraft NOS

[4th] **V93 Other injury due to accident on board watercraft, without accident to watercraft**
- [EXCLUDES1] *civilian water transport accident involving military watercraft (V94.81-)*
- *other injury due to accident to watercraft (V91.-)*
- *military watercraft accident in military or war operations (Y36, Y37.-)*
- [EXCLUDES2] *drowning and submersion due to accident on board watercraft, without accident to watercraft (V92.-)*

The appropriate 7th character is to be added to each code from category V93
- **A = initial encounter**
- **D = subsequent encounter**
- **S = sequela**

[5th] **V93.0 Burn due to localized fire on board watercraft**
- [EXCLUDES1] *burn due to watercraft on fire (V91.0-)*

[7th] **V93.00 Burn due to localized fire on board merchant vessel** [POA]

[7th] **V93.01 Burn due to localized fire on board passenger vessel** [POA]
- Burn due to localized fire on board Ferry-boat
- Burn due to localized fire on board Liner

[7th] **V93.02 Burn due to localized fire on board fishing boat** [POA]

[7th] **V93.03 Burn due to localized fire on board other powered watercraft** [POA]

Burn due to localized fire on board Hovercraft
Burn due to localized fire on board Jet ski

[7th] **V93.04 Burn due to localized fire on board sailboat** [POA]

[7th] **V93.09 Burn due to localized fire on board unspecified watercraft** [POA]
Burn due to localized fire on board boat NOS
Burn due to localized fire on board ship NOS
Burn due to localized fire on board watercraft NOS

[5th] **V93.1 Other burn on board watercraft**
Burn due to source other than fire on board watercraft
[EXCLUDES1] *burn due to watercraft on fire (V91.0-)*

[7th] **V93.10 Other burn on board merchant vessel** [POA]

[7th] **V93.11 Other burn on board passenger vessel** [POA]
Other burn on board Ferry-boat
Other burn on board Liner

[7th] **V93.12 Other burn on board fishing boat** [POA]

[7th] **V93.13 Other burn on board other powered watercraft** [POA]
Other burn on board Hovercraft
Other burn on board Jet ski

[7th] **V93.14 Other burn on board sailboat** [POA]

[7th] **V93.19 Other burn on board unspecified watercraft** [POA]
Other burn on board boat NOS
Other burn on board ship NOS
Other burn on board watercraft NOS

[5th] **V93.2 Heat exposure on board watercraft**
[EXCLUDES1] *exposure to man-made heat not aboard watercraft (W92)*
exposure to natural heat while on board watercraft (X30)
exposure to sunlight while on board watercraft (X32)
[EXCLUDES2] *burn due to fire on board watercraft (V93.0-)*

[7th] **V93.20 Heat exposure on board merchant ship** [POA]

[7th] **V93.21 Heat exposure on board passenger ship** [POA]
Heat exposure on board Ferry-boat
Heat exposure on board Liner

[7th] **V93.22 Heat exposure on board fishing boat** [POA]

[7th] **V93.23 Heat exposure on board other powered watercraft** [POA]
Heat exposure on board hovercraft

[7th] **V93.24 Heat exposure on board sailboat** [POA]

[7th] **V93.29 Heat exposure on board unspecified watercraft** [POA]
Heat exposure on board boat NOS
Heat exposure on board ship NOS
Heat exposure on board watercraft NOS

[5th] **V93.3 Fall on board watercraft**
[EXCLUDES1] *fall due to collision of watercraft (V91.2-)*

[7th] **V93.30 Fall on board merchant ship** [POA]

[7th] **V93.31 Fall on board passenger ship** [POA]
Fall on board Ferry-boat
Fall on board Liner

[7th] **V93.32 Fall on board fishing boat** [POA]

[7th] **V93.33 Fall on board other powered watercraft** [POA]
Fall on board Hovercraft (on open water)
Fall on board Jet ski

[7th] **V93.34 Fall on board sailboat** [POA]

[7th] **V93.35 Fall on board canoe or kayak** [POA]

[7th] **V93.36 Fall on board (nonpowered) inflatable craft** [POA]

[7th] **V93.38 Fall on board other unpowered watercraft** [POA]

[7th] **V93.39 Fall on board unspecified watercraft** [POA]
Fall on board boat NOS
Fall on board ship NOS
Fall on board watercraft NOS

[5th] **V93.4 Struck by falling object on board watercraft**
Hit by falling object on board watercraft
[EXCLUDES1] *struck by falling object due to accident to watercraft (V91.3)*

[7th] **V93.40 Struck by falling object on merchant ship** [POA]

[7th] **V93.41 Struck by falling object on passenger ship** [POA]
Struck by falling object on Ferry-boat
Struck by falling object on Liner

[7th] **V93.42 Struck by falling object on fishing boat** [POA]

[7th] **V93.43 Struck by falling object on other powered watercraft** [POA]
Struck by falling object on Hovercraft

[7th] **V93.44 Struck by falling object on sailboat** [POA]

[7th] **V93.48 Struck by falling object on other unpowered watercraft** [POA]

[7th] **V93.49 Struck by falling object on unspecified watercraft** [POA]

[5th] **V93.5 Explosion on board watercraft**
Boiler explosion on steamship
[EXCLUDES2] *fire on board watercraft (V93.0-)*

[7th] **V93.50 Explosion on board merchant ship** [POA]

[7th] **V93.51 Explosion on board passenger ship** [POA]
Explosion on board Ferry-boat
Explosion on board Liner

[7th] **V93.52 Explosion on board fishing boat** [POA]

[7th] **V93.53 Explosion on board other powered watercraft** [POA]
Explosion on board Hovercraft
Explosion on board Jet ski

[7th] **V93.54 Explosion on board sailboat** [POA]

[7th] **V93.59 Explosion on board unspecified watercraft** [POA]
Explosion on board boat NOS
Explosion on board ship NOS
Explosion on board watercraft NOS

[5th] **V93.6 Machinery accident on board watercraft**
[EXCLUDES1] *machinery explosion on board watercraft (V93.4-)*
machinery fire on board watercraft (V93.0-)

[7th] **V93.60 Machinery accident on board merchant ship** [POA]

[7th] **V93.61 Machinery accident on board passenger ship** [POA]
Machinery accident on board Ferry-boat
Machinery accident on board Liner

[7th] **V93.62 Machinery accident on board fishing boat** [POA]

[7th] **V93.63 Machinery accident on board other powered watercraft** [POA]
Machinery accident on board Hovercraft

[7th] **V93.64 Machinery accident on board sailboat** [POA]

[7th] **V93.69 Machinery accident on board unspecified watercraft** [POA]
Machinery accident on board boat NOS
Machinery accident on board ship NOS
Machinery accident on board watercraft NOS

[5th] **V93.8 Other injury due to other accident on board watercraft**
Accidental poisoning by gases or fumes on watercraft

[7th] **V93.80 Other injury due to other accident on board merchant ship** [POA]

[7th] **V93.81 Other injury due to other accident on board passenger ship** [POA]
Other injury due to other accident on board Ferry-boat
Other injury due to other accident on board Liner

[7th] **V93.82 Other injury due to other accident on board fishing boat** [POA]

[7th] **V93.83 Other injury due to other accident on board other powered watercraft** [POA]
Other injury due to other accident on board Hovercraft
Other injury due to other accident on board Jet ski

[7th] **V93.84 Other injury due to other accident on board sailboat** [POA]

[7th] **V93.85 Other injury due to other accident on board canoe or kayak** [POA]

[7th] **V93.86 Other injury due to other accident on board (nonpowered) inflatable craft** [POA]

[7th] **V93.87 Other injury due to other accident on board water-skis** [POA]
Hit or struck by object while waterskiing

[7th] **V93.88 Other injury due to other accident on board other unpowered watercraft** [POA]
Hit or struck by object while surfing
Hit or struck by object while on board windsurfer

[7th] **V93.89 Other injury due to other accident on board unspecified watercraft** [POA]
Other injury due to other accident on board boat NOS

[PDx] Unacceptable principal diagnosis symbol per Medicare code edits [POA] Code exempt from diagnosis present on admission requirement
[?] Questionable admission [CC] Complication or comorbidity [CC/MCC Exc] CC/MCC exclusion [MCC] Major complication or comorbidity
[PDx CC] Principal diagnosis as its own CC [PDx MCC] Principal diagnosis as its own MCC [HCC] HCC diagnosis code [RxHCC] RxHCC diagnosis code
MACRA code [Z1] Z code as first-listed diagnosis

Other injury due to other accident on board ship NOS
Other injury due to other accident on board watercraft NOS

[4th] **V94 Other and unspecified water transport accidents**

[EXCLUDES1] *military watercraft accidents in military or war operations (Y36, Y37)*

The appropriate 7th character is to be added to each code from category V94
- **A = initial encounter**
- **D = subsequent encounter**
- **S = sequela**

[7th] **V94.0 Hitting object or bottom of body of water due to fall from watercraft** [POA]
[EXCLUDES2] *drowning and submersion due to fall from watercraft (V92.0-)*

[5th] **V94.1 Bather struck by watercraft**
Swimmer hit by watercraft
[7th] **V94.11 Bather struck by powered watercraft** [POA]
[7th] **V94.12 Bather struck by nonpowered watercraft** [POA]

[5th] **V94.2 Rider of nonpowered watercraft struck by other watercraft**
[7th] **V94.21 Rider of nonpowered watercraft struck by other nonpowered watercraft** [POA]
Canoer hit by other nonpowered watercraft
Surfer hit by other nonpowered watercraft
Windsurfer hit by other nonpowered watercraft
[7th] **V94.22 Rider of nonpowered watercraft struck by powered watercraft** [POA]
Canoer hit by motorboat
Surfer hit by motorboat
Windsurfer hit by motorboat

[5th] **V94.3 Injury to rider of (inflatable) watercraft being pulled behind other watercraft**
[7th] **V94.31 Injury to rider of (inflatable) recreational watercraft being pulled behind other watercraft** [POA]
Injury to rider of inner-tube pulled behind motor boat
[7th] **V94.32 Injury to rider of non-recreational watercraft being pulled behind other watercraft** [POA]
Injury to occupant of dingy being pulled behind boat or ship
Injury to occupant of life-raft being pulled behind boat or ship

[7th] **V94.4 Injury to barefoot water-skier** [POA]
Injury to person being pulled behind boat or ship

[5th] **V94.8 Other water transport accident**
[6th] **V94.81 Water transport accident involving military watercraft**
[7th] **V94.810 Civilian watercraft involved in water transport accident with military watercraft** [POA]
Passenger on civilian watercraft injured due to accident with military watercraft
[7th] **V94.811 Civilian in water injured by military watercraft** [POA]
[7th] **V94.818 Other water transport accident involving military watercraft** [POA]
[7th] **V94.89 Other water transport accident** [POA]

[7th] **V94.9 Unspecified water transport accident** [POA]
Water transport accident NOS

Air and space transport accidents (V95-V97)

[EXCLUDES1] *military aircraft accidents in military or war operations (Y36, Y37)*

[4th] **V95 Accident to powered aircraft causing injury to occupant**

The appropriate 7th character is to be added to each code from category V95
- **A = initial encounter**
- **D = subsequent encounter**
- **S = sequela**

[5th] **V95.0 Helicopter accident injuring occupant**
[7th] **V95.00 Unspecified helicopter accident injuring occupant** [POA]
[7th] **V95.01 Helicopter crash injuring occupant** [POA]
[7th] **V95.02 Forced landing of helicopter injuring occupant** [POA]
[7th] **V95.03 Helicopter collision injuring occupant** [POA]
Helicopter collision with any object, fixed, movable or moving
[7th] **V95.04 Helicopter fire injuring occupant** [POA]
[7th] **V95.05 Helicopter explosion injuring occupant** [POA]
[7th] **V95.09 Other helicopter accident injuring occupant** [POA]

[5th] **V95.1 Ultralight, microlight or powered-glider accident injuring occupant**
[7th] **V95.10 Unspecified ultralight, microlight or powered-glider accident injuring occupant** [POA]
[7th] **V95.11 Ultralight, microlight or powered-glider crash injuring occupant** [POA]
[7th] **V95.12 Forced landing of ultralight, microlight or powered-glider injuring occupant** [POA]
[7th] **V95.13 Ultralight, microlight or powered-glider collision injuring occupant** [POA]
Ultralight, microlight or powered-glider collision with any object, fixed, movable or moving
[7th] **V95.14 Ultralight, microlight or powered-glider fire injuring occupant** [POA]
[7th] **V95.15 Ultralight, microlight or powered-glider explosion injuring occupant** [POA]
[7th] **V95.19 Other ultralight, microlight or powered-glider accident injuring occupant** [POA]

[5th] **V95.2 Other private fixed-wing aircraft accident injuring occupant**
[7th] **V95.20 Unspecified accident to other private fixed-wing aircraft, injuring occupant** [POA]
[7th] **V95.21 Other private fixed-wing aircraft crash injuring occupant** [POA]
[7th] **V95.22 Forced landing of other private fixed-wing aircraft injuring occupant** [POA]
[7th] **V95.23 Other private fixed-wing aircraft collision injuring occupant** [POA]
Other private fixed-wing aircraft collision with any object, fixed, movable or moving
[7th] **V95.24 Other private fixed-wing aircraft fire injuring occupant** [POA]
[7th] **V95.25 Other private fixed-wing aircraft explosion injuring occupant** [POA]
[7th] **V95.29 Other accident to other private fixed-wing aircraft injuring occupant** [POA]

[5th] **V95.3 Commercial fixed-wing aircraft accident injuring occupant**
[7th] **V95.30 Unspecified accident to commercial fixed-wing aircraft injuring occupant** [POA]
[7th] **V95.31 Commercial fixed-wing aircraft crash injuring occupant** [POA]
[7th] **V95.32 Forced landing of commercial fixed-wing aircraft injuring occupant** [POA]
[7th] **V95.33 Commercial fixed-wing aircraft collision injuring occupant** [POA]
Commercial fixed-wing aircraft collision with any object, fixed, movable or moving
[7th] **V95.34 Commercial fixed-wing aircraft fire injuring occupant** [POA]
[7th] **V95.35 Commercial fixed-wing aircraft explosion injuring occupant** [POA]
[7th] **V95.39 Other accident to commercial fixed-wing aircraft injuring occupant** [POA]

[5th] **V95.4 Spacecraft accident injuring occupant**
[7th] **V95.40 Unspecified spacecraft accident injuring occupant** [POA]
[7th] **V95.41 Spacecraft crash injuring occupant** [POA]
[7th] **V95.42 Forced landing of spacecraft injuring occupant** [POA]
[7th] **V95.43 Spacecraft collision injuring occupant** [POA]
Spacecraft collision with any object, fixed, moveable or moving
[7th] **V95.44 Spacecraft fire injuring occupant** [POA]
[7th] **V95.45 Spacecraft explosion injuring occupant** [POA]
[7th] **V95.49 Other spacecraft accident injuring occupant** [POA]

[7th] **V95.8 Other powered aircraft accidents injuring occupant** [POA]

[7th] **V95.9 Unspecified aircraft accident injuring occupant** [POA]
Aircraft accident NOS
Air transport accident NOS

Unspecified Code Other Specified Code Manifestation Code [N] Newborn [P] Pediatric [M] Maternity [A] Adult ♂ Male ♀ Female
● New Code ▲ Revised Code Title ►◄ Revised Text [NOTES] [INCLUDES] [EXCLUDES1] Not coded here [EXCLUDES2] Not included here
[4th] 4th character required [5th] 5th character required [6th] 6th character required [7th] 7th character required
[x] Extension 'X' Alert [HAC] Hospital-acquired condition (HAC) alert AHA AHA Coding Clinic©

When symbols appear on a code that requires a 7th character extension, refer to Appendix B to identify applicable 7th character codes.

V96 Accident to nonpowered aircraft **causing injury to occupant**

The appropriate 7th character is to be added to each code from category V96

A = initial encounter
D = subsequent encounter
S = sequela

V96.0 Balloon **accident injuring occupant**

V96.00 Unspecified balloon accident injuring occupant POA

V96.01 Balloon crash **injuring occupant** POA

V96.02 Forced landing of balloon injuring occupant POA

V96.03 Balloon collision **injuring occupant** POA
Balloon collision with any object, fixed, moveable or moving

V96.04 Balloon fire **injuring occupant** POA

V96.05 Balloon explosion **injuring occupant** POA

V96.09 Other balloon accident injuring occupant POA

V96.1 Hang-glider **accident injuring occupant**

V96.10 Unspecified hang-glider accident injuring occupant POA

V96.11 Hang-glider crash **injuring occupant** POA

V96.12 Forced landing of hang-glider injuring occupant POA

V96.13 Hang-glider collision **injuring occupant** POA
Hang-glider collision with any object, fixed, moveable or moving

V96.14 Hang-glider fire **injuring occupant** POA

V96.15 Hang-glider explosion **injuring occupant** POA

V96.19 Other hang-glider accident injuring occupant POA

V96.2 Glider (nonpowered) **accident injuring occupant**

V96.20 Unspecified glider (nonpowered) accident injuring occupant POA

V96.21 Glider (nonpowered) crash **injuring occupant** POA

V96.22 Forced landing of glider (nonpowered) injuring occupant POA

V96.23 Glider (nonpowered) collision **injuring occupant** POA
Glider (nonpowered) collision with any object, fixed, moveable or moving

V96.24 Glider (nonpowered) fire **injuring occupant** POA

V96.25 Glider (nonpowered) explosion **injuring occupant** POA

V96.29 Other glider (nonpowered) accident injuring occupant POA

V96.8 Other nonpowered-aircraft accidents injuring occupant POA
Kite carrying a person accident injuring occupant

V96.9 Unspecified nonpowered-aircraft accident injuring occupant POA
Nonpowered-aircraft accident NOS

V97 Other specified air transport accidents

The appropriate 7th character is to be added to each code from category V97

A = initial encounter
D = subsequent encounter
S = sequela

V97.0 Occupant of aircraft injured in other specified air transport accidents
Fall in, on or from aircraft in air transport accident
EXCLUDES1 accident while boarding or alighting aircraft (V97.1)

V97.1 Person injured while boarding or alighting **from aircraft** POA

V97.2 Parachutist accident

V97.21 Parachutist entangled in object POA
Parachutist landing in tree

V97.22 Parachutist injured on landing POA

V97.29 Other parachutist accident

V97.3 Person on ground injured in air transport accident

V97.31 Hit by object falling from **aircraft** POA
Hit by crashing aircraft
Injured by aircraft hitting house
Injured by aircraft hitting car

V97.32 Injured by rotating propeller POA

V97.33 Sucked into jet engine POA

V97.39 Other injury to person on ground due to air transport accident POA

V97.8 Other air transport accidents, not elsewhere classified
EXCLUDES1 aircraft accident NOS (V95.9)
exposure to changes in air pressure during ascent or descent (W94.-)

V97.81 Air transport accident involving military **aircraft**

V97.810 Civilian aircraft involved in air transport accident with military aircraft POA
Passenger in civilian aircraft injured due to accident with military aircraft

V97.811 Civilian injured by military aircraft POA

V97.818 Other air transport accident involving military aircraft POA

V97.89 Other air transport accidents, not elsewhere classified POA
Injury from machinery on aircraft

Other and unspecified transport accidents (V98-V99)

EXCLUDES1 vehicle accident, type of vehicle unspecified (V89.-)

V98 Other specified transport accidents

The appropriate 7th character is to be added to each code from category V98

A = initial encounter
D = subsequent encounter
S = sequela

V98.0 Accident to, on or involving cable-car, not on rails POA
Caught or dragged by cable-car, not on rails
Fall or jump from cable-car, not on rails
Object thrown from or in cable-car, not on rails

V98.1 Accident to, on or involving land-yacht POA

V98.2 Accident to, on or involving ice yacht POA

V98.3 Accident to, on or involving ski lift POA
Accident to, on or involving ski chair-lift
Accident to, on or involving ski-lift with gondola

V98.8 Other specified transport accidents POA

V99 Unspecified transport accident POA

The appropriate 7th character is to be added to code V99

A = initial encounter
D = subsequent encounter
S = sequela

Other external causes of accidental injury (W00-X58)

Slipping, tripping, stumbling and falls (W00-W19)

EXCLUDES1 assault involving a fall (Y01-Y02)
fall from animal (V80.-)
fall (in) (from) machinery (in operation) (W28-W31)
fall (in) (from) transport vehicle (V01-V99)
intentional self-harm involving a fall (X80-X81)

EXCLUDES2 at risk for fall (history of fall) Z91.81
fall (in) (from) burning building (X00.-)
fall into fire ▶(X00-X04, X08)◄

W00 Fall due to ice and snow

INCLUDES pedestrian on foot falling (slipping) on ice and snow

EXCLUDES1 fall on (from) ice and snow involving pedestrian conveyance (V00.-)
fall from stairs and steps not due to ice and snow (W10.-)

The appropriate 7th character is to be added to each code from category W00

A = initial encounter
D = subsequent encounter
S = sequela

W00.0 Fall on same level **due to ice and snow**

W00.1 Fall from stairs and steps **due to ice and snow**

W00.2 Other fall from one level to another due to ice and snow

W00.9 Unspecified fall due to ice and snow

W01 Fall on same level from slipping, tripping and stumbling
INCLUDES fall on moving sidewalk

POA Unacceptable principal diagnosis symbol per Medicare code edits   POA Code exempt from diagnosis present on admission requirement
❓ Questionable admission   CC Complication or comorbidity   CC/MCC Exo CC/MCC exclusion   MCC Major complication or comorbidity
Principal diagnosis as its own CC   Principal diagnosis as its own MCC   HCC HCC diagnosis code   RxHCC RxHCC diagnosis code
MACRA code   Z1 Z code as first-listed diagnosis

EXCLUDES1 *fall due to bumping (striking) against object (W18.0-)*

fall in shower or bathtub (W18.2-)

fall on same level NOS (W18.30)

fall on same level from slipping, tripping and stumbling due to ice or snow (W00.0)

fall off or from toilet (W18.1-)

slipping, tripping and stumbling NOS (W18.40)

slipping, tripping and stumbling without falling (W18.4-)

The appropriate 7th character is to be added to each code from category W01
A = initial encounter
D = subsequent encounter
S = sequela

W01.0 **Fall on same level from slipping, tripping and stumbling** without subsequent striking against object
Falling over animal

W01.1 **Fall on same level from slipping, tripping and stumbling** with subsequent striking against object

W01.10 **Fall on same level from slipping, tripping and stumbling with subsequent striking against** unspecified object

W01.11 **Fall on same level from slipping, tripping and stumbling with subsequent striking against** sharp object

W01.110 **Fall on same level from slipping, tripping and stumbling with subsequent striking against** sharp glass

W01.111 **Fall on same level from slipping, tripping and stumbling with subsequent striking against** power tool or machine

W01.118 **Fall on same level from slipping, tripping and stumbling with subsequent striking against** other sharp object

W01.119 **Fall on same level from slipping, tripping and stumbling with subsequent striking against unspecified sharp object**

W01.19 **Fall on same level from slipping, tripping and stumbling with subsequent striking against** other object

W01.190 **Fall on same level from slipping, tripping and stumbling with subsequent striking against** furniture

W01.198 **Fall on same level from slipping, tripping and stumbling with subsequent striking against other object**

W03 **Other fall on same level due to collision with another person**
Fall due to non-transport collision with other person

EXCLUDES1 *collision with another person without fall (W51)*

crushed or pushed by a crowd or human stampede (W52)

fall involving pedestrian conveyance (V00-V09)

fall due to ice or snow (W00)

fall on same level NOS (W18.30)

The appropriate 7th character is to be added to code W03
A = initial encounter
D = subsequent encounter
S = sequela

W04 **Fall while being carried or supported by other persons**
Accidentally dropped while being carried
The appropriate 7th character is to be added to code W04
A = initial encounter
D = subsequent encounter
S = sequela

W05 **Fall from** non-moving **wheelchair, nonmotorized scooter and motorized mobility scooter**

EXCLUDES1 *fall from moving wheelchair (powered) (V00.811)*

fall from moving motorized mobility scooter (V00.831)

fall from nonmotorized scooter (V00.141)

The appropriate 7th character is to be added to each code from category W05
A = initial encounter
D = subsequent encounter
S = sequela

W05.0 **Fall from non-moving** wheelchair

W05.1 **Fall from non-moving** nonmotorized scooter

W05.2 **Fall from non-moving** motorized mobility scooter

W06 **Fall from** bed
The appropriate 7th character is to be added to code W06
A = initial encounter
D = subsequent encounter
S = sequela

W07 **Fall from** chair
The appropriate 7th character is to be added to code W07
A = initial encounter
D = subsequent encounter
S = sequela

W08 **Fall from other furniture**
The appropriate 7th character is to be added to code W08
A = initial encounter
D = subsequent encounter
S = sequela

W09 **Fall on and from playground equipment**

EXCLUDES1 *fall involving recreational machinery (W31)*

The appropriate 7th character is to be added to each code from category W09
A = initial encounter
D = subsequent encounter
S = sequela

W09.0 **Fall on or from playground slide**   POA

W09.1 **Fall from playground swing**   POA

W09.2 **Fall on or from jungle gym**   POA

W09.8 **Fall on or from other playground equipment**   POA

W10 **Fall on and from stairs and steps**

EXCLUDES1 *Fall from stairs and steps due to ice and snow (W00.1)*

The appropriate 7th character is to be added to each code from category W10
A = initial encounter
D = subsequent encounter
S = sequela

W10.0 **Fall (on)(from)** escalator

W10.1 **Fall (on)(from)** sidewalk curb

W10.2 **Fall (on)(from)** incline
Fall (on) (from) ramp

W10.8 **Fall (on) (from) other stairs and steps**

W10.9 **Fall (on) (from) unspecified stairs and steps**

W11 **Fall on and from** ladder
The appropriate 7th character is to be added to code W11
A = initial encounter
D = subsequent encounter
S = sequela

W12 **Fall on and from** scaffolding
The appropriate 7th character is to be added to code W12
A = initial encounter
D = subsequent encounter
S = sequela

W13 **Fall from, out of or through** building or structure
The appropriate 7th character is to be added to each code from category W13
A = initial encounter
D = subsequent encounter
S = sequela

W13.0 **Fall from, out of or through** balcony
Fall from, out of or through railing

W13.1 **Fall from, out of or through** bridge

W13.2 **Fall from, out of or through** roof

W13.3 **Fall through** floor

W13.4 **Fall from, out of or through** window

Unspecified Code   Other Specified Code   Manifestation Code   N Newborn   P Pediatric   M Maternity   A Adult   ♂ Male   ♀ Female
● New Code   ▲ Revised Code Title   ►◄ Revised Text   NOTES   INCLUDES   EXCLUDES1 Not coded here   EXCLUDES2 Not included here
4th character required   5th character required   6th character required   7th character required
Extension 'X' Alert   HAC Hospital-acquired condition (HAC) alert   AHA AHA Coding Clinic©

EXCLUDES2 fall with subsequent striking against sharp glass (W01.110)

W13.8 Fall from, out of or through other building or structure
Fall from, out of or through viaduct
Fall from, out of or through wall
Fall from, out of or through flag-pole

W13.9 Fall from, out of or through building, not otherwise specified
EXCLUDES1 collapse of a building or structure (W20.-)
fall or jump from burning building or structure (X00.-)

W14 Fall from tree
The appropriate 7th character is to be added to code W14
A = initial encounter
D = subsequent encounter
S = sequela

W15 Fall from cliff
The appropriate 7th character is to be added to code W15
A = initial encounter
D = subsequent encounter
S = sequela

W16 Fall, jump or diving into water
EXCLUDES1 accidental non-watercraft drowning and submersion not involving fall (W65-W74)
effects of air pressure from diving (W94.-)
fall into water from watercraft (V90-V94)
hitting an object or against bottom when falling from watercraft (V94.0)
EXCLUDES2 striking or hitting diving board (W21.4)
The appropriate 7th character is to be added to each code from category W16
A = initial encounter
D = subsequent encounter
S = sequela

W16.0 Fall into swimming pool
Fall into swimming pool NOS
EXCLUDES1 fall into empty swimming pool (W17.3)

W16.01 Fall into swimming pool striking water surface

W16.011 Fall into swimming pool striking water surface causing drowning and submersion
EXCLUDES1 drowning and submersion while in swimming pool without fall (W67)

W16.012 Fall into swimming pool striking water surface causing other injury

W16.02 Fall into swimming pool striking bottom

W16.021 Fall into swimming pool striking bottom causing drowning and submersion
EXCLUDES1 drowning and submersion while in swimming pool without fall (W67)

W16.022 Fall into swimming pool striking bottom causing other injury

W16.03 Fall into swimming pool striking wall

W16.031 Fall into swimming pool striking wall causing drowning and submersion
EXCLUDES1 drowning and submersion while in swimming pool without fall (W67)

W16.032 Fall into swimming pool striking wall causing other injury

W16.1 Fall into natural body of water
Fall into lake
Fall into open sea
Fall into river
Fall into stream

W16.11 Fall into natural body of water striking water surface

W16.111 Fall into natural body of water striking water surface causing drowning and submersion
EXCLUDES1 drowning and submersion while in natural body of water without fall (W69)

W16.112 Fall into natural body of water striking water surface causing other injury

W16.12 Fall into natural body of water striking bottom

W16.121 Fall into natural body of water striking bottom causing drowning and submersion
EXCLUDES1 drowning and submersion while in natural body of water without fall (W69)

W16.122 Fall into natural body of water striking bottom causing other injury

W16.13 Fall into natural body of water striking side

W16.131 Fall into natural body of water striking side causing drowning and submersion
EXCLUDES1 drowning and submersion while in natural body of water without fall (W69)

W16.132 Fall into natural body of water striking side causing other injury

W16.2 Fall in (into) filled bathtub or bucket of water

W16.21 Fall in (into) filled bathtub
EXCLUDES1 fall into empty bathtub (W18.2)

W16.211 Fall in (into) filled bathtub causing drowning and submersion
EXCLUDES1 drowning and submersion while in filled bathtub without fall (W65)

W16.212 Fall in (into) filled bathtub causing other injury

W16.22 Fall in (into) bucket of water

W16.221 Fall in (into) bucket of water causing drowning and submersion

W16.222 Fall in (into) bucket of water causing other injury

W16.3 Fall into other water
Fall into fountain
Fall into reservoir

W16.31 Fall into other water striking water surface

W16.311 Fall into other water striking water surface causing drowning and submersion
EXCLUDES1 drowning and submersion while in other water without fall (W73)

W16.312 Fall into other water striking water surface causing other injury

W16.32 Fall into other water striking bottom

W16.321 Fall into other water striking bottom causing drowning and submersion
EXCLUDES1 drowning and submersion while in other water without fall (W73)

W16.322 Fall into other water striking bottom causing other injury

W16.33 Fall into other water striking wall

W16.331 Fall into other water striking wall causing drowning and submersion
EXCLUDES1 drowning and submersion while in other water without fall (W73)

W16.332 Fall into other water striking wall causing other injury

W16.4 Fall into unspecified water

W16.41 Fall into unspecified water causing drowning and submersion

W16.42 Fall into unspecified water causing other injury

W16.5 Jumping or diving into swimming pool

W16.51 Jumping or diving into swimming pool striking water surface

W16.511 Jumping or diving into swimming pool striking water surface causing drowning and submersion
EXCLUDES1 drowning and submersion while in swimming pool without jumping or diving (W67)

PDx Unacceptable principal diagnosis symbol per Medicare code edits   Code exempt from diagnosis present on admission requirement
❓ Questionable admission   Complication or comorbidity   CC/MCC exclusion   Major complication or comorbidity
Principal diagnosis as its own CC   Principal diagnosis as its own MCC   HCC diagnosis code   RxHCC diagnosis code
MACRA code   Z code as first-listed diagnosis

1218   When symbols appear on a code that requires a 7th character extension, refer to Appendix B to identify applicable 7th character codes.   **2018 ICD-10-CM**

(7ᵗʰ) **W16.512** Jumping or diving into swimming pool striking water surface causing other injury ᴾᴼᴬ

(6ᵗʰ) **W16.52** Jumping or diving into swimming pool striking bottom

  (7ᵗʰ) **W16.521** Jumping or diving into swimming pool striking bottom causing drowning and submersion ᴾᴼᴬ

    EXCLUDES1 *drowning and submersion while in swimming pool without jumping or diving (W67)*

  (7ᵗʰ) **W16.522** Jumping or diving into swimming pool striking bottom causing other injury ᴾᴼᴬ

(6ᵗʰ) **W16.53** Jumping or diving into swimming pool striking wall

  (7ᵗʰ) **W16.531** Jumping or diving into swimming pool striking wall causing drowning and submersion ᴾᴼᴬ

    EXCLUDES1 *drowning and submersion while in swimming pool without jumping or diving (W67)*

  (7ᵗʰ) **W16.532** Jumping or diving into swimming pool striking wall causing other injury ᴾᴼᴬ

(5ᵗʰ) **W16.6** Jumping or diving into natural body of water
Jumping or diving into lake
Jumping or diving into open sea
Jumping or diving into river
Jumping or diving into stream

(6ᵗʰ) **W16.61** Jumping or diving into natural body of water striking water surface

  (7ᵗʰ) **W16.611** Jumping or diving into natural body of water striking water surface causing drowning and submersion ᴾᴼᴬ

    EXCLUDES1 *drowning and submersion while in natural body of water without jumping or diving (W69)*

  (7ᵗʰ) **W16.612** Jumping or diving into natural body of water striking water surface causing other injury ᴾᴼᴬ

(6ᵗʰ) **W16.62** Jumping or diving into natural body of water striking bottom

  (7ᵗʰ) **W16.621** Jumping or diving into natural body of water striking bottom causing drowning and submersion ᴾᴼᴬ

    EXCLUDES1 *drowning and submersion while in natural body of water without jumping or diving (W69)*

  (7ᵗʰ) **W16.622** Jumping or diving into natural body of water striking bottom causing other injury ᴾᴼᴬ

(5ᵗʰ) **W16.7** Jumping or diving from boat

  EXCLUDES1 *Fall from boat into water-see watercraft accident (V90-V94)*

(6ᵗʰ) **W16.71** Jumping or diving from boat striking water surface

  (7ᵗʰ) **W16.711** Jumping or diving from boat striking water surface causing drowning and submersion ᴾᴼᴬ

  (7ᵗʰ) **W16.712** Jumping or diving from boat striking water surface causing other injury ᴾᴼᴬ

(6ᵗʰ) **W16.72** Jumping or diving from boat striking bottom

  (7ᵗʰ) **W16.721** Jumping or diving from boat striking bottom causing drowning and submersion ᴾᴼᴬ

  (7ᵗʰ) **W16.722** Jumping or diving from boat striking bottom causing other injury ᴾᴼᴬ

(5ᵗʰ) **W16.8** Jumping or diving into other water
Jumping or diving into fountain
Jumping or diving into reservoir

(6ᵗʰ) **W16.81** Jumping or diving into other water striking water surface

  (7ᵗʰ) **W16.811** Jumping or diving into other water striking water surface causing drowning and submersion

    EXCLUDES1 *drowning and submersion while in other water without jumping or diving (W73)*

  (7ᵗʰ) **W16.812** Jumping or diving into other water striking water surface causing other injury ᴾᴼᴬ

(6ᵗʰ) **W16.82** Jumping or diving into other water striking bottom

  (7ᵗʰ) **W16.821** Jumping or diving into other water striking bottom causing drowning and submersion ᴾᴼᴬ

    EXCLUDES1 *drowning and submersion while in other water without jumping or diving (W73)*

  (7ᵗʰ) **W16.822** Jumping or diving into other water striking bottom causing other injury ᴾᴼᴬ

(6ᵗʰ) **W16.83** Jumping or diving into other water striking wall

  (7ᵗʰ) **W16.831** Jumping or diving into other water striking wall causing drowning and submersion ᴾᴼᴬ

    EXCLUDES1 *drowning and submersion while in other water without jumping or diving (W73)*

  (7ᵗʰ) **W16.832** Jumping or diving into other water striking wall causing other injury ᴾᴼᴬ

(5ᵗʰ) **W16.9** Jumping or diving into unspecified water

(7ᵗʰ) **W16.91** Jumping or diving into unspecified water causing drowning and submersion ᴾᴼᴬ

(7ᵗʰ) **W16.92** Jumping or diving into unspecified water causing other injury ᴾᴼᴬ

(4ᵗʰ) **W17** Other fall from one level to another

The appropriate 7th character is to be added to each code from category W17
  A = initial encounter
  D = subsequent encounter
  S = sequela

(7ᵗʰ) **W17.0** Fall into well ᴾᴼᴬ

(7ᵗʰ) **W17.1** Fall into storm drain or manhole ᴾᴼᴬ

(7ᵗʰ) **W17.2** Fall into hole
Fall into pit

(7ᵗʰ) **W17.3** Fall into empty swimming pool ᴾᴼᴬ

  EXCLUDES1 *fall into filled swimming pool (W16.0-)*

(7ᵗʰ) **W17.4** Fall from dock ᴾᴼᴬ

(5ᵗʰ) **W17.8** Other fall from one level to another

(7ᵗʰ) **W17.81** Fall down embankment (hill) ᴾᴼᴬ

(7ᵗʰ) **W17.82** Fall from (out of) grocery cart ᴾᴼᴬ
Fall due to grocery cart tipping over

(7ᵗʰ) **W17.89** Other fall from one level to another ᴾᴼᴬ
Fall from cherry picker
Fall from lifting device
Fall from mobile elevated work platform [MEWP]
Fall from sky lift

(4ᵗʰ) **W18** Other slipping, tripping and stumbling and falls

The appropriate 7th character is to be added to each code from category W18
  A = initial encounter
  D = subsequent encounter
  S = sequela

(5ᵗʰ) **W18.0** Fall due to bumping against object
Striking against object with subsequent fall

  EXCLUDES1 *fall on same level due to slipping, tripping, or stumbling with subsequent striking against object (W01.1-)*

(7ᵗʰ) **W18.00** Striking against unspecified object with subsequent fall ᴾᴼᴬ

(7ᵗʰ) **W18.01** Striking against sports equipment with subsequent fall ᴾᴼᴬ

(7ᵗʰ) **W18.02** Striking against glass with subsequent fall ᴾᴼᴬ

(7ᵗʰ) **W18.09** Striking against other object with subsequent fall ᴾᴼᴬ

(5ᵗʰ) **W18.1** Fall from or off toilet

(7ᵗʰ) **W18.11** Fall from or off toilet without subsequent striking against object ᴾᴼᴬ
Fall from (off) toilet NOS

Unspecified Code Other Specified Code Manifestation Code N Newborn P Pediatric M Maternity A Adult ♂ Male ♀ Female
● New Code ▲ Revised Code Title ►◄ Revised Text **NOTES** *INCLUDES* *EXCLUDES 1* Not coded here *EXCLUDES 2* Not included here
(4ᵗʰ) 4ᵗʰ character required (5ᵗʰ) 5ᵗʰ character required (6ᵗʰ) 6ᵗʰ character required (7ᵗʰ) 7ᵗʰ character required
(7ᵡ) Extension 'X' Alert **HAC** Hospital-acquired condition (HAC) alert **AHA** AHA Coding Clinic©

W18.12 **Fall from or off toilet** with subsequent striking against object POA

7️⃣ W18.2 **Fall in (into)** shower or empty bathtub POA

EXCLUDES1 fall in full bathtub causing drowning or submersion (W16.21-)

5️⃣ W18.3 Other and unspecified **fall on same level**

7️⃣ W18.30 **Fall on same level, unspecified** POA

7️⃣ W18.31 **Fall on same level due to** stepping on an object POA

Fall on same level due to stepping on an animal

EXCLUDES1 slipping, tripping and stumbling without fall due to stepping on animal (W18.41)

7️⃣ W18.39 **Other fall on same level** POA

5️⃣ W18.4 **Slipping, tripping and stumbling** without falling

EXCLUDES1 collision with another person without fall (W51)

7️⃣ W18.40 **Slipping, tripping and stumbling without falling, unspecified** POA

7️⃣ W18.41 **Slipping, tripping and stumbling without falling due to** stepping on object POA

Slipping, tripping and stumbling without falling due to stepping on animal

EXCLUDES1 slipping, tripping and stumbling with fall due to stepping on animal (W18.31)

7️⃣ W18.42 **Slipping, tripping and stumbling without falling due to** stepping into hole or opening POA

7️⃣ W18.43 **Slipping, tripping and stumbling without falling due to** stepping from one level to another POA

7️⃣ W18.49 **Other slipping, tripping and stumbling without falling** POA

7️⃣ W19 **Unspecified fall**

Accidental fall NOS

The appropriate 7th character is to be added to code W19

A = initial encounter

D = subsequent encounter

S = sequela

Exposure to inanimate mechanical forces (W20-W49)

EXCLUDES1 assault (X92-Y09)

contact or collision with animals or persons (W50-W64)

exposure to inanimate mechanical forces involving military or war operations (Y36.-, Y37.-)

intentional self-harm (X71-X83)

4️⃣ W20 **Struck by thrown, projected or falling object**

Code first any associated:

cataclysm (X34-X39)

lightning strike (T75.00)

EXCLUDES1 falling object in machinery accident (W24, W28-W31)

falling object in transport accident (V01-V99)

object set in motion by explosion (W35-W40)

object set in motion by firearm (W32-W34)

struck by thrown sports equipment (W21.-)

The appropriate 7th character is to be added to each code from category W20

A = initial encounter

D = subsequent encounter

S = sequela

7️⃣ W20.0 **Struck by falling object in cave-in**

EXCLUDES2 asphyxiation due to cave-in (T71.21)

7️⃣ W20.1 **Struck by object due to collapse of building**

EXCLUDES1 struck by object due to collapse of burning building (X00.2, X02.2)

7️⃣ W20.8 **Other cause of strike by thrown, projected or falling object**

EXCLUDES1 struck by thrown sports equipment (W21.-)

4️⃣ W21 **Striking against or struck by** sports equipment

EXCLUDES1 assault with sports equipment (Y08.0-)

striking against or struck by sports equipment with subsequent fall (W18.01)

The appropriate 7th character is to be added to each code from category W21

A = initial encounter

D = subsequent encounter

S = sequela

5️⃣ W21.0 **Struck by** hit or thrown ball

7️⃣ W21.00 **Struck by hit or thrown ball, unspecified type** POA

7️⃣ W21.01 **Struck by** football POA

7️⃣ W21.02 **Struck by** soccer ball POA

7️⃣ W21.03 **Struck by** baseball POA

7️⃣ W21.04 **Struck by** golf ball POA

7️⃣ W21.05 **Struck by** basketball POA

7️⃣ W21.06 **Struck by** volleyball POA

7️⃣ W21.07 **Struck by** softball POA

7️⃣ W21.09 **Struck by other hit or thrown ball** POA

5️⃣ W21.1 **Struck by** bat, racquet or club

7️⃣ W21.11 **Struck by** baseball bat POA

7️⃣ W21.12 **Struck by** tennis racquet POA

7️⃣ W21.13 **Struck by** golf club POA

7️⃣ W21.19 **Struck by other bat, racquet or club** POA

5️⃣ W21.2 **Struck by** hockey stick or puck

6️⃣ W21.21 **Struck by** hockey stick

7️⃣ W21.210 **Struck by** ice hockey stick POA

7️⃣ W21.211 **Struck by** field hockey stick POA

6️⃣ W21.22 **Struck by** hockey puck

7️⃣ W21.220 **Struck by** ice hockey puck POA

7️⃣ W21.221 **Struck by** field hockey puck POA

5️⃣ W21.3 **Struck by** sports foot wear

7️⃣ W21.31 **Struck by** shoe cleats POA

Stepped on by shoe cleats

7️⃣ W21.32 **Struck by** skate blades POA

Skated over by skate blades

7️⃣ W21.39 **Struck by other sports foot wear** POA

7️⃣ W21.4 **Striking against** diving board POA

Use additional code for subsequent falling into water, if applicable (W16.-)

5️⃣ W21.8 **Striking against or struck by** other sports equipment

7️⃣ W21.81 **Striking against or struck by** football helmet POA

7️⃣ W21.89 **Striking against or struck by other sports equipment** POA

7️⃣ W21.9 **Striking against or struck by unspecified sports equipment** POA

4️⃣ W22 **Striking against or struck by** other objects

EXCLUDES1 striking against or struck by object with subsequent fall (W18.09)

The appropriate 7th character is to be added to each code from category W22

A = initial encounter

D = subsequent encounter

S = sequela

5️⃣ W22.0 **Striking against** stationary object

EXCLUDES1 striking against stationary sports equipment (W21.8)

7️⃣ W22.01 **Walked into** wall POA

7️⃣ W22.02 **Walked into** lamppost POA

7️⃣ W22.03 **Walked into** furniture POA

6️⃣ W22.04 **Striking against** wall of swimming pool

7️⃣ W22.041 **Striking against wall of swimming pool causing** drowning and submersion POA

EXCLUDES1 drowning and submersion while swimming without striking against wall (W67)

7️⃣ W22.042 **Striking against wall of swimming pool causing other injury** POA

7️⃣ W22.09 **Striking against other stationary object** POA

5️⃣ W22.1 **Striking against or struck by** automobile airbag

7️⃣ W22.10 **Striking against or struck by unspecified automobile airbag** POA

7️⃣ W22.11 **Striking against or struck by** driver side automobile airbag POA

POA Unacceptable principal diagnosis symbol per Medicare code edits POA Code exempt from diagnosis present on admission requirement
❓ Questionable admission cc Complication or comorbidity CC/MCC CC/MCC exclusion MCC Major complication or comorbidity
Principal diagnosis as its own CC Principal diagnosis as its own MCC HCC HCC diagnosis code RxHCC RxHCC diagnosis code
MACRA code Z1 Z code as first-listed diagnosis

W22.12 **Striking against or struck by** front passenger side automobile airbag

W22.19 **Striking against or struck by other automobile airbag**

W22.8 **Striking against or struck by** other objects

Striking against or struck by object NOS

EXCLUDES1 struck by thrown, projected or falling object (W20.-)

W23 **Caught, crushed, jammed or pinched in or between objects**

EXCLUDES1 injury caused by cutting or piercing instruments (W25-W27)

injury caused by firearms malfunction (W32.1, W33.1-, W34.1-)

injury caused by lifting and transmission devices (W24.-)

injury caused by machinery (W28-W31)

injury caused by nonpowered hand tools (W27.-)

injury caused by transport vehicle being used as a means of transportation (V01-V99)

injury caused by struck by thrown, projected or falling object (W20.-)

The appropriate 7th character is to be added to each code from category W23

A = initial encounter

D = subsequent encounter

S = sequela

W23.0 **Caught, crushed, jammed, or pinched between** moving objects

W23.1 **Caught, crushed, jammed, or pinched between** stationary objects

W24 **Contact with lifting and transmission devices, not elsewhere classified**

EXCLUDES1 transport accidents (V01-V99)

The appropriate 7th character is to be added to each code from category W24

A = initial encounter

D = subsequent encounter

S = sequela

W24.0 **Contact with** lifting **devices, not elsewhere classified**

Contact with chain hoist

Contact with drive belt

Contact with pulley (block)

W24.1 **Contact with** transmission **devices, not elsewhere classified**

Contact with transmission belt or cable

W25 **Contact with** sharp glass

Code first any associated:

injury due to flying glass from explosion or firearm discharge (W32-W40)

transport accident (V00-V99)

EXCLUDES1 fall on same level due to slipping, tripping and stumbling with subsequent striking against sharp glass (W01.10)

striking against sharp glass with subsequent fall (W18.02)

EXCLUDES2 glass embedded in skin (W45)

The appropriate 7th character is to be added to code W25

A = initial encounter

D = subsequent encounter

S = sequela

W26 **Contact with other sharp objects**

EXCLUDES2 sharp object(s) embedded in skin (W45)

The appropriate 7th character is to be added to each code from category W26

A = initial encounter

D = subsequent encounter

S = sequela

W26.0 **Contact with** knife

EXCLUDES1 contact with electric knife (W29.1)

W26.1 **Contact with** sword or dagger

W26.2 **Contact with** edge of stiff paper

AHA: Q4 2016

Paper cut

W26.8 **Contact with other sharp object(s),** not elsewhere classified

AHA: Q4 2016

Contact with tin can lid

W26.9 **Contact with** unspecified **sharp object(s)**

AHA: Q4 2016

W27 **Contact with** nonpowered hand tool

The appropriate 7th character is to be added to each code from category W27

A = initial encounter

D = subsequent encounter

S = sequela

W27.0 **Contact with** workbench tool

Contact with auger

Contact with axe

Contact with chisel

Contact with handsaw

Contact with screwdriver

W27.1 **Contact with** garden tool

Contact with hoe

Contact with nonpowered lawn mower

Contact with pitchfork

Contact with rake

W27.2 **Contact with** scissors

W27.3 **Contact with** needle (sewing)

EXCLUDES1 contact with hypodermic needle (W46.-)

W27.4 **Contact with** kitchen utensil

Contact with fork

Contact with ice-pick

Contact with can-opener NOS

W27.5 **Contact with** paper-cutter

W27.8 **Contact with other nonpowered hand tool**

Contact with nonpowered sewing machine

Contact with shovel

W28 **Contact with** powered lawn mower

Powered lawn mower (commercial) (residential)

EXCLUDES1 contact with nonpowered lawn mower (W27.1)

EXCLUDES2 exposure to electric current (W86.-)

The appropriate 7th character is to be added to code W28

A = initial encounter

D = subsequent encounter

S = sequela

W29 **Contact with other powered** hand tools and household machinery

EXCLUDES1 contact with commercial machinery (W31.82)

contact with hot household appliance (X15)

contact with nonpowered hand tool (W27.-)

exposure to electric current (W86)

The appropriate 7th character is to be added to each code from category W29

A = initial encounter

D = subsequent encounter

S = sequela

W29.0 **Contact with** powered kitchen appliance

Contact with blender

Contact with can-opener

Contact with garbage disposal

Contact with mixer

W29.1 **Contact with** electric knife

W29.2 **Contact with other powered household machinery**

Contact with electric fan

Contact with powered dryer (clothes) (powered) (spin)

Contact with washing-machine

Contact with sewing machine

W29.3 **Contact with powered** garden and outdoor hand tools and machinery

Contact with chainsaw

Contact with edger

Contact with garden cultivator (tiller)

Contact with hedge trimmer

Contact with other powered garden tool

EXCLUDES1 contact with powered lawn mower (W28)

Unspecified Code　Other Specified Code　Manifestation Code　N Newborn　P Pediatric　M Maternity　A Adult　♂ Male　♀ Female

● New Code　▲ Revised Code Title　▶◀ Revised Text　NOTES　INCLUDES　EXCLUDES 1 Not coded here　EXCLUDES 2 Not included here

4th character required　5th character required　6th character required　7th character required

Extension 'X' Alert　HAC Hospital-acquired condition (HAC) alert　AHA AHA Coding Clinic©

W29.4 **Contact with** nail gun

▲ W29.8 **Contact with** other powered hand tools and household machinery

Contact with do-it-yourself tool NOS

W30 **Contact with** agricultural machinery

INCLUDES   animal-powered farm machine

EXCLUDES1   agricultural transport vehicle accident (V01-V99)

explosion of grain store (W40.8)

exposure to electric current (W86.-)

The appropriate 7th character is to be added to each code from category W30

A = initial encounter

D = subsequent encounter

S = sequela

W30.0 **Contact with** combine harvester

Contact with reaper

Contact with thresher

W30.1 **Contact with** power take-off devices (PTO)

W30.2 **Contact with** hay derrick

W30.3 **Contact with** grain storage elevator

EXCLUDES1 explosion of grain store (W40.8)

W30.8 **Contact with** other specified agricultural machinery

W30.81 **Contact with agricultural transport vehicle in stationary use**

Contact with agricultural transport vehicle under repair, not on public roadway

EXCLUDES1 agricultural transport vehicle accident (V01-V99)

W30.89 **Contact with other specified agricultural machinery**

W30.9 **Contact with** unspecified agricultural machinery

Contact with farm machinery NOS

W31 **Contact with** other and unspecified machinery

EXCLUDES1 contact with agricultural machinery (W30.-)

contact with machinery in transport under own power or being towed by a vehicle (V01-V99)

exposure to electric current (W86)

The appropriate 7th character is to be added to each code from category W31

A = initial encounter

D = subsequent encounter

S = sequela

W31.0 **Contact with** mining and earth-drilling machinery

Contact with bore or drill (land) (seabed)

Contact with shaft hoist

Contact with shaft lift

Contact with undercutter

W31.1 **Contact with** metalworking machines

Contact with abrasive wheel

Contact with forging machine

Contact with lathe

Contact with mechanical shears

Contact with metal drilling machine

Contact with milling machine

Contact with power press

Contact with rolling-mill

Contact with metal sawing machine

W31.2 **Contact with** powered woodworking and forming machines

Contact with band saw

Contact with bench saw

Contact with circular saw

Contact with molding machine

Contact with overhead plane

Contact with powered saw

Contact with radial saw

Contact with sander

EXCLUDES1 nonpowered woodworking tools (W27.0)

W31.3 **Contact with** prime movers

Contact with gas turbine

Contact with internal combustion engine

Contact with steam engine

Contact with water driven turbine

W31.8 **Contact with** other specified machinery

W31.81 **Contact with** recreational machinery

Contact with roller coaster

W31.82 **Contact with other commercial machinery**

Contact with commercial electric fan

Contact with commercial kitchen appliances

Contact with commercial powered dryer (clothes) (powered) (spin)

Contact with commercial washing-machine

Contact with commercial sewing machine

EXCLUDES1 contact with household machinery (W29.-)

contact with powered lawn mower (W28)

W31.83 **Contact with** special construction vehicle in stationary use

Contact with special construction vehicle under repair, not on public roadway

EXCLUDES1 special construction vehicle accident (V01-V99)

W31.89 **Contact with other specified machinery**

W31.9 **Contact with** unspecified machinery

Contact with machinery NOS

W32 **Accidental** handgun **discharge and malfunction**

INCLUDES   accidental discharge and malfunction of gun for single hand use

accidental discharge and malfunction of pistol

accidental discharge and malfunction of revolver

Handgun discharge and malfunction NOS

EXCLUDES1 accidental airgun discharge and malfunction (W34.010, W34.110)

accidental BB gun discharge and malfunction (W34.010, W34.110)

accidental pellet gun discharge and malfunction (W34.010, W34.110)

accidental shotgun discharge and malfunction (W33.01, W33.11)

assault by handgun discharge (X93)

handgun discharge involving legal intervention (Y35.0-)

handgun discharge involving military or war operations (Y36.4-)

intentional self-harm by handgun discharge (X72)

Very pistol discharge and malfunction (W34.09, W34.19)

The appropriate 7th character is to be added to each code from category W32

A = initial encounter

D = subsequent encounter

S = sequela

W32.0 **Accidental handgun** discharge

W32.1 **Accidental handgun** malfunction

Injury due to explosion of handgun (parts)

Injury due to malfunction of mechanism or component of handgun

Injury due to recoil of handgun

Powder burn from handgun

W33 **Accidental** rifle, shotgun and larger firearm **discharge and malfunction**

INCLUDES   rifle, shotgun and larger firearm discharge and malfunction NOS

EXCLUDES1 accidental airgun discharge and malfunction (W34.010, W34.110)

accidental BB gun discharge and malfunction (W34.010, W34.110)

accidental handgun discharge and malfunction (W32.-)

accidental pellet gun discharge and malfunction (W34.010, W34.110)

assault by rifle, shotgun and larger firearm discharge (X94)

firearm discharge involving legal intervention (Y35.0-)

firearm discharge involving military or war operations (Y36.4-)

ᴘᴏᴡ Unacceptable principal diagnosis symbol per Medicare code edits   ᴘᴏᴀ Code exempt from diagnosis present on admission requirement

❓ Questionable admission   ᴄᶜ Complication or comorbidity   ᴄᴄ/ᴍᴄᴄ ᴇˣ CC/MCC exclusion   ᴍᴄᴄ Major complication or comorbidity

ᴄᴄ Principal diagnosis as its own CC   ᴍᴄᴄ Principal diagnosis as its own MCC   ʜᴄᴄ HCC diagnosis code   ʀˣʜᴄᴄ RxHCC diagnosis code

MACRA code   ᴢ Z code as first-listed diagnosis

intentional self-harm by rifle, shotgun and larger firearm discharge (X73)

The appropriate 7th character is to be added to each code from category W33

A = initial encounter
D = subsequent encounter
S = sequela

W33.0 Accidental rifle, shotgun and larger firearm discharge

W33.00 Accidental discharge of unspecified larger firearm POA
Discharge of unspecified larger firearm NOS

W33.01 Accidental discharge of shotgun POA
Discharge of shotgun NOS

W33.02 Accidental discharge of hunting rifle POA
Discharge of hunting rifle NOS

W33.03 Accidental discharge of machine gun POA
Discharge of machine gun NOS

W33.09 Accidental discharge of other larger firearm POA
Discharge of other larger firearm NOS

W33.1 Accidental rifle, shotgun and larger firearm malfunction

Injury due to explosion of rifle, shotgun and larger firearm (parts)
Injury due to malfunction of mechanism or component of rifle, shotgun and larger firearm
Injury due to piercing, cutting, crushing or pinching due to (by) slide trigger mechanism, scope or other gun part
Injury due to recoil of rifle, shotgun and larger firearm
Powder burn from rifle, shotgun and larger firearm

W33.10 Accidental malfunction of unspecified larger firearm POA
Malfunction of unspecified larger firearm NOS

W33.11 Accidental malfunction of shotgun POA
Malfunction of shotgun NOS

W33.12 Accidental malfunction of hunting rifle POA
Malfunction of hunting rifle NOS

W33.13 Accidental malfunction of machine gun POA
Malfunction of machine gun NOS

W33.19 Accidental malfunction of other larger firearm POA
Malfunction of other larger firearm NOS

W34 Accidental discharge and malfunction from other and unspecified firearms and guns

The appropriate 7th character is to be added to each code from category W34

A = initial encounter
D = subsequent encounter
S = sequela

W34.0 Accidental discharge from other and unspecified firearms and guns

W34.00 Accidental discharge from unspecified firearms or gun POA
Discharge from firearm NOS
Gunshot wound NOS
Shot NOS

W34.01 Accidental discharge of gas, air or spring-operated guns

W34.010 Accidental discharge of airgun POA
Accidental discharge of BB gun
Accidental discharge of pellet gun

W34.011 Accidental discharge of paintball gun POA
Accidental injury due to paintball discharge

W34.018 Accidental discharge of other gas, air or spring-operated gun POA

W34.09 Accidental discharge from other specified firearms POA
Accidental discharge from Very pistol [flare]

W34.1 Accidental malfunction from other and unspecified firearms and guns

W34.10 Accidental malfunction from unspecified firearms or gun POA
Firearm malfunction NOS

W34.11 Accidental malfunction of gas, air or spring-operated guns

W34.110 Accidental malfunction of airgun POA
Accidental malfunction of BB gun
Accidental malfunction of pellet gun

W34.111 Accidental malfunction of paintball gun POA
Accidental injury due to paintball gun malfunction

W34.118 Accidental malfunction of other gas, air or spring-operated gun POA

W34.19 Accidental malfunction from other specified firearms POA
Accidental malfunction from Very pistol [flare]

W35 Explosion and rupture of boiler POA
EXCLUDES1 explosion and rupture of boiler on watercraft (V93.4)
The appropriate 7th character is to be added to code W35
A = initial encounter
D = subsequent encounter
S = sequela

W36 Explosion and rupture of gas cylinder
The appropriate 7th character is to be added to each code from category W36
A = initial encounter
D = subsequent encounter
S = sequela

W36.1 Explosion and rupture of aerosol can POA
W36.2 Explosion and rupture of air tank POA
W36.3 Explosion and rupture of pressurized-gas tank POA
W36.8 Explosion and rupture of other gas cylinder POA
W36.9 Explosion and rupture of unspecified gas cylinder POA

W37 Explosion and rupture of pressurized tire, pipe or hose
The appropriate 7th character is to be added to each code from category W37
A = initial encounter
D = subsequent encounter
S = sequela

W37.0 Explosion of bicycle tire POA
W37.8 Explosion and rupture of other pressurized tire, pipe or hose POA

W38 Explosion and rupture of other specified pressurized devices POA
The appropriate 7th character is to be added to code W38
A = initial encounter
D = subsequent encounter
S = sequela

W39 Discharge of firework POA
The appropriate 7th character is to be added to code W39
A = initial encounter
D = subsequent encounter
S = sequela

W40 Explosion of other materials
EXCLUDES1 assault by explosive material (X96)
explosion involving legal intervention (Y35.1-)
explosion involving military or war operations (Y36.0-, Y36.2-)
intentional self-harm by explosive material (X75)
The appropriate 7th character is to be added to each code from category W40
A = initial encounter
D = subsequent encounter
S = sequela

W40.0 Explosion of blasting material POA
Explosion of blasting cap
Explosion of detonator
Explosion of dynamite
Explosion of explosive (any) used in blasting operations

W40.1 Explosion of explosive gases POA
Explosion of acetylene
Explosion of butane
Explosion of coal gas
Explosion in mine NOS
Explosion of explosive gas
Explosion of fire damp
Explosion of gasoline fumes

Unspecified Code   Other Specified Code   Manifestation Code   N Newborn   P Pediatric   M Maternity   A Adult   ♂ Male   ♀ Female
● New Code   ▲ Revised Code Title   ►◄ Revised Text   NOTES   INCLUDES   EXCLUDES 1 Not coded here   EXCLUDES 2 Not included here
4th character required   5th character required   6th character required   7th character required
Extension 'X' Alert   HAC Hospital-acquired condition (HAC) alert   AHA AHA Coding Clinic©

Explosion of methane

Explosion of propane

W40.8 **Explosion of other specified explosive materials** POA

Explosion in dump NOS

Explosion in factory NOS

Explosion in grain store

Explosion in munitions

EXCLUDES1 *explosion involving legal intervention (Y35.1-)*

explosion involving military or war operations (Y36.0-, Y36.2-)

W40.9 **Explosion of unspecified explosive materials** POA

Explosion NOS

W42 **Exposure to** noise

The appropriate 7th character is to be added to each code from category W42

A = initial encounter

D = subsequent encounter

S = sequela

W42.0 **Exposure to** supersonic waves POA

W42.9 **Exposure to other noise** POA

Exposure to sound waves NOS

W45 **Foreign body or object** entering through skin

INCLUDES *foreign body or object embedded in skin*

nail embedded in skin

EXCLUDES2 *contact with hand tools (nonpowered) (powered) (W27-W29)*

contact with other sharp object(s) (W26.-)

contact with sharp glass (W25.-)

struck by objects (W20-W22)

The appropriate 7th character is to be added to each code from category W45

A = initial encounter

D = subsequent encounter

S = sequela

W45.0 **Nail** entering through skin POA

W45.8 **Other foreign body or object entering through skin**

Splinter in skin NOS

W46 **Contact with hypodermic needle**

The appropriate 7th character is to be added to each code from category W46

A = initial encounter

D = subsequent encounter

S = sequela

W46.0 **Contact with** hypodermic **needle**

Hypodermic needle stick NOS

W46.1 **Contact with** contaminated hypodermic **needle**

W49 **Exposure to** other inanimate mechanical forces

INCLUDES *exposure to abnormal gravitational [G] forces*

exposure to inanimate mechanical forces NEC

EXCLUDES1 *exposure to inanimate mechanical forces involving military or war operations (Y36.-, Y37.-)*

The appropriate 7th character is to be added to each code from category W49

A = initial encounter

D = subsequent encounter

S = sequela

W49.0 **Item** causing external constriction

W49.01 **Hair** causing external constriction POA

W49.02 **String or thread** causing external constriction POA

W49.03 **Rubber band** causing external constriction POA

W49.04 **Ring or other jewelry** causing external constriction POA

W49.09 **Other specified item causing external constriction** POA

W49.9 **Exposure to other inanimate mechanical forces** POA

Exposure to animate mechanical forces (W50-W64)

EXCLUDES1 *Toxic effect of contact with venomous animals and plants (T63.-)*

W50 **Accidental hit, strike, kick, twist, bite or scratch by another person**

INCLUDES *hit, strike, kick, twist, bite, or scratch by another person NOS*

EXCLUDES1 *assault by bodily force (Y04)*

struck by objects (W20-W22)

The appropriate 7th character is to be added to each code from category W50

A = initial encounter

D = subsequent encounter

S = sequela

W50.0 **Accidental** hit or strike **by another person**

Hit or strike by another person NOS

W50.1 **Accidental** kick **by another person**

Kick by another person NOS

W50.2 **Accidental** twist **by another person**

Twist by another person NOS

W50.3 **Accidental** bite **by another person**

Human bite

Bite by another person NOS

W50.4 **Accidental** scratch **by another person**

Scratch by another person NOS

W51 **Accidental** striking against or bumped **into by another person**

EXCLUDES1 *assault by striking against or bumping into by another person (Y04.2)*

fall due to collision with another person (W03)

The appropriate 7th character is to be added to code W51

A = initial encounter

D = subsequent encounter

S = sequela

W52 **Crushed, pushed or stepped on by crowd or human stampede** POA

Crushed, pushed or stepped on by crowd or human stampede with or without fall

The appropriate 7th character is to be added to code W52

A = initial encounter

D = subsequent encounter

S = sequela

W53 **Contact with** rodent

INCLUDES *contact with saliva, feces or urine of rodent*

The appropriate 7th character is to be added to each code from category W53

A = initial encounter

D = subsequent encounter

S = sequela

W53.0 **Contact with** mouse

W53.01 **Bitten** by mouse POA

W53.09 **Other contact with mouse** POA

W53.1 **Contact with** rat

W53.11 **Bitten** by rat POA

W53.19 **Other contact with rat** POA

W53.2 **Contact with** squirrel

W53.21 **Bitten** by squirrel POA

W53.29 **Other contact with squirrel** POA

W53.8 **Contact with** other rodent

W53.81 **Bitten** by other rodent POA

W53.89 **Other contact with other rodent** POA

W54 **Contact with** dog

INCLUDES *contact with saliva, feces or urine of dog*

The appropriate 7th character is to be added to each code from category W54

A = initial encounter

D = subsequent encounter

S = sequela

W54.0 **Bitten** by dog POA

W54.1 **Struck** by dog POA

Knocked over by dog

W54.8 **Other contact with dog** POA

W55 **Contact with** other mammals

INCLUDES *contact with saliva, feces or urine of mammal*

EXCLUDES1 *animal being ridden- see transport accidents*

bitten or struck by dog (W54)

bitten or struck by rodent (W53.-)

contact with marine mammals (W56.-)

PDx Unacceptable principal diagnosis symbol per Medicare code edits   POA Code exempt from diagnosis present on admission requirement

❓ Questionable admission   CC Complication or comorbidity   CC/MCC Exc CC/MCC exclusion   MCC Major complication or comorbidity

Principal diagnosis as its own CC   Principal diagnosis as its own MCC   HCC HCC diagnosis code   RxHCC RxHCC diagnosis code

MACRA code   Z Z code as first-listed diagnosis

The appropriate 7th character is to be added to each code from category W55
- A = initial encounter
- D = subsequent encounter
- S = sequela

🄔 W55.0 **Contact with** cat
- 🄥 W55.01 Bitten **by cat** POA
- 🄥 W55.03 Scratched **by cat** POA
- 🄥 W55.09 Other contact **with cat** POA

🄔 W55.1 **Contact with** horse
- 🄥 W55.11 Bitten **by horse** POA
- 🄥 W55.12 Struck **by horse** POA
- 🄥 W55.19 Other contact **with horse** POA

🄔 W55.2 **Contact with** cow
  Contact with bull
- 🄥 W55.21 Bitten **by cow** POA
- 🄥 W55.22 Struck **by cow** POA
    Gored by bull
- 🄥 W55.29 Other contact **with cow** POA

🄔 W55.3 **Contact with** other hoof stock
  Contact with goats
  Contact with sheep
- 🄥 W55.31 Bitten **by other hoof stock** POA
- 🄥 W55.32 Struck **by other hoof stock** POA
    Gored by goat
    Gored by ram
- 🄥 W55.39 Other contact **with other hoof stock** POA

🄔 W55.4 **Contact with** pig
- 🄥 W55.41 Bitten **by pig** POA
- 🄥 W55.42 Struck **by pig** POA
- 🄥 W55.49 Other contact **with pig** POA

🄔 W55.5 **Contact with** raccoon
- 🄥 W55.51 Bitten **by raccoon** POA
- 🄥 W55.52 Struck **by raccoon** POA
- 🄥 W55.59 Other contact **with raccoon** POA

🄔 W55.8 **Contact with** other mammals
- 🄥 W55.81 Bitten **by other mammals** POA
- 🄥 W55.82 Struck **by other mammals** POA
- 🄥 W55.89 Other contact **with other mammals** POA

🄓 W56 **Contact with** nonvenomous marine animal
  EXCLUDES1 contact with venomous marine animal (T63.-)
  The appropriate 7th character is to be added to each code from category W56
- A = initial encounter
- D = subsequent encounter
- S = sequela

🄔 W56.0 **Contact with** dolphin
- 🄥 W56.01 Bitten **by dolphin** POA
- 🄥 W56.02 Struck **by dolphin** POA
- 🄥 W56.09 Other contact **with dolphin** POA

🄔 W56.1 **Contact with** sea lion
- 🄥 W56.11 Bitten **by sea lion** POA
- 🄥 W56.12 Struck **by sea lion** POA
- 🄥 W56.19 Other contact **with sea lion** POA

🄔 W56.2 **Contact with** orca
  Contact with killer whale
- 🄥 W56.21 Bitten **by orca** POA
- 🄥 W56.22 Struck **by orca** POA
- 🄥 W56.29 Other contact **with orca** POA

🄔 W56.3 **Contact with** other marine mammals
- 🄥 W56.31 Bitten **by other marine mammals** POA
- 🄥 W56.32 Struck **by other marine mammals** POA
- 🄥 W56.39 Other contact **with other marine mammals** POA

🄔 W56.4 **Contact with** shark
- 🄥 W56.41 Bitten **by shark** POA
- 🄥 W56.42 Struck **by shark** POA
- 🄥 W56.49 Other contact **with shark** POA

🄔 W56.5 **Contact with other fish**
- 🄥 W56.51 Bitten **by other fish** POA

🄥 W56.52 Struck **by other fish** POA
🄥 W56.59 Other contact **with other fish** POA

🄔 W56.8 **Contact with** other nonvenomous marine animals
- 🄥 W56.81 Bitten **by other nonvenomous marine animals** POA
- 🄥 W56.82 Struck **by other nonvenomous marine animals** POA
- 🄥 W56.89 Other contact **with other nonvenomous marine animals** POA

🄓 W57 **Bitten or stung by nonvenomous** insect and other nonvenomous arthropods
  EXCLUDES1 contact with venomous insects and arthropods (T63.2-, T63.3-, T63.4-)
  The appropriate 7th character is to be added to code W57
- A = initial encounter
- D = subsequent encounter
- S = sequela

🄓 W58 **Contact with** crocodile or alligator
  The appropriate 7th character is to be added to each code from category W58
- A = initial encounter
- D = subsequent encounter
- S = sequela

🄔 W58.0 **Contact with** alligator
- 🄥 W58.01 Bitten **by alligator** POA
- 🄥 W58.02 Struck **by alligator** POA
- 🄥 W58.03 Crushed **by alligator** POA
- 🄥 W58.09 Other contact **with alligator** POA

🄔 W58.1 **Contact with** crocodile
- 🄥 W58.11 Bitten **by crocodile** POA
- 🄥 W58.12 Struck **by crocodile** POA
- 🄥 W58.13 Crushed **by crocodile** POA
- 🄥 W58.19 Other contact **with crocodile** POA

🄓 W59 **Contact with** other nonvenomous reptiles
  EXCLUDES1 contact with venomous reptile (T63.0-, T63.1-)
  The appropriate 7th character is to be added to each code from category W59
- A = initial encounter
- D = subsequent encounter
- S = sequela

🄔 W59.0 **Contact with** nonvenomous lizards
- 🄥 W59.01 Bitten **by nonvenomous lizards** POA
- 🄥 W59.02 Struck **by nonvenomous lizards** POA
- 🄥 W59.09 Other contact **with nonvenomous lizards** POA
    Exposure to nonvenomous lizards

🄔 W59.1 **Contact with** nonvenomous snakes
- 🄥 W59.11 Bitten **by nonvenomous snake** POA
- 🄥 W59.12 Struck **by nonvenomous snake** POA
- 🄥 W59.13 Crushed **by nonvenomous snake** POA
- 🄥 W59.19 Other contact **with nonvenomous snake** POA

🄔 W59.2 **Contact with** turtles
  EXCLUDES1 contact with tortoises (W59.8-)
- 🄥 W59.21 Bitten **by turtle** POA
- 🄥 W59.22 Struck **by turtle** POA
- 🄥 W59.29 Other contact **with turtle** POA
    Exposure to turtles

🄔 W59.8 **Contact with** other nonvenomous reptiles
- 🄥 W59.81 Bitten **by other nonvenomous reptiles** POA
- 🄥 W59.82 Struck **by other nonvenomous reptiles** POA
- 🄥 W59.83 Crushed **by other nonvenomous reptiles** POA
- 🄥 W59.89 Other contact **with other nonvenomous reptiles** POA

🄥 W60 **Contact with** nonvenomous plant thorns and spines and sharp leaves POA
  EXCLUDES1 Contact with venomous plants (T63.7-)
  The appropriate 7th character is to be added to code W60
- A = initial encounter
- D = subsequent encounter
- S = sequela

🄓 W61 **Contact with** birds (domestic) (wild)
  INCLUDES contact with excreta of birds

Unspecified Code   Other Specified Code   Manifestation Code   N Newborn   P Pediatric   M Maternity   A Adult   ♂ Male   ♀ Female
● New Code   ▲ Revised Code Title   ►◄ Revised Text   NOTES   INCLUDES   EXCLUDES 1 Not coded here   EXCLUDES 2 Not included here
🄓 4th character required   🄔 5th character required   🄖 6th character required   🄦 7th character required
🄥 Extension 'X' Alert   HAC Hospital-acquired condition (HAC) alert   AHA AHA Coding Clinic©

The appropriate 7th character is to be added to each code from category W61
- A = initial encounter
- D = subsequent encounter
- S = sequela

5ᵗʰ W61.0 Contact with parrot
- 7ᵗʰ W61.01 Bitten by parrot
- 7ᵗʰ W61.02 Struck by parrot
- 7ᵗʰ W61.09 Other contact with parrot
  - Exposure to parrots

5ᵗʰ W61.1 Contact with macaw
- 7ᵗʰ W61.11 Bitten by macaw
- 7ᵗʰ W61.12 Struck by macaw
- 7ᵗʰ W61.19 Other contact with macaw
  - Exposure to macaws

5ᵗʰ W61.2 Contact with other psittacines
- 7ᵗʰ W61.21 Bitten by other psittacines
- 7ᵗʰ W61.22 Struck by other psittacines
- 7ᵗʰ W61.29 Other contact with other psittacines
  - Exposure to other psittacines

5ᵗʰ W61.3 Contact with chicken
- 7ᵗʰ W61.32 Struck by chicken
- 7ᵗʰ W61.33 Pecked by chicken
- 7ᵗʰ W61.39 Other contact with chicken
  - Exposure to chickens

5ᵗʰ W61.4 Contact with turkey
- 7ᵗʰ W61.42 Struck by turkey
- 7ᵗʰ W61.43 Pecked by turkey
- 7ᵗʰ W61.49 Other contact with turkey

5ᵗʰ W61.5 Contact with goose
- 7ᵗʰ W61.51 Bitten by goose
- 7ᵗʰ W61.52 Struck by goose
- 7ᵗʰ W61.59 Other contact with goose

5ᵗʰ W61.6 Contact with duck
- 7ᵗʰ W61.61 Bitten by duck
- 7ᵗʰ W61.62 Struck by duck
- 7ᵗʰ W61.69 Other contact with duck

5ᵗʰ W61.9 Contact with other birds
- 7ᵗʰ W61.91 Bitten by other birds
- 7ᵗʰ W61.92 Struck by other birds
- 7ᵗʰ W61.99 Other contact with other birds
  - Contact with bird NOS

4ᵗʰ **W62 Contact with nonvenomous amphibians**

EXCLUDES1 contact with venomous amphibians (T63.81-R63.83)

The appropriate 7th character is to be added to each code from category W62
- A = initial encounter
- D = subsequent encounter
- S = sequela

7ᵗʰ W62.0 Contact with nonvenomous frogs
7ᵗʰ W62.1 Contact with nonvenomous toads
7ᵗʰ W62.9 Contact with other nonvenomous amphibians

7ᵗʰ **W64 Exposure to other animate mechanical forces**

INCLUDES exposure to nonvenomous animal NOS

EXCLUDES1 contact with venomous animal (T63.-)

The appropriate 7th character is to be added to code W64
- A = initial encounter
- D = subsequent encounter
- S = sequela

Accidental non-transport drowning and submersion (W65-W74)

EXCLUDES1 accidental drowning and submersion due to fall into water (W16.-)

accidental drowning and submersion due to water transport accident (V90.-, V92.-)

EXCLUDES2 accidental drowning and submersion due to cataclysm (X34-X39)

7ᵗʰ **W65 Accidental drowning and submersion while in bath-tub**

EXCLUDES1 accidental drowning and submersion due to fall in (into) bathtub (W16.211)

The appropriate 7th character is to be added to code W65
- A = initial encounter
- D = subsequent encounter
- S = sequela

7ᵗʰ **W67 Accidental drowning and submersion while in swimming-pool**

EXCLUDES1 accidental drowning and submersion due to fall into swimming pool (W16.011, W16.021, W16.031)

accidental drowning and submersion due to striking into wall of swimming pool (W22.041)

The appropriate 7th character is to be added to code W67
- A = initial encounter
- D = subsequent encounter
- S = sequela

7ᵗʰ **W69 Accidental drowning and submersion while in natural water**

Accidental drowning and submersion while in lake
Accidental drowning and submersion while in open sea
Accidental drowning and submersion while in river
Accidental drowning and submersion while in stream

EXCLUDES1 accidental drowning and submersion due to fall into natural body of water (W16.111, W16.121, W16.131)

The appropriate 7th character is to be added to code W69
- A = initial encounter
- D = subsequent encounter
- S = sequela

7ᵗʰ **W73 Other specified cause of accidental non-transport drowning and submersion**

Accidental drowning and submersion while in quenching tank
Accidental drowning and submersion while in reservoir

EXCLUDES1 accidental drowning and submersion due to fall into other water (W16.311, W16.321, W16.331)

The appropriate 7th character is to be added to code W73
- A = initial encounter
- D = subsequent encounter
- S = sequela

7ᵗʰ **W74 Unspecified cause of accidental drowning and submersion**

Drowning NOS

The appropriate 7th character is to be added to code W74
- A = initial encounter
- D = subsequent encounter
- S = sequela

Exposure to electric current, radiation and extreme ambient air temperature and pressure (W85-W99)

EXCLUDES1 exposure to:

failure in dosage of radiation or temperature during surgical and medical care (Y63.2-Y63.5)

lightning (T75.0-)

natural cold (X31)

natural heat (X30)

natural radiation NOS (X39)

radiological procedure and radiotherapy (Y84.2)

sunlight (X32)

7ᵗʰ **W85 Exposure to electric transmission lines**

Broken power line

The appropriate 7th character is to be added to code W85
- A = initial encounter
- D = subsequent encounter
- S = sequela

4ᵗʰ **W86 Exposure to other specified electric current**

The appropriate 7th character is to be added to each code from category W86
- A = initial encounter
- D = subsequent encounter
- S = sequela

7ᵗʰ W86.0 Exposure to domestic wiring and appliances

POA Unacceptable principal diagnosis symbol per Medicare code edits   POA Code exempt from diagnosis present on admission requirement
❓ Questionable admission   CC Complication or comorbidity   CC/MCC EXC CC/MCC exclusion   MCC Major complication or comorbidity
Principal diagnosis as its own CC   Principal diagnosis as its own MCC   HCC HCC diagnosis code   RxHCC RxHCC diagnosis code
MACRA code   Z1 Z code as first-listed diagnosis

When symbols appear on a code that requires a 7th character extension, refer to Appendix B to identify applicable 7th character codes.   **2018 ICD-10-CM**

7️⃣ **W86.1 Exposure to** industrial **wiring, appliances and electrical machinery** POA
Exposure to conductors
Exposure to control apparatus
Exposure to electrical equipment and machinery
Exposure to transformers

7️⃣ **W86.8 Exposure to other electric current** POA
Exposure to wiring and appliances in or on farm (not farmhouse)
Exposure to wiring and appliances outdoors
Exposure to wiring and appliances in or on public building
Exposure to wiring and appliances in or on residential institutions
Exposure to wiring and appliances in or on schools

4️⃣ **W88 Exposure to** ionizing radiation
EXCLUDES1 *exposure to sunlight (X32)*
The appropriate 7th character is to be added to each code from category W88
A = initial encounter
D = subsequent encounter
S = sequela

7️⃣ **W88.0 Exposure to** X-rays POA
7️⃣ **W88.1 Exposure to** radioactive isotopes POA
7️⃣ **W88.8 Exposure to other ionizing radiation** POA

4️⃣ **W89 Exposure to** man-made visible and ultraviolet light
INCLUDES *exposure to welding light (arc)*
EXCLUDES1 *exposure to sunlight (X32)*
The appropriate 7th character is to be added to each code from category W89
A = initial encounter
D = subsequent encounter
S = sequela

7️⃣ **W89.0 Exposure to** welding light (arc) POA
7️⃣ **W89.1 Exposure to** tanning bed POA
7️⃣ **W89.8 Exposure to other man-made visible and ultraviolet light** POA
7️⃣ **W89.9 Exposure to unspecified man-made visible and ultraviolet light** POA

4️⃣ **W90 Exposure to** other nonionizing radiation
EXCLUDES1 *exposure to sunlight (X32)*
The appropriate 7th character is to be added to each code from category W90
A = initial encounter
D = subsequent encounter
S = sequela

7️⃣ **W90.0 Exposure to** radiofrequency POA
7️⃣ **W90.1 Exposure to** infrared radiation POA
7️⃣ **W90.2 Exposure to** laser radiation POA
7️⃣ **W90.8 Exposure to other nonionizing radiation** POA

7️⃣ **W92 Exposure to** excessive heat of man-made origin POA
The appropriate 7th character is to be added to code W92
A = initial encounter
D = subsequent encounter
S = sequela

4️⃣ **W93 Exposure to** excessive cold of man-made origin
The appropriate 7th character is to be added to each code from category W93
A = initial encounter
D = subsequent encounter
S = sequela

5️⃣ **W93.0 Contact with or inhalation of** dry ice
7️⃣ **W93.01 Contact with dry ice** POA
7️⃣ **W93.02** Inhalation **of dry ice** POA

5️⃣ **W93.1 Contact with or inhalation of** liquid air
7️⃣ **W93.11** Contact **with liquid air** POA
Contact with liquid hydrogen
Contact with liquid nitrogen
7️⃣ **W93.12** Inhalation **of liquid air** POA
Inhalation of liquid hydrogen
Inhalation of liquid nitrogen

7️⃣ **W93.2 Prolonged exposure in deep freeze unit or refrigerator** POA

7️⃣ **W93.8 Exposure to other excessive cold of man-made origin** POA

4️⃣ **W94 Exposure to high and low air pressure and changes in air pressure**
The appropriate 7th character is to be added to each code from category W94
A = initial encounter
D = subsequent encounter
S = sequela

7️⃣ **W94.0 Exposure to prolonged** high air pressure POA
5️⃣ **W94.1 Exposure to prolonged** low air pressure
7️⃣ **W94.11 Exposure to residence or prolonged visit at** high altitude POA
7️⃣ **W94.12 Exposure to other prolonged low air pressure** POA

5️⃣ **W94.2 Exposure to rapid changes in air pressure during** ascent
7️⃣ **W94.21 Exposure to reduction in atmospheric pressure while surfacing from** deep-water diving POA
7️⃣ **W94.22 Exposure to reduction in atmospheric pressure while surfacing from** underground POA
7️⃣ **W94.23 Exposure to sudden change in air pressure in** aircraft **during ascent** POA
7️⃣ **W94.29 Exposure to other rapid changes in air pressure during ascent** POA

5️⃣ **W94.3 Exposure to rapid changes in air pressure during** descent
7️⃣ **W94.31 Exposure to sudden change in air pressure in** aircraft **during descent** POA
7️⃣ **W94.32 Exposure to high air pressure from rapid descent in** water POA
7️⃣ **W94.39 Exposure to other rapid changes in air pressure during descent** POA

7️⃣ **W99 Exposure to** other man-made environmental factors POA
The appropriate 7th character is to be added to code W99
A = initial encounter
D = subsequent encounter
S = sequela

Exposure to smoke, fire and flames (X00-X08)

EXCLUDES1 *arson (X97)*
EXCLUDES2 *explosions (W35-W40)*
lightning (T75.0-)
transport accident (V01-V99)

4️⃣ **X00 Exposure to** uncontrolled fire **in building or structure**
INCLUDES *conflagration in building or structure*
Code first any associated cataclysm
EXCLUDES2 *Exposure to ignition or melting of nightwear (X05)*
Exposure to ignition or melting of other clothing and apparel (X06.-)
Exposure to other specified smoke, fire and flames (X08.-)
The appropriate 7th character is to be added to each code from category X00
A = initial encounter
D = subsequent encounter
S = sequela

5️⃣ **X00.0 Exposure to** flames **in uncontrolled fire in building or structure**
5️⃣ **X00.1 Exposure to** smoke **in uncontrolled fire in building or structure**
5️⃣ **X00.2** Injury due to collapse **of burning building or structure in uncontrolled fire**
EXCLUDES1 *injury due to collapse of building not on fire (W20.1)*
5️⃣ **X00.3** Fall from **burning building or structure in uncontrolled fire**
5️⃣ **X00.4** Hit by object **from burning building or structure in uncontrolled fire**
5️⃣ **X00.5** Jump from **burning building or structure in uncontrolled fire**
X00.8 Other exposure to uncontrolled fire in building or structure

4️⃣ **X01 Exposure to uncontrolled fire,** not in building or structure
INCLUDES *exposure to forest fire*
The appropriate 7th character is to be added to each code from category X01
A = initial encounter

| Unspecified Code | Other Specified Code | Manifestation Code | Ⓝ Newborn | Ⓟ Pediatric | Ⓜ Maternity | Ⓐ Adult | ♂ Male | ♀ Female |

● New Code ▲ Revised Code Title ▶◀ Revised Text **NOTES** *INCLUDES* *EXCLUDES 1* Not coded here *EXCLUDES 2* Not included here
4️⃣ 4th character required 5️⃣ 5th character required 6️⃣ 6th character required 7️⃣ 7th character required
Ⓧ Extension 'X' Alert **HAC** Hospital-acquired condition (HAC) alert **AHA** AHA Coding Clinic©

D = subsequent encounter

S = sequela

- X01.0 Exposure to flames in uncontrolled fire, not in building or structure
- X01.1 Exposure to smoke in uncontrolled fire, not in building or structure
- X01.3 Fall due to uncontrolled fire, not in building or structure
- X01.4 Hit by object due to uncontrolled fire, not in building or structure
- X01.8 Other exposure to uncontrolled fire, not in building or structure

X02 **Exposure to controlled fire in building or structure**

INCLUDES   exposure to fire in fireplace

exposure to fire in stove

The appropriate 7th character is to be added to each code from category X02

A = initial encounter

D = subsequent encounter

S = sequela

- X02.0 Exposure to flames in controlled fire in building or structure
- X02.1 Exposure to smoke in controlled fire in building or structure
- X02.2 Injury due to collapse of burning building or structure in controlled fire

EXCLUDES1 injury due to collapse of building not on fire (W20.1)

- X02.3 Fall from burning building or structure in controlled fire
- X02.4 Hit by object from burning building or structure in controlled fire
- X02.5 Jump from burning building or structure in controlled fire
- X02.8 Other exposure to controlled fire in building or structure

X03 **Exposure to controlled fire, not in building or structure**

INCLUDES   exposure to bon fire

exposure to camp-fire

exposure to trash fire

The appropriate 7th character is to be added to each code from category X03

A = initial encounter

D = subsequent encounter

S = sequela

- X03.0 Exposure to flames in controlled fire, not in building or structure
- X03.1 Exposure to smoke in controlled fire, not in building or structure
- X03.3 Fall due to controlled fire, not in building or structure
- X03.4 Hit by object due to controlled fire, not in building or structure
- X03.8 Other exposure to controlled fire, not in building or structure

X04 **Exposure to ignition of highly flammable material**

Exposure to ignition of gasoline

Exposure to ignition of kerosene

Exposure to ignition of petrol

EXCLUDES2 exposure to ignition or melting of nightwear (X05)

exposure to ignition or melting of other clothing and apparel (X06)

The appropriate 7th character is to be added to code X04

A = initial encounter

D = subsequent encounter

S = sequela

X05 **Exposure to ignition or melting of nightwear**

EXCLUDES2 exposure to uncontrolled fire in building or structure (X00.-)

exposure to uncontrolled fire, not in building or structure (X01.-)

exposure to controlled fire in building or structure (X02.-)

exposure to controlled fire, not in building or structure (X03.-)

exposure to ignition of highly flammable materials (X04.-)

The appropriate 7th character is to be added to code X05

A = initial encounter

D = subsequent encounter

S = sequela

X06 **Exposure to ignition or melting of other clothing and apparel**

EXCLUDES2 exposure to uncontrolled fire in building or structure (X00.-)

exposure to uncontrolled fire, not in building or structure (X01.-)

exposure to controlled fire in building or structure (X02.-)

exposure to controlled fire, not in building or structure (X03.-)

exposure to ignition of highly flammable materials (X04.-)

The appropriate 7th character is to be added to each code from category X06

A = initial encounter

D = subsequent encounter

S = sequela

- X06.0 Exposure to ignition of plastic jewelry
- X06.1 Exposure to melting of plastic jewelry
- X06.2 Exposure to ignition of other clothing and apparel
- X06.3 Exposure to melting of other clothing and apparel

X08 **Exposure to other specified smoke, fire and flames**

The appropriate 7th character is to be added to each code from category X08

A = initial encounter

D = subsequent encounter

S = sequela

- X08.0 Exposure to bed fire

Exposure to mattress fire

- X08.00 Exposure to bed fire due to unspecified burning material
- X08.01 Exposure to bed fire due to burning cigarette
- X08.09 Exposure to bed fire due to other burning material
- X08.1 Exposure to sofa fire
- X08.10 Exposure to sofa fire due to unspecified burning material
- X08.11 Exposure to sofa fire due to burning cigarette
- X08.19 Exposure to sofa fire due to other burning material
- X08.2 Exposure to other furniture fire
- X08.20 Exposure to other furniture fire due to unspecified burning material
- X08.21 Exposure to other furniture fire due to burning cigarette
- X08.29 Exposure to other furniture fire due to other burning material
- X08.8 Exposure to other specified smoke, fire and flames

Contact with heat and hot substances (X10-X19)

EXCLUDES1 exposure to excessive natural heat (X30)

exposure to fire and flames ▶(X00-X08)◀

X10 **Contact with hot drinks, food, fats and cooking oils**

The appropriate 7th character is to be added to each code from category X10

A = initial encounter

D = subsequent encounter

S = sequela

- X10.0 Contact with hot drinks
- X10.1 Contact with hot food
- X10.2 Contact with fats and cooking oils

X11 **Contact with hot tap-water**

INCLUDES   contact with boiling tap-water

contact with boiling water NOS

EXCLUDES1 contact with water heated on stove (X12)

The appropriate 7th character is to be added to each code from category X11

A = initial encounter

D = subsequent encounter

S = sequela

- X11.0 Contact with hot water in bath or tub

EXCLUDES1 contact with running hot water in bath or tub (X11.1)

POA Unacceptable principal diagnosis symbol per Medicare code edits   Code exempt from diagnosis present on admission requirement

? Questionable admission   Complication or comorbidity   CC/MCC exclusion   MCC Major complication or comorbidity

Principal diagnosis as its own CC   Principal diagnosis as its own MCC   HCC HCC diagnosis code   RxHCC RxHCC diagnosis code

MACRA code   Z code as first-listed diagnosis

X11.1 **Contact with** running hot water
Contact with hot water running out of hose
Contact with hot water running out of tap

X11.8 **Contact with other hot tap-water**
Contact with hot water in bucket
Contact with hot tap-water NOS

X12 **Contact with** other hot fluids
Contact with water heated on stove
EXCLUDES1 *hot (liquid) metals (X18)*
The appropriate 7th character is to be added to code X12
A = initial encounter
D = subsequent encounter
S = sequela

X13 **Contact with** steam and other hot vapors
The appropriate 7th character is to be added to each code from category X13
A = initial encounter
D = subsequent encounter
S = sequela

X13.0 **Inhalation of steam and other hot vapors**

X13.1 **Other contact with steam and other hot vapors**

X14 **Contact with** hot air and other hot gases
The appropriate 7th character is to be added to each code from category X14
A = initial encounter
D = subsequent encounter
S = sequela

X14.0 Inhalation of hot air and gases

X14.1 **Other contact with hot air and other hot gases**

X15 **Contact with** hot household appliances
EXCLUDES1 *contact with heating appliances (X16)*
contact with powered household appliances (W29.-)
exposure to controlled fire in building or structure due to household appliance (X02.8)
exposure to household appliances electrical current (W86.0)
The appropriate 7th character is to be added to each code from category X15
A = initial encounter
D = subsequent encounter
S = sequela

X15.0 **Contact with hot** stove (kitchen)

X15.1 **Contact with hot** toaster

X15.2 **Contact with** hotplate

X15.3 **Contact with hot** saucepan or skillet

X15.8 **Contact with other hot household appliances**
Contact with cooker
Contact with kettle
Contact with light bulbs

X16 **Contact with** hot heating appliances, radiators and pipes
EXCLUDES1 *contact with powered appliances (W29.-)*
exposure to controlled fire in building or structure due to appliance (X02.8)
exposure to industrial appliances electrical current (W86.1)
The appropriate 7th character is to be added to code X16
A = initial encounter
D = subsequent encounter
S = sequela

X17 **Contact with** hot engines, machinery and tools
EXCLUDES1 *contact with hot heating appliances, radiators and pipes (X16)*
contact with hot household appliances (X15)
The appropriate 7th character is to be added to code X17
A = initial encounter
D = subsequent encounter
S = sequela

X18 **Contact with** other hot metals
Contact with liquid metal
The appropriate 7th character is to be added to code X18
A = initial encounter

D = subsequent encounter
S = sequela

X19 **Contact with** other heat and hot substances
EXCLUDES1 *objects that are not normally hot, e.g., an object made hot by a house fire ▶(X00-X08)◀*
The appropriate 7th character is to be added to code X19
A = initial encounter
D = subsequent encounter
S = sequela

Exposure to forces of nature (X30-X39)

X30 **Exposure to** excessive natural heat
Exposure to excessive heat as the cause of sunstroke
Exposure to heat NOS
EXCLUDES1 *excessive heat of man-made origin (W92)*
exposure to man-made radiation (W89)
exposure to sunlight (X32)
exposure to tanning bed (W89)
The appropriate 7th character is to be added to code X30
A = initial encounter
D = subsequent encounter
S = sequela

X31 **Exposure to** excessive natural cold
Excessive cold as the cause of chilblains NOS
Excessive cold as the cause of immersion foot or hand
Exposure to cold NOS
Exposure to weather conditions
EXCLUDES1 *cold of man-made origin (W93.-)*
contact with or inhalation of dry ice (W93.-)
contact with or inhalation of liquefied gas (W93.-)
The appropriate 7th character is to be added to code X31
A = initial encounter
D = subsequent encounter
S = sequela

X32 **Exposure to** sunlight
EXCLUDES1 *man-made radiation (tanning bed) (W89)*
EXCLUDES2 *radiation-related disorders of the skin and subcutaneous tissue (L55-L59)*
The appropriate 7th character is to be added to code X32
A = initial encounter
D = subsequent encounter
S = sequela

X34 **Earthquake**
EXCLUDES2 *tidal wave (tsunami) due to earthquake (X37.41)*
The appropriate 7th character is to be added to code X34
A = initial encounter
D = subsequent encounter
S = sequela

X35 **Volcanic eruption**
EXCLUDES2 *tidal wave (tsunami) due to volcanic eruption (X37.41)*
The appropriate 7th character is to be added to code X35
A = initial encounter
D = subsequent encounter
S = sequela

X36 **Avalanche, landslide and other earth movements**
INCLUDES *victim of mudslide of cataclysmic nature*
EXCLUDES1 *earthquake (X34)*
EXCLUDES2 *transport accident involving collision with avalanche or landslide not in motion (V01-V99)*
The appropriate 7th character is to be added to each code from category X36
A = initial encounter
D = subsequent encounter
S = sequela

X36.0 **Collapse of dam or man-made structure causing** earth movement

X36.1 Avalanche, landslide, or mudslide

Unspecified Code   Other Specified Code   Manifestation Code   N Newborn   P Pediatric   M Maternity   A Adult   ♂ Male   ♀ Female
● New Code   ▲ Revised Code Title   ▶◀ Revised Text   **NOTES**   *INCLUDES*   *EXCLUDES 1* Not coded here   *EXCLUDES 2* Not included here
4th character required   5th character required   6th character required   7th character required
Extension 'X' Alert   **HAC** Hospital-acquired condition (HAC) alert   **AHA** AHA Coding Clinic©

X37-X73 CHAPTER 20: EXTERNAL CAUSES OF MORBIDITY (V00-Y99)

X37 **Cataclysmic storm**
The appropriate 7th character is to be added to each code from category X37
A = initial encounter
D = subsequent encounter
S = sequela

X37.0 **Hurricane**
Storm surge
Typhoon

X37.1 **Tornado**
Cyclone
Twister

X37.2 **Blizzard (snow)(ice)**

X37.3 **Dust storm**

X37.4 **Tidalwave**

X37.41 **Tidal wave due to** earthquake or volcanic eruption
Tidal wave NOS
Tsunami

X37.42 **Tidal wave due to** storm

X37.43 **Tidal wave due to** landslide

X37.8 **Other cataclysmic storms**
Cloudburst
Torrential rain
EXCLUDES2 *flood (X38)*

X37.9 **Unspecified cataclysmic storm**
Storm NOS
EXCLUDES1 *collapse of dam or man-made structure causing earth movement (X39.0)*

X38 **Flood**
Flood arising from remote storm
Flood of cataclysmic nature arising from melting snow
Flood resulting directly from storm
EXCLUDES1 *collapse of dam or man-made structure causing earth movement (X39.0)*
tidal wave NOS (X37.41)
tidal wave caused by storm (X37.2)
The appropriate 7th character is to be added to code X38
A = initial encounter
D = subsequent encounter
S = sequela

X39 **Exposure to** other forces of nature
The appropriate 7th character is to be added to each code from category X39
A = initial encounter
D = subsequent encounter
S = sequela

X39.0 **Exposure to** natural radiation
EXCLUDES1 *contact with and (suspected) exposure to radon and other naturally occuring radiation (Z77.123)*
exposure to man-made radiation (W88-W90)
exposure to sunlight (X32)

X39.01 **Exposure to** radon

X39.08 **Exposure to other natural radiation**

X39.8 **Other exposure to forces of nature**

Overexertion and strenuous or repetitive movements (X50)

X50 **Overexertion and strenuous or repetitive movements**
The appropriate 7th character is to be added to each code from category X50
A = initial encounter
D = subsequent encounter
S = sequela

X50.0 **Overexertion** from strenuous movement or load
Lifting heavy objects
Lifting weights

X50.1 **Overexertion from** prolonged static or awkward postures
Prolonged bending
Prolonged kneeling
Prolonged reaching

Prolonged sitting
Prolonged standing
Prolonged twisting
Static bending
Static kneeling
Static reaching
Static sitting
Static standing
Static twisting

X50.3 **Overexertion from** repetitive movements
Use of hand as hammer
EXCLUDES2 *Overuse from prolonged static or awkward postures (X50.1)*

X50.9 **Other and unspecified** overexertion or strenuous movements or postures
Contact pressure
Contact stress

Accidental exposure to other specified factors (X52-X58)

X52 **Prolonged stay in weightless environment**
Weightlessness in spacecraft (simulator)
The appropriate 7th character is to be added to code X52
A = initial encounter
D = subsequent encounter
S = sequela

X58 **Exposure to other specified factors**
Accident NOS
Exposure NOS
The appropriate 7th character is to be added to code X58
A = initial encounter
D = subsequent encounter
S = sequela

Intentional self-harm (X71-X83)

Purposely self-inflicted injury
Suicide (attempted)

X71 **Intentional self-harm by** drowning and submersion
The appropriate 7th character is to be added to each code from category X71
A = initial encounter
D = subsequent encounter
S = sequela

X71.0 **Intentional self-harm by drowning and submersion** while in bathtub   HCC

X71.1 **Intentional self-harm by drowning and submersion** while in swimming pool   HCC

X71.2 **Intentional self-harm by drowning and submersion** after jump into swimming pool   HCC

X71.3 **Intentional self-harm by drowning and submersion in** natural water   HCC

X71.8 **Other intentional self-harm by drowning and submersion** HCC

X71.9 **Intentional self-harm by drowning and submersion, unspecified**   HCC

X72 **Intentional self-harm by** handgun discharge   HCC
Intentional self-harm by gun for single hand use
Intentional self-harm by pistol
Intentional self-harm by revolver
EXCLUDES1 *Very pistol (X74.8)*
The appropriate 7th character is to be added to code X72
A = initial encounter
D = subsequent encounter
S = sequela

X73 **Intentional self-harm by rifle, shotgun and larger firearm discharge**
EXCLUDES1 *airgun (X74.01)*
The appropriate 7th character is to be added to each code from category X73
A = initial encounter
D = subsequent encounter
S = sequela

PDₓ Unacceptable principal diagnosis symbol per Medicare code edits   POA Code exempt from diagnosis present on admission requirement
? Questionable admission   CC Complication or comorbidity   CC-MCC EXC CC/MCC exclusion   MCC Major complication or comorbidity
Pcc Principal diagnosis as its own CC   Pmcc Principal diagnosis as its own MCC   HCC HCC diagnosis code   RxHCC RxHCC diagnosis code
MACRA code   Z1 Z code as first-listed diagnosis

[5th] X73.0 Intentional self-harm by shotgun discharge [HCC]
[5th] X73.1 Intentional self-harm by hunting rifle discharge [HCC]
[5th] X73.2 Intentional self-harm by machine gun discharge [HCC]
[5th] X73.8 Intentional self-harm by other larger firearm discharge [HCC]
[5th] X73.9 Intentional self-harm by unspecified larger firearm discharge [HCC]

[4th] X74 Intentional self-harm by other and unspecified firearm and gun discharge
The appropriate 7th character is to be added to each code from category X74
A = initial encounter
D = subsequent encounter
S = sequela
[5th] X74.0 Intentional self-harm by gas, air or spring-operated guns
[6th] X74.01 Intentional self-harm by airgun [HCC]
Intentional self-harm by BB gun discharge
Intentional self-harm by pellet gun discharge
[6th] X74.02 Intentional self-harm by paintball gun [HCC]
[6th] X74.09 Intentional self-harm by other gas, air or spring-operated gun [HCC]
[5th] X74.8 Intentional self-harm by other firearm discharge [HCC]
Intentional self-harm by Very pistol [flare] discharge
[5th] X74.9 Intentional self-harm by unspecified firearm discharge [HCC]

[4th] X75 Intentional self-harm by explosive material [HCC]
The appropriate 7th character is to be added to code X75
A = initial encounter
D = subsequent encounter
S = sequela

[4th] X76 Intentional self-harm by smoke, fire and flames [HCC]
The appropriate 7th character is to be added to code X76
A = initial encounter
D = subsequent encounter
S = sequela

[4th] X77 Intentional self-harm by steam, hot vapors and hot objects
The appropriate 7th character is to be added to each code from category X77
A = initial encounter
D = subsequent encounter
S = sequela
[5th] X77.0 Intentional self-harm by steam or hot vapors [HCC]
[5th] X77.1 Intentional self-harm by hot tap water [HCC]
[5th] X77.2 Intentional self-harm by other hot fluids [HCC]
[5th] X77.3 Intentional self-harm by hot household appliances [HCC]
[5th] X77.8 Intentional self-harm by other hot objects [HCC]
[5th] X77.9 Intentional self-harm by unspecified hot objects [HCC]

[4th] X78 Intentional self-harm by sharp object
The appropriate 7th character is to be added to each code from category X78
A = initial encounter
D = subsequent encounter
S = sequela
[5th] X78.0 Intentional self-harm by sharp glass [HCC]
[5th] X78.1 Intentional self-harm by knife [HCC]
[5th] X78.2 Intentional self-harm by sword or dagger [HCC]
[5th] X78.8 Intentional self-harm by other sharp object [HCC]
[5th] X78.9 Intentional self-harm by unspecified sharp object [HCC]

[4th] X79 Intentional self-harm by blunt object [HCC]
The appropriate 7th character is to be added to code X79
A = initial encounter
D = subsequent encounter
S = sequela

[4th] X80 Intentional self-harm by jumping from a high place [HCC]
Intentional fall from one level to another
The appropriate 7th character is to be added to code X80
A = initial encounter
D = subsequent encounter
S = sequela

[4th] X81 Intentional self-harm by jumping or lying in front of moving object
The appropriate 7th character is to be added to each code from category X81
A = initial encounter
D = subsequent encounter
S = sequela
[5th] X81.0 Intentional self-harm by jumping or lying in front of motor vehicle [HCC]
[5th] X81.1 Intentional self-harm by jumping or lying in front of (subway) train [HCC]
[5th] X81.8 Intentional self-harm by jumping or lying in front of other moving object [HCC]

[4th] X82 Intentional self-harm by crashing of motor vehicle
The appropriate 7th character is to be added to each code from category X82
A = initial encounter
D = subsequent encounter
S = sequela
[5th] X82.0 Intentional collision of motor vehicle with other motor vehicle [HCC]
[5th] X82.1 Intentional collision of motor vehicle with train [HCC]
[5th] X82.2 Intentional collision of motor vehicle with tree [HCC]
[5th] X82.8 Other intentional self-harm by crashing of motor vehicle [HCC]

[4th] X83 Intentional self-harm by other specified means
[EXCLUDES1] *intentional self-harm by poisoning or contact with toxic substance- See Table of Drugs and Chemicals*
The appropriate 7th character is to be added to each code from category X83
A = initial encounter
D = subsequent encounter
S = sequela
[5th] X83.0 Intentional self-harm by crashing of aircraft [HCC]
[5th] X83.1 Intentional self-harm by electrocution [HCC]
[5th] X83.2 Intentional self-harm by exposure to extremes of cold [HCC]
[5th] X83.8 Intentional self-harm by other specified means [HCC]

Assault (X92-Y09)

[INCLUDES] *homicide*
injuries inflicted by another person with intent to injure or kill, by any means
[EXCLUDES1] *injuries due to legal intervention (Y35.-)*
injuries due to operations of war (Y36.-)
injuries due to terrorism (Y38.-)

[4th] X92 Assault by drowning and submersion
The appropriate 7th character is to be added to each code from category X92
A = initial encounter
D = subsequent encounter
S = sequela
[5th] X92.0 Assault by drowning and submersion while in bathtub
[5th] X92.1 Assault by drowning and submersion while in swimming pool
[5th] X92.2 Assault by drowning and submersion after push into swimming pool
[5th] X92.3 Assault by drowning and submersion in natural water
[5th] X92.8 Other assault by drowning and submersion
[5th] X92.9 Assault by drowning and submersion, unspecified

[4th] X93 Assault by handgun discharge
Assault by discharge of gun for single hand use
Assault by discharge of pistol
Assault by discharge of revolver
[EXCLUDES1] *Very pistol (X95.8)*
The appropriate 7th character is to be added to code X93
A = initial encounter
D = subsequent encounter
S = sequela

[4th] X94 Assault by rifle, shotgun and larger firearm discharge
[EXCLUDES1] *airgun (X95.01)*

Unspecified Code Other Specified Code Manifestation Code [N] Newborn [P] Pediatric [M] Maternity [A] Adult ♂ Male ♀ Female
● New Code ▲ Revised Code Title ►◄ Revised Text [NOTES] [INCLUDES] [EXCLUDES1] Not coded here [EXCLUDES2] Not included here
[4th] 4th character required [5th] 5th character required [6th] 6th character required [7th] 7th character required
[7th] Extension 'X' Alert [HAC] Hospital-acquired condition (HAC) alert AHA AHA Coding Clinic©

The appropriate 7th character is to be added to each code from category X94

   A = initial encounter

   D = subsequent encounter

   S = sequela

X94.0 Assault by shotgun

X94.1 Assault by hunting rifle

X94.2 Assault by machine gun

X94.8 Assault by other larger firearm discharge

X94.9 Assault by unspecified larger firearm discharge

X95 Assault by other and unspecified firearm and gun discharge

The appropriate 7th character is to be added to each code from category X95

   A = initial encounter

   D = subsequent encounter

   S = sequela

X95.0 Assault by gas, air or spring-operated guns

   X95.01 Assault by airgun discharge

   Assault by BB gun discharge

   Assault by pellet gun discharge

   X95.02 Assault by paintball gun discharge

   X95.09 Assault by other gas, air or spring-operated gun

X95.8 Assault by other firearm discharge

   Assault by very pistol [flare] discharge

X95.9 Assault by unspecified firearm discharge

X96 Assault by explosive material

   EXCLUDES1 incendiary device (X97)

   terrorism involving explosive material (Y38.2-)

The appropriate 7th character is to be added to each code from category X96

   A = initial encounter

   D = subsequent encounter

   S = sequela

X96.0 Assault by antipersonnel bomb

   EXCLUDES1 antipersonnel bomb use in military or war (Y36.2-)

X96.1 Assault by gasoline bomb

X96.2 Assault by letter bomb

X96.3 Assault by fertilizer bomb

X96.4 Assault by pipe bomb

X96.8 Assault by other specified explosive

X96.9 Assault by unspecified explosive

X97 Assault by smoke, fire and flames

   Assault by arson

   Assault by cigarettes

   Assault by incendiary device

The appropriate 7th character is to be added to code X97

   A = initial encounter

   D = subsequent encounter

   S = sequela

X98 Assault by steam, hot vapors and hot objects

The appropriate 7th character is to be added to each code from category X98

   A = initial encounter

   D = subsequent encounter

   S = sequela

X98.0 Assault by steam or hot vapors

X98.1 Assault by hot tap water

X98.2 Assault by hot fluids

X98.3 Assault by hot household appliances

X98.8 Assault by other hot objects

X98.9 Assault by unspecified hot objects

X99 Assault by sharp object

   EXCLUDES1 assault by strike by sports equipment (Y08.0-)

The appropriate 7th character is to be added to each code from category X99

   A = initial encounter

   D = subsequent encounter

   S = sequela

X99.0 Assault by sharp glass

X99.1 Assault by knife

X99.2 Assault by sword or dagger

X99.8 Assault by other sharp object

X99.9 Assault by unspecified sharp object

   Assault by stabbing NOS

Y00 Assault by blunt object

   EXCLUDES1 assault by strike by sports equipment (Y08.0-)

The appropriate 7th character is to be added to code Y00

   A = initial encounter

   D = subsequent encounter

   S = sequela

Y01 Assault by pushing from high place

The appropriate 7th character is to be added to code Y01

   A = initial encounter

   D = subsequent encounter

   S = sequela

Y02 Assault by pushing or placing victim in front of moving object

The appropriate 7th character is to be added to each code from category Y02

   A = initial encounter

   D = subsequent encounter

   S = sequela

Y02.0 Assault by pushing or placing victim in front of motor vehicle

Y02.1 Assault by pushing or placing victim in front of (subway) train

Y02.8 Assault by pushing or placing victim in front of other moving object

Y03 Assault by crashing of motor vehicle

The appropriate 7th character is to be added to each code from category Y03

   A = initial encounter

   D = subsequent encounter

   S = sequela

Y03.0 Assault by being hit or run over by motor vehicle

Y03.8 Other assault by crashing of motor vehicle

Y04 Assault by bodily force

   EXCLUDES1 assault by:

   submersion (X92.-)

   use of weapon (X93-X95, X99, Y00)

The appropriate 7th character is to be added to each code from category Y04

   A = initial encounter

   D = subsequent encounter

   S = sequela

Y04.0 Assault by unarmed brawl or fight

Y04.1 Assault by human bite

Y04.2 Assault by strike against or bumped into by another person

Y04.8 Assault by other bodily force

   Assault by bodily force NOS

Y07 Perpetrator of assault, maltreatment and neglect

   NOTES Codes from this category are for use only in cases of confirmed abuse (T74.-)

   Selection of the correct perpetrator code is based on the relationship between the perpetrator and the victim

   INCLUDES perpetrator of abandonment

   perpetrator of emotional neglect

   perpetrator of mental cruelty

   perpetrator of physical abuse

   perpetrator of physical neglect

   perpetrator of sexual abuse

   perpetrator of torture

Y07.0 Spouse or partner, perpetrator of maltreatment and neglect

   Spouse or partner, perpetrator of maltreatment and neglect against spouse or partner

   Y07.01 Husband, perpetrator of maltreatment and neglect

   Y07.02 Wife, perpetrator of maltreatment and neglect

POAⁱ Unacceptable principal diagnosis symbol per Medicare code edits   POA Code exempt from diagnosis present on admission requirement
❓ Questionable admission   cc Complication or comorbidity   cc/mcc exⁱ CC/MCC exclusion   mcc Major complication or comorbidity
cc Principal diagnosis as its own CC   mcc Principal diagnosis as its own MCC   HCC HCC diagnosis code   RxHCC RxHCC diagnosis code
MACRA code   Z Z code as first-listed diagnosis

Y07.03 Male partner, **perpetrator of maltreatment and neglect** POA

Y07.04 Female partner, **perpetrator of maltreatment and neglect** POA

Y07.1 Parent (adoptive) (biological), **perpetrator of maltreatment and neglect**

Y07.11 Biological father, **perpetrator of maltreatment and neglect** POA

Y07.12 Biological mother, **perpetrator of maltreatment and neglect** POA

Y07.13 Adoptive father, **perpetrator of maltreatment and neglect** POA

Y07.14 Adoptive mother, **perpetrator of maltreatment and neglect** POA

Y07.4 Other family member, **perpetrator of maltreatment and neglect**

Y07.41 Sibling, **perpetrator of maltreatment and neglect**

EXCLUDES1 *stepsibling, perpetrator of maltreatment and neglect (Y07.435, Y07.436)*

Y07.410 Brother, **perpetrator of maltreatment and neglect** POA

Y07.411 Sister, **perpetrator of maltreatment and neglect** POA

Y07.42 Foster parent, **perpetrator of maltreatment and neglect**

Y07.420 Foster father, **perpetrator of maltreatment and neglect** POA

Y07.421 Foster mother, **perpetrator of maltreatment and neglect** POA

Y07.43 Stepparent or stepsibling, **perpetrator of maltreatment and neglect**

Y07.430 Stepfather, **perpetrator of maltreatment and neglect** POA

Y07.432 Male friend of parent (co-residing in household), **perpetrator of maltreatment and neglect** POA

Y07.433 Stepmother, **perpetrator of maltreatment and neglect** POA

Y07.434 Female friend of parent (co-residing in household), **perpetrator of maltreatment and neglect** POA

Y07.435 Stepbrother, **perpetrator or maltreatment and neglect** POA

Y07.436 Stepsister, **perpetrator of maltreatment and neglect** POA

Y07.49 Other family member, **perpetrator of maltreatment and neglect**

Y07.490 Male cousin, **perpetrator of maltreatment and neglect** POA

Y07.491 Female cousin, **perpetrator of maltreatment and neglect** POA

Y07.499 Other family member, **perpetrator of maltreatment and neglect** POA

Y07.5 Non-family member, **perpetrator of maltreatment and neglect**

Y07.50 Unspecified **non-family member, perpetrator of maltreatment and neglect**

Y07.51 Daycare provider, **perpetrator of maltreatment and neglect**

Y07.510 At-home childcare provider, **perpetrator of maltreatment and neglect** POA

Y07.511 Daycare center childcare provider, **perpetrator of maltreatment and neglect** POA

Y07.512 At-home adultcare provider, **perpetrator of maltreatment and neglect** POA

Y07.513 Adultcare center provider, **perpetrator of maltreatment and neglect** POA

Y07.519 Unspecified **daycare provider, perpetrator of maltreatment and neglect** POA

Y07.52 Healthcare provider, **perpetrator of maltreatment and neglect**

Y07.521 Mental health provider, **perpetrator of maltreatment and neglect** POA

Y07.528 Other therapist or healthcare provider, **perpetrator of maltreatment and neglect** POA

Nurse perpetrator of maltreatment and neglect

Occupational therapist perpetrator of maltreatment and neglect

Physical therapist perpetrator of maltreatment and neglect

Speech therapist perpetrator of maltreatment and neglect

Y07.529 Unspecified healthcare provider, **perpetrator of maltreatment and neglect** POA

Y07.53 Teacher or instructor, **perpetrator of maltreatment and neglect** POA

Coach, perpetrator of maltreatment and neglect

Y07.59 Other **non-family member, perpetrator of maltreatment and neglect** POA

Y07.9 Unspecified **perpetrator of maltreatment and neglect** POA

Y08 Assault by other specified means

The appropriate 7th character is to be added to each code from category Y08

A = initial encounter
D = subsequent encounter
S = sequela

Y08.0 **Assault by** strike by sport equipment

Y08.01 **Assault by strike by** hockey stick POA

Y08.02 **Assault by strike by** baseball bat POA

Y08.09 Assault by strike by other specified type of sport equipment POA

Y08.8 **Assault by** other specified means

Y08.81 **Assault by** crashing of aircraft POA

Y08.89 Assault by other specified means POA

Y09 **Assault by unspecified means**

AHA: Q4 2016

Assassination (attempted) NOS
Homicide (attempted) NOS
Manslaughter (attempted) NOS
Murder (attempted) NOS

Event of undetermined intent (Y21-Y33)

Undetermined intent is only for use when there is specific documentation in the record that the intent of the injury cannot be determined. If no such documentation is present, code to accidental (unintentional)

Y21 Drowning and submersion, undetermined intent

The appropriate 7th character is to be added to each code from category Y21

A = initial encounter
D = subsequent encounter
S = sequela

Y21.0 Drowning and submersion while in bathtub, **undetermined intent** POA

Y21.1 Drowning and submersion after fall into bathtub, undetermined intent POA

Y21.2 Drowning and submersion while in swimming pool, undetermined intent POA

Y21.3 Drowning and submersion after fall into swimming pool, undetermined intent POA

Y21.4 Drowning and submersion in natural water, **undetermined intent** POA

Y21.8 Other drowning and submersion, undetermined intent POA

Y21.9 Unspecified drowning and submersion, undetermined intent POA

Y22 Handgun discharge, undetermined intent POA

Discharge of gun for single hand use, undetermined intent
Discharge of pistol, undetermined intent
Discharge of revolver, undetermined intent

Unspecified Code	Other Specified Code	Manifestation Code	N Newborn	P Pediatric	M Maternity	A Adult	♂ Male ♀ Female

● New Code ▲ Revised Code Title ►◄ Revised Text **NOTES** *INCLUDES* *EXCLUDES 1* Not coded here *EXCLUDES 2* Not included here

4th character required 5th character required 6th character required 7th character required

Extension 'X' Alert HAC Hospital-acquired condition (HAC) alert **AHA** AHA Coding Clinic©

EXCLUDES2 *very pistol (Y24.8)*

The appropriate 7th character is to be added to code Y22
- A = initial encounter
- D = subsequent encounter
- S = sequela

4ᵗʰ Y23 Rifle, shotgun and larger firearm discharge, undetermined intent

EXCLUDES2 *airgun (Y24.0)*

The appropriate 7th character is to be added to each code from category Y23
- A = initial encounter
- D = subsequent encounter
- S = sequela

7ᵗʰ Y23.0 Shotgun discharge, undetermined intent POA

7ᵗʰ Y23.1 Hunting rifle discharge, undetermined intent POA

7ᵗʰ Y23.2 Military firearm discharge, undetermined intent POA

7ᵗʰ Y23.3 Machine gun discharge, undetermined intent POA

7ᵗʰ Y23.8 Other larger firearm discharge, undetermined intent POA

7ᵗʰ Y23.9 Unspecified larger firearm discharge, undetermined intent POA

4ᵗʰ Y24 Other and unspecified firearm discharge, undetermined intent

The appropriate 7th character is to be added to each code from category Y24
- A = initial encounter
- D = subsequent encounter
- S = sequela

7ᵗʰ Y24.0 Airgun discharge, undetermined intent POA
BB gun discharge, undetermined intent
Pellet gun discharge, undetermined intent

7ᵗʰ Y24.8 Other firearm discharge, undetermined intent POA
Paintball gun discharge, undetermined intent
Very pistol [flare] discharge, undetermined intent

7ᵗʰ Y24.9 Unspecified firearm discharge, undetermined intent POA

7ᵗʰ Y25 Contact with explosive material, undetermined intent
The appropriate 7th character is to be added to code Y25
- A = initial encounter
- D = subsequent encounter
- S = sequela

7ᵗʰ Y26 Exposure to smoke, fire and flames, undetermined intent
The appropriate 7th character is to be added to code Y26
- A = initial encounter
- D = subsequent encounter
- S = sequela

4ᵗʰ Y27 Contact with steam, hot vapors and hot objects, undetermined intent
The appropriate 7th character is to be added to each code from category Y27
- A = initial encounter
- D = subsequent encounter
- S = sequela

7ᵗʰ Y27.0 Contact with steam and hot vapors, undetermined intent

7ᵗʰ Y27.1 Contact with hot tap water, undetermined intent

7ᵗʰ Y27.2 Contact with hot fluids, undetermined intent

7ᵗʰ Y27.3 Contact with hot household appliance, undetermined intent

7ᵗʰ Y27.8 Contact with other hot objects, undetermined intent

7ᵗʰ Y27.9 Contact with unspecified hot objects, undetermined intent

4ᵗʰ Y28 Contact with sharp object, undetermined intent
The appropriate 7th character is to be added to each code from category Y28
- A = initial encounter
- D = subsequent encounter
- S = sequela

7ᵗʰ Y28.0 Contact with sharp glass, undetermined intent

7ᵗʰ Y28.1 Contact with knife, undetermined intent

7ᵗʰ Y28.2 Contact with sword or dagger, undetermined intent

7ᵗʰ Y28.8 Contact with other sharp object, undetermined intent

7ᵗʰ Y28.9 Contact with unspecified sharp object, undetermined intent

7ᵗʰ Y29 Contact with blunt object, undetermined intent
The appropriate 7th character is to be added to code Y29
- A = initial encounter

- D = subsequent encounter
- S = sequela

7ᵗʰ Y30 Falling, jumping or pushed from a high place, undetermined intent POA
Victim falling from one level to another, undetermined intent
The appropriate 7th character is to be added to code Y30
- A = initial encounter
- D = subsequent encounter
- S = sequela

7ᵗʰ Y31 Falling, lying or running before or into moving object, undetermined intent
The appropriate 7th character is to be added to code Y31
- A = initial encounter
- D = subsequent encounter
- S = sequela

7ᵗʰ Y32 Crashing of motor vehicle, undetermined intent POA
The appropriate 7th character is to be added to code Y32
- A = initial encounter
- D = subsequent encounter
- S = sequela

7ᵗʰ Y33 Other specified events, undetermined intent
The appropriate 7th character is to be added to code Y33
- A = initial encounter
- D = subsequent encounter
- S = sequela

Legal intervention, operations of war, military operations, and terrorism (Y35-Y38)

4ᵗʰ Y35 Legal intervention

INCLUDES *any injury sustained as a result of an encounter with any law enforcement official, serving in any capacity at the time of the encounter, whether on-duty or off-duty. Includes: injury to law enforcement official, suspect and bystander*

The appropriate 7th character is to be added to each code from category Y35
- A = initial encounter
- D = subsequent encounter
- S = sequela

5ᵗʰ Y35.0 Legal intervention involving firearm discharge

6ᵗʰ Y35.00 Legal intervention involving unspecified firearm discharge
Legal intervention involving gunshot wound
Legal intervention involving shot NOS

7ᵗʰ Y35.001 Legal intervention involving unspecified firearm discharge, law enforcement official injured POA

7ᵗʰ Y35.002 Legal intervention involving unspecified firearm discharge, bystander injured POA

7ᵗʰ Y35.003 Legal intervention involving unspecified firearm discharge, suspect injured POA

6ᵗʰ Y35.01 Legal intervention involving injury by machine gun

7ᵗʰ Y35.011 Legal intervention involving injury by machine gun, law enforcement official injured POA

7ᵗʰ Y35.012 Legal intervention involving injury by machine gun, bystander injured POA

7ᵗʰ Y35.013 Legal intervention involving injury by machine gun, suspect injured POA

6ᵗʰ Y35.02 Legal intervention involving injury by handgun

7ᵗʰ Y35.021 Legal intervention involving injury by handgun, law enforcement official injured POA

7ᵗʰ Y35.022 Legal intervention involving injury by handgun, bystander injured POA

7ᵗʰ Y35.023 Legal intervention involving injury by handgun, suspect injured POA

6ᵗʰ Y35.03 Legal intervention involving injury by rifle pellet

7ᵗʰ Y35.031 Legal intervention involving injury by rifle pellet, law enforcement official injured POA

PDₓ Unacceptable principal diagnosis symbol per Medicare code edits   POA Code exempt from diagnosis present on admission requirement
? Questionable admission   CC Complication or comorbidity   CC/MCC Exc CC/MCC exclusion   MCC Major complication or comorbidity
CC Principal diagnosis as its own CC   MCC Principal diagnosis as its own MCC   HCC HCC diagnosis code   RxHCC RxHCC diagnosis code
MACRA code   Z1 Z code as first-listed diagnosis

1234   When symbols appear on a code that requires a 7th character extension, refer to Appendix B to identify applicable 7th character codes.   2018 ICD-10-CM

- [7th] Y35.032 Legal intervention involving injury by rifle pellet, bystander injured [POA]
- [7th] Y35.033 Legal intervention involving injury by rifle pellet, suspect injured [POA]
- [6th] Y35.04 Legal intervention involving injury by rubber bullet
  - [7th] Y35.041 Legal intervention involving injury by rubber bullet, law enforcement official injured [POA]
  - [7th] Y35.042 Legal intervention involving injury by rubber bullet, bystander injured [POA]
  - [7th] Y35.043 Legal intervention involving injury by rubber bullet, suspect injured [POA]
- [6th] Y35.09 Legal intervention involving other firearm discharge
  - [7th] Y35.091 Legal intervention involving other firearm discharge, law enforcement official injured [POA]
  - [7th] Y35.092 Legal intervention involving other firearm discharge, bystander injured [POA]
  - [7th] Y35.093 Legal intervention involving other firearm discharge, suspect injured [POA]

[5th] Y35.1 Legal intervention involving explosives
- [6th] Y35.10 Legal intervention involving unspecified explosives
  - [7th] Y35.101 Legal intervention involving unspecified explosives, law enforcement official injured [POA]
  - [7th] Y35.102 Legal intervention involving unspecified explosives, bystander injured [POA]
  - [7th] Y35.103 Legal intervention involving unspecified explosives, suspect injured [POA]
- [6th] Y35.11 Legal intervention involving injury by dynamite
  - [7th] Y35.111 Legal intervention involving injury by dynamite, law enforcement official injured [POA]
  - [7th] Y35.112 Legal intervention involving injury by dynamite, bystander injured [POA]
  - [7th] Y35.113 Legal intervention involving injury by dynamite, suspect injured [POA]
- [6th] Y35.12 Legal intervention involving injury by explosive shell
  - [7th] Y35.121 Legal intervention involving injury by explosive shell, law enforcement official injured [POA]
  - [7th] Y35.122 Legal intervention involving injury by explosive shell, bystander injured [POA]
  - [7th] Y35.123 Legal intervention involving injury by explosive shell, suspect injured [POA]
- [6th] Y35.19 Legal intervention involving other explosives
  Legal intervention involving injury by grenade
  Legal intervention involving injury by mortar bomb
  - [7th] Y35.191 Legal intervention involving other explosives, law enforcement official injured [POA]
  - [7th] Y35.192 Legal intervention involving other explosives, bystander injured [POA]
  - [7th] Y35.193 Legal intervention involving other explosives, suspect injured [POA]

[5th] Y35.2 Legal intervention involving gas
Legal intervention involving asphyxiation by gas
Legal intervention involving poisoning by gas
- [6th] Y35.20 Legal intervention involving unspecified gas
  - [7th] Y35.201 Legal intervention involving unspecified gas, law enforcement official injured [POA]
  - [7th] Y35.202 Legal intervention involving unspecified gas, bystander injured [POA]
  - [7th] Y35.203 Legal intervention involving unspecified gas, suspect injured [POA]
- [6th] Y35.21 Legal intervention involving injury by tear gas
  - [7th] Y35.211 Legal intervention involving injury by tear gas, law enforcement official injured [POA]
  - [7th] Y35.212 Legal intervention involving injury by tear gas, bystander injured [POA]
  - [7th] Y35.213 Legal intervention involving injury by tear gas, suspect injured [POA]
- [6th] Y35.29 Legal intervention involving other gas
  - [7th] Y35.291 Legal intervention involving other gas, law enforcement official injured [POA]
  - [7th] Y35.292 Legal intervention involving other gas, bystander injured [POA]
  - [7th] Y35.293 Legal intervention involving other gas, suspect injured [POA]

[5th] Y35.3 Legal intervention involving blunt objects
Legal intervention involving being hit or struck by blunt object
- [6th] Y35.30 Legal intervention involving unspecified blunt objects
  - [7th] Y35.301 Legal intervention involving unspecified blunt objects, law enforcement official injured [POA]
  - [7th] Y35.302 Legal intervention involving unspecified blunt objects, bystander injured [POA]
  - [7th] Y35.303 Legal intervention involving unspecified blunt objects, suspect injured [POA]
- [6th] Y35.31 Legal intervention involving baton
  - [7th] Y35.311 Legal intervention involving baton, law enforcement official injured [POA]
  - [7th] Y35.312 Legal intervention involving baton, bystander injured [POA]
  - [7th] Y35.313 Legal intervention involving baton, suspect injured [POA]
- [6th] Y35.39 Legal intervention involving other blunt objects
  - [7th] Y35.391 Legal intervention involving other blunt objects, law enforcement official injured [POA]
  - [7th] Y35.392 Legal intervention involving other blunt objects, bystander injured [POA]
  - [7th] Y35.393 Legal intervention involving other blunt objects, suspect injured [POA]

[5th] Y35.4 Legal intervention involving sharp objects
Legal intervention involving being cut by sharp objects
Legal intervention involving being stabbed by sharp objects
- [6th] Y35.40 Legal intervention involving unspecified sharp objects
  - [7th] Y35.401 Legal intervention involving unspecified sharp objects, law enforcement official injured [POA]
  - [7th] Y35.402 Legal intervention involving unspecified sharp objects, bystander injured [POA]
  - [7th] Y35.403 Legal intervention involving unspecified sharp objects, suspect injured [POA]
- [6th] Y35.41 Legal intervention involving bayonet
  - [7th] Y35.411 Legal intervention involving bayonet, law enforcement official injured [POA]
  - [7th] Y35.412 Legal intervention involving bayonet, bystander injured [POA]
  - [7th] Y35.413 Legal intervention involving bayonet, suspect injured [POA]
- [6th] Y35.49 Legal intervention involving other sharp objects
  - [7th] Y35.491 Legal intervention involving other sharp objects, law enforcement official injured [POA]
  - [7th] Y35.492 Legal intervention involving other sharp objects, bystander injured [POA]
  - [7th] Y35.493 Legal intervention involving other sharp objects, suspect injured [POA]

[5th] Y35.8 Legal intervention involving other specified means
- [6th] Y35.81 Legal intervention involving manhandling
  - [7th] Y35.811 Legal intervention involving manhandling, law enforcement official injured [POA]
  - [7th] Y35.812 Legal intervention involving manhandling, bystander injured [POA]
  - [7th] Y35.813 Legal intervention involving manhandling, suspect injured [POA]
- [6th] Y35.89 Legal intervention involving other specified means

7️⃣ **Y35.891 Legal intervention involving other specified means, law enforcement official injured** POA

7️⃣ **Y35.892 Legal intervention involving other specified means, bystander injured** POA

7️⃣ **Y35.893 Legal intervention involving other specified means, suspect injured** POA

5️⃣ Y35.9 **Legal intervention, means** unspecified

7️⃣ **Y35.91 Legal intervention, means unspecified, law enforcement official injured** POA

7️⃣ **Y35.92 Legal intervention, means unspecified, bystander injured** POA

7️⃣ **Y35.93 Legal intervention, means unspecified, suspect injured** POA

4️⃣ Y36 **Operations of war**

INCLUDES *injuries to military personnel and civilians caused by war, civil insurrection, and peacekeeping missions*

EXCLUDES1 *injury to military personnel occurring during peacetime military operations (Y37.-)*

military vehicles involved in transport accidents with non-military vehicle during peacetime (V09.01, V09.21, V19.81, V29.81, V39.81, V49.81, V59.81, V69.81, V79.81)

The appropriate 7th character is to be added to each code from category Y36

A = initial encounter
D = subsequent encounter
S = sequela

5️⃣ Y36.0 **War operations involving** explosion of marine weapons

5️⃣ Y36.00 **War operations involving explosion of** unspecified **marine weapon**

War operations involving underwater blast NOS

7️⃣ **Y36.000 War operations involving explosion of unspecified marine weapon, military personnel** POA

7️⃣ **Y36.001 War operations involving explosion of unspecified marine weapon, civilian** POA

6️⃣ Y36.01 **War operations involving explosion of** depth-charge

7️⃣ **Y36.010 War operations involving explosion of depth-charge, military personnel** POA

7️⃣ **Y36.011 War operations involving explosion of depth-charge, civilian** POA

6️⃣ Y36.02 **War operations involving explosion of** marine mine

War operations involving explosion of marine mine, at sea or in harbor

7️⃣ **Y36.020 War operations involving explosion of marine mine, military personnel** POA

7️⃣ **Y36.021 War operations involving explosion of marine mine, civilian** POA

6️⃣ Y36.03 **War operations involving explosion of** sea-based artillery shell

7️⃣ **Y36.030 War operations involving explosion of sea-based artillery shell, military personnel** POA

7️⃣ **Y36.031 War operations involving explosion of sea-based artillery shell, civilian** POA

6️⃣ Y36.04 **War operations involving explosion of** torpedo

7️⃣ **Y36.040 War operations involving explosion of torpedo, military personnel** POA

7️⃣ **Y36.041 War operations involving explosion of torpedo, civilian** POA

6️⃣ Y36.05 **War operations involving** accidental detonation of onboard marine weapons

7️⃣ **Y36.050 War operations involving accidental detonation of onboard marine weapons, military personnel** POA

7️⃣ **Y36.051 War operations involving accidental detonation of onboard marine weapons, civilian** POA

6️⃣ Y36.09 **War operations involving explosion of** other marine weapons

7️⃣ **Y36.090 War operations involving explosion of other marine weapons, military personnel** POA

7️⃣ **Y36.091 War operations involving explosion of other marine weapons, civilian** POA

5️⃣ Y36.1 **War operations involving destruction of aircraft**

6️⃣ Y36.10 **War operations involving** unspecified **destruction of aircraft**

7️⃣ **Y36.100 War operations involving unspecified destruction of aircraft, military personnel** POA

7️⃣ **Y36.101 War operations involving unspecified destruction of aircraft, civilian** POA

6️⃣ Y36.11 **War operations involving destruction of aircraft due to** enemy fire or explosives

War operations involving destruction of aircraft due to air to air missile

War operations involving destruction of aircraft due to explosive placed on aircraft

War operations involving destruction of aircraft due to rocket propelled grenade [RPG]

War operations involving destruction of aircraft due to small arms fire

War operations involving destruction of aircraft due to surface to air missile

7️⃣ **Y36.110 War operations involving destruction of aircraft due to enemy fire or explosives, military personnel** POA

7️⃣ **Y36.111 War operations involving destruction of aircraft due to enemy fire or explosives, civilian** POA

6️⃣ Y36.12 **War operations involving destruction of aircraft due to** collision with other aircraft

7️⃣ **Y36.120 War operations involving destruction of aircraft due to collision with other aircraft, military personnel** POA

7️⃣ **Y36.121 War operations involving destruction of aircraft due to collision with other aircraft, civilian** POA

6️⃣ Y36.13 **War operations involving destruction of aircraft due to** onboard fire

7️⃣ **Y36.130 War operations involving destruction of aircraft due to onboard fire, military personnel** POA

7️⃣ **Y36.131 War operations involving destruction of aircraft due to onboard fire, civilian** POA

6️⃣ Y36.14 **War operations involving destruction of aircraft due to** accidental detonation of onboard munitions and explosives

7️⃣ **Y36.140 War operations involving destruction of aircraft due to accidental detonation of onboard munitions and explosives, military personnel** POA

7️⃣ **Y36.141 War operations involving destruction of aircraft due to accidental detonation of onboard munitions and explosives, civilian** POA

6️⃣ Y36.19 **War operations involving** other **destruction of aircraft**

7️⃣ **Y36.190 War operations involving other destruction of aircraft, military personnel** POA

7️⃣ **Y36.191 War operations involving other destruction of aircraft, civilian** POA

5️⃣ Y36.2 **War operations involving** other **explosions and fragments**

EXCLUDES1 *war operations involving explosion of aircraft (Y36.1-)*

war operations involving explosion of marine weapons (Y36.0-)

war operations involving explosion of nuclear weapons (Y36.5-)

war operations involving explosion occurring after cessation of hostilities (Y36.8-)

6️⃣ Y36.20 **War operations involving** unspecified **explosion and fragments**

War operations involving air blast NOS

War operations involving blast NOS

PDx❌ Unacceptable principal diagnosis symbol per Medicare code edits   POA Code exempt from diagnosis present on admission requirement

❓ Questionable admission   «c» Complication or comorbidity   CC/MCC Exc CC/MCC exclusion   MCC Major complication or comorbidity

PDx CC Principal diagnosis as its own CC   Ab Principal diagnosis as its own MCC   HCC HCC diagnosis code   RHCC RxHCC diagnosis code

MACRA code   Z1 Z code as first-listed diagnosis

War operations involving blast fragments NOS
War operations involving blast wave NOS
War operations involving blast wind NOS
War operations involving explosion NOS
War operations involving explosion of bomb NOS

[7th] **Y36.200 War operations involving unspecified explosion and fragments, military personnel** POA

[7th] **Y36.201 War operations involving unspecified explosion and fragments, civilian** POA

[6th] **Y36.21 War operations involving explosion of aerial bomb**

[7th] **Y36.210 War operations involving explosion of aerial bomb, military personnel** POA

[7th] **Y36.211 War operations involving explosion of aerial bomb, civilian** POA

[6th] **Y36.22 War operations involving explosion of guided missile**

[7th] **Y36.220 War operations involving explosion of guided missile, military personnel** POA

[7th] **Y36.221 War operations involving explosion of guided missile, civilian** POA

[6th] **Y36.23 War operations involving explosion of improvised explosive device [IED]**

War operations involving explosion of person-borne improvised explosive device [IED]
War operations involving explosion of vehicle-borne improvised explosive device [IED]
War operations involving explosion of roadside improvised explosive device [IED]

[7th] **Y36.230 War operations involving explosion of improvised explosive device [IED], military personnel** POA

[7th] **Y36.231 War operations involving explosion of improvised explosive device [IED], civilian** POA

[6th] **Y36.24 War operations involving explosion due to accidental detonation and discharge of own munitions or munitions launch device**

[7th] **Y36.240 War operations involving explosion due to accidental detonation and discharge of own munitions or munitions launch device, military personnel** POA

[7th] **Y36.241 War operations involving explosion due to accidental detonation and discharge of own munitions or munitions launch device, civilian** POA

[6th] **Y36.25 War operations involving fragments from munitions**

[7th] **Y36.250 War operations involving fragments from munitions, military personnel** POA

[7th] **Y36.251 War operations involving fragments from munitions, civilian** POA

[6th] **Y36.26 War operations involving fragments of improvised explosive device [IED]**

War operations involving fragments of person-borne improvised explosive device [IED]
War operations involving fragments of vehicle-borne improvised explosive device [IED]
War operations involving fragments of roadside improvised explosive device [IED]

[7th] **Y36.260 War operations involving fragments of improvised explosive device [IED], military personnel** POA

[7th] **Y36.261 War operations involving fragments of improvised explosive device [IED], civilian** POA

[6th] **Y36.27 War operations involving fragments from weapons**

[7th] **Y36.270 War operations involving fragments from weapons, military personnel** POA

[7th] **Y36.271 War operations involving fragments from weapons, civilian** POA

[6th] **Y36.29 War operations involving other explosions and fragments**

War operations involving explosion of grenade
War operations involving explosions of land mine
War operations involving shrapnel NOS

[7th] **Y36.290 War operations involving other explosions and fragments, military personnel** POA

[7th] **Y36.291 War operations involving other explosions and fragments, civilian** POA

[5th] **Y36.3 War operations involving fires, conflagrations and hot substances**

War operations involving smoke, fumes, and heat from fires, conflagrations and hot substances

EXCLUDES1 *war operations involving fires and conflagrations aboard military aircraft (Y36.1-)*
war operations involving fires and conflagrations aboard military watercraft (Y36.0-)
war operations involving fires and conflagrations caused indirectly by conventional weapons (Y36.2-)
war operations involving fires and thermal effects of nuclear weapons (Y36.53-)

[6th] **Y36.30 War operations involving unspecified fire, conflagration and hot substance**

[7th] **Y36.300 War operations involving unspecified fire, conflagration and hot substance, military personnel** POA

[7th] **Y36.301 War operations involving unspecified fire, conflagration and hot substance, civilian** POA

[6th] **Y36.31 War operations involving gasoline bomb**

War operations involving incendiary bomb
War operations involving petrol bomb

[7th] **Y36.310 War operations involving gasoline bomb, military personnel** POA

[7th] **Y36.311 War operations involving gasoline bomb, civilian** POA

[6th] **Y36.32 War operations involving incendiary bullet**

[7th] **Y36.320 War operations involving incendiary bullet, military personnel** POA

[7th] **Y36.321 War operations involving incendiary bullet, civilian** POA

[6th] **Y36.33 War operations involving flamethrower**

[7th] **Y36.330 War operations involving flamethrower, military personnel** POA

[7th] **Y36.331 War operations involving flamethrower, civilian** POA

[6th] **Y36.39 War operations involving other fires, conflagrations and hot substances**

[7th] **Y36.390 War operations involving other fires, conflagrations and hot substances, military personnel** POA

[7th] **Y36.391 War operations involving other fires, conflagrations and hot substances, civilian** POA

[5th] **Y36.4 War operations involving firearm discharge and other forms of conventional warfare**

[6th] **Y36.41 War operations involving rubber bullets**

[7th] **Y36.410 War operations involving rubber bullets, military personnel** POA

[7th] **Y36.411 War operations involving rubber bullets, civilian** POA

[6th] **Y36.42 War operations involving firearms pellets**

[7th] **Y36.420 War operations involving firearms pellets, military personnel** POA

[7th] **Y36.421 War operations involving firearms pellets, civilian** POA

[6th] **Y36.43 War operations involving other firearms discharge**

War operations involving bullets NOS

EXCLUDES1 *war operations involving munitions fragments (Y36.25-)*
war operations involving incendiary bullets (Y36.32-)

[7th] **Y36.430 War operations involving other firearms discharge, military personnel** POA

[7th] **Y36.431 War operations involving other firearms discharge, civilian** POA

6ᵗʰ **Y36.44** **War operations involving** unarmed hand to hand combat

    EXCLUDES1 *war operations involving combat using blunt or piercing object (Y36.45-)*

    war operations involving intentional restriction of air and airway (Y36.46-)

    war operations involving unintentional restriction of air and airway (Y36.47-)

7ᵗʰ **Y36.440** **War operations involving unarmed hand to hand combat,** military personnel

7ᵗʰ **Y36.441** **War operations involving unarmed hand to hand combat,** civilian

5ᵗʰ **Y36.45** **War operations involving combat using blunt or piercing object**

7ᵗʰ **Y36.450** **War operations involving combat using blunt or piercing object,** military personnel

7ᵗʰ **Y36.451** **War operations involving combat using blunt or piercing object,** civilian

6ᵗʰ **Y36.46** **War operations involving intentional restriction of air and airway**

7ᵗʰ **Y36.460** **War operations involving intentional restriction of air and airway, military personnel**

7ᵗʰ **Y36.461** **War operations involving intentional restriction of air and airway, civilian**

6ᵗʰ **Y36.47** **War operations involving** unintentional restriction of air and airway

7ᵗʰ **Y36.470** **War operations involving unintentional restriction of air and airway,** military personnel

7ᵗʰ **Y36.471** **War operations involving unintentional restriction of air and airway,** civilian

6ᵗʰ **Y36.49** **War operations involving** other forms of conventional warfare

7ᵗʰ **Y36.490** **War operations involving other forms of conventional warfare, military personnel**

7ᵗʰ **Y36.491** **War operations involving other forms of conventional warfare, civilian**

5ᵗʰ **Y36.5** **War operations involving** nuclear weapons

    War operations involving dirty bomb NOS

6ᵗʰ **Y36.50** **War operations involving** unspecified **effect of nuclear weapon**

7ᵗʰ **Y36.500** **War operations involving unspecified effect of nuclear weapon, military personnel**

7ᵗʰ **Y36.501** **War operations involving unspecified effect of nuclear weapon, civilian**

6ᵗʰ **Y36.51** **War operations involving** direct blast **effect of nuclear weapon**

    War operations involving blast pressure of nuclear weapon

7ᵗʰ **Y36.510** **War operations involving direct blast effect of nuclear weapon,** military personnel

7ᵗʰ **Y36.511** **War operations involving direct blast effect of nuclear weapon,** civilian

6ᵗʰ **Y36.52** **War operations involving** indirect blast **effect of nuclear weapon**

    War operations involving being thrown by blast of nuclear weapon

    War operations involving being struck or crushed by blast debris of nuclear weapon

7ᵗʰ **Y36.520** **War operations involving indirect blast effect of nuclear weapon,** military personnel

7ᵗʰ **Y36.521** **War operations involving indirect blast effect of nuclear weapon,** civilian

6ᵗʰ **Y36.53** **War operations involving** thermal radiation **effect of nuclear weapon**

    War operations involving direct heat from nuclear weapon

    War operation involving fireball effects from nuclear weapon

7ᵗʰ **Y36.530** **War operations involving thermal radiation effect of nuclear weapon,** military personnel

7ᵗʰ **Y36.531** **War operations involving thermal radiation effect of nuclear weapon,** civilian

6ᵗʰ **Y36.54** **War operation involving** nuclear radiation **effects of nuclear weapon**

    War operation involving acute radiation exposure from nuclear weapon

    War operation involving exposure to immediate ionizing radiation from nuclear weapon

    War operation involving fallout exposure from nuclear weapon

    War operation involving secondary effects of nuclear weapons

7ᵗʰ **Y36.540** **War operation involving nuclear radiation effects of nuclear weapon,** military personnel

7ᵗʰ **Y36.541** **War operation involving nuclear radiation effects of nuclear weapon,** civilian

6ᵗʰ **Y36.59** **War operation involving** other **effects of nuclear weapons**

7ᵗʰ **Y36.590** **War operation involving other effects of nuclear weapons, military personnel**

7ᵗʰ **Y36.591** **War operation involving other effects of nuclear weapons, civilian**

5ᵗʰ **Y36.6** **War operations involving biological weapons**

6ᵗʰ **Y36.6X** **War operations involving** biological weapons

7ᵗʰ **Y36.6X0** **War operations involving biological weapons,** military personnel

7ᵗʰ **Y36.6X1** **War operations involving biological weapons,** civilian

5ᵗʰ **Y36.7** **War operations involving chemical weapons and other forms of unconventional warfare**

    EXCLUDES1 *war operations involving incendiary devices (Y36.3-, Y36.5-)*

6ᵗʰ **Y36.7X** **War operations involving chemical weapons and other forms of** unconventional warfare

7ᵗʰ **Y36.7X0** **War operations involving chemical weapons and other forms of unconventional warfare, military personnel**

7ᵗʰ **Y36.7X1** **War operations involving chemical weapons and other forms of unconventional warfare, civilian**

5ᵗʰ **Y36.8** **War operations occurring** after cessation of hostilities

    War operations classifiable to categories Y36.0-Y36.8 but occurring after cessation of hostilities

6ᵗʰ **Y36.81** **Explosion of** mine **placed during war operations but exploding after cessation of hostilities**

7ᵗʰ **Y36.810** **Explosion of mine placed during war operations but exploding after cessation of hostilities,** military personnel

7ᵗʰ **Y36.811** **Explosion of mine placed during war operations but exploding after cessation of hostilities,** civilian

6ᵗʰ **Y36.82** **Explosion of** bomb **placed during war operations but exploding after cessation of hostilities**

7ᵗʰ **Y36.820** **Explosion of bomb placed during war operations but exploding after cessation of hostilities,** military personnel

7ᵗʰ **Y36.821** **Explosion of bomb placed during war operations but exploding after cessation of hostilities,** civilian

6ᵗʰ **Y36.88** Other **war operations occurring after cessation of hostilities**

PDxₓ: Unacceptable principal diagnosis symbol per Medicare code edits   POA: Code exempt from diagnosis present on admission requirement

❓ Questionable admission   cc Complication or comorbidity   CC/MCC Exc CC/MCC exclusion   MCC Major complication or comorbidity

Principal diagnosis as its own CC   Principal diagnosis as its own MCC   HCC HCC diagnosis code   RxHCC RxHCC diagnosis code

MACRA code   Z code as first-listed diagnosis

1238

When symbols appear on a code that requires a 7th character extension, refer to Appendix B to identify applicable 7th character codes.

2018 ICD-10-CM

[7th] Y36.880 Other war operations occurring after cessation of hostilities, military personnel [POA]
[7th] Y36.881 Other war operations occurring after cessation of hostilities, civilian [POA]
[6th] Y36.89 Unspecified war operations occurring after cessation of hostilities
[7th] Y36.890 Unspecified war operations occurring after cessation of hostilities, military personnel [POA]
[7th] Y36.891 Unspecified war operations occurring after cessation of hostilities, civilian [POA]
[5th] Y36.9 Other and unspecified war operations
[7th] Y36.90 War operations, unspecified [POA]
[7th] Y36.91 War operations involving unspecified weapon of mass destruction [WMD] [POA]
[7th] Y36.92 War operations involving friendly fire [POA]

[4th] Y37 Military operations

[INCLUDES] *injuries to military personnel and civilians occurring during peacetime on military property and during routine military exercises and operations*

[EXCLUDES1] *military aircraft involved in aircraft accident with civilian aircraft (V97.81-)*
military vehicles involved in transport accident with civilian vehicle (V09.01, V09.21, V19.81, V29.81, V39.81, V49.81, V59.81, V69.81, V79.81)
military watercraft involved in water transport accident with civilian watercraft (V94.81-)
war operations (Y36.-)

The appropriate 7th character is to be added to each code from category Y37
A = initial encounter
D = subsequent encounter
S = sequela

[5th] Y37.0 Military operations involving explosion of marine weapons
[6th] Y37.00 Military operations involving explosion of unspecified marine weapon
Military operations involving underwater blast NOS
[7th] Y37.000 Military operations involving explosion of unspecified marine weapon, military personnel [POA]
[7th] Y37.001 Military operations involving explosion of unspecified marine weapon, civilian [POA]
[6th] Y37.01 Military operations involving explosion of depth-charge
[7th] Y37.010 Military operations involving explosion of depth-charge, military personnel [POA]
[7th] Y37.011 Military operations involving explosion of depth-charge, civilian [POA]
[6th] Y37.02 Military operations involving explosion of marine mine
Military operations involving explosion of marine mine, at sea or in harbor
[7th] Y37.020 Military operations involving explosion of marine mine, military personnel [POA]
[7th] Y37.021 Military operations involving explosion of marine mine, civilian [POA]
[6th] Y37.03 Military operations involving explosion of sea-based artillery shell
[7th] Y37.030 Military operations involving explosion of sea-based artillery shell, military personnel [POA]
[7th] Y37.031 Military operations involving explosion of sea-based artillery shell, civilian [POA]
[6th] Y37.04 Military operations involving explosion of torpedo
[7th] Y37.040 Military operations involving explosion of torpedo, military personnel [POA]
[7th] Y37.041 Military operations involving explosion of torpedo, civilian [POA]
[6th] Y37.05 Military operations involving accidental detonation of onboard marine weapons
[7th] Y37.050 Military operations involving accidental detonation of onboard marine weapons, military personnel [POA]
[7th] Y37.051 Military operations involving accidental detonation of onboard marine weapons, civilian [POA]
[6th] Y37.09 Military operations involving explosion of other marine weapons
[7th] Y37.090 Military operations involving explosion of other marine weapons, military personnel [POA]
[7th] Y37.091 Military operations involving explosion of other marine weapons, civilian [POA]

[5th] Y37.1 Military operations involving destruction of aircraft
[6th] Y37.10 Military operations involving unspecified destruction of aircraft
[7th] Y37.100 Military operations involving unspecified destruction of aircraft, military personnel [POA]
[7th] Y37.101 Military operations involving unspecified destruction of aircraft, civilian [POA]
[6th] Y37.11 Military operations involving destruction of aircraft due to enemy fire or explosives
Military operations involving destruction of aircraft due to air to air missile
Military operations involving destruction of aircraft due to explosive placed on aircraft
Military operations involving destruction of aircraft due to rocket propelled grenade [RPG]
Military operations involving destruction of aircraft due to small arms fire
Military operations involving destruction of aircraft due to surface to air missile
[7th] Y37.110 Military operations involving destruction of aircraft due to enemy fire or explosives, military personnel [POA]
[7th] Y37.111 Military operations involving destruction of aircraft due to enemy fire or explosives, civilian [POA]
[6th] Y37.12 Military operations involving destruction of aircraft due to collision with other aircraft
[7th] Y37.120 Military operations involving destruction of aircraft due to collision with other aircraft, military personnel [POA]
[7th] Y37.121 Military operations involving destruction of aircraft due to collision with other aircraft, civilian [POA]
[6th] Y37.13 Military operations involving destruction of aircraft due to onboard fire
[7th] Y37.130 Military operations involving destruction of aircraft due to onboard fire, military personnel [POA]
[7th] Y37.131 Military operations involving destruction of aircraft due to onboard fire, civilian [POA]
[6th] Y37.14 Military operations involving destruction of aircraft due to accidental detonation of onboard munitions and explosives
[7th] Y37.140 Military operations involving destruction of aircraft due to accidental detonation of onboard munitions and explosives, military personnel [POA]
[7th] Y37.141 Military operations involving destruction of aircraft due to accidental detonation of onboard munitions and explosives, civilian [POA]
[6th] Y37.19 Military operations involving other destruction of aircraft
[7th] Y37.190 Military operations involving other destruction of aircraft, military personnel [POA]
[7th] Y37.191 Military operations involving other destruction of aircraft, civilian [POA]

Y37.2 Military operations involving other explosions and fragments

EXCLUDES1 *military operations involving explosion of aircraft (Y37.1-)*

military operations involving explosion of marine weapons (Y37.0-)

military operations involving explosion of nuclear weapons (Y37.5-)

Y37.20 Military operations involving unspecified explosion and fragments

Military operations involving air blast NOS
Military operations involving blast NOS
Military operations involving blast fragments NOS
Military operations involving blast wave NOS
Military operations involving blast wind NOS
Military operations involving explosion NOS
Military operations involving explosion of bomb NOS

Y37.200 Military operations involving unspecified explosion and fragments, military personnel

Y37.201 Military operations involving unspecified explosion and fragments, civilian

Y37.21 Military operations involving explosion of aerial bomb

Y37.210 Military operations involving explosion of aerial bomb, military personnel

Y37.211 Military operations involving explosion of aerial bomb, civilian

Y37.22 Military operations involving explosion of guided missile

Y37.220 Military operations involving explosion of guided missile, military personnel

Y37.221 Military operations involving explosion of guided missile, civilian

Y37.23 Military operations involving explosion of improvised explosive device [IED]

Military operations involving explosion of person-borne improvised explosive device [IED]
Military operations involving explosion of vehicle-borne improvised explosive device [IED]
Military operations involving explosion of roadside improvised explosive device [IED]

Y37.230 Military operations involving explosion of improvised explosive device [IED], military personnel

Y37.231 Military operations involving explosion of improvised explosive device [IED], civilian

Y37.24 Military operations involving explosion due to accidental detonation and discharge of own munitions or munitions launch device

Y37.240 Military operations involving explosion due to accidental detonation and discharge of own munitions or munitions launch device, military personnel

Y37.241 Military operations involving explosion due to accidental detonation and discharge of own munitions or munitions launch device, civilian

Y37.25 Military operations involving fragments from munitions

Y37.250 Military operations involving fragments from munitions, military personnel

Y37.251 Military operations involving fragments from munitions, civilian

Y37.26 Military operations involving fragments of improvised explosive device [IED]

Military operations involving fragments of person-borne improvised explosive device [IED]
Military operations involving fragments of vehicle-borne improvised explosive device [IED]
Military operations involving fragments of roadside improvised explosive device [IED]

Y37.260 Military operations involving fragments of improvised explosive device [IED], military personnel

Y37.261 Military operations involving fragments of improvised explosive device [IED], civilian

Y37.27 Military operations involving fragments from weapons

Y37.270 Military operations involving fragments from weapons, military personnel

Y37.271 Military operations involving fragments from weapons, civilian

Y37.29 Military operations involving other explosions and fragments

Military operations involving explosion of grenade
Military operations involving explosions of land mine
Military operations involving shrapnel NOS

Y37.290 Military operations involving other explosions and fragments, military personnel

Y37.291 Military operations involving other explosions and fragments, civilian

Y37.3 Military operations involving fires, conflagrations and hot substances

Military operations involving smoke, fumes, and heat from fires, conflagrations and hot substances

EXCLUDES1 *military operations involving fires and conflagrations aboard military aircraft (Y37.1-)*

military operations involving fires and conflagrations aboard military watercraft (Y37.0-)

military operations involving fires and conflagrations caused indirectly by conventional weapons (Y37.2-)

military operations involving fires and thermal effects of nuclear weapons (Y36.53-)

Y37.30 Military operations involving unspecified fire, conflagration and hot substance

Y37.300 Military operations involving unspecified fire, conflagration and hot substance, military personnel

Y37.301 Military operations involving unspecified fire, conflagration and hot substance, civilian

Y37.31 Military operations involving gasoline bomb

Military operations involving incendiary bomb
Military operations involving petrol bomb

Y37.310 Military operations involving gasoline bomb, military personnel

Y37.311 Military operations involving gasoline bomb, civilian

Y37.32 Military operations involving incendiary bullet

Y37.320 Military operations involving incendiary bullet, military personnel

Y37.321 Military operations involving incendiary bullet, civilian

Y37.33 Military operations involving flamethrower

Y37.330 Military operations involving flamethrower, military personnel

Y37.331 Military operations involving flamethrower, civilian

Y37.39 Military operations involving other fires, conflagrations and hot substances

Y37.390 Military operations involving other fires, conflagrations and hot substances, military personnel

Y37.391 Military operations involving other fires, conflagrations and hot substances, civilian

Y37.4 Military operations involving firearm discharge and other forms of conventional warfare

Y37.41 Military operations involving rubber bullets

Y37.410 Military operations involving rubber bullets, military personnel

---

POA Unacceptable principal diagnosis symbol per Medicare code edits · Code exempt from diagnosis present on admission requirement · ? Questionable admission · CC Complication or comorbidity · CC/MCC CC/MCC exclusion · MCC Major complication or comorbidity · Principal diagnosis as its own CC · Principal diagnosis as its own MCC · HCC HCC diagnosis code · RxHCC RxHCC diagnosis code · MACRA code · Z code as first-listed diagnosis

1240

When symbols appear on a code that requires a 7th character extension, refer to Appendix B to identify applicable 7th character codes.

2018 ICD-10-CM

7️⃣ **Y37.411** Military operations involving rubber bullets, civilian POA

6️⃣ **Y37.42** Military operations involving firearms pellets
  7️⃣ **Y37.420** Military operations involving firearms pellets, military personnel POA
  7️⃣ **Y37.421** Military operations involving firearms pellets, civilian POA

6️⃣ **Y37.43** Military operations involving other firearms discharge
  Military operations involving bullets NOS
  EXCLUDES1 *military operations involving munitions fragments (Y37.25-)*
  military operations involving incendiary bullets (Y37.32-)
  7️⃣ **Y37.430** Military operations involving other firearms discharge, military personnel POA
  7️⃣ **Y37.431** Military operations involving other firearms discharge, civilian POA

6️⃣ **Y37.44** Military operations involving unarmed hand to hand combat
  EXCLUDES1 *military operations involving combat using blunt or piercing object (Y37.45-)*
  military operations involving intentional restriction of air and airway (Y37.46-)
  military operations involving unintentional restriction of air and airway (Y37.47-)
  7️⃣ **Y37.440** Military operations involving unarmed hand to hand combat, military personnel POA
  7️⃣ **Y37.441** Military operations involving unarmed hand to hand combat, civilian POA

6️⃣ **Y37.45** Military operations involving combat using blunt or piercing object
  7️⃣ **Y37.450** Military operations involving combat using blunt or piercing object, military personnel POA
  7️⃣ **Y37.451** Military operations involving combat using blunt or piercing object, civilian POA

6️⃣ **Y37.46** Military operations involving intentional restriction of air and airway
  7️⃣ **Y37.460** Military operations involving intentional restriction of air and airway, military personnel POA
  7️⃣ **Y37.461** Military operations involving intentional restriction of air and airway, civilian POA

6️⃣ **Y37.47** Military operations involving unintentional restriction of air and airway
  7️⃣ **Y37.470** Military operations involving unintentional restriction of air and airway, military personnel POA
  7️⃣ **Y37.471** Military operations involving unintentional restriction of air and airway, civilian POA

6️⃣ **Y37.49** Military operations involving other forms of conventional warfare
  7️⃣ **Y37.490** Military operations involving other forms of conventional warfare, military personnel POA
  7️⃣ **Y37.491** Military operations involving other forms of conventional warfare, civilian POA

5️⃣ **Y37.5** Military operations involving nuclear weapons
  Military operation involving dirty bomb NOS
6️⃣ **Y37.50** Military operations involving unspecified effect of nuclear weapon
  7️⃣ **Y37.500** Military operations involving unspecified effect of nuclear weapon, military personnel POA
  7️⃣ **Y37.501** Military operations involving unspecified effect of nuclear weapon, civilian POA
6️⃣ **Y37.51** Military operations involving direct blast effect of nuclear weapon

Military operations involving blast pressure of nuclear weapon
  7️⃣ **Y37.510** Military operations involving direct blast effect of nuclear weapon, military personnel POA
  7️⃣ **Y37.511** Military operations involving direct blast effect of nuclear weapon, civilian POA

6️⃣ **Y37.52** Military operations involving indirect blast effect of nuclear weapon
  Military operations involving being thrown by blast of nuclear weapon
  Military operations involving being struck or crushed by blast debris of nuclear weapon
  7️⃣ **Y37.520** Military operations involving indirect blast effect of nuclear weapon, military personnel POA
  7️⃣ **Y37.521** Military operations involving indirect blast effect of nuclear weapon, civilian POA

6️⃣ **Y37.53** Military operations involving thermal radiation effect of nuclear weapon
  Military operations involving direct heat from nuclear weapon
  Military operation involving fireball effects from nuclear weapon
  7️⃣ **Y37.530** Military operations involving thermal radiation effect of nuclear weapon, military personnel POA
  7️⃣ **Y37.531** Military operations involving thermal radiation effect of nuclear weapon, civilian POA

6️⃣ **Y37.54** Military operation involving nuclear radiation effects of nuclear weapon
  Military operation involving acute radiation exposure from nuclear weapon
  Military operation involving exposure to immediate ionizing radiation from nuclear weapon
  Military operation involving fallout exposure from nuclear weapon
  Military operation involving secondary effects of nuclear weapons
  7️⃣ **Y37.540** Military operation involving nuclear radiation effects of nuclear weapon, military personnel POA
  7️⃣ **Y37.541** Military operation involving nuclear radiation effects of nuclear weapon, civilian POA

6️⃣ **Y37.59** Military operation involving other effects of nuclear weapons
  7️⃣ **Y37.590** Military operation involving other effects of nuclear weapons, military personnel POA
  7️⃣ **Y37.591** Military operation involving other effects of nuclear weapons, civilian POA

5️⃣ **Y37.6** Military operations involving biological weapons
6️⃣ **Y37.6X** Military operations involving biological weapons
  7️⃣ **Y37.6X0** Military operations involving biological weapons, military personnel POA
  7️⃣ **Y37.6X1** Military operations involving biological weapons, civilian POA

5️⃣ **Y37.7** Military operations involving chemical weapons and other forms of unconventional warfare
  EXCLUDES1 *military operations involving incendiary devices (Y36.3-, Y36.5-)*
6️⃣ **Y37.7X** Military operations involving chemical weapons and other forms of unconventional warfare
  7️⃣ **Y37.7X0** Military operations involving chemical weapons and other forms of unconventional warfare, military personnel POA
  7️⃣ **Y37.7X1** Military operations involving chemical weapons and other forms of unconventional warfare, civilian POA

5️⃣ **Y37.9** Other and unspecified military operations
  7️⃣ **Y37.90** **Military operations, unspecified** POA

Unspecified Code   Other Specified Code   Manifestation Code   N Newborn   P Pediatric   M Maternity   A Adult   ♂ Male   ♀ Female
● New Code   ▲ Revised Code Title   ▶◀ Revised Text   NOTES   *INCLUDES*   EXCLUDES 1 Not coded here   EXCLUDES 2 Not included here
4️⃣ 4th character required   5️⃣ 5th character required   6️⃣ 6th character required   7️⃣ 7th character required
7️⃣ Extension 'X' Alert   HAC Hospital-acquired condition (HAC) alert   **AHA** AHA Coding Clinic©

Y37.91 Military operations involving unspecified weapon of mass destruction [WMD] POA

Y37.92 Military operations involving friendly fire POA

Y38 Terrorism

These codes are for use to identify injuries resulting from the unlawful use of force or violence against persons or property to intimidate or coerce a Government, the civilian population, or any segment thereof, in furtherance of political or social objective

Use additional code for place of occurrence (Y92.-)

The appropriate 7th character is to be added to each code from category Y38

A = initial encounter
D = subsequent encounter
S = sequela

Y38.0 Terrorism involving explosion of marine weapons

Terrorism involving depth-charge
Terrorism involving marine mine
Terrorism involving mine NOS, at sea or in harbor
Terrorism involving sea-based artillery shell
Terrorism involving torpedo
Terrorism involving underwater blast

Y38.0X Terrorism involving explosion of marine weapons

Y38.0X1 Terrorism involving explosion of marine weapons, public safety official injured POA

Y38.0X2 Terrorism involving explosion of marine weapons, civilian injured POA

Y38.0X3 Terrorism involving explosion of marine weapons, terrorist injured POA

Y38.1 Terrorism involving destruction of aircraft

Terrorism involving aircraft burned
Terrorism involving aircraft exploded
Terrorism involving aircraft being shot down
Terrorism involving aircraft used as a weapon

Y38.1X Terrorism involving destruction of aircraft

Y38.1X1 Terrorism involving destruction of aircraft, public safety official injured POA

Y38.1X2 Terrorism involving destruction of aircraft, civilian injured POA

Y38.1X3 Terrorism involving destruction of aircraft, terrorist injured POA

Y38.2 Terrorism involving other explosions and fragments

Terrorism involving antipersonnel (fragments) bomb
Terrorism involving blast NOS
Terrorism involving explosion NOS
Terrorism involving explosion of breech block
Terrorism involving explosion of cannon block
Terrorism involving explosion (fragments) of artillery shell
Terrorism involving explosion (fragments) of bomb
Terrorism involving explosion (fragments) of grenade
Terrorism involving explosion (fragments) of guided missile
Terrorism involving explosion (fragments) of land mine
Terrorism involving explosion of mortar bomb
Terrorism involving explosion of munitions
Terrorism involving explosion (fragments) of rocket
Terrorism involving explosion (fragments) of shell
Terrorism involving shrapnel
Terrorism involving mine NOS, on land

EXCLUDES1 terrorism involving explosion of nuclear weapon (Y38.5)

terrorism involving suicide bomber (Y38.81)

Y38.2X Terrorism involving other explosions and fragments

Y38.2X1 Terrorism involving other explosions and fragments, public safety official injured POA

Y38.2X2 Terrorism involving other explosions and fragments, civilian injured POA

Y38.2X3 Terrorism involving other explosions and fragments, terrorist injured POA

Y38.3 Terrorism involving fires, conflagration and hot substances

Terrorism involving conflagration NOS
Terrorism involving fire NOS
Terrorism involving petrol bomb

EXCLUDES1 terrorism involving fire or heat of nuclear weapon (Y38.5)

Y38.3X Terrorism involving fires, conflagration and hot substances

Y38.3X1 Terrorism involving fires, conflagration and hot substances, public safety official injured POA

Y38.3X2 Terrorism involving fires, conflagration and hot substances, civilian injured POA

Y38.3X3 Terrorism involving fires, conflagration and hot substances, terrorist injured POA

Y38.4 Terrorism involving firearms

Terrorism involving carbine bullet
Terrorism involving machine gun bullet
Terrorism involving pellets (shotgun)
Terrorism involving pistol bullet
Terrorism involving rifle bullet
Terrorism involving rubber (rifle) bullet

Y38.4X Terrorism involving firearms

Y38.4X1 Terrorism involving firearms, public safety official injured POA

Y38.4X2 Terrorism involving firearms, civilian injured POA

Y38.4X3 Terrorism involving firearms, terrorist injured POA

Y38.5 Terrorism involving nuclear weapons

Terrorism involving blast effects of nuclear weapon
Terrorism involving exposure to ionizing radiation from nuclear weapon
Terrorism involving fireball effect of nuclear weapon
Terrorism involving heat from nuclear weapon

Y38.5X Terrorism involving nuclear weapons

Y38.5X1 Terrorism involving nuclear weapons, public safety official injured POA

Y38.5X2 Terrorism involving nuclear weapons, civilian injured POA

Y38.5X3 Terrorism involving nuclear weapons, terrorist injured POA

Y38.6 Terrorism involving biological weapons

Terrorism involving anthrax
Terrorism involving cholera
Terrorism involving smallpox

Y38.6X Terrorism involving biological weapons

Y38.6X1 Terrorism involving biological weapons, public safety official injured POA

Y38.6X2 Terrorism involving biological weapons, civilian injured POA

Y38.6X3 Terrorism involving biological weapons, terrorist injured POA

Y38.7 Terrorism involving chemical weapons

Terrorism involving gases, fumes, chemicals
Terrorism involving hydrogen cyanide
Terrorism involving phosgene
Terrorism involving sarin

Y38.7X Terrorism involving chemical weapons

Y38.7X1 Terrorism involving chemical weapons, public safety official injured POA

Y38.7X2 Terrorism involving chemical weapons, civilian injured POA

Y38.7X3 Terrorism involving chemical weapons, terrorist injured POA

Y38.8 Terrorism involving other and unspecified means

Y38.80 Terrorism involving unspecified means POA

Terrorism NOS

Y38.81 Terrorism involving suicide bomber

Y38.811 Terrorism involving suicide bomber, public safety official injured POA

Y38.812 Terrorism involving suicide bomber, civilian injured POA

Y38.89 Terrorism involving other means

Terrorism involving drowning and submersion
Terrorism involving lasers
Terrorism involving piercing or stabbing instruments

Y38.891 Terrorism involving other means, public safety official injured POA

PDNR Unacceptable principal diagnosis symbol per Medicare code edits   POA Code exempt from diagnosis present on admission requirement
☑ Questionable admission   cc Complication or comorbidity   CC·MCC Excl CC/MCC exclusion   MCC Major complication or comorbidity
Lcc Principal diagnosis as its own CC   Lmcc Principal diagnosis as its own MCC   HCC HCC diagnosis code   RxHCC RxHCC diagnosis code
MACRA code   Z1 Z code as first-listed diagnosis

(7ᵗʰ) Y38.892 Terrorism involving other means, civilian injured ⊘POA

(7ᵗʰ) Y38.893 Terrorism involving other means, terrorist injured ⊘POA

(5ᵗʰ) Y38.9 Terrorism, secondary effects

NOTES This code is for use to identify conditions occurring subsequent to a terrorist attack not those that are due to the initial terrorist attack

(6ᵗʰ) Y38.9X Terrorism, secondary effects

(7ᵗʰ) Y38.9X1 Terrorism, secondary effects, public safety official injured ⊘POA

(7ᵗʰ) Y38.9X2 Terrorism, secondary effects, civilian injured ⊘POA

Complications of medical and surgical care (Y62-Y84)

INCLUDES complications of medical devices

surgical and medical procedures as the cause of abnormal reaction of the patient, or of later complication, without mention of misadventure at the time of the procedure

Misadventures to patients during surgical and medical care (Y62-Y69)

EXCLUDES1 surgical and medical procedures as the cause of abnormal reaction of the patient, without mention of misadventure at the time of the procedure (Y83-Y84)

EXCLUDES2 breakdown or malfunctioning of medical device (during procedure) (after implantation) (ongoing use) (Y70-Y82)

(4ᵗʰ) Y62 Failure of sterile precautions during surgical and medical care

Y62.0 Failure of sterile precautions during surgical operation

Y62.1 Failure of sterile precautions during infusion or transfusion

Y62.2 Failure of sterile precautions during kidney dialysis and other perfusion HCC RHCC

Y62.3 Failure of sterile precautions during injection or immunization

Y62.4 Failure of sterile precautions during endoscopic examination

Y62.5 Failure of sterile precautions during heart catheterization

Y62.6 Failure of sterile precautions during aspiration, puncture and other catheterization

Y62.8 Failure of sterile precautions during other surgical and medical care

Y62.9 Failure of sterile precautions during unspecified surgical and medical care

(4ᵗʰ) Y63 Failure in dosage during surgical and medical care

EXCLUDES2 accidental overdose of drug or wrong drug given in error (T36-T50)

Y63.0 Excessive amount of blood or other fluid given during transfusion or infusion

Y63.1 Incorrect dilution of fluid used during infusion

Y63.2 Overdose of radiation given during therapy

Y63.3 Inadvertent exposure of patient to radiation during medical care

Y63.4 Failure in dosage in electroshock or insulin-shock therapy

Y63.5 Inappropriate temperature in local application and packing

Y63.6 Underdosing and nonadministration of necessary drug, medicament or biological substance

Y63.8 Failure in dosage during other surgical and medical care

Y63.9 Failure in dosage during unspecified surgical and medical care

(4ᵗʰ) Y64 Contaminated medical or biological substances

Y64.0 Contaminated medical or biological substance, transfused or infused

Y64.1 Contaminated medical or biological substance, injected or used for immunization

Y64.8 Contaminated medical or biological substance administered by other means

Y64.9 Contaminated medical or biological substance administered by unspecified means

Administered contaminated medical or biological substance NOS

(4ᵗʰ) Y65 Other misadventures during surgical and medical care

Y65.0 Mismatched blood in transfusion

Y65.1 Wrong fluid used in infusion

Y65.2 Failure in suture or ligature during surgical operation

Y65.3 Endotracheal tube wrongly placed during anesthetic procedure

Y65.4 Failure to introduce or to remove other tube or instrument

(5ᵗʰ) Y65.5 Performance of wrong procedure (operation)

Y65.51 Performance of wrong procedure (operation) on correct patient

Wrong device implanted into correct surgical site

EXCLUDES1 performance of correct procedure (operation) on wrong side or body part (Y65.53)

Y65.52 Performance of procedure (operation) on patient not scheduled for surgery

Performance of procedure (operation) intended for another patient

Performance of procedure (operation) on wrong patient

Y65.53 Performance of correct procedure (operation) on wrong side or body part

Performance of correct procedure (operation) on wrong side

Performance of correct procedure (operation) on wrong site

Y65.8 Other specified misadventures during surgical and medical care

Y66 Nonadministration of surgical and medical care

Premature cessation of surgical and medical care

EXCLUDES1 DNR status (Z66)

palliative care (Z51.5)

Y69 Unspecified misadventure during surgical and medical care

Medical devices associated with adverse incidents in diagnostic and therapeutic use (Y70-Y82)

INCLUDES breakdown or malfunction of medical devices (during use) (after implantation) (ongoing use)

EXCLUDES2 breakdown or malfunctioning of medical device (after implantation) (during procedure) (ongoing use) (Y70-Y82)

later complications following use of medical devices without breakdown or malfunctioning of device (Y83-Y84)

misadventure to patients during surgical and medical care, classifiable to (Y62-Y69)

surgical and other medical procedures as the cause of abnormal reaction of the patient, or of later complication, without mention of misadventure at the time of the procedure (Y83-Y84)

(4ᵗʰ) Y70 Anesthesiology devices associated with adverse incidents

Y70.0 Diagnostic and monitoring anesthesiology devices associated with adverse incidents

Y70.1 Therapeutic (nonsurgical) and rehabilitative anesthesiology devices associated with adverse incidents

Y70.2 Prosthetic and other implants, materials and accessory anesthesiology devices associated with adverse incidents

Y70.3 Surgical instruments, materials and anesthesiology devices (including sutures) associated with adverse incidents

Y70.8 Miscellaneous anesthesiology devices associated with adverse incidents, not elsewhere classified

(4ᵗʰ) Y71 Cardiovascular devices associated with adverse incidents

Y71.0 Diagnostic and monitoring cardiovascular devices associated with adverse incidents

Y71.1 Therapeutic (nonsurgical) and rehabilitative cardiovascular devices associated with adverse incidents

Y71.2 Prosthetic and other implants, materials and accessory cardiovascular devices associated with adverse incidents

Y71.3 Surgical instruments, materials and cardiovascular devices (including sutures) associated with adverse incidents

Y71.8 Miscellaneous cardiovascular devices associated with adverse incidents, not elsewhere classified

---

Unspecified Code   Other Specified Code   Manifestation Code   Ⓝ Newborn   Ⓟ Pediatric   Ⓜ Maternity   Ⓐ Adult   ♂ Male   ♀ Female
● New Code   ▲ Revised Code Title   ▶◀ Revised Text   NOTES   INCLUDES   EXCLUDES 1 Not coded here   EXCLUDES 2 Not included here
(4ᵗʰ) 4ᵗʰ character required   (5ᵗʰ) 5ᵗʰ character required   (6ᵗʰ) 6ᵗʰ character required   (7ᵗʰ) 7ᵗʰ character required
(X) Extension 'X' Alert   HAC Hospital-acquired condition (HAC) alert   AHA AHA Coding Clinic©

Y72 Otorhinolaryngological devices associated with adverse incidents

Y72.0 Diagnostic and monitoring otorhinolaryngological devices associated with adverse incidents

Y72.1 Therapeutic (nonsurgical) and rehabilitative otorhinolaryngological devices associated with adverse incidents

Y72.2 Prosthetic and other implants, materials and accessory otorhinolaryngological devices associated with adverse incidents

Y72.3 Surgical instruments, materials and otorhinolaryngological devices (including sutures) associated with adverse incidents

Y72.8 Miscellaneous otorhinolaryngological devices associated with adverse incidents, not elsewhere classified

Y73 Gastroenterology and urology devices associated with adverse incidents

Y73.0 Diagnostic and monitoring gastroenterology and urology devices associated with adverse incidents

Y73.1 Therapeutic (nonsurgical) and rehabilitative gastroenterology and urology devices associated with adverse incidents

Y73.2 Prosthetic and other implants, materials and accessory gastroenterology and urology devices associated with adverse incidents

Y73.3 Surgical instruments, materials and gastroenterology and urology devices (including sutures) associated with adverse incidents

Y73.8 Miscellaneous gastroenterology and urology devices associated with adverse incidents, not elsewhere classified

Y74 General hospital and personal-use devices associated with adverse incidents

Y74.0 Diagnostic and monitoring general hospital and personal-use devices associated with adverse incidents

Y74.1 Therapeutic (nonsurgical) and rehabilitative general hospital and personal-use devices associated with adverse incidents

Y74.2 Prosthetic and other implants, materials and accessory general hospital and personal-use devices associated with adverse incidents

Y74.3 Surgical instruments, materials and general hospital and personal-use devices (including sutures) associated with adverse incidents

Y74.8 Miscellaneous general hospital and personal-use devices associated with adverse incidents, not elsewhere classified

Y75 Neurological devices associated with adverse incidents

Y75.0 Diagnostic and monitoring neurological devices associated with adverse incidents

Y75.1 Therapeutic (nonsurgical) and rehabilitative neurological devices associated with adverse incidents

Y75.2 Prosthetic and other implants, materials and neurological devices associated with adverse incidents

Y75.3 Surgical instruments, materials and neurological devices (including sutures) associated with adverse incidents

Y75.8 Miscellaneous neurological devices associated with adverse incidents, not elsewhere classified

Y76 Obstetric and gynecological devices associated with adverse incidents

Y76.0 Diagnostic and monitoring obstetric and gynecological devices associated with adverse incidents ♀

Y76.1 Therapeutic (nonsurgical) and rehabilitative obstetric and gynecological devices associated with adverse incidents ♀

Y76.2 Prosthetic and other implants, materials and accessory obstetric and gynecological devices associated with adverse incidents ♀

Y76.3 Surgical instruments, materials and obstetric and gynecological devices (including sutures) associated with adverse incidents ♀

Y76.8 Miscellaneous obstetric and gynecological devices associated with adverse incidents, not elsewhere classified ♀

Y77 Ophthalmic devices associated with adverse incidents

Y77.0 Diagnostic and monitoring ophthalmic devices associated with adverse incidents

Y77.1 Therapeutic (nonsurgical) and rehabilitative ophthalmic devices associated with adverse incidents

Y77.2 Prosthetic and other implants, materials and accessory ophthalmic devices associated with adverse incidents

Y77.3 Surgical instruments, materials and ophthalmic devices (including sutures) associated with adverse incidents

Y77.8 Miscellaneous ophthalmic devices associated with adverse incidents, not elsewhere classified

Y78 Radiological devices associated with adverse incidents

Y78.0 Diagnostic and monitoring radiological devices associated with adverse incidents

Y78.1 Therapeutic (nonsurgical) and rehabilitative radiological devices associated with adverse incidents

Y78.2 Prosthetic and other implants, materials and accessory radiological devices associated with adverse incidents

Y78.3 Surgical instruments, materials and radiological devices (including sutures) associated with adverse incidents

Y78.8 Miscellaneous radiological devices associated with adverse incidents, not elsewhere classified

Y79 Orthopedic devices associated with adverse incidents

Y79.0 Diagnostic and monitoring orthopedic devices associated with adverse incidents

Y79.1 Therapeutic (nonsurgical) and rehabilitative orthopedic devices associated with adverse incidents

Y79.2 Prosthetic and other implants, materials and accessory orthopedic devices associated with adverse incidents

Y79.3 Surgical instruments, materials and orthopedic devices (including sutures) associated with adverse incidents

Y79.8 Miscellaneous orthopedic devices associated with adverse incidents, not elsewhere classified

Y80 Physical medicine devices associated with adverse incidents

Y80.0 Diagnostic and monitoring physical medicine devices associated with adverse incidents

Y80.1 Therapeutic (nonsurgical) and rehabilitative physical medicine devices associated with adverse incidents

Y80.2 Prosthetic and other implants, materials and accessory physical medicine devices associated with adverse incidents

Y80.3 Surgical instruments, materials and physical medicine devices (including sutures) associated with adverse incidents

Y80.8 Miscellaneous physical medicine devices associated with adverse incidents, not elsewhere classified

Y81 General- and plastic-surgery devices associated with adverse incidents

Y81.0 Diagnostic and monitoring general- and plastic-surgery devices associated with adverse incidents

Y81.1 Therapeutic (nonsurgical) and rehabilitative general- and plastic-surgery devices associated with adverse incidents

Y81.2 Prosthetic and other implants, materials and accessory general- and plastic-surgery devices associated with adverse incidents

Y81.3 Surgical instruments, materials and general- and plastic-surgery devices (including sutures) associated with adverse incidents

Y81.8 Miscellaneous general- and plastic-surgery devices associated with adverse incidents, not elsewhere classified

Y82 Other and unspecified medical devices associated with adverse incidents

Y82.8 Other medical devices associated with adverse incidents

Y82.9 Unspecified medical devices associated with adverse incidents

Surgical and other medical procedures as the cause of abnormal reaction of the patient, or of later complication, without mention of misadventure at the time of the procedure (Y83-Y84)

EXCLUDES1 misadventures to patients during surgical and medical care, classifiable to (Y62-Y69)

EXCLUDES2 breakdown or malfunctioning of medical device (after implantation) (during procedure) (ongoing use) (Y70-Y82)

PDx Unacceptable principal diagnosis symbol per Medicare code edits   PDx Code exempt from diagnosis present on admission requirement

❓ Questionable admission   CC Complication or comorbidity   CC/MCC CC/MCC exclusion   MCC Major complication or comorbidity

PDx CC Principal diagnosis as its own CC   PDx MCC Principal diagnosis as its own MCC   HCC HCC diagnosis code   RxHCC RxHCC diagnosis code

MACRA code   Z1 Z code as first-listed diagnosis

Ⓐ Y83 Surgical operation and other surgical procedures as the cause of abnormal reaction of the patient, or of later complication, without mention of misadventure at the time of the procedure

Y83.0 Surgical operation with transplant of whole organ as the cause of abnormal reaction of the patient, or of later complication, without mention of misadventure at the time of the procedure

Y83.1 Surgical operation with implant of artificial internal device as the cause of abnormal reaction of the patient, or of later complication, without mention of misadventure at the time of the procedure

Y83.2 Surgical operation with anastomosis, bypass or graft as the cause of abnormal reaction of the patient, or of later complication, without mention of misadventure at the time of the procedure

Y83.3 Surgical operation with formation of external stoma as the cause of abnormal reaction of the patient, or of later complication, without mention of misadventure at the time of the procedure

Y83.4 Other reconstructive surgery as the cause of abnormal reaction of the patient, or of later complication, without mention of misadventure at the time of the procedure

Y83.5 Amputation of limb(s) as the cause of abnormal reaction of the patient, or of later complication, without mention of misadventure at the time of the procedure

Y83.6 Removal of other organ (partial) (total) as the cause of abnormal reaction of the patient, or of later complication, without mention of misadventure at the time of the procedure

Y83.8 Other surgical procedures as the cause of abnormal reaction of the patient, or of later complication, without mention of misadventure at the time of the procedure

Y83.9 Surgical procedure, unspecified as the cause of abnormal reaction of the patient, or of later complication, without mention of misadventure at the time of the procedure

Ⓐ Y84 Other medical procedures as the cause of abnormal reaction of the patient, or of later complication, without mention of misadventure at the time of the procedure

Y84.0 Cardiac catheterization as the cause of abnormal reaction of the patient, or of later complication, without mention of misadventure at the time of the procedure

Y84.1 Kidney dialysis as the cause of abnormal reaction of the patient, or of later complication, without mention of misadventure at the time of the procedure

Y84.2 Radiological procedure and radiotherapy as the cause of abnormal reaction of the patient, or of later complication, without mention of misadventure at the time of the procedure
AHA: Q1 2017

Y84.3 Shock therapy as the cause of abnormal reaction of the patient, or of later complication, without mention of misadventure at the time of the procedure

Y84.4 Aspiration of fluid as the cause of abnormal reaction of the patient, or of later complication, without mention of misadventure at the time of the procedure

Y84.5 Insertion of gastric or duodenal sound as the cause of abnormal reaction of the patient, or of later complication, without mention of misadventure at the time of the procedure

Y84.6 Urinary catheterization as the cause of abnormal reaction of the patient, or of later complication, without mention of misadventure at the time of the procedure

Y84.7 Blood-sampling as the cause of abnormal reaction of the patient, or of later complication, without mention of misadventure at the time of the procedure

Y84.8 Other medical procedures as the cause of abnormal reaction of the patient, or of later complication, without mention of misadventure at the time of the procedure

Y84.9 Medical procedure, unspecified as the cause of abnormal reaction of the patient, or of later complication, without mention of misadventure at the time of the procedure

Supplementary factors related to causes of morbidity classified elsewhere (Y90-Y99)

NOTES These categories may be used to provide supplementary information concerning causes of morbidity. They are not to be used for single-condition coding.

Ⓐ Y90 Evidence of alcohol involvement determined by blood alcohol level
Code first any associated alcohol related disorders (F10)

Y90.0 Blood alcohol level of less than 20 mg/100 ml
Y90.1 Blood alcohol level of 20-39 mg/100 ml
Y90.2 Blood alcohol level of 40-59 mg/100 ml
Y90.3 Blood alcohol level of 60-79 mg/100 ml
Y90.4 Blood alcohol level of 80-99 mg/100 ml
Y90.5 Blood alcohol level of 100-119 mg/100 ml
Y90.6 Blood alcohol level of 120-199 mg/100 ml
Y90.7 Blood alcohol level of 200-239 mg/100 ml
Y90.8 Blood alcohol level of 240 mg/100 ml or more
Y90.9 Presence of alcohol in blood, level not specified

Ⓐ Y92 Place of occurrence of the external cause
The following category is for use, when relevant, to identify the place of occurrence of the external cause. Use in conjunction with an activity code.
Place of occurrence should be recorded only at the initial encounter for treatment

Ⓢ Y92.0 Non-institutional (private) residence as the place of occurrence of the external cause
EXCLUDES1 abandoned or derelict house (Y92.89)
home under construction but not yet occupied (Y92.6-)
institutional place of residence (Y92.1-)

Ⓐ Y92.00 Unspecified non-institutional (private) residence as the place of occurrence of the external cause

Y92.000 Kitchen of unspecified non-institutional (private) residence as the place of occurrence of the external cause POA

Y92.001 Dining room of unspecified non-institutional (private) residence as the place of occurrence of the external cause POA

Y92.002 Bathroom of unspecified non-institutional (private) residence single-family (private) house as the place of occurrence of the external cause POA

Y92.003 Bedroom of unspecified non-institutional (private) residence as the place of occurrence of the external cause POA

Y92.007 Garden or yard of unspecified non-institutional (private) residence as the place of occurrence of the external cause POA

Y92.008 Other place in unspecified non-institutional (private) residence as the place of occurrence of the external cause POA

Y92.009 Unspecified place in unspecified non-institutional (private) residence as the place of occurrence of the external cause POA
Home (NOS) as the place of occurrence of the external cause

Ⓐ Y92.01 Single-family non-institutional (private) house as the place of occurrence of the external cause
Farmhouse as the place of occurrence of the external cause
EXCLUDES1 barn (Y92.71)
chicken coop or hen house (Y92.72)
farm field (Y92.73)
orchard (Y92.74)
single family mobile home or trailer (Y92.02-)
slaughter house (Y92.86)

Unspecified Code   Other Specified Code   Manifestation Code   Ⓝ Newborn   Ⓟ Pediatric   Ⓜ Maternity   Ⓐ Adult   ♂ Male   ♀ Female
● New Code   ▲ Revised Code Title   ►◄ Revised Text   NOTES   INCLUDES   EXCLUDES 1 Not coded here   EXCLUDES 2 Not included here
Ⓐ 4th character required   Ⓢ 5th character required   Ⓐ 6th character required   Ⓐ 7th character required
Ⓧ Extension 'X' Alert   HAC Hospital-acquired condition (HAC) alert   AHA AHA Coding Clinic©

Y92.010   Kitchen of single-family (private) house as the place of occurrence of the external cause POA

Y92.011   Dining room of single-family (private) house as the place of occurrence of the external cause POA

Y92.012   Bathroom of single-family (private) house as the place of occurrence of the external cause POA

Y92.013   Bedroom of single-family (private) house as the place of occurrence of the external cause POA

Y92.014   Private driveway to single-family (private) house as the place of occurrence of the external cause POA

Y92.015   Private garage of single-family (private) house as the place of occurrence of the external cause POA

Y92.016   Swimming-pool in single-family (private) house or garden as the place of occurrence of the external cause POA

Y92.017   Garden or yard in single-family (private) house as the place of occurrence of the external cause POA

Y92.018   Other place in single-family (private) house as the place of occurrence of the external cause POA

Y92.019   Unspecified place in single-family (private) house as the place of occurrence of the external cause POA

6ᵗʰ Y92.02 Mobile home as the place of occurrence of the external cause

Y92.020   Kitchen in mobile home as the place of occurrence of the external cause POA

Y92.021   Dining room in mobile home as the place of occurrence of the external cause POA

Y92.022   Bathroom in mobile home as the place of occurrence of the external cause POA

Y92.023   Bedroom in mobile home as the place of occurrence of the external cause POA

Y92.024   Driveway of mobile home as the place of occurrence of the external cause POA

Y92.025   Garage of mobile home as the place of occurrence of the external cause POA

Y92.026   Swimming-pool of mobile home as the place of occurrence of the external cause POA

Y92.027   Garden or yard of mobile home as the place of occurrence of the external cause POA

Y92.028   Other place in mobile home as the place of occurrence of the external cause POA

Y92.029   Unspecified place in mobile home as the place of occurrence of the external cause POA

6ᵗʰ Y92.03 Apartment as the place of occurrence of the external cause

Condominium as the place of occurrence of the external cause

Co-op apartment as the place of occurrence of the external cause

Y92.030   Kitchen in apartment as the place of occurrence of the external cause POA

Y92.031   Bathroom in apartment as the place of occurrence of the external cause POA

Y92.032   Bedroom in apartment as the place of occurrence of the external cause POA

Y92.038   Other place in apartment as the place of occurrence of the external cause POA

Y92.039   Unspecified place in apartment as the place of occurrence of the external cause POA

6ᵗʰ Y92.04 Boarding-house as the place of occurrence of the external cause

Y92.040   Kitchen in boarding-house as the place of occurrence of the external cause POA

Y92.041   Bathroom in boarding-house as the place of occurrence of the external cause POA

Y92.042   Bedroom in boarding-house as the place of occurrence of the external cause POA

Y92.043   Driveway of boarding-house as the place of occurrence of the external cause POA

Y92.044   Garage of boarding-house as the place of occurrence of the external cause POA

Y92.045   Swimming-pool of boarding-house as the place of occurrence of the external cause POA

Y92.046   Garden or yard of boarding-house as the place of occurrence of the external cause POA

Y92.048   Other place in boarding-house as the place of occurrence of the external cause POA

Y92.049   Unspecified place in boarding-house as the place of occurrence of the external cause POA

6ᵗʰ Y92.09 Other non-institutional residence as the place of occurrence of the external cause

Y92.090   Kitchen in other non-institutional residence as the place of occurrence of the external cause POA

Y92.091   Bathroom in other non-institutional residence as the place of occurrence of the external cause POA

Y92.092   Bedroom in other non-institutional residence as the place of occurrence of the external cause POA

Y92.093   Driveway of other non-institutional residence as the place of occurrence of the external cause POA

Y92.094   Garage of other non-institutional residence as the place of occurrence of the external cause POA

Y92.095   Swimming-pool of other non-institutional residence as the place of occurrence of the external cause POA

Y92.096   Garden or yard of other non-institutional residence as the place of occurrence of the external cause POA

Y92.098   Other place in other non-institutional residence as the place of occurrence of the external cause POA
   AHA: Q2 2017

Y92.099   Unspecified place in other non-institutional residence as the place of occurrence of the external cause POA
   AHA: Q2 2017

5ᵗʰ Y92.1 Institutional (nonprivate) residence as the place of occurrence of the external cause

Y92.10   Unspecified residential institution as the place of occurrence of the external cause POA

6ᵗʰ Y92.11 Children's home and orphanage as the place of occurrence of the external cause

Y92.110   Kitchen in children's home and orphanage as the place of occurrence of the external cause POA

Y92.111   Bathroom in children's home and orphanage as the place of occurrence of the external cause POA

Y92.112   Bedroom in children's home and orphanage as the place of occurrence of the external cause POA

Y92.113   Driveway of children's home and orphanage as the place of occurrence of the external cause POA

POA Unacceptable principal diagnosis symbol per Medicare code edits   POA Code exempt from diagnosis present on admission requirement
? Questionable admission   CC Complication or comorbidity   CC/MCC Exc CC/MCC exclusion   MCC Major complication or comorbidity
Principal diagnosis as its own CC   Principal diagnosis as its own MCC   HCC HCC diagnosis code   RxHCC RxHCC diagnosis code
MACRA code   Z Z code as first-listed diagnosis

Y92.114   Garage of children's home and orphanage as the place of occurrence of the external cause   POA

Y92.115   Swimming-pool of children's home and orphanage as the place of occurrence of the external cause   POA

Y92.116   Garden or yard of children's home and orphanage as the place of occurrence of the external cause   POA

Y92.118   Other place in children's home and orphanage as the place of occurrence of the external cause   POA

Y92.119   Unspecified place in children's home and orphanage as the place of occurrence of the external cause   POA

6ᵗʰ Y92.12   Nursing home as the place of occurrence of the external cause

Home for the sick as the place of occurrence of the external cause

Hospice as the place of occurrence of the external cause

Y92.120   Kitchen in nursing home as the place of occurrence of the external cause   POA

Y92.121   Bathroom in nursing home as the place of occurrence of the external cause   POA

Y92.122   Bedroom in nursing home as the place of occurrence of the external cause   POA

Y92.123   Driveway of nursing home as the place of occurrence of the external cause   POA

Y92.124   Garage of nursing home as the place of occurrence of the external cause   POA

Y92.125   Swimming-pool of nursing home as the place of occurrence of the external cause   POA

Y92.126   Garden or yard of nursing home as the place of occurrence of the external cause   POA

Y92.128   Other place in nursing home as the place of occurrence of the external cause   POA

Y92.129   Unspecified place in nursing home as the place of occurrence of the external cause   POA

AHA: Q2 2017

6ᵗʰ Y92.13   Military base as the place of occurrence of the external cause

EXCLUDES1 military training grounds (Y92.83)

Y92.130   Kitchen on military base as the place of occurrence of the external cause   POA

Y92.131   Mess hall on military base as the place of occurrence of the external cause   POA

Y92.133   Barracks on military base as the place of occurrence of the external cause   POA

Y92.135   Garage on military base as the place of occurrence of the external cause   POA

Y92.136   Swimming-pool on military base as the place of occurrence of the external cause   POA

Y92.137   Garden or yard on military base as the place of occurrence of the external cause   POA

Y92.138   Other place on military base as the place of occurrence of the external cause   POA

Y92.139   Unspecified place military base as the place of occurrence of the external cause   POA

6ᵗʰ Y92.14   Prison as the place of occurrence of the external cause

Y92.140   Kitchen in prison as the place of occurrence of the external cause   POA

Y92.141   Dining room in prison as the place of occurrence of the external cause   POA

Y92.142   Bathroom in prison as the place of occurrence of the external cause   POA

Y92.143   Cell of prison as the place of occurrence of the external cause   POA

Y92.146   Swimming-pool of prison as the place of occurrence of the external cause   POA

Y92.147   Courtyard of prison as the place of occurrence of the external cause   POA

Y92.148   Other place in prison as the place of occurrence of the external cause   POA

Y92.149   Unspecified place in prison as the place of occurrence of the external cause   POA

6ᵗʰ Y92.15   Reform school as the place of occurrence of the external cause

Y92.150   Kitchen in reform school as the place of occurrence of the external cause   POA

Y92.151   Dining room in reform school as the place of occurrence of the external cause   POA

Y92.152   Bathroom in reform school as the place of occurrence of the external cause   POA

Y92.153   Bedroom in reform school as the place of occurrence of the external cause   POA

Y92.154   Driveway of reform school as the place of occurrence of the external cause   POA

Y92.155   Garage of reform school as the place of occurrence of the external cause   POA

Y92.156   Swimming-pool of reform school as the place of occurrence of the external cause   POA

Y92.157   Garden or yard of reform school as the place of occurrence of the external cause   POA

Y92.158   Other place in reform school as the place of occurrence of the external cause   POA

Y92.159   Unspecified place in reform school as the place of occurrence of the external cause   POA

6ᵗʰ Y92.16   School dormitory as the place of occurrence of the external cause

EXCLUDES1 reform school as the place of occurrence of the external cause (Y92.15-)

school buildings and grounds as the place of occurrence of the external cause (Y92.2-)

school sports and athletic areas as the place of occurrence of the external cause (Y92.3-)

Y92.160   Kitchen in school dormitory as the place of occurrence of the external cause   POA

Y92.161   Dining room in school dormitory as the place of occurrence of the external cause   POA

Y92.162   Bathroom in school dormitory as the place of occurrence of the external cause   POA

Y92.163   Bedroom in school dormitory as the place of occurrence of the external cause   POA

Y92.168   Other place in school dormitory as the place of occurrence of the external cause   POA

Y92.169   Unspecified place in school dormitory as the place of occurrence of the external cause   POA

6ᵗʰ Y92.19   Other specified residential institution as the place of occurrence of the external cause

Y92.190   Kitchen in other specified residential institution as the place of occurrence of the external cause   POA

Y92.191   Dining room in other specified residential institution as the place of occurrence of the external cause   POA

Y92.192   Bathroom in other specified residential institution as the place of occurrence of the external cause   POA

Y92.193   Bedroom in other specified residential institution as the place of occurrence of the external cause   POA

Unspecified Code   Other Specified Code   Manifestation Code   N Newborn   P Pediatric   M Maternity   A Adult   ♂ Male   ♀ Female
● New Code   ◄ Revised Code Title   ►◄ Revised Text   NOTES   INCLUDES   EXCLUDES1 Not coded here   EXCLUDES2 Not included here
4ᵗʰ character required   5ᵗʰ character required   6ᵗʰ character required   7ᵗʰ character required
7ᵗʰ Extension 'X' Alert   HAC Hospital-acquired condition (HAC) alert   AHA AHA Coding Clinic©

Y92.194 Driveway of other specified residential institution as the place of occurrence of the external cause POA

Y92.195 Garage of other specified residential institution as the place of occurrence of the external cause POA

Y92.196 Pool of other specified residential institution as the place of occurrence of the external cause POA

Y92.197 Garden or yard of other specified residential institution as the place of occurrence of the external cause POA

Y92.198 Other place in other specified residential institution as the place of occurrence of the external cause POA

Y92.199 Unspecified place in other specified residential institution as the place of occurrence of the external cause POA
    AHA: Q2 2017

Y92.2 School, other institution and public administrative area as the place of occurrence of the external cause
    Building and adjacent grounds used by the general public or by a particular group of the public
    EXCLUDES1 building under construction as the place of occurrence of the external cause (Y92.6)
        residential institution as the place of occurrence of the external cause (Y92.1)
        school dormitory as the place of occurrence of the external cause (Y92.16-)
        sports and athletics area of schools as the place of occurrence of the external cause (Y92.3-)

Y92.21 School (private) (public) (state) as the place of occurrence of the external cause

Y92.210 Daycare center as the place of occurrence of the external cause POA

Y92.211 Elementary school as the place of occurrence of the external cause POA
    Kindergarten as the place of occurrence of the external cause

Y92.212 Middle school as the place of occurrence of the external cause POA

Y92.213 High school as the place of occurrence of the external cause POA
    AHA: Q4 2012

Y92.214 College as the place of occurrence of the external cause POA
    University as the place of occurrence of the external cause

Y92.215 Trade school as the place of occurrence of the external cause POA

Y92.218 Other school as the place of occurrence of the external cause POA

Y92.219 Unspecified school as the place of occurrence of the external cause POA

Y92.22 Religious institution as the place of occurrence of the external cause POA
    Church as the place of occurrence of the external cause
    Mosque as the place of occurrence of the external cause
    Synagogue as the place of occurrence of the external cause

Y92.23 Hospital as the place of occurrence of the external cause
    EXCLUDES1 ambulatory (outpatient) health services establishments (Y92.53-)
        home for the sick as the place of occurrence of the external cause (Y92.12-)
        hospice as the place of occurrence of the external cause (Y92.12-)
        nursing home as the place of occurrence of the external cause (Y92.12-)

Y92.230 Patient room in hospital as the place of occurrence of the external cause

Y92.231 Patient bathroom in hospital as the place of occurrence of the external cause

Y92.232 Corridor of hospital as the place of occurrence of the external cause

Y92.233 Cafeteria of hospital as the place of occurrence of the external cause

Y92.234 Operating room of hospital as the place of occurrence of the external cause

Y92.238 Other place in hospital as the place of occurrence of the external cause

Y92.239 Unspecified place in hospital as the place of occurrence of the external cause

Y92.24 Public administrative building as the place of occurrence of the external cause

Y92.240 Courthouse as the place of occurrence of the external cause POA

Y92.241 Library as the place of occurrence of the external cause POA

Y92.242 Post office as the place of occurrence of the external cause POA

Y92.243 City hall as the place of occurrence of the external cause POA

Y92.248 Other public administrative building as the place of occurrence of the external cause POA

Y92.25 Cultural building as the place of occurrence of the external cause

Y92.250 Art Gallery as the place of occurrence of the external cause POA

Y92.251 Museum as the place of occurrence of the external cause POA

Y92.252 Music hall as the place of occurrence of the external cause POA

Y92.253 Opera house as the place of occurrence of the external cause POA

Y92.254 Theater (live) as the place of occurrence of the external cause POA

Y92.258 Other cultural public building as the place of occurrence of the external cause POA

Y92.26 Movie house or cinema as the place of occurrence of the external cause POA

Y92.29 Other specified public building as the place of occurrence of the external cause POA
    Assembly hall as the place of occurrence of the external cause
    Clubhouse as the place of occurrence of the external cause

Y92.3 Sports and athletics area as the place of occurrence of the external cause

Y92.31 Athletic court as the place of occurrence of the external cause
    EXCLUDES1 tennis court in private home or garden (Y92.09)

Y92.310 Basketball court as the place of occurrence of the external cause POA

Y92.311 Squash court as the place of occurrence of the external cause POA

Y92.312 Tennis court as the place of occurrence of the external cause POA

Y92.318 Other athletic court as the place of occurrence of the external cause POA

Y92.32 Athletic field as the place of occurrence of the external cause

Y92.320 Baseball field as the place of occurrence of the external cause POA

Y92.321 Football field as the place of occurrence of the external cause POA

Y92.322 Soccer field as the place of occurrence of the external cause POA

PDMR Unacceptable principal diagnosis symbol per Medicare code edits   POA Code exempt from diagnosis present on admission requirement
? Questionable admission   CC Complication or comorbidity   CC-MCC ExC CC/MCC exclusion   MCC Major complication or comorbidity
CC Principal diagnosis as its own CC   MCC Principal diagnosis as its own MCC   HCC HCC diagnosis code   RxHCC RxHCC diagnosis code
MACRA code   Z1 Z code as first-listed diagnosis

1248   When symbols appear on a code that requires a 7th character extension, refer to Appendix B to identify applicable 7th character codes.   2018 ICD-10-CM

Y92.328 Other athletic field as the place of occurrence of the external cause
Cricket field as the place of occurrence of the external cause
Hockey field as the place of occurrence of the external cause

Y92.33 Skating rink as the place of occurrence of the external cause
  Y92.330 Ice skating rink (indoor) (outdoor) as the place of occurrence of the external cause
  Y92.331 Roller skating rink as the place of occurrence of the external cause

Y92.34 Swimming pool (public) as the place of occurrence of the external cause
  EXCLUDES1 swimming pool in private home or garden (Y92.016)

Y92.39 Other specified sports and athletic area as the place of occurrence of the external cause
Golf-course as the place of occurrence of the external cause
Gymnasium as the place of occurrence of the external cause
Riding-school as the place of occurrence of the external cause
Stadium as the place of occurrence of the external cause

Y92.4 Street, highway and other paved roadways as the place of occurrence of the external cause
  EXCLUDES1 private driveway of residence (Y92.014, Y92.024, Y92.043, Y92.093, Y92.113, Y92.123, Y92.154, Y92.194)

Y92.41 Street and highway as the place of occurrence of the external cause
  Y92.410 Unspecified street and highway as the place of occurrence of the external cause
Road NOS as the place of occurrence of the external cause
  Y92.411 Interstate highway as the place of occurrence of the external cause
Freeway as the place of occurrence of the external cause
Motorway as the place of occurrence of the external cause
  Y92.412 Parkway as the place of occurrence of the external cause
  Y92.413 State road as the place of occurrence of the external cause
  Y92.414 Local residential or business street as the place of occurrence of the external cause
  Y92.415 Exit ramp or entrance ramp of street or highway as the place of occurrence of the external cause

Y92.48 Other paved roadways as the place of occurrence of the external cause
  Y92.480 Sidewalk as the place of occurrence of the external cause
  Y92.481 Parking lot as the place of occurrence of the external cause
  Y92.482 Bike path as the place of occurrence of the external cause
  Y92.488 Other paved roadways as the place of occurrence of the external cause

Y92.5 Trade and service area as the place of occurrence of the external cause
  EXCLUDES1 garage in private home (Y92.015)
    schools and other public administration buildings (Y92.2-)

Y92.51 Private commercial establishments as the place of occurrence of the external cause
  Y92.510 Bank as the place of occurrence of the external cause

Y92.511 Restaurant or café as the place of occurrence of the external cause
Y92.512 Supermarket, store or market as the place of occurrence of the external cause
Y92.513 Shop (commercial) as the place of occurrence of the external cause

Y92.52 Service areas as the place of occurrence of the external cause
  Y92.520 Airport as the place of occurrence of the external cause
  Y92.521 Bus station as the place of occurrence of the external cause
  Y92.522 Railway station as the place of occurrence of the external cause
  Y92.523 Highway rest stop as the place of occurrence of the external cause
  Y92.524 Gas station as the place of occurrence of the external cause
Petroleum station as the place of occurrence of the external cause
Service station as the place of occurrence of the external cause

Y92.53 Ambulatory health services establishments as the place of occurrence of the external cause
  Y92.530 Ambulatory surgery center as the place of occurrence of the external cause
Outpatient surgery center, including that connected with a hospital as the place of occurrence of the external cause
Same day surgery center, including that connected with a hospital as the place of occurrence of the external cause
  Y92.531 Health care provider office as the place of occurrence of the external cause
Physician office as the place of occurrence of the external cause
  Y92.532 Urgent care center as the place of occurrence of the external cause
  Y92.538 Other ambulatory health services establishments as the place of occurrence of the external cause

Y92.59 Other trade areas as the place of occurrence of the external cause
Office building as the place of occurrence of the external cause
Casino as the place of occurrence of the external cause
Garage (commercial) as the place of occurrence of the external cause
Hotel as the place of occurrence of the external cause
Radio or television station as the place of occurrence of the external cause
Shopping mall as the place of occurrence of the external cause
Warehouse as the place of occurrence of the external cause

Y92.6 Industrial and construction area as the place of occurrence of the external cause
  Y92.61 Building [any] under construction as the place of occurrence of the external cause
  Y92.62 Dock or shipyard as the place of occurrence of the external cause
Dockyard as the place of occurrence of the external cause
Dry dock as the place of occurrence of the external cause
Shipyard as the place of occurrence of the external cause
  Y92.63 Factory as the place of occurrence of the external cause
Factory building as the place of occurrence of the external cause
Factory premises as the place of occurrence of the external cause

Unspecified Code   Other Specified Code   Manifestation Code   N Newborn   P Pediatric   M Maternity   A Adult   ♂ Male   ♀ Female
● New Code   ▲ Revised Code Title   ►◄ Revised Text   NOTES   INCLUDES   EXCLUDES 1 Not coded here   EXCLUDES 2 Not included here
4ᵗʰ character required   5ᵗʰ character required   6ᵗʰ character required   7ᵗʰ character required
Extension 'X' Alert   HAC Hospital-acquired condition (HAC) alert   AHA AHA Coding Clinic©

Industrial yard as the place of occurrence of the external cause

Y92.64 Mine or pit as the place of occurrence of the external cause POA

Mine as the place of occurrence of the external cause

Y92.65 Oil rig as the place of occurrence of the external cause POA

Pit (coal) (gravel) (sand) as the place of occurrence of the external cause

Y92.69 Other specified industrial and construction area as the place of occurrence of the external cause POA

Gasworks as the place of occurrence of the external cause

Power-station (coal) (nuclear) (oil) as the place of occurrence of the external cause

Tunnel under construction as the place of occurrence of the external cause

Workshop as the place of occurrence of the external cause

5ᵗʰ Y92.7 Farm as the place of occurrence of the external cause

Ranch as the place of occurrence of the external cause

EXCLUDES1 farmhouse and home premises of farm (Y92.01-)

Y92.71 Barn as the place of occurrence of the external cause POA

Y92.72 Chicken coop as the place of occurrence of the external cause POA

Hen house as the place of occurrence of the external cause

Y92.73 Farm field as the place of occurrence of the external cause POA

Y92.74 Orchard as the place of occurrence of the external cause POA

Y92.79 Other farm location as the place of occurrence of the external cause POA

5ᵗʰ Y92.8 Other places as the place of occurrence of the external cause

6ᵗʰ Y92.81 Transport vehicle as the place of occurrence of the external cause

EXCLUDES1 transport accidents (V00-V99)

Y92.810 Car as the place of occurrence of the external cause POA

Y92.811 Bus as the place of occurrence of the external cause POA

Y92.812 Truck as the place of occurrence of the external cause POA

Y92.813 Airplane as the place of occurrence of the external cause POA

Y92.814 Boat as the place of occurrence of the external cause POA

Y92.815 Train as the place of occurrence of the external cause POA

Y92.816 Subway car as the place of occurrence of the external cause POA

Y92.818 Other transport vehicle as the place of occurrence of the external cause POA

5ᵗʰ Y92.82 Wilderness area

Y92.820 Desert as the place of occurrence of the external cause POA

Y92.821 Forest as the place of occurrence of the external cause POA

Y92.828 Other wilderness area as the place of occurrence of the external cause POA

Swamp as the place of occurrence of the external cause

Mountain as the place of occurrence of the external cause

Marsh as the place of occurrence of the external cause

Prairie as the place of occurrence of the external cause

5ᵗʰ Y92.83 Recreation area as the place of occurrence of the external cause

Y92.830 Public park as the place of occurrence of the external cause POA

Y92.831 Amusement park as the place of occurrence of the external cause POA

Y92.832 Beach as the place of occurrence of the external cause POA

Seashore as the place of occurrence of the external cause

Y92.833 Campsite as the place of occurrence of the external cause POA

Y92.834 Zoological garden (Zoo) as the place of occurrence of the external cause POA

Y92.838 Other recreation area as the place of occurrence of the external cause POA

Y92.84 Military training ground as the place of occurrence of the external cause POA

Y92.85 Railroad track as the place of occurrence of the external cause POA

Y92.86 Slaughter house as the place of occurrence of the external cause POA

Y92.89 Other specified places as the place of occurrence of the external cause POA

Derelict house as the place of occurrence of the external cause

Y92.9 Unspecified place or not applicable POA

4ᵗʰ Y93 Activity codes

NOTES Category Y93 is provided for use to indicate the activity of the person seeking healthcare for an injury or health condition, such as a heart attack while shoveling snow, which resulted from, or was contributed to, by the activity. These codes are appropriate for use for both acute injuries, such as those from chapter 19, and conditions that are due to the long-term, cumulative effects of an activity, such as those from chapter 13. They are also appropriate for use with external cause codes for cause and intent if identifying the activity provides additional information on the event. These codes should be used in conjunction with codes for external cause status (Y99) and place of occurrence (Y92). This section contains the following broad activity categories:

Y93.0 Activities involving walking and running

Y93.1 Activities involving water and water craft

Y93.2 Activities involving ice and snow

Y93.3 Activities involving climbing, rappelling, and jumping off

Y93.4 Activities involving dancing and other rhythmic movement

Y93.5 Activities involving other sports and athletics played individually

Y93.6 Activities involving other sports and athletics played as a team or group

Y93.7 Activities involving other specified sports and athletics

Y93.A Activities involving other cardiorespiratory exercise

Y93.B Activities involving other muscle strengthening exercises

Y93.C Activities involving computer technology and electronic devices

Y93.D Activities involving arts and handcrafts

Y93.E Activities involving personal hygiene and interior property and clothing maintenance

Y93.F Activities involving caregiving

Y93.G Activities involving food preparation, cooking and grilling

Y93.H Activities involving exterior property and land maintenance, building and construction

Y93.I Activities involving roller coasters and other types of external motion

Y93.J Activities involving playing musical instrument

Y93.K Activities involving animal care

Y93.8 Activities, other specified

Y93.9 Activity, unspecified

POA Unacceptable principal diagnosis symbol per Medicare code edits   POA Code exempt from diagnosis present on admission requirement
? Questionable admission   cc Complication or comorbidity   CC/MCC CC/MCC exclusion   MCC Major complication or comorbidity
Principal diagnosis as its own CC   Principal diagnosis as its own MCC   HCC HCC diagnosis code   RxHCC RxHCC diagnosis code
MACRA code   Z code as first-listed diagnosis

1250   When symbols appear on a code that requires a 7th character extension, refer to Appendix B to identify applicable 7th character codes.   2018 ICD-10-CM

[5th] **Y93.0 Activities involving walking and running**
[EXCLUDES1] *activity, walking an animal (Y93.K1)*
activity, walking or running on a treadmill (Y93.A1)
Y93.01 Activity, walking, marching and hiking
Activity, walking, marching and hiking on level or elevated terrain
[EXCLUDES1] *activity, mountain climbing (Y93.31)*
Y93.02 Activity, running

[5th] **Y93.1 Activities involving water and water craft**
[EXCLUDES1] *activities involving ice (Y93.2-)*
Y93.11 Activity, swimming
Y93.12 Activity, springboard and platform diving [POA]
Y93.13 Activity, water polo [POA]
Y93.14 Activity, water aerobics and water exercise [POA]
Y93.15 Activity, underwater diving and snorkeling [POA]
Activity, SCUBA diving
Y93.16 Activity, rowing, canoeing, kayaking, rafting and tubing [POA]
Activity, canoeing, kayaking, rafting and tubing in calm and turbulent water
Y93.17 Activity, water skiing and wake boarding [POA]
Y93.18 Activity, surfing, windsurfing and boogie boarding [POA]
Activity, water sliding
Y93.19 Activity, other involving water and watercraft [POA]
Activity involving water NOS
Activity, parasailing
Activity, water survival training and testing

[5th] **Y93.2 Activities involving ice and snow**
[EXCLUDES1] *activity, shoveling ice and snow (Y93.H1)*
Y93.21 Activity, ice skating [POA]
Activity, figure skating (singles) (pairs)
Activity, ice dancing
[EXCLUDES1] *activity, ice hockey (Y93.22)*
Y93.22 Activity, ice hockey [POA]
Y93.23 Activity, snow (alpine) (downhill) skiing, snow boarding, sledding, tobogganing and snow tubing [POA]
[EXCLUDES1] *activity, cross country skiing (Y93.24)*
Y93.24 Activity, cross country skiing [POA]
Activity, nordic skiing
Y93.29 Activity, other involving ice and snow [POA]
Activity involving ice and snow NOS

[5th] **Y93.3 Activities involving climbing, rappelling and jumping off**
[EXCLUDES1] *activity, hiking on level or elevated terrain (Y93.01)*
activity, jumping rope (Y93.56)
activity, trampoline jumping (Y93.44)
Y93.31 Activity, mountain climbing, rock climbing and wall climbing [POA]
Y93.32 Activity, rappelling [POA]
Y93.33 Activity, BASE jumping [POA]
Activity, Building, Antenna, Span, Earth jumping
Y93.34 Activity, bungee jumping [POA]
Y93.35 Activity, hang gliding [POA]
Y93.39 Activity, other involving climbing, rappelling and jumping off [POA]

[5th] **Y93.4 Activities involving dancing and other rhythmic movement**
[EXCLUDES1] *activity, martial arts (Y93.75)*
Y93.41 Activity, dancing [POA]
AHA: Q4 2012
Y93.42 Activity, yoga [POA]
Y93.43 Activity, gymnastics [POA]
Activity, rhythmic gymnastics
[EXCLUDES1] *activity, trampolining (Y93.44)*
Y93.44 Activity, trampolining [POA]
Y93.45 Activity, cheerleading [POA]
Y93.49 Activity, other involving dancing and other rhythmic movements [POA]

[5th] **Y93.5 Activities involving other sports and athletics played individually**
[EXCLUDES1] *activity, dancing (Y93.41)*
activity, gymnastic (Y93.43)
activity, trampolining (Y93.44)
activity, yoga (Y93.42)
Y93.51 Activity, roller skating (inline) and skateboarding [POA]
Y93.52 Activity, horseback riding [POA]
Y93.53 Activity, golf [POA]
Y93.54 Activity, bowling [POA]
Y93.55 Activity, bike riding [POA]
Y93.56 Activity, jumping rope [POA]
Y93.57 Activity, non-running track and field events [POA]
[EXCLUDES1] *activity, running (any form) (Y93.02)*
Y93.59 Activity, other involving other sports and athletics played individually [POA]
[EXCLUDES1] *activities involving climbing, rappelling, and jumping (Y93.3-)*
activities involving ice and snow (Y93.2-)
activities involving walking and running (Y93.0-)
activities involving water and watercraft (Y93.1-)

[5th] **Y93.6 Activities involving other sports and athletics played as a team or group**
[EXCLUDES1] *activity, ice hockey (Y93.22)*
activity, water polo (Y93.13)
Y93.61 Activity, american tackle football [POA]
Activity, football NOS
Y93.62 Activity, american flag or touch football [POA]
Y93.63 Activity, rugby [POA]
Y93.64 Activity, baseball [POA]
Activity, softball
Y93.65 Activity, lacrosse and field hockey [POA]
AHA: Q1 2015
Y93.66 Activity, soccer [POA]
Y93.67 Activity, basketball [POA]
Y93.68 Activity, volleyball (beach) (court) [POA]
Y93.6A Activity, physical games generally associated with school recess, summer camp and children [POA]
Activity, capture the flag
Activity, dodge ball
Activity, four square
Activity, kickball
Y93.69 Activity, other involving other sports and athletics played as a team or group [POA]
Activity, cricket

[5th] **Y93.7 Activities involving other specified sports and athletics**
Y93.71 Activity, boxing [POA]
Y93.72 Activity, wrestling [POA]
Y93.73 Activity, racquet and hand sports [POA]
Activity, handball
Activity, racquetball
Activity, squash
Activity, tennis
Y93.74 Activity, frisbee [POA]
Activity, ultimate frisbee
Y93.75 Activity, martial arts [POA]
Activity, combatives
Y93.79 Activity, other specified sports and athletics [POA]
[EXCLUDES1] *sports and athletics activities specified in categories Y93.0-Y93.6*

[5th] **Y93.A Activities involving other cardiorespiratory exercise**
Activities involving physical training
Y93.A1 Activity, exercise machines primarily for cardiorespiratory conditioning [POA]
Activity, elliptical and stepper machines
Activity, stationary bike
Activity, treadmill

Unspecified Code | Other Specified Code | Manifestation Code | [N] Newborn | [P] Pediatric | [M] Maternity | [A] Adult | ♂ Male | ♀ Female
● New Code | ▲ Revised Code Title | ►◄ Revised Text | [NOTES] | [INCLUDES] | [EXCLUDES1] Not coded here | [EXCLUDES2] Not included here
[4th] 4th character required | [5th] 5th character required | [6th] 6th character required | [7th] 7th character required
[x7th] Extension 'X' Alert | [HAC] Hospital-acquired condition (HAC) alert | AHA AHA Coding Clinic©

Y93.A2 **Activity,** calisthenics `POA`
　　　Activity, jumping jacks
　　　Activity, warm up and cool down
Y93.A3 **Activity,** aerobic and step exercise `POA`
Y93.A4 **Activity,** circuit training `POA`
Y93.A5 **Activity,** obstacle course `POA`
　　　Activity, challenge course
　　　Activity, confidence course
Y93.A6 **Activity,** grass drills `POA`
　　　Activity, guerilla drills
Y93.A9 **Activity, other** involving cardiorespiratory exercise `POA`
　　　　EXCLUDES1 *activities involving cardiorespiratory exercise specified in categories Y93.0-Y93.7*

🔵 **Y93.B** **Activities involving other muscle strengthening exercises**
Y93.B1 **Activity,** exercise machines **primarily for muscle strengthening** `POA`
Y93.B2 **Activity,** push-ups, pull-ups, sit-ups `POA`
Y93.B3 **Activity,** free weights `POA`
　　　Activity, barbells
　　　Activity, dumbbells
Y93.B4 **Activity,** pilates `POA`
Y93.B9 **Activity, other** involving muscle strengthening exercises `POA`
　　　　EXCLUDES1 *activities involving muscle strengthening specified in categories Y93.0-Y93.A*

🔵 **Y93.C** **Activities involving computer technology and electronic devices**
　　　EXCLUDES1 *activity, electronic musical keyboard or instruments (Y93.J-)*
Y93.C1 **Activity,** computer keyboarding `POA`
　　　Activity, electronic game playing using keyboard or other stationary device
Y93.C2 **Activity,** hand held interactive electronic device `POA`
　　　Activity, cellular telephone and communication device
　　　Activity, electronic game playing using interactive device
　　　　EXCLUDES1 *activity, electronic game playing using keyboard or other stationary device (Y93.C1)*
Y93.C9 **Activity, other** involving computer technology and electronic devices `POA`

🔵 **Y93.D** **Activities involving arts and handcrafts**
　　　EXCLUDES1 *activities involving playing musical instrument (Y93.J-)*
Y93.D1 **Activity,** knitting and crocheting `POA`
Y93.D2 **Activity,** sewing `POA`
Y93.D3 **Activity,** furniture building and finishing `POA`
　　　Activity, furniture repair
Y93.D9 **Activity, other** involving arts and handcrafts `POA`

🔵 **Y93.E** **Activities involving personal hygiene and interior property and clothing maintenance**
　　　EXCLUDES1 *activities involving cooking and grilling (Y93.G-)*
　　　　　activities involving exterior property and land maintenance, building and construction (Y93.H-)
　　　　　activities involving caregiving (Y93.F-)
　　　　　activity, dishwashing (Y93.G1)
　　　　　activity, food preparation (Y93.G1)
　　　　　activity, gardening (Y93.H2)
Y93.E1 **Activity,** personal bathing and showering `POA`
Y93.E2 **Activity,** laundry `POA`
Y93.E3 **Activity,** vacuuming `POA`
Y93.E4 **Activity,** ironing `POA`
Y93.E5 **Activity,** floor mopping and cleaning `POA`
Y93.E6 **Activity,** residential relocation `POA`
　　　Activity, packing up and unpacking involved in moving to a new residence
Y93.E8 **Activity, other** personal hygiene `POA`
Y93.E9 **Activity, other** interior property and clothing maintenance `POA`

🔵 **Y93.F** **Activities involving caregiving**

Activity involving the provider of caregiving
Y93.F1 **Activity, caregiving,** bathing `POA`
Y93.F2 **Activity, caregiving,** lifting `POA`
　　　AHA: Q4 2016
Y93.F9 **Activity, other** caregiving `POA`

🔵 **Y93.G** **Activities involving food preparation, cooking and grilling**
Y93.G1 **Activity,** food preparation and clean up `POA`
　　　Activity, dishwashing
Y93.G2 **Activity,** grilling and smoking food `POA`
Y93.G3 **Activity,** cooking and baking `POA`
　　　Activity, use of stove, oven and microwave oven
Y93.G9 **Activity, other** involving cooking and grilling `POA`

🔵 **Y93.H** **Activities involving exterior property and land maintenance, building and construction**
Y93.H1 **Activity,** digging, shoveling and raking `POA`
　　　Activity, dirt digging
　　　Activity, raking leaves
　　　Activity, snow shoveling
Y93.H2 **Activity,** gardening and landscaping `POA`
　　　Activity, pruning, trimming shrubs, weeding
Y93.H3 **Activity,** building and construction `POA`
Y93.H9 **Activity, other** involving exterior property and land maintenance, building and construction `POA`

🔵 **Y93.I** **Activities involving roller coasters and other types of external motion**
Y93.I1 **Activity,** roller coaster riding `POA`
Y93.I9 **Activity, other** involving external motion `POA`

🔵 **Y93.J** **Activities involving playing** musical instrument
Activity involving playing electric musical instrument
Y93.J1 **Activity,** piano playing `POA`
　　　Activity, musical keyboard (electronic) playing
Y93.J2 **Activity,** drum and other percussion instrument playing `POA`
Y93.J3 **Activity,** string instrument **playing** `POA`
Y93.J4 **Activity,** winds and brass instrument **playing** `POA`

🔵 **Y93.K** **Activities involving animal care**
　　　EXCLUDES1 *activity, horseback riding (Y93.52)*
Y93.K1 **Activity,** walking an animal `POA`
Y93.K2 **Activity,** milking an animal `POA`
Y93.K3 **Activity,** grooming and shearing an animal `POA`
Y93.K9 **Activity, other** involving animal care `POA`

🔵 **Y93.8** **Activities,** other specified
Y93.81 **Activity,** refereeing a sports activity `POA`
Y93.82 **Activity,** spectator at an event `POA`
Y93.83 **Activity,** rough housing and horseplay `POA`
　　　AHA: Q1 2015
Y93.84 **Activity,** sleeping `POA`
Y93.85 **Activity,** choking game `POA`
　　　AHA: Q4 2016
　　　Activity, blackout game
　　　Activity, fainting game
　　　Activity, pass out game
Y93.89 **Activity, other specified** `POA`
Y93.9 **Activity, unspecified** `POA`

Y95 **Nosocomial condition**
　　　AHA: Q4 2013

🔵 **Y99** **External cause status**
　　　NOTES A single code from category Y99 should be used in conjunction with the external cause code(s) assigned to a record to indicate the status of the person at the time the event occurred.
Y99.0 Civilian **activity done for income or pay** `POA`
　　　Civilian activity done for financial or other compensation
　　　EXCLUDES1 *military activity (Y99.1)*
　　　　　volunteer activity (Y99.2)
Y99.1 Military **activity** `POA`
　　　EXCLUDES1 *activity of off duty military personnel (Y99.8)*
Y99.2 Volunteer **activity** `POA`
　　　EXCLUDES1 *activity of child or other family member assisting in compensated work of other family member (Y99.8)*

`POA` Unacceptable principal diagnosis symbol per Medicare code edits　`POA` Code exempt from diagnosis present on admission requirement
❓ Questionable admission　©© Complication or comorbidity　CC/MCC ex. CC/MCC exclusion　MCC© Major complication or comorbidity
🔲 Principal diagnosis as its own CC　🔲 Principal diagnosis as its own MCC　HCC HCC diagnosis code　RHCC RxHCC diagnosis code
MACRA code　Z1 Z code as first-listed diagnosis

Y99.8 **Other external cause status** POA

Activity NEC

Activity of child or other family member assisting in compensated work of other family member

Hobby not done for income

Leisure activity

Off-duty activity of military personnel

Recreation or sport not for income or while a student

Student activity

EXCLUDES1 *civilian activity done for income or compensation (Y99.0)*

military activity (Y99.1)

Y99.9 **Unspecified external cause status** POA

Unspecified Code   Other Specified Code   Manifestation Code   N Newborn   P Pediatric   M Maternity   A Adult   ♂ Male   ♀ Female
● New Code   ▲ Revised Code Title   ▶◀ Revised Text   NOTES   INCLUDES   EXCLUDES 1 Not coded here   EXCLUDES 2 Not included here
4th character required   5th character required   6th character required   7th character required
Extension 'X' Alert   HAC Hospital-acquired condition (HAC) alert   AHA AHA Coding Clinic©

2018 ICD-10-CM   When symbols appear on a code that requires a 7th character extension, refer to Appendix B to identify applicable 7th character codes.   **1253**

NOTES

Chapter 21: Factors Influencing Health Status and Contact with Health Services (Z00-Z99)

Factors influencing health status and contact with health services (Z00-Z99)

NOTES Z codes represent reasons for encounters. A corresponding procedure code must accompany a Z code if a procedure is performed. Categories Z00-Z99 are provided for occasions when circumstances other than a disease, injury or external cause classifiable to categories A00-Y89 are recorded as 'diagnoses' or 'problems'. This can arise in two main ways:

(a) When a person who may or may not be sick encounters the health services for some specific purpose, such as to receive limited care or service for a current condition, to donate an organ or tissue, to receive prophylactic vaccination (immunization), or to discuss a problem which is in itself not a disease or injury.

(b) When some circumstance or problem is present which influences the person's health status but is not in itself a current illness or injury.

This chapter contains the following blocks:

Z00-Z13	Persons encountering health services for examinations
Z14-Z15	Genetic carrier and genetic susceptibility to disease
Z16	Resistance to antimicrobial drugs
Z17	Estrogen receptor status
Z18	Retained foreign body fragments
Z19	Hormone sensitivity malignancy status

Editor's Note: At press time, CMS deleted this block for 2018 even though there are valid codes within the block. The block has been left here because it includes valid codes. Check www.cms.gov for further updates.

Z20-Z29	Persons with potential health hazards related to communicable diseases
Z30-Z39	Persons encountering health services in circumstances related to reproduction
Z40-Z53	Encounters for other specific health care
Z55-Z65	Persons with potential health hazards related to socioeconomic and psychosocial circumstances
Z66	Do not resuscitate status
Z67	Blood type
Z68	Body mass index (BMI)
Z69-Z76	Persons encountering health services in other circumstances
Z77-Z99	Persons with potential health hazards related to family and personal history and certain conditions influencing health status

Persons encountering health services for examinations (Z00-Z13)

NOTES Nonspecific abnormal findings disclosed at the time of these examinations are classified to categories R70-R94.

EXCLUDES1 *examinations related to pregnancy and reproduction (Z30-Z36, Z39.-)*

Z00 Encounter for general examination without complaint, suspected or reported diagnosis

EXCLUDES1 *encounter for examination for administrative purposes (Z02.-)*

EXCLUDES2 *encounter for pre-procedural examinations (Z01.81-)*

special screening examinations (Z11-Z13)

Z00.0 Encounter for general adult medical examination

Encounter for adult periodic examination (annual) (physical) and any associated laboratory and radiologic examinations

EXCLUDES1 *encounter for examination of sign or symptom- code to sign or symptom*

general health check-up of infant or child (Z00.12.-)

Z00.00 Encounter for general adult medical examination without abnormal findings Ⓐ ⬛ ⬛ ⬛

AHA: Q1 2016

Encounter for adult health check-up NOS

Z00.01 Encounter for general adult medical examination with abnormal findings Ⓐ ⬛ ⬛ ⬛

AHA: Q1 2016

Use additional code to identify abnormal findings

Z00.1 Encounter for newborn, infant and child health examinations

Z00.11 Newborn health examination

Health check for child under 29 days old

Use additional code to identify any abnormal findings

EXCLUDES1 *health check for child over 28 days old (Z00.12-)*

Z00.110 Health examination for newborn under 8 days old Ⓝ ⬛ ⬛ ⬛

Health check for newborn under 8 days old

Z00.111 Health examination for newborn 8 to 28 days old Ⓝ ⬛ ⬛ ⬛

Health check for newborn 8 to 28 days old

Newborn weight check

Z00.12 Encounter for routine child health examination

Encounter for development testing of infant or child

Health check (routine) for child over 28 days old

EXCLUDES1 *health check for child under 29 days old (Z00.11-)*

health supervision of foundling or other healthy infant or child (Z76.1-Z76.2)

newborn health examination (Z00.11-)

Z00.121 Encounter for routine child health examination with abnormal findings Ⓟ ⬛ ⬛ ⬛

AHA: Q1 2016

Use additional code to identify abnormal findings

Z00.129 Encounter for routine child health examination without abnormal findings Ⓟ ⬛ ⬛ ⬛

AHA: Q1 2016

Encounter for routine child health examination NOS

Z00.2 Encounter for examination for period of rapid growth in childhood ⬛ ⬛ ⬛

Z00.3 Encounter for examination for adolescent development state Ⓟ ⬛ ⬛ ⬛

Encounter for puberty development state

Z00.5 Encounter for examination of potential donor of organ and tissue ⬛ ⬛ ⬛

Z00.6 Encounter for examination for normal comparison and control in clinical research program ⬛

Examination of participant or control in clinical research program

Z00.7 Encounter for examination for period of delayed growth in childhood

Z00.70 Encounter for examination for period of delayed growth in childhood without abnormal findings Ⓟ ⬛ ⬛ ⬛

Z00.71 Encounter for examination for period of delayed growth in childhood with abnormal findings Ⓟ ⬛ ⬛ ⬛

Use additional code to identify abnormal findings

Z00.8 Encounter for other general examination ⬛ ⬛ ⬛

Encounter for health examination in population surveys

Z01 Encounter for other special examination without complaint, suspected or reported diagnosis

INCLUDES *routine examination of specific system*

NOTES Codes from category Z01 represent the reason for the encounter. A separate procedure code is required to identify any examinations or procedures performed

---

Unspecified Code	Other Specified Code	Manifestation Code	Ⓝ Newborn	Ⓟ Pediatric	Ⓜ Maternity	Ⓐ Adult	♂ Male	♀ Female

● New Code ▲ Revised Code Title ▶◀ Revised Text **NOTES** *INCLUDES* *EXCLUDES 1* Not coded here *EXCLUDES 2* Not included here

4th character required 5th character required 6th character required 7th character required

Extension 'X' Alert **HAC** Hospital-acquired condition (HAC) alert **AHA** AHA Coding Clinic©

EXCLUDES1 *encounter for examination for administrative purposes (Z02.-)*

encounter for examination for suspected conditions, proven not to exist (Z03.-)

encounter for laboratory and radiologic examinations as a component of general medical examinations (Z00.0-)

encounter for laboratory, radiologic and imaging examinations for sign(s) and symptom(s) - code to the sign(s) or symptom(s)

EXCLUDES2 *screening examinations (Z11-Z13)*

Z01.0 Encounter for examination of eyes and vision

EXCLUDES1 *examination for driving license (Z02.4)*

Z01.00 Encounter for examination of eyes and vision without abnormal findings

Encounter for examination of eyes and vision NOS

Z01.01 Encounter for examination of eyes and vision with abnormal findings

AHA: Q4 2016

Use additional code to identify abnormal findings

Z01.1 Encounter for examination of ears and hearing

Z01.10 Encounter for examination of ears and hearing without abnormal findings

AHA: Q4 2016

Encounter for examination of ears and hearing NOS

Z01.11 Encounter for examination of ears and hearing with abnormal findings

Z01.110 Encounter for hearing examination following failed hearing screening

AHA: Q3 2016

Z01.118 Encounter for examination of ears and hearing with other abnormal findings

AHA: Q3 2016

Use additional code to identify abnormal findings

Z01.12 Encounter for hearing conservation and treatment

Z01.2 Encounter for dental examination and cleaning

Z01.20 Encounter for dental examination and cleaning without abnormal findings

Encounter for dental examination and cleaning NOS

Z01.21 Encounter for dental examination and cleaning with abnormal findings

Use additional code to identify abnormal findings

Z01.3 Encounter for examination of blood pressure

Z01.30 Encounter for examination of blood pressure without abnormal findings

Encounter for examination of blood pressure NOS

Z01.31 Encounter for examination of blood pressure with abnormal findings

Use additional code to identify abnormal findings

Z01.4 Encounter for gynecological examination

EXCLUDES2 *pregnancy examination or test (Z32.0-)*

routine examination for contraceptive maintenance (Z30.4-)

Z01.41 Encounter for routine **gynecological examination**

Encounter for general gynecological examination with or without cervical smear

Encounter for gynecological examination (general) (routine) NOS

Encounter for pelvic examination (annual) (periodic)

Use additional code:

for screening for human papillomavirus, if applicable, (Z11.51)

for screening vaginal pap smear, if applicable (Z12.72)

to identify acquired absence of uterus, if applicable (Z90.71-)

EXCLUDES1 *gynecologic examination status-post hysterectomy for malignant condition (Z08)*

screening cervical pap smear not a part of a routine gynecological examination (Z12.4)

Z01.411 Encounter for gynecological examination (general) (routine) with abnormal findings

Use additional code to identify abnormal findings

Z01.419 Encounter for gynecological examination (general) (routine) without abnormal findings

Z01.42 Encounter for cervical smear to confirm findings of recent normal smear following initial abnormal smear

Z01.8 Encounter for other specified special examinations

Z01.81 Encounter for preprocedural examinations

Encounter for preoperative examinations

Encounter for radiological and imaging examinations as part of preprocedural examination

Z01.810 Encounter for preprocedural cardiovascular examination

Z01.811 Encounter for preprocedural respiratory **examination**

Z01.812 Encounter for preprocedural laboratory **examination**

Blood and urine tests prior to treatment or procedure

Z01.818 Encounter for other preprocedural examination

Encounter for preprocedural examination NOS

Encounter for examinations prior to antineoplastic chemotherapy

Z01.82 Encounter for allergy testing

EXCLUDES1 *encounter for antibody response examination (Z01.84)*

Z01.83 Encounter for blood typing

Encounter for Rh typing

Z01.84 Encounter for antibody response examination

Encounter for immunity status testing

EXCLUDES1 *encounter for allergy testing (Z01.82)*

Z01.89 Encounter for other specified special examinations

Z02 Encounter for administrative examination

Z02.0 Encounter for examination for admission to educational institution

Encounter for examination for admission to preschool (education)

Encounter for examination for re-admission to school following illness or medical treatment

Z02.1 Encounter for pre-employment examination

Z02.2 Encounter for examination for admission to residential institution

EXCLUDES1 *examination for admission to prison (Z02.89)*

Z02.3 Encounter for examination for recruitment to armed forces

Z02.4 Encounter for examination for driving license

Z02.5 Encounter for examination for participation in sport

EXCLUDES1 *blood-alcohol and blood-drug test (Z02.83)*

Z02.6 Encounter for examination for insurance purposes

Z02.7 Encounter for issue of medical certificate

EXCLUDES1 *encounter for general medical examination (Z00-Z01, Z02.0-Z02.6, Z02.8-Z02.9,)*

Z02.71 Encounter for disability determination

Encounter for issue of medical certificate of incapacity

Encounter for issue of medical certificate of invalidity

Z02.79 Encounter for issue of other medical certificate

Z02.8 Encounter for other administrative examinations

Z02.81 Encounter for paternity testing

Z02.82 Encounter for adoption services

PDxIR Unacceptable principal diagnosis symbol per Medicare code edits   POA Code exempt from diagnosis present on admission requirement
❓ Questionable admission   CC Complication or comorbidity   CC-MCC Excl CC/MCC exclusion   MCC Major complication or comorbidity
CC Principal diagnosis as its own CC   MCC Principal diagnosis as its own MCC   HCC HCC diagnosis code   RxHCC RxHCC diagnosis code
MACRA code   Z1 Z code as first-listed diagnosis

1256   When symbols appear on a code that requires a 7th character extension, refer to Appendix B to identify applicable 7th character codes.   **2018 ICD-10-CM**

Z02.83 **Encounter for blood-alcohol and blood-drug test** POA Z1

Use additional code for findings of alcohol or drugs in blood (R78.-)

Z02.89 **Encounter for other administrative examinations** POA PDxIn Z1

Encounter for examination for admission to prison

Encounter for examination for admission to summer camp

Encounter for immigration examination

Encounter for naturalization examination

Encounter for premarital examination

EXCLUDES1 *health supervision of foundling or other healthy infant or child (Z76.1-Z76.2)*

Z02.9 **Encounter for administrative examinations, unspecified** POA PDxIn Z1

Z03 **Encounter for medical observation for suspected diseases and conditions ruled out**

This category is to be used when a person without a diagnosis is suspected of having an abnormal condition, without signs or symptoms, which requires study, but after examination and observation, is ruled out. This category is also for use for administrative and legal observation status.

EXCLUDES1 *contact with and (suspected) exposures hazardous to health (Z77.-)*

encounter for observation and evaluation of newborn for suspected diseases and conditions ruled out (Z05.0-)

person with feared complaint in whom no diagnosis is made (Z71.1)

signs or symptoms under study- code to signs or symptoms

Z03.6 **Encounter for observation for suspected toxic effect from ingested substance ruled out** POA Z1

Encounter for observation for suspected adverse effect from drug

Encounter for observation for suspected poisoning

Z03.7 **Encounter for suspected maternal and fetal conditions ruled out**

Encounter for suspected maternal and fetal conditions not found

EXCLUDES1 *known or suspected fetal anomalies affecting management of mother, not ruled out (O26.-, O35.-, O36.-, O40.-, O41.-)*

Z03.71 **Encounter for suspected problem with amniotic cavity and membrane ruled out** M POA ♀ PDxIn Z1

Encounter for suspected oligohydramnios ruled out

Encounter for suspected polyhydramnios ruled out

Z03.72 **Encounter for suspected placental problem ruled out** M POA ♀ PDxIn Z1

Z03.73 **Encounter for suspected fetal anomaly ruled out** M POA ♀ PDxIn Z1

AHA: Q4 2016

Z03.74 **Encounter for suspected problem with fetal growth ruled out** M POA ♀ PDxIn Z1

Z03.75 **Encounter for suspected cervical shortening ruled out** M POA ♀ PDxIn Z1

Z03.79 **Encounter for other suspected maternal and fetal conditions ruled out** M POA ♀ PDxIn Z1

Z03.8 **Encounter for observation for other suspected diseases and conditions ruled out**

Z03.81 **Encounter for observation for suspected exposure to biological agents ruled out**

Z03.810 **Encounter for observation for suspected exposure to anthrax ruled out** POA Z1

Z03.818 **Encounter for observation for suspected exposure to other biological agents ruled out** POA Z1

Z03.89 **Encounter for observation for other suspected diseases and conditions ruled out** POA Z1

Z04 **Encounter for examination and observation for other reasons**

INCLUDES *encounter for examination for medicolegal reasons*

This category is to be used when a person without a diagnosis is suspected of having an abnormal condition, without signs or symptoms, which requires study, but after examination

and observation, is ruled-out. This category is also for use for administrative and legal observation status.

Z04.1 **Encounter for examination and observation following transport accident** Z1

EXCLUDES1 *encounter for examination and observation following work accident (Z04.2)*

Z04.2 **Encounter for examination and observation following work accident**

Z04.3 **Encounter for examination and observation following other accident** Z1

Z04.4 **Encounter for examination and observation following alleged rape**

Encounter for examination and observation of victim following alleged rape

Encounter for examination and observation of victim following alleged sexual abuse

Z04.41 **Encounter for examination and observation following alleged adult rape** A Z1

AHA: Q4 2016

Suspected adult rape, ruled out

Suspected adult sexual abuse, ruled out

Z04.42 **Encounter for examination and observation following alleged child rape** P Z1

AHA: Q4 2016

Suspected child rape, ruled out

Suspected child sexual abuse, ruled out

Z04.6 **Encounter for general psychiatric examination, requested by authority** Z1

Z04.7 **Encounter for examination and observation following alleged physical abuse**

Z04.71 **Encounter for examination and observation following alleged adult physical abuse** A Z1

Suspected adult physical abuse, ruled out

EXCLUDES1 *confirmed case of adult physical abuse (T74.-)*

encounter for examination and observation following alleged adult sexual abuse (Z04.41)

suspected case of adult physical abuse, not ruled out (T76.-)

Z04.72 **Encounter for examination and observation following alleged child physical abuse** P Z1

Suspected child physical abuse, ruled out

EXCLUDES1 *confirmed case of child physical abuse (T74.-)*

encounter for examination and observation following alleged child sexual abuse (Z04.42)

suspected case of child physical abuse, not ruled out (T76.-)

Z04.8 **Encounter for examination and observation for other specified reasons** PDxIn Z1

Encounter for examination and observation for request for expert evidence

Z04.9 **Encounter for examination and observation for unspecified reason** PDxIn Z1

Encounter for observation NOS

▲ Z05 **Encounter for observation and evaluation of newborn for suspected diseases and conditions ruled out**

This category is to be used for newborns, within the neonatal period (the first 28 days of life), who are suspected of having an abnormal condition, ▶but without signs or symptoms, and which,◀ after examination and observation, is ruled out.

Z05.0 **Observation and evaluation of newborn for suspected cardiac condition ruled out** POA PDxIn

AHA: Q4 2016

Z05.1 **Observation and evaluation of newborn for suspected infectious condition ruled out** POA PDxIn

AHA: Q4 2016

Z05.2 **Observation and evaluation of newborn for suspected neurological condition ruled out** POA PDxIn

AHA: Q4 2016

Z05.3 **Observation and evaluation of newborn for suspected respiratory condition ruled out** POA PDxIn

AHA: Q4 2016

Unspecified Code   Other Specified Code   Manifestation Code   N Newborn   P Pediatric   M Maternity   A Adult   ♂ Male   ♀ Female
● New Code   ▲ Revised Code Title   ▶◀ Revised Text   **NOTES** *INCLUDES* *EXCLUDES 1* Not coded here   *EXCLUDES 2* Not included here
4th character required   5th character required   6th character required   7th character required
Extension 'X' Alert   HAC Hospital-acquired condition (HAC) alert   **AHA** AHA Coding Clinic©

Z05.4 Observation and evaluation of newborn for suspected genetic, metabolic or immunologic condition ruled out

Z05.41 Observation and evaluation of newborn for suspected genetic condition ruled out POA PDxIn
AHA: Q4 2016

Z05.42 Observation and evaluation of newborn for suspected metabolic condition ruled out POA PDxIn
AHA: Q4 2016

Z05.43 Observation and evaluation of newborn for suspected immunologic condition ruled out POA PDxIn
AHA: Q4 2016

Z05.5 Observation and evaluation of newborn for suspected gastrointestinal condition ruled out POA PDxIn
AHA: Q4 2016

Z05.6 Observation and evaluation of newborn for suspected genitourinary condition ruled out POA PDxIn
AHA: Q4 2016

Z05.7 Observation and evaluation of newborn for suspected skin, subcutaneous, musculoskeletal and connective tissue condition ruled out

Z05.71 Observation and evaluation of newborn for suspected skin and subcutaneous tissue condition ruled out POA PDxIn
AHA: Q4 2016

Z05.72 Observation and evaluation of newborn for suspected musculoskeletal condition ruled out POA PDxIn
AHA: Q4 2016

Z05.73 Observation and evaluation of newborn for suspected connective tissue condition ruled out POA PDxIn
AHA: Q4 2016

Z05.8 Observation and evaluation of newborn for other specified suspected condition ruled out POA PDxIn
AHA: Q4 2016

Z05.9 Observation and evaluation of newborn for unspecified suspected condition ruled out POA PDxIn
AHA: Q4 2016

Z08 Encounter for follow-up examination after completed treatment for malignant neoplasm POA PDxIn
Medical surveillance following completed treatment
Use additional code to identify any acquired absence of organs (Z90.-)
Use additional code to identify the personal history of malignant neoplasm (Z85.-)
EXCLUDES1 aftercare following medical care (Z43-Z49, Z51)

Z09 Encounter for follow-up examination after completed treatment for conditions other than malignant neoplasm POA PDxIn
AHA: Q1 2017, Q1 2015
Medical surveillance following completed treatment
Use additional code to identify any applicable history of disease code (Z86.-. Z87.-)
EXCLUDES1 aftercare following medical care (Z43-Z49, Z51)
surveillance of contraception (Z30.4-)
surveillance of prosthetic and other medical devices (Z44-Z46)

Z11 Encounter for screening for infectious and parasitic diseases
Screening is the testing for disease or disease precursors in asymptomatic individuals so that early detection and treatment can be provided for those who test positive for the disease.
EXCLUDES1 encounter for diagnostic examination-code to sign or symptom

Z11.0 Encounter for screening for intestinal infectious diseases POA PDxIn

Z11.1 Encounter for screening for respiratory tuberculosis POA PDxIn

Z11.2 Encounter for screening for other bacterial diseases POA PDxIn

Z11.3 Encounter for screening for infections with a predominantly sexual mode of transmission POA PDxIn
EXCLUDES2 encounter for screening for human immunodeficiency virus [HIV] (Z11.4)
encounter for screening for human papillomavirus (Z11.51)

Z11.4 Encounter for screening for human immunodeficiency virus [HIV] POA PDxIn

Z11.5 Encounter for screening for other viral diseases
EXCLUDES2 encounter for screening for viral intestinal disease (Z11.0)

Z11.51 Encounter for screening for human papillomavirus (HPV) POA PDxIn

Z11.59 Encounter for screening for other viral diseases POA PDxIn

Z11.6 Encounter for screening for other protozoal diseases and helminthiases POA PDxIn
EXCLUDES2 encounter for screening for protozoal intestinal disease (Z11.0)

Z11.8 Encounter for screening for other infectious and parasitic diseases POA PDxIn
Encounter for screening for chlamydia
Encounter for screening for rickettsial
Encounter for screening for spirochetal
Encounter for screening for mycoses

Z11.9 Encounter for screening for infectious and parasitic diseases, unspecified POA PDxIn

Z12 Encounter for screening for malignant neoplasms
Screening is the testing for disease or disease precursors in asymptomatic individuals so that early detection and treatment can be provided for those who test positive for the disease.
Use additional code to identify any family history of malignant neoplasm (Z80.-)
EXCLUDES1 encounter for diagnostic examination-code to sign or symptom

Z12.0 Encounter for screening for malignant neoplasm of stomach POA PDxIn

Z12.1 Encounter for screening for malignant neoplasm of intestinal tract

Z12.10 Encounter for screening for malignant neoplasm of intestinal tract, unspecified POA PDxIn

Z12.11 Encounter for screening for malignant neoplasm of colon POA PDxIn
AHA: Q1 2017
Encounter for screening colonoscopy NOS

Z12.12 Encounter for screening for malignant neoplasm of rectum POA PDxIn

Z12.13 Encounter for screening for malignant neoplasm of small intestine POA PDxIn

Z12.2 Encounter for screening for malignant neoplasm of respiratory organs POA PDxIn

Z12.3 Encounter for screening for malignant neoplasm of breast

Z12.31 Encounter for screening mammogram for malignant neoplasm of breast POA PDxIn
AHA: Q1 2015
EXCLUDES1 inconclusive mammogram (R92.2)

Z12.39 Encounter for other screening for malignant neoplasm of breast POA PDxIn

Z12.4 Encounter for screening for malignant neoplasm of cervix POA ♀
Encounter for screening pap smear for malignant neoplasm of cervix
EXCLUDES1 when screening is part of general gynecological examination (Z01.4-)
EXCLUDES2 encounter for screening for human papillomavirus (Z11.51)

Z12.5 Encounter for screening for malignant neoplasm of prostate POA ♂

Z12.6 Encounter for screening for malignant neoplasm of bladder POA PDxIn

Z12.7 Encounter for screening for malignant neoplasm of other genitourinary organs

Z12.71 Encounter for screening for malignant neoplasm of testis POA ♂ PDxIn

Z12.72 Encounter for screening for malignant neoplasm of vagina POA ♀ PDxIn
Vaginal pap smear status-post hysterectomy for non-malignant condition

PDxIn Unacceptable principal diagnosis symbol per Medicare code edits   POA Code exempt from diagnosis present on admission requirement
? Questionable admission   CC Complication or comorbidity   CC-MCC Exc CC/MCC exclusion   MCC Major complication or comorbidity
Principal diagnosis as its own CC   Principal diagnosis as its own MCC   HCC HCC diagnosis code   RxHCC RxHCC diagnosis code
MACRA code   Z code as first-listed diagnosis

1258   When symbols appear on a code that requires a 7th character extension, refer to Appendix B to identify applicable 7th character codes.   2018 ICD-10-CM

Use additional code to identify acquired absence of uterus (Z90.71-)

EXCLUDES1 *vaginal pap smear status-post hysterectomy for malignant conditions (Z08)*

Z12.73 Encounter for screening for malignant neoplasm of ovary POA ♀ PDxIn

Z12.79 Encounter for screening for malignant neoplasm of other genitourinary organs POA PDxIn

⑤ᵗʰ Z12.8 Encounter for screening for malignant neoplasm of other sites

Z12.81 Encounter for screening for malignant neoplasm of oral cavity POA PDxIn

Z12.82 Encounter for screening for malignant neoplasm of nervous system POA PDxIn

Z12.83 Encounter for screening for malignant neoplasm of skin POA PDxIn

Z12.89 Encounter for screening for malignant neoplasm of other sites POA PDxIn

Z12.9 Encounter for screening for malignant neoplasm, site unspecified POA PDxIn

④ᵗʰ Z13 Encounter for screening for other diseases and disorders

Screening is the testing for disease or disease precursors in asymptomatic individuals so that early detection and treatment can be provided for those who test positive for the disease.

EXCLUDES1 *encounter for diagnostic examination-code to sign or symptom*

Z13.0 Encounter for screening for diseases of the blood and blood-forming organs and certain disorders involving the immune mechanism POA PDxIn

Z13.1 Encounter for screening for diabetes mellitus POA PDxIn

⑤ᵗʰ Z13.2 Encounter for screening for nutritional, metabolic and other endocrine disorders

Z13.21 Encounter for screening for nutritional disorder POA PDxIn

⑥ᵗʰ Z13.22 Encounter for screening for metabolic disorder

Z13.220 Encounter for screening for lipoid disorders POA PDxIn

Encounter for screening for cholesterol level

Encounter for screening for hypercholesterolemia

Encounter for screening for hyperlipidemia

Z13.228 Encounter for screening for other metabolic disorders POA PDxIn

Z13.29 Encounter for screening for other suspected endocrine disorder POA PDxIn

EXCLUDES1 *encounter for screening for diabetes mellitus (Z13.1)*

Z13.4 Encounter for screening for certain developmental disorders in childhood P POA PDxIn

Encounter for screening for developmental handicaps in early childhood

EXCLUDES1 *routine development testing of infant or child (Z00.1-)*

Z13.5 Encounter for screening for eye and ear disorders POA PDxIn

AHA: Q3 2016

EXCLUDES2 *encounter for general hearing examination (Z01.1-)*

encounter for general vision examination (Z01.0-)

Z13.6 Encounter for screening for cardiovascular disorders POA PDxIn

⑤ᵗʰ Z13.7 Encounter for screening for genetic and chromosomal anomalies

EXCLUDES1 *genetic testing for procreative management (Z31.4-)*

Z13.71 Encounter for nonprocreative screening for genetic disease carrier status POA PDxIn

Z13.79 Encounter for other screening for genetic and chromosomal anomalies POA PDxIn

⑤ᵗʰ Z13.8 Encounter for screening for other specified diseases and disorders

EXCLUDES2 *screening for malignant neoplasms (Z12.-)*

⑥ᵗʰ Z13.81 Encounter for screening for digestive system disorders

Z13.810 Encounter for screening for upper gastrointestinal disorder POA PDxIn

Z13.811 Encounter for screening for lower gastrointestinal disorder POA PDxIn

EXCLUDES1 *encounter for screening for intestinal infectious disease (Z11.0)*

Z13.818 Encounter for screening for other digestive system disorders POA PDxIn

⑥ᵗʰ Z13.82 Encounter for screening for musculoskeletal disorder

Z13.820 Encounter for screening for osteoporosis POA PDxIn

Z13.828 Encounter for screening for other musculoskeletal disorder POA PDxIn

Z13.83 Encounter for screening for respiratory disorder NEC POA PDxIn

EXCLUDES1 *encounter for screening for respiratory tuberculosis (Z11.1)*

Z13.84 Encounter for screening for dental disorders POA PDxIn

⑥ᵗʰ Z13.85 Encounter for screening for nervous system disorders

Z13.850 Encounter for screening for traumatic brain injury POA PDxIn

Z13.858 Encounter for screening for other nervous system disorders POA PDxIn

Z13.88 Encounter for screening for disorder due to exposure to contaminants POA PDxIn

EXCLUDES1 *those exposed to contaminants without suspected disorders (Z57.-, Z77.-)*

Z13.89 Encounter for screening for other disorder POA PDxIn

Encounter for screening for genitourinary disorders

Z13.9 Encounter for screening, unspecified POA PDxIn

Genetic carrier and genetic susceptibility to disease (Z14-Z15)

④ᵗʰ Z14 Genetic carrier

⑤ᵗʰ Z14.0 Hemophilia A carrier

Z14.01 Asymptomatic hemophilia A carrier POA PDxIn

Z14.02 Symptomatic hemophilia A carrier POA PDxIn

Z14.1 Cystic fibrosis carrier POA PDxIn

Z14.8 Genetic carrier of other disease POA PDxIn

④ᵗʰ Z15 Genetic susceptibility to disease

INCLUDES *confirmed abnormal gene*

Use additional code, if applicable, for any associated family history of the disease (Z80-Z84)

EXCLUDES1 *chromosomal anomalies (Q90-Q99)*

⑤ᵗʰ Z15.0 Genetic susceptibility to malignant neoplasm

Code first, if applicable, any current malignant neoplasm (C00-C75, C81-C96)

Use additional code, if applicable, for any personal history of malignant neoplasm (Z85.-)

Z15.01 Genetic susceptibility to malignant neoplasm of breast POA PDxIn

Z15.02 Genetic susceptibility to malignant neoplasm of ovary POA ♀ PDxIn

Z15.03 Genetic susceptibility to malignant neoplasm of prostate POA ♂ PDxIn

Z15.04 Genetic susceptibility to malignant neoplasm of endometrium POA ♀ PDxIn

Z15.09 Genetic susceptibility to other malignant neoplasm POA PDxIn

⑤ᵗʰ Z15.8 Genetic susceptibility to other disease

Z15.81 Genetic susceptibility to multiple endocrine neoplasia [MEN] POA PDxIn

EXCLUDES1 *multiple endocrine neoplasia [MEN] syndromes (E31.2-)*

Z15.89 Genetic susceptibility to other disease POA PDxIn

Unspecified Code	Other Specified Code	Manifestation Code Ⓝ Newborn Ⓟ Pediatric Ⓜ Maternity Ⓐ Adult ♂ Male ♀ Female

● New Code ▲ Revised Code Title ►◄ Revised Text **NOTES** *INCLUDES* *EXCLUDES 1* Not coded here *EXCLUDES 2* Not included here

④ᵗʰ 4ᵗʰ character required ⑤ᵗʰ 5ᵗʰ character required ⑥ᵗʰ 6ᵗʰ character required ⑦ᵗʰ 7ᵗʰ character required

⑦ˣ Extension 'X' Alert **HAC** Hospital-acquired condition (HAC) alert **AHA** AHA Coding Clinic©

Resistance to antimicrobial drugs (Z16)

Z16 Resistance to antimicrobial drugs

NOTES   The codes in this category are provided for use as additional codes to identify the resistance and non-responsiveness of a condition to antimicrobial drugs.

Code first the infection

EXCLUDES1 *Methicillin resistant Staphylococcus aureus infection (A49.02)*

Methicillin resistant Staphylococcus aureus pneumonia (J15.212)

Sepsis due to Methicillin resistant Staphylococcus aureus (A41.02)

Z16.1 Resistance to beta lactam antibiotics

   Z16.10 Resistance to unspecified beta lactam antibiotics PDxIn

   Z16.11 Resistance to penicillins
      Resistance to amoxicillin
      Resistance to ampicillin

   Z16.12 Extended spectrum beta lactamase (ESBL) resistance PDxIn
      EXCLUDES2 *Methicillin resistant Staphylococcus aureus infection in diseases classified elsewhere (B95.62)*

   Z16.19 Resistance to other specified beta lactam antibiotics PDxIn
      Resistance to cephalosporins

Z16.2 Resistance to other antibiotics

   Z16.20 Resistance to unspecified antibiotic PDxIn
      Resistance to antibiotics NOS

   Z16.21 Resistance to vancomycin PDxIn

   Z16.22 Resistance to vancomycin related antibiotics PDxIn

   Z16.23 Resistance to quinolones and fluoroquinolones PDxIn

   Z16.24 Resistance to multiple antibiotics PDxIn

   Z16.29 Resistance to other single specified antibiotic PDxIn
      Resistance to aminoglycosides
      Resistance to macrolides
      Resistance to sulfonamides
      Resistance to tetracyclines

Z16.3 Resistance to other antimicrobial drugs
   EXCLUDES1 *resistance to antibiotics (Z16.1-, Z16.2-)*

   Z16.30 Resistance to unspecified antimicrobial drugs PDxIn
      Drug resistance NOS

   Z16.31 Resistance to antiparasitic drug(s) PDxIn
      Resistance to quinine and related compounds

   Z16.32 Resistance to antifungal drug(s) PDxIn

   Z16.33 Resistance to antiviral drug(s) PDxIn

   Z16.34 Resistance to antimycobacterial drug(s)
      Resistance to tuberculostatics

      Z16.341 Resistance to single antimycobacterial drug PDxIn
         Resistance to antimycobacterial drug NOS

      Z16.342 Resistance to multiple antimycobacterial drugs PDxIn

   Z16.35 Resistance to multiple antimicrobial drugs PDxIn
      EXCLUDES1 *Resistance to multiple antibiotics only (Z16.24)*

   Z16.39 Resistance to other specified antimicrobial drug PDxIn

Estrogen receptor status (Z17)

Z17 Estrogen receptor status
   Code first malignant neoplasm of breast (C50.-)

   Z17.0 Estrogen receptor positive status [ER+] POA PDxIn

   Z17.1 Estrogen receptor negative status [ER-] POA PDxIn

Retained foreign body fragments (Z18)

Z18 Retained foreign body fragments
   INCLUDES *embedded fragment (status)*
      embedded splinter (status)
      retained foreign body status

EXCLUDES1 *artificial joint prosthesis status (Z96.6-)*

foreign body accidentally left during a procedure (T81.5-)

foreign body entering through orifice (T15-T19)

in situ cardiac device (Z95.-)

organ or tissue replaced by means other than transplant (Z96.-, Z97.-)

organ or tissue replaced by transplant (Z94.-)

personal history of retained foreign body fully removed Z87.821

superficial foreign body (non-embedded splinter) - code to superficial foreign body, by site

Z18.0 Retained radioactive fragments

   Z18.01 Retained depleted uranium fragments POA PDxIn

   Z18.09 Other retained radioactive fragments POA PDxIn
      Other retained depleted isotope fragments
      Retained nontherapeutic radioactive fragments

Z18.1 Retained metal fragments
   EXCLUDES1 *retained radioactive metal fragments (Z18.01-Z18.09)*

   Z18.10 Retained metal fragments, unspecified POA PDxIn
      Retained metal fragment NOS

   Z18.11 Retained magnetic metal fragments POA PDxIn

   Z18.12 Retained nonmagnetic metal fragments POA PDxIn

Z18.2 Retained plastic fragments
   Acrylics fragments
   Diethylhexylphthalates fragments
   Isocyanate fragments

Z18.3 Retained organic fragments

   Z18.31 Retained animal quills or spines POA PDxIn

   Z18.32 Retained tooth POA PDxIn

   Z18.33 Retained wood fragments POA PDxIn

   Z18.39 Other retained organic fragments POA PDxIn

Z18.8 Other specified retained foreign body

   Z18.81 Retained glass fragments POA PDxIn

   Z18.83 Retained stone or crystalline fragments POA PDxIn
      Retained concrete or cement fragments

   Z18.89 Other specified retained foreign body fragments POA PDxIn
      AHA: Q3 2016

   Z18.9 Retained foreign body fragments, unspecified material POA PDxIn

Hormone sensitivity malignancy status (Z19)

Z19 Hormone sensitivity malignancy status
   Code first malignant neoplasm -see Table of Neoplasms, by site, malignant

   Z19.1 Hormone sensitive malignancy status POA PDxIn
      AHA: Q4 2016

   Z19.2 Hormone resistant malignancy status POA PDxIn
      AHA: Q4 2016
      Castrate resistant prostate malignancy status

Persons with potential health hazards related to communicable diseases (Z20-Z29)

Z20 Contact with and (suspected) exposure to communicable diseases
   EXCLUDES1 *carrier of infectious disease (Z22.-)*
      diagnosed current infectious or parasitic disease -see Alphabetic Index
   EXCLUDES2 *personal history of infectious and parasitic diseases (Z86.1-)*

   Z20.0 Contact with and (suspected) exposure to intestinal infectious diseases

      Z20.01 Contact with and (suspected) exposure to intestinal infectious diseases due to Escherichia coli (E. coli)

      Z20.09 Contact with and (suspected) exposure to other intestinal infectious diseases PDxIn

   Z20.1 Contact with and (suspected) exposure to tuberculosis PDxIn

   Z20.2 Contact with and (suspected) exposure to infections with a predominantly sexual mode of transmission PDxIn

   Z20.3 Contact with and (suspected) exposure to rabies PDxIn

   Z20.4 Contact with and (suspected) exposure to rubella PDxIn

---

PDxIn Unacceptable principal diagnosis symbol per Medicare code edits   POA Code exempt from diagnosis present on admission requirement
? Questionable admission   CC Complication or comorbidity   CC-MCC Exc CC/MCC exclusion   MCC Major complication or comorbidity
Principal diagnosis as its own CC   Principal diagnosis as its own MCC   HCC HCC diagnosis code   RxHCC RxHCC diagnosis code
MACRA code   Z Z code as first-listed diagnosis

When symbols appear on a code that requires a 7th character extension, refer to Appendix B to identify applicable 7th character codes.

Z20.5 Contact with and (suspected) exposure to viral hepatitis

Z20.6 Contact with and (suspected) exposure to human immunodeficiency virus [HIV]

EXCLUDES1 asymptomatic human immunodeficiency virus [HIV] HIV infection status (Z21)

Z20.7 Contact with and (suspected) exposure to pediculosis, acariasis and other infestations PDxIn

5ᵗʰ Z20.8 Contact with and (suspected) exposure to other communicable diseases

6ᵗʰ Z20.81 Contact with and (suspected) exposure to other bacterial communicable diseases

Z20.810 Contact with and (suspected) exposure to anthrax PDxIn

Z20.811 Contact with and (suspected) exposure to meningococcus

Z20.818 Contact with and (suspected) exposure to other bacterial communicable diseases PDxIn

6ᵗʰ Z20.82 Contact with and (suspected) exposure to other viral communicable diseases

Z20.820 Contact with and (suspected) exposure to varicella

Z20.828 Contact with and (suspected) exposure to other viral communicable diseases

AHA: Q4 2016

Z20.89 Contact with and (suspected) exposure to other communicable diseases PDxIn

Z20.9 Contact with and (suspected) exposure to unspecified communicable disease PDxIn

Z21 Asymptomatic human immunodeficiency virus [HIV] infection status HCC ? RxHCC

HIV positive NOS

Code first Human immunodeficiency virus [HIV] disease complicating pregnancy, childbirth and the puerperium, if applicable (O98.7-)

EXCLUDES1 acquired immunodeficiency syndrome (B20)

contact with human immunodeficiency virus [HIV] (Z20.6)

exposure to human immunodeficiency virus [HIV] (Z20.6)

human immunodeficiency virus [HIV] disease (B20)

inconclusive laboratory evidence of human immunodeficiency virus [HIV] (R75)

4ᵗʰ Z22 Carrier of infectious disease

INCLUDES colonization status

suspected carrier

EXCLUDES2 carrier of viral hepatitis (B18.-)

Z22.0 Carrier of typhoid POA PDxIn

Z22.1 Carrier of other intestinal infectious diseases POA PDxIn

Z22.2 Carrier of diphtheria POA PDxIn

5ᵗʰ Z22.3 Carrier of other specified bacterial diseases

Z22.31 Carrier of bacterial disease due to meningococci POA PDxIn

6ᵗʰ Z22.32 Carrier of bacterial disease due to staphylococci

Z22.321 Carrier or suspected carrier of Methicillin susceptible Staphylococcus aureus POA PDxIn

MSSA colonization

Z22.322 Carrier or suspected carrier of Methicillin resistant Staphylococcus aureus POA PDxIn

MRSA colonization

6ᵗʰ Z22.33 Carrier of bacterial disease due to streptococci

Z22.330 Carrier of Group B streptococcus POA PDxIn

EXCLUDES1 Carrier of streptococcus group B (GBS) complicating pregnancy, childbirth and the puerperium (O99.82-)

Z22.338 Carrier of other streptococcus POA PDxIn

Z22.39 Carrier of other specified bacterial diseases POA PDxIn

Z22.4 Carrier of infections with a predominantly sexual mode of transmission POA PDxIn

Z22.6 Carrier of human T-lymphotropic virus type-1 [HTLV-1] infection POA PDxIn

Z22.8 Carrier of other infectious diseases POA PDxIn

Z22.9 Carrier of infectious disease, unspecified POA PDxIn

Z23 Encounter for immunization

Code first any routine childhood examination

NOTES procedure codes are required to identify the types of immunizations given

4ᵗʰ Z28 Immunization not carried out and underimmunization status

INCLUDES vaccination not carried out

5ᵗʰ Z28.0 Immunization not carried out because of contraindication

Z28.01 Immunization not carried out because of acute illness of patient POA PDxIn

Z28.02 Immunization not carried out because of chronic illness or condition of patient POA PDxIn

Z28.03 Immunization not carried out because of immune compromised state of patient POA PDxIn

Z28.04 Immunization not carried out because of patient allergy to vaccine or component POA PDxIn

Z28.09 Immunization not carried out because of other contraindication POA PDxIn

Z28.1 Immunization not carried out because of patient decision for reasons of belief or group pressure POA PDxIn

Immunization not carried out because of religious belief

5ᵗʰ Z28.2 Immunization not carried out because of patient decision for other and unspecified reason

Z28.20 Immunization not carried out because of patient decision for unspecified reason POA PDxIn

Z28.21 Immunization not carried out because of patient refusal POA PDxIn

Z28.29 Immunization not carried out because of patient decision for other reason POA PDxIn

Z28.3 Underimmunization status POA PDxIn

Delinquent immunization status

Lapsed immunization schedule status

5ᵗʰ Z28.8 Immunization not carried out for other reason

Z28.81 Immunization not carried out due to patient having had the disease POA PDxIn

Z28.82 Immunization not carried out because of caregiver refusal POA PDxIn

Immunization not carried out because of guardian refusal

Immunization not carried out because of parent refusal

EXCLUDES1 immunization not carried out because of caregiver refusal because of religious belief (Z28.1)

Z28.89 Immunization not carried out for other reason POA PDxIn

Z28.9 Immunization not carried out for unspecified reason POA PDxIn

4ᵗʰ Z29 Encounter for other prophylactic measures

Excludes 1: desensitization to allergens (Z51.6)

prophylactic surgery (Z40.-)

5ᵗʰ Z29.1 Encounter for prophylactic immunotherapy

Encounter for administration of immunoglobulin

Z29.11 Encounter for prophylactic immunotherapy for respiratory syncytial virus (RSV) POA PDxIn

AHA: Q4 2016

Z29.12 Encounter for prophylactic antivenin POA PDxIn

AHA: Q4 2016

Z29.13 Encounter for prophylactic Rho(D) immune globulin POA PDxIn

AHA: Q4 2016

Z29.14 Encounter for prophylactic rabies immune globin POA PDxIn

AHA: Q4 2016

Z29.3 Encounter for prophylactic fluoride administration POA PDxIn

AHA: Q4 2016

Z29.8 Encounter for other specified prophylactic measures POA PDxIn

AHA: Q4 2016

Z29.9 Encounter for prophylactic measures, unspecified POA PDxIn

AHA: Q4 2016

Unspecified Code   Other Specified Code   Manifestation Code   N Newborn   P Pediatric   M Maternity   A Adult   ♂ Male   ♀ Female
● New Code   ▲ Revised Code Title   ▶◀ Revised Text   NOTES   INCLUDES   EXCLUDES 1 Not coded here   EXCLUDES 2 Not included here
4ᵗʰ 4ᵗʰ character required   5ᵗʰ 5ᵗʰ character required   6ᵗʰ 6ᵗʰ character required   7ᵗʰ 7ᵗʰ character required
Extension 'X' Alert   HAC Hospital-acquired condition (HAC) alert   AHA AHA Coding Clinic©

Persons encountering health services in circumstances related to reproduction (Z30-Z39)

Z30 Encounter for contraceptive management

Z30.0 Encounter for general counseling and advice on contraception

Z30.01 Encounter for initial prescription of contraceptives

EXCLUDES1 encounter for surveillance of contraceptives (Z30.4-)

Z30.011 Encounter for initial prescription of contraceptive pills

Z30.012 Encounter for prescription of emergency contraception

Encounter for postcoital contraception

Z30.013 Encounter for initial prescription of injectable contraceptive

Z30.014 Encounter for initial prescription of intrauterine contraceptive device

EXCLUDES1 encounter for insertion of intrauterine contraceptive device (Z30.430, Z30.432)

Z30.015 Encounter for initial prescription of vaginal ring hormonal contraceptive

AHA: Q4 2016

Z30.016 Encounter for initial prescription of transdermal patch hormonal contraceptive device

AHA: Q4 2016

Z30.017 Encounter for initial prescription of implantable subdermal contraceptive

AHA: Q4 2016

Z30.018 Encounter for initial prescription of other contraceptives

Encounter for initial prescription of barrier contraception

Encounter for initial prescription of diaphragm

Z30.019 Encounter for initial prescription of contraceptives, unspecified

Z30.02 Counseling and instruction in natural family planning to avoid pregnancy

Z30.09 Encounter for other general counseling and advice on contraception

Encounter for family planning advice NOS

Z30.2 Encounter for sterilization

Z30.4 Encounter for surveillance of contraceptives

Z30.40 Encounter for surveillance of contraceptives, unspecified

Z30.41 Encounter for surveillance of contraceptive pills

Encounter for repeat prescription for contraceptive pill

Z30.42 Encounter for surveillance of injectable contraceptive

Z30.43 Encounter for surveillance of intrauterine contraceptive device

Z30.430 Encounter for insertion of intrauterine contraceptive device

Z30.431 Encounter for routine checking of intrauterine contraceptive device

Z30.432 Encounter for removal of intrauterine contraceptive device

Z30.433 Encounter for removal and reinsertion of intrauterine contraceptive device

Encounter for replacement of intrauterine contraceptive device

Z30.44 Encounter for surveillance of vaginal ring hormonal contraceptive device

AHA: Q4 2016

Z30.45 Encounter for surveillance of transdermal patch hormonal contraceptive device

AHA: Q4 2016

Z30.46 Encounter for surveillance of implantable subdermal contraceptive

AHA: Q4 2016

Encounter for checking, reinsertion or removal of implantable subdermal contraceptive

Z30.49 Encounter for surveillance of other contraceptives

Encounter for surveillance of barrier contraception

Encounter for surveillance of diaphragm

Z30.8 Encounter for other contraceptive management

Encounter for postvasectomy sperm count

Encounter for routine examination for contraceptive maintenance

EXCLUDES1 sperm count following sterilization reversal (Z31.42)

sperm count for fertility testing (Z31.41)

Z30.9 Encounter for contraceptive management, unspecified

Z31 Encounter for procreative management

EXCLUDES1 complications associated with artificial fertilization (N98.-)

female infertility (N97.-)

male infertility (N46.-)

Z31.0 Encounter for reversal of previous sterilization

Z31.4 Encounter for procreative investigation and testing

EXCLUDES1 postvasectomy sperm count (Z30.8)

Z31.41 Encounter for fertility testing

Encounter for fallopian tube patency testing

Encounter for sperm count for fertility testing

Z31.42 Aftercare following sterilization reversal

Sperm count following sterilization reversal

Z31.43 Encounter for genetic testing of female for procreative management

Use additional code for recurrent pregnancy loss, if applicable (N96, O26.2-)

EXCLUDES1 nonprocreative genetic testing (Z13.7-)

Z31.430 Encounter of female for testing for genetic disease carrier status for procreative management

Z31.438 Encounter for other genetic testing of female for procreative management

Z31.44 Encounter for genetic testing of male for procreative management

EXCLUDES1 nonprocreative genetic testing (Z13.7-)

Z31.440 Encounter of male for testing for genetic disease carrier status for procreative management

Z31.441 Encounter for testing of male partner of patient with recurrent pregnancy loss

Z31.448 Encounter for other genetic testing of male for procreative management

Z31.49 Encounter for other procreative investigation and testing

▲ **Z31.5** Encounter for ▶procreative◀ genetic counseling

Z31.6 Encounter for general counseling and advice on procreation

Z31.61 Procreative counseling and advice using natural family planning

Z31.62 Encounter for fertility preservation counseling

Encounter for fertility preservation counseling prior to cancer therapy

Encounter for fertility preservation counseling prior to surgical removal of gonads

Z31.69 Encounter for other general counseling and advice on procreation

Z31.7 Encounter for procreative management and counseling for gestational carrier

AHA: Q4 2016

EXCLUDES1 pregnant state, gestational carrier (Z33.3)

Z31.8 Encounter for other procreative management

Z31.81 Encounter for male factor infertility in female patient

1st 1st trimester   2nd 2nd trimester   3rd 3rd trimester   PDx Unacceptable principal diagnosis symbol per Medicare code edits

POA Code exempt from diagnosis present on admission requirement   ? Questionable admission   cc Complication or comorbidity

cc/mcc excl CC/MCC exclusion   mcc Major complication or comorbidity   Principal diagnosis as its own CC   Principal diagnosis as its own MCC

HCC HCC diagnosis code   RxHCC RxHCC diagnosis code   MACRA code   Z1 Z code as first-listed diagnosis

1262   When symbols appear on a code that requires a 7th character extension, refer to Appendix B to identify applicable 7th character codes.   **2018 ICD-10-CM**

Z31.82 Encounter for Rh incompatibility **status** POA ♀ PDxIn Z1
AHA: Q3 2015

Z31.83 Encounter for assisted reproductive fertility procedure cycle POA ♀ PDxIn Z1
Patient undergoing in vitro fertilization cycle
Use additional code to identify the type of infertility
EXCLUDES1 pre-cycle diagnosis and testing -code to reason for encounter

Z31.84 Encounter for fertility preservation procedure POA PDxIn Z1
Encounter for fertility preservation procedure prior to cancer therapy
Encounter for fertility preservation procedure prior to surgical removal of gonads

Z31.89 Encounter for other procreative management POA PDxIn

Z31.9 Encounter for procreative management, unspecified POA PDxIn

4th⃝ Z32 Encounter for pregnancy test and childbirth and childcare instruction

5th⃝ Z32.0 Encounter for pregnancy test

Z32.00 Encounter for pregnancy test, result unknown ♀
Encounter for pregnancy test NOS

Z32.01 Encounter for pregnancy test, result positive M ♀

Z32.02 Encounter for pregnancy test, result negative ♀

Z32.2 Encounter for childbirth instruction PDxIn

Z32.3 Encounter for childcare instruction PDxIn
Encounter for prenatal or postpartum childcare instruction

4th⃝ Z33 Pregnant state

Z33.1 Pregnant state, incidental *patient seen for something unrelated to pregnancy but code pregnant as well* M ♀ PDxIn
Pregnant state NOS
EXCLUDES1 complications of pregnancy (O00-O9A)
pregnant state, gestational carrier (Z33.3)

Z33.2 Encounter for elective termination of pregnancy M ♀ Z1
EXCLUDES1 early fetal death with retention of dead fetus (O02.1)
late fetal death (O36.4)
spontaneous abortion (O03)

Z33.3 Pregnant state, gestational carrier M POA ♀ PDxIn
AHA: Q4 2016
EXCLUDES1 encounter for procreative management and counseling for gestational carrier (Z31.7)

4th⃝ Z34 Encounter for supervision of normal pregnancy *Can only use by itself*
EXCLUDES1 any complication of pregnancy (O00-O9A)
encounter for pregnancy test (Z32.0-)
encounter for supervision of high risk pregnancy (O09.-)

5th⃝ Z34.0 Encounter for supervision of normal first **pregnancy**

Z34.00 Encounter for supervision of normal first pregnancy, unspecified trimester M POA ♀ PDxIn Z1

Z34.01 Encounter for supervision of normal first pregnancy, first trimester 1st M POA ♀ PDxIn Z1

Z34.02 Encounter for supervision of normal first pregnancy, second trimester 2nd M POA ♀ PDxIn Z1

Z34.03 Encounter for supervision of normal first pregnancy, third trimester 3rd M POA ♀ PDxIn Z1

5th⃝ Z34.8 Encounter for supervision of other **normal pregnancy**

Z34.80 Encounter for supervision of other normal pregnancy, unspecified trimester M POA ♀ PDxIn Z1

Z34.81 Encounter for supervision of other normal pregnancy, first **trimester** 1st M POA ♀ PDxIn Z1

Z34.82 Encounter for supervision of other normal pregnancy, second **trimester** 2nd M POA ♀ PDxIn Z1

Z34.83 Encounter for supervision of other normal pregnancy, third **trimester** 3rd M POA ♀ PDxIn Z1

5th⃝ Z34.9 Encounter for supervision of normal pregnancy, unspecified

Z34.90 Encounter for supervision of normal pregnancy, unspecified trimester M POA ♀ PDxIn Z1

Z34.91 Encounter for supervision of normal pregnancy, first trimester 1st M POA ♀ PDxIn Z1

Z34.92 Encounter for supervision of normal pregnancy, second trimester 2nd M POA ♀ PDxIn Z1

Z34.93 Encounter for supervision of normal pregnancy, third trimester 3rd M POA ♀ PDxIn Z1

4th⃝ Z36 Encounter for antenatal screening of mother
INCLUDES Encounter for placental sample (taken vaginally)
Screening is the testing for disease or disease precursors in asymptomatic individuals so that early detection and treatment can be provided for those who test positive for the disease.
EXCLUDES1 diagnostic examination- code to sign or symptom
encounter for suspected maternal and fetal conditions ruled out (Z03.7-)
suspected fetal condition affecting management of pregnancy - code to condition in Chapter 15
EXCLUDES2 abnormal findings on antenatal screening of mother (O28.-)
genetic counseling and testing (Z31.43-, Z31.5)
routine prenatal care (Z34)

● **Z36.0 Encounter for antenatal screening for** chromosomal anomalies M ♀

● **Z36.1 Encounter for antenatal screening for** raised alphafetoprotein level M ♀
Encounter for antenatal screening for elevated maternal serum alphafetoprotein level

● **Z36.2 Encounter for other antenatal screening** follow-up M ♀
Non-visualized anatomy on a previous scan

● **Z36.3 Encounter for antenatal screening for** malformations M ♀
Screening for a suspected anomaly

● **Z36.4 Encounter for antenatal screening for** fetal growth retardation M ♀
Intrauterine growth restriction (IUGR)/small-for-dates

● **Z36.5 Encounter for antenatal screening for** isoimmunization M ♀

● **5th⃝ Z36.8 Encounter for** other **antenatal screening**

● **Z36.81 Encounter for antenatal screening for** hydrops fetalis M ♀

● **Z36.82 Encounter for antenatal screening for** nuchal translucency M ♀

● **Z36.83 Encounter for fetal screening for** congenital cardiac abnormalities M ♀

● **Z36.84 Encounter for antenatal screening for** fetal lung maturity M ♀

● **Z36.85 Encounter for antenatal screening for** Streptococcus B M ♀

● **Z36.86 Encounter for antenatal screening for** cervical length M ♀
Screening for risk of pre-term labor

● **Z36.87 Encounter for antenatal screening for** uncertain dates M ♀

● **Z36.88 Encounter for antenatal screening for** fetal macrosomia M ♀
Screening for large-for-dates

● **Z36.89 Encounter for other specified** antenatal screening M ♀

Z36.8A Encounter for antenatal screening for other genetic defects M ♀

● **Z36.9 Encounter for antenatal screening,** unspecified M ♀

4th⃝ Z3A Weeks of gestation
NOTES Codes from category Z3A are for use, only on the maternal record, to indicate the weeks of gestation of the pregnancy, if known.
Code first complications of pregnancy, childbirth and the puerperium ▶(O09-O9A)◀

5th⃝ Z3A.0 Weeks of gestation of pregnancy, unspecified or less than 10 weeks

Z3A.00 Weeks of gestation of pregnancy not specified M POA ♀ PDxIn

Z3A.01 Less than 8 weeks **gestation of pregnancy** 1st M POA ♀ PDxIn

Z3A.08 8 weeks **gestation of pregnancy** 1st M POA ♀ PDxIn

Z3A.09 9 weeks **gestation of pregnancy** 1st M POA ♀ PDxIn

5th⃝ Z3A.1 Weeks of gestation of pregnancy, weeks 10-19

Z3A.10 10 weeks **gestation of pregnancy** 1st M POA ♀ PDxIn

Z3A.11 11 weeks **gestation of pregnancy** 1st M POA ♀ PDxIn

Z3A.12 12 weeks **gestation of pregnancy** 1st M POA ♀ PDxIn

Z3A.13 13 weeks **gestation of pregnancy** 2nd M POA ♀ PDxIn

Unspecified Code   Other Specified Code   Manifestation Code   N Newborn   P Pediatric   M Maternity   A Adult   ♂ Male   ♀ Female
● New Code   ▲ Revised Code Title   ▶◀ Revised Text   NOTES   INCLUDES   EXCLUDES 1 Not coded here   EXCLUDES 2 Not included here
4th⃝ 4th character required   5th⃝ 5th character required   6th⃝ 6th character required   7th⃝ 7th character required
Extension 'X' Alert   HAC Hospital-acquired condition (HAC) alert   AHA AHA Coding Clinic©

Z3A.14 14 weeks **gestation of pregnancy** 2nd M PDx ♀ PDxIn
Z3A.15 15 weeks **gestation of pregnancy** 2nd M PDx ♀ PDxIn
Z3A.16 16 weeks **gestation of pregnancy** 2nd M PDx ♀ PDxIn
  AHA: Q4 2016
Z3A.17 17 weeks **gestation of pregnancy** 2nd M PDx ♀ PDxIn
Z3A.18 18 weeks **gestation of pregnancy** 2nd M PDx ♀ PDxIn
Z3A.19 19 weeks **gestation of pregnancy** 2nd M PDx ♀ PDxIn

5ᵗʰ **Z3A.2 Weeks of gestation of pregnancy, weeks** 20-29
Z3A.20 20 weeks **gestation of pregnancy** 2nd M PDx ♀ PDxIn
  AHA: Q4 2016
Z3A.21 21 weeks **gestation of pregnancy** 2nd M PDx ♀ PDxIn
Z3A.22 22 weeks **gestation of pregnancy** 2nd M PDx ♀ PDxIn
  AHA: Q4 2016
Z3A.23 23 weeks **gestation of pregnancy** 2nd M PDx ♀ PDxIn
Z3A.24 24 weeks **gestation of pregnancy** 2nd M PDx ♀ PDxIn
Z3A.25 25 weeks **gestation of pregnancy** 2nd M PDx ♀ PDxIn
Z3A.26 26 weeks **gestation of pregnancy** 2nd M PDx ♀ PDxIn
Z3A.27 27 weeks **gestation of pregnancy** 2nd M PDx ♀ PDxIn
Z3A.28 28 weeks **gestation of pregnancy** 3rd M PDx ♀ PDxIn
Z3A.29 29 weeks **gestation of pregnancy** 3rd M PDx ♀ PDxIn

5ᵗʰ **Z3A.3 Weeks of gestation of pregnancy, weeks** 30-39
Z3A.30 30 weeks **gestation of pregnancy** 3rd M PDx ♀ PDxIn
Z3A.31 31 weeks **gestation of pregnancy** 3rd M PDx ♀ PDxIn
Z3A.32 32 weeks **gestation of pregnancy** 3rd M PDx ♀ PDxIn
  AHA: Q4 2016
Z3A.33 33 weeks **gestation of pregnancy** 3rd M PDx ♀ PDxIn
Z3A.34 34 weeks **gestation of pregnancy** 3rd M PDx ♀ PDxIn
Z3A.35 35 weeks **gestation of pregnancy** 3rd M PDx ♀ PDxIn
Z3A.36 36 weeks **gestation of pregnancy** 3rd M PDx ♀ PDxIn
Z3A.37 37 weeks **gestation of pregnancy** 3rd M PDx ♀ PDxIn
Z3A.38 38 weeks **gestation of pregnancy** 3rd M PDx ♀ PDxIn
  AHA: Q2 2016
Z3A.39 39 weeks **gestation of pregnancy** 3rd M PDx ♀ PDxIn

5ᵗʰ **Z3A.4 Weeks of gestation of pregnancy, weeks** 40 or greater
Z3A.40 40 weeks **gestation of pregnancy** 3rd M PDx ♀ PDxIn
Z3A.41 41 weeks **gestation of pregnancy** 3rd M PDx ♀ PDxIn
Z3A.42 42 weeks **gestation of pregnancy** 3rd M PDx ♀ PDxIn
Z3A.49 Greater than 42 weeks **gestation of pregnancy** 3rd M PDx ♀ PDxIn

4ᵗʰ **Z37 Outcome of delivery**
  This category is intended for use as an additional code to identify the outcome of delivery on the mother's record. It is not for use on the newborn record.
  EXCLUDES1 stillbirth (P95)
Z37.0 **Single live birth** M PDx ♀ PDxIn
  AHA: Q2 2016
Z37.1 **Single stillbirth** M PDx ♀ PDxIn
Z37.2 **Twins, both liveborn** M PDx ♀ PDxIn
Z37.3 **Twins, one liveborn and one stillborn** M PDx ♀ PDxIn
Z37.4 **Twins, both stillborn** M PDx ♀ PDxIn
5ᵗʰ **Z37.5 Other** multiple births, all liveborn
Z37.50 **Multiple births, unspecified, all liveborn** M PDx ♀ PDxIn
Z37.51 **Triplets, all liveborn** M PDx ♀ PDxIn
Z37.52 **Quadruplets, all liveborn** M PDx ♀ PDxIn
Z37.53 **Quintuplets, all liveborn** M PDx ♀ PDxIn
Z37.54 **Sextuplets, all liveborn** M PDx ♀ PDxIn
Z37.59 **Other multiple births, all liveborn** M PDx ♀ PDxIn
5ᵗʰ **Z37.6 Other** multiple births, some liveborn
Z37.60 **Multiple births, unspecified, some liveborn** M PDx ♀ PDxIn
Z37.61 **Triplets, some liveborn** M PDx ♀ PDxIn
Z37.62 **Quadruplets, some liveborn** M PDx ♀ PDxIn
Z37.63 **Quintuplets, some liveborn** M PDx ♀ PDxIn
Z37.64 **Sextuplets, some liveborn** M PDx ♀ PDxIn
Z37.69 **Other multiple births, some liveborn** M PDx ♀ PDxIn
Z37.7 **Other multiple births, all stillborn** M PDx ♀ PDxIn
Z37.9 **Outcome of delivery, unspecified** M PDx ♀ PDxIn
  Multiple birth NOS
  Single birth NOS

4ᵗʰ **Z38 Liveborn infants according to place of birth and type of delivery**
  This category is for use as the principal code on the initial record of a newborn baby. It is to be used for the initial birth record only. It is not to be used on the mother's record. *[handwritten: Always primary diagnosis code for newborn]*
5ᵗʰ **Z38.0 Single liveborn infant,** born in hospital
  Single liveborn infant, born in birthing center or other health care facility
Z38.00 **Single liveborn infant, delivered vaginally** N PDx Z1
  AHA: Q2 2017, Q4 2016
Z38.01 **Single liveborn infant, delivered by cesarean** N PDx Z1
  AHA: Q2 2017, Q3 2016
Z38.1 **Single liveborn infant, born** outside hospital N PDx Z1
Z38.2 **Single liveborn infant, unspecified as to place of birth** N PDx Z1
  Single liveborn infant NOS
5ᵗʰ **Z38.3 Twin liveborn infant,** born in hospital
Z38.30 **Twin liveborn infant, delivered vaginally** N PDx Z1
Z38.31 **Twin liveborn infant, delivered by cesarean** N PDx Z1
Z38.4 **Twin liveborn infant, born outside hospital** N PDx Z1
Z38.5 **Twin liveborn infant, unspecified as to place of birth** N PDx Z1
5ᵗʰ **Z38.6 Other** multiple liveborn infant, born in hospital
Z38.61 **Triplet** liveborn infant, delivered vaginally N PDx Z1
Z38.62 **Triplet** liveborn infant, delivered by cesarean N PDx Z1
Z38.63 **Quadruplet** liveborn infant, delivered vaginally N PDx Z1
Z38.64 **Quadruplet** liveborn infant, delivered by cesarean N PDx Z1
Z38.65 **Quintuplet** liveborn infant, delivered vaginally N PDx Z1
Z38.66 **Quintuplet** liveborn infant, delivered by cesarean N PDx Z1
Z38.68 **Other multiple** liveborn infant, delivered vaginally N PDx Z1
Z38.69 **Other multiple** liveborn infant, delivered by cesarean N PDx Z1
Z38.7 **Other multiple liveborn infant, born outside hospital** N PDx Z1
Z38.8 **Other multiple liveborn infant, unspecified as to place of birth** N PDx Z1
4ᵗʰ **Z39 Encounter for maternal postpartum care and examination**
Z39.0 **Encounter for care and examination of mother** immediately after delivery M PDx ♀ Z1
  Care and observation in uncomplicated cases when the delivery occurs outside a healthcare facility
  EXCLUDES1 care for postpartum complication- see Alphabetic index
Z39.1 **Encounter for care and examination of** lactating mother M PDx ♀ PDxIn Z1
  Encounter for supervision of lactation
  EXCLUDES1 disorders of lactation (O92.-)
Z39.2 **Encounter for** routine postpartum **follow-up** M PDx ♀ PDxIn Z1

Encounters for other specific health care (Z40-Z53)

  Categories Z40-Z53 are intended for use to indicate a reason for care. They may be used for patients who have already been treated for a disease or injury, but who are receiving aftercare or prophylactic care, or care to consolidate the treatment, or to deal with a residual state
  EXCLUDES2 follow-up examination for medical surveillance after treatment (Z08-Z09)
4ᵗʰ **Z40 Encounter for prophylactic surgery**
  EXCLUDES1 organ donations (Z52.-)
    therapeutic organ removal-code to condition
5ᵗʰ **Z40.0 Encounter for prophylactic surgery for** risk factors related to malignant neoplasms
  Admission for prophylactic organ removal
  Use additional code to identify risk factor
Z40.00 **Encounter for prophylactic removal of unspecified organ**
Z40.01 **Encounter for prophylactic removal of** breast

1st 1st trimester 2nd 2nd trimester 3rd 3rd trimester PDx Unacceptable principal diagnosis symbol per Medicare code edits
PDxIn Code exempt from diagnosis present on admission requirement ❓ Questionable admission cᶜ Complication or comorbidity
cc/Mcc CC/MCC exclusion Mcc Major complication or comorbidity PDxCC Principal diagnosis as its own CC PDxM Principal diagnosis as its own MCC
HCC HCC diagnosis code RxHCC RxHCC diagnosis code MACRA code Z1 Z code as first-listed diagnosis

When symbols appear on a code that requires a 7th character extension, refer to Appendix B to identify applicable 7th character codes. **2018 ICD-10-CM**

▲ **Z40.02** Encounter for prophylactic removal of ►ovary(s)◄ ♀
Encounter for prophylactic removal of ovary(s) and fallopian tube(s)

● **Z40.03** Encounter for prophylactic removal of fallopian tube(s) ♀

Z40.09 Encounter for prophylactic removal of other organ

Z40.8 Encounter for other prophylactic surgery PDxIn

Z40.9 Encounter for prophylactic surgery, unspecified PDxIn

Z41 Encounter for procedures for purposes other than remedying health state

Z41.1 Encounter for cosmetic surgery POA
Encounter for cosmetic breast implant
Encounter for cosmetic procedure
EXCLUDES1 encounter for plastic and reconstructive surgery following medical procedure or healed injury (Z42.-)
encounter for post-mastectomy breast implantation (Z42.1)

Z41.2 Encounter for routine and ritual male circumcision POA ♂

Z41.3 Encounter for ear piercing POA PDxExc

Z41.8 Encounter for other procedures for purposes other than remedying health state POA

Z41.9 Encounter for procedure for purposes other than remedying health state, unspecified POA PDxIn

Z42 Encounter for plastic and reconstructive surgery following medical procedure or healed injury
EXCLUDES1 encounter for cosmetic plastic surgery (Z41.1)
encounter for plastic surgery for treatment of current injury - code to relevent injury

Z42.1 Encounter for breast reconstruction following mastectomy A POA Z1
EXCLUDES1 deformity and disproportion of reconstructed breast (N65.1-)

Z42.8 Encounter for other plastic and reconstructive surgery following medical procedure or healed injury POA Z1
AHA: Q1 2017

Z43 Encounter for attention to artificial openings
INCLUDES closure of artificial openings
passage of sounds or bougies through artificial openings
reforming artificial openings
removal of catheter from artificial openings
toilet or cleansing of artificial openings
EXCLUDES1 complications of external stoma (J95.0-, K94.-, N99.5-)
EXCLUDES2 fitting and adjustment of prosthetic and other devices (Z44-Z46)

Z43.0 Encounter for attention to tracheostomy POA HCC

Z43.1 Encounter for attention to gastrostomy CC POA HCC CC/MCC Exc
EXCLUDES2 artificial opening status only, without need for care (Z93.-)

Z43.2 Encounter for attention to ileostomy POA HCC
AHA: Q3 2016

Z43.3 Encounter for attention to colostomy POA HCC

Z43.4 Encounter for attention to other artificial openings of digestive tract POA HCC

Z43.5 Encounter for attention to cystostomy POA HCC

Z43.6 Encounter for attention to other artificial openings of urinary tract POA HCC
Encounter for attention to nephrostomy
Encounter for attention to ureterostomy
Encounter for attention to urethrostomy

Z43.7 Encounter for attention to artificial vagina POA

Z43.8 Encounter for attention to other artificial openings POA HCC

Z43.9 Encounter for attention to unspecified artificial opening POA HCC PDxIn

Z44 Encounter for fitting and adjustment of external prosthetic device
INCLUDES removal or replacement of external prosthetic device
EXCLUDES1 malfunction or other complications of device - see Alphabetical Index
presence of prosthetic device (Z97.-)

Z44.0 Encounter for fitting and adjustment of artificial arm

Z44.00 Encounter for fitting and adjustment of unspecified artificial arm

Z44.001 Encounter for fitting and adjustment of unspecified right artificial arm POA

Z44.002 Encounter for fitting and adjustment of unspecified left artificial arm POA

Z44.009 Encounter for fitting and adjustment of unspecified artificial arm, unspecified arm POA

Z44.01 Encounter for fitting and adjustment of complete artificial arm

Z44.011 Encounter for fitting and adjustment of complete right artificial arm POA

Z44.012 Encounter for fitting and adjustment of complete left artificial arm POA

Z44.019 Encounter for fitting and adjustment of complete artificial arm, unspecified arm POA

Z44.02 Encounter for fitting and adjustment of partial artificial arm

Z44.021 Encounter for fitting and adjustment of partial artificial right arm POA

Z44.022 Encounter for fitting and adjustment of partial artificial left arm POA

Z44.029 Encounter for fitting and adjustment of partial artificial arm, unspecified arm POA

Z44.1 Encounter for fitting and adjustment of artificial leg

Z44.10 Encounter for fitting and adjustment of unspecified artificial leg

Z44.101 Encounter for fitting and adjustment of unspecified right artificial leg POA HCC

Z44.102 Encounter for fitting and adjustment of unspecified left artificial leg POA HCC

Z44.109 Encounter for fitting and adjustment of unspecified artificial leg, unspecified leg POA HCC

Z44.11 Encounter for fitting and adjustment of complete artificial leg

Z44.111 Encounter for fitting and adjustment of complete right artificial leg POA HCC

Z44.112 Encounter for fitting and adjustment of complete left artificial leg POA HCC

Z44.119 Encounter for fitting and adjustment of complete artificial leg, unspecified leg POA HCC

Z44.12 Encounter for fitting and adjustment of partial artificial leg

Z44.121 Encounter for fitting and adjustment of partial artificial right leg POA HCC

Z44.122 Encounter for fitting and adjustment of partial artificial left leg POA HCC

Z44.129 Encounter for fitting and adjustment of partial artificial leg, unspecified leg POA HCC

Z44.2 Encounter for fitting and adjustment of artificial eye
EXCLUDES1 mechanical complication of ocular prosthesis (T85.3)

Z44.20 Encounter for fitting and adjustment of artificial eye, unspecified POA

Z44.21 Encounter for fitting and adjustment of artificial right eye POA

Z44.22 Encounter for fitting and adjustment of artificial left eye POA

Z44.3 Encounter for fitting and adjustment of external breast prosthesis
EXCLUDES1 complications of breast implant (T85.4-)
encounter for adjustment or removal of breast implant (Z45.81-)
encounter for initial breast implant insertion for cosmetic breast augmentation (Z41.1)
encounter for breast reconstruction following mastectomy (Z42.1)

Unspecified Code   Other Specified Code   Manifestation Code   Ⓝ Newborn   Ⓟ Pediatric   Ⓜ Maternity   Ⓐ Adult   ♂ Male   ♀ Female
● New Code   ▲ Revised Code Title   ►◄ Revised Text   NOTES   INCLUDES   EXCLUDES 1 Not coded here   EXCLUDES 2 Not included here
4th character required   5th character required   6th character required   7th character required
Extension 'X' Alert   HCC Hospital-acquired condition (HAC) alert   AHA AHA Coding Clinic©

Z44.30 Encounter for fitting and adjustment of external breast prosthesis, unspecified breast ⃠POA

Z44.31 Encounter for fitting and adjustment of external right breast prosthesis ⃠POA

Z44.32 Encounter for fitting and adjustment of external left breast prosthesis ⃠POA

Z44.8 Encounter for fitting and adjustment of other external prosthetic devices ⃠POA

Z44.9 Encounter for fitting and adjustment of unspecified external prosthetic device ⃠POA PDxIn

Z45 Encounter for adjustment and management of implanted device

INCLUDES removal or replacement of implanted device

EXCLUDES1 malfunction or other complications of device - see Alphabetical Index

EXCLUDES2 encounter for fitting and adjustment of non-implanted device (Z46.-)

Z45.0 Encounter for adjustment and management of cardiac device

Z45.01 Encounter for adjustment and management of cardiac pacemaker

Encounter for adjustment and management of cardiac resynchronization therapy pacemaker (CRT-P)

EXCLUDES1 encounter for adjustment and management of automatic implantable cardiac defibrillator with synchronous cardiac pacemaker (Z45.02)

Z45.010 Encounter for checking and testing of cardiac pacemaker pulse generator [battery] ⃠POA ❓

Encounter for replacing cardiac pacemaker pulse generator [battery]

Z45.018 Encounter for adjustment and management of other part of cardiac pacemaker ⃠POA ❓

EXCLUDES2 presence of prosthetic and other devices (Z95-Z97)

Z45.02 Encounter for adjustment and management of automatic implantable cardiac defibrillator ⃠POA ❓

Encounter for adjustment and management of automatic implantable cardiac defibrillator with synchronous cardiac pacemaker

Encounter for adjustment and management of cardiac resynchronization therapy defibrillator (CRT-D)

Z45.09 Encounter for adjustment and management of other cardiac device ⃠POA ❓

Z45.1 Encounter for adjustment and management of infusion pump ⃠POA

Z45.2 Encounter for adjustment and management of vascular access device ⃠POA

Encounter for adjustment and management of vascular catheters

EXCLUDES1 encounter for adjustment and management of renal dialysis catheter (Z49.01)

Z45.3 Encounter for adjustment and management of implanted devices of the special senses

Z45.31 Encounter for adjustment and management of implanted visual substitution device ⃠POA

Z45.32 Encounter for adjustment and management of implanted hearing device

EXCLUDES1 Encounter for fitting and adjustment of hearing aide (Z46.1)

Z45.320 Encounter for adjustment and management of bone conduction device ⃠POA

Z45.321 Encounter for adjustment and management of cochlear device ⃠POA

Z45.328 Encounter for adjustment and management of other implanted hearing device ⃠POA

Z45.4 Encounter for adjustment and management of implanted nervous system device

Z45.41 Encounter for adjustment and management of cerebrospinal fluid drainage device ⃠POA

Encounter for adjustment and management of cerebral ventricular (communicating) shunt

Z45.42 Encounter for adjustment and management of neuropacemaker (brain) (peripheral nerve) (spinal cord) ⃠POA

Z45.49 Encounter for adjustment and management of other implanted nervous system device ⃠POA

Z45.8 Encounter for adjustment and management of other implanted devices

Z45.81 Encounter for adjustment or removal of breast implant

Encounter for elective implant exchange (different material) (different size)

Encounter removal of tissue expander without synchronous insertion of permanent implant

EXCLUDES1 complications of breast implant (T85.4-)

encounter for initial breast implant insertion for cosmetic breast augmentation (Z41.1)

encounter for breast reconstruction following mastectomy (Z42.1)

Z45.811 Encounter for adjustment or removal of right breast implant ⃠POA

Z45.812 Encounter for adjustment or removal of left breast implant ⃠POA

Z45.819 Encounter for adjustment or removal of unspecified breast implant ⃠POA

Z45.82 Encounter for adjustment or removal of myringotomy device (stent) (tube) ⃠POA PDxIn

Z45.89 Encounter for adjustment and management of other implanted devices ⃠POA PDxIn

Z45.9 Encounter for adjustment and management of unspecified implanted device ⃠POA PDxIn

Z46 Encounter for fitting and adjustment of other devices

INCLUDES removal or replacement of other device

EXCLUDES1 malfunction or other complications of device - see Alphabetical Index

EXCLUDES2 encounter for fitting and management of implanted devices (Z45.-)

issue of repeat prescription only (Z76.0)

presence of prosthetic and other devices (Z95-Z97)

Z46.0 Encounter for fitting and adjustment of spectacles and contact lenses ⃠POA PDxIn

Z46.1 Encounter for fitting and adjustment of hearing aid ⃠POA PDxIn

EXCLUDES1 encounter for adjustment and management of implanted hearing device (Z45.32-)

Z46.2 Encounter for fitting and adjustment of other devices related to nervous system and special senses ⃠POA

EXCLUDES2 encounter for adjustment and management of implanted nervous system device (Z45.4-)

encounter for adjustment and management of implanted visual substitution device (Z45.31)

Z46.3 Encounter for fitting and adjustment of dental prosthetic device ⃠POA

Encounter for fitting and adjustment of dentures

Z46.4 Encounter for fitting and adjustment of orthodontic device ⃠POA PDxIn

Z46.5 Encounter for fitting and adjustment of other gastrointestinal appliance and device

EXCLUDES1 encounter for attention to artificial openings of digestive tract (Z43.1-Z43.4)

Z46.51 Encounter for fitting and adjustment of gastric lap band ⃠POA PDxIn

Z46.59 Encounter for fitting and adjustment of other gastrointestinal appliance and device ⃠POA PDxIn

Z46.6 Encounter for fitting and adjustment of urinary device ⃠POA PDxIn

EXCLUDES2 attention to artificial openings of urinary tract (Z43.5, Z43.6)

PDxIn Unacceptable principal diagnosis symbol per Medicare code edits   POA Code exempt from diagnosis present on admission requirement
❓ Questionable admission   CC Complication or comorbidity   CC/MCC ExC CC/MCC exclusion   MCC Major complication or comorbidity
Principal diagnosis as its own CC   Principal diagnosis as its own MCC   HCC HCC diagnosis code   RxHCC RxHCC diagnosis code
MACRA code   Z Z code as first-listed diagnosis

5ᵗʰ Z46.8 Encounter for fitting and adjustment of other **specified devices**

Z46.81 Encounter for fitting and adjustment of insulin pump   POA PDxIn
Encounter for insulin pump instruction and training
Encounter for insulin pump titration

Z46.82 Encounter for fitting and adjustment of non-vascular catheter   POA

Z46.89 Encounter for fitting and adjustment of other specified devices   POA PDxIn
Encounter for fitting and adjustment of wheelchair

Z46.9 Encounter for fitting and adjustment of unspecified device   POA PDxIn

4ᵗʰ Z47 Orthopedic aftercare

EXCLUDES1 *aftercare for healing fracture-code to fracture with 7th character D*

Z47.1 Aftercare following joint replacement surgery   POA
Use additional code to identify the joint (Z96.6-)

Z47.2 Encounter for removal of internal fixation device   POA

EXCLUDES1 *encounter for adjustment of internal fixation device for fracture treatment- code to fracture with appropriate 7th character*

encounter for removal of external fixation device- code to fracture with 7th character D

infection or inflammatory reaction to internal fixation device (T84.6-)

mechanical complication of internal fixation device (T84.1-)

5ᵗʰ Z47.3 Aftercare following explantation of joint prosthesis
Aftercare following explantation of joint prosthesis, staged procedure
Encounter for joint prosthesis insertion following prior explantation of joint prosthesis

Z47.31 Aftercare following explantation of shoulder **joint prosthesis**   POA

EXCLUDES1 *acquired absence of shoulder joint following prior explantation of shoulder joint prosthesis (Z89.23-)*

shoulder joint prosthesis explantation status (Z89.23-)

Z47.32 Aftercare following explantation of hip **joint prosthesis**   POA
AHA: Q1 2015

EXCLUDES1 *acquired absence of hip joint following prior explantation of hip joint prosthesis (Z89.62-)*

hip joint prosthesis explantation status (Z89.62-)

Z47.33 Aftercare following explantation of knee **joint prosthesis**   POA

EXCLUDES1 *acquired absence of knee joint following prior explantation of knee prosthesis (Z89.52-)*

knee joint prosthesis explantation status (Z89.52-)

5ᵗʰ Z47.8 Encounter for other **orthopedic aftercare**

Z47.81 Encounter for orthopedic aftercare following surgical amputation   POA
Use additional code to identify the limb amputated (Z89.-)

Z47.82 Encounter for orthopedic aftercare following scoliosis surgery   POA

Z47.89 Encounter for other orthopedic aftercare   POA
AHA: Q1 2015

4ᵗʰ Z48 Encounter for other postprocedural aftercare

EXCLUDES1 *encounter for follow-up examination after completed treatment (Z08-Z09)*

encounter for aftercare following injury - code to Injury, by site, with appropriate 7th character for subsequent encounter

EXCLUDES2 *encounter for attention to artificial openings (Z43.-)*

encounter for fitting and adjustment of prosthetic and other devices (Z44-Z46)

5ᵗʰ Z48.0 Encounter for attention to dressings, sutures and drains

EXCLUDES1 *encounter for planned postprocedural wound closure (Z48.1)*

Z48.00 Encounter for change or removal of nonsurgical wound dressing   POA PDxIn
Encounter for change or removal of wound dressing NOS

Z48.01 Encounter for change or removal of surgical wound dressing   POA PDxIn
AHA: Q4 2015

Z48.02 Encounter for removal of sutures   POA PDxIn
AHA: Q1 2015
Encounter for removal of staples

Z48.03 Encounter for change or removal of drains   POA

Z48.1 Encounter for planned postprocedural wound closure   POA

EXCLUDES1 *encounter for attention to dressings and sutures (Z48.0-)*

5ᵗʰ Z48.2 Encounter for aftercare following organ transplant

Z48.21 Encounter for aftercare following heart transplant   CC⊘ POA HCC 🔲 RxHCC CC/MCC Exc

Z48.22 Encounter for aftercare following kidney transplant   CC⊘ POA 🔲 RxHCC CC/MCC Exc

Z48.23 Encounter for aftercare following liver transplant   CC⊘ POA 🔲 RxHCC CC/MCC Exc

Z48.24 Encounter for aftercare following lung transplant   CC⊘ POA HCC 🔲 RxHCC CC/MCC Exc

6ᵗʰ Z48.28 Encounter for aftercare following multiple organ transplant

Z48.280 Encounter for aftercare following heart-lung **transplant**   CC⊘ POA HCC 🔲 RxHCC CC/MCC Exc

Z48.288 Encounter for aftercare following multiple organ **transplant**   POA

6ᵗʰ Z48.29 Encounter for aftercare following other **organ transplant**

Z48.290 Encounter for aftercare following bone marrow **transplant**   CC⊘ POA HCC 🔲 RxHCC CC/MCC Exc

Z48.298 Encounter for aftercare following other organ transplant   POA

Z48.3 Aftercare following surgery for neoplasm   POA
Use additional code to identify the neoplasm

5ᵗʰ Z48.8 Encounter for other specified **postprocedural aftercare**

6ᵗʰ Z48.81 Encounter for surgical aftercare following surgery on specified body systems
These codes identify the body system requiring aftercare. They are for use in conjunction with other aftercare codes to fully explain the aftercare encounter. The condition treated should also be coded if still present.

EXCLUDES1 *aftercare for injury- code the injury with 7th character D*

aftercare following surgery for neoplasm (Z48.3)

EXCLUDES2 *aftercare following organ transplant (Z48.2-)*

orthopedic aftercare (Z47.-)

Z48.810 Encounter for surgical aftercare following surgery on the sense organs   POA

Z48.811 Encounter for surgical aftercare following surgery on the nervous system   POA

EXCLUDES2 *encounter for surgical aftercare following surgery on the sense organs (Z48.810)*

Z48.812 Encounter for surgical aftercare following surgery on the circulatory system   POA
AHA: Q4 2012

Z48.813 Encounter for surgical aftercare following surgery on the respiratory system   POA

Z48.814 Encounter for surgical aftercare following surgery on the teeth or oral cavity   POA

Z48.815 Encounter for surgical aftercare following surgery on the digestive system   POA
AHA: Q4 2015

Unspecified Code   Other Specified Code   Manifestation Code   Ⓝ Newborn   Ⓟ Pediatric   Ⓜ Maternity   Ⓐ Adult   ♂ Male   ♀ Female
● New Code   ▲ Revised Code Title   ►◄ Revised Text   **NOTES**   *INCLUDES*   *EXCLUDES 1* Not coded here   *EXCLUDES 2* Not included here
4ᵗʰ 4ᵗʰ character required   5ᵗʰ 5ᵗʰ character required   6ᵗʰ 6ᵗʰ character required   7ᵗʰ 7ᵗʰ character required
Ⓧ Extension 'X' Alert   HAC Hospital-acquired condition (HAC) alert   AHA AHA Coding Clinic©

Z48.816 Encounter for surgical aftercare following surgery on the genitourinary system [POA]
[EXCLUDES1] *encounter for aftercare following sterilization reversal (Z31.42)*

Z48.817 Encounter for surgical aftercare following surgery on the skin and subcutaneous tissue [POA]
AHA: Q1 2015

Z48.89 Encounter for other specified surgical aftercare [POA]

[4th] **Z49 Encounter for care involving renal dialysis**
Code also associated end stage renal disease (N18.6)

[5th] **Z49.0 Preparatory care for renal dialysis**
Encounter for dialysis instruction and training

Z49.01 Encounter for fitting and adjustment of extracorporeal dialysis catheter [POA] [HCC] [RxHCC]
Removal or replacement of renal dialysis catheter
Toilet or cleansing of renal dialysis catheter

Z49.02 Encounter for fitting and adjustment of peritoneal dialysis catheter [POA] [HCC] [RxHCC] [PDx]

[5th] **Z49.3 Encounter for adequacy testing for dialysis**

Z49.31 Encounter for adequacy testing for hemodialysis [POA] [HCC] [RxHCC] [PDx]

Z49.32 Encounter for adequacy testing for peritoneal dialysis [POA] [HCC] [RxHCC] [PDx]
Encounter for peritoneal equilibration test

[4th] **Z51 Encounter for other aftercare and medical care**
Code also condition requiring care
[EXCLUDES1] *follow-up examination after treatment (Z08-Z09)*

Z51.0 Encounter for antineoplastic radiation therapy [POA] [Z1]

[5th] **Z51.1 Encounter for antineoplastic chemotherapy and immunotherapy**
[EXCLUDES2] *encounter for chemotherapy and immunotherapy for nonneoplastic condition - code to condition*

Z51.11 Encounter for antineoplastic chemotherapy [POA] [Z1]
AHA: Q3 2015

Z51.12 Encounter for antineoplastic immunotherapy [POA] [Z1]

Z51.5 Encounter for palliative care [PDx]
AHA: Q1 2017

Z51.6 Encounter for desensitization to allergens [POA] [PDx]
AHA: Q4 2016

[5th] **Z51.8 Encounter for other specified aftercare**
[EXCLUDES1] *holiday relief care (Z75.5)*

Z51.81 Encounter for therapeutic drug level monitoring [POA]
Code also any long-term (current) drug therapy (Z79.-)
[EXCLUDES1] *encounter for blood-drug test for administrative or medicolegal reasons (Z02.83)*

Z51.89 Encounter for other specified aftercare [POA]
AHA: Q4 2012

[4th] **Z52 Donors of organs and tissues**
[INCLUDES] *autologous and other living donors*
[EXCLUDES1] *cadaveric donor - omit code*
examination of potential donor (Z00.5)

[5th] **Z52.0 Blood donor**

[6th] **Z52.00 Unspecified blood donor**
Z52.000 Unspecified donor, whole blood [POA] [PDx] [Z1]
Z52.001 Unspecified donor, stem cells [POA] [PDx] [Z1]
Z52.008 Unspecified donor, other blood [POA] [PDx] [Z1]

[6th] **Z52.01 Autologous blood donor**
Z52.010 Autologous donor, whole blood [POA] [PDx] [Z1]
Z52.011 Autologous donor, stem cells [POA] [PDx] [Z1]
Z52.018 Autologous donor, other blood [POA] [PDx] [Z1]

[6th] **Z52.09 Other blood donor**
Volunteer donor
Z52.090 Other blood donor, whole blood [POA] [PDx] [Z1]
Z52.091 Other blood donor, stem cells [POA] [PDx] [Z1]
Z52.098 Other blood donor, other blood [POA] [PDx] [Z1]

[5th] **Z52.1 Skin donor**
Z52.10 Skin donor, unspecified [POA] [Z1]
Z52.11 Skin donor, autologous [POA] [Z1]
Z52.19 Skin donor, other [POA] [Z1]

[5th] **Z52.2 Bone donor**
Z52.20 Bone donor, unspecified [POA] [Z1]
Z52.21 Bone donor, autologous [POA] [Z1]
Z52.29 Bone donor, other [POA] [Z1]

Z52.3 Bone marrow donor [POA] [Z1]
Z52.4 Kidney donor [POA] [Z1]
Z52.5 Cornea donor [POA] [Z1]
Z52.6 Liver donor [POA] [Z1]

[5th] **Z52.8 Donor of other specified organs or tissues**

[6th] **Z52.81 Egg (Oocyte) donor**
Z52.810 Egg (Oocyte) donor under age 35, anonymous recipient [POA] ♀ [PDx] [Z1]
Egg donor under age 35 NOS
Z52.811 Egg (Oocyte) donor under age 35, designated recipient [POA] ♀ [PDx] [Z1]
Z52.812 Egg (Oocyte) donor age 35 and over, anonymous recipient [POA] ♀ [PDx] [Z1]
Egg donor age 35 and over NOS
Z52.813 Egg (Oocyte) donor age 35 and over, designated recipient [POA] ♀ [PDx] [Z1]
Z52.819 Egg (Oocyte) donor, unspecified [POA] ♀ [PDx] [Z1]

Z52.89 Donor of other specified organs or tissues [POA] [Z1]

Z52.9 Donor of unspecified organ or tissue [POA] [Z1]
Donor NOS

[4th] **Z53 Persons encountering health services for specific procedures and treatment, not carried out**

[5th] **Z53.0 Procedure and treatment not carried out because of contraindication**
Z53.01 Procedure and treatment not carried out due to patient smoking [PDx]
Z53.09 Procedure and treatment not carried out because of other contraindication [PDx]

Z53.1 Procedure and treatment not carried out because of patient's decision for reasons of belief and group pressure [PDx]

[5th] **Z53.2 Procedure and treatment not carried out because of patient's decision for other and unspecified reasons**
Z53.20 Procedure and treatment not carried out because of patient's decision for unspecified reasons [PDx]
Z53.21 Procedure and treatment not carried out due to patient leaving prior to being seen by health care provider [PDx]
Z53.29 Procedure and treatment not carried out because of patient's decision for other reasons [PDx]

[5th] **Z53.3 Procedure converted to open procedure**
Z53.31 Laparoscopic surgical procedure converted to open procedure [POA] [PDx]
AHA: Q4 2016
Z53.32 Thoracoscopic surgical procedure converted to open procedure [POA] [PDx]
AHA: Q4 2016
Z53.33 Arthroscopic surgical procedure converted to open procedure [POA] [PDx]
AHA: Q4 2016
Z53.39 Other specified procedure converted to open procedure [POA] [PDx]
AHA: Q4 2016

Z53.8 Procedure and treatment not carried out for other reasons [PDx]

Z53.9 Procedure and treatment not carried out, unspecified reason [PDx]

[PDx] Unacceptable principal diagnosis symbol per Medicare code edits [POA] Code exempt from diagnosis present on admission requirement
[?] Questionable admission [CC] Complication or comorbidity [CC/MCC Exc] CC/MCC exclusion [MCC] Major complication or comorbidity
[PDx CC] Principal diagnosis as its own CC [PDx MCC] Principal diagnosis as its own MCC [HCC] HCC diagnosis code [RxHCC] RxHCC diagnosis code
MACRA code [Z1] Z code as first-listed diagnosis

When symbols appear on a code that requires a 7th character extension, refer to Appendix B to identify applicable 7th character codes.

Persons with potential health hazards related to socioeconomic and psychosocial circumstances (Z55-Z65)

Z55 Problems related to education and literacy
EXCLUDES1 *disorders of psychological development (F80-F89)*

Z55.0 Illiteracy and low-level literacy

Z55.1 Schooling unavailable and unattainable

Z55.2 Failed school examinations

Z55.3 Underachievement in school

Z55.4 Educational maladjustment and discord with teachers and classmates

Z55.8 Other problems related to education and literacy
Problems related to inadequate teaching

Z55.9 Problems related to education and literacy, unspecified
Academic problems NOS

Z56 Problems related to employment and unemployment
EXCLUDES2 *occupational exposure to risk factors (Z57.-)*
problems related to housing and economic circumstances (Z59.-)

Z56.0 Unemployment, unspecified

Z56.1 Change of job

Z56.2 Threat of job loss

Z56.3 Stressful work schedule

Z56.4 Discord with boss and workmates

Z56.5 Uncongenial work environment
Difficult conditions at work

Z56.6 Other physical and mental strain related to work

Z56.8 Other problems related to employment

Z56.81 Sexual harassment on the job

Z56.82 Military deployment status
Individual (civilian or military) currently deployed in theater or in support of military war, peacekeeping and humanitarian operations

Z56.89 Other problems related to employment

Z56.9 Unspecified problems related to employment
Occupational problems NOS

Z57 Occupational exposure to risk factors

Z57.0 Occupational exposure to noise

Z57.1 Occupational exposure to radiation

Z57.2 Occupational exposure to dust

Z57.3 Occupational exposure to other air contaminants

Z57.31 Occupational exposure to environmental tobacco smoke
EXCLUDES2 *exposure to environmental tobacco smoke (Z77.22)*

Z57.39 Occupational exposure to other air contaminants

Z57.4 Occupational exposure to toxic agents in agriculture
Occupational exposure to solids, liquids, gases or vapors in agriculture

Z57.5 Occupational exposure to toxic agents in other industries
Occupational exposure to solids, liquids, gases or vapors in other industries

Z57.6 Occupational exposure to extreme temperature

Z57.7 Occupational exposure to vibration

Z57.8 Occupational exposure to other risk factors

Z57.9 Occupational exposure to unspecified risk factor

Z59 Problems related to housing and economic circumstances
EXCLUDES2 *problems related to upbringing (Z62.-)*

Z59.0 Homelessness

Z59.1 Inadequate housing
Lack of heating
Restriction of space
Technical defects in home preventing adequate care
Unsatisfactory surroundings
EXCLUDES1 *problems related to the natural and physical environment (Z77.1-)*

Z59.2 Discord with neighbors, lodgers and landlord

Z59.3 Problems related to living in residential institution
Boarding-school resident
EXCLUDES1 *institutional upbringing (Z62.2)*

Z59.4 Lack of adequate food and safe drinking water
Inadequate drinking water supply
EXCLUDES1 *effects of hunger (T73.0)*
inappropriate diet or eating habits (Z72.4)
malnutrition (E40-E46)

Z59.5 Extreme poverty

Z59.6 Low income

Z59.7 Insufficient social insurance and welfare support

Z59.8 Other problems related to housing and economic circumstances
Foreclosure on loan
Isolated dwelling
Problems with creditors

Z59.9 Problem related to housing and economic circumstances, unspecified

Z60 Problems related to social environment

Z60.0 Problems of adjustment to life-cycle transitions
Empty nest syndrome
Phase of life problem
Problem with adjustment to retirement [pension]

Z60.2 Problems related to living alone

Z60.3 Acculturation difficulty
Problem with migration
Problem with social transplantation

Z60.4 Social exclusion and rejection
Exclusion and rejection on the basis of personal characteristics, such as unusual physical appearance, illness or behavior.
EXCLUDES1 *target of adverse discrimination such as for racial or religious reasons (Z60.5)*

Z60.5 Target of (perceived) adverse discrimination and persecution
EXCLUDES1 *social exclusion and rejection (Z60.4)*

Z60.8 Other problems related to social environment

Z60.9 Problem related to social environment, unspecified

Z62 Problems related to upbringing
INCLUDES *current and past negative life events in childhood*
current and past problems of a child related to upbringing
EXCLUDES2 *maltreatment syndrome (T74.-)*
problems related to housing and economic circumstances (Z59.-)

Z62.0 Inadequate parental supervision and control

Z62.1 Parental overprotection

Z62.2 Upbringing away from parents
EXCLUDES1 *problems with boarding school (Z59.3)*

Z62.21 Child in welfare custody
Child in care of non-parental family member
Child in foster care
EXCLUDES2 *problem for parent due to child in welfare custody (Z63.5)*

Z62.22 Institutional upbringing
Child living in orphanage or group home

Z62.29 Other upbringing away from parents

Z62.3 Hostility towards and scapegoating of child

Z62.6 Inappropriate (excessive) parental pressure

Z62.8 Other specified problems related to upbringing

Z62.81 Personal history of abuse in childhood

Z62.810 Personal history of physical and sexual abuse in childhood
EXCLUDES1 *current child physical abuse (T74.12, T76.12)*
current child sexual abuse (T74.22, T76.22)

Z62.811 Personal history of psychological abuse in childhood
EXCLUDES1 *current child psychological abuse (T74.32, T76.32)*

Unspecified Code   Other Specified Code   Manifestation Code   N Newborn   P Pediatric   M Maternity   A Adult   ♂ Male   ♀ Female
● New Code   ▲ Revised Code Title   ►◄ Revised Text   NOTES   INCLUDES   EXCLUDES1 Not coded here   EXCLUDES2 Not included here
4th character required   5th character required   6th character required   7th character required
Extension 'X' Alert   HAC Hospital-acquired condition (HAC) alert   AHA AHA Coding Clinic©

2018 ICD-10-CM   When symbols appear on a code that requires a 7th character extension, refer to Appendix B to identify applicable 7th character codes.   **1269**

Z62.812 Personal history of neglect in childhood PDxIn
> EXCLUDES1 current child neglect (T74.02, T76.02)

Z62.819 Personal history of unspecified abuse in childhood PDxIn
> EXCLUDES1 current child abuse NOS (T74.92, T76.92)

Z62.82 Parent-child conflict

Z62.820 Parent-biological child conflict PDxIn
Parent-child problem NOS

Z62.821 Parent-adopted child conflict PDxIn

Z62.822 Parent-foster child conflict PDxIn

Z62.89 Other specified problems related to upbringing

Z62.890 Parent-child estrangement NEC PDxIn

Z62.891 Sibling rivalry PDxIn

Z62.898 Other specified problems related to upbringing PDxIn

Z62.9 Problem related to upbringing, unspecified PDxIn

Z63 Other problems related to primary support group, including family circumstances
> EXCLUDES2 maltreatment syndrome (T74.-, T76)
> parent-child problems (Z62.-)
> problems related to negative life events in childhood (Z62.-)
> problems related to upbringing (Z62.-)

Z63.0 Problems in relationship with spouse or partner PDxIn
Relationship distress with spouse or intimate partner
> EXCLUDES1 counseling for spousal or partner abuse problems (Z69.1)
> counseling related to sexual attitude, behavior, and orientation (Z70.-)

Z63.1 Problems in relationship with in-laws PDxIn

Z63.3 Absence of family member
> EXCLUDES1 absence of family member due to disappearance and death (Z63.4)
> absence of family member due to separation and divorce (Z63.5)

Z63.31 Absence of family member due to military deployment PDxIn
Individual or family affected by other family member being on military deployment
> EXCLUDES1 family disruption due to return of family member from military deployment (Z63.71)

Z63.32 Other absence of family member PDxIn

Z63.4 Disappearance and death of family member PDxIn
Assumed death of family member
Bereavement

Z63.5 Disruption of family by separation and divorce PDxIn
Marital estrangement

Z63.6 Dependent relative needing care at home PDxIn

Z63.7 Other stressful life events affecting family and household

Z63.71 Stress on family due to return of family member from military deployment PDxIn
Individual or family affected by family member having returned from military deployment (current or past conflict)

Z63.72 Alcoholism and drug addiction in family PDxIn

Z63.79 Other stressful life events affecting family and household PDxIn
Anxiety (normal) about sick person in family
Health problems within family
Ill or disturbed family member
Isolated family

Z63.8 Other specified problems related to primary support group PDxIn
Family discord NOS
Family estrangement NOS
High expressed emotional level within family
Inadequate family support NOS
Inadequate or distorted communication within family

Z63.9 Problem related to primary support group, unspecified PDxIn
Relationship disorder NOS

Z64 Problems related to certain psychosocial circumstances

Z64.0 Problems related to unwanted pregnancy POA ♀ PDxIn

Z64.1 Problems related to multiparity POA ♀ PDxIn

Z64.4 Discord with counselors POA PDxIn
Discord with probation officer
Discord with social worker

Z65 Problems related to other psychosocial circumstances

Z65.0 Conviction in civil and criminal proceedings without imprisonment POA PDxIn

Z65.1 Imprisonment and other incarceration POA PDxIn

Z65.2 Problems related to release from prison POA PDxIn

Z65.3 Problems related to other legal circumstances POA PDxIn
Arrest
Child custody or support proceedings
Litigation
Prosecution

Z65.4 Victim of crime and terrorism POA PDxIn
Victim of torture

Z65.5 Exposure to disaster, war and other hostilities POA PDxIn
> EXCLUDES1 target of perceived discrimination or persecution (Z60.5)

Z65.8 Other specified problems related to psychosocial circumstances POA PDxIn
Religious or spiritual problem

Z65.9 Problem related to unspecified psychosocial circumstances POA PDxIn

Do not resuscitate status (Z66)

Z66 Do not resuscitate PDxIn
DNR status

Blood type (Z67)

Z67 Blood type

Z67.1 Type A blood

Z67.10 Type A blood, Rh positive POA PDxIn

Z67.11 Type A blood, Rh negative POA PDxIn

Z67.2 Type B blood

Z67.20 Type B blood, Rh positive POA PDxIn

Z67.21 Type B blood, Rh negative POA PDxIn

Z67.3 Type AB blood

Z67.30 Type AB blood, Rh positive POA PDxIn

Z67.31 Type AB blood, Rh negative POA PDxIn

Z67.4 Type O blood

Z67.40 Type O blood, Rh positive POA PDxIn

Z67.41 Type O blood, Rh negative POA PDxIn

Z67.9 Unspecified blood type

Z67.90 Unspecified blood type, Rh positive POA PDxIn

Z67.91 Unspecified blood type, Rh negative POA PDxIn
AHA: Q3 2015

Body mass index [BMI] (Z68)

Z68 Body mass index [BMI]
Kilograms per meters squared
> NOTES BMI adult codes are for use for persons 21 years of age or older
> BMI pediatric codes are for use for persons 2-20 years of age. These percentiles are based on the growth charts published by the Centers for Disease Control and Prevention (CDC)

▲ **Z68.1** Body mass index (BMI) ►19.9◄ or less, adult A CC POA PDxIn CC/MCC Exc

Z68.2 Body mass index (BMI) 20-29, adult

Z68.20 Body mass index (BMI) 20.0-20.9, adult A POA PDxIn

Z68.21 Body mass index (BMI) 21.0-21.9, adult A POA PDxIn

Z68.22 Body mass index (BMI) 22.0-22.9, adult A POA PDxIn

Z68.23 Body mass index (BMI) 23.0-23.9, adult A POA PDxIn

Z68.24 Body mass index (BMI) 24.0-24.9, adult A POA PDxIn

Z68.25 Body mass index (BMI) 25.0-25.9, adult A POA PDxIn

POA Unacceptable principal diagnosis symbol per Medicare code edits   POA Code exempt from diagnosis present on admission requirement
❓ Questionable admission   CC Complication or comorbidity   CC/MCC Exc CC/MCC exclusion   MCC Major complication or comorbidity
Principal diagnosis as its own CC   Principal diagnosis as its own MCC   HCC HCC diagnosis code   RxHCC RxHCC diagnosis code
MACRA code   Z Z code as first-listed diagnosis

Z68.26 Body mass index (BMI) 26.0-26.9, adult [A] POA PDx
Z68.27 Body mass index (BMI) 27.0-27.9, adult [A] POA PDx
Z68.28 Body mass index (BMI) 28.0-28.9, adult [A] POA PDx
Z68.29 Body mass index (BMI) 29.0-29.9, adult [A] POA PDx

[5th] Z68.3 Body mass index (BMI) 30-39, adult
Z68.30 Body mass index (BMI) 30.0-30.9, adult [A] POA PDx
Z68.31 Body mass index (BMI) 31.0-31.9, adult [A] POA PDx
Z68.32 Body mass index (BMI) 32.0-32.9, adult [A] POA PDx
Z68.33 Body mass index (BMI) 33.0-33.9, adult [A] POA PDx
Z68.34 Body mass index (BMI) 34.0-34.9, adult [A] POA PDx
Z68.35 Body mass index (BMI) 35.0-35.9, adult [A] POA PDx
Z68.36 Body mass index (BMI) 36.0-36.9, adult [A] POA PDx
Z68.37 Body mass index (BMI) 37.0-37.9, adult [A] POA PDx
Z68.38 Body mass index (BMI) 38.0-38.9, adult [A] POA PDx
Z68.39 Body mass index (BMI) 39.0-39.9, adult [A] POA PDx

[5th] Z68.4 Body mass index (BMI) 40 or greater, adult
Z68.41 Body mass index (BMI) 40.0-44.9, adult [A] CC POA [HCC] [RxHCC] PDx CC/MCC Exc
Z68.42 Body mass index (BMI) 45.0-49.9, adult [A] CC POA [HCC] [RxHCC] PDx CC/MCC Exc
Z68.43 Body mass index (BMI) 50-59.9, adult [A] CC POA [HCC] [RxHCC] PDx CC/MCC Exc
Z68.44 Body mass index (BMI) 60.0-69.9, adult [A] CC POA [HCC] [RxHCC] PDx CC/MCC Exc
Z68.45 Body mass index (BMI) 70 or greater, adult [A] CC POA [HCC] [RxHCC] PDx CC/MCC Exc

[5th] Z68.5 Body mass index (BMI) pediatric
Z68.51 Body mass index (BMI) pediatric, less than 5th percentile for age POA PDx
Z68.52 Body mass index (BMI) pediatric, 5th percentile to less than 85th percentile for age POA PDx
Z68.53 Body mass index (BMI) pediatric, 85th percentile to less than 95th percentile for age POA PDx
Z68.54 Body mass index (BMI) pediatric, greater than or equal to 95th percentile for age POA PDx

Persons encountering health services in other circumstances (Z69-Z76)

[4th] Z69 Encounter for mental health services for victim and perpetrator of abuse

INCLUDES *counseling for victims and perpetrators of abuse*

[5th] Z69.0 Encounter for mental health services for child abuse problems

[6th] Z69.01 Encounter for mental health services for parental child abuse

Z69.010 Encounter for mental health services for victim of parental child abuse [P] POA
Encounter for mental health services for victim of child abuse by parent
Encounter for mental health services for victim of child neglect by parent
Encounter for mental health services for victim of child psychological abuse by parent
Encounter for mental health services for victim of child sexual abuse by parent

Z69.011 Encounter for mental health services for perpetrator of parental child abuse POA PDx
Encounter for mental health services for perpetrator of parental child neglect
Encounter for mental health services for perpetrator of parental child psychological abuse
Encounter for mental health services for perpetrator of parental child sexual abuse
EXCLUDES1 *encounter for mental health services for non-parental child abuse (Z69.02-)*

[6th] Z69.02 Encounter for mental health services for non-parental child abuse

Z69.020 Encounter for mental health services for victim of non-parental child abuse [P] POA
Encounter for mental health services for victim of non-parental child neglect
Encounter for mental health services for victim of non-parental child psychological abuse
Encounter for mental health services for victim of non-parental child sexual abuse

Z69.021 Encounter for mental health services for perpetrator of non-parental child abuse POA PDx
Encounter for mental health services for perpetrator of non-parental child neglect
Encounter for mental health services for perpetrator of non-parental child psychological abuse
Encounter for mental health services for perpetrator of non-parental child sexual abuse

[5th] Z69.1 Encounter for mental health services for spousal or partner abuse problems

Z69.11 Encounter for mental health services for victim of spousal or partner abuse POA PDx
Encounter for mental health services for victim of spouse or partner neglect
Encounter for mental health services for victim of spouse or partner psychological abuse
Encounter for mental health services for victim of spouse or partner violence, physical

Z69.12 Encounter for mental health services for perpetrator of spousal or partner abuse POA PDx
Encounter for mental health services for perpetrator of spouse or partner neglect
Encounter for mental health services for perpetrator of spouse or partner psychological abuse
Encounter for mental health services for perpetrator of spouse or partner violence, physical
Encounter for mental health services for perpetrator of spouse or partner violence, sexual

[5th] Z69.8 Encounter for mental health services for victim or perpetrator of other abuse

Z69.81 Encounter for mental health services for victim of other abuse POA PDx
Encounter for mental health services for perpetrator of non-spousal adult abuse
Encounter for mental health services for victim of non-spousal adult abuse
Encounter for mental health services for victim of spouse or partner violence, sexual
Encounter for rape victim counseling

Z69.82 Encounter for mental health services for perpetrator of other abuse POA PDx

[4th] Z70 Counseling related to sexual attitude, behavior and orientation

INCLUDES *encounter for mental health services for sexual attitude, behavior and orientation*

EXCLUDES2 *contraceptive or procreative counseling (Z30-Z31)*

Z70.0 Counseling related to sexual attitude POA PDx

Z70.1 Counseling related to patient's sexual behavior and orientation POA PDx
Patient concerned regarding impotence
Patient concerned regarding non-responsiveness
Patient concerned regarding promiscuity
Patient concerned regarding sexual orientation

Z70.2 Counseling related to sexual behavior and orientation of third party POA PDx
Advice sought regarding sexual behavior and orientation of child
Advice sought regarding sexual behavior and orientation of partner
Advice sought regarding sexual behavior and orientation of spouse

Z70.3 Counseling related to combined concerns regarding sexual attitude, behavior and orientation

Z70.8 Other sex counseling

Encounter for sex education

Z70.9 Sex counseling, unspecified

Z71 Persons encountering health services for other counseling and medical advice, not elsewhere classified

EXCLUDES2 *contraceptive or procreation counseling (Z30-Z31)*

sex counseling (Z70.-)

Z71.0 Person encountering health services to consult on behalf of another person

Person encountering health services to seek advice or treatment for non-attending third party

EXCLUDES2 *anxiety (normal) about sick person in family (Z63.7)*

expectant (adoptive) parent(s) pre-birth pediatrician visit (Z76.81)

Z71.1 Person with feared health complaint in whom no diagnosis is made

AHA: Q4 2016

Person encountering health services with feared condition which was not demonstrated

Person encountering health services in which problem was normal state

'Worried well'

EXCLUDES1 *medical observation for suspected diseases and conditions proven not to exist (Z03.-)*

Z71.2 Person consulting for explanation of examination or test findings

Z71.3 Dietary counseling and surveillance

Use additional code for any associated underlying medical condition

Use additional code to identify body mass index (BMI), if known (Z68.-)

Z71.4 Alcohol abuse counseling and surveillance

Use additional code for alcohol abuse or dependence (F10.-)

Z71.41 Alcohol abuse counseling and surveillance of alcoholic

Z71.42 Counseling for family member of alcoholic

Counseling for significant other, partner, or friend of alcoholic

Z71.5 Drug abuse counseling and surveillance

Use additional code for drug abuse or dependence (F11-F16, F18-F19)

Z71.51 Drug abuse counseling and surveillance of drug abuser

Z71.52 Counseling for family member of drug abuser

Counseling for significant other, partner, or friend of drug abuser

Z71.6 Tobacco abuse counseling

Use additional code for nicotine dependence (F17.-)

Z71.7 Human immunodeficiency virus [HIV] counseling

Z71.8 Other specified counseling

EXCLUDES2 *counseling for contraception (Z30.0-)*

Z71.81 Spiritual or religious counseling

● **Z71.82** Exercise counseling

● **Z71.83** Encounter for nonprocreative genetic counseling

EXCLUDES1 *counseling for procreative genetics (Z31.5)*

counseling for procreative management (Z31.6)

Z71.89 Other specified counseling

Z71.9 Counseling, unspecified

Encounter for medical advice NOS

Z72 Problems related to lifestyle

EXCLUDES2 *problems related to life-management difficulty (Z73.-)*

problems related to socioeconomic and psychosocial circumstances (Z55-Z65)

Z72.0 Tobacco use

Tobacco use NOS

EXCLUDES1 *history of tobacco dependence (Z87.891)*

nicotine dependence (F17.2-)

tobacco dependence (F17.2-)

tobacco use during pregnancy (O99.33-)

Z72.3 Lack of physical exercise

Z72.4 Inappropriate diet and eating habits

EXCLUDES1 *behavioral eating disorders of infancy or childhood (F98.2.-F98.3)*

eating disorders (F50.-)

lack of adequate food (Z59.4)

malnutrition and other nutritional deficiencies (E40-E64)

Z72.5 High risk sexual behavior

Promiscuity

EXCLUDES1 *paraphilias (F65)*

Z72.51 High risk heterosexual behavior

Z72.52 High risk homosexual behavior

Z72.53 High risk bisexual behavior

Z72.6 Gambling and betting

EXCLUDES1 *compulsive or pathological gambling (F63.0)*

Z72.8 Other problems related to lifestyle

Z72.81 Antisocial behavior

EXCLUDES1 *conduct disorders (F91.-)*

Z72.810 Child and adolescent antisocial behavior

Antisocial behavior (child) (adolescent) without manifest psychiatric disorder

Delinquency NOS

Group delinquency

Offenses in the context of gang membership

Stealing in company with others

Truancy from school

Z72.811 Adult antisocial behavior

Adult antisocial behavior without manifest psychiatric disorder

Z72.82 Problems related to sleep

Z72.820 Sleep deprivation

Lack of adequate sleep

EXCLUDES1 *insomnia (G47.0-)*

Z72.821 Inadequate sleep hygiene

Bad sleep habits

Irregular sleep habits

Unhealthy sleep wake schedule

EXCLUDES1 *insomnia (F51.0-, G47.0-)*

Z72.89 Other problems related to lifestyle

Self-damaging behavior

Z72.9 Problem related to lifestyle, unspecified

Z73 Problems related to life management difficulty

EXCLUDES2 *problems related to socioeconomic and psychosocial circumstances (Z55-Z65)*

Z73.0 Burn-out

Z73.1 Type A behavior pattern

Z73.2 Lack of relaxation and leisure

Z73.3 Stress, not elsewhere classified

Physical and mental strain NOS

EXCLUDES1 *stress related to employment or unemployment (Z56.-)*

Z73.4 Inadequate social skills, not elsewhere classified

Z73.5 Social role conflict, not elsewhere classified

Z73.6 Limitation of activities due to disability

EXCLUDES1 *care-provider dependency (Z74.-)*

Z73.8 Other problems related to life management difficulty

Z73.81 Behavioral insomnia of childhood

Z73.810 Behavioral insomnia of childhood, sleep-onset association type

---

PDx Unacceptable principal diagnosis symbol per Medicare code edits   POA Code exempt from diagnosis present on admission requirement

? Questionable admission   CC Complication or comorbidity   CC-MCC Excl CC/MCC exclusion   MCC Major complication or comorbidity

PDx CC Principal diagnosis as its own CC   PDx MCC Principal diagnosis as its own MCC   HCC HCC diagnosis code   RxHCC RxHCC diagnosis code

MACRA code   Z1 Z code as first-listed diagnosis

Z73.811 Behavioral insomnia of childhood, limit setting type **P** **POA** **PDxIn**

Z73.812 Behavioral insomnia of childhood, combined type **P** **POA** **PDxIn**

Z73.819 Behavioral insomnia of childhood, unspecified type **P** **POA** **PDxIn**

Z73.82 Dual sensory impairment **POA** **PDxIn**

Z73.89 Other problems related to life management difficulty **POA** **PDxIn**

Z73.9 **Problem related to life management difficulty, unspecified** **POA** **PDxIn**

Z74 Problems related to care provider dependency

EXCLUDES2 *dependence on enabling machines or devices NEC (Z99.-)*

Z74.0 Reduced mobility

Z74.01 **Bed confinement status** **POA** **PDxIn**
Bedridden

Z74.09 **Other reduced mobility** **PDxIn**
Chairridden
Reduced mobility NOS
EXCLUDES2 *wheelchair dependence (Z99.3)*

Z74.1 Need for assistance with personal care **PDxIn**

Z74.2 Need for assistance at home and no other household member able to render care **PDxIn**

Z74.3 Need for continuous supervision **PDxIn**

Z74.8 Other problems related to care provider dependency **PDxIn**

Z74.9 **Problem related to care provider dependency, unspecified** **PDxIn**

Z75 Problems related to medical facilities and other health care

Z75.0 **Medical services** not available in home **POA** **PDxIn**
EXCLUDES1 *no other household member able to render care (Z74.2)*

Z75.1 **Person** awaiting admission to adequate facility elsewhere **POA** **PDxIn**

Z75.2 **Other** waiting period for investigation and treatment **POA** **PDxIn**

Z75.3 Unavailability and inaccessibility of health-care facilities **POA** **PDxIn**
EXCLUDES1 *bed unavailable (Z75.1)*

Z75.4 Unavailability and inaccessibility of other helping agencies **POA** **PDxIn**

Z75.5 Holiday relief care

Z75.8 **Other problems related to medical facilities and other health care** **POA** **PDxIn**

Z75.9 **Unspecified problem related to medical facilities and other health care** **POA** **PDxIn**

Z76 Persons encountering health services in other circumstances

Z76.0 **Encounter for issue of repeat prescription** **POA** **PDxIn**
Encounter for issue of repeat prescription for appliance
Encounter for issue of repeat prescription for medicaments
Encounter for issue of repeat prescription for spectacles
EXCLUDES2 *issue of medical certificate (Z02.7)*
repeat prescription for contraceptive (Z30.4-)

Z76.1 **Encounter for health supervision and care of foundling** **POA** **Z4.1**

Z76.2 **Encounter for health supervision and care of other healthy infant and child** **P** **POA** **PDxIn** **Z4.1**
Encounter for medical or nursing care or supervision of healthy infant under circumstances such as adverse socioeconomic conditions at home
Encounter for medical or nursing care or supervision of healthy infant under circumstances such as awaiting foster or adoptive placement
Encounter for medical or nursing care or supervision of healthy infant under circumstances such as maternal illness
Encounter for medical or nursing care or supervision of healthy infant under circumstances such as number of children at home preventing or interfering with normal care

Z76.3 **Healthy person accompanying sick person** **POA**

Z76.4 **Other boarder to healthcare facility** **POA**
EXCLUDES1 *homelessness (Z59.0)*

Z76.5 **Malingerer [conscious simulation]** **POA**
Person feigning illness (with obvious motivation)
EXCLUDES1 *factitious disorder (F68.1-)*
peregrinating patient (F68.1-)

Z76.8 Persons encountering health services in other specified circumstances

Z76.81 **Expectant parent(s) prebirth pediatrician visit** **POA** **PDxIn**
Pre-adoption pediatrician visit for adoptive parent(s)

Z76.82 **Awaiting organ transplant status** **POA** **PDxIn**
Patient waiting for organ availability

Z76.89 Persons encountering health services in other specified circumstances **POA** **PDxIn**
Persons encountering health services NOS

Persons with potential health hazards related to family and personal history and certain conditions influencing health status (Z77-Z99)

Code also any follow-up examination (Z08-Z09)

Z77 **Other contact with and (suspected) exposures hazardous to health**

INCLUDES *contact with and (suspected) exposures to potential hazards to health*

EXCLUDES2 *contact with and (suspected) exposure to communicable diseases (Z20.-)*
exposure to (parental) (environmental) tobacco smoke in the perinatal period (P96.81)
newborn affected by noxious substances transmitted via placenta or breast milk (P04.-)
occupational exposure to risk factors (Z57.-)
retained foreign body (Z18.-)
retained foreign body fully removed (Z87.821)
toxic effects of substances chiefly nonmedicinal as to source (T51-T65)

Z77.0 Contact with and (suspected) exposure to hazardous, chiefly nonmedicinal, chemicals

Z77.01 **Contact with and (suspected) exposure to hazardous** metals

Z77.010 **Contact with and (suspected) exposure to arsenic** **PDxIn**

Z77.011 **Contact with and (suspected) exposure to lead** **PDxIn**

Z77.012 **Contact with and (suspected) exposure to uranium** **PDxIn**
EXCLUDES1 *retained depleted uranium fragments (Z18.01)*

Z77.018 **Contact with and (suspected) exposure to other hazardous metals** **PDxIn**
Contact with and (suspected) exposure to chromium compounds
Contact with and (suspected) exposure to nickel dust

Z77.02 **Contact with and (suspected) exposure to hazardous** aromatic compounds

Z77.020 **Contact with and (suspected) exposure to aromatic amines** **PDxIn**

Z77.021 **Contact with and (suspected) exposure to benzene** **PDxIn**

Z77.028 **Contact with and (suspected) exposure to other hazardous aromatic compounds** **PDxIn**
Aromatic dyes NOS
Polycyclic aromatic hydrocarbons

Z77.09 Contact with and (suspected) exposure to other hazardous, chiefly nonmedicinal, chemicals

Z77.090 **Contact with and (suspected) exposure to asbestos** **PDxIn**

Z77.098 **Contact with and (suspected) exposure to other hazardous, chiefly nonmedicinal, chemicals** **PDxIn**
Dyes NOS

Z77.1 Contact with and (suspected) exposure to environmental pollution and hazards in the physical environment

Z77.11 **Contact with and (suspected) exposure to** environmental pollution

Z77.110 **Contact with and (suspected) exposure to air pollution** **POA** **PDxIn**

Unspecified Code   Other Specified Code   Manifestation Code   **N** Newborn   **P** Pediatric   **M** Maternity   **A** Adult   ♂ Male   ♀ Female
● New Code   ▲ Revised Code Title   ▶◀ Revised Text   **NOTES**   INCLUDES   EXCLUDES 1   Not coded here   EXCLUDES 2   Not included here
4th character required   5th character required   6th character required   7th character required
Extension 'X' Alert   **HAC** Hospital-acquired condition (HAC) alert   **AHA** AHA Coding Clinic©

Z77.111　Contact with and (suspected) exposure to water pollution POA PDxIn

Z77.112　Contact with and (suspected) exposure to soil pollution POA PDxIn

Z77.118　Contact with and (suspected) exposure to other environmental pollution POA PDxIn

Z77.12　Contact with and (suspected) exposure to hazards in the physical environment

Z77.120　Contact with and (suspected) exposure to mold (toxic) POA PDxIn

Z77.121　Contact with and (suspected) exposure to harmful algae and algae toxins POA PDxIn

Contact with and (suspected) exposure to (harmful) algae bloom NOS

Contact with and (suspected) exposure to blue-green algae bloom

Contact with and (suspected) exposure to brown tide

Contact with and (suspected) exposure to cyanobacteria bloom

Contact with and (suspected) exposure to Florida red tide

Contact with and (suspected) exposure to pfiesteria piscicida

Contact with and (suspected) exposure to red tide

Z77.122　Contact with and (suspected) exposure to noise POA PDxIn

Z77.123　Contact with and (suspected) exposure to radon and other naturally occuring radiation POA PDxIn

EXCLUDES2 radiation exposure as the cause of a confirmed condition (W88-W90, X39.0-)

radiation sickness NOS (T66)

Z77.128　Contact with and (suspected) exposure to other hazards in the physical environment POA PDxIn

Z77.2　Contact with and (suspected) exposure to other hazardous substances

Z77.21　Contact with and (suspected) exposure to potentially hazardous body fluids PDxIn

Z77.22　Contact with and (suspected) exposure to environmental tobacco smoke (acute) (chronic) PDxIn

Exposure to second hand tobacco smoke (acute) (chronic)

Passive smoking (acute) (chronic)

EXCLUDES1 nicotine dependence (F17.-)

tobacco use (Z72.0)

EXCLUDES2 occupational exposure to environmental tobacco smoke (Z57.31)

Z77.29　Contact with and (suspected) exposure to other hazardous substances PDxIn

AHA: Q2 2016

Z77.9　Other contact with and (suspected) exposures hazardous to health PDxIn

Z78　Other specified health status

EXCLUDES2 asymptomatic human immunodeficiency virus [HIV] infection status (Z21)

postprocedural status (Z93-Z99)

sex reassignment status (Z87.890)

Z78.0　Asymptomatic menopausal state A POA ♀ PDxIn

Menopausal state NOS

Postmenopausal status NOS

EXCLUDES2 symptomatic menopausal state (N95.1)

Z78.1　Physical restraint status POA PDxIn

EXCLUDES1 physical restraint due to a procedure - omit code

Z78.9　Other specified health status POA PDxIn

Z79　Long term (current) drug therapy

INCLUDES long term (current) drug use for prophylactic purposes

Code also any therapeutic drug level monitoring (Z51.81)

EXCLUDES2 drug abuse and dependence (F11-F19)

drug use complicating pregnancy, childbirth, and the puerperium (O99.32-)

long term (current) use of oral antidiabetic drugs (Z79.84)

long term (current) use of oral hypoglycemic drugs (Z79.84)

Z79.0　Long term (current) use of anticoagulants and antithrombotics/antiplatelets

EXCLUDES2 long term (current) use of aspirin (Z79.82)

Z79.01　Long term (current) use of anticoagulants POA

Z79.02　Long term (current) use of antithrombotics/antiplatelets POA PDxIn

Z79.1　Long term (current) use of non-steroidal anti-inflammatories (NSAID) POA PDxIn

EXCLUDES2 long term (current) use of aspirin (Z79.82)

Z79.2　Long term (current) use of antibiotics POA PDxIn

Z79.3　Long term (current) use of hormonal contraceptives POA

Long term (current) use of birth control pill or patch

Z79.4　Long term (current) use of insulin POA HCC RxHCC

AHA: Q4 2016

Z79.5　Long term (current) use of steroids

Z79.51　Long term (current) use of inhaled steroids POA PDxIn

Z79.52　Long term (current) use of systemic steroids POA PDxIn

Z79.8　Other long term (current) drug therapy

Z79.81　Long term (current) use of agents affecting estrogen receptors and estrogen levels

Code first, if applicable:

malignant neoplasm of breast (C50.-)

malignant neoplasm of prostate (C61)

Use additional code, if applicable, to identify:

estrogen receptor positive status (Z17.0)

family history of breast cancer (Z80.3)

genetic susceptibility to malignant neoplasm (cancer) (Z15.0-)

personal history of breast cancer (Z85.3)

personal history of prostate cancer (Z85.46)

postmenopausal status (Z78.0)

EXCLUDES1 hormone replacement therapy (Z79.890)

Z79.810　Long term (current) use of selective estrogen receptor modulators (SERMs) POA PDxIn

Long term (current) use of raloxifene (Evista)

Long term (current) use of tamoxifen (Nolvadex)

Long term (current) use of toremifene (Fareston)

Z79.811　Long term (current) use of aromatase inhibitors POA PDxIn

Long term (current) use of anastrozole (Arimidex)

Long term (current) use of exemestane (Aromasin)

Long term (current) use of letrozole (Femara)

Z79.818　Long term (current) use of other agents affecting estrogen receptors and estrogen levels POA PDxIn

Long term (current) use of estrogen receptor downregulators

Long term (current) use of fulvestrant (Faslodex)

Long term (current) use of gonadotropin-releasing hormone (GnRH) agonist

Long term (current) use of goserelin acetate (Zoladex)

Long term (current) use of leuprolide acetate (leuprorelin) (Lupron)

Long term (current) use of megestrol acetate (Megace)

POA Unacceptable principal diagnosis symbol per Medicare code edits　POA Code exempt from diagnosis present on admission requirement
? Questionable admission　CC Complication or comorbidity　CC/MCC Excl CC/MCC exclusion　MCC Major complication or comorbidity
CC Principal diagnosis as its own CC　MCC Principal diagnosis as its own MCC　HCC HCC diagnosis code　RxHCC RxHCC diagnosis code
MACRA code　Z1 Z code as first-listed diagnosis

Z79.82 Long term (current) use of aspirin [POA]

Z79.83 Long term (current) use of bisphosphonates [POA] [PDx]
AHA: Q4 2016

Z79.84 Long term (current) use of oral hypoglycemic drugs [POA] [PDx]
AHA: Q4 2016
Long term (current) use of oral antidiabetic drugs
EXCLUDES2 *long term (current) use of insulin (Z79.4)*

[6th] Z79.89 Other long term (current) drug therapy

▲ Z79.890 Hormone replacement therapy [POA] [PDx]

Z79.891 Long term (current) use of opiate analgesic [POA]
Long term (current) use of methadone for pain management
EXCLUDES1 *methodone use NOS (F11.9-)*
use of methodone for treatment of heroin addiction (F11.2-)

Z79.899 Other long term (current) drug therapy [POA]
AHA: Q3 2015, Q4 2015

[4th] Z80 Family history of primary malignant neoplasm

Z80.0 Family history of malignant neoplasm of digestive organs [POA] [PDx]
Conditions classifiable to C15-C26

Z80.1 Family history of malignant neoplasm of trachea, bronchus and lung [POA] [PDx]
Conditions classifiable to C33-C34

Z80.2 Family history of malignant neoplasm of other respiratory and intrathoracic organs [POA] [PDx]
Conditions classifiable to C30-C32, C37-C39

Z80.3 Family history of malignant neoplasm of breast [POA] [PDx]
Conditions classifiable to C50.-

[5th] Z80.4 Family history of malignant neoplasm of genital organs
Conditions classifiable to C51-C63

Z80.41 Family history of malignant neoplasm of ovary [POA] [PDx]

Z80.42 Family history of malignant neoplasm of prostate [POA] [PDx]

Z80.43 Family history of malignant neoplasm of testis [POA] [PDx]

Z80.49 Family history of malignant neoplasm of other genital organs [POA] [PDx]

[5th] Z80.5 Family history of malignant neoplasm of urinary tract
Conditions classifiable to C64-C68

Z80.51 Family history of malignant neoplasm of kidney [POA] [PDx]

Z80.52 Family history of malignant neoplasm of bladder [POA] [PDx]

Z80.59 Family history of malignant neoplasm of other urinary tract organ [POA] [PDx]

Z80.6 Family history of leukemia [POA] [PDx]
Conditions classifiable to C91-C95

Z80.7 Family history of other malignant neoplasms of lymphoid, hematopoietic and related tissues [POA] [PDx]
Conditions classifiable to C81-C90, C96.-

Z80.8 Family history of malignant neoplasm of other organs or systems [POA] [PDx]
Conditions classifiable to C00-C14, C40-C49, C69-C79

Z80.9 Family history of malignant neoplasm, unspecified [POA] [PDx]
Conditions classifiable to C80.1

[4th] Z81 Family history of mental and behavioral disorders

Z81.0 Family history of intellectual disabilities [POA] [PDx]
Conditions classifiable to F70-F79

Z81.1 Family history of alcohol abuse and dependence [POA] [PDx]
Conditions classifiable to F10.-

Z81.2 Family history of tobacco abuse and dependence [POA] [PDx]
Conditions classifiable to F17.-

Z81.3 Family history of other psychoactive substance abuse and dependence [POA] [PDx]
Conditions classifiable to F11-F16, F18-F19

Z81.4 Family history of other substance abuse and dependence [POA] [PDx]
Conditions classifiable to F55

Z81.8 Family history of other mental and behavioral disorders [POA] [PDx]
Conditions classifiable elsewhere in F01-F99

[4th] Z82 Family history of certain disabilities and chronic diseases (leading to disablement)

Z82.0 Family history of epilepsy and other diseases of the nervous system [POA] [PDx]
Conditions classifiable to G00-G99

Z82.1 Family history of blindness and visual loss [POA] [PDx]
Conditions classifiable to H54.-

Z82.2 Family history of deafness and hearing loss [POA] [PDx]
Conditions classifiable to H90-H91

Z82.3 Family history of stroke [POA] [PDx]
Conditions classifiable to I60-I64

[5th] Z82.4 Family history of ischemic heart disease and other diseases of the circulatory system
Conditions classifiable to I00-I52, I65-I99

Z82.41 Family history of sudden cardiac death [POA] [PDx]

Z82.49 Family history of ischemic heart disease and other diseases of the circulatory system [POA] [PDx]

Z82.5 Family history of asthma and other chronic lower respiratory diseases [POA] [PDx]
Conditions classifiable to J40-J47
EXCLUDES2 *family history of other diseases of the respiratory system (Z83.6)*

[5th] Z82.6 Family history of arthritis and other diseases of the musculoskeletal system and connective tissue
Conditions classifiable to M00-M99

Z82.61 Family history of arthritis [POA] [PDx]

Z82.62 Family history of osteoporosis [POA] [PDx]

Z82.69 Family history of other diseases of the musculoskeletal system and connective tissue [POA] [PDx]

[5th] Z82.7 Family history of congenital malformations, deformations and chromosomal abnormalities
Conditions classifiable to Q00-Q99

Z82.71 Family history of polycystic kidney [POA] [PDx]

Z82.79 Family history of other congenital malformations, deformations and chromosomal abnormalities [POA] [PDx]

Z82.8 Family history of other disabilities and chronic diseases leading to disablement, not elsewhere classified [POA] [PDx]

[4th] Z83 Family history of other specific disorders
EXCLUDES2 *contact with and (suspected) exposure to communicable disease in the family (Z20.-)*

Z83.0 Family history of human immunodeficiency virus [HIV] disease [POA] [PDx]
Conditions classifiable to B20

Z83.1 Family history of other infectious and parasitic diseases [POA] [PDx]
Conditions classifiable to A00-B19, B25-B94, B99

Z83.2 Family history of diseases of the blood and blood-forming organs and certain disorders involving the immune mechanism [POA] [PDx]
Conditions classifiable to D50-D89

Z83.3 Family history of diabetes mellitus [POA] [PDx]
Conditions classifiable to E08-E13

[5th] Z83.4 Family history of other endocrine, nutritional and metabolic diseases
Conditions classifiable to E00-E07, E15-E88

Z83.41 Family history of multiple endocrine neoplasia [MEN] syndrome [POA] [PDx]

Z83.42 Family history of familial hypercholesterolemia [POA] [PDx]
AHA: Q4 2016

Z83.49 Family history of other endocrine, nutritional and metabolic diseases [POA] [PDx]

[5th] Z83.5 Family history of eye and ear disorders

[6th] Z83.51 Family history of eye disorders
Conditions classifiable to H00-H53, H55-H59
EXCLUDES2 *family history of blindness and visual loss (Z82.1)*

Z83.511 Family history of glaucoma [POA] [PDx]

Z83.518 Family history of other specified eye disorder [POA] [PDx]

Unspecified Code | Other Specified Code | Manifestation Code | [N] Newborn | [P] Pediatric | [M] Maternity | [A] Adult | ♂ Male | ♀ Female
● New Code | ▲ Revised Code Title | ►◄ Revised Text | NOTES | INCLUDES | EXCLUDES1 Not coded here | EXCLUDES2 Not included here
[4th] 4th character required | [5th] 5th character required | [6th] 6th character required | [7th] 7th character required
[7th] Extension 'X' Alert | [HAC] Hospital-acquired condition (HAC) alert | AHA AHA Coding Clinic©

When symbols appear on a code that requires a 7th character extension, refer to Appendix B to identify applicable 7th character codes.

Z83.52 Family history of ear disorders
Conditions classifiable to H60-H83, H92-H95
EXCLUDES2 family history of deafness and hearing loss (Z82.2)

Z83.6 Family history of other diseases of the respiratory system
Conditions classifiable to J00-J39, J60-J99
EXCLUDES2 family history of asthma and other chronic lower respiratory diseases (Z82.5)

Z83.7 Family history of diseases of the digestive system
Conditions classifiable to K00-K93

Z83.71 Family history of colonic polyps
EXCLUDES2 family history of malignant neoplasm of digestive organs (Z80.0)

Z83.79 Family history of other diseases of the digestive system

Z84 Family history of other conditions

Z84.0 Family history of diseases of the skin and subcutaneous tissue
Conditions classifiable to L00-L99

Z84.1 Family history of disorders of kidney and ureter
Conditions classifiable to N00-N29

Z84.2 Family history of other diseases of the genitourinary system
Conditions classifiable to N30-N99

Z84.3 Family history of consanguinity

Z84.8 Family history of other specified conditions

Z84.81 Family history of carrier of genetic disease

Z84.82 Family history of sudden infant death syndrome
AHA: Q4 2016
Family history of SIDS

Z84.89 Family history of other specified conditions

Z85 Personal history of malignant neoplasm
Code first any follow-up examination after treatment of malignant neoplasm (Z08)
Use additional code to identify:
alcohol use and dependence (F10.-)
exposure to environmental tobacco smoke (Z77.22)
history of tobacco dependence (Z87.891)
occupational exposure to environmental tobacco smoke (Z57.31)
tobacco dependence (F17.-)
tobacco use (Z72.0)
EXCLUDES2 personal history of benign neoplasm (Z86.01-)
personal history of carcinoma-in-situ (Z86.00-)

Z85.0 Personal history of malignant neoplasm of digestive organs

Z85.00 Personal history of malignant neoplasm of unspecified digestive organ

Z85.01 Personal history of malignant neoplasm of esophagus
Conditions classifiable to C15

Z85.02 Personal history of malignant neoplasm of stomach

Z85.020 Personal history of malignant carcinoid tumor of stomach
Conditions classifiable to C7A.092

Z85.028 Personal history of other malignant neoplasm of stomach
Conditions classifiable to C16

Z85.03 Personal history of malignant neoplasm of large intestine

Z85.030 Personal history of malignant carcinoid tumor of large intestine
Conditions classifiable to C7A.022-C7A.025, C7A.029

Z85.038 Personal history of other malignant neoplasm of large intestine
Conditions classifiable to C18

Z85.04 Personal history of malignant neoplasm of rectum, rectosigmoid junction, and anus

Z85.040 Personal history of malignant carcinoid tumor of rectum
Conditions classifiable to C7A.026

Z85.048 Personal history of other malignant neoplasm of rectum, rectosigmoid junction, and anus
Conditions classifiable to C19-C21

Z85.05 Personal history of malignant neoplasm of liver
Conditions classifiable to C22

Z85.06 Personal history of malignant neoplasm of small intestine

Z85.060 Personal history of malignant carcinoid tumor of small intestine
Conditions classifiable to C7A.01-

Z85.068 Personal history of other malignant neoplasm of small intestine
Conditions classifiable to C17

Z85.07 Personal history of malignant neoplasm of pancreas
Conditions classifiable to C25

Z85.09 Personal history of malignant neoplasm of other digestive organs

Z85.1 Personal history of malignant neoplasm of trachea, bronchus and lung

Z85.11 Personal history of malignant neoplasm of bronchus and lung

Z85.110 Personal history of malignant carcinoid tumor of bronchus and lung
Conditions classifiable to C7A.090

Z85.118 Personal history of other malignant neoplasm of bronchus and lung
Conditions classifiable to C34

Z85.12 Personal history of malignant neoplasm of trachea
Conditions classifiable to C33

Z85.2 Personal history of malignant neoplasm of other respiratory and intrathoracic organs

Z85.20 Personal history of malignant neoplasm of unspecified respiratory organ

Z85.21 Personal history of malignant neoplasm of larynx
Conditions classifiable to C32

Z85.22 Personal history of malignant neoplasm of nasal cavities, middle ear, and accessory sinuses
Conditions classifiable to C30-C31

Z85.23 Personal history of malignant neoplasm of thymus

Z85.230 Personal history of malignant carcinoid tumor of thymus
Conditions classifiable to C7A.091

Z85.238 Personal history of other malignant neoplasm of thymus
Conditions classifiable to C37

Z85.29 Personal history of malignant neoplasm of other respiratory and intrathoracic organs

Z85.3 Personal history of malignant neoplasm of breast
Conditions classifiable to C50.-

Z85.4 Personal history of malignant neoplasm of genital organs
Conditions classifiable to C51-C63

Z85.40 Personal history of malignant neoplasm of unspecified female genital organ

Z85.41 Personal history of malignant neoplasm of cervix uteri

Z85.42 Personal history of malignant neoplasm of other parts of uterus

Z85.43 Personal history of malignant neoplasm of ovary

Z85.44 Personal history of malignant neoplasm of other female genital organs

Z85.45 Personal history of malignant neoplasm of unspecified male genital organ

Z85.46 Personal history of malignant neoplasm of prostate

Z85.47 Personal history of malignant neoplasm of testis

Z85.48 Personal history of malignant neoplasm of epididymis

PDxIn Unacceptable principal diagnosis symbol per Medicare code edits   Code exempt from diagnosis present on admission requirement
? Questionable admission   Complication or comorbidity   CC/MCC exclusion   Major complication or comorbidity
Principal diagnosis as its own CC   Principal diagnosis as its own MCC   HCC HCC diagnosis code   RxHCC diagnosis code
MACRA code   Z code as first-listed diagnosis

1276   When symbols appear on a code that requires a 7th character extension, refer to Appendix B to identify applicable 7th character codes.   **2018 ICD-10-CM**

Z85.49   Personal history of malignant neoplasm of other male genital organs   POA ♂ PDxIn

5ᵈ Z85.5   Personal history of malignant neoplasm of urinary tract
Conditions classifiable to C64-C68

Z85.50   Personal history of malignant neoplasm of unspecified urinary tract organ   POA PDxIn

Z85.51   Personal history of malignant neoplasm of bladder   POA PDxIn

6ᵈ Z85.52   Personal history of malignant neoplasm of kidney
EXCLUDES1 personal history of malignant neoplasm of renal pelvis (Z85.53)

Z85.520   Personal history of malignant carcinoid tumor of kidney   POA PDxIn
Conditions classifiable to C7A.093

Z85.528   Personal history of other malignant neoplasm of kidney   POA PDxIn
Conditions classifiable to C64

Z85.53   Personal history of malignant neoplasm of renal pelvis   POA PDxIn

Z85.54   Personal history of malignant neoplasm of ureter   POA PDxIn

Z85.59   Personal history of malignant neoplasm of other urinary tract organ   POA PDxIn

Z85.6   Personal history of leukemia
Conditions classifiable to C91-C95
EXCLUDES1 leukemia in remission C91.0-C95.9 with 5th character 1

5ᵈ Z85.7   Personal history of other malignant neoplasms of lymphoid, hematopoietic and related tissues

Z85.71   Personal history of Hodgkin lymphoma   POA PDxIn
Conditions classifiable to C81

Z85.72   Personal history of non-Hodgkin lymphomas   POA PDxIn
Conditions classifiable to C82-C85

Z85.79   Personal history of other malignant neoplasms of lymphoid, hematopoietic and related tissues   POA PDxIn
Conditions classifiable to C88-C90, C96
EXCLUDES1 multiple myeloma in remission (C90.01)
plasma cell leukemia in remission (C90.11)
plasmacytoma in remission (C90.21)

5ᵈ Z85.8   Personal history of malignant neoplasms of other organs and systems
Conditions classifiable to C00-C14, C40-C49, C69-C75, C7A.098, C76-C79

6ᵈ Z85.81   Personal history of malignant neoplasm of lip, oral cavity, and pharynx

Z85.810   Personal history of malignant neoplasm of tongue   POA PDxIn

Z85.818   Personal history of malignant neoplasm of other sites of lip, oral cavity, and pharynx   POA PDxIn

Z85.819   Personal history of malignant neoplasm of unspecified site of lip, oral cavity, and pharynx   POA PDxIn

6ᵈ Z85.82   Personal history of malignant neoplasm of skin

Z85.820   Personal history of malignant melanoma of skin   POA PDxIn
Conditions classifiable to C43

Z85.821   Personal history of Merkel cell carcinoma   POA PDxIn
Conditions classifiable to C4A

Z85.828   Personal history of other malignant neoplasm of skin   POA PDxIn
Conditions classifiable to C44

6ᵈ Z85.83   Personal history of malignant neoplasm of bone and soft tissue

Z85.830   Personal history of malignant neoplasm of bone   POA PDxIn

Z85.831   Personal history of malignant neoplasm of soft tissue   POA PDxIn
EXCLUDES2 personal history of malignant neoplasm of skin (Z85.82-)

6ᵈ Z85.84   Personal history of malignant neoplasm of eye and nervous tissue

Z85.840   Personal history of malignant neoplasm of eye   POA PDxIn

Z85.841   Personal history of malignant neoplasm of brain   POA PDxIn

Z85.848   Personal history of malignant neoplasm of other parts of nervous tissue   POA PDxIn

6ᵈ Z85.85   Personal history of malignant neoplasm of endocrine glands

Z85.850   Personal history of malignant neoplasm of thyroid   POA PDxIn

Z85.858   Personal history of malignant neoplasm of other endocrine glands   POA PDxIn

Z85.89   Personal history of malignant neoplasm of other organs and systems   POA PDxIn

Z85.9   Personal history of malignant neoplasm, unspecified   POA PDxIn
Conditions classifiable to C7A.00, C80.1

4ᵈ Z86   Personal history of certain other diseases
Code first any follow-up examination after treatment (Z09)

5ᵈ Z86.0   Personal history of in-situ and benign neoplasms and neoplasms of uncertain behavior
EXCLUDES2 personal history of malignant neoplasms (Z85.-)

6ᵈ Z86.00   Personal history of in-situ neoplasm
Conditions classifiable to D00-D09

Z86.000   Personal history of in-situ neoplasm of breast   POA PDxIn

Z86.001   Personal history of in-situ neoplasm of cervix uteri   POA ♀ PDxIn
Personal history of cervical intraepithelial neoplasia III [CIN III]

Z86.008   Personal history of in-situ neoplasm of other site   POA PDxIn
Personal history of vaginal intraepithelial neoplasia III [VAIN III]
Personal history of vulvar intraepithelial neoplasia III [VIN III]

6ᵈ Z86.01   Personal history of benign neoplasm

Z86.010   Personal history of colonic polyps   POA PDxIn
AHA: Q1 2017

Z86.011   Personal history of benign neoplasm of the brain   POA PDxIn

Z86.012   Personal history of benign carcinoid tumor   POA PDxIn

Z86.018   Personal history of other benign neoplasm   POA PDxIn
AHA: Q1 2017

Z86.03   Personal history of neoplasm of uncertain behavior   POA PDxIn

5ᵈ Z86.1   Personal history of infectious and parasitic diseases
Conditions classifiable to A00-B89, B99
EXCLUDES1 personal history of infectious diseases specific to a body system
sequelae of infectious and parasitic diseases (B90-B94)

Z86.11   Personal history of tuberculosis   POA PDxIn

Z86.12   Personal history of poliomyelitis   POA PDxIn

Z86.13   Personal history of malaria   POA PDxIn

Z86.14   Personal history of Methicillin resistant Staphylococcus aureus infection   POA PDxIn
Personal history of MRSA infection

Z86.19   Personal history of other infectious and parasitic diseases   POA PDxIn

Z86.2   Personal history of diseases of the blood and blood-forming organs and certain disorders involving the immune mechanism   POA PDxIn
Conditions classifiable to D50-D89

5ᵈ Z86.3   Personal history of endocrine, nutritional and metabolic diseases
Conditions classifiable to E00-E88

Z86.31   Personal history of diabetic foot ulcer   POA PDxIn
EXCLUDES2 current diabetic foot ulcer (E08.621, E09.621, E10.621, E11.621, E13.621)

Unspecified Code   Other Specified Code   Manifestation Code   Ⓝ Newborn   Ⓟ Pediatric   Ⓜ Maternity   Ⓐ Adult   ♂ Male   ♀ Female
● New Code   ▲ Revised Code Title   ►◄ Revised Text   NOTES   INCLUDES   EXCLUDES 1 Not coded here   EXCLUDES 2 Not included here
4ᵈ 4ᵗʰ character required   5ᵈ 5ᵗʰ character required   6ᵈ 6ᵗʰ character required   7ᵈ 7ᵗʰ character required
7ᵈ Extension 'X' Alert   HAC Hospital-acquired condition (HAC) alert   AHA AHA Coding Clinic©

Z86.32 Personal history of gestational diabetes POA ♀ PDx
Personal history of conditions classifiable to O24.4-
[EXCLUDES1] *gestational diabetes mellitus in current pregnancy (O24.4-)*

Z86.39 Personal history of other endocrine, nutritional and metabolic disease POA PDx

[5th] **Z86.5 Personal history of mental and behavioral disorders**
Conditions classifiable to F40-F59

Z86.51 Personal history of combat and operational stress reaction [A] POA PDx

Z86.59 Personal history of other mental and behavioral disorders POA PDx

[5th] **Z86.6 Personal history of diseases of the nervous system and sense organs**
Conditions classifiable to G00-G99, H00-H95

Z86.61 Personal history of infections of the central nervous system POA PDx
Personal history of encephalitis
Personal history of meningitis

Z86.69 Personal history of other diseases of the nervous system and sense organs POA PDx
AHA: Q4 2016

[5th] **Z86.7 Personal history of diseases of the circulatory system**
Conditions classifiable to I00-I99
[EXCLUDES2] *old myocardial infarction (I25.2)*
personal history of anaphylactic shock (Z87.892)
postmyocardial infarction syndrome (I24.1)

[6th] **Z86.71 Personal history of venous thrombosis and embolism**

Z86.711 Personal history of pulmonary embolism POA PDx

Z86.718 Personal history of other venous thrombosis and embolism POA PDx

Z86.72 Personal history of thrombophlebitis POA PDx

Z86.73 Personal history of transient ischemic attack (TIA), and cerebral infarction without residual deficits POA PDx
Personal history of prolonged reversible ischemic neurological deficit (PRIND)
Personal history of stroke NOS without residual deficits
[EXCLUDES1] *personal history of traumatic brain injury (Z87.820)*
sequelae of cerebrovascular disease (I69.-)

Z86.74 Personal history of sudden cardiac arrest POA PDx
Personal history of sudden cardiac death successfully resuscitated

Z86.79 Personal history of other diseases of the circulatory system POA PDx

[4th] **Z87 Personal history of other diseases and conditions**
Code first any follow-up examination after treatment (Z09)

[5th] **Z87.0 Personal history of diseases of the respiratory system**
Conditions classifiable to J00-J99

Z87.01 Personal history of pneumonia (recurrent) POA PDx

Z87.09 Personal history of other diseases of the respiratory system POA PDx

[5th] **Z87.1 Personal history of diseases of the digestive system**
Conditions classifiable to K00-K93

Z87.11 Personal history of peptic ulcer disease POA PDx

Z87.19 Personal history of other diseases of the digestive system POA PDx
AHA: Q1 2017

Z87.2 Personal history of diseases of the skin and subcutaneous tissue POA PDx
Conditions classifiable to L00-L99
[EXCLUDES2] *personal history of diabetic foot ulcer (Z86.31)*

[5th] **Z87.3 Personal history of diseases of the musculoskeletal system and connective tissue**
Conditions classifiable to M00-M99
[EXCLUDES2] *personal history of (healed) traumatic fracture (Z87.81)*

[6th] **Z87.31 Personal history of (healed) nontraumatic fracture**

Z87.310 Personal history of (healed) osteoporosis fracture POA PDx
Personal history of (healed) fragility fracture
Personal history of (healed) collapsed vertebra due to osteoporosis

Z87.311 Personal history of (healed) other pathological fracture POA PDx
Personal history of (healed) collapsed vertebra NOS
[EXCLUDES2] *personal history of osteoporosis fracture (Z87.310)*

Z87.312 Personal history of (healed) stress fracture POA PDx
Personal history of (healed) fatigue fracture

Z87.39 Personal history of other diseases of the musculoskeletal system and connective tissue POA PDx

[5th] **Z87.4 Personal history of diseases of genitourinary system**
Conditions classifiable to N00-N99

[6th] **Z87.41 Personal history of dysplasia of the female genital tract**
[EXCLUDES1] *personal history of intraepithelial neoplasia III of female genital tract ►(Z86.001, Z86.008)◄*
personal history of malignant neoplasm of female genital tract (Z85.40-Z85.44)

Z87.410 Personal history of cervical dysplasia POA ♀ PDx

Z87.411 Personal history of vaginal dysplasia POA ♀ PDx

Z87.412 Personal history of vulvar dysplasia POA ♀ PDx

Z87.42 Personal history of other diseases of the female genital tract POA ♀ PDx

[6th] **Z87.43 Personal history of diseases of male genital organs**

Z87.430 Personal history of prostatic dysplasia POA ♂ PDx
[EXCLUDES1] *personal history of malignant neoplasm of prostate (Z85.46)*

Z87.438 Personal history of other diseases of male genital organs POA ♂ PDx

[6th] **Z87.44 Personal history of diseases of urinary system**
[EXCLUDES1] *personal history of malignant neoplasm of cervix uteri (Z85.41)*

Z87.440 Personal history of urinary (tract) infections POA PDx

Z87.441 Personal history of nephrotic syndrome POA PDx

Z87.442 Personal history of urinary calculi POA PDx
Personal history of kidney stones

Z87.448 Personal history of other diseases of urinary system POA PDx

[5th] **Z87.5 Personal history of complications of pregnancy, childbirth and the puerperium**
Conditions classifiable to O00-O9A
[EXCLUDES2] *recurrent pregnancy loss (N96)*

Z87.51 Personal history of pre-term labor POA ♀ PDx
[EXCLUDES1] *current pregnancy with history of pre-term labor (O09.21-)*

Z87.59 Personal history of other complications of pregnancy, childbirth and the puerperium POA ♀ PDx
Personal history of trophoblastic disease

[5th] **Z87.7 Personal history of (corrected) congenital malformations**
Conditions classifiable to Q00-Q89 that have been repaired or corrected
[EXCLUDES1] *congenital malformations that have been partially corrected or repair but which still require medical treatment - code to condition*
[EXCLUDES2] *other postprocedural states (Z98.-)*
personal history of medical treatment (Z92.-)
presence of cardiac and vascular implants and grafts (Z95.-)

PDx Unacceptable principal diagnosis symbol per Medicare code edits · POA Code exempt from diagnosis present on admission requirement
[A] Questionable admission · CC Complication or comorbidity · CC/MCC Exc CC/MCC exclusion · MCC Major complication or comorbidity
PDx CC Principal diagnosis as its own CC · PDx MCC Principal diagnosis as its own MCC · [HCC] HCC diagnosis code · [RxHCC] RxHCC diagnosis code
MACRA code · [Z1] Z code as first-listed diagnosis

presence of other devices (Z97.-)
presence of other functional implants (Z96.-)
transplanted organ and tissue status (Z94.-)

[6th] Z87.71 Personal history of (corrected) congenital malformations of genitourinary system
- Z87.710 Personal history of (corrected) hypospadias POA ♂ PDx
- Z87.718 Personal history of other specified (corrected) congenital malformations of genitourinary system POA PDx

[6th] Z87.72 Personal history of (corrected) congenital malformations of nervous system and sense organs
- Z87.720 Personal history of (corrected) congenital malformations of eye
- Z87.721 Personal history of (corrected) congenital malformations of ear POA PDx
- Z87.728 Personal history of other specified (corrected) congenital malformations of nervous system and sense organs POA PDx

[6th] Z87.73 Personal history of (corrected) congenital malformations of digestive system
- Z87.730 Personal history of (corrected) cleft lip and palate POA PDx
- Z87.738 Personal history of other specified (corrected) congenital malformations of digestive system POA PDx

Z87.74 Personal history of (corrected) congenital malformations of heart and circulatory system POA PDx

Z87.75 Personal history of (corrected) congenital malformations of respiratory system POA PDx

Z87.76 Personal history of (corrected) congenital malformations of integument, limbs and musculoskeletal system POA PDx

[6th] Z87.79 Personal history of other (corrected) congenital malformations
- Z87.790 Personal history of (corrected) congenital malformations of face and neck POA PDx
- Z87.798 Personal history of other (corrected) congenital malformations POA PDx

[5th] Z87.8 Personal history of other specified conditions

EXCLUDES2 *personal history of self harm (Z91.5)*

Z87.81 Personal history of (healed) traumatic fracture POA PDx

EXCLUDES2 *personal history of (healed) nontraumatic fracture (Z87.31-)*

[6th] Z87.82 Personal history of other (healed) physical injury and trauma

Conditions classifiable to S00-T88, except traumatic fractures

- Z87.820 Personal history of traumatic brain injury POA PDx

  EXCLUDES1 *personal history of transient ischemic attack (TIA), and cerebral infarction without residual deficits (Z86.73)*
- Z87.821 Personal history of retained foreign body fully removed POA PDx
- Z87.828 Personal history of other (healed) physical injury and trauma POA PDx

[6th] Z87.89 Personal history of other specified conditions
- Z87.890 Personal history of sex reassignment POA
- Z87.891 Personal history of nicotine dependence POA PDx

  AHA: Q2 2017

  EXCLUDES1 *current nicotine dependence (F17.2-)*
- Z87.892 Personal history of anaphylaxis POA PDx

  Code also allergy status such as:
  - allergy status to drugs, medicaments and biological substances (Z88.-)
  - allergy status, other than to drugs and biological substances (Z91.0-)
- Z87.898 Personal history of other specified conditions POA PDx

  AHA: Q1 2013

[4th] Z88 Allergy status to drugs, medicaments and biological substances

EXCLUDES2 *Allergy status, other than to drugs and biological substances (Z91.0-)*

- Z88.0 Allergy status to penicillin POA PDx
- Z88.1 Allergy status to other antibiotic agents status POA PDx
- Z88.2 Allergy status to sulfonamides status POA PDx

  AHA: Q3 2015
- Z88.3 Allergy status to other anti-infective agents status POA PDx
- Z88.4 Allergy status to anesthetic agent status POA PDx
- Z88.5 Allergy status to narcotic agent status POA PDx
- Z88.6 Allergy status to analgesic agent status POA PDx
- Z88.7 Allergy status to serum and vaccine status POA PDx
- Z88.8 Allergy status to other drugs, medicaments and biological substances status POA PDx
- Z88.9 Allergy status to unspecified drugs, medicaments and biological substances status POA PDx

[4th] Z89 Acquired absence of limb

INCLUDES *amputation status*
postprocedural loss of limb
post-traumatic loss of limb

EXCLUDES1 *acquired deformities of limbs (M20-M21)*
congenital absence of limbs (Q71-Q73)

[5th] Z89.0 Acquired absence of thumb and other finger(s)

[6th] Z89.01 Acquired absence of thumb
- Z89.011 Acquired absence of right thumb POA PDx
- Z89.012 Acquired absence of left thumb POA PDx
- Z89.019 Acquired absence of unspecified thumb POA PDx

[6th] Z89.02 Acquired absence of other finger(s)

EXCLUDES2 *acquired absence of thumb (Z89.01-)*
- Z89.021 Acquired absence of right finger(s) POA PDx
- Z89.022 Acquired absence of left finger(s) POA PDx
- Z89.029 Acquired absence of unspecified finger(s) POA PDx

[5th] Z89.1 Acquired absence of hand and wrist

[6th] Z89.11 Acquired absence of hand
- Z89.111 Acquired absence of right hand POA PDx
- Z89.112 Acquired absence of left hand POA PDx
- Z89.119 Acquired absence of unspecified hand POA PDx

[6th] Z89.12 Acquired absence of wrist

Disarticulation at wrist
- Z89.121 Acquired absence of right wrist POA PDx
- Z89.122 Acquired absence of left wrist POA PDx
- Z89.129 Acquired absence of unspecified wrist POA PDx

[5th] Z89.2 Acquired absence of upper limb above wrist

[6th] Z89.20 Acquired absence of upper limb, unspecified level
- Z89.201 Acquired absence of right upper limb, unspecified level POA PDx
- Z89.202 Acquired absence of left upper limb, unspecified level POA PDx
- Z89.209 Acquired absence of unspecified upper limb, unspecified level POA PDx

  Acquired absence of arm NOS

[6th] Z89.21 Acquired absence of upper limb below elbow
- Z89.211 Acquired absence of right upper limb below elbow POA PDx
- Z89.212 Acquired absence of left upper limb below elbow POA PDx
- Z89.219 Acquired absence of unspecified upper limb below elbow POA PDx

[6th] Z89.22 Acquired absence of upper limb above elbow

Disarticulation at elbow
- Z89.221 Acquired absence of right upper limb above elbow POA PDx

Unspecified Code | Other Specified Code | Manifestation Code | [N] Newborn | [P] Pediatric | [M] Maternity | [A] Adult | ♂ Male | ♀ Female
● New Code | ▲ Revised Code Title | ►◄ Revised Text | NOTES | INCLUDES | EXCLUDES1 Not coded here | EXCLUDES2 Not included here
[4th] 4th character required | [5th] 5th character required | [6th] 6th character required | [7th] 7th character required
[x7] Extension 'X' Alert | [HAC] Hospital-acquired condition (HAC) alert | AHA AHA Coding Clinic©

When symbols appear on a code that requires a 7th character extension, refer to Appendix B to identify applicable 7th character codes.

Z89.222 Acquired absence of left upper limb above elbow

Z89.229 Acquired absence of unspecified upper limb above elbow POA PDxIn

Z89.23 Acquired absence of shoulder
Acquired absence of shoulder joint following explantation of shoulder joint prosthesis, with or without presence of antibiotic-impregnated cement spacer

Z89.231 Acquired absence of right shoulder POA PDxIn

Z89.232 Acquired absence of left shoulder POA PDxIn

Z89.239 Acquired absence of unspecified shoulder POA PDxIn

Z89.4 Acquired absence of toe(s), foot, and ankle

Z89.41 Acquired absence of great toe

Z89.411 Acquired absence of right great toe POA HCC PDxIn

Z89.412 Acquired absence of left great toe POA HCC PDxIn

Z89.419 Acquired absence of unspecified great toe POA HCC PDxIn

Z89.42 Acquired absence of other toe(s)

EXCLUDES2 acquired absence of great toe (Z89.41-)

Z89.421 Acquired absence of other right toe(s) POA HCC PDxIn

Z89.422 Acquired absence of other left toe(s) POA HCC PDxIn

Z89.429 Acquired absence of other toe(s), unspecified side POA HCC PDxIn

Z89.43 Acquired absence of foot

Z89.431 Acquired absence of right foot POA HCC PDxIn

Z89.432 Acquired absence of left foot POA HCC PDxIn

Z89.439 Acquired absence of unspecified foot POA HCC PDxIn

Z89.44 Acquired absence of ankle
Disarticulation of ankle

Z89.441 Acquired absence of right ankle POA HCC PDxIn

Z89.442 Acquired absence of left ankle POA HCC PDxIn

Z89.449 Acquired absence of unspecified ankle POA HCC PDxIn

Z89.5 Acquired absence of leg below knee

Z89.51 Acquired absence of leg below knee

Z89.511 Acquired absence of right leg below knee POA HCC PDxIn

Z89.512 Acquired absence of left leg below knee POA HCC PDxIn

Z89.519 Acquired absence of unspecified leg below knee POA HCC PDxIn

Z89.52 Acquired absence of knee
Acquired absence of knee joint following explantation of knee joint prosthesis, with or without presence of antibiotic-impregnated cement spacer

Z89.521 Acquired absence of right knee POA PDxIn

Z89.522 Acquired absence of left knee POA PDxIn

Z89.529 Acquired absence of unspecified knee POA PDxIn

Z89.6 Acquired absence of leg above knee

Z89.61 Acquired absence of leg above knee
Acquired absence of leg NOS
Disarticulation at knee

Z89.611 Acquired absence of right leg above knee POA HCC PDxIn

Z89.612 Acquired absence of left leg above knee POA HCC PDxIn

Z89.619 Acquired absence of unspecified leg above knee POA HCC PDxIn

Z89.62 Acquired absence of hip
Acquired absence of hip joint following explantation of hip joint prosthesis, with or without presence of antibiotic-impregnated cement spacer
Disarticulation at hip

Z89.621 Acquired absence of right hip joint POA PDxIn

Z89.622 Acquired absence of left hip joint POA PDxIn

Z89.629 Acquired absence of unspecified hip joint POA PDxIn

Z89.9 Acquired absence of limb, unspecified

Z90 Acquired absence of organs, not elsewhere classified
INCLUDES postprocedural or post-traumatic loss of body part NEC
EXCLUDES1 congenital absence - see Alphabetical Index
EXCLUDES2 postprocedural absence of endocrine glands (E89.-)

Z90.0 Acquired absence of part of head and neck

Z90.01 Acquired absence of eye POA PDxIn

Z90.02 Acquired absence of larynx POA PDxIn

Z90.09 Acquired absence of other part of head and neck POA PDxIn
Acquired absence of nose
EXCLUDES2 teeth (K08.1)

Z90.1 Acquired absence of breast and nipple

Z90.10 Acquired absence of unspecified breast and nipple POA

Z90.11 Acquired absence of right breast and nipple POA

Z90.12 Acquired absence of left breast and nipple POA

Z90.13 Acquired absence of bilateral breasts and nipples POA

Z90.2 Acquired absence of lung [part of] POA PDxIn

Z90.3 Acquired absence of stomach [part of] POA PDxIn

Z90.4 Acquired absence of other specified parts of digestive tract

Z90.41 Acquired absence of pancreas
Code also exocrine pancreatic insufficiency (K86.81)
Use additional code to identify any associated:
insulin use (Z79.4)
diabetes mellitus, postpancreatectomy (E13.-)

Z90.410 Acquired total absence of pancreas POA PDxIn
Acquired absence of pancreas NOS

Z90.411 Acquired partial absence of pancreas POA PDxIn

Z90.49 Acquired absence of other specified parts of digestive tract POA PDxIn

Z90.5 Acquired absence of kidney POA PDxIn

Z90.6 Acquired absence of other parts of urinary tract POA PDxIn
Acquired absence of bladder

Z90.7 Acquired absence of genital organ(s)
EXCLUDES1 personal history of sex reassignment (Z87.890)
EXCLUDES2 female genital mutilation status (N90.81-)

Z90.71 Acquired absence of cervix and uterus

Z90.710 Acquired absence of both cervix and uterus POA ♀ PDxIn
Acquired absence of uterus NOS
Status post total hysterectomy

Z90.711 Acquired absence of uterus with remaining cervical stump POA ♀ PDxIn
Status post partial hysterectomy with remaining cervical stump

Z90.712 Acquired absence of cervix with remaining uterus POA ♀ PDxIn

Z90.72 Acquired absence of ovaries

Z90.721 Acquired absence of ovaries, unilateral POA ♀ PDxIn

Z90.722 Acquired absence of ovaries, bilateral POA ♀ PDxIn

Z90.79 Acquired absence of other genital organ(s) POA PDxIn

Z90.8 Acquired absence of other organs

Z90.81 Acquired absence of spleen POA PDxIn

Z90.89 Acquired absence of other organs POA PDxIn

Z91 Personal risk factors, not elsewhere classified
EXCLUDES2 contact with and (suspected) exposures hazardous to health (Z77.-)
exposure to pollution and other problems related to physical environment (Z77.1-)
female genital mutilation status (N90.81-)
personal history of physical injury and trauma (Z87.81, Z87.82-)
occupational exposure to risk factors (Z57.-)

Z91.0 Allergy status, other than to drugs and biological substances
EXCLUDES2 Allergy status to drugs, medicaments, and biological substances (Z88.-)

POA̲ Unacceptable principal diagnosis symbol per Medicare code edits POA̲ Code exempt from diagnosis present on admission requirement
❓ Questionable admission ↩ Complication or comorbidity CC/MCC EXC CC/MCC exclusion MCC Major complication or comorbidity
🅲 Principal diagnosis as its own CC 🅼 Principal diagnosis as its own MCC HCC HCC diagnosis code RXHCC RxHCC diagnosis code
MACRA code Z1 Z code as first-listed diagnosis

1280   When symbols appear on a code that requires a 7th character extension, refer to Appendix B to identify applicable 7th character codes.   2018 ICD-10-CM

6ᵖ **Z91.01** Food **allergy status**

EXCLUDES2 *food additives allergy status (Z91.02)*

Z91.010 Allergy to peanuts   POA PDxIn

Z91.011 Allergy to milk products   POA PDxIn

EXCLUDES1 *lactose intolerance (E73.-)*

Z91.012 Allergy to eggs   POA PDxIn

Z91.013 Allergy to seafood   POA PDxIn

Allergy to shellfish

Allergy to octopus or squid ink

Z91.018 Allergy to other foods   POA PDxIn

Allergy to nuts other than peanuts

Z91.02 Food additives allergy status

6ᵖ **Z91.03** Insect **allergy status**

Z91.030 Bee **allergy status**   POA PDxIn

Z91.038 Other insect allergy status   POA PDxIn

6ᵖ **Z91.04 Nonmedicinal substance allergy status**

Z91.040 Latex **allergy status**   POA PDxIn

Latex sensitivity status

Z91.041 Radiographic dye **allergy status**   POA PDxIn

Allergy status to contrast media used for diagnostic X-ray procedure

Z91.048 Other nonmedicinal substance allergy status   POA PDxIn

Z91.09 Other allergy status, other than to drugs and biological substances   POA PDxIn

5ᵖ **Z91.1 Patient's noncompliance with medical treatment and regimen**

Z91.11 Patient's noncompliance with dietary regimen   POA PDxIn

6ᵖ **Z91.12 Patient's** intentional underdosing of medication **regimen**

Code first underdosing of medication (T36-T50) with fifth or sixth character 6

EXCLUDES1 *adverse effect of prescribed drug taken as directed- code to adverse effect*

poisoning (overdose) -code to poisoning

Z91.120 Patient's intentional underdosing of medication regimen due to financial hardship   POA PDxIn

Z91.128 Patient's intentional underdosing of medication regimen for other reason   POA PDxIn

6ᵖ **Z91.13 Patient's** unintentional underdosing of medication **regimen**

Code first underdosing of medication (T36-T50) with fifth or sixth character 6

EXCLUDES1 *adverse effect of prescribed drug taken as directed- code to adverse effect*

poisoning (overdose) -code to poisoning

Z91.130 Patient's unintentional underdosing of medication regimen due to age-related debility   POA PDxIn

Z91.138 Patient's unintentional underdosing of medication regimen for other reason   POA PDxIn

Z91.14 Patient's other noncompliance with medication regimen

Patient's underdosing of medication NOS

Z91.15 Patient's noncompliance with renal dialysis   POA HCC RxHCC PDxIn

Z91.19 Patient's noncompliance with other medical treatment and regimen   POA PDxIn

Nonadherence to medical treatment

5ᵖ **Z91.4 Personal history of psychological trauma, not elsewhere classified**

6ᵖ **Z91.41 Personal history of** adult abuse

EXCLUDES2 *personal history of abuse in childhood (Z62.81-)*

Z91.410 Personal history of adult physical and sexual **abuse**   A POA PDxIn

EXCLUDES1 *current adult physical abuse (T74.11, T76.11)*

current adult sexual abuse (T74.21, T76.11)

Z91.411 Personal history of adult psychological abuse   A POA PDxIn

Z91.412 Personal history of adult neglect   A POA PDxIn

EXCLUDES1 *current adult neglect (T74.01, T76.01)*

Z91.419 Personal history of unspecified adult abuse   A POA PDxIn

Z91.49 Other personal history of psychological trauma, not elsewhere classified   POA PDxIn

Z91.5 Personal history of self-harm

Personal history of parasuicide

Personal history of self-poisoning

Personal history of suicide attempt

5ᵖ **Z91.8 Other specified personal risk factors, not elsewhere classified**

Z91.81 History of falling   POA PDxIn

At risk for falling

Z91.82 Personal history of military deployment   A POA PDxIn

Individual (civilian or military) with past history of military war, peacekeeping and humanitarian deployment (current or past conflict)

Returned from military deployment

Z91.83 Wandering in diseases classified elsewhere   POA

Code first underlying disorder such as:

Alzheimer's disease (G30.-)

autism or pervasive developmental disorder (F84.-)

intellectual disabilities (F70-F79)

unspecified dementia with behavioral disturbance (F03.9-)

● 6ᵖ **Z91.84** Oral health **risk factors**

● **Z91.841 Risk for dental caries,** low

● **Z91.842 Risk for dental caries,** moderate

● **Z91.843 Risk for dental caries,** high

● **Z91.849 Unspecified risk for dental caries**

Z91.89 Other specified **personal risk factors, not elsewhere classified**   POA PDxIn

AHA: Q1 2017

4ᵖ **Z92 Personal history of medical treatment**

EXCLUDES2 *postprocedural states (Z98.-)*

Z92.0 Personal history of contraception   POA PDxIn

EXCLUDES1 *counseling or management of current contraceptive practices (Z30.-)*

long term (current) use of contraception (Z79.3)

presence of (intrauterine) contraceptive device (Z97.5)

5ᵖ **Z92.2 Personal history of** drug therapy

EXCLUDES2 *long term (current) drug therapy (Z79.-)*

Z92.21 Personal history of antineoplastic chemotherapy   POA PDxIn

Z92.22 Personal history of monoclonal drug **therapy**   POA PDxIn

Z92.23 Personal history of estrogen **therapy**   POA PDxIn

6ᵖ **Z92.24 Personal history of** steroid **therapy**

Z92.240 Personal history of inhaled steroid **therapy**   POA PDxIn

Z92.241 Personal history of systemic steroid **therapy**   POA PDxIn

Personal history of steroid therapy NOS

Z92.25 Personal history of immunosuppression therapy   POA PDxIn

EXCLUDES2 *personal history of steroid therapy (Z92.24)*

Z92.29 Personal history of other drug therapy   POA PDxIn

Z92.3 Personal history of irradiation   POA PDxIn

Personal history of exposure to therapeutic radiation

EXCLUDES1 *exposure to radiation in the physical environment (Z77.12)*

occupational exposure to radiation (Z57.1)

5ᵖ **Z92.8 Personal history of other medical treatment**

Z92.81 Personal history of extracorporeal membrane oxygenation (ECMO)   POA PDxIn

Unspecified Code   Other Specified Code   Manifestation Code   N Newborn   P Pediatric   M Maternity   A Adult   ♂ Male   ♀ Female

● New Code   ▲ Revised Code Title   ▶◀ Revised Text   NOTES   INCLUDES   EXCLUDES1 Not coded here   EXCLUDES2 Not included here

4ᵖ 4ᵗʰ character required   5ᵖ 5ᵗʰ character required   6ᵖ 6ᵗʰ character required   7ᵖ 7ᵗʰ character required

Extension 'X' Alert   HAC Hospital-acquired condition (HAC) alert   AHA AHA Coding Clinic©

2018 ICD-10-CM   When symbols appear on a code that requires a 7th character extension, refer to Appendix B to identify applicable 7th character codes.   **1281**

Z92.82 Status post administration of tPA (rtPA) in a different facility within the last 24 hours prior to admission to current facility [POA] [PDx]
AHA: Q4 2013
Code first condition requiring tPA administration, such as:
acute cerebral infarction (I63.-)
acute myocardial infarction (I21.-, I22.-)

Z92.83 Personal history of failed moderate sedation [POA] [PDx]
Personal history of failed conscious sedation
[EXCLUDES2] *failed moderate sedation during procedure (T88.52)*

Z92.84 Personal history of unintended awareness under general anesthesia [POA] [PDx]
AHA: Q4 2016
[EXCLUDES2] *unintended awareness under general anesthesia during procedure (T88.53)*

Z92.89 Personal history of other medical treatment [POA] [PDx]

[4th] **Z93 Artificial opening status**
[EXCLUDES1] *artificial openings requiring attention or management (Z43.-)*
complications of external stoma (J95.0-, K94.-, N99.5-)

Z93.0 Tracheostomy status [POA] [HCC] [PDx]
AHA: Q4 2013
Z93.1 Gastrostomy status [POA] [HCC] [PDx]
Z93.2 Ileostomy status [POA] [HCC] [PDx]
Z93.3 Colostomy status [POA] [HCC] [PDx]
Z93.4 Other artificial openings of gastrointestinal tract status [POA] [HCC] [PDx]
[5th] **Z93.5 Cystostomy status**
Z93.50 Unspecified cystostomy status [POA] [HCC] [PDx]
Z93.51 Cutaneous-vesicostomy status [POA] [HCC] [PDx]
Z93.52 Appendico-vesicostomy status [POA] [HCC] [PDx]
Z93.59 Other cystostomy status [POA] [HCC] [PDx]
Z93.6 Other artificial openings of urinary tract status [POA] [HCC] [PDx]
Nephrostomy status
Ureterostomy status
Urethrostomy status
Z93.8 Other artificial opening status [POA] [HCC] [PDx]
Z93.9 Artificial opening status, unspecified [POA] [HCC] [PDx]

[4th] **Z94 Transplanted organ and tissue status**
[INCLUDES] *organ or tissue replaced by heterogenous or homogenous transplant*
[EXCLUDES1] *complications of transplanted organ or tissue - see Alphabetical Index*
[EXCLUDES2] *presence of vascular grafts (Z95.-)*

Z94.0 Kidney transplant status [CC] [POA] [RxHCC] [PDx] [CC/MCC Exc]
Z94.1 Heart transplant status [CC] [POA] [HCC] [RxHCC] [PDx] [CC/MCC Exc]
[EXCLUDES1] *artificial heart status (Z95.812)*
heart-valve replacement status (Z95.2-Z95.4)
Z94.2 Lung transplant status [CC] [POA] [HCC] [RxHCC] [PDx] [CC/MCC Exc]
Z94.3 Heart and lungs transplant status [CC] [POA] [HCC] [PDx CC] [RxHCC] [PDx] [CC/MCC Exc]
Z94.4 Liver transplant status [CC] [POA] [HCC] [RxHCC] [PDx] [CC/MCC Exc]
Z94.5 Skin transplant status [POA] [PDx]
Autogenous skin transplant status
Z94.6 Bone transplant status [POA] [PDx]
Z94.7 Corneal transplant status [POA] [PDx]
[5th] **Z94.8 Other transplanted organ and tissue status**
Z94.81 Bone marrow transplant status [CC] [POA] [HCC] [RxHCC] [PDx] [CC/MCC Exc]
Z94.82 Intestine transplant status [CC] [POA] [HCC] [RxHCC] [PDx] [CC/MCC Exc]
Z94.83 Pancreas transplant status [CC] [POA] [HCC] [RxHCC] [PDx] [CC/MCC Exc]
Z94.84 Stem cells transplant status [CC] [POA] [HCC] [RxHCC] [PDx] [CC/MCC Exc]
Z94.89 Other transplanted organ and tissue status [POA] [PDx]
Z94.9 Transplanted organ and tissue status, unspecified [POA] [PDx]

[4th] **Z95 Presence of cardiac and vascular implants and grafts**
[EXCLUDES2] *complications of cardiac and vascular devices, implants and grafts (T82.-)*

Z95.0 Presence of cardiac pacemaker [POA] [PDx]
Presence of cardiac resynchronization therapy (CRT-P) pacemaker
[EXCLUDES1] *adjustment or management of cardiac device (Z45.0-)*
adjustment or management of cardiac pacemaker (Z45.0)
presence of automatic (implantable) cardiac defibrillator with synchronous cardiac pacemaker (Z95.810)
Z95.1 Presence of aortocoronary bypass graft [POA] [PDx]
Presence of coronary artery bypass graft
Z95.2 Presence of prosthetic heart valve [POA] [PDx]
Presence of heart valve NOS
Z95.3 Presence of xenogenic heart valve [POA] [PDx]
Z95.4 Presence of other heart-valve replacement [POA] [PDx]
Z95.5 Presence of coronary angioplasty implant and graft [POA] [PDx]
[EXCLUDES1] *coronary angioplasty status without implant and graft (Z98.61)*
[5th] **Z95.8 Presence of other cardiac and vascular implants and grafts**
[6th] **Z95.81 Presence of other cardiac implants and grafts**
Z95.810 Presence of automatic (implantable) cardiac defibrillator [POA] [PDx]
Presence of automatic (implantable) cardiac defibrillator with synchronous cardiac pacemaker
Presence of cardiac resynchronization therapy defibrillator (CRT-D)
Presence of cardioverter-defibrillator (ICD)
Z95.811 Presence of heart assist device [CC] [POA] [HCC] [PDx] [CC/MCC Exc]
Z95.812 Presence of fully implantable artificial heart [CC] [POA] [HCC] [PDx] [CC/MCC Exc]
Z95.818 Presence of other cardiac implants and grafts [POA] [PDx]
[6th] **Z95.82 Presence of other vascular implants and grafts**
Z95.820 Peripheral vascular angioplasty status with implants and grafts [POA] [PDx]
[EXCLUDES1] *peripheral vascular angioplasty without implant and graft (Z98.62)*
Z95.828 Presence of other vascular implants and grafts [POA] [PDx]
Presence of intravascular prosthesis NEC
Z95.9 Presence of cardiac and vascular implant and graft, unspecified [POA] [PDx]

[4th] **Z96 Presence of other functional implants**
[EXCLUDES2] *complications of internal prosthetic devices, implants and grafts (T82-T85)*
fitting and adjustment of prosthetic and other devices (Z44-Z46)

Z96.0 Presence of urogenital implants [PDx]
Z96.1 Presence of intraocular lens [PDx]
Presence of pseudophakia
[5th] **Z96.2 Presence of otological and audiological implants**
Z96.20 Presence of otological and audiological implant, unspecified [PDx]
Z96.21 Cochlear implant status [PDx]
Z96.22 Myringotomy tube(s)status [PDx]
Z96.29 Presence of other otological and audiological implants [PDx]
Presence of bone-conduction hearing device
Presence of eustachian tube stent
Stapes replacement
Z96.3 Presence of artificial larynx [PDx]
[5th] **Z96.4 Presence of endocrine implants**
Z96.41 Presence of insulin pump (external) (internal) [PDx]
Z96.49 Presence of other endocrine implants [PDx]
Z96.5 Presence of tooth-root and mandibular implants [PDx]
[5th] **Z96.6 Presence of orthopedic joint implants**
Z96.60 Presence of unspecified orthopedic joint implant [PDx]
[6th] **Z96.61 Presence of artificial shoulder joint**

[PDx] Unacceptable principal diagnosis symbol per Medicare code edits [POA] Code exempt from diagnosis present on admission requirement
[Q] Questionable admission [CC] Complication or comorbidity [CC/MCC Exc] CC/MCC exclusion [MCC] Major complication or comorbidity
[PDx CC] Principal diagnosis as its own CC [PDx MCC] Principal diagnosis as its own MCC [HCC] HCC diagnosis code [RxHCC] RxHCC diagnosis code
MACRA code [Z1] Z code as first-listed diagnosis

Z96.611 Presence of right artificial shoulder joint PDxIn

Z96.612 Presence of left artificial shoulder joint PDxIn

Z96.619 Presence of unspecified artificial shoulder joint PDxIn

6ᵗʰ Z96.62 Presence of artificial elbow joint

Z96.621 Presence of right artificial elbow joint PDxIn

Z96.622 Presence of left artificial elbow joint PDxIn

Z96.629 Presence of unspecified artificial elbow joint PDxIn

6ᵗʰ Z96.63 Presence of artificial wrist joint

Z96.631 Presence of right artificial wrist joint PDxIn

Z96.632 Presence of left artificial wrist joint PDxIn

Z96.639 Presence of unspecified artificial wrist joint PDxIn

6ᵗʰ Z96.64 Presence of artificial hip joint

Hip-joint replacement (partial) (total)

Z96.641 Presence of right artificial hip joint PDxIn

AHA: Q3 2016

Z96.642 Presence of left artificial hip joint PDxIn

AHA: Q1 2015

Z96.643 Presence of artificial hip joint, bilateral PDxIn

Z96.649 Presence of unspecified artificial hip joint PDxIn

6ᵗʰ Z96.65 Presence of artificial knee joint

Z96.651 Presence of right artificial knee joint PDxIn

Z96.652 Presence of left artificial knee joint PDxIn

Z96.653 Presence of artificial knee joint, bilateral PDxIn

Z96.659 Presence of unspecified artificial knee joint PDxIn

6ᵗʰ Z96.66 Presence of artificial ankle joint

Z96.661 Presence of right artificial ankle joint PDxIn

Z96.662 Presence of left artificial ankle joint PDxIn

Z96.669 Presence of unspecified artificial ankle joint PDxIn

6ᵗʰ Z96.69 Presence of other orthopedic joint implants

Z96.691 Finger-joint replacement of right hand PDxIn

Z96.692 Finger-joint replacement of left hand PDxIn

Z96.693 Finger-joint replacement, bilateral PDxIn

Z96.698 Presence of other orthopedic joint implants PDxIn

Z96.7 Presence of other bone and tendon implants PDxIn

Presence of skull plate

5ᵗʰ Z96.8 Presence of other specified functional implants

Z96.81 Presence of artificial skin PDxIn

Z96.89 Presence of other specified functional implants PDxIn

Z96.9 Presence of functional implant, unspecified PDxIn

4ᵗʰ Z97 Presence of other devices

EXCLUDES1 complications of internal prosthetic devices, implants and grafts (T82-T85)

fitting and adjustment of prosthetic and other devices (Z44-Z46)

EXCLUDES2 presence of cerebrospinal fluid drainage device (Z98.2)

Z97.0 Presence of artificial eye POA PDxIn

5ᵗʰ Z97.1 Presence of artificial limb (complete) (partial)

Z97.10 Presence of artificial limb (complete) (partial), unspecified POA PDxIn

Z97.11 Presence of artificial right arm (complete) (partial) POA PDxIn

Z97.12 Presence of artificial left arm (complete) (partial) POA PDxIn

Z97.13 Presence of artificial right leg (complete) (partial) POA PDxIn

Z97.14 Presence of artificial left leg (complete) (partial) POA PDxIn

Z97.15 Presence of artificial arms, bilateral (complete) (partial) POA PDxIn

Z97.16 Presence of artificial legs, bilateral (complete) (partial) POA PDxIn

Z97.2 Presence of dental prosthetic device (complete) (partial) POA PDxIn

Presence of dentures (complete) (partial)

Z97.3 Presence of spectacles and contact lenses POA PDxIn

Z97.4 Presence of external hearing-aid

Z97.5 Presence of (intrauterine) contraceptive device POA ♀

EXCLUDES1 checking, reinsertion or removal of implantable subdermal contraceptive (Z30.46)

checking, reinsertion or removal of intrauterine contraceptive device (Z30.43-)

Z97.8 Presence of other specified devices POA PDxIn

4ᵗʰ Z98 Other postprocedural states

EXCLUDES2 aftercare (Z43-Z49, Z51)

follow-up medical care (Z08-Z09)

postprocedural complication - see Alphabetical Index

Z98.0 Intestinal bypass and anastomosis status POA PDxIn

EXCLUDES2 bariatric surgery status (Z98.84)

gastric bypass status (Z98.84)

obesity surgery status (Z98.84)

Z98.1 Arthrodesis status POA PDxIn

Z98.2 Presence of cerebrospinal fluid drainage device POA PDxIn

Presence of CSF shunt

Z98.3 Post therapeutic collapse of lung status POA PDxIn

Code first underlying disease

5ᵗʰ Z98.4 Cataract extraction status

Use additional code to identify intraocular lens implant status (Z96.1)

EXCLUDES1 aphakia (H27.0)

Z98.41 Cataract extraction status, right eye POA PDxIn

Z98.42 Cataract extraction status, left eye POA PDxIn

Z98.49 Cataract extraction status, unspecified eye POA PDxIn

5ᵗʰ Z98.5 Sterilization status

EXCLUDES1 female infertility (N97.-)

male infertility (N46.-)

Z98.51 Tubal ligation status POA ♀ PDxIn

Z98.52 Vasectomy status A POA ♂ PDxIn

5ᵗʰ Z98.6 Angioplasty status

Z98.61 Coronary angioplasty status POA PDxIn

EXCLUDES1 coronary angioplasty status with implant and graft (Z95.5)

Z98.62 Peripheral vascular angioplasty status POA PDxIn

EXCLUDES1 peripheral vascular angioplasty status with implant and graft (Z95.820)

5ᵗʰ Z98.8 Other specified postprocedural states

6ᵗʰ Z98.81 Dental procedure status

Z98.810 Dental sealant status POA PDxIn

Z98.811 Dental restoration status POA PDxIn

Dental crown status

Dental fillings status

Z98.818 Other dental procedure status POA PDxIn

Z98.82 Breast implant status POA PDxIn

EXCLUDES1 breast implant removal status (Z98.86)

Z98.83 Filtering (vitreous) bleb after glaucoma surgery status POA PDxIn

EXCLUDES1 Inflammation (infection) of postprocedural bleb (H59.4-)

Z98.84 Bariatric surgery status POA PDxIn

Gastric banding status

Gastric bypass status for obesity

Obesity surgery status

EXCLUDES1 bariatric surgery status complicating pregnancy, childbirth, or the puerperium (O99.84)

EXCLUDES2 intestinal bypass and anastomosis status (Z98.0)

Unspecified Code   Other Specified Code   Manifestation Code   Ⓝ Newborn   Ⓟ Pediatric   Ⓜ Maternity   Ⓐ Adult   ♂ Male   ♀ Female
● New Code   ▲ Revised Code Title   ▶◀ Revised Text   NOTES   INCLUDES   EXCLUDES 1 Not coded here   EXCLUDES 2 Not included here
4ᵗʰ character required   5ᵗʰ 5ᵗʰ character required   6ᵗʰ 6ᵗʰ character required   7ᵗʰ 7ᵗʰ character required
7ᵖ Extension 'X' Alert   HAC Hospital-acquired condition (HAC) alert   AHA AHA Coding Clinic©

2018 ICD-10-CM   When symbols appear on a code that requires a 7th character extension, refer to Appendix B to identify applicable 7th character codes.   1283

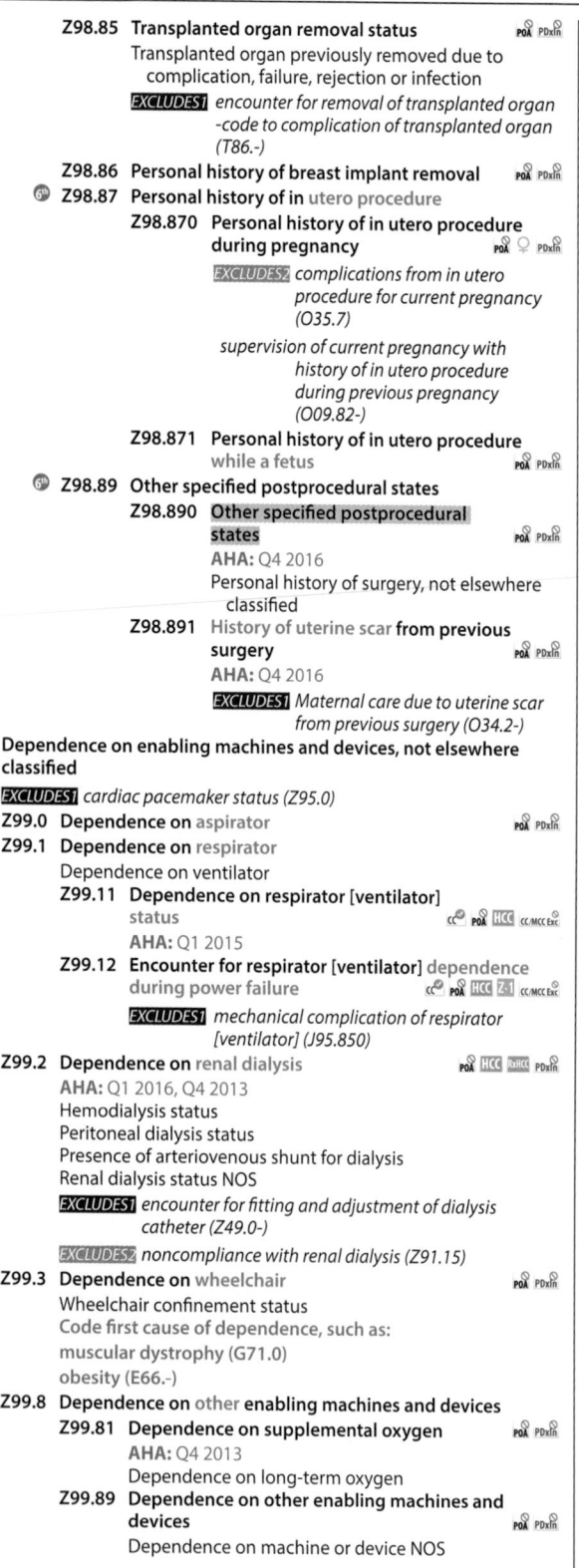

Z98.85 Transplanted organ removal status POA PDxIn

Transplanted organ previously removed due to complication, failure, rejection or infection

EXCLUDES1 *encounter for removal of transplanted organ -code to complication of transplanted organ (T86.-)*

Z98.86 Personal history of breast implant removal POA PDxIn

Z98.87 Personal history of in utero procedure

Z98.870 Personal history of in utero procedure during pregnancy POA ♀ PDxIn

EXCLUDES2 *complications from in utero procedure for current pregnancy (O35.7)*

supervision of current pregnancy with history of in utero procedure during previous pregnancy (O09.82-)

Z98.871 Personal history of in utero procedure while a fetus POA PDxIn

Z98.89 Other specified postprocedural states

Z98.890 Other specified postprocedural states POA PDxIn

AHA: Q4 2016

Personal history of surgery, not elsewhere classified

Z98.891 History of uterine scar from previous surgery POA PDxIn

AHA: Q4 2016

EXCLUDES1 *Maternal care due to uterine scar from previous surgery (O34.2-)*

Z99 Dependence on enabling machines and devices, not elsewhere classified

EXCLUDES1 *cardiac pacemaker status (Z95.0)*

Z99.0 Dependence on aspirator POA PDxIn

Z99.1 Dependence on respirator

Dependence on ventilator

Z99.11 Dependence on respirator [ventilator] status CC POA HCC CC/MCC Exc

AHA: Q1 2015

Z99.12 Encounter for respirator [ventilator] dependence during power failure CC POA HCC Z-1 CC/MCC Exc

EXCLUDES1 *mechanical complication of respirator [ventilator] (J95.850)*

Z99.2 Dependence on renal dialysis POA HCC RxHCC PDxIn

AHA: Q1 2016, Q4 2013

Hemodialysis status

Peritoneal dialysis status

Presence of arteriovenous shunt for dialysis

Renal dialysis status NOS

EXCLUDES1 *encounter for fitting and adjustment of dialysis catheter (Z49.0-)*

EXCLUDES2 *noncompliance with renal dialysis (Z91.15)*

Z99.3 Dependence on wheelchair POA PDxIn

Wheelchair confinement status

Code first cause of dependence, such as:

muscular dystrophy (G71.0)

obesity (E66.-)

Z99.8 Dependence on other enabling machines and devices

Z99.81 Dependence on supplemental oxygen POA PDxIn

AHA: Q4 2013

Dependence on long-term oxygen

Z99.89 Dependence on other enabling machines and devices POA PDxIn

Dependence on machine or device NOS

PDxIn Unacceptable principal diagnosis symbol per Medicare code edits   POA Code exempt from diagnosis present on admission requirement

? Questionable admission   CC Complication or comorbidity   CC/MCC Exc CC/MCC exclusion   MCC Major complication or comorbidity

POA Principal diagnosis as its own CC   MCC Principal diagnosis as its own MCC   HCC HCC diagnosis code   RxHCC RxHCC diagnosis code

MACRA code   Z-1 Z code as first-listed diagnosis

When symbols appear on a code that requires a 7th character extension, refer to Appendix B to identify applicable 7th character codes.

2018 ICD-10-CM

NOTES

NOTES

Appendix A: Z Codes for Long-term Use of Drugs

The following Z codes/categories may only be reported as the principal/first-listed diagnosis, except when there are multiple encounters on the same day and the medical records for the encounters are combined:

Drug Name	Code	Code Descriptor
acarbose	Z79.84	Long term (current) use of oral hypoglycemic drugs
Achromycin V®	Z79.2	Long term (current) use of antibiotics
Aclasta®	Z79.83	Long term (current) use of bisphosphonates
Acova®	Z79.02	Long term (current) use of antithrombotics/antiplatelets
Actiprofen®	Z79.1	Long term (current) use of non-steroidal anti-inflammatories (NSAID)
Activella®	Z79.890	Hormone replacement therapy (postmenopausal)
Actonel®	Z79.83	Long term (current) use of bisphosphonates
Actos®	Z79.84	Long term (current) use of oral hypoglycemic drugs
Addaprin®	Z79.1	Long term (current) use of non-steroidal anti-inflammatories (NSAID)
Advil Children's®	Z79.1	Long term (current) use of non-steroidal anti-inflammatories (NSAID)
Advil Infant's Concentrated Drops®	Z79.1	Long term (current) use of non-steroidal anti-inflammatories (NSAID)
Advil Liqui-Gels®	Z79.1	Long term (current) use of non-steroidal anti-inflammatories (NSAID)
Advil®	Z79.1	Long term (current) use of non-steroidal anti-inflammatories (NSAID)
Aerospan HFA®	Z79.51	Long term (current) use of inhaled steroids
Aflaxen®	Z79.1	Long term (current) use of non-steroidal anti-inflammatories (NSAID)
Afrezza®	Z79.4	Long term (current) use of insulin
A-G Profen®	Z79.1	Long term (current) use of non-steroidal anti-inflammatories (NSAID)
Akne-Mycin®	Z79.2	Long term (current) use of antibiotics
alendronate	Z79.83	Long term (current) use of bisphosphonates
Aleve®	Z79.1	Long term (current) use of non-steroidal anti-inflammatories (NSAID)
All Day Pain Relief®	Z79.1	Long term (current) use of non-steroidal anti-inflammatories (NSAID)
All Day Relief®	Z79.1	Long term (current) use of non-steroidal anti-inflammatories (NSAID)
Alora®	Z79.890	Hormone replacement therapy (postmenopausal)
Altabax®	Z79.2	Long term (current) use of antibiotics
Altavera®	Z79.3	Long term (current) use of hormonal contraceptives
Alvesco®	Z79.51	Long term (current) use of inhaled steroids
Alyacen 1 / 35®	Z79.3	Long term (current) use of hormonal contraceptives
Alyacen 1 / 35®	Z79.890	Hormone replacement therapy (postmenopausal)
Amaryl®	Z79.84	Long term (current) use of oral hypoglycemic drugs
Amethia Lo®	Z79.3	Long term (current) use of hormonal contraceptives
Amethia®	Z79.3	Long term (current) use of hormonal contraceptives
Amethyst®	Z79.3	Long term (current) use of hormonal contraceptives
amoxicillin	Z79.2	Long term (current) use of antibiotics
ampicillin/sulbactam	Z79.2	Long term (current) use of antibiotics
Anaprox®	Z79.1	Long term (current) use of non-steroidal anti-inflammatories (NSAID)
Anaprox-DS®	Z79.1	Long term (current) use of non-steroidal anti-inflammatories (NSAID)
anastrozole	Z79.811	Long term (current) use of aromatase inhibitors
Angeliq®	Z79.890	Hormone replacement therapy (postmenopausal)
Angiomax®	Z79.02	Long term (current) use of antithrombotics/antiplatelets
Antibiotic Plus Pain Relief®	Z79.2	Long term (current) use of antibiotics
Apidra Solostar®	Z79.4	Long term (current) use of insulin
Apidra®	Z79.4	Long term (current) use of insulin
apixaban	Z79.01	Long term (current) use of anticoagulants
Apri®	Z79.3	Long term (current) use of hormonal contraceptives
Aranelle®	Z79.3	Long term (current) use of hormonal contraceptives
Aranelle®	Z79.890	Hormone replacement therapy (postmenopausal)
Aredia®	Z79.83	Long term (current) use of bisphosphonates

Drug Name	Code	Code Descriptor
argatroban	Z79.02	Long term (current) use of antithrombotics/antiplatelets
Arimidex®	Z79.811	Long term (current) use of aromatase inhibitors
Aristospan®	Z79.52	Long term (current) use of systemic steroids
Arixtra®	Z79.01	Long term (current) use of anticoagulants
Arnuity Ellipta®	Z79.51	Long term (current) use of inhaled steroids
Aromasin®	Z79.811	Long term (current) use of aromatase inhibitors
Arthrotec®	Z79.1	Long term (current) use of non-steroidal anti-inflammatories (NSAID)
Ascriptin®	Z79.82	Long term (current) use of aspirin
Ashlyna®	Z79.3	Long term (current) use of hormonal contraceptives
Asmanex HFA®	Z79.51	Long term (current) use of inhaled steroids
Asmanex Twisthaler®	Z79.51	Long term (current) use of inhaled steroids
Aspir 81®	Z79.82	Long term (current) use of aspirin
aspirin	Z79.82	Long term (current) use of aspirin
Aspir-Low®	Z79.82	Long term (current) use of aspirin
Atelvia®	Z79.83	Long term (current) use of bisphosphonates
atovaquone	Z79.2	Long term (current) use of antibiotics
Aubra®	Z79.3	Long term (current) use of hormonal contraceptives
Avandia®	Z79.84	Long term (current) use of oral hypoglycemic drugs
Avar Cleanser®	Z79.2	Long term (current) use of antibiotics
Avar LS Cleanser®	Z79.2	Long term (current) use of antibiotics
Avar®	Z79.2	Long term (current) use of antibiotics
Avar-E Green®	Z79.2	Long term (current) use of antibiotics
Avar-E LS®	Z79.2	Long term (current) use of antibiotics
Avar-E®	Z79.2	Long term (current) use of antibiotics
Aviane®	Z79.3	Long term (current) use of hormonal contraceptives
Aygestin®	Z79.3	Long term (current) use of hormonal contraceptives
azithromycin	Z79.2	Long term (current) use of antibiotics
Azurette®	Z79.3	Long term (current) use of hormonal contraceptives
Baci-IM®	Z79.2	Long term (current) use of antibiotics
bacitracin	Z79.2	Long term (current) use of antibiotics
bacitracin/neomycin/polymyxin B	Z79.2	Long term (current) use of antibiotics
bacitracin/polymyxin b	Z79.2	Long term (current) use of antibiotics
Bactroban Nasal®	Z79.2	Long term (current) use of antibiotics
Bactroban®	Z79.2	Long term (current) use of antibiotics
Balziva®	Z79.890	Hormone replacement therapy (postmenopausal)
Basaglar®	Z79.4	Long term (current) use of insulin
Baycadron®	Z79.52	Long term (current) use of systemic steroids
Bayer Children's Aspirin®	Z79.82	Long term (current) use of aspirin
bazedoxifene/conjugated estrogens	Z79.890	Hormone replacement therapy (postmenopausal)
beclomethasone	Z79.51	Long term (current) use of inhaled steroids
Bekyree®	Z79.3	Long term (current) use of hormonal contraceptives
betamethasone	Z79.52	Long term (current) use of systemic steroids
Beyaz®	Z79.3	Long term (current) use of hormonal contraceptives
Binosto®	Z79.83	Long term (current) use of bisphosphonates
bivalirudin	Z79.02	Long term (current) use of antithrombotics/antiplatelets
Boniva®	Z79.83	Long term (current) use of bisphosphonates
BP 10-Wash®	Z79.2	Long term (current) use of antibiotics
Brevicon 28®	Z79.890	Hormone replacement therapy (postmenopausal)
Briellyn®	Z79.3	Long term (current) use of hormonal contraceptives
Briellyn®	Z79.890	Hormone replacement therapy (postmenopausal)
budesonide	Z79.52	Long term (current) use of systemic steroids
Bufferin Low Dose®	Z79.82	Long term (current) use of aspirin

Drug Name	Code	Code Descriptor
buprenorphine	Z79.891	Long term (current) use of opiate analgesic
Butrans®	Z79.891	Long term (current) use of opiate analgesic
Caldolor®	Z79.1	Long term (current) use of non-steroidal anti-inflammatories (NSAID)
Cambia®	Z79.1	Long term (current) use of non-steroidal anti-inflammatories (NSAID)
Camila®	Z79.3	Long term (current) use of hormonal contraceptives
Camrese®	Z79.3	Long term (current) use of hormonal contraceptives
CamreseLo®	Z79.3	Long term (current) use of hormonal contraceptives
Carmol Scalp Treatment Kit®	Z79.2	Long term (current) use of antibiotics
Carmol Scalp®	Z79.2	Long term (current) use of antibiotics
Caziant®	Z79.3	Long term (current) use of hormonal contraceptives
cefaclor	Z79.2	Long term (current) use of antibiotics
cefazolin	Z79.2	Long term (current) use of antibiotics
cefdinir	Z79.2	Long term (current) use of antibiotics
cefepime	Z79.2	Long term (current) use of antibiotics
cefixime	Z79.2	Long term (current) use of antibiotics
cefoxitin sodium	Z79.2	Long term (current) use of antibiotics
cefpodoxime	Z79.2	Long term (current) use of antibiotics
ceftaroline	Z79.2	Long term (current) use of antibiotics
ceftazidime	Z79.2	Long term (current) use of antibiotics
ceftolozane/tazobactam	Z79.2	Long term (current) use of antibiotics
ceftriaxone	Z79.2	Long term (current) use of antibiotics
cefuroxime	Z79.2	Long term (current) use of antibiotics
Celestone Soluspan®	Z79.52	Long term (current) use of systemic steroids
Centany AT Kit®	Z79.2	Long term (current) use of antibiotics
Centany®	Z79.2	Long term (current) use of antibiotics
cephalexin	Z79.2	Long term (current) use of antibiotics
Cerisa Wash®	Z79.2	Long term (current) use of antibiotics
Cesia®	Z79.3	Long term (current) use of hormonal contraceptives
Chateal®	Z79.3	Long term (current) use of hormonal contraceptives
Children's Motrin®	Z79.1	Long term (current) use of non-steroidal anti-inflammatories (NSAID)
chlorpropamide	Z79.84	Long term (current) use of oral hypoglycemic drugs
ciclesonide	Z79.51	Long term (current) use of inhaled steroids
cilastatin/imipenem	Z79.2	Long term (current) use of antibiotics
Clarifoam EF®	Z79.2	Long term (current) use of antibiotics
Clenia Emollient Cream®	Z79.2	Long term (current) use of antibiotics
Climara Pro®	Z79.890	Hormone replacement therapy (postmenopausal)
Climara®	Z79.890	Hormone replacement therapy (postmenopausal)
Clinacort®	Z79.52	Long term (current) use of systemic steroids
Colocort®	Z79.52	Long term (current) use of systemic steroids
CombiPatch®	Z79.890	Hormone replacement therapy (postmenopausal)
conjugated estrogens	Z79.890	Hormone replacement therapy (postmenopausal)
conjugated estrogens/medroxyprogesterone	Z79.890	Hormone replacement therapy (postmenopausal)
Cortef®	Z79.52	Long term (current) use of systemic steroids
Cortenema®	Z79.52	Long term (current) use of systemic steroids
Cortifoam®	Z79.52	Long term (current) use of systemic steroids
cortisone	Z79.52	Long term (current) use of systemic steroids
Coumadin®	Z79.01	Long term (current) use of anticoagulants
Covaryx HS®	Z79.890	Hormone replacement therapy (postmenopausal)
Covaryx®	Z79.890	Hormone replacement therapy (postmenopausal)
Cryselle®	Z79.3	Long term (current) use of hormonal contraceptives
Cyclafem 1 / 35®	Z79.3	Long term (current) use of hormonal contraceptives
Cyclafem 1 / 35®	Z79.890	Hormone replacement therapy (postmenopausal)

Drug Name	Code	Code Descriptor
Cyclafem 7 / 7 / 7®	Z79.3	Long term (current) use of hormonal contraceptives
Cyclafem 7 / 7 / 7®	Z79.890	Hormone replacement therapy (postmenopausal)
Cyclessa®	Z79.3	Long term (current) use of hormonal contraceptives
cycloserine	Z79.2	Long term (current) use of antibiotics
Cyred®	Z79.3	Long term (current) use of hormonal contraceptives
dabigatran	Z79.02	Long term (current) use of antithrombotics/antiplatelets
dalfopristin/quinupristin	Z79.2	Long term (current) use of antibiotics
dalteparin	Z79.01	Long term (current) use of anticoagulants
Dasetta 1 / 35®	Z79.3	Long term (current) use of hormonal contraceptives
Dasetta 1 / 35®	Z79.890	Hormone replacement therapy (postmenopausal)
Dasetta 7 / 7 / 7®	Z79.3	Long term (current) use of hormonal contraceptives
Dasetta 7 / 7 / 7®	Z79.890	Hormone replacement therapy (postmenopausal)
Daypro®	Z79.1	Long term (current) use of non-steroidal anti-inflammatories (NSAID)
Daysee®	Z79.3	Long term (current) use of hormonal contraceptives
Delestrogen®	Z79.890	Hormone replacement therapy (postmenopausal)
Delyla®	Z79.3	Long term (current) use of hormonal contraceptives
Depo-Medrol®	Z79.52	Long term (current) use of systemic steroids
Depo-Provera Contraceptive®	Z79.3	Long term (current) use of hormonal contraceptives
Depo-Provera®	Z79.3	Long term (current) use of hormonal contraceptives
Depo-subQ provera 104®	Z79.3	Long term (current) use of hormonal contraceptives
desirudin	Z79.02	Long term (current) use of antithrombotics/antiplatelets
Desogen®	Z79.3	Long term (current) use of hormonal contraceptives
desogestrel/ethinyl estradiol	Z79.3	Long term (current) use of hormonal contraceptives
De-Sone LA®	Z79.52	Long term (current) use of systemic steroids
Dexacen-4®	Z79.52	Long term (current) use of systemic steroids
dexamethasone	Z79.52	Long term (current) use of systemic steroids
Dexamethasone Intensol®	Z79.52	Long term (current) use of systemic steroids
Dexasone LA®	Z79.52	Long term (current) use of systemic steroids
Dexasone®	Z79.52	Long term (current) use of systemic steroids
Dexpak Taperpak®	Z79.52	Long term (current) use of systemic steroids
DiaBeta ®	Z79.84	Long term (current) use of oral hypoglycemic drugs
Diabinese ®	Z79.84	Long term (current) use of oral hypoglycemic drugs
diclofenac	Z79.1	Long term (current) use of non-steroidal anti-inflammatories (NSAID)
diclofenac/misoprostol	Z79.1	Long term (current) use of non-steroidal anti-inflammatories (NSAID)
dicloxacillin	Z79.2	Long term (current) use of antibiotics
Didronel®	Z79.83	Long term (current) use of bisphosphonates
dienogest/estradiol	Z79.3	Long term (current) use of hormonal contraceptives
Dolophine®	Z79.891	Long term (current) use of opiate analgesic
doxycycline	Z79.2	Long term (current) use of antibiotics
drospirenone/estradiol	Z79.890	Hormone replacement therapy (postmenopausal)
drospirenone/ethinyl estradiol	Z79.3	Long term (current) use of hormonal contraceptives
drospirenone/ethinyl estradiol/levomefolate calcium	Z79.3	Long term (current) use of hormonal contraceptives
Duavee®	Z79.890	Hormone replacement therapy (postmenopausal)
Duexis®	Z79.1	Long term (current) use of non-steroidal anti-inflammatories (NSAID)
Duospore®	Z79.2	Long term (current) use of antibiotics
Duragesic®	Z79.891	Long term (current) use of opiate analgesic
Durlaza®	Z79.82	Long term (current) use of aspirin
Dyloject®	Z79.1	Long term (current) use of non-steroidal anti-inflammatories (NSAID)
Dynacin®	Z79.2	Long term (current) use of antibiotics
E.E.S. Granules®	Z79.2	Long term (current) use of antibiotics
E.E.S.-400 Filmtab®	Z79.2	Long term (current) use of antibiotics
E.E.S.-400®	Z79.2	Long term (current) use of antibiotics

APPENDIX A: Z CODES FOR LONG-TERM USE OF DRUGS

Drug Name	Code	Code Descriptor
EC-Naprosyn®	Z79.1	Long term (current) use of non-steroidal anti-inflammatories (NSAID)
Ecotrin®	Z79.82	Long term (current) use of aspirin
Ecpirin®	Z79.82	Long term (current) use of aspirin
edoxaban	Z79.01	Long term (current) use of anticoagulants
EEMT DS®	Z79.890	Hormone replacement therapy (postmenopausal)
EEMT HS®	Z79.890	Hormone replacement therapy (postmenopausal)
EEMT®	Z79.890	Hormone replacement therapy (postmenopausal)
Eligard®	Z79.818	Long term (current) use of other agents affecting estrogen receptors and estrogen levels
Elinest®	Z79.3	Long term (current) use of hormonal contraceptives
Eliquis®	Z79.01	Long term (current) use of anticoagulants
Embeda®	Z79.891	Long term (current) use of opiate analgesic
Emcin Clear®	Z79.2	Long term (current) use of antibiotics
Emoquette®	Z79.3	Long term (current) use of hormonal contraceptives
Ena®	Z79.890	Hormone replacement therapy (postmenopausal)
Enjuvia®	Z79.890	Hormone replacement therapy (postmenopausal)
enoxaparin	Z79.01	Long term (current) use of anticoagulants
Enpresse®	Z79.3	Long term (current) use of hormonal contraceptives
Enskyce®	Z79.3	Long term (current) use of hormonal contraceptives
Entocort EC®	Z79.52	Long term (current) use of systemic steroids
Errin®	Z79.3	Long term (current) use of hormonal contraceptives
ertapenem	Z79.2	Long term (current) use of antibiotics
Ery Pads®	Z79.2	Long term (current) use of antibiotics
Eryc®	Z79.2	Long term (current) use of antibiotics
Erygel®	Z79.2	Long term (current) use of antibiotics
EryPed®	Z79.2	Long term (current) use of antibiotics
Ery-Tab®	Z79.2	Long term (current) use of antibiotics
Erythrocin Stearate Filmtab®	Z79.2	Long term (current) use of antibiotics
Erythrocin®	Z79.2	Long term (current) use of antibiotics
erythromycin	Z79.2	Long term (current) use of antibiotics
esomeprazole/naproxen	Z79.1	Long term (current) use of non-steroidal anti-inflammatories (NSAID)
Essian H.S.®	Z79.890	Hormone replacement therapy (postmenopausal)
Essian®	Z79.890	Hormone replacement therapy (postmenopausal)
Estarylla®	Z79.3	Long term (current) use of hormonal contraceptives
esterified estrogens/methyltestosterone	Z79.890	Hormone replacement therapy (postmenopausal)
Estraderm®	Z79.890	Hormone replacement therapy (postmenopausal)
estradiol	Z79.890	Hormone replacement therapy (postmenopausal)
estradiol acetate vaginal ring	Z79.890	Hormone replacement therapy (postmenopausal)
estradiol topical emulsion	Z79.890	Hormone replacement therapy (postmenopausal)
estradiol valerate	Z79.890	Hormone replacement therapy (postmenopausal)
estradiol/levonorgestrel	Z79.890	Hormone replacement therapy (postmenopausal)
estradiol/norethindrone	Z79.890	Hormone replacement therapy (postmenopausal)
Estrasorb®	Z79.890	Hormone replacement therapy (postmenopausal)
Estratest H.S.®	Z79.890	Hormone replacement therapy (postmenopausal)
Estratest®	Z79.890	Hormone replacement therapy (postmenopausal)
Estrostep Fe®	Z79.3	Long term (current) use of hormonal contraceptives
Estrostep Fe®	Z79.890	Hormone replacement therapy (postmenopausal)
ethinyl estradiol/ethynodiol	Z79.3	Long term (current) use of hormonal contraceptives
ethinyl estradiol/etonogestrel	Z79.3	Long term (current) use of hormonal contraceptives
ethinyl estradiol/levonorgestrel	Z79.3	Long term (current) use of hormonal contraceptives
ethinyl estradiol/norethindrone	Z79.3	Long term (current) use of hormonal contraceptives
ethinyl estradiol/norethindrone	Z79.890	Hormone replacement therapy (postmenopausal)
ethinyl estradiol/norgestimate	Z79.3	Long term (current) use of hormonal contraceptives

Drug Name	Code	Code Descriptor
ethinyl estradiol/norgestrel	Z79.3	Long term (current) use of hormonal contraceptives
etidronate	Z79.83	Long term (current) use of bisphosphonates
etonogestrel	Z79.3	Long term (current) use of hormonal contraceptives
Evista®	Z79.810	Long term (current) use of selective estrogen receptor modulators (SERMs)
Exalgo®	Z79.891	Long term (current) use of opiate analgesic
exemestane	Z79.811	Long term (current) use of aromatase inhibitors
Falmina®	Z79.3	Long term (current) use of hormonal contraceptives
famotidine/ibuprofen	Z79.1	Long term (current) use of non-steroidal anti-inflammatories (NSAID)
Fareston®	Z79.810	Long term (current) use of selective estrogen receptor modulators (SERMs)
Faslodex®	Z79.818	Long term (current) use of other agents affecting estrogen receptors and estrogen levels
Fasprin®	Z79.82	Long term (current) use of aspirin
Feldene®	Z79.1	Long term (current) use of non-steroidal anti-inflammatories (NSAID)
Femara®	Z79.811	Long term (current) use of aromatase inhibitors
Femcon Fe®	Z79.890	Hormone replacement therapy (postmenopausal)
femhrt	Z79.3	Long term (current) use of hormonal contraceptives
femhrt	Z79.890	Hormone replacement therapy (postmenopausal)
Femring®	Z79.890	Hormone replacement therapy (postmenopausal)
Femynor®	Z79.3	Long term (current) use of hormonal contraceptives
fenoprofen	Z79.1	Long term (current) use of non-steroidal anti-inflammatories (NSAID)
Fenortho®	Z79.1	Long term (current) use of non-steroidal anti-inflammatories (NSAID)
fentanyl	Z79.891	Long term (current) use of opiate analgesic
Flagyl 375®	Z79.2	Long term (current) use of antibiotics
Flagyl ER®	Z79.2	Long term (current) use of antibiotics
Flagyl®	Z79.2	Long term (current) use of antibiotics
Flanax Pain Reliever®	Z79.1	Long term (current) use of non-steroidal anti-inflammatories (NSAID)
Flovent Diskus®	Z79.51	Long term (current) use of inhaled steroids
Flovent HFA®	Z79.51	Long term (current) use of inhaled steroids
Flovent Rotadisk®	Z79.51	Long term (current) use of inhaled steroids
flunisolide	Z79.51	Long term (current) use of inhaled steroids
flurbiprofen sodium	Z79.1	Long term (current) use of non-steroidal anti-inflammatories (NSAID)
fluticasone	Z79.51	Long term (current) use of inhaled steroids
fondaparinux	Z79.01	Long term (current) use of anticoagulants
Fortamet®	Z79.84	Long term (current) use of oral hypoglycemic drugs
Fortaz®	Z79.2	Long term (current) use of antibiotics
Fosamax®	Z79.83	Long term (current) use of bisphosphonates
fosfomycin	Z79.2	Long term (current) use of antibiotics
Fragmin®	Z79.01	Long term (current) use of anticoagulants
fulvestrant	Z79.818	Long term (current) use of other agents affecting estrogen receptors and estrogen levels
Garimide®	Z79.2	Long term (current) use of antibiotics
Generess Fe®	Z79.3	Long term (current) use of hormonal contraceptives
Generess Fe®	Z79.890	Hormone replacement therapy (postmenopausal)
Genpril®	Z79.1	Long term (current) use of non-steroidal anti-inflammatories (NSAID)
Gianvi®	Z79.3	Long term (current) use of hormonal contraceptives
Gildagia®	Z79.890	Hormone replacement therapy (postmenopausal)
Gildess 1 / 20®	Z79.3	Long term (current) use of hormonal contraceptives
Gildess 1 / 20®	Z79.890	Hormone replacement therapy (postmenopausal)
Gildess 1.5 / 30®	Z79.3	Long term (current) use of hormonal contraceptives
Gildess 1.5 / 30®	Z79.890	Hormone replacement therapy (postmenopausal)
Gildess Fe 1 / 20®	Z79.3	Long term (current) use of hormonal contraceptives
Gildess Fe 1 / 20®	Z79.890	Hormone replacement therapy (postmenopausal)
Gildess Fe 1.5 / 30®	Z79.3	Long term (current) use of hormonal contraceptives
Gildess Fe 1.5 / 30®	Z79.890	Hormone replacement therapy (postmenopausal)

Drug Name	Code	Code Descriptor
glimepiride	Z79.84	Long term (current) use of oral hypoglycemic drugs
glipizide	Z79.84	Long term (current) use of oral hypoglycemic drugs
GlipiZIDE XL®	Z79.84	Long term (current) use of oral hypoglycemic drugs
Glucophage XR®	Z79.84	Long term (current) use of oral hypoglycemic drugs
Glucophage®	Z79.84	Long term (current) use of oral hypoglycemic drugs
Glucotrol XL®	Z79.84	Long term (current) use of oral hypoglycemic drugs
Glucotrol®	Z79.84	Long term (current) use of oral hypoglycemic drugs
Glumetza®	Z79.84	Long term (current) use of oral hypoglycemic drugs
glyburide	Z79.84	Long term (current) use of oral hypoglycemic drugs
Glycron®	Z79.84	Long term (current) use of oral hypoglycemic drugs
Glynase PresTab®	Z79.84	Long term (current) use of oral hypoglycemic drugs
Glynase®	Z79.84	Long term (current) use of oral hypoglycemic drugs
Glyset®	Z79.84	Long term (current) use of oral hypoglycemic drugs
goserelin	Z79.818	Long term (current) use of other agents affecting estrogen receptors and estrogen levels
Halfprin®	Z79.82	Long term (current) use of aspirin
Haltran®	Z79.1	Long term (current) use of non-steroidal anti-inflammatories (NSAID)
heparin	Z79.01	Long term (current) use of anticoagulants
Heparin Sodium®	Z79.01	Long term (current) use of anticoagulants
histrelin	Z79.818	Long term (current) use of other agents affecting estrogen receptors and estrogen levels
Humalog KwikPen®	Z79.4	Long term (current) use of insulin
Humalog Mix 50 / 50 KwikPen®	Z79.4	Long term (current) use of insulin
Humalog Mix 50 / 50®	Z79.4	Long term (current) use of insulin
Humalog Mix 75 / 25 KwikPen®	Z79.4	Long term (current) use of insulin
Humalog Mix 75 / 25®	Z79.4	Long term (current) use of insulin
Humalog®	Z79.4	Long term (current) use of insulin
Humulin 70 / 30 Pen®	Z79.4	Long term (current) use of insulin
Humulin 70 / 30®	Z79.4	Long term (current) use of insulin
Humulin N®	Z79.4	Long term (current) use of insulin
Humulin R®	Z79.4	Long term (current) use of insulin
hydrocortisone	Z79.52	Long term (current) use of systemic steroids
hydromorphone hydrochloride extended-release	Z79.891	Long term (current) use of opiate analgesic
ibandronate	Z79.83	Long term (current) use of bisphosphonates
Ibu-4®	Z79.1	Long term (current) use of non-steroidal anti-inflammatories (NSAID)
Ibu-6®	Z79.1	Long term (current) use of non-steroidal anti-inflammatories (NSAID)
Ibu-8®	Z79.1	Long term (current) use of non-steroidal anti-inflammatories (NSAID)
ibuprofen	Z79.1	Long term (current) use of non-steroidal anti-inflammatories (NSAID)
Ibu-Tab®	Z79.1	Long term (current) use of non-steroidal anti-inflammatories (NSAID)
Indocin IV®	Z79.1	Long term (current) use of non-steroidal anti-inflammatories (NSAID)
Indocin®	Z79.1	Long term (current) use of non-steroidal anti-inflammatories (NSAID)
indomethacin	Z79.1	Long term (current) use of non-steroidal anti-inflammatories (NSAID)
insulin aspart	Z79.4	Long term (current) use of insulin
insulin aspart/insulin aspart protamine	Z79.4	Long term (current) use of insulin
insulin aspart/insulin degludec	Z79.4	Long term (current) use of insulin
insulin degludec	Z79.4	Long term (current) use of insulin
insulin detemir	Z79.4	Long term (current) use of insulin
insulin glargine	Z79.4	Long term (current) use of insulin
insulin inhalation, rapid acting	Z79.4	Long term (current) use of insulin
insulin isophane	Z79.4	Long term (current) use of insulin
insulin isophane/insulin regular	Z79.4	Long term (current) use of insulin
insulin lispro	Z79.4	Long term (current) use of insulin
insulin lispro/insulin lispro protamine	Z79.4	Long term (current) use of insulin
insulin regular	Z79.4	Long term (current) use of insulin

Drug Name	Code	Code Descriptor
Introvale®	Z79.3	Long term (current) use of hormonal contraceptives
Invanz®	Z79.2	Long term (current) use of antibiotics
Iprivask®	Z79.02	Long term (current) use of antithrombotics/antiplatelets
Isoject Permapen®	Z79.2	Long term (current) use of antibiotics
Jantoven®	Z79.01	Long term (current) use of anticoagulants
Jencycla®	Z79.3	Long term (current) use of hormonal contraceptives
Jevantique®	Z79.3	Long term (current) use of hormonal contraceptives
Jevantique®	Z79.890	Hormone replacement therapy (postmenopausal)
Jinteli®	Z79.3	Long term (current) use of hormonal contraceptives
Jinteli®	Z79.890	Hormone replacement therapy (postmenopausal)
Jolessa®	Z79.3	Long term (current) use of hormonal contraceptives
Jolivette®	Z79.3	Long term (current) use of hormonal contraceptives
Juleber®	Z79.3	Long term (current) use of hormonal contraceptives
Junel 1 / 20®	Z79.3	Long term (current) use of hormonal contraceptives
Junel 1 / 20®	Z79.890	Hormone replacement therapy (postmenopausal)
Junel 1.5 / 30®	Z79.3	Long term (current) use of hormonal contraceptives
Junel 1.5 / 30®	Z79.890	Hormone replacement therapy (postmenopausal)
Kadian ®	Z79.891	Long term (current) use of opiate analgesic
Kariva®	Z79.3	Long term (current) use of hormonal contraceptives
Keflex®	Z79.2	Long term (current) use of antibiotics
Kefzol®	Z79.2	Long term (current) use of antibiotics
Kelnor 1 / 35®	Z79.3	Long term (current) use of hormonal contraceptives
Kenalog-10®	Z79.52	Long term (current) use of systemic steroids
Kenalog-40®	Z79.52	Long term (current) use of systemic steroids
Ketek Pak®	Z79.2	Long term (current) use of antibiotics
ketoprofen	Z79.1	Long term (current) use of non-steroidal anti-inflammatories (NSAID)
ketorolac	Z79.1	Long term (current) use of non-steroidal anti-inflammatories (NSAID)
Kimidess®	Z79.3	Long term (current) use of hormonal contraceptives
Kisqali Femara Co-pack®	Z79.811	Long term (current) use of aromatase inhibitors
Kitabis Pak®	Z79.2	Long term (current) use of antibiotics
Klaron®	Z79.2	Long term (current) use of antibiotics
Kurvelo®	Z79.3	Long term (current) use of hormonal contraceptives
Lantus Solostar®	Z79.4	Long term (current) use of insulin
Lantus®	Z79.4	Long term (current) use of insulin
Larin Fe 1 / 20®	Z79.3	Long term (current) use of hormonal contraceptives
Larin Fe 1 / 20®	Z79.890	Hormone replacement therapy (postmenopausal)
Larin Fe 1.5 / 30®	Z79.3	Long term (current) use of hormonal contraceptives
Larin Fe 1.5 / 30®	Z79.890	Hormone replacement therapy (postmenopausal)
Larissia®	Z79.3	Long term (current) use of hormonal contraceptives
Leader Naproxen Sodium®	Z79.1	Long term (current) use of non-steroidal anti-inflammatories (NSAID)
Leena®	Z79.3	Long term (current) use of hormonal contraceptives
Leena®	Z79.890	Hormone replacement therapy (postmenopausal)
Lessina®	Z79.3	Long term (current) use of hormonal contraceptives
letrozole	Z79.811	Long term (current) use of aromatase inhibitors
leuprolide	Z79.818	Long term (current) use of other agents affecting estrogen receptors and estrogen levels
Levemir®	Z79.4	Long term (current) use of insulin
Levlen®	Z79.3	Long term (current) use of hormonal contraceptives
Levonest®	Z79.3	Long term (current) use of hormonal contraceptives
Levonest-28®	Z79.3	Long term (current) use of hormonal contraceptives
levonorgestrel	Z79.3	Long term (current) use of hormonal contraceptives
Levora®	Z79.3	Long term (current) use of hormonal contraceptives
Liletta®	Z79.3	Long term (current) use of hormonal contraceptives

Drug Name	Code	Code Descriptor
Lincocin®	Z79.2	Long term (current) use of antibiotics
lincomycin	Z79.2	Long term (current) use of antibiotics
linezolid	Z79.2	Long term (current) use of antibiotics
Lo Loestrin Fe®	Z79.3	Long term (current) use of hormonal contraceptives
Lo Loestrin Fe®	Z79.890	Hormone replacement therapy (postmenopausal)
Lo Minastrin Fe®	Z79.3	Long term (current) use of hormonal contraceptives
Lo Minastrin Fe®	Z79.890	Hormone replacement therapy (postmenopausal)
Loestrin 1 / 20®	Z79.3	Long term (current) use of hormonal contraceptives
Loestrin 1 / 20®	Z79.890	Hormone replacement therapy (postmenopausal)
Loestrin 21 1.5 / 30®	Z79.3	Long term (current) use of hormonal contraceptives
Loestrin 21 1.5 / 30®	Z79.890	Hormone replacement therapy (postmenopausal)
Loestrin 24 Fe®	Z79.3	Long term (current) use of hormonal contraceptives
Loestrin 24 Fe®	Z79.890	Hormone replacement therapy (postmenopausal)
Loestrin Fe 1 / 20®	Z79.890	Hormone replacement therapy (postmenopausal)
Loryna®	Z79.3	Long term (current) use of hormonal contraceptives
LoSeasonique®	Z79.3	Long term (current) use of hormonal contraceptives
Lovenox®	Z79.01	Long term (current) use of anticoagulants
Lupron Depot 11.25 mg®	Z79.818	Long term (current) use of other agents affecting estrogen receptors and estrogen levels
Lupron Depot 3.75 mg®	Z79.818	Long term (current) use of other agents affecting estrogen receptors and estrogen levels
Lupron Depot®	Z79.818	Long term (current) use of other agents affecting estrogen receptors and estrogen levels
Lupron Depot-PED®	Z79.818	Long term (current) use of other agents affecting estrogen receptors and estrogen levels
Lutera®	Z79.3	Long term (current) use of hormonal contraceptives
Lyza®	Z79.3	Long term (current) use of hormonal contraceptives
mafenide	Z79.2	Long term (current) use of antibiotics
Marlissa®	Z79.3	Long term (current) use of hormonal contraceptives
Maxipime®	Z79.2	Long term (current) use of antibiotics
meclofenamate	Z79.1	Long term (current) use of non-steroidal anti-inflammatories (NSAID)
Meclomen®	Z79.1	Long term (current) use of non-steroidal anti-inflammatories (NSAID)
Medi-Quik®	Z79.2	Long term (current) use of antibiotics
Medrol Dosepak®	Z79.52	Long term (current) use of systemic steroids
Medrol®	Z79.52	Long term (current) use of systemic steroids
medroxyprogesterone	Z79.3	Long term (current) use of hormonal contraceptives
mefenamic acid	Z79.1	Long term (current) use of non-steroidal anti-inflammatories (NSAID)
Mefoxin®	Z79.2	Long term (current) use of antibiotics
Megace ES®	Z79.818	Long term (current) use of other agents affecting estrogen receptors and estrogen levels
megestrol	Z79.818	Long term (current) use of other agents affecting estrogen receptors and estrogen levels
meloxicam	Z79.1	Long term (current) use of non-steroidal anti-inflammatories (NSAID)
Menogen®	Z79.890	Hormone replacement therapy (postmenopausal)
Mepron®	Z79.2	Long term (current) use of antibiotics
meropenem	Z79.2	Long term (current) use of antibiotics
Merrem®	Z79.2	Long term (current) use of antibiotics
mestranol/norethindrone	Z79.3	Long term (current) use of hormonal contraceptives
metformin	Z79.84	Long term (current) use of oral hypoglycemic drugs
methadone hydrochloride	Z79.891	Long term (current) use of opiate analgesic
methylprednisolone	Z79.52	Long term (current) use of systemic steroids
MethylPREDNISolone Dose Pack®	Z79.52	Long term (current) use of systemic steroids
metronidazole	Z79.2	Long term (current) use of antibiotics
Mexar®	Z79.2	Long term (current) use of antibiotics
Microgestin 1 / 20®	Z79.890	Hormone replacement therapy (postmenopausal)
Microgestin 1.5 / 30®	Z79.890	Hormone replacement therapy (postmenopausal)
Microgestin Fe 1 / 20®	Z79.3	Long term (current) use of hormonal contraceptives
Microgestin Fe 1 / 20®	Z79.890	Hormone replacement therapy (postmenopausal)

Drug Name	Code	Code Descriptor
Midol Extended Relief®	Z79.1	Long term (current) use of non-steroidal anti-inflammatories (NSAID)
Midol IB®	Z79.1	Long term (current) use of non-steroidal anti-inflammatories (NSAID)
miglitol	Z79.84	Long term (current) use of oral hypoglycemic drugs
Millipred DP®	Z79.52	Long term (current) use of systemic steroids
Millipred®	Z79.52	Long term (current) use of systemic steroids
Mimvey®	Z79.890	Hormone replacement therapy (postmenopausal)
Minastrin 24 Fe®	Z79.890	Hormone replacement therapy (postmenopausal)
Miniprin®	Z79.82	Long term (current) use of aspirin
Minocin®	Z79.2	Long term (current) use of antibiotics
minocycline	Z79.2	Long term (current) use of antibiotics
Mirena®	Z79.3	Long term (current) use of hormonal contraceptives
Mobic®	Z79.1	Long term (current) use of non-steroidal anti-inflammatories (NSAID)
Modicon®	Z79.890	Hormone replacement therapy (postmenopausal)
mometasone	Z79.51	Long term (current) use of inhaled steroids
Monodox®	Z79.2	Long term (current) use of antibiotics
Mono-Linyah®	Z79.3	Long term (current) use of hormonal contraceptives
Mononessa®	Z79.3	Long term (current) use of hormonal contraceptives
Monurol®	Z79.2	Long term (current) use of antibiotics
Morgidox®	Z79.2	Long term (current) use of antibiotics
morphine sulfate and naltrexone extended-release	Z79.891	Long term (current) use of opiate analgesic
morphine sulfate controlled-release	Z79.891	Long term (current) use of opiate analgesic
morphine sulfate extended-release	Z79.891	Long term (current) use of opiate analgesic
Motrin Childrens®	Z79.1	Long term (current) use of non-steroidal anti-inflammatories (NSAID)
Motrin IB®	Z79.1	Long term (current) use of non-steroidal anti-inflammatories (NSAID)
Motrin Junior Strength®	Z79.1	Long term (current) use of non-steroidal anti-inflammatories (NSAID)
Moxatag®	Z79.2	Long term (current) use of antibiotics
Moxilin®	Z79.2	Long term (current) use of antibiotics
MS Contin®	Z79.891	Long term (current) use of opiate analgesic
mupirocin	Z79.2	Long term (current) use of antibiotics
My Way®	Z79.3	Long term (current) use of hormonal contraceptives
Mycobutin®	Z79.2	Long term (current) use of antibiotics
Myrac®	Z79.2	Long term (current) use of antibiotics
Myzilra®	Z79.3	Long term (current) use of hormonal contraceptives
nabumetone	Z79.1	Long term (current) use of non-steroidal anti-inflammatories (NSAID)
nafarelin	Z79.818	Long term (current) use of other agents affecting estrogen receptors and estrogen levels
nafcillin sodium	Z79.2	Long term (current) use of antibiotics
Nalfon®	Z79.1	Long term (current) use of non-steroidal anti-inflammatories (NSAID)
Nallpen®	Z79.2	Long term (current) use of antibiotics
Naprelan®	Z79.1	Long term (current) use of non-steroidal anti-inflammatories (NSAID)
Naprosyn®	Z79.1	Long term (current) use of non-steroidal anti-inflammatories (NSAID)
naproxen	Z79.1	Long term (current) use of non-steroidal anti-inflammatories (NSAID)
Natazia®	Z79.3	Long term (current) use of hormonal contraceptives
nateglinide	Z79.84	Long term (current) use of oral hypoglycemic drugs
Nebupent®	Z79.2	Long term (current) use of antibiotics
Necon 1 / 35®	Z79.890	Hormone replacement therapy (postmenopausal)
Necon 1 / 50®	Z79.3	Long term (current) use of hormonal contraceptives
Necon 7 / 7 / 7®	Z79.3	Long term (current) use of hormonal contraceptives
Necon 7 / 7 / 7®	Z79.890	Hormone replacement therapy (postmenopausal)
neomycin	Z79.2	Long term (current) use of antibiotics
neomycin/polymyxin b/pramoxine	Z79.2	Long term (current) use of antibiotics
NeoProfen®	Z79.1	Long term (current) use of non-steroidal anti-inflammatories (NSAID)
Neosporin®	Z79.2	Long term (current) use of antibiotics

Drug Name	Code	Code Descriptor
Neo-Tab®	Z79.2	Long term (current) use of antibiotics
Nexplanon®	Z79.3	Long term (current) use of hormonal contraceptives
Next Choice®	Z79.3	Long term (current) use of hormonal contraceptives
Nora-Be®	Z79.3	Long term (current) use of hormonal contraceptives
norethindrone	Z79.3	Long term (current) use of hormonal contraceptives
Norinyl 1+50®	Z79.3	Long term (current) use of hormonal contraceptives
Nor-QD®	Z79.3	Long term (current) use of hormonal contraceptives
Nortrel 1 / 35®	Z79.3	Long term (current) use of hormonal contraceptives
Nortrel 1 / 35®	Z79.890	Hormone replacement therapy (postmenopausal)
Novolin 70 / 30®	Z79.4	Long term (current) use of insulin
Novolin N®	Z79.4	Long term (current) use of insulin
Novolin R®	Z79.4	Long term (current) use of insulin
NovoLog FlexPen®	Z79.4	Long term (current) use of insulin
NovoLog Mix 70 / 30 FlexPen®	Z79.4	Long term (current) use of insulin
NovoLog Mix 70 / 30®	Z79.4	Long term (current) use of insulin
NovoLog PenFill®	Z79.4	Long term (current) use of insulin
Novolog®	Z79.4	Long term (current) use of insulin
Nucynta ER®	Z79.891	Long term (current) use of opiate analgesic
NuvaRing®	Z79.3	Long term (current) use of hormonal contraceptives
Ocella®	Z79.3	Long term (current) use of hormonal contraceptives
Ocudox®	Z79.2	Long term (current) use of antibiotics
Ocufen®	Z79.1	Long term (current) use of non-steroidal anti-inflammatories (NSAID)
Ogestrel®	Z79.3	Long term (current) use of hormonal contraceptives
Ogestrel-28®	Z79.3	Long term (current) use of hormonal contraceptives
Omnicef Omni-Pac®	Z79.2	Long term (current) use of antibiotics
Omnipen-N®	Z79.2	Long term (current) use of antibiotics
Opana ER®	Z79.891	Long term (current) use of opiate analgesic
Oracea®	Z79.2	Long term (current) use of antibiotics
Orapred ODT®	Z79.52	Long term (current) use of systemic steroids
Oraxyl®	Z79.2	Long term (current) use of antibiotics
Orbactiv®	Z79.2	Long term (current) use of antibiotics
oritavancin	Z79.2	Long term (current) use of antibiotics
Orsythia®	Z79.3	Long term (current) use of hormonal contraceptives
Ortho Cyclen®	Z79.3	Long term (current) use of hormonal contraceptives
Ortho Micronor®	Z79.3	Long term (current) use of hormonal contraceptives
Ortho Tri-Cyclen Lo®	Z79.3	Long term (current) use of hormonal contraceptives
Ortho Tri-Cyclen®	Z79.3	Long term (current) use of hormonal contraceptives
Ortho-Novum 1 / 35®	Z79.3	Long term (current) use of hormonal contraceptives
Ortho-Novum 1 / 35®	Z79.890	Hormone replacement therapy (postmenopausal)
Ortho-Novum 7 / 7 / 7®	Z79.890	Hormone replacement therapy (postmenopausal)
ospemifene	Z79.810	Long term (current) use of selective estrogen receptor modulators (SERMs)
Osphena®	Z79.810	Long term (current) use of selective estrogen receptor modulators (SERMs)
Ovace Plus®	Z79.2	Long term (current) use of antibiotics
Ovace®	Z79.2	Long term (current) use of antibiotics
oxaprozin	Z79.1	Long term (current) use of non-steroidal anti-inflammatories (NSAID)
oxycodone hydrochloride controlled-release	Z79.891	Long term (current) use of opiate analgesic
OxyContin®	Z79.891	Long term (current) use of opiate analgesic
oxymorphone hydrochloride extended-release	Z79.891	Long term (current) use of opiate analgesic
pamidronate	Z79.83	Long term (current) use of bisphosphonates
Panixine®	Z79.2	Long term (current) use of antibiotics
paromomycin	Z79.2	Long term (current) use of antibiotics
Paromycin®	Z79.2	Long term (current) use of antibiotics

Drug Name	Code	Code Descriptor
PCE Dispertab®	Z79.2	Long term (current) use of antibiotics
PediaPred®	Z79.52	Long term (current) use of systemic steroids
penicillin G benzathine	Z79.2	Long term (current) use of antibiotics
penicillin G potassium	Z79.2	Long term (current) use of antibiotics
penicillin V potassium	Z79.2	Long term (current) use of antibiotics
Penicillin VK®	Z79.2	Long term (current) use of antibiotics
Pentam 300®	Z79.2	Long term (current) use of antibiotics
Pentam®	Z79.2	Long term (current) use of antibiotics
pentamidine	Z79.2	Long term (current) use of antibiotics
Pfizerpen®	Z79.2	Long term (current) use of antibiotics
Philith®	Z79.3	Long term (current) use of hormonal contraceptives
Philith®	Z79.890	Hormone replacement therapy (postmenopausal)
Pimtrea®	Z79.3	Long term (current) use of hormonal contraceptives
pioglitazone hydrochloride	Z79.84	Long term (current) use of oral hypoglycemic drugs
piperacillin/tazobactam	Z79.2	Long term (current) use of antibiotics
Pirmella 1 / 35®	Z79.3	Long term (current) use of hormonal contraceptives
Pirmella 1 / 35®	Z79.890	Hormone replacement therapy (postmenopausal)
Pirmella 7 / 7 / 7®	Z79.3	Long term (current) use of hormonal contraceptives
Pirmella 7 / 7 / 7®	Z79.890	Hormone replacement therapy (postmenopausal)
piroxicam	Z79.1	Long term (current) use of non-steroidal anti-inflammatories (NSAID)
Plan B One-Step®	Z79.3	Long term (current) use of hormonal contraceptives
Plexion Cleansing Cloths®	Z79.2	Long term (current) use of antibiotics
Plexion SCT®	Z79.2	Long term (current) use of antibiotics
Plexion TS®	Z79.2	Long term (current) use of antibiotics
Plexion®	Z79.2	Long term (current) use of antibiotics
Ponstel®	Z79.1	Long term (current) use of non-steroidal anti-inflammatories (NSAID)
Portia®	Z79.3	Long term (current) use of hormonal contraceptives
Pradaxa®	Z79.02	Long term (current) use of antithrombotics/antiplatelets
Prandin®	Z79.84	Long term (current) use of oral hypoglycemic drugs
Prascion Cleanser®	Z79.2	Long term (current) use of antibiotics
Prascion FC Cloths®	Z79.2	Long term (current) use of antibiotics
Prascion RA®	Z79.2	Long term (current) use of antibiotics
Precose®	Z79.84	Long term (current) use of oral hypoglycemic drugs
prednisolone	Z79.52	Long term (current) use of systemic steroids
prednisone	Z79.52	Long term (current) use of systemic steroids
Prelone®	Z79.52	Long term (current) use of systemic steroids
Premarin Intravenous®	Z79.890	Hormone replacement therapy (postmenopausal)
Premarin Vaginal Cream®	Z79.890	Hormone replacement therapy (postmenopausal)
Premarin®	Z79.890	Hormone replacement therapy (postmenopausal)
Premphase®	Z79.890	Hormone replacement therapy (postmenopausal)
Prempro®	Z79.890	Hormone replacement therapy (postmenopausal)
Previfem®	Z79.3	Long term (current) use of hormonal contraceptives
Priftin®	Z79.2	Long term (current) use of antibiotics
Primaxin IV®	Z79.2	Long term (current) use of antibiotics
procaine penicillin	Z79.2	Long term (current) use of antibiotics
Proprinal®	Z79.1	Long term (current) use of non-steroidal anti-inflammatories (NSAID)
Provera®	Z79.3	Long term (current) use of hormonal contraceptives
Pulmicort Flexhaler®	Z79.51	Long term (current) use of inhaled steroids
Pulmicort Nebuamp®	Z79.51	Long term (current) use of inhaled steroids
Pulmicort Respules®	Z79.51	Long term (current) use of inhaled steroids
Pulmicort Turbuhaler®	Z79.51	Long term (current) use of inhaled steroids
Q-Profen®	Z79.1	Long term (current) use of non-steroidal anti-inflammatories (NSAID)

PCE Dispertab® - Q-Profen®

APPENDIX A: Z CODES FOR LONG-TERM USE OF DRUGS

Drug Name	Code	Code Descriptor
Quartette®	Z79.3	Long term (current) use of hormonal contraceptives
Quasense®	Z79.3	Long term (current) use of hormonal contraceptives
Qvar®	Z79.51	Long term (current) use of inhaled steroids
raloxifene	Z79.810	Long term (current) use of selective estrogen receptor modulators (SERMs)
Rayos®	Z79.52	Long term (current) use of systemic steroids
Rebetol®	Z79.2	Long term (current) use of antibiotics
Reclast®	Z79.83	Long term (current) use of bisphosphonates
Reclipsen®	Z79.3	Long term (current) use of hormonal contraceptives
Relenza®	Z79.2	Long term (current) use of antibiotics
Relion Novolin 70 / 30 Innolet®	Z79.4	Long term (current) use of insulin
repaglinide	Z79.84	Long term (current) use of oral hypoglycemic drugs
retapamulin	Z79.2	Long term (current) use of antibiotics
RibaPak®	Z79.2	Long term (current) use of antibiotics
Ribasphere®	Z79.2	Long term (current) use of antibiotics
RibaTab®	Z79.2	Long term (current) use of antibiotics
ribavirin	Z79.2	Long term (current) use of antibiotics
ribociclib succinate	Z79.811	Long term (current) use of aromatase inhibitors
rifabutin	Z79.2	Long term (current) use of antibiotics
Rifadin IV®	Z79.2	Long term (current) use of antibiotics
Rifadin®	Z79.2	Long term (current) use of antibiotics
rifampin	Z79.2	Long term (current) use of antibiotics
rifapentine	Z79.2	Long term (current) use of antibiotics
rifaximin	Z79.2	Long term (current) use of antibiotics
Rimactane®	Z79.2	Long term (current) use of antibiotics
Riomet®	Z79.84	Long term (current) use of oral hypoglycemic drugs
risedronate	Z79.83	Long term (current) use of bisphosphonates
rivaroxaban	Z79.01	Long term (current) use of anticoagulants
Rosac®	Z79.2	Long term (current) use of antibiotics
Rosaderm Cleanser®	Z79.2	Long term (current) use of antibiotics
Rosanil Cleanser®	Z79.2	Long term (current) use of antibiotics
rosiglitazone maleate	Z79.84	Long term (current) use of oral hypoglycemic drugs
Rosula Cleanser®	Z79.2	Long term (current) use of antibiotics
Rosula CLK®	Z79.2	Long term (current) use of antibiotics
Rosula NS®	Z79.2	Long term (current) use of antibiotics
Rosula Wash®	Z79.2	Long term (current) use of antibiotics
Rosula®	Z79.2	Long term (current) use of antibiotics
Ryzodeg 70 / 30®	Z79.4	Long term (current) use of insulin
Safyral®	Z79.3	Long term (current) use of hormonal contraceptives
Savaysa®	Z79.01	Long term (current) use of anticoagulants
Seasonale®	Z79.3	Long term (current) use of hormonal contraceptives
Seasonique®	Z79.3	Long term (current) use of hormonal contraceptives
Sebizon®	Z79.2	Long term (current) use of antibiotics
Seb-Prev®	Z79.2	Long term (current) use of antibiotics
Septra DS®	Z79.2	Long term (current) use of antibiotics
Septra®	Z79.2	Long term (current) use of antibiotics
Seromycin®	Z79.2	Long term (current) use of antibiotics
Setlakin®	Z79.3	Long term (current) use of hormonal contraceptives
Silvadene®	Z79.2	Long term (current) use of antibiotics
silver sulfadiazine	Z79.2	Long term (current) use of antibiotics
Sivextro®	Z79.2	Long term (current) use of antibiotics
Skyla®	Z79.3	Long term (current) use of hormonal contraceptives
SMZ-TMP DS®	Z79.2	Long term (current) use of antibiotics

Drug Name	Code	Code Descriptor
Solia®	Z79.3	Long term (current) use of hormonal contraceptives
Solodyn®	Z79.2	Long term (current) use of antibiotics
Soltamox®	Z79.810	Long term (current) use of selective estrogen receptor modulators (SERMs)
Solu-Cortef®	Z79.52	Long term (current) use of systemic steroids
Solu-Medrol®	Z79.52	Long term (current) use of systemic steroids
Solurex LA®	Z79.52	Long term (current) use of systemic steroids
Solurex®	Z79.52	Long term (current) use of systemic steroids
Sprintec®	Z79.3	Long term (current) use of hormonal contraceptives
Sprix®	Z79.1	Long term (current) use of non-steroidal anti-inflammatories (NSAID)
Sronyx®	Z79.3	Long term (current) use of hormonal contraceptives
SSD AF®	Z79.2	Long term (current) use of antibiotics
SSD®	Z79.2	Long term (current) use of antibiotics
Starlix®	Z79.84	Long term (current) use of oral hypoglycemic drugs
sulfacetamide sodium	Z79.2	Long term (current) use of antibiotics
sulfacetamide sodium/sulfur	Z79.2	Long term (current) use of antibiotics
sulfacetamide sodium/sulfur/urea	Z79.2	Long term (current) use of antibiotics
sulfacetamide sodium/urea	Z79.2	Long term (current) use of antibiotics
Sulfacleanse 8 / 4®	Z79.2	Long term (current) use of antibiotics
sulfamethoxazole/trimethoprim	Z79.2	Long term (current) use of antibiotics
Sulfamylon®	Z79.2	Long term (current) use of antibiotics
Sulfatol C®	Z79.2	Long term (current) use of antibiotics
Sulfatol Cleanser®	Z79.2	Long term (current) use of antibiotics
Sulfatol SS®	Z79.2	Long term (current) use of antibiotics
Sulfatol®	Z79.2	Long term (current) use of antibiotics
Sulfatrim Pediatric®	Z79.2	Long term (current) use of antibiotics
sulindac	Z79.1	Long term (current) use of non-steroidal anti-inflammatories (NSAID)
Sumadan®	Z79.2	Long term (current) use of antibiotics
Sumaxin Cleansing Pads®	Z79.2	Long term (current) use of antibiotics
Sumaxin TS®	Z79.2	Long term (current) use of antibiotics
Sumaxin®	Z79.2	Long term (current) use of antibiotics
Suphera®	Z79.2	Long term (current) use of antibiotics
Supprelin LA®	Z79.818	Long term (current) use of other agents affecting estrogen receptors and estrogen levels
Suprax®	Z79.2	Long term (current) use of antibiotics
Syeda®	Z79.3	Long term (current) use of hormonal contraceptives
Synarel®	Z79.818	Long term (current) use of other agents affecting estrogen receptors and estrogen levels
Synercid®	Z79.2	Long term (current) use of antibiotics
synthetic conjugated estrogens, B	Z79.890	Hormone replacement therapy (postmenopausal)
tamoxifen	Z79.810	Long term (current) use of selective estrogen receptor modulators (SERMs)
tapentadol extended-release	Z79.891	Long term (current) use of opiate analgesic
Tazicef®	Z79.2	Long term (current) use of antibiotics
tedizolid	Z79.2	Long term (current) use of antibiotics
Teflaro®	Z79.2	Long term (current) use of antibiotics
telavancin	Z79.2	Long term (current) use of antibiotics
telithromycin	Z79.2	Long term (current) use of antibiotics
Teslac®	Z79.811	Long term (current) use of aromatase inhibitors
testolactone	Z79.811	Long term (current) use of aromatase inhibitors
tetracycline hydrochloride	Z79.2	Long term (current) use of antibiotics
Theramycin Z®	Z79.2	Long term (current) use of antibiotics
Thermazene®	Z79.2	Long term (current) use of antibiotics
tigecycline	Z79.2	Long term (current) use of antibiotics
Tilia Fe®	Z79.3	Long term (current) use of hormonal contraceptives
Tilia Fe®	Z79.890	Hormone replacement therapy (postmenopausal)

Drug Name	Code	Code Descriptor
Tivorbex®	Z79.1	Long term (current) use of non-steroidal anti-inflammatories (NSAID)
Tobi Podhaler®	Z79.2	Long term (current) use of antibiotics
Tobi®	Z79.2	Long term (current) use of antibiotics
tobramycin	Z79.2	Long term (current) use of antibiotics
tolmetin	Z79.1	Long term (current) use of non-steroidal anti-inflammatories (NSAID)
Topisulf®	Z79.2	Long term (current) use of antibiotics
toremifene	Z79.810	Long term (current) use of selective estrogen receptor modulators (SERMs)
Toujeo Solostar®	Z79.4	Long term (current) use of insulin
Toujeo®	Z79.4	Long term (current) use of insulin
Trelstar Depot®	Z79.818	Long term (current) use of other agents affecting estrogen receptors and estrogen levels
Trelstar LA®	Z79.818	Long term (current) use of other agents affecting estrogen receptors and estrogen levels
Trelstar®	Z79.818	Long term (current) use of other agents affecting estrogen receptors and estrogen levels
Tresiba®	Z79.4	Long term (current) use of insulin
triamcinolone	Z79.52	Long term (current) use of systemic steroids
Tri-Estarylla®	Z79.3	Long term (current) use of hormonal contraceptives
Tri-Legest Fe®	Z79.3	Long term (current) use of hormonal contraceptives
Tri-Legest Fe®	Z79.890	Hormone replacement therapy (postmenopausal)
Tri-Legest®	Z79.890	Hormone replacement therapy (postmenopausal)
Tri-Linyah®	Z79.3	Long term (current) use of hormonal contraceptives
Tri-Lo-Estarylla®	Z79.3	Long term (current) use of hormonal contraceptives
Tri-Lo-Marzia®	Z79.3	Long term (current) use of hormonal contraceptives
Tri-Lo-Sprintec®	Z79.3	Long term (current) use of hormonal contraceptives
TriNessa Lo®	Z79.3	Long term (current) use of hormonal contraceptives
TriNessa®	Z79.3	Long term (current) use of hormonal contraceptives
Tri-Norinyl®	Z79.3	Long term (current) use of hormonal contraceptives
Tri-Norinyl®	Z79.890	Hormone replacement therapy (postmenopausal)
Triphasil®	Z79.3	Long term (current) use of hormonal contraceptives
Triple Antibiotic®	Z79.2	Long term (current) use of antibiotics
Tri-Previfem®	Z79.3	Long term (current) use of hormonal contraceptives
triptorelin	Z79.818	Long term (current) use of other agents affecting estrogen receptors and estrogen levels
Tri-Sprintec®	Z79.3	Long term (current) use of hormonal contraceptives
Trivora-28®	Z79.3	Long term (current) use of hormonal contraceptives
Tygacil®	Z79.2	Long term (current) use of antibiotics
Uceris®	Z79.52	Long term (current) use of systemic steroids
Unasyn®	Z79.2	Long term (current) use of antibiotics
Vancocin HCl Pulvules®	Z79.2	Long term (current) use of antibiotics
Vancocin HCl®	Z79.2	Long term (current) use of antibiotics
Vancocin®	Z79.2	Long term (current) use of antibiotics
vancomycin	Z79.2	Long term (current) use of antibiotics
Vantas®	Z79.818	Long term (current) use of other agents affecting estrogen receptors and estrogen levels
Velivet®	Z79.3	Long term (current) use of hormonal contraceptives
Veripred 20®	Z79.52	Long term (current) use of systemic steroids
Vestura®	Z79.3	Long term (current) use of hormonal contraceptives
Vibativ®	Z79.2	Long term (current) use of antibiotics
Vibramycin®	Z79.2	Long term (current) use of antibiotics
Vienva®	Z79.3	Long term (current) use of hormonal contraceptives
Vimovo®	Z79.1	Long term (current) use of non-steroidal anti-inflammatories (NSAID)
Viorele®	Z79.3	Long term (current) use of hormonal contraceptives
Virazole®	Z79.2	Long term (current) use of antibiotics
Virti-Sulf®	Z79.2	Long term (current) use of antibiotics
Vivelle®	Z79.890	Hormone replacement therapy (postmenopausal)
Vivelle-Dot®	Z79.890	Hormone replacement therapy (postmenopausal)

Drug Name	Code	Code Descriptor
Voltaren®	Z79.1	Long term (current) use of non-steroidal anti-inflammatories (NSAID)
warfarin	Z79.01	Long term (current) use of anticoagulants
Wera®	Z79.3	Long term (current) use of hormonal contraceptives
Wera®	Z79.890	Hormone replacement therapy (postmenopausal)
Wycillin®	Z79.2	Long term (current) use of antibiotics
Wymzya Fe®	Z79.3	Long term (current) use of hormonal contraceptives
Xarelto®	Z79.01	Long term (current) use of anticoagulants
Xifaxan®	Z79.2	Long term (current) use of antibiotics
Ximino®	Z79.2	Long term (current) use of antibiotics
Yasmin®	Z79.3	Long term (current) use of hormonal contraceptives
Yaz®	Z79.3	Long term (current) use of hormonal contraceptives
zanamivir	Z79.2	Long term (current) use of antibiotics
Zarah®	Z79.3	Long term (current) use of hormonal contraceptives
Zema Pak®	Z79.52	Long term (current) use of systemic steroids
Zenchent Fe®	Z79.3	Long term (current) use of hormonal contraceptives
Zenchent Fe®	Z79.890	Hormone replacement therapy (postmenopausal)
Zenchent®	Z79.3	Long term (current) use of hormonal contraceptives
Zenchent®	Z79.890	Hormone replacement therapy (postmenopausal)
Zencia Wash®	Z79.2	Long term (current) use of antibiotics
Zeosa®	Z79.3	Long term (current) use of hormonal contraceptives
Zeosa®	Z79.890	Hormone replacement therapy (postmenopausal)
Zerbaxa®	Z79.2	Long term (current) use of antibiotics
Zetacet®	Z79.2	Long term (current) use of antibiotics
Zinacef®	Z79.2	Long term (current) use of antibiotics
Zipsor®	Z79.1	Long term (current) use of non-steroidal anti-inflammatories (NSAID)
Zithromax®	Z79.2	Long term (current) use of antibiotics
Zmax®	Z79.2	Long term (current) use of antibiotics
Zoladex®	Z79.818	Long term (current) use of other agents affecting estrogen receptors and estrogen levels
zoledronic acid	Z79.83	Long term (current) use of bisphosphonates
Zometa®	Z79.83	Long term (current) use of bisphosphonates
Zorvolex®	Z79.1	Long term (current) use of non-steroidal anti-inflammatories (NSAID)
Zosyn®	Z79.2	Long term (current) use of antibiotics
Zovia 1 / 35®	Z79.3	Long term (current) use of hormonal contraceptives
Zovia®	Z79.3	Long term (current) use of hormonal contraceptives
Zyvox®	Z79.2	Long term (current) use of antibiotics
N/A	Z79.899	Other long term (current) drug therapy

Note: This list of brand name and generic drugs correspond by drug class to Z codes for long-term use of drugs. This comprehensive but not exhaustive list is provided solely as a reference and does not imply a guarantee of reimbursement. Check with individual payers to determine their billing, coding, and reimbursement guidelines.

Appendix B: Symbols for 7th-character Codes

Adult - Age range is 18–124 years inclusive (e.g., senile delirium, mature cataract); based on Medicare's Outpatient Code Editor (OCE).

H35.3110	H35.3190	H35.3232	M80.011K	M80.021A	M80.029K	M80.039A	M80.042K	M80.052A	M80.061K	M80.071A	M80.079K	T74.21XA	T76.21XA
H35.3111	H35.3191	H35.3233	M80.011P	M80.021D	M80.029P	M80.039D	M80.042P	M80.052D	M80.061P	M80.071D	M80.079P	T74.21XD	T76.21XD
H35.3112	H35.3192	H35.3290	M80.011S	M80.021G	M80.029S	M80.039G	M80.042S	M80.052G	M80.061S	M80.071G	M80.079S	T74.21XS	T76.21XS
H35.3113	H35.3193	H35.3291	M80.012A	M80.021K	M80.031A	M80.039K	M80.049A	M80.052K	M80.062A	M80.071K	M80.08XA	T74.31XA	T76.31XA
H35.3114	H35.3194	H35.3292	M80.012D	M80.021P	M80.031D	M80.039P	M80.049D	M80.052P	M80.062D	M80.071P	M80.08XD	T74.31XD	T76.31XD
H35.3120	H35.3210	H35.3293	M80.012G	M80.021S	M80.031G	M80.039S	M80.049G	M80.052S	M80.062G	M80.071S	M80.08XG	T74.31XS	T76.31XS
H35.3121	H35.3211	M80.00XA	M80.012K	M80.022A	M80.031K	M80.041A	M80.049K	M80.059A	M80.062K	M80.072A	M80.08XK	T74.91XA	T76.91XA
H35.3122	H35.3212	M80.00XD	M80.012P	M80.022D	M80.031P	M80.041D	M80.049P	M80.059D	M80.062P	M80.072D	M80.08XP	T74.91XD	T76.91XD
H35.3123	H35.3213	M80.00XG	M80.012S	M80.022G	M80.031S	M80.041G	M80.049S	M80.059G	M80.062S	M80.072G	M80.08XS	T74.91XS	T76.91XS
H35.3124	H35.3220	M80.00XK	M80.019A	M80.022K	M80.032A	M80.041K	M80.051A	M80.059K	M80.069A	M80.072K		T74.01XA	T76.01XA
H35.3130	H35.3221	M80.00XP	M80.019D	M80.022P	M80.032D	M80.041P	M80.051D	M80.059P	M80.069D	M80.072P		T74.01XD	T76.01XD
H35.3131	H35.3222	M80.00XS	M80.019G	M80.022S	M80.032G	M80.041S	M80.051G	M80.059S	M80.069G	M80.072S		T74.01XS	T76.01XS
H35.3132	H35.3223	M80.011A	M80.019K	M80.029A	M80.032K	M80.042A	M80.051K	M80.061A	M80.069K	M80.079A		T74.11XA	T76.11XA
H35.3133	H35.3230	M80.011D	M80.019P	M80.029D	M80.032P	M80.042D	M80.051P	M80.061D	M80.069P	M80.079D		T74.11XD	T76.11XD
H35.3134	H35.3231	M80.011G	M80.019S	M80.029G	M80.032S	M80.042G	M80.051S	M80.061G	M80.069S	M80.079G		T74.11XS	T76.11XS

AHA Coding Clinic®

H35.3112	O60.14X1	S01.411A	S31.613A	S53.031D	S72.141D	T20.25XS	T24.392A	T45.615A	T81.4XXD	T88.53XA	W03.XXXA	X00.0XXD	X95.9XXA
H35.3121	O60.14X2	S01.411D	S36.029A	S53.114A	S72.401A	T20.312S	T36.8X5A	T45.8X5A	T82.7XXA	V00.321A	W03.XXXD	X00.0XXS	
M84.454A	S01.02XA	S06.1X0A	S39.012A	S62.002A	S81.841A	T21.31XD	T39.015A	T50.901S	T84.50XA	V43.61XA	W19.XXXD	X03.0XXS	
M97.01XA	S01.02XD	S06.340A	S51.001A	S62.102D	S82.234A	T23.301S	T40.5X1A	T59.811A	T84.51XA	V43.61XD	W34.00XS	X04.XXXA	
O35.3XX0	S01.21XA	S06.5X0A	S52.532D	S72.002D	S82.234D	T23.302S	T43.592A	T71.191A	T84.52XA	V49.9XXA	W50.2XXA	X08.01XS	
O60.14X0	S01.21XD	S06.6X0A	S53.031A	S72.002S	S83.511D	T24.391A	T45.525A	T81.31XA	T85.628A	W00.0XXD	W50.2XXD	X50.0XXA	

Complication or Comorbidity (CC) - Based on CMS data

H34.8110	M80.031P	M80.08XK	M80.852A	M84.331P	M84.372P	M84.433A	M84.461P	M84.50XK	M84.550A	M84.575P	M84.641K	M84.673A	M84.759P
H34.8111	M80.032A	M80.08XP	M80.852K	M84.332K	M84.373K	M84.433K	M84.462A	M84.50XP	M84.550K	M84.576A	M84.641P	M84.673K	M97.01XA
H34.8112	M80.032K	M80.80XA	M80.852P	M84.332P	M84.373P	M84.433P	M84.462K	M84.511A	M84.550P	M84.576K	M84.642A	M84.673P	M97.02XA
H34.8120	M80.032P	M80.80XK	M80.859A	M84.333K	M84.374K	M84.434A	M84.462P	M84.511K	M84.551A	M84.576P	M84.642K	M84.674A	M97.11XA
H34.8121	M80.039A	M80.80XP	M80.859K	M84.333P	M84.374P	M84.434K	M84.463A	M84.511P	M84.551K	M84.58XA	M84.642P	M84.674K	M97.12XA
H34.8122	M80.039K	M80.811A	M80.859P	M84.334K	M84.375K	M84.434P	M84.463K	M84.512A	M84.551P	M84.58XK	M84.649A	M84.674P	M97.21XA
H34.8130	M80.039P	M80.811K	M80.861A	M84.334P	M84.375P	M84.439A	M84.463P	M84.512K	M84.552A	M84.58XP	M84.649K	M84.675A	M97.22XA
H34.8131	M80.041A	M80.811P	M80.861K	M84.339K	M84.376K	M84.439K	M84.464A	M84.512P	M84.552K	M84.60XA	M84.649P	M84.675K	M97.31XA
H34.8132	M80.041K	M80.812A	M80.861P	M84.339P	M84.376P	M84.439P	M84.464K	M84.519A	M84.552P	M84.60XK	M84.650A	M84.675P	M97.32XA
H34.8190	M80.041P	M80.812K	M80.862A	M84.341K	M84.377K	M84.441A	M84.464P	M84.519K	M84.553A	M84.60XP	M84.650K	M84.676A	M97.41XA
H34.8191	M80.042A	M80.812P	M80.862K	M84.341P	M84.377P	M84.441K	M84.469A	M84.519P	M84.553K	M84.611A	M84.650P	M84.676K	M97.42XA
H34.8192	M80.042K	M80.819A	M80.862P	M84.342K	M84.378K	M84.441P	M84.469K	M84.521A	M84.553P	M84.611K	M84.651A	M84.676P	M97.8XXA
M48.50XA	M80.042P	M80.819K	M80.869A	M84.342P	M84.378P	M84.442A	M84.469P	M84.521K	M84.559A	M84.611P	M84.651K	M84.68XA	M97.9XXA
M48.51XA	M80.049A	M80.819P	M80.869K	M84.343K	M84.379K	M84.442K	M84.471A	M84.521P	M84.559K	M84.612A	M84.651P	M84.68XK	O31.8X10
M48.52XA	M80.049K	M80.821A	M80.869P	M84.343P	M84.379P	M84.442P	M84.471K	M84.522A	M84.559P	M84.612K	M84.652A	M84.68XP	O31.8X11
M48.53XA	M80.049P	M80.821K	M80.871A	M84.344K	M84.38XK	M84.443A	M84.471P	M84.522K	M84.561A	M84.612P	M84.652K	M84.750A	O31.8X12
M48.54XA	M80.051A	M80.821P	M80.871K	M84.344P	M84.38XP	M84.443K	M84.472A	M84.522P	M84.561K	M84.619A	M84.652P	M84.750K	O31.8X13
M48.55XA	M80.051K	M80.822A	M80.871P	M84.345K	M84.40XA	M84.443P	M84.472K	M84.529A	M84.561P	M84.619K	M84.653A	M84.750P	O31.8X14
M48.56XA	M80.051P	M80.822K	M80.872A	M84.345P	M84.40XK	M84.444A	M84.472P	M84.529K	M84.562A	M84.619P	M84.653K	M84.751A	O31.8X15
M48.57XA	M80.052A	M80.822P	M80.872K	M84.346K	M84.40XP	M84.444K	M84.473A	M84.529P	M84.562K	M84.621A	M84.653P	M84.751K	O31.8X19
M48.58XA	M80.052K	M80.829A	M80.872P	M84.346P	M84.411A	M84.444P	M84.473K	M84.531A	M84.562P	M84.621K	M84.659A	M84.751P	O31.8X20
M80.00XA	M80.052P	M80.829K	M80.879A	M84.350K	M84.411K	M84.445A	M84.473P	M84.531K	M84.563A	M84.621P	M84.659K	M84.752A	O31.8X21
M80.00XK	M80.059A	M80.829P	M80.879K	M84.350P	M84.411P	M84.445K	M84.474A	M84.531P	M84.563K	M84.622A	M84.659P	M84.752K	O31.8X22
M80.00XP	M80.059K	M80.831A	M80.879P	M84.351K	M84.412A	M84.445P	M84.474K	M84.532A	M84.563P	M84.622K	M84.661A	M84.752P	O31.8X23
M80.011A	M80.059P	M80.831K	M80.88XA	M84.351P	M84.412K	M84.446A	M84.474P	M84.532K	M84.564A	M84.622P	M84.661K	M84.753A	O31.8X24
M80.011K	M80.061A	M80.831P	M80.88XK	M84.352K	M84.412P	M84.446K	M84.475A	M84.532P	M84.564K	M84.629A	M84.661P	M84.753K	O31.8X25
M80.011P	M80.061K	M80.832A	M80.88XP	M84.352P	M84.419A	M84.446P	M84.475K	M84.533A	M84.564P	M84.629K	M84.662A	M84.753P	O31.8X29
M80.012A	M80.061P	M80.832K	T83.518A	M84.353K	M84.419K	M84.451A	M84.475P	M84.533K	M84.569A	M84.629P	M84.662K	M84.754A	O31.8X30
M80.012K	M80.062A	M80.832P	T83.598A	M84.353P	M84.419P	M84.451K	M84.476A	M84.533P	M84.569K	M84.631A	M84.662P	M84.754K	O31.8X31
M80.012P	M80.062K	M80.839A	M84.30XK	M84.359K	M84.421A	M84.451P	M84.476K	M84.534A	M84.569P	M84.631K	M84.663A	M84.754P	O31.8X32
M80.019A	M80.062P	M80.839K	M84.30XP	M84.359P	M84.421K	M84.452A	M84.476P	M84.534K	M84.571A	M84.631P	M84.663K	M84.755A	O31.8X33
M80.019K	M80.069A	M80.839P	M84.311K	M84.361K	M84.421P	M84.452K	M84.477A	M84.534P	M84.571K	M84.632A	M84.663P	M84.755K	O31.8X34
M80.019P	M80.069K	M80.841A	M84.311P	M84.361P	M84.422A	M84.452P	M84.477K	M84.539A	M84.571P	M84.632K	M84.664A	M84.755P	O31.8X35
M80.021A	M80.069P	M80.841K	M84.312A	M84.362K	M84.422K	M84.453A	M84.477P	M84.539K	M84.572A	M84.632P	M84.664K	M84.756A	O31.8X39
M80.021K	M80.071A	M80.841P	M84.312K	M84.362P	M84.422P	M84.453K	M84.478A	M84.539P	M84.572K	M84.633A	M84.664P	M84.756K	O36.0110
M80.021P	M80.071K	M80.842A	M84.312P	M84.363K	M84.429A	M84.453P	M84.478K	M84.541A	M84.572P	M84.633K	M84.669A	M84.756P	O36.0111
M80.022A	M80.071P	M80.842K	M84.319K	M84.363P	M84.429K	M84.454A	M84.478P	M84.541K	M84.573A	M84.633P	M84.669K	M84.757A	O36.0112
M80.022K	M80.072A	M80.842P	M84.319P	M84.364K	M84.429P	M84.454K	M84.479A	M84.541P	M84.573K	M84.634A	M84.669P	M84.757K	O36.0113
M80.022P	M80.072K	M80.849A	M84.321K	M84.364P	M84.431A	M84.454P	M84.479K	M84.542A	M84.573P	M84.634K	M84.671A	M84.757P	O36.0114
M80.029A	M80.072P	M80.849K	M84.321P	M84.369K	M84.431K	M84.459A	M84.479P	M84.542K	M84.574A	M84.634P	M84.671K	M84.758A	O36.0115
M80.029K	M80.079A	M80.849P	M84.322A	M84.369P	M84.431P	M84.459K	M84.48XA	M84.542P	M84.574K	M84.639A	M84.671P	M84.758K	O36.0119
M80.029P	M80.079K	M80.851A	M84.322K	M84.371K	M84.432A	M84.459P	M84.48XK	M84.549A	M84.574P	M84.639K	M84.672A	M84.758P	O36.0120
M80.031A	M80.079P	M80.851K	M84.322P	M84.371P	M84.432K	M84.461A	M84.48XP	M84.549K	M84.575A	M84.639P	M84.672K	M84.759A	O36.0121
M80.031K	M80.08XA	M80.851P	M84.331K	M84.372K	M84.432P	M84.461K	M84.50XA	M84.549P	M84.575K	M84.641A	M84.672P	M84.759K	O36.0122

Complication or Comorbidity (CC) (cont.) - Based on CMS data

O36.0123	S01.101A	S02.40EB	S02.652K	S05.40XA	S09.309A	S12.231A	S12.64XA	S15.321A	S22.039K	S22.49XK	S32.008K	S32.131K	S32.461K
O36.0124	S01.102A	S02.40EK	S02.66XA	S05.41XA	S09.311A	S12.231K	S12.64XK	S15.322A	S22.040A	S22.5XXK	S32.009A	S32.132A	S32.462K
O36.0125	S01.109A	S02.40FA	S02.66XB	S05.42XA	S09.312A	S12.24XA	S12.650A	S15.329A	S22.040K	S22.9XXA	S32.009K	S32.132K	S32.463K
O36.0129	S02.0XXA	S02.40FB	S02.66XK	S05.50XA	S09.313A	S12.24XK	S12.650K	S15.391A	S22.041A	S22.9XXK	S32.010A	S32.139A	S32.464K
O36.0130	S02.0XXK	S02.40FK	S02.670A	S05.51XA	S09.319A	S12.250A	S12.651A	S15.392A	S22.041K	S25.501A	S32.010K	S32.139K	S32.465K
O36.0131	S02.101A	S02.411A	S02.670B	S05.52XA	S09.391A	S12.250K	S12.651K	S15.399A	S22.042A	S25.502A	S32.011A	S32.14XA	S32.466K
O36.0132	S02.101K	S02.411B	S02.670K	S05.70XA	S09.392A	S12.251A	S12.690A	S15.8XXA	S22.042K	S25.509A	S32.011K	S32.14XK	S32.471K
O36.0133	S02.102A	S02.411K	S02.671A	S05.71XA	S09.399A	S12.251K	S12.690K	S15.9XXA	S22.048A	S25.511A	S32.012A	S32.15XA	S32.472K
O36.0134	S02.102K	S02.412A	S02.671B	S05.72XA	S11.10XA	S12.290A	S12.691A	S17.0XXA	S22.048K	S25.512A	S32.012K	S32.15XK	S32.473K
O36.0135	S02.109A	S02.412B	S02.671K	S05.8X1A	S11.11XA	S12.290K	S12.691K	S17.8XXA	S22.049A	S25.519A	S32.018A	S32.16XA	S32.474K
O36.0136	S02.109K	S02.412K	S02.672A	S05.8X2A	S11.12XA	S12.291A	S12.9XXA	S17.9XXA	S22.049K	S25.591A	S32.018K	S32.16XK	S32.475K
O36.0910	S02.110A	S02.413A	S02.672B	S05.8X9A	S11.13XA	S12.291K	S13.0XXA	S21.101A	S22.050A	S25.592A	S32.019A	S32.17XA	S32.476K
O36.0911	S02.110K	S02.413B	S02.672K	S05.91XA	S11.14XA	S12.300A	S13.100A	S21.102A	S22.050K	S25.599A	S32.019K	S32.17XK	S32.481K
O36.0912	S02.111A	S02.413K	S02.69XA	S05.92XA	S11.15XA	S12.300K	S13.101A	S21.109A	S22.051A	S25.801A	S32.020A	S32.19XA	S32.482K
O36.0913	S02.111K	S02.42XA	S02.69XB	S06.0X1A	S11.20XA	S12.301A	S13.110A	S21.111A	S22.051K	S25.802A	S32.020K	S32.19XK	S32.483K
O36.0914	S02.112A	S02.42XB	S02.69XK	S06.0X9A	S11.21XA	S12.301K	S13.111A	S21.112A	S22.052A	S25.809A	S32.021A	S32.2XXA	S32.484K
O36.0915	S02.112K	S02.42XK	S02.80XA	S06.2X1A	S11.22XA	S12.330A	S13.120A	S21.119A	S22.052K	S25.811A	S32.021K	S32.2XXK	S32.485K
O36.0919	S02.113A	S02.5XXX	S02.80XB	S06.2X2A	S11.23XA	S12.330K	S13.121A	S21.121A	S22.058A	S25.812A	S32.022A	S32.301A	S32.486K
O36.0920	S02.113K	S02.600A	S02.80XK	S06.2X3A	S11.24XA	S12.331A	S13.130A	S21.122A	S22.058K	S25.819A	S32.022K	S32.301K	S32.491K
O36.0921	S02.118A	S02.600B	S02.81XA	S06.2X4A	S11.25XA	S12.331K	S13.131A	S21.129A	S22.059A	S25.891A	S32.028A	S32.302A	S32.492K
O36.0922	S02.118K	S02.600K	S02.81XB	S06.2X5A	S12.000A	S12.34XA	S13.140A	S21.131A	S22.059K	S25.892A	S32.028K	S32.302K	S32.499K
O36.0923	S02.119A	S02.601A	S02.81XK	S06.2X9A	S12.000K	S12.34XK	S13.141A	S21.132A	S22.060A	S25.899A	S32.029A	S32.309A	S32.501A
O36.0924	S02.119K	S02.601B	S02.82XA	S06.301A	S12.001A	S12.350A	S13.150A	S21.139A	S22.060K	S25.90XA	S32.029K	S32.309K	S32.501K
O36.0925	S02.11AA	S02.601K	S02.82XB	S06.302A	S12.001K	S12.350K	S13.151A	S21.141A	S22.061A	S25.91XA	S32.030A	S32.311A	S32.502A
O36.0929	S02.11AK	S02.602A	S02.82XK	S06.303A	S12.01XA	S12.351A	S13.160A	S21.142A	S22.061K	S25.99XA	S32.030K	S32.311K	S32.502K
O36.0930	S02.11BA	S02.602B	S02.91XA	S06.304A	S12.01XK	S12.351K	S13.161A	S21.149A	S22.062A	S26.00XA	S32.031A	S32.312A	S32.509A
O36.0931	S02.11BK	S02.602K	S02.91XK	S06.305A	S12.02XA	S12.390A	S13.170A	S21.151A	S22.062K	S26.01XA	S32.031K	S32.312K	S32.509K
O36.0932	S02.11CA	S02.609A	S02.92XA	S06.309A	S12.02XK	S12.390K	S13.171A	S21.152A	S22.068A	S26.09XA	S32.032A	S32.313A	S32.511A
O36.0933	S02.11CK	S02.609B	S02.92XB	S06.371A	S12.030A	S12.391A	S13.180A	S21.159A	S22.068K	S26.10XA	S32.032K	S32.313K	S32.511K
O36.0934	S02.11DA	S02.609K	S02.92XK	S06.372A	S12.030K	S12.391K	S13.181A	S21.90XA	S22.069A	S26.11XA	S32.038A	S32.314A	S32.512A
O36.0935	S02.11DK	S02.610A	S04.011A	S06.373A	S12.031A	S12.400A	S13.20XA	S21.91XA	S22.069K	S26.19XA	S32.038K	S32.314K	S32.512K
O36.0939	S02.11EA	S02.610B	S04.012A	S06.374A	S12.031K	S12.400K	S13.29XA	S21.92XA	S22.070A	S26.90XA	S32.039A	S32.315A	S32.519A
O36.4XX0	S02.11EK	S02.610K	S04.019A	S06.375A	S12.040A	S12.401A	S15.001A	S21.93XA	S22.070K	S26.91XA	S32.039K	S32.315K	S32.519K
O36.4XX1	S02.11FA	S02.611A	S04.02XA	S06.379A	S12.040K	S12.401K	S15.002A	S21.94XA	S22.071A	S26.99XA	S32.040A	S32.316A	S32.591A
O36.4XX2	S02.11FK	S02.611B	S04.031A	S06.381A	S12.041A	S12.430A	S15.009A	S21.95XA	S22.071K	S27.0XXA	S32.040K	S32.316K	S32.591K
O36.4XX3	S02.11GA	S02.611K	S04.032A	S06.382A	S12.041K	S12.430K	S15.011A	S22.000A	S22.072A	S27.301A	S32.041A	S32.391A	S32.592A
O36.4XX4	S02.11GK	S02.612A	S04.039A	S06.383A	S12.090A	S12.431A	S15.012A	S22.000K	S22.072K	S27.302A	S32.041K	S32.391K	S32.592K
O36.4XX5	S02.11HA	S02.612B	S04.041A	S06.384A	S12.090K	S12.431K	S15.019A	S22.001A	S22.078A	S27.309A	S32.042A	S32.392A	S32.599A
O36.4XX9	S02.11HK	S02.612K	S04.042A	S06.385A	S12.091A	S12.44XA	S15.021A	S22.001K	S22.078K	S27.311A	S32.042K	S32.392K	S32.599K
O41.01X0	S02.19XA	S02.620A	S04.049A	S06.389A	S12.091K	S12.44XK	S15.022A	S22.002A	S22.079A	S27.312A	S32.048A	S32.399A	S32.601A
O41.01X1	S02.19XK	S02.620B	S04.10XA	S06.811A	S12.100A	S12.450A	S15.029A	S22.002K	S22.079K	S27.319A	S32.048K	S32.399K	S32.601K
O41.01X2	S02.2XXB	S02.620K	S04.11XA	S06.812A	S12.100K	S12.450K	S15.091A	S22.008A	S22.080A	S27.321A	S32.049A	S32.401K	S32.602A
O41.01X3	S02.2XXK	S02.621A	S04.12XA	S06.813A	S12.101A	S12.451A	S15.092A	S22.008K	S22.080K	S27.322A	S32.049K	S32.402K	S32.602K
O41.01X4	S02.30XA	S02.621B	S04.20XA	S06.814A	S12.101K	S12.451K	S15.099A	S22.009A	S22.081A	S27.329A	S32.050A	S32.409K	S32.609A
O41.01X5	S02.30XB	S02.621K	S04.21XA	S06.815A	S12.110A	S12.490A	S15.101A	S22.009K	S22.081K	S27.391A	S32.050K	S32.411K	S32.609K
O41.01X9	S02.30XK	S02.622A	S04.22XA	S06.819A	S12.110K	S12.490K	S15.102A	S22.010A	S22.082A	S27.392A	S32.051A	S32.412K	S32.611A
O41.02X0	S02.31XA	S02.622B	S04.30XA	S06.821A	S12.111A	S12.491A	S15.109A	S22.010K	S22.082K	S27.399A	S32.051K	S32.413K	S32.611K
O41.02X1	S02.31XB	S02.622K	S04.31XA	S06.822A	S12.111K	S12.491K	S15.111A	S22.011A	S22.088A	S27.50XA	S32.052A	S32.414K	S32.612A
O41.02X2	S02.31XK	S02.630A	S04.32XA	S06.823A	S12.112A	S12.500A	S15.112A	S22.011K	S22.088K	S27.51XA	S32.052K	S32.415K	S32.612K
O41.02X3	S02.32XA	S02.630B	S04.40XA	S06.824A	S12.112K	S12.500K	S15.119A	S22.012A	S22.089A	S27.52XA	S32.058A	S32.416K	S32.613A
O41.02X4	S02.32XB	S02.630K	S04.41XA	S06.825A	S12.120A	S12.501A	S15.121A	S22.012K	S22.089K	S27.53XA	S32.058K	S32.421K	S32.613K
O41.02X5	S02.32XK	S02.631A	S04.42XA	S06.829A	S12.120K	S12.501K	S15.122A	S22.018A	S22.20XA	S27.59XA	S32.059A	S32.422K	S32.614A
O41.02X9	S02.400A	S02.631B	S04.50XA	S06.891A	S12.121A	S12.530A	S15.129A	S22.018K	S22.20XK	S27.60XA	S32.059K	S32.423K	S32.614K
O41.03X0	S02.400B	S02.631K	S04.51XA	S06.892A	S12.121K	S12.530K	S15.191A	S22.019A	S22.21XA	S27.63XA	S32.10XA	S32.424K	S32.615A
O41.03X1	S02.400K	S02.632A	S04.52XA	S06.893A	S12.130A	S12.531A	S15.192A	S22.019K	S22.21XK	S27.69XA	S32.10XK	S32.425K	S32.615K
O41.03X2	S02.401A	S02.632B	S04.60XA	S06.894A	S12.130K	S12.531K	S15.199A	S22.020A	S22.22XA	S27.802A	S32.110A	S32.426K	S32.616A
O41.03X3	S02.401B	S02.632K	S04.61XA	S06.895A	S12.131A	S12.54XA	S15.201A	S22.020K	S22.22XK	S27.803A	S32.110K	S32.431K	S32.616K
O41.03X4	S02.401K	S02.640A	S04.62XA	S06.899A	S12.131K	S12.54XK	S15.202A	S22.021A	S22.23XA	S27.808A	S32.111A	S32.432K	S32.691A
O41.03X5	S02.402A	S02.640B	S04.70XA	S06.9X1A	S12.14XA	S12.550A	S15.209A	S22.021K	S22.23XK	S27.809A	S32.111K	S32.433K	S32.691K
O41.03X9	S02.402B	S02.640K	S04.71XA	S06.9X2A	S12.14XK	S12.550K	S15.211A	S22.022A	S22.24XA	S27.892A	S32.112A	S32.434K	S32.692A
O60.10X0	S02.402K	S02.641A	S04.72XA	S06.9X3A	S12.150A	S12.551A	S15.212A	S22.022K	S22.24XK	S27.893A	S32.112K	S32.435K	S32.692K
O60.10X1	S02.40AA	S02.641B	S04.811A	S06.9X4A	S12.150K	S12.551K	S15.219A	S22.028A	S22.31XA	S27.898A	S32.119A	S32.436K	S32.699A
O60.10X2	S02.40AB	S02.641K	S04.812A	S06.9X5A	S12.151A	S12.590A	S15.221A	S22.028K	S22.31XK	S27.899A	S32.119K	S32.441K	S32.699K
O60.10X3	S02.40AK	S02.642A	S04.819A	S06.9X9A	S12.151K	S12.590K	S15.222A	S22.029A	S22.32XA	S27.9XXA	S32.120A	S32.442K	S32.810A
O60.10X4	S02.40BA	S02.642B	S04.891A	S07.0XXA	S12.190A	S12.591A	S15.229A	S22.029K	S22.32XK	S28.1XXA	S32.120K	S32.443K	S32.810K
O60.10X5	S02.40BB	S02.642K	S04.892A	S07.1XXA	S12.190K	S12.591K	S15.291A	S22.030A	S22.39XA	S29.021A	S32.121A	S32.444K	S32.811A
O60.10X9	S02.40BK	S02.650A	S04.899A	S07.8XXA	S12.191A	S12.600A	S15.292A	S22.030K	S22.39XK	S29.029A	S32.121K	S32.445K	S32.811K
O60.20X0	S02.40CA	S02.650B	S04.9XXA	S07.9XXA	S12.191K	S12.600K	S15.299A	S22.031A	S22.41XA	S32.000A	S32.122A	S32.446K	S32.82XA
O60.20X1	S02.40CB	S02.650K	S05.20XA	S09.0XXA	S12.200A	S12.601A	S15.301A	S22.031K	S22.41XK	S32.000K	S32.122K	S32.451K	S32.82XK
O60.20X2	S02.40CK	S02.651A	S05.21XA	S09.20XA	S12.200K	S12.601K	S15.302A	S22.032A	S22.42XA	S32.001A	S32.129A	S32.452K	S32.89XA
O60.20X3	S02.40DA	S02.651B	S05.22XA	S09.21XA	S12.201A	S12.630A	S15.309A	S22.032K	S22.42XK	S32.001K	S32.129K	S32.453K	S32.89XK
O60.20X4	S02.40DB	S02.651K	S05.30XA	S09.22XA	S12.201K	S12.630K	S15.311A	S22.038A	S22.43XA	S32.002A	S32.130A	S32.454K	S32.9XXA
O60.20X5	S02.40DK	S02.652A	S05.31XA	S09.301A	S12.230A	S12.631A	S15.312A	S22.038K	S22.43XK	S32.002K	S32.130K	S32.455K	S32.9XXK
O60.20X9	S02.40EA	S02.652B	S05.32XA	S09.302A	S12.230K	S12.631K	S15.319A	S22.039A	S22.49XA	S32.008A	S32.131A	S32.456K	S35.531A

Complication or Comorbidity (CC) (cont.) - Based on CMS data

S35.532A	S36.499A	S37.39XA	S42.032B	S42.135P	S42.216K	S42.271A	S42.334P	S42.402K	S42.446A	S42.489P	S45.802A	S49.022A	S49.142P
S35.533A	S36.500A	S37.60XA	S42.032K	S42.136B	S42.216P	S42.271K	S42.335A	S42.402P	S42.446K	S42.491A	S45.809A	S49.022K	S49.149A
S35.534A	S36.501A	S37.62XA	S42.032P	S42.136K	S42.221A	S42.271P	S42.335K	S42.409A	S42.446P	S42.491K	S45.811A	S49.022P	S49.149K
S35.535A	S36.502A	S37.63XA	S42.033B	S42.136P	S42.221K	S42.272A	S42.335P	S42.409K	S42.447A	S42.491P	S45.812A	S49.029A	S49.149P
S35.536A	S36.503A	S37.69XA	S42.033K	S42.141B	S42.221P	S42.272K	S42.336A	S42.409P	S42.447K	S42.492A	S45.819A	S49.029P	S49.191A
S35.8X1A	S36.508A	S37.812A	S42.033P	S42.141K	S42.222A	S42.272P	S42.336K	S42.411A	S42.447P	S42.492K	S45.891A	S49.031A	S49.191K
S35.8X8A	S36.509A	S37.813A	S42.034B	S42.141P	S42.222K	S42.279A	S42.336P	S42.411K	S42.448A	S42.492P	S45.892A	S49.031K	S49.191P
S35.8X9A	S36.510A	S37.818A	S42.034K	S42.142B	S42.222P	S42.279K	S42.341A	S42.411P	S42.448K	S42.493A	S45.899A	S49.031P	S49.192A
S35.90XA	S36.511A	S37.819A	S42.034P	S42.142K	S42.223A	S42.279P	S42.341K	S42.412A	S42.448P	S42.493K	S45.901A	S49.032A	S49.192K
S35.91XA	S36.512A	S37.892A	S42.035B	S42.142P	S42.223K	S42.291A	S42.341P	S42.412K	S42.449A	S42.493P	S45.902A	S49.032K	S49.192P
S35.99XA	S36.513A	S37.893A	S42.035K	S42.143B	S42.223P	S42.291K	S42.342A	S42.412P	S42.449K	S42.494A	S45.909A	S49.032P	S49.199A
S36.00XA	S36.518A	S37.898A	S42.035P	S42.143K	S42.224A	S42.291P	S42.342K	S42.413A	S42.449P	S42.494K	S45.911A	S49.039A	S49.199K
S36.020A	S36.519A	S37.899A	S42.036B	S42.143P	S42.224K	S42.292A	S42.342P	S42.413K	S42.451A	S42.494P	S45.912A	S49.039K	S49.199P
S36.021A	S36.520A	S37.90XA	S42.036K	S42.144B	S42.224P	S42.292K	S42.343A	S42.413P	S42.451K	S42.495A	S45.919A	S49.039P	S52.001K
S36.029A	S36.521A	S37.92XA	S42.036P	S42.144K	S42.225A	S42.292P	S42.343K	S42.414A	S42.451P	S42.495K	S45.991A	S49.041A	S52.001M
S36.030A	S36.522A	S37.93XA	S42.101B	S42.144P	S42.225K	S42.293A	S42.343P	S42.414K	S42.452A	S42.495P	S45.992A	S49.041K	S52.001N
S36.039A	S36.523A	S37.99XA	S42.101K	S42.145B	S42.225P	S42.293K	S42.344A	S42.414P	S42.452K	S42.496A	S45.999A	S49.041P	S52.001P
S36.09XA	S36.528A	S42.001B	S42.101P	S42.145K	S42.226A	S42.293P	S42.344K	S42.415A	S42.452P	S42.496K	S46.021A	S49.042A	S52.001Q
S36.112A	S36.529A	S42.001K	S42.102B	S42.145P	S42.226K	S42.294A	S42.344P	S42.415K	S42.453A	S42.496P	S46.022A	S49.042K	S52.001R
S36.113A	S36.530A	S42.001P	S42.102K	S42.146B	S42.226P	S42.294K	S42.345A	S42.415P	S42.453K	S42.90XA	S46.029A	S49.042P	S52.002K
S36.114A	S36.531A	S42.002B	S42.102P	S42.146K	S42.231A	S42.294P	S42.345K	S42.416A	S42.453P	S42.90XK	S46.121A	S49.049A	S52.002M
S36.118A	S36.532A	S42.002K	S42.109B	S42.146P	S42.231K	S42.295A	S42.345P	S42.416K	S42.454A	S42.90XP	S46.122A	S49.049K	S52.002N
S36.119A	S36.533A	S42.002P	S42.109K	S42.151B	S42.231P	S42.295K	S42.346A	S42.416P	S42.454K	S42.91XA	S46.129A	S49.049P	S52.002P
S36.122A	S36.538A	S42.009B	S42.109P	S42.151K	S42.232A	S42.295P	S42.346K	S42.421A	S42.454P	S42.91XK	S46.221A	S49.091A	S52.002Q
S36.123A	S36.539A	S42.009K	S42.111B	S42.151P	S42.232K	S42.296A	S42.346P	S42.421K	S42.455A	S42.91XP	S46.222A	S49.091K	S52.002R
S36.128A	S36.590A	S42.009P	S42.111K	S42.152B	S42.232P	S42.296K	S42.351A	S42.421P	S42.455K	S42.92XA	S46.229A	S49.091P	S52.009K
S36.129A	S36.591A	S42.011B	S42.111P	S42.152K	S42.239A	S42.296P	S42.351K	S42.422A	S42.455P	S42.92XK	S46.321A	S49.092A	S52.009M
S36.13XA	S36.592A	S42.011K	S42.112B	S42.152P	S42.239K	S42.301A	S42.351P	S42.422K	S42.456A	S42.92XP	S46.322A	S49.092K	S52.009N
S36.200A	S36.593A	S42.011P	S42.112K	S42.153B	S42.239P	S42.301K	S42.352A	S42.422P	S42.456K	S43.201A	S46.329A	S49.092P	S52.009P
S36.201A	S36.598A	S42.012B	S42.112P	S42.153K	S42.241A	S42.301P	S42.352K	S42.423A	S42.456P	S43.202A	S46.821A	S49.099A	S52.009Q
S36.202A	S36.599A	S42.012K	S42.113B	S42.153P	S42.241K	S42.302A	S42.352P	S42.423K	S42.461A	S43.203A	S46.822A	S49.099K	S52.009R
S36.209A	S36.60XA	S42.012P	S42.113K	S42.154B	S42.241P	S42.302K	S42.353A	S42.423P	S42.461K	S43.204A	S46.829A	S49.099P	S52.011A
S36.220A	S36.61XA	S42.013B	S42.113P	S42.154K	S42.242A	S42.302P	S42.353K	S42.424A	S42.461P	S43.205A	S46.921A	S49.101A	S52.011K
S36.221A	S36.62XA	S42.013K	S42.114B	S42.154P	S42.242K	S42.309A	S42.353P	S42.424K	S42.462A	S43.206A	S46.922A	S49.101K	S52.011P
S36.222A	S36.63XA	S42.013P	S42.114K	S42.155B	S42.242P	S42.309K	S42.354A	S42.424P	S42.462K	S43.211A	S46.929A	S49.101P	S52.012A
S36.229A	S36.69XA	S42.014B	S42.114P	S42.155K	S42.249A	S42.309P	S42.354K	S42.425A	S42.462P	S43.212A	S48.011A	S49.102A	S52.012K
S36.230A	S36.81XA	S42.014K	S42.115B	S42.155P	S42.249K	S42.311A	S42.354P	S42.425K	S42.463A	S43.213A	S48.012A	S49.102K	S52.012P
S36.231A	S36.892A	S42.014P	S42.115K	S42.156B	S42.249P	S42.311K	S42.355A	S42.425P	S42.463K	S43.214A	S48.019A	S49.102P	S52.019A
S36.232A	S36.893A	S42.015B	S42.115P	S42.156K	S42.251A	S42.311P	S42.355K	S42.426A	S42.463P	S43.215A	S48.021A	S49.109A	S52.019K
S36.239A	S36.898A	S42.015K	S42.116B	S42.156P	S42.251K	S42.312A	S42.355P	S42.426K	S42.464A	S43.216A	S48.022A	S49.109K	S52.019P
S36.240A	S36.899A	S42.015P	S42.116K	S42.191A	S42.251P	S42.312K	S42.356A	S42.426P	S42.464K	S43.221A	S48.029A	S49.109P	S52.021K
S36.241A	S36.90XA	S42.016B	S42.116P	S42.191K	S42.252A	S42.312P	S42.356K	S42.431A	S42.464P	S43.222A	S48.111A	S49.111A	S52.021M
S36.242A	S36.92XA	S42.016K	S42.121B	S42.191P	S42.252K	S42.319A	S42.356P	S42.431K	S42.465A	S43.223A	S48.112A	S49.111K	S52.021N
S36.249A	S36.93XA	S42.016P	S42.121K	S42.192B	S42.252P	S42.319K	S42.361A	S42.431P	S42.465K	S43.224A	S48.119A	S49.111P	S52.021P
S36.250A	S36.99XA	S42.017B	S42.121P	S42.192K	S42.253A	S42.319P	S42.361K	S42.432A	S42.465P	S43.225A	S48.121A	S49.112A	S52.021Q
S36.251A	S37.001A	S42.017K	S42.122B	S42.192P	S42.253K	S42.321A	S42.361P	S42.432K	S42.466A	S43.226A	S48.122A	S49.112K	S52.021R
S36.252A	S37.002A	S42.017P	S42.122K	S42.199B	S42.253P	S42.321K	S42.362A	S42.432P	S42.466K	S45.101A	S48.129A	S49.112P	S52.022K
S36.259A	S37.009A	S42.018B	S42.122P	S42.199K	S42.254A	S42.321P	S42.362K	S42.433A	S42.466P	S45.102A	S48.911A	S49.119A	S52.022M
S36.260A	S37.011A	S42.018K	S42.123B	S42.199P	S42.254K	S42.322A	S42.362P	S42.433K	S42.471A	S45.109A	S48.912A	S49.119K	S52.022N
S36.261A	S37.012A	S42.018P	S42.123K	S42.201A	S42.254P	S42.322K	S42.363A	S42.433P	S42.471K	S45.111A	S48.919A	S49.119P	S52.022P
S36.262A	S37.019A	S42.019B	S42.123P	S42.201K	S42.255A	S42.322P	S42.363K	S42.434A	S42.471P	S45.112A	S48.921A	S49.121A	S52.022Q
S36.269A	S37.021A	S42.019K	S42.124B	S42.201P	S42.255K	S42.323A	S42.363P	S42.434K	S42.472A	S45.119A	S48.922A	S49.121K	S52.022R
S36.290A	S37.022A	S42.019P	S42.124K	S42.202A	S42.255P	S42.323K	S42.364A	S42.434P	S42.472K	S45.191A	S48.929A	S49.121P	S52.023K
S36.291A	S37.029A	S42.021B	S42.124P	S42.202K	S42.256A	S42.323P	S42.364K	S42.435A	S42.472P	S45.192A	S49.001A	S49.122A	S52.023M
S36.292A	S37.031A	S42.021K	S42.125B	S42.202P	S42.256K	S42.324A	S42.364P	S42.435K	S42.473A	S45.199A	S49.001K	S49.122K	S52.023N
S36.299A	S37.032A	S42.021P	S42.125K	S42.209A	S42.256P	S42.324K	S42.365A	S42.435P	S42.473K	S45.201A	S49.001P	S49.122P	S52.023P
S36.30XA	S37.039A	S42.022B	S42.125P	S42.209K	S42.261A	S42.324P	S42.365K	S42.436A	S42.473P	S45.202A	S49.002A	S49.129A	S52.023Q
S36.32XA	S37.041A	S42.022K	S42.126B	S42.209P	S42.261K	S42.325A	S42.365P	S42.436K	S42.474A	S45.209A	S49.002P	S49.129K	S52.023R
S36.33XA	S37.042A	S42.022P	S42.126K	S42.211A	S42.261P	S42.325K	S42.366A	S42.436P	S42.474K	S45.211A	S49.009A	S49.129P	S52.024K
S36.39XA	S37.049A	S42.023B	S42.126P	S42.211K	S42.262A	S42.325P	S42.366K	S42.441A	S42.474P	S45.212A	S49.009K	S49.131A	S52.024M
S36.400A	S37.051A	S42.023K	S42.131B	S42.211P	S42.262K	S42.326A	S42.366P	S42.441K	S42.475A	S45.219A	S49.009P	S49.131K	S52.024N
S36.408A	S37.052A	S42.023P	S42.131K	S42.212A	S42.262P	S42.326K	S42.391A	S42.441P	S42.475K	S45.291A	S49.011A	S49.131P	S52.024P
S36.409A	S37.059A	S42.024B	S42.131P	S42.212K	S42.263A	S42.326P	S42.391K	S42.442A	S42.475P	S45.292A	S49.011K	S49.132A	S52.024Q
S36.410A	S37.10XA	S42.024K	S42.132B	S42.212P	S42.263K	S42.331A	S42.391P	S42.442K	S42.476A	S45.299A	S49.011P	S49.132K	S52.024R
S36.418A	S37.12XA	S42.024P	S42.132K	S42.213A	S42.263P	S42.331K	S42.392A	S42.442P	S42.476K	S45.301A	S49.012A	S49.132P	S52.025K
S36.419A	S37.13XA	S42.025B	S42.132P	S42.213K	S42.264A	S42.331P	S42.392K	S42.443A	S42.476P	S45.302A	S49.012K	S49.139A	S52.025M
S36.420A	S37.19XA	S42.025K	S42.133B	S42.213P	S42.264K	S42.332A	S42.392P	S42.443K	S42.481A	S45.309A	S49.012P	S49.139K	S52.025N
S36.428A	S37.20XA	S42.025P	S42.133K	S42.214A	S42.264P	S42.332K	S42.399A	S42.443P	S42.481K	S45.311A	S49.019A	S49.139P	S52.025P
S36.429A	S37.22XA	S42.026B	S42.133P	S42.214K	S42.265A	S42.332P	S42.399K	S42.444A	S42.481P	S45.312A	S49.019K	S49.141A	S52.025Q
S36.430A	S37.23XA	S42.026K	S42.134B	S42.214P	S42.265K	S42.333A	S42.399P	S42.444K	S42.482A	S45.319A	S49.019P	S49.141K	S52.025R
S36.438A	S37.29XA	S42.026P	S42.134K	S42.215A	S42.265P	S42.333K	S42.401A	S42.444P	S42.482K	S45.391A	S49.021A	S49.141P	S52.026K
S36.439A	S37.30XA	S42.031B	S42.134P	S42.215K	S42.266A	S42.333P	S42.401K	S42.445A	S42.482P	S45.392A	S49.021K	S49.142A	S52.026M
S36.490A	S37.32XA	S42.031K	S42.135B	S42.215P	S42.266K	S42.334A	S42.401P	S42.445K	S42.489A	S45.399A	S49.021P	S49.142K	S52.026N
S36.498A	S37.33XA	S42.031P	S42.135K	S42.216A	S42.266P	S42.334K	S42.402A	S42.445P	S42.489K	S45.801A	S49.022A		S52.026P

Complication or Comorbidity (CC) (cont.) – Based on CMS data

S52.026Q	S52.091K	S52.125R	S52.202R	S52.233K	S52.251Q	S52.266M	S52.302M	S52.332P	S52.351K	S52.365Q	S52.501M	S52.531P	S52.569K
S52.026R	S52.091M	S52.126K	S52.209A	S52.233M	S52.251R	S52.266N	S52.302N	S52.332Q	S52.351M	S52.365R	S52.501N	S52.531Q	S52.569M
S52.031K	S52.091N	S52.126M	S52.209K	S52.233N	S52.252A	S52.266P	S52.302P	S52.332R	S52.351N	S52.366A	S52.501P	S52.531R	S52.569N
S52.031M	S52.091P	S52.126N	S52.209M	S52.233P	S52.252K	S52.266Q	S52.302Q	S52.333A	S52.351P	S52.366K	S52.501Q	S52.532A	S52.569P
S52.031N	S52.091Q	S52.126P	S52.209N	S52.233Q	S52.252M	S52.266R	S52.302R	S52.333K	S52.351Q	S52.366M	S52.501R	S52.532K	S52.569Q
S52.031P	S52.091R	S52.126Q	S52.209P	S52.233R	S52.252N	S52.271K	S52.309A	S52.333M	S52.351R	S52.366N	S52.502A	S52.532M	S52.569R
S52.031Q	S52.092K	S52.131K	S52.209Q	S52.234A	S52.252Q	S52.271N	S52.309K	S52.333N	S52.352A	S52.366P	S52.502K	S52.532N	S52.571A
S52.031R	S52.092M	S52.131M	S52.209R	S52.234K	S52.252R	S52.271P	S52.309M	S52.333Q	S52.352K	S52.366Q	S52.502M	S52.532P	S52.571K
S52.032K	S52.092N	S52.131N	S52.211A	S52.234M	S52.253A	S52.271Q	S52.309N	S52.333R	S52.352M	S52.366R	S52.502N	S52.532Q	S52.571M
S52.032M	S52.092P	S52.131P	S52.211K	S52.234N	S52.253K	S52.271R	S52.309P	S52.334A	S52.352N	S52.371A	S52.502P	S52.532R	S52.571N
S52.032N	S52.092Q	S52.131Q	S52.211P	S52.234P	S52.253M	S52.272K	S52.309Q	S52.334K	S52.352P	S52.371K	S52.502Q	S52.539A	S52.571P
S52.032P	S52.092R	S52.131R	S52.212A	S52.234Q	S52.253P	S52.272M	S52.309R	S52.334M	S52.352Q	S52.371M	S52.502R	S52.539K	S52.571Q
S52.032Q	S52.099K	S52.132K	S52.212K	S52.234R	S52.253Q	S52.272P	S52.311A	S52.334P	S52.352R	S52.371N	S52.509A	S52.539M	S52.571R
S52.032R	S52.099M	S52.132M	S52.212P	S52.235A	S52.253R	S52.272Q	S52.311K	S52.334Q	S52.353A	S52.371P	S52.509K	S52.539N	S52.572A
S52.033K	S52.099N	S52.132N	S52.219A	S52.235K	S52.254A	S52.272R	S52.311P	S52.334R	S52.353K	S52.371Q	S52.509N	S52.539P	S52.572K
S52.033M	S52.099P	S52.132P	S52.219K	S52.235M	S52.254K	S52.279K	S52.312A	S52.335A	S52.353M	S52.371R	S52.509P	S52.539Q	S52.572M
S52.033N	S52.099Q	S52.132Q	S52.219P	S52.235N	S52.254M	S52.279M	S52.312K	S52.335K	S52.353N	S52.372A	S52.509Q	S52.539R	S52.572P
S52.033P	S52.099R	S52.132R	S52.221A	S52.235P	S52.254P	S52.279N	S52.312P	S52.335M	S52.353P	S52.372K	S52.509R	S52.541A	S52.572Q
S52.033Q	S52.101K	S52.133K	S52.221K	S52.235Q	S52.254Q	S52.279P	S52.319A	S52.335N	S52.353Q	S52.372M	S52.511A	S52.541K	S52.572R
S52.033R	S52.101M	S52.133M	S52.221M	S52.235R	S52.254R	S52.279Q	S52.319K	S52.335P	S52.353R	S52.372N	S52.511K	S52.541M	S52.579A
S52.034K	S52.101N	S52.133N	S52.221N	S52.236A	S52.255A	S52.279R	S52.319P	S52.335Q	S52.354A	S52.372Q	S52.511M	S52.541N	S52.579K
S52.034M	S52.101P	S52.133P	S52.221P	S52.236K	S52.255K	S52.281A	S52.321A	S52.335R	S52.354K	S52.372R	S52.511N	S52.541P	S52.579M
S52.034N	S52.101Q	S52.133Q	S52.221Q	S52.236M	S52.255M	S52.281K	S52.321K	S52.336A	S52.354M	S52.379A	S52.511P	S52.541Q	S52.579N
S52.034P	S52.101R	S52.133R	S52.221R	S52.236N	S52.255P	S52.281M	S52.321M	S52.336K	S52.354N	S52.379K	S52.511Q	S52.541R	S52.579P
S52.034Q	S52.102K	S52.134K	S52.222A	S52.236P	S52.255Q	S52.281N	S52.321N	S52.336M	S52.354P	S52.379M	S52.511R	S52.542A	S52.579Q
S52.034R	S52.102M	S52.134M	S52.222K	S52.236Q	S52.255R	S52.281P	S52.321P	S52.336P	S52.354Q	S52.379N	S52.512A	S52.542K	S52.579R
S52.035K	S52.102N	S52.134N	S52.222N	S52.236R	S52.256A	S52.281R	S52.321Q	S52.336Q	S52.354R	S52.379P	S52.512K	S52.542M	S52.591A
S52.035M	S52.102P	S52.134P	S52.222P	S52.241A	S52.256K	S52.282A	S52.321R	S52.336R	S52.355A	S52.379R	S52.512M	S52.542N	S52.591K
S52.035N	S52.102Q	S52.134Q	S52.222Q	S52.241K	S52.256M	S52.282K	S52.322A	S52.341A	S52.355K	S52.381A	S52.512N	S52.542P	S52.591M
S52.035P	S52.102R	S52.134R	S52.222R	S52.241M	S52.256N	S52.282M	S52.322K	S52.341K	S52.355M	S52.381K	S52.512P	S52.542Q	S52.591N
S52.035Q	S52.109K	S52.135K	S52.223A	S52.241N	S52.256P	S52.282N	S52.322M	S52.341M	S52.355N	S52.381M	S52.512Q	S52.542R	S52.591P
S52.035R	S52.109M	S52.135M	S52.223K	S52.241P	S52.256Q	S52.282P	S52.322N	S52.341P	S52.355P	S52.381N	S52.512R	S52.549A	S52.591Q
S52.036K	S52.109N	S52.135N	S52.223M	S52.241Q	S52.256R	S52.282Q	S52.322P	S52.341Q	S52.355Q	S52.381P	S52.513A	S52.549K	S52.591R
S52.036M	S52.109P	S52.135P	S52.223N	S52.241R	S52.261A	S52.282R	S52.322Q	S52.341R	S52.355R	S52.381Q	S52.513K	S52.549M	S52.592A
S52.036N	S52.109Q	S52.135Q	S52.223P	S52.242A	S52.261K	S52.283A	S52.322R	S52.342A	S52.356A	S52.381R	S52.513M	S52.549N	S52.592K
S52.036P	S52.109R	S52.135R	S52.223Q	S52.242K	S52.261M	S52.283K	S52.323A	S52.342K	S52.356K	S52.382A	S52.513P	S52.549P	S52.592M
S52.036Q	S52.111A	S52.136K	S52.223R	S52.242M	S52.261N	S52.283M	S52.323K	S52.342M	S52.356M	S52.382K	S52.513Q	S52.549R	S52.592N
S52.036R	S52.111K	S52.136M	S52.224A	S52.242N	S52.261P	S52.283N	S52.323M	S52.342N	S52.356N	S52.382M	S52.513R	S52.551A	S52.592P
S52.041K	S52.111P	S52.136N	S52.224K	S52.242P	S52.261Q	S52.283Q	S52.323N	S52.342P	S52.356P	S52.382N	S52.514A	S52.551K	S52.592Q
S52.041M	S52.112A	S52.136P	S52.224M	S52.242Q	S52.261R	S52.283R	S52.323P	S52.342Q	S52.356Q	S52.382Q	S52.514K	S52.551M	S52.592R
S52.041N	S52.112K	S52.136Q	S52.224N	S52.243A	S52.262A	S52.291A	S52.323Q	S52.342R	S52.356R	S52.382R	S52.514M	S52.551N	S52.599A
S52.041P	S52.112P	S52.136R	S52.224P	S52.243K	S52.262K	S52.291K	S52.324A	S52.343A	S52.361A	S52.389A	S52.514P	S52.551P	S52.599K
S52.041Q	S52.119A	S52.181K	S52.224Q	S52.243M	S52.262M	S52.291M	S52.324K	S52.343K	S52.361K	S52.389K	S52.514Q	S52.551R	S52.599M
S52.041R	S52.119K	S52.181M	S52.224R	S52.243N	S52.262N	S52.291N	S52.324M	S52.343M	S52.361M	S52.389M	S52.514R	S52.552A	S52.599N
S52.042K	S52.119P	S52.181N	S52.225A	S52.243P	S52.262P	S52.291P	S52.324N	S52.343N	S52.361N	S52.389N	S52.515A	S52.552K	S52.599P
S52.042M	S52.121K	S52.181P	S52.225K	S52.243Q	S52.262Q	S52.291Q	S52.324P	S52.343P	S52.361P	S52.389P	S52.515K	S52.552M	S52.599Q
S52.042N	S52.121M	S52.181Q	S52.225M	S52.243R	S52.262R	S52.291R	S52.324Q	S52.343Q	S52.361Q	S52.389R	S52.515M	S52.552N	S52.599R
S52.042P	S52.121N	S52.181R	S52.225N	S52.244A	S52.263A	S52.292A	S52.324R	S52.343R	S52.361R	S52.391A	S52.515P	S52.552Q	S52.601A
S52.042Q	S52.121P	S52.182K	S52.225P	S52.244K	S52.263K	S52.292K	S52.325A	S52.344A	S52.362A	S52.391K	S52.515Q	S52.552R	S52.601K
S52.042R	S52.121Q	S52.182M	S52.225Q	S52.244M	S52.263M	S52.292M	S52.325K	S52.344K	S52.362K	S52.391M	S52.515R	S52.559A	S52.601M
S52.043K	S52.121R	S52.182N	S52.225R	S52.244N	S52.263N	S52.292N	S52.325M	S52.344M	S52.362M	S52.391N	S52.516A	S52.559K	S52.601P
S52.043M	S52.122K	S52.182P	S52.226A	S52.244P	S52.263P	S52.292P	S52.325N	S52.344N	S52.362N	S52.391P	S52.516K	S52.559M	S52.601Q
S52.043N	S52.122M	S52.182Q	S52.226K	S52.244Q	S52.263Q	S52.292Q	S52.325P	S52.344Q	S52.362P	S52.391Q	S52.516M	S52.559N	S52.601R
S52.043P	S52.122P	S52.182R	S52.226M	S52.245A	S52.263R	S52.292R	S52.325R	S52.344R	S52.362Q	S52.391R	S52.516N	S52.559P	S52.602A
S52.043Q	S52.122Q	S52.189K	S52.226N	S52.245K	S52.264A	S52.299A	S52.326A	S52.345A	S52.363A	S52.392A	S52.516P	S52.559Q	S52.602K
S52.043R	S52.122R	S52.189M	S52.226P	S52.245M	S52.264K	S52.299K	S52.326K	S52.345K	S52.363K	S52.392K	S52.516Q	S52.559R	S52.602M
S52.044K	S52.123K	S52.189P	S52.226Q	S52.245N	S52.264M	S52.299M	S52.326M	S52.345M	S52.363M	S52.392M	S52.516R	S52.561A	S52.602N
S52.044M	S52.123M	S52.189Q	S52.226R	S52.245P	S52.264N	S52.299N	S52.326N	S52.345N	S52.363N	S52.392N	S52.521A	S52.561K	S52.602P
S52.044N	S52.123N	S52.189R	S52.231A	S52.245Q	S52.264P	S52.299P	S52.326P	S52.345P	S52.363P	S52.392P	S52.521K	S52.561M	S52.602Q
S52.044P	S52.123P	S52.201A	S52.231K	S52.245R	S52.264Q	S52.299Q	S52.326Q	S52.345Q	S52.363Q	S52.392Q	S52.522A	S52.561N	S52.602R
S52.044Q	S52.123Q	S52.201K	S52.231N	S52.246A	S52.264R	S52.299R	S52.326R	S52.345R	S52.363R	S52.392R	S52.522K	S52.561P	S52.609A
S52.044R	S52.123R	S52.201M	S52.231P	S52.246K	S52.265A	S52.301A	S52.331A	S52.346A	S52.364A	S52.399A	S52.522P	S52.561R	S52.609K
S52.045K	S52.124K	S52.201N	S52.231Q	S52.246M	S52.265K	S52.301K	S52.331K	S52.346K	S52.364K	S52.399K	S52.529A	S52.562A	S52.609M
S52.045M	S52.124M	S52.201P	S52.231R	S52.246N	S52.265M	S52.301M	S52.331M	S52.346M	S52.364M	S52.399M	S52.529K	S52.562K	S52.609Q
S52.045N	S52.124N	S52.201Q	S52.232A	S52.246P	S52.265N	S52.301N	S52.331N	S52.346N	S52.364N	S52.399N	S52.529P	S52.562M	S52.609R
S52.045P	S52.124P	S52.201R	S52.232M	S52.251A	S52.265P	S52.301P	S52.331P	S52.346P	S52.364P	S52.399P	S52.531A	S52.562N	S52.611A
S52.045Q	S52.124Q	S52.202A	S52.232N	S52.251K	S52.265Q	S52.301Q	S52.331Q	S52.346Q	S52.364Q	S52.399Q	S52.531K	S52.562P	S52.611K
S52.045R	S52.124R	S52.202K	S52.232P	S52.251M	S52.265R	S52.301R	S52.331R	S52.346R	S52.364R	S52.399R	S52.531M	S52.562R	S52.611M
S52.046K	S52.125K	S52.202M	S52.232Q	S52.251N	S52.266A	S52.302A	S52.332A	S52.351A	S52.365K	S52.501A	S52.531N	S52.569A	S52.611N
S52.046M	S52.125M	S52.202N	S52.232R	S52.251P	S52.266K	S52.302K	S52.332K		S52.365M	S52.501K			S52.611P
S52.046N	S52.125N	S52.202P					S52.332M		S52.365N				
S52.046P	S52.125P	S52.202Q					S52.332N		S52.365P				
S52.046Q	S52.125Q												
S52.046R													

Complication or Comorbidity (CC) (cont.) - Based on CMS data

S52.611Q	S52.91XA	S56.321A	S59.039P	S59.221K	S62.025B	S62.132P	S62.173K	S62.234B	S62.306P	S62.331K	S62.356B	S62.501P	S62.610K
S52.611R	S52.91XK	S56.322A	S59.041A	S59.221P	S62.025K	S62.133B	S62.173P	S62.234K	S62.307B	S62.331P	S62.356K	S62.502B	S62.610P
S52.612A	S52.91XM	S56.329A	S59.041K	S59.222A	S62.025P	S62.133K	S62.174B	S62.234P	S62.307K	S62.332B	S62.356P	S62.502K	S62.611B
S52.612K	S52.91XN	S56.421A	S59.041P	S59.222K	S62.026B	S62.133P	S62.174K	S62.235B	S62.307P	S62.332K	S62.357B	S62.502P	S62.611K
S52.612M	S52.91XP	S56.422A	S59.042A	S59.222P	S62.026K	S62.134B	S62.174P	S62.235K	S62.308B	S62.332P	S62.357K	S62.509B	S62.611P
S52.612N	S52.91XQ	S56.423A	S59.042K	S59.229A	S62.026P	S62.134K	S62.175B	S62.235P	S62.308K	S62.333B	S62.357P	S62.509K	S62.612B
S52.612P	S52.91XR	S56.424A	S59.042P	S59.229K	S62.031B	S62.134P	S62.175K	S62.236B	S62.308P	S62.333K	S62.358B	S62.509P	S62.612K
S52.612Q	S52.92XA	S56.425A	S59.049A	S59.229P	S62.031K	S62.135B	S62.175P	S62.236K	S62.309B	S62.333P	S62.358K	S62.511B	S62.612P
S52.612R	S52.92XK	S56.426A	S59.049K	S59.231A	S62.031P	S62.135K	S62.176B	S62.236P	S62.309K	S62.334B	S62.358P	S62.511K	S62.613B
S52.613A	S52.92XM	S56.427A	S59.049P	S59.231K	S62.032B	S62.135P	S62.176K	S62.241B	S62.309P	S62.334K	S62.359B	S62.511P	S62.613K
S52.613K	S52.92XN	S56.428A	S59.091A	S59.231P	S62.032K	S62.136B	S62.176P	S62.241K	S62.310B	S62.334P	S62.359K	S62.512B	S62.613P
S52.613M	S52.92XP	S56.429A	S59.091K	S59.232A	S62.032P	S62.136K	S62.181B	S62.241P	S62.310K	S62.335B	S62.359P	S62.512K	S62.614B
S52.613N	S52.92XQ	S56.521A	S59.091P	S59.232K	S62.033B	S62.136P	S62.181K	S62.242B	S62.310P	S62.335K	S62.360B	S62.512P	S62.614K
S52.613P	S52.92XR	S56.522A	S59.092A	S59.232P	S62.033K	S62.141B	S62.181P	S62.242K	S62.311B	S62.335P	S62.360K	S62.513B	S62.614P
S52.613Q	S55.001A	S56.529A	S59.092K	S59.239A	S62.033P	S62.141K	S62.182B	S62.242P	S62.311K	S62.336B	S62.360P	S62.513K	S62.615B
S52.613R	S55.002A	S56.821A	S59.092P	S59.239K	S62.034B	S62.141P	S62.182K	S62.243B	S62.311P	S62.336K	S62.361B	S62.513P	S62.615K
S52.614A	S55.009A	S56.822A	S59.099A	S59.239P	S62.034K	S62.142B	S62.182P	S62.243K	S62.312B	S62.336P	S62.361K	S62.514B	S62.615P
S52.614K	S55.011A	S56.829A	S59.099K	S59.241A	S62.034P	S62.142K	S62.183B	S62.243P	S62.312K	S62.337B	S62.361P	S62.514K	S62.616B
S52.614M	S55.012A	S56.921A	S59.099P	S59.241K	S62.035B	S62.142P	S62.183K	S62.244B	S62.312P	S62.337K	S62.362B	S62.514P	S62.616K
S52.614N	S55.019A	S56.922A	S59.101K	S59.241P	S62.035K	S62.143B	S62.183P	S62.244K	S62.313B	S62.337P	S62.362K	S62.515B	S62.616P
S52.614P	S55.091A	S56.929A	S59.101P	S59.242A	S62.035P	S62.143K	S62.184B	S62.244P	S62.313K	S62.338B	S62.362P	S62.515K	S62.617B
S52.614Q	S55.092A	S58.011A	S59.102K	S59.242K	S62.036B	S62.143P	S62.184K	S62.245B	S62.313P	S62.338K	S62.363B	S62.515P	S62.617K
S52.614R	S55.099A	S58.012A	S59.102P	S59.242P	S62.036K	S62.144B	S62.184P	S62.245K	S62.314B	S62.338P	S62.363K	S62.516B	S62.617P
S52.615A	S55.101A	S58.019A	S59.109K	S59.249A	S62.036P	S62.144K	S62.185B	S62.245P	S62.314K	S62.339B	S62.363P	S62.516K	S62.618B
S52.615K	S55.102A	S58.021A	S59.109P	S59.249K	S62.101B	S62.144P	S62.185K	S62.246B	S62.314P	S62.339K	S62.364B	S62.516P	S62.618K
S52.615M	S55.109A	S58.022A	S59.111K	S59.249P	S62.101K	S62.145B	S62.185P	S62.246K	S62.315B	S62.339P	S62.364K	S62.521B	S62.618P
S52.615N	S55.111A	S58.029A	S59.111P	S59.291A	S62.101P	S62.145K	S62.186B	S62.246P	S62.315K	S62.340B	S62.364P	S62.521K	S62.619B
S52.615P	S55.112A	S58.111A	S59.112K	S59.291K	S62.102B	S62.145P	S62.186K	S62.251B	S62.315P	S62.340K	S62.365B	S62.521P	S62.619K
S52.615Q	S55.119A	S58.112A	S59.112P	S59.291P	S62.102K	S62.146B	S62.186P	S62.251K	S62.316B	S62.340P	S62.365K	S62.522B	S62.619P
S52.615R	S55.191A	S58.119A	S59.119K	S59.292A	S62.102P	S62.146K	S62.201B	S62.251P	S62.316K	S62.341B	S62.365P	S62.522K	S62.620B
S52.616A	S55.192A	S58.121A	S59.119P	S59.292K	S62.109B	S62.146P	S62.201K	S62.252B	S62.316P	S62.341K	S62.366B	S62.522P	S62.620K
S52.616K	S55.199A	S58.122A	S59.121K	S59.292P	S62.109K	S62.151B	S62.201P	S62.252K	S62.317B	S62.341P	S62.366K	S62.523B	S62.620P
S52.616M	S55.201A	S58.129A	S59.121P	S59.299A	S62.109P	S62.151K	S62.202B	S62.252P	S62.317K	S62.342B	S62.366P	S62.523K	S62.621B
S52.616N	S55.202A	S58.911A	S59.122K	S59.299K	S62.111B	S62.151P	S62.202K	S62.253B	S62.317P	S62.342K	S62.367B	S62.523P	S62.621K
S52.616P	S55.209A	S58.912A	S59.122P	S59.299P	S62.111K	S62.152B	S62.202P	S62.253K	S62.318B	S62.342P	S62.367K	S62.524B	S62.621P
S52.616Q	S55.211A	S58.919A	S59.129K	S62.001B	S62.111P	S62.152K	S62.209B	S62.253P	S62.318K	S62.343B	S62.367P	S62.524K	S62.622B
S52.616R	S55.212A	S58.921A	S59.129P	S62.001K	S62.112B	S62.152P	S62.209K	S62.254B	S62.318P	S62.343K	S62.368B	S62.524P	S62.622K
S52.621A	S55.219A	S58.922A	S59.131K	S62.001P	S62.112K	S62.153B	S62.209P	S62.254K	S62.319B	S62.343P	S62.368K	S62.525B	S62.622P
S52.621K	S55.291A	S58.929A	S59.131P	S62.002B	S62.112P	S62.153K	S62.211B	S62.254P	S62.319K	S62.344B	S62.368P	S62.525K	S62.623B
S52.621P	S55.292A	S59.001A	S59.132K	S62.002K	S62.113B	S62.153P	S62.211K	S62.255B	S62.319P	S62.344K	S62.369B	S62.525P	S62.623K
S52.622A	S55.299A	S59.001K	S59.132P	S62.002P	S62.113K	S62.154B	S62.211P	S62.255K	S62.320B	S62.344P	S62.369K	S62.526B	S62.623P
S52.622K	S55.801A	S59.001P	S59.139K	S62.009B	S62.113P	S62.154K	S62.212B	S62.255P	S62.320K	S62.345B	S62.369P	S62.526K	S62.624B
S52.622P	S55.802A	S59.002A	S59.139P	S62.009K	S62.114B	S62.154P	S62.212K	S62.256B	S62.320P	S62.345K	S62.390B	S62.526P	S62.624K
S52.629A	S55.809A	S59.002K	S59.141K	S62.009P	S62.114K	S62.155B	S62.212P	S62.256K	S62.321B	S62.345P	S62.390K	S62.600B	S62.624P
S52.629K	S55.811A	S59.002P	S59.141P	S62.011B	S62.114P	S62.155K	S62.213B	S62.256P	S62.321K	S62.346B	S62.390P	S62.600K	S62.625B
S52.629P	S55.812A	S59.009A	S59.142K	S62.011K	S62.115B	S62.155P	S62.213K	S62.291B	S62.321P	S62.346K	S62.391B	S62.600P	S62.625K
S52.691A	S55.819A	S59.009K	S59.142P	S62.011P	S62.115K	S62.156B	S62.213P	S62.291K	S62.322B	S62.346P	S62.391K	S62.601B	S62.625P
S52.691K	S55.891A	S59.009P	S59.149K	S62.012B	S62.115P	S62.156K	S62.221B	S62.291P	S62.322K	S62.347B	S62.391P	S62.601K	S62.626B
S52.691M	S55.892A	S59.011A	S59.149P	S62.012K	S62.116B	S62.156P	S62.221K	S62.292B	S62.322P	S62.347K	S62.392B	S62.601P	S62.626K
S52.691N	S55.899A	S59.011K	S59.191K	S62.012P	S62.116K	S62.161B	S62.221P	S62.292K	S62.323B	S62.347P	S62.392K	S62.602B	S62.626P
S52.691P	S55.901A	S59.011P	S59.191P	S62.013B	S62.116P	S62.161K	S62.222B	S62.292P	S62.323K	S62.348B	S62.392P	S62.602K	S62.627B
S52.691Q	S55.902A	S59.012A	S59.192K	S62.013K	S62.121B	S62.161P	S62.222K	S62.299B	S62.323P	S62.348K	S62.393B	S62.602P	S62.627K
S52.691R	S55.909A	S59.012K	S59.192P	S62.013P	S62.121K	S62.162B	S62.222P	S62.299K	S62.324B	S62.348P	S62.393K	S62.603B	S62.627P
S52.692A	S55.911A	S59.012P	S59.199K	S62.014B	S62.121P	S62.162K	S62.223B	S62.299P	S62.324K	S62.349B	S62.393P	S62.603K	S62.628B
S52.692K	S55.912A	S59.019A	S59.199P	S62.014K	S62.122B	S62.162P	S62.223K	S62.300B	S62.324P	S62.349K	S62.394B	S62.603P	S62.628K
S52.692M	S55.919A	S59.019K	S59.201A	S62.014P	S62.122K	S62.163B	S62.223P	S62.300K	S62.325B	S62.349P	S62.394K	S62.604B	S62.628P
S52.692N	S55.991A	S59.019P	S59.201K	S62.015B	S62.122P	S62.163K	S62.224B	S62.300P	S62.325K	S62.350B	S62.394P	S62.604K	S62.629B
S52.692P	S55.992A	S59.021A	S59.201P	S62.015K	S62.123B	S62.163P	S62.224K	S62.301B	S62.325P	S62.350K	S62.395B	S62.604P	S62.629K
S52.692Q	S55.999A	S59.021K	S59.202A	S62.015P	S62.123K	S62.164B	S62.224P	S62.301K	S62.326B	S62.350P	S62.395K	S62.605B	S62.629P
S52.692R	S56.021A	S59.021P	S59.202K	S62.016B	S62.123P	S62.164K	S62.225B	S62.301P	S62.326K	S62.351B	S62.395P	S62.605K	S62.630B
S52.699A	S56.022A	S59.022A	S59.202P	S62.016K	S62.124B	S62.164P	S62.225K	S62.302B	S62.326P	S62.351K	S62.396B	S62.605P	S62.630K
S52.699K	S56.029A	S59.022K	S59.209A	S62.016P	S62.124K	S62.165B	S62.225P	S62.302K	S62.327B	S62.351P	S62.396K	S62.606B	S62.630P
S52.699M	S56.121A	S59.022P	S59.209K	S62.021B	S62.124P	S62.165K	S62.226B	S62.302P	S62.327K	S62.352B	S62.396P	S62.606K	S62.631B
S52.699N	S56.122A	S59.029A	S59.209P	S62.021K	S62.125B	S62.165P	S62.226K	S62.303B	S62.327P	S62.352K	S62.397B	S62.606P	S62.631K
S52.699P	S56.123A	S59.029K	S59.211A	S62.021P	S62.125K	S62.166B	S62.226P	S62.303K	S62.328B	S62.352P	S62.397K	S62.607B	S62.631P
S52.699Q	S56.124A	S59.029P	S59.211K	S62.022B	S62.125P	S62.166K	S62.231B	S62.303P	S62.328K	S62.353B	S62.397P	S62.607K	S62.632B
S52.699R	S56.125A	S59.031A	S59.211P	S62.022K	S62.126B	S62.166P	S62.231K	S62.304B	S62.328P	S62.353K	S62.398B	S62.607P	S62.632K
S52.90XA	S56.126A	S59.031K	S59.212A	S62.022P	S62.126K	S62.171B	S62.231P	S62.304K	S62.329B	S62.353P	S62.398K	S62.608B	S62.632P
S52.90XK	S56.127A	S59.031P	S59.212K	S62.023B	S62.126P	S62.171K	S62.232B	S62.304P	S62.329K	S62.354B	S62.398P	S62.608K	S62.633B
S52.90XM	S56.128A	S59.032A	S59.212P	S62.023K	S62.131B	S62.171P	S62.232K	S62.305B	S62.329P	S62.354K	S62.399B	S62.608P	S62.633K
S52.90XN	S56.129A	S59.032K	S59.219A	S62.023P	S62.131K	S62.172B	S62.232P	S62.305K	S62.330B	S62.354P	S62.399K	S62.609B	S62.633P
S52.90XP	S56.221A	S59.032P	S59.219K	S62.024B	S62.131P	S62.172K	S62.233B	S62.305P	S62.330K	S62.355B	S62.399P	S62.609K	S62.634B
S52.90XQ	S56.222A	S59.039A	S59.219P	S62.024K	S62.132B	S62.172P	S62.233K	S62.306B	S62.330P	S62.355K	S62.501B	S62.609P	S62.634K
S52.90XR	S56.229A	S59.039K	S59.221A	S62.024P	S62.132K	S62.173B	S62.233P	S62.306K	S62.331B	S62.355P	S62.501K	S62.610B	S62.634P

Complication or Comorbidity (CC) (cont.) - Based on CMS data

S62.635B	S62.659P	S65.392A	S66.229A	S72.019N	S72.036Q	S72.064K	S72.114N	S72.134Q	S72.25XK	S72.332N	S72.352Q	S72.399K	S72.421Q
S62.635K	S62.660B	S65.399A	S66.320A	S72.019P	S72.036R	S72.064M	S72.114P	S72.134R	S72.25XM	S72.332P	S72.352R	S72.399M	S72.421R
S62.635P	S62.660K	S65.401A	S66.321A	S72.019Q	S72.041K	S72.064N	S72.114Q	S72.135K	S72.25XN	S72.332Q	S72.353M	S72.399N	S72.422A
S62.636B	S62.660P	S65.402A	S66.322A	S72.019R	S72.041M	S72.064P	S72.114R	S72.135M	S72.25XP	S72.332R	S72.353N	S72.399P	S72.422M
S62.636K	S62.661B	S65.409A	S66.323A	S72.021K	S72.041N	S72.064Q	S72.115K	S72.135N	S72.25XQ	S72.333K	S72.353P	S72.399Q	S72.422N
S62.636P	S62.661K	S65.411A	S66.324A	S72.021M	S72.041P	S72.064R	S72.115M	S72.135P	S72.25XR	S72.333M	S72.353Q	S72.399R	S72.422P
S62.637B	S62.661P	S65.412A	S66.325A	S72.021N	S72.041Q	S72.065K	S72.115N	S72.135Q	S72.26XK	S72.333N	S72.353R	S72.401A	S72.422Q
S62.637K	S62.662B	S65.419A	S66.326A	S72.021P	S72.042K	S72.065N	S72.115P	S72.135R	S72.26XM	S72.333P	S72.354K	S72.401K	S72.422R
S62.637P	S62.662K	S65.491A	S66.327A	S72.021Q	S72.042M	S72.065P	S72.115Q	S72.136K	S72.26XN	S72.333R	S72.354N	S72.401M	S72.423A
S62.638B	S62.662P	S65.492A	S66.328A	S72.021R	S72.042N	S72.065Q	S72.115R	S72.136M	S72.26XP	S72.334K	S72.354P	S72.401N	S72.423N
S62.638K	S62.663B	S65.499A	S66.329A	S72.022K	S72.042P	S72.065R	S72.116K	S72.136N	S72.26XQ	S72.334M	S72.354Q	S72.401P	S72.423P
S62.638P	S62.663K	S65.500A	S66.421A	S72.022M	S72.042Q	S72.066K	S72.116M	S72.136P	S72.26XR	S72.334N	S72.354R	S72.401Q	S72.423Q
S62.639B	S62.663P	S65.501A	S66.422A	S72.022N	S72.042R	S72.066M	S72.116N	S72.136Q	S72.301K	S72.334P	S72.355K	S72.401R	S72.423R
S62.639K	S62.664B	S65.502A	S66.429A	S72.022P	S72.043K	S72.066N	S72.116P	S72.136R	S72.301M	S72.334Q	S72.355M	S72.402A	S72.424A
S62.639P	S62.664K	S65.503A	S66.520A	S72.022Q	S72.043M	S72.066Q	S72.116Q	S72.141K	S72.301N	S72.334R	S72.355N	S72.402K	S72.424K
S62.640B	S62.664P	S65.504A	S66.521A	S72.022R	S72.043N	S72.066R	S72.116R	S72.141M	S72.301P	S72.335K	S72.355P	S72.402M	S72.424M
S62.640K	S62.665B	S65.505A	S66.522A	S72.023K	S72.043P	S72.091K	S72.121K	S72.141N	S72.301Q	S72.335M	S72.355Q	S72.402N	S72.424N
S62.640P	S62.665K	S65.506A	S66.523A	S72.023M	S72.043Q	S72.091M	S72.121M	S72.141P	S72.301R	S72.335N	S72.355R	S72.402P	S72.424P
S62.641B	S62.665P	S65.507A	S66.524A	S72.023N	S72.043R	S72.091N	S72.121N	S72.141Q	S72.302K	S72.335P	S72.356K	S72.402Q	S72.424Q
S62.641K	S62.666B	S65.508A	S66.525A	S72.023P	S72.044K	S72.091P	S72.121P	S72.141R	S72.302M	S72.335Q	S72.356M	S72.402R	S72.424R
S62.641P	S62.666K	S65.509A	S66.526A	S72.023Q	S72.044N	S72.091R	S72.121Q	S72.142K	S72.302N	S72.335R	S72.356N	S72.409A	S72.425A
S62.642B	S62.666P	S65.510A	S66.527A	S72.023R	S72.044P	S72.092K	S72.121R	S72.142M	S72.302P	S72.336K	S72.356Q	S72.409K	S72.425K
S62.642K	S62.667B	S65.511A	S66.528A	S72.024K	S72.044Q	S72.092M	S72.122K	S72.142P	S72.302Q	S72.336M	S72.356R	S72.409M	S72.425M
S62.642P	S62.667K	S65.512A	S66.529A	S72.024M	S72.044R	S72.092N	S72.122M	S72.142Q	S72.302R	S72.336N	S72.361K	S72.409P	S72.425N
S62.643B	S62.667P	S65.513A	S66.821A	S72.024N	S72.045K	S72.092P	S72.122N	S72.142R	S72.309K	S72.336P	S72.361M	S72.409Q	S72.425P
S62.643K	S62.668B	S65.514A	S66.822A	S72.024P	S72.045N	S72.092Q	S72.122P	S72.143K	S72.309M	S72.336Q	S72.361N	S72.409R	S72.425Q
S62.643P	S62.668K	S65.515A	S66.829A	S72.024Q	S72.045P	S72.092R	S72.122Q	S72.143M	S72.309N	S72.336R	S72.361P	S72.411A	S72.425R
S62.644B	S62.668P	S65.516A	S66.921A	S72.024R	S72.045Q	S72.099K	S72.122R	S72.143N	S72.309P	S72.341K	S72.361Q	S72.411K	S72.426A
S62.644K	S62.669B	S65.517A	S66.922A	S72.025K	S72.045R	S72.099M	S72.123K	S72.143P	S72.309Q	S72.341M	S72.361R	S72.411M	S72.426K
S62.644P	S62.669K	S65.518A	S66.929A	S72.025M	S72.046K	S72.099N	S72.123M	S72.143Q	S72.321K	S72.341N	S72.362K	S72.411N	S72.426M
S62.645B	S62.669P	S65.519A	S68.411A	S72.025N	S72.046M	S72.099P	S72.123N	S72.143R	S72.321M	S72.341P	S72.362M	S72.411P	S72.426N
S62.645K	S62.90XB	S65.590A	S68.412A	S72.025P	S72.046P	S72.099Q	S72.123P	S72.144K	S72.321N	S72.341Q	S72.362N	S72.411Q	S72.426P
S62.645P	S62.90XK	S65.591A	S68.419A	S72.025Q	S72.046Q	S72.099R	S72.123Q	S72.144M	S72.321P	S72.341R	S72.362P	S72.411R	S72.426Q
S62.646B	S62.90XP	S65.592A	S68.421A	S72.025R	S72.046R	S72.101K	S72.123R	S72.144N	S72.321Q	S72.342K	S72.362Q	S72.412A	S72.426R
S62.646K	S62.91XB	S65.593A	S68.422A	S72.026K	S72.051K	S72.101M	S72.124K	S72.144P	S72.321R	S72.342M	S72.362R	S72.412K	S72.431A
S62.646P	S62.91XK	S65.594A	S68.429A	S72.026M	S72.051M	S72.101N	S72.124M	S72.144Q	S72.322K	S72.342N	S72.363K	S72.412M	S72.431K
S62.647B	S62.91XP	S65.595A	S68.711A	S72.026N	S72.051N	S72.101P	S72.124N	S72.144R	S72.322M	S72.342P	S72.363M	S72.412N	S72.431M
S62.647K	S62.92XB	S65.596A	S68.712A	S72.026P	S72.051P	S72.101Q	S72.124P	S72.145K	S72.322N	S72.342Q	S72.363N	S72.412P	S72.431N
S62.647P	S62.92XK	S65.597A	S68.719A	S72.026Q	S72.051Q	S72.101R	S72.124Q	S72.145M	S72.322P	S72.343K	S72.363P	S72.412Q	S72.431P
S62.648B	S62.92XP	S65.598A	S68.721A	S72.026R	S72.051R	S72.102K	S72.124R	S72.145N	S72.322Q	S72.343M	S72.363Q	S72.412R	S72.431Q
S62.648K	S65.001A	S65.599A	S68.722A	S72.031K	S72.052K	S72.102M	S72.125K	S72.145P	S72.322R	S72.343N	S72.363R	S72.413A	S72.431R
S62.648P	S65.002A	S65.801A	S68.729A	S72.031M	S72.052M	S72.102N	S72.125M	S72.145Q	S72.323K	S72.343P	S72.364K	S72.413K	S72.432A
S62.649B	S65.009A	S65.802A	S72.001K	S72.031N	S72.052N	S72.102P	S72.125N	S72.145R	S72.323M	S72.343Q	S72.364M	S72.413M	S72.432K
S62.649K	S65.011A	S65.809A	S72.001M	S72.031P	S72.052P	S72.102Q	S72.125P	S72.146K	S72.323N	S72.343R	S72.364N	S72.413N	S72.432M
S62.649P	S65.012A	S65.811A	S72.001N	S72.031Q	S72.052Q	S72.109K	S72.125Q	S72.146M	S72.323P	S72.344K	S72.364P	S72.413P	S72.432N
S62.650B	S65.019A	S65.812A	S72.001P	S72.031R	S72.052R	S72.109M	S72.125R	S72.146N	S72.323Q	S72.344M	S72.364Q	S72.413Q	S72.432P
S62.650K	S65.091A	S65.819A	S72.001Q	S72.032K	S72.059K	S72.109P	S72.126K	S72.146P	S72.323R	S72.344N	S72.365K	S72.413R	S72.432Q
S62.650P	S65.092A	S65.891A	S72.001R	S72.032M	S72.059M	S72.109Q	S72.126M	S72.146Q	S72.324K	S72.344P	S72.365M	S72.414A	S72.432R
S62.651B	S65.099A	S65.892A	S72.002K	S72.032N	S72.059N	S72.109R	S72.126N	S72.21XK	S72.324M	S72.344Q	S72.365N	S72.414K	S72.433A
S62.651K	S65.101A	S65.899A	S72.002M	S72.032P	S72.059P	S72.111K	S72.126P	S72.21XM	S72.324N	S72.345K	S72.365P	S72.414M	S72.433M
S62.651P	S65.102A	S65.901A	S72.002N	S72.032Q	S72.059Q	S72.111M	S72.126Q	S72.21XN	S72.324P	S72.345M	S72.365Q	S72.414N	S72.433N
S62.652B	S65.109A	S65.902A	S72.002P	S72.032R	S72.059R	S72.111P	S72.126R	S72.21XP	S72.324Q	S72.345N	S72.365R	S72.414P	S72.433P
S62.652K	S65.111A	S65.909A	S72.002Q	S72.033K	S72.061K	S72.111Q	S72.131K	S72.21XQ	S72.324R	S72.345P	S72.366K	S72.414Q	S72.433Q
S62.652P	S65.112A	S65.911A	S72.002R	S72.033M	S72.061M	S72.111R	S72.131M	S72.21XR	S72.325K	S72.345Q	S72.366M	S72.414R	S72.433R
S62.653B	S65.119A	S65.912A	S72.009K	S72.033N	S72.061N	S72.112K	S72.131N	S72.22XK	S72.325M	S72.346K	S72.366N	S72.415A	S72.434A
S62.653K	S65.191A	S65.919A	S72.009M	S72.033P	S72.061P	S72.112M	S72.131P	S72.22XM	S72.325N	S72.346M	S72.366P	S72.415K	S72.434K
S62.653P	S65.192A	S65.991A	S72.009N	S72.033Q	S72.061Q	S72.112P	S72.131Q	S72.22XN	S72.325P	S72.346N	S72.366Q	S72.415M	S72.434M
S62.654B	S65.199A	S65.992A	S72.009P	S72.033R	S72.061R	S72.112Q	S72.131R	S72.22XP	S72.325Q	S72.346P	S72.366R	S72.415N	S72.434N
S62.654K	S65.201A	S65.999A	S72.009Q	S72.034K	S72.062K	S72.112R	S72.132K	S72.22XQ	S72.325R	S72.346Q	S72.391K	S72.415P	S72.434P
S62.654P	S65.202A	S66.021A	S72.009R	S72.034M	S72.062M	S72.113K	S72.132M	S72.22XR	S72.326K	S72.351K	S72.391M	S72.415Q	S72.434Q
S62.655B	S65.209A	S66.022A	S72.011K	S72.034N	S72.062N	S72.113M	S72.132N	S72.23XK	S72.326M	S72.351M	S72.391N	S72.415R	S72.434R
S62.655K	S65.211A	S66.029A	S72.011M	S72.034P	S72.062P	S72.113N	S72.132P	S72.23XM	S72.326N	S72.351N	S72.391P	S72.416A	S72.435A
S62.655P	S65.212A	S66.120A	S72.011P	S72.034Q	S72.062Q	S72.113P	S72.133K	S72.23XN	S72.326P	S72.351P	S72.391Q	S72.416K	S72.435K
S62.656B	S65.219A	S66.121A	S72.011Q	S72.034R	S72.062R	S72.113Q	S72.133M	S72.23XP	S72.326Q	S72.351Q	S72.391R	S72.416M	S72.435M
S62.656K	S65.291A	S66.122A	S72.011R	S72.035K	S72.063K	S72.113R	S72.133N	S72.23XQ	S72.326R	S72.351R	S72.392K	S72.416P	S72.435N
S62.656P	S65.292A	S66.123A	S72.012K	S72.035M	S72.063M	S72.114K	S72.133P	S72.23XR	S72.331K	S72.352K	S72.392M	S72.416Q	S72.435P
S62.657B	S65.299A	S66.124A	S72.012M	S72.035N	S72.063N	S72.114M	S72.133Q	S72.24XK	S72.331M	S72.352M	S72.392N	S72.416R	S72.435Q
S62.657K	S65.301A	S66.125A	S72.012P	S72.035P	S72.063P		S72.133R	S72.24XM	S72.331N	S72.352N	S72.392P	S72.421A	S72.435R
S62.657P	S65.302A	S66.126A	S72.012Q	S72.035Q	S72.063Q		S72.134K	S72.24XN	S72.331P	S72.352P	S72.392Q	S72.421K	S72.436A
S62.658B	S65.309A	S66.127A	S72.012R	S72.036K	S72.063R		S72.134M	S72.24XP			S72.392R	S72.421M	S72.436K
S62.658K	S65.311A	S66.128A	S72.019K	S72.036M			S72.134N					S72.421N	
S62.658P	S65.312A	S66.129A	S72.019M	S72.036N			S72.134P					S72.421P	
S62.659B	S65.319A	S66.221A		S72.036P									
S62.659K	S65.391A	S66.222A											

Appendix B: Symbols for 7th-character Codes

Complication or Comorbidity (CC) (cont.) - Based on CMS data

S72.436M	S72.454R	S72.492K	S73.042A	S78.921A	S79.199P	S82.016B	S82.032K	S82.044N	S82.111P	S82.126K	S82.144Q	S82.192A	S82.226P
S72.436N	S72.455A	S72.492M	S73.043A	S78.922A	S82.001A	S82.016C	S82.032M	S82.044P	S82.111Q	S82.126M	S82.144R	S82.192K	S82.226Q
S72.436P	S72.455K	S72.492N	S73.044A	S78.929A	S82.001B	S82.016K	S82.032N	S82.044Q	S82.111R	S82.126N	S82.145A	S82.192M	S82.226R
S72.436Q	S72.455M	S72.492P	S73.045A	S79.001K	S82.001C	S82.016M	S82.032P	S82.044R	S82.112A	S82.126P	S82.145K	S82.192N	S82.231A
S72.436R	S72.455N	S72.492Q	S73.046A	S79.001P	S82.001K	S82.016N	S82.032Q	S82.045A	S82.112K	S82.126Q	S82.145M	S82.192P	S82.231K
S72.441A	S72.455P	S72.492R	S75.201A	S79.002K	S82.001M	S82.016P	S82.032R	S82.045B	S82.112M	S82.131A	S82.145P	S82.192Q	S82.231N
S72.441K	S72.455Q	S72.499A	S75.202A	S79.002P	S82.001N	S82.016Q	S82.033A	S82.045C	S82.112N	S82.131K	S82.145Q	S82.192R	S82.231P
S72.441M	S72.455R	S72.499M	S75.209A	S79.009K	S82.001P	S82.016R	S82.033B	S82.045K	S82.112P	S82.131M	S82.145R	S82.199A	S82.231Q
S72.441N	S72.456A	S72.499N	S75.211A	S79.009P	S82.001Q	S82.021A	S82.033C	S82.045M	S82.112Q	S82.131N	S82.146A	S82.199K	S82.231R
S72.441P	S72.456K	S72.499P	S75.212A	S79.011K	S82.001R	S82.021B	S82.033K	S82.045N	S82.112R	S82.131P	S82.146K	S82.199M	S82.232A
S72.441Q	S72.456M	S72.499Q	S75.219A	S79.011P	S82.002A	S82.021C	S82.033M	S82.045P	S82.113A	S82.131Q	S82.146M	S82.199N	S82.232M
S72.441R	S72.456N	S72.499R	S75.221A	S79.012K	S82.002B	S82.021K	S82.033N	S82.045Q	S82.113K	S82.131R	S82.146N	S82.199P	S82.232N
S72.442A	S72.456P	S72.8X1K	S75.222A	S79.012P	S82.002C	S82.021M	S82.033P	S82.045R	S82.113M	S82.132A	S82.146P	S82.199Q	S82.232P
S72.442K	S72.456Q	S72.8X1M	S75.229A	S79.019K	S82.002K	S82.021N	S82.033Q	S82.046A	S82.113N	S82.132K	S82.146Q	S82.199R	S82.232Q
S72.442M	S72.456R	S72.8X1N	S75.291A	S79.019P	S82.002M	S82.021P	S82.033R	S82.046B	S82.113P	S82.132M	S82.146R	S82.201A	S82.232R
S72.442N	S72.461A	S72.8X1P	S75.292A	S79.091K	S82.002N	S82.021Q	S82.034A	S82.046C	S82.113Q	S82.132N	S82.151A	S82.201K	S82.233A
S72.442P	S72.461K	S72.8X1Q	S75.299A	S79.091P	S82.002P	S82.021R	S82.034B	S82.046K	S82.113R	S82.132P	S82.151K	S82.201M	S82.233K
S72.442Q	S72.461M	S72.8X1R	S75.801A	S79.092K	S82.002Q	S82.022A	S82.034C	S82.046M	S82.114A	S82.132Q	S82.151M	S82.201N	S82.233N
S72.442R	S72.461N	S72.8X2K	S75.802A	S79.092P	S82.002R	S82.022B	S82.034K	S82.046N	S82.114K	S82.133A	S82.151N	S82.201P	S82.233P
S72.443A	S72.461P	S72.8X2M	S75.809A	S79.099K	S82.009A	S82.022C	S82.034M	S82.046Q	S82.114M	S82.133K	S82.151P	S82.201Q	S82.233Q
S72.443K	S72.461Q	S72.8X2N	S75.811A	S79.099P	S82.009B	S82.022K	S82.034N	S82.046R	S82.114N	S82.133M	S82.151Q	S82.201R	S82.233R
S72.443M	S72.461R	S72.8X2P	S75.812A	S79.101A	S82.009C	S82.022M	S82.034P	S82.091A	S82.114P	S82.133N	S82.151R	S82.202A	S82.234A
S72.443N	S72.462A	S72.8X2Q	S75.819A	S79.101K	S82.009K	S82.022N	S82.034Q	S82.091B	S82.114Q	S82.133P	S82.152A	S82.202K	S82.234K
S72.443P	S72.462K	S72.8X2R	S75.891A	S79.101P	S82.009M	S82.022P	S82.034R	S82.091C	S82.114R	S82.133Q	S82.152K	S82.202M	S82.234N
S72.443Q	S72.462M	S72.8X9K	S75.892A	S79.102A	S82.009N	S82.022Q	S82.035A	S82.091K	S82.115A	S82.133R	S82.152M	S82.202N	S82.234P
S72.443R	S72.462N	S72.8X9M	S75.899A	S79.102K	S82.009P	S82.022R	S82.035B	S82.091M	S82.115K	S82.134A	S82.152N	S82.202P	S82.234Q
S72.444A	S72.462P	S72.8X9N	S75.901A	S79.102P	S82.009Q	S82.023A	S82.035C	S82.091N	S82.115M	S82.134K	S82.152P	S82.202Q	S82.234R
S72.444K	S72.462Q	S72.8X9N	S75.902A	S79.109A	S82.009R	S82.023B	S82.035K	S82.091P	S82.115N	S82.134M	S82.152Q	S82.202R	S82.235A
S72.444M	S72.462R	S72.8X9P	S75.909A	S79.109K	S82.011A	S82.023C	S82.035M	S82.091Q	S82.115P	S82.134N	S82.152R	S82.209A	S82.235K
S72.444N	S72.463A	S72.8X9Q	S75.911A	S79.109P	S82.011B	S82.023K	S82.035N	S82.091R	S82.115Q	S82.134P	S82.153A	S82.209K	S82.235M
S72.444P	S72.463K	S72.8X9R	S75.912A	S79.111A	S82.011C	S82.023M	S82.035P	S82.092A	S82.115R	S82.134Q	S82.153K	S82.209M	S82.235N
S72.444Q	S72.463M	S72.90XK	S75.919A	S79.111K	S82.011K	S82.023N	S82.035Q	S82.092B	S82.116A	S82.134R	S82.153M	S82.209N	S82.235P
S72.444R	S72.463N	S72.90XM	S75.991A	S79.111P	S82.011M	S82.023P	S82.035R	S82.092C	S82.116K	S82.135A	S82.153N	S82.209P	S82.235Q
S72.445A	S72.463P	S72.90XN	S75.992A	S79.112A	S82.011N	S82.023Q	S82.036A	S82.092M	S82.116M	S82.135K	S82.153P	S82.209Q	S82.235R
S72.445K	S72.463Q	S72.90XP	S75.999A	S79.112K	S82.011P	S82.023R	S82.036B	S82.092N	S82.116N	S82.135M	S82.153Q	S82.209R	S82.236A
S72.445M	S72.463R	S72.90XQ	S76.021A	S79.112P	S82.011Q	S82.024A	S82.036C	S82.092P	S82.116P	S82.135N	S82.153R	S82.221A	S82.236K
S72.445N	S72.464A	S72.90XR	S76.022A	S79.119A	S82.011R	S82.024B	S82.036K	S82.092Q	S82.116Q	S82.135P	S82.154A	S82.221K	S82.236M
S72.445P	S72.464K	S72.91XK	S76.029A	S79.119K	S82.012A	S82.024C	S82.036M	S82.092R	S82.116R	S82.135Q	S82.154K	S82.221M	S82.236N
S72.445Q	S72.464M	S72.91XM	S76.121A	S79.119P	S82.012B	S82.024K	S82.036N	S82.099A	S82.121A	S82.135R	S82.154M	S82.221N	S82.236P
S72.445R	S72.464N	S72.91XN	S76.122A	S79.121A	S82.012C	S82.024M	S82.036P	S82.099B	S82.121K	S82.136A	S82.154N	S82.221P	S82.236Q
S72.446A	S72.464P	S72.91XP	S76.129A	S79.121K	S82.012K	S82.024N	S82.036Q	S82.099C	S82.121M	S82.136K	S82.154P	S82.221Q	S82.236R
S72.446K	S72.464Q	S72.91XQ	S76.221A	S79.121P	S82.012M	S82.024P	S82.036R	S82.099K	S82.121N	S82.136M	S82.154Q	S82.221R	S82.241A
S72.446M	S72.464R	S72.91XR	S76.222A	S79.122A	S82.012N	S82.024Q	S82.041A	S82.099M	S82.121P	S82.136N	S82.154R	S82.222A	S82.241K
S72.446N	S72.465A	S72.92XK	S76.229A	S79.122K	S82.012P	S82.024R	S82.041B	S82.099N	S82.121Q	S82.136P	S82.155A	S82.222K	S82.241M
S72.446P	S72.465K	S72.92XM	S76.321A	S79.122P	S82.012Q	S82.025A	S82.041C	S82.099P	S82.121R	S82.136Q	S82.155K	S82.222M	S82.241N
S72.446Q	S72.465M	S72.92XN	S76.322A	S79.129A	S82.012R	S82.025B	S82.041K	S82.099Q	S82.122A	S82.136R	S82.155M	S82.222N	S82.241P
S72.446R	S72.465N	S72.92XP	S76.329A	S79.129K	S82.013A	S82.025C	S82.041M	S82.099R	S82.122K	S82.141A	S82.155N	S82.222Q	S82.241Q
S72.451A	S72.465P	S72.92XQ	S76.821A	S79.129P	S82.013B	S82.025K	S82.041N	S82.101A	S82.122M	S82.141K	S82.155P	S82.222R	S82.241R
S72.451K	S72.465Q	S72.92XR	S76.822A	S79.131A	S82.013C	S82.025M	S82.041P	S82.101K	S82.122N	S82.141M	S82.155Q	S82.223A	S82.242A
S72.451M	S72.465R	S73.001A	S76.829A	S79.131K	S82.013K	S82.025N	S82.041Q	S82.101M	S82.122P	S82.141N	S82.155R	S82.223K	S82.242K
S72.451N	S72.466A	S73.002A	S76.921A	S79.131P	S82.013M	S82.025P	S82.041R	S82.101N	S82.122Q	S82.141P	S82.156A	S82.223M	S82.242M
S72.451P	S72.466K	S73.003A	S76.922A	S79.132A	S82.013N	S82.025Q	S82.042A	S82.101P	S82.122R	S82.141Q	S82.156K	S82.223N	S82.242N
S72.451Q	S72.466M	S73.004A	S76.929A	S79.132K	S82.013P	S82.025R	S82.042B	S82.101Q	S82.123A	S82.141R	S82.156M	S82.223P	S82.242P
S72.451R	S72.466N	S73.005A	S77.00XA	S79.132P	S82.013Q	S82.026A	S82.042C	S82.101R	S82.123K	S82.141Q	S82.156N	S82.223Q	S82.242Q
S72.452A	S72.466P	S73.006A	S77.01XA	S79.139A	S82.013R	S82.026B	S82.042K	S82.102A	S82.123M	S82.141R	S82.156P	S82.223R	S82.242R
S72.452K	S72.466Q	S73.011A	S77.02XA	S79.139K	S82.014A	S82.026C	S82.042M	S82.102K	S82.123N	S82.142A	S82.156Q	S82.224A	S82.243A
S72.452M	S72.466R	S73.012A	S77.10XA	S79.139P	S82.014B	S82.026K	S82.042N	S82.102M	S82.123P	S82.142K	S82.156R	S82.224K	S82.243K
S72.452N	S72.471A	S73.013A	S77.11XA	S79.141A	S82.014C	S82.026M	S82.042P	S82.102N	S82.123Q	S82.142M	S82.161A	S82.224M	S82.243M
S72.452P	S72.471K	S73.014A	S77.12XA	S79.141K	S82.014K	S82.026N	S82.042Q	S82.102P	S82.123R	S82.142N	S82.161K	S82.224N	S82.243N
S72.452Q	S72.471P	S73.015A	S78.011A	S79.141P	S82.014M	S82.026P	S82.042R	S82.102Q	S82.124A	S82.142P	S82.161P	S82.224P	S82.243P
S72.452R	S72.472A	S73.016A	S78.012A	S79.142A	S82.014N	S82.026Q	S82.043A	S82.102R	S82.124K	S82.142Q	S82.162A	S82.224Q	S82.243Q
S72.453A	S72.472K	S73.021A	S78.019A	S79.142K	S82.014P	S82.026R	S82.043B	S82.109A	S82.124M	S82.142R	S82.162K	S82.224R	S82.243R
S72.453K	S72.472P	S73.022A	S78.021A	S79.142P	S82.014Q	S82.031A	S82.043C	S82.109K	S82.124N	S82.143A	S82.162P	S82.225A	S82.244A
S72.453M	S72.479A	S73.023A	S78.022A	S79.149A	S82.014R	S82.031B	S82.043K	S82.109M	S82.124P	S82.143K	S82.169A	S82.225K	S82.244K
S72.453N	S72.479K	S73.024A	S78.029A	S79.149K	S82.015A	S82.031C	S82.043M	S82.109N	S82.124Q	S82.143M	S82.169K	S82.225M	S82.244M
S72.453P	S72.479P	S73.025A	S78.111A	S79.149P	S82.015B	S82.031K	S82.043N	S82.109P	S82.124R	S82.143N	S82.169P	S82.225N	S82.244N
S72.453Q	S72.491A	S73.026A	S78.112A	S79.191A	S82.015C	S82.031M	S82.043P	S82.109Q	S82.125A	S82.143P	S82.191A	S82.225P	S82.244P
S72.453R	S72.491K	S73.031A	S78.119A	S79.191K	S82.015K	S82.031N	S82.043Q	S82.109Q	S82.125K	S82.143Q	S82.191K	S82.225Q	S82.244Q
S72.454A	S72.491M	S73.032A	S78.121A	S79.191P	S82.015M	S82.031P	S82.043R	S82.109R	S82.125M	S82.143R	S82.191M	S82.225R	S82.244R
S72.454K	S72.491N	S73.033A	S78.122A	S79.192A	S82.015N	S82.031Q	S82.044A	S82.111A	S82.125N	S82.144A	S82.191N	S82.226A	S82.244P
S72.454M	S72.491P	S73.034A	S78.129A	S79.192K	S82.015P	S82.031R	S82.044B	S82.111K	S82.125P	S82.144K	S82.191P	S82.226K	S82.244Q
S72.454N	S72.491Q	S73.035A	S78.911A	S79.192P	S82.015Q	S82.032A	S82.044C	S82.111M	S82.125Q	S82.144M	S82.191Q	S82.226M	S82.244R
S72.454P	S72.491R	S73.036A	S78.912A	S79.199A	S82.015R	S82.032B	S82.044K	S82.111N	S82.125R	S82.144N	S82.191R	S82.226N	S82.245A
S72.454Q	S72.492A	S73.041A	S78.919A	S79.199K	S82.016A	S82.032C	S82.044M		S82.126A	S82.144P			

Complication or Comorbidity (CC) (cont.) - Based on CMS data

S82.245K	S82.263Q	S82.319A	S82.425R	S82.446M	S82.466P	S82.61XP	S82.841C	S82.854M	S82.873C	S82.92XM	S85.991A	S89.039P	S89.291P
S82.245M	S82.263R	S82.319K	S82.426K	S82.446N	S82.466Q	S82.61XQ	S82.841K	S82.854N	S82.873K	S82.92XN	S85.992A	S89.041A	S89.292K
S82.245N	S82.264A	S82.319P	S82.426M	S82.446P	S82.466R	S82.61XR	S82.841M	S82.854P	S82.873M	S82.92XP	S85.999A	S89.041K	S89.292P
S82.245P	S82.264K	S82.391B	S82.426N	S82.446Q	S82.491K	S82.62XB	S82.841N	S82.854Q	S82.873N	S82.92XQ	S86.021A	S89.041P	S89.299K
S82.245Q	S82.264M	S82.391C	S82.426P	S82.446R	S82.491M	S82.62XC	S82.841P	S82.854R	S82.873P	S82.92XR	S86.022A	S89.042A	S89.299P
S82.245R	S82.264N	S82.391K	S82.426Q	S82.451K	S82.491N	S82.62XK	S82.841Q	S82.855B	S82.873Q	S85.101A	S86.029A	S89.042K	S89.301K
S82.246A	S82.264P	S82.391M	S82.426R	S82.451M	S82.491P	S82.62XM	S82.841R	S82.855C	S82.873R	S85.102A	S86.121A	S89.042P	S89.301P
S82.246K	S82.264Q	S82.391N	S82.431K	S82.451N	S82.491Q	S82.62XN	S82.842B	S82.855K	S82.874B	S85.109A	S86.122A	S89.049A	S89.302K
S82.246M	S82.264R	S82.391P	S82.431M	S82.451P	S82.491R	S82.62XP	S82.842C	S82.855N	S82.874C	S85.111A	S86.129A	S89.049K	S89.302P
S82.246N	S82.265A	S82.391Q	S82.431N	S82.451Q	S82.492K	S82.62XQ	S82.842K	S82.855P	S82.874K	S85.112A	S86.221A	S89.049P	S89.309K
S82.246P	S82.265K	S82.391R	S82.431P	S82.451R	S82.492M	S82.62XR	S82.842M	S82.855Q	S82.874M	S85.119A	S86.222A	S89.091A	S89.309P
S82.246Q	S82.265M	S82.392B	S82.431Q	S82.452K	S82.492N	S82.63XB	S82.842N	S82.855R	S82.874N	S85.121A	S86.229A	S89.091K	S89.311K
S82.246R	S82.265N	S82.392C	S82.431R	S82.452M	S82.492P	S82.63XC	S82.842P	S82.856B	S82.874P	S85.122A	S86.321A	S89.091P	S89.311P
S82.251A	S82.265P	S82.392K	S82.432K	S82.452N	S82.492Q	S82.63XK	S82.842Q	S82.856C	S82.874Q	S85.129A	S86.322A	S89.092A	S89.312K
S82.251K	S82.265Q	S82.392M	S82.432M	S82.452P	S82.492R	S82.63XM	S82.843B	S82.856M	S82.874R	S85.131A	S86.329A	S89.092K	S89.312P
S82.251M	S82.265R	S82.392N	S82.432N	S82.452Q	S82.499K	S82.63XN	S82.843C	S82.856N	S82.875B	S85.132A	S86.821A	S89.092P	S89.319K
S82.251N	S82.266A	S82.392P	S82.432P	S82.452R	S82.499M	S82.63XP	S82.843K	S82.856P	S82.875C	S85.139A	S86.822A	S89.099A	S89.319P
S82.251P	S82.266K	S82.392Q	S82.432Q	S82.453K	S82.499N	S82.63XQ	S82.843M	S82.856Q	S82.875K	S85.141A	S86.829A	S89.099K	S89.321K
S82.251Q	S82.266M	S82.392R	S82.432R	S82.453N	S82.499P	S82.63XR	S82.843N	S82.856R	S82.875M	S85.142A	S86.921A	S89.099P	S89.321P
S82.251R	S82.266N	S82.399B	S82.433K	S82.453P	S82.499Q	S82.64XB	S82.843P	S82.861B	S82.875N	S85.149A	S86.922A	S89.101K	S89.322K
S82.252A	S82.266P	S82.399C	S82.433M	S82.453Q	S82.499R	S82.64XC	S82.843Q	S82.861M	S82.875P	S85.151A	S86.929A	S89.101P	S89.322P
S82.252K	S82.266Q	S82.399K	S82.433N	S82.453R	S82.51XB	S82.64XK	S82.844B	S82.861N	S82.875R	S85.152A	S88.011A	S89.102K	S89.329K
S82.252M	S82.266R	S82.399M	S82.433P	S82.454K	S82.51XC	S82.64XM	S82.844C	S82.861P	S82.876B	S85.159A	S88.012A	S89.102P	S89.329P
S82.252N	S82.291A	S82.399N	S82.433Q	S82.454M	S82.51XK	S82.64XN	S82.844K	S82.861Q	S82.876C	S85.161A	S88.019A	S89.109K	S89.391K
S82.252P	S82.291K	S82.399P	S82.433R	S82.454N	S82.51XM	S82.64XP	S82.844M	S82.861R	S82.876K	S85.162A	S88.021A	S89.109P	S89.391P
S82.252Q	S82.291M	S82.399Q	S82.434K	S82.454P	S82.51XN	S82.64XQ	S82.844N	S82.862K	S82.876M	S85.169A	S88.029A	S89.111K	S89.392K
S82.252R	S82.291N	S82.401K	S82.434M	S82.454Q	S82.51XP	S82.64XR	S82.844P	S82.862M	S82.876N	S85.171A	S88.111A	S89.111P	S89.392P
S82.253A	S82.291P	S82.401M	S82.434N	S82.454R	S82.51XQ	S82.65XB	S82.844Q	S82.862N	S82.876P	S85.172A	S88.112A	S89.112K	S89.399K
S82.253K	S82.291Q	S82.401N	S82.434P	S82.455K	S82.51XR	S82.65XC	S82.844R	S82.862P	S82.876Q	S85.179A	S88.121A	S89.112P	S89.399P
S82.253M	S82.291R	S82.401P	S82.434Q	S82.455M	S82.52XB	S82.65XK	S82.845B	S82.862Q	S82.876R	S85.181A	S88.122A	S89.119K	S92.001K
S82.253N	S82.292A	S82.401Q	S82.434R	S82.455N	S82.52XC	S82.65XM	S82.845C	S82.862R	S82.891B	S85.182A	S88.129A	S89.119P	S92.001M
S82.253P	S82.292K	S82.401R	S82.435K	S82.455P	S82.52XK	S82.65XN	S82.845K	S82.863K	S82.891C	S85.189A	S88.911A	S89.121K	S92.001P
S82.253Q	S82.292M	S82.402M	S82.435M	S82.455Q	S82.52XM	S82.65XP	S82.845M	S82.863M	S82.891K	S85.201A	S88.912A	S89.121P	S92.002B
S82.253R	S82.292N	S82.402N	S82.435N	S82.455R	S82.52XN	S82.65XQ	S82.845N	S82.863N	S82.891M	S85.202A	S88.919A	S89.122K	S92.002K
S82.254A	S82.292P	S82.402P	S82.435P	S82.456K	S82.52XP	S82.65XR	S82.845P	S82.863P	S82.891N	S85.209A	S88.921A	S89.122P	S92.002P
S82.254K	S82.292Q	S82.402Q	S82.435Q	S82.456M	S82.52XQ	S82.66XB	S82.845Q	S82.863Q	S82.891P	S85.211A	S88.922A	S89.129K	S92.009B
S82.254M	S82.292R	S82.402R	S82.435R	S82.456N	S82.52XR	S82.66XC	S82.845R	S82.863R	S82.891Q	S85.212A	S88.929A	S89.129P	S92.009K
S82.254N	S82.299A	S82.409K	S82.436K	S82.456P	S82.53XB	S82.66XK	S82.846B	S82.864K	S82.891R	S85.219A	S89.001A	S89.131K	S92.009P
S82.254P	S82.299K	S82.409N	S82.436M	S82.456Q	S82.53XC	S82.66XM	S82.846C	S82.864M	S82.892B	S85.291A	S89.001K	S89.131P	S92.011B
S82.254Q	S82.299M	S82.409P	S82.436N	S82.456R	S82.53XK	S82.66XN	S82.846K	S82.864N	S82.892C	S85.292A	S89.001P	S89.132K	S92.011K
S82.254R	S82.299N	S82.409Q	S82.436P	S82.461K	S82.53XM	S82.66XP	S82.846M	S82.864P	S82.892K	S85.299A	S89.002A	S89.132P	S92.011P
S82.255A	S82.299P	S82.409R	S82.436Q	S82.461M	S82.53XN	S82.66XR	S82.846N	S82.864Q	S82.892M	S85.301A	S89.002K	S89.139K	S92.012B
S82.255K	S82.299Q	S82.421K	S82.436R	S82.461N	S82.53XP	S82.811K	S82.846P	S82.864R	S82.892N	S85.302A	S89.002P	S89.139P	S92.012K
S82.255M	S82.299R	S82.421M	S82.441K	S82.461P	S82.53XQ	S82.811P	S82.846Q	S82.865K	S82.892P	S85.309A	S89.009A	S89.141K	S92.012P
S82.255N	S82.301B	S82.421N	S82.441M	S82.461Q	S82.53XR	S82.812K	S82.846R	S82.865M	S82.892Q	S85.311A	S89.009K	S89.141P	S92.013B
S82.255P	S82.301C	S82.421P	S82.441N	S82.461R	S82.54XB	S82.812P	S82.851B	S82.865N	S82.892R	S85.312A	S89.009P	S89.142K	S92.013K
S82.255Q	S82.301K	S82.421Q	S82.441P	S82.462K	S82.54XC	S82.819K	S82.851C	S82.865P	S82.899B	S85.319A	S89.011A	S89.142P	S92.013P
S82.255R	S82.301M	S82.421R	S82.441Q	S82.462M	S82.54XK	S82.819P	S82.851K	S82.865Q	S82.899C	S85.391A	S89.011K	S89.149K	S92.014B
S82.256A	S82.301N	S82.422K	S82.441R	S82.462N	S82.54XM	S82.821K	S82.851M	S82.865R	S82.899M	S85.392A	S89.011P	S89.149P	S92.014K
S82.256K	S82.301P	S82.422M	S82.442K	S82.462P	S82.54XN	S82.821P	S82.851N	S82.866K	S82.899N	S85.399A	S89.012A	S89.191K	S92.014P
S82.256M	S82.301Q	S82.422N	S82.442M	S82.462Q	S82.54XP	S82.822K	S82.851P	S82.866M	S82.899P	S85.401A	S89.012K	S89.191P	S92.015B
S82.256N	S82.301R	S82.422P	S82.442N	S82.462R	S82.54XQ	S82.822P	S82.851Q	S82.866N	S82.899Q	S85.402A	S89.012P	S89.192K	S92.015K
S82.256P	S82.302B	S82.422Q	S82.442P	S82.463K	S82.54XR	S82.829K	S82.851R	S82.866P	S82.899R	S85.409A	S89.019A	S89.192P	S92.015P
S82.256Q	S82.302C	S82.422R	S82.442Q	S82.463M	S82.55XB	S82.829P	S82.852B	S82.866Q	S82.90XB	S85.411A	S89.019K	S89.199K	S92.016B
S82.256R	S82.302K	S82.423K	S82.442R	S82.463N	S82.55XC	S82.831K	S82.852C	S82.866R	S82.90XK	S85.412A	S89.019P	S89.199P	S92.016K
S82.261A	S82.302M	S82.423M	S82.443K	S82.463P	S82.55XM	S82.831M	S82.852K	S82.871B	S82.90XM	S85.419A	S89.021A	S89.201K	S92.016P
S82.261K	S82.302N	S82.423N	S82.443M	S82.463Q	S82.55XN	S82.831N	S82.852M	S82.871C	S82.90XN	S85.491A	S89.021K	S89.201P	S92.021B
S82.261M	S82.302P	S82.423P	S82.443N	S82.463R	S82.55XP	S82.831P	S82.852N	S82.871K	S82.90XP	S85.492A	S89.021P	S89.202K	S92.021K
S82.261N	S82.302Q	S82.423Q	S82.443P	S82.464K	S82.55XQ	S82.831Q	S82.852P	S82.871M	S82.90XQ	S85.499A	S89.022A	S89.202P	S92.021P
S82.261P	S82.302R	S82.423R	S82.443Q	S82.464M	S82.55XR	S82.831R	S82.852Q	S82.871N	S82.90XR	S85.801A	S89.022K	S89.209K	S92.022B
S82.261Q	S82.309B	S82.424K	S82.443R	S82.464N	S82.56XB	S82.832K	S82.852R	S82.871P	S82.91XC	S85.802A	S89.022P	S89.209P	S92.022K
S82.261R	S82.309C	S82.424M	S82.444K	S82.464P	S82.56XC	S82.832M	S82.853B	S82.871Q	S82.91XK	S85.809A	S89.029A	S89.211K	S92.022P
S82.262A	S82.309K	S82.424N	S82.444M	S82.464Q	S82.56XK	S82.832N	S82.853C	S82.871R	S82.91XM	S85.811A	S89.029K	S89.211P	S92.023B
S82.262K	S82.309M	S82.424P	S82.444N	S82.464R	S82.56XM	S82.832P	S82.853K	S82.872B	S82.91XN	S85.812A	S89.029P	S89.212K	S92.023K
S82.262M	S82.309N	S82.424Q	S82.444P	S82.465K	S82.56XN	S82.832Q	S82.853M	S82.872C	S82.91XP	S85.819A	S89.031A	S89.212P	S92.023P
S82.262N	S82.309P	S82.424R	S82.444Q	S82.465M	S82.56XP	S82.832R	S82.853N	S82.872K	S82.91XQ	S85.891A	S89.031K	S89.219K	S92.024B
S82.262P	S82.309Q	S82.425K	S82.444R	S82.465N	S82.56XQ	S82.839K	S82.853P	S82.872M	S82.91XR	S85.892A	S89.031P	S89.219P	S92.024K
S82.262Q	S82.309R	S82.425M	S82.445K	S82.465P	S82.56XR	S82.839M	S82.853Q	S82.872N	S82.92XB	S85.899A	S89.032A	S89.221K	S92.024P
S82.262R	S82.311A	S82.425N	S82.445M	S82.465Q	S82.61XB	S82.839N	S82.853R	S82.872P	S82.92XC	S85.901A	S89.032K	S89.221P	S92.025B
S82.263A	S82.311K	S82.425P	S82.445P	S82.465R	S82.61XC	S82.839P	S82.854B	S82.872Q	S82.92XK	S85.902A	S89.032P	S89.222K	S92.025K
S82.263K	S82.311P	S82.425Q	S82.445Q	S82.466K	S82.61XK	S82.839Q	S82.854C	S82.872R	S85.901A	S85.909A	S89.039A	S89.222P	S92.025P
S82.263M	S82.312A		S82.445R	S82.466M	S82.61XM	S82.839R	S82.854K	S82.873B	S85.912A	S85.911A	S89.039K	S89.229K	S92.026B
S82.263N	S82.312K		S82.446K	S82.466N	S82.61XN	S82.841B				S85.919A		S89.291K	S92.026K
S82.263P	S82.312P												S92.026P

Complication or Comorbidity (CC) (cont.) - Based on CMS data

S92.031B	S92.101P	S92.145K	S92.226B	S92.313P	S92.354K	S92.521K	S95.209A	T17.800A	T22.721A	T24.309A	T33.09XA	T70.3XXA	T79.A11A
S92.031K	S92.102B	S92.145P	S92.226K	S92.314B	S92.354P	S92.521P	S95.211A	T17.808A	T22.722A	T24.311A	T33.1XXA	T71.111A	T79.A12A
S92.031P	S92.102K	S92.146B	S92.226P	S92.314K	S92.355B	S92.522K	S95.212A	T17.810A	T22.729A	T24.312A	T33.2XXA	T71.112A	T79.A19A
S92.032B	S92.102P	S92.146K	S92.231B	S92.314P	S92.355K	S92.522P	S95.219A	T17.818A	T22.731A	T24.319A	T33.3XXA	T71.113A	T79.A21A
S92.032K	S92.109B	S92.146P	S92.231K	S92.315B	S92.355P	S92.523K	S95.291A	T17.820A	T22.732A	T24.321A	T33.40XA	T71.114A	T79.A22A
S92.032P	S92.109K	S92.151B	S92.231P	S92.315K	S92.356B	S92.523P	S95.292A	T17.828A	T22.739A	T24.322A	T33.41XA	T71.121A	T79.A29A
S92.033B	S92.109P	S92.151K	S92.232B	S92.315P	S92.356K	S92.524K	S95.299A	T17.890A	T22.741A	T24.329A	T33.42XA	T71.122A	T79.A3XA
S92.033K	S92.111B	S92.151P	S92.232K	S92.316B	S92.356P	S92.524P	S95.801A	T17.898A	T22.742A	T24.331A	T33.511A	T71.123A	T79.A9XA
S92.033P	S92.111K	S92.152B	S92.232P	S92.316K	S92.401K	S92.525K	S95.802A	T20.30XA	T22.749A	T24.332A	T33.512A	T71.124A	T80.1XXA
S92.034B	S92.111P	S92.152K	S92.233B	S92.316P	S92.401P	S92.525P	S95.809A	T20.311A	T22.751A	T24.339A	T33.519A	T71.131A	T80.211A
S92.034K	S92.112B	S92.152P	S92.233K	S92.321B	S92.402K	S92.526K	S95.811A	T20.312A	T22.752A	T24.391A	T33.521A	T71.132A	T80.212A
S92.034P	S92.112K	S92.153B	S92.233P	S92.321K	S92.402P	S92.526P	S95.812A	T20.319A	T22.759A	T24.392A	T33.522A	T71.133A	T80.218A
S92.035B	S92.112P	S92.153K	S92.234B	S92.321P	S92.403K	S92.531K	S95.819A	T20.32XA	T22.761A	T24.399A	T33.529A	T71.134A	T80.219A
S92.035K	S92.113B	S92.153P	S92.234K	S92.322B	S92.403P	S92.531P	S95.891A	T20.33XA	T22.762A	T24.701A	T33.531A	T71.141A	T80.22XA
S92.035P	S92.113K	S92.154B	S92.234P	S92.322K	S92.404K	S92.532K	S95.892A	T20.34XA	T22.769A	T24.702A	T33.532A	T71.143A	T80.29XA
S92.036B	S92.113P	S92.154K	S92.235B	S92.322P	S92.404P	S92.532P	S95.899A	T20.35XA	T22.791A	T24.709A	T33.539A	T71.144A	T80.30XA
S92.036K	S92.114B	S92.154P	S92.235K	S92.323B	S92.405K	S92.533K	S95.901A	T20.36XA	T22.792A	T24.711A	T33.60XA	T71.151A	T80.310A
S92.036P	S92.114K	S92.155B	S92.235P	S92.323K	S92.405P	S92.533P	S95.902A	T20.37XA	T22.799A	T24.712A	T33.61XA	T71.152A	T80.311A
S92.041B	S92.114P	S92.155K	S92.236B	S92.323P	S92.406K	S92.534K	S95.909A	T20.39XA	T23.301A	T24.719A	T33.62XA	T71.153A	T80.319A
S92.041K	S92.115B	S92.155P	S92.236K	S92.324B	S92.406P	S92.534P	S95.911A	T20.70XA	T23.302A	T24.721A	T33.70XA	T71.154A	T80.39XA
S92.041P	S92.115K	S92.156B	S92.236P	S92.324K	S92.411K	S92.535K	S95.912A	T20.711A	T23.309A	T24.722A	T33.71XA	T71.161A	T80.40XA
S92.042B	S92.115P	S92.156K	S92.241B	S92.324P	S92.411P	S92.535P	S95.919A	T20.712A	T23.311A	T24.729A	T33.72XA	T71.162A	T80.410A
S92.042K	S92.116B	S92.156P	S92.241K	S92.325B	S92.412K	S92.536K	S95.991A	T20.719A	T23.312A	T24.731A	T33.811A	T71.163A	T80.411A
S92.042P	S92.116K	S92.191B	S92.241P	S92.325K	S92.412P	S92.536P	S95.992A	T20.72XA	T23.319A	T24.732A	T33.812A	T71.164A	T80.419A
S92.043B	S92.116P	S92.191K	S92.242B	S92.325P	S92.413K	S92.591K	S95.999A	T20.73XA	T23.321A	T24.739A	T33.819A	T71.191A	T80.49XA
S92.043K	S92.121B	S92.191P	S92.242K	S92.326B	S92.413P	S92.591P	S96.021A	T20.74XA	T23.322A	T24.791A	T33.821A	T71.192A	T80.51XA
S92.043P	S92.121K	S92.192B	S92.242P	S92.326K	S92.414K	S92.592K	S96.022A	T20.75XA	T23.329A	T24.792A	T33.822A	T71.193A	T80.52XA
S92.044B	S92.121P	S92.192K	S92.243B	S92.326P	S92.414P	S92.592P	S96.029A	T20.76XA	T23.331A	T24.799A	T33.829A	T71.194A	T80.59XA
S92.044K	S92.122B	S92.192P	S92.243K	S92.331B	S92.415K	S92.599K	S96.121A	T20.77XA	T23.332A	T25.311A	T33.831A	T71.20XA	T80.61XA
S92.044P	S92.122K	S92.199B	S92.243P	S92.331K	S92.415P	S92.599P	S96.122A	T20.79XA	T23.339A	T25.312A	T33.832A	T71.21XA	T80.62XA
S92.045B	S92.122P	S92.199K	S92.244B	S92.331P	S92.416K	S92.811B	S96.129A	T21.30XA	T23.341A	T25.319A	T33.839A	T71.221A	T80.69XA
S92.045K	S92.123B	S92.199P	S92.244K	S92.332B	S92.416P	S92.811K	S96.221A	T21.31XA	T23.342A	T25.321A	T33.90XA	T71.222A	T80.810A
S92.045P	S92.123K	S92.201B	S92.244P	S92.332K	S92.421K	S92.811P	S96.222A	T21.32XA	T23.349A	T25.322A	T33.99XA	T71.223A	T80.818A
S92.046B	S92.123P	S92.201K	S92.245B	S92.332P	S92.421P	S92.812B	S96.229A	T21.33XA	T23.351A	T25.329A	T34.011A	T71.224A	T80.910A
S92.046K	S92.124B	S92.201P	S92.245K	S92.333B	S92.422K	S92.812K	S96.821A	T21.34XA	T23.352A	T25.331A	T34.012A	T71.231A	T80.911A
S92.046P	S92.124K	S92.202B	S92.245P	S92.333K	S92.422P	S92.812P	S96.822A	T21.35XA	T23.359A	T25.332A	T34.019A	T71.232A	T80.919A
S92.051B	S92.124P	S92.202K	S92.246B	S92.333P	S92.423K	S92.819B	S96.829A	T21.36XA	T23.361A	T25.339A	T34.02XA	T71.233A	T80.A0XA
S92.051K	S92.125B	S92.202P	S92.246K	S92.334B	S92.423P	S92.819K	S96.921A	T21.37XA	T23.362A	T25.391A	T34.09XA	T71.234A	T80.A10A
S92.051P	S92.125K	S92.209B	S92.246P	S92.334K	S92.424K	S92.819P	S96.922A	T21.39XA	T23.369A	T25.392A	T34.1XXA	T71.29XA	T80.A11A
S92.052B	S92.125P	S92.209K	S92.251B	S92.334P	S92.424P	S92.901B	S96.929A	T21.70XA	T23.371A	T25.399A	T34.2XXA	T71.9XXA	T80.A19A
S92.052K	S92.126B	S92.209P	S92.251K	S92.335B	S92.425K	S92.901K	S98.011A	T21.71XA	T23.372A	T25.711A	T34.3XXA	T74.01XA	T80.A9XA
S92.052P	S92.126K	S92.211B	S92.251P	S92.335K	S92.425P	S92.901P	S98.012A	T21.72XA	T23.379A	T25.712A	T34.40XA	T74.02XA	T81.10XA
S92.053B	S92.126P	S92.211K	S92.252B	S92.335P	S92.426K	S92.902B	S98.019A	T21.73XA	T23.391A	T25.719A	T34.41XA	T74.11XA	T81.30XA
S92.053K	S92.131B	S92.211P	S92.252K	S92.336B	S92.426P	S92.902K	S98.021A	T21.74XA	T23.392A	T25.721A	T34.42XA	T74.12XA	T81.31XA
S92.053P	S92.131K	S92.212B	S92.252P	S92.336K	S92.491K	S92.902P	S98.022A	T21.75XA	T23.399A	T25.722A	T34.511A	T74.21XA	T81.32XA
S92.054B	S92.131P	S92.212K	S92.253B	S92.336P	S92.491P	S92.909B	S98.029A	T21.76XA	T23.701A	T25.729A	T34.512A	T74.22XA	T81.33XA
S92.054K	S92.132B	S92.212P	S92.253K	S92.341B	S92.492K	S92.909K	S98.311A	T21.77XA	T23.702A	T25.731A	T34.519A	T74.32XA	T81.4XXA
S92.054P	S92.132K	S92.213B	S92.253P	S92.341K	S92.492P	S92.909P	S98.312A	T21.79XA	T23.709A	T25.732A	T34.521A	T74.4XXA	T81.500A
S92.055B	S92.132P	S92.213K	S92.254B	S92.341P	S92.499K	S92.911B	S98.319A	T22.30XA	T23.711A	T25.739A	T34.522A	T74.91XA	T81.501A
S92.055K	S92.133B	S92.213P	S92.254K	S92.342B	S92.499P	S92.911P	S98.321A	T22.311A	T23.712A	T25.791A	T34.529A	T74.92XA	T81.502A
S92.055P	S92.133K	S92.214B	S92.254P	S92.342K	S92.501K	S92.912K	S98.322A	T22.312A	T23.719A	T25.792A	T34.531A	T75.1XXA	T81.503A
S92.056B	S92.133P	S92.214K	S92.255B	S92.342P	S92.501P	S92.912P	S98.329A	T22.319A	T23.721A	T25.799A	T34.532A	T76.01XA	T81.504A
S92.056K	S92.134B	S92.214P	S92.255K	S92.343B	S92.502K	S92.919K	S98.911A	T22.321A	T23.722A	T26.20XA	T34.539A	T76.02XA	T81.505A
S92.056P	S92.134K	S92.215B	S92.255P	S92.343K	S92.502P	S92.919P	S98.912A	T22.322A	T23.729A	T26.21XA	T34.611A	T76.11XA	T81.506A
S92.061B	S92.134P	S92.215K	S92.256B	S92.343P	S92.503K	S95.001A	S98.919A	T22.329A	T23.731A	T26.22XA	T34.612A	T76.12XA	T81.507A
S92.061K	S92.135B	S92.215P	S92.256K	S92.344B	S92.503P	S95.002A	S98.921A	T22.331A	T23.732A	T26.70XA	T34.619A	T76.21XA	T81.508A
S92.061P	S92.135K	S92.216B	S92.256P	S92.344K	S92.504K	S95.009A	S98.922A	T22.332A	T23.739A	T26.71XA	T34.62XA	T76.22XA	T81.509A
S92.062B	S92.135P	S92.216K	S92.301B	S92.344P	S92.504P	S95.011A	S98.929A	T22.339A	T23.741A	T26.72XA	T34.70XA	T76.32XA	T81.510A
S92.062K	S92.136B	S92.216P	S92.301K	S92.345B	S92.505K	S95.012A	T17.400A	T22.341A	T23.742A	T27.0XXA	T34.71XA	T76.91XA	T81.511A
S92.062P	S92.136K	S92.221B	S92.301P	S92.345K	S92.505P	S95.019A	T17.408A	T22.342A	T23.749A	T27.1XXA	T34.72XA	T76.92XA	T81.512A
S92.063B	S92.136P	S92.221K	S92.302B	S92.345P	S92.506K	S95.091A	T17.410A	T22.349A	T23.751A	T27.2XXA	T34.811A	T78.00XA	T81.513A
S92.063K	S92.141B	S92.221P	S92.302K	S92.346B	S92.506P	S95.092A	T17.418A	T22.351A	T23.752A	T27.3XXA	T34.812A	T78.01XA	T81.514A
S92.063P	S92.141K	S92.222B	S92.302P	S92.346K	S92.511K	S95.099A	T17.420A	T22.352A	T23.759A	T27.4XXA	T34.819A	T78.02XA	T81.515A
S92.064B	S92.141P	S92.222K	S92.309B	S92.346P	S92.511P	S95.101A	T17.428A	T22.359A	T23.761A	T27.5XXA	T34.821A	T78.03XA	T81.516A
S92.064K	S92.142B	S92.222P	S92.309K	S92.351B	S92.512K	S95.102A	T17.490A	T22.361A	T23.762A	T27.6XXA	T34.822A	T78.04XA	T81.517A
S92.064P	S92.142K	S92.223B	S92.309P	S92.351K	S92.512P	S95.109A	T17.498A	T22.362A	T23.769A	T27.7XXA	T34.829A	T78.05XA	T81.518A
S92.065B	S92.142P	S92.223K	S92.311B	S92.351P	S92.513K	S95.111A	T17.500A	T22.369A	T23.771A	T28.1XXA	T34.831A	T78.06XA	T81.519A
S92.065K	S92.143B	S92.223P	S92.311K	S92.352B	S92.513P	S95.112A	T17.508A	T22.391A	T23.772A	T28.2XXA	T34.832A	T78.07XA	T81.520A
S92.065P	S92.143K	S92.224B	S92.311P	S92.352K	S92.514K	S95.119A	T17.510A	T22.392A	T23.779A	T28.6XXA	T34.839A	T78.08XA	T81.521A
S92.066B	S92.143P	S92.224K	S92.312B	S92.352P	S92.514P	S95.191A	T17.518A	T22.399A	T23.791A	T28.7XXA	T34.99XA	T78.09XA	T81.522A
S92.066K	S92.144B	S92.224P	S92.312K	S92.353B	S92.515K	S95.192A	T17.520A	T22.70XA	T23.792A	T33.011A	T67.0XXA	T78.2XXA	T81.523A
S92.066P	S92.144K	S92.225B	S92.312P	S92.353K	S92.515P	S95.199A	T17.528A	T22.711A	T23.799A	T33.012A	T69.021A	T79.2XXA	T81.524A
S92.101B	S92.144P	S92.225K	S92.313B	S92.353P	S92.516K	S95.201A	T17.590A	T22.712A	T24.301A	T33.019A	T69.022A	T79.7XXA	T81.525A
S92.101K	S92.145B	S92.225P	S92.313K	S92.354B	S92.516P	S95.202A	T17.598A	T22.719A	T24.302A	T33.02XA	T69.029A	T79.A0XA	T81.526A

Complication or Comorbidity (CC) (cont.) - Based on CMS data

T81.527A	T81.72XA	T82.319A	T82.522A	T82.847A	T83.21XA	T83.722A	T84.038A	T84.121A	T84.318A	T84.625A	T85.193A	T85.615A	T85.79XA
T81.528A	T81.83XA	T82.320A	T82.523A	T82.848A	T83.22XA	T83.723A	T84.039A	T84.122A	T84.320A	T84.629A	T85.199A	T85.618A	T85.810A
T81.529A	T82.01XA	T82.321A	T82.524A	T82.855A	T83.23XA	T83.724A	T84.050A	T84.123A	T84.328A	T84.63XA	T85.21XA	T85.620A	T85.810D
T81.530A	T82.02XA	T82.322A	T82.525A	T82.856A	T83.24XA	T83.728A	T84.051A	T84.124A	T84.390A	T84.69XA	T85.22XA	T85.621A	T85.820A
T81.531A	T82.03XA	T82.328A	T82.528A	T82.857A	T83.25XA	T83.729A	T84.052A	T84.125A	T84.398A	T84.7XXA	T85.29XA	T85.622A	T85.820D
T81.532A	T82.09XA	T82.329A	T82.529A	T82.858A	T83.29XA	T83.79XA	T84.053A	T84.126A	T84.410A	T84.81XA	T85.310A	T85.623A	T85.830A
T81.533A	T82.110A	T82.330A	T82.530A	T82.867A	T83.410A	T83.81XA	T84.058A	T84.127A	T84.418A	T84.82XA	T85.311A	T85.624A	T85.830D
T81.534A	T82.111A	T82.331A	T82.531A	T82.868A	T83.411A	T83.82XA	T84.059A	T84.129A	T84.420A	T84.83XA	T85.320A	T85.625A	T85.840A
T81.535A	T82.118A	T82.332A	T82.532A	T82.897A	T83.418A	T83.83XA	T84.060A	T84.190A	T84.428A	T84.84XA	T85.321A	T85.628A	T85.840D
T81.536A	T82.119A	T82.338A	T82.533A	T82.898A	T83.420A	T83.84XA	T84.061A	T84.191A	T84.490A	T84.85XA	T85.390A	T85.630A	T85.850A
T81.537A	T82.120A	T82.339A	T82.534A	T82.9XXA	T83.421A	T83.85XA	T84.062A	T84.192A	T84.498A	T84.86XA	T85.391A	T85.631A	T85.850D
T81.538A	T82.121A	T82.390A	T82.535A	T83.010A	T83.428A	T83.86XA	T84.063A	T84.193A	T84.50XA	T84.89XA	T85.41XA	T85.633A	T85.860A
T81.539A	T82.128A	T82.391A	T82.538A	T83.020A	T83.490A	T83.89XA	T84.068A	T84.194A	T84.51XA	T84.9XXA	T85.42XA	T85.635A	T85.860D
T81.590A	T82.129A	T82.392A	T82.539A	T83.030A	T83.491A	T83.9XXA	T84.069A	T84.195A	T84.52XA	T85.01XA	T85.43XA	T85.638A	T85.890A
T81.591A	T82.190A	T82.398A	T82.590A	T83.090A	T83.498A	T84.010A	T84.090A	T84.196A	T84.53XA	T85.02XA	T85.44XA	T85.690A	T85.890D
T81.592A	T82.191A	T82.399A	T82.591A	T83.110A	T83.510A	T84.011A	T84.091A	T84.197A	T84.54XA	T85.03XA	T85.49XA	T85.691A	T88.0XXA
T81.593A	T82.198A	T82.41XA	T82.592A	T83.111A	T83.511A	T84.012A	T84.092A	T84.199A	T84.59XA	T85.09XA	T85.510A	T85.692A	T88.1XXA
T81.594A	T82.199A	T82.42XA	T82.593A	T83.112A	T83.512A	T84.013A	T84.093A	T84.210A	T84.60XA	T85.110A	T85.511A	T85.693A	T88.2XXA
T81.595A	T82.211A	T82.43XA	T82.594A	T83.113A	T83.590A	T84.018A	T84.098A	T84.213A	T84.610A	T85.111A	T85.518A	T85.694A	T88.3XXA
T81.596A	T82.212A	T82.49XA	T82.595A	T83.118A	T83.591A	T84.019A	T84.099A	T84.216A	T84.611A	T85.112A	T85.520A	T85.695A	T88.6XXA
T81.597A	T82.213A	T82.510A	T82.598A	T83.120A	T83.592A	T84.020A	T84.110A	T84.218A	T84.612A	T85.113A	T85.521A	T85.698A	
T81.598A	T82.218A	T82.511A	T82.599A	T83.121A	T83.593A	T84.021A	T84.111A	T84.220A	T84.613A	T85.118A	T85.528A	T85.71XA	
T81.599A	T82.221A	T82.512A	T82.6XXA	T83.122A	T83.61XA	T84.022A	T84.112A	T84.223A	T84.614A	T85.120A	T85.590A	T85.72XA	
T81.60XA	T82.222A	T82.513A	T82.7XXA	T83.123A	T83.62XA	T84.023A	T84.113A	T84.226A	T84.615A	T85.121A	T85.591A	T85.730A	
T81.61XA	T82.223A	T82.514A	T82.817A	T83.128A	T83.69XA	T84.028A	T84.114A	T84.228A	T84.619A	T85.122A	T85.598A	T85.731A	
T81.69XA	T82.228A	T82.515A	T82.818A	T83.190A	T83.712A	T84.029A	T84.115A	T84.290A	T84.620A	T85.123A	T85.610A	T85.732A	
T81.710A	T82.310A	T82.518A	T82.827A	T83.191A	T83.713A	T84.030A	T84.116A	T84.293A	T84.621A	T85.128A	T85.611A	T85.733A	
T81.711A	T82.311A	T82.519A	T82.828A	T83.192A	T83.714A	T84.031A	T84.117A	T84.296A	T84.622A	T85.190A	T85.612A	T85.734A	
T81.718A	T82.312A	T82.520A	T82.837A	T83.193A	T83.718A	T84.032A	T84.119A	T84.298A	T84.623A	T85.191A	T85.613A	T85.735A	
T81.719A	T82.318A	T82.521A	T82.838A	T83.198A	T83.719A	T84.033A	T84.120A	T84.310A	T84.624A	T85.192A	T85.614A	T85.738A	

Complications or Comorbidities/Major Complications or Comorbidities (CC/MCC) Exclusions - Based on CMS data

H34.8110	M80.029P	M80.072K	M80.842A	M84.312P	M84.361K	M84.419P	M84.446K	M84.474A	M84.529P	M84.561K	M84.612A	M84.650P	M84.675K
H34.8111	M80.031A	M80.072P	M80.842K	M84.319K	M84.361P	M84.421A	M84.446P	M84.474K	M84.531A	M84.561P	M84.612K	M84.651A	M84.675P
H34.8112	M80.031K	M80.079A	M80.842P	M84.319P	M84.362K	M84.421K	M84.451A	M84.474P	M84.531K	M84.562A	M84.612P	M84.651K	M84.676A
H34.8120	M80.031P	M80.079K	M80.849A	M84.321K	M84.362P	M84.421P	M84.451K	M84.475A	M84.531P	M84.562K	M84.619A	M84.651P	M84.676K
H34.8121	M80.032A	M80.079P	M80.849K	M84.321P	M84.363K	M84.422A	M84.451P	M84.475K	M84.532A	M84.562P	M84.619K	M84.652A	M84.676P
H34.8122	M80.032K	M80.08XA	M80.849P	M84.322K	M84.363P	M84.422K	M84.452A	M84.475P	M84.532K	M84.563A	M84.619P	M84.652K	M84.68XA
H34.8130	M80.032P	M80.08XK	M80.851A	M84.322P	M84.364K	M84.422P	M84.452K	M84.476A	M84.532P	M84.563K	M84.621A	M84.652P	M84.68XK
H34.8131	M80.039A	M80.08XP	M80.851K	M84.329K	M84.364P	M84.429A	M84.452P	M84.476K	M84.533A	M84.563P	M84.621K	M84.653A	M84.68XP
H34.8132	M80.039K	M80.80XA	M80.851P	M84.329P	M84.369K	M84.429K	M84.453A	M84.476P	M84.533K	M84.564A	M84.621P	M84.653K	M84.750A
H34.8190	M80.039P	M80.80XK	M80.852A	M84.331K	M84.369P	M84.429P	M84.453K	M84.477A	M84.533P	M84.564K	M84.622A	M84.653P	M84.750K
H34.8191	M80.041A	M80.80XP	M80.852K	M84.331P	M84.371K	M84.431A	M84.453P	M84.477K	M84.534A	M84.564P	M84.622K	M84.659A	M84.750P
H34.8192	M80.041K	M80.811A	M80.852P	M84.332K	M84.371P	M84.431K	M84.454A	M84.477P	M84.534K	M84.569A	M84.622P	M84.659K	M84.751A
M48.50XA	M80.041P	M80.811K	M80.859A	M84.332P	M84.372K	M84.431P	M84.454K	M84.478A	M84.534P	M84.569K	M84.629A	M84.659P	M84.751K
M48.51XA	M80.042A	M80.811P	M80.859K	M84.333K	M84.372P	M84.432A	M84.454P	M84.478K	M84.539A	M84.569P	M84.629K	M84.661A	M84.751P
M48.52XA	M80.042K	M80.812A	M80.859P	M84.333P	M84.373K	M84.432K	M84.459A	M84.478P	M84.539K	M84.571A	M84.629P	M84.661K	M84.752A
M48.53XA	M80.042P	M80.812K	M80.861A	M84.334K	M84.373P	M84.432P	M84.459K	M84.479A	M84.539P	M84.571K	M84.631A	M84.661P	M84.752K
M48.54XA	M80.049A	M80.812P	M80.861K	M84.334P	M84.374K	M84.433A	M84.459P	M84.479K	M84.541A	M84.571P	M84.631K	M84.662A	M84.752P
M48.55XA	M80.049K	M80.819A	M80.861P	M84.339K	M84.374P	M84.433K	M84.461A	M84.479P	M84.541K	M84.572A	M84.631P	M84.662K	M84.753A
M48.56XA	M80.049P	M80.819K	M80.862A	M84.339P	M84.375K	M84.433P	M84.461K	M84.48XA	M84.541P	M84.572K	M84.632A	M84.662P	M84.753K
M48.57XA	M80.051A	M80.819P	M80.862K	M84.341K	M84.375P	M84.434A	M84.461P	M84.48XK	M84.542A	M84.572P	M84.632K	M84.663A	M84.753P
M48.58XA	M80.051K	M80.821A	M80.862P	M84.341P	M84.376K	M84.434K	M84.462A	M84.48XP	M84.542K	M84.573A	M84.632P	M84.663K	M84.754A
M80.00XA	M80.051P	M80.821K	M80.869A	M84.342K	M84.376P	M84.434P	M84.462K	M84.50XA	M84.542P	M84.573K	M84.633A	M84.663P	M84.754K
M80.00XK	M80.052A	M80.821P	M80.869K	M84.342P	M84.377K	M84.439A	M84.462P	M84.50XK	M84.549A	M84.573P	M84.633K	M84.664A	M84.754P
M80.00XP	M80.052K	M80.822A	M80.869P	M84.343K	M84.377P	M84.439K	M84.463A	M84.50XP	M84.549K	M84.574A	M84.633P	M84.664K	M84.755A
M80.011A	M80.052P	M80.822K	M80.871A	M84.343P	M84.378K	M84.439P	M84.463K	M84.511A	M84.549P	M84.574K	M84.634A	M84.664P	M84.755K
M80.011K	M80.059A	M80.822P	M80.871K	M84.344K	M84.378P	M84.441A	M84.463P	M84.511K	M84.550A	M84.574P	M84.634K	M84.669A	M84.755P
M80.011P	M80.059K	M80.829A	M80.871P	M84.344P	M84.379K	M84.441K	M84.464A	M84.511P	M84.550K	M84.575A	M84.634P	M84.669K	M84.756A
M80.012A	M80.059P	M80.829K	M80.872A	M84.345K	M84.379P	M84.441P	M84.464K	M84.512A	M84.550P	M84.575K	M84.639A	M84.669P	M84.756K
M80.012K	M80.061A	M80.829P	M80.872K	M84.345P	M84.38XK	M84.442A	M84.464P	M84.512K	M84.551A	M84.575P	M84.639K	M84.671A	M84.756P
M80.012P	M80.061K	M80.831A	M80.872P	M84.346K	M84.38XP	M84.442K	M84.469A	M84.512P	M84.551K	M84.576A	M84.639P	M84.671K	M84.757A
M80.019A	M80.061P	M80.831K	M80.879A	M84.346P	M84.40XA	M84.442P	M84.469K	M84.519A	M84.551P	M84.576K	M84.641A	M84.671P	M84.757K
M80.019K	M80.062A	M80.831P	M80.879K	M84.350K	M84.40XK	M84.443A	M84.469P	M84.519K	M84.552A	M84.576P	M84.641K	M84.672A	M84.757P
M80.019P	M80.062K	M80.832A	M80.879P	M84.350P	M84.40XP	M84.443K	M84.471A	M84.519P	M84.552K	M84.58XA	M84.641P	M84.672K	M84.758A
M80.021A	M80.062P	M80.832K	M80.88XA	M84.351K	M84.411A	M84.443P	M84.471K	M84.521A	M84.552P	M84.58XK	M84.642A	M84.672P	M84.758K
M80.021K	M80.069A	M80.832P	M80.88XK	M84.351P	M84.411K	M84.444A	M84.471P	M84.521K	M84.553A	M84.58XP	M84.642K	M84.673A	M84.758P
M80.021P	M80.069K	M80.839A	M80.88XP	M84.352K	M84.411P	M84.444K	M84.472A	M84.521P	M84.553K	M84.60XA	M84.642P	M84.673K	M84.759A
M80.022A	M80.069P	M80.839K	M84.30XA	M84.352P	M84.412A	M84.444P	M84.472K	M84.522A	M84.553P	M84.60XK	M84.649A	M84.673P	M84.759K
M80.022K	M80.071A	M80.839P	M84.30XK	M84.353K	M84.412K	M84.445A	M84.472P	M84.522K	M84.559A	M84.60XP	M84.649K	M84.674A	M84.759P
M80.022P	M80.071K	M80.841A	M84.311K	M84.353P	M84.412P	M84.445K	M84.473A	M84.522P	M84.559K	M84.611A	M84.649P	M84.674K	M97.01XA
M80.029A	M80.071P	M80.841K	M84.311P	M84.359K	M84.419A	M84.445P	M84.473K	M84.529A	M84.559P	M84.611K	M84.650A	M84.674P	M97.02XA
M80.029K	M80.072A	M80.841P	M84.312K	M84.359P	M84.419K	M84.446A	M84.473P	M84.529K	M84.561A	M84.611P	M84.650K	M84.675A	M97.11XA

Complications or Comorbidities/Major Complications or Comorbidities (CC/MCC) Exclusions (cont.) - Based on CMS data

M97.12XA	O36.4XX2	O41.1419	R40.2210	S02.11FB	S02.610A	S02.92XK	S06.2X4A	S06.369A	S06.896A	S12.030B	S12.250A	S12.530A	S14.105A
M97.21XA	O36.4XX3	O41.1420	R40.2211	S02.11FK	S02.610B	S04.011A	S06.2X5A	S06.370A	S06.897A	S12.030K	S12.250B	S12.531A	S14.106A
M97.22XA	O36.4XX4	O41.1421	R40.2212	S02.11GA	S02.610K	S04.012A	S06.2X6A	S06.371A	S06.898A	S12.031A	S12.250K	S12.531B	S14.107A
M97.31XA	O36.4XX5	O41.1422	R40.2213	S02.11GB	S02.611A	S04.019A	S06.2X7A	S06.372A	S06.899A	S12.031B	S12.251A	S12.531K	S14.108A
M97.32XA	O36.4XX9	O41.1423	R40.2214	S02.11GK	S02.611B	S04.02XA	S06.2X8A	S06.373A	S06.9X1A	S12.031K	S12.251B	S12.54XA	S14.111A
M97.41XA	O41.01X0	O41.1424	R40.2220	S02.11HA	S02.611K	S04.031A	S06.2X9A	S06.374A	S06.9X2A	S12.040A	S12.251K	S12.54XB	S14.112A
M97.42XA	O41.01X1	O41.1425	R40.2221	S02.11HB	S02.612A	S04.032A	S06.301A	S06.375A	S06.9X3A	S12.040B	S12.290A	S12.54XK	S14.113A
M97.8XXA	O41.01X2	O41.1429	R40.2222	S02.11HK	S02.612B	S04.039A	S06.302A	S06.376A	S06.9X4A	S12.040K	S12.290B	S12.550A	S14.114A
M97.9XXA	O41.01X3	O41.1430	R40.2223	S02.19XA	S02.612K	S04.041A	S06.303A	S06.377A	S06.9X5A	S12.041A	S12.290K	S12.550B	S14.115A
O31.8X10	O41.01X4	O41.1431	R40.2224	S02.19XB	S02.620A	S04.042A	S06.304A	S06.378A	S06.9X6A	S12.041B	S12.291A	S12.550K	S14.116A
O31.8X11	O41.01X5	O41.1432	R40.2310	S02.19XK	S02.620B	S04.049A	S06.305A	S06.379A	S06.9X7A	S12.041K	S12.291B	S12.551A	S14.117A
O31.8X12	O41.01X9	O41.1433	R40.2311	S02.2XXB	S02.620K	S04.10XA	S06.306A	S06.380A	S06.9X8A	S12.090A	S12.291K	S12.551B	S14.118A
O31.8X13	O41.02X0	O41.1434	R40.2312	S02.2XXK	S02.621A	S04.11XA	S06.307A	S06.381A	S06.9X9A	S12.090B	S12.300A	S12.551K	S14.121A
O31.8X14	O41.02X1	O41.1435	R40.2313	S02.30XA	S02.621B	S04.12XA	S06.308A	S06.382A	S07.0XXA	S12.090K	S12.300B	S12.590A	S14.122A
O31.8X15	O41.02X2	O41.1439	R40.2314	S02.30XB	S02.621K	S04.20XA	S06.309A	S06.383A	S07.1XXA	S12.091A	S12.300K	S12.590B	S14.123A
O31.8X19	O41.02X3	O60.10X0	R40.2320	S02.30XK	S02.622A	S04.21XA	S06.310A	S06.384A	S07.8XXA	S12.091B	S12.301A	S12.590K	S14.124A
O31.8X20	O41.02X4	O60.10X1	R40.2321	S02.31XA	S02.622B	S04.22XA	S06.311A	S06.385A	S07.9XXA	S12.091K	S12.301B	S12.591A	S14.125A
O31.8X21	O41.02X5	O60.10X2	R40.2322	S02.31XB	S02.622K	S04.30XA	S06.312A	S06.386A	S09.0XXA	S12.100A	S12.301K	S12.591B	S14.126A
O31.8X22	O41.02X9	O60.10X3	R40.2323	S02.31XK	S02.630A	S04.31XA	S06.313A	S06.387A	S09.20XA	S12.100B	S12.330A	S12.591K	S14.127A
O31.8X23	O41.03X0	O60.10X4	R40.2324	S02.32XA	S02.630B	S04.32XA	S06.314A	S06.388A	S09.21XA	S12.100K	S12.330B	S12.600A	S14.128A
O31.8X24	O41.03X1	O60.10X5	R40.2340	S02.32XB	S02.630K	S04.40XA	S06.315A	S06.389A	S09.22XA	S12.101A	S12.330K	S12.600B	S14.131A
O31.8X25	O41.03X2	O60.10X9	R40.2341	S02.32XK	S02.631A	S04.41XA	S06.316A	S06.4X0A	S09.301A	S12.101B	S12.331A	S12.600K	S14.132A
O31.8X29	O41.03X3	O60.12X0	R40.2342	S02.400A	S02.631B	S04.42XA	S06.317A	S06.4X1A	S09.302A	S12.101K	S12.331B	S12.601A	S14.133A
O31.8X30	O41.03X4	O60.12X1	R40.2343	S02.400B	S02.631K	S04.50XA	S06.318A	S06.4X2A	S09.309A	S12.110A	S12.331K	S12.601B	S14.134A
O31.8X31	O41.03X5	O60.12X2	R40.2344	S02.400K	S02.632A	S04.51XA	S06.319A	S06.4X3A	S09.311A	S12.110B	S12.34XA	S12.601K	S14.135A
O31.8X32	O41.03X9	O60.12X3	S01.101A	S02.401A	S02.632B	S04.52XA	S06.320A	S06.4X4A	S09.312A	S12.110K	S12.34XB	S12.630A	S14.136A
O31.8X33	O41.1010	O60.12X4	S01.102A	S02.401B	S02.632K	S04.60XA	S06.321A	S06.4X5A	S09.313A	S12.111A	S12.34XK	S12.630B	S14.137A
O31.8X34	O41.1011	O60.12X5	S01.109A	S02.401K	S02.640A	S04.61XA	S06.322A	S06.4X6A	S09.319A	S12.111B	S12.350A	S12.630K	S14.138A
O31.8X35	O41.1012	O60.12X9	S02.0XXA	S02.402A	S02.640B	S04.62XA	S06.323A	S06.4X7A	S09.391A	S12.111K	S12.350B	S12.631A	S14.141A
O31.8X39	O41.1013	O60.13X0	S02.0XXB	S02.402B	S02.640K	S04.70XA	S06.324A	S06.4X8A	S09.392A	S12.112A	S12.350K	S12.631B	S14.142A
O36.0110	O41.1014	O60.13X1	S02.0XXK	S02.402K	S02.641A	S04.71XA	S06.325A	S06.4X9A	S09.399A	S12.112B	S12.351A	S12.631K	S14.143A
O36.0111	O41.1015	O60.13X2	S02.101A	S02.40AA	S02.641B	S04.72XA	S06.326A	S06.5X0A	S11.011A	S12.112K	S12.351B	S12.64XA	S14.144A
O36.0112	O41.1019	O60.13X3	S02.101B	S02.40AB	S02.641K	S04.811A	S06.327A	S06.5X1A	S11.012A	S12.120A	S12.351K	S12.64XB	S14.145A
O36.0113	O41.1020	O60.13X4	S02.101K	S02.40AK	S02.642A	S04.812A	S06.328A	S06.5X2A	S11.013A	S12.120B	S12.390A	S12.64XK	S14.146A
O36.0114	O41.1021	O60.13X5	S02.102A	S02.40BA	S02.642B	S04.819A	S06.329A	S06.5X3A	S11.014A	S12.120K	S12.390B	S12.650A	S14.147A
O36.0115	O41.1022	O60.13X9	S02.102B	S02.40BB	S02.642K	S04.891A	S06.330A	S06.5X4A	S11.015A	S12.121A	S12.390K	S12.650B	S14.148A
O36.0119	O41.1023	O60.14X0	S02.102K	S02.40BK	S02.650A	S04.892A	S06.331A	S06.5X5A	S11.019A	S12.121B	S12.391A	S12.650K	S14.151A
O36.0120	O41.1024	O60.14X1	S02.109A	S02.40CA	S02.650B	S04.899A	S06.332A	S06.5X6A	S11.021A	S12.121K	S12.391B	S12.651A	S14.152A
O36.0121	O41.1025	O60.14X2	S02.109B	S02.40CB	S02.650K	S04.9XXA	S06.333A	S06.5X7A	S11.022A	S12.130A	S12.391K	S12.651B	S14.153A
O36.0122	O41.1029	O60.14X3	S02.109K	S02.40CK	S02.651A	S05.20XA	S06.334A	S06.5X8A	S11.023A	S12.130B	S12.400A	S12.651K	S14.154A
O36.0123	O41.1030	O60.14X4	S02.110A	S02.40DA	S02.651B	S05.21XA	S06.335A	S06.5X9A	S11.024A	S12.130K	S12.400B	S12.690A	S14.155A
O36.0124	O41.1031	O60.14X5	S02.110B	S02.40DB	S02.651K	S05.22XA	S06.336A	S06.6X0A	S11.025A	S12.131A	S12.400K	S12.690B	S14.156A
O36.0125	O41.1032	O60.14X9	S02.110K	S02.40DK	S02.652A	S05.30XA	S06.337A	S06.6X1A	S11.029A	S12.131B	S12.401A	S12.690K	S14.157A
O36.0129	O41.1033	O60.20X0	S02.111A	S02.40EA	S02.652B	S05.31XA	S06.338A	S06.6X2A	S11.031A	S12.131K	S12.401B	S12.691A	S14.158A
O36.0130	O41.1034	O60.20X1	S02.111B	S02.40EB	S02.652K	S05.32XA	S06.339A	S06.6X3A	S11.032A	S12.14XA	S12.401K	S12.691B	S15.001A
O36.0131	O41.1035	O60.20X2	S02.111K	S02.40EK	S02.66XA	S05.40XA	S06.340A	S06.6X4A	S11.033A	S12.14XB	S12.430A	S12.691K	S15.002A
O36.0132	O41.1039	O60.20X3	S02.112A	S02.40FA	S02.66XB	S05.41XA	S06.341A	S06.6X5A	S11.034A	S12.14XK	S12.430B	S12.8XXA	S15.009A
O36.0133	O41.1210	O60.20X4	S02.112B	S02.40FB	S02.66XK	S05.42XA	S06.342A	S06.6X6A	S11.035A	S12.150A	S12.430K	S12.9XXA	S15.011A
O36.0134	O41.1211	O60.20X5	S02.112K	S02.40FK	S02.670A	S05.50XA	S06.343A	S06.6X7A	S11.039A	S12.150B	S12.431A	S13.0XXA	S15.012A
O36.0135	O41.1212	O60.20X9	S02.113A	S02.411A	S02.670B	S05.51XA	S06.344A	S06.6X8A	S11.10XA	S12.150K	S12.431B	S13.100A	S15.019A
O36.0139	O41.1213	O60.22X0	S02.113B	S02.411B	S02.670K	S05.52XA	S06.345A	S06.6X9A	S11.11XA	S12.151A	S12.431K	S13.101A	S15.021A
O36.0910	O41.1214	O60.22X1	S02.113K	S02.411K	S02.671A	S05.70XA	S06.346A	S06.811A	S11.12XA	S12.151B	S12.44XA	S13.110A	S15.022A
O36.0911	O41.1215	O60.22X2	S02.118A	S02.412A	S02.671B	S05.71XA	S06.347A	S06.812A	S11.13XA	S12.151K	S12.44XB	S13.111A	S15.029A
O36.0912	O41.1219	O60.22X3	S02.118B	S02.412B	S02.671K	S05.72XA	S06.348A	S06.813A	S11.14XA	S12.190A	S12.44XK	S13.120A	S15.091A
O36.0913	O41.1220	O60.22X4	S02.118K	S02.412K	S02.672A	S05.8X1A	S06.349A	S06.814A	S11.15XA	S12.190B	S12.450A	S13.121A	S15.092A
O36.0914	O41.1221	O60.22X5	S02.119A	S02.413A	S02.672B	S05.8X2A	S06.350A	S06.815A	S11.20XA	S12.190K	S12.450B	S13.130A	S15.099A
O36.0915	O41.1222	O60.22X9	S02.119B	S02.413B	S02.672K	S05.8X9A	S06.351A	S06.816A	S11.21XA	S12.191A	S12.450K	S13.131A	S15.101A
O36.0919	O41.1223	O60.23X0	S02.119K	S02.413K	S02.69XA	S05.91XA	S06.352A	S06.817A	S11.22XA	S12.191B	S12.451A	S13.140A	S15.102A
O36.0920	O41.1224	O60.23X1	S02.11AA	S02.42XA	S02.69XB	S05.92XA	S06.353A	S06.818A	S11.23XA	S12.191K	S12.451B	S13.141A	S15.109A
O36.0921	O41.1225	O60.23X2	S02.11AB	S02.42XB	S02.69XK	S06.0X1A	S06.354A	S06.819A	S11.24XA	S12.200A	S12.451K	S13.150A	S15.111A
O36.0922	O41.1229	O60.23X3	S02.11AK	S02.42XK	S02.80XA	S06.0X9A	S06.355A	S06.821A	S11.25XA	S12.200B	S12.490A	S13.151A	S15.112A
O36.0923	O41.1230	O60.23X4	S02.11BA	S02.5XXA	S02.80XB	S06.1X0A	S06.356A	S06.822A	S12.000A	S12.200K	S12.490B	S13.160A	S15.119A
O36.0924	O41.1231	O60.23X5	S02.11BB	S02.600A	S02.80XK	S06.1X1A	S06.357A	S06.823A	S12.000B	S12.201A	S12.490K	S13.161A	S15.121A
O36.0925	O41.1232	O60.23X9	S02.11BK	S02.600B	S02.81XA	S06.1X2A	S06.358A	S06.824A	S12.000K	S12.201B	S12.491A	S13.170A	S15.122A
O36.0929	O41.1233	R40.2110	S02.11CA	S02.600K	S02.81XB	S06.1X3A	S06.359A	S06.825A	S12.001A	S12.201K	S12.491B	S13.171A	S15.129A
O36.0930	O41.1234	R40.2111	S02.11CB	S02.601A	S02.81XK	S06.1X4A	S06.360A	S06.826A	S12.001B	S12.230A	S12.491K	S13.180A	S15.191A
O36.0931	O41.1235	R40.2112	S02.11CK	S02.601B	S02.82XA	S06.1X5A	S06.361A	S06.827A	S12.001K	S12.230B	S12.500A	S13.181A	S15.192A
O36.0932	O41.1239	R40.2113	S02.11DA	S02.601K	S02.82XB	S06.1X6A	S06.362A	S06.828A	S12.01XA	S12.230K	S12.500B	S13.20XA	S15.199A
O36.0933	O41.1410	R40.2114	S02.11DB	S02.602A	S02.82XK	S06.1X7A	S06.363A	S06.829A	S12.01XB	S12.231A	S12.500K	S13.29XA	S15.201A
O36.0934	O41.1411	R40.2120	S02.11DK	S02.602B	S02.91XA	S06.1X8A	S06.364A	S06.891A	S12.01XK	S12.231B	S12.501A	S14.0XXA	S15.202A
O36.0935	O41.1412	R40.2121	S02.11EA	S02.602K	S02.91XB	S06.1X9A	S06.365A	S06.892A	S12.02XA	S12.231K	S12.501B	S14.101A	S15.209A
O36.0939	O41.1413	R40.2122	S02.11EB	S02.609A	S02.91XK	S06.2X1A	S06.366A	S06.893A	S12.02XB	S12.24XA	S12.501K	S14.102A	S15.211A
O36.4XX0	O41.1414	R40.2123	S02.11EK	S02.609B	S02.92XA	S06.2X2A	S06.367A	S06.894A	S12.02XK	S12.24XB	S12.530A	S14.103A	S15.212A
O36.4XX1	O41.1415	R40.2124	S02.11FA	S02.609K	S02.92XB	S06.2X3A	S06.368A	S06.895A	S12.030A	S12.24XK	S12.530B	S14.104A	S15.219A

Complications or Comorbidities/Major Complications or Comorbidities (CC/MCC) Exclusions (cont.) - Based on CMS data

S15.221A	S21.451A	S22.041K	S22.21XB	S25.199A	S27.322A	S31.630A	S32.032K	S32.139B	S32.414A	S32.454K	S32.502B	S34.01XA	S35.493A
S15.222A	S21.452A	S22.042A	S22.21XK	S25.20XA	S27.329A	S31.631A	S32.038A	S32.139K	S32.414B	S32.455A	S32.502K	S34.02XA	S35.494A
S15.229A	S21.459A	S22.042B	S22.22XA	S25.21XA	S27.331A	S31.632A	S32.038B	S32.14XA	S32.414K	S32.455B	S32.509A	S34.101A	S35.495A
S15.291A	S21.90XA	S22.042K	S22.22XB	S25.22XA	S27.332A	S31.633A	S32.038K	S32.14XB	S32.415A	S32.455K	S32.509B	S34.102A	S35.496A
S15.292A	S21.91XA	S22.048A	S22.22XK	S25.29XA	S27.339A	S31.634A	S32.039A	S32.14XK	S32.415B	S32.456A	S32.509K	S34.103A	S35.50XA
S15.299A	S21.92XA	S22.048B	S22.23XA	S25.301A	S27.391A	S31.635A	S32.039B	S32.15XA	S32.415K	S32.456B	S32.511A	S34.104A	S35.511A
S15.301A	S21.93XA	S22.048K	S22.23XB	S25.302A	S27.392A	S31.639A	S32.039K	S32.15XB	S32.416A	S32.456K	S32.511B	S34.105A	S35.512A
S15.302A	S21.94XA	S22.049A	S22.23XK	S25.309A	S27.399A	S31.640A	S32.040A	S32.15XK	S32.416B	S32.461A	S32.511K	S34.109A	S35.513A
S15.309A	S21.95XA	S22.049B	S22.24XA	S25.311A	S27.401A	S31.641A	S32.040B	S32.16XA	S32.416K	S32.461B	S32.512A	S34.111A	S35.514A
S15.311A	S22.000A	S22.049K	S22.24XB	S25.312A	S27.402A	S31.642A	S32.040K	S32.16XB	S32.421A	S32.461K	S32.512B	S34.112A	S35.515A
S15.312A	S22.000B	S22.050A	S22.24XK	S25.319A	S27.409A	S31.643A	S32.041A	S32.16XK	S32.421B	S32.462A	S32.512K	S34.113A	S35.516A
S15.319A	S22.000K	S22.050B	S22.31XA	S25.321A	S27.411A	S31.644A	S32.041B	S32.17XA	S32.421K	S32.462B	S32.519A	S34.114A	S35.531A
S15.321A	S22.001A	S22.050K	S22.31XB	S25.322A	S27.412A	S31.645A	S32.041K	S32.17XB	S32.422A	S32.462K	S32.519B	S34.115A	S35.532A
S15.322A	S22.001B	S22.051A	S22.31XK	S25.329A	S27.419A	S31.649A	S32.042A	S32.17XK	S32.422B	S32.463A	S32.519K	S34.119A	S35.533A
S15.329A	S22.001K	S22.051B	S22.32XA	S25.391A	S27.421A	S31.650A	S32.042B	S32.19XA	S32.422K	S32.463B	S32.591A	S34.121A	S35.534A
S15.391A	S22.002A	S22.051K	S22.32XB	S25.392A	S27.422A	S31.651A	S32.042K	S32.19XB	S32.423A	S32.463K	S32.591B	S34.122A	S35.535A
S15.392A	S22.002B	S22.052A	S22.32XK	S25.399A	S27.429A	S31.652A	S32.048A	S32.19XK	S32.423B	S32.464A	S32.591K	S34.123A	S35.536A
S15.399A	S22.002K	S22.052B	S22.39XA	S25.401A	S27.431A	S31.653A	S32.048B	S32.2XXA	S32.423K	S32.464B	S32.592A	S34.124A	S35.59XA
S15.8XXA	S22.008A	S22.052K	S22.39XB	S25.402A	S27.432A	S31.654A	S32.048K	S32.2XXB	S32.424A	S32.464K	S32.592B	S34.125A	S35.8X1A
S15.9XXA	S22.008B	S22.058A	S22.39XK	S25.409A	S27.439A	S31.655A	S32.049A	S32.2XXK	S32.424B	S32.465A	S32.592K	S34.129A	S35.8X8A
S17.0XXA	S22.008K	S22.058B	S22.41XA	S25.411A	S27.491A	S31.659A	S32.049B	S32.301A	S32.424K	S32.465B	S32.599A	S34.131A	S35.8X9A
S17.8XXA	S22.009A	S22.058K	S22.41XB	S25.412A	S27.492A	S32.000A	S32.049K	S32.301B	S32.425A	S32.465K	S32.599B	S34.132A	S35.90XA
S17.9XXA	S22.009B	S22.059A	S22.41XK	S25.419A	S27.499A	S32.000B	S32.050A	S32.301K	S32.425B	S32.466A	S32.599K	S34.139A	S35.91XA
S21.101A	S22.009K	S22.059B	S22.42XA	S25.421A	S27.50XA	S32.000K	S32.050B	S32.302A	S32.425K	S32.466B	S32.601A	S34.3XXA	S35.99XA
S21.102A	S22.010A	S22.059K	S22.42XB	S25.422A	S27.51XA	S32.001A	S32.050K	S32.302B	S32.426A	S32.466K	S32.601B	S35.00XA	S36.00XA
S21.109A	S22.010B	S22.060A	S22.42XK	S25.429A	S27.52XA	S32.001B	S32.051A	S32.302K	S32.426B	S32.471A	S32.601K	S35.01XA	S36.020A
S21.111A	S22.010K	S22.060B	S22.43XA	S25.491A	S27.53XA	S32.001K	S32.051B	S32.309A	S32.426K	S32.471B	S32.602A	S35.02XA	S36.021A
S21.112A	S22.011A	S22.060K	S22.43XB	S25.492A	S27.59XA	S32.002A	S32.051K	S32.309B	S32.431A	S32.471K	S32.602B	S35.09XA	S36.029A
S21.119A	S22.011B	S22.061A	S22.43XK	S25.499A	S27.60XA	S32.002B	S32.052A	S32.309K	S32.431B	S32.472A	S32.602K	S35.10XA	S36.030A
S21.121A	S22.011K	S22.061B	S22.49XA	S25.501A	S27.63XA	S32.002K	S32.052B	S32.311A	S32.431K	S32.472B	S32.609A	S35.11XA	S36.031A
S21.122A	S22.012A	S22.061K	S22.49XB	S25.502A	S27.69XA	S32.008A	S32.052K	S32.311B	S32.432A	S32.472K	S32.609B	S35.12XA	S36.032A
S21.129A	S22.012B	S22.062A	S22.49XK	S25.509A	S27.802A	S32.008B	S32.058A	S32.311K	S32.432B	S32.473A	S32.609K	S35.19XA	S36.039A
S21.131A	S22.012K	S22.062B	S22.5XXA	S25.511A	S27.803A	S32.008K	S32.058B	S32.312A	S32.432K	S32.473B	S32.611A	S35.211A	S36.09XA
S21.132A	S22.018A	S22.062K	S22.5XXB	S25.512A	S27.808A	S32.009A	S32.058K	S32.312B	S32.433A	S32.473K	S32.611B	S35.212A	S36.112A
S21.139A	S22.018B	S22.068A	S22.5XXK	S25.519A	S27.809A	S32.009B	S32.059A	S32.312K	S32.433B	S32.474A	S32.611K	S35.218A	S36.113A
S21.141A	S22.018K	S22.068B	S22.9XXA	S25.591A	S27.812A	S32.009K	S32.059B	S32.313A	S32.433K	S32.474B	S32.612A	S35.219A	S36.114A
S21.142A	S22.019A	S22.068K	S22.9XXB	S25.592A	S27.813A	S32.010A	S32.059K	S32.313B	S32.434A	S32.474K	S32.612B	S35.221A	S36.115A
S21.149A	S22.019B	S22.069A	S22.9XXK	S25.599A	S27.818A	S32.010B	S32.10XA	S32.313K	S32.434B	S32.475A	S32.612K	S35.222A	S36.116A
S21.151A	S22.019K	S22.069B	S24.0XXA	S25.801A	S27.819A	S32.010K	S32.10XB	S32.314A	S32.434K	S32.475B	S32.613A	S35.228A	S36.118A
S21.152A	S22.020A	S22.069K	S24.101A	S25.802A	S27.892A	S32.011A	S32.10XK	S32.314B	S32.435A	S32.475K	S32.613B	S35.229A	S36.119A
S21.159A	S22.020B	S22.070A	S24.102A	S25.809A	S27.893A	S32.011B	S32.110A	S32.314K	S32.435B	S32.476A	S32.613K	S35.231A	S36.122A
S21.301A	S22.020K	S22.070B	S24.103A	S25.811A	S27.898A	S32.011K	S32.110B	S32.315A	S32.435K	S32.476B	S32.614A	S35.232A	S36.123A
S21.302A	S22.021A	S22.070K	S24.104A	S25.812A	S27.899A	S32.012A	S32.110K	S32.315B	S32.436A	S32.476K	S32.614B	S35.238A	S36.128A
S21.309A	S22.021B	S22.071A	S24.111A	S25.819A	S27.9XXA	S32.012B	S32.111A	S32.315K	S32.436B	S32.481A	S32.614K	S35.239A	S36.129A
S21.311A	S22.021K	S22.071B	S24.112A	S25.891A	S28.1XXA	S32.012K	S32.111B	S32.316A	S32.436K	S32.481B	S32.615A	S35.291A	S36.13XA
S21.312A	S22.022A	S22.071K	S24.113A	S25.892A	S29.021A	S32.018A	S32.111K	S32.316B	S32.441A	S32.481K	S32.615B	S35.292A	S36.200A
S21.319A	S22.022B	S22.072A	S24.114A	S25.899A	S29.029A	S32.018B	S32.112A	S32.316K	S32.441B	S32.482A	S32.615K	S35.298A	S36.201A
S21.321A	S22.022K	S22.072B	S24.131A	S25.90XA	S31.001A	S32.018K	S32.112B	S32.391A	S32.441K	S32.482B	S32.616A	S35.299A	S36.202A
S21.322A	S22.028A	S22.072K	S24.132A	S25.91XA	S31.011A	S32.019A	S32.112K	S32.391B	S32.442A	S32.482K	S32.616B	S35.311A	S36.209A
S21.329A	S22.028B	S22.078A	S24.133A	S25.99XA	S31.021A	S32.019B	S32.119A	S32.391K	S32.442B	S32.483A	S32.616K	S35.318A	S36.220A
S21.331A	S22.028K	S22.078B	S24.134A	S26.00XA	S31.031A	S32.019K	S32.119B	S32.392A	S32.442K	S32.483B	S32.691A	S35.319A	S36.221A
S21.332A	S22.029A	S22.078K	S24.141A	S26.01XA	S31.041A	S32.020A	S32.119K	S32.392B	S32.443A	S32.483K	S32.691B	S35.321A	S36.222A
S21.339A	S22.029B	S22.079A	S24.142A	S26.020A	S31.051A	S32.020B	S32.120A	S32.392K	S32.443B	S32.484A	S32.691K	S35.328A	S36.229A
S21.341A	S22.029K	S22.079B	S24.143A	S26.021A	S31.600A	S32.020K	S32.120B	S32.399A	S32.443K	S32.484B	S32.692A	S35.329A	S36.230A
S21.342A	S22.030A	S22.079K	S24.144A	S26.022A	S31.601A	S32.021A	S32.120K	S32.399B	S32.444A	S32.484K	S32.692B	S35.331A	S36.231A
S21.349A	S22.030B	S22.080A	S24.151A	S26.09XA	S31.602A	S32.021B	S32.121A	S32.399K	S32.444B	S32.485A	S32.692K	S35.338A	S36.232A
S21.351A	S22.030K	S22.080B	S24.152A	S26.10XA	S31.603A	S32.021K	S32.121B	S32.401A	S32.444K	S32.485B	S32.699A	S35.339A	S36.239A
S21.352A	S22.031A	S22.080K	S24.153A	S26.11XA	S31.604A	S32.022A	S32.121K	S32.401B	S32.445A	S32.485K	S32.699B	S35.341A	S36.240A
S21.359A	S22.031B	S22.081A	S24.154A	S26.12XA	S31.605A	S32.022B	S32.122A	S32.401K	S32.445B	S32.486A	S32.699K	S35.348A	S36.241A
S21.401A	S22.031K	S22.081B	S25.00XA	S26.19XA	S31.609A	S32.022K	S32.122B	S32.402A	S32.445K	S32.486B	S32.810A	S35.349A	S36.242A
S21.402A	S22.032A	S22.081K	S25.01XA	S26.90XA	S31.610A	S32.028A	S32.122K	S32.402B	S32.446A	S32.486K	S32.810B	S35.401A	S36.249A
S21.409A	S22.032B	S22.082A	S25.02XA	S26.91XA	S31.611A	S32.028B	S32.129A	S32.402K	S32.446B	S32.491A	S32.810K	S35.402A	S36.250A
S21.411A	S22.032K	S22.082B	S25.09XA	S26.92XA	S31.612A	S32.028K	S32.129B	S32.409A	S32.446K	S32.491B	S32.811A	S35.403A	S36.251A
S21.412A	S22.038A	S22.082K	S25.101A	S26.99XA	S31.613A	S32.029A	S32.129K	S32.409B	S32.451A	S32.491K	S32.811B	S35.404A	S36.252A
S21.419A	S22.038B	S22.088A	S25.102A	S27.0XXA	S31.614A	S32.029B	S32.130A	S32.409K	S32.451B	S32.492A	S32.811K	S35.405A	S36.259A
S21.421A	S22.038K	S22.088B	S25.109A	S27.1XXA	S31.615A	S32.029K	S32.130B	S32.411A	S32.451K	S32.492B	S32.82XA	S35.406A	S36.260A
S21.422A	S22.039A	S22.088K	S25.111A	S27.2XXA	S31.619A	S32.030A	S32.130K	S32.411B	S32.452A	S32.492K	S32.82XB	S35.411A	S36.261A
S21.429A	S22.039B	S22.089A	S25.112A	S27.301A	S31.620A	S32.030B	S32.131A	S32.411K	S32.452B	S32.499A	S32.82XK	S35.412A	S36.262A
S21.431A	S22.039K	S22.089B	S25.119A	S27.302A	S31.621A	S32.030K	S32.131B	S32.412A	S32.452K	S32.499B	S32.89XA	S35.413A	S36.269A
S21.432A	S22.040A	S22.089K	S25.121A	S27.309A	S31.622A	S32.031A	S32.131K	S32.412B	S32.453A	S32.499K	S32.89XB	S35.414A	S36.290A
S21.439A	S22.040B	S22.20XA	S25.122A	S27.311A	S31.623A	S32.031B	S32.132A	S32.412K	S32.453B	S32.501A	S32.89XK	S35.415A	S36.291A
S21.441A	S22.040K	S22.20XB	S25.129A	S27.312A	S31.624A	S32.031K	S32.132B	S32.413A	S32.453K	S32.501B	S32.9XXA	S35.416A	S36.292A
S21.442A	S22.041A	S22.20XK	S25.191A	S27.319A	S31.625A	S32.032A	S32.132K	S32.413B	S32.454A	S32.501K	S32.9XXB	S35.491A	S36.299A
S21.449A	S22.041B	S22.21XA	S25.192A	S27.321A	S31.629A	S32.032B	S32.139A	S32.413K	S32.454B	S32.502A	S32.9XXK	S35.492A	S36.30XA

Complications or Comorbidities/Major Complications or Comorbidities (CC/MCC) Exclusions (cont.) - Based on CMS data

S36.32XA	S37.041A	S42.019K	S42.124B	S42.201K	S42.242A	S42.293A	S42.334K	S42.365A	S42.425K	S42.453A	S42.491B	S45.211A	S49.002P
S36.33XA	S37.042A	S42.019P	S42.124K	S42.201P	S42.242B	S42.293B	S42.334P	S42.365B	S42.425P	S42.453B	S42.491K	S45.212A	S49.009A
S36.39XA	S37.049A	S42.021B	S42.124P	S42.202A	S42.242K	S42.293K	S42.335A	S42.365K	S42.426A	S42.453K	S42.491P	S45.219A	S49.009K
S36.400A	S37.051A	S42.021K	S42.125B	S42.202B	S42.242P	S42.293P	S42.335B	S42.365P	S42.426B	S42.453P	S42.492A	S45.291A	S49.009P
S36.408A	S37.052A	S42.021P	S42.125K	S42.202K	S42.249A	S42.294A	S42.335K	S42.366A	S42.426K	S42.454A	S42.492B	S45.292A	S49.011A
S36.409A	S37.059A	S42.022B	S42.125P	S42.202P	S42.249B	S42.294B	S42.335P	S42.366B	S42.426P	S42.454B	S42.492K	S45.299A	S49.011K
S36.410A	S37.061A	S42.022K	S42.126B	S42.209A	S42.249K	S42.294K	S42.336A	S42.366K	S42.431A	S42.454K	S42.492P	S45.301A	S49.011P
S36.418A	S37.062A	S42.022P	S42.126K	S42.209B	S42.249P	S42.294P	S42.336B	S42.366P	S42.431B	S42.454P	S42.493A	S45.302A	S49.012A
S36.419A	S37.069A	S42.023B	S42.126P	S42.209P	S42.251A	S42.295A	S42.336K	S42.391A	S42.431K	S42.455A	S42.493B	S45.309A	S49.012K
S36.420A	S37.091A	S42.023K	S42.131B	S42.211A	S42.251B	S42.295B	S42.336P	S42.391B	S42.431P	S42.455B	S42.493K	S45.311A	S49.012P
S36.428A	S37.092A	S42.023P	S42.131K	S42.211B	S42.251K	S42.295K	S42.341A	S42.391K	S42.432A	S42.455K	S42.493P	S45.312A	S49.019A
S36.429A	S37.099A	S42.024B	S42.131P	S42.211K	S42.251P	S42.295P	S42.341B	S42.391P	S42.432B	S42.455P	S42.494A	S45.319A	S49.019K
S36.430A	S37.10XA	S42.024K	S42.132B	S42.211P	S42.252A	S42.296A	S42.341K	S42.392A	S42.432K	S42.456A	S42.494B	S45.391A	S49.019P
S36.438A	S37.12XA	S42.024P	S42.132K	S42.212A	S42.252B	S42.296B	S42.341P	S42.392B	S42.432P	S42.456B	S42.494K	S45.392A	S49.021A
S36.439A	S37.13XA	S42.025B	S42.132P	S42.212B	S42.252K	S42.296P	S42.342A	S42.392K	S42.433A	S42.456K	S42.494P	S45.399A	S49.021K
S36.490A	S37.19XA	S42.025K	S42.133B	S42.212K	S42.252P	S42.301A	S42.342B	S42.392P	S42.433B	S42.456P	S42.495A	S45.801A	S49.021P
S36.498A	S37.20XA	S42.025P	S42.133K	S42.212P	S42.253A	S42.301B	S42.342K	S42.399A	S42.433K	S42.461A	S42.495B	S45.802A	S49.022A
S36.499A	S37.22XA	S42.026B	S42.133P	S42.213A	S42.253B	S42.301K	S42.342P	S42.399B	S42.433P	S42.461B	S42.495K	S45.809A	S49.022K
S36.500A	S37.23XA	S42.026K	S42.134B	S42.213B	S42.253K	S42.301P	S42.343A	S42.399K	S42.434A	S42.461K	S42.495P	S45.811A	S49.022P
S36.501A	S37.29XA	S42.026P	S42.134K	S42.213K	S42.253P	S42.302A	S42.343B	S42.399P	S42.434B	S42.461P	S42.496A	S45.812A	S49.029A
S36.502A	S37.30XA	S42.031B	S42.134P	S42.214A	S42.254A	S42.302B	S42.343K	S42.401A	S42.434K	S42.462A	S42.496B	S45.819A	S49.029K
S36.503A	S37.32XA	S42.031K	S42.135B	S42.214B	S42.254B	S42.302K	S42.343P	S42.401B	S42.434P	S42.462B	S42.496K	S45.891A	S49.029P
S36.508A	S37.33XA	S42.031P	S42.135K	S42.214K	S42.254K	S42.302P	S42.344A	S42.401K	S42.435A	S42.462K	S42.496P	S45.892A	S49.031A
S36.509A	S37.39XA	S42.032B	S42.135P	S42.214P	S42.254P	S42.309A	S42.344B	S42.401P	S42.435B	S42.462P	S42.90XA	S45.899A	S49.031K
S36.510A	S37.60XA	S42.032K	S42.136B	S42.215A	S42.255A	S42.309B	S42.344K	S42.402A	S42.435K	S42.463A	S42.90XB	S45.901A	S49.031P
S36.511A	S37.62XA	S42.032P	S42.136K	S42.215B	S42.255B	S42.309K	S42.344P	S42.402B	S42.436A	S42.463B	S42.90XK	S45.902A	S49.032A
S36.512A	S37.63XA	S42.033B	S42.136P	S42.215K	S42.255K	S42.309P	S42.345A	S42.402K	S42.436B	S42.463K	S42.90XP	S45.909A	S49.032K
S36.513A	S37.69XA	S42.033K	S42.141B	S42.215P	S42.255P	S42.311A	S42.345B	S42.402P	S42.436P	S42.463P	S42.91XA	S45.911A	S49.039A
S36.518A	S37.812A	S42.033P	S42.141K	S42.216A	S42.256A	S42.311K	S42.345K	S42.409A	S42.441A	S42.464A	S42.91XB	S45.912A	S49.039K
S36.519A	S37.813A	S42.034B	S42.141P	S42.216B	S42.256B	S42.311P	S42.345P	S42.409B	S42.441B	S42.464B	S42.91XK	S45.919A	S49.039P
S36.520A	S37.818A	S42.034K	S42.142B	S42.216K	S42.256K	S42.312A	S42.346A	S42.409K	S42.441K	S42.464K	S42.91XP	S45.991A	S49.041A
S36.521A	S37.819A	S42.034P	S42.142K	S42.216P	S42.256P	S42.312B	S42.346B	S42.409P	S42.441P	S42.464P	S42.92XA	S45.992A	S49.041K
S36.522A	S37.892A	S42.035B	S42.142P	S42.221A	S42.261A	S42.312P	S42.346K	S42.411A	S42.442A	S42.465A	S42.92XB	S45.999A	S49.041P
S36.523A	S37.893A	S42.035K	S42.143B	S42.221B	S42.261B	S42.319A	S42.346P	S42.411B	S42.442B	S42.465B	S42.92XK	S46.021A	S49.042A
S36.528A	S37.898A	S42.035P	S42.143K	S42.221K	S42.261K	S42.319K	S42.351A	S42.411K	S42.442K	S42.465K	S42.92XP	S46.022A	S49.042K
S36.529A	S37.899A	S42.036B	S42.143P	S42.221P	S42.261P	S42.321A	S42.351B	S42.411P	S42.442P	S42.466A	S43.201A	S46.029A	S49.042P
S36.530A	S37.90XA	S42.036K	S42.144B	S42.222A	S42.262A	S42.321B	S42.351K	S42.412A	S42.443A	S42.466B	S43.202A	S46.121A	S49.049A
S36.531A	S37.92XA	S42.036P	S42.144K	S42.222B	S42.262B	S42.321K	S42.351P	S42.412B	S42.443B	S42.466K	S43.203A	S46.122A	S49.049K
S36.532A	S37.93XA	S42.101B	S42.144P	S42.222K	S42.262K	S42.321P	S42.352A	S42.412K	S42.443K	S42.466P	S43.204A	S46.129A	S49.049P
S36.533A	S37.99XA	S42.101K	S42.145B	S42.222P	S42.262P	S42.322A	S42.352B	S42.412P	S42.443P	S42.471A	S43.205A	S46.221A	S49.091A
S36.538A	S42.001B	S42.101P	S42.145K	S42.223A	S42.263A	S42.322B	S42.352K	S42.413A	S42.444A	S42.471B	S43.206A	S46.222A	S49.091K
S36.539A	S42.001K	S42.102B	S42.145P	S42.223B	S42.263B	S42.322P	S42.352P	S42.413B	S42.444B	S42.471K	S43.211A	S46.229A	S49.091P
S36.590A	S42.001P	S42.102K	S42.146B	S42.223K	S42.263K	S42.323A	S42.353A	S42.413K	S42.444K	S42.471P	S43.212A	S46.321A	S49.092A
S36.591A	S42.002B	S42.102P	S42.146K	S42.223P	S42.263P	S42.323B	S42.353B	S42.413P	S42.444P	S42.472A	S43.213A	S46.322A	S49.092K
S36.592A	S42.002K	S42.109B	S42.146P	S42.224A	S42.264A	S42.323K	S42.353K	S42.414A	S42.445A	S42.472B	S43.214A	S46.329A	S49.092P
S36.593A	S42.002P	S42.109K	S42.151B	S42.224B	S42.264B	S42.323P	S42.353P	S42.414B	S42.445B	S42.472K	S43.215A	S46.821A	S49.099A
S36.598A	S42.009B	S42.109P	S42.151K	S42.224K	S42.264K	S42.324A	S42.354A	S42.414K	S42.445K	S42.472P	S43.216A	S46.822A	S49.099K
S36.599A	S42.009K	S42.111B	S42.151P	S42.224P	S42.264P	S42.324B	S42.354B	S42.414P	S42.445P	S42.473A	S43.221A	S46.829A	S49.099P
S36.60XA	S42.009P	S42.111K	S42.152B	S42.225A	S42.265A	S42.324K	S42.354K	S42.415A	S42.446A	S42.473B	S43.222A	S46.921A	S49.101A
S36.61XA	S42.011B	S42.111P	S42.152K	S42.225B	S42.265B	S42.324P	S42.354P	S42.415B	S42.446B	S42.473K	S43.223A	S46.922A	S49.101K
S36.62XA	S42.011K	S42.112B	S42.152P	S42.225K	S42.265K	S42.325A	S42.355A	S42.415K	S42.446K	S42.473P	S43.224A	S46.929A	S49.101P
S36.63XA	S42.012B	S42.112K	S42.153B	S42.225P	S42.265P	S42.325B	S42.355B	S42.415P	S42.446P	S42.474A	S43.225A	S48.011A	S49.102A
S36.69XA	S42.012K	S42.112P	S42.153K	S42.226A	S42.266A	S42.325K	S42.355K	S42.416A	S42.447A	S42.474B	S43.226A	S48.012A	S49.102K
S36.81XA	S42.012P	S42.113B	S42.153P	S42.226B	S42.266B	S42.325P	S42.355P	S42.416B	S42.447B	S42.474K	S45.001A	S48.019A	S49.102P
S36.892A	S42.013B	S42.113K	S42.154B	S42.226K	S42.266K	S42.326A	S42.356A	S42.416K	S42.447K	S42.474P	S45.002A	S48.021A	S49.109A
S36.893A	S42.013K	S42.113P	S42.154K	S42.226P	S42.266P	S42.326B	S42.356B	S42.416P	S42.447P	S42.475A	S45.009A	S48.022A	S49.109K
S36.898A	S42.013P	S42.114B	S42.154P	S42.231A	S42.271A	S42.326K	S42.356K	S42.421A	S42.448A	S42.475B	S45.011A	S48.029A	S49.109P
S36.899A	S42.014B	S42.114K	S42.155B	S42.231B	S42.271K	S42.326P	S42.356P	S42.421B	S42.448B	S42.475K	S45.012A	S48.111A	S49.111A
S36.90XA	S42.014K	S42.114P	S42.155K	S42.231K	S42.271P	S42.331A	S42.361A	S42.421K	S42.448K	S42.476A	S45.019A	S48.112A	S49.111K
S36.92XA	S42.014P	S42.115B	S42.155P	S42.231P	S42.272A	S42.331B	S42.361B	S42.421P	S42.448P	S42.476B	S45.091A	S48.119A	S49.111P
S36.93XA	S42.015B	S42.115K	S42.156B	S42.232A	S42.272K	S42.331K	S42.361K	S42.422A	S42.449A	S42.476K	S45.092A	S48.121A	S49.112A
S36.99XA	S42.015K	S42.115P	S42.156K	S42.232B	S42.272P	S42.331P	S42.361P	S42.422B	S42.449B	S42.476P	S45.099A	S48.122A	S49.112K
S37.001A	S42.015P	S42.116B	S42.156P	S42.232K	S42.279A	S42.332A	S42.362A	S42.422K	S42.449K	S42.481A	S45.101A	S48.129A	S49.112P
S37.002A	S42.016B	S42.116K	S42.191B	S42.232P	S42.279K	S42.332B	S42.362B	S42.422P	S42.449P	S42.481K	S45.102A	S48.911A	S49.119A
S37.009A	S42.016K	S42.116P	S42.191K	S42.239A	S42.279P	S42.332K	S42.362K	S42.423A	S42.451A	S42.481P	S45.109A	S48.912A	S49.119K
S37.011A	S42.016P	S42.121B	S42.191P	S42.239B	S42.291A	S42.332P	S42.362P	S42.423B	S42.451B	S42.482A	S45.111A	S48.919A	S49.119P
S37.012A	S42.017B	S42.121K	S42.192B	S42.239K	S42.291B	S42.333A	S42.363A	S42.423K	S42.451K	S42.482K	S45.112A	S48.921A	S49.121A
S37.019A	S42.017K	S42.121P	S42.192K	S42.239P	S42.291K	S42.333B	S42.363B	S42.423P	S42.451P	S42.482P	S45.119A	S48.922A	S49.121K
S37.021A	S42.017P	S42.122B	S42.192P	S42.241A	S42.291P	S42.333K	S42.363K	S42.424A	S42.452A	S42.489A	S45.191A	S48.929A	S49.121P
S37.022A	S42.018B	S42.122K	S42.199B	S42.241B	S42.292A	S42.333P	S42.363P	S42.424B	S42.452B	S42.489K	S45.192A	S49.001A	S49.122A
S37.029A	S42.018K	S42.122P	S42.199K	S42.241K	S42.292B	S42.334A	S42.364A	S42.424K	S42.452K	S42.489P	S45.199A	S49.001K	S49.122K
S37.031A	S42.018P	S42.123B	S42.199P	S42.241P	S42.292P	S42.334B	S42.364B	S42.424P	S42.452P	S42.491A	S45.201A	S49.001P	S49.129A
S37.032A	S42.019B	S42.123K	S42.201A				S42.364K	S42.425A			S45.202A	S49.002A	
S37.039A		S42.123P	S42.201B				S42.364P	S42.425B			S45.209A	S49.002K	

Complications or Comorbidities/Major Complications or Comorbidities (CC/MCC) Exclusions (cont.) - Based on CMS data

S49.129K	S52.022N	S52.035Q	S52.099B	S52.125C	S52.182M	S52.223Q	S52.236A	S52.252C	S52.264M	S52.291A	S52.322C	S52.334M	S52.346P
S49.129P	S52.022P	S52.035R	S52.099C	S52.125K	S52.182N	S52.223R	S52.236B	S52.252K	S52.264N	S52.291B	S52.322K	S52.334N	S52.346Q
S49.131A	S52.022Q	S52.036B	S52.099K	S52.125M	S52.182P	S52.224A	S52.236C	S52.252N	S52.264P	S52.291C	S52.322M	S52.334P	S52.346R
S49.131K	S52.022R	S52.036C	S52.099M	S52.125N	S52.182Q	S52.224B	S52.236K	S52.252P	S52.264Q	S52.291K	S52.322P	S52.334Q	S52.351A
S49.131P	S52.023B	S52.036K	S52.099N	S52.125P	S52.182R	S52.224C	S52.236M	S52.252Q	S52.264R	S52.291M	S52.322Q	S52.335A	S52.351B
S49.132A	S52.023C	S52.036M	S52.099P	S52.125Q	S52.189B	S52.224K	S52.236N	S52.252R	S52.265A	S52.291N	S52.322R	S52.335B	S52.351C
S49.132K	S52.023K	S52.036N	S52.099Q	S52.125R	S52.189C	S52.224M	S52.236P	S52.253A	S52.265B	S52.291P	S52.323A	S52.335C	S52.351K
S49.132P	S52.023N	S52.036P	S52.099R	S52.126B	S52.189K	S52.224N	S52.236Q	S52.253B	S52.265C	S52.291Q	S52.323B	S52.335K	S52.351M
S49.139A	S52.023P	S52.036Q	S52.101B	S52.126C	S52.189M	S52.224P	S52.236R	S52.253K	S52.265K	S52.291R	S52.323C	S52.335M	S52.351N
S49.139K	S52.023Q	S52.036R	S52.101C	S52.126K	S52.189N	S52.224Q	S52.241A	S52.253M	S52.265N	S52.292A	S52.323M	S52.335P	S52.351P
S49.139P	S52.023R	S52.041B	S52.101K	S52.126M	S52.189P	S52.224R	S52.241B	S52.253N	S52.265P	S52.292B	S52.323N	S52.335Q	S52.351Q
S49.141A	S52.024B	S52.041C	S52.101M	S52.126N	S52.189Q	S52.225A	S52.241C	S52.253P	S52.265Q	S52.292C	S52.323P	S52.335R	S52.351R
S49.141K	S52.024C	S52.041K	S52.101N	S52.126P	S52.189R	S52.225B	S52.241K	S52.253Q	S52.265R	S52.292K	S52.323Q	S52.336A	S52.352A
S49.141P	S52.024K	S52.041M	S52.101P	S52.126Q	S52.201A	S52.225C	S52.241M	S52.253R	S52.266A	S52.292M	S52.323R	S52.336B	S52.352B
S49.142A	S52.024M	S52.041P	S52.101Q	S52.126R	S52.201B	S52.225K	S52.241N	S52.254A	S52.266B	S52.292N	S52.324A	S52.336C	S52.352C
S49.142K	S52.024N	S52.041Q	S52.101R	S52.131B	S52.201C	S52.225M	S52.241P	S52.254B	S52.266K	S52.292P	S52.324B	S52.336M	S52.352K
S49.142P	S52.024P	S52.041R	S52.102B	S52.131C	S52.201K	S52.225N	S52.241Q	S52.254C	S52.266M	S52.292Q	S52.324C	S52.336N	S52.352M
S49.149A	S52.024Q	S52.042B	S52.102C	S52.131K	S52.201M	S52.225P	S52.241R	S52.254K	S52.266N	S52.299A	S52.324K	S52.336P	S52.352P
S49.149K	S52.024R	S52.042C	S52.102K	S52.131M	S52.201N	S52.225Q	S52.242A	S52.254M	S52.266P	S52.299B	S52.324M	S52.336Q	S52.352Q
S49.149P	S52.025B	S52.042K	S52.102M	S52.131N	S52.201P	S52.225R	S52.242B	S52.254N	S52.266Q	S52.299C	S52.324N	S52.336R	S52.352R
S49.191A	S52.025C	S52.042M	S52.102N	S52.131P	S52.201Q	S52.226A	S52.242C	S52.254Q	S52.266R	S52.299K	S52.324P	S52.341A	S52.353A
S49.191K	S52.025K	S52.042P	S52.102P	S52.131Q	S52.201R	S52.226B	S52.242K	S52.254R	S52.271B	S52.299M	S52.324Q	S52.341B	S52.353B
S49.191P	S52.025M	S52.042Q	S52.102Q	S52.131R	S52.202A	S52.226K	S52.242M	S52.255A	S52.271C	S52.299N	S52.324R	S52.341C	S52.353C
S49.192A	S52.025N	S52.042R	S52.102R	S52.132B	S52.202B	S52.226M	S52.242N	S52.255B	S52.271K	S52.299P	S52.325A	S52.341K	S52.353M
S49.192K	S52.025P	S52.043B	S52.109B	S52.132C	S52.202C	S52.226N	S52.242P	S52.255C	S52.271M	S52.299Q	S52.325B	S52.341M	S52.353N
S49.192P	S52.025Q	S52.043C	S52.109C	S52.132K	S52.202K	S52.226P	S52.242Q	S52.255K	S52.271N	S52.299R	S52.325C	S52.341N	S52.353P
S49.199A	S52.025R	S52.043M	S52.109K	S52.132M	S52.202M	S52.226Q	S52.242R	S52.255M	S52.271P	S52.301A	S52.325K	S52.341P	S52.353Q
S49.199K	S52.026B	S52.043N	S52.109M	S52.132N	S52.202N	S52.226R	S52.243A	S52.255P	S52.271Q	S52.301B	S52.325M	S52.341Q	S52.353R
S49.199P	S52.026C	S52.043P	S52.109N	S52.132P	S52.202P	S52.231A	S52.243B	S52.255Q	S52.271R	S52.301C	S52.325N	S52.341R	S52.354B
S52.001B	S52.026K	S52.043Q	S52.109P	S52.132Q	S52.202Q	S52.231B	S52.243C	S52.255R	S52.272B	S52.301M	S52.325Q	S52.342A	S52.354C
S52.001C	S52.026M	S52.043R	S52.109Q	S52.132R	S52.202R	S52.231C	S52.243K	S52.256A	S52.272C	S52.301N	S52.325R	S52.342B	S52.354K
S52.001K	S52.026N	S52.044B	S52.109R	S52.133B	S52.209A	S52.231K	S52.243M	S52.256B	S52.272K	S52.301P	S52.326A	S52.342C	S52.354M
S52.001M	S52.026P	S52.044C	S52.111A	S52.133C	S52.209B	S52.231M	S52.243N	S52.256C	S52.272M	S52.301Q	S52.326B	S52.342K	S52.354Q
S52.001N	S52.026Q	S52.044M	S52.111K	S52.133K	S52.209C	S52.231N	S52.243P	S52.256M	S52.272N	S52.301R	S52.326C	S52.342M	S52.354R
S52.001P	S52.026R	S52.044N	S52.111P	S52.133M	S52.209K	S52.231P	S52.243Q	S52.256N	S52.272P	S52.302A	S52.326M	S52.342N	S52.355A
S52.001Q	S52.031B	S52.044P	S52.112A	S52.133N	S52.209M	S52.231Q	S52.243R	S52.256P	S52.272Q	S52.302B	S52.326N	S52.342P	S52.355C
S52.001R	S52.031C	S52.044Q	S52.112K	S52.133P	S52.209N	S52.231R	S52.244A	S52.256Q	S52.272R	S52.302C	S52.326P	S52.342Q	S52.355K
S52.002B	S52.031K	S52.044R	S52.112P	S52.133Q	S52.209P	S52.232A	S52.244B	S52.256R	S52.279B	S52.302K	S52.326Q	S52.342R	S52.355M
S52.002C	S52.031M	S52.045C	S52.119A	S52.133R	S52.209Q	S52.232B	S52.244C	S52.261A	S52.279C	S52.302M	S52.326R	S52.343A	S52.355N
S52.002K	S52.031N	S52.045K	S52.119K	S52.134B	S52.209R	S52.232C	S52.244K	S52.261B	S52.279K	S52.302N	S52.331A	S52.343B	S52.355P
S52.002M	S52.031P	S52.045M	S52.119P	S52.134C	S52.211A	S52.232K	S52.244M	S52.261C	S52.279M	S52.302P	S52.331B	S52.343C	S52.355Q
S52.002N	S52.031Q	S52.045N	S52.121B	S52.134K	S52.211K	S52.232M	S52.244N	S52.261K	S52.279N	S52.302Q	S52.331C	S52.343M	S52.356A
S52.002P	S52.031R	S52.045P	S52.121C	S52.134M	S52.211P	S52.232N	S52.244P	S52.261M	S52.279P	S52.302R	S52.331K	S52.343N	S52.356B
S52.002Q	S52.032B	S52.045Q	S52.121K	S52.134N	S52.212A	S52.232P	S52.244R	S52.261N	S52.279Q	S52.309A	S52.331M	S52.343P	S52.356C
S52.002R	S52.032C	S52.046B	S52.121M	S52.134P	S52.212K	S52.232Q	S52.245A	S52.261P	S52.279R	S52.309B	S52.331N	S52.343Q	S52.356K
S52.009B	S52.032K	S52.046C	S52.121N	S52.134Q	S52.212P	S52.232R	S52.245B	S52.261Q	S52.281A	S52.309C	S52.331P	S52.343R	S52.356M
S52.009C	S52.032M	S52.046K	S52.121P	S52.134R	S52.219A	S52.233A	S52.245C	S52.261R	S52.281B	S52.309K	S52.331Q	S52.344A	S52.356N
S52.009K	S52.032N	S52.046M	S52.121Q	S52.135B	S52.219K	S52.233B	S52.245K	S52.262A	S52.281C	S52.309M	S52.331R	S52.344B	S52.356P
S52.009M	S52.032P	S52.046N	S52.121R	S52.135C	S52.219P	S52.233C	S52.245M	S52.262B	S52.281K	S52.309N	S52.332B	S52.344C	S52.356Q
S52.009N	S52.032Q	S52.046P	S52.122B	S52.135K	S52.221A	S52.233M	S52.245N	S52.262C	S52.281M	S52.309P	S52.332C	S52.344K	S52.361A
S52.009P	S52.033B	S52.046Q	S52.122C	S52.135M	S52.221B	S52.233N	S52.245P	S52.262K	S52.281N	S52.309Q	S52.332K	S52.344M	S52.361B
S52.009Q	S52.033C	S52.046R	S52.122K	S52.135N	S52.221C	S52.233P	S52.245Q	S52.262M	S52.281P	S52.309R	S52.332M	S52.344N	S52.361K
S52.009R	S52.033K	S52.091B	S52.122M	S52.135P	S52.221K	S52.233Q	S52.245R	S52.262P	S52.281Q	S52.311A	S52.332N	S52.344P	S52.361M
S52.011A	S52.033M	S52.091C	S52.122N	S52.135Q	S52.221M	S52.233R	S52.246A	S52.262Q	S52.281R	S52.311K	S52.332P	S52.344Q	S52.361N
S52.011K	S52.033N	S52.091K	S52.122P	S52.135R	S52.221N	S52.234A	S52.246B	S52.262R	S52.282A	S52.311P	S52.332R	S52.344R	S52.361P
S52.011P	S52.033P	S52.091M	S52.122Q	S52.136B	S52.221P	S52.234B	S52.246C	S52.263A	S52.282B	S52.312A	S52.333A	S52.345A	S52.361Q
S52.012A	S52.033Q	S52.091N	S52.122R	S52.136C	S52.221Q	S52.234C	S52.246K	S52.263B	S52.282C	S52.312K	S52.333B	S52.345B	S52.361R
S52.012K	S52.033R	S52.091P	S52.123B	S52.136K	S52.222A	S52.234K	S52.246M	S52.263C	S52.282K	S52.312P	S52.333C	S52.345C	S52.362A
S52.012P	S52.034B	S52.091Q	S52.123C	S52.136M	S52.222B	S52.234M	S52.246N	S52.263M	S52.282M	S52.319A	S52.333K	S52.345K	S52.362B
S52.019A	S52.034C	S52.091R	S52.123K	S52.136N	S52.222C	S52.234N	S52.246P	S52.263N	S52.282N	S52.319K	S52.333M	S52.345M	S52.362C
S52.019K	S52.034K	S52.092B	S52.123M	S52.136P	S52.222K	S52.234P	S52.246Q	S52.263P	S52.282P	S52.319P	S52.333N	S52.345N	S52.362K
S52.019P	S52.034M	S52.092C	S52.123N	S52.136Q	S52.222M	S52.234Q	S52.246R	S52.263Q	S52.282Q	S52.321A	S52.333P	S52.345P	S52.362N
S52.021B	S52.034N	S52.092K	S52.123P	S52.136R	S52.222N	S52.234R	S52.251A	S52.263R	S52.282R	S52.321B	S52.333Q	S52.345Q	S52.362Q
S52.021C	S52.034P	S52.092M	S52.123R	S52.181B	S52.222P	S52.235A	S52.251B	S52.264A	S52.283A	S52.321C	S52.333R	S52.345R	
S52.021K	S52.034Q	S52.092N	S52.124B	S52.181C	S52.222Q	S52.235B	S52.251C	S52.264C	S52.283B	S52.321K	S52.334A	S52.346A	
S52.021M	S52.034R	S52.092P	S52.124C	S52.181K	S52.222R	S52.235C	S52.251K	S52.264K	S52.283C	S52.321M	S52.334B	S52.346B	
S52.021N	S52.035B	S52.092Q	S52.124K	S52.181M	S52.223A	S52.235K	S52.251M		S52.283K	S52.321N	S52.334C	S52.346C	
S52.021P	S52.035C	S52.092R	S52.124M	S52.181N	S52.223B	S52.235M	S52.251N		S52.283M	S52.321P	S52.334K	S52.346K	
S52.021Q	S52.035K		S52.124N	S52.181P	S52.223C	S52.235N	S52.251P		S52.283N	S52.321Q		S52.346M	
S52.021R	S52.035M		S52.124P	S52.181Q	S52.223K	S52.235P	S52.251Q		S52.283P	S52.321R		S52.346N	
S52.022C	S52.035N		S52.124R	S52.181R	S52.223N	S52.235Q	S52.251R		S52.283Q	S52.322A			
S52.022K	S52.035P		S52.125B	S52.182B	S52.223P	S52.235R	S52.252A		S52.283R	S52.322B			
S52.022M				S52.182C			S52.252B						

Complications or Comorbidities/Major Complications or Comorbidities (CC/MCC) Exclusions (cont.) – Based on CMS data

S52.362R	S52.382B	S52.511K	S52.532N	S52.561Q	S52.601A	S52.616C	S55.012A	S56.921A	S59.099P	S59.241K	S62.035B	S62.142P	S62.183K
S52.363A	S52.382C	S52.511M	S52.532P	S52.561R	S52.601B	S52.616K	S55.019A	S56.922A	S59.101K	S59.241P	S62.035K	S62.143B	S62.183P
S52.363B	S52.382K	S52.511N	S52.532Q	S52.562A	S52.601C	S52.616M	S55.091A	S56.929A	S59.101P	S59.242A	S62.035P	S62.143K	S62.184B
S52.363C	S52.382M	S52.511P	S52.532R	S52.562B	S52.601K	S52.616N	S55.092A	S58.011A	S59.102K	S59.242K	S62.036B	S62.143P	S62.184K
S52.363K	S52.382N	S52.511Q	S52.539A	S52.562C	S52.601M	S52.616P	S55.099A	S58.012A	S59.102P	S59.242P	S62.036K	S62.144B	S62.184P
S52.363M	S52.382P	S52.511R	S52.539B	S52.562K	S52.601N	S52.616Q	S55.101A	S58.019A	S59.109A	S59.249A	S62.036P	S62.144K	S62.185B
S52.363N	S52.382Q	S52.512A	S52.539C	S52.562M	S52.601P	S52.616R	S55.102A	S58.021A	S59.109P	S59.249K	S62.101B	S62.144P	S62.185K
S52.363P	S52.382R	S52.512B	S52.539K	S52.562N	S52.601Q	S52.621A	S55.109A	S58.022A	S59.111A	S59.249P	S62.101K	S62.145B	S62.185P
S52.363Q	S52.389A	S52.512C	S52.539M	S52.562P	S52.601R	S52.621K	S55.111A	S58.029A	S59.111P	S59.291A	S62.101P	S62.145K	S62.186B
S52.363R	S52.389B	S52.512K	S52.539N	S52.562Q	S52.602A	S52.621P	S55.112A	S58.111A	S59.112A	S59.291K	S62.102B	S62.145P	S62.186K
S52.364A	S52.389C	S52.512M	S52.539P	S52.562R	S52.602B	S52.622A	S55.119A	S58.112A	S59.112P	S59.291P	S62.102K	S62.146B	S62.186P
S52.364B	S52.389K	S52.512N	S52.539Q	S52.569A	S52.602C	S52.622K	S55.191A	S58.119A	S59.119K	S59.292A	S62.102P	S62.146K	S62.201B
S52.364C	S52.389M	S52.512P	S52.539R	S52.569B	S52.602K	S52.622P	S55.192A	S58.121A	S59.119P	S59.292K	S62.109B	S62.146P	S62.201K
S52.364K	S52.389N	S52.512Q	S52.541A	S52.569C	S52.602M	S52.629A	S55.199A	S58.122A	S59.121K	S59.292P	S62.109K	S62.151B	S62.201P
S52.364M	S52.389P	S52.512R	S52.541B	S52.569K	S52.602N	S52.629K	S55.201A	S58.129A	S59.121P	S59.299A	S62.109P	S62.151K	S62.202B
S52.364N	S52.389Q	S52.513A	S52.541C	S52.569M	S52.602P	S52.629P	S55.202A	S58.911A	S59.122K	S59.299K	S62.111B	S62.151P	S62.202K
S52.364P	S52.389R	S52.513B	S52.541K	S52.569N	S52.602Q	S52.691A	S55.209A	S58.912A	S59.122P	S59.299P	S62.111K	S62.152B	S62.202P
S52.364Q	S52.391A	S52.513C	S52.541M	S52.569P	S52.602R	S52.691B	S55.211A	S58.919A	S59.129K	S62.001B	S62.111P	S62.152K	S62.209B
S52.364R	S52.391B	S52.513K	S52.541N	S52.569Q	S52.609A	S52.691C	S55.212A	S58.921A	S59.129P	S62.001K	S62.112B	S62.152P	S62.209K
S52.365A	S52.391C	S52.513M	S52.541P	S52.569R	S52.609B	S52.691K	S55.219A	S58.922A	S59.131K	S62.001P	S62.112K	S62.153B	S62.209P
S52.365B	S52.391K	S52.513N	S52.541Q	S52.571A	S52.609C	S52.691M	S55.291A	S58.929A	S59.131P	S62.002B	S62.112P	S62.153K	S62.211B
S52.365C	S52.391M	S52.513P	S52.541R	S52.571B	S52.609K	S52.691N	S55.292A	S59.001A	S59.132K	S62.002K	S62.113B	S62.153P	S62.211K
S52.365K	S52.391N	S52.513Q	S52.542A	S52.571C	S52.609M	S52.691P	S55.299A	S59.001K	S59.132P	S62.002P	S62.113K	S62.154B	S62.211P
S52.365M	S52.391P	S52.513R	S52.542B	S52.571K	S52.609N	S52.691Q	S55.801A	S59.001P	S59.139K	S62.009B	S62.113P	S62.154K	S62.212B
S52.365N	S52.391Q	S52.514A	S52.542C	S52.571M	S52.609P	S52.691R	S55.802A	S59.002A	S59.139P	S62.009K	S62.114B	S62.154P	S62.212K
S52.365P	S52.391R	S52.514B	S52.542K	S52.571N	S52.609Q	S52.692A	S55.809A	S59.002K	S59.141K	S62.009P	S62.114K	S62.155B	S62.212P
S52.365Q	S52.392A	S52.514C	S52.542M	S52.571P	S52.609R	S52.692B	S55.811A	S59.002P	S59.141P	S62.011B	S62.114P	S62.155K	S62.213B
S52.365R	S52.392B	S52.514K	S52.542N	S52.571Q	S52.611A	S52.692C	S55.812A	S59.009A	S59.142K	S62.011K	S62.115B	S62.155P	S62.213K
S52.366A	S52.392C	S52.514M	S52.542P	S52.571R	S52.611B	S52.692K	S55.819A	S59.009K	S59.142P	S62.011P	S62.115K	S62.156B	S62.213P
S52.366B	S52.392K	S52.514N	S52.542Q	S52.572A	S52.611C	S52.692M	S55.891A	S59.009P	S59.149K	S62.012B	S62.115P	S62.156K	S62.221B
S52.366C	S52.392M	S52.514P	S52.542R	S52.572B	S52.611K	S52.692N	S55.892A	S59.011A	S59.149P	S62.012K	S62.116B	S62.156P	S62.221K
S52.366K	S52.392N	S52.514Q	S52.549A	S52.572C	S52.611M	S52.692P	S55.899A	S59.011K	S59.191K	S62.012P	S62.116K	S62.161B	S62.221P
S52.366M	S52.392P	S52.514R	S52.549B	S52.572K	S52.611N	S52.692Q	S55.901A	S59.011P	S59.191P	S62.013B	S62.116P	S62.161K	S62.222B
S52.366N	S52.392Q	S52.515A	S52.549C	S52.572M	S52.611P	S52.692R	S55.902A	S59.012A	S59.192K	S62.013K	S62.121B	S62.161P	S62.222K
S52.366P	S52.392R	S52.515B	S52.549K	S52.572N	S52.611Q	S52.699A	S55.909A	S59.012K	S59.192P	S62.013P	S62.121K	S62.162B	S62.222P
S52.366Q	S52.399A	S52.515C	S52.549M	S52.572P	S52.611R	S52.699B	S55.911A	S59.012P	S59.199K	S62.014B	S62.121P	S62.162K	S62.223B
S52.366R	S52.399B	S52.515K	S52.549N	S52.572Q	S52.612A	S52.699C	S55.912A	S59.019A	S59.199P	S62.014K	S62.122B	S62.162P	S62.223K
S52.371A	S52.399C	S52.515M	S52.549P	S52.572R	S52.612B	S52.699K	S55.919A	S59.019K	S59.201A	S62.014P	S62.122K	S62.163B	S62.223P
S52.371B	S52.399K	S52.515N	S52.549Q	S52.579A	S52.612C	S52.699M	S55.991A	S59.019P	S59.201K	S62.015B	S62.122P	S62.163K	S62.224B
S52.371C	S52.399M	S52.515P	S52.549R	S52.579B	S52.612K	S52.699N	S55.992A	S59.021A	S59.201P	S62.015K	S62.123B	S62.163P	S62.224K
S52.371K	S52.399N	S52.515Q	S52.551A	S52.579C	S52.612M	S52.699P	S55.999A	S59.021K	S59.202A	S62.015P	S62.123K	S62.164B	S62.224P
S52.371M	S52.399P	S52.515R	S52.551B	S52.579K	S52.612N	S52.699Q	S56.021A	S59.021P	S59.202K	S62.016B	S62.123P	S62.164K	S62.225B
S52.371N	S52.399Q	S52.516A	S52.551C	S52.579M	S52.612P	S52.699R	S56.022A	S59.022A	S59.202P	S62.016K	S62.124B	S62.164P	S62.225K
S52.371P	S52.399R	S52.516B	S52.551K	S52.579N	S52.612Q	S52.90XA	S56.029A	S59.022K	S59.209A	S62.016P	S62.124K	S62.165B	S62.225P
S52.371Q	S52.501A	S52.516C	S52.551M	S52.579P	S52.612R	S52.90XB	S56.121A	S59.022P	S59.209K	S62.021B	S62.124P	S62.165K	S62.226B
S52.371R	S52.501B	S52.516K	S52.551N	S52.579Q	S52.613A	S52.90XC	S56.122A	S59.029A	S59.209P	S62.021K	S62.125B	S62.165P	S62.226K
S52.372A	S52.501C	S52.516M	S52.551P	S52.579R	S52.613B	S52.90XK	S56.123A	S59.029K	S59.211A	S62.021P	S62.125K	S62.166B	S62.226P
S52.372B	S52.501K	S52.516N	S52.551Q	S52.591A	S52.613C	S52.90XM	S56.124A	S59.029P	S59.211K	S62.022B	S62.125P	S62.166K	S62.231B
S52.372C	S52.501M	S52.516P	S52.551R	S52.591B	S52.613K	S52.90XN	S56.125A	S59.031A	S59.211P	S62.022K	S62.126B	S62.171B	S62.231K
S52.372K	S52.501N	S52.516Q	S52.552A	S52.591C	S52.613M	S52.90XP	S56.126A	S59.031K	S59.212A	S62.022P	S62.126K	S62.171K	S62.231P
S52.372M	S52.501P	S52.516R	S52.552B	S52.591K	S52.613N	S52.90XQ	S56.127A	S59.031P	S59.212K	S62.023B	S62.126P	S62.171P	S62.232B
S52.372N	S52.501Q	S52.521A	S52.552C	S52.591M	S52.613P	S52.90XR	S56.128A	S59.032A	S59.212P	S62.023K	S62.131B	S62.172B	S62.232K
S52.372P	S52.501R	S52.521K	S52.552K	S52.591N	S52.613Q	S52.91XA	S56.129A	S59.032K	S59.219A	S62.023P	S62.131K	S62.172K	S62.232P
S52.372Q	S52.502A	S52.521P	S52.552M	S52.591P	S52.613R	S52.91XB	S56.221A	S59.032P	S59.219K	S62.024B	S62.131P	S62.172P	S62.233B
S52.372R	S52.502B	S52.522A	S52.552N	S52.591Q	S52.614A	S52.91XC	S56.222A	S59.039A	S59.219P	S62.024K	S62.132B	S62.173B	S62.233K
S52.379A	S52.502C	S52.522K	S52.552P	S52.591R	S52.614B	S52.91XK	S56.229A	S59.039K	S59.221A	S62.024P	S62.132K	S62.173K	S62.233P
S52.379B	S52.502K	S52.522P	S52.552Q	S52.592A	S52.614C	S52.91XM	S56.321A	S59.039P	S59.221K	S62.025B	S62.132P	S62.173P	S62.234B
S52.379C	S52.502M	S52.529A	S52.552R	S52.592B	S52.614K	S52.91XN	S56.322A	S59.041A	S59.221P	S62.025K	S62.133B	S62.174B	S62.234K
S52.379K	S52.502N	S52.529K	S52.559A	S52.592C	S52.614M	S52.91XP	S56.329A	S59.041K	S59.222A	S62.025P	S62.133K	S62.174K	S62.234P
S52.379M	S52.502P	S52.529P	S52.559B	S52.592K	S52.614N	S52.91XQ	S56.421A	S59.041P	S59.222K	S62.026B	S62.133P	S62.174P	S62.235B
S52.379N	S52.502Q	S52.531A	S52.559C	S52.592M	S52.614P	S52.91XR	S56.422A	S59.042A	S59.222P	S62.026K	S62.134B	S62.175B	S62.235K
S52.379P	S52.502R	S52.531B	S52.559K	S52.592N	S52.614Q	S52.92XA	S56.423A	S59.042K	S59.229A	S62.026P	S62.134K	S62.175K	S62.235P
S52.379Q	S52.509A	S52.531C	S52.559M	S52.592P	S52.614R	S52.92XB	S56.424A	S59.042P	S59.229K	S62.031B	S62.134P	S62.175P	S62.236B
S52.379R	S52.509B	S52.531K	S52.559N	S52.592Q	S52.615A	S52.92XC	S56.425A	S59.049A	S59.229P	S62.031K	S62.135B	S62.176B	S62.236K
S52.381A	S52.509C	S52.531M	S52.559P	S52.592R	S52.615B	S52.92XK	S56.426A	S59.049K	S59.231A	S62.031P	S62.135K	S62.176K	S62.236P
S52.381B	S52.509K	S52.531N	S52.559Q	S52.599A	S52.615C	S52.92XM	S56.427A	S59.049P	S59.231K	S62.032B	S62.135P	S62.176P	S62.241B
S52.381C	S52.509M	S52.531P	S52.559R	S52.599B	S52.615K	S52.92XN	S56.428A	S59.091A	S59.231P	S62.032K	S62.136B	S62.181B	S62.241K
S52.381K	S52.509N	S52.531Q	S52.561A	S52.599C	S52.615M	S52.92XP	S56.429A	S59.091K	S59.232A	S62.032P	S62.136K	S62.181K	S62.241P
S52.381M	S52.509P	S52.531R	S52.561B	S52.599K	S52.615N	S52.92XQ	S56.521A	S59.091P	S59.232K	S62.033B	S62.136P	S62.181P	S62.242B
S52.381N	S52.509Q	S52.532A	S52.561C	S52.599M	S52.615P	S52.92XR	S56.522A	S59.092A	S59.232P	S62.033K	S62.141B	S62.182B	S62.242K
S52.381P	S52.509R	S52.532B	S52.561K	S52.599N	S52.615Q	S55.001A	S56.529A	S59.092K	S59.239A	S62.033P	S62.141K	S62.182K	S62.242P
S52.381Q	S52.511A	S52.532C	S52.561M	S52.599P	S52.615R	S55.002A	S56.821A	S59.092P	S59.239K	S62.034B	S62.141P	S62.182P	S62.243B
S52.381R	S52.511B	S52.532K	S52.561N	S52.599Q	S52.616A	S55.009A	S56.822A	S59.099A	S59.239P	S62.034K	S62.142B	S62.183B	S62.243K
S52.382A	S52.511C	S52.532M	S52.561P	S52.599R	S52.616B	S55.011A	S56.829A	S59.099K	S59.241A	S62.034P	S62.142K	S62.183K	S62.243P

Complications or Comorbidities/Major Complications or Comorbidities (CC/MCC) Exclusions (cont.) - Based on CMS data

S62.244B	S62.312P	S62.337K	S62.362B	S62.514P	S62.616K	S62.641B	S62.665P	S65.507A	S66.524A	S72.019N	S72.032Q	S72.045A	S72.064C
S62.244K	S62.313B	S62.337P	S62.362K	S62.515B	S62.616P	S62.641K	S62.666B	S65.508A	S66.525A	S72.019P	S72.032R	S72.045B	S72.064K
S62.244P	S62.313K	S62.338B	S62.362P	S62.515K	S62.617B	S62.641P	S62.666K	S65.509A	S66.526A	S72.019Q	S72.033A	S72.045C	S72.064M
S62.245B	S62.313P	S62.338K	S62.363B	S62.515P	S62.617K	S62.642B	S62.666P	S65.510A	S66.527A	S72.019R	S72.033B	S72.045K	S72.064N
S62.245K	S62.314B	S62.338P	S62.363K	S62.516B	S62.617P	S62.642K	S62.667B	S65.511A	S66.528A	S72.021A	S72.033C	S72.045M	S72.064P
S62.245P	S62.314K	S62.339B	S62.363P	S62.516K	S62.618B	S62.642P	S62.667K	S65.512A	S66.529A	S72.021B	S72.033K	S72.045N	S72.064R
S62.246B	S62.314P	S62.339K	S62.364B	S62.516P	S62.618K	S62.643B	S62.667P	S65.513A	S66.821A	S72.021C	S72.033M	S72.045P	S72.065A
S62.246K	S62.315B	S62.339P	S62.364K	S62.521B	S62.618P	S62.643K	S62.668B	S65.514A	S66.822A	S72.021K	S72.033N	S72.045Q	S72.065B
S62.246P	S62.315K	S62.340B	S62.364P	S62.521K	S62.619B	S62.643P	S62.668K	S65.515A	S66.829A	S72.021M	S72.033P	S72.045R	S72.065C
S62.251B	S62.315P	S62.340K	S62.365B	S62.521P	S62.619K	S62.644B	S62.668P	S65.516A	S66.921A	S72.021N	S72.033Q	S72.046A	S72.065M
S62.251K	S62.316B	S62.340P	S62.365K	S62.522B	S62.619P	S62.644K	S62.669B	S65.517A	S66.922A	S72.021P	S72.033R	S72.046B	S72.065N
S62.251P	S62.316K	S62.341B	S62.365P	S62.522K	S62.620B	S62.644P	S62.669K	S65.518A	S66.929A	S72.021Q	S72.034A	S72.046C	S72.065P
S62.252B	S62.316P	S62.341K	S62.366B	S62.522P	S62.620K	S62.645B	S62.669P	S65.519A	S68.411A	S72.021R	S72.034B	S72.046K	S72.065Q
S62.252K	S62.317B	S62.341P	S62.366K	S62.523B	S62.620P	S62.645K	S62.90XB	S65.590A	S68.412A	S72.022A	S72.034C	S72.046M	S72.065R
S62.252P	S62.317K	S62.342B	S62.366P	S62.523K	S62.621B	S62.645P	S62.90XK	S65.591A	S68.419A	S72.022B	S72.034K	S72.046N	S72.066A
S62.253B	S62.317P	S62.342K	S62.367B	S62.523P	S62.621K	S62.646B	S62.90XP	S65.592A	S68.421A	S72.022C	S72.034M	S72.046P	S72.066B
S62.253K	S62.318B	S62.342P	S62.367K	S62.524B	S62.621P	S62.646K	S62.91XB	S65.593A	S68.422A	S72.022K	S72.034N	S72.046Q	S72.066C
S62.253P	S62.318K	S62.343B	S62.367P	S62.524K	S62.622B	S62.646P	S62.91XK	S65.594A	S68.429A	S72.022M	S72.034P	S72.046R	S72.066M
S62.254B	S62.318P	S62.343K	S62.368B	S62.524P	S62.622K	S62.647B	S62.91XP	S65.595A	S68.711A	S72.022N	S72.034Q	S72.051A	S72.066N
S62.254K	S62.319B	S62.343P	S62.368K	S62.525B	S62.622P	S62.647K	S62.92XB	S65.596A	S68.712A	S72.022P	S72.034R	S72.051B	S72.066P
S62.254P	S62.319K	S62.344B	S62.368P	S62.525K	S62.623B	S62.647P	S62.92XK	S65.597A	S68.719A	S72.022Q	S72.035A	S72.051C	S72.066Q
S62.255B	S62.319P	S62.344K	S62.369B	S62.525P	S62.623K	S62.648B	S62.92XP	S65.598A	S68.721A	S72.022R	S72.035B	S72.051K	S72.066R
S62.255K	S62.320B	S62.344P	S62.369K	S62.526B	S62.623P	S62.648K	S65.001A	S65.599A	S68.722A	S72.023A	S72.035C	S72.051M	S72.091A
S62.255P	S62.320K	S62.345B	S62.369P	S62.526K	S62.624B	S62.648P	S65.002A	S65.801A	S68.729A	S72.023B	S72.035K	S72.051N	S72.091B
S62.256B	S62.320P	S62.345K	S62.390B	S62.526P	S62.624K	S62.649B	S65.009A	S65.802A	S72.001A	S72.023C	S72.035M	S72.051P	S72.091C
S62.256K	S62.321B	S62.345P	S62.390K	S62.600B	S62.624P	S62.649K	S65.011A	S65.809A	S72.001B	S72.023K	S72.035N	S72.051Q	S72.091K
S62.256P	S62.321K	S62.346B	S62.390P	S62.600K	S62.625B	S62.649P	S65.012A	S65.811A	S72.001C	S72.023M	S72.035P	S72.051R	S72.091M
S62.291B	S62.321P	S62.346K	S62.391B	S62.600P	S62.625K	S62.650B	S65.019A	S65.812A	S72.001K	S72.023N	S72.035Q	S72.052A	S72.091N
S62.291K	S62.322B	S62.346P	S62.391K	S62.601B	S62.625P	S62.650K	S65.091A	S65.819A	S72.001M	S72.023P	S72.035R	S72.052B	S72.091P
S62.291P	S62.322K	S62.347B	S62.391P	S62.601K	S62.626B	S62.650P	S65.092A	S65.891A	S72.001N	S72.023Q	S72.036A	S72.052C	S72.091Q
S62.292B	S62.322P	S62.347K	S62.392B	S62.601P	S62.626K	S62.651B	S65.099A	S65.892A	S72.001P	S72.023R	S72.036B	S72.052K	S72.091R
S62.292K	S62.323B	S62.347P	S62.392K	S62.602B	S62.626P	S62.651K	S65.101A	S65.899A	S72.001Q	S72.024A	S72.036C	S72.052M	S72.092A
S62.292P	S62.323K	S62.348B	S62.392P	S62.602K	S62.627B	S62.651P	S65.102A	S65.901A	S72.001R	S72.024B	S72.036K	S72.052N	S72.092B
S62.299B	S62.323P	S62.348K	S62.393B	S62.602P	S62.627K	S62.652B	S65.109A	S65.902A	S72.002A	S72.024C	S72.036M	S72.052P	S72.092C
S62.299K	S62.324B	S62.348P	S62.393K	S62.603B	S62.627P	S62.652K	S65.111A	S65.909A	S72.002B	S72.024K	S72.036N	S72.052Q	S72.092K
S62.299P	S62.324K	S62.349B	S62.393P	S62.603K	S62.628B	S62.652P	S65.112A	S65.911A	S72.002C	S72.024M	S72.036P	S72.052R	S72.092M
S62.300B	S62.324P	S62.349K	S62.394B	S62.603P	S62.628K	S62.653B	S65.119A	S65.912A	S72.002K	S72.024N	S72.036Q	S72.059A	S72.092N
S62.300K	S62.325B	S62.349P	S62.394K	S62.604B	S62.628P	S62.653K	S65.191A	S65.919A	S72.002M	S72.024P	S72.036R	S72.059B	S72.092P
S62.300P	S62.325K	S62.350B	S62.394P	S62.604K	S62.629B	S62.653P	S65.192A	S65.991A	S72.002N	S72.024Q	S72.041A	S72.059C	S72.092Q
S62.301B	S62.325P	S62.350K	S62.395B	S62.604P	S62.629K	S62.654B	S65.199A	S65.992A	S72.002P	S72.024R	S72.041B	S72.059K	S72.092R
S62.301K	S62.326B	S62.350P	S62.395K	S62.605B	S62.629P	S62.654K	S65.201A	S65.999A	S72.002Q	S72.025A	S72.041C	S72.059M	S72.099A
S62.301P	S62.326K	S62.351B	S62.395P	S62.605K	S62.630B	S62.654P	S65.202A	S66.021A	S72.002R	S72.025B	S72.041K	S72.059N	S72.099B
S62.302B	S62.326P	S62.351K	S62.396B	S62.605P	S62.630K	S62.655B	S65.209A	S66.022A	S72.009A	S72.025C	S72.041M	S72.059P	S72.099C
S62.302K	S62.327B	S62.351P	S62.396K	S62.606B	S62.630P	S62.655K	S65.211A	S66.029A	S72.009B	S72.025K	S72.041N	S72.059Q	S72.099K
S62.302P	S62.327K	S62.352B	S62.396P	S62.606K	S62.631B	S62.655P	S65.212A	S66.120A	S72.009C	S72.025M	S72.041P	S72.059R	S72.099M
S62.303B	S62.327P	S62.352K	S62.397B	S62.606P	S62.631K	S62.656B	S65.219A	S66.121A	S72.009K	S72.025N	S72.041Q	S72.061A	S72.099N
S62.303K	S62.328B	S62.352P	S62.397K	S62.607B	S62.631P	S62.656K	S65.291A	S66.122A	S72.009M	S72.025P	S72.041R	S72.061B	S72.099P
S62.303P	S62.328K	S62.353B	S62.397P	S62.607K	S62.632B	S62.656P	S65.292A	S66.123A	S72.009N	S72.025Q	S72.042A	S72.061C	S72.099Q
S62.304B	S62.328P	S62.353K	S62.398B	S62.607P	S62.632K	S62.657B	S65.299A	S66.124A	S72.009P	S72.025R	S72.042B	S72.061K	S72.099R
S62.304K	S62.329B	S62.353P	S62.398K	S62.608B	S62.632P	S62.657K	S65.301A	S66.125A	S72.009Q	S72.026A	S72.042C	S72.061M	S72.101A
S62.304P	S62.329K	S62.354B	S62.398P	S62.608K	S62.633B	S62.657P	S65.302A	S66.126A	S72.009R	S72.026B	S72.042K	S72.061N	S72.101B
S62.305B	S62.329P	S62.354K	S62.399B	S62.608P	S62.633K	S62.658B	S65.309A	S66.127A	S72.011A	S72.026C	S72.042M	S72.061P	S72.101C
S62.305K	S62.330B	S62.354P	S62.399K	S62.609B	S62.633P	S62.658K	S65.311A	S66.128A	S72.011B	S72.026K	S72.042N	S72.061Q	S72.101M
S62.305P	S62.330K	S62.355B	S62.399P	S62.609K	S62.634B	S62.658P	S65.312A	S66.129A	S72.011C	S72.026M	S72.042P	S72.061R	S72.101N
S62.306B	S62.330P	S62.355K	S62.501B	S62.609P	S62.634K	S62.659B	S65.319A	S66.221A	S72.011K	S72.026N	S72.042Q	S72.062A	S72.101P
S62.306K	S62.331B	S62.355P	S62.501K	S62.610B	S62.634P	S62.659K	S65.391A	S66.222A	S72.011M	S72.026P	S72.042R	S72.062B	S72.101Q
S62.306P	S62.331K	S62.356B	S62.501P	S62.610K	S62.635B	S62.659P	S65.392A	S66.229A	S72.011N	S72.026Q	S72.043A	S72.062C	S72.101R
S62.307B	S62.331P	S62.356K	S62.502B	S62.610P	S62.635K	S62.660B	S65.399A	S66.320A	S72.011P	S72.026R	S72.043B	S72.062K	S72.102A
S62.307K	S62.332B	S62.356P	S62.502K	S62.611B	S62.635P	S62.660K	S65.401A	S66.321A	S72.011Q	S72.031A	S72.043C	S72.062M	S72.102B
S62.307P	S62.332K	S62.357B	S62.502P	S62.611K	S62.636B	S62.660P	S65.402A	S66.322A	S72.011R	S72.031B	S72.043K	S72.062N	S72.102C
S62.308B	S62.332P	S62.357K	S62.509B	S62.611P	S62.636K	S62.661B	S65.409A	S66.323A	S72.012A	S72.031C	S72.043M	S72.062P	S72.102M
S62.308K	S62.333B	S62.357P	S62.509K	S62.612B	S62.636P	S62.661K	S65.411A	S66.324A	S72.012B	S72.031K	S72.043N	S72.062Q	S72.102N
S62.308P	S62.333K	S62.358B	S62.509P	S62.612K	S62.637B	S62.661P	S65.412A	S66.325A	S72.012C	S72.031M	S72.043P	S72.062R	S72.102P
S62.309B	S62.333P	S62.358K	S62.511B	S62.612P	S62.637K	S62.662B	S65.419A	S66.326A	S72.012K	S72.031N	S72.043Q	S72.063A	S72.102Q
S62.309K	S62.334B	S62.358P	S62.511K	S62.613B	S62.637P	S62.662K	S65.491A	S66.327A	S72.012M	S72.031P	S72.043R	S72.063B	S72.102R
S62.309P	S62.334K	S62.359B	S62.511P	S62.613K	S62.638B	S62.662P	S65.492A	S66.328A	S72.012N	S72.031Q	S72.044A	S72.063C	S72.109A
S62.310B	S62.334P	S62.359K	S62.512B	S62.613P	S62.638K	S62.663B	S65.499A	S66.329A	S72.012P	S72.031R	S72.044B	S72.063K	S72.109B
S62.310K	S62.335B	S62.359P	S62.512K	S62.614B	S62.638P	S62.663K	S65.500A	S66.421A	S72.012Q	S72.032A	S72.044C	S72.063M	S72.109C
S62.310P	S62.335K	S62.360B	S62.512P	S62.614K	S62.639B	S62.663P	S65.501A	S66.422A	S72.012R	S72.032B	S72.044K	S72.063N	S72.109K
S62.311B	S62.335P	S62.360K	S62.513B	S62.614P	S62.639K	S62.664B	S65.502A	S66.429A	S72.019A	S72.032C	S72.044M	S72.063P	
S62.311K	S62.336B	S62.360P	S62.513K	S62.615B	S62.639P	S62.664K	S65.503A	S66.520A	S72.019B	S72.032K	S72.044N	S72.063Q	
S62.311P	S62.336K	S62.361B	S62.513P	S62.615K	S62.640B	S62.664P	S65.504A	S66.521A	S72.019C	S72.032M	S72.044P	S72.063R	
S62.312B	S62.336P	S62.361K	S62.514B	S62.615P	S62.640K	S62.665B	S65.505A	S66.522A	S72.019K	S72.032N	S72.044Q	S72.064A	
S62.312K	S62.337B	S62.361P	S62.514K	S62.616B	S62.640P	S62.665K	S65.506A	S66.523A	S72.019M	S72.032P	S72.044R	S72.064B	

Complications or Comorbidities/Major Complications or Comorbidities (CC/MCC) Exclusions (cont.) – Based on CMS data

S72.109M	S72.122P	S72.134R	S72.21XB	S72.309K	S72.332N	S72.344Q	S72.361A	S72.399C	S72.415M	S72.431P	S72.443R	S72.456B	S72.491K
S72.109N	S72.122Q	S72.135A	S72.21XC	S72.309M	S72.332P	S72.344R	S72.361B	S72.399K	S72.415N	S72.431Q	S72.444A	S72.456C	S72.491M
S72.109P	S72.122R	S72.135B	S72.21XK	S72.309N	S72.332Q	S72.345A	S72.361C	S72.399M	S72.415P	S72.431R	S72.444B	S72.456K	S72.491N
S72.109R	S72.123A	S72.135C	S72.21XM	S72.309P	S72.332R	S72.345B	S72.361K	S72.399N	S72.415Q	S72.432A	S72.444C	S72.456M	S72.491P
S72.111A	S72.123B	S72.135K	S72.21XN	S72.309Q	S72.333A	S72.345C	S72.361M	S72.399P	S72.415R	S72.432B	S72.444K	S72.456N	S72.491Q
S72.111B	S72.123C	S72.135M	S72.21XP	S72.309R	S72.333B	S72.345K	S72.361N	S72.399Q	S72.416A	S72.432C	S72.444M	S72.456P	S72.491R
S72.111C	S72.123K	S72.135N	S72.21XQ	S72.321A	S72.333C	S72.345M	S72.361P	S72.399R	S72.416B	S72.432K	S72.444P	S72.456Q	S72.492A
S72.111K	S72.123M	S72.135P	S72.21XR	S72.321B	S72.333K	S72.345N	S72.361Q	S72.401A	S72.416C	S72.432M	S72.444Q	S72.456R	S72.492C
S72.111M	S72.123N	S72.135R	S72.22XA	S72.321C	S72.333M	S72.345P	S72.361R	S72.401B	S72.416K	S72.432N	S72.444R	S72.461A	S72.492K
S72.111N	S72.123P	S72.136A	S72.22XB	S72.321K	S72.333N	S72.345Q	S72.362A	S72.401C	S72.416M	S72.432P	S72.445A	S72.461B	S72.492M
S72.111P	S72.123Q	S72.136B	S72.22XC	S72.321M	S72.333P	S72.345R	S72.362B	S72.401M	S72.416N	S72.432Q	S72.445B	S72.461C	S72.492N
S72.111Q	S72.123R	S72.136C	S72.22XK	S72.321N	S72.333Q	S72.346A	S72.362C	S72.401N	S72.416P	S72.432R	S72.445C	S72.461K	S72.492P
S72.111R	S72.124A	S72.136K	S72.22XM	S72.321P	S72.333R	S72.346B	S72.362K	S72.401P	S72.416Q	S72.433A	S72.445K	S72.461M	S72.492Q
S72.112A	S72.124B	S72.136M	S72.22XN	S72.321Q	S72.334A	S72.346C	S72.362M	S72.401Q	S72.421A	S72.433B	S72.445M	S72.461N	S72.492R
S72.112B	S72.124C	S72.136N	S72.22XP	S72.321R	S72.334B	S72.346M	S72.362P	S72.401R	S72.421B	S72.433C	S72.445N	S72.461P	S72.499A
S72.112C	S72.124K	S72.136P	S72.22XQ	S72.322A	S72.334C	S72.346N	S72.362Q	S72.402A	S72.421C	S72.433K	S72.445P	S72.461Q	S72.499B
S72.112K	S72.124M	S72.136Q	S72.22XR	S72.322B	S72.334K	S72.346P	S72.362R	S72.402B	S72.421K	S72.433M	S72.445Q	S72.461R	S72.499C
S72.112M	S72.124N	S72.136R	S72.23XA	S72.322C	S72.334M	S72.346Q	S72.363A	S72.402C	S72.421M	S72.433N	S72.445R	S72.462A	S72.499K
S72.112N	S72.124P	S72.141A	S72.23XB	S72.322K	S72.334N	S72.346R	S72.363B	S72.402K	S72.421N	S72.433P	S72.446A	S72.462B	S72.499N
S72.112P	S72.124Q	S72.141B	S72.23XC	S72.322M	S72.334P	S72.351A	S72.363C	S72.402M	S72.421P	S72.433Q	S72.446B	S72.462C	S72.499P
S72.112Q	S72.124R	S72.141C	S72.23XK	S72.322N	S72.334Q	S72.351B	S72.363K	S72.402N	S72.421Q	S72.433R	S72.446C	S72.462K	S72.499Q
S72.112R	S72.125A	S72.141K	S72.23XM	S72.322P	S72.334R	S72.351C	S72.363M	S72.402P	S72.421R	S72.434A	S72.446K	S72.462M	S72.499R
S72.113A	S72.125B	S72.141M	S72.23XN	S72.322Q	S72.335A	S72.351K	S72.363N	S72.402Q	S72.422A	S72.434B	S72.446M	S72.462N	S72.8X1A
S72.113B	S72.125C	S72.141N	S72.23XP	S72.322R	S72.335B	S72.351M	S72.363P	S72.402R	S72.422B	S72.434C	S72.446N	S72.462P	S72.8X1B
S72.113C	S72.125K	S72.141P	S72.23XQ	S72.323A	S72.335C	S72.351N	S72.363Q	S72.409A	S72.422C	S72.434K	S72.446P	S72.462Q	S72.8X1C
S72.113K	S72.125M	S72.141Q	S72.23XR	S72.323B	S72.335K	S72.351P	S72.363R	S72.409B	S72.422K	S72.434M	S72.446Q	S72.463A	S72.8X1K
S72.113M	S72.125N	S72.141R	S72.24XA	S72.323C	S72.335M	S72.351Q	S72.364A	S72.409C	S72.422M	S72.434N	S72.446R	S72.463B	S72.8X1M
S72.113P	S72.125P	S72.142A	S72.24XB	S72.323K	S72.335N	S72.351R	S72.364B	S72.409K	S72.422N	S72.434Q	S72.451A	S72.463C	S72.8X1N
S72.113Q	S72.125Q	S72.142B	S72.24XC	S72.323M	S72.335P	S72.352A	S72.364C	S72.409M	S72.422P	S72.434R	S72.451B	S72.463K	S72.8X1P
S72.113R	S72.125R	S72.142C	S72.24XK	S72.323N	S72.335Q	S72.352B	S72.364K	S72.409N	S72.422Q	S72.435A	S72.451C	S72.463M	S72.8X1Q
S72.114A	S72.126A	S72.142K	S72.24XM	S72.323P	S72.335R	S72.352C	S72.364M	S72.409P	S72.422R	S72.435B	S72.451K	S72.463N	S72.8X1R
S72.114B	S72.126B	S72.142M	S72.24XN	S72.323Q	S72.336A	S72.352K	S72.364N	S72.409Q	S72.423A	S72.435C	S72.451M	S72.463Q	S72.8X2A
S72.114C	S72.126C	S72.142N	S72.24XP	S72.323R	S72.336B	S72.352M	S72.364P	S72.409R	S72.423B	S72.435K	S72.451N	S72.463R	S72.8X2B
S72.114K	S72.126K	S72.142P	S72.24XQ	S72.324A	S72.336C	S72.352N	S72.364Q	S72.411A	S72.423C	S72.435M	S72.451P	S72.464A	S72.8X2C
S72.114M	S72.126M	S72.142Q	S72.24XR	S72.324B	S72.336K	S72.352P	S72.364R	S72.411B	S72.423M	S72.435N	S72.451Q	S72.464B	S72.8X2K
S72.114N	S72.126N	S72.142R	S72.25XA	S72.324C	S72.336M	S72.352Q	S72.365A	S72.411C	S72.423N	S72.435P	S72.451R	S72.464C	S72.8X2M
S72.114P	S72.126P	S72.143A	S72.25XB	S72.324M	S72.336N	S72.352R	S72.365B	S72.411K	S72.423P	S72.435Q	S72.452A	S72.464K	S72.8X2N
S72.114Q	S72.126R	S72.143B	S72.25XC	S72.324N	S72.336P	S72.353A	S72.365C	S72.411M	S72.423Q	S72.435R	S72.452B	S72.464M	S72.8X2P
S72.114R	S72.131A	S72.143C	S72.25XK	S72.324P	S72.336Q	S72.353B	S72.365K	S72.411N	S72.423R	S72.436A	S72.452C	S72.464N	S72.8X2Q
S72.115A	S72.131B	S72.143K	S72.25XM	S72.324Q	S72.336R	S72.353C	S72.365M	S72.411P	S72.424A	S72.436B	S72.452K	S72.464P	S72.8X2R
S72.115B	S72.131C	S72.143M	S72.25XN	S72.324R	S72.341A	S72.353K	S72.365N	S72.411Q	S72.424B	S72.436C	S72.452M	S72.464Q	S72.8X9A
S72.115C	S72.131K	S72.143N	S72.25XP	S72.325A	S72.341B	S72.353N	S72.365Q	S72.411R	S72.424C	S72.436K	S72.452N	S72.464R	S72.8X9B
S72.115K	S72.131M	S72.143P	S72.25XQ	S72.325B	S72.341C	S72.353P	S72.365R	S72.412A	S72.424K	S72.436M	S72.452P	S72.465A	S72.8X9C
S72.115M	S72.131N	S72.143Q	S72.25XR	S72.325C	S72.341K	S72.353Q	S72.366A	S72.412B	S72.424M	S72.436N	S72.452Q	S72.465B	S72.8X9K
S72.115N	S72.131P	S72.143R	S72.26XA	S72.325K	S72.341M	S72.353R	S72.366B	S72.412C	S72.424N	S72.436P	S72.452R	S72.465C	S72.8X9M
S72.115P	S72.131Q	S72.144A	S72.26XB	S72.325M	S72.341N	S72.354A	S72.366C	S72.412K	S72.424P	S72.436Q	S72.453A	S72.465K	S72.8X9N
S72.115Q	S72.131R	S72.144B	S72.26XC	S72.325N	S72.341P	S72.354B	S72.366K	S72.412M	S72.424Q	S72.436R	S72.453B	S72.465N	S72.8X9P
S72.115R	S72.132A	S72.144C	S72.26XK	S72.325P	S72.341R	S72.354K	S72.366M	S72.412P	S72.424R	S72.441A	S72.453C	S72.465P	S72.8X9Q
S72.116A	S72.132B	S72.144K	S72.26XM	S72.325Q	S72.342A	S72.354M	S72.366N	S72.412Q	S72.425A	S72.441B	S72.453K	S72.465Q	S72.8X9R
S72.116B	S72.132K	S72.144M	S72.26XP	S72.326A	S72.342B	S72.354N	S72.366P	S72.412R	S72.425B	S72.441C	S72.453M	S72.465R	S72.90XA
S72.116C	S72.132M	S72.144N	S72.26XQ	S72.326B	S72.342C	S72.354P	S72.366Q	S72.413A	S72.425C	S72.441K	S72.453N	S72.466A	S72.90XB
S72.116K	S72.132N	S72.144P	S72.26XR	S72.326C	S72.342K	S72.354Q	S72.366R	S72.413B	S72.425K	S72.441M	S72.453P	S72.466B	S72.90XC
S72.116M	S72.132P	S72.144Q	S72.301A	S72.326K	S72.342M	S72.354R	S72.391A	S72.413C	S72.425M	S72.441N	S72.453Q	S72.466C	S72.90XM
S72.116N	S72.132Q	S72.144R	S72.301B	S72.326M	S72.342N	S72.355A	S72.391B	S72.413K	S72.425N	S72.441P	S72.454A	S72.466K	S72.90XN
S72.116P	S72.132R	S72.145A	S72.301C	S72.326N	S72.342P	S72.355B	S72.391C	S72.413M	S72.425P	S72.441Q	S72.454B	S72.466M	S72.90XP
S72.116Q	S72.133A	S72.145B	S72.301K	S72.326P	S72.342R	S72.355C	S72.391K	S72.413N	S72.425Q	S72.441R	S72.454C	S72.466N	S72.90XQ
S72.116R	S72.133B	S72.145C	S72.301M	S72.326Q	S72.343A	S72.355K	S72.391M	S72.413P	S72.425R	S72.442A	S72.454K	S72.466P	S72.90XR
S72.121A	S72.133C	S72.145K	S72.301N	S72.326R	S72.343B	S72.355M	S72.391N	S72.413Q	S72.426A	S72.442B	S72.454M	S72.466Q	S72.91XA
S72.121B	S72.133K	S72.145M	S72.301P	S72.331A	S72.343C	S72.355N	S72.391P	S72.413R	S72.426B	S72.442C	S72.454N	S72.466R	S72.91XB
S72.121C	S72.133M	S72.145N	S72.301Q	S72.331B	S72.343K	S72.355P	S72.391Q	S72.414A	S72.426C	S72.442K	S72.454Q	S72.471A	S72.91XC
S72.121K	S72.133N	S72.145P	S72.301R	S72.331C	S72.343M	S72.355Q	S72.391R	S72.414B	S72.426K	S72.442M	S72.454R	S72.471K	S72.91XK
S72.121M	S72.133P	S72.145Q	S72.302A	S72.331K	S72.343P	S72.355R	S72.392A	S72.414C	S72.426M	S72.442N	S72.455A	S72.471P	S72.91XM
S72.121N	S72.133R	S72.145R	S72.302B	S72.331M	S72.343Q	S72.356A	S72.392B	S72.414K	S72.426N	S72.442P	S72.455B	S72.472A	S72.91XN
S72.121P	S72.134A	S72.146A	S72.302K	S72.331N	S72.343R	S72.356B	S72.392C	S72.414M	S72.426P	S72.442Q	S72.455C	S72.472K	S72.91XP
S72.121Q	S72.134B	S72.146B	S72.302M	S72.331P	S72.344A	S72.356C	S72.392K	S72.414N	S72.426Q	S72.442R	S72.455K	S72.472P	S72.91XQ
S72.121R	S72.134C	S72.146C	S72.302N	S72.331Q	S72.344B	S72.356K	S72.392M	S72.414P	S72.426R	S72.443A	S72.455M	S72.479A	S72.91XR
S72.122A	S72.134K	S72.146K	S72.302P	S72.331R	S72.344C	S72.356M	S72.392N	S72.414Q	S72.431A	S72.443B	S72.455N	S72.479K	S72.92XA
S72.122B	S72.134M	S72.146N	S72.302Q	S72.332A	S72.344K	S72.356N	S72.392P	S72.415A	S72.431B	S72.443C	S72.455P	S72.479P	S72.92XB
S72.122C	S72.134N	S72.146P	S72.309A	S72.332B	S72.344M	S72.356P	S72.392Q	S72.415B	S72.431C	S72.443K	S72.455Q	S72.491A	S72.92XC
S72.122M	S72.134P	S72.146R	S72.309B	S72.332K	S72.344N	S72.356Q	S72.399A	S72.415C	S72.431M	S72.443P	S72.455R	S72.491B	S72.92XK
S72.122N	S72.134Q	S72.21XA	S72.309C	S72.332M	S72.344P	S72.356R	S72.399B	S72.415K	S72.431N	S72.443Q	S72.456A	S72.491C	S72.92XM

Complications or Comorbidities/Major Complications or Comorbidities (CC/MCC) Exclusions (cont.) - Based on CMS data

S72.92XN	S75.812A	S79.091A	S82.002C	S82.021M	S82.033P	S82.046A	S82.112B	S82.124K	S82.136N	S82.152Q	S82.201A	S82.226C	S82.242M
S72.92XP	S75.819A	S79.091K	S82.002K	S82.021N	S82.033Q	S82.046B	S82.112C	S82.124M	S82.136P	S82.152R	S82.201B	S82.226K	S82.242N
S72.92XQ	S75.891A	S79.091P	S82.002M	S82.021P	S82.033R	S82.046C	S82.112M	S82.124N	S82.136R	S82.153A	S82.201C	S82.226M	S82.242P
S72.92XR	S75.892A	S79.092A	S82.002N	S82.021Q	S82.034A	S82.046K	S82.112N	S82.124P	S82.141A	S82.153C	S82.201K	S82.226N	S82.242Q
S73.001A	S75.899A	S79.092K	S82.002P	S82.021R	S82.034B	S82.046M	S82.112P	S82.124R	S82.141B	S82.153K	S82.201M	S82.226P	S82.243A
S73.002A	S75.901A	S79.092P	S82.002Q	S82.022A	S82.034C	S82.046N	S82.112Q	S82.125A	S82.141C	S82.153M	S82.201N	S82.226Q	S82.243B
S73.003A	S75.902A	S79.099A	S82.002R	S82.022B	S82.034K	S82.046P	S82.112R	S82.125B	S82.141K	S82.153N	S82.201P	S82.226R	S82.243C
S73.004A	S75.909A	S79.099K	S82.009A	S82.022C	S82.034M	S82.046Q	S82.113A	S82.125C	S82.141M	S82.153P	S82.201Q	S82.231A	S82.243K
S73.005A	S75.911A	S79.099P	S82.009B	S82.022K	S82.034N	S82.091A	S82.113B	S82.125K	S82.141N	S82.153Q	S82.201R	S82.231B	S82.243M
S73.006A	S75.912A	S79.101A	S82.009C	S82.022M	S82.034P	S82.091B	S82.113C	S82.125M	S82.141P	S82.153R	S82.202A	S82.231C	S82.243N
S73.011A	S75.919A	S79.101K	S82.009K	S82.022N	S82.034Q	S82.091C	S82.113K	S82.125N	S82.141Q	S82.154A	S82.202B	S82.231K	S82.243Q
S73.012A	S75.991A	S79.101P	S82.009M	S82.022P	S82.034R	S82.091K	S82.113M	S82.125P	S82.141R	S82.154B	S82.202C	S82.231M	S82.243R
S73.013A	S75.992A	S79.102A	S82.009N	S82.022Q	S82.035A	S82.091M	S82.113N	S82.125Q	S82.142A	S82.154C	S82.202K	S82.231N	S82.244A
S73.014A	S75.999A	S79.102K	S82.009P	S82.022R	S82.035B	S82.091N	S82.113P	S82.125R	S82.142B	S82.154K	S82.202M	S82.231P	S82.244B
S73.015A	S76.021A	S79.102P	S82.009Q	S82.023A	S82.035C	S82.091P	S82.113Q	S82.126A	S82.142C	S82.154M	S82.202N	S82.231Q	S82.244C
S73.016A	S76.022A	S79.109A	S82.009R	S82.023B	S82.035K	S82.091Q	S82.113R	S82.126B	S82.142K	S82.154P	S82.202P	S82.231R	S82.244K
S73.021A	S76.029A	S79.109K	S82.011A	S82.023C	S82.035M	S82.091R	S82.114A	S82.126C	S82.142M	S82.154Q	S82.202Q	S82.232A	S82.244N
S73.022A	S76.121A	S79.109P	S82.011B	S82.023K	S82.035N	S82.092A	S82.114B	S82.126K	S82.142N	S82.154R	S82.202R	S82.232B	S82.244P
S73.023A	S76.122A	S79.111A	S82.011C	S82.023M	S82.035P	S82.092B	S82.114C	S82.126M	S82.142P	S82.155A	S82.209A	S82.232C	S82.244Q
S73.024A	S76.129A	S79.111K	S82.011K	S82.023N	S82.035Q	S82.092C	S82.114K	S82.126N	S82.142Q	S82.155B	S82.209B	S82.232K	S82.245A
S73.025A	S76.221A	S79.111P	S82.011M	S82.023P	S82.035R	S82.092K	S82.114M	S82.126P	S82.142R	S82.155C	S82.209C	S82.232M	S82.245B
S73.026A	S76.222A	S79.112A	S82.011N	S82.023Q	S82.036A	S82.092M	S82.114N	S82.126Q	S82.143A	S82.155M	S82.209K	S82.232N	S82.245C
S73.031A	S76.229A	S79.112K	S82.011P	S82.023R	S82.036B	S82.092N	S82.114P	S82.131A	S82.143B	S82.155N	S82.209M	S82.232P	S82.245K
S73.032A	S76.321A	S79.112P	S82.011Q	S82.024A	S82.036C	S82.092P	S82.114R	S82.131B	S82.143C	S82.155P	S82.209N	S82.232Q	S82.245M
S73.033A	S76.322A	S79.119A	S82.011R	S82.024B	S82.036K	S82.092Q	S82.115A	S82.131C	S82.143K	S82.155Q	S82.209P	S82.232R	S82.245N
S73.034A	S76.329A	S79.119K	S82.012A	S82.024C	S82.036M	S82.092R	S82.115B	S82.131K	S82.143M	S82.155R	S82.209Q	S82.233A	S82.245P
S73.035A	S76.821A	S79.119P	S82.012B	S82.024K	S82.036N	S82.099A	S82.115C	S82.131M	S82.143N	S82.156A	S82.209R	S82.233B	S82.245Q
S73.036A	S76.822A	S79.121A	S82.012C	S82.024M	S82.036P	S82.099B	S82.115K	S82.131N	S82.143P	S82.156B	S82.221A	S82.233C	S82.246A
S73.041A	S76.829A	S79.121K	S82.012K	S82.024N	S82.036Q	S82.099C	S82.115M	S82.131P	S82.143Q	S82.156C	S82.221B	S82.233K	S82.246B
S73.042A	S76.921A	S79.121P	S82.012M	S82.024P	S82.036R	S82.099K	S82.115N	S82.131R	S82.143R	S82.156K	S82.221C	S82.233M	S82.246C
S73.043A	S76.922A	S79.122A	S82.012N	S82.024Q	S82.041A	S82.099M	S82.115P	S82.132A	S82.144A	S82.156M	S82.221K	S82.233N	S82.246K
S73.044A	S76.929A	S79.122K	S82.012P	S82.024R	S82.041B	S82.099N	S82.115Q	S82.132B	S82.144B	S82.156N	S82.221N	S82.233Q	S82.246M
S73.045A	S77.00XA	S79.122P	S82.012Q	S82.025A	S82.041C	S82.099P	S82.115R	S82.132C	S82.144C	S82.156P	S82.221P	S82.233R	S82.246N
S73.046A	S77.01XA	S79.129A	S82.012R	S82.025B	S82.041K	S82.099Q	S82.116A	S82.132K	S82.144K	S82.156Q	S82.221Q	S82.234A	S82.246P
S75.001A	S77.02XA	S79.129K	S82.013A	S82.025C	S82.041M	S82.099R	S82.116B	S82.132M	S82.144M	S82.156R	S82.221R	S82.234B	S82.246Q
S75.002A	S77.10XA	S79.129P	S82.013B	S82.025K	S82.041N	S82.101A	S82.116C	S82.132N	S82.144N	S82.161A	S82.222A	S82.234C	S82.251A
S75.009A	S77.11XA	S79.131A	S82.013C	S82.025M	S82.041Q	S82.101B	S82.116K	S82.132P	S82.144P	S82.161K	S82.222B	S82.234K	S82.251B
S75.011A	S77.12XA	S79.131K	S82.013K	S82.025N	S82.041R	S82.101C	S82.116M	S82.132Q	S82.144Q	S82.161P	S82.222K	S82.234N	S82.251C
S75.012A	S78.011A	S79.131P	S82.013M	S82.025P	S82.042A	S82.101K	S82.116N	S82.132R	S82.144R	S82.162A	S82.222M	S82.234P	S82.251K
S75.019A	S78.012A	S79.132A	S82.013N	S82.025Q	S82.042B	S82.101M	S82.116P	S82.133A	S82.145A	S82.162K	S82.222N	S82.234Q	S82.251M
S75.021A	S78.019A	S79.132K	S82.013P	S82.025R	S82.042C	S82.101N	S82.116Q	S82.133B	S82.145B	S82.162P	S82.222P	S82.234R	S82.251N
S75.022A	S78.021A	S79.132P	S82.013Q	S82.026A	S82.042K	S82.101P	S82.116R	S82.133C	S82.145C	S82.169A	S82.222Q	S82.235A	S82.251P
S75.029A	S78.022A	S79.139A	S82.013R	S82.026B	S82.042M	S82.101Q	S82.121A	S82.133K	S82.145K	S82.169K	S82.222R	S82.235B	S82.251Q
S75.091A	S78.029A	S79.139K	S82.014A	S82.026C	S82.042N	S82.101R	S82.121B	S82.133M	S82.145M	S82.169P	S82.223A	S82.235C	S82.251R
S75.092A	S78.111A	S79.139P	S82.014B	S82.026K	S82.042P	S82.102A	S82.121C	S82.133N	S82.145N	S82.191A	S82.223B	S82.235K	S82.252A
S75.099A	S78.112A	S79.141A	S82.014C	S82.026M	S82.042Q	S82.102B	S82.121K	S82.133P	S82.145P	S82.191B	S82.223C	S82.235M	S82.252B
S75.101A	S78.119A	S79.141K	S82.014K	S82.026N	S82.042R	S82.102C	S82.121M	S82.133Q	S82.145Q	S82.191C	S82.223K	S82.235N	S82.252C
S75.102A	S78.121A	S79.141P	S82.014M	S82.026P	S82.043A	S82.102K	S82.121N	S82.133R	S82.145R	S82.191K	S82.223M	S82.235P	S82.252K
S75.109A	S78.122A	S79.142A	S82.014N	S82.026Q	S82.043B	S82.102M	S82.121P	S82.134A	S82.146A	S82.191N	S82.223N	S82.235Q	S82.252M
S75.111A	S78.129A	S79.142K	S82.014P	S82.026R	S82.043C	S82.102N	S82.121Q	S82.134B	S82.146B	S82.191P	S82.223P	S82.235R	S82.252N
S75.112A	S78.911A	S79.142P	S82.014Q	S82.031A	S82.043M	S82.102P	S82.121R	S82.134C	S82.146C	S82.191Q	S82.223R	S82.236A	S82.252P
S75.119A	S78.912A	S79.149A	S82.014R	S82.031B	S82.043N	S82.102Q	S82.122A	S82.134K	S82.146K	S82.191R	S82.224A	S82.236B	S82.252Q
S75.121A	S78.919A	S79.149K	S82.015A	S82.031C	S82.043P	S82.102R	S82.122B	S82.134M	S82.146M	S82.192A	S82.224B	S82.236C	S82.252R
S75.122A	S78.921A	S79.149P	S82.015B	S82.031K	S82.043Q	S82.109A	S82.122C	S82.134N	S82.146N	S82.192B	S82.224C	S82.236K	S82.253B
S75.129A	S78.922A	S79.191A	S82.015C	S82.031M	S82.043R	S82.109B	S82.122K	S82.134P	S82.146P	S82.192C	S82.224K	S82.236M	S82.253C
S75.191A	S78.929A	S79.191K	S82.015K	S82.031N	S82.044A	S82.109C	S82.122M	S82.134R	S82.146Q	S82.192K	S82.224N	S82.236N	S82.253K
S75.192A	S79.001A	S79.191P	S82.015N	S82.031P	S82.044B	S82.109K	S82.122N	S82.135A	S82.146R	S82.192M	S82.224P	S82.236P	S82.253M
S75.199A	S79.001K	S79.192A	S82.015P	S82.031Q	S82.044C	S82.109M	S82.122P	S82.135B	S82.151A	S82.192N	S82.224Q	S82.236R	S82.253P
S75.201A	S79.001P	S79.192K	S82.015Q	S82.031R	S82.044K	S82.109N	S82.122Q	S82.135C	S82.151B	S82.192P	S82.224R	S82.241A	S82.253Q
S75.202A	S79.002A	S79.192P	S82.015R	S82.032A	S82.044M	S82.109P	S82.122R	S82.135K	S82.151C	S82.192Q	S82.225A	S82.241B	S82.253R
S75.209A	S79.002K	S79.199A	S82.016A	S82.032B	S82.044N	S82.109Q	S82.123A	S82.135M	S82.151K	S82.192R	S82.225B	S82.241C	S82.254A
S75.211A	S79.002P	S79.199K	S82.016B	S82.032C	S82.044P	S82.109R	S82.123B	S82.135P	S82.151M	S82.199A	S82.225C	S82.241K	S82.254B
S75.212A	S79.009A	S79.199P	S82.016C	S82.032K	S82.044Q	S82.111B	S82.123C	S82.135Q	S82.151N	S82.199B	S82.225K	S82.241M	S82.254K
S75.219A	S79.009K	S82.001A	S82.016K	S82.032M	S82.045A	S82.111C	S82.123K	S82.135R	S82.151P	S82.199C	S82.225M	S82.241N	S82.254M
S75.221A	S79.009P	S82.001B	S82.016M	S82.032N	S82.045B	S82.111K	S82.123M	S82.136A	S82.151Q	S82.199K	S82.225N	S82.241P	S82.254N
S75.222A	S79.011A	S82.001C	S82.016N	S82.032P	S82.045C	S82.111M	S82.123N	S82.136B	S82.151R	S82.199M	S82.225P	S82.241Q	
S75.229A	S79.011K	S82.001K	S82.016P	S82.032Q	S82.045K	S82.111N	S82.123P	S82.136C	S82.152A	S82.199N	S82.225Q	S82.241R	
S75.291A	S79.011P	S82.001M	S82.016Q	S82.032R	S82.045M	S82.111P	S82.123Q	S82.136K	S82.152B	S82.199P	S82.225R	S82.242A	
S75.292A	S79.012A	S82.001N	S82.016R	S82.033A	S82.045N	S82.111Q	S82.123R	S82.136M	S82.152C	S82.199Q	S82.226A	S82.242B	
S75.299A	S79.012K	S82.001P	S82.021A	S82.033B	S82.045P	S82.111R	S82.124A		S82.152K	S82.199R	S82.226B	S82.242C	
S75.801A	S79.012P	S82.001Q	S82.021B	S82.033C	S82.045Q	S82.112A	S82.124B		S82.152M			S82.242K	
S75.802A	S79.019A	S82.001R	S82.021C	S82.033K			S82.124C		S82.152N				
S75.809A	S79.019K	S82.002A	S82.021K	S82.033M					S82.152P				
S75.811A	S79.019P	S82.002B		S82.033N									

Complications or Comorbidities/Major Complications or Comorbidities (CC/MCC) Exclusions (cont.) - Based on CMS data

S82.254P	S82.266R	S82.392P	S82.425R	S82.443C	S82.456M	S82.499P	S82.63XR	S82.842P	S82.855R	S82.873C	S82.92XM	S85.591A	S89.019P
S82.254Q	S82.291A	S82.392Q	S82.426B	S82.443K	S82.456N	S82.499Q	S82.64XB	S82.842Q	S82.856B	S82.873K	S82.92XN	S85.592A	S89.021A
S82.254R	S82.291B	S82.392R	S82.426C	S82.443M	S82.456P	S82.499R	S82.64XC	S82.842R	S82.856C	S82.873M	S82.92XP	S85.599A	S89.021K
S82.255A	S82.291C	S82.399B	S82.426K	S82.443N	S82.456Q	S82.51XB	S82.64XK	S82.843B	S82.856K	S82.873N	S82.92XQ	S85.801A	S89.021P
S82.255B	S82.291K	S82.399C	S82.426M	S82.443P	S82.456R	S82.51XC	S82.64XM	S82.843C	S82.856M	S82.873P	S82.92XR	S85.802A	S89.022A
S82.255C	S82.291M	S82.399K	S82.426N	S82.443Q	S82.461B	S82.51XK	S82.64XP	S82.843K	S82.856N	S82.873Q	S85.001A	S85.809A	S89.022K
S82.255K	S82.291N	S82.399M	S82.426P	S82.444B	S82.461C	S82.51XM	S82.64XQ	S82.843M	S82.856P	S82.873R	S85.002A	S85.811A	S89.022P
S82.255M	S82.291P	S82.399N	S82.426R	S82.444C	S82.461K	S82.51XN	S82.64XR	S82.843N	S82.856Q	S82.874B	S85.009A	S85.812A	S89.029A
S82.255N	S82.291Q	S82.399P	S82.431B	S82.444K	S82.461M	S82.51XP	S82.65XB	S82.843P	S82.856R	S82.874C	S85.011A	S85.819A	S89.029K
S82.255P	S82.291R	S82.399Q	S82.431C	S82.444M	S82.461N	S82.51XQ	S82.65XC	S82.843Q	S82.861B	S82.874K	S85.012A	S85.891A	S89.029P
S82.255Q	S82.292A	S82.399R	S82.431K	S82.444N	S82.461P	S82.51XR	S82.65XK	S82.843R	S82.861C	S82.874M	S85.019A	S85.892A	S89.031A
S82.255R	S82.292B	S82.401B	S82.431M	S82.444P	S82.461Q	S82.52XB	S82.65XN	S82.844B	S82.861K	S82.874N	S85.091A	S85.899A	S89.031K
S82.256A	S82.292C	S82.401C	S82.431N	S82.444R	S82.461R	S82.52XC	S82.65XP	S82.844C	S82.861M	S82.874P	S85.092A	S85.901A	S89.031P
S82.256B	S82.292K	S82.401K	S82.431P	S82.445B	S82.462B	S82.52XK	S82.65XQ	S82.844K	S82.861N	S82.874Q	S85.099A	S85.902A	S89.032A
S82.256C	S82.292M	S82.401N	S82.431Q	S82.445C	S82.462C	S82.52XM	S82.65XR	S82.844M	S82.861P	S82.874R	S85.101A	S85.909A	S89.032K
S82.256K	S82.292N	S82.401P	S82.431R	S82.445K	S82.462K	S82.52XN	S82.66XB	S82.844N	S82.861Q	S82.875B	S85.102A	S85.911A	S89.032P
S82.256M	S82.292P	S82.401Q	S82.432B	S82.445M	S82.462M	S82.52XP	S82.66XC	S82.844P	S82.861R	S82.875C	S85.109A	S85.912A	S89.039A
S82.256N	S82.292Q	S82.401R	S82.432C	S82.445N	S82.462N	S82.52XQ	S82.66XM	S82.844Q	S82.862B	S82.875K	S85.111A	S85.919A	S89.039K
S82.256P	S82.292R	S82.402B	S82.432K	S82.445P	S82.462P	S82.52XR	S82.66XN	S82.844R	S82.862C	S82.875M	S85.112A	S85.991A	S89.039P
S82.256Q	S82.299A	S82.402C	S82.432N	S82.445R	S82.462Q	S82.53XB	S82.66XP	S82.845B	S82.862M	S82.875P	S85.119A	S85.992A	S89.041A
S82.256R	S82.299B	S82.402K	S82.432P	S82.446B	S82.462R	S82.53XC	S82.66XQ	S82.845C	S82.862N	S82.875Q	S85.121A	S85.999A	S89.041K
S82.261A	S82.299C	S82.402M	S82.432Q	S82.446C	S82.463B	S82.53XK	S82.66XR	S82.845K	S82.862P	S82.875R	S85.122A	S86.021A	S89.041P
S82.261B	S82.299K	S82.402N	S82.432R	S82.446K	S82.463C	S82.53XM	S82.811K	S82.845M	S82.862Q	S82.876B	S85.129A	S86.022A	S89.042A
S82.261C	S82.299M	S82.402P	S82.433B	S82.446M	S82.463K	S82.53XN	S82.811P	S82.845N	S82.862R	S82.876C	S85.131A	S86.029A	S89.042K
S82.261K	S82.299N	S82.402Q	S82.433C	S82.446P	S82.463M	S82.53XP	S82.812K	S82.845P	S82.863B	S82.876K	S85.132A	S86.121A	S89.042P
S82.261M	S82.299P	S82.402R	S82.433M	S82.446Q	S82.463N	S82.53XQ	S82.812P	S82.845Q	S82.863C	S82.876M	S85.139A	S86.122A	S89.049A
S82.261N	S82.299Q	S82.409B	S82.433N	S82.446R	S82.463P	S82.53XR	S82.819K	S82.845R	S82.863M	S82.876P	S85.141A	S86.129A	S89.049K
S82.261P	S82.299R	S82.409C	S82.433P	S82.451B	S82.463Q	S82.54XB	S82.819P	S82.846B	S82.863N	S82.876Q	S85.142A	S86.221A	S89.049P
S82.261Q	S82.301B	S82.409K	S82.433Q	S82.451C	S82.463R	S82.54XC	S82.821K	S82.846C	S82.863P	S82.876R	S85.149A	S86.222A	S89.091A
S82.261R	S82.301C	S82.409M	S82.433R	S82.451K	S82.464B	S82.54XK	S82.821P	S82.846K	S82.863Q	S82.891B	S85.151A	S86.229A	S89.091K
S82.262A	S82.301K	S82.409N	S82.434B	S82.451M	S82.464C	S82.54XM	S82.822K	S82.846M	S82.863R	S82.891C	S85.152A	S86.321A	S89.091P
S82.262B	S82.301M	S82.409P	S82.434C	S82.451N	S82.464K	S82.54XN	S82.822P	S82.846N	S82.864B	S82.891K	S85.159A	S86.322A	S89.092A
S82.262C	S82.301N	S82.409Q	S82.434K	S82.451P	S82.464M	S82.54XP	S82.829K	S82.846P	S82.864K	S82.891M	S85.161A	S86.329A	S89.092K
S82.262K	S82.301P	S82.409R	S82.434M	S82.451Q	S82.464N	S82.54XR	S82.829P	S82.846R	S82.864M	S82.891N	S85.162A	S86.821A	S89.092P
S82.262M	S82.301R	S82.421B	S82.434N	S82.451R	S82.464P	S82.55XB	S82.831B	S82.851B	S82.864N	S82.891P	S85.169A	S86.822A	S89.099A
S82.262N	S82.302B	S82.421C	S82.434P	S82.452B	S82.464Q	S82.55XC	S82.831C	S82.851C	S82.864P	S82.891Q	S85.171A	S86.829A	S89.099K
S82.262P	S82.302C	S82.421K	S82.434Q	S82.452C	S82.464R	S82.55XK	S82.831K	S82.851K	S82.864Q	S82.891R	S85.172A	S86.921A	S89.099P
S82.262Q	S82.302K	S82.421M	S82.434R	S82.452M	S82.465B	S82.55XM	S82.831N	S82.851M	S82.864R	S82.892B	S85.179A	S86.922A	S89.101K
S82.262R	S82.302M	S82.421N	S82.435C	S82.452N	S82.465C	S82.55XN	S82.831P	S82.851N	S82.865B	S82.892C	S85.181A	S86.929A	S89.101P
S82.263A	S82.302N	S82.421P	S82.435K	S82.452P	S82.465K	S82.55XP	S82.831Q	S82.851P	S82.865C	S82.892K	S85.182A	S88.011A	S89.102K
S82.263B	S82.302P	S82.421Q	S82.435M	S82.452Q	S82.465M	S82.55XR	S82.831R	S82.851Q	S82.865K	S82.892M	S85.189A	S88.012A	S89.102P
S82.263C	S82.302Q	S82.421R	S82.435N	S82.452R	S82.465N	S82.56XB	S82.832B	S82.851R	S82.865M	S82.892N	S85.201A	S88.019A	S89.109K
S82.263K	S82.302R	S82.422B	S82.435P	S82.453B	S82.465P	S82.56XC	S82.832C	S82.852B	S82.865N	S82.892P	S85.202A	S88.021A	S89.109P
S82.263M	S82.309B	S82.422C	S82.435Q	S82.453C	S82.465Q	S82.56XK	S82.832K	S82.852C	S82.865P	S82.892Q	S85.209A	S88.022A	S89.111K
S82.263N	S82.309C	S82.422K	S82.435R	S82.453K	S82.465R	S82.56XM	S82.832M	S82.852K	S82.865R	S82.892R	S85.211A	S88.029A	S89.111P
S82.263P	S82.309K	S82.422M	S82.436B	S82.453M	S82.466B	S82.56XN	S82.832N	S82.852M	S82.866B	S82.899B	S85.212A	S88.111A	S89.112K
S82.263Q	S82.309M	S82.422N	S82.436C	S82.453N	S82.466C	S82.56XP	S82.832P	S82.852P	S82.866C	S82.899C	S85.219A	S88.112A	S89.112P
S82.263R	S82.309P	S82.422P	S82.436K	S82.453P	S82.466K	S82.56XQ	S82.832Q	S82.852Q	S82.866K	S82.899K	S85.291A	S88.119A	S89.119K
S82.264A	S82.309Q	S82.422Q	S82.436M	S82.453Q	S82.466M	S82.56XR	S82.832R	S82.852R	S82.866M	S82.899M	S85.292A	S88.121A	S89.119P
S82.264B	S82.309R	S82.422R	S82.436N	S82.453R	S82.466N	S82.61XB	S82.839B	S82.853B	S82.866P	S82.899N	S85.299A	S88.122A	S89.121K
S82.264C	S82.311A	S82.423B	S82.436P	S82.454B	S82.466P	S82.61XC	S82.839C	S82.853C	S82.866Q	S82.899P	S85.301A	S88.129A	S89.121P
S82.264K	S82.311K	S82.423C	S82.436R	S82.454C	S82.466Q	S82.61XK	S82.839K	S82.853K	S82.866R	S82.899Q	S85.302A	S88.911A	S89.122K
S82.264M	S82.311P	S82.423K	S82.441B	S82.454K	S82.466R	S82.61XN	S82.839M	S82.853M	S82.871B	S82.899R	S85.309A	S88.912A	S89.122P
S82.264N	S82.312A	S82.423M	S82.441C	S82.454M	S82.491B	S82.61XP	S82.839N	S82.853N	S82.871C	S82.90XB	S85.311A	S88.919A	S89.129K
S82.264P	S82.312K	S82.423P	S82.441K	S82.454N	S82.491C	S82.61XQ	S82.839P	S82.853P	S82.871K	S82.90XC	S85.312A	S88.921A	S89.129P
S82.264Q	S82.312P	S82.423Q	S82.441M	S82.454P	S82.491K	S82.61XR	S82.839Q	S82.853Q	S82.871M	S82.90XK	S85.319A	S88.922A	S89.131K
S82.264R	S82.319A	S82.423R	S82.441N	S82.454Q	S82.491M	S82.62XB	S82.839R	S82.853R	S82.871N	S82.90XM	S85.391A	S88.929A	S89.131P
S82.265A	S82.319K	S82.424B	S82.441P	S82.454R	S82.491N	S82.62XC	S82.841B	S82.854B	S82.871P	S82.90XN	S85.392A	S89.001A	S89.132K
S82.265B	S82.319P	S82.424C	S82.441Q	S82.455B	S82.491P	S82.62XK	S82.841C	S82.854C	S82.871Q	S82.90XP	S85.399A	S89.001K	S89.132P
S82.265C	S82.391B	S82.424K	S82.441R	S82.455C	S82.491Q	S82.62XM	S82.841K	S82.854K	S82.871R	S82.90XQ	S85.401A	S89.001P	S89.139K
S82.265K	S82.391C	S82.424M	S82.442B	S82.455K	S82.491R	S82.62XN	S82.841M	S82.854M	S82.872B	S82.90XR	S85.402A	S89.002A	S89.139P
S82.265M	S82.391K	S82.424N	S82.442C	S82.455M	S82.492B	S82.62XP	S82.841N	S82.854N	S82.872C	S82.91XB	S85.409A	S89.002K	S89.141K
S82.265N	S82.391M	S82.424P	S82.442K	S82.455N	S82.492C	S82.62XQ	S82.841P	S82.854P	S82.872K	S82.91XC	S85.411A	S89.002P	S89.141P
S82.265P	S82.391N	S82.424Q	S82.442M	S82.455P	S82.492K	S82.62XR	S82.842B	S82.854Q	S82.872M	S82.91XK	S85.412A	S89.009A	S89.142K
S82.265Q	S82.391P	S82.424R	S82.442P	S82.455Q	S82.492M	S82.63XB	S82.842C	S82.855B	S82.872N	S82.91XM	S85.419A	S89.009K	S89.142P
S82.265R	S82.391Q	S82.425B	S82.442Q	S82.455R	S82.492N	S82.63XK	S82.842K	S82.855K	S82.872P	S82.91XN	S85.491A	S89.009P	S89.149K
S82.266A	S82.391R	S82.425C	S82.442R	S82.456B	S82.492P	S82.63XM	S82.842M	S82.855M	S82.872Q	S82.91XP	S85.492A	S89.011A	S89.149P
S82.266B	S82.392C	S82.425K	S82.443B	S82.456C	S82.492Q	S82.63XN	S82.842N	S82.855N	S82.872R	S82.91XQ	S85.499A	S89.011K	S89.191K
S82.266C	S82.392K	S82.425M		S82.456K	S82.492R	S82.63XP		S82.855P	S82.873B	S82.91XR	S85.501A	S89.011P	S89.191P
S82.266K	S82.392M	S82.425N			S82.499B	S82.63XQ		S82.855Q		S82.92XB	S85.502A	S89.012A	S89.192K
S82.266M	S82.392N	S82.425P			S82.499C					S82.92XC	S85.509A	S89.012P	S89.192P
S82.266N		S82.425Q			S82.499K					S82.92XK	S85.511A	S89.019A	S89.199K
S82.266P					S82.499M						S85.512A	S89.019K	S89.199P
S82.266Q					S82.499N						S85.519A		S89.201K

Complications or Comorbidities/Major Complications or Comorbidities (CC/MCC) Exclusions (cont.) - Based on CMS data

S89.201P	S92.021B	S92.061P	S92.135K	S92.216B	S92.256P	S92.344K	S92.504K	S95.009A	S98.922A	T22.332A	T23.739A	T26.71XA	T34.70XA
S89.202K	S92.021K	S92.062B	S92.135P	S92.216K	S92.301B	S92.344P	S92.504P	S95.011A	S98.929A	T22.339A	T23.741A	T26.72XA	T34.71XA
S89.202P	S92.021P	S92.062K	S92.136B	S92.216P	S92.301K	S92.345B	S92.505K	S95.012A	T17.400A	T22.341A	T23.742A	T27.0XXA	T34.72XA
S89.209K	S92.022B	S92.062P	S92.136K	S92.221B	S92.301P	S92.345K	S92.505P	S95.019A	T17.408A	T22.342A	T23.749A	T27.1XXA	T34.811A
S89.209P	S92.022K	S92.063B	S92.136P	S92.221K	S92.302B	S92.345P	S92.506K	S95.091A	T17.410A	T22.349A	T23.751A	T27.2XXA	T34.812A
S89.211K	S92.022P	S92.063K	S92.141B	S92.221P	S92.302K	S92.346B	S92.506P	S95.092A	T17.418A	T22.351A	T23.752A	T27.3XXA	T34.819A
S89.211P	S92.023B	S92.063P	S92.141K	S92.222B	S92.302P	S92.346K	S92.511K	S95.099A	T17.420A	T22.352A	T23.759A	T27.4XXA	T34.821A
S89.212K	S92.023K	S92.064B	S92.141P	S92.222K	S92.309B	S92.346P	S92.511P	S95.101A	T17.428A	T22.359A	T23.761A	T27.5XXA	T34.822A
S89.212P	S92.023P	S92.064K	S92.142B	S92.222P	S92.309K	S92.351B	S92.512K	S95.102A	T17.490A	T22.361A	T23.762A	T27.6XXA	T34.829A
S89.219K	S92.024B	S92.064P	S92.142K	S92.223B	S92.309P	S92.351K	S92.512P	S95.109A	T17.498A	T22.362A	T23.769A	T27.7XXA	T34.831A
S89.219P	S92.024K	S92.065B	S92.142P	S92.223K	S92.311B	S92.351P	S92.513K	S95.111A	T17.500A	T22.369A	T23.771A	T28.1XXA	T34.832A
S89.221K	S92.024P	S92.065K	S92.143B	S92.223P	S92.311K	S92.352B	S92.513P	S95.112A	T17.508A	T22.391A	T23.772A	T28.2XXA	T34.839A
S89.221P	S92.025B	S92.065P	S92.143K	S92.224B	S92.311P	S92.352K	S92.514K	S95.119A	T17.510A	T22.392A	T23.779A	T28.6XXA	T34.90XA
S89.222K	S92.025K	S92.066B	S92.143P	S92.224K	S92.312B	S92.352P	S92.514P	S95.191A	T17.518A	T22.399A	T23.791A	T28.7XXA	T34.99XA
S89.222P	S92.025P	S92.066K	S92.144B	S92.224P	S92.312K	S92.353B	S92.515K	S95.192A	T17.520A	T22.70XA	T23.792A	T33.011A	T67.0XXA
S89.229K	S92.026B	S92.066P	S92.144K	S92.225B	S92.312P	S92.353K	S92.515P	S95.199A	T17.528A	T22.711A	T23.799A	T33.012A	T69.021A
S89.229P	S92.026K	S92.101B	S92.144P	S92.225K	S92.313B	S92.353P	S92.516K	S95.201A	T17.590A	T22.712A	T24.301A	T33.019A	T69.022A
S89.291K	S92.026P	S92.101K	S92.145B	S92.225P	S92.313K	S92.354B	S92.516P	S95.202A	T17.598A	T22.719A	T24.302A	T33.02XA	T69.029A
S89.291P	S92.031B	S92.101P	S92.145K	S92.226B	S92.313P	S92.354K	S92.521K	S95.209A	T17.800A	T22.721A	T24.309A	T33.09XA	T70.3XXA
S89.292K	S92.031K	S92.102B	S92.145P	S92.226K	S92.314B	S92.354P	S92.521P	S95.211A	T17.808A	T22.722A	T24.311A	T33.1XXA	T71.111A
S89.292P	S92.031P	S92.102K	S92.146B	S92.226P	S92.314K	S92.355B	S92.522K	S95.212A	T17.810A	T22.729A	T24.312A	T33.2XXA	T71.112A
S89.299K	S92.032B	S92.102P	S92.146K	S92.231B	S92.314P	S92.355K	S92.522P	S95.219A	T17.818A	T22.731A	T24.319A	T33.3XXA	T71.113A
S89.299P	S92.032K	S92.109B	S92.146P	S92.231K	S92.315B	S92.355P	S92.523K	S95.291A	T17.820A	T22.732A	T24.321A	T33.40XA	T71.114A
S89.301K	S92.032P	S92.109K	S92.151B	S92.231P	S92.315K	S92.356B	S92.523P	S95.292A	T17.828A	T22.739A	T24.322A	T33.41XA	T71.121A
S89.301P	S92.033B	S92.109P	S92.151K	S92.232B	S92.315P	S92.356K	S92.524K	S95.299A	T17.890A	T22.741A	T24.329A	T33.42XA	T71.122A
S89.302K	S92.033K	S92.111B	S92.151P	S92.232K	S92.316B	S92.356P	S92.524P	S95.801A	T17.898A	T22.742A	T24.331A	T33.511A	T71.123A
S89.302P	S92.033P	S92.111K	S92.152B	S92.232P	S92.316K	S92.401K	S92.525K	S95.802A	T20.30XA	T22.749A	T24.332A	T33.512A	T71.124A
S89.309K	S92.034B	S92.111P	S92.152K	S92.233B	S92.316P	S92.401P	S92.525P	S95.809A	T20.311A	T22.751A	T24.339A	T33.519A	T71.131A
S89.309P	S92.034K	S92.112B	S92.152P	S92.233K	S92.321B	S92.402K	S92.526K	S95.811A	T20.312A	T22.752A	T24.391A	T33.521A	T71.132A
S89.311K	S92.034P	S92.112K	S92.153B	S92.233P	S92.321K	S92.402P	S92.526P	S95.812A	T20.319A	T22.759A	T24.392A	T33.522A	T71.133A
S89.311P	S92.035B	S92.112P	S92.153K	S92.234B	S92.321P	S92.403K	S92.531K	S95.819A	T20.32XA	T22.761A	T24.399A	T33.529A	T71.134A
S89.312K	S92.035K	S92.113B	S92.153P	S92.234K	S92.322B	S92.403P	S92.531P	S95.891A	T20.33XA	T22.762A	T24.701A	T33.531A	T71.141A
S89.312P	S92.035P	S92.113K	S92.154B	S92.234P	S92.322K	S92.404K	S92.532K	S95.892A	T20.34XA	T22.769A	T24.702A	T33.532A	T71.143A
S89.319K	S92.036B	S92.113P	S92.154K	S92.235B	S92.322P	S92.404P	S92.532P	S95.899A	T20.35XA	T22.791A	T24.709A	T33.539A	T71.144A
S89.319P	S92.036K	S92.114B	S92.154P	S92.235K	S92.323B	S92.405K	S92.533K	S95.901A	T20.36XA	T22.792A	T24.711A	T33.60XA	T71.151A
S89.321K	S92.036P	S92.114K	S92.155B	S92.235P	S92.323K	S92.405P	S92.533P	S95.902A	T20.37XA	T22.799A	T24.712A	T33.61XA	T71.152A
S89.321P	S92.041B	S92.114P	S92.155K	S92.236B	S92.323P	S92.406K	S92.534K	S95.909A	T20.39XA	T23.301A	T24.719A	T33.62XA	T71.153A
S89.322K	S92.041K	S92.115B	S92.155P	S92.236K	S92.324B	S92.406P	S92.534P	S95.911A	T20.70XA	T23.302A	T24.721A	T33.70XA	T71.154A
S89.322P	S92.041P	S92.115K	S92.156B	S92.236P	S92.324K	S92.411K	S92.535K	S95.912A	T20.711A	T23.309A	T24.722A	T33.71XA	T71.161A
S89.329K	S92.042B	S92.115P	S92.156K	S92.241B	S92.324P	S92.411P	S92.535P	S95.919A	T20.712A	T23.311A	T24.729A	T33.72XA	T71.162A
S89.329P	S92.042K	S92.116B	S92.156P	S92.241K	S92.325B	S92.412K	S92.536K	S95.991A	T20.719A	T23.312A	T24.731A	T33.811A	T71.163A
S89.391K	S92.042P	S92.116K	S92.191B	S92.241P	S92.325K	S92.412P	S92.536P	S95.992A	T20.72XA	T23.319A	T24.732A	T33.812A	T71.164A
S89.391P	S92.043B	S92.116P	S92.191K	S92.242B	S92.325P	S92.413K	S92.591K	S95.999A	T20.73XA	T23.321A	T24.739A	T33.819A	T71.191A
S89.392K	S92.043K	S92.121B	S92.191P	S92.242K	S92.326B	S92.413P	S92.591P	S96.021A	T20.74XA	T23.322A	T24.791A	T33.821A	T71.192A
S89.392P	S92.043P	S92.121K	S92.192B	S92.242P	S92.326K	S92.414K	S92.592K	S96.022A	T20.75XA	T23.329A	T24.792A	T33.822A	T71.193A
S89.399K	S92.044B	S92.121P	S92.192K	S92.243B	S92.326P	S92.414P	S92.592P	S96.029A	T20.76XA	T23.331A	T24.799A	T33.829A	T71.194A
S89.399P	S92.044K	S92.122B	S92.192P	S92.243K	S92.331B	S92.415K	S92.599K	S96.121A	T20.77XA	T23.332A	T25.311A	T33.831A	T71.20XA
S92.001B	S92.044P	S92.122K	S92.199B	S92.243P	S92.331K	S92.415P	S92.599P	S96.122A	T20.79XA	T23.339A	T25.312A	T33.832A	T71.21XA
S92.001K	S92.045B	S92.122P	S92.199K	S92.244B	S92.331P	S92.416K	S92.811B	S96.129A	T21.30XA	T23.341A	T25.319A	T33.839A	T71.221A
S92.001P	S92.045K	S92.123B	S92.199P	S92.244K	S92.332B	S92.416P	S92.811K	S96.221A	T21.31XA	T23.342A	T25.321A	T33.90XA	T71.222A
S92.002B	S92.045P	S92.123K	S92.201B	S92.244P	S92.332K	S92.421K	S92.811P	S96.222A	T21.32XA	T23.349A	T25.322A	T33.99XA	T71.223A
S92.002K	S92.046B	S92.123P	S92.201K	S92.245B	S92.332P	S92.421P	S92.812B	S96.229A	T21.33XA	T23.351A	T25.329A	T34.011A	T71.224A
S92.002P	S92.046K	S92.124B	S92.201P	S92.245K	S92.333B	S92.422K	S92.812K	S96.821A	T21.34XA	T23.352A	T25.331A	T34.012A	T71.231A
S92.009B	S92.046P	S92.124K	S92.202B	S92.245P	S92.333K	S92.422P	S92.812P	S96.822A	T21.35XA	T23.359A	T25.332A	T34.019A	T71.232A
S92.009K	S92.051B	S92.124P	S92.202K	S92.246B	S92.333P	S92.423K	S92.819B	S96.829A	T21.36XA	T23.361A	T25.339A	T34.02XA	T71.233A
S92.009P	S92.051K	S92.125B	S92.202P	S92.246K	S92.334B	S92.423P	S92.819K	S96.921A	T21.37XA	T23.362A	T25.391A	T34.09XA	T71.234A
S92.011B	S92.051P	S92.125K	S92.209B	S92.246P	S92.334K	S92.424K	S92.819P	S96.929A	T21.39XA	T23.369A	T25.392A	T34.1XXA	T71.29XA
S92.011K	S92.052B	S92.125P	S92.209K	S92.251B	S92.334P	S92.424P	S92.901B	S98.011A	T21.70XA	T23.371A	T25.399A	T34.2XXA	T71.9XXA
S92.011P	S92.052K	S92.126B	S92.209P	S92.251K	S92.335B	S92.425K	S92.901K	S98.012A	T21.71XA	T23.372A	T25.711A	T34.3XXA	T74.01XA
S92.012B	S92.052P	S92.126K	S92.211B	S92.251P	S92.335K	S92.425P	S92.901P	S98.019A	T21.72XA	T23.379A	T25.712A	T34.40XA	T74.02XA
S92.012K	S92.053B	S92.126P	S92.211K	S92.252B	S92.335P	S92.426K	S92.902B	S98.021A	T21.73XA	T23.391A	T25.719A	T34.41XA	T74.11XA
S92.012P	S92.053K	S92.131B	S92.211P	S92.252K	S92.336B	S92.426P	S92.902K	S98.022A	T21.74XA	T23.392A	T25.721A	T34.42XA	T74.12XA
S92.013B	S92.053P	S92.131K	S92.212B	S92.252P	S92.336K	S92.491K	S92.902P	S98.029A	T21.75XA	T23.399A	T25.722A	T34.511A	T74.21XA
S92.013K	S92.054B	S92.131P	S92.212K	S92.253B	S92.336P	S92.491P	S92.909B	S98.311A	T21.76XA	T23.701A	T25.729A	T34.512A	T74.22XA
S92.013P	S92.054K	S92.132B	S92.212P	S92.253K	S92.341B	S92.492K	S92.909K	S98.312A	T21.77XA	T23.702A	T25.731A	T34.519A	T74.32XA
S92.014B	S92.054P	S92.132K	S92.213B	S92.253P	S92.341K	S92.492P	S92.909P	S98.319A	T21.79XA	T23.709A	T25.732A	T34.521A	T74.4XXA
S92.014K	S92.055B	S92.132P	S92.213K	S92.254B	S92.341P	S92.499K	S92.911K	S98.321A	T22.30XA	T23.711A	T25.739A	T34.522A	T74.91XA
S92.014P	S92.055K	S92.133B	S92.213P	S92.254K	S92.342B	S92.499P	S92.911P	S98.322A	T22.311A	T23.712A	T25.791A	T34.529A	T74.92XA
S92.015B	S92.055P	S92.133K	S92.214B	S92.254P	S92.342K	S92.501K	S92.912K	S98.329A	T22.312A	T23.719A	T25.792A	T34.531A	T75.1XXA
S92.015K	S92.056B	S92.133P	S92.214K	S92.255B	S92.342P	S92.501P	S92.912P	S98.911A	T22.319A	T23.721A	T25.799A	T34.532A	T76.01XA
S92.015P	S92.056K	S92.134B	S92.214P	S92.255K	S92.343B	S92.502K	S92.919K	S98.912A	T22.321A	T23.722A	T26.20XA	T34.539A	T76.02XA
S92.016B	S92.056P	S92.134K	S92.215B	S92.255P	S92.343K	S92.502P	S92.919P	S98.919A	T22.322A	T23.729A	T26.21XA	T34.60XA	T76.11XA
S92.016K	S92.061B	S92.134P	S92.215K	S92.256B	S92.343P	S92.503K	S95.001A	S98.921A	T22.329A	T23.731A	T26.22XA	T34.61XA	T76.12XA
S92.016P	S92.061K	S92.135B	S92.215P	S92.256K	S92.344B	S92.503P	S95.002A		T22.331A	T23.732A	T26.70XA	T34.62XA	T76.21XA

Complications or Comorbidities/Major Complications or Comorbidities (CC/MCC) Exclusions (cont.) - Based on CMS data

T76.22XA	T80.29XA	T81.501A	T81.538A	T82.211A	T82.515A	T82.855A	T83.420A	T84.010A	T84.111A	T84.298A	T84.81XA	T85.42XA	T85.695A
T76.32XA	T80.30XA	T81.502A	T81.539A	T82.212A	T82.518A	T82.856A	T83.421A	T84.011A	T84.112A	T84.310A	T84.82XA	T85.43XA	T85.698A
T76.91XA	T80.310A	T81.503A	T81.590A	T82.213A	T82.519A	T82.857A	T83.428A	T84.012A	T84.113A	T84.318A	T84.83XA	T85.44XA	T85.71XA
T76.92XA	T80.311A	T81.504A	T81.591A	T82.218A	T82.520A	T82.858A	T83.490A	T84.013A	T84.114A	T84.320A	T84.84XA	T85.49XA	T85.72XA
T78.00XA	T80.319A	T81.505A	T81.592A	T82.221A	T82.521A	T82.867A	T83.491A	T84.018A	T84.115A	T84.328A	T84.85XA	T85.510A	T85.730A
T78.01XA	T80.39XA	T81.506A	T81.593A	T82.222A	T82.522A	T82.868A	T83.498A	T84.019A	T84.116A	T84.390A	T84.86XA	T85.511A	T85.731A
T78.02XA	T80.40XA	T81.507A	T81.594A	T82.223A	T82.523A	T82.897A	T83.510A	T84.020A	T84.117A	T84.398A	T84.89XA	T85.518A	T85.732A
T78.03XA	T80.410A	T81.508A	T81.595A	T82.228A	T82.524A	T82.898A	T83.511A	T84.021A	T84.119A	T84.410A	T84.9XXA	T85.520A	T85.733A
T78.04XA	T80.411A	T81.509A	T81.596A	T82.310A	T82.525A	T82.9XXA	T83.512A	T84.022A	T84.120A	T84.418A	T85.01XA	T85.521A	T85.734A
T78.05XA	T80.419A	T81.510A	T81.597A	T82.311A	T82.528A	T83.010A	T83.518A	T84.023A	T84.121A	T84.420A	T85.02XA	T85.528A	T85.735A
T78.06XA	T80.49XA	T81.511A	T81.598A	T82.312A	T82.529A	T83.020A	T83.590A	T84.028A	T84.122A	T84.428A	T85.03XA	T85.590A	T85.738A
T78.07XA	T80.51XA	T81.512A	T81.599A	T82.318A	T82.530A	T83.030A	T83.591A	T84.029A	T84.123A	T84.490A	T85.09XA	T85.591A	T85.79XA
T78.08XA	T80.52XA	T81.513A	T81.60XA	T82.319A	T82.531A	T83.090A	T83.592A	T84.030A	T84.124A	T84.498A	T85.110A	T85.598A	T85.810A
T78.09XA	T80.59XA	T81.514A	T81.61XA	T82.320A	T82.532A	T83.110A	T83.593A	T84.031A	T84.125A	T84.50XA	T85.111A	T85.610A	T85.810D
T78.2XXA	T80.61XA	T81.515A	T81.69XA	T82.321A	T82.533A	T83.111A	T83.598A	T84.032A	T84.126A	T84.51XA	T85.112A	T85.611A	T85.820A
T79.0XXA	T80.62XA	T81.516A	T81.710A	T82.322A	T82.534A	T83.112A	T83.61XA	T84.033A	T84.127A	T84.52XA	T85.113A	T85.612A	T85.820D
T79.1XXA	T80.69XA	T81.517A	T81.711A	T82.328A	T82.535A	T83.113A	T83.62XA	T84.038A	T84.129A	T84.53XA	T85.118A	T85.613A	T85.830A
T79.2XXA	T80.810A	T81.518A	T81.718A	T82.329A	T82.538A	T83.118A	T83.69XA	T84.039A	T84.190A	T84.54XA	T85.120A	T85.614A	T85.830D
T79.4XXA	T80.818A	T81.519A	T81.719A	T82.330A	T82.539A	T83.120A	T83.712A	T84.050A	T84.191A	T84.59XA	T85.121A	T85.615A	T85.840A
T79.5XXA	T80.910A	T81.520A	T81.72XA	T82.331A	T82.590A	T83.121A	T83.713A	T84.051A	T84.192A	T84.60XA	T85.122A	T85.618A	T85.840D
T79.7XXA	T80.911A	T81.521A	T81.83XA	T82.332A	T82.591A	T83.122A	T83.714A	T84.052A	T84.193A	T84.610A	T85.123A	T85.620A	T85.850A
T79.A0XA	T80.919A	T81.522A	T82.01XA	T82.338A	T82.592A	T83.123A	T83.718A	T84.053A	T84.194A	T84.611A	T85.128A	T85.621A	T85.850D
T79.A11A	T80.A0XA	T81.523A	T82.02XA	T82.339A	T82.593A	T83.128A	T83.719A	T84.058A	T84.195A	T84.612A	T85.190A	T85.622A	T85.860A
T79.A12A	T80.A10A	T81.524A	T82.03XA	T82.390A	T82.594A	T83.190A	T83.722A	T84.059A	T84.196A	T84.613A	T85.191A	T85.623A	T85.860D
T79.A19A	T80.A11A	T81.525A	T82.09XA	T82.391A	T82.595A	T83.191A	T83.723A	T84.060A	T84.197A	T84.614A	T85.192A	T85.624A	T85.890A
T79.A21A	T80.A19A	T81.526A	T82.110A	T82.392A	T82.598A	T83.192A	T83.724A	T84.061A	T84.199A	T84.615A	T85.193A	T85.625A	T85.890D
T79.A22A	T80.A9XA	T81.527A	T82.111A	T82.398A	T82.599A	T83.193A	T83.728A	T84.062A	T84.210A	T84.619A	T85.199A	T85.628A	T88.0XXA
T79.A29A	T81.10XA	T81.528A	T82.118A	T82.399A	T82.6XXA	T83.198A	T83.729A	T84.063A	T84.213A	T84.620A	T85.21XA	T85.630A	T88.1XXA
T79.A3XA	T81.11XA	T81.529A	T82.119A	T82.41XA	T82.7XXA	T83.21XA	T83.79XA	T84.068A	T84.216A	T84.621A	T85.22XA	T85.631A	T88.2XXA
T79.A9XA	T81.12XA	T81.530A	T82.120A	T82.42XA	T82.817A	T83.22XA	T83.81XA	T84.069A	T84.218A	T84.622A	T85.29XA	T85.633A	T88.3XXA
T80.0XXA	T81.19XA	T81.531A	T82.121A	T82.43XA	T82.818A	T83.23XA	T83.82XA	T84.090A	T84.220A	T84.623A	T85.310A	T85.635A	T88.6XXA
T80.1XXA	T81.30XA	T81.532A	T82.128A	T82.49XA	T82.827A	T83.24XA	T83.83XA	T84.091A	T84.223A	T84.624A	T85.311A	T85.638A	
T80.211A	T81.31XA	T81.533A	T82.129A	T82.510A	T82.828A	T83.25XA	T83.84XA	T84.092A	T84.226A	T84.625A	T85.320A	T85.690A	
T80.212A	T81.32XA	T81.534A	T82.190A	T82.511A	T82.837A	T83.29XA	T83.85XA	T84.093A	T84.228A	T84.629A	T85.321A	T85.691A	
T80.218A	T81.33XA	T81.535A	T82.191A	T82.512A	T82.838A	T83.410A	T83.86XA	T84.098A	T84.290A	T84.63XA	T85.390A	T85.692A	
T80.219A	T81.4XXA	T81.536A	T82.198A	T82.513A	T82.847A	T83.411A	T83.89XA	T84.099A	T84.293A	T84.69XA	T85.391A	T85.693A	
T80.22XA	T81.500A	T81.537A	T82.199A	T82.514A	T82.848A	T83.418A	T83.9XXA	T84.110A	T84.296A	T84.7XXA	T85.41XA	T85.694A	

Female - Based on Medicare's Outpatient Code Editor (OCE)

O31.00X0	O31.10X9	O31.21X5	O31.32X4	O31.8X93	O32.4XX2	O33.4XX1	O35.1XX0	O35.5XX9	O36.0115	O36.0924	O36.1133	O36.1992	O36.4XX1
O31.00X1	O31.11X0	O31.21X9	O31.32X5	O31.8X94	O32.4XX3	O33.4XX2	O35.1XX1	O35.6XX0	O36.0119	O36.0925	O36.1134	O36.1993	O36.4XX2
O31.00X2	O31.11X1	O31.22X0	O31.32X9	O31.8X95	O32.4XX4	O33.4XX3	O35.1XX2	O35.6XX1	O36.0120	O36.0929	O36.1135	O36.1994	O36.4XX3
O31.00X3	O31.11X2	O31.22X1	O31.33X0	O31.8X99	O32.4XX5	O33.4XX4	O35.1XX3	O35.6XX2	O36.0121	O36.0930	O36.1139	O36.1995	O36.4XX4
O31.00X4	O31.11X3	O31.22X2	O31.33X1	O32.0XX0	O32.4XX9	O33.4XX5	O35.1XX4	O35.6XX3	O36.0122	O36.0931	O36.1190	O36.1999	O36.4XX5
O31.00X5	O31.11X4	O31.22X3	O31.33X2	O32.0XX1	O32.6XX0	O33.4XX9	O35.1XX5	O35.6XX4	O36.0123	O36.0932	O36.1191	O36.20X0	O36.4XX9
O31.00X9	O31.11X5	O31.22X4	O31.33X3	O32.0XX2	O32.6XX1	O33.5XX0	O35.1XX9	O35.6XX5	O36.0124	O36.0933	O36.1192	O36.20X1	O36.5110
O31.01X0	O31.11X9	O31.22X5	O31.33X4	O32.0XX3	O32.6XX2	O33.5XX1	O35.2XX0	O36.0115	O36.0125	O36.0934	O36.1193	O36.20X2	O36.5111
O31.01X1	O31.12X0	O31.22X9	O31.33X5	O32.0XX4	O32.6XX3	O33.5XX2	O35.2XX1	O35.7XX0	O36.0129	O36.0935	O36.1194	O36.20X3	O36.5112
O31.01X2	O31.12X1	O31.23X0	O31.33X9	O32.0XX5	O32.6XX4	O33.5XX3	O35.2XX2	O35.7XX1	O36.0130	O36.0939	O36.1195	O36.20X4	O36.5113
O31.01X3	O31.12X2	O31.23X1	O31.8X10	O32.0XX9	O32.6XX5	O33.5XX4	O35.2XX3	O35.7XX2	O36.0131	O36.0990	O36.1199	O36.20X5	O36.5114
O31.01X4	O31.12X3	O31.23X2	O31.8X11	O32.1XX0	O32.6XX9	O33.5XX5	O35.2XX4	O35.7XX3	O36.0132	O36.0991	O36.1910	O36.20X9	O36.5115
O31.01X5	O31.12X4	O31.23X3	O31.8X12	O32.1XX1	O32.8XX0	O33.5XX9	O35.2XX5	O35.7XX4	O36.0133	O36.0992	O36.1911	O36.21X0	O36.5119
O31.01X9	O31.12X5	O31.23X4	O31.8X13	O32.1XX2	O32.8XX1	O33.6XX0	O35.2XX9	O35.7XX5	O36.0134	O36.0993	O36.1912	O36.21X1	O36.5120
O31.02X0	O31.12X9	O31.23X5	O31.8X14	O32.1XX3	O32.8XX2	O33.6XX1	O35.3XX0	O35.9XX0	O36.0135	O36.0994	O36.1913	O36.21X2	O36.5121
O31.02X1	O31.13X0	O31.23X9	O31.8X15	O32.1XX4	O32.8XX3	O33.6XX2	O35.3XX1	O35.8XX0	O36.0139	O36.0995	O36.1914	O36.21X3	O36.5122
O31.02X2	O31.13X1	O31.30X0	O31.8X19	O32.1XX5	O32.8XX4	O33.6XX3	O35.3XX2	O35.8XX1	O36.0190	O36.0999	O36.1915	O36.21X4	O36.5123
O31.02X3	O31.13X2	O31.30X1	O31.8X20	O32.1XX9	O32.8XX5	O33.6XX4	O35.3XX3	O35.8XX2	O36.0191	O36.1110	O36.1919	O36.21X5	O36.5124
O31.02X4	O31.13X3	O31.30X2	O31.8X21	O32.2XX0	O32.8XX9	O33.6XX5	O35.3XX4	O35.8XX3	O36.0192	O36.1111	O36.1920	O36.21X9	O36.5125
O31.02X5	O31.13X4	O31.30X3	O31.8X22	O32.2XX1	O32.9XX0	O33.6XX9	O35.3XX5	O35.8XX4	O36.0193	O36.1112	O36.1921	O36.22X0	O36.5129
O31.02X9	O31.13X5	O31.30X4	O31.8X23	O32.2XX2	O32.9XX1	O33.7XX0	O35.3XX9	O35.8XX5	O36.0194	O36.1113	O36.1922	O36.22X1	O36.5130
O31.03X0	O31.13X9	O31.30X5	O31.8X24	O32.2XX3	O32.9XX2	O33.7XX1	O35.4XX0	O35.9XX0	O36.0195	O36.1114	O36.1923	O36.22X2	O36.5131
O31.03X1	O31.20X0	O31.31X0	O31.8X25	O32.2XX4	O32.9XX3	O33.7XX2	O35.4XX1	O35.9XX1	O36.0199	O36.1115	O36.1924	O36.22X3	O36.5132
O31.03X2	O31.20X1	O31.31X0	O31.8X28	O32.2XX5	O32.9XX4	O33.7XX3	O35.4XX2	O35.9XX2	O36.0910	O36.1119	O36.1925	O36.22X4	O36.5133
O31.03X3	O31.20X2	O31.31X1	O31.8X29	O32.2XX9	O32.9XX5	O33.7XX4	O35.4XX3	O35.9XX3	O36.0911	O36.1120	O36.1929	O36.22X5	O36.5134
O31.03X4	O31.20X3	O31.31X2	O31.8X30	O32.3XX0	O32.9XX9	O33.7XX5	O35.4XX4	O35.9XX4	O36.0912	O36.1121	O36.1930	O36.22X9	O36.5135
O31.03X5	O31.20X4	O31.31X3	O31.8X31	O32.3XX1	O33.3XX0	O33.7XX9	O35.4XX5	O35.9XX5	O36.0913	O36.1122	O36.1931	O36.23X0	O36.5139
O31.03X9	O31.20X5	O31.31X4	O31.8X32	O32.3XX3	O33.3XX1	O35.0XX0	O35.4XX9	O35.9XX9	O36.0914	O36.1123	O36.1932	O36.23X1	O36.5190
O31.10X0	O31.20X9	O31.31X5	O31.8X33	O32.3XX3	O33.3XX2	O35.0XX1	O35.5XX0	O35.9XX9	O36.0915	O36.1124	O36.1933	O36.23X2	O36.5191
O31.10X1	O31.21X0	O31.32X0	O31.8X34	O32.3XX4	O33.3XX3	O35.0XX2	O35.5XX1	O36.0110	O36.0919	O36.1125	O36.1934	O36.23X3	O36.5192
O31.10X2	O31.21X1	O31.32X0	O31.8X35	O32.3XX5	O33.3XX4	O35.0XX3	O35.5XX2	O36.0111	O36.0920	O36.1129	O36.1935	O36.23X4	O36.5193
O31.10X3	O31.21X2	O31.32X1	O31.8X90	O32.3XX9	O33.3XX5	O35.0XX4	O35.5XX3	O36.0112	O36.0921	O36.1130	O36.1939	O36.23X5	O36.5194
O31.10X4	O31.21X3	O31.32X2	O31.8X91	O32.4XX0	O33.3XX9	O35.0XX5	O35.5XX4	O36.0113	O36.0922	O36.1131	O36.1990	O36.23X9	O36.5195
O31.10X5	O31.21X4	O31.32X3	O31.8X92	O32.4XX1	O33.4XX0	O35.0XX9	O35.5XX5	O36.0114	O36.0923	O36.1132	O36.1991	O36.4XX0	O36.5199

Female (cont.) - Based on Medicare's Outpatient Code Editor (OCE)

O36.5910	O36.70X5	O36.8223	O36.8931	O40.3XX9	O41.1094	O41.8X12	O60.12X0	O64.2XX5	O69.3XX3	S30.826A	S31.532D	S37.499S	S38.03XA
O36.5911	O36.70X9	O36.8224	O36.8932	O40.9XX0	O41.1095	O41.8X13	O60.12X1	O64.2XX9	O69.3XX4	S30.826D	S31.532S	S37.501A	S38.03XD
O36.5912	O36.71X0	O36.8225	O36.8933	O40.9XX1	O41.1099	O41.8X14	O60.12X2	O64.3XX0	O69.3XX5	S30.826S	S31.542A	S37.501D	S38.03XS
O36.5913	O36.71X1	O36.8229	O36.8934	O40.9XX2	O41.1210	O41.8X15	O60.12X3	O64.3XX1	O69.3XX9	S30.844A	S31.542D	S37.501S	S38.211A
O36.5914	O36.71X2	O36.8230	O36.8935	O40.9XX3	O41.1211	O41.8X19	O60.12X4	O64.3XX2	O69.4XX0	S30.844D	S31.542S	S37.502A	S38.211D
O36.5915	O36.71X3	O36.8231	O36.8939	O40.9XX4	O41.1212	O41.8X20	O60.12X5	O64.3XX3	O69.4XX1	S30.844S	S31.552A	S37.502D	S38.211S
O36.5919	O36.71X4	O36.8232	O36.8990	O40.9XX9	O41.1213	O41.8X21	O60.13X0	O64.3XX4	O69.4XX2	S30.846A	S31.552D	S37.502S	S38.212A
O36.5920	O36.71X5	O36.8233	O36.8991	O41.00X0	O41.1214	O41.8X22	O60.13X1	O64.3XX5	O69.4XX3	S30.846D	S31.552S	S37.509A	S38.212D
O36.5921	O36.71X9	O36.8234	O36.8992	O41.00X1	O41.1215	O41.8X23	O60.13X2	O64.3XX9	O69.4XX4	S30.846S	S35.531A	S37.509D	S38.212S
O36.5922	O36.72X0	O36.8235	O36.8993	O41.00X2	O41.1219	O41.8X24	O60.13X3	O64.4XX0	O69.4XX5	S30.854A	S35.531D	S37.509S	T19.2XXA
O36.5923	O36.72X1	O36.8239	O36.8994	O41.00X3	O41.1220	O41.8X25	O60.13X4	O64.4XX1	O69.4XX9	S30.854D	S35.531S	S37.511A	T19.2XXD
O36.5924	O36.72X2	O36.8290	O36.8995	O41.00X4	O41.1221	O41.8X29	O60.13X5	O64.4XX2	O69.5XX0	S30.854S	S35.532A	S37.511D	T19.2XXS
O36.5925	O36.72X3	O36.8291	O36.8999	O41.00X5	O41.1222	O41.8X30	O60.13X9	O64.4XX3	O69.5XX1	S30.856A	S35.532D	S37.511S	T19.3XXA
O36.5929	O36.72X4	O36.8292	O36.90X0	O41.00X9	O41.1223	O41.8X31	O60.14X0	O64.4XX4	O69.5XX2	S30.856D	S35.532S	S37.512A	T19.3XXD
O36.5930	O36.72X5	O36.8293	O36.90X1	O41.01X0	O41.1224	O41.8X32	O60.14X1	O64.4XX5	O69.5XX3	S30.856S	S35.533A	S37.512D	T19.3XXS
O36.5931	O36.72X9	O36.8294	O36.90X2	O41.01X1	O41.1225	O41.8X33	O60.14X2	O64.4XX9	O69.5XX4	S30.864A	S35.533D	S37.512S	T21.07XA
O36.5932	O36.73X0	O36.8295	O36.90X3	O41.01X2	O41.1229	O41.8X34	O60.14X3	O64.5XX0	O69.5XX5	S30.864D	S35.533S	S37.519A	T21.07XD
O36.5933	O36.73X1	O36.8299	O36.90X4	O41.01X3	O41.1230	O41.8X35	O60.14X4	O64.5XX1	O69.5XX9	S30.864S	S35.534A	S37.519D	T21.07XS
O36.5934	O36.73X2	O36.8310	O36.90X5	O41.01X4	O41.1231	O41.8X39	O60.14X5	O64.5XX2	O69.81X0	S30.866A	S35.534D	S37.519S	T21.17XA
O36.5935	O36.73X3	O36.8311	O36.90X9	O41.01X5	O41.1232	O41.8X90	O60.14X9	O64.5XX3	O69.81X1	S30.866D	S35.534S	S37.521A	T21.17XD
O36.5939	O36.73X4	O36.8312	O36.91X0	O41.01X9	O41.1233	O41.8X91	O60.20X0	O64.5XX4	O69.81X2	S30.866S	S35.535A	S37.521D	T21.17XS
O36.5990	O36.73X5	O36.8313	O36.91X1	O41.02X0	O41.1234	O41.8X92	O60.20X1	O64.5XX5	O69.81X4	S30.874A	S35.535D	S37.521S	T21.27XA
O36.5991	O36.73X9	O36.8314	O36.91X2	O41.02X1	O41.1235	O41.8X93	O60.20X2	O64.5XX9	O69.81X5	S30.874D	S35.535S	S37.522A	T21.27XD
O36.5992	O36.80X0	O36.8315	O36.91X3	O41.02X2	O41.1239	O41.8X94	O60.20X3	O64.8XX0	O69.81X9	S30.874S	S35.536A	S37.522D	T21.27XS
O36.5993	O36.80X1	O36.8319	O36.91X4	O41.02X3	O41.1290	O41.8X95	O60.20X4	O64.8XX1	O69.82X0	S30.876A	S35.536D	S37.522S	T21.37XA
O36.5994	O36.80X2	O36.8320	O36.91X5	O41.02X4	O41.1291	O41.8X99	O60.20X5	O64.8XX3	O69.82X1	S30.876D	S35.536S	S37.529A	T21.37XD
O36.5995	O36.80X3	O36.8321	O36.91X9	O41.02X5	O41.1292	O41.90X0	O60.22X0	O64.8XX4	O69.82X2	S30.876S	S37.401A	S37.529D	T21.37XS
O36.5999	O36.80X4	O36.8322	O36.92X0	O41.02X9	O41.1293	O41.90X1	O60.22X1	O64.8XX5	O69.82X3	S30.95XA	S37.401D	S37.529S	T21.47XA
O36.60X0	O36.80X5	O36.8323	O36.92X1	O41.03X0	O41.1294	O41.90X2	O60.22X2	O64.8XX9	O69.82X4	S30.95XD	S37.401S	S37.531A	T21.47XD
O36.60X1	O36.80X9	O36.8324	O36.92X2	O41.03X1	O41.1295	O41.90X3	O60.22X3	O64.9XX0	O69.82X5	S30.95XS	S37.402A	S37.531D	T21.47XS
O36.60X2	O36.8120	O36.8325	O36.92X3	O41.03X2	O41.1299	O41.90X4	O60.22X4	O64.9XX1	O69.82X9	S30.97XA	S37.402D	S37.531S	T21.57XA
O36.60X3	O36.8121	O36.8329	O36.92X4	O41.03X3	O41.1410	O41.90X5	O60.22X5	O64.9XX3	O69.89X0	S30.97XD	S37.402S	S37.532A	T21.57XD
O36.60X4	O36.8122	O36.8330	O36.92X5	O41.03X4	O41.1411	O41.90X9	O60.23X0	O64.9XX4	O69.89X1	S30.97XS	S37.409A	S37.532D	T21.57XS
O36.60X5	O36.8123	O36.8331	O36.92X9	O41.03X5	O41.1412	O41.91X0	O60.23X1	O64.9XX5	O69.89X2	S31.40XA	S37.409D	S37.532S	T21.67XA
O36.60X9	O36.8124	O36.8332	O36.93X0	O41.03X9	O41.1413	O41.91X1	O60.23X2	O64.9XX9	O69.89X3	S31.40XD	S37.409S	S37.539A	T21.67XD
O36.61X0	O36.8125	O36.8333	O36.93X1	O41.1010	O41.1414	O41.91X2	O60.23X3	O69.0XX0	O69.89X4	S31.40XS	S37.421A	S37.539D	T21.67XS
O36.61X1	O36.8129	O36.8334	O36.93X2	O41.1011	O41.1415	O41.91X3	O60.23X4	O69.0XX1	O69.89X5	S31.41XA	S37.421D	S37.539S	T21.77XA
O36.61X2	O36.8130	O36.8335	O36.93X3	O41.1012	O41.1419	O41.91X4	O60.23X5	O69.0XX2	O69.89X9	S31.41XD	S37.421S	S37.591A	T21.77XD
O36.61X3	O36.8131	O36.8339	O36.93X4	O41.1013	O41.1420	O41.91X5	O64.0XX0	O69.0XX3	O69.9XX0	S31.41XS	S37.422A	S37.591D	T21.77XS
O36.61X4	O36.8132	O36.8390	O36.93X5	O41.1014	O41.1421	O41.91X9	O64.0XX1	O69.0XX4	O69.9XX1	S31.42XA	S37.422D	S37.591S	T83.31XA
O36.61X5	O36.8133	O36.8391	O36.93X9	O41.1015	O41.1422	O41.92X0	O64.0XX2	O69.0XX5	O69.9XX2	S31.42XD	S37.422S	S37.592A	T83.31XD
O36.61X9	O36.8134	O36.8392	O40.1XX0	O41.1019	O41.1423	O41.92X1	O64.0XX3	O69.0XX9	O69.9XX3	S31.42XS	S37.429A	S37.592D	T83.31XS
O36.62X0	O36.8135	O36.8393	O40.1XX1	O41.1020	O41.1424	O41.92X2	O64.0XX4	O69.1XX0	O69.9XX4	S31.43XA	S37.429D	S37.592S	T83.32XA
O36.62X1	O36.8139	O36.8394	O40.1XX2	O41.1021	O41.1425	O41.92X3	O64.0XX5	O69.1XX1	O69.9XX5	S31.43XD	S37.429S	S37.599A	T83.32XD
O36.62X2	O36.8190	O36.8395	O40.1XX3	O41.1022	O41.1429	O41.92X4	O64.1XX0	O69.1XX2	O69.9XX9	S31.43XS	S37.431A	S37.599D	T83.32XS
O36.62X3	O36.8191	O36.8399	O40.1XX4	O41.1023	O41.1430	O41.92X5	O64.1XX1	O69.1XX3	S30.202A	S31.44XA	S37.431D	S37.599S	T83.39XA
O36.62X4	O36.8192	O36.8910	O40.1XX5	O41.1024	O41.1431	O41.92X9	O64.1XX2	O69.1XX4	S30.202D	S31.44XD	S37.431S	S37.60XA	T83.39XD
O36.62X5	O36.8193	O36.8911	O40.1XX9	O41.1025	O41.1432	O41.93X0	O64.1XX3	O69.1XX5	S30.202S	S31.44XS	S37.432A	S37.60XD	T83.39XS
O36.62X9	O36.8194	O36.8912	O40.2XX0	O41.1029	O41.1433	O41.93X1	O64.1XX4	O69.1XX9	S30.23XA	S31.45XA	S37.432D	S37.60XS	T83.711A
O36.63X0	O36.8195	O36.8913	O40.2XX1	O41.1030	O41.1434	O41.93X2	O64.1XX5	O69.2XX0	S30.23XD	S31.45XD	S37.432S	S37.62XA	T83.711D
O36.63X1	O36.8199	O36.8914	O40.2XX2	O41.1031	O41.1435	O41.93X3	O64.2XX0	O69.2XX1	S30.23XS	S31.45XS	S37.439A	S37.62XD	T83.711S
O36.63X2	O36.8210	O36.8915	O40.2XX3	O41.1032	O41.1439	O41.93X4	O64.2XX1	O69.2XX2	S30.814A	S31.502A	S37.439D	S37.62XS	T83.721A
O36.63X3	O36.8211	O36.8919	O40.2XX4	O41.1033	O41.1490	O41.93X5	O64.2XX2	O69.2XX3	S30.814D	S31.502D	S37.439S	S37.63XA	T83.721D
O36.63X4	O36.8212	O36.8920	O40.2XX5	O41.1034	O41.1491	O41.93X9	O64.2XX3	O69.2XX4	S30.814S	S31.502S	S37.491A	S37.63XD	T83.721S
O36.63X5	O36.8213	O36.8921	O40.3XX0	O41.1035	O41.1492	O60.10X0	O64.2XX4	O69.2XX5	S30.816A	S31.512A	S37.491D	S37.63XS	
O36.63X9	O36.8214	O36.8922	O40.3XX1	O41.1039	O41.1493	O60.10X1		O69.2XX9	S30.816D	S31.512D	S37.491S	S37.69XA	
O36.70X0	O36.8215	O36.8923	O40.3XX2	O41.1090	O41.1494	O60.10X2		O69.3XX0	S30.816S	S31.512S	S37.492A	S37.69XD	
O36.70X1	O36.8219	O36.8924	O40.3XX3	O41.1091	O41.1495	O60.10X3		O69.3XX1	S30.824A	S31.522A	S37.492D	S37.69XS	
O36.70X2	O36.8220	O36.8925	O40.3XX4	O41.1092	O41.1499	O60.10X4		O69.3XX2	S30.824D	S31.522D	S37.492S	S38.002A	
O36.70X3	O36.8221	O36.8929	O40.3XX5	O41.1093	O41.8X10	O60.10X5			S30.824S	S31.522S	S37.499A	S38.002D	
O36.70X4	O36.8222	O36.8930			O41.8X11	O60.10X9				S31.532A	S37.499D	S38.002S	

Hospital-acquired Condition (HAC) - Based on CMS data

S02.0XXA	S02.118A	S02.401B	S02.42XB	S02.91XB	S06.1X6A	S06.2X7A	S06.308A	S06.318A	S06.328A	S06.338A	S06.348A	S06.358A	S06.368A
S02.0XXB	S02.118B	S02.402A	S02.600A	S02.92XA	S06.1X7A	S06.2X8A	S06.309A	S06.319A	S06.329A	S06.339A	S06.349A	S06.359A	S06.369A
S02.110A	S02.119A	S02.402B	S02.600B	S02.92XB	S06.1X8A	S06.2X9A	S06.310A	S06.320A	S06.330A	S06.340A	S06.350A	S06.360A	S06.370A
S02.110B	S02.119B	S02.411A	S02.609A	S06.0X1A	S06.1X9A	S06.301A	S06.311A	S06.321A	S06.331A	S06.341A	S06.351A	S06.361A	S06.371A
S02.111A	S02.19XA	S02.411B	S02.609B	S06.0X9A	S06.2X1A	S06.302A	S06.312A	S06.322A	S06.332A	S06.342A	S06.352A	S06.362A	S06.372A
S02.111B	S02.19XB	S02.412A	S02.66XA	S06.1X1A	S06.2X2A	S06.303A	S06.313A	S06.323A	S06.333A	S06.343A	S06.353A	S06.363A	S06.373A
S02.112A	S02.2XXB	S02.412B	S02.66XB	S06.1X2A	S06.2X3A	S06.304A	S06.314A	S06.324A	S06.334A	S06.344A	S06.354A	S06.364A	S06.374A
S02.112B	S02.400A	S02.413A	S02.69XA	S06.1X3A	S06.2X4A	S06.305A	S06.315A	S06.325A	S06.335A	S06.345A	S06.355A	S06.365A	S06.375A
S02.113A	S02.400B	S02.413B	S02.69XB	S06.1X4A	S06.2X5A	S06.306A	S06.316A	S06.326A	S06.336A	S06.346A	S06.356A	S06.366A	S06.376A
S02.113B	S02.401A	S02.42XA	S02.91XA	S06.1X5A	S06.2X6A	S06.307A	S06.317A	S06.327A	S06.337A	S06.347A	S06.357A	S06.367A	S06.377A

Hospital-acquired Condition (HAC) (cont.) - Based on CMS data

S06.378A	S06.9X6A	S12.300A	S13.0XXA	S22.012A	S22.089A	S32.028B	S32.302B	S32.446B	S32.601B	S42.032B	S42.232B	S42.333B	S42.424B
S06.379A	S06.9X7A	S12.300B	S13.100A	S22.012B	S22.089B	S32.029A	S32.309A	S32.451A	S32.602A	S42.033B	S42.239A	S42.334A	S42.425A
S06.380A	S06.9X8A	S12.301A	S13.101A	S22.018A	S22.20XA	S32.029B	S32.309B	S32.451B	S32.602B	S42.034B	S42.239B	S42.334B	S42.425B
S06.381A	S06.9X9A	S12.301B	S13.110A	S22.018B	S22.20XB	S32.030A	S32.311A	S32.452A	S32.609A	S42.035B	S42.241A	S42.335A	S42.426A
S06.382A	S07.0XXA	S12.330A	S13.111A	S22.019A	S22.21XA	S32.030B	S32.311B	S32.452B	S32.609B	S42.036B	S42.241B	S42.335B	S42.426B
S06.383A	S07.1XXA	S12.330B	S13.120A	S22.019B	S22.21XB	S32.031A	S32.312A	S32.453A	S32.611A	S42.101B	S42.242A	S42.336A	S42.431A
S06.384A	S07.8XXA	S12.331A	S13.121A	S22.020A	S22.22XA	S32.031B	S32.312B	S32.453B	S32.611B	S42.102B	S42.242B	S42.336B	S42.431B
S06.385A	S07.9XXA	S12.331B	S13.130A	S22.020B	S22.22XB	S32.032A	S32.313A	S32.454A	S32.612A	S42.109B	S42.249A	S42.341A	S42.432A
S06.386A	S12.000A	S12.34XA	S13.131A	S22.021A	S22.23XA	S32.032B	S32.313B	S32.454B	S32.612B	S42.111B	S42.249B	S42.341B	S42.432B
S06.387A	S12.000B	S12.34XB	S13.140A	S22.021B	S22.23XB	S32.038A	S32.314A	S32.455A	S32.613A	S42.112B	S42.251A	S42.342A	S42.433A
S06.388A	S12.001A	S12.350A	S13.141A	S22.022A	S22.24XA	S32.038B	S32.314B	S32.455B	S32.613B	S42.113B	S42.251B	S42.342B	S42.433B
S06.389A	S12.001B	S12.350B	S13.150A	S22.022B	S22.24XB	S32.039A	S32.315A	S32.456A	S32.614A	S42.114B	S42.252A	S42.343A	S42.434A
S06.4X0A	S12.01XA	S12.351A	S13.151A	S22.028A	S22.31XA	S32.039B	S32.315B	S32.456B	S32.614B	S42.115B	S42.252B	S42.343B	S42.434B
S06.4X1A	S12.01XB	S12.351B	S13.160A	S22.028B	S22.31XB	S32.040A	S32.316A	S32.461A	S32.615A	S42.116B	S42.253A	S42.344A	S42.435A
S06.4X2A	S12.02XA	S12.390A	S13.161A	S22.029A	S22.32XA	S32.040B	S32.316B	S32.461B	S32.615B	S42.121B	S42.253B	S42.344B	S42.435B
S06.4X3A	S12.02XB	S12.390B	S13.170A	S22.029B	S22.32XB	S32.041A	S32.391A	S32.462A	S32.616A	S42.122B	S42.254A	S42.345A	S42.436A
S06.4X4A	S12.030A	S12.391A	S13.171A	S22.030A	S22.39XA	S32.041B	S32.391B	S32.462B	S32.616B	S42.123B	S42.254B	S42.345B	S42.436B
S06.4X5A	S12.030B	S12.391B	S13.180A	S22.030B	S22.39XB	S32.042A	S32.392A	S32.463A	S32.691A	S42.124B	S42.255A	S42.346A	S42.441A
S06.4X6A	S12.031A	S12.400A	S13.181A	S22.031A	S22.41XA	S32.042B	S32.392B	S32.463B	S32.691B	S42.125B	S42.255B	S42.346B	S42.441B
S06.4X7A	S12.031B	S12.400B	S13.20XA	S22.031B	S22.41XB	S32.048A	S32.399A	S32.464A	S32.692A	S42.126B	S42.256A	S42.351A	S42.442A
S06.4X8A	S12.040A	S12.401A	S13.29XA	S22.032A	S22.42XA	S32.048B	S32.399B	S32.464B	S32.692B	S42.131B	S42.256B	S42.351B	S42.442B
S06.4X9A	S12.040B	S12.401B	S14.101A	S22.032B	S22.42XB	S32.049A	S32.401A	S32.465A	S32.699A	S42.132B	S42.261A	S42.352A	S42.443A
S06.5X0A	S12.041A	S12.430A	S14.102A	S22.038A	S22.43XA	S32.049B	S32.401B	S32.465B	S32.699B	S42.133B	S42.261B	S42.352B	S42.443B
S06.5X1A	S12.041B	S12.430B	S14.103A	S22.038B	S22.43XB	S32.050A	S32.402A	S32.466A	S32.810A	S42.134B	S42.262A	S42.353A	S42.444A
S06.5X2A	S12.090A	S12.431A	S14.104A	S22.039A	S22.49XA	S32.050B	S32.402B	S32.466B	S32.810B	S42.135B	S42.262B	S42.353B	S42.444B
S06.5X3A	S12.090B	S12.431B	S14.105A	S22.039B	S22.49XB	S32.051A	S32.409A	S32.471A	S32.811A	S42.136B	S42.263A	S42.354A	S42.445A
S06.5X4A	S12.091A	S12.44XA	S14.106A	S22.040A	S22.5XXA	S32.051B	S32.409B	S32.471B	S32.811B	S42.141B	S42.263B	S42.354B	S42.445B
S06.5X5A	S12.091B	S12.44XB	S14.107A	S22.040B	S22.5XXB	S32.052A	S32.411A	S32.472A	S32.82XA	S42.142B	S42.264A	S42.355A	S42.446A
S06.5X6A	S12.100A	S12.450A	S14.109A	S22.041A	S22.9XXA	S32.052B	S32.411B	S32.472B	S32.82XB	S42.143B	S42.264B	S42.355B	S42.446B
S06.5X7A	S12.100B	S12.450B	S14.111A	S22.041B	S22.9XXB	S32.058A	S32.412A	S32.473A	S32.89XA	S42.144B	S42.265A	S42.356A	S42.447A
S06.5X8A	S12.101A	S12.451A	S14.112A	S22.042A	S24.101A	S32.058B	S32.412B	S32.473B	S32.89XB	S42.145B	S42.265B	S42.356B	S42.447B
S06.5X9A	S12.101B	S12.451B	S14.113A	S22.042B	S24.102A	S32.059A	S32.413A	S32.474A	S32.9XXA	S42.146B	S42.266A	S42.361A	S42.448A
S06.6X0A	S12.110A	S12.490A	S14.114A	S22.048A	S24.103A	S32.059B	S32.413B	S32.474B	S32.9XXB	S42.151B	S42.266B	S42.361B	S42.448B
S06.6X1A	S12.110B	S12.490B	S14.115A	S22.048B	S24.104A	S32.10XA	S32.414A	S32.475A	S34.101A	S42.152B	S42.271A	S42.362A	S42.449A
S06.6X2A	S12.111A	S12.491A	S14.116A	S22.049A	S24.109A	S32.10XB	S32.414B	S32.475B	S34.102A	S42.153B	S42.272A	S42.362B	S42.449B
S06.6X3A	S12.111B	S12.491B	S14.117A	S22.049B	S24.111A	S32.110A	S32.415A	S32.476A	S34.103A	S42.154B	S42.279A	S42.363A	S42.451A
S06.6X4A	S12.112A	S12.500A	S14.121A	S22.050A	S24.112A	S32.110B	S32.415B	S32.476B	S34.104A	S42.155B	S42.291A	S42.363B	S42.451B
S06.6X5A	S12.112B	S12.500B	S14.122A	S22.050B	S24.113A	S32.111A	S32.416A	S32.481A	S34.105A	S42.156B	S42.291B	S42.364A	S42.452A
S06.6X6A	S12.120A	S12.501A	S14.123A	S22.051A	S24.114A	S32.111B	S32.416B	S32.481B	S34.109A	S42.191B	S42.292A	S42.364B	S42.452B
S06.6X7A	S12.120B	S12.501B	S14.124A	S22.051B	S24.131A	S32.112A	S32.421A	S32.482A	S34.111A	S42.192B	S42.292B	S42.365A	S42.453A
S06.6X8A	S12.121A	S12.530A	S14.125A	S22.052A	S24.132A	S32.112B	S32.421B	S32.482B	S34.112A	S42.199B	S42.293A	S42.365B	S42.453B
S06.6X9A	S12.121B	S12.530B	S14.126A	S22.052B	S24.133A	S32.119A	S32.422A	S32.483A	S34.113A	S42.201A	S42.293B	S42.366A	S42.454A
S06.811A	S12.130A	S12.531A	S14.127A	S22.058A	S24.134A	S32.119B	S32.422B	S32.483B	S34.114A	S42.201B	S42.294A	S42.366B	S42.454B
S06.812A	S12.130B	S12.531B	S14.131A	S22.058B	S24.151A	S32.120A	S32.423A	S32.484A	S34.115A	S42.202A	S42.294B	S42.391A	S42.455A
S06.813A	S12.131A	S12.54XA	S14.132A	S22.059A	S24.152A	S32.120B	S32.423B	S32.484B	S34.119A	S42.202B	S42.295A	S42.391B	S42.455B
S06.814A	S12.131B	S12.54XB	S14.133A	S22.059B	S24.153A	S32.121A	S32.424A	S32.485A	S34.121A	S42.209A	S42.295B	S42.392A	S42.456A
S06.815A	S12.14XA	S12.550A	S14.134A	S22.060A	S24.154A	S32.121B	S32.424B	S32.485B	S34.122A	S42.209B	S42.296A	S42.392B	S42.456B
S06.816A	S12.14XB	S12.550B	S14.135A	S22.060B	S32.000A	S32.122A	S32.425A	S32.486A	S34.123A	S42.211A	S42.296B	S42.399A	S42.461A
S06.817A	S12.150A	S12.551A	S14.136A	S22.061A	S32.000B	S32.122B	S32.425B	S32.486B	S34.124A	S42.211B	S42.301A	S42.399B	S42.461B
S06.818A	S12.150B	S12.551B	S14.137A	S22.061B	S32.001A	S32.129A	S32.426A	S32.491A	S34.125A	S42.212A	S42.301B	S42.401A	S42.462A
S06.819A	S12.151A	S12.590A	S14.151A	S22.062A	S32.001B	S32.129B	S32.426B	S32.491B	S34.129A	S42.212B	S42.302A	S42.401B	S42.462B
S06.821A	S12.151B	S12.590B	S14.152A	S22.062B	S32.002A	S32.130A	S32.431A	S32.492A	S34.131A	S42.213A	S42.302B	S42.402A	S42.463A
S06.822A	S12.190A	S12.591A	S14.153A	S22.068A	S32.002B	S32.130B	S32.431B	S32.492B	S34.132A	S42.213B	S42.309A	S42.402B	S42.463B
S06.823A	S12.190B	S12.591B	S14.154A	S22.068B	S32.008A	S32.131A	S32.432A	S32.499A	S34.139A	S42.214A	S42.309B	S42.409A	S42.464A
S06.824A	S12.191A	S12.600A	S14.155A	S22.069A	S32.008B	S32.131B	S32.432B	S32.499B	S34.3XXA	S42.214B	S42.311A	S42.409B	S42.464B
S06.825A	S12.191B	S12.600B	S14.156A	S22.069B	S32.009A	S32.132A	S32.433A	S32.501A	S42.001B	S42.215A	S42.312A	S42.411A	S42.465A
S06.826A	S12.200A	S12.601A	S14.157A	S22.070A	S32.009B	S32.132B	S32.433B	S32.501B	S42.002B	S42.215B	S42.319A	S42.411B	S42.465B
S06.827A	S12.200B	S12.601B	S17.0XXA	S22.070B	S32.010A	S32.139A	S32.434A	S32.502A	S42.009B	S42.216A	S42.321A	S42.412A	S42.466A
S06.828A	S12.201A	S12.630A	S17.8XXA	S22.071A	S32.010B	S32.139B	S32.434B	S32.502B	S42.011B	S42.216B	S42.321B	S42.412B	S42.466B
S06.829A	S12.201B	S12.630B	S17.9XXA	S22.071B	S32.011A	S32.14XA	S32.435A	S32.509A	S42.012B	S42.221A	S42.322A	S42.413A	S42.471A
S06.891A	S12.230A	S12.631A	S22.000A	S22.072A	S32.011B	S32.14XB	S32.435B	S32.509B	S42.013B	S42.221B	S42.322B	S42.413B	S42.471B
S06.892A	S12.230B	S12.631B	S22.000B	S22.072B	S32.012A	S32.15XA	S32.436A	S32.511A	S42.014B	S42.222A	S42.323A	S42.414A	S42.472A
S06.893A	S12.231A	S12.64XA	S22.001A	S22.078A	S32.012B	S32.15XB	S32.436B	S32.511B	S42.015B	S42.222B	S42.323B	S42.414B	S42.472B
S06.894A	S12.231B	S12.64XB	S22.001B	S22.078B	S32.018A	S32.16XA	S32.441A	S32.512A	S42.016B	S42.223A	S42.324A	S42.415A	S42.473A
S06.895A	S12.24XA	S12.650A	S22.002A	S22.079A	S32.018B	S32.16XB	S32.441B	S32.512B	S42.017B	S42.223B	S42.324B	S42.415B	S42.473B
S06.896A	S12.24XB	S12.650B	S22.002B	S22.079B	S32.019A	S32.17XA	S32.442A	S32.519A	S42.018B	S42.224A	S42.325A	S42.416A	S42.474A
S06.897A	S12.250A	S12.651A	S22.008A	S22.080A	S32.019B	S32.17XB	S32.442B	S32.519B	S42.019B	S42.224B	S42.325B	S42.416B	S42.474B
S06.898A	S12.250B	S12.651B	S22.008B	S22.080B	S32.020A	S32.19XA	S32.443A	S32.591A	S42.021B	S42.225A	S42.326A	S42.421A	S42.475A
S06.899A	S12.251A	S12.690A	S22.009A	S22.081A	S32.020B	S32.19XB	S32.443B	S32.591B	S42.022B	S42.225B	S42.326B	S42.421B	S42.475B
S06.9X1A	S12.251B	S12.690B	S22.009B	S22.081B	S32.021A	S32.2XXA	S32.444A	S32.592A	S42.023B	S42.226A	S42.331A	S42.422A	S42.476A
S06.9X2A	S12.290A	S12.691A	S22.010A	S22.082A	S32.021B	S32.2XXB	S32.444B	S32.592B	S42.024B	S42.226B	S42.331B	S42.422B	S42.476B
S06.9X3A	S12.290B	S12.691B	S22.010B	S22.082B	S32.022A	S32.301A	S32.445A	S32.599A	S42.025B	S42.231A	S42.332A	S42.423A	S42.481A
S06.9X4A	S12.291A	S12.8XXA	S22.011A	S22.088A	S32.022B	S32.301B	S32.445B	S32.599B	S42.026B	S42.231B	S42.332B	S42.423B	S42.482A
S06.9X5A	S12.291B	S12.9XXA	S22.011B	S22.088B	S32.028A	S32.302A	S32.446A	S32.601A	S42.031B	S42.232A	S42.333A	S42.424A	S42.489A

Hospital-acquired Condition (HAC) (cont.) - Based on CMS data

S42.491A	S52.002B	S52.133B	S52.245A	S52.309C	S52.356B	S52.521A	S52.613C	S62.015B	S62.224B	S62.350B	S62.629B	S72.025A	S72.092C
S42.491B	S52.002C	S52.133C	S52.245B	S52.311A	S52.356C	S52.522A	S52.614A	S62.016B	S62.225B	S62.351B	S62.630B	S72.025B	S72.099A
S42.492A	S52.009B	S52.134B	S52.245C	S52.312A	S52.361A	S52.529A	S52.614B	S62.021B	S62.226B	S62.352B	S62.631B	S72.025C	S72.099B
S42.492B	S52.009C	S52.134C	S52.246A	S52.319A	S52.361B	S52.531A	S52.614C	S62.022B	S62.231B	S62.353B	S62.632B	S72.026A	S72.099C
S42.493A	S52.011A	S52.135B	S52.246B	S52.321A	S52.361C	S52.531B	S52.615A	S62.023B	S62.232B	S62.354B	S62.633B	S72.026B	S72.101A
S42.493B	S52.012A	S52.135C	S52.246C	S52.321B	S52.362A	S52.531C	S52.615B	S62.024B	S62.233B	S62.355B	S62.634B	S72.026C	S72.101B
S42.494A	S52.019A	S52.136B	S52.251A	S52.321C	S52.362B	S52.532A	S52.615C	S62.025B	S62.234B	S62.356B	S62.635B	S72.031A	S72.101C
S42.494B	S52.021B	S52.136C	S52.251B	S52.322A	S52.362C	S52.532B	S52.616A	S62.026B	S62.235B	S62.357B	S62.636B	S72.031B	S72.102A
S42.495A	S52.021C	S52.181B	S52.251C	S52.322B	S52.363A	S52.532C	S52.616B	S62.031B	S62.236B	S62.358B	S62.637B	S72.031C	S72.102B
S42.495B	S52.022B	S52.181C	S52.252A	S52.322C	S52.363B	S52.539A	S52.616C	S62.032B	S62.241B	S62.359B	S62.638B	S72.032A	S72.102C
S42.496A	S52.022C	S52.182B	S52.252B	S52.323A	S52.363C	S52.539B	S52.621A	S62.033B	S62.242B	S62.360B	S62.639B	S72.032B	S72.109A
S42.496B	S52.023B	S52.182C	S52.252C	S52.323B	S52.364A	S52.539C	S52.622A	S62.034B	S62.243B	S62.361B	S62.640B	S72.032C	S72.109B
S42.90XA	S52.023C	S52.189B	S52.253A	S52.323C	S52.364B	S52.541A	S52.629A	S62.035B	S62.244B	S62.362B	S62.641B	S72.033A	S72.109C
S42.90XB	S52.024B	S52.189C	S52.253B	S52.324A	S52.364C	S52.541B	S52.691A	S62.036B	S62.245B	S62.363B	S62.642B	S72.033B	S72.111A
S42.91XA	S52.024C	S52.201A	S52.253C	S52.324B	S52.365A	S52.541C	S52.691B	S62.101B	S62.246B	S62.364B	S62.643B	S72.033C	S72.111B
S42.91XB	S52.025B	S52.201B	S52.254A	S52.324C	S52.365B	S52.542A	S52.691C	S62.102B	S62.251B	S62.365B	S62.644B	S72.034A	S72.111C
S42.92XA	S52.025C	S52.201C	S52.254B	S52.325A	S52.365C	S52.542B	S52.692A	S62.109B	S62.252B	S62.366B	S62.645B	S72.034B	S72.112A
S42.92XB	S52.026B	S52.202A	S52.254C	S52.325B	S52.366A	S52.542C	S52.692B	S62.111B	S62.253B	S62.367B	S62.646B	S72.034C	S72.112B
S43.201A	S52.026C	S52.202B	S52.255A	S52.325C	S52.366B	S52.549A	S52.692C	S62.112B	S62.254B	S62.368B	S62.647B	S72.035A	S72.112C
S43.202A	S52.031B	S52.202C	S52.255B	S52.326A	S52.366C	S52.549B	S52.699A	S62.113B	S62.255B	S62.369B	S62.648B	S72.035B	S72.113A
S43.203A	S52.031C	S52.209A	S52.255C	S52.326B	S52.371A	S52.549C	S52.699B	S62.114B	S62.256B	S62.390B	S62.649B	S72.035C	S72.113B
S43.204A	S52.032B	S52.209B	S52.256A	S52.326C	S52.371B	S52.551A	S52.699C	S62.115B	S62.291B	S62.391B	S62.650B	S72.036A	S72.113C
S43.205A	S52.032C	S52.209C	S52.256B	S52.331A	S52.371C	S52.551B	S52.90XA	S62.116B	S62.292B	S62.392B	S62.651B	S72.036B	S72.114A
S43.206A	S52.033B	S52.211A	S52.256C	S52.331B	S52.372A	S52.551C	S52.90XB	S62.121B	S62.299B	S62.393B	S62.652B	S72.036C	S72.114B
S43.211A	S52.033C	S52.212A	S52.261A	S52.331C	S52.372B	S52.552A	S52.90XC	S62.122B	S62.300B	S62.394B	S62.653B	S72.041A	S72.114C
S43.212A	S52.034B	S52.219A	S52.261B	S52.332A	S52.372C	S52.552B	S52.91XA	S62.123B	S62.301B	S62.395B	S62.654B	S72.041B	S72.115A
S43.213A	S52.034C	S52.221A	S52.261C	S52.332B	S52.379A	S52.552C	S52.91XB	S62.124B	S62.302B	S62.396B	S62.655B	S72.041C	S72.115B
S43.214A	S52.035B	S52.221B	S52.262A	S52.332C	S52.379B	S52.559A	S52.91XC	S62.125B	S62.303B	S62.397B	S62.656B	S72.042A	S72.115C
S43.215A	S52.035C	S52.221C	S52.262B	S52.333A	S52.379C	S52.559B	S52.92XA	S62.126B	S62.304B	S62.398B	S62.657B	S72.042B	S72.116A
S43.216A	S52.036B	S52.222A	S52.262C	S52.333B	S52.381A	S52.559C	S52.92XB	S62.131B	S62.305B	S62.399B	S62.658B	S72.042C	S72.116B
S43.221A	S52.036C	S52.222B	S52.263A	S52.333C	S52.381B	S52.561A	S52.92XC	S62.132B	S62.306B	S62.501B	S62.659B	S72.043A	S72.116C
S43.222A	S52.041B	S52.222C	S52.263B	S52.334A	S52.381C	S52.561B	S59.001A	S62.133B	S62.307B	S62.502B	S62.660B	S72.043B	S72.121A
S43.223A	S52.041C	S52.223A	S52.263C	S52.334B	S52.382A	S52.561C	S59.002A	S62.134B	S62.308B	S62.509B	S62.661B	S72.043C	S72.121B
S43.224A	S52.042B	S52.223B	S52.264A	S52.334C	S52.382B	S52.562A	S59.009A	S62.135B	S62.309B	S62.511B	S62.662B	S72.044A	S72.121C
S43.225A	S52.042C	S52.223C	S52.264B	S52.335A	S52.382C	S52.562B	S59.011A	S62.136B	S62.310B	S62.512B	S62.663B	S72.044B	S72.122A
S43.226A	S52.043B	S52.224A	S52.264C	S52.335B	S52.389A	S52.562C	S59.012A	S62.141B	S62.311B	S62.513B	S62.664B	S72.044C	S72.122B
S49.001A	S52.043C	S52.224B	S52.265A	S52.335C	S52.389B	S52.569A	S59.019A	S62.142B	S62.312B	S62.514B	S62.665B	S72.045A	S72.122C
S49.002A	S52.044B	S52.224C	S52.265B	S52.336A	S52.389C	S52.569B	S59.021A	S62.143B	S62.313B	S62.515B	S62.666B	S72.045B	S72.123A
S49.009A	S52.044C	S52.225A	S52.265C	S52.336B	S52.391A	S52.569C	S59.022A	S62.144B	S62.314B	S62.516B	S62.667B	S72.045C	S72.123B
S49.011A	S52.045B	S52.225B	S52.266A	S52.336C	S52.391B	S52.571A	S59.029A	S62.145B	S62.315B	S62.521B	S62.668B	S72.046A	S72.123C
S49.012A	S52.045C	S52.225C	S52.266B	S52.341A	S52.391C	S52.571B	S59.031A	S62.146B	S62.316B	S62.522B	S62.669B	S72.046B	S72.124A
S49.019A	S52.046B	S52.226A	S52.266C	S52.341B	S52.392A	S52.571C	S59.032A	S62.151B	S62.317B	S62.523B	S62.90XB	S72.046C	S72.124B
S49.021A	S52.046C	S52.226B	S52.271B	S52.341C	S52.392B	S52.572A	S59.039A	S62.152B	S62.318B	S62.524B	S62.91XB	S72.051A	S72.124C
S49.022A	S52.091B	S52.226C	S52.271C	S52.342A	S52.392C	S52.572B	S59.041A	S62.153B	S62.319B	S62.525B	S62.92XB	S72.051B	S72.125A
S49.029A	S52.091C	S52.231A	S52.272B	S52.342B	S52.399A	S52.572C	S59.042A	S62.154B	S62.320B	S62.526B	S72.001A	S72.051C	S72.125B
S49.031A	S52.092B	S52.231B	S52.272C	S52.342C	S52.399B	S52.579A	S59.049A	S62.155B	S62.321B	S62.600B	S72.001B	S72.052A	S72.125C
S49.032A	S52.092C	S52.231C	S52.279B	S52.343A	S52.399C	S52.579B	S59.091A	S62.156B	S62.322B	S62.601B	S72.001C	S72.052B	S72.126A
S49.039A	S52.099B	S52.232A	S52.279C	S52.343B	S52.501A	S52.579C	S59.092A	S62.161B	S62.323B	S62.602B	S72.002A	S72.052C	S72.126B
S49.041A	S52.099C	S52.232B	S52.281A	S52.343C	S52.501B	S52.591A	S59.099A	S62.162B	S62.324B	S62.603B	S72.002B	S72.059A	S72.126C
S49.042A	S52.101B	S52.232C	S52.281B	S52.344A	S52.501C	S52.591B	S59.201A	S62.163B	S62.325B	S62.604B	S72.002C	S72.059B	S72.131A
S49.049A	S52.101C	S52.233A	S52.281C	S52.344B	S52.502A	S52.591C	S59.202A	S62.164B	S62.326B	S62.605B	S72.009A	S72.059C	S72.131B
S49.091A	S52.102B	S52.233B	S52.282A	S52.344C	S52.502B	S52.592A	S59.209A	S62.165B	S62.327B	S62.606B	S72.009B	S72.061A	S72.131C
S49.092A	S52.102C	S52.233C	S52.282B	S52.345A	S52.502C	S52.592B	S59.211A	S62.166B	S62.328B	S62.607B	S72.009C	S72.061B	S72.132A
S49.099A	S52.109B	S52.234A	S52.282C	S52.345B	S52.509A	S52.592C	S59.212A	S62.171B	S62.329B	S62.608B	S72.011A	S72.061C	S72.132B
S49.101A	S52.109C	S52.234B	S52.283A	S52.345C	S52.509B	S52.599A	S59.219A	S62.172B	S62.330B	S62.609B	S72.011B	S72.062A	S72.132C
S49.102A	S52.111A	S52.234C	S52.283B	S52.346A	S52.509C	S52.599B	S59.221A	S62.173B	S62.331B	S62.610B	S72.011C	S72.062B	S72.133A
S49.109A	S52.112A	S52.235A	S52.283C	S52.346B	S52.511A	S52.599C	S59.222A	S62.174B	S62.332B	S62.611B	S72.012A	S72.062C	S72.133B
S49.111A	S52.119A	S52.235B	S52.291A	S52.346C	S52.511B	S52.601A	S59.229A	S62.175B	S62.333B	S62.612B	S72.012B	S72.063A	S72.133C
S49.112A	S52.121B	S52.235C	S52.291B	S52.351A	S52.511C	S52.601B	S59.231A	S62.176B	S62.334B	S62.613B	S72.012C	S72.063B	S72.134A
S49.119A	S52.121C	S52.236A	S52.291C	S52.351B	S52.512A	S52.601C	S59.232A	S62.181B	S62.335B	S62.614B	S72.019A	S72.063C	S72.134B
S49.121A	S52.122B	S52.236B	S52.292A	S52.351C	S52.512B	S52.602A	S59.239A	S62.182B	S62.336B	S62.615B	S72.019B	S72.064A	S72.134C
S49.122A	S52.122C	S52.236C	S52.292B	S52.352A	S52.512C	S52.602B	S59.241A	S62.183B	S62.337B	S62.616B	S72.019C	S72.064B	S72.135A
S49.129A	S52.123B	S52.241A	S52.292C	S52.352B	S52.513A	S52.602C	S59.242A	S62.184B	S62.338B	S62.617B	S72.021A	S72.064C	S72.135B
S49.131A	S52.123C	S52.241B	S52.299A	S52.352C	S52.513B	S52.609A	S59.249A	S62.185B	S62.339B	S62.618B	S72.021B	S72.065A	S72.135C
S49.132A	S52.124B	S52.241C	S52.299B	S52.353A	S52.513C	S52.609B	S59.291A	S62.186B	S62.340B	S62.619B	S72.021C	S72.065B	S72.136A
S49.139A	S52.124C	S52.242A	S52.299C	S52.353B	S52.514A	S52.609C	S59.292A	S62.201B	S62.341B	S62.620B	S72.022A	S72.065C	S72.136B
S49.141A	S52.125B	S52.242B	S52.301A	S52.353C	S52.514B	S52.611A	S59.299A	S62.202B	S62.342B	S62.621B	S72.022B	S72.066A	S72.136C
S49.142A	S52.125C	S52.242C	S52.301B	S52.354A	S52.514C	S52.611B	S62.001B	S62.209B	S62.343B	S62.622B	S72.022C	S72.066B	S72.141A
S49.149A	S52.126B	S52.243A	S52.301C	S52.354B	S52.515A	S52.611C	S62.002B	S62.211B	S62.344B	S62.623B	S72.023A	S72.066C	S72.141B
S49.191A	S52.126C	S52.243B	S52.302A	S52.354C	S52.515B	S52.612A	S62.009B	S62.212B	S62.345B	S62.624B	S72.023B	S72.091A	S72.141C
S49.192A	S52.131B	S52.243C	S52.302B	S52.355A	S52.515C	S52.612B	S62.011B	S62.213B	S62.346B	S62.625B	S72.023C	S72.091B	S72.142A
S49.199A	S52.131C	S52.244A	S52.302C	S52.355B	S52.516A	S52.612C	S62.012B	S62.221B	S62.347B	S62.626B	S72.024A	S72.091C	S72.142B
S52.001B	S52.132B	S52.244B	S52.309A	S52.355C	S52.516B	S52.613A	S62.013B	S62.222B	S62.348B	S62.627B	S72.024B	S72.092A	S72.142C
S52.001C	S52.132C	S52.244C	S52.309B	S52.356A	S52.516C	S52.613B	S62.014B	S62.223B	S62.349B	S62.628B	S72.024C	S72.092B	S72.143A

Hospital-acquired Condition (HAC) (cont.) - Based on CMS data

S72.143B	S72.341A	S72.411C	S72.452B	S73.021A	S82.015C	S82.109B	S82.151A	S82.236C	S82.391C	S82.492C	S82.873C	S92.065B	S92.311B
S72.143C	S72.341B	S72.412A	S72.452C	S73.022A	S82.016A	S82.109C	S82.151B	S82.241A	S82.392B	S82.499B	S82.874B	S92.066B	S92.312B
S72.144A	S72.341C	S72.412B	S72.453A	S73.023A	S82.016B	S82.111A	S82.151C	S82.241B	S82.392C	S82.499C	S82.874C	S92.101B	S92.313B
S72.144B	S72.342A	S72.412C	S72.453B	S73.024A	S82.016C	S82.111B	S82.152A	S82.241C	S82.399B	S82.51XB	S82.875B	S92.102B	S92.314B
S72.144C	S72.342B	S72.413A	S72.453C	S73.025A	S82.021A	S82.111C	S82.152B	S82.242A	S82.399C	S82.51XC	S82.875C	S92.109B	S92.315B
S72.145A	S72.342C	S72.413B	S72.454A	S73.026A	S82.021B	S82.112A	S82.152C	S82.242B	S82.401B	S82.52XB	S82.876B	S92.111B	S92.316B
S72.145B	S72.343A	S72.413C	S72.454B	S73.031A	S82.021C	S82.112B	S82.153A	S82.242C	S82.401C	S82.52XC	S82.876C	S92.112B	S92.321B
S72.145C	S72.343B	S72.414A	S72.454C	S73.032A	S82.022A	S82.112C	S82.153B	S82.243A	S82.402B	S82.53XB	S82.891B	S92.113B	S92.322B
S72.146A	S72.343C	S72.414B	S72.455A	S73.033A	S82.022B	S82.113A	S82.153C	S82.243B	S82.402C	S82.53XC	S82.891C	S92.114B	S92.323B
S72.146B	S72.344A	S72.414C	S72.455B	S73.034A	S82.022C	S82.113B	S82.154A	S82.243C	S82.409B	S82.54XB	S82.892B	S92.115B	S92.324B
S72.146C	S72.344B	S72.415A	S72.455C	S73.035A	S82.023A	S82.113C	S82.154B	S82.244A	S82.409C	S82.54XC	S82.892C	S92.116B	S92.325B
S72.21XA	S72.344C	S72.415B	S72.456A	S73.036A	S82.023B	S82.114A	S82.154C	S82.244B	S82.421B	S82.55XB	S82.899B	S92.121B	S92.326B
S72.21XB	S72.345A	S72.415C	S72.456B	S73.041A	S82.023C	S82.114B	S82.155A	S82.244C	S82.421C	S82.55XC	S82.899C	S92.122B	S92.331B
S72.21XC	S72.345B	S72.416A	S72.456C	S73.042A	S82.024A	S82.114C	S82.155B	S82.245A	S82.422B	S82.56XB	S82.90XB	S92.123B	S92.332B
S72.22XA	S72.345C	S72.416B	S72.461A	S73.043A	S82.024B	S82.115A	S82.155C	S82.245B	S82.422C	S82.56XC	S82.90XC	S92.124B	S92.333B
S72.22XB	S72.346A	S72.416C	S72.461B	S73.044A	S82.024C	S82.115B	S82.156A	S82.245C	S82.423B	S82.61XB	S82.91XB	S92.125B	S92.334B
S72.22XC	S72.346B	S72.421A	S72.461C	S73.045A	S82.025A	S82.115C	S82.156B	S82.246A	S82.423C	S82.61XC	S82.91XC	S92.126B	S92.335B
S72.23XA	S72.346C	S72.421B	S72.462A	S73.046A	S82.025B	S82.116A	S82.156C	S82.246B	S82.424B	S82.62XB	S82.92XB	S92.131B	S92.336B
S72.23XB	S72.351A	S72.421C	S72.462B	S77.00XA	S82.025C	S82.116B	S82.161A	S82.246C	S82.424C	S82.62XC	S82.92XC	S92.132B	S92.341B
S72.23XC	S72.351B	S72.422A	S72.462C	S77.01XA	S82.026A	S82.116C	S82.162A	S82.251A	S82.425B	S82.63XB	S89.001A	S92.133B	S92.342B
S72.24XA	S72.351C	S72.422B	S72.463A	S77.02XA	S82.026B	S82.121A	S82.169A	S82.251B	S82.425C	S82.63XC	S89.002A	S92.134B	S92.343B
S72.24XB	S72.352A	S72.422C	S72.463B	S77.10XA	S82.026C	S82.121B	S82.191A	S82.251C	S82.426B	S82.64XB	S89.009A	S92.135B	S92.344B
S72.24XC	S72.352B	S72.423A	S72.463C	S77.11XA	S82.031A	S82.121C	S82.191B	S82.252A	S82.426C	S82.64XC	S89.011A	S92.136B	S92.345B
S72.25XA	S72.352C	S72.423B	S72.464A	S77.12XA	S82.031B	S82.122A	S82.191C	S82.252B	S82.431B	S82.65XB	S89.012A	S92.141B	S92.346B
S72.25XB	S72.353A	S72.423C	S72.464B	S79.001A	S82.031C	S82.122B	S82.192A	S82.252C	S82.431C	S82.65XC	S89.019A	S92.142B	S92.351B
S72.25XC	S72.353B	S72.424A	S72.464C	S79.002A	S82.032A	S82.122C	S82.192B	S82.253A	S82.432B	S82.66XB	S89.021A	S92.143B	S92.352B
S72.26XA	S72.353C	S72.424B	S72.465A	S79.009A	S82.032B	S82.123A	S82.192C	S82.253B	S82.432C	S82.66XC	S89.022A	S92.144B	S92.353B
S72.26XB	S72.354A	S72.424C	S72.465B	S79.011A	S82.032C	S82.123B	S82.199A	S82.253C	S82.433B	S82.831B	S89.029A	S92.145B	S92.354B
S72.26XC	S72.354B	S72.425A	S72.465C	S79.012A	S82.033A	S82.123C	S82.199B	S82.254A	S82.433C	S82.831C	S89.031A	S92.146B	S92.355B
S72.301A	S72.354C	S72.425B	S72.466A	S79.019A	S82.033B	S82.124A	S82.199C	S82.254B	S82.434B	S82.832B	S89.032A	S92.151B	S92.356B
S72.301B	S72.355A	S72.425C	S72.466B	S79.091A	S82.033C	S82.124B	S82.201A	S82.254C	S82.434C	S82.832C	S89.039A	S92.152B	S92.901B
S72.301C	S72.355B	S72.426A	S72.466C	S79.092A	S82.034A	S82.124C	S82.201B	S82.255A	S82.435B	S82.839B	S89.041A	S92.153B	S92.902B
S72.302A	S72.355C	S72.426B	S72.471A	S79.099A	S82.034B	S82.125A	S82.201C	S82.255B	S82.435C	S82.839C	S89.042A	S92.154B	S92.909B
S72.302B	S72.356A	S72.426C	S72.472A	S79.101A	S82.034C	S82.125B	S82.202A	S82.255C	S82.436B	S82.841B	S89.049A	S92.155B	T20.30XA
S72.302C	S72.356B	S72.431A	S72.479A	S79.102A	S82.035A	S82.125C	S82.202B	S82.256A	S82.436C	S82.841C	S89.091A	S92.156B	T20.311A
S72.309A	S72.356C	S72.431B	S72.491A	S79.109A	S82.035B	S82.126A	S82.202C	S82.256B	S82.441B	S82.842B	S89.092A	S92.191B	T20.312A
S72.309B	S72.361A	S72.431C	S72.491B	S79.111A	S82.035C	S82.126B	S82.209A	S82.256C	S82.441C	S82.842C	S89.099A	S92.192B	T20.319A
S72.309C	S72.361B	S72.432A	S72.491C	S79.112A	S82.036A	S82.126C	S82.209B	S82.261A	S82.442B	S82.843B	S92.001B	S92.199B	T20.32XA
S72.321A	S72.361C	S72.432B	S72.492A	S79.119A	S82.036B	S82.131A	S82.209C	S82.261B	S82.442C	S82.843C	S92.002B	S92.201B	T20.33XA
S72.321B	S72.362A	S72.432C	S72.492B	S79.121A	S82.036C	S82.131B	S82.221A	S82.261C	S82.443B	S82.844B	S92.009B	S92.202B	T20.34XA
S72.321C	S72.362B	S72.433A	S72.492C	S79.122A	S82.041A	S82.131C	S82.221B	S82.262A	S82.443C	S82.844C	S92.011B	S92.209B	T20.35XA
S72.322A	S72.362C	S72.433B	S72.499A	S79.129A	S82.041B	S82.132A	S82.221C	S82.262B	S82.444B	S82.845B	S92.012B	S92.211B	T20.36XA
S72.322B	S72.363A	S72.433C	S72.499B	S79.131A	S82.041C	S82.132B	S82.222A	S82.262C	S82.444C	S82.845C	S92.013B	S92.212B	T20.37XA
S72.322C	S72.363B	S72.434A	S72.499C	S79.132A	S82.042A	S82.132C	S82.222B	S82.263A	S82.445B	S82.846B	S92.014B	S92.213B	T20.39XA
S72.323A	S72.363C	S72.434B	S72.8X1A	S79.139A	S82.042B	S82.133A	S82.222C	S82.263B	S82.445C	S82.846C	S92.015B	S92.214B	T20.70XA
S72.323B	S72.364A	S72.434C	S72.8X1B	S79.141A	S82.042C	S82.133B	S82.223A	S82.263C	S82.446B	S82.851B	S92.016B	S92.215B	T20.711A
S72.323C	S72.364B	S72.435A	S72.8X1C	S79.142A	S82.043A	S82.133C	S82.223B	S82.264A	S82.446C	S82.851C	S92.021B	S92.216B	T20.712A
S72.324A	S72.364C	S72.435B	S72.8X2A	S79.149A	S82.043B	S82.134A	S82.223C	S82.264B	S82.451B	S82.852B	S92.022B	S92.221B	T20.719A
S72.324B	S72.365A	S72.435C	S72.8X2B	S79.191A	S82.043C	S82.134B	S82.224A	S82.264C	S82.451C	S82.852C	S92.023B	S92.222B	T20.72XA
S72.324C	S72.365B	S72.436A	S72.8X2C	S79.192A	S82.044A	S82.134C	S82.224B	S82.265A	S82.452B	S82.853B	S92.024B	S92.223B	T20.73XA
S72.325A	S72.365C	S72.436B	S72.8X9A	S79.199A	S82.044B	S82.135A	S82.224C	S82.265B	S82.452C	S82.853C	S92.025B	S92.224B	T20.74XA
S72.325B	S72.366A	S72.436C	S72.8X9B	S82.001A	S82.044C	S82.135B	S82.225A	S82.265C	S82.453B	S82.854B	S92.026B	S92.225B	T20.75XA
S72.325C	S72.366B	S72.441A	S72.8X9C	S82.001B	S82.045A	S82.135C	S82.225B	S82.266A	S82.453C	S82.854C	S92.031B	S92.226B	T20.76XA
S72.326A	S72.366C	S72.441B	S72.90XA	S82.001C	S82.045B	S82.136A	S82.225C	S82.266B	S82.454B	S82.855B	S92.032B	S92.231B	T20.77XA
S72.326B	S72.391A	S72.441C	S72.90XB	S82.002A	S82.045C	S82.136B	S82.226A	S82.266C	S82.454C	S82.855C	S92.033B	S92.232B	T20.79XA
S72.326C	S72.391B	S72.442A	S72.90XC	S82.002B	S82.046A	S82.136C	S82.226B	S82.291A	S82.455B	S82.856B	S92.034B	S92.233B	T21.30XA
S72.331A	S72.391C	S72.442B	S72.91XA	S82.002C	S82.046B	S82.141A	S82.226C	S82.291B	S82.455C	S82.856C	S92.035B	S92.234B	T21.31XA
S72.331B	S72.392A	S72.442C	S72.91XB	S82.009A	S82.046C	S82.141B	S82.231A	S82.291C	S82.456B	S82.861B	S92.036B	S92.235B	T21.32XA
S72.331C	S72.392B	S72.443A	S72.91XC	S82.009B	S82.091A	S82.141C	S82.231B	S82.292A	S82.456C	S82.861C	S92.041B	S92.236B	T21.33XA
S72.332A	S72.392C	S72.443B	S72.92XA	S82.009C	S82.091B	S82.142A	S82.231C	S82.292B	S82.461B	S82.862B	S92.042B	S92.241B	T21.34XA
S72.332B	S72.399A	S72.443C	S72.92XB	S82.011A	S82.091C	S82.142B	S82.232A	S82.292C	S82.461C	S82.862C	S92.043B	S92.242B	T21.35XA
S72.332C	S72.399B	S72.444A	S72.92XC	S82.011B	S82.092A	S82.142C	S82.232B	S82.299A	S82.462B	S82.863B	S92.044B	S92.243B	T21.36XA
S72.333A	S72.399C	S72.444B	S73.001A	S82.011C	S82.092B	S82.143A	S82.232C	S82.299B	S82.462C	S82.863C	S92.045B	S92.244B	T21.37XA
S72.333B	S72.401A	S72.444C	S73.002A	S82.012A	S82.092C	S82.143B	S82.233A	S82.299C	S82.463B	S82.864B	S92.046B	S92.245B	T21.39XA
S72.333C	S72.401B	S72.445A	S73.003A	S82.012B	S82.099A	S82.143C	S82.233B	S82.301B	S82.463C	S82.864C	S92.051B	S92.246B	T21.70XA
S72.334A	S72.401C	S72.445B	S73.004A	S82.012C	S82.099B	S82.144A	S82.233C	S82.301C	S82.464B	S82.865B	S92.052B	S92.251B	T21.71XA
S72.334B	S72.402A	S72.445C	S73.005A	S82.013A	S82.099C	S82.144B	S82.234A	S82.302B	S82.464C	S82.865C	S92.053B	S92.252B	T21.72XA
S72.334C	S72.402B	S72.446A	S73.006A	S82.013B	S82.101A	S82.144C	S82.234B	S82.302C	S82.465B	S82.866B	S92.054B	S92.253B	T21.73XA
S72.335A	S72.402C	S72.446B	S73.011A	S82.013C	S82.101B	S82.145A	S82.234C	S82.309B	S82.465C	S82.866C	S92.055B	S92.254B	T21.74XA
S72.335B	S72.409A	S72.446C	S73.012A	S82.014A	S82.101C	S82.145B	S82.235A	S82.309C	S82.466B	S82.871B	S92.056B	S92.255B	T21.75XA
S72.335C	S72.409B	S72.451A	S73.013A	S82.014B	S82.102A	S82.145C	S82.235B	S82.311A	S82.466C	S82.871C	S92.061B	S92.256B	T21.76XA
S72.336A	S72.409C	S72.451B	S73.014A	S82.014C	S82.102B	S82.146A	S82.235C	S82.312A	S82.491B	S82.872B	S92.062B	S92.301B	T21.77XA
S72.336B	S72.411A	S72.451C	S73.015A	S82.015A	S82.102C	S82.146B	S82.236A	S82.319A	S82.491C	S82.872C	S92.063B	S92.302B	T21.79XA
S72.336C	S72.411B	S72.452A	S73.016A	S82.015B	S82.109A	S82.146C	S82.236B	S82.391B	S82.492B	S82.873B	S92.064B	S92.309B	T22.30XA

Hospital-acquired Condition (HAC) (cont.) - Based on CMS data

T22.311A	T22.722A	T23.331A	T23.729A	T24.322A	T25.321A	T26.72XA	T33.519A	T34.019A	T34.819A	T71.141A	T80.310A	T81.521A	T81.597A
T22.312A	T22.729A	T23.332A	T23.731A	T24.329A	T25.322A	T27.0XXA	T33.521A	T34.02XA	T34.821A	T71.143A	T80.311A	T81.522A	T81.598A
T22.319A	T22.731A	T23.339A	T23.732A	T24.331A	T25.329A	T27.1XXA	T33.522A	T34.09XA	T34.822A	T71.144A	T80.319A	T81.523A	T81.599A
T22.321A	T22.732A	T23.341A	T23.739A	T24.332A	T25.331A	T27.2XXA	T33.529A	T34.1XXA	T34.829A	T71.151A	T80.39XA	T81.524A	T81.60XA
T22.322A	T22.739A	T23.342A	T23.741A	T24.339A	T25.332A	T27.3XXA	T33.531A	T34.2XXA	T34.831A	T71.152A	T81.4XXA	T81.525A	T81.61XA
T22.329A	T22.741A	T23.349A	T23.742A	T24.391A	T25.339A	T27.4XXA	T33.532A	T34.3XXA	T34.832A	T71.153A	T81.500A	T81.526A	T81.69XA
T22.331A	T22.742A	T23.351A	T23.749A	T24.392A	T25.391A	T27.5XXA	T33.539A	T34.40XA	T34.839A	T71.154A	T81.501A	T81.527A	T82.6XXA
T22.332A	T22.749A	T23.352A	T23.751A	T24.399A	T25.392A	T27.6XXA	T33.60XA	T34.41XA	T34.90XA	T71.161A	T81.502A	T81.528A	T82.7XXA
T22.339A	T22.751A	T23.359A	T23.752A	T24.701A	T25.399A	T27.7XXA	T33.61XA	T34.42XA	T34.99XA	T71.162A	T81.503A	T81.529A	T84.60XA
T22.341A	T22.752A	T23.361A	T23.759A	T24.702A	T25.711A	T28.1XXA	T33.62XA	T34.511A	T67.0XXA	T71.163A	T81.504A	T81.530A	T84.610A
T22.342A	T22.759A	T23.362A	T23.761A	T24.709A	T25.712A	T28.2XXA	T33.70XA	T34.512A	T69.021A	T71.164A	T81.505A	T81.531A	T84.611A
T22.349A	T22.761A	T23.369A	T23.762A	T24.711A	T25.719A	T28.6XXA	T33.71XA	T34.519A	T69.022A	T71.191A	T81.506A	T81.532A	T84.612A
T22.351A	T22.762A	T23.371A	T23.769A	T24.712A	T25.721A	T28.7XXA	T33.72XA	T34.521A	T69.029A	T71.192A	T81.507A	T81.533A	T84.613A
T22.352A	T22.769A	T23.372A	T23.771A	T24.719A	T25.722A	T33.011A	T33.811A	T34.522A	T70.3XXA	T71.193A	T81.508A	T81.534A	T84.614A
T22.359A	T22.791A	T23.379A	T23.772A	T24.721A	T25.729A	T33.012A	T33.812A	T34.529A	T71.111A	T71.194A	T81.509A	T81.535A	T84.615A
T22.361A	T22.792A	T23.391A	T23.779A	T24.722A	T25.731A	T33.019A	T33.819A	T34.531A	T71.112A	T71.20XA	T81.510A	T81.536A	T84.619A
T22.362A	T22.799A	T23.392A	T23.791A	T24.729A	T25.732A	T33.02XA	T33.821A	T34.532A	T71.113A	T71.21XA	T81.511A	T81.537A	T84.63XA
T22.369A	T23.301A	T23.399A	T23.792A	T24.731A	T25.739A	T33.09XA	T33.822A	T34.539A	T71.114A	T71.29XA	T81.512A	T81.538A	T84.69XA
T22.391A	T23.302A	T23.701A	T23.799A	T24.732A	T25.791A	T33.1XXA	T33.829A	T34.60XA	T71.121A	T71.9XXA	T81.513A	T81.539A	T84.7XXA
T22.392A	T23.309A	T23.702A	T24.301A	T24.739A	T25.792A	T33.2XXA	T33.831A	T34.61XA	T71.122A	T75.1XXA	T81.514A	T81.590A	
T22.399A	T23.311A	T23.709A	T24.302A	T24.791A	T25.799A	T33.3XXA	T33.832A	T34.62XA	T71.123A	T80.0XXA	T81.515A	T81.591A	
T22.70XA	T23.312A	T23.711A	T24.309A	T24.792A	T26.20XA	T33.40XA	T33.839A	T34.70XA	T71.124A	T80.211A	T81.516A	T81.592A	
T22.711A	T23.319A	T23.712A	T24.311A	T24.799A	T26.21XA	T33.41XA	T33.90XA	T34.71XA	T71.131A	T80.212A	T81.517A	T81.593A	
T22.712A	T23.321A	T23.719A	T24.312A	T25.311A	T26.22XA	T33.42XA	T33.99XA	T34.72XA	T71.132A	T80.218A	T81.518A	T81.594A	
T22.719A	T23.322A	T23.721A	T24.319A	T25.312A	T26.70XA	T33.511A	T34.011A	T34.811A	T71.133A	T80.219A	T81.519A	T81.595A	
T22.721A	T23.329A	T23.722A	T24.321A	T25.319A	T26.71XA	T33.512A	T34.012A	T34.812A	T71.134A	T80.30XA	T81.520A	T81.596A	

HCC - Based on CMS data

E08.3211	E08.3592	E09.3543	E10.3529	E11.3511	E13.3412	H35.3232	R40.2112	S02.0XXS	S02.11FS	S02.40FS	S02.630S	S02.81XS	S06.300A
E08.3212	E08.3593	E09.3549	E10.3531	E11.3512	E13.3413	H35.3233	R40.2113	S02.101A	S02.11GA	S02.411A	S02.631A	S02.82XA	S06.300S
E08.3213	E08.3599	E09.3551	E10.3532	E11.3513	E13.3419	H35.3290	R40.2114	S02.101B	S02.11GB	S02.411B	S02.631B	S02.82XB	S06.301A
E08.3219	E08.37X1	E09.3552	E10.3533	E11.3519	E13.3491	H35.3291	R40.2120	S02.101S	S02.11GS	S02.411S	S02.631S	S02.82XS	S06.301S
E08.3291	E08.37X2	E09.3553	E10.3539	E11.3521	E13.3492	H35.3292	R40.2121	S02.102A	S02.11HA	S02.412A	S02.632A	S02.91XA	S06.302A
E08.3292	E08.37X3	E09.3559	E10.3541	E11.3522	E13.3493	H35.3293	R40.2122	S02.102B	S02.11HB	S02.412B	S02.632B	S02.91XB	S06.302S
E08.3293	E08.37X9	E09.3591	E10.3542	E11.3523	E13.3499	M48.50XA	R40.2123	S02.102S	S02.11HS	S02.412S	S02.632S	S02.91XS	S06.303A
E08.3299	E09.3211	E09.3592	E10.3543	E11.3529	E13.3511	M48.51XA	R40.2124	S02.109A	S02.19XA	S02.413A	S02.640A	S02.92XA	S06.303S
E08.3311	E09.3212	E09.3593	E10.3549	E11.3531	E13.3512	M48.52XA	R40.2210	S02.109B	S02.19XB	S02.413B	S02.640B	S02.92XB	S06.304A
E08.3312	E09.3213	E09.3599	E10.3551	E11.3532	E13.3513	M48.53XA	R40.2211	S02.109S	S02.19XS	S02.413S	S02.640S	S02.92XS	S06.304S
E08.3313	E09.3219	E09.37X1	E10.3552	E11.3533	E13.3519	M48.54XA	R40.2212	S02.110A	S02.30XA	S02.42XA	S02.641A	S06.0X0S	S06.305A
E08.3319	E09.3291	E09.37X2	E10.3553	E11.3539	E13.3521	M48.55XA	R40.2213	S02.110B	S02.30XB	S02.42XB	S02.641B	S06.0X1S	S06.305S
E08.3391	E09.3292	E09.37X3	E10.3559	E11.3541	E13.3522	M48.56XA	R40.2214	S02.110S	S02.30XS	S02.42XS	S02.641S	S06.0X9S	S06.306A
E08.3392	E09.3293	E09.37X9	E10.3591	E11.3542	E13.3523	M48.57XA	R40.2220	S02.111A	S02.31XA	S02.600A	S02.642A	S06.1X0A	S06.306S
E08.3393	E09.3299	E10.3211	E10.3592	E11.3543	E13.3529	M48.58XA	R40.2221	S02.111B	S02.31XB	S02.600B	S02.642B	S06.1X0S	S06.309A
E08.3399	E09.3311	E10.3212	E10.3593	E11.3549	E13.3531	M80.051A	R40.2222	S02.111S	S02.31XS	S02.600S	S02.642S	S06.1X1A	S06.309S
E08.3411	E09.3312	E10.3213	E10.3599	E11.3551	E13.3532	M80.052A	R40.2223	S02.112A	S02.32XA	S02.601A	S02.650A	S06.1X1S	S06.310A
E08.3412	E09.3313	E10.3219	E10.37X1	E11.3552	E13.3533	M80.059A	R40.2224	S02.112B	S02.32XB	S02.601B	S02.650B	S06.1X2A	S06.310S
E08.3413	E09.3319	E10.3291	E10.37X2	E11.3553	E13.3539	M80.08XA	R40.2310	S02.112S	S02.32XS	S02.601S	S02.650S	S06.1X2S	S06.311A
E08.3419	E09.3391	E10.3292	E10.37X3	E11.3559	E13.3541	M80.851A	R40.2311	S02.113A	S02.400A	S02.602A	S02.651A	S06.1X3A	S06.311S
E08.3491	E09.3392	E10.3293	E10.37X9	E11.3591	E13.3542	M80.852A	R40.2312	S02.113B	S02.400B	S02.602B	S02.651B	S06.1X3S	S06.312A
E08.3492	E09.3393	E10.3299	E11.3211	E11.3592	E13.3543	M80.859A	R40.2313	S02.113S	S02.400S	S02.602S	S02.651S	S06.1X4A	S06.312S
E08.3493	E09.3399	E10.3311	E11.3212	E11.3593	E13.3549	M80.88XA	R40.2314	S02.118A	S02.401A	S02.609A	S02.652A	S06.1X4S	S06.313A
E08.3499	E09.3411	E10.3312	E11.3213	E11.3599	E13.3551	M84.451A	R40.2320	S02.118B	S02.401B	S02.609B	S02.652B	S06.1X5A	S06.313S
E08.3511	E09.3412	E10.3313	E11.3219	E11.37X1	E13.3552	M84.452A	R40.2321	S02.118S	S02.401S	S02.609S	S02.652S	S06.1X5S	S06.314A
E08.3512	E09.3413	E10.3319	E11.3291	E11.37X2	E13.3553	M84.453A	R40.2322	S02.119A	S02.402A	S02.610A	S02.66XA	S06.1X6A	S06.314S
E08.3513	E09.3419	E10.3391	E11.3292	E11.37X3	E13.3559	M84.459A	R40.2323	S02.119B	S02.402B	S02.610B	S02.66XB	S06.1X6S	S06.315A
E08.3519	E09.3491	E10.3392	E11.3293	E11.37X9	E13.3591	M84.551A	R40.2324	S02.119S	S02.402S	S02.610S	S02.66XS	S06.1X9A	S06.315S
E08.3521	E09.3492	E10.3393	E11.3299	E13.3211	E13.3592	M84.552A	R40.2340	S02.11AA	S02.40AA	S02.611A	S02.670A	S06.1X9S	S06.316A
E08.3522	E09.3493	E10.3399	E11.3311	E13.3212	E13.3593	M84.553A	R40.2341	S02.11AB	S02.40AB	S02.611B	S02.670B	S06.2X0A	S06.316S
E08.3523	E09.3499	E10.3411	E11.3312	E13.3213	E13.3599	M84.559A	R40.2342	S02.11AS	S02.40AS	S02.611S	S02.670S	S06.2X0S	S06.319A
E08.3529	E09.3511	E10.3412	E11.3313	E13.3219	E13.37X1	M84.651A	R40.2343	S02.11BA	S02.40BA	S02.612A	S02.671A	S06.2X1A	S06.319S
E08.3531	E09.3512	E10.3413	E11.3319	E13.3291	E13.37X2	M84.652A	R40.2344	S02.11BB	S02.40BB	S02.612B	S02.671B	S06.2X1S	S06.320A
E08.3532	E09.3513	E10.3419	E11.3391	E13.3292	E13.37X3	M84.653A	R40.2430	S02.11BS	S02.40BS	S02.612S	S02.671S	S06.2X2A	S06.320S
E08.3533	E09.3519	E10.3491	E11.3392	E13.3293	E13.37X9	M84.659A	R40.2431	S02.11CA	S02.40CA	S02.620A	S02.672A	S06.2X2S	S06.321A
E08.3539	E09.3521	E10.3492	E11.3393	E13.3299	H35.3210	M84.754A	R40.2432	S02.11CB	S02.40CB	S02.620B	S02.672B	S06.2X3A	S06.321S
E08.3541	E09.3522	E10.3493	E11.3399	H35.3210	H35.3211	M84.755A	R40.2433	S02.11CS	S02.40CS	S02.620S	S02.672S	S06.2X3S	S06.322A
E08.3542	E09.3523	E10.3499	E11.3411	H35.3211	H35.3212	M84.756A	R40.2434	S02.11DA	S02.40DA	S02.621A	S02.69XA	S06.2X4A	S06.322S
E08.3543	E09.3529	E10.3511	E11.3412	H35.3212	H35.3213	M84.757A	R40.2440	S02.11DB	S02.40DB	S02.621B	S02.69XB	S06.2X4S	S06.323A
E08.3549	E09.3531	E10.3512	E11.3413	H35.3213	H35.3220	M84.758A	R40.2441	S02.11DS	S02.40DS	S02.621S	S02.69XS	S06.2X5A	S06.323S
E08.3551	E09.3532	E10.3513	E11.3419	H35.3391	H35.3221	M84.759A	R40.2442	S02.11EA	S02.40EA	S02.622A	S02.80XA	S06.2X5S	S06.324A
E08.3552	E09.3533	E10.3519	E11.3491	H35.3392	H35.3222	M97.01XA	R40.2443	S02.11EB	S02.40EB	S02.622B	S02.80XB	S06.2X6A	S06.324S
E08.3553	E09.3539	E10.3521	E11.3492	H35.3393	H35.3223	M97.02XA	R40.2444	S02.11ES	S02.40ES	S02.622S	S02.80XS	S06.2X6S	S06.325A
E08.3559	E09.3541	E10.3522	E11.3493	H35.3399	H35.3230	R40.2110	S02.0XXA	S02.11FA	S02.40FA	S02.630A	S02.81XA	S06.2X9A	S06.325S
E08.3591	E09.3542	E10.3523	E11.3499	E13.3411	H35.3231	R40.2111	S02.0XXB	S02.11FB	S02.40FB	S02.630B	S02.81XB	S06.2X9S	S06.326A

HCC (cont.) - Based on CMS data

S06.326S	S06.373S	S06.810S	S12.031B	S12.400B	S14.106D	S14.134A	S22.001A	S22.078A	S24.149A	S32.058A	S32.412A	S32.473A	S32.89XA
S06.329A	S06.374A	S06.811A	S12.040A	S12.401A	S14.106S	S14.134D	S22.001B	S22.078B	S24.149D	S32.058B	S32.412B	S32.473B	S32.89XB
S06.329S	S06.374S	S06.811S	S12.040B	S12.401B	S14.107A	S14.134S	S22.002A	S22.079A	S24.149S	S32.059A	S32.413A	S32.474A	S32.9XXA
S06.330A	S06.375A	S06.812A	S12.041A	S12.430A	S14.107D	S14.135A	S22.002B	S22.079B	S24.151A	S32.059B	S32.413B	S32.474B	S32.9XXB
S06.330S	S06.375S	S06.812S	S12.041B	S12.430B	S14.107S	S14.135D	S22.008A	S22.080A	S24.151D	S32.10XA	S32.414A	S32.475A	S34.01XA
S06.331A	S06.376A	S06.813A	S12.090A	S12.431A	S14.108A	S14.135S	S22.008B	S22.080B	S24.151S	S32.10XB	S32.414B	S32.475B	S34.01XD
S06.331S	S06.376S	S06.813S	S12.090B	S12.431B	S14.108D	S14.136A	S22.009A	S22.081A	S24.152A	S32.110A	S32.415A	S32.476A	S34.01XS
S06.332A	S06.379A	S06.814A	S12.091A	S12.44XA	S14.108S	S14.136D	S22.009B	S22.081B	S24.152D	S32.110B	S32.415B	S32.476B	S34.02XA
S06.332S	S06.379S	S06.814S	S12.091B	S12.44XB	S14.109A	S14.136S	S22.010A	S22.082A	S24.152S	S32.111A	S32.416A	S32.481A	S34.02XD
S06.333A	S06.380A	S06.815A	S12.100A	S12.450A	S14.109D	S14.137A	S22.010B	S22.082B	S24.153A	S32.111B	S32.416B	S32.481B	S34.02XS
S06.333S	S06.380S	S06.815S	S12.100B	S12.450B	S14.109S	S14.137D	S22.011A	S22.088A	S24.153D	S32.112A	S32.421A	S32.482A	S34.101A
S06.334A	S06.381A	S06.816A	S12.101A	S12.451A	S14.111A	S14.137S	S22.011B	S22.088B	S24.153S	S32.112B	S32.421B	S32.482B	S34.101D
S06.334S	S06.381S	S06.816S	S12.101B	S12.451B	S14.111D	S14.138A	S22.012A	S22.089A	S24.154A	S32.119A	S32.422A	S32.483A	S34.101S
S06.335A	S06.382A	S06.819A	S12.110A	S12.490A	S14.111S	S14.138D	S22.012B	S22.089B	S24.154D	S32.119B	S32.422B	S32.483B	S34.102A
S06.335S	S06.382S	S06.819S	S12.110B	S12.490B	S14.112A	S14.138S	S22.018A	S24.0XXA	S24.154S	S32.120A	S32.423A	S32.484A	S34.102D
S06.336A	S06.383A	S06.820A	S12.111A	S12.491A	S14.112D	S14.139A	S22.018B	S24.0XXD	S24.159A	S32.120B	S32.423B	S32.484B	S34.102S
S06.336S	S06.383S	S06.820S	S12.111B	S12.491B	S14.112S	S14.139D	S22.019A	S24.0XXS	S24.159D	S32.121A	S32.424A	S32.485A	S34.103A
S06.339A	S06.384A	S06.821A	S12.112A	S12.500A	S14.113A	S14.139S	S22.019B	S24.101A	S24.159S	S32.121B	S32.424B	S32.485B	S34.103D
S06.339S	S06.384S	S06.821S	S12.112B	S12.500B	S14.113D	S14.141A	S22.020A	S24.101D	S32.000A	S32.122A	S32.425A	S32.486A	S34.103S
S06.340A	S06.385A	S06.822A	S12.120A	S12.501A	S14.113S	S14.141D	S22.020B	S24.101S	S32.000B	S32.122B	S32.425B	S32.486B	S34.104A
S06.340S	S06.385S	S06.822S	S12.120B	S12.501B	S14.114A	S14.141S	S22.021A	S24.102A	S32.001A	S32.129A	S32.426A	S32.491A	S34.104D
S06.341A	S06.386A	S06.823A	S12.121A	S12.530A	S14.114D	S14.142A	S22.021B	S24.102D	S32.001B	S32.129B	S32.426B	S32.491B	S34.104S
S06.341S	S06.386S	S06.823S	S12.121B	S12.530B	S14.114S	S14.142D	S22.022A	S24.102S	S32.002A	S32.130A	S32.431A	S32.492A	S34.105A
S06.342A	S06.389A	S06.824A	S12.130A	S12.531A	S14.115A	S14.142S	S22.022B	S24.103A	S32.002B	S32.130B	S32.431B	S32.492B	S34.105D
S06.342S	S06.389S	S06.824S	S12.130B	S12.531B	S14.115D	S14.143A	S22.028A	S24.103D	S32.008A	S32.131A	S32.432A	S32.499A	S34.105S
S06.343A	S06.4X0A	S06.825A	S12.131A	S12.54XA	S14.115S	S14.143D	S22.028B	S24.103S	S32.008B	S32.131B	S32.432B	S32.499B	S34.109A
S06.343S	S06.4X0S	S06.825S	S12.131B	S12.54XB	S14.116A	S14.143S	S22.029A	S24.104A	S32.009A	S32.132A	S32.433A	S32.501A	S34.109D
S06.344A	S06.4X1A	S06.826A	S12.14XA	S12.550A	S14.116D	S14.144A	S22.029B	S24.104D	S32.009B	S32.132B	S32.433B	S32.501B	S34.109S
S06.344S	S06.4X1S	S06.826S	S12.14XB	S12.550B	S14.116S	S14.144D	S22.030A	S24.104S	S32.010A	S32.139A	S32.434A	S32.502A	S34.111A
S06.345A	S06.4X2A	S06.829A	S12.150A	S12.551A	S14.117A	S14.144S	S22.030B	S24.109A	S32.010B	S32.139B	S32.434B	S32.502B	S34.111D
S06.345S	S06.4X2S	S06.829S	S12.150B	S12.551B	S14.117D	S14.145A	S22.031A	S24.109D	S32.011A	S32.14XA	S32.435A	S32.509A	S34.111S
S06.346A	S06.4X3A	S06.890A	S12.151A	S12.590A	S14.117S	S14.145D	S22.031B	S24.109S	S32.011B	S32.14XB	S32.435B	S32.509B	S34.112A
S06.346S	S06.4X3S	S06.890S	S12.151B	S12.590B	S14.118A	S14.145S	S22.032A	S24.111A	S32.012A	S32.15XA	S32.436A	S32.511A	S34.112D
S06.349A	S06.4X4A	S06.891A	S12.190A	S12.591A	S14.118D	S14.146A	S22.032B	S24.111D	S32.012B	S32.15XB	S32.436B	S32.511B	S34.112S
S06.349S	S06.4X4S	S06.891S	S12.190B	S12.591B	S14.118S	S14.146D	S22.038A	S24.111S	S32.018A	S32.16XA	S32.441A	S32.512A	S34.113A
S06.350A	S06.4X5A	S06.892A	S12.191A	S12.600A	S14.119A	S14.146S	S22.038B	S24.112A	S32.018B	S32.16XB	S32.441B	S32.512B	S34.113D
S06.350S	S06.4X5S	S06.892S	S12.191B	S12.600B	S14.119D	S14.147A	S22.039A	S24.112D	S32.019A	S32.17XA	S32.442A	S32.519A	S34.113S
S06.351A	S06.4X6A	S06.893A	S12.200A	S12.601A	S14.119S	S14.147D	S22.039B	S24.112S	S32.019B	S32.17XB	S32.442B	S32.519B	S34.114A
S06.351S	S06.4X6S	S06.893S	S12.200B	S12.601B	S14.121A	S14.147S	S22.040A	S24.113A	S32.020A	S32.19XA	S32.443A	S32.591A	S34.114D
S06.352A	S06.4X9A	S06.894A	S12.201A	S12.630A	S14.121D	S14.148A	S22.040B	S24.113D	S32.020B	S32.19XB	S32.443B	S32.591B	S34.114S
S06.352S	S06.4X9S	S06.894S	S12.201B	S12.630B	S14.121S	S14.148D	S22.041A	S24.113S	S32.021A	S32.2XXA	S32.444A	S32.592A	S34.115A
S06.353A	S06.5X0A	S06.895A	S12.230A	S12.631A	S14.122A	S14.148S	S22.041B	S24.114A	S32.021B	S32.2XXB	S32.444B	S32.592B	S34.115D
S06.353S	S06.5X0S	S06.895S	S12.230B	S12.631B	S14.122D	S14.149A	S22.042A	S24.114D	S32.022A	S32.301A	S32.445A	S32.599A	S34.115S
S06.354A	S06.5X1A	S06.896A	S12.231A	S12.64XA	S14.122S	S14.149D	S22.042B	S24.114S	S32.022B	S32.301B	S32.445B	S32.599B	S34.119A
S06.354S	S06.5X1S	S06.896S	S12.231B	S12.64XB	S14.123A	S14.149S	S22.048A	S24.119A	S32.028A	S32.302A	S32.446A	S32.601A	S34.119D
S06.355A	S06.5X2A	S06.899A	S12.24XA	S12.650A	S14.123D	S14.151A	S22.048B	S24.119D	S32.028B	S32.302B	S32.446B	S32.601B	S34.119S
S06.355S	S06.5X2S	S06.899S	S12.24XB	S12.650B	S14.123S	S14.151D	S22.049A	S24.119S	S32.029A	S32.309A	S32.451A	S32.602A	S34.121A
S06.356A	S06.5X3A	S06.9X0A	S12.250A	S12.651A	S14.124A	S14.151S	S22.049B	S24.131A	S32.029B	S32.309B	S32.451B	S32.602B	S34.121D
S06.356S	S06.5X3S	S06.9X0S	S12.250B	S12.651B	S14.124D	S14.152A	S22.050A	S24.131D	S32.030A	S32.311A	S32.452A	S32.609A	S34.121S
S06.359A	S06.5X4A	S06.9X1A	S12.251A	S12.690A	S14.124S	S14.152D	S22.050B	S24.131S	S32.030B	S32.311B	S32.452B	S32.609B	S34.122A
S06.359S	S06.5X4S	S06.9X1S	S12.251B	S12.690B	S14.125A	S14.152S	S22.051A	S24.132A	S32.031A	S32.312A	S32.453A	S32.611A	S34.122D
S06.360A	S06.5X5A	S06.9X2A	S12.290A	S12.691A	S14.125D	S14.153A	S22.051B	S24.132D	S32.031B	S32.312B	S32.453B	S32.611B	S34.122S
S06.360S	S06.5X5S	S06.9X2S	S12.290B	S12.691B	S14.125S	S14.153D	S22.052A	S24.132S	S32.032A	S32.313A	S32.454A	S32.612A	S34.123A
S06.361A	S06.5X6A	S06.9X3A	S12.291A	S12.8XXA	S14.126A	S14.153S	S22.052B	S24.133A	S32.032B	S32.313B	S32.454B	S32.612B	S34.123D
S06.361S	S06.5X6S	S06.9X3S	S12.291B	S12.9XXA	S14.126D	S14.154A	S22.058A	S24.133D	S32.038A	S32.314A	S32.455A	S32.613A	S34.123S
S06.362A	S06.5X9A	S06.9X4A	S12.300A	S14.0XXA	S14.126S	S14.154D	S22.058B	S24.133S	S32.038B	S32.314B	S32.455B	S32.613B	S34.124A
S06.362S	S06.5X9S	S06.9X4S	S12.300B	S14.0XXD	S14.127A	S14.154S	S22.059A	S24.134A	S32.039A	S32.315A	S32.456A	S32.614A	S34.124D
S06.363A	S06.6X0A	S06.9X5A	S12.301A	S14.0XXS	S14.127D	S14.155A	S22.059B	S24.134D	S32.039B	S32.315B	S32.456B	S32.614B	S34.124S
S06.363S	S06.6X0S	S06.9X5S	S12.301B	S14.101A	S14.127S	S14.155D	S22.060A	S24.134S	S32.040A	S32.316A	S32.461A	S32.615A	S34.125A
S06.364A	S06.6X1A	S06.9X6A	S12.330A	S14.101D	S14.128A	S14.155S	S22.060B	S24.139A	S32.040B	S32.316B	S32.461B	S32.615B	S34.125D
S06.364S	S06.6X1S	S06.9X6S	S12.330B	S14.101S	S14.128D	S14.156A	S22.061A	S24.139D	S32.041A	S32.391A	S32.462A	S32.616A	S34.125S
S06.365A	S06.6X2A	S06.9X9A	S12.331A	S14.102A	S14.128S	S14.156D	S22.061B	S24.139S	S32.041B	S32.391B	S32.462B	S32.616B	S34.129A
S06.365S	S06.6X2S	S06.9X9S	S12.331B	S14.102D	S14.129A	S14.156S	S22.062A	S24.141A	S32.042A	S32.392A	S32.463A	S32.691A	S34.129D
S06.366A	S06.6X3A	S12.000A	S12.34XA	S14.102S	S14.129D	S14.157A	S22.062B	S24.141D	S32.042B	S32.392B	S32.463B	S32.691B	S34.129S
S06.366S	S06.6X3S	S12.000B	S12.34XB	S14.103A	S14.129S	S14.157D	S22.068A	S24.141S	S32.048A	S32.399A	S32.464A	S32.692A	S34.131A
S06.369A	S06.6X4A	S12.001A	S12.350A	S14.103D	S14.131A	S14.157S	S22.068B	S24.142A	S32.048B	S32.399B	S32.464B	S32.692B	S34.131D
S06.369S	S06.6X4S	S12.001B	S12.350B	S14.103S	S14.131D	S14.158A	S22.069A	S24.142D	S32.049A	S32.401A	S32.465A	S32.699A	S34.131S
S06.370A	S06.6X5A	S12.01XA	S12.351A	S14.104A	S14.131S	S14.158D	S22.069B	S24.142S	S32.049B	S32.401B	S32.465B	S32.699B	S34.132A
S06.370S	S06.6X5S	S12.01XB	S12.351B	S14.104D	S14.132A	S14.158S	S22.070A	S24.143A	S32.050A	S32.402A	S32.466A	S32.810A	S34.132D
S06.371A	S06.6X6A	S12.02XA	S12.390A	S14.104S	S14.132D	S14.159A	S22.070B	S24.143D	S32.050B	S32.402B	S32.466B	S32.810B	S34.132S
S06.371S	S06.6X6S	S12.02XB	S12.390B	S14.105A	S14.132S	S14.159D	S22.071A	S24.143S	S32.051A	S32.409A	S32.471A	S32.811A	S34.139A
S06.372A	S06.6X9A	S12.030A	S12.391A	S14.105D	S14.133A	S14.159S	S22.071B	S24.144A	S32.051B	S32.409B	S32.471B	S32.811B	S34.139D
S06.372S	S06.6X9S	S12.030B	S12.391B	S14.105S	S14.133D	S22.000A	S22.072A	S24.144D	S32.052A	S32.411A	S32.472A	S32.82XA	S34.139S
S06.373A	S06.810A	S12.031A	S12.400A	S14.106A	S14.133S	S22.000B	S22.072B	S24.144S	S32.052B	S32.411B	S32.472B	S32.82XB	S34.3XXA

HCC (cont.) - Based on CMS data

S48.011A	S68.019S	S72.001A	S72.051C	S72.125B	S72.323A	S72.363C	S72.434B	S72.8X1A	S78.119S	S88.111D	S98.132A	T36.2X2S	T39.92XS
S48.011S	S68.021S	S72.001B	S72.052A	S72.125C	S72.323B	S72.364A	S72.434C	S72.8X1B	S78.121A	S88.111S	S98.132D	T36.3X2A	T40.0X2A
S48.012A	S68.022S	S72.001C	S72.052B	S72.126A	S72.323C	S72.364B	S72.435A	S72.8X1C	S78.121D	S88.112A	S98.132S	T36.3X2S	T40.0X2S
S48.012S	S68.029S	S72.002A	S72.052C	S72.126B	S72.324A	S72.364C	S72.435B	S72.8X2A	S78.121S	S88.112D	S98.139A	T36.4X2A	T40.1X2A
S48.019A	S68.110S	S72.002B	S72.059A	S72.126C	S72.324B	S72.365A	S72.435C	S72.8X2B	S78.122A	S88.112S	S98.139D	T36.4X2S	T40.1X2S
S48.019S	S68.111S	S72.002C	S72.059B	S72.131A	S72.324C	S72.365B	S72.436A	S72.8X2C	S78.122D	S88.119A	S98.139S	T36.5X2A	T40.2X2A
S48.021A	S68.112S	S72.009A	S72.059C	S72.131B	S72.325A	S72.365C	S72.436B	S72.8X9A	S78.122S	S88.119D	S98.141A	T36.5X2S	T40.2X2S
S48.021S	S68.113S	S72.009B	S72.061A	S72.131C	S72.325B	S72.366A	S72.436C	S72.8X9B	S78.129A	S88.119S	S98.141D	T36.6X2A	T40.3X2A
S48.022A	S68.114S	S72.009C	S72.061B	S72.132A	S72.325C	S72.366B	S72.441A	S72.8X9C	S78.129D	S88.121A	S98.141S	T36.6X2S	T40.3X2S
S48.022S	S68.115S	S72.011A	S72.061C	S72.132B	S72.326A	S72.366C	S72.441B	S72.90XA	S78.129S	S88.121D	S98.142A	T36.7X2A	T40.4X2A
S48.029A	S68.116S	S72.011B	S72.062A	S72.132C	S72.326B	S72.391A	S72.441C	S72.90XB	S78.911A	S88.121S	S98.142D	T36.7X2S	T40.4X2S
S48.029S	S68.117S	S72.011C	S72.062B	S72.133A	S72.326C	S72.391B	S72.442A	S72.90XC	S78.911D	S88.122A	S98.142S	T36.8X2A	T40.5X2A
S48.111A	S68.118S	S72.012A	S72.062C	S72.133B	S72.331A	S72.391C	S72.442B	S72.91XA	S78.911S	S88.122D	S98.149A	T36.8X2S	T40.5X2S
S48.111S	S68.119S	S72.012B	S72.063A	S72.133C	S72.331B	S72.392A	S72.442C	S72.91XB	S78.912A	S88.122S	S98.149D	T36.92XA	T40.602A
S48.112A	S68.120S	S72.012C	S72.063B	S72.134A	S72.331C	S72.392B	S72.443A	S72.91XC	S78.912D	S88.129A	S98.149S	T36.92XS	T40.602S
S48.112S	S68.121S	S72.019A	S72.063C	S72.134B	S72.332A	S72.392C	S72.443B	S72.92XA	S78.912S	S88.129D	S98.211A	T37.0X2A	T40.692A
S48.119A	S68.122S	S72.019B	S72.064A	S72.134C	S72.332B	S72.399A	S72.443C	S72.92XB	S78.919A	S88.129S	S98.211D	T37.0X2S	T40.692S
S48.119S	S68.123S	S72.019C	S72.064B	S72.135A	S72.332C	S72.399B	S72.444A	S72.92XC	S78.919D	S88.911A	S98.211S	T37.1X2A	T40.7X2A
S48.121A	S68.124S	S72.021A	S72.064C	S72.135B	S72.333A	S72.399C	S72.444B	S73.001A	S78.919S	S88.911D	S98.212A	T37.1X2S	T40.7X2S
S48.121S	S68.125S	S72.021B	S72.065A	S72.135C	S72.333B	S72.401A	S72.444C	S73.002A	S78.921A	S88.911S	S98.212D	T37.2X2A	T40.8X2A
S48.122A	S68.126S	S72.021C	S72.065B	S72.136A	S72.333C	S72.401B	S72.445A	S73.003A	S78.921D	S88.912A	S98.212S	T37.2X2S	T40.8X2S
S48.122S	S68.127S	S72.022A	S72.065C	S72.136B	S72.334A	S72.401C	S72.445B	S73.004A	S78.921S	S88.912D	S98.219A	T37.3X2A	T40.902A
S48.129A	S68.128S	S72.022B	S72.066A	S72.136C	S72.334B	S72.402A	S72.445C	S73.005A	S78.922A	S88.912S	S98.219D	T37.3X2S	T40.902S
S48.129S	S68.129S	S72.022C	S72.066B	S72.141A	S72.334C	S72.402B	S72.446A	S73.006A	S78.922D	S88.919A	S98.219S	T37.4X2A	T40.992A
S48.911A	S68.411A	S72.023A	S72.066C	S72.141B	S72.335A	S72.402C	S72.446B	S73.011A	S78.922S	S88.919D	S98.221A	T37.4X2S	T40.992S
S48.911S	S68.411S	S72.023B	S72.091A	S72.141C	S72.335B	S72.409A	S72.446C	S73.012A	S78.929A	S88.919S	S98.221D	T37.5X2A	T41.0X2A
S48.912A	S68.412A	S72.023C	S72.091B	S72.142A	S72.335C	S72.409B	S72.451A	S73.013A	S78.929D	S88.921A	S98.221S	T37.5X2S	T41.0X2S
S48.912S	S68.412S	S72.024A	S72.091C	S72.142B	S72.336A	S72.409C	S72.451B	S73.014A	S78.929S	S88.921D	S98.222A	T37.8X2A	T41.1X2A
S48.919A	S68.419A	S72.024B	S72.092A	S72.142C	S72.336B	S72.411A	S72.451C	S73.015A	S79.001A	S88.921S	S98.222D	T37.8X2S	T41.1X2S
S48.919S	S68.419S	S72.024C	S72.092B	S72.143A	S72.336C	S72.411B	S72.452A	S73.016A	S79.002A	S88.922A	S98.222S	T37.92XA	T41.202A
S48.921A	S68.421A	S72.025A	S72.092C	S72.143B	S72.341A	S72.411C	S72.452B	S73.021A	S79.009A	S88.922D	S98.229A	T37.92XS	T41.202S
S48.921S	S68.421S	S72.025B	S72.099A	S72.143C	S72.341B	S72.412A	S72.452C	S73.022A	S79.011A	S88.922S	S98.229D	T38.0X2A	T41.292A
S48.922A	S68.422A	S72.025C	S72.099B	S72.144A	S72.341C	S72.412B	S72.453A	S73.023A	S79.012A	S88.929A	S98.229S	T38.0X2S	T41.292S
S48.922S	S68.422S	S72.026A	S72.099C	S72.144B	S72.342A	S72.412C	S72.453B	S73.024A	S79.019A	S88.929D	S98.311A	T38.1X2A	T41.3X2A
S48.929A	S68.429A	S72.026B	S72.101A	S72.144C	S72.342B	S72.413A	S72.453C	S73.025A	S79.091A	S88.929S	S98.311D	T38.1X2S	T41.3X2S
S48.929S	S68.429S	S72.026C	S72.101B	S72.145A	S72.342C	S72.413B	S72.454A	S73.026A	S79.092A	S98.011A	S98.311S	T38.2X2A	T41.42XA
S58.011A	S68.511S	S72.031A	S72.101C	S72.145B	S72.343A	S72.413C	S72.454B	S73.031A	S79.099A	S98.011D	S98.312A	T38.2X2S	T41.42XS
S58.011S	S68.512S	S72.031B	S72.102A	S72.145C	S72.343B	S72.414A	S72.454C	S73.032A	S79.101A	S98.011S	S98.312D	T38.3X2A	T41.5X2A
S58.012A	S68.519S	S72.031C	S72.102B	S72.146A	S72.343C	S72.414B	S72.455A	S73.033A	S79.102A	S98.012A	S98.312S	T38.3X2S	T41.5X2S
S58.012S	S68.521S	S72.032A	S72.102C	S72.146B	S72.344A	S72.414C	S72.455B	S73.034A	S79.109A	S98.012D	S98.319A	T38.4X2A	T42.0X2A
S58.019A	S68.522S	S72.032B	S72.109A	S72.146C	S72.344B	S72.415A	S72.455C	S73.035A	S79.111A	S98.012S	S98.319D	T38.4X2S	T42.0X2S
S58.019S	S68.529S	S72.032C	S72.109B	S72.21XA	S72.344C	S72.415B	S72.456A	S73.036A	S79.112A	S98.019A	S98.319S	T38.5X2A	T42.1X2A
S58.021A	S68.610S	S72.033A	S72.109C	S72.21XB	S72.345A	S72.415C	S72.456B	S73.041A	S79.119A	S98.019D	S98.321A	T38.5X2S	T42.1X2S
S58.021S	S68.611S	S72.033B	S72.111A	S72.21XC	S72.345B	S72.416A	S72.456C	S73.042A	S79.121A	S98.019S	S98.321D	T38.6X2A	T42.2X2A
S58.022A	S68.612S	S72.033C	S72.111B	S72.22XA	S72.345C	S72.416B	S72.461A	S73.043A	S79.122A	S98.021A	S98.321S	T38.6X2S	T42.2X2S
S58.022S	S68.613S	S72.034A	S72.111C	S72.22XB	S72.346A	S72.416C	S72.461B	S73.044A	S79.129A	S98.021D	S98.322A	T38.7X2A	T42.3X2A
S58.029A	S68.614S	S72.034B	S72.112A	S72.22XC	S72.346B	S72.421A	S72.461C	S73.045A	S79.131A	S98.021S	S98.322D	T38.7X2S	T42.3X2S
S58.029S	S68.615S	S72.034A	S72.112B	S72.23XA	S72.346C	S72.421B	S72.462A	S73.046A	S79.132A	S98.022A	S98.322S	T38.802A	T42.4X2A
S58.111A	S68.616S	S72.035A	S72.112C	S72.23XB	S72.351A	S72.421C	S72.462B	S78.011A	S79.139A	S98.022D	S98.329A	T38.802S	T42.4X2S
S58.111S	S68.617S	S72.035B	S72.113A	S72.23XC	S72.351B	S72.422A	S72.462C	S78.011D	S79.141A	S98.022S	S98.329D	T38.812A	T42.5X2A
S58.112A	S68.618S	S72.035C	S72.113B	S72.24XA	S72.351C	S72.422B	S72.463A	S78.011S	S79.142A	S98.029A	S98.329S	T38.812S	T42.5X2S
S58.112S	S68.619S	S72.036A	S72.113C	S72.24XB	S72.352A	S72.422C	S72.463B	S78.012A	S79.149A	S98.029D	S98.911A	T38.892A	T42.6X2A
S58.119A	S68.620S	S72.036B	S72.114A	S72.24XC	S72.352B	S72.423A	S72.463C	S78.012D	S79.191A	S98.029S	S98.911D	T38.892S	T42.6X2S
S58.119S	S68.621S	S72.036C	S72.114B	S72.25XA	S72.352C	S72.423B	S72.464A	S78.012S	S79.192A	S98.111A	S98.911S	T38.902A	T42.72XA
S58.121A	S68.622S	S72.041A	S72.114C	S72.25XB	S72.353A	S72.423C	S72.464B	S78.019A	S79.199A	S98.111D	S98.912A	T38.902S	T42.72XS
S58.121S	S68.623S	S72.041B	S72.115A	S72.25XC	S72.353B	S72.424A	S72.464C	S78.019D	S88.011A	S98.111S	S98.912S	T38.992A	T42.8X2A
S58.122A	S68.624S	S72.041C	S72.115B	S72.26XA	S72.353C	S72.424B	S72.465A	S78.019S	S88.011D	S98.112A	S98.919A	T38.992S	T42.8X2S
S58.122S	S68.625S	S72.042A	S72.115C	S72.26XB	S72.354A	S72.424C	S72.465B	S78.021A	S88.011S	S98.112D	S98.919D	T39.012A	T43.012A
S58.129A	S68.626S	S72.042B	S72.116A	S72.26XC	S72.354B	S72.425A	S72.465C	S78.021D	S88.012A	S98.112S	S98.919S	T39.012S	T43.012S
S58.129S	S68.627S	S72.042C	S72.116B	S72.301A	S72.354C	S72.425B	S72.466A	S78.021S	S88.012D	S98.119A	S98.921A	T39.092A	T43.022A
S58.911A	S68.628S	S72.043A	S72.116C	S72.301B	S72.355A	S72.425C	S72.466B	S78.022A	S88.012S	S98.119D	S98.921S	T39.092S	T43.022S
S58.911S	S68.629S	S72.043B	S72.121A	S72.301C	S72.355B	S72.426A	S72.466C	S78.022D	S88.019A	S98.119S	S98.921D	T39.1X2A	T43.1X2A
S58.912A	S68.711A	S72.043C	S72.121B	S72.302A	S72.355C	S72.426B	S72.471A	S78.022S	S88.019D	S98.121A	S98.921S	T39.1X2S	T43.1X2S
S58.912S	S68.711S	S72.044A	S72.121C	S72.302B	S72.356A	S72.426C	S72.472A	S78.029A	S88.019S	S98.121D	S98.922A	T39.2X2A	T43.202A
S58.919A	S68.712A	S72.044B	S72.122A	S72.302C	S72.356B	S72.431A	S72.479A	S78.029D	S88.021A	S98.121S	S98.922D	T39.2X2S	T43.202S
S58.919S	S68.712S	S72.044C	S72.122B	S72.309A	S72.356C	S72.431B	S72.491A	S78.029S	S88.021D	S98.122A	S98.922S	T39.312A	T43.212A
S58.921A	S68.719A	S72.045A	S72.122C	S72.309B	S72.361A	S72.431C	S72.491B	S78.111A	S88.021S	S98.122D	S98.929A	T39.312S	T43.212S
S58.921S	S68.719S	S72.045B	S72.123A	S72.309C	S72.361B	S72.432A	S72.491C	S78.111D	S88.022A	S98.122S	S98.929D	T39.392A	T43.222A
S58.922A	S68.721A	S72.045C	S72.123B	S72.321A	S72.361C	S72.432B	S72.492A	S78.111S	S88.022D	S98.129A	S98.929S	T39.392S	T43.222S
S58.922S	S68.721S	S72.046A	S72.123C	S72.321B	S72.362A	S72.432C	S72.492B	S78.112A	S88.022S	S98.129D	T36.0X2A	T39.4X2A	T43.292A
S58.929A	S68.722A	S72.046B	S72.124A	S72.321C	S72.362B	S72.433A	S72.492C	S78.112D	S88.029A	S98.129S	T36.0X2S	T39.4X2S	T43.292S
S58.929S	S68.722S	S72.046C	S72.124B	S72.322A	S72.362C	S72.433B	S72.499A	S78.112S	S88.029D	S98.131A	T36.1X2A	T39.8X2A	T43.3X2A
S68.011S	S68.729A	S72.051A	S72.124C	S72.322B	S72.363A	S72.433C	S72.499B	S78.119A	S88.029S	S98.131D	T36.1X2S	T39.8X2S	T43.3X2S
S68.012S	S68.729S	S72.051B	S72.125A	S72.322C	S72.363B	S72.434A	S72.499C	S78.119D	S88.111A	S98.131S	T36.2X2A	T39.92XA	T43.4X2A

HCC (cont.) - Based on CMS data

T43.4X2S	T46.0X2A	T49.3X2S	T52.4X2A	T57.8X2S	T62.92XA	T63.812S	T79.A19A	T82.533A	T83.518A	T84.113A	T84.63XA	X71.1XXD	X77.9XXD
T43.502A	T46.0X2S	T49.4X2A	T52.4X2S	T57.92XA	T62.92XS	T63.822A	T79.A21A	T82.534A	T83.590A	T84.114A	T84.69XA	X71.1XXS	X77.9XXS
T43.502S	T46.1X2A	T49.4X2S	T52.8X2A	T57.92XS	T63.002A	T63.822S	T79.A22A	T82.535A	T83.591A	T84.115A	T84.7XXA	X71.2XXA	X78.0XXA
T43.592A	T46.1X2S	T49.5X2A	T52.8X2S	T58.02XA	T63.002S	T63.832A	T79.A29A	T82.538A	T83.592A	T84.116A	T84.81XA	X71.2XXD	X78.0XXD
T43.592S	T46.2X2A	T49.5X2S	T52.92XA	T58.02XS	T63.012A	T63.832S	T79.A3XA	T82.590A	T83.593A	T84.117A	T84.82XA	X71.2XXS	X78.0XXS
T43.602A	T46.2X2S	T49.6X2A	T52.92XS	T58.12XA	T63.012S	T63.892A	T79.A9XA	T82.591A	T83.598A	T84.119A	T84.83XA	X71.3XXA	X78.1XXA
T43.602S	T46.3X2A	T49.6X2S	T53.0X2A	T58.12XS	T63.022A	T63.892S	T81.11XA	T82.593A	T83.61XA	T84.120A	T84.84XA	X71.3XXD	X78.1XXD
T43.612A	T46.3X2S	T49.7X2A	T53.0X2S	T58.2X2A	T63.022S	T63.92XA	T81.12XA	T82.594A	T83.62XA	T84.121A	T84.85XA	X71.3XXS	X78.1XXS
T43.612S	T46.4X2A	T49.7X2S	T53.1X2A	T58.2X2S	T63.032A	T63.92XS	T81.502A	T82.595A	T83.69XA	T84.122A	T84.86XA	X71.8XXA	X78.2XXA
T43.622A	T46.4X2S	T49.8X2A	T53.1X2S	T58.8X2A	T63.032S	T64.02XA	T81.502D	T82.598A	T83.711A	T84.123A	T84.89XA	X71.8XXD	X78.2XXD
T43.622S	T46.5X2A	T49.8X2S	T53.2X2A	T58.8X2S	T63.042A	T64.02XS	T81.502S	T82.6XXA	T83.712A	T84.124A	T84.9XXA	X71.8XXS	X78.2XXS
T43.632A	T46.5X2S	T49.92XA	T53.2X2S	T58.92XA	T63.042S	T64.82XA	T81.512A	T82.7XXA	T83.713A	T84.125A	T85.01XA	X71.9XXA	X78.8XXA
T43.632S	T46.6X2A	T49.92XS	T53.3X2A	T58.92XS	T63.062A	T64.82XS	T81.512D	T82.818A	T83.714A	T84.126A	T85.02XA	X71.9XXD	X78.8XXD
T43.692A	T46.6X2S	T50.0X2A	T53.3X2S	T59.0X2A	T63.062S	T65.0X2A	T81.512S	T82.828A	T83.718A	T84.127A	T85.03XA	X71.9XXS	X78.8XXS
T43.692S	T46.7X2A	T50.0X2S	T53.4X2A	T59.0X2S	T63.072A	T65.0X2S	T81.522A	T82.838A	T83.719A	T84.129A	T85.09XA	X72.XXXA	X78.9XXA
T43.8X2A	T46.7X2S	T50.1X2A	T53.4X2S	T59.1X2A	T63.072S	T65.1X2A	T81.522D	T82.848A	T83.721A	T84.190A	T85.110A	X72.XXXD	X78.9XXD
T43.8X2S	T46.8X2A	T50.1X2S	T53.5X2A	T59.1X2S	T63.082A	T65.1X2S	T81.522S	T82.856A	T83.722A	T84.191A	T85.111A	X72.XXXS	X78.9XXS
T43.92XA	T46.8X2S	T50.2X2A	T53.5X2S	T59.2X2A	T63.082S	T65.212A	T81.532A	T82.858A	T83.723A	T84.192A	T85.112A	X73.0XXA	X79.XXXA
T43.92XS	T46.902A	T50.2X2S	T53.6X2A	T59.2X2S	T63.092A	T65.212S	T81.532D	T82.868A	T83.724A	T84.193A	T85.113A	X73.0XXD	X79.XXXD
T44.0X2A	T46.902S	T50.3X2A	T53.6X2S	T59.3X2A	T63.092S	T65.222A	T81.532S	T82.898A	T83.728A	T84.194A	T85.118A	X73.0XXS	X79.XXXS
T44.0X2S	T46.992A	T50.3X2S	T53.7X2A	T59.3X2S	T63.112A	T65.222S	T81.592A	T83.010A	T83.729A	T84.195A	T85.120A	X73.1XXA	X80.XXXA
T44.1X2A	T46.992S	T50.4X2A	T53.7X2S	T59.4X2A	T63.112S	T65.292A	T81.592D	T83.011A	T83.79XA	T84.196A	T85.121A	X73.1XXD	X80.XXXD
T44.1X2S	T47.0X2A	T50.4X2S	T53.92XA	T59.4X2S	T63.122A	T65.292S	T81.592S	T83.012A	T83.81XA	T84.197A	T85.122A	X73.1XXS	X80.XXXS
T44.2X2A	T47.0X2S	T50.5X2A	T53.92XS	T59.5X2A	T63.122S	T65.3X2A	T82.310A	T83.018A	T83.82XA	T84.199A	T85.123A	X73.2XXA	X81.0XXA
T44.2X2S	T47.1X2A	T50.5X2S	T54.0X2A	T59.5X2S	T63.192A	T65.3X2S	T82.311A	T83.020A	T83.83XA	T84.210A	T85.128A	X73.2XXD	X81.0XXD
T44.3X2A	T47.1X2S	T50.6X2A	T54.0X2S	T59.6X2A	T63.192S	T65.4X2A	T82.312A	T83.021A	T83.84XA	T84.213A	T85.190A	X73.2XXS	X81.0XXS
T44.3X2S	T47.2X2A	T50.6X2S	T54.1X2A	T59.6X2S	T63.2X2A	T65.4X2S	T82.318A	T83.022A	T83.85XA	T84.216A	T85.191A	X73.8XXA	X81.1XXA
T44.4X2A	T47.2X2S	T50.7X2A	T54.1X2S	T59.7X2A	T63.2X2S	T65.5X2A	T82.319A	T83.028A	T83.86XA	T84.218A	T85.192A	X73.8XXD	X81.1XXD
T44.4X2S	T47.3X2A	T50.7X2S	T54.2X2A	T59.7X2S	T63.302A	T65.5X2S	T82.320A	T83.030A	T83.89XA	T84.220A	T85.193A	X73.8XXS	X81.1XXS
T44.5X2A	T47.3X2S	T50.8X2A	T54.2X2S	T59.812A	T63.302S	T65.6X2A	T82.321A	T83.031A	T83.9XXA	T84.223A	T85.199A	X73.9XXA	X81.8XXA
T44.5X2S	T47.4X2A	T50.8X2S	T54.3X2A	T59.812S	T63.312A	T65.6X2S	T82.322A	T83.032A	T84.010A	T84.226A	T85.611A	X73.9XXD	X81.8XXD
T44.6X2A	T47.4X2S	T50.902A	T54.3X2S	T59.892A	T63.312S	T65.812A	T82.328A	T83.038A	T84.011A	T84.228A	T85.611D	X74.01XA	X82.0XXA
T44.6X2S	T47.5X2A	T50.902S	T54.92XA	T59.892S	T63.322A	T65.812S	T82.329A	T83.090A	T84.012A	T84.290A	T85.611S	X74.01XD	X82.0XXD
T44.7X2A	T47.5X2S	T50.992A	T54.92XS	T59.92XA	T63.322S	T65.822A	T82.330A	T83.091A	T84.013A	T84.293A	T85.615A	X74.01XS	X82.0XXS
T44.7X2S	T47.6X2A	T50.992S	T55.0X2A	T59.92XS	T63.332A	T65.822S	T82.331A	T83.092A	T84.018A	T84.296A	T85.621A	X74.02XA	X82.1XXA
T44.8X2A	T47.6X2S	T50.A12A	T55.0X2S	T60.0X2A	T63.332S	T65.832A	T82.332A	T83.098A	T84.019A	T84.298A	T85.621D	X74.02XD	X82.1XXD
T44.8X2S	T47.7X2A	T50.A12S	T55.1X2A	T60.0X2S	T63.392A	T65.832S	T82.338A	T83.110A	T84.020A	T84.310A	T85.621S	X74.02XS	X82.1XXS
T44.902A	T47.7X2S	T50.A22A	T55.1X2S	T60.1X2A	T63.392S	T65.892A	T82.339A	T83.111A	T84.021A	T84.318A	T85.625A	X74.09XA	X82.2XXA
T44.902S	T47.8X2A	T50.A22S	T56.0X2A	T60.1X2S	T63.412A	T65.892S	T82.390A	T83.112A	T84.022A	T84.320A	T85.631A	X74.09XD	X82.2XXD
T44.992A	T47.8X2S	T50.A92A	T56.0X2S	T60.2X2A	T63.412S	T65.92XA	T82.391A	T83.113A	T84.023A	T84.328A	T85.631D	X74.09XS	X82.2XXS
T44.992S	T47.92XA	T50.A92S	T56.1X2A	T60.2X2S	T63.422A	T65.92XS	T82.392A	T83.118A	T84.028A	T84.390A	T85.631S	X74.8XXA	X82.8XXA
T45.0X2A	T47.92XS	T50.B12A	T56.1X2S	T60.3X2A	T63.422S	T71.112A	T82.398A	T83.120A	T84.029A	T84.398A	T85.635A	X74.8XXD	X82.8XXD
T45.0X2S	T48.0X2A	T50.B12S	T56.2X2A	T60.3X2S	T63.432A	T71.112S	T82.399A	T83.121A	T84.030A	T84.410A	T85.691A	X74.8XXS	X82.8XXS
T45.1X2A	T48.0X2S	T50.B92A	T56.2X2S	T60.4X2A	T63.432S	T71.122A	T82.41XA	T83.122A	T84.031A	T84.418A	T85.691D	X74.9XXA	X83.0XXA
T45.1X2S	T48.1X2A	T50.B92S	T56.3X2A	T60.4X2S	T63.442A	T71.122S	T82.41XD	T83.123A	T84.032A	T84.420A	T85.691S	X74.9XXD	X83.0XXD
T45.2X2A	T48.1X2S	T50.Z12A	T56.3X2S	T60.8X2A	T63.442S	T71.132A	T82.41XS	T83.128A	T84.033A	T84.428A	T85.71XA	X74.9XXS	X83.0XXS
T45.2X2S	T48.202A	T50.Z12S	T56.4X2A	T60.8X2S	T63.452A	T71.132S	T82.42XA	T83.190A	T84.038A	T84.490A	T85.71XD	X75.XXXA	X83.1XXA
T45.3X2A	T48.202S	T50.Z92A	T56.4X2S	T60.92XA	T63.452S	T71.152A	T82.42XD	T83.191A	T84.039A	T84.498A	T85.71XS	X75.XXXD	X83.1XXD
T45.3X2S	T48.292A	T50.Z92S	T56.5X2A	T60.92XS	T63.462A	T71.152S	T82.42XS	T83.192A	T84.050A	T84.50XA	T85.72XA	X75.XXXS	X83.1XXS
T45.4X2A	T48.292S	T51.0X2A	T56.5X2S	T61.02XA	T63.462S	T71.162A	T82.43XA	T83.193A	T84.051A	T84.51XA	T85.730A	X76.XXXA	X83.2XXA
T45.4X2S	T48.3X2A	T51.0X2S	T56.6X2A	T61.02XS	T63.482A	T71.162S	T82.43XD	T83.198A	T84.052A	T84.52XA	T85.731A	X76.XXXD	X83.2XXD
T45.512A	T48.3X2S	T51.1X2A	T56.6X2S	T61.12XA	T63.482S	T71.192A	T82.43XS	T83.21XA	T84.053A	T84.53XA	T85.732A	X76.XXXS	X83.2XXS
T45.512S	T48.4X2A	T51.1X2S	T56.7X2A	T61.12XS	T63.512A	T71.192S	T82.49XA	T83.22XA	T84.058A	T84.54XA	T85.733A	X77.0XXA	X83.8XXA
T45.522A	T48.4X2S	T51.2X2A	T56.7X2S	T61.772A	T63.512S	T71.222A	T82.49XD	T83.23XA	T84.059A	T84.59XA	T85.734A	X77.0XXD	X83.8XXD
T45.522S	T48.5X2A	T51.2X2S	T56.812A	T61.772S	T63.592A	T71.222S	T82.49XS	T83.24XA	T84.060A	T84.60XA	T85.735A	X77.0XXS	X83.8XXS
T45.602A	T48.5X2S	T51.3X2A	T56.812S	T61.782A	T63.592S	T71.232A	T82.510A	T83.25XA	T84.061A	T84.610A	T85.738A	X77.1XXA	
T45.602S	T48.6X2A	T51.3X2S	T56.892A	T61.782S	T63.612A	T71.232S	T82.511A	T83.29XA	T84.062A	T84.611A	T85.79XA	X77.1XXD	
T45.612A	T48.6X2S	T51.8X2A	T56.892S	T61.8X2A	T63.612S	T79.0XXA	T82.513A	T83.410A	T84.063A	T84.612A	T85.810A	X77.1XXS	
T45.612S	T48.902A	T51.8X2S	T56.92XA	T61.8X2S	T63.622A	T79.1XXA	T82.514A	T83.411A	T84.068A	T84.613A	T85.820A	X77.2XXA	
T45.622A	T48.902S	T51.92XA	T56.92XS	T61.92XA	T63.622S	T79.2XXA	T82.515A	T83.418A	T84.069A	T84.614A	T85.830A	X77.2XXD	
T45.622S	T48.992A	T51.92XS	T57.0X2A	T61.92XS	T63.632A	T79.4XXA	T82.518A	T83.420A	T84.090A	T84.615A	T85.840A	X77.2XXS	
T45.692A	T48.992S	T52.0X2A	T57.0X2S	T62.0X2A	T63.632S	T79.5XXA	T82.520A	T83.421A	T84.091A	T84.619A	T85.850A	X77.3XXA	
T45.692S	T49.0X2A	T52.0X2S	T57.1X2A	T62.0X2S	T63.692A	T79.6XXA	T82.521A	T83.428A	T84.092A	T84.620A	T85.860A	X77.3XXD	
T45.7X2A	T49.0X2S	T52.1X2A	T57.1X2S	T62.1X2A	T63.692S	T79.7XXA	T82.523A	T83.490A	T84.093A	T84.621A	T85.890A	X77.3XXS	
T45.7X2S	T49.1X2A	T52.1X2S	T57.2X2A	T62.1X2S	T63.712A	T79.8XXA	T82.524A	T83.491A	T84.098A	T84.622A	X71.0XXA	X77.8XXA	
T45.8X2A	T49.1X2S	T52.2X2A	T57.2X2S	T62.2X2A	T63.712S	T79.9XXA	T82.525A	T83.498A	T84.099A	T84.623A	X71.0XXD	X77.8XXD	
T45.8X2S	T49.2X2A	T52.2X2S	T57.3X2A	T62.2X2S	T63.792A	T79.A0XA	T82.528A	T83.510A	T84.110A	T84.624A	X71.0XXS	X77.8XXS	
T45.92XA	T49.2X2S	T52.3X2A	T57.3X2S	T62.8X2A	T63.792S	T79.A11A	T82.530A	T83.511A	T84.111A	T84.625A	X71.1XXA	X77.9XXA	
T45.92XS	T49.3X2A	T52.3X2S	T57.8X2A	T62.8X2S	T63.812A	T79.A12A	T82.531A	T83.512A	T84.112A	T84.629A			

MACRA - Based on CMS data

E08.3211	E08.3541	E09.3511	E10.3391	E10.37X1	E11.3531	E13.3411	H35.3110	H40.10X4	H40.1290	S02.32XA	S02.672A	S06.352A	S06.822A
E08.3212	E08.3542	E09.3512	E10.3392	E10.37X2	E11.3532	E13.3412	H35.3111	H40.1110	H40.1291	S02.400A	S02.69XA	S06.353A	S06.823A
E08.3213	E08.3543	E09.3513	E10.3393	E10.37X3	E11.3533	E13.3413	H35.3112	H40.1111	H40.1292	S02.401A	S02.80XA	S06.354A	S06.824A
E08.3219	E08.3549	E09.3519	E10.3399	E10.37X9	E11.3539	E13.3419	H35.3113	H40.1112	H40.1293	S02.402A	S02.81XA	S06.359A	S06.829A
E08.3291	E08.3551	E09.3521	E10.3411	E11.3211	E11.3541	E13.3491	H35.3114	H40.1113	H40.1294	S02.40AA	S02.82XA	S06.360A	S06.890A
E08.3292	E08.3552	E09.3522	E10.3412	E11.3212	E11.3542	E13.3492	H35.3120	H40.1114	S00.03XA	S02.40BA	S02.91XA	S06.361A	S06.891A
E08.3293	E08.3553	E09.3523	E10.3413	E11.3213	E11.3543	E13.3493	H35.3121	H40.1120	S00.33XA	S02.40CA	S02.92XA	S06.362A	S06.892A
E08.3299	E08.3559	E09.3529	E10.3419	E11.3219	E11.3549	E13.3499	H35.3122	H40.1121	S00.431A	S02.40DA	S06.0X0A	S06.363A	S06.893A
E08.3311	E08.3591	E09.3531	E10.3491	E11.3291	E11.3551	E13.3511	H35.3123	H40.1122	S00.432A	S02.40EA	S06.0X1A	S06.364A	S06.894A
E08.3312	E08.3592	E09.3532	E10.3492	E11.3292	E11.3552	E13.3512	H35.3124	H40.1123	S00.439A	S02.40FA	S06.0X9A	S06.369A	S06.899A
E08.3313	E08.3593	E09.3533	E10.3493	E11.3293	E11.3553	E13.3513	H35.3130	H40.1124	S00.531A	S02.411A	S06.1X0A	S06.4X0A	S06.9X0A
E08.3319	E08.3599	E09.3539	E10.3499	E11.3299	E11.3559	E13.3519	H35.3131	H40.1130	S00.532A	S02.412A	S06.1X1A	S06.4X1A	S06.9X1A
E08.3391	E09.3211	E09.3541	E10.3511	E11.3311	E11.3591	E13.3521	H35.3132	H40.1131	S00.83XA	S02.413A	S06.1X2A	S06.4X2A	S06.9X2A
E08.3392	E09.3212	E09.3542	E10.3512	E11.3312	E11.3592	E13.3522	H35.3133	H40.1132	S00.93XA	S02.42XA	S06.1X3A	S06.4X3A	S06.9X3A
E08.3393	E09.3213	E09.3543	E10.3513	E11.3313	E11.3593	E13.3523	H35.3134	H40.1133	S02.0XXA	S02.600A	S06.1X4A	S06.4X4A	S06.9X4A
E08.3399	E09.3219	E09.3549	E10.3519	E11.3319	E11.3599	E13.3529	H35.3190	H40.1134	S02.101A	S02.601A	S06.1X9A	S06.4X9A	S06.9X9A
E08.3411	E09.3291	E09.3551	E10.3521	E11.3391	E11.37X1	E13.3531	H35.3191	H40.1190	S02.102A	S02.602A	S06.2X0A	S06.5X0A	S09.10XA
E08.3412	E09.3292	E09.3552	E10.3522	E11.3392	E11.37X2	E13.3532	H35.3192	H40.1191	S02.109A	S02.609A	S06.2X1A	S06.5X1A	S09.11XA
E08.3413	E09.3293	E09.3553	E10.3523	E11.3393	E11.37X3	E13.3533	H35.3193	H40.1192	S02.110A	S02.610A	S06.2X2A	S06.5X2A	S09.19XA
E08.3419	E09.3299	E09.3559	E10.3529	E11.3399	E11.37X9	E13.3539	H35.3194	H40.1193	S02.111A	S02.611A	S06.2X3A	S06.5X3A	S09.8XXA
E08.3491	E09.3311	E09.3591	E10.3531	E11.3411	E13.3211	E13.3541	H35.3210	H40.1194	S02.112A	S02.612A	S06.2X4A	S06.5X4A	S09.90XA
E08.3492	E09.3312	E09.3592	E10.3532	E11.3412	E13.3212	E13.3542	H35.3211	H40.1210	S02.113A	S02.620A	S06.2X9A	S06.5X9A	S09.92XA
E08.3493	E09.3313	E09.3593	E10.3533	E11.3413	E13.3213	E13.3543	H35.3212	H40.1211	S02.118A	S02.621A	S06.300A	S06.6X0A	S09.93XA
E08.3499	E09.3319	E09.3599	E10.3539	E11.3419	E13.3219	E13.3549	H35.3213	H40.1212	S02.119A	S02.622A	S06.301A	S06.6X1A	S10.0XXA
E08.3511	E09.3391	E10.3211	E10.3541	E11.3491	E13.3291	E13.3551	H35.3220	H40.1213	S02.11AA	S02.630A	S06.302A	S06.6X2A	S10.83XA
E08.3512	E09.3392	E10.3212	E10.3542	E11.3492	E13.3292	E13.3552	H35.3221	H40.1214	S02.11BA	S02.631A	S06.303A	S06.6X3A	S10.93XA
E08.3513	E09.3393	E10.3213	E10.3543	E11.3493	E13.3293	E13.3553	H35.3222	H40.1220	S02.11CA	S02.632A	S06.304A	S06.6X4A	
E08.3519	E09.3399	E10.3219	E10.3549	E11.3499	E13.3299	E13.3559	H35.3223	H40.1221	S02.11DA	S02.640A	S06.309A	S06.6X9A	
E08.3521	E09.3411	E10.3291	E10.3551	E11.3511	E13.3311	E13.3591	H35.3230	H40.1222	S02.11EA	S02.641A	S06.340A	S06.810A	
E08.3522	E09.3412	E10.3292	E10.3552	E11.3512	E13.3312	E13.3592	H35.3231	H40.1223	S02.11FA	S02.642A	S06.341A	S06.811A	
E08.3523	E09.3413	E10.3293	E10.3553	E11.3513	E13.3313	E13.3593	H35.3232	H40.1224	S02.11GA	S02.650A	S06.342A	S06.812A	
E08.3529	E09.3419	E10.3299	E10.3559	E11.3519	E13.3319	E13.3599	H35.3233	H40.1230	S02.11HA	S02.651A	S06.343A	S06.813A	
E08.3531	E09.3491	E10.3311	E10.3591	E11.3521	E13.3391	E13.37X1	H40.10X0	H40.1231	S02.19XA	S02.652A	S06.344A	S06.814A	
E08.3532	E09.3492	E10.3312	E10.3592	E11.3522	E13.3392	E13.37X2	H40.10X1	H40.1232	S02.2XXA	S02.66XA	S06.349A	S06.819A	
E08.3533	E09.3493	E10.3313	E10.3593	E11.3523	E13.3393	E13.37X3	H40.10X2	H40.1233	S02.30XA	S02.670A	S06.350A	S06.820A	
E08.3539	E09.3499	E10.3319	E10.3599	E11.3529	E13.3399	E13.37X9	H40.10X3	H40.1234	S02.31XA	S02.671A	S06.351A	S06.821A	

Major Complication or Comorbidity (MCC) - Based on CMS data

O41.1010	O41.1230	O60.13X0	R40.2122	S02.113B	S06.316A	S06.351A	S06.4X8A	S11.012A	S12.131B	S12.530B	S14.122A	S21.312A	S22.008B
O41.1011	O41.1231	O60.13X1	R40.2123	S02.118B	S06.317A	S06.352A	S06.4X9A	S11.013A	S12.14XB	S12.531B	S14.123A	S21.319A	S22.009B
O41.1012	O41.1232	O60.13X2	R40.2124	S02.119B	S06.318A	S06.353A	S06.5X0A	S11.014A	S12.150B	S12.54XB	S14.124A	S21.321A	S22.010B
O41.1013	O41.1233	O60.13X3	R40.2210	S02.11AB	S06.319A	S06.354A	S06.5X1A	S11.015A	S12.151B	S12.550B	S14.125A	S21.322A	S22.011B
O41.1014	O41.1234	O60.13X4	R40.2211	S02.11BB	S06.320A	S06.355A	S06.5X2A	S11.019A	S12.190B	S12.551B	S14.126A	S21.329A	S22.012B
O41.1015	O41.1235	O60.13X5	R40.2212	S02.11CB	S06.321A	S06.356A	S06.5X3A	S11.021A	S12.191B	S12.590B	S14.127A	S21.331A	S22.018B
O41.1019	O41.1239	O60.13X9	R40.2213	S02.11DB	S06.322A	S06.357A	S06.5X4A	S11.022A	S12.200B	S12.591B	S14.128A	S21.332A	S22.019B
O41.1020	O41.1410	O60.14X0	R40.2214	S02.11EB	S06.323A	S06.358A	S06.5X5A	S11.023A	S12.201B	S12.600B	S14.131A	S21.339A	S22.020B
O41.1021	O41.1411	O60.14X1	R40.2220	S02.11FB	S06.324A	S06.359A	S06.5X6A	S11.024A	S12.230B	S12.601B	S14.132A	S21.341A	S22.021B
O41.1022	O41.1412	O60.14X2	R40.2221	S02.11GB	S06.325A	S06.360A	S06.5X7A	S11.025A	S12.231B	S12.630B	S14.133A	S21.342A	S22.022B
O41.1023	O41.1413	O60.14X3	R40.2222	S02.11HB	S06.326A	S06.361A	S06.5X8A	S11.029A	S12.24XB	S12.631B	S14.134A	S21.349A	S22.028B
O41.1024	O41.1414	O60.14X4	R40.2223	S02.19XB	S06.327A	S06.362A	S06.5X9A	S11.031A	S12.250B	S12.64XB	S14.135A	S21.351A	S22.029B
O41.1025	O41.1415	O60.14X5	R40.2224	S02.91XB	S06.328A	S06.363A	S06.6X0A	S11.032A	S12.251B	S12.650B	S14.136A	S21.352A	S22.030B
O41.1029	O41.1419	O60.14X9	R40.2310	S06.1X0A	S06.329A	S06.364A	S06.6X1A	S11.033A	S12.290B	S12.651B	S14.137A	S21.359A	S22.031B
O41.1030	O41.1420	O60.22X0	R40.2311	S06.1X1A	S06.330A	S06.365A	S06.6X2A	S11.034A	S12.291B	S12.690B	S14.138A	S21.401A	S22.032B
O41.1031	O41.1421	O60.22X1	R40.2312	S06.1X2A	S06.331A	S06.366A	S06.6X3A	S11.035A	S12.300B	S12.691B	S14.141A	S21.402A	S22.038B
O41.1032	O41.1422	O60.22X2	R40.2313	S06.1X3A	S06.332A	S06.367A	S06.6X4A	S11.039A	S12.301B	S12.8XXA	S14.142A	S21.409A	S22.039B
O41.1033	O41.1423	O60.22X3	R40.2314	S06.1X4A	S06.333A	S06.368A	S06.6X5A	S12.000B	S12.330B	S14.0XXA	S14.143A	S21.411A	S22.040B
O41.1034	O41.1424	O60.22X4	R40.2320	S06.1X5A	S06.334A	S06.369A	S06.6X6A	S12.001B	S12.331B	S14.101A	S14.144A	S21.412A	S22.041B
O41.1035	O41.1425	O60.22X5	R40.2321	S06.1X6A	S06.335A	S06.370A	S06.6X7A	S12.01XB	S12.34XB	S14.102A	S14.145A	S21.419A	S22.042B
O41.1039	O41.1429	O60.22X9	R40.2322	S06.1X7A	S06.336A	S06.376A	S06.6X8A	S12.02XB	S12.350B	S14.103A	S14.146A	S21.421A	S22.048B
O41.1210	O41.1430	O60.23X0	R40.2323	S06.1X8A	S06.337A	S06.377A	S06.6X9A	S12.030B	S12.351B	S14.104A	S14.147A	S21.422A	S22.049B
O41.1211	O41.1431	O60.23X1	R40.2324	S06.1X9A	S06.338A	S06.378A	S06.816A	S12.031B	S12.390B	S14.105A	S14.148A	S21.429A	S22.050B
O41.1212	O41.1432	O60.23X2	R40.2340	S06.2X6A	S06.339A	S06.380A	S06.817A	S12.040B	S12.391B	S14.106A	S14.151A	S21.431A	S22.051B
O41.1213	O41.1433	O60.23X3	R40.2341	S06.2X7A	S06.340A	S06.386A	S06.818A	S12.041B	S12.400B	S14.107A	S14.152A	S21.432A	S22.052B
O41.1214	O41.1434	O60.23X4	R40.2342	S06.2X8A	S06.341A	S06.387A	S06.826A	S12.090B	S12.401B	S14.108A	S14.153A	S21.439A	S22.058B
O41.1215	O41.1435	O60.23X5	R40.2343	S06.306A	S06.342A	S06.388A	S06.827A	S12.091B	S12.430B	S14.111A	S14.154A	S21.441A	S22.059B
O41.1219	O41.1439	O60.23X9	R40.2344	S06.307A	S06.343A	S06.4X0A	S06.828A	S12.100B	S12.431B	S14.112A	S14.155A	S21.442A	S22.060B
O41.1220	O60.12X0	R40.2110	S02.0XXB	S06.308A	S06.344A	S06.4X1A	S06.896A	S12.101B	S12.44XB	S14.113A	S14.156A	S21.449A	S22.061B
O41.1221	O60.12X1	R40.2111	S02.101B	S06.310A	S06.345A	S06.4X2A	S06.897A	S12.110B	S12.450B	S14.114A	S14.157A	S21.451A	S22.062B
O41.1222	O60.12X2	R40.2112	S02.102B	S06.311A	S06.346A	S06.4X3A	S06.898A	S12.111B	S12.451B	S14.115A	S14.158A	S21.452A	S22.068B
O41.1223	O60.12X3	R40.2113	S02.109B	S06.312A	S06.347A	S06.4X4A	S06.9X6A	S12.112B	S12.490B	S14.116A	S21.301A	S21.459A	S22.069B
O41.1224	O60.12X4	R40.2114	S02.110B	S06.313A	S06.348A	S06.4X5A	S06.9X7A	S12.120B	S12.491B	S14.117A	S21.302A	S22.000B	S22.070B
O41.1225	O60.12X5	R40.2120	S02.111B	S06.314A	S06.349A	S06.4X6A	S06.9X8A	S12.121B	S12.500B	S14.118A	S21.309A	S22.001B	S22.071B
O41.1229	O60.12X9	R40.2121	S02.112B	S06.315A	S06.350A	S06.4X7A	S11.011A	S12.130B	S12.501B	S14.121A	S21.311A	S22.002B	S22.072B

Major Complication or Comorbidity (MCC) (cont.) - Based on CMS data

S22.078B	S25.399A	S31.635A	S32.391B	S32.463B	S34.114A	S35.59XA	S42.354B	S45.019A	S52.133B	S52.264B	S52.355B	S52.569B	S72.025A
S22.079B	S25.401A	S31.639A	S32.392B	S32.464A	S34.115A	S36.031A	S42.355B	S45.091A	S52.133C	S52.264C	S52.355C	S52.569C	S72.025B
S22.080B	S25.402A	S31.640A	S32.399B	S32.464B	S34.119A	S36.032A	S42.356B	S45.092A	S52.134B	S52.265B	S52.356B	S52.571B	S72.025C
S22.081B	S25.409A	S31.641A	S32.401A	S32.465A	S34.121A	S36.115A	S42.361B	S45.099A	S52.134C	S52.265C	S52.356C	S52.571C	S72.026A
S22.082B	S25.411A	S31.642A	S32.401B	S32.465B	S34.122A	S36.116A	S42.362B	S52.001B	S52.135B	S52.266B	S52.361B	S52.572B	S72.026B
S22.088B	S25.412A	S31.643A	S32.402A	S32.466A	S34.123A	S37.061A	S42.363B	S52.001C	S52.135C	S52.266C	S52.361C	S52.572C	S72.026C
S22.089B	S25.419A	S31.644A	S32.402B	S32.466B	S34.124A	S37.062A	S42.364B	S52.002B	S52.136B	S52.271B	S52.362B	S52.579B	S72.031A
S22.20XB	S25.421A	S31.645A	S32.409A	S32.471A	S34.125A	S37.069A	S42.365B	S52.002C	S52.136C	S52.271C	S52.362C	S52.579C	S72.031B
S22.21XB	S25.422A	S31.649A	S32.409B	S32.471B	S34.129A	S37.091A	S42.366B	S52.009B	S52.181B	S52.272B	S52.363B	S52.591B	S72.031C
S22.22XB	S25.429A	S31.650A	S32.411A	S32.472A	S34.131A	S37.092A	S42.391B	S52.009C	S52.181C	S52.272C	S52.363C	S52.591C	S72.032A
S22.23XB	S25.491A	S31.651A	S32.411B	S32.472B	S34.132A	S37.099A	S42.392B	S52.021B	S52.182B	S52.279B	S52.364B	S52.592B	S72.032B
S22.24XB	S25.492A	S31.652A	S32.412A	S32.473A	S34.139A	S42.201B	S42.399B	S52.021C	S52.182C	S52.279C	S52.364C	S52.592C	S72.032C
S22.31XB	S25.499A	S31.653A	S32.412B	S32.473B	S34.3XXA	S42.202B	S42.401B	S52.022B	S52.189B	S52.281B	S52.365B	S52.599B	S72.033A
S22.32XB	S26.020A	S31.654A	S32.413A	S32.474A	S35.00XA	S42.209B	S42.402B	S52.022C	S52.189C	S52.281C	S52.365C	S52.599C	S72.033B
S22.39XB	S26.021A	S31.655A	S32.413B	S32.474B	S35.01XA	S42.211B	S42.409B	S52.023B	S52.201B	S52.282B	S52.366B	S52.601B	S72.033C
S22.41XB	S26.022A	S31.659A	S32.414A	S32.475A	S35.02XA	S42.212B	S42.411B	S52.023C	S52.201C	S52.282C	S52.366C	S52.601C	S72.034A
S22.42XB	S26.12XA	S32.000B	S32.414B	S32.475B	S35.09XA	S42.213B	S42.412B	S52.024B	S52.202B	S52.283B	S52.371B	S52.602B	S72.034B
S22.43XB	S26.92XA	S32.001B	S32.415A	S32.476A	S35.10XA	S42.214B	S42.413B	S52.024C	S52.202C	S52.283C	S52.371C	S52.602C	S72.034C
S22.49XB	S27.1XXA	S32.002B	S32.415B	S32.476B	S35.11XA	S42.215B	S42.414B	S52.025B	S52.209B	S52.291B	S52.372B	S52.609B	S72.035A
S22.5XXA	S27.2XXA	S32.008B	S32.416A	S32.481A	S35.12XA	S42.216B	S42.415B	S52.025C	S52.209C	S52.291C	S52.372C	S52.609C	S72.035B
S22.5XXB	S27.331A	S32.009B	S32.416B	S32.481B	S35.19XA	S42.221B	S42.416B	S52.026B	S52.221B	S52.292B	S52.379B	S52.611B	S72.035C
S22.9XXB	S27.332A	S32.010B	S32.421A	S32.482A	S35.211A	S42.222B	S42.421B	S52.026C	S52.221C	S52.292C	S52.379C	S52.611C	S72.036A
S24.0XXA	S27.339A	S32.011B	S32.421B	S32.482B	S35.212A	S42.223B	S42.422B	S52.031B	S52.222B	S52.299B	S52.381B	S52.612B	S72.036B
S24.101A	S27.401A	S32.012B	S32.422A	S32.483A	S35.218A	S42.224B	S42.423B	S52.031C	S52.222C	S52.299C	S52.381C	S52.612C	S72.036C
S24.102A	S27.402A	S32.018B	S32.422B	S32.483B	S35.219A	S42.225B	S42.424B	S52.032B	S52.223B	S52.301B	S52.382B	S52.613B	S72.041A
S24.103A	S27.409A	S32.019B	S32.423A	S32.484A	S35.221A	S42.226B	S42.425B	S52.032C	S52.223C	S52.301C	S52.382C	S52.613C	S72.041B
S24.104A	S27.411A	S32.020B	S32.423B	S32.484B	S35.222A	S42.231B	S42.426B	S52.033B	S52.224B	S52.302B	S52.389B	S52.614B	S72.041C
S24.111A	S27.412A	S32.021B	S32.424A	S32.485A	S35.228A	S42.232B	S42.431B	S52.033C	S52.224C	S52.302C	S52.389C	S52.614C	S72.042A
S24.112A	S27.419A	S32.022B	S32.424B	S32.485B	S35.229A	S42.239B	S42.432B	S52.034B	S52.225B	S52.309B	S52.391B	S52.615B	S72.042B
S24.113A	S27.421A	S32.028B	S32.425A	S32.486A	S35.231A	S42.241B	S42.433B	S52.034C	S52.225C	S52.309C	S52.391C	S52.615C	S72.042C
S24.114A	S27.422A	S32.029B	S32.425B	S32.486B	S35.232A	S42.242B	S42.434B	S52.035B	S52.226B	S52.321B	S52.392B	S52.616B	S72.043A
S24.131A	S27.429A	S32.030B	S32.426A	S32.491A	S35.238A	S42.249B	S42.435B	S52.035C	S52.226C	S52.321C	S52.392C	S52.616C	S72.043B
S24.132A	S27.431A	S32.031B	S32.426B	S32.491B	S35.239A	S42.251B	S42.436B	S52.036B	S52.231B	S52.322B	S52.399B	S52.691B	S72.044A
S24.133A	S27.432A	S32.032B	S32.431A	S32.492A	S35.291A	S42.252B	S42.441B	S52.036C	S52.231C	S52.322C	S52.399C	S52.691C	S72.044B
S24.134A	S27.439A	S32.038B	S32.431B	S32.492B	S35.292A	S42.253B	S42.442B	S52.041B	S52.232B	S52.323B	S52.501B	S52.692B	S72.044C
S24.141A	S27.491A	S32.039B	S32.432A	S32.499A	S35.298A	S42.254B	S42.443B	S52.041C	S52.232C	S52.323C	S52.501C	S52.692C	S72.045A
S24.142A	S27.492A	S32.040B	S32.432B	S32.499B	S35.299A	S42.255B	S42.444B	S52.042B	S52.233B	S52.324B	S52.502B	S52.699B	S72.045B
S24.143A	S27.499A	S32.041B	S32.433A	S32.501B	S35.311A	S42.256B	S42.445B	S52.042C	S52.233C	S52.324C	S52.502C	S52.699C	S72.045C
S24.144A	S27.812A	S32.042B	S32.433B	S32.502B	S35.318A	S42.261B	S42.446B	S52.043B	S52.234B	S52.325B	S52.509B	S52.90XB	S72.046A
S24.151A	S27.813A	S32.048B	S32.434A	S32.509B	S35.319A	S42.262B	S42.447B	S52.043C	S52.234C	S52.325C	S52.509C	S52.90XC	S72.046B
S24.152A	S27.818A	S32.049B	S32.434B	S32.511B	S35.321A	S42.263B	S42.448B	S52.044B	S52.235B	S52.326B	S52.511B	S52.91XB	S72.046C
S24.153A	S27.819A	S32.050B	S32.435A	S32.512B	S35.328A	S42.264B	S42.449B	S52.044C	S52.235C	S52.326C	S52.511C	S52.91XC	S72.051A
S24.154A	S31.001A	S32.051B	S32.435B	S32.519B	S35.329A	S42.265B	S42.451B	S52.045B	S52.236B	S52.331B	S52.512B	S52.92XB	S72.051B
S25.00XA	S31.011A	S32.052B	S32.436A	S32.591B	S35.331A	S42.266B	S42.452B	S52.045C	S52.236C	S52.331C	S52.512C	S52.92XC	S72.051C
S25.01XA	S31.021A	S32.058B	S32.436B	S32.592B	S35.338A	S42.291B	S42.453B	S52.046B	S52.241B	S52.332B	S52.513B	S72.001A	S72.052A
S25.02XA	S31.031A	S32.059B	S32.441A	S32.599B	S35.339A	S42.292B	S42.454B	S52.046C	S52.241C	S52.332C	S52.513C	S72.001B	S72.052B
S25.09XA	S31.041A	S32.10XB	S32.441B	S32.601B	S35.341A	S42.293B	S42.455B	S52.091B	S52.242B	S52.333B	S52.514B	S72.001C	S72.052C
S25.101A	S31.051A	S32.110B	S32.442A	S32.602B	S35.348A	S42.294B	S42.456B	S52.091C	S52.242C	S52.333C	S52.514C	S72.002A	S72.059A
S25.102A	S31.600A	S32.111B	S32.442B	S32.609B	S35.349A	S42.295B	S42.461B	S52.092B	S52.243B	S52.334B	S52.515B	S72.002B	S72.059B
S25.109A	S31.601A	S32.112B	S32.443A	S32.611B	S35.401A	S42.296B	S42.462B	S52.092C	S52.243C	S52.334C	S52.515C	S72.002C	S72.059C
S25.111A	S31.602A	S32.119B	S32.443B	S32.612B	S35.402A	S42.301B	S42.463B	S52.099B	S52.244B	S52.335B	S52.516B	S72.009A	S72.061A
S25.112A	S31.603A	S32.120B	S32.444A	S32.613B	S35.403A	S42.302B	S42.464B	S52.099C	S52.244C	S52.335C	S52.516C	S72.009B	S72.061B
S25.119A	S31.604A	S32.121B	S32.444B	S32.614B	S35.404A	S42.309B	S42.465B	S52.101B	S52.245B	S52.336B	S52.531B	S72.009C	S72.061C
S25.121A	S31.605A	S32.122B	S32.445A	S32.615B	S35.405A	S42.321B	S42.466B	S52.101C	S52.245C	S52.336C	S52.531C	S72.011A	S72.062A
S25.122A	S31.609A	S32.129B	S32.445B	S32.616B	S35.406A	S42.322B	S42.471B	S52.102B	S52.246B	S52.341B	S52.532B	S72.011B	S72.062B
S25.129A	S31.610A	S32.130B	S32.446A	S32.691B	S35.411A	S42.323B	S42.472B	S52.102C	S52.246C	S52.341C	S52.532C	S72.011C	S72.062C
S25.191A	S31.611A	S32.131B	S32.446B	S32.692B	S35.412A	S42.324B	S42.473B	S52.109B	S52.251B	S52.342B	S52.539B	S72.012A	S72.063A
S25.192A	S31.612A	S32.132B	S32.451A	S32.699B	S35.413A	S42.325B	S42.474B	S52.109C	S52.251C	S52.342C	S52.539C	S72.012B	S72.063B
S25.199A	S31.613A	S32.139B	S32.451B	S32.810B	S35.414A	S42.326B	S42.475B	S52.121B	S52.252B	S52.343B	S52.541B	S72.012C	S72.063C
S25.20XA	S31.614A	S32.14XB	S32.452A	S32.811B	S35.415A	S42.331B	S42.476B	S52.121C	S52.252C	S52.343C	S52.541C	S72.019A	S72.064A
S25.21XA	S31.615A	S32.15XB	S32.452B	S32.82XB	S35.416A	S42.332B	S42.491B	S52.122B	S52.253B	S52.344B	S52.542B	S72.019B	S72.064B
S25.22XA	S31.619A	S32.16XB	S32.453A	S32.89XB	S35.491A	S42.333B	S42.492B	S52.122C	S52.253C	S52.344C	S52.542C	S72.019C	S72.064C
S25.29XA	S31.620A	S32.17XB	S32.453B	S32.9XXB	S35.492A	S42.334B	S42.493B	S52.123B	S52.254B	S52.345B	S52.549B	S72.021A	S72.065A
S25.301A	S31.621A	S32.19XB	S32.454A	S34.01XA	S35.493A	S42.335B	S42.494B	S52.123C	S52.254C	S52.345C	S52.549C	S72.021B	S72.065B
S25.302A	S31.622A	S32.2XXB	S32.454B	S34.02XA	S35.494A	S42.336B	S42.495B	S52.124B	S52.255B	S52.346B	S52.551B	S72.021C	S72.065C
S25.309A	S31.623A	S32.301B	S32.455A	S34.101A	S35.495A	S42.341B	S42.496B	S52.124C	S52.255C	S52.346C	S52.551C	S72.022A	S72.066A
S25.311A	S31.624A	S32.302B	S32.455B	S34.102A	S35.496A	S42.342B	S42.90XB	S52.125B	S52.256B	S52.351B	S52.552B	S72.022B	S72.066B
S25.312A	S31.625A	S32.309B	S32.456A	S34.103A	S35.50XA	S42.343B	S42.91XB	S52.125C	S52.256C	S52.351C	S52.552C	S72.022C	S72.066C
S25.319A	S31.629A	S32.311B	S32.456B	S34.104A	S35.511A	S42.344B	S42.92XB	S52.126B	S52.261B	S52.352B	S52.559B	S72.023A	S72.091A
S25.321A	S31.630A	S32.312B	S32.461A	S34.105A	S35.512A	S42.345B	S45.001A	S52.126C	S52.261C	S52.352C	S52.559C	S72.023B	S72.091B
S25.322A	S31.631A	S32.313B	S32.461B	S34.109A	S35.513A	S42.346B	S45.002A	S52.131B	S52.262B	S52.353B	S52.561B	S72.023C	S72.091C
S25.329A	S31.632A	S32.314B	S32.462A	S34.111A	S35.514A	S42.351B	S45.009A	S52.131C	S52.262C	S52.353C	S52.561C	S72.024A	S72.092A
S25.391A	S31.633A	S32.315B	S32.462B	S34.112A	S35.515A	S42.352B	S45.011A	S52.132B	S52.263B	S52.354B	S52.562B	S72.024B	S72.092B
S25.392A	S31.634A	S32.316B	S32.463A	S34.113A	S35.516A	S42.353B	S45.012A	S52.132C	S52.263C	S52.354C	S52.562C	S72.024C	

Major Complication or Comorbidity (MCC) (cont.) - Based on CMS data

S72.092C	S72.125B	S72.22XA	S72.331C	S72.354B	S72.412C	S72.446C	S72.91XB	S82.111B	S82.145B	S82.233B	S82.291B	S82.445B	S82.863B
S72.099A	S72.125C	S72.22XB	S72.332A	S72.354C	S72.413B	S72.451B	S72.91XC	S82.111C	S82.145C	S82.233C	S82.291C	S82.445C	S82.863C
S72.099B	S72.126A	S72.22XC	S72.332B	S72.355A	S72.413C	S72.451C	S72.92XA	S82.112B	S82.146B	S82.234B	S82.292B	S82.446B	S82.864B
S72.099C	S72.126B	S72.23XA	S72.332C	S72.355B	S72.414B	S72.452B	S72.92XB	S82.112C	S82.146C	S82.234C	S82.292C	S82.446C	S82.864C
S72.101A	S72.126C	S72.23XB	S72.333A	S72.355C	S72.414C	S72.452C	S72.92XC	S82.113B	S82.151B	S82.235B	S82.299B	S82.451B	S82.865B
S72.101B	S72.131A	S72.23XC	S72.333B	S72.356A	S72.415B	S72.453B	S75.001A	S82.113C	S82.151C	S82.235C	S82.299C	S82.451C	S82.865C
S72.101C	S72.131B	S72.24XA	S72.333C	S72.356B	S72.415C	S72.453C	S75.002A	S82.114B	S82.152B	S82.236B	S82.401B	S82.452B	S82.866B
S72.102A	S72.131C	S72.24XB	S72.334A	S72.356C	S72.416B	S72.454B	S75.009A	S82.114C	S82.152C	S82.236C	S82.401C	S82.452C	S82.866C
S72.102B	S72.132A	S72.24XC	S72.334B	S72.361A	S72.416C	S72.454C	S75.011A	S82.115B	S82.153B	S82.241B	S82.402B	S82.453B	S85.001A
S72.102C	S72.132B	S72.25XA	S72.334C	S72.361B	S72.421B	S72.455B	S75.012A	S82.115C	S82.153C	S82.241C	S82.402C	S82.453C	S85.002A
S72.109A	S72.132C	S72.25XB	S72.335A	S72.361C	S72.421C	S72.455C	S75.019A	S82.116B	S82.154B	S82.242B	S82.409B	S82.454B	S85.009A
S72.109B	S72.133A	S72.25XC	S72.335B	S72.362A	S72.422B	S72.456B	S75.021A	S82.116C	S82.154C	S82.242C	S82.409C	S82.454C	S85.011A
S72.109C	S72.133B	S72.26XA	S72.335C	S72.362B	S72.422C	S72.456C	S75.022A	S82.121B	S82.155B	S82.243B	S82.421B	S82.455B	S85.012A
S72.111A	S72.133C	S72.26XB	S72.336A	S72.362C	S72.423B	S72.461B	S75.029A	S82.121C	S82.155C	S82.243C	S82.421C	S82.455C	S85.019A
S72.111B	S72.134A	S72.26XC	S72.336B	S72.363A	S72.423C	S72.461C	S75.091A	S82.122B	S82.156B	S82.244B	S82.422B	S82.456B	S85.091A
S72.111C	S72.134B	S72.301A	S72.336C	S72.363B	S72.424B	S72.462B	S75.092A	S82.122C	S82.156C	S82.244C	S82.422C	S82.456C	S85.092A
S72.112A	S72.134C	S72.301B	S72.341A	S72.363C	S72.424C	S72.462C	S75.099A	S82.123B	S82.191B	S82.245B	S82.423B	S82.461B	S85.099A
S72.112B	S72.135A	S72.301C	S72.341B	S72.364A	S72.425B	S72.463B	S75.101A	S82.123C	S82.191C	S82.245C	S82.423C	S82.461C	S85.501A
S72.112C	S72.135B	S72.302A	S72.341C	S72.364B	S72.425C	S72.463C	S75.102A	S82.124B	S82.192B	S82.246B	S82.424B	S82.462B	S85.502A
S72.113A	S72.135C	S72.302B	S72.342A	S72.364C	S72.426B	S72.464B	S75.109A	S82.124C	S82.192C	S82.246C	S82.424C	S82.462C	S85.509A
S72.113B	S72.136A	S72.302C	S72.342B	S72.365A	S72.426C	S72.464C	S75.111A	S82.125B	S82.199B	S82.251B	S82.425B	S82.463B	S85.511A
S72.113C	S72.136B	S72.309A	S72.342C	S72.365B	S72.431B	S72.465B	S75.112A	S82.125C	S82.199C	S82.251C	S82.425C	S82.463C	S85.512A
S72.114A	S72.136C	S72.309B	S72.343A	S72.365C	S72.431C	S72.465C	S75.119A	S82.126B	S82.201B	S82.252B	S82.426B	S82.464B	S85.519A
S72.114B	S72.141A	S72.309C	S72.343B	S72.366A	S72.432B	S72.466B	S75.121A	S82.126C	S82.201C	S82.252C	S82.426C	S82.464C	S85.591A
S72.114C	S72.141B	S72.321A	S72.343C	S72.366B	S72.432C	S72.466C	S75.122A	S82.131B	S82.202B	S82.253B	S82.431B	S82.465B	S85.592A
S72.115A	S72.141C	S72.321B	S72.344A	S72.366C	S72.433B	S72.491B	S75.129A	S82.131C	S82.202C	S82.253C	S82.431C	S82.465C	S85.599A
S72.115B	S72.142A	S72.321C	S72.344B	S72.391A	S72.433C	S72.491C	S75.191A	S82.132B	S82.209B	S82.254B	S82.432B	S82.466B	T79.0XXA
S72.115C	S72.142B	S72.322A	S72.344C	S72.391B	S72.434B	S72.492B	S75.192A	S82.132C	S82.209C	S82.254C	S82.432C	S82.466C	T79.1XXA
S72.116A	S72.142C	S72.322B	S72.345A	S72.391C	S72.434C	S72.492C	S75.199A	S82.133B	S82.221B	S82.255B	S82.433B	S82.491B	T79.4XXA
S72.116B	S72.143A	S72.322C	S72.345B	S72.392A	S72.435B	S72.499B	S79.001A	S82.133C	S82.221C	S82.255C	S82.433C	S82.491C	T79.5XXA
S72.116C	S72.143B	S72.323A	S72.345C	S72.392B	S72.435C	S72.499C	S79.002A	S82.134B	S82.222B	S82.256B	S82.434B	S82.492B	T80.0XXA
S72.121A	S72.143C	S72.323B	S72.346A	S72.392C	S72.436B	S72.8X1A	S79.009A	S82.134C	S82.222C	S82.256C	S82.434C	S82.492C	T81.11XA
S72.121B	S72.144A	S72.323C	S72.346B	S72.399B	S72.436C	S72.8X1B	S79.011A	S82.135B	S82.223B	S82.261B	S82.435B	S82.499B	T81.12XA
S72.121C	S72.144B	S72.324A	S72.346C	S72.399C	S72.441B	S72.8X1C	S79.012A	S82.135C	S82.223C	S82.261C	S82.435C	S82.499C	T81.19XA
S72.122A	S72.144C	S72.324B	S72.351A	S72.401B	S72.441C	S72.8X2A	S79.019A	S82.136B	S82.224B	S82.262B	S82.436B	S82.831B	
S72.122B	S72.145A	S72.324C	S72.351B	S72.401C	S72.442B	S72.8X2B	S79.091A	S82.136C	S82.224C	S82.262C	S82.436C	S82.831C	
S72.122C	S72.145B	S72.325A	S72.351C	S72.402B	S72.442C	S72.8X2C	S79.092A	S82.141B	S82.225B	S82.263B	S82.441B	S82.832B	
S72.123A	S72.145C	S72.325B	S72.352A	S72.402C	S72.443B	S72.8X9A	S79.099A	S82.141C	S82.225C	S82.263C	S82.441C	S82.832C	
S72.123B	S72.146A	S72.325C	S72.352B	S72.409B	S72.443C	S72.8X9B	S82.101B	S82.142B	S82.226B	S82.264B	S82.442B	S82.839B	
S72.123C	S72.146B	S72.326A	S72.352C	S72.409C	S72.444B	S72.8X9C	S82.101C	S82.142C	S82.226C	S82.264C	S82.442C	S82.839C	
S72.124A	S72.146C	S72.326B	S72.353A	S72.411B	S72.444C	S72.90XA	S82.102B	S82.143B	S82.231B	S82.265B	S82.443B	S82.861B	
S72.124B	S72.21XA	S72.326C	S72.353B	S72.411C	S72.445B	S72.90XB	S82.102C	S82.143C	S82.231C	S82.265C	S82.443C	S82.861C	
S72.124C	S72.21XB	S72.331A	S72.353C	S72.412B	S72.445C	S72.90XC	S82.109B	S82.144B	S82.232B	S82.266B	S82.444B	S82.862B	
S72.125A	S72.21XC	S72.331B	S72.354A		S72.446B	S72.91XA	S82.109C	S82.144C	S82.232C	S82.266C	S82.444C	S82.862C	

Male - Based on Medicare's Outpatient Code Editor (OCE)

S30.201A	S30.815A	S30.843A	S30.862A	S30.875A	S31.21XA	S31.30XA	S31.35XA	S31.541A	S37.829A	S38.222A	T21.06XA	T21.56XA	T83.490A
S30.201D	S30.815D	S30.843D	S30.862D	S30.875D	S31.21XD	S31.30XD	S31.35XD	S31.541D	S37.829D	S38.222D	T21.06XD	T21.56XD	T83.490D
S30.201S	S30.815S	S30.843S	S30.862S	S30.875S	S31.21XS	S31.30XS	S31.35XS	S31.541S	S37.829S	S38.222S	T21.06XS	T21.56XS	T83.490S
S30.21XA	S30.822A	S30.845A	S30.863A	S30.93XA	S31.22XA	S31.31XA	S31.501A	S31.551A	S38.001A	S38.231A	T21.16XA	T21.66XA	
S30.21XD	S30.822D	S30.845D	S30.863D	S30.93XD	S31.22XD	S31.31XD	S31.501D	S31.551D	S38.001D	S38.231D	T21.16XD	T21.66XD	
S30.21XS	S30.822S	S30.845S	S30.863S	S30.93XS	S31.22XS	S31.31XS	S31.501S	S31.551S	S38.001S	S38.231S	T21.16XS	T21.66XS	
S30.22XA	S30.823A	S30.852A	S30.865A	S30.94XA	S31.23XA	S31.32XA	S31.511A	S37.822A	S38.01XA	S38.232A	T21.26XA	T21.76XA	
S30.22XD	S30.823D	S30.852D	S30.865D	S30.94XD	S31.23XD	S31.32XD	S31.511D	S37.822D	S38.01XD	S38.232D	T21.26XD	T21.76XD	
S30.22XS	S30.823S	S30.852S	S30.865S	S30.94XS	S31.23XS	S31.32XS	S31.511S	S37.822S	S38.01XS	S38.232S	T21.26XS	T21.76XS	
S30.812A	S30.825A	S30.853A	S30.872A	S30.96XA	S31.24XA	S31.33XA	S31.521A	S37.823A	S38.02XA	S39.840A	T21.36XA		
S30.812D	S30.825D	S30.853D	S30.872D	S30.96XD	S31.24XD	S31.33XD	S31.521D	S37.823D	S38.02XD	S39.840D	T21.36XD		
S30.812S	S30.825S	S30.853S	S30.872S	S30.96XS	S31.24XS	S31.33XS	S31.521S	S37.823S	S38.02XS	S39.840S	T21.36XS		
S30.813A	S30.842A	S30.855A	S30.873A	S31.20XA	S31.25XA	S31.34XA	S31.531A	S37.828A	S38.221A	T19.4XXA	T21.46XA		
S30.813D	S30.842D	S30.855D	S30.873D	S31.20XD	S31.25XD	S31.34XD	S31.531D	S37.828D	S38.221D	T19.4XXD	T21.46XD		
S30.813S	S30.842S	S30.855S	S30.873S	S31.20XS	S31.25XS	S31.34XS	S31.531S	S37.828S	S38.221S	T19.4XXS	T21.46XS		

Manifestation - Based on CMS data

E08.3211	E08.3291	E08.3311	E08.3391	E08.3411	E08.3491	E08.3511	E08.3521	E08.3531	E08.3541	E08.3551	E08.3591	E08.37X1
E08.3212	E08.3292	E08.3312	E08.3392	E08.3412	E08.3492	E08.3512	E08.3522	E08.3532	E08.3542	E08.3552	E08.3592	E08.37X2
E08.3213	E08.3293	E08.3313	E08.3393	E08.3413	E08.3493	E08.3513	E08.3523	E08.3533	E08.3543	E08.3553	E08.3593	E08.37X3
E08.3219	E08.3299	E08.3319	E08.3399	E08.3419	E08.3499	E08.3519	E08.3529	E08.3539	E08.3549	E08.3559	E08.3599	E08.37X9

Maternity - Based on Medicare's Outpatient Code Editor (OCE)

O31.00X0	O31.23X0	O32.2XX0	O35.0XX0	O36.0120	O36.1910	O36.5130	O36.71X0	O36.8310	O36.93X0	O41.1030	O41.8X20	O60.20X0	O69.0XX0
O31.00X1	O31.23X1	O32.2XX1	O35.0XX1	O36.0121	O36.1911	O36.5131	O36.71X1	O36.8311	O36.93X1	O41.1031	O41.8X21	O60.20X1	O69.0XX1
O31.00X2	O31.23X2	O32.2XX2	O35.0XX2	O36.0122	O36.1912	O36.5132	O36.71X2	O36.8312	O36.93X2	O41.1032	O41.8X22	O60.20X2	O69.0XX2
O31.00X3	O31.23X3	O32.2XX3	O35.0XX3	O36.0123	O36.1913	O36.5133	O36.71X3	O36.8313	O36.93X3	O41.1033	O41.8X23	O60.20X3	O69.0XX3
O31.00X4	O31.23X4	O32.2XX4	O35.0XX4	O36.0124	O36.1914	O36.5134	O36.71X4	O36.8314	O36.93X4	O41.1034	O41.8X24	O60.20X4	O69.0XX4
O31.00X5	O31.23X5	O32.2XX5	O35.0XX5	O36.0125	O36.1915	O36.5135	O36.71X5	O36.8315	O36.93X5	O41.1035	O41.8X25	O60.20X5	O69.0XX5
O31.00X9	O31.23X9	O32.2XX9	O35.0XX9	O36.0129	O36.1919	O36.5139	O36.71X9	O36.8319	O36.93X9	O41.1039	O41.8X29	O60.20X9	O69.0XX9
O31.01X0	O31.30X0	O32.3XX0	O35.1XX0	O36.0130	O36.1920	O36.5190	O36.72X0	O36.8320	O40.1XX0	O41.1090	O41.8X30	O60.22X0	O69.1XX0
O31.01X1	O31.30X1	O32.3XX1	O35.1XX1	O36.0131	O36.1921	O36.5191	O36.72X1	O36.8321	O40.1XX1	O41.1091	O41.8X31	O60.22X1	O69.1XX1
O31.01X2	O31.30X2	O32.3XX2	O35.1XX2	O36.0132	O36.1922	O36.5192	O36.72X2	O36.8322	O40.1XX2	O41.1092	O41.8X32	O60.22X2	O69.1XX2
O31.01X3	O31.30X3	O32.3XX3	O35.1XX3	O36.0133	O36.1923	O36.5193	O36.72X3	O36.8323	O40.1XX3	O41.1093	O41.8X33	O60.22X3	O69.1XX3
O31.01X4	O31.30X4	O32.3XX4	O35.1XX4	O36.0134	O36.1924	O36.5194	O36.72X4	O36.8324	O40.1XX4	O41.1094	O41.8X34	O60.22X4	O69.1XX4
O31.01X5	O31.30X5	O32.3XX5	O35.1XX5	O36.0135	O36.1925	O36.5195	O36.72X5	O36.8325	O40.1XX5	O41.1095	O41.8X35	O60.22X5	O69.1XX5
O31.01X9	O31.30X9	O32.3XX9	O35.1XX9	O36.0139	O36.1929	O36.5199	O36.72X9	O36.8329	O40.1XX9	O41.1099	O41.8X39	O60.22X9	O69.1XX9
O31.02X0	O31.31X0	O32.4XX0	O35.2XX0	O36.0190	O36.1930	O36.5910	O36.73X0	O36.8330	O40.2XX0	O41.1210	O41.8X90	O60.23X0	O69.2XX0
O31.02X1	O31.31X1	O32.4XX1	O35.2XX1	O36.0191	O36.1931	O36.5911	O36.73X1	O36.8331	O40.2XX1	O41.1211	O41.8X91	O60.23X1	O69.2XX1
O31.02X2	O31.31X2	O32.4XX2	O35.2XX2	O36.0192	O36.1932	O36.5912	O36.73X2	O36.8332	O40.2XX2	O41.1212	O41.8X92	O60.23X2	O69.2XX2
O31.02X3	O31.31X3	O32.4XX3	O35.2XX3	O36.0193	O36.1933	O36.5913	O36.73X3	O36.8333	O40.2XX3	O41.1213	O41.8X93	O60.23X3	O69.2XX3
O31.02X4	O31.31X4	O32.4XX4	O35.2XX4	O36.0194	O36.1934	O36.5914	O36.73X4	O36.8334	O40.2XX4	O41.1214	O41.8X94	O60.23X4	O69.2XX4
O31.02X5	O31.31X5	O32.4XX5	O35.2XX5	O36.0195	O36.1935	O36.5915	O36.73X5	O36.8335	O40.2XX5	O41.1215	O41.8X95	O60.23X5	O69.2XX5
O31.02X9	O31.31X9	O32.4XX9	O35.2XX9	O36.0199	O36.1939	O36.5919	O36.73X9	O36.8339	O40.2XX9	O41.1219	O41.8X99	O60.23X9	O69.2XX9
O31.03X0	O31.32X0	O32.6XX0	O35.3XX0	O36.0910	O36.1990	O36.5920	O36.80X0	O36.8390	O40.3XX0	O41.1220	O41.90X0	O64.0XX0	O69.3XX0
O31.03X1	O31.32X1	O32.6XX1	O35.3XX1	O36.0911	O36.1991	O36.5921	O36.80X1	O36.8391	O40.3XX1	O41.1221	O41.90X1	O64.0XX1	O69.3XX1
O31.03X2	O31.32X2	O32.6XX2	O35.3XX2	O36.0912	O36.1992	O36.5922	O36.80X2	O36.8392	O40.3XX2	O41.1222	O41.90X2	O64.0XX2	O69.3XX2
O31.03X3	O31.32X3	O32.6XX3	O35.3XX3	O36.0913	O36.1993	O36.5923	O36.80X3	O36.8393	O40.3XX3	O41.1223	O41.90X3	O64.0XX3	O69.3XX3
O31.03X4	O31.32X4	O32.6XX4	O35.3XX4	O36.0914	O36.1994	O36.5924	O36.80X4	O36.8394	O40.3XX4	O41.1224	O41.90X4	O64.0XX4	O69.3XX4
O31.03X5	O31.32X5	O32.6XX5	O35.3XX5	O36.0915	O36.1995	O36.5925	O36.80X5	O36.8395	O40.3XX5	O41.1225	O41.90X5	O64.0XX5	O69.3XX5
O31.03X9	O31.32X9	O32.6XX9	O35.3XX9	O36.0919	O36.1999	O36.5929	O36.80X9	O36.8399	O40.3XX9	O41.1229	O41.90X9	O64.0XX9	O69.3XX9
O31.10X0	O31.33X0	O32.8XX0	O35.4XX0	O36.0920	O36.20X0	O36.5930	O36.8120	O36.8910	O40.9XX0	O41.1230	O41.91X0	O64.1XX0	O69.4XX0
O31.10X1	O31.33X1	O32.8XX1	O35.4XX1	O36.0921	O36.20X1	O36.5931	O36.8121	O36.8911	O40.9XX1	O41.1231	O41.91X1	O64.1XX1	O69.4XX1
O31.10X2	O31.33X2	O32.8XX2	O35.4XX2	O36.0922	O36.20X2	O36.5932	O36.8122	O36.8912	O40.9XX2	O41.1232	O41.91X2	O64.1XX2	O69.4XX2
O31.10X3	O31.33X3	O32.8XX3	O35.4XX3	O36.0923	O36.20X3	O36.5933	O36.8123	O36.8913	O40.9XX3	O41.1233	O41.91X3	O64.1XX3	O69.4XX3
O31.10X4	O31.33X4	O32.8XX4	O35.4XX4	O36.0924	O36.20X4	O36.5934	O36.8124	O36.8914	O40.9XX4	O41.1234	O41.91X4	O64.1XX4	O69.4XX4
O31.10X5	O31.33X5	O32.8XX5	O35.4XX5	O36.0925	O36.20X5	O36.5935	O36.8125	O36.8915	O40.9XX5	O41.1235	O41.91X5	O64.1XX5	O69.4XX5
O31.10X9	O31.33X9	O32.8XX9	O35.4XX9	O36.0929	O36.20X9	O36.5939	O36.8129	O36.8919	O40.9XX9	O41.1239	O41.91X9	O64.1XX9	O69.4XX9
O31.11X0	O31.8X10	O32.9XX0	O35.5XX0	O36.0930	O36.21X0	O36.5990	O36.8130	O36.8920	O41.00X0	O41.1290	O41.92X0	O64.2XX0	O69.5XX0
O31.11X1	O31.8X11	O32.9XX1	O35.5XX1	O36.0931	O36.21X1	O36.5991	O36.8131	O36.8921	O41.00X1	O41.1291	O41.92X1	O64.2XX1	O69.5XX1
O31.11X2	O31.8X12	O32.9XX2	O35.5XX2	O36.0932	O36.21X2	O36.5992	O36.8132	O36.8922	O41.00X2	O41.1292	O41.92X2	O64.2XX2	O69.5XX2
O31.11X3	O31.8X13	O32.9XX3	O35.5XX3	O36.0933	O36.21X3	O36.5993	O36.8133	O36.8923	O41.00X3	O41.1293	O41.92X3	O64.2XX3	O69.5XX3
O31.11X4	O31.8X14	O32.9XX4	O35.5XX4	O36.0934	O36.21X4	O36.5994	O36.8134	O36.8924	O41.00X4	O41.1294	O41.92X4	O64.2XX4	O69.5XX4
O31.11X5	O31.8X15	O32.9XX5	O35.5XX5	O36.0935	O36.21X5	O36.5995	O36.8135	O36.8925	O41.00X5	O41.1295	O41.92X5	O64.2XX5	O69.5XX5
O31.11X9	O31.8X19	O32.9XX9	O35.5XX9	O36.0939	O36.21X9	O36.5999	O36.8139	O36.8929	O41.00X9	O41.1299	O41.92X9	O64.2XX9	O69.5XX9
O31.12X0	O31.8X20	O33.3XX0	O35.6XX0	O36.0990	O36.22X0	O36.60X0	O36.8190	O36.8930	O41.01X0	O41.1410	O41.93X0	O64.3XX0	O69.81X0
O31.12X1	O31.8X21	O33.3XX1	O35.6XX1	O36.0991	O36.22X1	O36.60X1	O36.8191	O36.8931	O41.01X1	O41.1411	O41.93X1	O64.3XX1	O69.81X1
O31.12X2	O31.8X22	O33.3XX2	O35.6XX2	O36.0992	O36.22X2	O36.60X2	O36.8192	O36.8932	O41.01X2	O41.1412	O41.93X2	O64.3XX2	O69.81X2
O31.12X3	O31.8X23	O33.3XX3	O35.6XX3	O36.0993	O36.22X3	O36.60X3	O36.8193	O36.8933	O41.01X3	O41.1413	O41.93X3	O64.3XX3	O69.81X3
O31.12X4	O31.8X24	O33.3XX4	O35.6XX4	O36.0994	O36.22X4	O36.60X4	O36.8194	O36.8934	O41.01X4	O41.1414	O41.93X4	O64.3XX4	O69.81X4
O31.12X5	O31.8X25	O33.3XX5	O35.6XX5	O36.0995	O36.22X5	O36.60X5	O36.8195	O36.8935	O41.01X5	O41.1415	O41.93X5	O64.3XX5	O69.81X5
O31.12X9	O31.8X29	O33.3XX9	O35.6XX9	O36.0999	O36.22X9	O36.60X9	O36.8199	O36.8939	O41.01X9	O41.1419	O41.93X9	O64.3XX9	O69.81X9
O31.13X0	O31.8X30	O33.4XX0	O35.7XX0	O36.1110	O36.23X0	O36.61X0	O36.8210	O36.8990	O41.02X0	O41.1420	O60.10X0	O64.4XX0	O69.82X0
O31.13X1	O31.8X31	O33.4XX1	O35.7XX1	O36.1111	O36.23X1	O36.61X1	O36.8211	O36.8991	O41.02X1	O41.1421	O60.10X1	O64.4XX1	O69.82X1
O31.13X2	O31.8X32	O33.4XX2	O35.7XX2	O36.1112	O36.23X2	O36.61X2	O36.8212	O36.8992	O41.02X2	O41.1422	O60.10X2	O64.4XX2	O69.82X2
O31.13X3	O31.8X33	O33.4XX3	O35.7XX3	O36.1113	O36.23X3	O36.61X3	O36.8213	O36.8993	O41.02X3	O41.1423	O60.10X3	O64.4XX3	O69.82X3
O31.13X4	O31.8X34	O33.4XX4	O35.7XX4	O36.1114	O36.23X4	O36.61X4	O36.8214	O36.8994	O41.02X4	O41.1424	O60.10X4	O64.4XX4	O69.82X4
O31.13X5	O31.8X35	O33.4XX5	O35.7XX5	O36.1115	O36.23X5	O36.61X5	O36.8215	O36.8995	O41.02X5	O41.1425	O60.10X5	O64.4XX5	O69.82X5
O31.13X9	O31.8X39	O33.4XX9	O35.7XX9	O36.1119	O36.23X9	O36.61X9	O36.8219	O36.8999	O41.02X9	O41.1429	O60.10X9	O64.4XX9	O69.82X9
O31.20X0	O31.8X90	O33.5XX0	O35.8XX0	O36.1120	O36.4XX0	O36.62X0	O36.8220	O36.90X0	O41.03X0	O41.1430	O60.12X0	O64.5XX0	O69.89X0
O31.20X1	O31.8X91	O33.5XX1	O35.8XX1	O36.1121	O36.4XX1	O36.62X1	O36.8221	O36.90X1	O41.03X1	O41.1431	O60.12X1	O64.5XX1	O69.89X1
O31.20X2	O31.8X92	O33.5XX2	O35.8XX2	O36.1122	O36.4XX2	O36.62X2	O36.8222	O36.90X2	O41.03X2	O41.1432	O60.12X2	O64.5XX2	O69.89X2
O31.20X3	O31.8X93	O33.5XX3	O35.8XX3	O36.1123	O36.4XX3	O36.62X3	O36.8223	O36.90X3	O41.03X3	O41.1433	O60.12X3	O64.5XX3	O69.89X3
O31.20X4	O31.8X94	O33.5XX4	O35.8XX4	O36.1124	O36.4XX4	O36.62X4	O36.8224	O36.90X4	O41.03X4	O41.1434	O60.12X4	O64.5XX4	O69.89X4
O31.20X5	O31.8X95	O33.5XX5	O35.8XX5	O36.1125	O36.4XX5	O36.62X5	O36.8225	O36.90X5	O41.03X5	O41.1435	O60.12X5	O64.5XX5	O69.89X5
O31.20X9	O31.8X99	O33.5XX9	O35.8XX9	O36.1129	O36.4XX9	O36.62X9	O36.8229	O36.90X9	O41.03X9	O41.1439	O60.12X9	O64.5XX9	O69.89X9
O31.21X0	O32.0XX0	O33.6XX0	O35.9XX0	O36.1130	O36.5110	O36.63X0	O36.8230	O36.91X0	O41.1010	O41.1490	O60.13X0	O64.8XX0	O69.9XX0
O31.21X1	O32.0XX1	O33.6XX1	O35.9XX1	O36.1131	O36.5111	O36.63X1	O36.8231	O36.91X1	O41.1011	O41.1491	O60.13X1	O64.8XX1	O69.9XX1
O31.21X2	O32.0XX2	O33.6XX2	O35.9XX2	O36.1132	O36.5112	O36.63X2	O36.8232	O36.91X2	O41.1012	O41.1492	O60.13X2	O64.8XX2	O69.9XX2
O31.21X3	O32.0XX3	O33.6XX3	O35.9XX3	O36.1133	O36.5113	O36.63X3	O36.8233	O36.91X3	O41.1013	O41.1493	O60.13X3	O64.8XX3	O69.9XX3
O31.21X4	O32.0XX4	O33.6XX4	O35.9XX4	O36.1134	O36.5114	O36.63X4	O36.8234	O36.91X4	O41.1014	O41.1494	O60.13X4	O64.8XX4	O69.9XX4
O31.21X5	O32.0XX5	O33.6XX5	O35.9XX5	O36.1135	O36.5115	O36.63X5	O36.8235	O36.91X5	O41.1015	O41.1495	O60.13X5	O64.8XX5	O69.9XX5
O31.21X9	O32.0XX9	O33.6XX9	O35.9XX9	O36.1139	O36.5119	O36.63X9	O36.8239	O36.91X9	O41.1019	O41.1499	O60.13X9	O64.8XX9	O69.9XX9
O31.22X0	O32.1XX0	O33.7XX0	O36.0110	O36.1190	O36.5120	O36.70X0	O36.8290	O36.92X0	O41.1020	O41.8X10	O60.14X0	O64.9XX0	
O31.22X1	O32.1XX1	O33.7XX1	O36.0111	O36.1191	O36.5121	O36.70X1	O36.8291	O36.92X1	O41.1021	O41.8X11	O60.14X1	O64.9XX1	
O31.22X2	O32.1XX2	O33.7XX2	O36.0112	O36.1192	O36.5122	O36.70X2	O36.8292	O36.92X2	O41.1022	O41.8X12	O60.14X2	O64.9XX2	
O31.22X3	O32.1XX3	O33.7XX3	O36.0113	O36.1193	O36.5123	O36.70X3	O36.8293	O36.92X3	O41.1023	O41.8X13	O60.14X3	O64.9XX3	
O31.22X4	O32.1XX4	O33.7XX4	O36.0114	O36.1194	O36.5124	O36.70X4	O36.8294	O36.92X4	O41.1024	O41.8X14	O60.14X4	O64.9XX4	
O31.22X5	O32.1XX5	O33.7XX5	O36.0115	O36.1195	O36.5125	O36.70X5	O36.8295	O36.92X5	O41.1025	O41.8X15	O60.14X5	O64.9XX5	
O31.22X9	O32.1XX9	O33.7XX9	O36.0119	O36.1199	O36.5129	O36.70X9	O36.8299	O36.92X9	O41.1029	O41.8X19	O60.14X9	O64.9XX9	

PDx as MCC - Based on CMS data

S06.1X0A	S06.1X1A	S06.1X2A	S06.1X3A	S06.1X4A	S06.1X5A	S06.1X6A	S06.1X7A	S06.1X8A	S06.1X9A

Pediatrics - For patients 0-17 years of age; based on Medicare's Outpatient Code Editor (OCE)

T74.02XA	T74.12XA	T74.22XA	T74.32XA	T74.4XXA	T74.92XA	T76.02XA	T76.12XA	T76.22XA	T76.32XA	T76.92XA
T74.02XD	T74.12XD	T74.22XD	T74.32XD	T74.4XXD	T74.92XD	T76.02XD	T76.12XD	T76.22XD	T76.32XD	T76.92XD
T74.02XS	T74.12XS	T74.22XS	T74.32XS	T74.4XXS	T74.92XS	T76.02XS	T76.12XS	T76.22XS	T76.32XS	T76.92XS

RxHCC - Based on CMS data

E08.3211	E08.3543	E09.3511	E10.3313	E10.37X1	E11.3533	E13.3491	H40.1111	H40.1294	M80.032A	M84.40XA	M84.50XA	M84.629A	T81.592A
E08.3212	E08.3549	E09.3512	E10.3319	E10.37X2	E11.3539	E13.3492	H40.1112	H40.1310	M80.039A	M84.411A	M84.511A	M84.631A	T81.592D
E08.3213	E08.3551	E09.3513	E10.3391	E10.37X3	E11.3541	E13.3493	H40.1113	H40.1311	M80.041A	M84.412A	M84.512A	M84.632A	T81.592S
E08.3219	E08.3552	E09.3519	E10.3392	E10.37X9	E11.3542	E13.3499	H40.1114	H40.1312	M80.042A	M84.419A	M84.519A	M84.633A	T82.41XA
E08.3291	E08.3553	E09.3521	E10.3393	E11.3211	E11.3543	E13.3511	H40.1120	H40.1313	M80.049A	M84.421A	M84.521A	M84.634A	T82.41XD
E08.3292	E08.3559	E09.3522	E10.3399	E11.3212	E11.3549	E13.3512	H40.1121	H40.1314	M80.051A	M84.422A	M84.522A	M84.639A	T82.41XS
E08.3293	E08.3591	E09.3523	E10.3411	E11.3213	E11.3551	E13.3513	H40.1122	H40.1320	M80.052A	M84.429A	M84.529A	M84.641A	T82.42XA
E08.3299	E08.3592	E09.3529	E10.3412	E11.3219	E11.3552	E13.3519	H40.1123	H40.1321	M80.059A	M84.431A	M84.531A	M84.642A	T82.42XD
E08.3311	E08.3593	E09.3531	E10.3413	E11.3291	E11.3553	E13.3521	H40.1124	H40.1322	M80.061A	M84.432A	M84.532A	M84.649A	T82.42XS
E08.3312	E08.3599	E09.3532	E10.3419	E11.3292	E11.3559	E13.3522	H40.1130	H40.1323	M80.062A	M84.433A	M84.533A	M84.650A	T82.43XA
E08.3313	E08.37X1	E09.3533	E10.3491	E11.3293	E11.3591	E13.3523	H40.1131	H40.1324	M80.069A	M84.434A	M84.534A	M84.651A	T82.43XD
E08.3319	E08.37X2	E09.3539	E10.3492	E11.3299	E11.3592	E13.3529	H40.1132	H40.1330	M80.071A	M84.439A	M84.539A	M84.652A	T82.43XS
E08.3391	E08.37X3	E09.3541	E10.3493	E11.3311	E11.3593	E13.3531	H40.1133	H40.1331	M80.072A	M84.441A	M84.541A	M84.659A	T82.49XA
E08.3392	E08.37X9	E09.3542	E10.3499	E11.3312	E11.3599	E13.3532	H40.1134	H40.1332	M80.079A	M84.442A	M84.542A	M84.661A	T82.49XD
E08.3393	E09.3211	E09.3543	E10.3511	E11.3313	E11.37X1	E13.3533	H40.1190	H40.1333	M80.08XA	M84.443A	M84.549A	M84.662A	T82.49XS
E08.3399	E09.3212	E09.3549	E10.3512	E11.3319	E11.37X2	E13.3539	H40.1191	H40.1334	M80.80XA	M84.444A	M84.550A	M84.663A	T85.611A
E08.3411	E09.3213	E09.3551	E10.3513	E11.3391	E11.37X3	E13.3541	H40.1192	H40.1390	M80.811A	M84.445A	M84.551A	M84.664A	T85.611D
E08.3412	E09.3219	E09.3552	E10.3519	E11.3392	E11.37X9	E13.3542	H40.1193	H40.1391	M80.812A	M84.446A	M84.552A	M84.669A	T85.611S
E08.3413	E09.3291	E09.3553	E10.3521	E11.3393	E13.3211	E13.3543	H40.1194	H40.1392	M80.819A	M84.451A	M84.553A	M84.671A	T85.621A
E08.3419	E09.3292	E09.3559	E10.3522	E11.3399	E13.3212	E13.3549	H40.1210	H40.1393	M80.821A	M84.452A	M84.559A	M84.672A	T85.621D
E08.3491	E09.3293	E09.3591	E10.3523	E11.3411	E13.3213	E13.3551	H40.1211	H40.1394	M80.822A	M84.453A	M84.561A	M84.673A	T85.621S
E08.3492	E09.3299	E09.3592	E10.3529	E11.3412	E13.3219	E13.3552	H40.1212	M48.50XA	M80.829A	M84.454A	M84.562A	M84.674A	T85.631A
E08.3493	E09.3311	E09.3593	E10.3531	E11.3413	E13.3291	E13.3553	H40.1213	M48.51XA	M80.831A	M84.459A	M84.563A	M84.675A	T85.631D
E08.3499	E09.3312	E09.3599	E10.3532	E11.3419	E13.3292	E13.3559	H40.1214	M48.52XA	M80.832A	M84.461A	M84.564A	M84.676A	T85.631S
E08.3511	E09.37X1	E10.3533	E10.3533	E11.3491	E13.3293	E13.3591	H40.1220	M48.53XA	M80.839A	M84.462A	M84.569A	M84.68XA	T85.691A
E08.3512	E09.37X2	E10.3539	E10.3539	E11.3492	E13.3299	E13.3592	H40.1221	M48.54XA	M80.841A	M84.463A	M84.571A	M84.68XA	T85.691D
E08.3513	E09.37X3	E09.3391	E10.3541	E11.3493	E13.3311	E13.3593	H40.1222	M48.55XA	M80.842A	M84.464A	M84.572A	T81.502A	T85.691S
E08.3519	E09.37X9	E09.3392	E10.3542	E11.3499	E13.3312	E13.3599	H40.1223	M48.56XA	M80.849A	M84.469A	M84.573A	T81.502D	T85.71XA
E08.3521	E09.3393	E10.3211	E10.3543	E11.3511	E13.3313	E13.37X1	H40.1224	M48.57XA	M80.851A	M84.471A	M84.574A	T81.502S	T85.71XD
E08.3522	E09.3399	E10.3212	E10.3549	E11.3512	E13.3319	E13.37X2	H40.1230	M48.58XA	M80.852A	M84.472A	M84.575A	T81.512A	T85.71XS
E08.3523	E09.3411	E10.3213	E10.3551	E11.3513	E13.3391	E13.37X3	H40.1231	M80.00XA	M80.859A	M84.473A	M84.576A	T81.512D	
E08.3529	E09.3412	E10.3219	E10.3552	E11.3519	E13.3392	E13.37X9	H40.1232	M80.011A	M80.861A	M84.474A	M84.58XA	T81.512S	
E08.3531	E09.3413	E10.3291	E10.3553	E11.3521	E13.3393	H40.10X0	H40.1233	M80.012A	M80.862A	M84.475A	M84.60XA	T81.522A	
E08.3532	E09.3419	E10.3292	E10.3559	E11.3522	E13.3399	H40.10X1	H40.1234	M80.019A	M80.869A	M84.476A	M84.611A	T81.522D	
E08.3533	E09.3491	E10.3293	E10.3591	E11.3523	E13.3411	H40.10X2	H40.1290	M80.021A	M80.871A	M84.477A	M84.612A	T81.522S	
E08.3539	E09.3492	E10.3299	E10.3592	E11.3529	E13.3412	H40.10X3	H40.1291	M80.022A	M80.872A	M84.478A	M84.619A	T81.532A	
E08.3541	E09.3493	E10.3311	E10.3593	E11.3531	E13.3413	H40.10X4	H40.1292	M80.029A	M80.879A	M84.479A	M84.621A	T81.532D	
E08.3542	E09.3499	E10.3312	E10.3599	E11.3532	E13.3419	H40.1110	H40.1293	M80.031A	M80.88XA	M84.48XA	M84.622A	T81.532S	

Unacceptable Principal Diagnosis - Based on Medicare code edits

H40.1210	H40.1313	O36.80X9	R40.2212	R40.2310	R40.2353	R40.2441	T36.3X5D	T36.7X5A	T37.0X6S	T37.4X6D	T38.0X6A	T38.4X5S	T38.805D
H40.1211	H40.1314	R40.2110	R40.2213	R40.2311	R40.2354	R40.2442	T36.3X5S	T36.7X5D	T37.1X5A	T37.4X6S	T38.0X6D	T38.4X6A	T38.805S
H40.1212	H40.1320	R40.2111	R40.2214	R40.2312	R40.2360	R40.2443	T36.3X6A	T36.7X5S	T37.1X5D	T37.5X5A	T38.0X6S	T38.4X6D	T38.806A
H40.1213	H40.1321	R40.2112	R40.2220	R40.2313	R40.2361	R40.2444	T36.3X6D	T36.7X6A	T37.1X5S	T37.5X5D	T38.1X5A	T38.4X6S	T38.806D
H40.1214	H40.1322	R40.2113	R40.2221	R40.2314	R40.2362	T36.0X5A	T36.3X6S	T36.7X6D	T37.1X6A	T37.5X5S	T38.1X5D	T38.5X5A	T38.806S
H40.1220	H40.1323	R40.2114	R40.2222	R40.2320	R40.2363	T36.0X5D	T36.4X5A	T36.7X6S	T37.1X6D	T37.5X6A	T38.1X5S	T38.5X5D	T38.815A
H40.1221	H40.1324	R40.2120	R40.2223	R40.2321	R40.2364	T36.0X5S	T36.4X5D	T36.8X5A	T37.1X6S	T37.5X6D	T38.1X6A	T38.5X5S	T38.815D
H40.1222	H40.1330	R40.2121	R40.2224	R40.2322	R40.2410	T36.0X6A	T36.4X5S	T36.8X5D	T37.2X5A	T37.5X6S	T38.1X6D	T38.5X6A	T38.815S
H40.1223	H40.1331	R40.2122	R40.2230	R40.2323	R40.2411	T36.0X6D	T36.4X6A	T36.8X5S	T37.2X5D	T37.8X5A	T38.1X6S	T38.5X6D	T38.816A
H40.1224	H40.1332	R40.2123	R40.2231	R40.2324	R40.2412	T36.0X6S	T36.4X6D	T36.8X6A	T37.2X5S	T37.8X5D	T38.2X5A	T38.5X6S	T38.816D
H40.1230	H40.1333	R40.2124	R40.2232	R40.2330	R40.2413	T36.1X5A	T36.4X6S	T36.8X6D	T37.2X6A	T37.8X5S	T38.2X5D	T38.6X5A	T38.816S
H40.1231	H40.1334	R40.2130	R40.2233	R40.2331	R40.2414	T36.1X5D	T36.5X5A	T36.8X6S	T37.2X6D	T37.8X6A	T38.2X5S	T38.6X5D	T38.895A
H40.1232	H40.1390	R40.2131	R40.2234	R40.2332	R40.2420	T36.1X5S	T36.5X5D	T36.95XA	T37.2X6S	T37.8X6D	T38.2X6A	T38.6X5S	T38.895D
H40.1233	H40.1391	R40.2132	R40.2240	R40.2333	R40.2421	T36.1X6A	T36.5X5S	T36.95XD	T37.3X5A	T37.8X6S	T38.2X6D	T38.6X6A	T38.895S
H40.1234	H40.1392	R40.2133	R40.2241	R40.2334	R40.2422	T36.1X6D	T36.5X6A	T36.95XS	T37.3X5D	T37.95XA	T38.2X6S	T38.6X6D	T38.896A
H40.1290	H40.1393	R40.2134	R40.2242	R40.2340	R40.2423	T36.1X6S	T36.5X6D	T36.96XA	T37.3X5S	T37.95XD	T38.3X5A	T38.6X6S	T38.896D
H40.1291	H40.1394	R40.2140	R40.2243	R40.2341	R40.2424	T36.2X5A	T36.5X6S	T36.96XD	T37.3X6A	T37.95XS	T38.3X5D	T38.7X5A	T38.896S
H40.1292	O36.80X0	R40.2141	R40.2244	R40.2342	R40.2430	T36.2X5D	T36.6X5A	T36.96XS	T37.3X6D	T37.96XA	T38.3X5S	T38.7X5D	T38.905A
H40.1293	O36.80X1	R40.2142	R40.2250	R40.2343	R40.2431	T36.2X5S	T36.6X5D	T37.0X5A	T37.3X6S	T37.96XD	T38.3X6A	T38.7X5S	T38.905D
H40.1294	O36.80X2	R40.2143	R40.2251	R40.2344	R40.2432	T36.2X6A	T36.6X5S	T37.0X5D	T37.4X5A	T37.96XS	T38.3X6D	T38.7X6A	T38.905S
H40.1310	O36.80X3	R40.2144	R40.2252	R40.2350	R40.2433	T36.2X6D	T36.6X6A	T37.0X5S	T37.4X5D	T38.0X5A	T38.3X6S	T38.7X6D	T38.906A
H40.1311	O36.80X4	R40.2210	R40.2253	R40.2351	R40.2434	T36.2X6S	T36.6X6D	T37.0X6A	T37.4X5S	T38.0X5D	T38.4X5A	T38.7X6S	T38.906D
H40.1312	O36.80X5	R40.2211	R40.2254	R40.2352	R40.2440	T36.3X5A	T36.6X6S	T37.0X6D	T37.4X6A	T38.0X5S	T38.4X5D	T38.805A	T38.906S

Unacceptable Principal Diagnosis (cont.) - Based on Medicare code edits

T38.995A	T39.96XS	T40.996D	T42.2X6A	T43.205S	T43.625D	T44.5X5A	T45.3X6S	T45.96XD	T46.906A	T47.8X5S	T48.905D	T49.8X5A	T50.7X6S
T38.995D	T40.0X5A	T40.996S	T42.2X6D	T43.206A	T43.625S	T44.5X5D	T45.4X5A	T45.96XS	T46.906D	T47.8X6A	T48.905S	T49.8X5D	T50.8X5A
T38.995S	T40.0X5D	T41.0X5A	T42.2X6S	T43.206D	T43.626A	T44.5X5S	T45.4X5D	T46.0X5A	T46.906S	T47.8X6D	T48.906A	T49.8X5S	T50.8X5D
T38.996A	T40.0X5S	T41.0X5D	T42.3X5A	T43.206S	T43.626D	T44.5X6A	T45.4X5S	T46.0X5D	T46.995A	T47.8X6S	T48.906D	T49.8X6A	T50.8X5S
T38.996D	T40.0X6A	T41.0X5S	T42.3X5D	T43.215A	T43.626S	T44.5X6D	T45.4X6A	T46.0X5S	T46.995D	T47.95XA	T48.906S	T49.8X6D	T50.8X6A
T38.996S	T40.0X6D	T41.0X6A	T42.3X5S	T43.215D	T43.635A	T44.6X5A	T45.4X6D	T46.0X6A	T46.995S	T47.95XS	T48.995A	T49.8X6S	T50.8X6D
T39.015A	T40.2X5A	T41.0X6D	T42.3X6A	T43.215S	T43.635D	T44.6X5D	T45.4X6S	T46.0X6D	T46.996A	T47.96XA	T48.995D	T49.95XA	T50.8X6S
T39.015D	T40.2X5D	T41.0X6S	T42.3X6D	T43.216A	T43.635S	T44.6X5S	T45.515A	T46.0X6S	T46.996D	T47.96XD	T48.995S	T49.95XD	T50.A15A
T39.015S	T40.2X5S	T41.1X5A	T42.3X6S	T43.216D	T43.636A	T44.6X6A	T45.515D	T46.1X5A	T46.996S	T47.96XS	T48.996A	T49.95XS	T50.A15D
T39.016A	T40.2X6A	T41.1X5D	T42.4X5A	T43.216S	T43.636D	T44.6X6D	T45.515S	T46.1X5D	T47.0X5A	T48.0X5A	T48.996D	T49.96XA	T50.A15S
T39.016D	T40.2X6D	T41.1X5S	T42.4X5D	T43.225A	T43.636S	T44.6X6S	T45.516A	T46.1X5S	T47.0X5D	T48.0X5D	T48.996S	T49.96XD	T50.A16A
T39.016S	T40.2X6S	T41.1X6A	T42.4X5S	T43.225D	T43.695A	T44.7X5A	T45.516D	T46.1X6A	T47.0X5S	T48.0X5S	T49.0X5A	T49.96XS	T50.A16D
T39.095A	T40.3X5A	T41.1X6D	T42.4X6A	T43.225S	T43.695D	T44.7X5D	T45.516S	T46.1X6D	T47.0X6A	T48.0X6A	T49.0X5D	T50.0X5A	T50.A16S
T39.095D	T40.3X5D	T41.1X6S	T42.4X6D	T43.226A	T43.695S	T44.7X5S	T45.525A	T46.1X6S	T47.0X6D	T48.0X6D	T49.0X5S	T50.0X5D	T50.A25A
T39.095S	T40.3X5S	T41.205A	T42.4X6S	T43.226D	T43.696A	T44.7X6A	T45.525D	T46.2X5A	T47.0X6S	T48.0X6S	T49.0X6D	T50.0X5S	T50.A25D
T39.096A	T40.3X6A	T41.205D	T42.5X5A	T43.226S	T43.696D	T44.7X6D	T45.525S	T46.2X5D	T47.1X5A	T48.1X5A	T49.0X6S	T50.0X6A	T50.A25S
T39.096D	T40.3X6D	T41.205S	T42.5X5D	T43.295A	T43.696S	T44.7X6S	T45.526A	T46.2X5S	T47.1X5D	T48.1X5D	T49.1X5A	T50.0X6D	T50.A26A
T39.096S	T40.3X6S	T41.206A	T42.5X5S	T43.295D	T43.8X5A	T44.8X5A	T45.526D	T46.2X6A	T47.1X5S	T48.1X5S	T49.1X5D	T50.0X6S	T50.A26D
T39.1X5A	T40.4X5A	T41.206D	T42.5X6A	T43.295S	T43.8X5D	T44.8X5D	T45.526S	T46.2X6D	T47.1X6A	T48.1X6A	T49.1X5S	T50.1X5A	T50.A26S
T39.1X5D	T40.4X5D	T41.206S	T42.5X6D	T43.296A	T43.8X5S	T44.8X5S	T45.605A	T46.2X6S	T47.1X6D	T48.1X6D	T49.1X6A	T50.1X5D	T50.A95A
T39.1X5S	T40.4X5S	T41.295A	T42.5X6S	T43.296D	T43.8X6A	T44.8X6A	T45.605D	T46.3X5A	T47.1X6S	T48.1X6S	T49.1X6D	T50.1X5S	T50.A95D
T39.1X6A	T40.4X6A	T41.295D	T42.6X5A	T43.296S	T43.8X6D	T44.8X6D	T45.605S	T46.3X5D	T47.2X5A	T48.205A	T49.1X6S	T50.1X6A	T50.A95S
T39.1X6D	T40.4X6D	T41.295S	T42.6X5D	T43.3X5A	T43.8X6S	T44.8X6S	T45.606A	T46.3X5S	T47.2X5D	T48.205D	T49.2X5A	T50.1X6D	T50.A96A
T39.1X6S	T40.4X6S	T41.296A	T42.6X5S	T43.3X5D	T43.95XA	T44.905A	T45.606D	T46.3X6A	T47.2X5S	T48.205S	T49.2X5D	T50.1X6S	T50.A96D
T39.2X5A	T40.5X5A	T41.296D	T42.6X6A	T43.3X5S	T43.95XD	T44.905D	T45.606S	T46.3X6D	T47.2X6A	T48.206A	T49.2X5S	T50.2X5A	T50.A96S
T39.2X5D	T40.5X5D	T41.296S	T42.6X6D	T43.3X6A	T43.95XS	T44.905S	T45.615A	T46.3X6S	T47.2X6D	T48.206D	T49.2X6A	T50.2X5D	T50.B15A
T39.2X5S	T40.5X5S	T41.3X5A	T42.6X6S	T43.3X6D	T43.96XA	T44.906A	T45.615D	T46.4X5A	T47.2X6S	T48.206S	T49.2X6S	T50.2X5S	T50.B15D
T39.2X6A	T40.5X6A	T41.3X5D	T42.75XA	T43.3X6S	T43.96XD	T44.906D	T45.615S	T46.4X5D	T47.3X5A	T48.295A	T49.3X5A	T50.2X6A	T50.B15S
T39.2X6D	T40.5X6D	T41.3X5S	T42.75XD	T43.4X5A	T43.96XS	T44.906S	T45.616A	T46.4X5S	T47.3X5D	T48.295D	T49.3X5D	T50.2X6D	T50.B16A
T39.2X6S	T40.5X6S	T41.3X6A	T42.75XS	T43.4X5D	T44.0X5A	T44.995A	T45.616D	T46.4X6A	T47.3X5S	T48.295S	T49.3X5S	T50.2X6S	T50.B16D
T39.315A	T40.605A	T41.3X6D	T42.76XA	T43.4X5S	T44.0X5D	T44.995D	T45.616S	T46.4X6D	T47.3X6A	T48.296A	T49.3X6A	T50.3X5A	T50.B16S
T39.315D	T40.605D	T41.3X6S	T42.76XD	T43.4X6A	T44.0X5S	T44.995S	T45.625A	T46.4X6S	T47.3X6D	T48.296D	T49.3X6D	T50.3X5D	T50.B95A
T39.315S	T40.605S	T41.45XA	T42.76XS	T43.4X6D	T44.0X6A	T44.996A	T45.625D	T46.5X5A	T47.3X6S	T48.296S	T49.3X6S	T50.3X5S	T50.B95D
T39.316A	T40.606A	T41.45XD	T42.8X5A	T43.4X6S	T44.0X6D	T44.996D	T45.625S	T46.5X5D	T47.4X5A	T48.3X5A	T49.4X5A	T50.3X6D	T50.B95S
T39.316D	T40.606D	T41.45XS	T42.8X5D	T43.505A	T44.0X6S	T44.996S	T45.626A	T46.5X5S	T47.4X5D	T48.3X5D	T49.4X5D	T50.3X6S	T50.B96A
T39.316S	T40.606S	T41.46XA	T42.8X5S	T43.505D	T44.1X5A	T45.0X5A	T45.626D	T46.5X6A	T47.4X5S	T48.3X5S	T49.4X5S	T50.4X5A	T50.B96D
T39.395A	T40.695A	T41.46XD	T42.8X6A	T43.505S	T44.1X5D	T45.0X5D	T45.626S	T46.5X6D	T47.4X6A	T48.3X6A	T49.4X6A	T50.4X5D	T50.B96S
T39.395D	T40.695D	T41.46XS	T42.8X6D	T43.506A	T44.1X5S	T45.0X5S	T45.695A	T46.5X6S	T47.4X6D	T48.3X6D	T49.4X6S	T50.4X5S	T50.Z15A
T39.395S	T40.695S	T41.5X5A	T42.8X6S	T43.506D	T44.1X6A	T45.0X6A	T45.695D	T46.6X5A	T47.4X6S	T48.3X6S	T49.5X5D	T50.4X6D	T50.Z15D
T39.396A	T40.696A	T41.5X5D	T43.015A	T43.506S	T44.1X6D	T45.0X6D	T45.695S	T46.6X5D	T47.5X5A	T48.4X5A	T49.5X5S	T50.4X6S	T50.Z15S
T39.396D	T40.696D	T41.5X5S	T43.015D	T43.595A	T44.1X6S	T45.0X6S	T45.696A	T46.6X5S	T47.5X5D	T48.4X5D	T49.5X6A	T50.5X5A	T50.Z16A
T39.396S	T40.696S	T41.5X6A	T43.015S	T43.595D	T44.2X5A	T45.1X5A	T45.696D	T46.6X6A	T47.5X5S	T48.4X5S	T49.5X6D	T50.5X5D	T50.Z16D
T39.4X5A	T40.7X5A	T41.5X6D	T43.016A	T43.595S	T44.2X5D	T45.1X5D	T45.696S	T46.6X6D	T47.5X6A	T48.4X6A	T49.5X6S	T50.5X5S	T50.Z16S
T39.4X5D	T40.7X5D	T41.5X6S	T43.016D	T43.596A	T44.2X5S	T45.1X5S	T45.7X5A	T46.6X6S	T47.5X6D	T48.4X6D	T49.6X5A	T50.5X6A	T50.Z95A
T39.4X5S	T40.7X5S	T42.0X5A	T43.016S	T43.596D	T44.2X6A	T45.1X6A	T45.7X5D	T46.7X5A	T47.5X6S	T48.4X6S	T49.6X5D	T50.5X6D	T50.Z95D
T39.4X6A	T40.7X6A	T42.0X5D	T43.025A	T43.596S	T44.2X6D	T45.1X6D	T45.7X5S	T46.7X5D	T47.6X5A	T48.5X5A	T49.6X5S	T50.6X5A	T50.Z95S
T39.4X6D	T40.7X6D	T42.0X5S	T43.025D	T43.605A	T44.2X6S	T45.1X6S	T45.7X6A	T46.7X5S	T47.6X5D	T48.5X5D	T49.6X6D	T50.6X5D	T50.Z96A
T39.4X6S	T40.7X6S	T42.0X6A	T43.025S	T43.605D	T44.3X5A	T45.2X5A	T45.7X6D	T46.7X6A	T47.6X5S	T48.5X5S	T49.6X6S	T50.6X5S	T50.Z96D
T39.8X5A	T40.905A	T42.0X6D	T43.026A	T43.605S	T44.3X5D	T45.2X5D	T45.7X6S	T46.7X6D	T47.6X6A	T48.5X6A	T49.7X5A	T50.6X6A	T50.Z96S
T39.8X5D	T40.905D	T42.0X6S	T43.026D	T43.606A	T44.3X5S	T45.2X5S	T45.8X5A	T46.7X6S	T47.6X6D	T48.5X6D	T49.7X5D	T50.6X6D	T81.12XA
T39.8X5S	T40.905S	T42.1X5A	T43.026S	T43.606D	T44.3X6A	T45.2X6A	T45.8X5D	T46.8X5A	T47.6X6S	T48.6X5A	T49.7X5S	T50.6X6S	
T39.8X6A	T40.906A	T42.1X5D	T43.1X5A	T43.606S	T44.3X6D	T45.2X6D	T45.8X5S	T46.8X5D	T47.7X5D	T48.6X5D	T49.7X6A	T50.7X5A	
T39.8X6D	T40.906D	T42.1X5S	T43.1X5D	T43.615A	T44.3X6S	T45.2X6S	T45.8X6A	T46.8X5S	T47.7X5S	T48.6X5S	T49.7X6D	T50.7X5D	
T39.8X6S	T40.906S	T42.1X6A	T43.1X5S	T43.615D	T44.4X5A	T45.3X5A	T45.8X6D	T46.8X6A	T47.7X6A	T48.6X6A	T49.7X6S	T50.7X5S	
T39.95XA	T40.995A	T42.1X6D	T43.1X6A	T43.615S	T44.4X5D	T45.3X5D	T45.8X6S	T46.8X6D	T47.7X6D	T48.6X6D		T50.7X6A	
T39.95XD	T40.995D	T42.1X6S	T43.1X6D	T43.616A	T44.4X5S	T45.3X5S	T45.95XA	T46.8X6S	T47.7X6S	T48.6X6S			
T39.95XS	T40.995S	T42.2X5A	T43.1X6S	T43.616D	T44.4X6A	T45.3X6A	T45.95XD	T46.905A	T47.8X5A	T48.905A			
T39.96XA	T40.996A	T42.2X5D	T43.205A	T43.616S	T44.4X6D	T45.3X6D	T45.95XS	T46.905D	T47.8X5D				
T39.96XD		T42.2X5S	T43.205D	T43.625A	T44.4X6S		T45.96XA	T46.905S					

1st Trimester - Based on CMS data

O31.01X0	O31.11X9	O31.31X5	O36.0114	O36.1113	O36.21X2	O36.5911	O36.71X0	O36.8219	O36.8915	O40.1XX4	O41.1013	O41.1412	O41.91X1
O31.01X1	O31.21X0	O31.31X9	O36.0115	O36.1114	O36.21X3	O36.5912	O36.71X1	O36.8310	O36.8919	O40.1XX5	O41.1014	O41.1413	O41.91X2
O31.01X2	O31.21X1	O31.8X10	O36.0119	O36.1115	O36.21X4	O36.5913	O36.71X2	O36.8311	O36.91X0	O40.1XX9	O41.1015	O41.1414	O41.91X3
O31.01X3	O31.21X2	O31.8X11	O36.0910	O36.1119	O36.21X5	O36.5914	O36.71X3	O36.8312	O36.91X1	O41.01X0	O41.1019	O41.1415	O41.91X4
O31.01X4	O31.21X3	O31.8X12	O36.0911	O36.1910	O36.21X9	O36.5915	O36.71X4	O36.8313	O36.91X3	O41.01X1	O41.1210	O41.1419	O41.91X5
O31.01X5	O31.21X4	O31.8X13	O36.0912	O36.1911	O36.5110	O36.5919	O36.71X5	O36.8314	O36.91X4	O41.01X2	O41.1211	O41.8X10	
O31.01X9	O31.21X5	O31.8X14	O36.0913	O36.1912	O36.5111	O36.61X0	O36.71X9	O36.8315	O36.91X5	O41.01X3	O41.1212	O41.8X11	
O31.11X0	O31.21X9	O31.8X15	O36.0914	O36.1913	O36.5112	O36.61X1	O36.8210	O36.8319	O36.91X9	O41.01X4	O41.1213	O41.8X12	
O31.11X1	O31.31X0	O31.8X19	O36.0915	O36.1914	O36.5113	O36.61X2	O36.8211	O36.8910	O40.1XX0	O41.01X5	O41.1214	O41.8X13	
O31.11X2	O31.31X1	O36.0110	O36.0919	O36.1915	O36.5114	O36.61X3	O36.8212	O36.8911	O40.1XX1	O41.01X9	O41.1215	O41.8X14	
O31.11X3	O31.31X2	O36.0111	O36.1110	O36.1919	O36.5115	O36.61X4	O36.8213	O36.8912	O40.1XX2	O41.1010	O41.1219	O41.8X15	
O31.11X4	O31.31X3	O36.0112	O36.1111	O36.21X0	O36.5119	O36.61X5	O36.8214	O36.8913	O40.1XX3	O41.1011	O41.1410	O41.8X19	
O31.11X5	O31.31X4	O36.0113	O36.1112	O36.21X1	O36.5910	O36.61X9	O36.8215	O36.8914		O41.1012	O41.1411	O41.91X0	

2nd Trimester - Based on CMS data

O31.02X0	O31.22X1	O31.8X22	O36.0923	O36.1924	O36.5125	O36.62X9	O36.8220	O36.8921	O40.2XX2	O41.1023	O41.1424	O41.92X5	O60.13X9
O31.02X1	O31.22X2	O31.8X23	O36.0924	O36.1925	O36.5129	O36.72X0	O36.8221	O36.8922	O40.2XX3	O41.1024	O41.1425	O41.92X9	O60.22X0
O31.02X2	O31.22X3	O31.8X24	O36.0925	O36.1929	O36.5920	O36.72X1	O36.8222	O36.8923	O40.2XX4	O41.1025	O41.1429	O60.12X0	O60.22X1
O31.02X3	O31.22X4	O31.8X25	O36.0929	O36.22X0	O36.5921	O36.72X2	O36.8223	O36.8924	O40.2XX5	O41.1029	O41.8X20	O60.12X1	O60.22X2
O31.02X4	O31.22X5	O31.8X29	O36.1120	O36.22X1	O36.5922	O36.72X3	O36.8224	O36.8925	O40.2XX9	O41.1220	O41.8X21	O60.12X2	O60.22X3
O31.02X5	O31.22X9	O36.0120	O36.1121	O36.22X2	O36.5923	O36.72X4	O36.8225	O36.8929	O41.02X0	O41.1221	O41.8X22	O60.12X3	O60.22X4
O31.02X9	O31.32X0	O36.0121	O36.1122	O36.22X3	O36.5924	O36.72X5	O36.8229	O36.92X0	O41.02X1	O41.1222	O41.8X23	O60.12X4	O60.22X5
O31.12X0	O31.32X1	O36.0122	O36.1123	O36.22X4	O36.5925	O36.72X9	O36.8320	O36.92X1	O41.02X2	O41.1223	O41.8X24	O60.12X5	O60.22X9
O31.12X1	O31.32X2	O36.0123	O36.1124	O36.22X5	O36.5929	O36.8120	O36.8321	O36.92X2	O41.02X3	O41.1224	O41.8X25	O60.12X9	
O31.12X2	O31.32X3	O36.0124	O36.1125	O36.22X9	O36.62X0	O36.8121	O36.8322	O36.92X3	O41.02X4	O41.1225	O41.8X29	O60.13X0	
O31.12X3	O31.32X4	O36.0125	O36.1129	O36.5120	O36.62X1	O36.8122	O36.8323	O36.92X4	O41.02X5	O41.1229	O41.92X0	O60.13X1	
O31.12X4	O31.32X5	O36.0129	O36.1920	O36.5121	O36.62X2	O36.8123	O36.8324	O36.92X5	O41.02X9	O41.1420	O41.92X1	O60.13X2	
O31.12X5	O31.32X9	O36.0920	O36.1921	O36.5122	O36.62X3	O36.8124	O36.8325	O36.92X9	O41.1020	O41.1421	O41.92X2	O60.13X3	
O31.12X9	O31.8X20	O36.0921	O36.1922	O36.5123	O36.62X4	O36.8125	O36.8329	O40.2XX0	O41.1021	O41.1422	O41.92X3	O60.13X4	
O31.22X0	O31.8X21	O36.0922	O36.1923	O36.5124	O36.62X5	O36.8129	O36.8920	O40.2XX1	O41.1022	O41.1423	O41.92X4	O60.13X5	

3rd Trimester - Based on CMS data

O31.03X0	O31.23X1	O31.8X32	O36.0933	O36.1934	O36.5135	O36.63X9	O36.8230	O36.8931	O40.3XX2	O41.1033	O41.1434	O41.93X5	O60.14X9
O31.03X1	O31.23X2	O31.8X33	O36.0934	O36.1935	O36.5139	O36.73X0	O36.8231	O36.8932	O40.3XX3	O41.1034	O41.1435	O41.93X9	O60.23X0
O31.03X2	O31.23X3	O31.8X34	O36.0935	O36.1939	O36.5930	O36.73X1	O36.8232	O36.8933	O40.3XX4	O41.1035	O41.1439	O60.13X0	O60.23X1
O31.03X3	O31.23X4	O31.8X35	O36.0939	O36.23X0	O36.5931	O36.73X2	O36.8233	O36.8934	O40.3XX5	O41.1039	O41.8X30	O60.13X1	O60.23X2
O31.03X4	O31.23X5	O31.8X39	O36.1130	O36.23X1	O36.5932	O36.73X3	O36.8234	O36.8935	O40.3XX9	O41.1230	O41.8X31	O60.13X2	O60.23X3
O31.03X5	O31.23X9	O36.0130	O36.1131	O36.23X2	O36.5933	O36.73X4	O36.8235	O36.8939	O41.03X0	O41.1231	O41.8X32	O60.13X3	O60.23X4
O31.03X9	O31.33X0	O36.0131	O36.1132	O36.23X3	O36.5934	O36.73X5	O36.8239	O36.93X0	O41.03X1	O41.1232	O41.8X33	O60.13X4	O60.23X5
O31.13X0	O31.33X1	O36.0132	O36.1133	O36.23X4	O36.5935	O36.73X9	O36.8330	O36.93X1	O41.03X2	O41.1233	O41.8X34	O60.13X5	O60.23X9
O31.13X1	O31.33X2	O36.0133	O36.1134	O36.23X5	O36.5939	O36.8130	O36.8331	O36.93X2	O41.03X3	O41.1234	O41.8X35	O60.13X9	
O31.13X2	O31.33X3	O36.0134	O36.1135	O36.23X9	O36.63X0	O36.8131	O36.8332	O36.93X3	O41.03X4	O41.1235	O41.8X39	O60.14X0	
O31.13X3	O31.33X4	O36.0135	O36.1139	O36.5130	O36.63X1	O36.8132	O36.8333	O36.93X4	O41.03X5	O41.1239	O41.93X0	O60.14X1	
O31.13X4	O31.33X5	O36.0139	O36.1930	O36.5131	O36.63X2	O36.8133	O36.8334	O36.93X5	O41.03X9	O41.1430	O41.93X1	O60.14X2	
O31.13X5	O31.33X9	O36.0930	O36.1931	O36.5132	O36.63X3	O36.8134	O36.8335	O36.93X9	O41.1030	O41.1431	O41.93X2	O60.14X3	
O31.13X9	O31.8X30	O36.0931	O36.1932	O36.5133	O36.63X4	O36.8135	O36.8339	O40.3XX0	O41.1031	O41.1432	O41.93X3	O60.14X4	
O31.23X0	O31.8X31	O36.0932	O36.1933	O36.5134	O36.63X5	O36.8139	O36.8930	O40.3XX1	O41.1032	O41.1433	O41.93X4	O60.14X5	

Code exempt from diagnosis present on admission requirement

CMS includes over 36,000 codes that are exempt. Please go to the CMS site for the most updated Present on Admission (POA) Exempt List (https://www.cms.gov/Medicare/Medicare-Fee-for-Service-Payment/HospitalAcqCond/Coding.html - Go to downloads).

Editor's Note: At press time, the most updated list on the CMS site was FY 2017.

ICD-10-CM Official Guidelines for Coding and Reporting FY 2018

Narrative changes appear in bold text

Items <u>underlined</u> have been moved within the guidelines since the FY 2017 version

Italics are used to indicate revisions to heading changes

The Centers for Medicare and Medicaid Services (CMS) and the National Center for Health Statistics (NCHS), two departments within the U.S. Federal Government's Department of Health and Human Services (DHHS) provide the following guidelines for coding and reporting using the International Classification of Diseases, 10th Revision, Clinical Modification (ICD-10-CM). These guidelines should be used as a companion document to the official version of the ICD-10-CM as published on the NCHS website. The ICD-10-CM is a morbidity classification published by the United States for classifying diagnoses and reason for visits in all health care settings. The ICD-10-CM is based on the ICD-10, the statistical classification of disease published by the World Health Organization (WHO).

These guidelines have been approved by the four organizations that make up the Cooperating Parties for the ICD-10-CM: the American Hospital Association (AHA), the American Health Information Management Association (AHIMA), CMS, and NCHS.

These guidelines are a set of rules that have been developed to accompany and complement the official conventions and instructions provided within the ICD-10-CM itself. The instructions and conventions of the classification take precedence over guidelines. These guidelines are based on the coding and sequencing instructions in the Tabular List and Alphabetic Index of ICD-10-CM, but provide additional instruction. Adherence to these guidelines when assigning ICD-10-CM diagnosis codes is required under the Health Insurance Portability and Accountability Act (HIPAA). The diagnosis codes (Tabular List and Alphabetic Index) have been adopted under HIPAA for all healthcare settings. A joint effort between the healthcare provider and the coder is essential to achieve complete and accurate documentation, code assignment, and reporting of diagnoses and procedures. These guidelines have been developed to assist both the healthcare provider and the coder in identifying those diagnoses that are to be reported. The importance of consistent, complete documentation in the medical record cannot be overemphasized. Without such documentation accurate coding cannot be achieved. The entire record should be reviewed to determine the specific reason for the encounter and the conditions treated.

The term encounter is used for all settings, including hospital admissions. In the context of these guidelines, the term provider is used throughout the guidelines to mean physician or any qualified health care practitioner who is legally accountable for establishing the patient's diagnosis. Only this set of guidelines, approved by the Cooperating Parties, is official.

The guidelines are organized into sections. Section I includes the structure and conventions of the classification and general guidelines that apply to the entire classification, and chapter-specific guidelines that correspond to the chapters as they are arranged in the classification. Section II includes guidelines for selection of principal diagnosis for non-outpatient settings. Section III includes guidelines for reporting additional diagnoses in non-outpatient settings. Section IV is for outpatient coding and reporting. It is necessary to review all sections of the guidelines to fully understand all of the rules and instructions needed to code properly.

Section I. Conventions, general coding guidelines and chapter specific guidelines

The conventions, general guidelines and chapter-specific guidelines are applicable to all health care settings unless otherwise indicated. The conventions and instructions of the classification take precedence over guidelines.

A. Conventions for the ICD-10-CM

The conventions for the ICD-10-CM are the general rules for use of the classification independent of the guidelines. These conventions are incorporated within the Alphabetic Index and Tabular List of the ICD-10-CM as instructional notes.

1. The Alphabetic Index and Tabular List

The ICD-10-CM is divided into the Alphabetic Index, an alphabetical list of terms and their corresponding code, and the Tabular List, a structured list of codes divided into chapters based on body system or condition. The Alphabetic Index consists of the following parts: the Index of Diseases and Injury, the Index of External Causes of Injury, the Table of Neoplasms and the Table of Drugs and Chemicals.

See Section I.C2. General guidelines

See Section I.C.19. Adverse effects, poisoning, underdosing and toxic effects

2. Format and Structure:

The ICD-10-CM Tabular List contains categories, subcategories and codes. Characters for categories, subcategories and codes may be either a letter or a number. All categories are 3 characters. A three-character category that has no further subdivision is equivalent to a code. Subcategories are either 4 or 5 characters. Codes may be 3, 4, 5, 6 or 7 characters. That is, each level of subdivision after a category is a subcategory. The final level of subdivision is a code. Codes that have applicable 7th characters are still referred to as codes, not subcategories. A code that has an applicable 7th character is considered invalid without the 7th character.

The ICD-10-CM uses an indented format for ease in reference.

3. Use of codes for reporting purposes

For reporting purposes only codes are permissible, not categories or subcategories, and any applicable 7th character is required.

4. Placeholder character

The ICD-10-CM utilizes a placeholder character "X". The "X" is used as a placeholder at certain codes to allow for future expansion. An example of this is at the poisoning, adverse effect and underdosing codes, categories T36-T50.

Where a placeholder exists, the X must be used in order for the code to be considered a valid code.

5. 7th Characters

Certain ICD-10-CM categories have applicable 7th characters. The applicable 7th character is required for all codes within the category, or as the notes in the Tabular List instruct. The 7th character must always be the 7th character in the data field. If a code that requires a 7th character is not 6 characters, a placeholder X must be used to fill in the empty characters.

6. Abbreviations

a. Alphabetic Index abbreviations

NEC "Not elsewhere classifiable"

This abbreviation in the Alphabetic Index represents "other specified." When a specific code is not available for a condition, the Alphabetic Index directs the coder to the "other specified" code in the Tabular List.

NOS "Not otherwise specified"

This abbreviation is the equivalent of unspecified.

b. Tabular List abbreviations

NEC "Not elsewhere classifiable"

This abbreviation in the Tabular List represents "other specified". When a specific code is not available for a condition, the Tabular List includes an NEC entry under a code to identify the code as the "other specified" code.

NOS "Not otherwise specified"

This abbreviation is the equivalent of unspecified.

7. Punctuation

[ ] Brackets are used in the Tabular List to enclose synonyms, alternative wording or explanatory phrases. Brackets are used in the Alphabetic Index to identify manifestation codes.

( ) Parentheses are used in both the Alphabetic Index and Tabular List to enclose supplementary words that may be present or absent in the statement of a disease or procedure without affecting the code number to which it is assigned. The terms within the parentheses are referred to as nonessential modifiers. The nonessential modifiers in the Alphabetic

Index to Diseases apply to subterms following a main term except when a nonessential modifier and a subentry are mutually exclusive, the subentry takes precedence. For example, in the ICD-10-CM Alphabetic Index under the main term Enteritis, "acute" is a nonessential modifier and "chronic" is a subentry. In this case, the nonessential modifier "acute" does not apply to the subentry "chronic".

: Colons are used in the Tabular List after an incomplete term which needs one or more of the modifiers following the colon to make it assignable to a given category.

8. Use of "and".

See Section I.A.14. Use of the term "And"

9. Other and Unspecified codes

a. "Other" codes

Codes titled "other" or "other specified" are for use when the information in the medical record provides detail for which a specific code does not exist. Alphabetic Index entries with NEC in the line designate "other" codes in the Tabular List. These Alphabetic Index entries represent specific disease entities for which no specific code exists so the term is included within an "other" code.

b. "Unspecified" codes

Codes titled "unspecified" are for use when the information in the medical record is insufficient to assign a more specific code. For those categories for which an unspecified code is not provided, the "other specified" code may represent both other and unspecified.

See Section I.B.18 Use of Signs/Symptom/Unspecified Codes

10. Includes Notes

This note appears immediately under a three character code title to further define, or give examples of, the content of the category.

11. Inclusion terms

List of terms is included under some codes. These terms are the conditions for which that code is to be used. The terms may be synonyms of the code title, or, in the case of "other specified" codes, the terms are a list of the various conditions assigned to that code. The inclusion terms are not necessarily exhaustive. Additional terms found only in the Alphabetic Index may also be assigned to a code.

12. Excludes Notes

The ICD-10-CM has two types of excludes notes. Each type of note has a different definition for use but they are all similar in that they indicate that codes excluded from each other are independent of each other.

a. Excludes1

A type 1 Excludes note is a pure excludes note. It means "NOT CODED HERE!" An Excludes1 note indicates that the code excluded should never be used at the same time as the code above the Excludes1 note. An Excludes1 is used when two conditions cannot occur together, such as a congenital form versus an acquired form of the same condition.

An exception to the Excludes1 definition is the circumstance when the two conditions are unrelated to each other. If it is not clear whether the two conditions involving an Excludes1 note are related or not, query the provider. For example, code F45.8, Other somatoform disorders, has an Excludes1 note for "sleep related teeth grinding (G47.63)," because "teeth grinding" is an inclusion term under F45.8. Only one of these two codes should be assigned for teeth grinding. However psychogenic dysmenorrhea is also an inclusion term under F45.8, and a patient could have both this condition and sleep related teeth grinding. In this case, the two conditions are clearly unrelated to each other, and so it would be appropriate to report F45.8 and G47.63 together.

b. Excludes2

A type 2 Excludes note represents "Not included here." An excludes2 note indicates that the condition excluded is not part of the condition represented by the code, but a patient may have both conditions at the same time. When an Excludes2 note appears under a code, it is acceptable to use both the code and the excluded code together, when appropriate.

13. Etiology/manifestation convention ("code first", "use additional code" and "in diseases classified elsewhere" notes)

Certain conditions have both an underlying etiology and multiple body system manifestations due to the underlying etiology. For such conditions, the ICD-10-CM has a coding convention that requires the underlying condition be sequenced first, if applicable, followed by the manifestation. Wherever such a combination exists, there is a "use additional code" note at the etiology code, and a "code first" note at the manifestation code. These instructional notes indicate the proper sequencing order of the codes, etiology followed by manifestation.

In most cases the manifestation codes will have in the code title, "in diseases classified elsewhere." Codes with this title are a component of the etiology/manifestation convention. The code title indicates that it is a manifestation code. "In diseases classified elsewhere" codes are never permitted to be used as first-listed or principal diagnosis codes. They must be used in conjunction with an underlying condition code and they must be listed following the underlying condition. See category F02, Dementia in other diseases classified elsewhere, for an example of this convention.

There are manifestation codes that do not have "in diseases classified elsewhere" in the title. For such codes, there is a "use additional code" note at the etiology code and a "code first" note at the manifestation code, and the rules for sequencing apply.

In addition to the notes in the Tabular List, these conditions also have a specific Alphabetic Index entry structure. In the Alphabetic Index both conditions are listed together with the etiology code first followed by the manifestation codes in brackets. The code in brackets is always to be sequenced second.

An example of the etiology/manifestation convention is dementia in Parkinson's disease. In the Alphabetic Index, code G20 is listed first, followed by code F02.80 or F02.81 in brackets. Code G20 represents the underlying etiology, Parkinson's disease, and must be sequenced first, whereas code F02.80 and F02.81 represent the manifestation of dementia in diseases classified elsewhere, with or without behavioral disturbance.

"Code first" and "Use additional code" notes are also used as sequencing rules in the classification for certain codes that are not part of an etiology/ manifestation combination.

See Section I.B.7. Multiple coding for a single condition.

14. "And"

The word "and" should be interpreted to mean either "and" or "or" when it appears in a title.

For example, cases of "tuberculosis of bones", "tuberculosis of joints" and "tuberculosis of bones and joints" are classified to subcategory A18.0, Tuberculosis of bones and joints.

15. "With"

The word "with" **or "in"** should be interpreted to mean "associated with" or "due to" when it appears in a code title, the Alphabetic Index, or an instructional note in the Tabular List. The classification presumes a causal relationship between the two conditions linked by these terms in the Alphabetic Index or Tabular List.

These conditions should be coded as related even in the absence of provider documentation explicitly linking them, unless the documentation clearly states the conditions are unrelated **or when another guideline exists that specifically requires a documented linkage between two conditions (e.g., sepsis guideline for "acute organ dysfunction that is not clearly associated with the sepsis").**

For conditions not specifically linked by these relational terms in the classification **or when a guideline requires that a linkage between two conditions be explicitly documented**, provider documentation must link the conditions in order to code them as related.

The word "with" in the Alphabetic Index is sequenced immediately following the main term, not in alphabetical order.

16. "See" and "See Also"

The "see" instruction following a main term in the Alphabetic Index indicates that another term should be referenced. It is necessary to go to the main term referenced with the "see" note to locate the correct code.

A "see also" instruction following a main term in the Alphabetic Index instructs that there is another main term that may also be referenced that may provide additional Alphabetic Index entries that may be useful. It is not necessary to follow the "see also" note when the original main term provides the necessary code.

17. "Code also" note

A "code also" note instructs that two codes may be required to fully describe a condition, but this note does not provide sequencing direction. **The sequencing depends on the circumstances of the encounter.**

18. Default codes

A code listed next to a main term in the ICD-10-CM Alphabetic Index is referred to as a default code. The default code represents that condition that is most commonly associated with the main term, or is the unspecified code for the condition. If a condition is documented in a medical record (for example, appendicitis) without any additional information, such as acute or chronic, the default code should be assigned.

19. Code assignment and Clinical Criteria

The assignment of a diagnosis code is based on the provider's diagnostic statement that the condition exists. The provider's statement that the patient has a particular condition is sufficient. Code assignment is not based on clinical criteria used by the provider to establish the diagnosis.

B. General Coding Guidelines

1. Locating a code in the ICD-10-CM

To select a code in the classification that corresponds to a diagnosis or reason for visit documented in a medical record, first locate the term in the Alphabetic Index, and then verify the code in the Tabular List. Read and be guided by instructional notations that appear in both the Alphabetic Index and the Tabular List.

It is essential to use both the Alphabetic Index and Tabular List when locating and assigning a code. The Alphabetic Index does not always provide the full code. Selection of the full code, including laterality and any applicable 7th character can only be done in the Tabular List. A dash (-) at the end of an Alphabetic Index entry indicates that additional characters are required. Even if a dash is not included at the Alphabetic Index entry, it is necessary to refer to the Tabular List to verify that no 7th character is required.

2. Level of Detail in Coding

Diagnosis codes are to be used and reported at their highest number of characters available.

ICD-10-CM diagnosis codes are composed of codes with 3, 4, 5, 6 or 7 characters. Codes with three characters are included in ICD-10-CM as the heading of a category of codes that may be further subdivided by the use of fourth and/or fifth characters and/or sixth characters, which provide greater detail.

A three-character code is to be used only if it is not further subdivided. A code is invalid if it has not been coded to the full number of characters required for that code, including the 7th character, if applicable.

3. Code or codes from A00.0 through T88.9, Z00-Z99.8

The appropriate code or codes from A00.0 through T88.9, Z00-Z99.8 must be used to identify diagnoses, symptoms, conditions, problems, complaints or other reason(s) for the encounter/visit.

4. Signs and symptoms

Codes that describe symptoms and signs, as opposed to diagnoses, are acceptable for reporting purposes when a related definitive diagnosis has not been established (confirmed) by the provider. Chapter 18 of ICD-10-CM, Symptoms, Signs, and Abnormal Clinical and Laboratory Findings, Not Elsewhere Classified (codes R00.0-R99) contains many, but not all, codes for symptoms.

See Section I.B.18 Use of Signs/Symptom/Unspecified Codes

5. Conditions that are an integral part of a disease process

Signs and symptoms that are associated routinely with a disease process should not be assigned as additional codes, unless otherwise instructed by the classification.

6. Conditions that are not an integral part of a disease process

Additional signs and symptoms that may not be associated routinely with a disease process should be coded when present.

7. Multiple coding for a single condition

In addition to the etiology/manifestation convention that requires two codes to fully describe a single condition that affects multiple body systems, there are other single conditions that also require more than one code. "Use additional code" notes are found in the Tabular List at codes that are not part of an etiology/manifestation pair where a secondary code is useful to fully describe a condition. The sequencing rule is the same as the etiology/ manifestation pair, "use additional code" indicates that a secondary code should be added, **if known.**

For example, for bacterial infections that are not included in chapter 1, a secondary code from category B95, Streptococcus, Staphylococcus, and Enterococcus, as the cause of diseases classified elsewhere, or B96, Other bacterial agents as the cause of diseases classified elsewhere, may be required to identify the bacterial organism causing the infection. A "use additional code" note will normally be found at the infectious disease code, indicating a need for the organism code to be added as a secondary code.

"Code first" notes are also under certain codes that are not specifically manifestation codes but may be due to an underlying cause. When there is a "code first" note and an underlying condition is present, the underlying condition should be sequenced first, **if known.**

"Code, if applicable, any causal condition first" notes indicate that this code may be assigned as a principal diagnosis when the causal condition is unknown or not applicable. If a causal condition is known, then the code for that condition should be sequenced as the principal or first-listed diagnosis.

Multiple codes may be needed for sequela, complication codes and obstetric codes to more fully describe a condition. See the specific guidelines for these conditions for further instruction.

8. Acute and Chronic Conditions

If the same condition is described as both acute (subacute) and chronic, and separate subentries exist in the Alphabetic Index at the same indentation level, code both and sequence the acute (subacute) code first.

9. Combination Code

A combination code is a single code used to classify: Two diagnoses, or

A diagnosis with an associated secondary process (manifestation)

A diagnosis with an associated complication

Combination codes are identified by referring to subterm entries in the Alphabetic Index and by reading the inclusion and exclusion notes in the Tabular List.

Assign only the combination code when that code fully identifies the diagnostic conditions involved or when the Alphabetic Index so directs. Multiple coding should not be used when the classification provides a combination code that clearly identifies all of the elements documented in the diagnosis. When the combination code lacks necessary specificity in describing the manifestation or complication, an additional code should be used as a secondary code.

10. Sequela (Late Effects)

A sequela is the residual effect (condition produced) after the acute phase of an illness or injury has terminated. There is no time limit on when a sequela code can be used. The residual may be apparent early, such as in cerebral infarction, or it may occur months or years later, such as that due to a previous injury. Examples of sequela include: scar formation resulting from a burn, deviated septum due to a nasal fracture, and infertility due to tubal occlusion from old tuberculosis. Coding of sequela generally requires two codes sequenced in the following order: the condition or nature of the sequela is sequenced first. The sequela code is sequenced second.

An exception to the above guidelines are those instances where the code for the sequela is followed by a manifestation code identified in the Tabular List and title, or the sequela code has been expanded (at the fourth, fifth or sixth character levels) to include the manifestation(s). The code for the acute phase of an illness or injury that led to the sequela is never used with a code for the late effect.

See Section I.C.9. Sequelae of cerebrovascular disease

See Section I.C.15. Sequelae of complication of pregnancy, childbirth and the puerperium

See Section I.C.19. Application of 7th characters for Chapter 19

11. Impending or Threatened Condition

Code any condition described at the time of discharge as "impending" or "threatened" as follows:

If it did occur, code as confirmed diagnosis.

If it did not occur, reference the Alphabetic Index to determine if the condition has a subentry term for "impending" or "threatened" and also reference main term entries for "Impending" and for "Threatened."

If the subterms are listed, assign the given code.

If the subterms are not listed, code the existing underlying condition(s) and not the condition described as impending or threatened.

12. Reporting Same Diagnosis Code More than Once

Each unique ICD-10-CM diagnosis code may be reported only once for an encounter. This applies to bilateral conditions when there are no distinct codes identifying laterality or two different conditions classified to the same ICD-10-CM diagnosis code.

13. Laterality

Some ICD-10-CM codes indicate laterality, specifying whether the condition occurs on the left, right or is bilateral. If no bilateral code is provided and the condition is bilateral, assign separate codes for both the left and right side. If the side is not identified in the medical record, assign the code for the unspecified side.

When a patient has a bilateral condition and each side is treated during separate encounters, assign the "bilateral" code (as the condition still exists on both sides), including for the encounter to treat the first side. For the second encounter for treatment after one side has previously been treated and the condition no longer exists on that side, assign the appropriate unilateral code for the side where the condition still exists (e.g., cataract surgery performed on each eye in separate encounters). The bilateral code would not be assigned for the subsequent encounter, as the patient no longer has the condition in the previously-treated site. If the treatment on the first side did not completely resolve the condition, then the bilateral code would still be appropriate.

14. Documentation for BMI, Depth of Non-pressure ulcers, Pressure Ulcer Stages, Coma Scale, and NIH Stroke Scale

For the Body Mass Index (BMI), depth of non-pressure chronic ulcers, pressure ulcer stage, coma scale, and NIH stroke scale (NIHSS) codes, code assignment may be based on medical record documentation from clinicians who are not the patient's provider (i.e., physician or other qualified healthcare practitioner legally accountable for establishing the patient's diagnosis), since this information is typically documented by other clinicians involved in the care of the patient (e.g., a dietitian often documents the BMI, a nurse often documents the pressure ulcer stages, and an emergency medical technician

often documents the coma scale). However, the associated diagnosis (such as overweight, obesity, acute stroke, or pressure ulcer) must be documented by the patient's provider. If there is conflicting medical record documentation, either from the same clinician or different clinicians, the patient's attending provider should be queried for clarification.

The BMI, coma scale, and NIHSS codes should only be reported as secondary diagnoses.

15. Syndromes

Follow the Alphabetic Index guidance when coding syndromes. In the absence of Alphabetic Index guidance, assign codes for the documented manifestations of the syndrome. Additional codes for manifestations that are not an integral part of the disease process may also be assigned when the condition does not have a unique code.

16. Documentation of Complications of Care

Code assignment is based on the provider's documentation of the relationship between the condition and the care or procedure, unless otherwise instructed by the classification. The guideline extends to any complications of care, regardless of the chapter the code is located in. It is important to note that not all conditions that occur during or following medical care or surgery are classified as complications. There must be a cause-and-effect relationship between the care provided and the condition, and an indication in the documentation that it is a complication. Query the provider for clarification, if the complication is not clearly documented.

17. Borderline Diagnosis

If the provider documents a "borderline" diagnosis at the time of discharge, the diagnosis is coded as confirmed, unless the classification provides a specific entry (e.g., borderline diabetes). If a borderline condition has a specific index entry in ICD-10-CM, it should be coded as such. Since borderline conditions are not uncertain diagnoses, no distinction is made between the care setting (inpatient versus outpatient). Whenever the documentation is unclear regarding a borderline condition, coders are encouraged to query for clarification.

18. Use of Sign/Symptom/Unspecified Codes

Sign/symptom and "unspecified" codes have acceptable, even necessary, uses. While specific diagnosis codes should be reported when they are supported by the available medical record documentation and clinical knowledge of the patient's health condition, there are instances when signs/symptoms or unspecified codes are the best choices for accurately reflecting the healthcare encounter. Each healthcare encounter should be coded to the level of certainty known for that encounter.

If a definitive diagnosis has not been established by the end of the encounter, it is appropriate to report codes for sign(s) and/or symptom(s) in lieu of a definitive diagnosis. When sufficient clinical information isn't known or available about a particular health condition to assign a more specific code, it is acceptable to report the appropriate "unspecified" code (e.g., a diagnosis of pneumonia has been determined, but not the specific type). Unspecified codes should be reported when they are the codes that most accurately reflect what is known about the patient's condition at the time of that particular encounter. It would be inappropriate to select a specific code that is not supported by the medical record documentation or conduct medically unnecessary diagnostic testing in order to determine a more specific code.

C. Chapter-Specific Coding Guidelines

In addition to general coding guidelines, there are guidelines for specific diagnoses and/or conditions in the classification. Unless otherwise indicated, these guidelines apply to all health care settings. Please refer to Section II for guidelines on the selection of principal diagnosis.

1. Chapter 1: Certain Infectious and Parasitic Diseases (A00-B99)

a. Human Immunodeficiency Virus (HIV) Infections

1) Code only confirmed cases

Code only confirmed cases of HIV infection/illness. This is an exception to the hospital inpatient guideline Section II, H.

In this context, "confirmation" does not require documentation of positive serology or culture for HIV; the provider's diagnostic statement that the patient is HIV positive, or has an HIV-related illness is sufficient.

2) Selection and sequencing of HIV codes

(a) Patient admitted for HIV-related condition

If a patient is admitted for an HIV-related condition, the principal diagnosis should be B20, Human immunodeficiency virus [HIV] disease followed by additional diagnosis codes for all reported HIV-related conditions.

(b) Patient with HIV disease admitted for unrelated condition

If a patient with HIV disease is admitted for an unrelated condition (such as a traumatic injury), the code for the unrelated condition (e.g., the nature of injury code) should be the principal diagnosis. Other diagnoses would be B20 followed by additional diagnosis codes for all reported HIV-related conditions.

(c) Whether the patient is newly diagnosed

Whether the patient is newly diagnosed or has had previous admissions/encounters for HIV conditions is irrelevant to the sequencing decision.

(d) Asymptomatic human immunodeficiency virus

Z21, Asymptomatic human immunodeficiency virus [HIV] infection status, is to be applied when the patient without any documentation of symptoms is listed as being "HIV positive," "known HIV," "HIV test positive," or similar terminology. Do not use this code if the term "AIDS" is used or if the patient is treated for any HIV-related illness or is described as having any condition(s) resulting from his/her HIV positive status; use B20 in these cases.

(e) Patients with inconclusive HIV serology

Patients with inconclusive HIV serology, but no definitive diagnosis or manifestations of the illness, may be assigned code R75, Inconclusive laboratory evidence of human immunodeficiency virus [HIV].

(f) Previously diagnosed HIV-related illness

Patients with any known prior diagnosis of an HIV-related illness should be coded to B20. Once a patient has developed an HIV-related illness, the patient should always be assigned code B20 on every subsequent admission/encounter. Patients previously diagnosed with any HIV illness (B20) should never be assigned to R75 or Z21, Asymptomatic human immunodeficiency virus [HIV] infection status.

(g) HIV Infection in Pregnancy, Childbirth and the Puerperium

During pregnancy, childbirth or the puerperium, a patient admitted (or presenting for a health care encounter) because of an HIV-related illness should receive a principal diagnosis code of O98.7-, Human immunodeficiency [HIV] disease complicating pregnancy, childbirth and the puerperium, followed by B20 and the code(s) for the HIV-related illness(es). Codes from Chapter 15 always take sequencing priority.

Patients with asymptomatic HIV infection status admitted (or presenting for a health care encounter) during pregnancy, childbirth, or the puerperium should receive codes of O98.7- and Z21.

(h) Encounters for testing for HIV

If a patient is being seen to determine his/her HIV status, use code Z11.4, Encounter for screening for human immunodeficiency virus [HIV]. Use additional codes for any associated high risk behavior.

If a patient with signs or symptoms is being seen for HIV testing, code the signs and symptoms. An additional counseling code Z71.7, Human immunodeficiency virus [HIV] counseling, may be used if counseling is provided during the encounter for the test.

When a patient returns to be informed of his/her HIV test results and the test result is negative, use code Z71.7, Human immunodeficiency virus [HIV] counseling.

If the results are positive, see previous guidelines and assign codes as appropriate.

b. Infectious agents as the cause of diseases classified to other chapters

Certain infections are classified in chapters other than Chapter 1 and no organism is identified as part of the infection code. In these instances, it is necessary to use an additional code from Chapter 1 to identify the organism. A code from category B95, Streptococcus, Staphylococcus, and Enterococcus as the cause of diseases classified to other chapters, B96, Other bacterial agents as the cause of diseases classified to other chapters, or B97, Viral agents as the cause of diseases classified to other chapters, is to be used as an additional code to identify the organism. An instructional note will be found at the infection code advising that an additional organism code is required.

c. Infections resistant to antibiotics

Many bacterial infections are resistant to current antibiotics. It is necessary to identify all infections documented as antibiotic resistant. Assign a code from category Z16, Resistance to antimicrobial drugs, following the infection code only if the infection code does not identify drug resistance.

d. Sepsis, Severe Sepsis, and Septic Shock

1) Coding of Sepsis and Severe Sepsis

(a) Sepsis

For a diagnosis of sepsis, assign the appropriate code for the underlying systemic infection. If the type of infection or causal organism is not further specified, assign code A41.9, Sepsis, unspecified organism.

A code from subcategory R65.2, Severe sepsis, should not be assigned unless severe sepsis or an associated acute organ dysfunction is documented.

(i) Negative or inconclusive blood cultures and sepsis

Negative or inconclusive blood cultures do not preclude a diagnosis of sepsis in patients with clinical evidence of the condition; however, the provider should be queried.

(ii) Urosepsis

The term urosepsis is a nonspecific term. It is not to be considered synonymous with sepsis. It has no default code in the Alphabetic Index.

Should a provider use this term, he/she must be queried for clarification.

(iii) Sepsis with organ dysfunction

If a patient has sepsis and associated acute organ dysfunction or multiple organ dysfunction (MOD), follow the instructions for coding severe sepsis.

(iv) Acute organ dysfunction that is not clearly associated with the sepsis

If a patient has sepsis and an acute organ dysfunction, but the medical record documentation indicates that the acute organ dysfunction is related to a medical condition other than the sepsis, do not assign a code from subcategory R65.2, Severe sepsis. An acute organ dysfunction must be associated with the sepsis in order to assign the severe sepsis code. If the documentation is not clear as to whether an acute organ dysfunction is related to the sepsis or another medical condition, query the provider.

(b) Severe sepsis

The coding of severe sepsis requires a minimum of 2 codes: first a code for the underlying systemic infection, followed by a code from subcategory R65.2, Severe sepsis. If the causal organism is not documented, assign code A41.9, Sepsis, unspecified organism, for the infection. Additional code(s) for the associated acute organ dysfunction are also required.

Due to the complex nature of severe sepsis, some cases may require querying the provider prior to assignment of the codes.

2) Septic shock

(a) Septic shock generally refers to circulatory failure associated with severe sepsis, and therefore, it represents a type of acute organ dysfunction.

For cases of septic shock, the code for the systemic infection should be sequenced first, followed by code R65.21, Severe sepsis with septic shock or code T81.12, Postprocedural septic shock. Any additional codes for the other acute organ dysfunctions should also be assigned. As noted in the sequencing instructions in the Tabular List, the code for septic shock cannot be assigned as a principal diagnosis.

3) Sequencing of severe sepsis

If severe sepsis is present on admission, and meets the definition of principal diagnosis, the underlying systemic infection should be assigned as principal diagnosis followed by the appropriate code from subcategory R65.2 as required by the sequencing rules in the Tabular List. A code from subcategory R65.2 can never be assigned as a principal diagnosis.

When severe sepsis develops during an encounter (it was not present on admission), the underlying systemic infection and the appropriate code from subcategory R65.2 should be assigned as secondary diagnoses.

Severe sepsis may be present on admission, but the diagnosis may not be confirmed until sometime after admission. If the documentation is not clear whether severe sepsis was present on admission, the provider should be queried.

4) Sepsis and severe sepsis with a localized infection

If the reason for admission is both sepsis or severe sepsis and a localized infection, such as pneumonia or cellulitis, a code(s) for the underlying systemic infection should be assigned first and the code for the localized infection should be assigned as a secondary diagnosis. If the patient has severe sepsis, a code from subcategory R65.2 should also be assigned as a secondary diagnosis. If the patient is admitted with a localized infection, such as pneumonia, and sepsis/severe sepsis doesn't develop until after admission, the localized infection should be assigned first, followed by the appropriate sepsis/severe sepsis codes.

5) Sepsis due to a postprocedural infection

(a) Documentation of causal relationship

As with all postprocedural complications, code assignment is based on the provider's documentation of the relationship between the infection and the procedure.

(b) Sepsis due to a postprocedural infection

For such cases, the postprocedural infection code, such as T80.2, Infections following infusion, transfusion, and therapeutic injection, T81.4, Infection following a procedure, T88.0, Infection following immunization, or O86.0, Infection of obstetric surgical wound, should be coded first, followed by the code for the specific infection. If the patient has severe sepsis, the appropriate code from subcategory R65.2 should also be assigned with the additional code(s) for any acute organ dysfunction.

(c) Postprocedural infection and postprocedural septic shock

In cases where a postprocedural infection has occurred and has resulted in severe sepsis the code for the precipitating complication such as code T81.4, Infection following a procedure, or O86.0, Infection of obstetrical surgical wound should be coded first followed by code R65.20, Severe sepsis without septic shock. A code for the systemic infection should also be assigned.

If a postprocedural infection has resulted in postprocedural septic shock, the code for the precipitating complication such as code T81.4, Infection following a procedure, or O86.0, Infection of obstetrical surgical wound should be coded first followed by code T81.12-, Postprocedural septic shock. A code for the systemic infection should also be assigned.

6) Sepsis and severe sepsis associated with a noninfectious process (condition)

In some cases a noninfectious process (condition), such as trauma, may lead to an infection which can result in sepsis or severe sepsis. If sepsis or severe sepsis is documented as associated with a noninfectious condition, such as a burn or serious injury, and this condition meets the definition for principal diagnosis, the code for the noninfectious condition should be sequenced first, followed by the code for the resulting infection. If severe sepsis is present, a code from subcategory R65.2 should also be assigned with any associated organ dysfunction(s) codes. It is not necessary to assign a code from subcategory R65.1, Systemic inflammatory response syndrome (SIRS) of non-infectious origin, for these cases.

If the infection meets the definition of principal diagnosis, it should be sequenced before the non-infectious condition. When both the associated non-infectious condition and the infection meet the definition of principal diagnosis, either may be assigned as principal diagnosis.

Only one code from category R65, Symptoms and signs specifically associated with systemic inflammation and infection, should be assigned. Therefore, when a non-infectious condition leads to an infection resulting in severe sepsis, assign the appropriate code from subcategory R65.2, Severe sepsis. Do not additionally assign a code from subcategory R65.1, Systemic inflammatory response syndrome (SIRS) of non-infectious origin.

See Section I.C.18. SIRS due to non-infectious process

7) Sepsis and septic shock complicating abortion, pregnancy, childbirth, and the puerperium

See Section I.C.15. Sepsis and septic shock complicating abortion, pregnancy, childbirth and the puerperium

8) Newborn sepsis

See Section I.C.16. f. Bacterial sepsis of Newborn

e. Methicillin Resistant Staphylococcus Aureus (MRSA) Conditions

1) Selection and sequencing of MRSA codes

(a) Combination codes for MRSA infection

When a patient is diagnosed with an infection that is due to methicillin resistant *Staphylococcus aureus* (MRSA), and that infection has a combination code that includes the causal organism (e.g., sepsis, pneumonia) assign the appropriate combination code for the condition (e.g., code A41.02, Sepsis due to Methicillin resistant Staphylococcus aureus or code J15.212, Pneumonia due to Methicillin resistant Staphylococcus aureus). Do not assign code B95.62, Methicillin resistant Staphylococcus aureus infection as the cause of diseases classified elsewhere, as an additional code, because the combination code includes the type of infection and the MRSA organism. Do not assign a code from subcategory Z16.11, Resistance to penicillins, as an additional diagnosis.

See Section C.1. for instructions on coding and sequencing of sepsis and severe sepsis.

(b) Other codes for MRSA infection

When there is documentation of a current infection (e.g., wound infection, stitch abscess, urinary tract infection) due to MRSA, and that infection does not have a combination code that includes the causal organism, assign the appropriate code to identify the condition along with code B95.62, Methicillin resistant

Staphylococcus aureus infection as the cause of diseases classified elsewhere for the MRSA infection. Do not assign a code from subcategory Z16.11, Resistance to penicillins.

(c) Methicillin susceptible Staphylococcus aureus (MSSA) and MRSA colonization

The condition or state of being colonized or carrying MSSA or MRSA is called colonization or carriage, while an individual person is described as being colonized or being a carrier.

Colonization means that MSSA or MSRA is present on or in the body without necessarily causing illness. A positive MRSA colonization test might be documented by the provider as "MRSA screen positive" or "MRSA nasal swab positive".

Assign code Z22.322, Carrier or suspected carrier of Methicillin resistant Staphylococcus aureus, for patients documented as having MRSA colonization. Assign code Z22.321, Carrier or suspected carrier of Methicillin susceptible Staphylococcus aureus, for patient documented as having MSSA colonization. Colonization is not necessarily indicative of a disease process or as the cause of a specific condition the patient may have unless documented as such by the provider.

(d) MRSA colonization and infection

If a patient is documented as having both MRSA colonization and infection during a hospital admission, code Z22.322, Carrier or suspected carrier of Methicillin resistant Staphylococcus aureus, and a code for the MRSA infection may both be assigned.

f. Zika virus infections

1) Code only confirmed cases

Code only a confirmed diagnosis of Zika virus (A92.5, Zika virus disease) as documented by the provider. This is an exception to the hospital inpatient guideline Section II, H. In this context, "confirmation" does not require documentation of the type of test performed; the physician's diagnostic statement that the condition is confirmed is sufficient. This code should be assigned regardless of the stated mode of transmission.

If the provider documents "suspected", "possible" or "probable" Zika, do not assign code A92.5. Assign a code(s) explaining the reason for encounter (such as fever, rash, or joint pain) or Z20.828, Contact with and (suspected) exposure to other viral communicable diseases.

2. Chapter 2: Neoplasms (C00-D49)

General guidelines

Chapter 2 of the ICD-10-CM contains the codes for most benign and all malignant neoplasms. Certain benign neoplasms, such as prostatic adenomas, may be found in the specific body system chapters. To properly code a neoplasm it is necessary to determine from the record if the neoplasm is benign, in-situ, malignant, or of uncertain histologic behavior. If malignant, any secondary (metastatic) sites should also be determined.

Primary malignant neoplasms overlapping site boundaries

A primary malignant neoplasm that overlaps two or more contiguous (next to each other) sites should be classified to the subcategory/code .8 ('overlapping lesion'), unless the combination is specifically indexed elsewhere. For multiple neoplasms of the same site that are not contiguous such as tumors in different quadrants of the same breast, codes for each site should be assigned.

Malignant neoplasm of ectopic tissue

Malignant neoplasms of ectopic tissue are to be coded to the site of origin mentioned, e.g., ectopic pancreatic malignant neoplasms involving the stomach are coded to **malignant neoplasm of** pancreas, unspecified (C25.9).

The neoplasm table in the Alphabetic Index should be referenced first. However, if the histological term is documented, that term should be referenced first, rather than going immediately to the Neoplasm Table, in order to determine which column in the Neoplasm Table is appropriate. For example, if the documentation indicates "adenoma," refer to the term in the Alphabetic Index to review the entries under this term and the instructional note to "see also neoplasm, by site, benign." The table provides the proper code based on the type of neoplasm and the site. It is important to select the proper column in the table that corresponds to the type of neoplasm. The Tabular List should then be referenced to verify that the correct code has been selected from the table and that a more specific site code does not exist.

See Section I.C.21. Factors influencing health status and contact with health services, Status, for information regarding Z15.0, codes for genetic susceptibility to cancer.

a. Treatment directed at the malignancy

If the treatment is directed at the malignancy, designate the malignancy as the principal diagnosis.

The only exception to this guideline is if a patient admission/encounter is solely for the administration of chemotherapy, immunotherapy or

external beam radiation therapy, assign the appropriate Z51.-- code as the first-listed or principal diagnosis, and the diagnosis or problem for which the service is being performed as a secondary diagnosis.

b. Treatment of secondary site

When a patient is admitted because of a primary neoplasm with metastasis and treatment is directed toward the secondary site only, the secondary neoplasm is designated as the principal diagnosis even though the primary malignancy is still present.

c. Coding and sequencing of complications

Coding and sequencing of complications associated with the malignancies or with the therapy thereof are subject to the following guidelines:

1) Anemia associated with malignancy

When admission/encounter is for management of an anemia associated with the malignancy, and the treatment is only for anemia, the appropriate code for the malignancy is sequenced as the principal or first-listed diagnosis followed by the appropriate code for the anemia (such as code D63.0, Anemia in neoplastic disease**).**

2) Anemia associated with chemotherapy, immunotherapy and radiation therapy

When the admission/encounter is for management of an anemia associated with an adverse effect of the administration of chemotherapy or immunotherapy and the only treatment is for the anemia, the anemia code is sequenced first followed by the appropriate codes for the neoplasm and the adverse effect (T45.1X5-, Adverse effect of antineoplastic and immunosuppressive drugs).

When the admission/encounter is for management of an anemia associated with an adverse effect of radiotherapy, the anemia code should be sequenced first, followed by the appropriate neoplasm code and code Y84.2, Radiological procedure and radiotherapy as the cause of abnormal reaction of the patient, or of later complication, without mention of misadventure at the time of the procedure.

3) Management of dehydration due to the malignancy

When the admission/encounter is for management of dehydration due to the malignancy and only the dehydration is being treated (intravenous rehydration), the dehydration is sequenced first, followed by the code(s) for the malignancy.

4) Treatment of a complication resulting from a surgical procedure

When the admission/encounter is for treatment of a complication resulting from a surgical procedure, designate the complication as the principal or first-listed diagnosis if treatment is directed at resolving the complication.

d. Primary malignancy previously excised

When a primary malignancy has been previously excised or eradicated from its site and there is no further treatment directed to that site and there is no evidence of any existing primary malignancy, a code from category Z85, Personal history of malignant neoplasm, should be used to indicate the former site of the malignancy. Any mention of extension, invasion, or metastasis to another site is coded as a secondary malignant neoplasm to that site. The secondary site may be the principal or first-listed with the Z85 code used as a secondary code.

e. Admissions/Encounters involving chemotherapy, immunotherapy and radiation therapy

1) Episode of care involves surgical removal of neoplasm

When an episode of care involves the surgical removal of a neoplasm, primary or secondary site, followed by adjunct chemotherapy or radiation treatment during the same episode of care, the code for the neoplasm should be assigned as principal or first-listed diagnosis**.**

2) Patient admission/encounter solely for administration of chemotherapy, immunotherapy and radiation therapy

If a patient admission/encounter is solely for the administration of chemotherapy, immunotherapy or **external beam** radiation therapy assign code Z51.0, Encounter for antineoplastic radiation therapy, or Z51.11, Encounter for antineoplastic chemotherapy, or Z51.12, Encounter for antineoplastic immunotherapy as the first-listed or principal diagnosis. If a patient receives more than one of these therapies during the same admission more than one of these codes may be assigned, in any sequence.

The malignancy for which the therapy is being administered should be assigned as a secondary diagnosis.

If a patient admission/encounter is for the insertion or implantation of radioactive elements (e.g., brachytherapy) the appropriate code for the malignancy is sequenced as the principal or first-listed diagnosis. Code Z51.0 should not be assigned.

3) Patient admitted for radiation therapy, chemotherapy or immunotherapy and develops complications

When a patient is admitted for the purpose of **external beam** radiotherapy, immunotherapy or chemotherapy and develops complications such as uncontrolled nausea and vomiting or dehydration, the principal or first-listed diagnosis is Z51.0, Encounter for antineoplastic radiation therapy, or Z51.11, Encounter for antineoplastic chemotherapy, or Z51.12, Encounter for antineoplastic immunotherapy followed by any codes for the complications.

When a patient is admitted for the purpose of insertion or implantation of radioactive elements (e.g., brachytherapy) and develops complications such as uncontrolled nausea and vomiting or dehydration, the principal or first-listed diagnosis is the appropriate code for the malignancy followed by any codes for the complications.

f. Admission/encounter to determine extent of malignancy

When the reason for admission/encounter is to determine the extent of the malignancy, or for a procedure such as paracentesis or thoracentesis, the primary malignancy or appropriate metastatic site is designated as the principal or first-listed diagnosis, even though chemotherapy or radiotherapy is administered.

g. Symptoms, signs, and abnormal findings listed in Chapter 18 associated with neoplasms

Symptoms, signs, and ill-defined conditions listed in Chapter 18 characteristic of, or associated with, an existing primary or secondary site malignancy cannot be used to replace the malignancy as principal or first-listed diagnosis, regardless of the number of admissions or encounters for treatment and care of the neoplasm.

See section I.C.21. Factors influencing health status and contact with health services, Encounter for prophylactic organ removal.

h. Admission/encounter for pain control/management

See Section I.C.6. for information on coding admission/encounter for pain control/management.

i. Malignancy in two or more noncontiguous sites

A patient may have more than one malignant tumor in the same organ. These tumors may represent different primaries or metastatic disease, depending on the site. Should the documentation be unclear, the provider should be queried as to the status of each tumor so that the correct codes can be assigned.

j. Disseminated malignant neoplasm, unspecified

Code C80.0, Disseminated malignant neoplasm, unspecified, is for use only in those cases where the patient has advanced metastatic disease and no known primary or secondary sites are specified. It should not be used in place of assigning codes for the primary site and all known secondary sites.

k. Malignant neoplasm without specification of site

Code C80.1, Malignant (primary) neoplasm, unspecified, equates to Cancer, unspecified. This code should only be used when no determination can be made as to the primary site of a malignancy. This code should rarely be used in the inpatient setting.

l. Sequencing of neoplasm codes

1) Encounter for treatment of primary malignancy

If the reason for the encounter is for treatment of a primary malignancy, assign the malignancy as the principal/first-listed diagnosis. The primary site is to be sequenced first, followed by any metastatic sites.

2) Encounter for treatment of secondary malignancy

When an encounter is for a primary malignancy with metastasis and treatment is directed toward the metastatic (secondary) site(s) only, the metastatic site(s) is designated as the principal/first-listed diagnosis. The primary malignancy is coded as an additional code.

3) Malignant neoplasm in a pregnant patient

When a pregnant woman has a malignant neoplasm, a code from subcategory O9A.1-, Malignant neoplasm complicating pregnancy, childbirth, and the puerperium, should be sequenced first, followed by the appropriate code from Chapter 2 to indicate the type of neoplasm.

4) Encounter for complication associated with a neoplasm

When an encounter is for management of a complication associated with a neoplasm, such as dehydration, and the treatment is only for the complication, the complication is coded first, followed by the appropriate code(s) for the neoplasm.

The exception to this guideline is anemia. When the admission/encounter is for management of an anemia associated with the malignancy, and the treatment is only for anemia, the appropriate code for the malignancy is sequenced as the principal or first-listed diagnosis followed by code D63.0, Anemia in neoplastic disease.

5) Complication from surgical procedure for treatment of a neoplasm

When an encounter is for treatment of a complication resulting from a surgical procedure performed for the treatment of the neoplasm, designate the complication as the principal/first-listed diagnosis. See guideline regarding the coding of a current malignancy versus personal history to determine if the code for the neoplasm should also be assigned.

6) Pathologic fracture due to a neoplasm

When an encounter is for a pathological fracture due to a neoplasm, and the focus of treatment is the fracture, a code from subcategory M84.5, Pathological fracture in neoplastic disease, should be sequenced first, followed by the code for the neoplasm.

If the focus of treatment is the neoplasm with an associated pathological fracture, the neoplasm code should be sequenced first, followed by a code from M84.5 for the pathological fracture.

m. Current malignancy versus personal history of malignancy

When a primary malignancy has been excised but further treatment, such as an additional surgery for the malignancy, radiation therapy or chemotherapy is directed to that site, the primary malignancy code should be used until treatment is completed.

When a primary malignancy has been previously excised or eradicated from its site, there is no further treatment (of the malignancy) directed to that site, and there is no evidence of any existing primary malignancy, a code from category Z85, Personal history of malignant neoplasm, should be used to indicate the former site of the malignancy.

See Section I.C.21. Factors influencing health status and contact with health services, History (of)

n. Leukemia, Multiple Myeloma, and Malignant Plasma Cell Neoplasms in remission versus personal history

The categories for leukemia, and category C90, Multiple myeloma and malignant plasma cell neoplasms, have codes indicating whether or not the leukemia has achieved remission. There are also codes Z85.6, Personal history of leukemia, and Z85.79, Personal history of other malignant neoplasms of lymphoid, hematopoietic and related tissues. If the documentation is unclear as to whether the leukemia has achieved remission, the provider should be queried.

See Section I.C.21. Factors influencing health status and contact with health services, History (of)

o. Aftercare following surgery for neoplasm

See Section I.C.21. Factors influencing health status and contact with health services, Aftercare

p. Follow-up care for completed treatment of a malignancy

See Section I.C.21. Factors influencing health status and contact with health services, Follow-up

q. Prophylactic organ removal for prevention of malignancy

See Section I.C. 21, Factors influencing health status and contact with health services, Prophylactic organ removal

r. Malignant neoplasm associated with transplanted organ

A malignant neoplasm of a transplanted organ should be coded as a transplant complication. Assign first the appropriate code from category T86.-, Complications of transplanted organs and tissue, followed by code C80.2, Malignant neoplasm associated with transplanted organ. Use an additional code for the specific malignancy.

3. Chapter 3: Disease of the blood and blood-forming organs and certain disorders involving the immune mechanism (D50-D89)

Reserved for future guideline expansion

4. Chapter 4: Endocrine, Nutritional, and Metabolic Diseases (E00-E89)

a. Diabetes mellitus

The diabetes mellitus codes are combination codes that include the type of diabetes mellitus, the body system affected, and the complications affecting that body system. As many codes within a particular category as are necessary to describe all of the complications of the disease may be used. They should be sequenced based on the reason for a particular encounter. Assign as many codes from categories E08–E13 as needed to identify all of the associated conditions that the patient has.

1) Type of diabetes

The age of a patient is not the sole determining factor, though most type 1 diabetics develop the condition before reaching puberty. For this reason type 1 diabetes mellitus is also referred to as juvenile diabetes.

2) Type of diabetes mellitus not documented

If the type of diabetes mellitus is not documented in the medical record the default is E11.-, Type 2 diabetes mellitus.

3) Diabetes mellitus and the use of insulin and oral hypoglycemics

If the documentation in a medical record does not indicate the type of diabetes but does indicate that the patient uses insulin, code E11.-, Type 2 diabetes mellitus, should be assigned. **An additional code should be assigned from category Z79 to identify the long-term (current) use of insulin or oral hypoglycemic drugs. If the patient is treated with both oral medications and insulin, only the code for long-term (current) use of insulin should be assigned. Code Z79.4 should not be assigned if insulin is given temporarily to bring a type 2 patient's blood sugar under control during an encounter.**

4) Diabetes mellitus in pregnancy and gestational diabetes

See Section I.C.15. Diabetes mellitus in pregnancy.

See Section I.C.15. Gestational (pregnancy induced) diabetes

5) Complications due to insulin pump malfunction

(a) Underdose of insulin due to insulin pump failure

An underdose of insulin due to an insulin pump failure should be assigned to a code from subcategory T85.6, Mechanical complication of other specified internal and external prosthetic devices, implants and grafts, that specifies the type of pump malfunction, as the principal or first-listed code, followed by code T38.3X6-, Underdosing of insulin and oral hypoglycemic [antidiabetic] drugs. Additional codes for the type of diabetes mellitus and any associated complications due to the underdosing should also be assigned.

(b) Overdose of insulin due to insulin pump failure

The principal or first-listed code for an encounter due to an insulin pump malfunction resulting in an overdose of insulin, should also be T85.6-, Mechanical complication of other specified internal and external prosthetic devices, implants and grafts, followed by code T38.3X1-, Poisoning by insulin and oral hypoglycemic [antidiabetic] drugs, accidental (unintentional).

6) Secondary diabetes mellitus

Codes under categories E08, Diabetes mellitus due to underlying condition, E09, Drug or chemical induced diabetes mellitus, and E13, Other specified diabetes mellitus, identify complications/manifestations associated with secondary diabetes mellitus. Secondary diabetes is always caused by another condition or event (e.g., cystic fibrosis, malignant neoplasm of pancreas, pancreatectomy, adverse effect of drug, or poisoning).

(a) Secondary diabetes mellitus and the use of insulin or *oral hypoglycemic drugs*

For patients with secondary diabetes mellitus who routinely use insulin or oral hypoglycemic drugs, an additional code from category Z79 should be assigned to identify the long-term (current) use of insulin or oral hypoglycemic drugs. If the patient is treated with both oral medications and insulin, only the code for long-term (current) use of insulin should be assigned. Code Z79.4 should not be assigned if insulin is given temporarily to bring a type 2 patient's blood sugar under control during an encounter.

(b) Assigning and sequencing secondary diabetes codes and its causes

The sequencing of the secondary diabetes codes in relationship to codes for the cause of the diabetes is based on the Tabular List instructions for categories E08, E09 and E13.

(i) Secondary diabetes mellitus due to pancreatectomy

For postpancreatectomy diabetes mellitus (lack of insulin due to the surgical removal of all or part of the pancreas), assign code E89.1, Postprocedural hypoinsulinemia. Assign a code from category E13 and a code from subcategory Z90.41, Acquired absence of pancreas, as additional codes.

(ii) Secondary diabetes due to drugs

Secondary diabetes may be caused by an adverse effect of correctly administered medications, poisoning or sequela of poisoning.

See section I.C.19.e for coding of adverse effects and poisoning, and section I.C.20 for external cause code reporting.

5. **Chapter 5: Mental, Behavioral and Neurodevelopmental disorders (F01–F99)**

   a. **Pain disorders related to psychological factors**

   Assign code F45.41, for pain that is exclusively related to psychological disorders. As indicated by the Excludes 1 note under category G89, a code from category G89 should not be assigned with code F45.41.

   Code F45.42, Pain disorders with related psychological factors, should be used with a code from category G89, Pain, not elsewhere classified, if there is documentation of a psychological component for a patient with acute or chronic pain.

   See Section I.C.6. Pain

   b. **Mental and behavioral disorders due to psychoactive substance use**

      1) **In Remission**

      Selection of codes for "in remission" for categories F10-F19, Mental and behavioral disorders due to psychoactive substance use (categories F10-F19 with **-11**, -.21) requires the provider's clinical judgment. The appropriate codes for "in remission" are assigned only on the basis of provider documentation (as defined in the Official Guidelines for Coding and Reporting), **unless otherwise instructed by the classification.**

      Mild substance use disorders in early or sustained remission are classified to the appropriate codes for substance abuse in remission, and moderate or severe substance use disorders in early or sustained remission are classified to the appropriate codes for substance dependence in remission.

      2) **Psychoactive Substance Use, Abuse and Dependence**

      When the provider documentation refers to use, abuse and dependence of the same substance (e.g., alcohol, opioid, cannabis, etc.), only one code should be assigned to identify the pattern of use based on the following hierarchy:

      ❑ If both use and abuse are documented, assign only the code for abuse

      ❑ If both abuse and dependence are documented, assign only the code for dependence

      ❑ If use, abuse and dependence are all documented, assign only the code for dependence

      ❑ If both use and dependence are documented, assign only the code for dependence.

      3) **Psychoactive Substance Use *Disorders***

      As with all other diagnoses, the codes for psychoactive substance use **disorders** (F10.9-, F11.9-, F12.9-, F13.9-, F14.9-, F15.9-, F16.9-) should only be assigned based on provider documentation and when they meet the definition of a reportable diagnosis (see Section III, Reporting Additional Diagnoses). The codes are to be used only when the psychoactive substance use is associated with a **physical,** mental or behavioral disorder, and such a relationship is documented by the provider.

6. **Chapter 6: Diseases of the Nervous System (G00-G99)**

   a. **Dominant/nondominant side**

   Codes from category G81, Hemiplegia and hemiparesis, and subcategories G83.1, Monoplegia of lower limb, G83.2, Monoplegia of upper limb, and G83.3, Monoplegia, unspecified, identify whether the dominant or nondominant side is affected. Should the affected side be documented, but not specified as dominant or nondominant, and the classification system does not indicate a default, code selection is as follows:

   ❑ For ambidextrous patients, the default should be dominant.

   ❑ If the left side is affected, the default is non-dominant.

   ❑ If the right side is affected, the default is dominant.

   b. **Pain - Category G89**

      1) **General coding information**

      Codes in category G89, Pain, not elsewhere classified, may be used in conjunction with codes from other categories and chapters to provide more detail about acute or chronic pain and neoplasm-related pain, unless otherwise indicated below.

      If the pain is not specified as acute or chronic, post-thoracotomy, postprocedural, or neoplasm-related, do not assign codes from category G89.

      A code from category G89 should not be assigned if the underlying (definitive) diagnosis is known, unless the reason for the encounter is pain control/management and not management of the underlying condition.

      When an admission or encounter is for a procedure aimed at treating the underlying condition (e.g., spinal fusion, kyphoplasty), a code for the underlying condition (e.g., vertebral fracture, spinal stenosis)

should be assigned as the principal diagnosis. No code from category G89 should be assigned.

   (a) **Category G89 Codes as Principal or First-Listed Diagnosis**

   Category G89 codes are acceptable as principal diagnosis or the first-listed code:

   ❑ When pain control or pain management is the reason for the admission/encounter (e.g., a patient with displaced intervertebral disc, nerve impingement and severe back pain presents for injection of steroid into the spinal canal). The underlying cause of the pain should be reported as an additional diagnosis, if known.

   ❑ When a patient is admitted for the insertion of a neurostimulator for pain control, assign the appropriate pain code as the principal or first-listed diagnosis. When an admission or encounter is for a procedure aimed at treating the underlying condition and a neurostimulator is inserted for pain control during the same admission/encounter, a code for the underlying condition should be assigned as the principal diagnosis and the appropriate pain code should be assigned as a secondary diagnosis.

   (b) **Use of Category G89 Codes in Conjunction with Site Specific Pain Codes**

      (i) **Assigning Category G89 and Site-Specific Pain Codes**

      Codes from category G89 may be used in conjunction with codes that identify the site of pain (including codes from chapter 18) if the category G89 code provides additional information. For example, if the code describes the site of the pain, but does not fully describe whether the pain is acute or chronic, then both codes should be assigned.

      (ii) **Sequencing of Category G89 Codes with Site-Specific Pain Codes**

      The sequencing of category G89 codes with site-specific pain codes (including chapter 18 codes), is dependent on the circumstances of the encounter/admission as follows:

      ❑ If the encounter is for pain control or pain management, assign the code from category G89 followed by the code identifying the specific site of pain (e.g., encounter for pain management for acute neck pain from trauma is assigned code G89.11, Acute pain due to trauma, followed by code M54.2, Cervicalgia, to identify the site of pain).

      ❑ If the encounter is for any other reason except pain control or pain management, and a related definitive diagnosis has not been established (confirmed) by the provider, assign the code for the specific site of pain first, followed by the appropriate code from category G89.

      2) **Pain due to devices, implants and grafts**

      See Section I.C.19. Pain due to medical devices

      3) **Postoperative Pain**

      The provider's documentation should be used to guide the coding of postoperative pain, as well as *Section III. Reporting Additional Diagnoses* and *Section IV. Diagnostic Coding and Reporting in the Outpatient Setting*.

      The default for post-thoracotomy and other postoperative pain not specified as acute or chronic is the code for the acute form.

      Routine or expected postoperative pain immediately after surgery should not be coded.

      (a) **Postoperative pain not associated with specific postoperative complication**

      Postoperative pain not associated with a specific postoperative complication is assigned to the appropriate postoperative pain code in category G89.

      (b) **Postoperative pain associated with specific postoperative complication**

      Postoperative pain associated with a specific postoperative complication (such as painful wire sutures) is assigned to the appropriate code(s) found in Chapter 19, Injury, poisoning, and certain other consequences of external causes. If appropriate, use additional code(s) from category G89 to identify acute or chronic pain (G89.18 or G89.28).

      4) **Chronic pain**

      Chronic pain is classified to subcategory G89.2. There is no time frame defining when pain becomes chronic pain. The provider's documentation should be used to guide use of these codes.

      5) **Neoplasm Related Pain**

      Code G89.3 is assigned to pain documented as being related, associated or due to cancer, primary or secondary malignancy, or tumor. This code is assigned regardless of whether the pain is acute or chronic.

This code may be assigned as the principal or first-listed code when the stated reason for the admission/encounter is documented as pain control/pain management. The underlying neoplasm should be reported as an additional diagnosis.

When the reason for the admission/encounter is management of the neoplasm and the pain associated with the neoplasm is also documented, code G89.3 may be assigned as an additional diagnosis. It is not necessary to assign an additional code for the site of the pain.

See Section I.C.2 for instructions on the sequencing of neoplasms for all other stated reasons for the admission/encounter (except for pain control/pain management).

6) Chronic pain syndrome

Central pain syndrome (G89.0) and chronic pain syndrome (G89.4) are different than the term "chronic pain," and therefore codes should only be used when the provider has specifically documented this condition.

See Section I.C.5. Pain disorders related to psychological factors

7. Chapter 7: Diseases of the Eye and Adnexa (H00-H59)

a. Glaucoma

1) Assigning Glaucoma Codes

Assign as many codes from category H40, Glaucoma, as needed to identify the type of glaucoma, the affected eye, and the glaucoma stage.

2) Bilateral glaucoma with same type and stage

When a patient has bilateral glaucoma and both eyes are documented as being the same type and stage, and there is a code for bilateral glaucoma, report only the code for the type of glaucoma, bilateral, with the seventh character for the stage.

When a patient has bilateral glaucoma and both eyes are documented as being the same type and stage, and the classification does not provide a code for bilateral glaucoma (i.e., subcategories H40.10, H40.11 and H40.20) report only one code for the type of glaucoma with the appropriate seventh character for the stage.

3) Bilateral glaucoma stage with different types or stages

When a patient has bilateral glaucoma and each eye is documented as having a different type or stage, and the classification distinguishes laterality, assign the appropriate code for each eye rather than the code for bilateral glaucoma.

When a patient has bilateral glaucoma and each eye is documented as having a different type, and the classification does not distinguish laterality (i.e., subcategories H40.10, H40.11 and H40.20), assign one code for each type of glaucoma with the appropriate seventh character for the stage.

When a patient has bilateral glaucoma and each eye is documented as having the same type, but different stage, and the classification does not distinguish laterality (i.e., subcategories H40.10, H40.11 and H40.20), assign a code for the type of glaucoma for each eye with the seventh character for the specific glaucoma stage documented for each eye.

4) Patient admitted with glaucoma and stage evolves during the admission

If a patient is admitted with glaucoma and the stage progresses during the admission, assign the code for highest stage documented.

5) Indeterminate stage glaucoma

Assignment of the seventh character "4" for "indeterminate stage" should be based on the clinical documentation. The seventh character "4" is used for glaucomas whose stage cannot be clinically determined. This seventh character should not be confused with the seventh character "0", unspecified, which should be assigned when there is no documentation regarding the stage of the glaucoma.

b. Blindness

If "blindness" or "low vision" of both eyes is documented but the visual impairment category is not documented, assign code H54.3, Unqualified visual loss, both eyes. If "blindness" or "low vision" in one eye is documented but the visual impairment category is not documented, assign a code from H54.6-, Unqualified visual loss, one eye. If "blindness" or "visual loss" is documented without any information about whether one or both eyes are affected, assign code H54.7, Unqualified visual loss.

8. Chapter 8: Diseases of the Ear and Mastoid Process (H60-H95)

Reserved for future guideline expansion

9. Chapter 9: Diseases of the Circulatory System (I00-I99)

a. Hypertension

The classification presumes a causal relationship between hypertension and heart involvement and between hypertension and kidney involvement, as the two conditions are linked by the term "with" in the Alphabetic Index. These conditions should be coded as related even in the absence of provider documentation explicitly linking them, unless the documentation clearly states the conditions are unrelated.

For hypertension and conditions not specifically linked by relational terms such as "with," "associated with" or "due to" in the classification, provider documentation must link the conditions in order to code them as related.

1) Hypertension with Heart Disease

Hypertension with heart conditions classified to I50.- or I51.4-I51.9, are assigned to a code from category I11, Hypertensive heart disease. Use additional code(s) from category I50, Heart failure, to identify the type(s) of heart failure in those patients with heart failure.

The same heart conditions (I50.-, I51.4-I51.9) with hypertension are coded separately if the provider has specifically documented a different cause. Sequence according to the circumstances of the admission/encounter.

2) Hypertensive Chronic Kidney Disease

Assign codes from category I12, Hypertensive chronic kidney disease, when both hypertension and a condition classifiable to category N18, Chronic kidney disease (CKD), are present. CKD should not be coded as hypertensive if the physician has specifically documented a different cause.

The appropriate code from category N18 should be used as a secondary code with a code from category I12 to identify the stage of chronic kidney disease.

See Section I.C.14. Chronic kidney disease.

If a patient has hypertensive chronic kidney disease and acute renal failure, an additional code for the acute renal failure is required.

3) Hypertensive Heart and Chronic Kidney Disease

Assign codes from combination category I13, Hypertensive heart and chronic kidney disease, when there is hypertension with both heart and kidney involvement. If heart failure is present, assign an additional code from category I50 to identify the type of heart failure.

The appropriate code from category N18, Chronic kidney disease, should be used as a secondary code with a code from category I13 to identify the stage of chronic kidney disease.

See Section I.C.14. Chronic kidney disease.

The codes in category I13, Hypertensive heart and chronic kidney disease, are combination codes that include hypertension, heart disease and chronic kidney disease. The Includes note at I13 specifies that the conditions included at I11 and I12 are included together in I13. If a patient has hypertension, heart disease and chronic kidney disease, then a code from I13 should be used, not individual codes for hypertension, heart disease and chronic kidney disease, or codes from I11 or I12.

For patients with both acute renal failure and chronic kidney disease, an additional code for acute renal failure is required.

4) Hypertensive Cerebrovascular Disease

For hypertensive cerebrovascular disease, first assign the appropriate code from categories I60-I69, followed by the appropriate hypertension code.

5) Hypertensive Retinopathy

Subcategory H35.0, Background retinopathy and retinal vascular changes, should be used with a code from category I10–I15, Hypertensive disease to include the systemic hypertension. The sequencing is based on the reason for the encounter.

6) Hypertension, Secondary

Secondary hypertension is due to an underlying condition. Two codes are required: one to identify the underlying etiology and one from category I15 to identify the hypertension. Sequencing of codes is determined by the reason for admission/encounter.

7) Hypertension, Transient

Assign code R03.0, Elevated blood pressure reading without diagnosis of hypertension, unless patient has an established diagnosis of hypertension. Assign code O13.-, Gestational [pregnancy-induced] hypertension without significant proteinuria, or O14.-, Pre-eclampsia, for transient hypertension of pregnancy.

8) Hypertension, Controlled

This diagnostic statement usually refers to an existing state of hypertension under control by therapy. Assign the appropriate code from categories I10-I15, Hypertensive diseases.

9) Hypertension, Uncontrolled

Uncontrolled hypertension may refer to untreated hypertension or hypertension not responding to current therapeutic regimen. In either case, assign the appropriate code from categories I10-I15, Hypertensive diseases.

10) Hypertensive Crisis

Assign a code from category I16, Hypertensive crisis, for documented hypertensive urgency, hypertensive emergency or unspecified hypertensive crisis. Code also any identified hypertensive disease (I10-I15). The sequencing is based on the reason for the encounter.

11) Pulmonary Hypertension

Pulmonary hypertension is classified to category I27, Other pulmonary heart diseases. For secondary pulmonary hypertension (I27.1, I27.2-), code also any associated conditions or adverse effects of drugs or toxins. The sequencing is based on the reason for the encounter.

b. Atherosclerotic Coronary Artery Disease and Angina

ICD-10-CM has combination codes for atherosclerotic heart disease with angina pectoris. The subcategories for these codes are I25.11, Atherosclerotic heart disease of native coronary artery with angina pectoris and I25.7, Atherosclerosis of coronary artery bypass graft(s) and coronary artery of transplanted heart with angina pectoris.

When using one of these combination codes it is not necessary to use an additional code for angina pectoris. A causal relationship can be assumed in a patient with both atherosclerosis and angina pectoris, unless the documentation indicates the angina is due to something other than the atherosclerosis.

If a patient with coronary artery disease is admitted due to an acute myocardial infarction (AMI), the AMI should be sequenced before the coronary artery disease.

See Section I.C.9. Acute myocardial infarction (AMI)

c. Intraoperative and Postprocedural Cerebrovascular Accident

Medical record documentation should clearly specify the cause-and-effect relationship between the medical intervention and the cerebrovascular accident in order to assign a code for intraoperative or postprocedural cerebrovascular accident.

Proper code assignment depends on whether it was an infarction or hemorrhage and whether it occurred intraoperatively or postoperatively. If it was a cerebral hemorrhage, code assignment depends on the type of procedure performed.

d. Sequelae of Cerebrovascular Disease

1) Category I69, Sequelae of Cerebrovascular disease

Category I69 is used to indicate conditions classifiable to categories I60-I67 as the causes of sequela (neurologic deficits), themselves classified elsewhere. These "late effects" include neurologic deficits that persist after initial onset of conditions classifiable to categories I60-I67. The neurologic deficits caused by cerebrovascular disease may be present from the onset or may arise at any time after the onset of the condition classifiable to categories I60-I67.

Codes from category I69, Sequelae of cerebrovascular disease, that specify hemiplegia, hemiparesis and monoplegia identify whether the dominant or nondominant side is affected. Should the affected side be documented, but not specified as dominant or nondominant, and the classification system does not indicate a default, code selection is as follows:

❑ For ambidextrous patients, the default should be dominant.

❑ If the left side is affected, the default is non-dominant.

❑ If the right side is affected, the default is dominant.

2) Codes from category I69 with codes from I60-I67

Codes from category I69 may be assigned on a health care record with codes from I60-I67, if the patient has a current cerebrovascular disease and deficits from an old cerebrovascular disease.

3) Codes from category I69 and Personal history of transient ischemic attack (TIA) and cerebral infarction (Z86.73)

Codes from category I69 should not be assigned if the patient does not have neurologic deficits.

See Section I.C.21. 4. History (of) for use of personal history codes

e. Acute myocardial infarction (AMI)

1) Type 1 ST elevation myocardial infarction (STEMI) and non-ST elevation myocardial infarction (NSTEMI)

The ICD-10-CM codes for **type 1** acute myocardial infarction (AMI) identify the site, such as anterolateral wall or true posterior wall. Subcategories I21.0-I21.2 and code I21.3 are used for **type 1** ST elevation myocardial infarction (STEMI). Code I21.4, Non-ST elevation (NSTEMI) myocardial infarction, is used for **type 1** non ST elevation myocardial infarction (NSTEMI) and nontransmural MIs.

If **a type 1** NSTEMI evolves to STEMI, assign the STEMI code. If **a type 1** STEMI converts to NSTEMI due to thrombolytic therapy, it is still coded as STEMI.

For encounters occurring while the myocardial infarction is equal to, or less than, four weeks old, including transfers to another acute setting or a postacute setting, and the myocardial infarction meets the definition for "other diagnoses" (see Section III, Reporting Additional Diagnoses), codes from category I21 may continue to be reported. For encounters after the 4 week time frame and the patient is still receiving care related to the myocardial infarction, the appropriate aftercare code should be assigned, rather than a code from category I21. For old or healed myocardial infarctions not requiring further care, code I25.2, Old myocardial infarction, may be assigned.

2) Acute myocardial infarction, unspecified

Code **I21.9, Acute myocardial infarction, unspecified,** is the default for unspecified acute myocardial infarction **or unspecified type**. If only **type 1** STEMI or transmural MI without the site is documented, assign code I21.3, **ST elevation (STEMI) myocardial infarction of unspecified site**.

3) AMI documented as nontransmural or subendocardial but site provided

If an AMI is documented as nontransmural or subendocardial, but the site is provided, it is still coded as a subendocardial AMI.

See Section I.C.21.3 for information on coding status post administration of tPA in a different facility within the last 24 hours.

4) Subsequent acute myocardial infarction

A code from category I22, Subsequent ST elevation (STEMI) and non-ST elevation (NSTEMI) myocardial infarction, is to be used when a patient who has suffered **a type 1 or unspecified** AMI has a new AMI within the 4 week time frame of the initial AMI. A code from category I22 must be used in conjunction with a code from category I21. The sequencing of the I22 and I21 codes depends on the circumstances of the encounter.

Do not assign code I22 for subsequent myocardial infarctions other than type 1 or unspecified. For subsequent type 2 AMI assign only code I21.A1. For subsequent type 4 or type 5 AMI, assign only code I21.A9.

5) Other Types of Myocardial Infarction

The ICD-10-CM provides codes for different types of myocardial infarction. Type 1 myocardial infarctions are assigned to codes I21.0-I21.4.

Type 2 myocardial infarction, and myocardial infarction due to demand ischemia or secondary to ischemic balance, is assigned to code I21.A1, Myocardial infarction type 2 with a code for the underlying cause. Do not assign code I24.8,

Other forms of acute ischemic heart disease for the demand ischemia. Sequencing of type 2 AMI or the underlying cause is dependent on the circumstances of admission. When a type 2 AMI code is described as NSTEMI or STEMI, only assign code I21.A1. Codes I21.01-I21.4 should only be assigned for type 1 AMIs.

Acute myocardial infarctions type 3, 4a, 4b, 4c and 5 are assigned to code I21.A9, Other myocardial infarction type.

The "Code also" and "Code first" notes should be followed related to complications, and for coding of postprocedural myocardial infarctions during or following cardiac surgery.

10. Chapter 10: Diseases of the Respiratory System (J00-J99)

a. Chronic Obstructive Pulmonary Disease [COPD] and Asthma

1) Acute exacerbation of chronic obstructive bronchitis and asthma

The codes in categories J44 and J45 distinguish between uncomplicated cases and those in acute exacerbation. An acute exacerbation is a worsening or a decompensation of a chronic condition. An acute exacerbation is not equivalent to an infection superimposed on a chronic condition, though an exacerbation may be triggered by an infection.

b. Acute Respiratory Failure

1) Acute respiratory failure as principal diagnosis

A code from subcategory J96.0, Acute respiratory failure, or subcategory J96.2, Acute and chronic respiratory failure, may be assigned as a principal diagnosis when it is the condition established after study to be chiefly responsible for occasioning the admission to the hospital, and the selection is supported by the Alphabetic Index and Tabular List. However, chapter-specific coding guidelines (such as obstetrics, poisoning, HIV, newborn) that provide sequencing direction take precedence.

2) Acute respiratory failure as secondary diagnosis

Respiratory failure may be listed as a secondary diagnosis if it occurs after admission, or if it is present on admission, but does not meet the definition of principal diagnosis.

3) Sequencing of acute respiratory failure and another acute condition

When a patient is admitted with respiratory failure and another acute condition, (e.g., myocardial infarction, cerebrovascular accident, aspiration pneumonia), the principal diagnosis will not be the same in every situation. This applies whether the other acute condition is a respiratory or nonrespiratory condition. Selection of the principal diagnosis will be dependent on the circumstances of admission. If both the respiratory failure and the other acute condition are equally responsible for occasioning the admission to the hospital, and there are no chapter-specific sequencing rules, the guideline regarding two or more diagnoses that equally meet the definition for principal diagnosis (Section II, C.) may be applied in these situations.

If the documentation is not clear as to whether acute respiratory failure and another condition are equally responsible for occasioning the admission, query the provider for clarification.

c. Influenza due to certain identified influenza viruses

Code only confirmed cases of influenza due to certain identified influenza viruses (category J09), and due to other identified influenza virus (category J10). This is an exception to the hospital inpatient guideline Section II, H. (Uncertain Diagnosis).

In this context, "confirmation" does not require documentation of positive laboratory testing specific for avian or other novel influenza A or other identified influenza virus. However, coding should be based on the provider's diagnostic statement that the patient has avian influenza, or other novel influenza A, for category J09, or has another particular identified strain of influenza, such as H1N1 or H3N2, but not identified as novel or variant, for category J10.

If the provider records "suspected" or "possible" or "probable" avian influenza, or novel influenza, or other identified influenza, then the appropriate influenza code from category J11, Influenza due to unidentified influenza virus, should be assigned. A code from category J09, Influenza due to certain identified influenza viruses, should not be assigned nor should a code from category J10, Influenza due to other identified influenza virus.

d. Ventilator associated Pneumonia

1) Documentation of Ventilator associated Pneumonia

As with all procedural or postprocedural complications, code assignment is based on the provider's documentation of the relationship between the condition and the procedure.

Code J95.851, Ventilator associated pneumonia, should be assigned only when the provider has documented ventilator associated pneumonia (VAP). An additional code to identify the organism (e.g., Pseudomonas aeruginosa, code B96.5) should also be assigned. Do not assign an additional code from categories J12-J18 to identify the type of pneumonia.

Code J95.851 should not be assigned for cases where the patient has pneumonia and is on a mechanical ventilator and the provider has not specifically stated that the pneumonia is ventilator-associated pneumonia. If the documentation is unclear as to whether the patient has a pneumonia that is a complication attributable to the mechanical ventilator, query the provider.

2) Ventilator associated Pneumonia Develops after Admission

A patient may be admitted with one type of pneumonia (e.g., code J13, Pneumonia due to Streptococcus pneumonia) and subsequently develop VAP. In this instance, the principal diagnosis would be the appropriate code from categories J12-J18 for the pneumonia diagnosed at the time of admission. Code J95.851, Ventilator associated pneumonia, would be assigned as an additional diagnosis when the provider has also documented the presence of ventilator associated pneumonia.

11. Chapter 11: Diseases of the Digestive System (K00-K95)

Reserved for future guideline expansion

12. Chapter 12: Diseases of the Skin and Subcutaneous Tissue (L00-L99)

a. Pressure ulcer stage codes

1) Pressure ulcer stages

Codes from category L89, Pressure ulcer, identify the site of the pressure ulcer as well as the stage of the ulcer.

The ICD-10-CM classifies pressure ulcer stages based on severity, which is designated by stages 1-4, unspecified stage and unstageable.

Assign as many codes from category L89 as needed to identify all the pressure ulcers the patient has, if applicable.

2) Unstageable pressure ulcers

Assignment of the code for unstageable pressure ulcer (L89.--0) should be based on the clinical documentation. These codes are used for pressure ulcers whose stage cannot be clinically determined (e.g., the ulcer is covered by eschar or has been treated with a skin or muscle graft) and pressure ulcers that are documented as deep tissue injury but not documented as due to trauma. This code should not be confused with the codes for unspecified stage (L89.--9). When there is no documentation regarding the stage of the pressure ulcer, assign the appropriate code for unspecified stage (L89.--9).

3) Documented pressure ulcer stage

Assignment of the pressure ulcer stage code should be guided by clinical documentation of the stage or documentation of the terms found in the Alphabetic Index. For clinical terms describing the stage that are not found in the Alphabetic Index, and there is no documentation of the stage, the provider should be queried.

4) Patients admitted with pressure ulcers documented as healed

No code is assigned if the documentation states that the pressure ulcer is completely healed.

5) Patients admitted with pressure ulcers documented as healing

Pressure ulcers described as healing should be assigned the appropriate pressure ulcer stage code based on the documentation in the medical record. If the documentation does not provide information about the stage of the healing pressure ulcer, assign the appropriate code for unspecified stage.

If the documentation is unclear as to whether the patient has a current (new) pressure ulcer or if the patient is being treated for a healing pressure ulcer, query the provider.

For ulcers that were present on admission but healed at the time of discharge, assign the code for the site and stage of the pressure ulcer at the time of admission.

6) Patient admitted with pressure ulcer evolving into another stage during the admission

If a patient is admitted to an inpatient hospital with a pressure ulcer at one stage and it progresses to a higher stage, two separate codes should be assigned: one code for the site and stage of the ulcer on admission and a second code for the same ulcer site and the highest stage reported during the stay.

b. Non-Pressure Chronic Ulcers

1) Patients admitted with non-pressure ulcers documented as healed

No code is assigned if the documentation states that the non-pressure ulcer is completely healed.

2) Patients admitted with non-pressure ulcers documented as healing

Non-pressure ulcers described as healing should be assigned the appropriate non-pressure ulcer code based on the documentation in the medical record. If the documentation does not provide information about the severity of the healing non-pressure ulcer, assign the appropriate code for unspecified severity.

If the documentation is unclear as to whether the patient has a current (new) non-pressure ulcer or if the patient is being treated for a healing non-pressure ulcer, query the provider.

For ulcers that were present on admission but healed at the time of discharge, assign the code for the site and severity of the non-pressure ulcer at the time of admission.

3) Patient admitted with non-pressure ulcer that progresses to another severity level during the admission

If a patient is admitted to an inpatient hospital with a non-pressure ulcer at one severity level and it progresses to a higher severity level, two separate codes should be assigned: one code for the site and severity level of the ulcer on admission and a second code for the same ulcer site and the highest severity level reported during the stay.

13. Chapter 13: Diseases of the Musculoskeletal System and Connective Tissue (M00-M99)

a. Site and laterality

Most of the codes within Chapter 13 have site and laterality designations. The site represents the bone, joint or the muscle involved. For some conditions where more than one bone, joint or muscle is usually involved, such as osteoarthritis, there is a "multiple sites" code available. For categories where no multiple site code is provided and more than one bone, joint or muscle is involved, multiple codes should be used to indicate the different sites involved.

1) Bone versus joint

For certain conditions, the bone may be affected at the upper or lower end, (e.g., avascular necrosis of bone, M87, Osteoporosis, M80, M81). Though the portion of the bone affected may be at the joint, the site designation will be the bone, not the joint.

b. Acute traumatic versus chronic or recurrent musculoskeletal conditions

Many musculoskeletal conditions are a result of previous injury or trauma to a site, or are recurrent conditions. Bone, joint or muscle conditions that are the result of a healed injury are usually found in chapter 13. Recurrent bone, joint or muscle conditions are also usually found in chapter 13. Any current, acute injury should be coded to the appropriate injury code from chapter 19. Chronic or recurrent conditions should generally be coded with a code from chapter 13. If it is difficult to determine from the documentation in the record which code is best to describe a condition, query the provider.

c. Coding of Pathologic Fractures

7th character A is for use as long as the patient is receiving active treatment for the fracture. While the patient may be seen by a new or different provider over the course of treatment for a pathological fracture, assignment of the 7th character is based on whether the patient is undergoing active treatment and not whether the provider is seeing the patient for the first time.

7th character D is to be used for encounters after the patient has completed active treatment **for the fracture and is receiving routine care for the fracture during the healing or recovery phase**. The other 7th characters, listed under each subcategory in the Tabular List, are to be used for subsequent encounters for treatment of problems associated with the healing, such as malunions, nonunions, and sequelae.

Care for complications of surgical treatment for fracture repairs during the healing or recovery phase should be coded with the appropriate complication codes.

See Section I.C.19. Coding of traumatic fractures.

d. Osteoporosis

Osteoporosis is a systemic condition, meaning that all bones of the musculoskeletal system are affected. Therefore, site is not a component of the codes under category M81, Osteoporosis without current pathological fracture. The site codes under category M80, Osteoporosis with current pathological fracture, identify the site of the fracture, not the osteoporosis.

1) Osteoporosis without pathological fracture

Category M81, Osteoporosis without current pathological fracture, is for use for patients with osteoporosis who do not currently have a pathologic fracture due to the osteoporosis, even if they have had a fracture in the past. For patients with a history of osteoporosis fractures, status code Z87.310, Personal history of (healed) osteoporosis fracture, should follow the code from M81.

2) Osteoporosis with current pathological fracture

Category M80, Osteoporosis with current pathological fracture, is for patients who have a current pathologic fracture at the time of an encounter. The codes under M80 identify the site of the fracture. A code from category M80, not a traumatic fracture code, should be used for any patient with known osteoporosis who suffers a fracture, even if the patient had a minor fall or trauma, if that fall or trauma would not usually break a normal, healthy bone.

14. Chapter 14: Diseases of Genitourinary System (N00-N99)

a. Chronic kidney disease

1) Stages of chronic kidney disease (CKD)

The ICD-10-CM classifies CKD based on severity. The severity of CKD is designated by stages 1-5. Stage 2, code N18.2, equates to mild CKD; stage 3, code N18.3, equates to moderate CKD; and stage 4, code N18.4, equates to severe CKD. Code N18.6, End stage renal disease (ESRD), is assigned when the provider has documented end-stage-renal disease (ESRD).

If both a stage of CKD and ESRD are documented, assign code N18.6 only.

2) Chronic kidney disease and kidney transplant status

Patients who have undergone kidney transplant may still have some form of chronic kidney disease (CKD) because the kidney transplant may not fully restore kidney function. Therefore, the presence of CKD alone does not constitute a transplant complication. Assign the appropriate N18 code for the patient's stage of CKD and code Z94.0, Kidney transplant status. If a transplant complication such as failure or rejection or other transplant complication is documented, see section I.C.19.g for information on coding complications of a kidney transplant. If the documentation is unclear as to whether the patient has a complication of the transplant, query the provider.

3) Chronic kidney disease with other conditions

Patients with CKD may also suffer from other serious conditions, most commonly diabetes mellitus and hypertension. The sequencing of the CKD code in relationship to codes for other contributing conditions is based on the conventions in the Tabular List.

See I.C.9. Hypertensive chronic kidney disease.

See I.C.19. Chronic kidney disease and kidney transplant complications.

15. Chapter 15: Pregnancy, Childbirth, and the Puerperium (O00-O9A)

a. General Rules for Obstetric Cases

1) Codes from chapter 15 and sequencing priority

Obstetric cases require codes from chapter 15, codes in the range O00-O9A, Pregnancy, Childbirth, and the Puerperium. Chapter 15 codes have sequencing priority over codes from other chapters. Additional codes from other chapters may be used in conjunction with chapter 15 codes to further specify conditions. Should the provider document that the pregnancy is incidental to the encounter, then code Z33.1, Pregnant state, incidental, should be used in place of any chapter 15 codes. It is the provider's responsibility to state that the condition being treated is not affecting the pregnancy.

2) Chapter 15 codes used only on the maternal record

Chapter 15 codes are to be used only on the maternal record, never on the record of the newborn.

3) Final character for trimester

The majority of codes in Chapter 15 have a final character indicating the trimester of pregnancy. The timeframes for the trimesters are indicated at the beginning of the chapter. If trimester is not a component of a code, it is because the condition always occurs in a specific trimester, or the concept of trimester of pregnancy is not applicable. Certain codes have characters for only certain trimesters because the condition does not occur in all trimesters, but it may occur in more than just one.

Assignment of the final character for trimester should be based on the provider's documentation of the trimester (or number of weeks) for the current admission/encounter. This applies to the assignment of trimester for pre-existing conditions as well as those that develop during or are due to the pregnancy. The provider's documentation of the number of weeks may be used to assign the appropriate code identifying the trimester.

Whenever delivery occurs during the current admission, and there is an "in childbirth" option for the obstetric complication being coded, the "in childbirth" code should be assigned.

4) Selection of trimester for inpatient admissions that encompass more than one trimester

In instances when a patient is admitted to a hospital for complications of pregnancy during one trimester and remains in the hospital into a subsequent trimester, the trimester character for the antepartum complication code should be assigned on the basis of the trimester when the complication developed, not the trimester of the discharge. If the condition developed prior to the current admission/encounter or represents a pre-existing condition, the trimester character for the trimester at the time of the admission/encounter should be assigned.

5) Unspecified trimester

Each category that includes codes for trimester has a code for "unspecified trimester." The "unspecified trimester" code should rarely be used, such as when the documentation in the record is insufficient to determine the trimester and it is not possible to obtain clarification.

6) 7th character for Fetus Identification

Where applicable, a 7th character is to be assigned for certain categories (O31, O32, O33.3-O33.6, O35, O36, O40, O41, O60.1, O60.2, O64, and O69) to identify the fetus for which the complication code applies.

Assign 7th character "0":

❑ For single gestations

❑ When the documentation in the record is insufficient to determine the fetus affected and it is not possible to obtain clarification.

❑ When it is not possible to clinically determine which fetus is affected.

b. Selection of OB Principal or First-listed Diagnosis

1) Routine outpatient prenatal visits

For routine outpatient prenatal visits when no complications are present, a code from category Z34, Encounter for supervision of normal pregnancy, should be used as the first-listed diagnosis. These codes should not be used in conjunction with chapter 15 codes.

2) Supervision of High-Risk Pregnancy

Codes from category O09, Supervision of high-risk pregnancy, are intended for use only during the prenatal period. For complications during the labor or delivery episode as a result of a high-risk pregnancy, assign the applicable complication codes from Chapter 15. If there are no complications during the labor or delivery episode, assign code O80, Encounter for full-term uncomplicated delivery.

For routine prenatal outpatient visits for patients with high-risk pregnancies, a code from category O09, Supervision of high-risk pregnancy, should be used as the first-listed diagnosis. Secondary chapter 15 codes may be used in conjunction with these codes if appropriate.

3) Episodes when no delivery occurs

In episodes when no delivery occurs, the principal diagnosis should correspond to the principal complication of the pregnancy which necessitated the encounter. Should more than one complication exist, all of which are treated or monitored, any of the complications codes may be sequenced first.

4) When a delivery occurs

When an obstetric patient is admitted and delivers during that admission, the condition that prompted the admission should be sequenced as the principal diagnosis. If multiple conditions prompted the admission, sequence the one most related to the delivery as the principal diagnosis. A code for any complication of the delivery should be assigned as an additional diagnosis. In cases of cesarean delivery, if the patient was admitted with a condition that resulted in the performance of a cesarean procedure, that condition should be selected as the principal diagnosis. If the reason for the admission was unrelated to the condition resulting in the cesarean delivery, the condition related to the reason for the admission should be selected as the principal diagnosis.

5) Outcome of delivery

A code from category Z37, Outcome of delivery, should be included on every maternal record when a delivery has occurred. These codes are not to be used on subsequent records or on the newborn record.

c. Pre-existing conditions versus conditions due to the pregnancy

Certain categories in Chapter 15 distinguish between conditions of the mother that existed prior to pregnancy (pre-existing) and those that are a direct result of pregnancy. When assigning codes from Chapter 15, it is important to assess if a condition was pre-existing prior to pregnancy or developed during or due to the pregnancy in order to assign the correct code.

Categories that do not distinguish between pre-existing and pregnancy-related conditions may be used for either. It is acceptable to use codes specifically for the puerperium with codes complicating pregnancy and childbirth if a condition arises postpartum during the delivery encounter.

d. Pre-existing hypertension in pregnancy

Category O10, Pre-existing hypertension complicating pregnancy, childbirth and the puerperium, includes codes for hypertensive heart and hypertensive chronic kidney disease. When assigning one of the O10 codes that includes hypertensive heart disease or hypertensive chronic kidney disease, it is necessary to add a secondary code from the appropriate hypertension category to specify the type of heart failure or chronic kidney disease.

See Section I.C.9. Hypertension.

e. Fetal Conditions Affecting the Management of the Mother

1) Codes from categories O35 and O36

Codes from categories O35, Maternal care for known or suspected fetal abnormality and damage, and O36, Maternal care for other fetal problems, are assigned only when the fetal condition is actually responsible for modifying the management of the mother, i.e., by requiring diagnostic studies, additional observation, special care, or termination of pregnancy. The fact that the fetal condition exists does not justify assigning a code from this series to the mother's record.

2) In utero surgery

In cases when surgery is performed on the fetus, a diagnosis code from category O35, Maternal care for known or suspected fetal abnormality and damage, should be assigned identifying the fetal condition. Assign the appropriate procedure code for the procedure performed.

No code from Chapter 16, the perinatal codes, should be used on the mother's record to identify fetal conditions. Surgery performed in utero on a fetus is still to be coded as an obstetric encounter.

f. HIV Infection in Pregnancy, Childbirth and the Puerperium

During pregnancy, childbirth or the puerperium, a patient admitted because of an HIV-related illness should receive a principal diagnosis from subcategory O98.7-, Human immunodeficiency [HIV] disease complicating pregnancy, childbirth and the puerperium, followed by the code(s) for the HIV-related illness(es).

Patients with asymptomatic HIV infection status admitted during pregnancy, childbirth, or the puerperium should receive codes of O98.7- and Z21, Asymptomatic human immunodeficiency virus [HIV] infection status.

g. Diabetes mellitus in pregnancy

Diabetes mellitus is a significant complicating factor in pregnancy. Pregnant women who are diabetic should be assigned a code from category O24, Diabetes mellitus in pregnancy, childbirth, and the puerperium, first, followed by the appropriate diabetes code(s) (E08-E13) from Chapter 4.

h. Long term use of insulin and oral hypoglycemics

See section I.C.4.a.3 for information on the long term use of insulin and oral hypoglycemic.

i. Gestational (pregnancy induced) diabetes

Gestational (pregnancy induced) diabetes can occur during the second and third trimester of pregnancy in women who were not diabetic prior to pregnancy. Gestational diabetes can cause complications in the pregnancy similar to those of pre-existing diabetes mellitus. It also puts the woman at greater risk of developing diabetes after the pregnancy. Codes for gestational diabetes are in subcategory O24.4, Gestational diabetes mellitus. No other code from category O24, Diabetes mellitus in pregnancy, childbirth, and the puerperium, should be used with a code from O24.4.

The codes under subcategory O24.4 include diet controlled, insulin controlled, and controlled by oral hypoglycemic drugs. If a patient with gestational diabetes is treated with both diet and insulin, only the code for insulin-controlled is required. If a patient with gestational diabetes is treated with both diet and oral hypoglycemic medications, only the code for "controlled by oral hypoglycemic drugs" is required. Code Z79.4, Long-term (current) use of insulin or code Z79.84, Long-term (current) use of oral hypoglycemic drugs, should not be assigned with codes from subcategory O24.4.

An abnormal glucose tolerance in pregnancy is assigned a code from subcategory O99.81, Abnormal glucose complicating pregnancy, childbirth, and the puerperium.

j. Sepsis and septic shock complicating abortion, pregnancy, childbirth and the puerperium

When assigning a chapter 15 code for sepsis complicating abortion, pregnancy, childbirth, and the puerperium, a code for the specific type of infection should be assigned as an additional diagnosis. If severe sepsis is present, a code from subcategory R65.2, Severe sepsis, and code(s) for associated organ dysfunction(s) should also be assigned as additional diagnoses.

k. Puerperal sepsis

Code O85, Puerperal sepsis, should be assigned with a secondary code to identify the causal organism (e.g., for a bacterial infection, assign a code from category B95-B96, Bacterial infections in conditions classified elsewhere). A code from category A40, Streptococcal sepsis, or A41, Other sepsis, should not be used for puerperal sepsis. If applicable, use additional codes to identify severe sepsis (R65.2-) and any associated acute organ dysfunction.

l. Alcohol and tobacco use during pregnancy, childbirth and the puerperium

1) Alcohol use during pregnancy, childbirth and the puerperium

Codes under subcategory O99.31, Alcohol use complicating pregnancy, childbirth, and the puerperium, should be assigned for any pregnancy case when a mother uses alcohol during the pregnancy or postpartum. A secondary code from category F10, Alcohol related disorders, should also be assigned to identify manifestations of the alcohol use.

2) Tobacco use during pregnancy, childbirth and the puerperium

Codes under subcategory O99.33, Smoking (tobacco) complicating pregnancy, childbirth, and the puerperium, should be assigned for any pregnancy case when a mother uses any type of tobacco product during the pregnancy or postpartum. A secondary code from category F17, Nicotine dependence, should also be assigned to identify the type of nicotine dependence.

m. Poisoning, toxic effects, adverse effects and underdosing in a pregnant patient

A code from subcategory O9A.2, Injury, poisoning and certain other consequences of external causes complicating pregnancy, childbirth, and the puerperium, should be sequenced first, followed by the appropriate injury, poisoning, toxic effect, adverse effect or underdosing code, and then the additional code(s) that specifies the condition caused by the poisoning, toxic effect, adverse effect or underdosing.

See Section I.C.19. Adverse effects, poisoning, underdosing and toxic effects.

n. Normal Delivery, Code O80

1) Encounter for full term uncomplicated delivery

Code O80 should be assigned when a woman is admitted for a full-term normal delivery and delivers a single, healthy infant without any complications antepartum, during the delivery, or postpartum during the delivery episode. Code O80 is always a principal diagnosis. It is not to be used if any other code from chapter 15 is needed to describe a current complication of the antenatal, delivery, or perinatal period. Additional codes from other chapters may be used with code O80 if they are not related to or are in any way complicating the pregnancy.

2) Uncomplicated delivery with resolved antepartum complication

Code O80 may be used if the patient had a complication at some point during the pregnancy, but the complication is not present at the time of the admission for delivery.

3) Outcome of delivery for O80

Z37.0, Single live birth, is the only outcome of delivery code appropriate for use with O80.

o. The Peripartum and Postpartum Periods

1) Peripartum and Postpartum periods

The postpartum period begins immediately after delivery and continues for six weeks following delivery. The peripartum period is defined as the last month of pregnancy to five months postpartum.

2) Peripartum and postpartum complication

A postpartum complication is any complication occurring within the six-week period.

3) Pregnancy-related complications after 6 week period

Chapter 15 codes may also be used to describe pregnancy-related complications after the peripartum or postpartum period if the provider documents that a condition is pregnancy related.

4) Admission for routine postpartum care following delivery outside hospital

When the mother delivers outside the hospital prior to admission and is admitted for routine postpartum care and no complications are noted, code Z39.0, Encounter for care and examination of mother immediately after delivery, should be assigned as the principal diagnosis.

5) Pregnancy associated cardiomyopathy

Pregnancy associated cardiomyopathy, code O90.3, is unique in that it may be diagnosed in the third trimester of pregnancy but may continue to progress months after delivery. For this reason, it is referred to as peripartum cardiomyopathy. Code O90.3 is only for use when the cardiomyopathy develops as a result of pregnancy in a woman who did not have pre-existing heart disease.

p. Code O94, Sequelae of complication of pregnancy, childbirth, and the puerperium

1) Code O94

Code O94, Sequelae of complication of pregnancy, childbirth, and the puerperium, is for use in those cases when an initial complication of a pregnancy develops a sequelae requiring care or treatment at a future date.

2) After the initial postpartum period

This code may be used at any time after the initial postpartum period.

3) Sequencing of Code O94

This code, like all sequela codes, is to be sequenced following the code describing the sequelae of the complication.

q. Termination of Pregnancy and Spontaneous abortions

1) Abortion with Liveborn Fetus

When an attempted termination of pregnancy results in a liveborn fetus, assign code Z33.2, Encounter for elective termination of pregnancy and a code from category Z37, Outcome of Delivery.

2) Retained Products of Conception following an abortion

Subsequent encounters for retained products of conception following a spontaneous abortion or elective termination of pregnancy, **without complications** are assigned O03.**4, Incomplete spontaneous,** abortion **without complication**, or codes O07.4, Failed attempted termination of pregnancy without complication. This advice is appropriate even when the patient was discharged previously with a discharge diagnosis of complete abortion. **If the patient has a specific complication associated with the spontaneous abortion or elective termination of pregnancy in addition to retained products of conception, assign the appropriate complication in category O03 or O07 instead of code O03.4 or O07.4**

3) Complications leading to abortion

Codes from Chapter 15 may be used as additional codes to identify any documented complications of the pregnancy in conjunction with codes in categories in **O04**, O07 and O08.

r. Abuse in a pregnant patient

For suspected or confirmed cases of abuse of a pregnant patient, a code(s) from subcategories O9A.3, Physical abuse complicating pregnancy, childbirth, and the puerperium, O9A.4, Sexual abuse complicating pregnancy, childbirth, and the puerperium, and O9A.5, Psychological abuse complicating pregnancy, childbirth, and the puerperium, should be sequenced first, followed by the appropriate codes (if applicable) to identify any associated current injury due to physical abuse, sexual abuse, and the perpetrator of abuse.

See Section I.C.19. Adult and child abuse, neglect and other maltreatment.

16. Chapter 16: Certain Conditions Originating in the Perinatal Period (P00-P96)

For coding and reporting purposes the perinatal period is defined as before birth through the 28th day following birth. The following guidelines are provided for reporting purposes.

a. General Perinatal Rules

1) Use of Chapter 16 Codes

Codes in this chapter are never for use on the maternal record. Codes from Chapter 15, the obstetric chapter, are never permitted on the newborn record. Chapter 16 codes may be used throughout the life of the patient if the condition is still present.

2) Principal Diagnosis for Birth Record

When coding the birth episode in a newborn record, assign a code from category Z38, Liveborn infants according to place of birth and type of delivery, as the principal diagnosis. A code from category Z38 is assigned only once, to a newborn at the time of birth. If a newborn is transferred to another institution, a code from category Z38 should not be used at the receiving hospital.

A code from category Z38 is used only on the newborn record, not on the mother's record.

3) Use of Codes from other Chapters with Codes from Chapter 16

Codes from other chapters may be used with codes from chapter 16 if the codes from the other chapters provide more specific detail. Codes for signs and symptoms may be assigned when a definitive diagnosis has not been established. If the reason for the encounter is a perinatal condition, the code from chapter 16 should be sequenced first.

4) Use of Chapter 16 Codes after the Perinatal Period

Should a condition originate in the perinatal period, and continue throughout the life of the patient, the perinatal code should continue to be used regardless of the patient's age.

5) Birth process or community acquired conditions

If a newborn has a condition that may be either due to the birth process or community acquired and the documentation does not indicate which it is, the default is due to the birth process and the code from Chapter 16 should be used. If the condition is community-acquired, a code from Chapter 16 should not be assigned.

6) Code all clinically significant conditions

All clinically significant conditions noted on routine newborn examination should be coded. A condition is clinically significant if it requires:

❑ clinical evaluation; or

❑ therapeutic treatment; or

❑ diagnostic procedures; or

❑ extended length of hospital stay; or

❑ increased nursing care and/or monitoring; or

❑ has implications for future health care needs

Note: The perinatal guidelines listed above are the same as the general coding guidelines for "additional diagnoses", except for the final point regarding implications for future health care needs. Codes should be assigned for conditions that have been specified by the provider as having implications for future health care needs.

b. Observation and Evaluation of Newborns for Suspected Conditions not Found

1) *Use of Z05 codes*

Assign a code from category Z05, Observation and evaluation of newborns and infants for suspected conditions ruled out, to identify those instances when a healthy newborn is evaluated for a suspected condition that is determined after study not to be present. Do not use a code from category Z05 when the patient has identified signs or symptoms of a suspected problem; in such cases code the sign or symptom.

2) Z05 on Other than the Birth Record

A code from category Z05 may also be assigned as a principal or first-listed code for readmissions or encounters when the code from category Z38 code no longer applies. Codes from category Z05 are for use only for healthy newborns and infants for which no condition after study is found to be present.

3) Z05 on a birth record

A code from category Z05 is to be used as a secondary code after the code from category Z38, Liveborn infants according to place of birth and type of delivery.

c. Coding Additional Perinatal Diagnoses

1) Assigning codes for conditions that require treatment

Assign codes for conditions that require treatment or further investigation, prolong the length of stay, or require resource utilization.

2) Codes for conditions specified as having implications for future health care needs

Assign codes for conditions that have been specified by the provider as having implications for future health care needs.

Note: This guideline should not be used for adult patients.

d. Prematurity and Fetal Growth Retardation

Providers utilize different criteria in determining prematurity. A code for prematurity should not be assigned unless it is documented.

Assignment of codes in categories P05, Disorders of newborn related to slow fetal growth and fetal malnutrition, and P07, Disorders of newborn related to short gestation and low birth weight, not elsewhere classified, should be based on the recorded birth weight and estimated gestational age.

When both birth weight and gestational age are available, two codes from category P07 should be assigned, with the code for birth weight sequenced before the code for gestational age.

e. Low birth weight and immaturity status

Codes from category P07, Disorders of newborn related to short gestation and low birth weight, not elsewhere classified, are for use for a child or adult who was premature or had a low birth weight as a newborn and this is affecting the patient's current health status.

See Section I.C.21. Factors influencing health status and contact with health services, Status.

f. Bacterial Sepsis of Newborn

Category P36, Bacterial sepsis of newborn, includes congenital sepsis. If a perinate is documented as having sepsis without documentation of congenital or community acquired, the default is congenital and a code from category P36 should be assigned. If the P36 code includes the causal organism, an additional code from category B95, Streptococcus, Staphylococcus, and Enterococcus as the cause of diseases classified elsewhere, or B96, Other bacterial agents as the cause of diseases classified elsewhere, should not be assigned. If the P36 code does not include the causal organism, assign an additional code from category B96. If applicable, use additional codes to identify severe sepsis (R65.2-) and any associated acute organ dysfunction.

g. Stillbirth

Code P95, Stillbirth, is only for use in institutions that maintain separate records for stillbirths. No other code should be used with P95. Code P95 should not be used on the mother's record.

17. Chapter 17: Congenital malformations, deformations, and chromosomal abnormalities (Q00-Q99)

Assign an appropriate code(s) from categories Q00-Q99, Congenital malformations, deformations, and chromosomal abnormalities when a malformation/deformation or chromosomal abnormality is documented. A malformation/deformation/or chromosomal abnormality may be the principal/first-listed diagnosis on a record or a secondary diagnosis.

When a malformation/deformation or chromosomal abnormality does not have a unique code assignment, assign additional code(s) for any manifestations that may be present.

When the code assignment specifically identifies the malformation/ deformation or chromosomal abnormality, manifestations that are an inherent component of the anomaly should not be coded separately. Additional codes should be assigned for manifestations that are not an inherent component.

Codes from Chapter 17 may be used throughout the life of the patient. If a congenital malformation or deformity has been corrected, a personal history code should be used to identify the history of the malformation or deformity. Although present at birth, malformation/deformation/or chromosomal abnormality may not be identified until later in life. Whenever the condition is diagnosed by the physician, it is appropriate to assign a code from codes Q00-Q99. For the birth admission, the appropriate code from category Z38,

Liveborn infants, according to place of birth and type of delivery, should be sequenced as the principal diagnosis, followed by any congenital anomaly codes, Q00-Q99.

18. Chapter 18: Symptoms, signs, and abnormal clinical and laboratory findings, not elsewhere classified (R00-R99)

Chapter 18 includes symptoms, signs, abnormal results of clinical or other investigative procedures, and ill-defined conditions regarding which no diagnosis classifiable elsewhere is recorded. Signs and symptoms that point to a specific diagnosis have been assigned to a category in other chapters of the classification.

a. Use of symptom codes

Codes that describe symptoms and signs are acceptable for reporting purposes when a related definitive diagnosis has not been established (confirmed) by the provider.

b. Use of a symptom code with a definitive diagnosis code

Codes for signs and symptoms may be reported in addition to a related definitive diagnosis when the sign or symptom is not routinely associated with that diagnosis, such as the various signs and symptoms associated with complex syndromes. The definitive diagnosis code should be sequenced before the symptom code.

Signs or symptoms that are associated routinely with a disease process should not be assigned as additional codes, unless otherwise instructed by the classification.

c. Combination codes that include symptoms

ICD-10-CM contains a number of combination codes that identify both the definitive diagnosis and common symptoms of that diagnosis.

When using one of these combination codes, an additional code should not be assigned for the symptom.

d. Repeated falls

Code R29.6, Repeated falls, is for use for encounters when a patient has recently fallen and the reason for the fall is being investigated.

Code Z91.81, History of falling, is for use when a patient has fallen in the past and is at risk for future falls. When appropriate, both codes R29.6 and Z91.81 may be assigned together.

e. Coma scale

The coma scale codes (R40.2-) can be used in conjunction with traumatic brain injury codes, acute cerebrovascular disease or sequelae of cerebrovascular disease codes. These codes are primarily for use by trauma registries, but they may be used in any setting where this information is collected. The coma scale may also be used to assess the status of the central nervous system for other non-trauma conditions, such as monitoring patients in the intensive care unit regardless of medical condition. The coma scale codes should be sequenced after the diagnosis code(s).

These codes, one from each subcategory, are needed to complete the scale. The 7th character indicates when the scale was recorded. The 7th character should match for all three codes.

At a minimum, report the initial score documented on presentation at your facility. This may be a score from the emergency medicine technician (EMT) or in the emergency department. If desired, a facility may choose to capture multiple coma scale scores.

Assign code R40.24, Glasgow coma scale, total score, when only the total score is documented in the medical record and not the individual score(s).

f. Functional quadriplegia

GUIDELINE HAS BEEN DELETED EFFECTIVE OCTOBER 1, 2017

g. SIRS due to Non-Infectious Process

The systemic inflammatory response syndrome (SIRS) can develop as a result of certain non-infectious disease processes, such as trauma, malignant neoplasm, or pancreatitis. When SIRS is documented with a noninfectious condition, and no subsequent infection is documented, the code for the underlying condition, such as an injury, should be assigned, followed by code R65.10, Systemic inflammatory response syndrome (SIRS) of non-infectious origin without acute organ dysfunction, or code R65.11, Systemic inflammatory response syndrome (SIRS) of non-infectious origin with acute organ dysfunction. If an associated acute organ dysfunction is documented, the appropriate code(s) for the specific type of organ dysfunction(s) should be assigned in addition to code R65.11. If acute organ dysfunction is documented, but it cannot be determined if the acute organ dysfunction is associated with SIRS or due to another condition (e.g., directly due to the trauma), the provider should be queried.

h. Death NOS

Code R99, Ill-defined and unknown cause of mortality, is only for use in the very limited circumstance when a patient who has already died is brought into an emergency department or other healthcare facility and is pronounced dead upon arrival. It does not represent the discharge disposition of death.

i. NIHSS Stroke Scale

The NIH stroke scale (NIHSS) codes (R29.7--) can be used in conjunction with acute stroke codes (I63) to identify the patient's neurological status and the severity of the stroke. The stroke scale codes should be sequenced after the acute stroke diagnosis code(s).

At a minimum, report the initial score documented. If desired, a facility may choose to capture multiple stroke scale scores.

See Section I.B.14. for information concerning the medical record documentation that may be used for assignment of the NIHSS codes.

19. Chapter 19: Injury, poisoning, and certain other consequences of external causes (S00-T88)

a. Application of 7th Characters in Chapter 19

Most categories in chapter 19 have a 7th character requirement for each applicable code. Most categories in this chapter have three 7th character values (with the exception of fractures): A, initial encounter, D, subsequent encounter and S, sequela. Categories for traumatic fractures have additional 7th character values. While the patient may be seen by a new or different provider over the course of treatment for an injury, assignment of the 7th character is based on whether the patient is undergoing active treatment and not whether the provider is seeing the patient for the first time.

For complication codes, active treatment refers to treatment for the condition described by the code, even though it may be related to an earlier precipitating problem. For example, code T84.50XA, Infection and inflammatory reaction due to unspecified internal joint prosthesis, initial encounter, is used when active treatment is provided for the infection, even though the condition relates to the prosthetic device, implant or graft that was placed at a previous encounter.

7th character "A", initial encounter is used for each encounter where the patient is receiving active treatment for the condition.

7th character "D" subsequent encounter is used for encounters after the patient has completed active treatment of the condition and is receiving routine care for the condition during the healing or recovery phase.

The aftercare Z codes should not be used for aftercare for conditions such as injuries or poisonings, where 7th characters are provided to identify subsequent care. For example, for aftercare of an injury, assign the acute injury code with the 7th character "D" (subsequent encounter).

7th character "S", sequela, is for use for complications or conditions that arise as a direct result of a condition, such as scar formation after a burn. The scars are sequelae of the burn. When using 7th character "S", it is necessary to use both the injury code that precipitated the sequela and the code for the sequela itself. The "S" is added only to the injury code, not the sequela code. The 7th character "S" identifies the injury responsible for the sequela. The specific type of sequela (e.g., scar) is sequenced first, followed by the injury code.

See Section I.B.10 Sequelae, (Late Effects)

b. Coding of Injuries

When coding injuries, assign separate codes for each injury unless a combination code is provided, in which case the combination code is assigned. **Codes from category** T07, Unspecified multiple injuries should not be assigned in the inpatient setting unless information for a more specific code is not available. Traumatic injury codes (S00-T14.9) are not to be used for normal, healing surgical wounds or to identify complications of surgical wounds.

The code for the most serious injury, as determined by the provider and the focus of treatment, is sequenced first.

1) Superficial injuries

Superficial injuries such as abrasions or contusions are not coded when associated with more severe injuries of the same site.

2) Primary injury with damage to nerves/blood vessels

When a primary injury results in minor damage to peripheral nerves or blood vessels, the primary injury is sequenced first with additional code(s) for injuries to nerves and spinal cord (such as category S04), and/or injury to blood vessels (such as category S15). When the primary injury is to the blood vessels or nerves, that injury should be sequenced first.

c. Coding of Traumatic Fractures

The principles of multiple coding of injuries should be followed in coding fractures. Fractures of specified sites are coded individually by site in accordance with both the provisions within categories S02, S12, S22, S32, S42, S49, S52, S59, S62, S72, S79, S82, S89, S92 and the level of detail furnished by medical record content.

A fracture not indicated as open or closed should be coded to closed. A fracture not indicated whether displaced or not displaced should be coded to displaced.

More specific guidelines are as follows:

1) Initial vs. Subsequent Encounter for Fractures

Traumatic fractures are coded using the appropriate 7th character for initial encounter (A, B, C) for each encounter where the patient is receiving active treatment for the fracture. The appropriate 7th character for initial encounter should also be assigned for a patient who delayed seeking treatment for the fracture or nonunion.

Fractures are coded using the appropriate 7th character for subsequent care for encounters after the patient has completed active treatment of the fracture and is receiving routine care for the fracture during the healing or recovery phase.

Care for complications of surgical treatment for fracture repairs during the healing or recovery phase should be coded with the appropriate complication codes.

Care of complications of fractures, such as malunion and nonunion, should be reported with the appropriate 7th character for subsequent care with nonunion (K, M, N,) or subsequent care with malunion (P, Q, R).

Malunion/nonunion: The appropriate 7th character for initial encounter should also be assigned for a patient who delayed seeking treatment for the fracture or nonunion.

The open fracture designations in the assignment of the 7th character for fractures of the forearm, femur and lower leg, including ankle are based on the Gustilo open fracture classification. When the Gustilo classification type is not specified for an open fracture, the 7th character for open fracture type I or II should be assigned (B, E, H, M, Q).

A code from category M80, not a traumatic fracture code, should be used for any patient with known osteoporosis who suffers a fracture, even if the patient had a minor fall or trauma, if that fall or trauma would not usually break a normal, healthy bone.

See Section I.C.13. Osteoporosis.

The aftercare Z codes should not be used for aftercare for traumatic fractures. For aftercare of a traumatic fracture, assign the acute fracture code with the appropriate 7th character.

2) Multiple fractures sequencing

Multiple fractures are sequenced in accordance with the severity of the fracture.

d. Coding of Burns and Corrosions

The ICD-10-CM makes a distinction between burns and corrosions. The burn codes are for thermal burns, except sunburns, that come from a heat source, such as a fire or hot appliance. The burn codes are also for burns resulting from electricity and radiation. Corrosions are burns due to chemicals. The guidelines are the same for burns and corrosions.

Current burns (T20-T25) are classified by depth, extent and by agent (X code). Burns are classified by depth as first degree (erythema), second degree (blistering), and third degree (full-thickness involvement). Burns of the eye and internal organs (T26-T28) are classified by site, but not by degree.

1) Sequencing of burn and related condition codes

Sequence first the code that reflects the highest degree of burn when more than one burn is present.

a. When the reason for the admission or encounter is for treatment of external multiple burns, sequence first the code that reflects the burn of the highest degree.

b. When a patient has both internal and external burns, the circumstances of admission govern the selection of the principal diagnosis or first-listed diagnosis.

c. When a patient is admitted for burn injuries and other related conditions such as smoke inhalation and/or respiratory failure, the circumstances of admission govern the selection of the principal or first-listed diagnosis.

2) Burns of the same local site

Classify burns of the same local site (three-character category level, T20-T28) but of different degrees to the subcategory identifying the highest degree recorded in the diagnosis.

3) Non-healing burns

Non-healing burns are coded as acute burns.

Necrosis of burned skin should be coded as a non-healed burn.

4) Infected Burn

For any documented infected burn site, use an additional code for the infection.

5) Assign separate codes for each burn site

When coding burns, assign separate codes for each burn site. Category T30, Burn and corrosion, body region unspecified is extremely vague and should rarely be used.

6) Burns and Corrosions Classified According to Extent of Body Surface Involved

Assign codes from category T31, Burns classified according to extent of body surface involved, or T32, Corrosions classified according to extent of body surface involved, when the site of the burn is not specified or when there is a need for additional data. It is advisable to use category T31 as additional coding when needed to provide data for evaluating burn mortality, such as that needed by burn units. It is also advisable to use category T31 as an additional code for reporting purposes when there is mention of a third-degree burn involving 20 percent or more of the body surface.

Categories T31 and T32 are based on the classic "rule of nines" in estimating body surface involved: head and neck are assigned nine percent, each arm nine percent, each leg 18 percent, the anterior trunk 18 percent, posterior trunk 18 percent, and genitalia one percent. Providers may change these percentage assignments where necessary to accommodate infants and children who have proportionately larger heads than adults, and patients who have large buttocks, thighs, or abdomen that involve burns.

7) Encounters for treatment of sequela of burns

Encounters for the treatment of the late effects of burns or corrosions (i.e., scars or joint contractures) should be coded with a burn or corrosion code with the 7th character "S" for sequela.

8) Sequelae with a late effect code and current burn

When appropriate, both a code for a current burn or corrosion with 7th character "A" or "D" and a burn or corrosion code with 7th character "S" may be assigned on the same record (when both a current burn and sequelae of an old burn exist). Burns and corrosions do not heal at the same rate and a current healing wound may still exist with sequela of a healed burn or corrosion.

See Section I.B.10 Sequela (Late Effects)

9) Use of an external cause code with burns and corrosions

An external cause code should be used with burns and corrosions to identify the source and intent of the burn, as well as the place where it occurred.

e. Adverse Effects, Poisoning, Underdosing and Toxic Effects

Codes in categories T36-T65 are combination codes that include the substance that was taken as well as the intent. No additional external cause code is required for poisonings, toxic effects, adverse effects and underdosing codes.

1) Do not code directly from the Table of Drugs

Do not code directly from the Table of Drugs and Chemicals. Always refer back to the Tabular List.

2) Use as many codes as necessary to describe

Use as many codes as necessary to describe completely all drugs, medicinal or biological substances.

3) If the same code would describe the causative agent

If the same code would describe the causative agent for more than one adverse reaction, poisoning, toxic effect or underdosing, assign the code only once.

4) If two or more drugs, medicinal or biological substances

If two or more drugs, medicinal or biological substances are reported, code each individually unless a combination code is listed in the Table of Drugs and Chemicals.

5) The occurrence of drug toxicity is classified in ICD-10-CM as follows:

(a) Adverse Effect

When coding an adverse effect of a drug that has been correctly prescribed and properly administered, assign the appropriate code for the nature of the adverse effect followed by the appropriate code for the adverse effect of the drug (T36-T50). The code for the drug should have a 5th or 6th character "5" (for example T36.0X5-) Examples of the nature of an adverse effect are tachycardia, delirium, gastrointestinal hemorrhaging, vomiting, hypokalemia, hepatitis, renal failure, or respiratory failure.

(b) Poisoning

When coding a poisoning or reaction to the improper use of a medication (e.g., overdose, wrong substance given or taken in error, wrong route of administration), first assign the appropriate code from categories T36-T50. The poisoning codes have an associated intent as their 5th or 6th character (accidental,

intentional self-harm, assault and undetermined. If the intent of the poisoning is unknown or unspecified, code the intent as accidental intent. The undetermined intent is only for use if the documentation in the record specifies that the intent cannot be determined. Use additional code(s) for all manifestations of poisonings.

If there is also a diagnosis of abuse or dependence of the substance, the abuse or dependence is assigned as an additional code.

Examples of poisoning include:

(i) Error was made in drug prescription Errors made in drug prescription or in the administration of the drug by provider, nurse, patient, or other person.

(ii) Overdose of a drug intentionally taken

If an overdose of a drug was intentionally taken or administered and resulted in drug toxicity, it would be coded as a poisoning.

(iii) Nonprescribed drug taken with correctly prescribed and properly administered drug

If a nonprescribed drug or medicinal agent was taken in combination with a correctly prescribed and properly administered drug, any drug toxicity or other reaction resulting from the interaction of the two drugs would be classified as a poisoning.

(iv) Interaction of drug(s) and alcohol

When a reaction results from the interaction of a drug(s) and alcohol, this would be classified as poisoning.

See Section I.C.4. if poisoning is the result of insulin pump malfunctions.

(c) Underdosing

Underdosing refers to taking less of a medication than is prescribed by a provider or a manufacturer's instruction. For underdosing, assign the code from categories T36-T50 (fifth or sixth character "6").

Codes for underdosing should never be assigned as principal or first-listed codes. If a patient has a relapse or exacerbation of the medical condition for which the drug is prescribed because of the reduction in dose, then the medical condition itself should be coded.

Noncompliance (Z91.12-, Z91.13-) or complication of care (Y63.6-Y63.9) codes are to be used with an underdosing code to indicate intent, if known.

(d) Toxic Effects

When a harmful substance is ingested or comes in contact with a person, this is classified as a toxic effect. The toxic effect codes are in categories T51-T65.

Toxic effect codes have an associated intent: accidental, intentional self-harm, assault and undetermined.

f. Adult and child abuse, neglect and other maltreatment

Sequence first the appropriate code from categories T74, Adult and child abuse, neglect and other maltreatment, confirmed) or T76, Adult and child abuse, neglect and other maltreatment, suspected) for abuse, neglect and other maltreatment, followed by any accompanying mental health or injury code(s).

If the documentation in the medical record states abuse or neglect it is coded as confirmed (T74.-). It is coded as suspected if it is documented as suspected (T76.-).

For cases of confirmed abuse or neglect an external cause code from the assault section (X92-Y09) should be added to identify the cause of any physical injuries. A perpetrator code (Y07) should be added when the perpetrator of the abuse is known. For suspected cases of abuse or neglect, do not report external cause or perpetrator code.

If a suspected case of abuse, neglect or mistreatment is ruled out during an encounter code Z04.71, Encounter for examination and observation following alleged physical adult abuse, ruled out, or code Z04.72, Encounter for examination and observation following alleged child physical abuse, ruled out, should be used, not a code from T76.

If a suspected case of alleged rape or sexual abuse is ruled out during an encounter code Z04.41, Encounter for examination and observation following alleged adult rape or code Z04.42, Encounter for examination and observation following alleged child rape, should be used, not a code from T76.

See Section I.C.15. Abuse in a pregnant patient.

g. Complications of care

1) General guidelines for complications of care

(a) Documentation of complications of care

See Section I.B.16. for information on documentation of complications of care.

2) Pain due to medical devices

Pain associated with devices, implants or grafts left in a surgical site (for example painful hip prosthesis) is assigned to the appropriate code(s) found in Chapter 19, Injury, poisoning, and certain other consequences of external causes. Specific codes for pain due to medical devices are found in the T code section of the ICD-10-CM. Use additional code(s) from category G89 to identify acute or chronic pain due to presence of the device, implant or graft (G89.18 or G89.28).

3) Transplant complications

(a) Transplant complications other than kidney

Codes under category T86, Complications of transplanted organs and tissues, are for use for both complications and rejection of transplanted organs. A transplant complication code is only assigned if the complication affects the function of the transplanted organ. Two codes are required to fully describe a transplant complication: the appropriate code from category T86 and a secondary code that identifies the complication.

Pre-existing conditions or conditions that develop after the transplant are not coded as complications unless they affect the function of the transplanted organs.

See I.C.21. for transplant organ removal status See I.C.2. for malignant neoplasm associated with transplanted organ.

(b) Kidney transplant complications

Patients who have undergone kidney transplant may still have some form of chronic kidney disease (CKD) because the kidney transplant may not fully restore kidney function. Code T86.1- should be assigned for documented complications of a kidney transplant, such as transplant failure or rejection or other transplant complication. Code T86.1- should not be assigned for post kidney transplant patients who have chronic kidney (CKD) unless a transplant complication such as transplant failure or rejection is documented. If the documentation is unclear as to whether the patient has a complication of the transplant, query the provider.

Conditions that affect the function of the transplanted kidney, other than CKD, should be assigned a code from subcategory T86.1, Complications of transplanted organ, Kidney, and a secondary code that identifies the complication.

For patients with CKD following a kidney transplant, but who do not have a complication such as failure or rejection, *see section I.C.14. Chronic kidney disease and kidney transplant status.*

4) Complication codes that include the external cause

As with certain other T codes, some of the complications of care codes have the external cause included in the code. The code includes the nature of the complication as well as the type of procedure that caused the complication. No external cause code indicating the type of procedure is necessary for these codes.

5) Complications of care codes within the body system chapters

Intraoperative and postprocedural complication codes are found within the body system chapters with codes specific to the organs and structures of that body system. These codes should be sequenced first, followed by a code(s) for the specific complication, if applicable.

20. Chapter 20: Chapter 20: External Causes of Morbidity (V00-Y99)

The external causes of morbidity codes should never be sequenced as the first-listed or principal diagnosis.

External cause codes are intended to provide data for injury research and evaluation of injury prevention strategies. These codes capture how the injury or health condition happened (cause), the intent (unintentional or accidental; or intentional, such as suicide or assault), the place where the event occurred the activity of the patient at the time of the event, and the person's status (e.g., civilian, military).

There is no national requirement for mandatory ICD-10-CM external cause code reporting. Unless a provider is subject to a state-based external cause code reporting mandate or these codes are required by a particular payer, reporting of ICD-10-CM codes in Chapter 20, External Causes of Morbidity, is not required. In the absence of a mandatory reporting requirement, providers are encouraged to voluntarily report external cause codes, as they provide valuable data for injury research and evaluation of injury prevention strategies.

a. General External Cause Coding Guidelines

1) Used with any code in the range of A00.0-T88.9 Z00-Z99

An external cause code may be used with any code in the range of A00.0-T88.9, Z00-Z99, classification that **represents** a health condition due to an external cause. Though they are most applicable to injuries, they are also valid for use with such things as infections or diseases due to an external source, and other health conditions, such as a heart attack that occurs during strenuous physical activity.

2) External cause code used for length of treatment

Assign the external cause code, with the appropriate 7th character (initial encounter, subsequent encounter or sequela) for each encounter for which the injury or condition is being treated.

Most categories in chapter 20 have a 7th character requirement for each applicable code. Most categories in this chapter have three 7th character values: A, initial encounter, D, subsequent encounter and S, sequela. While the patient may be seen by a new or different provider over the course of treatment for an injury or condition, assignment of the 7th character for external cause should match the 7th character of the code assigned for the associated injury or condition for the encounter.

3) Use the full range of external cause codes

Use the full range of external cause codes to completely describe the cause, the intent, the place of occurrence, and if applicable, the activity of the patient at the time of the event, and the patient's status, for all injuries, and other health conditions due to an external cause.

4) Assign as many external cause codes as necessary

Assign as many external cause codes as necessary to fully explain each cause. If only one external code can be recorded, assign the code most related to the principal diagnosis.

5) The selection of the appropriate external cause code

The selection of the appropriate external cause code is guided by the Alphabetic Index of External Causes and by Inclusion and Exclusion notes in the Tabular List.

6) External cause code can never be a principal diagnosis

An external cause code can never be a principal (first-listed) diagnosis.

7) Combination external cause codes

Certain of the external cause codes are combination codes that identify sequential events that result in an injury, such as a fall which results in striking against an object. The injury may be due to either event or both. The combination external cause code used should correspond to the sequence of events regardless of which caused the most serious injury.

8) No external cause code needed in certain circumstances

No external cause code from Chapter 20 is needed if the external cause and intent are included in a code from another chapter (e.g., T36.0X1- Poisoning by penicillins, accidental (unintentional)).

b. Place of Occurrence Guideline

Codes from category Y92, Place of occurrence of the external cause, are secondary codes for use after other external cause codes to identify the location of the patient at the time of injury or other condition.

Generally, a place of occurrence code is assigned only once, at the initial encounter for treatment. However, in the rare instance that a new injury occurs during hospitalization, an additional place of occurrence code may be assigned. No 7th characters are used for Y92.

Do not use place of occurrence code Y92.9 if the place is not stated or is not applicable.

c. Activity Code

Assign a code from category Y93, Activity code, to describe the activity of the patient at the time the injury or other health condition occurred.

An activity code is used only once, at the initial encounter for treatment. Only one code from Y93 should be recorded on a medical record.

The activity codes are not applicable to poisonings, adverse effects, misadventures or sequela.

Do not assign Y93.9, Unspecified activity, if the activity is not stated.

A code from category Y93 is appropriate for use with external cause and intent codes if identifying the activity provides additional information about the event.

d. Place of Occurrence, Activity, and Status Codes Used with other External Cause Code

When applicable, place of occurrence, activity, and external cause status codes are sequenced after the main external cause code(s). Regardless of the number of external cause codes assigned, generally there should be only one place of occurrence code, one activity code, and one external cause status code assigned to an encounter. However, in the rare instance that a new injury occurs during hospitalization, an additional place of occurrence code may be assigned.

e. If the Reporting Format Limits the Number of External Cause Codes

If the reporting format limits the number of external cause codes that can be used in reporting clinical data, report the code for the cause/intent most related to the principal diagnosis. If the format permits capture of additional external cause codes, the cause/intent, including medical misadventures, of the additional events should be reported rather than the codes for place, activity, or external status.

f. Multiple External Cause Coding Guidelines

More than one external cause code is required to fully describe the external cause of an illness or injury. The assignment of external cause codes should be sequenced in the following priority:

If two or more events cause separate injuries, an external cause code should be assigned for each cause. The first-listed external cause code will be selected in the following order:

External codes for child and adult abuse take priority over all other external cause codes.

See Section I.C.19., Child and Adult abuse guidelines.

External cause codes for terrorism events take priority over all other external cause codes except child and adult abuse.

External cause codes for cataclysmic events take priority over all other external cause codes except child and adult abuse and terrorism.

External cause codes for transport accidents take priority over all other external cause codes except cataclysmic events, child and adult abuse and terrorism.

Activity and external cause status codes are assigned following all causal (intent) external cause codes.

The first-listed external cause code should correspond to the cause of the most serious diagnosis due to an assault, accident, or self-harm, following the order of hierarchy listed above.

g. Child and Adult Abuse Guideline

Adult and child abuse, neglect and maltreatment are classified as assault. Any of the assault codes may be used to indicate the external cause of any injury resulting from the confirmed abuse.

For confirmed cases of abuse, neglect and maltreatment, when the perpetrator is known, a code from Y07, Perpetrator of maltreatment and neglect, should accompany any other assault codes.

See Section I.C.19. Adult and child abuse, neglect and other maltreatment

h. Unknown or Undetermined Intent Guideline

If the intent (accident, self-harm, assault) of the cause of an injury or other condition is unknown or unspecified, code the intent as accidental intent. All transport accident categories assume accidental intent.

1) Use of undetermined intent

External cause codes for events of undetermined intent are only for use if the documentation in the record specifies that the intent cannot be determined.

i. Sequelae (Late Effects) of External Cause Guidelines

1) Sequelae external cause codes

Sequela are reported using the external cause code with the 7th character "S" for sequela. These codes should be used with any report of a late effect or sequela resulting from a previous injury.

See Section I.B.10 Sequela (Late Effects)

2) Sequela external cause code with a related current injury

A sequela external cause code should never be used with a related current nature of injury code.

3) Use of sequela external cause codes for subsequent visits

Use a late effect external cause code for subsequent visits when a late effect of the initial injury is being treated. Do not use a late effect external cause code for subsequent visits for follow-up care (e.g., to assess healing, to receive rehabilitative therapy) of the injury when no late effect of the injury has been documented.

j. Terrorism Guidelines

1) Cause of injury identified by the Federal Government (FBI) as terrorism

When the cause of an injury is identified by the Federal Government (FBI) as terrorism, the first-listed external cause code should be a code from category Y38, Terrorism. The definition of terrorism employed by the FBI is found at the inclusion note at the beginning of category Y38. Use additional code for place of occurrence (Y92.-). More than one Y38 code may be assigned if the injury is the result of more than one mechanism of terrorism.

2) Cause of an injury is suspected to be the result of terrorism

When the cause of an injury is suspected to be the result of terrorism a code from category Y38 should not be assigned. Suspected cases should be classified as assault.

3) Code Y38.9, Terrorism, secondary effects

Assign code Y38.9, Terrorism, secondary effects, for conditions occurring subsequent to the terrorist event. This code should not be assigned for conditions that are due to the initial terrorist act.

It is acceptable to assign code Y38.9 with another code from Y38 if there is an injury due to the initial terrorist event and an injury that is a subsequent result of the terrorist event.

k. External cause status

A code from category Y99, External cause status, should be assigned whenever any other external cause code is assigned for an encounter, including an Activity code, except for the events noted below. Assign a code from category Y99, External cause status, to indicate the work status of the person at the time the event occurred. The status code indicates whether the event occurred during military activity, whether a non-military person was at work, whether an individual including a student or volunteer was involved in a non-work activity at the time of the causal event.

A code from Y99, External cause status, should be assigned, when applicable, with other external cause codes, such as transport accidents and falls. The external cause status codes are not applicable to poisonings, adverse effects, misadventures or late effects.

Do not assign a code from category Y99 if no other external cause codes (cause, activity) are applicable for the encounter.

An external cause status code is used only once, at the initial encounter for treatment. Only one code from Y99 should be recorded on a medical record.

Do not assign code Y99.9, Unspecified external cause status, if the status is not stated.

21. Chapter 21: Factors influencing health status and contact with health services (Z00-Z99)

Note: The chapter specific guidelines provide additional information about the use of Z codes for specified encounters.

a. Use of Z codes in any healthcare setting

Z codes are for use in any healthcare setting. Z codes may be used as either a first-listed (principal diagnosis code in the inpatient setting) or secondary code, depending on the circumstances of the encounter.

Certain Z codes may only be used as first-listed or principal diagnosis.

b. Z Codes indicate a reason for an encounter

Z codes are not procedure codes. A corresponding procedure code must accompany a Z code to describe any procedure performed.

c. Categories of Z Codes

1) Contact/Exposure

Category Z20 indicates contact with, and suspected exposure to, communicable diseases. These codes are for patients who do not show any sign or symptom of a disease but are suspected to have been exposed to it by close personal contact with an infected individual or are in an area where a disease is epidemic.

Category Z77, Other contact with and (suspected) exposures hazardous to health, indicates contact with and suspected exposures hazardous to health.

Contact/exposure codes may be used as a first-listed code to explain an encounter for testing, or, more commonly, as a secondary code to identify a potential risk.

2) Inoculations and vaccinations

Code Z23 is for encounters for inoculations and vaccinations. It indicates that a patient is being seen to receive a prophylactic inoculation against a disease. Procedure codes are required to identify the actual administration of the injection and the type(s) of immunizations given. Code Z23 may be used as a secondary code if the inoculation is given as a routine part of preventive health care, such as a well-baby visit.

3) Status

Status codes indicate that a patient is either a carrier of a disease or has the sequelae or residual of a past disease or condition. This includes such things as the presence of prosthetic or mechanical devices resulting from past treatment. A status code is informative, because the status may affect the course of treatment and its outcome. A status code is distinct from a history code. The history code indicates that the patient no longer has the condition.

A status code should not be used with a diagnosis code from one of the body system chapters, if the diagnosis code includes the information provided by the status code. For example, code Z94.1, Heart transplant status, should not be used with a code from subcategory T86.2, Complications of heart transplant. The status code does not provide additional information. The complication code indicates that the patient is a heart transplant patient.

For encounters for weaning from a mechanical ventilator, assign a code from subcategory J96.1, Chronic respiratory failure, followed by code Z99.11, Dependence on respirator [ventilator] status.

The status Z codes/categories are:

Z14   Genetic carrier

Genetic carrier status indicates that a person carries a gene, associated with a particular disease, which may be passed to offspring who may develop that disease. The person does not have the disease and is not at risk of developing the disease.

Z15   Genetic susceptibility to disease

Genetic susceptibility indicates that a person has a gene that increases the risk of that person developing the disease.

Codes from category Z15 should not be used as principal or first-listed codes. If the patient has the condition to which he/she is susceptible, and that condition is the reason for the encounter, the code for the current condition should be sequenced first. If the patient is being seen for follow-up after completed treatment for this condition, and the condition no longer exists, a follow-up code should be sequenced first, followed by the appropriate personal history and genetic susceptibility codes. If the purpose of the encounter is genetic counseling associated with procreative management, code Z31.5, Encounter for genetic counseling, should be assigned as the first-listed code, followed by a code from category Z15. Additional codes should be assigned for any applicable family or personal history.

Z16   Resistance to antimicrobial drugs

This code indicates that a patient has a condition that is resistant to antimicrobial drug treatment. Sequence the infection code first.

Z17   Estrogen receptor status

Z18   Retained foreign body fragments

Z19   Hormone sensitivity malignancy status

Z21   Asymptomatic HIV infection status

This code indicates that a patient has tested positive for HIV but has manifested no signs or symptoms of the disease.

Z22   Carrier of infectious disease

Carrier status indicates that a person harbors the specific organisms of a disease without manifest symptoms and is capable of transmitting the infection.

Z28.3   Underimmunization status

Z33.1   Pregnant state, incidental

This code is a secondary code only for use when the pregnancy is in no way complicating the reason for visit. Otherwise, a code from the obstetric chapter is required.

Z66   Do not resuscitate

This code may be used when it is documented by the provider that a patient is on do not resuscitate status at any time during the stay.

Z67   Blood type

Z68   Body mass index (BMI)

As with all other secondary diagnosis codes, the BMI codes should only be assigned when they meet the definition of a reportable diagnosis (see Section III, Reporting Additional Diagnoses).

Z74.01   Bed confinement status

Z76.82   Awaiting organ transplant status

Z78   Other specified health status

Code Z78.1, Physical restraint status, may be used when it is documented by the provider that a patient has been put in restraints during the current encounter. Please note that this code should not be reported when it is documented by the provider that a patient is temporarily restrained during a procedure.

Z79   Long-term (current) drug therapy

Codes from this category indicate a patient's continuous use of a prescribed drug (including such things as aspirin therapy) for the long-term treatment of a condition or for prophylactic use. It is not for use for patients who have

addictions to drugs. This subcategory is not for use of medications for detoxification or maintenance programs to prevent withdrawal symptoms in patients with drug dependence (e.g., methadone maintenance for opiate dependence). Assign the appropriate code for the drug dependence instead.

Assign a code from Z79 if the patient is receiving a medication for an extended period as a prophylactic measure (such as for the prevention of deep vein thrombosis) or as treatment of a chronic condition (such as arthritis) or a disease requiring a lengthy course of treatment (such as cancer). Do not assign a code from category Z79 for medication being administered for a brief period of time to treat an acute illness or injury (such as a course of antibiotics to treat acute bronchitis).

Z88   Allergy status to drugs, medicaments and biological substances

Except: Z88.9, Allergy status to unspecified drugs, medicaments and biological substances status

Z89   Acquired absence of limb

Z90   Acquired absence of organs, not elsewhere classified

Z91.0-   Allergy status, other than to drugs and biological substances

Z92.82   Status post administration of tPA (rtPA) in a different facility within the last 24 hours prior to admission to a current facility

Assign code Z92.82, Status post administration of tPA (rtPA) in a different facility within the last 24 hours prior to admission to current facility, as a secondary diagnosis when a patient is received by transfer into a facility and documentation indicates they were administered tissue plasminogen activator (tPA) within the last 24 hours prior to admission to the current facility.

This guideline applies even if the patient is still receiving the tPA at the time they are received into the current facility.

The appropriate code for the condition for which the tPA was administered (such as cerebrovascular disease or myocardial infarction) should be assigned first.

Code Z92.82 is only applicable to the receiving facility record and not to the transferring facility record.

Z93   Artificial opening status

Z94   Transplanted organ and tissue status

Z95   Presence of cardiac and vascular implants and grafts

Z96   Presence of other functional implants

Z97   Presence of other devices

Z98   Other postprocedural states

Assign code Z98.85, Transplanted organ removal status, to indicate that a transplanted organ has been previously removed. This code should not be assigned for the encounter in which the transplanted organ is removed. The complication necessitating removal of the transplant organ should be assigned for that encounter.

See section I.C19. for information on the coding of organ transplant complications.

Z99   Dependence on enabling machines and devices, not elsewhere classified

Note: Categories Z89-Z90 and Z93-Z99 are for use only if there are no complications or malfunctions of the organ or tissue replaced, the amputation site or the equipment on which the patient is dependent.

4) **History (of)**

There are two types of history Z codes, personal and family. Personal history codes explain a patient's past medical condition that no longer exists and is not receiving any treatment, but that has the potential for recurrence, and therefore may require continued monitoring.

Family history codes are for use when a patient has a family member(s) who has had a particular disease that causes the patient to be at higher risk of also contracting the disease.

Personal history codes may be used in conjunction with follow-up codes and family history codes may be used in conjunction with screening codes to explain the need for a test or procedure. History codes are also acceptable on any medical record regardless of the reason for visit. A history of an illness, even if no longer present, is important information that may alter the type of treatment ordered.

The history Z code categories are:

Z80   Family history of primary malignant neoplasm

Z81   Family history of mental and behavioral disorders

Z82   Family history of certain disabilities and chronic diseases (leading to disablement)

Z83   Family history of other specific disorders

Z84   Family history of other conditions

Z85   Personal history of malignant neoplasm

Z86   Personal history of certain other diseases

Z87   Personal history of other diseases and conditions

Z91.4-   Personal history of psychological trauma, not elsewhere classified

Z91.5   Personal history of self-harm

Z91.81   History of falling

Z91.82   Personal history of military deployment

Z92   Personal history of medical treatment

Except: Z92.0, Personal history of contraception Except: Z92.82, Status post administration of tPA (rtPA) in a different facility within the last 24 hours prior to admission to a current facility

5) Screening

Screening is the testing for disease or disease precursors in seemingly well individuals so that early detection and treatment can be provided for those who test positive for the disease (e.g., screening mammogram).

The testing of a person to rule out or confirm a suspected diagnosis because the patient has some sign or symptom is a diagnostic examination, not a screening. In these cases, the sign or symptom is used to explain the reason for the test.

A screening code may be a first-listed code if the reason for the visit is specifically the screening exam. It may also be used as an additional code if the screening is done during an office visit for other health problems. A screening code is not necessary if the screening is inherent to a routine examination, such as a pap smear done during a routine pelvic examination.

Should a condition be discovered during the screening then the code for the condition may be assigned as an additional diagnosis.

The Z code indicates that a screening exam is planned. A procedure code is required to confirm that the screening was performed.

The screening Z codes/categories:

Z11   Encounter for screening for infectious and parasitic diseases

Z12   Encounter for screening for malignant neoplasms

Z13   Encounter for screening for other diseases and disorders

Except: Z13.9, Encounter for screening, unspecified

Z36   Encounter for antenatal screening for mother

6) Observation

There are three observation Z code categories. They are for use in very limited circumstances when a person is being observed for a suspected condition that is ruled out. The observation codes are not for use if an injury or illness or any signs or symptoms related to the suspected condition are present. In such cases the diagnosis/symptom code is used with the corresponding external cause code.

The observation codes are to be used as principal diagnosis only. The only exception to this is when the principal diagnosis is required to be a code from category Z38, Liveborn infants according to place of birth and type of delivery. Then a code from category Z05, Encounter for observation and evaluation of newborn for suspected diseases and conditions ruled out, is sequenced after the Z38 code. Additional codes may be used in addition to the observation code, but only if they are unrelated to the suspected condition being observed.

Codes from subcategory Z03.7, Encounter for suspected maternal and fetal conditions ruled out, may either be used as a first-listed or as an additional code assignment depending on the case. They are for use in very limited circumstances on a maternal record when an encounter is for a suspected maternal or fetal condition that is ruled out during that encounter (for example, a maternal or fetal condition may be suspected due to an abnormal test result). These codes should not be used when the condition is confirmed. In those cases, the confirmed condition should be coded. In addition, these codes are not for use if an illness or any signs or symptoms related to the suspected condition or problem are present. In such cases the diagnosis/symptom code is used.

Additional codes may be used in addition to the code from subcategory Z03.7, but only if they are unrelated to the suspected condition being evaluated.

Codes from subcategory Z03.7 may not be used for encounters for antenatal screening of mother. *See Section I.C.21. Screening.*

For encounters for suspected fetal condition that are inconclusive following testing and evaluation, assign the appropriate code from category O35, O36, O40 or O41.

The observation Z code categories:

Z03   Encounter for medical observation for suspected diseases and conditions ruled out

Z04   Encounter for examination and observation for other reasons

Except: Z04.9, Encounter for examination and observation for unspecified reason

Z05   Encounter for observation and evaluation of newborn for suspected diseases and conditions ruled out

7) Aftercare

Aftercare visit codes cover situations when the initial treatment of a disease has been performed and the patient requires continued care during the healing or recovery phase, or for the long-term consequences of the disease. The aftercare Z code should not be used if treatment is directed at a current, acute disease. The diagnosis code is to be used in these cases. Exceptions to this rule are codes Z51.0, Encounter for antineoplastic radiation therapy, and codes from subcategory Z51.1, Encounter for antineoplastic chemotherapy and immunotherapy. These codes are to be first-listed, followed by the diagnosis code when a patient's encounter is solely to receive radiation therapy, chemotherapy, or immunotherapy for the treatment of a neoplasm. If the reason for the encounter is more than one type of antineoplastic therapy, code Z51.0 and a code from subcategory Z51.1 may be assigned together, in which case one of these codes would be reported as a secondary diagnosis.

The aftercare Z codes should also not be used for aftercare for injuries. For aftercare of an injury, assign the acute injury code with the appropriate 7th character (for subsequent encounter).

The aftercare codes are generally first-listed to explain the specific reason for the encounter. An aftercare code may be used as an additional code when some type of aftercare is provided in addition to the reason for admission and no diagnosis code is applicable. An example of this would be the closure of a colostomy during an encounter for treatment of another condition.

Aftercare codes should be used in conjunction with other aftercare codes or diagnosis codes to provide better detail on the specifics of an aftercare encounter visit, unless otherwise directed by the classification. Should a patient receive multiple types of antineoplastic therapy during the same encounter, code Z51.0, Encounter for antineoplastic radiation therapy, and codes from subcategory Z51.1, Encounter for antineoplastic chemotherapy and immunotherapy, may be used together on a record. The sequencing of multiple aftercare codes depends on the circumstances of the encounter.

Certain aftercare Z code categories need a secondary diagnosis code to describe the resolving condition or sequelae. For others, the condition is included in the code title.

Additional Z code aftercare category terms include fitting and adjustment, and attention to artificial openings.

Status Z codes may be used with aftercare Z codes to indicate the nature of the aftercare. For example code Z95.1, Presence of aortocoronary bypass graft, may be used with code Z48.812, Encounter for surgical aftercare following surgery on the circulatory system, to indicate the surgery for which the aftercare is being performed. A status code should not be used when the aftercare code indicates the type of status, such as using Z43.0, Encounter for attention to tracheostomy, with Z93.0, Tracheostomy status.

The aftercare Z category/codes:

Z42   Encounter for plastic and reconstructive surgery following medical procedure or healed injury

Z43   Encounter for attention to artificial openings

Z44   Encounter for fitting and adjustment of external prosthetic device

Z45   Encounter for adjustment and management of implanted device

Z46   Encounter for fitting and adjustment of other devices

Z47   Orthopedic aftercare

Z48   Encounter for other postprocedural aftercare

Z49   Encounter for care involving renal dialysis

Z51   Encounter for other aftercare and medical care

8) Follow-up

The follow-up codes are used to explain continuing surveillance following completed treatment of a disease, condition, or injury. They imply that the condition has been fully treated and no longer exists. They should not be confused with aftercare codes, or injury codes with a 7th character for subsequent encounter, that explain ongoing care of a healing condition or its sequelae. Follow-up codes may be used in conjunction with history codes to provide the full picture of the healed condition and its treatment. The follow-up code is sequenced first, followed by the history code.

A follow-up code may be used to explain multiple visits. Should a condition be found to have recurred on the follow-up visit, then the diagnosis code for the condition should be assigned in place of the follow-up code.

The follow-up Z code categories:

Z08   Encounter for follow-up examination after completed treatment for malignant neoplasm

Z09   Encounter for follow-up examination after completed treatment for conditions other than malignant neoplasm

Z39   Encounter for maternal postpartum care and examination

9) Donor

Codes in category Z52, Donors of organs and tissues, are used for living individuals who are donating blood or other body tissue. These codes are only for individuals donating for others, not for self-donations. They are not used to identify cadaveric donations.

10) Counseling

Counseling Z codes are used when a patient or family member receives assistance in the aftermath of an illness or injury, or when support is required in coping with family or social problems.

The counseling Z codes/categories:

Z30.0-   Encounter for general counseling and advice on contraception

Z31.5   Encounter for **procreative** genetic counseling

Z31.6-   Encounter for general counseling and advice on procreation

Z32.2   Encounter for childbirth instruction

Z32.3   Encounter for childcare instruction

Z69   Encounter for mental health services for victim and perpetrator of abuse

Z70   Counseling related to sexual attitude, behavior and orientation

Z71   Persons encountering health services for other counseling and medical advice, not elsewhere classified

Z76.81   Expectant mother prebirth pediatrician visit

11) Encounters for Obstetrical and Reproductive Services

See Section I.C.15. Pregnancy, Childbirth, and the Puerperium, for further instruction on the use of these codes.

Z codes for pregnancy are for use in those circumstances when none of the problems or complications included in the codes from the Obstetrics chapter exist (a routine prenatal visit or postpartum care). Codes in category Z34, Encounter for supervision of normal pregnancy, are always first-listed and are not to be used with any other code from the OB chapter.

Codes in category Z3A, Weeks of gestation, may be assigned to provide additional information about the pregnancy. Category Z3A codes should not be assigned for pregnancies with abortive outcomes (categories O00-O08), elective termination of pregnancy (code **Z33.2**), nor for postpartum conditions, as category Z3A is not applicable to these conditions. The date of the admission should be used to determine weeks of gestation for inpatient admissions that encompass more than one gestational week.

The outcome of delivery, category Z37, should be included on all maternal delivery records. It is always a secondary code. Codes in category Z37 should not be used on the newborn record.

Z codes for family planning (contraceptive) or procreative management and counseling should be included on an obstetric record either during the pregnancy or the postpartum stage, if applicable.

Z codes/categories for obstetrical and reproductive services:

Z30   Encounter for contraceptive management

Z31   Encounter for procreative management

Z32.2   Encounter for childbirth instruction

Z32.3   Encounter for childcare instruction

Z33   Pregnant state

Z34   Encounter for supervision of normal pregnancy

Z36   Encounter for antenatal screening of mother

Z3A   Weeks of gestation

Z37   Outcome of delivery

Z39   Encounter for maternal postpartum care and examination

Z76.81   Expectant mother prebirth pediatrician visit

12) Newborns and Infants

See Section I.C.16. Newborn (Perinatal) Guidelines, for further instruction on the use of these codes.

Newborn Z codes/categories:

Z76.1   Encounter for health supervision and care of foundling

Z00.1-   Encounter for routine child health examination

Z38   Liveborn infants according to place of birth and type of delivery

13) Routine and administrative examinations

The Z codes allow for the description of encounters for routine examinations, such as, a general check-up, or, examinations for administrative purposes, such as, a pre-employment physical. The codes are not to be used if the examination is for diagnosis of a suspected condition or for treatment purposes. In such cases the diagnosis code is used. During a routine exam, should a diagnosis or condition be discovered, it should be coded as an additional code. Pre-existing and chronic conditions and history codes may also be included as additional codes as long as the examination is for administrative purposes and not focused on any particular condition.

Some of the codes for routine health examinations distinguish between "with" and "without" abnormal findings. Code assignment depends on the information that is known at the time the encounter is being coded. For example, if no abnormal findings were found during the examination, but the encounter is being coded before test results are back, it is acceptable to assign the code for "without abnormal findings." When assigning a code for "with abnormal findings," additional code(s) should be assigned to identify the specific abnormal finding(s).

Pre-operative examination and pre-procedural laboratory examination Z codes are for use only in those situations when a patient is being cleared for a procedure or surgery and no treatment is given.

The Z codes/categories for routine and administrative examinations:

Z00   Encounter for general examination without complaint, suspected or reported diagnosis

Z01   Encounter for other special examination without complaint, suspected or reported diagnosis

Z02   Encounter for administrative examination Except: Z02.9, Encounter for administrative examinations, unspecified

Z32.0-   Encounter for pregnancy test

14) Miscellaneous Z codes

The miscellaneous Z codes capture a number of other health care encounters that do not fall into one of the other categories. Certain of these codes identify the reason for the encounter; others are for use as additional codes that provide useful information on circumstances that may affect a patient's care and treatment.

Prophylactic Organ Removal

For encounters specifically for prophylactic removal of an organ (such as prophylactic removal of breasts due to a genetic susceptibility to cancer or a family history of cancer), the principal or first-listed code should be a code from category Z40, Encounter for prophylactic surgery, followed by the appropriate codes to identify the associated risk factor (such as genetic susceptibility or family history).

If the patient has a malignancy of one site and is having prophylactic removal at another site to prevent either a new primary malignancy or metastatic disease, a code for the malignancy should also be assigned in addition to a code from subcategory Z40.0, Encounter for prophylactic surgery for risk factors related to malignant neoplasms. A Z40.0 code should not be assigned if the patient is having organ removal for treatment of a malignancy, such as the removal of the testes for the treatment of prostate cancer.

Miscellaneous Z codes/categories:

Z28   Immunization not carried out

     Except: Z28.3, Underimmunization status

Z29   Encounter for other prophylactic measures

Z40   Encounter for prophylactic surgery

Z41   Encounter for procedures for purposes other than remedying health state

     Except: Z41.9, Encounter for procedure for purposes other than remedying health state, unspecified

Z53   Persons encountering health services for specific procedures and treatment, not carried out

Z55   Problems related to education and literacy

Z56	Problems related to employment and unemployment
Z57	Occupational exposure to risk factors
Z58	Problems related to physical environment
Z59	Problems related to housing and economic circumstances
Z60	Problems related to social environment
Z62	Problems related to upbringing
Z63	Other problems related to primary support group, including family circumstances
Z64	Problems related to certain psychosocial circumstances
Z65	Problems related to other psychosocial circumstances
Z72	Problems related to lifestyle

Note: These codes should be assigned only when the documentation specifies that the patient has an associated problem

Z73	Problems related to life management difficulty
Z74	Problems related to care provider dependency

Except: Z74.01, Bed confinement status

Z75	Problems related to medical facilities and other health care
Z76.0	Encounter for issue of repeat prescription
Z76.3	Healthy person accompanying sick person
Z76.4	Other boarder to healthcare facility
Z76.5	Malingerer [conscious simulation]
Z91.1-	Patient's noncompliance with medical treatment and regimen
Z91.83	Wandering in diseases classified elsewhere
Z91.84 -	**Oral health risk factors**
Z91.89	Other specified personal risk factors, not elsewhere classified

15) Nonspecific Z codes

Certain Z codes are so non-specific, or potentially redundant with other codes in the classification, that there can be little justification for their use in the inpatient setting. Their use in the outpatient setting should be limited to those instances when there is no further documentation to permit more precise coding. Otherwise, any sign or symptom or any other reason for visit that is captured in another code should be used.

Nonspecific Z codes/categories:

Z02.9	Encounter for administrative examinations, unspecified
Z04.9	Encounter for examination and observation for unspecified reason
Z13.9	Encounter for screening, unspecified
Z41.9	Encounter for procedure for purposes other than remedying health state, unspecified
Z52.9	Donor of unspecified organ or tissue
Z86.59	Personal history of other mental and behavioral disorders
Z88.9	Allergy status to unspecified drugs, medicaments and biological substances status
Z92.0	Personal history of contraception

16) Z Codes That May Only be Principal/First-Listed Diagnosis

The following Z codes/categories may only be reported as the principal/first-listed diagnosis, except when there are multiple encounters on the same day and the medical records for the encounters are combined:

Z00	Encounter for general examination without complaint, suspected or reported diagnosis Except: Z00.6
Z01	Encounter for other special examination without complaint, suspected or reported diagnosis
Z02	Encounter for administrative examination
Z03	Encounter for medical observation for suspected diseases and conditions ruled out
Z04	Encounter for examination and observation for other reasons
Z33.2	Encounter for elective termination of pregnancy
Z31.81	Encounter for male factor infertility in female patient
Z31.83	Encounter for assisted reproductive fertility procedure cycle
Z31.84	Encounter for fertility preservation procedure
Z34	Encounter for supervision of normal pregnancy
Z39	Encounter for maternal postpartum care and examination
Z38	Liveborn infants according to place of birth and type of delivery

Z40	**Encounter for prophylactic surgery**
Z42	Encounter for plastic and reconstructive surgery following medical procedure or healed injury
Z51.0	Encounter for antineoplastic radiation therapy
Z51.1-	Encounter for antineoplastic chemotherapy and immunotherapy
Z52	Donors of organs and tissues
	Except: Z52.9, Donor of unspecified organ or tissue
Z76.1	Encounter for health supervision and care of foundling
Z76.2	Encounter for health supervision and care of other healthy infant and child
Z99.12	Encounter for respirator [ventilator] dependence during power failure

Section II. Selection of Principal Diagnosis

The circumstances of inpatient admission always govern the selection of principal diagnosis. The principal diagnosis is defined in the Uniform Hospital Discharge Data Set (UHDDS) as "that condition established after study to be chiefly responsible for occasioning the admission of the patient to the hospital for care."

The UHDDS definitions are used by hospitals to report inpatient data elements in a standardized manner. These data elements and their definitions can be found in the July 31, 1985, Federal Register (Vol. 50, No, 147), pp. 31038-40.

Since that time the application of the UHDDS definitions has been expanded to include all non-outpatient settings (acute care, short term, long term care and psychiatric hospitals; home health agencies; rehab facilities; nursing homes, etc). The UHDDS definitions also apply to hospice services (all levels of care).

In determining principal diagnosis, coding conventions in the ICD-10-CM, the Tabular List and Alphabetic Index take precedence over these official coding guidelines.

(See Section I.A., Conventions for the ICD-10-CM)

The importance of consistent, complete documentation in the medical record cannot be overemphasized. Without such documentation the application of all coding guidelines is a difficult, if not impossible, task.

A. Codes for symptoms, signs, and ill-defined conditions

Codes for symptoms, signs, and ill-defined conditions from Chapter 18 are not to be used as principal diagnosis when a related definitive diagnosis has been established.

B. Two or more interrelated conditions, each potentially meeting the definition for principal diagnosis.

When there are two or more interrelated conditions (such as diseases in the same ICD-10-CM chapter or manifestations characteristically associated with a certain disease) potentially meeting the definition of principal diagnosis, either condition may be sequenced first, unless the circumstances of the admission, the therapy provided, the Tabular List, or the Alphabetic Index indicate otherwise.

C. Two or more diagnoses that equally meet the definition for principal diagnosis

In the unusual instance when two or more diagnoses equally meet the criteria for principal diagnosis as determined by the circumstances of admission, diagnostic workup and/or therapy provided, and the Alphabetic Index, Tabular List, or another coding guidelines does not provide sequencing direction, any one of the diagnoses may be sequenced first.

D. Two or more comparative or contrasting conditions

In those rare instances when two or more contrasting or comparative diagnoses are documented as "either/or" (or similar terminology), they are coded as if the diagnoses were confirmed and the diagnoses are sequenced according to the circumstances of the admission. If no further determination can be made as to which diagnosis should be principal, either diagnosis may be sequenced first.

E. A symptom(s) followed by contrasting/comparative diagnoses

GUIDELINE HAS BEEN DELETED EFFECTIVE OCTOBER 1, 2014

F. Original treatment plan not carried out

Sequence as the principal diagnosis the condition, which after study occasioned the admission to the hospital, even though treatment may not have been carried out due to unforeseen circumstances.

G. Complications of surgery and other medical care

When the admission is for treatment of a complication resulting from surgery or other medical care, the complication code is sequenced as the principal diagnosis. If the complication is classified to the T80-T88 series and the code lacks the necessary specificity in describing the complication, an additional code for the specific complication should be assigned.

H. Uncertain Diagnosis

If the diagnosis documented at the time of discharge is qualified as "probable", "suspected", "likely", "questionable", "possible", or "still to be ruled out", or other similar terms indicating uncertainty, code the condition as if it existed or was established. The bases for these guidelines are the diagnostic workup, arrangements for further workup or observation, and initial therapeutic approach that correspond most closely with the established diagnosis.

Note: This guideline is applicable only to inpatient admissions to short-term, acute, long-term care and psychiatric hospitals.

I. Admission from Observation Unit

1. Admission Following Medical Observation

When a patient is admitted to an observation unit for a medical condition, which either worsens or does not improve, and is subsequently admitted as an inpatient of the same hospital for this same medical condition, the principal diagnosis would be the medical condition which led to the hospital admission.

2. Admission Following Post-Operative Observation

When a patient is admitted to an observation unit to monitor a condition (or complication) that develops following outpatient surgery, and then is subsequently admitted as an inpatient of the same hospital, hospitals should apply the Uniform Hospital Discharge Data Set (UHDDS) definition of principal diagnosis as "that condition established after study to be chiefly responsible for occasioning the admission of the patient to the hospital for care."

J. Admission from Outpatient Surgery

When a patient receives surgery in the hospital's outpatient surgery department and is subsequently admitted for continuing inpatient care at the same hospital, the following guidelines should be followed in selecting the principal diagnosis for the inpatient admission:

❑ If the reason for the inpatient admission is a complication, assign the complication as the principal diagnosis.

❑ If no complication, or other condition, is documented as the reason for the inpatient admission, assign the reason for the outpatient surgery as the principal diagnosis.

❑ If the reason for the inpatient admission is another condition unrelated to the surgery, assign the unrelated condition as the principal diagnosis.

K. Admissions/Encounters for Rehabilitation

When the purpose for the admission/encounter is rehabilitation, sequence first the code for the condition for which the service is being performed. For example, for an admission/encounter for rehabilitation for right-sided dominant hemiplegia following a cerebrovascular infarction, report code I69.351, Hemiplegia and hemiparesis following cerebral infarction affecting right dominant side, as the first-listed or principal diagnosis.

If the condition for which the rehabilitation service is no longer present, report the appropriate aftercare code **as the first-listed or principal diagnosis, unless the rehabilitation service is being provided following an injury. For rehabilitation services following active treatment of an injury, assign the injury code with the appropriate seventh character for subsequent encounter** as the first-listed or principal diagnosis. For example, if a patient with severe degenerative osteoarthritis of the hip, underwent hip replacement and the current encounter/admission is for rehabilitation, report code Z47.1, Aftercare following joint replacement surgery, as the first-listed or principal diagnosis. **If the patient requires rehabilitation post hip replacement for right intertrochanteric femur fracture, report code S72.141D, Displaced intertrochanteric fracture of right femur, subsequent encounter for closed fracture with routine healing, as the first-listed or principal diagnosis.**

See Section I.C.21.c.7, Factors influencing health states and contact with health services, Aftercare.

See Section I.C.19.a for additional information about the use of 7th characters for injury codes.

Section III. Reporting Additional Diagnoses

GENERAL RULES FOR OTHER (ADDITIONAL) DIAGNOSES

For reporting purposes the definition for "other diagnoses" is interpreted as additional conditions that affect patient care in terms of requiring:

clinical evaluation; or

therapeutic treatment; or

diagnostic procedures; or

extended length of hospital stay; or

increased nursing care and/or monitoring.

The UHDDS item #11-b defines Other Diagnoses as "all conditions that coexist at the time of admission, that develop subsequently, or that affect the treatment received and/or the length of stay. Diagnoses that relate to an earlier episode which have no

bearing on the current hospital stay are to be excluded." UHDDS definitions apply to inpatients in acute care, short-term, long term care and psychiatric hospital setting. The UHDDS definitions are used by acute care short-term hospitals to report inpatient data elements in a standardized manner. These data elements and their definitions can be found in the July 31, 1985, Federal Register (Vol. 50, No, 147), pp. 31038-40.

Since that time the application of the UHDDS definitions has been expanded to include all non-outpatient settings (acute care, short term, long term care and psychiatric hospitals; home health agencies; rehab facilities; nursing homes, etc). The UHDDS definitions also apply to hospice services (all levels of care).

The following guidelines are to be applied in designating "other diagnoses" when neither the Alphabetic Index nor the Tabular List in ICD-10-CM provide direction. The listing of the diagnoses in the patient record is the responsibility of the attending provider.

A. Previous conditions

If the provider has included a diagnosis in the final diagnostic statement, such as the discharge summary or the face sheet, it should ordinarily be coded. Some providers include in the diagnostic statement resolved conditions or diagnoses and status-post procedures from previous admission that have no bearing on the current stay. Such conditions are not to be reported and are coded only if required by hospital policy.

However, history codes (categories Z80-Z87) may be used as secondary codes if the historical condition or family history has an impact on current care or influences treatment.

B. Abnormal findings

Abnormal findings (laboratory, x-ray, pathologic, and other diagnostic results) are not coded and reported unless the provider indicates their clinical significance. If the findings are outside the normal range and the attending provider has ordered other tests to evaluate the condition or prescribed treatment, it is appropriate to ask the provider whether the abnormal finding should be added.

Please note: This differs from the coding practices in the outpatient setting for coding encounters for diagnostic tests that have been interpreted by a provider.

C. Uncertain Diagnosis

If the diagnosis documented at the time of discharge is qualified as "probable", "suspected", "likely", "questionable", "possible", or "still to be ruled out" or other similar terms indicating uncertainty, code the condition as if it existed or was established. The bases for these guidelines are the diagnostic workup, arrangements for further workup or observation, and initial therapeutic approach that correspond most closely with the established diagnosis.

Note: This guideline is applicable only to inpatient admissions to short-term, acute, long-term care and psychiatric hospitals.

Section IV. Diagnostic Coding and Reporting Guidelines for Outpatient Services

These coding guidelines for outpatient diagnoses have been approved for use by hospitals/providers in coding and reporting hospital-based outpatient services and provider-based office visits. Guidelines in Section I, Conventions, general coding guidelines and chapter-specific guidelines, should also be applied for outpatient services and office visits.

Information about the use of certain abbreviations, punctuation, symbols, and other conventions used in the ICD-10-CM Tabular List (code numbers and titles), can be found in Section IA of these guidelines, under "Conventions Used in the Tabular List." Section I.B. contains general guidelines that apply to the entire classification. Section I.C. contains chapter-specific guidelines that correspond to the chapters as they are arranged in the classification. Information about the correct sequence to use in finding a code is also described in Section I.

The terms encounter and visit are often used interchangeably in describing outpatient service contacts and, therefore, appear together in these guidelines without distinguishing one from the other.

Though the conventions and general guidelines apply to all settings, coding guidelines for outpatient and provider reporting of diagnoses will vary in a number of instances from those for inpatient diagnoses, recognizing that:

The Uniform Hospital Discharge Data Set (UHDDS) definition of principal diagnosis does not apply to hospital-based outpatient services and provider-based office visits.

Coding guidelines for inconclusive diagnoses (probable, suspected, rule out, etc.) were developed for inpatient reporting and do not apply to outpatients.

A. Selection of first-listed condition

In the outpatient setting, the term first-listed diagnosis is used in lieu of principal diagnosis.

In determining the first-listed diagnosis the coding conventions of ICD-10-CM, as well as the general and disease specific guidelines take precedence over the outpatient guidelines.

Diagnoses often are not established at the time of the initial encounter/visit. It may take two or more visits before the diagnosis is confirmed.

The most critical rule involves beginning the search for the correct code assignment through the Alphabetic Index. Never begin searching initially in the Tabular List as this will lead to coding errors.

1. Outpatient Surgery

When a patient presents for outpatient surgery (same day surgery), code the reason for the surgery as the first-listed diagnosis (reason for the encounter), even if the surgery is not performed due to a contraindication.

2. Observation Stay

When a patient is admitted for observation for a medical condition, assign a code for the medical condition as the first-listed diagnosis.

When a patient presents for outpatient surgery and develops complications requiring admission to observation, code the reason for the surgery as the first reported diagnosis (reason for the encounter), followed by codes for the complications as secondary diagnoses.

Codes from A00.0 through T88.9, Z00-Z99

The appropriate code(s) from A00.0 through T88.9, Z00-Z99 must be used to identify diagnoses, symptoms, conditions, problems, complaints, or other reason(s) for the encounter/visit.

Accurate reporting of ICD-10-CM diagnosis codes

For accurate reporting of ICD-10-CM diagnosis codes, the documentation should describe the patient's condition, using terminology which includes specific diagnoses as well as symptoms, problems, or reasons for the encounter. There are ICD-10-CM codes to describe all of these.

Codes that describe symptoms and signs

Codes that describe symptoms and signs, as opposed to diagnoses, are acceptable for reporting purposes when a diagnosis has not been established (confirmed) by the provider. Chapter 18 of ICD-10-CM, Symptoms, Signs, and Abnormal Clinical and Laboratory Findings Not Elsewhere Classified (codes R00-R99) contain many, but not all codes for symptoms.

Encounters for circumstances other than a disease or injury

ICD-10-CM provides codes to deal with encounters for circumstances other than a disease or injury. The Factors Influencing Health Status and Contact with Health Services codes (Z00-Z99) are provided to deal with occasions when circumstances other than a disease or injury are recorded as diagnosis or problems.

See Section I.C.21. Factors influencing health status and contact with health services.

Level of Detail in Coding

1. ICD-10-CM codes with 3, 4, 5, 6 or 7 characters

ICD-10-CM is composed of codes with 3, 4, 5, 6 or 7 characters. Codes with three characters are included in ICD-10-CM as the heading of a category of codes that may be further subdivided by the use of fourth, fifth, sixth or seventh characters to provide greater specificity.

2. Use of full number of characters required for a code

A three-character code is to be used only if it is not further subdivided. A code is invalid if it has not been coded to the full number of characters required for that code, including the 7th character, if applicable.

ICD-10-CM code for the diagnosis, condition, problem, or other reason for encounter/visit

List first the ICD-10-CM code for the diagnosis, condition, problem, or other reason for encounter/visit shown in the medical record to be chiefly responsible for the services provided. List additional codes that describe any coexisting conditions. In some cases the first-listed diagnosis may be a symptom when a diagnosis has not been established (confirmed) by the physician.

Uncertain diagnosis

Do not code diagnoses documented as "probable", "suspected," "questionable," "rule out," or "working diagnosis" or other similar terms indicating uncertainty. Rather, code the condition(s) to the highest degree of certainty for that encounter/visit, such as symptoms, signs, abnormal test results, or other reason for the visit.

Please note: This differs from the coding practices used by short-term, acute care, long-term care and psychiatric hospitals.

Chronic diseases

Chronic diseases treated on an ongoing basis may be coded and reported as many times as the patient receives treatment and care for the condition(s)

Code all documented conditions that coexist

Code all documented conditions that coexist at the time of the encounter/visit, and require or affect patient care treatment or management. Do not code conditions that were previously treated and no longer exist. However, history

codes (categories Z80-Z87) may be used as secondary codes if the historical condition or family history has an impact on current care or influences treatment.

K. Patients receiving diagnostic services only

For patients receiving diagnostic services only during an encounter/visit, sequence first the diagnosis, condition, problem, or other reason for encounter/visit shown in the medical record to be chiefly responsible for the outpatient services provided during the encounter/visit. Codes for other diagnoses (e.g., chronic conditions) may be sequenced as additional diagnoses.

For encounters for routine laboratory/radiology testing in the absence of any signs, symptoms, or associated diagnosis, assign Z01.89, Encounter for other specified special examinations. If routine testing is performed during the same encounter as a test to evaluate a sign, symptom, or diagnosis, it is appropriate to assign both the Z code and the code describing the reason for the non-routine test.

For outpatient encounters for diagnostic tests that have been interpreted by a physician, and the final report is available at the time of coding, code any confirmed or definitive diagnosis(es) documented in the interpretation. Do not code related signs and symptoms as additional diagnoses.

Please note: This differs from the coding practice in the hospital inpatient setting regarding abnormal findings on test results.

L. Patients receiving therapeutic services only

For patients receiving therapeutic services only during an encounter/visit, sequence first the diagnosis, condition, problem, or other reason for encounter/visit shown in the medical record to be chiefly responsible for the outpatient services provided during the encounter/visit. Codes for other diagnoses (e.g., chronic conditions) may be sequenced as additional diagnoses.

The only exception to this rule is that when the primary reason for the admission/encounter is chemotherapy or radiation therapy, the appropriate Z code for the service is listed first, and the diagnosis or problem for which the service is being performed listed second.

M. Patients receiving preoperative evaluations only

For patients receiving preoperative evaluations only, sequence first a code from subcategory Z01.81, Encounter for pre-procedural examinations, to describe the pre-op consultations. Assign a code for the condition to describe the reason for the surgery as an additional diagnosis. Code also any findings related to the pre-op evaluation.

N. Ambulatory surgery

For ambulatory surgery, code the diagnosis for which the surgery was performed. If the postoperative diagnosis is known to be different from the preoperative diagnosis at the time the diagnosis is confirmed, select the postoperative diagnosis for coding, since it is the most definitive.

O. Routine outpatient prenatal visits

See Section I.C.15. Routine outpatient prenatal visits.

P. Encounters for general medical examinations with abnormal findings

The subcategories for encounters for general medical examinations, Z00.0- **and encounter for routine child health examination, Z00.12-,** provide codes for with and without abnormal findings. Should a general medical examination result in an abnormal finding, the code for general medical examination with abnormal finding should be assigned as the first-listed diagnosis. An examination with abnormal findings refers to a condition/diagnosis that is newly identified or a change in severity of a chronic condition (such as uncontrolled hypertension, or an acute exacerbation of chronic obstructive pulmonary disease) during a routine physical examination. A secondary code for the abnormal finding should also be coded.

Q. Encounters for routine health screenings

See Section I.C.21. Factors influencing health status and contact with health services, Screening

Appendix I: Present on Admission Reporting Guidelines

Introduction

These guidelines are to be used as a supplement to the *ICD-10-CM Official Guidelines for Coding and Reporting* to facilitate the assignment of the Present on Admission (POA) indicator for each diagnosis and external cause of injury code reported on claim forms (UB-04 and 837 Institutional).

These guidelines are not intended to replace any guidelines in the main body of the *ICD-10-CM Official Guidelines for Coding and Reporting*. The POA guidelines are not intended to provide guidance on when a condition should be coded, but rather, how to apply the POA indicator to the final set of diagnosis codes that have been assigned in accordance with Sections I, II, and III of the official coding guidelines. Subsequent to the assignment of the ICD-10-CM codes, the POA indicator should then be assigned to those conditions that have been coded.

As stated in the Introduction to the ICD-10-CM Official Guidelines for Coding and Reporting, a joint effort between the healthcare provider and the coder is essential to achieve complete and accurate documentation, code assignment, and reporting of diagnoses and procedures. The importance of consistent, complete documentation in the medical record cannot be overemphasized. Medical record documentation from any provider involved in the care and treatment of the patient may be used to support the determination of whether a condition was present on admission or not. In the context of the official coding guidelines, the term "provider" means a physician or any qualified healthcare practitioner who is legally accountable for establishing the patient's diagnosis.

These guidelines are not a substitute for the provider's clinical judgment as to the determination of whether a condition was/was not present on admission. The provider should be queried regarding issues related to the linking of signs/symptoms, timing of test results, and the timing of findings.

Please see the CDC website for the detailed list of ICD-10-CM codes that do not require the use of a POA indicator (https://www.cms.gov/Medicare/Coding/ICD10/2018-ICD-10-CM-and-GEMs.html). The **codes and categories** on this exempt list **are** for circumstances regarding the healthcare encounter or factors influencing health status that do not represent a current disease or injury or **that describe conditions that** are always present on admission.

General Reporting Requirements

All claims involving inpatient admissions to general acute care hospitals or other facilities that are subject to a law or regulation mandating collection of present on admission information.

Present on admission is defined as present at the time the order for inpatient admission occurs -- conditions that develop during an outpatient encounter, including emergency department, observation, or outpatient surgery, are considered as present on admission.

POA indicator is assigned to principal and secondary diagnoses (as defined in Section II of the Official Guidelines for Coding and Reporting) and the external cause of injury codes.

Issues related to inconsistent, missing, conflicting or unclear documentation must still be resolved by the provider.

If a condition would not be coded and reported based on UHDDS definitions and current official coding guidelines, then the POA indicator would not be reported.

Reporting Options

Y - Yes

N - No

U - Unknown

W – Clinically undetermined

Unreported/Not used – (Exempt from POA reporting)

Reporting Definitions

Y = present at the time of inpatient admission

N = not present at the time of inpatient admission

U = documentation is insufficient to determine if condition is present on admission

W = provider is unable to clinically determine whether condition was present on admission or not

Timeframe for POA Identification and Documentation

There is no required timeframe as to when a provider (per the definition of "provider" used in these guidelines) must identify or document a condition to be present on admission. In some clinical situations, it may not be possible for a provider to make a definitive diagnosis (or a condition may not be recognized or reported by the patient) for a period of time after admission. In some cases it may be several days before the provider arrives at a definitive diagnosis. This does not mean that the condition was not present on admission. Determination of whether the condition was present on admission or not will be based on the applicable POA guideline as identified in this document, or on the provider's best clinical judgment.

If at the time of code assignment the documentation is unclear as to whether a condition was present on admission or not, it is appropriate to query the provider for clarification.

Assigning the POA Indicator

Condition is on the "Exempt from Reporting" list

Leave the "present on admission" field blank if the condition is on the list of ICD-10-CM codes for which this field is not applicable. This is the only circumstance in which the field may be left blank.

POA Explicitly Documented

Assign Y for any condition the provider explicitly documents as being present on admission.

Assign N for any condition the provider explicitly documents as not present at the time of admission.

Conditions diagnosed prior to inpatient admission

Assign "Y" for conditions that were diagnosed prior to admission (example: hypertension, diabetes mellitus, asthma)

Conditions diagnosed during the admission but clearly present before admission

Assign "Y" for conditions diagnosed during the admission that were clearly present but not diagnosed until after admission occurred.

Diagnoses subsequently confirmed after admission are considered present on admission if at the time of admission they are documented as suspected, possible, rule out, differential diagnosis, or constitute an underlying cause of a symptom that is present at the time of admission.

Condition develops during outpatient encounter prior to inpatient admission

Assign Y for any condition that develops during an outpatient encounter prior to a written order for inpatient admission.

Documentation does not indicate whether condition was present on admission

Assign "U" when the medical record documentation is unclear as to whether the condition was present on admission. "U" should not be routinely assigned and used only in very limited circumstances. Coders are encouraged to query the providers when the documentation is unclear.

Documentation states that it cannot be determined whether the condition was or was not present on admission

Assign "W" when the medical record documentation indicates that it cannot be clinically determined whether or not the condition was present on admission.

Chronic condition with acute exacerbation during the admission

If a single code identifies both the chronic condition and the acute exacerbation, see POA guidelines pertaining to codes that contain multiple clinical concepts.

If a single code only identifies the chronic condition and not the acute exacerbation (e.g., acute exacerbation of chronic leukemia), assign "Y."

Conditions documented as possible, probable, suspected, or rule out at the time of discharge

If the final diagnosis contains a possible, probable, suspected, or rule out diagnosis, and this diagnosis was based on signs, symptoms or clinical findings suspected at the time of inpatient admission, assign "Y."

If the final diagnosis contains a possible, probable, suspected, or rule out diagnosis, and this diagnosis was based on signs, symptoms or clinical findings that were not present on admission, assign "N".

Conditions documented as impending or threatened at the time of discharge

If the final diagnosis contains an impending or threatened diagnosis, and this diagnosis is based on symptoms or clinical findings that were present on admission, assign "Y".

If the final diagnosis contains an impending or threatened diagnosis, and this diagnosis is based on symptoms or clinical findings that were not present on admission, assign "N".

Acute and Chronic Conditions

Assign "Y" for acute conditions that are present at time of admission and N for acute conditions that are not present at time of admission.

Assign "Y" for chronic conditions, even though the condition may not be diagnosed until after admission.

If a single code identifies both an acute and chronic condition, see the POA guidelines for codes that contain multiple clinical concepts.

Codes That Contain Multiple Clinical Concepts

Assign "N" if at least one of the clinical concepts included in the code was not present on admission (e.g., COPD with acute exacerbation and the exacerbation was not present on admission; gastric ulcer that does not start bleeding until after admission; asthma patient develops status asthmaticus after admission).

Assign "Y" if all of the clinical concepts included in the code were present on admission (e.g., duodenal ulcer that perforates prior to admission).

For infection codes that include the causal organism, assign "Y" if the infection (or signs of the infection) were present on admission, even though the culture results may not be known until after admission (e.g., patient is admitted with pneumonia and the provider documents Pseudomonas as the causal organism a few days later).

Same Diagnosis Code for Two or More Conditions

When the same ICD-10-CM diagnosis code applies to two or more conditions during the same encounter (e.g., two separate conditions classified to the same ICD-10-CM diagnosis code):

Assign "Y" if all conditions represented by the single ICD-10-CM code were present on admission (e.g., bilateral unspecified age-related cataracts).

Assign "N" if any of the conditions represented by the single ICD-10-CM code was not present on admission (e.g., traumatic secondary and recurrent hemorrhage and seroma is assigned to a single code T79.2, but only one of the conditions was present on admission).

Obstetrical conditions

Whether or not the patient delivers during the current hospitalization does not affect assignment of the POA indicator. The determining factor for POA assignment is whether the pregnancy complication or obstetrical condition described by the code was present at the time of admission or not.

If the pregnancy complication or obstetrical condition was present on admission (e.g., patient admitted in preterm labor), assign "Y".

If the pregnancy complication or obstetrical condition was not present on admission (e.g., 2nd degree laceration during delivery, postpartum hemorrhage that occurred during current hospitalization, fetal distress develops after admission), assign "N".

If the obstetrical code includes more than one diagnosis and any of the diagnoses identified by the code were not present on admission assign "N".

(e.g., Category O11, Pre-existing hypertension with pre-eclampsia)

Perinatal conditions

Newborns are not considered to be admitted until after birth. Therefore, any condition present at birth or that developed in utero is considered present at admission and should be assigned "Y". This includes conditions that occur during delivery (e.g., injury during delivery, meconium aspiration, exposure to streptococcus B in the vaginal canal).

Congenital conditions and anomalies

Assign "Y" for congenital conditions and anomalies except for categories Q00-Q99, Congenital anomalies, which are on the exempt list. Congenital conditions are always considered present on admission.

External cause of injury codes

Assign "Y" for any external cause code representing an external cause of morbidity that occurred prior to inpatient admission (e.g., patient fell out of bed at home, patient fell out of bed in emergency room prior to admission).

Assign "N" for any external cause code representing an external cause of morbidity that occurred during inpatient hospitalization (e.g., patient fell out of hospital bed during hospital stay, patient experienced an adverse reaction to a medication administered after inpatient admission).

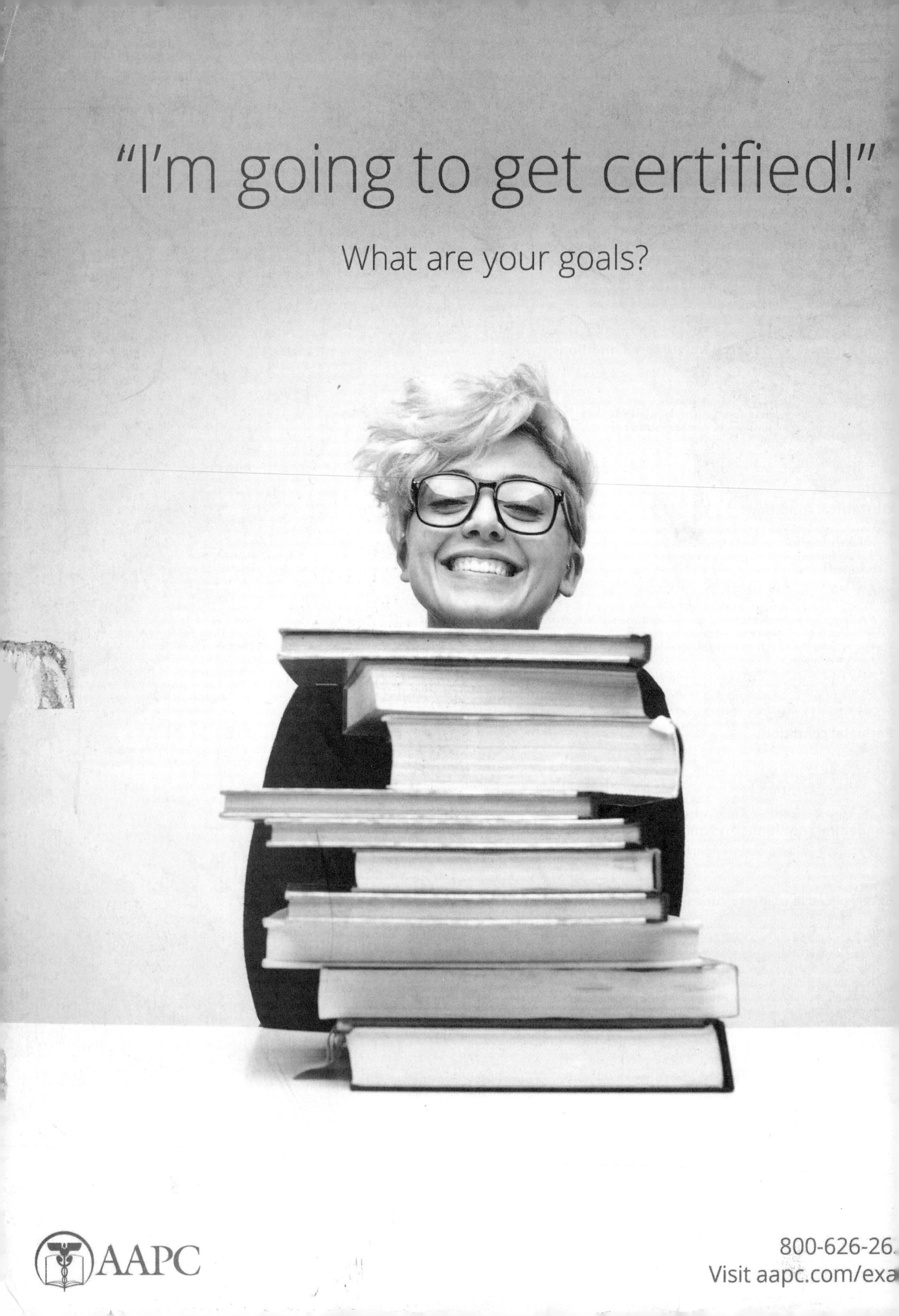

"I'm going to get certified!"

What are your goals?

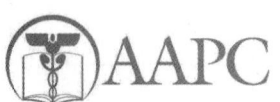
AAPC

800-626-26

Visit aapc.com/exa